Expert CONSULT

Online + Print

Online access activation instructions

This Expert Consult title comes with access to the complete contents online. **Activate your access today** by following these simple instructions:

1. Gently scratch off the surface of the sticker below, using the edge of a coin, to reveal your **activation code.**
2. Visit **www.expertconsultbook.com** and click on the **"Register"** button.
3. **Enter your activation code** along with the other information requested...and begin enjoying your access.

It's that easy! For technical assistance, email **online.help@elsevier.com** or **call 800-401-9962** (inside the US) or **+1-314-995-3200** (outside the US).

To download your PDA software for **Ferri's Clinical Advisor 2009,** go to: http://www.us.elsevierhealth.com/ferri2009pda

Please enter the following serial number when prompted:
SCRATCH OFF BELOW

Scratch off Below

Ferri – PDA

INFECTIOUS DISEASES

MISCELLANEOUS

NEPHROLOGY

Ferri's CLINICAL ADVISOR

2009

Ferri's CLINICAL ADVISOR

Instant Diagnosis and Treatment

FRED F. FERRI, M.D., F.A.C.P.

Clinical Professor
Alpert Medical School
Brown University
Providence, Rhode Island

MOSBY
ELSEVIER

MOSBY
ELSEVIER

1600 John F. Kennedy Blvd.
Suite 1800
Philadelphia, PA 19103-2899

FERRI'S CLINICAL ADVISOR 2009: INSTANT DIAGNOSIS AND TREATMENT

ISBN-13: 978-0-323-04134-8

Notice

Knowledge and best practice in this field are constantly changing. As new research and experience broaden our knowledge, changes in practice, treatment and drug therapy may become necessary or appropriate. Readers are advised to check the most current information provided (i) on procedures featured or (ii) by the manufacturer of each product to be administered, to verify the recommended dose or formula, the method and duration of administration, and contraindications. It is the responsibility of the practitioner, relying on their own experience and knowledge of the patient, to make diagnoses, to determine dosages and the best treatment for each individual patient, and to take all appropriate safety precautions. To the fullest extent of the law, neither the Publisher nor the Editors assume any liability for any injury and/or damage to persons or property arising out of or related to any use of the material contained in this book.

The Publisher

International Standard Serial Number (ISSN) 1541-4515

ISBN-13: 978-0-323-04134-8

Acquisitions Editor: Druanne Martin
Developmental Editor: Mary Beth Murphy
Editorial Assistant: John Ingram
Design Direction: Teresa McBryan
Marketing Manager: Bill Veltre

Printed in the United States of America
Last digit is the print number: 9 8 7 6 5 4 3 2 1

Section Editors

RUBEN ALVERO, M.D.
Associate Professor
Obstetrics and Gynecology
University of Colorado Health Sciences Center
Aurora, Colorado
SECTION I

MICHAEL G. BENATAR, M.B.Ch.B., D.Phil.
Assistant Professor of Neurology
Department of Neurology
Emory University
Atlanta, Georgia
SECTION I

JEFFREY M. BORKAN, M.D., Ph.D.
Professor and Chair
Department of Family Medicine
Physician-in-Chief
Alpert Medical School
Brown University
Memorial Hospital of Rhode Island
Pawtucket and Providence, Rhode Island
SECTION I

MITCHELL D. FELDMAN, M.D., M.Phil.
Professor of Medicine
Director of Faculty Mentoring
University of California, San Francisco
Division of General Internal Medicine
San Francisco, California
SECTION I

FRED F. FERRI, M.D., F.A.C.P.
Clinical Professor
Alpert Medical School
Brown University
Providence, Rhode Island
SECTIONS I-V

GLENN G. FORT, M.D., M.P.H.
Clinical Associate Professor of Medicine
Alpert Medical School
Brown University
Chief
Infectious Diseases
Our Lady of Fatima Hospital
North Providence, Rhode Island
SECTION I

LONNIE R. MERCIER, M.D.
Clinical Instructor
Department of Orthopedic Surgery
Creighton University School of Medicine
Omaha, Nebraska
SECTION I

DENNIS J. MIKOLICH, M.D., F.A.C.P., F.C.C.P.
Chief
Division of Infectious Diseases
VA Medical Center
Clinical Associate Professor of Medicine
Alpert Medical School
Brown University
Providence, Rhode Island
SECTION I

IRIS TONG, M.D.
Clinical Assistant Professor
Alpert Medical School
Brown University
Division of Ambulatory General Internal Medicine
Rhode Island Hospital
Providence, Rhode Island
SECTION I

WEN-CHIH WU, M.D.
Assistant Professor of Medicine
Alpert Medical School
Brown University
Cardiologist
Providence VA Medical Center
Providence, Rhode Island
SECTION I

Contributors

SONYA S. ABDEL-RAZEQ, M.D.
Clinical Assistant Instructor
Department of Obstetrics and Gynecology/Resident Education
State University of New York at Buffalo
Women's and Children's Hospital
Buffalo, New York

ABDULBAKI ABDULRAHMAN, M.D.
Department of Internal Medicine
Memorial Hospital of Rhode Island
Alpert Medical School
Brown University
Providence, Rhode Island

PURVA AGARWAL, M.D.
Department of Internal Medicine
Memorial Hospital of Rhode Island
Alpert Medical School
Brown University
Providence, Rhode Island

TANYA ALI, M.D.
Clinical Assistant Professor of Medicine
Department of Medicine
Alpert Medical School
Brown University
Providence, Rhode Island

PHILIP J. ALIOTTA, M.D., M.S.H.A., F.A.C.S.
Clinical Instructor
Department of Urology
School of Medicine and Biomedical Sciences
State University of New York at Buffalo
Buffalo, New York
Medical Director
Center for Urologic Research of Western New York
Williamsville, New York

GEORGE O. ALONSO, M.D.
Director
Department of Infection Control
Elmhurst Hospital Center
Elmhurst, New York
Instructor in Medicine
Mount Sinai School of Medicine
New York, New York

RUBEN ALVERO, M.D.
Associate Professor
Obstetrics and Gynecology
University of Colorado Health Sciences Center
Aurora, Colorado

SRIVIDYA ANANDAN, M.D.
Attending Physician
Internal Medicine
Harvard Vanguard Medical Associates
Quincy, Massachusetts

GOWRI ANANDARAJAH, M.D.
Clinical Associate Professor
Department of Family Medicine
Alpert Medical School
Brown University
Providence, Rhode Island

MEL L. ANDERSON, M.D., F.A.C.P
Assistant Professor of Medicine
University of Colorado School of Medicine
Denver Veterans Affairs Medical Center
Denver, Colorado

MICHELLE STOZEK ANVAR, M.D.
Clinical Instructor
Division of General Internal Medicine
Rhode Island Hospital
Clinical Instructor
Alpert Medical School
Brown University
Providence, Rhode Island

ETSUKO AOKI, M.D., Ph.D
Fellow
Leukemia Department
University of Texas
M.D. Anderson Cancer Center
Houston, Texas

PATRICIA AREAN, Ph.D.
Associate Professor
Department of Psychiatry
University of California, San Francisco
San Francisco, California

VASANTHI ARUMUGAM, M.D.
Assistant Professor
Department of Medicine
Mount Sinai School of Medicine
New York, New York
Attending Physician
Division of Infectious Diseases/Department of Medicine
Elmhurst Hospital Center
Elmhurst, New York

AMAAR ASHRAF, M.D.
Assistant Professor
Department of Medicine
Mount Sinai School of Medicine
New York, New York
Attending Physician
Division of Infectious Diseases
Elmhurst Hospital Center
Elmhurst, New York

SUDEEP KAUR AULAKH, M.D., C.M., F.R.C.P.C.
Associate Professor of Medicine
Albany Medical College
Albany, New York

MICHAEL G. BENATAR, M.B.Ch.B., D.Phil.
Assistant Professor of Neurology
Department of Neurology
Emory University
Atlanta, Georgia

AGNIESZKA K. BIALIKIEWICZ, M.D.
Assistant Clinical Instructor
Department of Family Medicine
Alpert Medical School
Brown University
Providence, Rhode Island

NIRALI BORA, M.D.
Family Medicine Resident
Department of Family Medicine
Memorial Hospital of Rhode Island
Alpert Medical School
Brown University
Pawtucket, Rhode Island

JEFFREY M. BORKAN, M.D., Ph.D.
Professor and Chair
Department of Family Medicine
Physician-in-Chief
Alpert Medical School
Brown University
Memorial Hospital of Rhode Island
Pawtucket and Providence, Rhode Island

KELLY BOSSENBROK, M.D.
Assistant Clinical Instructor
Alpert Medical School
Brown University
Providence, Rhode Island

LYNN BOWLBY, M.D.
Attending Physician
Division of General Internal Medicine
Rhode Island Hospital
Clinical Instructor of Medicine
Alpert Medical School
Brown University
Providence, Rhode Island

MANDEEP K. BRAR, M.D.
Clinical Assistant Professor
Department of Obstetrics and Gynecology
State University of New York at Buffalo
Buffalo, New York

JOANNA BROWN, M.D.
Fellow
Adolescent/Young Adult Program
Children's Hospital
Boston, Massachusetts

JONATHAN BURNS, M.A., M.D.
Assistant Clinical Instructor
Department of Family Medicine
Alpert Medical School
Brown University
Providence, Rhode Island

STEVEN BUSSELEN, M.D.
Assistant Clinical Instructor
Department of Family Medicine
Alpert Medical School
Brown University
Pawtucket, Rhode Island

BRIAN CASSERLY, M.D.
Reading Internal Medicine
Reading, Massachusetts

GAURAV CHAUDHARY, M.D.
Assistant Professor of Medicine
Alpert Medical School
Brown University
Providence, Rhode Island

KARA CHEW, M.D.
Department of Medicine
University of California, San Francisco
San Francisco, California

MARIA A. CORIGLIANO, M.D., F.A.C.O.G.
Clinical Assistant Professor
Department of Obstetrics and Gynecology
State University of New York at Buffalo
Buffalo, New York

BRIAN J. COWLES, Pharm.D.
Clinical Assistant Professor
Department of Pharmacy Practice
College of Pharmacy
University of Rhode Island
Kingston, Rhode Island

JOHN E. CROOM, M.D., Ph.D.
Co-Director
Comprehensive Epilepsy Center
Saint Luke's Mid America Brain and Stroke Institute
Neurological Consultants of Kansas City, Inc.
Kansas City, Missouri

ALICIA J. CURTIN, Ph.D., G.N.P.
Assistant Professor
Division of Geriatrics
Alpert Medical School
Brown University
Providence, Rhode Island

CLAUDIA L. DADE, M.D.
Attending Physician
Division of Infectious Diseases
Elmhurst Hospital Center
Elmhurst, New York
Instructor in Medicine
Mount Sinai School of Medicine
New York, New York

GEORGE T. DANAKAS, M.D., F.A.C.O.G.
Clinical Assistant Professor
Department of Obstetrics and Gynecology
State University of New York at Buffalo
Buffalo, New York

ALEXANDRA DEGENHARDT, M.D.
Director
Multiple Sclerosis Center
New York Methodist Hospital
Brooklyn, New York

JOSEPH DIAZ, M.D.
Assistant Professor of Medicine
Division of General Internal Medicine
Memorial Hospital of Rhode Island
Alpert Medical School
Brown University
Providence, Rhode Island

CHRISTINE M. DUFFY, M.D., M.P.H.
Fellow
Center for Gerontology and Health Care Research
Alpert Medical School
Brown University
Providence, Rhode Island

JEFFREY S. DURMER, M.D., Ph.D., D.ABSM.
Chief Medical Officer
Fusion Sleep Center
Johns Creek, Georgia

JANE V. EASON, M.D.
Attending Physician
Division of Infectious Diseases
Elmhurst Hospital Center
Elmhurst, New York
Instructor in Medicine
Mount Sinai School of Medicine
New York, New York

STUART EISENDRATH, M.D.
Professor of Clinical Psychiatry
University of California, San Francisco
San Francisco, California

PAMELA ELLSWORTH, M.D.
Associate Professor of Urology
Alpert Medical School
Brown University
Providence, Rhode Island

RAMI ELTIBI, M.D.
Department of Internal Medicine
Memorial Hospital of Rhode Island
Alpert Medical School
Brown University
Providence, Rhode Island

GREGORY J. ESPER, M.D.
Director
General Neurology
Emory University
Atlanta, Georgia

MARILYN FABBRI, M.D.
Instructor
Department of Medicine
Mount Sinai School of Medicine
New York, New York
Attending Physician
Division of Infectious Diseases/Department of Medicine
Elmhurst Hospital Center
Elmhurst, New York

MARK J. FAGAN, M.D.
Director
Medical Primary Care Unit
Rhode Island Hospital
Associate Professor of Medicine
Alpert Medical School
Brown University
Providence, Rhode Island

GIL M. FARKASH, M.D.
Assistant Clinical Professor
State University of New York at Buffalo
School of Medicine
Buffalo, New York

TIMOTHY W. FARRELL, M.D.
Clinical Assistant Instructor
Department of Family Medicine
Alpert Medical School
Brown University
Providence, Rhode Island

MITCHELL D. FELDMAN, M.D., M.Phil.
Professor of Medicine
Director of Faculty Mentoring
University of California, San Francisco
Division of General Internal Medicine
San Francisco, California

FRED F. FERRI, M.D., F.A.C.P.
Clinical Professor
Alpert Medical School
Brown University
Providence, Rhode Island

STACI A. FISCHER, M.D., F.A.C.P.
Assistant Professor of Medicine
Division of Infectious Diseases
Alpert Medical School
Brown University
Rhode Island Hospital
Providence, Rhode Island

TAMARA G. FONG, M.D., Ph.D.
Instructor in Neurology
Beth Israel Deaconess Medical Center
Harvard Medical School
Boston, Massachusetts

GLENN G. FORT, M.D., M.P.H.
Clinical Associate Professor of Medicine
Alpert Medical School
Brown University
Chief
Infectious Diseases
Our Lady of Fatima Hospital
North Providence, Rhode Island

GENNA GEKHT, M.D.
Chief Resident in Neurology
Department of Neurology
Emory University
Atlanta, Georgia

PAUL F. GEORGE, M.D.
Assistant Clinical Instructor
Department of Family Medicine
Alpert Medical School
Brown University
Pawtucket, Rhode Island

DAVID R. GIFFORD, M.D., M.P.H.
Assistant Physician
Division of Geriatrics
Rhode Island Hospital
Assistant Professor of Community Health and Medicine
Alpert Medical School
Brown University
Providence, Rhode Island

ANNGENE A. GIUSTOZZI, M.D., M.P.H.
Assistant Professor
Department of Family Medicine
Alpert Medical School
Brown University
Providence, Rhode Island

CINDY GLEIT, M.D.
Assistant Clinical Instructor
Department of Family Medicine
Alpert Medical School
Brown University
Providence, Rhode Island

GEETHA GOPALAKRISHNAN, M.D.
Assistant Professor of Medicine
Alpert Medical School
Brown University
Providence, Rhode Island

NANCY R. GRAFF, M.D.
Associate Clinical Professor
Department of Pediatrics
University of California, San Diego
San Diego, California

REBECCA A. GRIFFITH, M.D.
Attending Physician
Department of Medicine
Morristown Memorial Hospital
Morristown, New Jersey

JOSEPH GRILLO, M.D.
Fellow
Department of Infectious Diseases
Roger Williams Medical Center
Providence, Rhode Island

LAWRENCE HABER, M.D.
Department of Medicine
University of California, San Francisco
San Francisco. California

MOHAMMED HAJJIRI, M.D.
Internal Medicine Resident
Memorial Hospital of Rhode Island
Alpert Medical School
Brown University
Providence, Rhode Island

MICHELE HALPERN, M.D.
Attending Physician
Division of Infectious Diseases
Sound Shore Medical Center of Westchester
New Rochelle, New York
Clinical Assistant Professor of Medicine
New York Medical College
Valhalla, New York

MUSTAFA A. HAMMAD, M.D.
Clinical Neurophysiology Fellow
Department of Neurology
Emory University
Atlanta, Georgia

SAJEEV HANDA, M.D.
Director
Division of Hospitalist Medicine
Rhode Island Hospital
Clinical Instructor of Medicine
Alpert Medical School
Brown University
Providence, Rhode Island

MIKE HARPER, M.D.
Associate Professor of Medicine
Division of Geriatrics
Department of Medicine
San Francisco Veterans Affairs Medical Center
University of California, San Diego
San Diego, California

TAYLOR HARRISON, M.D.
Assistant Professor of Neurology
Department of Neurology
Emory University
Atlanta, Georgia

CHRISTINE HARTLEY, M.D.
Assistant Clinical Instructor
Department of Family Medicine
Memorial Hospital of Rhode Island
Alpert Medical School
Brown University
Providence, Rhode Island

ANNE L. HUME, Pharm.D.
Professor of Pharmacy
Department of Pharmacy Practice
University of Rhode Island
Kingston, Rhode Island
Adjunct Professor of Family Medicine
Memorial Hospital of Rhode Island
Pawtucket, Rhode Island

JENNIFER ROH HUR, M.D.
Assistant Professor of Clinical Medicine
Indiana University School of Medicine
Indianapolis, Indiana

RICHARD S. ISAACSON, M.D.
Resident in Neurology
Beth Israel Deaconess Medical Center
Harvard Medical School
Boston, Massachusetts

JENNIFER JEREMIAH, M.D.
Clinical Associate Professor of Medicine
Alpert Medical School
Brown University
Providence, Rhode Island

MICHAEL P. JOHNSON, M.D.
Staff Physician
Division of General Internal Medicine
Rhode Island Hospital
Assistant Professor of Medicine
Alpert Medical School
Brown University
Providence, Rhode Island

KOHAR JONES, M.D.
Assistant Clinical Instructor
Department of Family Medicine
Alpert Medical School
Brown University
Memorial Hospital of Rhode Island
Pawtucket, Rhode Island

LUCY KALANITHI, M.D.
Internal Medicine/Primary
University of California, San Francisco
San Francisco, California

BHARAT K. KANTHARIA, M.D.
Division of Cardiology
Albert Einstein Medical Center
Philadelphia, Pennsylvania

DANIEL KAPLON, M.D.
Associate Professor of Surgery (Urology)
Division of Urology
Alpert Medical School
Brown University
Providence, Rhode Island

WAN J. KIM, M.D.
Clinical Instructor
Department of Obstetrics and Gynecology
State University of New York at Buffalo
Buffalo, New York

MELVYN KOBY, M.D.
Associate Clinical Professor of Medicine
Department of Ophthalmology
University of Louisville School of Medicine
Louisville, Kentucky

DAVID KURSS, M.D., F.A.C.O.G.
Clinical Assistant Professor
Department of Obstetrics and Gynecology
State University of New York at Buffalo
Buffalo, New York

CINDY LAI, M.D.
Department of Medicine
University of California, San Francisco
San Francisco, California

SUZETTE M. LAROCHE, M.D.
Assistant Professor of Neurology
Emory University
Atlanta, Georgia

JOSEPH J. LIEBER, M.D.
Associate Director of Medicine
Chief
Medical Consultation Service
Elmhurst Hospital Center
Clinical Associate Professor of Medicine
Mount Sinai School of Medicine
New York, New York

CHUN LIM, M.D., Ph.D.
Department of Neurology
Beth Israel Deaconess Medical Center
Boston, Massachusetts

MARA LINSCOTT, M.D.
Department of Medicine
Women and Infants Hospital of Rhode Island
Providence, Rhode Island

ZEENA LOBO, M.D.
Attending Physician
Division of Infectious Diseases
Elmhurst Medical Center
Elmhurst, New York

RICHARD LONG, M.D.
Clinical Associate Professor
Department of Family Medicine
Alpert Medical School
Brown University
Providence, Rhode Island

MICHAEL MAHER, M.D.
Assistant Professor of Internal Medicine
Alpert Medical School
Brown University
Rhode Island Hospital
Providence, Rhode Island

ACHRAF A. MAKKI, M.D., M.Sc.
Resident
Department of Neurology
Emory University
Atlanta, Georgia

JOSEPH R. MASCI, M.D.
Director of Medicine
Elmhurst Hospital Center
Professor of Medicine
Mount Sinai School of Medicine
Elmhurst, New York

DANIEL T. MATTSON, M.D., M.S.C. (Med.)
St. Louis Neurological Institute
St. Louis, Missouri

JEFFREY MAZER, M.D.
Department of Medicine
Alpert Medical School
Brown University
Providence, Rhode Island

MAITREYI MAZUMDAR, M.D., M.P.H., M.Sc.
Instructor in Neurology
Harvard Medical School
Children's Hospital Boston
Department of Neurology
Boston, Massachusetts

KELLY A. McGARRY, M.D.
Associate Program Director
General Internal Medicine Residency Program
Rhode Island Hospital
Assistant Professor of Medicine
Alpert Medical School
Brown University
Providence, Rhode Island

CRAIG J. McMACKIN, M.D.
Fellow
Cardiovascular Diseases
Alpert Medical School
Brown University
Rhode Island Hospital
Providence, Rhode Island

LYNN McNICOLL, M.D.
Assistant Professor of Medicine
Alpert Medical School
Brown University
Geriatrician
Division of Geriatrics
Rhode Island Hospital
Providence, Rhode Island

LONNIE R. MERCIER, M.D.
Clinical Instructor
Department of Orthopedic Surgery
Creighton University School of Medicine
Omaha, Nebraska

DENNIS J. MIKOLICH, M.D., F.A.C.P., F.C.C.P.
Chief
Division of Infectious Diseases
VA Medical Center
Clinical Associate Professor of Medicine
Alpert Medical School
Brown University
Providence, Rhode Island

MICHELE MONTANDON, M.D.
University of California, San Francisco
San Francisco, California

TAKUMA NEMOTO, M.D.
Research Associate Professor of Surgery
State University of New York at Buffalo
Buffalo, New York

JAMES J. NG, M.D.
Staff Physician
The Vancouver Clinic
Vancouver, Washington

MELISSA NOTHNAGLE, M.D.
Assistant Professor of Family Medicine
Alpert Medical School
Brown University
Providence, Rhode Island

ELIZABETH NOWAK, D.O.
Clinical Instructor of Family Medicine
Department of Family Medicine
Memorial Hospital of Rhode Island
Pawtucket, Rhode Island

JUDITH NUDELMAN, M.D.
Clinical Assistant Professor
Department of Family Medicine
Alpert Medical School
Brown University
Providence, Rhode Island

GAIL M. O'BRIEN, M.D.
Medical Director
Adult Ambulatory Services
Rhode Island Hospital
Clinical Associate Professor of Medicine
Alpert Medical School
Brown University
Providence, Rhode Island

CAROLYN J. O'CONNOR, M.D.
Assistant Clinical Professor
Yale University School of Medicine
Department of Medicine
St. Mary's Hospital
Waterbury, Connecticut

ALEXANDER B. OLAWAIYE, M.D.
Fellow
Division of Gynecologic Oncology
Vincent Department of Obstetrics, Gynecology and Reproductive Biology
Massachusetts General Hospital
Harvard Medical School
Boston, Massachusetts

MICHAEL K. ONG, M.D., Ph.D.
Assistant Professor
UCLA Division of General Internal Medicine/Health Services Research
UCLA School of Medicine
Los Angeles, California

STEVEN M. OPAL, M.D.
Professor of Medicine
Infectious Disease Division
Alpert Medical School
Brown University
Providence, Rhode Island

CRISTINA A. PACHECO, M.D.
Clinical Assistant Professor
Department of Family Medicine
Alpert Medical School
Brown University
Providence, Rhode Island

MINA B. PANTCHEVA, M.D.
Internal Medicine
Roger Williams Medical Center
Providence, Rhode Island

JANICE PATACSIL-TRULL, M.D.
Clinical Instructor of Family Medicine
Department of Family Medicine
Memorial Hospital of Rhode Island
Pawtucket, Rhode Island

PRANAV M. PATEL, M.D.
Assistant Professor of Medicine
Division of Cardiology
University of California
Irvine Medical Center
Orange, California

SHALINI PATEL, M.D.
Associate Physician
Department of Medicine
University of California, San Francisco
San Francisco, California

ELENI PATROZOU, M.D.
Division of Infectious Diseases
Alpert Medical School
Brown University
Rhode Island Hospital
Providence, Rhode Island

STEVEN PELIGIAN, D.O.
Medical Director
CODAC Behavioral Healthcare
Providence, Rhode Island

PETER PETROPOULOS, M.D., F.A.C.C.
Clinical Assistant Professor
Alpert Medical School
Brown University
Department of Veterans Affairs
Providence, Rhode Island

PAUL A. PIRRAGLIA, M.D., M.P.H.
Assistant Professor of Medicine
Alpert Medical School
Brown University
Rhode Island Hospital
Providence, Rhode Island

SHARON S. HARTMAN POLENSEK, M.D., Ph.D.
Clinical Associate
Department of Neurology
Emory University
Atlanta, Georgia

MAURICE POLICAR, M.D.
Chief of Infectious Diseases
Elmhurst Hospital Center
Elmhurst, New York
Assistant Professor of Medicine
Mount Sinai School of Medicine
New York, New York

ARUNDATHI G. PRASAD, M.D.
Clinical Instructor
Department of Obstetrics and Gynecology/Resident Education
State University of New York at Buffalo
Women's and Children's Hospital
Buffalo, New York

KITTICHAI PROMRAT, M.D.
Assistant Professor
Division of Gastroenterology
Department of Medicine
Alpert Medical School
Brown University
Chief
Gastroenterology Section
Providence Veterans Affairs Medical Center
Providence, Rhode Island

JOHN RAGSDALE, M.D.
Clinical Assistant Professor of Family Medicine
Alpert Medical School
Brown University
Providence, Rhode Island

CHAITANYA V. REDDY, D.O.
Assistant Clinical Instructor
Department of Family Medicine
Alpert Medical School
Brown University
Providence, Rhode Island

VICTOR I. REUS, M.D.
Professor of Psychiatry
Department of Psychiatry
Langley Porter Psychiatric Institute
University of California, San Francisco
San Francisco, California

HARLAN G. RICH, M.D.
Director of Endoscopy
Rhode Island Hospital
Associate Professor of Medicine
Alpert Medical School
Brown University
Providence, Rhode Island

LUTHER K. ROBINSON, M.D.
Associate Professor of Pediatrics
Director
Dysmorphology and Clinical Genetics
State University of New York at Buffalo
Buffalo, New York

HEMANT K. SATPATHY, M.D.
Assistant Professor
Department of Family Medicine
Chief Resident
Department of OBGYN
Creighton University Medical Center
Omaha, Nebraska

RUBY SATPATHY, M.D.
Fellow, Cardiology
Department of Internal Medicine
Creighton University
Omaha, Nebraska

JASON M. SATTERFIELD, Ph.D.
Director
Behavioral Medicine
Associate Professor of Clinical Medicine
University of California, San Francisco
San Francisco, California

SEAN I. SAVITZ, M.D.
Assistant Professor of Neurology
University of Texas
Houston, Texas

JACK L. SCHWARTZWALD, M.D.
Clinical Assistant Professor of Medicine
Rhode Island Hospital
Providence, Rhode Island

CATHERINE SHAFTS, D.O.
Assistant Clinical Instructor
Alpert Medical School
Brown University
Providence, Rhode Island

MADHAVI SHAH, M.D.
Assistant Clinical Instructor
Department of Family Medicine
Alpert Medical School
Brown University
Providence, Rhode Island

HARVEY M. SHANIES, M.D., Ph.D.
Director of Critical Care Medicine
Vassar Brothers Medical Center
Poughkeepsie, New York

DEBORAH L. SHAPIRO, M.D.
Chief
Division of Rheumatology
Elmhurst Hospital Center
Elmhurst, New York
Clinical Assistant Professor of Medicine
Mount Sinai School of Medicine
New York, New York

GRACE SHIH, M.D.
Assistant Clinical Instructor
Department of Family Medicine
Alpert Medical School
Brown University
Providence, Rhode Island

MARK SIGMAN, M.D.
Associate Professor of Surgery (Urology)
Division of Urology
Alpert Medical School
Brown University
Providence, Rhode Island

JOANNE M. SILVIA, M.D.
Assistant Clinical Instructor
Department of Family Medicine
Alpert Medical School
Brown University
Providence, Rhode Island

CLIFFORD MILO SINGER, M.D.
Associate Professor of Psychiatry
Director
Insomnia and Chronobiology Clinic
Vermont Regional Sleep Center
University of Vermont College of Medicine
Burlington, Vermont

NICOLE SIROTIN, M.D.
Division of General Internal Medicine
Department of Medicine
University of California, San Francisco
San Francisco, California

U. SHIVRAJ SOHUR, M.D., Ph.D.
Assistant Professor of Neurology
Harvard Medical School
Boston, Massachusetts

JENNIFER SOUTHER, M.D.
Attending Physician
Department of Family Practice
Memorial Hospital of Rhode Island
Pawtucket, Rhode Island

JULIE ANNE SZUMIGALA, M.D.
Clinical Instructor
Department of Obstetrics and Gynecology
State University of New York at Buffalo
Buffalo, New York

DOMINICK TAMMARO, M.D.
Associate Director
Categorical Internal Medicine Residency
Co-Director
Medicine-Pediatrics Residency
Division of General Internal Medicine
Rhode Island Hospital
Associate Professor of Medicine
Alpert Medical School
Brown University
Providence, Rhode Island

IRIS TONG, M.D.
Clinical Assistant Professor
Alpert Medical School
Brown University
Division of Ambulatory General Internal Medicine
Rhode Island Hospital
Providence, Rhode Island

MARGARET TRYFOROS, M.D.
Clinical Assistant Professor
Department of Family Medicine
Alpert Medical School
Brown University
Providence, Rhode Island

EROBOGHENE E. UBOGU, M.B.B.S. (Hons.)
Assistant Professor of Neurology
Case Western Reserve University School of Medicine
Staff Neurologist
Louis Stokes Cleveland Veterans Affairs Medical Center
Cleveland, Ohio

SEAN H. UITERWYK, M.D.
Clinical Assistant Professor
Department of Family Medicine
Alpert Medical School
Brown University
Providence, Rhode Island

NICOLE J. ULLRICH, M.D., Ph.D.
Clinical Fellow in Neurology/Neurooncology
Children's Hospital Boston
Boston, Massachusetts

JORGE A. VILLAFUERTE, M.D.
Attending Orthopedic Surgeon
VA Medical Center
West Roxbury, Massachusetts

HANNAH VU, D.O.
Assistant Clinical Instructor
Department of Family Medicine
Alpert Medical School
Brown University
Providence, Rhode Island

TOM J. WACHTEL, M.D.
Physician-in-Charge
Division of Geriatrics
Rhode Island Hospital
Professor of Community Health and Medicine
Alpert Medical School
Brown University
Providence, Rhode Island

DENNIS M. WEPPNER, M.D., F.A.C.O.G.
Associate Professor of Clinical Gynecology/Obstetrics
State University of New York at Buffalo
Clinical Chief
Department of Gynecology/Obstetrics
Millard Fillmore Hospital
Buffalo, New York

LAUREL M. WHITE, M.D.
Clinical Assistant Professor
Department of Obstetrics and Gynecology
Division of Maternal Fetal Medicine
State University of New York at Buffalo
Buffalo, New York

DAVID P. WILLIAMS, M.D.
Neurologist
Peachtree Neurological Clinics, PC
Atlanta, Georgia

MARIE ELIZABETH WONG, M.D.
Physician
Family Medicine
Baystate Brightwood Health Center
Springfield, Massachusetts

WEN-CHIH WU, M.D.
Assistant Professor of Medicine
Alpert Medical School
Brown University
Cardiologist
Providence VA Medical Center
Providence, Rhode Island

WEN Y. (HELENA) WU-CHEN, M.D.
Department of Neurology
Temple University Hospital
Philadelphia, Pennsylvania

AMANDA WULFSTAT, M.D.
Department of Medicine
University of California, San Francisco
San Francisco, California

BETH J. WUTZ, M.D.
Clinical Assistant Professor of Medicine
Division of Internal Medicine/Pediatrics
Kajeida Health–Buffalo General Hospital
State University of New York at Buffalo
Buffalo, New York

JOHN Q. YOUNG, M.D., M.P.P.
Assistant Director
Adult Psychiatry Clinic
Associate Director
Residency Training Program
Langley Porter Psychiatric Hospitals and Clinics
Department of Psychiatry
University of California, San Francisco
San Francisco, California

CINDY ZADIKOFF, M.D., F.R.C.P.C.
Assistant Professor of Neurology
Parkinson's Disease and Movement Disorders Center
Davee Department of Neurology and Clinical Neurological Sciences
Feinberg School of Medicine
Northwestern University
Chicago, Illinois

SCOTT J. ZUCCALA, D.O., F.A.C.O.G.
Staff Physician
Mercy Hospital of Buffalo
Buffalo, New York

To our families.

Their constant support and encouragement made this book a reality.

Preface

This book is intended to be a clear and concise reference for physicians and allied health professionals. Its user-friendly format was designed to provide a fast and efficient way to identify important clinical information and to offer practical guidance in patient management. The book is divided into five sections and an appendix, each with emphasis on clinical information.

The tremendous success of the previous editions and the enthusiastic comments from numerous colleagues have brought about several positive changes. Each section has also been significantly expanded from prior editions, bringing the total number of medical topics covered in this book to more than 1000. Illustrations have been added to several topics to enhance recollection of clinically important facts. The use of ICD-9CM codes in all the topics will expedite claims submission and reimbursement.

Section I describes in detail over 700 medical disorders. Several new topics have been added to the 2009 edition. Medical topics in this section are arranged alphabetically, and the material in each topic is presented in outline format for ease of retrieval. Topics with an accompanying algorithm in Section III are identified with an algorithm symbol (ALG). Similarly, if topics also have a Patient Teaching Guide (PTG) available online, this has been noted. Key, quick-access information is consistently highlighted; clinical photographs are used to further illustrate selected medical conditions; and relevant ICD-9CM codes are listed. Most references focus on current peer-reviewed journal articles rather than outdated textbooks and old review articles. Evidence-based medicine data have been added to relevant topics.

Topics in this section use the following structured approach:

1. Basic Information (Definition, Synonyms, ICD-9CM Codes, Epidemiology & Demographics, Physical Findings & Clinical Presentation, Etiology)
2. Diagnosis (Differential Diagnosis, Workup, Laboratory Tests, Imaging Studies)
3. Treatment (Nonpharmacologic Therapy, Acute General Rx, Chronic Rx, Disposition, Referral)
4. Pearls and Considerations (Comments, Suggested Readings)
5. Evidence-Based Data and References

Section II includes the differential diagnosis, etiology, and classification of signs and symptoms. This section has been significantly expanded for the 2009 edition. It is a practical section that allows the user investigating a physical complaint or abnormal laboratory value to follow a "workup" leading to a diagnosis. The physician can then easily look up the presumptive diagnosis in Section I for the information specific to that illness.

Section III includes clinical algorithms to guide and expedite the patient's workup and therapy. For the 2009 edition, several new algorithms have been added and many others have been revised. Many physicians describe this section as particularly valuable in today's managed-care environment.

Section IV includes normal laboratory values and interpretation of results of commonly ordered laboratory tests. By providing interpretation of abnormal results, this section facilitates the diagnosis of medical disorders and further adds to the comprehensive, "one-stop" nature of our text.

Section V focuses on preventive medicine and offers essential guidelines from the U.S. Preventive Services Task Force. It has been significantly expanded for the 2009 edition. Information in this section includes recommendations for the periodic health examination, screening for major diseases and disorders, patient counseling, and immunization and chemoprophylaxis recommendations.

The **Appendix** contains extensive information on complementary and alternative medicine (CAM). It has been completely revised in the 2009 edition. With the material in this appendix, we hope to lessen the current lack of exposure of allopathic and osteopathic physicians to the diversity of CAM therapies. Another important addition to the Appendix for the 2009 edition is an extensive section on primary care procedures.

As clinicians, we all realize the importance of patient education and the need for clear communication with our patients. Toward that end, practical patient instruction sheets, organized alphabetically and covering the majority of the topics in this book, are available online and can be easily customized and printed from any computer. Most of them have been updated and over 100 new instruction sheets have been added to the 2009 edition. They represent a valuable addition to patient care and are useful for improving physician-patient communication, patient satisfaction, and quality of care.

I believe that we have produced a state-of-the-art information system with significant differences from existing texts. It contains five sections and patient education guides that could be sold separately based on their content, yet are available under a single cover, offering the reader a tremendous value. I hope that the *Clinical Advisor*'s user-friendly approach, numerous unique features, and yearly updates will make this book a valuable medical reference, not only to primary care physicians but also to physicians in other specialties, medical students, and allied health professionals.

Fred F. Ferri, M.D., F.A.C.P.

EVALUATION OF EVIDENCE

Ferri's Clinical Advisor evaluates all evidence based on a rating system published by the American Academy of Family Physicians. In order to indicate the strength of the supporting evidence, each summary statement is accorded one of three levels:

LEVEL A

- Systematic reviews of randomized controlled trials, including meta-analyses
- Good-quality randomized controlled trials

LEVEL B

- Good-quality nonrandomized clinical trials
- Systematic reviews not in Level A
- Lower-quality randomized controlled trials not in Level A
- Other types of study: case-control studies, clinical cohort studies, cross-sectional studies, retrospective studies, and uncontrolled studies

LEVEL C

- Evidence-based consensus statements and expert guidelines

SOURCES OF EVIDENCE

Evidence is summarized principally from three critically evaluated, very highly regarded sources:

- **Cochrane Systematic Reviews** are respected throughout the world as one of the most rigorous searches of medical journals for randomized controlled trials. They provide highly structured systematic reviews, with evidence included or excluded on the basis of explicit quality-related criteria, and they often use meta-analyses to increase the power of the findings of numerous studies.
- ***Clinical Evidence*** is produced by the BMJ Publishing Group. It provides synopses of the best currently available evidence on the treatment and prevention of many clinical conditions, based on searches and appraisals of the available literature.
- **The National Guideline Clearinghouse** is a comprehensive database of evidence-based clinical practicc guidelines and related documents produced by the Agency for Healthcare Research and Quality in partnership with the American Medical Association and the American Association of Health Plans.

In addition, where evidence exists that has not yet been critically reviewed in one of the three sites listed here, the evidence is summarized briefly, categorized, and fully referenced. Guidelines are also sourced from governmental and professional bodies.

Contents

Detailed Contents

SECTION I Diseases and Disorders

PTG indicates that a Patient Teaching Guide is available at: www.expertconsult.com.

SECTION II **Differential Diagnosis**

SECTION III Clinical Algorithms

SECTION IV Laboratory Tests and Interpretation of Results

SECTION V Clinical Preventive Services

APPENDIX I Complementary and Alternative Medicine

APPENDIX II Primary Care Procedures

Additional PTGs Available at www.expertconsult.com Not Linked to Topics in Section I

Section I

Diseases and Disorders

BASIC INFORMATION

DEFINITION

Abruptio placentae is the separation of placenta from the uterine wall before delivery of the fetus. There are three classes of abruption based on maternal and fetal status, including an assessment of uterine contractions, quantity of bleeding, fetal heart rate monitoring, and abnormal coagulation studies (fibrinogen, PT, PTT).

- Grade I: mild vaginal bleeding, uterine irritability, stable vital signs, reassuring fetal heart rate, normal coagulation profile (fibrinogen 450 mg %)
- Grade II: moderate vaginal bleeding, hypertonic uterine contractions, orthostatic blood pressure measurements, unfavorable fetal status, fibrinogen 150 mg % to 250 mg %
- Grade III: severe bleeding (may be concealed), hypertonic uterine contractions, overt signs of hypovolemic shock, fetal death, thrombocytopenia, fibrinogen <150 mg %

SYNONYMS

Premature separation of placenta

ICD-9CM CODES
641.2 Premature separation of placenta

EPIDEMIOLOGY & DEMOGRAPHICS

INCIDENCE (IN U.S.): 1/86-206 births; incidence by grade: I = 40%, II = 45%, III = 15%; 80% occur before the onset of labor

RISK FACTORS: Hypertension (greatest association), trauma, polyhydramnios, multifetal gestation, smoking, use of crack cocaine, chorioamnionitis, preterm premature rupture of membranes

RECURRENCE RATE: 5% to 17%; with two prior episodes, 25%

PHYSICAL FINDINGS & CLINICAL PRESENTATION

- Triad of uterine bleeding (concealed or per vagina), hypertonic uterine contractions or signs of preterm labor, and evidence of fetal compromise exists.
- More than 80% of cases have external bleeding; 20% of cases have no bleeding but have indirect evidence of abruption, such as failed tocolysis for preterm labor.
- Tetanic uterine contractions are found in only 17% of cases, unless grade II or III abruption.

ETIOLOGY

- Primary etiology: unknown
- Hypertension: found in 40% to 50% of grade III abruptions
- Rapid decompression of uterine cavity, as can occur in polyhydramnios or multifetal gestation
- Blunt external trauma (motor vehicle accident, spousal abuse)

DIAGNOSIS

DIFFERENTIAL DIAGNOSIS

- Placenta previa
- Cervical or vaginal trauma
- Labor
- Cervical cancer
- Rupture of membranes
- The differential diagnosis of vaginal bleeding in pregnancy is described in Section II

WORKUP

- Initial assessment should evaluate for the source of bleeding, ruling out placenta previa and associated conditions that contraindicate any type of vaginal examination (e.g., pelvic speculum examination).
- Continuous fetal heart monitoring is indicated for all viable gestations (60% incidence of fetal distress in labor); may show early signs of maternal hypovolemia (late decelerations or fetal tachycardia) before overt maternal vital sign changes.
- Actual amount of blood loss is often greater than initially perceived because of the possibility of concealed retroplacental bleeding and apparent "normal" vital signs. The relative hypervolemia of pregnancy initially protects the patient until late in the course of bleeding, when abrupt and sudden cardiovascular collapse can occur.

LABORATORY TESTS

- Baseline Hgb and HCT help quantify blood loss and establish baseline values for serious comparisons during expectant management.
- Coagulation profile: platelets, fibrinogen, prothrombin, and partial thromboplastin time. DIC can develop with severe abruption. If fibrinogen is <150 mg %, estimated blood loss is approximately 2000 ml, and if fibrinogen is <100 mg %, consider FFP to prevent further bleeding.
- Type and antibody screen is important to identify Rh-negative patients who may need Rh immune globulin.

IMAGING STUDIES

Ultrasound should include fetal presentation and status, amniotic fluid volume, placental location, as well as any evidence of hematoma (retroplacental, subchorionic, or preplacental).

TREATMENT

ACUTE GENERAL Rx

- Stabilization of the mother is the first priority.
- Treatment is dependent on gestational age of the fetus, severity of the abruption, and maternal status.
- Initial assessment for signs of maternal hemodynamic compromise or hemorrhagic shock; large-bore intravenous access, with crystalloid fluid resuscitation using a replacement of 3 ml LR solution for every 1 ml estimated blood loss.
- Indwelling Foley catheter to monitor urine output and maternal volume status, with a goal of 30 ml/hr urine output.
- Assess fetal status and gestational age using sonogram and continuous fetal heart rate monitoring.
- Because of the unpredictable nature of abruptions, cross-matched blood should be made available during the initial resuscitation period.

CHRONIC Rx

- In the term fetus or when lung maturity has been documented, delivery is indicated.
- In the preterm fetus or a fetus with an immature lung profile, consider betamethasone 12.5 mg IM q24h for two doses and then delivery, depending on the severity of the abruption and the likelihood of fetal complications from preterm birth.
- C-section should be reserved for cases of fetal distress or for standard obstetric indications.
- In select cases, such as severe prematurity with a stable mother and mild contractions, magnesium sulfate can be used for tocolysis, 6 g IV loading dose then 3 g/hr maintenance, to allow for course of steroids.

DISPOSITION

Because of the unpredictable nature of abruptions, expectant management should occur only under controlled circumstances.

REFERRAL

Abruptio placentae places mother and fetus in a high-risk situation and should be managed by a qualified obstetrician in a facility with capability for neonatal and maternal resuscitation and ability to perform emergency C-sections.

AUTHORS: **SCOTT J. ZUCCALA, D.O.,** and **RUBEN ALVERO, M.D.**

Section I
DISEASES AND DISORDERS

BASIC INFORMATION

DEFINITION

A brain abscess is a focal, intracerebral infection that begins as a localized area of cerebritis and develops into a collection of pus surrounded by a well-vascularized capsule.

ICD-9CM CODES
324.0 Brain abscess

EPIDEMIOLOGY & DEMOGRAPHICS

INCIDENCE: Quite uncommon (occurs about 2% as commonly as brain tumors)
PEAK INCIDENCE: Preadolescence and middle age
PREDOMINANT AGE: Occurs at any age
PREDOMINANT SEX: Men affected more than women

- Most common source of underlying infection: Contiguous spread from the paranasal sinuses, middle ear, or teeth.

PHYSICAL FINDINGS & CLINICAL PRESENTATION

- Classic triad: fever, headache, and focal neurologic deficit are present in 50% of cases.
- Fever is present in only 50% of patients.
- Headache is usually localized to the side of the abscess, onset can be gradual or severe; present in 70% of cases.
- Focal neurologic findings (e.g., seizures, hemiparesis, aphasia, ataxia) depend on the location of the abscess and are seen in 30% to 50% of cases.
- Papilledema is present in 25% of cases.
- Presence of adjacent infections (dental abscess, otitis media, and sinusitis) may be a clue to the underlying diagnosis and should be sought in any suspected case.
- Time course from symptom onset to presentation ranges from hours in fulminant cases to more than 1 mo; 75% present in the first 2 wk.
- The nonspecific presentation of a brain abscess warrants that clinicians maintain a high index of suspicion.

ETIOLOGY

- Brain abscesses arise from:
  Contiguous infection
  Hematogenous spread from a remote site
- They are classified based on the likely portal of entry.

Likely source of abscess:

A. Contiguous focus or primary infection (55% of all brain abscesses):
   1. Paranasal sinus: occur in frontal lobe; streptococci, *Bacteroides, Haemophilus,* and *Fusobacterium* species
   2. Otitis media/mastoiditis: occur in temporal lobe and cerebellum; streptococci, Enterobacteriaceae, *Bacteroides,* and *Pseudomonas* species
   3. Dental sepsis: occur in frontal lobe; mixed *Fusobacterium, Bacteroides,* and *Streptococcus* species
   4. Penetrating head injury: site of abscess depends on site of wound; *Staphylococcus aureus, Clostridium* species, Enterobacteriaceae species
   5. Postoperative: *Staphylococcus epidermidis* and *S. aureus,* Enterobacteriaceae, and Pseudomonadaceae

B. Hematogenous spread/distant site of infection (25% of all brain abscesses): abscesses most commonly multiple, especially in middle cerebral artery distribution; infecting organisms depend on source.
   1. Congenital heart disease: streptococci, *Haemophilus* species
   2. Endocarditis: *S. aureus,* viridans streptococci
   3. Urinary tract: Enterobacteriaceae, Pseudomonadaceae
   4. Intraabdominal: streptococci, Enterobacteriaceae, anaerobes
   5. Lung: streptococci, *Actinomyces* species, *Fusobacterium* species
   6. Immunocompromised host: *Toxoplasma* species, fungi, Enterobacteriaceae, *Nocardia* species, tuberculosis, listeriosis

C. Cryptogenic (unknown source): 20% of all brain abscesses

DIAGNOSIS (Dx)

DIFFERENTIAL DIAGNOSIS

- Other parameningeal infections: subdural empyema, epidural abscess, thrombophlebitis of the major dural venous sinuses and cortical veins
- Embolic strokes in patients with bacterial endocarditis
- Mycotic aneurysms with leakage
- Viral encephalitis (usually resulting from herpes simplex)
- Acute hemorrhagic leukoencephalitis
- Parasitic infections: toxoplasmosis, echinococcosis, cysticercosis
- Metastatic or primary brain tumors
- Cerebral infarction
- CNS vasculitis
- Chronic subdural hematoma

WORKUP

Physical examination, laboratory tests, and imaging studies

LABORATORY TESTS

- WBC counts are elevated in 60% of patients.
- ESR is usually elevated, but may be normal.
- Blood cultures are most often negative (10% positive).
- Lumbar puncture is contraindicated in patients with suspected abscess (20% die or suffer neurologic decline).
- The yield of Gram stain and culture of material aspirated at time of surgical drainage approaches 100%.

IMAGING STUDIES

- MRI is the diagnostic procedure of choice; provides superior detail compared with CT scan (higher sensitivity and specificity than CT scan, but not always immediately available).
- CT scan (Fig. 1-1) with intravenous contrast is still an excellent test (sensitivity 95% to 99%).

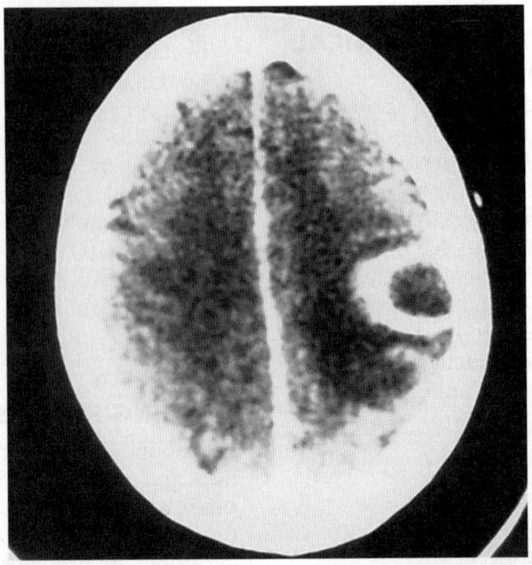

FIGURE 1-1 Computed tomography (CT) scan showing a brain abscess. A woman presented to physicians after a focal seizure followed by headache and weakness of the arm. Dental work had been performed several weeks before. CT scan revealed a contrast-enhanced, ringlike mass surrounded by edema. It is not possible on this scan to differentiate tumor from abscess. At surgery a well-encapsulated abscess was encountered. (From Andreoli TE [ed]: *Cecil essentials of medicine,* ed 4, Philadelphia, 1997, WB Saunders.)

- Serial CT or MRI scanning is recommended to follow the response to therapy.

TREATMENT

ACUTE GENERAL Rx

- Effective treatment involves a combination of empiric antibiotic therapy and timely excision or aspiration of the abscess.
- If evidence of edema or mass effect, treatment of elevated intracranial pressure is paramount.
  - Hyperventilation of mechanically ventilated patient.
  - Dexamethasone initially in a dosage of 10 mg IV followed by 4 mg IV q6h until symptoms of cerebral edema subside. Dosage may be reduced after 2 to 4 days and gradually discontinued over a period of 5 to 7 days.
  - Mannitol 0.25 to 1 gram/kg IV over 20 to 30 min q6 to 8h; Maximum of 6 g/kg in 24 hr.
- Medical therapy is never a substitute for surgical intervention to relieve increased intracranial pressure. Neurologic deterioration usually mandates surgery.
- Steroids should be limited to patients with severe cerebral edema or midline shift.

MEDICAL Rx

If abscess <2.5 cm and patient is neurologically stable and conscious, may start antibiotics and observe. Empiric antibiotic therapy guided by:

- Abscess location
- Suspicion of primary source
- Presence of single or multiple abscesses
- Patient's underlying medical conditions (e.g., HIV, immunocompromised)

Selection of empiric antibiotic therapy:

- Primary infection or contiguous source:
  1. Otitis media/mastoiditis, sinusitis, dental infection: third-generation cephalosporin (cefotaxime 2 g q6h IV or ceftriaxone 2 g q12h IV) plus metronidazole 15 mg/kg IV as a loading dose, then 7.5 mg/kg q6h IV or 15 mg/kg q12h IV
  2. Dental infection: penicillin G 6 million units q6° plus metronidazole 15 mg/kg IV as a loading dose, then 7.5 mg/kg IV q6h or 15 mg/kg IV q12h
  3. Head trauma or postcranial surgery: third-generation cephalosporin (cefotaxime 2 g IV q6h or ceftriaxone 2 g IV q12h) plus metronidazole 7.5 mg/kg IV q6h or 15 mg/kg IV q12h and nafcillin 2 g IV q4h or vancomycin (30 mg/kg IV in two divided doses adjusted for renal function)
- Hematogenous spread (congenital heart disease, endocarditis, urinary tract, lung, intraabdominal): nafcillin or vancomycin plus metronidazole plus third-generation cephalosporin (cefotaxime 2 g IV q6h or ceftriaxone 2 g IV q12h)

Duration of antibiotic therapy is unclear. Most recommend parenteral treatment for 4 to 8 wk, with repeated neuroimaging to ensure adequate treatment. (Imaging suggested every wk for first 2 wk of therapy, then every 2 wk until antibiotics finished, and then every 2 to 4 mo for 1 yr to monitor for disease recurrence.)

SURGICAL Rx

- Two indications for surgical intervention:
  1. Collect specimens for culture and sensitivity
  2. Reduce mass effect
- Stereotactic biopsy or aspirate of the abscess if surgically feasible
- Essential to selection of targeted antimicrobial coverage
- Timing and choice of surgery depends on:
  - Primary infection source
  - Number and location of the abscesses
  - Whether the procedure is diagnostic or therapeutic
  - Neurologic status of the patient

DISPOSITION

- Prompt diagnostic consideration, early institution of appropriate antimicrobial therapy, and advanced neuroradiologic imaging have reduced the mortality resulting from brain abscesses from 40% to 80% in the preantibiotic era to 10% to 20% at present.
- Morbidity is usually manifest as persistent neurologic sequelae (seizures, intellectual or behavioral impairment, motor deficits) seen in 20% to 60% of patients.

REFERRAL

Consultation with a neurosurgeon is mandatory.

PEARLS & CONSIDERATIONS

COMMENTS

- It is important to maintain a high index of suspicion because a brain abscess often presents with nonspecific symptoms.
- Rapid imaging and early institution of appropriate antimicrobial therapy improves patient morbidity and mortality.
- Neurosurgical consultation is mandatory.

PREVENTION

Because brain abscesses arise from either contiguous infections or hematogenously from a remote site, early and appropriate treatment of inciting infections is paramount to prevention of brain abscess.

EVIDENCE

Although antimicrobial therapy and surgical drainage are the mainstays of the clinical management of brain abscess, evidence for these therapies is limited.

SUGGESTED READINGS

Bhand AA: Brain abscess—diagnosis and management, *J Coll Physicians Surg Pak* 14:7, 2004.

Carpenter J et al: Retrospective analysis of 49 cases of brain abscess and review of the literature, *Eur J Clin Microbiol Infect Dis* 26:1, 2007.

Gomes JA et al: Glucocorticoid therapy in neurologic critical care, *Crit Care Med* 33(6).1211, 2005.

Kao PT et al: Brain abscess: clinical analysis of 53 cases, *J Microbiol Immunol Infect* 36:2, 2003.

McClelland S 3rd et al: Postoperative central nervous system infections: incidence and associated factors in 2111 neurosurgical procedures, *Clin Infect Dis* 45;1, 2007.

Tattevin P et al: Bacterial brain abscesses: a retrospective study of 94 patients admitted to an intensive care unit (1980–1999), *Am J Med* 115:143, 2003.

The rational use of antibiotics in the treatment of brain abscess: Report by the "Infection in Neurosurgery" Working Party of the British Society for Antimicrobial Chemotherapy, *Br J Neurosurg* 14(6):525, 2000.

AUTHOR: **KELLY MCGARRY, M.D.**

BASIC INFORMATION

DEFINITION

Breast abscess is an acute inflammatory process resulting in the formation of a collection of pus. Typically there is painful erythematous mass formation in the breast, occasionally draining through the overlying skin or nipple duct.

SYNONYMS

Subareolar abscess
Lactational or puerperal abscess

ICD-9CM CODES
6.110 Abscess of the breast
675.0 Abscess of the nipple related to childbirth
675.1 Abscess of the breast related to childbirth

EPIDEMIOLOGY & DEMOGRAPHICS

INCIDENCE: 10% to 30% of all breast abscesses are lactational; acute mastitis occurs in 2.5% of nursing mothers, with 1 in 15 of these women developing abscess.

PHYSICAL FINDINGS & CLINICAL PRESENTATION

Painful erythematous induration involving breast and leading to fluctuant abscess

ETIOLOGY

- Lactational abscess: milk stasis and bacterial infection leading to mastitis and then abscess, with *Staphylococcus aureus* the most common causative agent
- Subareolar abscess:
  1. Central ducts involved, with obstructive nipple duct changes leading to bacterial infection
  2. Cultured organisms mixed, including anaerobes, staphylococci, streptococci, and others

DIAGNOSIS

DIFFERENTIAL DIAGNOSIS

- Inflammatory carcinoma
- Advanced carcinoma with erythema, edema, and/or ulceration
- Tuberculous abscess (rare in the United States)
- Hydradenitis of breast skin
- Sebaceous cyst with infection

WORKUP

- Clinical examination sufficient
- If abscess suspected, referral to surgeon for incision, drainage, and biopsy
- If possible abscess or advanced carcinoma, referral for workup required

LABORATORY TESTS

- Perform C&S test of abscess contents.
- If mammogram or ultrasound required and prevented by discomfort, perform after resolution of abscess.

TREATMENT

NONPHARMACOLOGIC THERAPY

- Established abscess: incision and drainage, preferably with general anesthesia
- Biopsy of abscess cavity wall to exclude carcinoma

ACUTE GENERAL Rx

- Antibiotics: generally staphylococci in lactational abscess. Recommended initial antibiotic therapy is nafcillin or oxacillin 2 g q4h IV or cefazolin 1 g q8h IV for 10 to 14 days. Alternative includes vancomycin 1 g IV q12h.
- If acute mastitis is treated early, resolution without drainage is possible.
- Subareolar abscess: broad-spectrum antibiotic treatment (e.g., cephalexin 500 mg PO qid or cefazolin 1 g q8h IV for 10 to 14 days for more severe infection) and drainage are needed to control acute phase.

CHRONIC Rx

Further surgical treatment for recurrences or fistula

DISPOSITION

- Lactational abscess: possible to continue breast-feeding without apparent risk of infection to the infant
- Subareolar abscess:
  1. Notorious for recurrence or complication of fistula formation
  2. Patient informed and referred for subsequent care

REFERRAL

- If abscess drainage required
- For surgical consultation if subareolar abscess involved

SUGGESTED READINGS

Schwarz RJ, Shrestha R: Needle aspiration of breast abscesses, *Am J Surg* 182(2):117, 2001.

Tan YM, Yeo A, Chia KH, Wong CY: Breast abscess as the initial presentation of squamous cell of the breast, *Eur J Surg Oncol* 28(1):91, 2002.

AUTHORS: **TAKUMA NEMOTO, M.D.,** and **RUBEN ALVERO, M.D.**

BASIC INFORMATION

DEFINITION

Liver abscess is a necrotic infection of the liver usually classified as pyogenic or amebic.

SYNONYMS

Pyogenic hepatic abscess
Amebic hepatic abscess

ICD-9CM CODES
572.0 Abscess of liver

EPIDEMIOLOGY & DEMOGRAPHICS

INCIDENCE: Incidence of pyogenic liver abscess is 2.3 cases per 100,000 population.

PREVALANCE (WORLDWIDE): Amebic liver abscess is more common than pyogenic liver abscess.

PREVALENCE (IN U.S.): Pyogenic liver abscess is more common than amebic liver abscess.

PREDOMINANT SEX AND AGE: More common in men than women; Male:female ratio, 2:1; most common in fourth to sixth decade of life.

PHYSICAL FINDINGS & CLINICAL PRESENTATION

- Fever, chills, and sweats
- Weakness/Malaise
- Anorexia with weight loss
- Nausea, vomiting, and diarrhea
- Cough with pleuritic chest pain
- Right upper quadrant abdominal pain
- Hepatomegaly
- Splenomegaly
- Jaundice
- Pleural effusions, rales, and friction rubs may be present
- Most abscesses occur on the right lobe of the liver

ETIOLOGY

- Pyogenic liver abscess is usually polymicrobial (*K. pneumoniae* [43%], *E. coli* [33%], *Streptococcal Sp* [37%], *P. aeruginosa, Proteus, Bacteroides* [24%], *Fusobacterium, Actinomyces,* gram-positive anaerobes, and *S. aureus).*
- Amebic hepatic abscess is caused by the parasite *Entamoeba histolytica.*
- Pyogenic liver abscess occurs from:
  1. Biliary disease with cholangitis (accounts for approximately 40% to 60%)
  2. Gallbladder disease with contiguous spread to the liver
  3. Diverticulitis or appendicitis with spread via the portal circulation
  4. Hematogenous spread via the hepatic artery, though uncommon; if a solitary organism is isolated, a distant source of hematogenous seeding should be sought.
  5. Penetrating wounds
  6. Cryptogenic
  7. Infection via portal system (portal pyemia)
  8. No causes found in approximately half of cases
  9. Incidence increased in patients with diabetes and metastatic cancer
- Amebiasis is usually due to fecal-oral contamination and invades the intestinal mucosa gaining entry into the portal system to reach the liver.

DIAGNOSIS

The diagnosis of liver abscess requires a high index of suspicion after a detailed history and physical examination. Imaging studies, microbiologic, serologic, and percutaneous techniques (e.g., aspiration) confirm the presence of a liver abscess.

DIFFERENTIAL DIAGNOSIS

- Cholangitis
- Cholecystitis
- Diverticulitis
- Appendicitis
- Perforated viscus
- Mesentery ischemia
- Pulmonary embolism
- Pancreatitis

WORKUP

- The workup of a liver abscess should focus on differentiating between amebic and pyogenic causes.
- Features suggesting an amebic cause include travel to an endemic area, single abscess rather than multiple abscesses, subacute onset of symptoms, and absence of conditions predisposing to pyogenic liver abscess as highlighted under "Etiology."
- Laboratory studies are not specific but useful as adjunctive tests.
- Imaging studies cannot differentiate between the two, and bacteriologic cultures may be sterile in 50% of the cases.

LABORATORY TESTS

- CBC showing leukocytosis
- Liver function tests: alkaline phosphatase is most commonly elevated (95% to 100%); AST and ALT elevated in 50% of cases; elevated bilirubin (28% to 30%); decreased albumin
- PT (INR) prolonged (70%)
- Blood cultures positive in 50% of cases
- Aspiration (50% sterile)
- Stool samples for *E. histolytica* trophozoites (positive in 10% to 15% of amebic liver abscess cases)
- Serologic testing for *E. histolytica* does not differentiate acute from old infections

IMAGING STUDIES

- Ultrasound (80% to 100% sensitivity in detecting abscesses) seen as round or oval hypoechogenic mass.
- CT scans more sensitive in detecting hepatic abscesses and contiguous organ extension (Fig. 1-2). Imaging study of choice.
- Chest x-ray examination abnormal in 50% of the cases: showing elevated right hemidiaphragm, subdiaphragmatic air-fluid levels, pleural effusions, and consolidating infiltrates.
- Most liver abscesses are single; however, multiple liver abscesses are seen with systemic bacteremia.

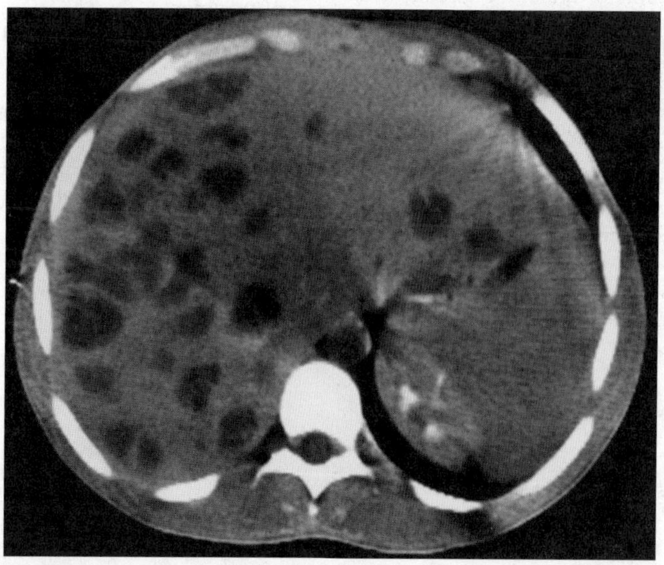

FIGURE 1-2 CT scan demonstrating multiple pyogenic liver abscesses in a 25-year-old man. (From Goldman L, Bennett JC [ed]: *Cecil textbook of medicine,* ed 21, Philadelphia, 2000, WB Saunders.)

TREATMENT

Rx

NONPHARMACOLOGIC THERAPY

- The management of pyogenic liver abscess differs from that of amebic liver abscess.
- Medical management is the cornerstone of therapy in amebic liver abscess, whereas early intervention in the form of surgical therapy or catheter drainage and parenteral antibiotics is the rule in pyogenic liver abscess.

ACUTE GENERAL Rx

- Percutaneous drainage under CT or ultrasound guidance is essential in the treatment of pyogenic liver abscesses.
- Aspiration of hepatic amebic abscesses is not required unless there is no response to treatment or a pyogenic cause is being considered.
- Empiric broad spectrum antibiotics are recommended initially until culture results are available. Common choices include:
  1. Metronidazole (500 mg IV q8h) plus a fluoroquinolone (ciprofloxacin 400 mg IV q12h or levofloxacin 500 mg IV daily).
  2. Monotherapy with a beta-lactam/beta-lactamase inhibitor, such as piperacillin/tazobactam (4.5 g q6h), ticarcillin-clavulanate (3.1 g q4h), or ampicillin-sulbactam (3 g q6h).
  3. Monotherapy with a carbapenem, such as imipenem (500 mg IV q6h), meropenem (1 g q8h), or ertapenem (1 g daily).
  4. In patients with penicillin allergy, clindamycin 600 to 900 mg IV q8h with an aminoglycoside can be considered.
  5. Duration of antibiotic treatment is usually 4 to 6 wk with IV antibiotics used for the first 1 to 2 wk or until a favorable clinical response, followed thereafter with PO antibiotics (e.g., metronidazole 500 mg PO q8h plus cipro 500 mg PO q12h).
  6. Third-generation cephalosporins should not be used for empiric therapy for risk of the emergence of extended-spectrum beta-lactamase-producing bacteria.
- Antibiotic coverage for amebic liver abscesses includes:
  1. Metronidazole 750 mg PO tid for 10 days
  2. Dehydroemetine 1 mg/kg/day IM for 5 days followed by chloroquine 1 g/day for 2 days; then 500 mg/day for 2 to 3 wk can be used as an alternative to metronidazole

CHRONIC Rx

- If fever persists for 2 wk despite percutaneous drainage and antibiotic therapy as outlined under "Acute General Rx," or if there is failure of aspiration or failure of percutaneous drainage, surgery is indicated.
- In patients failing intravenous antibiotics and percutaneous drainage, hepatic artery antibiotic infusion can be considered.
- In patients with evidence of metastatic disease that is causing biliary obstruction, a gastroenterology consultation for ERCP and stenting should be considered.

DISPOSITION

- Most patients with pyogenic liver abscesses defervesce within 2 wk of treatment with antibiotics and drainage.
- No randomized controlled studies have evaluated the optimal duration of antibiotic therapy for pyogenic liver abscess. Typical duration of antibiotic therapy is at least 4 to 6 wk.
- Pyogenic liver abscess cure rates using percutaneous drainage and antibiotics have been reported to be between 88% and 100%.
- Mortality of untreated pyogenic liver abscess is nearly 100%.
- Most patients with amebic liver abscesses defervesce within 4 to 5 days of treatment.
- Amebic liver abscess mortality rate is <1% unless complications occur (see under Comments).
- Follow-up imaging to monitor response to therapy: continue treatment until CT scan shows complete or near complete resolution of cavity.

REFERRAL

Infectious disease, gastroenterology, interventional radiology, and general surgical consultations are recommended in any patient with a single hepatic abscess or multiple abscesses.

PEARLS & CONSIDERATIONS

!

COMMENTS

- Complications of pyogenic and amebic liver abscesses include:
  1. Pleuropulmonary extension resulting in empyema, abscess, and fistula formation
  2. Peritonitis
  3. Purulent pericarditis
  4. Sepsis
- Amebic liver abscesses complicate amebic colitis in nearly 10% of cases.

SUGGESTED READINGS

Blessman J et al: Treatment of amoebic liver abscess with metronidazole alone or in combination with ultrasound guided needle aspiration: a comparative, prospective and randomized study, *Trop Med Int Health* 8(11):1030, 2003.

Kaplan GG et al: Population-based study of the epidemiology of and the risk factors for pyogenic liver abscess, *Clin Gastroenterol Hepatol* 2(11):1032, 2004.

Kurland JE et al: Pyogenic and amebic liver abscess, *Curr Gastroenterol Rep* 6(4):273, 2004.

Lederman ER et al: Pyogenic liver abscess with a focus on *Klebsiella pneumonae* as a primary pathogen: an emerging disease with unique clinical characteristics, *Am J Gastroenterol* 100:322, 2005.

Lodhi S et al: Features distinguishing amebic from pyogenic liver abscess: a review of 577 adult cases, *Trop Med Int Health* 9(6):718, 2004.

Yu SC et al: Treatment of pyogenic liver abscess: prospective randomized comparison of catheter drainage and needle aspiration, *Hepatology* 39(9):932, 2004.

AUTHOR: **TANYA ALI, M.D.**

BASIC INFORMATION

DEFINITION

A lung abscess is an infection of the lung parenchyma resulting in a necrotic cavity containing pus.

SYNONYMS

Pulmonary abscess

ICD-9CM CODES
513.0 Abscess of lung

EPIDEMIOLOGY & DEMOGRAPHICS

INCIDENCE: Has decreased over the last 30 years as a result of antibiotic therapy.

- Lung abscess in patients age 50 and over is associated with primary lung neoplasia in 30% of the cases.
- Lung abscesses commonly coexist with empyemas.

RISK FACTORS:

1. Alcohol-related problems
2. Seizure disorders
3. Cerebrovascular disorders with dysphagia
4. Drug abuse
5. Esophageal disorders (e.g., scleroderma, esophageal carcinoma, etc.)
6. Poor oral hygiene
7. Obstructive malignant lung disease
8. Bronchiectasis

PHYSICAL FINDINGS & CLINICAL PRESENTATION

- Symptoms are generally insidious and prolonged, occurring for weeks to months
- Fever, chills, and sweats
- Cough
- Sputum production (purulent with foul odor)
- Pleuritic chest pain
- Hemoptysis
- Dyspnea
- Malaise, fatigue, and weakness
- Tachycardia and tachypnea
- Dullness to percussion, whispered pectoriloquy, and bronchophony
- Amphoric breath sounds (low pitched sound of air moving across a large open cavity)

ETIOLOGY

- The most important factor predisposing to lung abscess is aspiration.
- Following aspiration as a major predisposing factor is periodontal disease.
- Lung abscess is rare in an edentulous person.
- Approximately 90% of lung abscesses are caused by anaerobic microorganisms (*Bacteroides fragilis, Fusobacterium nucleatum,* peptostreptococci, microaerophilic streptococci). Pulmonary actinomycosis will also generate lung abscess.
- In most cases anaerobic infection is mixed with aerobic or facultative anaerobic organisms *(S. aureus, E. coli, K. pneumoniae, P. aeruginosa).*
- Parasitic organisms including Paragonimus westermani and Entamoeba histolytica.
- Fungi including *Aspergillus, Cryptococcus, Histoplasma, Blastomyces,* and *Coccidioides spp.*
- Immunocompromised hosts may become infected with *Aspergillus,* mycobacteria, *Nocardia, Legionella micdadei,* and *Rhodococcus equi.*

DIAGNOSIS (Dx)

Lung abscess may be primary or secondary.

- Primary lung abscess refers to infection from normal host organisms within the lung (e.g., aspiration, pneumonia).
- Secondary lung abscess results from other preexisting conditions (e.g., endocarditis, underlying lung cancer, pulmonary emboli).

Lung abscess may be acute or chronic.

- Acute lung abscess is present if symptoms are of less than 4 to 6 wk.
- Chronic lung abscess is present if symptoms are greater than 6 wk.

DIFFERENTIAL DIAGNOSIS

The differential diagnosis is similar to that for cavitary lung lesions:

- Bacterial (anaerobic, aerobic, infected bulla, empyema, actinomycosis, tuberculosis)
- Fungal (histoplasmosis, coccidioidomycosis, blastomycosis, aspergillosis, cryptococcosis)
- Parasitic (amebiasis, echinococcosis)
- Malignancy (primary lung carcinoma, metastatic lung disease, lymphoma, Hodgkin's disease)
- Wegener's granulomatosis, sarcoidosis, endocarditis, and septic pulmonary emboli

WORKUP

- The workup of a patient with lung abscess attempts to elicit a primary or a secondary cause.
- Blood tests are not specific in diagnosing lung abscesses.
- Most diagnoses are made from imaging studies; however, to diagnose a specific cause bacteriologic studies are needed.

LABORATORY TESTS

- CBC with leukocytosis
- Bacteriologic studies
  1. Sputum Gram stain and culture (commonly contaminated by oral flora)
  2. Percutaneous transtracheal aspiration
  3. Percutaneous transthoracic aspiration
  4. Fiberoptic bronchoscopy using bronchial brushings or bronchoalveolar lavage is the most widely used intervention when trying to obtain diagnostic bacteriologic cultures
- Blood cultures on some occasions may be positive
- If an empyema is present, obtaining empyema fluid via thoracentesis may isolate the organism

IMAGING STUDIES

- Chest x-ray examination makes the diagnosis of lung abscess showing the cavitary lesion with an air fluid level.
- Lung abscesses are most commonly found in the posterior segment of the right upper lobe.
- Chest CT scan can localize and size the lesion and assist in differentiating lung abscesses from other pathologic processes (e.g., tumor, empyema, infected bulla, etc.) (Fig. 1-3).

TREATMENT (Rx)

NONPHARMACOLOGIC THERAPY

- Oxygen therapy
- Postural drainage
- Respiratory therapy maneuvers

ACUTE GENERAL Rx

- Penicillin 1 to 2 million units IV q4h until improvement (e.g., afebrile, decrease in sputum production, etc.) followed by penicillin VK 500 mg PO qid for the next 2 to 3 wk but usually requiring longer 6- to 8-wk courses.
- Metronidazole is given with penicillin at doses of 7.5 mg/kg IV q6h followed by PO 500 mg bid to qid dosing.
- Clindamycin is an alternative choice if concerned about penicillin-resistant organisms. The dose is 600 mg IV q8h until improvement followed by 300 mg PO q6h.

CHRONIC Rx

- Bronchoscopy to assist with drainage and/or diagnosis is indicated in patients who fail to respond to antibiotics or if there is suspected underlying malignancy.
- Surgery is indicated on rare occasions (<10%) in patients with complications of lung abscess (see "Comments").

DISPOSITION

- More than 95% of patients are cured with the use of antibiotics alone.
- Complications of lung abscesses include:
  1. Empyema
  2. Massive hemoptysis

3. Pneumothorax
4. Bronchopleural fistula

- Mortality is low in community-acquired lung abscess (2.5%).
- Hospital-acquired lung abscess carries a high mortality rate (65%).

REFERRAL

If lung abscess is present, consultation with pulmonary and infectious disease specialist is recommended.

PEARLS & CONSIDERATIONS

COMMENTS

- Complications of lung abscesses include:
  1. Empyema
  2. Bronchopleural fistula
  3. Hepatobronchial fistula
  4. Brain abscess
  5. Bronchiectasis
- Refractory cases are usually the result of:
  1. Large cavity size (>6 cm)
  2. Recurrent aspiration
  3. Thick-walled cavities
  4. Underlying lung carcinoma
  5. Empyema formation
- Necrotizing pneumonia is similar to a lung abscess but differs in size (<2 cm in diameter) and number (usually multiple suppurative cavitary lesions).

SUGGESTED READINGS

Finegold SM: Lung abscess. In *Mandell, Douglas, and Bennett's principles and practice of infectious diseases,* ed 5, New York, 2000, Churchill Livingstone.

Herth F et al: Endoscopic drainage of lung abscesses: technique and outcome, *Chest* 127(4):1378, 2005.

Levison J et al: The value of a CT-guided fine needle aspirate in infants with lung abscess, *J Paediatr Child Health* 40(8):474, 2004.

Mansharamani NG, Koziel H: Chronic lung sepsis: lung abscess, bronchiectasis, and empyema, *Curr Opin Pulm Med* 9(3):181, 2003.

Mansharamani N et al: Lung abscess in adults: clinical comparison of immunocompromised to non-immunocompromised patients, *Respir Med* 96(3):178, 2002.

Schiza S, Siafakas NM: Clinical presentation and management of empyema, lung abscess and pleural effusion, *Curr Opin Pulm Med* 12(3):205, 2006.

AUTHORS: **GLENN G. FORT, M.D., M.P.H.,** and **DENNIS J. MIKOLICH, M.D.**

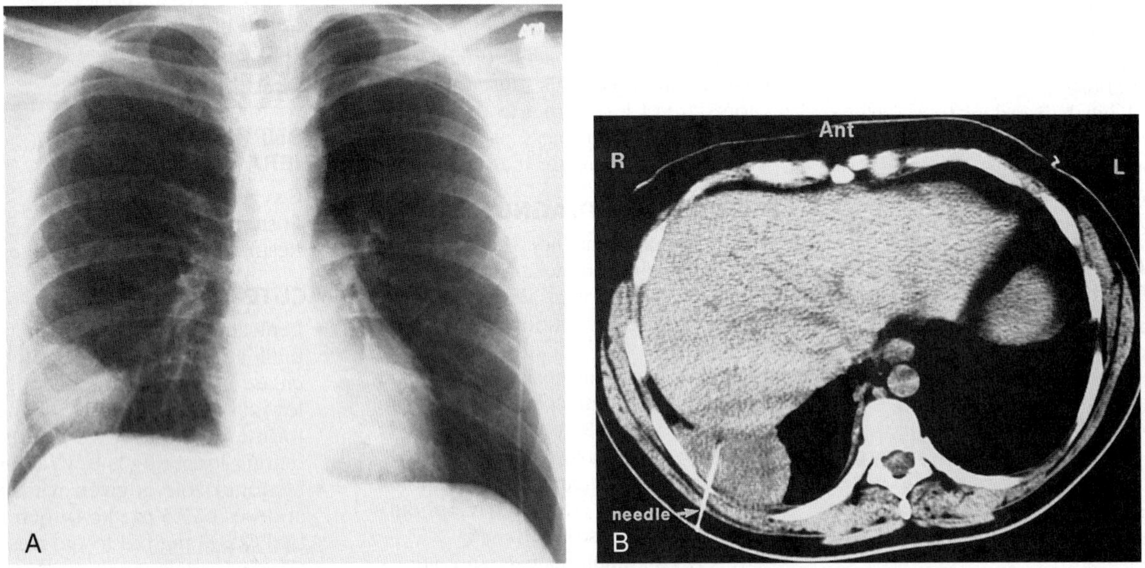

FIGURE 1-3 Lung abscess. On a chest radiograph, a lung abscess may look to be a solid rounded lesion **(A),** or, if it has a connection with the bronchus, there may be an air fluid level in a thick-walled cavitary lesion. CT scanning **(B)** can be used to localize the lesion and to place a needle for drainage and aspiration of contents for culture. (From Mettler FA [ed]: *Primary care radiology,* Philadelphia, 2000, WB Saunders.)

BASIC INFORMATION

DEFINITION

Pelvic abscess is an acute or chronic infection, most commonly involving the pelvic viscera, initially localized and creating its own unique environment so that treatment and possible cure require directed therapy. There are four categories based on etiologic factors:

- Ascending infection, spreading from cervix through endometrial cavity to adnexa, forming a tuboovarian complex
- Infection occurring in the puerperium, which spreads to the adnexa from the endometrium or myometrium via hematogenous or lymphatic route
- Abscess complicating pelvic surgery
- Involvement of the pelvic viscera secondary to spread from contiguous organs, such as appendicitis or diverticulitis

SYNONYMS

Tuboovarian abscess (TOA)
Vaginal cuff abscess

ICD-9CM CODES
614.2 Salpingitis and oophoritis not specified as acute, subacute, or chronic

EPIDEMIOLOGY & DEMOGRAPHICS

INCIDENCE:

- 34% of hospitalized patients with PID
- 1% to 2% of patients undergoing hysterectomy, most with vaginal approach
- Peak incidence third to fourth decade
- 25% to 50% are nulliparous

RISK FACTORS: Same risk factors as for PID, although in 30% to 50% of patients there is no prior history of salpingitis before abscess forms.

PHYSICAL FINDINGS & CLINICAL PRESENTATION

- Abdominal or pelvic pain (90%)
- Fever or chills (50%)
- Abnormal bleeding (21%)
- Vaginal discharge (28%)
- Nausea (26%)
- Up to 60% to 80% present in the absence of fever or leukocytosis; absence of these findings should not rule out diagnosis

ETIOLOGY

- Mixed flora of anaerobes, aerobes, and facultative anaerobes, such as *E. coli, B. fragilis, Prevotella* species, aerobic streptococci, *Peptococcus,* and *Peptostreptococcus.*
- *N. gonorrhoeae* and *Chlamydia* are the major etiologic factors in cervicitis and salpingitis but are rarely found in abscess cavity cultures.
- In elderly patients, consider diverticular disease.

DIAGNOSIS

DIFFERENTIAL DIAGNOSIS

- Pelvic neoplasms, such as ovarian tumors and leiomyomas.
- Inflammatory masses involving adjacent bowel or omentum, such as ruptured appendicitis or diverticulitis.
- Pelvic hematomas, as may occur after C-section or hysterectomy.
- Section III describes the diagnostic approach to patients with a pelvic mass; the differential diagnosis of pelvic mass is described in Section II.
- The differential diagnosis of pelvic pain is described in Section II.
- Physical examination.
- Sonogram or CT scan: commonly employed because, owing to associated pain and guarding, a suboptimal abdominal or pelvic examination is the rule rather than the exception.
- Most common cause of preventable death: physician delay in diagnosis.

LABORATORY TESTS

- CBC including WBC with differential, Hgb, and HCT
- Aerobic, as well as anaerobic, cultures of cervix, blood, urine, sputum, peritoneal cavity (if entered), and abscess cavity before starting antibiotics
- Pregnancy test in patients of reproductive age if the possibility of pregnancy exists

IMAGING STUDIES

- Sonogram: noninvasive, inexpensive study to confirm diagnosis, estimate size of abscess, and monitor response to therapy; sensitivity >90%
- CT scan: used for both diagnosis and therapy (CT-guided drainage)
  1. Useful where sonogram provides insufficient information, as with intraabdominal abscesses
  2. Success rate with CT-guided abscess drainage: unilocular, 90%; multilocular, 40%

TREATMENT

Major concerns:

1. Desire for future fertility
2. Likelihood of rupture of abscess, with resulting peritonitis, septic shock, and morbid sequelae

ACUTE GENERAL Rx

- Clinical quandary is whether patient requires immediate surgery (uncertain diagnosis or suspicion of rupture) or management with IV antibiotics, reserving surgery for those with inadequate clinical response (e.g., 48 to 72 hr of therapy, with persistent fever or leukocytosis, increasing size of mass, or suspicion of rupture)
- Surgery indicated in poor response to medical therapy in those with large adnexal masses (>8 cm) or immunocompromised patients
- Antibiotic combinations:
  1. Clindamycin 900 mg IV q8h or metronidazole 500 mg IV q6 to 8h plus gentamicin either 5 to 7 mg/kg q24h or 1.5 mg/kg q8h
  2. Alternatives: ampicillin sulbactam 3 g IV q6h or cefoxitin 2 g IV q6h or cefotetan 2 g IV q12h plus doxycycline 100 mg IV q12h
- During medical management, high index of suspicion for acute rupture, such as acute worsening of abdominal pain or new-onset tachycardia and hypotension, mandating immediate surgical intervention after patient stabilization
- Surgical options:
  1. Laparoscopy with drainage and irrigation
  2. Transvaginal colpotomy (abscess must be midline, dissect rectovaginal septum, and be adherent to vaginal fornix)
  3. Laparotomy, including total abdominal hysterectomy with bilateral salpingo-oophorectomy or unilateral salpingo-oophorectomy
  4. Evidence of ruptured TOA is a surgical emergency

DISPOSITION

- Of patients treated with medical therapy, response in 75%, with a 50% pregnancy rate
- No response in 30% to 40%; can be treated with either CT-guided drainage or surgical intervention, keeping in mind that unilateral adnexectomy may give equal chance of cure vs. hysterectomy, yet preserve reproductive potential

REFERRAL

If patient has a TOA, refer to gynecologist.

PEARLS & CONSIDERATIONS

COMMENTS

If *Actinomyces* species is isolated from culture, treatment with penicillin is required for an extended period (6 wk to 3 mo).

SUGGESTED READINGS

Aimakhu CO, Olayemi O, Odukogbe AA: Surgical management of pelvic abscess: laparotomy versus colpotomy, *J Obstet Gynaecol* 23(1):71, 2003.

Sudakoff GS, Lundeen SJ, Otterson MF: Transrectal and transvaginal sonographic intervention of infected pelvic fluid collections: a complete approach, *Ultrasound Q* 21(3): 175, 2005.

AUTHORS: **SCOTT J. ZUCCALA, D.O.,** and **RUBEN ALVERO, M.D.**

BASIC INFORMATION

DEFINITION

A perirectal abscess is a localized inflammatory process that can be associated with infections of soft tissue and anal glands based on anatomic location. Perianal and perirectal abscesses may be simple or complex, causing suppuration. Infections in these spaces may be classified as superficial perianal or perirectal with involvement in the following anatomic spaces: ischiorectal, intersphincteric, perianal, and supralevator (Fig. 1-4).

SYNONYMS

Rectal abscess
Perianal abscess
Anorectal abscess

ICD-9CM CODES
566 Perirectal abscess

EPIDEMIOLOGY & DEMOGRAPHICS

INCIDENCE (IN U.S.): Commonly encountered
PREDOMINANT SEX: Male > female
PREDOMINANT AGE: All ages
PEAK INCIDENCE: Not seasonal; common
GENETICS: None known

PHYSICAL FINDINGS & CLINICAL PRESENTATION

- Localized perirectal or anal pain—often worsened with movement or straining
- Perirectal erythema or cellulitis
- Perirectal mass by inspection or palpation

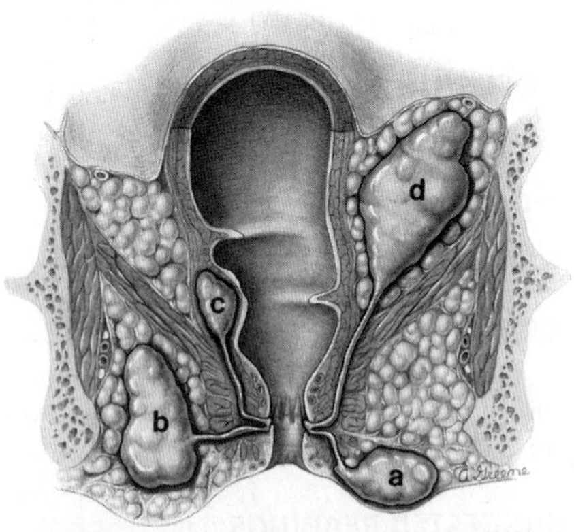

FIGURE 1-4 Common sites of anorectal abscesses: perianal **(a)**, ischiorectal **(b)**, intersphincteric **(c)**, and supralevator **(d)**. (From Noble J [ed]: *Textbook of primary care medicine,* ed 2, St Louis, 1996, Mosby.)

- Fever and signs of sepsis with deep abscess
- Urinary retention

ETIOLOGY

- Polymicrobial aerobic and anaerobic bacteria involving one of the anatomic spaces (see "Definition"), often associated with localized trauma
- Microbiology: most bacteria are polymicrobial, mixed enteric and skin flora
- Predominant anaerobic bacteria:
  1. *Bacteroides fragilis*
  2. *Peptostreptococcus spp.*
  3. *Prevotella spp.*
  4. *Porphyromonas spp.*
  5. *Clostridium spp.*
  6. *Fusobacterium spp.*
- Predominant aerobic bacteria:
  1. *Staphylococcus aureus*
  2. *Streptococcus spp.*
  3. *Escherichia coli*
  4. *Enterococcus spp.*

DIAGNOSIS

Many patients will have predisposing underlying conditions including:
- Malignancy or leukemia
- Immune deficiency
- Diabetes mellitus
- Recent surgery
- Steroid therapy

DIFFERENTIAL DIAGNOSIS

- Neutropenic enterocolitis
- Crohn's disease (inflammatory bowel disease)
- Pilonidal disease
- Hidradenitis suppurativa
- Tuberculosis or actinomycosis; Chagas' disease
- Cancerous lesions
- Chronic anal fistula
- Rectovaginal fistula
- Proctitis—often STD-associated, including: syphilis, gonococcal, chlamydia, chancroid, condylomata acuminata
- AIDS-associated: Kaposi's sarcoma, lymphoma, CMV

WORKUP

- Examination of rectal, perirectal/perineal areas
- Rule out necrotic process and crepitance suggesting deep tissue involvement
- Local aerobic and anaerobic culture
- Blood cultures if toxic, febrile, or compromised
- Possible sigmoidoscopy

IMAGING STUDIES

Usually not indicated unless extensive disease abscess

TREATMENT

ACUTE GENERAL Rx

- Incision and drainage of abscess
- Debridement if necrotic tissue
- Rule out need for fistulectomy
- Local wound care—packing
- Sitz baths

Antibiotic treatment: Directed toward coverage for mixed skins and enteric flora
Outpatient—oral:
Amoxicillin/clavulanic acid 875 to 1000 mg bid
Ciprofloxacin 750 mg by mouth every 12 hr plus metronidazole 500 to 750 mg by mouth every 8 hr *or*
Clindamycin 150 to 300 mg by mouth every 8 hr
Inpatient—intravenous:
Ampicillin/sulbactam (Unasyn) 1.5 to 3 gm IV every 6 hr
Cefotetan 1 to 2 gm IV every 8 hr
Piperacillin/Tazobactam 3.375 gm IV every 6 to 8 hr
Imipenem 500 to 1000 mg IV every 8 hr

DISPOSITION

Follow-up with a general surgeon or infectious disease physician is often warranted.

REFERRAL

- General surgeon or colorectal surgeon for drainage.
- AIDS specialist may be needed for perirectal complications of HIV infection.
- Gastroenterologist follow-up may be warranted in Crohn's disease with perirectal fistula and other complications.

PEARLS & CONSIDERATIONS

Perirectal abscess may be a presenting manifestation of type 2 diabetes mellitus in older adults. Check the blood sugar in patients to exclude the possibility of unrecognized diabetes mellitus.

AUTHORS: **GLENN G. FORT, M.D., M.P.H.,** and **DENNIS J. MIKOLICH, M.D.**

BASIC INFORMATION

DEFINITION

Definition from the Federal Child Abuse Prevention and Treatment Act (CAPTA): any recent act or failure to act on the part of a parent or caretaker which results in death, serious physical or emotional harm, sexual abuse or exploitation of a child; or an act or failure to act which presents an imminent risk of serious harm to a child.

- Neglect: failure to provide for the basic needs of a child (e.g., food, shelter, supervision)
  1. Medical neglect: failure to provide basic medical or mental health care
  2. Educational neglect: failure to meet educational needs
  3. Emotional neglect: failure to attend to emotional needs, exposure to domestic violence
- Physical abuse: injury inflicted by an adult intentionally or in the course of excessive discipline
- Sexual abuse: sexual act inflicted by parent or caretaker, includes exploitation and pornography
- Emotional abuse: pattern of behavior of caretaker toward a child that impairs emotional development, such as verbal abuse or cruelty

SYNONYMS

Child maltreatment
Physical abuse
Sexual abuse
Battered child syndrome
Shaken baby syndrome
Shaken impact syndrome
Abusive head trauma

ICD-9CM CODES
995.5 Child maltreatment
995.50 Child abuse, unspecified
995.51 Child abuse, emotional or psychological
995.52 Child neglect
995.53 Child abuse, sexual
995.54 Child abuse, physical
995.55 Shaken infant syndrome
995.59 Multiple forms of child abuse

EPIDEMIOLOGY & DEMOGRAPHICS

INCIDENCE (IN U.S.): Any reports of incidence are underestimates because many cases are never recognized or reported. These are collected based on Child Protective Services (CPS) state aggregates. Roughly 899,000 children were determined to be victims of abuse or neglect.

- Types of abuse by percentage. Note that the following amounts add to greater than 100% because many children are subject to more than one type of victimization:
  1. Neglect 62.8%
  2. Physical abuse 16.6%
  3. Sexual abuse 9.3%
  4. Emotional abuse 7.1%
  5. Medical neglect 2%
  6. Other 14.3% (e.g., abandonment, threats of harm, congenital drug addiction)
- For 2005, an estimated 1460 child deaths were caused by abuse or neglect.
  - Overall annual death rate resulting from abuse or neglect is estimated to be 2 deaths/100,000 children.
  - More than 40% of these deaths are due to neglect.
  - 77% of these children are <4 yr of age.
  - Most fatalities are suffered at the hand of one or both parents (77%).
  - Many child abuse fatalities are underreported because of misdiagnosis or variations in state definitions and coding.
- More than 83% of abused children were victimized by one or both of their parents.
- One fifth of adult women report history of molestation or sexual assault as a child or adolescent.

PREDOMINANT SEX:
- There is a slight predominance of females as victims.
- Infant boys (<1 yr) have the highest death rate: 17 per 100,000 boys of the same age vs. 14 per 100,000 infant girls of the same age.

PREDOMINANT AGE: Youngest children (0 to 3 years old) have the highest rates of victimization (16.5 victims/1000 children of the same age).

GENETICS: No known genetic factors.

ETIOLOGY

Multiple factors contribute to the incidence. No factor or combination of factors can definitively predict which children will be victimized. Factors contributing to risk of abuse or neglect include the following:

- Parent
  1. Substance abuse
  2. Mental illness
  3. Intellectual impairment
  4. Parental history of being abused as a child
  5. Domestic violence
- Child
  1. Low birth weight or prematurity
  2. Chronic physical disability
- Family
  1. Social isolation
  2. Poor parent-child bonding
  3. Stress: unemployment, chronic illness, eviction, arrest, poverty
- Community/society
  1. Limited transportation
  2. Limited day care
  3. Unsafe neighborhoods
  4. Poverty

DIAGNOSIS

Careful history and physical exam are the most important aspects of the evaluation. Careful documentation of any statements regarding origin of injuries or history of abuse are crucial. Chart and photographic documentation of injuries is also essential. The following are keys to the final diagnosis:

- Patterned bruising (e.g., loop-shaped, square, oval) is indicative of being struck with an object.
- Injury observed is incompatible with the history provided.
- History of injury provided is incompatible with the developmental capabilities of the child.
- There is delay in seeking care for a significant injury (e.g., callus formation on a fracture, eschar formation on a burn).
- Bruising is rare in healthy precruising infants and warrants further investigation.
- There are multiple significant injuries of different ages.
- Infant with clinically significant head trauma attributed to a trivial cause (e.g., a short fall). Often associated with retinal hemorrhages and skeletal fractures is indicative of shaken baby syndrome or abusive head trauma.
- Certain fractures in infants without a history of significant trauma (e.g., MVA) are characteristic of abuse: metaphyseal, rib, sternum, scapula, vertebral body.
- Inflicted contact burns are indicated by an impression of the burning object: lighter, iron, cigarette.
- Inflicted immersion burns are indicated by "stocking" burns of the feet or "glove" burns of the hands. Stocking burns are often associated with buttocks/perineal burns from immersion of a minor in a flexed position.
- Most sexual abuse victims will have a normal or nonspecific genital examination. A normal genital examination does not mean the child was not abused. History is the most important part of the diagnosis. Examination by an experienced health care provider is essential for child and adolescent victims of sexual abuse.
- The identification of a sexually transmitted disease in a prepubertal child who is beyond the neonatal period is suggestive of sexual abuse. Reporting and further careful investigation are warranted. Consult current CDC guidelines for further guidance.

DIFFERENTIAL DIAGNOSIS

In all categories, accidental injury is the most common entity to be distinguished from abuse. Accidental injuries are most common over bony prominences: forehead, elbows, knees, shins; soft, fleshy areas are more common for inflicted injury: buttocks, thighs, upper arms.

Bruising
- Bleeding disorder (ITP, hemophilia, leukemia, hemorrhagic disease of the newborn, von Willebrand's disease)
- Connective tissue disorder (Ehlers-Danlos syndrome, vasculitis)
- Pigments (Mongolian spots)
- Dermatitis (phytophotodermatitis, nickel allergy)
- Folk treatment (coining, cupping)

Burns
- Chemical burn
- Impetigo
- Folk treatment (moxibustion)
- Dermatitis (phytophotodermatitis)

Intracranial hemorrhage
- Bleeding disorder
- Perinatal trauma (should resolve by 4 wk)
- AVM rupture
- Glutaric aciduria

Fractures
- Osteogenesis imperfecta
- Ricketts
- Congenital syphilis
- Very low birth weight (osteopenia of prematurity)

Sexual abuse
- Normal variants
- Lichen sclerosis et atrophicus
- Congenital abnormalities
- Urethral prolapse
- Hemangioma
- Nonsexually acquired infection (group A *Streptococcus, Shigella*)

WORKUP

History and physical
- Careful history from all caretakers and child.
- Scene investigation may be necessary.
- Complete physical examination.
- Sexual abuse: forensic interview and magnified examinations by trained professionals is the standard for evaluation and evidence collection.

Laboratory tests for physical abuse
- Tests performed may vary depending on the severity of abuse and clinical presentation of the child.
- CBC with differential and platelets.
- PT, aPTT.
- Consider closure time (PFA-100), VWB panel.
- SGPT, amylase, UA.

Laboratory tests for sexual abuse
- If within 72 hr of acute sexual assault/abuse, swabs are obtained for sperm, acid phosphatase, P30, MHS-5 antigen, blood group typing, DNA testing. Also collect samples of foreign hair, blood, saliva, or other tissue if present.
- Per current CDC recommendations, adolescent victims of acute assault should have appropriate specimens collected from sites of penetration for *Neisseria gonorrhea* and *Chlamydia*. Nucleic acid amplification tests (NAATs) may be used and are preferred. In females, wet mount for bacterial vaginosis and trichomonas should also be done. Serum should be obtained for HIV, hepatitis B, and syphilis testing acutely. If negative, HIV and syphilis testing should be repeated 6, 12, and 24 wk after the assault.
- Child victims (i.e., prepubertal) should have specimens collected if considered high risk for a sexually transmitted disease (STD) per current CDC recommendations. Cervical specimens are not collected and vaginal specimens must be collected with care to avoid further traumatizing the child. *Gonorrhea* and *Chlamydia* culture are the gold standard for diagnosis and legal purposes. However, some providers analyze specimens via NAAT followed by culture confirmation if any positive results are obtained. Specimens should be collected for *Gonorrhea* and *Chlamydia,* wet mount, and blood for serologic testing (HIV, hepatitis B, syphilis) in the following cases:
  1. Presence of vaginal discharge or genital ulcer
  2. Alleged assailant is known to have an STD or be at high risk for an STD
  3. A sibling or adult in the same household has a known STD
  4. High prevalence of STDs in the community
  5. Evidence of ejaculation or penetration is present on the examination
  6. Child or parent requests testing

IMAGING STUDIES

Physical abuse
- Radiographic skeletal survey for all children <2 yr; for 2- to 5-yr-olds, done only for severe abuse. Consider repeat skeletal survey in 2 wk if severe physical injury is present.
- Noncontrast head CT scan or MRI for all children <1 yr; for children >1 yr, clinical judgment should be used.
- Head MRI for children with significant abusive head trauma. This is used as an adjunct a few days after initial head CT.
- Abdominal CT scan if indicated by clinical examination or laboratory evaluation.

TREATMENT (Rx)

ACUTE GENERAL Rx

- Stabilize and treat acute medical injuries.
- Report to Child Protective Services. HIPAA allows reports for suspected child abuse without parental authorization.
- Early report to law enforcement for suspected physical abuse or sexual abuse. This allows for scene investigation.
- Disposition, once medically stable, is dependent on CPS. The child cannot be returned home if the environment is not safe.
- Physician should remain available to discuss with investigators. This is often critical to determining the outcome of the case and placement of the child.
- For adolescent victims of acute sexual assault, empirically treat for *Gonorrhea, Chlamydia,* trichomonas, and bacterial vaginosis. Pregnancy prophylaxis should also be offered. Hepatitis B immunization should be offered if not previously given. HIV prophylaxis is offered in certain situations depending on local epidemiology and risk. Consult local infectious disease experts for current recommendations. Repeat examination should be done in 2 weeks for all victims of sexual assault, especially if they declined empiric treatment.
- Empiric treatment of child victims of sexual abuse is generally not recommended. This is especially important if NAATs are used for screening for STDs because culture confirmation is necessary for any positive results. Careful follow-up within 2 weeks and treatment based on culture results is indicated. HIV prophylaxis is offered in certain circumstances according to local epidemiology and risk. Consult with a local ID expert for further recommendations.

CHRONIC Rx

- Often dependent on CPS and court-ordered interventions
- Treatment of parental mental illness
- Treatment of parental substance abuse, including requirements for random drug testing
- Instruction for parents in behavior management skills including appropriate limit setting and discipline
- Anger management classes for parents
- Trauma-focused cognitive-behavioral therapy (CBT) for victims of sexual abuse and exposure to domestic violence; useful to include nonoffending parent/caregiver
- Ongoing individual and family therapy
- May need long-term placement in foster care before it is safe to return home

DISPOSITION

- Victims of chronic abuse and neglect have more mental illness (depression, suicide, PTSD, eating disorders)
- Victims have more cognitive difficulties and often have impaired academic performance

- Victims are more likely to become aggressive
- Victims, as adults, are more likely to have adverse physical health outcomes (cardiovascular disease, cancer, STDs)
- Victims of abusive head trauma:
  1. One third die.
  2. One third have severe disability.
  3. One third appear normal in the short term.

PEARLS & CONSIDERATIONS

PREVENTION

- Home visitation to high-risk families during pregnancy and infancy has shown positive outcomes.
- Anticipatory guidance at health visits to teach normal developmental expectations and appropriate discipline.
- Screening to identify at-risk or abused children.
- Targeted education in the newborn nursery for shaken baby prevention has been shown to be effective.
- Substance abuse prevention and treatment.
- Identification and intervention for domestic violence before children are born.

EVIDENCE

EBM

A systematic review studied randomized controlled trials of psychological treatments for children who had been sexually abused. It found that cognitive-behavioral therapy, particularly for young children, had the strongest evidence for improving psychological symptoms.[1] (B)

Evidence-Based Reference

1. Ramchandani P, Jones DP: Treating psychological symptoms in sexually abused children: from research findings to service provision, *Br J Psychiatry* 183:484, 2003. (B)

SUGGESTED READINGS

Adams JA et al: Guidelines for medical care of children who may have been sexually abused, *J Pediatric Adolesc Gynecol* 10:163, 2007.

Kos L, Shwayder T: Cutaneous manifestations of child abuse, *Pediatr Dermatol* 23:311, 2006.

Maguire S et al: Are there patterns of bruising in childhood which are diagnostic or suggestive of abuse? a systematic review, *Arch Dis Child* 90:182, 2005.

MMWR: Sexually Transmitted Diseases Treatment Guidelines 55(RR11):1, 2006.

Sirotnak AP et al: Physical abuse of children, *Pediatr Rev* 25:264, 2004.

United States Department of Health and Human Services: Child Maltreatment 2005. Available at http://www.acf.hhs.gov/programs/cb/pubs/cm05/index.htm.

United States Department of Health and Human Services: What is child abuse and neglect? 2006. Available at http://www.childwelfare.gov/pubs/factsheets/whatiscan.pdf.

AUTHOR: **NANCY R. GRAFF, M.D.**

BASIC INFORMATION

DEFINITION

Drug abuse is a recurring pattern of harmful use of a substance despite adverse consequences in work, school, relationships, the legal system, or personal health. This may occur concurrently with or independently from *substance dependence,* in which the impairment or distress is more pervasive and that often (though not necessarily) includes physical dependence and withdrawal symptoms (Table 1-1).

SYNONYMS

Substance abuse
Addiction

ICD-9CM CODES
Defined by specific substance F10-F19 (DSM-IV code is also defined by specific substance 291-292, 303-305)

EPIDEMIOLOGY & DEMOGRAPHICS

INCIDENCE (IN U.S.): Alcohol or drug dependence: 5% to 10% of population
PREVALENCE (IN U.S.): 15% of patients in primary care practice have "at-risk" pattern of drug and/or alcohol use; lifetime prevalence of any alcohol use disorder: 30%
PREDOMINANT SEX: Males > females
PREDOMINANT AGE:

- Problematic use of substances may begin in early life (8 to 10 yr).
- The mean age of onset of problem drinking is about 25 yr for men and 30 yr for women.

PEAK INCIDENCE:

- For most substances: age 15 to 30 yr
- Men: average >20 yr of heavy drinking
- Women: average 15 yr of heavy drinking

GENETICS: There is evidence of nonspecific genetic factors.

PHYSICAL FINDINGS & CLINICAL PRESENTATION

- Polysubstance use is common.
- Anxiety, depression, insomnia, cognitive and memory dysfunction, and behavioral problems are frequent.
- Alcohol and cocaine abuse associated with violence and accidents (more than half of all murderers and their victims are intoxicated at the time of the crime).
- Alcohol withdrawal can present with seizures and delirium.

ETIOLOGY

Two models of addiction:

- Conditioning: Substance use is paired with enforcing and triggering stimuli.
- Homeostatic: Either preexisting abnormalities or drug-induced abnormalities lead to initial or continued use of the drug.

DIAGNOSIS

DIFFERENTIAL DIAGNOSIS

- Psychiatric disorders such as depression, mania, social phobia, or other anxiety disorders that coexist or occur as a consequence of substance abuse.
- Rule out seizure disorder and underlying illness in persons presenting with substance use.

WORKUP

- A thorough history is crucial for diagnosis of any substance abuse disorder.
- The physician's history-taking style and techniques strongly affect patient's willingness to participate in future treatment activities.
- A structured approach is generally preferable. Possibilities include the following:
  1. Ask about alcohol or drug use in the past year.
  2. Use a short screening instrument such as the two-item screen ("In the last year, have you ever consumed alcohol or used drugs more than you meant to? Have you felt you wanted or needed to cut down on your drinking or drug use in the last year?").
  3. Ask about quantity and frequency. For example, the National Institute on Alcohol and Alcoholism declares that problem drinking for men is defined as more than 14 drinks/wk or more than 4 drinks on any one occasion; for women and anyone older than 65 yr, the limits are 7 drinks and no more than 3 on any one occasion.
- Observation of problematic behavior during intoxication or withdrawal is diagnostic.
- Physical examination findings are limited. Odor of alcohol or intoxication is worrisome and indicates a high likelihood of drug or alcohol disorder.

LABORATORY TESTS

- Consider toxicology screen or blood alcohol level.
- Elevated mean corpuscular volume and γ-glutamyltransferase are most sensitive indicators of alcohol intake.

IMAGING STUDIES

Not helpful in routine diagnosis and management of substance abuse, but possibly useful in the management of sequelae of substance abuse (e.g., brain imaging to evaluate the alcohol abuse–associated increased risk of subdural hematomas or increased evidence of cerebral atrophy).

TREATMENT

NONPHARMACOLOGIC THERAPY

- Nonpharmacologic strategies have greatest documented efficacy. Effective nonpharmacologic interventions generally include advice, feedback,

TABLE 1-1 Diagnostic Criteria for Dependence and Drug Abuse

Dependence (>3 needed)	Abuse (>1 for 12 mo)
1. Tolerance 2. Withdrawal 3. The substance is often taken in larger amounts over a longer period than intended 4. Any unsuccessful effort or a persistent desire to cut down or control substance use 5. A great deal of time is spent in activities necessary to obtain the substance or recover from its effects 6. Important social, occupational, or recreational activities given up or reduced because of substance use 7. Continued substance use despite knowledge of having had persistent or recurrent physical or psychological problems that are likely to be caused or exacerbated by the substance	1. Recurrent substance use resulting in failure to fulfill major role obligations at work, school, or home 2. Recurrent substance use in situations in which it is physically hazardous 3. Recurrent substance-related legal problems 4. Continued substance use despite having persistent or recurrent social or interpersonal problems caused or exacerbated by the effects of the substance Never met criteria for dependence

From Goldman L, Bennett JC (eds): *Cecil textbook of medicine,* ed 21, Philadelphia, 2000, WB Saunders.

goal setting, and additional contacts for further assistance and support.
- Relapse prevention by avoidance of trigger stimuli or by uncoupling trigger stimuli from substance ingestion.
- Self-help groups such as Alcoholics Anonymous, Narcotics Anonymous, and Al-Anon.

ACUTE GENERAL Rx

- Detoxification is an important first step in substance abuse treatment. Its goals are to facilitate withdrawal and reduce symptoms, initiate abstinence, and refer the patient into ongoing treatment.
- Benzodiazepines, particularly long-acting ones, are safe and effective in acute alcohol withdrawal. One strategy is to give the patient a loading dose of a long-acting benzodiazepine (e.g., 20 mg of diazepam), and then follow the patient clinically. An alternative "symptom driven" strategy is to follow the patient closely with serial assessments such as with the Clinical Institute Withdrawal Assessment for Alcohol scale and to dose with 5 to 10 mg of diazepam as needed to treat withdrawal symptoms.
- Beta-blockers and clonidine generally should be avoided in alcohol withdrawal; they may mask markers of the severity of the withdrawal (blood pressure and pulse rate).
- Clonidine alleviates the discomfort of opiate and nicotine withdrawal. For treatment of opiate withdrawal, prescribe 0.2 mg q8h for 10 to 14 days.
- "Rapid" detoxification in opioid dependence uses opioid antagonists (naloxone, naltrexone) to induce withdrawal and prevent relapse. More recent "ultra-rapid" (anesthesia-assisted) detoxification methods are associated with increased risk and are no more effective.
- Buprenorphine is a partial μ-opioid receptor agonist that may be used for both detoxification and maintenance in treatment of opioid dependence (see dosing in next section).

CHRONIC Rx

- Naltrexone helps reduce craving for alcohol. Naltrexone 50 mg once daily for 12 wk can be a useful adjunct to substance abuse counseling or rehabilitation programs. Randomized treatment studies are equivocal for long-term outcomes. Naltrexone reduces relapse and the intensity or frequency of any drinking that does occur. It can be hepatotoxic. Intramuscular naltrexone (380 mg monthly) may be considered if adherence to treatment is an issue.
- Acamprosate also helps reduce craving for alcohol. Acamprosate 666 mg three times daily may be an effective adjunct to counseling. Most randomized trials have shown benefit in reducing relapse rates; one recent large trial has shown no benefit compared to placebo.
- Disulfiram (Antabuse) provokes acetaldehyde accumulation after alcohol ingestion, producing a toxic state manifested by nausea, headache, flushing, and respiratory distress. Studies have shown limited efficacy.
- Methadone maintenance for opiate addiction is effective and involves once daily dosing of methadone in a controlled setting.
- Buprenorphine is as effective as low-dose methadone and may be prescribed by physicians who have completed approved training. For induction, initiate 12 to 24 hr after short-acting opioid use and 24 to 48 hr after long-acting opioid use. Use buprenorphine/naloxone tablets in most patients; buprenorphine only on day 1 for patients with dependence on long-acting opioids. Maximum first-day dosage is 8 to 12 mg of buprenorphine (2 mg buprenorphine q2h for signs of withdrawal). Titrate buprenorphine dose up to 16 mg on day 2 for signs of withdrawal and up to 32 mg daily by end of week 1. Then adjust dosage to minimum needed for maintenance. Naltrexone (oral) may also be used for maintenance in opioid dependence treatment, though evidence of effectiveness is limited.
- Always combine pharmacotherapy with counseling.
- Adjunctive use of antidepressants or lithium is helpful when substance use is associated with anxiety and mood symptoms.
- The effect of any intervention wanes after discontinuation of the intervention.

DISPOSITION

- Substance abuse is a chronic relapsing illness.
- The goal of treatment is always abstinence, but success of treatment is measured by return of function and increasing duration between relapses.

REFERRAL

Physicians should refer any patients who do not make good progress on changing substance use patterns.

PEARLS & CONSIDERATIONS

- Withdrawal from opioids can resemble a severe case of the flu.
- A brief intervention (providing information and advising the patient to reduce consumption of alcohol) by the primary care doctor has been demonstrated in randomized trials to reduce drinking in at-risk patients.
- Treatment rates for alcohol use disorders remain low despite available effective treatments.

EVIDENCE

EBM

Naltrexone reduces short-term relapse rates for alcohol dependence when combined with psychosocial treatment.[1] Evidence suggests equivalent efficacy of naltrexone compared to behavioral therapy, without added benefit by combining the two, in the presence of medical management.[2]

Naltrexone is safe and acceptably tolerated.[3]

Brief motivational interviewing is an effective intervention for excessive drinking.[4]

Buprenorphine is significantly superior to placebo in treatment of opiate dependence, but has no significant benefit compared to methadone in terms of treatment retention and suppression of heroin use.[5]

Evidence-Based References

1. Srisurapanont M, Jarusuraisin N: Opioid antagonists for alcohol dependence, *Cochrane Database Syst Rev* 1:CD001867, 2005.
2. Anton RF et al: Combined pharmacotherapies and behavioral interventions for alcohol dependence: the COMBINE study: a randomized controlled trial, *JAMA* 295(17):2003-2017, 2006.
3. Bouza C et al: Efficacy and safety of naltrexone and acamprosate in the treatment of alcohol dependence: a systematic review, *Addiction* 99:811, 2004. Ⓐ
4. Vasilaki EI et al: The efficacy of motivational interviewing as a brief intervention for excessive drinking: a meta-analytic review, *Alcohol* 41(3):328, 2006. Ⓐ
5. Mattick RP et al: Buprenorphine maintenance versus placebo or methadone maintenance for opioid dependence, *Cochrane Database Syst Rev* 2:CD002207, 2003. Ⓐ

SUGGESTED READINGS

Center for Substance Abuse Treatment, U.S. Department of Health and Human Services: www.csat.samhsa.gov.

Reiff-Hekking S et al: Brief physician and nurse practitioner-delivered counseling for high-risk drinking: results at 12-month follow-up, *J Gen Intern Med* 20:7, 2005.

Ricaurte GA, McCann UD: Recognition and management of complications of new recreational drug use, *Lancet* 365:2137, 2005.

Whitlock EP et al: Behavioral counseling interventions in primary care to reduce risky/harmful alcohol use by adults: a summary of the evidence for the U.S. Preventive Services Task Force, *Ann Intern Med* 140(7):557, 2004.

AUTHORS: **MITCHELL D. FELDMAN, M.D., M.PHIL.**, and **KARA CHEW, M.D.**

BASIC INFORMATION

DEFINITION

Elder abuse is the willful infliction of physical pain or injury; emotional pain, humiliation, or intimidation; exploitation or misappropriation of money or property; or neglect of an elder by a designated caregiver. In general, three basic categories of elder abuse exist: domestic elder abuse (or abuse in the home), institutional elder abuse (abuse that occurs in nursing homes, foster homes, group homes, board and care facilities), and self-neglect.

Seven types of abuse are described:

- Physical abuse: inflicting of physical pain or injury
- Sexual abuse: inflicting of nonconsensual sexual activity of any kind
- Psychological abuse: inflicting mental anguish, including intimidation, humiliation, ridicule, or threats
- Financial abuse: improper use of the resources of any older person without the elder's consent for another's benefit
- Abandonment: desertion of an elderly person by the responsible caregiver
- Neglect: failure to fulfill a caretaking obligation, including provision of food, a safe living environment, health care, hygiene, or basic custodial care
- Self-neglect: behavior that threatens the elder's health or safety

SYNONYMS

Battered elder syndrome
Elder mistreatment
Domestic violence in the elderly

ICD-9CM CODES
995.80 Adult maltreatment, unspecified
995.81 Physical abuse
995.82 Emotional/psychological abuse
995.83 Sexual abuse
995.84 Adult maltreatment, neglect (nutritional)
995.85 Other abuse and neglect—multiple forms of abuse and neglect

EPIDEMIOLOGY & DEMOGRAPHICS

U.S. INCIDENCE & PREVALENCE: There were estimated to be 1 million victims of elder abuse in 1996; if self-neglect is included, that number increases to more than 2 million (National Center on Elder Abuse).

- Most epidemiologic studies estimate a prevalence rate of 2% to 5% in those older than 65, but rates vary with the definition of abuse that is used.
- In 2004 there were over 500,000 cases of possible elder abuse reported to Adult Protective Service Agencies in the United States and Guam, of which almost half were substantiated (National Center on Elder Abuse).
- Neglect is the most common form of elder mistreatment, representing about 27% of all cases.

PREDOMINANT AGE: Risk increases as level of disability increases

PEAK INCIDENCE: >80 yr of age

RISK FACTORS (VICTIM):

- Impaired cognition
- Shared living situation
- Social isolation

RISK FACTORS (PERPETRATOR):

- Substance abuse
- Mental illness, particularly depression
- Dependence on the victim
- Being an involuntary or ill-equipped caregiver
- History of violence

PHYSICAL FINDINGS & CLINICAL PRESENTATION

- Physical abuse with multiple injuries at various stages with implausible or inconsistent descriptions of their origins; injuries are usually to head, neck, chest, breast, and abdomen.
- Fear, hypervigilance, or withdrawal.
- Evidence of poor nutrition, poor hygiene, multiple or neglected pressure ulcers, neglected medical conditions, or evidence of restraint use (bruises around wrists or ankles).
- Toxicologic evidence of unprescribed medications.
- Poor adherence, frequent no-shows, or little contact with health care system.

DIAGNOSIS

DIFFERENTIAL DIAGNOSIS

- Advancing dementia
- Depression or other psychiatric disorders
- Malnutrition due to intrinsic causes
- Conscious nonadherence
- Financial hardship
- Falling
- Diogenes syndrome

WORKUP

- Interview patient separately from the suspected abuser.
- Build trust; patients may be reticent or scared to report on their perpetrator.
- Ask direct specific questions such as "Do you ever feel unsafe where you live?" or "Do you ever felt threatened by anyone close to you?"
- There is no ideal screening instrument; studies suggest that instruments that identify specific indicators of abuse will reveal more cases than abuse disclosure questionnaires.
- Be aware that physical findings are usually unexplained injuries or burns.
- Pelvic examination if sexual abuse suspected.

LABORATORY TESTS

- If sexual abuse suspected, screening for sexually transmitted diseases.
- Toxicology screens or therapeutic drug monitoring are sometimes helpful.

IMAGING STUDIES

X-rays as indicated by physical presentation

TREATMENT

NONPHARMACOLOGIC THERAPY

- Reporting abuse to Adult Protective Services is mandatory in most states. This also provides the physician access to specialized personnel who can aid in evaluation and disposition.
- Separate patient and abuser.
- If the burden of care appears to be the major factor in contributing to abuse, referral to respite services or other support services may allow the patient to remain with the caregiver in some instances.
- Patient and caregiver may benefit from screening and treatment for depression, substance abuse, anxiety, mental illness, or cognitive impairment.

ACUTE GENERAL Rx

As indicated for injury or pain relief

DISPOSITION

If the patient's level of disability does not allow for independent living, institutionalization may be required. Guidelines vary at the state and county levels regarding guardianship and conservatorship requirements.

REFERRAL

Adult Protective Services (mandatory in most states in the U.S.)

PEARLS & CONSIDERATIONS

COMMENTS

- A home visit may be useful if abuse, neglect, or self-neglect is suspected.
- Care should be taken in interacting with the alleged abuser so that access to the victim is not lost.

PREVENTION

- Offer social services (e.g., respite care) for stressed caregivers.
- Make financial arrangements and arrange durable power of attorney for health care and finances while patient still cognitively intact.

PATIENT/FAMILY EDUCATION

The National Center on Elder Abuse: http://www.elderabusecenter.org/default.cfm?p=worried.cfm.

SUGGESTED READINGS

Cohen M et al: Elder abuse: disparities between older people's disclosure of abuse, evident signs of abuse, and high risk of abuse, *J Am Geriatr Soc* 55:1224, 2007.
Lachs MS, Pillemer K: Elder abuse, *Lancet* 364(9441):1263, 2004.

AUTHORS: **BREE JOHNSTON, M.D., M.P.H.,** and **MIKE HARPER, M.D.**

BASIC INFORMATION

DEFINITION

Acetaminophen poisoning is a disorder manifested by hepatic necrosis, jaundice, somnolence, and potential death if not treated appropriately. Pathologically there is hepatic necrosis.

SYNONYMS

Paracetamol poisoning

ICD-9CM CODES
965.4 Acetaminophen poisoning

EPIDEMIOLOGY & DEMOGRAPHICS

- Potentially toxic ingestions of acetaminophen-containing medications exceed 100,000 cases annually.
- Death rate is approximately 1/1000 persons. Nearly 50% of exposures occur in children <6 yr.
- Hepatic necrosis is most likely to occur in people who are chronically malnourished, who regularly abuse alcohol, and who are using other potentially hepatotoxic medications.

PHYSICAL FINDINGS & CLINICAL PRESENTATION

- The physical examination may vary depending on the number of hours lapsed from the ingestion of acetaminophen.
- Initially, symptoms may be mild or absent and may consist of diaphoresis, malaise, nausea, and vomiting.
- After the initial 12 to 24 hr, patient may complain of right upper quadrant pain with associated vomiting, diaphoresis, and subsequent somnolence.
- In massive overdoses, jaundice may occur within the initial 72 hr.
- Subsequent coma, somnolence, and confusion follow and can ultimately lead to death if not treated appropriately.

ETIOLOGY

- The amount of acetaminophen necessary for hepatic toxicity varies with the patient's body size and hepatic function.
- Using standardized nomograms calculating the acetaminophen plasma level and the number of hours after ingestion, the clinician can determine potential hepatic toxicity. See acetaminophen ingestion algorithm in Section III.

DIAGNOSIS

DIFFERENTIAL DIAGNOSIS

- Liver disease from alcohol abuse or hepatitis
- Ingestion of other hepatotoxic substances

WORKUP

Initial workup is aimed at confirming acetaminophen overdose with plasma acetaminophen level and assessment of hepatic damage and potential damage to other organ systems, such as kidneys, pancreas, and heart (see "Laboratory Tests").

LABORATORY TESTS

- Initial laboratory evaluation consists of plasma acetaminophen level with a second level drawn approximately 4 to 6 hr after the initial level. Subsequent levels can be obtained q2 to 4h until the levels stabilize or decline. These levels can be plotted using the Rumack-Matthew nomogram (see acetaminophen ingestion algorithm [Fig. 3-3] in Section III) to calculate potential hepatic toxicity.
- Transaminases (AST, ALT), bilirubin level, PT (INR), BUN, and creatinine should be initially obtained on all patients.
- Serum and urine toxicology screen for other potential toxic substances is also recommended on admission.

TREATMENT

NONPHARMACOLOGIC THERAPY

Consultation with Poison Control Center for management recommendations is recommended in patients with large ingestions of acetaminophen and/or ingestion of other toxic substances. A toxic dose of acetaminophen usually exceeds 7.5 g in the adult or 140 mg/kg.

ACUTE GENERAL Rx

- Perform gastric lavage and administer activated charcoal if the patient is seen within 1 hr of ingestion or the clinician suspects polydrug ingestion.
- Determine blood levels 4 hr after ingestion; if in the toxic range, start *N*-acetylcysteine either IV (Acetadote) or PO (Mucomyst). Acetylcysteine IV loading dose is 150 mg/kg over 15 min ×1. Maintenance dose is 50 mg/kg over 4 hr, followed by 100 mg/kg over 16 hr. Oral administration consists of 140 mg/kg PO as a loading dose, followed by 70 mg/kg PO q4h for 48 hr. *N*-Acetylcysteine therapy should be started within 24 hr of acetaminophen overdose. If charcoal therapy was initially instituted, lavage the stomach and recover as much charcoal as possible; then instill *N*-acetylcysteine, increasing the loading dose by 40%. Advantages of IV administration include more reliable absorption, fewer doses, and shorter duration of treatment (1 day vs. 3 days).
- Monitor acetaminophen level; use graph to plot possible hepatic toxicity.
- Provide adequate IV hydration (e.g., $D_5$1/2NS at 150 ml/hr).
- If acetaminophen level is nontoxic, acetylcysteine therapy may be discontinued.

DISPOSITION

Most patients will recover fully without persisting hepatic abnormalities. Hepatic failure is particularly unusual in children <6 yr.

REFERRAL

Psychiatric referral is recommended following intentional ingestions.

EVIDENCE

A systematic review found that activated charcoal, gastric lavage, and ipecac are able to reduce absorption of acetaminophen but the clinical benefits are unclear.[1] B

Intravenous N-acetylcysteine may reduce mortality in patients with established acetaminophen-induced liver failure.[2] B

Methionine appears to reduce rates of hepatotoxicity compared with supportive care.[2] B

Evidence-Based References

1. Brok J, Buckley N, Gluud C: Interventions for paracetamol (acetaminophen) overdoses, *Cochrane Database of Syst Rev* (3):CD003328, 2002. B
2. Brok J, Buckley N, Gluud C: Interventions for paracetamol (acetaminophen) overdoses, *Cochrane Database of Syst Rev* 12:1951, 2004. B

AUTHOR: **FRED F. FERRI, M.D.**

BASIC INFORMATION

DEFINITION

Achalasia is a motility disorder of the esophagus characterized by incomplete relaxation of the lower esophageal sphincter (LES) and aperistalsis of esophageal smooth muscle. The result is functional obstruction of the esophagus.

SYNONYMS

Achalasia and cardiospasm
Achalasia (of cardia)
Aperistalsis of esophagus
Megaesophagus
Esophageal achalasia
Esophageal cardiospasm

ICD-9CM CODES
530.0 Achalasia

EPIDEMIOLOGY & DEMOGRAPHICS

- Annual incidence is about 0.5 in 100,000 persons.
- Prevalence is <10 per 100,000 persons.
- Although the onset of symptoms may occur at any age, incidence is typically bimodal, 20 to 40 yr, then after 60 yr, with greater incidence in the older group.
- Men and women are affected equally.

PHYSICAL FINDINGS & CLINICAL PRESENTATION

Symptoms:
- Dysphagia to both solids and liquids
- Difficulty belching
- Regurgitation
- Chest pain and/or heartburn
- Globus
- Frequent hiccups
- Vomiting of undigested food
- Symptoms of aspiration such as nocturnal cough; possible dyspnea and pneumonia

Physical findings:
- Focal lung examination abnormalities and wheezing also possible

ETIOLOGY

- Etiology is poorly understood.
- Loss of myenteric nerve fibers in the lower esophageal sphincter and smooth muscle portion of the esophagus.
- Loss of nitric oxide synthase (NOS) producing neurons in the myenteric plexus of the lower esophageal sphincter is the cause of incomplete relaxation.
- This motility disorder may be due to autoimmune degeneration of the esophageal myenteric plexus because association with the HLA class II antigen, DQw1, has been noted. Antimyenteric plexus antibodies have also been described.
- Varicella zoster, herpes simplex type I, and measles viruses have been implicated, but the association has not been confirmed.
- Achalasia is also seen in the rare autosomal recessive disorder Allgrove's syndrome (achalasia, alacrima, autonomic disturbance, and ACTH insensitivity), which has been linked to a gene mutation on chromosome 12q13.

DIAGNOSIS

DIFFERENTIAL DIAGNOSIS

- Primary achalasia:
  Idiopathic
- Secondary achalasia:
  Chagas' disease
  Vagal injury/surgery
- Pseudoachalasia:
  Esophageal cancer
  Infiltrating gastric cancer
  Oat cell and bronchogenic lung cancer
  Lymphoma
  Amyloidosis
  Paraneoplastic syndrome
- Angina
- Bulimia
- Anorexia nervosa
- Gastric bezoar
- Gastritis
- Peptic ulcer disease
- Postvagotomy dysmotility
- Esophageal disease:
  Gastroesophageal reflux disease (GERD)
  Sarcoidosis
  Amyloidosis
  Esophageal stricture
  Esophageal webs and rings
  Scleroderma
  Barrett's esophagus
  Esophagitis
  Diffuse esophageal spasm

WORKUP

- Physical examination and laboratory analyses to rule out other causes and assess complications
- Imaging studies, manometry, and endoscopy

LABORATORY TESTS

- Assessment of nutritional status with albumin and prealbumin if indicated
- CBC, ECG, stress test, stool and emesis for occult blood if diagnosis is in doubt

IMAGING STUDIES

Barium swallow with fluoroscopy may demonstrate:
- Uncoordinated or absent esophageal contractions
- An acutely tapered contrast column ("bird's beak," Fig. 1-5)
- Dilation of the distal (smooth muscle portion) esophagus
- Esophageal air fluid level

Manometry is generally required to confirm the diagnosis. Characteristic abnormalities are as follows:
- Low-amplitude disorganized contractions
- High LES pressure
- Inadequate LES relaxation after swallow
- A subset of patients with vigorous achalasia may have high-amplitude, long-duration, simultaneous esophageal contractions
- Direct visualization by endoscopy should be performed to exclude other causes of dysphagia including secondary causes of achalasia

TREATMENT

NONPHARMACOLOGIC THERAPY

- Pneumatic dilation may benefit up to 90% of patients. Esophageal rupture or perforation is a rare complication (2% to 3%) that can be managed conservatively in some stable patients.
- Surgical: Laparoscopic or, now less commonly, open esophagomyotomy is effective (90%). This approach currently offers the most durable symptom relief. About 35% of patients undergoing surgery will develop reflux disease. As a result, some surgeons will perform a "loose" antireflux repair as part of the surgical procedure. An observational study has suggested that

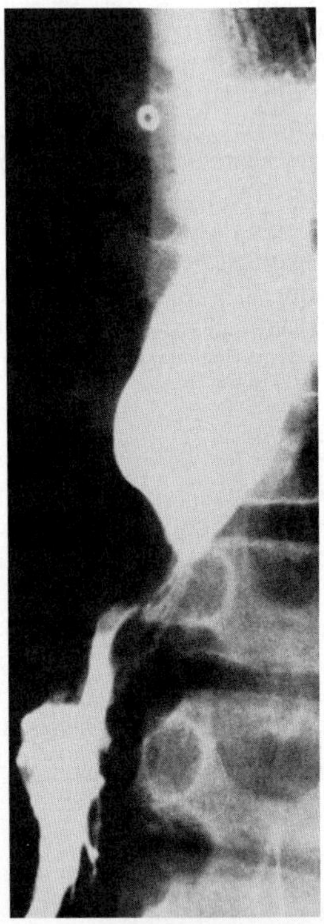

FIGURE 1-5 Classic appearance of achalasia of the esophagus. The dilated esophagus ends in a narrow segment. (From Hoekelman R [ed]: *Primary pediatric care,* ed 3, St Louis, 1997, Mosby.)

those who have had prior endoscopic treatment before myotomy may not do as well as those who have a primary myotomy.

GENERAL Rx

- Medications may be useful when the only goal is short-term symptom relief. Lower esophageal sphincter pressure may be lowered by 50% through sublingual use of long-acting nitrates (e.g., isosorbide dinitrate 5 to 20 mg) or calcium channel blockers (e.g., nifedipine 10 to 30 mg). However, side effects are common and duration of relief tends to be short.
- Botulinum toxin injection will benefit up to 85% of patients, but up to half of these patients will require repeat injections by 6 months.

PEARLS & CONSIDERATIONS

COMMENTS

- Medication has a limited role in treatment.
- Chemical paralysis with botulinum toxin is effective but not permanent.
- Mechanical dilation or surgical myotomy are treatments of choice.
- Patients with achalasia may be at long-term risk of squamous cell carcinoma of the esophagus and non–reflux associated esophagitis. Treated patients may be at long-term risk for reflux esophagitis, Barrett's esophagus, and adenocarcinoma.

SUGGESTED READINGS

Kraichely RE et al: Achalasia: physiology and etiopathogenesis, *Dis Esophagus* 19:213, 2006.

Leyden JE et al: Endoscopic pneumatic dilation versus botulinum toxin injection in the management of primary achalasia, *Cochrane Database Syst Rev* 4:CD005046, 2006. DOI: 10.1002/14651858.CD005046.pub2.

Smith CD et al: Endoscopic therapy for achalasia before Heller myotomy results in worse outcomes than Heller myotomy alone, *Ann Surg* 243(5):579, 2006.

AUTHOR: **HARLAN G. RICH, M.D.**

BASIC INFORMATION

DEFINITION

Achilles tendon rupture refers to the loss of continuity of the *tendo Achillis,* usually from attrition.

ICD-9CM CODES
845.09 Achilles tendon rupture

EPIDEMIOLOGY & DEMOGRAPHICS

PREDOMINANT AGE: 30 to 55 yr

PHYSICAL FINDINGS & CLINICAL PRESENTATION

Injury often occurs during an activity that puts great stress on the tendon. Sudden "pop" is often felt followed by weakness and swelling. Sometimes the patient feels like he or she has been shot in the calf.

- Patient walks flat-footed and is unable to stand on the ball of the foot.
- Tenderness and hemorrhage are present at the site of injury, and a sulcus is usually palpable but may be obscured by an organizing clot if the examination is delayed.
- Although active plantar flexion is usually lost, some plantar flexion occasionally remains because of the activity of the other posterior compartment muscles.
- Thompson's test is usually positive. Test measures plantar flexion of the foot when the calf is squeezed with the patient kneeling on a chair; normal foot plantar flexes with calf compression, but movement is absent when *tendo Achillis* is ruptured.
- Excessive passive dorsiflexion of the foot is also present on the injured side (Fig. 1-6).

ETIOLOGY

- Relative hypovascularity predisposing to tendon rupture in several tendons (Achilles, biceps, and supraspinatus)
- With advancing age, vascular supply to the tendon further compromised
- Repetitive trauma leading to degeneration of this critical area and weakness
- Rupture of *tendo Achillis* usually 2.5 to 5 cm from the insertion of the tendon into the os calcis
- Most common causative event leading to rupture: sudden dorsiflexion of the plantar flexed foot (landing from a height) or sudden pushing off with the weight on the forefoot
- The tendon may be adversely affected by the use of fluoroquinolone antibiotics

DIAGNOSIS

DIFFERENTIAL DIAGNOSIS

- Incomplete (partial) *tendo Achillis* rupture
- Partial rupture of gastrocnemius muscle, often medial head (previously thought to be "plantaris tendon rupture")

WORKUP

- Clinical diagnosis of complete *tendo Achillis* rupture is usually obvious.
- MRI helpful in partial ruptures.

TREATMENT

- Early referral is necessary for open, end-to-end surgical repair.
- If surgery is contraindicated, a short leg cast applied with the foot in equinus may allow healing.
- In cases of neglected rupture, reconstruction is usually indicated.
- Physical therapy is helpful after repair to restore strength and flexibility.
- Bracing for partial rupture.

DISPOSITION

- Prognosis for recovery after surgical repair of the acute rupture is good, but recurrence is not uncommon regardless of treatment.
- *Tendo Achillis* must be protected from excessive activity for up to 1 yr.
- Results of reconstruction for neglected cases are worse than with primary repair.
- Return to work with limited weight-bearing is possible in 2 to 4 wk.

SUGGESTED READINGS

Bhandari M et al: Treatment of acute Achilles tendon rupture: a systematic overview and metaanalysis, *Clin Orthop* (400):190, 2002.

Khan RJ et al: Treatment of acute achilles tendon ruptures: a meta-analysis of randomized controlled trials, *J Bone Joint Surg* 87A:2202, 2005.

Lawrence SJ, Grau GF: Management of acute Achilles tendon ruptures, *Orthopedics* 27:579, 2004.

Maffulli N et al: Chronic rupture of tendo Achilles, *Foot Ankle Clin* 12:583, 2007.

Rettig AC et al: Potential risk of rerupture in primary Achilles tendon repair in athletes younger than 30 years of age, *Am J Sports Med* 33:119, 2005.

Roberts C, Deliss L: Acute rupture of tendo Achillis, *J Bone Joint Surg Br* 84(4):620, 2002.

Smigielski R: Management of partial tears of the gastro-soleus complex, *Clin Sports Med* 27:219, 2008.

Wallace RG, Traynor IE et al: Combined conservative and orthotic management of acute ruptures of the Achiles tendon, *J Bone Joint Surg* 86A:1198, 2004.

Worth N et al: Management of acute Achilles tendon ruptures in the United Kingdom, *J Orthop Surg* (Hong Kong) 15:311, 2007.

AUTHOR: **LONNIE R. MERCIER, M.D.**

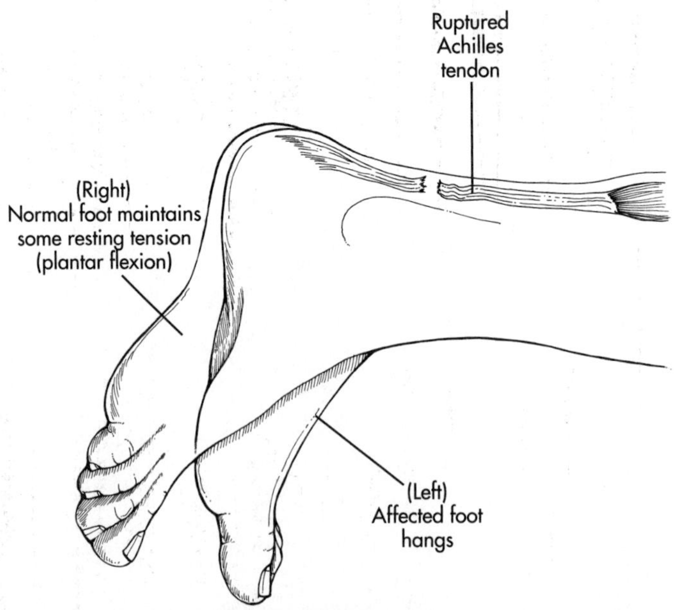

FIGURE 1-6 Observation of Achilles tendon rupture. The patient is asked to lie prone on the examining table with feet hanging off the end. The intact leg retains inherent plantar flexion, whereas on the injured side, the foot hangs straight down with gravity. (From Scudieri G [ed]: *Sports medicine: principles of primary care,* St Louis, 1997, Mosby.)

BASIC INFORMATION

DEFINITION

Acne vulgaris is a chronic disorder of the pilosebaceous apparatus caused by abnormal desquamation of follicular epithelium leading to obstruction of the pilosebaceous canal, resulting in inflammation and subsequent formation of papules, pustules, nodules, comedones, and scarring. Acne can be classified by the type of lesion (comedonal, papulopustular, and nodulocystic). The American Academy of Dermatology classification scheme for acne denotes the following three levels:

1. Mild acne: characterized by the presence of comedomes (noninflammatory lesions), few papules and pustules (generally <10) but no nodules.
2. Moderate acne: presence of several to many papules and pustules (10 to 40) along with comedomes (10 to 40). The presence of >40 papules and pustules along with larger, deeper nodular inflamed lesions (up to 5) denotes moderately severe acne (Fig. 1-7).
3. Severe acne: presence of numerous or extensive papules and pustules as well as many nodular lesions.

SYNONYMS

Acne

ICD-9CM CODES
706.1 Acne vulgaris

EPIDEMIOLOGY & DEMOGRAPHICS

- Acne is the most common skin disease in the U.S.
- It is most common in teenagers (highest incidence between ages of 16 and 18 yr).

PHYSICAL FINDINGS & CLINICAL PRESENTATION

- Open comedones (blackheads), closed comedones (whiteheads)
- Greasiness (oily skin)
- Presence of scars from prior acne cysts
- Various stages of development and severity may be present concomitantly
- Common distribution of acne: face, back, and upper chest
- Inflammatory papules, pustules, and ectatic pores

ETIOLOGY

- Overactivity of the sebaceous glands and blockage in the ducts. The obstruction leads to the formation of comedones, which can become inflamed because of overgrowth of *Propionibacterium acnes.*
- Exacerbated by environmental factors (hot, humid, tropical climate), medications (e.g., iodine in cough mixtures, hair greases), industrial exposure to halogenated hydrocarbons.

DIAGNOSIS

DIFFERENTIAL DIAGNOSIS

- Gram-negative folliculitis
- Staphylococcal pyoderma
- Acne rosacea
- Drug eruption
- Sebaceous hyperplasia
- Angiofibromas, basal cell carcinomas, osteoma cutis
- Occupational exposures to oils or grease
- Steroid acne

WORKUP

History and physical examination:
- Inquire about previous treatment
- Careful drug history
- Family history, history of cyclic menstrual flares
- History of use of cosmetics and cleansers
- Oral contraceptive use

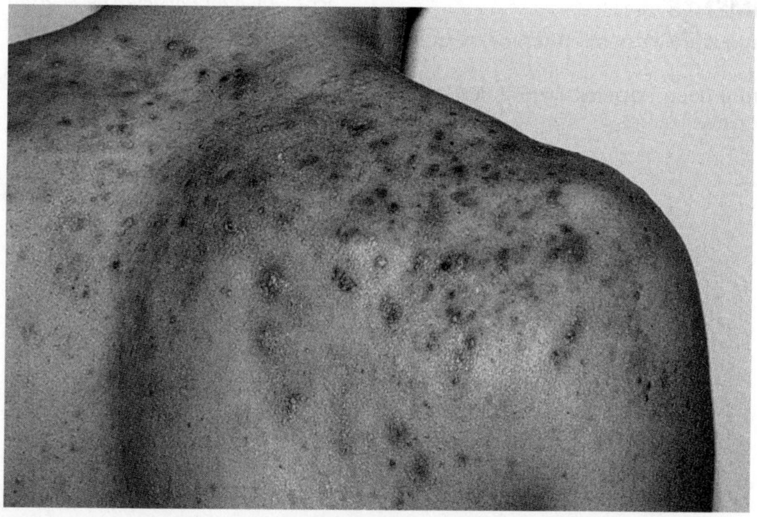

FIGURE 1-7 Acne on back and shoulders. This acne is typically inflammatory and usually needs oral antibiotics or possibly isoretinoin, but the patient may apply topical medication as well. Heat and sweat may aggravate. (From White GM, Cox NH [eds]: *Diseases of the skin,* a color atlas and text, ed 2, St. Louis, 2006, Mosby.)

LABORATORY TESTS

- Laboratory evaluation is generally not helpful.
- Patients who are candidates for therapy with isotretinoin (Accutane) should have baseline liver enzymes, cholesterol, and triglycerides checked, because this medication may result in elevation of lipids and liver enzymes.
- A negative serum pregnancy test or two negative urine pregnancy tests should also be obtained in females 1 wk before initiation of isotretinoin; it is also imperative to maintain effective contraception during and 1 mo after therapy with isotretinoin ends because of its teratogenic effects. Pregnancy status should be rechecked at monthly visits.
- In female patients if hyperandrogenism is suspected, levels of dehydroepiandrosterone sulfate (DHEAS), testosterone (total and free), and androstenedione should be measured. Generally for women with regular menstrual cycles, serum androgen measurements are not necessary.

TREATMENT

NONPHARMACOLOGIC THERAPY

- Blue light (ClearLight therapy system) can be used for treatment of moderate inflammatory acne vulgaris. Light in the violet/blue range can cause bacterial death by a photoreaction in which porphyrins react with oxygen to generate reactive oxygen species, which damage the cell membranes of *P. acnes.* Treatment usually consists of 15 min exposures twice weekly for 4 wk.

ACUTE GENERAL Rx

Treatment generally varies with the type of lesions (comedones, papules, pustules, cystic lesions) and the severity of acne.

- Comedones can be treated with retinoids or retinoid analogs. Topical retinoids are comedolytic and work by normalizing follicular keratinization. Commonly available agents are Adapalene (Differin, 0.1% gel or cream, applied once or twice daily), Tazarotene (Tazorac 0.1% cream or gel applied daily), tretinoin (Retin-A 0.1% cream or 0.025 gel applied once qhs), tretinoin microsphere (Retin-A Micro, 0.1% gel, applied at hs). Tretinoin is inactivated by UV light and oxydized by benzoyl peroxide, therefore it should only be applied at night and not used concomitantly with benzoyl peroxide.

Tretinoin is pregnancy category C, tazarotene is pregnancy category X. Salicylic acid preparations (e.g., Neutrogena 2% wash) have keratolytic and anti-inflammatory properties and are also useful in the treatment of comedones. Large open comedones (blackheads) should be expressed.

- Patients should be reevaluated after 4 to 6 wk. Benzoyl peroxide gel (2.5% or 5%) may be added if the comedones become inflamed or form pustules. The most common adverse effects are dryness, erythema, and peeling. Topical antibiotics (erythromycin, clindamycin lotions or pads) can also be used in patients with significant inflammation. They reduce *P. acnes* in the pilosebaceous follicle and have some anti-inflammatory effects. The combination of 5% benzoyl peroxide and 3% erythromycin (Benzamycin) or 1% clindamycin with 5% benzoyl peroxide (Benzaclin) are highly effective in patients who have a mixture of comedonal and inflammatory acne lesions.
- Pustular acne can be treated with tretinoin and benzoyl peroxide gel applied on alternate evenings; drying agents (sulfacetamide-sulfa lotions [Novacet, Sulfacet]) are also effective when used in combination with benzoyl peroxide; oral antibiotics (doxycycline 100 mg qd or erythromycin 1 g qd given in 2 to 3 divided doses) are effective in patients with moderate to severe pustular acne; patients not responding well to these antibiotics can be switched over to minocycline 50 to 100 mg bid; however, this medication is more expensive.
- Patients with nodular cystic acne can be treated with systemic agents: antibiotics (erythromycin, tetracycline, doxycycline, minocycline), isotretinoin (Accutane), or oral contraceptives. Periodic intralesional triamcinolone (Kenalog) injections by a dermatologist are also effective. The possibility of endocrinopathy should be considered in patients responding poorly to therapy.
- Isotretinoin is indicated for acne resistant to antibiotic therapy and severe acne; dosage is 0.5 to 1 mg/kg/day in 2 divided doses (maximum of 2 mg/kg/day); duration of therapy is generally 20 wk for a cumulative dose ≥120 mg/kg for severe cystic acne; before using this medication patients should undergo baseline laboratory evaluation (see "Laboratory Tests"). This drug is absolutely contraindicated during pregnancy because of its teratogenicity. It should be used with caution in patients with history of depression. In order to prescribe this drug, physicians must be registered members of the manufacturer's System to Manage Accutane-Related Teratogenicity (SMART) program.
- Azelaic acid is a bacteriostatic dicarboxylic acid used to normalize keratinization and reduce inflammation.
- Oral contraceptives reduce androgen levels and therefore sebum production. They represent a useful adjunctive therapy for all types of acne in women and adolescent girls. Commonly used agents are norgestimate/ethinyl estradiol (Ortho Tri-Cyclen) and drospirenone/ethinyl estradiol (Yasmin).

REFERRAL

Referral for intralesional injection and dermabrasion should be considered in patients with severe acne unresponsive to conventional therapy.

PEARLS & CONSIDERATIONS

- Gram-negative folliculitis should be suspected if inflammatory acne worsens after several months of oral antibiotic therapy.
- Acne may worsen during the first 3 to 4 wk of retinoid therapy before improving.

COMMENTS

Indications for systemic therapy of acne are:

- Painful deep papules or nodules
- Extensive lesions
- Active acne with severe scarring or hyperpigmentation
- Patient's morale

Patients should be educated that in most cases acne can be controlled but not cured and that at least 4 to 6 wk of initial therapy should be required before significant improvement is noted.

EVIDENCE

EBM

Out of 250 comparisons of treatment for acne studied, only 14 had evidence of high quality. This severely limits the number of meaningful conclusions that can be drawn.[1] Ⓑ

Of the 14 trials considered to provide higher quality evidence, several treatments were considered to be beneficial when compared with placebo. These were aluminum chlorhydroxide/sulfur, topical clindamycin, topical erythromycin, benzoyl peroxide, topical isotretinoin, tretinoin, oral tetracycline, and norgestimate/ethinyl estradiol.[1] Ⓑ

Again, considering the higher quality data, the systematic review found evidence that certain treatments were equally effective. It found benzoyl peroxide at various strengths was equally efficacious in mild/moderate acne; adapalene and tretinoin were equally efficacious in unspecified severity; motretinide and tretinoin were equally effective; adding vitamin A to oxytetracycline conferred no added efficacy; and cyproterone was equally effective at two different doses.[1] Ⓑ

Evidence-Based Reference

1. Evidence Report/Technology Assessment, Number 17: Management of Acne, AHRQ Publication No. 01-E019, 2001. Ⓑ

SUGGESTED READINGS

Feldman S et al: Diagnosis and treatment of acne, *Am Fam Physician* 69:2123, 2004.

Haider A, Shaw JC: Treatment of acne vulgaris, *JAMA* 292:726, 2004.

James WD: Acne, *N Engl J Med* 352:1463, 2005.

AUTHOR: **FRED F. FERRI, M.D.**

BASIC INFORMATION

DEFINITION

Acoustic neuroma is a benign proliferation of the Schwann cells that cover the vestibular branch of the eighth cranial nerve (CN VIII). Symptoms are commonly a result of compression of the acoustic branch of CN VIII, the facial nerve (CN VII), and the trigeminal nerve (CN V). The glossopharyngeal nerve (CN IX) and vagus nerve (CN X) are less commonly involved. In extreme cases, compression of the brainstem may lead to obstruction of cerebrospinal fluid (CSF) outflow and elevated intracranial pressure (ICP).

SYNONYMS

Vestibular schwannoma

ICD-9CM CODES
225.1 Acoustic neuroma

EPIDEMIOLOGY & DEMOGRAPHICS

Annual incidence is about 1 in 100,000 patients per year. There may be a slight female predominance. The tumor most commonly presents in the fifth and sixth decades.

PHYSICAL FINDINGS & CLINICAL PRESENTATION

- Most frequently unilateral hearing loss and/or tinnitus. Also balance problems, vertigo, facial pain (trigeminal neuralgia) and weakness, difficulty swallowing, fullness or pain of the involved ear. Headache may occur.
- With elevated ICP, patients may also suffer from vomiting, fever, and visual changes.
- Hearing loss is the most common presenting complaint and is usually high frequency.

ETIOLOGY

The etiology is incompletely understood, but long-term exposure to acoustic trauma has been implicated. Bilateral acoustic neuromas may be inherited in an autosomal dominant manner as part of neurofibromatosis type 2. This disease is associated with a defect on chromosome 22q1.

DIAGNOSIS

DIFFERENTIAL DIAGNOSIS

- Benign positional vertigo
- Meniere's disease
- Trigeminal neuralgia
- Cerebellar disease
- Normal-pressure hydrocephalus
- Presbycusis
- Glomus tumors
- Vertebrobasilar insufficiency
- Ototoxicity from medications
- Other tumors:
  - Meningioma, glioma
  - Facial nerve schwannoma
  - Cavernous hemangioma
  - Metastatic tumors

WORKUP

- A detailed neurologic examination with special attention to the cranial nerves is crucial.
- Otoscopic evaluation may help to rule out other causes of hearing loss.

LABORATORY TESTS

- Audiometry is useful, often shows asymmetric, sensorineural, high frequency hearing loss.
- CSF protein may be elevated.

IMAGING STUDIES

- MRI with gadolinium is the preferred test. It can detect tumors as small as 2 mm in diameter.
- CT scan with contrast can detect tumors 1 cm in diameter or larger.
- Treatment decisions should be based on the size of the tumor, rate of growth (older patients tend to have slower-growing tumors), degree of neurologic deficit, desire to preserve hearing, life expectancy, age of the patient, and surgical risk. A combination of treatments can also be employed.

TREATMENT

NONPHARMACOLOGIC THERAPY

- Surgery is the definitive treatment. Choice of approach (middle cranial fossa, translabyrinthine, or retromastoid suboccipital) may vary depending on the size of the tumor, amount of residual hearing desired, and degree of surgical risk that can be tolerated. Partial resection is sometimes undertaken to minimize the risk of injury to nearby structures. Intraoperative facial nerve monitoring is recommended.
- Radiation therapy (stereotactic radiotherapy, stereotactic radiosurgery, or proton beam radiotherapy) is useful for tumors <3 cm in diameter or for those in whom surgery is not an option. Radiotherapy following partial resection has also been used to minimize complications.
- Age alone is not a contraindication to surgery.

ACUTE GENERAL Rx

Not applicable

CHRONIC Rx

- Observation with MRI every 6 to 12 mo may be appropriate for frail patients with small tumors, but risk of unrecoverable hearing loss may increase if surgery is delayed.

DISPOSITION

Hearing can be preserved at near preoperative levels in more than two thirds of patients with small- to medium-sized tumors.

REFERRAL

Prompt referral to an ENT specialist or neurosurgeon who is facile with all three surgical approaches is recommended.

PEARLS & CONSIDERATIONS

COMMENTS

- Presents most commonly as unilateral, sensorineural hearing loss.
- Treatment outcomes are generally good, with cure rates approaching 90% at 5 years.
- Of those who are managed with observation only, about half have continued enlargement and about a fifth eventually have a surgical intervention.

PATIENT/FAMILY EDUCATION

Acoustic Neuroma Association: http://anausa.org

EVIDENCE

EBM

There is some evidence from randomized controlled trials (RCTs) for the use of masking devices for the treatment of tinnitus.

A systematic review found one RCT assessing two tinnitus-masking devices versus a nonblinded control. There was a significant improvement in symptoms with either device.[1]

One systematic review and an RCT found little evidence to support the use of ginkgo biloba in tinnitus.[1]

Evidence-Based Reference

1. Waddell A, Canter R: Tinnitus, *Clin Evid* 10:634, 2003.

SUGGESTED READINGS

Kondziolka D et al: Long-term outcomes after radiosurgery for acoustic neuromas, *N Engl J Med* 339:1426, 1999.

Mendenhall WM et al: Management of acoustic schwannoma, *Am J Otolaryngol* 25(1):38, 2004.

Pitts LH, Jackler RK: Treatment of acoustic neuromas, *N Engl J Med* 339:1471, 1998.

Yoshimoto Y: Systematic review of the natural history of vestibular schwannoma, *J Neurosurg* 103(1):59, 2005.

AUTHORS: **SRIVIDYA ANANDAN, M.D.,** and **PAUL PIRRAGLIA, M.D., M.P.H.**

BASIC INFORMATION

DEFINITION

Acquired immunodeficiency syndrome (AIDS) is a disorder caused by infection with the human immunodeficiency virus, type 1 (HIV-1) and marked by progressive deterioration of the cellular immune system, leading to secondary infections or malignancies.

SYNONYMS

AIDS

ICD-9CM CODES
042.9 AIDS, unspecified

EPIDEMIOLOGY & DEMOGRAPHICS

INCIDENCE (IN U.S.):
- 27.1 cases/100,000 persons
- Varies widely by location
- 85% of cases in large cities

PREVALENCE (IN U.S.): 62 cases/100,000 persons
PREDOMINANT SEX: Males 84%, females 16% (through 1998); 40% of newly reported U.S. cases in 1999 were in females
PREDOMINANT AGE: 80% between ages 20 and 40 yr
PEAK INCIDENCE: See "Incidence"
GENETICS:
- Familial disposition: Although there is no proven genetic predisposition, individuals with deletions in the CCR5 gene are immune from infection with macrophage tropic virus (the predominant virus in sexual transmission).
- Congenital infection:
  1. Transmittable from an infected mother to the fetus in utero in as many as 30% of pregnancies.
  2. No specific congenital malformations associated with infection; low birth weight and spontaneous abortion are possible.
- Neonatal infection: transmission possible to the neonate intrapartum or postpartum through breast-feeding.

PHYSICAL FINDINGS & CLINICAL PRESENTATION

- Nonspecific findings: fever, weight loss, anorexia
- Specific syndromes:
  1. Seen in association with opportunistic infection and malignancies, so-called indicator diseases; these include:
     a. Opportunistic infections:
        Disseminated strongyloidiasis
        Disseminated toxoplasmosis, cryptococcosis, histoplasmosis, CMV, herpes simplex, or mycobacterial disease
        Candida esophagitis or bronchopulmonary disease
        Chronic *Cryptosporidia spp.* diarrhea
        Pneumocystis jiroveci pneumonia
        Extensive pulmonary and extrapulmonary tuberculosis
        Recurrent bacterial pneumonia
        Progressive multifocal leukoencephalopathy
     b. AIDS-related neoplasms:
        Kaposi's sarcoma in a person <60 yr of age
        Primary brain lymphoma
        Invasive cervical carcinoma
        High grade B cell non-Hodgkin's lymphoma, Burkitt's lymphoma, undifferentiated non-Hodgkin's lymphoma, or immunoblastic lymphoma
  2. Most common:
     Respiratory infections (*Pneumocystis jiroveci* [formerly known as *Pneumocystis carinii*] pneumonia, TB, bacterial pneumonia, fungal infection)
     CNS infections (toxoplasmosis, cryptococcal meningitis, TB)
     GI (cryptosporidiosis, isosporiasis, cytomegalovirus); Sections II and III describe organisms associated with diarrhea in patients with AIDS
     Eye infections (cytomegalovirus, toxoplasmosis)
     Kaposi's sarcoma (cutaneous or visceral) or lymphoma (nodal or extranodal)
- Possibly asymptomatic
- Diagnosis of AIDS if T-lymphocyte subset analysis demonstrating CD4 cell count <200 or <14% of total lymphocyte in the presence of proven HIV infection even in the absence of other infections
- The various manifestations of HIV infection are described in Section II

ETIOLOGY

- Caused by infection with human immunodeficiency virus, type 1 (HIV-1)
- Transmitted by heterosexual or male homosexual contact, needle-sharing (during IV drug use), transfusion of contaminated blood or blood products, and from infected mother to fetus or neonate as described previously

DIAGNOSIS

DIFFERENTIAL DIAGNOSIS

- Other wasting illnesses mimicking the nonspecific features of AIDS:
  1. TB
  2. Neoplasms
  3. Disseminated fungal infection
  4. Malabsorption syndromes
  5. Depression
- Other disorders associated with dementia or demyelination producing encephalopathy, myelopathy, or neuropathy

WORKUP

Prompt evaluation of respiratory, CNS, GI complaints

LABORATORY TESTS

- HIV antibody testing
- T-lymphocyte subset analysis: performed to determine the degree of immunodeficiency
- Viral load assay: to plan long-term antiviral therapy consider genotype or phenotype sensitivity testing for patients failing therapy
- CSF examination: for meningitis
- Serologic tests for syphilis, hepatitis B, hepatitis C, and toxoplasmosis
- Genotypic resistance testing: used to assess for primary resistance in naïve patients and secondary resistance in patients failing a regimen
- Eye exam: to evaluate for CMV retinitis in patients with CD4 counts <50 cells/mm^3
- Cryptococcal antigen: part of the evaluation in AIDS patients with CD4 <100 cells/mm^3 who have fever, diffuse pneumonia, or symptoms of meningitis

IMAGING STUDIES

- Cerebral CT for encephalopathy or focal CNS complications (e.g., toxoplasmosis, lymphoma)
- Pulmonary gallium scanning to aid in the diagnosis of *Pneumocystis jiroveci* (*P. carinii*) pneumonia
- Baseline chest x-ray

TREATMENT

NONPHARMACOLOGIC THERAPY

- Maintain adequate caloric intake.
- Encourage good oral hygiene, regular dental care.
- Avoid high risk behaviors that increase the risk of repeated exposure to HIV and other potential pathogens—safer sexual practices, avoid sharing needles, etc.
- Update vaccines—particularly the pneumococcal and hepatitis B vaccine along with annual influenza vaccines.
- Avoid administration of any live attenuated vaccines that may be a risk to these immunocompromised patients.
- When feasible, avoid activities that might increase risk of exposure to opportunistic infections (i.e., cleaning out a cat litter box [toxoplasmosis], getting scratched by a cat [*Bartonella* infections], exposure to pet reptiles [salmonellosis], traveling to developing countries [cryptosporidiosis, tuberculosis], eating undercooked foods and drinking from unsafe water supplies, etc.)

ACUTE GENERAL Rx

Acute management of opportunistic infections and malignancies is reviewed elsewhere in this text under specific AIDS-related disorders.

CHRONIC Rx

For all HIV-infected patients, particularly those meeting the case definition of AIDS:

- Preventive therapy for *Pneumocystis jiroveci* pneumonia and TB (see specific chapters elsewhere in this text). With the advent of modern antiretroviral therapy many patients have experienced substantial restoration of cellular immune function. It has become clear that preventive therapy for *Pneumocystis jiroveci* and *Mycobacterium avium* complex as well as suppressive therapy for cytomegaloviral and cryptococcal infection can often be safely withdrawn if the CD4 cell count rises above 200 for at least 6 mo.
- Begin HAART (highly active antiretroviral therapy) when any of the following are present:
  1. Symptomatic HIV infection is associated with any opportunistic infection
  2. CD4 count <200 cells/mm^3
  3. CD4 count <350 cells/mm^3 and before it reaches 200 cells/mm^3, especially if the viral load >30,000 copies/ml
  4. Consider therapy if CD4 count is rapidly decreasing and viral load >100,000 copies/ml
- Antiretroviral therapy employing combinations of nucleoside reverse transcriptase inhibitor (NRTI) agents: zidovudine (AZT), didanosine (DDI), zalcitabine (DDC), lamivudine (3TC), Emtricitabine (FTC), stavudine (D4T), abacavir in addition to protease inhibitors (PI) (saquinavir, indinavir, nelfinavir, agenerase, ritonavir/lopinavir, atazanavir) nonnucleoside reverse transcriptase inhibitors (NNRTI) (nevirapine, delavirdine, efavirenz) or the nucleotide agent tenofovir according to current recommendations based on clinical stage and viral load studies. The protease inhibitor ritonavir should be used, in low dose, in combination with other protease inhibitors to obtain more sustained drug levels. Usual initial dosing regimen consists of two NRTIs and a NNRTI (or a PI). Common regimens include:
  1. Combivir (AZT and 3TC) one tablet by mouth twice a day and efavirenz 600 mg by mouth once daily
  2. Combivir (AZT and 3TC) one tablet by mouth twice a day and ritonavir/lopinavir 3 tablets by mouth twice daily with food
  3. Truvada (tenofovir plus Emtricitabine [FTC]) one tablet once daily and efavirenz 600 mg by mouth once daily

  All these drugs have unique and class-specific side effects and require careful and expert follow up to achieve optimal antiviral effects, assure compliance, and maintain efficacy. Antiviral response should be monitored by baseline HIV viral load and CD4 count and repeat measurement at 2 wk and 4 wk into treatment and then periodically (every 3 mo) to assure viral suppression.
- An approach to evaluating chronic diarrhea in patients with HIV infection, the approach to the acutely ill HIV-infected patient, and the evaluation of respiratory complaints are described in Section III. Approach to a patient with a suspected CNS lesion is also described in Section III.
- Genotypic resistance testing should be strongly considered for any patient failing antiretroviral therapy. Poor adherence to therapy, however, often underlies virologic failure.

DISPOSITION

The outlook for AIDS has changed radically in the last decade from an essentially uniformly fatal disease to a chronic medical illness compatible with long term survival and remarkably good quality of life. Patients should be aggressively supported in the presence of severe illness as outcomes following ICU admissions remain good. This is accomplished through expert and continuous follow up, use of highly active antiretroviral drugs, and careful detail to compliance to medications and lifestyle modification.

REFERRAL

All patients with AIDS: to a physician knowledgeable and experienced in the management of the disease and its complications

EVIDENCE

EBM

Three-drug regimens are associated with significantly improved clinical outcomes after 2 years of follow-up compared with two-drug regimens.[1] Ⓐ

Maintenance therapies with fewer antiretrovirals are associated with a higher risk of resistance and of loss of HIV suppression. Maintenance with zidovudine/lamivudine/indinavir is superior to zidovudine/lamivudine. Maintenance therapy that has been modified by discontinuing one or more of the protease inhibitors that were used in the induction phase is also associated with a significantly increased risk of failure.[2] Ⓐ

A multicenter randomized controlled trial (RCT) compared pairs of sequential three-drug regimens. People with HIV-1 who had not previously received antiretroviral therapy were followed for a median of 2.3 yr. The combination of zidovudine, lamivudine, and efavirenz was found to be superior to the other antiretroviral regimens used as initial therapy (didanosine and stavudine in combination with either nelfinavir or efavirenz).[3] Ⓑ

The same group compared initial therapy involving a four-drug regimen with therapy involving two consecutive three-drug regimens, the first of which contained either efavirenz or nelfinavir, in combination with either didanosine and stavudine or zidovudine and lamivudine. There was no significant difference in the duration of successful HIV-1 treatment between a single four-drug regimen and two consecutive three-drug regimens; initiating therapy with the three-drug regimen of zidovudine, lamivudine, and efavirenz was the optimal choice.[4] Ⓑ

Another multicenter RCT compared the effect of alternating antiretroviral regimens while patients' viral load remains suppressed in order to minimize HIV resistance mutations. Patients were treated by continuous stavudine, didanosine, efavirenz (regimen A), or zidovudine, lamivudine, nelfinavir (regimen B) until virologic failure, or by alternating between the two regimens every 3 mo. It was found that, over 48 wk, virologic failure was delayed in the alternating regimen group (incidence rate 1.2 events/1000 person-wk) compared with the pooled standard-of-care groups (4.8).[5] Ⓑ

A systematic review found one controlled study comparing a pharmacist-led program of educational and supportive counseling (for promoting adherence to HAART) versus conventional dispensing of HAART medication. Adherence to HAART was significantly improved in the intervention group, but there was less evidence that viral load was subsequently reduced due to participation in the program.[6] Ⓑ

Immediate use of zidovudine, compared with waiting until the early signs of AIDS appear, significantly reduces the rate of disease progression during the first year. However, this effect is not sustained, and there is no improvement in survival in the short or long term compared with deferred administration.[7] Ⓐ

There is evidence to support the use of pharmacotherapy for the prevention of opportunistic infections in patients with HIV and AIDS.[8,9] Ⓐ

There is evidence that the use of antituberculous prophylaxis in patients with HIV will reduce the risk of active tuberculosis in people with a positive tuberculin skin test.[10] Ⓐ

A systematic review has found that performing constant or interval aerobic exercise, or a combination of aerobic and progressive resistive exercise for at least 20 min, three times a wk for 4 wk appears to be safe and may lead to clinically significant improvements in fitness. Furthermore, it may improve psychological well-being.[11] Ⓐ

Evidence-Based References

1. Jordan R et al: Systematic review and meta-analysis of evidence for increasing numbers of drugs in antiretroviral therapy, *BMJ* 324:757, 2002. Ⓐ
2. Rutherford GW et al: Three- or four- versus two-drug antiretroviral maintenance regimens for HIV infection, *Cochrane Database Syst Rev* (4):CD002037, 2003. Ⓐ
3. Robbins GK et al: Comparison of sequential three-drug regimens as initial therapy for HIV-1 infection, *N Engl J Med* 349:2293, 2003. Ⓑ
4. Shafer RW et al: Comparison of four-drug regimens and pairs of sequential three-drug regimens as initial therapy for HIV-1 infection, *N Engl J Med* 349:2304, 2003. Ⓑ
5. Martinez-Picado J et al: Alternation of antiretroviral drug regimens for HIV infection. A randomized, controlled trial, *Ann Intern Med* 139:81, 2003. Ⓑ
6. Haddad M et al: Patient support and education for promoting adherence to highly active antiretroviral therapy for HIV/AIDS, *Cochrane Database Syst Rev* (3):CD001442, 2000. Ⓑ
7. Darbyshire J et al: Immediate versus deferred zidovudine (AZT) in asymptomatic or mildly symptomatic HIV infected adults, *Cochrane Database Syst Rev* (3):CD002039, 2000. Ⓐ
8. Ioannidis J, Wilkinson D: HIV: prevention of opportunistic infections, *Clin Evid* 11:913, 2004.
9. Grimwade K, Swingler, G: Cotrimoxazole prophylaxis for opportunistic infections in adults with HIV, *Cochrane Database Syst Rev* (3):CD003108, 2003. Ⓐ
10. Woldehanna S, Volmink J: Treatment of latent tuberculosis infection in HIV infected persons, *Cochrane Database Syst Rev* (1):CD000171, 2004.
11. Nixon S et al: Aerobic exercise interventions for adults living with HIV/AIDS, *Cochrane Database Syst Rev* (2):CD001796, 2005. Ⓐ

SUGGESTED READINGS

d'Arminio Monforte A et al: The changing incidence of AIDS events in patients receiving highly active antiretroviral therapy, *Arch Intern Med* 165(4):416, 2005.

Hammer SM et al: Treatment for adult HIV infection: 2006 recommendations of the International AIDS Society—USA panel, *JAMA* 296(7):827, 2006.

Hermsen ED, Wynn HE, McNabb J: Discontinuation of prophylaxis for HIV-associated opportunistic infections in the era of highly active antiretroviral therapy, *Am J Health Syst Pharm* 61(3):245, 2004.

Huang L et al: Intensive care of patients with HIV infection, *N Engl J Med* 355(2):173, 2006.

Kantor R et al: Evolution of resistance to drugs in HIV-1-infected patients failing antiretroviral therapy, *AIDS* 18(11):1503, 2004.

Monier PL, Wilcox R: Metabolic complications associated with the use of highly active antiretroviral therapy in HIV-1-infected adults, *Am J Med Sci* 328(1):48, 2004.

Olsen CH et al: Risk of AIDS and death at given HIV-RNA and CD4 cell count, in relation to specific antiretroviral drugs in regimen, *AIDS* 19(3):319, 2005.

AUTHORS: **STEVEN M. OPAL, M.D.**, and **JOSEPH R. MASCI, M.D.**

BASIC INFORMATION

DEFINITION

Acromegaly is a chronic debilitating disease with an insidious onset, resulting from the effects of either hypersecretion of growth hormone (GH) or increased amounts of an insulin-like growth factor I (IGF-I).

SYNONYMS

Marie's disease

ICD-9CM CODES
253.0 Acromegaly

EPIDEMIOLOGY & DEMOGRAPHICS

INCIDENCE: 3 to 4 new cases/1,000,000 persons annually

PREVALENCE: 50 to 60 cases/1 million persons, with some estimates as high as 90 cases/1 million persons

PREDOMINANT SEX: No sexual predominance

MEAN AGE AT DIAGNOSIS: Males: 40 yr; females: 45 yr

RISK FACTORS
- Increased mortality, primarily from cardiovascular and respiratory causes
- Death in 50% of untreated patients by age 50 yr
- Increased prevalence of colon carcinoma and other malignancies

PHYSICAL FINDINGS & CLINICAL PRESENTATION

- Coarse features resulting from growth of soft tissue
- Coarse, oily skin
- Hands and feet that are spadelike, fleshy, and moist
- Prognathism, which can give an underbite
- Carpal tunnel syndrome
- Excessive sweating
- Arthralgias and severe osteoarthritis
- History of increased hat, glove, and/or shoe size
- Hypertension
- Skin tags
- Muscle weakness and decreased exercise capacity
- Headache, often severe
- Diabetes mellitus
- Visual field defects

ETIOLOGY

Cause is usually a pituitary adenoma affecting the anterior lobe.

DIAGNOSIS

DIFFERENTIAL DIAGNOSIS

Ectopic production of growth hormone–releasing hormone (GHRH) from a carcinoid or other neuroendocrine tumor

WORKUP

1. First screening test: measure serum IGF-I level.
   a. Direct measurement of the GH level is not as useful, because it is secreted in a pulsatile fashion and a random level may be falsely normal.
   b. Upper limits of a normal IGF-I level, depending on the assay: >380 ng/ml or 2.5 U/ml.
2. Failure to suppress serum GH to less than 2 ng/ml after 100 g oral glucose is considered conclusive.
   a. Patients may show suppression of GH (paradoxical response).
   b. Patients will not suppress GH to 2 ng/ml or less (typical response in patients with acromegaly).
   c. GHRH level >300 ng/ml is indicative of an ectopic source of GH.

LABORATORY TESTS

- Elevated serum phosphate
- Elevated urine calcium

IMAGING STUDIES

- Imaging studies of choice: MRI of the pituitary and hypothalamus
- CT of the pituitary and hypothalamus used initially

TREATMENT

SURGERY

Treatment of choice: transsphenoidal microsurgical adenomectomy
- Surgical failure rate: about 13.3% for microadenomas (tumors <10 mm) and 11.1% for macroadenomas (tumors >10 mm confined to the sella)
- Preoperative IGF-I level: indicator of surgical outcome with higher levels associated with surgical failure

RADIOTHERAPY

- Irradiation to reduce further growth of the tumor in most patients
- Major complication: hypopituitarism, which may occur in up to 50% of patients; this complication is more likely in patients who had surgery irradiation

ACUTE GENERAL Rx

- Indicated when patients have failed surgical therapy, when surgery is contraindicated, and in patients waiting for the effects of radiotherapy to begin
- Octreotide
  1. A somatostatin analog given tid at a dose of 100 mg subcutaneously
  2. Important side effects: biliary sludge and gallstones; nausea, cramps, and steatorrhea; suppression of GH levels to about 5 mg/L in 52% of patients; IGF-I levels normalized in about 53%
  3. Important in the preoperative shrinkage of pituitary tumors and softening of adenomatous tissue
- Bromocriptine
  1. A dopamine analog given at a dosage of 10 to 60 mg PO tid to qid
  2. Less effective than octreotide
  3. Important advantages: less expensive than octreotide and taken orally
  4. Important side effects: orthostatic hypotension, lightheadedness, nausea, constipation, and nasal stuffiness
  5. Suppresses GH levels to <5 mg/L in about 20% of patients; normalizes GH levels in approximately 10%, and shrinks pituitary adenomas in 10% to 20%; IGF-I levels normalized in about 10%
- Pegvisomant is a growth hormone receptor antagonist that has shown promising results in the treatment of acromegaly.

CHRONIC Rx

Combination of bromocriptine and octreotide may be synergistic, allowing a lower combination dosage than alone.

DISPOSITION

- Patients receiving radiotherapy need long-term follow-up to monitor the potential development of hypopituitarism.
- Continuation of medical therapy should be based on the normalization of IGF-I levels.

EVIDENCE

A 12-wk randomized controlled trial compared three daily doses of subcutaneous pegvisomant (10 mg, 15 mg, and 20 mg) with placebo in patients with acromegaly. All groups benefitted compared with placebo, the greatest benefit being seen with 15 and 20 mg doses.[1] B

Evidence-Based Reference

1. Trainer PJ et al: Treatment of acromegaly with the growth hormone-receptor antagonist pegvisomant, *N Engl J Med* 342:1171, 2000. B

SUGGESTED READINGS

Doga M et al: Diagnostic and therapeutic consensus on acromegaly, *J Endocrinol Invest* 28(5 Suppl):56, 2005.

Ezzat S: Pharmacological options in the treatment of acromegaly, *Cur Opin Invest Drugs* 6(10):1023, 2005.

Ketznelson L: Diagnosis and treatment of acromegaly, *Growth Horm IGF Res* 15 Suppl A:S31, 2005.

Melmad S et al: Current status and future opportunities for controlling acromegaly, *Pituitary* 5(3):185, 2002.

Trainer PJ et al: Treatment of acromegaly with the growth hormone-receptor antagonist pegvisomant, *N Engl J Med* 342:1172, 2000.

AUTHORS: **BETH J. WUTZ, M.D.,** and **RUBEN ALVERO, M.D.**

BASIC INFORMATION

DEFINITION

Actinomycosis is an indolent, slowly progressive infection caused by both anaerobic or microaerophilic bacteria that normally colonize the mouth, vagina, and colon. Actinomycosis is characterized by the formation of painful abscesses, soft tissue infiltration, and draining sinuses.

SYNONYMS

Actinomyces infection
Lumpy jaw

ICD-9CM CODES

039.9 Actinomycosis

EPIDEMIOLOGY & DEMOGRAPHICS

Geographic distribution:
- Actinomycosis is worldwide in distribution.
- Commonly found as normal flora of the oral cavity (within gingival crevices, tonsillar crypts, periodontal pockets, dental plaques, and carious teeth), pharynx, tracheobronchial tree, gastrointestinal tract, and female urogenital tract.

Incidence and prevalence:
- Incidence 1:300,000.
- Males infected more often than females 3:1.
- Can occur at any age but commonly seen in midlife.
- Incidence has decreased since the 1950s and is attributed to better oral hygiene and antibiotics.

PHYSICAL FINDINGS & CLINICAL PRESENTATION

Actinomycosis can affect any organ. Although not typically considered as opportunistic pathogens, *Actinomyces* species capitalize on tissue injury or mucosal breach to invade adjacent structures in the head and neck regions. As a result, dental infections and oromaxillofacial trauma are common antecedent events. Characteristic manifestations include:
- Cervicofacial disease (most common site):
  1. Occurs in the setting of poor dental hygiene, recent dental surgery, or minor oral trauma
  2. Painful soft tissue swelling commonly seen at the angle of the mandible
  3. Fever, chills, and weight loss
  4. Trismus
  5. Soft tissue facial infection with sinus tract or fistula formation
- Thoracic disease:
  1. Can involve the lungs, pleura, mediastinum, or chest wall.
  2. Presumed secondary to aspiration of *Actinomyces* organisms in patients with poor oral hygiene.
  3. Fever, cough, weight loss, and pleuritic chest pains are common symptoms.
  4. Signs of pneumonia or pleural effusion may be present.
  5. With extension beyond the lungs to mediastinal structures and the chest wall, signs and symptoms of pericarditis, empyema, chest wall sinus drainage, and tracheoesophageal fistula can all occur (Fig. 1-8).
- Abdominal disease:
  1. Occurs most commonly after appendectomy, perforated bowel, diverticulitis, or surgery to the gastrointestinal tract.
  2. Lesions develop most commonly in the ileocecal valve, causing abdominal pain, fever, weight loss, and a palpable mass.
  3. Extension may occur to the liver, causing jaundice and abscess formation.
  4. Sinus tracts to the abdominal wall can occur.
- Pelvic disease:
  1. Commonly occurs by extension from abdominal disease of the ileocecal valve to the right adnexa (80% of cases).
  2. Endometritis.

ETIOLOGY

- Actinomycosis is most commonly caused by *Actinomyces israelii*. Other causes are *A. naeslundii, A. odontolyticus, A. viscosus,* and *A. meyeri*.
- *Actinomyces* are gram-positive, non-spore-forming, filamentous, anaerobic or microaerophilic rods.
- Actinomycosis infections are polymicrobial, usually associated with *Streptococcus, Bacteroides, Eikenella corrodens, Enterococcus,* and *Fusobacterium* spp.
- Infects individuals only after entry into disrupted mucosa or tissue injury.

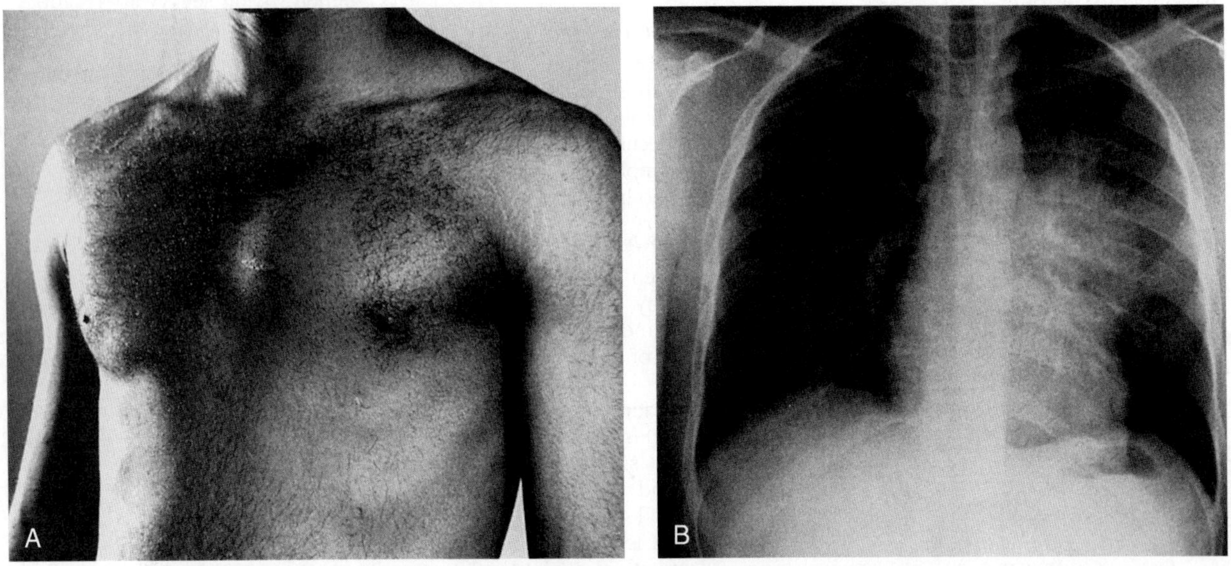

FIGURE 1-8 Thoracic actinomycosis. A, Initial presentation with a bulging mass lesion in the chest wall with a central sinus tract. **B,** The chest radiograph with the associated pulmonary infiltrate. (From Gorbach SL: *Infectious diseases,* ed 2, Philadelphia, 1998, WB Saunders.)

DIAGNOSIS

Dx

Isolating the bacteria in the proper clinical setting makes the diagnosis of actinomycosis.

DIFFERENTIAL DIAGNOSIS

- Cervicofacial disease: odontogenic abscesses, brachial cleft cyst
- Pulmonary disease: nocardiosis, botryomycosis, chromomycosis, fungal disease of the lung, tuberculosis
- Intestinal disease: intestinal tuberculosis, ameboma, Crohn's disease, colon cancer
- Pelvic disease: chronic pelvic inflammatory disease, Crohn's disease
- CNS disease: other forms of brain abscess, brain tumors, toxoplasmosis, intracranial hematoma

WORKUP

The workup includes obtaining specimens either by aspirating abscesses, excising sinus tracts, or tissue biopsies.

LABORATORY TESTS

- Isolating "sulfur granules" from tissue specimens or draining sinuses confirms the diagnosis of actinomycosis. *Actinomyces* are noted for forming characteristic sulfur granules in infected tissue but not in vitro. The term *sulfur granule* is a misnomer, reflecting only the yellow color of the granule in pus, because the granules are not composed of any sulfur at all.
  1. Sulfur granules are nests of *Actinomyces* species. Sulfur granules may be macroscopic or microscopic (Fig. 1-9).
  2. Sulfur granules are crushed and stained for identification of *Actinomyces* organisms and may take up to 3 wk to grow in culture media.

IMAGING STUDIES

Imaging studies are useful adjunctive tests in localizing the site and spread of infection.

1. Chest x-ray examination
2. CT scan of the head, chest, abdomen, and pelvic areas is useful

TREATMENT

Rx

NONPHARMACOLOGIC THERAPY

- Incision and drainage of abscesses
- Excision of sinus tract

ACUTE GENERAL Rx

- Penicillin 10 to 20 million units per day in 4 divided doses for 4 to 6 wk.
- In penicillin-allergic patients, erythromycin, tetracycline, clindamycin, or cephalosporins (depending on the type of penicillin allergy) are reasonable alternatives.
- Chloramphenicol 50 to 60 mg/kg/day can be used for CNS actinomycosis.

CHRONIC Rx

- Following 4 to 6 wk IV penicillin, oral penicillin V 500 mg PO qid for 6 to 12 mo.
- Treatment of associated microorganisms is not needed.

DISPOSITION

- Clinical actinomycosis, if not treated, spreads to contiguous tissues and structures ignoring tissue planes. Hematogenous spread, although possible, is rare.
- Actinomycosis is very sensitive to antibiotics but requires chronic long-term treatment to prevent relapse.

REFERRAL

If the diagnosis of actinomycosis is suspected, consultation with an infectious disease specialist is suggested. General surgical consultation for excision of sinus tracts and abscess incision and drainage is recommended.

PEARLS & CONSIDERATIONS

!

COMMENTS

- There is no person-to-person transmission of *Actinomyces*.
- Isolation of the organism in an asymptomatic individual does not mean the person has actinomycosis. Active symptoms must be present to make the diagnosis.
- Pelvic actinomycosis has been associated with use of an intrauterine device (IUD).
- Actinomycosis can also involve the CNS, causing multiple brain abscesses.

SUGGESTED READINGS

Choi J: Optimal duration of IV and oral antibiotics in the treatment of thoracic actinomycosis, *Chest* 128(4):2211, 2005.

Jacobs RF, Schutze GE: Actinomycosis. In Behrman RE (Ed), *Nelson Textbook of Pediatrics*, ed 16, Philadelphia, 2000, WB Saunders, p. 823.

Russo TA: Agents of actinomycosis. In *Mandell, Douglas, and Bennett's principles and practice of infectious diseases,* ed 5, New York, 2000, Churchill Livingstone.

AUTHORS: **GLENN G. FORT, M.D., M.P.H.,** and **DENNIS J. MIKOLICH, M.D.**

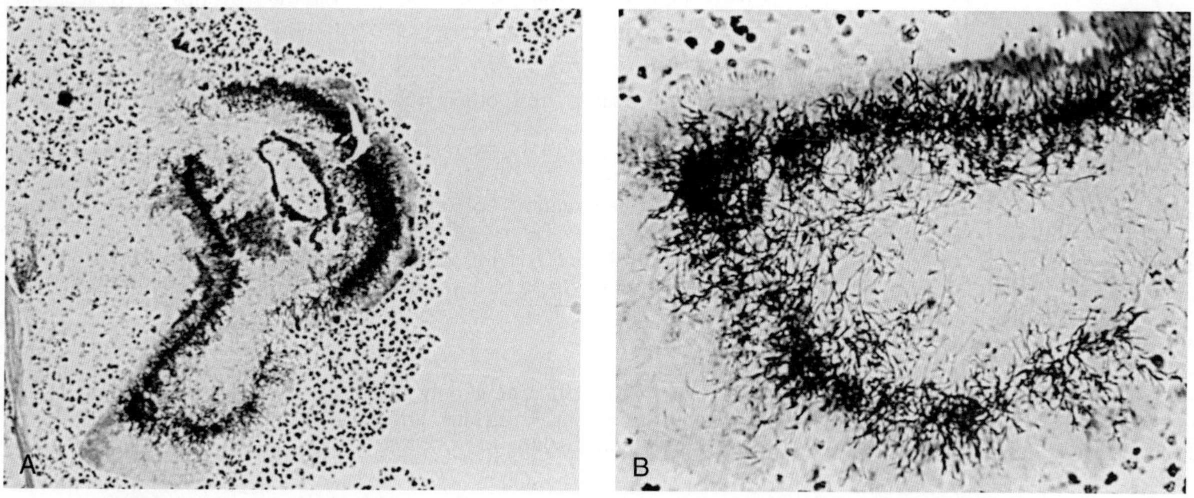

FIGURE 1-9 **A,** Actinomycotic sulfur granule surrounded by inflammatory cells (Brown-Brenn stain, ×250). **B,** Increased magnification (×1000) demonstrates the delicate, branched filaments of *Actinomyces.* (From Mandell GL [ed]: *Mandell, Douglas, and Bennett's principles and practice of infectious diseases,* ed 5, New York, 2000, Churchill Livingstone.)

BASIC INFORMATION

DEFINITION

Acute bronchitis is the inflammation of trachea and bronchi.

SYNONYMS

Chest cold

ICD-9CM CODES
466.0 Acute bronchitis

EPIDEMIOLOGY & DEMOGRAPHICS

- Highest incidence in smokers, older adults, young children, and in winter months.
- In the U.S. there are nearly 30 million ambulatory visits annually for cough, leading to more than 12 million diagnoses of "bronchitis."
- Acute lower respiratory tract infection is the most common condition treated in primary care.

PHYSICAL FINDINGS & CLINICAL PRESENTATION

- Cough, usually worse in the morning, often productive. Mainly caused by transient bronchial hyperresponsiveness
- Low-grade fever
- Substernal discomfort worsened by coughing
- Postnasal drip, pharyngeal injection
- Rhonchi that may clear after cough, occasional wheezing

ETIOLOGY

- Viral infections are the leading cause of bronchitis (rhinovirus, influenza virus, adenovirus, respiratory syncytial virus)
- Atypical organisms (*Mycoplasma, Chlamydia pneumoniae*)
- Bacterial infections (*Haemophilus influenzae, Moraxella, Streptococcus pneumoniae*)

DIAGNOSIS

DIFFERENTIAL DIAGNOSIS

- Pneumonia
- Asthma
- Sinusitis
- Bronchiolitis
- Aspiration
- Cystic fibrosis
- Pharyngitis
- Cough secondary to medications
- Neoplasm (elderly patients)
- Influenza
- Allergic aspergillosis
- GERD
- CHF (in elderly patients)
- Bronchogenic neoplasm

WORKUP

Seldom necessary (e.g., to rule out pneumonia, neoplasm)

LABORATORY TESTS

Lab tests are generally not necessary.

IMAGING STUDIES

Chest x-ray examination is usually reserved for patients with suspected pneumonia, influenza, or underlying COPD and no improvement with therapy.

TREATMENT

NONPHARMACOLOGIC THERAPY

- Avoidance of tobacco and other pulmonary irritants
- Increased fluid intake
- Use of vaporizer to increase room humidity

ACUTE GENERAL Rx

- Inhaled bronchodilators (e.g., albuterol, metaproterenol) prn for 1 to 2 wk in patients with wheezing or troublesome cough. Inhaled albuterol has been proven effective in reducing the duration of cough in adults with uncomplicated acute bronchitis.
- Cough suppression with dextromethorphan and guaifenesin is commonly recommended; addition of codeine for cough suppression if cough is severe and is significantly interrupting patient's sleep pattern.
- Use of antibiotics (TMP-SMX, amoxicillin, doxycycline, cefuroxime) for acute bronchitis is generally not indicated; should be considered only in patients with concomitant COPD and purulent sputum or in patients unresponsive to prolonged conservative treatment.
- Antibiotics are overused in patients with acute bronchitis (70% to 90% of office visits for acute bronchitis result in treatment with antibiotics); this practice pattern is contributing to increases in resistant organisms.

CHRONIC Rx

Avoidance of tobacco and other pulmonary irritants

DISPOSITION

- Complete recovery within 7 to 10 days in most patients.
- Patients should be informed to expect to have a cough for 10 to 14 days after the visit.

REFERRAL

For pulmonary function testing only in patients with recurrent bronchitis and suspected underlying asthma

PEARLS & CONSIDERATIONS

COMMENTS

- Intervention studies reveal that patient and physician education are effective in reducing the use of antibiotic therapy. No offer or delayed offer of antibiotics for acute uncomplicated lower respiratory tract infection is acceptable, is associated with little difference in symptom resolution, and is likely to reduce antibiotic use and beliefs in the effectiveness of antibiotics.
- It is helpful to refer to acute bronchitis as a "chest cold." Patients should be informed that antibiotics are probably not going to be beneficial and may result in significant side effects.

EVIDENCE

Overall, the evidence for the use of beta-2 agonists in acute bronchitis is not strong, especially for those with no evidence of airflow obstruction.[1] (A)

Antibiotics for the treatment of acute bronchitis may produce modest benefits, but these must be weighed against the increased risk of adverse effects; moreover, most cases of acute bronchitis are viral and so will be unaffected by antibiotic therapy. Patients with other typical symptoms of an upper respiratory tract infection who have been ill for less than 1 week may be the least likely to benefit from antibiotics.[2] (A)

There is little evidence that one antibiotic is preferred over any other.[3] (A)

Even though physicians may be more likely to prescribe antibiotics for smokers suffering from acute bronchitis rather than nonsmokers, seven trials in a systematic review found no evidence that there was a difference between the two groups in their response to treatment.[2] (A)

There is no good evidence that dextromethorphan is effective in acute bronchitis.[4] (A)

Evidence-Based References

1. Smucny J et al: Beta2-agonists for acute bronchitis, *Cochrane Database Syst Rev* 1:2004. (A)
2. Smucny J et al: Antibiotics for acute bronchitis, *Cochrane Database Syst Rev* 4:2004. (A)
3. Wark P: Acute bronchitis, *Clin Evid* 13:1844, 2005, London, BMJ Publishing Group. (A)
4. Schroeder K, Fahey T: Over-the-counter medications for acute cough in children and adults in ambulatory settings, *Cochrane Database Syst Rev* 4:2004. (B)

SUGGESTED READING

Wenzel R, Fowler A: Acute bronchitis. *N Engl J Med* 355:2125, 2006.

AUTHOR: **FRED F. FERRI, M.D.**

BASIC INFORMATION

DEFINITION

Acute respiratory distress syndrome (ARDS) is a form of noncardiogenic pulmonary edema that results from acute damage to the alveoli. It is characterized by acute diffuse infiltrative lung lesions with resulting interstitial and alveolar edema, severe hypoxemia, and respiratory failure. The definition of ARDS includes the following three components:

1. A ratio of Pao_2 to Fio_2 $\leq$200 regardless of the level of positive end respiratory pressure (PEEP)
2. The detection of bilateral pulmonary infiltrates on frontal chest x-ray
3. Absence of congestive heart failure (pulmonary artery wedge pressure [PAWP] $\leq$18 mm Hg or no clinical evidence of elevated left atrial pressure on the basis of chest radiograph or other clinical data)

The cardinal feature of ARDS, refractory hypoxemia, is caused by formation of protein-rich alveolar edema after damage to the integrity of the lung's aveolar-capillary barrier.

SYNONYMS

ARDS

Adult respiratory distress syndrome

ICD-9CM CODES

518.82 Acute respiratory distress syndrome

EPIDEMIOLOGY & DEMOGRAPHICS

In the U.S. there are >150,000 ARDS cases/yr.

Incidence is 1.5 to 8.3 cases/100,000/yr.

About 50% of patients who develop ARDS do so within 24 hours of the inciting event. Mortality is 40% to 50%.

PHYSICAL FINDINGS & CLINICAL PRESENTATION

- Signs and symptoms
  1. Dyspnea
  2. Chest discomfort
  3. Cough
  4. Anxiety
- Physical examination
  1. Tachypnea
  2. Tachycardia
  3. Hypertension
  4. Coarse crepitations of both lungs
  5. Fever may be present if infection is the underlying etiology

ETIOLOGY

- Sepsis (>40% of cases)
- Aspiration: near drowning, aspiration of gastric contents (>30% of cases)
- Trauma (>20% of cases)
- Multiple transfusions, blood products
- Drugs (e.g., overdose of morphine, methadone, heroin; reaction to nitrofurantoin)
- Noxious inhalation (e.g., chlorine gas, high O_2 concentration)
- Post-resuscitation
- Cardiopulmonary bypass
- Pneumonia
- Burns
- Pancreatitis
- A history of chronic alcohol abuse significantly increases the risk of developing ARDS in critically ill patients

DIAGNOSIS

DIFFERENTIAL DIAGNOSIS

- Cardiogenic pulmonary edema
- Viral pneumonitis
- Lymphangitic carcinomatosis

WORKUP

The search for an underlying cause should focus on treatable causes (e.g., infections such as sepsis or pneumonia)

- ABGs
- Hemodynamic monitoring
- Bronchoalveolar lavage (selected patients)

LABORATORY TESTS

- ABGs:
  1. Initially: varying degrees of hypoxemia, generally resistant to supplemental oxygen
  2. Respiratory alkalosis, decreased Pco_2
  3. Widened alveolar-arterial gradient
  4. Hypercapnia as the disease progresses
- Bronchoalveolar lavage:
  1. The most prominent finding is an increased number of polymorphonucleocytes.
  2. The presence of eosinophilia has therapeutic implications, because these patients respond to corticosteroids.
- Blood and urine cultures

IMAGING STUDIES

Chest x-ray (Fig. 1-10).

- The initial chest radiogram might be normal in the initial hours after the precipitating event.
- Bilateral interstitial infiltrates are usually seen within 24 hr; they often are more prominent in the bases and periphery.
- "White out" of both lung fields can be seen in advanced stages.
- CT scan of chest: diffuse consolidation with air bronchograms, bullae, pleural effusions. Pneumomediastinum and pneumathoraces may also be present.

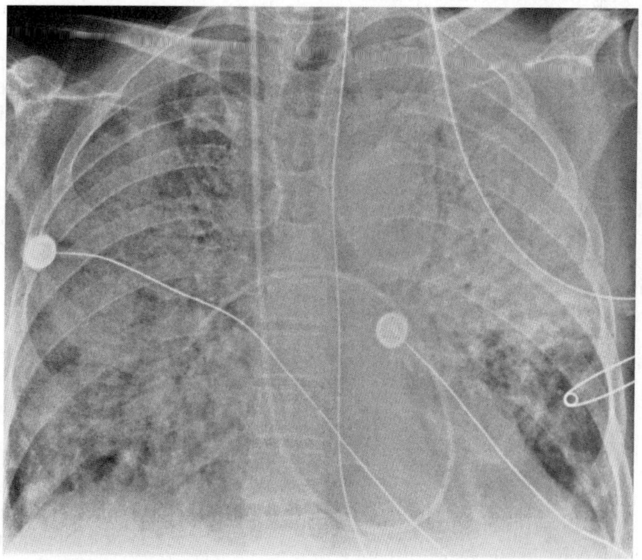

FIGURE 1-10 ARDS. AP radiograph in an elderly woman reveals widespread consolidation with air bronchograms. The heart size is normal. There are no pleural effusions. (From McLoud TC: *Thoracic radiology: the requisites,* St Louis, 1998, Mosby.)

TREATMENT

Rx

NONPHARMACOLOGIC THERAPY

Hemodynamic monitoring:

- Hemodynamic monitoring can be used for the initial evaluation of ARDS (in ruling out cardiogenic pulmonary edema) and its subsequent management. Recent studies, however, have shown that clinical management involving the early use of pulmonary artery catheters in patients with ARDS did not significantly affect mortality and morbidity.
- Although no dynamic profile is diagnostic of ARDS, the presence of pulmonary edema, a high cardiac output and a low pulmonary capillary wedge pressures (PCWP) is characteristic of ARDS.
- It is important to remember that partially treated intravascular volume overload and flash pulmonary edema can have the hemodynamic features of ARDS; filling pressures can also be elevated by increased intrathoracic pressures or with fluid administration; cardiac function can be depressed by acidosis, hypoxemia, or other factors associated with sepsis.

Ventilatory support: mechanical ventilation is generally necessary to maintain adequate gas exchange (see Section III). A low tidal volume and low plateau pressure ventilator strategy is recommended to avoid ventilator-induced injury. Assist-control is generally preferred initially with the following ventilator settings:

- Fio_2 1.0 (until a lower value can be used to achieve adequate oxygenation). When possible, minimize oxygen toxicity by maintaining Fio_2 at <60%.
- Tidal volume: Set initial tidal volume at 6 ml/kg of predicted body weight (PBW = 50.0 + 0.91 [height in cm − 152.4] for men, PBW = 45.5 + 0.91 [height in cm − 152.4] for women). The concept of using PBW is that because lung size depends most strongly on height and sex, PBW normalizes the tidal volume to lung size. Aim to maintain plateau pressure (Pplat) at <30 mm Hg.
- PEEP 5 cm H_2O or greater (to increase lung volume and keep alveoli open). PEEP should be applied in small increments of 3 to 5 cm H_2O (up to a maximum of 15 cm H_2O) to achieve acceptable arterial saturation (>0.9) with nontoxic FiO_2 values (<0.6) and acceptable airway plateau pressures (>30 to 35 cm H_2O). It is important to remember that an increase in PEEP may lower cardiac output and, despite improvement in PaO_2, may actually have a negative effect on tissue oxygenation (the major determinants of tissue oxygenation are Hb, percent saturation, and cardiac output).
- Inspiratory flow: 60 L/min.
- Ventilatory rate: high ventilatory rates of 18 to 24 breaths/min are often necessary in patients with ARDS because of their increased physiologic dead-space and smaller lung volumes. Patients must be monitored for excessive intrathoracic gas trapping ("auto-PEEP" or "intrinsic-PEEP") that can depress cardiac output.

ACUTE GENERAL Rx

Identify and treat precipitating conditions:

- Blood and urine cultures and trial of antibiotics in presumed sepsis (routine administration of antibiotics in all cases of ARDS is not recommended).
- Prompt repair of bone fractures in patients with major trauma.
- Bowel rest and crystalloid resuscitation in pancreatitis.
- Fluid management: optimal fluid and hemodynamic management of patients with ARDS is patient specific; generally, administration of crystalloids is recommended if a downward trend in PCWP is associated with diminished cardiac index, resulting in prerenal azotemia, oliguria, and relative tachycardia; on the other hand, if PCWP increases with little or no change in cardiac index, one should begin diuretic therapy and use low-dose dopamine (2 to 4 μg/kg/min) to maintain natriuresis and support adequate renal flow.
- Positioning the patient: changes in position can improve oxygenation by improving the distribution of perfusion to ventilated lung regions; repositioning (lateral decubitus positioning) should be attempted in patients with hypoxemia that is not responsive to other medical interventions. Placing patients with acute respiratory failure in a prone position improves their oxygenation but does not improve their survival.
- Corticosteroids: routine use of corticosteroids in ARDS is not recommended; corticosteroids may be beneficial in patients with many eosinophils in the bronchoalveolar lavage fluid; systemic infections should be ruled out or adequately treated before administration of corticosteroids. Use of methylprednisolone has not been shown to increase the rate of infectious complications but is associated with a higher rate of neuromuscular weakness. In addition, starting methylprednisolone therapy more than 2 wk after the onset of ARDS may increase the risk of death.
- Nutritional support: nutritional support, preferably administered by the enteral route, is necessary to maintain adequate colloid oncotic pressure and intravascular volume. The inclusion of eicosapentaenoic acid from fish oil may be beneficial in improving ventilation requirements and length of stay in patients with ARDS.
- Tracheostomy: tracheostomy is warranted in patients requiring >2 wk of mechanical ventilation; discussion regarding tracheostomy should begin with patient (if alert and oriented) and family members/legal guardian, after 5 to 7 days of ventilatory support.
- Some form of DVT prophylaxis is indicated in all patients with ARDS.
- Stress ulcer prophylaxis with sucralfate suspension (via NG tube), or IV proton pump inhibitors (PPIs) or IV H_2 blockers.
- The use of surfactant remains controversial. Patients who receive surfactant have a greater improvement in gas exchange in the initial 24-hour period than patients who receive standard therapy alone; however, the use of exogenous surfactant does not improve survival.

DISPOSITION

- Prognosis for ARDS varies with the underlying cause. Prognosis is worse in patients with chronic liver disease, nonpulmonary organ dysfunction, sepsis, and advanced age.
- Elevated values of dead space fraction ($[Paco_2\text{-}Peco_2]/Paco_2$) (normal is <0.3) is associated with an increased risk of death.
- In ARDS, the percentage of potentially recruitable lung is variable and associated with the response to PEEP.
- Overall mortality varies between 32% and 45%. The majority of deaths are attributable to sepsis or multiorgan dysfunction rather than primary respiratory causes.

REFERRAL

Surgical referral for tracheostomy (see "Acute General Rx").

SUGGESTED READINGS

Gattinoni L et al: Lung recruitment in patients with acute respiratory distress syndrome, *N Engl J Med* 354:1775, 2006.

Malhotra A: Low tidal volume ventilation in the acute respiratory distress syndrome, *N Engl J Med* 357:1113, 2007.

Mercat A et al: Positive end-respiratory pressure setting in adults with acute lung injury and acute respiratory distress syndrome, *JAMA* 299(6):646-655, 2008.

The National Heart, Lung, and Blood Institute ARDS Clinical Trials Network: Efficacy and safety of corticosteroids for persistent acute respiratory distress syndrome, *N Engl J Med* 354:1671, 2006.

The National Heart, Lung, and Blood Institute ARDS Clinical Trials Network, Higher versus Lower Positive End-Expiratory pressures in patients with the Acute Respiratory Distress Syndrome, *N Engl J Med* 351:327, 2004.

Wheeler AP: Acute lung injury and the acute respiratory distress syndrome, *Lancet* 369:1553, 2007.

AUTHOR: **FRED F. FERRI, M.D.**

BASIC INFORMATION

DEFINITION

Addison's disease is characterized by inadequate secretion of corticosteroids resulting from partial or complete destruction of the adrenal glands.

SYNONYMS

Primary adrenocortical insufficiency
Adrenal insufficiency

ICD-9CM CODES
255.4 Addison's disease

EPIDEMIOLOGY & DEMOGRAPHICS

PREVALENCE: 5 cases/100,000 persons
PREDOMINANT SEX: Female:male ratio of 2:1

PHYSICAL FINDINGS & CLINICAL PRESENTATION

- Hyperpigmentation: more prominent in palmar creases, buccal mucosa, pressure points (elbows, knees, knuckles), perianal mucosa, and around areolas of nipples
- Hypotension
- Generalized weakness
- Amenorrhea and loss of axillary hair in females

ETIOLOGY

- Autoimmune destruction of the adrenal glands (80% of cases)
- Tuberculosis (15% of cases)
- Carcinomatous destruction of the adrenal glands
- Adrenal hemorrhage (anticoagulants, trauma, coagulopathies, pregnancy, sepsis)
- Adrenal infarction (arteritis, thrombosis)
- AIDS (adrenal insufficiency develops in 30% of patients with AIDS)
- Other: sarcoidosis, amyloidosis, postoperative, fungal infections

DIAGNOSIS

DIFFERENTIAL DIAGNOSIS

Sepsis, hypovolemic shock, acute abdomen, apathetic hyperthyroidism in the elderly, myopathies, GI malignancy, major depression, anorexia nervosa, hemochromatosis, salt-losing nephritis, chronic infection

WORKUP

- If the clinical picture is highly suggestive of adrenocortical insufficiency, the diagnosis can be made with the rapid ACTH (Cortrosyn) test:
  1. Give 250 mg ACTH by IV push and measure cortisol levels at 0 and 30 min.
  2. Cortisol level <18 mg/dl at 30 or 60 min is suggestive of adrenal insufficiency.
  3. Measure plasma ACTH. A high ACTH level confirms primary adrenal insufficiency.
- Secondary adrenocortical insufficiency (caused by pituitary dysfunction) can be distinguished from primary adrenal insufficiency by the following:
  1. Normal or low plasma ACTH level following rapid ACTH (Cortrosyn test)
  2. Absence of hyperpigmentation
  3. No significant impairment of aldosterone secretion (because aldosterone secretion is under control of the renin-angiotensin system)
  4. Additional evidence of hypopituitarism (e.g., hypogonadism, hypothyroidism)

LABORATORY TESTS

- Increased potassium, decreased sodium and chloride
- Decreased glucose
- Increased BUN/creatinine ratio (prerenal azotemia)
- Mild normocytic, normochromic anemia, neutropenia, lymphocytosis, eosinophilia (significant dehydration may mask hyponatremia and anemia)
- PPD and antiadrenal antibodies

IMAGING STUDIES

- Chest x-ray examination may reveal a small heart.
- Abdominal x-ray film: adrenal calcifications may be noted if the adrenocortical insufficiency is secondary to TB or fungus.
- Abdominal CT scan: small adrenal glands generally indicate either idiopathic atrophy or long-standing TB, whereas enlarged glands are suggestive of early TB or potentially treatable diseases.

TREATMENT

NONPHARMACOLOGIC THERAPY

- Perform periodic monitoring of serum electrolytes, vital signs, and body weight; liberal sodium intake is suggested.
- Periodic measurement of bone density may be helpful in identifying patients at risk for the development of osteoporosis.
- Patients should carry a Medic Alert bracelet and an emergency pack containing hydrocortisone 100 mg ampule, syringe, and needle.
- Patients and partners should be educated on how to give IM injection in case of vomiting or coma.

ACUTE GENERAL Rx

- Addisonian crisis is an acute complication of adrenal insufficiency characterized by circulatory collapse, dehydration, nausea, vomiting, hypoglycemia, and hyperkalemia.
  1. Draw plasma cortisol level; do not delay therapy while waiting for confirming laboratory results.
  2. Administer hydrocortisone 50 to 100 mg IV q6h for 24 hr; if patient shows good clinical response, gradually taper dosage and change to oral maintenance dose (usually prednisone 7.5 mg/day).
  3. Provide adequate volume replacement with D_5NS solution until hypotension, dehydration, and hypoglycemia are completely corrected. Large volumes (2 to 3 L) may be necessary in the first 2 to 3 hr to correct the volume deficit and hypoglycemia and to avoid further hyponatremia.
- Identify and correct any precipitating factor (e.g., sepsis, hemorrhage).

CHRONIC Rx

- Give hydrocortisone 15 to 20 mg PO every morning and 5 to 10 mg in late afternoon or prednisone 5 mg in morning and 2.5 mg hs.
- Give oral fludrocortisone 0.05 mg/day to 0.20 mg/day: this mineralocorticoid is necessary if the patient has primary adrenocortical insufficiency. The dose is adjusted based on the serum sodium level and the presence of postural hypotension or marked orthostasis.
- Instruct patients to increase glucocorticoid replacement in times of stress and to receive parenteral glucocorticoids if diarrhea or vomiting occurs. Typical supplementation varies from 25 mg PO qd of hydrocortisone for minor medical and surgical stress to 50-100 mg IV hydrocortisone every 8 hr for sepsis-induced hypotension or shock.
- The administration of dehydroepiandrosterone 50 mg PO qd improves well-being and sexuality in women with adrenal insufficiency.

SUGGESTED READINGS

Cooper MS, Stewart PM: Corticosteroid insufficiency in acutely ill patients, *N Engl J Med* 348:727, 2003.

Dorin RI et al: Diagnosis of adrenal insufficiency, *Ann Intern Med* 139:194, 2003.

Salvadori R: Adrenal insufficiency, *JAMA* 294:2481, 2005.

AUTHOR: **FRED F. FERRI, M.D.**

BASIC INFORMATION

DEFINITION

Although it is impossible to define alcoholism precisely, among the commonly used screening instruments for this disorder are the CAGE questionnaire, short Michigan Alcoholism Screening Test (SMAST), National Council on Alcoholism criteria, and DSM-IV-R criteria. Moderate drinking has been defined as two standard drinks (e.g., 12 oz of beer) per day and one drink per day for women and persons older than 65 years of age.

Although not generally included under the alcoholism topic, hazardous or at-risk drinking should also be considered. For men, *at-risk drinking* is defined as greater than 14 drinks/week or more than 4 drinks/occasion. For women, at-risk drinking is defined as about half that given for men.

The American Psychiatric Association defines diagnostic criteria for *alcohol withdrawal* as follows:

A. Cessation of (or reduction in) alcohol use that has been heavy and prolonged.
B. Two (or more) of the following, developing within several hours to a few days after criterion A:
   1. Autonomic hyperactivity (e.g., sweating or pulse rate >100 beats/min)
   2. Increased hand tremor
   3. Insomnia
   4. Nausea and vomiting
   5. Transient visual, tactile, or auditory hallucinations or illusions
   6. Psychomotor agitation
   7. Anxiety
   8. Grand mal seizures
C. The symptoms in criterion B cause clinically significant distress or impairment in social, occupational, or other important areas of functioning.

The symptoms are not due to a general medical condition and are not better accounted for by another mental disorder.

SYNONYMS

Alcohol abuse
Substance abuse

ICD-9CM CODES
303.9 Alcoholism

EPIDEMIOLOGY & DEMOGRAPHICS

INCIDENCE (IN U.S.):
- The clinical history suggests alcohol problems in 15% to 20% of patients in primary care and patients that are hospitalized. In the U.S. alcohol abuse generates nearly $185 billion in annual economic costs. An estimated 8 million adults in the U.S. have alcohol dependence.
- 20% achieve abstinence without help, 70% achieve sobriety for 1 yr.

PREVALENCE (IN U.S.): 7% of population 18 yr or older

PREDOMINANT SEX:
- Lifetime risk for males 8% to 10%
- Lifetime risk for females 3% to 5%

PEAK INCIDENCE: 20 to 40 yr

GENETICS: More common with a family history of alcoholism and in patients of Irish, Scandinavian, and Native American descent

PHYSICAL FINDINGS & CLINICAL PRESENTATION

- Recurring minor trauma
- GI bleeding from gastritis and/or varices
- Pancreatitis (acute and chronic)
- Liver disease
- Odor of alcohol on breath
- Tremulousness
- Tachycardia
- Peripheral neuropathy
- Recent memory loss

ETIOLOGY

- Social and genetic factors important
- Risk factors:
  1. Broken homes
  2. Unemployment
  3. Divorce
  4. Recurrent depression
  5. Addiction to another substance, including tobacco

DIAGNOSIS

WORKUP

- Several screening tests (CAGE, AUDIT, TWEAK, CRAFFT, SMAST) are available. The four-item CAGE (feeling need to Cut down, Annoyed by criticism, Guilty about drinking, and need for an Eye-opener in the morning) is the most popular screening test in primary care. A positive response should lead to further questioning. The sensitivity of the CAGE ranges from 43% to 94% and its specificity ranges from 70% to 97%. The five-item TWEAK scale (Tolerance, Worry, Eye-openers, Amnesia, [K] cut down) and the T-ACE questionnaire (Tolerance, Annoyance, Cut down, Eye-opener) are designed to screen pregnant women for alcohol misuse. They detect lower levels of alcohol consumption that may pose risks during pregnancy. The CRAFFT questionnaire (riding in Car with someone who was drinking, using alcohol to Relax, using alcohol while Alone, Forgetfulness, criticism from Friends and Family, Trouble) is useful as a screening tool for adolescents. Its sensitivity is 92% and specificity 64% for alcohol abuse. Single question screening about alcohol consumption in a day ("When was the last time you had more than x drinks in a day?" [where $x = 5$ for men and 4 for women]) with the threshold set at "in the past 3 months" is 85% sensitive and 70% specific in men and 82% and 70% in women for unhealthy alcohol use. Screening tools are available at the National Institute on Alcohol Abuse and Alcoholism website: http://www.niaaa.nih.gov/publications/niaaa-guide.
- Blood studies (see "Laboratory Tests")

LABORATORY TESTS

- γ-Glutamyltransferase (GGTP), generally elevated
- Liver transaminases (ALT, AST), often elevated, may be normal or low in advanced liver disease
- Low albumin level, hypophosphatemia, hypomagnesemia from malnutrition
- CBC reveals elevated mean corpuscular volume (MCV) from toxic effect of alcohol on erythrocyte development on nutritional deficiencies
- Stool for occult blood may be positive secondary to gastritis, or variceal bleeding

IMAGING STUDIES

Indicated only if there is a history of trauma. CT or ultrasound of abdomen may reveal fatty liver or cirrhosis in advanced stages.

TREATMENT

NONPHARMACOLOGIC THERAPY

- Complete abstinence
- Depression, if present, should be treated at same time ETOH is withdrawn

ACUTE GENERAL Rx

Alcohol withdrawal syndrome occurs when a person stops ingesting alcohol after prolonged consumption. It can result in four possible clinical patterns depending on the severity of the patient's alcohol abuse and the time interval from the patient's previous alcohol ingestion. Blood ethanol level decreases by 20 mg/dL/hr in a normal person. Although discussed separately in the text, these alcohol withdrawal states blend together in real life.

1. **Tremulous state** (early alcohol withdrawal, "impending DTs," "shakes," "jitters")
   a. Time interval: usually occurs 6 to 8 hr after the last drink or 12 to 48 hr after reduction of alcohol intake; becomes most pronounced at 24 to 36 hr
   b. Manifestation: tremors, mild agitation, insomnia, tachycardia; symptoms are relieved by alcohol

c. Detoxification can be in the outpatient (ambulatory) or inpatient setting. Candidates for outpatient detoxification should have a reasonable support system (e.g., reliable contact person) that can monitor progress, and lack of any significant comorbid conditions (e.g., suicide risk, seizure disorder, coexisting benzodiazepine dependence, prior unsuccessful outpatient detoxification, pregnancy, cirrhosis) or risk factors for severe withdrawal (age >40, drinking >100 g of ethanol daily [e.g., 1 pint of liquor or eight 12-oz cans of beer, random blood alcohol concentration >200 mg/dL]).

d. Inpatient treatment
   (1) Admit to medical floor (private room); monitor vital signs q4h; institute seizure precautions; maintain adequate sedation.
   (2) Administer lorazepam as follows:
      (a) Day 1: 2 mg PO q4h while awake and not lethargic
      (b) Day 2: 1 mg PO q4h while awake and not lethargic
      (c) Day 3: 0.5 mg PO q4h while awake and not lethargic
      (d) NOTE: Hold sedation for lethargy or abnormal vital or neurologic signs. The preceding doses are only guidelines; it is best to titrate the dose case by case
   (3) In patients with mild to moderate withdrawal and without history of seizures, individualized benzodiazepine administration (rather than a fixed-dose regimen) results in lower benzodiazepine administration and avoids unnecessary sedation. The Clinical Institute Withdrawal Assessment-Alcohol (CIWA-A) scale can be used to measure the severity of alcohol withdrawal. It consists of 10 items: nausea; tremor; autonomic hyperactivity; anxiety; agitation; tactile, visual, and auditory disturbances; headache; and disorientation. Each item is assigned a score from 0 to 7. For example in the "agitation" category 0 indicates normal activity, 7 indicates that the patient constantly thrashes about, for the category of "tremor," 0 indicates that tremor is not present, 7 tremor is severe, even with arms not extended. The maximum total score is 67. When the CIWA-A score is ≥8, patients are usually given 2 to 4 mg of lorazepam hourly.
   (4) β-Adrenergic blockers: β-blockers are useful for controlling BP and tachyarrhythmias. However, they do not prevent progression to more serious symptoms of withdrawal and if used, should not be administered alone but in conjunction with benzodiazepines. β-Blockers should be avoided in patients with contraindications to their use (e.g., bronchospasm, bradycardia, or severe CHF). Centrally acting α-adrenergic agonists such as clonidine ameliorate symptoms in patients with mild-to-moderate withdrawal but do not reduce delirium or seizures.
   (5) Vitamin replacement: thiamine 100 mg IV or IM for at least 5 days, plus PO multivitamins. The IV administration of glucose can precipitate Wernicke's encephalopathy in alcoholics with thiamine deficiency; therefore thiamine administration should precede IV dextrose
   (6) Hydration PO or IV (high-caloric solution): if IV, glucose with Na^+, K^+, Mg^{2+}, and phosphate replacement prn
   (7) Laboratory studies
      (a) CBC, platelet count, INR
      (b) Electrolytes, glucose, BUN, creatinine
      (c) GGTP, ALT, AST
      (d) Phosphorus and magnesium
      (e) Serum vitamin B_{12} and folic acid (if megaloblastic features in blood smear)
   (8) Diagnostic imaging: generally not necessary; if subdural hematoma is suspected (evidence of trauma, persistent lethargy), a CT scan should be ordered.
   (9) Social rehabilitation: group therapy such as Alcoholics Anonymous; identification and treatment of social and family problems should be initiated during the patient's hospital stay.

2. **Alcoholic hallucinosis**
   a. Manifestations: usually hallucinations are auditory, but occasionally hallucinations are visual, tactile, or olfactory; usually there is no clouding of sensorium as in delirium (clinical presentation may be mistaken for an acute schizophrenic episode). Disordered perceptions become most pronounced after 24 to 36 hr of abstinence.
   b. Treatment: same as for DTs (see Withdrawal seizures).

3. **Withdrawal seizures** ("rum fits")
   a. Time interval: usually occurs 7 to 30 hr after cessation of drinking, with a peak incidence between 13 and 24 hr.
   b. Manifestations: generalized convulsions with loss of consciousness; focal signs are usually absent; consider further investigation with CT scan of head and EEG if clearly indicated (e.g., presence of focal neurologic deficits, prolonged postictal confusion state). In addition, in a febrile patient who is having a seizure or altered mental state, a lumbar puncture is necessary.
   c. Treatment
      (1) Diazepam 2.5 mg/min IV until seizure is controlled (check for respiratory depression or hypotension) may be beneficial for prolonged seizure activity; IV lorazepam 1 to 2 mg every 2 hr can be used in place of diazepam. Generally withdrawal seizures are self-limited and treatment is not required; the use of phenytoin or other anticonvulsants for short-term treatment of alcohol withdrawal seizures is not recommended.
      (2) Thiamine 100 mg IV, followed by IV dextrose, should also be administered.
      (3) Electrolyte imbalances (↑ Mg^{2+}, ↓ K^+, ↑/↓ Na^+, ↓ PO_4^{-3}) that may exacerbate seizures should be corrected.

4. **DTs**
   a. Time interval: variable; usually occurs within 1 wk after reduction or cessation of heavy alcohol intake and persists for 1 to 3 days. Peak incidence is 72 hr and 96 hr after the cessation of alcohol consumption.
   b. Manifestations: profound confusion, tremors, vivid visual and tactile hallucinations, autonomic hyperactivity; this is the most serious clinical presentation of alcohol withdrawal (mortality is approximately 15% in untreated patients).
   c. Treatment
      (1) Admission to a detoxification unit where patient can be observed closely
      (2) Vital signs q30min (neurologic signs, if necessary)
      (3) Use of lateral decubitus or prone position if restraints are necessary
      (4) NPO: NG tube for abdominal distention may be necessary

but should not be routinely used
(5) Laboratory studies: same as for early alcohol withdrawal
(6) Vigorous hydration (4 to 6 L/day): IV with glucose (Na^+, K^+, PO_4^{-3}, and Mg^{2+} replacement)
(7) Vitamins: thiamine, 100 mg IV qd. The initial dose of thiamine should precede the administration of IV dextrose; multivitamins (may be added to the hydrating solution)
(8) Sedation: Control of agitation should be achieved using rapid-acting sedative-hypnotic agents in adequate doses to maintain light somnolence for the duration of delirium.
  (a) Initially: lorazepam 2 to 5 mg IM/IV repeated prn
  (b) Maintenance (individualized dosage): chlordiazepoxide, 50 to 100 mg PO q4 to 6h, lorazepam 2 mg PO q4h, or diazepam 5 to 10 mg PO tid; withhold doses or decrease subsequent doses if signs of oversedation are apparent
  (c) Midazolam is also effective for managing DTs. Its rapid onset (sedation within 2 to 4 min of IV injection) and short duration of action (approximately 30 min) make it an ideal agent for titration in continuous infusion.
(9) Treatment of seizures (as previously described)
(10) Diagnosis and treatment of concomitant medical, surgical, or psychiatric conditions

CHRONIC Rx

- See "Referral."
- Pharmacotherapies for alcoholism include:
  - Acamprosate is a synthetic compound with a chemical structure similar to the neurotransmitter gamma-aminobutyric acid and the amino acid neuromodulator taurine. Its mechanism of action is not completely understood. It is indicated for the maintenance of abstinence from alcohol in patients with alcohol dependence who are abstinent at treatment initiation. It should be used only as part of a comprehensive psychosocial treatment program. It does not cause a disulfiram-like reaction as a result of ethanol ingestion. Dose is two 333-mg tablets tid. Treatment should be initiated as soon as possible after the period of alcohol withdrawal, when the patient has achieved abstinence, and should be maintained if the patient relapses.
  - The long-acting opiate antagonist naltrexone (Vivitrol). It inhibits the rewarding effects of alcohol. Dosage is 50 mg PO qd. An extended-release, once monthly injection of naltrexone is also available and can be used along with psychosocial support to maintain alcohol abstinence. In patients with opioid dependence, naltrexone can precipitate acute withdrawal syndrome and should not be used at least 7 days from last opioid use.
  - Disulfiram (Antabuse). Dosage is 500 mg max once/day for 1 to 2 wk, then 125 to 500 mg once/day. It interferes with the metabolism of alcohol and produces unpleasant symptoms when it is ingested. It is an older drug that is now rarely used.

DISPOSITION

See "Referral."

REFERRAL

- To Alcoholics Anonymous or Adult Children of Alcoholics
- Family members to Al-Anon or Al-A-Teen
- Many cities have Salvation Army Adult Rehabilitation centers; all patients accepted, regardless of ability to pay

PEARLS & CONSIDERATIONS

COMMENTS

- Relative indications for inpatient alcohol detoxification are as follows: history of DTs or withdrawal seizures, severe withdrawal symptoms, concomitant psychiatric or medical illness, pregnancy, multiple previous detoxifications, recent high levels of alcohol consumption, and lack of reliable support network.
- Detoxification is not a stand-alone treatment but should serve as a bridge to a formal treatment program for alcohol dependence.
- The cure rate for alcoholism is very disappointing, regardless of the modality. Only those who want to be helped will be helped. An effective strategy for the primary care physician is a prominently displayed sign in the office that states, "If you think you consume too much alcoholic beverage, please discuss it with me." Those who do open up the discussion can be given the facts in a nonjudgmental way and often can be helped. All too often, problem drinkers lie on the questionnaire until they face a life-threatening health issue—and even then denial often reigns supreme.
- In a recent clinical trial, patients receiving medical management with naltrexone (100 mg/day), combined behavioral intervention (CBI), or both fared better on drinking outcomes, whereas acamprosate showed no evidence of efficacy, with or without CBI. No combination produced better efficacy than naltrexone or CBI alone in the presence of medical management.

SUGGESTED READINGS

Anton RF et al: Combined pharmacotherapies and behavioral interventions for alcohol dependence, the COMBINE study: A randomized clinical trial, *JAMA* 295:2003, 2006.

Bayard M et al: Alcohol withdrawal syndrome, *Am Fam Physician* 69:1443, 2004.

Blondell RD: Ambulatory detoxification of patients with alcohol dependence, *Am Fam Physician* 71:495-510, 2005.

Conagasaby A, Vinson DC: Screening for hazardous or harmful drinking using one or two quantity-frequency questions, *Alcohol Alcohol* (May/June)40:208-13, 2005.

Johnson B et al: Topiramate for treating alcohol dependence, a randomized controlled trial, *JAMA* 298(14):1641-1651, 2007.

Kosten TR, O'Connor PG: Management of drug and alcohol withdrawal, *N Engl J Med* 348:1786, 2003.

Mayo-Smith MF et al: Management of alcohol withdrawal delirium, *Arch Intern Med* 164:1405, 2004.

Moss M, Burnham EL: Alcohol abuse in the critically ill patient, *Lancet* 368:2231, 2006.

U.S. Preventive Services Task Force: Screening and behavioral counseling interventions in primary care to reduce alcohol misuse: recommendation statement, *Ann Intern Med* 140:554, 2004.

AUTHOR: **FRED F. FERRI, M.D.**

BASIC INFORMATION

DEFINITION

Primary aldosteronism is a clinical syndrome characterized by hypokalemia, hypertension, low plasma renin activity (PRA), and excessive aldosterone secretion.

SYNONYMS

Hyperaldosteronism
Conn's syndrome

ICD-9CM CODES
255.1 Primary aldosteronism

EPIDEMIOLOGY & DEMOGRAPHICS

INCIDENCE: 1% to 2% of patients with hypertension
PREVALENCE: More common in females

PHYSICAL FINDINGS & CLINICAL PRESENTATION

- Generally asymptomatic
- If significant hypokalemia is present, possible muscle cramping, weakness, paresthesias
- Hypertension
- Polyuria, polydipsia

ETIOLOGY

- Aldosterone-producing adenoma (>60%)
- Idiopathic hyperaldosteronism (>30%)
- Glucocorticoid-suppressible hyperaldosteronism (<1%)
- Aldosterone-producing carcinoma (<1%)

DIAGNOSIS

DIFFERENTIAL DIAGNOSIS

- Diuretic use
- Hypokalemia from vomiting, diarrhea
- Renovascular hypertension
- Other endocrine neoplasm (pheochromocytoma, deoxycorticosterone-producing tumor, renin-secreting tumor)

WORKUP

In patients with hypokalemia and a low PRA, confirming tests for primary hyperaldosteronism include the following:

- 24-hr urine test for aldosterone and potassium levels (potassium >40 mEq and aldosterone >15 μg).
- Captopril test: administer 25 to 50 mg of captopril (ACE inhibitor) and measure plasma renin and aldosterone levels 1 to 2 hr later. A plasma aldosterone level >15 ng/dl confirms the diagnosis of primary aldosteronism. This test is more expensive and is best reserved for situations in which the 24-hr urine for aldosterone is ambiguous.
- 24-hr urinary tetrahydroaldosterone (<65 μg/24 hr) and saline infusion test (plasma aldosterone >10 ng/dl) can also be used in ambiguous cases.
- The renin-aldosterone stimulation test (posture test) is helpful in differentiating IHA from aldosterone-producing adenoma (APA). Patients with APA have a decrease in aldosterone levels at 4 hr, whereas patients with IHA have an increase in their aldosterone levels.
- As a screening test for primary aldosteronism, an elevated plasma aldosterone-renin ratio (ARR), drawn randomly from patients on hypertensive drugs, is predictive of primary aldosteronism (positive predictive value 100% in a recent study). ARR is calculated by dividing plasma aldosterone (mg/dl) by plasma renin activity (mg/ml/hour). ARR >100 is considered elevated.
- Bilateral adrenal venous sampling may be done to localize APA when adrenal CT scan is equivocal. In APA, ipsilateral/contralateral aldosterone level is >10:1, and ipsilateral venous aldosterone concentration is very high (>1000 ng/dl).
- A diagnostic evaluation of hypertensive patients with suspected aldosteronism is described in Section III, Hyperaldosteronism.

LABORATORY TESTS

Routine laboratory tests can be suggestive but are not diagnostic of primary aldosteronism. Common abnormalities are:

- Spontaneous hypokalemia or moderately severe hypokalemia while receiving conventional doses of diuretics
- Possible alkalosis and hypernatremia

IMAGING STUDIES

- Adrenal CT scans (with 3-mm cuts) may be used to localize neoplasm.
- Adrenal scanning with iodocholesterol (NP-59) or 6-beta-iodomethyl-19-norcholesterol after dexamethasone suppression. The uptake of tracer is increased in those with aldosteronoma and absent in those with idiopathic aldosteronism and adrenal carcinoma.

TREATMENT

NONPHARMACOLOGIC THERAPY

- Regular monitoring and control of blood pressure
- Low-sodium diet, tobacco avoidance, maintenance of ideal body weight, and regular exercise program

ACUTE GENERAL Rx

- Control of blood pressure and hypokalemia with spironolactone, amiloride, or ACE inhibitors
- Surgery (unilateral adrenalectomy) for APA

CHRONIC Rx

Chronic medical therapy with spironolactone, amiloride, or ACE inhibitors to control blood pressure and hypokalemia is necessary in all patients with bilateral idiopathic hyperaldosteronism.

DISPOSITION

- Unilateral adrenalectomy normalizes hypertension and hypokalemia in 70% of patients with APA after 1 yr. After 5 yr, 50% of patients remain normotensive.
- Experimental animal studies have suggested that long-term exposure to increased aldosterone levels in untreated aldosteronism may result in renal structural damage. However, clinical trials have shown that primary aldosteronism is characterized by partially reversible renal dysfunction in which elevated albuminuria is a marker of a dynamic rather than structural renal defect.

REFERRAL

Surgical referral for unilateral adrenalectomy following confirmation of unilateral APA or carcinoma

PEARLS & CONSIDERATIONS

COMMENTS

Frequent monitoring of blood pressure and electrolytes postoperatively is necessary, because normotension after unilateral adrenalectomy may take up to 4 mo.

- Recent investigations regarding serum aldosterone and the incidence of hypertension in nonhypertensive persons indicate that increased aldosterone levels within the physiologic range predispose to the development of hypertension.

SUGGESTED READINGS

Sechi L et al: Long-term renal outcomes in patients with primary aldosteronism, *JAMA* 295:2638, 2006.
Vasan RS et al: Serum aldosterone and the incidence of hypertension in nonhypertensive persons, *N Engl J Med* 351:33, 2004.

AUTHOR: **FRED F. FERRI, M.D.**

BASIC INFORMATION

DEFINITION

Allergic rhinitis is an IgE-mediated hypersensitivity response to nasally inhaled allergens that causes sneezing, rhinorrhea, nasal pruritus, and congestion.

SYNONYMS

Hay fever
IgE-mediated rhinitis

ICD-9CM CODES
477.9 Allergic rhinitis

EPIDEMIOLOGY & DEMOGRAPHICS

- Allergic rhinitis affects approximately 10% to 20% of the U.S. population.
- Mean age of onset is 8 to 12 yr.
- The prevalence of allergic rhinitis in patients presenting to their primary care provider with nasal symptoms is estimated to be 30% to 60%.

PHYSICAL FINDINGS & CLINICAL PRESENTATION

- Pale or violaceous mucosa of the turbinates caused by venous engorgement (this can distinguish it from erythema present in viral rhinitis)
- Nasal polyps
- Lymphoid hyperplasia in the posterior oropharynx with cobblestone appearance
- Erythema of the throat, conjunctival and scleral injection
- Clear nasal discharge
- Clinical presentation: usually consists of sneezing, nasal congestion, cough, postnasal drip, loss of or alteration of smell, and sensation of plugged ears

ETIOLOGY

- Pollens in the springtime, ragweed in fall, grasses in the summer
- Dust, mites, animal allergens
- Smoke or any irritants
- Perfumes, detergents, soaps
- Emotion, changes in atmospheric pressure or temperature

DIAGNOSIS

DIFFERENTIAL DIAGNOSIS

- Infections (sinusitis; viral, bacterial, or fungal rhinitis)
- Rhinitis medicamentosa (cocaine, sympathomimetic nasal drops)
- Vasomotor rhinitis (e.g., secondary to air pollutants)
- Septal obstruction (e.g., deviated septum), nasal polyps, nasal neoplasms
- Systemic diseases (e.g., Wegener's granulomatosis, hypothyroidism [rare])

WORKUP

- The initial strategy should be to determine whether patients should undergo diagnostic testing or receive empirical treatment.
- Workup is often unnecessary if the diagnosis is apparent. A detailed medical history is useful in identifying the culprit allergen.
- Selected patients with allergic rhinitis that is not controlled with standard therapy may benefit from allergy testing to target allergen avoidance measures or guide immunotherapy. Allergy testing can be performed using skin testing or radioallergosorbent (RAST) testing. Immunoglobulin E (IgE) testing using newest generation assays is also an excellent tool for diagnosing the cause of symptoms related to rhinitis. Allergy testing should generally be reserved for ambiguous or complicated cases.
- Examination of nasal smears for the presence of neutrophils to rule out infectious causes and the presence of eosinophils (suggestive of allergy) may be useful in selected patients.
- Peripheral blood eosinophil counts are not useful in allergy diagnosis.

TREATMENT

NONPHARMACOLOGIC THERAPY

- Maintain allergen-free environment by covering mattresses and pillows with allergen-proof casings, eliminating carpeting, eliminating animal products, and removing dust-collecting fixtures.
- Use of air purifiers and dust filters is helpful.
- Maintain humidity in the environment below 50% to prevent dust mites and mold.
- Use air conditioners, especially in the bedroom.
- Remove pets from homes of patients with suspected sensitivity to animal allergens.

ACUTE GENERAL Rx

- Determine if the patient is troubled by swollen turbinates (best treated with decongestants) or blockages secondary to mucus (effectively treated by antihistamines).
- Most first-generation antihistamines can cause considerable sedation and anticholinergic symptoms. The second-generation antihistamines (loratadine, fexofenadine, cetirizine, desloratadine) are preferred because they do not have any significant anticholinergic or sedative effects.
- Montelukast (Singulair), a leukotriene receptor antagonist commonly used for asthma, is also effective for allergic rhinitis. Usual adult dose is 10 mg qd.
- Azelastine (Astelin) is an antihistamine nasal spray effective for seasonal allergic rhinitis.
- Topical nasal steroids are very effective and are preferred by many as first-line treatment for allergic rhinitis in adults. Patients should be instructed on proper use and informed that improvement might not occur for at least 1 wk after initiation of therapy. Commonly available inhalers are:
  1. Beclomethasone dipropionate (Beconase AQ): one to two sprays in each nostril bid
  2. Fluticasone (Flonase): initially two sprays in each nostril qd or one spray in each nostril bid, decreasing to one spray in each nostril qd based on response
  3. Flunisolide (Nasalide): initially two sprays in each nostril bid
  4. Budesonide (Rhinocort): two sprays in each nostril bid or four sprays in each nostril qam

CHRONIC Rx

- Cromolyn sodium (Nasalcrom): one spray to each nostril three to four times daily can be used for prophylaxis (mast cell stabilizer).
- Immunotherapy is generally reserved for patients responding poorly to the above treatments.

DISPOSITION

Most patients experience significant relief with avoidance of allergens and proper use of medications.

REFERRAL

Allergy testing in patients with severe symptoms that are unresponsive to therapy or when the diagnosis is uncertain

EVIDENCE

A meta-analysis found that intranasal steroids are more effective for the treatment of nasal blockage and discharge, sneezing, postnasal drip, and nasal itch than antihistamines.[1] (B)

Evidence-Based Reference

1. Weiner JM, Abramson MJ, Puy RM: Intranasal corticosteroids versus oral H1 receptor antagonists in allergic rhinitis: systematic review of randomized controlled trials, *BMJ* 317:1624, 1998. (B)

SUGGESTED READING

Quillen DM, Feller DB: Diagnosing rhinitis: allergic vs. nonallergic, *Am Fam Physician* 73:1583, 2006.

AUTHOR: **FRED F. FERRI, M.D.**

BASIC INFORMATION

DEFINITION

Alpha-1-antitrypsin deficiency is a genetic deficiency of the protease inhibitor, alpha-1-antitrypsin, that results in a predisposition to pulmonary emphysema and hepatic cirrhosis.

SYNONYMS

AAT

ICD-9CM CODES

277.6 Alpha-1-antitrypsin deficiency

EPIDEMIOLOGY & DEMOGRAPHICS

- Accounts for approximately 2% of COPD cases in Americans
- Inherited as an autosomal codominant disorder
- Most frequent mutation is in the SERPINA 1 gene (previously known as PI)
- Most common alleles are:
  - normal "M" allele (95% frequency in the U.S.)
  - deficient variant "Z" allele (1% to 2%)
  - deficient variant "S" allele (2% to 3%)
- Severe deficiency is most commonly due to homozygotes ZZ
- Risk of lung disease in heterozygotes (MZ) is uncertain
- One in 10 individuals of European descent carry one of two mutations that may result in partial alpha-1-antitrypsin deficiency

PHYSICAL FINDINGS & CLINICAL PRESENTATION

- Physical findings and clinical presentation are varied and dependent upon phenotype (see "Etiology")
- Most often affects the lungs but can also involve liver and skin
- Classically associated with early-onset, severe, lower-lobe predominant emphysema; bronchiectasis may also be seen
- Symptoms are similar to "typical" COPD presentation (dyspnea, cough, sputum production)
- Liver involvement includes neonatal cholestasis, cirrhosis in children and adults, and primary carcinoma of the liver
- Panniculitis is the major dermatologic manifestation

ETIOLOGY

- Degree of alpha-1-antitrypsin deficiency is dependent on phenotype.
- "MM" represents the normal genotype and is associated with alpha-1-antitrypsin levels in the normal range.
- Mutation most commonly associated with emphysema is Z, with homozygote (ZZ) resulting in approximately 85% deficit in plasma alpha-1-antitrypsin concentrations.
- Development of emphysema is believed to be a result from an imbalance between the proteolytic enzyme, elastase, produced by neutrophils, and alpha-1-antitrypsin, which normally protects lung elastin by inhibiting elastase.
- Deficiency of alpha-1-antitrypsin increases risk of early-onset emphysema, but not all alpha-1-antitrypsin deficient individuals will develop lung disease.
- Smoking increases risk and accelerates onset of COPD.
- Liver disease is caused by pathologic accumulation of alpha-1-antitrypsin in hepatocytes.
- Similar to lung disease, skin involvement is thought to be secondary to unopposed proteolysis in skin.

DIAGNOSIS

DIFFERENTIAL DIAGNOSIS

See "COPD"
See "Cirrhosis"

WORKUP

- Suspicion for alpha-1-antitrypsin deficiency usually results from emphysema developing at an early age and with basilar predominance of disease.
- Suspicion for alpha-1-antitrypsin deficiency resulting in liver disease or skin involvement may arise when other more common etiologies are excluded.

LABORATORY TESTS

- Serum level of alpha-1-antitrypsin is decreased or not detected in lung disease.
- Investigate possibility of abnormal alleles with genotyping.
- Pulmonary function testing is generally consistent with "typical" COPD.

IMAGING STUDIES

- Chest x-ray examination shows characteristic emphysematous changes at lung bases.
- High-resolution chest CT usually confirms the lower-lobe predominant emphysema and may also show significant bronchiectasis.

TREATMENT

NONPHARMACOLOGIC THERAPY

- Avoidance of smoking is paramount
- Avoidance of other environmental and occupational exposures that may increase risk of COPD

ACUTE GENERAL Rx

Acute exacerbations of COPD secondary to alpha-1-antitrypsin deficiency are treated in a similar fashion to "typical" COPD exacerbations.

CHRONIC Rx

- The goal of treatment in alpha-1-antitrypsin deficiency is to increase serum alpha-1-antitrypsin levels above a minimum, "protective" threshold.
- Although there are several therapeutic options under investigation, IV administration of pooled human alpha-1-antitrypsin is currently the only approved method to raise serum alpha-1-antitrypsin levels.
- Organ transplantation for patients with end-stage lung or liver disease is also an option.

DISPOSITION

- Prognosis of patients with alpha-1-antitrypsin deficiency will depend on phenotype and level of deficiency.
- Among patients with severe alpha-1-antitrypsin deficiency, the most common underlying causes of death are emphysema (72%) and cirrhosis (10%).

REFERRAL

- Pulmonary and hepatology referrals for advanced lung and liver disease, or if replacement therapy is contemplated (e.g., moderate-severe lung disease)
- Lung and liver transplantation in suitable cases

PEARLS & CONSIDERATIONS

- The liver damage arising from the mutation is not from a deficiency in alpha-1-antitrypsin but from a pathologic accumulation of alpha-1-antitrypsin in hepatocytes.
- Consider alpha-1-antitrypsin deficiency in patients presenting with lower-lobe predominant emphysema; in most smokers without alpha-1-antitrypsin deficiency, emphysema predominates in the upper lobes.
- Alpha-1-antitrypsin deficiency is felt to be under recognized.

EVIDENCE

Observational data demonstrate that in patients with AAT, augmentation therapy with human plasma α1 antitrypsin lowers the decline in FEV1 and improves overall mortality compared to patients who received no such therapy.[1]

Evidence-Based Reference

1. Alpha-1 Antitrypsin Deficiency Registry Study Group: Survival and FEV1 decline in individuals with severe deficiency of alpha1-antitrypsin, *Am J Respir Crit Care Med* 158:49, 1998. Ⓑ

SUGGESTED READINGS

American Thoracic Society/European Respiratory Society Statement: Standards for the diagnosis and management of individuals with alpha-1 antitrypsin deficiency, *Am J Respir Crit Care Med* 168:818, 2003.

Hersh CP et al: Chronic obstructive pulmonary disease in alpha1-antitrypsin PI MZ herterozygotes: a meta-analysis, *Thorax* 59(10):843, 2004.

Kohnlgin T, Welte T: Alpha-1-antitrypsin deficiency: pathogenesis, clinical presentation, diagnosis, and treatment, *Am J Med* 121:3-9, 2008.

Stoller J, Aboussouan L: Alpha 1-antitrypsin deficiency, *Lancet* 365:2225, 2005.

Stoller JK et al: Mortality in individuals with severe deficiency of α1-antitrypsin, *Chest* 127:1196, 2005.

AUTHOR: **JOSEPH A. DIAZ, M.D.**

BASIC INFORMATION

DEFINITION

Altitude sickness refers to a spectrum of illnesses related to hypoxia occurring in people rapidly ascending to high altitudes. Common acute syndromes occurring at high altitudes include acute mountain sickness (AMS), high-altitude pulmonary edema (HAPE), and high-altitude cerebral edema (HACE).

SYNONYMS

Acute mountain sickness
High-altitude pulmonary edema
High-altitude cerebral edema

ICD-9CM CODES
289 Mountain sickness, acute
993.2 High altitude, effects

EPIDEMIOLOGY & DEMOGRAPHICS

- More than 30 million people are at risk of developing altitude sickness.
- AMS is the most common of the altitude diseases.
  - Approximately 40% to 50% of people ascending to 14,000 ft (4200 m) from lowland living develop AMS.
- HAPE generally arises in people who rapidly ascend to 12,000 to 13,000 ft (3600 to 3900 m), but it has been reported at altitudes as low as 8000 ft.
- Men are 5 times more likely to develop HAPE than women.
- AMS and HACE affect men and women equally.

PHYSICAL FINDINGS & CLINICAL PRESENTATION

Acute mountain sickness
- Occurs within hours to a few days after rapid ascent over 8000 ft (2500 m)
- Headache is the most common symptom
- Dizziness and lightheadedness
- Nausea, vomiting, and loss of appetite
- Fatigue
- Sleep disturbance resulting from an exaggerated hyperventilatory phase of Cheynes-Stokes respiration in response to hypoxia and alkalosis.
- AMS can evolve into HAPE and HACE

Pulmonary edema (Fig. 1-11 and Section III, "High-Altitude Pulmonary Edema")
- Occurs typically 2 to 4 days after ascent over 8000 ft (2500 m)
- Dyspnea
- Dry cough or cough with frothy rust- or pink-tinged sputum
- Chest tightness
- Tachycardia, tachypnea, rales, cyanosis

High-altitude cerebral edema
- Usually presents several days after AMS
- Confusion, irritability, drowsiness, stupor, hallucinations
- Headache, nausea, vomiting
- Ataxia, paralysis, and seizures
- Coma and death may develop within hours of the first symptoms

ETIOLOGY

- As one ascends to altitudes above sea level, the atmospheric pressure decreases. Although the percentage of oxygen in the air remains the same, the partial pressure of oxygen decreases with altitude.
- Thus, the cause of altitude sickness is primarily hypoxia resulting from low partial pressures of oxygen.
- The body responds to low oxygen partial pressures through a process of acclimatization (see "Comments").

DIAGNOSIS

The diagnosis of altitude sickness is made by clinical presentation and physical findings described previously.

DIFFERENTIAL DIAGNOSIS

- Dehydration
- Carbon monoxide poisoning
- Hypothermia
- Infection
- Substance abuse
- Congestive heart failure
- Pulmonary embolism
- Cerebrovascular accident

WORKUP

Typically the diagnosis is self-evident after history and physical examination. Laboratory tests and imaging studies help monitor cardiopulmonary and CNS status in patients admitted to the intensive care unit for pulmonary and/or cerebral edema. In patients with HAPE occurring at lower altitudes (<8000 ft), an evaluation of preexisting pulmonary hypertension or a left-to-right shunt should be considered.

LABORATORY TESTS

Laboratory tests are not very useful in diagnosing altitude sickness.

IMAGING STUDIES

CXR showing Kerley B-lines and patchy edema (see Fig. 1-11)
CT scan of the head showing diffuse or patchy edema

TREATMENT

NONPHARMACOLOGIC THERAPY

- Stop the ascent to allow acclimatization or start to descend until symptoms have resolved.
- Oxygen 4 to 6 L/min is used for severe AMS, HAPE, and HACE.
- Portable hyperbaric bags are useful if available at the site.
- Avoid dehydration.

ACUTE PHARMACOLOGIC Rx

- NSAIDs or aspirin are effective in treating headaches in AMS.
- Acetazolamide 125 mg to 250 mg PO bid has been shown in randomized controlled trials to be both a preventa-

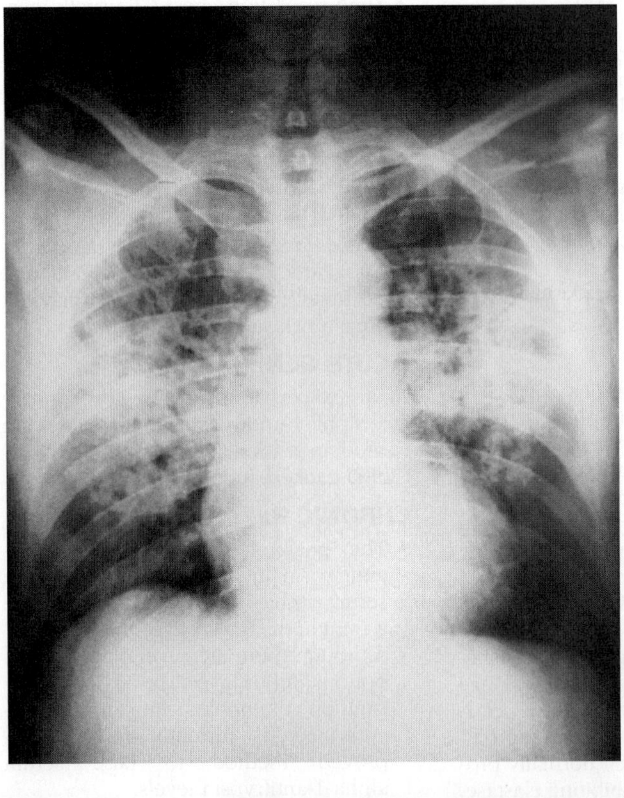

FIGURE 1-11 Chest radiograph showing high-altitude pulmonary edema. (From Strauss RH [ed]: *Sports medicine,* ed 2, Philadelphia, 1991, WB Saunders.)

tive and acute therapy for patients with AMS and HAPE.

- Nifedipine 10 mg sublingual followed by long-acting nifedipine 30 mg bid is used for patients with HAPE who cannot descend immediately.
- Dexamethasone 4 mg PO every 6 hr is used in patients with severe AMS, HAPE, and HACE.

CHRONIC Rx

- Prevention therapy is the most prudent therapy.
  1. Slow, staged ascent to avoid altitude sickness.
  2. Start the ascent below 8000 ft.
  3. Ascend 1000 ft/day (300 m/day).
  4. Spend 2 nights at the same altitude every 3 days.
  5. Sleep at lower heights than the altitude climbed ("climb high, sleep low").
  6. Prophylactic therapy with acetazolamide 750 mg daily and/or dexamethasone 8 to 16 mg daily decreases the risk of developing AMS. (In combination, the drugs may have an additive benefit.) The drugs are used until acclimatization occurs.
  7. Prophylactic inhalation of a β-adrenergic agonist, salmeterol 125 μg every 12 hr, or the use of slow-release nifedipine 20 mg bid have both been shown to reduce the risk of HAPE in susceptible individuals.
  8. Tadalafil, a long-acting phosphodiesterase inhibitor, has recently been shown to decrease the incidence of HAPE in susceptible individuals.

DISPOSITION

- AMS improves over a period of 2 to 3 days.
- HAPE is the most common cause of death among the altitude illnesses.
- More than 60% of patients with HAPE will have recurrence of symptoms on subsequent climbs.
- Neurologic deficits may persist for weeks but eventually resolve. If coma occurs, prognosis is poor.

REFERRAL

Cardiology and neurology referrals are made in patients with pulmonary edema and CNS findings, respectively.

PEARLS & CONSIDERATIONS

COMMENTS

- Acclimatization is the process in which individuals who normally reside at low altitude adapt to hypobaric hypoxia to improve their tolerance and performance at a higher altitude. These mechanisms include:
  1. An increase in respiratory rates and tidal volume. This hyperventilation allows for lowering of arterial carbon dioxide to preserve oxygen delivery even at extreme altitudes.
  2. An early increase in heart rate and stroke volume to improve oxygen delivery, which within 1 week both drop off because of diuresis and lower catecholamine levels.
  3. Pulmonary hypertension develops in response to hypoxemia and results in an improved ventilation-perfusion mismatch. This may be maladaptive and lead to the development of HAPE.
  4. Cerebral vasodilation to increase blood flow to the brain.
  5. Rise in hemoglobin and hematocrit. This is a chronic process that takes up to a week to occur. It occurs in response to the need for improved oxygen delivery.
- Adaptation to altitude is different from acclimatization; adaption refers to physiologic differences in persons who reside permanently at high altitude (e.g., an increased diffusion capacity).
- Risk factors for the development of altitude sicknesses are:
  1. Rapid ascent
  2. Previous history of altitude sickness
  3. Strenuous exertion on arrival
  4. Obesity
  5. Male gender
- Physical fitness is not protective against high-altitude illness.
- HAPE is characterized by elevated pulmonary pressures resulting in protein-rich, hemorrhagic exudates into the lung alveoli.

SUGGESTED READINGS

Basnyat B, Murcoch DR: High-altitude illness, *Lancet* 361:1967, 2003.

Gallagher SA, Hackett PH: High-altitude illness, *Emer Med Clin Am* 22:329, 2004.

Hachett PH, Roach RC: High-altitude illness, *N Engl J Med* 345:107, 2001.

Hackett P, Rennie D: High altitude pulmonary edema, *JAMA* 287:2275, 2002.

Rodway GW et al: High-altitude related disorders. Part 1. Pathophysiology, differential diagnosis and treatment, *Heart Lung* 32:353, 2003.

Swenson ER et al: Pathogenesis of high-altitude pulmonary edema, *JAMA* 287:2228, 2002.

West, JB: The physiologic basis of high-altitude diseases, *Ann Int Med* 141:789, 2004

AUTHORS: **JEFFREY MAZER, M.D.**, and **GAURAV CHOUDHARY, M.D.**

BASIC INFORMATION

DEFINITION

Dementia is a syndrome characterized by progressive loss of previously acquired cognitive skills including memory, language, insight, and judgment. Alzheimer's disease (AD) accounts for the majority (50% to 75%) of all cases of dementia.

ICD-9CM CODES
331.0 Alzheimer's disease
290.0 Senile dementia, uncomplicated

EPIDEMIOLOGY & DEMOGRAPHICS

INCIDENCE: Risk doubles every 5 yr after the age of 65; above the age of 85 the incidence is about 8%.

PREVALENCE: Currently an estimated 4 million Americans have AD; 7% between the ages of 65 and 74, 53% between the ages of 75 and 84, and 40% over the age of 85.

PREDOMINANT SEX: Female.

PHYSICAL FINDINGS & CLINICAL PRESENTATION

- Spouse or other family member, not the patient, often notes insidious memory impairment.
- Patients have difficulties learning and retaining new information, handling complex tasks (e.g., balancing the checkbook), and have impairments in reasoning, judgment, spatial ability, and orientation (e.g., difficulty driving, getting lost away from home).
- Behavioral changes, such as mood changes and apathy, may accompany memory impairment. In later stages patients may develop agitation and psychosis.
- Atypical presentations include early and severe behavioral changes, focal findings on examination, parkinsonism, hallucinations, falls, or onset of symptoms younger than the age of 65.

DIAGNOSIS

There is no definitive imaging or laboratory test for the diagnosis of dementia; rather, diagnosis is dependent on clinical history, a thorough physical and neurologic examination, and use of reliable and valid diagnostic criteria (i.e., DSM-IV or NINDCS-ADRDA) such as the following:

- Loss of memory and one or more additional cognitive abilities (aphasia, apraxia, agnosia, or other disturbance in executive functioning)
- Impairment in social or occupational functioning that represents a decline from a previous level of functioning and results in significant disability
- Deficits that do not occur exclusively during the course of delirium
- Insidious onset and gradual progression of symptoms
- Cognitive loss documented by neuropsychologic tests
- No physical signs, neuroimaging, or laboratory evidence of other diseases that can cause dementia (i.e., metabolic abnormalities, medication or toxin effects, infection, stroke, Parkinson's disease, subdural hematoma, or tumors)

Patients with isolated memory loss who lack functional impairment at home or work do not meet criteria for dementia but may have a mild cognitive impairment (MCI). Identifying patients with MCI is important because patients with MCI may have a slightly higher rate of progression to dementia.

DIFFERENTIAL DIAGNOSIS

- Cancer (brain tumor, meningeal neoplasia)
- Infection (AIDS, neurosyphilis, progressive multifocal leucoencephalopathy)
- Metabolic (EtOH, hypothyroidism, B_{12} deficiency)
- Organ failure (dialysis dementia, Wilson's disease)
- Vascular disorder (chronic subdural hematoma)
- Depression

WORKUP

HISTORY & GENERAL PHYSICAL EXAMINATION:

- Medication use should always be reviewed for drugs that may cause mental status changes.
- Patients should be screened for depression, because it can sometimes mimic dementia but also often occurs as a coexisting condition and should be treated.
- On examination, look for signs of metabolic disturbance, presence of psychiatric features, or focal neurologic deficits.

MENTAL STATUS TESTING:

Brief mental status testing can be done easily and quickly in the office. Most commonly used is the Folstein Mini-Mental Status Examination (MMSE). The MMSE is widely available in many reference books and on the Internet. An MMSE score <24 (scores range from 0 to 30, with lower scores reflecting poorer performance) suggests dementia; however, the MMSE is not sensitive enough to detect mild dementia, or dementia in patients with high baseline IQ. Scores may be spuriously low in patients with limited education, poor motor function, African American or Hispanic ethnicity, poor language skills, or impaired vision.

If the MMSE is not available, mental status testing should include tests that assess the following cognitive functions:

- *Orientation:* Ask the patient to give the day, date, month, year, and place, and to name the current president.
- *Attention:* Ask patient to recite the months of the year forwards and in reverse.
- *Verbal recall:* Ask the patient to remember four items; test for recall after a 1-min and a 5-min delay.
- *Language:* Ask patient to write and then read a sentence; have the patient name both common and less common objects.
- *Visual-Spatial:* Ask the patient to draw a clock and to set the hands of the clock at 11:10.

Patients with AD typically have trouble with verbal recall, plus visual-spatial and/or language deficits. Attention is usually preserved until the late stages of AD, so consider alternate diagnoses in patients who do poorly on tests of attention.

LABORATORY TESTS

- CBC
- Serum electrolytes
- Glucose
- BUN/creatinine
- Liver and thyroid function tests
- Serum vitamin B_{12} and methylmalonic acid
- Syphilis serology, if high clinical suspicion
- Lumbar puncture if history or signs of cancer, infectious process, or when the clinical presentation is unusual (i.e., rapid progression of symptoms)
- EEG if there is history of seizures, episodic confusion, rapid clinical decline, or suspicion of Creutzfeldt-Jakob disease
- Measurement of apolipoprotein E genotyping, CSF tau and amyloid, and functional imaging including positron emission tomography (PET) or scanning proton emission computed tomography (SPECT) are not routinely indicated

IMAGING STUDIES

CT scan or MRI to rule out hydrocephalus and mass lesions, including subdural hematoma.

TREATMENT

NONPHARMACOLOGIC THERAPY

- Patient safety, including risks associated with impaired driving, wandering behavior, leaving stoves unattended, and accidents, must be addressed with the patient and family early and appropriate measures implemented.
- Wandering, hoarding or hiding objects, repetitive questioning, withdrawal, and social inappropriateness often respond to behavioral therapies.

ACUTE GENERAL Rx

None

CHRONIC Rx

1. Symptomatic treatment of memory disturbance (Table 1-2):
   a. Cholinesterase inhibitors (ChEI): FDA approved for the treatment of mild to moderate AD (MMSE 10-26). Common side effects include nausea, diarrhea, and anorexia and may be bothersome enough to require a slower escalation of dosage, or switching to another agent.
   b. NMDA receptor antagonist: Memantine (Namenda). FDA-approved for the treatment of moderate to severe AD. Common side effects include constipation, dizziness, or headache. Memantine is contraindicated in patients with renal insufficiency or history of seizures.
2. Symptomatic treatment of neuropsychiatric and behavioral disturbances (Table 1-3):
   Depression, agitation, delusions, or hallucinations may respond to medications.

DISPOSITION AND REFERRAL

- Patients with complex or atypical presentations or challenging management issues should be referred to a specialist with expertise in dementia.
- Family education and support may help reduce need for skilled nursing facility, and reduce caregiver stress, depression, and burnout.

PEARLS & CONSIDERATIONS

The physician must make a thorough search for the treatable causes of dementia.

Current American Academy of Neurology practice parameters recommend:

- Treat cognitive symptoms of AD with cholinesterase inhibitors and vitamin E.
- Treat agitation, psychosis, and depression.
- Encourage caregivers to participate in educational programs and support groups.

COMMENTS

For additional information for patients, families, and clinicians:

- Alzheimer's Association (www.alzheimers.org; 800-272-3900)
- Alzheimer's Disease Education and Referral Center (www.alzheimers. org; 800-438-4380)

EVIDENCE

EBM

Cholinesterase inhibitors have been shown to be effective in the treatment of dementia. Clinical studies have demonstrated small improvements in memory, language, and ability to perform activities of daily living. Treatment with ChEI may also help to reduce symptoms of agitation and aggressiveness, slow functional decline, and lessen caregiver stress. At present there are no data supporting superiority of one cholinesterase inhibitor over another. Recent data suggest ChEI may be of some benefit in moderate to severe AD.[1-3]

There is evidence that memantine, a noncompetetive NMDA antagonist, is also effective in the treatment of dementia.[4] Clinical studies have demonstrated improvement in function and cognition, and possibly a delay in disease progression.

Combination therapy of memantine with ChEI has added benefits in moderate to severe AD patients compared to use of ChEI alone. There may be symptomatic benefit of monotherapy in mild AD but additional studies are still needed.

The use of vitamin E 1000 IU given twice daily was shown to delay progression in patients with moderate disease in a single randomized controlled study. However, newer data show no benefit for patients with MCI, and patients taking high-dose vitamin E may have a slightly increased risk of mortality.

The Women's Health Initiative Memory Study (WHIMS) demonstrated that estrogen alone or in combination with progestin does not prevent cognitive decline and may increase the risk of dementia.

Gingko biloba has been shown in some trials to have a small but statistically significant effect compared to placebo. Further evidence is necessary before routine use is recommended.

Evidence-Based References

1. Raskind MA et al: Galantamine in AD—a 6-month randomized, placebo-controlled trial with a 6-month extension, *Neurology* 54:2261, 2000.
2. Rogers SL et al: A 24-week, double-blind, placebo-controlled trial of donepezil in patients with Alzheimer's disease, *Neurology* 50:136, 1998.
3. Rösler M et al: Efficacy and safety of rivastigmine in patients with Alzheimer's disease: international randomised controlled trial, *BMJ* 318:633, 1999.
4. Reisberg B et al: Memantine in moderate-to-severe Alzheimer's disease, *N Engl J Med* 348:1333, 2003.

SUGGESTED READINGS

Cummings JL: Alzheimer's disease, *N Engl J Med* 351:56, 2004.

Doody RS et al: Management of dementia (an evidence-based review): report of the Quality Standards Subcommittee of the American Academy of Neurology, *Neurology* 56:1154, 2001.

DSM-IV: Diagnostic and statistical manual of mental disorders, ed 4, Washington, DC, 1994, American Psychiatric Association.

Folstein MF et al: "Mini-mental state": a practical method for grading the cognitive state of patients for the clinician, *J Psychiatr Res* 12:189, 1975.

Kawas CH: Early Alzheimer's disease, *N Engl J Med* 349(11):1056, 2003.

AUTHOR: **TAMARA G. FONG, M.D., PH.D.**

TABLE 1-2 Symptomatic Treatment of Memory Disturbance

	Initial Dose	Target Dose
Donepezil (Aricept)	5 mg PO qd for 4-6 weeks	10 mg PO qd
Rivastigmine (Exelon)	1.5 mg PO bid with food, increase by 1.5 mg bid weekly	3-6 mg PO bid
	or	
	4.6 mg/24 hr transdermal patch daily	9.5 mg/24 hr transdermal patch daily
Galantamine (Reminyl)	4 mg PO bid with food, increase by 4 mg bid every 4 weeks	8-12 mg bid
Memantine (Namenda)	5 mg PO qd, increase by 5 mg weekly	10 mg bid

TABLE 1-3 Treatment of Behavioral and Neuropsychiatric Symptoms

	Initial Dose	Maximum Dose
	ATYPICAL ANTIPSYCHOTICS	
Olanzapine (Zyprexa)	2.5 mg qd to bid, may increase by 2.5 mg as needed	7.5 mg bid
Quetiapine (Seroquel)	25 mg bid, may increase by 25 mg every 2 days	250 mg tid
	ANTIDEPRESSANTS	
Sertraline (Zoloft)	25-50 mg qd, may increase by 25 mg every week	200 mg qd
Citalopram (Celexa)	10 mg qd, may increase after 1 week	20 mg qd

BASIC INFORMATION

DEFINITION

Amaurosis fugax (AF) is a temporary loss of monocular vision caused by transient retinal ischemia.

ICD-9CM CODES
362.34 Amaurosis fugax

EPIDEMIOLOGY & DEMOGRAPHICS

INCIDENCE (IN U.S.): An uncommon presentation of carotid artery disease
PEAK INCIDENCE: 55 yr and older

PHYSICAL FINDINGS & CLINICAL PRESENTATION

- Onset is sudden, typically lasting seconds to minutes, and often accompanied by scotomas such as a shade or curtain being pulled over the front of the eye (usually downward, but also upward).
- Vision loss may involve the entire or half the visual field or be quadrantic.
- There are usually no physical findings.
- Acute stage: cholesterol emboli may be seen in retinal artery (Hollenhorst plaque): carotid bruits or other evidence of generalized atherosclerosis.
- If embolus is cardiac in origin, atrial fibrillation is often present.

ETIOLOGY

- Usually embolic from the internal carotid artery or the heart: embolic occlusion of the central retinal artery or a branch vessel of the retinal artery feeding the upper or lower retina
- May also be due to vasculitis, such as giant cell arteritis (GCA), or hyperviscosity syndromes, such as sickle cell disease, that cause ischemia in the vascular territory of the ophthalmic artery

DIAGNOSIS

DIFFERENTIAL DIAGNOSIS

The differential diagnosis of transient monocular visual loss includes the following:

- Retinal migraine: in contrast to amaurosis, the onset of visual loss develops more slowly, usually over a period of 15 to 20 min.
- Transient visual obscurations (TVOs) occur in the setting of papilledema; intermittent rises in intracranial pressure briefly compromise optic disc perfusion and cause transient visual loss lasting 1 to 2 sec and the episodes may be binocular. If the visual loss persists at the time of evaluation (i.e., vision has not yet recovered), then the differential diagnosis should be broadened to include:
- Anterior ischemic optic neuropathy—arteritic (classically GCA) or nonarteritic
- Central retinal vein occlusion

WORKUP

- Workup should focus on embolic sources but GCA should always be considered.
- Careful examination of retina; embolus may be visible and confirm the diagnosis (Fig. 1-12).
- Auscultation of arteries for carotid bruits.
- Examination of all pulses and for temporal artery tenderness.
- Inquire about symptoms of GCA (scalp tenderness, jaw claudication).
- Examine for signs of hemispheric stroke resulting from ICA disease (contralateral limb and face weakness or sensory loss, aphasia, etc.).

LABORATORY TESTS

- CBC with ESR and CRP.
- Serum chemistries, including lipid profile.
- ECG and consider cycling cardiac enzymes.
- Hypercoagulable workup is discretionary based on younger age and history.

IMAGING STUDIES

- Carotid Dopplers followed by MR or CT angiography as indicated.
- Transthoracic echocardiography (TTE) is indicated to screen for embolization in patients with evidence of heart disease and in patients without an evident source for their transient neurologic deficit. Transesophageal echocardiography (TEE) is more sensitive for detecting cardiac sources of embolization (ventricular mural thrombus, atrial appendage, patent foramen ovale, aortic arch).
- Consider MRI of the brain with diffusion-weighted imaging to look for infarcts.

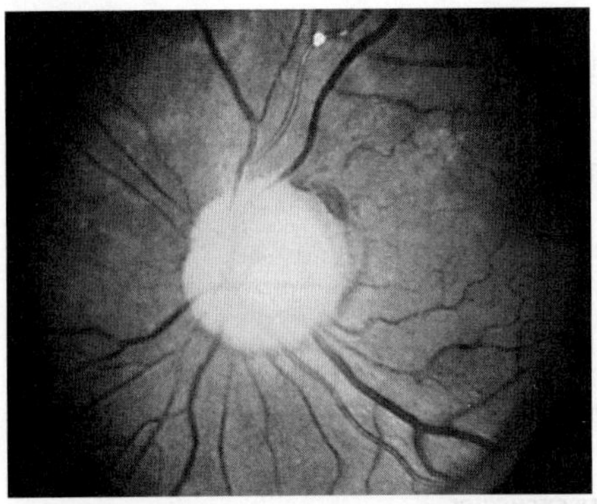

FIGURE 1-12 A cholesterol crystal embolus lodged at an arterial bifurcation. (From Stein JH [ed]: *Internal medicine*, ed 5, St Louis, 1998, Mosby.)

TREATMENT

NONPHARMACOLOGIC THERAPY

- Diet (decrease saturated fatty acids and high-cholesterol foods)
- Exercise
- Cessation of tobacco use

ACUTE GENERAL Rx

- Investigate as an emergency.
- Give aspirin if etiology is presumed embolic.
- If GCA is suspected, start prednisone and refer for temporal artery biopsy within 48 hr (see Section I, "Giant Cell Arteritis").

CHRONIC Rx

- Reduce risks by carotid endarterectomy or stent if stenosis >70%.
- Control hypertension and manage vascular risk factors.
- Antiplatelet therapy.
- Consider starting an HMG CoA reductase inhibitor.

DISPOSITION

Among patients with >50% carotid stenosis who do not undergo carotid endarterectomy, those who present with transient monocular blindness have about a 10% risk of stroke in 3 yr compared with a 20% risk in patients who present with a hemispheric transient ischemic attack (TIA).

REFERRAL

- Recommend referral to a neurologist for an evaluation and workup.
- If significant carotid stenosis, consider carotid endarterectomy or carotid stenting for the following:
  1. High-grade (≥70%) stenosis
  2. Multiple TIAs despite medical therapy, in the setting of high-grade or ulcerative disease

PEARLS & CONSIDERATIONS

- Cholesterol emboli in retinal arteries on funduscopy confirms the diagnosis.
- Permanent visual loss should raise concern for anterior ischemic optic neuropathy and is not amaurosis fugax.
- Recognize that transient visual loss has multiple other causes.

SUGGESTED READING

Murtha T, Stasheff SF: Visual dysfunction in retinal and optic nerve disease, *Neurol Clin* 21:445, 2003.

AUTHOR: **SEAN I. SAVITZ, M.D.**

BASIC INFORMATION

DEFINITION

Amblyopia refers to a decrease in vision in one or both eyes in the presence of an otherwise normal ophthalmologic examination.

SYNONYMS

Deprivation amblyopia
Occlusion amblyopia
Strabismus amblyopia
Refractive amblyopia
Organic or toxic amblyopias
Lazy eye

ICD-9CM CODES
368.00 Amblyopia

EPIDEMIOLOGY & DEMOGRAPHICS

INCIDENCE (IN U.S.): 1% to 4% of the general population
PREVALENCE (IN U.S.): High incidence in premature infants with drug-dependent mothers and in neurologically impaired children
PREDOMINANT SEX: None
PREDOMINANT AGE: Childhood
PEAK INCIDENCE: Childhood

PHYSICAL FINDINGS & CLINICAL PRESENTATION

Decreased vision using best refraction in the presence of normal corneal, lens, retinal, and optic nerve appearance (Fig. 1-13)

ETIOLOGY

- Visual deprivation
- Strabismus
- Occlusion with patching
- Refractive error organic lesions in the nervous system
- Toxins

DIAGNOSIS

DIFFERENTIAL DIAGNOSIS

- Central nervous system (CNS) disease (brainstem)
- Optic nerve disorders
- Corneal or other eye diseases
- Retinal disorders

WORKUP

- Complete eye examination to find cause of amblyopia or deprivation of vision
- Motility evaluation

LABORATORY TESTS

Usually none

IMAGING STUDIES

Usually not necessary unless CNS lesion suspected

TREATMENT

NONPHARMACOLOGIC THERAPY

- Glasses or prisms to align eyes with minor deviations and improve vision.
- Patches, mechanical vs. atropine—Patching and atropine both work. Atropine 1% is used daily for 6 months; patching is used 6 hr/day for 6 months. Patching may be more effective. Fifty percent get best vision improvement by 16 weeks.
- Removal of the cause of the amblyopia if possible.
- Surgery to align the eyes or remove obstruction to vision.

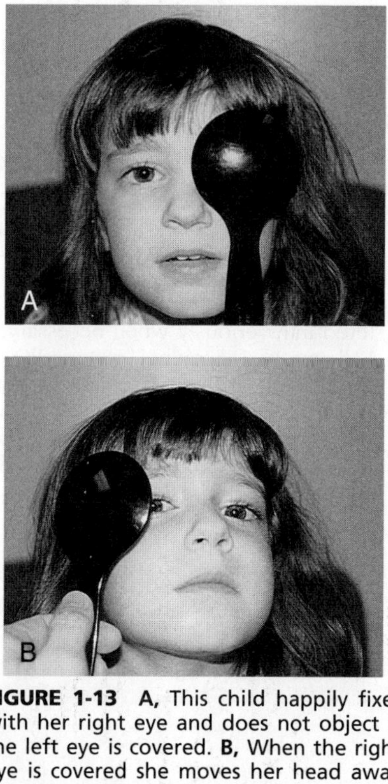

FIGURE 1-13 **A,** This child happily fixes with her right eye and does not object if the left eye is covered. **B,** When the right eye is covered she moves her head away and tries to remove the cover, demonstrating a fixation preference for the right eye and amblyopia of the left eye. (From Hoekelman R [ed]: *Primary pediatric care,* ed 3, St Louis, 1997, Mosby.)

CHRONIC Rx

Patching or optics, including prisms and atropine most effective in 3 to 7 yr olds only; minimal or no help after 7 yrs old

DISPOSITION

Immediate patching, alternating eyes daily

REFERRAL

To ophthalmologist if vision is compromised

PEARLS & CONSIDERATIONS

COMMENTS

- The earlier the referral, the better the outcome.
- Amblyopia causes unilateral vision loss in 2% to 4% of the population.

EVIDENCE

A randomized controlled trial assessed whether full treatment with glasses and patching, compared with glasses only or no treatment, was effective in 177 children aged 3 to 5 yr with mild to moderate unilateral impairment of acuity (6/9 to 6/36) detected by screening. Effects of treatment depended on initial acuity: full treatment showed a substantial effect in moderate acuity (6/36 to 6/18 at recruitment) and no significant effect in mild acuity (6/9 to 6/12 at recruitment). Children in the treatment groups had better visual acuity at follow-up than those in the no treatment group.[1] Ⓑ

A randomized controlled trial compared atropine sulfate eye drops versus patching in the treatment of moderate amblyopia in children younger than 7. Both therapies were equally effective in improving visual acuity after 6 months of treatment.[2] Ⓑ

Evidence-Based References

1. Clarke MP et al: Randomized controlled trial of treatment of unilateral visual impairment detected at preschool vision screening, *BMJ* 327:1251, 2003. Ⓑ
2. Pediatric Eye Disease Investigator Group: A randomized trial of atropine vs. patching for treatment of moderate amblyopia in children, *Arch Ophthalmol* 120:268, 2002. Ⓑ

SUGGESTED READING

Doshi NR, Rodriguez ML: Amblyopia, *Am Fam Physician* 75:361, 2007.

AUTHOR: **MELVYN KOBY, M.D.**

BASIC INFORMATION

DEFINITION

Amebiasis is an infection caused by the protozoal parasite *Entamoeba histolytica*. Although primarily an infection of the colon, amebiasis may cause extraintestinal disease, particularly liver abscess.

SYNONYMS

Amebic dysentery (when severe intestinal infection)

ICD-9CM CODES
006.9 Amebiasis

EPIDEMIOLOGY & DEMOGRAPHICS

INCIDENCE (IN U.S.): Highest in institutionalized patients, sexually active homosexual men

PREVALENCE (IN U.S.): 4% (80% of infections asymptomatic)

PREDOMINANT SEX:
- Equal sex distribution in general
- Striking male predominance of liver abscess

PREDOMINANT AGE: Second through sixth decades

PEAK INCIDENCE: Peaks at age 2 to 3 yr and >40 yr

GENETICS: Infection more likely to be fulminant in young infants

PHYSICAL FINDINGS & CLINICAL PRESENTATION

- Often nonspecific
- Approximately 20% of cases symptomatic
  1. Diarrhea, which may be bloody
  2. Abdominal and back pain
- Abdominal tenderness in 83% of severe cases
- Fever in 38% of severe cases
- Hepatomegaly, RUQ tenderness, and fever in almost all patients with liver abscess (may be absent in fulminant cases)

ETIOLOGY

- Caused by the protozoal parasite *E. histolytica* (Fig. 1-14)
- Transmission by the fecal-oral route
- Infection usually localized to the large bowel, particularly the cecum where a localized mass lesion (ameboma) may form
- Extraintestinal infection in which the organism invades the bowel mucosa and gains access to the portal circulation

DIAGNOSIS

DIFFERENTIAL DIAGNOSIS

- Severe intestinal infection possibly confused with ulcerative colitis or other infectious enterocolitis syndromes, such as those caused by *Shigella, Salmonella, Campylobacter,* or invasive *Escherichia coli*
- In elderly patients: ischemic bowel possibly producing a similar picture

WORKUP

- Three stool specimens over a period of 7 to 10 days to exclude the diagnosis (sensitivity 50% to 80%)
- Concentration and staining the specimen with Lugol's iodine or methylene blue to increase the diagnostic yield
- Available culture (rarely necessary in routine cases)

LABORATORY TESTS

- Stool examination is generally reliable.
- Mucosal biopsy is occasionally necessary.
- Serum antibody may be detected and is particularly sensitive and specific for extraintestinal infection or severe intestinal disease.
- Aspiration of abscess fluid is used to distinguish amebic from bacterial abscesses.

IMAGING STUDIES

Abdominal imaging studies (sonography or CT scan) to diagnose liver abscess

TREATMENT

ACUTE GENERAL Rx

- Metronidazole (750 mg PO tid for 10 days) is used in the treatment of mild to severe intestinal infection and amebic liver abscess; it may be administered intravenously when necessary.
- Follow with iodoquinol (650 mg PO tid for 20 days) to eradicate persistent cysts.
- For asymptomatic patients with amebic cysts on stool examination, use iodoquinol or paromomycin (500 mg PO tid for 7 days).
- Avoid antiperistaltic agents in severe intestinal infections to avoid risk of toxic megacolon.
- Liver abscess is generally responsive to medical management but surgical intervention indicated for extension of liver abscess into pericardium or for toxic megacolon.

DISPOSITION

Host immunity incomplete and reinfection rate high for patients remaining at risk

REFERRAL

- For consultation with infectious diseases specialist for extraintestinal infection or persistent or relapsing intestinal infection
- For surgical consultation:
  1. For toxic megacolon
  2. For impending rupture of or extension of liver abscess into adjacent structures

PEARLS & CONSIDERATIONS

COMMENTS

Infection with other intestinal parasites, particularly *Giardia lamblia,* may coexist with amebiasis.

SUGGESTED READINGS

Haque R et al: Entamoeba histolytica infection in children and protection from subsequent amebiasis, *Infect Immun* 74(2):904, 2006.
Hung CC et al: Invasive amebiasis as an emerging parasitic disease in patients with human immunodeficiency virus type 1 infection in Taiwan, *Arch Intern Med* 165(4):409, 2005.

AUTHORS: **GLENN G. FORT, M.D., M.P.H., JOSEPH R. MASCI, M.D.,** and **DENNIS J. MIKOLICH, M.D.**

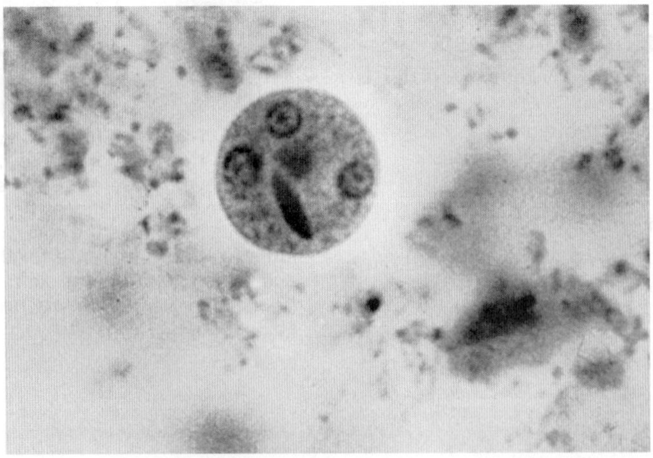

FIGURE 1-14 Mature cyst of *Entamoeba histolytica*. Three of the four nuclei are seen in the plane of focus of this photomicrograph. (From Mandell GL [ed]: *Mandell, Douglas, and Bennett's principles and practice of infectious diseases,* ed 5, New York, 2000, Churchill Livingstone.)

BASIC INFORMATION

DEFINITION

The acquired inability to learn new information or recall new information. The impairment compromises personal, social, or occupational functioning. Disorder is not secondary to delirium or dementia.

SYNONYMS

Korsakoff's syndrome
Amnesia

ICD-9CM CODES
780.9 Amnesia (retrograde); memory disturbance, loss or lack
DSM-IV-TR codes
294 Amnestic disorder due to . . . [indicate the general medical condition]
294.8 Amnestic disorder NOS

EPIDEMIOLOGY & DEMOGRAPHICS

INCIDENCE: Data not available on true incidence or lifetime risk.
PREDOMINANT AGE: Transient global amnesia onset usually over age 50.
GENETICS: Genetic defect for thiamine metabolism has been described in some patients.

PHYSICAL FINDINGS & CLINICAL PRESENTATION

History
- Diagnosis dependent upon history.
- The inability to learn or recall new information is the key feature of this disorder.
- Mini mental status examination useful. Patients unable to recall events that transpire during the interview but may have a normal digit span and be able to follow the conversation.
- Patients unable to recall events subsequent to the onset of the amnesia.
- Individuals may learn new motor tasks but are unable to recall those learning experiences.
- Amnesia generally has both anterograde and retrograde components.

ETIOLOGY

- Traumatic brain injury
- Focal tumors or infarction
- Herpes simplex encephalitis
- Cerebral anoxia
- Korsakoff's syndrome (thiamine deficiency)
- Carbon monoxide poisoning
- Transient amnesia may arise from concussion, acute intoxications, anasthesia, seizures, transient global amnesia, and post-ECT

DIAGNOSIS

DIFFERENTIAL DIAGNOSIS

- Dementia
- Delirium
- Major depression
- Benign senescent forgetfulness

WORKUP

- Complete medical history and mental status testing
- Neuropsychologic testing

LABORATORY TESTS

No current role in diagnosis of amnestic disorders.

IMAGING STUDIES

- No specific or diagnostic features of amnestic disorder are detectable on imaging.
- Brain MRI indicates specific atrophy in diencephalic structures in Korsakoff's syndrome.

TREATMENT

NONPHARMACOLOGIC THERAPY

- Cognitive rehabilitation to promote recovery from brain injury may be helpful.
- Supervised living to ensure appropriate long-term care.

ACUTE GENERAL Rx

Initial treatment directed to the underlying etiology

CHRONIC Rx

No known effective treatments to reverse or ameliorate memory deficits.

DISPOSITION

Amnesias may be chronic or transient, depending upon etiology.

REFERRAL

Refer for neuropsychological testing.

PEARLS & CONSIDERATIONS

COMMENTS

In Korsakoff's syndrome, anterograde amnesia (disturbance in acquisition of new information) is more prominent than retrograde amnesia (problems remembering old information).

PREVENTION

High-dose thiamine for prevention of Korsakoff's syndrome

PATIENT/FAMILY EDUCATION

Respite care and in-home services for family caregivers

SUGGESTED READINGS

Butler CR et al: The syndrome of transient epileptic amnesia, *Ann Neurol* 61:587, 2007.
Uttner I et al: Transient global amnesia—full recovery without persistent cognitive impairment, *Eur Neurol* 58(3):146, 2007.

AUTHOR: **MITCHELL D. FELDMAN, M.D., M.PHIL.**

BASIC INFORMATION

DEFINITION

Amyloidosis is a generic term describing the deposition of amyloid fibrils in body tissues. *Amyloid* is an amorphous, eosinophilic material; it is birefringent and usually extracellular. Electron microscopy reveals nonbranching fibrils that are soluble and relatively resistant to proteolytic digestion. There are two major forms of acquired systemic amyloidosis:

- AA, associated with chronic inflammatory diseases (e.g., rheumatoid arthritis) and amyloid deposits in kidneys, liver, and spleen. Deposition of amyloid fibrils derived from circulating acute-phase reactant serum amyloid A protein (SAA) causes systemic AA amyloidosis.
- AL (formerly known as primary amyloidosis) affecting the kidneys, heart, liver, intestines, skin, peripheral sensory nervous system, spleen, and lungs.

ICD-9CM CODES
277.3 Amyloidosis

EPIDEMIOLOGY & DEMOGRAPHICS

INCIDENCE (IN U.S): There are between 1500 and 3500 new cases annually. The most common type is immunoglobulin light chain related (AL), occurring in 5 to 12 persons/yr.

PREVALANCE: Amyloidosis affects primarily males between the ages of 60 and 70 yr.

PHYSICAL FINDINGS & CLINICAL PRESENTATION

- Findings are variable with organ system involvement. Symmetric polyarthritis, peripheral neuropathy, and carpal tunnel syndrome may be present with joint involvement.
- Signs and symptoms of nephrotic syndrome may be present with renal involvement.
- Fatigue and dyspnea may occur with pulmonary involvement.
- Diarrhea, macroglossia (20% of patients), malabsorption, hepatomegaly, and weight loss may occur with GI involvement.
- Cardiac involvement is common and can lead to predominantly right-sided CHF, JVD, peripheral edema, and hepatomegaly.
- Vascular involvement can result in easy bleeding and periorbital purpura ("raccoon eyes").

ETIOLOGY

In patients with amyloidosis, a soluble circulating protein (serum amyloid P [SAP]) is deposited in tissues as insoluble β-pleated sheets. The source of amyloid protein is a population of monoclonal plasma cells in the bone marrow. There are several chemically documented amyloidoses that can be principally subdivided into:

1. Acquired systemic amyloidosis (immunoglobulin light chain, multiple myeloma, hemodialysis amyloidosis)
2. Heredofamilial systemic (polyneuropathy, familial Mediterranean fever)
3. Organ-limited (Alzheimer's disease)
4. Localized endocrine (pancreatic islet, medullary thyroid carcinoma)

DIAGNOSIS

DIFFERENTIAL DIAGNOSIS

Variable, depending on the organ involvement:

- Renal involvement (toxin- or drug-induced necrosis, glomerulonephritis, renal vein thrombosis)
- Interstitial lung disease (sarcoidosis, connective tissue disease, infectious etiologies)
- Restrictive cardiomyopathy (endomyocardial fibrosis, viral myocarditis)
- Carpal tunnel (rheumatoid arthritis, hypothyroidism, overuse)
- Mental status changes (multiinfarct dementia)
- Peripheral neuropathy (alcohol abuse, vitamin deficiencies, diabetes mellitus)

WORKUP

Diagnostic approach is aimed at demonstration of amyloid deposits in tissues. This may be accomplished with rectal biopsy (positive in >60% of cases). Renal, myocardial, and bone marrow biopsy are other options. Abdominal fat pad biopsy can also be diagnostic; however, its yield is low and it should generally be reserved for evaluation of patients with peripheral neuropathy who also have findings associated with systemic amyloidosis.

LABORATORY TESTS

- Initial laboratory evaluation should include CBC, TSH, renal functions studies, ALT, AST, alkaline phosphatase, bilirubin, uric acid, urinalysis, and serum and urine protein immunoelectrophoresis.
- Various laboratory abnormalities include proteinuria (found in >70% of cases), anemia, renal insufficiency, liver function abnormalities, hypothyroidism (10% to 20% of patients), and elevated monoclonal proteins. The finding of a monoclonal light chain in the serum or urine is very useful for diagnosis. Measurement of blood SAA has prognostic value in AA amyloidosis.
- DNA analysis is necessary for the diagnosis of hereditary amyloidosis.

IMAGING STUDIES

- Chest x-ray may reveal hilar adenopathy and mediastinal adenopathy.
- Two-dimensional Doppler echocardiography to study diagnostic filling is useful to evaluate for cardiac involvement.
- Nuclear imaging with technetium-labeled aprotinin may detect cardiac amyloidosis. SAP scintigraphy has high sensitivity for the detection of amyloid deposits in liver, spleen, kidneys, adrenal glands, and bones.

TREATMENT

ACUTE GENERAL Rx

- Therapy is variable, depending on the type of amyloidosis. Amyloidosis associated with plasma cell disorders may be treated with melphalan and prednisone, along with colchicine. Colchicine may also be effective in renal amyloidosis.
- Treatment of AL amyloidosis with high-dose melphalan plus autologous stem-cell rescue is not superior to the outcome with standard-dose melphalan plus dexamethasone.
- Promising results have been found with the use of a molecule known as CPHPC given IV or SC in amyloidosis. This molecule has been shown effective in reducing circulating levels of SAP.
- Renal transplantation is needed in patients with renal amyloidosis. Peritoneal dialysis in place of hemodialysis in patients with renal failure may improve hemodialysis amyloidosis by clearing β-2 microglobulin.

DISPOSITION

Prognosis is determined primarily by the presence or absence of cardiac involvement and with the form of amyloidosis:

- In reactive amyloidosis, eradication of the predisposing disease slows and can occasionally reverse the progression of amyloid disease. Median survival after diagnosis is 133 months. Renal dysfunction is the predominant disease manifestation of AA amyloidosis. This form is associated with a more favorable outcome in patients with blood samples showing SAA concentrations that remain in the low to normal range (<4 mg/L).
- Patients with familial amyloidotic polyneuropathy generally have a prolonged course lasting 10 to 15 yr.
- Amyloidosis associated with immunocytic processes carries the worst prognosis (life expectancy <1 yr).
- The progression of amyloidosis associated with renal hemodialysis can be improved with newer dialysis membranes that can pass β-2 microglobulin.
- Median survival in patients with overt CHF is approximately 6 mo, 30 mo without CHF.
- Serum uric acid has a prognostic value in primary systemic amyloidosis. Patients with uric acid levels >8 mg/dl have a median overall survival of 9 mo from diagnosis compared to 20.3 mo for those with lower levels.

SUGGESTED READING

Kumar S et al: Serum uric acid: novel prognostic factor in primary systemic amyloidosis, *Mayo Clin Proc* 83(3):297-303, 2008.

AUTHOR: **FRED F. FERRI, M.D.**

BASIC INFORMATION

DEFINITION

Amyotrophic lateral sclerosis (ALS) is a progressive, degenerative neuromuscular condition of undetermined etiology affecting corticospinal tracts and anterior horn cells resulting in dysfunction of both upper motor neurons (UMN) and lower motor neurons (LMN), respectively.

ICD-9CM CODES
335.20 Amyotrophic lateral sclerosis

EPIDEMIOLOGY & DEMOGRAPHICS

INCIDENCE: 0.5 to 2 cases/100,000 persons. Onset is usually between the ages of 50 and 70 years. The male:female ratio is 2:1.

PREVALENCE: 5 in 100,000 persons

PHYSICAL FINDINGS & CLINICAL PRESENTATION

- Lower motor neuron signs (weakness, hypotonia, wasting, fasciculations, hypoflexia or areflexia).
- Upper motor neuron signs (loss of fine motor dexterity, spasticity, extensor plantar responses, hyperreflexia, clonus).
- Preservation of extraocular movements, sensation, bowel and bladder function.
- Dysarthria, dysphagia, pseudobulbar affect, frontal lobe dysfunction.
- ALS comprises approximately 90% of adult-onset motor neuron disease. Other presentations of motor neuron disease include progressive muscular atrophy, primary lateral sclerosis, progressive bulbar palsy, progressive pseudobulbar palsy, and ALS parkinsonism-dementia complex.

ETIOLOGY

90% to 95% of all cases are sporadic; of the familial cases, approximately 20% are associated with a genetic defect in the copper-zinc superoxide dismutase enzyme (SOD1).

DIAGNOSIS

DIFFERENTIAL DIAGNOSIS

- Multifocal motor neuropathy with conduction block (MMN)
- Cervical spondylotic myelopathy with polyradiculopathy
- Spinal stenosis with compression of lumbosacral nerve roots
- Chronic inflammatory demyelinating polyneuropathy with CNS lesions
- Syringomyelia
- Syringobulbia
- Foramen magnum tumor
- Spinal muscular atrophy (SMA)
- Late-onset hexosaminidase A deficiency
- Polyglucosan body disease
- Bulbospinal muscular atrophy (Kennedy's disease)
- Monomyelic amyotrophy
- ALS-like syndromes have been reported in the setting of lead intoxication, HIV, hyperparathyroidism, hyperthyroidism, lymphoma, and B_{12} deficiency.

WORKUP

- EMG and nerve conduction studies
- Lumbar puncture to assess protein
- Serum GM-1 Ab if MMN suspected
- Assessment of respiratory function (FVC, NIF)

LABORATORY TESTS

- B_{12}, thyroid function, PTH, HIV may be considered.
- Serum protein and immunofixation electrophoresis.
- DNA studies for SMA or bulbospinal atrophy, hexosaminidase levels in pure LMN syndrome.
- 24-hour urine for lead if indicated.

IMAGING STUDIES

- Craniospinal neuroimaging contingent upon clinical scenario
- Modified barium swallow to evaluate aspiration risk

TREATMENT

NONPHARMACOLOGIC THERAPY

- Noninvasive positive pressure ventilation may improve quality of life and may increase tracheostomy-free survival.
- PEG placement improves nutritional intake, promotes weight stabilization, and eases medication administration. Some studies suggest PEG placement may prolong life on the order of 1-4 mo, particularly when placed prior to an FVC ≤50% of predicted value.
- Nutrition, speech therapy, physical and occupational therapy services.
- Suction device for sialorrhea.
- Communication may be eased with computerized assistive devices.
- Early discussion of living will, resuscitation orders, desire for PEG and tracheostomy, potential long-term care options.
- Encourage contact with local support groups.

ACUTE GENERAL Rx

Riluzole (Rilutek), a glutamate antagonist, is the only FDA-approved medication known to extend tracheostomy-free survival in patients with ALS. Dosage is 50 mg q12h, at least 1 hr before or 2 hr after meals. Manufacturer recommends checking ALT at an initial frequency of once a month for 3 months, followed by once every 3 months until the first year of therapy is completed. ALT should be checked periodically thereafter.

CHRONIC Rx

- Sialorrhea may respond to either glycopyrrolate or amitriptyline (consider either propranolol or metoprolol if secretions are thick).
- Spasticity may be treated pharmacologically with baclofen, tizanidine, clonazepam.
- Pseudobulbar affect may improve with amitriptyline, sertraline (Zoloft), or dextromethorphan.

DISPOSITION

- Mean duration of symptoms is 3 to 5 yr.
- About 20% of patients survive >5 yr.

REFERRAL

- Referral to a neurologist experienced in neuromuscular disease is recommended to confirm the diagnosis. One prospective, population-based study suggested improved survival in subjects treated in a multidisciplinary clinic.
- GI referral for PEG placement is recommended while forced vital capacity (FVC) remains > 50% to minimize morbidity secondary to risks inherent to the procedure.

PEARLS & CONSIDERATIONS

- Patient-physician communication is an integral and essential part in both the initial diagnosis and subsequent treatment of ALS.
- A multidisciplinary approach to supportive care may lead to an improved level of daily functioning and foster increased sense of independence.

EVIDENCE

The use of riluzole has a modest impact on survival, approximately 2 to 3 mo.[1,2] Noninvasive ventilation may improve survival up to 6 mo in patients without severe bulbar involvement, with an additional benefit on health-related quality of life.[3]

Evidence-Based References

1. Bensimon G et al: A controlled trial of riluzole in amyotrophic lateral sclerosis, ALS/Riluzole Study Group, *N Engl J Med* 330:585, 1994.
2. Bensimon G et al: Riluzole/ALS Study Group, A study of riluzole in the treatment of advanced stage or elderly patients with amyotrophic lateral sclerosis, *J Neurol* 249:609, 2002.
3. Bourke SC et al: Effects of non-invasive ventilation on survival and quality of life in patients with amyotrophic lateral sclerosis: a randomized controlled trial, *Lancet Neurol* 5:140, 2006.

SUGGESTED READINGS

American Academy of Neurology, Practice parameter: the care of the patient with amyotrophic lateral sclerosis (an evidence-based review), *Muscle Nerve* 22:1104, 1999.

Miller RG et al: Riluzole for amyotrophic lateral sclerosis/motor neuron disease (MND), *Cochrane Database Syst Rev* 3, 2007.

AUTHOR: **TAYLOR HARRISON, M.D.**

BASIC INFORMATION

DEFINITION

An anaerobic infection is caused by one of a group of bacteria that requires a reduced oxygen tension for growth.

ICD-9CM CODES
See specific condition.

PHYSICAL FINDINGS & CLINICAL PRESENTATION

- May occur at any site, but most are anatomically related to mucosal surfaces
- Should be suspected when there is foul-smelling tissue, soft tissue gas, necrotic tissue, or abscesses
- Head and neck
  1. Odontogenic infections from dental or soft tissue possibly progressing to periapical abscesses, at times extending to bone
  2. Both anaerobic and aerobic pathogens in chronic sinusitis, chronic mastoiditis, peritonsillar abscess, and chronic otitis media
  3. Complications: deep neck space infections, brain abscesses, mediastinitis
- Pleuropulmonary
  1. May involve anaerobes present in the oropharynx
  2. Aspiration more common in persons with altered mental status or seizures
  3. Anaerobic bacteria more likely in those with gingivitis or periodontitis
  4. Manifestations: necrotizing pneumonia, empyema, lung abscess
- Intraabdominal
  1. Disruption of intestinal integrity leading to infection involving anaerobic bacteria
  2. Bacteria from colonic neoplasm, perforated appendicitis, diverticulitis, or bowel surgery, causing bacteremia, peritonitis, at times intraabdominal abscesses
  3. Resulting infections usually mixed, containing both anaerobes and aerobes
- Female genital tract
  1. Anaerobes in bacterial vaginosis, salpingitis, endometritis, pelvic abscesses, septic abortion; infections tend to be mixed
  2. Possible pelvic thrombophlebitis when resolving pelvic infection is accompanied by new or persistent fever
- Other anaerobic infections
  1. Skin and soft tissue infection at any site
  2. More commonly associated infections: synergistic gangrene, bite wound infections, infected decubitus ulcers
  3. Clinical significance of anaerobes in diabetic foot infections unclear
  4. Anaerobic bacteremia uncommon with source usually intraabdominal, followed by female genital tract, pleuropulmonary, and head and neck infections
  5. Osteomyelitis especially when associated with decubitus ulcers or vascular insufficiency
  6. Facial bone osteomyelitis from adjacent infections of the teeth or sinuses

ETIOLOGY

- Most commonly endogenous, arising from bacteria that normally line mucosal surfaces
- Disruption of mucosal barriers resulting from various conditions (trauma, ischemia, surgery, perforation), with infection occurring when organisms gain access to normally sterile sites, causing tissue destruction and abscess formation
- Synergy between different anaerobes or between anaerobes and aerobes important

DIAGNOSIS

DIFFERENTIAL DIAGNOSIS

- Primary differential possibility is an aerobic bacterial infection without the presence of anaerobic bacteria.
- Ischemic necrosis without accompanying anaerobic infection (or "dry" gangrene [noninfected necrosis] vs. "wet" gangrene [infected tissue with anaerobic infection]).

WORKUP

- Specimens submitted for culture processed within 30 min
- Large volume of material more likely to have significant growth; swabs less efficient for transporting infected material
- Blood cultures—preferably before antibiotic administration

LABORATORY TESTS

- Elevated WBC count, with extremely high WBC counts sometimes seen with pseudomembranous colitis
- Positive stool *C. difficile* toxin assay
- Increased lactate levels in ischemia or perforation
- Possible positive blood or wound cultures, but failure to grow anaerobes in culture may be common, attributed to inadequate culturing techniques or fastidious organisms

IMAGING STUDIES

- Plain film of an affected area to show gas in tissues, free air resulting from a perforated viscus, or an air/fluid level inside an abscess
- Ultrasound, CT scan, or MRI to reveal abscesses or tissue destruction

TREATMENT

NONPHARMACOLOGIC THERAPY

- Removal of necrotic tissue
- Drainage of abscesses (accomplished by CT scan–guided percutaneous drainage)

ACUTE GENERAL RX

Oral antibiotics with anaerobic activity: clindamycin, metronidazole, and chloramphenicol

- Broader spectrum of activity with amoxicillin/clavulanate
- Penicillin VK in odontogenic infections
- Oral metronidazole for *C. difficile*–associated diarrhea, with oral vancomycin reserved for severe, recurrent, or recalcitrant infections

Parenteral antibiotics for more serious illness

- IV clindamycin, metronidazole, and chloramphenicol
- Cephalosporins (anaerobic or mixed infections): cefoxitin and cefotetan
- Extended-spectrum penicillins (e.g., piperacillin) and combination beta-lactamase plus beta-lactamase inhibitor drugs (e.g., clavulanic acid, sulbactam, tazobactam)
  1. Significant anaerobic activity, plus various degrees of broad-spectrum coverage
  2. Include ampicillin/sulbactam, ticarcillin/clavulanate, and piperacillin/tazobactam
- Imipenem or other carbapenem such as meropenem or ertapenem: broad-spectrum agents with extensive anaerobic activity
- Actinomycosis treated with penicillin for 6 to 12 mo
- SMX/TMP and fluoroquinolones are generally ineffective, but some newer quinolones (e.g., moxifloxacin) have inhibitory activity against anaerobes

DISPOSITION

It is essential that all necrotic debris be removed when treating an anaerobic infection or it will recur; follow-up is critically important to assure resolution of the process.

REFERRAL

Refer to a surgeon if drainage is required; infectious disease consultation may be useful in complicated patients or if treatment regimen is failing or slow to respond.

SUGGESTED READING

Stein GE, Goldstein EJ: Fluoroquinolones and anaerobes, *Clin Infect Dis* 42(11):1598, 2006.

AUTHORS: **GLENN G. FORT, M.D., M.P.H., DENNIS J. MIKOLICH, M.D.,** and **MAURICE POLICAR, M.D.**

BASIC INFORMATION

DEFINITION

A fissure is a tear in the epithelial lining of the anal canal (i.e., from the dentate line to the anal verge).

SYNONYMS

Anorectal fissure
Anal ulcer

ICD-9CM CODES
565.0 Anal fissure

EPIDEMIOLOGY & DEMOGRAPHICS

PREDOMINANT SEX: Occurs in men > women. Women are more likely to have anterior fissure than men (10% vs. 1%, respectively). Common in women before and after childbirth.

PREDOMINANT AGE: Can occur at any age. Most common in young and middle-aged adults. Most common cause of rectal bleeding in infants.

PHYSICAL FINDINGS & CLINICAL PRESENTATION

With separation of the buttocks will see a tear in the posterior midline or, less frequently, in the anterior midline (Fig. 1-15)

- Acute anal fissure:
  1. Sharp burning or tearing pain exacerbated by bowel movements
  2. Bright-red blood on toilet paper, a streak of blood on the stool or in the water
- Chronic anal fissure:
  1. Pruritus ani
  2. Pain seldom present
  3. Intermittent bleeding
  4. Sentinel tag at the caudal aspect of the fissure, hypertrophied anal papilla at the proximal end
- Underlying disease possible if the fissure:
  1. Is ectopically located
  2. Extends proximal to the dentate line
  3. Is broad-based or deep
  4. Is especially purulent

ETIOLOGY

- Most initiated after passage of a large, hard stool
- May result from frequent defecation and diarrhea
- Bacterial infections: TB, syphilis, gonorrhea, chancroid, lymphogranuloma venereum
- Viral infections: herpes simplex virus, cytomegalovirus, human immunodeficiency virus
- Inflammatory bowel disease (IBD): Crohn's disease, ulcerative colitis
- Trauma: surgery (hemorrhoidectomy), foreign bodies, anal intercourse
- Malignancy: carcinoma, lymphoma, Kaposi's sarcoma

DIAGNOSIS

DIFFERENTIAL DIAGNOSIS

- Proctalgia fugax
- Thrombosed hemorrhoid

WORKUP

- Digital rectal examination after lubricating the entire anus with anesthetic jelly (i.e., 2% lidocaine) and waiting 5 to 10 min
- Anoscopy
- Proctosigmoidoscopy to exclude inflammatory or neoplastic disease
- Biopsy if doubt exists about the etiology of the condition
- All studies done under adequate anesthesia

IMAGING STUDIES

- Colonoscopy or barium enema if diagnosis of IBD or malignancy is suspected
- Small bowel series occasionally obtained for similar reasons
- Biopsy to reveal caseating granuloma if TB is suspected
- Wet prep with darkfield examination to demonstrate treponemes if syphilis is suspected

TREATMENT

NONPHARMACOLOGIC THERAPY

- Sitz baths
- High-fiber diet
- Increased oral fluid intake

ACUTE GENERAL Rx

- Bulk-producing agent (e.g., Metamucil)/stool softener
- Local anesthetic jelly (may exacerbate pruritus ani)
- Nitroglycerin ointment
- Suppositories *not* recommended
- Surgery

CHRONIC Rx

- Surgery: lateral internal anal sphincterotomy
- Topical glyceryl trinitrate ointment
- Injection of botulinum toxin (an injection into each side of the internal anal sphincter) is effective in healing chronic anal fissures in more than 90% of patients.

DISPOSITION

Outpatient surgery

REFERRAL

- If fissure does not resolve with conservative therapy in 4 to 6 wk
- If patient prefers surgery for acute fissure
- If patient has chronic fissure

PEARLS & CONSIDERATIONS

COMMENTS

HIV-positive patients should be referred to clinicians who are well versed in the myriad infectious and neoplastic conditions that masquerade as anal ulcers in these patients.

SUGGESTED READINGS

Brisinda G et al: Treating chronic anal fissure with botulinum neurotoxin, *Nat Clin Pract Gastroenterol & Hepatol* 1(2):82, 2004.

Brisinda G et al: A comparison of injection of botulinum toxin and topical nitroglycerin ointment for the treatment of chronic anal fissure, *N Engl J Med* 341:65, 1999.

Dwarkasing S, Hussain SM, Krestin GP: Magnetic resonance imaging of perianal fistulas, *Semin Ultrasound CT MR* 26(4):247, 2005.

Pfenninger JL, Zainea GG: Common anorectal conditions, *Am Fam Physician* 64:77, 2001.

AUTHORS: **GEORGE T. DANAKAS, M.D.**, and **RUBEN ALVERO, M.D.**

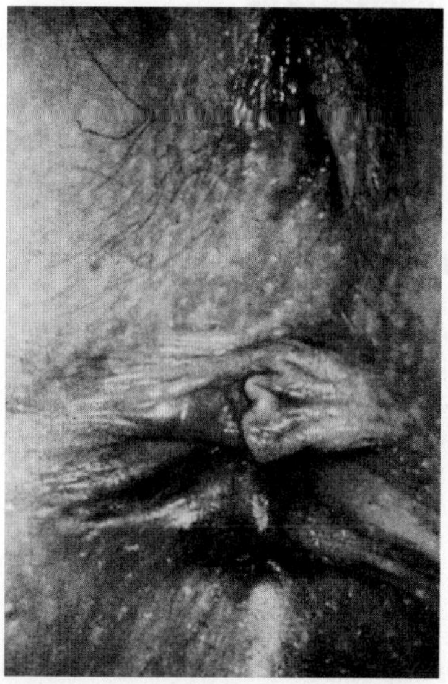

FIGURE 1-15 Lateral anal fissure. (In Seidel HM et al: *Mosby's guide to physical examination,* ed 3, St Louis, 1995, Mosby. Courtesy Gershon Efron, MD, Sinai Hospital of Baltimore.)

BASIC INFORMATION

DEFINITION

Anaphylaxis is a sudden-onset, life-threatening event characterized by bronchial contractions in conjunction with hemodynamic changes. Its clinical presentation may include respiratory, cardiovascular, cutaneous, or gastrointestinal manifestations.

SYNONYMS

Anaphylactoid reaction is closely related to anaphylaxis. It is caused by release of mast cells and basophil mediators triggered by non-IgE-mediated events.

ICD-9CM CODES
995.0 Anaphylactic shock
995.60 Anaphylaxis due to food
999.4 Anaphylaxis due to immunization
977.9 Anaphylaxis due to drugs
989.5 Anaphylaxis following stings

EPIDEMIOLOGY & DEMOGRAPHICS

INCIDENCE: 20,000 to 50,000 persons/yr in the U.S. Anaphylaxis rates are 0.0004% for food, 0.7% to 10% for penicillin, 0.22% to 1% for radiocontrast media, and 0.5% to 5% after insect stings. It is estimated that 1 in every 3000 inpatients in U.S. hospitals develops an anaphylactic reaction.

PHYSICAL FINDINGS & CLINICAL PRESENTATION

- Urticaria, pruritus, skin flushing, angioedema, weakness, dizziness
- Dyspnea, cough, malaise, difficulty swallowing
- Wheezing, tachycardia, diarrhea
- Hypotension, vascular collapse

ETIOLOGY

Anaphylaxis results from sudden release into the systemic circulation of histamine, tryptase, and other inflammation mediators from basophils and mast cells. Virtually any substance may induce anaphylaxis in a given individual.

- Commonly implicated medications are antibiotics, insulin, allergen extracts, opiates, vaccines, NSAIDs, contrast media, streptokinase
- Foods and food additives, nuts, egg whites, shellfish, fish, milk, fruits, and berries
- Blood products, plasma, immunoglobulin, cryoprecipitate, whole blood
- Venoms such as snake venom, fire ant venom, bee sting (*Hymenoptera* stings)
- Latex

DIAGNOSIS

DIFFERENTIAL DIAGNOSIS

- Endocrine disorders (carcinoid, pheochromocytoma)
- Globus hystericus, anxiety disorder
- Systemic mastocytosis
- Pulmonary embolism, serum sickness, vasovagal reactions
- Severe asthma (the key clinical difference is the abrupt onset of symptoms in anaphylaxis without a history of progressive worsening of symptoms)
- Septic shock or other form of shock
- Airway foreign body

WORKUP

Workup is aimed mainly at eliminating other conditions that may mimic anaphylaxis (e.g., vasovagal syncope may be differentiated by the presence of bradycardia as opposed to the tachycardia seen in anaphylaxis; the absence of hypoxemia in ABG analysis may be useful to exclude pulmonary embolism or foreign body aspiration).

LABORATORY TESTS

- Laboratory evaluation is generally not helpful, because the diagnosis of anaphylaxis is a clinical one.
- ABG analysis may be useful to exclude pulmonary embolism, status asthmaticus, and foreign body aspiration.
- Elevated serum and urine histamine levels can be useful for diagnosis of anaphylaxis, but these tests are not commonly available.

IMAGING STUDIES

Generally not helpful.

- Chest x-ray is indicated in patients presenting with acute respiratory compromise.
- Radiologic evaluation for epiglottitis is useful in patients with acute respiratory compromise.
- ECG should be considered in all patients with sudden loss of consciousness or complaints of chest pains or dyspnea and in any elderly patient.

TREATMENT

NONPHARMACOLOGIC THERAPY

- IV access should be rapidly established, and intravenous fluids (i.e., saline) should be administered. The patient should be placed supine or in Trendelenburg position.
- Supplemental oxygen and cardiac monitoring are also recommended.

ACUTE GENERAL Rx

- Epinephrine should be rapidly administered as an SC or IM injection at a dose of 0.01 ml/kg of aqueous epinephrine 1:1000 (maximum adult dose 0.3 to 0.5 ml). The dose may be repeated approximately q5 to 10min if there is persistence or recurrence of symptoms. Endotracheal epinephrine should be considered if IV access is not possible during life-threatening reactions.
- Administration of H_1- and H_2-receptor antagonists is also recommended in the initial treatment of anaphylaxis.
  1. Administer diphenhydramine 50 to 75 mg IV or IM.
  2. Cimetidine 300 mg IV over 3 to 5 min, or ranitidine 50 mg IV, should be given initially; subsequent doses of H_1- and H_2-blockers can be given orally q6h for 48 hr.
- Corticosteroids are not useful in the acute episode because of their slow onset of action; however, they should be administered in most cases to prevent prolonged or recurrent anaphylaxis. Commonly used agents are hydrocortisone sodium succinate 250 to 500 mg IV q4 to 6h in adults (4 to 8 mg/kg for children) or methylprednisolone 60 to 125 mg IV in adults (1 to 2 mg/kg in children).
- Aerosolized β-agonists (i.e., albuterol, 2.5 mg, repeat prn 20 min) are useful to control bronchospasm.
- Additional useful agents in specific circumstances: atropine for refractory bradycardia, dopamine for refractory hypotension (despite volume expansion), and glucagon in patients on β-blocking drugs.

PEARLS & CONSIDERATIONS

COMMENTS

- Patient education regarding the nature of the illness and preventive measures is recommended. A documented history of previous anaphylactic episodes or known anaphylaxis triggers is the most reliable method of identifying individuals at risk.
- Prescription for prefilled epinephrine syringe (EpiPen) should be given, and the patient should be instructed on the use of this emergency epinephrine kit in case of recurrent anaphylactic episodes.
- Patients should also be advised to carry or wear Medic Alert ID describing substances that have caused anaphylaxis.
- Avoidance of radiologic contrast is also recommended.
- Venom immunotherapy immediately after a sting is effective and recommended for up to 5 yr after the anaphylactic incident.

SUGGESTED READING

Tang AW: A practical guide to anaphylaxis, *Am Fam Physician* 68:1325, 2003.

AUTHOR: **FRED F. FERRI, M.D.**

BASIC INFORMATION

DEFINITION

Aplastic anemia is a bone marrow failure resulting from a variety of causes and characterized by stem cell destruction or suppression leading to pancytopenia.

SYNONYMS

Refractory anemia
Hypoplastic anemia

ICD-9CM CODES
284.9 Aplastic anemia
284.8 Acquired aplastic anemia
284.0 Congenital aplastic anemia

EPIDEMIOLOGY & DEMOGRAPHICS

INCIDENCE (IN U.S.): The annual incidence of aplastic anemia is 3 to 9 cases/1 million persons.

PREDOMINANT SEX AND AGE: There is no predominant sex or age for the acquired form.

PHYSICAL FINDINGS & CLINICAL PRESENTATION

- Skin pallor, ecchymosis, petechiae, retinal hemorrhage
- Possible fever, mouth and tongue ulceration, pharyngitis
- Possible short stature or skeletal and nail anomalies in the congenital form
- Possible audible systolic ejection murmur with profound anemia

ETIOLOGY

- In most patients with acquired aplastic anemia, bone marrow failure results from immunologically mediated, active destruction of blood-forming cells by lymphocytes.
- Mutations in TERT, the gene for the RNA component of telomerase, cause short telomerases in congenital aplastic anemia and in some cases of apparently acquired hematopoietic failure.
- Common etiologic factors in aplastic anemia:
  Toxins (e.g., benzene, insecticides)
  Drugs (e.g., Felbatol, cimetidine, busulfan and other myelosuppressive drugs, gold salts, chloramphenicol, sulfonamides, trimethadione, quinacrine, phenylbutazone)
  Ionizing irradiation
  Infections (e.g., hepatitis C, HIV, EB virus, parvovirus B_{19})
  Idiopathic
  Inherited (Fanconi's anemia)
  Other: immunologic, pregnancy

DIAGNOSIS

DIFFERENTIAL DIAGNOSIS

- Bone marrow infiltration from lymphoma, carcinoma, myelofibrosis
- Severe infection
- Hypoplastic acute lymphoblastic leukemia in children
- Hypoplastic myelodysplastic syndrome or hypoplastic acute myeloid leukemia in adults
- Hypersplenism
- Hairy cell leukemia

WORKUP

- Diagnostic workup consists primarily of bone marrow aspiration and biopsy and laboratory evaluation (CBC and examination of blood film).
- Bone marrow examination generally reveals paucity or absence of erythropoietic and myelopoietic precursor cells; patients with pure red cell aplasia demonstrate only absence of RBC precursors in the marrow.

LABORATORY TESTS

- CBC reveals pancytopenia. Macrocytosis and toxic granulation of neutrophils may also be present. Isolated cytopenias may occur in the early stages.
- Reticulocyte count reveals reticulocytopenia.
- Additional initial laboratory evaluation should include Ham test to exclude paroxysmal nocturnal hemoglobinuria (PNH) and testing for hepatitis C.

IMAGING STUDIES

- Chest x-ray
- Abdominal sonogram or CT scan to evaluate for splenomegaly
- Radiography of hand and forearm in patients with constitutional anemia
- CT scan of thymus region if thymoma-associated RBC aplasia is suspected

TREATMENT

NONPHARMACOLOGIC THERAPY

- Discontinuation of any offending drugs or agents
- Evaluation for bone marrow transplantation

ACUTE GENERAL Rx

- Aggressive treatment of neutropenic fevers with parenteral broad-spectrum antibiotics.
- Platelet and RBC transfusions prn; however, avoidance of transfusions in patients who are candidates for bone marrow transplantation.
- Immunosuppressive therapy with antithymocyte globulin (ATG) and/or cyclosporine (CSP); ATG in combination with prednisone (1 to 2 mg/kg/day initially) to avoid complications of serum sickness.
- Transplantation of allogeneic marrow or peripheral blood stem cell transplantation from a histocompatible sibling usually cures the underlying bone marrow failure.
- The humanized monoclonal antibody to the interleukin-2 receptor Daclizumab has been reported effective in moderate aplastic anemia, producing durable responses in >50% of patients.

CHRONIC Rx

- Long-term patient monitoring with physical examination and routine laboratory evaluation to screen for relapse.
- ATG with CSP restore hematopoiesis in approximately two thirds of patients; however, recovery of blood cell count is often incomplete, recurrent pancytopenia requires retreatment. In some patients, myelodysplasia is a late complication of immunosuppressive therapy.
- Patients refractory to immunosuppression have a poor long-term outlook and should consider unrelated stem cell transplantation.
- There is little justification for either a therapeutic trial of corticosteroids as primary treatment or for their long-term use to prevent bleeding.

DISPOSITION

- Patients with severe aplastic anemia who have marrow transplants before the onset of transfusion-induced sensitization have an excellent probability of long-term survival and normal life; age is a significant factor; the incidence of graft vs. host disease increases with age and is >90% in patients >30 yr of age.
- Following bone marrow transplantation from an HLA-identical sibling, >70% of patients are long-term survivors and can be considered cured.
- Response to immunosuppression in aplastic anemia is independent of age, but treatment is associated with increased mortality in older patients.
- Overall 5-yr survival rate for aplastic anemia is now 70% to 90%.

REFERRAL

Hematology referral is indicated in all patients with aplastic anemia.

SUGGESTED READING

Sloand EM et al: Brief communication: Successful treatment of pure red-cell aplasia with an anti-interleukin-2 receptor antibody (Daclizumab), *Ann Int Med* 144:181, 2006.

AUTHOR: **FRED F. FERRI, M.D.**

BASIC INFORMATION

DEFINITION

Autoimmune hemolytic anemia (AIHA) is anemia secondary to premature destruction of red blood cells caused by the binding of autoantibodies and/or complement to red blood cells.

ICD-9CM CODES
283.0 Autoimmune hemolytic anemia

EPIDEMIOLOGY & DEMOGRAPHICS

PREDOMINANT SEX AND AGE: Most common in women <50 yr.

PHYSICAL FINDINGS & CLINICAL PRESENTATION

- Pallor, jaundice
- Tachycardia with a flow murmur may be present if anemia is pronounced
- Most common presentation is dyspnea and fatigue
- Patients with intravascular hemolysis may present with dark urine and back pain
- The presence of hepatomegaly, and/or lymphadenopathy suggests an underlying lymphoproliferative disorder or malignancy; splenomegaly may indicate hypersplenism as a cause of hemolysis

ETIOLOGY

- Warm antibody mediated: IgG (often idiopathic or associated with leukemia, lymphoma, thymoma, myeloma, viral infections, and collagen-vascular disease)
- Cold antibody mediated: IgM and complement in majority of cases (often idiopathic, at times associated with infections, lymphoma, or cold agglutinin disease)
- Drug induced: three major mechanisms:
  1. Antibody directed against Rh complex (e.g., methyldopa)
  2. Antibody directed against RBC-drug complex (hapten induced, e.g., penicillin)
  3. Antibody directed against complex formed by drug and plasma proteins; the drug-plasma protein-antibody complex causes destruction of RBCs (innocent bystander, e.g., quinidine)

DIAGNOSIS

DIFFERENTIAL DIAGNOSIS

- Hemolytic anemia caused by membrane defects (paroxysmal nocturnal hemoglobinuria, spur-cell anemia, Wilson's disease)
- Non–immune mediated (microangiopathic hemolytic anemia, hypersplenism, cardiac valve prosthesis, giant cavernous hemangiomas, march hemoglobinuria, physical agents, infections, heavy metals, certain drugs [nitrofurantoin, sulfonamides])

WORKUP

Evaluation consists primarily of laboratory evaluation to confirm hemolysis and to exclude other causes of the anemia. Although most cases of AIHA are idiopathic, potential causes should always be sought. Section III describes an algorithm for evaluation of suspected hemolytic anemia.

LABORATORY TESTS

- Initial laboratory tests: CBC (anemia), reticulocyte count (elevated), liver function studies (elevated indirect bilirubin, LDH), evaluation of peripheral smear, Coombs' test (positive direct Coombs' test indicates presence of antibodies or complement on the surface of RBC, positive indirect Coombs' test implies presence of anti-RBC antibodies freely circulating in the patient's serum), haptoglobin level (decreased)
- IgG antibody and IgM antibody
- Hepatitis serology, ANA
- Urinary tests may reveal hemosiderinuria or hemoglobinuria

IMAGING STUDIES

- Chest x-ray
- CT scan of chest and abdomen to rule out lymphoma should also be considered

TREATMENT

NONPHARMACOLOGIC THERAPY

- Discontinuation of any potentially offensive drugs
- Plasmapheresis-exchange transfusion for severe life-threatening cases only
- Avoid cold exposure in patients with cold antibody

ACUTE GENERAL Rx

- Prednisone 1 to 2 mg/kg/day in divided doses initially in warm antibody autoimmune hemolytic anemia. Corticosteroids are generally ineffective in cold antibody autoimmune hemolytic anemia
- Splenectomy in patients responding inadequately to corticosteroids when RBC sequestration studies indicate splenic sequestration
- Immunosuppressive drugs and/or immunoglobulins only after both corticosteroids and splenectomy (unless surgery is contraindicated) have failed to produce an adequate remission
- Danazol, usually used in conjunction with corticosteroids (may be useful in warm antibody autoimmune hemolytic anemia)
- Immunosuppressive drugs (azathioprine, cyclophosphamide) may be useful in warm antibody autoimmune hemolytic anemia but are indicated only after both corticosteroids and splenectomy (unless surgery is contraindicated) have failed to produce an adequate remission

DISPOSITION

Prognosis is generally good unless anemia is associated with underlying disorder with a poor prognosis (e.g., leukemia, myeloma).

REFERRAL

- Hematology referral in all cases of AIHA
- Surgical referral for splenectomy in refractory cases

PEARLS & CONSIDERATIONS

COMMENTS

- The direct Coombs' test (also known as the direct antiglobulin test [DAT]) demonstrates the presence of antibodies or complement on the surface of RBCs and is the hallmark of autoimmune hemolysis.
- Warm AIHA is often associated with autoimmune diseases whereas cold AIHA often follows viral infections (e.g., mononucleosis) and *Mycoplasma pneumoniae* infections.
- HIV can induce both warm and cold AIHA.

SUGGESTED READINGS

Dhaliwal G et al: Hemolytic anemia, *Am Fam Physician* 69:2599, 2004.

Gehrs BC, Friedberg RC: Autoimmune hemolytic anemia, *Am J Hematol* 69:258, 2002.

AUTHOR: **FRED F. FERRI, M.D.**

BASIC INFORMATION

DEFINITION

Iron deficiency anemia is anemia secondary to inadequate iron supplementation or excessive blood loss.

ICD-9CM CODES
280.9 Iron deficiency anemia
648.2 Iron deficiency anemia complicating pregnancy

EPIDEMIOLOGY & DEMOGRAPHICS

- Dietary iron deficiency occurs often in infants as a result of unsupplemented milk diets. It is also commonly seen in women during their reproductive years, as a result of heavy menstrual periods, and during pregnancy (increased demand).
- Iron deficiency is the most common nutritional deficiency worldwide.
- The prevalence of iron deficiency is greatest among toddlers ages 1 to 2 yr (7%) from inadequate intake and females ages 12 to 49 yr (9% to 16%) from menstrual losses.
- The prevalence of iron deficiency is 2% in adult men, 9% to 12% in non-Hispanic white women, and 20% in black and Mexican American women.
- GI cancer is diagnosed in 10% of elderly patients with iron deficiency anemia.

PHYSICAL FINDINGS & CLINICAL PRESENTATION

- Most patients have a normal examination.
- Skin pallor and conjunctival pallor may be present.

ETIOLOGY

- Blood loss from GI or menstrual bleeding (GU blood loss less often the cause)
- Dietary iron deficiency (rare in adults)
- Poor iron absorption in patients with gastric or small bowel surgery
- Repeated phlebotomy
- Increased requirements (e.g., during pregnancy)
- Other: traumatic hemolysis (abnormally functioning cardiac valves), idiopathic pulmonary hemosiderosis (iron sequestration in pulmonary macrophages), paroxysmal nocturnal hemoglobinuria (intravascular hemolysis)

DIAGNOSIS

DIFFERENTIAL DIAGNOSIS

- Anemia of chronic disease
- Sideroblastic anemia
- Thalassemia trait
- Lead poisoning

WORKUP

Diagnostic workup consists primarily of laboratory evaluation. Most patients with iron deficiency anemia are asymptomatic in the early stages. With progressive anemia, the major complaints are fatigue, dizziness, exertional dyspnea, pagophagia (ice eating), and pica. Patient's history may also suggest GI blood loss (melena, hematochezia, hemoptysis).

LABORATORY TESTS

- Laboratory results vary with the stage of deficiency.
- Absent iron marrow stores and decreased serum ferritin are the initial abnormalities.
- Decreased serum iron and increased TIBC are the next abnormalities.
- Hypochromic microcytic anemia is present with significant iron deficiency.
- Peripheral smear in patients with iron deficiency generally reveals microcytic hypochromic RBCs with a wide area of central pallor, anisocytosis, and poikilocytosis when severe.
- Laboratory abnormalities consistent with iron deficiency are low serum ferritin level, elevated RBC distribution width (RDW) with values generally >15, low MCV, elevated TIBC, and low serum iron.
- The reticulocyte hemoglobin content (CHr) may be a good screening test for iron deficiency. It can be measured on an automated hematology analyzer and represents a relatively inexpensive and fast way to detect iron deficiency.

TREATMENT

NONPHARMACOLOGIC THERAPY

Patients should be instructed to consume foods containing large amounts of iron, such as liver, red meat, and legumes.

ACUTE GENERAL Rx

- Treatment consists of ferrous sulfate 325 mg PO qd for at least 6 mo. Calcium supplements can decrease iron absorption; therefore, these two medications should be staggered.
- Parenteral iron therapy is reserved for patients with poor tolerance, noncompliance with oral preparations, or malabsorption.
- Transfusion of packed RBCs is indicated in patients with severe symptomatic anemia (e.g., angina) or life-threatening anemia.

CHRONIC Rx

Patients should be instructed to continue their iron supplements for at least 6 mo or longer to correct depleted body iron stores.

DISPOSITION

Most patients respond rapidly to iron supplementation with improvement in CBC and general well-being. GI side effects from oral iron therapy are common and may require decreased dose to once every other day.

REFERRAL

GI referral for evaluation of GI malignancy is recommended in all patients with iron deficiency and suspected GI blood loss.

PEARLS & CONSIDERATIONS

COMMENTS

If the diagnosis of iron deficiency anemia is made, it is mandatory to try to locate the suspected site of iron loss.

EVIDENCE

A systematic review found that iron supplementation in pregnancy appears to prevent low hemoglobin at birth or 6 weeks postpartum.[1] Ⓐ

Another systematic review found inconclusive evidence on the effects of treatment for iron deficiency anemia in pregnancy due to a shortage of good-quality trials.[2] Ⓑ

Evidence-Based References

1. Mahomed K: Iron supplementation in pregnancy, *Cochrane Database Syst Rev* (2):CD001135, 2000. Ⓐ
2. Cuervo LG, Mahomed K: Treatments for iron deficiency anaemia in pregnancy, *Cochrane Database Syst Rev* (2):CD003094, 2001. Ⓑ

SUGGESTED READINGS

Killip S et al: Iron deficiency anemia, *Am Fam Physician* 75:671, 2007.
Tefferi A: Anemia in adults: a contemporary approach to diagnosis, *Mayo Clin Proc* 78:1274, 2004.

AUTHOR: **FRED F. FERRI, M.D.**

BASIC INFORMATION

DEFINITION

Pernicious anemia is an autoimmune disease resulting from antibodies against intrinsic factor and gastric parietal cells.

SYNONYMS

Megaloblastic anemia resulting from vitamin B_{12} deficiency

ICD-9CM CODES
281.0 Pernicious anemia

EPIDEMIOLOGY & DEMOGRAPHICS

- Increased incidence in females and older adults (diagnosis is unusual before age 35 yr)
- The overall prevalence of undiagnosed PA over age 60 yr is 1.9%
- Prevalence is highest in women (2.7%), particularly in black women (4.3%)
- Increased incidence of autoimmune disease (e.g., type 1 DM, Graves' disease, Addison's disease), *Helicobacter pylori* infection

PHYSICAL FINDINGS & CLINICAL PRESENTATION

- Mucosal pallor, glossitis
- Peripheral sensory neuropathy with paresthesias initially and absent reflexes in advanced cases
- Loss of joint position sense, pyramidal or long track signs
- Possible splenomegaly and mild hepatomegaly
- Generalized weakness and delirium/dementia

ETIOLOGY

- Antigastric parietal cell antibodies in >70% of patients, antiintrinsic factor antibodies in >50% of patients
- Atrophic gastric mucosa

DIAGNOSIS

DIFFERENTIAL DIAGNOSIS

- Nutritional vitamin B_{12} deficiency
- Malabsorption
- Chronic alcoholism (multifactorial)
- Chronic gastritis related to *H. pylori* infection
- Folic acid deficiency
- Myelodysplasia

WORKUP

- The clinical presentation of pernicious anemia varies with the stage. Initially, patients may be asymptomatic. In advanced stages, patients may present with impaired memory, depression, gait disturbances, paresthesias, and complaints of generalized weakness.
- Investigation consists primarily of laboratory evaluation.
- Endoscopy and biopsy for atrophic gastritis may be performed in selected cases.
- Diagnosis is crucial because failure to treat may result in irreversible neurologic deficits.

LABORATORY TESTS

- CBC generally reveals macrocytic anemia and leukopenia with hypersegmented neutrophils.
- MCV is generally significantly elevated in the advanced stages.
- Reticulocyte count is low/normal.
- Falsely low serum cobalamin levels can occur in patients with severe folate deficiency, in patients using high doses of ascorbic acid, and when cobalamin levels are measured following nuclear medicine studies (radioactivity interferes with cobalamin RIA measurement).
- Falsely high normal levels in patients with cobalamin deficiency can occur in severe liver disease or chronic granulocytic leukemia.
- The absence of anemia or macrocytosis does not exclude the diagnosis of cobalamin deficiency. Anemia is absent in 20% of patients with cobalamin deficiency, and macrocytosis is absent in >30% of patients at the time of diagnosis. It can be blocked by concurrent iron deficiency or anemia of chronic disease and may be masked by thalassemia trait.
- Schilling test is abnormal in part I; part II corrects to normal after administration of intrinsic factor.
- Laboratory tests used for detecting cobalamin deficiency in patients with normal vitamin B_{12} levels include serum and urinary methylmalonic acid level (elevated), total homocysteine level (elevated), intrinsic factor antibody (positive).
- An increased concentration of plasma methylmalonic acid (P-MMA) does not predict clinical manifestations of vitamin B_{12} deficiency and should not be used as the only marker for diagnosis of B_{12} deficiency.
- Additional laboratory abnormalities can include elevated LDH, direct hyperbilirubinemia, and decreased haptoglobin.

TREATMENT

NONPHARMACOLOGIC THERAPY

Avoid folic acid supplementation without proper vitamin B_{12} supplementation.

ACUTE GENERAL Rx

Traditional therapy of a cobalamin deficiency consists of IM injections of vitamin B_{12} 1000 μg/wk for the initial 4 to 6 wk followed by 1000 μg/mo IM indefinitely. When hematologic parameters have returned to normal range, intranasal cyanocobalamin may be used in place of IM cyanocobalamin. The initial dose of intranasal cyanocobalamin (Nascobal) is one spray (500 μg) in one nostril once per week. Cost generally exceeds $120/mo. Monitor response and increase dose if serum B_{12} levels decline. Consider return to intramuscular vitamin B_{12} supplementation if decline persists.

CHRONIC Rx

Parenteral vitamin B_{12} 1000 μg/mo or intranasal cyanocobalamin 500 μg/wk (see "Acute General Rx") for the remainder of life

DISPOSITION

Anemia generally resolves with appropriate treatment. Neurologic deficits, if present at diagnosis, may be permanent.

REFERRAL

GI referral for endoscopy upon diagnosis of pernicious anemia and surveillance endoscopy every 5 yr to rule out gastric carcinoma

PEARLS & CONSIDERATIONS

COMMENTS

- Patients must understand that therapy is lifelong.
- Self-injection of vitamin B_{12} may be taught in selected patients. Cost of monthly injection is <$5.
- Oral cobalamin (1000 to 2000 mcg/day) has been reported as also being effective in mild cases of pernicious anemia because about 1% of an oral dose is absorbed by passive diffusion, a pathway that does not require intrinsic factor. Cost for 1 mo of therapy is approximately $5.

AUTHOR: **FRED F. FERRI, M.D.**

BASIC INFORMATION

DEFINITION

Sideroblastic anemias are blood disorders resulting from defective heme synthesis and are classified as hereditary, acquired, and reversible.

SYNONYMS

- Primary hereditary sideroblastic anemia
- Primary acquired refractory anemia with ringed sideroblasts (RARS)
- Reversible sideroblastic anemias

ICD-9CM CODES
285.0 Sideroblastic anemia

EPIDEMIOLOGY & DEMOGRAPHICS

- Sex-linked, primarily affects males.
- Primary acquired sideroblastic anemia is usually a disease of the elderly.

PHYSICAL FINDINGS & CLINICAL PRESENTATION

The symptoms for sideroblastic anemia are the same for any anemia:

- Fatigue, weakness, palpitations, shortness of breath, headaches, irritability, and chest pain.
- Physical findings may include pallor, tachycardia, hepatosplenomegaly, S_3 gallop, jugular vein distension, and rales.

ETIOLOGY

- The exact cause in many cases of hereditary and primary acquired sideroblastic anemias remains unknown. In some cases, the molecular defect may involve genes encoding for:
  - 5-aminolevulinate synthase enzyme (ALAS2)
  - Mitochondrial iron transporter (ABC7)
  - Ferrochelatase
  - Cytochrome oxidase
  - Mitochondrial proteins (e.g., Pearson Marrow-Pancrease Syndrome)
- Primary hereditary sideroblastic anemia may be inherited as a sex-linked recessive disease.
- Secondary acquired sideroblastic anemia can be caused by alcohol, isoniazid, pyrazinamide, cycloserine, chloramphenicol, and copper deficiency.

DIAGNOSIS

DIFFERENTIAL DIAGNOSIS

- Sideroblastic anemia must be differentiated from other causes of microcytic hypochromic anemia: iron deficiency anemia, thalassemia, anemia of chronic disease, and lead poisoning.
- Tissue iron overload from sideroblastic anemia may act similar to hereditary hemochromatosis with liver cirrhosis, diabetes, congestive heart failure, and cardiac arrhythmias.

WORKUP

Laboratory evaluation and bone marrow aspiration and biopsy

LABORATORY TESTS

- Hypochromic anemia (low Hgb, low Hct, low MCV, high RDW).
- High serum iron levels, low transferrin, along with increased transferrin saturation and serum ferritin.
- Free erythrocyte protoporphyrin (FEP) is generally low in hereditary sideroblastic anemia and characteristically increased in acquired sideroblastic anemia.
- Serum copper and zinc levels may assist in the diagnosis of sideroblastic anemias.
- Peripheral smear: dimorphic large and small cells revealing "Pappenheimer bodies" or siderocytes when stained for iron.
- Bone marrow shows the classic ringed sideroblasts not seen in normal bone marrow tissue (Fig. 1-16). The ringed sideroblasts represent iron storage in the mitochondria of normoblasts.

TREATMENT

Treatment is directed at controlling symptoms of anemia and preventing organ damage from iron overload.

NONPHARMACOLOGIC THERAPY

Avoid alcohol.

ACUTE GENERAL Rx

- Hereditary sideroblastic anemia:
  1. Nearly 35% of patients receiving vitamin B_6 (50 to 200 mg/day) will improve their red blood cell to near normal values.
  2. The remainder of patients will require blood transfusions to treat symptoms of anemia.
- Primary acquired sideroblastic anemia:
  1. Most patients do not respond to vitamin B_6.
  2. Erythropoietin and granulocyte colony-stimulating factor (G-CSF) have shown some success in improving the anemia.
  3. Blood transfusions are indicated for patients with symptomatic anemia.
- Secondary sideroblastic anemia due to isoniazid, pyrazinamide, and cycloserine can expect a full recovery by withdrawing the medication and by the use of vitamin B_6 (50 to 200 mg/day).

CHRONIC Rx

- Hereditary sideroblastic anemia:
  1. Organ dysfunction resulting from iron overload will require periodic phlebotomies.
  2. In advanced cases, deferoxamine 40 mg/kg/day IV is given with the goal to maintain serum ferritin levels <500 μg/L.
- Primary acquired sideroblastic anemia:
  1. As in the hereditary form, periodic phlebotomies are indicated when serum ferritin levels increase to >500 μg/L and deferoxamine is used in patients refractory to therapeutic phlebotomy and those requiring frequent blood transfusions.

DISPOSITION

- Hereditary sideroblastic anemia:
  1. With previously mentioned treatment, prognosis is good for a normal life expectancy.
- Primary acquired sideroblastic anemia:
  1. In patients with anemia alone, life expectancy is normal. In patients dependent on blood transfusions, one can expect morbidity from iron overload.
  2. Some patients with acquired sideroblastic anemia can go on to develop leukemia.

REFERRAL

Hematology

PEARLS & CONSIDERATIONS

Sideroblastic anemia can be thought of as an iron-loading anemia secondary to defective heme synthesis.

COMMENTS

Vitamin B_6, pyridoxal phosphate, is a required cofactor in heme synthesis, and drugs such as isoniazid, cycloserine, and pyrazinamide can inhibit its function.

SUGGESTED READINGS

Alcindor T, Bridges KR: Sideroblastic anemias, *Br J Hematol* 116(4):733, 2002.

Bottomley SS: Congenital sideroblastic anemias, *Current Hematol Rep* 5(1):41, 2006.

AUTHOR: **PETER PETROPOULOS, M.D.**

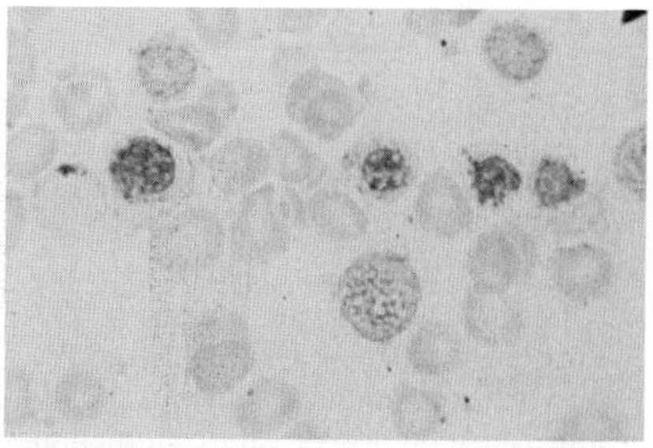

FIGURE 1-16 Prussian blue iron stain of the bone marrow shows ringed sideroblasts. (From Goldman L, Ausiello D [eds]: *Cecil textbook of medicine,* ed 22, Philadelphia, 2004, WB Saunders.)

BASIC INFORMATION

DEFINITION

An abdominal aortic aneurysm (AAA) is a permanent localized dilation of the abdominal aortic artery to at least 50% when compared with the normal diameter. Generally, an AAA is considered present when the minimal anteroposterior diameter reaches 3.0 cm.

SYNONYMS

AAA

ICD-9CM CODES
441.4 Aneurysm, abdominal (aorta)
441.3 Ruptured abdominal aortic aneurysm

EPIDEMIOLOGY & DEMOGRAPHICS

- AAA is predominantly a disease of older adults, affecting men > women (4:1).
- The prevalence in men ranges from 1% to 2% at age 50, up to 5% to 10% at age 80.
- Rupture of an abdominal aortic aneurysm is the tenth leading cause of death in men >55 yr (15,000 deaths/yr in the U.S.).
- Risk factors for AAA are similar to other cardiovascular diseases, including smoking, hypertension, hyperlipidemia, male sex, and family history of AAA.

PHYSICAL FINDINGS & CLINICAL PRESENTATION

- Most aneurysms are asymptomatic and incidentally discovered on imaging studies.
- Physical exam has a sensitivity of 76% for detecting AAA >5 cm and only 29% for AAA 3.0-3.9 cm.
- Pulsatile epigastric mass that may or may not be tender.
- Abdominal pain radiating to the back, flank, and groin.
- Early satiety, nausea, and vomiting caused by compression of adjacent bowel.
- Venous thrombosis from iliocaval venous compression.
- Discoloration and pain of the feet from distal embolization of the thrombus within the aneurysm.
- Flank and groin pain from ureteral obstruction and hydronephrosis.
- Rupture presents as shock, organ hypoperfusion, and abdominal distention.
- Rare presentations include hematemesis or melena associated with abdominal and back pain, in patients with aortoenteric fistulas.
- Aortocaval fistulas may also form and produce loud abdominal bruits.

ETIOLOGY

- Atherosclerotic (degenerative or nonspecific)
- Genetic (e.g., Ehlers-Danlos syndrome)
- Traumatic
- Cystic medial necrosis (Marfan's syndrome)
- Arteritis, inflammatory
- Mycotic, infected (syphilis)

DIAGNOSIS

DIFFERENTIAL DIAGNOSIS

Almost 75% of AAAs are asymptomatic and are discovered on routine examination or serendipitously when ordering studies for other complaints. Diagnosis of AAA should be considered in the differential of:

- Abdominal pain
- Back pain

IMAGING STUDIES

- Abdominal ultrasound is nearly 100% accurate in identifying an aneurysm and estimating the size to within 0.3 to 0.4 cm. It is not very good in estimating the extension to the renal arteries or the iliac arteries.
- CT scan is recommended for preoperative aneurysm imaging and estimates the size of the AAA to within 0.3 mm. There are no false-negatives, and the CT scan can localize the extent to renal vessels with more precision than ultrasound, detect the integrity of the wall, and exclude rupture.
- Angiography gives detailed arterial anatomy, localizing the aneurysm relative to the renal and visceral arteries. This is the definitive preoperative study prior to surgery.
- MRI may also be used, but it is more expensive and not as readily available.

TREATMENT

NONPHARMACOLOGIC THERAPY

- Despite lack of data substantiating reduction in expansion rate through treatment of cardiac risk factors, nonpharmacologic treatment continues to focus on risk factor modification (most importantly smoking cessation, diet, and exercise).
- Serial studies have shown that expansion rates are faster in current smokers than former smokers.
- Definitive treatment depends on the size of the aneurysm (see "Chronic Rx").

ACUTE GENERAL Rx

- AAA rupture is an emergency.
- Emergent open repair is the traditional method of treatment. However, more centers are increasingly using endovascular repair for patients who fit certain anatomic and physiologic criteria.

CHRONIC Rx

- Blood pressure and fasting lipids should be monitored and controlled as recommended for patients with atherosclerotic disease.
- The most commonly used predictor of rupture is the maximum diameter of the AAA.
- Monitoring by ultrasound or CT scan should be performed every 6 to 12 months for AAA measuring 4.0 to 5.4 cm. In patients with AAA smaller than 4.0 cm, every 2 to 3 years is reasonable.
- Surgical repair to eliminate the risk of rupture should be performed for patients with infrarenal or juxtarenal AAA of 5.5 cm or larger. Repair is possibly beneficial for AAAs of 5.0 to 5.4 cm.
- Intervention is not recommended for asymptomatic infrarenal or juxtarenal AAAs less than 5.0 cm in men or 4.5 cm in women.
- For the high-risk patient, percutaneous endovascular stent-anchored grafts under local anesthesia have provided an alternative approach.
- Research is ongoing to determine the appropriate low or average surgical risk patients for which the endovascular approach may be an elective option.

DISPOSITION

- The 5-year rupture rate of incidentally is about 25% to 40% for diagnosed aneurysms larger than 5.0 cm, 1% to 7% for AAAs of 4.0 to 5.0 cm, and nearly 0% for AAAs less than 4.0 cm.
- Mortality after rupture is >90% since most patients do not reach the hospital in time for surgical repair. Of those patients who reach the hospital, the mortality rate is still 50%, compared with the 1% to 4% mortality rate for elective repair of a nonruptured AAA.

REFERRAL

Vascular surgical referral should be made in asymptomatic patients with AAA 4.0 cm or greater or in rapidly expanding aneurysms of 0.6 to 0.8 cm/yr, especially if symptoms are present.

PEARLS & CONSIDERATIONS

Screening by physical exam and ultrasound should be performed for men 60 years or older who are either the siblings or offspring of patients with AAA and for men age 65 to 75 who have ever smoked.

COMMENTS

- Most AAAs are infrarenal.
- Surgical risk is increased in patients with coexisting coronary artery disease, pulmonary disease, liver cirrhosis, and chronic renal failure. Evaluation for ischemia and aggressive perioperative hemodynamic monitoring help identify high-risk patients and decrease postoperative complications.
- It is estimated that AAAs <5 cm expand at a rate of 0.4 cm/yr.

EVIDENCE

The results of endovascular aneurysm repair trial (EVAR) (156 patients underwent open operation and 122 underwent endovascular aneurysm repair) suggest that there is no significant difference in mortality between the two groups.

There is limited evidence for the effectiveness of beta-blockade in reducing the rate of expansion of large aneurysms. Patients receiving propanolol have significantly better quality-of-life scores. Ⓑ

A prospective study following 519 patients who had survived 30 days postelective repair of their AAAs, concluded after a median of 4.7 years follow-up, that long-term statin use is associated with a reduced all-cause and cardiovascular mortality, irrespective of clinical risk factors and beta-blocker use. Ⓑ

SUGGESTED READINGS

Fleming C et al: Screening for abdominal aortic aneurysm: a best-evidence systematic review for the U.S. Preventive Services Task Force, *Ann Intern Med* 142(3):203, 2005.

Hirsch AT et al: ACC/AHA 2005 practice guidelines for the management of patients with peripheral arterial disease (lower extremity, renal, mesenteric, and abdominal aortic): a collaborative report, *Circulation,* 113(11):e463-e465, 2006.

Upchurch GR, Schaub TA: Abdominal aortic aneurysm, *Am Fam Physician* 73:1198, 2006.

AUTHORS: **CRAIG J. McMACKIN, M.D.,** and **WEN-CHIH WU, M.D.**

BASIC INFORMATION

DEFINITION

Angina pectoris is characterized by discomfort that occurs when myocardial oxygen demand exceeds the supply. Myocardial ischemia can be asymptomatic (silent ischemia), particularly in diabetics. Angina can be classified as follows:

1. Chronic (stable):
   - Usually follows a precipitating event (e.g., climbing stairs, sexual intercourse, a heavy meal, emotional stress, cold weather).
   - Generally same severity as previous attacks; relieved by rest or by the customary dose of nitroglycerin.
   - Caused by a fixed coronary artery obstruction secondary to atherosclerosis. The presence of one or more obstructions in major coronary arteries is likely; the severity of stenosis is usually >70%.
2. Unstable (rest or crescendo, coronary syndrome):
   - Recent onset
   - Increasing severity, duration, or frequency of chronic angina
   - Occurs at rest or with minimal exertion
3. Prinzmetal's variant:
   - Occurs at rest
   - Manifests electrocardiographically as episodic ST-segment elevations
   - Caused by coronary artery spasms with or without superimposed coronary artery disease
   - Patients also more likely to develop ventricular arrhythmias
4. Microvascular angina (syndrome X):
   - Refers to patients with normal coronary angiograms and no coronary spasm but chest pain resembling angina and positive exercise test.
   - Defective endothelium-dependent dilation in the coronary microcirculation contributing to the altered regulation of myocardial perfusion and the ischemic manifestations in these patients.
   - Patients with chest pain and normal or nonobstructive coronary angiograms are predominantly women, and many have a prognosis that is not as benign as commonly thought (2% risk of death or MI at 30 days of follow-up).
   - Useful therapeutic agents for symptom relief are beta blockers, ACE inhibitors, and tricyclic agents. Aggressive antiatherosclerotic therapy with statins should also be undertaken.
5. Other:
   - Angina due to aortic stenosis and idiopathic hypertrophic subaortic stenosis, cocaine-induced coronary vasoconstriction.
6. Refractory angina:
   - Refers to patients who despite optimal medical therapy have both angina and objective evidence of ischemia and are not considered candidates for revascularization.
   - Current FDA-approved therapies consist of enhanced external counterpulsation (EECP), transcutaneous electrical nerve stimulation (TENS), and invasive therapies such as spinal cord stimulation, transmyocardial revascularization, and percutaneous myocardial revascularization. Although some of these therapies may improve symptoms and quality of life, they have not been shown to improve mortality.

FUNCTIONAL CLASSIFICATION

- New York Heart Association Functional Classification of angina:
  - Class I—Angina only with unusually strenuous activity.
  - Class II—Angina with slightly more prolonged or rigorous activity than usual.
  - Class III—Angina with usual daily activity.
  - Class IV—Angina at rest.
- Grading of Angina by the Canadian Cardiovascular Society Classification System:
  - Class I—Ordinary physical activity does not cause angina, such as walking, climbing stairs. Angina (occurs) with strenuous, rapid, or prolonged exertion at work or recreation.
  - Class II—Slight limitation of ordinary activity. Angina occurs on walking or climbing stairs rapidly; walking uphill; walking or stair climbing after meals, in cold, in wind, or under emotional stress; or only during the few hours after awakening. Angina occurs on walking more than two blocks on the level and climbing more than one flight of ordinary stairs at a normal pace and in normal condition.
  - Class III—Marked limitations of ordinary physical activity. Angina occurs on walking one to two blocks on the level and climbing one flight of stairs in normal conditions and at a normal pace.
  - Class IV—Inability to carry on any physical activity without discomfort—anginal symptoms may be present at rest.

ICD-9CM CODES

411.1 Angina, stable
413 Angina pectoris
413.1 Prinzmetal's angina
413.9 Angina, unspecified

EPIDEMIOLOGY & DEMOGRAPHICS

- Angina is most common in middle-aged and elderly males.
- Females are usually affected after menopause.
- Prevalence of angina pectoris in people older than 30 yr is >3%.
- Within 12 mo of initial diagnosis, 10% to 20% of patients with diagnosis of stable angina progress to MI or unstable angina.

PHYSICAL FINDINGS & CLINICAL PRESENTATION

- Although there is significant individual variation, most patients complain of substernal chest pain (pressure, tightness, heaviness, sharp pain, sensation similar to intestinal gas or dysphagia).
- The pain is of short duration (30 sec to 30 min), nonpleuritic, and often accompanied by shortness of breath, nausea, diaphoresis, and numbness or pain in the left arm, jaw, or shoulder.
- Women are significantly less likely to report chest pain or discomfort compared with men.

ETIOLOGY

UNCONTROLLABLE RISK FACTORS FOR ANGINA:

- Advanced age
- Male sex
- Genetic predisposition

MODIFIABLE RISK FACTORS FOR ANGINA:

- Smoking (risk is almost double).
- Hypertension (risk is double if systolic blood pressure is >180 mm Hg).
- Hyperlipidemia.
- Impaired glucose tolerance or diabetes mellitus.
- Obesity (weight >30% over ideal). A higher body mass index (BMI) during childhood is also associated with an increased risk of CHD in adulthood.
- Hypothyroidism.
- Left ventricular hypertrophy (LVH).
- Sedentary lifestyle.
- Oral contraceptive use.
- Cocaine use (Cocaine is used by >5,000,000 Americans regularly and is responsible for >64,000 ER evaluations yearly to rule out myocardial ischemia.)
- Low serum folate levels. (Folate is required for conversion of homocysteine to methionine. Hyperhomocysteinemia has a toxic effect on vascular endothelium and interferes with proliferation of arterial wall smooth muscle cells. Folate deficiencies are associated with an increased risk of fatal coronary heart disease.)
- Elevated homocysteine levels. Elevated plasma homocysteine level is a strong and independent risk factor for CHD events especially in patients with type 2 DM. Trials lowering homocysteine lev-

els have however been disappointing because lowering therapy with folate did not prevent cardiovascular events among patients with coronary disease.
- Elevated levels of highly sensitive C-reactive protein (hs-CRP, cardio CRP)
- Elevated levels of lipoprotein-associated phospholipase A2.
- Elevated fibrinogen levels.
- Elevated levels of glycosylated hemoglobin.
- Depression.
- Vasculitis.
- Low level of RBC glutathione peroxidase 1 activity.
- The development of coronary artery calcium (CAC) is associated with an increased risk of myocardial infarction.
- Chronic use of NSAIDs is associated with increased cardiovascular risk.
- Exposure to air pollution from traffic (dilute diesel exhaust) promotes myocardial ischemia and is associated with adverse cardiovascular events.

DIAGNOSIS Dx

DIFFERENTIAL DIAGNOSIS

Noncardiac pain mimicking angina may be caused by:
- Pulmonary diseases (pulmonary hypertension, pulmonary embolism, pleurisy, pneumothorax, pneumonia)
- GI disorders (peptic ulcer disease, pancreatitis, esophageal spasm or spontaneous esophageal muscle contraction, esophageal reflux, cholecystitis, cholelithiasis)
- Musculoskeletal conditions (costochondritis, chest wall trauma, cervical arthritis with radiculopathy, muscle strain, myositis)
- Acute aortic dissection
- Herpes zoster
- Anxiety disorder

WORKUP

- In patients presenting with chest pain, the probability of CAD should be estimated on the basis of patient age, sex, cardiovascular risk factors, and pain characteristics.
- The most important diagnostic factor is the history. Chest pain or left arm pain or discomfort reproducing previously documented angina and a known history of CAD or MI are indicative of high likelihood of acute coronary syndrome.
- The physical examination is of little diagnostic help and may be totally normal in many patients, although the presence of an S_4 gallop is suggestive of ischemic chest pain. Transient mitral regurgitation, hypotension, diaphoresis, and rales indicate a high likelihood of acute coronary syndrome.
- An ECG taken during the acute episode may show transient T-wave inversion or ST-segment depression or elevation, but more than 50% of patients with chronic stable angina have normal results on resting ECG.
- Patients with intermediate or high probability should undergo risk stratification through further testing. Treadmill exercise tolerance test is useful to identify patients with coronary artery disease who would benefit from cardiac catheterization. Stress echocardiogram or radionuclide testing (e.g., thallium, Persantine, dobutamine) are useful and sensitive in the detection of myocardial ischemia.
- Although invasive, coronary angiography remains the gold standard for the identification of clinically significant coronary artery disease. Coronary magnetic resonance angiography can also detect coronary artery disease of the proximal and middle segments. This noninvasive approach, where available, can be used to reliably identify (or rule out) left main coronary artery or three-vessel disease.
- Multidetector computed tomography (MDCT) is a newer screening modality for coronary artery disease. Its advantages are its speed, safety, and low cost when compared to angiography. It has high sensitivity and negative predictive value. Its limitations are as follows: limited to patients with a regular rhythm and slow rates, poor image in morbidly obese patients, inaccurate visualization of the coronary artery within a stent, decreased diagnostic accuracy in older patients due to the prevalence and severity of coronary calcifications with increasing age. Its routine use in clinical practice is not justified. However, it may be useful in excluding coronary disease in selected patients in whom a false-positive or inconclusive stress test is suspected.

LABORATORY TESTS

- Initial laboratory tests in patients with chronic stable angina should include hemoglobin, fasting glucose, and fasting lipid panel.
- Cardiac isoenzymes (CK-MB q8h × 2) should be obtained to rule out MI in patients presenting with acute chest pain.
- Cardiac troponin I and T are specific markers of myocardial necrosis and are useful in evaluating patients with acute chest pain. Elevation of either of these proteins in the setting of an acute coronary syndrome identifies patients with a several-fold increased risk of death in subsequent weeks. Patients with negative troponin assays on arrival in the ER and repeated 4 hr later are at a low level of risk for cardiac events within the following 30 days, and most of these patients can be safely discharged from the ER. Troponin T tests can be false-positive in patients with renal failure, sepsis, rhabdomyolysis, fibrin clots, and heterophile antibodies. The presence of jaundice or the concurrent use of heparin can result in underestimation of troponin.
- Cardio-CRP (hs-CRP)—elevation of cardio-CRP is a relatively moderate predictor of coronary heart disease and it adds prognostic information to that conveyed by the Framingham risk score. However, based on current data, it may be premature to adapt widespread assessment of cardio-CRP.
- Measurement of total cholesterol, LDL cholesterol (LDL-C), high-density lipoprotein cholesterol (HDL-C), and fasting serum triglycerides are recommended for cardiovascular screening. Non-HDL-C and the ratio of total cholesterol to HDL-C and measurements of apolipoprotein fractions (e.g., apolipoprotein B100, apolipoprotein A1) can also be used to estimate cardiovascular risk.
- A single measurement of B-type natriuretic peptide, a natriuretic and vasodilative peptide regulated by ventricular wall tension and stored mainly in the ventricular myocardium, obtained in the first few days after the onset of ischemic symptoms, provides predictive information for risk stratification in acute coronary syndromes. NT-pro-BNP is also a marker of long-term mortality in patients with stable coronary disease and provides prognostic information beyond that provided by conventional cardiovascular risk factors and the degree of left ventricular systolic dysfunction.

IMAGING STUDIES

- Echocardiography is indicated in patients with systolic murmur suggestive of aortic stenosis, mitral valve prolapse, or hypertrophic cardiomyopathy. It is also useful in the detection of ischemia-induced regional wall motion abnormalities or mitral regurgitation. Echocardiography combined with treadmill exercise (stress echo) or pharmacologic stress with dobutamine can be used to detect regional wall abnormalities that occur during myocardial ischemia associated with CAD.
- Coronary angiography is performed to define the location and extent of coronary disease; this is indicated in selected patients who are candidates for CABG surgery or angioplasty.
- Noninvasive methods for assessing myocardial viability to predict which patients will have increased LVEF and improved survival after revascularization include positron-emission tomography, dobutamine echocardiography, multidetector computed tomography, and contrast-enhanced MRI. Additional studies are needed to determine the cost effectiveness of these studies in patients with ischemic cardiomyopathy.

TREATMENT

Rx

NONPHARMACOLOGIC THERAPY

- Aggressive modification of preventable risk factors (weight reduction in obese patients, regular aerobic exercise program, correction of folate deficiency, low-cholesterol and low-sodium diet, cessation of tobacco use).
- Diets using nonhydrogenated unsaturated fats as the predominant form of dietary fat, whole grains as the main form of carbohydrates, an abundance of fruits and vegetables, and adequate omega-3 fatty acids are optimal for prevention of coronary heart disease.
- Correction of possible aggravating factors (e.g., anemia, hypertension, diabetes mellitus, hyperlipidemia, thyrotoxicosis, hypothyroidism). Blood transfusion in the setting of acute coronary syndromes is associated with higher mortality. Use caution regarding the routine use of blood transfusion to maintain arbitrary hematocrit levels in stable patients with ischemic heart disease.

ACUTE GENERAL Rx

The major classes of antiischemic agents are nitrates, beta-adrenergic blockers, calcium channel blockers, aspirin, and heparin; they can be used alone or in combination.

- Nitrates cause venodilation and relaxation of vascular smooth muscle; the decreased venous return from venodilation decreases diastolic ventricular wall tension (preload) and thereby reduces mechanical activity (and myocardial oxygen consumption) during systole. Relaxation of vascular smooth muscle increases coronary blood flow and reduces systemic pressure. Tolerance to nitrates can be minimized by avoiding sustained blood levels with a daily nitrate-free period (e.g., omission of bedtime dose of oral isosorbide dinitrate or 12 hr on/12 hr off transdermal nitroglycerin therapy). Nitrates are relatively contraindicated in patients with hypertrophic obstructive cardiomyopathy, and should also be avoided in patients with severe aortic stenosis. Nitrates should not be used within 24 hr of sildenafil (Viagra) or vardenafil (Levitra) or within 48 hr of tadafil (Cialis) because of the potential for hypotension.
- Beta-adrenergic blockers achieve their major antianginal effect by decreasing myocardial oxygen consumption by reducing heart rate and systolic blood pressure. Absent contraindications, they should be regarded as initial therapy for stable angina for all patients. Their dose should generally be adjusted to reduce the resting heart rate to 50 to 60 beats/min.
- Calcium channel blockers dilate coronary and systemic arteries, increase coronary blood flow, and decrease myocardial oxygen consumption. They play a major role in preventing and terminating myocardial ischemia induced by coronary artery spasm. They are particularly effective in treating microvascular angina. Short-acting calcium channel blockers should be avoided. Calcium channel blockers should generally also be avoided after complicated MI (CHF) and in patients with CHF secondary to systolic dysfunction (unless necessary to control heart rate).
- Aspirin: use of aspirin reduces cardiovascular mortality and morbidity by 20% to 25% among patients with coronary artery disease. Initial dose is at least 160 mg/day followed by 81 to 325 mg/day. Aspirin inhibits cyclooxygenics and synthesis of thromboxane A_2 and reduces the risk of adverse cardiovascular events by 33% in patients with unstable angina. Patients intolerant to aspirin can be treated with the antiplatelet agent clopidogrel. Clopidogrel acts by irreversibly blocking the P2Y12 adenosine diphosphate receptor on the platelet surface, thereby interrupting platelet activation and aggregation.
- Heparin is useful in patients with unstable angina and reduces the frequency of MI and refractory angina. Patients with unstable angina treated with aspirin plus heparin have a 32% reduction in the risk of MI and death compared with those treated with aspirin alone; therefore, unless heparin is contraindicated, most hospitalized patients with unstable angina should be treated with both aspirin and heparin. Enoxaparin (low molecular weight heparin) 1 mg bid SC is as effective as continuous unfractionated heparin in reducing the incidence of unstable angina. It is usually given for 3 to 8 days, or until coronary revascularization is performed. Longer administration does not provide additional cardiac benefits and may increase risk of hemorrhage.
- Early administration of platelet glycoprotein IIb/IIIa receptor antagonists is useful in addition to aspirin and heparin in patients with unstable angina, in high-risk patients with positive troponin tests, or those undergoing percutaneous revascularization. Abciximab, the first GP IIb/IIa inhibitor, is an important component of percutaneous revascularization. Started in the catheterization lab, it reduces the incidence of ischemic events. Abciximab is contraindicated in patients for whom an early invasive strategy is not planned. Contraindications to the use of GP IIb/IIa inhibitors are: severe hypertension (>180/110), internal bleeding within 30 days, history of intracranial hemorrhage, neoplasm, NVM, aneurysm, CVA within 30 days or history of hemorrhagic CVA, thrombocytopenin (<100 k), acute pericarditis, history or symptoms suggestive of aortic dissection, and major surgical procedures or severe physical trauma within previous month.

CHRONIC Rx

- Use of lipid-lowering drugs is recommended in patients with coronary heart disease and in patients with hyperlipidemia refractory to diet and exercise. Among patients who have recently had an acute coronary syndrome, an intensive lipid-lowering statin regimen to reduce LDL cholesterol to <70 mg/dL is a reasonable treatment objective. Statins also decrease the level of the inflammatory marker hs-CRP independently of the magnitude of change in lipid parameters.
- ACE inhibition (e.g., ramipril 10 mg/day) has been shown to be effective in reducing cardiovascular death, MI, and stroke in patients who are at risk for or who had vascular disease (without heart failure). Currently evidence for routine use of ACEs in chronic stable angina is insufficient.
- Ranolazine is a newer agent indicated for treatment of chronic angina that is inadequately controlled with other antianginals. It represents a new class of drugs known as metabolic modulators. Its exact mechanism of action is unknown. It seems to increase the efficiency of energy production in the heart, maintaining cardiac function. Its antianginal and antiischemic effects do not depend upon reductions in heart rate or blood pressure. It is labeled for use in combination with beta-blockers, amlodipine, or nitrates in patients without an adequate antianginal response to those agents. Side effects include prolongation of QT interval.

REFERRAL

Revascularization:

- Revascularization includes either percutaneous coronary intervention (balloon angioplasty and stenting) or coronary artery bypass surgery.
- *CABG surgery* is recommended for patients with left main coronary disease, for those with symptomatic three-vessel disease, and for those with left ventricular EF <40% and critical (>70% stenosis) in all three major coronary arteries. Surgical therapy improves prognosis, particularly in diabetic patients with multivessel disease.

Angioplasty and coronary stents:

- *Percutaneous coronary intervention (PCI)* should be considered for patients with one- or two-vessel disease that does not involve the main left coronary artery and in whom ventricular function is normal or near normal. PCI has an established place in treating angina but is not superior to intensive medical therapy to prevent MI and death in symptomatic or asymptomatic patients. Patients selected for PCI should also be candidates for CABG. The types of lesions best suited for angioplasty are proximal lesions, noncalcified, concentric, and preferably shorter than 5 mm (should not exceed 10 mm). Approximately 80% of patients show immediate benefit after PCI. The frequency of abrupt closure postangioplasty can be reduced by pretreatment with IV glycoprotein IIb/IIIa receptor inhibitors, which block the final common pathway of platelet aggregation. In patients with clinically documented acute coronary syndrome who are treated with GP IIb/IIa inhibitors, even small elevations in cTmI and cTmT identify high-risk patients who derive a large clinical benefit from an early invasive strategy. Abciximab (ReoPro) and eptifibatide (Integrilin) are approved for use before and during percutaneous coronary interventions. They are expensive and can cause thrombocytopenia in 0.5% to 1% of patients. Platelet counts should be monitored for 24 hours after starting glycoprotein IIb/IIIa inhibitors. Reversal of thrombocytopenia (e.g., patients undergoing emergency CABG) can be achieved with platelet transfusions. Optimal long-term care after PCI requires aggressive systemic pharmacotherapy (antiplatelet agents [aspirin plus clopidogrel], statins, beta blockers, and ACE inhibitors) and therapeutic lifestyle to minimize the risk of future atherothrombotic events.

- The development of *coronary stents* has broadened the number of patients who can be treated in the cardiac laboratory. Cardiac stents are currently used in nearly 95% of all percutaneous interventional lesions. The rate of restenosis may be reduced by placing a stent electively in primary atheromatous lesions. In patients with symptomatic isolated stenosis of the proximal left anterior descending artery, stenting has advantages over standard coronary angioplasty in that it is associated with both a lower rate of restenosis and a better clinical outcome. The major limitations of stenting are subacute thrombosis, restenosis within the stent, bleeding complications when anticoagulants are used post stenting, and higher cost. The combination of aspirin and clopidogrel is effective in preventing coronary stent thrombosis. Vitamin therapy to lower homocysteine levels has been recommended by some for the prevention of restenosis after coronary angioplasty, however, recent reports indicate that the administration of folate, vitamin B_6, and vitamin B_{12} after coronary stenting may increase the risk of in-stent restenosis and the need for target-vessel revascularization. Stents coated with sirolimus have been reported to dramatically reduce the incidence of stent restenosis by inhibiting the growth of endothelium and fibrosis within the lumen of the stent on the short term. However, in a pooled analysis of data from four trials comparing sirolimus-eluting stents and bare-metal stents, no significant differences were found between the two treatments in rates of death, myocardial infarction, or stent thrombosis (Spaulding et al).

PEARLS & CONSIDERATIONS

COMMENTS

- Although nitrate responsiveness is usually an integral part of a diagnostic strategy for chronic stable chest pain, recent reports question its value and conclude that in a general population admitted for chest pain, relief of pain after nitroglycerin treatment does not predict active coronary artery disease and should not be used to guide diagnosis in the acute care setting.
- CABG is associated with higher long-term survival rates and lower rates of repeat revascularization than PCI and stenting; however, patients often prefer stenting because it is less invasive, has a shorter hospital stay, and has lower in-hospital mortality.
- Section III describes an algorithm for the surgical management of ischemic cardiomyopathy.

EVIDENCE

EBM

Percutaneous transluminal coronary intervention (PCI) appears to reduce the angina symptoms of patients with moderate to severe stable angina more effectively than medical therapy, but it is associated with a higher rate of subsequent need for CABG. It does not reduce the rate of subsequent myocardial infarction, the need for later PCI, or death.[1-3] Ⓐ

CABG is more effective than medical therapy at reducing mortality rates, particularly in patients with more severe CHD.[4] Ⓐ

Evidence-Based References

1. Bucher HC et al: Percutaneous transluminal coronary angioplasty versus medical treatment for non-acute coronary heart disease: meta-analysis of randomised controlled trials, *BMJ* 321:73-77, 2000. Reviewed in: Clinical Evidence 11:197-239, 2004. Ⓐ
2. Pocock SJ et al: Quality of life after coronary angioplasty or continued medical treatment for angina: three-year follow-up in the RITA-2 trial. Randomized Intervention Treatment of Angina, *J Am Coll Cardiol* 35:907-914, 2000. Reviewed in: Clinical Evidence 11:197-239, 2004. Ⓐ
3. Coronary angioplasty versus medical therapy for angina: the second Randomised Intervention Treatment of Angina (RITA-2) trial. RITA-2 trial participants, *Lancet* 350:461-468, 1997. Reviewed in: Clinical Evidence 11:197-239, 2004. Ⓐ
4. Yusuf S et al: Effect of coronary artery bypass graft surgery on survival: overview of 10-year results from randomized trials by the coronary artery bypass surgery trialists collaboration, *Lancet* 244:565-570, 1994. Reviewed in: Clinical Evidence 11:197-239, 2004. Ⓐ

SUGGESTED READINGS

Abrams J: Chronic stable angina, *N Engl J Med* 352:2524-2533, 2005.

Bibbins-Domingo K et al: N-terminal fragment of the prohormone brain-type natriuretic peptide 9NT-proBNP, cardiovascular events, and mortality in patients with stable coronary heart disease, *JAMA* 297:169, 2007.

Garcia MJ et al: Accuracy of 16-row multidetector computed tomography for the assessment of coronary artery stenosis, *JAMA* 296:403, 2006.

Hilas O: Ranolazine for chronic angina, *Am Fam Physician* 75:544, 2007.

Hochman JS et al: Coronary intervention for persistent occlusion after myocardial infarction, *N Engl J Med* 355:2395, 2007.

Hurst T et al: Cardiac syndrome X and endothelial dysfunction: New concepts in prognosis and treatment, *Am J Med* 119:560, 2006.

Kragelund C et al: N-Terminal pro-B-type natriuretic peptide and long-term mortality in stable coronary heart disease, *N Engl J Med* 352:666-675, 2005.

Mills NL et al: Ischemic and thrombotic effects of dilute diesel exhaust inhalation in men with coronary heart disease, *N Engl J Med* 357:1075, 2007.

Smith SC et al: AHA/ACC guidelines for secondary prevention for patients with coronary and other atherosclerotic vascular disease: 2006 update, *Circulation* 113:2363, 2006.

Snow V et al: Evaluation of primary care patients with chronic stable angina: guidelines from the American College of Physicians, *Ann Intern Med* 141:57 and 562, 2004.

Spaulding C et al: A pooled analysis of data comparing sirolimus-eluting stents with bare-metal stents, *N Engl J Med* 356:989, 2007.

Stone GW, Aronow HD: Long-term care after percutaneous coronary intervention: focus on the role of antiplatelet therapy, *Mayo Clin Proc* 81(5):641, 2006.

AUTHOR: **FRED F. FERRI, M.D.**

BASIC INFORMATION

DEFINITION

- The mucocutaneous swelling caused by the release of vasoactive mediators is called urticaria and angioedema.
- Urticaria causes edema of the superficial dermis.
- Angioedema involves the deep layers of the dermis and the subcutaneous tissue.

SYNONYMS

Angioneurotic edema

ICD-9CM CODES
995.1 Angioedema (allergic)
277.6 Angioedema (hereditary)

EPIDEMIOLOGY & DEMOGRAPHICS

INCIDENCE: 100 to 3000/100,000 persons (for urticaria and angioedema).

LIFETIME PREVALENCE: Approximately 20% of the population experiences urticaria and/or angioedema at some time during life.

DEMOGRAPHICS: Race: Slightly more common among African Americans. Sex: More occurrences in women than men. Angioedema commonly occurs after adolescence in the third decade of life. Angioedema can occur together with urticaria (40%) or alone (20%); the remaining 40% have urticaria alone.

PHYSICAL FINDINGS & CLINICAL PRESENTATION

- Angioedema may be acute or chronic.
  1. Acute angioedema is defined as symptoms lasting 6 wk.
  2. Chronic angioedema is defined as symptoms lasting >6 wk.
- Urticaria is commonly known as "hives" and is:
  1. Pruritic
  2. Palpable and well demarcated
  3. Erythematous
  4. Millimeters to centimeters in size
  5. Multiple in number
  6. Fades within 12 to 24 hr
  7. Reappears at other sites
- Angioedema is characterized by the following:
  1. Nonpruritic
  2. Burning
  3. Not well demarcated
  4. Involves eyelids (Fig. 1-17), lips, tongue, and extremities
  5. Can involve the upper airway causing respiratory distress
  6. Can involve the GI tract leading to cyclic abdominal pain
  7. Resolves slowly

ETIOLOGY

- Angioedema, with or without urticaria, is classified as acquired (allergic or idiopathic) or hereditary.
- Angioedema is primarily due to mast cell activation and degranulation with release of vasoactive mediators (e.g., histamine, serotonin, bradykinins) resulting in postcapillary venule inflammation, vascular leakage, and edema in the deep layers of the dermis and subcutaneous tissue.
- Pathologically angioedema has both immunological and nonimmunological mediated mechanisms.
  1. Immunoglobulin E (Ig E)-mediated angioedema may result from antigen exposure (e.g., foods [milk, eggs, peanuts, shell fish, tomatoes, chocolate, sulfites] or drugs [penicillin, aspirin, NSAIDs, phenytoin, sulfonamides, rt-PA]).
  2. Complement-mediated angioedema involving immune complex mechanisms can also lead to mast cell activation that manifests as serum sickness.
  3. Hereditary angioedema is an autosomal dominant disease caused by a deficiency of C1 esterase inhibitor (C1-INH). C1-INH is a protease inhibitor that is normally present in high concentrations in the plasma. C1-INH serves many functions, one of which is to inhibit plasma kallikrein, a protease that cleaves kininogen and releases bradykinin. A deficiency in C1-INH results in excess concentration of kininogen and the subsequent release of kinin mediators.
  4. Acquired angioedema is usually associated with other diseases, most commonly B-cell lympho-proliferative disorders, but may also result from the formation of autoantibodies directed against C1 inhibitor protein.
  5. Other causes of angioedema include infection (e.g., herpes simplex, hepatitis B, coxsackie A and B, streptococcus, candida, ascaris, and strongyloides), insect bites and stings, stress, physical factors (e.g., cold, exercise, pressure, and vibration), connective tissue diseases (e.g., SLE, Henoch-Schönlein purpura), and idiopathic causes. ACE inhibitors can increase kinin activity and lead to angioedema.

DIAGNOSIS

A detailed history and physical examination usually establishes the diagnosis of angioedema. Extensive lab testing is of limited value.

DIFFERENTIAL DIAGNOSIS

- Cellulitis
- Arthropod bite
- Hypothyroidism
- Contact dermatitis
- Atopic dermatitis
- Mastocytosis
- Granulomatous cheilitis
- Bullous pemphigoid
- Urticaria pigmentosa
- Anaphylaxis
- Erythema multiforme
- Epiglottitis
- Peritonsillar abscess

WORKUP

- An extensive workup searching for the cause of angioedema is often unrevealing (90%).
- Workup including diagnostic blood tests and allergy testing is performed based on the history and physical examination.

LABORATORY TESTS

- CBC, ESR, and urinalysis are sometimes helpful as part of the initial evaluation
- Stools for ova and parasites
- Serology testing
- C4 levels are reduced in acquired and hereditary angioedema (occuring without urticaria). If C4 levels are low, C1-INH levels and activity should be obtained. There are isolated reports of hereditary angioedema with normal C4 levels but reduced C1-INH levels

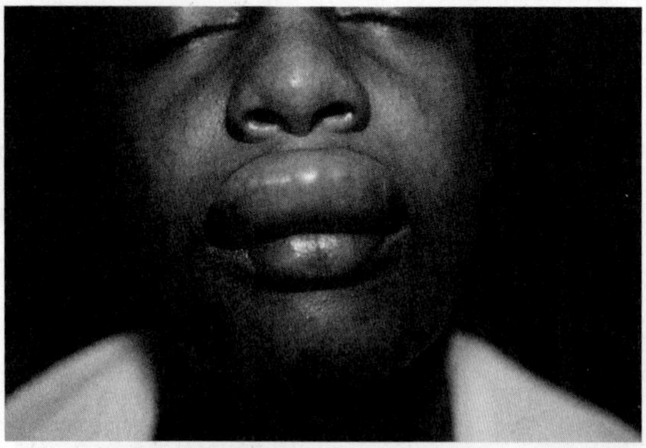

FIGURE 1-17 Angioedema of the upper lip, with severe swelling of deeper tissues. (From Goldstein BG, Goldstein AO: *Practical dermatology,* ed 2, St Louis, 1997, Mosby.)

- Skin and radioallergosorbent (RAST) testing may be done if food allergies are suspected
- Skin biopsy is usually done in patients with chronic angioedema refractory to corticosteroid treatment

TREATMENT

NONPHARMACOLOGIC THERAPY

- Eliminate the offending agent
- Avoid triggering factors (e.g., cold, stress)
- Cold compresses to affected areas

ACUTE GENERAL Rx

- Acute life-threatening angioedema involving the larynx is treated with:
  1. Epinephrine 0.3 mg in a solution of 1:1000 given SC
  2. Diphenhydramine 25 to 50 mg IV or IM
  3. Cimetidine 300 mg IV or ranitidine 50 mg IV
  4. Methylprednisolone 125 mg IV
- Mainstay therapy in angioedema is H1 antihistamines.
  1. Diphenhydramine 25 to 50 mg q6h
  2. Chlorpheniramine 4 mg q6h
  3. Hydroxyzine 10 to 25 mg q6h
  4. Cetirizine 5 to 10 mg qd
  5. Loratadine 10 mg qd
  6. Fexofenadine 60 mg qd
- H2 antihistamines can be added to H1 antihistamines.
  1. Ranitidine 150 mg bid
  2. Cimetidine 400 mg bid
  3. Famotidine 20 mg bid
- Tricyclic antidepressants
  1. Doxepin 25 to 50 mg qd can be tried.
- Corticosteroids are rarely required for symptomatic relief of acute angioedema.

CHRONIC Rx

- Chronic angioedema is treated as described under "Acute General Rx."
- Corticosteroids are used more often in chronic angioedema.
- Prednisone 1 mg/kg/day for 5 days and then tapered over a period of weeks.
- Androgens are used for the treatment of hereditary angioedema, which does not respond to antihistamines or corticosteroids. C1-INH replacement therapy is available in some countries.

DISPOSITION

- Antihistamines achieve symptomatic relief in more than 80% of patients with angioedema.
- In chronic angioedema, corticosteroids are given in addition to antihistamines.
- A small percentage of people will have recurrence of symptoms after steroid treatment.
- Chronic angioedema can last for months and even years.

REFERRAL

Dermatology consultation is recommended in patients with chronic angioedema, hereditary angioedema, and recurring angioedema.

PEARLS & CONSIDERATIONS

ACE inhibitors can cause angioedema up to many months after initiation. There are multiple case reports and case series of Angiotensin Receptor Blocker (ARB) induced angioedema, although the risk is substantially less than that of ACEIs.

COMMENTS

- Identifying a cause for angioedema in patients is often difficult and met with frustration.
- Chronic angioedema, unlike acute angioedema, is rarely caused by an allergic reaction.

SUGGESTED READINGS

Baxi S, Dinakar C: Urticaria and angioedema, *Immunol Allergy Clin North Am,* 25(2):353, 2005.

Bowen T et al: Canadian 2003 international concensus algorithm for the diagnosis, therapy, and management of hereditary angioedema, *J Allergy Clin Immunol* 114(3):629, 2004.

Frigas E, Park M: Idiopathic recurrent angioedema, *Immunol and Allergy Clin North Am* 26(4):739, 2006.

Kaplan AP: Clinical practice: chronic urticaria and angioedema, *N Engl J Med* 346(3):175, 2002.

Muller B: Urticaria and angioedema: a practical approach, *Am Fam Physician,* 69(5):1123, 2004.

AUTHOR: **MEL ANDERSON, M.D.**

BASIC INFORMATION

DEFINITION

Ankle fractures involve the lateral, medial, or posterior malleolus of the ankle and may occur either alone or in some combination. Associated ligamentous injuries are included.

ICD-9CM CODES
824.8 Ankle fracture (malleolus) (closed)
824.2 Lateral malleolus fracture (fibular)
824.0 Medial malleolus fracture (tibial)

PHYSICAL FINDINGS & CLINICAL PRESENTATION

- Deformity usually dependent on extent of displacement
- Pain, tenderness, and hemorrhage at the site of injury
- Gentle palpation of ligamentous structures (especially deltoid ligament) to determine the extent of soft tissue injury
- Evaluation of distal neurovascular status; results recorded

ETIOLOGY

- The ankle depends on its ligamentous and bony support for stability. The joint, or *mortise,* is an inverted U with the dome of the talus fitting into the medial and lateral malleoli. The posterior margin of the tibia is often called the *third* or *posterior malleolus.*
- Most common ankle fractures are the result of eversion or lateral rotation forces on the talus (in contrast to common sprains, which are caused usually by inversion).

DIAGNOSIS

The diagnosis is usually established on the basis of the nature of the injury, the presence of typical findings of bony tenderness with swelling, and abnormal imaging studies.

DIFFERENTIAL DIAGNOSIS

- Ankle sprain
- Avulsion fracture of hindfoot or metatarsal

IMAGING STUDIES

Standard AP and lateral views accompanied by an AP taken 15° internally rotated. The last view is taken to properly visualize the mortise.

TREATMENT

All fractures: elevation and ice to control swelling for 48 to 72 hr.

ACUTE GENERAL Rx

- Clinical and roentgenographic assessment of the status of the ankle mortise and stability of the injury is mandatory to determine treatment.
- There is potential for displacement if both sides of the joint are significantly injured (e.g., fracture of the lateral malleolus with deltoid ligament injury).
- Deviation of the position of the talus in the mortise could lead to traumatic arthritis.
- If there is no widening of the ankle mortise, many injuries can be safely treated with simple casting without reduction:
  1. Undisplaced or avulsion fractures of either malleolus below the ankle joint line:
     a. Stability of the joint is not compromised and a short leg walking cast or ankle support is sufficient.
     b. Weight bearing is allowed as tolerated.
     c. In 4 to 6 wk, protection may be discontinued.
  2. Isolated undisplaced fractures of the medial, lateral, or posterior malleolus:
     a. Usually stable and require only the application of a short leg walking cast with the ankle in the neutral position or fracture cast boot.
     b. Immobilization should be continued for 8 wk.
     c. Fracture line of lateral malleolus may persist roentgenographically for several months, but immobilization beyond 8 wk is usually unnecessary.
     d. Undisplaced bimalleolar fractures are treated with a long leg cast flexed 30 degrees at the knee to prevent motion and displacement of the fracture fragments. In 4 wk, a short leg walking cast may be applied for an additional 4 wk.
  3. Isolated fractures of the lateral malleolus that are slightly displaced:
     a. May be treated with casting if no medial injury is present.
     b. A below-knee walking cast is applied with ankle in the neutral position and weight bearing is allowed as tolerated.
     c. Six weeks of immobilization is sufficient.
     d. If medial tenderness is present, suggesting deltoid ligament rupture, a carefully molded cast may suffice if weight bearing is not allowed and the patient is followed closely for signs of instability, especially after swelling recedes. If significant widening of the medial ankle mortise (increase in the "medial clear space") develops as a result of lateral displacement of the talus, referral for possible reduction is indicated.
     e. If signs of instability are already present at initial examination (widening of the medial clear space with medial tenderness), referral is indicated.
  4. Undisplaced fracture of the distal fibular epiphysis:
     a. Often diagnosed clinically.
     b. There is tenderness over the epiphyseal plate.
     c. Roentgenographic findings are often negative.
     d. A short leg walking cast or fracture boot is applied for 4 wk.
     e. Growth disturbance is rare.
  5. Isolated posterior malleolar fractures involving less than 25% of the joint surface on the lateral roentgenogram: Safely treated by applying a short leg walking cast or fracture brace. (Fractures involving >25% of the weight-bearing surface should be referred because of the potential for instability and subsequent traumatic arthritis.)

CHRONIC Rx

- Early motion is encouraged through a home exercise program.
- Protection from reinjury is appropriate for 4 to 6 wk following cast or brace removal.
- Temporary increase in lower extremity swelling that frequently occurs after short leg cast removal may benefit from the use of support hose.

DISPOSITION

Significant factors involved in the development of traumatic arthritis:

- Amount of joint trauma at the time of injury
- Eventual position of the talus in the mortise

Fracture nonunion is uncommon unless displacement is significant.

REFERRAL

Orthopedic consultation for:

- Unstable ankle joint
- Widened ankle mortise
- Posterior malleolar fracture over 25% of joint with incongruity
- Marked displacement of fracture fragment

SUGGESTED READINGS

Bachmann LM et al: Accuracy of Ottawa rules to exclude fractures of the ankle and mid-foot, *BMJ* 326:417, 2003.

Chaudhary SB et al: Complications of ankle fracture in patients with diabetes, *J Am Acad Orthop Surg* 16:159, 2008.

Egol KA et al: Predictors of short-term functional outcome following ankle fracture surgery, *J Bone Joint Surg* 88A:974, 2006.

Haraguchi N et al: Pathoanatomy of posterior malleolar fractures of the ankle, *J Bone Joint Surg* 88A:1085, 2006.

Schnetzler KA, Hoernschemeyer D: The pediatric triplane fracture, *J Am Acad Orthop Surg* 15:738, 2007.

Tejwani NC et al: Are outcomes of bimalleolar fractures poorer than those of lateral malleolar fractures with medial ligamentous injury? *J Bone Joint Surg Am* 89:1438, 2007.

AUTHOR: **LONNIE R. MERCIER, M.D.**

BASIC INFORMATION

DEFINITION

An ankle sprain is an injury to the ligamentous support of the ankle. Most (85%) involve the lateral ligament complex (Fig. 1-18). The anterior inferior tibiofibular (AITF) ligament, deltoid ligament, and interosseous membrane may also be injured. Damage to the tibiofibular syndesmosis is sometimes called a *high sprain* because of pain above the ankle.

ICD-9CM CODES
845.00 Sprain, ankle or foot

EPIDEMIOLOGY & DEMOGRAPHICS

PREVALENCE: 1 case/10,000 people each day

PREDOMINANT SEX: Varies according to age and level of physical activity

PHYSICAL FINDINGS & CLINICAL PRESENTATION

- Often a history of a "pop"
- Variable amounts of tenderness and hemorrhage
- Possible abnormal anterior drawer test (pulling the plantar flexed foot forward to determine if there is any abnormal increase in forward movement of the talus in the ankle mortise) (Fig. 1-19)
- Inversion sprains: tender laterally; syndesmotic injuries: area of tenderness is more anterior and proximal
- Evaluation of motor function (Fig. 1-20)

ETIOLOGY

- Lateral injuries usually result from inversion and plantar flexion injuries.
- Eversion and rotational forces may injure the deltoid or AITF ligament or the interosseous membrane.

DIAGNOSIS

DIFFERENTIAL DIAGNOSIS

- Fracture of the ankle or foot, particularly involving the distal fibular growth plate in the immature patient
- Avulsion fracture of the fifth metatarsal base

WORKUP

- History and clinical examination are usually sufficient to establish the diagnosis.
- Plain radiographs are always needed.

IMAGING STUDIES

Roentgenographic evaluation
1. Usually normal but always performed
2. Should include the fifth metatarsal base
3. All minor avulsion fractures noted

Varying opinions on the usefulness of arthrograms, tenograms, and stress films

TREATMENT

ACUTE GENERAL Rx

Ankle sprains are often graded I, II, or III, according to severity, with Grade III injury implying complete rupture. The first line of treatment is described by the mnemonic device, *RICE:*
- Rest
- Ice
- Compression
- Elevation
- Varying opinions regarding the initial use of NSAIDs
- In 48 to 72 hr, active range of motion and weight bearing as tolerated
- In 4 to 5 days, exercise against resistance added
- Possible cast immobilization for some patients who require early independent walking; short leg orthoses also available for the same purpose

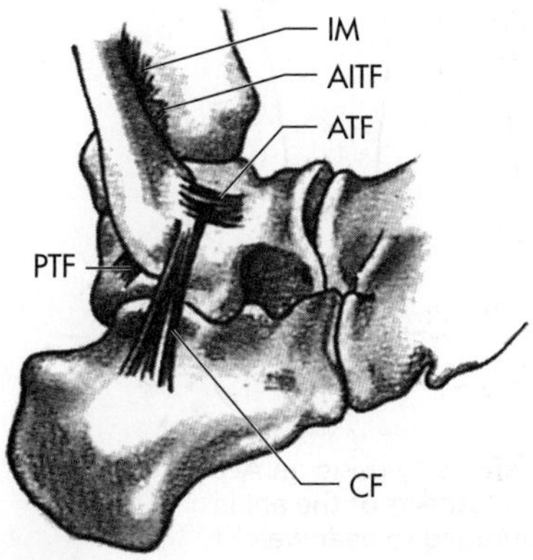

FIGURE 1-18 The lateral ankle ligaments, anterior and posterior talofibular *(ATF, PTF)* and calcaneofibular *(CF)*. Also shown are the anterior inferior tibiofibular ligament *(AITF)* and the beginning of the interosseous membrane *(IM)*. (From Mercier LR [ed]: *Practical orthopaedics,* ed 4, St Louis, 1995, Mosby.)

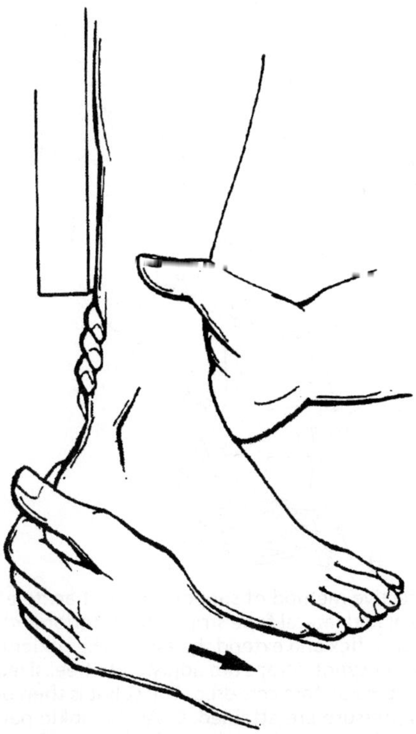

FIGURE 1-19 Anterior drawer test of the ankle (tests the integrity of the anterior talofibular ligament). (From Brinker MR, Miller MD: *Fundamentals of orthopaedics,* Philadelphia, 1999, WB Saunders.)

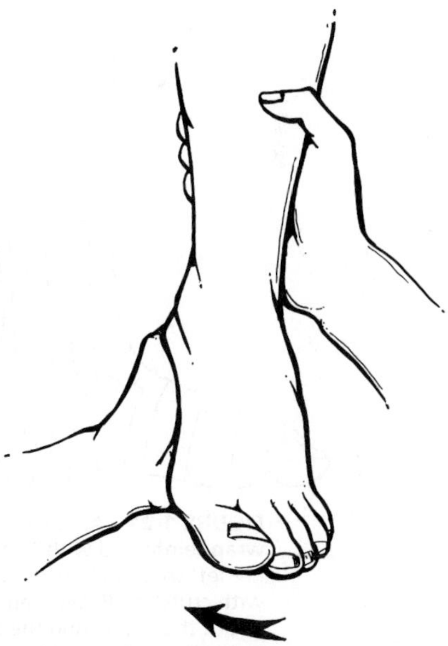

FIGURE 1-20 Talar tilt test (inversion stress) of the ankle (tests the integrity of the anterior talofibular ligament and the calcaneofibular ligament). (From Brinker MR, Miller MD: *Fundamentals of orthopaedics,* Philadelphia, 1999, WB Saunders.)

- Surgery is rarely recommended, even for Grade III sprains; reports of equally satisfactory outcomes with nonsurgical treatment

CHRONIC Rx

- Lateral heel and sole wedge to prevent inversion
- Protective taping or bracing during vigorous activities (Fig. 1-21)
- Strengthening exercises

DISPOSITION

- Lateral sprains of any severity may cause lingering symptoms for weeks and months.
  1. Some syndesmotic sprains take even longer to heal.
  2. Heterotopic ossification may even develop in the interosseous membrane, but long-term results do not seem to be affected by such ossification.
- Continuing lateral symptoms may require surgical reconstruction, although late traumatic arthritis or chronic instability is rare regardless of treatment.

REFERRAL

For orthopedic consultation for cases that fail to respond to conservative treatment

PEARLS & CONSIDERATIONS

COMMENTS

If healing seems delayed (more than 6 wk), the following conditions should be considered:

1. Talar dome fracture
2. Reflex sympathetic dystrophy
3. Chronic tendinitis
4. Peroneal tendon subluxation
5. Other occult fracture
6. Peroneal weakness (poor rehabilitation)
7. A "high" (syndesmotic) sprain

Repeat plain roentgenograms, bone scan, or MRI may be indicated.

SUGGESTED READINGS

Bachman LM, Kolb E et al: Accuracy of Ottawa ankle rules to exclude fractures of the ankle and mid-foot: systematic review, *BMJ* 326:417, 2003.

Berkowitz MJ, Kim DH: Process and tubercule fractures of the hindfoot, *J Am Acad Orthop Surg* 13:492, 2005.

Dahners LE, Mullis BH: Effects of nonsteroidal anti-inflammatory drugs on bone formation and soft tissue healing, *J Am Acad Orthop Surg* 12:139, 2004.

Hale SA et al: The effect of a 4-week comprehensive rehabilitation program on postural control and lower extremity function in individuals with chronic ankle instability, *J Orthop Sports Phys Ther* 37:303, 2007.

Judd DB, Kim DH: Foot fractures misdiagnosed as ankle sprains, *Am Fam Physician* 66:785, 2002.

Le Gall F et al: Injuries in young elite female soccer players: an 8-season prospective study, *Am J Sports Med* 36:276, 2008.

Mizel MS, Hecht PJ et al: Evaluation and treatment of chronic ankle pain, *J Bone Joint Surg* 86A:622, 2004.

O'Neill PJ et al: Excursion and strain of the superficial peroneal nerve during inversion ankle sprain, *J Bone Joint Surg* 89A:979, 2007.

Pedowtiz DI et al: Prophylactic bracing decreases ankle injuries in collegiate female volleyball players, *Am J Sports Med* 36:324, 2008.

Zalavras C, Thordarson D: Ankle syndesmotic injury, *J Am Acad Orthop Surg* 15:330, 2007.

AUTHOR: **LONNIE R. MERCIER, M.D.**

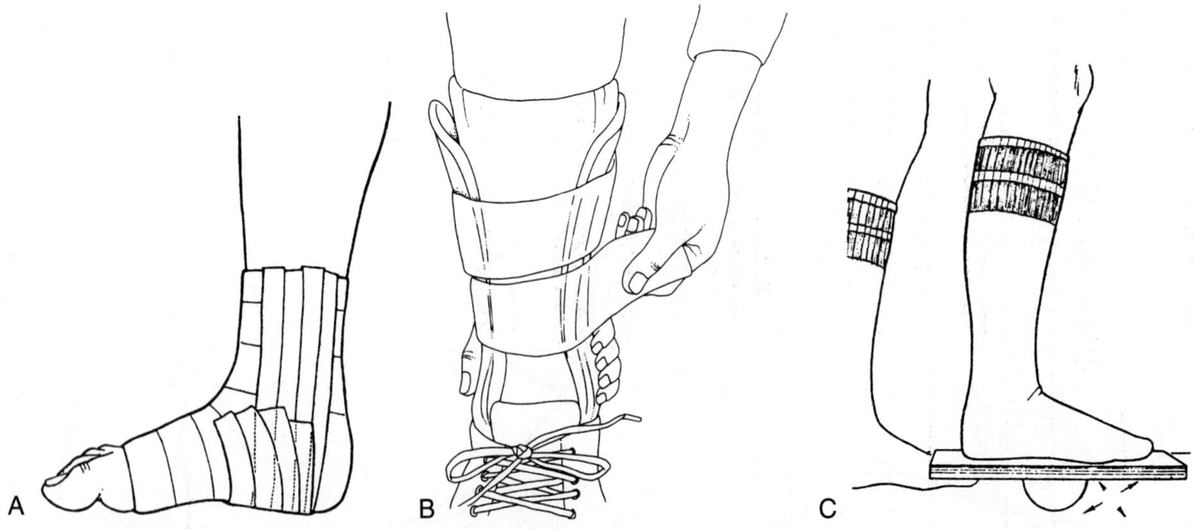

FIGURE 1-21 **A,** The most effective method of supporting most acute ankle sprains is by using an Ace wrap reinforced with 1-in medial and lateral tape strips. The anterior and posterior aspects of the ankle are left free to allow the patient to flex and extend the ankle. The patient is encouraged to bear weight with crutches. **B,** Diagram of an air splint. Straps are adjusted to heel size, the lower straps are wrapped about the ankle, and the side extensions are centered. The splint is then pressurized and straps adjusted until comfortable support and pressure are attained. **C,** As the ankle pain subsides, about the third to fifth day, balancing exercises can begin to allow the patient to regain ankle proprioception and avoid recurrent instability problems. (From Jardon OM, Mathews MS: Orthopedics. In Rakel RE [ed]: *Textbook of family practice,* ed 5, Philadelphia, 1995, WB Saunders.)

BASIC INFORMATION

DEFINITION

Ankylosing spondylitis is a chronic inflammatory condition involving the sacroiliac joints and axial skeleton characterized by ankylosis and enthesitis (inflammation at tendon insertions). It is one of a group of several overlapping syndromes, including spondylitis associated with Reiter's syndrome, psoriasis, and IBD. Patients are typically seronegative for the rheumatoid factor, and these disorders are now commonly called *rheumatoid variants* or *seronegative spondyloarthropathies*.

SYNONYMS

Marie-Strümpell disease

ICD-9CM CODES
720.0 Ankylosing spondylitis

EPIDEMIOLOGY & DEMOGRAPHICS

PREVALENCE: 0.15% of male population (rare in blacks)

PREDOMINANT AGE AT ONSET: 15 to 35 yr

PREDOMINANT SEX: Male:female ratio of 10:1

PHYSICAL FINDINGS & CLINICAL PRESENTATION

- Morning stiffness
- Fatigue, weight loss, anorexia, and other systemic complaints in more severe forms
- Bilateral sacroiliac tenderness (sacroiliitis)
- Limited lumbar spine motion (Fig. 1-22)
- Loss of chest expansion measured at the nipple line <2.5 cm, reflecting rib cage involvement

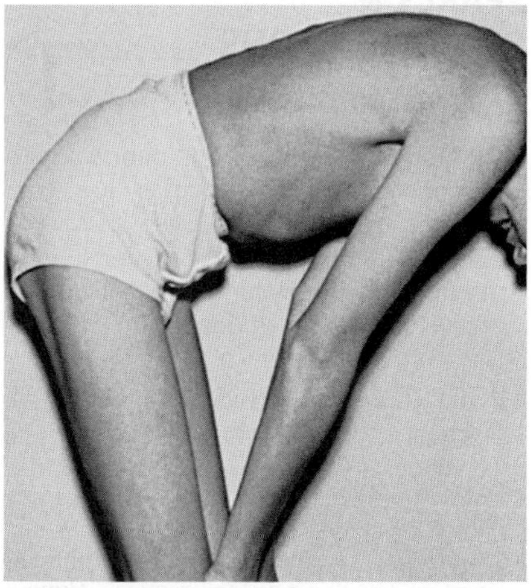

FIGURE 1-22 Loss of lumbodorsal spine mobility in a boy with ankylosing spondylitis: the lower spine remains straight when the patient bends forward. (From Behrman RE: *Nelson textbook of pediatrics,* Philadelphia, 1996, WB Saunders.)

- Occasionally, peripheral joint involvement (large joints are more commonly affected)
- Possible extraskeletal manifestations affecting the cardiovascular system (aortic insufficiency, heart block, cardiomegaly), lungs (pulmonary fibrosis), and eye (uveitis)
- Tenderness at tendon insertion sites, especially the Achilles tendons, plantar fascia
- Radiation below the knee is rare

ETIOLOGY

Unknown. Genetic factors play an important role. Destructive changes probably due to release of cytokines and tumor necrosis factor.

DIAGNOSIS

DIFFERENTIAL DIAGNOSIS

- Diffuse idiopathic skeletal hyperostosis (DISH, Forestier's disease)
- Other spondyloarthropathies
- A clinical algorithm for the evaluation of back pain is described in Section III

WORKUP

The modified New York criteria are often used for diagnosis:
- Low back pain of at least 3 mo duration improved by exercise and not relieved by rest
- Limitation of lumbar spine movement in sagittal and frontal planes
- Decreased chest expansion below normal values for age and sex
- Bilateral sacroiliitis of minimal grade or greater
- Unilateral sacroiliitis of moderate grade or greater

LABORATORY TESTS

- Elevated sedimentation rate, CRP
- Absence of rheumatoid factor and ANA
- Possible mild hyperchromic anemia
- Presence of HLA/B27 antigen in >90% of patients (although this antigen is often present in the general population)

IMAGING STUDIES

- Early roentgenographic features are those of bilateral sacroiliitis on plain films.
- Vertebral bodies may become demineralized and a typical "squaring off" occurs.
- With progression, calcification of the annulus fibrosus and paravertebral ligaments develop, giving rise to the so-called bamboo spine appearance.
- End result may be a forward protruding cervical spine and fixed dorsal kyphosis.
- MRI may be helpful in detecting early inflammatory lesions and is especially helpful when the history is suggestive but plain films are normal.

TREATMENT

NONPHARMACOLOGIC THERAPY

- Exercises primarily to maintain flexibility; general aerobic activity also important
- Postural training
  1. Patients must be instructed to sit in the erect position and to avoid stooping; otherwise, a flexion contracture of the spine may develop, which can become so severe that the patient cannot see forward.
  2. Sleeping should be in the supine position on a firm mattress; pillows should not be placed under the head or knees.

CHRONIC Rx

- NSAIDs: indomethacin is often successful in relieving symptoms; newer nonsteroidal agents may be tried as well.
- New research into the use of tumor necrosis factor antagonists such as etanercept appears promising.

DISPOSITION

- Most patients have a normal life span.
- The usual course of the disease is not life-threatening, but death may occur as a result of aortic insufficiency or secondary amyloidosis with renal disease.

REFERRAL

- Orthopedic consultation for pain or deformity
- Ophthalmologic consultation for ocular complications
- Rheumatology consultation for uncontrolled symptoms

PEARLS & CONSIDERATIONS

COMMENTS

Years may pass between the onset of symptoms and the ultimate diagnosis because of the frequency of nonspecific low back pain.

SUGGESTED READINGS

Davis JC Jr et al: Health-related quality of life outcomes in patients with active ankylosing spondylitis treated with adalimumab: results from a randomized controlled study, *Arthritis Rheum* 57(6):1050, 2007.

Heiberg MS et al: The comparative one-year performance of anti-tumor necrosis factor alpha drugs in patients with rheumatoid arthritis, psoriatic arthritis, and ankylosing spondylitis: results from a longitudinal, observational, multicenter study, *Arthritis Rheum* 59:234, 2008.

Zochling J, Braun J: Assessments in ankylosing spondylitis, *Best Pract Res Clin Rheumatol* 21(4):699, 2007.

AUTHOR: **LONNIE R. MERCIER, M.D.**

BASIC INFORMATION

DEFINITION

A fistula is an inflammatory tract with a secondary (external) opening in the perianal skin and a primary (internal) opening in the anal canal at the dentate line. It originates in an abscess in the intersphincteric space of the anal canal. Fistulas can be classified as follows:

1. Intersphincteric: fistula track passes within the intersphincteric plane to the perianal skin (most common)
2. Transsphincteric: fistula track passes from the internal opening, through the internal and external sphincter, and into the ischiorectal fossa to the perianal skin (frequent)
3. Suprasphincteric: after passing through the internal sphincter, fistula tract passes above the puborectalis and then tracts downward, lateral to the external sphincter, into the ischiorectal space to the perianal skin; uncommon; if abscess cavity extends cephalad, a supralevator abscess possibly palpable on rectal examination
4. Extrasphincteric: fistula tract passes from the rectum, above the levators, through the levator muscles to the ischiorectal space and perianal skin (rare)

With a horseshoe fistula, the tract passes from one ischiorectal fossa to the other behind the rectum.

SYNONYMS

Fistula-in-ano

ICD-9CM CODES
565.1 Anal fistula

EPIDEMIOLOGY & DEMOGRAPHICS

- Common in all ages
- Occurs equally in men and women
- Associated with constipation
- Pediatric age group: more common in infants; boys > girls

PHYSICAL FINDINGS & CLINICAL PRESENTATION

- Acute stage: perianal swelling, pain, and fever
- Chronic stage: history of rectal drainage or bleeding; previous abscess with drainage
- Tender external fistulous opening, with 2 to 3 cm of the anal verge, with purulent or serosanguineous drainage on compression; the greater the distance from the anal margin, the greater the probability of a complicated upward extension
- Goodsall's rule:
  1. Location of the internal opening related to the location of the external opening.
  2. With external opening anterior to an imaginary line drawn horizontally across the midpoint of the anus: fistulous tract runs radially into the anal canal.
  3. With opening posterior to the transanal line: tract is usually curvilinear, entering the anal canal in the posterior midline.
  4. Exception to this rule: an external, anterior opening that is >3 cm from the anus. In this case the tract may curve posteriorly and end in the posterior midline.
- If perianal abscess recurs, presence of a fistula is suggested

ETIOLOGY

- Most common: nonspecific cryptoglandular infection (skin or intestinal flora)
- Fistulas more common when intestinal microorganisms are cultured from the anorectal abscess
- Tuberculosis
- Lymphogranuloma venereum
- Actinomycosis
- Inflammatory bowel disease (IBD): Crohn's disease, ulcerative colitis
- Trauma: surgery (episiotomy, prostatectomy), foreign bodies, anal intercourse
- Malignancy: carcinoma, leukemia, lymphoma
- Treatment of malignancy: surgery, radiation

DIAGNOSIS

DIFFERENTIAL DIAGNOSIS

- Hidradenitis suppurativa
- Pilonidal sinus
- Bartholin's gland abscess or sinus
- Infected perianal sebaceous cysts

WORKUP

- Digital rectal examination:
  1. Assess sphincter tone and voluntary squeeze pressure
  2. Determine the presence of an extraluminal mass
  3. Identify an indurated track
  4. Palpate an internal opening or pit
- Gentle probing of external orifice to avoid creating a false tract; 50% do not have clinically detectable opening
- Anoscopy
- Proctosigmoidoscopy to exclude inflammatory or neoplastic disease
- All studies done under adequate anesthesia

LABORATORY TESTS

- CBC
- Rectal biopsy if diagnosis of IBD or malignancy suspected; biopsy of external orifice is useless

IMAGING STUDIES

- Colonoscopy or barium enema if:
  1. Diagnosis of IBD or malignancy is suspected
  2. History of recurrent or multiple fistulas
  3. Patient <25 yr old
- Small bowel series: occasionally obtained for reasons similar to above
- Fistulography: unreliable but may be helpful in complicated fistulas

TREATMENT

NONPHARMACOLOGIC THERAPY

Sitz baths

ACUTE GENERAL Rx

- Treatment of choice: surgery
- Broad-spectrum antibiotic given if:
  1. Cellulitis present
  2. Patient is immunocompromised
  3. Valvular heart disease present
  4. Prosthetic devices present
- Stool softener/laxative

CHRONIC Rx

- Surgery
- Surgical goals are as follows:
  1. Cure the fistula
  2. Prevent recurrence
  3. Preserve sphincter function
  4. Minimize healing time
- Methods for the management of anal fistulas: fistulotomy, setons, rectal advancement flaps, colostomy

DISPOSITION

Outpatient surgery

REFERRAL

Refer to a surgeon with expertise in this area.

PEARLS & CONSIDERATIONS

COMMENTS

- HIV-positive and diabetic patients with perirectal abscesses/fistulas are true surgical emergencies.
- Risk of septicemia, Fournier's gangrene, and other septic complications make immediate drainage imperative.

SUGGESTED READINGS

Pfenninger JL, Zainea GG: Common anorectal condition, *Am Fam Physician,* 64:22, 2001.

Rickard MJ: Anal abscesses and fistulas, *ANZ J Surg* 75(1–2):64, 2005.

Schwartz DA, Herdman CR: The medical treatment of Crohn's perianal fistulas, *Aliment Pharmacol Ther* 19(9):953, 2004.

AUTHORS: **GEORGE T. DANAKAS, M.D.,** and **RUBEN ALVERO, M.D.**

BASIC INFORMATION

DEFINITION

Anorexia nervosa is a psychiatric disorder characterized by abnormal eating behavior, severe self-induced weight loss, and a specific psychopathology (see "Workup").

ICD-9CM CODES
307.1 Anorexia nervosa

EPIDEMIOLOGY & DEMOGRAPHICS

INCIDENCE/PREVALENCE (IN U.S.):

- Anorexia nervosa occurs in 0.2% to 1.3% of the general population, with an annual incidence of 5 to 10 cases/100,000 persons.
- Participation in activities that promote thinness (athletics, modeling) is associated with a higher incidence of anorexia nervosa.

PREDOMINANT SEX: Female:male ratio is 9:1. Approximately 0.5% to 1% of women between the ages of 15 and 30 yr have anorexia nervosa.

PREDOMINANT AGE: Adolescence to young adulthood is the predominant age. Mean age of onset is 17 yr. Approximately 0.5% to 1% of college-aged women have anorexia nervosa.

PHYSICAL FINDINGS & CLINICAL PRESENTATION

Primary care physicians must be skilled at recognizing this disorder because patients with mild cases usually present with nonspecific symptoms such as asthenia, cold intolerance, lack of energy, or dizziness. The physical examination may be normal in the early stages or in mild cases. Patients with moderate to severe anorexia have the following physical characteristics:

- Patient is emaciated and bundled in clothing.
- Skin is dry and has excessive growth of lanugo. Skin may also be yellow-tinged from carotenodermia.
- Brittle nails, thinning scalp hair are present.
- Bradycardia, hypotension, hypothermia, and bradypnea are common.
- Female fat distribution pattern is no longer evident.
- Axillary and pubic hair is preserved.
- Peripheral edema may be present.

ETIOLOGY

- Etiology is unknown, but probably multifactorial (sociocultural, psychologic, familial, and genetic factors).
- A history of sexual abuse has been reported in as many as 50% of patients with anorexia nervosa.
- Psychologic factors: anorexics often have an incompletely developed personal identity. They struggle to maintain a sense of control over their environment, they usually have a low self-esteem, and they lack the sense that they are valued and loved for themselves.

DIAGNOSIS

DIFFERENTIAL DIAGNOSIS

- Depression with loss of appetite
- Schizophrenia
- Conversion disorder
- Occult carcinoma, lymphoma
- Endocrine disorders: Addison's disease, diabetes mellitus, hypothyroidism or hyperthyroidism, panhypopituitarism
- GI disorders: celiac disease, Crohn's disease, intestinal parasitosis
- Infectious disorders: AIDS, TB
- A clinical algorithm for the evaluation of anorexia is described in Section III

WORKUP

- A diagnosis can be made using the following DSM-IV diagnostic criteria for anorexia nervosa:
  1. Refusal to maintain body weight (BW) at or above a minimally normal weight for age and height (e.g., weight loss leading to maintenance of BW <85% of that expected or failure to make expected weight gain during a period of growth, leading to BW <85% of that expected)
  2. Intense fear of gaining weight or becoming fat, even though underweight
  3. Disturbance in the way in which BW or shape is experienced, undue influence of BW or shape on self-evaluation, or denial of the seriousness of the current low BW
  4. In postmenarchal females, amenorrhea, that is, the absence of at least three consecutive menstrual cycles (A woman is considered to have amenorrhea if her periods occur only following hormone, [e.g., estrogen] administration.)

Specify type:

Restricting type: During the current episode of anorexia nervosa, the person has not regularly engaged in binge-eating or purging behavior (i.e., self-induced vomiting or the misuse of laxatives, diuretics, or enemas).

Binge-eating/purging type: During the current episode of anorexia nervosa, the person has regularly engaged in binge-eating or purging behavior (i.e., self-induced vomiting or the misuse of laxatives, diuretics, or enemas).

- The SCOFF questionnaire is a useful screening tool used in England for eating disorders. It consists of the following five questions:
  1. Do you make yourself Sick because you feel full?
  2. Have you lost Control over how much you eat?
  3. Have you lost more than One stone (about 6 kg) recently?
  4. Do you believe yourself to be Fat when others say you are thin?
  5. Does Food dominate your life?
- A positive response to two or more questions has a reported sensitivity of 100% for anorexia and bulimia, and an overall specificity of 87.5%.
- In college-aged females a positive response to any of the following screening questions also warrants further evaluation:
  1. How many diets have you been on in the past year?
  2. Do you think you should be dieting?
  3. Are you dissatisfied with your body size?
  4. Does your weight affect the way you think about yourself?
- Baseline ECG should be performed on all patients with anorexia nervosa. Routine monitoring of patients with prolonged QT interval is necessary; sudden death in these patients is often caused by ventricular arrhythmias related to QT interval prolongation.
- A DEXA scan to screen for osteopenia should be considered after 6 months of amenorrhea in patients suspected of anorexia nervosa.

LABORATORY TESTS

- In mild cases, laboratory findings might be completely normal.
- Endocrine abnormalities:
  1. Decreased FSH, LH, T_4, T_3, estrogens, urinary 17-OH steroids, estrone, and estradiol
  2. Normal free T_4, TSH

3. Increased cortisol, GH, rT_3, T_3RU
4. Absence of cyclic surge of LH

- Leukopenia, thrombocytopenia, anemia, reduced ESR, reduced complement levels, and reduced CD4 and CD8 cells may be present.
- Metabolic alkalosis, hypocalcemia, hypokalemia, hypomagnesemia, hypercholesterolemia, and hypophosphatemia may be present.
- Increased plasma β-carotene levels are useful to distinguish these patients from others on starvation diets.

TREATMENT (Rx)

NONPHARMACOLOGIC THERAPY

- A multidisciplinary approach with psychologic, medical, and nutritional support is necessary.
- A goal weight should be set and the patient should be initially monitored at least once a week in the office setting. The target weight is 100% of ideal BW for teenagers and 90% to 100% for older patients.
- Weight gain should be gradual (1 to 3 lb/wk) to prevent gastric dilation. Begin with 800 to 1200 kcal in frequent small meals (to avoid bloating sensation), then increase calories to 1500 to 3000 depending on height and age.
- Add, as necessary, vitamin and mineral supplements.
- In severe cases, total parenteral nutrition must be used (starting at 800 to 1200 kcal/day).
- Electrolyte levels should be strictly monitored.
- Mealtime should be a time for social interaction, not confrontation.
- Postprandially, sedentary activities are recommended. The patient's access to a bathroom should be monitored to prevent purging.

ACUTE GENERAL Rx

- Criteria to decide on the appropriate initial course of treatment for patients with anorexia nervosa are usually based on the presence of complications, percentage of ideal body weight, and severity of body image distortion.
- Outpatient treatment is adequate for most patients.
- Indications for hospitalization are described in the "Referral" section.
- Medically stable patients who are within 85% of ideal body weight can be followed up by the primary care physician at 3- or 4-wk intervals, which can be lengthened as the patient improves.
- Pharmacologic treatment generally has no role in anorexia nervosa unless major depression or another psychiatric disorder is present. SSRIs can be used to alleviate the depressed mood and moderate obsessive-compulsive behavior in some individuals.

CHRONIC Rx

- Psychotherapy continued for years and focused specifically on self-image, family and peer interactions, and relapse prevention is an integral part of a successful recovery.
- Family therapy is also recommended, especially in younger patients.

DISPOSITION

- The long-term prognosis is generally poor and marked by recurrent exacerbations. The percentage of patients with anorexia nervosa who fully recover is modest. Most patients continue to suffer from a distorted body image, disordered eating habits, and psychic difficulties.
- Most patients with anorexia nervosa will recover menses within 6 months of reaching 90% of their ideal body weight. It is important to note that patients with anorexia nervosa can become pregnant despite amenorrhea.
- Mortality rates vary from 5% to 20% and are six times that of peers without anorexia. Frequent causes of death are electrolyte abnormalities, starvation, or suicide.
- Factors that predict improved outcome in patients with eating disorders include early age at diagnosis, brief interval before initiation of treatment, good parent-child relationships, and having other healthy relationships with friends or therapists.
- A prolonged QT interval is a marker for risk of sudden death.

REFERRAL

Hospitalization should be considered in the following situations:

1. Severe dehydration or electrolyte imbalance
2. ECG abnormalities (prolonged QT interval, arrhythmias)
3. Significant physiologic instability (hypotension, orthostatic changes)
4. Intractable vomiting, purging, or bingeing
5. Patient having suicidal thoughts
6. Weight loss exceeds 30% of ideal BW and is unresponsive to outpatient treatment
7. Rapidly progressing weight loss (>2 lbs in a week)
8. Failure to progress in nutritional rehabilitation in outpatient treatment

EVIDENCE (EBM)

A small randomized clinical trial (RCT) found limited evidence that fluoxetine reduced relapse in women discharged from hospital.[1] Ⓐ

Another RCT aimed to compare psychotherapy with dietary advice. Cognitive therapy led to significant improvements compared with baseline. There was a 100% withdrawal rate with dietary advice, thus making comparison between the groups impossible.[2] Ⓐ

Several small RCTs found no overall significant difference between different types of psychotherapy.[3] Ⓐ

Evidence-Based References

1. Kaye WH et al: Double-blind placebo-controlled administration of fluoxetine in restricting- and restricting-purging-type anorexia nervosa, *Soc Biol Psych* 49:644, 2001. Ⓐ
2. Serfaty MA: Cognitive therapy versus dietary counselling in the outpatient treatment of anorexia nervosa: effects of the treatment phase, *Eur Eat Dis Rev* 7:334, 1999. Ⓐ
3. Treasure J, Schmidt U: Anorexia nervosa. In *Clinical Evidence,* London, 2005, BMJ Publishing Group, p. 13. Ⓐ

SUGGESTED READINGS

American Psychiatric Association: Practice guideline for the treatment of patients with eating disorders, *Am J Psychiatry* 157(suppl):4, 2000 (revision).

Anstine D, Grinenko D: Rapid screening for disordered eating in college-aged females in the primary care setting, *J Adolesc Health* 26:338, 2000.

Mehler PS: Diagnosis and care of patients with anorexia nervosa in primary care setting, *Ann Intern Med* 134:1048, 2001.

Miller KK et al: Medical findings in outpatients with anorexia nervosa, *Arch Intern Med* 165:561, 2005.

Morgan JF et al: The SCOFF questionnaire: assessment of a new screening tool for eating disorders, *BMJ* 319:1467, 1999.

Pritts SD, Susman J: Diagnosis of eating disorders in primary care, *Am Fam Physician* 67:297, 2003.

Williams PM et al: Treating eating disorders in primary care, *Am Fam Physician* 77(2):187-195, 2008.

Yager J, Andersen AE: Anorexia nervosa, *N Engl J Med* 353:1481, 2005.

AUTHOR: **FRED F. FERRI, M.D.**

BASIC INFORMATION

DEFINITION

Anthrax is an acute infectious disease caused by the spore-forming bacterium *Bacillus anthracis*.

ICD-9CM CODES
022.0 Cutaneous anthrax
022.1 Inhalation anthrax
022.2 Gastrointestinal anthrax
022.3 Sepsis from anthrax

EPIDEMIOLOGY & DEMOGRAPHICS

- Anthrax most commonly occurs in hoofed animals and can only incidentally infect humans who come in contact with infected animals or animal products. Between 20,000 and 100,000 cases of cutaneous anthrax occur worldwide annually. In the U.S. the annual incidence was about 130 cases before 2001.
- Until the recent bioterrorism attack in 2001, most cases of anthrax occurred in industrial environments (contaminated raw materials used in manufacturing process) or in agriculture.
- In 2001 there were more than 20 confirmed cases of anthrax resulting from bioterrorism, most of which were associated with handling of contaminated mail. Inhalation anthrax is the most lethal form of anthrax and results from inspiration of 8000-50,000 spores of *Bacillus anthracis*. Before 2001 there had not been a case of inhalation anthrax in the U.S. for 20 years.
- Direct person-to-person spread of anthrax is extremely unlikely, if it occurs at all; therefore, there is no need to immunize or treat contacts of persons ill with anthrax, such as household contacts, friends, or co-workers, unless they also were exposed to the same source of infection.

PHYSICAL FINDINGS & CLINICAL PRESENTATION

Symptoms of disease vary depending on how the disease was contracted, but usually occur within 7 days after exposure. The serious forms of human anthrax are inhalation anthrax, cutaneous anthrax, and intestinal anthrax.

- **Inhalation anthrax** begins with a brief prodrome resembling a viral respiratory illness followed by development of hypoxia and dyspnea, with radiographic evidence of mediastinal widening. Host factors, dose of exposure, and chemoprophylaxis may affect the duration of the incubation period. Initial symptoms include mild fever, muscle aches, and malaise and may progress to respiratory failure and shock; meningitis often develops.
- **Cutaneous anthrax** is characterized by a skin lesion evolving from a papule, through a vesicular stage, to a depressed black eschar. The incubation period ranges from 1 to 12 days. The lesion is usually painless, but patients also may have fever, malaise, headache, and regional lymphadenopathy. The eschar dries and falls off in 1 to 2 wk with little scarring.
- **Gastrointestinal anthrax** is characterized by severe abdominal pain followed by fever and signs of septicemia. Bloody diarrhea and signs of acute abdomen may occur. This form of anthrax usually follows after eating raw or undercooked contaminated meat and can have an incubation period of 1 to 7 days. Gastric ulcers may occur and may be associated with hematemesis. An oropharyngeal and an abdominal form of the disease have been described. Involvement of the pharynx is usually characterized by lesions at the base of the tongue, dysphagia, fever, and regional lymphadenopathy. Lower bowel inflammation typically causes nausea, loss of appetite, and fever followed by abdominal pain, hematemesis, and bloody diarrhea.

ETIOLOGY

The disease is caused by *Bacillus anthracis,* a gram-positive, spore-forming bacillus. It is aerobic, nonmotile, nonhemolytic on sheep's blood agar, and grows readily at temperature of 37° C, forming large colonies with irregularly tapered outgrowths (a Medusa's head appearance). In the host it appears as single organisms or chains of two or three bacilli.

DIAGNOSIS

DIFFERENTIAL DIAGNOSIS

- Inhalation anthrax must be distinguished from influenza-like illness (ILI) and tularemia. Most cases of ILI are associated with nasal congestion and rhinorrhea, which are unusual in inhalation anthrax. Additional distinguishing factors are the usual absence of abnormal chest x-ray in ILI (see below).
- Cutaneous anthrax should be distinguished from staphylococcal disease, ecthyma, ecthyma gangrenosum, plague, brown recluse spider bite, and tularemia.
- The differential diagnosis of gastrointestinal anthrax includes viral gastroenteritis, shigellosis, and yersiniosis.

LABORATORY TESTS

- Presumptive identification is based on Gram stain of material from skin lesion, CSF, or blood showing encapsulated gram-positive bacilli.
- Confirmatory tests are performed at specialized labs. Virulent strains grow on nutrient agar in the presence of 5% CO_2. Susceptibility to lysis by gamma phage or DFA staining of cell-wall polysaccharide antigen are also useful confirmatory tests.
- Nasal swab culture to determine inhalation exposure is of limited diagnostic value. A negative result does not exclude the possibility of exposure. It may be used by public health officials to assist in epidemiologic investigations of exposed persons to evaluate the dispersion of spores.
- Serologic testing by enzyme-linked immunosorbent assay (ELISA) can confirm the diagnosis.
- A skin test (Anthracin Test) that detects anthrax cell-mediated immunity is also available in specialized labs.

IMAGING STUDIES

Chest x-ray usually reveals mediastinal widening. Additional findings include infiltrates and pleural effusion.

TREATMENT

NONPHARMACOLOGIC THERAPY

IV hydration and ventilator support may be necessary in inhalation anthrax

ACUTE GENERAL THERAPY

- Most naturally occurring *B. anthracis* strains are sensitive to penicillin. The FDA has approved penicillin, doxycycline, and ciprofloxacin for the treatment of inhalational anthrax infection.
- Table 1-4 describes a treatment protocol for inhalation anthrax.

- Initial postexposure prophylaxis therapy in adults is with ciprofloxacin, 500 mg PO bid or doxycycline 100 mg bid. The total duration of treatment is 60 days.

DISPOSITION

- Case fatality estimates for inhalation anthrax are extremely high (>90%).
- The case fatality rate for cutaneous anthrax is 20% without and <1% with antibiotic treatment.
- The case fatality rate for gastrointestinal anthrax is estimated to be 25% to 60%.

REFERRAL

Consultation with an infectious disease specialist is recommended in all cases of anthrax. Local and state authorities should also be notified of suspected cases of anthrax.

PEARLS & CONSIDERATIONS

COMMENTS

- Postexposure prophylaxis: If the exposure to *B. anthracis* is confirmed and anthrax vaccine is available, 3 doses of the vaccine should be given at 0, 2, and 4 wk, and antibiotics should be continued throughout the 4-wk period. If vaccine is not available, antibiotics should be continued for 60 days.
- Preexposure vaccination is limited to groups at risk for repeated exposures to *B. anthracis* spores, such as bioterrorism level-B laboratories and workers who will be making repeated entries into known *B. anthracis* spore-contaminated areas.
- The U.S. anthrax vaccine is an inactivated cellfree product licensed to be given in a 6-dose series.

SUGGESTED READINGS

Holty JE et al: Systematic review: A century of inhalational anthrax cases from 1900 to 2005, *Ann Intern Med* 144:270, 2006.

Hupert N et al: Accuracy of screening for inhalational anthrax after a bioterrorist attack, *Ann Intern Med* 139:337, 2003.

Inglesby TV et al: Anthrax as a biological weapon, 2002, *JAMA* 287:2236, 2002.

Interim guidelines for investigation of and response to *Bacillus anthracis* exposures, *MMWR* 50:987, 2001.

Post-exposure anthrax prophylaxis, *Med Lett Drugs Ther* 43:91, 2001.

Swartz MN: Recognition and management of anthrax: an update, *N Engl J Med* 345:1621, 2001.

Use of anthrax vaccine for pre-exposure vaccination, *MMWR Morb Mortal Wkly Rep* 51:1024, 2002.

AUTHOR: **FRED F. FERRI, M.D.**

TABLE 1-4 Inhalation Anthrax Treatment Protocol[a,b]

Category	Initial Therapy (Intravenous)[c,d]	Duration
Adults	Ciprofloxacin 400 mg every 12 hr[a] **or** Doxycycline 100 mg every 12 hr[f] **and** One or two additional antimicrobials[d]	IV treatment initially.[e] Switch to oral antimicrobial therapy when clinically appropriate: Ciprofloxacin 500 mg PO bid **or** Doxycycline 100 mg PO bid Continue for 60 days (IV and PO combined)[g]
Children	Ciprofloxacin 10-15 mg/kg every 12 hr[h,i] **or** Doxycycline[f,j]: >8 yr and >45 kg: 100 mg every 12 hr >8 yr and ≤45 kg: 2.2 mg/kg every 12 hr ≤8 yr: 2.2 mg/kg every 12 hr **and** One or two additional antimicrobials[d]	IV treatment initially.[e] Switch to oral antimicrobial therapy when clinically appropriate: Ciprofloxacin 10-15 mg/kg PO every 12 hr[i] **or** Doxycycline[j]: >8 yr and >45 kg: 100 mg PO bid >8 yr and ≤45 kg: 2.2 mg/kg PO bid ≤8 yr: 2.2 mg/kg PO bid Continue for 60 days (IV and PO combined)[g]
Pregnant women[k]	Same for nonpregnant adults (the high death rate from the infection outweighs the risk posed by the antimicrobial agent)	IV treatment initially. Switch to oral antimicrobial therapy when clinically appropriate.[b] Oral therapy regimens same for nonpregnant adults
Immunocompromised persons	Same for nonimmunocompromised persons and children	Same for nonimmunocompromised persons and children

MMRW 5:987, 2001.

[a]For gastrointestinal and oropharyngeal anthrax, use regimens recommended for inhalational anthrax.

[b]Ciprofloxacin or doxycycline should be considered an essential part of first-line therapy for inhalational anthrax.

[c]Steroids may be considered as an adjunct therapy for patients with severe edema and for meningitis based on experience with bacterial meningitis of other etiologies.

[d]Other agents with in vitro activity include rifampin, vancomycin, penicillin, ampicillin, chloramphenicol, imipenem, clindamycin, and clarithromycin. Because of concerns of constitutive and inducible beta-lactamases in *Bacillus anthracis,* penicillin and ampicillin should not be used alone. Consultation with an infectious disease specialist is advised.

[e]Initial therapy may be altered based on clinical course of the patient; one or two antimicrobial agents (e.g., ciprofloxacin or doxycycline) may be adequate as the patient improves.

[f]If meningitis is suspected, doxycycline may be less optimal because of poor central nervous system penetration.

[g]Because of the potential persistence of spores after an aerosol exposure, antimicrobial therapy should be continued for 60 days.

[h]If intravenous ciprofloxacin is not available, oral ciprofloxacin may be acceptable because it is rapidly and well absorbed from the gastrointestinal tract with no substantial loss by first-pass metabolism. Maximum serum concentrations are attained 1-2 hours after oral dosing but may not be achieved if vomiting or ileus are present.

[i]In children, ciprofloxacin dosage should not exceed 1 g/day.

[j]The American Academy of Pediatrics recommends treatment of young children with tetracyclines for serious infections (e.g., Rocky Mountain spotted fever).

[k]Although tetracyclines are not recommended during pregnancy, their use may be indicated for life-threatening illness. Adverse effects on developing teeth and bones are dose related; therefore, doxycycline might be used for a short time (7-14 days) before 6 months of gestation.

BASIC INFORMATION

DEFINITION

The antiphospholipid antibody syndrome (APS) is characterized by arterial or venous thrombosis and/or pregnancy loss *and* the presence of antiphospholipid antibodies (aPL). APL are antibodies directed against either phospholipids or proteins bound to anionic phospholipids. Three types of aPL have been characterized:

- Lupus anticoagulants
- Anticardiolipin antibodies
- Anti-β2 glycoprotein-1 antibodies

The syndrome is referred to as primary APS when it occurs alone and as secondary APS when in association with systemic lupus erythematosus (SLE), other rheumatic disorders, or certain infections or medications. APS can affect all organ systems and includes venous and arterial thrombosis, recurrent fetal losses, and thrombocytopenia.

ICD-9CM CODES
795.79 Antiphospholipid antibody syndrome

EPIDEMIOLOGY & DEMOGRAPHICS

PREVALENCE:

- 1% to 5% of healthy individuals have anticardiolipin (ACL) and lupus anticoagulant (LA) antibodies.
- 12% to 30% of patients with systemic lupus erythematosus have ACL and 15% to 34% have LA antibodies.

PREDOMINANT AGE: Young to middle-age adults.

RISK FACTORS:

- Underlying SLE and collagen-vascular diseases; other autoimmune disorders including rheumatoid arthritis, Sjögren's syndrome, Behçet's syndrome, and ITP; AIDS.
- Most individuals are otherwise healthy and have no underlying medical condition.
- Several studies assessing presence of aPL in patients with cardiovascular and cerebrovascular disease have found a higher than expected prevalence of antibody.

GENETICS: Some APS-positive families exist, and human leukocyte antigen (HLA) studies have suggested associations with HLA DR7, DR4, and Dqw7 plus Drw53.

PHYSICAL FINDINGS & CLINICAL PRESENTATION

- **Thrombosis:** Patients with APS are at risk for both venous and arterial thromboses. Venous thromboses are more common, occurring as the initial manifestation of APS in approximately 30% of APS patients. Of all patients with venous thrombosis, 5% to 20% have aPL. The most common site for deep vein thrombosis is the calf, but thromboses may also occur in the renal, hepatic, axillary, subclavian, vena cava, and retinal veins. The most common site of arterial thrombosis is the cerebral vessels. Other common sites are the coronary, renal, mesenteric, and bypass arteries. Recurrent thrombosis is common with APS.
- **Central nervous system:** stroke, TIA, migraine, multiinfarct dementia, epilepsy, movement disorders, transverse myelopathy, depression, and Guillain-Barré syndrome.
- **Pulmonary:** pulmonary embolism and infarction, pulmonary HTN, ARDS, intraalveolar pulmonary hemorrhage, a postpartum syndrome characterized by fever, pleuritic chest pain, dyspnea, and patchy infiltrates with pleural effusion on CXR.
- **Cardiology:** Libman-Sacks endocarditis, intracardiac thrombosis, CAD, MI
- **Gastrointestinal:** abdominal pain, GI bleed secondary to ischemia, splenic or pancreatic infarction, hepatic vein thrombosis, Budd-Chiari syndrome (second most common cause of BCS).
- **Renal:** proteinuria, acute renal failure, HTN, renal infarct, renal artery or vein thrombosis, postpartum hemolytic-uremic syndrome.
- **Hematology:** thrombocytopenia, hemolytic anemia.
- **Endocrine:** Addison's disease secondary to adrenal hemorrhage and less frequently thrombosis.
- **Cutaneous:** livedo reticularis, cutaneous necrosis, skin ulcerations, gangrene of digits.
- **Obstetrics:** recurrent spontaneous abortion (secondary to placental vessel thrombosis and ischemia).
- **Catastrophic APS:** widespread thrombotic disease with visceral damage. To make the diagnosis of catastrophic APS, four criteria must be satisfied:
  1. Evidence of involvement of ≥3 organs, systems, and/or tissues
  2. Development of manifestations simultaneously or in ≤1 week
  3. Confirmation by histopathology of small vessel occlusion in at least one organ or tissue
  4. Laboratory confirmation of the presence of aPL

ETIOLOGY

- APL react with negatively charged phospholipids.
- Possible mechanisms of thrombosis include effects of aPL on platelet membranes, endothelial cells, and clotting components such as prothrombin, protein C or S.
- Recently shown that prephospholipids are not immunogenic and that a binding protein (β_2-glycoprotein I) may be the key immunogen in the APS.

DIAGNOSIS

DIFFERENTIAL DIAGNOSIS

Other hypercoagulable states (inherited or acquired)

- Inherited: ATIII, protein C, S deficiences, Factor V Leiden, prothrombin gene mutation
- Acquired: heparin-induced thrombocytopenia, myeloproliferative syndromes, cancer, hyperviscosity
- Hyperhomocysteinemia
- Nephrotic syndrome

WORKUP

Diagnostic criteria of APS include at least one clinical criterion and at least one laboratory criterion.

- *Clinical:*
  1. venous, arterial, or small vessel thrombosis *or*
  2. morbidity with pregnancy defined as
     - fetal death at ≥10 wk gestation *or*
     - ≥1 premature births before 34 wk gestation secondary to eclampsia, preeclampsia, or severe placental insufficiency *or*
     - ≥3 unexplained consecutive spontaneous abortions at <10 wk gestation
- *Laboratory:*
  1. IgG and/or IgM anticardiolipin antibody in medium or high titers *or*
  2. Lupus anticoagulant activity found *or*
  3. Anti-β2 glycoprotein-1 IgM or IgG antibodies found on ≥2 occasions, at least 12 wk apart

LABORATORY TESTS

Laboratory testing of ACL and LA antibodies indicated in:

- Patient with underlying SLE or collagen-vascular disease with thrombosis
- Patient with recurrent, familial, or juvenile DVT or thrombosis in an unusual location (mesenteric or cerebral)
- Possibly in patients with lupus or lupus-like disorders in high-risk situations (e.g., surgery, prolonged immobilization, pregnancy)

Abnormal tests include:

- False-positive test for syphilis (RPR/VDRL)
- Lupus anticoagulant activity, demonstrated by prolongation of aPTT that does not correct with 1:1 mixing study
- Presence of anticardiolipin antibodies (ELISA for anticardiolipin is most sensitive and specific test [>80%])
- Presence of anti β_2-glycoprotein I antibody

TREATMENT

Rx

ACUTE GENERAL Rx

- For positive aPL and venous thrombosis:
  - Initial anticoagulation with heparin, then lifelong warfarin treatment, INR 2.0 to 3.0
- For positive aPL with arterial thrombosis:
  - Cerebral arterial thrombosis: ASA 325 mg daily or warfarin therapy (INR 1.4 to 2.8)
  - Noncerebral arterial thrombosis: Warfarin therapy (INR 2.0 to 3.0)
- For pregnant women with previously diagnosed APS:
  - Warfarin should be discontinued secondary to its teratogenic effects.
  - ASA, 81 mg, and heparin SQ to PTT of 1.5 to 2 times control value.
  - IVIG and prednisone have also been used with success if aspirin and heparin fail.
- For pregnant women with (+) aPL antibodies and a history of <3 spontaneous abortions:
  - ASA 81 mg daily at conception and SQ heparin 5,000 to 10,000 IU q12h at time of documented viable intrauterine pregnancy (approximately 7 wk gestation) until 6 wk postpartum.
  - A mid-interval PTT should be checked and should be normal or similar to baseline before therapy.
- For pregnant women with (+) aPL antibodies without a history of DVT or pregnancy loss:
  - Consider low-dose SQ heparin, ASA 81 mg, or surveillance.
- For catastrophic APS:
  - Highest survival rate achieved with the combination of anticoagulation, corticosteroids, and IVIG or plasma exchange.
  - Case reports of Rituximab as successful therapy for patients with life-threatening thrombosis refractory to anticoagulation.

CHRONIC Rx

- Anticoagulation with warfarin therapy.
- Immunosuppressive agents such as corticosteriods and cyclophosphamide not effective.
- Limited data suggest that hydroxychloroquine may be effective.

DISPOSITION

- APS patients have a 20% to 70% risk for recurrent thrombosis.
- Initial arterial thrombosis tends to be followed by arterial events, and initial venous thrombosis tends to be followed by venous events.
- Catastrophic APS is associated with a high mortality rate, approaching 50%.
- Incidence of developing catastrophic APS is approximately 0.8% among APS patients.

REFERRAL

To hematology and/or obstetric medicine when diagnosis is made

PEARLS & CONSIDERATIONS

!

COMMENTS

Cerebral features of lupus may be more related to thrombosis than inflammation and may respond better to anticoagulants than immunosuppression.

PREVENTION

Prophylaxis for asymptomatic patients with (+) aPL without previous thrombosis:

- No routine prophylaxis is recommended.
- Questionable whether ASA 81 mg daily is effective.
- Antithrombotic prophylaxis for major surgery, prolonged immobilization, and pregnancy.
- Avoid oral contraceptive pills in women with (+) aPL.

EVIDENCE

EBM

Target INR of 2.0 to 3.0 for warfarin therapy in patients with APS:

- One prospective analysis of 147 patients comparing warfarin therapy (INR >3.0) to warfarin therapy (INR <3.0) to aspirin demonstrated the following:
  - Aspirin alone appears to be of no benefit for the thrombotic manifestations of APS.
  - Low-intensity warfarin (INR <3.0), with or without low-dose aspirin, reduced the rate of thrombosis from 30% to 23% per year.
  - High-intensity warfarin (INR >3.0) reduced the risk of thrombosis from 30% to 1.3% per year.[1]
- Two recent randomized, double blind trials comparing warfarin therapy (INR 2.0 to 3.0) vs. warfarin therapy (INR 3.0 to 4.0) in patients with APS demonstrated the following:
  - No difference in thrombosis rate or bleeding events and therefore target INR of 2.0 to 3.0 may be appropriate for patients with APS.[2,3]
- Treatment of arterial cerebral thrombosis:
  - A large randomized controlled trial comparing adjusted-dose warfarin (target INR 1.4 to 2.8) to aspirin 325 mg/day for prevention of recurrent ischemia demonstrated similar rates of recurrence in patients with or without antiphospholipid antibodies.[4]

Evidence-Based References

1. Khamashta MA: The management of thrombosis in the antiphospholipid-antibody syndrome, *N Engl J Med* 332:993, 1995.
2. Crowther MA et al: A comparison of two intensities of warfarin for the prevention of recurrent thrombosis in patients with the antiphospholipid antibody syndrome, *N Engl J Med* 359(12):1133, 2003.
3. Finazzi G et al: A randomized clinical trial of high-intensity warfarin vs. conventional antithrombotic therapy for the prevention of recurrent thrombosis in patients with the antiphospholipid antibody syndrome, *J Thromb Haemost* 3:848, 2005.
4. Levine SR et al: APASS Investigators. Antiphospholipid antibodies and subsequent thrombo-occlusive events in patients with ischemic stroke, *JAMA* 291:576, 2004.

SUGGESTED READINGS

Ahn ER et al: Long-term remission from life-threatening hypercoagulable state associated with lupus anticoagulant (LA) following rituximab therapy, *Am J Hematol* 78(2): 127, 2005.

Asherson RA et al: Catastrophic antiphospholipid syndrome: international consensus statement on classification criteria and treatment guidelines, *Lupus* 12:530, 2003.

Erkan D and Lockshin MD: New treatments for antiphospholipid syndrome, *Rheumatic Disease Clinics of North America* 32:129, 2006.

Lim W et al: Management of antiphospholipid antibody syndrome: a systematic review, *JAMA* 295(9):1050, 2006.

Miyakis S et al: International consensus statement on an update of the classification criteria for definite antiphospholipid syndrome, *J Thromb Haemost* 4:295, 2006.

Rubenstein E et al: Rituximab treatment for resistant antiphospholipid syndrome, *J Rheumatol* 33(2):355, 2006.

AUTHOR: **IRIS TONG, M.D.**

BASIC INFORMATION

DEFINITION

Generalized anxiety disorder (GAD) is most likely to present in combination with other psychiatric and medical conditions. GAD commonly presents with excessive anxiety, fear, and worry for most of the time, continuously for at least 6 mo. The subjective anxiety must be accompanied by at least three somatic symptoms (e.g., restlessness, irritability, sleep disturbance, muscle tension, difficulty concentrating, or fatigability). Because worry is also a symptom of depression, officially, GAD is not present if there is a concurrent major depression. However, the field is recognizing that the two conditions can coexist, and research on the commonalities is being conducted.

SYNONYMS

Anxiety neurosis
Chronic anxiety
GAD

ICD-9CM CODES
F41.1 (DSM-IV Code 300.02)

EPIDEMIOLOGY & DEMOGRAPHICS

INCIDENCE (IN U.S.): 31% in 1 yr
PEAK INCIDENCE: Chronic condition with onset in early life
PREVALENCE (IN U.S.):
- In general population: prevalence of 5% lifetime
- In primary care setting: 3% (It is the most common anxiety disorder in this setting.)

PREDOMINANT SEX: Females are more frequently affected (2:1 ratio), but they present for treatment less frequently (3:2 female:male).
PREDOMINANT AGE:
- 30% of patients report onset of symptoms before age 11 yr.
- 50% of patients have onset before age 18 yr.

GENETICS: Concordance rates in dizygotic twins and monozygotic twins are not different (0% to 5%), but detailed analysis of 1033 female twin pairs finds that heredity contributes about 30% of the factors that may cause GAD.

PHYSICAL FINDINGS & CLINICAL PRESENTATION

- Report of being "anxious" all of their lives.
- Excessive worry, usually regarding family, finances, work, or health.
- Sleep disturbance, particularly early insomnia.
- Muscle tension (typically in the muscles of neck and shoulders).
- Headaches (muscle tension).
- Difficulty concentrating.
- Day form of fatigue.
- Gastrointestinal symptoms compatible with IBD (one third of patients).
- Physical consequences of anxiety are the driving force for patients seeking medical attention.
- Comorbid psychiatric illness (e.g., dysthymia or major depression) and substance abuse (e.g., alcohol abuse) are frequent.

ETIOLOGY

- There is no clear etiology.
- Several hypotheses centering on neurotransmitter (catecholamines, indolamines) and developmental psychology are used as framework for treatment recommendations.
- Risk factors include a family history, increase in stress, history of physical or emotional trauma, and medical illness.

DIAGNOSIS

DIFFERENTIAL DIAGNOSIS

- Wide range of psychiatric and medical conditions; however, for a diagnosis of GAD to be made a person must experience anxiety with coexisting physical symptoms the majority of the time continuously for at least 6 mo.
- Cardiovascular and pulmonary disease.
- Hyperthyroidism.
- Parkinson's disease.
- Myasthenia gravis.
- Consequence of recreational drug use (e.g., cocaine, amphetamine, and PCP) or withdrawal (e.g., alcohol or benzodiazepines).

WORKUP

- History: required for diagnosis.
- Physical examination: confirm the patient's physical complaints.
- Exclusion of organic basis for the complaints possibly requiring additional workup.
- Physical cause should be suspected if anxiety follows recent changes in medication.

TREATMENT

NONPHARMACOLOGIC THERAPY

- Cognitive-behavioral therapy
- Relaxation training
- Biofeedback
- Psychodynamic psychotherapy

PHARMACOLOGIC THERAPY

- Benzodiazepines
- Azapirones
- SSRIs

ACUTE GENERAL Rx

- Acute treatment is rarely indicated because GAD is a chronic condition.
- Occasionally, patients are in acute distress, requiring physician to respond quickly; benzodiazepines are given under these conditions as drug of choice for both daytime anxiety and initial insomnia.

NOTE: Caution should be taken in prescribing benzodiazepines because of the propensity for misuse and dependence in this population. If provided, the patient should be educated about the use of other medications and the risks in using benzodiazepines.

CHRONIC Rx

- SSRIs, venlafaxine, and duloxetine are also effective in generalized anxiety disorders and are typically given as a first line treatment. These are particularly useful if comorbid depression is present. A recent, 4-week double blind trial indicates that 300 mg pregabalin (Lyrica) may be superior to venlafaxine, the standard medication treatment for GAD.
- If used and prescribed with supervision, benzodiazepines can provide long-term symptom control with only occasional problems with tolerance or abuse; however, tolerance to benzodiazepines is common and for this reason they have fallen from a first line treatment to second line treatment for GAD. Further, the rate of relapse after discontinuation of benzodiazepines may be twice the rate after discontinuation of the available nonbenzodiazepine anxiolytic buspirone.
- Buspirone is effective without any potential for tolerance or abuse.
- Sedating antidepressants are also useful in ameliorating initial insomnia.

DISPOSITION

- This condition is chronic with periodic exacerbations.
- Treatment is given to provide a significant degree of improvement, but symptoms and dysfunction may persist.
- The risk for suicide is higher than general population.

REFERRAL

- If the symptoms are refractory to treatment
- If the case is complicated with a comorbid psychiatric condition
- If treatment response is suboptimal with residual dysfunction

PEARLS & CONSIDERATIONS

One recent study found that escitalopram (Lexapro) had fewer side effects and better outcomes for GAD than paroxetine (Paxil).

EVIDENCE

A recent Cochrane review of Azapirones (e.g. Buspirone) concluded that while they are a useful intervention, particularly for those who have never been treated with benzodiazepines, they are potentially not as acceptable as benzodiazepines.[1]

Kava kava has also been investigated as an intervention for GAD, but recent research finds no affect on symptoms.[2]

Studies directly comparing medications with psychotherapy are not available, but the general clinical impression is that the psychotherapies are probably superior to pharmacotherapies. The only exception is in the treatment of GAD in late life; research suggests that selective serotonin reuptake inhibitors (SSRIs) are superior to cognitive behavior therapy (CBT) for late life GAD.[3]

Buspirone is an effective treatment for GAD.[4,5] There is evidence for the efficacy of benzodiazepines in the management of anxiety.[4] There is evidence for the efficacy of antidepressants in the management of anxiety, in particular duloxetine.[6,7] Further research is needed to determine which agents are likely to be most beneficial for which type of patient.[7]

There is evidence that cognitive therapy is effective for the management of generalized anxiety disorder but that relaxation therapy alone is as good as CBT in treating GAD.[4,8]

Evidence-Based References

1. Chessick et al: Azapirones for generalized anxiety disorder, *Cochrane Database Syst Rev* 3:CD006115, 2006.
2. Connor et al: Kava in generalized anxiety disorder: three placebo-controlled trials, *Int Clin Psychpharmacol* 21(5):249, 2006.
3. Schuurmans et al: A randomized, controlled trial of the effectiveness of cognitive-behavioral therapy and sertraline versus a waitlist control group for anxiety disorders in older adults, *Am J Geriatr Psychiatry* 14(3):255, 2006.
4. Gould RA et al: Cognitive behavioural and pharmacological treatment of generalised anxiety disorder: a preliminary meta-analysis, *Behav Res Ther* 28:285, 1997. Ⓐ
5. Sramek JJ et al: Efficacy of buspirone in generalized anxiety disorder with coexisting mild depressive symptoms, *J Clin Psychiatry* 57:287-291, 1996. Reviewed in: Clinical Evidence 12:1435-1457, 2004. Ⓐ
6. Kapczinski F et al: Antidepressants for generalized anxiety disorder, *Cochrane Database Syst Rev* 2:2003. Ⓐ
7. Davidson JR et al: Efficacy, safety and tolerability of venlafaxine extended release and buspirone in outpatients with generalised anxiety disorder, *J Clin Psychiatry* 60:528, 1999. Reviewed in: Clinical Evidence 12:1435-1457, 2004. Ⓐ
8. Westen D, Morrison K: A multidimensional meta-analysis of treatments for depression, panic and generalized anxiety disorder: an empirical examination of the status of empirically supported therapies, *J Consult Clin Psychol* 69:875-689, 2001. Reviewed in: Clinical Evidence 12:1435-1457, 2004. Ⓐ

SUGGESTED READINGS

Fricchione G: Clinical practice. Generalized anxiety disorder, *N Engl J Med* 351(7):675, 2004.

Lang AJ: Treating generalized anxiety disorder with cognitive-behavioral therapy, *J Clin Psychiatry* 65(suppl 13):14, 2004.

Nutt D et al: Generalized anxiety disorder: A comorbid disease, *Eur Neuropsychopharmacol* 16(2):S109, 2006.

Rickels K et al: Pregabalin for treatment of generalized anxiety disorder: a 4-week, multicenter, double-blind, placebo-controlled trial of pregabalin and alprazolam, *Arch Gen Psychiatry* 62(9):1022, 2005.

AUTHORS: **PATRICIA AREAN, PH.D.,** and **MITCHELL D. FELDMAN, M.D., M.PHIL.**

BASIC INFORMATION

DEFINITION

Aortic dissection occurs when blood passes through an intimal tear, separating the intima from the medial layers and creating a false lumen.

SYNONYMS Dissecting aortic aneurysm

ICD-9CM CODES
441.00 Aortic dissection
444.01 Aortic dissection, thoracic

EPIDEMIOLOGY & DEMOGRAPHICS

PREDOMINANT SEX: Males > females
PEAK INCIDENCE: Ages 60 to 80; mean 63
RISK FACTORS:

- Hypertension
- Atherosclerosis
- Family history of aortic aneurysms/dissection
- History of cardiac surgery, intraaortic catheterization
- Disorders of collagen (Marfan syndrome, Ehlers-Danlos syndrome)
- Vascular inflammation (giant cell arteritis, Takayasu arteritis, rheumatoid arthritis, syphillitic aortitis)
- Aortic coarctation, bicuspid aortic valve
- Turner's syndrome
- Cocaine abuse
- Trauma

CLASSIFICATION

Two main classification schemes based on the location of dissection (Fig. 1-23):

- DeBakey: type I ascending and descending aorta, II ascending aorta, III descending aorta
- Stanford: type A ascending aorta (proximal), type B descending aorta (distal)

PHYSICAL FINDINGS & CLINICAL PRESENTATION

- Sudden onset of severe sharp, tearing, or ripping chest pain
- Anterior chest pain (ascending dissection)
- Back pain, abdominal pain (descending dissection)

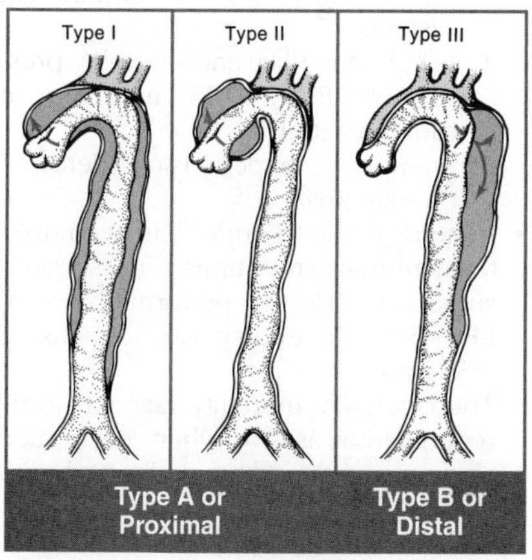

FIGURE 1-23 Classification systems for aortic dissection. (From Isselbacher EM, Eagle KA, DeSanctis RW: Disease of the aorta. In Braunwald E [ed]: *Heart disease: a textbook of cardiovascular medicine,* ed 5, Philadelphia, 1997, WB Saunders.)

- Syncope, congestive heart failure (CHF), malperfusion may occur
- Most present with severe hypertension, 25% with hypotension (systolic blood pressure <100), which can indicate bleeding, cardiac tamponade, or severe aortic regurgitation
- Pulse and blood pressure differentials (>20 mm Hg between arms) in 9% to 30% of cases, caused by partial compression of subclavian arteries
- Aortic regurgitation in 18% to 50% of cases of proximal dissection, often with diastolic decrescendo murmur
- Myocardial ischemia caused by coronary artery occlusion
- Stroke in 5% to 10% of patients

ETIOLOGY

- Degeneration or alteration of the intimal and medial layers seems to be the common pathology involved with acquired (e.g., hypertension, vascular inflammation) and genetic (e.g., collagen vascular disease) risk factors for dissection.
- Aortic dissection reflects systemic illness of vasculature.

DIAGNOSIS

DIFFERENTIAL DIAGNOSIS

- Known as the great imitator: PE, ACS, aortic stenosis/insufficiency, nondissecting aneurysm, pericarditis, cholecystitis, peptic ulcer disease, pancreatitis.
- Acute MI needs to be ruled out.
- Consider aortic dissection in patients with unexplained stroke, chest pain, syncope, acute onset CHF, abdominal pain, back pain, malperfusion of extremities or internal organs.

LABORATORY TESTS

- ECG: helpful to rule out MI, although dissection can lead to coronary ischemia
- Currently no readily available, reliable serum biomarker
- Smooth muscle myosin heavy chain protein (released from damaged medial smooth muscle), CRP, fibrinogen, D-dimer, and elastin fragments under investigation

IMAGING STUDIES

- Chest x-ray may show widened mediastinum (62%) and displacement of aortic intimal calcium.
- Transesophageal echocardiography (TEE) is study of choice in unstable patients, but operator dependent.
- MRI has the highest sensitivity and specificity but limited availability; not suitable for unstable patients; contraindicated with pacemakers, metal devices.
- Helical CT is least operator dependent, but involves intravenous contrast.
- TEE, MRI, helical CT are imaging modalities of choice. Sensitivities (98% to 100%) and specificities (95% to 98%) nearly equal in skilled hands. Test of choice depends on clinical circumstances and availability.
- With medium or high pretest probability, a second diagnostic test should be done if the first is negative.
- Transthoracic echocardiography has poor sensitivity
- Aortography rarely done now.

TREATMENT

ACUTE GENERAL Rx

- Admit to ICU for monitoring.
- Target SBP 100 to 120, heart rate <60 to reduce aortic wall stress.
- IV beta-blockers are cornerstones of treatment.
- Propanolol 1 mg every 3 to 5 min; metoprolol 5 mg IV every 5 min; or labetalol 20 mg IV, then 20 to 80 mg every 10 min, followed by nitroprusside 0.3 to 10 mg/kg/min.
- Nitroprusside should not be used without beta-blockade because vasodilation can induce reflex sympathetic stimulation and increased aortic sheer stress.
- IV calcium channel blockers with negative inotropy may be used.
- Pain control, often with morphine.
- Multiple medications may be needed.
- Proximal dissections require emergent surgery to prevent rupture or pericardial effusion.
- Distal dissections are treated medically unless distal organ involvement or impending rupture occurs.
- Evolving role for endovascular stent placement as less invasive treatment for high-risk surgical patients.

CHRONIC Rx

- Chronic aortic dissection (>2 wk) managed with aggressive BP control: target <120/80 in most patients.
- Target LDL <70 mg/dl.
- Statins can directly modulate the biology of the aorta.
- Serial imaging of the aorta at 1, 3, 6, 9, and 12 months and every 6 to 12 months thereafter, usually with contrast CT.
- Ongoing research on role of endovascular stents in chronic dissection.

DISPOSITION

- 85% mortality within 2 wk if untreated.
- Proximal dissection is a surgical emergency. Time is critical; mortality is 1% to 3% per hr.
- Overall, in-hospital mortality is 30% with proximal dissections and 10% with distal dissections.

REFERRAL

For ICU management and surgery

PEARLS & CONSIDERATIONS

- Blood pressure control is essential; beta-blocker is first-line medication.
- Proximal dissection is a surgical emergency.

SUGGESTED READINGS

Mukherjee D, Eagle KA: Aortic dissection—an update, *Curr Probl Cardiol* 30(6):287, 2005.
Shiga T et al: Diagnostic accuracy of TEE, helical CT, and MRI for suspected thoracic aortic dissection *Arch Intern Med* 166:1350, 2006.
Tsai TT et al: Acute aortic syndromes, *Circulation* 112:3802, 2005.

AUTHORS: **MARA LINSCOTT, M.D.,** and **LYNN BOWLBY, M.D.**

BASIC INFORMATION

DEFINITION

Aortic regurgitation is retrograde blood flow into the left ventricle from the aorta secondary to incompetent aortic valve.

SYNONYMS

Aortic insufficiency
AI
AR

ICD-9CM CODES
424.1 Aortic valve disorders

EPIDEMIOLOGY & DEMOGRAPHICS

- Prevalence ranges from 4.9% to 10% and increases with age.
- The most common cause of isolated severe aortic regurgitation is aortic root dilation.
- Infectious endocarditis is the most frequent cause of acute aortic regurgitation.

PHYSICAL FINDINGS & CLINICAL PRESENTATION

The clinical presentation varies depending on whether aortic insufficiency is acute or chronic. Chronic aortic insufficiency is well tolerated (except when secondary to infective endocarditis), and the patients remain asymptomatic for years. Common manifestations after significant deterioration of left ventricular function are dyspnea on exertion, syncope, chest pain, and CHF. Acute aortic insufficiency manifests primarily with hypotension caused by a sudden fall in cardiac output. A rapid rise in left ventricular diastolic pressure results in a further decrease in coronary blood flow.

Physical findings in chronic aortic insufficiency include the following:

- Widened pulse pressure (markedly increased systolic blood pressure, decreased diastolic blood pressure) is present.
- Bounding pulses, head "bobbing" with each systole (de Musset's sign) are present; "water hammer" or collapsing pulse (Corrigan's pulse) can be palpated at the wrist or on the femoral arteries ("pistol shot" femorals) and is caused by rapid rise and sudden collapse of the arterial pressure during late systole; capillary pulsations (Quincke's pulse) may occur at the base of the nail beds.
- A to-and-fro "double Duroziez" murmur may be heard over femoral arteries with slight compression.
- Popliteal systolic pressure is increased over brachial systolic pressure ≥40 mm Hg (Hill's sign).
- Cardiac auscultation reveals:
  1. Displacement of cardiac impulse downward and to the patient's left
  2. S_3 heard over the apex
  3. Decrescendo, blowing diastolic murmur heard along left sternal border
  4. Low-pitched apical diastolic rumble (Austin-Flint murmur) caused by contrast of the aortic regurgitant jet with the left ventricular wall
  5. Early systolic apical ejection murmur

In patients with acute aortic insufficiency both the wide pulse pressure and the large stroke volume are absent. A short blowing diastolic murmur may be the only finding on physical examination.

ETIOLOGY

- Infective endocarditis
- Rheumatic fibrosis (most common cause in developing countries)
- Trauma with valvular rupture
- Congenital bicuspid aortic valve (most common cause in U.S.)
- Myxomatous degeneration
- Annuloaortic ectasia
- Syphilitic aortitis
- Rheumatic spondylitis
- SLE
- Aortic dissection
- Fenfluramine, dexfenfluramine, pergolide, cabergoline
- Takayasu's arteritis, granulomatous arteritis

DIAGNOSIS

DIFFERENTIAL DIAGNOSIS

- Patent ductus arteriosus, pulmonary regurgitation, and other valvular abnormalities
- The differential diagnosis of cardiac murmurs is described in Section II

WORKUP

- Echocardiogram, chest x-ray, ECG, and cardiac catheterization (selected patients)
- Medical history and physical examination focused on the following clinical manifestations:
  1. Dyspnea on exertion
  2. Syncope
  3. Chest pain
  4. CHF

IMAGING STUDIES

- Chest x-ray
  1. Left ventricular hypertrophy (chronic aortic regurgitation)
  2. Aortic dilation
  3. Normal cardiac silhouette with pulmonary edema: possible in patients with acute aortic regurgitation
- ECG: left ventricular hypertrophy
- Echocardiography: coarse diastolic fluttering of the anterior mitral leaflet; LVH in patients with chronic aortic regurgitation. Use of Doppler echo can quantify regurgitant orifice (severe if >0.30 cm^2) and regurgitant volume (severe if >60 ml per beat).
- Cardiac catheterization in selected patients to assess degree of left ventricular dysfunction, confirm the presence of a wide pulse pressure, assess surgical risk, and determine if there is coexistent coronary artery disease.

TREATMENT

NONPHARMACOLOGIC THERAPY

- Avoidance of competitive sports and strenuous activity
- Salt restriction

ACUTE GENERAL Rx

MEDICAL:

- ACE inhibitors, diuretics, and sodium restriction for CHF; nitroprusside in patients with acute aortic regurgitation
- Long-term vasodilator therapy with ACE inhibitors or nifedipine for reducing or delaying the need for aortic valve replacement in asymptomatic patients with severe aortic regurgitation and normal left ventricular function
- Bacterial endocarditis prophylaxis for surgical and dental procedures

SURGICAL: Reserved for:

- Symptomatic patients with chronic aortic regurgitation despite optimal medical therapy
- Patients with acute aortic regurgitation (i.e., infective endocarditis) producing left ventricular failure
- Evidence of systolic failure:
  1. Echocardiographic fractional shortening <25%
  2. Echocardiographic and diastolic dimension >55 mm
  3. Angiographic ejection fraction <50% or end-systolic volume index (ESVI) >60 ml/m2
- Evidence of diastolic failure:
  1. Pulmonary pressure >45 mm Hg systolic
  2. Left ventricular end-diastolic pressure (LVEDP) >15 mm Hg at catheterization
  3. Pulmonary hypertension detected on examination
- In general, the "55 rule" has been used to determine the timing of surgery: surgery should be performed before EF <55% or end-systolic dimension >55 mm
- The operative mortality rate for aortic regurgitation is 4% when performed alone and 6.8% when performed with CABG

SUGGESTED READING

Enriquez-Sarano M, Tajik J: Aortic regurgitation, *N Engl J Med* 351:1539, 2004.

AUTHOR: **FRED F. FERRI, M.D.**

BASIC INFORMATION

DEFINITION

Aortic stenosis is obstruction to systolic left ventricular outflow across the aortic valve. Symptoms appear when the valve orifice decreases to <1 cm^2 (normal orifice is 3 cm^2). The stenosis is considered severe when the orifice is <0.5 cm^2/m^2 or the pressure gradient is 50 mm Hg or higher.

SYNONYMS

Aortic valvular stenosis
AS

ICD-9CM CODES
424.1 Aortic valvular stenosis

EPIDEMIOLOGY & DEMOGRAPHICS

- Aortic stenosis is the most common valve lesion in adults in Western countries.
- Calcific stenosis (most common cause in patients >60 yr old) occurs in 75% of patients.

PHYSICAL FINDINGS & CLINICAL PRESENTATION

- Rough, loud systolic diamond-shaped murmur, best heard at base of heart and transmitted into neck vessels; often associated with a thrill or ejection click; may also be heard well at the apex
- Absence or diminished intensity of sound of aortic valve closure (in severe aortic stenosis)
- Late, slow-rising carotid upstroke with decreased amplitude
- Strong apical pulse
- Narrowing of pulse pressure in later stages of aortic stenosis
- Some patients with aortic stenosis experience bleeding into their GI tract or skin. This is caused by an acquired defect in von Willebrandt factor. Aortic valve replacement restores normal hemostasis.

ETIOLOGY

- Rheumatic inflammation of aortic valve
- Progressive stenosis of congenital bicuspid valve (found in 1% to 2% of population)
- Idiopathic calcification of the aortic valve
- Congenital (major cause of aortic stenosis in patients <30 yr)

DIAGNOSIS

DIFFERENTIAL DIAGNOSIS

- Hypertrophic cardiomyopathy
- Mitral regurgitation
- Ventricular septal defect
- Aortic sclerosis. Aortic stenosis is distinguished from aortic sclerosis by the degree of valve impairment. In aortic sclerosis, the valve leaflets are abnormally thickened but obstruction to outflow is minimal.

WORKUP

- Echocardiography
- Chest x-ray, ECG
- Lab: B-Type natriuretic peptide or N-terminal pro-B-type natriuretic peptide (NT-proBNP) correlates with the mean pressure gradient, aortic valve area, and functional status. It is a useful biochemical marker to evaluate severity of AS, monitor disease progression at an early stage, and decide on the optimal time for aortic valve replacement. An increased level of B-type natriuretic peptide correlates with severity of AS and New York Heart Association functional class.
- Cardiac catheterization in selected patients (see "Imaging Studies")
- Medical history focusing on symptoms and potential complications:
  1. Angina
  2. Syncope (particularly with exertion)
  3. CHF
  4. GI bleeding: in patients with associated hemorrhagic telangiectasia (AVM)
- Section III describes an algorithm for evaluation of suspected aortic stenosis.

IMAGING STUDIES

- Chest x-ray examination
  1. Poststenotic dilation of the ascending aorta
  2. Calcification of aortic cusps
  3. Pulmonary congestion (in advanced stages of aortic stenosis)
- ECG:
  1. Left ventricular hypertrophy (found in >80% of patients)
  2. ST-T wave changes
  3. Atrial fibrillation: frequent
- Doppler echocardiography: thickening of the left ventricular wall; if the patient has valvular calcifications, multiple echoes may be seen from within the aortic root and there is poor separation of the aortic cusps during systole. Gradient across the valve can be estimated but is less precise than with cardiac catheterization. Section III describes an algorithm for the management of patients with aortic stenosis detected by echocardiography.
- Cardiac catheterization: indicated in symptomatic patients; it confirms the diagnosis and estimates the severity of the disease by measuring the gradient across the valve, allowing calculation of the valve area. It also detects coexisting coronary artery stenosis that may need bypass at the same time as aortic valve replacement.

TREATMENT

NONPHARMACOLOGIC THERAPY

- Strenuous activity should be avoided.
- Sodium restriction if CHF is present.

GENERAL Rx

MEDICAL:

- Diuretics and sodium restriction are needed if CHF is present; digoxin is used only to control rate of atrial fibrillation.
- ACE inhibitors are relatively contraindicated.
- Calcium channel blocker verapamil may be useful only to control rate of atrial fibrillation.
- Antibiotic prophylaxis is necessary for surgical and dental procedures.

SURGICAL:

- Valve replacement is the treatment of choice in symptomatic patients because the 5-yr mortality rate after onset of symptoms is extremely high, even with optimal medical therapy; valve replacement is indicated if cardiac catheterization establishes a pressure gradient >50 mm Hg and valve area <1 cm^2.
- Balloon aortic valvotomy for adult acquired aortic stenosis is useful only for palliation.

DISPOSITION

- 15% to 20% of patients with severe aortic stenosis die before age 20 yr.
- The 5-yr survival rate in adults is 40%.
- The average duration of symptoms before death is as follows: angina, 60 mo; syncope, 36 mo; CHF, 24 mo.
- About 75% of patients with symptomatic aortic stenosis will be dead 3 yr after onset of symptoms unless the aortic valve is replaced.

REFERRAL

- Surgical referral for valve replacement in symptomatic patients. However, the presence of moderate or severe valvular calcification, together with a rapid increase in aortic-jet velocity and elevated B-type natriuretic peptide, identifies patients with a very poor prognosis who should be considered for early valve replacement rather than have surgery delayed until symptoms develop.
- Surgical mortality rate for valve replacement is 3% to 5%; however, it varies with patient's age (>8% in patients >75 yr old).
- Balloon valvuloplasty is useful in infants and children or poor surgical candidates who do not have calcified valve apparatus; it can be done as an intermediate procedure to stabilize high-risk patients before surgery.
- When performed in adults who have calcified valves, balloon valvuloplasty is useful only for short-term reduction in severity of aortic stenosis when surgery is contraindicated, because restenosis occurs rapidly.

AUTHOR: **FRED F. FERRI, M.D.**

BASIC INFORMATION

DEFINITION

Appendicitis is the acute inflammation of the appendix.

ICD-9CM CODES
540.9 Appendicitis
540.0 Appendicitis with generalized peritonitis

EPIDEMIOLOGY & DEMOGRAPHICS

- Appendicitis occurs in 10% of the population, most commonly between the ages of 10 and 30 yr.
- More than 250,000 appendectomies are performed in the U.S. each year.
- It is the most common abdominal surgical emergency.
- Incidence of appendicitis has declined over the past 30 yr.
- Male:female ratio is 3:2 until mid-20s; it equalizes after age 30 yr.

PHYSICAL FINDINGS & CLINICAL PRESENTATION

- In children with abdominal pain, fever is the single most useful sign associated with appendicitis.
- Abdominal pain: initially the pain may be epigastric or periumbilical in nearly 50% of patients; it subsequently localizes to the right lower quadrant within 12 to 18 hr. Pain can be found in back or right flank if appendix is retrocecal or in other abdominal locations if there is malrotation of the appendix.
- Pain with right thigh extension (psoas sign), low-grade fever: temperature may be >38° C if there is appendiceal perforation.
- Pain with internal rotation of the flexed right thigh (obturator sign) is present.
- RLQ pain on palpation of the LLQ (Rovsing's sign): physical examination may reveal right-sided tenderness in patients with pelvic appendix.
- Point of maximum tenderness is in the RLQ (McBurney's point).
- Nausea, vomiting, tachycardia, cutaneous hyperesthesias at the level of T12 can be present.

ETIOLOGY

Obstruction of the appendiceal lumen with subsequent vascular congestion, inflammation, and edema; common causes of obstruction are:

- Fecaliths: 30% to 35% of cases (most common in adults)
- Foreign body: 4% (fruit seeds, pinworms, tapeworms, roundworms, calculi)
- Inflammation: 50% to 60% of cases (submucosal lymphoid hyperplasia [most common etiology in children, teens])
- Neoplasms: 1% (carcinoids, metastatic disease, carcinoma)

DIAGNOSIS

DIFFERENTIAL DIAGNOSIS

- Intestinal: regional cecal enteritis, incarcerated hernia, cecal diverticulitis, intestinal obstruction, perforated ulcer, perforated cecum, Meckel's diverticulitis
- Reproductive: ectopic pregnancy, ovarian cyst, torsion of ovarian cyst, salpingitis, tuboovarian abscess, Mittelschmerz endometriosis, seminal vesiculitis
- Renal: renal and ureteral calculi, neoplasms, pyelonephritis
- Vascular: leaking aortic aneurysm
- Psoas abscess
- Trauma
- Cholecystitis
- Mesenteric adenitis

WORKUP

Patients presenting with RLQ pain, nausea, vomiting, anorexia, and RLQ rebound tenderness should undergo prompt clinical and laboratory evaluation. Imaging studies are generally not necessary in typical appendicitis. They are useful when the diagnosis is uncertain. Laparoscopy may be useful as both a diagnostic and a therapeutic modality.

LABORATORY TESTS

- CBC with differential reveals leukocytosis with a left shift in 90% of patients with appendicitis. Total WBC count is generally lower than 20,000/mm^3. Higher counts may be indicative of perforation. Less than 4% have a normal WBC and differential. A WBC count <10,000/mm^3 decreases the likelihood of appendicitis. A low Hgb and Hct in an older patient should raise suspicion for GI tract carcinoma.
- Microscopic hematuria and pyuria may occur in <20% of patients.

IMAGING STUDIES

- Spiral CT of the right lower quadrant of the abdomen has a sensitivity of >90% and an accuracy >94% for acute appendicitis. A distended appendix, periappendiceal inflammation, and a thickened appendiceal wall are indicative of appendicitis.
- Ultrasonography has a sensitivity of 75% to 90% for the diagnosis of acute appendicitis, although it is highly operator dependent and difficult in patients with large body habitus. Ultrasound is useful, especially in younger women when diagnosis is unclear. Normal ultrasonographic findings should not deter surgery if the history and physical examination are indicative of appendicitis.

TREATMENT

NONPHARMACOLOGIC THERAPY

- NPO
- Do not administer analgesics or antibiotics until the diagnosis is made (may mask signs of peritonitis).

ACUTE GENERAL Rx

- Urgent appendectomy (laparoscopic or open), correction of fluid and electrolyte imbalance with vigorous IV hydration and electrolyte replacement
- IV antibiotic prophylaxis to cover gram-negative bacilli and anaerobes (ampicillin-sulbactam [Unasyn] 3 g IV q6h or piperacillin-tazobactam [Zosyn] 4.5 g IV q8h in adults)

PEARLS & CONSIDERATIONS

COMMENTS

- Perforation is common (20% in adult patients). Indicators of perforation are pain lasting >24 hr, leukocytosis >20,000/mm^3, temperature >102° F, palpable abdominal mass, and peritoneal findings.
- In general, prognosis is excellent. Mortality is <1% in young adults without complications; however, it exceeds 10% in elderly patients with ruptured appendix.
- In approximately 20% of patients who undergo exploratory laparatomy because of suspected appendicitis, the appendix is normal.

SUGGESTED READINGS

Bundy DG et al: Does this child have appendicitis? *JAMA* 298(4):438, 2007.

Old JL et al: Imaging for suspected appendicitis, *Am Fam Physician* 71:71, 2005.

Paulson EK et al: Suspected appendicitis, *N Engl J Med* 348:236, 2003.

Teresawa T et al: Systematic review: Computed tomography and ultrasonography to detect acute appendicitis in adults and adolescents, *Ann Intern Med* 141:537, 2004.

AUTHOR: **FRED F. FERRI, M.D.**

BASIC INFORMATION

DEFINITION

The prototype of granulomatous arthritis is tuberculous arthritis. Atypical mycobacteria, sarcoidosis, and sporotrichosis can cause granulomatous involvement of the synovium, but these entities are much less common.

SYNONYMS

Tuberculous arthritis
Pott's disease

ICD-9CM CODES
711.40 Arthropathy associated with other bacterial disease
730.88 Other infection involving bone

EPIDEMIOLOGY & DEMOGRAPHICS

INCIDENCE (IN U.S.): Unknown
PEAK INCIDENCE: No seasonal predilection
PREVALENCE (IN U.S.): Unknown
PREDOMINANT SEX: Male = female
PREDOMINANT AGE: Rare in childhood

PHYSICAL FINDINGS AND CLINICAL PRESENTATION

- Often no constitutional symptoms (fever and weight loss)
- Possibly no clinical or radiographic evidence of pulmonary TB
- Spinal infection most often in the thoracic or upper lumbar area, with back pain as the most common symptom
- Considerable local muscle spasm possible
- Kyphosis and neurologic symptoms resulting from spinal cord compression in advanced disease
- Chronic monoarticular arthritis in the peripheral joints
- Single joint involved in 85% of patients
- Pain, swelling, limitation of motion, and joint stiffness less dramatic than in acute bacterial arthritis; possibly present for months to years
- Seen more often in persons from developing countries, elderly patients, and hemodialysis patients

ETIOLOGY

- Hematogenous spread of organisms from a distant site of infection or by direct spread from bone
- Most commonly affected area: 50% of cases in the spine; next most commonly affected area: large joints (knee and hip)
- Primary infection beginning in the lungs and spreading to the highly vascular synovium
- Tuberculous osteomyelitis commonly involving an adjacent joint
- In peripheral joints, a granulomatous reaction in the synovium causing joint effusion and eventual destruction of underlying bone
- In the spine, infection of the intervertebral disk spreading to adjacent vertebrae
- Osteomyelitis of vertebrae causing collapse, kyphosis, or gibbous deformity, and possibly paraspinal "cold" abscess

DIAGNOSIS

DIFFERENTIAL DIAGNOSIS

- Sarcoidosis
- Fungal arthritis
- Metastatic cancer
- Primary or metastatic synovial tumors

WORKUP

- High index of suspicion needed
- Gold standard: synovial biopsy
- Joint aspiration and culture of the synovial fluid performed while awaiting biopsy
- Positive synovial fluid smear for acid-fast bacilli in 20% of cases; positive culture in 80%
- Elevated synovial fluid protein, low glucose
- Considerable variation in synovial fluid WBC count, but values of 10,000 to 20,000 cells/mm^3 typical; may be predominantly polymorphonuclear leukocytes
- Usually positive tuberculin skin test
- Anergy in elderly patients or in advanced disease
- In spinal infections, percutaneous or open biopsy to obtain accurate C&S data

LABORATORY TESTS

Peripheral WBC count and ESR are elevated but nonspecific.

IMAGING STUDIES

- Plain radiographs of the affected joint
  1. Typically demonstrate bony destruction with little new bone formation
  2. Osteopenia and soft tissue swelling in early infections
  3. Later, erosions at the joint margins
  4. In the spine, disk space narrowing with vertebral collapse (wedging) causing characteristic kyphosis
- CT scan: useful in early diagnosis of infections of the spine and to detect paraspinal abscess
- Technetium and gallium scintigraphic scans: may be positive, but do not permit differentiation from inflammation or osteoarthritis

TREATMENT

NONPHARMACOLOGIC THERAPY

Encourage range-of-motion exercises of the affected joint to prevent contractures.

ACUTE GENERAL Rx

- Combination chemotherapy
  1. If sensitive TB suspected, give isoniazid 5 mg/kg/day (maximum 300 mg/day) plus rifampin 10 mg/kg/day (maximum 600 mg/day) for at least 6 mo and pyrazinamide 15 to 30 mg/kg/day (maximum 2 g/day) for at least the first 2 mo plus ethambutol 15 to 25 mg/kg/day until sensitivity results are available.
  2. Most patients are treated successfully with chemotherapy alone.
  3. Urgent surgical intervention is necessary if spinal cord compression causes neurologic changes.
- Surgical debridement in cases of extensive bone involvement

CHRONIC Rx

In long-standing extensive disease, arthrodesis of weight-bearing joints

DISPOSITION

Loss of cartilage and destruction of underlying bone if treatment is not initiated promptly

REFERRAL

- To a physician experienced in the management of TB
- For consultation with an infectious diseases specialist if drug resistance is suspected or documented
- For neurosurgical and/or orthopedic consultation if neurologic impairment suspected

PEARLS & CONSIDERATIONS

COMMENTS

As TB has become less prevalent in the U.S. in the last 10 yr, TB arthritis and osteomyelitis have also become less common.

SUGGESTED READINGS

Crowson AN, Magro C: Interstitial granulomatous dermatitis with arthritis, *Hum Pathol* 35(7):779, 2004.

Emery P et al: Detection of *Mycobacterium tuberculosis* group organisms in human and mouse joint tissue by reverse transcriptase PCR: prevalence in diseased synovial tissue suggests lack of specific association with rheumatoid arthritis, *Infect Immun* 69(30):1821, 2001.

Rose CD et al: Blau syndrome mutation of CARD15/NOD2 in sporadic early onset granulomatous arthritis, *J Rheumatol* 32(2):373, 2005.

van de Loo FA et al: Deficiency of NADPH oxidase components p47phox and gp91phox caused granulomatous synovitis and increased connective tissue destruction in experimental arthritis models, *Am J Pathol* 163(4):1525, 2003.

AUTHORS: **STEVEN M. OPAL, M.D.,** and **DEBORAH L. SHAPIRO, M.D.**

BASIC INFORMATION

DEFINITION

Bacterial arthritis is a highly destructive form of joint disease most often caused by hematogenous spread of organisms from a distant site of infection. Direct penetration of the joint as a result of trauma or surgery and spread from adjacent osteomyelitis may also cause bacterial arthritis. Any joint in the body may be affected.

SYNONYMS

Septic arthritis
Pyogenic arthritis

ICD-9CM CODES
711 Pyogenic arthritis, site unspecified

EPIDEMIOLOGY & DEMOGRAPHICS

INCIDENCE (IN U.S.): Unknown
PEAK INCIDENCE:
- Gonococcal arthritis: young adults
- Other bacterial causes: all ages

PREVALENCE (IN U.S.): Unknown
PREDOMINANT SEX: Gonococcal arthritis in females
PREDOMINANT AGE: Gonococcal arthritis in sexually active adults

PHYSICAL FINDINGS & CLINICAL PRESENTATION

- Hallmark: acute onset of a swollen, painful joint
- Limited range of motion of the joint
- Effusion, with varying degrees of erythema and increased warmth around the joint
- Single joint affected in 80% to 90% of cases of nongonococcal arthritis
- Gonococcal dermatitis-arthritis syndrome
  1. Typical pattern is a migratory polyarthritis or tenosynovitis
  2. Small pustules on the trunk or extremities
- Febrile patient at presentation
- Most commonly affected joints in adult: knee and hip, but any joint may be involved; in children: hip

ETIOLOGY

- Bacteria spread from another locus of infection
  1. Highly vascular synovium is invaded by hematogenously spread bacteria.
  2. WBC enzymes cause necrosis of synovium, cartilage, and bone.
  3. Extensive joint destruction is rapid if infection is not treated with appropriate IV antibiotics and drainage of necrotic material.
- Predisposing factors: rheumatoid arthritis, prosthetic joints, advanced age, immunodeficiency
- The most common nongonococcal organisms are *Staphylococcus aureus,* β-hemolytic streptococci, and gram-negative bacilli

DIAGNOSIS

DIFFERENTIAL DIAGNOSIS

- Gout
- Pseudogout
- Trauma
- Hemarthrosis
- Rheumatic fever
- Adult or juvenile rheumatoid arthritis
- Spondyloarthropathies such as reactive arthritis (Reiter's syndrome)
- Osteomyelitis
- Viral arthritides
- Septic bursitis

WORKUP

- Joint aspiration, Gram stain, and culture of the synovial fluid
- Immediate arthrocentesis before other studies are undertaken or antibiotics instituted

LABORATORY TESTS

- Joint fluid analysis
  1. Synovial fluid leukocyte count is usually elevated >50,000 cells/mm^3 with >80% polymorphonuclear cells.
  2. Counts are highly variable, with similar findings in gout, pseudogout, or rheumatoid arthritis.
  3. The differential diagnosis of synovial fluid abnormalities is described in Section II.
- Blood cultures
- Culture of possible extraarticular sources of infection
- Elevated peripheral WBC count and ESR (nonspecific)

IMAGING STUDIES

- X-ray examination of the affected joint to rule out osteomyelitis
- CT scan for early diagnosis of infections of the spine, hips, and sternoclavicular and sacroiliac joints
- Technetium and gallium scintigraphic scans (positive, but do not permit differentiation of infection from inflammation)
- Indium-labeled WBC scans (less sensitive, but more specific)

TREATMENT

NONPHARMACOLOGIC THERAPY

- Affected joints aspirated daily to remove necrotic material and to follow serial WBC counts and cultures
- If no resolution with IV antibiotics and closed drainage: open debridement and lavage, particularly in nongonococcal infections
- Prevention of contractures:
  1. After acute stage of inflammation, range-of-motion exercises of the affected joint
  2. Physical therapy helpful

ACUTE GENERAL Rx

- IV antibiotics immediately after joint aspiration and Gram stain of the synovial fluid
- For infections caused by gram-positive cocci: penicillinase-resistant penicillin, such as nafcillin (2 g IV q4h), unless there is clinical suspicion of methicillin-resistant *Staphylococcus aureus,* in which case vancomycin (1 g IV q12h)
- Infections caused by gram-negative bacilli: treated with a third-generation cephalosporin or an antipseudomonal penicillin plus an aminoglycoside, pending C&S results
- For suspected gonococcal infection, including young adults when the synovial fluid Gram stain is nondiagnostic: ceftriaxone 1 g IV q24h

CHRONIC Rx

See indications for surgical drainage.

DISPOSITION

- With prompt treatment, complete resolution is expected.
- Delay in treatment may result in permanent destruction of cartilage and loss of function of the affected joint.

REFERRAL

To an orthopedist for open drainage if the infected joint fails to improve on appropriate antibiotics and closed aspiration

PEARLS & CONSIDERATIONS

COMMENTS

Any patient with an acute monoarticular arthritis should undergo an urgent joint aspiration to rule out septic arthritis, even if there is a history of gout.

SUGGESTED READINGS

Berendt T, Byren I: Bone and joint infection, *Clin Med* 4(6):510, 2004.

García-De La Torre I et al: Advances in the management of septic arthritis, *Rheum Dis Clin North Am* 29(1):61, 2003.

Weisfelt M et al: Arthritis in adults with community-acquired bacterial meningitis: a prospective cohort study, *BMC Infect Dis* 6:64, 2006.

Yagupsky P: Differentiation between septic arthritis and transient synovitis of the hip in children, *J Bone Joint Surg Am* 87(2):459, 2005.

AUTHORS: **STEVEN M. OPAL, M.D.,** and **DEBORAH L. SHAPIRO, M.D.**

BASIC INFORMATION

DEFINITION

Psoriatic arthritis is an inflammatory spondyloarthritis occurring in patients with psoriasis who are usually seronegative for rheumatoid factor. It is often included in a class of disorders called *rheumatoid variants* or *seronegative spondyloarthropathies.*

ICD-9CM CODES
696.0 Psoriatic arthritis

EPIDEMIOLOGY & DEMOGRAPHICS

PREVALENCE: 5% to 10% of patients with psoriasis (psoriasis affects 1% to 1.5% of general population)
PREDOMINANT SEX: Males = females
PREDOMINANT AGE: 30 to 55 yr

PHYSICAL FINDINGS & CLINICAL PRESENTATION

- Usually gradual clinical onset
- Asymmetric involvement of scattered joints
- Selective involvement of the DIP joints (described in "classic" cases but present in only 5% of patients; Fig. 1-24)
- Symmetric arthritis similar to RA in 15% of patients
- Possible development of predominant sacroiliitis in a small number of cases
- Advanced form of hand involvement (arthritis mutilans) in some patients
- Dystrophic changes in the nails (pitting, ridging) in many patients with DIP involvement
- Fingers often assume a "sausage" appearance (dactylitis)

ETIOLOGY

Unknown. Destructive changes probably due to release of cytokines and tumor necrosis factor.

DIAGNOSIS

DIFFERENTIAL DIAGNOSIS

- Rheumatoid arthritis
- Erosive osteoarthritis
- Gouty arthritis
- Ankylosing spondylitis
- The differential diagnosis of spondyloarthropathies is described in Section II

WORKUP

- Early diagnosis may be difficult to establish because the arthritis may develop before skin lesions appear.
- Laboratory studies show no specific abnormalities in most cases.

LABORATORY TESTS

- Slight elevation of ESR
- Possible mild anemia
- Possible HLA-B27 antigen (especially in patients with sacroiliitis)

IMAGING STUDIES

- Peripheral joint findings similar to those in rheumatoid arthritis but erosive changes in the distal phalangeal tufts characteristic of psoriatic arthritis
- Bony osteolysis; periosteal new bone formation
- Changes in axial skeleton: sacroiliitis, development of vertebral syndesmophytes (osteophytes) that often bridge adjacent vertebral bodies
- Paravertebral ossification
- Spinal changes: do not have same appearance as ankylosing spondylitis; however, spine abnormalities are less common than sacroiliitis

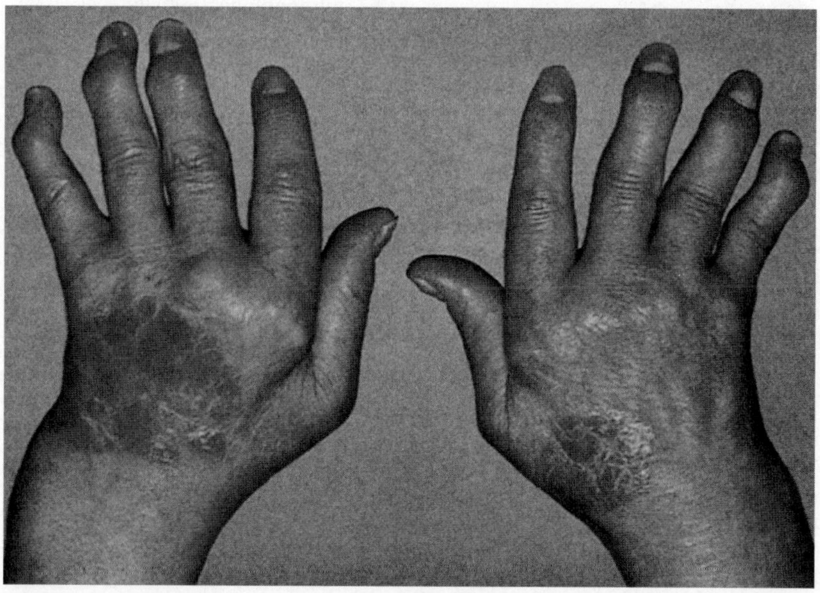

FIGURE 1-24 The hands of a woman with symmetric polyarthritis. Initially, this was indistinguishable from rheumatoid disease, but note the distal interphalangeal joint involvement, which is uncommon in rheumatoid arthritis, as well as the skin psoriasis. (From Klippel J, Dieppe P, Ferri F [eds]: *Primary care rheumatology,* London, 1999, Mosby.)

TREATMENT

NONPHARMACOLOGIC THERAPY

- Rest
- Splinting
- Joint protection
- PT

ACUTE GENERAL Rx

- NSAIDs
- Occasional intraarticular steroid injections
- DMARDs: rarely are required

DISPOSITION

- Different from rheumatoid arthritis in both prognosis and response to treatment.
- Generally, mild joint symptoms in psoriatic arthritis although some patients develop a more severe form which requires intensive treatment.
- Disease-free intervals lasting for several years in many patients.

REFERRAL

- Orthopedic surgery consultation for painful joint deformity.
- Rheumatology for uncontrolled symptoms.

PEARLS & CONSIDERATIONS

- There is often a strong family history of psoriasis in patients who develop psoriatic arthritis.
- Enthesitis (inflammation of tendon and fascial attachments) is a common feature of the spondyloarthropathies typically involving the plantar fascia and tendo Achilles.

SUGGESTED READINGS

Ali Y et al: Improved survival in psoriatic arthritis with calendar time, *Arthritis Rheum* 56(8):2708, 2007.

Griffiths CE, Barker JN: Pathogenesis and clinical features of psoriasis, *Lancet* 370(9583):263, 2007.

Heiberg MS et al: The comparative one-year performance of anti-tumor necrosis factor alpha drugs in patients with rheumatoid arthritis, psoriatic arthritis, and ankylosing spondylitis: results from a longitudinal, observational, multicenter study, *Arthritis Rheum* 59:234, 2008.

Kataria RK, Brent LH: Spondyloarthiopathies, *Am Fam Phys* 69:2853, 2004.

Liu Y, Cortinovis D, Stone MA: Recent advances in the treatment of the spondyloarthropathies, *Curr Opin Rheumatol* 16:357, 2004.

Scarpa R et al: Early psoriatic arthritis: the clinical spectrum, *J Rheumatol* 57(8):1560, 2007.

Taylor WJ: Assessment of outcome in psoriatic arthritis, *Curr Opin Rheumatol* 16:350, 2004.

AUTHOR: **LONNIE R. MERCIER, M.D.**

BASIC INFORMATION

DEFINITION

Asbestosis is a slowly progressive diffuse interstitial fibrosis resulting from dose-related inhalation exposure to fibers of asbestos.

ICD-9CM CODES
501 Asbestosis

EPIDEMIOLOGY & DEMOGRAPHICS

- In U.S.: 5 to 10 new cases/100,000 persons/yr
- Prolonged interval (20 to 30 yr) between exposures to inhaled fibers and clinical manifestations of disease
- Most common in workers involved in the primary extraction of asbestos from rock deposits and in those involved in the fabrication and installation of products containing asbestos (e.g., naval shipyards in World War II, installation of floor tiles, ceiling tiles, acoustic ceiling coverings, wall insulation, and pipe coverings in public buildings)

PHYSICAL FINDINGS & CLINICAL PRESENTATION

- Insidious onset of shortness of breath with exertion is usually the first sign of asbestosis.
- Dyspnea becomes more severe as the disease advances; with time, progressively less exertion is tolerated.
- Cough is frequent and usually paroxysmal, dry, and nonproductive.
- Scant mucoid sputum may accompany the cough in the later stages of the disease.
- Fine end respiratory crackles (rales, crepitations) are heard more predominantly in the lung bases.
- Digital clubbing, edema, jugular venous distention are present.

ETIOLOGY

Inhalation of asbestos fibers

DIAGNOSIS

DIFFERENTIAL DIAGNOSIS

- Silicosis
- Siderosis, other pneumonoconioses
- Lung cancer
- Atelectasis

WORKUP

Documentation of exposure history, diagnostic imaging, pulmonary function testing

LABORATORY TESTS

- Generally not helpful
- Possible mild elevation of ESR, positive ANA and RF (These tests are nonspecific and do not correlate with disease severity or activity.)
- Pulmonary function testing: decreased vital capacity, decreased total lung capacity, decreased carbon monoxide gas transfer
- ABGs: hypoxemia, hypercarbia in advanced stages

IMAGING STUDIES

Chest x-ray (Fig. 1-25):
- Small, irregular shadows in lower lung zones
- Thickened pleural, calcified plaques (present under diaphragms and lateral chest wall)

CT scan of chest confirms the diagnosis. Typical findings on high-resolution CT of the chest include increased interstitial markings found mainly at the bases. As the disease progresses, honeycombing is noted.

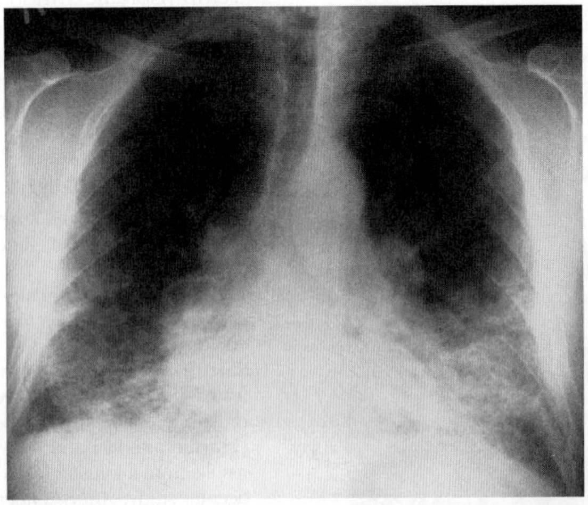

FIGURE 1-25 Asbestosis. PA radiograph shows coarse linear opacities at both lung bases obscuring the cardiac borders. (From McLoud TC: *Thoracic radiology: the requisites,* St Louis, 1998, Mosby.)

TREATMENT

NONPHARMACOLOGIC THERAPY

- Smoking cessation, proper nutrition, exercise program to maximize available lung function
- Home oxygen therapy prn
- Removal of patient from further asbestos fiber exposure

GENERAL Rx

- Prompt identification and treatment of respiratory infections
- Supplemental oxygen on a prn basis
- Annual influenza vaccination, pneumococcal vaccination

DISPOSITION

- There is no specific treatment for asbestosis.
- Death is usually secondary to respiratory failure from cor pulmonale.
- Patients with asbestosis have increased risk for mesotheliomas, lung cancer, and TB. Recent reports indicate that the risk of asbestos-induced lung cancer may be overestimated.
- Survival in patients following development of mesothelioma is 4 to 6 yr.

REFERRAL

To pulmonologist initially

PEARLS & CONSIDERATIONS

COMMENTS

Patient information on asbestosis can be obtained from the American Lung Association, 1740 Broadway, New York, NY 10019.

SUGGESTED READINGS

American Thoracic Society: Diagnosis and initial management of nonmalignant diseases related to asbestos, *Am J Resp Crit Care Med* 170:691, 2004.

O'Reilly K et al: Asbestos-related lung disease, *Am Fam Physician* 75:683, 2007.

AUTHOR: **FRED F. FERRI, M.D.**

BASIC INFORMATION

DEFINITION

Ascariasis is a parasitic infection caused by the nematode *Ascaris lumbricoides.* The majority of those infected are asymptomatic; however, clinical disease may arise from pulmonary hypersensitivity, intestinal obstruction, and secondary complications.

SYNONYMS

round worms
worms

ICD-9CM CODES
127.0 Ascariasis

EPIDEMIOLOGY & DEMOGRAPHICS

INCIDENCE (IN U.S.):
- Unknown
- Three times the infection rates found in blacks as in whites

PEAK INCIDENCE: Unknown
PREVALENCE (IN U.S.): Estimated at 4,000,000, the majority of which live in the rural southeastern part of the country
PREDOMINANT SEX: Both sexes probably equally affected, with a possible slight female preponderance
PREDOMINANT AGE: Most common in children, with estimated mean age of approximately 5 yr based on surveys in highly endemic areas
NEONATAL INFECTION:
Probable transmission, though not specifically studied

PHYSICAL FINDINGS & CLINICAL PRESENTATION

- Occurs approximately 9 to 12 days after ingestion of eggs (corresponding to the larva migration through the lungs)
- Nonproductive cough
- Substernal chest discomfort
- Fever
- In patients with large worm burdens, especially children, intestinal obstruction associated with perforation, volvulus, and intussusception
- Migration of worms into the biliary tree giving clinical appearance of biliary colic and pancreatitis as well as acute appendicitis with movement into that appendage
- Rarely, infection with *A. lumbricoides* producing interstitial nephritis and acute renal failure
- In endemic areas in Asia and Africa, malabsorption of dietary proteins and vitamins as a consequence of chronic worm intestinal carriage

ETIOLOGY

- Transmission is usually hand to mouth, but eggs may be ingested via transported vegetables grown in contaminated soil.
- Eggs are hatched in the small intestine, with larvae penetrating intestinal mucosa and migrating via the circulation to the lungs.
- Larval forms proceed through the alveoli, ascend the bronchial tree, and return to the intestines after swallowing, where they mature into adult worms.
- Estimated time until the female adult worm begins producing eggs is 2 to 3 mo.
- Eggs are passed out of the intestines with feces.
- Within human host, adult worm lifespan is 1 to 2 yr.

DIAGNOSIS

DIFFERENTIAL DIAGNOSIS

- Radiologic manifestations and eosinophilia to be distinguished from drug hypersensitivity and Löffler's syndrome
- The differential diagnosis of intestinal helminths is described in Section II

LABORATORY TESTS

- Examination of the stool for *Ascaris* ova
- Expectoration or fecal passage of adult worm
- Eosinophilia: most prominent early in the infection and subsides as the adult worm infestation established in the intestines
- Anti-ascaris IgG4 blood levels by ELISA is a sensitive and specific marker of infection and may be useful in the evaluation of treatment
- Malondialdehyde levels clearly increase in patients infected with *A. lumbricoides*

IMAGING STUDIES

- Chest x-ray examination to reveal bilateral oval or round infiltrates of varying size (Löffler's syndrome); NOTE: infiltrates are transient and eventually resolve.
- Plain films of the abdomen and contrast studies to reveal worm masses in loops of bowel.
- Ultrasonography and endoscopic retrograde cholangiopancreatography (ERCP) to identify worms in the pancreaticobiliary tract.

TREATMENT

NONPHARMACOLOGIC THERAPY

Aggressive IV hydration, especially in children with fever, severe vomiting, and resultant dehydration

ACUTE GENERAL Rx

- Mebendazole (Vermox)
  1. Drug of choice for intestinal infection with *A. lumbricoides*
  2. 100 mg PO tid given for 3 days or 500 mg as a single dose
- Albendazole, given as a single 400-mg dose PO
- Both mebendazole and albendazole are contraindicated in pregnancy
- Pyrantel pamoate (Antiminth)
  1. Given at a dose of 11 mg/kg PO (maximum dose of 1 g/day)
  2. Considered safe for use in pregnant women
- Piperazine citrate
  1. Recommended in cases of intestinal or biliary obstruction
  2. Administered as a syrup, given via nasogastric tube, a 150 mg/kg loading dose, followed by six doses of 65 mg/kg q12h
  3. Considered safe in pregnancy, but cannot be given concurrently with chlorpromazine
- Complete obstruction should be managed surgically

DISPOSITION

Overall prognosis is good. Patients should be reevaluated in 2 to 3 months. Reinfection is common.

REFERRAL

- To gastroenterologist in cases of visualized pancreaticobiliary tract or appendiceal obstruction
- To surgeon in cases of complete obstruction or suspected secondary complication (e.g., perforation or volvulus)

PEARLS & CONSIDERATIONS

COMMENTS

- Hepatic abscess, containing both viable and dead worms, complicating *Ascaris*-induced biliary duct disease has been documented.
- Given the known transmission of the parasite, routine hand washing and proper disposal of human waste would significantly decrease the prevalence of this disease.

SUGGESTED READINGS

Bradley JE, Jackson JA: Immunity, immunoregulation, and the ecology of trichuriasis and ascariasis, *Parasite Immunol* 26(11-12):429, 2004.

Kilic E et al: Serum malondialdehyde level in patients infected with *Ascaris lumbricoides, World J Gastroenterol* 9(10):2332, 2003.

Legesse M, Erko B, Medhin G: Comparative efficacy of albendazole and three brands of mebendazole in the treatment of ascariasis and trichuriasis, *East Afr Med J* 81(3):134, 2004.

Sangkhathat S et al: Massive gastrointestinal bleeding in infants with ascariasis, *J Pediatr Surg* 38(11):1696, 2003.

Shah OJ et al: Biliary ascariasis: a review, *World J Surg* 30(8):1500, 2006.

AUTHORS: **GLENN G. FORT, M.D., M.P.H., DENNIS J. MIKOLICH, M.D.,** and **GEORGE O. ALONSO, M.D.**

BASIC INFORMATION

DEFINITION

Ascites is the accumulation of excess fluid in the peritoneal cavity, most commonly caused by liver cirrhosis.

SYNONYMS

Fluid in peritoneal cavity, hydroperitoneum, hydroperitonia, hydrops abdominis

ICD-9CM CODES
789.5 Ascites

EPIDEMIOLOGY & DEMOGRAPHICS

Ascites is the most common complication of cirrhosis. Ascites occurs in 50% of individuals with cirrhosis within 10 years of diagnosis. Cirrhosis is the cause of 75% of cases of ascites. Other causes include malignancy (10%), cardiac failure (3%), tuberculosis (3%), and pancreatitis (5%).

CLINICAL PRESENTATION

- Important information to elicit within history:
  - Viral hepatitis
  - Alcoholism
  - Increasing abdominal girth
  - Increasing lower extremity edema
  - Intravenous drug use
  - Sexual history (i.e., men who have sex with men)
  - History of transfusions
- Important physical exam findings:
  - Bulging flanks
  - Flank dullness to percussion
  - Fluid wave on abdominal exam
  - Lower extremity edema
  - Shifting dullness on abdominal exam
  - Physical signs associated with liver cirrhosis: spider angiomas, jaundice, loss of body hair, Dupuytren's contracture, muscle wasting, bruising, palmar erythema, gynecomastia, testicular atrophy, hemorrhoids, caput medusae

ETIOLOGY

Pathophysiology of ascites: increased hepatic resistance to portal flow leads to portal hypertension. The splanchnic vessels respond by increased secretion of nitric oxide causing splanchnic artery vasodilation. Early in the disease increased plasma volume and increased cardiac output compensate for this vasodilation. However, as disease progresses the effective arterial blood volume decreases causing sodium and fluid retention through activation of the renin-angiotensin system. The change in capillary pressure causes increased permeability and retention of fluid in the abdomen.

DIAGNOSIS

DIFFERENTIAL DIAGNOSIS

- Chronic parenchymal liver disease, leading to portal hypertension
- Peritoneal carcinomatosis
- Congestive heart failure
- Peritoneal tuberculosis
- Nephrotic syndrome
- Pancreatitis

LABORATORY TESTS

- Initial evaluation should always include:
  - Diagnostic paracentesis. Laboratory tests on this fluid should include a CBC with differential, albumin, total protein, culture and a gram stain. Optional tests on paracentesis fluid include amylase, LDH, acid-fast bacilli and glucose levels
  - AST, ALT, total and direct bilirubin, albumin, alkaline phosphatase, GGTP
  - CBC, coagulation studies
  - Electrolytes, BUN, creatinine
- A serum to ascites albumin gradient should be calculated in all patients. If the SAAG is greater than 1.1, the cause of ascites can be attributed to portal hypertension. If SAAG is less than 1.1, a nonportal hypertension etiology of ascites must be sought.

IMAGING STUDIES

- Endoscopy of the upper GI tract to evaluate for esophageal varices if ascites secondary to portal hypertension.
- Abdominal ultrasound is the most sensitive measure for detecting ascitic fluid; a CT scan is a viable alternative.
- Liver biopsy in selected patients (i.e., those with portal hypertension of uncertain etiology).

TREATMENT

NONPHARMACOLOGIC THERAPY

- Sodium-restricted diet (maximum 60 to 90 milliequivalents per day).
- Fluid restriction to 1 liter per day in patients with hyponatremia.

ACUTE GENERAL Rx

- Patients with moderate-volume ascites causing only moderate discomfort may be treated on an outpatient basis with the following diuretic regimen: spironolactone 50 to 200 mg daily or amiloride 5 to 10 mg daily. Add Lasix 20 to 40 mg per day in the first several days of treatment, monitoring renal functions carefully for signs of prerenal azotemia (in patients without edema goal weight loss is 300 to 500 grams/day, in patients with edema 800 to 1000 grams/day).
- Patients with large-volume ascites causing marked discomfort or decrease in activities of daily living may also be treated as outpatients if there are no complications. There are two options for treatment in these patients: (1) large-volume paracentesis or (2) diuretic therapy until loss of fluid is noted (maximum spironolactone 400 mg daily and Lasix 160 mg daily). No difference in long-term mortality was found; however paracentesis is faster, more effective, and associated with fewer adverse effects.

CHRONIC Rx

5% to 10% of patients with large-volume ascites will be refractory to high-dose diuretic treatment. Treatment strategies include repeated large-volume paracentesis with infusion of albumin every 2 to 4 weeks or placement of a transjugular intrahepatic portosystemic shunt (TIPS).

DISPOSITION

Monitor closely for worsening liver function, development of SBP.

REFERRAL

Referral to gastroenterology for endoscopy in patients with ascites secondary to cirrhosis

PEARLS & CONSIDERATIONS

COMMENTS

Prevalence of spontaneous bacterial peritonitis (SBP) in patients with ascites ranges between 10% and 30%. Presence of at least 250 neutrophils per cubic millimeter of ascitic fluid is diagnostic. Gram-negatives such as E. coli are the most common isolates. Third-generation cephalosporins are the treatment of choice. By 1 year, 70% of patients have recurrence of SBP and may be prophylaxed with quinolones.

PREVENTION

Prevention of liver cirrhosis through avoidance of long-term use of alcohol, immunization against hepatitis B, and treatment of hepatitis C

SUGGESTED READINGS

Bickley L: *Bates' Guide to Physical Examination and History Taking.* Philadelphia, 1999, Lippincott, Williams and Wilkins, pp 374-375, 53.

Gines P et al: Management of cirrhosis and ascites, *N Engl J Med* 350:1646-1654, 2004.

Moore et al: The management of ascites in cirrhosis. Report on the Consensus Conference of the International Ascites Club, *Hepatology* 38:258-266, 2003.

AUTHORS: **JOANNE M. SILVIA, M.D.,** and **PAUL F. GEORGE, M.D.**

BASIC INFORMATION

DEFINITION

Aseptic necrosis is cell death in components of bone: hematopoietic fat marrow and mineralized tissue. Osteonecrosis is not a specific disease entity but a final common pathway to several disorders that impair blood supply to the femoral head and other locations.

SYNONYMS

Osteonecrosis
Avascular necrosis

ICD-9CM CODES

733.40 Aseptic necrosis
733.43 Aseptic necrosis of femoral condyle
733.42 Aseptic necrosis of femoral head
733.41 Aseptic necrosis of humeral head
733.44 Aseptic necrosis of talus

EPIDEMIOLOGY & DEMOGRAPHICS

- 15,000 new cases per year in the U.S.
- Associated conditions:
  1. Corticosteroid treatment: 35%
  2. Alcohol abuse: 22%
  3. Idiopathic and other: 43%
- Common sites involved
  1. Femoral head
  2. Femoral condyle
  3. Humeral head
  4. Navicular and lunate wrist bones
  5. Talus

PHYSICAL FINDINGS & CLINICAL PRESENTATION

- May be asymptomatic
- Pain in the involved area exacerbated by movement or weight bearing
- Decreased range of motion as the disease progresses
- Functional limitation

ETIOLOGY

Final common pathway of conditions that lead to impairment of the blood supply to the involved bone.
Stages:
Stage 0
- Asymptomatic
- Normal imaging
- Histologic findings only (i.e., silent osteonecrosis)

Stage 1
- Asymptomatic or symptomatic
- Normal x-ray and CT scan
- Abnormal bone scan or MRI

Stage 2
- Abnormal x-rays or CT scan including linear sclerosis, focal bead mineralization, cysts; however, the overall architecture of the involved bone is normal

Stage 3
- Early evidence of mechanical bone failure (subchondral fracture), but the overall shape of the bone is still intact

Stage 4
- Flattening or collapse of the bone

Stage 5
- Joint space narrowing

Stage 6
- Extensive joint destruction

DIAGNOSIS

DIFFERENTIAL DIAGNOSIS

- None in late stages
- Early: any condition causing focal musculoskeletal pain including arthritis, bursitis, tendinitis, myopathy, neoplastic bone and joint diseases, traumatic injuries, pathologic fractures

IMAGING STUDIES (Fig. 1-26)

1. X-ray: insensitive early in the course. The earliest changes include diffuse osteopenia, areas of radiolucency with sclerotic border, and linear sclerosis. Later a subchondral lucency (crescent sign) indicates subchondral fracture. More advanced cases reveal flattening, collapsed bone, and abnormal bone contour. In late disease, osteoarthritic changes are seen.
2. Bone scan:
   - Early: "cold" area.
   - Later: increased radionuclide uptake as a result of remodeling.
   - Sensitivity in early disease is only 70% and specificity is poor.
3. CT scan: may reveal central necrosis and area of collapse before those are visible in x-ray.
4. MRI: the most sensitive technology to diagnose early aseptic necrosis. The first sign is a margin of low signal. An inner border of high signal associated with a low-signal line is specific of aseptic necrosis ("double line sign"). Sensitivity is 75% to 100%.

TREATMENT

PREVENTION

- Management of etiologic conditions
- Minimize corticosteroid use

NONPHARMACOLOGIC THERAPY

- Core decompression: effectiveness 35% to 95% in early phases
- Bone grafting
- Osteotomies
- Joint replacement

ACUTE GENERAL Rx

- Decrease weight bearing of affected area.
- Pulsing electromagnetic fields applied externally (still experimental).
- Peripheral vasodilators (e.g., dihydrogotamine) (unproven).

PROGNOSIS

- When diagnosed at an early stage treatment is appropriate in all cases because 85% to 90% can be expected to progress to a more advanced stage.
- Contralateral joint involvement is common (30% to 70%).

SUGGESTED READINGS

Glesby MJ et al: Osteonecrosis in patients infected with HIV, *J Infect Dis* 184:519-523, 2001.

Mont MA et al: Atraumatic osteonecrosis of the knee, *J Bone Joint Surg* 82A:1279-1290, 2000.

AUTHORS: **FRED F. FERRI, M.D.**, and **TOM J. WACHTEL, M.D.**

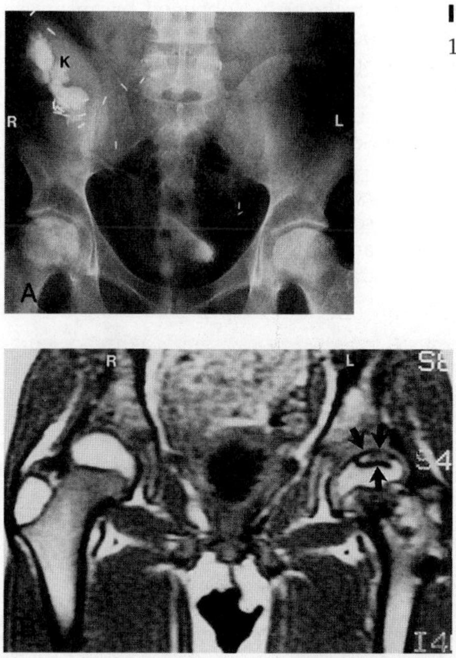

FIGURE 1-26 Aseptic necrosis of the hips. A, Aseptic necrosis can occur from a number of causes, including trauma and steroid use. In this patient, an anteroposterior view of the pelvis shows a transplanted kidney (K) in the right iliac fossa. Use of steroids has caused this patient to have bilateral aseptic necrosis. The femoral heads are somewhat flattened, irregular, and increased in density. **B,** Aseptic necrosis in a different patient is demonstrated on an MRI scan as an area of decreased signal (*arrows*) in the left femoral head. This is the most sensitive method for detection of early aseptic necrosis. (From Mettler FA [ed]: *Primary care radiology,* Philadelphia, 2000, WB Saunders).

BASIC INFORMATION

DEFINITION

Aspergillosis refers to several forms of a broad range of illnesses caused by infection with *Aspergillus* species.

ICD-9CM CODES
117.3 Aspergillosis
117.3 Aspergillosis with pneumonia
117.3 *Aspergillus* infection *(flavus, fumigatus, terreus)*

EPIDEMIOLOGY & DEMOGRAPHICS

INCIDENCE & PREVALENCE:
- *Aspergillus* species are ubiquitous in the environment internationally and occur as a mold found in soil.
- Cause a variety of illness from hypersensitivity pneumonitis to disseminated overwhelming infection in immunosuppressed patients.
- Frequently cultured from hospital wards from unfiltered outside air circulating through open windows as well as water sources.
- Reaches the patient by airborne conidia (spores) that are small enough (2.5 to 3 μm) to reach the alveoli on inhalation.
- Can invade the nose, paranasal sinuses, external ear, or traumatized skin.

RISK FACTORS:
- The clinical syndrome is dependent on the underlying lung architecture, the host's immune response, and the degree of inoculum.
- Incidence of invasive aspergillosis is increasing with advances in the treatment of life-threatening diseases: aggressive chemotherapy; bone marrow and organ transplantation, although it rarely can occur in normal hosts especially associated with influenza A. Liver and lung transplant recipients are at highest risk for pulmonary disease.
- Patients with AIDS and a CD4 <50 mm^3 have an increased susceptibility to invasive aspergillosis.

ETIOLOGY

- *Aspergillus fumigatus* is the usual cause.
- *A. flavus* is the second most important species, particularly in invasive disease of immunosuppressed patients and in lesions beginning in the nose and paranasal sinuses. *A. niger* can also cause invasive human infection.

ALLERGIC ASPERGILLOSIS
- Is a hypersensitivity pneumonitis.
- Presents as cough, dyspnea, fever, chills, malaise typically 4 to 8 hr after exposure.
- Repeated attacks can lead to granulomatous disease and pulmonary fibrosis.

ALLERGIC BRONCHOPULMONARY ASPERGILLOSIS (ABPA):
- Symptoms occur most commonly in atopic individuals during the third and fourth decades of life.
- Hypersensitivity reaction to *Aspergillus* fungal antigens present in the bronchial tree.
- Results from an initial type I (immediate hypersensitivity) and type III reaction (immune complexes).
- Underdiagnosed pulmonary disorder in patients with asthma and cystic fibrosis.

ASPERGILLOMAS ("FUNGUS BALLS"):
- In the absence of invasion or significant immune response, *Aspergillus* can colonize a preexisting cavity, causing pulmonary aspergilloma.
- Forms masses of tangled hyphal elements, fibrin, and mucus.
- Patients typically have a history of chronic lung disease, tuberculosis, sarcoidosis, or emphysema.
- Manifests commonly as hemoptysis.
- Many are asymptomatic.

INVASIVE ASPERGILLOSIS:
- Patients with prolonged and profound granulocytopenia or impaired phagocytic function are predisposed to rapidly progressive *Aspergillus* pneumonia.
- Typically a necrotizing bronchopneumonia, ranging from small areas of infiltrate to intensive bilateral hemorrhagic infarction.
- Most common presentation: unremitting fever and a new pulmonary infiltrate despite broad-spectrum antibiotic therapy in an immunosuppressed patient.
- Dyspnea and nonproductive cough are common; sudden pleuritic pain and tachycardia, sometimes with a pleural rub, may mimic pulmonary embolism; hemoptysis is uncommon.
- CXR may reveal patchy bronchopneumonic, nodular densities, consolidation, or cavitation.
- Immunocompromised patients: invasive pulmonary *Aspergillus* (IPA) generally is acute and evolves over days to weeks; less commonly, patients with normal or only mild abnormalities of their immune systems may develop a more chronic, slowly progressive form of IPA.

EXTRAPULMONARY DISSEMINATION:
- Cerebral infarction from hematogenous dissemination may occur in immunosuppressed individuals.
- Abscess formation from direct extension or invasive disease in the sinuses.
- Esophageal or gastrointestinal ulcerations may occur in the immunosuppressed host.
- Fatal perforation of the viscus or bowel infarction may occur.
- Necrotizing skin ulcers involving the extremities (Fig. 1-27).
- Osteomyelitis.
- Endocarditis in patients who have recently undergone open heart surgery.
- Infection of an implantable cardioverter-defibrillator has been reported.

DIAGNOSIS

DIFFERENTIAL DIAGNOSIS

- Tuberculosis
- Cystic fibrosis
- Carcinoma of the lung
- Eosinophilic pneumonia
- Bronchiectasis
- Sarcoidosis
- Lung abscess

WORKUP

Physical exam and laboratory data

LABORATORY TESTS

ABPA:
- Peripheral blood eosinophilia and an elevated total serum IgE level.
- Skin test with *Aspergillus* antigenic extract is usually positive but nonspecific.
- *Aspergillus* serum precipitating antibody is present in 70% to 100% of cases.
- Sputum cultures may be positive for *Aspergillus* spp. but are nonspecific.

ASPERGILLOMAS:
- Sputum culture
- Serum precipitating antibody

INVASIVE ASPERGILLOSIS: Definitive diagnosis requires the demonstration of tissue invasion (i.e., septate, acute angle branching hyphae) or a positive culture from the tissue obtained by an invasive procedure such as transbronchial biopsy.
- Sputum and nasal cultures: in high-risk patients a positive culture is strongly suggestive of invasive aspergillosis.
- Serology: the *Platelia Aspergillus* ELISA assay detects a circulating fungal antigen, galactomannan, and is used in some centers in neutropenic patients and for those undergoing stem cell transplantation.

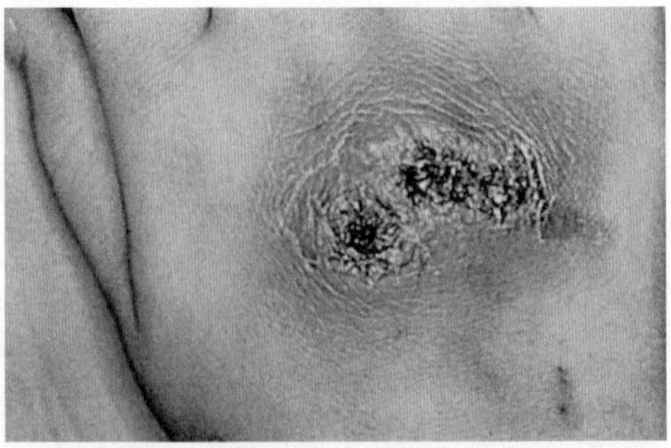

FIGURE 1-27 Cutaneous aspergillosis in a patient with acute leukemia and marked neutropenia. The lesion developed at the site where a steel needle had been left for several days of intravenous infusion. (From Mandell GL [ed]: *Mandell, Douglas, and Bennett's principles and practice of infectious diseases,* ed 6, New York, 2005, Churchill Livingstone.)

- Blood cultures: usually negative.
- Lung biopsy is necessary for definitive diagnosis.
- Biopsy and culture of extrapulmonary lesions.
- Real-time polymerase chain reaction tests are investigational.

IMAGING STUDIES

ABPA:

- CXR show a variety of abnormalities from small, patchy, fleeting infiltrates (commonly in the upper lobes) to lobar consolidation or cavitation.
- A majority of patients eventually develop central bronchiectasis.

ASPERGILLOMAS: CXR or CT scans usually show the characteristic intracavity mass partially surrounded by a crescent of air (Fig. 1-28).

INVASIVE ASPERGILLOSIS: CXR and CT scanning may reveal cavity formation.

TREATMENT

Rx

ACUTE GENERAL Rx

ABPA:

- Prednisone (0.5 to 1 mg/kg po) until the CXR has cleared, followed by alternate-day therapy at 0.5 mg/kg po (3 to 6 mo).
- If a patient is corticosteroid dependent, prophylaxis for the prevention of *Pneumocystis jiroveci* infection and maintenance of bone mineralization should be considered.
- Bronchodilators and physiotherapy.
- Serial CXR and serum IgE useful in guiding treatment.
- Itraconazole 200 mg po bid for 4 to 6 mo, then taper over 4 to 6 mo may be considered as a steroid-sparing agent or if steroids are ineffective.

ASPERGILLOMAS:

- Controversial and problematic; the optimal treatment strategy is unknown.
- Up to 10% of aspergillomas may resolve clinically without overt pharmacologic or surgical intervention.
- Observation for asymptomatic patients.
- Surgical resection/arterial embolization for those patients with severe hemoptysis or life-threatening hemorrhage.
- For those patients at risk for marked hemoptysis with inadequate pulmonary reserve, consider itraconazole 200 to 400 mg/day po.

INVASIVE ASPERGILLOSIS:

- Amphotericin B 0.8 to 1.2 mg/kg IV qd to total dose of 2 to 2.5 g; itraconazole 200 to 400 mg/d po × 1 yr.
- Amphotericin B lipid complex (ABLC) 5 mg/kg IV qd in those intolerant of or refractory to amphotericin B.
- Amphotericin B colloidal dispersion (ABCD) 3 to 6 mg/kg IV qd; stepwise approach in those who have failed amphotericin B.
- Liposomal amphotericin B (L-AMB) 3 to 5 mg/kg IV q day; stepwise approach is indicated as empiric therapy for presumed fungal infection in febrile neutropenic patients who are refractory to or intolerant of amphotericin B.
- Itraconazole 200 mg IV bid × 4 doses followed by 200 mg IV qd or 200 mg tid for 4 days, then 200 mg po bid—first line therapy if not taking p450 inducers. Levels may be obtained to ensure compliance and adequate absorption.
- Voriconazole 6 mg/kg IV bid followed by 4 mg/kg IV q 12 or 200 mg po q 12 for body weight >40 kg but 100 mg po q 12 for body weight <40 kg.
- Posaconazole 200 mg po tid with food or liquid nutritional supplement to enhance absorption; ravuconazole is currently under investigation.
- Caspofungin (Candigas) is the first of a new class of antifungals, the echinocandins, approved for the treatment of invasive aspergillosis in patients who fail or are unable to tolerate other antifungal drugs. Starting dose 70 mg IV over 1 hr on day 1, then 50 mg IV daily thereafter (reduce to 35 mg IV daily in cases with moderate hepatic insufficiency). Can switch to oral voriconazole after 2 to 3 weeks if the response is favorable. Micafungin 150 mg IV daily is another alternative.
- Because azoles and echinocandins target different cellular sites, combination therapy may have additive activity against *Aspergillus sp*. Although still under investigation, some bone marrow transplant units use caspofungin and voriconazole as the preferred initial treatment especially in patients receiving high dose corticosteroids.
- Cytokine therapy may offer future treatment options in conjunction with the currently available antifungals.

REFERRAL

To an infectious diseases specialist

PEARLS & CONSIDERATIONS

!

- Unlike fluconazole, the potential for drug-drug interactions with voriconazole is high.
- Agitation of hospital buildings by renovations or repairs may increase the incidence of *Aspergillus* infections in immunosuppressed individuals.
- Breakthrough zygomycosis infection may occur with voriconazole treatment.

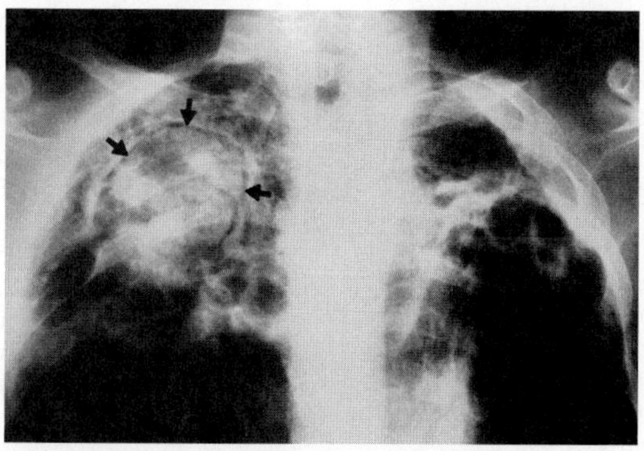

FIGURE 1-28 Fungus ball or mycetoma caused by *Aspergillus*. Coned-down PA view of the chest of a patient with biapical fibrocavitary tuberculosis accompanied by volume loss. There is a mass in a large right upper-lobe cavity with air dissecting into the cavity producing "air crescents" (*arrows*). (From McLoud TC: *Thoracic radiology: the requisites*, St Louis, 1998, Mosby.)

SUGGESTED READINGS

Cook RJ et al: Aspergillus infection of implantable cardioverter defibrillator, *Mayo Clinic Proc* 79(4):549-552, 2005.

Hasejima N et al: Invasive pulmonary aspergillosis associated with influenza B, *Respirology* 10(1):116-119, 2005.

Herbrecht R et al: Voriconazole versus amphotericin B for primary therapy of invasive aspergillosis, *N Engl J Med* 347:408, 2002.

Marr KA et al: Combination antifungal therapy for invasive aspergillosis, *CID* 39:797, 2004.

Pfaller MA: Anidulafungin: an echinocandin antifungal, *Expert Opin Investig Drugs* 13(9): 1183-1197, 2004.

Steinbach WJ, Stevens DA: Review of newer antifungal and immunomodulatory strategies for invasive aspergillosis, *Clin Infect Dis* 37(supp 3):S157, 2003.

AUTHOR: **SAJEEV HANDA, M.D.**

BASIC INFORMATION

DEFINITION

The American Thoracic Society defines asthma as a "disease characterized by an increased responsiveness of the trachea and bronchi to various stimuli and manifested by a widespread narrowing of the airways that changes in severity either spontaneously or as a result of treatment." *Status asthmaticus* can be defined as a severe continuous bronchospasm.

SYNONYMS

Bronchospasm
Reactive airway disease
Bronchial asthma

ICD-9CM CODES
493.9 Asthma, unspecified
493.1 Intrinsic asthma
493.0 Extrinsic asthma

EPIDEMIOLOGY & DEMOGRAPHICS

- Asthma affects 5% to 12% of the population and accounts for over 450,000 hospitalizations and nearly 2 million emergency department visits yearly in the U.S.
- It is more common in children (10% of children, 5% of adults).
- 50% to 80% of children with asthma develop symptoms before 5 yr of age.
- Overall asthma mortality in the U.S. is 20 per 1 million persons.

PHYSICAL FINDINGS & CLINICAL PRESENTATION

Physical examination varies with the stage and severity of asthma and may reveal only increased inspiratory and expiratory phases of respiration. Physical examination during status asthmaticus may reveal:

- Tachycardia and tachypnea
- Use of accessory respiratory muscles
- Pulsus paradoxus (inspiratory decline in systolic blood pressure >10 mm Hg)
- Wheezing: absence of wheezing (silent chest) or decreased wheezing can indicate worsening obstruction
- Mental status changes: generally secondary to hypoxia and hypercapnia and constitute an indication for urgent intubation
- Paradoxic abdominal and diaphragmatic movement on inspiration (detected by palpation over the upper part of the abdomen in a semirecumbent position): important sign of impending respiratory crisis, indicates diaphragmatic fatigue
- The following abnormalities in vital signs are indicative of severe asthma:
  1. Pulsus paradoxus >18 mm Hg
  2. Respiratory rate >30 breaths/min
  3. Tachycardia with heart rate >120 beats/min

ETIOLOGY

- Intrinsic asthma: occurs in patients who have no history of allergies; may be triggered by upper respiratory infections or psychologic stress.
- Extrinsic asthma (allergic asthma): brought on by exposure to allergens (e.g., dust mites, cat allergen, industrial chemicals).
- Exercise-induced asthma: seen most frequently in adolescents; manifests with bronchospasm following initiation of exercise and improves with discontinuation of exercise.
- Drug-induced asthma: often associated with use of NSAIDs, beta blockers, sulfites, certain foods and beverages.
- There is a strong association of the ADAM 33 gene with asthma and bronchial hyperresponsiveness.

DIAGNOSIS

DIFFERENTIAL DIAGNOSIS

- CHF
- COPD
- Pulmonary embolism (in adult and elderly patients)
- Foreign body aspiration (most frequent in younger patients)
- Pneumonia and other upper respiratory infections
- Rhinitis with postnasal drip
- TB
- Hypersensitivity pneumonitis
- Anxiety disorder
- Wegener's granulomatosis
- Diffuse interstitial lung disease

WORKUP

- For symptomatic adults and children aged >5 years who can perform spirometry, asthma can be diagnosed after a medical history and physical examination documenting an episodic pattern of respiratory symptoms and from spirometry that indicates partially reversible airflow obstruction (>12% increase and 200 ml in forced expiratory volume in 1 second [FEV_1] after inhaling a short bronchodilator or receiving a short [2 to 3 week] course of oral corticosteroids). For children aged <5, spirometry is generally not feasible. Young children with asthma symptoms should be treated as having suspected asthma once alternative diagnoses are ruled out.
- Section III describes an algorithm for diagnosing asthma.
- Following diagnosis, it is necessary to classify severity of asthma and monitor at every visit. The following questions are important in assessing patients with asthma:

In the past 2 weeks, how many times have you:

- Had problems with coughing, wheezing, shortness of breath, or chest tightness during the day?
- Awakened at night from sleep because of coughing or other asthma symptoms?
- Awakened in the morning with asthma symptoms?
- Had asthma symptoms that did not improve within 15 min of inhaling a short-acting beta-2 agonist?
- Missed days from school/work?
- Had symptoms while exercising or playing?

What is your highest and lowest peak flow rate since your last visit?
Has your peak flow dropped below ___ L/min (80% of personal best) since your last visit?

LABORATORY TESTS

Laboratory tests are usually not necessary and can be normal if obtained during a stable period. The following laboratory abnormalities may be present during an acute bronchospasm:

- ABGs can be used in staging the severity of an asthmatic attack:
  - Mild: decreased Pao_2 and $Paco_2$, increased pH
  - Moderate: decreased Pao_2, normal $Paco_2$, normal pH
  - Severe: marked decreased Pao_2, increased $Paco_2$, and decreased pH
- CBC, leukocytosis with "left shift" may indicate the existence of bacterial infection.
- Spirometry is recommended at the initial assessment and at least every 1 to 2 years after treatment is initiated and when the symptoms and peak expiratory flow have stabilized. Spirometry as a monitoring measure may be performed more frequently, if indicated, based on severity of symptoms and the disease's lack of response to treatment.
- Pulmonary function studies: during acute severe bronchospasm, FEV_1 is <1 L and peak expiratory flow rate (PEFR) <80 L/min.

IMAGING STUDIES

- Chest x-ray: usually normal, may show evidence of thoracic hyperinflation (e.g., flattening of the diaphragm, increased volume over the retrosternal air space).
- ECG: tachycardia, nonspecific ST-T wave changes are common during an asthmatic attack; may also show cor pulmonale, right bundle-branch block, right axial deviation, counter-clockwise rotation.

TREATMENT

NONPHARMACOLOGIC THERAPY

- Avoidance of triggering factors (e.g., salicylates, sulfites), environmental or occupational triggers
- Encouragement of regular exercise (e.g., swimming)

- Patient education regarding warning signs of an attack and proper use of medications (e.g., correct use of inhalers)

GENERAL Rx

The Expert Panel of the National Asthma Education and Prevention Program (NAEPP) based on the classification of asthma severity recommends the following stepwise approach in the pharmacologic management of asthma in adults and children older than 5 yr:

STEP 1 (MILD INTERMITTENT ASTHMA): No daily medications are needed.

- Short-acting inhaled beta-2 agonists as needed (e.g., albuterol [Ventolin, Proventil], terbutaline [Brethaire], bitolterol [Tornalate], pirbuterol [Maxair]).

STEP 2 (MILD PERSISTENT ASTHMA):

- Low-dose inhaled corticosteroid (e.g., beclomethasone [Beclovent, Vanceril], flunisolide [AeroBid], triamcinolone [Azmacort]) can be used.
- Cromolyn (Intal) or nedocromil (Tilade) can also be used.
- Additional considerations for long-term control are the use of the leukotriene receptor antagonist montelukast (Singulair).
- Quick relief of asthma can be achieved with short-acting inhaled beta-2 agonists (see step 1).
- Although guidelines recommend daily treatment in patients with mild persistent asthma, recent trials have shown that it may be possible to treat mild persistent asthma with short, intermittent courses of inhaled or oral corticosteroids when symptoms worsen thus maintaining control with the least amount of medication without adverse effect on clinical outcome.

STEP 3 (MODERATE PERSISTENT ASTHMA): Daily medication is recommended.

- Low-dose or medium-dose inhaled corticosteroids (see step 2) plus long-acting inhaled beta-2 agonist (salmeterol [Serevent]), or long-acting oral beta-2 agonists (e.g., albuterol, sustained-release tablets). Salmeterol is also available as a dry powder inhaler (Discus) that does not require a spacer device; the dosage is one puff bid. A salmeterol-fluticasone combination for the Discus inhaler (Advair) is now available and simplifies therapy for patients with asthma. It generally should be reserved for patients with at least moderately severe asthma not controlled by an inhaled corticosteroid alone.
- Use short-acting inhaled beta-2 agonists on a prn basis for quick relief.

STEP 4 (SEVERE PERSISTENT ASTHMA):

- Daily treatment with high-dose inhaled corticosteroids plus long-acting inhaled beta-2 agonists (e.g., long-acting oral beta-2 agonist plus long-term systemic corticosteroids [e.g., methylprednisolone, prednisolone, prednisone]) can be used.
- Short-acting beta-2 agonists can be used on a prn basis for quick relief.

Treatment of *status asthmaticus* is as follows:

- Oxygen generally started at 2 to 4 L/min via nasal cannula or Venti-Mask at 40% Fio_2; further adjustments are made according to the ABGs.
- Bronchodilators: various agents and modalities are available. Inhaled bronchodilators are preferred when they can be administered quickly. Parenteral administration of sympathomimetics (e.g., SC epinephrine) when necessary should be accompanied by electrocardiographic monitoring.
- Albuterol (Proventil, Ventolin): 0.5 to 1 ml (2.5 to 5 mg) in 3 ml of saline solution tid or qid via nebulizer is effective. Other useful medications are levalbuterol (R-albuterol, Xopenex) nebulizer solution (0.31 mg/3 mL, 0.63 mg/3mL, 1.25 mg/3 mL), and ipratoprium (Atrovent) nebulizer solution (0.25/mL [0.025%]).
- Corticosteroids
  1. Early administration is advised, particularly in patients using steroids at home.
  2. Patients may be started on methylprednisolone (Solu-Medrol) 0.5 to 1 mg/kg IV loading dose, then q6h prn; higher doses may be necessary in selected patients (particularly those receiving steroids at home); steroids given by inhalation (e.g., beclomethasone 2 inhalations qid, maximum 20 inhalations/day) are also useful for controlling bronchospasm and tapering oral steroids and should be used in all patients with severe asthma. However, inhaled steroids are less effective than oral steroids in mild to moderate and severe acute asthma.
  3. Rapid but judicious tapering of corticosteroids will eliminate serious steroid toxicity; long-term low-dose methotrexate may be an effective means of reducing the systemic corticosteroid requirement in some patients with severe refractory asthma.
  4. The most common errors regarding steroid therapy in acute bronchospasms are the use of "too little, too late" and too rapid tapering with return of bronchospasm.
- IV hydration: judicious use is necessary to avoid CHF in elderly patients.
- IV antibiotics are indicated when there is suspicion of bacterial infection (e.g., infiltrate on chest x-ray, fever, or leukocytosis).
- Intubation and mechanical ventilation are indicated when previous measures fail to produce significant improvement.
- General anesthesia: halothane may reverse bronchospasm in a severe asthmatic who cannot be ventilated adequately by mechanical means.
- IV magnesium sulfate supplementation in children with low or borderline-low magnesium levels may improve acute bronchospasm. Several reports in recent literature point to the beneficial effect on bronchospasm with a 20-min infusion of 40 mg/kg, up to a maximum of 2 g of magnesium sulfate in patients with acute asthma attack.

REFERRAL

Box 1-1 describes indications for referral to an asthma specialist.

BOX 1-1 Possible Indications for Referral to an Asthma Specialist

Severe, acute asthma that has caused loss of consciousness, hypoxia, respiratory failure, convulsions, or near death
Poorly controlled asthma as indicated by admission to a hospital, frequent need for emergency care, need for oral corticosteroids, absence from school or work, disruption of sleep, interference with quality of life
Severe, persistent asthma requiring step 4 care (consider for patients who require step 3 care)
Patient less than 3 years old who requires step 3 or 4 care (consider for patient less than 3 years old who requires step 2 care)
Requirement for continuous oral corticosteroids or high-dose inhaled corticosteroids or more than two short courses of oral corticosteroids within 1 year
Need for additional diagnostic testing such as allergy skin testing, rhinoscopy, provocative challenge, complete pulmonary function testing, bronchoscopy
Consideration for immunotherapy
Need for additional education regarding asthma, complications of asthma and treatment of asthma, problems with adherence to management recommendations, or allergen avoidance
Uncertainty of diagnosis
Complications of asthma, including sinusitis, nasal polyposis, aspergillosis, severe rhinitis, vocal cord dysfunction, gastroesophageal reflux

Modified from National Asthma Education and Prevention Program, National Heart, Lung, and Blood Institute, Expert Panel Report 2: Guidelines for the diagnosis and management of asthma. Washington, DC, NIH Pub No 97-4051, July 1997.

PEARLS & CONSIDERATIONS

COMMENTS

- The differentiation of asthma from COPD can be challenging. A history of atopy and intermittent, reactive symptoms points toward a diagnosis of asthma, whereas smoking and advanced age are more indicative of COPD. Spirometry is very useful to distinguish asthma from COPD.
- In all asthma patients, it is important to treat or prevent comorbid conditions (e.g., rhinosinusitis, vocal cord dysfunction, GERD).
- Inhaled low-dose corticosteroids are the single most effective therapy for adult patients with asthma who require more than an occasional use of short-acting beta-2 agonists to control their asthma.
- Leukotriene modifiers/receptor agonists represent a reasonable alternative in adults unable or unwilling to use corticosteroids; however, these agents are less effective than monotherapy with inhaled corticosteroids.
- Patients who remain symptomatic despite inhaled corticosteroids benefit from the addition of long-acting beta-2 agonists.
- In patients with allergies and elevated serum IgE levels use of anti-IgE therapy is beneficial.
- Omalizumab (Xolair) is a recombinant DNA-derived humanized iGG monoclonal antibody that selectively binds to IgE. It is FDA approved for children 12 years and older with moderate to severe persistent asthma who have a positive skin test or in vitro reactivity to a perennial aeroallergen and whose symptoms are inadequately controlled with inhaled corticosteroids. Its excessive cost (>$10,000 per patient per year) limits its use.

EVIDENCE

Adults

Inhaled and oral corticosteroids have similar efficacy in the treatment of asthma. A systematic review of randomized controlled trials (RCTs) that compared inhaled corticosteroids with oral corticosteroids found that a daily oral dose of prednisolone 7.5 to 10 mg appears to be equivalent to a moderate-to-high inhaled dose. The reviewers note that if there is no alternative to the use of oral corticosteroids for asthma, the lowest possible dose should be used to avoid side effects.[1] Ⓐ

Inhaled corticosteroids lead to clinical improvement and a reduction in oral corticosteroid requirements for asthma patients. There is evidence that antimediators are effective in reducing asthma symptoms, including exercise-induced bronchoconstriction. In general, nedocromil and cromolyn appear to be equally effective. Cromolyn or zafirlukast vs. placebo have been shown to be effective in reducing symptoms and improving lung function in patients with peak expiratory flow variability of 10% or more.[2] Ⓑ

There is no benefit from regular inhaled beta-agonists compared with as needed use in patients with mild to moderate asthma. A systematic review showed little advantage from regular as opposed to as needed use of inhaled beta-agonists. The reviewers note that the findings support the current recommendations to use short-acting beta-2 agonists only for relief of symptoms on an as needed basis, while at the same time giving reassuring evidence against concerns over regular use of inhaled short-acting beta-2 agonists.[3] Ⓐ

Patients with asthma that is poorly controlled on inhaled corticosteroids benefit from the addition of a long-acting beta-2 agonist. A systematic review has found that the addition of a long-acting beta-2 agonist to inhaled corticosteroid therapy results in a 26% reduction in exacerbations over that achieved by steroid monotherapy, and that combination therapy is associated with fewer exacerbations than is achieved by increasing the dose of inhaled corticosteroids.[4] Ⓑ

Evidence-Based References

1. Mash B, Bheekie A, Jones PW: Inhaled versus oral steroids for adults with chronic asthma, *Cochrane Database Syst Rev* 1:2001. Ⓐ
2. Nathan RA, Minkwitz MC, Bonuccelli CM: Two first-line therapies in the treatment of mild asthma: use of peak flow variability as a predictor of effectiveness, *Ann Allergy Asthma Immunol* 82:497-503, 1999. Ⓑ
3. Walters EH et al: Inhaled short acting beta2-agonist use in asthma: regular versus as needed treatment, *Cochrane Database Syst Rev* 1:2003. Ⓐ
4. Sin DD et al: Pharmacological management to reduce exacerbations in adults with asthma: a systematic review and meta-analysis, *JAMA* 292:367-376, 2004. Ⓑ

Children

Systemic and inhaled corticosteroids are both effective in the management of acute asthma in children. Three systematic reviews have demonstrated the effectiveness of systemic corticosteroids in the treatment of acute asthma in children.[1-3] Ⓐ

The first of these reviews found that significantly more children treated with systemic steroids were discharged from hospital early and had fewer relapses in the subsequent 1-3 months compared with placebo.[1] Ⓐ

The second review found that where oral corticosteroids were given early (within 1 h of presentation to the emergency department), there were significantly reduced hospital admission rates vs. placebo.[2] Ⓐ

The third systematic review concluded it was not clear whether there was a benefit with inhaled corticosteroids when used in addition to systemic corticosteroids. There was insufficient evidence that inhaled corticosteroids alone were as effective as systemic therapy.[3] Ⓐ

Evidence-Based References

1. Smith M et al: Corticosteroids for hospitalised children with acute asthma, *Cochrane Database Syst Rev* 1:2003. Ⓐ
2. Rowe BH et al: Early emergency department treatment of acute asthma with systemic corticosteroids, *Cochrane Database Syst Rev* 1:2001. Ⓐ
3. Edmonds ML et al: Early use of inhaled corticosteroids in the emergency department treatment of acute asthma, *Cochrane Database Syst Rev* 3:2003. Ⓐ

SUGGESTED READINGS

American Lung Association Asthma Clinical Research Centers: Randomized comparison of strategies for reducing treatment in mild persistent asthma, *N Engl J Med* 356:2027, 2007.

Boushey HA et al: Daily versus as-needed corticosteroids for mild persistent asthma, *N Engl J Med* 352:1519-1528, 2005.

Courtney AU, McCarter DF, Pollart SM: Childhood asthma: treatment update, *Am Fam Physician* 71:1959-1969, 2005.

Mintz M: Asthma update: part I. Diagnosis, monitoring, and prevention of disease progression, *Am Fam Physician* 70:893, 2004.

National Asthma Education and Prevention Program: *Expert panel report 2: guidelines for diagnosis and management of asthma*, Bethesda, Md, 1997, National Institutes of Health.

National Asthma Education and Prevention Program (NAEPP): Expert panel report: guidelines for the diagnosis and management of asthma—update on selected topics 2002, *J Allergy Clin Immunol* 110(suppl 5):5161, 2002.

Schub S et al: High-dose inhaled fluticasone does not replace oral prednisolone in children with mild to moderate acute asthma, *Pediatrics* 118:644, 2006.

Sin DD et al: Pharmacological management to reduce exacerbations in adults with asthma, *JAMA* 292:367, 2004.

AUTHOR: **FRED F. FERRI, M.D.**

BASIC INFORMATION

DEFINITION

Astrocytoma is a type of neuroepithelial tumor that arises from glial precursor cells (i.e., astrocytes, oligodendrocytes, ependymal cells, choroids plexus and others). Astrocytoma arises from astrocytes within the CNS. They are commonly graded by the World Health Organization (WHO) or the Saint Anne–Mayo grading system.

WHO grades astrocytomas as follows:

- Grade I: juvenile pilocytic astrocytoma, subependymal giant cell astrocytoma, and pleomorphic xanthoastrocytoma
- Grade II: low-grade astrocytoma (LGA), fibrillary infiltrating astrocytoma
- Grade III: anaplastic astrocytoma
- Grade IV: glioblastoma multiforme (GBM)

Grades III and IV are considered high-grade or malignant.

The Saint Anne–Mayo system grades astrocytomas according to the presence or absence of four histologic features: nuclear atypia, mitoses, endothelial proliferation, and necrosis.

- Grade I tumors have none of the features.
- Grade II tumors have one feature.
- Grade III tumors have two features.
- Grade IV tumors have three or more features.

SYNONYMS

Astroglial neoplasms

ICD-9CM CODES
191.9 Astrocytoma, unspecified site

EPIDEMIOLOGY & DEMOGRAPHICS

- Incidence for intracranial astrocytomas is 5 to 10 cases/100,000 persons.
- Astrocytomas can be found at all ages, with an early peak from birth to 4 years of age, followed by a trough between the ages of 15 to 24, and then a steady rise in incidence.
- Male:female ratio is 2:1.
- In adults, glioblastoma is the most common brain tumor, while low-grade astrocytomas represent about 15% of gliomas in adults.
- In children, astrocytomas are the second most common primary brain tumor, and medulloblastoma is the most common.
- Low-grade astrocytomas represent about 25% of all CNS gliomas in children.
- Peak age incidence for juvenile pilocytic astrocytomas is 5 to 14 yr.
- Peak age incidence of anaplastic astrocytoma is 41 yr.
- Peak age incidence for glioblastoma is 45 to 70 yr.

GENETICS:

- Genetic abnormalities that lead to inactivation of tumor-suppressing genes, such as *p53* on chromosome 17p, have been proposed as a predisposing factor.
- Genetic heterogeneity is common within these tumors, suggesting accumulation of genetic abnormalities and a multistep mechanism of progression to higher grades.
- Loss of the *CDKN2* gene on chromosome 9p has been associated with progression to higher grades in patients with low-grade astrocytomas.
- Overexpression of platelet-derived growth factor ligands has been found in most glioblastomas.

PHYSICAL FINDINGS & CLINICAL PRESENTATION

The presenting symptoms of astrocytoma depend, in part, on the location of the lesion and its rate of growth. Astrocytomas classically present with any one or more of the following features:

- Headache (less frequent)
- New-onset partial or generalized seizures (>50%)
- Nausea and vomiting
- Focal neurologic deficit (cranial nerve palsy, hemiplegia, ataxia)
- Change in mental status
- Papilledema (rare)

ETIOLOGY

- The specific etiology of astrocytoma is unknown.
- The only proven risk factor for development of astrocytoma has been significant exposure to ionizing radiation.
- Other risk factors, such as increased exposure to certain chemicals (petroleum, solvents, lead, pesticides and herbicides) have been proposed, but not proven.

DIAGNOSIS

A provisional diagnosis of astrocytoma is made on clinical grounds and radiographic imaging studies. Tissue pathology is needed to establish the diagnosis and to grade the astrocytoma.

DIFFERENTIAL DIAGNOSIS

The differential diagnosis is vast and includes any cause of headache, seizures, change in mental status, and focal neurologic deficits.

WORKUP

- A CT scan or MRI of the head makes the diagnosis of an intracranial brain tumor. However, tissue is needed to establish a diagnosis of astrocytoma.
- Electroencephalography (EEG) is sometimes useful to localize the lesion in patients who present with seizures.
- Stereotactic biopsy under CT or MRI guidance has been shown to be a relatively safe and accurate method for diagnosis of LGA.
- In the presence of mass effect, either clinically or radiologically, craniotomy with open biopsy and tumor debulking is more appropriate than stereotactic biopsy to establish a tissue diagnosis.
- Lumbar puncture (LP) is useful for detection of microscopic leptomeningeal dissemination in malignant astrocytomas. It should be avoided for most patients who are thought to have spinal tumor because the withdrawal of CSF may decompensate spinal mass effect.

LABORATORY TESTS

Blood tests are not very specific.

IMAGING STUDIES

- MRI is the diagnostic imaging study of choice. MRI and magnetic resonance angiography (MRA) are used to locate the margins of the tumor, distinguish vascular masses from tumors, detect low-grade astrocytomas not seen by CT scan, and provide clear views of the posterior fossa.
- Low-grade astrocytomas usually show mass effect and blurring of anatomic boundaries due to their infiltrative nature. Cystic change, focal calcification, or extension into contralateral structures may also be seen.
- High-grade astrocytomas are typically more associated with enhancement after IV contrast administration due to disruption of the blood brain barrier. Only about 8% to 15% of LGAs enhance.
- PET scanning and MR spectroscopy are newer imaging modalities that may be indicated in some patients to assess metabolic and vascular features of a tumor.

ACUTE GENERAL Rx

- When there is evidence of increased intracranial pressure, initiation of intravenous mannitol followed by IV dexamethasone is indicated while waiting for surgical intervention.
- Mechanical ventilation with hyperventilation may be considered if there is depressed consciousness.
- Surgery remains the initial treatment of almost all astrocytomas, particularly if the tumor is in an anatomically accessible location. Surgery helps in:
  1. Establishing a pathologic diagnosis
  2. Debulking the tumor
  3. Alleviating intracranial pressure
  4. Offering complete excision with hope for a cure
- Before surgery, dexamethasone 10 mg IV is given followed by 4 to 6 mg IV q6h.

- Surgical morbidity and mortality is related to tumor location. Patients with deep tumors or tumors in eloquent cortex are at high risk for neurologic deterioration from surgical resection or biopsy.
- Stereotactic radiosurgery is reserved for nonresectable lesions.
- Observation is one option that may be justified if risks of surgical or radiation treatment are greater than risks of medical treatment of presenting symptoms.
- Single or recurrent seizures should be treated with anticonvulsants. Common choices are phenytoin, valproate, carbamazepine, or levetiracetam. The latter has no drug interactions as compared with the older antiepileptic medications.

CHRONIC Rx

- Postoperative radiation therapy is controversial in patients with LGA, but standard in high-grade astrocytoma. Some authorities recommend waiting for symptoms to occur after surgery in patients with LGA before using radiation therapy.
- A randomized controlled trial has shown no survival benefit in treating LGA with adjuvant chemotherapy.
- Chemotherapeutic drugs have been used with some effect in patients with *high-grade astrocytoma*. The addition of adjuvant chemotherapy in these patients has been shown to increase the proportion of long-term survivors from less than 5% to approximately 15% to 20%.
- Current options for adjuvant chemotherapy include single agent carmustine or temozolomide, the PCV regimen (procarbazine/lomustine/vincristine), or placement of Gliadel wafers into the resection cavity at the time of surgery.
- High-dose chemotherapy followed by autologous bone marrow transplantation is a consideration.

DISPOSITION

- Approximately 10% to 35% of astrocytomas (usually grade I pilocytic astrocytomas) are amenable to complete surgical excision and cure. WHO grade I astrocytomas do not usually progress to higher-grade tumors.
- In LGAs, the tumor is more infiltrative and therefore not amenable to complete excision. Nevertheless, most studies recommend surgery to remove as much of the tumor burden as possible.
- The prognosis of patients with LGA is highly variable. A median of 7 yr survival is cited.
- Most LGAs typically progress to higher-grade tumors, and progression occurs more rapidly in older patients.
- Young age at diagnosis is by far the most important prognostic factor correlating with long survival. Other factors associated with a more favorable prognosis include good clinical condition at the time of diagnosis, seizure as a presenting symptom, and small preoperative tumor volume.
- Patient presentation with focal neurologic deficit or changes in personality/mental status is indicative of worse prognosis. Large preoperative tumor volume and high mitotic activity index are associated with a poorer prognosis.
- Malignant astrocytomas, grades III and IV, usually require surgery for debulking. It is not known from prospective studies if surgery improves survival; however, retrospective studies suggest a survival benefit in the surgically treated group.
- Median survival for patients with high-grade astrocytomas is 2 yr for anaplastic type and 1 yr for GBM. Median survival of patients with GBM treated with supportive care is approximately 14 wk. This increases to 20 wk with surgical resection alone, 36 wk with surgery plus XRT, and 40 to 50 wk with the addition of adjuvant chemotherapy.

REFERRAL

A team of specialty consultations is indicated in patients diagnosed with astrocytoma. A neurosurgeon, radiation oncologist, and neurooncologist are all needed to assist in establishing the diagnosis and to provide immediate and follow-up treatment.

PEARLS & CONSIDERATIONS

- Astrocytomas should be resected if possible.
- Approximately two thirds of LGAs will progress to higher-grade lesions, but it is not possible to predict which tumors will progress.
- Other treatment modalities include stereotactic radiosurgery using a gamma knife, and interstitial brachytherapy.

COMMENTS

Controversy exists as to proper management of LGA. It has not been proven that earlier treatment of LGA produces an increase in patient survival as measured from the time of diagnosis.

SUGGESTED READINGS

Claus, EB, Black, PM: Survival rates and patterns of care for patients diagnosed with supratentorial low-grade gliomas: data from the SEER program, 1973-2001, *Cancer* 106:1358, 2006.

Grossman SA, Batara JF: Current management of glioblastoma multiforme, *Semin Oncol* 31(5):635, 2004.

Reardon DA et al: Recent advances in the treatment of malignant astrocytoma, *J Clin Oncol* 24:8, 2006.

See SJ, Gilbert MR: Anaplastic astrocytoma: diagnosis, prognosis, and management, *Semin Oncol* 31(5):618, 2004.

Siker ML et al: Should concomitant and adjuvant treatment with temozolomide be used as standard therapy in patients with anaplastic glioma? *Crit Rev Oncol Hematol* 60:2, 2006.

AUTHOR: **WEN-Y. WU-CHEN, M.D.**

BASIC INFORMATION

DEFINITION

Ataxia telangiectasia (A-T) is a rare autosomal recessive disorder of childhood that results from defective DNA damage repair. A-T is a multisystemic disease characterized by progressive cerebellar ataxia, choreoathetosis, telangiectasias of the skin and conjunctiva (see Fig. 1-29), frequent infections, increased sensitivity to ionizing radiation, and predisposition to malignancies, particularly leukemia and lymphoma.

ICD-9CM CODES
334.8 Ataxia telangiectasia

EPIDEMIOLOGY & DEMOGRAPHICS

INCIDENCE: 1/40,000 live births. A-T is the most common cause of progressive cerebellar ataxia in childhood in most countries. It is estimated that 1% to 2% of the U.S. population may be carriers of A-T.
PEAK INCIDENCE: Childhood
PREDOMINANT SEX: Males = Females
GENETICS: AR, chromosome 11q22-q23. Gene product is *ATM,* which encodes a protein kinase.

PHYSICAL FINDINGS & CLINICAL PRESENTATION

- Children show normal early development until they start to walk, when gait and truncal ataxia become apparent. They soon develop polyneuropathy, progressive apraxia of eye movements and slurred speech, choreoathetosis, mild diabetes mellitus, delayed physical and sexual development, and signs of premature aging (graying of the hair).
- Children with A-T experience deterioration of motor skills; by the second decade of life, most patients rely on wheelchairs for at least part of the day. Progressive oromotor difficulties also develop over time, placing patients at risk for aspiration.

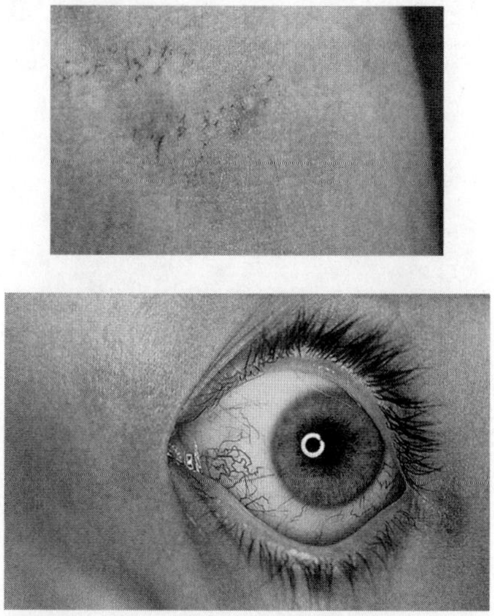

FIGURE 1-29 Ataxia telangiectasia. (From Callen JP [ed]: *Color atlas of dermatology,* ed 2, Philadelphia, 2000, WB Saunders.)

- Telangiectasias, which are characteristic of the disease but not always present, occur in the outer parts of the bulbar conjunctivae, over the surface of the ears and cheeks, on exposed parts of the neck, on the bridge of the nose, and in the flexor creases of the forearms.
- Immunodeficiencies occur in 60% to 80% of individuals with A-T. Impaired humoral and cellular immunity lead to recurrent sinopulmonary infections in about 70% of children.
- Cancer risk in individuals with A-T is 38%, of which leukemia and lymphoma account for about 95% of malignancies. As individuals begin to have longer life span, other malignancies are observed, such as melanoma, sarcomas, and cancers of the ovary, breast, stomach, brain, larynx, liver, and parotid gland. Multicenter trials are investigating the interaction between *ATM* and mutations in breast cancer susceptibility genes (BRCA 1 and 2).
- Typically, individuals with A-T have normal intelligence. Deterioration of speech is typically noted after the age of 5 to 8 years.
- Heterozygotes/carriers of the *ATM* gene are thought to have none of the classical manifestations of A-T.

DIAGNOSIS

Diagnosis relies on the constellation of clinical findings, including ataxia and speech changes, as well as family history and neuroimaging studies. A clinical diagnosis can now be confirmed by radiosensitivity testing (colony survival assay), immunoblotting, and mutation analysis.

DIFFERENTIAL DIAGNOSIS (OF EARLY ONSET ATAXIAS)

- Friedreich's ataxia
- Abetalipoproteinemia
- Acquired vitamin E deficiency
- Early-onset cerebellar ataxia with retained reflexes (EOCA)
- Ataxia-ocular apraxia type 1 (AOA1)
- Ataxia with metabolic abnormalities: associated with ceroid lipofuscinosis, xeroderma pigmentosa, Cockayne's syndrome, adrenoleukodystrophy, metachromatic leukodystrophy, mitochondrial disease, sialidosis, Niemann-Pick

WORKUP

- Patients should be evaluated for immunoglobulin (IgA, IgG, IgE, and IgG subclasses) deficiency, and alpha fetoprotein, which is elevated in more than 95% of patients.
- Cytogenetics show a 7;14 translocation in 5% to 15% of individuals with A-T. The result is a defective protein kinase. This delays accumulation of the tumor suppressor p53 in response to DNA damage, thereby increasing the risk of cancer. Cells are susceptible to damage by ionizing radiation or chemotherapeutic agents that cause double-stranded DNA breakages. Prenatal testing is available. Fibroblasts can be screened for abnormal sensitivity to ionizing radiation.
- CT or MRI scans will show cerebellar atrophy, but may not be obvious in very young children.
- Immunoblotting for ATM protein. This determines whether ATM protein is present in cells; approximately 90% of individuals will have no detectable ATM protein.
- Pathology shows cerebellar degeneration, loss of pigmented neurons, and posterior column degeneration in the spinal cord.

TREATMENT

- There is no proven treatment available to delay the progressive ataxia, dysarthria and oculomotor apraxia. Treatment remains supportive.
- Surveillance for infections and neoplasms. Individuals with frequent and severe infections may benefit from intravenous immunoglobulin to supplement immune system.
- Antioxidant treatment with Vitamin E is often given empirically, though it has not been formally tested.
- Minimize radiation. Even diagnostic x-rays should be limited.
- Physical and occupational therapy to maintain flexibility and minimize contractures.

DISPOSITION

- The expected life span has increased considerably; most individuals now live beyond 25 years of age and some into the fourth and fifth decades.

REFERRAL

Immunology, neurology, physical and occupational therapy, genetic counselor

PEARLS & CONSIDERATIONS

- Most common cause of hereditary ataxia
- Defect in DNA repair
- Predisposition to frequent infections, malignancies and sensitivity to ionizing radiation

SUGGESTED READINGS

Butch AW et al: Immunoassay to measure ataxia-telangiectasia mutated protein in cellular lysates, *Clin Chem* 50:2302-2308, 2004.

Nowak-Wegrzyn A: Immunodeficiency and infections in ataxia-telangiectasia, *J Pediatr* 144:505, 2004.

Sun X et al: Early diagnosis of ataxia-telangiectasia using radiosensitivity testing, *J Pediatr* 140:724-731, 2002.

Taylor AMR, Byrd, PJ: Molecular pathology of ataxia telangiectasia, *J Clin Pathol* 58(10): 1009-1015, 2005.

AUTHOR: **NICOLE J. ULLRICH, M.D., PH.D.**

BASIC INFORMATION

DEFINITION

Atelectasis is the collapse of lung volume.

ICD-9CM CODES
518.0 Atelectasis

EPIDEMIOLOGY & DEMOGRAPHICS

- Occurs frequently in patients receiving mechanical ventilation with higher Fio_2
- Dependent regions of the lung are more prone to atelectasis: they are partially compressed, they are not as well ventilated, and there is no spontaneous drainage of secretions with gravity

PHYSICAL FINDINGS & CLINICAL PRESENTATION

- Decreased or absent breath sounds
- Abnormal chest percussion
- Cough, dyspnea, decreased vocal fremitus and vocal resonance
- Diminished chest expansion, tachypnea, tachycardia

ETIOLOGY

- Mechanical ventilation with higher Fio_2
- Chronic bronchitis
- Cystic fibrosis
- Endobronchial neoplasms
- Foreign bodies
- Infections (e.g., TB, histoplasmosis)
- Extrinsic bronchial compression from neoplasms, aneurysms of ascending aorta, enlarged left atrium
- Sarcoidosis
- Silicosis
- Anterior chest wall injury, pneumothorax
- Alveolar injury (e.g., toxic fumes, aspiration of gastric contents)
- Pleural effusion, expanding bullae
- Chest wall deformity (e.g., scoliosis)
- Muscular weaknesses or abnormalities (e.g., neuromuscular disease)
- Mucus plugs from asthma, allergic bronchopulmonary aspergillosis, postoperative state

DIAGNOSIS

DIFFERENTIAL DIAGNOSIS

- Neoplasm
- Pneumonia
- Encapsulated pleural effusion
- Abnormalities of brachiocephalic vein and of the left pulmonary ligament

WORKUP

- Chest x-ray (Fig. 1-30)
- CT scan and fiberoptic bronchoscopy (selected patients)

IMAGING STUDIES

- Chest x-ray will confirm diagnosis.
- CT scan is useful in patients with suspected endobronchial neoplasm or extrinsic bronchial compression.
- Fiberoptic bronchoscopy (selected patients) is useful for removal of foreign body or evaluation of endobronchial and peribronchial lesions.

TREATMENT

NONPHARMACOLOGIC THERAPY

- Deep breathing, mobilization of the patient
- Incentive spirometry
- Tracheal suctioning
- Humidification
- Chest physiotherapy with percussion and postural drainage

ACUTE GENERAL Rx

- Positive-pressure breathing (CPAP by face mask, positive end-expiratory pressure [PEEP] for patients on mechanical ventilation)
- Use of mucolytic agents (e.g., acetylcysteine [Mucomyst])
- Recombinant human DNase (dornase alpha) in patients with cystic fibrosis
- Bronchodilator therapy in selected patients

CHRONIC Rx

- Chest physiotherapy
- Humidification of inspired air
- Frequent nasotracheal suctioning

DISPOSITION

Prognosis varies with the underlying etiology.

REFERRAL

- Bronchoscopy for removal of foreign body or plugs unresponsive to conservative treatment
- Surgical referral for removal of obstructing neoplasms

PEARLS & CONSIDERATIONS

COMMENTS

Patients should be educated that frequent changes of position are helpful in clearing secretions. Sitting the patient upright in a chair is recommended to increase both volume and vital capacity relative to the supine position.

AUTHOR: **FRED F. FERRI, M.D.**

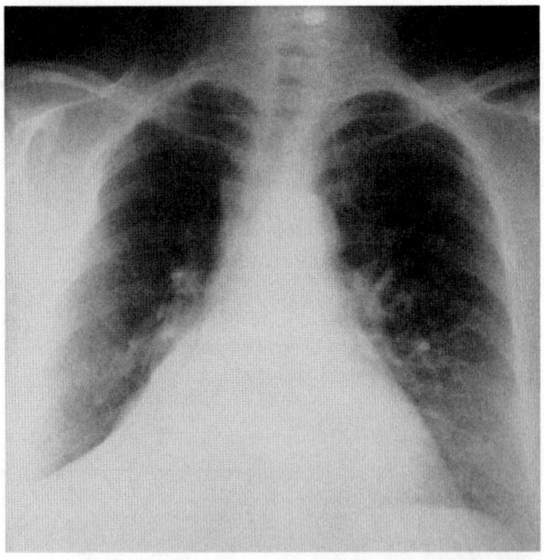

FIGURE 1-30 Right middle and right lower lobe atelectasis that silhouettes the diaphram and the right heart border. (From Specht N [ed]: *Practical guide to diagnostic imaging,* St Louis, 1998, Mosby.)

BASIC INFORMATION

DEFINITION

Atopic dermatitis is a genetically determined eczematous eruption that is pruritic, symmetric, and associated with personal family history of allergic manifestations (atopy).

SYNONYMS

Eczema
Atopic neurodermatitis
Atopic eczema

ICD-9CM CODES
691.8 Atopic dermatitis

EPIDEMIOLOGY & DEMOGRAPHICS

- Incidence is between 5 and 25 cases/1000 persons.
- Highest incidence is among children (5% to 10%). It accounts for 4% of acute care pediatric visits.
- Onset of disease before age 5 yr in 85% of patients.
- More than 50% of children with generalized atopic dermatitis develop asthma and allergic rhinitis by age 13 yr.
- Concordance in monozygotic twins is 86%.

PHYSICAL FINDINGS & CLINICAL PRESENTATION

- There are no specific cutaneous signs for atopic dermatitis, and there is a wide spectrum of presentations ranging from minimal flexural eczema to erythroderma.
- The primary lesions are a result of itching caused by severe and chronic pruritus. The repeated scratching modifies the skin surface, producing lichenification, dry and scaly skin, and redness.
- The lesions are typically on the neck, face, upper trunk, and bends of elbows and knees (symmetric on flexural surfaces of extremities).
- There is dryness, thickening of the involved areas, discoloration, blistering, and oozing.
- Papular lesions are frequently found in the antecubital and popliteal fossae.
- In children, red scaling plaques are often confined to the cheeks and the perioral and perinasal areas.
- Inflammation in the flexural areas and lichenified skin is a very common presentation in children.
- Constant scratching may result in areas of hypopigmentation or hyperpigmentation (more common in blacks).
- In adults, redness and scaling in the dorsal aspect of the hands or about the fingers are the most common expression of atopic dermatitis; oozing and crusting may be present.
- Secondary skin infections may be present (*Staphylococcus aureus,* dermatophytosis, herpes simplex).

ETIOLOGY

Unknown; elevated T-lymphocyte activation, defective cell immunity, and B cell IgE overproduction may play a significant role.

DIAGNOSIS

DIFFERENTIAL DIAGNOSIS

- Scabies
- Psoriasis
- Dermatitis herpetiform
- Contact dermatitis
- Photosensitivity
- Seborrheic dermatitis
- Candidiasis
- Lichen simplex chronicus
- Other: Wiskott-Aldrich syndrome, PKU, mycosis fungoides, ichthyosis, HIV dermatitis, nonnummular eczema, histiocytosis X

WORKUP

Diagnosis is based on the presence of three of the following major features and three minor features.

MAJOR FEATURES:
- Pruritus
- Personal or family history of atopy: asthma, allergic rhinitis, atopic dermatitis
- Facial and extensor involvement in infants and children
- Flexural lichenification in adults

MINOR FEATURES:
- Elevated IgE
- Eczema-perifollicular accentuation
- Recurrent conjunctivitis
- Ichthyosis
- Nipple dermatitis
- Wool intolerance
- Cutaneous *S. aureus* infections or herpes simplex infections
- Food intolerance
- Hand dermatitis (nonallergic irritant)
- Facial pallor, facial erythema
- Cheilitis
- White dermographism
- Early age of onset (after 2 mo of age)

LABORATORY TESTS

- Lab tests are generally not helpful.
- Elevated IgE levels are found in 80% to 90% of atopic dermatitis.
- Blood eosinophilia correlates with disease severity.

TREATMENT

NONPHARMACOLOGIC THERAPY

Avoidance of triggering factors:
- Sudden temperature changes, sweating, low humidity in the winter
- Contact with irritating substance (e.g., wool, cosmetics, some soaps and detergents, tobacco)
- Foods that provoke exacerbations (e.g., eggs, peanuts, fish, soy, wheat, milk)
- Stressful situations
- Allergens and dust
- Excessive hand washing
- Clip nails to decrease abrasion of skin

GENERAL Rx

- Emollients can be used to prevent dryness. Severely affected skin can be optimally hydrated by occlusion in addition to application of emollients.
- Topical corticosteroids (e.g., 1% to 2.5% hydrocortisone) may be helpful and are generally considered first line therapy. Use intermediate-potency steroids (e.g., triamcinolone, fluocinolone) for more severe cases and limit potent corticosteroids (e.g., betamethasone, desoximetasone, clobetasol) to severe cases.
- The topical immunomodulators pimecrolimus and tacrolimus are especially useful for treatment of the face and intertriginous sites, where steroid-induced atrophy may occur. However, due to concerns about carcinogenic potential, the FDA recommends limiting their use for short periods in patients who are intolerant or unresponsive to other treatments. Pimecrolimus cream (Elidel) 1% is applied bid and has antiinflammatory effects secondary to blockage of activated T-cell cytokine production. Tacrolimus (Protopic) ointment (0.03% or 0.1%) applied bid is a macrolide that suppresses humoral and cell-mediated immune responses.
- Oral antihistamines (e.g., hydroxyzine, diphenhydramine) are effective in controlling pruritus and inducing sedation, restful sleep, and prevention of scratching during sleep. Doxepin and other tricyclic antidepressants also have antihistamine effect, induce sleep, and reduce pruritus.
- Oral prednisone, IM triamcinolone, Goeckerman regimen, PUVA are generally reserved for severe cases.
- Methotrexate, cyclosporine azathioprine, and systemic corticosteroids are sometimes tried for recalcitrant disease in adults.

DISPOSITION

- Resolution occurs in approximately 40% of patients by adulthood.
- Most patients have a course characterized by remissions and intermittent flares.

SUGGESTED READING

Buys LM: Treatment options for atopic dermatitis, *Am Fam Physician* 75:523-528, 2007.

AUTHOR: **FRED F. FERRI, M.D.**

BASIC INFORMATION

DEFINITION

Atrial fibrillation is totally chaotic atrial activity caused by simultaneous discharge of multiple atrial foci.

SYNONYMS

AF
A-fib

ICD-9CM CODES
427.31 Atrial fibrillation

EPIDEMIOLOGY & DEMOGRAPHICS

- The prevalence of atrial fibrillation increases with age, from 2% in the general population, to 5% in patients older than 60 yr, to 9% of those aged 80 years or older.
- Atrial fibrillation affects 2.3 million people in the U.S. and is a major cause of stroke (fivefold increased risk of stroke).
- Chronic atrial fibrillation develops in 25% 5 years after paroxysmal atrial fibrillation.

PHYSICAL FINDINGS & CLINICAL PRESENTATION

Clinical presentation is variable:
- Most common complaint: palpitations
- Fatigue, dizziness, light-headedness in some patients
- A few completely asymptomatic patients
- Cardiac auscultation revealing irregularly irregular rhythm

ETIOLOGY

- Coronary artery disease
- MS, MR, AS, AR
- Thyrotoxicosis
- Pulmonary embolism, COPD
- Pericarditis
- Myocarditis, cardiomyopathy
- Tachycardia-bradycardia syndrome
- Alcohol abuse
- MI
- WPW syndrome
- Obesity (The excess risk of AF associated with obesity appears to be mediated by left atrial dilation.)
- Other causes: left atrial myxoma, atrial septal defect, carbon monoxide poisoning, pheochromocytoma, idiopathic, hypoxia, hypokalemia, sepsis, pneumonia
- Arterial stiffness as measured by an elevated pulse pressure (the difference between systolic and diastolic pressure) is a risk factor for incident AF

DIAGNOSIS

DIFFERENTIAL DIAGNOSIS

- Multifocal atrial tachycardia
- Atrial flutter
- Frequent atrial premature beats

WORKUP

New-onset atrial fibrillation: ECG, echocardiogram, Holter monitor (selected patients), and laboratory evaluation

LABORATORY TESTS

- TSH, free T_4
- Serum electrolytes

IMAGING STUDIES

- ECG (see Fig. 1-31 for "Atrial flutter and atrial fibrillation")
  1. Irregular, nonperiodic wave forms (best seen in V1) reflecting continuous atrial reentry
  2. Absence of P waves
  3. Conducted QRS complexes showing no periodicity
- Echocardiography to evaluate left atrial size and detect valvular disorders
- Holter monitor: useful only in selected patients to evaluate paroxysmal atrial fibrillation

TREATMENT

NONPHARMACOLOGIC THERAPY

- Avoidance of alcohol in patients with suspected excessive alcohol use
- Avoidance of caffeine and nicotine

ACUTE GENERAL Rx

New-onset atrial fibrillation
- If the patient is hemodynamically unstable, perform synchronized cardioversion following immediate conscious sedation with a rapid short-acting sedative (e.g., midazolam).
- If the patient is hemodynamically stable, treatment options include the following:
  1. Diltiazem 0.25 mg/kg given over 2 min followed by a second dose of 0.35 mg/kg 15 min later if the rate is not slowed. May then follow with IV infusion 10 mg/hr (range 5 to 15 mg/hr). Onset of action following IV administration is usually within 3 min, with peak effect most often occurring within 10 min. After the ventricular rate is slowed, the patient can be changed to oral diltiazem 60 to 90 mg q 6 hr.
  2. Verapamil 2.5 to 5 mg IV initially, then 5 to 10 mg IV 10 min later if the rate is still not slowed. After the ventricular rate is slowed, the patient can be changed to oral verapamil 80 to 120 mg q6 to 8h.
  3. Esmolol, metoprolol, atenolol are beta blockers that are available in IV preparations that can be used in atrial fibrillation.
  4. Other medications useful for converting atrial fibrillation to sinus rhythm are ibutilide, flecainide, propafenone, disopyramide, amiodarone, and quinidine.
  5. Digoxin is not a very potent AV nodal blocking agent and cannot be relied on for acute control of the ventricular response. When used, give 0.5 mg IV loading dose (slow), then 0.25 mg IV 6 hr later. A third dose may be needed after 6 to 8 hr; daily dose varies from 0.125 to 0.25 mg (decrease dosage in patients with renal insufficiency and elderly patients). Digoxin should be avoided in Wolff-Parkinson-White patients with atrial fibrillation. Procainamide is the preferred pharmacologic agent in these patients.
- IV heparin or SC low molecular weight heparin.
- Cardioversion is indicated if the ventricular rate is >140 bpm and the patient is symptomatic (particularly in acute MI, chest pain, dyspnea, CHF) or when there is no conversion to normal sinus rhythm after 3 days of pharmacologic therapy. The likelihood of cardioversion-related clinical thromboembolism is low in patients with atrial fibrillation lasting <48 hr. Patients with atrial fibrillation lasting >2 days have a 5% to 7% risk of clinical thromboembolism if cardioversion is not preceded by several weeks of warfarin therapy. However, if transesophageal echocardiography reveals no atrial thrombus, cardioversion may be performed safely after only a short period of anticoagulant therapy. Anticoagulant therapy should be continued for at least 1 mo after cardioversion to minimize the incidence of adverse thromboembolic events following conversion from atrial fibrillation to sinus rhythm.
- Anticoagulate with warfarin (unless patient has specific contraindications).
- Long-term anticoagulation with warfarin (adjusted to maintain an INR of 2 to 3) is indicated in all patients with atrial fibrillation and associated cardiovascular disease, including the following:
  1. Rheumatic valvular disease (MS, MR, AI)
  2. Aortic stenosis
  3. Prostatic heart valves
  4. History of previous embolism
  5. Persistent atrial thrombus on transesophageal echocardiography
  6. CHF
  7. Cardiomyopathy with poor left ventricular function
  8. Nonrheumatic heart disease (e.g., hypertensive cardiovascular disease, coronary artery disease, ASD)
- Anticoagulation with warfarin is generally not recommended in patients <60

yr with lone atrial fibrillation (no associated cardiovascular disease or diabetes). Aspirin at a dose of 325 mg/day is appropriate therapy in these patients.
- Aspirin 325 mg/day may also be a suitable alternative to warfarin in patients 60 to 75 yr and no risk factors and in those who refuse warfarin or have contraindications to its use.
- Medical cardioversion:
  1. Attempts at medical (pharmacologic) intervention should be considered only after proper anticoagulation because cardioversion can lead to systemic emboli. Following successful cardioversion, anticoagulation with warfarin should be continued for 4 wk.
  2. Useful agents for medical cardioversion are quinidine, flecainide, propafenone, amiodarone, ibutilide, sotalol, dofetilide, and procainamide. Procainamide (total dose of 15 mg/kg given IV at 15 to 20 mg/kg) will restore sinus rhythm in 60% of patients with AF of <1 wk duration. AV nodal blocking agents should be administered before using procainamide or any other primary antiarrhythmic agent to prevent conversion of atrial fibrillation into atrial flutter.
  3. Amiodarone appears to be the most effective agent for converting to sinus rhythm in patients who do not respond to other agents. Amiodarone therapy should be considered for patients with recent atrial fibrillation and structural heart disease, particularly those with left ventricular dysfunction. Amiodarone should also be considered for patients with refractory conditions who do not have heart disease, before therapies with irreversible effects such as AV nodal ablation are attempted. Amiodarone is also effective in maintaining sinus rhythm in atrial fibrillation but is associated with potentially serious toxic effects. Dronedarone is a new antiarrhythmic agent, pharmacologically related to amiodarone, which appears to be effective with less side effects in early trials.
  4. Anticoagulant therapy should be continued for at least 1 mo after cardioversion with antiarrhythmic drugs because patients may remain at risk, in the short term, for atrial clot formation even after restoration of sinus rhythm.

CHRONIC Rx

- Anticoagulation with warfarin (see "Acute General Rx")
- Rate control with atenolol, metoprolol, verapamil, or diltiazem

DISPOSITION

Factors associated with maintenance of sinus rhythm following cardioversion:
- Left atrium diameter <60 mm
- Absence of mitral valve disease
- Short duration of atrial fibrillation

REFERRAL

Surgical treatment of atrial fibrillation:
- The maze procedure with its recent modifications creating electrical barriers to the macroreentrant circuits that are thought to underlie atrial fibrillation is being performed with good results in several medical centers (preservation of sinus rhythm in >95% of patients without the use of long-term antiarrhythmic medication). Clear indications for its use remain undefined. Generally surgery is reserved for patients with rapid heart rate refractory to pharmacologic therapy or who cannot tolerate pharmacologic therapy.
- Catheter-based radiofrequency ablation procedures designed to eliminate atrial fibrillation represent newer approaches to atrial fibrillation. Restoration and maintenance of sinus rhythm by catheter ablation without the use of drugs in patients with congestive heart failure and atrial fibrillation significantly improves cardiac function, symptoms, exercise capacity, and quality of life.
- Pulmonary vein ablation for chronic atrial fibrillation: Sinus rhythm can be maintained long term in the majority of patients with chronic atrial fibrillation by means of circumferential pulmonary vein ablation, independently of the effects of antiarrhythmic drug therapy, cardioversion, or both.
- Implantable pacemakers and defibrillators that combine pacing and cardioversion therapies to both prevent and treat atrial defibrillation are likely to have an increasing role in the future management of atrial fibrillation.

PEARLS & CONSIDERATIONS

COMMENTS

The American Academy of Family Physicians and the American College of Physicians provide the following recommendations for the management of newly detected atrial fibrillation:
- Rate control with chronic anticoagulation is the recommended strategy for the majority of patients with atrial fibrillation. Rhythm control has not been shown to be superior to rate control (with chronic anticoagulation) in reducing morbidity and mortality and may be inferior in some patient subgroups to rate control. Rhythm control is appropriate when based on other special considerations, such as patient symptoms, exercise tolerance, and patient preference.
- Patients with atrial fibrillation should receive chronic anticoagulation with adjusted-dose warfarin, unless they are at low risk of stroke or have a specific contraindication to the use of warfarin (thrombocytopenia, recent trauma or surgery, alcoholism).
- For patients with atrial fibrillation, the following drugs are recommended for their demonstrated efficacy in rate control during exercise and while at rest: atenolol, metoprolol, diltiazem, and verapamil (drugs listed alphabetically by class). Digoxin is only effective for rate control at rest and therefore should only be used as a second-line agent for rate control in atrial fibrillation.
- For those patients who elect to undergo acute cardioversion to achieve sinus rhythm in atrial fibrillation, both direct-current cardioversion and pharmacologic conversion are appropriate options.
- Both transesophageal echocardiography with short-term prior anticoagulation followed by early acute cardioversion (in absence of intracardiac thrombus) with postcardioversion anticoagulation versus delayed cardioversion with pre- and postanticoagulation are appropriate management strategies for those patients who elect to undergo cardioversion.
- Most patients converted to sinus rhythm from atrial fibrillation should not be placed on rhythm maintenance therapy since the risks outweigh the benefits. In a selected group of patients whose quality of life is compromised by atrial fibrillation, the recommended pharmacologic agents for rhythm maintenance are amiodarone, disopyramide, propafenone, and sotalol (drugs listed in alphabetical order). The choice of agent depends on specific risk of side effects based on patient characteristics.

EVIDENCE

EBM

There is evidence for similar mortality and cardiovascular morbidity in older patients with atrial fibrillation treated with either a rate-controlling therapy or rhythm-controlling therapy.

Five randomized controlled trials (RCTs) have recently found similar mortality rates between patients with rate-controlled atrial fibrillation and rhythm control.[1] The largest of these trials used a beta blocker, a calcium channel blocker, digoxin, or a combination of these for rate-control therapy. The rhythm-control therapies consisted of a wide range of antiarrhythmic drugs (most often amiodarone, followed by sotalol and propafenone), and 18% of that group underwent cardioversion. Patients included were at least 65 years old and had at least one other risk factor for stroke or death. After an average of 3.5 years follow-up there was no difference between the two groups in rates of death, disabling stroke, disabling encephalopathy, major bleeding, or cardiac arrest. It also found that more patients in the rhythm-control group required hospitalization and had adverse drug effects. These results may not apply to younger, healthier patients.[2] Ⓑ

However, a recent systematic review has questioned the validity of previous reviews and RCTs and suggests that benefits of long-term anticoagulation have yet to be established in patients with nonrheumatic atrial fibrillation.[3] Ⓐ

Digoxin is ineffective during exercise and may be more useful in patients with chronic atrial fibrillation when rate control during exercise is less important. Intravenous digoxin has been shown to reduce the ventricular rate in patients with acute atrial fibrillation in the short term.[4,5] Ⓐ

Digoxin was not shown to be more effective than placebo for converting patients in acute atrial fibrillation to sinus rhythm in three RCTs.[4-6] Ⓐ

In patients with chronic atrial fibrillation, control of the ventricular rate during exercise with digoxin was poor unless a beta blocker or rate-limiting calcium channel blocker was added.[7]

There is evidence that verapamil is effective at controlling rate at rest and during exercise. A systematic review included five RCTs comparing verapamil with placebo. It found that the heart rate was reduced significantly both at rest and with exercise, compared with placebo.[8] Ⓑ

In selected patients rhythm control may be more appropriate, however studies of pharmacologic rhythm control have only produced limited evidence due to their small size and short follow-up. A meta-analysis of 60 RCTs found ibutilide, flecainide, dofetilide, propafenone, and amiodarone to be the most effective of the eight drugs evaluated.[9] Ⓑ

Two RCTs that compared oral flecainide vs intravenous amiodarone in people with atrial fibrillation found that flecainide was associated with a higher rate of conversion to sinus rhythm at 8h.[10,11] Ⓐ

A study of 172 patients with nonvalvular atrial fibrillation treated with transesophageal echocardiographic guided early cardioversion found that short-term low molecular weight heparin treatment was as safe as standard unfractionated heparin for the prevention of thromboembolic events after cardioversion.[12] Ⓑ

Evidence-Based References

1. Cadwallader K, Jankowski TA: Other than anticoagulation, what is the best therapy for those with atrial fibrillation? *J Fam Pract* 53:581-583, 2004.
2. AFFIRM Investigators: A comparison of rate control and rhythm control in patients with atrial fibrillation, *N Engl J Med* 347:1825-1833, 2002. Ⓑ
3. Taylor F, Cohen H, Ebrahim S: Systematic review of long term anticoagulation or antiplatelet treatment in patients with non-rheumatic atrial fibrillation, *BMJ* 322:321-326, 2001. Reviewed in: Clinical Evidence 11:257-283, 2004. Ⓐ
4. DAAF trial group: Intravenous digoxin in acute atrial fibrillation. Results of a randomized, placebo-controlled multicentre trial in 239 patients. The Digitalis in Acute AF (DAAF) Trial Group, *Eur Heart J* 18:649-654, 1997. Reviewed in: Clinical Evidence 11:76-97, 2004. Ⓐ
5. Jordaens L et al: Conversion of atrial fibrillation to sinus rhythm and rate control by digoxin in comparison to placebo, *Eur Heart J* 18:643-648, 1997. Reviewed in: Clinical Evidence 11:76-97, 2004. Ⓐ
6. Falk RH et al: Digoxin for converting recent-onset atrial fibrillation to sinus rhythm, *Ann Intern Med* 106:503-506, 1987. Reviewed in: Clinical Evidence 11:76-97, 2004. Ⓐ
7. Lip GYH, Kamath S, Freestone B: Atrial fibrillation (acute). In: Clinical Evidence 11:76-97, 2004. London: BMJ Publishing Group.
8. Segal JB et al: The evidence regarding the drugs used for ventricular rate control, *J Fam Pract* 49:47-59, 2000. Ⓑ
9. McNamara RL et al: Management of atrial fibrillation: a review of the evidence for the role of pharmacologic therapy, electrical cardioversion, and echocardiography, *Ann Intern Med* 139:1018-1033, 2003. Ⓑ
10. Boriani G et al: Conversion of recent-onset atrial fibrillation to sinus rhythm: effects of different drug protocols, *Pacing Clin Electrophysiol* 21:2470-2474, 1998. Reviewed in: Clinical Evidence 11:76-97, 2004. Ⓐ
11. Capucci A et al: Effectiveness of loading oral flecainide for converting recent-onset atrial fibrillation to sinus rhythm in patients without organic heart disease or with only systemic hypertension, *Am J Cardiol* 70:69-70, 1992. Reviewed in: Clinical Evidence 11:76-97, 2004. Ⓐ
12. Yigit Z et al: The safety of low-molecular weight heparins for the prevention of thromboembolic events after cardioversion of atrial fibrillation, *Jpn Heart J* 44:369-377, 2003. Ⓑ

SUGGESTED READINGS

Cooper JM et al: Implantable devices for the treatment of atrial fibrillation, *N Engl J Med* 346:2062, 2002.

Ezekowitz M, Falk RH: The increasing need for anticoagulation therapy to prevent stroke in patients with atrial fibrillation, *Mayo Clin Proc* 79(7):904, 2004.

Hart RG: Atrial fibrillation and stroke prevention, *N Engl J Med* 349:1015, 2003.

Hart RG et al: Meta-analysis: antithrombotic therapy to prevent stroke in patients who have non-valvular atrial fibrillation, *Ann Intern Med* 146:857, 2007.

Hilek E et al: Effect of intensity of oral anticoagulation on stroke severity and mortality in atrial fibrillation. *N Engl J Med* 349:1019, 2003.

Hsu LF et al: Catheter ablation for atrial fibrillation in congestive heart failure, *N Engl J Med* 351:2373-2383, 2004.

Klein AL et al: Use of transesophageal echocardiography to guide cardioversions in patients with atrial fibrillation, *N Engl J Med* 344:1411, 2001.

Lip G, Tse H: Management of atrial fibrillation, *Lancet* 370:604, 2007.

Mitchell GF et al: Pulse pressure and risk of new-onset atrial fibrillation, *JAMA* 297:709, 2007.

Oral H et al: Circumferential pulmonary-vein ablation for chronic atrial fibrillation, *N Engl J Med* 354:934, 2006.

Page RL: Newly diagnosed atrial fibrillation, *N Engl J Med* 351:2408-2416, 2004.

Singh B et al: Dronedarone for maintenance of sinus rhythm in atrial fibrillation or flutter, *N Engl J Med* 357:987, 2007.

Snow V et al: Management of newly detected atrial fibrillation: a clinical practice guideline from the Academy of Family Physicians and the American College of Physicians, *Ann Intern Med* 139:1009, 2003.

SPORTIF Executive Steering Committee for the Sportif V Investigators: ximelagatran vs warfarin for stroke prevention in patients with nonvalvular atrial fibrillation, *JAMA* 293:690-698, 2005.

Wang TJ et al: Obesity and the risk of new-onset atrial fibrillation, *JAMA* 292:2471-2477, 2004.

Zimetbaum P: Amiodarone for atrial fibrillation, *N Engl J Med* 356:935, 2007.

AUTHOR: **FRED F. FERRI, M.D.**

BASIC INFORMATION

DEFINITION

Atrial flutter is a rapid atrial rate of 280 to 340 bpm with varying degrees of intraventricular block. It is a macrorentrant tachycardia, most often involving right atrial tissue.

ICD-9CM CODES
427.32 Atrial flutter

EPIDEMIOLOGY & DEMOGRAPHICS

- Atrial flutter is the second most common atrial tachyarrhythmia after atrial fibrillation, with an estimated 200,000 new cases annually in the U.S.
- Atrial flutter is common during the first week after open heart surgery.

PHYSICAL FINDINGS & CLINICAL PRESENTATION

- Approximately 150 bpm
- Symptoms of cardiac failure, lightheadedness, and angina pectoris

ETIOLOGY

- Atherosclerotic heart disease
- MI
- Thyrotoxicosis
- Pulmonary embolism
- Mitral valve disease
- Cardiac surgery
- COPD
- Atrial flutter can also occur spontaneously or as a result of organization of atrial fibrillation from antiarrhythmic therapy

DIAGNOSIS

DIFFERENTIAL DIAGNOSIS

- Atrial fibrillation
- Paroxysmal atrial tachycardia

WORKUP

- ECG
- Laboratory evaluation

LABORATORY TESTS

- Thyroid function studies
- Serum electrolytes

IMAGING STUDIES

ECG (Fig. 1-31)

- Regular, "sawtooth," or "F" wave pattern, best seen in II, III, and AVF and secondary to atrial depolarization
- AV conduction block (2:1, 3:1, or varying)
- The criteria of F waves in the frontal plane and a partially or completely regular ventricular response has a sensitivity of 90% and a specificity of 100% for atrial flutter

TREATMENT

NONPHARMACOLOGIC THERAPY

- Valsalva maneuver or carotid sinus massage usually slows the ventricular rate (increases grade of AV block) and may make flutter waves more evident.
- DC cardioversion is the treatment of choice for acute management of atrial flutter. Electrical cardioversion is given at low energy levels (20 to 25 J). Sedation of a conscious patient is highly recommended before cardioversion is performed. The use of external defibrillators having biphasic waveforms decreases the amount of energy required for cardioversion and improves cardioversion success rate.
- Overdrive pacing in the atrium may also terminate atrial flutter. This method is especially useful in patients who have recently undergone cardiac surgery and still have temporary atrial pacing wires.

ACUTE GENERAL Rx

- In absence of cardioversion, IV diltiazem or digitalization may be tried to slow the ventricular rate and convert flutter to fibrillation. Esmolol, verapamil, and adenosine may also be effective. In patients with atrial flutter it is essential to preadminister AV nodal blocking agents prior to using procainamide or ibutilide.
- Atrial flutter is frequently associated with intermittent atrial fibrillation. It may be prudent to anticoagulate patients with atrial flutter and coexisting medical disorders (e.g., diabetes mellitus, hypertension, cardiac disease) before cardioversion. Anticoagulation should also be considered for all patients with atrial flutter who are older than 65 years of age.

CHRONIC Rx

- Chronic atrial flutter may respond to amiodarone.
- Radiofrequency ablation to interrupt the atrial flutter is very effective for patients with chronic or recurring atrial flutter and is generally considered first-line therapy in those with recurrent episodes of atrial flutter.

DISPOSITION

More than 85% of patients convert to regular sinus rhythm following cardioversion with as little as 25 to 50 J.

REFERRAL

For radiofrequency ablation in patients with chronic or recurring atrial flutter

PEARLS & CONSIDERATIONS

COMMENTS

- Lone atrial flutter has a stroke risk at least as high as lone atrial fibrillation and carries a higher risk for subsequent development of atrial fibrillation than in the general population.
- Anticoagulation should be considered for all patients with atrial flutter who are older than 65 years of age.

SUGGESTED READINGS

Halligan SC et al: The natural history of long atrial flutter, *Ann Int Med* 140:265, 2004.

Weinberg KM et al: Criteria for the electrocardiographic diagnosis of atrial flutter improve diagnostic accuracy, *Am J Med* 120:814, 2007.

AUTHOR: **FRED F. FERRI, M.D.**

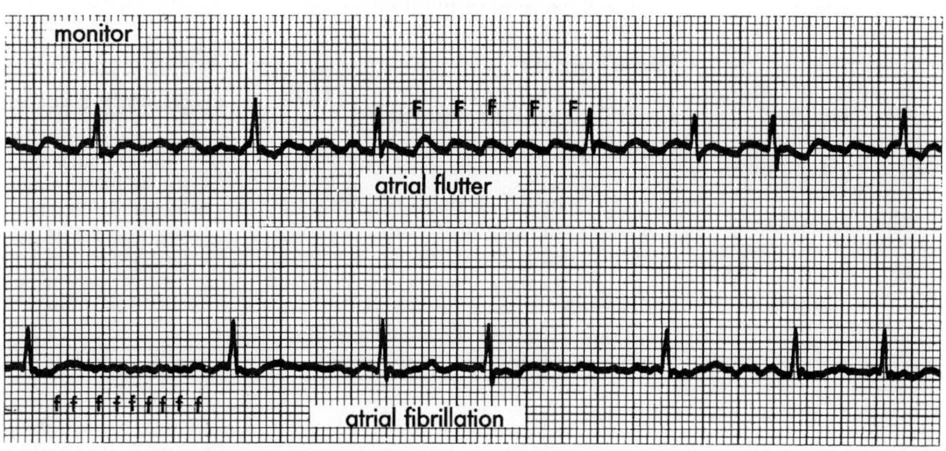

FIGURE 1-31 Atrial flutter and fibrillation. Notice the sawtooth waves with atrial flutter *(F)* and the irregular fibrillatory waves with atrial fibrillation *(f)*. (From Goldberger AL [ed]: *Clinical electrocardiography,* ed 5, St Louis, 1994, Mosby.)

BASIC INFORMATION

DEFINITION

Atrial myxoma is a benign neoplasm of mesenchymal origin and is the most common primary tumor of the heart.

SYNONYMS

Cardiac myxoma

ICD-9CM CODES
212.7 Benign neoplasm, heart

EPIDEMIOLOGY & DEMOGRAPHICS

- Primary cardiac tumors are extremely rare, with an autopsy frequency of 0.001% to 0.03%. (The most frequent cardiac tumors are metastases.)
- Benign atrial myxomas account for 75% of all primary tumors of the heart. (The remaining 25% are aggressive malignant angiosarcomas that usually occur in the ventricles.)
- 70% of sporadic cases occur in females.
- Average age of incidence of sporadic cases is 30 to 60 years but can occur at any age.
- Average age of incidence of familial cases is 25 yr.

PHYSICAL FINDINGS & CLINICAL PRESENTATION

Patients with atrial myxomas characteristically present in one of three ways:

- Atrioventricular valve obstruction (e.g., mitral or tricuspid valve): dyspnea, orthopnea, paroxysmal nocturnal dyspnea, edema, dizziness, syncope, elevated jugular venous pressure, loud S1, secondary pulmonary hypertension, murmurs of regurgitation (holosystolic) or stenosis (rumbles), third heart sound "tumor plop," atrial fibrillation
- Systemic embolization: leading to cerebrovascular accidents, pulmonary embolism, paradoxical embolism
- Constitutional symptoms: fever, weight loss, arthralgias, Raynaud's phenomenon

ETIOLOGY

- Most cases (90%) of atrial myxomas are sporadic with no known cause.
- In the remaining 10% of cases, a familial pattern occurs having an autosomal dominant transmission known as the Carney complex (myxomas of the heart, skin, and breast; skin pigmentation; endocrine tumors; and schwanomas).

DIAGNOSIS

DIFFERENTIAL DIAGNOSIS

- Primary valvular diseases: mitral stenosis, mitral regurgitaiton, tricuspid stenosis, tricuspid regurgitation
- Pulmonary hypertension
- Endocarditis
- Vasculitis
- Atrial thrombus
- Pulmonary embolism
- Cerebrovascular accidents
- Collagen-vascular disease
- Carcinoid heart disease
- Ebstein's anomaly

WORKUP

A high index of suspicion is needed because the clinical manifestations are nonspecific and similar to many common cardiovascular and pulmonary diseases.

LABORATORY TESTS

Although not very specific, the following laboratory findings may be abnormal in patients with atrial myxomas:

- CBC: anemia, polycythemia, thrombocytopenia may occur
- Erythrocyte sedimentation rate, C-reactive protein, and serum immunoglobulins are commonly elevated
- ECG: left or right atrial enlargement, atrial fibrillation, premature ventricular depolarizations, or ventricular tachycardia

IMAGING STUDIES

- Echocardiography: initial test of choice in suspected cases of atrial myxoma
- Chest x-ray examination: altered cardiac contour and chamber enlargement
- Transesophageal echocardiography: may better define cardiac masses not clearly visualized by transthoracic echocardiography
- MRI: delineates size, shape, and tumor characterizations
- Cardiac catheterization: may be required to rule out concomitant coronary artery disease in anticipation to surgical excision of the tumor

TREATMENT

ACUTE GENERAL THERAPY

- Surgical excision is the treatment of choice.
- Surgery should be done promptly because systemic embolization and/or sudden death can occur while waiting for the procedure (see "Disposition").
- Treatment of constitutional and cardiac symptoms: diuresis, heart rate and blood pressure control, and fever control.

CHRONIC Rx

Postoperative arrhythmias and conductions abnormalities were present in 26% of patients and can be treated according to convention.

DISPOSITION

- Surgical results have reported a 95% survival rate after a follow-up of 3 yr.
- Careful follow-up is necessary since up to 5% of sporadic cases and 20% of familial cases of atrial myxoma may recur within the first 6 yr after surgery.
- Sudden death in untreated patients may occur in up to 15%, resulting from coronary or systemic embolization, or by obstruction of the mitral or tricuspid valve.

REFERRAL

- Consultation with a cardiologist is recommended.
- Once the presence of cardiac tumor is confirmed, consultation with a cardiovascular surgeon is needed for prompt surgical excision.

PEARLS & CONSIDERATIONS

- Approximately 75% of myxomas arise from the left atrium close to the fossa ovalis.
- Approximately two thirds of patients present with cardiovascular symptoms, specifically dyspnea, often suggestive of valvular obstruction.
- Nearly one third of patients have evidence of systemic embolization.

COMMENTS

Annual echocardiograms should be performed to monitor for recurrence of atrial myxomas following surgical excision.

EVIDENCE

As far as research is concerned, there are simply too few cardiac tumors to merit major investigations. Most data are obtained through clinical series and case reports.

SUGGESTED READINGS

Ipek G et al: Surgical management of cardiac myxoma, *J Card Surg* 20(3):300, 2005.

Swartz MF et al: Atrial myxomas: pathologic types, tumor location, and presenting symptoms, *J Card Surg* 21(4):435, 2006.

Vasquez A et al: Atrial myxomas in the elderly: a case report and review of the literature, *Am J Geriatr Cardiol* 13(1):39, 2004.

AUTHORS: **CRAIG McMACKIN, M.D.**, and **WEN-CHIH WU, M.D.**

BASIC INFORMATION

DEFINITION

Atrial septal defect (ASD) is an abnormal opening in the atrial septum that allows for blood flow between the atria. There are several forms (Fig. 1-32):
- Ostium primum: defect low in the septum
- Ostium secundum: occurs mainly in the region of the fossa ovalis
- Sinus venous defect: less common form, involves the upper part of the septum

SYNONYMS

ASD

ICD-9CM CODES
429.71 Atrial septal defect

EPIDEMIOLOGY & DEMOGRAPHICS

- 80% of cases of ASD involve persistence of ostium secundum.
- Incidence is higher in females.
- ASD accounts for 8% to 10% of congenital heart abnormalities.

PHYSICAL FINDINGS & CLINICAL PRESENTATION

- Pansystolic murmur best heard at apex secondary to mitral regurgitation (ostium primum defect)
- Widely split S_2
- Visible and palpable pulmonary artery pulsations
- Ejection systolic flow murmur
- Prominent right ventricular impulse
- Cyanosis and clubbing (severe cases)
- Exertional dyspnea
- Patients with small defects: generally asymptomatic

ETIOLOGY

Unknown

DIAGNOSIS

DIFFERENTIAL DIAGNOSIS

- Primary pulmonary hypertension
- Pulmonary stenosis
- Rheumatic heart disease
- Mitral valve prolapse
- Cor pulmonale

WORKUP

- ECG
- Chest x-ray examination
- Echocardiography
- Cardiac catheterization

IMAGING STUDIES

- ECG
  1. Ostium primum defect: left axis deviation, RBBB, prolongation of PR interval
  2. Sinus venous defect: leftward deviation of P axis
  3. Ostium secundum defect: right axis deviation, right bundle-branch block
- Chest x-ray: cardiomegaly, enlargement of right atrium and ventricle, increased pulmonary vascularity, small aortic knob
- Echocardiography with saline bubble contrast and Doppler flow studies: may demonstrate the defect and the presence of shunting. Transesophageal echocardiography is much more sensitive than transthoracic echocardiography in identifying sinus venous defects and is preferred by some for the initial diagnostic evaluation
- Cardiac catheterization: confirms the diagnosis in patients who are candidates for surgery. It is useful if the patient has some anatomic finding on echocardiography that is not completely clear or has significant elevation of pulmonary artery pressures

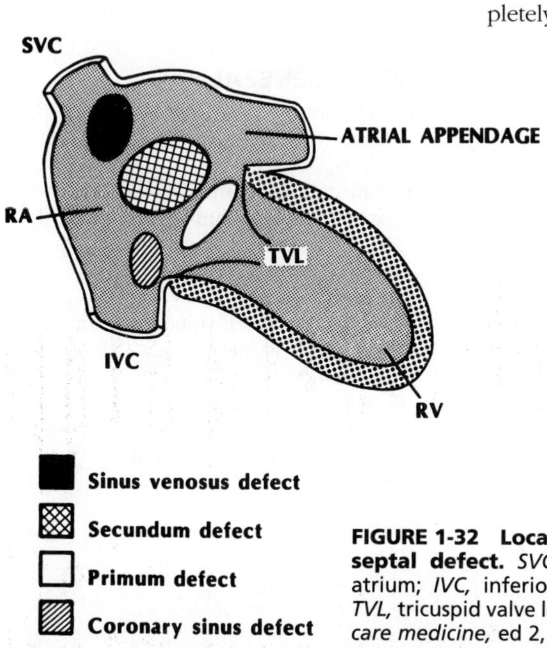

FIGURE 1-32 Location of the four types of atrial septal defect. *SVC,* Superior vena cava; *RA,* right atrium; *IVC,* inferior vena cava; *RV,* right ventricle; *TVL,* tricuspid valve leaflet. (From Noble J [ed]: *Primary care medicine,* ed 2, St Louis, 1996, Mosby.)

TREATMENT

NONPHARMACOLOGIC THERAPY

Avoidance of strenuous activity in symptomatic patients

GENERAL Rx

- Children and infants: closure of ASD before age 10 yr is indicated if pulmonary:systemic flow ratio is >1.5:1.
- Adults: closure is indicated in symptomatic patients with shunts >2:1.
- Surgery should be avoided in patients with pulmonary hypertension with reversed shunting (Eisenmenger's syndrome) because of increased risk of right heart failure.
- Transcatheter closure is advocated in children when feasible.
- Prophylactic β-blocker therapy to prevent atrial arrhythmias should be considered in adults with ASD.
- Surgical closure is indicated in all patients with ostium primum defect and significant shunting unless patient has significant pulmonary vascular disease.

DISPOSITION

- Mortality is high in patients with significant ostium primum defect.
- Patients with small shunts have a normal life expectancy.
- Surgical mortality varies with the age of the patient and the presence of cardiac failure and systolic pulmonary artery hypertension; mortality ranges from <1% in young patients (<45 yr old) to >10% in elderly patients with presence of heart failure and systolic pulmonary hypertension.
- Preoperative atrial fibrillation is a risk factor for immediate postoperative and long-term atrial fibrillation. Patients with a repaired ASD still have an increased risk of developing atrial fibrillation that directly correlates with the age at which the defect is corrected (later correction = higher risk).
- Thromboembolism after surgical repair of an ASD in an adult can occur in the early postoperative period. Giving early postoperative anticoagulation in patients >35 yr of age at the time of ASD repair and continuing it for at least 6 mo will decrease the risk.

EVIDENCE

One randomized controlled trial of 400 patients over age 40 years, assessed whether surgical treatment of secundum ASDs improves their long-term outcome. After a median follow-up of 7.3 years, surgical closure was associated with lower rates of mortality and cardiovascular events.[1] (B)

Evidence-Based Reference

1. Attie F et al: Surgical treatment for secundum atrial septal defects in patients >40 years old. A randomized clinical trial, *J Am Coll Cardiol* 38:2035, 2001. (B)

SUGGESTED READING

Krasuski RA: When and how to fix a "hole in the heart": approach to ASD and PFO, *Cleve Clin J Med* 74:137, 2007.

AUTHOR: **FRED F. FERRI, M.D.**

BASIC INFORMATION

DEFINITION

Attention deficit hyperactivity disorder (AD/HD) is a chronic disorder of attention/concentration and/or hyperactivity/impulsivity. Symptoms must be present in early childhood, last at least 6 mo, and cause functional impairment in multiple settings.

SYNONYMS

Hyperactivity, attention deficit disorder (ADD)

ICD-9CM CODES
ICD-9: 314.XX; ICD-10: F90.X

EPIDEMIOLOGY & DEMOGRAPHICS

PEAK INCIDENCE: Diagnosis is usually first made in school-aged children (6 to 9 years).

PREVALENCE: 3% to 9% of school-aged children and 2% to 5% of adults.

PREDOMINANT SEX: Among children, male predominance with ratio of 3:1 to 9:1. Among adults, ratio is closer to 1:1. (Sex difference may reflect referral bias.)

PREDOMINANT AGE: Some symptoms must occur before age 7. Symptoms (especially hyperactivity) tend to diminish with age. Greater than 70% continue to meet criteria in adolescence and an estimated 40% to 65% have some symptoms in adulthood.

GENETICS: Strong polygenetic component. First-degree relatives of AD/HD patients have 5 times greater risk of AD/HD relative to controls. Studies suggest potential involvement of several genes including those associated with dopamine metabolism/transmission.

RISK FACTORS: Possible environmental/epidemiologic risk factors include in utero tobacco/drug exposure or hypoxia, low birth weight, prematurity, pregnancy complications, lead exposure, family dysfunction, low SES.

PHYSICAL FINDINGS & CLINICAL PRESENTATION

- Three types:
  1. Predominantly inattentive: difficulty organizing, planning, remembering, concentrating, starting/completing tasks; symptoms may not be present during preferred activities.
  2. Predominantly hyperactive-impulsive: edgy/restless, talkative, disruptive/intrusive, disinhibited, impatient.
  3. Combined.
- Usually diagnosed in elementary school when achievement is compromised and behavioral problems are not tolerated. Children with academic underproductivity, problems with peer and family relations, or discipline issues are often referred for evaluation.
- Adults with substance abuse or other addictions, multiple traffic violations, or frequent life failures should be screened.
- Up to 50% may have associated disorders such as psychiatric diagnoses (oppositional defiant disorder, conduct disorder, depression, anxiety), learning disabilities, substance abuse, and criminal behavior.

ETIOLOGY

Strongest evidence exists for genetic inheritance. Other theories include abnormal metabolism of brain catecholamines, structural brain abnormalities, and environmental factors (see earlier).

DIAGNOSIS

DIFFERENTIAL DIAGNOSIS

- Medical: visual/hearing impairment, seizure disorder, head injury, sleep disorder, medication interactions, mental retardation, developmental delay, thyroid abnormalities, lead toxicity.
- Psychiatric: depression, bipolar disorder, anxiety, obsessive-compulsive disorder, conduct disorder, posttraumatic stress disorder, substance abuse, antisocial personality disorder, Tourette syndrome, tics.
- Psychosocial: mismatch of learning environment with ability, family dysfunction, abuse/neglect.

WORKUP

- Clinical interview should include assessment of symptoms and impact on work/school and relationships; developmental history; personal and family psychiatric history including substance abuse; social history including family dysfunction; medical history.
- Thorough physical examination should be performed to investigate medical causes for symptoms, coexisting conditions, and contraindications to treatment.
- Many patients will not display symptoms during an office visit and may under- or over-report symptoms. Therefore, information from collateral sources (parents, partners, teachers) is crucial to diagnosis.
- Self-rating scales and standardized symptom-specific questionnaires from collateral sources can aid in diagnosis and in assessing response to treatment.
- Laboratory or imaging studies should be undertaken only if indicated by history or physical examination.
- Ancillary testing (e.g., IQ/achievement testing, language evaluation, and mental health assessment) may be indicated based on clinical findings and may require referral.

TREATMENT

NONPHARMACOLOGIC THERAPY

- Data comparing the efficacy of behavioral or educational therapy versus pharmacologic management are limited. Prevailing opinion favors a multimodal approach in which nonpharmacologic therapies can be used to target comorbid conditions or behaviors that have not responded to medication.
- Educational interventions are recommended, particularly in the setting of learning disabilities. Children with AD/HD are entitled to reasonable educational accommodations under a 504 Plan or the Individuals with Disabilities Education Act.
- Behavioral interventions (e.g., goal setting and rewards systems) show short-term efficacy and are endorsed by most national organizations (e.g., American Academy of Pediatrics, American Medical Association). Time management and organizational skills appear useful.
- Psychotherapy (cognitive behavioral, group, social skills, and parent training) may be beneficial, particularly when there is coexisting psychiatric disease.
- Many support/advocacy groups provide education and other resources (e.g., Children and Adolescents with AD/HD, National ADD Association, American Academy of Child and Adolescent Psychiatry).

ACUTE GENERAL Rx

- Most studies on treatment of AD/HD performed in children. Limited data on adults.
- Mainstay of treatment is drug therapy, particularly stimulants. Second-line therapies include antidepressants and alpha-agonists.
- Stimulants:
  1. Release/block uptake of dopamine and norepinephrine.
  2. Include short- and long-acting methylphenidate (Ritalin, Concerta), dextroamphetamine/amphetamine combinations (Adderall).

3. Do not cause euphoria or lead to addiction when taken as directed.
4. Improve cognition, inattention, impulsiveness/hyperactivity, and driving skills. Limited impact on academic performance, learning, and emotional problems.
5. Side effects are mild, reversible, and dose dependent. Include anorexia, weight loss, sleep disturbances, increased heart rate/blood pressure, nervousness/irritability, headache, onset or worsening of motor tics, reduction of growth velocity (but not adult height). Do not worsen seizures in patients on adequate anticonvulsant therapy. Rebound of symptoms can occur with withdrawal of medication.
6. All equally effective; however, not all patients improve with stimulants. Patients who do not respond well to one stimulant may respond to another.

- Atomoxetine (Strattera):
  1. Selective norepinephrine reuptake inhibitor.
  2. Efficacy/safety of long-term use has not been studied. Reports of behavioral abnormalities and increased suicidality in children.
  3. Side effects: gastrointestinal upset, sleep disturbance, decreased appetite, dizziness, sexual side effects in men.
  4. Monitor liver function as there have been reports of severe liver injury in adults and children.
- Antidepressants (bupropion, imipramine, nortriptyline):
  1. May be useful in patients with coexisting psychiatric disorders.
  2. Studies comparing efficacy versus stimulants are inconclusive.
  3. Side effects: arrhythmias, anticholinergic effects, lowering of seizure threshold.
- Use of medications, particularly stimulants (which are monitored under the Controlled Substance Act), require frequent monitoring.
- Stimulants have been associated with cardiovascular events and mortality. Patients should be carefully evaluated for cardiovascular disease prior to initiation of therapy and be periodically monitored, including blood pressure checks, while they are treated.

DISPOSITION

- While symptoms may change over time, for many patients, AD/HD represents a chronic condition that requires lifelong management.
- Patients are at higher risk for academic underachievement, lower SES, work and relationship difficulties, high-risk behavior, and psychiatric comorbidities.

REFERRAL

- Diagnosis complicated by difficult-to-treat comorbid psychiatric conditions, developmental disorders, or mental retardation.
- Lack of adequate response to stimulants/atomoxetine.

PEARLS & CONSIDERATIONS

The World Health Organization's Adult Self-Report Scale (ASRS) v1.1 has good sensitivity and adaptability to the primary care setting.

EVIDENCE

EBM

Systematic review found that methylphenidate plus behavioral treatment was superior to behavioral treatment alone. Symptoms and behaviors associated with ADHD and academic achievements were significantly improved with combination therapy, but no significant difference was noted in social skills or parent-child relationships.[1] (A)

A randomized controlled trial (RCT) found that children with ADHD had a significant improvement in measures of core symptoms when treated with intensive behavioral treatment plus medication vs. behavioral treatment alone.[2] (A)

A systematic review and several RCTs found that methylphenidate reduced core symptoms of ADHD in the short term.[1,3] (A)

Another systematic review of longer-term studies found limited evidence that dextroamphetamine improved concentration and hyperactivity compared with placebo. The RCTs included in the review had methodological problems.[4] (A)

A crossover RCT compared slow-release dextroamphetamine with placebo in children with ADHD. Dextroamphetamine was associated with significant improvement on two rating scales.[5] (A)

RCTs found that atomoxetine was more effective than placebo in treating children with ADHD.[6-8] (B)

Evidence-Based References

1. Lord J, Paisley S: The clinical effectiveness and cost-effectiveness of methylphenidate for hyperactivity in childhood, National Institute for Clinical Excellence, Version 2, August 2000. (A)
2. Jensen PS et al: A 14-month randomized clinical trial of treatment strategies for attention-deficit/hyperactivity disorder. The MTA Cooperative Group. Multimodal Treatment Study of Children with ADHD, *Arch Gen Psychiatry* 56:1073, 1999. (A)
3. Ramchandani P, Joughin C, Zwi M: Attention deficit hyperactivity disorder in children, *Clin Evid* 9:318, 2003. (A)
4. Jadad AR et al: Treatment of attention-deficit/hyperactivity disorder. Evidence report/technology assessment No 11, Rockville MD: Agency for Health Care Policy and Research and Quality, 1999. Reviewed in: *Clinical Evidence* 9:318, 2003. (A)
5. James RS et al: Double-blind, placebo-controlled study of single-dose amphetamine formulations in ADHD, *J Am Acad Child Adolesc Psychiatry* 40:1268, 2001. (A)
6. Michelson D et al: Atomoxetine ADHD study group. Atomoxetine in the treatment of children and adolescents with attention-deficit/hyperactivity disorder: a randomized, placebo-controlled, dose-response study, *Pediatrics* 108:E83, 2001. (B)
7. Spencer T et al: Results from 2 proof-of-concept, placebo-controlled studies of atomoxetine in children with attention-deficit/hyperactivity disorder, *J Clin Psychiatry* 63:1140, 2002. (B)
8. Michelson D et al: Once-daily atomoxetine treatment for children and adolescents with attention deficit hyperactivity disorder: a randomized, placebo-controlled study, *Am J Psychiatry* 159:1896, 2002. (B)

SUGGESTED READINGS

Culpetter L: Primary care treatment of attention-deficit/hyperactivity disorder, *J Clin Psychiatry* 67(8):51, 2006.

Polayczyk G et al: The worldwide prevalence of ADHD: a systematic review and metaregression analysis, *Am J Psychiatry* 164(6):942, 2007.

Rappley MD: Attention deficit–hyperactivity disorder, *N Engl J Med* 352:(2):165, 2005.

AUTHOR: **MITCHELL D. FELDMAN, M.D., M.PHIL.**

BASIC INFORMATION

DEFINITION

Autistic spectrum disorders (ASD) encompass a spectrum of developmental disorders characterized by impairment in several behavioral domains. There is usually impairment in the development of language, communication, and reciprocal social interaction along with a restricted behavioral repertoire. Onset is typically before age 3 yr.

SYNONYMS

Autism
Early infantile autism
Childhood autism
Kanner's autism
Pervasive developmental disorder

ICD-9CM CODES
F84.0 Autistic disorder (DSM-IV coded 299.0 Autistic disorder)

EPIDEMIOLOGY & DEMOGRAPHICS

INCIDENCE (IN U.S.): 3 to 6/1000 of ASD (2 to 5/10,000 if restricted to autism alone)
PEAK INCIDENCE: Before age 3 yr
PREVALENCE: 3.3 to 10.6/100 (mean 6.6)
PREDOMINANT SEX: Male:female ratio of 3.4 to 6.5:1.0
PREDOMINANT AGE: Lifelong
GENETICS:
- Unknown genetic component, though recent linkage analyses have identified chromosomal abnormalities in multiple genetic loci, including glutamate-related genes
- 3% risk for sibling of affected individual
- 60% to 92% concordance for classic autism in monozygotic twins, and 0% to 10% for dizygotic pairs

PHYSICAL FINDINGS & CLINICAL PRESENTATION

- Marked impairment in the understanding and use of both verbal and nonverbal communication (probably underlies the profound impairment in social interaction)
- Stereotypic behavior or language
- Sensory overload and avoidance of novel stimuli is typical.

ETIOLOGY

- Majority of cases are not associated with a medical condition.
- Significant increase in comorbid seizure disorder (25%) and developmental delay (45% to 60%).
- Autism is sometimes associated with other neurologic conditions (e.g., encephalitis, tuberous sclerosis, phenylketonuria, fragile X, and others), suggesting that it may result from nonspecific neuronal injury.

DIAGNOSIS

DIFFERENTIAL DIAGNOSIS

- Rett's syndrome: occurs in females, characterized by head growth deceleration, loss of previously acquired motor skills, and incoordination
- Childhood disintegration disorder: normal development until age 2 yr, followed by regression
- Childhood-onset schizophrenia: follows period of normal development
- Asperger's syndrome: lacks the language developmental abnormalities of autism
- Isolated symptoms of autism: when occurring in isolation, defined as disorders (i.e., selective mutism, expressive language disorder, mixed receptive-expressive language disorder, or stereotypic movement disorder)

WORKUP

- Rule out underlying medical condition.
- Diagnostic instruments based on questionnaires and observation noting scales (e.g., Autism Diagnostic Interview) may be helpful.

LABORATORY TESTS

- PKU screen (usually done at birth in the U.S.)
- Chromosome analysis to rule out fragile X in both boys and girls (carrier girls may exhibit mild symptoms)
- IQ testing to help determine functional level of child

IMAGING STUDIES

- EEG to diagnose coexisting seizure disorder (a normal EEG does not rule out a seizure disorder)
- Head CT or MRI to rule out tuberous sclerosis
- Consider BAER to rule out hearing deficit

TREATMENT

NONPHARMACOLOGIC THERAPY

- A behavioral training program that is consistent in both the home and school environments.
- Educational program focused on language and social development.
- A highly structured environment benefits most children.
- Education for parents and teachers is of great value.

ACUTE GENERAL Rx

- Haloperidol or other high-potency neuroleptics are helpful in reducing aggression and stereotypy. Atypical neuroleptics, such as risperidone, also reduce aggression and irritability and improve overall behavioral symptoms.
- Selective serotonin reuptake inhibitors may be useful in children with coexisting depression or with marked obsessive or ritualistic behaviors.
- Buspirone reported to reduce aggression, hyperactivity and repetitive behaviors.
- Valproic acid and carbamazepine are preferred for seizure control.

CHRONIC Rx

- Extended use of medications used for acute management
- Pharmacotherapy is palliative only, not curative.

DISPOSITION

- Most children (70%) will require some degree of assistance as adults, will not be able to work, and will not achieve proper social adjustment.
- Some 10% (particularly if IQ is in the normal range and speech is achieved by age 5 yr) may have a reasonable outcome.
- Children with Asperger's syndrome may have a very good outcome despite ongoing symptoms.

REFERRAL

Assistance may be needed in diagnosis, management, parental teaching, or intervention with the school system.

PEARLS & CONSIDERATIONS

- Researchers are examining the relationship between childhood vaccination and the development of autism.
- A center devoted to the study of autism: http://www.ucdmc.ucdavis.edu/mindinstitute/.

EVIDENCE

Clomipramine may be superior to desipramine and to placebo for obsessive-compulsive and stereotyped motor behaviors in autistic disorder.[1] Ⓑ

Small but significant reductions in hyperactivity ratings may be seen in response to stimulants such as methylphenidate and dextroamphetamine.[2,3] Ⓑ

Clonidine reduced irritability, hyperactivity, and impulsivity in the short term compared with placebo, and improved social relationships in two randomized controlled trials (RCTs).[4,5] Ⓑ

Clomipramine and haloperidol have been shown to be equally effective and more effective than placebo. However, 60% of those receiving clomipramine discontinued the trial early because of side effects, and haloperidol was better tolerated.[6] Ⓑ

A long-term prospective study of autistic children who responded to initial haloperidol therapy found several factors increase the risk of dyskinesias, including cumulative dose and length of exposure to haloperidol, female sex, and perinatal complications. The most common dyskinesias were withdrawal dyskinesias, which developed in about one-third of patients; about half of these had more than one episode.[7] Ⓑ

Risperidone was shown to be effective in children with autistic disorder who have serious behavioral disturbances, and the benefit was maintained at 6 mo in some.[8] Ⓑ

Naltrexone appears to reduce hyperactivity in children with autism, but produces a more rapid clinical progression of the condition in children with Rett's syndrome.[9-11] Ⓑ

A systematic review found no evidence to warrant recommendation of the use of pyridoxine and magnesium as a treatment for autism.[12] Ⓐ

There is limited evidence for an improvement in aberrant behavior scores at 3 months in children with autism spectrum disorders treated with auditory integration training.[13] Ⓑ

A 30-wk, double-blind RCT examining the effects of (8 g/70 kg/day) ascorbic acid on autistic children in residential school found a reduction in symptom severity with ascorbic acid treatment.[14] Ⓑ

Many other therapies appear to be effective in autism according to anecdotal evidence and case reports, but the trials do not reach our criteria for evidence. We are unable to cite evidence that meets our criteria for other therapies that may be used successfully in autism.

Evidence-Based References

1. Gordon C et al: A double-blind comparison of clomipramine, desipramine, and placebo in the treatment of autistic disorder, *Arch Gen Psychiatry* 50:44, 1993. Ⓑ
2. Quintana H et al: Use of methylphenidate in the treatment of children with autistic disorder, *J Autism Dev Disord* 25:283, 1995. Ⓑ
3. Handen BL, Johnson CR, Lubetsky M: Efficacy of methylphenidate among children with autism and symptoms of attention-deficit hyperactivity disorder, *J Autism Dev Disord* 30:245, 2000. Ⓑ
4. Jaselskis CA et al: Clonidine treatment of hyperactive and impulsive children with autistic disorder, *J Clin Psychopharmacol* 12:322, 1992. Ⓑ
5. Fankhauser MP et al: A double-blind, placebo-controlled study of the efficacy of transdermal clonidine in autism, *J Clin Psychiatry* 53:77, 1992. Ⓑ
6. Remington G et al: Clomipramine versus haloperidol in the treatment of autistic disorder: a double-blind, placebo-controlled, crossover study, *J Clin Psychopharmacol* 21:440, 2001. Ⓑ
7. Campbell M et al: Neuroleptic-related dyskinesias in autistic children: a prospective, longitudinal study, *J Am Acad Child Adolesc Psychiatry* 36:835, 1997. Ⓑ
8. McCracken JT et al: Risperidone in children with autism and serious behavioral problems, *N Engl J Med* 347:314, 2002. Ⓑ
9. Campbell M et al: Naltrexone in autistic children: behavioral symptoms and attentional learning, *J Am Acad Child Adolesc Psychiatry* 32:1283, 1993. Ⓑ
10. Kolmen BK: Naltrexone in young autistic children: a double-blind, placebo-controlled crossover study, *J Am Acad Child Adolesc Psychiatry* 34:223, 1995. Ⓑ
11. Percy AK et al: Rett's syndrome: controlled study of an oral opiate antagonist, naltrexone, *Ann Neurol* 35:464, 1994. Ⓑ
12. Nye C, Brice A: Combined vitamin B6-magnesium treatment in autism spectrum disorder, *Cochrane Database Syst Rev* (4):CD003497, 2005. Ⓐ
13. Sinha Y et al: Auditory integration training and other sound therapies for autism spectrum disorders, *Cochrane Database Syst Rev* (1):CD003681, 2004. Ⓑ
14. Dolske MC et al: A preliminary trial of ascorbic acid as a supplement therapy for autism, *Prog Neuropsychopharmacol Biol Psychiatry* 17:765, 1993. Ⓑ

SUGGESTED READINGS

Autism Genome Project Consortium: Mapping autism risk loci using genetic linkage and chromosomal rearrangements, *Nat Genet* 39:319, 2007.

Prevalence of Autism Spectrum Disorders—Autism and Developmental Disabilities Monitoring Network, 14 Sites, United States, 2002. *MMWR Morb Mortal Wkly Rep* 56(SS-1):1, 2007.

Weiss LA et al: Association between microdeletion and microduplication at 16p4.2 and autism, *N Engl J Med* 358:667-675, 2008.

AUTHOR: **MITCHELL D. FELDMAN, M.D., M.PHIL.**

BASIC INFORMATION

DEFINITION

Babesiosis is a tick-transmitted protozoan disease of animals, caused by intraerythrocytic parasites of the genus *Babesia*. Humans are incidentally infected, resulting in a nonspecific febrile illness. The disease can be severe in immunocompromised hosts.

ICD-9CM CODES
088.82 Babesiosis

EPIDEMIOLOGY & DEMOGRAPHICS

INCIDENCE (IN U.S.): Unknown
PREVALENCE (IN U.S.):

- In areas of high endemicity, seropositivity ranging from 9% (Rhode Island) to 21% (Connecticut)
- Highest number of reported cases in New York

PREDOMINANT SEX: Males (most likely through increased exposure to vectors during recreational or occupational activities)
PREDOMINANT AGE: Severity apparently increasing with age >40 yr
PEAK INCIDENCE: Spring and summer months, May through September
GENETICS: None known
CONGENITAL INFECTION: At least one case of probable vertical transmission
NEONATAL INFECTION: At least two cases of perinatal transmission

PHYSICAL FINDINGS & CLINICAL PRESENTATION

- Incubation period 1 to 4 wk, or 6 to 9 wk in transfusion-associated disease
- Gradual onset of irregular fever, chills, diaphoresis, headache, myalgia, arthralgia, fatigue, and dark urine
- On physical examination: petechiae, frank or mild hepatosplenomegaly, and jaundice
- Infection with *B. divergens* producing a more severe illness with a rapid onset of symptoms and increasing parasitemia progressing to massive intravascular hemolysis and renal failure

ETIOLOGY

- Vector: Deer tick, *Ixodes scapularis* (also known as *I. dammini*)
  1. Feeds on rodents during the spring and summer while in its larval and nymphal stages and on deer as an adult
  2. During the warmer months in endemic areas, humans are readily infected while engaging in outdoor activities
- *B. microti,* along with *B. divergens* and *B. bovis,* account for most human infections.
- In the U.S., cases caused by *B. microti* are acquired on offshore islands of the northeastern coast, including Nantucket Island, Cape Cod, and Martha's Vineyard in Massachusetts; Block Island in Rhode Island; and Long Island, Fire Island, and Shelter Island in New York; as well as the nearby mainland including Connecticut and New Jersey.
- Sporadic cases reported from California, Georgia, Maryland, Minnesota, Virginia, Wisconsin, and most recently the WA-1 strain from Washington State and the MO-1 strain from Missouri.
- *B. divergens* and *B. bovis* are implicated in human disease in Europe, where the disease remains rare and predominantly associated with asplenia.
- Majority of cases are asymptomatic.
- May be transmissible by transfusion, through platelets and erythrocytes.
- Mixed infections (*B. microti* and *Borrelia burgdorferi,* the causative agent of Lyme disease) are estimated to occur in 10% (Rhode Island and Connecticut) to 60% (New York) of cases.

DIAGNOSIS

DIFFERENTIAL DIAGNOSIS

- Amebiasis
- Ehrlichiosis
- Hepatic abscess
- Leptospirosis
- Malaria
- Salmonellosis, including typhoid fever
- Acute viral hepatitis
- Hemorrhagic fevers

WORKUP

Should be suspected in any febrile patient living or traveling in an endemic area, irrespective of exposure history to ticks or tick bites, especially if asplenic

LABORATORY TESTS

- CBC to reveal mild to moderate pancytopenia
- Abnormally elevated serum chemistries, including creatinine, liver function profile, lactate dehydrogenase, and direct and total bilirubin levels
- Urinalysis to reveal proteinuria and hemoglobinuria
- Examination of Giemsa- or Wright-stained thick and thin blood films for intraerythrocytic parasites
  1. In its classic, though infrequently seen, form a "tetrad" or "Maltese Cross" composed of four daughter cells attached by cytoplasmic strands is observed.
  2. More commonly, smaller forms composed of a single chromatin dot are eccentrically located within bluish cytoplasm.
  3. Parasitized erythrocytes may be multiply infected but not enlarged, or they may show evidence of pigment deposition, seen with Plasmodium species.
- Diagnosis achieved serologically by indirect immunofluorescence assay (IFA) is specific for *B. microti.*
  1. Titer of ≥1:64 is indicative of seropositivity, whereas one ≥1:256 is considered diagnostic of acute infection.
  2. Assay is hampered by the inability to distinguish between exposed patients and those who are actively infected.
  3. Immunoglobulin M indirect immunofluorescent-antibody test may be highly sensitive and specific for diagnosis.
  4. Babesial DNA by polymerase chain reaction (PCR) has comparable sensitivity and specificity to microscopic analysis of thin blood smears.

TREATMENT

NONPHARMACOLOGIC THERAPY

Supportive care with adequate hydration

ACUTE GENERAL Rx

- In patients with intact spleens: predominantly asymptomatic or if symptomatic, generally self-limited
- Therapy reserved for the severely ill patient, especially if asplenic, elderly, or immunosuppressed
- Combination of quinine sulfate 650 mg PO tid plus clindamycin 600 mg PO tid (1.2 g parenterally bid) taken for 7 to 10 days: effective but may not eliminate parasites
- Combination of atovaquone 750 mg every 12 hr and azithromycin 500 mg on day 1 and 250 mg per day thereafter for 7 days appears to be as effective as a regimen of clindamycin and quinine with fewer adverse reactions
- Exchange transfusions in addition to antimicrobial therapy: successful treatment for severe infections in asplenic patients associated with high levels of *B. microti* or *B. divergens* parasitemia

DISPOSITION

Prognosis is usually good and fatal outcomes are rare.

REFERRAL

- For prompt consultation with an infectious disease specialist if the diagnosis is acutely suspected, especially in the asplenic, elderly, or immunocompromised patient

- For hospitalization for the severely ill patient who may require exchange transfusions in addition to antibiotic therapy

PEARLS & CONSIDERATIONS

COMMENTS

- Prevention of babesiosis in asplenic or immunocompromised hosts is best achieved by avoidance of areas where the vector is endemic, especially during the months of May through September.
- If residence or travel in endemic areas is unavoidable, advise patients to perform daily cutaneous self-examination, wear light-colored clothing (to facilitate removal of ticks), and apply tick repellent (diethyltoluamide and dimethylphthalate) to skin or clothing.
- Advise a daily inspection for ticks in family pets (e.g., cats and dogs).
- Infection with *B. divergens,* especially in the asplenic patient, is often fatal.
- Concurrent babesiosis and Lyme disease has been documented—check for combined infection in severely ill patients.
- Clindamycin and quinine has been successfully used to treat Babesiosis during the third trimester of pregnancy without incurring apparent adverse effect on the fetus.

EVIDENCE

Combination therapy with clindamycin and quinine is as effective as the atovaquone and azithromycin combination. Adverse effects from medication may be more common with clindamycin and quinine. Both combinations are effective in eradicating babesiosis parasites at 3 mo after the treatment course.[1] Ⓑ

Silent infection may persist for months or years when left untreated. Treatment of babesiosis with clindamycin and quinine may reduce the duration of parasitemia.[2] Ⓑ

Evidence-Based References

1. Krause PJ et al: Atovaquone and azithromycin for the treatment of babesiosis, *N Engl J Med* 343:1454, 2000. Ⓑ
2. Krause PJ et al: Persistent parasitemia after acute babesiosis, *N Engl J Med* 339:160, 1998. Ⓑ

SUGGESTED READINGS

Cable RG, Leiby DA: Risk and prevention of transfusion-transmitted babesiosis and other tick-borne diseases, *Curr Opin Hematol* 10(6):405, 2003.

Gelfand JA, Callahan MV: Babesiosis: an update on epidemiology and treatment, *Curr Infect Dis Rep* 5(1):53, 2003.

Krause PJ: Babesiosis diagnosis and treatment, *Vector Borne Zoonotic Dis* 3(1):45, 2003.

AUTHORS: **GLENN G. FORT, M.D., M.P.H., DENNIS J. MIKOLICH, M.D.,** and **GEORGE O. ALONSO, M.D.**

Section I

DISEASES AND DISORDERS

BASIC INFORMATION

DEFINITION

Baker's cyst refers to a fluid-filled popliteal bursa located along the medial border of the popliteal fossa.

SYNONYMS

Popliteal cyst

ICD-9CM CODES
727.51 Baker's cyst (knee)

EPIDEMIOLOGY & DEMOGRAPHICS

- Occurs at all ages.
- Incidence is unknown.
- Between 2% to 6% of all patients thought to have clinical DVT turn out to have symptomatic Baker's cysts.
- Approximately 5% of MRIs of the knees reveal popliteal cysts.

PHYSICAL FINDINGS & CLINICAL PRESENTATION

- Pain in the popliteal space
- Knee swelling
- Leg edema
- Prominence of the popliteal fossa
- Decreased range of motion of the knee
- Locking of the knee
- Foucher's sign: The cyst becomes hard with knee extension and soft with knee flexion.
- Neuropathic lancinating pains radiating from the knee down the back of the leg.
- Deep vein thrombosis (DVT)

ETIOLOGY

- Believed to represent fluid distention of the bursal sac separating the semimembranous tendon from the medial head of the gastrocnemius.
- In children, Baker's cysts are thought to be secondary to trauma and irritation of the knee.
- In adults, Baker's cysts are usually associated with pathologic changes of the knee joint:
  1. Rheumatoid arthritis
  2. Osteoarthritis of the knee
  3. Meniscal tears
  4. Patellofemoral chondromalacia
  5. Fracture
  6. Gout
  7. Pseudogout
  8. Infection (tuberculosis)

DIAGNOSIS

Baker's cyst frequently mimics a DVT and is sometimes called *pseudothrombo-phlebitis syndrome.*

DIFFERENTIAL DIAGNOSIS

- DVT
- Popliteal aneurysms
- Abscess
- Tumors
- Lymphadenopathy
- Varicosities
- Ganglion

WORKUP

Anyone suspected of having a popliteal cyst should undergo imaging studies to exclude other causes.

LABORATORY TESTS

Blood tests are not very specific in the diagnosis of Baker's cysts.

IMAGING STUDIES

- Plain x-ray (AP and lateral views) may show calcification in a solid tumor or in the posterior meniscal area.
- Ultrasound is easy, cost effective, and excludes other causes of popliteal fossa pathology.
- MRI of the knee identifies coexisting joint pathology (e.g., osteoarthritis, torn meniscus).
- Noninvasive venous studies to rule out DVT.

TREATMENT

NONPHARMACOLOGIC THERAPY

- Rest
- Strenuous activity avoidance
- Knee immobilization necessary in some cases

ACUTE GENERAL Rx

- NSAIDs, ibuprofen 400 to 800 mg PO tid, or naproxen 250 to 500 mg PO bid can be used to treat Baker's cyst caused by RA, gout, and pseudogout.
- Intraarticular injection or injection of the cyst with corticosteroids, triamcinolone acetonide 40 mg is sometimes tried.

CHRONIC Rx

Surgical procedures addressing the underlying cause include:

1. Arthroscopic surgery to remove loose cartilaginous fragment
2. Partial or total meniscectomy
3. Open excision of the cyst (Fig. 1-33)

DISPOSITION

- Baker's cyst may spontaneously resolve without treatment.
- Complications of Baker's cysts are:
  1. Rupture
  2. DVT
  3. Nerve impingement

REFERRAL

Rheumatology or orthopedics if surgery is contemplated

PEARLS & CONSIDERATIONS

- Popliteal cysts were first described in 1877 by Baker in connection with disease of the knee joint.
- In the setting of meniscus injury, Baker's cysts commonly originate from the posterior horn of the medial meniscus with or without a tear.

COMMENTS

Baker's cyst and DVT can coexist. It is imperative to exclude the diagnosis of DVT before discharging the patient.

SUGGESTED READINGS

Fritshy D et al: The popliteal cyst, *Knee Surg Sports Traumatol Arthrosc* 14(7):623, 2006.

Handy JR: Popliteal cysts in adults: a review, *Semin Arthritis Rheum* 31(2):108, 2001.

Torreggiani WC et al: The imaging spectrum of Baker's (Popliteal) cysts, *Clin Radiol* 57(8):681, 2002.

AUTHOR: **PETER PETROPOULOS, M.D.**

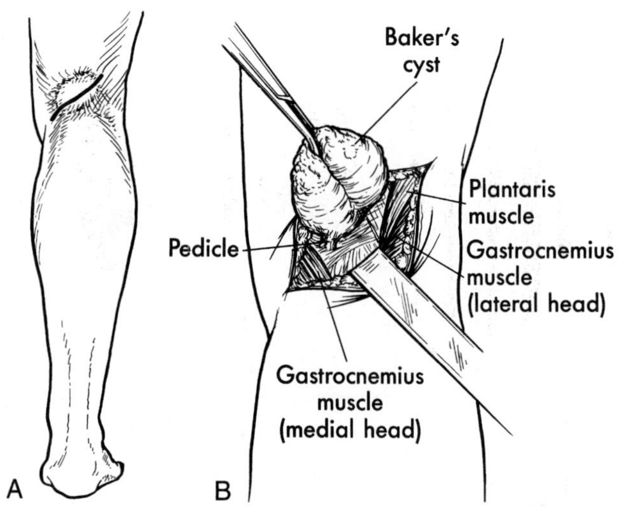

FIGURE 1-33 Removal of midline Baker's cyst. A, Skin incision. **B,** After being exposed, pedicle is clamped, ligated, divided, and inverted. (Redrawn and modified from Meyerding HW, Van Demark GE: *JAMA* 122:858, 1943.)

BASIC INFORMATION

DEFINITION

Balanitis is an inflammation of the superficial tissues of the penile head (Fig. 1-34).

ICD-9CM CODES
112.2 Balanitis

EPIDEMIOLOGY & DEMOGRAPHICS

INCIDENCE (IN U.S.): Unknown
PREVALENCE (IN U.S.): Unknown
PREDOMINANT SEX: Exclusive to males
PEAK INCIDENCE: All ages, especially in sexually active men

PHYSICAL FINDINGS & CLINICAL PRESENTATION

- Itching and tenderness
- Pain, dysuria, and local edema
- Rarely, ulceration and lymph node enlargement
- Severe ulcerations leading to superimposed bacterial infections
- Inability to void: unusual, but a more distressing and serious complication

ETIOLOGY

- Poor hygiene, causing erosion of tissue with erythema and promoting growth of *Candida albicans*
- Sexual contact, urinary catheters, and trauma
- Allergic reactions to condoms or medications

DIAGNOSIS

DIFFERENTIAL DIAGNOSIS

- Leukoplakia
- Reiter's syndrome
- Lichen planus
- Balanitis xerotica obliterans
- Psoriasis
- Carcinoma of the penis
- Erythroplasia of Queyrat
- Nodular scabies

WORKUP

- Sexually active males: assessment for evidence of other sexually transmitted diseases
- Biopsy if lesions do not heal

LABORATORY TESTS

- VDRL
- Serum glucose
- Wet mount
- KOH prep
- Microbial culture

TREATMENT

NONPHARMACOLOGIC THERAPY

- Maintenance of meticulous hygiene
- Retraction and bathing of prepuce several times a day
- Warm sitz baths to ease edema and erythema
- Consideration of circumcision, especially when symptoms are severe or recurrent
- With Foley catheters, strict catheter care strongly advised

ACUTE GENERAL Rx

- Analgesics, such as acetaminophen and/or codeine
- Clotrimazole 1% cream applied topically twice daily to affected areas
- Bacitracin or Neosporin ointment applied topically 4 times daily
- With more severe bacterial superinfection: cephalexin 500 mg PO qid
- Topical corticosteroids added 4 times daily if dermatitis severe
- Patients with suspected urinary tract infections: trimethoprim-sulfa DS twice daily or ciprofloxacin 500 mg PO bid after obtaining appropriate cultures

DISPOSITION

Balanitis is often self-limited and usually responds to conservative therapy; if it does not improve, consider circinate balanitis (Reiter's Syndrome), nodular scabies, primary skin lesions including skin carcinoma.

PEARLS & CONSIDERATIONS

Don't forget about nodular scabies involving the prepubic area—examine the region carefully for burrows and tracks of *Sarcoptes scabiei*.

REFERRAL

- For surgical evaluation for circumcision if symptoms are recurrent, especially if phimosis or meatitis occurs (NOTE: Severe phimosis with an inability to void may require prompt slit drainage.)
- For biopsy to rule out other diagnosis such as premalignant or malignant lesions if lesions are not healing

SUGGESTED READINGS

Buechner SA: Common skin disorders of the penis, *BJU Int* 90(5):498, 2002.

Bunker CB: Topics in penile dermatology, *Clin Exp Dermatol* 26(6):469, 2001.

Huntley JS et al: Troubles with the foreskin: one hundred consecutive referrals to paediatric surgeons, *J R Soc Med* 96(9):449, 2003.

Pandher BS et al: Treatment of balanitis xerotica obliterans with topical tacrolimus, *J Urol* 170(3):923, 2003.

Thiruchelvan M et al: Emergency dorsal slit for balanitis with retention, *J R Soc Med* 97(4):206, 2004.

AUTHORS: **GLENN G. FORT, M.D., M.P.H., JOSEPH J. LIEBER, M.D.,** and **DENNIS J. MIKOLICH, M.D.**

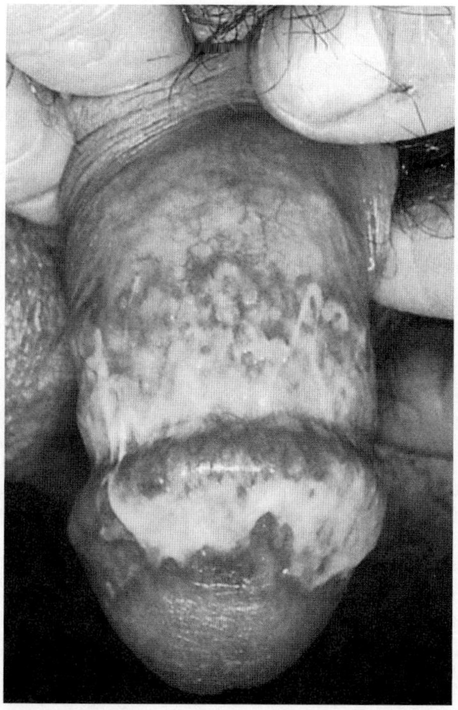

FIGURE 1-34 ***Candida* balanitis.** The moist space between the skin surfaces of the uncircumcised penis is an ideal environment for *Candida* infection. This thick white exudate is typical of a severe acute infection. (From Habif TP: *Clinical dermatology: a color guide to diagnosis and therapy,* ed 3, St Louis, 1996, Mosby.)

BASIC INFORMATION

DEFINITION

Barrett's esophagus occurs when the squamous lining of the lower esophagus is replaced by metaplastic, intestinalized columnar epithelium. The condition is associated with an increased risk of adenocarcinoma of the esophagus.

SYNONYMS

Intestinal metaplasia of lower esophagus

ICD-9CM CODES

530.85 Barrett's esophagus

EPIDEMIOLOGY & DEMOGRAPHICS

- 4:1 ratio of men to women
- Mean age of onset is 40 yr with a mean age of diagnosis of 55 to 60 yr
- Occurs more frequently in Caucasians and Hispanics than in African Americans with a ratio of 10 to 20:1
- Mean prevalence of 5% to 15% in patients undergoing endoscopy (EGD) for symptoms of GERD
- Prevalence in asymptomatic cohorts ranges from 5% to 25%

CLINICAL PRESENTATION

Symptoms:

- Chronic heartburn
- Dysphagia for solid food
- May be an incidental finding on EGD in patients without reflux symptoms
- Less frequent: chest pain, hematemesis, or melena

Physical findings:

- Nonspecific; can be completely normal
- Epigastric tenderness on palpation

ETIOLOGY

- Metaplasia is thought to result from reepithelialization of esophageal tissue injured secondary to chronic GERD.
- Patients with Barrett's tend to have more severe esophageal motility disturbances (decreased lower esophageal sphincter pressure, ineffective peristalsis) and greater esophageal acid exposure on 24-hour pH monitoring.
- Intraesophageal bile reflux may also play a role in the pathogenesis.
- Familial clustering of GERD and Barrett's suggests a genetic predisposition, but no gene has yet been identified.
- Progression from metaplasia to carcinoma is associated with changes in gene structure and expression.

DIAGNOSIS

DIFFERENTIAL DIAGNOSIS

- GERD, uncomplicated
- Erosive esophagitis
- Gastritis
- Peptic ulcer disease
- Angina
- Malignancy
- Stricture or Schatzki's ring

WORKUP

- EGD with biopsy for diagnosis.
- Diagnosis requires the presence of intestinal metaplasia in columnar epithelium proximal to the gastroesophageal junction. Longer segment Barrett's is more readily diagnosed.
- Intestinal metaplasia of the gastric cardia is not Barrett's and does not have the same risk of malignancy.
- Imaging studies are nonspecific and insensitive for the diagnosis.
- The Practice Parameters Committee of the American College of Gastroenterology (ACG) has recommended that patients with chronic GERD symptoms be considered for EGD to exclude Barrett's. General population screening is not currently recommended. Although screening has become standard of practice in some communities, the effectiveness of screening using current techniques is controversial because it may not improve mortality from adenocarcinoma or be cost effective.
- Screening for *H. pylori* infection in patients with GERD and Barrett's esophagus is not recommended.

TREATMENT

Goal is to control GERD symptoms and maintain healed mucosa.

NONPHARMACOLOGIC THERAPY

- Lifestyle modifications, elevating head of bed, avoiding chocolate, tobacco, caffeine, mints, and certain drugs (see "Gastroesophageal Reflux Disease").
- Chronic acid suppression is often necessary to control symptoms and promote healing.

ACUTE GENERAL Rx

- Proton pump inhibitors (PPIs) are most effective.
- Adequate control of GERD symptoms in patients with Barrett's may or may not completely control intraesophageal acid exposure. Some studies suggest that normalization of intraesophageal acid exposure may either lead to regression of Barrett's or reduce the risk of dysplasia.
- If asymptomatic and incidentally found to have Barrett's esophagus, medication use may be considered.

CHRONIC Rx

- Thermal ablation techniques, photodynamic therapy, and endoscopic mucosal resection are all possible approaches in patients with Barrett's and high-grade dysplasia, either in conjunction with aggressive surveillance or as an alternate to surgery in poor operative candidates. All these options run the risk of residual intestinal metaplasia. As only a minority of patients with Barrett's progress to high-grade dysplasia or carcinoma, these techniques cannot be currently recommended in patients with Barrett's alone. Studies will need to show that they reduce or eliminate the need for surveillance endoscopy and/or the risk of cancer, and that they are cost effective.
- Antireflux surgery may be considered for management of GERD and associated sequelae. Patients should still have EGD surveillance of their Barrett's. Surgical resection is offered for multifocal high-grade dysplasia or carcinoma.

DISPOSITION

- Overall, 30 to 50× increased risk of adenocarcinoma of the esophagus.
- Corresponds to 500 cancers per yr per 100,000 persons with Barrett's.
- Frequency of monitoring is controversial; no studies have proven that surveillance increases life expectancy.
- ACG recommends that patients with Barrett's undergo surveillance EGD and systematic four-quadrant biopsy at intervals determined by the presence and grade of dysplasia. All mucosal abnormalities should be biopsied. Patients who have had two EGDs showing no dysplasia should have follow-up every 3 years. Patients with low-grade dysplasia should have extensive mucosal sampling and follow-up every year. Patients with high-grade dysplasia should have expert confirmation and extensive mucosal sampling. Consider intensive surveillance every 3 months for patients with focal high-grade dysplasia. Patients with multifocal high-grade dysplasia or carcinoma should be considered for resection, or ablation if not an operative candidate.
- Patients should be treated aggressively for GERD before surveillance.

REFERRAL

- For EGD with biopsy in patients with chronic GERD who have not had previous EGD.
- For surveillance in those with biopsy-proven Barrett's.
- For those with high-grade dysplasia, refer for intensive surveillance or esophageal resection; ablative therapy may be considered as part of a research protocol or if not an operative candidate.

SUGGESTED READINGS

Bonino JA, Sharma P: Barrett's esophagus, *Curr Opin Gastroenterol* 22:406, 2006.

Dellon ES, Shaheen NJ: Does screening for Barrett's esophagus and adenocarcinoma of the esophagus prolong survival? *J Clin Oncol* 23:4478, 2005.

Shaheen NJ: Advances in Barrett's esophagus and esophageal adenocarcinoma, *Gastroenterology* 128:1554, 2005.

Sharma P et al: A critical review of the diagnosis and management of Barrett's esophagus: the AGA Chicago workshop, *Gastroenterology* 127:310, 2004.

Spechler SJ, Barr B: Review article: screening and surveillance of Barrett's esophagus: what is a cost-effective framework? *Aliment Pharmacol Ther* 19(Suppl 1):49, 2004.

AUTHOR: **HARLAN G. RICH, M.D.**

BASIC INFORMATION

DEFINITION

Bartter's syndrome is a group of renal tubular disorders characterized by metabolic alkalosis, hypokalemia, hyperplasia of the juxtaglomerular apparatus, hyperreninemic hyperaldosteronism, and hypercalciuria.

SYNONYMS

Hypokalemic alkalosis with hypercalciuria

ICD-9CM CODES
255.13 Bartter's Syndrome

EPIDEMIOLOGY & DEMOGRAPHICS

Classic Bartter's syndrome can present with symptoms at 2 years of age or younger.

Neonatal Bartter's syndrome can be diagnosed at birth.

The true incidence in the U.S. is not known.

Incidence is similar in males and in females.

CLINICAL PRESENTATION

- Neonatal Bartter's syndrome involves maternal polyhydramnios, frequent preterm delivery, fetal polyuria, and FTT.
- Classic Bartter's syndrome may include a history of maternal polyhydramnios and premature delivery. The following features are characteristic:
  - Polyuria.
  - Polydipsia.
  - Hypokalemia.
  - Metabolic alkalosis.
  - Hypercalciuria.
  - Plasma magnesium is normal or mildly reduced.
  - Patients are normotensive.
  - Patients do not have edema.

ETIOLOGY

- Disorder of chloride reabsorption in the thick ascending loop of Henle.
- A couple of defects manifest the same phenotype.
- Tubular pathophysiology is identical to loop diuretic mechanism of action.

DIAGNOSIS

DIFFERENTIAL DIAGNOSIS

- Diuretic abuse
- Surreptitious vomiting
- Gitelman's syndrome
- Autosomal dominant hypocalcemia
- Hyperprostaglandin E syndrome

WORKUP

- Classic Bartter's syndrome is usually a diagnosis of exclusion.
- Vomiting associated with a low urine chloride and scarring of the dorsum of the hand and dental erosions suggests bulimia nervosa.
- Diuretic abuse can only be excluded by a urinary assay for diuretics.

LABORATORY TESTS

- Serum sodium, potassium, chloride, bicarbonate, calcium, magnesium, phosphorus.
- Urine calcium, chloride, assay for diuretics as above.
- Serum pH can be confirmed by performing ABG.

IMAGING STUDIES

- Renal ultrasonography may show nephrocalcinosis, hydronephrosis, and hydroureter in neonatal Bartter's syndrome.
- Classic signs of hypokalemia may be present on ECG.

TREATMENT

NONPHARMACOLOGIC THERAPY

None

ACUTE GENERAL Rx

Neonatal Bartter's syndrome requires correction of electrolyte imbalance and volume depletion.

CHRONIC Rx

- Usual treatment includes oral potassium and magnesium supplementation though achievement of normal serum potassium and magnesium levels is often difficult.
- Potassium-sparing diuretics such as spironolactone/amiloride have also been used effectively in the treatment of Bartter's.

REFERRAL

Consultation with nephrology facilitates diagnosis and management of this condition.

PEARLS & CONSIDERATIONS

COMMENTS

- Just as Bartter's looks like loop diuretic use from the point of view of laboratory testing, Gitelman's syndrome appears identical to thiazide use.
- High urine calcium is the best way to distinguish Bartter's from Gitelman's syndrome.
- Serum magnesium differences have been described but are likely to be low in both syndromes and are probably not useful in distinguishing these syndromes.

PREVENTION

None

PATIENT/FAMILY EDUCATION

- Foods with high potassium content should be emphasized in dietary education.
- Patients with Bartter's syndrome are more vulnerable to volume depletion due to potassium derangement during exercise and exposure.

SUGGESTED READINGS

Hebert SC: Bartter syndrome, *Curr Opin Nephrol Hypertens* 12(5):527-532, 2003.

Kurtz I: Molecular pathogenesis of Bartter's and Gitelman's syndromes, *Kidney Int* 54:1396, 1998.

AUTHOR: **JONATHAN BURNS, M.A., M.D.**

BASIC INFORMATION

DEFINITION

Basal cell carcinoma (BCC) is a malignant tumor of the skin arising from basal cells of the lower epidermis and adnexal structures. It may be classified as one of six types (nodular, superficial, pigmented, cystic, sclerosing or morpheaform, and nevoid). The most common type is nodular (21%); the least common is morpheaform (1%); a mixed pattern is present in approximately 40% of cases. Basal cell carcinoma advances by direct expansion and destroys normal tissue.

SYNONYMS

BCC

ICD-9CM CODES

179.9 Basal cell carcinoma, site unspecified
173.3 Basal cell carcinoma, face
173.4 Basal cell carcinoma, neck, scalp
173.5 Basal cell carcinoma, trunk
173.6 Basal cell carcinoma of the limb
173.7 Basal cell carcinoma, lower limb

EPIDEMIOLOGY & DEMOGRAPHICS

- Most common cutaneous neoplasm
- 85% appear on the head and neck region
- Most common site: nose (30%)
- Increased incidence with age >40 yr
- Increased incidence in men
- Risk factors: fair skin, increased sun exposure, use of tanning salons with ultraviolet A or B radiation, history of irradiation (e.g., Hodgkin's disease), personal or family history of skin cancer, impaired immune system

PHYSICAL FINDINGS & CLINICAL PRESENTATION

Variable with the histologic type:

- Nodular: dome-shaped, painless lesion that may become multilobular and frequently ulcerates (rodent ulcer); prominent telangiectatic vessels are noted on the surface; border is translucent, elevated, pearly white (Fig. 1-35); some nodular basal cell carcinomas may contain pigmentation, giving an appearance similar to a melanoma.
- Superficial: circumscribed scaling black appearance with a thin raised pearly white border; a crust and erosions may be present; occurs most frequently on the trunk and extremities.
- Morpheaform: flat or slightly raised yellowish or white appearance (similar to localized scleroderma); appearance similar to scars, surface has a waxy consistency.

DIAGNOSIS

DIFFERENTIAL DIAGNOSIS

- Keratoacanthoma
- Melanoma (pigmented basal cell carcinoma)
- Xeroderma pigmentosa
- Basal cell nevus syndrome
- Molluscum contagiosum
- Sebaceous hyperplasia
- Psoriasis

WORKUP

Biopsy to confirm diagnosis

TREATMENT

Variable with tumor size, location, and cell type:

- Excision surgery: preferred method for large tumors with well-defined borders on the legs, cheeks, forehead, and trunk.
- Mohs' micrographic surgery: preferred for lesions in high-risk areas (e.g., nose, eyelid), very large primary tumors, recurrent basal cell carcinomas, and tumors with poorly defined clinical margins.
- Electrodesiccation and curettage: useful for small (<6 mm) nodular basal cell carcinomas.
- Cryosurgery with liquid nitrogen: useful in basal cell carcinomas of the superficial and nodular types with clearly definable margins; no clear advantages over the other forms of therapy; generally reserved for uncomplicated tumors.
- Radiation therapy: generally used for basal cell carcinomas in areas requiring preservation of normal surround tissues for cosmetic reasons (e.g., around lips); also useful in patients who cannot tolerate surgical procedures or for large lesions and surgical failures.
- Imiquimod (Aldara) 5% cream can be used for treatment of small, superficial BCCs of the trunk and extremities. Efficacy rate is approximately 80%. Its main advantage is lack of scarring, which must be weighed against higher cure rates with surgical intervention.

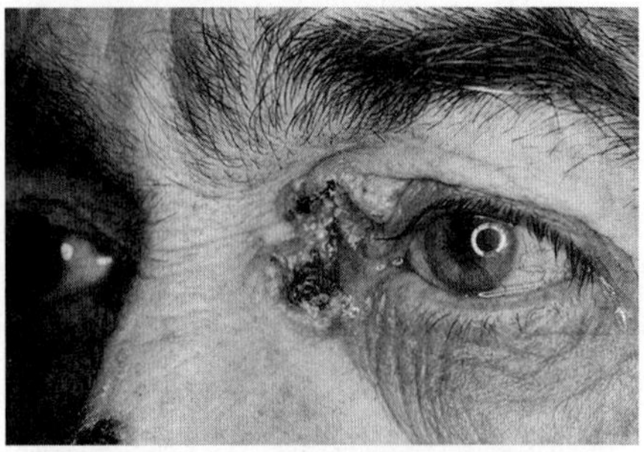

FIGURE 1-35 Basal cell carcinoma. Note rolled translucent border and central ulceration in typical facial location. (From Noble J et al: *Textbook of primary care medicine,* ed 3, St Louis, 2001, Mosby.)

DISPOSITION

- More than 90% of patients are cured, however, periodic evaluation for at least 5 yr is necessary because of increased risk of recurrence of another basal cell carcinoma (>40% risk within 5 yr of treatment).
- A lesion is considered low risk if it is <1.5 cm in diameter, is nodular or cystic, is not in a difficult-to-treat area (H zone of face), and has not been previously treated.
- Nodular and superficial basal cell carcinomas are the least aggressive.
- Morpheaform lesions have the highest incidence of positive tumor margins (>30%) and the greatest recurrence rate.

EVIDENCE

Surgical treatment of primary facial basal cell carcinomas results in a significantly lower treatment failure rate at 4 yr compared with radiotherapy, in addition to a significantly superior cosmetic result.[1] (A)

In the treatment of primary superficial and nodular BCCs of the head and neck, both surgery and cryotherapy give equivalent recurrence rates at 12 mo, but cosmetic results favor surgery.[1] (B)

Radiotherapy treatment of primary basal cell carcinoma results in significantly fewer recurrences at 1 yr vs. cryotherapy. Such short-term results, however, should be interpreted with caution. Cosmetic results, at 1 yr, do not significantly differ between the two groups.[1] (B)

A randomized phase III study compared imiquimod or vehicle cream once daily 5 or 7 times per wk for 6 wk on superficial basal cell carcinoma. Combined clinical and histological assessments produced clearance rates for the 5 and 7 times per week imiquimod groups of 75% and 73%, respectively. The researchers concluded that imiquimod appears to be safe and effective for the treatment of BCC compared with vehicle cream.[2] (B)

Evidence-Based References

1. Bath FJ et al: Interventions for basal cell carcinoma of the skin, *Cochrane Database Sys Rev* Issue 2, 2003. (A) (B)
2. Geisse J et al: Imiquimod 5% cream for the treatment of superficial basal cell carcinoma: results from two phase III, randomized, vehicle-controlled studies, *J Am Acad Dermatol* 50:722, 2004. (B)

AUTHOR: **FRED F. FERRI, M.D.**

BASIC INFORMATION

DEFINITION

Behçet's disease is a chronic, relapsing, inflammatory disorder characterized by the presence of recurrent oral aphthous ulcers, genital ulcers, uveitis, and skin lesions (Figs. 1-36 and 1-37).

SYNONYMS

Behçet's syndrome

ICD-9CM CODES

136.1 Behçet's syndrome

EPIDEMIOLOGY & DEMOGRAPHICS

Behçet's disease is observed in two different geographic locations.

- One region consists of Japan, Korea, Turkey, and the Mediterranean basin.
  1. Prevalence ranges from 1:7000 to 1:10,000.
  2. Turkey has the highest prevalence at 80 to 370 cases per 100,000.
- The second region consists of North America and Northern Europe.
  1. Prevalence ranges from 1:20,000 to 1:100,000.
  2. Prevalence of Behçet's disease in the U.S. is 0.12 to 0.33 cases per 100,000.
- In these regions the prevalence of HLA-B51 is higher in patients with Behçet's disease.
- Males = females.

PHYSICAL FINDINGS & CLINICAL PRESENTATION

- Behçet's disease typically affects individuals in the third to fourth decade of life and primarily presents with painful aphthous oral ulcers. The ulcers occur in crops measuring 2 to 10 mm in size and are found on the mucous membrane of the cheek, gingiva, tongue, pharynx, and soft palate
- Genital ulcers are similar to the oral ulcers
- Decreased vision secondary to uveitis, keratitis, or vitreous hemorrhage, or occlusion of the retinal artery or vein may occur
- Skin findings include nodular lesions, which are histologically equally divided to erythema nodosum-like lesions, superficial thrombophlebitis, and acne lesions, which are also presented at sites uncommon for ordinary acne (arms and legs)
- Arthritis and arthralgias
- CNS: meningeal findings including headache, fever, and stiff neck can occur. Cerebellar ataxia and pseudobulbar palsy occur with involvement of the brainstem
- Vasculitis leading to both arterial and venous inflammation or occlusion can result in signs and symptoms of a myocardial infarction, intermittent claudication, deep vein thrombosis, hemoptysis, and aneurysm formation

ETIOLOGY

The etiology of Behçet's disease is unknown. An immune-related vasculitis is thought to lead to many of the manifestations of Behçet's disease. What triggers the immune response and activation is not yet known.

DIAGNOSIS

According to the International Study Group for Behçet's disease, the diagnosis of Behçet's disease is established when recurrent oral ulceration is present along with at least two of the following in the absence of other systemic diseases:

- Recurrent genital ulceration
- Eye lesions
- Skin lesions
- Positive pathergy test (enlarging papules at sterile needle injection sites)

DIFFERENTIAL DIAGNOSIS

- Ulcerative colitis
- Crohn's disease
- Lichen planus
- Pemphigoid
- Herpes simplex infection
- Benign aphthous stomatitis
- SLE
- Reiter's syndrome
- Ankylosing spondylitis
- AIDS
- Hypereosinophilic syndrome.
- Sweet's syndrome

WORKUP

The diagnosis of Behçet's disease is a clinical diagnosis. Laboratory tests and x-ray imaging may be helpful in working up the complications of Behçet's disease or excluding other diseases in the differential.

LABORATORY TESTS

There are no diagnostic laboratory tests for Behçet's disease.

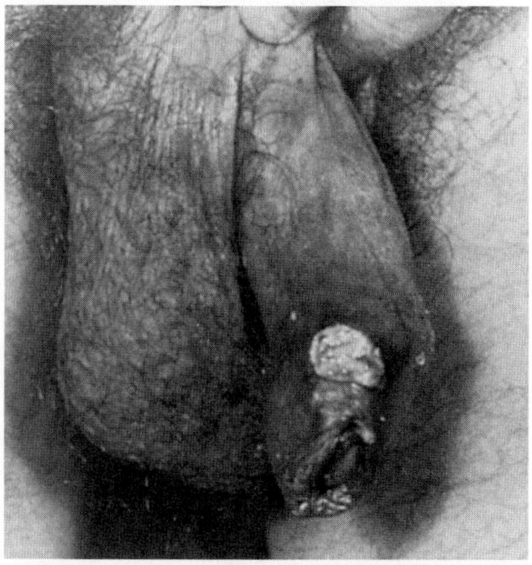

FIGURE 1-36 Behçet's syndrome. Painful prepuceal ulcer in a male with superficial thrombophlebitis, oral ulcers, and bowel vasculitis. (From Canoso J: *Rheumatology in primary care,* Philadelphia, 1997, WB Saunders.)

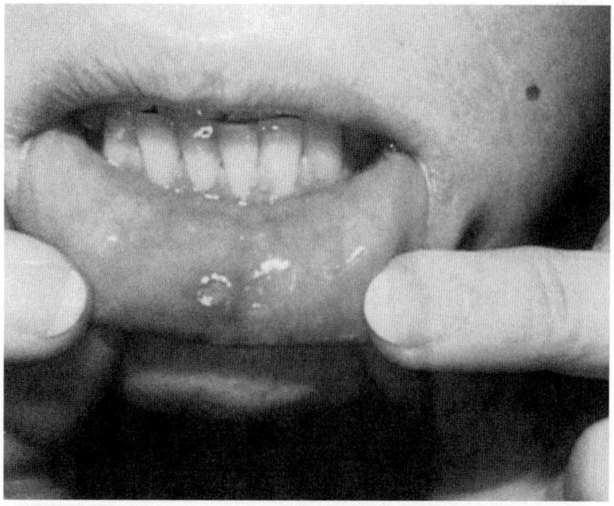

FIGURE 1-37 Behçet's syndrome. Painful aphthous inner lower lip ulcer in a 30-year-old Chinese woman with relapsing oral and genital ulcers and uveitis. She did well on low-dose prednisone plus colchicine. (From Canoso J: *Rheumatology in primary care,* Philadelphia, 1997, WB Saunders.)

IMAGING STUDIES

CT scan, MRI, and angiography are useful for detecting CNS and vascular lesions.

TREATMENT

Rx

Treatment is directed at the patient's clinical presentation (e.g., mucocutaneous lesions, ocular lesions, arthritis, GI, CNS, or vascular lesions).

NONPHARMACOLOGIC THERAPY

Supportive care

ACUTE GENERAL Rx

- Oral and genital ulcers
  1. Topical corticosteroids (e.g., triamcinolone acetonide ointment applied tid)
  2. Tetracycline tablets 250 mg dissolved in 5 cc water and applied to the ulcer for 2 to 3 min
  3. Colchicine 0.5 to 1.5 mg/kg/day PO
  4. Thalidomide 100 to 300 mg PO daily
  5. Dapsone 100 mg PO daily
  6. Pentoxifylline 300 mg/day PO
  7. Azathioprine 1 to 2.5 mg/kg/day PO
  8. Methotrexate 7.5 to 25 mg/wk PO or IV
- Ocular lesions
  1. Anterior uveitis is treated by an ophthalmologist with topical corticosteroids (e.g., betamethasone drops 1 to 2 drops tid). Topical injection with dexamethasone 1 to 1.5 mg has also been tried
  2. Infliximab 5 mg/kg single dose
- CNS disease
  1. Chlorambucil 0.1 mg/kg/day is used in the treatment of posterior uveitis, retinal vasculitis, or CNS disease. Patients not responding to chlorambucil can be tried on cyclosporine 5 to 7 mg/kg/day.
  2. In CNS vasculitis, cyclophosphamide 2 to 3 mg/kg/day is used. Prednisone can be used as an alternative.
- Arthritis
  1. NSAIDs (e.g., ibuprofen 400 to 800 mg tid PO or indomethacin 50 to 75 mg/day PO)
  2. Sulfasalazine 1 to 3 g/day PO is an alternative treatment
- GI lesions
  1. Sulfasalazine 1 to 3 g/day PO
  2. Prednisone 40 to 60 mg/day PO
- Vascular lesions
  1. Prednisone 40 to 60 mg/day PO
  2. Cytotoxic agents as mentioned previously
  3. Heparin 5000 to 20,000 U/day followed by oral warfarin

CHRONIC Rx

- Chronic therapy is usually continued for approximately 1 yr after remission.
- Surgery may be indicated in patients with complications of bowel perforation, vascular occlusive disease, and aneurysm formation.

DISPOSITION

- The aphthous oral ulcers last 1 to 2 wk, recurring more frequently than genital ulcers.
- Approximately 25% of patients with ocular lesions become blind.
- The disease course is unpredictable.
- Complications include:
  1. Meningitis
  2. Cerebrovascular accident (stroke)
  3. Aneurysm rupture
  4. Peripheral lower-extremity ischemia
  5. Mesenteric ischemia
  6. Myocardial infarction

REFERRAL

If the diagnosis of Behçet's disease is suspected, a referral to both rheumatology and ophthalmology is indicated because the disease is so rare.

PEARLS & CONSIDERATIONS

!

COMMENTS

- The pathergy test refers to the formation of a papule or pustule of 2 mm or more in size after oblique insertion of a sterile 20- or 25-gauge needle into the skin.
- Due to rarity of this disease, data from controlled, prospective, randomized clinical trials are lacking.

SUGGESTED READINGS

Al-Otaibi LM, Porter SR, Poate TW: Behcet's disease: a review, *J Dent Res* 84(3):209, 2005.

Bonfioli AA, Orefice F: Behcet's disease, *Semin Ophthalmol* 20(3):199, 2005.

Evereklioglu C: Managing the symptoms of Behcet's disease, *Expert Opin Pharmacother* 5(2):317, 2004.

Kurokawa MS, Yoshikawa H, Suzuki N: Behcet's disease, *Semin Respir Crit Care Med* 25(5):557, 2004.

Yazici H: Behçet's syndrome: an update, *Curr Rheumatol Rep* (5):195, 2003.

AUTHORS: **GLENN G. FORT, M.D., M.P.H., DENNIS J. MIKOLICH, M.D.,** and **JOSEPH GRILLO, M.D.**

BASIC INFORMATION

DEFINITION

Bell's palsy is an idiopathic, isolated, usually unilateral facial weakness in the distribution of the seventh cranial nerve (<1% are bilateral).

SYNONYMS

Idiopathic facial paralysis

ICD-9CM CODES
351.0 Bell's palsy

EPIDEMIOLOGY & DEMOGRAPHICS

INCIDENCE: 20 to 30 cases/100,000; occurs at any age, median age 45

RISK FACTORS:

- Pregnancy (especially third trimester/first postpartum week)
- Diabetes (5% to 10% of patients)
- Travel to area endemic for Lyme disease

PHYSICAL FINDINGS & CLINICAL PRESENTATION

- Unilateral paralysis of the upper and lower facial muscles (asymmetric eye closure, brow, and smile).
- Ipsilateral loss of taste
- Ipsilateral ear pain, usually 2 to 3 days before presentation
- Increased or decreased unilateral eye tearing
- Hyperacusis
- Subjective ipsilateral facial numbness
- In about 8% of cases, other cranial neuropathies may occur

ETIOLOGY

- Most cases are idiopathic although the cause is often viral (herpes simplex).
- Herpes zoster can cause Bell's palsy in association with herpetic blisters affecting the outer ear canal or the area behind the ear (Ramsay-Hunt syndrome).
- Bell's palsy can also be one of the manifestations of Lyme disease and less commonly has been associated with hepatitis and post-smallpox vaccination.

DIAGNOSIS

DIFFERENTIAL DIAGNOSIS

- Neoplasms affecting the base of the skull or the parotid gland
- Infectious process (meningitis, otitis media, osteomyelitis of the skull base)
- Brainstem stroke
- Multiple sclerosis
- Head trauma/temporal bone fracture
- Other: sarcoidosis, Guillain-Barré, carcinomatous or leukemic meningitis, leprosy, Melkersson-Rosenthal syndrome

WORKUP

Bell's palsy is a clinical diagnosis. A focused history and neurologic examination confirms the diagnosis.

LABORATORY TESTS

- Consider CBC, fasting glucose, VDRL, ESR, ACE in selected patients.
- Lyme titer in endemic areas.

IMAGING STUDIES

- Contrast-enhanced MRI to exclude neoplasms is indicated only in patients with atypical features or course.
- Chest x-ray may be useful to exclude sarcoidosis or rule out TB in selected patients before treating with steroids.

TREATMENT

NONPHARMACOLOGIC THERAPY

- Reassure patient that the prognosis is usually good and the disease is most likely a result of a virus attacking the nerve, not a stroke.
- Avoid corneal drying by patching the eye. Lacri-Lube ophthalmic ointment at night and artificial tears during the day are also useful to prevent excessive drying.

ACUTE GENERAL Rx

- A short course of oral prednisone is commonly used and may improve the chances of complete recovery at 3 and 9 mo.
- If used, prednisone therapy should be started within 24 to 48 hr of symptom onset. Optimal steroid dose is unknown.
- Combination therapy with acyclovir and prednisone is not effective in improving clinical recovery.
- Surgical decompression remains controversial and data from randomized trials are lacking to compare medical vs. surgical therapy.
- There are some data that suggest that methylcobalamin (active form of vitamin B_{12}) and hyperbaric oxygen may be of benefit, but these have not yet received widespread acceptance.
- Botulinum toxin may be helpful for treatment of synkinesis and hemifacial spasm, two late sequelae of Bell's palsy.

CHRONIC Rx

Patients should be monitored for evidence of corneal abrasion and ulceration. Physical therapy including moist heat and massage may be beneficial.

DISPOSITION

- 71% of patients should recover completely. Prognosis is better for those with less severity of symptoms at onset and clinical improvement within 3 wk. Diabetes may confer a worse prognosis.
- Recovery begins within 3 wk in 85% of patients. The remainder have some improvement within 3 to 6 months.
- Recurrence occurs in 5% of cases.

REFERRAL

- Persistent eye irritation or redness requires referral to ophthalmology.
- Neurology referral is recommended if diagnosis is unclear or if clinical course is atypical.

PEARLS & CONSIDERATIONS

Assure that both upper and lower aspects of the face are involved (as this suggests a peripheral lesion). Lower facial asymmetry alone is more likely central (e.g., stroke) and further workup is necessary.

EVIDENCE

There is no unequivocal evidence favoring the use of corticosteroids, either alone or in combination with acyclovir, for patients with Bell's palsy.

The available evidence from randomized controlled trials is conflicting and meta-analysis of the data from these trials suggests that steroids are probably beneficial.[1,2]

The available evidence suggests that acyclovir given alone or in combination with steroids offers any additional benefit.[3]

Evidence-Based References

1. Grogan PM: Practice parameter: steroids, acyclovir, and surgery for Bell's Palsy (an evidence-based review): report of the Quality Standards Subcommittee of the American Academy of Neurology. *Neurology* 57(7):830, 2001.
2. Salinas RA et al: Corticosteroids for Bell's palsy (idiopathic facial paralysis), *Cochrane Database Syst Rev* 4:CD001942, 2004.
3. Sullivan FM et al: Early treatment with prednisone or acyclovir in Bell's palsy, *N Eng J Med* 357:1598-1607, 2009.

SUGGESTED READINGS

Alberton DL, Zed PJ: Bell's palsy: a review of treatment using antiviral agents, *Ann Pharmacother* 40(10):1838, 2006. Epub ahead of print.

Austin JR et al: Idiopathic facial nerve paralysis: a randomized double blind controlled study of placebo versus prednisone, *Laryngoscope* 103:1326, 1993.

Benatar M, Edlow JA: The spectrum of cranial neuropathy in patients with Bell's palsy, *Arch Intern Med* 164:2283, 2004.

Gilden D: Bell's palsy, *N Engl J Med* 351:1323, 2004.

Holland NJ, Weiner GM: Recent developments in Bell's palsy, *BMJ* 329:553, 2004.

Kanazawa A et al: Prognosis for Bell's palsy: a comparison of diabetic and nondiabetic patients. *Acta Otolaryngol* 127(8):888, 2007.

Sipe J, Dunn L: Acyclovir for Bell's palsy (idiopathic facial paralysis), *Cochrane Database Syst Rev* 3:CD001869, 2004.

Tigmstra JD, Khatkhate N: Bell's palsy: diagnosis and management, *Am Fam Physician* 76:997-1002, 2004.

AUTHOR: **RICHARD ISAACSON, M.D.**

BASIC INFORMATION

DEFINITION

Bipolar disorder is an episodic, recurrent, and frequently progressive condition in which the afflicted individual experiences at least one episode of mania, characterized by at least 1 week of continuous symptoms of elevated, expansive, or irritable mood in association with three or four of the following:

- Decreased need for sleep
- Grandiosity
- Pressured speech
- Subjective or objective flight of ideas
- Distractibility
- Increased level of goal-directed activity
- Problematic behavior

Most individuals with bipolar disorder will also experience one or more episodes of major depression over their lifetime or have symptoms of a depressive episode commingled with those of mania (mixed episode).

SYNONYMS

Manic-depression
Cycloid psychosis

ICD-9CM CODES
296.4-6 Circular manic, circular depressed, circular type mixed

EPIDEMIOLOGY & DEMOGRAPHICS

INCIDENCE: 0.016% to 0.021%
PREVALENCE (IN U.S.): 0.7% to 1.6%; bipolar spectrum disorders 2.8% to 6.5%
PREDOMINANT SEX: Equal distribution among male and female
PREDOMINANT AGE: Lifelong condition with symptoms present 50% of the time and depression 3 times more frequent than mania
PEAK INCIDENCE: Onset of symptoms between ages 15 and 19 yr
GENETICS:

- Concordance rates for monozygotic twins: 0.7 to 0.8; for dizygotic twins: 0.2
- Risk of affective disorder in offspring with one affected parent with bipolar disorder: 27% to 29%; with two affected parents: 50% to 74%
- Heritability estimate of 0.85
- Although no specific causal mutations have been identified, candidate gene loci have been reported on chromosomes 4, 5, 8, 18, and 21, as well as others; a recent whole genome association study of 2000 patients and 3000 controls found a signal at 16p12, but this was not supported in a replication sample.

PHYSICAL FINDINGS & CLINICAL PRESENTATION

- Mania associated with psychomotor activation that is usually goal directed but not necessarily productive; increase in goal-directed activity and excessive involvement in activities leading to unexpected adverse outcomes
- Elevated, euphoric, and frequently labile mood
- Decreased need for sleep
- Flight of ideas with rapid, loud, pressured speech
- Psychosis may occur, with delusions, hallucinations, and formal thought disorder
- Depressive episodes resembling major depressive disorder (see "Depression, Major"); however, atypical features (hypersomnia, weight gain) may be present
- Mixed states, characterized by activation, irritability, and dysphoria also possible

ETIOLOGY

- Hypotheses:
  1. Abnormalities of receptor and membrane function and of circadian regulation
  2. Alteration of cAMP, MAP kinase, protein kinase C, and glycogen synthase kinase-3 signal transduction pathways
  3. Alteration in cell survival pathways

DIAGNOSIS

DIFFERENTIAL DIAGNOSIS

- Secondary manias caused by medical disorders (e.g., hyperthyroidism, AIDS, TBI, stroke, Cushing's syndrome) or drug treatment (stimulants, steroids) are frequent.
- First onset of mania after age 50 yr is suggestive of secondary mania.
- Less severe, and possibly distinct, conditions of bipolar type II and cyclothymia are possible.
- Comorbidity with substance abuse or dependency is common and may confound diagnostic assessment and treatment.
- Cross-sectional examination of acutely manic patient can be confused with schizophrenia or a paranoid psychosis.

WORKUP

- History
- Physical examination
- Mental status examination
- Mood disorder questionnaire (MDQ)

LABORATORY TESTS

Because of high rate of secondary manias, initial evaluation to confirm health of all major organ systems (routine chemistries, complete blood count, urinalysis, sedimentation rate)

IMAGING STUDIES

- Consider brain imaging if late onset or if neurologic exam is abnormal.
- Neuroimaging may show evidence of ventricular enlargement or increased white matter hyperintensities; changes in amygdala, frontal cortex, and striatal volume have also been reported.

TREATMENT

NONPHARMACOLOGIC THERAPY

- Cognitive-behavioral and family-focused psychoeducational psychotherapy to help patients cope with consequences of the disease, improve adherence with medications, and identify possible environmental triggers
- Bright light therapy in the northern latitudes in individuals exhibiting a seasonal pattern of winter depression
- Lifestyle "regularization"

ACUTE GENERAL RX

- First-line agents for acute mania: lithium 1500 to 1800 mg/day (0.8 to 1.2 meq/L), valproate 1000 to 1500 mg/day (50 to 125 mg/ml), carbamazepine 600 to 800 mg/day (4 to 12 μg/ml), oxcarbazepine 900 to 2400 mg/day, olanzapine 10 to 20 mg/day, risperidone 2 to 4 mg/day, quetiapine 350 to 800 mg/day, ziprasidone 80 to 120 mg/day, and aripiprazole 10 to 30 mg/day.
- Useful adjuncts to acute treatment: Benzodiazepines: lorazepam 1 to 2 mg/q4h, clonazepam 1 to 2 mg/q4h.
- Traditional antidepressants are effective in bipolar depression but can induce manic episodes and exacerbate mania in mixed episodes.
- Lamotrigine can have acute antidepressant benefit; monotherapy with quetiapine or a combination of olanzapine and fluoxetine are secondary options in bipolar depression.

CHRONIC RX

- Goal of long-term treatment: prevention of relapse or episode recurrence
- Best agents for prophylaxis of mania: lithium, valproate, and olanzapine (carbamazepine/oxcarbazepine possibly beneficial)
- Best agents for prophylaxis of depression: lamotrigine and lithium
- Role of atypical antipsychotics in maintenance unclear; combination therapy with a mood stabilizer is more effective than monotherapy
- Long-term use of antidepressants: frequently destabilizes patient and leads to more frequent relapses

DISPOSITION

- Course is variable.
- More than 90% of patients having a single manic episode are likely to experience others.

- Uncontrolled manic or depressive episodes can lead to additional episodes ("illness begets illness").
- Lithium treatment is shown to specifically decrease suicidal risk.
- Psychosocioeconomic consequences of both mania and depression can be severe and disabling.

REFERRAL

- If use of antidepressant contemplated
- If patient is severely manic, rapid cycling, or suicidal or is in a bipolar, mixed episode

PEARLS & CONSIDERATIONS

COMMENTS

- All patients presenting with depression should be asked about past personal and family history of mania and hypomania; 70% of bipolar patients have previously been misdiagnosed.
- Denial of illness is common in mania and often necessitates more assertive therapeutic interventions.
- Prompt recognition of the earliest signs of mania in a given individual (e.g., decreased need for sleep, increased rate of speech) allows earlier intervention and a better likelihood of preventing a full episode.
- Bipolar disorder in children frequently manifests as behavioral disinhibition and impulsive aggression.
- Life charting helps identify environmental triggers and drug efficacy.

PATIENT/FAMILY EDUCATION

Information available at www.NMHA.org and www.dbsalliance.org.

EVIDENCE

EBM

Lithium and valproate are effective in the treatment of acute mania.[1,2] Systematic reviews of randomized clinical trials (RCTs) of lithium and valproate have found that both drugs are significantly more effective than placebo in therapeutic response measured after 3 to 4 weeks. Ⓐ

Lithium is also effective in the long-term prevention of recurrence of mania,[3] as shown in a systematic review of RCTs comparing lithium to placebo and assessing relapse over 2 years. Lamotrigine also delayed time to treatment of depression, as well as mania, in a pooled analysis of two RCTs.[4] A beneficial effect of helping people to recognize early warning signs of recurrence in bipolar disorder on rate of recurrence and risk of hospitalization has also been shown in a review of eleven RCTs.[5] Ⓐ

Evidence-Based References

1. Poolsup N et al: Systematic overview of lithium treatment in acute mania, *J Clin Pharm Ther* 25:139, 2000. Reviewed in: *Clin Evid* 13:1158, 2005. Ⓐ
2. Macritchie K et al: Valproate for acute mood episodes in bipolar disorder, *Cochrane Database Syst Rev* 1:CD004052, 2003.
3. Burgess S et al: Lithium for maintenance treatment of mood disorders, *Cochrane Database Syst Rev* 3:CD003013, 2001.
4. Goodwin GM et al: A pooled analysis of 2 placebo-controlled 18-month trials of Lamotrigine and lithium maintenance in bipolar I disorder, *J Clin Psychiatry* 65(3):432-441, 2004. Ⓐ
5. Morriss RK et al: Interventions for helping people recognize early signs of recurrence in bipolar disorder, *Cochrane Database Syst Rev* 1:CD004854, 2007. Ⓐ

SUGGESTED READINGS

Arora M et al: Mania in the medically ill, *Curr Psychiatry Rep* 9(3):232-235, 2007.

Cousins DA et al: The armamentarium of treatments for bipolar disorder: a review of the literature, *Int J Neuropsychopharmacol* 10(3):411-431, 2007.

Farmer A et al: The genetics of bipolar affective disorder, *Curr Opin Psychiatry* 20(1):8-12, 2007.

Goodwin FK, Redfield JK: *Manic-depressive illness: bipolar disorders and recurrent depression,* ed 2, New York, 2007, Oxford University Press.

Keck PE: Long-term management strategies to achieve optimal function in patients with bipolar disorder, *J Clin Psychiatry* 67(12): e17, 2006.

McClellan J et al: Practice parameter for the assessment and treatment of children and adolescents with bipolar disorder, *J Am Acad Child Adolesc Psychiatry* 46(1):107, 2007.

Miklowitz DJ: A review of evidence-based psychosocial interventions for bipolar disorder, *J Clin Psychiatry* 67(Suppl 11):28-33, 2006.

Rouget BW et al: Efficacy of psychoeducational approaches on bipolar disorders: a review of the literature, *J Affect Disor,* 98(1-2):11-27, 2007.

Sachs GS et al: Effectiveness of adjunctive antidepressant treatment for bipolar depression, *N Engl J Med,* 356(17):1711-1722, 2007.

Scherk H et al: Second-generation antipsychotic agents in the treatment of acute mania: a systematic review and meta-analysis of randomized controlled trials, *Arch Gen Psychiatry* 64(4):442-455, 2007.

Vieta E et al: Evolving trends in the long-term treatment of bipolar disorder, *World J Biol Psychiatry* 8(1):4-11, 2007.

AUTHOR: **VICTOR I. REUS, M.D.**

BASIC INFORMATION

DEFINITION

A bite wound can be animal or human, accidental or intentional.

ICD-9CM CODES
879.8 Bite wound, unspecified site

EPIDEMIOLOGY & DEMOGRAPHICS

- Bite wounds account for 1% of emergency department visits.
- More than 1 million bites occur in humans annually in the U.S.
- Dog bites account for 85% to 90% of all bites and result in 10 to 20 fatalities yearly in the U.S.; cat bites, 10% to 20%. Typically the animal is owned by the victim.
- Infection rates are highest for cat bites (30% to 50%), followed by human bites (15% to 30%) and dog bites (5%).
- The extremities are involved in 75% of bites.

PHYSICAL FINDINGS & CLINICAL PRESENTATION

- The appearance of the bite wound is variable (e.g., puncture wound, tear, avulsion).
- Cellulitis, lymphangitis, and focal adenopathy may be present in infected bite wounds.
- Patient may experience fever and chills.

ETIOLOGY

- Increased risk of infection: human and cat bites, closed fist injuries, wounds involving joints, puncture wounds, face and lip bites, bites with skull penetration, bites in immunocompromised hosts
- Most frequent infecting organisms:
  1. *Pasteurella* spp.: responsible for majority of infections within 24 hr of dog *(P. canis)* and cat *(P. multocida, P. septica)* bites
  2. *Capnocytophaga canimorsus* (formerly DF-2 bacillus): a gram-negative organism responsible for late infection, usually following dog bites
  3. Gram-negative organisms *(Pseudomonas, Haemophilus)*: often found in human bites
  4. *Streptococcus* spp., *Staphylococcus aureus*
  5. *Eikenella corrodens* in human bites

DIAGNOSIS

DIFFERENTIAL DIAGNOSIS

- Bite from a rabid animal (often the attack is unprovoked)
- Factitious injury

WORKUP

- Determination of the time elapsed since the patient was bitten, status of rabies immunization of the animal, and underlying medical conditions that might predispose the patient to infection (e.g., DM, immunodeficiency)
- Documentation of bite site, notification of appropriate authorities (e.g., police department, animal officer)

LABORATORY TESTS

- Generally not necessary
- Hct if there has been significant blood loss
- Wound cultures (aerobic and anaerobic) if there is evidence of sepsis or victim is immunocompromised patient; cultures should be obtained before irrigation of the wound but after superficial cleaning

IMAGING STUDIES

X-rays are indicated when bony penetration is suspected or if there is suspicion of fracture or significant trauma; x-rays are also useful for detecting presence of foreign bodies (when suspected).

TREATMENT

NONPHARMACOLOGIC THERAPY

- Local care with debridement, vigorous cleansing, and saline irrigation of the wound; debridement of devitalized tissue
- High-pressure irrigation to clean bite wound and ensure removal of contaminants (e.g., use saline solution with a 30- to 35-ml syringe equipped with a 20-gauge needle or catheter with tip of syringe placed 2 to 3 cm above the wound)
- Avoid blunt probing of wounds (increased risk of infection)
- If the animal is suspected to be rabid: infiltrate wound edges with 1% procaine hydrochloride, swab wound surface vigorously with cotton swabs and 1% benzalkoronium solution or other soap, and rinse wound with normal saline

ACUTE GENERAL Rx

- Avoid suturing of hand wounds and any wounds that appear infected
- Puncture wounds should be left open
- Give antirabies therapy and tetanus immune globulin (250 to 500 units IM in limb controlateral to toxoid) and toxoid (adult or child older than 5 years: 0.5 ml DT given IM, child less than 5 years 0.5 ml DPT IM) as needed
- Use empiric antibiotic therapy in high-risk wounds (e.g., cat bite, hand bites, face bites, genital area bites, bites with joint or bone penetration, human bites, immunocompromised host): amoxicillin-clavulanate 875 to 1000 mg bid for 7 days or cefuroxime 500 mg bid for 7 days
- In hospitalized patients, IV antibiotics of choice are cefoxitin 1 to 2 g q6h, ampicillin-sulbactam 1.5 to 3 g q6h, ticarcillin-clavulanate 3 g q6h, or ceftriaxone 1 to 2 g q24h
- Prophylactic therapy for persons bitten by others with HIV and hepatitis B (see Section V)

DISPOSITION

- Prognosis is favorable with proper treatment.
- Important prognostic factors are type and depth of wound, which compartments are entered, and pathogenicity of inoculated bacteria.
- Punctures that are difficult to irrigate adequately, carnivore bites over vital structures (arteries, nerves, joints), and tissue crushing that cannot be debrided have a worse prognosis.
- In general, human bites have a higher complication and infection rate than do animal bites.
- Nearly 50% of the anaerobic gram-negative bacilli isolated from human bite wounds may be penicillin resistant and beta-lactamase positive.

REFERRAL

- Hospitalization and IV antibiotic therapy for infected human bites; bites with injury to joints, nerves, or tendons; or any animal bites unresponsive to oral therapy.
- In the outpatient setting, bite wounds should be reevaluated within 48 hr to assess for signs of infection.

SUGGESTED READING

Broder J et al: Human bites, *Am J Med* 22:10, 2004.

AUTHOR: **FRED F. FERRI, M.D.**

BASIC INFORMATION

DEFINITION

There are two major classes of arthropods: insects and arachnida. This chapter will focus on the class arachnida. Arachnid bites consist of bites caused by:

- Spiders
- Scorpions
- Ticks

ICD-9CM CODES
E905.1 Venomous spiders (black widow spider, brown spider, tarantula)
E905.2 Scorpion
989.5 Bites of venomous snakes, lizards, and spiders; tick paralysis
E906.4 Bite of nonvenomous arthropod; insect bite NOS

EPIDEMIOLOGY & DEMOGRAPHICS

- Spiders: ubiquitous; only three types potentially significantly harmful:
  1. Sydney funnel web spider—Australia
  2. Black widow—worldwide (not Alaska)
  3. Brown recluse—most common (South Central U.S.)
- Scorpions: various warm climates: Africa, Central South America, Middle East, India; in U.S.: Texas, New Mexico, California, Nevada
- Ticks: woodlands

PHYSICAL FINDINGS & CLINICAL PRESENTATION

Spiders:

- Sydney funnel web—atrataxin toxin
  1. Piloerection, muscle spasms leading to tachycardia, HTN, increased intracranial pressure, coma
- Black widow—females toxic
  1. Initial reaction: local swelling, redness (two fang marks) leading to local piloerection, edema, urticaria, diaphoresis, lymphangitis
  2. Pain in limb leading to rest of body (chest pain, abdominal pain)
- Brown recluse
  1. Minor sting or burn.
  2. Wound may become pruritic and red with a blanched center with vesicle. Can necrose, especially in fatty areas. Leaves eschar, which sloughs and leaves ulcer, can take months to heal.
  3. Systemic symptoms: headache, fever, chills, GI upset, hemolysis, renal tubular necrosis, disseminated intravascular coagulation (DIC) possible.

Scorpions:

- Sting leading to sympathetic and parasympathetic stimulation: HTN, bradycardia, vasoconstriction, pulmonary edema, reduced coronary blood flow, priapism, inhibition of insulin
- Also possible: tachycardia, arrhythmia, vasodilation, bronchial relaxation, excessive salivation, vomiting, sweating, bronchoconstriction

Ticks: U.S., Europe, Asia

- Very small (<1 mm). Must be attached >36 hours to transmit disease.
- Lyme disease—most common
  1. Early: erythema migrans 60% to 80% of cases
  2. 7 to 10 days: mild to moderate constitutional symptoms—disseminated—secondary skin lesions, fever, adenopathy, constitutional symptoms, facial palsy, peripheral neuropathy, lymphocytic meningitis, meningoencephalitis, cardiac manifestations (heart block)
  3. Late: chronic arthritis, dermatitis, neuropathy, keratitis

DIAGNOSIS

DIFFERENTIAL DIAGNOSIS

Cellulitis
Urticaria
Other tick-borne illnesses:

- Babesiosis
- Tick-borne relapsing fever
- Tularemia
- Rocky Mountain spotted fever
- Ehrlichiosis
- Colorado tick fever
- Tick paralysis
- Community-acquired cutaneous MRSA

WORKUP

Physical examination: thorough skin examination may reveal fang marks, attached ticks, black eschar.

TREATMENT

ACUTE GENERAL Rx

Spiders:

- Sydney funnel web
  1. Pressure, immobilization immediately, supportive care, antivenin
- Black widow
  1. Treatment based on severity of symptoms. Bite is rarely fatal.
  2. All should get on oxygen, IV, cardiac monitor, tetanus prophylaxis.
  3. Symptomatic/supportive therapy.
  4. 10% calcium gluconate for muscle cramps (controversial).
  5. Antivenin only for more severe reactions. Antivenin carries risk of anaphylaxis.
     - Dose: one vial in 100 ml 0.9% saline over 20 to 30 minutes.
     - Skin test before use.
     - Give antihistamines with use.
- Brown recluse
  1. Pain management, tetanus, supportive treatment.
  2. No consensus regarding best treatment. Some evidence for hyperbaric oxygen.

Scorpions:

- Fluids, supportive care, species-specific antivenin (equine based, risk of serum sickness)—controversial.

Ticks:

- Prophylactic: tick >36 hours: single dose of doxycycline 200 mg
- Early localized disease
  1. Treatment of choice in children: amoxicillin × 14 days.
  2. Doxycycline preferred in patients with possible concurrent ehrlichiosis.
  3. Early disseminated: treatment depends on manifestation.
  4. Late disease: may require longer-term/IV therapy. Controversial for neurologic disease. (See "Lyme Disease" for further details.)

DISPOSITION

- For patients with systemic reactions, send home with emergency epinephrine kit.
- If severe or anaphylactic reaction, admit and observe for 48 hours for cardiac, renal, or neurologic problems.

REFERRAL

For patients with systemic reactions, refer to allergist for immunotherapy; 95% to 98% effective in preventing anaphylaxis.

PEARLS & CONSIDERATIONS

Identification of spider should not be based on patient history (many look-alikes); spider should be brought into medical facility to be identified.

SUGGESTED READINGS

Bolgiano EB, Sexton J: Tick-borne illnesses. In *Rosen's emergency medicine,* ed 6, Philadelphia, 2006, Mosby.
Hayes P: Current concepts: how can we prevent Lyme disease? *N Engl J Med* 348(24): 2424, 2003.
Otten E: Venomous animal injuries. In *Rosen's emergency medicine,* ed 6, Philadelphia, 2006, Mosby.

AUTHOR: **GAIL O'BRIEN, M.D.**

BASIC INFORMATION

DEFINITION

Most stinging insects belong to the Hymenoptera order and include yellow jackets (most common cause of reactions), hornets, bumble bees, sweat bees, wasps, harvester ants, fire ants, and the Africanized honey bee "killer bee." Brown recluse spiders, although they are not insects, are another common cause of bites (see Bites and Stings, Arachnids). The usual effect of a sting is intense local pain, some immediate erythema, and often a small area of edema by injecting venom. Allergic reactions can be either local or generalized leading to anaphylactic shock. The majority of reactions occur within the first 6 hr after the sting or bite, but a delayed presentation may occur up to 24 hr.

SYNONYMS Venom allergy

ICD-9CM CODES
989.5 Stings (bees, wasps)
989.5 Bites (fire ant, brown recluse spider)

EPIDEMIOLOGY & DEMOGRAPHICS

PREVALENCE (OF BEE STINGS AND INSECT BITES):

- Unknown
- Between 0.4% and 4% of the population is allergic to the venom of one or more stinging insects
- Most anaphylactic reactions occur during summer months in those most likely to be exposed including children, males, outdoor workers
- About one half of fatal reactions occur without prior allergic response
- Bites by fire ants and brown recluse spiders are less likely to cause systemic disease

INCIDENCE (IN U.S.): About 45 people die each year from insect sting anaphylaxis; anaphylaxis occurs more often within 10 to 30 min of a sting. Delayed reactions are rare occurring only in <0.3% of stings.

PHYSICAL FINDINGS & CLINICAL PRESENTATION

Stings:

- Cutaneous: the skin is the most common site of an allergic reaction. Manifestations include flushing, urticaria, pruritus, and angioedema.
- Respiratory: hoarseness, difficulty speaking, choking, throat tightness or tingling may progress to stridor, laryngeal edema, laryngospasm, and bronchoconstriction. This is the leading cause of anaphylactic death.
- Cardiovascular: tachycardia, hypotension, arrhythmia, can progress to profound hypovolemic shock. Myocardial infarction is rare. Cardiac manifestations are the second leading cause of death from anaphylaxis.
- Other symptoms: abdominal pain, nausea, vomiting, and diarrhea.

Fire ant bites:

- Initial wheal and flare response.
- Subsequent development of circularly arrayed blisters within 24 hr.
- Blisters may develop appearance of pustules, but they are not infected.

ETIOLOGY

Stings:

- Most systemic reactions to insect stings are classic IgE-mediated reactions.
- Reactions occur in previously sensitized patients who have produced high titers of IgE antibody to insect venom antigens.
- Sensitization to wasp venom requires only a few stings and can occur after a single sting.
- Sensitization to bee venom occurs mainly in people who have been stung frequently by bees.

Bites: Fire ant venom contains proteins toxic to the skin.

DIAGNOSIS

DIFFERENTIAL DIAGNOSIS

- Stings: cellulitis, bites
- Bites: stings, cellulitis

WORKUP

History is essential for accurate diagnosis including timing of sting or bite and type of insect (bee, wasp, spider, or ant) if known.

LABORATORY TESTS

- Skin test: either skin prick test or intradermal method with fire ant or hymenoptera venom.
- Venom skin tests and occasionally radioallergosorbent tests (RAST) to provide additional information.

TREATMENT

ACUTE GENERAL Rx

Sting:

- Removal of the stinger most readily performed with a flat tool like a credit card, cleansing, and application of ice
- Treatment with oral antihistamines and nonsteroidal anti-inflammatory medications for limited reactions. Topical corticosteroids may provide some relief of inflammation
- Patients with previous reactions or multiple stings to the mouth or neck should be evaluated in an emergency department
- Larger swellings may benefit from oral steroids
- Generalized reactions should be treated with epinephrine. Antihistamines, oxygen, intravenous corticosteroids, beta-agonists, pressors, and IV fluids may also be beneficial for anaphylaxis

Bite:

- Supportive care
- Application of ice
- Surveillance for secondary infection

DISPOSITION

Sting:

- Prognosis for a limited reaction is excellent.
- Subsequent anaphylaxis may occur in 35% to 65% of patients stung again.
- There is no evidence that the next sting will necessarily cause a more severe reaction. The reasons for the variable outcome include patient's immune status at the time of sting, dose of venom injected, and site of sting.
- Patients with a history of sting allergies should carry syringes preloaded with epinephrine (EpiPen) and oral antihistamines to take if they are stung again.
- Patients should seek additional medical care after using an autoinjector.
- Patients at risk should wear shoes and socks outdoors, remove nests near homes, keep food containers closed, and avoid wearing perfume or flower print clothing.

Bite.

- Prognosis for fire ant bite is excellent.
- Large lesions from brown recluse spider bites may take months to heal.

REFERRAL

- Consider a referral to an allergist for venom immunotherapy (VIT).
- Risk of subsequent anaphylaxis with immunotherapy falls to <3%.
- VIT for 3 to 5 yr induces long-term protection in most patients.

PEARLS & CONSIDERATIONS

Hypersensitivity to stings is common. Reactions range from local nonallergic reaction to venom to life-threatening anaphylaxis. Venom-specific immunotherapy is highly effective in decreasing subsequent reactions.

EVIDENCE

EBM

Venom immunotherapy can significantly reduce risk of subsequent sting reactions. Those patients who would benefit from venom immunotherapy should undergo immediate hypersensitivity skin tests with stinging insect venoms.

Evidence-Based Reference

Clark S: Multicenter study of emergency department visits for insect sting allergies, *J Allergy Clin Immunol* 116(3):643, 2005.

SUGGESTED READINGS

Annila I: Bee venom allergy, *Clin Exp Allergy* 30(12):1682, 2000.

Ewan PW: ABC of allergies: venom allergy, *BMJ* 316(7141):1365, 1998.

Freeman TM: Hypersensitivity to hymenoptera stings, *N Eng J Med* 351(19):1978, 2004.

Graft D: Insect sting allergy, *Med Clin N Am* 1(90): 211-232, 2006.

Greco LK: Hymenoptera stings, *Top Emerg Med* 22(2):37, 2000.

Neugut AI et al: Anaphylaxis in the United States: an investigation into its epidemiology, *Arch Intern Med* 161(1):15, 2001.

Youlton L: Insect sting reactions, *Clin Exp Dermatol* 24(4):338, 2000.

AUTHOR: **JENNIFER JEREMIAH, M.D.**

BASIC INFORMATION

DEFINITION

Injury resulting from snake biting a human.

ICD-9CM CODES
989.5 Venomous poisoning

EPIDEMIOLOGY & DEMOGRAPHICS

- 45,000 snakebites occur annually in the U.S. Of the 8000 caused by poisonous snakes, approximately 5 to 12 result in fatality (i.e., ~ 1%-2%). Children, the elderly, and those in whom treatment has been delayed are at highest risk.
- In the U.S. at least one species of poisonous snake has been identified in every state except Alaska, Hawaii, and Maine. The majority of venomous snakes are members of the family Crotalidae, which includes rattlesnakes, copperheads, and cottonmouths. The Elapidae family, which includes the coral snake, accounts for the remainder.

PHYSICAL FINDINGS & CLINICAL PRESENTATION

In addition to local tissue injury, envenomation may affect the renal, neurologic, gastrointestinal, vascular, and coagulation systems. Species-specific signs and symptoms include:

CROTALIDAE (PIT VIPERS): Signs and symptoms:

- Fang punctures (see "Diagnosis")
- Pain within 5 min
- Edema within 30 min
- Erythema of site and adjacent tissues/serous or hemorrhagic bullae, ecchymosis and/or lymphangitis over the ensuing hours

If no edema or erythema is manifested within 8 hr after a confirmed Crotalid snakebite, it is safe to assume envenomation did not occur. (Roughly 25% of cases do not involve envenomation.)

Systemic manifestations may include:

- Mild to moderate manifestations: nausea/vomiting, perioral paresthesias, metallic taste, tingling of fingers or toes (especially with rattlesnake bites) and/or fasciculations (local or generalized).
- Severe manifestations: hypotension (due to increased vascular permeability), mental status change, respiratory distress, tachycardia, acute renal failure, rhabdomyolysis, intravascular hemolysis, disseminated intravascular coagulation.

ELAPIDAE (CORAL SNAKES): Signs and symptoms:

- Local symptoms are far less pronounced (little or no pain/swelling immediately after the bite).
- Systemic symptoms predominate, but onset may be delayed for up to 12 hr. Examples include:
  - Cranial nerve palsies featuring ptosis, dysphagia, or dysarthria
  - Tremors
  - Intense salivation
  - Loss of DTRs and respiratory depression (late manifestations)

ETIOLOGY

- The majority of victims are young men who purposefully attempt to handle or harm a snake that formerly had no intention of biting them.
- Victims are frequently intoxicated at the time of the bite.

DIAGNOSIS

DIFFERENTIAL DIAGNOSIS

- Harmless snakebite
- Scorpion bite
- Insect bite
- Cellulitis
- Laceration or puncture wound

NOTE: Harmless snakebites are usually characterized by four rows of small scratches (teeth in upper jaw) separated from two rows of scratches (teeth in lower jaw). This is in distinction to venomous snakebites, which should have puncture wounds produced by the snake's fangs, whether other teeth marks are noted.

WORKUP

An estimated 25% of venomous snakebites do not result in envenomation, but observation is critical in all suspected cases:

- Clinical and laboratory evaluation are used to assess the severity of envenomation.
- A nonstandardized classification system for grading envenomations was developed by Russell in 1964:
  - Minimal: confined to the site of the bite, no significant systemic symptoms or signs, no laboratory abnormalities
  - Moderate: manifestations extend beyond the site of the bite, but no life-threatening systemic symptoms
  - Severe: extensive limb involvement, severe systemic symptoms and signs, or significant laboratory abnormalities (including abnormal coagulation studies)

Determination of severity is based on the most severe symptom, sign, or laboratory result. Continual reassessment is indicated throughout the observation period because grading may change.

LABORATORY TESTS

- For all suspected envenomations, obtain CBC (with peripheral smear and platelet count), DIC screen (PT/INR, PTT, fibrinogen, fibrin degradation products, D-dimer), ECG, serum electrolytes, BUN, Cr, and urinalysis.
- For more severe bites, consider LFTs, sedimentation rate, creatine kinase (r/o rhabdomyolysis), ABG, and type and cross-match.
- Other: consider CXR in cases with severe envenomation or in patients >40 yr with underlying cardiopulmonary disease; x-ray of bite site for retained fangs (poor sensitivity); head CT if concern is raised for intracranial hemorrhage.

TREATMENT

ACUTE GENERAL Rx

IN THE FIELD: For a suspected snakebite:

- Immobilize affected part below level of the heart.
- Remove any constricting items. Local pressure has been advocated for elapid bites, particularly in Australia, as a means of delaying absorption of neurotoxins. However, crotalid bites are far more common in the U.S., and these frequently have tissue-necrosing venom, which will yield more damage with local pressure. Thus, as with incision and suction techniques, use by those without specialized training in snakebite management is discouraged.
- *Do not* apply ice; keep victim warm.
- Avoid alcohol, stimulants (caffeine), or agents that can suppress mental status.
- Transport immediately to nearest medical facility and contact poison control center.

IN THE HOSPITAL:

- Establish intravenous access.
- Initiate reconstitution of appropriate antivenom. (Antivenoms are typically supplied in powder form and must be reconstituted before administration. The process can take up to 1 hr, so it is recommended that it be initiated as soon as the patient arrives in the ED). While this is being done:
  - Obtain time of bite and description of snake if possible.
  - Obtain past medical history; ask about allergies to horse serum in those previously treated for snakebite.
  - Record vital signs: BP, HR, T, RR.
  - Inspect site of bite for fang marks, local symptoms.
  - Delineate margins of erythema/edema with a marker.
  - Measure circumference of bitten part at two or more proximal sites and compare with unaffected limb; repeat every 15 to 20 min; assess for extension of erythema/edema.
  - Neurologic examination.

- Gauge the severity of the bite and decide whether administration of antivenom is necessary.
- For minimal envenomation without progressive manifestations:
  1. Clean and immobilize affected part.
  2. Immunize against tetanus.
  3. Observe patient for at least 8 hr. If, at the end of this interval, local and systemic sequelae are absent and lab values remain normal, the likelihood of significant envenomation is low, and the patient can be discharged from the acute setting.

- Patients who have progressive symptoms (local or systemic) or moderate to severe envenomation should be considered for antivenom. The high incidence of allergic reactions argues against its use in less severe cases.
- Since the introduction of antivenoms in the U.S. in the 1950s, mortality rates from snakebites have dropped from as high as 25% (when no treatment was available) to 0.5% in patients who receive timely administration of antivenom.
- Antivenom is most effective when given within 4 hr of the bite and least effective if delayed beyond 12 hr. Systemic symptoms (coagulopathy, CNS effects, etc.) respond better to treatment than local symptoms (erythema/edema, bullae, etc.).
- It is recommended that patients be monitored in an ICU setting during administration of antivenom.

Once the decision is made to use antivenom:

- Prepare epinephrine 0.5 to 1.0 ml of a 0.1% solution to be administered in case of a hypersensitivity reaction to the antivenom. (Prophylactic antihistamines are not efficacious.)

TREATMENT OF CROTALID (PIT VIPER) BITES WITH SHEEP IMMUNOGLOBULIN–BASED ANTIVENOM:

- Most centers now have sheep immunoglobulin-based antivenom (Crofab) for crotalid bites. (A potent, safe, sheep-based antivenom for elapid bites exists but is not yet approved in the U.S.) Sheep-based antivenoms are very safe, but repeat administration may be necessary owing to a short half-life. An initial IV loading dose of 4 to 6 vials (depending on the size and age of the patient and the severity of the bite) is infused over 60 min. If the patient has not responded after 1 hr, a repeat dose of 4 to 6 vials is indicated.
- Because of the short half-life of sheep-based antivenom, relapse may occur in up to two thirds of patients after an initial response. Consequently, it is recommended that three maintenance doses—each consisting of 2 vials—be given at 6, 12, and 18 hours following the patient's initial response to the loading dose.
- Help in using the antivenom is available 24/7 by calling (877) 377-3784.

TREATMENT OF CROTALID (PIT VIPER) OR ELAPID (CORAL SNAKE) BITES WITH HORSE SERUM–BASED ANTIVENOM:

- Horse serum–based antivenoms are available for both crotalid and elapid (coral snake), but it runs a much higher risk of hypersensitivity reactions such as anaphylaxis and serum sickness. (Skin testing is available, but it is not recommended because it is not completely reliable and may delay time to administration beyond the most effective period.) For treatment considerations, see "Complications." Guidelines to dosage of horse serum–based antivenom are as follows:
- For pit viper bites
  - Mild 5 vials
  - Moderate 10 vials
  - Severe 15 vials
  - Shock 20 vials
- For confirmed coral snake bites, antivenom (different formulation) should be administered immediately. If coral snake bite is only suspected, the patient should be monitored for 12 hr for evidence of envenomation, and treated if it occurs.
- If there are no systemic symptoms at the time of administration, start with 3 vials. If symptoms evolve, repeat with 5 vials.
- If systemic symptoms are already present, an initial dose of 6 to 10 vials is recommended.

TREATMENT OF NONNATIVE (EXOTIC) SNAKE BITES:

- For bites by exotic or nonnative snakes, contact a poison control center or your local zoo. (Zoos with exotic snakes are required to maintain a supply of snake-specific antivenom on their premises.)

Other considerations:

- Initial dose of antivenom should be repeated until progression of symptoms has abated, but observation of bitten part should be continued for another 48 hr.
- Children require more antivenom; increase dose by 50%.
- Pregnancy is not a contraindication to antivenom.
- Immunize against tetanus if no booster within past 5 yr; if never immunized, give immunoglobulin as well as toxoid.
- Manage pain as needed (acetaminophen, codeine, meperidine).
- Avoid sedation in Mojave rattlesnake, eastern diamondback rattlesnake, and coral snake bites.
- Antibiotics reserved for moderate to severe cases; use those with broad-spectrum coverage (which includes gram-negatives, i.e., quinolone derivatives).

DISPOSITION

Prognosis is good with prompt evaluation and treatment.

REFERRAL

To medical facility with ICU for administration of antivenom

PEARLS & CONSIDERATIONS

COMPLICATIONS

Most frequent complication of treated envenomations is serum sickness; occurs 7 to 14 days after antivenom administration and is characterized by fever, rash, arthralgias, and lymphadenopathy. It can be treated with po prednisone 60 mg/day, tapered over 7 to 10 days. Acutely, there is the risk of anaphylaxis to antivenom as mentioned previously. This occurs within 30 min and is treated with:

- IV epinephrine
- IV diphenhydramine
- IV hydrocortisone

Injuries also result from:

- Tourniquet placement
- Cryotherapy

National poison control hotline: (800) 222-1222

EVIDENCE

EBM

For snakebites in the U.S. there are few controlled clinical trials, but, internationally, some studies document routine administration of antivenin many hours after the first doses. This is thought to represent an initial underdosing of the first administration of antivenin. (Fab molecules have a shorter half-life than IgG molecules and may allow recurrence of venom effects, if additional doses are not administered.)

SUGGESTED READINGS

Dart RC: Efficacy, safety and use of snake antivenoms in the United States, *Ann Emerg Med* 37:181-188, 2001.

Gold BS et al: Bites of venomous snakes, *N Engl J Med* 347:347, 2002.

Juckett G, Honcox JG: Venomous snakebites in the United States: management review and update, *Am Fam Physician* 65:1367, 2002.

LoVecchio F et al: Antibiotics after rattlesnake envenomation, *J Emerg Med* 23:327-328, 2002.

The Medical Letter: a new snake antivenom, *Med Lett Drugs Ther* 43:55, 2001.

Offerman SR et al: Crotaline Fab antivenom for the treatment of children with rattlesnake envenomation, *Pediatrics* 110:968-971, 2002.

Ries NL, Dart RC: New developments in antidotes, *Med Clin North Am* 89(6):1379, 2005.

AUTHORS: **JACK SCHWARTZWALD, M.D.,** and **REBECCA A. GRIFFITH, M.D.**

BASIC INFORMATION

DEFINITION

Bladder cancer is a heterogeneous spectrum of neoplasms ranging from non–life-threatening, low-grade, superficial papillary lesions to high-grade invasive tumors, which often have metastasized at the time of presentation. It is a field change disease in which the entire urothelium from the renal pelvis to the urethra may be susceptible to malignant transformation. *Types:* Transitional cell carcinoma (TCCa), squamous cell carcinoma, and adenocarcinoma.

ICD-9CM CODES
Primary: 188.9
Secondary: 198.1
CIS: 233.7
Benign: 223.3
Uncertain behavior: 236.7
Unspecified: 239.4

EPIDEMIOLOGY & DEMOGRAPHICS

Each year approximately 54,000 new cases are diagnosed and more than 12,000 deaths are attributed to bladder cancer.

Until 1990, the incidence of bladder cancer in the U.S. was rising. Since 1990, the incidence of bladder cancer is decreasing at a rate of 0.8% per year (1.2% among men and 0.4% among women).

PREDOMINANT SEX: In males, it is the fourth most common cancer, accounting for 10% of all cancers. In females, it is the eighth most common cancer, accounting for 4% of all cancers.

RISK: The lifetime risk of developing bladder cancer is 2.8% in white males, 0.9% in black males, 1% in white females, and 0.6% in black females.

Smoking:
- Users of "black" tobacco in place of "blond" tobacco have a twofold to threefold increase in developing bladder cancer.
- Smoking risk is based on consumption: With a twofold to threefold increase for subjects smoking at least 10 cigarettes per day

The risk increases again when the daily consumption rises above 40 to 60 cigarettes per day
- Smokers of low-tar and nicotine cigarettes have a lower risk when compared with higher tar and nicotine cigarettes.
- Unfiltered cigarettes have a 50% increased risk of bladder cancer compared with those who smoke filtered cigarettes.
- Pipe smokers have a lower risk of bladder cancer compared with cigarette smokers.
- Cigar smoking, snuff, and chewing tobacco, although implicated in nonurologic cancers, are not believed to influence bladder cancer risk.

Diet:
- Diets rich in beef, pork, and animal fat consumption increase risk of bladder cancer.
- There is no indication that consumption of nonbeer alcoholic drinks contributes to bladder cancer development.
- Beer consumption has been linked to bladder cancer development as a result of the presence of nitrosamines in the beer. Similarly, these nitrosamines have been implicated in the development of rectal cancer.
- Drinking coffee is not believed to contribute to bladder cancer risk. There is additional evidence that coffee consumption is protective for colorectal cancers, possibly by diminishing fecal transit time.

PEAK INCIDENCE: Incidence increases with age, high >60 yr, uncommon <40 yr.

GENETICS: It is thought to be multifactorial in etiology, involving both genetic and environmental interactions. Overall, it is estimated that approximately 20% to 25% of the male population in the U.S. with bladder cancer has the disease as a result of occupational exposure.

DISTRIBUTION: In North America, transitional cell carcinomas comprise 93%, squamous cell carcinomas comprise 6%, and adenocarcinomas account for 1% of bladder cancers.

PATHOGENESIS: Two pathways exist for bladder cancer (TCCa):
1. Papillary superficial disease occasionally leading to invasive cancer (75%)
2. Carcinoma-in-situ (CIS) and solid invasive cancer with high risk of disease progression (25%)

Two distinct forms of "Superficial Cancer" exist:

T_a Papillary low-grade tumor. High rate of recurrence. Disease progression occurs 5%

T_1 Higher-grade papillary tumors that infiltrate the lamina propria. Often associated with flat CIS that may involve the urothelium diffusely. Disease progression occurs between 30% to 50%

Subdivided into:

T_{1a} Penetration of tumor up to the muscularis mucosae. Disease progression 5.3%

T_{1b} Penetration of tumor through the muscularis mucosae. Disease progression 53%

Flat CIS:

Entirely different and separate pathway of cancer development whose mechanism is manifested by dysplasia, which leads to the occurrence of poorly differentiated malignant cells that replace or undermine the normal urothelium and extend along the plane of the bladder wall. It penetrates the basement membrane and lamina propria in 20% to 30% of the cases and is associated with the development of solid tumor growth. A defect in chromosome 17p53 occurs in 50% of the cases.

At presentation, 72% of cancers are localized to the bladder, 20% of the cancers extend to the regional lymph nodes, and 3% present with distant metastases. 80% of superficial TCCa recur with up to 30% progressing to a higher stage or grade. Younger patients most commonly develop low-grade papillary noninvasive TCCa and are less likely to have recurrences when compared with older patients with similar lesions. Involvement of the upper tracts with tumor occurs in 25% to 50% of the cases.

STAGING (BASED ON THE TNM SYSTEM):

T_0 No tumor in specimen
T_{is} CIS
T_a Papillary TCCa noninvasive
T_1 Papillary TCCa into lamina propria
T_2 TCCa invasive of superficial muscle
T_{3a} Invasive of deep muscle
T_{3b} Invasive of perivesical fat
T_{4a} Invasive of adjacent pelvic organ
T_{4b} Invasive of pelvic wall with fixation

Invasive of nodal status:
N_0 No nodal involvement
$N_{1\text{-}3}$ Pelvic nodes
N_4 Nodes above bifurcation
N_x Unknown

Invasive of metastatic status:
M_0 No distant metastases
M_1 Distant metastases
M_x Unknown

MOLECULAR EPIDEMIOLOGY: TCCa is usually a field change disease with tumors arising at different times and sites in the urothelium, suggesting a polyclonal etiology of bladder cancer. Bladder cancers have been associated with abnormalities on chromosomes 1, 4, 11, 5, 7, 3, 9, 21, 18, 13, 8; with alterations in suppressor genes *P53,* retinoblastoma gene, and *P16;* and with alterations in oncogenes H-ras and epidermal growth factor receptor.

PHYSICAL FINDINGS & CLINICAL PRESENTATION

- Gross painless hematuria
- Microhematuria
- Frequency, urgency, occasional dysuria

With locally invasive to distant metastatic disease, the presentation can include:
- Abdominal pain
- Flank pain
- Lymphedema
- Renal failure
- Anorexia
- Bone pain

ETIOLOGY

Bladder cancer is a potentially preventable disease associated with specific etiologic factors:

- Cigarette smoking is associated with 25% to 65% of the cases. The risk of developing a TCCa is 2 to 4 times higher in smokers than in nonsmokers, and that risk persists for many years, being equal to nonsmokers only after 12 to 15 yr of smoking abstinence. Smoking tobacco is associated with tumors that are characterized by higher histologic grade, increased tumor stage, increase in the numbers of tumor present, and increased tumor size.
- Occupational exposures: dye workers, textile workers, tire and rubber workers, petroleum workers.
- Chemical exposure: O-toluidine, 2-naphthylamine, benzidine, 4-aminobiphenyl, and nitrosamines
- Exposure to HPV type 16.

Squamous carcinomas are associated with:

- Schistosomiasis
- Urinary calculi
- Indwelling catheters
- Bladder diverticula

Miscellaneous causes:

- Phenacetin abuse
- Cyclophosphamide
- Pelvic irradiation
- Tuberculosis

Adenocarcinomas are associated with:

- Exstrophy
- Endometriosis
- Neurogenic bladder
- Urachal abnormalities
- As a secondary site for distant metastases from other organs (e.g., colon cancer)

DIAGNOSIS (Dx)

- History and physical examination.
- Urinalysis.
- Cystoscopy with bladder barbotage and biopsy.
- Transurethral resection of bladder tumor(s).
- There is insufficient evidence to determine whether a decrease in mortality from bladder cancer occurs with hematuria testing, urinary cytology, or a variety of other tests on exfoliated urinary cells or other substances.
- In addition to urinary cytologies and bladder barbotage, BTA, NMP22, and Fibrin Degradation Products (FDP) have been approved by the FDA as bladder cancer tumor markers. No marker has general, widespread acceptance because the results are affected by the presence of stents, recent urologic manipulation, stones, infection, bowel interposition, and prostatitis creating false-positive results.

DIFFERENTIAL DIAGNOSIS

- Urinary tract infection
- Frequency-urgency syndrome
- Interstitial cystitis
- Stone disease
- Endometriosis
- Neurogenic bladder

LABORATORY TESTS

- Urine cytology.
- Urine telomerase: telomerase activity in voided urine or bladder washings determined by the telomeric repeat amplification protocol (TRAP) assay. This test has been reported to accurately detect the presence of bladder tumors in men. It represents a potentially useful noninvasive diagnostic innovation for bladder cancer detection in high-risk groups such as habitual smokers or in symptomatic patients.

RADIOLOGIC TESTS:

- IVP, renal ultrasound, retrograde pyelography, CT scan, and MRI.
- One or a combination of studies can be used. In the absence of skeletal symptoms, bone scan is not recommended.

TREATMENT (Rx)

NONPHARMACOLOGIC THERAPY

- Initially, transurethral resection of bladder tumor (TURBT)
- Loop biopsy of the prostatic urethra if high-grade TCCa is suspected
- If superficial disease, follow-up protocol with repeat TURBT and/or the use of intravesical agents is recommended
- For advanced bladder cancer, radical cystectomy with urethrectomy (unless orthotopic diversion is planned) and either ileal loop conduit or orthotopic diversion

BLADDER PRESERVATION APPROACHES: Following cystectomy for muscle invasive disease, 50% or more of the patients will develop metastases. Most patients develop metastases at distant sites, a third relapse locally. Bladder preservation management is offered in those individuals who refuse surgery or who might not be suitable radical cystectomy patients. Bladder-sparing protocols include extensive TURBT or partial cystectomy with external beam or interstitial radiotherapy and systemic chemotherapy. Radiotherapy as a single treatment modality is not effective. The best predictor of successful bladder preservation is a complete response following the combination of initial TURBT and two cycles of CMV (cisplatin, methotrexate, vinblastine) chemotherapy used with stages T2 to T3a.

INDICATIONS FOR PARTIAL CYSTECTOMY:

- Tumor within a bladder diverticulum
- Solitary, primary, and muscle-invasive or high-grade lesion of a region of the bladder that allows complete excision with adequate surgical margins
- Inability to adequately resect tumor by TURBT alone because of size or location
- Tumor overlying a ureteral orifice requiring ureteral reimplantation
- Biopsy of a radiation-induced ulceration
- Palliation of severe local symptoms
- Patient refusal of urinary diversion
- Poor-risk patient who is not a diversion candidate

CONTRAINDICATIONS:

- Multiple tumors
- CIS
- Cellular atypia on biopsy
- Prostatic invasion
- Invasion of the trigone
- Inability to achieve adequate surgical margins
- Prior radiotherapy
- Inability to maintain adequate bladder volume after resection
- Evidence of extravesical tumor extension
- Poor surgical risk

ACUTE GENERAL Rx

INDICATIONS FOR INTRAVESICAL CHEMOTHERAPY:

- High-grade tumor
- Tumor size >5 cm
- Tumor multiplicity
- Presence of CIS
- Positive urinary cytologies following a resection
- Incomplete tumor resection

Intravesical agents: thiotepa, Adriamycin, mitomycin C, AD-32, BCG, interferon, bropirimine, Epodyl, interleukin-2, and keyhole-limpet hemocyanin. Photodynamic therapy with hematoporphyrin derivatives has also been used.

INDICATIONS FOR CYSTECTOMY:

- Large tumors not amenable to complete TURBT
- High-grade tumor
- Multiple tumors with frequent recurrences
- Diffuse CIS not responsive to intravesical chemotherapy
- Prostatic urethra involvement
- Irritative bladder symptoms with upper tract deterioration
- Muscle-invasive disease
- Disease outside of the bladder

SYSTEMIC CHEMOTHERAPY: Used as neoadjuvant and adjuvant therapy for systemic disease. The most effective agents are cisplatin, methotrexate, vinblastine, Adriamycin (MVAC). Other agents include mitoxantrone, vincristine, etoposide (VP16), 5FU, ifosfamide,

Taxol, gemcitabine, Piritrexim, and gallium nitrate. Chemotherapy in combination can provide palliation and modest survival benefit.

RADIOTHERAPY: Conflicting reports suggest that superficial bladder cancer is more sensitive to radiotherapy. Squamous changes within the tumor and secretion of human chorionic gonadotropin by the lesion are associated with poor response to radiotherapy. Only 20% to 30% of patients with invasive bladder cancer can be cured by external beam radiation therapy alone. It is used in combination with surgery or with systemic agents to treat bladder cancer primarily in those patients who are not surgical candidates or who refuse surgery.

CHRONIC Rx

FOLLOW-UP RECOMMENDATIONS FOR SUPERFICIAL BLADDER CANCER:

- Cystoscopy, bladder barbotage, and bimanual examination every 3 mo for 2 yr, then every 6 mo for 2 yr, and annually thereafter.
- Upper tract studies are based on the risk of upper tract tumor development, generally every 2 to 5 yr.

FOLLOW-UP RECOMMENDATIONS FOR ADVANCED DISEASE:

Bladder preservation:

- Cystoscopy, barbotage, bimanual examination, biopsy (when indicated), every 3 mo for 2 yr, then every 6 mo for 2 yr, yearly thereafter.
- CT scan of abdomen and pelvis every 6 mo for 2 yr in addition to chest x-ray examination, liver function testing, and serum creatinine.

Cystectomy with ileal loop/orthotopic bladder:

- Neobladder endoscopy and IVP yearly.
- CT scan of abdomen and pelvis every 6 mo for 2 yr in addition to chest x-ray examination, liver function tests, and serum creatinine.
- Loopogram every 6 mo for 2 yr, then yearly.

PEARLS & CONSIDERATIONS

COMMENTS

- The most useful prognostic parameters for bladder tumor recurrence and subsequent cancer progression are tumor grade, depth of tumor penetration, multifocal tumors, frequency of recurrence, tumor size, CIS, lymphatic invasion, papillary or solid tumor configuration.
- Box 1-2 describes the American Urological Association Guideline Recommendations for bladder cancer.

BOX 1-2 American Urological Association Guideline Recommendations

1. Undiagnosed bladder tumor: obtain a histologic diagnosis of the tumor: Transurethral resection of the tumor is the most common method.
2. Stage Ta or T1 cancer: Complete surgical eradication of all visible tumors. The lesion can be treated with electrocautery resection, fulguration, or laser ablation. Adjuvant intravesical therapy is recommended for patients with carcinoma-in-situ, T1, or high-grade Ta tumors. The agent recommended is BCG or mitomycin C. Cystectomy is an option for this set of tumors because of risk of progression to muscle-invasive disease even after intravesical chemotherapy.
   An increased risk of disease progression is associated with large tumor, high-grade tumor, location of the tumor in a site that is poorly accessible to complete resection, diffuse disease, infiltration of lymphatic or vascular spaces, and prostatic urethral involvement.
3. Carcinoma-in-situ or high-grade T1 cancer and prior intravesical chemotherapy: Cystectomy is the recommendation based on the panel's expert opinion rather than evidence from outcomes data. The data show a substantial risk of progression to muscle-invasive cancer in patients with diffuse carcinoma-in-situ and high-grade T1 tumors. The response to intravesical chemotherapy in terms of altering this disease progression is unknown, and as a result of this, cystectomy is an option for the afflicted patient.

American Urological Association, Guideline Division, 1120 North Charles Street, Baltimore, MD 21201.

EVIDENCE

EBM

Superficial bladder tumors

Immunotherapy with intravesical BCG following transurethral tumor resection appears to provide a significant advantage over resection alone in delaying tumor recurrence.[1] (A)

Recurrence following transurethral tumor resection is less likely with intravesical BCG than with mitomycin C, although only the subgroup of patients at high risk of recurrence benefit. There is no difference in terms of disease progression or survival.[2] (A)

Muscle-invasive bladder tumors

There appears to be an overall survival benefit from radical surgery compared with radical radiotherapy. However, it should be noted that only three trials could be included in a systematic review, that patients numbers were small, that many patients did not receive the treatment that they had been randomized to receive, and that there have been improvements in both surgery and radiotherapy since the initiation of the included trials.[3] (A)

A systematic review and meta-analysis found neoadjuvant, platinum-based combination chemotherapy was beneficial for the treatment of biopsy proven invasive (i.e., stage T2 to T4a) transitional cell carcinoma of the bladder, with a 5% improvement in survival at five years.[4] (A)

Evidence-Based References

1. Shelley MD: Intravesical bacillus calmette-guerin in Ta and T1 bladder cancer, *Cochrane Database Sys Rev* Issue 4, 2000. (A)
2. Shelley MD et al: Intravesical bacillus calmette-guerin versus mitomycin C for Ta and T1 bladder cancer, *Cochrane Database Sys Rev* Issue 3, 2003. (A)
3. Shelley MD et al: Surgery versus radiotherapy for muscle invasive bladder cancer, *Cochrane Database Sys Rev* Issue 4, 2001. (A)
4. Advanced Bladder Cancer Overview Collaboration: Neoadjuvant chemotherapy for invasive bladder cancer, *Cochrane Database Sys Rev* Issue 1, 2004. (A)

SUGGESTED READINGS

Lamm DL et al: Megadose vitamins in bladder cancer: a double-blind clinical trial, *J Urol* 151:21, 1994.

Sanchini MA et al: Relevance of urine telomerase in the diagnosis of bladder cancer, *JAMA* 294:2052, 2005.

AUTHORS: **PHILIP J. ALIOTTA, M.D., M.S.H.A.,** and **RUBEN ALVERO, M.D.**

Section I

DISEASES AND DISORDERS

BASIC INFORMATION

DEFINITION

Blastomycosis is a systemic pyogranulomatous disease caused by a dimorphic fungus, *Blastomyces dermatitidis*.

ICD-9CM CODES
116.0 Blastomycosis

EPIDEMIOLOGY & DEMOGRAPHICS

INCIDENCE & PREVALENCE:
- Most patients reside in the southeastern and south central states, especially those bordering the Mississippi and Ohio River valleys, the Midwestern states, and Canadian provinces bordering the Great Lakes.
- Rare cases reported outside the U.S.

RISK FACTORS:
- Widely disseminated disease is most common in immunocompromised hosts, especially those with acquired immunodeficiency syndrome (AIDS).
- Initial infections result from inhalation of conidia into the lungs, although primary cutaneous blastomycosis has been reported after dog bites.

PHYSICAL FINDINGS & CLINICAL PRESENTATION

- Acute infection: <50% symptomatic, median incubation 30 to 45 days, symptoms are nonspecific: mimic influenza or bacterial infection with abrupt onset of myalgias, arthralgias, chills and fever; transient pleuritic pain, cough that is initially nonproductive; resolution within 4 wk is usual
- Chronic or recurrent infection: indolent, progressive; includes pulmonary or extrapulmonary disease

Pulmonary manifestations: Symptoms and signs of chronic pneumonia: productive cough, hemoptysis, pleuritic chest pain, weight loss, low-grade pyrexia

Extrapulmonary manifestations:
1. Cutaneous: most common; may occur with or without pulmonary disease. Two different lesions:
   Verrucous: beginning as a small papulopustular lesion on exposed body areas that may develop into an eschar with peripheral microabscesses
   Ulcerative: Subcutaneous nodules (cold abscesses), and rarely cutaneous inoculation blastomycosis may occur
2. Bone and joint: 10% to 50% have osteolytic lesions; affects long bones, vertebrae, and ribs; lesions may present with contiguous soft-tissue abscess or draining sinus that spreads to a joint, resulting in pyarthrosis
3. Genitourinary: 10% to 30%; prostatic involvement is most common and may present as obstruction; epididymis and testes may also be affected
4. Central nervous system: 5% normal host; 40% AIDS patients; meningitis and abscess formation

ETIOLOGY

Blastomyces dermatitidis exists in warm, moist soil that is rich in organic material. When these microfoci are disturbed, the aerosolized spores or conidia are inhaled into the lungs. Disease at other sites is a result of dissemination from the initial pulmonary infection; the latter may be acute or chronic.

DIAGNOSIS

DIFFERENTIAL DIAGNOSIS

PULMONARY INFECTION:
- Tuberculosis
- Bronchogenic carcinoma
- Histoplasmosis
- Bacterial pneumonia

CUTANEOUS INFECTION:
- Bromoderma
- Pyoderma gangrenosum
- *Mycobacterium marinum* infection
- Squamous cell carcinoma
- Giant keratoacanthoma

WORKUP

- Physical exam and laboratory data
- Definitive diagnosis established by culture

LABORATORY TESTS

- Presumptive diagnosis can be made by visualizing the distinctive yeast forms in clinical specimens
- Culture: on Sabouraud's or more enriched media
  1. Aspirated material from abscesses
  2. Skin scrapings
  3. Prostatic secretions (urine culture with prostatic massage)
- Direct examination of specimens
  1. Wet preparation with 10% KOH
  2. Histopathology: typically demonstrates pyogranulomas; yeast identification requires special stains
- Serologic tests: a negative test cannot exclude blastomycosis, nor should a positive titer be an indication to start treatment

IMAGING STUDIES

In chronic disease, chest radiographic findings are nonspecific, but lobar or segmental alveolar infiltrates, especially of the upper lobes, are most common and may progress to cavitation.

TREATMENT

ACUTE BLASTOMYCOSIS GENERAL Rx

- Treatment remains controversial for acute pulmonary blastomycosis.
- Because the acute form may be benign and self-limited, patients may be closely observed.
- Some patients progress to chronic infection with significant morbidity and therefore may require treatment.
- Patients who are immunocompromised, have extrapulmonary disease, or progressive pulmonary disease should be treated.

CHRONIC BLASTOMYCOSIS

- Itraconazole 200 mg IV bid × 4 doses + 200 mg IV qd or itraconazole 200 to 400 mg/day for 6 mo is the drug of choice except for patients with CNS disease or with fulminant illness who require amphotericin B.
- Amphotericin B: total dose of 1.5 to 2.5 g IV is recommended in immunocompromised patients, those with life-threatening disease or CNS disease, or those who have failed azole treatment. Only drug approved for treating blastomycosis in pregnant women.
- Amphotericin B lipid complex (ABLC) 5 mg/kg/day IV may be considered in patients who are intolerant of or refractory to amphotericin.
- Fluconazole 400 to 800 mg/day PO for 6 mo if unable to tolerate itraconazole or amphotericin B.
- Ketoconazole 400 mg/day PO × 6 mo is an option in mild-moderate disease.
- Surgery may be indicated for drainage of large abscesses.

DISPOSITION

- Before antifungal therapy, the disease had a progressive course with eventual extrapulmonary disease and a mortality >60%.
- Relapse rate for patients treated with amphotericin B is 5%; relapse is more common in AIDS patients.

PEARLS & CONSIDERATIONS

- *Blastomyces dermatitidis* may mimic other diseases.
- Colonization does not occur as with Candida and Aspergillus species.

SUGGESTED READINGS

Bradsher RW et al: Blastomycosis, *Infect Dis Clin N Am* 17:21, 2003.

Martynowicz MA et al: Pulmonary blastomycosis: an appraisal of diagnostic techniques, *Chest* 121(3):768, 2002.

AUTHOR: **SAJEEV HANDA, M.D.**

BASIC INFORMATION

DEFINITION

Blepharitis is an acute or, most often, chronic inflammation of the eyelid margins that is often refractory to treatment.

SYNONYMS

Eyelid infection or inflammation
Eczema of the eyelids
Dermatoblepharitis
Angular blepharitis

ICD-9CM CODES
373.0 Blepharitis

EPIDEMIOLOGY & DEMOGRAPHICS

- Common in children, particularly those with atopic dermatitis and eczema
- Adults with seborrhea involving the eyelids

PHYSICAL FINDINGS & CLINICAL PRESENTATION

- Chronically infected lids are usually diffusely erythematous, with collarettes (fibrin exudate) at the base of the lashes (Fig. 1-38).
- Lid margins thicken over time, with associated loss of eyelashes (madarosis), misdirected growth of lashes (trichiasis), and overflow or inspissation of the meibomian glands.
- Associated conjunctivitis with erythema, edema but no discharge.
- Chalazia may develop.
- Superficial punctate erosions of the inferior corneal epithelium are common.
- More severe findings, such as corneal pannus, ulcerative keratitis, or lid ectropion, are less common.

ETIOLOGY

Multiple: bacterial and nonbacterial causes

- Staphylococcal infection most common but streptococcal, Moraxella, and other bacterial infections; viral infections (e.g., herpes simplex, herpes zoster, *Molluscum contagiosum*); and a number of ectoparasites, including pediculosis, may cause blepharitis
- Seborrheic dermatitis
- Rosacea
- Dry eye (keratoconjunctivitis sicca): decrease in tear volume
- Meibomian gland dysfunction
- Two categories of blepharitis:
  1. Anterior blepharitis, most often associated with staphylococcal infection or seborrheic dermatitis
  2. Posterior blepharitis, associated with meibomian gland dysfunction

NOTE: Blepharitis patients have normal skin microflora in greater amounts (mostly *S. epidermidis* and *P. acnes*). (*S. aureus* and *S. epidermidis* can be cultured in 10% to 35% and 90% to 95% of healthy persons, respectively.)

DIAGNOSIS

DIFFERENTIAL DIAGNOSIS

- Keratoconjunctivitis sicca
- Eyelid malignancies
- Herpes simplex blepharitis
- Molluscum contagiosum
- Phthiriasis palpebrarum
- Phthirus pubis (pubic lice)
- Demodex folliculorum (transparent mites)
- Allergic blepharitis

WORKUP

Scrapings of the eyelids to show polymorphonuclear leukocytes and gram-positive cocci

LABORATORY TESTS

Eyelid cultures and antibiotic sensitivity testing (usually not done unless patient fails to respond to initial treatment regimen)

TREATMENT

NONPHARMACOLOGIC THERAPY

- Alkaline soaps may be beneficial; alcohol and some detergents remove surface lipids and microflora.
- Hot compresses applied to closed lids for 5 to 10 min: heat loosens debris from lid margins and increases meibomian gland fluidity.
- Firm massage of the lid margins to enhance the flow of secretions from glands, followed by cleansing of the lids with cotton-tipped applicators dipped in a 50:50 mixture of baby shampoo and water.
- Lashes and lid margins scrubbed vigorously while the eyelids are closed, followed by thorough rinsing.
- Following local massage and cleansing, the mainstay of treatment is application of topical antibiotic ointment to the eyelid margins.
  1. Most effective topical antibiotics include bacitracin, erythromycin, aminoglycoside and fluoroquinolone ophthalmic ointments.
  2. Ointment is applied 1 to 4 times daily, depending on the severity, for 1 to 2 wk, followed by once daily, at bedtime, for another 4 to 8 wk until all signs of inflammation have disappeared.

For patients with rosacea:

1. Tetracycline 250 mg orally 4 times daily or doxycycline 100 mg orally bid along with local treatment for several months

Recalcitrant cases with antibiotic resistance:

1. Vancomycin eye drops 1%
2. Ciprofloxacin or ofloxacin eyedrops

CHRONIC Rx

By definition, this is a chronic condition for which there is frequently no cure.

Some newer agents being evaluated are antioxidant flavonoid-type compounds (resveratrol, silymarin); azelaic acid and glycolic acid (antikeratinizing effects); and adapalene gel (anti-inflammatory properties and an antiproliferative effect on keratinocytes).

DISPOSITION

This condition may be refractory to treatment.

REFERRAL

To an ophthalmologist if patient fails to respond to local therapy.

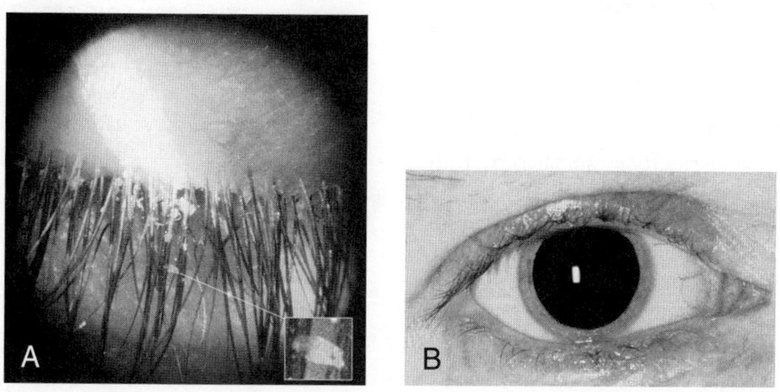

FIGURE 1-38 **A,** Seborrheic blepharitis. The typical scales (scurf) are translucent and easily removed. **B,** Staphylococcal blepharitis showing the typical lid margin erythema and discharge. (From Palay D [ed]: *Ophthalmology for the primary care physician,* St Louis, 1997, Mosby.)

SUGGESTED READINGS

Mathers WD, Choi D: Cluster analysis of patients with ocular surface disease, blepharitis and dry eye, *Arch Ophthalmol* 122:1700, 2004.

McCulley JP, Shine WB: Eyelid disorders, the meibomian gland, blepharitis and contact lens, *Eye Contact Lens* 29:S93, 2003.

Saccà SC: Prevalence and treatment of *Helicobacter pylori* in patients with blepharitis, *Invest Ophthalmol Vis Sci* 47(2):501, 2006.

AUTHORS: **GLENN G. FORT, M.D., M.P.H., DENNIS J. MIKOLICH, M.D., JANE V. EASON, M.D.,** and **JOSEPH R. MASCI, M.D.**

BASIC INFORMATION

DEFINITION

Body dysmorphic disorder (BDD) is a somatoform disorder characterized by a preoccupation with minor or imagined defects in physical appearance that causes significant impairment in social and/or occupational functioning. Other psychiatric conditions such as anorexia nervosa or depression may occur with body dysmorphic disorder, diagnosis of this condition requires a preoccupation not otherwise explained by another mental disorder.

SYNONYMS

Dysmorphophobia
Dysmorphic syndrome
Body dysmorphia

ICD-9CM CODES
306.9 Unspecified psychophysiologic malfunction
DSM-IV: 300.7

EPIDEMIOLOGY & DEMOGRAPHICS

- Affects about 1% to 2% of the general population.
- Incidence among cosmetic surgery patients, 2% to 15%.
- Onset is generally adolescence and young adulthood.
- Equal prevalence among males and females.
- No known genetic predisposition.

PHYSICAL FINDINGS & CLINICAL PRESENTATION

- Patients have an excessive preoccupation (obsession) with a perceived or minor defect in their appearance. Any part of the body may be a focus of concern, although skin, hair, body odor, and nose shape and size are the most common.
- The patient usually appears physically normal; if a defect is present, the patient's reaction to it is disproportionate to its severity.
- Most patients have poor insight or are delusional.
- Many patients engage in compulsive behaviors such as frequent mirror checking, excess grooming, camouflaging, skin picking, and repeatedly measuring or feeling the perceived defect, and seek constant reassurance about the perceived defect.
- Most patients experience some impairment in functioning.

ETIOLOGY

- Cognitive-behavioral models of BDD suggest that these individuals exhibit perfectionistic thinking and maladaptive attractiveness beliefs.
- Unknown, though comorbid mental disorders associated with BDD include major depression, obsessive-compulsive disorder (OCD), generalized anxiety disorder, agoraphobia, trichotillomania, eating disorders.

DIAGNOSIS

- Psychiatric interview
- Ask: (1) Have you ever been worried about your appearance in any way? (2) Did this concern preoccupy you? (3) What effect did this have on your life?

DIFFERENTIAL DIAGNOSIS

- Often goes unrecognized and undiagnosed because of patient's reluctance to divulge symptoms.
- BDD has many features in common with OCD.
- Anorexia nervosa.
- Obsessive-compulsive disorder.
- Anxiety disorder.
- Social phobia.
- Hypochondriasis.
- Many patients have comorbid personality disorder.

WORKUP

- Organic etiology should be assessed with Mini Mental Status Exam (MMSE).
- Body Dysmorphic Disorder Examination Self-Report used in clinical trials.

TREATMENT

NONPHARMACOLOGIC THERAPY

- Cognitive behavioral therapy (particularly exposure and response prevention).
- Do not try to talk patients out of their concern—it is ineffective.
- Avoid cosmetic procedures.

ACUTE GENERAL Rx

Precautions/hospitalization if actively suicidal

CHRONIC Rx

- High-dose selective serotonin reuptake inhibitors (SSRIs).
- Other agents (neuroleptic, TCAs, anticonvulsants) not as beneficial.
- Cognitive behavioral therapy highly recommended as stand-alone or along with SSRIs.
- Support groups, if available, can help.

DISPOSITION

- If untreated, BDD tends to be chronic and can lead to social isolation, school dropout, major depression, unnecessary surgery, and even suicide.
- With early diagnosis and treatment patients appear to have a favorable course (though prospective trials not completed).

REFERRAL

Refer for psychiatric evaluation and treatment if diagnosis is suspected.

PEARLS & CONSIDERATIONS

- In clinical settings, up to 60% of patients with BDD have major depression.
- Compliments and reassurance rarely lessen the patient's fear or dislike of his or her appearance.
- Patients often have an unrealistic expectation of improvement regarding plastic surgery, and surgery itself provides little to no relief.
- Almost one third of patients with BDD attempt suicide.

PATIENT/FAMILY EDUCATION

- Family behavioral treatment can be useful, especially if the affected individual is an adolescent.
- Consider therapy with family members, spouse, significant others.
- Body Dysmorphic Disorder Central: www.BDDCentral.com.

SUGGESTED READINGS

Allen LA et al: Cognitive-behavioral therapy for somatization disorder: a randomized controlled trial, *Arch Intern Med* 166(14):1512, 2006.

Buhlman U et al: Facial attractiveness ratings and perfectionism in body dysmorphic disorder and obsessive-compulsive disorder, *J Anxiety Disord* 22(3):540-547, 2008.

Mackley CL: Body dysmorphic disorder, *Dermatol Surg* 31(5):553-558, 2005.

Phillips KA: Body dysmorphic disorder: a guide for primary care physicians, *Prim Care* 29(1):99-111, 2002.

AUTHOR: **MITCHELL D. FELDMAN, M.D., M.PHIL.**

BASIC INFORMATION

DEFINITION

Primary malignant bone tumors are invasive, anaplastic, and have the ability to metastasize. Most arise from the marrow (myeloma), but tumors may develop from bone, cartilage, fat, and fibrous tissues. Leukemia and lymphoma are excluded from this discussion.

FIBROSARCOMA AND LIPOSARCOMA: Extremely rare. They are similar to those tumors arising in soft tissue.

OSTEOSARCOMA: A rare primary malignant tumor of bone characterized by malignant tumor cells that produce osteoid or bone. Several variants have been described: parosteal sarcoma, periosteal sarcoma, multicentric, and telangiectatic forms.

CHONDROSARCOMA: A malignant cartilage tumor that may develop primarily or secondarily from transformation of a benign osteocartilaginous exostosis or enchondroma.

EWING'S SARCOMA: A malignant tumor of unknown histogenesis.

MULTIPLE MYELOMA: A neoplastic proliferation of plasma cells.

SYNONYMS

Multiple myeloma:
1. Plasma cell myeloma
2. Plasmacytoma

ICD-9CM CODES
203.0 Multiple myeloma
170.9 Neoplasma, bone (periosteum), primary malignant
M9180/3 Osteosarcoma
N9220/3 Chondrosarcoma
M9260/3 Ewing's sarcoma

EPIDEMIOLOGY & DEMOGRAPHICS

MULTIPLE MYELOMA:
- The most common tumor in bone
- Age at onset: usually >40 yr
- Male:female ratio of 2:1

OSTEOGENIC SARCOMA:
- Average age at onset: 10 to 20 yr
- Males > females
- Parosteal sarcoma in older patients

CHONDROSARCOMA:
- Age at onset: 40 to 60 yr
- Male:female ratio of 2:1

EWING'S SARCOMA: Age at onset: 10 to 15 yr

PHYSICAL FINDINGS & CLINICAL PRESENTATION

MULTIPLE MYELOMA:
- May present as a systemic process or, less commonly, as a "solitary" lesion
- Early manifestations: anorexia, weight loss, and bone pain; majority of cases present initially with back pain that often leads to the detection of a destructive skeletal lesion
- Other organ systems eventually become involved, resulting in more bone pain, anemia, renal insufficiency, and/or bacterial infections, usually as a result of the dysproteinemia typical of this disorder
- Possible secondary amyloidosis, leading to cardiac failure or nephrotic syndrome

OSTEOSARCOMA:
- Most originating in the metaphysis
- 50% to 60% around the knee
- Possible pain and swelling, but otherwise healthy patient
- Osteosarcoma in conjunction with Paget's disease, manifested primarily as a sudden increase in bone pain

CHONDROSARCOMA:
- Tumor most commonly involving the pelvis, upper femur, and shoulder girdle
- Painful swelling

EWING'S SARCOMA:
- Painful soft tissue mass often present
- Possibly increased local heat
- Midshaft of a long bone usually affected (in contrast to other tumors)
- Weight loss, fever, and lethargy

DIAGNOSIS

DIFFERENTIAL DIAGNOSIS

- Osteomyelitis
- Metastatic bone disease

LABORATORY TESTS

- Slightly elevated alkaline phosphatase in osteosarcoma
- In Ewing's sarcoma: reflective of systemic reaction; include anemia, an increase in WBC count, and an elevated sedimentation rate
- In multiple myeloma:
  1. Bence Jones protein in the urine
  2. Anemia and elevated sedimentation rate
  3. Characteristic dysproteinemia on serum protein electrophoresis
  4. Diagnostic feature: peak in the electrophoretic pattern suggestive of a monoclonal gammopathy
  5. Rouleaux formation in the peripheral blood smear
  6. Often, presence of hypercalcemia, but alkaline phosphatase levels usually normal

IMAGING STUDIES

- Classic osteogenic sarcoma penetrates the cortex early in many cases.
  1. A blastic (dense), lytic (lucent), or mixed response may be seen in the affected bone.
  2. An aggressive perpendicular sunburst pattern may be present as a result of periosteal reaction, and peripheral Codman's triangles are often noted.
  3. Margins of the tumor are poorly defined.
- Speckled calcifications in a destructive radiolucent lesion are usually suggestive of chondrosarcoma.
- Ewing's sarcoma is characterized radiographically by mottled, irregular destructive changes with periosteal new bone formation. The latter may be multilayered, producing the typical "onion skin" appearance.
- Typical roentgenographic finding in multiple myeloma is the "punched out" lesion with sharply demarcated edges.
  1. Multiple lesions are usual.
  2. Diffuse osteoporosis may be the only finding in many cases.
  3. Pathologic fractures are common.

TREATMENT

The evaluation and treatment of malignant bone tumors are complicated. Diagnostic studies and treatment should be supervised by an orthopedic cancer specialist and oncologist.

DISPOSITION

- In the past 20 yr, dramatic improvements have been made in the treatment protocols for osteosarcoma with the use of adjuvant multidrug regimens and limb-sparing surgery.
- Prognosis of multiple myeloma remains poor despite new therapies.
- Prognosis for Ewing's sarcoma has improved with a combination of chemotherapy, local resection, and radiation therapy.
- Chondrosarcomas are not sensitive to chemotherapy or radiation, and prognosis will depend on the grade of the tumor and the ability to obtain an adequate resection.

PEARLS & CONSIDERATIONS

Early diagnosis is important because most tumors have not metastasized at the time of initial presentation.

SUGGESTED READINGS

Dormans JP, Moroz L: Infection and tumors of the spine in children, *J Bone Joint Surg* 89A:79, 2007.

Futani H et al: Long-term follow-up after limb salvage in skeletally immature children with a primary malignant tumor of the distal end of the femur, *J Bone Joint Surg* 88A:595, 2006.

Hoffmann C et al: Functional results and quality of life after treatment of pelvic sarcomas involving the acetabulum, *J Bone Joint Surg* 88A:575, 2006.

Lewis VO: What's new in musculoskeletal oncology? *J Bone Joint Surg* 89:1399, 2007.

Plate AM et al: Malignant tumors of the hand and wrist, *J Am Acad Orthop Surg* 14:680, 2006.

Staals EL et al: Dedifferentiated chondrosarcomas arising in preexisting osteochondromas, *J Bone Joint Surg* 89A:987, 2007.

AUTHOR: **LONNIE R. MERCIER, M.D.**

BASIC INFORMATION

DEFINITION

Borderline personality disorder (BPD) is characterized by a pervasive pattern of instability in interpersonal relationships, self-image, affect regulation, and impulse control that causes significant subjective distress or impairment of functioning. The individual must meet five or more of the following criteria:

1. Frantic efforts to avoid real or imagined abandonment
2. Unstable and intense personal relationships characterized by alternating between extremes of idealization and devaluation
3. Identity disturbance characterized by an unstable self-image
4. Impulsivity in at least two areas that are potentially self-damaging (e.g., overspending, sex, substance abuse, binge eating, reckless driving)
5. Recurrent suicidal behavior, gestures, threats, or self-mutilating behavior
6. Affective instability due to a marked reactivity of mood
7. Chronic feelings of emptiness
8. Inappropriate, intense anger, or difficulty controlling anger
9. Transient, stress-related paranoid ideation or severe dissociative symptoms

ICD-9CM CODES
301.83 Borderline personality

EPIDEMIOLOGY & DEMOGRAPHICS

PREVALENCE: Affects about 1% to 2% of the general population and up to 10% of psychiatric outpatients
PREDOMINANT SEX: Female (3:1)
PREDOMINANT AGE: 20s
GENETICS: Five times as likely if BPD is present in first-degree relative. An increased prevalence of mood disorders and substance abuse disorders is also found in first-degree relatives of persons with BPD.
RISK FACTORS: Association with childhood physical, sexual, or emotional abuse and/or neglect

PHYSICAL FINDINGS & CLINICAL PRESENTATION

- There are no specific physical findings associated with BPD.
- Mental status examination may reveal affective lability.

Clinical presentation may reveal the following:

- Patients experience a pervasive sense of loneliness and emptiness. In addition to affective instability, persons with BPD often demonstrate an underlying negative affect with dysphoria.
- Intense emotions with difficulty returning to emotional baseline.
- All-or-nothing, either-or cognitive style that is represented by a phenomenon known as "splitting," in which patient sees situations or people as all good or all bad.
- Difficulty in maintaining commitment to long-term goals; history of numerous stormy relationships and multiple jobs.
- Reacts with rage, panic, despair to actual or perceived abandonment; may present with suicidality or self-mutilating behavior in response to recent stressor.
- Attempts to block the experience of pain, which may induce feelings of de realization, depersonalization, changes in consciousness, and/or brief psychotic reactions with delusions and hallucinations.
- Substance use, gambling, overspending, eating binges, and/or self-mutilation as a way to escape intensely painful affect.
- Some patients may display psychotic symptoms.

ETIOLOGY

- Interaction of psychosocial adversity plus genetic factors
- Hypotheses:
  1. Genetic: increased risk if first-degree relative with BPD.
  2. Biologic: abnormalities in limbic system and other areas of the brain cause emotional dysregulation. Serotonergic functioning appears to be disturbed.
  3. Environmental: history of childhood abuse or neglect.

DIAGNOSIS

DIFFERENTIAL DIAGNOSIS

- Histrionic and narcissistic personality disorders share some common features.
- Dysthymia and other depressive disorders: requires a stability of affective symptoms not seen in BPD.
- Bipolar disorder: mood changes in BPD are often triggered by stressors and are less sustained than in bipolar disorder.
- Substance abuse or dependence: often induces impulsive, emotionally labile behavior.
- Posttraumatic stress disorder: individuals with BPD often have history of trauma but do not avoid the feared stimulus or reexperience the trauma as do individuals with PTSD.
- Mild cases of schizophrenia may superficially resemble BPD.

WORKUP

- History (often helpful to gather collateral information from family and friends)
- Physical examination
- Mental status examination

LABORATORY TESTS

- Toxicology screen. Substance use is common and can mimic features of personality disorders.
- Screen for HIV and other sexually transmitted illnesses. Patients with personality disorders often exhibit poor impulse control.

IMAGING STUDIES

Structural and functional MRI demonstrate abnormalities in the amygdala and hippocampus. PET scans reveal altered metabolism in prefrontal cortex. Imaging is not recommended as part of routine evaluation.

TREATMENT

NONPHARMACOLOGIC THERAPY

- Few randomized trials have assessed psychosocial interventions for BPD.
- Dialectical behavior therapy (DBT), a variation of cognitive behavior therapy (CBT), and transference-focused psychotherapy, a type of psychodynamic therapy, have the most empirical support from randomized trials. The goal of DBT is to help patients control impulses and angry outbursts and to develop social skills, and the focus of transference-focused psychotherapy is on examining the affect-laden themes that emerge in the relationship between patient and therapist.

ACUTE GENERAL Rx

Low-dose antipsychotics to control impulsivity, brief psychotic episodes.

CHRONIC Rx

- Medications have low to moderate effectiveness and are most effective in improving symptoms of impulsivity, mood instability, and self-destructive behavior. Effectiveness of medications for BPD has only been studied within the first 3 mo of treatment.
- SSRIs if concurrent mood disorder. Higher doses of antidepressants may be required than for patients with major depression alone.
- Low-dose antipsychotics.
- Mood stabilizers (lithium, valproate, carbamazepine, topiramate).
- In preliminary studies, daily omega-3 fatty acids improve symptoms of irritability.

DISPOSITION

- Course is variable. The most unstable period is typically in early adulthood; the majority of patients achieve greater stability in social/occupational functioning later in life but often continue to have difficulty maintaining intimate relationships.

- There is no evidence of progression to schizophrenia, but patients have a high incidence of episodes of major depressive disorder and other Axis I disorders. This highlights the importance of evaluating for Axis I pathology in patients with BPD to identify potentially treatable illness.

REFERRAL

- Referral to mental health specialty care advised to confirm diagnosis and assist in management.
- Referral recommended if:
  - Use of pharmacotherapy contemplated
  - Patient is severely impaired in daily function or suicidal

PEARLS & CONSIDERATIONS

COMMENTS

Guidelines for physician management of patients with BPD:

- Consider frequent, brief, scheduled visits for needy, demanding, or somaticizing patients with BPD.
- Validate the patient's feelings while stating the expectation of behavior control.
- Be matter-of-fact; avoid expressing extreme emotions.
- Be alert to the risk of suicide and assess suicide risk often.
- Convey a demeanor of competence but openly acknowledge minor errors.
- Have a low threshold for seeking psychiatric consultation.

PREVENTION

There are no known ways to prevent BPD and other personality disorders. Attempts may be made to prevent the deleterious consequences of personality disorders:

- Suicidality should be actively and consistently monitored.
- Benzodiazepines, narcotic analgesics, and other drugs with potential for dependency should be used rarely and with great caution. Nearly all personality disorders are marked by impaired impulse control and consequent risk of addictive behavior.
- Patients with personality disorder who have children should be asked frequently and in detail about their parenting practices. Their low frustration tolerance, externalization of blame for psychological distress, and impaired impulse control put the children of these patients at risk for neglect or abuse.

PATIENT/FAMILY EDUCATION

National Alliance for the Mentally Ill (NAMI), http://www.nami.org, provides patient information, on-line chat groups, and information on support groups throughout the U.S. for people with borderline personality disorder and their families.

SUGGESTED READINGS

American Psychiatric Association practice guidelines for the treatment of patients with BPD: http://www.psych.org/psych_pract/treatg/pg/borderline_revisebook_index.cfm.

Clarkin JF et al: Evaluating three treatments for BPD: a multiwave study, *Am J Psychiatry* 164:922, 2007.

Conklin C, Westin D: Borderline personality disorder in clinical practice, *Am J Psychiatry* 162:867, 2005.

Zanarini MC et al: Prediction of the 10-year course of borderline personality disorder, *Am J Psychiatry* 163(5):827, 2006.

AUTHORS: **MICHELE MONTANDON, M.D.**, and **MITCHELL D. FELDMAN, M.D., M.PHIL.**

BASIC INFORMATION

DEFINITION

Botulism is an illness caused by a neurotoxin produced by *Clostridium botulinum.* Three types of disease can occur: foodborne botulism, wound botulism, and infant intestinal botulism. Recent concern has increased about a possible fourth type of disease: inhalational botulism, which does not occur naturally, but may occur as a result of bioterrorism.

SYNONYMS

Clostridium botulinum food poisoning
Botulinum toxin food poisoning
Wound botulism
Infantile botulism

ICD-9CM CODE
005.1 Botulism

EPIDEMIOLOGY & DEMOGRAPHICS

INCIDENCE (IN U.S.): Approximately 24 cases/yr of foodborne illness, 3 cases/yr of wound botulism, and 71 cases/yr of infant botulism

PHYSICAL FINDINGS & CLINICAL PRESENTATION

- Symptoms usually begin 12 to 36 hr following ingestion.
- Severity of illness is related to the quantity of toxin ingested.
- Significant findings:
  1. Cranial nerve palsies, with ocular and bulbar manifestations being most frequent (diplopia, ophthalmoplegia, ptosis, dysphagia, dysarthria, fixed and dilated pupils, and dry mouth)
  2. Usually bilateral nerve involvement that may progress to a descending flaccid paralysis
  3. Typically, absence of sensory findings; sensorium intact
  4. GI symptoms (nausea, vomiting, diarrhea, or cramps)
  5. Usually no fever
- Wound botulism
  1. Occurs mostly in injecting drug users (subcutaneous heroin injection—"skin popping") or with traumatic injury.
  2. Presentation is similar to that of foodborne disease, except for a longer incubation period and the absence of GI symptoms.
  3. Wound infection is not always apparent, but injection sites frequently reveal cellulitis, draining pus, or abscess formation.

ETIOLOGY

- Cause is one of several types of neurotoxins (usually A, B, or E) produced by *C. botulinum,* an anaerobic, gram-positive bacillus. Spore production guarantees survival of the organism in extreme conditions. Botulinum toxin is the most powerful neurotoxin known.
- Disease results from absorption of toxin into the circulation from a mucosal surface or wound. Botulinum toxin does not penetrate intact skin.
- In foodborne variety, disease is caused by ingestion of preformed toxin. Although rapidly inactivated by heat, the toxin can survive the proteolytic environment of the stomach.
- In wound botulism, toxin is elaborated by organisms that contaminate a wound. Most cases reported are from California.
- In infant botulism, toxin is produced by organisms in the GI tract.
- Inhalational botulism has been demonstrated experimentally in primates. This manufactured form results from aerosolized toxin, and has been attempted by bioterrorists.

DIAGNOSIS (Dx)

DIFFERENTIAL DIAGNOSIS

- Myasthenia gravis
- Guillain-Barré syndrome
- Tick paralysis
- CVA

WORKUP

- Search made for toxin and the organism (see "Laboratory Tests")
- Electrophysiologic studies (EMG) may aid in the diagnosis

LABORATORY TESTS

- Samples of food and stool are cultured for the organism.
- Food, serum, and stool are sent for toxin assay.

TREATMENT (Rx)

NONPHARMACOLOGIC THERAPY

- Supportive care with intubation if respiratory failure occurs
- Debridement of the wound in wound botulism

ACUTE GENERAL Rx

- Give trivalent equine serum botulinum antitoxin as early as possible. Once a clinical diagnosis is made, antitoxin should be administered before laboratory confirmation.
  1. Give one vial by IM injection and one vial IV.
  2. The antitoxin is available from the Centers for Disease Control and Prevention [(404) 639-2206 or (404) 639-2888]; it is derived from horse serum, so there is a significant incidence of serum sickness. A human-derived antitoxin immunoglobin is now available for infants less than 1 yr of age (BIG-IV).
  3. Skin testing (conjunctival instillation and observation for 15 min), and possible desensitization, is recommended before treatment.
- Give wound botulism patients penicillin 2 million U IV q4h.
- Babies with infantile intestinal botulism may benefit from a cathartic to mechanically clear the number of *C. botulinum* vegetative forms and spores residing in the gastrointestinal tract.

CHRONIC Rx

- Supportive
- Rehabilitation/physical therapy

DISPOSITION

- Highest mortality in the first case in an outbreak, with subsequent cases receiving rapid treatment
- Complete recovery for most individuals (this may take several weeks in severely affected individuals)

REFERRAL

Immediate for all cases to an ER and an infectious disease consultant

PEARLS & CONSIDERATIONS (!)

COMMENTS

- Routine cooking inactivates the toxin, but spores are resistant to environmental factors. At room temperature, spores can germinate and produce toxin.
- Most outbreaks are associated with home-canned foods, especially vegetables.
- Patients must be closely monitored for progression to respiratory paralysis.
- There is increasing concern over the potential use of botulinum toxin as a biologic weapon, either by the enteric route or by aerosolization.
- Notify public health authorities immediately to alert other health care services of possible additional cases and to initiate investigation into cause and scope of outbreak.
- Recent botulism food recalls have involved canned chili, cut green beans, and olives.

SUGGESTED READINGS

Amon SS et al: Botulinum toxin as a biological weapon, *JAMA* 285(8):1059, 2001.

Arnon SS et al: Human botulism immune globulin for the treatment of infant botulism, *N Engl J Med* 354(5):462, 2006.

Bleck TP: *Clostridium botulinum* (botulism). In Mandell GL, Bennett JE, Dolin R (eds): *Principles and practice of infectious diseases,* ed 5, New York, 2000, Churchill Livingstone.

Cherington M: Botulism: update and review, *Semin Neurol* 24:155, 2004.

Sobel J: Botulism, *Clin Infect Dis* 41(8):1167, 2005.

AUTHORS: **GLENN G. FORT, M.D., M.P.H., DENNIS J. MIKOLICH, M.D.,** and **MAURICE POLICAR, M.D.**

BASIC INFORMATION

DEFINITION

Brain neoplasms are a diverse group of primary (nonmetastatic) tumors arising from one of many different cell types within the central nervous system (CNS). Specific tumors' subtypes and prognosis depend on the tumor cell of origin and pattern of growth.

SYNONYMS

Brain tumors
Primary tumors of the central nervous system

ICD-9CM CODES
225.0 Brain neoplasm (benign)
239.2 Brain neoplasm (unspecified)

EPIDEMIOLOGY & DEMOGRAPHICS

INCIDENCE (IN U.S.): Approximately 8 cases/100,000 persons/yr. In 2002, the Central Brian Tumor Registry data estimated approximately 41,130 new cases of both malignant and benign brain tumors in the U.S. in 2004. Primary brain neoplasms account for ~2% of all cancers, ~20% of all cancers in children >15 yr. Most common cause of cancer death in children up to 15 yr.

PREDOMINANT SEX: Male:female = 3:2; except for meningiomas: female:male = 3:1.

PREDOMINANT AGE: Male: 75+ yr; female: 65 to 74 yr.

GENETICS: Most primary CNS neoplasms are sporadic; 5% are associated with hereditary syndromes that predispose to neoplasia. The most common of these include:

- Li-Fraumeni syndrome: *p53* mutation on chromosome 17q13, gliomas
- Von Hippel-Lindau: VHL, chromosome 3p25, hemangioblastoma
- Tuberous sclerosis: *TSC1/TSC2* (chromosome 9q34/16p13), subependymal giant cell astrocytoma
- Neurofibromatosis type 1: *NF1,* chromosome 17q11, neurofibroma, optic nerve glioma, meningioma
- Neurofibromatosis type 2: *NF2,* chromosome 22q12, schwannoma, meningioma, ependymoma
- Retinoblastoma: *pRB,* chromosome 13q, retinoblastoma
- Gorlin's syndrome: chromosome 9q31, desmoplastic medulloblastoma

PHYSICAL FINDINGS & CLINICAL PRESENTATION

- In general, the location, size, and rate of growth will determine the symptoms and signs. Even within a tumor subtype, clinical presentation may vary. Brain tumors can produce signs and symptoms related to local invasion, compression of adjacent structures, and increased intracranial pressure.
- Headache is a common problem; this may be a presenting symptom in 20% and develops later in 60%. The headache can be localizing or may result from increased intracranial pressure, and may worsen with change in body position, such as bending over, or coughing/sneezing/Valsalva-type maneuvers. Concerning features of headaches include nausea and vomiting, change in typical headache pattern, worsening with position, and vertex location. Headaches with brain tumors tend to be worse during the night and may awaken the patient. The nocturnal pattern may be related to increased pCO_2 levels during sleep, which acts as a potent vasodilator.
- Seizures occur in 33% of patients, and are among the most common symptoms, particularly with brain metastases and low-grade gliomas. The type of seizure and clinical presentation depends on location. Seizures are more common in low-grade compared to high-grade gliomas. Tumor-related seizures are often repetitive and stereotypical in a given patient. It is thought that patients who present with seizures typically have smaller tumors at time of diagnosis compared to those who present with other symptoms, because the onset of seizures prompts an imaging study, leading to an earlier diagnosis.
- Symptoms and signs of hydrocephalus and raised intracranial pressure (headache, vomiting [particularly in children], clouding of consciousness, papilledema). Extremity weakness or sensory changes are common complaints in patients with brain tumors. These symptoms often respond to high-dose steroids, meaning that the weakness is caused by edema more likely than direct tumor involvement.
- Patients may also present with subtle behavioral changes or cognitive and visual-spatial dysfunction. These symptoms are often recognized in retrospect and may be quite subtle. The pattern of these symptoms can be confused with depression.

ETIOLOGY

- Most cases are idiopathic, though specific chromosomal abnormalities have been implicated in some tumor types.
- Exposure to ionizing radiation has been implicated in meningiomas, gliomas, and nerve sheath tumors. No convincing evidence has shown a link with trauma, occupation, diet, or electromagnetic fields.

DIAGNOSIS

- Most common tumors in children: astrocytoma, medulloblastoma, ependymoma
- Most common adult tumors: glioblastoma multiforma, anaplastic astrocytoma, meningioma

DIFFERENTIAL DIAGNOSIS

- Stroke
- Abscess/parasitic cyst
- Demyelinating disease—multiple sclerosis, postinfectious encephalomyelitis
- Metastatic tumors
- Primary CNS lymphoma

LABORATORY TESTS

- Cerebrospinal fluid (CSF) analysis for measurement of tumor markers and cytology may yield tumor cells for histology.
- Lumbar puncture must never be performed if there is concern for increased intracranial pressure.

IMAGING STUDIES (Fig. 1-39)

- MRI with gadolinium enhancement is highly sensitive, though CT scan is useful if calcification or hemorrhage suspected. MRI imaging permits visualization of the tumor as well as the relationship to the surrounding tissue. Enhancing tumor can be distinguished from surrounding edema. Low-grade tumors often present as an infiltrating lesion without mass effect. MRI is superior to CT scan to evaluate the meninges, subarachnoid space, and

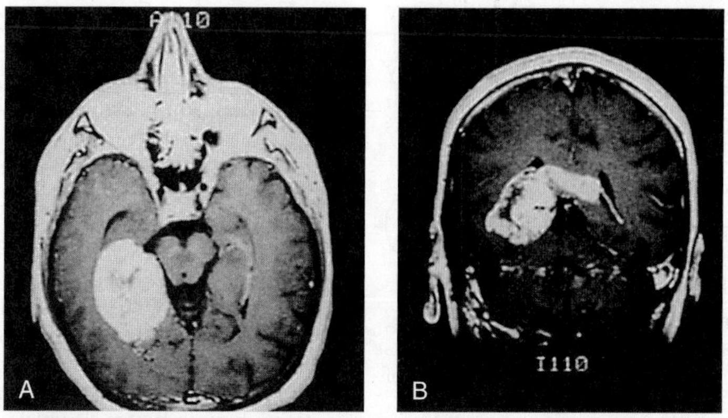

FIGURE 1-39 Glioblastoma multiforme. Axial **(A)** and coronal **(B)** postcontrast enhanced T1-weighted image showing a large homogenously contrast-enhancing mass in the right medial temporal lobe with extension across the midline. (From Specht N [ed]: *Practical guide to diagnostic imaging,* St Louis, 1998, Mosby.)

posterior fossa, and for defining relationship to major intracranial vessels.
- MR spectroscopy is increasingly being used as a diagnostic tool to define metabolic composition of an area of interest and may be useful to contrast areas of tumor progression from radiation necrosis. N-acetylaspartate is often decreased in brain tumors, whereas choline, a component of cell membranes, is increased due to high cellular turnover.
- PET scan is helpful to distinguish neoplastic lesions (with high rate of metabolism) from other lesions such as demyelination or radiation necrosis (with a much lower metabolic rate). Such lesions take up greater amounts of glucose than surrounding tissues or tumors with slower metabolic rates. May be useful to help map functional areas of the brain before surgery or radiation.
- Functional MRI is now used as an adjunct to perioperative planning for patients whose lesion is in vital regions, such as those responsible for speech, language, and motor control.

PATHOLOGY

- Ultimately, only a histologic examination can provide the exact diagnosis. Information may also be gleaned from additional features such as proliferative index, immunohistochemical stains, and electron microscopy.
- The present classification schema for gliomas is based on pathologic and microscopic criteria.
- Molecular classification: Different subtypes of gliomas have distinct gene-expression profiles, which can be distinguished from one another and from normal tissue; these differences typically involve pathways of cell proliferation, energy metabolism, and signal transduction. In adults, global expression profiling identified differences in 360 genes between low-grade and high-grade tumors. Epidermal growth factor receptor gene (EGFR) amplification is the most frequent genetic change in adult high-grade glioma and is considered a negative prognostic marker. Mutation of the *P53* and *PTEN* pathways are also relatively frequent.
- Genetic analysis of tumors is rapidly becoming important for genetic classification and stratification of treatments and for predicting outcome.

TREATMENT (Rx)

NONPHARMACOLOGIC THERAPY

- Maximal surgical removal or debulking is the initial treatment of choice. Outcome is often dependent on extent of resection.
- Biopsy alone is performed if the tumor is located in eloquent regions of brain or is inaccessible; this is essential for histopathologic diagnosis. Biopsy can be performed under CT or MRI guidance using stereotactic localization.
- If the tumor is benign (e.g., meningioma, acoustic neuroma), no further therapy is usually required.

ACUTE GENERAL Rx

- Steroids are used to reduce edema and may also be used perioperatively or during radiation therapy.
- Antiseizure medications have been used perioperatively and to control seizures resulting from focal lesions. Prophylactic use of anticonvulsants is not typically recommended without clear history of seizures.

CHRONIC Rx

- Current standard-of-care therapies include surgery, radiation, and palliative chemotherapy, which have significant side effects and limited efficacy.
- Chemotherapy (combination or single agent) may be used before, during, or after surgery and radiation therapy. (In children, chemotherapy is often used to delay radiation therapy.) Radiosensitizers may help increase the therapeutic effect of radiation therapy.
- Radiation is useful for certain types of tumors: Conventional radiation uses external beams over a period of weeks, whereas stereotactic radiosurgery delivers a single, high dose of radiation to a well-defined area (usually <1 cm). Long-term effects of radiation therapy include radiation necrosis (particularly of white matter), blood vessel hyalinization, secondary tumors (usually meningiomas, sarcomas, and malignant astrocytomas).
- Experimental therapies are continually in development and are typically based on molecular characterization of tumors and small molecule blockers of signal transduction cascades. Some of these therapies involve antisense molecules, biologic agents, immunotherapies, or angiogenesis inhibitors. Intratumoral drug infusions and convection-enhanced delivery of novel agents are currently under study.

DISPOSITION/PROGNOSTIC FACTORS

- Tumor histology/histologic diagnosis (WHO grading system), including number of mitoses, capillary endothelial proliferation, and necrosis. (NOTE: There can be a high degree of morbidity based on tumor location, even with more benign histology.)
- In general, younger age, high-performance status, and lower pathologic grade have more favorable prognosis. For all histologic subtypes of brain tumors, pediatric and young adult patients have a better survival.
- Terminal events typically result from raised intracranial pressure.

REFERRAL

- All cases warrant evaluation by an oncologist and neurosurgeon.
- Patients should be evaluated for physical and occupational therapy.
- Children should undergo neuropsychologic evaluations and screening for learning disabilities.

EVIDENCE (EBM)

The use of prophylactic anticonvulsants in patients with newly diagnosed brain tumors remains controversial; because of the lack of defined efficacy and potential for serious side effects, anticonvulsants are not recommended prophylactically in this population.[1] (C)

Evidence-Based Reference

1. Glantz MJ et al: Practice parameter: anticonvulsant prophylaxis in patients with newly diagnosed brain tumors. Report of the Quality Standards Subcommittee of the American Academy of Neurology, *Neurology* 54:1886, 2000. (C)

SUGGESTED READINGS

Bogomolny DL et al: Functional MRI in the brain tumor patient, *Top Magn Reson Imaging* 15(5):325-335, 2004.

Bradley KA, Mehta MP: Management of brain metastases, *Semin Oncol* 31(5):693-701, 2004.

Chao ST: The sensitivity and specificity of FDG PET in distinguishing recurrent brain tumor from radionecrosis in patients treated with stereotactic radiosurgery, *Int J Cancer* 96:191, 2001.

Glantz MJ et al: Practice parameter: anticonvulsant prophylaxis in patients with newly diagnosed brain tumors. Report of the Quality Standards Subcommittee of the American Academy of Neurology, *Neurology* 54:1886, 2000.

Jemel A et al: Cancer statistics, 2007, *CA Cancer J Clin* 57:43, 2007.

Kesari S et al: Targeted molecular therapy of malignant gliomas, *Curr Neurol Neurosci Rep* 5(3):186-197, 2005.

Kleihues P: Pathology and genetics of tumors of the nervous system. In Kleihues P, Cavenee WK (eds): *International agency for research on cancer,* Lyon, 2000, Harcourt, p. 22.

Mischel PS, Cloughesy TF, Nelson SF: DNA-microarray analysis of brain cancer: molecular classification for therapy, *Nat Rev Neurosci* 5(10):782-792, 2004.

Pietsch T, Taylor MD, Rutka JT: Molecular pathogenesis of childhood brain tumors, *J Neuro-oncol* 70(2):203-215, 2004.

Purow B, Fine HA: Progress report on the potential of angiogenesis inhibitors for neuro-oncology, *Cancer Invest* 22(4):577-587, 2004.

Riva M: Brain tumoral epilepsy: a review, *Neurol Sci* 26(Suppl 1):S40-S42, 2005.

Ullrich NJ, Pomeroy SL: Pediatric brain tumors, *Neurol Clin NA* 21:897-913, 2003.

Wen PY, Marks PW: Medical management of patients with brain tumors, *Curr Opin Oncol* 14:299, 2002.

Wrensch M: Epidemiology of primary brain tumors: current concepts and review of the literature, *Neuro-oncol* 4:278, 2002.

AUTHOR: **NICOLE J. ULLRICH, M.D., PH.D.**

BASIC INFORMATION

DEFINITION

The term *breast cancer* refers to invasive carcinoma of the breast, whether ductal or lobular.

SYNONYMS

Carcinoma of the breast

ICD-9CM CODES
174.9 Malignant neoplasm female breast

EPIDEMIOLOGY & DEMOGRAPHICS

- Nearly exclusively the disease of women, with only 1% of breast cancers in males
- Steady increase in its incidence in the U.S., with 205,000 new patients annually
- Annual mortality of 40,000
- Risk steadily increases with age
- Genetically defined group of women with BRCA-1 or BRCA-2 identified to carry lifetime risk as high as 85%

PHYSICAL FINDINGS & CLINICAL PRESENTATION

- Increasing number of small breast cancers found by mammograms
- Patients usually completely free of physical findings
- Palpable tumors possibly as small as 1 cm or even smaller
- Size of the mass and its location measured and documented
- Skin and/or nipple retraction and skin edema/erythema/ulcer/satellite nodule
- Nodal enlargement in axilla and supraclavicular areas
- Advanced disease: clinical signs of pleural effusion and/or hepatomegaly
- Rare instances: clear, serous, or bloody discharge only symptom
- Nipple evaluation (see "Paget's Disease of the Breast")

ETIOLOGY

- Precise mechanism of carcinogenesis not understood
- Possibly interaction of ovarian estrogen, nonovarian estrogen, estrogens of exogenous origin with breast tissue of varied carcinogenic susceptibility to develop cancer
- Other known or suspected variables: childbearing, breast-feeding practice, diet, physical activities, body mass, alcoholic intake
- Have identified families with known high risk
- Women with BRCA-1 and BRCA-2 associated with high risk

DIAGNOSIS

DIFFERENTIAL DIAGNOSIS

The following nonmalignant breast lesions can simulate breast cancer on both physical and mammogram examinations:

1. Fibrocystic changes
2. Fibroadenoma
3. Hamartoma

WORKUP

- Physical examination:
  1. Mass detected by patient or medical professional: workup required
  2. Negative mammogram: breast cancer not ruled out
  3. Sonogram: to demonstrate mass to be cyst, usually eliminating need for further workup
- To establish diagnosis:
  1. Positive aspiration cytology on a clinically and mammographically malignant mass—highly accurate but still requires open biopsy confirmation
  2. Stereotactic core needle biopsy diagnosis: reliable with invasive carcinoma identified, but negative or equivocal results require careful evaluation
  3. Atypical hyperplasia or in situ carcinoma found by core needle biopsy: open surgical biopsy confirmation still required
  4. Excisional or incisional biopsy: establishes diagnosis
- NOTE: Do not rely on negative mammogram or negative aspiration cytology to exclude malignancy. Make appropriate referral. Obtain imaging studies such as bone scan, chest x-ray examination, CT scan of abdomen, or CT scan of liver.
- Breast radiologic evaluation and an algorithm for breast cancer screening and evaluation are described in Section III. The differential diagnosis of breast lumps is described in Section II.

IMAGING STUDIES

Mammograms: 30% to 50% of breast cancers detected by screening mammograms only as a spiculated mass, a mass with or without microcalcifications, or a cluster of microcalcifications. MRI is an excellent modality, particularly useful in patients with breast implants and when there is a strong family history of breast cancer.

TREATMENT

NONPHARMACOLOGIC THERAPY

- Early breast cancer: primarily surgical or surgical and radiotherapeutic
- Choice in 60% to 70% of women between modified mastectomy and breast-conserving treatment, which consists of lumpectomy, axillary staging with sentinel node biopsy or axillary dissection, and breast irradiation

ACUTE GENERAL Rx

- May require adjuvant chemotherapy or endocrine therapy
- Evaluation and treatment by medical oncologist

CHRONIC Rx

Follow-up required after proper treatment of primary breast cancer includes:

1. Periodic clinical evaluations as delineated by medical oncologist or surgeon
2. Annual mammograms
3. Other tests as indicated
4. Patient instruction in monthly breast self-examination technique

DISPOSITION

- Prognosis after curative therapy: depends on size of tumor, extent of nodal metastasis, and pathologic grade of tumor
  1. Patient with 1-cm tumor with no axillary node metastasis: 10-yr disease-free survival rate of 90%
  2. Patient with 3-cm tumor with metastasis in four nodes: 10-yr disease-free survival rate of 15% if no systemic adjuvant therapy given
  3. Outlook for most patients is between these extremes
- Systemic adjuvant therapy: improves prognosis significantly

REFERRAL

Referral is necessary as soon as breast cancer is even remotely suspected.

PEARLS & CONSIDERATIONS

Breast cancer in pregnancy and lactation:

1. Frequency in women 40 yr or younger reported to be 15%
2. May carry worse prognosis because disease discovery delayed by engorged and nodular breast changes and/or because disease progression more rapid in pregnancy
3. Survival rates similar to those for nonpregnant early-stage breast cancer patients in same age group
4. Mass usually found by patient or obstetrician
5. Expedient workup recommended, including mammography and sonography
6. Diagnosis to be made without delay
7. Choice of mastectomy or lumpectomy with axillary dissection for treatment
8. Adjuvant chemotherapy delayed until third trimester or after delivery
9. Irradiation to breast after lumpectomy delayed until after delivery

Duct carcinoma in situ (DCIS, intraductal carcinoma):

1. "New" disease mostly found by mammogram as cluster of microcalcification and/or density
2. Less often, presents as palpable mass or nipple discharge
3. Before mammogram screening, DCIS accounted for 1% of all breast cancers
4. Now, 15% to 20% or even higher proportion present with DCIS
5. Formerly treated with mastectomy, now lumpectomy
6. Cure rates 98% to 99%
7. No axillary dissection required
8. With radiation, breast recurrences reduced
9. Mastectomy possibly required with extensive and/or high-grade DCIS
10. Systemic adjuvant treatment is not indicated

Inflammatory carcinoma:

1. Rare but rapidly progressive and often lethal form of breast cancer
2. Presents as erythematous and edematous breast resembling mastitis
3. Biopsy required, including skin
4. Treatment with combination chemotherapy followed by surgery and radiation therapy
5. Prognosis once dismal, now 5-yr disease-free survival in 50% of patients

COMMENTS

- Patient education material can be obtained from the following:
  1. SHARE: Self-Help for Women with Breast Cancer, 19 W 44th Street, No 415, New York, NY 10036-5902.
  2. Y-ME National Organization of Breast Cancer Information and Support, 18220 Harwood Avenue, Homewood, IL 80430.
- Breast radiologic evaluation, evaluation of nipple discharge, and evaluation of palpable mass are described in Section III.

EVIDENCE

EBM

Nonmetastatic breast cancer

Tamoxifen therapy substantially improves survival and reduces recurrence rate in nonmetastatic breast cancer. The effects are most marked, or limited to, women with estrogen receptor-positive tumors.[1,2] Ⓐ

Although tamoxifen therapy for 5 yr is associated with significantly greater reductions in recurrence rate, the effect of treatment for longer than 5 yr is not clear.[2] Ⓐ

A large randomized trial showed that goserelin-tamoxifen combination gave a relapse-free survival that was significantly better than cyclophosphamide, methotrexate, and fluorouracil treatment in women with hormone-responsive disease. Overall survival was also better with the goserelin-tamoxifen combination.[3] Ⓑ

Breast-conserving therapy in early breast cancer appears to be as effective as mastectomy in suitable patients. More extensive mastectomy is not associated with better outcomes provided that all local disease is excised.[4,5] Ⓐ

The 20- and 25-yr follow-up results from three randomized controlled trials (RTCs) comparing different types of surgery (plus irradiation) for invasive breast cancer found no significant difference in survival between radical mastectomy and total mastectomy, between radical mastectomy and quadrantectomy, and between lumpectomy and total mastectomy.[6] Ⓐ

A metaanalysis of 10- and 20-yr results from randomized trials of radiotherapy for early breast cancer concluded that it reduces local recurrence by about two thirds. Mortality from breast cancer was significantly reduced, although other mortality was increased. Radiotherapy is likely to be favorable for younger patients with a relatively high risk of local recurrence.[7] Ⓐ

Radiotherapy given after breast-conserving surgery for DCIS reduces the risk of local recurrence and invasive carcinoma, although there is no evidence of an effect on survival.[8,9] Ⓐ

The addition of tamoxifen to radiotherapy treatment following breast-conserving surgery for DCIS confers no overall survival advantage over radiotherapy alone.[10-12] Ⓐ

Radiotherapy reduces the risk of local recurrence when used after breast-conserving surgery.[5] Ⓐ

Radiotherapy to the chest wall after mastectomy reduces the risk of local recurrence by two thirds and also reduces the risk of mortality from breast cancer at 10 yr.[5] Ⓐ

Radiotherapy plus tamoxifen significantly reduces the risk of breast and axillary recurrence after lumpectomy in women with small, node-negative, hormone-receptor-positive breast cancers when compared with tamoxifen alone but does not improve overall survival.[13,14]

Adjuvant polychemotherapy improves 10-yr survival rates in patients with nonmetastatic breast cancer. The benefit is most marked in younger women.[15] Ⓐ

Chemotherapy reduces the rate of any kind of recurrence.[16] Ⓐ

There is no evidence that longer chemotherapy regimens (8 to 12 mo) are more beneficial than shorter regimens (4 to 6 mo).[16] Ⓐ

High-dose chemotherapy with autograft may improve early progression-free survival compared with conventional chemotherapy, but the side effects are significant, and there is no evidence of benefit in overall survival.[17] Ⓐ

Metastatic breast cancer

Two nonsystematic reviews of 86 RCTs of patients with metastatic breast cancer found the overall objective response rate to tamoxifen to be 34%. A further 20% achieved disease stabilization. The overall median duration of response was 12 to 18 mo.[18,19] Ⓐ

Progestins, such as megestrol, appear to be as effective as tamoxifen as first-line hormonal therapy in metastatic breast cancer, although they are not so well tolerated.[20] Ⓐ

Progestins, such as megestrol, appear to be less effective than selective aromatase inhibitors as second-line therapy in patients whose cancers are unresponsive to tamoxifen.[20] Ⓐ

Aromatase inhibitors have been shown to be at least as effective as tamoxifen as first-line therapy in metastatic breast disease, and in certain patient groups they may be more effective.[20] Ⓐ

Aromatase inhibitors have been shown to be more effective than progestins and aminoglutethimide as non-first-line therapy in metastatic breast disease.[20] Ⓐ

Combined therapy with goserelin plus tamoxifen in metastatic breast cancer is associated with significant improvement in progression-free survival and overall survival compared with therapy with goserelin alone.[21] Ⓐ

Gonadorelin analogs and surgical oophorectomy appear to be equally effective as first-line treatment in premenopausal patients with metastatic breast cancer.[22,23] Ⓐ

First-line chemotherapy in patients with metastatic breast cancer has been found to be associated with an objective tumor response in 40% to 60% of women. Complete remission may be achieved in a small proportion of women.[20] Ⓐ

First-line nontaxane combination chemotherapy provides no survival advantage over hormonal treatment with tamoxifen or progestins in women with metastatic breast cancer.[24] Ⓐ

Taxane-containing combination chemotherapy appears more effective than non-taxane-containing regimens in women with metastatic disease.[25] Ⓐ

High-dose chemotherapy with autograft provides a significant improvement in early progression-free survival compared with conventional chemotherapy but no benefit in overall survival.[26] Ⓐ

In women with bone metastases, bisphosphonates reduce the risk of developing a skeletal event and also the skeletal event rate. They increase the time to a skeletal event. They may reduce bone pain.[27] Ⓐ

Evidence-Based References

1. Early Breast Cancer Trialists' Collaborative Group: Tamoxifen for early breast cancer, *Cochrane Database Sys Rev* Issue 1, 2001. Ⓐ
2. Early Breast Cancer Trialists' Collaborative Group: Tamoxifen for early breast cancer: an overview of the randomized trials, *Lancet* 351:1451, 1998. Ⓐ
3. Jakesz R et al: Randomized adjuvant trial of tamoxifen and goserelin versus cyclophosphamide, methotrexate, and fluorouracil: evidence for the superiority of treatment with endocrine blockade in premenopausal patients with hormone-responsive breast cancer. Austrian Breast and Colorectal Cancer Study Group Trial 5, *J Clin Oncol* 20:4621, 2002. Ⓑ
4. Early Breast Cancer Trialists' Collaborative Group: Effects of radiotherapy and surgery in early breast cancer: an overview of the randomized trials, *N Engl J Med* 333:1444, 1995. Ⓐ
5. Morris AD et al: Breast conserving therapy versus mastectomy in early stage breast cancer: a meta-analysis of 10 year survival, *Cancer J Sci Am* 3:6, 1997. Ⓐ
6. Dixon JM et al: Breast cancer (non-metastatic), *Clin Evid* 11:2300, 2004. Ⓐ
7. Early Breast Cancer Trialists' Collaborative Group: Radiotherapy for early breast cancer, *Cochrane Database Sys Rev* Issue 2, 2002. Ⓐ
8. Fisher B et al: Lumpectomy and radiation therapy for the treatment of intraductal breast cancer: findings of the National Surgical Adjuvant Breast and Bowel Project B-17, *J Clin Oncol* 16:441, 1998. Ⓐ
9. Julien JP et al: Radiotherapy in breast-conserving treatment for ductal carcinoma in situ; first results of EORTC randomized phase III trial 10853, *Lancet* 355:528, 2000. Ⓐ
10. Fisher B et al: Tamoxifen in treatment of intraductal breast cancer: National Surgical Adjuvant Breast and Bowel Project B-24 randomized controlled trial, *Lancet* 353:1993, 1999. Ⓐ
11. Allred D et al: Estrogen receptor expression as a positive marker of the effectiveness of tamoxifen in the treatment of DCIS: findings from NSABP Protocol B-24, San Antonio Breast Cancer Symposium, 2002. Reviewed in: *Clin Evid* 11:2300, 2004. Ⓐ
12. Houghton J et al: Radiotherapy and tamoxifen in women with completely excised ductal carcinoma in situ of the breast in the UK, Australia, and New Zealand: randomized controlled trial, *Lancet* 362:95, 2003. Ⓐ
13. Hughes KS et al: Lumpectomy plus tamoxifen with or without irradiation in women 70 years of age or older with early breast cancer, *N Engl J Med* 351:971, 2004.
14. Fyles AW et al: Tamoxifen with or without breast irradiation in women 50 years of age or older with early breast cancer, *N Engl J Med* 351:963, 2004.
15. Early Breast Cancer Trialists' Collaborative Group: Multi-agent chemotherapy for early breast cancer, *Cochrane Database Sys Rev* Issue 4, 2001. Ⓐ
16. Early Breast Cancer Trialists' Collaborative Group: Polychemotherapy for early breast cancer: an overview of the randomized trials, *Lancet* 352:930, 1998. Ⓐ
17. Farquhar C et al: High dose chemotherapy and autologous bone marrow or stem cell transplantation versus conventional chemotherapy for women with early poor prognosis breast cancer, *Cochrane Database Sys Rev* Issue 1, 2003.
18. Jackson IM, Litherland S, Wakeling AE: Tamoxifen and other antioestrogens. In: Powels TJ, Smith IE (Eds), *Medical Management of Breast Cancer*, London, 1991, Martin Dunitz. Ⓐ
19. Arafah BM, Pearson OH: Endocrine treatment of advanced breast cancer. In: Jordan VC, (ed), *Estrogen/Antiestrogen Action and Breast Cancer Therapy*, Madison, 1986, University of Wisconsin Press. Ⓐ
20. Stebbing J, Glassman R: Breast cancer (metastatic), *Clin Evid* 11:2266, 2004. Ⓐ
21. Klijn JGN et al: Combined tamoxifen and luteinising hormone (LHRH) agonist versus LHRH agonist alone in premenopausal advanced breast cancer; a meta-analysis of four randomized trials, *J Clin Oncol* 19:343, 2001. Ⓐ
22. Taylor CW et al: Multicenter randomized clinical trial of goserelin versus surgical ovariectomy in premenopausal patients with receptor-positive metastatic breast cancer: an intergroup study, *J Clin Oncol* 16:994, 1998. Ⓐ
23. Boccardo F et al: Ovarian ablation versus goserelin with or without tamoxifen in pre-perimenopausal patients with advanced breast cancer: results of a multicentric Italian study, *Ann Oncol* 5:337, 1994. Ⓐ
24. Wilcken N, Hornbuckle J, Ghersi D: Chemotherapy alone versus endocrine therapy alone for metastatic breast cancer, *Cochrane Database Sys Rev* Issue 2, 2003. Ⓐ
25. Ghersi D et al: Taxane containing regimens for metastatic breast cancer, *Cochrane Database Sys Rev* Issue 3, 2003. Ⓐ
26. Farquhar C et al: High dose chemotherapy and autologous bone marrow or stem cell transplantation versus conventional chemotherapy for women with metastatic breast cancer, *Cochrane Database Sys Rev* Issue 4, 2002. Ⓐ
27. Pavlakis N, Stockler M: Bisphosphonates for breast cancer, *Cochrane Database Sys Rev* Issue 1, 2002. Ⓐ

SUGGESTED READINGS

Boyd NF et al: Heritability of mammographic density, a risk factor for breast cancer, *N Engl J Med* 347:886, 2002.

Graham J et al: Stressful life experiences and risk of relapse of breast cancer: observational cohort study, *BMJ* 324:1420, 2002.

Hellekson KL: NIH statement on adjuvant therapy for breast cancer, *Am Fam Physician* 63:1857, 2001.

Humphrey LL et al: Breast cancer screening: a summary of the evidence for the U.S. Preventive Services Task Force, *Ann Intern Med* 137:347, 2002.

Kinsinger LS et al: Chemoprevention of breast cancer: a summary of the evidence for U.S. Preventive Services Task Force, *Ann Intern Med* 137:59, 2002.

Marchbanks PA et al: Oral contraceptives and the risk of breast cancer, *N Engl J Med* 346:2025, 2002.

Miller AB et al: The Canadian National Breast Screening Study—1: breast cancer mortality after 11 to 16 years of follow-up, *Ann Intern Med* 137:305, 2002.

Pruthi S: Detection and evaluation of palpable breast mass, *Mayo Clin Proc* 76:641, 2001.

Rebbeck TR et al: Prophylactic oophorectomy in carriers of BRCA1 or BRCA2 mutations, *N Engl J Med* 346:1616, 2002.

Slamon DJ et al: Use of chemotherapy plus a monoclonal antibody against HER2 for metastatic breast cancer that overexpresses HER2, *N Engl J Med* 344(11):783, 2001.

The ATAC Trialists' Group: Anastrozole alone or in combination with tamoxifen versus tamoxifen alone for adjuvant treatment of postmenopausal women with early breast cancer: first results of the ATAC randomized trial, *Lancet* 359:2131, 2002.

U.S. Preventive Services Task Force: Chemoprevention of breast cancer. Recommendations and rationale, *Ann Intern Med* 137:56, 2002.

Van 't Veer LJ et al: Gene expression profiling predicts clinical outcome of breast cancer, *Nature* 415:530, 2002.

AUTHORS: **TAKUMA NEMOTO, M.D.**, and **RUBEN ALVERO, M.D.**

BASIC INFORMATION

DEFINITION

Breech presentation exists when the fetal longitudinal axis is such that the cephalic pole occupies the uterine fundus. Three types exist, with respective percentages at term, frank (48% to 73%, flexed hips, extended thighs), complete (4.6% to 11.5%, flexed hips and knees), and footling (12% to 38%, hips extended).

ICD-9CM CODES
652.2 Breech presentation without mention of version

EPIDEMIOLOGY & DEMOGRAPHICS

INCIDENCE: Gestational age dependent: 3% to 4% overall, 14% at 29 to 32 wk, 33% at 21 to 24 wk

PERINATAL MORTALITY: 9% to 25% or 3 to 5 times increase over vertex presentation at term. If one corrects for the associated increase in congenital anomalies and complications of prematurity, the morbidity and mortality approach that of the vertex presentation at term regardless of route of delivery.

PHYSICAL FINDINGS & CLINICAL PRESENTATION

- Lack of presenting part on vaginal examination
- Fetal heart tones heard above the umbilicus
- Leopold maneuvers revealing mobile fetal part in the uterine fundus

ETIOLOGY

- Abnormal placentation (fundal), uterine anomalies (fibroids, septa), pelvic or adnexal masses, alterations in fetal muscular tone, or fetal malformations
- Associated conditions: trisomy 13, 18, 21; Potter syndrome; myotonic dystrophy; prematurity

DIAGNOSIS

DIFFERENTIAL DIAGNOSIS

Vertex, oblique, or transverse lie

WORKUP

- Determine reason for breech presentation, history of uterine anomalies, gestational age, or associated fetal congenital anomalies.
- Assess fetal status, by either continuous fetal heart rate monitoring or ultrasound.
- Assess pelvis to determine feasibility of vaginal delivery.
- Assess risk for safety of vaginal vs. abdominal delivery.

IMAGING STUDIES

Ultrasound to evaluate for:

- Fetal anomalies, such as hydrocephalus
- Placental location
- Position of fetal head relative to spine (check for hyperextension)
- Estimated fetal weight (2500 to 3800 g)
- Type of breech (frank, complete, footling)

TREATMENT

ACUTE GENERAL Rx

- Vaginal delivery in selected patient (see Comments section): allow maternal expulsive forces to deliver fetus until scapula visible (avoiding traction); with flexion and/or Piper forceps, deliver fetal head
- Perform C-section (see "Comments")
- External cephalic version, success 60% to 75%, after 37 wk, contraindicated with placental abruption, low-lying placenta, maternal hypertension, previous uterine incision, multiple gestation, nonreassuring fetal status
- Adequate pelvic/cervical relaxation essential for vaginal breech (i.e., need anesthesia in-room during birth [delivery] with uterine relaxants on hand [NTG, terbutaline])

COMPLICATIONS

- Head entrapment: leading cause of death (with the exception of anomalous fetuses), 88 cases/1000 deliveries, avoid by maintaining flexion of fetal head, use of Piper forceps or Dührssen's incisions. Before 36 wk, HC > AC, thus fetal predisposition. Tentorial tears secondary to hyperextended head. Association with trisomy 21 in 3% to 5% of cases. Avoid hyperextension of head during delivery.
- Cord prolapse: usually occurs late in the course of labor. Incidence depends on type of breech—frank (0.5%), complete (4% to 5%), footling (10%).
- Nuchal arm: arm extended above fetal head, occurs when there is undue traction before delivery of fetal scapulas. Treatment depends on bringing trapped arm across infant's face.

DISPOSITION

If confounding variables are corrected for, such as prematurity and associated congenital anomalies (6.3% of breeches vs. 2.4% in general population), route of delivery plays a less important role in fetal outcome than previously thought.

REFERRAL

An obstetrician trained in delivery of the vaginal breech is a prerequisite for attempting vaginal route, although it must be explained to the patient that with C-section certain risks (such as hyperextension of the fetal head with resultant spinal cord injury) may be minimized but not eliminated.

PEARLS & CONSIDERATIONS

COMMENTS

For breech presentation, in general, mortality is increased thirteenfold and morbidity sevenfold. The main reasons are an increase in congenital anomalies, perinatal hypoxia, birth injury, and prematurity.

There is no contraindication to induction of labor in the breech presentation, nor is labor prohibited in a primigravida.

CRITERIA FOR TRIAL OF LABOR:

- Estimated fetal weight 2000 to 3800 g
- Frank breech
- Adequate pelvis
- Flexed fetal head
- Continuous fetal monitoring
- Normal progress of labor
- Bedside availability of anesthesia and capability for immediate C-section
- Informed consent
- Obstetrician trained in vaginal breech delivery

CRITERIA FOR C-SECTION:

- Estimated fetal weight <1500 g or >4000 g
- Footling presentation (20% risk of cord prolapse, usually late in course of labor)
- Inadequate pelvis
- Hyperextended fetal head (21% risk of spinal cord injury)
- Nonreassuring fetal status
- Abnormal progress of labor
- Lack of trained obstetrician

AUTHORS: **SCOTT J. ZUCCALA, D.O.,** and **RUBEN ALVERO, M.D.**

BASIC INFORMATION

DEFINITION

Bronchiectasis is the abnormal dilation and destruction of bronchial walls, which may be congenital or acquired.

ICD-9CM CODES
494.0 Bronchiectasis

EPIDEMIOLOGY & DEMOGRAPHICS

- Cystic fibrosis is responsible for nearly 50% of all cases of bronchiectasis.
- Acquired primary bronchiectasis is uncommon because of rapid diagnosis of pulmonary infections and frequent use of antibiotics.
- Effective childhood immunizations have led to a significant decrease in the incidence of bronchiectasis resulting from pertussis.

PHYSICAL FINDINGS & CLINICAL PRESENTATION

- Moist crackles at lung bases
- Cough with expectoration of large amount of purulent sputum
- Fever, night sweats, generalized malaise, weight loss
- Hemoptysis
- Halitosis, skin pallor
- Clubbing (infrequent)

ETIOLOGY

- Cystic fibrosis
- Lung infections (pneumonia, lung abscess, TB, fungal infections, viral infections)
- Abnormal host defense (panhypogammaglobulinemia, Kartagener's syndrome, AIDS, chemotherapy)
- Localized airway obstruction (congenital structural defects, foreign bodies, neoplasms)
- Inflammation (inflammatory pneumonitis, granulomatous lung disease, allergic aspergillosis)

DIAGNOSIS

DIFFERENTIAL DIAGNOSIS

- TB
- Asthma
- Chronic bronchitis or chronic sinusitis
- Interstitial fibrosis
- Chronic lung abscess
- Foreign body aspiration
- Cystic fibrosis
- Lung carcinoma

LABORATORY TESTS

- Sputum for Gram stain, C&S, and acid-fast bacteria (AFB)
- CBC with differential (leukocytosis with left shift, anemia)
- Serum protein electrophoresis to evaluate for hypogammaglobulinemia
- Antibody test for aspergillosis
- Sweat test in patients with suspected cystic fibrosis

IMAGING STUDIES

- Chest x-ray: hyperinflation, crowded lung markings, small cystic spaces at the base of the lungs.
- High-resolution CT scan of the chest has become the best tool to detect cystic lesions and exclude underlying obstruction from neoplasm. The CT study should be a noncontrast study with the use of 1 to 1.5 mm window every 1 cm with acquisition time of 1 sec. Typical findings on CT include dilation of airway lumen, lack of tapering of an airway toward periphery, ballooned cysts at the end of bronchus, and varicose constrictions along airways.
- Bronchoscopy may be helpful to evaluate hemoptysis, rule out obstructive lesions, and remove mucus plugs.

TREATMENT

NONPHARMACOLOGIC THERAPY

- Postural drainage (reclining prone on a bed with the head down on the side) and chest percussion with use of inflatable vests or mechanical vibrators applied to the chest may enhance removal of respiratory secretions
- Adequate hydration
- Supplemental oxygen for hypoxemia

ACUTE GENERAL Rx

- Antibiotic therapy is based on the results of sputum, Gram stain, and C&S; in patients with inadequate or inconclusive results, empiric therapy with amoxicillin/clavulanate 500 mg to 875 mg q12h, TMP-SMX q12h, doxycycline 100 mg bid, or cefuroxime 250 mg bid for 10 to 14 days is recommended.
- Bronchodilators are useful in patients with demonstrable airflow obstruction.

CHRONIC Rx

- Avoidance of tobacco
- Maintenance of proper nutrition and hydration
- Prompt identification and treatment of infections
- Pneumococcal vaccination and annual influenza vaccination

DISPOSITION

Prognosis is variable with severity of the disease and underlying etiology of bronchiectasis.

REFERRAL

Surgical referral for partial lung resection in patients with localized severe disease unresponsive to medical therapy or in patients with massive hemoptysis

EVIDENCE

There is evidence that inspiratory muscle training vs. placebo improves endurance exercise capacity in patients with bronchiectasis.[1] Ⓐ

A systematic review found a small benefit for the use of prolonged antibiotics (given with prophylactic intent) in the treatment of bronchiectasis compared with placebo. Response rates showed a significant benefit but exacerbation rates and lung function showed no difference to placebo.[2] Ⓑ

Inhaled tobramycin may result in bacterial eradication and clinical improvement for patients infected with *Pseudomonas aeruginosa.* Further studies are required to evaluate the use of inhaled tobramycin.[3] Ⓑ

Although there is no clear evidence sufficient to guide clinical practice, regular inhaled corticosteroids may improve lung function in patients with bronchiectasis. Further studies are required.[4] Ⓐ

There is not enough evidence to evaluate the routine use of mucolytics for bronchiectasis.[5]

We are unable to cite any evidence that meets our criteria for the effectiveness of long-acting bronchodilator or short-acting bronchodilator therapy in the management of bronchiectasis.

The evidence for bronchopulmonary hygiene physical therapy is insufficient. No effect on pulmonary function was seen in most comparison studies apart from improved sputum clearance.[6]

We were unable to cite any evidence that meets our criteria concerning the efficacy of surgical intervention for bronchiectasis.

Evidence-Based References

1. Bradley J, Moran F, Greenstone M: Physical training for bronchiectasis, *Cochrane Database Sys Rev* Issue 1, 2000. Ⓐ
2. Evans DJ, Bara AI, Greenstone M: Prolonged antibiotics for purulent bronchiectasis, *Cochrane Database Sys Rev* Issue 2, 2002. Ⓑ
3. Barker AF et al: Tobramycin solution for inhalation reduces sputum *Pseudomonas aeruginosa* density in bronchiectasis, *Am J Respir Crit Care Med* 162:481, 2000. Ⓑ
4. Ram FSF, Wells A, Kolbe J: Inhaled steroids for bronchiectasis, *Cochrane Database Sys Rev* Issue 2, 2000. Ⓐ
5. Crockett AJ et al: Mucolytics for bronchiectasis, *Cochrane Database Sys Rev* Issue 1, 2001.
6. Jones AP, Rowe BH: Bronchopulmonary hygiene physical therapy for chronic obstructive pulmonary disease and bronchiectasis, *Cochrane Database Sys Rev* Issue 4, 1998. Ⓑ

SUGGESTED READING

Barker AF: Bronchiectasis, *N Engl J Med* 346:1383, 2002.

AUTHOR: **FRED F. FERRI, M.D.**

BASIC INFORMATION

DEFINITION

Brucellosis is a zoonotic infection caused by one of four species of *Brucella*. It commonly presents as a nondescript febrile illness.

SYNONYMS

Malta fever, ungulate fever
Bang's disease

ICD-9CM CODES
023.9 Brucellosis

EPIDEMIOLOGY & DEMOGRAPHICS

INCIDENCE (IN U.S.): About 100 cases/yr (may be underreported)
PREDOMINANT SEX: Male
PREDOMINANT AGE: Adult
CONGENITAL INFECTION: Recent evidence suggests a high rate of spontaneous abortions in untreated pregnant women during the first and second trimesters.
NEONATAL INFECTION: Can occur if mother is infected during pregnancy.

PHYSICAL FINDINGS & CLINICAL PRESENTATION

- Incubation period is 1 wk to 3 mo.
- Patients may be asymptomatic or have nonspecific symptoms such as fever, sweats, malaise, weight loss, depression, arthralgia, and arthritis.
- Fever is the most common finding.
- Hepatomegaly, splenomegaly, or lymphadenopathy is possible.
- Localized disease includes endocarditis, meningitis, spondylitis, sacroiliitis, and osteomyelitis (especially vertebral).

Chronic hepatosplenic suppurative brucellosis (CHSB) presents with hepatic or splenic abscesses. This form is thought to be a reactivation and can occur years after the acute infection.

ETIOLOGY

- Caused by infection with *Brucella* species:
  1. Most commonly *B. melitensis,* but also *suis, abortus,* or *canis*
  2. A small, gram-negative coccobacillus
- Acquired through ingestion of organisms (unpasteurized goat or cow's milk), breaks in the skin, or by inhalation.
- Most cases occur after exposure to animals (sheep, goats, swine, cattle, or dogs), or animal products (i.e., milk, hides, tissue).
- Most cases (in U.S.) occur in men with occupational exposure to animals (farmers, ranchers, laboratory workers, veterinarians, abattoir workers).

DIAGNOSIS

DIFFERENTIAL DIAGNOSIS

Many febrile conditions without localizing manifestations (i.e., TB, endocarditis, typhoid fever, malaria, autoimmune diseases)

WORKUP

- Cultures of blood, bone marrow, or other tissue (lymph node, liver) should be sent and held for 4 wk, because *Brucella* spp. grow slowly in vitro.
- Granulomas on biopsy are suggestive of diagnosis.

LABORATORY TESTS

- WBC count: normal or low
- Serology:
  1. Serum agglutination test (SAT) to detect antibodies to *B. abortus, melitensis,* and *suis.*
  2. Specific antibody test to identify antibodies to *B. canis.*
  3. False-negative SAT possibly resulting from a prozone effect.
  4. PCR (polymerase chain reaction) for *Brucella* spp. specific 16S rRNA or DNA sequences are increasingly used for the diagnosis of brucellosis from blood, tissue samples, and bone marrow.

IMAGING STUDIES

- Radiographs to show splenic or hepatic calcifications in chronic disease
- Bone scan, MRI, and radiographs of the spine to suggest osteomyelitis
- Ultrasound or CT scan of the abdomen to show an enlarged liver or spleen
- Echocardiogram to reveal vegetations in endocarditis

TREATMENT

NONPHARMACOLOGIC THERAPY

- Drainage of abscesses
- Valve replacement for endocarditis

ACUTE GENERAL Rx

Combination antibiotics required:

- Doxycycline 100 mg po bid plus streptomycin 15 mg/kg IM qd for 6 wk
- Less effective: doxycycline 100 mg po bid plus rifampin 600 mg po qd or sulfamethoxazole 800 mg/trimethoprim 160 mg one DS tablet po qid, ciprofloxacin 500 mg bid for 6 weeks along with doxycycline or rifampin as an alternative regimen

Courses <6 wk are associated with higher relapse rates; longer courses are recommended for complicated disease (e.g., osteomyelitis, endocarditis, and neurobrucellosis).

DISPOSITION

- Relapse is possible weeks to months after the completion of therapy.
- Reactivation with CHSB has been reported up to 35 yr after initial illness.

REFERRAL

For all cases to an infectious disease specialist

PEARLS & CONSIDERATIONS

COMMENTS

- Alert the microbiology laboratory to the possibility of *Brucella* spp. (prolonged incubation needed and biohazard for laboratory personnel).
- Do not use doxycycline in children or pregnant women.
- Avoid aminoglycosides in pregnant women.

EVIDENCE

A doxycycline-rifampin combination therapy for 45 days is as effective as the classic doxycycline-streptomycin combination in most patients with brucellosis.[1]

Doxycycline-rifampin therapy may be less effective in patients with spondylitis.[1]

Streptomycin plus doxycycline therapy is associated with higher success rates (judged by the frequency of treatment failure and relapse following therapy) than combinations of rifampin and doxycycline.[2]

Oral rifampin plus oral doxycycline for 45 days has a high cure rate, as does oral doxycycline for 45 days plus intramuscular streptomycin for 21 days.[3]

Regimens containing streptomycin yielded favorable results in clinical study.[4]

Rifampin plus trimethoprim-sulfamethoxazole is associated with low relapse rates ranging from 4% to 8% in patients receiving therapy for 3 or 5 weeks and no relapses in patients treated for 8 weeks.[5]

Evidence-Based References

1. Ariza J et al: Treatment of human brucellosis with doxycycline plus rifampin or doxycycline plus streptomycin, *Ann Intern Med* 117:25-30, 1992.
2. Luzzi GA et al: Brucellosis: imported and laboratory acquired cases, and an overview of treatment trials, *Trans R Soc Trop Med Hyg* 87:138-141, 1993.
3. Acocella G et al: Comparison of three different regimens in the treatment of acute brucellosis: a multinational study, *J Antimicrob Agents Chemother* 23:433-439, 1989.
4. Montejo JM et al: Open, randomized therapeutic trial of six antimicrobial regimens in the treatment of human brucellosis, *Clin Infect Dis* 16:671-676, 1993.
5. Lubani et al: A multicenter therapeutic study of 1100 children with brucellosis, *Ped Infect Dis J* 8:75-78, 1989.

SUGGESTED READING

Pappas et al: Brucellosis, *N Engl J Med* 352:2335, 2005.

AUTHORS: **GLENN G. FORT, M.D., M.P.H., DENNIS J. MIKOLICH, M.D.,** and **MAURICE POLICAR, M.D.**

BASIC INFORMATION

DEFINITION

Forcible clenching or grinding of the teeth during sleep or wakefulness, often leading to damage of the teeth.

ICD-9CM CODES
306.8 Bruxism

EPIDEMIOLOGY & DEMOGRAPHICS

- Occurs in 15% of children and 75% of adults
- Occasionally familial cases have been described.
- Bruxism often presents between 10 and 20 yr of age but may persist throughout life.
- Nocturnal bruxism is noted most often during stages I and II NREM sleep and REM sleep.

PHYSICAL FINDINGS & CLINICAL PRESENTATION

Complaints of grinding of teeth from sleep partner or members of the family. In many cases, the masticatory system will adapt to the phenomenon, but in severe cases nearly every part of the masticatory system may be damaged. Excessive wearing of dentition is the most common physical finding. Tender or hypoatrophied masticatory muscles may also be observed.

ETIOLOGY

- Cause is quite controversial.
- Possible causes in the literature include occlusal discrepancies, anatomy of the bony structures of the orofacial region, part of the sleep arousal response, disturbances of the central dopaminergic system, smoking, alcohol, drugs, stress, and personality.

DIAGNOSIS

DIFFERENTIAL DIAGNOSIS

- Dental compression syndrome
- Temporomandibular joint disorders
- Chronic orofacial pain disorders
- Oral motor disorders
- Malocclusion

WORKUP

- History should have an emphasis on sleep habits, including excessive snoring, pain in the temporal mandibular region, interview with close family members, health habits, personality quirks.
- Physical examination of the teeth and masticatory muscles is mandatory.
- Sleep studies in selected cases may be helpful.

LABORATORY TESTS

None indicated unless a systemic disease suspected (e.g., infection, autoimmune)

IMAGING STUDIES

X-ray studies of teeth and temporomandibular joints

TREATMENT

NONPHARMACOLOGIC THERAPY

Biofeedback, psychological counseling, and elimination of harmful health habits have been used with limited success.

GENERAL Rx

- Oral splints (Fig. 1-40); a nightguard to protect teeth may be useful
- Correction of malocclusion
- Pain management (e.g., gabapentin, ibuprofen)
- Medication to relieve anxiety and improve sleep (e.g., benzodiazepine or trazodone at hs)
- Local injections of botulinum toxin into masseter muscles may be used to prevent dental and temporomandibular joint complications.

DISPOSITION

Referral to dentist mandatory if damage to teeth evident.

PEARLS & CONSIDERATIONS

- Like any poorly understood disease, treatment is often unsatisfactory and subject to quackery.
- Both diurnal and nocturnal bruxism may be associated with various movement and degenerative disorders (e.g., Huntington's disease, oromandibular dystonia) and are very common in children with cerebral palsy and mental retardation.

SUGGESTED READINGS

Attansio R: An overview of bruxism and its management, *Dent Clin North Am* 41(2):229, 1997.

Dae TT, Lavigne EJ: Oral splints: the crutches for temporomandibular disorders and bruxism, *Crit Rev Oral Biol Med* 9(3):345, 1998.

Lopbezoo F, Naeije M: Bruxism is mainly regulated centrally, not peripherally, *J Oral Rehabil* 28(12):1085, 2001.

Tan EK, Jankovic J: Treating severe bruxism with botulinum toxin, *J Am Dent Assoc* 131:211, 2000.

AUTHOR: **FRED F. FERRI, M.D.**

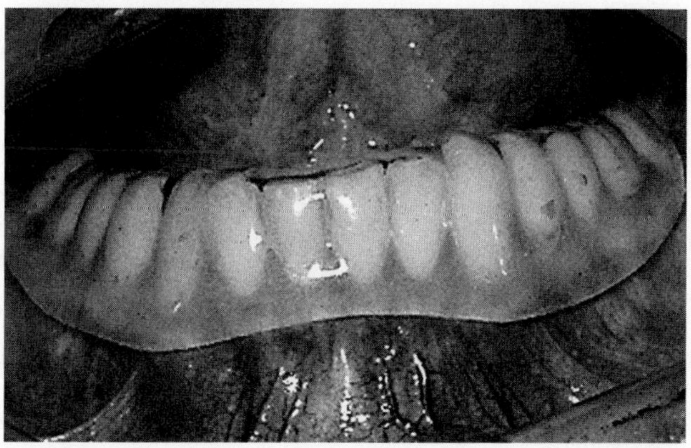

FIGURE 1-40 Occlusal splint. (From Hochberg MC, Silman AJ, Smolen JS, Weinblatt ME, Weisman MH [eds]: *Rheumatology,* ed 3, St. Louis, 2003, Mosby.)

BASIC INFORMATION

DEFINITION

Budd-Chiari syndrome (BCS) is a rare disease defined by the obstruction of hepatic venous outflow anywhere from the small hepatic veins to the junction of the inferior vena cava (IVC) and the right atrium. Primary BCS is defined by endoluminal obstruction as seen in thromboses or webs. Secondary BCS is when the obstruction is caused by nonvascular invasion (malignancy or parasitic masses) or extrinsic compression (tumor, abscess, cysts).

SYNONYMS

Hepatic vein thrombosis
Obliterative endophlebitis of the hepatic veins
Obliterative hepatocavopathy

ICD-9CM CODES
453.0 Budd-Chiari syndrome

EPIDEMIOLOGY & DEMOGRAPHICS

BCS is a rare disorder. Women are more commonly affected and presentation is usually in the third and fourth decades of life. Clinical presentation and characteristics vary with geography. IVC thrombosis in Africa and South Asia is more often associated with intravascular webs, and 45% to 50% ultimately develop hepatocellular carcinoma even in the absence of cirrhosis. In the U.S., BCS is more commonly associated with primary myeloproliferative disorders, underlying hypercoagulable states, although IVC membranes and tumors are also seen. Underlying factors contributing to BCS can be identified in approximately 75% of cases, and the finding of multiple causes in the same patient is quite common.

CLINICAL PRESENTATION

Variable according to the degree, location, acuity of obstruction, and presence of collateral circulation:

- Fulminant/Acute: (20%) severe right upper quadrant abdominal pain, fever, nausea, vomiting, jaundice, hepatomegaly, ascites, marked elevation in serum aminotransferases, elevation of alkaline phosphatase to 300 to 400 IU/L, decrease in coagulation factors, and encephalopathy. Early recognition and treatment are essential to survival.
- Subacute/Chronic: (60%) vague abdominal discomfort, gradual progression to caudate lobe hypertrophy with atrophy of the rest of the liver, portal hypertension with or without cirrhosis and its sequelae, ascites, lower extremity edema, esophageal varices, splenomegaly, coagulopathy, hepatorenal syndrome in up to half of patients, hepatopulmonary syndrome in up to 28% of patients and, rarely, encephalopathy.
- Asymptomatic: (5% to 20%) usually discovered incidentally by abnormal liver function tests.

ETIOLOGY

Myeloproliferative disease—often discovered in cases of initially idiopathic BCS, 20% to 53%

- Polycythemia vera, responsible for 10% to 40% of cases
- Essential thrombocytosis
- Myelofibrosis
- *JAK2* mutations associated with many myeloproliferative disorders are now being implicated in cases of idiopathic BCS

Hypercoagulable states—often coexist with other causes, up to 31%

- Protein C deficiency
- Protein S deficiency
- Antithrombin III deficiency
- Prothrombin gene mutation
- Methylene-tetrahydrofolate reductase mutation
- Antiphospholipid antibody syndrome
- Hyperhomocysteinemia
- Activated protein C resistance/Factor V Leiden mutation—in as many as 30% of all BCS cases and usually in cases of:
  - Pregnancy
  - Oral contraceptive pills
- Sickle cell anemia
- Infection:
  - Liver abscess (amebic)
  - Filariasis
  - Schistosomiasis
  - Hydatid cyst (echinococcosis)
  - Syphilis
  - Tuberculosis
  - Aspergillosis
- Malignancy (<5%)
  - Adrenal carcinoma
  - Ovarian
  - Bronchogenic
  - Renal cell carcinoma
  - Hepatocellular carcinoma
  - Intrahepatic cholangiocarcinoma
  - Leiomyosarcoma
  - Metastatic cancer
- Other:
  - Sarcoid
  - Behçet's disease
  - Paroxysmal nocturnal hemoglobinuria (PNH)—hepatic vein thrombosis in up to 12% of patients; leading cause of mortality in PNH
  - IVC membrane/congenital web
  - Abdominal trauma
  - Ulcerative colitis
  - Celiac disease
  - Dacarbazine therapy
  - Idiopathic

DIAGNOSIS

DIFFERENTIAL DIAGNOSIS

- Shock liver/ischemic hepatitis
- Viral hepatitis
- Toxic hepatitis
- Alcoholic hepatitis
- Cholecystitis
- Hepatic venoocclusive disease (sinusoidal obstruction syndrome)
- Congestive hepatopathy, also known as cardiac cirrhosis
  - Tricuspid regurgitation
  - Right atrial myxoma
  - Constrictive pericarditis
- Cirrhosis of other etiologies:
  - Alcoholic cirrhosis
  - Wilson's disease
  - Hemochromatosis
  - Alpha-1-antitrypsin deficiency
  - Autoimmune

LABORATORY TESTS

- Assessment of liver injury and function: serum aminotransferases, prothrombin time, albumin, bilirubin.
- Diagnostic tests (directed by history): CBC, bone marrow biopsy, viral hepatitis panel, alpha-1 antitrypsin, serum iron, transferrin saturation, alkaline phosphatase, ceruloplasmin, toxicology screen, antismooth muscle antibody, antimitochondrial antibody, and double-stranded DNA antibody. Tests for hypercoagulable states (particularly protein C, protein S, and antithrombin deficiencies) may be difficult to interpret in the setting of liver dysfunction but levels <20% of normal are suggestive of a true deficiency. Evaluation of ascitic fluid reveals a high serum-ascitic fluid albumin gradient (SAAG), mimicking the ascitic fluid in patients with cardiac disease.

IMAGING STUDIES

- Diagnosis of BCS is made by radiographic imaging.
- Ultrasound, color and pulsed Doppler, is the first-line test. Diagnostic sensitivity and specificity of 85% to 90%. Findings include nonvisualization of or abnormal flow in the hepatic veins; large intrahepatic collateral vessels; enlarged, stenotic, or tortuous hepatic veins; and caudate lobe hypertrophy.
- MRI with gadolinium contrast—better than contrast-enhanced CT, with a sensitivity/specificity of about 90%—is the second-line test. Findings include large, intrahepatic, comma-shaped collaterals, and caudate lobe hypertrophy.
- CT image reconstruction of vasculature is becoming available.
- Venography—not essential for diagnosis but when done with measurement of pressure gradients is mainly indi-

cated to predict success of percutaneous or surgical shunt intervention. Confirms the classic spider web pattern caused by collateral venous flow.

- Liver biopsy—not necessary to diagnose BCS but may be helpful in patients with cirrhosis in whom the diagnosis remains uncertain and the differential still includes sinusoidal obstruction syndrome, cirrhosis of other origins, and malignancy. Findings include hepatic congestion, hepatocyte necrosis and fibrosis in centrilobular areas, and compensatory nodular regenerative hyperplasia with progression to fibrosis and cirrhosis. In advanced BCS, may also see infarction owing to concomitant thrombosis of the intrahepatic, extrahepatic, and portal veins.

TREATMENT

Rx

NONPHARMACOLOGIC THERAPY

- Goal of therapy is decompression of hepatic congestion.
- In general, therapeutic procedures should be introduced by order of increasing invasiveness based on response/failure to therapy rather than disease severity.

ACUTE GENERAL Rx

- Anticoagulation, first with low-molecular-weight heparin (LMWH), followed by coumadin, even in the absence of an underlying hypercoagulable disorder.
- In-situ thrombolysis.
- Balloon angioplasty—complicated by 50% restenosis rate.
- Stenting—may improve long-term patency rates to 90%, but if placed above the intrahepatic IVC, may complicate future liver transplantation.
- Transjugular intrahepatic portosystemic shunt (TIPS) has been used successfully in the emergent setting of fulminant hepatic failure and is growing in use despite 50% long-term patency rates.
- Surgical portal systemic shunts—may be difficult to find a surgeon experienced enough to perform these.
- Liver transplant may be indicated for patients that fail the previous therapies or have advanced liver dysfunction.
- Supportive measures.

CHRONIC Rx

- Lifelong anticoagulation. Warfarin therapy with a target INR 2 to 3. Lessens, but does not completely prevent, recurrence.
- Treatment of underlying myeloproliferative or other disorders.
- Treatment of liver dysfunction and complications related to portal hypertension, such as ascites.
- Invasive interventions should be reserved for symptomatic patients who do not improve with medical therapy.
- Management of shunt thrombosis, which is a common complication.
- Liver transplantation.

DISPOSITION

Prognosis is variable and dependent on multiple factors including time to recognition and treatment, etiology, acuity, the type of intervention, and the condition of the patient at the time of treatment. Overall mortality rates are decreasing with the use of anticoagulation and early diagnosis of asymptomatic cases. Survival has been reported as 77%, 65%, and 57% at 1, 5, and 10 years from diagnosis. A prognostic index called the Rotterdam BCS Index has been described: 1.27× encephalopathy + 1.04× ascites + 0.72× PT + 0.004× bilirubin. Encephalopathy and ascites are scored as 1 for present or 0 as absent, and PT is scored as greater (1) or less than (0) an INR of 2.3. An index of <1.1 correlates to low risk (5-yr survival of 89%); 1.1 to 1.5 with intermediate risk (5-yr survival of 74%); and >1.5 with high risk (5-yr survival of 42%).

REFERRAL

Fulminant presentations should immediately be referred to a center capable of liver transplantation. All cases benefit from referral to a hepatologist, hematologist, an interventional radiologist, and a surgeon specializing in hepatobiliary disease.

PEARLS & CONSIDERATIONS

!

COMMENTS

- Look for one or more underlying causes, especially hypercoagulable or hematologic disorders.
- Diagnosis relies on imaging, beginning with Doppler ultrasound.
- Treatment with anticoagulation comes first, followed by invasive interventions as needed.
- Referral for liver transplantation may be necessary.
- Prognosis is dependent on presence of ascites, encephalopathy, prothrombin time, and serum bilirubin levels.

PREVENTION

In the setting of known risk factors such as a hypercoagulable state or myeloproliferative disorder, any additional risks, such as smoking or oral contraceptive therapy, should be avoided.

SUGGESTED READINGS

Bayraktar UD et al: Hepatic outflow obstruction: three similar syndromes, *World J Gastroenterol* 13(13):1912-1927, 2007.

Bogin V et al: Budd-Chiari syndrome: in evolution, *Eur J Gastroenterol Hepatol* 17:33-35, 2005.

Janssen HLA et al: Budd Chiari syndrome: a review by an expert panel, *J Hepatol* 38(3):364, 2003.

Menon KVN et al: The Budd-Chiari syndrome, *N Engl J Med* 350(6):578, 2004.

Murad SD et al: Determinants of survival and the effects of portosystemic shunting in patients with Budd-Chiari Syndrome, *Hepatology* 39:500-508, 2004.

Valla DC: The diagnosis and management of the Budd-Chiari syndrome: consensus and controversies, *Hepatology* 38(4):793, 2003.

AUTHOR: **JENNIFER ROH HUR, M.D.**

BASIC INFORMATION

DEFINITION

Bulimia nervosa is a prolonged illness characterized by a specific psychopathology.

ICD-9CM CODES
783.6 Bulimia

EPIDEMIOLOGY & DEMOGRAPHICS

INCIDENCE/PREVALENCE: Affects 1% to 3% of female adolescents and young adults

PREDOMINANT SEX: Female:male ratio of 10:1

PREDOMINANT AGE: Adolescence to young adulthood; mean age of onset: 17 yr

PHYSICAL FINDINGS & CLINICAL PRESENTATION

- Parotid and salivary gland swelling
- Scars on the back of the hand and knuckles (Russell's sign) from rubbing against the upper incisors when inducing vomiting
- Eroded enamel, particularly on the lingual surface of the upper teeth; pyorrhea and other gum disorders possible
- Petechial hemorrhages of the cornea, soft palate, or face possibly noted after vomiting
- Loss of gag reflex, well-developed abdominal musculature
- Usually no emaciation; normal physical examination possible

ETIOLOGY

- Etiology is unknown but likely multifactorial (sociocultural, psychologic, familial factors).
- Bulimia is much more common in Western societies where there is a strong cultural pressure to be slender.
- According to the American Psychiatric Association, patients with eating disorders display a broad range of symptoms that occur along a continuum between those of anorexia nervosa and bulimia.

DIAGNOSIS

DIFFERENTIAL DIAGNOSIS

- Schizophrenia
- GI disorders
- Neurologic disorders (seizures, Kleine-Levin syndrome, Klüver-Bucy syndrome)
- Brain neoplasms
- Psychogenic vomiting

WORKUP

- The following questions are useful to screen patients for bulimia:
  1. "Are you satisfied with your eating habits?"
  2. "Do you ever eat in secret?"
- Answering "no" to the first question and/or "yes" to the second question has 100% sensitivity and 90% specificity for bulimia. The SCOFF questionnaire can also be used as a screening tool for eating disorders (see "Anorexia Nervosa").
- A diagnosis can be made using the following DSM-IV diagnostic criteria for bulimia nervosa:
  1. Recurrent episodes of binge eating (rapid consumption of a large amount of food in a discrete period)
  2. A feeling of lack of control over eating behavior during the eating binges
  3. Self-induced vomiting, use of laxatives or diuretics, strict dieting or fasting, or rigorous exercise to prevent weight gain
  4. A minimum of two binge-eating episodes a week for at least 3 mo
  5. Persistent overconcern with body shape and weight

LABORATORY TESTS

- Electrolyte abnormalities secondary to vomiting (hypokalemia and metabolic alkalosis) or to diarrhea from laxative abuse (hypokalemia and hyperchloremic metabolic acidosis)
- Hyponatremia, hypocalcemia, hypomagnesemia (caused by laxative abuse)
- Elevated cortisol, decreased LH, decreased FSH

TREATMENT

NONPHARMACOLOGIC THERAPY

- Cognitive behavioral therapy to control abnormal behaviors
- Use of food diaries, nutritional counseling, and planning meals at least a day in advance is useful to counter abnormal eating behaviors
- Correction of electrolyte abnormalities

ACUTE GENERAL Rx

- SSRIs are generally considered to be the safest medication option in these patients. They are useful in severely depressed patients and in those who fail to benefit from cognitive behavioral therapy.
- Prompt recognition and treatment of complications:
  1. Ipecac cardiotoxicity from laxative abuse
  2. Electrolyte abnormalities (see "Laboratory Tests")
  3. Esophagitis and Mallory-Weiss tears; esophageal rupture from repeated vomiting
  4. Aspiration pneumonia and pneumomediastinum
  5. Menstrual irregularities (including amenorrhea)
  6. GI abnormalities: acute gastric dilatation, pancreatitis, abdominal pain, constipation

CHRONIC Rx

- Psychotherapy continued for years and focused specifically on self-image and family and peer interactions is an integral part of successful recovery.
- Family therapy is also recommended, especially in younger patients.

DISPOSITION

Course is variable and marked by frequent recurrence of exacerbations.

REFERRAL

- In addition to the primary care physician, the multidisciplinary team should include a dietician, a psychiatrist, and a family therapist.
- Hospitalization should be considered for patients with severe electrolyte abnormalities or those with suicidal thoughts.

PEARLS & CONSIDERATIONS

COMMENTS

- Bulimia has a close association with depression, bipolar disorder, obsessive-compulsive disorder, alcoholism, and substance abuse.
- Bulimia should be considered in all patients (especially adolescents) with unexplained hypokalemia and metabolic alkalosis.

EVIDENCE

A systematic review, which currently includes six trials with tricyclics, five with fluoxetine, five with monoamine oxidase inhibitors, and three with other classes of drugs (mianserin, trazodone and bupropion), found that antidepressants were associated with a more frequent remission of bulimic episodes. There was no significant difference between different classes of antidepressants.[1] Ⓐ

Evidence-Based Reference

1. Bacaltchuk J, Hay P: Antidepressants versus placebo for people with bulimia nervosa, *Cochrane Database Sys Rev* Issue 4, 2003. Ⓐ

SUGGESTED READINGS

American Psychiatric Association: Practice guideline for the treatment of patients with eating disorders, *Am J Psychiatry* 157(suppl): 4, 2000.

Mehler PS: Bulimia nervosa, *N Engl J Med* 349:875, 2003.

Prits SD, Susman J: Diagnosis of eating disorders in primary care, *Am Fam Physician* 67:297, 2003.

AUTHOR: **FRED F. FERRI, M.D.**

BASIC INFORMATION

DEFINITION

Bullous pemphigoid refers to an autoimmune, subepidermal blistering disease that is commonly seen in the elderly.

SYNONYMS

Subepidermal autoimmune bullous dermatoses

ICD-9CM CODES
694.5 Pemphigoid

EPIDEMIOLOGY & DEMOGRAPHICS

- Commonly seen in people over age 70 yr
- Incidence 10 cases/1 million persons/yr
- Equal prevalence in males and females
- No racial predilection
- Most common of the autoimmune bullous dermatoses

PHYSICAL FINDINGS & CLINICAL PRESENTATION

History:
- Bullous pemphigoid typically starts as an eczematous or urticarial rash on the extremities.
- Blisters form between 1 week and several months.

Physical findings:
- Anatomic distribution
  1. Flexor surfaces of the arms, legs, groin, axilla, and lower abdomen
  2. Spares the head and neck
  3. Rare involvement of mucous membranes

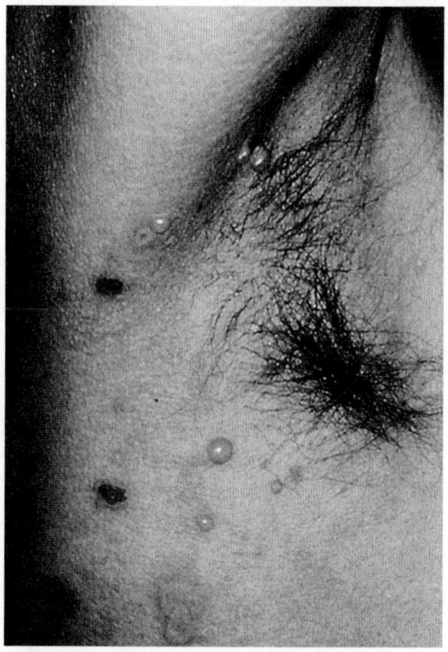

FIGURE 1-41 Bullous pemphigoid. Note intact bullae with erosions in aflexural distribution. (From Goldstein BG, Goldstein AO: *Practical dermatology,* ed 2, St Louis, 1997, Mosby.)

- Lesion configuration
  1. May be localized to the extremities or generalized
  2. Lesions irregularly grouped but sometimes can be serpiginous (Fig. 1-41)
- Lesion morphology
  1. Blistering bullae are characteristic findings, measuring anywhere from 5 mm to 2 cm in diameter
  2. Contains clear or bloody fluid
  3. Arises from normal skin or from an erythematous base
  4. Heals without scarring if denuded

ETIOLOGY

- Autoimmune disease with IgG and/or C3 complement components reacting with antigens located in the epidermal basement membrane zone.
- Drug-induced pemphigoid, although rare, can occur in patients taking penicillamine, furosemide, captopril, penicillin, and sulfasalazine.

DIAGNOSIS

A skin biopsy is required to make the diagnosis. Biopsies are characteristically sent for staining and immunofluorescence.

DIFFERENTIAL DIAGNOSIS

- Cicatricial pemphigoid
- Epidermolysis bullosa acquisita
- Pemphigus
- Pemphigoid nodularis

LABORATORY TESTS

- Antibodies to the basement membrane zone are detected in the serum in 70% of patients with bullous pemphigoid.
- Skin biopsy staining with hematoxylin and eosin reveals subepidermal blisters.
- Direct and indirect immunofluorescence studies to detect the presence of IgG and C3 immune complexes.
- Immunoelectron microscopy also reveals immune deposits on the basement membrane zone.

TREATMENT

Is a self-limited disease, but may last from months to years. Treatment is based on the degree of involvement and rate of disease progression.

NONPHARMACOLOGIC THERAPY

- Avoid scratching.
- Use mild soaps and emollients after bathing to prevent dryness of the skin.

ACUTE GENERAL Rx

- Systemic disease: prednisone, alone or in combination with a steroid-sparing agents such as azathioprine, mycophenolate mofetil, or a tetracycline. They can be started simultaneously, followed by a gradual tapering of the prednisone and continuation of the steroid-sparing agent until clinical remission is achieved. A minimal dose of prednisone of 1 mg/kg/day is usually recommended and is continued until new blister formation ceases. The dose is gradually tapered according to the clinical findings.
- Localized disease: Topical steroids in general have been used in localized bullous pemphigoid. Clobetasol 40 g/day divided in twice daily application is continued until 15 days after disease containment, at which time the dose is tapered to 20 g/day × 1 mo, 10 g/day × 2 mo, followed by 10 g every other day × 4 mo, and then 10 g twice weekly × 4 mo.
- Methotrexate may be used in patients with severe disease who are unable to tolerate prednisone.

CHRONIC Rx

- Combination prednisone and azathioprine protocols are available in the treatment of bullous pemphigoid.
- Cyclophosphamide can be considered in attempt to reduce chronic long-term use of corticosteroids.

DISPOSITION

Mortality rates are estimated at 19% at 1 year and 28% to 30% at 3 years.

REFERRAL

Dermatology

PEARLS & CONSIDERATIONS

COMMENTS

- Bullous pemphigoid has been associated with diabetes, multiple sclerosis, pernicious anemia, rheumatoid arthritis, lichen planus, psoriasis, and vitiligo.
- Not known to transform into malignancies or to represent a dermatologic manifestation of harboring malignancies.

SUGGESTED READINGS

Bickle KM, Roark TR: Autoimmune bullous dermatoses: a review, *Am Fam Physician* 65:1861-1870, 2002.

Kolanko E et al: Subepidermal blistering disorders: a clinical and histopathologic review, *Semin Cutan Med Surg* 23(1): 10-18, 2004.

Walsh SR et al: Bullous pemphigoid: from bench to bedside, *Drugs* 65(7):905, 2005.

Wojnarowska F et al: Guidelines for the management of bullous pemphigoid, *Br J Dermatol* 147:214-221, 2002.

AUTHOR: **MOHAMMAD HAJJIRI, M.D.**

BASIC INFORMATION

DEFINITION

Burning mouth syndrome (BMS) is characterized by burning pain in the tongue or oral mucous membranes, usually occurring without any identifiable precipitating factor. Patients may also have the sensation of dryness, or a bitter or metallic taste in their mouth.

SYNONYMS

Scalded mouth syndrome
Glossodynia
Glossopyrosis

ICD-9CM CODES
529.6 Glossodynia

EPIDEMIOLOGY & DEMOGRAPHICS

- Most prevalent in postmenopausal women, reported in 10% to 40% of women presenting for treatment of menopausal symptoms.
- Epidemiologic studies report 0.7% to 2.6% in the general population of both men and women.
- Typically occurs in middle-aged or older adults.

PHYSICAL FINDINGS & CLINICAL PRESENTATION

- For the majority of patients, the onset of pain is spontaneous without an identifiable precipitating factor.
- One third of patients relate the time of onset to a dental procedure, recent illness, or medication.
- Often persists for many years.
- The burning sensation often occurs in more than one oral site, most frequently in the anterior two thirds of the tongue, the anterior hard palate, and the lower lip mucosa.
- Pain is often absent at night, but will increase in severity progressively throughout the day.
- Associated with sleep disturbances as well as difficulty falling asleep.
- Also associated with mood changes, such as irritability, anxiety, and depression.
- Up to two thirds of patients report a spontaneous partial recovery within 6 to 7 years from onset, with the pain changing from constant to intermittent.

ETIOLOGY

Because of its complex clinical picture, many different hypotheses have been suggested for its etiology. Possible causes include:

- Psychologic dysfunction—many patients concomitantly have personality or mood changes.
- Chronic pain conditions, such as headaches.
- High blood glucose levels, although this has not been consistently proven.
- Dry mouth—however most salivary flow rate studies in affected patients have not shown a decrease in unstimulated or stimulated salivary flow.
- Oral candidal infections.
- Medications—angiotensin-converting enzyme (ACE) inhibitors.
- Nerve damage.
- Nutritional deficiencies—iron, zinc, folate and vitamin B.

There may be an association between supertasters (those with enhanced ability to taste) and those with BMS, due to their increased density of taste buds that are surrounded by bundles of trigeminal nerve neurons.

DIAGNOSIS

DIFFERENTIAL DIAGNOSIS

- Mucosal disease such as lichen planus or candidiasis
- Nutritional deficiency in zinc, iron, folate, or vitamins B_1, B_2, B_6, B_9, B_{12}
- Dry mouth from Sjögren's syndrome or after chemo/radiation therapy
- Cranial nerve injury
- Medication effect

WORKUP

- Clinical history is the most important in diagnosing BMS.
- Very important to rule out other pathologic conditions first.

LABORATORY TESTS

There is no test for BMS but consider testing for vitamin B or zinc deficiency.

TREATMENT

NONPHARMACOLOGIC THERAPY

Capsaicin (hot pepper powder) can be used as a topical desensitizing agent.

- Rinse mouth with 1 tsp of a 1:2 solution of hot pepper and water; increase strength of capsaicin as tolerated to a maximum 1:1 dilution.

ACUTE GENERAL Rx

- Low-dose benzodiazepines
  - Clonazepam (Klonopin) 0.25 to 2 mg/day—start with 0.25 mg qhs and increase dose q4 to 7 days until oral burning is relieved or side effects
  - Chlordiazepoxide (Librium) 10 to 30 mg/day—start with 5 mg qhs and increase dose q4 to 7 days until oral burning is relieved or side effects
- Low-dose tricyclic antidepressants
  - Amitriptyline (Elavil) or nortriptyline (Pamelor) 10 to 150 mg/day—start with 10 mg qhs and increase dose by 10 mg q4 to 7 days.
- Low-dose gabapentin (Neurontin) 300 to 1600 mg/day—start with 100 mg qhs and increase dose by 100 mg q4 to 7 days (take in divided doses).

REFERRAL

To a subspecialist in this area if initial therapy fails to resolve symptoms, such as a dentist or ENT

PEARLS & CONSIDERATIONS

COMMENTS

Burning mouth syndrome is a rare but possibly debilitating disease. Other diseases should be ruled out, such as vitamin deficiency.

SUGGESTED READINGS

Grushka M et al: Burning mouth syndrome, *Am Fam Physician* 65:615, 2002.

Grushka M et al: Burning mouth syndrome: evolving concepts, *Oral Maxillofac Surg Clin North Am* 12:287, 2000.

MayoClinic.com: www.mayoclinic.com/invoke.cfm?id=DS00462

AUTHOR: **MADHAVI SHAH, M.D.**

BASIC INFORMATION

DEFINITION

Burn injuries include thermal injuries (flames, scalds, cigarettes), as well as chemical, electrical, and radiation burns.

SYNONYMS Thermal injury

ICD-9CM CODES
942-949 (by region, % burn)

EPIDEMIOLOGY & DEMOGRAPHICS

PREVALENCE (IN U.S.): Burn injuries account for about 500,000 emergency room visits, 40,000 hospitalizations, and 4500 deaths annually.

PREDOMINANT SEX: Male:female ratio of 2:1

PHYSICAL FINDINGS & CLINICAL PRESENTATION

- Burns are defined based on surface area and depth of skin involved.
- *First-degree burns (superficial)* involve the epidermis only and appear painful and red.
- *Second-degree burns* involve the dermis and appear blistered, moist, and red with two-point discrimination intact *(superficial partial-thickness)* or red and blanched white with only sensation of pressure intact *(deep partial thickness)*.
- *Third-degree burns (full-thickness)* extend through the dermis with associated destruction of hair follicles and sweat glands. The skin is charred, pale, *painless,* and leathery. These burns are caused by flames, immersion scalds, chemical and high voltage injuries.

DIAGNOSIS

CLASSIFICATION

Burns are classified based on extent of the burn or total burn surface area (TBSA). The TBSA is best classified using age-specific burn charts.

Major burns: Partial-thickness burns >25% TBSA (or 20% if younger than 10 or older than 50 yr); full-thickness burns >10% TBSA; burns crossing major joints or involving the hands, face, feet, or perineum; electrical or chemical burns; those complicated by inhalation injury, or involving high-risk patients (extremes of age/comorbid diseases)

Moderate burns: Partial-thickness burns >15% to 25% TBSA (or 10% in children and older adults); full-thickness burns >2% to 10% TBSA and not involving the specific conditions of major burns

Minor burns: Partial-thickness burns <15% TBSA or full-thickness burns <2% TBSA

WORKUP

Diagnosis is based on clinical findings.

LABORATORY STUDIES

- CBC, electrolytes, BUN, creatinine, and glucose
- Serial ABG and carboxyhemoglobin if smoke inhalation suspected
- Urinalysis, urine myoglobin, and CPK levels if concern for rhabdomyolysis

IMAGING STUDIES

Chest x-ray and bronchoscopy if smoke inhalation suspected

TREATMENT

ACUTE GENERAL Rx

- Establish airway: inspect for inhalation injury and intubate for suspected airway edema (often seen 12 to 24 hr later); supplemental O_2
- Remove jewelry and clothing and place one or two large-bore peripheral IVs (if TBSA >20%)
- Fluid resuscitation with Ringer's lactate at 2 to 4 ml/kg per %TBSA per 24 hr with half the calculated fluid given in the first 8 hr
- Foley catheter and NG tube (20% of patients develop an ileus)
- Tetanus update
- Pain control
- Stress ulcer prophylaxis in high-risk patients
- Address adequate nutritional support
- Prophylactic antibiotics are not recommended; however, burn victims should be considered immunosuppressed
- High-voltage burn patients should have ECG monitoring because they are at increased risk for arrhythmias

BURN WOUND Rx

First-degree burns (e.g., sunburns) can be treated with cool compresses, antihistamines, emollients, and at times, a rapidly tapering dose of steroids.

Second-degree and third-degree burns:

- Wash burned skin with cool tap water or saline (15° to 25° C; immerse approximately 30 min if able) and cleanse with mild soap. Ice or ice water may increase tissue injury and should not be used.
- Sharp debridement of ruptured blisters (except palms and soles). Leave unruptured blisters intact.
- There are several approaches to burn dressings after cleansing and debriding:
  1. Apply thin layer of antibiotic ointment (silver sulfadiazine can be used unless sulfa allergy or facial burn) and cover with a nonadherent dressing (e.g., Telfa or petroleum-soaked gauze) followed by a sterile gauze wrap. Wash wound and change dressing when dressing soaked.
  2. Apply saline-soaked gauze (Xeroform, Owen's), cover with 4 × 4 dressing and a bulky absorbent dressing such as Kerlex. Reevaluate in 5 to 7 days.
  3. Apply occlusive dressing (Duoderm, Tegasorb), remove in 7 to 10 days.
- Specialized care, such as excision and auto grafting, is required for some deep second-degree and most third-degree burns.

DISPOSITION

- Respiratory injury, sepsis, and multiorgan failure may complicate severe burns.
- Scarring can be expected in many second-degree and all third-degree burns.

REFERRAL

Major and some moderate burns require referral to specialized burn centers for surgical debridement, grafting evaluation and rehabilitation.

PEARLS & CONSIDERATIONS

COMMENTS

Burn victims need to be reassessed frequently because the examination can change significantly in the first 24 to 72 hr.

EVIDENCE

In the management of critically ill patients, including patients with burns, there is no evidence that the use of colloids reduces the risk of death compared with crystalloids, nor is there any evidence that albumin reduces mortality in critically ill burn patients or those with hypoalbuminemia.[1,2] There is no clear consensus regarding the optimal timing for initiation of enteral nutritional support in these patients.[3] There is evidence to show that hydrocolloid dressing reduces wound healing time and pain when compared with silver sulfadiazene in the treatment of minor burns.[4]

Evidence-Based References

1. Albumin Reviewers (Alderson P et al): Human albumin solution for resuscitation and volume expansion in critically ill patients, *Cochrane Database Syst Rev* 18(4):CD001208, 2004. Ⓐ
2. Roberts I et al: Colloids versus crystalloids for fluid resuscitation in critically ill patients, *Cochrane Database Syst Rev* 4:CD000567, 2004. Ⓐ
3. Wasiak J et al: Early versus delayed enteral nutrition support for burn injuries, *Cochrane Database Syst Rev* 3:CD005489, 2006.
4. Wyatt D et al: Comparison of a hydrocolloid dressing and silver sulfadiazine cream in the outpatient management of second-degree burns, *J Trauma* 30:857, 1990. Reviewed in: *Clin Evidence* 14:2388, 2005.

SUGGESTED READINGS

Sheridan R: Burn care: results of technical and organizational progress, *JAMA* 290(6):719, 2003.

Sheridan R: Burns, *Crit Care Med* 30(11)S:S500, 2002.

Singer AJ: Management of local burn wounds in the ED, *Am J Emerg Med* 25(6):666, 2007.

AUTHORS: **SRIVIDYA ANANDAN, M.D.,** and **MICHELLE STOZEK, M.D.**

BASIC INFORMATION

DEFINITION

Bursitis is an inflammation of a bursa and is usually aseptic. A *bursa* is a closed sac lined with a synovial-like membrane that sometimes contains fluid that is found or that develops in an area subject to pressure or friction.

SYNONYMS

Housemaid's knee (prepatellar bursitis)
Weaver's bottom (ischial gluteal bursitis)
Baker's cyst (gastrocnemius-semimembranosus bursa)

ICD-9CM CODES
726.19 Subacromial bursitis
726.33 Olecranon bursitis
726.5 Ischiogluteal bursitis (hip)
726.5 Iliopsoas bursitis (hip)
726.61 Anserine bursitis
726.5 Trochanteric bursitis
726.65 Prepatellar bursitis
727.51 Baker's cyst
726.79 Retrocalcaneal bursitis

PHYSICAL FINDINGS & CLINICAL PRESENTATION

- Swelling, especially if bursa is superficial (olecranon, prepatellar)
- Local tenderness with pain on pressure against bursa
- Pain with joint movement
- Referred pain
- Palpable occasional fibrocartilaginous bodies (most common in olecranon and prepatellar bursae)

ETIOLOGY

- Acute trauma
- Repetitive trauma
- Sepsis
- Crystalline deposit disease
- Rheumatoid arthritis

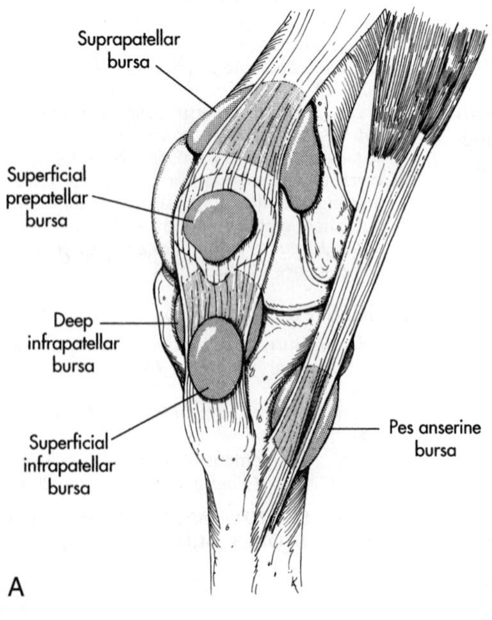

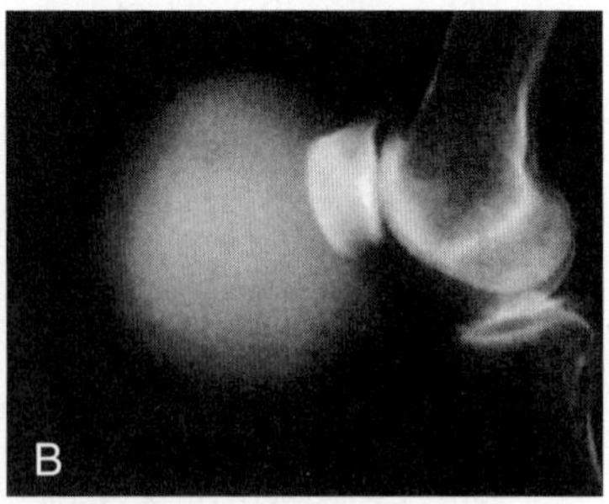

FIGURE 1-42 **A,** Bursae around the knee. **B,** Markedly swollen prepatellar bursa. (From Scudieri G [ed]: *Sports medicine principles of primary care,* St Louis, 1997, Mosby.)

DIAGNOSIS

DIFFERENTIAL DIAGNOSIS

- Degenerative joint disease
- Tendinitis (sometimes occurs in conjunction with bursitis)
- Cellulitis (if bursitis is septic)
- Infectious arthritis

WORKUP

Aspiration with Gram stain and C&S

IMAGING STUDIES

- Plain radiography to rule out other potential or coexisting bone or joint problems (Fig. 1-42)
- MRI

TREATMENT

NONPHARMACOLOGIC THERAPY

- If chronic, elimination of cause of pressure or irritation
- Use of relief pads, avoidance of direct pressure
- Rest
- Elevation
- Ice for acute trauma

ACUTE GENERAL Rx

- Septic:
  1. Appropriate antibiotic coverage and drainage
  2. Aspiration of purulent fluid with a large-bore needle (if there is no rapid clinical response, incision and drainage are indicated)
- Nonseptic:
  1. Aspiration of blood from acute trauma
  2. Application of compression dressing

CHRONIC Rx

- Aspiration if excessive fluid volume present, followed by application of compression dressing to prevent fluid reaccumulation (repeat aspiration may be required)
- Steroid injection into bursa (1 ml of triamcinolone, 40 mg, mixed with 1 to 3 ml of Xylocaine depending on size of bursa)
- NSAIDs

DISPOSITION

- Many bursal sacs "dry up" eventually.
- Nonsurgical treatment is effective in most cases.

REFERRAL

For orthopedic consultation to assist in treatment of sepsis or for excision of chronic enlarged bursa when indicated

PEARLS & CONSIDERATIONS

COMMENTS

- Injection of trochanteric bursa may require spinal needle in large patient.
- Sterile bursae should not be incised and drained because a chronic draining sinus tract may develop.
- Involvement of the iliopsoas bursa may cause groin pain, although the diagnosis is difficult to make because of the inaccessibility of the area to direct examination. (This also makes steroid injection impossible even if the diagnosis could be established.)

SUGGESTED READINGS

Beaman FD, Peterson JJ: MR imaging of cysts, ganglia and bursae about the knee, *Radiol Clin North Am* 45:969, 2007.
Floemer F, Morrison WB et al: MRI characteristics of olecranon bursitis, *Am J Roentgenol* 183:29, 2004.
Pateder DB et al: Masquerade: nonspinal musculoskeletal disorders that mimic spinal conditions, *Cleve Clin J Med* 75:50, 2008.
Sofka CM, Adler RS: Sonography of cubital bursitis, *Am J Roengenol* 183:51, 2004.
Tortolani PJ, Carbone JJ, Quartaro LG: Greater trochanteric pain syndrome in patients referred to orthopedic spine specialists, *Spine* 2:251, 2002.
Van Mieghem IM, Boets A et al: Ischiogluteal bursitis: an uncommon type of bursitis, *Skeletal Radiol* 33:413, 2004.
Webner D, Drezner JA: Lesser trochanteric bursitis: a rare cause of anterior hip pain, *Clin J Sport Med* 14:242, 2004.
Woodley SJ et al: Morphology of the bursae associated with the greater trochanter of the femur, *J Bone Joint Surg* 90:284, 2008.

AUTHOR: **LONNIE R. MERCIER, M.D.**

BASIC INFORMATION

DEFINITION

Candidiasis is an inflammatory process involving the vulva or the vagina and is caused by superficial invasion of epithelial cells by *Candida* species.

SYNONYMS

Moniliasis
Thrush

ICD-9CM CODES
112.1 Moniliasis
112.0 Thrush
112 Candidosis

EPIDEMIOLOGY & DEMOGRAPHICS

- This is the second most common form of vaginitis in the U.S. 75% of women will have at least one episode of vulvovaginal candidiasis (VVC) during their childbearing years and about 45% will have a second attack. A small subpopulation of probably <5% of adult women has recurrent, often intractable episodes. *Candida* may be isolated in up to 20% of asymptomatic women of childbearing age.
- Factors that predispose to development of symptomatic VVC include pregnancy, antibiotic use, and diabetes. Antibiotic use disturbs normal vaginal flora and allows overgrowth of fungi; pregnancy and diabetes are associated with decrease in cell-mediated immunity.
- Factors associated with increased rates of asymptomatic vaginal colonization: pregnancy, high-estrogen oral contraceptives, uncontrolled diabetes mellitus, attendance at STD clinics.

UNCOMPLICATED VVC

- Infrequent VVC
- Mild-to-moderate vaginitis and candida
- Likely to be *C. albicans*
- Nonimmunocompromised women (HIV)

COMPLICATED VVC

- Recurrent VVC
- Severe VVC
- Non-*albicans* candidiasis
- Women with uncontrolled diabetes, immunosuppression, or those who are pregnant

PHYSICAL FINDINGS & CLINICAL PRESENTATION

Symptoms of VVC consist of:

- Vulvar pruritus with vaginal discharge that typically resembles cottage cheese.
- Erythema and edema of labia and vulvar skin; possible discrete pustulopapular peripheral lesions (satellite lesions) (Fig. 1-43).
- Vagina may be erythematous with an adherent, whitish discharge.
- Cervix may appear normal.
- Symptoms characteristically exacerbated in the week preceding menses with some relief after onset of menstrual flow.

ETIOLOGY

- *Candida* are dimorphic fungi (spores and mycelial forms).
- *C. albicans* is responsible for 85% to 90% of vaginal yeast infections.
- *C. glabrata, C. tropicalis* (non-*albicans* species) also cause vaginitis and may be more resistant to conventional therapy.

DIAGNOSIS

DIFFERENTIAL DIAGNOSIS

- Bacterial vaginosis
- Trichomoniasis

WORKUP

- Usually normal vaginal pH (<4.5).
- Budding yeast forms or mycelia will appear in as many as 80% of cases. Saline wet prep of vaginal secretions usually is normal; may be increased in inflammatory cells in severe cases.
- Whiff test negative (KOH).
- 10% KCl useful and more sensitive than wet mount for microscopic identification.

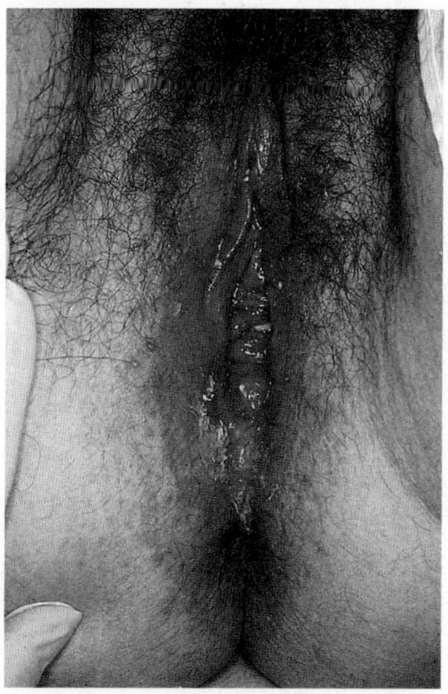

FIGURE 1-43 Candidiasis. Vaginal candidiasis is common, and lesions often spread to the vulva. Peeling and erosions are seen in tertriginous areas, and satellite pustules are scattered at the periphery. In contrast, tinea infections do not have satellite lesions; tiny vesiculopustules occur along the lesional border. (From Black M, McKay M: *Obstetrics and gynecological dermatology,* ed 2, St Louis, 2002, Mosby.)

- Can make a presumptive diagnosis based on symptomatology in the absence of microscopy-proven fungal elements if the pH and wet prep are normal. Fungal culture is recommended to confirm diagnosis.
- In chronic/recurrent, burning replaces itching as prominent symptom. Confirm diagnosis with direct microscopy and culture. Many may actually have chronic or atrophic dermatitis. Test for HIV.

LABORATORY TESTS

If sending cultures, send on Nickerson's media or semiquantitative slide-stix cultures. There is no reliable serologic technique for diagnosis.

TREATMENT

ACUTE GENERAL Rx (UNCOMPLICATED VVC)

TOPICAL BUTOCONAZOLE:

- 2% vaginal cream 5 g intravaginally for 3 days
- Butoconazole (sustained release) 5 gm intravaginally for 1 dose

TOPICAL CLOTRIMAZOLE

- 1% cream 5 g intravaginally for 7 to 14 days
- 100-mg vaginal tablet for 7 days
- 100-mg vaginal tablets, 2 tablets for 3 days
- 500-mg vaginal tablet, single dose

TOPICAL MICONAZOLE:

- 2% cream 5 g intravaginally for 7 days
- 200-mg vaginal suppository for 3 days
- 100-mg vaginal suppository for 7 days

TOPICAL TIOCONAZOLE: 6.5% ointment 5 g intravaginally, single dose

TOPICAL TERCONAZOLE:

- 0.4% cream 5 g intravaginally for 7 days
- 0.8% cream 5 g intravaginally for 3 days
- 80-mg suppository for 3 days

ORAL FLUCONAZOLE: 150-mg single po dose

(COMPLICATED VVC)

- Recurrent VVC: 7 to 14 days of topical therapy
- 150 mg fluconazole po, repeat in 3 days
- Maintenance regimen
  1. Clotrimazole: 500-mg vaginal suppositories once weekly
  2. Ketoconazole: 100 mg once daily
  3. Fluconazole: 100 to 150 mg po once weekly
  4. Itraconazole 400 mg/mo or 100 mg/day
  5. Continue one of the above regimens for 6 mo

(COMPROMISED HOST)

- Treat with traditional antimycotics for at least 7 to 14 days
- Pregnancy: topical azoles recommended for 7 days

- Women with HIV: fluconazole 200 mg/wk
- Not usually an STD

CHRONIC Rx

Ketoconazole 400 mg po qd or fluconazole 200 mg po qd until symptoms resolve. Then maintenance on prophylactic doses of these agents for 6 mo (ketoconazole 100 mg/day, fluconazole 150 mg/wk).

DISPOSITION

If chronic or recurrent, consider screening for diabetes, HIV, or other immune deficiencies.

PEARLS & CONSIDERATIONS

COMMENTS

- Azoles are more effective than nystatin. Symptoms usually take 2 to 3 days to resolve. Adjunctive treatment with weak topical steroid such as 1% hydrocortisone cream may help with relief of symptoms.
- Creams and suppositories are oil based and may weaken latex condoms and diaphragms.

EVIDENCE

Vulvovaginal candidiasis

Several randomized controlled trials (RCTs) found that topical imidazoles were more effective than placebo for the treatment of vulvovaginal candidiasis in nonpregnant women.[1] (A)

An RCT compared intravaginal nystatin vs. placebo in nonpregnant women with symptomatic vulvovaginal candidiasis. Nystatin significantly reduced the number of patients reporting a poor symptomatic response after 2 weeks.[2] (A)

A systematic review found that topical imidazole therapy was more effective than nystatin in the management of vaginal candidiasis in pregnancy. Treatment for 7 days may be necessary during pregnancy.[3] (A)

An RCT compared intravaginal imidazoles vs. nystatin for the treatment of vaginal candidiasis in nonpregnant women. There was a significantly lower relapse rate over 6 months in patients treated with imidazoles.[4] (A)

A systematic review compared oral vs. topical azoles in nonpregnant women with vulvovaginal candidiasis. Both routes of administration were found to be equally effective in terms of clinical and mycologic cure.[5] (A)

An RCT compared itraconazole vs. placebo in women with vaginal candidiasis. Significantly fewer women treated with itraconazole had persistent symptoms 7 days after treatment.[6] (A)

Another RCT (single blind) found that itraconazole was significantly more effective than placebo in reducing recurrent symptoms over 6 months in women with recurrent vulvovaginal candidiasis. Recurrence rates were similar once itraconazole was discontinued.[7] (A)

Evidence-Based References

1. Spence D: Candidiasis (vulvovaginal). Reviewed in: Clinical Evidence 10:2044-2054, 2004. London, BMJ Publishing Group. (A)
2. Isaacs JH: Nystatin vaginal cream in monilial vaginitis, *Illinois Med J* 3:240-241, 1973. Reviewed in: *Clin Evid* 13:2268, 2005. (A)
3. Young GL, Jewell D: Topical treatment for vaginal candidiasis (thrush) in pregnancy, *Cochrane Database Syst Rev* 3:2001. (A)
4. Dennerstein GJ, Langley R: Vulvovaginal candidiasis: treatment and recurrence, *Aust N Z J Obstet Gynaecol* 22:231-233, 1982. Reviewed in: *Clin Evid* 10:2044-2054, 2003. (A)
5. Watson MC et al: Oral versus intra-vaginal imidazole and triazole anti-fungal treatment of uncomplicated vulvovaginal candidiasis (thrush). Reviewed in: Cochrane Library, 1, Chichester, UK, 2004, John Wiley. (A)
6. Stein GE, Mummaw N: Placebo-controlled trial of itraconazole for treatment of acute vaginal candidiasis, *Antimicrob Agents Chemother* 37:89-92, 1993. Reviewed in: *Clin Evid* 10:2044-2054, 2003. (A)
7. Spinillo A et al: Managing recurrent vulvovaginal candidiasis. Intermittent prevention with itraconazole, *J Reprod Med* 42:83-87, 1997. Reviewed in: *Clin Evid* 10:2044-2054, 2003. (A)

SUGGESTED READINGS

Centers for Disease Control and Prevention: 2006 sexually transmitted diseases treatment guidelines, *MMWR Morb Mortal Wkly Rep* 55(RR-11), 2006.

Sheary B, Dayan L: Recurrent vulvovaginal candidiasis, *Aust Fam Physician* 34(3):147-150, 2005.

Spence D: Candidiasis (vulvovaginal), *Clin Evid* (12):2493-2511, 2004.

AUTHORS: **MARIA A. CORIGLIANO, M.D.,** and **RUBEN ALVERO, M.D.**

BASIC INFORMATION

DEFINITION

Carbon monoxide (CO) is a colorless, odorless, tasteless, nonirritating gas. When inhaled it produces toxicity by causing cellular hypoxia and damage.

ICD-9CM CODES
986 Carbon monoxide poisoning

EPIDEMIOLOGY & DEMOGRAPHICS

- A leading cause of lethal poisoning in the U.S.
- CO poisoning is seen more frequently during the fall and winter months in cold climates. It is now recognized with increasing frequency after storm-related power outages, mostly because of the use of portable gasoline-powered generators.
- In adults, 20% of CO poisonings occur in occupational settings.

PHYSICAL FINDINGS & CLINICAL PRESENTATION

Depends on the severity and duration of exposure. The brain and heart are most sensitive to CO poisoning.

- Presentation is often nonspecific and may be mistaken for a flulike illness.
- Mild to moderate poisoning may present with headache, fatigue, dizziness, nausea, dyspnea, difficulty concentrating, confusion, and blurred vision. Patients may have tachypnea and tachycardia.
- Severe poisoning may present with hypotension, arrhythmias, myocardial ischemia, pulmonary edema, lethargy, ataxia, syncope, seizure, coma, or rarely, cherry-red skin.
- Severity of symptoms does not correlate with carboxyhemoglobin (COHgb) levels.
- Delayed neurologic sequelae can occur days to weeks after recovery from acute poisoning. Patients may present with neurologic or psychiatric symptoms (cognitive deficits, memory loss, personality disorders, movement disorders, Parkinson's, psychosis, neurologic deficits).

ETIOLOGY

- CO results from the incomplete combustion of carbon-containing compounds. CO poisoning occurs from inhaling smoke from fires, motor vehicle exhaust, or the burning of fuel (oil, wood, coal, natural gas) in poorly functioning or improperly ventilated devices (heating systems, stoves, etc.). Methylene chloride (paint stripper) fumes are converted to CO by the liver.
- CO toxicity results from tissue hypoxia and direct CO-mediated damage at the cellular level. This may explain why COHgb levels alone are not predictive of clinical toxicity.
- CO interferes with oxygen transportation and release. CO binds to hemoglobin with an affinity 200 to 250 times greater than oxygen, displacing oxygen from hemoglobin and decreasing the oxygen-carrying capacity of blood. By binding to hemoglobin, CO changes the structure of the hemoglobin molecule and decreases oxygen release to tissue.
- CO binds to other heme-containing proteins. Cellular respiration is depressed by inhibition of the mitochondrial cytochrome oxidase system. Cardiac function is depressed by direct binding to cardiac myoglobin.
- Neurologic toxicity is not explained by hypoxia alone and is related to the complex intracellular actions of CO, its effect on nitric oxide, cerebral vasodilation, oxidative damage, and lipid peroxidation of brain tissue.

DIAGNOSIS

DIFFERENTIAL DIAGNOSIS

- Viral syndromes
- Cyanide, hydrogen sulfide
- Methemoglobinemia
- Amphetamines and derivatives
- Cocaine, phencyclidine (PCP)
- Cyclic antidepressants
- Phenothiazines
- Theophylline

WORKUP

History, physical examination (detailed neurologic exam), laboratory and imaging tests

LABORATORY TESTS

- COHgb level: COHgb level > 3% in nonsmokers confirms exposure. Heavy smokers may have baseline levels of up to 10%. Levels may be low if the patient has already received supplemental oxygen or if there is a delay between exposure and testing.
- Direct measurement of arterial oxyhemoglobin (by co-oximetry): Pulse oximetry and arterial blood gas (ABG) may be falsely normal because neither measures oxygen saturation of hemoglobin directly. Pulse oximetry is inaccurate because of the similar absorption characteristics of oxyhemoglobin and COHgb. An ABG is inaccurate because it measures oxygen dissolved in plasma (which is not affected by CO) and then calculates oxygen saturation of hemoglobin.
- Electrolytes, glucose, BUN, creatinine, cardiac biomarkers, ABG (lactic acidosis and rhabdomyolysis may develop), CBC (polycythemia due to hypoxia in chronic CO poisoning).
- ECG (ischemia, arrhythmia).
- Pregnancy test (fetus at high risk).
- Consider toxicology screen.
- Imaging studies.
  - Chest x-ray (noncardiogenic edema)
  - CT, MRI if neurologic abnormalities are present

TREATMENT

ACUTE GENERAL Rx

- Remove from site of CO exposure.
- Ensure adequate airway.
- Continuous ECG monitor.
- Fetal monitoring if pregnant.
- 100% oxygen by tight-fitting nonrebreather mask or endotracheal tube for 6 to 12 hr (decreases half-life of COHgb from 4 to 6 hr to 60 to 90 min).
- Hyperbaric oxygen (2.5 to 3 ATM).
  - Decreases half-life of COHgb to 20 to 30 min, increases amount of oxygen dissolved in plasma
  - Questionable if there is any beneficial effect over normobaric oxygen
  - May prevent the delayed neurologic sequelae of CO poisoning by decreasing cellular hypoxia and toxicity
  - Consider for individuals with:
    1. Severe intoxication (COHgb > 25%, history of loss of consciousness, neurologic symptoms or signs, cardiovascular compromise, severe metabolic acidosis)
    2. Persistent symptoms after 2 to 4 hr of normobaric oxygen
    3. Pregnant women with COHgb >15% or signs of fetal distress: CO elimination slower in fetus than mother, fetal Hgb has greater affinity for CO than adult Hgb
  - Should be instituted quickly if deemed necessary
- Consider concomitant poisoning with other toxic/irritant gases that may be present in smoke (e.g., cyanide) or thermal injury to airway. Toxic effects of CO and cyanide are synergistic.
- Identify source of exposure and determine if poisoning was accidental.

DISPOSITION

- Patients with mild poisoning can be treated in an ambulatory setting. Those with moderate/severe poisoning or coexisting illness require hospitalization.
- Survivors of severe poisoning are at 14% to 40% risk for neurologic sequelae.
  - Deficits usually apparent within 3 wk of poisoning but may present months later.
  - Risk of developing sequelae is greater if there was loss of consciousness during acute poisoning and with older age.
  - Brain MRI may show changes in the white matter and basal ganglia.
  - Recovery may occur over months to years.

- CO-mediated cardiac damage is associated with increased long-term mortality.
- High risk of fetal demise.

REFERRAL

- Poison control center
- Medical toxicologist
- Hyperbaric unit

PEARLS & CONSIDERATIONS

- Severity of poisoning and prognosis do not correlate with COHgb levels.
- Neuropsychometric testing is an objective measure of cognitive function but is not universally used.
- Contact Fire Department to assess environment.

EVIDENCE

Hyperbaric oxygen

A systematic review compared normobaric oxygen vs. hyperbaric oxygen for the treatment of acute CO poisoning. The review found no evidence from randomized controlled trials (RCTs) that unselected use of hyperbaric oxygen reduces the frequency of neurological symptoms at 1 mo and that the evidence is insufficient to provide clear guidelines for practice.[1] Ⓐ

An RCT compared 100 min of hyperbaric oxygen treatment vs. 100 min of normobaric oxygen treatment given in a hyperbaric oxygen chamber daily for 3 days. This was extended for 6 days for patients who were clinically abnormal or had poor neuropsychological outcome after three treatments. Both groups received continuous high-flow oxygen between treatments. A greater percentage of severely poisoned patients in the group receiving hyperbaric oxygen had a poor outcome at completion of treatment.[2] Ⓑ

In contrast, an RCT assessing the effect of hyperbaric oxygen treatment on cognitive sequelae after acute (<24 hr), symptomatic CO poisoning found that patients treated with three hyperbaric oxygen sessions within 24 hr had lower rates of cognitive sequelae at 6 wk and 12 mo compared with those treated with normobaric oxygen.[3] Ⓑ

Evidence-Based References

1. Juurlink DN, Stanbrook MB, McGuigan MA: Hyperbaric oxygen for carbon monoxide poisoning, *Cochrane Database Syst Rev* 1:CD002041, 2005. Ⓐ
2. Scheinkestel CD et al: Hyperbaric or normobaric oxygen for acute carbon monoxide poisoning: a randomised controlled clinical trial, *Med J Aust* 170:20310, 1999. Ⓑ
3. Weaver LK et al: Hyperbaric oxygen for acute carbon monoxide poisoning, *N Engl J Med* 347:1057, 2002. Reviewed in: The *PedsCCM Evidence-Based Journal Club*, 2003. Ⓑ

SUGGESTED READINGS

Domachevsky L et al: Hyperbaric oxygen in the treatment of carbon monoxide poisoning, *Clin Toxicol* 43(3):181, 2005.

Graber J et al: Results from a state-based surveillance system for carbon monoxide poisoning, *Public Health Reports* 122(2):145, 2007.

Kao LW et al: Toxicity associated with carbon monoxide, *Clin Lab Med* 26:99, 2006.

Hampson N: Storm-related carbon monoxide poisoning: lessons learned from recent epidemics, *Undersea Hyperb Med* 33(4):257, 2006.

Henry CR et al: Myocardial injury and long-term mortality following moderate to severe carbon monoxide poisoning, *JAMA* 295(4):398, 2006.

AUTHOR: **SUDEEP K. AULAKH, M.D., F.R.C.P.C.**

BASIC INFORMATION

DEFINITION

Carcinoid syndrome is a symptom complex characterized by paroxysmal vasomotor disturbances, diarrhea, and bronchospasm. It is caused by the action of amines and peptides (serotonin, bradykinin, histamine) produced by tumors arising from neuroendocrine cells.

SYNONYMS

Flush syndrome
Argentaffinoma syndrome

ICD-9CM CODES
259.2 Carcinoid syndrome

EPIDEMIOLOGY & DEMOGRAPHICS

INCIDENCE:

- Carcinoid tumors are found incidentally in 0.5% to 0.75% of autopsies.
- Carcinoid tumors are principally found in the following organs: appendix (40%); small bowel (20%; 15% in the ileum); rectum (15%); bronchi (12%); esophagus, stomach, colon (10%); ovary, biliary tract, pancreas (3%).

PHYSICAL FINDINGS & CLINICAL PRESENTATION

- Cutaneous flushing (75% to 90%)
  1. The patient usually has red-purple flushes starting in the face, then spreading to the neck and upper trunk.
  2. The flushing episodes last from a few minutes to hours (longer-lasting flushes may be associated with bronchial carcinoids).
  3. Flushing may be triggered by emotion, alcohol, or foods, or it may occur spontaneously.
  4. Dizziness, tachycardia, and hypotension may be associated with the cutaneous flushing.
- Diarrhea (>70%): often associated with abdominal bloating and audible peristaltic rushes
- Intermittent bronchospasm (25%): characterized by severe dyspnea and wheezing
- Facial telangiectasia
- Tricuspid regurgitation from carcinoid heart lesions

ETIOLOGY

- The carcinoid syndrome is caused by neoplasms originating from neuroendocrine cells.
- Carcinoid tumors do not usually produce the syndrome unless liver metastases are present or the primary tumor does not involve the GI tract.

DIAGNOSIS

DIFFERENTIAL DIAGNOSIS

The carcinoid syndrome must be distinguished from idiopathic flushing (IF); patients with IF more often are females, younger, and with a longer duration of symptoms; palpitations, syncope, and hypotension occur primarily in patients with IF.

LABORATORY TESTS

- The biochemical marker for carcinoid syndrome is increased 24-hr urinary 5-hydroxyindoleacetic acid (5-HIAA), a metabolite of serotonin (5-hydroxytryptamine).
- False elevations can be seen with ingestion of certain foods (bananas, pineapples, eggplant, avocados, walnuts) and certain medications (acetaminophen, caffeine, guaifenesin, reserpine); therefore patients should be on a restricted diet and should avoid these medications when the test is ordered.
- Liver function studies are an unreliable indicator of liver involvement.

IMAGING STUDIES

- Chest x-ray is useful to detect bronchial carcinoids.
- CT scan of abdomen or a liver and spleen radionuclide scan are useful to detect liver metastases (palpable in >50% of cases).
- Iodine-123 labeled somatostatin (123-ISS) can detect carcinoid endocrine tumors with somatostatin receptors.
- Scanning with radiolabeled octreotide can visualize previously undetected or metastatic lesions.

TREATMENT

NONPHARMACOLOGIC THERAPY

Avoidance of ethanol ingestion (may precipitate flushing)

GENERAL Rx

- Surgical resection of the tumor can be curative if the tumor is localized or palliative and results in prolonged asymptomatic periods if metastases are present. Surgical manipulation of the tumor can, however, cause severe vasomotor abnormalities and bronchospasm (carcinoid crisis).
- Percutaneous embolization and ligation of the hepatic artery can decrease the bulk of the tumor in the liver and provide palliative treatment of tumors with hepatic metastases.
- Cytotoxic chemotherapy: combination chemotherapy with 5-fluorouracil and streptozotocin can be used in patients with unresectable or recurrent carcinoid tumors; however, it has only limited success.
- Control of clinical manifestations:
  1. Diarrhea usually responds to diphenoxylate with atropine (Lomotil).
  2. Flushing can be controlled by the combination of H_1- and H_2-receptor antagonists (e.g., diphenhydramine 25 to 50 mg PO q6h and ranitidine 150 mg bid).
  3. Somatostatin analogue (SMS 201-995) is effective for both flushing and diarrhea in most patients.
  4. Bronchospasm can be treated with aminophylline and/or albuterol.
- Nutritional support: supplemental niacin therapy may be useful to prevent pellagra, because the tumor uses dietary tryptophan for serotonin synthesis, resulting in a nutritional deficiency in some patients.
- Subcutaneous somatostatin analogues (octreotide, lanreotide) have been used successfully for long-term control of symptoms in patients with unresectable neoplasms.
- Echocardiography and monitoring for right-sided CHF are recommended for patients with unresectable disease because endocardial fibrosis, involving predominantly the endocardium, chordae, and valves of the right side of the heart, can occur.

DISPOSITION

Carcinoids of the appendix and rectum have a low malignancy potential and rarely produce the clinical syndrome; metastases are also uncommon if the size of the primary lesion is <2 cm in diameter.

EVIDENCE

Treatment with octreotide and lanreotide have been shown to be equally effective with regard to improving quality of life, symptom control (flushing and diarrhea), and reduction of tumor marker levels in patients with carcinoid syndrome. Lanreotide is preferred, however, due to its simplicity of administration.[1] B

Limited evidence suggests that the combination of interferon (IFN) alpha and octreotide may slow tumor growth compared with octreotide alone in patients with midgut carcinoid tumors that have metastasized to the liver.[2] B

We are unable to cite evidence that meets our criteria for the other therapies for carcinoid syndrome.

Evidence-Based References

1. O'Toole D et al: Treatment of carcinoid syndrome: a prospective crossover evaluation of lanreotide versus octreotide in terms of efficacy, patient acceptability, and tolerance, *Cancer* 88:770, 2000. B
2. Kolby L et al: Randomized clinical trial of the effect of interferon alpha on survival in patients with disseminated midgut carcinoid tumours, *Br J Surg* 90:687, 2003. B

AUTHOR: **FRED F. FERRI, M.D.**

BASIC INFORMATION

DEFINITION

Cardiac tamponade is a life-threatening compression of the heart within the pericardial sac that impairs filling of the ventricles during diastole.

SYNONYMS None

ICD-9CM CODES
423.9 Unspecified diseases of the pericardium

PHYSICAL FINDINGS & CLINICAL PRESENTATION

- Chest pain
- Tachypnea
- Beck's triad
  - Absolute or relative hypotension
  - Jugular venous distention (with prominent x descent and blunted y descent) from elevated central venous pressure
  - Quiet heart sounds
- Tachycardia (except in uremia or hypothyroid patients)
- Pulsus paradoxus (an inspiratory fall in systolic arterial pressure of 10 mm Hg or more during normal breathing)
- Pericardial friction rub may be present

ETIOLOGY

Acute (rapidly accumulating pericardial effusion leading to cardiac tamponade): does not need a large amount of effusion to cause tamponade
- Penetrating trauma
- Aortic dissection
- Following treatment of MI with thrombolytics and/or heparin due to myocardial rupture and/or hemorrhagic pericarditis
- Iatrogenic (central line and pacemaker insertions, post–coronary bypass surgery)

Subacute or chronic (effusion is usually large)
- Malignancy (e.g., lung, breast, lymphoma)
- Viral pericarditis (e.g., coxsackie, HIV)
- Bacterial, fungal, or tuberculous pericarditis
- Uremia
- Myxedema (rare)
- Collagen-vascular disease (e.g., systemic lupus erythematosus, rheumatoid arthritis, scleroderma)
- Radiation
- Idiopathic

DIAGNOSIS

Cardiac tamponade is a clinical diagnosis made at the bedside by history and physical examination. The echocardiogram will help confirm or reject the clinical diagnosis, and can be confirmed by the measurement of intrapericardial pressures and its response to pericardial fluid drainage. Thereafter, one must pursue the underlying etiology with specific laboratory work (see "Laboratory Tests").

DIFFERENTIAL DIAGNOSIS

Other conditions that can also lead to elevated jugular venous pressure, decreased systemic pressure, and pulsus paradoxus include:
- COPD
- Constrictive pericarditis
- Restrictive cardiomyopathy
- Right ventricular infarction
- Pulmonary embolism

LABORATORY TESTS

- Electrolytes, BUN, creatinine, ESR, thyroid function tests, ANA, RF, PPD, blood cultures, viral titers, and pericardial fluid analysis and cultures.
- 12-lead ECG:
  - Sinus tachycardia
  - PR depression and/or diffuse ST elevations if acute pericarditis is present
  - Electrical alternans
  - Low voltage, if massive effusion is present

IMAGING STUDIES

- Chest x-ray.
- Echocardiogram (collapse of the right atrium and right ventricle during diastole, respiratory variation in transvalvular blood flow).
- Right-side heart catheterization and intrapericardial pressure measurements confirm the diagnosis.
- Typical findings are diastolic equalization of pressures usually from 15 to 30 mm Hg (diastolic pulmonary artery pressure = right ventricular diastolic pressure = right atrial pressure = intrapericardial pressure).

TREATMENT

NONPHARMACOLOGIC THERAPY

- Cardiac tamponade should be treated urgently.
- Avoid drugs that reduce preload (e.g., nitrates, diuretics).
- Large pericardial effusions without hemodynamic compromise can be managed conservatively with careful monitoring, treatment of the underlying cause, and surveillance echocardiography.

ACUTE GENERAL RX

- The acute causes of tamponade as mentioned earlier (see "Etiology") usually require emergency pericardial fluid removal either via pericardiocentesis or surgical pericardiotomy.
- Pericardiocentesis should be performed under echocardiographic guidance when available.
- Intravascular volume expansion (blood, saline, or dextran).
- Inotropic or vasopressor support.

CHRONIC RX

- Depends on etiology.
- Pericardiocentesis with draining catheter: The catheter can be left inside the pericardium for 48 hr to allow for continued drainage. If residual fluid still persists with hemodynamic compromise, surgical drainage should be sought for. In absence of hemodynamic compromise or significant residual fluid, discontinuation of the draining catheter can be done with periodic postprocedure echocardiographic monitoring of reaccumulation (e.g., at 24 hr, 7 days, 30 days, 3 mo, 6 mo, and 12 mo) depending on the etiology and rate of reaccumulation.
- Other surgical drainage procedures include:
  - Subxiphoid pericardiotomy drainage
  - Limited pericardiectomy draining the pericardial fluid into the left hemithorax
  - Complete pericardiectomy

DISPOSITION

The prognosis of cardiac tamponade depends on the underlying cause.

REFERRAL

- Cardiology consultation should be made if cardiac tamponade is suspected.
- Cardiothoracic surgery consultation should also be considered if surgical pericardial drainage is indicated.

PEARLS & CONSIDERATIONS

- Cardiac tamponade should always be considered during pulseless electrical activity (PEA) arrest and may require urgent subxiphoid pericardiocentesis.
- Evaluation for pulsus paradoxus should always be performed during normal respiration because deep inspiration will elevate the difference.

COMMENTS

As little as 200 ml of fluid can lead to acute cardiac tamponade, whereas with gradual accumulation, the pericardial sac can hold up to 5 L of fluid before tamponade occurs.

SUGGESTED READINGS

Meltser H, Kalaria VG: Cardiac tamponade, *Catheter Cardiovasc Interv* 64(2):245; 2005.

Roy CL et al: Does this patient with pericardial effusion have cardiac tamponade? *JAMA* 297(16):1810, 2007.

Sagrista-Sauleda J et al: Effusive, constrictive pericarditis, *N Eng J Med* 350(5):469, 2004.

Spodick DH: Acute cardiac tamponade, *N Engl J Med* 349(7):684, 2003.

AUTHORS: **CRAIG J. MCMACKIN, M.D.,** and **WEN-CHIH WU, M.D.**

BASIC INFORMATION

DEFINITION

Cardiomyopathies are a group of diseases primarily involving the myocardium and characterized by myocardial dysfunction that is not the result of hypertension, coronary atherosclerosis, valvular dysfunction, or pericardial abnormalities. In dilated cardiomyopathy, the heart is enlarged, and both ventricles are dilated.

SYNONYMS

Congestive cardiomyopathy

ICD-9CM CODES
425.4 Other primary cardiomyopathies

EPIDEMIOLOGY & DEMOGRAPHICS

- The prevalence of dilated cardiomyopathy in the general adult population is approximately 1%.
- Incidence increases with age and approaches 10% at age 80 yr.

PHYSICAL FINDINGS & CLINICAL PRESENTATION

- Increased jugular venous pressure
- Small pulse pressure
- Pulmonary rales, hepatomegaly, peripheral edema
- S_3, S_4
- Mitral regurgitation, tricuspid regurgitation (less common)

ETIOLOGY

- Idiopathic
- Alcoholism (15% to 40% of all cases in Western countries)
- Collagen-vascular disease (SLE, RA, polyarteritis, dermatomyositis)
- Postmyocarditis
- Peripartum (last trimester of pregnancy or 6 mo postpartum)
- Heredofamilial neuromuscular disease
- Toxins (cobalt, lead, phosphorus, carbon monoxide, mercury, doxorubicin, daunorubicin)
- Nutritional (beriberi, selenium deficiency, carnitine deficiency, thiamine deficiency)
- Cocaine, heroin, organic solvents ("glue-sniffer's heart")
- Irradiation
- Acromegaly, osteogenesis imperfecta, myxedema, thyrotoxicosis, diabetes
- Hypocalcemia
- Antiretroviral agents (zidovudine, didanosine, zalcitabine)
- Phenothiazines
- Infections (viral [HIV], rickettsial, mycobacterial, toxoplasmosis, trichinosis, Chagas' disease)
- Hematologic (e.g., sickle cell anemia)

DIAGNOSIS

DIFFERENTIAL DIAGNOSIS

- Frank pulmonary disease
- Valvular dysfunction
- Pericardial abnormalities
- Coronary atherosclerosis
- Psychogenic dyspnea

WORKUP

- Chest x-ray, ECG, echocardiogram.
- Medical history with emphasis on the following symptoms:
  1. Dyspnea on exertion, orthopnea, PND
  2. Palpitations
  3. Systemic and pulmonary embolism
- Cardiac troponin T levels: Persistently elevated troponin T levels are a marker of poor outcome in cardiomyopathy patients.

IMAGING STUDIES

CHEST X-RAY:
- Massive cardiac enlargement
- Interstitial pulmonary edema

ECG:
- Left ventricular hypertrophy with ST-T wave changes
- RBBB or LBBB
- Arrhythmias (atrial fibrillation, PVC, PAC, ventricular tachycardia)

ECHOCARDIOGRAM:
Low ejection fraction with global akinesia

TREATMENT

NONPHARMACOLOGIC THERAPY

- Limit activity when CHF is present
- Treatment of underlying disease (SLE, alcoholism)

ACUTE GENERAL Rx

- Treat CHF (cause of death in 70% of patients) with sodium restriction, diuretics, ACE inhibitors, β-blockers, spironolactone, and digitalis.
- Vasodilators (combined with nitrates and ACE inhibitors) are effective agents in all symptomatic patients with left ventricular dysfunction.
- Prevent thromboembolism with oral anticoagulants in all patients with atrial fibrillation and in patients with moderate or severe failure.
- Low-dose β-blockade with carvedilol or other β-blockers may improve ventricular function by interrupting the cycle of reflex sympathetic activity and controlling tachycardia.
- Diltiazem and ACE inhibitors have also been reported to have a long-term beneficial effect in idiopathic dilated cardiomyopathy.
- Use antiarrhythmic treatment as appropriate. Empiric pharmacologic suppression of asymptomatic ventricular ectopy does not reduce risk of sudden death or improve long-term survival. In patients with severe left ventricular dysfunction and/or symptomatic and sustained ventricular tachycardia, the use of an automatic implantable cardioverter-defibrillator should be considered.
- Growth hormone administration has been shown to increase myocardial mass and reduce the size of the left ventricular chamber, resulting in improvement in hemodynamics and clinical status. This therapeutic approach remains controversial.
- Patients with dilated cardiomyopathy (LVEF <25%) and associated coronary atherosclerosis (angina, ECG changes, reversible defects on thallium scan) may benefit from surgical revascularization.

DISPOSITION

- Annual mortality is 20% in patients with moderate heart failure, and it exceeds 50% in patients with severe heart failure.
- The implantation of a cardioverter-defibrillator in patients with severe, nonischemic dilated cardiomyopathy already being treated with ACE inhibitors and β-blockers significantly reduces the risk of sudden death from arrhythmia.

REFERRAL

Consider heart transplant for young patients (<60 yr old) who are no longer responsive to medical therapy. Dilated cardiomyopathy is the cause of 45% of heart transplantations.

PEARLS & CONSIDERATIONS

COMMENTS

- Patients should be encouraged to restrict or eliminate alcohol and decrease sodium intake.
- Vulnerability to cardiomyopathy among chronic alcohol abusers is partially genetic and is related to the presence of angiotensin-converting-enzyme (ACE) DD genotype.
- Idiopathic dilated cardiomyopathy is often familial, and apparently, healthy relatives may have latent, early, or undiagnosed established disease. Echocardiographic evaluation of family members is recommended.

SUGGESTED READINGS

Kadish A et al: Prophylactic defibrillator implantation in patients with non-ischemic dilated cardiomyopathy, *N Engl J Med* 350:2151, 2004.

Mahon NG et al: Echocardiographic evaluation in asymptomatic relatives of patients with dilated cardiomyopathy reveals preclinical disease, *Ann Intern Med* 143:108, 2005.

AUTHOR: **FRED F. FERRI, M.D.**

BASIC INFORMATION

DEFINITION

Cardiomyopathies are a group of diseases primarily involving the myocardium and characterized by myocardial dysfunction that is not the result of hypertension, coronary atherosclerosis, valvular dysfunction, or pericardial abnormalities. In hypertrophic cardiomyopathy (HCM) there is marked hypertrophy of the myocardium and disproportionally greater thickening of the intraventricular septum than that of the free wall of the left ventricle (asymmetric septal hypertrophy [ASH]).

SYNONYMS

Idiopathic hypertrophic subaortic stenosis (IHSS)
Hypertrophic obstructive cardiomyopathy (HOCM)
ASH
HCM

ICD-9CM CODES
425.4 Cardiomyopathy, hypertrophic nonobstructive
425.1 Cardiomyopathy, hypertrophic obstructive
746.84 Cardiomyopathy, hypertrophic congenital

EPIDEMIOLOGY & DEMOGRAPHICS

- The disease occurs in two major forms:
  1. A familial form, usually diagnosed in young patients and gene mapped to chromosome 14q. It is caused by a missense mutation in 1 of at least 10 genes that encode the proteins of the cardiac sarcomere (0% of cases of hypertrophic cardiomyopathy are familial).
  2. A sporadic form, usually found in elderly patients.
- The prevalence of phenotypically expressed HCM in the adult general population is 0.2% (most common genetic cardiovascular disease) and manifests with massive hypertrophy involving primarily the ventricular septum.
- To date, more than 200 different hypertrophic cardiomyopathy–causing mutations have been reported.

PHYSICAL FINDINGS & CLINICAL PRESENTATION

- Hypertrophic cardiomyopathy may be suspected on the basis of abnormalities found on physical examination. Classic findings include:
  1. Harsh, systolic, diamond-shaped murmur at the left sternal border or apex that increases with Valsalva maneuver and decreases with squatting
  2. Paradoxic splitting of S_2 (if left ventricular obstruction is present)
  3. S_4
  4. Double or triple apical impulse
- Increased obstruction can occur with:
  1. Drugs: digitalis, β-adrenergic stimulators (isoproterenol, dopamine, epinephrine), nitroglycerin, vasodilators, diuretics, alcohol
  2. Hypovolemia
  3. Tachycardia
  4. Valsalva maneuver
  5. Standing position
- Decreased obstruction is seen with:
  1. Drugs: β-adrenergic blockers, calcium channel blockers, disopyramide, α-adrenergic stimulators
  2. Volume expansion
  3. Bradycardia
  4. Hand grip exercise
  5. Squatting position
- Clinical manifestations are as follows:
  1. Dyspnea
  2. Syncope (usually seen with exercise)
  3. Angina (decreased angina in recumbent position)
  4. Palpitations

ETIOLOGY

- Autosomal dominant trait with variable penetrance caused by mutations in any of 1 to 10 genes, each encoding proteins of cardiac sarcomere
- Sporadic occurrence

DIAGNOSIS

DIFFERENTIAL DIAGNOSIS

- Coronary atherosclerosis
- Valvular dysfunction
- Pericardial abnormalities
- Chronic pulmonary disease
- Psychogenic dyspnea

WORKUP

- The diagnosis can be confirmed by two-dimensional echocardiography. Continuous-wave Doppler echocardiography can be used to diagnose obstruction.
- ECG is abnormal in 75% to 95% of patients: left ventricular hypertrophy, abnormal Q waves in anterolateral and inferior leads.
- 24-hr Holter monitor to screen for potential lethal arrhythmias (principal cause of syncope or sudden death in obstructive cardiomyopathy) should be performed initially and annually.
- Exercise testing is indicated and can also provide prognostic information and should also be considered on an annual basis.

IMAGING STUDIES

- Chest x-ray: may be normal or may show cardiomegaly.
- Two-dimensional echocardiography is used to establish the diagnosis. Findings include: ventricular hypertrophy, ratio of septum thickness to left ventricular wall thickness >1.3:1, increased ejection fraction.
- Magnetic resonance imaging may be of diagnostic value when echocardiographic studies are technically inadequate. MRI is also useful in identifying segmental LVH undetectable by echocardiography.

TREATMENT

NONPHARMACOLOGIC THERAPY

Advise avoidance of alcohol; alcohol use (even in small amounts) results in increased obstruction of the left ventricular outflow tract. Patients should also be advised on avoidance of dehydration and strenuous exertion.

GENERAL Rx

- Therapy for hypertrophic cardiomyopathy is directed at blocking the effect of catecholamines that can exacerbate dynamic left ventricular outflow tract obstruction and avoidance of certain agents (e.g., vasodilator or diuretic agents), which can worsen the obstruction.
- Propranolol 160 to 240 mg/day. The beneficial effects of β-blockers on symptoms (principally dyspnea and chest pain) and exercise tolerance appear to be largely a result of a decrease in the heart rate with consequent prolongation of diastole and increased passive ventricular filling. By reducing the inotropic response, β-blockers may also lessen myocardial oxygen demand and decrease the outflow gradient during exercise, when sympathetic tone is increased.
- Verapamil also decreases left ventricular outflow obstruction by improving filling and probably reducing myocardial ischemia. It is used mainly as a second line agent in patients who cannot tolerate β-blockers. It should be used with caution in patients with symptomatic obstruction. Administration in the hospital setting is recommended in these patients.
- IV saline infusion in addition to propranolol or verapamil is indicated in patients with CHF.
- Disopyramide is a useful antiarrhythmic because it is also a negative inotrope resulting in further decrease in outflow gradient.
- Use antibiotic prophylaxis for surgical procedures.
- Avoid use of digitalis, diuretics, nitrates, and vasodilators.

- Encouraging results have been reported on the use of DDD pacing for hemodynamic and symptomatic benefit in patients with drug-resistant hypertrophic obstructive cardiomyopathy. Implantation of a dual-chamber pacemaker has not been shown to result in significant improvement in objective measures of exercise capacity.
- Implantable cardiac defibrillators (ICD) are a safe and effective therapy in HCM patients prone to ventricular arrhythmias. Their use is strongly warranted for patients with prior cardiac arrest or sustained spontaneous ventricular tachycardia. The use of ICD to prevent sudden death in HCM has been advocated by some cardiologists not only for patients with HCM who are at high risk but also in others with a single risk factor.

DISPOSITION

HCM is not a static disease. Some adults may experience subtle regression in wall thickness while others (approximately 5% to 10%) paradoxically evolve into an end stage resembling dilated cardiomyopathy and characterized by cavity enlargement, LV wall thinning, and diastolic dysfunction. Patients with HCM are at increased risk of sudden death, especially if there is onset of symptoms during childhood. Left ventricular outflow at rest is also a strong, independent predictor of severe symptoms of heart failure and of death. Adult patients can be considered low risk if they have no symptoms or mild symptoms and also if they have none of the following:

- A family history of premature death caused by hypertrophic cardiomyopathy
- Nonsustained ventricular tachycardia during Holter monitoring
- A marked outflow tract gradient
- Substantial hypertrophy (>20 mm)
- Marked left atrial enlargement
- Abnormal blood pressure response during exercise

REFERRAL

- Surgical treatment (myotomy-myectomy involving resection of the basal septum) is reserved for patients who have both a large outflow gradient (≥50 mm Hg) and severe symptoms of heart failure that are unresponsive to medical therapy. The risk of sudden death from arrhythmias is not altered by surgery. When this operation is performed by experienced surgeons in tertiary referral centers the operative mortality is <2% and many patients are able to achieve near normal exercise capacity postoperatively.
- Nonsurgical reduction of interventricular septum represents a controversial therapeutic approach that can be used in patients with HCM refractory to pharmacologic treatment. This technique involves the injection of ethanol in the septal perforator branch of the left anterior descending coronary artery, producing a controlled myocardial infarction of the interventricular septum and thereby reducing the left ventricular outflow tract gradient. This method may lead to improvement in both subjective and objective measures of exercise capacity but is associated with a high incidence of heart block, often requiring permanent pacing in about one fourth of patients.

PEARLS & CONSIDERATIONS

COMMENTS

- Screening of first-degree relatives with two-dimensional echocardiography and electrocardiography is indicated, particularly if adverse HCM-related events have occurred in the family. Annual screening is recommended for all adolescents from age 12 to 18. Periodic screening of all first-degree adult family members at 5-year intervals is recommended since hypertrophy may not be detected until the sixth decade of life. It is advisable to have a trained clinical genetic counselor see the patient and obtain consent before genetic testing.
- Future screening techniques may involve identification of mutations in the gene encoding the sarcomeric proteins. The most common sarcomeric subtype is MYBPC3-HCM affecting 1 in 5 patients. Clinical predictors of positive genotype, such as the presence of an implantable cardioverter-defibrillator, age at diagnosis, degree of left ventricular wall hypertrophy, and family history of HCM, may aid in patient selection for genetic testing and increase the yield of cardiac sarcomere gene screening.
- Mortality rate in HCM is approximately 1% to 2%.
- It is important to remember that HCM is predominantly a non-obstructive disease (75% of patients do not have a sizable resting outflow tract gradient).
- Patients should be instructed on need for bacterial endocarditis prophylaxis.
- Section III describes an algorithm for the management of symptoms and risk in patients with hypertrophic cardiomyopathy.

SUGGESTED READINGS

Maron BJ: Hypertrophic cardiomyopathy, a systematic review, *JAMA* 287:1308, 2002.

Maron BJ et al: Implantable cardioverter-defibrillators and prevention of sudden cardiac death in hypertrophic cardiomyopathy, *JAMA* 298(4):405, 2007.

Maron MS et al: Effect of left ventricular outflow tract obstruction on clinical outcome in hypertrophic cardiomyopathy, *N Engl J Med* 348:295, 2003.

Nishimura RA, Holmes DR: Hypertrophic obstructive cardiomyopathy, *N Engl J Med* 350:1320, 2004.

Shamim W et al: Nonsurgical reduction of the interventricular septum in patients with hypertrophic cardiomyopathy, *N Engl J Med* 347:1326, 2002.

VanDriest SL et al: Yield of genetic testing in hypertrophic cardiomyopathy, *Mayo Clin Proc* 80(6):739, 2005.

AUTHOR: **FRED F. FERRI, M.D.**

BASIC INFORMATION

DEFINITION

Cardiomyopathies are a group of diseases primarily involving the myocardium and characterized by myocardial dysfunction that is not the result of hypertension, coronary atherosclerosis, valvular dysfunction, or pericardial abnormalities. Restrictive cardiomyopathies are characterized by decreased ventricular compliance, usually secondary to infiltration of the myocardium. These patients have impaired ventricular filling and reduced diastolic volume, normal systolic function, and normal or near-normal myocardial thickness.

ICD-9CM CODES
425.4 Other primary cardiomyopathies

EPIDEMIOLOGY & DEMOGRAPHICS

- Relatively uncommon cardiomyopathy that is most frequently caused by amyloidosis (Fig. 1-44), myocardial fibrosis (after open heart surgery), and radiation.
- Many patients classified as having "idiopathic" restrictive cardiomiopathy may have mutations in the gene for cardiac troponin I, and restrictive cardiomyopathy may represent an overlap with hypertrophic cardiomyopathy in many familial cases.

PHYSICAL FINDINGS & CLINICAL PRESENTATION

Restrictive cardiomyopathy presents with symptoms of progressive left-sided and right-sided heart failure:

- Edema, ascites, hepatomegaly, distended neck veins
- Fatigue, weakness (secondary to low output)
- Kussmaul's sign: may be present
- Regurgitant murmurs
- Possible prominent apical impulse

ETIOLOGY

- Infiltrative and storage disorders (glycogen storage disease, amyloidosis, sarcoidosis, hemochromatosis)
- Scleroderma
- Radiation
- Endocardial fibroelastosis
- Endomyocardial fibrosis
- Idiopathic
- Toxic effects of anthracycline
- Carcinoid heart disease, metastatic cancers
- Diabetic cardiomyopathy
- Eosinophilic cardiomyopathy (Löffler's endocarditis)

DIAGNOSIS

DIFFERENTIAL DIAGNOSIS

- Coronary atherosclerosis
- Valvular dysfunction
- Pericardial abnormalities
- Chronic lung disease
- Psychogenic dyspnea

WORKUP

- Chest x-ray, ECG, echocardiogram
- Cardiac catheterization, MRI (selected cases)

IMAGING STUDIES

- Chest x-ray:
  1. Moderate cardiomegaly
  2. Possible evidence of CHF (pulmonary vascular congestion, pleural effusion)
- ECG:
  1. Low voltage with ST-T wave changes
  2. Possible frequent arrhythmias, left axis deviation, and atrial fibrillation
- Echocardiogram: increased wall thickness and thickened cardiac valves (especially in patients with amyloidosis)
- Cardiac catheterization to distinguish restrictive cardiomyopathy from constrictive pericarditis
  1. Constrictive pericarditis: usually involves both ventricles and produces a plateau of elevated filling pressures
  2. Restrictive cardiomyopathy: impairs the left ventricle more than the right (PCWP $>$ RAP, PASP >50 mm Hg)
- MRI may also be useful to distinguish restrictive cardiomyopathy from constrictive pericarditis (thickness of the pericardium >5 mm in the latter)

TREATMENT

NONPHARMACOLOGIC THERAPY

Control CHF by restricting salt.

ACUTE GENERAL Rx

- Cardiomyopathy caused by hemochromatosis may respond to repeated phlebotomies to decrease iron deposition in the heart.
- Sarcoidosis may respond to corticosteroid therapy.
- Corticosteroid and cytotoxic drugs may improve survival in patients with eosinophilic cardiomyopathy.
- There is no effective therapy for other causes of restrictive cardiomyopathy.

CHRONIC Rx

Death usually results from CHF or arrhythmias; therefore therapy should be aimed at controlling CHF by restricting salt, administering diuretics, and treating potentially fatal arrhythmias.

DISPOSITION

Prognosis varies with the etiology of the cardiomyopathy.

REFERRAL

Cardiac transplantation can be considered in patients with refractory symptoms and idiopathic or familial restrictive cardiomyopathies.

AUTHOR: **FRED F. FERRI, M.D.**

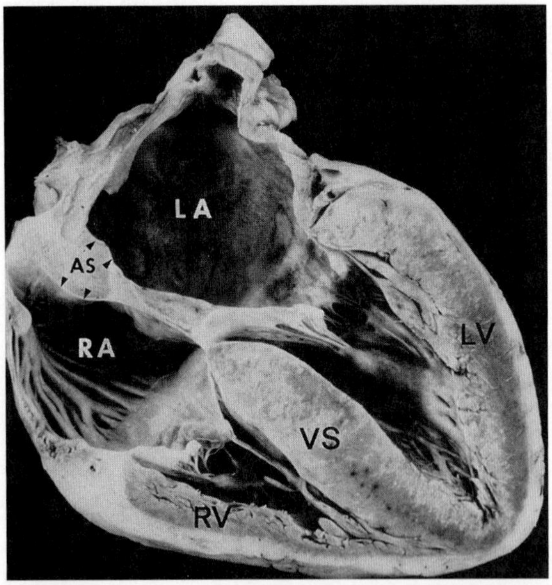

FIGURE 1-44 A necropsy specimen of an amyloid heart demonstrating the thickened ventricular septum *(VS)*, atrial septum *(AS)*, and free wall of the left ventricle *(LV)* and right ventricle *(RV)*, and the dilated left atrium *(LA)*. *RA*, Right atrium. (Courtesy Dr. William Edwards, Mayo Clinic, Rochester, MN. In Goldman L, Ausiello D [eds]: *Cecil textbook of medicine,* ed 22, Philadelphia, 2004, WB Saunders.)

BASIC INFORMATION

DEFINITION

Light-headedness, dizziness, presyncope, or syncope in a patient with carotid sinus hypersensitivity is defined as carotid sinus syndrome (CSS). Carotid sinus hypersensitivity is the exaggerated response to carotid stimulation resulting in bradycardia, hypotension, or both.

SYNONYMS

Carotid sinus syncope
CSS
Carotid sinus hypersensitivity

ICD-9CM CODES
337.0 Idiopathic peripheral autonomic neuropathy
780.2 Syncope or collapse

EPIDEMIOLOGY & DEMOGRAPHICS

- Carotid sinus hypersensitivity accounts for 10% to 20% of presyncopal and syncopal episodes.
- Carotid sinus hypersensitivity is frequently associated with atherosclerosis and diabetes mellitus.
- The incidence increases with age, with an average age of 61 to 74 yr.
- Men are affected more often than women (2:1).
- Carotid sinus syndrome is rarely found in patients younger than 50 yr of age.

PHYSICAL FINDINGS & CLINICAL PRESENTATION

- Usually associated with sudden neck movements or tight-fitting collars
- Usually associated with prodrome of nausea, warmth, pallor, or diaphoresis
- Light-headedness or presyncopal symptoms
- Syncope

Properly performed carotid sinus massage (CSM) at the bedside is diagnostic. This maneuver can elicit three types of responses in patients with carotid sinus hypersensitivity (see "Diagnosis").

1. CSM should be performed in the supine and upright positions while monitoring the patient's blood pressure by cuff and heart rate by ECG.
2. CSM should be performed on only one artery at a time.
3. CSM should be applied for approximately 5 to 10 seconds and repeated on the opposite side if no effect is produced.
4. Contraindications to CSM include the presence of carotid artery bruits, documented carotid artery stenosis >70%, history of stroke or transient ischemic attack <3 months, history of myocardial infarction <6 months, history of serious cardiac arrhythmias, or prior carotid endarterectomy.
5. Complications of visual disturbance and transient paresis from CSM occur in less than 1% of patients.

ETIOLOGY

- Idiopathic
- Head and neck tumors (e.g., thyroid)
- Significant lymphadenopathy
- Carotid body tumors
- Prior neck surgery

DIAGNOSIS

- Screening must be performed by doctors experienced with the maneuver and monitoring of the patient.
- The diagnosis of CSS is made when carotid sinus hypersensitivity is demonstrated by CSM and no other cause of syncope is identified.
- CSM can elicit three types of responses that are diagnostic of carotid sinus hypersensitivity:
  1. Cardioinhibitory type: CSM producing (1) asystole for at least 3 seconds in the absence of symptoms or (2) reproduction of symptoms occurring with a decline in heart rate of 30% to 40% or asystole of up to 2 seconds in duration. Symptoms should not recur when CSM is repeated after atropine infusion.
  2. Vasodepressor type: CSM producing (1) a decrease in systolic blood pressure of 50 mm Hg in absence of symptoms, or 30 mm Hg in the presence of neurologic symptoms; (2) no evidence of asystole; and (3) neurologic symptoms that persist after infusion of atropine.
  3. Mixed type: CSM producing both types of responses.

DIFFERENTIAL DIAGNOSIS

All causes of syncope

WORKUP

- It is a diagnosis of exclusion.
- Exclude other causes of syncope or presyncope: history and physical examination. Other tests should be ordered depending on the clinical setting.

TREATMENT

NONPHARMACOLOGIC THERAPY

Avoid applying neck pressure from tight collars, shaving, or rapid head turning.

ACUTE GENERAL Rx

Treatment will vary according to the type of carotid hypersensitivity response and symptoms present (see "Chronic Rx").

CHRONIC Rx

Therapy is divided into three classes: medical, surgical (carotid denervation), and cardiac pacing. Surgical therapy has been largely abandoned except in cases of compressing tumors or masses that are responsible for CSS.

For infrequent and mildly symptomatic carotid sinus hypersensitivity of either the cardioinhibitory or vasodepressor type, treatment is generally not necessary.

For symptomatic patients with a cardioinhibitory response to CSM:

- A dual-chamber permanent pacemaker is a class I indication.

For symptomatic patients with a vasodepressor response to CSM:

- Sympathomimetics: midodrine 2.5 to 10 mg tid
- Serotonin reuptake inhibitors
- Fludrocortisone
- Elastic knee-high or thigh-high stockings
- Carotid sinus denervation

For symptomatic patients with CSS with a mixed response to CSM:

- Combination of dual-chamber permanent pacemaker, atropine, and agents used to treat vasodepressor response.

DISPOSITION

- Up to 50% of the patients will have recurrent symptoms.
- No increased mortality of patients with idiopathic CSS when compared with the general population.

REFERRAL

Cardiology referral is indicated if a pacemaker is considered.

PEARLS & CONSIDERATIONS

The most common type is cardioinhibitory, followed by mixed and vasodepressor responses.

COMMENTS

Prognosis depends on the underlying cause.

SUGGESTED READINGS

AHA/ACCF scientific statement on the evaluation of syncope, *J Am Coll Cardiol* 47(2):473, 2006.

Brignole M et al: Task Force on Syncope, European Society of Cardiology, Guidelines on management (diagnosis and treatment) of syncope—update 2004, *Europace* 6:467, 2004.

Grubb BP: Clinical practice: neurocardiogenic syncope, *N Engl J Med* 352:1004, 2005.

Kerr SR et al: Carotid sinus hypersensitivity in asymptomatic older persons: implications for diagnosis of syncope and falls, *Arch Intern Med* 166(5):515, 2006.

AUTHORS: **RAMI ELTIBI, M.D.,** and **WEN-CHIH WU, M.D.**

BASIC INFORMATION

DEFINITION

Carpal tunnel syndrome is an entrapment neuropathy involving the median nerve at the wrist (Fig. 1-45). It is the most common entrapment neuropathy in the upper extremity.

ICD-9CM CODES
354.0 Carpal tunnel syndrome

EPIDEMIOLOGY & DEMOGRAPHICS

PREVALENT AGE: 30 to 60 yr (bilateral up to 50%)
PREVALENT SEX: Females are affected two to five times as often as males

PHYSICAL FINDINGS & CLINICAL PRESENTATION

- Nocturnal pain
- Occasional median nerve sensory impairment (often only index and long fingers)
- Positive Tinel's sign at wrist (tapping over the median nerve on the flexor surface of the wrist produces a tingling sensation radiating from the wrist to the hand)
- Positive Phalen's test (reproduction of symptoms after 1 min of gentle, unforced wrist flexion)
- Carpal compression test: Pressure with the examiner's thumb over the patient's carpal tunnel for 30 sec elicits symptoms
- Thenar atrophy in long-standing cases

ETIOLOGY

- Idiopathic in most cases
- Space-occupying lesions in carpal tunnel (tenosynovitis, ganglia, aberrant muscles)
- Often associated with hypothyroidism, hormonal changes of pregnancy
- Job-related mechanical overuse may be a risk factor
- Traumatic injuries to wrist

DIAGNOSIS

DIFFERENTIAL DIAGNOSIS

- Cervical radiculopathy
- Chronic tendinitis
- Vascular occlusion
- Reflex sympathetic dystrophy
- Osteoarthritis
- Other arthritides
- Other entrapment neuropathies

IMAGING STUDIES

Routine roentgenograms may be helpful in establishing cause or ruling out other conditions.

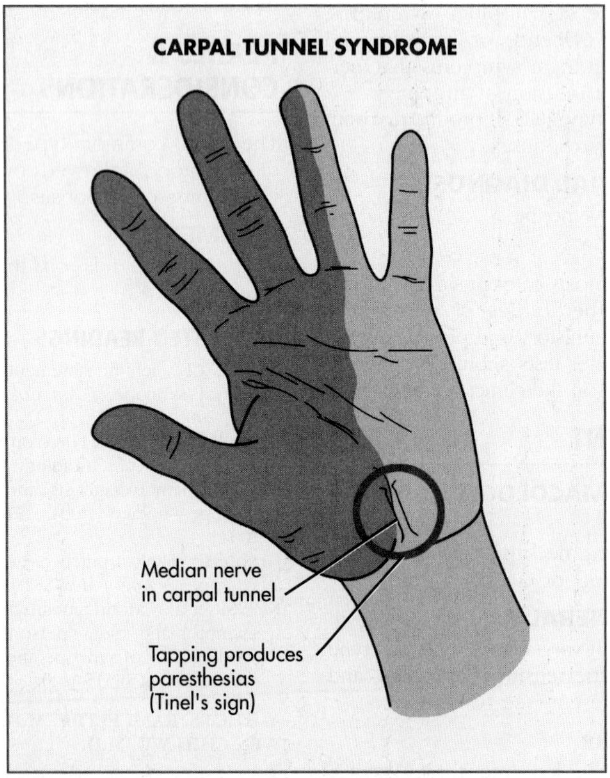

FIGURE 1-45 Distribution of pain and/or paresthesias *(dark-shaded area)* when the median nerve is compressed by swelling in the wrist (carpal tunnel). (From Arnett FC: Rheumatoid arthritis. In Andreoli TE [ed]: *Cecil essentials of medicine,* ed 4, Philadelphia, 1997, WB Saunders.)

ELECTRODIAGNOSTIC STUDIES

Nerve conduction velocity tests and electromyography are useful in establishing the diagnosis and ruling out other syndromes.

TREATMENT

ACUTE GENERAL Rx

- Elimination of repetitive trauma
- Occupational splints or braces
- NSAIDs
- Injection of carpal canal on ulnar side of palmaris longus tendon at wrist flexor crease (avoiding median nerve)
- Low-dose oral corticosteroids (e.g., prednisolone 20 mg qd for 2 wk, followed by 10 mg qd for 2 more wk) are also effective for symptom relief in selected patients
- Stretching exercises

DISPOSITION

Prognosis is variable. Some cases resolve spontaneously. Relief from local injection appears transient and symptoms recur in the majority of cases following injection. Carpal tunnel syndrome is common in the third trimester of pregnancy, but symptoms subside after delivery in most cases, often dramatically. Symptoms may recur with subsequent pregnancies. Surgery is not recommended in pregnant patients because of the likelihood of spontaneous recovery.

REFERRAL

Surgical referral in cases of failed medical management or signs of motor weakness. Results of surgery usually excellent with return to full activity in 4 to 6 weeks.

PEARLS & CONSIDERATIONS

- Carpal tunnel syndrome may occur in conjunction with cervical nerve root compression, a situation sometimes termed "double-crush syndrome." It has been suggested that compression at a more proximal level may decrease the ability of the nerve to tolerate distal compression.
- Whether computer keyboard use is a risk factor is controversial.

EVIDENCE

Local corticosteroid injections have been shown to be effective for the treatment of carpal tunnel syndrome in the short term.[1,2] Ⓐ

A single injection of methylprednisolone is no more effective than an oral anti-inflammatory plus nocturnal neutral wrist splints in relieving symptoms at 2 weeks.[1] Ⓐ

A single local methylprednisolone injection reduces symptoms at 8 and 12 weeks compared with oral prednisolone given for 10 days.[3] Ⓐ

Full time use of a neutral-angle wrist splint has not been shown to be superior to nighttime only use for improving mean symptom severity score[4] Ⓐ

Ultrasound plus nocturnal wrist splints and chiropractic manipulation were compared with nocturnal wrist splints and NSAIDs in an RCT of patients with carpal tunnel syndrome. After 9 weeks there was no significant difference in symptom severity between the groups.[5] Ⓐ

Vitamin B6 does not significantly improve overall symptoms compared with placebo.[6] Ⓐ

Evidence-Based References

1. Marshall S, Tardif G, Ashworth N: Local corticosteroid injection for carpal tunnel syndrome, *Cochrane Database Syst Rev* 4:CD001554, 2002. Ⓐ
2. O'Gradiagh D, Merry P: Corticosteroid injection for the treatment of carpal tunnel syndrome, *Ann Rheum Dis* 59:918, 2000. Ⓐ
3. Wong SM et al: Local vs systemic corticosteroids in the treatment of carpal tunnel syndrome, *Neurology* 56:1565, 2001. Reviewed in: *Clin Evid* 10:1271, 2003. Ⓐ
4. Walker WC et al: Neutral wrist splinting in carpal tunnel syndrome: a comparison of night-only versus full-time wear instructions, *Arch Phys Med Rehabil* 81:424, 2000. Reviewed in: *Clin Evid* 10:1271, 2003. Ⓐ
5. Davis PT et al: Comparative efficacy of conservative medical and chiropractic treatments for carpal tunnel syndrome: a randomized clinical trial, *J Manipulative Physiol Ther* 21:317, 1998. Reviewed in: *Clin Evid* 10:1271, 2003. Ⓐ
6. Gerritsen AAM et al: Conservative treatment options for carpal tunnel syndrome: a systematic review of randomised controlled trials, *J Neurol* 249:272, 2002. Reviewed in: *Clin Evid*10;1271, 2003. Ⓐ

SUGGESTED READINGS

Atroshi I et al: Carpal tunnel syndrome and keyboard use at work: a population-based study, *Arthritis Rheum* 56:3620, 2007.

Burke FD et al: Primary care management of patients with carpal tunnel syndrome referred to surgeons: are non-operative interventions effectively utilized? *Postgrad Med J* 83:498, 2007.

Cranford CS et al: Carpal tunnel syndrome, *J Am Acad Orthop Surg* 15:537, 2007.

Dias JJ, Burke FD et al: Carpal Tunnel Syndrome and work, *J Hand Surg* 29:329, 2004.

Geoghegan JM, Clark DI et al: Risk factors in carpal tunnel syndrome, *J Hand Surg* 29:315, 2004.

Gerritsen AM et al: Splinting vs surgery in the treatment of carpal tunnel syndrome, *JAMA* 288:1245, 2002.

Goodyear-Smith F, Arroll B: What can family physicians offer patients with carpal tunnel syndrome other than surgery? A systematic review of nonsurgical management, *Ann Fam Med* 2:267, 2004.

Hui AC, Wong SM et al: Long-term outcome of carpal tunnel syndrome after conservative treatment, *Int J Clin Pract* 58:337, 2004.

Katz JN, Simmons BP: Carpal tunnel syndrome, *N Engl J Med* 346:1807, 2002.

Lee DH, Claussen GC, Oh S: Clinical nerve conduction and needle electromyography studies, *J Am Acad Orthop Surg* 12:276, 2004.

Piszzini DB et al: A systematic review of conservative treatment of carpal tunnel syndrome, *Clin Rehabil* 21:299, 2007.

Rich JT et al: Carpal tunnel syndrome due to tophaceous gout, *Orthopedics* 27:862, 2004.

Vjera AJ: Management of carpal tunnel syndrome, *Am Fam Physician* 68:265, 2003.

AUTHOR: **LONNIE R. MERCIER, M.D.**

BASIC INFORMATION

DEFINITION

Cataracts are the clouding and opacification of the normally clear crystalline lens of the eye. The opacity may occur in the cortex, the nucleus of the lens, or the posterior subcapsular region, but it is usually in a combination of areas.

SYNONYMS

Congenital cataracts (e.g., from rubella)
Metabolic cataracts (e.g., caused by diabetes)
Collagen-vascular disease cataracts (caused by lupus)
Hereditary cataracts
Age-related senile cataracts
Traumatic cataracts
Toxic or drug-induced cataracts (e.g., caused by steroids)
Lenticular opacities

ICD-9CM CODES
366 Cataract

EPIDEMIOLOGY & DEMOGRAPHICS

INCIDENCE (IN U.S.): Highest cause of treatable blindness; cataract removal is the most frequent surgical procedure in patients >65 yr old (1.3 million operations/yr, with an annual cost of approximately $3 billion). By year 2020 expect over 30 million Americans to have cataracts. Of Americans >40, 20.5 million (17.2%) have cataracts. Of these, 5% have had surgery.

PEAK INCIDENCE:

- In early life: congenital and hereditary causes predominant; consider drug related and trauma
- In older age group: senile cataracts (after 40 yr of age)

PREDOMINANT AGE: Elderly; some stage of cataract development is present in >50% of persons 65 to 74 yr old and in 65% of those >75 yr old. Lens clouding begins at 39 to 40 yr old and then usually progresses either slowly or rapidly depending on individual and health.

GENETICS: Hereditary with such syndromes as galactosemia, homocystinuria, diabetes

PHYSICAL FINDINGS & CLINICAL PRESENTATION

Cloudiness and opacification of the crystalline lens of the eye (Fig. 1-46)

ETIOLOGY

- Heredity
- Trauma
- Toxins
- Age related
- Drug related
- Congenital
- Inflammatory
- Diabetes
- Collagen vascular disease

DIAGNOSIS

DIFFERENTIAL DIAGNOSIS

- Corneal lesions
- Retinal lesions, detached retina, tumors
- Vitreous disease, chronic inflammation

WORKUP

- Complete eye examination, including slit lamp examination, funduscopic examination, and brightness acuity testing
- Complete physical exam for other underlying causes

LABORATORY TESTS

- Rarely, urinary amino acid screening and CNS imaging studies with congenital cataracts
- Fasting glucose in young adults with cataracts
- Diabetes, collagen vascular, other metabolic diseases in younger patients
- Genetic and hereditary evaluation

TREATMENT

There is no evidence that antioxidants or drugs will slow down or help cataracts.

NONPHARMACOLOGIC THERAPY

- Wait until vision is compromised before doing surgery.
- Surgery is indicated when corrected visual acuity in the affected eye is >20/30 in the absence of other ocular disease; however, surgery may be justified when visual acuity is better in specific situations (especially disabling glare, monocular diplopia). Surgery indicated when vision in one eye is greatly different from the other and affects patient's life.

ACUTE GENERAL Rx

None necessary except when acute glaucoma or inflammation occurs

CHRONIC Rx

- Change glasses as cataracts develop.
- Myopia is common, and glasses can be adjusted until surgery is contemplated.

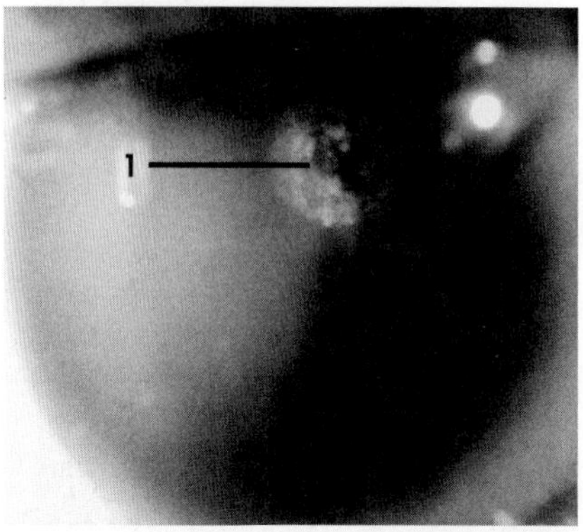

FIGURE 1-46 The central location of a posterior subcapsular cataract *(1).* (From Palay D [ed]: *Ophthalmology for the primary care physician,* St Louis, 1997, Mosby.)

DISPOSITION

Refer if sight compromised or inflamed red eye.

REFERRAL

Refer to ophthalmologist for evaluation extraction when vision is compromised (see "Nonpharmacologic Therapy").

PEARLS & CONSIDERATIONS

Patients want to know five things about cataracts:

1. Chance for vision improvement
2. When vision will improve
3. Risk from surgery
4. Effect of surgery
5. Types of complications

EVIDENCE

Phacoemulsification has been shown to give a better visual outcome than extracapsular extraction with sutures.[1] (B)

Extracapsular surgery with posterior chamber lens implant gives acceptable visual outcomes at 1 to 2 years after surgery.[1] (A)

Extracapsular cataract extraction with a posterior chamber lens implant provides a better visual outcome and quality of life, with fewer complications, than intracapsular extraction with aphakic glasses.[1] (A)(B)

Lensectomy and lens aspiration with primary capsulotomy are both effective treatments in children with bilateral, symmetrical, congential cataracts, but lens aspiration is associated with a significantly greater risk of secondary opacification.[2] (B)

Multifocal or bifocal intraocular lenses are very promising and successful in properly selected and qualifying patients.

Evidence-Based References

1. Snellingen T et al: Surgical interventions for age-related cataract. Reviewed in: Cochrane Library, 3, Chichester, UK, 2004, John Wiley. (A)(B)
2. Long V, Chen S: Surgical interventions for bilateral congenital cataract. Reviewed in: Cochrane Library, 3, Chichester, UK, 2004, John Wiley. (B)

SUGGESTED READINGS

Congdon N et al: Prevalence of cataract and pseudophakia/aphakia among adults in the US, *Arch Ophthalmol* 122(4):487, 2004.

Solomon R, Donninfeld ED: Recent advances and future frontiers in treating age-related cataracts, *JAMA* 290:248, 2003.

AUTHOR: **MELVYN KOBY, M.D.**

BASIC INFORMATION

DEFINITION

Cat-scratch disease (CSD) is a syndrome consisting of gradually enlarging regional lymphadenopathy occurring after contact with a feline. Atypical presentations are characterized by a variety of neurologic manifestations as well as granulomatous involvement of the eye, liver, spleen, and bone. The disease is usually self-limiting, and recovery is complete; however, patients with atypical presentations, especially if immunocompromised, may suffer significant morbidity and mortality.

SYNONYMS

Cat-scratch fever
Benign inoculation lymphoreticulosis
Nonbacterial regional lymphadenitis

ICD-9CM CODES
078.3 Cat-scratch disease

EPIDEMIOLOGY & DEMOGRAPHICS

PREVALENCE: Unknown

INCIDENCE (IN U.S.):
- Unknown
- Majority of reported cases in children

PEAK INCIDENCE: August through January

GENETICS: Unknown

PHYSICAL FINDINGS & CLINICAL PRESENTATION

- Classic, most common finding: regional lymphadenopathy occurring within 2 wk of a scratch or contact with felines; usually a new kitten in the household
- Tender, swollen lymph nodes most commonly found in the head and neck, followed by the axilla and the epitrochlear, inguinal, and femoral areas
- Erythematous overlying skin, showing signs of suppuration from involved lymph nodes
- On careful examination; evidence of cutaneous inoculation in the form of a nonpruritic, slightly tender pustule or papule (Fig. 1-47)
- Fever in most patients
- Malaise and headache in fewer than a third of patients
- Atypical presentations in fewer than 15% of cases
  1. Usually in association with lymphadenopathy and a low-grade or frank fever (>101° F, >38.3° C)
  2. Include granulomatous involvement of the conjunctiva (Parinaud's oculoglandular syndrome) and focal masses in the liver, spleen, and mesenteric nodes
- CNS involvement: neuroretinitis, encephalopathy, encephalitis, transverse myelitis, seizure activity, and coma
- Osteomyelitis in adults and children

ETIOLOGY

- Major cause: *Bartonella (Rochalimaea) henselae*
- Mode of transmission: predominantly by direct inoculation through the scratch, bite, or lick of a cat, especially a kitten
- Limited evidence in support of an arthropod (flea) as an alternative vector of infection arising from bacteremic felines
- Rarely, associated with dogs, monkeys, and inanimate objects with which a feline has been in recent contact
- Approximately 2 wk after introduction of the bacteria into the host, regional lymphatic tissues displaying granulomatous infiltration associated with gradual hypertrophy
- Possible dissemination to distant sites (e.g., liver, spleen, and bone), usually characterized by focal masses or discrete parenchymal lesions

DIAGNOSIS

DIFFERENTIAL DIAGNOSIS

Granulomas of this syndrome must be differentiated from those associated with:
- tularemia
- tuberculosis or other myobacterial infections
- brucellosis
- sarcoidosis
- sporotrichosis or other fungal diseases
- toxoplasmosis
- lymphogranuloma venerum
- benign and malignant tumors such as lymphoma

WORKUP

Diagnosis should be considered in patients who present with a predominant complaint of gradually enlarging regional (focal) lymphadenopathy, often with fever and a recent history of having contact with a cat. A primary ulcer at the site of the cat scratch may or may not be present at the time lymphadenopathy becomes manifest.

LABORATORY TESTS

- CSD skin test is no longer used for clinical purposes.
- Biopsied lymph node histology consistent with CSD.
- Enhanced culture techniques and serologies augment establishment of the diagnosis. An IFA *Bartonella* serology is commercially available. A PCR is used in research settings.
- Histopathologically, Warthin-Starry silver stain has been used to identify the bacillus.
- Routine laboratory findings:
  1. Mild leukocytosis or leukopenia
  2. Infrequent eosinophilia
  3. Elevated ESR or CRP
- Abnormalities of bilirubin excretion and elevated hepatic transaminases are usually secondary to hepatic obstruction by granuloma, mass, or lymph node.
- In patients with neurologic manifestations, lumbar puncture usually reveals normal CSF, although there may be a mild pleocytosis and modest elevation in protein.

TREATMENT

NONPHARMACOLOGIC THERAPY

- Warm compresses to the affected nodes
- In cases of encephalitis or coma: supportive care

ACUTE GENERAL Rx

- There is no consensus over therapy, especially as the disease is self-limited in a majority of cases.
- It would be prudent to treat severely ill patients, especially if immunocompromised, with antibiotic therapy, because these patients tend to suffer dissemination of infection and increased morbidity.

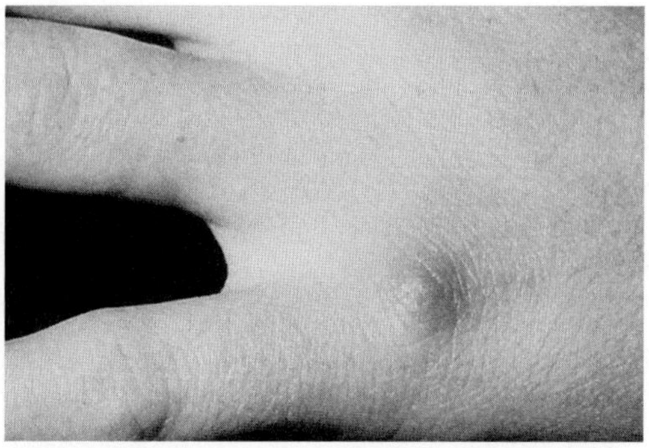

FIGURE 1-47 Primary lesion of cat-scratch disease is a tender papule occurring 3 to 10 days after a scratch. (From Noble J [ed]: *Primary care medicine*, ed 2, St Louis, 1996, Mosby.)

- *Bartonella* is usually sensitive to a 5-day course of azithromycin, or alternatively aminoglycosides, tetracycline, and the quinolones can be used.
- When the isolate is proven by culture, the patient should receive antibiotic therapy as directed by the obtained susceptibilities.
- Antipyretics and NSAIDs may also be used.

DISPOSITION

Overall prognosis is good.

REFERRAL

- To an appropriate subspecialist to evaluate specific lesions
- For diagnostic aspiration or excision in presence of regional lymphadenopathy, bone lesions, and mesenteric lymph nodes and organs
- To ophthalmologist for ocular granulomas
  1. Usually diagnosed clinically
  2. Rarely require excision

PEARLS & CONSIDERATIONS

COMMENTS

- A presentation of this syndrome, especially in patients with HIV infection or impaired cellular immunity, may be fever of unknown origin.
- Hepatic and splenic granulomas, coronary valve infections may offer few physical clues to diagnosis, emphasizing the need for a complete history.
- CSD should be considered in the differential diagnosis of school-aged children presenting with status epilepticus.
- Chronically immunocompromised patients considering the acquisition of a young feline should be made aware of the possible risk of infection.
- No signs of illness may be apparent in bacteremic kittens.

SUGGESTED READINGS

Arvand M, Schäd SG: Isolation of Bartonella henselae DNA from the peripheral blood of a patient with cat scratch disease up to 4 months after the cat scratch injury, *J Clin Microbiol* 44(6):2288, 2006.

Batts S, Demers DM: Spectrum and treatment of cat-scratch disease, *Pediatr Infect Dis J* 23(12):1161, 2004.

Koehler JE et al: Prevalence of Bartonella infection among human immunodeficiency virus-infected patients with fever, *Clin Infect Dis* 37(4):559, 2003.

Manfredi R, Sabbatani S, Chiodo F: Bartonellosis: light and shoadows in diagnostic and therapeutic issues, *Clin Microbiol Infect* 11(3):167, 2005.

Tsuneoka H, Isukahara M: Analysis of data in 30 patients with cat scratch disease without lymphadenopathy, *J Infect Chemother* 12(4):224, 2006.

AUTHORS: **GLENN G. FORT, M.D., M.P.H., DENNIS J. MIKOLICH, M.D.,** and **GEORGE O. ALONSO, M.D.**

BASIC INFORMATION

DEFINITION

Cavernous sinus thrombosis (CST) is a late complication of face or paranasal sinuses infection, resulting in thrombosis of the cavernous sinus and inflammation of its surrounding anatomic structures, including cranial nerves III, IV, V (ophthalmic and maxillary branch), and VI, and the internal carotid artery.

SYNONYMS

Intracranial venous sinus thrombosis or thrombophlebitis

ICD-9CM CODES
325 Phlebitis and thrombophlebitis of intracranial venous sinus

EPIDEMIOLOGY & DEMOGRAPHICS

- Cavernous sinus thrombosis is rare in the postantibiotic era.
- Before antibiotics the mortality rate was 80% to 100%.
- With antibiotics and early diagnosis, mortality rates have fallen to <20%.
- Reported morbidity rates have also declined from between 50% and 70% to only 22% with advances in imaging modalities, and aggressive medical care.

PHYSICAL FINDINGS & CLINICAL PRESENTATION

- Can be either an acute and fulminant disease or an indolent and subacute presentation.
- Most common signs are related to the anatomic structures affected within the cavernous sinus, notably cranial nerves III to VI, as well as symptoms resulting from impaired venous drainage from the orbit and the eye.
- A classic presentation is abrupt onset of unilateral periorbital edema, headache, photophobia, and proptosis. Headache is usually the presenting complaint and may precede fever and periorbital edema by several days. Elderly patients may present only with alteration in mental status without antecedent headache.

Other common signs and symptoms include:

- Ptosis
- Chemosis
- Cranial nerve palsies (III, IV, V, VI)
  1. Sixth nerve palsy is the most common.
  2. Hypoesthesia or hyperesthesia of the ophthalmic and maxillary branch of the fifth nerve are common. Periorbital sensory loss and impaired corneal reflex may be noted.

Papilledema, retinal hemorrhages, and decreased visual acuity and blindness may occur from venous congestion within the retina.

- Pupil may be dilated and sluggishly reactive.
- Fever, tachycardia, sepsis may be present.
- Headache with nuchal rigidity and changes in mental status may occur.

Infection can spread to the contralateral cavernous sinus through the intercavernous sinuses within 24 to 48 hr of initial presentation.

ETIOLOGY

- CST most commonly results from contiguous spread of an infection from the sinuses (sphenoid, ethmoid, or frontal) or the middle third region of the face. Nasal furuncles are the most common facial infection to produce this complication. Less common primary sites of infection include dental abscess, tonsils, soft palate, middle ear, or orbit (orbital cellulitis).
- It also can result from hematogenous spread of infection to the cavernous sinus via the superior and inferior ophthalmic veins. This venous system has a predisposition to impaired drainage because it is valveless, where the direction of blood flow depends on the venous pressure gradient.
- *Staphylococcus aureus* is the most common infectious microbe, found in 60% to 70% of the cases.
- *Streptococcus* is the second leading cause.
- Gram-negative rods and anaerobes may also lead to cavernous sinus thrombosis.
- Rarely, *Aspergillus fumigatus* and mucormycosis cause CST.

DIAGNOSIS

- The diagnosis of cavernous sinus thrombosis is made by clinical suspicion and confirmed by appropriate imaging studies.
- Proptosis, ptosis, chemosis, and cranial nerve palsy beginning in one eye and progressing to the other eye establish the diagnosis.

DIFFERENTIAL DIAGNOSIS

- Orbital or periorbital cellulitis
- Internal carotid artery aneurysm or fistula
- CVA
- Migraine headache
- Allergic blepharitis
- Thyroid ophthalmopathy
- Orbital neoplasm
- Meningitis
- Epidural and subdural infections
- Epidural and subdural hematoma
- Subarachnoid hemorrhage
- Acute angle-closure glaucoma
- Trauma

WORKUP

Cavernous sinus thrombosis is a clinical diagnosis with laboratory tests and imaging studies confirming the clinical impression.

LABORATORY TESTS

- CBC, ESR, blood cultures, and sinus cultures help establish and identify an infectious primary source.
- Lumbar puncture (LP) is necessary in distinguishing CST from more localized processes (e.g., sinusitis, orbital cellulites). LP reveals inflammatory cells in 75% of cases. The CSF profile is typically that of a parameningeal focus (high WBC, normal glucose, normal protein, culture negative) but may be similar to that of a bacterial meningitis.

IMAGING STUDIES

- Historically, sinus films are helpful in the diagnosis of sphenoid sinusitis. Opacification, sclerosis, and air-fluid levels are typical findings.
- Noncontrast CT can demonstrate an increase density in the region of the cavernous sinus. Contrast-enhanced CT scan may reveal underlying sinusitis, thickening of the superior ophthalmic vein, and irregular filling defects within the cavernous sinus; however, findings may be normal early in the disease course.
- MRI with gadolinium including MR angiography is more sensitive than CT scan and is the imaging study of choice to diagnose cavernous sinus thrombosis. Findings may include deformity of the internal carotid artery within the cavernous sinus, and an obvious signal hyperintensity within thrombosed vascular sinuses on all pulse sequences.
- Cerebral angiography can be performed, but it is invasive and not very sensitive.
- Orbital venography is difficult to perform, but it is excellent in diagnosing occlusion of the cavernous sinus.

TREATMENT

NONPHARMACOLOGIC THERAPY

Recognizing the primary source of infection (i.e., facial cellulitis, middle ear, and sinus infections) and treating the primary source expeditiously is the best way to prevent cavernous sinus thrombosis.

ACUTE GENERAL Rx

- Appropriate therapy should take into account the primary source of infection as well as possible associated complications such as brain abscess, meningitis, or subdural empyema.
- Broad-spectrum intravenous antibiotics are used as empiric therapy until a definite pathogen is found. Treatment should include a penicillinase-resistant penicillin at maximum dose plus a third- or fourth-generation cephalosporin:
  1. Nafcillin (or oxacillin) 2 g IV q4h plus either ceftriaxone (2 g q12h) or cefipime (2 g q6h).
  2. Metronidazole 500 mg IV q6h should be added if anaerobic bacterial infection is suspected (dental or sinus infection).
- Vancomycin (1 g q12h with normal renal function) may be substituted for nafcillin if significant concern exists for infection by methicillin-resistant *Staphylococcus aureus* or resistant *Streptococcus pneumoniae.*
- Anticoagulation with heparin is controversial. Cerebral infarction or intracranial hemorrhage should first be ruled out by noncontrast CT scan before initiating heparin therapy. Current recommendation is for early heparinization in patients with unilateral cavernous sinus thrombosis to prevent clot propagation and to reduce the incidence of septic emboli. Coumadin therapy should be avoided in the acute phase of the illness, but should ultimately be instituted to achieve an INR of 2 to 3, and continued until the infection, symptoms, and signs of cavernous thrombosis have resolved or significantly improved.
- Steroid therapy is also controversial but may prove helpful in reducing cranial nerve dysfunction or when progression to pituitary insufficiency occurs. Corticosteroids should only be instituted after appropriate antibiotic coverage. Dexamethasone 10 mg q6h is the treatment of choice.

CHRONIC Rx

- Emergent surgical drainage with sphenoidotomy is indicated if the primary site of infection is thought to be the sphenoid sinus.
- All patients with CST are usually treated with prolonged courses (3 to 4 wk) of IV antibiotics. If there is evidence of complications such as intracranial suppuration, 6 to 8 wk of total therapy may be warranted.
- All patients should be monitored for signs of complicated infection, continued sepsis, or septic emboli while antibiotic therapy is being administered.

DISPOSITION

- Cavernous sinus thrombosis can be a life-threatening, rapidly progressive infectious disease with high morbidity and mortality rates (30%) despite antibiotic use. Morbidity and mortality are increased in cases of sphenoid sinus infection.
- Complications of untreated CST include extension of thrombus to other dural venous sinuses, carotid thrombosis with concomitant strokes, subdural empyema, brain abscess, or meningitis. Septic embolization may also occur to the lungs, resulting in ARDS, pulmonary abscess, empyema, and pneumothorax.
- 30% of treated patients develop long-term sequelae, which include cranial nerve palsies, blindness, pituitary insufficiency, and hemiparesis.

REFERRAL

If the diagnosis is suspected, this should be considered a medical emergency. Depending on the primary site of infection, appropriate consultation should be made (i.e., ENT, ophthalmology, and infectious disease).

PEARLS & CONSIDERATIONS

COMMENTS

Realizing the cavernous sinus lies just above and lateral to the sphenoid sinus and drains the middle portion of the face via the superior and inferior ophthalmic veins and knowing that cranial nerves III, IV, V, and VI pass alongside or through the cavernous sinus make the clinical findings and diagnosis easier to understand.

EVIDENCE

EBM

We were unable to cite any evidence that meets our criteria regarding the use of antibiotics in cavernous sinus thrombosis.

A systematic review concluded that heparin treatment appeared safe and was associated with an important reduction in the risk of death or dependency, which did not reach statistical significance in cases of cerebral sinus thrombosis.[1] A

Evidence-Based Reference

1. Stam J, de Bruijn SFTM, DeVeber G: Anticoagulation for cerebral sinus thrombosis. In: Cochrane Library, 3, Chichester, UK, 2004, John Wiley. A

SUGGESTED READINGS

Bhatia K, Jones NS: Septic cavernous sinus thrombosis secondary to sinusitis: are anticoagulants indicated? A review of the literature, *J Laryngol Otol* 116(9):667-676, 2002.

Ferro JM et al: Cerebral vein and dural sinus thrombosis in elderly patients, *Stroke* 36:1927, 2005.

Hoshino CH et al: Septic cavernous sinus thrombosis complicated by narrowing of the internal carotid artery, subarachnoid abcess and multiple pulmonary septic emboli, *Intern Med* 46:317, 2007.

Lee JH et al: Cavernous sinus syndrome: clinical features and differential diagnosis with MR imaging, *AJR* 181:583, 2003.

AUTHOR: **WEN-Y WU-CHEN, M.D.**

BASIC INFORMATION

DEFINITION

Celiac disease is a chronic disease characterized by malabsorption and diarrhea precipitated by ingestion of food products containing gluten.

SYNONYMS

Gluten-sensitive enteropathy
Celiac sprue
Nontropical sprue

ICD-9CM CODES
579.0 Celiac disease

EPIDEMIOLOGY & DEMOGRAPHICS

- The prevalence of celiac disease is 1% in the general population in North America and Western Europe and 5% in high-risk groups such as first-degree relatives of persons with the disease.
- Incidence is highest during infancy and the initial 36 mo (secondary to the introduction of foods containing gluten), in the third decade (frequently associated with pregnancy and severe anemia during pregnancy), and in the seventh decade.
- There is a slight female predominance.

PHYSICAL FINDINGS & CLINICAL PRESENTATION

- Physical examination may be entirely within normal limits.
- Weight loss, dyspepsia, short stature, and failure to thrive may be noted in children and infants.
- Weight loss, fatigue, and diarrhea are common in adults.
- Abdominal pain, nausea, and vomiting are unusual.
- Pallor as a result of iron deficiency anemia is common.
- Atypical forms of the disease are being increasingly recognized and include osteoporosis, short stature, anemia, infertility, and neurologic problems. Manifestations of calcium deficiency, such as tetany and seizures, are rare and can be exacerbated by coexistent magnesium deficiency.
- Angular cheilitis, aphthous ulcers, atopic dermatitis, and dermatitis herpetiformis are frequently associated with celiac disease.

ETIOLOGY

- Celiac sprue is considered an autoimmune-type disease with tissue transglutaminase (tTG) suggested as a major autoantigen. It results from an inappropriate T-cell-mediated immune response against ingested gluten in genetically predisposed individuals who carry either HLA-DQ2 or HLA-DQ8 genes. There is sensitivity to gliadin, a protein fraction of gluten found in wheat, rye, and barley.
- Timing of introduction of gluten into the infant diet is associated with the appearance of celiac disease in children at risk. Children initially exposed to gluten in the first 3 mo of life have a fivefold increased risk.

DIAGNOSIS

DIFFERENTIAL DIAGNOSIS

- IBD
- Laxative abuse
- Intestinal parasitic infestations
- Other: irritable bowel syndrome, tropical sprue, chronic pancreatitis, Zollinger-Ellison syndrome, cystic fibrosis (children), lymphoma, eosinophilic gastroenteritis, short bowel syndrome, Whipple's disease

LABORATORY TESTS

- Iron deficiency anemia (microcytic anemia, low ferritin level)
- Folic acid deficiency
- Vitamin B_{12} deficiency, hypomagnesemia, hypocalcemia
- IgA antiendomysium antibodies (EMA) are a good screening test for celiac disease, except in the case of patients with IgA deficiency. IgA tissue transglutaminase (TTG) antibody by ELISA is a newer and very accurate serologic test for celiac sprue.
- Biopsy of the small bowel is helpful in confirming a suspected diagnosis when positive, but a negative result does not rule out the diagnosis. It may be reasonable in children with significant elevations of TTG levels (>100U) to first try a gluten-free diet and consider biopsy in those who do not improve with diet.
- Human leukocyte antigen DQ2DQ8 testing is highly sensitive (90% to 95%) for celiac disease but not very specific. Its greatest diagnostic value is in its negative predictive value, making it useful when negative in ruling out the disease.

IMAGING STUDIES

Capsule endoscopy can be used to evaluate the small-intestinal mucosa, especially if future innovations will allow mucosal biopsy.

TREATMENT

NONPHARMACOLOGIC THERAPY

Patients should be instructed on gluten-free diet (avoidance of wheat, rye, and barley). Recent studies show that oats do not damage the mucosa in celiac disease.

GENERAL Rx

- Correct nutritional deficiencies with iron, folic acid, calcium, vitamin B_{12} as needed.
- Prednisone 20 to 60 mg qd gradually tapered is useful in refractory cases.
- Lifelong gluten-free diet is necessary.

DISPOSITION

- Prognosis is good with adherence to gluten-free diet. Rapid improvement is usually seen within a few days of treatment.
- Serial antigliadin or antiendomysial antibody tests can be used to monitor the patient's adherence to a gluten-free diet.
- Repeat small bowel biopsy following treatment generally reveals significant improvement. It is also useful to evaluate for increased risk of small bowel T-cell lymphoma in these patients, especially in untreated patients.

PEARLS & CONSIDERATIONS

COMMENTS

- Some experts recommend a repeat biopsy only in selected patients who have an unsatisfactory response to a strict gluten-free diet.
- Celiac disease should be considered in patients with unexplained metabolic bone disease, osteoporosis, or hypocalcemia, especially because GI symptoms may be absent or mild. Clinicians should also consider testing children and young adults for celiac disease if unexplained weight loss, abdominal pain or distention, or chronic diarrhea is present.
- The prevalence of celiac disease in patients with dyspepsia is twice that of the general population. Screening for celiac disease should be considered in all patients with persistent dyspepsia.
- Celiac disease is associated with an increased risk for non-Hodgkin's lymphoma, especially of T-cell type and primarily localized in the gut. Lymphoma is 4 to 40 times more common and death from lymphoma is 11 to 70 times more common in patients with celiac disease.

SUGGESTED READINGS

Alaedini A, Green PH: Narrative review: celiac disease: understanding a complex autoimmune disorder, *Ann Intern Med* 142:289-298, 2005.
Green PH, Cellier C: Celiac disease, *N Engl J Med* 357:1731-1743, 2007.
Hadithi M et al: Accuracy of serologic tests and HLA-DQ typing for diagnosing celiac disease, *Am Intern Med* 147:294-302, 2007.
Norris JM et al: Risk of celiac disease autoimmunity and timing of gluten introduction in the diet of infants at increased risk of disease, *JAMA* 293:2343-2351, 2005.

AUTHOR: **FRED F. FERRI, M.D.**

BASIC INFORMATION

DEFINITION

Cellulitis is a superficial inflammatory condition of the skin. It is characterized by erythema, warmth, and tenderness of the area involved.

SYNONYMS

Erysipelas (cellulitis generally secondary to group A β-hemolytic streptococci)

ICD-9CM CODES
682.9 Cellulitis

EPIDEMIOLOGY & DEMOGRAPHICS

- Occurs most frequently in diabetics, immunocompromised hosts, and patients with venous and lymphatic compromise.
- Frequently found near skin breaks (trauma, surgical wounds, ulcerations, tinea infections). Edema, animal or human bites, subadjacent osteomyelitis, and bacteremia are potential sources of cellulitis.

PHYSICAL FINDINGS & CLINICAL PRESENTATION

Variable with the causative organism

- Erysipelas: superficial-spreading, warm, erythematous lesion distinguished by its indurated and elevated margin; lymphatic involvement and vesicle formation are common.
- Staphylococcal cellulitis: area involved is erythematous, hot, and swollen; differentiated from erysipelas by nonelevated, poorly demarcated margin; local tenderness and regional adenopathy are common; up to 85% of cases occur on the legs and feet.
- *H. influenzae* cellulitis: area involved is a blue-red/purple-red color; occurs mainly in children; generally involves the face in children and the neck or upper chest in adults.
- *Vibrio vulnificus:* larger hemorrhagic bullae, cellulitis, lymphadenitis, myositis; often found in critically ill patients in septic shock.

ETIOLOGY

- Group A β-hemolytic streptococci (may follow a streptococcal infection of the upper respiratory tract)
- Staphylococcal cellulitis
- *H. influenzae*
- *Vibrio vulnificus:* higher incidence in patients with liver disease (75%) and in immunocompromised hosts (corticosteroid use, diabetes mellitus, leukemia, renal failure)
- *Erysipelothrix rhusiopathiae:* common in people handling poultry, fish, or meat
- *Aeromonas hydrophila:* generally occurring in contaminated open wound in fresh water
- Fungi *(Cryptococcus neoformans):* immunocompromised granulopenic patients
- Gram-negative rods *(Serratia, Enterobacter, Proteus, Pseudomonas):* immunocompromised or granulopenic patients

DIAGNOSIS

DIFFERENTIAL DIAGNOSIS

- Necrotizing fasciitis
- DVT
- Peripheral vascular insufficiency
- Paget's disease of the breast
- Thrombophlebitis
- Acute gout
- Psoriasis
- Candida intertrigo
- Pseudogout
- Osteomyelitis
- Insect bite
- Fixed drug eruption
- Lymphedema
- Rare causes: Vaccinia vaccination, Kawasaki disease, pyoderma gangrenosa, Sweet's syndrome, carcinoma erysipeloides, anaerobic myonecrosis, erythromelalgia, eosinophilic cellulitis (Well's syndrome), familial Mediterranean Fever

LABORATORY TESTS

- Gram stain and culture (aerobic and anaerobic)
  1. Aspirated material from:
     a. Advancing edge of cellulitis
     b. Any vesicles
  2. Swab of any drainage material
  3. Punch biopsy (in selected patients)
- Blood cultures in hospitalized patients, in patients who have cellulitis superimposed on lymphedema, in patients with buccal or periorbital cellulitis, and in patients suspected of having a salt-water or fresh-water source of infection. Bacteremia is uncommon in cellulitis (positive blood cultures in only 4% of patients)
- ALOS titer (in suspected streptococcal disease)

Despite the previous measures, the cause of cellulitis remains unidentified in most patients.

IMAGING STUDIES

CT or MRI in patients with suspected necrotizing fasciitis (deep-seated infection of the subcutaneous tissue that results in the progressive destruction of fascia and fat).

TREATMENT

NONPHARMACOLOGIC THERAPY

Immobilization and elevation of the involved limb. Cool sterile saline dressings to remove purulence from any open lesion. Support stockings in patients with peripheral edema.

ACUTE GENERAL Rx

Erysipelas
- PO: dicloxacillin 500 mg PO q6h
- IV: cefazolin 1 g q6 to 8h or nafcillin 1.0 or 1.5 g IV q4 to 6h

NOTE: Use erythromycin, clindamycin, or vancomycin in patients allergic to penicillin.

Staphylococcus cellulitis
- PO: dicloxacillin 250 to 500 mg qid
- IV: nafcillin, 1 to 2 g q4 to 6h
- Cephalosporins (cephalothin, cephalexin, cephradine) also provide adequate antistaphylococcal coverage except for MRSA
- Use vancomycin 1.0 to 2.0 g IV qd or linezolid 0.6 g IV q12h in patients allergic to penicillin or cephalosporins and in patients with methicillin-resistant *S. aureus* (MRSA). Daptomycin (Cubicin), a cyclic lipopeptide can be used as an alternative to vancomycin for complicated skin and skin structure infections. Usual dose is 4 mg/kg IV given over 30 min every 24 hr

H. influenzae cellulitis
- PO: cefixime or cefuroxime
- IV: cefuroxime or ceftriaxone

Vibrio vulnificus
- Doxycycline 100 mg IV or PO bid +/− third-generation cephalosporin. Ciprofloxacin is an alternative antibiotic
- IV support and admission into ICU (mortality rate >50% in septic shock)

Erysipelothrix
- Penicillin

Aeromonas hydrophila
- Aminoglycosides
- Chloramphenicol
- Complicated skin and skin structure infections in hospitalized patients can be treated with daptomycin (cubicin) 4 mg/kg IV every 24 hr

DISPOSITION

Prognosis is good with prompt treatment.

REFERRAL

For surgical debridement in addition to antibiotics in patients with suspected necrotizing fasciitis

SUGGESTED READINGS

Swartz MN: Cellulitis, *N Engl J Med* 350:904, 2004.

Falagas M, Vergidis PI: Narrative review: diseases that masquerade as infectious cellulitis, *Ann Intern Med* 142:47, 2005.

AUTHOR: **FRED F. FERRI, M.D.**

BASIC INFORMATION

DEFINITION

Cerebral palsy (CP) is a group of disorders of the central nervous system characterized by aberrant control of movement or posture, present since early in life and not the result of a progressive or degenerative disease.

SYNONYMS

Little's disease
Congenital static encephalopathy
Congenital spastic paralysis

ICD-9CM CODES
343 Infantile cerebral palsy

EPIDEMIOLOGY & DEMOGRAPHICS

INCIDENCE (IN U.S.): 2 to 2.5 per 1000 live births
PREDOMINANT SEX: Male = female
PREDOMINANT AGE: Diagnosis made at 3 to 5 yr

PHYSICAL FINDINGS & CLINICAL PRESENTATION

- Monoplegia, diplegia, quadriplegia, hemiplegia
- Often hypotonic in newborn period, followed by development of hypertonia
- Spasticity
- Athetosis
- Delay in motor milestones
- Hyperreflexia
- Seizures
- Mental retardation

ETIOLOGY

Mulitfactorial, including low birthweight, congenital malformation, asphyxia, multiple gestations, intrauterine exposure to infection, neonatal stroke, and hyperbilirubinemia

DIAGNOSIS

A motor deficit is always present.
The usual presenting complaint is that child is not reaching motor milestones at the appropriate age. Medical history establishes that the child is not losing function. This history, combined with a neurologic examination establishing that motor deficit is due to a cerebral abnormality, establishes the diagnosis of CP. Serial examinations may be necessary if the history is unreliable.

DIFFERENTIAL DIAGNOSIS

Other causes of neonatal hypotonia include: muscular dystrophies, spinal muscular atrophy, Down's syndrome, spinal cord injuries

WORKUP

- Laboratory tests are not necessary to establish the diagnosis.
- Workup is helpful for assessment of recurrence risk, implementation of prevention programs, and medicolegal purposes.

LABORATORY TESTS

- Metabolic and genetic testing should be considered if on follow-up the child has (1) evidence of deterioration or episodes of metabolic decompensation, (2) no etiology determined by neuroimaging, (3) family history of childhood neurologic disorder associated with CP, (4) developmental malformation on neuroimaging.
- If previous stroke seen on neuroimaging, consider evaluation for coagulopathy.
- An EEG should be obtained when a child with CP has a history suggestive of seizures.
- Children with CP should be screened for ophthalmologic and hearing impairments, speech and language disorders. Nutrition, growth, and swallowing function should be monitored.

IMAGING STUDIES

- Neuroimaging is recommended if the etiology has not been established previously; for example, by perinatal imaging.
- MRI, when available, is preferred to CT scanning because of higher yield in suggesting an etiology, and timing of the insult leading to CP.

TREATMENT

NONPHARMACOLOGIC THERAPY

- Physical therapy, occupational therapy, and speech therapy.
- Orthotics and casting are used to increase musculotendinous length.

ACUTE GENERAL Rx

If present, treatment of seizures

CHRONIC Rx

- Treatment of seizures, as directed by seizure type.
- Medical treatment of spasticity includes baclofen (oral and intrathecal) and botulinum toxin A.
- Surgical treatments of spasticity include dorsal rhizotomy, tendon lengthening, and osteotomy.

DISPOSITION

Most children with cerebral palsy live at home. Those children with severely impaired mobility or other disabilities often live in chronic-care nursing facilities.

REFERRAL

If the child has difficulty with spasticity, physical medicine and rehabilitation referrals are especially helpful.

PEARLS & CONSIDERATIONS

In full-term infants, history of traumatic delivery is usually not present.

EVIDENCE

Intensive (weekly) neurodevelopmental therapy has been demonstrated to lead to improved motor and functional outcomes after 6 months when compared with monthly therapy in children under age 18 months.[1] Speech and language therapy might help children with cerebral palsy communicate more effectively,[2] but more research is needed.

Continuous administration of intrathecal baclofen has been shown to improve motor function in a small series of children with spasticity due to cerebral palsy.[3]

Studies have shown that children who receive botulinum toxin or selective dorsal rhizotomy have improvement in some objective measures of spasticity, but the effect of these therapies on functional ability is still unclear.[4-6]

Evidence-Based References

1. Mayo NE: The effect of physical therapy for children with motor delay and cerebral palsy. A randomized clinical trial, *Am J Phys Med Rehabil* 70(5):258-267, 1991.
2. Pennington L et al: Speech and language therapy to improve the communication skills of children with cerebral palsy, *Cochrane Database Syst Rev* 2, 2004.
3. Van Schaeybroeck P et al: Intrathecal baclofen for intractable cerebral spasticity: a prospective placebo-controlled, double-blind study, *Neurosurgery* 46(3):603-609; discussion 609-612, 2000.
4. Ade-Hall RA, Moore AP: Botulinum toxin type A in the treatment of lower limb spasticity in cerebral palsy, *Cochrane Database Syst Rev* 1, 2000.
5. Wasiak J, Hoare B, Wallen M: Botulinum toxin A as an adjunct to treatment in the management of the upper limb in children with spastic cerebral palsy, *Cochrane Database Syst Rev* 4, 2004.
6. Graubert C et al: Changes in gait at 1 year post-selective dorsal rhizotomy: results of a prospective randomized study, *J Pediatr Orthop* 20(4):496-500, 2000.

SUGGESTED READINGS

Ashwal S et al: Practice parameter: diagnostic assessment of the child with cerebral palsy: report of the Quality Standards Subcommittee of the American Academy of Neurology and the Practice Committee of the Child Neurology Society, *Neurology* 62(6):851, 2004.

Nelson KB: The epidemiology of cerebral palsy in term infants, *Ment Retard Dev Disabil Res Rev* 8(3):146, 2002.

AUTHOR: **MAITREYI MAZUMDAR, M.D., M.P.H.**

BASIC INFORMATION

DEFINITION

Cervical cancer is penetration of the basement membrane and infiltration of the stroma of the uterine cervix by malignant cells.

ICD-9CM CODES
180 Malignant neoplasm of cervix uteri

EPIDEMIOLOGY & DEMOGRAPHICS

INCIDENCE: There are approximately 15,000 new cases annually, with 4000 to 5000 associated deaths. The U.S. has an age-adjusted mortality of 2.6 cases/100,000 persons for cervical cancer.
PREDOMINANCE: Higher incidence rates occur in developing countries. Among the U.S. population, Hispanics have a higher incidence than African Americans, who likewise have a higher incidence than whites.
RISK FACTORS: Smoking, early age at first intercourse, multiple sexual partners, immunocompromised state, nonbarrier methods of birth control, infection with high-risk HPV (types 16 and 18), and multiparity.

PHYSICAL FINDINGS & CLINICAL PRESENTATION

- Unusual vaginal bleeding, particularly postcoital
- Vaginal discharge and/or odor
- Advanced cases may present with lower extremity edema or renal failure
- In early stages there may be little or no obvious cervical lesion, more advanced cases may present with large, bulky, friable lesions encompassing the majority of the vagina (Fig. 1-48)

ETIOLOGY

- Dysplastic cells progress to invasive carcinoma.
- Thought to be linked to the presence of HPV types 16, 18, 45, and 56 via interaction of E6 oncoproteins on p53 gene product.
- There may be an association with past infection with *Chlamydia trachomatis*.

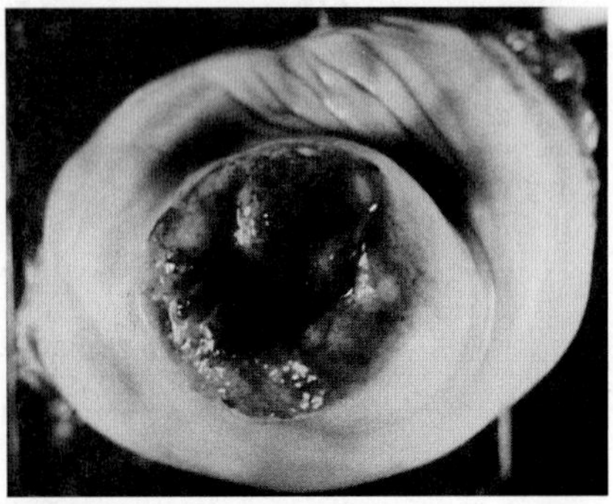

FIGURE 1-48 Carcinoma of cervix (gross specimen). (From Mishell D [ed]: *Comprehensive gynecology,* ed 3, St Louis, 1997, Mosby.)

DIAGNOSIS

DIFFERENTIAL DIAGNOSIS

- Cervical polyp or prolapsed uterine fibroid
- Preinvasive cervical lesions
- Neoplasia metastatic from a separate primary

WORKUP

- Thorough history and physical examination.
- Pelvic examination with careful rectovaginal examination.
- As compared with PAP testing, HPV testing has a greater sensitivity for the detection of cervical intraepithelial neoplasia. The addition of an HPV test to the PAP test to screen women in their mid-30s for cervical cancer reduces the incidence of grade 2 or 3 cervical intraepithelial neoplasia or cancer detected by subsequent screening examinations.
- Colposcopy with directed biopsy and endocervical curettage.
- Clinically staged, not surgically staged.

LABORATORY TESTS

- CBC, chemistry profile
- Squamous cell carcinoma (SCC) antigen in research setting
- Carcinoembryonic antigen (CEA)

IMAGING STUDIES

- Chest x-ray examination
- IVP
- Depending on stage, may need cystoscopy, sigmoidoscopy or BE, CT scan or MRI, lymphangiography

TREATMENT

NONPHARMACOLOGIC THERAPY

- FIGO stage Ia: cone biopsy or simple hysterectomy
- FIGO stage Ib or IIa: type III radical hysterectomy and pelvic lymphadenectomy *or* pelvic radiation therapy
- Advanced or bulky disease: multimodality therapy (radiation, chemotherapy, and/or surgery); platinum use before radiation therapy

ACUTE GENERAL Rx

Cervical cancer may present with massive and acute vaginal bleeding requiring volume and blood replacement, vaginal packing or other hemostatic modalities, and/or high-dose local radiotherapy.

CHRONIC Rx

- Physical examination with Pap smear every 3 mo for 2 yr, every 6 mo during the third to fifth year, and annually thereafter
- Chest x-ray examination annually

DISPOSITION

Five-year survival varies by stage:
- Stage I 60% to 90%
- Stage II 40% to 80%
- Stage III <60%
- Stage IV <15%

Early detection by Pap smear imperative to long-term improvements in survival.

REFERRAL

Gynecologic oncologist for all invasive disease

PEARLS & CONSIDERATIONS

Gardasil is a vaccine indicated in girls and women 9 to 26 yr of age for the prevention of cervical cancer caused by human papilloma virus types 6, 11, 16, and 18.

EVIDENCE

There is little evidence that is available and that meets rigorous criteria for the management of cervical malignancy/dysplasia.

Concomitant chemotherapy and radiotherapy appears to improve overall survival and progression-free survival in patients with locally advanced cervical cancer. Local and distant recurrence rates are also reduced with chemoradiation.[1] Ⓐ

Evidence-Based Reference

1. Green J et al: Concomitant chemotherapy and radiation therapy for cancer of the uterine cervix, *Cochrane Database Sys Rev* Issue 4, 2001. Ⓐ

SUGGESTED READINGS

Long HJ et al: Prevention, diagnoisis, and treatment of cervical cancer, *Mayo Clin Proc* 82(12):1566-1574, 2007.

Mayrand MH et al: Human papillomavirus DNA versus Papanicolaou screening tests for cervical cancer, *N Eng J Med* 357:1579-1588, 2007.

McCreath S: Cervical cancer: current management of early/late disease, *Surg Oncol Clin N Am*, 14(2):249, 2005.

Naucler P et al: Human papillomavirus and Papanicolaou tests to screen for cervical cancer, *N Eng J Med* 357:1589-1597, 2007.

AUTHORS: **GIL FARKASH, M.D.,** and **RUBEN ALVERO, M.D.**

BASIC INFORMATION

DEFINITION

Cervical disk syndromes refer to diseases of the cervical spine resulting from disk disorder, either herniation or degenerative change (spondylosis). When posterior osteophytes compress the anterior spinal cord, lower extremity symptoms may result, a condition termed *cervical spondylotic myelopathy*.

ICD-9CM CODES
722.4 Degenerative intervertebral cervical disk
722.71 Degenerative cervical disk with myelopathy

EPIDEMIOLOGY & DEMOGRAPHICS

PREVALENCE: 10% of general adult population (symptoms in 50% of population at some time in their life)
PREDOMINANT SEX: Male = female
PREDOMINANT AGE: 30 to 60 yr

PHYSICAL FINDINGS & CLINICAL PRESENTATION

- Neck pain, radicular symptoms, or myelopathy, either alone or in combination
- Limited neck movement
- Pain with neck motion, especially extension
- Referred unilateral interscapular pain, resulting in a local trigger point
- Radicular arm pain (usually unilateral), numbness, and tingling possible, most commonly involving the C6 (C5-C6 disk) or C7 (C6-C7 disk) nerve root
- Weakness and reflex changes (C6—biceps, C7—triceps)
- Myelopathy possibly resulting in gait disturbance, weakness, and even spasticity
- Sensory examination usually not helpful

ETIOLOGY

Unknown

DIAGNOSIS

DIFFERENTIAL DIAGNOSIS

- Rotator cuff tendinitis
- Carpal tunnel syndrome
- Thoracic outlet syndrome
- Brachial neuritis

A differential diagnosis for evaluation of neck pain is described in Section II.

WORKUP

In most cases, the diagnosis can be established on a clinical basis alone.

Section III, "Cervical Disk Syndrome," describes an algorithm for a workup of suspected cases.

IMAGING STUDIES

- Plain roentgenograms within the first few weeks
  1. Usually normal in soft disk herniation
  2. With chronic degenerative disk disease, usually loss of height of the disk space, anterior and posterior osteophyte formation, and encroachment on the intervertebral foramen by osteophytes
- Myelography, CT scanning, and MRI indicated in patients whose symptoms do not resolve or when other spinal pathology suspected
- Electrodiagnostic studies to confirm the diagnosis or rule out peripheral nerve disorders

TREATMENT

NONPHARMACOLOGIC THERAPY

- Rest and cervical collar if needed
- Local modalities such as heat
- Physical therapy (Fig. 1-49)
- Avoid extreme range of motion exercises in degenerative disk disease

ACUTE GENERAL Rx

- NSAIDs
- "Muscle relaxants" for their sedative effect
- Analgesics as needed
- Epidural steroid injection for radicular pain

DISPOSITION

- Usually improve with time
- Surgical intervention in <5%

REFERRAL

Orthopedic or neurosurgical consultation for intractable pain or neurologic deficit

PEARLS & CONSIDERATIONS

Myelopathy from cervical spondylosis is the most common cause of acquired spastic paralysis in the adult and is usually progressive. Whether to intervene surgically is a complicated decision.

COMMENTS

- Pain relief with physical therapy seems anecdotal and short-lived; any overall improvement usually parallels what would have probably occurred naturally.
- Sometimes carpal tunnel syndrome and cervical radiculopathy occur together; this is termed the *double-crush syndrome* and results from nerve compression at two separate levels. Proximal compression may decrease the ability of the nerve to tolerate a second, more distal compression.
- Surgical intervention is indicated primarily for relief of radicular pain caused by nerve root compression or for the treatment of myelopathy; it is generally not helpful when chief complaint is neck pain alone.
- In many cases of cervical spondylosis with myelopathy, the lower-extremity symptoms are much more disabling than the neck symptoms, a situation that can cause some difficulty in determining their etiology.

SUGGESTED READINGS

Gorski JM, Schwartz LH: Shoulder impingement presenting as neck pain, *J Bone Joint Surg* 85A:635, 2003.
King JT et al: Preference-based quality of life measurement in patients with cervical spondylotic myelopathy, *Spine* 29:1271, 2004.
Rao RD et al: Operative treatment of cervical spondylotic myelopathy, *J Bone Joint Surg* 88A:1619, 2006.
Rao RD et al: Degenerative cervical spondylosis: clinical syndromes, pathogenesis, and management, *J Bone Joint Surg* 89A:1360, 2007.
Rhee JM, Yoou T, Riew KD: Cervical radiculopathy, *J Am Acad Orthop Surg* 15:486, 2007.

AUTHOR: **LONNIE R. MERCIER, M.D.**

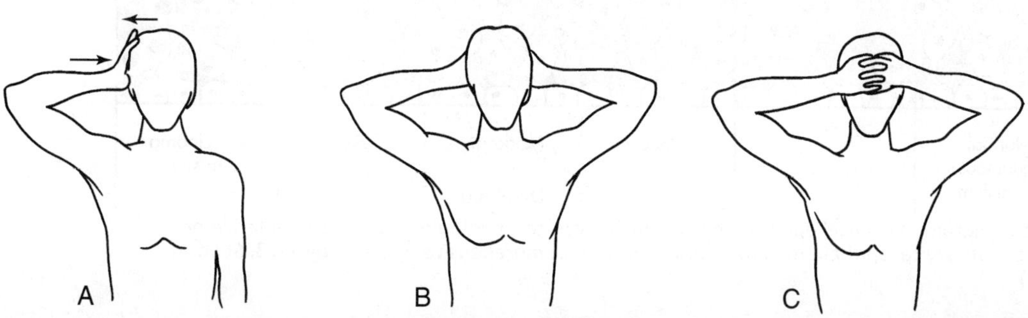

FIGURE 1-49 Isometric neck exercises. A, The hand is placed against the side of the head slightly above the ear, and pressure is gradually increased while resisting with the neck muscles and keeping the head in the same position. The position is held 5 sec, relaxed, and repeated five times. **B,** The exercise is performed on the other side and then from the back and front **(C).** The exercise should be performed three to four times daily. (From Mercier LR [ed]: *Practical orthopedics,* ed 4, St Louis, 1995, Mosby.)

BASIC INFORMATION

DEFINITION

Cervical dysplasia refers to atypical development of immature squamous epithelium that does not penetrate the basement epithelial membrane. Characteristics include increased cellularity, nuclear abnormalities, and increased nuclear to cytoplasm ratio. A progressive polarized loss of squamous differentiation exists beginning adjacent to the basement membrane and progressing to the most advanced stage (severe dysplasia), which encompasses the complete squamous epithelial layer thickness (Fig. 1-50).

BETHESDA 2001 UPDATED CLASSIFICATION: Interpretation/result (including specimen adequacy)

- Negative for intraepithelial lesion or malignancy
- Organisms (i.e., *Trichomonas vaginalis, Candida* sp., bacterial vaginosis), reactive cellular changes (inflammation), atrophy
- Epithelial cell abnormalities: atypical squamous cells (ASC), of undetermined significance (ASC-US), cannot exclude HSIL (ASC-H), LSIL (CIN 1 and HPV), HSIL (CIN 2 & 3, CIS), squamous cell carcinoma
- Glandular cell abnormalities: atypical glandular cells (AGC): *(specify endocervical, endometrial,* or *NOS),* atypical glandular cells, favor neoplastic *(specify endocervical, endometrial,* or *NOS)* endocervical adenocarcinoma in situ (AIS), adenocarcinoma
- Other: endometrial cells in a woman 40 yr of age

SYNONYMS

Class III or class IV Pap smear
Cervical intraepithelial neoplasia (CIN)
Low-grade or high-grade squamous intraepithelial lesion (LGSIL or HGSIL)

ICD-9CM CODES
622.1 Dysplasia of cervix (uteri)

EPIDEMIOLOGY & DEMOGRAPHICS

PEAK INCIDENCE:

- Age 35 yr
- Abnormal Pap smear rate revealing dysplasia approximates 2% to 5%, depending on population risk factors and false-negative rate variance
- False-negative rate approaching 40%
- Average age-adjusted incidence of severe dysplasia 35 cases/100,000 persons

PREVALENCE:

- Dysplasia: peak age, 26 yr (3600 cases/100,000 persons)
- CIS: peak age, 32 yr (1100 cases/100,000 persons)
- Invasive cancer: peak age, >60 yr (800 cases/100,000 persons)

PHYSICAL FINDINGS & CLINICAL PRESENTATION

- Cervical lesions associated with dysplasia usually are not visible to the naked eye; therefore physical findings are best viewed by colposcopy of a 3% acetic acid–prepared cervix.
- Patients evaluated by colposcopy are identified by abnormal cervical cytology screening from Pap smear screening.
- Colposcopic findings:
  1. Leukoplakia (white lesion seen by the unaided eye that may represent condyloma, dysplasia, or cancer)
  2. Acetowhite epithelium with or without associated punctation, mosaicism, abnormal vessels
  3. Abnormal transformation zone (abnormal iodine uptake, “cuffed” gland openings)

ETIOLOGY

- Not clearly elucidated
- May be caused by abnormal reserve cell hyperplasia resulting in atypical metaplasia and dysplastic epithelium
- Strongly associated and initiated by oncogenic HPV infection (high-risk HPV types 16, 18, 31, 33, 35, 45, 51, 52, 56, and 58; low-risk HPV types 6, 11, 42, 43, and 44)
- Risk factors:
  1. Any heterosexual coitus
  2. Coitus during puberty (Transformation-zone metaplasia peak)
  3. DES exposure
  4. Multiple sexual partners
  5. Lack of prior Pap smear screening
  6. History of STD
  7. Other genital tract neoplasia
  8. HIV
  9. TB
  10. Substance abuse
  11. “High-risk” male partner (HPV)
  12. Low socioeconomic status

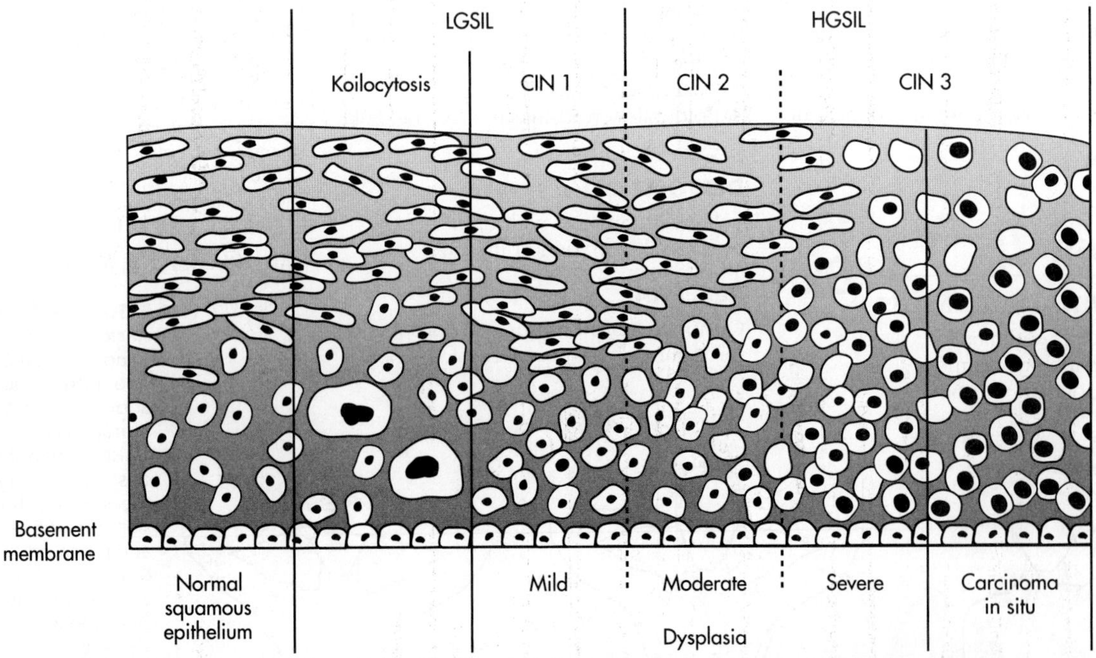

FIGURE 1-50 Diagram of cervical epithelium showing various terminologies used to characterize progressive degrees of cervical epithelium. (From Mishell D [ed]: *Comprehensive gynecology,* ed 3, St Louis, 1997, Mosby.)

13. Early first pregnancy
14. Tobacco use
15. HPV

DIAGNOSIS

DIFFERENTIAL DIAGNOSIS

- Metaplasia
- Hyperkeratosis
- Condyloma
- Microinvasive carcinoma
- Glandular epithelial abnormalities
- Adenocarcinoma in situ
- VIN
- VAIN
- Metastatic tumor involvement of the cervix

WORKUP

Periodic history and physical examination (including cytologic screening), depending on age, risk factors, and history of preinvasive cervical lesions

- Consider screening for sexually transmitted disease (GC, *Chlamydia,* VDRL, HIV, HPV)
- Abnormal cytology (HSIL/LSIL, initial ASC/ASC-US/ASC-H in high-risk patients, recurrent in low-risk/postmenopausal patients) and grossly evident suspicious lesions; refer for colposcopy and possible directed biopsy/ECC (examination should include cervix, vagina, vulva, and anus)
- For glandular cell abnormalities (AGC): refer for colposcopy and possible directed biopsy/ECC, and consider endometrial sampling
- In pregnancy: abnormal cytology followed by colposcopy in the first trimester and at 28 to 32 wk; only high-grade lesions suspect for cancer biopsied; ECC contraindicated

LABORATORY TESTS

- GC, *Chlamydia* to rule out STD
- Pap cytology screening (requires appropriate sampling, preparation, cytologist interpretation and reporting)
- Colposcopy and directed biopsy, ECC for indications (see "Workup")
- HPV-DNA typing if identified abnormal cytology

IMAGING STUDIES

- Cervicography
- Computer-enhanced Pap cytology screening (e.g., PAPNET)

TREATMENT

NONPHARMACOLOGIC THERAPY

- Superficial ablative techniques (cryosurgery, CO_2 laser, and electrocoagulation diathermy) considered for colposcopy-identified dysplasia (moderate to severe dysplasia or CIS) and negative ECC; mild dysplasia followed conservatively in a compliant patient
- Cone biopsy (LEEP, CO_2 laser, "cold knife" cone biopsy) considered for colposcopy-identified dysplasia (moderate to severe dysplasia or CIS) and positive ECC or if there is a two-grade or more discrepancy between the Pap smear, colposcopy, and biopsy or ECC findings
- Hysterectomy if patient has completed child bearing and has persistent or recurrent severe dysplasia or CIS
- In pregnancy: treatment for cervical dysplasia deferred until after delivery

ACUTE GENERAL Rx

Topical 5-fluorouracil (5-FU) is rarely used for recurrent cervicovaginal lesions.

CHRONIC Rx

- Because of the risk for persistent and recurrent dysplasia, long-term follow-up is individualized based on patient risk factors, Pap smear and colposcopy results, treatment history, and presence of high-risk HPV (e.g., Pap smear q3 to 4mo/yr, then q6mo/1 yr, then annually [if all normal], or repeat colposcopy examination and treat as indicated).
- Mild dysplasia with negative ECC should be followed conservatively in a compliant patient as a majority of these lesions regress.

DISPOSITION

- Because of the large numbers of women in high-risk groups, the prevalence of HPV, and the high false-negative Pap smear rate, routine Pap smear screening should be strongly encouraged for all women, especially those with a history of cervical dysplasia. The addition of an HPV test to the PAP test reduces the incidence of grade 2 or 3 cervical intraepithelial neoplasia or cancer detected by subsequent screening.
- Success rates for treatment approach 80% to 90%.
- Detection of persistence of recurrence requires careful follow-up.
- Cervical treatment possibly results in infertility (cervical stenosis or incompetence), which requires careful consideration and discretion for use of LEEP and cone biopsy.
- Appropriate counseling and informed consent needed when considering any form of management of cervical dysplasia.

REFERRAL

- Patients with abnormal Pap cytology should not be followed by repeat Pap smear screening.
- Patients with identified abnormal cytology should be evaluated by a skilled colposcopist (defined as documented didactic and preceptorship training including 50 cases of identified pathology, ongoing colposcopy activity with a minimum of 2 cases/wk, QA log, and periodic CME).
- If treatment is required, patient should be referred to a gynecologist or gynecologic oncologist skilled in the diagnosis and treatment of preinvasive cervical disease.

PEARLS & CONSIDERATIONS

COMMENTS

- Patient education material available from American College of Obstetricians and Gynecologists.
- Gardasil is a vaccine indicated in girls and women 9 to 26 yr of age for the prevention of CIN caused by human papillomavirus (HPV) types 6, 11, 16, and 18.

EVIDENCE

There is little evidence that is available and that meets our criteria for the management of cervical malignancy/dysplasia.

The available evidence suggests that there is no obviously superior surgical technique for the treatment of cervical intraepithelial neoplasia.[1] Ⓐ

Evidence-Based Reference

1. Martin-Hirsch PL, Paraskevaidis E, Kitchener H: Surgery for cervical intraepithelial neoplasia, *Cochrane Database Sys Rev* Issue 3, 1999. Ⓐ

SUGGESTED READINGS

Apgar BS, Brotzman G: Management of cervical cytologic abnormalities, *Am Fam Physician* 70(10):1905, 2004.

Naucler P et al: Human papillomavirus and Papanicolaou tests to screen for cervical cancer, *N Eng J Med* 357:1589-1597, 2007.

Schlecht NF et al: Persistent human papillomavirus infection as a predictor of cervical intraepithelial neoplasia, *JAMA* 286:3106, 2001.

Solomon D et al: The 2001 Bethesda system terminology for reporting results of cervical cytology, *JAMA* 287:2114, 2002.

Stoler MH: New Bethesda terminology and evidence-based management guidelines for cervical cytology findings, *JAMA* 287:2140, 2002.

Wright TC et al: 2001 consensus guidelines for the management of women with cervical cytological abnormalities, *JAMA* 287:2120, 2002.

AUTHORS: **DENNIS M. WEPPNER, M.D.,** and **RUBEN ALVERO, M.D.**

BASIC INFORMATION

DEFINITION

A cervical polyp is a growth protruding from the cervix or endocervical canal. Polyps that arise from the endocervical canal are called *endocervical polyps*. If they arise from the ectocervix, they are called *cervical polyps*.

ICD-9CM CODES
622.7 Mucous polyp of cervix

EPIDEMIOLOGY & DEMOGRAPHICS

Cervical polyps are common. Found in approximately 4% of all gynecologic patients. Most commonly present in perimenopausal and multigravid women between the ages of 30 and 50 yr. Endocervical polyps are more common than cervical polyps and are almost always benign (Fig. 1-51). Malignant degeneration is extremely rare.

PHYSICAL FINDINGS & CLINICAL PRESENTATION

Polyps may be single or multiple and vary in size from being extremely small (a few mm) to large (4 cm). They are soft, smooth, reddish-purple to cherry-red in color. They bleed easily when touched. Very large polyps can cause some cervical dilation. There may be vaginal discharge associated with cervical polyps if the polyp has become infected.

ETIOLOGY

- Most unknown
- Inflammatory
- Traumatic
- Pregnancy

DIAGNOSIS

DIFFERENTIAL DIAGNOSIS

- Endometrial polyp
- Prolapsed myoma
- Retained products of conception
- Squamous papilloma
- Sarcoma
- Cervical malignancy

WORKUP

Polyps are most commonly asymptomatic and are usually found at the time of annual gynecologic pelvic examination. Polyps are also found in women who present for evaluation of intermenstrual or postcoital bleeding and for profuse vaginal discharge. Polyps are painless. Unless a patient has a bleeding abnormality that necessitates her being evaluated by a physician, polyps would go undiagnosed until her next Pap smear was obtained.

TREATMENT

NONPHARMACOLOGIC THERAPY

Simple surgical excision can be done in the office. The physician should be prepared for bleeding, which can easily be controlled with silver nitrate or Monsel's solution. Most commonly, a polyp is excised by grasping it at the stalk and twisting it off. Polyps can also be excised by electrocautery or, in the case of very large polyps, in an outpatient surgical suite. Sexual intercourse and tampon usage are to be avoided until the patient's follow-up visit. Also, douching is not to be performed.

ACUTE GENERAL Rx

Generally, no medication is needed.

CHRONIC Rx

Patient is followed up in 2 wk for recheck of the surgical excision site unless there is active bleeding, in which case she would be seen immediately. The cervix should be checked at the patient's routine gynecologic visits.

DISPOSITION

Because these are almost always benign, usually no further treatment is needed. Annual gynecologic examinations should be performed to check for any regrowths.

REFERRAL

To a gynecologist for removal of polyps

PEARLS & CONSIDERATIONS

COMMENTS

A Pap smear should be obtained before removing the polyp. If an abnormal Pap smear is obtained, more than likely the cause will be secondary to the polyp. If a colposcopic evaluation is needed, this should also be performed. During pregnancy, the cervix is highly vascularized. If the polyps are stable and benign-appearing, they should just be observed during the pregnancy and removed only if they are causing bleeding.

SUGGESTED READINGS

Endo H et al: Cervical polyp with eccrine syringofibroadenoma-like features, *Histopathology* 42(3):301, 2003.

Rupke S: Family practice forum: clinical medicine. Evaluation and management of cervical polyps, *Hosp Pract* 33(6):81, 1998.

Scott PM: Procedures in family practice. Performing cervical polypectomy, *JAAPA* 12(6):81, 1999.

Spiewankiewicz B: Hysteroscopy in cases of cervical polyps, *Eur J Gynaecol Oncol* 24(1):67, 2003.

AUTHORS: **GEORGE T. DANAKAS, M.D.,** and **RUBEN ALVERO, M.D.**

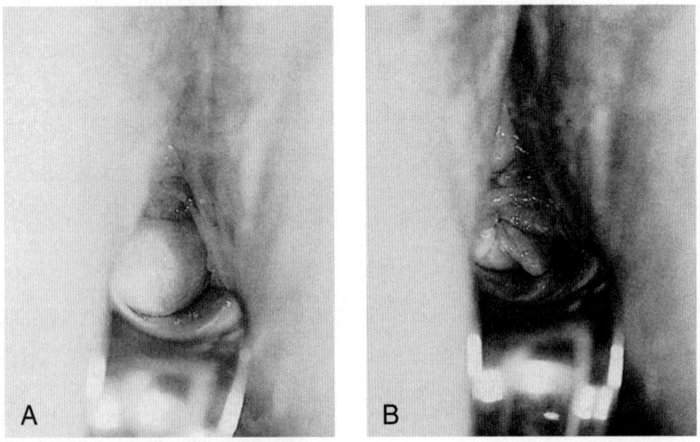

FIGURE 1-51 **A,** Fibroid polyp protruding through the external cervical os. **B,** Small endocervical polyp. (From Symonds EM, Macpherson MBA: *Color atlas of obstetrics and gynecology,* St Louis, 1994, Mosby.)

BASIC INFORMATION

DEFINITION

Cervicitis is an infection of the cervix. It may result from direct infection of the cervix, or it may be secondary to uterine or vaginal infection.

SYNONYMS

Endocervicitis
Ectocervicitis
Mucopurulent cervicitis

ICD-9CM CODES
616.0 Cervicitis
098.15 Acute gonococcal cervicitis
079.8 Chlamydia infection

EPIDEMIOLOGY & DEMOGRAPHICS

Cervicitis accounts for 20% to 25% of patients presenting with abnormal vaginal discharge, and this affects women only. It is most common in adolescents, but it can be found in any sexually active woman. Practicing unsafe sex with multiple sexual partners increases the risk of developing cervicitis, as well as other sexually transmitted diseases.

PHYSICAL FINDINGS & CLINICAL PRESENTATION

Cervicitis is usually asymptomatic or associated with mild symptoms. Copious purulent or mucopurelence in vaginal discharge (Fig. 1-52), pelvic pain, and dyspareunia may be present if cervicitis is severe. The cervix can be erythematous and tender on palpation during bimanual examination. The cervix may also bleed easily when obtaining cultures or a Pap smear. May have postcoital bleeding.

ETIOLOGY

- *Chlamydia*
- *Trichomonas*
- *Neisseria gonorrhoeae*
- Herpes simplex
- *Trichomonas vaginalis*
- Human papillomavirus

DIAGNOSIS

DIFFERENTIAL DIAGNOSIS

- Carcinoma of the cervix
- Cervical erosion
- Cervical metaplasia

WORKUP

The patient usually presents with a vaginal discharge or history of postcoital bleeding. Otherwise the patient is asymptomatic and diagnosed during routine examination. On examination there is gross visualization of yellow, mucopurulent material on the cotton swab.

LABORATORY TESTS

On a smear there will be ten or more polymorphonuclear leukocytes per microscopic field. Positive Gram stain is found. Cultures should be obtained for *Chlamydia* and *N. gonorrhoeae*. Use a wet mount to look for trichomonads. Obtain a Pap smear.

TREATMENT

NONPHARMACOLOGIC THERAPY

Cervicitis is treated in an outpatient setting. Cryosurgery is an option for treatment of cervicitis with negative cultures and negative biopsies. Safe sex should be practiced with the use of condoms. Partners should be treated in all cases of infection proven by culture.

ACUTE GENERAL Rx

Because *Chlamydia* and *N. gonorrhoeae* make up >50% of the cause of infectious cervicitis, if it is suspected, treat without waiting for culture results. Administer ceftriaxone 125-mg IM single dose followed by doxycycline 100 mg PO bid for 7 days. If the patient is pregnant, treat with azithromycin (Zithromax) 1-g single dose instead of using doxycycline, which is contraindicated in pregnant or nursing mothers. Alternative treatments include: erythromycin base 500 mg PO qid for 7 days, erythromycin ethylsuccinate 800 mg PO qid for 7 days, ofloxacin 300 mg PO bid for 7 days, or levofloxacin 500 mg PO qd for 7 days. If *Trichomonas* is the etiologic agent, treat with metronidazole 2-g single dose. For herpes, treat with acyclovir 200 mg PO five times daily for 7 days.

DISPOSITION

Cervicitis responds well to antibiotics. Possible complications to watch for are a subsequent PID and infertility (found in 5% to 10% of patients). Repeat cultures should be performed after treatment. Sexual relations can be resumed after negative cultures.

REFERRAL

If subsequent PID develops, consider hospital admission for IV antibiotics.

PEARLS & CONSIDERATIONS

COMMENTS

Patient educational material can be obtained from local health clinics and clinics for sexually transmitted diseases.

SUGGESTED READINGS

Centers for Disease Control and Prevention: 2006 sexually transmitted diseases treatment guidelines, *MMWR Morb Mortal Wkly Rep* 55(RR-11), 2006.

Marrazzo JM: Mucopurulent cervicitis: no longer ignored, but still misunderstood, *Infect Dis Clin of N Am* 19(2):333, 2005.

Simpson T: Urethritis and cervicitis in adolescents, *Adolesc Med Clin* 15(2):253, 2004.

AUTHORS: **GEORGE T. DANAKAS, M.D.,** and **RUBEN ALVERO, M.D.**

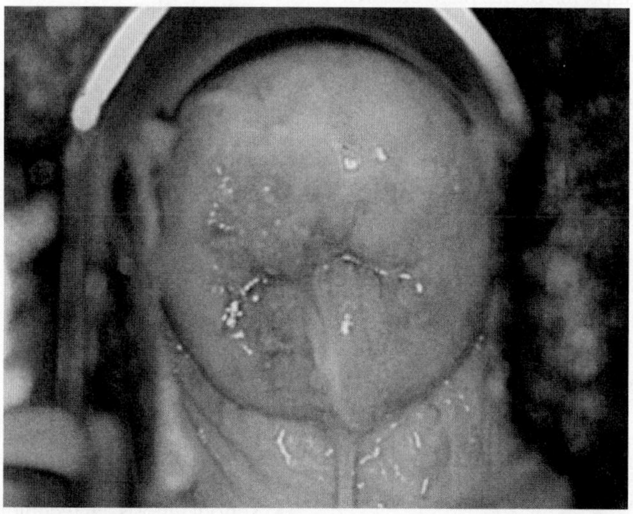

FIGURE 1-52 Colposcopy of a woman with mucopurulent cervicitis and purulent discharge from endocervical os. (Courtesy Dr. David Soper, Richmond, VA. From Mandell GL [ed]: *Mandell, Douglas, and Bennett's principles and practice of infectious diseases,* ed 5, New York, 2000, Churchill Livingstone.)

BASIC INFORMATION

DEFINITION

Chagas' disease is an infection caused by the protozoan parasite *Trypanosoma cruzi.* This is a vector-borne disease transmitted by reduviid bugs from multiple wild and domesticated animal reservoirs. The disease is characterized by an acute nonspecific febrile illness that may be followed, after a variable latency period, by chronic cardiac, GI, and neurologic sequelae.

SYNONYMS

American trypanosomiasis

ICD-9CM CODES
086.2 Chagas' disease

EPIDEMIOLOGY & DEMOGRAPHICS

INCIDENCE (IN U.S.):

- Four cases of autochthonous transmission in California and Texas
- In the last 2 decades, six cases of laboratory-acquired infection, three cases of transfusion-associated transmission, and nine cases of imported disease reported to the Centers for Disease Control and Prevention (none of the imported cases involving returning tourists)

PREVALENCE (IN U.S.): Based on regional seroprevalence studies in Hispanic blood donors, it is estimated that between 50,000 and 100,000 persons infected with *T. cruzi* are currently residing in the U.S.

PREDOMINANT SEX: Male = female

PREDOMINANT AGE:

- In highly endemic areas, mean age of acute infection: approximately 4 yr
- Variable age distribution for both types of chronic disease, depending on geography
- Mean age of onset: usually between 35 and 45 yr

PEAK INCIDENCE: Unknown

GENETICS:

Congenital infection: Congenital transmission has been documented with attendant high fetal mortality and morbidity in surviving infants.

Neonatal infection: In rural areas, within substandard housing, transmission is likely to occur.

PHYSICAL FINDINGS & CLINICAL PRESENTATION

- Inflammatory lesion that develops about 1 wk after contamination of a break in the skin with infected insect feces (chagoma)
  1. Area of induration and erythema
  2. Usually accompanied by local lymphadenopathy
- Presence of Romaña's sign, which consists of unilateral painless palpebral and periocular edema, when conjunctiva is portal of entry
- Constitutional symptoms of fever, fatigue, and anorexia, along with edema of the face and lower extremities, generalized lymphadenopathy, and mild hepatosplenomegaly after the appearance of local signs of disease
- Myocarditis in a small portion of patients, sometimes with resultant CHF
- Uncommonly, CNS disease, such as meningoencephalitis, which carries a poor prognosis
- Symptoms and signs of disease persisting for weeks to months, followed by spontaneous resolution of the acute illness; patient then in the indeterminate phase of the disease (asymptomatic with attendant subpatent parasitemia and reactive antibodies to *T. cruzi* antigens)
- Chronic disease may become manifest years to decades after the initial infection:
  1. Most common organ involved: heart, followed by GI tract, and to a much lesser extent the CNS
     a. Cardiac involvement takes the form of arrhythmias or cardiomyopathy, but rarely both.
     b. Cardiomyopathy is bilateral but predominantly affects the right ventricle and is often accompanied by apical aneurysms and mural thrombi.
     c. Arrhythmias are a consequence of involvement of the bundle of His and have been implicated as the leading cause of sudden death in adults in highly endemic areas.
     d. Right-sided heart failure, thromboembolization, and rhythm disturbances associated with symptoms of dizziness and syncope are characteristic.
  2. Patients with megaesophagus: dysphasia, odynophagia, chronic cough, and regurgitation, frequently resulting in aspiration pneumonitis
  3. Megacolon: abdominal pain and chronic constipation, which, when severe, may lead to obstruction and perforation
  4. CNS symptoms: most often secondary to embolization from the heart or varying degrees of peripheral neuropathy

ETIOLOGY

- *T. cruzi*
  1. Found only in the Americas, ranging from the southern U.S. to southern Argentina
  2. Transmitted to humans by various species of bloodsucking reduviid ("kissing") insects, primarily those of the genera *Triatoma, Panstrongylus,* and *Rhodnius*
  3. Usually found in burrows and trees where infected insects transmit the parasite to natural reservoirs (e.g., opossums and armadillos)
  4. Intrusion into enzootic areas for farmland, allowing insects to take up residence in rural dwellings, thus including humans and domestic animals in the cycle of transmission
  5. Initial infection of insects by ingesting blood from animals or humans that have circulating flagellated trypanosomes (trypomastigotes)
  6. Multiplication in the insect midgut as epimastigotes, then differentiation into metacyclic trypomastigotes discharged with the feces during subsequent blood meals
  7. Transmission to the second mammalian host through contamination of mucous membranes, conjunctivae, or wounds with insect feces containing infected forms
- In the vertebrate host
  1. Movement of parasites into various cell types, intracellular transformation into amastigotes, and thereafter differentiation into trypomastigotes
  2. Following rupture of the cell membrane, parasitic invasion of local tissues or hematogenous spread to distant sites, maintaining a parasitemia infective for vectors
- In addition to insect vectors, *T. cruzi* is transmitted through blood transfusions, transplacentally, and, occasionally, secondary to laboratory accidents

DIAGNOSIS

DIFFERENTIAL DIAGNOSIS

Acute disease

- Early African trypanosomiasis
- New World cutaneous and mucocutaneous leishmaniasis

Chronic disease

- Idiopathic cardiomyopathy
- Idiopathic achalasia
- Congenital or acquired megacolon

WORKUP

Principal considerations in diagnosis:

- A history of residence where transmission is known to occur
- Recent receipt of a blood product while in an endemic area
- Occupational exposure in a laboratory

LABORATORY TESTS

For acute diagnosis:

- Demonstration of *T. cruzi* in wet preparations of blood, buffy coat, or Giemsa-stained smears
- Xenodiagnosis, a technique involving laboratory-reared insect vectors fed on subjects with suspected infection thereafter examined for parasites, and culture of body fluids in liquid media to establish diagnosis

1. Hampered by the length of time required for completion
2. Of limited use in clinical decision making with regard to drug therapy
3. Although xenodiagnosis and broth culture are considered to be more sensitive than microscopic examination of body fluids, sensitivities may not exceed 50%

- Recent advances in serologic testing include immunoblot assay, in situ indirect fluorescent antibody, PCR-based techniques, and an immunochromatographic assay (Chagas Stat Pak)

For chronic *T. cruzi* infection:

- Traditional serologic tests including: complement fixation (CF), indirect immunofluorescence (IIF), indirect hemagglutination, and enzyme-linked immunosorbent assay (ELISA)
- Serologic tests have variable sensitivity and specificity and frequent false-positive results
- Saliva ELISA may be useful as a screening diagnostic test in epidemiologic studies of chronic trypanosomiasis infection in endemic areas

TREATMENT

Rx

NONPHARMACOLOGIC THERAPY

- Chronic chagasic heart disease: mainly supportive
- Megaesophagus: symptoms usually amenable to dietary measures or pneumonic dilation of the esophagogastric junction
- Chagasic megacolon: in its early stages responsive to a high-fiber diet, laxatives, and enemas

ACUTE GENERAL Rx

Nifurtimox (Lampit, Bayer 2502):

- Only drug available in the U.S. for the treatment of acute, congenital, or laboratory-acquired infection
- Recommended oral dosage for adults: 8 to 10 mg/kg/day given in 4 divided daily doses and continued for 90 to 120 days
- Parasitologic cure in approximately 50% of those treated; should be begun as early as possible

Benznidazole, a nitroimidazole derivative:

- Has demonstrated similar efficacy as nifurtimox in limited trials
- Recommended oral dosage: 5 mg/kg/day for 60 days

CHRONIC Rx

- In patients with indeterminate phase or chronic disease: Some evidence of benefit in a recent uncontrolled trial with benznidazole in patients with chagasic cardiomyopathy
- In patients exhibiting bradyarrhythmias: pacemakers
- In individuals with congestive heart failure:
  1. Treat with standard modalities for dilated, right-sided, cardiomyopathic disease.
  2. Cardiac transplant is an option for end-stage cardiomyopathy; however, reactivation rate found to be low and amenable to therapy without subsequent infection of the allograft.
  3. Myotomy or esophageal resection is reserved for patients with advanced disease.
- In advanced chagasic megacolon associated with chronic fecal impaction, perforation, or, less commonly, volvulus: surgical resection

DISPOSITION

Based on few prospective studies, most patients infected with *T. cruzi* will not develop symptomatic Chagas' disease.

REFERRAL

- For consultation with an infectious disease specialist or communication with the Centers for Disease Control and Prevention when the disease is acutely suspected
- To a cardiologist for pacemaker implantation for patients with brady-arrhythmias
- To a surgeon for symptomatic disease with chagasic megaesophagus or megacolon

PEARLS & CONSIDERATIONS

!

COMMENTS

- In recipients of solid organ or bone marrow transplants, patients with AIDS, or those receiving chemotherapy, there may be reactivation of indeterminate phase disease.
- Mortality predictors associated with chagasic cardiomyopathy include CHF, QT-interval dispersion, left ventricular (LV) end-systolic dimension, the presence of pathological Q waves, frequent PVCs, and isolated LAFB on ECG.
- Chagasic esophageal disease has an increased incidence of esophageal malignancy.
- The use of pyrethroid-impregnated curtains may represent an option for the reduction or elimination of Chagas' disease transmission in certain endemic areas.

SUGGESTED READINGS

Garcia S et al: Treatment with benznidazole during the chronic phase of experimental Chagas' disease decreases cardiac alterations, *Antimicrob Agents Chemother* 49(4):1521, 2005.

Golgher D, Gazzinelli RT: Innate and acquired immunity in the pathogenesis of Chagas disease, *Autoimmunity* 37(5):399, 2004.

Kirchhoff LV et al: Transfusion-associated Chagas disease (American trypanosomiasis) in Mexico: implications for transfusion medicine in the United States, *Transfusion* 46(2):298, 2006.

Viotti R et al: Long-term cardiac outcomes of treating chronic Chagas disease with benznidazole versus no treatment: a nonrandomized trial, *Ann Intern Med* 144(10):724, 2006.

AUTHORS: **GEORGE O. ALONSO, M.D., GLENN G. FORT, M.D., M.P.H.,** and **DENNIS J. MIKOLICH, M.D.**

BASIC INFORMATION

DEFINITION

Chancroid is a sexually transmitted disease characterized by painful genital ulceration and inflammatory inguinal adenopathy.

SYNONYMS

Soft chancre
Ulcus molle

ICD-9CM CODES
099.0 Chancroid

EPIDEMIOLOGY & DEMOGRAPHICS

- Exact incidence is unknown.
- Occurs more frequently in men (male:female ratio of 10:1).
- Clinical infection is rare in women.
- There is a higher incidence in uncircumcised men and in tropical and subtropical regions.
- Incubation period is 4 to 7 days but may take up to 3 wk.
- High incidence of HIV infection associated with chancroid.

PHYSICAL FINDINGS & CLINICAL PRESENTATION

- One to three extremely painful ulcers (Fig. 1-53), accompanied by tender inguinal lymphadenopathy (especially if fluctuant)
- May present with inguinal bubo and several ulcers
- In women: initial lesion in the fourchette, labia minora, urethra, cervix, or anus; inflammatory pustule or papule that ruptures, leaving a shallow, nonindurated ulceration, usually 1- to 2-cm diameter with ragged, undermined edges
- Unilateral lymphadenopathy develops 1 wk later in 50% of patients

ETIOLOGY

Haemophilus ducreyi, a bacillus

DIAGNOSIS

DIFFERENTIAL DIAGNOSIS

- Other genitoulcerative diseases such as syphilis, herpes, LGV, granuloma inguinale
- A clinical algorithm for the initial management of genital ulcer disease is described in Section III

WORKUP

Diagnosis based on history and physical examination is often inadequate. Must rule out syphilis in women because of the consequences of inappropriate therapy in pregnant women. Base initial diagnosis and treatment recommendations on clinical impression of appearance of ulcer and most likely diagnosis for population. Definitive diagnosis is made by isolation of organism from ulcers by culture or Gram stain.

LABORATORY TESTS

Darkfield microscopy, RPR, HSV cultures, *H. ducreyi* culture, HIV testing recommended

TREATMENT

NONPHARMACOLOGIC THERAPY

Fluctuant nodes should be aspirated through healthy adjacent skin to prevent formation of draining sinus. I&D not recommended, delays healing. Use warm compresses to remove necrotic material.

ACUTE GENERAL Rx

- Azithromycin 1 g PO (single dose) *or*
- Ceftriaxone 250 mg IM (single dose) *or*
- Ciprofloxacin 500 mg PO bid for 3 days *or*
- Erythromycin 500 mg PO qid for 7 days

NOTE: Ciprofloxacin is contraindicated in patients who are pregnant, lactating, or <18 yr.

- HIV-infected patients may need more prolonged therapy

DISPOSITION

- All sexual partners should be treated with a 10-day course of one of the previous regimens (see "Acute General Rx").
- Patients should be reexamined 3 to 7 days after initiation of therapy. Ulcers should improve symptomatically within 3 days and objectively within 7 days after initiation of successful therapy.

PEARLS & CONSIDERATIONS

COMMENTS

In the U.S. HSV-1 and syphilis are the most common causes of genital ulcers, followed by chancroid, LGV, and granuloma inguinale.

EVIDENCE

EBM

Despite the absence of an extensive clinical trial data base, these therapies have gained acceptance and are in accordance with CDC guidelines.

The Centers for Disease Control and Prevention recommend oral azithromycin, intramuscular ceftriaxone sodium, oral ciprofloxacin, or oral erythromycin as first line therapies for treatment of chancroid caused by *H. ducreyi.*

All regimens are effective for treating chancroid in patients that are HIV-negative and HIV-positive.

Azithromycin and ceftriaxone are offered as single dose therapies.

Evidence-Based Reference

Centers for Disease Control and Prevention: Sexually transmitted diseases treatment guidelines *MMRW* 55(RR-11):1, 2006.

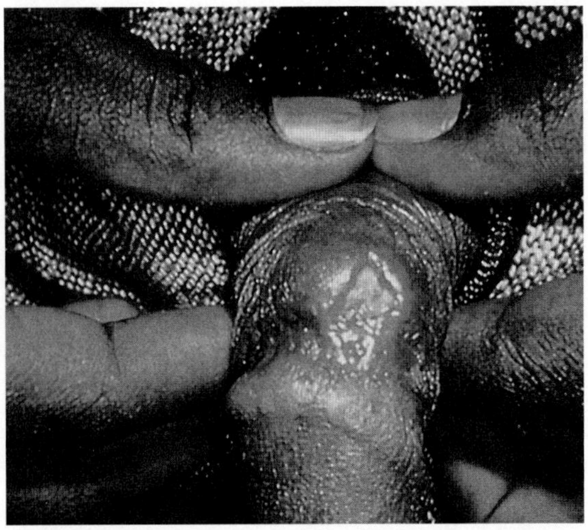

FIGURE 1-53 Chancroid. Note shaggy, ragged-edged ulcer with edema and exudative base. (Courtesy Beverly Sanders, M.D. From Goldstein B [ed]: *Practical dermatology,* ed 2, St Louis, 1997, Mosby.)

SUGGESTED READINGS

Sehgal VN, Srivastave G: Chancroid: contemporary appraisal, *Int J Dermatol* 42(3):182, 2003.
Lewis DA: Chancroid: clinical manifestations, diagnosis and management, *Sex Transm Infect* 79(1):68, 2003.

AUTHORS: **MARIA A. CORIGLIANO, M.D.,** and **RUBEN ALVERO, M.D.**

BASIC INFORMATION

DEFINITION

Charcot-Marie-Tooth disease is a heterogeneous group of noninflammatory inherited peripheral neuropathies. It is the most common inherited neuromuscular disorder. (See also "Neuropathy, Inherited Peripheral".)

SYNONYMS

Peroneal muscular atrophy
Hereditary motor and sensory neuropathy (HMSN)
Idiopathic dominantly inherited hypertrophic polyneuropathy

ICD-9CM CODES
356.1 Charcot-Marie-Tooth disease, paralysis, or syndrome

EPIDEMIOLOGY & DEMOGRAPHICS

PREDOMINANT AGE: Onset usually 10 to 20 yr but can be delayed to 50 to 60 yr
PREDOMINANT SEX: Male:female ratio of 3:1

PHYSICAL FINDINGS & CLINICAL PRESENTATION

- Variable presentation from family to family, but affected individuals in a family tend to have similar symptomatology
- Usually, gradual onset, with slowly progressive disorder
- Foot deformity producing a high arch (cavus) and hammertoes
- Atrophy of the lower legs producing a storklike appearance (muscle wasting does not involve the upper legs) (Fig. 1-54)
- Nerve enlargement
- Sensory loss or other neurologic signs, although the sensory involvement is usually mild
- Scoliosis
- Decreased proprioception that often interferes with balance and gait
- Painful paresthesias
- In late cases, possible involvement of hands
- Absence of DTRs in many cases
- Poorly healing foot ulcers in some patients

ETIOLOGY

Chronic segmental demyelination of peripheral nerves with hypertrophic changes caused by remyelination

DIAGNOSIS

DIFFERENTIAL DIAGNOSIS

- Other inherited neuropathies
- Toxic, metabolic, and nutritional polyneuropathies

WORKUP

- The early onset, slow progression, and familial nature of the disorder are usually sufficient to establish diagnosis.
- Electrophysiologic studies are often diagnostic and may also be helpful in defining various subtypes of this group of neuropathies.
- Occasionally, muscle and nerve (sural) biopsy may be required.

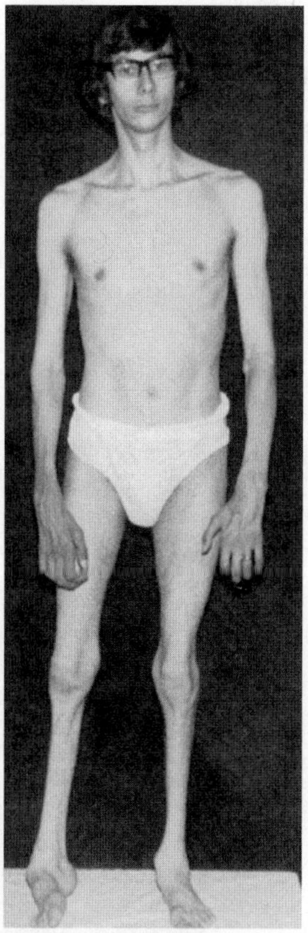

FIGURE 1-54 Patient with Charcot-Marie-Tooth disease showing marked wasting of calf muscles and intrinsic foot muscles. (From Dubowitz V: *Muscle disorders in childhood,* London, 1995, WB Saunders. In Goetz CG: *Textbook of clinical neurology,* Philadelphia, 1999, WB Saunders.)

TREATMENT

ACUTE GENERAL Rx

- Genetic counseling
- Supportive physical therapy and occupational therapy
- Prevention of injury to limbs with diminished sensibility
- Bracing

CHRONIC Rx

Occasionally, surgery to add stability and restore a plantigrade foot

DISPOSITION

- Disability is usually mild and compatible with a long life.
- 10% to 20% of patients are asymptomatic.
- A small number of cases are nonambulators by the sixth or seventh decade.
- The condition is usually not life threatening.

REFERRAL

- For orthopedic consultation for bracing and treatment of deformity
- For genetic counseling

PEARLS & CONSIDERATIONS

COMMENTS

Patient information on Charcot-Marie-Tooth disease is available from the Muscular Dystrophy Association, 3300 East Sunrise Drive, Tucson, Arizona 85718; phone: 1-800-572-1717.

SUGGESTED READINGS

Chetlin RD, Gutmann L et al: Resistance training exercise and creatine in patients with Charcot-Marie-Tooth disease, *Muscle Nerve* 30:69, 2004.

Gemignani F, Marbini A: Charcot-Marie-Tooth disease (CMT) distinctive phenotypic and genotypic features in CMT type 2, *J Neurol Sci* 184:1, 2001.

Karol LA, Elerson E: Scoliosis in patients with Charcot-Marie-Tooth disease, *J Bone Joint Surg* 89A:1504, 2007.

Nave KA et al: Mechanisms of disease: inherited demyelinating neuropathies—from basic to clinical research, *Nat Clin Pract Neurol* 3:453, 2007.

Pareyson D: Differential diagnosis of Charcot-Marie-Tooth disease and related neuropathies, *Neurol Sci* 25:72, 2004.

Parman Y: Hereditary neuropathies, *Curr Opin Neurol* 20:542, 2007.

AUTHOR: **LONNIE R. MERCIER, M.D.**

BASIC INFORMATION

DEFINITION

Charcot's joint is a chronic, progressive joint degeneration, often devastating, seen most commonly in peripheral weight-bearing joints and vertebrae, which develops as a result of the loss of normal sensory innervation of the joint. It was described by Charcot as a result of tabes dorsalis.

SYNONYMS

Neuropathic arthropathy

ICD-9CM CODES
094.0 Charcot's arthropathy

EPIDEMIOLOGY & DEMOGRAPHICS

PREVALENCE:

- 1 case/750 patients with diabetes mellitus; 5 cases/100 of those with peripheral neuropathy (foot is most commonly involved)
- 20% to 40% of patients with syringomyelia (shoulder most commonly involved)
- 5% to 10% of patients with tabes dorsalis; usually >60 yr (spine, hip, and knee most commonly involved)

PHYSICAL FINDINGS & CLINICAL PRESENTATION

Neuropathic joint disease is relatively painless, often in spite of considerable destruction

- Often, diffusely warm, swollen, and occasionally erythematous involved joint, the latter suggesting sepsis
- Possible progression of joint instability; palpable osseous debris; crepitus common
- Often, frank dislocation, leading to bony deformity, especially in more superficial joints

ETIOLOGY

The most widely accepted theory is the "neurotraumatic" theory:

- Impairment and loss of joint sensitivity decreases the protective mechanism about the joint.
- Rapid destruction occurs.
- Chronic inflammation and repetitive effusions develop, eventually contributing to joint instability and incongruity.

DIAGNOSIS

DIFFERENTIAL DIAGNOSIS

- Osteomyelitis, cellulitis, abscess
- Infectious arthritis
- Osteoarthritis
- Rheumatoid and other inflammatory arthritides

WORKUP

- An underlying neurologic disorder must always be present.
- Diabetes mellitus with peripheral neuropathy is the most common cause (Fig. 1-55).
- Syringomyelia, tabes dorsalis, Charcot-Marie-Tooth disease, congenital indifference to pain, alcoholism, and spinal dysraphism can all lead to the disorder.

LABORATORY TESTS

In questionable cases, aspiration, sometimes including biopsy, to rule out sepsis

IMAGING STUDIES

Plain roentgenography

- Sufficient to establish diagnosis in most cases, especially if etiology is known
- Findings: variable degrees of destruction and dislocation

TREATMENT

ACUTE GENERAL Rx

- Protection of effusions, sprains, and fractures until all hyperemic response has resolved
- Braces, special shoes with molded inserts, and elevation of the extremity
- Patient education with avoidance of weight bearing when lower extremity joints are involved
- Surgery: only limited value

DISPOSITION

Once the full-blown neuropathic joint has developed, treatment is difficult.

SUGGESTED READINGS

Choski P et al: Charcot arthropathy: an often overlooked complication of diabetes mellitus, *J Ark Med Soc* 103:229, 2007.

Guyton GP, Saltzman CL: The diabetic foot: basic mechanisms of disease, *Instr Course Lect* 51:169, 2002.

Herbst SA, Jones KB, Saltzman CL: Pattern of diabetic neuropathic arthropathy associated with peripheral bone mineral density, *J Bone Joint Surg* 86:378, 2004.

Neves FS et al: Syringomyelia, neuropathic arthropathy and rheumatoid arthritis as diagnostic dilemmas in two different cases: confounding factor and true coexistence, *Clin Rheumatol* 26:98, 2007.

Pakarinen TK et al: Charcot arthropathy of the diabetic foot: current concepts and review of 36 cases, *Scand J Surg* 91:195, 2002.

Pinzur MS: Current concepts review: Charcot arthropathy of the foot and ankle, *Foot Ankle Int* 28:952, 2007.

Slater RA et al: The diabetic Charcot foot, *1st Med Assoc J* 6:280, 2004.

AUTHOR: **LONNIE R. MERCIER, M.D.**

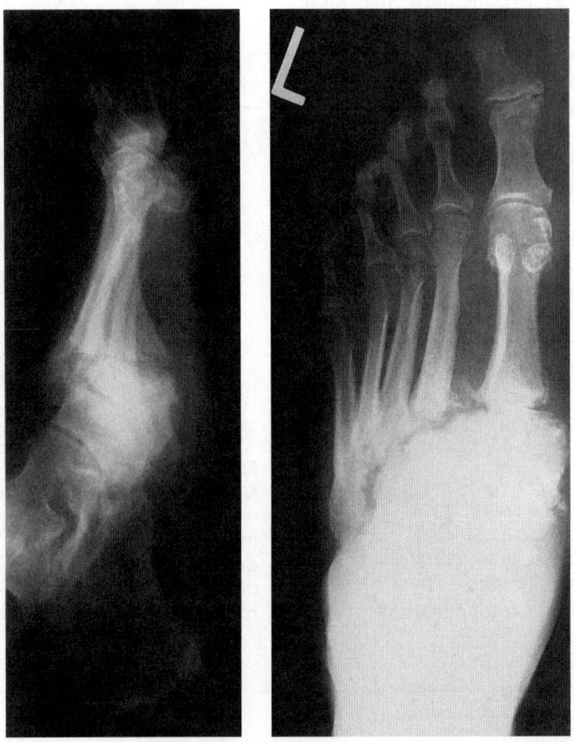

FIGURE 1-55 Diabetes mellitus and neuropathic arthritis. Note lateral displacement of metatarsals *(left)* and fragmentation and osseous debris *(right)*. (From Goldman L, Ausiello D [eds]: *Cecil textbook of medicine,* ed 22, Philadelphia, 2004, WB Saunders.)

BASIC INFORMATION

DEFINITION

Genital infection with *Chlamydia trachomatis* may result in urethritis, epididymitis, cervicitis, and acute salpingitis, but often it is asymptomatic in women (see "Pelvic Inflammatory Disease"). In men, urethritis, mucopurulent discharge, dysuria, urethral pruritus.

ICD-9CM CODES
597.80 Urethritis
604.0 Epididymitis
616.0 Cervicitis
381.51 Acute salpingitis

EPIDEMIOLOGY & DEMOGRAPHICS

- *Chlamydia trachomatis* is the most common cause of sexually transmitted disease in the U.S. More than 4 million infections occur annually, although the exact number is unknown because reporting is not required in all states. Occurrence is common worldwide and has been increasing steadily over the last 2 decades in the U.S., Canada, Australia, and Europe.
- Most women with endocervical or urethral infections are asymptomatic.
- Up to 45% of cases of gonococcal infection may have concomitant chlamydial infection.
- Infertility or ectopic pregnancy can result as a complication from symptomatic or asymptomatic chronic infections of the endometrium and fallopian tubes.
- Conjunctival and pneumonic infection of the newborn may result from infection in pregnancy.
- In men 15% to 55% of cases are of *C. trachomatis*. Complications of nongonococcal urethritis in men infected with *C. trachomatis* include epididymitis and Reiter's syndrome.

PHYSICAL FINDINGS & CLINICAL PRESENTATION

Clinical manifestations may be similar to those of gonorrhea: mucopurulent endocervical discharge, with edema, erythema, and easily induced endocervical bleeding caused by inflammation of endocervical columnar epithelium. Less frequent manifestations may include bartholinitis, urethral syndrome with dysuria and pyuria, perihepatitis (Fitz-Hugh–Curtis syndrome).

ETIOLOGY

- *Chlamydia trachomatis,* serotypes D through K
- Obligate, intracellular bacteria

DIAGNOSIS

DIFFERENTIAL DIAGNOSIS

Gonorrhea, nongonococcal urethritis (nonchlamydial etiologies)

WORKUP

Diagnosis based on laboratory demonstration of evidence of infection in intraurethral or endocervical swab by various tests. The intracellular organism is less readily recovered from the discharge.

LABORATORY TESTS

- Cell culture is the reference method for diagnosis (single culture sensitivity 80% to 90%), but it is labor intensive and takes 48 to 96 hr; it is not suited for large screening programs.
- Nonculture methods:
  Direct fluorescent antibody (DFA) tests
  Enzyme immunoassay (EIA)
  DNA probes
  Polymerase chain reaction (PCR)
- With the exception of PCR, the other tests are probably less specific than cell culture and may yield false-positive results.
- Because this is an intracellular organism, purulent discharge is not an appropriate specimen. An adequate sample of infected cells must be obtained.
- 10 WBCs per high-power field.

TREATMENT

ACUTE GENERAL Rx

Nongonococcal urethritis, urethritis, cervicitis, conjunctivitis (except for LGV):

- Azithromycin 1 g PO × 1 *or*
- Doxycycline 100 mg PO bid for 7 days
- Alternatives
  1. Erythromycin base 500 mg PO qid for 7 days *or*
  2. Erythromycin ethylsuccinate 800 mg PO qid for 7 days *or*
  3. Ofloxacin 300 mg PO bid for 7 days
  4. Levofloxacin 500 mg PO qd for 7 days

Infection in pregnancy:

- Erythromycin base 500 mg PO qid for 7 days *or*
- Amoxicillin 500 mg PO tid for 7 days

Alternatives:

1. Erythromycin base 250 mg PO qid for 7 days *or*
2. Erythromycin ethylsuccinate 800 mg PO qid for 7 days *or*
3. Erythromycin ethylsuccinate 400 mg PO qid for 14 days *or*
4. Azithromycin 1 g PO (single dose)

NOTE: Doxycycline and ofloxacin are contraindicated in pregnancy. Safety and efficacy of azithromycin are not established in pregnancy and lactation, although preliminary data indicate that it may be safe and effective. Erythromycin estolate is contraindicated in pregnancy because of drug-related hepatotoxicity.

FOLLOW-UP: Reculture after therapy completion and refer partners for evaluation and treatment.

RECURRENT AND PERSISTENT URETHRITIS: Retreat noncompliant patients with the above regimens. If patient was initially compliant, recommended regimens: metronidazole 2 g PO in single dose plus erythromycin base 500 mg PO qid for 7 days or erythromycin ethylsuccinate 800 mg PO qid for 7 days.

DISPOSITION

See "Gonorrhea."

REFFERAL

Refer to infectious disease specialist if persistant infection or to gynecologist if salpingitis is suspected.

EVIDENCE

Doxycycline is effective in the treatment of genital chlamydial infections in men and nonpregnant women. Small randomized controlled trials (RCTs) with short-term follow-up have found microbiological cure rates of at least 95%.[1] Ⓐ

Another systematic review found no significant difference between azithromycin and doxycycline in terms of microbiological cure rates in males and nonpregnant females with genital chlamydial infections.[2] Ⓐ

In small, short-term RCTs including men and nonpregnant women with genital chlamydial infection, cure rates achieved with erythromycin ranged from 77% to 100%.[1] Ⓐ

No significant difference was found in two unblinded RCTs between azithromycin and amoxicillin in terms of microbiological cure in pregnant women with chlamydial infections.[3] Ⓑ

Evidence-Based References

1. Low N: Chlamydia (uncomplicated, genital), *Clin Evid* 12:2203, 2004. Ⓐ
2. Lau CY, Qureshi AK: Azithromycin versus doxycycline for genital chlamydial infections: a meta-analysis of randomized clinical trials, *Sex Transm Dis* 29:497, 2002. Reviewed in: *Clin Evid* 12:2200, 2004. Ⓐ
3. Jacobson GF: A randomized controlled trial comparing amoxicillin and azithromycin for the treatment of *Chlamydia trachomatis* in pregnancy, *Am J Obstet Gynecol* 184:1352, 2001. Reviewed in: *Clin Evid* 12:2200, 2004. Ⓑ

SUGGESTED READINGS

Centers for Disease Control and Prevention: 2006 sexually transmitted diseases treatment guidelines, *MMWR Morb Mortal Wkly Rep* 55(RR-11), 2006.

Spiliopoulou et al: Chlamydia trachomatis: time for screening? *Clin Microbiol Infect* 11(9):687, 2005.

AUTHORS: **MARIA A. CORIGLIANO, M.D.,** and **RUBEN ALVERO, M.D.**

BASIC INFORMATION

DEFINITION

Cholangitis refers to an inflammation and/or infection of the hepatic and common bile ducts associated with obstruction of the common bile duct.

SYNONYMS

Biliary sepsis
Ascending cholangitis
Suppurative cholangitis

ICD-9CM CODES
576.1 Cholangitis

EPIDEMIOLOGY & DEMOGRAPHICS

INCIDENCE (IN U.S.): Complicates approximately 1% of cases of cholelithiasis
PEAK INCIDENCE: Seventh decade
PREVALENCE (IN U.S.): 2 cases/1000 hospital admissions
PREDOMINANT SEX:
- Females, for cholangitis secondary to gallstones
- Males, for cholangitis secondary to malignant obstruction and HIV infection

PREDOMINANT AGE: Seventh decade and older; unusual <50 yr of age

PHYSICAL FINDINGS & CLINICAL PRESENTATION

- Usually acute onset of fever, chills, abdominal pain, tenderness over the RUQ of the abdomen, and jaundice (Charcot's triad)
- All signs and symptoms in only 50% to 85% of patients
- Often, dark coloration of the urine resulting from bilirubinuria
- Complications:
  1. Bacteremia (50%) and septic shock
  2. Hepatic abscess and pancreatitis

ETIOLOGY

Obstruction of the common bile duct causing rapid proliferation of bacteria in the biliary tree
- Most common cause of common bile duct obstruction: stones, usually migrated from the gallbladder
- Other causes: prior biliary tract surgery with secondary stenosis, tumor (usually arising from the pancreas or biliary tree), and parasitic infections from *Ascaris lumbricoides* or *Fasciola hepatica*
- Iatrogenic after contamination of an obstructed biliary tree by endoscopic retrograde cholangiopancreatoscopy (ERCP) or percutaneous transhepatic cholangiography (PTC)
- Primary sclerosing cholangitis (PSC)
- HIV-associated sclerosing cholangitis: associated with infection by CMV, *Cryptosporidium,* Microsporidia, and *Mycobacterium avium* complex

DIAGNOSIS

DIFFERENTIAL DIAGNOSIS

- Biliary colic
- Acute cholecystitis
- Liver abscess
- Peptic ulcer disease (PUD)
- Pancreatitis
- Intestinal obstruction
- Right kidney stone
- Hepatitis
- Pyelonephritis

WORKUP

- Blood cultures
- CBC
- Liver function tests

LABORATORY TESTS

- Usually, elevated WBC count with a predominance of polymorphonuclear forms
- Elevated alkaline phosphatase and bilirubin in chronic obstruction
- Elevated transaminases in acute obstruction
- Positive blood cultures in 50% of cases, typically with enteric gram-negative aerobes (e.g., *E. coli, Klebsiella pneumoniae*), enterococci, or anaerobes

IMAGING STUDIES

- Ultrasound:
  1. Allows visualization of the gallbladder and bile ducts to differentiate extrahepatic obstruction from intrahepatic cholestasis
  2. Insensitive but specific for visualization of common duct stones
- CT scan:
  1. Less accurate for gallstones
  2. More sensitive than ultrasound for visualization of the distal part of the common bile duct
  3. Also allows better definition of neoplasm
- ERCP:
  1. Confirms obstruction and its level
  2. Allows collection of specimens for culture and cytology
  3. Indicated for diagnosis if ultrasound and CT scan are inconclusive
  4. May be indicated in therapy (see "Treatment")

TREATMENT

NONPHARMACOLOGIC THERAPY

Biliary decompression
- May be urgent in severely ill patients or those unresponsive to medical therapy within 12 to 24 hr
- May also be performed semielectively in patients who respond
- Options:
  1. ERCP with or without sphincterotomy or placement of a draining stent
  2. Percutaneous transhepatic biliary drainage for the acutely ill patient who is a poor surgical candidate
  3. Surgical exploration of the common bile duct

ACUTE GENERAL Rx

- Nothing by mouth
- Intravenous hydration
- Broad-spectrum antibiotics directed at gram-negative enteric organisms, anaerobes, and enterococcus: if infection is nosocomial, post-ERCP, or the patient is in shock, broaden antibiotic coverage.

CHRONIC Rx

Repeated decompression may be necessary, particularly when obstruction is related to neoplasm.

DISPOSITION

Excellent prognosis if obstruction is amenable to definitive surgical therapy; otherwise relapses are common.

REFERRAL

- To biliary endoscopist if obstruction is from stones or a stent needs to be placed
- To interventional radiologist if external drainage is necessary
- To a general surgeon in all other cases
- To an infectious disease specialist if blood cultures are positive or the patient is in shock or otherwise severely ill

PEARLS & CONSIDERATIONS

- Cholangitis is a life threatening form of intra-abdominal sepsis, though it may appear to be rather innocuous at its onset.
- Antibiotics alone will not resolve cholangitis in the presence of biliary obstruction because high intrabiliary pressures prevent antibiotic delivery. Decompression and drainage of the biliary tract to alleviate the obstruction with antimicrobial therapy is the therapy of choice.

SUGGESTED READINGS

Kumar R et al: Endoscopic biliary drainage for severe acute cholangitis in biliary obstruction as a result of malignant and benign diseases, *J Gastroenterol Hepatol* 19(9):994, 2004.
Ozden I et al: Endoscopic and radiologic interventions as the leading causes of severe cholangitis in a tertiary referral center, *Am J Surg* 189(6):702, 2005.
Yarze JC, Herlihy KJ, Scalia SV: Cholangiohepatoma presenting with recurrent cholangitis, *Dig Dis Sci* 50(3):552, 2005.

AUTHORS: **STEVEN M. OPAL, M.D.,** and **MICHELE HALPERN, M.D.**

BASIC INFORMATION

DEFINITION

Cholecystitis is an acute or chronic inflammation of the gallbladder generally secondary to gallstones (>95% of cases).

SYNONYMS

Gallbladder attack

ICD-9CM CODES
575.0 Acute cholecystitis
574.0 Calculus of the gallbladder with acute cholecystitis
575.1 Cholecystitis without mention of calculus

EPIDEMIOLOGY & DEMOGRAPHICS

- Acute cholecystitis occurs most commonly in females during the fifth and sixth decades.
- The incidence of gallstones is 0.6% in the general population and much higher in certain ethnic groups (>75% of Native Americans by age 60 yr).

PHYSICAL FINDINGS & CLINICAL PRESENTATION

- Pain and tenderness in the right hypochondrium or epigastrium; pain possibly radiating to the infrascapular region
- Palpation of the right upper quadrant (RUQ) eliciting marked tenderness and stoppage of inspired breath (Murphy's sign)
- Guarding
- Fever (33%)
- Jaundice (25% to 50% of patients)
- Palpable gallbladder (20% of cases)
- Nausea and vomiting (>70% of patients)
- Fever and chills (>25% of patients)
- Medical history often revealing ingestion of large, fatty meals before onset of pain in the epigastrium and RUQ

ETIOLOGY

- Gallstones (>95% of cases)
- Ischemic damage to the gallbladder, critically ill patient (acalculous cholecystitis)
- Infectious agents, especially in patients with AIDS (CMV, *Cryptosporidium*)
- Strictures of the bile duct
- Neoplasms, primary or metastatic

DIAGNOSIS

DIFFERENTIAL DIAGNOSIS

- Hepatic: hepatitis, abscess, hepatic congestion, neoplasm, trauma
- Biliary: neoplasm, stricture
- Gastric: pelvic ulcer disease (PUD), neoplasm, alcoholic gastritis, hiatal hernia
- Pancreatic: pancreatitis, neoplasm, stone in the pancreatic duct or ampulla
- Renal: calculi, infection, inflammation, neoplasm, ruptured kidney
- Pulmonary: pneumonia, pulmonary infarction, right-sided pleurisy
- Intestinal: retrocecal appendicitis, intestinal obstruction, high fecal impaction
- Cardiac: myocardial ischemia (particularly involving the inferior wall), pericarditis
- Cutaneous: herpes zoster
- Trauma
- Fitz-Hugh–Curtis syndrome (perihepatitis)
- Subphrenic abscess
- Dissecting aneurysm
- Nerve root irritation caused by osteoarthritis of the spine

WORKUP

Workup consists of detailed history and physical examination coupled with laboratory evaluation and imaging studies. No single clinical finding or laboratory test is sufficient to establish or exclude cholecystitis without further testing.

LABORATORY TESTS

- Leukocytosis (12,000 to 20,000) is present in >70% of patients.
- Elevated alkaline phosphatase, ALT, AST, bilirubin; bilirubin elevation >4 mg/dl is unusual and suggests presence of choledocholithiasis.
- Elevated amylase may be present (consider pancreatitis if serum amylase elevation exceeds 500 U).

IMAGING STUDIES

- Ultrasound of the gallbladder is the preferred initial test; it will demonstrate the presence of stones and also dilated gallbladder with thickened wall and surrounding edema in patients with acute cholecystitis.
- Nuclear imaging (HIDA scan) is useful for diagnosis of cholecystitis: sensitivity and specificity exceed 90% for acute cholecystis. This test is only reliable when bilirubin is <5 mg/dl. A positive test will demonstrate obstruction of the cystic or common hepatic duct; the test will not demonstrate the presence of stones.
- CT scan of abdomen is useful in cases of suspected abscess, neoplasm, or pancreatitis.
- Plain film of the abdomen generally is not useful, because <25% of stones are radiopaque.

TREATMENT

NONPHARMACOLOGIC THERAPY

Provide IV hydration; withhold oral feedings.

ACUTE GENERAL Rx

- Cholecystectomy (laparoscopic is preferred, open cholecystectomy is acceptable); conservative management with IV fluids and antibiotics (ampicillin-sulbactam [Unasyn] 3 g IV q6h *or* piperacillin-tazobactam [Zosyn] 4.5 g IV q8h) may be justified in some high-risk patients to convert an emergency procedure into an elective one with a lower mortality.
- Endoscopic retrograde cholangiopancreatoscopy (ERCP) with sphincterectomy and stone extraction can be performed in conjunction with laparoscopic cholecystectomy for patients with choledochal lithiasis; approximately 7% to 15% of patients with cholelithiasis also have stones in the common bile duct.
- IV fluids, broad-spectrum antibiotics, pain management (meperidine prn) should be used.

DISPOSITION

- Prognosis is good; elective laparoscopic cholecystectomy can be performed as outpatient procedure.
- Hospital stay (when necessary) varies from overnight with laparoscopic cholecystectomy to 4 to 7 days with open cholecystectomy.
- Complication rate is approximately 1% (hemorrhage and bile leak) for laparoscopic cholecystectomy and <0.5% (infection) with open cholecystectomy.

REFERRAL

Hospitalization and surgical referral in all patients with acute cholecystitis

PEARLS & CONSIDERATIONS

COMMENTS

- Patients should be instructed that stones may recur in bile ducts.
- Gallbladder aspiration in which all fluid visualized by ultrasound is aspirated represents a nonsurgical treatment when patients who are at high operative risk develop acute cholecystitis. Salvage cholecystectomy is reserved for nonresponders.

SUGGESTED READINGS

Cuschieri A: Management of patients with gallstones and ductal calculi, *Lancet* 360:739, 2002.
Trowbridge RL et al: Does this patient have acute cholecystitis? *JAMA* 289:80, 2003.

AUTHOR: **FRED F. FERRI, M.D.**

BASIC INFORMATION

DEFINITION

Cholelithiasis is the presence of stones in the gallbladder.

SYNONYMS

Gallstones

ICD-9CM CODES
574.2 Calculus of the gallbladder without mention of cholecystitis
574.0 Calculus of the gallbladder with acute cholecystitis

EPIDEMIOLOGY & DEMOGRAPHICS

- Gallstone disease can be found in 12% of the U.S. population. Of these, 2% to 3% (500,000 to 600,000) are treated with cholecystectomies each year.
- Annual medical expenditures for gallbladder surgeries in the U.S. exceed $5 billion.
- Incidence of gallbladder disease increases with age. Highest incidence is in the fifth and sixth decades. Predisposing factors for gallstones are female sex, pregnancy, age >40 yr, family history of gallstones, obesity, ileal disease, oral contraceptives, diabetes mellitus, rapid weight loss, estrogen replacement therapy.
- Patients with gallstones have a 20% chance of developing biliary colic or its complications at the end of a 20-yr period.

PHYSICAL FINDINGS & CLINICAL PRESENTATION

- Physical examination is entirely normal unless patient is having biliary colic; 80% of gallstones are asymptomatic.
- Typical symptoms of obstruction of the cystic duct include intermittent, severe, cramping pain affecting the right upper quadrant (RUQ).
- Pain occurs mostly at night and may radiate to the back or right shoulder. It can last from a few minutes to several hours.

ETIOLOGY

- 75% of gallstones contain cholesterol and are usually associated with obesity, female sex, diabetes mellitus; mixed stones are most common (80%), pure cholesterol stones account for only 10% of stones.
- 25% of gallstones are pigment stones (bilirubin, calcium, and variable organic material) associated with hemolysis and cirrhosis. These tend to be black pigment stones that are refractory to medical therapy.
- 50% of mixed-type stones are radiopaque.

DIAGNOSIS

DIFFERENTIAL DIAGNOSIS

- Pelvic ulcer disease (PUD)
- GERD
- IBD
- Pancreatitis
- Neoplasms
- Nonnuclear dyspepsia
- Inferior wall MI
- Hepatic abscess

LABORATORY TESTS

Generally normal unless patient has biliary obstruction (elevated alkaline phosphatase, bilirubin).

IMAGING STUDIES

- Ultrasound of the gallbladder will detect small stones and biliary sludge (sensitivity, 95%; specificity, 90%); the presence of dilated gallbladder with thickened wall is suggestive of acute cholecystitis.
- Nuclear imaging (HIDA scan) can confirm acute cholecystitis (>90% accuracy) if gallbladder does not visualize within 4 hr of injection and the radioisotope is excreted in the common bile duct.
- Common bile duct stones can be detected noninvasively by magnetic resonance cholangiopancreatography (MRCP) or invasively via endoscopic retrograde cholangiopancreatography (ERCP) and intraoperative cholangiography.

TREATMENT

NONPHARMACOLOGIC THERAPY

Lifestyle changes (avoidance of diets high in polyunsaturated fats, weight loss in obese patients—however, avoid rapid weight loss)

ACUTE GENERAL Rx

- The management of gallstones is affected by the clinical presentation.
- Asymptomatic patients do not require therapeutic intervention.
- Surgical intervention is generally the ideal approach for symptomatic patients. Laparoscopic cholecystectomy is generally preferred over open cholecystectomy because of the shorter recovery period and lower mortality. Between 5% and 26% of patients undergoing elective laparoscopic cholecystectomy will require conversion to an open procedure. Most common reason is inability to clearly identify the biliary anatomy.
- Laparoscopic cholecystectomy after endoscopic sphincterectomy is recommended for patients with common bile duct stones and residual gallbladder stones. Where possible, single-stage laparoscopic treatments with removal of duct stones and cholecystectomy during the same procedure are preferable.
- Patients who are not appropriate candidates for surgery because of coexisting illness or patients who refuse surgery can be treated with oral bile salts: ursodiol (Actigall) 8 to 10 mg/kg/day in 2 to 3 divided doses for 16 to 20 mo, or chenodiol (Chenix) 250 mg bid initially, increasing gradually to a dose of 60 mg/kg/day. Candidates for oral bile salts are patients with cholesterol stones (radiolucent, noncalcified stones), with a diameter of ≤15 mm and having three or fewer stones. Candidates for medical therapy must have a functioning gallbladder and must have absence of calcifications on CT scans.
- Direct solvent dissolution with methyl *tert*-butyl ether (MTBE) is rarely used. Administration of the solvent is either through percutaneous transhepatic placement of a catheter into the gallbladder or endoscopic retrograde catheter placement with subsequent continuous infusion and aspiration of the solvent either manually or by automatic pump system.
- Extracorporeal shock wave lithotripsy (ESWL) is another form of medical therapy. It can be used in patients with stone diameter of ≤3 cm and having three or fewer stones.

DISPOSITION

- Recurrence rate after bile acid treatment is approximately 50% in 5 yr. Periodic ultrasound is necessary to assess the effectiveness of treatment.
- Gallstones recur after dissolution therapy with MTBE in >40% of patients within 5 yr.
- Following extracorporeal shock wave lithotripsy, stones recur in approximately 20% of patients after 4 yr.
- Patients with at least one gallstone <5 mm in diameter have a greater than fourfold increased risk of presenting with acute biliary pancreatitis. A policy of watchful waiting in such cases is generally unwarranted.
- A potential serious complication of gallstones is acute cholangitis. ERCP and endoscopic sphincterectomy (EC) followed by interval laparoscopic cholecystectomy is effective in acute cholangitis.

SUGGESTED READINGS

Bellows CF et al: Management of gallstones, *Am Fam Physician* 72:637, 2005.
Moon JH et al: The detection of bile duct stones in suspected biliary pancreatitis: comparison of MRCP, ERCP, and intraductal US, *Am J Gastroenterol* 100:1051, 2005.

AUTHOR: **FRED F. FERRI, M.D.**

BASIC INFORMATION

DEFINITION

Cholera is an acute diarrheal illness caused by *Vibrio cholerae.*

SYNONYMS

None

ICD-9CM CODES
001.0 Cholera

EPIDEMIOLOGY & DEMOGRAPHICS

INCIDENCE (IN U.S.): Previously, approximately 50 cases per yr, mostly in travelers returning from endemic areas. From 1995 to 2000, 61 cases reported, 37 (61%) of which acquired outside the U.S.
PEAK INCIDENCE:
- None in the U.S.
- Summer and fall in endemic areas

PREDOMINANT SEX: None
PREDOMINANT AGE: In nonendemic areas, attack rates are equal in all age groups. In epidemic areas, children over the age of 2 yr are most commonly infected. Neonatal infection: illness is uncommon before the age of 2 yr, likely because of passive immunity.

PHYSICAL FINDINGS & CLINICAL PRESENTATION

Infection may result in asymptomatic illness or a mild diarrhea. The classic illness is described as the abrupt onset of voluminous watery diarrhea, which may lead to severe dehydration, acidosis, shock, and death. Vomiting may occur early in the illness, but fever and abdominal pain are usually absent. The typical "rice water" stools are pale with flecks of mucus and contain no blood. Muscle cramps may be prominent, and are the result of loss of fluid and electrolytes. Untreated illness results in hypovolemic shock, and death may occur in hours to days. With adequate fluid and electrolyte repletion, cholera is a self-limited illness that resolves in a few days. The use of antimicrobials can shorten the course of illness.

ETIOLOGY

The organism responsible for this illness is one of several strains of *V. cholerae.* Most infections result from the 01 serotype, the El Tor biotype. In the U.S., one outbreak occurred from the ingestion of illegally imported crab, and sporadic infection has been associated with the consumption of contaminated shellfish in Gulf Coast states. Most cases are seen in returning travelers. Transmission during epidemics is the result of the ingestion of contaminated water and, in some instances, contaminated food.

DIAGNOSIS

DIFFERENTIAL DIAGNOSIS

- Mild illness may mimic gastroenteritis resulting from a variety of etiologies.
- Sudden, voluminous diarrhea causing marked dehydration is uncommon in other illnesses.

WORKUP

Stool should be sent for culture and microscopy. Treatment should not be delayed while awaiting culture results.

LABORATORY TESTS

- WBC may be elevated, and hemoglobin may be increased as a result of hemoconcentration.
- Elevated bun and creatinine suggests prerenal azotemia. Hypoglycemia may occur. Stool cultures on appropriate media may grow the organism. Wet mount of stool under dark field or phase contrast microscopy shows organisms with characteristic darting motility.

TREATMENT

NONPHARMACOLOGIC THERAPY

The mainstay of therapy is adequate fluid and electrolyte replacement. This can usually be achieved using oral rehydration solutions containing salts and glucose. Some patients may require intravenous fluid and electrolyte replacement.

ACUTE GENERAL Rx

- Antimicrobial therapy can decrease shedding of fluid and organisms and can shorten the course of illness:
  1. Doxycycline 100 mg po bid for 5 days *or*
  2. SMX-TMP, one DS tablet po bid for 5 days *or*
  3. Azithromycin two 500 mg tablets po as a single dose
- Resistance to SMX-TMP is increasing in travel-associated infections.

CHRONIC Rx

It is likely that asymptomatic chronic carriers exist; however, because they are difficult to identify, and their role in transmission of disease appears to be rather limited, there is no recommendation for treatment of these individuals.

DISPOSITION

The mortality of adequately hydrated patients is less than 1%.

REFERRAL

If more than mild illness occurs

PEARLS & CONSIDERATIONS

COMMENTS

- There is currently no indication for vaccination of travelers to endemic areas. The risk of infection is small, protection from available vaccines is limited, and side effects are prominent and frequent.
- Doxycycline should not be used to treat children or pregnant women.
- A recent study indicates a single dose treatment strategy with azithromycin is significantly better than ciprofloxacin for the management of cholera.

EVIDENCE

Rice-based oral rehydration solution has been shown to be significantly more effective than standard oral rehydration solution for the reduction of stool volume in patients with cholera.[1,2] Ⓐ

Tetracycline has been shown to significantly reduce stool volume and duration of diarrhea compared with placebo in patients with severe cholera secondary to infection with *Vibrio cholerae* O139 Bengal.[3] Ⓑ

Clinical improvement and eradication of *V. cholerae* has been found to be similar with tetracycline and ciprofloxacin.[4] Ⓑ

Evidence-Based References

1. Rabbani GH et al: Antidiarrheal effects of L-histidine-supplemented rice-based oral rehydration solution in the treatment of male adults with severe cholera in Bangladesh: a double-blind, randomized trial, *J Infect Dis* 191(9):1507-1514, 2005.
2. Garcia L et al: The vaccine candidate *Vibrio cholerae* 638 is protective against cholera in healthy volunteers, *Infect Immun* 73(5):3018-3024, 2005.
3. Thiagarajah JR, Verkman AS: New drug targets for cholera therapy, *Trends Pharmacol Sci* 26(4):172-175, 2005.
4. Lucas ME et al: Effectiveness of mass oral cholera vaccination in Beira, Mozambique, *N Engl J Med* 352(8):757-767, 2005.

SUGGESTED READINGS

Hill DR et al: Oral cholera vaccines: use in clinical practice, *Lancet Infect Dis* 6(6):361, 2006.

Saha D et al: Single dose azithromycin for the treatment of cholera in adults, *N Engl J Med* 354(23):2452, 2006.

AUTHORS: **GLENN G. FORT, M.D., M.P.H., DENNIS J. MIKOLICH, M.D.,** and **MAURICE POLICAR, M.D.**

BASIC INFORMATION

DEFINITION

Chronic fatigue syndrome (CFS) is characterized by four or more of the following symptoms, present concurrently for at least 6 mo:

- Impaired memory or concentration
- Sore throat
- Tender cervical or axillary lymph nodes
- Muscle pain
- Multijoint pain
- New headaches
- Unrefreshing sleep
- Postexertion malaise

SYNONYMS

Yuppie flu
CFS
Chronic Epstein-Barr syndrome

ICD-9CM CODES
780.7 Chronic fatigue syndrome
300.8 Neurasthenia

EPIDEMIOLOGY & DEMOGRAPHICS

PREVALENCE IN U.S.: 100 to 300 cases/100,000 persons
PREDOMINANT AGE: Young adulthood and middle age
PREDOMINANT SEX: Female > male

PHYSICAL FINDINGS & CLINICAL PRESENTATION

- There are no physical findings specific for CFS.
- The physical examination may be useful to identify fibromyalgia and other rheumatologic conditions that may coexist with CFS.

ETIOLOGY

- The etiology of CFS is unknown.
- Many experts suspect that a viral illness may trigger certain immune responses leading to the various symptoms. Most patients often report the onset of their symptoms with a flulike illness.

DIAGNOSIS

DIFFERENTIAL DIAGNOSIS

- Psychosocial depression, dysthymia, anxiety-related disorders, and other psychiatric diseases
- Infectious diseases (SBE, Lyme disease, fungal diseases, mononucleosis, HIV, chronic hepatitis B or C, TB, chronic parasitic infections)
- Autoimmune diseases: SLE, myasthenia gravis, multiple sclerosis, thyroiditis, RA
- Endocrine abnormalities: hypothyroidism, hypopituitarism, adrenal insufficiency, Cushing's syndrome, diabetes mellitus, hyperparathyroidism, pregnancy, reactive hypoglycemia
- Occult malignant disease
- Substance abuse
- Systemic disorders: chronic renal failure, COPD, cardiovascular disease, anemia, electrolyte abnormalities, liver disease
- Other: inadequate rest, sleep apnea, narcolepsy, fibromyalgia, sarcoidosis, medications, toxic agent exposure, Wegener's granulomatosis

LABORATORY TESTS

- No specific laboratory tests exist for diagnosing CFS. Initial laboratory tests are useful to exclude other conditions that may mimic or may be associated with CFS.
  1. Screening laboratory tests: CBC, ESR, ALT, total protein, albumin, globulin, alkaline phosphatase, calcium, phosphorus, glucose, BUN, creatinine, electrolytes, TSH, and urinalysis are useful.
  2. Serologic tests for Epstein-Barr virus, *Candida albicans,* human herpesvirus 6, and other studies for immune cellular abnormalities are not useful; these tests are expensive and generally not recommended.
- Other tests may be indicated depending on the history and physical examination (e.g., ANA, RF in patients presenting with joint complaints or abnormalities on physical examination, Lyme titer in areas where Lyme disease is endemic).

IMAGING STUDIES

Generally not recommended unless history and physical examination indicate specific abnormalities (e.g., chest x-ray in any patient suspected of TB or sarcoidosis)

TREATMENT

NONPHARMACOLOGIC THERAPY

- Patients should be reassured that the illness is not fatal and that most patients improve over time.
- An initially supervised exercise program to preserve and increase strength is beneficial for most patients and can improve symptoms.

GENERAL Rx

Therapy is generally palliative. The following medications may be helpful:

- Antidepressants: The choice of antidepressant varies with the desired side effects. Patients with difficulty sleeping or fibromyalgia-like symptoms may benefit from low-dose tricyclics (doxepin 10 mg hs or amitriptyline 25 mg qhs). When sedation is not desirable, low-dose SSRIs (paroxetine 20 mg qd) often help alleviate fatigue and associated symptoms.
- NSAIDs can be used to relieve muscle and joint pain and headaches.

"Alternative" medications (herbs, multivitamins, nutritional supplements) are very popular with many CFS patients but are generally not very helpful.

PEARLS & CONSIDERATIONS

COMMENTS

- In CFS the symptoms are serious enough to reduce daily activities by >50% and in absence of any other medically identifiable disorders.
- Moderate to complete recovery at 1 yr occurs in 22% to 60% of patients with CFS.

EVIDENCE

Graded aerobic exercise has been shown to result in improvements in fatigue and physical functioning in patients with CFS.[1] Ⓐ

A randomized controlled trial compared graded exercise plus fluoxetine, graded exercise plus placebo, general advice to exercise plus fluoxetine, and general advice to exercise plus placebo. After 26 weeks, significantly fewer patients in the active exercise groups experienced fatigue.[2] Ⓐ

Cognitive behavioral therapy appears to be an effective treatment for adult outpatients with chronic fatigue syndrome (CFS). Physical functioning is significantly improved, and the treatment is highly acceptable to patients.[3] Ⓐ

There is insufficient evidence for the benefit of corticosteroids, nicotinamide adenine dinucleotide (NADH), immunoglobulins, prolonged rest, or antidepressants in the treatment of CFS.[4]

Evidence-Based References

1. Edmonds M, McGuire H, Price J: Exercise therapy for chronic fatigue syndrome, *Cochrane Database Syst Rev* 3:CD003200, 2004. Ⓐ
2. Wearden AJ et al: Randomised, double-blind, placebo controlled treatment trial of fluoxetine and a graded exercise programme for chronic fatigue syndrome, *Br J Psychiatry* 172:485-490, 1998. Ⓐ
3. Price JR, Couper J: Cognitive behaviour therapy for chronic fatigue syndrome in adults *Cochrane Database Syst Rev* 2:CD001027, 2000. Ⓐ
4. Reid S et al: Chronic fatigue syndrome. In: *Clinical Evidence*, 12, London, 2003, BMJ Publishing Group.

SUGGESTED READING

Hickie I et al: Post-infective and chronic fatigue syndromes precipitated by viral and non-viral pathogens: prospective cohort study, *BMJ* 333:575, 2006.

AUTHOR: **FRED F. FERRI, M.D.**

BASIC INFORMATION

DEFINITION

A chronic demyelinating disease of the spinal nerve roots and peripheral nerves that is characterized by weakness and sensory deficits.

SYNONYMS

CIDP

RELATED DISORDERS

- Multifocal motor neuropathy with conduction block
- Lewis-Sumner syndrome
- Multifocal acquired demyelinating sensory and motor (MADSAM) neuropathy

ICD-9CM CODES
357.8 Inflammatory and toxic neuropathy, other (use for chronic inflammatory demyelinating polyradiculoneuropathy)

EPIDEMIOLOGY & DEMOGRAPHICS

PREVALENCE: 1.0 to 1.9 per 100,000
PREDOMINANT SEX: Male predominance
PREDOMINANT AGE: Most common in the fifth to seventh decade, although may also occur in children

PHYSICAL FINDINGS & CLINICAL PRESENTATION

- Onset is over weeks, months, or years.
- Symptoms may be both sensory (paresthesias, neuropathic pain, and numbness of the hands and feet) and motor (weakness).
- Postural instability, gait abnormalities, and proximal muscle weakness may become prominent late in the disease.
- Sensory findings on examination include impaired vibration and joint position sense more commonly than impaired light touch, pinprick, and temperature sensation.
- Muscle weakness is usually distal and symmetric, although may occasionally be asymmetric and more proximal than distal.
- Reflexes are usually reduced or absent.
- Cranial nerve abnormalities as well as bowel and bladder dysfunction are highly unusual.
- Autonomic dysfunction is rare, but may occur.

ETIOLOGY

CIDP occurs as a primary (idiopathic) form and may also occur in association with a number of systemic disorders.
- The idiopathic variety is most common and an autoimmune process is likely.
- The most common systemic disorder associated with CIDP is a monoclonal gammopathy.
- Occasionally an underlying plasma cell dyscrasia such as Waldenstrom's macroglobulinemia, multiple myeloma, or osteosclerotic myeloma may be identified.
- An association with diabetes mellitus has been recognized more recently.
- CIDP may occasionally occur in the context of human immunodeficiency virus (HIV) and hepatitis B or C virus infection.

DIAGNOSIS

DIFFERENTIAL DIAGNOSIS

- Guillain-Barré syndrome (GBS)—the difference being that GBS evolves over a maximum of 4 wk and CIDP usually progresses over at least 8 wk.
- Diabetic neuropathy—the distinction can be made with electrodiagnostic studies, which show axonal physiology in diabetic neuropathy.
- Mononeuritis multiplex.
- Monoclonal gammopathy of undetermined significance, plasma cell dyscrasia, osteosclerotic myeloma, and HIV infection are not so much part of the differential diagnosis, but may coexist and so should always be sought.

WORKUP

Nerve conduction studies and electromyography—these should show evidence of primary demyelination (with or without secondary axonal loss). Nerve biopsy may occasionally be required.

LABORATORY TESTS

- Lumbar puncture
  1. Shows increased CSF protein (especially helpful if >100 mg/dl)
  2. There is little or no pleocytosis (<10 white cells)
- Serum protein electrophoresis and immunofixation electrophoresis to identify a small M-protein
- Urine protein electrophoresis
- Hepatitis and HIV serology
- Fasting blood sugar and/or glucose tolerance test
- Bone marrow biopsy if a monoclonal gammopathy is identified to exclude myeloma or other plasma cell dyscrasias

IMAGING STUDIES

Long bone skeletal survey to identify osteosclerotic myeloma

TREATMENT

NONPHARMACOLOGIC THERAPY

- Physical and occupational therapy
- Ankle foot orthoses if there is significant weakness of ankle dorsiflexion

ACUTE GENERAL Rx

- The three primary treatment modalities for CIDP include high-dose oral corticosteroids, intravenous immunoglobulin (IVIg), and plasma exchange (PE).
- The benefit of each of these primary treatment modalities has been proven in randomized controlled trials, but their relative efficacies have not been evaluated.
- These three options for therapy should be discussed with the patient and a decision made to initiate therapy with one modality based on patient preference, tolerability of potential side effects, and cost (IVIg and PE are extremely expensive).
- IVIg is usually administered at a dose of 2g/kg divided over 3 to 5 days. Initial improvement is observed in two thirds of patients. If there has been incomplete improvement or no major improvement, it is advised to repeat the course of IVIg in 1 to 2 months. If there continues to be further improvement of symptoms after repeated administration of IVIg, monthly infusions may be necessary to maintain a response.
- PE is usually performed every other day for approximately 4 to 6 weeks. Like IVIg, plasma exchanges may be repeated on regular basis if therapeutic benefit has been established.
- Oral prednisone is usually initiated at a dose of ~1 mg/kg/day. High-dose prednisone dosing should be maintained until a clinical response is achieved, typically within 4 to 8 weeks, after which the dose may be slowly tapered. The goal is to maintain a clinical response with the lowest possible dose administered on an alternate-day regimen.

CHRONIC Rx

- IVIg, PE, and/or prednisone are usually required on a chronic basis to maintain a clinical response. The frequency and dosing requirements must be determined on an individual basis.
- Steroid-sparing agents such as azathioprine, mycophenolate mofetil, methotrexate, cyclosporine, or cyclophosphamide may sometimes be necessary to reduce the maintenance dose of steroids or the frequency with which IVIg or PE is administered.

DISPOSITION

- Prognosis for functional recovery is quite variable, although most patients (70% to 80%) will be left with only minor disability (some difficulty with premorbid activities, but functionally independent) if treated aggressively with immunosuppressive therapy.
- Approximately 15% to 30% of patients will be left with moderate disability (i.e., require significant assistance

with activities of daily living or with ambulation).
- In terms of the neuropathy, there is no clear evidence that the prognosis differs for patients with idiopathic forms of CIDP compared with those with CIDP associated with monoclonal gammopathy.
- Overall prognosis (not related to the neuropathy) may be worse in patients with multiple myeloma.
- Younger age, female gender, and the presence of a relapsing-remitting (rather than a monophasic progressive) course may portend a better prognosis.

REFERRAL

- Neurologist (preferably with expertise in the management of patients with neuromuscular disease)
- Physical therapy
- Occupational therapy
- Hematologist for further evaluation and management of associated plasma cell dyscrasia

PEARLS & CONSIDERATIONS

COMMENTS

- Electrophysiology (nerve conduction studies) are essential as they offer the best combination of sensitivity and specificity for the diagnosis of CIDP.
- Lumbar puncture for CSF analysis is also extremely helpful, especially if a markedly elevated protein without associated pleocytosis is found.

PREVENTION

There is no known preventative therapy.

PATIENT/FAMILY EDUCATION

CIDP is a chronic and often lifelong illness. It is often punctuated by long periods of remission and significant improvement. With appropriate therapy, patients often return to previous baseline level of functioning. Relapses, however, do occur. Chronic steroid use is a major cause of morbidity in patients with CIDP.

EVIDENCE

EBM

The efficacy of corticosteroids in CIDP has been examined in a single quasi-randomized study.[1] This study showed a significant improvement in neurological disability scale scores, but the confidence in the conclusion that steroids are beneficial is limited by the methodological shortcomings of this study. Data from several large, uncontrolled case series support the conclusion that steroids are beneficial.

The results of two randomized, double-blind placebo controlled trials support the use of plasma exchange.[2,3]

There are data from several randomized controlled trials showing that IVIg is beneficial in patients with CIDP. Data from two randomized controlled trials suggest that IVIg, PE, and prednisone are equally effective.[4,5]

There have been a limited number of randomized controlled trials of other cytotoxic drugs in CIDP. One study of the combination of azathioprine and prednisone vs. prednisone alone and another study of interferon vs. placebo failed to show any benefit.

Evidence-Based References

1. Dyck PJ et al: Prednisone improves chronic inflammatory polyradiculoneuropathy more than no treatment, *Annals of Neurology* 11:136, 1982.
2. Dyck P et al: Plasma exchange in chronic inflammatory demyelinating polyradiculoneuropathy, *N Eng J Medicine* 314:461, 1986.
3. Hahn A et al: Plasma-exchange therapy in chronic inflammatory demyelinating polyneuropathy. A double-blind, sham-controlled, cross-over study, *Brain* 119:1055, 1996.
4. Hahn AF, et al: Intravenous immunoglobulin treatment (IVIg) in chronic inflammatory demyelinating polyneuropathy (CIDP): a double-blind, placebo-controlled, crossover study, *Neurology* 45(suppl 4):A416, 1995.
5. Van Doorn PA et al: Intravenous immunoglobulin treatment in patients with chronic inflammatory demyelinating polyneuropathy, *Arch Neurol* 48:217, 1991.

SUGGESTED READINGS

Adams R, Victor M: *Principles of neurology,* New York, 1993, McGraw-Hill.

Bouchard C et al: Clinicopathologic findings and prognosis of chronic inflammatory demyelinating polyneuropathy, *Neurology* 52:498, 1999.

Hughes RAC, Swan AV, van Doorn PA: Cytotoxic drugs and interferons for chronic inflammatory demyelinating polyraduculoneuropathy, *Cochrane Database Syst Rev* 3, 2005.

Koller H et al: Chronic inflammatory demyelinating polyneuropathy, *N Engl J Med* 352:1343, 2005.

Mehndriatta M, Hughes R: Corticosteroids for chronic inflammatory demyelinating polyradiculopathy, *Cochrane Database Syst Rev* 2, 2004.

Mehndriatta M, Hughes R, Agarwal P: Plasma exchange for chronic inflammatory demyelinating polyraduculoneuropathy, *Cochrane Database Syst Rev* 3:CD003906, 2004.

Noseworthy J et al: *Neurological therapeutics principles and practice,* London and New York, 2003, Martin Dunitz.

Van Schaik IN et al: Intravenous immunoglobulin for chronic inflammatory demyelinating polyraduculoneuropathy, *Cochrane Database Syst Rev* 3, 2005.

AUTHOR: **GENNA GEKHT, M.D.**

BASIC INFORMATION

DEFINITION

Chronic obstructive pulmonary disease (COPD) is a disorder characterized by the presence of airflow limitation that is not fully reversible. COPD encompasses *emphysema,* characterized by loss of lung elasticity and destruction of lung parenchyma with enlargement of air spaces, and *chronic bronchitis,* characterized by obstruction of small airways and productive cough greater than 3 months' duration for more than 2 successive years. Patients with COPD are classically subdivided in two major groups based on their appearance:

1. *Blue bloaters* are patients with chronic bronchitis; the name is derived from the bluish tinge of the skin (secondary to chronic hypoxemia and hypercapnia) and from the frequent presence of peripheral edema (secondary to cor pulmonale); chronic cough with production of large amounts of sputum is characteristic.
2. *Pink puffers* are patients with emphysema; they have a cachectic appearance but pink skin color (adequate oxygen saturation); shortness of breath is manifested by pursed-lip breathing and use of accessory muscles of respiration.

SYNONYMS

COPD
Emphysema
Chronic bronchitis

ICD 9CM CODES
496 COPD
492.8 Emphysema

EPIDEMIOLOGY & DEMOGRAPHICS

- COPD affects 16 million Americans and is responsible for >80,000 deaths/yr.
- COPD is the fourth leading cause of death in the U.S. and is expected to become the third leading cause of death by 2020.
- Highest incidence is in males >40 yr.
- 16 million office visits, 500,000 hospitalizations, and >$18 billion in direct health care costs annually can be attributed to COPD.

PHYSICAL FINDINGS & CLINICAL PRESENTATION

- Blue bloaters (chronic bronchitis): peripheral cyanosis, productive cough, tachypnea, tachycardia.
- Pink puffers (emphysema): dyspnea, pursed-lip breathing with use of accessory muscles for respiration, decreased breath sounds.
- Possible wheezing in both patients with chronic bronchitis and emphysema.
- Features of both chronic bronchitis and emphysema in many patients with COPD.
- Acute exacerbation of COPD is mainly a clinical diagnosis and generally manifests with worsening dyspnea, increase in sputum purulence, and increase in sputum volume.

ETIOLOGY

- Tobacco exposure
- Occupational exposure to pulmonary toxins (e.g., cadmium)
- Atmospheric pollution
- Alpha-1-antitrypsin deficiency (rare; <1% of COPD patients)

DIAGNOSIS

DIFFERENTIAL DIAGNOSIS

- CHF
- Asthma
- Respiratory infections
- Bronchiectasis
- Cystic fibrosis
- Neoplasm
- Pulmonary embolism
- Sleep apnea, obstructive
- Hypothyroidism

WORKUP

Chest x-ray, pulmonary function testing, blood gases (in selected patients with acute exacerbation)

LABORATORY TESTS

- CBC may reveal leukocytosis with "shift to the left" during acute exacerbation.
- Sputum may be purulent with bacterial respiratory tract infections. Sputum staining and cultures are usually reserved for cases that are refractory to antibiotic therapy.
- ABGs: normocapnia, mild to moderate hypoxemia may be present.
- Pulmonary function testing (PFT): the primary physiologic abnormality in COPD is an accelerated decline in forced expiratory volume in one second (FEV_1) from the normal rate in adults over 30 years of age of approximately 30 ml/yr to nearly 60 ml/yr. PFTs results in COPD reveal abnormal diffusing capacity, increased total lung capacity and/or residual volume, fixed reduction in FEV_1 in patients with emphysema; normal diffusing capacity, reduced FEV_1 in patients with chronic bronchitis. Patients with COPD can generally be distinguished from asthmatics by their incomplete response to albuterol (change in FEV_1 <200 ml and 12%) and absence of an abnormal bronchoconstrictor response to methacholine or other stimuli. However, nearly 40% of patients with COPD respond to bronchodilators.

IMAGING STUDIES

Chest x-ray:

- Hyperinflation with flattened diaphragm, tending of the diaphragm at the rib, and increased retrosternal chest space (Fig. 1-56)
- Decreased vascular markings and bullae in patients with emphysema

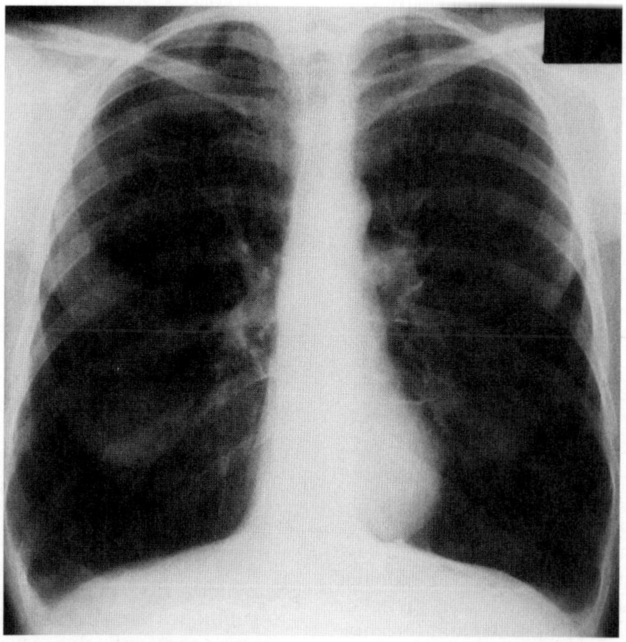

FIGURE 1-56 Severe diffuse emphysema. The PA chest radiograph shows the right hemidiaphragm to be flattened and located below the anterior aspect of the eighth rib. Left lung parenchyma is seen between the heart and the left hemidiaphragm. Arterial depletion is present in the lung bases. (From Grainger RG, Allison DJ, Adam A, Dixon AK [eds]: *Grainger & Allison's diagnostic radiology,* ed 4, Philadelphia, 2001, Churchill Livingstone.)

- Thickened bronchial markings and enlarged right side of the heart in patients with chronic bronchitis

TREATMENT

Rx

NONPHARMACOLOGIC THERAPY

- Weight loss in patients with chronic bronchitis.
- Avoidance of tobacco use and elimination of air pollutants.
- Supplemental oxygen, usually through a face mask to ensure oxygen saturation >90% measured by pulse oximetry.
- Pulmonary toilet: careful nasotracheal suction is indicated only in patients with excessive secretions and inability to expectorate. Mechanical percussion of the chest as applied by a physical or respiratory therapist is ineffective with acute exacerbations of COPD.

GENERAL Rx

- Pharmacologic treatment should be administered in a stepwise approach according to the severity of disease and patient's tolerance for specific drugs.
  1. Bronchodilators improve symptoms, quality of life, exercise tolerance, and decrease incidence of exacerbations.
  2. Short-acting beta-2 agonists (e.g., albuterol MDI 1 to 2 puffs q 4 to 6h prn) are acceptable in patients with mild, variable symptoms. Long-acting inhaled agents (e.g., salmeterol or formoterol 1 or 2 puffs bid) are preferred in patients with mild to moderate or continuous symptoms.
  3. Anticholinergics (e.g., ipratropium [Atrovent] inhaler 2 puffs qid) are also effective and are available in combination with albuterol (Combivent). Tiotropium (Spiriva handihaler) is a newer long-acting bronchodilator. It is very effective for the long-term, once-a-day maintenance treatment of bronchospasm.
  4. Addition of inhaled steroids and phosphodiesterase inhibitors (theophylline) is reserved for patients unresponsive to the above measures.
- Acute exacerbation of COPD can be treated with:
  1. Aerosolized beta-2 agonists (e.g., metaproterenol nebulizer solution 5% 0.3 ml or albuterol nebulized 5% solution 2.5 to 5 mg).
  2. Anticholinergic agents, which have equivalent efficacy to inhaled beta-adrenergic agonists. Inhalant solution of ipratropium bromide 0.5 mg can be administered every 4 to 8 hr.
  3. Short courses of systemic corticosteroids have been shown to improve spirometric and clinical outcomes. In the hospital setting give IV methylprednisolone 50- to 100-mg bolus, then 40 mg q6 to 8h; taper as soon as possible. In the outpatient setting, oral prednisone 40 mg/day initially, decreasing the dose by 10 mg every other day is generally effective.
  4. Use of noninvasive positive pressure ventilation (NIPPV) decreases the risk of endotracheal intubation and decreases ICU admission rates. Contraindications to its use are uncooperative patient, decreased level of consciousness, hemodynamic instability, inadequate mask fit, and severe respiratory acidosis. Increased airway pressure can be delivered by using inspiratory positive airway pressure, continuous positive airway pressure, or bilevel positive airway pressure (BiPAP), which combines the other modalities. When using NIPPV, the nasal mask is usually tolerated the best; however, patients must be instructed to keep their mouths closed while breathing with the nasal apparatus. Oxygen can be delivered at 10 to 15 L/min and started in spontaneous ventilation mode with an initial expiratory positive airway pressure setting of 3 to 5 cm H_2O and an inspiratory positive airway pressure setting of 8 to 10 cm H_2O. Adjustments in these settings should be made in 2-cm H_2O increments. It is important to monitor patients with frequent vital signs measurements, ABGs, or pulse oxymetry. Intubation and mechanical ventilation may be necessary if previous measures fail to provide improvement.
  5. The role of inhaled corticosteroids in COPD is controversial. Although some trials have demonstrated mild improvement in patients' symptoms and decreased frequency of exacerbations most pulmonologists believe that these drugs are ineffective in most patients with COPD but should be considered for patients with moderate to severe airflow limitation who have persistent symptoms despite optimal bronchodilator therapy.
  6. IV aminophylline administration is controversial and generally not recommended. When used, serum levels should be closely monitored (keep level 8 to 12 mcg/ml) to minimize risks of tachyarrhythmias.
- Antibiotics are indicated in suspected respiratory infection (e.g., increased purulence and volume of phlegm).
  1. *Haemophilus influenzae, Streptococcus pneumoniae* are frequent causes of acute bronchitis.
  2. Oral antibiotics of choice are azithromycin, levofloxacin, amoxicillin-clavulanate, and cefuroxime.
  3. The use of antibiotics is beneficial in exacerbations of COPD presenting with increased dyspnea and sputum purulence (especially if the patient is febrile).
- Guaifenesin may improve cough symptoms and mucus clearance; however, mucolytic medications are generally ineffective. Their benefits may be greatest in patients with more advanced disease.
- Lung volume reduction surgery has been proposed as a palliative treatment for severe emphysema. Overall it increases the chance of improved exercise capacity but does not confer a survival advantage over medical therapy. It is most beneficial in patients with both predominantly upper-lobe emphysema and low baseline exercise capacity.

In patients with end-stage emphysema who have an FEV_1 <25% of predicted normal value after administration of bronchodilator and additional complications such as severe hypoxemia, hypercapnia and pulmonary hypertension single lung transplantation should be considered a surgical option.

DISPOSITION

- Following the initial episode of respiratory failure, 5-yr survival is approximately 25%.
- Development of cor pulmonale or hypercapnia and persistent tachycardia are poor prognostic indicators.

PEARLS & CONSIDERATIONS

!

COMMENTS

- All patients with COPD should receive pneumococcal vaccine and yearly influenza vaccine.
- In assessing the severity of COPD, the FEV_1 is limited by the fact that it does not take into account the systemic manifestations of COPD. The BODE index (Body mass index [B], degree of obstruction [O], dyspnea [D], and exercise capacity [E]) has been proposed as a multidimensional scale to better assess the morbidity and mortality associated with COPD. It is better than the FEV_1 at predicting the risk of death from any cause and from respiratory causes among patients with COPD.

EVIDENCE

EBM

Management of stable COPD

None of the existing medications for COPD has been shown to modify the long-term decline in lung function that is the hallmark of the disease. The role of pharmacotherapy, therefore, is to decrease the symptoms and complications.[1] (C)

Bronchodilators are central to the symptomatic management of COPD

Short-acting anticholinergics are effective for the short-term management of stable COPD, significantly improving symptoms and FEV_1 compared with placebo.[2] (A)

Regular use of short-acting beta-2 agonists is associated with improvements in post bronchodilator lung function and a decrease in breathlessness.[3] (A)

Combination therapy with ipratropium bromide plus beta-2 agonists (short- and long-acting) may provide more benefit than either medication alone in the short-term treatment of patients with stable COPD.[2] (A)

The combination of ipratropium with the long-acting beta-2 agonist formoterol improves lung function significantly more than when it is combined with the short-acting agent, salbutamol.[4] (A)

Long-acting beta-2 agonists are effective in the short-term management of stable COPD: increasing FEV_1, quality of life, and the number of symptom-free days.[5-7] (A)

Long-acting beta-2 agonists produce small increases in FEV_1 in COPD patients who have low reversibility compared with short-acting bronchodilators.[8] (A)

Tiotropium, a long-acting anticholinergic, is an effective treatment of stable COPD.[9-11] (A)

Tiotropium has been shown to be more effective in improving trough FEV_1 than the short-acting agent, ipratropium, in both short-term and long-term RCTs. When used as long-term treatment it has been shown to significantly reduce exacerbation rates, compared with both placebo and ipratropium.[12,13] (A)

Tiotropium significantly improves predose FEV_1 compared with salmeterol. No differences exist between tiotropium and salmeterol with regards to the frequency of exacerbations, hospitalizations, or quality of life.[14] (A)

Corticosteroids

The addition of regular treatment with inhaled corticosteroids to bronchodilator treatment is appropriate for symptomatic COPD patients with an FEV_1 <50% predicted (stage III: severe COPD and stage IV: very severe COPD) and repeated exacerbations.[1] (C)

Long-term treatment with inhaled corticosteroids may have a positive effect on baseline lung function, but short-term treatment does not

In patients with stable COPD, short-term treatment (>10 wk) with inhaled corticosteroids is no more effective than placebo with regard to improving lung function.[15] (A)

The evidence regarding long-term treatment with inhaled corticosteroids vs. placebo is conflicting.[2,16-19] (A)

A systematic review has found that inhaled corticosteroids significantly reduce the rate of deterioration in pre bronchodilator FEV_1 compared with placebo. However, no significant difference in the rate of deterioration of post bronchodilator FEV_1 or in the frequency of exacerbations has been found between treatments.[16] (A)

Subsequent RCTs have found somewhat conflicting results. Some have shown that, compared with placebo, inhaled corticosteroids increase FEV_1 during the first 3 to 6 months of use but provide no ongoing effect on lung function.[2] (A)

A further RCT has shown no effect on decline in lung function between inhaled fluticasone and placebo.[17] (A)

More recent RCTs, however, have found that daily fluticasone vs. placebo significantly improves FEV_1 and dyspnea at 6 and 12 months.[18,19]

Long-term treatment with inhaled corticosteroids may reduce exacerbation rates

A systematic review has found that inhaled corticosteroids significantly reduce exacerbation rates compared with placebo.[20] (A)

Two RCTs not included in this review, however, have found conflicting results. The first compared fluticasone vs. placebo in patients with moderate to severe COPD over 3 years and found fluticasone significantly reduces the number of exacerbations, and the rate of deterioration in quality of life.[17] (A)

The second RCT, however, failed to find a reduction in exacerbation rates or improvement in quality of life, with inhaled budesonide twice daily for 12 months vs. placebo.[21] (A)

Combination therapy with inhaled corticosteroids and long-acting beta-2 agonists is an effective treatment in stable COPD, and significantly reduces exacerbation rates

With regard to reducing exacerbation rates, budesonide/formoterol has a modest benefit over component medication, but fluticasone/salmeterol does not significantly reduce exacerbations compared with either component. Both combinations reduce exacerbation rates compared with placebo.[22] (A)

There is insufficient evidence for the use of long-term oral corticosteroids

Short-term oral corticosteroids improve FEV_1 significantly more than placebo in patients with stable COPD.[23] (A)

No systematic review or RCT has compared long-term treatment with oral corticosteroids vs. placebo or oral vs. inhaled corticosteroids in the management of COPD.[2]

Three small crossover RCTs compared 2 weeks' treatment with oral prednisolone vs. inhaled beclomethasone. Results were conflicting, with the first finding no clinical difference between the treatments and the other two finding greater benefit from oral steroids. These results should be interpreted with caution, given the small size of the trials, the crossover design, and the short duration of treatment.[2]

Pulmonary rehabilitation

Rehabilitation relieves dyspnea and fatigue, and enhances the patient's sense of control over his or her condition.[24]

Home oxygen

Long-term home oxygen therapy improves survival in a select group of severely hypoxemic COPD patients.[25] (A)

Management of acute exacerbations

No significant difference exists between beta-2 agonists and ipratropium bromide with respect to degree of bronchodilation in patients with acute exacerbations of COPD. There is no evidence that combination therapy is more effective than either medication alone.[26] (A)

Systemic corticosteroids are beneficial in the management of exacerbations of COPD. They shorten recovery time and help restore lung function more quickly.[1] (C)

Systemic steroids increase the rate of lung function improvement over the first 72 hours of an acute exacerbation of COPD. However, there is no evidence that this benefit is maintained after 72 hours, or that other outcomes are improved.[27] (A)

Compared with placebo, treatment with 40 mg of prednisolone for 10 days (in addition to the standard treatment of an inhaled bronchodilator and oral antibiotics) has been shown to reduce relapse rates at 30 days, in outpatients following an exacerbation of COPD (43% vs. 27%).[28] (B)

There is evidence to suggest that noninvasive positive pressure ventilation as a first line treatment and an adjunct therapy to usual therapy is of benefit in the management of respiratory failure secondary to acute exacerbations of COPD.[29] (A)

Evidence-Based References

1. Workshop report, global strategy for diagnosis, management, and prevention of COPD. Bethesda, MD: Global Initiative for Chronic Obstructive Lung Disease (GOLD), World Health Organization (WHO), National Heart, Lung and Blood Institute (NHLBI), 2005. (A)
2. Kerstjens H, Postma D, ten Hacken N: Chronic obstructive pulmonary disease. In: *Clin Evid* 13:1923, 2005, London, BMJ Publishing Group. (A)

3. Sestini P et al: Short-acting beta 2 agonists for stable chronic obstructive pulmonary disease, *Cochrane Database Syst Rev* 3, 2002. Ⓐ
4. D'Urzo AD et al: In patients with COPD, treatment with a combination of formoterol and ipratropium is more effective than a combination of salbutamol and ipratropium: a 3-week randomized, double-blind, within-patient, multicenter study, *Chest* 119:1347-1356, 2001. Reviewed in: *Clin Evid* 11:2003-2030, 2004. Ⓐ
5. Rennard SI et al: Use of a long-acting inhaled beta2-adrenergic agonist, salmeterol xinafoate, in patients with chronic obstructive pulmonary disease, *Am J Respir Crit Care Med* 163:1087-1092, 2001. Reviewed in: *Clin Evid* 11:2003-2030, 2004. Ⓐ
6. Dahl R et al: Inhaled formoterol dry powder versus ipratropium bromide in chronic obstructive pulmonary disease, *Am J Respir Crit Care Med* 164:778-784, 2001. Reviewed in: *Clin Evid* 11:2003-2030, 2004. Ⓐ
7. Aalbers R et al: Formoterol in patients with chronic obstructive pulmonary disease: a randomized, controlled, 3-month trial, *Eur Respir J* 19:936-943, 2002. Reviewed in: *Clin Evid*11:2003-2030, 2004. Ⓐ
8. Appleton S et al: Long-acting beta2-agonists for chronic obstructive pulmonary disease patients with poorly reversible airflow limitation, *Cochrane Database Syst Rev* 4, 2001. Ⓐ
9. Littner MR et al: Long-acting bronchodilatation with once-daily dosing of tiotropium (Spiriva) in stable chronic obstructive pulmonary disease, *Am J Respir Crit Care Med* 161:1136-1142, 2000. Reviewed in: *Clin Evid* 11:2003-2030, 2004. Ⓐ
10. Casaburi R et al: The spirometric efficacy of once-daily dosing with tiotropium in stable COPD: a 13-week multicenter trial, *Chest*118:1294-1302, 2000. Reviewed in: *Clin Evid* 11:2003-2030, 2004 Ⓐ
11. Casaburi R et al: A long-term evaluation of once-daily inhaled tiotropium in chronic obstructive pulmonary disease. The Dutch Tiotropium Study Group, *Thorax* 55:289-294, 2000. Reviewed in: *Clin Evid* 11:2003-2030, 2004. Ⓐ
12. Van Noord JA et al: A randomised controlled comparison of tiotropium and ipratropium in the treatment of chronic obstructive pulmonary disease. The Dutch Tiotropium Study Group, *Thorax* 55:289-294, 2000. Reviewed in: *Clin Evid* 11:2003-2030, 2004. Ⓐ
13. Vincken W et al. Improved health outcomes in patients with COPD during 1 yr's treatment with tiotropium, *Eur Respir J* 19:209-216, 2002. Reviewed in: *Clin Evid* 11:2003-2030, 2004 Ⓐ
14. Brusasco V et al: Health outcomes following treatment for six months with once daily tiotropium compared with twice daily salmeterol in patients with COPD, *Thorax* 58:399-404, 2003. Reviewed in: *Clin Evid* 11:2003-2030, 2004. Ⓐ
15. Postma DS, Kerstjens HA: Are inhaled glucocorticosteroids effective in chronic obstructive pulmonary disease? *Am J Respir Crit Care Med*160:66-71, 1999. Reviewed in: *Clin Evid* 11:2003-2030, 2004. Ⓐ
16. Van Grunsven PM et al: Long term effects of inhaled corticosteroids in chronic obstructive pulmonary disease: a meta-analysis, *Thorax* 54:714-729, 1999. Reviewed in: *Clin Evid* 11:2003-2030, 2004. Ⓐ
17. Burge PS et al: Randomised, double blind, placebo controlled study of fluticasone propionate in patients with moderate to severe chronic obstructive pulmonary disease: the ISOLDE trial, *BMJ* 320:1297-1303, 2000. Reviewed in: *Clin Evid* 11:2003-2030, 2004. Ⓐ
18. Mahler DA et al: Effectiveness of fluticasone propionate and salmeterol combination delivered via the diskus device in the treatment of chronic obstructive pulmonary disease, *Am J Respir Crit Care Med* 166:1084-1091, 2002. Reviewed in: *Clin Evid* 11:2003-2030, 2004. Ⓐ
19. Calvery P et al: Combined salmeterol and fluticasone in the treatment of chronic obstructive pulmonary disease: a randomised controlled trial, *Lancet* 361:449-456, 2003. Reviewed in: *Clin Evid* 11:2003-2030, 2004. Ⓐ
20. Alsaeedi A, Sin DD, McAlister FA: The effects of inhaled corticosteroids in chronic obstructive pulmonary disease: a systematic review of randomized placebo-controlled trials, *Am J Med* 113:59-65, 2002. Reviewed in: *Clin Evid* 11:2003-2030, 2004. Ⓐ
21. Szafranski W et al: Efficacy and safety of budesonide/formoterol in the management of chronic obstructive pulmonary disease, *Eur Respir H*21:74-81, 2003. Reviewed in: *Clin Evid* 11:2003-2030, 2004. Ⓐ
22. Nannini L, Lasserson TJ, Poole P: Combined corticosteroid and longacting beta-agonist in one inhaler for chronic obstructive pulmonary disease, *Cochrane Database Syst Rev* 3, 2004. Ⓐ
23. Callahan CM, Dittus RS, Katz BP: Oral corticosteroid therapy for patients with stable chronic obstructive pulmonary disease: a meta-analysis, *Ann Intern Med* 114:216-223, 1991. Reviewed in: *Clin Evid* 11:2003-2030, 2004. Ⓐ
24. Lacasse Y et al: Pulmonary rehabilitation for chronic obstructive pulmonary disease, *Cochrane Database Syst Rev* 4, 2001. Ⓐ
25. Crockett AJ et al: Domiciliary oxygen for chronic obstructive pulmonary disease, *Cochrane Database Syst Rev* 4, 2000. Ⓐ
26. McCrory DC, Brown CD: Anti-cholinergic bronchodilators versus beta2-sympathomimetic agents for acute exacerbations of chronic obstructive pulmonary disease, *Cochrane Database Syst Rev* 3, 2002. Ⓐ
27. Wood-Baker R, Walters EH, Gibson P: Oral corticosteroids for acute exacerbations of chronic obstructive pulmonary disease. In: Cochrane Library, 3, Chichester, UK, 2004, John Wiley. Ⓐ
28. Aaron SD et al: Outpatient oral prednisone after emergency treatment of chronic obstructive pulmonary disease, *N Engl J Med* 348:2618-2625, 2003. Ⓑ
29. Ram FSF et al: Non-invasive positive pressure ventilation for treatment of respiratory failure due to exacerbations of chronic obstructive pulmonary disease, *Cochrane Database Syst Rev* 3, 2004. Ⓐ

SUGGESTED READINGS

Celli B et al: The body-mass index, airflow obstruction, dyspnea, and exercise capacity index in chronic obstructive pulmonary disease, *N Engl J Med* 350:1005, 2004.

Hersig M, Della-Giustina D, Younggren B: Managing acute exacerbations of COPD, part 2, *J Respir Dis* 26(2):69-72, 2005.

Hogg JC et al: The nature of small-airway obstruction in chronic obstructive pulmonary disease, *N Engl J Med* 350:2645, 2004.

Niewoehner DE et al: Prevention of exacerbations of chronic obstructive pulmonary disease with tiotropium, a once-daily inhaled anticholinergic bronchodilator, *Ann Intern Med* 143:317-326, 2005.

Sutherland ER, Cherniak RM: Management of chronic obstructive pulmonary disease, *N Engl J Med* 350:2689, 2004.

Tashkin DP et al: Comparing COPD treatment: nebulizer, metered dose inhaler, and concomitant therapy, *Am J Med* 120:435, 2007.

U.S. Preventive Services Task Force: Screening for chronic obstructive pulmonary disease using spirometry: U.S. Preventive Services Task Force recommendation statement, *Ann Intern Med* 148:529-534, 2008.

AUTHOR: **FRED F. FERRI, M.D.**

BASIC INFORMATION

DEFINITION

Chronic pain: pain that persists for longer than the expected time frame or that is associated with progressive, nonmalignant disease (Ashburn et al.). Chronic pain can be associated with ongoing tissue damage, occur after tissue damage has resolved, or without antecedent tissue damage or injury.

SYNONYMS Nonmalignant chronic pain

ICD9-CM CODES
Chronic pain v15.89
Opioid dependence 304.7x/304.8x

EPIDEMIOLOGY & DEMOGRAPHICS

The National Center for Health Statistics estimates that 32.8% of the U.S. population suffers from some form of chronic pain. Chronic pain is the third leading cause of physical impairment in the U.S. and related costs are estimated to be tens of billions annually. Patients with chronic pain may also experience changes in mood, depression, sleep disturbances, and fatigue and decreased overall physical functioning.

CLINICAL PRESENTATION

- History—it is important to clarify the features of the pain: due to an initial mishap vs. ongoing cause, trauma, location, timing, intensity, characteristics, exacerbating/relieving factors, triggers, therapies attempted in past and duration of attempts (both pharmacologic and nonpharmacologic), psychosocial factors and effect on daily activities, comorbidities, prior diagnostic studies. Patients should also be assessed for a history of depression, physical, and/or psychological abuse and chemical dependency.
- Physical exam—a thorough musculoskeletal, neurological, and psychological assessment should be performed to determine etiology, functional status, and contributing factors. Patients should be evaluated for the presence of muscle spasm and trigger points which are suggestive of musculoskeletal pain syndromes.

ETIOLOGY

Etiologies of chronic pain may include headache, low back pain, posttraumatic, arthritis, neurogenic (e.g., trigeminal neuralgia), psychogenic (related to depression or anxiety), fibromyalgia, reflex sympathetic dystrophy, myofascial pain syndrome, phantom limb pain, idiopathic or unknown.

DIAGNOSIS

DIFFERENTIAL DIAGNOSIS

- Based on proposed etiology.
- Depression and anxiety disorders can be both a cause and a result of chronic pain so temporal association of these disorders is important.

WORKUP

Laboratory testing and imaging studies should be used when etiology of chronic pain is unknown or unclear, when comorbidities are suspected, and as the H&P directs.

TREATMENT

NONPHARMACOLOGIC THERAPY

- Exercise
- Modalities: heat therapy, cold therapy, TENS units, cognitive behavioral therapy, psychologic counseling, physical therapy
- Electrostimulation therapy: TENS units
- Behavioral therapies: cognitive behavioral therapy, hypnosis, biofeedback, relaxation therapy
- Surgery

ACUTE GENERAL Rx

- Short-acting anti-inflammatory and analgesic medications (e.g., acetaminophen/NSAIDs/opioids)
- Trigger point or joint injections (immediate anesthetic + long-acting corticosteroids)
- Epidural steroid injections
- Nerve blocks

CHRONIC Rx

- Chronic pain management is considered a key aspect of therapy but often underused.
- Long-acting NSAIDs.
- Sustained-release opioids: oxycodone bid, morphine sr, methadone bid, or Duragesic patch with short-acting medications for breakthrough pain. Opiate medications are best utilized in a time-delineated fashion rather than PRN.
- Antidepressants (tricyclic and SSRI).
- Anticonvulsant medications: particularly helpful for neuropathic conditions.
- Implantable methods: epidural and intrathecal drug delivery systems, dorsal column stimulators (usually reserved for severe cases).
- Documentation of chronic pain management should include interval assessments of function, patient perception of pain severity, changes in physical functioning and daily activities, type of long-acting analgesic used and dosage, use of breakthrough analgesics, side effects and their management, use of nonpharmacologic therapies as well as adjunct medication use, and provider-patient agreement ("pain contract") indicating treatment goals and prescription dispensement guidelines.

COMPLEMENTARY & ALTERNATIVE MEDICINE

Acupuncture and massage (evidence based for some indications)

REFERRAL

- Pain medicine specialist or multidisciplinary pain clinic: useful when primary therapies fail, patients with complex pain conditions, or for invasive therapies.
- Consider referral to an addiction specialist if patient has a history of substance abuse or addiction.
- Psychiatry/psychologic services for counseling, if needed.

PEARLS & CONSIDERATIONS

COMMENTS

- Studies increasingly support the application of a multidisciplinary approach that addresses the multiple facets of pain (e.g., physical, psychologic, social aspects).
- It is important to determine the patient's expectations and goals related to pain. Patients often expect complete resolution of pain, which may not be possible.
- Therapeutic goal is the reduction of pain (elimination of chronic pain is generally unlikely and providers need to discuss these limitations with patients at outset) with improvement in physical functioning, decreased analgesic use, and decreased emergency department use.
- Chronic opiate therapy should include regular office visits to determine the effectiveness of treatment (degree of analgesia), presence of opioid-related side effects, functional status (physical and psychosocial), and screening for aberrant drug-related behaviors.
- Medication dependence and addiction should not be confused. Most patients receiving chronic opioid therapy can become dependent on these medications for pain relief but opioid addiction does not occur. Patients exhibiting signs of addiction often will seek escalating doses of medication, request refills of prescriptions earlier than planned, and engage in drug-seeking activities (e.g., ER visits between prescriptions, seeking multiple prescriptions).
- Side effects need not preclude use of opioid medications. Antiemetics can aid in controlling nausea. Constipation can be managed with increased fiber and water in diet, stool softeners, and laxatives.

PATIENT/FAMILY EDUCATION

- National Pain Foundation: www.painconnection.org
- American Pain Foundation: www.painfoundation.org
- National Institutes of Health website: www.nih.gov

SUGGESTED READINGS

American Academy of Pain Medicine: www.painmed.org

Ashburn MA et al: Management of chronic pain, *Lancet* 353:1865-1869, 1999.

Institute for Clinical Systems Improvement (ICSI). Assessment and management of chronic pain. Bloomington (MN). ICSI. November 2005.

Marcus D: Treatment of non-malignant chronic pain, *Am Fam Physician* 61:1331-1338, 2000.

AUTHOR: **ANNGENE A. GIUSTOZZI, M.D., M.P.H.**

BASIC INFORMATION

DEFINITION

Churg-Strauss syndrome (CSS) refers to a systemic vasculitis accompanied by severe asthma (core clinical feature), hypereosinophilia (HES), and necrotizing vasculitis with extravascular eosinophil granulomas.

SYNONYMS

Allergic angiitis
Allergic granulomatosis

ICD-9CM CODES
446.4 Angiitis, allergic granulomatous

EPIDEMIOLOGY & DEMOGRAPHICS

- Overall incidence of 1 to 3 cases/100,000 persons both in the U.S. and worldwide. Among asthma patients, the annual incidence of CSS is estimated to average 34.6 per million patients.
- Usually occurs between 14 and 75 years of age, with a mean age of 50 years, although cases have been reported as young as 4 years of age.
- There is no significant difference in incidence rate by gender.
- Prior to steroid therapy, 50% of untreated patients with CSS died within 3 months of the onset of vasculitis. Following treatment recommendations (see "Treatment"), 5-year survival exceeds 90%. The heart is involved in up to 60% of patients with CSS and represents major cause of mortality at 48%.

PHYSICAL FINDINGS & CLINICAL PRESENTATION

The clinical picture of CSS typically consists of three partially overlapping phases:

1. The prodromal phase or allergic phase occurs in the second and third decades of life. It is characterized by severe adult-onset asthma, with or without allergic rhinitis, sinusitis, headache, cough, and wheezing. This phase precedes full development of the syndrome usually by several years.
2. The eosinophilic phase, characterized by peripheral eosinophilia and eosinophilic infiltration of the lungs, myocardium, and GI tract, with or without granulomas, producing signs and symptoms of cough, fever, anorexia, weight loss, sweats, malaise, nausea, vomiting, abdominal pain, and diarrhea.
3. The systemic vasculitic phase, which appears approximately 3 to 8 years after asthma. This phase is characterized by the development of necrotizing vasculitis clinically apparent primarily in peripheral nerves, skin, and kidneys.

ETIOLOGY

- Exact cause is unknown. Believed to be an autoimmune disorder.
- Three distinct pathogenic mechanisms have been elucidated for various histological subtypes of the disease:
  - Asthma, involving T-helper lymphocytes
  - The role of antineutrophil cytoplasmic antibodies (ANCA) in the vasculitic manifestations of the disease such as glomerulonephritis
  - The role of eosinophil tissue infiltration with resultant cytotoxicity and cardiomyopathy
- Triggering factors implicated in CSS include inhaled allergens, vaccinations, infections, and drugs such as macrolides (see "Comments").

DIAGNOSIS

- Multiple systems used, mostly based on clinical findings and then confirmed by lung biopsy.
- Lanham et al. used for diagnosis the triad of asthma, eosinophilia exceeding 1.5×10^9 cells/L, and vasculitis involving at least two organs.
- The American College of Rheumatology has established the criteria for CSS diagnosis in patients without vasculitis:
  - Asthma
  - Eosinophilia >10% on WBC count
  - Mononeuropathy or polyneuropathy
  - Migratory pulmonary infiltrates
  - Paranasal sinus abnormalities
  - Extravascular eosinophils on biopsy

The presence of any four or more of the six criteria yields a sensitivity of 85% and a specificity of 99.7%. For patients with vasculitis, the presence of asthma and eosinophilia was 90% sensitive and 99% specific for CSS.

DIFFERENTIAL DIAGNOSIS

- Polyarteritis nodosa (PAN)
- Wegener's granulomatosis (WG)
- Sarcoidosis
- Loeffler syndrome
- Henoch-Schönlein purpura
- Allergic bronchopulmonary aspergillosis
- Rheumatoid arthritis
- Leukocytoclastic vasculitis

Although similar and at times grouped with patients with PAN or WG, CSS differs in that:

- CSS vasculitis involves not only small-sized arteries, but also veins and venules.
- CSS, unlike PAN, predominantly involves the lung. Other organs affected include heart, GI, CNS, kidney, and skin.
- Kidney involvement is much less common in CSS than in WG. Pulmonary lesions in WG usually involve the upper respiratory tract, vs. peripheral lung parenchyma in CSS.
- CSS shows necrotizing vasculitis along with a granulomatous extravascular reaction infiltrated by eosinophils.

In contrast to CSS, the eosinophilia in Loeffler syndrome is usually refractory to steroid therapy, systemic vasculitis and granulomas are absent on biopsy, and endomyocardial fibrosis is a typical finding.

WORKUP

History and physical exam, accompanied by laboratory tests, are suggestive. Tissue biopsy is confirmatory.

LABORATORY TESTS

- CBC with differential: eosinophilia.
- Erythrocyte sedimentation rate is usually elevated.
- BUN/creatinine may be elevated, suggesting renal involvement.
- Urinalysis may show hematuria and proteinuria.
- 24-hour urine for protein if greater than 1 g/day is a poor prognostic factor.
- ANCA is found in up to 70% of patients, usually with a perinuclear staining pattern.
- Stools may be positive for occult blood (enteric involvement during eosinophilic phase).
- AST, ALT, and CPK may indicate liver or muscle (skeletal or cardiac) involvement.
- RF and ANA may be positive.
- Biopsy confirms the diagnosis. Surgical lung biopsy is the gold standard. Transbronchial biopsy is rarely helpful. Necrotizing vasculitis and extravascular necrotizing granulomas, usually with eosinophilic infiltrates, are suggestive of CSS. The presence of eosinophils in extravascular tissues is most specific for CSS.

IMAGING STUDIES

- Chest x-ray is abnormal in 37% to 77% of the cases: asymmetrical patchy migratory infiltrates, interstitial lung disease, or nodular infiltrates (Fig. 1-57). Small pleural effusions are found in 29% of cases.
- Lung lesions in CSS are noncavitating, as opposed to WG.
- Paranasal sinus films may reveal sinus opacification.
- Angiography is sometimes done in patients with mesenteric ischemia or renal involvement.

TREATMENT

NONPHARMACOLOGIC THERAPY

Oxygen therapy in severe asthmatic exacerbations

PHARMACOLOGIC THERAPY

The following five factors suggest poor prognosis (five-factor score) and determines the aggressiveness of the immune suppressive therapy:

1. Proteinuria >1 g/day
2. Creatininemia >1.58 mg/dl
3. Cardiomyopathy
4. GI tract involvement
5. CNS involvement

ACUTE GENERAL Rx

- Corticosteroids are the treatment of choice if no poor prognostic factors are present. Prednisone 1 mg/kg/day is the starting dose and is continued for 6 to12 wk or until the disease has resolved. After clinically evident vasculitis resolves, prednisone is tapered progressively to 10 mg/day at 1 year.
- A drop in the eosinophil count and the ESR documents a response. ANCA does not reliably correspond with disease activity.

CHRONIC Rx

- In patients with one or more poor prognostic factors, addition of an immunosuppressant (cyclophosphamide) is a first-line therapy with corticosteroids.
- In patients who do not respond to corticosteroid treatment or in CSS relapse, cyclophosphamide therapy is indicated as a second-line therapy.
- Azathioprine or high-dose intravenous IG has shown benefit in patients with severe disease and in patients unresponsive to corticosteroids. Corticosteroids in combination with interferon-alpha have also been used in refractory cases.
- Patients with persistent symptoms of asthma will require long-term corticosteroids even if vasculitis is no longer present.

DISPOSITION

- Clinical remissions are obtained in more than 90% of patients after treatment.
- Relapse occurs in 26%.
- With treatment, long-term prognosis is good, with a 5-year survival rate of 90% and 50% at 7 years. Despite successful treatment of vasculitis, asthma generally remains persistent, and ischemic damage to peripheral nerves can be permanent.
- The 5-year survival of untreated CSS is 25%.
- Death usually occurs from progressive refractory vasculitis, myocardial involvement (approximately 50% of deaths), or severe GI involvement (mesenteric ischemia, pancreatitis).

REFERRAL

- A pulmonary referral for diagnosis and management is appropriate.
- Patients should be followed very closely at a rheumatology clinic. Patients usually need long-term immunosuppressive medications.

PEARLS & CONSIDERATIONS

COMMENTS

- First described by Churg and Strauss in 1951 after reviewing a number of autopsy cases previously classified as polyarteritis nodosa.
- CSS is distinguished from other vasculitides by the nearly universal presence of asthma that typically precedes all other symptoms.
- The asthma associated with CSS is distinct from common allergic asthma in that it typically has a late onset and a degree of eosinophilia that is much greater than typically seen in allergic asthma. Patients typically have no family history of allergies or asthma.
- Up to 77% of patients in the prodromal phase of CSS require oral steroids for asthma control.
- Nearly 50% of patients will experience improvement or dramatic remission of asthma symptoms shortly before or at the start of the vasculitic phase.
- Patients often experience constitutional symptoms of weight loss, fever, and malaise before specific organ involvement is clinically evident.
- Peripheral nerve involvement due to vasculitis of the vasa vasorum commonly manifests as mononeuritis multiplex. Patients may present with sudden foot or wrist drop, along with sensory deficits in the distribution of one or more distal nerves.
- Most patients with GI involvement are symptomatic. Gastroenteritis, acute abdomen, cholecystitis, hemorrhage, bowel perforation, and mesenteric ischemia have all been reported in patients with CSS.
- Cutaneous involvement is seen in 40% to 70% of cases of CSS, and manifests as palpable purpura, petechiae, and/or cutaneous nodules.
- Most patients with CSS respond to corticosteroid treatment and do not require cytotoxic therapy.
- Symptoms of CSS typically appear as oral corticosteroids are being decreased or discontinued for the treatment of asthma, and not triggered by leukotriene receptor-1 antagonists as previously reported.
- Reports of CSS developing in severe asthmatics after vaccination or desensitization therapy have led some authors to conclude that massive or nonspecific immunologic stimulation should be used with caution in patients with unstable asthma.

SUGGESTED READINGS

Masi A et al: American College of Rheumatology 1990 criteria for the classification of Churg-Strauss syndrome, *Arthritis Rheum* 33:1094, 1990.

Sable-Fourtassou R et al: Antineutrophil cytoplasmic antibodies and the Churg-Strauss syndrome, *Ann Intern Med* 143:632, 2005.

Pagnoux C et al: Churg Strauss syndrome, *Curr Opin Rheumatol* 19(1):25-32, 2007.

Kallenberg CG: Churg-Strauss syndrome: just one disease entity? *Arthritis Rheum* 52(9):2589-2593, 2005.

AUTHOR: **RAMI ELTIBI, M.D.**

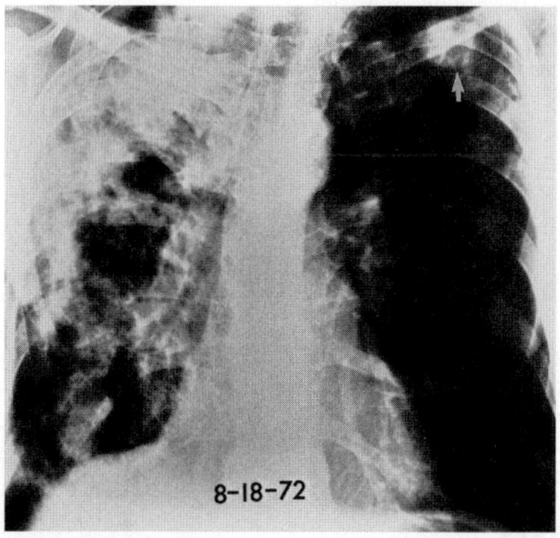

FIGURE 1-57 Allergic angiitis and granulomatosis. PA chest radiograph demonstrates peripheral air-space consolidation in the right lung and a nodule *(arrow)* in the left upper lobe in this asthmatic patient. (From McLoud TC [ed]: *Thoracic radiology: the requisites,* St Louis, 1998, Mosby.)

BASIC INFORMATION

DEFINITION

Cirrhosis is defined histologically as the presence of fibrosis and regenerative nodules in the liver. It can be classified as micronodular, macronodular, and mixed; however, each form may be seen in the same patient at different stages of the disease. Cirrhosis manifests clinically with portal hypertension, hepatic encephalopathy, and variceal bleeding.

ICD-9CM CODES
571.5 Cirrhosis of the liver
571.2 Cirrhosis of the liver secondary to alcohol

EPIDEMIOLOGY & DEMOGRAPHICS

- Cirrhosis is the eleventh leading cause of death in the U.S. (death rate 9 deaths/100,000 persons/yr).
- Alcohol abuse and viral hepatitis are the major causes of cirrhosis in the U.S.

PHYSICAL FINDINGS & CLINICAL PRESENTATION

SKIN: Jaundice, palmar erythema (alcohol abuse), spider angiomata, ecchymosis (thrombocytopenia or coagulation factor deficiency), dilated superficial periumbilical vein (caput medusae), increased pigmentation (hemochromatosis), xanthomas (primary biliary cirrhosis), needle tracks (viral hepatitis)
EYES: Kayser-Fleischer rings (corneal copper deposition seen in Wilson's disease; best diagnosed with slit lamp examination), scleral icterus
BREATH: Fetor hepaticus (musty odor of breath and urine found in cirrhosis with hepatic failure)
CHEST: Possible gynecomastia in men
ABDOMEN: Tender hepatomegaly (congestive hepatomegaly), small, nodular liver (cirrhosis), palpable, nontender gallbladder (neoplastic extrahepatic biliary obstruction), palpable spleen (portal hypertension), venous hum auscultated over periumbilical veins (portal hypertension), ascites (portal hypertension, hypoalbuminemia)
RECTAL EXAMINATION: Hemorrhoids (portal hypertension), guaiac-positive stools (alcoholic gastritis, bleeding esophageal varices, pelvic ulcer disease (PUD), bleeding hemorrhoids)
GENITALIA: Testicular atrophy in males (chronic liver disease, hemochromatosis)
EXTREMITIES: Pedal edema (hypoalbuminemia, failure of right side of the heart), arthropathy (hemochromatosis)
NEUROLOGIC: Flapping tremor, asterixis (hepatic encephalopathy), choreoathetosis, dysarthria (Wilson's disease)

ETIOLOGY

- Alcohol abuse
- Secondary biliary cirrhosis, obstruction of the common bile duct (stone, stricture, pancreatitis, neoplasm, sclerosing cholangitis)
- Drugs (e.g., acetaminophen, isoniazid, methotrexate, methyldopa)
- Hepatic congestion (e.g., CHF, constrictive pericarditis, tricuspid insufficiency, thrombosis of the hepatic vein, obstruction of the vena cava)
- Primary biliary cirrhosis
- Hemochromatosis
- Chronic hepatitis B or C
- Wilson's disease
- Alpha-1-antitrypsin deficiency
- Infiltrative diseases (amyloidosis, glycogen storage diseases, hemochromatosis)
- Nutritional: jejunoileal bypass
- Others: parasitic infections (schistosomiasis), idiopathic portal hypertension, congenital hepatic fibrosis, systemic mastocytosis, autoimmune hepatitis, hepatic steatosis, IBD

DIAGNOSIS

WORKUP

In addition to an assessment of liver function, the evaluation of patients with cirrhosis should also include an assessment of renal and circulatory function. Diagnostic workup is aimed primarily at identifying the most likely cause of cirrhosis. The history is extremely important:

- Alcohol abuse: alcoholic liver disease
- History of hepatitis B (chronic active hepatitis, primary hepatic neoplasm, or hepatitis C)
- History of IBD (primary sclerosing cholangitis)
- History of pruritus, hyperlipoproteinemia, and xanthomas in a middle-aged or elderly female (primary biliary cirrhosis)
- Impotence, diabetes mellitus, hyperpigmentation, arthritis (hemochromatosis)
- Neurologic disturbances (Wilson's disease, hepatolenticular degeneration)
- Family history of "liver disease" (hemochromatosis [positive family history in 25% of patients], alpha-1-antitrypsin deficiency)
- History of recurrent episodes of RUQ pain (biliary tract disease)
- History of blood transfusions, IV drug abuse (hepatitis C)
- History of hepatotoxic drug exposure
- Coexistence of other diseases with immune or autoimmune features (ITP, myasthenia gravis, thyroiditis, autoimmune hepatitis)

LABORATORY TESTS

- Decreased Hgb and Hct, elevated MCV, increased BUN and creatinine (the BUN may also be "normal" or low if the patient has severely diminished liver function), decreased sodium (dilutional hyponatremia), decreased potassium (as a result of secondary aldosteronism or urinary losses). Evaluation of renal function should also include measurement of urinary sodium and urinary protein from a 24-hr urine collection.
- Decreased glucose in a patient with liver disease indicating severe liver damage
- Other laboratory abnormalities:
  1. Alcoholic hepatitis and cirrhosis: there may be mild elevation of ALT and AST, usually <500 IU; AST > ALT (ratio >2:3).
  2. Extrahepatic obstruction: there may be moderate elevations of ALT and AST to levels <500 IU.
  3. Viral, toxic, or ischemic hepatitis: there are extreme elevations (>500 IU) of ALT and AST.
  4. Transaminases may be normal despite significant liver disease in patients with jejunoileal bypass operations or hemochromatosis or after methotrexate administration.
  5. Alkaline phosphatase elevation can occur with extrahepatic obstruction, primary biliary cirrhosis, and primary sclerosing cholangitis.
  6. Serum LDH is significantly elevated in metastatic disease of the liver; lesser elevations are seen with hepatitis, cirrhosis, extrahepatic obstruction, and congestive hepatomegaly.
  7. Serum γ-glutamyl transpeptidase (GGTP) is elevated in alcoholic liver disease and may also be elevated with cholestatic disease (primary biliary cirrhosis, primary sclerosing cholangitis).
  8. Serum bilirubin may be elevated; urinary bilirubin can be present in hepatitis, hepatocellular jaundice, and biliary obstruction.
  9. Serum albumin: significant liver disease results in hypoalbuminemia.
  10. Prothrombin time: an elevated PT in patients with liver disease indicates severe liver damage and poor prognosis.
  11. Presence of hepatitis B surface antigen implies acute or chronic hepatitis B.
  12. Presence of antimitochondrial antibody suggests primary biliary cirrhosis, chronic hepatitis.
  13. Elevated serum copper, decreased serum ceruloplasmin, and elevated 24-hr urine may be diagnostic of Wilson's disease.
  14. Protein immunoelectrophoresis may reveal decreased α-1 globulins (alpha-1-antitrypsin deficiency), increased IgA (alcoholic cirrhosis), increased IgM (primary biliary cirrhosis), increased IgG (chronic hepatitis, cryptogenic cirrhosis).

15. An elevated serum ferritin and increased transferrin saturation are suggestive of hemochromatosis.
16. An elevated blood ammonia suggests hepatocellular dysfunction; serial values, however, are generally not useful in following patients with hepatic encephalopathy because there is poor correlation between blood ammonia level and degree of hepatic encephalopathy.
17. Serum cholesterol is elevated in cholestatic disorders.
18. Antinuclear antibodies (ANA) may be found in autoimmune hepatitis.
19. Alpha fetoprotein: levels >1000 pg/ml are highly suggestive of primary liver cell carcinoma.
20. Hepatitis C viral testing identifies patients with chronic hepatitis C infection.
21. Elevated level of serum globulin (especially γ-globulins), positive ANA test may occur with autoimmune hepatitis.

IMAGING STUDIES

- Ultrasonography is the procedure of choice for detection of gallstones and dilation of common bile ducts.
- CT scan is useful for detecting mass lesions in liver and pancreas, assessing hepatic fat content, identifying idiopathic hemochromatosis, early diagnosing of Budd-Chiari syndrome, dilation of intrahepatic bile ducts, and detection of varices and splenomegaly.
- Technetium-99m sulfur colloid scanning is useful for diagnosing cirrhosis (there is a shift of colloid uptake to the spleen, bone marrow), identifying hepatic adenomas (cold defect is noted), diagnosing Budd-Chiari syndrome (there is increased uptake by the caudate lobe).
- ERCP is the procedure of choice for diagnosing periampullary carcinoma, common duct stones; it is also useful in diagnosing primary sclerosing cholangitis.
- Percutaneous transhepatic cholangiography (PTC) is useful when evaluating patients with cholestatic jaundice and dilated intrahepatic ducts by ultrasonography; presence of intrahepatic strictures and focal dilation is suggestive of PSC.
- Percutaneous liver biopsy is useful in evaluating hepatic filling defects, diagnosing hepatocellular disease or hepatomegaly, evaluating persistently abnormal liver function tests, and diagnosing hemachromatosis, primary biliary cirrhosis, Wilson's disease, glycogen storage diseases, chronic hepatitis, autoimmune hepatitis, infiltrative diseases, alcoholic liver disease, drug-induced liver disease, and primary or secondary carcinoma.

TREATMENT (Rx)

NONPHARMACOLOGIC THERAPY

Avoid any hepatotoxins (e.g., ethanol, acetaminophen); improve nutritional status.

GENERAL Rx

- Remove excess body iron with phlebotomy and deferoxamine in patients with hemochromatosis.
- Remove copper deposits with D-penicillamine in patients with Wilson's disease.
- Long-term ursodiol therapy will slow the progression of primary biliary cirrhosis. It is, however, ineffective in primary sclerosing cholangitis.
- Glucocorticoids (prednisone 20 to 30 mg/day initially or combination therapy or prednisone and azathioprine) is useful in autoimmune hepatitis.
- Liver transplantation may be indicated in otherwise healthy patients (age <65 yr) with sclerosing cholangitis, chronic hepatitis cirrhosis, or primary biliary cirrhosis with prognostic information suggesting <20% chance of survival without transplantation; contraindications to liver transplantation are AIDS, most metastatic malignancies, active substance abuse, uncontrolled sepsis, uncontrolled cardiac or pulmonary disease.
- Treatment of complications of portal hypertension (ascites, esophagogastric varices, hepatic encephalopathy, and hepatorenal syndrome).

DISPOSITION

- Prognosis varies with the etiology of the patient's cirrhosis and whether there is ongoing hepatic injury. Mortality rate exceeds 80% in patients with hepatorenal syndrome.
- If advanced cirrhosis is present and transplantation is not feasible, survival is 1 to 2 yr.

PEARLS & CONSIDERATIONS (!)

COMMENTS

Thrombocytopenia and advanced Child-Pugh cases are associated with the presence of varices. These factors are useful to identify cirrhotic patients who benefit most from referral for endoscopic screening for varices.

EVIDENCE (EBM)

Both neomycin plus sorbitol and lactulose plus placebo are effective in the treatment of patients with cirrhosis and chronic portal-systemic encephalopathy, but lactulose is more effective at reducing stool mean pH.[1] (B)

Antibiotic prophylaxis significantly reduces the incidence of bacterial infections and associated mortality in cirrhotic patients with gastrointestinal bleeding.[2] (A)

In people with cirrhosis, beta-blockers are more effective than placebo in preventing a first episode of variceal bleeding and in reducing the incidence of bleeding episodes.[3,4] (B)

When treating acute bleeding esophageal varices, treatment with somatostatin analogs does not significantly decrease mortality compared with placebo, but it is associated with fewer transfusions and a lower number of patients with failed hemostasis.[5] (A)

Current evidence does not support the use of emergency sclerotherapy over vasoactive agents as first line treatment of bleeding varices in cirrhotic patients.[6] (A)

In patients with cirrhosis and a recent esophageal variceal bleed, treatment with a beta-blocker with or without a nitrate is as effective as endoscopic banding of varices in preventing rebleeding or death.[7] (B)

Evidence-Based References

1. Conn HO et al: Comparison of lactulose and neomycin in the treatment of chronic portal-systemic encephalopathy. A double blind controlled trial, *Gastroenterology* 72:573, 1997. (B)
2. Soares-Weiser K et al: Antibiotic prophylaxis for cirrhotic patients with gastrointestinal bleeding, *Cochrane Database Syst Rev* 2:CD002907, 2002. (A)
3. Pagliaro L et al: Prevention of first bleeding in cirrhosis. A meta-analysis of randomized trials of nonsurgical treatment, *Ann Intern Med* 117:59, 1992. (B)
4. Pascal JP, Cales P: Propranolol in the prevention of first upper gastrointestinal tract hemorrhage in patients with cirrhosis of the liver and esophageal varices, *N Engl J Med* 317:856, 1987. (B)
5. Gotzsche PC: Somatostatin analogues for acute bleeding oesophageal varices, *Cochrane Database Syst Rev* 1:CD000193, 2002. (A)
6. D'Amico G et al: Emergency sclerotherapy versus medical interventions for bleeding oesophageal varices in cirrhotic patients, *Cochrane Database Syst Rev* 1:CD002233, 2002. (A)
7. Patch D et al: A randomized, controlled trial of medical therapy versus endoscopic ligation for the prevention of variceal rebleeding in patients with cirrhosis, *Gastroenterology* 123:1013, 2002. (B)

SUGGESTED READINGS

Gines P et al: Management of cirrhosis and ascites, *N Engl J Med* 350:1645, 2004.

Heidelbaugh JJ, Bruderly M: Cirrhosis and chronic liver failure, *Am Fam Physic* 74:756, 767, 2006.

AUTHOR: **FRED F. FERRI, M.D.**

BASIC INFORMATION

DEFINITION

Primary biliary cirrhosis (PBC) is a chronic, variably progressive disease most often affecting women and characterized by destruction of the small intrahepatic bile ducts leading to portal inflammation, fibrosis, cirrhosis, and ultimately liver failure.

SYNONYMS

Biliary cirrhosis
Nonsupparative destructive cholangitis
Autoimmune cholangiopathy

ICD-9CM CODES
571.6 Biliary cirrhosis

EPIDEMIOLOGY & DEMOGRAPHICS

- PBC affects all races and accounts for 0.6% to 2% of deaths from cirrhosis worldwide.
- Approximately 95% of patients are female.
- Annual incidence rates 0.7 to 49 cases per million.
- Prevalence highest in the U.K., Scandinavia, and the U.S. and varies tremendously by geographic areas, ranging from 67 to 402 cases per million.
- Although there are no clearly identified genetic factors affecting the occurrence of PBC, there is a clear familial occurrence. Prevalence among first-degree relatives is 5% to 6%, and 1% to 6% of all patients have at least one affected family member. The concordance rate among monozygotic twins is 63%.
- Onset typically occurs between the ages of 30 and 65, and it is uncommon before age 25.
- Up to 84% of patients with PBC have at least one other autoimmune disorder, such as thyroiditis, Sjögren's syndrome, rheumatoid arthritis (RA), Raynaud's phenomenon, or scleroderma. A variant form of PBC exists as an overlap syndrome with autoimmune hepatitis (AIH) and is referred to as autoimmune cholangiopathy (AIC).

ETIOLOGY

- Although the cause of PBC is still unknown, it is felt to be due to an environmental insult that modifies mitochondrial proteins triggering persistent T lymphocyte–mediated attack on intralobular bile duct epithelial cells in genetically susceptible individuals.
- Possible risk factors being examined include cigarette smoking, urinary tract infections (UTIs), Raynaud's phenomenon, autoimmune thyroid disease, history of tonsillectomy or cholecystectomy, multiple pregnancies, autoimmune thyroid disease, and family history of PBC, Sjögren's syndrome, and systemic lupus erythematosus (SLE).
- Recent studies have identified a peptide, an enzyme complex subunit (PDC-E2) in the mitochondrial membrane, as a major autoantigen in the early pathogenesis of PBC. Patients with PBC have a tenfold increased concentration of cytotoxic CD8 + lymphocytes recognizing this peptide in their livers as compared with their blood, and autoantibodies against mitochondria (AMA), especially the PDC-E2 subunit, are the serologic hallmark of this disease. In addition, bile duct epithelial cells handle PDC-E2 in a unique way that exposes them to immune-mediated attack by PDC-E2–oriented cytotoxic T cells. Future therapies may be specific immunomodulation directed at these peptides.
- In addition to the T lymphocyte–mediated direct destruction of small bile ducts, secondary damage to hepatocytes may result from the accumulation of noxious substances such as bile acids.

PHYSICAL FINDINGS & CLINICAL PRESENTATION

Clinical stages:
- Asymptomatic
- Symptomatic
- Cirrhotic
- Hepatic Failure

Symptoms:
- 48% to 60% of patients may be asymptomatic; 40% to 100% of these patients will go on to develop symptoms.
- Fatigue (78% of patients) and pruritus (20 to 70% of patients) are the usual presenting symptoms.
- Pruritus is worse at night, under constricting, coarse garments; in association with dry skin; and in hot, humid weather. The cause is unknown; it is no longer felt to be a result of the retention of bile acids in skin. Pruritus may first occur during pregnancy but is distinguished from pruritus of pregnancy because it persists into the postpartum period and beyond.
- Other common symptoms include hepatomegaly, jaundice, unexplained right upper quadrant pain (10%), splenomegaly, manifestations of portal hypertension, sicca symptoms, and scleroderma-like lesions.
- Musculoskeletal complaints caused by inflammatory arthropathy in 40% to 70% of patients: 5% to 10% develop chronic RA; 10% develop "arthritis of PBC."
- Steatorrhea may be seen in advanced disease.

Physical:
- Variable: dependent on stage of disease at time of presentation. Patients at early stage may be completely normal.
- 25% to 50% have hypopigmentation of skin.
- Excoriations may be present.
- Hepatomegaly (70%) and splenomegaly (initially 35%) may be present in more advanced disease.
- Xanthomas and jaundice appear in advanced disease. Kayser-Fleischer rings are rare and result from copper retention.
- Late physical findings mirror those of cirrhosis: spider nevi, temporal and proximal limb wasting, ascites, and edema.

DIAGNOSIS

- Based on three criteria:
  - Positive serum antimitochondrial antibodies (AMA), titer >1:40
  - Increased liver function tests (especially alkaline phosphatase) for >6 months
  - Characteristic liver histology: asymmetric destruction of the bile ducts within the portal triads
- Two criteria indicate a probable diagnosis and all three criteria are required for a definite diagnosis.

DIFFERENTIAL DIAGNOSIS

- Drug-induced cholestasis

Other etiologies of chronic liver disease and cirrhosis:
- Alcoholic cirrhosis
- Viral hepatitis (chronic)
- Primary sclerosing cholangitis
- Autoimmune chronic active hepatitis
- PBC-AIH overlap syndrome—reported in almost 10% of adults with AIH or PBC; transition from stable PBC to AIH and vice versa also seen
- Chemical/toxin-induced cirrhosis
- Other hereditary or familial disorders (e.g., CF, μ-1-antitrypsin deficiency)

WORKUP

- History, physical examination, laboratory evaluation, and liver biopsy

LABORATORY TESTS

- Antimitochondrial antibodies (AMA) found in 95% of patients with PBC and are 98% specific.
- Antinuclear antibodies (ANA) found in approximately 50%. Unlike AMA, these may correlate with disease severity and prognosis. Presence of anti-gp 210 antinuclear protein antibody seems to predict hepatic failure type progression, whereas an anticentromere pattern appears to be a risk factor for the development of portal hypertension.
- Markedly elevated alkaline phosphatase (of hepatic origin).
- Elevated GGTP.
- Elevated serum IgM levels or elevated IgG levels in AMA-negative PBC.
- Bilirubin normal early; increases with disease progression (direct and indirect) in 60% of patients. Elevated serum bilirubin is a poor prognostic sign.
- Normal or slightly elevated aminotransferases, rarely more than 5× the upper limit of normal, for more than 6 months. Degree of elevation has no prognostic significance.
- Markedly elevated serum lipids in more than 50% of patients. Total cholesterol may exceed 1000 mg/dl. No increased risk of death from athero-

sclerosis seen, possibly because of very high HDL levels and low serum levels of Lp(a) lipoprotein.

- Elevated ceruloplasmin.
- Percutaneous liver biopsy confirms or rules out the diagnosis, allows staging, and indicates response to therapy.
- Histology is not uniform and so histologic stage is based on the most advanced lesion present.
    - Stage I—lymphocytic infiltration of the epithelial cells of the small bile ducts with granuloma-like lesions, limited to portal triads.
    - Stage II—extension of inflammatory cells to periportal parenchyma, invasion by foamy macrophages, and development of biliary piecemeal necrosis.
    - Stage III—fibrous septa link portal triads.
    - Stage IV—frank cirrhosis. Hyaline deposits and accumulation of stainable copper are also seen.

IMAGING STUDIES

If history, physical examination, blood tests, and liver biopsy are all consistent with PBC, neither imaging nor cholangiography is necessary.

PROGNOSIS

- Median survival is 9 years.
- Mean time of progression from Stage I or II disease to cirrhosis with no medical treatment is 4 to 6 years.
- Neither presence nor titer of antimitochondrial antibodies predicts survival, disease progression, or response to therapy
- Unclear if presence of symptoms at time of diagnosis affects survival.
- Prognostic laboratory measures: serum bilirubin is most important, but also albumin and prothrombin time.
- Poor prognosis with jaundice, advanced histologic stage, advanced age, edema, coagulopathy, and ascites.
- Presence of cirrhosis confers increased risk for hepatocellular carcinoma.

TREATMENT

Rx

- Treatment is given according to the clinical stage of the disease.
- Asymptomatic stage—follow bilirubin every 3 to 4 months, and if begins to rise, start ursodeoxycholic acid (UDCA).
- No generally accepted treatment of underlying disease process.
- Treatment focuses on management of complications (pruritus, metabolic bone diseases, hyperlipidemia) because liver transplantation is the only definitive treatment for this disease.
- 20% of patients will not respond to medical therapy and proceed to liver transplantation.

ACUTE GENERAL Rx

- Goals of treatment: resolution of pruritus, decrease of alkaline phosphatase levels to <50% above normal, and improvement in liver biopsy histology.
- Ursodiol (12 to 15 mg/kg/day, divided or as one bedtime dose) significantly reduces ascites, jaundice, and levels of bilirubin and liver transaminases. Data are mixed as to whether ursodiol reduces mortality, need for liver transplantation, pruritus, fatigue, quality of life, liver histology, or portal blood pressures. Safe and well tolerated. Some reported side effects include weight gain, hair loss, diarrhea, and flatulence. May see decreased efficacy after 10 years. Ineffective and may actually worsen disease if started in advanced stages.
- Colchicine (0.6 mg twice daily) and methotrexate (15 mg/wk) yield less impressive results but may be helpful. Patients with PBC on methotrexate need to be monitored for the development of interstitial pneumonitis, which resolves with discontinuation of the drug.
- Prednisone, azathioprine, penicillamine, and cyclosporine are no longer used because of limited efficacy and significant toxicity.
- Experiments are ongoing to examine the use of budesonide in combination with ursodeoxycholic acid.
- For the pruritus of PBC, cholestyramine resin (8 to 24 g daily) reduces pruritus in most patients. Antihistamines at bedtime help nighttime symptoms. Rifampin (150 mg twice daily) is effective for those who do not respond to or tolerate resins. Naloxone and naltrexone are third-line agents and plasmapheresis is helpful when all other therapies fail.

CHRONIC Rx

- Diet low in neutral triglycerides and high in medium-chain triglycerides decreases steatorrhea and improves nutritional status.
- Treatment for acute bacterial cystitis, which occurs with greater frequency in these patients.
- Treatment for osteoporosis, including calcium and vitamin D, should be undertaken, although only liver transplantation results in improvement. Bisphosphonates may be helpful.
- Vitamin A, K, E deficiencies can be clinically important in advanced cases and respond to oral replacement.
- Esophageal variceal bleeding often happens earlier in the course of PBC than with other progressive liver diseases. These are best treated with endoscopic rubber-band ligation or TIPS shunt.
- Liver transplantation is the definitive cure and appropriate referral should be sought. Indications for transplant include unacceptable quality of life owing to pruritus and a Mayo (MELD) score of >10.
- Liver transplant recipients with PBC are more likely to develop chronic rejection and less likely to be weaned from immunosuppressive therapy. After transplant, antimitochondrial antibody levels persist and histologic changes of PBC are seen in up to 50% of liver transplant patients in 10 yr.
- With appropriate immunosuppression and despite histologic changes, patients who undergo transplant for PBC clinically do very well. Survival at 1 yr is 85% to 90%, and 70% survive at least 10 yr after transplantation; survival rates thereafter resemble age/sex-matched healthy persons.
- Other associated illnesses that should be detected and treated include hyperlipidemia (without increased risk of ASHD), Hashimoto's thyroiditis (20% of patients), interstitial pneumonitis, celiac disease, sarcoidosis, asymptomatic renal tubular acidosis (from copper deposition in the kidneys), hemolytic anemia, autoimmune thrombocytopenia, and coexisting autoimmune disease including Sjögren's syndrome, sicca syndrome, and scleroderma.

DISPOSITION

Definitive treatment requires liver transplantation; survival is 7 to 16 yr, dependent on symptoms at time of diagnosis.

REFERRAL

Gastroenterology and or hepatology referral for treatment, evaluation for liver transplantation, and potentially treatment of refractory variceal bleeding

PEARLS & CONSIDERATIONS

!

- Antimitochondrial antibodies are practically pathognomonic for PBC.
- Ursodiol can be an effective and well-tolerated treatment if started early in the course of the disease.
- Associated illnesses need to be detected and treated.
- Liver transplantation is the definitive treatment for PBC.

SUGGESTED READINGS

Gluud C, Christensen E: Ursodeoxycholic acid for primary biliary cirrhosis, *Cochrane Database Syst Rev* 4, 2001.

Kaplan M, Gershwin ME: Primary biliary cirrhosis (review), *N Engl J Med* 353:1261-1273, 2005.

Levy C, Lindor KD: Management of osteoporosis, fat-soluble vitamin deficiencies, and hyperlipidemia in primary biliary cirrhosis, *Clin Liver Dis* 7(4):901, 2003.

MacQuillan GC, Neuberger J: Liver transplantation for primary biliary cirrhosis, *Clin Liver Dis* 7(4):941, ix, 2003.

Selmi C et al: Epidemiology and pathogenesis of primary biliary cirrhosis, *J Clin Gastroenterol* 38(3):264, 2004.

AUTHOR: **JENNIFER ROH HUR, M.D.**

BASIC INFORMATION

DEFINITION

Claudication refers to leg pain brought on by exertion and relieved with rest.

SYNONYMS

Intermittent claudication

ICD-9CM CODES
443.9 Peripheral vascular disease, unspecified
440.21 Intermittent claudication due to atherosclerosis

EPIDEMIOLOGY & DEMOGRAPHICS

INCIDENCE: 3 to 8 cases/1000 persons
PREVALENCE: 2% to 4% in the general population
RISK FACTORS: Major risk factors of tobacco, hypertension, diabetes, and hypercholesterolemia increase the risk of developing claudication. Cigarette smoking is the major determinant of disease progression.

PHYSICAL FINDINGS & CLINICAL PRESENTATION

- Diminished pulses, cool skin temperature
- Bruits over the distal aorta, iliac or femoral arteries
- Pallor of the distal extremities on elevation
- Rubor with prolonged capillary refill on dependency
- Trophic changes of hair loss and muscle atrophy noted
- Nonhealing ulcers, necrotic tissue, and gangrene possible

ETIOLOGY

Primary cause of claudication is atherosclerosis.

DIAGNOSIS

History and physical findings make the diagnosis of claudication. Noninvasive studies help confirm the diagnosis.

DIFFERENTIAL DIAGNOSIS

- Spinal stenosis (neurogenic claudication)
- Muscle cramps
- Degenerative osteoarthritic joint disease, particularly of the lumbar spine and hips
- Compartment syndrome

WORKUP

- Ankle-brachial index (ABI): the ratio of ankle pressure to brachial pressure is usually about 1.
  1. In claudication, the ABI ranges from 0.5 to 0.8.
  2. In patients with rest pain or impending limb loss, ABI ≤0.3.
- Segmental systolic pressures usually are measured from the high thigh, above the knee, below the knee, and the ankle. Normally there should not be >20 mm Hg difference in pressures between adjacent segments. If the gradient is >20 mm Hg, significant narrowing is suspected in the intervening segment.
- Both ABI and segmental pressures can be done before and after exercise.

IMAGING STUDIES

- Duplex ultrasound can be used to locate the occluded areas and assess the patency of the distal arterial system or prior vein grafts.
- MRA and spiral CT angiography are further imaging techniques available.
- Angiography remains the gold standard for imaging peripheral arterial occlusion.

TREATMENT

NONPHARMACOLOGIC THERAPY

- Tobacco cessation is vital.
- Diet to control diabetes, blood pressure and cholesterol should be followed.
- Walking 30 to 60 min/day for 5 days at about 2 mi/hr is recommended.
- New prospective data point to intermittent pneumatic compression (IPC) as a promising adjunctive therapy.

ACUTE GENERAL Rx

Acute revascularization is usually reserved for patients with impending ischemic limb loss.

CHRONIC Rx

- Antiplatelet agents like aspirin or clopidogrel.
- Risk factor modification: pharmacologic treatment for hyperlipidemia, hypertension, and diabetes in particular.
- Pentoxifylline 400 mg tid or cilostazol 100 mg bid for 3 mo should be tried. If there is no improvement in symptoms, the medicine should be discontinued.
- Revascularization is indicated in patients with refractory rest pain or lifestyle altering pain, nonhealing ulcers, or gangrene and in a select group of patients with functional disability. Common procedures:
  1. Aortoiliofemoral reconstruction or bypass, or infrainguinal bypass (e.g., femoropopliteal, femorotibial).
  2. Angioplasty, often with stenting, is used primarily on short, discrete stenotic lesions in the iliac or femoropopliteal artery.

COMPLEMENTARY & ALTERNATIVE MEDICINE

- A systematic review found that over 12 to 24 wk, Gingko biloba increased pain-free walking distance by 33 meters compared to placebo.
- Systematic reviews have shown that chelation therapy is no better than placebo.

DISPOSITION

- Intermittent claudication progressing to an ischemic leg or limb loss is unusual, especially if maintaining the conservative treatment of exercise and abstaining from tobacco.
- The 5-yr risk for developing ischemic ulceration in patients treated for diabetes and with ABI <0.5 was 30% compared with only 5% in patients with neither characteristic.

REFERRAL

Consultation with an interventionalist is recommended in the patient with threatened limb loss, rest pain, nonhealing ulcers, functional disability from pain, and gangrene.

PEARLS & CONSIDERATIONS

- About 70% of patients with peripheral vascular disease will have concomitant coronary artery disease.
- Beta blockers may worsen claudication symptoms in some patients, although their underuse is associated with excess cardiovascular mortality.
- Patients with peripheral vascular disease may benefit from secondary cardiovascular prevention with clopidogrel versus aspirin more so than other high-risk patients (CAPRIE trial).

COMMENTS

- Claudication is a marker for generalized atherosclerosis. This group of patients has a higher risk of death from cardiovascular events than from limb loss.
- The ABI is more closely associated with leg function in persons with peripheral arterial disease than is intermittent claudication or other leg symptoms.

SUGGESTED READINGS

Abramson B, Huckell V: Canadian Cardiovascular Society Consensus Conference: peripheral arterial disease—executive summary, *Can J Cardiol* 21(12):997-1006, 2005.

ACC/AHA 2005 guidelines for the management of patients with peripheral arterial disease: www.acc.org/qualityandscience/clinical/topic/topic.htm (select Peripheral Arterial Disease).

Clagett G et al: Antithrombotic therapy in peripheral arterial occlusive disease: the Seventh ACCP Conference on Antithrombotic and Thrombolytic Therapy, *Chest* 126(suppl 3):609S-626S, 2004.

Kakkos S et al: Improvement of the walking ability in intermittent claudication due to superficial femoral artery occlusion with supervised exercise and pneumatic foot and calf compression: a randomized controlled trial, *Eur J Endovasc Surg* 302(2):164-175, 2005.

Simon RW et al: Intermittent claudication, *BMJ* 334:746, 2007.

White C: Clinical practice: intermittent claudication, *N Engl J Med* 356:1241-1250, 2007.

AUTHOR: **MEL ANDERSON, M.D.**

BASIC INFORMATION

DEFINITION

Cocaine is an alkaloid derived from the coca plant *Erythroxylon coca,* native to South America, which contains approximately 0.5% to 1% cocaine. The drug produces physiologic and behavioral effects when administered orally, intranasally, intravenously, or via inhalation following smoking. Cocaine has potent pharmacologic effects on dopamine, norepinephrine, and serotonin neurons in the central nervous system (CNS) involving alteration and blockade of cellular membrane transport and prevention of reuptake.

SYNONYMS

Cocaine hydrochloride: topical solution (FDA approved as a topical anesthetic)

Freebase: aqueous solution of cocaine hydrochloride converted to a more volatile base state by the addition of alkali, thereby extracting the cocaine base in a residue or precipitate

Crack: potent, purified smokable form; produces effects similar to those of intravenous administration

Street names include Bernice, Bernies, C, Cadillac or Champagne of drugs, Carrie, Cecil, Charlie, Coke, Dust, Dynamite, Flake, Gin, Girl, Gold dust, Green gold, Jet, Powder, Star dust, Paradise, Pimp's drug, Snowflake, Stardust, White girl

Liquid lady = alcohol + cocaine

Speedball = heroin + cocaine

Street measures: hit (2 to 200 mg), snort, line, dose, spoon (approximately 1 g)

ICD-9CM CODES
304.2 Cocainism

EPIDEMIOLOGY & DEMOGRAPHICS

The 1993 National Household Survey on Drug Abuse estimated that 4.5 million Americans used cocaine in 1992, with 1.3 million reporting use at least monthly. By 1998 this had not significantly changed.

Between 1993 and 1994, intravenous cocaine and heroin abusers accounted for a major new group of persons with human immunodeficiency virus (HIV) in several metropolitan areas.

In 1999 an estimated 25 million Americans admitted that they used cocaine at least once, 3.7 million the previous year, and 1.5 million were current users. It is the most frequent cause of drug-related deaths reported by medical examiners and is increasing more sharply in women than in men.

PHYSICAL FINDINGS & CLINICAL PRESENTATION

PHASE I:
- CNS: euphoria, agitation, headache, vertigo, twitching, bruxism, nonintentional tremor
- Nausea, vomiting, fever, hypertension, tachycardia

PHASE II:
- CNS: lethargy, hyperreactive deep tendon reflexes, seizures (status epilepticus)
- Sympathetic overdrive: tachycardia, hypertension, hyperthermia
- Incontinence

PHASE III:
- CNS: flaccid paralysis, coma, fixed dilated pupils, loss of reflexes
- Pulmonary edema
- Cardiopulmonary arrest

Psychologic dependence manifests with habituation, paranoia, hallucinations (cocaine "bugs").

Central nervous system: cerebral ischemia and infarction, cerebral arterial spasm, cerebral vasculitis, cerebral vascular thrombosis, subarachnoid hemorrhage, intraparenchymal hemorrhage, seizures, cerebral atrophy, movement disorders.

Cardiac: acute myocardial ischemia and infarction, arrhythmias and sudden death, dilated cardiomyopathy and myocarditis, infective endocarditis, aortic rupture.

Pulmonary: (secondary to smoking crack cocaine) inhalation injuries: cartilage and nasal septal perforation, oropharyngeal ulcers; immunologically mediated diseases: hypersensitivity pneumonitis, bronchiolitis obliterans; pulmonary vascular lesions and hemorrhage, pulmonary infarction, pulmonary edema secondary to left ventricular failure, pneumomediastinum, and pneumothorax.

Gastrointestinal: gastroduodenal ulceration and perforation; intestinal infarction or perforation, colitis.

Renal: acute renal failure secondary to rhabdomyolysis and myoglobinuria; renal infarction; focal segmental glomerulosclerosis.

Obstetric: placental abruption, low infant weight, prematurity, and microcephaly.

Psychiatric: anxiety, depression, paranoia, delirium, psychosis, and suicide.

ETIOLOGY

Cocaine may be absorbed through different routes with varying degrees of speed
- Nasal insufflation/snorting: 2.5 min
- Smoking: <30 sec
- Oral: 2 to 5 min
- Mucosal: <20 min
- Intravenous injection: <30 sec

DIAGNOSIS

DIFFERENTIAL DIAGNOSIS

- Methamphetamine ("speed") abuse
- Methylenedioxyamphetamine ("ecstasy") abuse
- Cathione ("khat") abuse
- Lysergic acid diethylamide (LSD) abuse

WORKUP

Physical examination and laboratory evaluation

LABORATORY TESTS

- Toxicology screen (urine): cocaine is metabolized within 2 hr by the liver to major metabolites, benzoylecgonine and ecgonine methylester, which are excreted in the urine. Metabolites can be identified in urine within 5 min of IV use and up to 48 hr after oral ingestion.
- Blood: CBC, electrolytes, glucose, BUN, creatinine, calcium.
- ABG analysis.
- ECG.
- Serum creatinine kinase and troponin concentration.

TREATMENT

There is no specific antidote and, at present, no drug therapy is uniquely effective in treating cocaine abuse and dependence. In addition, adulterants, contaminants, and other drugs may be admixed with street cocaine. Amantadine may provide effective treatment for cocaine-dependent patients with severe cocaine withdrawal symptoms, as well as the other dopamine agonist bromocriptine (1.5 mg po tid), which may alleviate some of the symptoms of craving associated with acute cocaine withdrawal.

ACUTE GENERAL Rx

Acute cocaine toxicity requires following advanced poisoning treatment and life support. A suspected "body-packer" should have an abdominal radiograph to detect the continued presence of cocaine-containing condoms in the intestinal tract. If present, gentle catharsis with charcoal and mineral oil should be performed with ICU admission and monitoring.

SPECIFIC TREATMENT

INHALATION: Wash nasal passages

AGITATION:
- Check STAT glucose.
- Diazepam 15 to 20 mg po or 2 to 10 mg IM or IV for severe agitation.

HYPERTHERMIA:
- Check rectal temperature, CK, electrolytes.

- Monitor with continuous rectal probe; bring temperature down to 101° F within 30 to 45 min.

RHABDOMYOLYSIS:
- Vigorous hydration with urine output at least 2 ml/kg
- Mannitol or bicarbonate for rhabdomyolysis resistant to hydration

SEIZURE MANAGEMENT (STATUS EPILEPTICUS):
- Diazepam 5 to 10 mg IV over 2 to 3 min, may be repeated every 10 to 15 min.
- Lorazepam 2 to 3 mg IV over 2 to 3 min, may be repeated.
- Phenytoin loading dose 15 to 18 mg/kg IV at a rate not to exceed 25 to 50 mg/min under cardiac monitoring.
- Phenobarbital loading dose 10 to 15 mg/kg IV at a rate of 25 mg/min; an additional 5 mg/kg may be given in 30 to 45 min if seizures are not controlled.
- Refractory seizures, consider:
  Pancuronium 0.1 mg/kg IV
  Halothane general anesthesia
  Both require EEG monitoring to determine brain seizure activity.

HYPERTENSION:
Cocaine-induced hypertension usually responds to benzodiazepines. If this fails:
- Consider arterial line for continuous BP monitoring
- Avoid the use of calcium channel blockers because they may potentiate the incidence of seizures and death, especially in body packers.
- The use of beta blockers may exacerbate cocaine-induced vasoconstriction
- Phentolamine (unopposed adrenergic effects) or nitroglycerin may be required.
- If diastolic pressure >120 mm Hg: hydralazine hydrochloride 25 mg IM or IV; may repeat q1h
- If hypertension uncontrolled or hypertensive encephalopathy is present: sodium nitroprusside initially at 0.5 μg/kg/min not to exceed 10 μg/kg/min

CHEST PAIN:
- CXR, ECG, cardiac enzymes.
- Benzodiazepines for agitation.
- ASA and nitroglycerin for ischemic pain.
- PTCA possibly better than thrombolysis for cocaine-associated MI.
- The use of beta-adrenergic blockers remains controversial because of the unopposed alpha-adrenergic effects of cocaine.
- The combination of nitroprusside and a beta-adrenergic blocking agent or phentolamine alone or in addition to a beta-adrenergic blocking agent may successfully treat myocardial ischemia and hypertension.

VENTRICULAR ARRHYTHMIAS:
- Antiarrhythmia agents should be used with caution during the early period after cocaine exposure as a result of their proarrhythmic and proconvulsant effects.
- Propranolol 1 mg/min IV for up to 6 mg.
- Lidocaine 1.5 mg/kg IV bolus followed by IV infusion (controversial: may be proarrhythmic and proconvulsant).
- Termination of ventricular arrhythmias may be resistant to lidocaine and even cardioversion.
- $NaHCO_3^-$ is under investigation in cocaine-mediated conduction abnormalities and rhythm disturbances.

DISPOSITION

Although many patients who use cocaine may not require any treatment because of the short half-life of the drug, others may require specific treatment for possible cocaine-related complications.

REFERRAL

Consider psychotherapy or behavioral therapy once stable.

PEARLS & CONSIDERATIONS

- Cocaine-induced vasoconstriction may be exacerbated by the use of selective and nonselective beta-adrenergic blocking agents.
- The use of lidocaine in treating ventricular arrhythmias may precipitate seizures and further arrhythmias.

SUGGESTED READINGS

Jones JH, Wier WB: Cocaine associated chest pain, *Med Clin North Am* 89(6):1323, 2005.

Lange RA, Hillis LD: Cardiovascular complications of cocaine use, *N Engl J Med* 345:351, 2001.

Mokhlesi B, Corbridge T: Adult toxicology in critical care: part II: Specific poisonings, *Clin Chest Med* 123(3):897, 2003.

AUTHOR: **SAJEEV HANDA, M.D.**

BASIC INFORMATION

DEFINITION

Coccidioidomycosis is an infectious disease caused by the fungus *Coccidioides immitis.* It is usually asymptomatic and characterized by a primary pulmonary focus with infrequent progression to chronic pulmonary disease and dissemination to other organs.

SYNONYMS

San Joaquin Valley fever

ICD-9CM CODES
114.0 Coccidioides pneumonia
114.1 Cutaneous or extrapulmonary (primary) coccidioidomycosis
114.3 Disseminated or prostate coccidioidomycosis
114.5 Pulmonary coccidioidomycosis
114.2 Coccidioidal meningitis
114.4 Chronic coccidioidomycosis

EPIDEMIOLOGY & DEMOGRAPHICS

INCIDENCE (IN U.S.): Estimated annual infection rate 100,000 persons, predominantly in southwest U.S.
PEAK INCIDENCE: Unknown
PREVALENCE: Unknown
PREDOMINANT SEX: Males, between the ages of 25 to 55 yr
Clinical disease more severe than in older children and adults

PHYSICAL FINDINGS & CLINICAL PRESENTATION

- Asymptomatic infections or illness consistent with a nonspecific upper respiratory tract infection in at least 60%.
- Symptoms of primary infection—cough, malaise, fever, chills, night sweats, anorexia, weakness, and arthralgias (desert rheumatism)—in remaining 40% within 3 wk of exposure.
- Erythema nodosum and erythema multiforme more common in women.
- Scattered rales and dullness on percussion.
- Spontaneous improvement within 2 wk of illness, with complete recovery usual.
- Pulmonary nodules and cavities in <10% of those patients with primary infection; half of these patients asymptomatic.
- In a small portion of these patients: a progressive pneumonitis, often with a fatal outcome.
- Immunocompromised or diabetic patients may progress to chronic pulmonary disease.
- Over many years, granulomas rupture, leading to new cavity formation and continued fibrosis, often accompanied by hemoptysis.
- Disseminated or extrapulmonary disease in approximately 0.5% of acutely infected patients.
  1. Early signs of probable dissemination: fever, malaise, hilar adenopathy, and elevated ESR persisting in the setting of primary infection.
  2. Most organs are susceptible to dissemination, with heart and GI tract generally spared.
- Musculoskeletal involvement: bone lesions often unifocal, ribs, long bones, and vertebral lesions are common.
  1. Joint lesions predominantly unifocal, most commonly involving the ankle and knee, and often accompanying adjacent sites of osteomyelitis.
- Meningeal involvement: headache, fever, weakness, confusion, lethargy, cranial nerve defects, seizures; meningeal signs often minimal or absent.
- Cutaneous involvement: variable lesions—pustules, papules, plaques, nodules, ulcers, abscesses, or verrucous proliferative lesions.
  1. Dissemination and fatal outcomes most common in men, pregnant women, neonates, immunocompromised hosts, and individuals of dark-skinned races, especially those of African, Filipino, Mexican, and Native American ancestry.

ETIOLOGY

- *Coccidioides immitis* is endemic to North and South America.
- In the U.S., endemic areas coincide with the Lower Sonoran Life Zone, with semiarid climate, sparse flora, and alkaline soil in Arizona, California, New Mexico, and Texas.
- Fungus exists in the mycelial phase in soil, having barrel-shaped hyphae (arthroconidia). Arthrospores are aerosolized and deposit in the alveoli, then fungus converts to thick-walled spherule.
- Internal spherical spores (endospores) are released through spherule rupture and mature into new spherules (parasitic cycle).
- Fungus incites a granulomatous reaction in host tissue, usually with caseation necrosis.

DIAGNOSIS

DIFFERENTIAL DIAGNOSIS

- Acute pulmonary coccidioidomycoses:
  1. Community-acquired pneumonias caused by *Mycoplasma* and *Chlamydia*
  2. Granulomatous diseases, such as *Mycobacterium tuberculosis* and sarcoidosis
  3. Other fungal diseases, such as *Blastomyces dermatitidis* and *Histoplasma capsulatum*
- Coccidioidomas: true neoplasms

WORKUP

Suspected in patients with a history of residence or travel in an endemic area, especially during periods favorable to spore dispersion (e.g., dust storms and drought followed by heavy rains)

LABORATORY TESTS

- CBC to reveal eosinophilia, especially with erythema nodosum
- Routine chemistries: usually normal but may reveal hyponatremia
- Elevated serum levels of IgE; associated with progressive disease
- CSF cell counts and chemistry: pleocytosis with mononuclear cell predominance associated with hypoglycorrhachia and elevated protein level
- Definitive diagnosis based on demonstration of the organism by culture from body fluids or tissues
  1. Greatest yield with pus, sputum, synovial fluid, and soft tissue aspirations, varying with the degree of dissemination
  2. Possible positive cultures of blood, gastric aspirate, pleural effusion, peritoneal fluid, and CSF, but less frequently obtained
- Serologic evaluations
  1. Latex agglutination and complement fixation
  2. Elevated serum complement-fixing antibody (CFA) titers ≥1:32 strongly correlated with disseminated disease, except with meningitis where lower titers seen
  3. In meningeal disease: CFA detected in CSF except with high serum CFA titers secondary to concurrent extraneural disease
  4. Enzyme-linked immunosorbent assay (ELISA) against a 33-kDa spherule antigen to detect and monitor CNS disease
- Skin test: coccidioidin, the mycelial phase antigen, and spherulin, the parasitic phase antigen
  1. Positive (>5 mm) 1 mo following onset of symptomatic primary infection
  2. Useful in assessing prior infection
  3. Negative skin test with primary infection: latent or future dissemination

IMAGING STUDIES

Chest x-ray examination:
- Reveals unilateral infiltrates, hilar adenopathy, or pleural effusion in primary infection
- Shows areas of fibrosis containing usually solitary, thin-walled cavities that persist as residua of primary infection
- Possible coccidioidoma, a coinlike lesion representing a healed area of previous pneumonitis

TREATMENT

NONPHARMACOLOGIC THERAPY

- Supportive care in mild symptomatic disease
- In patients with extrapulmonary manifestations involving draining skin, joint, and soft tissue infection: local wound care to avoid possible bacterial superinfection

ACUTE GENERAL Rx

- In general, drug therapy is not required for patients with asymptomatic pulmonary disease and most patients with mild symptomatic primary infection.
- Chemotherapy is indicated under the following circumstances:
  1. Severe symptomatic primary infection
  2. High serum CFA titers
  3. Persistent symptoms >6 wk
  4. Prostration
  5. Progressive pulmonary involvement
  6. Pregnancy
  7. Infancy
  8. Debilitation
  9. Concurrent illness (e.g., diabetes, asthma, COPD, malignancy)
  10. Acquired or induced immunosuppression
  11. Racial group with known predisposition for disseminated disease
- Fluconazole
  1. Most commonly, oral therapy with 400 mg/day up to 1.2 g/day appears to be the drug of choice for meningeal and deep-seated mycotic infections.
  2. In patients with AIDS, fluconazole may be considered the drug of choice for initial and maintenance therapy.
  3. All patients with coccidioidal meningitis should continue azole therapy indefinitely.
- Itraconazole
  1. 400 to 600 mg/day achieves 90% response rate in bone, joint, soft tissue, lymphatic, and genitourinary infections.
  2. Itraconazole may be more efficacious than fluconazole in the treatment of skeletal (bone) infections.
- Posaconazole is a new triazole that has recently been approved for use for systemic mycoses such as coccidioidomycosis; its relative efficacy compared to other agents will need additional clinical study.
- For pulmonary infections, treatment with either fluconazole or itraconazole, given for 6 to 12 wk, appears to be equal in efficacy.
- Amphotericin B is the classic therapy for disseminated extraneural disease, dose 1 to 1.5 mg/kg/day, qd for the first week and every other day, for a total dose of 1 to 2.5 g or until clinical and serologic remission is accomplished.
  1. Local instillation into body cavities such as sinuses, fistulae, and abscesses has been adjunct to therapy.
  2. Liposomal amphotericin B is probably equally effective, but further studies are needed.
  3. Duration of therapy for extraneural disease is undefined but probably about 1 yr.
- With meningeal disease:
  1. Intrathecal amphotericin B remains the traditional treatment modality, given alone or preceding the use of oral agents.
  2. Begin in doses of 0.01 to 0.025 mg/day, gradually increasing the dose as tolerated, to 0.5 mg/day with the patient in Trendelenburg's position.
  3. If given via Ommaya reservoir, as in ventriculitis, dose may be increased to 1.5 mg/day if tolerated.
  4. Concomitant parenteral therapy with amphotericin B is used for simultaneous extraneural disease as standard doses and with purely meningeal disease in smaller doses, although not strictly indicated.
  5. Intrathecal therapy is usually given three times a week for at least 3 mo, then discontinued or gradually tapered until once every 6 wk through 1 yr of therapy.
  6. Patients need routine monitoring of CSF, CFA, cell count, and chemistries for at least 2 yr following cessation of therapy.
- For osteomyelitis, soft tissue closed-space infections, and pulmonary fibrocavitary disease: surgical debridement, drainage, or resection, respectively, in addition to oral azole therapy or parenteral administration of amphotericin B.

CHRONIC Rx

For chronically immunocompromised patients, lifelong therapy with oral azoles or amphotericin B

DISPOSITION

- Prognosis for primary symptomatic infection is good.
- Immunocompromised patients are most likely to have disseminated disease and higher morbidity and mortality.

REFERRAL

- To surgeon for the evaluation of chronic hemoptysis, enlarging cavitary lesions despite chemotherapy and intrapleural rupture, osteomyelitis, and other synovial or soft tissue closed space infections
- For neurosurgical consultation in patients with meningeal disease to establish the delivery route of intrathecal drug therapy

PEARLS & CONSIDERATIONS

COMMENTS

- Infected body fluids contained within a closed moist environment (e.g., sputum in a specimen cup) provide the opportunity for the fungus to revert to its hyphal form whereby spores may be made airborne on opening of the container. This is a biohazard for laboratory personnel. Purulent drainage into a cast, allowing conversion of fungus to the saprophytic phase, has been responsible for acute disease when the cast was opened and the spores were unintentionally made airborne.
- Patients with a remote history of exposure, especially if immunosuppressed by medication or disease, may reactivate primary disease and suffer rapid dissemination.
- Although cardiac disease is rare, constrictive pericarditis in the setting of disseminated coccidioidomycosis has been documented and is potentially fatal.
- Organ transplant recipients may develop disease if the transplant donor has unrecognized active coccidioidomycosis at the time of death.

SUGGESTED READINGS

Ampel NM et al: The mannose receptor mediates the cellular immune response in human coccidioidomycosis, *Infect Immun* 73(4):2554-2555, 2005.

Blair JE, Smilack JD, Caples SM: Coccidioidomycosis in patients with hematologic malignancies, *Arch Intern Med* 165(1):113-117, 2005.

Parish JM, Blair JE: Coccidioidomycosis, *Mayo Clin Proc* 83(3):343-349, 2008.

Wang CY et al: Disseminated coccidioidomycosis, *Emerg Infect Dis* 11(1):177-179, 2005.

AUTHORS: **GEORGE O. ALONSO, M.D., GLENN G. FORT, M.D., M.P.H.,** and **DENNIS J. MIKOLICH, M.D.**

BASIC INFORMATION

DEFINITION

Acute self-limited febrile illness caused by infection with a Coltivirus

ICD-9CM CODES
066.1 Colorado Tick Fever

EPIDEMIOLOGY & DEMOGRAPHICS

- Incidence: approximately 330 cases reported per year in the U.S.
- Demographics: children and adults of both genders
- Geography: Rocky Mountains at elevations of 4000 to 10,000 feet. Sporadic cases have been reported from areas of California outside the range of *Dermacentor andersoni*
- Colorado has the highest incidence (Fig. 1-58)

PHYSICAL FINDINGS & CLINICAL PRESENTATION

- Incubation: 3 to 4 days is usual, but can be up to 14 days
- First symptoms: fever, chills, severe headache, severe myalgias, and hyperesthetic skin
- Initial signs and symptoms
  1. Tick bite
  2. Fever and chills
  3. Headache
  4. Myalgias
  5. Weakness
  6. Prostration and indifference
  7. Injected conjunctivae
  8. Erythematous pharyngitis
  9. Lymphadenopathy
  10. Maculopapular or petechial rash

These first symptoms last for 1 wk or less but 50% of the cases experience a febrile relapse 2 to 3 days following an initial remission. Weakness and fatigue may persist for several months after the acute phase(s). This chronic phase is more likely in older patients.

In children, 5% to 10% of cases are complicated by aseptic meningitis. In adults, rare complications include pneumonia, hepatitis, myocarditis, and epididymoorchitis. Vertically transmitted fetal infection is possible.

ETIOLOGY

- Infectious agent: Coltiviruses; 7 species, including 3 in the U.S.
- Vector: wood tick, *D. andersoni.*
- Pathogenesis: human transmission occurs via tick bite. Tick season spans from March to September. The virus infects marrow erythrocytic precursors, explaining the protracted disease course as viremia lasts for the lifespan of the infected RBC.

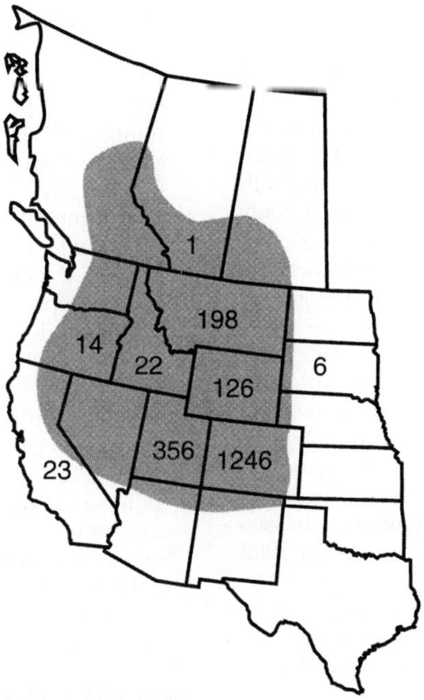

FIGURE 1-58 Geographic distribution of *Dermacentor andersoni* (wood ticks) and reported cases of Colorado tick fever, 1990-1996, United States and Canada. (From Mandell GL: *Mandell, Douglas, and Bennett's principles and practice of infectious diseases,* ed 6, New York, 2005, Churchill Livingstone.)

DIAGNOSIS

DIFFERENTIAL DIAGNOSIS

- Rocky Mountain spotted fever
- Influenza
- Leptospirosis
- Infectious mononucleosis
- CMV infection
- Pneumonia
- Hepatitis
- Meningitis
- Endocarditis
- Scarlet fever
- Measles
- Rubella
- Typhus
- Lyme disease
- Immune thrombocytopenic purpura (ITP)
- Thrombotic thrombocytopenic purpura (TTP)
- Kawasaki disease
- Toxic shock syndrome
- Vasculitis

WORKUP

Consider Colorado tick fever in the presence of the above symptoms associated with travel to an endemic area coupled with a history of tick exposure

LABORATORY TESTS

- CBC
  1. Leukopenia
  2. Atypical lymphocytes
  3. Moderate thrombocytopenia
- Virus identification in RBCs by indirect immunofluorescence
- Serology using ELISA, neutralization, or complement fixation

TREATMENT

- No specific therapy, although Coltiviruses are sensitive to ribavirin
- Bedrest, fluids, acetaminophen
- Avoid aspirin because of thrombocytopenia
- Prevention: tick avoidance measures

SUGGESTED READINGS

Jaffar FM et al: Recombinant VP-7-based enzyme-linked immunosorbent assay for detection of immunoglobulin G antibodies to Colorado tick fever virus, *J Clin Microbiology* 41:2102, 2003.

Tsai TF: Coltiviruses (Colorado tick fever). In Mandell GL, Bennett JF, Dolin R (eds): *Principles and practice of infectious diseases,* ed 6, Philadelphia, 2005, Churchill Livingstone.

AUTHORS: **FRED F. FERRI, M.D.,** and **TOM J. WACHTEL, M.D.**

BASIC INFORMATION

DEFINITION

Colorectal cancer (CRC) is a neoplasm arising from the luminal surface of the large bowel: descending colon (40% to 42%), rectosigmoid and rectum (30% to 33%), cecum and ascending colon (25% to 30%), transverse colon (10% to 13%).

ICD-9CM CODES
154.0 Colorectal cancer

EPIDEMIOLOGY & DEMOGRAPHICS

- CRC is the second leading cause of cancer deaths in the U.S. (>135,000 new cases and >50,000 deaths/yr).
- Peak incidence is in the seventh decade of life. The lifetime risk of developing CRC is 1 in 17, with 90% of cases occurring after the age of 50 years.
- 50% of rectal cancers are within reach of the examiner's finger, 50% of colon cancers are within reach of the flexible sigmoidoscope.
- CRC accounts for 14% of all cases of cancer (excluding skin malignancies) and 14% of all yearly cancer deaths.
- Risk factors:
  1. Hereditary polyposis syndromes
     a. Familial polyposis (high risk)
     b. Gardner's syndrome (high risk)
     c. Turcot's syndrome (high risk)
     d. Peutz-Jeghers syndrome (low to moderate risk)
  2. IBD, both ulcerative colitis and Crohn's disease
  3. Family history of "cancer family syndrome"
  4. Heredofamilial breast cancer and colon carcinoma
  5. History of previous colorectal carcinoma
  6. Women undergoing irradiation for gynecologic cancer
  7. First-degree relatives with colorectal carcinoma
  8. Age >40 yr
  9. Possible dietary factors (diet high in fat or meat, beer drinking, reduced vegetable consumption). Prolonged high consumption of red and processed meat may increase the risk of cancer of the large intestine.
  10. Hereditary nonpolyposis colon cancer (HNPCC): autosomal-dominant disorder characterized by early age of onset (mean age of 44 yr) and right-sided or proximal colon cancers, synchronous and metachronous colon cancers, mucinous and poorly differentiated colon cancers; it accounts for 1% to 5% of all cases of CRC
  11. Previous endometrial or ovarian cancer, particularly when diagnosed at an early age

PHYSICAL FINDINGS & CLINICAL PRESENTATION

- Physical examination may be completely unremarkable.
- Digital rectal examination can detect approximately 50% of rectal cancers.
- Palpable abdominal masses may indicate metastasis or complications of colorectal carcinoma (abscess, intussusception, volvulus).
- Abdominal distention and tenderness are suggestive of colonic obstruction.
- Hepatomegaly may be indicative of hepatic metastasis.

ETIOLOGY

CRC can arise through two mutational pathways: microsatellite instability or chromosomal instability. Germline genetic mutations are the basis of inherited colon cancer syndromes; an accumulation of somatic mutations in a cell is the basis of sporadic colon cancer.

DIAGNOSIS (Dx)

DIFFERENTIAL DIAGNOSIS

- Diverticular disease
- Strictures
- IBD
- Infectious or inflammatory lesions
- Adhesions
- Arteriovenous malformations
- Metastatic carcinoma (prostate, sarcoma)
- Extrinsic masses (cysts, abscesses)

WORKUP

- The clinical presentation of colorectal malignancies is initially vague and nonspecific (weight loss, anorexia, malaise). It is useful to divide colon cancer symptoms into those usually associated with right side of colon and those commonly associated with left side of colon, because the clinical presentation varies with the location of the carcinoma.
  1. Right side of colon
     a. Anemia (iron deficiency secondary to chronic blood loss).
     b. Dull, vague, and uncharacteristic abdominal pain may be present, or patient may be completely asymptomatic.
     c. Rectal bleeding is often missed because blood is mixed with feces.
     d. Obstruction and constipation are unusual because of large lumen and more liquid stools.
  2. Left side of colon
     a. Change in bowel habits (constipation, diarrhea, tenesmus, pencil-thin stools).
     b. Rectal bleeding (bright red blood coating the surface of the stool).
     c. Intestinal obstruction is frequent because of small lumen.
- Early diagnosis of patients with surgically curable disease (Dukes' A, B) is necessary, because survival time is directly related to the stage of the carcinoma at the time of diagnosis. Appropriate screening recommendations are discussed in Section V.

CLASSIFICATION AND STAGING: Dukes' and UICC classification for CRC:
A. Confined to the mucosa-submucosa (I)
B. Invasion of muscularis propria (II)
C. Local node involvement (III)
D. Distant metastasis (IV)
TNM Classification:

Stage	TNM classification
I	T1-2, N0, M0
IIA	T3, N0, M0
IIB	T4, N0, M0
IIIA	T1-2, N1, M0
IIIB	T3-4, N1, M0
IIIC	T(any), N2, M0
IV	T(any), N(any), M1

LABORATORY TESTS

- Positive fecal occult blood test. Many primary care physicians use single digital fecal occult blood test (FOBT) as their primary screening test for CRC. Single FOBT has low specificity for detecting human hemoglobin, is a poor screening method for CRC (sensitivity 4.9%), and is inappropriate as the only test because negative results do not decrease the odds of advanced neoplasia. The at-home 6-sample FOBT is more sensitive (sensitivity to 23.9%) and should be offered to patients who are unwilling to undergo screening colonoscopic evaluation or barium enema. Qualitative immunochemical FOBTs are specific for the detection of human hemoglobin and have better sensitivity and specificity for detection of clinically significant neoplasia.
- Newer modalities for early detection of colorectal neoplasms include the detection of mutations in the adenomatous polyposis coli (APC) gene from stool samples. Identification of abnormal fecal DNA has greater sensitivity for colorectal neoplasia than FOBT.
- Microcytic anemia.
- Elevated plasma carcinoembryonic antigen (CEA). CEA should not be used as a screening test for CRC because it can be elevated in patients with many other conditions (smoking, IBD, alcoholic liver disease). A normal CEA does not exclude the diagnosis of CRC.
- Liver function tests.

IMAGING STUDIES

- Colonoscopy with biopsy (primary assessment tool).
- Virtual colonoscopy (VC) uses helical (spiral) CT scan to generate a two- or three-dimensional virtual colorectal image. VC does not require sedation, but like optical colonoscopy, it requires some bowel preparation (either

bowel cathartics or ingestion of iodinated contrast medium with meals during the 48 hours before CT) and air insufflation. It also involves substantial exposure to radiation. In addition, patients with lesions detected by VC will require traditional colonoscopy.

- CT scan of abdomen/pelvis/chest to assist in preoperative staging.
- PET scanning can display functional information and is accurate in the detection of CRC and its distant metastases. Combined PET/CT scanners are increasingly more available and are useful to detect and characterize malignant lesions. Colonography composed of a combined modality of PET and CT is a newer diagnostic modality that can provide whole-body tumor staging in a single session.

TREATMENT

GENERAL Rx

- Surgical resection: 70% of CRC are resectable for cure at presentation; 45% of patients are cured by primary resection.
- The backbone of treatment of CRC is fluorouracil (FL). Leucovorin (folinic acid) enhances the effect of fluorouracil and is given together with it. Adjuvant chemotherapy with combination of 5-fluorouracil (5-FU) and levamisole substantially increases cure rates for patients with stage III colon cancer and should be considered standard treatment for all such patients and selected patients with high-risk stage II colon cancer (adherence of tumor to an adjacent organ, bowel perforation, or obstruction).
- Radiation therapy is a useful adjunct to fluorouracil and leucovorin therapy for stage II or III rectal cancers.
- When given as adjuvant therapy after a complete resection in stage III disease, FL increases overall 5-year survival from 51% to 64%. The use of adjuvant FL in stage II disease (no involvement of regional nodes) is controversial because 5-year overall survival is 80% for treated or untreated patients and the addition of FL only increases the probability of 5-year disease-free interval from 72% to 76%. For patients with standard-risk stage III tumors (e.g., involvement of one to three regional lymph nodes), both FL alone or FL with oxaliplatin (Eloxatin, an inhibitor of DNA synthesis) are reasonable choices. Generally reversible peripheral neuropathy is the main side effect of FL plus oxaliplatin. The oral fluoropyrimidine capecitabine (Xeloda) is a prodrug that undergoes enzymatic conversion to fluorouracil. It is an effective alternative to IV fluorouracil as adjuvant treatment for stage III colon cancer because it has a lower incidence of mouth sores and bone marrow suppression. It does however have an increased incidence of palmar-plantar erythrodysesthesia (hand-foot syndrome).
- Irinotecan (Camptosar), a potent inhibitor of topoisomerase I, a nuclear enzyme involved in the unwinding of DNA during replication, can be used to treat metastatic CRC refractory to other drugs, including 5-FU; it may offer a few months of palliation but is expensive and associated with significant toxicity.
- Oxaliplatin (Eloxatin), a third-generation platinum derivative, can be used in combination with fluorouracil and leucovorin (FL) for patients with metastatic CRC whose disease has recurred or progressed despite treatment with fluorouracil/leucovorin plus irinotecan. FL plus oxaliplatin should be considered for high-risk patients with stage III cancers (e.g., >3 involved regional nodes [N2] or tumor invasion beyond the serosa [T4 lesion]).
- Laboratory studies have identified molecular sites in tumor tissue that may serve as specific targets for treatment by using epidermal growth factor receptor antagonists and angiogenesis inhibitors. The monoclonal antibodies cetuximab (Erbitux), panitumumab (Vectibix), and bevacizumab (Avastatin) have been approved by the FDA for advanced CRC. Bevacizumab is an angiogenesis inhibitor that binds and inhibits the activity of human vascular endothelial growth factor (VEGF). Cetuximab and panitumumab are epidermal growth factor receptor [EGFR] blockers that inhibits the growth and survival of tumor cells that overexpress EGFR. Cetuximab has synergism with irinotecan and its addition to irinotecan in patients with advanced disease resistant to irinotecan increases response rate from 10% when cetuximab is used alone to 22% with combination of cetuximab and irinotecan. The addition of bevacizumab to FL in patients with advanced CRC has been reported to increase the response rate from 17% to 40%. Severe dermatologic toxicity can occur with both cetuximab and panitumumab.
- The liver is generally the initial and most common site of CRC metastases. Resection of metastases limited to the liver is curative in more than 30% of selected patients. In patients who undergo resection of liver metastases, postoperative treatment with a combination of hepatic arterial infusion of floxuridine and IV fluorouracil improves the outcome at 2 yr.

CHRONIC Rx

Follow-up is indicated with:

- Physician visits with a focus on the clinical and disease-related history, directed physical examination guided by this history, coordination of follow-up, and counseling every 3 to 6 mo for the first 3 yr then decreased frequency thereafter for 2 yr.
- Colonoscopy yearly for the initial 2 yr, then every 3 yr.
- CEA level should be obtained baseline; if elevated, it can be used postoperatively as a measure of completeness of tumor resection or to monitor tumor recurrence; if used to monitor tumor recurrence, CEA should be obtained every 3 to 6 mo for up to 5 yr. The role of CEA for monitoring patients with resected colon cancer has been questioned because of the small number of cures attributed to CEA monitoring despite the substantial cost in dollars and physical and emotional stress associated with monitoring.

DISPOSITION

- The 5-yr survival varies with the stage of the carcinoma:

Dukes':

1. Dukes' A 5-yr survival, >80%
2. Dukes' B 5-yr survival, 60%
3. Dukes' C 5-yr survival, 20%
4. Dukes' D 5-yr survival, 3%

TNM Classification:

Stage	TNM classification	5-year survival
I	T1-2, N0, M0	>90%
IIA	T3, N0, M0	60%-85%
IIB	T4, N0, M0	60%-85%
IIIA	T1-2, N1, M0	25%-65%
IIIB	T3-4, N1, M0	25%-65%
IIIC	T(any), N2, M0	25%-65%
IV	T(any), N(any), M1	5%-7%

- Overall 5-yr disease-free survival has increased from 50% to 63% during the past 2 decades.
- High-frequency microsatellite instability in CRC is independently predictive of a relatively favorable outcome and, in addition, reduces the likelihood of metastases.
- In patients with Dukes' C (stage III) CRC there is improved 5-year survival among women treated with adjuvant chemotherapy (53% with chemotherapy vs. 33% without) and among patients with right-sided tumors treated with adjuvant chemotherapy.
- Retention of 18q alleles in microsatellite-stable cancers and mutation of the gene for the type I receptor for TGF-B1 in cancers with high levels of microsatellite instability point to a favorable outcome after adjuvant chemotherapy with fluorouracil-based regimens for stage II colon cancer.

REFERRAL

- Surgical referral for resection
- Oncology referral for adjuvant chemotherapy in selected patients
- Radiation oncology referral for patients with stage II or III rectal cancers

PEARLS & CONSIDERATIONS

COMMENTS

- Decreased fat intake to 30% of total energy intake, increased fiber, and fruit and vegetable consumption may lower CRC risk. Recent literature reports, however, do not support a protective effect from dietary fiber against CRC in women.
- Chemoprophylaxis with aspirin (81 mg/day) reduces the incidence of colorectal adenomas in persons at risk.
- Statins inhibit the growth of colon cancer lines. Use of statins is associated with a 47% relative reduction in the risk of CRC. Additional trials are necessary to investigate the overall benefits of statins in preventing CRC.
- The National Cancer Institute has published consensus guidelines for universal screening for hereditary nonpolyposis colon cancer (HNPCC) in patients with newly diagnosed CRC. Tumors in mutation carriers of HNPCC typically exhibit microsatellite instability, a characteristic phenotype that is caused by expansions or contractions of short nucleotide repeat sequences. These guidelines (Bethesda Guidelines) are useful for selective patients for microsatellite instability testing. Screening patients with newly diagnosed CRC for HNPCC is cost effective, especially if the benefits to their immediate relatives are considered.
- Expression of guanylyl cyclase C mRNA in lymph nodes is associated with recurrence of CRC in patients with stage II disease. Analysis of guanylyl cyclase mRNA expression by RT-PCR may be useful for CRC staging.
- The use of either annual or biennial fecal occult-blood testing significantly reduces the incidence of CRC.
- The detection of mutations in the adenomatous polyposis coli (APC) gene from stool samples is a promising new modality for early detection of colorectal neoplasms.

EVIDENCE

Adjuvant systemic chemotherapy has been shown to significantly improve overall survival compared with no adjuvant chemotherapy in patients with Dukes' C colon cancer, and Dukes' B or C rectal cancer. The results were less clear with Dukes' B tumors.[1] (A)

Pooled analysis of three randomized controlled trials (RCTs) of adjuvant 5-fluorouracil and folinic acid found a significant increase in survival for patients with Dukes' C colon tumors at 3 years but no survival benefit for patients with Dukes' B tumors.[2] (A)

A significant survival advantage was seen at 6 years in patients treated with 1 week of continuing portal vein infusion chemotherapy commenced within 5 to 7 days of surgery vs. no additional treatment after surgery, in patients with Dukes' A, B, and C colorectal tumors. The benefit was only seen for patients with colon cancer.[3] (A)

A systematic review found that palliative chemotherapy was effective for prolonging time to disease progression in patients with advanced CRC. An absolute improvement in survival of 16% was seen at 6 and 12 months.[4] (A)

In a recent multiinstitutional study, 872 patients with adenocarcinoma of the colon were randomized into two groups receiving open or laparoscopically assisted colectomy performed by credentialed surgeons. At 3 years, the rates of recurrence were similar in the two groups.[5] (B)

Recently the FDA approved cetuximab (a monoclonal antibody that inhibits the epidermal growth factor receptor [EGFr] pathway) for the treatment of advanced CRC. A Phase II, open-label clinical trial found that in patients who had tumors with EGFr expression and who had also demonstrated clinical failure with irinotecanon, had modest results with a once-weekly cetuximab regime.[6] (B)

A recent randomized controlled clinical trial compared the addition of the monoclonal antibody against vascular endothelial growth factor, bevacizumab, to a fluorouracil-based combination chemotherapy regime vs. the addition of placebo to the same regime, in patients with untreated metastatic CRC. It found that the addition of bevacizumab resulted in a statistically significant and clinically meaningful improvement in survival.[7] (B)

Another recent randomized controlled clinical trial compared the addition of the platinum-containing chemotherapeutic agent oxaliplatin to the standard fluorouracil plus leucovorin (FL) regime vs. no additive treatment in patients who had undergone curative resection for stage II or III colon cancer. The researchers concluded that the group that had been treated with the addition of oxaliplatin to the FL regime had improved disease-free survival.[8] (B)

Evidence-Based References

1. Dube D, Heyen F, Jenicek M: Adjuvant chemotherapy in colorectal carcinoma. Results of a meta analysis, *Dis Colon Rectum* 40:35-41, 1997. Reviewed in: *Clin Evid* 11:562-570, 2003. (A)
2. International Multicenter Pooled Analysis of Colon Cancer Trials (IMPACT) Investigators: Efficacy of adjuvant fluorouracil and folinic acid in colon cancer, *Lancet* 348:939-944, 1995. Reviewed in: *Clin Evid* 11:562-570, 2003. (A)
3. Liver Infusion Meta-analysis Group: Portal vein chemotherapy for colorectal cancer: a meta-analysis of 4000 patients in 10 studies, *J Natl Cancer Inst* 89:497-505, 1997. Reviewed in: *Clin Evid* 11:562-570, 2003. (A)
4. Best L et al: Palliative chemotherapy for advanced or metastatic colorectal cancer (Cochrane Review). (A)
5. Clinical Outcomes of Surgical Therapy Study Group: A comparison of laparoscopically assisted and open colectomy for colon cancer, *N Engl J Med* 350(20):2050-2059, 2004. (B)
6. Saltz LB et al: Phase II trial of cetuximab in patients with refractory colorectal cancer that expresses the epidermal growth factor receptor, *J Clin Oncol* 22(7):1201-1208, 2004. (B)
7. Hurwitz H et al: Bevacizumab plus irinotecan, fluorouracil, and leucovorin for metastatic colorectal cancer, *N Engl J Med* 350(23):2335-2342, 2004. (B)
8. Andre T et al: Multicenter International Study of Oxaliplatin/5-Fluorouracil/Leucovorin in the Adjuvant Treatment of Colon Cancer (MOSAIC) Investigators. Oxaliplatin, fluorouracil, and leucovorin as adjuvant treatment for colon cancer, *N Engl J Med* 350(23):2343-2351, 2004. (B)

SUGGESTED READINGS

Gill S et al: Colorectal cancer, *Mayo Clin Proc* 82:114-129, 2007.

Jonker DJ et al: Cetuximab for the treatment of colorectal cancer, *N Eng J Med* 357:2040-2048, 2007.

Levi Z et al: A qualitative immunochemical fecal occult blood test for colorectal neoplasia, *Ann Intern Med* 146:244-255, 2007.

Meyerhardt JA, Mayer RJ: Systemic therapy for colorectal cancer, *N Engl J Med* 352:476-487, 2005.

Poynter JN et al: Statins and the risk of colorectal cancer, *N Engl J Med* 352:2184-2192, 2005.

Schetter AJ et al: MicroRNA expression profiles associated with prognosis and therapeutic outcome in colon adenocarcinoma, *JAMA* 299(4):425-436, 2008.

Twelves C et al: Capecitabine as adjuvant treatment for stage III colon cancer, *N Engl J Med* 352:2696-2704, 2005.

Veit-Haibach P et al: Diagnostic accuracy of colorectal cancer staging with whole-body PET/CT colonography, *JAMA* 296:2590-2600, 2006.

AUTHOR: **FRED F. FERRI, M.D.**

BASIC INFORMATION

DEFINITION

Condyloma acuminatum is a sexually transmitted viral disease of the vulva, vagina, and cervix that is caused by the human papillomavirus (HPV).

SYNONYMS

Genital warts
Venereal warts
Anogenital warts

ICD-9CM CODES
078.11 Condyloma acuminatum

EPIDEMIOLOGY & DEMOGRAPHICS

- Seen mostly in young adults with a mean age of onset of 16 to 25 yr
- A sexually transmitted disease spread by skin-to-skin contact
- Highly contagious, with 25% to 65% of sexual partners developing it
- Virus shed from both macroscopic and microscopic lesions
- Average incubation time 2 mo (range: 1 to 8 mo)
- Predisposing conditions: diabetes, pregnancy, local trauma, and immunosuppression (e.g., transplant patients, those with HIV infection)

PHYSICAL FINDINGS & CLINICAL PRESENTATION

- Usually found in genital area, but can be present elsewhere
- Lesions usually in similar positions on both sides of perineum
- Initial lesions pedunculated, soft papules about 2 to 3 mm in diameter, 10 to 20 mm long; may occur as single papule or in clusters
- Size of lesions varies from pinhead to large cauliflower-like masses
- Usually asymptomatic, but if infected, can cause pain, odor, or bleeding
- Vulvar condyloma more common than vaginal and cervical
- There are four morphologic types: condylomatous, keratotic, papular, and flat warts

ETIOLOGY

- HPV DNA types 6 and 11 usually found in exophytic warts and have no malignant potential
- HPV types 16 and 18 usually found in flat warts and are associated with increased risk of malignancy
- Recurrence associated with persisting viral infection of adjacent normal skin in 25% to 50% of cases

DIAGNOSIS

DIFFERENTIAL DIAGNOSIS

- Abnormal anatomic variants or skin tags around labia minora and introitus
- Dysplastic warts

WORKUP

- Colposcopic examination of lower genital tract from cervix to perianal skin with 3% to 5% acetic acid
- Biopsy of vulvar lesions that lack the classic appearance of warts and that become ulcerated or fail to respond to treatment
- Biopsy of flat white or ulcerated cervical lesions

LABORATORY TESTS

- Pap smear
- Cervical cultures for *N. gonorrhoeae* and *Chlamydia*
- Serologic test for syphilis
- HIV testing offered
- Wet mount for trichomoniasis, *Candida albicans,* and *Gardnerella vaginalis*
- Testing for diabetes (blood glucose)

TREATMENT

NONPHARMACOLOGIC THERAPY

- Keep genital area dry and clean.
- Keep diabetes, if present, well controlled.
- Advise use of condoms to prevent spread of infection to sexual partner.

ACUTE GENERAL Rx

Keratolytic agents:

- Podophyllin
  1. Acts by poisoning mitotic spindle and causing intense vasospasm
  2. Applied directly to lesion weekly and washed off in 6 hr
  3. Used in minimal vulvar or anal disease
  4. Applied cautiously to nonkeratinized epithelial surfaces
  5. Contraindicated in pregnancy
  6. Discontinued if lesions do not disappear in 6 wk; switch to other treatment
- Trichloroacetic acid (30% to 80% solution)
  1. Acts by precipitation of surface proteins
  2. Applied twice monthly to lesion
  3. Indicated for vulvar, anal, and vaginal lesions; can be used for cervical lesions
  4. Less painful and irritating to normal tissue than podophyllin
- Fluorouracil
  1. Causes necrosis and sloughing of growing tissue
  2. Can be used intravaginally or for vulvar, anal, or urethral lesions
  3. Better tolerated; 3 g (two thirds of vaginal applicator) applied weekly for 12 wk
  4. Possible vaginal ulceration and erythema
  5. Patient's vagina examined after four to six applications
  6. 80% cure rate

Physical agents:

- Cryotherapy
  1. Can be used weekly for 3 to 6 wk
  2. 62% to 79% success rate
  3. Not suitable for large warts
- Laser therapy
  1. Done by physician with necessary expertise and equipment
  2. Painful; requires anesthesia
- Electrocautery or excision
  1. For recurrent, very large lesions
  2. Local anesthesia needed

Immunotherapy:

- Interferon
  1. Injected intralesionally at a dose of 3 million U/m^2 three times weekly for 8 wk
  2. Side effects: fever, chills, malaise, headache
- Imiquimod 5% cream: increases wart clearance after 3 mo
- Interferon, topical: increases wart clearance at 4 wk

DISPOSITION

Follow-up exam every 6 to 12 months, as needed.

REFERRAL

Consult gynecologist in case of extensive lesions or lesions resistant to treatment with keratolytic agents (podophyllin and trichloroacetic acid).

EVIDENCE

Podofilox and imiquimod have been shown to be more effective than placebo.[1,2] Ⓐ

Trichloroacetic acid and cryotherapy appear to be equally effective at producing clearance of warts.[3,4] Ⓐ

Evidence-Based References

1. Wiley DJ. Genital warts, *Clin Evid* 8:1620, 2002. Ⓐ
2. Moore RA et al: Imiquimod for the treatment of genital warts: a quantitative systematic review, *BMC Infect Dis* 1:3, 2001. Reviewed in: *Clin Evid* 10, web version only, 2003. Ⓐ
3. Abdullah AN, Walzman M, Wade A: Treatment of external genital warts comparing cryotherapy (liquid nitrogen) and trichloroacetic acid, *Sex Transm Dis* 20:344, 1993. Reviewed in: *Clin Evid* 10, web version only, 2003. Ⓐ
4. Godley MJ et al: Cryotherapy compared with trichloroacetic acid in treating genital warts, *Genitourin Med* 63:390, 1987. Reviewed in: *Clin Evid* 10, web version only, 2003. Ⓐ

AUTHORS: **GEORGE T. DANAKAS, M.D.,** and **RUBEN ALVERO, M.D.**

BASIC INFORMATION

DEFINITION

Congenital adrenal hyperplasia (CAH) refers to several different genetic mutations in the enzymes responsible for cortisol synthesis, which are each inherited in an autosomal recessive fashion.

SYNONYMS

21-hydroxylase deficiency (equivalent to CYP21A2 deficiency)
11B-hydroxylase deficiency
3B-hydroxysteroid dehydrogenase deficiency
17-hydroxylase deficiency
Lipoid adrenal hyperplasia
CYP 17 deficiency

ICD-9-CM CODES
255.2 Adrenogenital disorders; hyperplasia, congenital adrenal

EPIDEMIOLOGY & DEMOGRAPHICS

- Between 90% and 95% of cases of CAH are caused by "classic" 21-hydroxylase deficiency, of which 75% of cases represent the salt-wasting form.
- Inheritance pattern is autosomal recessive.
- Prevalence of 21-hydroxylase deficiency is 1/16,000 infants in the U.S., but may be higher among other groups, such as Hispanics and Ashkenazi Jews (1% to 2%).
- The frequency of heterozygous carriers is controversial; estimates range between 1:5 and 1:80 persons.

CLINICAL PRESENTATION

"Classic" salt-wasting form (impaired cortisol and aldosterone synthesis):
- Infants are acutely ill with poor weight gain, hypovolemia, hyponatremia, hyperkalemia, and elevated plasma renin.
- If patients survive infancy, their overall life expectancy is not compromised.
- Females are born with ambiguous genitalia and may have irregular menses and infertility as adults.
- Males may have greater penile size and smaller testes than expected during childhood. Males may also develop adrenal rests, or ectopic islands of adrenal cortical tissue in the testes, in childhood and may experience infertility as adults.
- Both males and females may exhibit rapid growth in childhood (due to early epiphyseal closure, which then results in short stature in adulthood).
- Precocious puberty is common in both males and females.

"Classic" non-salt-wasting or simple virilizing form (impaired cortisol synthesis only):
- Females present with ambiguous genitalia at birth.
- The normal appearance of male genitalia in the simple virilizing form makes this a difficult diagnosis in male infants.
- Characterized by precocious puberty, short stature, and testicular adrenal rests as in the salt-wasting form.

"Nonclassic" or mild, late-onset form (varying degrees of androgen excess):
- Usually presents in adolescence or adulthood and is not detected on newborn screening.
- Often asymptomatic, but can be associated with mild virilization.
- PCOS-like symptoms occur in women (hirsutism, oligomenorrhea, acne, infertility, insulin resistance, abnormal menses).
- Associated with infertility in males.

ETIOLOGY

In 21-hydroxylase deficiency, the pathways for aldosterone production (from the conversion of progesterone to deoxycorticosterone) and cortisol production (from the conversion of 17-hydroxyprogesterone to 11-deoxycortisol) by the cP450 enzyme 21-hydroxylase are interrupted. The production of ACTH is thus stimulated by a negative feedback mechanism, leading to adrenal hyperplasia and mineralocorticoid deficiency as the intermediaries in aldosterone and cortisol synthesis are shunted to the androgen biosynthesis pathway (Fig. 1-59, *A* and *B*). A recombination event between the active CYP21A2 gene on chromosome 6p21.3 and the CYP21A1 pseudogene is thought to create the deficient 21-hydroxylase enzyme.

DIAGNOSIS

DIFFERENTIAL DIAGNOSIS

- Precocious puberty
- Polycystic ovarian syndrome (PCOS)
- Androgen resistance syndromes
- Pseudohermaphroditism
- Mixed gonadal dysgenesis
- Testicular carcinoma
- Leydig cell tumors
- Adrenocortical carcinoma

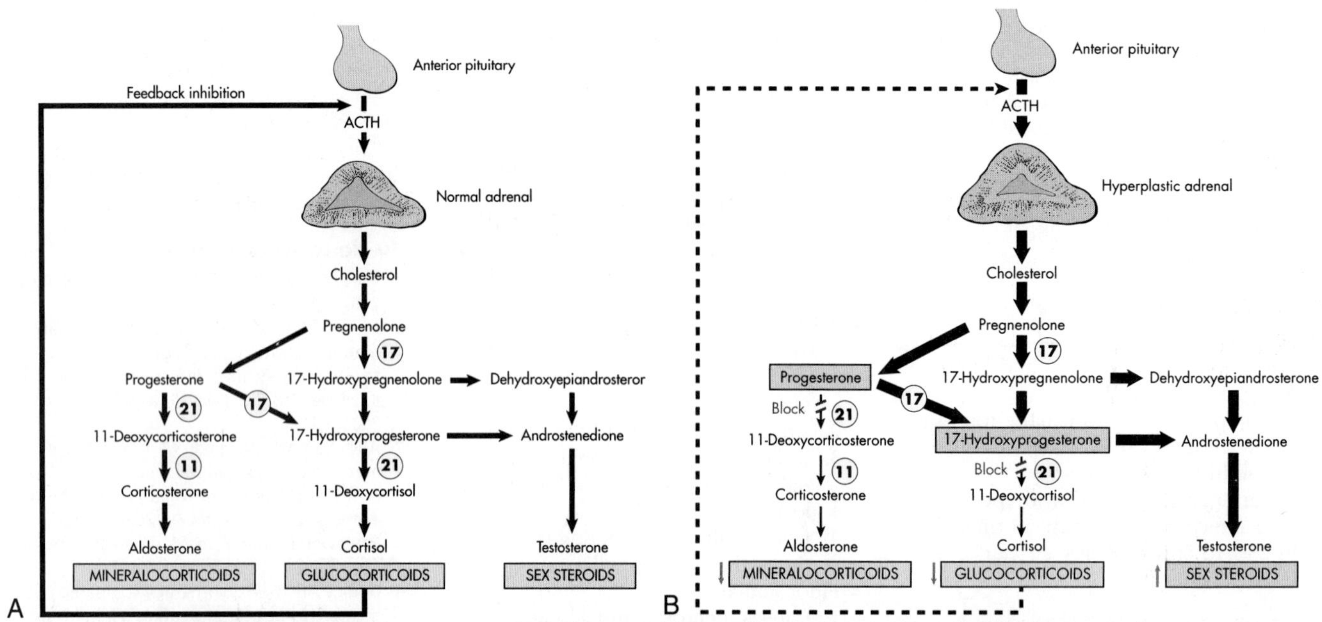

FIGURE 1-59 A, Normal adrenal steroidogenesis. **B,** Consequences of C-21 hydroxylase deficiency. (From Cotran R, Kumar V, Collins T [eds]: *Robbins pathologic basis of disease,* ed 6, Philadelphia, 1999, WB Saunders, p 1158.)

- Addison's disease
- Pituitary adenoma

LABORATORY TESTS

Laboratory tests (for 21-hydroxylase deficiency):

- Prenatal: chorionic villus sampling for genetic testing or measurement of 17-hydroxyprogesterone
- Neonates, children, and adults: screening for elevated 17-hydroxyprogesterone levels (not done by all states), high-dose cosyntropin stimulation test, and genotyping

IMAGING STUDIES

- Ultrasound to identify a uterus in cases of ambiguous genitalia.
- Ultrasound is preferred to rule out testicular adrenal rest tumors (found in classic and nonclassic forms) and should be done beginning in adolescence. MRI and color-flow Doppler may also be used for this purpose.

TREATMENT

Rx

NONPHARMACOLOGIC THERAPY

- Surgical correction of ambiguous genitalia is recommended by 6 months.
- Bilateral laparoscopic adrenalectomy with lifelong glucocorticoid and mineralocorticoid replacement (controversial).
- Gene therapy (hypothetical).

ACUTE GENERAL Rx

Overall goal is suppression of ACTH.

- Prenatal: dexamethasone 20 to 25 ug/kg/d in the first trimester in female fetuses only (controversial because long-term studies are unavailable).
- Infants: fludrocortisone 0.1 to 0.2 mg/d, hydrocortisone 5 to 15 mg/d, NaCl 1 to 2 gm/d.
- Stress states (e.g., major illness) require increased glucocorticoid dosing.

CHRONIC Rx

- Chronic Rx:
  - Children: hydrocortisone 10 to 30 mg/d (minimizes the risk of iatrogenic short stature found in other corticosteroids with longer half-lives).
  - Adolescents/Adults: dexamethasone 0.25 to 0.75 mg po QHS (also use to treat adrenal rests) or prednisone 5 to 7.5 mg/d.
  - Fludrocortisone: 0.1 to 0.2 mg/d (may decrease glucocorticoid requirement).
  - Experimental four-drug regimen: flutamide and testolactone in addition to hydrocortisone and fludrocortisone.
  - Psychologic counseling.
  - Monitoring: serum 17-hydroxyprogesterone and androstenedione, renin, electrolytes, blood pressure, bone age and density, Tanner staging, growth velocity, weight.
- Treatment of simple virilizing form: similar to salt-wasting form, but mineralocorticoid replacement is unnecessary.
- Treatment of nonclassic form:
  - In adolescent and adult women: oral contraceptives, glucocorticoids, and/or antiandrogens.
  - In children and adult males, usually no treatment is necessary.

PEARLS & CONSIDERATIONS

!

COMMENTS

- Consider the diagnosis of classic salt-wasting CAH in infants with failure to thrive.
- There is thought to be an increased prevalence of CAH in patients diagnosed with adrenal "incidentalomas"—adrenal gland lesions detected unexpectedly upon imaging, usually with MRI or CT scanning.
- Cushing's syndrome may result from overtreatment of CAH with glucocorticoids.
- Treatment of CAH in pregnancy with dexamethasone will confound newborn screening for 17-hydroxyprogesterone such that these infants should be screened 1 to 2 weeks postpartum.
- Patients with CAH may suffer from gender identity disorders and sexual dysfunction.

PREVENTION

- Early CVS sampling and maternal glucocorticoid administration (see above).
- Neonatal screening
- Genetic counseling

SUGGESTED READINGS

Levine L, DiGeorge A: Adrenal disorders and genital abnormalities: congenital adrenal hyperplasia. In Behrman R, Kliegman R, Jenson H (eds): *Nelson's Textbook of Pediatrics.* Philadelphia, 2000, WB Saunders, pp 1729-1737.

Merke DP et al: NIH conference: future directions in the study and management of congenital adrenal hyperplasia due to 21-hydroxylase deficiency, *Ann Intern Med* 136:320, 2002.

Speiser PW et al: Congenital adrenal hyperplasia, *N Engl J Med* 349:776, 2003.

AUTHOR: **NIRALI BORA, M.D.**

BASIC INFORMATION

DEFINITION

Congestive heart failure is a pathophysiologic state characterized by congestion in the pulmonary or systemic circulation. It is caused by the heart's inability to pump sufficient oxygenated blood to meet the metabolic needs of the tissues.

CLASSIFICATION:

The American College of Cardiology and the American Heart Association describe the following four stages of heart failure:

A. At high risk for heart failure, but without structural heart disease or symptoms of heart failure (e.g., CAD, hypertension)
B. Structural heart disease but without symptoms of heart failure
C. Structural heart disease with prior or current symptoms of heart failure
D. Refractory heart failure requiring specialized interventions

The New York Heart Association (NYHA) defines the following functional classes:

I. Asymptomatic
II. Symptomatic with moderate exertion
III. Symptomatic with minimal exertion
IV. Symptomatic at rest

SYNONYMS

CHF
Cardiac failure
Heart failure

ICD-9CM CODES
428.0 Congestive heart failure

EPIDEMIOLOGY & DEMOGRAPHICS

- CHF is the most common admission diagnosis (20%) in elderly patients.
- Heart failure occurs in 4.7 million persons in the U.S. and is the discharge diagnosis in 3.5 million hospitalizations annually.

PHYSICAL FINDINGS & CLINICAL PRESENTATION

The findings on physical examination in patients with CHF vary depending on the severity and whether the failure is right-sided or left-sided.

- Common clinical manifestations are:
  1. Dyspnea on exertion initially, then with progressively less strenuous activity, and eventually manifesting when patient is at rest; caused by increasing pulmonary congestion
  2. Orthopnea caused by increased venous return in the recumbent position
  3. Paroxysmal nocturnal dyspnea (PND) resulting from multiple factors (increased venous return in the recumbent position, decreased Pao_2, decreased adrenergic stimulation of myocardial function)
  4. Nocturnal angina resulting from increased cardiac work (secondary to increased venous return)
  5. Cheyne-Stokes respiration: alternating phases of apnea and hyperventilation caused by prolonged circulation time from lungs to brain
  6. Fatigue, lethargy resulting from low cardiac output
- Patients with failure of the left side of the heart will have the following abnormalities on physical examination: pulmonary rales, tachypnea, S_3 gallop, cardiac murmurs (AS, AR, MR), paradoxic splitting of S_2.
- Patients with failure of right side of the heart manifest with jugular venous distention, peripheral edema, perioral and peripheral cyanosis, congestive hepatomegaly, ascites, hepatojugular reflux.
- In patients with heart failure, elevated jugular venous pressure and a third heart sound are each independently associated with adverse outcomes.
- Acute precipitants of CHF exacerbations are: noncompliance with salt restriction, pulmonary infections, arrhythmias, medications (e.g., calcium channel blockers/antiarrhythmic agents), and inappropriate reductions in CHF therapy.

ETIOLOGY

LEFT VENTRICULAR FAILURE:

- Systemic hypertension
- Valvular heart disease (AS, AR, MR)
- Cardiomyopathy, myocarditis
- Bacterial endocarditis
- Myocardial infarction
- IHSS

Left ventricular failure is further differentiated according to systolic dysfunction (low ejection fraction) and diastolic dysfunction (normal or high ejection fraction), or "stiff ventricle." It is important to make this distinction because treatment is significantly different (see "Treatment"). Patients with heart failure and a normal ejection fraction have significant abnormalities in active relaxation and passive stiffness. In these patients, the pathophysiologic cause of elevated diastolic pressures and heart failure is abnormal diastolic function.

- Common causes of systolic dysfunction are post-MI, cardiomyopathy, myocarditis.
- Causes of diastolic dysfunction are hypertensive cardiovascular disease, valvular heart disease (AS, AR, MR, IHSS), restrictive cardiomyopathy.

RIGHT VENTRICULAR FAILURE:

- Valvular heart disease (mitral stenosis)
- Pulmonary hypertension
- Bacterial endocarditis (right-sided)
- Right ventricular infarction

BIVENTRICULAR FAILURE:

- Left ventricular failure
- Cardiomyopathy
- Myocarditis
- Arrhythmias
- Anemia
- Thyrotoxicosis
- AV fistula
- Paget's disease
- Beriberi

DIAGNOSIS

DIFFERENTIAL DIAGNOSIS

- Cirrhosis
- Nephrotic syndrome
- Venous occlusive disease
- COPD, asthma
- Pulmonary embolism
- ARDS
- Heroin overdose
- Pneumonia

WORKUP

- Echocardiography plays a critical diagnostic role in patients with heart failure. Doppler echocardiography, which measures the velocity of intracardiac blood flow, is also helpful in the assessment of diastolic function.
- Standard 12-lead ECG is useful to diagnose ischemic heart disease and obtain information about rhythm abnormalities. Over 25% of patients with CHF have some form of intraventricular conduction abnormality that is manifested as an increased QRS duration on ECG. The most common pattern is LBBB.
- Cardiac catheterization provides direct measurement of ventricular diastolic pressure and can demonstrate impaired relaxation and filling; however, it is invasive and indicated only in selected patients.

LABORATORY TESTS

- CBC (to rule out anemia, infections), BUN, creatinine, electrolytes, liver enzymes, TSH
- Beta-type natriuretic peptide (BNP) is a cardiac neurohormone specifically secreted from the ventricles in response to volume expansion and pressure overload. Elevated levels are indicative of left ventricular dysfunction. Bedside measurement of beta-type natriuretic peptide is useful in establishing or excluding the diagnosis of CHF in patients with acute dyspnea. Elevated BNP levels are also strong predictors of survival in patients with heart failure and possibly even in asymptomatic patients.

IMAGING STUDIES

- Chest x-ray:
  1. Pulmonary venous congestion
  2. Cardiomegaly with dilation of the involved heart chamber
  3. Pleural effusions

- Two-dimensional echocardiography is useful to assess global and regional left ventricular function and estimate ejection fraction.
- Exercise stress testing may be useful for evaluating concomitant coronary disease and assess degree of disability. The decision to perform exercise stress testing should be individualized.
- Cardiac catheterization remains an excellent method to evaluate ventricular diastolic properties, significant coronary artery disease, or valvular heart disease; however, it is invasive. The decision to perform cardiac catheterization should be individualized.

TREATMENT

NONPHARMACOLOGIC THERAPY

- Determine if CHF is secondary to systolic or diastolic dysfunction and treat accordingly.
- Identify and correct precipitating factors (i.e., anemia, thyrotoxicosis, infections, increased sodium load, medical noncompliance).
- Decrease cardiac workload in patients with systolic dysfunction: restrict patients' activity only during periods of acute decompensation; the risk of thromboembolism during this period can be minimized by using heparin 5000 U SC q12h in hospitalized patients. In patients with mild to moderate symptoms aerobic training may improve symptoms and exercise capacity.
- Restrict sodium intake to <2 g/day.
- Restricting fluid intake to 2 L or less may be useful in patients with hyponatremia.

ACUTE GENERAL Rx

TREATMENT OF CHF SECONDARY TO SYSTOLIC DYSFUNCTION:

1. ACE inhibitors:
   a. They cause dilation of the arteriolar resistance vessels and venous capacity vessels, thereby reducing both preload and afterload.
   b. They are associated with decreased mortality and improved clinical status when used in patients with CHF caused by systolic dysfunction. They are also indicated in patients with ejection fraction <40%.
   c. They can be used as first line therapy or they can be added to diuretics in patients with CHF poorly controlled with only diuretic therapy.
   d. Therapy with ACE inhibitors should be initiated at low dose (e.g., captopril 6.25 mg tid or enalapril 2.5 mg bid) to prevent hypotension and rapidly titrated up to high doses if tolerated.
   e. Contraindications to use of ACE inhibitors are renal insufficiency (creatinine >3.0 or creatinine clearance <30 ml/min), renal artery stenosis, persistent hyperkalemia (K^+ >5.5 mEQ/L), symptomatic hypotension, and history of adverse reactions (e.g., angioedema).
2. Diuretics: indicated in patients with systolic dysfunction and volume overload. The most useful approach to selecting the dose of, and monitoring the response to, diuretic therapy is by measuring body weight, preferably daily.
   a. Furosemide: 20 to 80 mg/day produces prompt venodilation and diuresis. IV therapy may produce diuresis when oral therapy has failed; when changing from IV to oral furosemide, doubling the dose is usually necessary to achieve an equal effect.
   b. Thiazides are not as powerful as furosemide but are useful in mild to moderate CHF.
   c. The addition of metolazone to furosemide enhances diuresis.
   d. Blockade of aldosterone receptors by spironolactone (12.5 to 25 mg qd) used in conjunction with ACE inhibitors reduces both mortality and morbidity in patients with severe CHF. It is generally not associated with hyperkalemia when used in low doses, however, serum electrolytes and renal function should be closely monitored after initiation of therapy and when changing doses. Spironolactone use should be considered in patients with recent or recurrent class IV (NYHA) symptoms.
   e. Frequent monitoring of renal function and electrolytes is recommended in all patients receiving diuretics.
3. Beta blockers: All patients with stable NYHA class II or III heart failure caused by left ventricular systolic dysfunction should receive a beta blocker unless they have a contraindication to its use or are intolerant to it. Beta blockers are especially useful in patients who remain symptomatic despite therapy with ACE inhibitors and diuretics. Carvedilol (Coreg) 3.125 mg bid initially, titrated upward as tolerated, is an effective agent.
4. Angiotensin II receptor blockers (ARBS) block the A-II type 1 (AT) receptor, which is responsible for many of the deleterious effects of angiotensin II. These receptors are potent vasoconstrictors that may contribute to the impairment of LV function. ARBS are useful in patients unable to tolerate ACE inhibitors because of angioedema or intractable cough. They can also be used in combination with a beta blocker.
5. Digitalis may be useful because of its positive inotropic and vagotonic effects in patients with CHF secondary to systolic dysfunction; it is of limited value in patients with mild CHF and normal sinus rhythm. It is more beneficial in patients with rapid atrial fibrillation, severe CHF, or ejection fraction of <30%; it can be added to diuretics and ACE inhibitors in patients with severe CHF. In patients with chronic heart failure and normal sinus rhythm, digoxin does not reduce mortality, but it does reduce the rate of hospitalization both overall and for worsening heart failure. Digoxin has a narrow therapeutic window. Its beneficial effects are found with a low dose that results in a serum concentration of approximately 0.7 ng/ml. Higher doses may be detrimental.
6. Direct vasodilating drugs (hydralazine and isosorbide) are useful in the therapy of systolic dysfunction with CHF because they can reduce the systemic vascular resistance and pulmonary venous pressure. Trials in black patients revealed that the combination of hydralazine and isosorbide is effective in advanced heart failure. Tolerability is an issue with over 20% of patients stopping the medications because of side effects.
7. Nesiritide (Natrecor): Usual nesiritide dosage is 2 mcg/kg IV bolus, then 0.01 mcg/kg/min. Use of nesiritide should be reserved for patients who present to the hospital with acutely decompensated heart failure and dyspnea at rest in whom standard combination therapy with diuretics and nitroglycerin has been inadequate. It should not be substituted for diuretics, used for intermittent outpatient infusion, or used repetitively.
8. Anticoagulants:
   a. Anticoagulation is not recommended for patients in sinus rhythm and no prior history of stroke, left ventricular thrombi, or arteriolar emboli.
   b. Anticoagulation therapy is appropriate for patients with heart failure and atrial fibrillation or a history of embolism.
9. Surgical revascularization should be considered in patients with both heart failure and severe limiting angina.
10. Antiarrhythmic therapy with amiodarone has a modest effect in reducing mortality in patients with CHF; however, it is not recommended for

general use in CHF. Its benefits must be weighed against the risk for adverse effects, especially potentially fatal pulmonary toxicity.

11. Atriobiventricular pacing significantly improves exercise tolerance and quality of life in patients with chronic heart failure and intraventricular conduction delay. Cardiac resynchronization therapy (CRT) reduces morbidity and mortality in patients with LV systolic dysfunction, prolonged QRS duration, and NYHA class 3 or 4 symptoms when combined with optimal pharmacotherapy.
12. Implantable cardioverter defibrillators are efficacious in reducing mortality for adult patients with LV systolic dysfunction.
13. The incremental benefits of combined CRT plus implantable cardioverter-defibrillator devices vs. CRT-alone devices remains to be determined.
14. Obstructive sleep apnea has an adverse effect on heart failure. Recognition and treatment of coexisting obstructive sleep apnea by continuous positive airway pressure reduces systolic blood pressure and improves left ventricular systolic function.
15. Tolvaptan, a new oral selective vasopressin V_2-receptor antagonist, has been reported beneficial in clinical trials when added to standard therapy in hospitalized patients with heart failure.

TREATMENT OF CHF SECONDARY TO DIASTOLIC DYSFUNCTION:

The initial treatment of diastolic heart failure should be directed at reducing the congestive state with the use of diuretics being careful not to avoid excessive diuresis. Long-term goals are to control hypertension, tachycardia, congestion, and ischemia. Therapeutic options are determined by the cause.

1. Hypertension
   a. Calcium channel blockers (verapamil)
   b. ACE inhibitors
   c. Beta blockers or verapamil to control heart rate and prolong diastolic filling
   d. Diuretics: vigorous diuresis should be avoided, because a higher filling pressure may be needed to maintain cardiac output in patients with diastolic dysfunction
   e. ARBs
2. Aortic stenosis
   a. Diuretics
   b. Contraindicated medications: ACE inhibitors, nitrates, digitalis (except to control rate of atrial fibrillation)
   c. Aortic valve replacement in patients with critical stenosis
3. Aortic insufficiency and mitral regurgitation
   a. ACE inhibitors increase cardiac output and decrease pulmonary wedge pressure. They are agents of choice along with diuretics.
   b. Hydralazine combined with nitrates can be used if ACE inhibitors are not tolerated.
   c. Surgery
4. IHSS
   a. Beta blockers or verapamil
   b. Contraindicated medications (they increase outlet obstruction by decreasing the size of the left ventricle in end systole): diuretics, digitalis, ACE inhibitors, hydralazine
   c. Restoration of intravascular volume with IV saline solution if necessary in acute pulmonary edema
   d. DDD pacing is useful in selected patients

TREATMENT OF CHF SECONDARY TO MITRAL STENOSIS:

1. Diuretics.
2. Control of the heart rate and atrial fibrillation with digitalis, verapamil, and/or beta blockers is critical to allow emptying of left atrium and relief of pulmonary congestion.
3. Repairing or replacing the mitral valve is indicated if CHF is not readily controlled by the above measures.
4. Balloon valvuloplasty is useful in selected patients.

DISPOSITION

- Annual mortality ranges from 10% in stable patients with mild symptoms to >50% in symptomatic patients with advanced disease.
- Sudden death secondary to ventricular arrhythmias occurs in >40% of patients with heart failure.
- Cardiac transplantation has a 5-yr survival rate of >70% in many centers and represents a viable option in selected patients.
- The use of a left ventricular assist device in patients with advanced heart failure can result in a clinically meaningful survival benefit and improve quality of life. It is an acceptable alternative therapy in selected patients who are not candidates for cardiac transplantation.
- In patients with advanced heart failure and a prolonged QRS interval, cardiac-resynchronization therapy decreases the combined risk of death from any cause or first hospitalization and, when combined with an implantable defibrillator, significantly reduces mortality.

COMMENTS

- Diabetes and obesity are established risk factors for CHF and both are associated with insulin resistance. Insulin resistance predicts CHF incidence independently of established risk factors, including diabetes.
- Sudden death from cardiac causes remains a leading cause of death among patients with CHF. In patients with NYHA class II or III CHF and LVEF ≤35% amiodarone has no favorable effect on survival, whereas single-lead, shock-only ICD therapy reduces overall mortality by 23%.

EVIDENCE

EBM

A large randomized controlled trial (RCT) compared patients with heart failure taking potassium-sparing diuretics and those that were not. It found that, after adjustment for covariates, the use of potassium-sparing diuretics was associated with a reduced risk of death from, or hospitalization for, progressive heart failure or all-cause or cardiovascular death, compared with patients taking only a non-potassium-sparing diuretic.[1] B

There is good evidence that ACE inhibitors reduce mortality rates in symptomatic left ventricular dysfunction or heart failure

A systematic review found that ACE inhibitors reduced mortality rates compared with placebo in patients with NYHA class III or IV heart failure.[2] A

Another systematic review found that ACE inhibitors significantly reduced rates of mortality, readmission for heart failure and reinfarction compared with placebo in patients with heart failure or left ventricular dysfunction.[3] A

There is evidence that angiotensin II receptor antagonists are effective as an alternative in patients with heart failure intolerant to ACE inhibitors

A systematic review compared angiotensin II receptor antagonists vs. placebo in people with NYHA class II to IV heart failure. There were nonsignificant trends for reductions in all-cause mortality and admissions for heart failure with angiotensin II receptor antagonists.[4] A

The review also compared angiotensin II receptor antagonists vs. ACE inhibitors in people with NYHA class II to IV heart failure. There was no significant difference between the drugs in terms of all-cause mortality or rate of admissions for heart failure. Combination therapy with angiotensin II receptor antagonists plus ACE inhibitors was found to be significantly more effective than ACE inhibitors alone in reducing admissions for heart failure, but there was no significant difference in all-cause mortality.[4] A

An RCT of patients with heart failure (NYHA class II to IV and LV ejection fraction of 40% or less) who were intolerant to ACE Inhibitors, compared candesartan vs. placebo. It found that there was a significant reduction in cardiovascular mortality and/or hospital admissions for chronic heart failure with candesartan compared with placebo.[5] Ⓐ

There is evidence that beta blockers, as an additive therapy, reduce death rates and hospital admission rates in patients with moderate and severe heart failure

Systematic reviews have found that beta blockers, when added to standard therapy with ACE inhibitors, are effective in reducing the rates of death and hospital admission in patients with moderate and severe heart failure.[6,7] Ⓐ

There is limited evidence, from a RCT of bucindolol vs. placebo in severe heart failure, that beta blockers do not have a significantly beneficial effect in African American people.[8] Ⓐ

There is evidence that the addition of spironolactone to existing medication in severe heart failure reduces mortality

An RCT found that spironolactone vs. placebo significantly reduced all-cause mortality at 2 years in patients with heart failure (NYHA class III to IV). Patients were also taking ACE inhibitors and loop diuretics, and most were also taking digoxin.[9] Ⓐ

Digoxin has been associated with lower rates of hospitalization in heart failure patients

A systematic review compared digitalis glycosides vs. placebo in patients with heart failure who were in sinus rhythm. Some patients were also receiving diuretics, ACE inhibitors, or beta blockers. There was no improvement in the mortality rate associated with digitalis, but lower rates of hospitalization and clinical deterioration were noted.[10] Ⓐ

There is limited evidence that implantation with cardiac resynchronization devices is associated with a reduction in mortality due to progressive heart failure but no long-term results are available as yet

A meta-analysis of four RCTs compared cardiac resynchronization vs control in patients with heart failure (NYHA class II to IV). Only trials that used implantable cardioverter defibrillators (ICDs) were included in the analysis. The control groups in the included studies had ICDs implanted, but the cardiac resynchronization was turned off. The authors concluded that cardiac resynchronization reduces mortality from progressive heart failure in patients with symptomatic left ventricular dysfunction. They also found a reduction in heart failure hospitalization.[11] Ⓑ

More evidence is required to define the benefit of anticoagulation in heart failure patients in sinus rhythm

An RCT (pilot study) included in a systematic review compared warfarin (international normalized ratio 2.5), aspirin (300 mg/day), and no antithrombotic treatment in patients with heart failure. It found no significant difference in the combined outcomes of death, myocardial infarction, and stroke between the warfarin and the no antithrombotic group after a mean of 27 months follow-up. It may be the case that this trial lacked power to detect a clinically important difference.[12,13] Ⓑ

The systematic review mentioned above, found evidence from a variety of study types for a reduction in mortality and cardiovascular events with anticoagulants compared with control. However, the authors conclude that although oral anticoagulation is indicated in certain groups of patients with heart failure (e.g., atrial fibrillation), the evidence available is not strong enough to advocate its routine use in heart failure patients in sinus rhythm.[13] Ⓑ

Evidence-Based References

1. Domanski M et al: Diuretic use, progressive heart failure, and death in patients in the studies of left ventricular dysfunction (SOLVD), *J Am Coll Cardiol* 42:705-708, 2003. Ⓑ
2. Garg R, Yusuf S: Overview of randomized trials of angiotensin-converting enzyme inhibitors on mortality and morbidity in patients with heart failure. Collaborative Group on ACE Inhibitor Trials, *JAMA* 273:1450-1456, 1995. Reviewed in: *Clin Evid* 12:115-143, 2004. Ⓐ
3. Flather M et al: Long-term ACE-inhibitor therapy in patients with heart failure or left-ventricular dysfunction: a systematic overview of data from individual patients. The ACE-inhibitor Myocardial Infarction Collaborative Group, *Lancet* 355:1575-1581, 2000. Reviewed in: *Clin Evid* 12:115-143, 2004. Ⓐ
4. Jong P et al: Angiotensin receptor blockers in heart failure: meta-analysis of randomized controlled trials, *J Am Coll Cardiol* 39:463-470, 2002. Reviewed in: *Clin Evid* 12:115-143, 2004. Ⓐ
5. Granger CB et al. (CHARM Investigators and Committees): Effects of candesartan in patients with chronic heart failure and reduced left-ventricular systolic function intolerant to angiotensin-converting-enzyme inhibitors: the CHARM-Alternative trial, *Lancet* 362:772-776, 2003. Reviewed in: *Clin Evid* 12:115-143, 2004. Ⓐ
6. Brophy JM, Joseph L, Rouleau JL: Beta-blockers in congestive heart failure: a Bayesian meta-analysis, *Ann Intern Med* 134:550-560, 2001. Reviewed in: *Clin Evid* 12:115-143, 2004. Ⓐ
7. Whorlow SL, Krum H: Meta-analysis of effect of β-blocker therapy on mortality in patients with New York Heart Association Class IV chronic congestive heart failure, *Am J Cardiol* 86:886-889, 2000. Reviewed in: *Clin Evid* 12:115-143, 2004. Ⓐ
8. The Beta-Blocker Evaluation of Survival Trial Investigators: A trial of the beta-blocker bucindolol in patients with advanced chronic heart failure, *N Engl J Med* 344:1659-1667, 2001. Reviewed in: *Clin Evid* 12:115-143, 2004. Ⓐ
9. Pitt B et al: Randomized Aldactone Evaluation Study Investigators. The effects of spironolactone on morbidity and mortality in patients with severe heart failure, *N Engl J Med* 341:709-717, 1999. Reviewed in: *Clin Evid* 12:115-143, 2004. Ⓐ
10. Hood WB et al: Digitalis for treatment of congestive heart failure in patients in sinus rhythm, *Cochrane Database Syst Rev* 2, 2004. Ⓐ
11. Bradley DJ et al: Cardiac resynchronization and death from progressive heart failure: a meta-analysis of randomized controlled trials, *JAMA* 289:730-740, 2003. Reviewed in: DARE Document 20038096. York, UK, Centre for Reviews and Dissemination.
12. Jones CG, Cleland JGF: Meeting report: the LIDO, HOPE, MOXCON, and WASH studies, *Eur J Heart Fail* 1:425-431, 1999. Reviewed in: *Clin Evid* 12:115-143, 2004. Ⓑ
13. Lip GYH, Gibbs CR: Anticoagulation for heart failure in sinus rhythm. *Cochrane Database Syst Rev* 2, 2000. Ⓑ

SUGGESTED READINGS

Aurigemma GP, Gaasch WH: Diastolic heart failure, *N Engl J Med* 351:1097, 2004.

Bardy GH et al: Amiodarone or an implantable cardioverter-defibrillator for congestive heart failure, *N Engl J Med* 352:225-237, 2005.

Bristow MR et al: Cardiac-resynchronization therapy with or without an implantable defibrillator in advanced chronic heart failure, *N Engl J Med* 350:2140, 2004.

Doust JA et al: How well does B-Type natriuretic peptide predict death and cardiac events in patients with heart failure: symptomatic review, *BMJ* 330:625-633, 2005.

Ezekowitz J et al: Systematic review: Implantable cardioverter defibrillators for adults with left ventricular systolic dysfunction, *Ann Intern Med* 147:251-262, 2007.

Gheorghiade M et al: Short-term clinical effects of tolvaptan, an oral vasopressin antagonist, in patients hospitalized for heart failure, *JAMA* 297:1332-1343, 2007.

Gutierrez C, Blanchard DG: Diastolic heart failure: challenges of diagnosis and treatment, *Am Fam Physician* 69:2609, 2004.

Ingelsson E et al: Insulin resistance and risk of congestive heart failure, *JAMA* 294:334-341, 2005.

McAlister FA et al: Cardiac resynchronization therapy for patients with left ventricular systolic dysfunction, *JAMA* 297:2502-2514, 2007.

Mueller C et al: Use of B-type natriuretic peptide in the evaluation and management of acute dyspnea, *N Engl J Med* 350:647, 2004.

Pfeffer MA et al: Valsartan, captopril, or both in myocardial infarction complicated by heart failure, left ventricular dysfunction, or both, *N Engl J Med* 349:1893, 2003.

Sackner-Bernstein DJ et al: Short-term risk of death after treatment with nesiritide for decompensated heart failure, *JAMA* 293:1900-1905, 2005.

Zile MR et al: Diastolic heart failure—abnormalities in active relaxation and passive stiffness of the left ventricle, *N Engl J Med* 350:1953, 2004.

AUTHOR: **FRED F. FERRI, M.D.**

BASIC INFORMATION

DEFINITION

The term *conjunctivitis* refers to an inflammation of the conjunctiva resulting from a variety of causes, including allergies and bacterial, viral, and chlamydial infections.

SYNONYMS

"Red eye"
Pink eye
Acute conjunctivitis
Subacute conjunctivitis
Chronic conjunctivitis
Purulent conjunctivitis
Pseudomembranous conjunctivitis
Papillary conjunctivitis
Follicular conjunctivitis
Newborn conjunctivitis

ICD-9CM CODES
372.30 Conjunctivitis, unspecified

EPIDEMIOLOGY & DEMOGRAPHICS

INCIDENCE (IN U.S.): Newborn 1.6% to 12%

PREVALENCE (IN U.S.):

- Allergic conjunctivitis, the most common form of ocular allergy, is usually associated with allergic rhinitis and may be seasonal or perennial
- Bacterial or viral conjunctivitis is often seasonal and can be extremely contagious

PREDOMINANT AGE: Occurs at any age

PEAK INCIDENCE: More common in the fall when viral infections and pollens increase

PHYSICAL FINDINGS & CLINICAL PRESENTATION

- Infection and chemosis of conjunctivae with discharge (Fig. 1-60)
- Cornea clear or can be involved
- Vision often normal, can be blurred

ETIOLOGY

- Bacterial
- Viral
- Chlamydial
- Allergic
- Traumatic

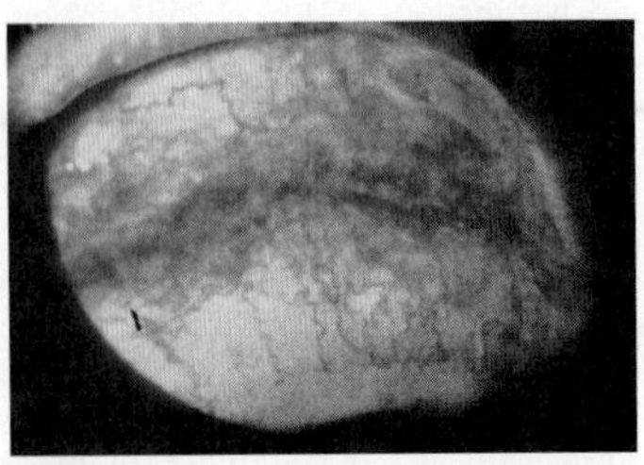

FIGURE 1-60 Conjunctival infection from viral conjunctivitis. (From Marx JA [ed]: *Rosen's emergency medicine,* ed 5, St Louis, 2002, Mosby.)

DIAGNOSIS

DIFFERENTIAL DIAGNOSIS

- Acute glaucoma
- Corneal lesions
- Acute iritis
- Episcleritis
- Scleritis
- Uveitis
- Canalicular obstruction
- The differential diagnosis of red eye is described in Section II

WORKUP

- History and physical examination
- Reports of itching, pain, visual changes

LABORATORY TESTS

Cultures are useful if not successfully treated with antibiotic medications; initial culture is usually not necessary.

TREATMENT

NONPHARMACOLOGIC THERAPY

- Warm compresses if infective conjunctivitis
- Cold compresses if irritative or allergic conjunctivitis

ACUTE GENERAL Rx

- Antibiotic drops (e.g., levofloxacin, ofloxin, ciprofloxacin, tobramycin, gentamicin ophthalmic solution one or two drops q2 to 4h) are indicated for suspected bacterial conjunctivitis.
- Caution: be careful with opthalmic corticosteroid treatment and avoid unless sure of diagnosis; corticosteroids can exacerbate infections and have been associated with increased intraocular pressure and cataract formation.
- An oral antihistamine (cetirizine, loratidine, desloratidine, or fexofenadine) is effective in relieving itching.
- Mast cell stabilizers (e.g., cromolyn [4%, 1 to 2 gtt q 4 to 6h], lodoxamine [Alomide, 0.1%, 1 to 2 gtt qid]) are effective on allergic conjunctivitis. Others include Elestat, Optivar, Patanol, etc.
- The topical NSAID ketorolac (Voltaren, 0.5%, 1 gtt qid) is also useful in allergic conjunctivitis but expensive.
- Antihistamine/decongestant combinations such as pheniramine/naphazoline (Visine A), available OTC, are more effective than either agent alone but have a short duration and can result in rebound vasodilatation with prolonged use. Others include Naphcon-A, Albacon-A, Opcon-A, etc.

CHRONIC Rx

- Depends on cause
- If allergic, nonsteroidals such as Voltaren, Acular, and Xibrom ophthalmic solution; mast cell stabilizers such as Alocril, Patanol, Zaditor are useful
- If infections, antibiotic drops (see "Acute General Rx")
- Dry eyes need artificial tears, ristasis, lacrameal duct plugs when indicated

DISPOSITION

Follow carefully for the first 2 wk to make sure secondary complications do not occur.

REFERRAL

To ophthalmologist if symptoms refractory to initial treatment

PEARLS & CONSIDERATIONS

COMMENTS

- Red eyes are not just conjunctivitis when there is significant pain or loss of sight. However, it is usually safe to treat pain-free eyes and the normal seeing red eye with lid hygene and topical treatment.
- Beware of patients wearing soft contact lenses and of babies and the elderly.
- Do not use steroids indiscriminately; use only when the diagnosis is certain.

EVIDENCE

Acute bacterial conjunctivitis is often self-limiting, but treatment with topical antibiotics improves the time to clinical recovery and rates of microbiological remission. The randomized controlled trials (RCTs) included in this systematic review were conducted in specialist centers, so the results may not be generalizable to a primary care population.[1] Ⓐ

An RCT found that combination treatment with naphazoline plus pheniramine and pheniramine alone were both effective in relieving symptoms associated with allergic conjunctivitis.[2] Ⓑ

Evidence-Based References

1. Sheikh A, Hurwitz B, Cave J: Antibiotics versus placebo for acute bacterial conjunctivitis, *Cochrane Database Syst Rev* 2:CD001211, 2000. Ⓐ
2. Dockhorn RJ, Duckett TG: Comparison of Naphcon-A and its components (naphazoline and pheniramine) in a provocative model of allergic conjunctivitis, *Curr Eye Res* 13:319, 1994. Ⓑ

AUTHOR: **MELVYN KOBY, M.D.**

BASIC INFORMATION

DEFINITION

Contact dermatitis is an acute or chronic skin inflammation, usually eczematous dermatitis resulting from exposure to substances in the environment. It can be subdivided into "irritant" contact dermatitis (nonimmunologic physical and chemical alteration of the epidermis) and "allergic" contact dermatitis (delayed hypersensitivity reaction).

SYNONYMS

Irritant contact dermatitis
Allergic contact dermatitis

ICD-9CM CODES
692 Contact dermatitis and other eczema

EPIDEMIOLOGY & DEMOGRAPHICS

- 20% of all cases of dermatitis in children are caused by allergic contact dermatitis.
- Rhus dermatitis (poison ivy, poison oak, and poison sumac) is responsible for most cases of contact dermatitis.
- Frequent causes of irritant contact dermatitis are soaps, detergents, and organic solvents.

PHYSICAL FINDINGS & CLINICAL PRESENTATION

IRRITANT CONTACT DERMATITIS:
- Mild exposure may result in dryness, erythema, and fissuring of the affected area (e.g., hand involvement in irritant dermatitis caused by exposure to soap, genital area involvement in irritant dermatitis caused by prolonged exposure to wet diapers).
- Eczematous inflammation may result from chronic exposure.

ALLERGIC CONTACT DERMATITIS:
- Poison ivy dermatitis can present with vesicles and blisters; linear lesions (as a result of dragging of the resins over the surface of the skin by scratching) are a classic presentation.
- The pattern of lesions is asymmetric; itching, burning, and stinging may be present.
- The involved areas are erythematous, warm to touch, swollen, and may be confused with cellulitis.

ETIOLOGY

- Irritant contact dermatitis: cement (construction workers), rubber, ragweed, malathion (farmers), orange and lemon peels (chefs, bartenders), hair tints, shampoos (beauticians), rubber gloves (medical, surgical personnel)
- Allergic contact dermatitis: poison ivy, poison oak, poison sumac, rubber (shoe dermatitis), nickel (jewelry), balsam of Peru (hand and face dermatitis), neomycin, formaldehyde (cosmetics)

DIAGNOSIS

DIFFERENTIAL DIAGNOSIS

- Impetigo
- Lichen simplex chronicus
- Atopic dermatitis
- Nummular eczema
- Seborrheic dermatitis
- Psoriasis
- Scabies

WORKUP

- Medical history: gradual onset vs. rapid onset, number of exposures, clinical presentation, occupational history
- Physical examination: contact dermatitis in the neck may be caused by necklaces, perfumes, after-shave lotion; involvement of the axillae is often secondary to deodorants, clothing; face involvement can occur with cosmetics, airborne allergens, aftershave lotion

LABORATORY TESTS

Patch testing is useful to confirm the diagnosis of contact dermatitis; it is indicated particularly when inflammation persists despite appropriate topical therapy and avoidance of suspected causative agent; patch testing should not be used for irritant contact dermatitis because this is a nonimmunologic-mediated inflammatory reaction.

TREATMENT

NONPHARMACOLOGIC THERAPY

Avoidance of suspected allergens

ACUTE GENERAL Rx

- Removal of the irritant substance by washing the skin with plain water or mild soap within 15 min of exposure is helpful in patients with poison ivy, poison oak, or poison sumac dermatitis.
- Cold or cool water compresses for 20 to 30 min five to six times a day for the initial 72 hr are effective during the acute blistering stage.
- Oral corticosteroids (e.g., prednisone 20 mg bid for 6 to 10 days) are generally reserved for severe, widespread dermatitis.
- IM steroids (e.g., Kenalog) are used for severe reactions and in patients requiring oral corticosteroids but unable to tolerate PO.
- Oral antihistamines (e.g., hydroxyzine 25 mg q6h) will control pruritus, especially at night; calamine lotion is also useful for pruritus; however, it can lead to excessive drying.
- Colloidal oatmeal (Aveeno) baths can also provide symptomatic relief.
- Patients with mild to moderate erythema may respond to topical steroid gels or creams.
- Patients with shoe allergy should change their socks at least once a day; use of aluminum chloride hexahydrate in a 20% solution (Drysol) qhs will also help control perspiration.
- Use hypoallergenic surgical gloves in patients with rubber and surgical glove allergy.

DISPOSITION

Allergic contact dermatitis generally resolves within 2 to 4 wk if reexposure to allergen is prevented.

REFERRAL

For patch testing in selected patients (see Laboratory Tests)

PEARLS & CONSIDERATIONS

COMMENTS

Commercially available corticosteroid dose packs should be avoided, because they generally provide an inadequate amount of medication.

EVIDENCE

A double-blind, intra-individual comparative study with 18 volunteers comparing 0.05% clobetasone butyrate vs its emollient carrier base alone vs 1% hydrocortisone cream vs no treatment in nickel-induced contact dermatitis found that 0.05% clobetasone butyrate had a significantly better response in terms of a physician's global assessment than hydrocortisone 1% cream or no treatment, though it was not significantly better than its emollient base alone.[1] Ⓑ

There is evidence that tacrolimus 0.1% ointment is significantly better than placebo in the treatment of nickel-induced contact dermatitis.

A double-blind, randomized, controlled, bilateral paired comparison study of topical 0.1% tacrolimus ointment in the treatment of nickel-induced allergic contact dermatitis found evidence that tacrolimus was significantly more effective than placebo in ameliorating the nickel reaction in volunteers and patient groups.[2] Ⓑ

Evidence-Based References

1. Parneix-Spake A et al: Eumovate (clobetasone butyrate) 0.05% cream with its moisturizing emollient base has better healing properties than hydrocortisone 1% cream: a study in nickel-induced contact dermatitis, *J Dermatol Treat* 12:191, 2001. Ⓑ
2. Saripalli YV et al: Tacrolimus ointment 0.1% in the treatment of nickel-induced allergic contact dermatitis, *J Am Acad Dermatol* 49:477, 2003. Ⓑ

AUTHOR: **FRED F. FERRI, M.D.**

BASIC INFORMATION

DEFINITION

Contraception refers to the various modalities that a sexually active couple use to prevent pregnancy. These options can be either medical or nonmedical and used by men or women or both. The options are as follows:

- No contraception: failure rate 85% both typical and perfect
- Abstinence
  1. 12.4% of unmarried men
  2. 13.2% of unmarried women
  3. More frequently practiced before age 17 yr
  4. No intercourse experienced by 13% of women ages 30 to 34 yr
  5. Failure rate 0%
- Withdrawal
  1. Used in only 2% of sexually active women
  2. Failure rate with perfect use, 4%; with typical use, 19%
- Rhythm method (natural family planning)
  1. Failure rate with perfect use, 1% to 9%; with typical use, 20%
  2. Symptothermal type: mucus method and ovulation pain combined with basal body temperature
  3. Ovulation (Billings' method): takes into account mucus quality
  4. Basal body temperature method: uses biphasic temperature chart
  5. Lactation amenorrhea method: effective in fully breast-feeding women, especially 70 to 100 days after delivery; depends on number of feedings per day
- Barriers
  1. Diaphragm and cervical cap: failure rate 5% to 9% in nulliparous women, 20% in multiparous women
  2. Female condom: failure rate with perfect use, 5.1%; with typical use, 12.4%; FDA labeling states 25% failure rate
  3. Male condom: failure rate with perfect use, 3%, with typical use, 12%
  4. Spermicides (aerosols, foam, jellies, creams, tabs): failure rate with perfect use, 3%; with typical use, 21%
- Oral contraceptives
  1. Failure rate with perfect use, <1%; with typical use, 3%
  2. Come in combinations of estrogen/progestin or as progestin only
- Hormonal implants and injectables
  1. Norplant
     a. Most typically used in U.S.
     b. Failure rate in first 5 yr: 1%
     c. Failure rate after 6 yr: 2%
     d. May be extended to 7 yr use
  2. Depo-Provera: failure rate 0.3% in first year of use
  3. Lunelle (approved October 2000): failure rate 0.2% in first year
  4. Etonogestrel implant: 2-yr cumulative pregnancy rate 0%
  5. Nestorone-releasing single implant: not yet available
  6. Jadelle implant
- Mini pill (progesterone only pill)
  1. Failure rate with typical use, 1.1% to 13.2%
  2. With perfect use, 5 pregnancies/1000 women
- Emergency postcoital contraception
  1. Decreases pregnancy rate by 75% with women treated immediately postcoitally
  2. Involves hormonal use or IUD insertion
- IUD (available OTC in some states)
  1. Progestasert: failure rate with perfect use, 2%; with typical use, 3%
  2. Copper T (380-A): failure rate with perfect use, 0.8%; with typical use, 3%
  3. Levonorgestrel Intrauterine System (Mirena)
     a. 1-yr failure rate, 1%
     b. 5-yr cumulative failure rate, 0.71/100 women
- Female sterilization (tubal ligation): failure rate with perfect use, 0.2%; with typical use, 3%
- Male sterilization (vasectomy): failure rate of 0.1% in first year
- Vaginal ring (Nuva ring): failure rate pearl index 0.77
- Contraceptive patch (Orthoevra): failure rate 0.4% to 0.7%

SYNONYMS

Birth control
Family planning

ICD-9CM CODES
V25.01 Oral contraceptives
V25.02 Other contraceptive measures
V25.09 Family planning
V25.1 IUD
V25.2 Sterilization

EPIDEMIOLOGY & DEMOGRAPHICS

For women at risk for pregnancy, ranges for USE of most commonly used birth control are age-dependent, as follows:

- Oral contraceptives: 3% (40 to 44 yr) to 60% (20 to 24 yr)
- Condoms: 9% (40 to 44 yr) to 26% (15 to 19 yr)
- Diaphragm: 0.8% (15 to 19 yr) to 8% (30 to 34 yr)
- Periodic abstinence: 0.7% (15 to 19 yr) to 3% (35 to 39 yr)
- Withdrawal: 1.1% (40 to 44 yr) to 3% (20 to 30 yr)
- IUD: 0% (15 to 19 yr) to 3% (30 to 34 yr)
- Spermicides: 0.8% (15 to 19 yr) to 2.7% (35 to 39 yr)
- No method: 6.3% (35 to 39 yr) to 19.8% (15 to 19 yr)
- Sterilization
  Female: 0.2% (15 to 19 yr) to 47% (40 to 44 yr)
  Male: 0.2% (15 to 19 yr) to 21% (40 to 44 yr)

Women are more likely to use contraception. The only two male forms available are condoms and vasectomy (sterilization).

DIAGNOSIS

WORKUP

- Thorough medical history
- Thorough surgical history
- Obstetric history (fertility desired?)
- Gynecologic history, including:
  1. History of previous sexually transmitted diseases
  2. Number of partners
  3. Previous difficulties with contraception
  4. Frequency of intercourse
- Family history

LABORATORY TESTS

- Pap smear
- Cultures, aerobic and *Chlamydia*
- Pregnancy test if suspected pregnancy
- Lipid profile if family history of premature vascular event

TREATMENT

NONPHARMACOLOGIC THERAPY

- Male condoms
  1. 95% latex (rubber), 5% skin or natural membrane
  2. Proper use: place on an erect penis and leave one-half-inch empty space at the tip of the condom; use with non-oil-based lubricants
  3. Effectiveness increased when used with spermicides
- Female condoms
  1. Composed of polyurethane, with one end open and one end closed
  2. Proper use: place closed end over cervix, open end hanging out of vagina to cover penis and scrotum
  3. Highly effective against HIV
- Spermicides
  1. Types: nonoxynol, octoxynol
  2. Forms: jellies, creams, foams, suppositories, tablets, soluble films
  3. Proper use: put in immediately before intercourse; may be used with other barrier methods
- Diaphragm and cervical cap
  1. Must be fitted by practitioner, used with contraceptive gels, and refitted with weight gain or loss
  2. Diaphragm sizes: 50 to 95 mm; cervical cap sizes: 22, 25, 28, and 31 mm
  3. Proper use of diaphragm: put in immediately before intercourse and

keep in for 6 hr after intercourse; must not remain in the vagina for longer than 24 hr
4. Proper use of cervical cap: fit over the cervix exactly; must not remain in place for longer than 48 hr

- Lactation amenorrhea method
  1. Depends on number of breast-feedings per day; effective as birth control for 6 mo if 15 or more feedings, lasting 10 min each, are accomplished daily
  2. Not a common practice in the U.S.
- Withdrawal
  1. Withdrawal of the penis from the vagina before ejaculation
  2. Dependent on self-control
- Rhythm method
  1. Dependent on awareness of physiology of male and female reproductive tracts
  2. Sperm viable in vagina for 2 to 7 days
  3. Ovum life span 24 hr
- Sterilization
  1. Male:
     a. Vasectomy to interrupt vas deferens and block passage of sperm to seminal ejaculate
     b. Scalpel and nonscalpel techniques available
     c. More easily performed procedure than female sterilization and does not require general anesthesia
  2. Female:
     a. Leading method of birth control in U.S. in women older than 30 yr
     b. Interrupts fallopian tubes, blocking passage of ovum proximally and sperm distally through tube
     c. Several types; modified Pomeroy done during cesarean section or laparoscopic done in nonpregnant females most common
     d. Essure-tubal occlusion through hysteroscopic placement of micro-inserts into the fallopian tubes.

ACUTE GENERAL Rx

- Combination oral contraceptives
  1. Taken daily for 21 days, pill-free interval of 7 days
  2. Less than 50 μg ethynyl estradiol in most common combination oral contraceptives; progestins most commonly used in combination pills are norethindrone, levonorgestrel, norgestrel, norethindrone acetate, ethynodiol diacetate, norgestimate, or desogestrel; triphasic combination oral contraceptives (give varying doses of progestin and estrogens throughout cycle); monophasic oral contraceptives: offer same dose of progestin and estrogen throughout cycle, taken daily at same time; estrophasic pill (constant progesterone with variation of estrogen throughout the cycle)
  3. If pill taken with antibiotics, efficacy affected by inadequate gastrointestinal absorption in most cases; only rifampin truly reduces pill's effectiveness
  4. Increased body weight decreases effectiveness
- Mini pill
  1. Progestin only; taken without a break
  2. Causes much irregular bleeding because of the lack of estrogen effect on the lining of the uterus
- Hormonal implants and injectables
  1. Norplant
     a. Progestin only; inserted under the skin
     b. Six levonorgestrel implants placed subcutaneously in upper inner arm effective for 5 yr
  2. Depo-Provera
     a. Medroxyprogesterone acetate given every 3 mo in IM injection form
     b. Major side effect: irregular bleeding
     c. Fertility return possibly delayed up to 18 mo after discontinuation
  3. Lunelle: monthly injectable administered intramuscularly. Contains 0.5 ml aqueous, 5 mg estradiol cypionate and 25 mg medroxyprogesterone acetate
  4. Etonogestrel implant: single-rod release etonogestrel for 3 yr placed subdermally
- Postcoital contraception
  1. Done on emergency basis, usually secondary to noncompliance with birth control or failure of birth control (e.g., condom breakage) at the time of ovulation
  2. Methods:
     a. IUD insertion within 7 days of coitus
     b. Hormonal methods (combination pills and danazol) given within 48 hr of coitus
- IUD
  1. Device inserted into uterus to prevent sperm and ovum from uniting in fallopian tube
  2. Types available in the U.S.:
     a. Progestasert: a T-shaped device that is an ethylene vinyl acetate copolymer T; vertical stem contains 38 mg progesterone and must be changed yearly
     b. ParaGard (Copper T/380-A): a polyethylene T wrapped with a fine copper wire that is effective for 10 yr of use
     c. Mirena Levonorgestrel Intrauterine System (LNGIUS): a T-shaped system with a chamber that contains LNG. Releases 20 μg per day; is effective for 5 yr
- Vaginal ring (brand name Nuvaring)
  1. Provides daily dose of 120 μg of etonogestrel and 15 μg ethinyl estradiol
  2. Stays in vagina 3 wk and removed the fourth
  3. Increased body weight decreases effectiveness
- Contraceptive patch (brand name Evra)
  1. Provides low daily dose of steroids
  2. Releases a progestin and estrogen (ethinyl estradiol)
  3. Patch size 20 cm^2
  4. Each patch contains 6 mg norelgestronin and delivers an estimated continuous systemic dose of 150 μg norelgestronin and 20 μg of ethinyl estradiol; common dose 250 μg/day progestin and 25 μg/day estrogen
  5. Worn 3 of 4 wk
  6. Increased body weight decreases effectiveness

CHRONIC Rx

- With all of the previously mentioned types of birth control, patient is followed at least yearly, or as necessary, if problems arise.
- Full history, physical examination, and Pap smear, including cultures when needed, are performed yearly.
- Patients with medical problems are followed about every 6 mo when taking hormonal therapy.

DISPOSITION

- Follow yearly or more frequently according to patient's side effects.
- Tailor birth control to patient according to different needs or side effects present at different times in life.

REFERRAL

With hormonal contraception, if neurologic or cardiac symptoms arise, stop method immediately, evaluate, and refer to internist when appropriate.

AUTHORS: **MARIA A. CORIGLIANO, M.D.,** and **RUBEN ALVERO, M.D.**

BASIC INFORMATION

DEFINITION

Conversion disorder is a form of somatization involving symptoms or deficits of the voluntary central nervous system that cannot be explained by known disease, usually in the setting of psychological stress. Patients do not willfully control their symptoms, distinguishing conversion disorder from factitious disorder and malingering.

SYNONYMS

Somatoform disorder (conversion disorder is a subset of this larger group)

ICD-9CM CODES
V61 10

EPIDEMIOLOGY & DEMOGRAPHICS

- Incidence estimated at 5 to 10/100,000 in general population, 20 to 100/100,000 in hospital inpatients
- All ages, including early childhood
- Women > men (ratios range from 2:1 to 5:1)
- Highest in rural areas, among under-educated, and in lower socioeconomic classes
- Associated with axis I disorders (depression > anxiety) and axis II disorders (most commonly histrionic, passive-dependent, and passive-aggressive)

PHYSICAL FINDINGS & CLINICAL PRESENTATION

- Presents with pseudoneurologic signs or symptoms.
- Signs or symptoms do not correlate with known organic disease patterns and instead reflect the patient's concept of the disease.
- Symptoms occur in isolation (as compared to multisystem involvement in somatization disorder).
- Motor symptoms may include weakness, paralysis, aphonia, and involuntary movements, including pseudoseizures.
- Sensory deficits may include anesthesia (especially of extremities), blindness, and deafness.
- Findings occur in the setting of marked psychological stress.
- The symptoms or signs persist whether the patient is observed or unobserved, though are typically worse when the patient is attentive to them.
- May last from hours to years.
- Classic features such as *la belle indifference* (patients seem undisturbed by their signs or symptoms) or secondary gain need not be present for diagnosis.

ETIOLOGY

- Complex interplay of neurologic and psychologic factors.
- Functional brain imaging studies suggest alterations in processing of sensory and motor signals.

DIAGNOSIS

DIFFERENTIAL DIAGNOSIS

- Broad differential diagnosis depending on presenting signs and symptoms
- Myasthenia gravis
- Neurologic disorders (multiple sclerosis, CNS neoplasm, Guillain-Barré syndrome, amyotrophic lateral sclerosis, Parkinson's disease, seizure disorder)
- Systemic lupus erythematosus
- Spinal cord compression
- Intracerebral hemorrhage
- Drug-induced dystonia
- HIV (or early manifestations of AIDS)

WORKUP

Thorough history and physical examination, including careful neurologic examination

LABORATORY TESTS

- No gold standard diagnostic tests exist; no single associated finding is pathognomonic.
- Laboratory tests or procedures may be needed to rule out other etiologies (e.g., EEG for seizures, EMG for lower motor neuron paralysis, optokinetic drum test in blindness).

IMAGING STUDIES

As indicated by presenting signs and symptoms

TREATMENT

NONPHARMACOLOGIC THERAPY

- Treatment success has been associated with a caring, long-term relationship between patient and physician and a safe, nonconfrontational approach.
- Physical and occupational therapy can help "retrain" the patient in normal behaviors.
- Psychotherapy (including cognitive-behavioral therapy) and addressing stress management may be effective in reducing symptoms.

ACUTE GENERAL Rx

- Studies have shown no additional benefit to hypnosis, although significant experience exists with barbiturate-induced hypnosis as a psychotherapeutic aid.
- Antidepressants may be helpful in treating underlying mood or anxiety disorders.
- Patients with long-standing symptoms may require inpatient treatment.

CHRONIC Rx

See "Nonpharmacologic Therapy" and "Acute General Rx."

DISPOSITION

Long-term follow-up is essential to address recurrent conversion reactions and underlying mood disorders.

REFERRAL

Refer to rule out other psychiatric disorders and for psychotherapy.

PEARLS & CONSIDERATIONS

COMMENTS

- Good prognostic factors: sudden onset, presence of psychologic stressors at onset of symptoms, short duration between diagnosis and treatment, high level of intelligence, absence of other psychiatric or medical disorders, and no ongoing compensation litigation.
- Poor prognostic factors: severe disability, long duration of symptoms, age >40 at symptom onset, and convulsions and paralysis as presenting symptoms.

EVIDENCE

A randomized controlled trial of cognitive-behavioral therapy in the treatment of medically unexplained symptoms found that, at 6-month follow-up, 82% of patients and 64% of controls had improved (a significant difference) and that this difference was largely maintained at 12 months.[1] Ⓑ

Evidence-Based Reference

1. Speckens AEM et al: Cognitive behavioural therapy for medically unexplained physical symptoms: a randomised controlled trial, *BMJ* 311:1328, 1995. Ⓑ

SUGGESTED READINGS

Hinson VK, Haren WB: Psychogenic movement disorders, *Lancet Neurol* 5:695, 2006.

Hurwitz TA: Somatization and conversion disorder, *Can J Psychiatry* 49(3):172, 2004.

Servan-Schreiber D et al: Somatizing patients: part II. Practical management, *Am Fam Physician* 61:1423, 2000.

AUTHOR: **KARA CHEW, M.D.**

BASIC INFORMATION

DEFINITION

Cor pulmonale is an alteration in the structure and function of the right ventricle due to pulmonary hypertension caused by diseases of the lungs or pulmonary vasculature. It is a state of cardiopulmonary dysfunction that may result from multiple etiologies rather than a specific disease state. Right-sided heart failure resulting from primary disease of the left heart or congenital heart disease are not considered in this disorder.

SYNONYMS

Acute cor pulmonale
Chronic cor pulmonale

ICD-9CM CODES
415.0 Cor pulmonale, acute
416.9 Cor pulmonale, chronic

ETIOLOGY

Most conditions that cause cor pulmonale are chronic. Acute cor pulmonales are often life threatening but transient. For example, acute pulmonary embolus may present with acute cor pulmonale, cardiogenic shock, or death, but if the patient survives the initial event, then the right ventricle often recovers and cor pulmonale is no longer existent after several weeks.

Mechanisms leading to pulmonary hypertension and predisposing to the development of cor pulmonale include:

- Pulmonary vasoconstriction resulting from any condition causing alveolar hypoxia and/or acidosis
- Anatomic reduction of the pulmonary vascular bed (e.g., emphysema, interstitial lung disease, pulmonary emboli)
- Increased blood viscosity (e.g., polycythemia vera, Waldenström's macroglobulinemia)

PHYSICAL FINDINGS & CLINICAL PRESENTATION

No symptoms are specific for cor pulmonale. Typically, the symptoms depend on the underlying disease process. They include:

- Dyspnea, fatigue, chest pain or syncope with exertion (secondary to pulmonary hypertension)
- Right upper quadrant abdominal pain and anorexia (secondary to passive hepatic congestion)
- Hoarseness (caused by compression of the left recurrent laryngeal nerve by dilation of the main pulmonary artery; known as Ortner's syndrome)
- Signs of right ventricular failure: jugular venous distention, peripheral edema, hepatic congestion, ascites, and a right ventricular third heart sound
- Signs of associated tricuspid regurgitation: holosystolic murmur heard best along the left parasternal border (augments during inspiration), prominent V-wave on jugular venous pulse, and pulsatile hepatomegaly (in severe tricuspid regurgitation)
- Pulmonary hypertension will increase the intensity of the pulmonic component of S2, which may be narrowly split
- Rarely, cough and hemoptysis

WORKUP

Search for an underlying pulmonary process resulting in pulmonary hypertension:

- Left ventricular dysfunction should be excluded in initial assessment.
- 80% to 90% of cor pulmonale cases are due to COPD.
- Consideration of alveolar hypoventilation, chronic thromboembolic disease, and neuromuscular disease should be given in the absence of parenchymal lung disease.

LABORATORY TESTS

- CBC may show erythrocytosis secondary to chronic hypoxia.
- Arterial blood gas (ABG) confirms hypoxemia and acidosis or hypercapnia.
- Pulmonary function tests.

IMAGING STUDIES

- Chest x-ray may show underlying pulmonary disease and evidence of pulmonary hypertension (e.g., enlargement of the pulmonary arteries or right atrium, and right ventricular dilation).
- Electrocardiogram may reveal right ventricular hypertrophy, right atrial enlargement (P-pulmonale), right-axis deviation, or incomplete/complete right bundle branch block.
- Echocardiogram to detect right ventricular enlargement and/or hypertrophy and estimate pulmonary artery pressure.
- Radionuclide ventriculography to measure right ventricular ejection fraction, which may be reduced.
- Cardiac MRI can accurately measure right ventricular dimensions and function.
- Right-sided heart catheterization measures pulmonary artery pressures and pulmonary vascular resistance. It can also determine response to oxygen or vasodilators.
- Chest CT can assess for pulmonary parenchymal disease and embolus in the pulmonary vasculature.

TREATMENT

The treatment of cor pulmonale is directed toward the underlying etiology while at the same time reversing hypoxemia, improving right ventricular contractility, decreasing pulmonary artery vascular resistance, and improving pulmonary hypertension

NONPHARMACOLOGIC THERAPY

- Continuous positive airway pressure (CPAP) is used in patients with obstructive sleep apnea.
- Phlebotomy is reserved as adjunctive therapy in patients with polycythemia (hematocrit >55%) who have acute decompensation of cor pulmonale or remain polycythemic despite long-term oxygen therapy. Phlebotomy has been shown to decrease mean pulmonary artery pressure and pulmonary vascular resistance.

ACUTE GENERAL Rx

- Pulmonary embolism is the most common cause of acute cor pulmonale (see "Pulmonary Embolism"). The treatment is anticoagulation, hemodynamic support, and consideration of thrombolytics
- In patients with preexisting cor pulmonale, acute pulmonary illnesses or hypoxia can increase pulmonary hypertension and worsen right ventricular function. The underlying exacerbating conditions should be treated.

CHRONIC Rx

- Long-term oxygen supplementation improves survival in hypoxemic patients with COPD.
- Right ventricular volume overload should be treated with diuretics (e.g., furosemide). However, over-diuresis can reduce right ventricular filling and decrease cardiac output
- Theophylline and sympathomimetic amines may improve diaphragmatic excursion, myocardial contraction, and pulmonary artery vasodilation.
- The long-term use of nonselective vasodilators including nitrates, calcium channel blockers, and angiotensin-converting enzyme inhibitors has not resulted in significant survival improvement. This is probably due to a lack of vasoreactivity in patients with COPD, as well as the risk of worsening of ventilation/perfusion mismatch and systemic vasodilation. Vasodilators to combat pulmonary hypertension should not be administered empirically in the absence of a right-sided heart catheterization.

DISPOSITION

The level of pulmonary artery pressure in COPD patients with cor pulmonale is a good indicator of prognosis. Right ventricular function may provide additional information.

REFERRAL

Patients with pulmonary disease that have progressed to cor pulmonale should be followed by a pulmonologist.

PEARLS & CONSIDERATIONS

- There is no differential diagnosis, but rather an evaluation of the patient to identify the underlying cause.
- Prognosis and treatment are related to the underlying cause, whereas the presence of cor pulmonale is merely a marker of the underlying disease severity

COMMENTS

There is increasing interest in selective pulmonary vasodilators to improve right ventricular heart function in patients with cor pulmonale.

EVIDENCE

EBM

A randomized controlled trial (RCT) found that domiciliary oxygen given at a rate of 2 L/min for at least 15 hr/day to patients with COPD who were very hypoxic significantly reduced mortality vs. no oxygen therapy over 5 years.[1] Ⓐ

A systematic review concluded that long-term oxygen therapy improved survival in those patients with COPD and severe hypoxemia, but not in those with moderate hypoxemia or only arterial desaturation at night. Four out of five of the RCTs included did not specifically include those diagnosed with cor pulmonale.[2] Ⓐ

Evidence-Based References

1. Medical Research Council Working Party: Long-term domiciliary oxygen therapy in chronic hypoxic cor pulmonale complicating chronic bronchitis and emphysema, *Lancet* 1:681, 1981. Ⓐ
2. Cranston JM et al: Domiciliary oxygen for chronic obstructive pulmonary disease, *Cochrane Database Syst Rev,* Issue 4, Chichester, UK, 2005, John Wiley & Sons, Ltd, pp. 27. Ⓐ

SUGGESTED READINGS

Lehrman S et al: Primary pulmonary hypertension and cor pulmonale, *Cardiol Rev* 10(5):265-278, 2002.

Weitzenblum E: Chronic cor pulmonale, *Heart* 89(2):225-230, 2003.

AUTHORS: **BRIAN CASSERLY, M.D.,** and **GAURAV CHOUDHARY, M.D.**

BASIC INFORMATION

DEFINITION

A corneal abrasion is a loss of surface epithelial tissue of the cornea caused by trauma.

SYNONYMS

Corneal erosion
Corneal contusion

ICD-9CM CODES
918.1 Corneal abrasion

EPIDEMIOLOGY & DEMOGRAPHICS

INCIDENCE (IN U.S.): A universal problem

PEAK INCIDENCE: Childhood through active adulthood and older and debilitated patients

PREDOMINANT AGE: Any age

PHYSICAL FINDINGS & CLINICAL PRESENTATION

- Haziness of the cornea
- Disruption of the corneal surface (Fig. 1-61)
- Redness and infection of the conjunctiva
- Pain
- Light sensitivity
- Tearing
- Foreign body sensation
- Gritty feeling
- Pain on opening or closing eyes
- Sensation of a foreign body

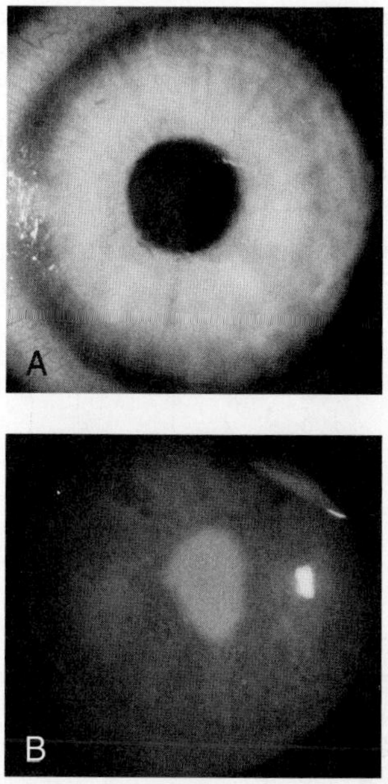

FIGURE 1-61 Corneal epithelial abrasion. A, Epithelial defect without fluorescein highlighting the defect. An irregularity in the otherwise smooth corneal surface is the key to identifying the defect if no fluorescein is available. **B,** Classic fluorescein staining of an epithelial defect. (From Palay D [ed]: *Ophthalmology for the primary care physician,* St Louis, 1997, Mosby.)

ETIOLOGY

- Trauma (direct mechanical event)
- Foreign body
- Contact lenses
- Unknown etiology

DIAGNOSIS

DIFFERENTIAL DIAGNOSIS

- Acute angle glaucoma
- Herpes ulcers and other corneal ulcers
- Foreign body in the cornea (be certain it is not a keratitis)

WORKUP

- Fluorescein staining, slit lamp evaluation
- Assessment of visual acuity
- Intraocular pressure
- Rule out corneal laceration
- Rule out other eye pathology

TREATMENT

NONPHARMACOLOGIC THERAPY

- Patching is controversial (see below).
- Bandage.
- Contact lenses.
- Warm compresses.
- Pressure dressing is controversial. Although eye patching traditionally has been recommended in the treatment of corneal abrasions, several studies show that patching does not help and may hinder healing.
- Removal of any foreign particles if present.

ACUTE GENERAL Rx

- Topical antibiotics such as 10% sulfacetamide or ofloxacin 0.3% solution 2 drops qid.
- Pressure patching of eye with eyelid closed is no longer recommended because it can result in decreased oxygen delivery, increased moisture, and a higher chance of infection.
- Cycloplegics such as 5% homatropine are often prescribed to relieve ciliary muscle spasm; however, their benefit has been questioned and they are no longer routinely recommended.
- Topical NSAIDs (e.g., diclofenac 0.1% or ketorolac 0.5%) 1 gtt qid.
- Topical antibiotics to prevent secondary infection.

DISPOSITION

Follow-up in 24 hr and then every 3 days until abrasion has cleared and vision has returned to normal

REFERRAL

To ophthalmologist if patient experiences no relief within 24 hr or for patients with deep eye injuries, foreign bodies that cannot be removed, or suspected recurrent corneal erosion (RCE)

PEARLS & CONSIDERATIONS

COMMENTS

- Never give patient topical anesthetic to use at home because these can cause decomposition of the cornea and permanent damage.
- Most corneal abrasions heal in 24 to 48 hours and rarely progress to corneal erosion or infection.

EVIDENCE

In patients with uncomplicated corneal abrasions, the application of an eye patch does not improve the rate of corneal healing, reduce pain, or reduce complications compared with wearing no patch.[1] B

Evidence-Based Reference

1. Flynn CA, D'Amico F, Smith G: Should we patch corneal abrasions? A meta-analysis, *J Fam Pract* 47:264-270, 1998. B

SUGGESTED READING

Wilson SA, Last A: Management of corneal abrasions, *Am Fam Physician* 70(1):123, 2004.

AUTHOR: **MELVYN KOBY, M.D.**

BASIC INFORMATION

DEFINITION

Corneal ulceration refers to the disruption of the corneal surface and/or deeper layers caused by trauma, contact lenses infection, degeneration, or other means.

SYNONYMS

Infectious keratitis with ulceration
Bacterial keratitis with ulceration
Viral keratitis with ulceration
Fungal keratitis with ulceration

ICD-9CM CODES
370.0 Corneal ulcer NOS

EPIDEMIOLOGY & DEMOGRAPHICS

INCIDENCE (IN U.S.): 4 to 6 cases/mo seen by average general ophthalmologist
PREVALENCE (IN U.S.): Common
PREDOMINANT SEX: Either
PREDOMINANT AGE: All ages

PHYSICAL FINDINGS & CLINICAL PRESENTATION

- Localized, well-demarcated, infiltrative lesion with corresponding focal ulcer (Fig. 1-62) or oval, yellow-white stromal suppuration with thick mucopurulent exudate and edema. Usually red, angry-looking eye with infiltration in surrounding area of cornea
- Eye possibly painful, with conjunctival edema and infection
- Sterile neurotrophic ulcers with tissue breakdown and no pain

ETIOLOGY

- Complication of contact lens wear, trauma, or diseases such as herpes simplex keratitis, keratoconjunctivitis sicca. Often associated with collagen vascular disease and severe exophthalmus and thyroid disease
- Viral causes often contagious

DIAGNOSIS

DIFFERENTIAL DIAGNOSIS

- *Pseudomonas* and pneumococcus and other bacterial infection—virulent
- *Moraxella, Staphylococcus, α-Streptococcus* infection—less virulent
- Herpes simplex infection or disease caused by other viruses
- Contact lens ulcers differ

WORKUP

- Fluorescein staining, slit lamp
- Appearance often typical
- Differentiate carefully with contact lens wearers
- Note previous eye surgery or laser vision correction

LABORATORY TESTS

Microscopic examination and culture of scrapings

TREATMENT

NONPHARMACOLOGIC THERAPY

- Warm compresses
- Bandage contact lenses
- Patching
- Stop contact lens wearing
- Remove eyelid crusting

ACUTE GENERAL Rx

- An ophthalmic emergency
- Intense antibiotic and antiviral Rx
- NSAIDs
- Viroptic/Zymar
- Bacterial infection: subconjunctival cefazolin or gentamicin (topical Zymar, Vigomax, etc.)
- Fungal infection: hospitalization and topical application of antifungal agents
- Herpes—Vioptic and oral Rx

DISPOSITION

Ideally treated by an ophthalmologist if the patient does not rapidly respond to antibiotics (within 24 hr)

PEARLS & CONSIDERATIONS

- Always stop contact lens wearing
- Always refer ulcers to ophthalmologist
- Never treat with topical anesthetics or steroids

COMMENTS

Do not use topical steroids because herpes, fungal, or other ulcers may be aggravated, leading to perforation of the cornea. Antibiotics may delay response and result in overgrowth of nonbacterial (fungal and amoebic) pathogens.

SUGGESTED READINGS

Price FW: New pieces for the puzzle: nonsteroidal anti-inflammatory drugs and corneal ulcers, *J Cataract Refract Surg* 26(9):1263, 2000.

Schaefer F et al: Bacterial keratitis: a prospective clinical and microbiological study, *Br J Ophthalmol,* 85(7):42, 2001.

Stretton S, Gopinathan U, Willcox MD: Corneal ulceration in pediatric patients: a brief overview of progress in topical treatment, *Paediatr Drugs* 4(2):95, 2002.

Varaprasathan G et al: Trends in the etiology of infectious corneal ulcers at the F. I. Proctor Foundation, *Cornea* 23(4):360, 2004.

AUTHOR: **MELVYN KOBY, M.D.**

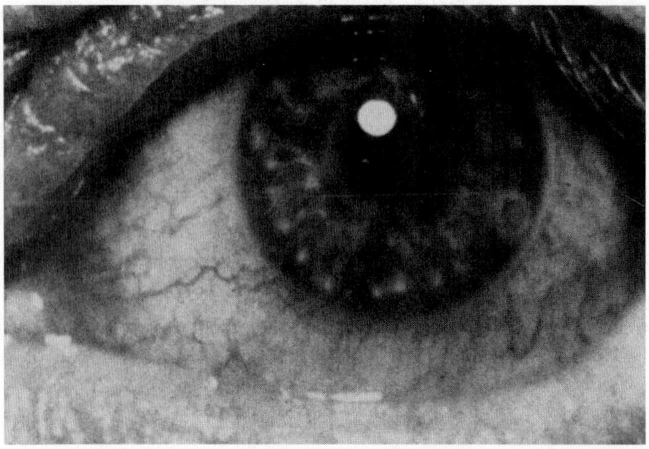

FIGURE 1-62 Peripherally located corneal ulcer. (From Marx JA [ed]: *Rosen's emergency medicine,* ed 5, St Louis, 2002, Mosby.)

BASIC INFORMATION

DEFINITION

Costochondritis is a poorly defined chest wall pain of uncertain cause.

SYNONYMS

Benign chest wall pain syndrome
Costosternal syndrome
Costosternal chondrodynia

ICD-9CM CODES
733.6 Costochondritis

EPIDEMIOLOGY & DEMOGRAPHICS

PREVALENCE: Unknown
PREDOMINANT SEX: Women > men
PREDOMINANT AGE: Over age 40 yr

PHYSICAL FINDINGS & CLINICAL PRESENTATION

- Tenderness of costochondral junctions (second through fifth) and/or sternum
- Pain with coughing and deep breathing
- Both sides of chest equal in frequency of involvement
- Often associated with anxiety, headache, and hyperventilation

ETIOLOGY

- Unknown
- May be a form of regional fibrositis
- May be referred pain from cervical or thoracic spine
- Emotional factors often involved

DIAGNOSIS

DIFFERENTIAL DIAGNOSIS

- Tietze's syndrome
- Cardiovascular disease
- GI disease
- Pulmonary disease
- Osteoarthritis (Table 1-5)
- Cervical disc syndrome

WORKUP

- There are no laboratory or radiographic abnormalities.
- Testing to rule out or rule in more serious disorders is performed on a case-by-case basis.

TREATMENT

ACUTE GENERAL Rx

- Explanation, reassurance
- Tricyclic antidepressants for sleep disturbance (amitriptyline 10 to 25 mg)
- Aerobic exercise program
- NSAIDs for analgesia

DISPOSITION

- The duration of the disorder is variable.
- Spontaneous remission is the rule.

REFERRAL

- Cardiology to rule out primary cardiac disease, when indicated.
- GI to rule out gastrointestinal disorders, when indicated.

PEARLS & CONSIDERATIONS

One of a large number of nonspecific musculoskeletal diagnoses based strictly on subjective symptoms and lacking any objective abnormalities.

COMMENTS

In spite of the name, no inflammation is present. After other, more serious conditions are ruled out, the treatment is strictly symptomatic and supportive.

EVIDENCE

EBM

Evidence supporting these treatments is lacking. However, clinical experience indicates that one or more of these treatments may be helpful for many patients.

SUGGESTED READINGS

Freeston J et al: Can early diagnosis and management of costochondritis reduce acute chest pain admissions? *J Rheumatol* 31:2269, 2004.

Gregory PL, Biswas AC, Batt ME: Musculoskeletal problems of the chest wall in athletes, *Sports Med* 32:325, 2002.

Hiramuro-Shoji F, Wirth MA, Rockwood CA: Atraumatic conditions of the sternoclavicular joint, *J Shoulder Elbow Surg* 12:79, 2003.

Jenson S: Musculoskeletal causes of chest pain, *Am Fam Physician* 30:834, 2001.

Rumball JS et al: Rowing injuries, *Sports Med* 35:537, 2005.

AUTHOR: **LONNIE R. MERCIER, M.D.**

TABLE 1-5 **Musculoskeletal Chest Pain**

Disorder	Clinical Features	Comments
Tietze's syndrome	Pain and swelling of sternoclavicular joint or second or third costochondral junctions (usually left). Worse with cough and deep breathing. Local tenderness.	Traumatic cause? Rare.
Costochondritis	Pain and tenderness but no swelling. Costochondral junctions of ribs 2-5. Increased pain with cough and sneeze.	Sometimes associated with headache and hyperventilation.
Seronegative spondyloarthropathy (ankylosing spondylitis)	Sternoclavicular or manubriosternal joint. Worse in am. Relieved by activity. May be associated with swelling.	Local chest findings usually associated with other symptoms of ankylosing spondylitis such as sacroilitis. May need HLA-B27 antigen testing.
Cervical, thoracic disc disease	Referred regional pain from affected area. No local swelling. Often aggravated by spine motion and may be accompanied by radicular pain into arm if cervical or along intercostal nerve if thoracic.	May mimic chest disease if spinal complaints are minimal and referred or radicular symptoms predominate.
Fibromyalgia	Widespread pain with other sites involved. Symptoms often change in location. Local "tender points" but no swelling or objective findings.	Female:male ratio of 9:1. Prevalent age 30-50 yr.
Osteoarthritis, sternoclavicular or manubriosternal joint	Dull, aching local pain with tenderness. Occasional bony joint enlargement with soft-tissue swelling.	Crepitus may rarely be present.

BASIC INFORMATION

DEFINITION

Craniopharyngiomas are tumors arising from squamous cell remnants of Rathke's pouch, located in the infundibulum or upper anterior hypophysis.

SYNONYMS

Subset of nonadenomatous pituitary tumors

ICD-9CM CODES
237.0 Craniopharyngioma

EPIDEMIOLOGY & DEMOGRAPHICS

PEAK INCIDENCE: Occurs at all ages; peak during the first 2 decades of life, with a second small peak occurring in the sixth decade.
PREDOMINANT SEX: Both sexes are usually equally affected.
Craniopharyngiomas are the most common nonglial tumors in children and account for 3% to 5% of all pediatric brain tumors.

PHYSICAL FINDINGS & CLINICAL PRESENTATION

- The typical onset is insidious and a 1- to 2-year history of slowly progressive symptoms is common.
- Presenting symptoms are usually related to the effects of a sella turcica mass. Approximately 75% of patients complain of headache and have visual disturbances.
- The usual visual defect is bitemporal hemianopsia. Optic nerve involvement with decreased visual acuity and scotomas and homonymous hemianopsia from optic tract involvement may also occur.
- Other symptoms include mental changes, nausea, vomiting, somnolence, or symptoms of pituitary failure. In adults, sexual dysfunction is the most common endocrine complaint, with impotence in males and primary or secondary amenorrhea in females. Diabetes insipidus is found in 25% of cases. In children, craniopharyngiomas may present with dwarfism.
- More than 70% of children at the time of diagnosis present with growth hormone deficiency, obstructive hydrocephalus, short-term memory deficits, and psychomotor slowing.

ETIOLOGY

Craniopharyngiomas are believed to arise from nests of squamous epithelial cells that are commonly found in the suprasellar area surrounding the pars tuberalis of the adult pituitary.

DIAGNOSIS

DIFFERENTIAL DIAGNOSIS

- Pituitary adenoma
- Empty sella syndrome
- Pituitary failure of any cause
- Primary brain tumors (e.g., meningiomas, astrocytomas)
- Metastatic brain tumors
- Other brain tumors
- Cerebral aneurysm

LABORATORY TESTS

- Hypothyroidism (low FT_4, FT_3 with high TSH).
- Hypercortisolism (low cortisol) with low ACTH.
- Low sex hormones (testosterone, estriol) with low FSH and LH.
- Diabetes insipidus (hypernatremia, low urine osmolarity, high plasma osmolarity).
- Prolactin may be normal or slightly elevated.
- Pituitary stimulation tests may be required in some cases.

IMAGING STUDIES

- Visual field testing for bitemporal hemianopsia.
- Skull film.
  - Enlarged or eroded sella turcica (50%)
  - Suprasellar calcification (50%)
- MRI (Fig. 1-63) or head CT. MRI features include a multicystic and solid enhancing suprasellar mass. Hydrocephalus may also be present if the mass is large. CT usually reveals intratumoral calcifications.

TREATMENT

GENERAL Rx

- Surgical resection (curative or palliative).
  - Transsphenoidal surgery for small intrasellar tumors
  - Subfrontal craniotomy for most patients
- Postoperative radiation.
- Intralesional ^{32}P irradiation or bleomycin for unresectable tumors. Long-term complications of radiation include secondary malignancies, optic neuropathy, and vascular injury.

PROGNOSIS

- Operative mortality: 3% to 16% (higher with large tumors).
- Postoperative recurrence rate: 30% of cases after total resection and 57% of cases after subtotal resection.
- 5-yr and 10-yr survival: 88% and 76%, respectively, with surgery and radiation.
- The most important factors that correlate with prognosis are the extent of resection and postoperative radiation.

AUTHORS: **FRED F. FERRI, M.D.,** and **TOM J. WACHTEL, M.D.**

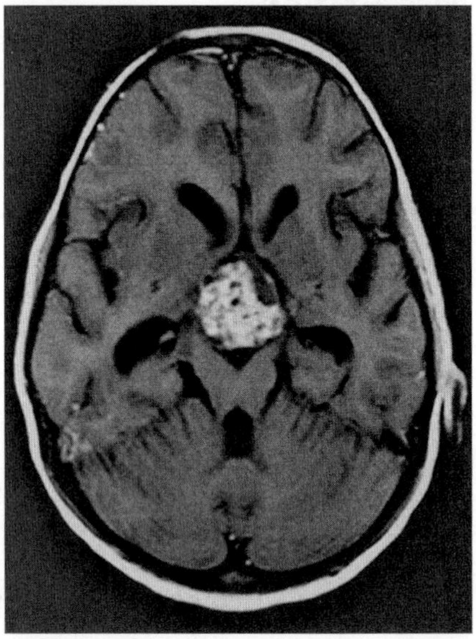

FIGURE 1-63 MRI scan of a craniopharyngioma, demonstrating a cystic contrast-enhancing mass in the suprasellar area extending upward and compressing the hypothalamus. (From Goetz CG: *Textbook of clinical neurology,* Philadelphia, 1999, WB Saunders.)

BASIC INFORMATION

DEFINITION

Creutzfeldt-Jakob disease (CJD) is a progressive, fatal, dementing illness caused by an infectious agent known as a *prion*.

SYNONYMS

Transmissible spongiform encephalopathy
Mad cow disease
Prion disease

ICD-9CM CODES
046.1 Creutzfeldt-Jakob disease

EPIDEMIOLOGY & DEMOGRAPHICS

- Incidence of 1 per 1,000,000 population per yr
- Peak age 60 yr (range 16 to 82 yr)
- 5% to 10% familial, remaining cases are sporadic; iatrogenic cases (corneal transplants, dura mater allograft, human pituitary extract) are very rare
- Normal prion protein gene found on human chromosome 20

PHYSICAL FINDINGS & CLINICAL PRESENTATION

- All patients present with cognitive deficits (dementing illness—memory loss, behavioral abnormalities, higher cortical function impairment).
- More than 80% will have myoclonus.
- Pyramidal tract signs (weakness), cerebellar signs (clumsiness), and extrapyramidal signs (parkinsonian features) are seen in more than 50% of the cases.
- Less common features include cortical visual abnormalities, abnormal eye movements, vestibular dysfunction, sensory disturbances, autonomic dysfunction, lower motor neuron signs, and seizures.

ETIOLOGY

Small proteinaceous infections particle (prion). Noninfectious prion protein (PrP) is a cellular protein found on the surfaces of neurons. Normal function is not known. Protein is converted to protease resistant and infectious agent (PrP^{sc}) by infectious prion protein (PrP^{sc}).

DIAGNOSIS

- Definite CJD: Neuropathologically confirmed spongiform encephalopathy in a case of progressive dementia.
- Probable CJD: History of rapidly progressive dementia (less than 2 yr) with typical EEG and with at least two of the following clinical features: myoclonus, visual or cerebellar dysfunction, pyramidal or extrapyramidal features, akinetic mutism.
- Possible CJD: Same as probable CJD without EEG findings.

DIFFERENTIAL DIAGNOSIS

- Primary CNS lymphoma
- Viral encephalitis
- CNS vasculitis
- Others (hydrocephalus, infectious, vitamin deficiency, endocrine)
- Other dementia (Alzheimer's, frontotemporal dementia, diffuse Lewy body disease, vascular)

A clinical algorithm for the evaluation of dementia is described in Section III, "Dementia."

WORKUP

- Evaluate for treatable causes of dementia (see "Alzheimer's Disease").
- Brain biopsy can be diagnostic, but it is usually not performed because there is no treatment or cure.

LABORATORY TESTS

- Presence of periodic sharp wave complexes on EEG in cases of rapidly progressive dementia has a sensitivity of 67% and a specificity of 86%.
- In cases of probable or possible CJD, presence of the 14,3,3 protein in CSF has a 95% positive predictive value with its absence having a 92% negative predictive value.

IMAGING STUDIES

MRI scan can show areas of restricted diffusion in the basal ganglia and cerebral cortex. MRI diffusion weighted imaging has a sensitivity of 92.3% and a specificity of 93.8% only in cases of rapidly progressive dementia.

TREATMENT

NONPHARMACOLOGIC THERAPY

Full time caregiver and/or nursing home. Social work can be helpful with end of life discussions, family counseling, and optimizing appropriate home services.

ACUTE GENERAL Rx

No known therapy

CHRONIC Rx

No known therapy

DISPOSITION

The disease is fatal. Mean duration of illness is 8 mo (range 1 to 130 mo). One in 7 survives to 1 yr and 1 in 30 survives to 2 yr. Better survival found in younger age at onset of disease and female gender.

REFERRAL

- Neurology for evaluation of any rapidly progressive dementia
- Social work

PEARLS & CONSIDERATIONS

COMMENTS

- Related diseases in humans: Kuru, Fatal familial insomnia, Gerstmann-Sträussler-Scheinker syndrome, new-variant Creutzfeldt-Jacob disease.
- Related diseases in animals: Scrapie, bovine spongiform encephalopathy (Mad cow disease).

EVIDENCE

No treatment is available to slow the inevitable decline.

SUGGESTED READINGS

Brown P et al: Human spongiform encephalopathy: the National Institutes of Health series of 300 cases of experimentally transmitted disease, *Ann Neurol* 35:513, 1994.

Hsich G et al: The 14-3-3 brain protein in cerebrospinal fluid as a marker for transmissible spongiform encephalopathies, *N Engl J Med* 335:924, 1996.

Knight RSG, Will RG: Prion disease, *J Neurol Neurosurg Psychiatry* 75:36, 2004.

Masters CL et al: Creutzfeldt-Jakob disease: patterns of worldwide occurrence and the significance of familial and sporadic clustering, *Ann Neurol* 5:177, 1979.

Shiga Y et al: Diffusion-weighted MRI abnormalities as an early diagnostic marker for Creutzfeldt-Jakob disease, *Neurology* 63:443, 2004.

Steinhoff BJ et al: Accuracy and reliability of periodic sharp wave complexes in Creutzfeldt-Jakob disease, *Arch Neurol* 53:162, 1996.

AUTHOR: **CHUN LIM, M.D., PH.D.**

BASIC INFORMATION

DEFINITION

Crohn's disease is an inflammatory disease of the bowel of unknown etiology, most commonly involving the terminal ileum and manifesting primarily with diarrhea, abdominal pain, fatigue, and weight loss.

SYNONYMS

Regional enteritis
Inflammatory bowel disease (IBD)

ICD-9CM CODES
555.9 Crohn's disease, unspecified site
555.0 Crohn's disease, small intestine
555.1 Crohn's disease involving large intestine

EPIDEMIOLOGY & DEMOGRAPHICS

PREVALENCE: 1 case/1000 persons; most common in Caucasians and Jews
- Crohn's disease affects approximately 380,000 to 480,000 persons in the U.S.
- Incidence: bimodal with a peak in the third decade of life and another one in the fifth decade

PHYSICAL FINDINGS & CLINICAL PRESENTATION

- Abdominal tenderness, mass, or distention
- Chronic or nocturnal diarrhea
- Weight loss, fever, night sweats
- Hyperactive bowel sounds in patients with partial obstruction, bloody diarrhea
- Delayed growth and failure of normal development in children
- Perianal and rectal abscesses, mouth ulcers, and atrophic glossitis
- Extraintestinal manifestations: joint swelling and tenderness, hepatosplenomegaly, erythema nodosum, clubbing, tenderness to palpation of the sacroiliac joints
- Symptoms may be intermittent with varying periods of remission

ETIOLOGY

Unknown. Pathophysiologically, Crohn's disease involves an immune system dysfunction.

DIAGNOSIS

DIFFERENTIAL DIAGNOSIS

- Ulcerative colitis
- Infectious diseases (TB, *Yersinia, Salmonella, Shigella, Campylobacter*)
- Parasitic infections (amebic infection)
- Pseudomembranous colitis
- Ischemic colitis in elderly patients
- Lymphoma
- Colon carcinoma
- Diverticulitis
- Radiation enteritis
- Collagenous colitis
- Fungal infections *(Histoplasma, Actinomyces)*
- Gay bowel syndrome (in homosexual patient)
- Carcinoid tumors
- Celiac sprue
- Mesenteric adenitis

LABORATORY TESTS

- Decreased Hgb and Hct from chronic blood loss, effect of inflammation on bone marrow, and malabsorption of vitamin B_{12}
- Hypokalemia, hypomagnesemia, hypocalcemia, and low albumin in patients with chronic diarrhea
- Vitamin B_{12} and folate deficiency
- Elevated ESR

ENDOSCOPIC EVALUATION

Endoscopic features of Crohn's disease include asymmetric and discontinued disease, deep longitudinal fissures, cobblestone appearance, presence of strictures. Crypt distortion and inflammation are also present. Granulomas may be present.

IMAGING STUDIES

- Barium imaging studies (when performed) reveal deep ulcerations (often longitudinal and transverse) and segmental lesions (skip lesions, strictures, fistulas, cobblestone appearance of mucosa caused by submucosal inflammation); "thumbprinting" is common, "string sign" in terminal ileum may be noted. Although the diagnosis may be suggested by radiographic studies, it should be confirmed by endoscopy and biopsy when possible.
- CT of abdomen is helpful in identifying abscesses and other complications.
- In 5% to 10% of patients with IBD, a clear distinction between ulcerative colitis and Crohn's disease cannot be made. Generally, Crohn's disease can be distinguished from ulcerative colitis by presence of transmural involvement and the frequent presence of noncaseating granulomas and lymphoid aggregates on biopsy.

TREATMENT

The medical management of Crohn's disease is based on disease activity. According to Hanauer and Sanborn, disease activity can be defined as follows:
- Mild to moderate disease: The patient is ambulatory and able to take oral alimentation. There is no dehydration, high fever, abdominal tenderness, painful mass, obstruction, or weight loss of >10%.
- Moderate to severe disease: Either the patient has failed treatment for mild to moderate disease OR has more pronounced symptoms including fever, significant weight loss, abdominal pain or tenderness, intermittent nausea and vomiting, or significant anemia.
- Severe fulminant disease: Either the patient has persistent symptoms despite outpatient steroid therapy OR has high fever, persistent vomiting, evidence of intestinal obstruction, rebound tenderness, cachexia, or evidence of an abscess.
- Remission: The patient is asymptomatic OR without inflammatory sequelae, including patients responding to acute medical intervention.

NONPHARMACOLOGIC THERAPY

- Nutritional supplementation is needed in patients with advanced disease. TPN may be necessary in selected patients.
- Low-residue diet is necessary when obstructive symptoms are present.
- If diarrhea is prominent, increased dietary fiber and lowering of fat in the diet are sometimes helpful.
- Psychotherapy is useful for situational adjustment crises. A trusting and mutually understanding relationship and referral to self-help groups are very important because of the chronicity of the disease and the relatively young age of the patients.
- Avoid oral feedings during acute exacerbation to decrease colonic activity: a low-roughage diet may be helpful in early relapse.

ACUTE GENERAL Rx

- Sulfasalazine, 500 mg PO qid initially, increased qd or qod by 1 g until therapeutic dosages of 4 to 6 g/day are achieved. The oral salicylates, mesalamine (Asacol, Rowasa) are as effective as sulfasalazine and better tolerated but more expensive; they may be useful in patients allergic to the sulfa moiety of sulfasalazine molecule. Individuals with sulfa allergies should avoid sulfasalazine. Folate supplementation is recommended because sulfasalazine inhibits folate absorption.
- Corticosteroids have been the mainstay for treating moderate to severe active Crohn's disease. Prednisone 40 to 60 mg/day are useful for acute exacerbation. Steroids are usually tapered over approximately 2 to 3 mo. Some patients require a low dose for prolonged period of maintenance.
- Steroid analogues are locally active corticosteroids that target specific areas of inflammation in the GI tract. Budesonide (Entocort EC) is available as a controlled-release formulation and is approved for mild to moderate active Crohn's disease involving the ileum

and/or ascending colon. The adult dose is 9 mg qd for a maximum of 8 wk.

- Immunosuppressants such as azathioprine (Imuran) 150 mg/day, methotrexate, or cyclosporine can be used for severe, progressive disease. In patients with Crohn's disease who enter remission after treatment with methotrexate, a low dose of methotrexate maintains remission.
- Metronidazole 500 mg qid may be useful for colonic fistulas and for treatment of mild to moderate active Crohn's disease. Ciprofloxacin 1 g qd has also been found effective in decreasing disease activity.
- Infliximab, a chimeric monoclonal antibody targeting tumor necrosis factor-α, is effective in the treatment of enterocutaneous fistulas. This medication can induce clinical improvement in 80% of patients with Crohn's disease refractory to other agents. Its mechanism of action is incompletely understood. It is very costly. A PPD test should be done before using this medication. Adalimumab, a fully human tumor necrosis factor (TNF), is also effective in inducing remissions and may be useful in adult patients with Crohn's disease who cannot tolerate infliximab or have symptoms despite receiving infliximab therapy.
- Natalizumab, a selective adhesion-molecule inhibitor, has been reported effective in increasing the rate of remission and response in patients with active Crohn's disease. Recent trials with pegylated antibody fragments in patients with moderate-to-severe Crohn's disease involving certolizumab pegol reveal a modest improvement in response rates but no significant improvement in remission rates.
- Hydrocortisone (Cortenema) enema bid or tid is useful for proctitis.
- Most patients who have anemia associated with Crohn's disease respond to iron supplementation. Erythropoietin is useful in patients with anemia refractory to treatment with iron and vitamins.

CHRONIC Rx

- Monitor disease activity with symptom review and laboratory evaluation (CBC and sedimentation rate)
- Liver tests and vitamin B_{12} levels monitored on a yearly basis

DISPOSITION

One tenth of patients have prolonged remission, three quarters have a chronic intermittent disease course, and one eighth have an unremitting course.

REFERRAL

- Surgical referral is needed for complications such as abscess formation, obstruction, fistulas, toxic megacolon, refractory disease, or severe hemorrhage. A conservative surgical approach is necessary, because surgery is not curative. Multiple surgeries may also result in short bowel syndrome.

EVIDENCE

There is evidence that corticosteroids are effective in the management of active Crohn's disease but are of limited benefit in the prevention of relapse.

Prednisone is effective in the management of moderate to severe, active Crohn's disease. Budesonide is comparable to prednisone in the management of active Crohn's disease and may be associated with fewer side effects than those encountered with prednisone use.[1] Ⓒ

However, systematic reviews have found little evidence for the use of either prednisone or budesonide in the maintenence of clinical remission in Crohn's disease.[2,3] Ⓐ

There is limited evidence that metronidazole is effective in the management of patients with Crohn's disease.

Metronidazole may be effective in a proportion of patients with mild to moderate active Crohn's disease.[1] Ⓒ

There is evidence that infliximab is of benefit in the treatment of a proportion of patients with Crohn's disease.

A systematic review identified one randomized controlled trial (RTC) that found that a single infusion of infliximab was effective in inducing remission in patients with active Crohn's disease.[4] Ⓐ

An RCT found that maintenance treatment with infliximab produced a significant improvement in clinical response, with maintained remission, compared with placebo.[5] Ⓑ

RCTs have shown that in patients with fistulizing Crohn's disease, infliximab significantly reduces the number of draining fistulas and promotes complete closure compared with placebo. Maintenance therapy with infliximab significantly improves clinical outcome in patients with fistulizing disease. [6,7] Ⓑ

There is some evidence that methotrexate is of benefit in some patients with refractory Crohn's disease.

A recent systematic review identified one RCT that compared intramuscular methotrexate (25 mg weekly) vs. placebo in patients with active Crohn's disease, refractory to treatment with steroids. The study found that the use of methotrexate in this patient group showed a substantial benefit compared with placebo.[8] Ⓐ

Clinical consensus supports the use of surgery in the management of Crohn's disease.

Guidelines from The American College of Gastroenterology state that, in patients with Crohn's disease, surgical resection, stricturoplasty, or drainage of abscesses are indicated to treat complications or medically refractory disease.[1] Ⓒ

Evidence-Based References

1. Hanauer SB, Sandborn W: Management of Crohn's disease in adults, *Am J Gastroenterol* 96:635, 2001. Ⓒ
2. Steinhart AH et al: Corticosteroids for maintenance of remission in Crohn's disease. *Cochrane Database Syst Rev* Issue 4, 2003. Ⓐ
3. Simms L, Steinhart AH: Budesonide for maintenance of remission in Crohn's disease, *Cochrane Database Syst Rev* Issue 1, 2001. Ⓐ
4. Akobeng AK, Zachos M: Tumor necrosis factor-alpha antibody for induction of remission in Crohn's disease, *Cochrane Database Syst Rev* Issue 4, 2003. Ⓐ
5. Hanauer SB et al: Maintenance infliximab for Crohn's disease: the ACCENT I randomised trial, *Lancet* 359:1541, 2002. Ⓑ
6. Present DH et al: Infliximab for the treatment of fistulas in patients with Crohn's disease, *N Engl J Med* 340:398, 1999. Ⓑ
7. Sands BE et al: Infliximab maintenance therapy for fistulizing Crohn's disease, *N Engl J Med* 350:876, 2004. Ⓑ
8. Alfadhli AAF, McDonald JWD, Feagan DG: Methotrexate for induction of remission in refractory Crohn's disease, *Cochrane Database Syst Rev* Issue 4, 2004. Ⓐ

SUGGESTED READINGS

Baumgart DC, Carding SR: Inflammatory bowel disease: cause and immunobiology, *Lancet* 369:1627, 2007.

Baumgart DC, Carding SR: Inflammatory bowel disease: clinical aspects and established and evolving therapies, *Lancet* 369:1641, 2007.

Sandborn WJ et al: Adalimumab induction therapy for Crohn disease previously treated with infliximab, *Ann Intern Med* 146:829, 2007.

Sandborn WJ et al: Certolizumab pegol for the treatment of Crohn's disease, *N Engl J Med* 357:228, 2007.

AUTHOR: **FRED F. FERRI, M.D.**

BASIC INFORMATION

DEFINITION

Cryptococcosis is an infection caused by the fungal organism *Cryptococcus neoformans.*

SYNONYMS

C. neoformans var. *neoformans* infection
C. neoformans var. *gatti* infection
C. neoformans var. *grubii* infection

ICD-9CM CODES
117.5 Cryptococcosis

EPIDEMIOLOGY & DEMOGRAPHICS

INCIDENCE (IN U.S.)

- 1 to 2 cases/1 million (non–HIV-infected) persons annually
- 6% to 7% in HIV-infected persons

PEAK INCIDENCE: 20 to 40 yr (parallel to AIDS epidemic)
PREDOMINANT SEX: Equal sex distribution when corrected for HIV status
PREDOMINANT AGE: Less than 2 yr of age; 20 to 40 yr of age
NEONATAL INFECTION: Very uncommon

PHYSICAL FINDINGS & CLINICAL PRESENTATION

- More than 90% present with meningitis; almost all have fever and headache.
- Meningismus, photophobia, mental status changes are seen in approximately 25%.
- Increased intracranial pressure.
- Most common infections outside the CNS:
  1. In the lungs (fever, cough, dyspnea)
  2. In the skin (cellulitis, papular eruption)
  3. In the lymph nodes (lymphadenitis)
  4. Potential involvement of virtually any organ

ETIOLOGY

- Caused by the fungal organism *C. neoformans*

There are 3 varieties of *Cryptococcus spp.* and 4 capsular serotypes: Serotype A is *Cryptococcus neoformans* var. *grubii* and Serotype D is known as *Cryptococcus neoformans* var. *neoformans.* Both cause disease primarily in immunocompromised patients. Serotype B and C are known as *C. neoformans* var. *gatti.* This organism causes disease primarily in normal hosts.

- Infection originates by inhalation into the respiratory tract followed by dissemination to the CNS in most cases, usually without recognizable lung involvement
- Almost always in the setting of AIDS or other disorders of cellular immune function
- Neutropenia alone poses a much lower risk of significant cryptococcal infection

DIAGNOSIS

DIFFERENTIAL DIAGNOSIS

- Subacute meningitis (caused by *Listeria monocytogenes, Mycobacterium tuberculosis, Histoplasma capsulatum,* viruses)
- Intracranial mass lesion (neoplasms, toxoplasmosis, TB)
- Pulmonary involvement confused with *Pneumocystis jiroveci* pneumonia when diffuse or confused with TB or bacterial pneumonia when focal or involving the pleura
- Skin lesions confused with bacterial cellulitis or molluscum contagiosum

WORKUP

- Lumbar puncture to exclude cryptococcal meningitis.
- CT scan of the head when focal lesion or increased intracranial pressure is suspected.
- Biopsy of enlarged lymph nodes and skin lesions if feasible.

LABORATORY TESTS

- Culture and India ink stain (60% to 80% sensitive in culture-proven cases [Fig. 1-64]) examination of the CSF in all cases when CNS involvement is suspected
- Blood and serum cryptococcal antigen assay (>90% sensitivity and specificity)
- Culture and histologic examination of biopsy material

IMAGING STUDIES

- CT scan or MRI of the head if focal neurologic involvement is suspected
- Chest x-ray examination to exclude pulmonary involvement

TREATMENT

ACUTE GENERAL Rx

- Therapy is initiated with IV amphotericin B (0.5 mg/kg/day) with or without flucytosine.
- After stabilization (usually several weeks), consider fluconazole (200 to 400 mg qd PO) for additional 6 to 8 wk. Voriconazole, a newer imidazole, also has activity against most isolates.
- Alternative: IV fluconazole for initial therapy in patients unable to tolerate amphotericin B.
- If symptomatic increased intracranial pressure, consider therapeutic lumbar taps or intraventricular shunt.

CHRONIC Rx

- Fluconazole (200 mg PO qd) is highly effective in preventing a relapse in HIV-infected patients; development of resistance may occur.
- Immune reconstitution syndrome following the institution of HARRT can cause transient worsening of meningitis and necessitate the use of a short course of corticosteroids.

DISPOSITION

Without maintenance therapy, relapse rate is >50% among AIDS patients.

REFERRAL

- For consultation with infectious diseases specialist in all cases
- For neurologic consultation if level of consciousness is depressed or focal lesion is present

PEARLS & CONSIDERATIONS

Cryptococcal meningitis can be remarkably insidious in nonimmunocomprised patients.

COMMENTS

Cryptococcosis is considered an AIDS-defining infection; thus all patients should be HIV tested.

SUGGESTED READINGS

Lortholary O et al: Incidence and risk factors of immune reconstitution inflammatory syndrome complicating HIV-associated cryptococcosis in France, *AIDS* 19(10):1043, 2005.
Lui G et al: Cryptococcosis in apparently immunocompetent patients, *QJM* 99(3):143, 2006.

AUTHORS: **STEVEN M. OPAL, M.D.,** and **JOSEPH R. MASCI, M.D.**

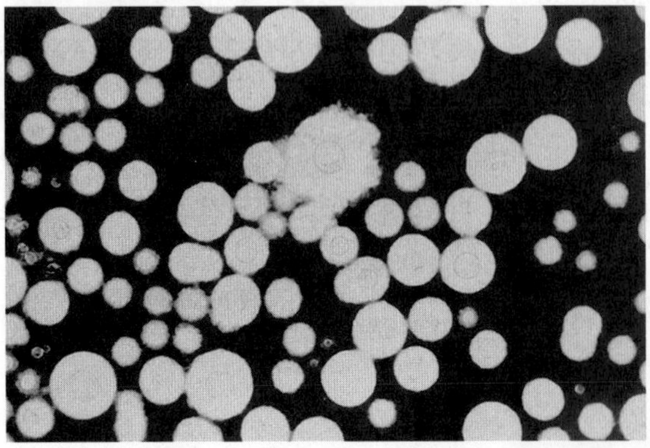

FIGURE 1-64 India ink preparation of cerebrospinal fluid revealing encapsulated cryptococci. Note the large capsules surrounding the smaller organisms. (From Andreoli TE [ed]: *Cecil essentials of medicine,* ed 4, Philadelphia, 1997, WB Saunders.)

BASIC INFORMATION

DEFINITION

Cryptorchidism is the incomplete or improper descent of the testis (testes) into the scrotum during fetal development. Testes that can be manually manipulated into the scrotum are called retractile. Testes previously located but are no longer palpable in the scrotum are called ascended testes.

SYNONYMS Undescended testis

ICD-9CM CODES
752.51 Cryptorchidism

EPIDEMIOLOGY & DEMOGRAPHICS

- Cryptorchidism is the most common genitourinary disorder of male children.
- Occurs in approximately 30% of premature and 5% of full-term males. In 10%, it can be bilateral.
- Within the first year of life, most cryptorchid testes descend into the scrotum so that incidence becomes approximately 1% in boys.
- Increased rates with premature birth, low birth weight, twins, and family history of cryptorchidism.
- Associated with Kallman's and Prader-Willi syndromes, pituitary hypoplasia, testicular feminization, prune belly syndrome, cystic fibrosis, myelomeningocele, and Reifenstein syndrome.

CLINICAL PRESENTATION

- Typically asymptomatic and is noted incidentally on screening examination. Undescended testes are at risk for testicular torsion.
- The testis may be nonpalpable or palpable in a location along the path of normal descent (Fig. 1-65), however, less commonly may be ectopic and located in the perineum, femoral canal, superficial inguinal pouch, suprapubic area, and contralateral hemiscrotum.
  - In 80%, the undescended testis is palpable in the inguinal canal.
- Associated with infertility and a sevenfold increased risk of testicular cancer. Risk of infertility is the greatest for a child with bilateral intra-abdominal testes and longer duration of cryptorchidism.

ETIOLOGY

Normal testicular descent is a complex interplay among mechanical (gubernaculums, vas deferens and testicular vessel length, cremasteric muscles, and abdominal pressure), hormonal (gonadotropin, testosterone, dihydrotestosterone, and mullerian inhibiting substance), and neural (ilioinguinal and genitofemoral nerves) factors.

DIAGNOSIS

DIFFERENTIAL DIAGNOSIS

- Retractile testis
- Ascended testis
- Atrophic testis
- Vanished testis

WORKUP

- Physical examination
  - When done in a warm room with warm hands, can identify presence, absence, and location of palpable testes.
  - Should be done in supine, sitting, and standing positions with adequate cremasteric relaxation to differentiate true cryptorchidism from retractile testes.
  - Often associated with an indirect inguinal hernia as the tunica vaginalis fails to close above the testis.
  - An enlarged contralateral testis in the presence of a nonpalpable undescended testis is suggestive of but not definitive for testicular atrophy/absence.
- Hormonal challenge
  - Human chorionic gonadotropin (hCG) will confirm the presence of functioning testicular tissue and is useful in the setting of bilateral nonpalpable undescended testes.
  - If the follicular stimulating hormone level is 3× normal and there is no increase in testosterone in response to hCG, functional testes are absent.

IMAGING

- Ultrasound: sensitivity of 76%, specificity of 100%, accuracy of 84%.
- MRI: sensitivity of 86% and specificity of 79%. CT results are inconsistent.

TREATMENT

- Repeat examination at 3 mo of age, because many testes will descend spontaneously. Spontaneous descent is rare after 3 mo of age.
- Treatment can be hormonal, surgical, or both.
- Treatment recommended as early as 6 mo and should be completed before 2 yr because histologic changes have been identified as early as 1.5 years of age.
- Earlier orchidopexy may improve testicular function and decrease the risk of testis cancer. Orchidopexy allows testicular self-examination and detection of testicular cancer should it occur.

HORMONAL Rx

- Results of hCG are variable for undescended testes but good for retractile testes.
- The International Health Foundation recommends biweekly injections of 250 IU for infants, 500 IU for children up to 6 yr, and 100 IU for children 6 yr and older, for a total of 5 wk. Therapy may induce precocious puberty.
- Administration of gonadotropin-releasing hormone before orchiopexy may improve fertility in adulthood.

SURGICAL Rx

- For the palpable undescended testis, orchiopexy, the surgical placement of an undescended testis into the scrotum, is the standard approach.
- In the setting of a nonpalpable undescended testis, laparoscopy is recommended to identify the presence/absence of a testis and the location of the testis if present and to determine the length of the testicular vessels.
- A two-stage approach is recommended for an intra-abdominal testis with short vessels. The testicular vessels are clipped laparoscopically in the first stage, and the testis is brought into the scrotum in the second stage.
- Although the risk of testicular cancer is higher, the removal of all intraabdominal testes is not warranted.

DISPOSITION

- Earlier orchidopexy may decrease the risk of malignancy and infertility.
- Lifelong testicular exam after puberty.

REFERRAL

Early referral to a pediatric urologist

PEARLS & CONSIDERATIONS

Regular testicular exams should be performed in infants and children, particularly those with retractile testes, as ascent of scrotal testis can occur.

SUGGESTED READINGS

Cortes D: *Scan J Nephrol* 9:54, 1998.
Dawson C, Whitfield H: *BMJ* 312(7041):1291, 1996.
Docimo S, Silver R, Cromie W: *Am Fam Physician* 62:2037, 2000.
Giannopoulos MD et al: *Horm Res* 55(1):33, 2001.
Lee P: *Urology* 66:427, 2005.
Leissner J et al: *Br J Urol Int* 83(8):885, 1999.
Patik K et al: *BJU* 95:704, 2005.
Schwentner C et al: *J Urol* 173:974, 2005.
Thayyil S et al: *Arch Dis Child* 89:890, 2004.

AUTHORS: **PAMELA ELLSWORTH, M.D.**, and **IRIS TONG, M.D.**

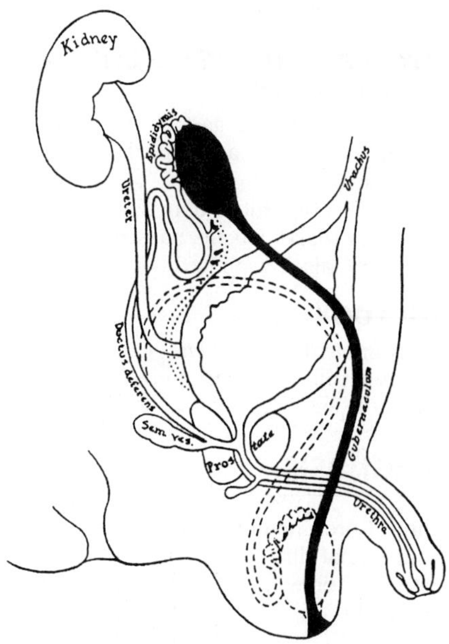

FIGURE 1-65 The path of testicular descent. (Reproduced with permission from Sarnat HB, Sarnat MS: Disorders of muscle in the newborn. In Moss AJ, Stern L [eds]: *Pediatrics update,* ed 4, New York, 1983, Elsevier-North Holland.)

BASIC INFORMATION

DEFINITION

The intracellular protozoan parasite *Cryptosporidium parvum* is associated with gastrointestinal disease and diarrhea, especially in AIDS patients or immunocompromised hosts. It is also associated with sporadic infections and waterborne outbreaks in immunocompetent hosts.

Other species, including *C. hominus, C. felis, C. muris,* and *C. meleagridis,* are now described to be pathogens as well.

SYNONYMS

Cryptosporidiosis

ICD-9CM CODES
007.4 Cryptosporidia infection

EPIDEMIOLOGY & DEMOGRAPHICS

INCIDENCE (IN U.S.):
- Approximately 2% in industrial countries, 5% to 10% in third world countries
- 10% to 20% of HIV patients in U.S. may excrete cyst

PREVALENCE: Worldwide, especially third world countries; associated with poor hygiene as a waterborne pathogen
PREDOMINANT SEX: Male = female
TRANSMISSION:
- Person to person (daycare, family members)
- Animal to person (pets, farm animals)
- Environmental (water-associated outbreaks, including travel associated with swimming in or drinking contaminated water)
- May be significant pathogen causing diarrhea in AIDS

PHYSICAL FINDINGS & CLINICAL PRESENTATION

- Usually limited to gastrointestinal tract
- Diarrhea, severe abdominal pain (2 to 28 days)
- Impaired digestion, dehydration
- Fever, malaise, fatigue, nausea, vomiting
- Pneumonia if aspirated

ETIOLOGY

Cryptosporidium hominis, Cryptosporidium parvum, C. felis, C. muris, C. meleagridis

DIAGNOSIS

Clinical presentation of acute gastrointestinal illness, especially associated with HIV or with travel and waterborne outbreaks.

DIFFERENTIAL DIAGNOSIS

- *Campylobacter*
- *Clostridium difficile*
- *Entamoeba histolytica*
- *Giardia lamblia*
- *Salmonella*
- *Shigella*
- Microsporidia
- Cytomegalovirus
- *Mycobacterium avium*

Disease may cause cholecystitis, reactive arthritis, hepatitis, pancreatitis, pneumonia in immunocompromised or HIV-infected patients.

WORKUP

- Stool evaluation looking for characteristic oocyst by modified acid-fast stain (Fig. 1-66).
- Direct immunofluorescence using monoclonal antibodies is the gold standard for stool exams.

TREATMENT

- May be self-limited in normal host—often requiring hydration. Antidiarrhea agents Pepto-Bismol, Kaopectate, or loperamide may give symptomatic relief.
- Pharmacologic treatment with antibiotics has been largely unsatisfactory in AIDS patients. Oocyst excretion reduction has been shown with nitazoxanide 500 mg po BID for 3 days. If treatment fails, consider a trial of paromomycin, metronidazole, or Bactrim.
- Nitazoxanide elixir has been approved for the treatment of cryptosporidiosis in children ages 1 to 11 yr.
- Biliary cryptosporidiosis can be treated with antiretroviral therapy in the HIV setting.

DISPOSITION

- A self-limited disease in immunocompetent patients with complete recovery over 2 to 3 weeks.
- Chronic arthralgia, headache, malaise, and weakness may persist after cryptosporidial infection even in immunologically normal people.
- If severe and prolonged (>30 days), testing for HIV and other immunocompromised states is appropriate along with a referral to an infectious disease specialist or gastroenterologist.

REFERRAL

- To an infectious disease specialist if symptoms persist and if HIV infection is found
- To a gastroenterologist if chronic malabsorption, or biliary or pancreatic complications occur

PEARLS & CONSIDERATIONS

- Chronic cryptosporidiosis (>30 days of diarrhea from *Cryptosporidium* spp. infection) in a patient with HIV is an AIDS-qualifying opportunistic infection.
- *Cryptosporidium hominis* has a limited host range (humans), whereas *Cryptosporidium parvum* has a wide host range including humans, horses, cattle, other domesticated animals, and wild animals—both species present a similar illness in humans.

SUGGESTED READINGS

Hunter PR et al: Health sequelae of human cryptosporidiosis in immunocompetent patients, *Clin Infect Dis* 39(4):504-510, 2004.

Smith HV, Corcoran GD: New drugs and treatment for cryptosporidiosis, *Curr Opin Infect Dis* 17(6):557, 2004.

AUTHORS: **GLENN G. FORT, M.D., M.P.H.,** and **DENNIS J. MIKOLICH, M.D.**

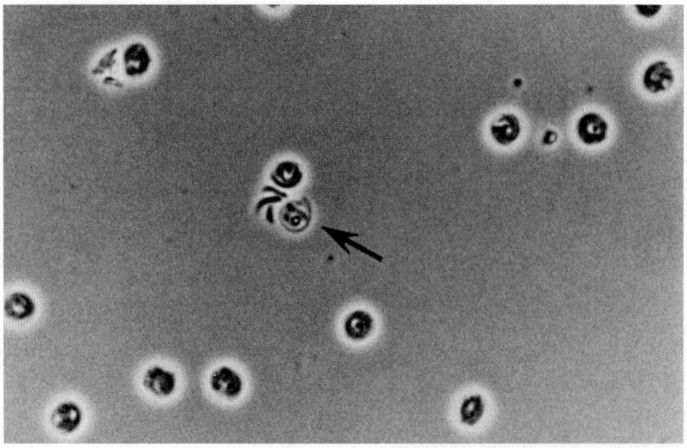

FIGURE 1-66 Human stool-derived *Cryptosporidium* oocysts. Excysting oocyst *(arrow)* is releasing three of its four sporozoites. (Phase-control microscopy ×630.) (From Gorbach SL: *Infectious diseases,* ed 2, Philadelphia, 1998, WB Saunders.)

BASIC INFORMATION

DEFINITION

Compression of the ulnar nerve behind the elbow (cubitus)

SYNONYMS

Tardy ulnar palsy

ICD-9CM CODES
354.2 Cubital tunnel syndrome

EPIDEMIOLOGY & DEMOGRAPHICS

Prevalent sex: Males = females

PHYSICAL FINDINGS & CLINICAL PRESENTATION

- Paresthesias and numbness along distribution of ulnar nerve (ulnar one and one-half fingers)
- Positive Tinel's sign at elbow
- Positive elbow flexion test (flexion of elbow with wrist extended for 30 sec may reproduce symptoms)
- May be diminished sensation to tip of small finger
- Ulnar nerve may be subluxable with elbow motion or by manipulation
- Cubitus valgus may be present if prior bony injury
- Interosseous weakness in long-standing cases with atrophy (Fig. 1-67)

ETIOLOGY

- Direct pressure
- Cubitus valgus deformity
- Subluxation of ulnar nerve
- Repeated stretching during throwing motion
- Elbow synovitis
- Local muscular hypertrophy

DIAGNOSIS

DIFFERENTIAL DIAGNOSIS

- Medial epicondylitis
- Medial elbow instability
- Carpal tunnel syndrome
- Cervical disc syndrome with radicular arm symptoms
- Ulnar nerve compression at wrist (Guyon's canal)

WORKUP

Diagnosis can usually be established clinically

IMAGING STUDIES

- Routine roentgenograms may be helpful in establishing cause or ruling out other conditions
- Electrodiagnostic studies: nerve conduction tests and electromyography are useful in establishing diagnosis and ruling out other syndromes

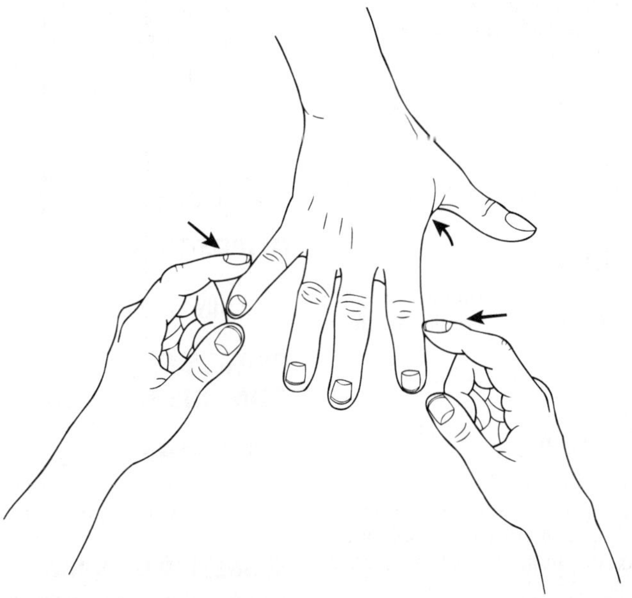

FIGURE 1-67 Testing for intrinsic (ulnar) motor weakness (fanning the fingers against resistance). Always look for atrophy of the first dorsal interosseus *(curved arrow)* when ulnar nerve lesions are suspected. (From Mercier LR: *Practical orthopedics,* ed 5, St Louis, 2000, Mosby.)

TREATMENT

ACUTE GENERAL Rx

- Protect nerve from pressure
- Elbow pads
- Avoid prolonged elbow flexion (talking on phone with elbow bent)

DISPOSITION

- Prognosis is variable.
- Mild to moderate cases recover well if offending activity can be eliminated. If muscle atrophy has developed, recovery of strength may be incomplete in spite of treatment.
- Medical management may be continued as long as symptoms are controlled and no motor deficit has developed.

REFERRAL

Surgical referral in cases of failed medical management or if signs of motor impairment are present

SUGGESTED READINGS

Creighton RA et al: Evaluation of the medial elbow in the throwing athlete, *Am J Orthop* 35:266, 2006.

Cutts S: Cubital tunnel syndrome, *Postgrad Med J* 83:28, 2007.

Elhassan B, Steinmann SP: Entrapment neuropathy of the ulnar nerve, *J Am Acad Orthop Surg* 15:672, 2007.

Grana W: Medial epicondylitis and cubital tunnel syndrome in the throwing athlete, *Clin Sports Med* 20(3):541, 2001.

Kato H et al: Cubital tunnel syndrome associated with medial elbow ganglia and osteoarthritis of the elbow, *J Bone Joint Surg* 84(A):1413, 2002.

Lee DH, Claussen GC, Oh S: Clinical nerve conduction and needle electroonyography studies, *J Am Acad Orthop Surg* 12:276, 2004.

Park GY, Kim JM, Lee SM: The ultrasonographic and electro-diagnostic findings of ulnar neuropathy at the elbow, *Arch Phys Med Rehabil* 85:1000, 2004.

Sasaki J et al: Ultrasonographic assessment of ulnar collateral ligament and medial elbow laxity in college baseball players, *J Bone Joint Surg* 84(A):525, 2002.

Shin R, Ring D: The ulnar nerve in elbow trauma, *J Bone Joint Surg* 89:1108, 2007.

Szabo RM, Kwak C: Natural history and conservative management of cubital tunnel syndrome, *Hand Clin* 23:311, 2007.

AUTHOR: **LONNIE R. MERCIER, M.D.**

BASIC INFORMATION

DEFINITION

- Cushing's syndrome is the occurrence of clinical abnormalities associated with glucocorticoid excess secondary to exaggerated adrenal cortisol production or chronic glucocorticoid therapy.
- Cushing's disease is Cushing's syndrome caused by pituitary ACTH excess.

ICD-9CM CODES
255.0 Cushing's disease or syndrome

PHYSICAL FINDINGS & CLINICAL PRESENTATION

- Hypertension
- Central obesity with rounding of the facies (moon facies); thin extremities
- Hirsutism, menstrual irregularities, hypogonadism
- Skin fragility, ecchymoses, red-purple abdominal striae, acne, poor wound healing, hair loss, facial plethora, hyperpigmentation (when there is ACTH excess)
- Psychosis, emotional lability, paranoia
- Muscle wasting with proximal myopathy

NOTE: The previous characteristics are not commonly present in Cushing's syndrome secondary to ectopic ACTH production. Many of these tumors secrete a biologically inactive ACTH that does not activate adrenal steroid synthesis. These patients may have only weight loss and weakness.

ETIOLOGY

- Iatrogenic from chronic glucocorticoid therapy (common)
- Pituitary ACTH excess (Cushing's disease; 60%)
- Adrenal neoplasms (30%)
- Ectopic ACTH production (neoplasms of lung, pancreas, kidney, thyroid, thymus; 10%)

DIAGNOSIS

DIFFERENTIAL DIAGNOSIS

- Alcoholic pseudo-Cushing's syndrome (endogenous cortisol overproduction)
- Obesity associated with diabetes mellitus
- Adrenogenital syndrome

WORKUP

- In patients with a clinical diagnosis of Cushing's syndrome the initial screening test is the overnight dexamethasone suppression test:
  1. Dexamethasone 1 mg PO given at 11 P.M.
  2. Plasma cortisol level measured 9 hr later (8 A.M.)
  3. Plasma cortisol level <5 μg/100 ml excludes Cushing's syndrome
- Serial measurements (two or three consecutive measurements) of 24-hr urinary free cortisol and creatinine (to ensure adequacy of collection) are undertaken if overnight dexamethasone test is suggestive of Cushing's syndrome. Persistent elevated cortisol excretion (>300 μg/24 hr) indicates Cushing's syndrome.
- The low-dose (2 mg) dexamethasone suppression test is useful to exclude pseudo-Cushing's syndrome if the previous results are equivocal. CRH stimulation after low-dose dexamethasone administration (dexamethasone-CRH test) is also used to distinguish patients with suspected Cushing's syndrome from those who have mildly elevated urinary free cortisol level and equivocal findings.
- The high-dose (8 mg) dexamethasone test and measurement of ACTH by RIA are useful to determine the etiology of Cushing's syndrome.
  1. ACTH undetectable or decreased and lack of suppression indicates adrenal etiology of Cushing's syndrome.
  2. ACTH normal or increased and lack of suppression indicate ectopic ACTH production.
  3. ACTH normal or increased and partial suppression suggest pituitary excess (Cushing's disease).
- A single midnight serum cortisol (normal diurnal variation leads to a nadir around midnight) >7.5 μg/dl has been reported as 96% sensitive and 100% specific for the diagnosis of Cushing's syndrome.

LABORATORY TESTS

- Hypokalemia, hypochloremia, metabolic alkalosis, hyperglycemia, hypercholesterolemia
- Increased 24-hr urinary free cortisol (>100 μg/24 hr)

IMAGING STUDIES

- CT scan or MRI of adrenal glands in suspected adrenal Cushing's syndrome
- MRI of pituitary gland with gadolinium in suspected pituitary Cushing's syndrome
- Additional imaging studies to localize neoplasms of the lung, pancreas, kidney, thyroid, or thymus in patients with ectopic ACTH production

TREATMENT

GENERAL Rx

The treatment of Cushing's syndrome varies with its cause:

- Pituitary adenoma: transsphenoidal microadenomectomy is the therapy of choice in adults. Pituitary irradiation is reserved for patients not cured by transsphenoidal surgery. In children, pituitary irradiation may be considered as initial therapy, because 85% of children are cured by radiation. Stereotactic radiotherapy (photon knife or gamma knife) is effective and exposes the surrounding neuronal tissues to less irradiation than conventional radiotherapy. Total bilateral adrenalectomy is reserved for patients not cured by transsphenoidal surgery or pituitary irradiation.
- Adrenal neoplasm:
  1. Surgical resection of the affected adrenal
  2. Glucocorticoid replacement for approximately 9 to 12 mo after the surgery to allow time for the contralateral adrenal to recover from its prolonged suppression
- Bilateral micronodular or macronodular adrenal hyperplasia: bilateral total adrenalectomy
- Ectopic ACTH:
  1. Surgical resection of the ACTH-secreting neoplasm
  2. Control of cortisol excess with metyrapone, aminoglutethimide, mifepristone, or ketoconazole
  3. Control of the mineralocorticoid effects of cortisol and 11-deoxycorticosteroid with spironolactone
  4. Bilateral adrenalectomy: a rational approach to patients with indolent, unresectable tumors

DISPOSITION

Prognosis is favorable in patients with surgically amenable disease.

PEARLS & CONSIDERATIONS

COMMENTS

Screening for MEN I should be considered in patients with Cushing's disease.

SUGGESTED READING

Boscaro M et al: The diagnosis of Cushing's syndrome, *Arch Intern Med* 160:3045, 2000.

AUTHOR: **FRED F. FERRI, M.D.**

BASIC INFORMATION

DEFINITION

Cystic fibrosis (CF) is an autosomal recessive disorder characterized by dysfunction of exocrine glands.

ICD-9CM CODES
277.0 Cystic fibrosis

EPIDEMIOLOGY & DEMOGRAPHICS

- It is the most common fatal hereditary disorder of caucasians in the U.S. (1 case/2500 caucasians) and second most common life-shortening childhood onset inherited disorder in the U.S., behind sickle cell disease.
- Median age at diagnosis is 5.3 months. Median survival is 30 yr.

PHYSICAL FINDINGS & CLINICAL PRESENTATION

- Failure to thrive in children
- Increased anterior/posterior chest diameter
- Basilar crackles and hyperresonance to percussion
- Digital clubbing
- Chronic cough
- Abdominal distention
- Greasy, smelly feces

ETIOLOGY

Chromosome 7 gene mutation (CFTR gene) resulting in abnormalities in chloride transport and water flux across the surface of epithelial cells; the abnormal secretions cause obstruction of glands and ducts in various organs and subsequent damage to exocrine tissue (recurrent pneumonia, atelectasis, bronchiectasis, diabetes mellitus, biliary cirrhosis, cholelithiasis, intestinal obstruction, increased risk of GI malignancies)

DIAGNOSIS

DIFFERENTIAL DIAGNOSIS

- Immunodeficiency states
- Celiac disease
- Asthma
- Recurrent pneumonia

WORKUP

A diagnosis of CF requires a positive quantitative pilocarpine iontophoresis test with one or more phenotypic features consistent with CF (e.g., chronic suppurative obstructive lung disease, pancreatic insufficiency) or documented CF in a sibling or first cousin.

LABORATORY TESTS

- Pilocarpine iontophoresis ("sweat test"): diagnostic of cystic fibrosis in children if sweat chloride is >60 mmol/L (>80 mmol/L in adults) on two separate tests on consecutive days. Repeat testing may be necessary because not all infants have sufficient quantities of sweat for reliable testing
- DNA testing may be useful for confirming the diagnosis and providing genetic information for family members
- Sputum C&S and Gram stain (frequent bacterial infections with *Staphylococcus aureus, Pseudomonas aeruginosa* [most common virulent respiratory pathogen], *Haemophilus influenzae*)
- Low albumin level, increased 72-hr fecal fat excretion
- Pulse oximetry or ABGs: hypoxemia
- Pulmonary function studies: decreased TLC, forced vital capacity, pulmonary diffusing capacity

IMAGING STUDIES

- Chest x-ray: may reveal focal atelectasis, peribronchial cuffing, bronchiectasis, increased interstitial markings, hyperinflation
- High-resolution chest CT scan: bronchial wall thickening, cystic lesions, ring shadows (bronchiectasis)

TREATMENT

NONPHARMACOLOGIC THERAPY

- Postural drainage and chest percussion
- Encouragement of regular exercise and proper nutrition
- Psychosocial evaluation and counseling of patient and family members

ACUTE GENERAL Rx

- Antibiotic therapy based on results of Gram stain and C&S of sputum (PO ciprofloxacin or floxacillin for *Pseudomonas*, cephalosporins for *S. aureus*, IV aminoglycosides plus ceftazidime for life-threatening *Pseudomonas* infections). Macrolides are also active against *pseudomona aeruginosa*. A recent study using azithromycin maintenance in children with CF for 6 mo found less use of additional antibiotics and improvement in some aspects of pulmonary function. Additional studies may be necessary to determine if azithromycin should be used as a primary therapy or rescue treatment
- Bronchodilators for patients with air flow obstruction
- Chronic pancreatic enzyme replacement
- Alternate-day prednisone (2 mg/kg) possibly beneficial in children with cystic fibrosis (decreased hospitalization rate, improved pulmonary function); routine use of corticosteroids not recommended in adults; among children with cystic fibrosis who have received alternate-day treatment with prednisone, boys, but not girls, have persistent growth impairment after treatment is discontinued
- Proper nutrition and vitamin supplementation
- Recombinant human deoxyribonuclease (DNase [Dornase alpha]) 2.5 mg qd or bid given by aerosol for patients with viscid sputum. It is useful to improve mucociliary clearance by liquefying difficult-to-clear pulmonary secretions. It is, however, very expensive (annual cost to the pharmacist is >$10,000); most beneficial in patients with FVC values >40% of predicted. Its cost can be decreased by using alternate-day rhDnase therapy
- Intermittent administration of inhaled tobramycin has been reported beneficial in CF
- Treatment of impaired glucose tolerance and diabetes mellitus

CHRONIC Rx Pneumococcal vaccination, yearly influenza vaccination

DISPOSITION

- More than 50% of children with cystic fibrosis live beyond age 20 yr.
- Lung transplantation is the only definitive treatment; 3-yr survival following transplantation exceeds 50%.
- Obstructive azoospermia is present in >98% of postpubertal males.

REFERRAL

- To regional ambulatory care cystic fibrosis center.
- For lung transplantation in selected patients. Indications for lung transplantation are: FEV in 1 sec <30% of predicted, rapidly progressive respiratory deterioration, increasing number of hospital admissions, massive hemoptysis, recurrent pneumothorax, arterial partial pressure of oxygen <55 mmHg, arterial partial pressure of carbon dioxide >50 mm Hg, multiresistant organisms, wasting. Young female patients should be referred earlier due to overall poor prognosis.
- For screening of family members with DNA analysis.

PEARLS & CONSIDERATIONS

COMMENTS

- Clinicians should think of cystic fibrosis in any patient with bronchiectasis plus any of the following: male infertility, recurrent idiopathic pancreatitis, recurrent nasal polyposis.
- Genetic testing for CF should be offered to adults with a positive family history of CF, to couples currently planning a pregnancy, and to couples seeking prenatal care.
- Inhalation of hypertonic saline (5 ml of 7% sodium chloride qid) has been reported to produce a sustained acceleration of mucus clearance and improved lung function.

SUGGESTED READINGS

Swiss Med Wkly 133:111, 2003.
JAMA 298(15):1787-1793, 2007.
N Engl J Med 354:241, 2006.
N Engl J Med 352:1992, 2005

AUTHOR: **FRED F. FERRI, M.D.**

BASIC INFORMATION

DEFINITION

Cysticercosis is an infection caused by the tissue deposition of larval forms of the pork tapeworm *Taenia solium*. *T. solium* cysts, or cysticerci, may accumulate in any tissue including the eyes, spinal cord, skin, muscle, heart, and brain.

Central nervous system involvement is common and is known as neurocysticercosis. Humans acquire cysticercosis via fecal-oral transmission of *T. solium* eggs from human tapeworm carriers, often by ingesting tapeworm eggs or cysts in contaminated food or water. Undercooked pork is the most commonly identified food source. The eggs hatch in the gastrointestinal tract, and larvae migrate hematogenously to tissues and then encyst, forming cysticerci.

SYNONYMS

Cysticerciasis
Taeniasis
Pork tapeworm

ICD-9CM CODES
123.1 Cysticercosis

EPIDEMIOLOGY & DEMOGRAPHICS

- *T. solium* infection is worldwide in distribution. Tapeworm infection and cysticercosis are endemic in rural, developing countries where pigs are raised as a food source.
- Serologic studies from endemic areas of Latin America have demonstrated seroprevalences of 4.9% to 24%.
- Neurocysticercosis is the most common cause of acquired epilepsy worldwide, and has become an important parasitic disease in the U.S., especially in states with large immigrant populations from countries where the disease is endemic.

PHYSICAL FINDINGS & CLINICAL PRESENTATION

- Following ingestion of *T. solium* eggs or cysts, humans may remain asymptomatic for several years.
- The symptoms are varied and depend on the location of cysticerci. Cysticerci in muscles and skin may form "cold" nodules, which are usually asymptomatic but may calcify.
- Neurocysticercosis, the presence of intraparenchymal cysts, may be asymptomatic. Symptoms stem from inflammation associated with the degeneration of cysts.
- Seizures are the most common manifestation of neurocysticercosis, occurring in 70% to 90% of symptomatic cases. Headache is also common.
- Inflammation around degenerating cysts may result in focal encephalitis, vasculitis, chronic meningitis, and cranial nerve palsies.
- When cysts lodge within the ventricular system (10% to 20% of neurocysticercosis cases), life-threatening acute intracranial hypertension, due to obstructive hydrocephalus, may occur. This syndrome is related to the location of the parasites in the cerebral ventricles or basal cisterns, blocking the circulation of the cerebrospinal fluid, and is caused by the presence of the parasite itself, ependymal inflammation, and/or fibrosis. Death may occur from progressive hydrocephalus, cerebral edema, or intractable seizures.

ETIOLOGY

- *T. solium* has a complex two-host life cycle.
- Humans are the only definitive host and harbor the adult worm in the intestine (taeniasis). However, both humans and pigs can serve as intermediate hosts and harbor the larvae or cysticerci (Fig. 1-68).

DIAGNOSIS Dx

DIFFERENTIAL DIAGNOSIS

- Idiopathic epilepsy
- Migraine
- Central nervous system (CNS) vasculitis
- Primary neoplasia of CNS
- Chronic CNS infections including toxoplasmosis, coccidioidomycosis, tuberculosis, cryptococcosis
- Brain abscess
- CNS sarcoidosis, systemic lupus erythematosus (SLE)

WORKUP

Comprehensive clinical history: Obtain information on area and sanitary conditions of residence, previous travel, and dietary habits, most importantly consumption of undercooked pork.

LABORATORY TESTS

- Definitive diagnosis is based on the histopathologic demonstration of cysticerci in the tissue involved.
- Peripheral eosinophilia is absent.
- Stool examination for ova and proglottids of *T. solium* is insensitive and not specific for the diagnosis of cysticercosis.
- Cerebrospinal fluid examination may demonstrate pleocytosis, with lymphocytic or eosinophilic predominance, low glucose, and elevated protein with neurocysticercosis. CSF is normal in most cases.
- An enzyme-linked immunoelectrotransfer blot (EITB) assay is the test of choice for detecting anticysticercal

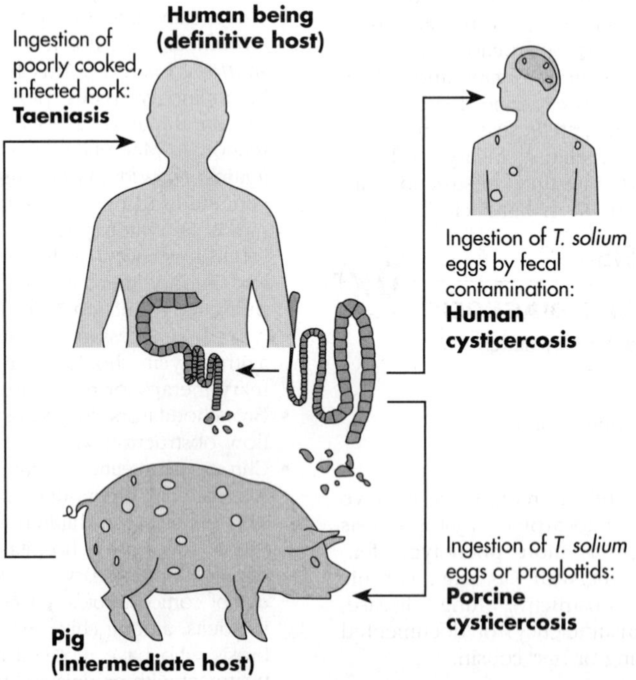

FIGURE 1-68 Cysticercosis is most commonly acquired by ingesting undercooked pork infected with *Taenia solium* cysticerci. Adult worms develop in the small intestine, forming proglottids that produce many fertilized eggs. Eggs and proglottids are intermittently shed in the stools of the persons infected with an adult tapeworm, where they can be ingested by pigs (the intermediate host) or transmitted via fecal-oral contamination to other humans. In the small intestine of the host, the eggs hatch and release larvae that travel through the bloodstream to various organs, where they develop into fluid-filled cystic larvae within months. Skeletal muscle, subcutaneous tissue, the eyes, and the central nervous system are most commonly invaded.

antibodies. This assay uses affinity purified glycoprotein antigens and has higher sensitivity (83% to 100%) and specificity (93% to 98%) than other enzyme-linked antibody (e.g., ELISA) tests. However, the diagnostic performance of the EITB can vary in different patient populations depending on the activity of the cysts and number of lesions. Single calcified lesions are more likely to be associated with a false negative assay result. Sensitivity is greater in serum than in CSF.
- There is no culture or nucleic acid (e.g., PCR) test available to diagnose active infection.

IMAGING STUDIES

- Plain radiographs of the extremities may reveal calcified cysts in patients with soft tissue or muscle involvement.
- For diagnosis of neurocysticercosis, CT and MRI are most commonly used.
  - Brain CT: Sensitivity and specificity of 95%. Can identify living cysticerci, which appear as hypodense lesions, as well as degenerating cysts, which appear as isodense or hyperdense lesions. It is considered the best method for detecting calcification associated with prior infection, which suggests inactivity.
  - Brain MRI: Most accurate technique to assess the extent of infection, location, and evolutionary stage of the parasites. Provides detailed images of living and degenerating cysts, perilesional edema, as well as small cysts or those located in the ventricles, brain stem, and cerebellum.

TREATMENT

Rx

Asymptomatic cysticercosis: There is no evidence that administering antiparasitic therapy is beneficial.

Symptomatic cysticercosis: Patients with active lesions, with evidence of surrounding edema and/or inflammation, generally warrant treatment with antiparasitics, corticosteroids, and anticonvulsants.

- *Anticonvulsant therapy:*
  - Patients who present with seizures or are considered to be at risk for recurrent seizures based on imaging should be treated with anticonvulsants.
- *Antiparasitic therapy:*
  - Pharmacologic therapy is indicated in the treatment of symptomatic patients with multiple viable brain parenchymal cysticerci.
  - Calcified cysticerci are inactive and do not warrant antiparasitic treatment.
  - Antiparasitic therapy is often unnecessary in patients with single cysts, because treatment does not alter the natural history of single-cyst disease.
- *Cysticidal therapy:*
  - Therapy hastens the disappearance of cysts and should initially be given in conjunction with corticosteroids to control the inflammation associated with dying organisms.
  - Patients with viable parenchymal or subarachnoid cysts should be treated with albendazole 15 mg/kg/day for 8 days or praziquantel 50 mg/kg/day for 15 days. Antiparasitics should be used cautiously in patients with massive cysticercal infection of the brain parenchyma (>50 cysts) or cysticercal encephalitis. These patients should be managed initially with corticosteroids, and perhaps mannitol, to control intracranial hypertension. Once the inflammation and the edema have resolved by MRI, antiparasitics can be administered.
  - Praziquantel may cause drug interactions with other agents metabolized via the cytochrome p450 systems, including phenytoin and phenobarbital.
  - Albendazole has no significant drug interactions with anticonvulsants.
- *Surgical therapy:*
  - Surgery may be indicated in patients with obstructive hydrocephalus or giant cysts with associated intracranial hypertension.
  - Surgical interventions may include craniotomy, with cyst extraction, stereotactic cyst aspiration, or ventriculoperitoneal shunt placement to control hydrocephalus.
  - Extraparenchymal cysticercosis, including ocular, subarachnoid, and intraventricular disease, carries poor prognosis and requires a more aggressive approach. When feasible, complete surgical excision of lesions remains the definitive therapy.

CHRONIC Rx

- Praziquantel and albendazole may not be a definitive cure for seizures, and antiepileptic medications may need to be continued indefinitely.
- Some patients with neurocysticercosis develop chronic or recurrent perilesional inflammation, requiring long-term, high-dose steroid therapy. Methotrexate has been reported to be of use as a steroid-sparing agent in this setting.

DISPOSITION

- In seizure-free, stable neurocysticercosis, outpatient management can be safely done. Long-term follow-up is warranted.
- In the U.S., law-enforced restriction of driving varies by state, and physicians have the duty to restrict or to release restriction of driving in patients with seizures.

REFERRAL

- Infectious diseases consultation
- Neurology consultation in patients with seizures
- Neurosurgical consultation if extraparenchymal neurocysticercosis or obstructive hydrocephalus is present

PREVENTION

Eradication of taeniasis/cysticercosis is possible. The disease disappears with implementation of meat inspection, improvement of pig husbandry, and improvement of socioeconomic conditions.

PATIENT/FAMILY EDUCATION

- Pork must be well cooked.
- Proper human excreta disposal and hand washing is of utmost importance to break the transmission cycle in households.

SUGGESTED READINGS

Cuetter AC et al: Neurocysticercosis: focus on intraventricular disease, *Clin Infect Dis* 24:157-164, 1997.

Del Brutto OH et al: Meta-analysis: cysticidal drugs for neurocysticercosis: albendazole and praziquantel, *Ann Intern Med* 145:43, 2006.

Garcia HH et al: New concepts in the diagnosis and management of neurocysticercosis *(Taenia solium), Am J Trop Med Hyg* 72:3, 2005.

Garcia HH et al: *Taenia solium* cysticercosis, *Lancet* 362:547-556, 2003.

Mitre E et al: Methotrexate as a corticosteroid-sparing agent in complicated neurocysticercosis, *Clin Infect Dis* 44:449-553, 2007.

Nash TE et al: Treatment of neurocysticercosis: current status and future research needs, *Neurology* 67:1120-1127, 2006.

Sorvillo FJ et al: Deaths from cysticercosis, United States, *Emerg Infect Dis* 13(2):230-235, 2007.

Takayanagui OM et al: Clinical aspects of neurocysticercosis, *Parasitology International* 55:S111-S115, 2006.

White AC: Neurocysticercosis: a major cause of neurological disease worldwide, *Clin Infect Dis* 24:101-115, 1997.

AUTHORS: **ELENI PATROZOU, M.D.,** and **STACI A. FISCHER, M.D., F.A.C.P.**

BASIC INFORMATION

DEFINITION

Infection with cytomegalovirus (CMV), a herpes virus, is common in the general population, with multiple mechanisms for transmission, often during childhood and adolescence. CMV is associated with pregnancy and can be a congenital disease. CMV is also associated with immunocompromised states and may be life threatening.

SYNONYMS

CMV
Heterophil-negative mononucleosis
Cytomegalic inclusion disease virus

ICD-9CM CODES
078.5 CMV infection
771.1 Congenital or perinatal CMV infection
V01.7 Exposure to CMV

EPIDEMIOLOGY & DEMOGRAPHICS

- Seroprevalence is widespread: 40% to 100% antibody positivity in adults.
- Increased infection develops perinatally, in day care exposure, and then during reproductive age, related to sexual activity.

ROUTES OF TRANSMISSION

- Blood transfusions
- Sexually (STDs) via uterus, cervix, and semen
- Perinatally via breast milk
- Transplant of organs—bone marrow, kidneys, liver, heart, or lung

PHYSICAL FINDINGS & CLINICAL PRESENTATION

Children: Congenital—25% of infected children with symptoms if congenital:
- Petechial rash
- Jaundice and/or hepatosplenomegaly
- Lethargy
- Respiratory distress
- CNS involvement, seizures

Postnatal acquisition:
- CMV mononucleosis
- Pharyngitis, croup, bronchitis, pneumonia

Healthy adults:
Common
- May be asymptomatic
- CMV mononucleosis similar to EBV mononucleosis
- Fever—lasting 9 to 30 days—mean of 19 days

Less common
- Exudative pharyngitis
- Lymphadenopathy, hepatitis, splenomegaly
- Interstitial pneumonia (rare)
- Nonspecific rash
- Thrombocytopenia/hemolytic anemia

Rare
- Guillain-Barré syndrome
- Meningoencephalitis
- Myocarditis

Immunosuppressed patients:
- Febrile mononucleosis
- GI ulcerations, hepatitis, pneumonitis, retinitis, encephalopathy, meningoencephalopathy
- HIV associated—dementia, demyelination, retinitis (Fig. 1-69), acalculous cholecystitis, adrenalitis, diarrhea, enterocolitis, esophagitis
- Diabetes associated with pancreatitis
- Adrenalitis associated with HIV

ETIOLOGY

Cytomegalovirus infection can remain latent, reactive with immunosuppression.

DIAGNOSIS

DIFFERENTIAL DIAGNOSIS

Congenital:
- Acute viral, bacterial, parasitic infections including other congenitally transmitted agents (toxoplasmosis, rubella, syphilis, pertussis, croup, bronchitis)

Acquired:
- EBV mononucleosis
- Viral hepatitis—A, B, C
- Cryptosporidiosis
- Toxoplasmosis
- *Mycobacterium avium* infections
- Human herpesvirus 6
- Acute HIV infection

WORKUP

- Laboratory confirmation combined with clinical findings often with leukopenia, thrombocytopenia, lymphocytosis

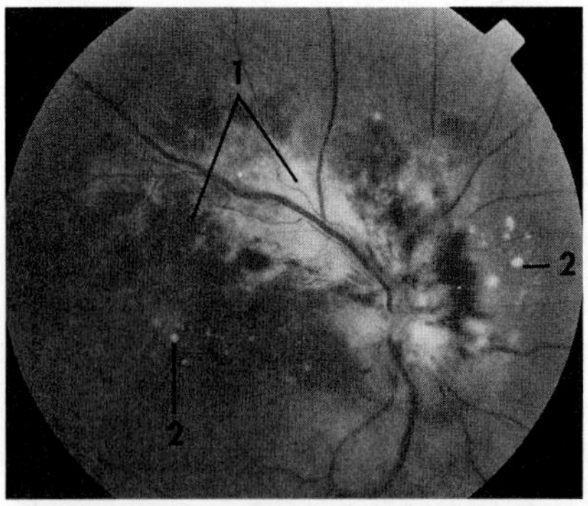

FIGURE 1-69 Sight-threatening CMV retinitis involves the macula and optic nerve of this HIV-positive young man. White, infected retina with intraretinal hemorrhage is present in the arcuate distribution of the nerve fiber layer *(1)*. A small amount of lipid exudation near the fovea and nasal to the optic nerve is also seen *(2)*. (From Palay D [ed]: *Ophthalmology for the primary care physician,* St Louis, 1997, Mosby.)

- Demonstration of virus in tissue or serologic testing including CMV IgM antibodies, rising titers of complement fixation (CF) and indirect fluorescent antibody (IFA) or anticomplement IFA
- Funduscopic—necrotic patches with white granular component of retina
- Cultures—(viral) human fibroblast from urine, cervical swab, tissue buffy coat
- Biopsy—"owl's eye" inclusion bodies on tissue sample

IMAGING STUDIES

- Chest x-ray—if pneumonitis suspected, consider bronchoscopy
- Endoscopy—if GI involvement
- CT scan/MRI—if CNS involvement

TREATMENT

NONPHARMACOLOGIC THERAPY

- Strict handwashing and standard precautions limit CMV transmission in health care facilities
- Highly active antiretroviral therapy (HAART) in patients with CD4 count $<50/mm^3$ for the goal of CD4 $>100/mm^3$ for a 3 to 6 mo period

ACUTE GENERAL Rx

For compromised hosts with CMV retinitis or pneumonitis:
- Ganciclovir 5 mg/kg bid IV × 21 days, then 5 mg/kg/day IV, or 1 g po tid or occular implant
- Foscarnet 60 mg/kg tid × 3 wk, then 90 mg/kg/day
- Cidofovir 5 mg/kg IV, repeat 1 wk later, then q2 wk IV
- Fomivirsen-salvage therapy for CMV retinitis 300 μg injected into vitreous

DISPOSITION

- CMV infection in patients who are immunocompromised (especially those with AIDS, bone marrow and solid organ transplant recipients, and disorders of cell-mediated immune function) will need expert, long-term follow-up by an infectious disease specialist or immunologist familiar with the care of such patients.
- CMV mononucleosis, hepatitis, pharyngitis, etc. in immunologically normal hosts are usually self-limiting infections requiring no special follow-up plans.

REFERRAL

- To an ophthalmologist if CMV retinitis is present
- To an infectious disease specialist or AIDS specialist for patients who are HIV-positive with CMV disease
- To a cellular immunologist or transplant specialist in the case of CMV infection in a transplant recipient

- To a pediatric infectious disease specialist for congenital CMV infection

PEARLS & CONSIDERATIONS

CMV is ubiquitous in the environment and is asymptomatically shed by latently infected persons with CMV infection, making it difficult to protect patients who are immunocompromised from acquiring this infection.

EVIDENCE

Ganciclovir is effective in preventing CMV disease and infections in recipients of solid organ transplants but has no effect on rate of graft loss, acute rejection, or death. It has been shown to be more effective than acyclovir in of kidney transplants.[1,2] Ⓐ Ⓑ

Uncertainty exists regarding the evidence for prophylactic oral ganciclovir in patients with advanced AIDS, and the benefits must be balanced with the serious side effects of treatment in this patient group.[3,4,5] Ⓐ Ⓑ

When deciding whether to institute prophylaxis in individual patients with advanced AIDS, ganciclovir-induced neutropenia, anemia, conflicting reports of efficacy, lack of proven survival benefit, risk for experiencing ganciclovir-resistant CMV, and cost are among the concerns that should be addressed.[6] Ⓒ

Evidence suggests that foscarnet may offer a survival advantage over ganciclovir for patients with AIDS and cytomegalovirus retinitis, but the rate of progression of retinitis is similar with both treatments.[5] Ⓑ

Intravenous cidofovir is as effective as oral ganciclovir plus the ganciclovir ocular implant in treating patients with acquired immunodeficiency syndrome (AIDS) and CMV retinitis.[7] Ⓑ

Intravenous cidofovir (low and high dose) delays progression of CMV retinitis in patients with AIDS, compared with deferred treatment, but is associated with some nephrotoxicity.[8,9] Ⓑ

A randomized controlled trial has shown a trend toward earlier mortality with valacyclovir vs. acyclovir in the treatment of CMV-seropositive patients with AIDS, and CD4 cell counts <100/mm3. This treatment is not recommended in this clinical setting.[10] Ⓑ

Prophylactic treatment with valacyclovir is an effective way to prevent CMV infection and delay the onset of CMV disease after renal transplantation.[11] Ⓑ

CMV immune globulin significantly reduces CMV-associated disease vs. placebo in CMV-seronegative patients who receive kidneys from CMV-seropositive donors.[12] Ⓑ

Compared with placebo, CMV immune globulin reduces severe CMV-associated disease in patients undergoing liver transplantation. This treatment, however, has no effect on rates of CMV infection, graft survival, or patient survival at 1 yr post transplant, nor is it beneficial in CMV donor-positive, recipient-negative liver transplant recipients.[13] Ⓑ

Evidence-Based References

1. Couchoud C: Cytomegalovirus prophylaxis with antiviral agents for solid organ transplantation, *Cochrane Database Sys Rev* Issue 4, 1998. Ⓐ
2. Flechner SM et al: A randomized prospective controlled trial of oral acyclovir versus oral ganciclovir for cytomegalovirus prophylaxis in high-risk kidney transplant recipients, *Transplantation* 66:1682, 1998. Ⓑ
3. Spector SA et al: Oral ganciclovir for the prevention of cytomegalovirus disease in persons with AIDS. Roche Cooperative Oral Ganciclovir Study Group, *N Engl J Med* 334:1491, 1996. Ⓐ
4. Brosqart CL et al: A randomized, placebo-controlled trial of the safety and efficacy of oral ganciclovir for prophylaxis of cytomegalovirus disease in HIV-infected individuals. Terry Beirn Community Programs for Clinical Research on AIDS, *AIDS* 12:269, 1998. Ⓐ
5. Studies of Ocular Complications of AIDS Research Group, in collaboration with the AIDS Clinical Trials Group: Mortality in patients with AIDS treated with either foscarnet or ganciclovir for CMV retinitis, *N Engl J Med* 326:213, 1992. Ⓑ
6. Kaplan JE et al: Guidelines for preventing opportunistic infections among HIV-infected persons—2002. Recommendations of the U.S. Public Health Service and the Infectious Diseases Society of America, *MMWR Recomm Rep* 51(RR-08):1, 2002. Ⓒ
7. Anon: The ganciclovir implant plus oral ganciclovir versus parenteral cidofovir for the treatment of CMV retinitis in patients with AIDS, *Am J Ophthalmol* 131:457, 2001. Ⓑ
8. The Studies of Ocular Complications of AIDS Research Group in Collaboration with ACTG. Cidofovir for the Rx. of CMV retinitis, *Ann Intern Med* 126:264, 1997. Ⓑ
9. Lalezari JP et al: Intravenous cidofovir for peripheral CMV retinitis in patients with AIDS. A randomized, controlled trial, *Ann Intern Med* 126:257, 1997. Ⓑ
10. Feinberg JE et al: A randomized, double-blind trial of valaciclovir prophylaxis for cytomegalovirus disease in patients with advanced human immunodeficiency virus infection. AIDS Clinical Trials Group Protocol 204/Glaxo Wellcome 123–014 International CMV Prophylaxis Study Group, *J Infect Dis* 177:48, 1998. Ⓑ
11. Lowance D et al: Valacyclovir for prevention of CMV disease after renal transplantation, *N Engl J Med* 340:1462, 1999. Ⓑ
12. Snydman DR et al: Use of CMVIG to prevent CMV disease in renal- transplant recipients, *N Engl J Med* 317:1049, 1987. Ⓑ
13. Snydman DR et al: CMVIG prophylaxis in liver transplantation, *Ann Intern Med* 119:984, 1993. Ⓑ

SUGGESTED READINGS

Burny W et al: Epidemiology, pathogenesis and prevention of congenital cytomegalovirus infection, *Expert Rev Anti Infect Ther* 2(6):881, 2004.

Fowler KB et al: Interval between births and risk of congenital cytomegalovirus infection, *Clin Infect Dis* 38(7):1035, 2004.

Fowler KB, Pass RF: Risk factors for congenital cytomegalovirus infection in the offspring of young women: exposure to young children and recent onset of sexual activity, *Pediatrics* 118(2):286, 2006.

Gao LH, Zheng SS: Cytomegalovirus and chronic allograft rejection in liver transplantation, *World J Gastroenterol* 10(13):1857, 2004.

AUTHORS: **STEVEN M. OPAL, M.D., MINA PANTCHEVA, M.D.,** and **DENNIS J. MIKOLICH, M.D.**

BASIC INFORMATION

DEFINITION

Decubitus ulcers (pressure ulcers) are any damage to the skin and the underlying tissue or both that results from pressure, friction, or shearing forces that usually occur over bony prominences.

SYNONYMS

Pressure ulcers
Pressure sores
Bedsores
Decubiti

ICD-9CM CODES
707.x Decubitus ulcers

EPIDEMIOLOGY & DEMOGRAPHICS

- Present in 5% to 10% of patients in all health care settings: hospitals, nursing homes, and home confined.
- Associated with significant morbidity and mortality. One-year mortality approaches 40%.
- Pain occurs in two thirds of patients with stage II or greater pressure ulcers.
- Complicated by cellulitis, osteomyelitis, abscesses, and sepsis.

CLINICAL PRESENTATION

All pressure ulcers should be staged according to depth and type of tissue damage.

Stage I	Nonblanchable erythema of intact skin or boggy mushy feeling of skin
Stage II	Partial-thickness skin loss involving the epidermis, dermis, or both
Stage III	Full-thickness skin loss involving damage or necrosis of subcutaneous tissue that may extend down to, but not through, underlying fascia or muscle
Stage IV	Full-thickness skin loss with extensive destruction and tissue damage to muscle, bone, or supporting structures (e.g., tendons, joint capsule)

ETIOLOGY

Decubitus ulcers are caused by constant, unrelieved pressure in tissues where circulation is diminished, leading to necrosis of the tissues. Shearing and friction forces can also contribute or cause damage to the tissues, leading to an ulcer.

DIAGNOSIS

DIFFERENTIAL DIAGNOSIS

- Venous stasis ulcers
- Arterial ulcers
- Diabetic ulcers
- Skin cancer
- Cellulitis

WORKUP

Describe ulcer, including the stage, location, and size, and for stages III and IV, describe the wound bed (i.e., epithelialization, granulation tissue, necrotic tissue, eschar); presence of any exudates, which includes type and amount; wound edges (i.e., undermining, sinus tracts, tunneling, or fistulas); any signs of infection; and pain. In addition, pressure ulcer risk factors and causes should be reassessed.

LABORATORY TESTS

- Directed at identifying cause of risk factors or any complications arising from the pressure ulcer (e.g., abscess or osteomyelitis).
- Cultures of wound bed are not helpful and should not be performed.
- Low prealbumin levels may reveal malnutrition.
- CBC if infection is suspected.

IMAGING STUDIES

- Ultrasound not proven to be effective.
- MRI or bone scans may help identify osteomyelitis when clinically suspected.

TREATMENT

PREVENTION

- Identify high-risk patients using standardized risk assessment scales such as the Braden scale.
- Routine skin inspection and good skin care for high-risk patients.
- Minimize prolonged skin exposure to moisture, urine, or stool.
- Treat dry, cracking skin.
- Use repositioning and pressure-reducing devices (e.g., foam mattresses, low-air-loss beds, pillows, or foam wedges when in bed or in a chair).
  - Patient repositioning
    1. Although there is clinical consensus that repositioning is critical, three randomized controlled trials (RCTs) found no evidence that regular manual repositioning prevented pressure ulcers.
  - Bed surface
    1. Air-fluidized beds
       a. Two RCTs found that use of air-fluidized beds healed a greater number of ulcers after 15 days compared with standard care.
       b. Systematic review revealed no differences in rate of pressure ulcer healing with use of either alternating-pressure mattresses or low-air-loss beds compared with standard care.
    2. Pressure-relieving overlays
       a. One RCT demonstrated that viscoelastic pad on the operating table significantly reduced incidence of postoperative pressure ulcers compared with standard operating table.
       b. An RCT found that sheepskin overlays plus standard care vs. standard care alone significantly reduced incidence of pressure sores in elderly patients recuperating from hip fracture.
    3. Foam alternatives
       a. Four RCTs revealed that foam alternatives vs. standard hospital mattresses reduced the incidence of pressure ulcer development in elderly patients in orthopedic hospital wards.
       b. Forty-one RCTs demonstrated that patients lying on standard hospital mattresses are more likely to develop pressure ulcers than those patients lying on higher specification foam mattresses.
- Use adequate support surfaces while in bed or in a chair to prevent "bottoming out" (defined as less than 1 inch between patient and support surface measured by putting hand under support surface and feeling thickness to patient).
- Recent systematic review of pressure ulcer prevention strategies showed poor methodology in most studies. Use of support surfaces, repositioning, optimizing nutrition, and moisturizing sacral skin were most appropriate.

NONPHARMACOLOGIC THERAPY

- Should be cleaned at each dressing change; necrotic tissue should be debrided quickly as it delays wound healing.
- Wound irrigation should not exceed 15 psi and is best done with an 18-gauge angiocatheter.
- No one dressing or product is superior; should be used to keep ulcer bed moist and protect it from urine/stool.
- Avoid agents that are cytotoxic to epithelial cells (e.g., iodine, iodophor, sodium hypochlorite, hydrogen peroxide, acetic acid, and alcohol).
- Reduce pressure by using foam mattress, dynamic support surface (e.g., low-air-loss bed), and frequent repositioning (e.g., q2h).
- Hyperbaric oxygen, ultrasound, ultraviolet and low-energy radiation either are ineffective or have not been extensively evaluated for efficacy.
- Negative pressure devices (Vac devices) may help for wounds that have significant drainage.

- Correct poor nutrition.
- Minimize urinary/fecal incontinence.
- Use standardized assessment tool (e.g., PUSH tool) to monitor wound healing on weekly basis.
- No RCTs comparing debridement vs. no debridement in the treatment of pressure ulcers.
- Thirty-two RCTs comparing different debridement agents, but there is insufficient evidence to promote the use of one particular agent.
- One RCT demonstrated ulcers treated with collagenase healed significantly more quickly than those treated with hydrocolloid.
- A meta-analysis and one RCT found significant benefit in rates of healing with use of hydrocolloid dressings vs. traditional saline gauze dressings.
- No benefit was found with nutritional supplements or ultrasound therapy.

ACUTE GENERAL Rx

- Pain medications may be necessary as 50% of decubitus ulcers are painful.
- Growth factors appear promising but are second line treatments if traditional approaches are ineffective.

CHRONIC Rx

Continue vigilance with pressure reduction as decubitus ulcers can recur with minimal trauma.

COMPLEMENTARY & ALTERNATIVE MEDICINE

Vitamin C, zinc, and multivitamin supplements may be of benefit to optimize nutrition.

DISPOSITION

- When systematic risk assessments are done and preventive measures are followed, most pressure ulcers can be prevented. Most heal when appropriate management strategies are followed.
- Stage IV ulcers in high-risk patients (e.g., paraplegics) can take months or years to heal.

REFERRAL

- Physical and occupational therapists to improve bed and chair mobility.
- Wounds with necrotic tissue need referral to persons trained in sharp debridement.
- To plastic surgeons for operative repair for large stage III or IV ulcers that do not respond to optimal care.
- To a specialty wound center for nonhealing ulcers.

PEARLS & CONSIDERATIONS

COMMENTS

- Up to 10% of older persons will have a pressure ulcer.
- Identify and reduce all risk factors for pressure ulcers.
- Treat the pain associated with pressure ulcers.
- Proper skin care, use of support surfaces, mobilization, and attention to nutrition are key for prevention and treatment.
- Clinical studies have not revealed if any one dressing product is superior.
- Nonhealing ulcers require assessment for debridement, infection, abscess, and/or referral to a wound center.

PATIENT/FAMILY EDUCATION

- Educate patient and family members on the risk factors for pressure ulcers.
- Encourage mobility, adequate nutritional intake, and avoid bedrest.

SUGGESTED READINGS

Lyder C: Pressure ulcer prevention and management, *JAMA* 289(2):223, 2003.

National Pressure Ulcer Advisory Panel 9 (NPUAP): Pressure Ulcer Scale for Healing (PUSH), PUSH tool version 3.0 http://www.npuap.org/push3-0.htm

Reddy M et al: Preventing pressure ulcers: a systematic review, *JAMA* 296(8):974, 2006.

AUTHORS: **DAVID R. GIFFORD, M.D., M.P.H.,** and **LYNN MCNICOLL, M.D., F.R.C.P.C.**

BASIC INFORMATION

DEFINITION

Deep venous thrombosis (DVT) is the development of thrombi in the deep veins of the extremities or pelvis.

SYNONYMS

DVT
Venous thromboembolism (VTE) (VTE includes DVT and pulmonary embolism (PE))
Deep vein thrombosis

ICD-9CM CODES
451.1 Thrombosis of deep vessels of lower extremities
451.83 Thrombosis of deep veins of upper extremities
541.9 Deep vein thrombosis of unspecified site

EPIDEMIOLOGY & DEMOGRAPHICS

- Annual incidence in urban population is 1.6 cases/1000 persons.
- The risk of recurrent thromboembolism is higher among men than women.

PHYSICAL FINDINGS & CLINICAL PRESENTATION

- Pain and swelling of the affected extremity
- In lower extremity DVT: leg pain on dorsiflexion of the foot (Homans' sign)
- Physical examination may be unremarkable in early DVT

ETIOLOGY

The etiology is often multifactorial (prolonged stasis, coagulation abnormalities, vessel wall trauma). The following are risk factors for DVT:
- Prolonged immobilization (≥3 days)
- Postoperative state
- Trauma to pelvis and lower extremities for lower extremity DVT; central line placement for upper extremity DVT
- Birth control pills, high-dose estrogen therapy; conjugated equine estrogen but not esterified estrogen is associated with increased risk of DVT; estrogen plus progestin is associated with doubling the risk of venous thrombosis
- Visceral cancer (lung, pancreas, alimentary tract, genitourinary tract)
- Age >60 yr
- History of thromboembolic disease
- Hematologic disorders (e.g., antithrombin III deficiency, protein C deficiency, protein S deficiency, heparin cofactor II deficiency, sticky platelet syndrome, G20210A prothrombin mutation, lupus anticoagulant, dysfibrinogenemias, anticardiolipin antibody, hyperhomocystinemia, concurrent homocystinuria, high levels of factors VIII, XI, and factor V Leiden mutation)
- Pregnancy and early puerperium
- Obesity (BMI >30)
- Congestive heart failure
- Surgery, fracture, or injury involving lower leg or pelvis
- Surgery requiring >30 min of anesthesia
- Gynecologic surgery (particularly gynecologic cancer surgery)
- Recent travel (within 2 wk, lasting >8 hours)
- Smoking and abdominal obesity
- Central venous catheter or pacemaker insertion
- Superficial vein thrombosis, varicose veins

DIAGNOSIS

DIFFERENTIAL DIAGNOSIS

- Postphlebitic syndrome
- Superficial thrombophlebitis
- Ruptured Baker's cyst
- Cellulitis, lymphangitis, Achilles tendinitis
- Hematoma
- Muscle or soft tissue injury, stress fracture
- Varicose veins, lymphedema
- Arterial insufficiency
- Abscess
- Claudication
- Venous stasis

WORKUP

- The clinical diagnosis of DVT is inaccurate. Pain, tenderness, swelling, or color changes are not specific for DVT.

  Clinical prediction rules can be used to establish pretest probability of DVT. The Wells prediction rules for DVT and for pulmonary embolism are described in Box 1-10 in "Pulmonary Embolism." These rules perform better in younger patients without a history of DVT and in those without comorbidities. In younger patients without associated comorbidities and a low pretest probability using Wells criteria and a negative high-sensitivity D-dimer test, the diagnosis of DVT can be reasonably excluded.
- Compression ultrasonography is preferred as the initial study to diagnose DVT in patients with intermediate to high pretest probability. An initial negative test should be repeated after 5 days (if the clinical suspicion of DVT persists) to detect propagation of any thrombosis to the proximal veins. Comprehensive ultrasonography is a more extensive test, which examines the deep veins from the inguinal ligament to the level of the malleolus. Recent literature reports indicate that it may be safe to withhold anticoagulation after negative results on comprehensive duplex ultrasonography in nonpregnant patients with a suspected first episode of symptomatic DVT of the leg.

LABORATORY TESTS

- Laboratory tests are not specific for DVT. Baseline prothrombin time (INR), partial thromboplastin time, and platelet count should be obtained on all patients before starting anticoagulation.
- Use of D-dimer assay by ELISA may be useful in the management of suspected DVT. The combination of a normal D-dimer study on presentation together with a normal compression venous ultrasound is useful to exclude DVT and generally eliminate the need to do repeat ultrasound at 5 to 7 days. Recent trials indicate that DVT can be ruled out in patients who are clinically unlikely to have DVT and who have a negative D-dimer test. Compressive ultrasonography can be safely omitted in such patients. See an algorithm for the diagnosis of deep vein thrombosis in Section III.
- Laboratory evaluation of young patients with DVT, patients with recurrent thrombosis without obvious causes, and those with a family history of thrombosis should include protein S, protein C, fibrinogen, antithrombin III level, lupus anticoagulant, anticardiolipin antibodies, factor V Leiden, factor VIII, factor IX, and plasma homocysteine levels.

IMAGING STUDIES

Compression ultrasonography is generally preferred as the initial study because it is noninvasive and can be repeated serially (useful to monitor suspected acute DVT); it offers good sensitivity for detecting proximal vein thrombosis (in the popliteal or femoral vein). Its disadvantages are poor visualization of deep iliac and pelvic veins and poor sensitivity in isolated or nonocclusive calf vein thrombi.

Contrast venography is the gold standard for evaluation of DVT of the lower extremity. It is, however, invasive and painful. Additional disadvantages are the increased risk of phlebitis, new thrombosis, renal failure, and hypersensitivity reaction to contrast media; it also gives poor visualization of deep femoral vein in the thigh and internal iliac vein and its tributaries.

Magnetic resonance direct thrombus imaging (MRDTI) is an accurate noninvasive test for diagnosis of DVT. Current limitations are its cost and lack of widespread availability.

TREATMENT

Rx

NONPHARMACOLOGIC THERAPY

- Gradual resumption of normal activity. Immobility promotes stasis and propagation of DVT. Patients should get up and walk as tolerated. The theoretical risk that ambulation may dislodge thrombi in the legs precipitating PE is unfounded.
- Patient education on anticoagulant therapy and associated risks.

ACUTE GENERAL Rx

- Low-molecular-weight heparin (LMWH) for 4 to 7 days followed by warfarin therapy. Recommended dose of enoxaparin is 1 mg/kg q12h SC and continued for a minimum of 5 days and until a therapeutic INR (2 to 3) has been achieved with warfarin. Once-daily fondaparinux, a synthetic analog of heparin, is also as effective and safe as twice daily enoxaparin in the initial treatment of patients with symptomatic DVT. Warfarin therapy should be initiated when appropriate (usually within 72 hr of initiation of heparin). A 5-mg loading dose of warfarin is recommended in inpatients because it produces less excess anticoagulation than does a 10-mg dose; the smaller dose also avoids the development of a potential hypercoagulable state caused by precipitous decreases in levels of protein C during the first 36 hr of warfarin therapy. In the outpatient setting, a warfarin nomogram using 10-mg loading doses may be more effective in reaching a therapeutic INR. Long term LMWH may be preferable to warfarin in patients with cancer or those whose INR is difficult to control.
- Outpatient treatment of DVT is appropriate for patients without prior DVT, thrombophilic conditions, or substantial comorbidity, but not for those who are pregnant or likely not to adhere to therapy.
- Exclusions from outpatient treatment of DVT include patients with potential high complication risk (e.g., hemoglobin <7, platelet count <75,000, guaiac-positive stool, recent cerebrovascular accident or noncutaneous surgery, noncompliance).
- Compression stockings are effective in reducing the incidence of postthrombotic syndrome and should be used starting within 1 month of proximal DVT and for at least 1 yr after diagnosis.
- Insertion of an inferior vena cava filter to prevent pulmonary embolism is recommended in patients with contraindications to anticoagulation.
- Thrombolytic therapy (streptokinase) can be used in rare cases (unless contraindicated) in patients with extensive iliofemoral venous thrombosis and a low risk of bleeding.
- Preliminary trials reveal that idraparinux, a long-acting inhibitor of activated factor X given once weekly SC as a fixed dose for 3 or 6 months has efficacy similar to that of heparin plus a vitamin K antagonist in the treatment of DVT and causes less bleeding. However, in patients with PE, idraparinux was less efficacious than standard therapy.

CHRONIC Rx

- Conventional-intensity warfarin therapy is more effective than low-intensity warfarin therapy for the long-term prevention of recurrent DVT. The low-intensity warfarin regimen does not reduce the risk of clinically important bleeding.
- The optimal duration of anticoagulant therapy varies with the cause of DVT and the patient's risk factors:
  - Therapy for 3 to 6 months is generally satisfactory in patients with reversible risk factors (low-risk group). A high D-dimer level measured after 3 months of anticoagulation in patients with unprovoked DVT should favor a longer duration of therapy.
  - Anticoagulation for at least 6 months is recommended for patients with idiopathic venous thrombosis or medical risk factors for DVT (intermediate-risk group).
  - Indefinite anticoagulation is necessary in patients with DVT associated with active cancer; long-term anticoagulation is also indicated in patients with inherited thrombophilia (e.g., deficiency of protein C or S antibody), antiphospholipid, and those with recurrent episodes of idiopathic DVT (high-risk group).
- Measurement of D-dimer after withdrawal of oral anticoagulation may be useful to estimate the risk of recurrence. Patients with a first spontaneous DVT and a D-dimer level <250 mg/ml after withdrawal of oral anticoagulation have a low risk of DVT recurrence.

PEARLS & CONSIDERATIONS

!

COMMENTS

- When using heparin, there is a risk of heparin-induced thrombocytopenia (with unfractionated more so than with LMWH). Platelet count should be obtained initially and repeated every 3 days while on heparin.
- Prophylaxis of DVT is recommended in all patients at risk (e.g., low-molecular-weight heparin [enoxaparin 30 mg SC bid] after major trauma, post surgery of hip and knee; enoxaparin 40 mg SC qd post–abdominal surgery in patients with moderate to high DVT risk; gradient elastic stockings alone or in combination with intermittent pneumatic compression [IPC] boots following neurosurgery). Graduated compression stockings are effective for preventing air-travel-related DVT.
- Fondaparinux, a synthetic analog of heparin, can also be used for prevention of DVT after hip fracture surgery, hip replacement, or knee replacement. Initial dose is 2.5 mg SC given 6 to 8 hr postoperatively and continued daily. Its bleeding risk is similar to enoxaparin; however, it is more effective in preventing DVT.
- The risk of recurrent venous thromboembolism in heterozygous carriers of factor V Leiden and a first spontaneous venous thromboembolism is similar to that of noncarriers of factor V Leiden; therefore, heterozygous patients should receive secondary thromboprophylaxis for a similar length of time as patients without factor V Leiden.
- Approximately 20% to 50% of patients with DVT develop postthrombotic syndrome characterized by leg edema, pain, venous ectasia, skin unduration, and ulceration.
- Exercise following DVT is reasonable because it improves flexibility of the affected leg and does not increase symptoms in patients with postthrombotic syndrome.

EVIDENCE

EBM

An RCT found that intravenous unfractionated heparin plus 3 months of warfarin was significantly more effective than heparin alone for reducing proximal extension of thrombus in patients with isolated calf vein thrombosis.[1] (A)

Two systematic reviews compared low-molecular-weight heparin (LMWH) vs. unfractionated heparin in patients with proximal DVT. Symptomatic thromboembolic complications, clinically important bleeding, and mortality rate were significantly reduced in patients treated with LMWH.[2] (A)

Subcutaneous fondaparinux has been compared with subcutaneous enoxaparin twice daily and intravenous unfractionated heparin in the initial management of deep venous thrombosis and pulmonary embolism, respectively. Fondaparinux was found to be as safe and effective as each comparator, with no significant difference in recurrent thromboembolism, major bleeding, or mortality rates observed.[3] (B)

Evidence-Based References

1. Lagerstedt C et al: Need for long term anticoagulant treatment in symptomatic calf vein thrombosis, *Lancet* 334:515, 1985. Reviewed in: *Clin Evid* 11:284, 2004. Ⓐ
2. van den Belt AGM et al: Fixed dose subcutaneous low molecular weight heparins versus adjusted dose unfractionated heparin for venous thromboembolism, *Cochrane Database Syst Rev* 4:2004. Ⓐ
3. Buller HR et al: Fondaparinux or enoxaparin for the initial treatment of symptomatic deep venous thrombosis: a randomized trial, *Ann Intern Med* 140:867, 2004. Ⓑ

SUGGESTED READINGS

Bates SM, Ginsberg JS: Treatment of deep-vein thrombosis, *N Engl J Med* 351:268, 2004.

Chan WS et al: A red blood cell agglutination D-dimer test to exclude deep venous thrombosis in pregnancy, *Ann Intern Med* 147:165-170, 2007.

Francis CW: Prophylaxis for thromboembolism in hospitalized medical patients, *N Engl J Med* 356:1438-1444, 2007.

Kovacs MJ et al: Comparison of 10-mg and 5-mg warfarin initiation nomograms together with low-molecular-weight heparin for outpatient treatment of acute venous thromboembolism: a randomized, double-blind, controlled trial, *Ann Intern Med* 138:714, 2003.

Polareti G et al: D-dimer testing to determine the duration of anticoagulation therapy, *N Engl J Med* 355:1780-1789, 2006

Qaseem A et al: Current diagnosis of venous thromboembolism in primary care: a clinical practice guideline from the American Academy of Family Physicians and the American College of Physicians, *Ann Intern Med* 146:454-458, 2007.

Segal JB et al: Management of venous thromboembolism: a systematic review for a practice guideline, *Ann Intern Med* 146:211-222, 2007.

Snow V et al: Management of venous thromboembolism: a clinical practice guideline from the American College of Physicians and the American Academy of Family Physicians, *Ann Intern Med* 146:204-210, 2007.

Stevens SM et al: Withholding anticoagulation after a negative result on duplex ultrasonography for suspected symptomatic deep venous thrombosis, *Ann Intern Med* 140:985, 2004.

The van Gogh investigators: Idraparinux versus standard therapy for venous thromboembolic disease, *N Engl J Med* 357:1094-1104, 2007.

Wells PS et al: Evaluation of D-dimer in the diagnosis of suspected deep vein thrombosis, *N Engl J Med* 349:1227, 2003.

AUTHOR: **FRED F. FERRI, M.D.**

BASIC INFORMATION

DEFINITION

The key to delirium is that it has an acute/subacute onset.

The American Psychiatric Association's *Diagnostic and Statistical Manual,* 4th edition, (DSM-IV) definition:

A. Disturbance of consciousness (i.e., reduced clarity of awareness about the environment) with reduced ability to focus, sustain, or shift attention.
B. A change in cognition (e.g., memory deficit, disorientation, language disturbance) or development of a perceptual disturbance that is not better accounted for by a pre-existing, established, or evolving dementia.
C. The disturbance develops over a short period of time (usually hours to days) and tends to fluctuate during the course of a day.
D. Evidence from the history, physical examination, or laboratory findings indicate that the disturbance is caused by direct physiologic consequences of a general medical condition.*

SYNONYMS

Acute confusional state
Acute brain syndrome
Toxic or metabolic encephalopathy

ICD-9CM CODES
780.09 Delirium

EPIDEMIOLOGY & DEMOGRAPHICS

Approximately 10% to 30% of hospitalized patients experience delirium during the course of their treatment, but the rates can be even higher especially in intensive care units where it can affect up to 60% to 80%. Risk factors include extremes of age, severe pain, illicit substance use, surgery, dementia, and kidney or liver failure.

PHYSICAL FINDINGS & CLINICAL PRESENTATION

- Pay particular attention to reversible causes for delirium.
- Start with a careful history including especially the time course of the symptoms. Symptomatology may differ both among and within one patient. Thus history from various caregivers may conflict as delirium implies a mental status that is frequently in flux. Symptoms may include poor attention, sleepiness, agitation, or psychosis. Take notice of new medications, recent surgeries/illnesses, or treatments.
- Next perform a physical exam focusing on signs of infection, dehydration, or chronic disease that may be exacerbated. Vital signs are key! Be sure to include Mini Mental Status Exam.

ETIOLOGY

Can be multifactorial; often falls into one of these categories:

- Drugs: psychiatric and neurologic, narcotics, anticholinergics, beta blockers, steroids, NSAIDs, digoxin, cimetidine
- Infection/inflammation: any, including abdominal processes
- Metabolic: renal or liver failure, thyroid, adrenal or glucose dysregulation, anemia, vitamin deficiency
- Stress: surgery, sleep problems, pain, fever, hypoxia, anesthesia, environmental changes, fecal/urinary retention
- FEN: dysregulation of Ca, Mg, K, Na, dehydration, volume overload, altered pH

DIAGNOSIS

DIFFERENTIAL DIAGNOSIS

- Psychosis
- Dementia
- Depression/mania

LABORATORY TEST(S)

- Complete blood count, BUN, creatinine, and electrolytes
- Toxicology screen, liver function tests, ammonia
- Thyroid function tests, B_{12}, and folate levels
- RPR for syphilis, blood, urine, and spinal culture
- Arterial blood gas measurement

IMAGING STUDIES

- Radiologic imaging to consider includes head CT (to look for bleed, trauma, tumor, atrophy/dementia, stroke)
- Chest x-ray (to look for tumor, infection)

TREATMENT

NONPHARMACOLOGIC THERAPY

- The most important consideration is to keep the patient safe using a variety of methods including frequent reorientation.
- A quiet, restful, simplified environment with cues to time and location such as clock or calendar are helpful, as well as consistent staff providing both personal and medical care.
- Physical restraints if necessary to ensure safety.

ACUTE GENERAL RX

- Reverse any treatable cause.
- Haloperidol can be used to control agitation, with dose range from 0.25 to 2 mg IM/IV twice daily, repeating the dose every 20 to 30 minutes until patient has calmed, using lower doses for elderly.
- Risperidone 0.5 mg twice daily can also be used with a slow increase to desired dose.

CHRONIC RX

Delirium is not a chronic condition; if assessing a more long-term mental status change, consider other diagnoses.

DISPOSITION

Requires frequent monitoring, often necessitating hospital level of care to ensure safety and assess etiology.

REFERRAL

Consider neurologic or psychiatric consultation if not improved in several days or in complicated cases.

PEARLS & CONSIDERATIONS

COMMENTS

Though benzodiazepines are frequently used in hospitalized patients for sedation, and are the mainstay of therapy for alcohol withdrawal, they must be used with caution in elderly as they can have a paradoxical effect on agitation.

PREVENTION

- Avoid polypharmacy as much as possible.
- Optimize chronic medical conditions.
- Provide frequent reorientation and a soothing environment for high-risk patients (i.e., lights on during the day, off at night; open curtains during the day so patient can see the weather).

PATIENT/FAMILY EDUCATION

Inform about the above preventative techniques, especially polypharmacy risks.

SUGGESTED READINGS

American Psychiatric Association: *Diagnostic and statistical manual of mental disorders,* ed 4, Washington DC, 2000, American Psychiatric Association Press.

Gleason O: Delirium, *Am Fam Physician* 67:5, 2003.

Pandharipande P et al: Delirium: acute cognitive dysfunction in the critically ill, *Curr Opin Crit Care* 11, 2005.

AUTHOR: **CRISTINA A. PACHECO, M.D.**

BASIC INFORMATION

DEFINITION

Delirium tremens refers to overactivity of the central nervous system after cessation of alcohol intake. The time interval is variable; it usually occurs within 1 wk after reduction or cessation of heavy alcohol intake and persists for 1 to 3 days.

SYNONYMS

Alcohol withdrawal syndrome
DTs
Alcoholic delirium

ICD-9CM CODES
291.00 Alcohol withdrawal delirium

EPIDEMIOLOGY & DEMOGRAPHICS

INCIDENCE (IN U.S.): Up to 500,000 cases annually
PEAK INCIDENCE: 30 yr and older
PREDOMINANT SEX: Male
PEAK AGE: Teenage years and older
GENETICS: More common with patients who have relatives who are alcoholics

PHYSICAL FINDINGS & CLINICAL PRESENTATION

- Initially: anxiety, insomnia, tremulousness
- Early: tachycardia, sweating, anorexia, agitation, headache, GI distress
- Late: seizures, visual hallucinations, delirium

ETIOLOGY

Alcoholism

DIAGNOSIS

DIFFERENTIAL DIAGNOSIS

- Coexisting illness
- Trauma
- Drug usage

WORKUP

- Frequent rating of symptoms (hallucinations, tremor, sweating, agitation, orientation).
- The Clinical Institute Withdrawal Assessment-Alcohol (CIWA-A) scale can be used to measure the severity of alcohol withdrawal. It consists of the 10 following items:
  1. Nausea
  2. Tremor
  3. Autonomic hyperactivity
  4. Anxiety
  5. Agitation
  6. Tactile disturbances
  7. Visual disturbances
  8. Auditory disturbances
  9. Headache
  10. Disorientation

The maximum score is 67. When the CIWA-A score is ≥8, patients are usually given 2 to 4 mg of lorazepam hourly.

LABORATORY TESTS

- Electrolytes
- Close monitoring of glucose levels
- Drug screen

IMAGING STUDIES

CT scan of head if there is a history of head trauma

TREATMENT

NONPHARMACOLOGIC THERAPY

Refer to drug rehabilitation program after patient recovers.

ACUTE GENERAL Rx

1. Admission to a detoxification unit where patient can be observed closely
2. Vital signs q30min initially (neurologic signs, if necessary)
3. Use of lateral decubitus or prone position if restraints are necessary
4. NPO: NG tube for abdominal distention may be necessary but should not be routinely used
5. Vigorous hydration (4 to 6 L/day): IV with glucose (Na^+, K^+, PO_4^{-3}, and Mg^{2+} replacement)
6. Vitamins: thiamine, 100 mg IV qd. The initial dose of thiamine should precede the administration of IV dextrose; multivitamins (may be added to the hydrating solution)
7. Sedation
   a. Initially: lorazepam 2 to 5 mg IM/IV repeated prn
   b. Maintenance (individualized dosage): chlordiazepoxide, 50 to 100 mg PO q4 to 6h, lorazepam 2 mg PO q4h, or diazepam 5 to 10 mg PO tid; withhold doses or decrease subsequent doses if signs of oversedation are apparent
   c. Midazolam is also effective for managing DTs. Its rapid onset (sedation within 2 to 4 min of IV injection) and short duration of action (approximately 30 min) make it an ideal agent for titration in continuous infusion
8. Treatment of seizures: Diazepam 2.5 mg/min IV until seizure is controlled (check for respiratory depression or hypotension) may be beneficial for prolonged seizure activity; IV lorazepam 1 to 2 mg every 2 hr can be used in place of diazepam; generally, withdrawal seizures are self-limited and treatment is not required; the use of phenytoin or other anticonvulsants for short-term treatment of alcohol withdrawal seizures is not recommended
9. Diagnosis and treatment of concomitant medical, surgical, or psychiatric conditions

CHRONIC Rx

Alcoholics Anonymous has the best record in breaking addiction, but the results are still disappointing.

DISPOSITION

Refer to drug rehabilitation program.

REFERRAL

If cardiac arrhythmias are prominent or respiratory distress develops

PEARLS & CONSIDERATIONS

COMMENTS

This is a potentially lethal disease if not carefully treated. Mortality is 15% in untreated patients.

SUGGESTED READING

Kosten TR, O'Connor PG: Management of drug and alcohol withdrawal, *N Engl J Med* 348:1786, 2003.

AUTHOR: **FRED F. FERRI, M.D.**

BASIC INFORMATION

DEFINITION

A progressive neurodegenerative disease with core features of dementia accompanied or followed by parkinsonism.

SYNONYMS

Diffuse Lewy body disease, dementia with parkinsonism

ICD-9CM CODES
331.82 Dementia with Lewy bodies (DLB)

EPIDEMIOLOGY & DEMOGRAPHICS

- Now thought to be the second most common primary degenerative dementia, accounting for 10% to 15% of cases at autopsy
- Prevalence at age 65 estimated at 0.7%; at age 85 rises to 5.0%

PHYSICAL FINDINGS & CLINICAL PRESENTATION

- Most often dementia precedes appearance of parkinsonism by months to years.
- Dementia is superficially quite similar to Alzheimer's disease. Early visual hallucinations (outside the setting of dopaminergic therapy) occur in up to 80% and are the major differentiating feature from AD. Typically the hallucinations are well formed and detailed.
- Fluctuations in performance, especially with regards to attention and alertness, are another key feature of the presentation. Can occur acutely, leading to misdiagnosis of vascular dementia presenting with stroke. These fluctuations may last hours or days.
- Parkinsonism is typically symmetrical and axially predominant, with little tremor but prominent gait impairment and postural instability.
- Parkinsonism is not ubiquitous; up to 25% of cases diagnosed by autopsy had mild or no reported parkinsonian features.
- Rapid eye movement (REM) sleep behavior disorder and other related sleep abnormalities are common.

ETIOLOGY

- Uncertain; it is felt that DLB probably results from abnormal handling of alpha-synuclein with resulting aggregation of the protein inside neurons.
- Lewy bodies are eosinophilic intracellular inclusions, which contain alpha-synuclein and ubiquitin; it is not clear whether they are pathogenic.

DIAGNOSIS

DIFFERENTIAL DIAGNOSIS

- Parkinson's disease dementia (PDD)—differentiated from DLB in which dementia usually precedes parkinsonism.
- Alzheimer's disease (AD)—differs from DLB in which visual hallucinations and parkinsonism are prominent.
- Atypical parkinsonian syndromes (multiple systems atrophy, progressive supranuclear palsy, corticobasal degeneration)—these syndromes have other features such as cerebellar degeneration, supranuclear gaze palsy, or asymmetrical limb apraxia that are not seen in DLB.
- Vascular dementia—differs from DLB in that despite the fluctuations in performance seen in DLB, there is no clear history of multiple strokes.
- Frontotemporal dementia (FTD, a.k.a. Pick's disease).
- Creutzfeldt-Jacob disease (CJD)—differs from DLB in that it is usually more rapidly progressive, can have cerebellar signs and symptoms, and often has distinctive EEG abnormalities.
- Toxic/metabolic/pharmacologic-related delirium.

WORKUP

- Diagnosis is largely clinical.
- Although dementia may be clinically similar to AD, detailed neuropsychologic testing can be helpful in bringing out prominent frontosubcortical and visuospatial deficits more typical of DLB.

LABORATORY TESTS

- Routine blood tests are normal but should be done to rule out treatable causes of dementia (e.g., B_{12}, TSH). In the setting of a fluctuation in performance, laboratory studies to rule out metabolic causes of delirium are appropriate.
- Spinal fluid analysis is normal; this may be helpful in more rapidly progressive cases if CJD is suspected.
- EEG may be helpful in the setting of fluctuations in performance to look for subclinical status epilepticus or other evidence of seizures, or if CJD is suspected.

IMAGING STUDIES

- Brain MRI is indicated mostly to look for multiple prior strokes suggestive of vascular dementia.
- Conventional neuroimaging is not diagnostic of DLB. Functional neuroimaging such as PET and SPECT show promise, but are not yet routinely indicated or available.

TREATMENT

NONPHARMACOLOGIC THERAPY

Dementia-care education with physical and occupational therapy may be of benefit to both patients and caregivers.

ACUTE GENERAL Rx

None available

CHRONIC Rx

- Treatment of parkinsonism with levodopa can be partially successful, but because of risk of hallucinations the lowest effective dose should be used. Anticholinergic medications (sometimes useful in Parkinson's disease) should be avoided.
- Cholinesterase inhibitors are modestly effective for treating cognitive impairment (possibly better than in AD), as well as hallucinations, sleep impairments, and anxiety.
- Antipsychotic medications are helpful in treating hallucinations; however, older neuroleptic agents should be avoided in favor of low doses of newer "atypical" antipsychotics.

DISPOSITION

Median survival similar to AD.

REFERRAL

Referral to a general neurologist, dementia specialist, or movement disorders center is appropriate.

PEARLS & CONSIDERATIONS

COMMENTS

- REM sleep behavior disorder is common in DLB (as it is in PD and multiple systems atrophy), but uncommon in Alzheimer's disease and frontotemporal dementia.
- DLB patients are unusually susceptible to extrapyramidal reactions to traditional neuroleptics, with sensitivity reactions in up to 50% of patients.

PREVENTION

None known

PATIENT/FAMILY EDUCATION

Comprehensive movement disorders website with disease information as well as links to support and discussion groups: http://www.wemove.org

EVIDENCE

A single, small, randomized, double-blinded controlled trial found that rivastigmine in doses 6 to 12 mg/day was safe and produced significant improvements compared with placebo in multiple domains such as apathy, anxiety, attention, hallucinations, and delusions.[1]

Evidence-Based Reference

1. McKeith I et al: Efficacy of rivastigmine in dementia with Lewy bodies: a randomised, double-blind, placebo-controlled international study, *Lancet* 356(9247):2031, 2000.

SUGGESTED READINGS

Burn DJ, McKeith IG: Current treatment of dementia with Lewy bodies and dementia associated with Parkinson's disease, *Mov Disord* 18(6):S72, 2003.

McKeith I et al: Diagnosis and management of dementia with Lewy bodies: third report of the DLB consortium, *Neurology* 65:1863, 2005.

Rossor M: Primary degenerative dementia. In Bradley W et al (eds): *Neurology in clinical practice,* ed 3, Boston, 2000, Butterworth-Heinemann.

AUTHOR: **DAVID P. WILLIAMS, M.D.**

BASIC INFORMATION

DEFINITION

Dependent personality disorder (DPD) is characterized by a pervasive and excessive need to be taken care of that leads to submissive and clinging behavior and fears of separation. DPD begins by early adulthood and causes significant distress or impairment in multiple domains of functioning. Individuals must meet five or more of the following criteria:

1. Difficulty making routine decisions without an excessive amount of advice and reassurance from others.
2. Need others to assume responsibility for most major areas of their life.
3. Difficulty expressing disagreement with others because of fear of loss of support or approval.
4. Difficulty initiating or completing projects on own because of a lack of self-confidence in abilities rather than lack of motivation or energy.
5. Excessive attempts to obtain nurturance and support from others.
6. Feel uncomfortable or helpless when alone because of exaggerated fears of being unable to care for self.
7. Urgently seek another relationship when a close relationship ends.
8. Unrealistically preoccupied with being left to take care of self.

SYNONYMS

None

ICD-9CM CODES
301.6

EPIDEMIOLOGY & DEMOGRAPHICS

PREVALENCE: 0.5% in general population. Dependent traits, as opposed to the disorder itself, among the most frequently reported in outpatient mental health clinics.

PREDOMINANT SEX: Female (2:1) in clinical settings.

CLINICAL PRESENTATION

- Early onset and chronic course. Impairment frequently mild.
- On interview, will defer excessively to partner or parent.
- Indecision in routine decisions.
- Depend on a parent or spouse to decide where they should live, work, and recreate and who they should befriend.
- Need for others to function for them goes beyond age-appropriate and situation-appropriate requests for assistance.
- Will agree with objectionable opinions, submit to unreasonable requests, and not express appropriate anger or disappointment for fear of alienating the person without whom they believe they cannot function.
- Convinced that they are not capable of independent function and present themselves as inept.
- Often do not develop independent living skills, perpetuating their dependency.
- Social relations tend to be limited to those few people on whom the person depends.

ETIOLOGY

Chronic physical illness or separation anxiety disorder may predispose for DPD.

DIAGNOSIS

DIFFERENTIAL DIAGNOSIS

- Dependency and personality changes arising as a consequence of an Axis I disorder.
- Dependency arising as a consequence of a general medical condition.
- Most common comorbid Axis I conditions are major depressive and other mood disorders, anxiety disorders, including social phobia, and adjustment disorder.
- Most common comorbid personality disorders are histrionic, avoidant, and borderline. Each of these disorders is characterized by dependent features. DPD distinguished by its predominantly submissive, reactive, and clinging behavior.

WORKUP

- History—collateral information essential to establishing presence of longstanding interpersonal pattern in multiple domains of the patient's life.
- Physical examination.
- Mental status examination.

LABORATORY TESTS

Those tests necessary to rule out medical causes of personality changes

IMAGING STUDIES

Those tests necessary to rule out medical causes of personality changes

TREATMENT

NONPHARMACOLOGIC THERAPY

- No randomized trials
- Cognitive behavioral and psychodynamic psychotherapy to diminish and better contain anxiety and to help patients develop sense of self as competent and requisite assertiveness skills

ACUTE GENERAL Rx

Benzodiazepines to control highly anxious states

CHRONIC Rx

- SSRIs and SNRIs for anxiety
- SSRIs and SNRIs for comorbid depression, social phobia, other anxiety disorders, and agoraphobia

DISPOSITION

- Chronic course, severity is variable.
- Impairments often mild.
- At increased risk for major depression, social phobia, and other anxiety disorders, including panic and agoraphobia.

REFERRAL

- If pharmacotherapy or psychotherapy contemplated.
- If patient's functioning impaired.

PEARLS & CONSIDERATIONS

COMMENTS

- DPD patients fear illness will lead to abandonment by others.
- This fear of simultaneous helplessness and abandonment intensifies neediness and may lead to dramatic demands for urgent medical attention.
- When physicians do not respond as wanted, angry outbursts may ensue.
- Medical care can also become a means by which dependency needs are met. As a result, some of these patients may unconsciously or consciously prolong their illness for primary gain.
- Physicians often react to the extreme neediness with avoidance or overengagement leading to burnout.
- Management guidelines:
  1. Overall strategy is to provide reassurance and allay fear of abandonment.
  2. Specific strategies include scheduling frequent visits, noncontingent care (i.e., scheduling visits regardless of whether ill or not).
  3. Establish firm and realistic limits to availability as early as possible in treatment.
  4. Enlist other members of health care team for support.
  5. Encourage patient to develop additional "outside" support systems.

SUGGESTED READINGS

Grant BF et al: Prevalence, correlates, and disability of personality disorders in the United States: results from the national epidemiologic survey on alcohol and related conditions, *J Clin Psychiatry* 65(7):948-958, 2004.

Shea MT et al: Associations in the course of personality disorders and Axis I disorders over time, *J Abnorm Psychol* 113(4):499-508, 2004.

Ward RK: Assessment and management of personality disorders, *Am Fam Physician* 15;70(8):1505-1512, 2004.

AUTHOR: **JOHN Q. YOUNG, M.D., M.P.P.**

BASIC INFORMATION

DEFINITION

Major depression is an episodic, frequently recurrent syndrome. Diagnosis of major depression requires that five of nine symptoms be present daily for 2 weeks. One of these nine symptoms must be either a persistent depressed mood and/or pervasive anhedonia (loss of interest or pleasure in living). Other symptoms include sleep disorder (insomnia or hypersomnia), appetite loss/gain or weight loss/gain, fatigue, psychomotor retardation or agitation, difficulty concentrating, feelings of guilt or low self-esteem, and recurrent thoughts of death or suicidal ideation.

SYNONYMS

Unipolar affective disorder
Melancholia
Manic-depressive illness, depressed type
Depressive episode

ICD-9CM CODES
296.2, 296.3, 311

EPIDEMIOLOGY & DEMOGRAPHICS

LIFETIME RISK (IN U.S.): 10% of men; 20% of women

PREVALENCE (in U.S.): Point prevalence in a community sample is 3% of men; 4.5% to 9.3% of women; prevalence of 20% to 50% in patients with comorbid medical conditions

PREDOMINANT SEX: Female:male ratio is 2:1

PREDOMINANT AGE: 25 to 44 yr; 5% of adolescents

PEAK INCIDENCE: 30 to 40 yr; 15% of postpartum women

GENETICS:
- Clear evidence of familial predominance.
- Prevalence is 2 to 3 times greater among first-degree relatives of patients with major depression.
- Concordance among monozygotic twins is about 50%.
- No established pattern of inheritance.

PHYSICAL FINDINGS & CLINICAL PRESENTATION

- Clinical evaluation can be facilitated by organizing the major symptoms into four hallmarks: (1) depressed mood, (2) anhedonia, (3) physical symptoms (sleep disorder, appetite problem, fatigue, psychomotor changes), and (4) psychologic symptoms (difficulty concentrating or indecisiveness, guilt or low self-esteem, and hopelessness).
- A stressful life event, typically a serious loss, may trigger a depressive episode; however, the presence or absence of identifiable precipitants is irrelevant to the diagnosis of major depression.
- Patients often present with somatic complaints such as pain, fatigue, insomnia, dizziness, headache, or gastrointestinal problems.
- May be associated with mood-congruent delusional thinking (paranoid and melancholic themes) in about 15% of individuals.
- May be associated with active or passive suicidal ideation.
- Among adolescents, serious misconduct may appear.
- Major depression may be misdiagnosed in elderly patients with signs and symptoms attributed to normal aging.

ETIOLOGY

- Major depression is a heterogeneous group of disorders probably arising from a variety of etiologic determinants.
- Genetic and family experiences both play roles though neither is a determining factor.
- Significant psychosocial stressors, especially involving loss, often trigger depression.
- Numerous biologic markers have been identified including endocrine and central nervous system factors, though none are considered causative.

DIAGNOSIS

DIFFERENTIAL DIAGNOSIS

- Other mental and behavioral disorders such as anxiety disorders, somatoform disorders, obsessive-compulsive disorder, substance abuse, and personality disorders often present with symptoms similar to depression.
- It is critical to distinguish between a depressive episode occurring as part of a major depression and a depressive episode that is part of bipolar disorder. Key to this distinction is whether the patient ever experienced clinical mania or hypomania. The Mood Disorder Questionnaire (MDQ) is a validated instrument that can be used, along with clinical interview, to screen for bipolar disorder.
- Approximately 10% to 15% of depression is caused by general medical illness. General medical conditions with high prevalence of depression include Alzheimer's disease and other dementia, Parkinson's disease, stroke, end-stage renal failure, cardiac disease, HIV infection, and cancer.
- Some medical conditions can present as depression; for example, hypothyroidism or hyperthyroidism, Cushing's syndrome, pancreatic cancer, and Parkinson's disease.
- Some exogenous medications can trigger depression (e.g., up to 50% of patients on interferon; antihypertensives, steroids, antineoplastic agents and others).
- Premenstrual dysphoric disorder.
- Elderly patients: depression often coexists with dementia.

WORKUP

- History: a careful medical history is required.
- Physical examination: there are no specific diagnostic signs of depression.
- Mental status examination.
- The Patient Health Questionnaire (PHQ-9) has documented high sensitivity and specificity for the diagnosis of depression and should be used for diagnosis and assessment of severity (see http://www.depression-primarycare.org).

LABORATORY TESTS

- No laboratory studies can definitively diagnose depression.
- The following can be done in selected patients to rule out other major organ system disease:
  - Routine chemistries
  - CBC with differential
  - Thyroid function studies
  - B_{12} levels

IMAGING STUDIES

With unusual presentations (e.g., associated with new-onset severe headache, focal neurologic signs, a cognitive or sensory disturbance), the following may be performed:
- EEG (diffuse slowing indicates metabolic encephalopathy)
- Lumbar puncture
- Anatomic brain imaging (CT scan or MRI)

TREATMENT

NONPHARMACOLOGIC THERAPY

- There is good evidence that cognitive-behavioral and interpersonal therapy is as effective as antidepressant medication in achieving a significant reduction or remission of depression.
- Problem-solving psychotherapy has efficacy rates of 50% to 60%.
- By 12 wk, psychotherapy and medication are equally effective in mild to moderate depression.
- Evidence suggests that combining pharmacologic and nonpharmacologic treatment is superior to either alone.

ACUTE GENERAL Rx

- In selecting an antidepressant medication, the patient's concurrent medical or psychiatric illnesses, history of prior response, cost, and side effects should be taken into account.

- Antidepressants are effective in about 60% to 70% of cases.
- Selective serotonin reuptake inhibitors (SSRIs) generally are first-line agents.
- The acute phase of treatment lasts about 6 to 12 weeks and has as its goal the reduction and removal of signs and symptoms of depression.
- Therapy should be continued for 4 to 9 months after the full remission of symptoms.
- Treatment-refractory patients should be switched to another medication or treated with an additional medication.
- Electroconvulsive therapy is the most effective means available for the treatment of severe, refractory depression.

CHRONIC Rx

The risk of recurrence exceeds 90% in individuals having experienced three or more depressive episodes; for these individuals continuous treatment is recommended.

DISPOSITION

- Major depression is a relapsing and remitting illness, characterized in most patients by recurrent episodes throughout life.
- Physical symptoms predict a favorable response to biologic intervention.
- Additional episodes are experienced by >60% of individuals having one depressive episode and >90% with three or more.
- Without treatment, episodes last an average of 6 to 12 months.

REFERRAL

- If treatment resistant or refractory
- If patient suicidal or psychotic
- For adjunctive psychotherapy in moderate to severe depression

PEARLS & CONSIDERATIONS

COMMENTS

- All threats of suicide should be taken very seriously. Clinicians can use the mnemonic SAL: Is the method Specific? Is it Available? Is it Lethal?
- It is imperative to rule out bipolar affective disorder before initiating treatment with an antidepressant medication.
- Many patients and families are reluctant to accept the diagnosis of depression because of associated stigma.
- A two-question screener is as effective as longer screening instruments. A positive answer to one of the following two questions should lead to a full diagnostic assessment for depression.
  1. Over the past 2 weeks have you ever felt down, depressed, or hopeless?
  2. Over the past 2 weeks, have you felt little interest or pleasure in doing things?

EVIDENCE

EBM

SSRIs are as effective as tricyclic antidepressants (TCAs) in the treatment of depression, and are better tolerated by patients.

Three systematic reviews compared SSRIs with TCAs and found no significant difference in efficacy overall. SSRIs appear to be slightly more acceptable, based on the number of patients who withdrew from clinical trials.[1-3] Ⓐ

One of the systematic reviews above was also conducted in a primary care setting, and found average response rates of 63% for newer agents, 35% for placebo, and 60% for TCAs.[4] Ⓐ

St. John's wort *(Hypericum perforatum)*

Two systematic reviews examined the effectiveness of St. John's wort *(Hypericum perforatum)* in the treatment of depression and found similar results. St. John's wort was more effective than placebo for the short-term treatment of mild to moderate depression, and there was no significant difference between St. John's wort and other antidepressants.[5,6] Ⓐ

Cognitive-behavioral therapy (CBT)

Four systematic reviews have found that cognitive therapy is effective in treating mild to moderate depression.[7-10] Ⓐ

One of these reviews also found limited evidence that cognitive therapy may result in fewer people with mild to moderate depression relapsing after treatment, compared with antidepressants or antidepressants plus cognitive therapy.[7] Ⓐ

Electroconvulsive therapy (ECT)

Severe and medication-resistant depression may be most effectively treated with electroconvulsive therapy (ECT).

A systematic review of ECT in younger and older adults with moderate to severe depression found that real ECT was more effective than simulated ECT, and that ECT was more effective than antidepressant medication for the short-term treatment of depression.[11] Ⓐ

Evidence-Based References

1. Geddes JR et al: Selective serotonin reuptake inhibitors (SSRIs) versus other antidepressants for depression, *Cochrane Database Syst Rev* 4, 1999. Ⓐ
2. Anderson IM: Selective serotonin reuptake inhibitors versus tricyclic antidepressants: a meta-analysis of efficacy and tolerability, *J Affect Disord* 58:19, 2000. Reviewed in: *Clin Evid* 13:1238, 2005. Ⓐ
3. Williams JW et al: A systematic review of newer pharmacotherapies for depression in adults: evidence report summary: clinical guidelines, part 2, *Ann Intern Med* 132:743, 2000. Reviewed in: *Clin Evid* 13:1238, 2005. Ⓐ
4. Mulrow CD et al: Efficacy of newer medications for treating depression in primary care patients, *Am Med J* 108:54, 2000. Reviewed in: *Clin Evid* 13:1238, 2005. Ⓐ
5. Linde K, Mulrow CD: St. John's wort for depression, *Cochrane Database Syst Rev* 4, 1998. Ⓐ
6. Whiskey A et al: A systematic review and meta-analysis of *Hypericum perforatum* in depression: a comprehensive clinical review, *Int Clin Psychopharmacol* 16:239, 2001. Reviewed in: *Clin Evid* 13:1238, 2005. Ⓐ
7. Gloaguen V et al: A meta-analysis of the effects of cognitive therapy in depressed patients, *J Affect Disord* 49:59, 1998. Reviewed in: *Clin Evid* 13:1238, 2005. Ⓐ
8. Cascalenda N et al: Remission in major depressive disorder: a comparison of pharmacotherapy, psychotherapy, and control conditions, *Am J Psychiatry* 159:1354, 2002. Reviewed in: *Clin Evid* 13:1238, 2005. Ⓐ
9. Churchill R et al: A systematic review of controlled trials of the effectiveness and cost-effectiveness of brief psychological treatments for depression, *Health Technol Assess* 5:1, 2001. Reviewed in: *Clin Evid* 13:1238, 2005. Ⓐ
10. van Schaik DJ et al: Effectiveness of psychotherapy for depression in primary care: a systematic review, *Tijdschrift voor Psychiatrie* 44:609, 2002. Reviewed in: *Clin Evid* 13:1238, 2005. Ⓐ
11. UK ECT Review Group: Efficacy and safety of electroconvulsive therapy in depressive disorders: a systematic review and meta-analysis, *Lancet* 361:799, 2003. Reviewed in: *Clin Evid* 13:1238, 2005. Ⓐ

SUGGESTED READINGS

Feldman MD et al: Let's not talk about it: suicide inquiry in primary care, *Ann Fam Medicine* 5(5):412, 2007.

Cole S et al: Depression. In Feldman MD, Christensen JF (eds): *Behavioral medicine: a guide for clinical practice,* ed 3, New York, 2008, Lange Medical Books/McGraw-Hill.

Trivedi MD et al: Medication augmentation after the failure of SSRIs for depression, *N Engl J Med* 354:1243, 2006.

AUTHOR: **MITCHELL D. FELDMAN, M.D., M.PHIL.**

BASIC INFORMATION

DEFINITION

De Quervain's tenosynovitis refers to a stenosing inflammatory process of the first dorsal retinacular compartment containing the tendons of the abductor pollicis longus (APL) and extensor pollicis brevis (EPB).

SYNONYMS

Stenosing tenosynovitis of the radial styloid process

Stenosing tenovaginitis of the first dorsal compartment

ICD-9CM CODES
727.04 Tenosynovitis radial styloid

EPIDEMIOLOGY & DEMOGRAPHICS

- More common in women than in men (10:1)
- Usually occurs between the ages of 30 to 50
- Associated with rheumatoid arthritis
- Seen in occupations (e.g., clerical, assembly, and manual labor)

PHYSICAL FINDINGS & CLINICAL PRESENTATION

- Pain over the styloid process of the radius
- Swelling
- Positive Finkelstein's test (Fig. 1-70)
- Crepitance

ETIOLOGY

- The cause is usually repetitive use or overuse of the hands (e.g., typing, writing, nailing, etc.)
- Acute trauma can also cause tenosynovitis of the radial styloid.

DIAGNOSIS

- The diagnosis of de Quervain's tenosynovitis is based on the clinical triad of:
  1. Tenderness over the radial styloid
  2. Swelling over the first dorsal retinacular compartment
  3. Positive Finkelstein's test (see Fig. 1-70)
- Sometimes 1.5 ml of 1% Xylocaine can be injected into the tenosynovial sac, and if all three physical signs resolve, the diagnosis is confirmed.

DIFFERENTIAL DIAGNOSIS

- Carpal tunnel syndrome
- Arithritis (e.g., degenerative osteoarthritis or rheumatoid arthritis)
- Gout
- Infiltrative tenosynovitis
- Radiculopathy
- Compression neuropathy (e.g., superficial branch of the radial nerve "bracelet syndrome")
- Infection (e.g., tuberculosis, bacterial)

LABORATORY TESTS

- Erythrocyte sedimentation rate (ESR) is usually normal in patients with de Quervain's tenosynovitis
- Aspiration to rule out gout
- Gram stain and culture of aspirate

IMAGING STUDIES

- X-ray studies of the hand

TREATMENT

NONPHARMACOLOGIC THERAPY

- Rest
- Splinting
- Physiotherapy

ACUTE GENERAL Rx

- Corticosteroid injection using 20 to 40 mg triamcinolone acetonide and 1% Xylocaine is effective in relieving pain.
- NSAIDs ibuprofen 800 mg tid or naproxen 500 mg bid.

CHRONIC Rx

Surgical release is generally reserved for patients not responding to NSAIDs and corticosteroid injection therapy.

DISPOSITION

- Approximately 90% of patients have relief of symptoms with either single or multiple steroid injections.
- Surgical control of symptoms occurs in 90% of cases.
- Complications of surgery include:
  1. Radial nerve damage
  2. Paresthesia (~10%)
  3. Neuroma

REFERRAL

Rheumatologist or orthopedist

PEARLS & CONSIDERATIONS

- Pain relief is usually noted within 48 hr with patient becoming asymptomatic by the first or second wk after corticosteroid injection.
- If there is no improvement by 6 wk post second corticosteroid injection, referral to an orthopedic hand surgeon is recommended.
- Avoid repetitive activities.

SUGGESTED READINGS

Chin DH, Jones NF: Repetitive motion hand disorder, *J Calif Dent Assoc* 30(2):149, 2002.

Jirarttanphochai K et al: Treatment of de Quervain disease with triamcinolone injection with or without nimesulide. A randomized, double-blind, placebo-controlled trial, *J.Bone Joint Surg Am* 86-A:2700, 2004.

Richie CA, Briner WW Jr: Corticosteroid injection for treatment of de Quervain's tenosynovitis: a pooled quantitative literature evaluation, *J Am Board Fam Pract* 16:102, 2003.

AUTHOR: **PETER PETROPOULOS, M.D.**

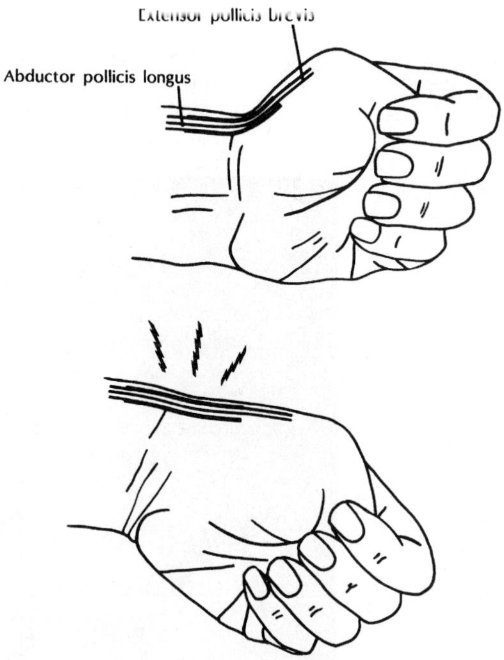

FIGURE 1-70 Finkelstein's test is positive in de Quervain's stenosing synovitis. Ulnar flexion of the wrist produces pain over the dorsal compartment containing the extensor policis brevis and abductor pollicis longus. (From Noble J [ed]: *Textbook of primary care medicine,* ed 2, St Louis, 1996, Mosby.)

BASIC INFORMATION

DEFINITION

Dermatitis herpetiformis (DH) is a rare, chronic skin disorder characterized by an intensely burning, pruritic, vesicular rash. It is strongly associated with gluten-sensitive enteropathy. Twenty to seventy percent of patients with DH will have gastrointestinal symptoms, whereas approximately 10% of patients with celiac sprue will have DH.

SYNONYMS

None

ICD-9CM CODES
694.0 Dermatitis herpetiformis

EPIDEMIOLOGY & DEMOGRAPHICS

PREVALENCE: 11.2 cases/100,000 persons in the U.S. The prevalence for celiac disease is 1 in 133 adults in the U.S.

PREDOMINANT SEX: Slight male predominance

PREDOMINANT AGE: Third and fourth decades

PREDOMINANT RACE: Rarely seen in blacks/African Americans or Asians

GENETICS: A specific HLA type, DQ2, is present in 90% of patients with celiac disease with or without DH. DQ8 is present in the remaining 10%. DQ2 is present in 16%-18% of the normal population. 11% of patients with DH have a first-degree relative with either DH or celiac disease.

PHYSICAL FINDINGS & CLINICAL PRESENTATION

- Pruritic, burning vesicles initially, frequently grouped (hence the name "herpetiform") (Fig. 1-71)
- Symmetrically distributed on extensor surfaces: elbows, knees, scalp, nuchal area, shoulder, and buttocks; rarely found in mouth
- May evolve in time to intensely burning urticarial papules, vesicles, and rarely bullae
- Celiac-type permanent-tooth enamel defects found in 53% of patients

DIAGNOSIS

Diagnosis is confirmed histologically by the demonstration of IgA deposits found along the subepidermal basement membrane, in the dermal papillary tips, which is specific to the diagnosis of DH.

DIFFERENTIAL DIAGNOSIS

- Linear IgA bullous dermatosis (not associated with gluten-sensitive enteropathy)
- Herpes simplex infection
- Herpes zoster infection
- Bullous erythema multiforme
- Bullous pemphigoid

WORKUP

History of chronic diarrhea and pruritic, vesicular rash highly suggestive of diagnosis

LABORATORY TESTS

- Skin biopsy for immunofluorescence studies. Diagnosis is confirmed by IgA deposits along the subepidermal basement membrane. >90% will have granular or fibrillar IgA deposits in the dermal papillae. Multiple specimens may be needed to obtain positive findings because of the focal nature of deposits. Biopsies are taken from adjacent normal skin because the diagnostic Ig deposits are usually destroyed by the blistering process.
- Circulating antibody levels
  1. IgA antiendomysial antibody is found
     a. In 70% of patients with rash and who are not on gluten-free diet and
     b. In 100% of patients with rash and grade 3 to 4 flattening of intestinal mucosa or with untreated celiac disease. Levels decrease to 0% when gluten is avoided for 3 mo.
  2. IgA antigliadin antibodies: found in 66% of patients with DH; also present in patients with pemphigus and pemphigoid
  3. IgA reticulin antibody: found in 36% of patients with DH
  4. IgA antitissue transglutaminase: elevated levels in 75% patients with DH and in 90% to 100% of patients with celiac disease

TREATMENT

- Spontaneous remission of DH in patients on a normal diet has been described in 10% to 15% of cases.
- Adherence to a gluten-free diet has been associated with sustained remission of DH.
- Patients may be given a trial of pharmacologic therapy if they are extremely uncomfortable. Symptoms are often dramatically relieved within hours or days of initiation of medical therapy.

NONPHARMACOLOGIC THERAPY

- Gluten-free diet: for at least 6 mo, which will allow most patients to begin to decrease or discontinue sulfone therapy (see "Acute General Rx"). The

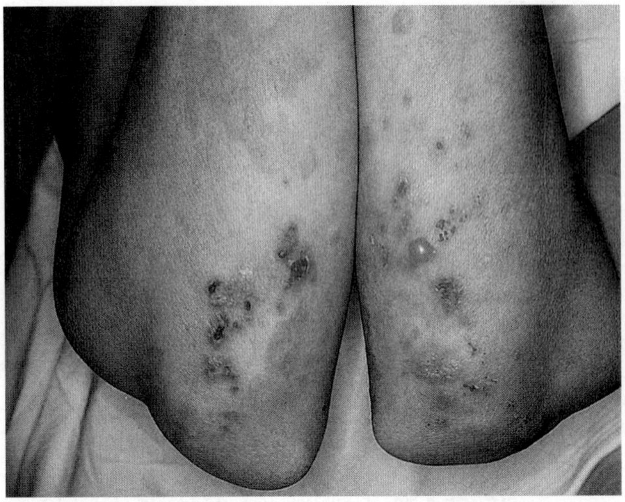

FIGURE 1-71 Dermatitis herpetiformis is an immunologically mediated blistering disease. There is a strong association of dermatitis herpetiformis with HLA-B8, DR3. Gluten-sensitive enteropathy is a common associated finding. The lesions are grouped (herpetiform) and extremely pruritic. (From Callen JP [ed]: *Color atlas of dermatology,* ed 2, Philadelphia, 2000, WB Saunders.)

diet usually needs to be followed for 2 yr before medications can be discontinued. Although intestinal villous architecture improves, symptoms and lesions recur in 1 to 3 wk if a normal diet is resumed. Most patients need to follow diet indefinitely. Gluten is found in all grains, such as wheat, barley, rye, and oats, except rice and corn.

A recent small study demonstrated that a gluten-free diet alone was comparable to a gluten-free diet plus dapsone in the treatment of DH.

- Elemental diet: Other dietary factors may also be important in dermatitis herpetiformis. Antigens stimulate the production of antibodies, leading to the formation of immune complexes. Most antigens that elicit a humoral immune response are proteins. Thus, a diet without full proteins, an elemental diet, is not likely to contain major antigens. A diet of amino acids, fat, and carbohydrates can produce a rapid benefit and allow a decrease in the dosage of dapsone within 2 wk.

ACUTE GENERAL Rx

- Dapsone:
  - Initial dose of 100 to 150 mg po qd. Itching and burning are controlled in 12 to 48 hr and new lesions stop appearing.
  - Adjust dose to the lowest level that provides adequate relief, which can range from 25 to 400 mg/day.
  - Peripheral motor neuropathy, such as paresthesias and weakness of the distal upper and lower extremities and footdrop, can occur in the first few months of therapy. Symptoms slowly improve over months to years after dapsone is discontinued.
  - Hemolysis, anemia, and methemoglobinemia occur to some degree in all patients receiving dapsone therapy. Patients at risk for having G6PD should have levels drawn before initiation as dapsone may cause severe hemolytic anemia in these patients.
  - Probenecid blocks the renal excretion of dapsone, and rifampin increases the rate of its clearance.
- Sulfapyridine:
  - Initial dosage 500 to 1500 mg/day.
  - Sulfapyridine is associated with agranulocytosis and aplastic anemia. It also may cause severe hemolysis in patients with G6PD.
- Sulfasalazine:
  - 500 to 1000 mg bid.
  - Sulfasalazine is metabolized to sulfapyridine and has been demonstrated to be effective in patients who are unable to tolerate dapsone in case reports.
- Tetracycline:
  - Successful treatment has been reported with tetracycline 500 mg po qd-tid and minocycline 100 mg po bid. Cessation resulted in a flare of the rash.
- Nicotinamide:
  - Successful treatment has been reported with nicotinamide 500 mg po bid-tid. Cessation resulted in a flare of the rash.
- Topical steroids: may help but can cause skin irritation and atrophy with prolonged use.
- Nonsteroidal anti-inflammatory drugs and iodide can worsen skin inflammation.

CHRONIC Rx

Gluten-free diet

DISPOSITION

- DH is considered to represent an intolerance to gluten, which requires lifelong avoidance of gluten.
- Some patients may be able to reintroduce gluten into their diet without experiencing a recurrence of DH.
  - A study of 38 patients demonstrated that 7 (18%) could resume a normal diet without relapse of cutaneous or gastrointestinal symptoms.
  - Patients who did not relapse after resumption of a normal diet were all diagnosed in childhood, had poor adherence to a gluten-free diet, and were more likely to have been treated with dapsone.
- There is an increased incidence of other autoimmune disorders, including thyroid disease, type 1 diabetes mellitus, systemic lupus erythematosus, vitiligo, and Sjögren's syndrome in patients with DH.
- Small bowel lymphoma and nonintestinal lymphoma have been reported in patients with DH and celiac disease. Patients adhering strictly to a gluten-free diet can reduce their risk of gut-related lymphomas within 5 years to that of the baseline population.

REFERRAL

To dermatologist for skin biopsy and to nutritionist to educate patients about gluten-free diet

PEARLS & CONSIDERATIONS

- Treatment with a gluten-free diet alone was found comparable to dapsone plus a gluten-free diet in a recent small study.
- Maintaining a gluten-free diet has been demonstrated to have a protective effect against the development of lymphoma in patients with celiac disease.

SUGGESTED READINGS

Bardella MT et al: Long-term remission in patients with dermatitis herpetiformis on a normal diet, *Br J Dermatol* 149:968-971, 2003.

Dieterich W et al: Antibodies to tissue transglutaminase as serologic markers in patients with dermatitis herpetiformis, *J Invest Dermatol* 113(1):133, 1999.

Eedy DJ et al: Updates from the British Association of Dermatologists 84th Annual Meeting, *Br J Dermatol* 152:13-28, 2005.

Nino M et al: A long-term gluten-free diet as an alternative treatment in severe forms of dermatitis herpetiformis, *J Dermatolog Treat* 13:10-12, 2007.

Turchin I, Barankin B: Dermatitis herpetiformi and gluten-free diet, *Dermotol Online J* 11(1):6, 2005.

Willsteed E et al: Sulfasalazine and dermatitis herpetiformis, *Australas J Dermatol* 26(2): 101, 2005.

Zone JJ et al: Warning: bread may be harmful to your health, *J Am Acad Dermatol* 51(suppl 1):S27, 2004.

AUTHOR: **IRIS L. TONG, M.D.**

BASIC INFORMATION

DEFINITION

Diabetes insipidus is a polyuric disorder resulting from insufficient production of antidiuretic hormone (ADH) (pituitary [neurogenic] diabetes insipidus) or unresponsiveness of the renal tubules to ADH (nephrogenic diabetes insipidus).

ICD-9CM CODES
253.5 Diabetes insipidus

EPIDEMIOLOGY & DEMOGRAPHICS

GENETICS:

- Nephrogenic diabetes insipidus can be inherited as sex-linked recessive.
- There is also a rare autosomal dominant form of neurogenic diabetes insipidus.

PHYSICAL FINDINGS & CLINICAL PRESENTATION

- Polyuria: urinary volumes ranging from 2.5 to 6 L/day
- Polydipsia (predilection for cold or iced drinks)
- Neurologic manifestations (seizures, headaches, visual field defects)
- Evidence of volume contractions

NOTE: The previous physical findings and clinical manifestations are generally not evident until vasopressin secretory capacity is reduced <20% of normal.

ETIOLOGY

NEUROGENIC DIABETES INSIPIDUS:

- Idiopathic
- Neoplasms of brain or pituitary fossa (craniopharyngiomas, metastatic neoplasms from breast or lung)
- Posttherapeutic neurosurgical procedures (e.g., hypophysectomy)
- Head trauma (e.g., basal skull fracture)
- Granulomatous disorders (sarcoidosis or TB)
- Histiocytosis (Hand-Schüller-Christian disease, eosinophilic granuloma)
- Familial (autosomal dominant)
- Other: interventricular hemorrhage, aneurysms, meningitis, postencephalitis, multiple sclerosis

NEPHROGENIC DIABETES INSIPIDUS:

- Drugs: lithium, amphotericin B, demeclocycline, methoxyflurane anesthesia
- Familial: X-linked
- Metabolic: hypercalcemia or hypokalemia
- Other: sarcoidosis, amyloidosis, pyelonephritis, polycystic disease, sickle cell disease, postobstructive

DIAGNOSIS

DIFFERENTIAL DIAGNOSIS

- Diabetes mellitus, nephropathies
- Primary polydipsia, medications (e.g., chlorpromazine)
- Osmotic diuresis (glucose, mannitol, anticholinergics)
- Psychogenic polydipsia, electrolyte disturbances

WORKUP

- The diagnostic workup is aimed at showing that the polyuria is caused by the inability to concentrate urine and determining whether the problem is secondary to decreased ADH or insensitivity to ADH. This is done with the water deprivation test:
  1. Following baseline measurement of weight, ADH, plasma sodium, and urine and plasma osmolarity, the patient is deprived of fluids under strict medical supervision.
  2. Frequent (q2h) monitoring of plasma and urine osmolarity follows.
  3. The test is generally terminated when plasma osmolarity is >295 or the patient loses ≥3.5% of initial body weight.
  4. Diabetes insipidus is confirmed if the plasma osmolarity is >295 and the urine osmolarity is <500.
  5. To distinguish nephrogenic from neurogenic diabetes insipidus, the patient is given 5 U of vasopressin (ADH) and the change in urine osmolarity is measured. A significant increase (>50%) in urine osmolarity following administration of ADH is indicative of neurogenic diabetes insipidus.
- A diagnostic algorithm for diabetes insipidus is described in Section III.

LABORATORY TESTS

- Decreased urinary specific gravity (≤1.005)
- Decreased urinary osmolarity (usually <200 mOsm/kg) even in the presence of high serum osmolality
- Hypernatremia, increased plasma osmolarity, hypercalcemia, hypokalemia

IMAGING STUDIES

MRI of the brain if neurogenic diabetes insipidus is confirmed

TREATMENT

NONPHARMACOLOGIC THERAPY

- Patient education regarding control of fluid balance and prevention of dehydration with adequate fluid intake
- Daily weight

ACUTE GENERAL Rx

Therapy varies with the degree and type of diabetes insipidus:

NEUROGENIC DIABETES INSIPIDUS:

1. Desmopressin acetate (DDAVP) 10 to 40 μg qd intranasally in one to three divided doses or in tablet form 0.1 or 0.2 mg. Usual oral dose is 0.1 to 1.2 mg/day in two to three divided doses Desmopressin is also available in injectable form given as 2 to 4 μg/day SC or IV in two divided doses
2. Vasopressin tannate in oil: 2.5 to 5 U IM q24 to 72h; useful for long-term management because of its long life
3. In mild cases of neurogenic diabetes insipidus, the polyuria may be controlled with HCTZ 50 mg qd (decreases urine volume by increasing proximal tubular reabsorption of glomerular infiltrate)

NEPHROGENIC DIABETES INSIPIDUS:

1. Adequate hydration
2. Low-sodium diet and chlorothiazide to induce mild sodium depletion
3. Polyuria of diabetes insipidus secondary to lithium can be ameliorated by using amiloride (5 mg PO bid initially, increased to 10 mg bid after 2 wk)

CHRONIC Rx

Patients should be aware of the danger of dehydration and the need for liberal water intake.

REFERRAL

Endocrinology evaluation for diagnostic testing

PEARLS & CONSIDERATIONS

COMMENTS

- Patients should be instructed to wear a medical identification tag or bracelet identifying their medical illness.
- In central diabetes insipidus, the use of DDAVP has become the standard of care. Extensive clinical experience has shown it to be both safe and effective in the treatment of this disorder.
- The treatment of nephrogenic diabetes insipidus is more complicated than the central form and varies among experts in the field. Consultation with a specialist is recommended in these settings.

SUGGESTED READING

Sands JM, Bichet DG: Nephrogenic diabetes insipidus, *Ann Intern Med* 144:186, 2006.

AUTHOR: **FRED F. FERRI, M.D.**

BASIC INFORMATION

DEFINITION

- Diabetes mellitus (DM) refers to a syndrome of hyperglycemia resulting from many different causes (see "Etiology"). It can be classified into type 1 (formerly IDDM) and type 2 (formerly NIDDM) DM. Because "insulin-dependent" and "non-insulin-dependent" refer to stage at diagnosis, when a type 2 diabetic needs insulin, he or she remains classified as type 2 and does not revert to type 1. Table 1-6 provides a general comparison of the two types of diabetes mellitus.
- The American Diabetes Association (ADA) defines DM as (1) a fasting plasma glucose ≥126 mg/dl, (2) a nonfasting plasma glucose ≥200 mg/dl, or (3) an oral glucose tolerance test (OGTT) ≥200 mg/dl in the 2-hr sample. Furthermore, the ADA also defines a value of 110 mg/dl on fasting blood sugar as the upper limit of normal for glucose. A fasting glucose between 110 mg/dl and 126 mg/dl is classified as "impaired fasting glucose" (IFG). When results of the oral glucose test are between 110 mg/dl and 200 mg/dl, the patient is also classified as having IFG.

SYNONYMS

IDDM (insulin-dependent diabetes mellitus)
NIDDM (non-insulin-dependent diabetes mellitus)
Type 1 diabetes mellitus (insulin-dependent diabetes mellitus)
Type 2 diabetes mellitus (non-insulin-dependent diabetes mellitus)

ICD-9CM CODES
250.0 Diabetes mellitus (NIDDM)
250.1 Insulin-dependent diabetes mellitus without complication (IDDM)

EPIDEMIOLOGY & DEMOGRAPHICS

- DM affects 5% to 7% of the U.S. population. Prevalence in Pima Indians is 35%.
- Incidence increases with age, with 2% in persons ages 20 to 44 yr to 18% in persons 65 to 74 yr.
- Diabetes accounts for 8% of all legal blindness and is the leading cause of end-stage renal disease in the U.S.
- Patients with diabetes are twice as likely as nondiabetic patients to develop cardiovascular disease.

PHYSICAL FINDINGS & CLINICAL PRESENTATION

1. Physical examination varies with the presence of complications and may be normal in early stages.
2. Diabetic retinopathy:
   a. Nonproliferative (background diabetic retinopathy):
      (1) Initially: microaneurysms, capillary dilation, waxy or hard exudates, dot and flame hemorrhages, AV shunts
      (2) Advanced stage: microinfarcts with cotton wool exudates, macular edema
   b. Proliferative retinopathy: characterized by formation of new vessels, vitreal hemorrhages, fibrous scarring, and retinal detachment
3. Cataracts and glaucoma occur with increased frequency in diabetics.
4. Peripheral neuropathy: patients often complain of paresthesias of extremities (feet more than hands); the symptoms are symmetric, bilateral, and associated with intense burning pain (particularly during the night).
   a. Mononeuropathies involving cranial nerves III, IV, and VI, intercostal nerves, and femoral nerves are also common.
   b. Physical examination may reveal:
      (1) Decreased pinprick sensation, sensation to light touch, and pain sensation
      (2) Decreased vibration sense
      (3) Loss of proprioception (leading to ataxia)
      (4) Motor disturbances (decreased deep tendon reflexes [DTR], weakness and atrophy of interossei muscles); when the hands are affected, the patient has trouble picking up small objects, dressing, and turning pages in a book
      (5) Diplopia, abnormalities of visual fields

TABLE 1-6 General Comparison of the Two Most Common Types of Diabetes Mellitus

	Type 1	Type 2
Previous terminology	Insulin-dependent diabetes mellitus (IDDM), type I, juvenile-onset diabetes	Non–insulin-dependent diabetes mellitus, type II, adult-onset diabetes
Age of onset	Usually <30 yr, particularly childhood and adolescence, but any age	Usually >40 yr, but any age
Genetic predisposition	Moderate; environmental factors required for expression; 35%-50% concordance in monozygotic twins; several candidate genes proposed	Strong; 60%-90% concordance in monozygotic twins; many candidate genes proposed; some genes identified in maturity-onset diabetes of the young
Human leukocyte antigen associations	Linkage to DQA and DQB, influenced by DRB (3 and 4) (DR2 protective)	None known
Other associations	Autoimmune; Graves' disease, Hashimoto's thyroiditis, vitiligo, Addison's disease, pernicious anemia	Heterogenous group, ongoing subclassification based on identification of specific pathogenic processes and genetic defects
Precipitating and risk factors	Largely unknown; microbial, chemical, dietary, other	Age, obesity (central), sedentary lifestyle, previous gestational diabetes
Findings at diagnosis	85%-90% of patients have one and usually more autoantibodies to ICA512/IA-2/IA-2β, GAD_{65}, insulin (IAA)	Possibly complications (microvascular and macrovascular) caused by significant preceeding asymptomatic period
Endogenous insulin levels	Low or absent	Usually present (relative deficiency), early hyperinsulinemia
Insulin resistance	Only with hyperglycemia	Mostly present
Prolonged fast	Hyperglycemia, ketoacidosis	Euglycemia
Stress, withdrawal of insulin	Ketoacidosis	Nonketotic hyperglycemia, occasionally ketoacidosis

From Andreoli TE (ed): *Cecil essentials of medicine,* ed 6, Philadelphia, 2005, WB Saunders.
GAD, Glutamic acid decarboxylase; *IA-2/IA-2β,* tyrosine phosphatases; *IAA,* insulin autoantibodies; *ICA,* islet cell antibody; *ICA512,* islet cell autoantigen 512 (fragment of IA-2).

5. Autonomic neuropathy:
   a. GI disturbances: esophageal motility abnormalities, gastroparesis, diarrhea (usually nocturnal)
   b. GU disturbances: neurogenic bladder (hesitancy, weak stream, and dribbling), impotence
   c. Orthostatic hypotension: postural syncope, dizziness, light-headedness
6. Nephropathy: pedal edema, pallor, weakness, uremic appearance.
7. Foot ulcers: occur in 15% of diabetics (annual incidence 2%) and are the leading causes of hospitalization. They are usually secondary to peripheral vascular insufficiency, repeated trauma (unrecognized because of sensory loss), and superimposed infections. If a diabetic foot ulcer has been present for weeks and foot pulses are palpable, neuropathy should be considered a major cause. Neuropathy can be detected with a simple exam of the lower extremities using a 10-g monofilament to test sensation. Prevention of foot ulcers in diabetics includes strict glucose control, patient education, prescription footwear, intensive podiatric care, and evaluation for surgical interventions.
8. Neuropathic arthropathy (Charcot's joints): bone or joint deformities from repeated trauma (secondary to peripheral neuropathy, see Fig. 1-72).
9. Necrobiosis lipoidica diabeticorum: plaquelike reddened areas with a central area that fades to white-yellow found on the anterior surfaces of the legs (Fig. 1-73); in these areas the skin becomes very thin and can ulcerate readily.

ETIOLOGY

IDIOPATHIC DIABETES:

Type 1 DM
- Hereditary factors:
  1. Islet cell antibodies (found in 90% of patients within the first year of diagnosis)
  2. Higher incidence of HLA types DR3, DR4
  3. 50% concordance in identical twins
- Environmental factors: viral infection (possibly coxsackie virus, mumps virus)

Type 2 DM
- Hereditary factors: 90% concordance in identical twins
- Environmental factor: obesity

DIABETES SECONDARY TO OTHER FACTORS:
- Hormonal excess: Cushing's syndrome, acromegaly, glucagonoma, pheochromocytoma
- Drugs: glucocorticoids, diuretics, oral contraceptives
- Insulin receptor unavailability (with or without circulating antibodies)
- Pancreatic disease: pancreatitis, pancreatectomy, hemochromatosis
- Genetic syndromes: hyperlipidemias, myotonic dystrophy, lipoatrophy
- Gestational diabetes

DIAGNOSIS (Dx)

DIFFERENTIAL DIAGNOSIS
- Diabetes insipidus
- Stress hyperglycemia
- Diabetes secondary to hormonal excess, drugs, pancreatic disease

LABORATORY TESTS
- Diagnosis is made on the basis of the following tests and should be confirmed by repeated testing on a different day:
  1. Fasting glucose ≥126 mg/dl (ADA criterion)
  2. Nonfasting plasma glucose ≥200 mg/dl
- Use of glycosylated hemoglobin (Hb A1c) level is not recommended for diagnosis at this time by the ADA because of lack of standardization of hemoglobin Alc values and the imperfect correlation between HbAlc and fasting plasma glucose levels. However, some physicians use this test to make the diagnosis of diabetes mellitus if the random plasma glucose is >200 mg/dl and the hemoglobin Alc level is ≥2 standard deviations above the laboratory mean.
- Screening for diabetic nephropathy by measuring microalbuminuria is recommended in all patients with diabetes. It can be accomplished by any of the following three methods:
  1. Measurement of the albumin-to-creatinine ratio in random spot urine collection. This is the easiest method to administer in the office setting because it is an easy assay to perform in most laboratories. To perform this test, the physician simply orders "Urine for microalbumin level."
  2. Measurement of a 24-hr urine collection for albumin, creatinine clearance.
  3. Timed (4-hr or overnight) urine collection.
- The diagnosis of microalbuminuria should be based on 2 to 3 elevated levels within a 3- to 6-month period because there is a marked variability in day-to-day albumin excretion and possible transient elevations in urine albumin from short-term hyperglycemia, exercise, severe hypertension, and other illnesses such as sepsis and CHF. Patients with overt nephropathy do not need screening for microalbumin-

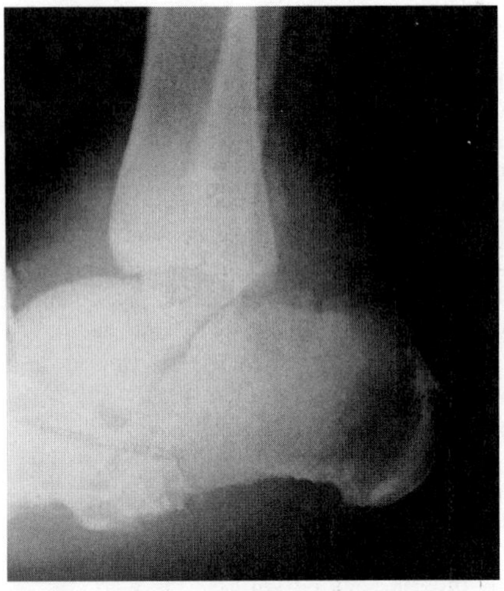

FIGURE 1-72 Diabetic neuropathy of the hindfoot. Destruction of the joint with collapse and fragmentation. (From Hochberg MC, Silman AJ, Smolen JS, Weinblatt ME, Weisman MH [eds]: *Rheumatology*, ed 3, St. Louis, 2003, Mosby.)

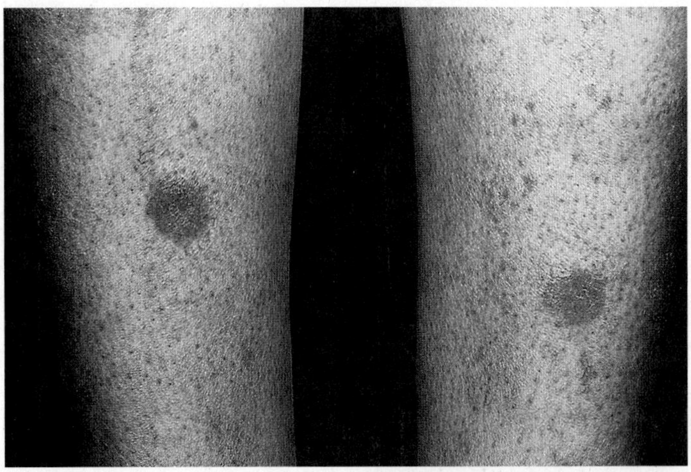

FIGURE 1-73 Necrobiosis lipoidica: symmetrical early lesions with erythema. (Courtesy the Institute of Dermatology. From McKee PH, Calonje E, Granter SR [eds]: *Pathology of the skin with clinical correlations*, ed 3, St. Louis, 2005, Mosby.)

uria because the level of protein in the urine is high enough to be detected on routine urinalysis.

- A fasting serum lipid panel, serum creatinine, and electrolytes should be obtained yearly on all adult diabetic patients.

TREATMENT

Rx

NONPHARMACOLOGIC THERAPY

1. Diet
   a. Calories
      (1) The diabetic patient can be started on 15 calories/lb of ideal body weight; this number can be increased to 20 calories/lb for an active person and 25 calories/lb if the patient does heavy physical labor.
      (2) The calories should be distributed as 50% to 60% carbohydrates, <30% fat, with saturated fat limited to <10% of total calories, and 15% to 20% protein.
      (3) The emphasis should be on complex carbohydrates rather than simple and refined starches and on polyunsaturated instead of saturated fats in a ratio of 2:1.
   b. Seven food groups
      (1) The exchange diet of the ADA includes protein, bread, fruit, milk, and low- and intermediate-carbohydrate vegetables.
      (2) The name of each exchange is meant to be all inclusive (e.g., cereal, muffins, spaghetti, potatoes, rice are in the bread group; meats, fish, eggs, cheese, peanut butter are in the protein group).
      (3) The *glycemic index* compares the rise in blood sugar after the ingestion of simple sugars and complex carbohydrates with the rise that occurs after the absorption of glucose; equal amounts of starches do not give the same rise in plasma glucose (pasta equal in calories to a baked potato causes less of a rise than the potato): thus it is helpful to know the glycemic index of a particular food product.
      (4) Fiber: insoluble fiber (bran, celery) and soluble globular fiber (pectin in fruit) delay glucose absorption and attenuate the postprandial serum glucose peak; they also appear to lower the elevated triglyceride level often present in uncontrolled diabetics. A diet high in fiber should be emphasized (20 to 35 g/day of soluble and insoluble fiber)
   c. Other principles
      (1) Modest sodium restriction to 2400 to 3000 mg/day. If hypertension is present, restrict to <2400 mg/day; if nephropathy and hypertension present, restrict to <2000 mg/day.
      (2) Moderation of alcohol intake (≤2 drinks/day in men, ≤1 drink/day in women).
      (3) Nonnutritive artificial sweeteners are acceptable in moderate amounts.
2. Exercise increases the cellular glucose uptake by increasing the number of cell receptors. The following points must be considered:
   a. Exercise program must be individualized and built up slowly.
   b. Insulin is more rapidly absorbed when injected into a limb that is then exercised, and this can result in hypoglycemia.
3. Weight loss: to ideal body weight if the patient is overweight.
4. Screening for nephropathy, neuropathy, and retinopathy.

GENERAL Rx

- When the previous measures fail to normalize the serum glucose, oral hypoglycemic agents (e.g., metformin or a sulfonylurea) should be added to the regimen in type 2 DM. Table 1-7 describes commonly used oral hypoglycemic agents. The sulfonamides and the biguanide metformin are the oldest and most commonly used classes of hypoglycemic drugs.
- Metformin's primary mechanism is to decrease hepatic glucose output. Because metformin does not produce hypoglycemia when used as a monotherapy, it is preferred for most patients. It is contraindicated in patients with renal insufficiency.
- Sulfonylureas and repaglinide work best when given before meals because they increase the postprandial output of insulin from the pancreas. All sulfonylureas are contraindicated in patients allergic to sulfa.
- Acarbose and miglitol work by competitively inhibiting pancreatic amylase and small intestinal glucosidases delay gastrointestinal absorption of carbohydrates, thereby reducing alimentary hyperglycemia. The major side effects are flatulence, diarrhea, and abdominal cramps.
- Pioglitazone and rosiglitazone increase insulin sensitivity and are useful in addition to other agents in type 2 diabetics whose hyperglycemia is inadequately controlled. Serum transaminase levels should be obtained before starting therapy and monitored periodically. A recent report suggested that rosiglitazone may increase the incidence of myocardial infarction and cardiovascular mortality.
- Sitagliptin (Januvia) inhibits the enzyme DPP-4, responsible for inactivation and degradation of glucagon-like peptide-1 (GLP-1) and glucose-dependent insulinotropic polypeptide (GIP), which potentiate insulin synthesis and release and decrease glucagon production. It is a weaker agent than metformin or thiazolidiones, with an average HbA1c decrease of 0.5% vs. 1.5% for metformin and 0.5% to 1.5% for thiazolidiones. Dose is 100 mg qd. It can be used as monotherapy or in combination with other agents and is well tolerated.
- Insulin is indicated for the treatment of all type 1 DM and type 2 DM patients who cannot be adequately controlled with diet and oral agents. Table 1-8 describes commonly used types of insulin. Inhaled insulin represents an alternative to SC insulin in the patient unwilling to consider injectable insulin. The risks of insulin therapy include weight gain, hypoglycemia, and, in rare cases, allergic or cutaneous reactions. Replacement insulin therapy should mimic normal release patterns. Approximately 50% to 60% of daily insulin should be a basal type consisting of a long-acting insulin (NPH, ultralente, glargine [Lantus], detemir [Levemir]) injected once or twice daily, the remaining 40% to 50% should be short-acting or rapid-acting insulin (regular, aspart, lispro) to cover mealtime carbohydrates and correct elevated current glucose levels. Among long-acting insulins, once-daily bedtime insulin glargine is as effective as once- or twice-daily NPH but has a lower risk of nocturnal hypoglycemia and less weight gain. Insulin detemir is a newer long-acting insulin analog approved as basal therapy for treatment of diabetes mellitus. It is indicated for use in adults and children in combination with short-acting insulin for type 1 diabetes and oral agents or short-acting insulin for adults with type 2 DM. Unlike NPH insulin, its use has not been associated with weight gain. When using short-acting insulins, insulin aspart and insulin lispro are more effective in lowering postprandial glucose levels than regular insulin.
- Pramlintide (Symlin), a synthetic analog of human amylin (a hormone synthesized by pancreatic beta cells and cosecreted with insulin in response to food intake) can be used as an adjunctive treatment for patients with type 1 or type 2 DM who inject insulin at meal-

time. In type 1 DM initial dose is 15 mcg SC before major meals. In type 2 DM initial dose is 60 mcg before major meals. Nausea is its major side effect.

- Exenatide (Byetta), a synthetic peptide that stimulates release of insulin from pancreatic beta cells, can be used as adjunctive therapy for patients with type 2 DM. It is an incretin mimetic. Incretins are endogenous proteins that modulate the glycemic response. Exenatide is not indicated in type 1 DM and is contraindicated in patients with severe renal impairment. Starting dose is 5 mcg SC bid before morning and evening meals.
- Combination therapy of various hypoglycemic agents is commonly used when monotherapy results in inadequate glycemic control.
- Continuous subcutaneous insulin infusion (CSII, or insulin pump) provides better glycemic control than does conventional therapy and comparable to or slightly better control than multiple daily injections. It should be considered for diabetes presenting in childhood or adolescence and during pregnancy.
- Low-dose aspirin (ASA; 81 mg/day) to decrease the risk of cerebrovascular disease is beneficial for diabetics over age 30 with other risk factors (hypertension, dyslipidemia, smoking, obesity).
- Strict lipid control (LDL <70 mg/dl) is indicated in all diabetics. Use of statins is usually necessary to achieve therapeutic goals.

DISPOSITION

The Diabetes Control and Complications Trial (DCCT) proved that intensive treatment decreases the development and progression of complications of DM. In this trial, the risks of retinopathy, nephropathy, and neuropathy were decreased by 35% to 90%. Each patient should be made aware of these findings.

- Diabetic retinopathy is the most severe of the several ocular complications of diabetes. It occurs in approximately 15% of diabetic patients after 15 yr and increases 1%/yr after diagnosis. Retinal laser photocoagulation and vitrectomy are effective treatment modalities. Prevention is best accomplished by strict glucose and blood pressure control.
- The frequency of neuropathy in type 2 diabetics approaches 70% to 80%. It

TABLE 1-7 Oral Antidiabetic Agents as Monotherapy

	Sulfonylureas	Biguanides	α-Glucosidase Inhibitors	Thiazolidinediones	Meglitinides
Generic name	Glimepiride, glyburide, glipizide, chlorpropamide, tolbutamide	Metformin	Acarbose, miglitol	Rosiglitazone, pioglitazone	Repaglinide, nateglinide
Mode of action	↑↑ Pancreatic insulin secretion chronically	↓↓ HGP; ↓ peripheral IR; ↓ intestinal glucose absorption	Delays PP digestion of carbohydrates and absorption of glucose	↓↓ Peripheral IR; ↑↑ glucose disposal; ↓ HGP	↑↑ Pancreatic insulin secretion acutely
Preferred patient type	Diagnosis age >30 yr, lean, diabetes <5 yr, insulinopenic	Overweight, IR, fasting hyperglycemia, dyslipidemia	PP hyperglycemia	Overweight, IR, dyslipidemia, renal dysfunction	PP hyperglycemia, insulinopenic
Therapeutic effects					
↓ HBA_{1c}* (%)	1-2	1-2	0.5-1	0.8-1	1-2
↓ FPG* (mg/dl)	50-70	50-80	15-30	25-50	40-80
↓ PPG* (mg/dl)	~90	80	40-50	—	30
Insulin levels	↑	—	—	—	↑
Weight	↑	–/↓	—	–/↑	↑
Lipids	—	↓ LDL ↓↓ TG		↑ Large "fluffy" LDL ↓↓ TG ↑ HDL	—
Side effects	Hypoglycemia	Diarrhea, lactic acidosis	Abdominal pain, flatulence, diarrhea	Idiosyncratic hepatotoxicity with troglitazone; edema	Hypoglycemia (low-risk)
Dose(s)/day	1-3	2-3	1-3	1	1-4+
Maximum daily dose (mg)	Depends on agent	2550	150 (<60-kg bw) 300 (>60-kg bw)	Depends on agent	16 (repaglinide), 360 (nateglinide)
Range/dose (mg)	Depends on agent	500-1000	25-50 (<60-kg bw) 25-100 (>60-kg bw)	Depends on agent	0.5-4 (repaglinide), 60, 120 (nateglinide)
Optimal administration time	~30 min premeal (some with food, others on empty stomach)	With meal	With first bite of meal	With meal (breakfast)	Preferably <15 (0-30 min) premeals (omit if no meal)
Main site of metabolism/excretion	Hepatic/renal, fecal	Not metabolized/renal	Only 2% absorbed/fecal	Hepatic/fecal	Hepatic/fecal

Modified from Andreoli TE (ed): *Cecil essentials of medicine,* ed 6, Philadelphia, 2005, WB Saunders.

↑, Increased; ↓, decreased; —, unchanged; *bw,* body weight; *FPG,* fasting plasma glucose; *HDL,* high-density lipoprotein; *HGP,* hepatic glucose production; *IR,* insulin resistance; *LDL,* low-density lipoprotein; *PP,* postprandial; *PPG,* postprandial plasma glucose; *TG,* triglyceride.

*Values combined from numerous studies; values are also dose dependent.

TABLE 1-8 Types of Insulin

Insulin Type	Generic Name	Preprandial Injection Timing* (hr)	Onset* (hr)	Peak* (hr)	Duration* (hr)	Blood Glucose (BG) Nadir* (hr)
Rapid acting	Lispro†	0-0.2	0.2-0.5	0.5-2	<5	2-4
Short acting	Regular	0.5-(1)	0.3-1	2-6	4-8 (≤16)	3-7 (Pre–next meal)
	Lente		1-2	4-12		
Intermediate acting	NPH	0.5-(1)	1-3	6-15	16-26	6-13
Long acting‡	Ultralente	0.5-(1)	4-6	8-30	24-36	10-28
	Insulin glargine (Lantus)	0.5-(1)	1.1	None	≥24	10-28
Mixed, short/intermediate acting	70/30					
	50/50	0.5-(1)	0.5-1	3-12	16-24	3-12

From Andreoli TE (ed): *Cecil essentials of medicine,* ed 6, Philadelphia, 2005, WB Saunders.

70/30, 70% NPH, 30% regular; *50/50,* 50% NPH, 50% regular; *NPH,* neutral protamine Hagedorn.

*Times depend on several factors including dose, anatomic site of injection, method (SQ, IM, IV), duration of diabetes, degree of insulin resistance, level of activity, and body temperature. Some time ranges are wide to include data from several separate studies. Preprandial injection depends on premeal BG values as well as insulin type. If BG is low, may need to inject insulin and eat immediately (carbohydrate portion of meal first). If BG is high, may delay meal after insulin injection and eat carbohydrate portion last.

†Insulin analogue with reversal of lysine and proline at positions 28 and 29 on the β chain.

‡Insulin glargine [rDNA origin] is a newer, once-daily insulin analog (Lantus) that provides 24-hour basal glucose-lowering with once-a-day bedtime dosing. Onset of action is 2 to 3 hr, duration of action is 24+ hr.

can be subdivided in sensorimotor neuropathy (distal symmetric polyneuropathy, focal neuropathy [diabetic mononeuropathy, mononeuropathy multiplex], diabetic amyotrophy) and autonomic neuropathy (abnormal pupillary function, vasomotor neuropathy, GI autonomic neuropathy [gastric atony, diabetic diarrhea or constipation, fecal incontinence], genitourinary autonomic neuropathy [bladder dysfunction, sexual dysfunction], hypoglycemic unawareness, sudomotor neuropathy). Duloxetine (Cymbalta), a selective serotonin and norepinephrine reuptake inhibitor is effective and FDA approved for relief of diabetic peripheral neuropathy. Pregabalin (Lyrica) and Gabapentin (900-3600 mg/day) are also effective for the symptomatic treatment of peripheral neuropathic pain. Topical capsaicin, 5% lidocaine transdermal patches, amitriptyline, and carbamazepine are also modestly effective.

- Diabetic gastroparesis is most often seen in patients who have had diabetes for at least 10 years and typically have retinopathy, neuropathy, and nephropathy. Major manifestations are postprandial fullness, nausea, vomiting, and bloating. Pharmacologic therapy involves prokinetic agents (metoclopramide). Endoscopic injection of botulinum toxin into the pylorus and gastric electrical stimulation with use of electrodes placed laparoscopically in the muscle wall of the stomach antrum and connected to a neurostimulator represent newer approaches to nonpharmacologic therapy.
- Nephropathy occurs in 35% to 45% of patients with type 1 DM and in 20% of type 2 DM. The first sign of renal involvement in patients with DM is most often microalbuminuria, which is classified as incipient nephropathy. Without specific intervention, 50% of patients with diabetes with type 1 DM and overt diabetic nephropathy (urine protein ≥300 mg/24 hr) progress to end-stage renal disease (ESRD) within 10 yr of onset, and >75% of type 1 DM and 20% of type 2 DM progress to ESRD over a 20-yr period. Angiotensin converting enzyme (ACE) inhibitors are effective in slowing the progression of renal disease in both type 1 and type 2 DM, independently of their reduction in blood pressure. Angiotensin receptor blockers (ARBs) are also effective in protecting against the progression of nephropathy in diabetics, especially in type 2 DM. Patients on ACEs or ARBs should have their serum potassium levels monitored for hyperkalemia. Nondihydropyridine calcium channel blockers (e.g., verapamil) may be useful in patients intolerant to ACEs or ARBs to reduce albuminuria; however, studies have failed to show a reduction in the rate of decrease in glomular filtration rate (GFR) with their use. Nephrology consultation is prudent when proteinuria is detected or when GFR has decreased to <30 ml/min per 1.73 m^2.
- Infections are generally more common in diabetics because of multiple factors, such as impaired leukocyte function, decreased tissue perfusion secondary to vascular disease, repeated trauma because of loss of sensation, and urinary retention secondary to neuropathy.
- Diabetic ketoacidosis and hyperosmolar coma are described in detail in Section I.

REFERRAL

- Diabetic patients should be advised to have annual ophthalmologic examination. In type 1 DM, ophthalmologic visits should begin within 3 to 5 yr, whereas type 2 DM patients should be seen from disease onset.
- Podiatric care can significantly reduce the rate of foot infections and amputations in patients with DM. Noninfected neuropathic foot ulcers require debridement and reduction of pressure.

PEARLS & CONSIDERATIONS

COMMENTS

- Because normalization of serum glucose level is the ultimate goal, every patient should measure his or her blood glucose unless contraindicated by senility or blindness.
- For blood glucose monitoring, glucose oxidase strips are used in conjunction with a meter to give a digital reading. The testing can be done once day, but the time should be varied each day so that over time the serum glucose level before meals and at bedtime can be assessed frequently without pricking the patient's fingers four times daily.
- Glycosylated hemoglobin should be measured at least twice yearly; measurement of microalbumin in the urine on a yearly basis is also recommended.

- Creatinine and serum-lipid panel should be obtained at least yearly in patients with diabetes.
- Underinsured children and those with psychiatric illness are at higher risk for acute complications in type 1 DM and require frequent monitoring and aggressive risk management with diet, exercise, and periodic laboratory evaluation.
- Vascular endothelial growth factor (VEGF) and erythropoietin have been identified as factors involved in angiogenesis in proliferative diabetic retinopathy. Tight glycemic and blood pressure control remains the cornerstone in the primary prevention of diabetic retinopathy.
- Trials involving islet transplantation with the use of the Edmonton protocol have been disappointing. Insulin independence after 2 yr remained in only 31% of subjects involved in the trial.

EVIDENCE

EBM

Type 1 in Adults

Intensive vs. conventional glycemic control therapy significantly reduces the risk of the development of retinopathy, nephropathy, and neuropathy in people with type 1 diabetes. This is the finding of a systematic review of randomized controlled trials (RCTs) and subsequent RCTs.[1-4] **A**

An RCT of the effects of intensive therapy vs. conventional therapy on complications of type 1 diabetes found that at 6.5 years intensive treatment significantly reduced the progression of retinopathy and neuropathy. After a further 4 years the benefit was maintained, regardless of whether patients stayed in the groups to which they had initially been randomized.[2,3] **A**

Long-term follow-up of people in the above RCT found that after 6 years, the rates of microalbuminuria and hypertension were significantly reduced in people who were originally randomized to intensive treatment.[4] **A**

A systematic review found that intensive insulin therapy was significantly more effective than conventional therapy in reducing the number of macrovascular events in people with type 1 diabetes. However, there was no significant difference in the number of people developing macrovascular disease, or in macrovascular mortality.[5] **A**

RCTs have shown that intensive treatment is associated with an increased risk of hypoglycemia and weight gain, although it does not seem to have an adverse effect on neuropsychologic function or quality of life.[6] **A**

Regular human insulin was compared with insulin analogues in patients with type 1 and type 2 diabetes mellitus. The short-acting insulin analogues showed only minor benefit over the regular human insulin, although most trials were of poor methodologic quality.[7] **B**

A meta-analysis of 12 RCTs comparing continuous subcutaneous insulin infusion (insulin infusion pump therapy) with optimized insulin injections in patients with type 1 diabetes found that mean blood glucose levels were lower in people receiving continuous subcutaneous insulin infusion. Blood glucose concentrations were also less variable during insulin infusion.[8] **B**

Evidence-Based References

1. Wang PH, Lau J, Chalmers TC: Meta-analysis of effects of intensive blood glucose control on late complications of type 1 diabetes, *Lancet* 341:1306-1309, 1993. Reviewed in: *Clin Evid* 12:844, 2004. **A**
2. The Diabetes Control and Complications Trial Research Group: The effect of intensive treatment of diabetes on the development and progression of long-term complications in insulin-dependent diabetes mellitus, *N Engl J Med* 329:977-986, 1993. Reviewed in: *Clin Evid* 11:753-761, 2004. **A**
3. The DCCT/Epidemiology of Diabetes Interventions and Complications Research Group: Retinopathy and nephropathy in patients with type 1 diabetes four years after a trial of intensive therapy, *N Engl J Med* 342:381-389, 2000. Reviewed in: *Clin Evid* 11:753-761, 2004 **A**
4. Genuth S et al: Effect of intensive therapy on the microvascular complications of type 1 diabetes mellitus, *JAMA* 287:2563-2569, 2002. Reviewed in: *Clin Evid* 11:753-761,2004. **A**
5. Lawson ML et al: Effect of intensive therapy on early macrovascular disease in young individuals with type 1 diabetes, *Diabetes Care*22:B35-B39, 1999. Reviewed in: *Clin Evid* 11:753-761, 2004. **A**
6. Bazian Ltd.: Glycaemic control in diabetes. In: *Clin Evid* 11:753-761, 2004. London, BMJ Publishing Group. **A**
7. Siebenhofer A et al: Short acting insulin analogues versus regular human insulin in patients with diabetes mellitus. Reviewed in: Cochrane Library, 2:2004, Chichester, UK, John Wiley. **B**
8. Pickup J, Mattock M, Kerry S: Glycemic control with continuous subcutaneous insulin infusion compared with intensive insulin injections in patients with type 1 diabetes: meta-analysis of randomised controlled trials, *BMJ* 324:705, 2002. **B**

Type 2 in Adults

A randomized controlled trial (RCT) compared intensive glycemic control with a sulfonylurea or insulin vs. conventional control using primarily diet in patients newly diagnosed with type 2 diabetes. It found no significant difference between the groups in rates of myocardial infarction or stroke over 5 years.[1] **A**

Tight glycemic control is, however, associated with sustained decreased rates of retinopathy, nephropathy, and neuropathy.

The trial did, however, find that intensive treatment was associated with a significant reduction in microvascular complications, including the need for retinal photocoagulation, compared with conventional treatment.[1] **A**

Intensive control increases the risk of severe hypoglycemia and weight gain.

Intensive treatment was associated with significantly more hypoglycemic episodes than conventional treatment. Intensive treatment was also associated with increased weight gain at 10 years, and weight gain was greater with the insulin regimen compared with the sulfonylurea regimen.[1,2] **A**

In overweight patients, regardless of the degree of glucose control, a large RCT found that treatment with metformin decreased diabetes-related mortality and diabetes-related complications.

Another RCT compared conventional therapy (primarily with diet alone) vs. intensive glucose control therapy (with metformin) in overweight people with newly diagnosed type 2 diabetes. Intensive treatment with metformin significantly reduced the risks of a diabetes-related complication and death. A similar change in body weight was noted in both groups.[3] **A**

Other trials have compared different insulin regimes.

A systematic review including 20 RCTs found that when bedtime NPH-insulin was combined with oral hypoglycemic agents as a daily regime in patients with type 2 diabetes, it resulted in comparable glycemic control to insulin monotherapy (given as twice daily or multiple daily injections). It was also associated with less weight gain if metformin was used.[4] **A**

An RCT compared a standard regime of one insulin injection daily with an intensive regime designed to attain near-normal blood glucose levels by stepping up insulin injections alone or with glipizide in patients with type 2 diabetes. It found no significant difference between the groups in the rates of new cardiovascular events over a mean follow-up of 27 months.[5] **A**

A small RCT of patients with type 2 diabetes given either conventional or intensive treatment (multiple insulin injection regimes) found that the number of major cerebrovascular, cardiovascular, and peripheral vascular events in the intensive treatment group was half that of the conventional treatment group. However, the results were not significant.[6] **B**

Limited research has found that the addition of pioglitazone to a sulfonylurea is effective and well tolerated.

A multicenter double-blind RCT compared the addition of pioglitazone to a sulfonylurea vs. metformin plus sulfonylurea in patients with poorly controlled type 2 diabetic. It found that both regimes resulted in equivalent improvements in glycemic control over 1 year.[7] Ⓑ

Control of other risk factors for cardiovascular disease is an important factor in the management of type 2 diabetes.

An RCT found a reduced rate of cardiovascular disease in patients with type 2 diabetes managed by intensive treatment of multiple risk factors compared with conventional treatment over 8 years of follow-up.[8] Ⓐ

An RCT of diabetic patients over 55 years old who had a previous cardiovascular event or at least one other cardiovascular risk factor compared ramipril 10 mg daily vs. placebo. It found that ramipril significantly reduced major cardiovascular events and death from any cause over 4.5 years. This result was independent of hypertensive status, type of diabetes, or type of diabetes treatment.[9] Ⓐ

A systematic review found that treatment with angiotensin-converting enzyme inhibitors in microalbuminuric normotensive diabetics (type 1 and 2 diabetes) resulted in a significant reduction in albumin excretion rate and a significantly greater lowering of blood pressure compared with placebo.[10] Ⓐ

Several trials have found that statins reduce cardiovascular morbidity and mortality in diabetic patients compared with placebo.[11] Ⓐ

Advice regarding dietary modifications are accepted as routine in the initial management of newly diagnosed diabetic patients.

A systematic review of various different diets used in the treatment of diabetes type 2 was unable to report any high-quality data on their efficacy. However, the available data indicated that exercise appears to improve glycated hemoglobin at 6 and 12 months.[12] Ⓐ

A systematic review found that fish oil supplementation significantly lowered triglycerides, and raised low-density lipoprotein cholesterol vs. placebo. These effects were most marked in hypertriglyceridemic patients on higher doses of fish oil. Fish oil had no significant effect on glycemic control.[13] Ⓐ

Evidence-Based References

1. UK Prospective Diabetes Study Group: Intensive blood-glucose control with sulphonylureas or insulin compared with conventional treatment and risk of complications in patients with type 2 diabetes, *Lancet* 352:837-853, 1998. Reviewed in: *Clin Evid* 12:844, 2004. Ⓐ
2. Abraira C et al: Cardiovascular events and correlates in the Veterans Affairs Diabetes Feasibility Trial: Veterans Affairs Cooperative Study on glycemic control and complications in type II diabetes, *Arch Intern Med* 157:181-188, 1997. Reviewed in: *Clin Evid* 11:777-806, 2004. Ⓐ
3. UK Prospective Diabetes Study Group: Effect of intensive blood-glucose control with metformin on complications in overweight patients with type 2 diabetes (UKPDS 34), *Lancet* 352:854-865, 1998. Reviewed in: *Clin Evid* 11:753-761,777-806, 2004. Ⓐ
4. Goudswaard AN et al: Insulin monotherapy versus combinations of insulin with oral hypoglycaemic agents in patients with type 2 diabetes mellitus, *Cochrane Database Syst Rev,* 4:2004. Ⓐ
5. Abraira C et al: Cardiovascular events and correlates in the Veterans Affairs Diabetes Feasibility Trial: Veterans Affairs Cooperative Study on glycemic control and complications in type II diabetes, *Arch Intern Med* 157:181-188, 1997. Reviewed in: *Clin Evid* 11:777-806, 2004. Ⓐ
6. Ohkubo Y et al: Intensive insulin therapy prevents the progression of diabetic microvascular complications in Japanese patients with non-insulin-dependent diabetes mellitus: a randomized prospective 6-year study, *Diabetes Res Clin Pract* 28:103-117, 1995. Reviewed in: *Clin Evid* 11:753-761, 2004. Ⓑ
7. Hanefeld M et al: QUARTET Study Group. One-year glycemic control with a sulfonylurea plus pioglitazone versus a sulfonylurea plus metformin in patients with type 2 diabetes, *Diabetes Care* 27:141-147, 2004. Ⓑ
8. Gaede P et al: Multifactorial intervention and cardiovascular disease in patients with type 2 diabetes, *N Engl J Med* 348:383-393, 2003. Reviewed in: *Clin Evid* 11:777-806, 2004. Ⓐ
9. Heart Outcomes Prevention Evaluation (HOPE) Study Investigators: Effects of ramipril on cardiovascular and microvascular outcomes in people with diabetes mellitus: results of the HOPE study and the MICRO-HOPE substudy, *Lancet* 355:253-259, 2000. Reviewed in: *Clin Evid* 11:777-806, 2004. Ⓐ
10. Lovell HG: Angiotensin converting enzyme inhibitors in normotensive diabetic patients with microalbuminuria, *Cochrane Database Syst Rev* 3,1999. Ⓐ
11. Malcolm J, Meggison H, Sigal R: Prevention of cardiovascular events in diabetes. Reviewed in: *Clin Evid* 11:777-806, 2004, London, BMJ Publishing Group .
12. Moore H et al: Dietary advice for treatment of type 2 diabetes mellitus in adults, *Cochrane Database Syst Rev* 2,2004. Ⓐ
13. Farmer A et al: Fish oil in people with type 2 diabetes mellitus, *Cochrane Database Syst Rev* 3,2001. Ⓐ

SUGGESTED READINGS

American Diabetes Association Position Statement: Standards of medical care for patients with diabetes mellitus, *Diabetes Care* 25:S33, 2002.

Aring AM et al: Evaluation and prevention of diabetic neuropathy, *Am Fam Physician,* 71:2123-2130, 2005.

Boulton AJM et al: Neuropathic diabetic foot ulcers, *N Engl J Med* 351:48, 2004.

Camilleri M: Diabetic gastroparesis, *N Engl J Med* 356:820-829, 2007.

Ceglia L et al: Meta-analysis: efficacy and safety of inhaled insulin therapy in adults with diabetes mellitus, *Ann Intern Med* 145:665-675, 2006.

Diabetes Control and Complications Trial (DCCT)/Epidemiology of Diabetes Interventions and Complications (EDIC) Research Group: Beneficial effects of intensive therapy of diabetes during adolescence: outcomes after the conclusion of the Diabetes Control and Complications Trial (DCCT), *J Pediatr* 139:804, 2001.

Diabetes Control and Complications Trial/ Epidemiology of Diabetes Interventions and Complications Research Group: Effect of intensive therapy on the microvascular complications of type 1 diabetes mellitus, *JAMA* 287:2563, 2002.

Hirsh IB: Insulin analogues, *N Engl J Med* 352:174-183, 2005.

Inzucchi SE: Management of hyperglycemia in the hospital setting, *N Engl J Med* 355:1903-1911, 2006.

Mayfield J, White R: Insulin therapy for type 2 DM: rescue, augmentation, and replacement of beta cell function, *Am Fam Physician* 70:489, 2004.

Mohamed Q et al: Management of diabetic retinopathy, *JAMA* 298(8):902-916, 2007.

Mooradian A et al: Narrative review: A rational approach to starting insulin therapy, *Ann Intern Med* 145:125, 2006.

Shapiro J et al: International trial of the Edmonton protocol for islet transplantatiion, *N Engl J Med* 355:1318, 2006.

Singh N et al: Preventing foot ulcers in patients with diabetes, *JAMA*, 293:217-228, 2005

Thorp ML: Diabetic nephropathy: Common questions, *Am Fam Physician* 72:96-99, 2005

U.S. Preventive Services Task Force: Screening for type 2 DM in adults: recommendations and rationale, *Ann Intern Med* 138:212, 2003.

Van den Berghe G et al: Intensive insulin therapy in the medical ICU, *N Engl J Med* 354:449, 2006.

Watanabe D et al: Erythropoietin as a retinal angiogenic factor in proliferative diabetic retinopathy, *N Engl J Med* 353:782-792, 2005.

Zandbergen AM et al: Effect of losartan on microalbuminuria in normotensive patients with type 2 DM, *Ann Intern Med* 139:90, 2003.

AUTHOR: **FRED F. FERRI, M.D.**

BASIC INFORMATION

DEFINITION

Diabetic ketoacidosis (DKA) is a life-threatening complication of diabetes mellitus resulting from severe insulin deficiency and manifested clinically by severe dehydration and alterations in the sensorium.

SYNONYMS

DKA

ICD-9CM CODES
250.1 Diabetic ketoacidosis

EPIDEMIOLOGY & DEMOGRAPHICS

INCIDENCE/PREVALENCE: 46 episodes/10,000 diabetics; cause of 14% of all hospital admissions of diabetic patients
PREDOMINANT AGE: 1 to 25 yr

PHYSICAL FINDINGS & CLINICAL PRESENTATION

- Evidence of dehydration (tachycardia, hypotension, dry mucous membranes, sunken eyeballs, poor skin turgor)
- Clouding of mental status
- Tachypnea with air hunger (Kussmaul's respiration)
- Fruity breath odor (caused by acetone)
- Lipemia retinalis in some patients
- Possible evidence of precipitating factors (infected wound, pneumonia)
- Abdominal or CVA tenderness in some patients

ETIOLOGY

Metabolic decompensation in diabetics usually precipitated by an infectious process (up to 40% of cases). Poor compliance with insulin therapy and severe medical illness (e.g., CVA, MI) are other common causes. Cocaine abuse has been reported as a risk factor for DKA in adult and teenage patients, particularly in patients with multiple admissions.

DIAGNOSIS

DIFFERENTIAL DIAGNOSIS

- Hyperosmolar nonketotic state (Table 1-9)
- Alcoholic ketoacidosis
- Uremic acidosis
- Metabolic acidosis secondary to methyl alcohol, ethylene glycol
- Salicylate poisoning

WORKUP

- Laboratory evaluation (see "Laboratory Tests") to confirm diagnosis and evaluate precipitating factors
- ECG to evaluate electrolyte abnormalities and rule out myocardial ischemia/infarction as a contributing factor

LABORATORY TESTS

- Glucose level reveals severe hyperglycemia (serum glucose generally >250 mg/dl); urine/serum ketones positive.
- ABGs reveal acidosis: arterial pH usually <7.30 with Pco_2 <40 mm Hg.
- Serum electrolytes:
  1. Serum bicarbonate is usually <18 mEq/L.
  2. Serum potassium may be low, normal, or high. There is always significant total body potassium depletion regardless of the initial potassium level.
  3. Serum sodium is usually decreased as a result of hyperglycemia, dehydration, and lipemia. Assume 1.6 mEq/L decrease in extracellular sodium for each 100 mg/dl increase in glucose concentration.
  4. Calculate the anion gap (AG):

$$AG = Na^+ - (Cl^- + HCO^{-3})$$

In DKA the anion gap is increased (generally >10); hyperchloremic metabolic acidosis may be present in unusual circumstances when both the glomerular filtration rate and the plasma volume are well maintained.

- CBC with differential, urinalysis, urine and blood cultures to rule out infectious precipitating factor.
- Serum calcium, magnesium, and phosphorus; the plasma phosphate and magnesium levels may be significantly depressed and should be rechecked within 24 hr because they may decrease further with correction of DKA.
- BUN and creatinine generally reveal significant dehydration.
- Amylase, liver enzymes should be checked in patients with abdominal pain.

IMAGING STUDIES

Chest x-ray is helpful to rule out infectious process. The initial chest x-ray may be negative if the patient has significant dehydration. Repeat chest x-ray examination after 24 hr if pulmonary infection is strongly suspected.

TREATMENT

NONPHARMACOLOGIC THERAPY

- Monitor mental status, vital signs, and urine output qh until improved, then monitor q2 to 4h.
- Monitor electrolytes, renal function, and glucose level (see "Acute General Rx").

ACUTE GENERAL Rx

FLUID REPLACEMENT (THE USUAL DEFICIT IS 6 TO 8 L):

1. Do not delay fluid replacement until laboratory results have been received. Fluid deficits are typically 100 ml/kg of body weight.
2. The initial fluid replacement should be with 0.9% NS until blood pressure and organ perfusion are restored (usually 1 L or more). In patients with severe hypernatremia (serum sodium >160 mEq/L), 0.45 % saline infusion can be used. Careful monitoring for fluid

TABLE 1-9 A Comparison of Diabetic Ketoacidosis (DKA) and Hyperosmolar Nonketotic Syndrome (HNKS)

Feature	DKA	HNKS
Age of patient	Usually <40 yr	Usually >60 yr
Duration of symptoms	Usually <2 days	Usually >5 days
Serum glucose concentration	Usually <800 mg/dl	Usually >800 mg/dl
Serum sodium concentration (Na^+)	More likely to be normal or low	More likely to be normal or high
Serum bicarbonate concentration (HCO_3^-)	Low	Normal
Ketone bodies	At least 4 + in 1:1 dilution	<2 + in 1:1 dilution
pH	Low	Normal
Serum osmolality	Usually <350 mOsm/kg	Usually >350 mOsm/kg
Cerebral edema	Occasionally clinical symptoms	Rarely (never?) clinical
Prognosis	3%-10% mortality	10%-20% mortality
Subsequent course	Insulin therapy required in almost all cases	Insulin therapy not required in most cases

From Andreoli TE (ed): *Cecil essentials of medicine,* ed 6, Philadelphia, 2005, WB Saunders.

overload is necessary in elderly patients and those with a history of CHF.

3. The rate of fluid replacement varies with the age of the patient and the presence of significant cardiac or renal disease.
   - The usual rate of infusion is 500 ml to 1 L over the first hour; 300 to 500 ml/hr for the next 12 hr.
   - Continue the infusion at a rate of 200 to 300 ml/hr, using 0.45% NS until the serum glucose level is <300 ml/dl, then change the hydrating solution to D_5W to prevent hypoglycemia, replenish free water, and introduce additional glucose substrate (necessary to suppress lipolysis and ketogenesis).

INSULIN ADMINISTRATION:

1. The patient should be given an initial loading IV bolus of 0.15 to 0.2 U/kg of regular insulin followed by a constant infusion at a rate of 0.1 U/kg/hr (e.g., 25 U of regular insulin in 250 ml of 0.9% saline solution at 70 ml/hr equals 7 U/hr for a 70-kg patient). Insulin replacement should generally not be started until serum potassium is >3.3 mEq/L to prevent life-threatening hypokalemia.
2. Monitor serum glucose qh for the first 2 hr, then monitor q2-4h.
3. The goal is to decrease serum glucose level by 80 mg/dl/hr (following an initial drop because of rehydration); if the serum glucose level is not decreasing at the expected rate, double the rate of insulin infusion.
4. When the serum glucose level approaches 250 mg/dl, decrease the rate of insulin infusion to 2 to 3 U/hr and continue this rate until the patient has received adequate fluid replacement, HCO^-_3 is close to normal, and ketones have cleared.
5. Approximately 30 to 60 min before stopping the IV insulin infusion, administer an SC dose of regular insulin (dose varies with the patient's demonstrated insulin sensitivity); this SC dose of regular insulin is necessary because of the extremely short life of the insulin in the IV infusion.
6. When the patient is able to eat, NPH insulin 10 to 15 U is given in the morning and regular insulin is administered before each meal and at bedtime by using a sliding scale. In newly diagnosed diabetics, the total daily dose to maintain metabolic control ranges from 0.5 to 0.8 U/kg/day. Split dose therapy with regular and NPH insulin may be given, with two thirds of the total daily dose administered in the morning and one third in the evening.

ELECTROLYTE REPLACEMENT:

Potassium Replacement: The average total potassium loss in DKA is 300 to 500 mEq.

- The rate of replacement varies with the patient's serum potassium level, degree of acidosis (decreased pH, increased potassium level), and renal function (potassium replacement should be used with caution in patients with renal failure).
- As a rule of thumb, potassium replacement may be started when there is no ECG evidence of hyperkalemia (tall, narrow, or tent-shaped T waves, decreased or absent P waves, short QT intervals, widening of QRS complex).
- In patients with normal renal function, potassium replacement can be started by adding 20 to 40 mEq KCl/L of IV hydrating solution if serum potassium is 4 to 5 mEq/L, more if serum potassium level is lower than 4 mEq/L. In patients with severe hypokalemia (potassium <3.3 mEq/L) give 40 mEq of potassium/hr until potassium is >3.3 mEq/L.
- Monitor serum potassium level qh for the first 2 hr, then monitor q2 to 4h.

Phosphate Replacement: If the serum PO_4 is <1.5 mEq/L, give 2.5 mg/kg IV over 6 hr of elemental phosphate. Routine replacement of phosphate (in absence of laboratory evidence of significant hypophosphatemia) is not indicated. Rapid IV phosphate administration can cause hypocalcemia.

Magnesium Replacement: Replacement indicated only in the presence of significant hypomagnesemia or refractory hypokalemia.

BICARBONATE THERAPY: Routine use of bicarbonate in DKA is contraindicated, because it can worsen hypokalemia and intracellular acidosis and cause cerebral edema. Bicarbonate therapy should be considered only if the arterial pH is <6.9 and HCO_3 is <5. In these patients 44 to 88 mEq of sodium bicarbonate can be added to a liter of 0.45% NS q2 to 4h until pH increases >7. Use of bicarbonate therapy is particularly dangerous in the pediatric population. Children with DKA who have low partial pressures of arterial carbon dioxide and high serum urea nitrogen concentration at presentation and who are treated with bicarbonate are at increased risk for cerebral edema. Bicarbonate therapy in children with DKA should be limited to those with severe circulatory failure and a high risk of cardiac decompensation resulting from profound acidosis.

DISPOSITION

- Average mortality in DKA is 5% to 10%.
- In children <10 yr of age, DKA causes 70% of diabetes-related deaths.
- Cerebral edema occurs in 1% of episodes of DKA in children and is associated with a mortality rate of 40% to 90%.

REFERRAL

Patients with DKA should be admitted to the ICU. Occasionally, alert patients who are able to take fluids orally and have mild DKA can be treated under observation and sent home. The ADA admission guidelines are a plasma glucose >250 mg/dl, with arterial pH <7.30, a serum bicarbonate <15 mEq/L, and a moderate or greater level of ketones in the serum or urine.

PEARLS & CONSIDERATIONS

COMMENTS

- Although DKA occurs more commonly in type 1 DM, a significant proportion (>20%) occurs in patients with type 2 DM.
- 20% of DKA admissions involve newly diagnosed diabetes.
- Potential complications of DKA therapy include hypoglycemia, cerebral edema, cardiac arrhythmias, shock, MI, and acute pancreatitis.
- Underinsured children and those with psychiatric illness are at higher risk for DKA.

SUGGESTED READINGS

Glaser N et al: Risk factor for cerebral edema in children with diabetic ketoacidosis, *N Engl J Med* 344:264, 2001.

Newton CA, Raskin P: Diabetic ketoacidosis in type 1 and type 2 diabetes mellitus, *N Engl J Med* 164:1925, 2004.

Trachtenbarg DE: Diabetic ketoacidosis, *Am Fam Physician* 71:1705, 2005.

AUTHOR: **FRED F. FERRI, M.D.**

BASIC INFORMATION

DEFINITION

Diabetic polyneuropathy (DPN) is an insidious and progressive length-dependent disorder of peripheral nerves (large, small, and autonomic fibers) that is secondary to diabetes and is characterized by distal and symmetric pain, numbness, tingling, or autonomic dysfunction. Other diabetic neuropathies may present with proximal or asymmetric pain and weakness.

SYNONYMS

Chronic distal symmetric polyneuropathy, diabetic neuropathy

ICD-9CM CODES
250.6 Diabetic polyneuropathy

EPIDEMIOLOGY & DEMOGRAPHICS

PREVELENCE (IN U.S.): 7.5% of diabetics at initial diagnosis and 40% (type 2 diabetics) after 10 years of diabetes. Overall, 10% to 64% of all diabetics.

PREDOMINANT SEX: Male diabetics have a higher incidence than females.

PREDOMINANT AGE: More common in patients older than 50 years of age.

RISK FACTORS:
- Hyperglycemia
- Older age
- Longer duration of diabetes
- Genetic predisposition
- Hypertension
- Smoking
- Other questionable risk factors (alcohol consumption, insulin use, and hyperlipidemia)

PHYSICAL FINDINGS & CLINICAL PRESENTATION

- Tingling, buzzing, numbness, tightness, electric shock-like, hot, cold, or burning sensations starting in the feet bilaterally and slowly progressing to involve the hands. The level of impairment in the legs usually reaches above the knees before the hands are affected and in severe cases the sensory disturbances may involve the anterior trunk and the head. Symptoms are typically worse at night.
- Some patients report difficulties in opening jars, turning keys, foot slapping, toe scuffing, difficulty with stairs, getting up from a sitting or lying position, raising their arms above the shoulders, and falling.
- Autonomic dysfunction presents as dry skin, lack of or excessive sweating, poor dark adaptation, sensitivity to bright lights, postural light-headedness, fainting, urinary urgency, incontinence, nocturnal diarrhea, constipation, vomiting, erectile and ejaculatory dysfunction in men, and loss of ability to reach sexual climax in women.
- Examination shows decreased pinprick, light touch, temperature, vibration, and proprioceptive sensations in a stocking or glove distribution with absent ankle reflexes. Gait abnormalities (sensory ataxia), anhidrosis, and unreactive pupils can be seen. Muscle weakness (of the distal muscles) can be seen in later stages.

OTHER DIABETIC NEUROPATHIES:

Generalized:
- *Hyperglycemic neuropathy:* tingling, pain, or hyperesthesia in the feet of a patient with poor glycemic control that rapidly resolves by improving hyperglycemia.
- *Insulin neuritis:* severe pain (worse at night) that is difficult to control, which is seen in patients who are on insulin.
- *Superimposed chronic inflammatory demyelinating polyneuropathy (CIDP):* more common in type 1 diabetics. DPN differs from CIDP in that patients with DPN are older, imbalance is more common, duration of symptoms at time of presentation is longer, and there is more prominent secondary axonal loss on nerve conduction studies and less response to therapy.

Focal:
- *Cranial neuropathies:* abrupt painless sixth or third nerve palsy. Third nerve palsy is less common than sixth and half of the patients complain of retroorbital pain and headache. The pupil is also spared due to central rather than peripheral ischemia of the nerve fascicle. Symptoms usually resolve within 6 months.
- *Somatic mononeuropathies:* focal neuropathies in the extremities caused by entrapment or compression of nerves including the median at the wrist (carpal tunnel syndrome), the ulnar at the elbow, or the common peroneal at the fibular head.
- *Diabetic truncal radiculoneuropathy (thoracoabdominal radiculopathy):* patients present with a unilateral (later becomes bilateral) focal contact hyperesthesia and stabbing, burning, beltlike pain in the same area (worse at night), focal weakness of the anterior abdominal wall muscles, and weight loss. Sensory deficits seen in a dermatomal distribution. Most recover within months.
- *Diabetic lumbosacral radiculoplexus neuropathy (Bruns-Garland syndrome or diabetic amyotrophy):* patients present with an abrupt onset of severe unilateral low back, hip, or anterior thigh pain. Asymmetric proximal weakness and muscle atrophy develop a few days to weeks later (initially unilateral then becomes bilateral) with marked weight loss.

ETIOLOGY

- Not fully understood.
- *The polyol pathway theory:* high blood glucose leads to high nerve glucose, which causes overactivity of the polyol pathway and a disturbance of axoplasmic transport.
- *Microvascular ischemia and hypoxia theory:* hyperglycemia causes endothelial cell hypertrophy of the blood vessel walls and capillary damage, which eventually causes ischemia of the central portion of the nerve fascicle.
- *Nonenzymatic glycosylation theory:* increased low-density lipoproteins (LDL) that promote smooth muscle proliferation and atheroma formation.
- *Immune theory:* immune-mediated attack on nerves or their vasa nervosa.

DIAGNOSIS (Dx)

DIFFERENTIAL DIAGNOSIS

- Idiopathic chronic inflammatory demyelinating polyneuropathy (CIDP)
- Amyloid neuropathy
- Vasculitic neuropathy
- Sarcoid neuropathy
- Alcoholic neuropathy
- Nutritional neuropathy
- Thyroid disease
- Toxic neuropathy
- Uremic neuropathy
- Idiopathic painful neuropathy

WORKUP

- A good history demonstrating the characteristic pattern of symmetric sensory complaints in a patient with established diabetes or with symptoms suggestive of diabetes
- A good physical examination showing absent ankle reflexes, sensory abnormalities (all or some modalities) in a stocking or glove distribution
- *Nerve conduction studies:* distal symmetric predominately sensory polyneuropathy with axonal features (reduced response amplitudes)
- *Electromyography:* denervation (positive sharp waves and fibrillations) and reinnervation (high-amplitude, long-duration, and polyphasic motor unit potentials) changes in the distal muscles
- Other diagnostic testing (MRI and CT of the spine and or brain) might be required if the patient has other diabetic neuropathy syndromes (listed above)
- Skin biopsy: checks intraepidermal nerve fiber density, which measures the sensory and sympathetic innervation to the skin. Used in some university centers and in drug trials to measure regenerative capacity of peripheral nerves (Herrmann et al)

LABORATORY TESTS

- Serum protein electrophoresis, immunofixation electrophoresis
- Antinuclear antigen (ANA), rheumatoid factor (RF), double-stranded DNA (ds-DNA), erythrocyte sedimentation rate (ESR), C-reactive protein (CRP), Rapid Plasma Reagin (RPR), scl-70, anti-SS-A (Ro), and anti-SS-B (La) to rule out other autoimmune diseases
- Thyroid function test to rule out thyroid disease
- Complete blood count, serum electrolytes, B_{12}, and folate
- Fasting blood sugar, hemoglobin A1c, or glucose tolerance test

TREATMENT

Rx

NONPHARMACOLOGIC THERAPY

- Tight glucose control from the time of diagnosis of diabetes is the most important measure taken (69% reduction in risk of developing neuropathy in type 1 diabetics). The same might be applied to type 2 diabetes, although it is not yet proven.
- Frequent follow-up visits.
- A rigorous foot-care program.

GENERAL Rx

- Treatment of pain and paresthesias
- Anticonvulsants:
  - Gabapentin (Neurontin): 100 to 2400 mg tid or qid
  - Pregabalin (Lyrica): 75 to 300 mg bid
  - Oxcarbazepine (Trileptal): 300 to 1800 mg bid
  - Carbamazepine (Tegritol): 100 to 200 mg bid or tid
  - Topiramate (Topamax): 25 to 200 mg bid
  - Lamitorigine (Lamical): 25 to 200 mg qd
- Antidepressants:
  - Duloxetine (Cymbalta): 30 to 60 mg qd
  - Nortriptyline (Pamelor): 25 to 150 mg qhs or bid
  - Amitriptyline (Elavil) 25 to 150 mg qhs or bid
  - Bupropion (Wellburtin): 150 to 300 mg qd
  - Venlafaxine (Effexor XR): 37.5 to 225 mg qd
  - Paroxitene (Paxil): 20 to 60 mg/day
  - Citalopram (Celexa): 20 to 60 mg/day
- Opioids:
  - Oxycodone CR: 40 to 160 mg/day
- Others:
  - Tramadol (Ultram): 50 to 400 mg qd-qid
  - Lidocaine patch: 5% 1 to 4 patches 12 hours on 12 hours off
  - Capsaicin extract: 7.5% 3 to 4 times per day
  - Anodyne therapy
  - Opiates as a last resort
- Diabetic autonomic neuropathy:
  - Treatments for autonomic dysfunction
  - Long-term intensive glucose control
  - Orthostatic hypotension: fludrocortisone and midodrine
  - Gastroparesis: dietary manipulation, prokinetic and antiemetic medications
  - Erectile dysfunction: sildenafil, tadalafil, or vardenafil
  - Bladder dysfunction: medications, catheterization, or surgery

DISPOSITION

Diabetes carries significant morbidity and complications. Patients with untreated diabetic peripheral neuropathy have higher morbidity and complication rates than those without neuropathy or those with treated neuropathy.

REFERRAL

- A neurologist or a neuromuscular specialist for neurophysiologic testing and assistance in managing pain and paresthesias
- Podiatrist for yearly foot examination
- Ophthalmologist for yearly eye examination

PEARLS & CONSIDERATIONS

!

COMMENTS

Nerve (sural) biopsy should be considered if there is prominent early autonomic neuropathy (amyloid) or rapid multifocal clinical pattern suggesting a mononeuritis multiplex that may be due to vasculitis.

EVIDENCE

EBM

Rigorous control of blood glucose levels reduces the risk of developing neuropathy in diabetic subjects (DCCT research group).

Pregabalin (Lyrica) and duloxetine (Cymbalta) are FDA approved for the treatment of pain in diabetic neuropathy.

Gabapentin (Neurontin) 3600 mg/day results in moderate pain relief in patients with diabetic neuropathy.[1]

Venlafaxin (Effexor) 150-225 mg was effective in reducing neuropathic pain in diabetic patients.[2,3]

Tricyclic antidepressants,[4] anticonvulsants,[4] capsaicin,[5] and tramadol[6] are significantly superior to placebo in alleviating the pain of DPN but not adequate enough to relieve the pain.

Evidence-Based References

1. Backonja M et al: Gabapentin for the symptomatic treatment of painful neuropathy in patients with diabetes mellitus: a randomized controlled trial, *JAMA* 280(21):1831-1836, 1998.
2. Kunz NR et al: Treating painful diabetic neuropathy with venlafaxine extended release, *Diabetes* 49(1 suppl):A, 2000.
3. Rowbotham MC et al: Venlafaxine extended release in the treatment of painful diabetic neuropathy: a double-blind, placebo-controlled study, *Pain* 110(3):697-706, 2004.
4. Collins SL et al: Antidepressants and anticonvulsants for diabetic neuropathy and postherpetic neuralgia: a quantitative systematic review, *J Pain Symptom Manage* 20:449-458, 2000.
5. Mason L et al: Systematic review of topical capsaicin for the treatment of chronic pain, *BMJ* 328:7446:991, 2004.
6. Duhmke R, Cornblath D, Hollingshead J: Tramadol for neuropathic pain, *Cochrane Database Syst Rev* 2:CD003726, 2004.

SUGGESTED READINGS

DCCT Research Group: The effect of intensive treatment of diabetes on the development and progression of long-term complications in insulin-dependent diabetes mellitus, *N Engl J Med* 329:14:977-986, 1993.

Herrmann DN et al: Epidermal nerve fiber density and sural nerve morphometry in peripheral neuropathies, *Neurology* 53:1634-1640, 1999.

Katirji B et al: *Neuromuscular disorders in clinical practice,* Boston, 2002, Butterworth-Heinemann, pp. 598-621.

Llewelyn G: The diabetic neuropathies: types, diagnosis and management, *J Neurol Neurosurg Psychiatry* 74:ii15, 2003.

Rosenstock J et al: Pregabalin for the treatment of painful diabetic peripheral neuropathy: a double-blind, placebo-controlled trial, *Pain* 110(3):628-638, 2004.

AUTHOR: **MUSTAFA A. HAMMAD, M.D.**

BASIC INFORMATION

DEFINITION

Digoxin, a cardiac glucoside, is used for the treatment of symptomatic heart failure and ventricular rate control in atrial fibrillation.

Acute or chronic consumption of digoxin can cause toxicity. Toxicity can occur even when serum levels are within the therapeutic range.

SYNONYMS

Digitalis overdose
Cardiac glycosides toxicity

ICD-9CM CODES
972.1 Digitalis overdose

PHARMACOKINETICS

Steady-state levels (not peak levels) correlate with toxicity; digoxin reaches steady state 6 to 8 hr after ingestion.
BIOAVAILABILITY: about 80%
VOLUME OF DISTRIBUTION: 5 to 7 L/kg
HALF-LIFE: 36 hr
EXCRETION: predominantly renal
THERAPEUTIC LEVEL: 0.8 to 2 ng/ml (0.5 to 1.0 ng/ml suggested in heart failure); check level 1 to 2 weeks after starting therapy

EPIDEMIOLOGY & DEMOGRAPHICS

- Digoxin toxicity occurs in up to 5% of individuals on therapy.
- Factors that potentiate toxicity: advanced age, female gender, renal insufficiency, cardiac or pulmonary disease, drugs that affect elimination (amiodarone, quinidine, verapamil, diltiazem, ACE inhibitors, spironolactone, cyclosporine, erythromycin, clarithromycin, tetracyclines, itraconazole, NSAIDs), coingestion of cardiotoxic drugs (beta blockers, calcium channel blockers, tricyclic antidepressants), hypokalemia, hypomagnesemia, hypercalcemia, acid-base disturbance, hypoxia, hypothyroidism, and volume depletion.

PHYSICAL FINDINGS & CLINICAL PRESENTATION

Cardiac, gastrointestinal, and central nervous systems are affected. Fatigue, malaise, and weakness are common complaints.

CARDIAC: Most common and often first finding is an increase in premature ventricular complexes. Can present with almost any dysrhythmia or conduction block.

GI: Anorexia, nausea, vomiting, diarrhea, abdominal pain.

CNS: Headache, dizziness, visual disturbance (flashing lights, halos, blurred vision, change in color perception, decreased visual acuity), confusion, hallucinations, delirium.

- Hyperkalemia often seen in acute poisoning, and hypokalemia more common in chronic toxicity.

ETIOLOGY

Digoxin reversibly inhibits the function of the Na-K ATPase, causing an increase in extracellular K+ and intracellular Na+. This affects the Na-Ca exchanger and leads to intracellular accumulation of calcium. This results in increased myocardial contractility and cardiac output, the positive inotropic effect associated with digoxin therapy. Cardiac glycosides also decrease the heart rate (effect on SA node) and slow conduction throughout the AV node by increasing parasympathetic tone. Sympathetic activity is decreased at therapeutic levels but increased in toxicity. These effects lead to the extrasystoles, tachyarrhythmias, bradyarrhythmias, and AV conduction delays seen in toxicity.

DIAGNOSIS

DIFFERENTIAL DIAGNOSIS

Medications:
- Beta blockers
- Calcium channel blockers
- Clonidine
- Cyclic antidepressants
- Encainide and flecainide
- Procainamide
- Propoxyphene
- Quinidine

Plants producing digitalis-like glycosides:
- Foxglove
- Oleander
- Lily of the valley

Cardiac conduction abnormalities:
- Sick sinus syndrome
- AV node dysfunction

Electrolyte abnormalities:
- Hyperkalemia

WORKUP

- History: medication changes, herbal supplements
- Physical examination

LABORATORY TESTS

- Stat digoxin level (in acute ingestion high levels may not be toxic as tissue redistribution will occur)
- Electrolytes, BUN, creatinine, magnesium, calcium
- ECG (Figs. 1-74 and 1-75)

Almost any dysrhythmia can occur but simultaneous increased automaticity of cardiac tissue and conduction delay in the AV node should raise suspicion. Findings suggestive of toxicity include:
- Frequent premature ventricular complexes

A

B

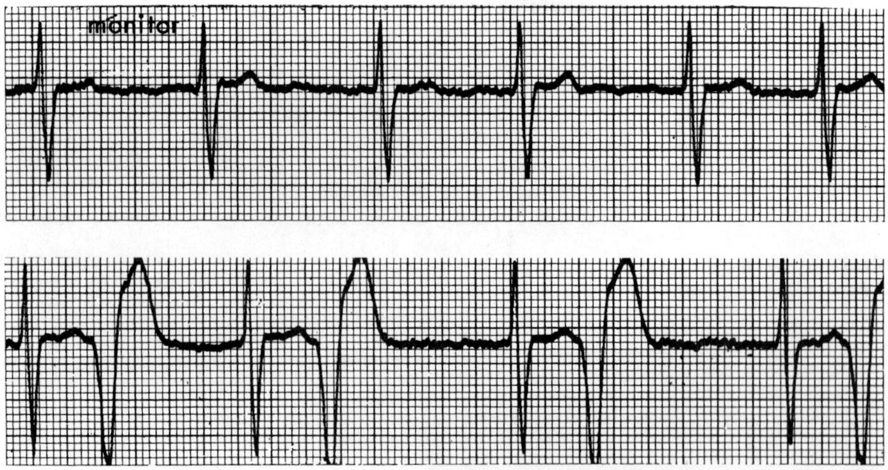

FIGURE 1-74 Ventricular bigeminy caused by digoxin toxicity. Ventricular ectopy is one of the most common signs of digoxin toxicity. The underlying rhythm in **(A)** is atrial fibrillation. In **(B)** each normal QRS is followed by a VPB. (From Goldberger AL [ed]: *Clinical electrocardiography,* ed 5, St Louis, 1994, Mosby.)

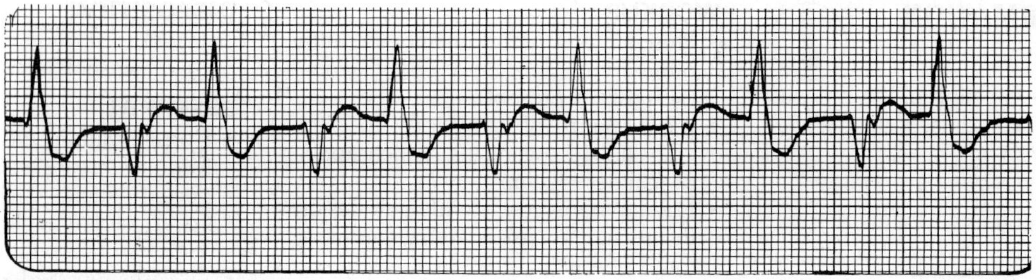

FIGURE 1-75 This digoxin-toxic arrhythmia is a special type of ventricular tachycardia (bidirectional tachycardia) with QRS complexes that alternate in direction from beat to beat. No P waves are present. (From Goldberger AL [ed]: *Clinical electrocardiography,* ed 5, St Louis, 1994, Mosby.)

- Bradydysrhythmias
- AV block (Mobitz type 1)
- Atrial tachycardia with AV block
- Junctional tachycardia
- Bidirectional ventricular tachycardia

TREATMENT

NONPHARMACOLOGIC THERAPY

- Ensure adequate airway
- Cardiac monitor

ACUTE GENERAL Rx

DECREASE TOXICITY:

- Acute toxicity: activated charcoal if within 1 hr of ingestion.
- Treat hyperkalemia, hypokalemia, and hypomagnesemia.
- Digoxin-specific Fab fragments (Digibind):
  1. Specific antibodies that bind to digoxin and to a lesser extent other cardiac glycosides.
  2. Initial response usually seen in 30 min, and complete reversal usually occurs within 4 hr.
  3. Indications: hyperkalemia (≥5 mEq/L), severe arrhythmias, massive overdose (acute ingestion of ≥10 mg digoxin or digoxin serum level ≥10 ng/ml), coingestion of cardiotoxic drugs or plants containing cardiac glycosides.
  4. Dosing: 1 vial (38 mg) of Fab fragments binds 0.5 mg of digoxin.
     a. Digoxin
        - Acute ingestion: number of vials = [ingested digoxin mg × 0.8]/0.5
        - Chronic ingestion: number of vials = [(serum digoxin level ng/ml) × weight kg]/100
     b. If neither the amount ingested nor serum level is known, treat empirically:
        - Acute intoxication—10 vials and repeat if needed
        - Chronic toxicity—6 vials

     NOTE: Underdosing of Fab fragments may result in rebound toxicity as free digoxin is released from tissue stores.
  5. After use of Fab fragments, the free digoxin level decreases, but the measured digoxin level may increase because most assays measure free and bound digoxin levels. Serum levels are unreliable for days.
  6. Inactive complexes are excreted in urine, half-life of complex is 15 to 20 hr. In renal failure, consider plasma exchange or plasmapheresis to remove Fab-digoxin complex; theoretically, complexes may dissociate before excretion and toxicity may reoccur.
  7. Class C for pregnancy.
  8. Adverse effects of treatment:
     a. May undo desirable action of drug and exacerbate heart failure or increase ventricular response in previously controlled atrial fibrillation,
     b. Hypokalemia: monitor potassium level hourly for several hours. The hyperkalemia seen in toxicity reflects a change in potassium distribution, not an increase in total body stores. As toxicity resolves, the potassium moves back into the cell and hypokalemia can occur.
     c. Allergic reactions (<1%)
- Hemodialysis and hemoperfusion: not useful because of extensive tissue binding and large volume of distribution.

COMPLICATIONS:

Hyperkalemia:

- Sodium bicarbonate.
- Glucose and insulin.
- Sodium polystyrene sulfonate (Kayexalate).
- Do not use calcium because it may worsen ventricular arrhythmias.

Bradycardia and heart block:

- Atropine.
- Temporary pacemaker if symptomatic.

Supraventricular and ventricular tachycardia:

- Lidocaine or phenytoin: decrease ventricular automaticity without slowing AV node conduction.
- Avoid quinidine, bretylium, procainamide, and verapamil; may increase ventricular arrhythmias/AV node block.
- Elective cardioversion is relatively contraindicated, because it may precipitate ventricular fibrillation.

DISPOSITION

- Good with prompt treatment.
- Chronic poisoning is associated with higher mortality than acute poisoning.

REFERRAL

Poison control

PEARLS & CONSIDERATIONS

- High index of suspicion helpful, often the signs and symptoms of toxicity are similar to those of the underlying disease.
- To minimize toxicity, digoxin levels should be checked if there is a change in patient's condition (e.g., weight loss, worsening renal function) or an interacting drug is started or stopped.
- Hyperkalemia in acute toxicity is suggestive of significant poisoning (reflects the amount of poisoning of the Na+-K+ ATPase) and is associated with increased mortality.
- Falsely elevated digoxin levels may be seen in pregnant women, renal failure, hepatobiliary disease, and CHF due to the presence of an endogenous digoxin-like substance.
- Severe toxicity from ingestion of nondigoxin cardiac glycosides (plants, etc.) may present with only mildly elevated digoxin levels due to low cross-reactivity between these substances and the digoxin assay.

SUGGESTED READINGS

Antman EM et al: Treatment of 150 cases of life-threatening digitalis intoxication with digoxin-specific Fab antibody fragments. Final report of a multicenter study, *Circulation* 81:1744, 1990.

Bauman JL et al: Mechanisms, manifestations, and management of digoxin toxicity in the modern era, *Am J Cardiovasc Drugs* 6(2):77, 2006.

AUTHOR: **SUDEEP K. AULAKH, M.D., F.R.C.P.C.**

BASIC INFORMATION

DEFINITION

Diphtheria is an infection of the mucous membranes or skin caused by *Corynebacterium diphtheriae.*

SYNONYMS

Pharyngeal diphtheria
Wound diphtheria
Diphtheric cardiomyopathy
Diphtheric polyneuropathy

ICD-9CM CODES
032.9 Diphtheria

EPIDEMIOLOGY & DEMOGRAPHICS

INCIDENCE (IN U.S.):

- Fewer than 5 cases/yr since 1980 (<0.002 cases/100,000 persons)
- Last culture-confirmed indigenous case in 1988

PREDOMINANT AGE: Adult years

PHYSICAL FINDINGS & CLINICAL PRESENTATION

RESPIRATORY DIPHTHERIA:

- Commonly presenting as pharyngitis, but any part of the respiratory tract may be involved, including the nasopharynx, larynx, trachea, or bronchi
- Areas of gray or white exudate coalescing to form a "pseudomembrane" that bleeds when removed
- Possible fever and dysphagia
- Complications: respiratory tract obstruction and pneumonia
- Systemic effects of the toxin: myocarditis and polyneuritis (frequently involving a bulbar distribution)
- Occurs mostly in nonimmune individuals; usually milder and less likely to be complicated in those adequately immunized

CUTANEOUS DIPHTHERIA:

- Usually complicates existing skin lesion (i.e., impetigo or scabies)
- Resembles the underlying condition

ETIOLOGY

- Caused by *C. diphtheriae,* an aerobic, gram-positive rod
- Transmitted by close contact through droplets of nasopharyngeal secretions
- Symptomatic disease of the respiratory system caused by toxin-producing strains (tox^+)
- Systemic effects of toxin: ranging from nausea and vomiting to polyneuropathy, myocarditis, and vascular collapse
- Presence of strains not producing toxin (tox^+) in the respiratory tract of asymptomatic carriers and in skin lesions of cutaneous diphtheria

DIAGNOSIS

DIFFERENTIAL DIAGNOSIS

- Streptococcal pharyngitis
- Viral pharyngitis
- Mononucleosis

WORKUP

- Presence of a pseudomembrane in the oropharynx suggestive of diagnosis (not always present)
- Gram stains of secretions to show club-shaped organisms, which appear as "Chinese letters"
- Nasolaryngoscopy to identify lesions in the nares, nasopharynx, larynx, or tracheobronchial tree

LABORATORY TESTS

- Cultures of mucosal lesions or of nasal discharge
  1. Positive culture for *C. diphtheriae* confirms the diagnosis.
  2. Laboratory is notified of the suspected diagnosis so that appropriate culture medium (Tinsdale agar) is used.
- Testing of all isolated organisms for toxin production

IMAGING STUDIES

Chest x-ray examination to rule out pneumonia

TREATMENT

NONPHARMACOLOGIC THERAPY

- Intubation or tracheostomy if signs of respiratory distress occur
- Nasogastric or parenteral nutrition in those with bulbar signs
- ICU monitoring for patients with signs of systemic toxicity
- Cardiac pacing in patients with heart block
- Respiratory isolation

ACUTE GENERAL Rx

- Administration of diphtheria antitoxin once a clinical diagnosis is made
- If tests for hypersensitivity to horse serum are negative: 50,000 U given for mild to moderate disease or 60,000 to 120,000 U for critically ill patients
- IV infusion of antitoxin over 60 min
- Serum sickness in 10% of treated individuals; those with hypersensitivity to horse serum should be desensitized before administration of antitoxin
- Antibiotics to eradicate the organism in carriers or patients
- For respiratory diphtheria:
  1. Erythromycin 500 mg qid PO or IV (clarithromycin and azithromycin are acceptable alternatives) or IM penicillin 600,000 U bid for 14 days
  2. Carriers or patients with cutaneous disease: erythromycin 500 mg PO qid or rifampin 600 mg PO qd for 7 days

CHRONIC Rx

Antibiotics to limit toxin production and eradicate carrier state, thereby preventing transmission

DISPOSITION

Complete recovery with adequate supportive measures and antitoxin

REFERRAL

- Hospitalization and referral to an infectious disease specialist for all suspected patients
- To an otolaryngologist for evaluation in cases of respiratory diphtheria
- All cases reported to the public health authorities

PEARLS & CONSIDERATIONS

COMMENTS

- Most cases are imported by travelers in epidemic areas, so recent epidemics in Eastern Europe are a cause for concern. A widespread epidemic of diphtheria began in 1990 in the former Soviet Union.
- Vaccination with diphtheria toxoid (attenuated toxin) is safe and effective in the form of DPT or Td; Td boosters should be given to adults every 10 yr. A new formulation of Tdap vaccine with reduced amounts of diphtheria toxoid and acellular pertussis antigens is available; it is well tolerated in clinical trials and provides excellent protection in adolescents and adults.
- According to serologic studies, 20% to 60% of U.S. adults >20 yr of age are susceptible to diphtheria.

EVIDENCE

Antiserum has been used for the treatment of diphtheria for over 100 years and has stood the test of time as an effective treatment strategy. It was tested in one of the first controlled trials in clinical medicine.[1] Ⓑ

Evidence-Based Reference

1. Fibiger JA: Om Serumbehandling af Difteri, *Hospitalstidende* 6:309, 1898. Reviewed in: The controlled clinical trial turns 100 years: Fibiger's trial of serum treatment of diphtheria, *BMJ* 317:1243, 1998. Ⓑ

SUGGESTED READINGS

Berrington J, Fenton A: Immunization responses in preterm infants who receive postnatal steroid treatment, *Pediatrics* 114(4):1127, 2004.

Bissumbhar B et al: Evaluation of diphtheria convalescent patients to serve as donors for the production of anti-diphtheria immunoglobulin preparations, *Vaccine* 22(15-16):1886, 2004.

Broder KR et al: Preventing tetanus, diphtheria, and pertussis among adolescents: use of tetanus toxoid, reduced diphtheria toxoid and acellular pertussis vaccines recommendations of the Advisory Committee on Immunization Practices (ACIP), *MMWR Recomm Rep* 55(RR-3):1, 2006.

AUTHORS: **STEVEN M. OPAL, M.D.,** and **MAURICE POLICAR, M.D.**

BASIC INFORMATION

DEFINITION

Discoid lupus erythematosus (DLE) refers to a chronic inflammatory autoimmune skin disorder. It is sometimes associated with systemic lupus erythematosus (SLE).

SYNONYMS

Chronic cutaneous lupus erythematosus

ICD-9CM CODES
695.4 Lupus erythematosus (local discoid)

EPIDEMIOLOGY & DEMOGRAPHICS

- More common in African Americans.
- More common in females, with peak incidence in the fourth decade of life.
- Approximately 10% to 20% of patients with SLE will also have discoid lupus skin lesions.

PHYSICAL FINDINGS & CLINICAL PRESENTATION

- Appearance of single or multiple asymptomatic plaque lesions (Fig. 1-76).
- Anatomic distribution: commonly involves the scalp, face, and ears, but is not limited to these areas.
- Lesion configuration: irregularly grouped.
- Lesion morphology:
  - Plaque lesions with scales
  - Follicular plugging
  - Atrophy
  - Scarring
  - Telangiectasia
- Color:
  - Erythematous
  - Red to violaceous
  - Hyperpigmentation or hypopigmentation
- Alopecia can occur and is permanent.
- Urticaria (5%).
- May be associated with other criteria for SLE (e.g., oral ulcers, arthritis, pleuritis, pericarditis).

ETIOLOGY

Immune complex mediated

DIAGNOSIS

Clinical inspection and skin biopsy establish the diagnosis of DLE.

DIFFERENTIAL DIAGNOSIS

Psoriasis, lichen planus, secondary syphilis, superficial fungal infections, photosensitivity eruption, sarcoidosis, subacute cutaneous lupus erythematosus, rosacea, keratoacanthoma, actinic keratosis, dermatomyositis

LABORATORY TESTS

- CBC is usually normal in isolated DLE.
- BUN/creatinine is normal.
- Erythrocyte sedimentation rate (ESR) is elevated in active disease.
- Urinalysis.
- Antinuclear antibody (ANA) positive in 20% of patients with isolated DLE.
- Anti-Ro (SS-A) autoantibodies are present in 1% to 3% of patients.
- dsDNA and antiSm antibodies are rarely present.
- Complement levels may be low in patients with SLE but not in DLE.
- Skin biopsy.

IMAGING STUDIES

Chest x-ray examination is not specific.

TREATMENT

NONPHARMACOLOGIC THERAPY

- Avoid sun exposure.
- Use sun protective factor (SPF) of at least 15.

ACUTE GENERAL Rx

1. Topical steroids: intermediate rather than high potency, steroids should be used on areas such as the face.
2. Intradermal steroids: Triamcinolone acetonide, 3 mg/ml with 1% Xylocaine.
3. Hydroxychloroquine 400 mg PO qd for 1 mo, then decrease the dose to 200 mg qd.

Treatment is continued for 3 to 6 mo.

CHRONIC Rx

- Dapsone: 100 mg/day can be used in patients who fail to respond to topical steroid or hydroxychloroquine.
- Other alternatives include:
  1. Chloroquine 250 to 500 mg PO qd
  2. Auranofin 6 mg/day PO qd or divided bid; after 3 mo, may increase to 9 mg/day divided tid
  3. Thalidomide 100 to 300 mg PO before sleep, with water, and >1 hr after meals
  4. Azathioprine 1 mg/kg/day PO for 6 to 8 wk, increase by 5 mg/kg q4 wk until response is seen or dose reaches 2.5 mg/kg/day
  5. If all of the previous treatments fail, mycophenolate 1 g PO bid or interferon α-2b (2 million units/m^2 subcutaneously 3 times/wk for 30 days) have been tried

DISPOSITION

- If untreated, DLE can lead to atrophy and scarring of the skin.
- A minority of patients with isolated cutaneous DLE progress to SLE.

REFERRAL

Dermatology, rheumatology

PEARLS & CONSIDERATIONS

- Cutaneous lesions account for 4 of the 11 criteria in the diagnosis of SLE (e.g., malar rash, discoid rash, photosensitivity, and oral ulcers).
- Rarely does DLE degenerate into a malignant nonmelanotic skin cancer.

EVIDENCE

A systematic review identified one randomized controlled trial comparing topical fluocinonide vs. hydrocortisone in 78 patients with DLE. Clinical improvement was low for both treatments, although improvement was seen in a greater number of patients treated with fluocinonide.[1] Ⓐ

A systematic review identified one randomized controlled trial that compared hydroxychloroquine vs. acitretin in 58 patients with DLE. Improvement was similar in both treatment groups (hydroxychloroquine 50% vs. 46% with acitretin), but patients treated with hydroxychloroquine had fewer adverse reactions.[1] Ⓐ

A recent study evaluated the efficacy of thalidomide in 48 patients with DLE ($n = 18$), subacute cutaneous lupus ($n = 6$), or systemic lupus erythematosus with skin involvement ($n = 24$)

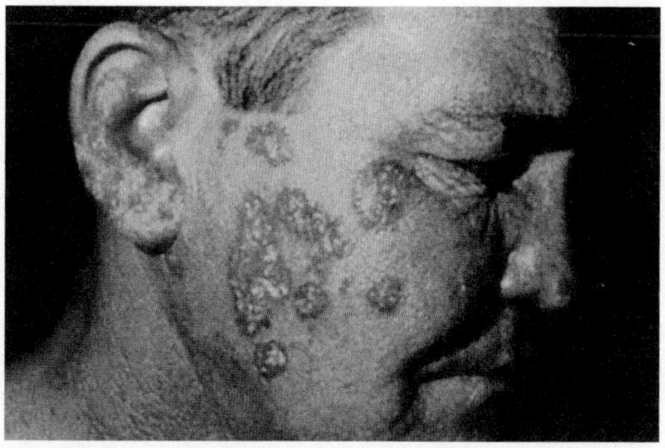

FIGURE 1-76 Scaling plaques with thick scales on the ear and face of a patient who has discoid lupus. (Courtesy Department of Dermatology, University of North Carolina at Chapel Hill. In Goldstein BG, Goldstein AO [eds]: *Practical dermatology,* ed 2, St Louis, 1977, Mosby.)

refractory to other therapies. Treatment with thalidomide resulted in complete remission in 60% of patients and partial remission in 21%. However, in patients with a complete/partial response, the relapse rate after stopping thalidomide was 67%.[2] Ⓑ

Evidence-Based References

1. Jessop S et al: Drugs for discoid lupus erythematosus, *Cochrane Database Syst Rev* 2, 2000. Ⓐ
2. Cuadrado MJ et al: Thalidomide for the treatment of resistant cutaneous lupus: efficacy and safety of different therapeutic regimens, *Am J Med* 118:246, 2005. Ⓑ
3. Ordi-Ros J et al: Thalidomide in the treatment of cutaneous lupus refractory to conventional therapy, *J Rheumatol* 27:1429, 2000. Ⓑ
4. Housman TS et al: Low-dose thalidomide therapy for refractory cutaneous lesions of lupus erythematosus, *Arch Dermatol* 139:50, 2003. Ⓑ

SUGGESTED READINGS

Callen JP: Lupus erythematosus, discoid, *e-Medicine Journal,* July 2, 2004. www.emedicine.com.

Fabri P et al: Cutaneous lupus erythematosus: diagnosis and management, *Am J Clin Dermatol* 4(7):449, 2003.

Pramatorov KD: Chronic cutaneous lupus erythematosus—clinical spectrum, *Clinical Dermatol* 22(2):113, 2004.

Werth V: Clinical manifestations of cutaneous lupus erythematosus, *Autoimmune Rev* 4(5):296, 2005. Epub 2005 Feb 10.

AUTHOR: **MOHAMMAD HAJJIRI, M.D.**

BASIC INFORMATION

DEFINITION

Disseminated intravascular coagulation (DIC) is an acquired thromboembolic disorder characterized by generalized activation of the clotting mechanism, which results in the intravascular formation of fibrin and ultimately thrombotic occlusion of small and midsize vessels.

SYNONYMS

Consumptive coagulopathy
DIC
Defibrination syndrome

ICD-9CM CODES
286.6 Disseminated intravascular coagulation

EPIDEMIOLOGY & DEMOGRAPHICS

Greater than 50% of cases are associated with gram-negative sepsis or other septicemic infections.

PHYSICAL FINDINGS & CLINICAL PRESENTATION

- Wound site bleeding, epistaxis, gingival bleeding, hemorrhagic bullae
- Petechiae, ecchymosis, purpura
- Dyspnea, localized rales, delirium
- Oliguria, anuria, GI bleeding, metrorrhagia

ETIOLOGY

- Infections (e.g., gram-negative sepsis, Rocky Mountain spotted fever, malaria, viral or fungal infection)
- Obstetric complications (e.g., dead fetus, amniotic fluid embolism, toxemia, abruptio placentae, septic abortion, eclampsia, placenta previa, uterine atony)
- Tissue trauma (e.g., burns, hypothermia-rewarming)
- Neoplasms (e.g., adenocarcinomas [GI, prostate, lung, breast], acute promyelocytic leukemia)
- Quinine, cocaine-induced rhabdomyolysis
- Liver failure
- Acute pancreatitis
- Transfusion reactions
- Respiratory distress syndrome
- Toxins (snake bites, amphetamine overdose)
- Other: SLE, vasculitis, aneurysms, polyarteritis, cavernous hemangiomas

DIAGNOSIS

DIFFERENTIAL DIAGNOSIS

- Hepatic necrosis: normal or elevated Factor VIII concentrations
- Vitamin K deficiency: normal platelet count
- Hemolytic uremic syndrome
- Thrombotic thrombocytopenic purpura (TTP)
- Renal failure, SLE, sickle cell crisis, dysfibrinogenemias
- HELLP syndrome (hemolysis, elevated liver function tests, and low platelets)
- Section III describes an algorithm for the differential diagnosis of DVT

WORKUP

Diagnostic workup includes laboratory screening to confirm the diagnosis and exclude conditions noted in the differential diagnosis. Workup is also aimed at distinguishing DIC progression (acute vs chronic), chief manifestations (thrombotic or hemorrhagic), and extent (localized or systemic).

LABORATORY TESTS

- Peripheral blood smear generally shows RBC fragments (schistocytes) and low platelet count.
- Coagulation factors are consumed at a rate in excess of the capacity of the liver to synthesize them, and platelets are consumed in excess of the capacity of the bone marrow megakaryocytes to release them. Diagnostic characteristics of DIC are increased PT, PTT, TT, fibrin split products, D-dimer; decreased fibrinogen level, thrombocytopenia.
- Coagulopathy secondary to DIC must be differentiated from that secondary to liver disease or vitamin K deficiency.
  1. Vitamin K deficiency manifests with prolonged PT and normal PTT, TT, platelet, and fibrinogen level; PTT may be elevated in severe cases.
  2. Patients with liver disease have abnormal PT and PTT; TT and fibrinogen are usually normal unless severe disease is present; platelets are usually normal unless splenomegaly is present.
  3. Factors V and VIII are low in DIC, but they are normal in liver disease with coagulopathy.

IMAGING STUDIES

Imaging studies are generally not useful. Chest x-ray may be helpful to exclude infectious processes in patients presenting with pulmonary symptoms such as dyspnea, cough, or hemoptysis.

TREATMENT

NONPHARMACOLOGIC THERAPY

No specific precautions regarding activity level are necessary unless thrombocytopenia is severe.

ACUTE GENERAL Rx

- Correct and eliminate underlying cause (e.g., antimicrobial therapy for infection, removal of necrotic bowel, evacuation of uterus in obstetric emergencies).
- Give replacement therapy with FFP and platelets in patients with significant hemorrhage:
  1. FFP 10 to 15 ml/kg can be given with a goal of normalizing INR.
  2. Platelet transfusions are given when platelet count is <10,000 (or higher if major bleeding is present).
  3. Cryoprecipitate 1 U/5 kg is reserved for hypofibrinogen states.
  4. Antithrombin III treatment may be considered as a supportive therapeutic option in patients with severe DIC. Its modest results and substantial cost are limiting factors.
- Heparin therapy at a dose lower than that used in venous thrombosis (300 to 500 U/hr) may be useful in selected cases to increase neutralization of thrombin (e.g., DIC associated with acute promyelocytic leukemia, purpura fulminans, acral ischemia).

CHRONIC Rx

Follow-up management includes coagulation screening to assess factor replacement therapy. Laboratory abnormalities generally correct with treatment of the underlying disorder. Chronic laboratory monitoring is not required.

DISPOSITION

Mortality in severe DIC exceeds 75%. Death generally results from progression of the underlying disease and complications such as acute renal failure, intracerebral hematoma, shock, or cardiac tamponade.

REFERRAL

Hematology consultation is recommended in all cases of DIC.

PEARLS & CONSIDERATIONS

COMMENTS

The treatment of chronic DIC is controversial. Low-dose SC heparin and/or combination antiplatelet agents such as aspirin and dipyridamole may be useful.

AUTHOR: **FRED F. FERRI, M.D.**

BASIC INFORMATION

DEFINITION

- Colonic diverticula are herniations of mucosa and submucosa through the muscularis. They are generally found along the colon's mesenteric border at the site where the vasa recta penetrates the muscle wall (anatomic weak point).
- *Diverticulosis* is the asymptomatic presence of multiple colonic diverticula.
- *Diverticulitis* is an inflammatory process or localized perforation of diverticulum.

ICD-9CM CODES
562.10 Diverticulosis of colon
562.11 Diverticulitis of colon

EPIDEMIOLOGY & DEMOGRAPHICS

- Incidence of diverticulosis in the general population is 35% to 50%.
- Diverticulosis is more common in Western countries, affecting >30% of people >40 yr and >50% of people >70 yr.

PHYSICAL FINDINGS & CLINICAL PRESENTATION

- Physical examination in patients with diverticulosis is generally normal.
- Painful diverticular disease can present with LLQ pain, often relieved by defecation; location of pain may be anywhere in the lower abdomen because of the redundancy of the sigmoid colon.
- Diverticulitis can cause muscle spasm, guarding, and rebound tenderness predominantly affecting the LLQ.

ETIOLOGY

Diverticular disease is believed to be secondary to low intake of dietary fiber.

DIAGNOSIS

DIFFERENTIAL DIAGNOSIS

- Irritable bowel syndrome
- IBD
- Carcinoma of colon
- Endometriosis
- Ischemic colitis
- Infections (pseudomembranous colitis, appendicitis, pyelonephritis, PID)
- Lactose intolerance

LABORATORY TESTS

- WBC count in diverticulitis reveals leukocytosis with left shift.
- Microcytic anemia can be present in patients with chronic bleeding from diverticular disease. MCV may be elevated in acute bleeding secondary to reticulocytosis.

IMAGING STUDIES

- Barium enema should only be considered in patients unwilling to undergo colonoscopy or with contraindications to the procedure. When perforated, barium enema will demonstrate multiple diverticula and muscle spasm ("sawtooth" appearance of the lumen) in patients with painful diverticular disease. Barium enema can be hazardous and should not be performed in the acute stage of diverticulitis because it may produce free perforation.
- A CT scan of the abdomen can be used to diagnose acute diverticulitis; typical findings are thickening of the bowel wall, fistulas, or abscess formation.
- Evaluation of suspected diverticular bleeding:
  1. Arteriography if the bleeding is faster than 1 ml/min (advantage: the possible infusion of vasopressin directly into the arteries supplying the bleeding, as well as selective arterial embolization; disadvantages: its cost and invasive nature)
  2. Technetium-99m sulfa colloid
  3. Technetium-99m labeled RBC (can detect bleeding rates as low as 0.12 to 5 ml/min)

TREATMENT

NONPHARMACOLOGIC THERAPY

- Increase in dietary fiber intake and regular exercise to improve bowel function
- NPO and IV hydration in severe diverticulitis; NG suction if ileus or small bowel obstruction is present

ACUTE GENERAL Rx

TREATMENT OF DIVERTICULITIS:

- Mild case: broad-spectrum PO antibiotics (e.g., Ciprofloxacin 500 mg bid to cover aerobic component of colonic flora and metronidazole 500 mg q6h for anaerobes) and liquid diet for 7 to 10 days
- Severe case: NPO and aggressive IV antibiotic therapy
  a. Ampicillin-sulbactam (Unasyn) 3 g IV q6h *or*
  b. Piperacillin-tazobactam (Zosyn) 4.5 g IV q8h *or*
  c. Ciprofloxacin 400 mg IV q12h plus metronidazole 500 mg IV q6h *or*
  d. Cefoxitin 2 g IV q8h plus metronidazole 500 mg IV q6h
- Life-threatening case: Imipenem 500 mg IV q6h *or* meropenem 1 g IV q8h
- Surgical treatment consisting of resection of involved areas and reanastomosis (if feasible); otherwise a diverting colostomy with reanastomosis performed when infection has been controlled; surgery should be considered in patients with:
  1. Repeated episodes of diverticulitis (two or more)
  2. Poor response to appropriate medical therapy (failure of conservative management)
  3. Abscess or fistula formation
  4. Obstruction
  5. Peritonitis
  6. Immunocompromised patients, first episode in young patient (<40 yr old)
  7. Inability to exclude carcinoma (10% to 20% of patients diagnosed with diverticulosis on clinical grounds are subsequently found to have carcinoma of the colon)

DIVERTICULAR HEMORRHAGE:

1. Bleeding is painless and stops spontaneously in the majority of patients (60%); it is usually caused by erosion of a blood vessel by a fecalith present within the diverticular sac.
2. Medical therapy consists of blood replacement and correction of volume and any clotting abnormalities.
3. Colonoscopic treatment with epinephrine injections, bipolar coagulation, or both may prevent recurrent bleeding and decrease the need for surgery.
4. Surgical resection is necessary if bleeding does not stop spontaneously after administration of 4 to 5 U of PRBCs or recurs with severity within a few days; if attempts at localization are unsuccessful, total abdominal colectomy with ileoproctostomy may be indicated (high incidence of rebleeding if segmental resection is performed without adequate localization).

CHRONIC Rx

Asymptomatic patients with diverticulosis can be treated with a high-fiber diet or fiber supplements.

DISPOSITION

- Most patients with diverticulitis respond well to antibiotic management and bowel rest. Up to 30% of patients with diverticulitis will eventually require surgical management.
- Diverticular bleeding can recur in 15% to 20% of patients within 5 yr.

REFERRAL

Surgical referral when considering resection (see "Acute General Rx")

AUTHOR: **FRED F. FERRI, M.D.**

BASIC INFORMATION

DEFINITION

Down syndrome is a disorder characterized by mental retardation and multiple organ defects that is caused by a chromosomal abnormality (trisomy 21).

SYNONYMS

Trisomy 21

ICD-9CM CODES
758.0 Down Syndrome

EPIDEMIOLOGY & DEMOGRAPHICS

INCIDENCE (IN U.S.): 1 in 800 births
PEAK INCIDENCE: Newborn
PREVALENCE (IN U.S.): 300,000 persons
PREDOMINANT SEX: Male:female ratio of 1.3:1.0
PREDOMINANT AGE: Newborn to early adulthood
GENETICS: Nondisjunction causing trisomy 21

PHYSICAL FINDINGS & CLINICAL PRESENTATION (Fig. 1-77)

- Microcephaly
- Flattening of occiput and face
- Upward slant to eyes with epicanthal folds
- Brushfield spots in iris
- Broad stocky neck
- Small feet, hands, digits
- Single palmar crease
- Hypotonia
- Short stature
- Associated with congenital heart disease, malformations of the GI tract, cataracts, hypothyroidism, hip dysplasia, obstructive sleep apnea, and myeloproliferative disorders
- About half of children with Down syndrome are born with congenital heart disease, with the most common lesions being atrial septal defect and ventricular septal defect
- Persistent primary congenital hypothyroidism is found in 1 in 141 newborns with Down syndrome, as compared with 1 in 4000 in the general population
- Ophthalmologic disorders increase in frequency with age. Over 80% of children aged 5 to 12 have disorders that need monitoring or intervention, such as refractive errors, strabismus, or cataracts
- Dermatologic issues such as folliculitis can become problematic in adolescents and require topical antibiotics and careful attention to hygiene.

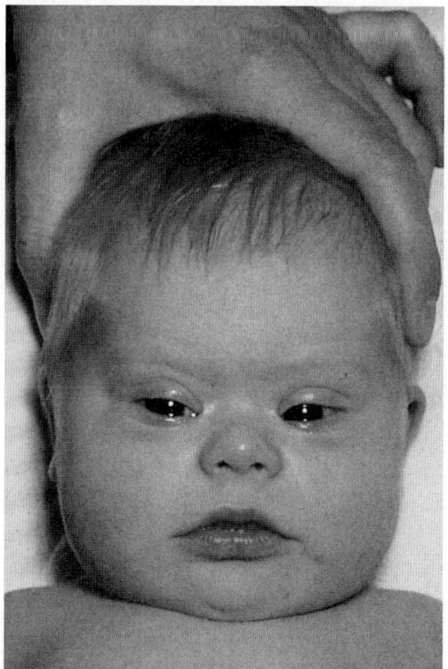

FIGURE 1-77 Down syndrome. Note depressed nasal bridge, epicanthal folds, mongoloid slant of eyes, low-set ears, and large tongue. (From Zitelli BJ, Davis HW: *Atlas of pediatric physical diagnosis,* ed 3, St Louis, 1997, Mosby.)

ETIOLOGY

Nondisjunction of chromosome 21

DIAGNOSIS

- Prenatal cytogenic diagnosis by amniocentesis or chorionic villus sampling
- Combined use of serum screening and fetal ultrasound testing for thickened nuchal fold has 85% detection rate with 5% false positives
- Postnatal chromosomal karyotype

DIFFERENTIAL DIAGNOSIS

- Congential hypothyroidism
- Other chromosomal abnormalities

WORKUP

Postnatal chromosomal karyotype

TREATMENT

- Thyroid screen at birth, at age 6 mo, and yearly thereafter
- Treatment consists of vigilant monitoring for comorbid states, such as obesity, hypothyroidism, leukemia, hearing loss, and valvular heart disease
- Echocardiogram in all newborns and cardiac assessment of adolescents for development of mitral valve prolapse
- Prevention of obesity with low-calorie, high-fiber diet
- Auditory brainstem responses in all newborns and aggressive testing for hearing loss in children with chronic otitis media
- Ophthalmologic assessment by age 6 mo for congenital cataracts and annual exams for monitoring of refractive errors and strabismus
- Regular dental care
- Pelvic examination of women who are sexually active or who have menstrual problems

DISPOSITION

Most children with Down syndrome live at home. As these individuals reach adulthood, those with higher functioning sometimes live in supervised settings away from their families.

REFERRAL

Down syndrome clinics use a preventive checklist to anticipate many clinical challenges.

PEARLS & CONSIDERATIONS

COMMENTS

- Screening for atlantoaxial subluxation is controversial.
- Most patients develop neuropathologic changes typical of Alzheimer disease. Presenting symptoms include seizures, focal neurologic signs, and apathy. If Alzheimer disease is suspected, screen for treatable diseases such as depression or hypothyroidism.
- This syndrome accounts for approximately one third of moderate to severe cases of mental retardation.
- Individuals with Down syndrome have a wide range of function, but all will have decrease in intelligence quotient in first decade of life.
- Deficiency of language production relative to other areas of development often causes substantial impairment.
- Individuals with Down syndrome have more behavioral and psychiatric problems than other children, but fewer than other individuals with mental retardation.
- Though increased maternal age is a risk factor, most children with Down syndrome are born to women under the age of 35 yr.

SUGGESTED READINGS

Ball RH et al: First- and second-trimester evaluation for Down syndrome, *Obstet Gynecol* 110(1):10-17, 2007.

Lott IT, Head E: Down syndrome and Alzheimer's disease: a link between development and aging, *Ment Retard Dev Disabil Res Rev* 7(3):172, 2001.

Patterson D, Costa AC: Down syndrome and genetics—a case of linked histories, *Nat Rev Genet* 6(2):137, 2005.

Roizen NJ: Medical care and monitoring for the adolescent with Down syndrome, *Adolesc Med* 13(2):345, 2002.

AUTHOR: **MAITREYI MAZUMDAR, M.D., M.P.H.**

BASIC INFORMATION

DEFINITION

Dumping syndrome refers to the constellation of postprandial symptoms as a result of rapid delivery of stomach contents into the small bowel seen after definitive surgery for peptic ulcer disease.

SYNONYMS

Early postgastrectomy syndrome

ICD-9CM CODES
564.2 Postgastric surgery syndromes

EPIDEMIOLOGY & DEMOGRAPHICS

Incidence is 10% of all patients having gastric surgery.

- Vagotomy and pyloroplasty (8.5% to 20%)
- Vagotomy and antrectomy (4% to 27%)
- Subtotal gastrectomy (10% to 40%)
- Parietal cell vagotomy (3% to 5%)
- Males and females are affected equally

PHYSICAL FINDINGS & CLINICAL PRESENTATION

1. Early dumping syndrome: symptoms start within 1 hr after eating food:
   - No symptoms in fasting state
   - Nausea, vomiting, and belching
   - Epigastric fullness, cramping, and diarrhea
   - Dizziness, flushing, diaphoresis, and syncope
   - Palpitations and tachycardia
2. Late dumping syndrome: symptoms occurring 1 to 3 hr after eating:
   - Diaphoresis
   - Irritability
   - Difficulty in concentration
   - Tremulousness

ETIOLOGY

Dumping syndrome occurs almost exclusively in patients who have had gastric surgery.

- Systemic symptoms are thought to be due to hypovolemia caused by rapid shifts of fluid from the intravascular space into the lumen of the bowel.
- Increase in vasoactive substances related to rapid gastric emptying is thought to play a role in dumping syndrome.
- Late dumping symptoms are thought to be due to reactive hypoglycemia.

DIAGNOSIS

A detailed clinical history and evidence of prior gastric surgery are necessary for the diagnosis.

DIFFERENTIAL DIAGNOSIS

- Pancreatic insufficiency
- Inflammatory bowel disease
- Afferent loop syndromes
- Bile acid reflux after surgery
- Bowel obstruction
- Gastroenteric fistula

WORKUP

Diagnosis is typically made on clinical grounds. In certain clinical settings, where patients exhibit symptoms with no prior history of gastric surgery, oral glucose challenge and imaging studies may be pursued and may aid in establishing the diagnosis.

LABORATORY TESTS

Oral glucose challenge test:

- Oral intake of 50 g of glucose is followed by serial measurements of heart rate, serum glucose, and hydrogen breath test every 15 min for 6 hr.
- An increase in the heart rate >12 beats/min and a rise in hydrogen breath excretion had a sensitivity of 94% and specificity >92%. A nadir blood glucose <3.3 mmol/L (<59 mg/dL) was present in 75% of late dumpers.

IMAGING STUDIES

- Upper GI series properly defines anatomy.
- Scintigraphic imaging documents rapid gastric emptying and may be useful in patients with dumping syndrome and no prior history of gastric surgery.

TREATMENT

NONPHARMACOLOGIC THERAPY

- Diet modification
  1. Divide calorie intake over six small meals
  2. Limit fluid intake with meals (try to avoid fluids 30 min before meals)
  3. Decrease carbohydrate intake and avoid simple sugars
  4. Increase/supplement dietary fibers
  5. Avoid milk/milk products

ACUTE GENERAL Rx

- Acarbose 50 mg PO daily can be tried if dietary modification does not help.
- Octreotide 25 to 50 μg SC 30 min before meals is effective in relieving symptoms of dumping syndrome.
- Pectin and Guar have been used to increase viscosity of intraluminal contents and relieving symptoms from rapid emptying and absorption.

CHRONIC Rx

- Surgery is considered in patients with severe symptoms refractory to the above mentioned dietary and acute general treatment.
- Surgical procedures include: reconstruction of the pylorus, converting Billroth II to a Billroth I anastomosis, and a Roux-en-Y reconstruction.
- In severe cases, can consider depot long acting release octreotide, given as 10 mg intramuscularly every 4 wk for symptom relief.

DISPOSITION

- Dumping syndrome improves with time. Approximately 1% to 2% of patients will continue to have significant symptoms several months after surgery.
- Dietary modification effectively treats the majority of patients.

REFERRAL

- A GI consult is recommended in patients suspected of having dumping syndrome.
- If medical management is unsuccessful, a general surgical consultation is warranted.

PEARLS & CONSIDERATIONS

COMMENTS

- The majority of patients usually manifest with early dumping symptoms or combination of early and late symptoms. Few have late dumping symptoms alone.
- Octreotide has an inhibitory effect on the release of insulin and other vasoactive substances released by the gut. It also works by decreasing gastric emptying.

SUGGESTED READINGS

Hasler WL: Dumping syndrome, *Current Treat Options Gastroenterol* 5(2):139, 2002.

Li-Ling J, Irving M: Therapeutic value of octreotide for patients with severe dumping syndrome: a review of randomized controlled trials, *Postgrad Med J* 77(909):441, 2001.

Ukleja A: Dumping syndrome: pathophysiology and treatment, *Nutr Clin Pract* 20(5):517, 2005.

AUTHOR: **MOHAMMAD HAJJIRI, M.D.**

BASIC INFORMATION

DEFINITION

Dupuytren's contracture is a disease of the palmar fascia characterized by nodular fibroblastic proliferation that often results in progressive contractures of the fascia and flexion deformity of the fingers.

ICD-9CM CODES
728.6 Dupuytren's contracture

EPIDEMIOLOGY & DEMOGRAPHICS

PREVALENCE: Varies depending on nationality
PREVALENT SEX: Male:female ratio of 10:1
PREVALENT AGE: 40 to 60 yr

PHYSICAL FINDINGS & CLINICAL PRESENTATION

- Usually asymptomatic
- Most common complaints: deformity and interference with the use of the hand by the flexed, contracted fingers (Fig. 1-78)
- Process usually begins in the ulnar side of the hand, often starting at the ring finger
- Isolated painless nodules that eventually harden and mature into a longitudinal cord that extends into the finger
- Lesion often begins in the distal palmar crease
- Overlying skin adherent to the fascia
- Later stages: fibrous cord begins to contract and pull the finger into flexion
- Possible involvement of other fingers, particularly small finger

ETIOLOGY

Unknown. Pathologically, the contracture consists of proliferating vascular tissue that later develops into mature collagen.

DIAGNOSIS

DIFFERENTIAL DIAGNOSIS

- Soft tissue tumor
- Tendon cyst

WORKUP

The typical case is easily diagnosed clinically. Plain radiographs may be useful to rule out bony abnormalities.

TREATMENT

NONPHARMACOLOGIC THERAPY

- Stretching exercises
- Local heat

DISPOSITION

Rate of development is variable.

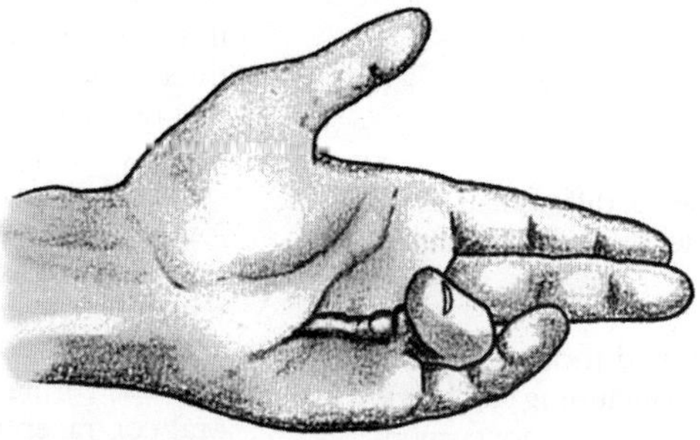

FIGURE 1-78 Dupuytren's contracture. A flexion deformity of the finger is present, with nodular thickening of the fascia to the ring finger.

REFERRAL

- If joint contracture begins to develop
- For excision of rare nodule that is painful (at any stage)

PEARLS & CONSIDERATIONS

COMMENTS

- Dupuytren's contracture develops earlier and more often in certain families.
- The disorder is more common in Scandinavians, and some Northern Europeans have a 25% prevalence over age 60 yr.
- About 5% of patients develop a similar condition elsewhere, such as Peyronie's disease or Ledderhose disease (involvement of the plantar fascia).
- Soft tissue "pads" in the knuckles may also be present.
- Individuals with these additional findings are considered to have Dupuytren's diathesis, and their disease is generally more severe and recurrent.

SUGGESTED READINGS

Frank PL: An update on Dupuytren's contracture, *Hosp Med* 62:678, 2001.

Khan AA et al: The role of manual occupation in the aetilogy of Dupuytren's disease in men in England and Wales, *J Hand Surg* 299(1):12, 2004.

McFarlane RM: On the origin and spread of Dupuytren's disease, *J Hand Surg* 27:385, 2002.

Ragsowansi RH, Britto JA: Genetic and epigenetic influence on the pathogenesis of Dupuytren's disease, *J Hand Surg* 26:1157, 2001.

Rayan GM: Dupuytren's disease: anatomy, pathology, presentation, and treatment, *J Bone Joint Surg* 89A:189, 2007.

Thurston AJ: Dupuytren's disease, *J Bone Joint Surg Br* 85(4):469, 2003.

Trojian TH, Chu SM: Dupuytren's disease: diagnosis and treatment, *Am Fam Physician* 76:86, 2007.

AUTHOR: **LONNIE R. MERCIER, M.D.**

Section I DISEASES AND DISORDERS

BASIC INFORMATION

DEFINITION

Dysfunctional uterine bleeding (DUB) describes abnormal uterine bleeding in the absence of disease in the pelvis, pregnancy, or medical illness. Specific types of abnormal bleeding include the following:

- Hypermenorrhea: excessive bleeding in amount during normal duration of regular menstrual cycles.
- Hypomenorrhea: decreased bleeding in amount in regular menstrual cycles.
- Menorrhagia: regular normal intervals, excessive flow and duration.
- Metrorrhagia: irregular intervals, excessive flow and duration.
- Menometrorrhagia: irregular or excessive bleeding during menstruation and between periods.
- Oligomenorrhea: intervals greater than 35 days.
- Polymenorrhea: intervals less than 21 days.

SYNONYMS

DUB

ICD-9CM CODES
626 Disorders of menstruation and other abnormal bleeding from female genital tract
626.2 Hypermenorrhea
626.1 Hypomenorrhea
626.2 Menorrhagia
626.6 Metrorrhagia
626.2 Menometrorrhagia
626.1 Oligomenorrhea
626.2 Polymenorrhea

EPIDEMIOLOGY & DEMOGRAPHICS

- Most cases of DUB occur in postmenarchal and perimenopausal age groups.
- During reproductive age, <20% of abnormal bleeding results from anovulatory DUB.

PHYSICAL FINDINGS & CLINICAL PRESENTATION

- A clinical diagnosis of exclusion
- Thorough physical and pelvic examination to exclude the other causes of abnormal bleeding
  1. Includes thyroid, breast, liver, presence or absence of ecchymotic lesions
  2. Patient possibly obese and hirsute (polycystic ovarian disease)
  3. No evidence of any vulvar, vaginal, cervical lesions, uterine (fibroid) or ovarian tumor, urethral caruncle, urethral diverticula, hemorrhoids, anal fissure, colorectal lesions
  4. Bimanual pelvic examination: normal-sized or slightly enlarged uterus

ETIOLOGY

- 90% is caused by anovulation.
- 10% is ovulatory in origin; can be caused by dysfunction of corpus luteum or midcycle bleeding.
- Section II describes the various causes of abnormal uterine bleeding.

DIAGNOSIS

DIFFERENTIAL DIAGNOSIS

- Pregnancy-related cause
- Anatomic uterine causes:
  1. Leiomyomas
  2. Adenomyosis
  3. Polyps
  4. Endometrial hyperplasia
  5. Cancer
  6. Sexually transmitted diseases
  7. Intrauterine contraceptive devices
- Anatomic nonuterine causes:
  1. Cervical neoplasia, cervicitis
  2. Vaginal neoplasia, adhesions, trauma, foreign body, atrophic vaginitis, infections, condyloma
  3. Vulvar trauma, infections, neoplasia, condyloma, dystrophy, varices
  4. Urinary tract: urethral caruncle, diverticulum, hematuria
  5. GI tract: hemorrhoids, anal fissure, colorectal lesions
- Systemic diseases:
  1. Exogenous hormone intake
  2. Coagulopathies: von Willebrand's disease, thrombocytopenia, hepatic failure
  3. Endocrinopathies: thyroid disorder, hypo- and hyperthyroidism, diabetes mellitus
  4. Renal diseases
- Section II describes a differential diagnosis of vaginal bleeding abnormalities.

WORKUP

- A detailed history and thorough physical examination, including a pelvic examination to exclude above mentioned causes.
- Clinical algorithms for the evaluation of vaginal bleeding are described in Section III, "Bleeding, Vaginal."

LABORATORY TESTS

- CBC with platelets; possible iron deficiency anemia or thrombocytopenia
- Prothrombin (PT); partial thromboplastin and bleeding time if coagulopathy is suspected
- Serum human chorionic gonadotropin (hCG)
- Chemistry profile, including liver function tests
- Thyroid profile
- Stool testing for occult blood
- Urinalysis for hematuria
- Pap smear
- Cultures for gonorrhea and *Chlamydia*
- Serum gonadotropins and prolactin
- Serum androgens
- Endometrial biopsy in women >35 yr, or earlier, if longstanding history of anovulatory bleeding
- Hysterogram and hysteroscopy

IMAGING STUDIES

- Pelvic ultrasound, including measurement of endometrial thickness
- Hydrosonogram (also known as fluid contrast ultrasound, saline sonogram)

TREATMENT

NONPHARMACOLOGIC THERAPY

Increase iron intake in the form of pills and in a diet rich in iron.

ACUTE GENERAL Rx

- Progestational agents
  1. Progesterone in oil, 100 to 200 mg
  2. Medroxyprogesterone acetate, 20 to 40 mg qd for 15 days
  3. Megestrol acetate, 40 to 120 mg daily in divided doses × 15 days
  4. Oral contraceptives: any oral contraceptive pill, 1 tablet qid for 5 to 7 days, followed by 1 tablet low-dose estrogen qd for 21 days; causes heavy withdrawal bleeding, should then be on cyclical Provera or continue on oral contraceptives
- Estrogens
  1. Conjugated estrogen (Premarin) 25 mg IV q4h until bleeding is under control (in cases of severe or life-threatening bleeding); maximum three doses
  2. For prolonged bleeding that is not life-threatening: Premarin 1.25 mg (Estrace 2 mg) q4h for 24 hr, followed by Provera to bring on withdrawal bleeding; then sequential regimen of estrogen and progestin (Premarin 1.25 mg qd for 24 days; Provera 10 mg for last 10 days) or oral contraceptives
- Surgical treatment
  1. Dilation and curettage (D&C) and hysteroscopy
  2. Endometrial ablation
  3. Hysterectomy

CHRONIC Rx

- Progestational agents
  1. Medroxyprogesterone acetate 10 mg qd for 12 days, then cyclically to induce monthly withdrawal bleeding
  2. Norethindrone 2.5 to 10 mg qd for 12 days
  3. Depo-Provera 150 mg IM and then 150 mg q3mo
  4. Oral contraceptives one tablet qd
- Clomiphene citrate: patients with anovulatory bleeding who want to become pregnant
- Others
  1. Antiprostaglandins
  2. Danazol

3. Gonadotropin-releasing hormone analogs (GNRH)
4. Human menopausal gonadotropin (HMG) (desire pregnancy)

- Surgical treatment
1. D&C and hysteroscopy
2. Endometrial ablation
3. Hysterectomy

DISPOSITION

Cyclical treatment on birth control pills or Provera for several cycles, then discontinue pill and watch patient for onset of regular menses

REFERRAL

To gynecologist in case of failure of treatment

PEARLS & CONSIDERATIONS

COMMENTS

Patient education material may be obtained from the American College of Obstetricians and Gynecologists, 409 12th Street SW, Washington, DC 20024-2188; phone (202) 638-5577.

EVIDENCE

Medical management

A systematic review of randomized controlled trials (RCTs) found luteal-phase progesterone (day 15 or 19 to 26) was less effective in reducing menstrual blood loss than danazol, tranexamic acid, and levonorgestrel intrauterine system (IUS). However, 21-day progesterone resulted in significant blood flow reduction, although women found this treatment less acceptable than the IUS.[1] Ⓐ

A systematic review found that levonorgestrel-releasing intrauterine device (LNG-IUS) was more effective than cyclical norethisterone (21 days) as a treatment for heavy menstrual bleeding. Women with an LNG-IUS were more satisfied and willing to continue with treatment but experienced more side effects such as intermenstrual bleeding and breast tenderness.[2] Ⓐ

A systematic review of 19 RCTs compared preoperative GnRH analogues with placebo for treatment of fibroids and found that preoperative and postoperative hemoglobin was improved and uterine volume and fibroid size were significantly reduced. Pelvic symptoms were also improved.[3] Ⓐ

A systematic review of antifibrinolytics (tranexamic acid) vs. placebo and vs. other medical therapies (mefenamic acid, norethisterone in luteal phase, and ethamsylate) has shown that in all cases there was a reduction in menstrual flow and improvement in quality of life measures.[4] Ⓐ

The same review found tranexamic acid was significantly better than luteal-phase progesterone.[4] Ⓐ

Surgical management

A systematic review comparing endometrial ablation (EA) with hysterectomy has concluded that endometrial destruction offers an alternative to hysterectomy, that both procedures are effective, and that satisfaction rates are high. However, retreatment is often necessary with ablation. There is some evidence of greater improvement in health for the hysterectomy patients and it offers permanent relief.[5] Ⓐ

A systematic review comparing hysteroscopic EA techniques for the management of heavy menstrual bleeding found the vaporizing electrode procedure was less difficult to perform and had less fluid deficit than transcervical resection of the endometrium (TCRE). However, odds of fluid overload and equipment failure were higher for laser treatment compared with TCRE. Overall, the newer techniques took less time to perform and were more likely to be performed under local anesthesia but had a greater chance of equipment failure.[6] Ⓐ

Medical vs. surgical management

A systematic review compared medical therapy (options included oral medications and a hormone-releasing intrauterine system, LNG-IUS) vs. surgery (options included uterine resection or ablation, and hysterectomy) in women with heavy menstrual bleeding. Surgery reduced menstrual bleeding at 1 year more than medical treatments, but LNG-IUS appeared equally beneficial in improving quality of life.[7] Ⓐ

Evidence-Based References

1. Lethaby A, Irvine G, Cameron I: Cyclical progestogens for heavy menstrual bleeding, *Cochrane Database Syst Rev* 4,1998. Ⓐ
2. Lethaby A, Farquhar C, Cooke I: Antifibrinolytics for heavy menstrual bleeding, *Cochrane Database Syst Rev* 4,2000. Ⓐ
3. Lethaby AE, Cooke I, Rees M: Progesterone/progestogen releasing intrauterine systems for heavy menstrual bleeding, *Cochrane Database Syst Rev* 4,2005. Ⓐ
4. Lethaby A, Vollenhoven B, Sowter M: Preoperative GnRH analogue therapy before hysterectomy or myomectomy for uterine fibroids, *Cochrane Database Syst Rev* 2,2001. Ⓐ
5. Lethaby A et al: Endometrial resection and ablation versus hysterectomy for heavy menstrual bleeding, *Cochrane Database Syst Rev* 2,1999. Ⓐ
6. Lethaby A, Hickey M, Garry R: Endometrial destruction techniques for heavy menstrual bleeding, *Cochrane Database Syst Rev* 4,2005. Ⓐ
7. Marjoribanks J, Lethaby A, Farquhar C: Surgery versus medical therapy for heavy menstrual bleeding, *Cochrane Database Syst Rev* 2,2003. Ⓐ

SUGGESTED READING

Mihm LM et al: The accuracy of endometrial biopsy and saline sonohysterography in the determination of the cause of abnormal uterine bleeding, *Am J Obstet Gynecol* 186:858, 2002.

AUTHORS: **MANDEEP K. BRAR, M.D.,** and **RUBEN ALVERO, M.D.**

BASIC INFORMATION

DEFINITION

Dysmenorrhea is pain with menstruation, usually as cramping and usually centered in the lower abdomen. It is defined as *primary dysmenorrhea* when there is no associated organic pathology and *secondary dysmenorrhea* when there is demonstrable organic pathology.

SYNONYMS

Menstrual cramps
Painful periods

ICD-9CM CODES
625.3 Dysmenorrhea

EPIDEMIOLOGY & DEMOGRAPHICS

Approximately 50% of menstruating women are affected by dysmenorrhea, with approximately 10% of them having severe dysmenorrhea with incapacitation for 1 to 3 days/mo. Dysmenorrhea is most common in the age group from 20 to 24 yr, and primary dysmenorrhea usually appears within 6 to 12 mo after menarche.

PHYSICAL FINDINGS & CLINICAL PRESENTATION

- Sharp, crampy, midline, lower abdomen pain without a lower quadrant or adnexal component but possible radiation to the lower back and upper thighs
- Unremarkable pelvic examination in nonmenstruating patient
- Accompanying symptoms: nausea, vomiting, headaches, anxiety, fatigue, diarrhea, fainting, and abdominal bloating
- Cramps usually lasting <24 hr and seldom lasting >2 to 3 days
- Secondary dysmenorrhea: dyspareunia is a common complaint, and bimanual pelvic-abdominal examination may demonstrate uterine or adnexal tenderness, fixed uterine retroflexion, uterosacral nodularity, a pelvic mass, or an enlarged, irregular uterus

ETIOLOGY

Prostaglandin $F_2\alpha$ (PG $F_2\alpha$) is the agent responsible for dysmenorrhea. It stimulates uterine contractions, cervical stenosis or narrowing, and increased vasopressin release. Behavior and psychologic factors have also been implicated in the etiology of primary dysmenorrhea. Primary dysmenorrhea only occurs in ovulatory cycles. Secondary dysmenorrhea is usually caused by endometriosis, adenomyosis, leiomyomas and, less commonly, chronic salpingitis, IUD use, or congenital or acquired outflow tract obstruction, including cervical stenosis.

DIAGNOSIS

DIFFERENTIAL DIAGNOSIS

- Adenomyosis
- Adhesions
- Allen-Masters syndrome
- Cervical structures or stenosis
- Congenital malformation of müllerian system
- Ectopic pregnancy
- Endometriosis, endometritis
- Imperforate hymen
- IUD use
- Leiomyomas
- Ovarian cysts
- Pelvic congestion syndrome, PID
- Polyps
- Transverse vaginal septum

WORKUP

- Primary dysmenorrhea: characteristic history, physical examination normal with the absence of an identifiable cause of pelvic pain
- Secondary dysmenorrhea: history of onset generally >2 yr after menarche, physical examination may reveal uterine irregularity, cul-de-sac tenderness, or nodularity or pelvic masses

LABORATORY TESTS

- No specific tests diagnostic for dysmenorrhea
- Elevated WBC count in the presence of infection
- hCG to rule out ectopic pregnancy

IMAGING STUDIES

- Ultrasound scan of the pelvis to evaluate the presence of leiomyomas, ovarian cysts, or ectopic pregnancy
- Hysterosalpingogram or saline ultrasonography to assess the uterine cavity to rule out endometrial polyps, submucosal or intraluminal leiomyomas

TREATMENT

NONPHARMACOLOGIC THERAPY

- Applying heat to the lower abdomen with hot compresses, heating pads, or hot water bottles seems to offer some relief.
- Other reassurance that this is a treatable condition.

ACUTE GENERAL Rx

- Nonsteroidal anti-inflammatory drugs such as ibuprofen 400 to 600 mg q4 to 6h or naproxen sodium 550 mg q12h, mefenamic acid 500 mg initial dose followed by 250 mg q6h prn, aspirin 650 mg q4 to 6h, or oral contraceptives
- Nifedipine 30 mg qd in difficult cases of dysmenorrhea
- Magnesium supplements have been found likely to be beneficial
- Thiamine supplements may reduce pain
- Secondary dysmenorrhea: treatment directed to the specific underlying condition; surgery plays a greater role

CHRONIC Rx

Acupuncture and transcutaneous electrical nerve stimulation (TENS) may be tried. In cases in which medical therapy has not worked, laparoscopy should be considered, as well as other surgical treatments depending on the secondary cause of the dysmenorrhea.

DISPOSITION

The majority of patients are satisfactorily treated with good outcomes. Possible chronic complications with primary dysmenorrhea that has not been adequately treated can lead to anxiety and depression. With certain causes of secondary dysmenorrhea infertility can become a problem.

REFERRAL

If a secondary cause of dysmenorrhea is revealed, refer to the appropriate specialist for further medical or surgical treatment (e.g., gynecologist, pain management center).

EVIDENCE

Nonsteroidal anti-inflammatory drugs are significantly more effective than placebo in providing pain relief in patients with primary dysmenorrhea.[1] Ⓐ

A systematic review found that high-frequency transcutaneous electrical nerve stimulation (TENS) was more effective than placebo for the treatment of dysmenorrhea.[2] Ⓐ

Limited evidence has shown that acupuncture is significantly more effective than placebo in the management of women with primary dysmenorrhea.[3] Ⓑ

Evidence-Based References

1. Marjoribanks J, Proctor ML, Farquhar C: Nonsteroidal anti-inflammatory drugs for primary dysmenorrhea, *Cochrane Database Syst Rev* 4,2003. Ⓐ
2. Proctor ML et al: Transcutaneous electrical nerve stimulation and acupuncture for primary dysmenorrhea, *Cochrane Database Syst Rev* 1,2002. Ⓐ
3. Helms JM: Acupuncture for the management of primary dysmenorrhea, *Obstet Gynecol* 69:51, 1987. Reviewed in: *Clin Evid* 12,2004. Ⓑ

AUTHORS: **GEORGE T. DANAKAS, M.D.,** and **RUBEN ALVERO, M.D.**

BASIC INFORMATION

DEFINITION

Persistent and/or recurrent sexual intercourse associated pain

SYNONYMS

Painful intercourse

ICD-9CM CODES
625.0 Pain associated with female genital organs
302.76 Sexual deviations and disorders with functional dyspareunia, psychogenic dyspareunia

EPIDEMIOLOGY & DEMOGRAPHICS

PREVALENCE: 7% to 60% depending on definition

PREDOMINANT SEX: Female

AT-RISK POPULATION:

No consistent findings regarding:
- Age
- Parity
- Educational status
- Race
- Income
- Marital status

RISK FACTORS:

Lower:
- Frequency of intercourse
- Levels of desire and arousal
- Orgasmic response
- Physical and emotional satisfaction
- General happiness

HISTORICAL FACTORS:
- Pain parameters
  1. Character
  2. Location (Introital/middle/deep)
  3. Onset
  4. Duration
  5. Timing
  6. Chronicity
  7. Cyclicity
  8. Recurrence
- Gynecologic history
  1. History of STD
  2. History of HSV or HPV
  3. Other sexual dysfunctions
  4. Prior abdominal or gynecologic surgery
  5. Prior pelvic or abdominal radiation
  6. History of endometriosis, fibroids
  7. History of genital/uterine prolapse
  8. History of gynecologic infection
  9. History of pelvic pain
  10. History of menopausal symptoms
  11. Sexual misinformation
- OB history
  1. Lacerations
  2. Episiotomy
- General medical causes
  1. History of chronic diseases
  2. GI or GU symptoms
  3. Medications
  4. History of psychological disorders
  5. History of dermatologic condition
  6. Religious beliefs
  7. Generalized anxiety

PHYSICAL FINDINGS & CLINICAL PRESENTATION

- Primary vs. secondary dyspareunia
  1. Latter with history of pain-free coitus
- Visual inspection
  1. Discoloration
  2. Ulcerations
  3. Discharge
  4. Prolapse
  5. Dysplastic changes
  6. Infestations
- Physical examination
  1. Sensitivity to light touch
  2. Tenderness to palpation
  3. Genital prolapse
     a. Uterus
     b. Bladder
     c. Cervix
     d. Vagina
     e. Adnexa
     f. Rectum
     g. Bowel
  4. Ridges/septum
  5. Levator muscle tone
  6. Evidence of previous surgery
  7. Vaginal length/depth/caliber constrictions

ETIOLOGY

- Pathology or alteration/reduction of genital-associated tissue
- Psychosocial factors
- Marital/relationship discord
- History of sexual abuse

DIAGNOSIS

DIFFERENTIAL DIAGNOSIS

(Not an exhaustive list)
- Congenital deformities (septa/agenesis)
- Imperforate hymen
- Menopausal changes
- Atrophic tissue
- Impaired lubrication
- Psychogenic
- Vaginismus
- Inadequate foreplay
- Endometriosis
- Levator ani myalgia
- Chronic pelvic pain
- Previous surgery (posterior colporrhaphy/perineorrhaphy)
  1. Alteration in vaginal length/depth/caliber
  2. Adhesions
- Infectious
  1. Human papilloma
  2. Herpes simplex
  3. Candidiasis
  4. Tinea cruris
  5. Acute/chronic salpingitis/endometritis
- Pelvic carcinoma
- Previous radiation
- Adnexal attachment or tubal prolapse
- Pelvic tumor
- Uterine prolapse/malpositions/enlargement/retroversion
- Genital prolapse
- Cystocele/rectocele/enterocele
- Urethral/bladder pathology
- Pelvic congestion
- Vulvar vestibulitis
- Postcoital cystitis
- Broad ligament pathology
- Neuroma at the site of previous episiotomy
- Previous sexual abuse
- Vulvodynia
- Contact or allergic dermatitis
- Vitamin A, B, or C deficiency
- Equestrian dyspareunia
- Interstitial cystitis
- Pudendal neuralgia
- Myofascial pain syndrome
- Rectal pathology
- Structural abnormalities/alterations
  1. Muscle
  2. Bone
  3. Ligament

WORKUP

- History and physical examination are key
- If needed
  1. Colposcopy
  2. Cystoscopy
  3. Consider laparoscopy for unexplained deep dyspareunia

LABORATORY TESTS

- ESR
- WBC
- Wet mount
- Cultures
  1. Cervical
     a. Gonorrhea
     b. Chlamydia
  2. Vaginal
  3. Lesions
  4. Urine
- Vulva/vaginal/cervical biopsy
- Pap smear
- Herpes simplex virus antibodies
- Gonadotropin levels

IMAGING STUDIES

Pelvic/abdominal ultrasonography

TREATMENT

NONPHARMACOLOGIC THERAPY

- Patient education
- Discontinue exacerbating activity and irritants
- Lubrication with coitus
- Coital position changes: female superior position
- Warm or cool soaks
- Reassurance to patient of nonmalignant condition

- Psychosocial interventions
    1. Systemic desensitization techniques
    2. Behavior modification
- Vaginal dilators
- Vaginal muscle exercises and relaxation techniques
- Excision of pathologic tissue
- Surgical correction of altered/reduced/deformed tissues

ACUTE GENERAL Rx

- Topical lidocaine
- Corticosteroids
- Antiinfective agents
- Trigger point injections
- Massage
- Acupuncture
- TENS
- Stress reduction techniques
- Safe sexual practices
- Hormonal replacement therapy
- Antiviral agents
- Intralesional interferon
- Mild analgesics
- Antidepressants

CHRONIC Rx

All the previous plus:

- Set supportive visits, as needed
- Oral contraceptives
- Regular sexual activity
- Balanced diet
- Vitamin supplementation
- Proper hygiene

DISPOSITION

Most patients will have a reduction and/or resolution of their symptoms by using the appropriate therapeutic approaches.

REFERRAL

A multidisciplinary approach using the expertise of psychologists, dermatologists, gynecologic surgeons, infectious disease specialists, or urologists is helpful.

PEARLS & CONSIDERATIONS

- Dyspareunia is a symptom complex resulting from a multitude of etiologies, some of which are acting simultaneously.
- Uncovering the etiology of dyspareunia is predominately based on a comprehensive history and physical examination.
- The differential diagnoses can be sorted into superficial, intermediate, and deep dyspareunia categories.
- As with the physical evaluation of any painful condition, attempt, by precise touching (moistened cotton swab), palpation, or applied pressure, to reproduce the patient's chief complaint.
- Performing a one-finger pelvic exam, without concurrent abdominal palpation, allows for a more precise assessment of the source of genital pain.
- Individualize therapy.
- Initiate and maintain an honest diagnosis and compassionate demeanor with the patient and her mate.
- Be open-minded, approachable, nonjudgmental, and diligent in your search for a solution to help these often silently suffering patients.

EVIDENCE

EBM

We are unable to cite evidence that meets our criteria for most of the recommended therapies.

Although the management recommendations are not evidence-based, they have been found to be successful clinically.

A Cochrane systematic review found that perineal repair with synthetic absorbable suture material vs catgut following childbirth was associated with less pain in the subsequent 3 days. However, there was no significant difference in long-term rates of dyspareunia experienced.[1] Ⓐ

Another Cochrane systematic review concluded that there is not enough evidence to evaluate the use of ultrasound in treating perineal pain and/or dyspareunia following childbirth.[2] Ⓐ

Evidence-Based References

1. Kettle C, Johanson RB: Absorbable synthetic versus catgut suture material for perineal repair, *Cochrane Database Syst Rev* 2:CD000006, 2000. Ⓐ
2. Hay-Smith EJC: Therapeutic ultrasound for postpartum perineal pain and dyspareunia, *Cochrane Database Syst Rev* 2:CD000495, 2000. Ⓐ

SUGGESTED READINGS

Hawton RL: Female dyspareunia, *BMJ* 328(7452):1357, 2004.

Helm LJ: Evaluation and differential diagnosis of dyspareunia, *Am Fam Physician* 63:1535, 2001.

Nichols D: *Reoperative gynecologic and obstetric surgery,* ed 2, St Louis, 1997, Mosby.

AUTHORS: **DAVID I. KURSS, M.D.,** and **RUBEN ALVERO, M.D.**

BASIC INFORMATION

DEFINITION

Nonulcerative dyspepsia is persistent or recurrent dyspepsia centered in the upper abdomen without evidence of organic disease.

SYNONYMS

Functional dyspepsia
Idiopathic dyspepsia

ICD-9CM CODES
536.8 Nonulcerative dyspepsia

EPIDEMIOLOGY & DEMOGRAPHICS

- Annual prevalence of dyspepsia approximately 25% of population.
- Dyspepsia, GERD, PUD account for 2% to 5% of all primary care visits.

CLINICAL PRESENTATION

An international committee of clinical investigators developed the Rome II criteria to define nonulcerative dyspepsia for both research purposes and clinical practice:

- Having at least 12 weeks (may be nonconsecutive) within preceding 12 months of:
  1. Persistent or recurrent dyspepsia
  2. No evidence of organic disease that is likely to explain symptoms
  3. No evidence that dyspepsia is exclusively relieved by defecation or associated with the onset of a change in stool frequency or form
- Additional symptoms include:
  - Bloating
  - Early satiety
  - Indigestion
  - Nausea, vomiting
  - Weight loss/anorexia

ETIOLOGY

Pathophysiology is still unclear but research is focused on the following factors:

- Abnormalities of gastric motor function—especially in delayed gastric emptying, antral hypomotility, the relationship between low fasting gastric volumes and faster gastric emptying, and lower gastric compliance
- Visceral hypersensitivity
- *Helicobacter pylori* infection
- Psychosocial factors—associated with anxiety and depression

DIAGNOSIS

DIFFERENTIAL DIAGNOSIS

Made from the exclusion of other causes of dyspepsia

Other possible etiologies for dyspepsia:

- Peptic ulcer disease
- Gastroesophageal reflux
- Gastric/esophageal/all abdominal cancers
- Biliary tract disease
- Gastroparesis
- Pancreatitis
- Medications (i.e., NSAIDs, erythromycin, steroids)
- Infiltrative diseases of the stomach (i.e., Crohn's or sarcoidosis)
- Metabolic disturbances (i.e., hypercalcemia or hyperkalemia)
- Ischemic bowel disease
- System disorders (i.e., diabetes, thyroid disorders, or connective tissue diseases)

LABORATORY TESTS

WORKUP:

- The pattern of symptoms overlap considerably for all types of dyspepsia; therefore, the history should focus on finding specific symptoms that help exclude other causes of dyspepsia.
- However, the specific etiology of dyspepsia often cannot be identified by history and physical exam alone and much controversy surrounds the optimal approach for further testing and treatment.

IMAGING STUDIES

ENDOSCOPY:

The American Gastroenterological Association as well as the Maastricht European consensus report both recommend:

- Patients older than age 45 or those with alarming symptoms (weight loss, bleeding, anemia, or dysphagia) should have early upper endoscopy for tissue sampling to evaluate for gastric malignancy, as well as *H. pylori* testing. Patients whose symptoms have failed to respond to empiric therapeutic approaches should also undergo endoscopy.
- AGA also recommends empiric trial of antisecretory therapy or prokinetic agent for 1 month in patients younger than 45 years without alarming symptoms who are *H. pylori* negative. *H. pylori* testing includes serology, stool antigen, or urea breath test.

TREATMENT

NONPHARMACOLOGIC THERAPY

Controversial and often disappointing. Goal should be to help patients accept, diminish, and cope with symptoms rather than eliminate them.

ACUTE GENERAL Rx

PHARMACOLOGIC THERAPY:

Treatment sometimes depends on the predominant symptoms.

Predominant Symptom	Possible Etiology	Medication Recommended
Nausea	Motility Dysfunction	Prokinetic Agent
Bloating	Motility Dysfunction	Prokinetic Agent
Pain	Mucosal Disease or *H. pylori* Infection	Trial of medications listed below or *H. pylori* regimen
Somatic Complaints	Psychosocial	Psychotropic Medication

Medication Categories

Antacids (i.e., aluminum hydroxide, calcium carbonate)
Proton pump inhibitors (PPIs) (i.e., omeprazole)
H2-receptor antagonists (i.e., cimetidine)
Prokinetic agents (i.e., metoclopramide)
Antidepressants (i.e., selective serotonin receptor inhibitors)
H. pylori therapy/antibiotic therapy (clarithromycin + amoxicillin or metronidazole + PPI)

REFERRAL

Gastroenterology if patient with alarming symptoms or when endoscopy is indicated

SUGGESTED READING

Dickerson LM et al: Evaluation and management of nonulcer dyspepsia, *Am Fam Physician* 70:1, 2004.

AUTHOR: **HANNAH VU, D.O.**

BASIC INFORMATION

DEFINITION

Dystonia is characterized by involuntary muscle contractions (sustained or spasmodic) that lead to abnormal body movements or postures. Dystonia can be generalized or focal; of early onset (<20 years of age) or late onset; and primary or secondary.

SYNONYMS

Blepharospasm
Oromandibular (orofacial) dystonia
Spasmodic (limb or axial) dystonia
Torticollis
Writer's cramp

ICD-9CM CODES
333.6 Dystonia musculorum deformans
335.7 Dystonia caused by drugs
333.7 Dystonia, torsion, symptomatic

EPIDEMIOLOGY & DEMOGRAPHICS

PREVALENCE: Estimated at 1 in 3000 persons.

PREDOMINANT SEX: Cervical dystonia has a 3:2 female preponderance.

PREDOMINANT AGE:

- Focal cervical dystonia usually has its onset in the fifth decade.
- Hereditary forms may have an onset in childhood or adulthood and tend to be more severe.

GENETICS: Autosomal dominant, autosomal recessive, and X-linked forms of dystonia have been identified. Ashkenazi Jews are particularly susceptible to primary early-onset dystonia.

CLINICAL PRESENTATION

Focal dystonias produce abnormal sustained muscle contractions in a single region of the body:

- Neck (torticollis): most commonly affected site with a tendency for the head to turn to one side
- Eyelids (blepharospasm): involuntary closure of the eyelids
- Mouth (oromandibular dystonia): involuntary contraction of muscles of the mouth, tongue, or face
- Hand (writer's cramp) (Fig. 1-79)

Generalized dystonia affects multiple areas of the body and can lead to marked joint deformities.

ETIOLOGY

- Exact pathophysiology of primary dystonia is unknown but thought to involve abnormalities of basal ganglia. Specifically, reduced and abnormal patterns of neuronal activity in the basal ganglia result in disinhibition of the motor thalamus and cortex leading to abnormal movement.
- Fifteen hereditary forms have been described, including the severe progressive form, dystonia musculorum deformans.
- Secondary dystonia occurs due to CNS disease of the basal ganglia (stroke, demyelination), hypoxia, severe head injury, kernicterus, Huntington's disease, Wilson's disease, Parkinson's disease, lysosomal storage diseases.
- Acute dystonia can occur following treatment with drugs that block dopamine receptors, such as phenothiazines or butyrophenones.
- Tardive dyskinesia can result from long-term treatment with certain medication classes: antiemetics (e.g., phenothiazines), antipsychotics (e.g., haloperidol), levodopa, anticonvulsants, or ergots.

DIAGNOSIS

DIFFERENTIAL DIAGNOSIS

- Parkinson's disease
- Progressive supranuclear palsy
- Wilson's disease
- Huntington's disease
- Drug effects

WORKUP

History (family history, birth history, trauma, medication use), physical examination

LABORATORY TESTS

- Usually not helpful for diagnosis
- Serum ceruloplasmin if Wilson's disease is suspected

IMAGING STUDIES

- Primary dystonias are generally not associated with structural CNS abnormalities. CT scan or MRI of brain if a CNS lesion is suspected as a cause of secondary dystonia.
- Electrophysiologic testing can provide diagnostic support for the diagnosis.

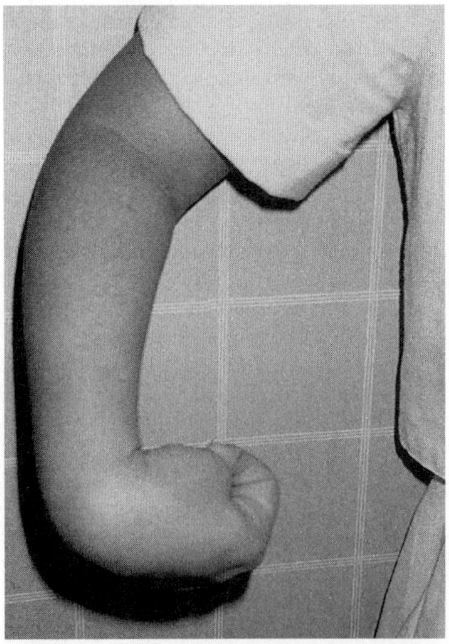

FIGURE 1-79 Focal dystonia of the distal right arm. (From Goldman L, Ausiello D [eds]: *Cecil textbook of medicine*, ed 22, Philadelphia, 2004, WB Saunders.)

TREATMENT

NONPHARMACOLOGIC THERAPY

- Heat, massage, physical therapy to relieve pain
- Splints to prevent contractures

ACUTE GENERAL Rx

For acute dystonic reactions to phenothiazines/butyrophenones, use diphenhydramine 50 mg IV or benztropine 2 mg IV.

CHRONIC Rx

- Treatment is often ineffective.
- Slowly withdraw offending agents.
- Diazepam, baclofen, or carbamazepine may be helpful.
- Intrathecal baclofen is most useful for spastic or truncal dystonia.
- Trihexyphenidyl or benztropine may be helpful in up to 50% of tardive dyskinesia or dystonia.
- For generalized dystonia, a trial of carbidopa/levodopa may be beneficial.
- Injections of botulinum toxin into the affected muscles is the standard treatment for focal dystonias.
- Surgical procedures including denervation, myectomy, rhizotomy, thalamotomy (pallidotomy), or deep brain stimulation may be helpful for severe, refractory cases.

DISPOSITION

Spontaneous remission of focal cervical dystonia can occur, but dystonia is generally progressive and pharmacologic therapy is often ineffective.

REFERRAL

Neurology for severe or refractory cases

PEARLS & CONSIDERATIONS

COMMENTS

- Avoid triggers/exacerbating factors.
- Early physical therapy and splinting to prevent contractures.
- Consider botulism injections or deep brain stimulation surgery for severe or refractory dystonia.
- Botulism injections remain the treatment of choice for focal dystonias.

SUGGESTED READINGS

Bhidaya Siri R: Dystonia: genetics and treatment update, *Neurologist* 12:74, 2006.
Defazio G et al: Epidemiology of primary dystonia, *Lancet Neurol* 3:673, 2004.
Tarsy D, Simon DK: Dystonia, *N Engl J Med* 355:818, 2006.

AUTHORS: **LYNN MCNICOLL, M.D., F.R.C.P.C.,** and **MARK FAGAN, M.D.**

BASIC INFORMATION

DEFINITION

Echinococcosis is a chronic infection caused by the larval stage of several animal cestodes (tapeworms) of the genus *Echinococcus.*

SYNONYMS

Hydatid disease

ICD-9CM CODES
122.9 *Echinococcus* infection

EPIDEMIOLOGY & DEMOGRAPHICS

INCIDENCE (IN U.S.): Seen primarily in immigrants.
PEAK INCIDENCE: Presumed to be acquired in childhood or early adulthood in most cases.
PREVALENCE (IN U.S.): See Incidence
PREDOMINANT SEX: Male = female
PREDOMINANT AGE: 20 to 50 yr of age

PHYSICAL FINDINGS & CLINICAL PRESENTATION

- Signs of an enlarging mass lesion in a visceral site such as the liver, lungs, kidneys, bone, or CNS
- Occasional cyst rupture causing allergic manifestations such as urticaria, angioedema, or anaphylaxis that bring the patient to medical attention
- Incidental discovery of cysts by abdominal or thoracic imaging studies performed for other reasons

ETIOLOGY

- Four species of *Echinococcus: E. granulosus, E. multilocularis, E. oligarthrus,* and *E. vogeli.*
  1. *E. granulosus* is the cause of cystic hydatid disease.
  2. *E. multilocularis* and *E. vogeli* are the causes of alveolar and polycystic disease.
- The disease is transmitted to humans by infected canines (domestic or wild dogs, wolves, foxes) and seen most commonly in livestock-producing areas of the Middle East, Africa, Australia, New Zealand, Europe, and the Americas, including the southwestern U.S.
- Eggs are present in the feces of infected canines; human infection occurs by ingestion of viable eggs in contaminated food.
- It is common in many areas of the world, especially the Middle East.

DIAGNOSIS

DIFFERENTIAL DIAGNOSIS

- Cystic neoplasms
- Abscess (amebic or bacterial)
- Congenital polycystic disease

WORKUP

- Antibody assay
- Imaging study (CT scan, ultrasonography)
- Histologic examination of cyst or contents obtained by aspiration or resection (if possible) to confirm diagnosis

LABORATORY TESTS

Antibody assays (ELISA, Latex agglutination, and Western blot): >90% sensitive and specific for liver cysts, but less accurate for cysts in other sites. A PCR assay is now available for problematic cases.

IMAGING STUDIES

Ultrasonography and/or CT scan:
- Both are extremely sensitive for the detection of cysts, especially in the liver (Fig. 1-80).
- Both lack specificity and are inadequate to establish the diagnosis of echinococcosis with certainty.

TREATMENT

NONPHARMACOLOGIC THERAPY

- Treatment of choice for echinococcal cysts is surgical resection, when feasible.
- If resection is not feasible, perform percutaneous drainage with instillation of 95% ethanol to prevent dissemination of viable larvae.
- Surgical therapy is followed by medical therapy with albendazole (see "Acute General Rx").

ACUTE GENERAL Rx

For echinococcosis confined to the liver:
- Albendazole (400 mg bid for 28 days followed by 14 days of rest for at least three cycles)
- Mebendazole (50 to 70 mg/kg qd) if albendazole not available

CHRONIC Rx

See "Acute General Rx."

DISPOSITION

- Long-term follow-up is necessary following surgical or medical therapy because of the high incidence of late relapse.
- Antibody assays and imaging studies are repeated every 6 to 12 mo for several years following successful surgical or medical therapy.

REFERRAL

All patients for evaluation for possible surgical resection of cysts

PEARLS & CONSIDERATIONS

COMMENTS

Cyst resection, if indicated, should be performed by surgeons experienced with this procedure.

SUGGESTED READINGS

Eckert J, Deplazes P: Biological, epidemiological, and clinical aspects of echinococcosis, a zoonosis of increasing concern, *Clin Microbiol Rev* 17(1):107, 2004.

Yang YR et al: A hospital-based retrospective survey of human cystic and alveolar echinococcosis in Ningxia Hui Autonomous Region, PR China, *Acta Trop* 97(3):284, 2006.

Zhang W, McManus DP: Recent advances in the immunology and diagnosis of echinococcosis, *FEMS Immunol Med Microbiol* 47(1):24, 2006.

AUTHORS: **GLENN G. FORT, M.D., M.P.H., JOSEPH R. MASCI, M.D.,** and **DENNIS J. MIKOLICH, M.D.**

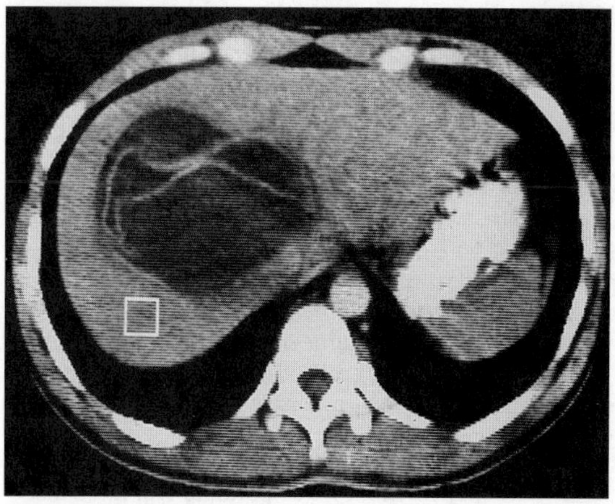

FIGURE 1-80 Computed tomography scan of an echinococcal cyst in a 25-year-old man, demonstrating the complex structure of the wall and the interior. (From Goldman L, Ausiello D [eds]: *Cecil textbook of medicine,* ed 22, Philadelphia, 2004, WB Saunders.)

BASIC INFORMATION

DEFINITION

Eclampsia is the occurrence of seizures or coma in a woman with preeclampsia, occurring at >20 wk gestation or <48 hr postpartum. Atypical eclampsia occurs at <20 wk gestation or as much as 14 days postpartum.

SYNONYMS

Toxemia
Seizures of pregnancy

ICD-9CM CODES
642.6 Eclampsia

EPIDEMIOLOGY & DEMOGRAPHICS

INCIDENCE: 1 case/150 to 3000 pregnancies; 2% to 4% of those with preeclampsia
GENETICS: Increased incidence with first-degree relatives (sister or mother) having had eclampsia
RISK FACTORS: Multifetal gestation (3.6% in twin gestation), molar pregnancy, nonimmune hydrops fetalis, uncontrolled hypertension, preexisting hypertension, or renal disease

PHYSICAL FINDINGS & CLINICAL PRESENTATION

- Seizure begins as facial twitching then spreads to generalized clonicotonic state, with cessation of respiration, followed by a postictal period of amnesia, agitation, and confusion.
- 40% have severe hypertension, 40% have mild to moderate hypertension, and 20% are normotensive.
- Generalized edema with rapid weight gain (>2 lb/wk) may be one of the earliest signs of eclampsia.
- Persistent occipital headache and hyperreflexia with clonus occur in 80% of patients with eclampsia; epigastric pain exists in 20% of these patients.

ETIOLOGY

- Exact etiology unknown.
- Common pathway relates to abnormalities in autoregulation of cerebral blood flow. This may involve transient vasospasm, ischemia, cerebral hemorrhage, and edema, occurring by a mechanism involving hypertensive encephalopathy, decreased colloid osmotic pressure, and prostaglandin imbalance.

DIAGNOSIS

DIFFERENTIAL DIAGNOSIS

- Preexisting seizure disorder
- Metabolic abnormalities (hypoglycemia, hyponatremia, hypocalcemia)
- Substance abuse
- Head trauma, infection (meningitis, encephalitis)
- Intracerebral bleeding or thrombosis
- Amniotic fluid embolism
- Space-occupying brain lesions or neoplasms
- Pseudoseizure

WORKUP

- Rule out other causes of seizures during pregnancy.
- Atypical presentations such as prolonged postictal state, status epilepticus, gestational age <20 wk or >48 hr postpartum, or signs of meningitis, substance abuse, or severe uncontrolled hypertension should prompt a search for other seizure etiologies.

LABORATORY TESTS

- Proteinuria: severe (49%), mild to moderate (29%), absent (22%)
- HCT: elevated secondary to hemoconcentration
- Platelet count: decreased; LFTs elevated in HELLP syndrome
- BUN and creatinine: elevated with renal involvement
- Serum electrolytes, glucose, calcium, toxicology profile: to rule out other causes of seizures
- Hyperuricemia: >6.9 mg/dl found in 70% of eclamptics
- ABG: maternal acidemia and hypoxia

IMAGING STUDIES

- CT scan or MRI indicated in atypical presentation, suspected intracerebral bleeding, focal neurologic deficit.
- There are abnormal findings, including cerebral edema, hemorrhage, and infarction, in 50% of patients.

TREATMENT

NONPHARMACOLOGIC THERAPY

- Airway protection (risk of aspiration)
- Supportive care during acute event

ACUTE GENERAL Rx

- Maintain airway, adequate oxygenation, and IV access.
- Fetal resuscitation, involving maternal oxygenation, left lateral positioning, and continuous fetal heart rate monitoring, is needed.
- Magnesium sulfate is drug of choice. Give magnesium sulfate 6 g IV load over 20 min, then 3 g/hr maintenance, for recurrent seizure prophylaxis. If repeated convulsion, may give an additional 2 g IV over 3 to 5 min. About 10% to 15% of patients will have a second seizure after initial loading dose. Check magnesium level 1 hr after loading dose, then q6h (therapeutic range 4 to 6 mg/dl). Antidote for toxicity is calcium gluconate 10 ml of 10% solution. Phenytoin has been used as an alternative in patients in whom magnesium sulfate is contraindicated (renal insufficiency, heart block, myasthenia gravis, hypoparathyroidism).
- Give sodium amobarbital 250 mg IV over 3 min for persistent seizures.
- Treat blood pressure if >160 mm Hg/110 mm Hg, with labetalol 20- to 40-mg IV bolus, hydralazine 10 mg IV, or nifedipine 10 to 20 mg sublingual q20min.
- Evaluate patient for delivery.

CHRONIC Rx

- The first priority is stabilization of the mother in terms of adequate oxygenation, hemodynamics, and laboratory abnormalities, such as associated coagulopathies.
- Cervical status and gestational age should be assessed. If unfavorable cervix and <30 wk consider C-section, otherwise consider induction.
- Controlled epidural is the anesthesia of choice for labor or C-section.
- Avoid general anesthesia in uncontrolled hypertension to minimize risk of catastrophic cerebral events.

DISPOSITION

The maternal mortality rate for eclampsia averages 5% to 6%. Morbidity is 25%, including placental abruption (10%), maternal apnea with fetal asphyxia, aspiration pneumonia, pulmonary edema (4%), renal failure, cardiopulmonary arrest, and coma.

REFERRAL

Because of the potential for serious permanent maternal and fetal sequelae, all cases should be managed by a team approach of obstetrician, neonatologist, and intensivist.

PEARLS & CONSIDERATIONS

COMMENTS

- Eclampsia antepartum, 50%; intrapartum, 20%; and postpartum, 30%.
- Postseizure there is an associated period of fetal bradycardia from 1 to 9 min; if there is evidence of fetal compromise beyond that time, consider alternative etiologies such as placental abruption (23% incidence).

SUGGESTED READINGS

Duley L: Evidence and practice: the magnesium sulphate story, *Best Pract Res Clin Obstet Gynaecol* 19(1):57, 2005.

Schroeder BM: ACOG practice bulletin on diagnosing and managing preeclampsia and eclampsia, *Am Fam Physician* 66:330, 2002.

Sibai BM: Diagnosis, prevention, and management of eclampsia, *Obstet Gynecol* 105(2):402, 2005.

AUTHORS: **SCOTT J. ZUCCALA, D.O.,** and **RUBEN ALVERO, M.D.**

BASIC INFORMATION

DEFINITION

An ectopic pregnancy (EP) is one in which a fertilized ovum implants outside the endometrial lining of the uterus.

SYNONYMS

Abdominal pregnancy (1% to 2%)
Cervical pregnancy (0.5%)
Interstitial pregnancy (2% to 3%)
Ovarian pregnancy (1%)
Tubal pregnancy (97%)

ICD-9CM CODES
633 Ectopic pregnancy

EPIDEMIOLOGY & DEMOGRAPHICS

- 1% to 2% of pregnancies
- 13% of maternal deaths

PREVALENCE (IN U.S.): Increasing number of EPs; 17,800 reported cases in 1970 and 108,000 reported cases in 1992.

RISK FACTORS: Previous salpingitis, previous EP, previous tubal ligation, previous tuboplasty, IUD use, progestin-only pill, and assisted reproductive techniques

PHYSICAL FINDINGS & CLINICAL PRESENTATION

- Abdominal tenderness: 95%
- Adnexal tenderness: 87% to 99%
- Peritoneal signs: 71% to 76%
- Adnexal mass: 33% to 53%
- Enlarged uterus: 6% to 30%
- Shock: 2% to 17%
- Amenorrhea or abnormal vaginal bleeding: 75%
- Shoulder pain: 10%
- Tissue passage: 6% to 7%

ETIOLOGY

- Anatomic obstruction to zygote passage
- Abnormalities in tubal motility
- Transperitoneal migration of the zygote

DIAGNOSIS

DIFFERENTIAL DIAGNOSIS

- Corpus luteum cyst
- Rupture or torsion of ovarian cyst
- Threatened or incomplete abortion
- PID
- Appendicitis
- Gastroenteritis
- Dysfunctional uterine bleeding
- Degenerating uterine fibroids
- Endometriosis

WORKUP

1. The classic presentation of EP includes the triad of abnormal vaginal bleeding, pelvic pain, and an adnexal mass. Consider in all women with abdominal-pelvic pain and a positive pregnancy test
2. Transvaginal ultrasound
3. Laparoscopy in equivocal situations and possibly for treatment

LABORATORY TESTS

- hCG: if normal IUP, 85% have doubling time of 2 days. If abnormal gestation, will show <66% increase of QhCG within 2 days. However, 13% of ectopic pregnancies have a normal doubling time (Section III, "Ectopic Pregnancy").
- Progesterone: decreased production in EP, <5 ng/ml strongly predictive of abnormal pregnancy. If >25 ng/ml, strongly predictive of normal IUP.
- Dropping HCT associated with tubal rupture, or resolving ectopic pregnancy or abnormal intrauterine pregnancy.
- Leukocytosis

IMAGING STUDIES

- Ultrasound: presence of an IUP rules out EP.
- If QhCG >6000 mIU/ml, should see IUP on abdominal scan, and QhCG >1500 mIU/ml for transvaginal scan.
- Findings on ultrasound in EP include:
  1. Empty uterus
  2. Adnexal mass
  3. Cul-de-sac fluid
  4. Fetal sac in tube
  5. Fetal cardiac activity in adnexa

TREATMENT

NONPHARMACOLOGIC THERAPY

Surgery: can be performed by laparoscopy if patient is stable or by laparotomy if patient is unstable. Salpingiosis: direct injection of chemotherapy into ectopic via laparoscopy, transvaginal ultrasound, or hysteroscopy.

- Conservative surgery-salpingostomy or segmental resection depends on tubal location and size of ectopic.
- Salpingectomy should be considered in the following circumstances:
  1. Ruptured tube
  2. Future fertility not desired
  3. Recurrent ectopic in the same tube
  4. Uncontrolled hemorrhage

ACUTE GENERAL Rx

- If the patient is stable and compliant may consider medical management with methotrexate. Patient should not have contraindications to methotrexate such as hepatic or renal disease, thrombocytopenia, leukopenia, or significant anemia. There should be no evidence of hemoperitoneum on transvaginal ultrasound. Ectopic should be <4 cm mass with QhCG <30,000 mIU/ml.
- Most common regimen is methotrexate 50 mg/m^2 body surface area. May require second dose or surgical intervention if QhCG increases or plateaus after 7 days.

CHRONIC Rx

Persistent EP results from residual trophoblastic tissue or secondary implantation after conservative surgery. There is a 5% incidence of persistent ectopic with conservative treatment.

DISPOSITION

If diagnosed and treated early (before rupture) prognosis is excellent for good recovery. Follow QhCG weekly until negative. Use reliable contraception until hCG negative. With subsequent pregnancies, follow QhCG and perform early ultrasound to confirm IUP. There is a 12% recurrence rate for EP.

REFERRAL

Should obtain gynecologic consultation if EP is suspected.

EVIDENCE

Open salpingostomy is significantly more successful than laparoscopic salpingostomy in eliminating ectopic pregnancy.[1] Ⓐ

Laparoscopy and open surgery have similar long-term tubal patency rates and subsequent intrauterine pregnancy rates, but laparoscopy has a tendency to reduce subsequent ectopic rates, is cheaper, and reduces operating, hospital stay and convalescent time.[1] Ⓐ

Systemic methotrexate as a single injection often requires subsequent medical or surgical intervention.[1] Ⓐ

Evidence-Based Reference

1. Hajenius PJ et al: Interventions for tubal ectopic pregnancy, *Cochrane Database Syst Rev* 1, 2000. Ⓐ

SUGGESTED READINGS

Della-Giustina D, Denny M: Ectopic pregnancy, *Emerg Med Clin North Am* 21(3):565, 2003.

Gracia CR, Barnhart KT: Diagnosing ectopic pregnancy: decision analysis comparing six strategies, *Obstet Gynecol* 97(3):464, 2001.

AUTHORS: **GEORGE T. DANAKAS, M.D.,** and **RUBEN ALVERO, M.D.**

BASIC INFORMATION

DEFINITION

Ehlers-Danlos syndrome (EDS) refers to a group of inherited, clinically variable, and genetically heterogeneous connective tissue disorders. EDS is characterized by skin hyperextensibility, skin fragility, joint laxity, and joint hyperextensibility.

ICD-9CM CODES
756.83 Ehlers-Danlos syndrome

EPIDEMIOLOGY & DEMOGRAPHICS

- The prevalence of EDS is estimated to be about 1 in 5000 births, although it is somewhat higher in African Americans.
- There are six distinct forms of EDS according to the revised classification system established at the Villefranche Consensus Conference, 1997 (see "Physical Findings & Clinical Presentation").
- Classic and hypermobility EDS are most prevalent. Classic EDS accounts for approximately 80% of reported cases.
- Vascular EDS is the most dangerous because it is associated with spontaneous rupture of medium and large arteries and hollow organs, especially large intestine and uterus; occurs in 4% of patients with EDS.
- In most cases, transmission is autosomal dominant except for some unclassified forms of EDS (previously known as type V and type IX, are x-linked; type X is autosomal recessive).

PHYSICAL FINDINGS & CLINICAL PRESENTATION

- Classic (previously types I and II): hyperextensibility ("Gorlin's sign": ability to touch tip of tongue to nose), easy scarring and bruising ("cigarette-paper scars"), smooth, velvety skin, subcutaneous spheroids (small, firm, cystlike nodules) along shins or forearms.
- Hypermobility (type III): joint hypermobility and some skin hypermobility with or without very smooth skin.
- Vascular (type IV): thin, translucent skin with visible veins; marked bruising; pinched nose; acrogeria; generalized tissue friability; spontaneous dissection and rupture of medium and large arteries; spontaneous rupture of organs, especially sigmoid colon, spleen, liver, and uterus.
- Kyphoscoliotic (type VI): characterized by joint hypermobility, progressive scoliosis, ocular fragility and possible globe rupture, mitral valve prolapse, and aortic dilation.
- Arthrochalasia (types VIIA and VIIB): prominent joint hypermobility with subluxations, congenital hip dislocation, skin hyperextensibility, and tissue fragility.
- Dermatosparaxis (type VIIC): severe skin fragility with decreased elasticity, bruising, hernias.
- Unclassified types: types V and IX: classic characteristics; type VIII: classic characteristics and periodontal disease; type X: mild classic characteristics, mitral valve prolapse; type XI: joint instability.

ETIOLOGY

- Defects of collagen in extracellular matrices of multiple tissues (skin, tendons, blood vessels, and viscera) underlie all forms of EDS.
- Classic EDS is associated with defects in type V collagen, corresponding to mutations of the *COL5A* genes.
- Vascular EDS involves a deficiency in type III collagen, and several studies suggest that mutations of gene *COL3A1* lead to this deficiency.
- Arthrochalasia EDS results from a defect in type I collagen, caused by mutations in the *COL1A1* and *COL1A2* genes.

DIAGNOSIS (Dx)

Diagnosis is based solely on clinical criteria. It is important to identify patients with vascular EDS because of the grave consequences of the disease.

- Clinical criteria for vascular EDS: 2 of 4 major diagnostic criteria establishes the diagnosis; ≥1 minor criteria supports but is not sufficient to establish the diagnosis.
- Major criteria:
  1. Easy bruising
  2. Arterial, intestinal, or uterine fragility
  3. Thin, translucent skin
  4. Characteristic facial features (thin, delicate, and pinched nose, hollow cheeks, prominent staring eyes): occur in <30% of patients with vascular EDS
- Minor criteria:
  - Small joint hypermobility
  - Skin hyperextensibility
  - Spontaneous pneumothorax/hemothorax
  - Tendon or muscle rupture
  - Early-onset varicose veins
  - Carotid-cavernous fistula
  - Talipes equinovarus (clubfoot)

DIFFERENTIAL DIAGNOSIS

- Marfan's syndrome
- Osteogensis imperfecta
- Autosomal dominant cutis laxa
- Familial joint hypermobility

WORKUP

Diagnosis is based solely on clinical criteria.

LABORATORY TESTS

- Biochemical and gene testing for known molecular defects recommended to confirm the diagnosis in vascular EDS.
- Plain radiographs may reveal calcified nodules along the shin or forearms, corresponding to the subcutaneous spheroids.
- Echocardiogram can identify MVP and aortic dilation.

TREATMENT (Rx)

- All patients should receive genetic counseling about the mode of inheritance of their EDS.
- Management of most skin and joint problems should be conservative and preventive. Joint hypermobility and pain in EDS usually does not require surgical intervention. Physical therapy to strengthen muscles is helpful. Surgical repair and tightening of joint ligaments can be performed but ligaments frequently will not hold sutures. Surgical intervention should be considered on an individual basis.
- For patients with vascular EDS:
  - Special surgical care is required because of increased tissue friability.
  - Patients should be advised to avoid contact sports.
  - Elevated blood pressure should be aggressively treated with beta-blockers given the risk of arterial dissection.

DISPOSITION

Prognosis varies according to type of EDS. For vascular EDS:

- 25% will have a complication by age 25; >80% will have a complication by age 40.
- Most vascular complications consist of arterial dissections.
- Median age of survival is 48 years. Most deaths are related to arterial rupture.

REFERRAL

Referral to dermatology for skin biopsy to confirm diagnosis of vascular EDS and to cardiology, orthopedic surgery, general surgery, and physical therapy as needed.

PEARLS & CONSIDERATIONS (!)

- Women with vascular EDS should be counseled about the risk of uterine, intestinal, and arterial rupture. Pregnancy is associated with an 11% mortality rate, and there is a 50% chance that the child will be affected.
- Family members of patients with EDS should be recommended for evaluation for EDS and genetic testing/counseling.

SUGGESTED READINGS

Oderich GS: Current concepts in the diagnosis and management of vascular Ehlers-Danlos syndrome, *Perspect Vasc Surg Endovasc Ther* 18(3):206, 2006.

Pepin M et al: Clinical and genetic features of Ehlers-Danlos syndrome type IV, the vascular type, *N Engl J Med* 342:673, 2000.

Prahlow JA: Death due to Ehlers-Danlos syndrome type IV, *Am J Forensic Med Pathol* 26(1):78, 2005.

Pyeritz R: Ehlers-Danlos syndrome, *N Engl J Med* 342(10):730, 2000.

Pyeritz RE: Ehlers-Danlos syndromes. In Goldman L, Bennett JC (eds): *Cecil textbook of medicine*, ed 21, vol 1, Philadelphia, 2000, WB Saunders.

Shapiro JR: Heritable disorders of structural proteins, *Kelley's textbook of rheumatology*, ed 6, Philadelphia, 2001, WB Saunders.

AUTHOR: **IRIS TONG, M.D.**

BASIC INFORMATION

DEFINITION

The clinically significant disorders of ejaculation are failure of emission, retrograde ejaculation, premature ejaculation, and anorgasmia. Failure of emission occurs when semen is not propulsed into the urethra during orgasm. This results in a dry ejaculate. Retrograde ejaculation is a backward flow of semen into the bladder. Premature ejaculation is the inability to control ejaculation for sufficient time to allow adequate penetration and intercourse. Anorgasmia is the inability to achieve orgasm in a timely manner.

SYNONYMS

Ejaculatory dysfunction
Retarded ejaculation
Early or rapid ejaculation
Inhibited ejaculation

ICD-9CM CODES
608.87 Ejaculation, retrograde
306.59 Ejaculation, psychogenic
302.75 Ejaculation, premature
302.74 Orgasm inhibited male (psychosexual)

EPIDEMIOLOGY & DEMOGRAPHICS

The prevalence of premature ejaculation is estimated to be approximately 20% in adult men.

CLINICAL PRESENTATION

- Failure of emission: no ejaculate is expelled either antegrade or retrograde during orgasm; physical findings may be normal or may reveal nervous system dysfunction (e.g., spinal cord injury); may present with infertility.
- Retrograde ejaculation: little or no ejaculate is expelled at orgasm (<1 cc). Patients may report cloudy postcoital urine. Physical exam is often normal but may reveal stigmata of underlying neurologic condition; may present with infertility.
- Premature ejaculation: ejaculation occurs sooner than desired, either before or shortly after penetration. Physical examination is normal. Assess sexual and psychologic history. Patients often incorrectly complain of erectile dysfunction because they lose the erection after orgasm.
- Anorgasmia: patient is not able to achieve orgasm despite appropriate stimulation.

ETIOLOGY

- Retrograde ejaculation may be caused by anatomic abnormalities of the bladder neck due to bladder neck surgery and transurethral resection of the prostate.
- Either retrograde ejaculation or failure of emission may result from functional abnormalities. These include spinal cord injury, diabetes mellitus, retroperitoneal surgery, alpha blocker therapy (for BPH), multiple sclerosis, peripheral neuropathies, or other neurologic abnormalities.
- The exact etiology of premature ejaculation is unknown, but there is evidence for psychological and biologic contributions.
- Anorgasmia may be due to medications, particularly serotonin reuptake inhibitors. Patients with spinal cord injuries may be unable to achieve orgasm. Additional causes include psychogenic factors and dysfunctional sexual techniques.

DIAGNOSIS

DIFFERENTIAL DIAGNOSIS

Erectile dysfunction
Low seminal volume due to hypogonadism or ejaculatory duct obstruction

LABORATORY TESTS

- In the case of a dry or very low volume ejaculate, a postejaculate urine should be evaluated for spermatozoa to differentiate failure of emission from retrograde ejaculation.
- A fasting blood glucose may be considered if diabetes is suspected as a cause of lack of emission or retrograde ejaculation.

IMAGING STUDIES

Transrectal ultrasonography to rule out ejaculatory duct obstruction or absence of the seminal vesicles only if these diagnoses are suspected as a cause of low volume ejaculate.

TREATMENT

NONPHARMACOLOGIC THERAPY

- Retrograde ejaculation and failure of emission do not usually require treatment unless fertility is desired. Retrograde ejaculation may rarely be converted to antegrade ejaculation if intercourse occurs when the bladder is full. Viable sperm can be recovered from the postejaculate urine or from the bladder via catheterization and used for intrauterine insemination or in vitro fertilization.
- Premature ejaculation can improve with sex therapy (e.g., coronal squeeze technique or start-and-stop technique) and effective partner communication. These approaches are often more effective when combined with pharmacologic therapy.
- Anorgasmia due to serotonin reuptake inhibitors usually improves with withdrawal of the medication or by changing to another medication. Sexual therapy and counseling can improve anorgasmia due to dysfunctional sexual techniques or psychological issues. Vibratory or electrical stimulation of emission may be used in selected cases.

ACUTE GENERAL Rx

- Therapy varies with underlying disorder. Treatment of retrograde ejaculation and failure of emission is usually not necessary unless fertility is desired. Most evidence is expert opinion and not from clinical trial.
- Retrograde ejaculation: it is crucial to distinguish between anatomic and functional causes because pharmacologic treatment is only likely to be effective in patients that do not have an anatomic disturbance of the bladder neck. Sympathomimetic medications (phenylpropanolamine, ephedrine, pseudoephedrine) and imipramine may be useful in converting retrograde ejaculation to antegrade ejaculation.
- Failure of emission may be converted to retrograde ejaculation by oral sympathomimetic therapy.
- Premature ejaculation: selective serotonin reuptake inhibitors (sertraline, fluoxetine) and clomipramine have shown success in delaying premature ejaculation. Initially these are taken only on the days of intercourse. If no improvement occurs, they may be taken daily. Topical anesthetics such as lidocaine cream have also been used.

SURGICAL THERAPY

There is currently no role for surgery for ejaculatory disorders.

DISPOSITION

Prognosis varies with etiology. Ejaculatory dysfunction due to sexual techniques or psychological issues can improve with therapy and counseling.

REFERRAL

All fertility issues and suspected anatomic problems should be referred to a urologist. Professional psychotherapy and sex therapy should be considered for some patients. Endocrine input should be considered for diabetes.

SUGGESTED READINGS

Lue TF, Broderick GA: Evaluation and nonsurgical management of erectile dysfunction and premature ejaculation. In Wein AJ, Kavoussi LR, Novick AC, Partin AW, Peters CA (eds): *Campbell-Walsh urology,* ed 9, Philadelphia, 2007, Saunders Elsevier, pp. 784-787.

Master VA, Turek PJ: Ejaculation physiology and dysfunction, *Urol Clin North Am* 28(2):363, 2001.

Montague DK et al: American Urological Association guideline on the pharmacologic management of premature ejaculation, *J Urol* 172(1):290, 2004.

AUTHORS: **DANIEL KAPLON, M.D.,** and **MARK SIGMAN, M.D.**

BASIC INFORMATION

DEFINITION

Premature ejaculation is a persistent or recurrent problem in which a male experiences orgasm or ejaculation in the early phases of sexual contact and before he and his partner wish it. Other definitions have emphasized elapsed time after intromission (with durations of 30 sec to several min), number of thrusts, or rate of partner satisfaction. However, no absolute measure is applicable to the diverse numbers of men with this problem.

SYNONYMS

Rapid ejaculation
Early ejaculation
Inadequate ejaculatory control

ICD-9CM CODES
F52.4 Premature ejaculation
(DSM-IV Code 302.75)

EPIDEMIOLOGY & DEMOGRAPHICS

PEAK INCIDENCE: Adolescence and young adulthood

PREVALENCE (IN U.S.):

- 7% to 40% of adult men, most with no underlying physical condition
- Often present more or less since start of sexual life
- Most prevalent sexual disorder in men; more common than low libido and erectile dysfunction

PREDOMINANT AGE: None defined

GENETICS: No identifiable genetic factors

PHYSICAL FINDINGS & CLINICAL PRESENTATION

- Complaint of ejaculation before, upon, or shortly after penetration
- Frequently associated with anxiety related to either sexual activity or more generalized anxiety disorder
- Premature ejaculation secondary to a medical condition frequently associated with low anxiety, low desire, and/or erectile insufficiency

ETIOLOGY

- Increasingly thought to be a neurobiological phenomenon, particularly related to serotonergic pathway
- Different theoretical frameworks emphasizing anxiety related to performance or personal interactions, behavioral concepts of learned expectations related to early experience, or heightened penile sensitivity
- Organic factors are contributory in some individuals (e.g., abdominal or pelvic trauma or surgery, neuropathies, or urologic pathology such as prostatic urethritis)
- Biological causes include penile hypersensitivity, hyperexcitable ejaculatory reflex, increased sexual arousability, possible endocrinopathy, a genetic predisposition, and central 5-hydroxytryptamine (5-HT) receptor dysfunction

DIAGNOSIS

DIFFERENTIAL DIAGNOSIS

- In as many as 25% of men with complaints of premature ejaculation, partner is anorgasmic.
- In young adolescents, premature ejaculation may be normally experienced as a consequence of heightened excitation.

WORKUP

- History with a specific emphasis on sexual activities and beliefs
- Factors to be assessed include patient's subjective evaluation, degree of sexual satisfaction, and sense of control
- Collateral information from sexual partner when possible
- Additional history regarding surgery, trauma, and mycologic symptoms
- History of prescribed and recreational drugs (e.g., antidepressants, alcohol, opiates)

LABORATORY TESTS

Urinalysis and urine culture after prostatic massage to rule out prostatic infection

IMAGING STUDIES

None routinely indicated

TREATMENT

NONPHARMACOLOGIC THERAPY

- Behavioral and psychotherapeutic interventions: strongly guided by a specific theoretical framework; often inadequate data to suggest the superiority of any particular approach
- Use of condoms may reduce penile sensitivity
- Use of "pause-squeeze" technique (in which 4 sec of moderate pressure is applied to the frenulum to reduce ejaculatory urge) or "stop-start" technique may be helpful for some patients

ACUTE GENERAL Rx

- Topical anesthetic, such as lidocaine-prilocaine cream (EMLA), increases ejaculatory latency if applied <20 minutes prior to intercourse.
- Anxiolytics (benzodiazepines) may be useful in individuals with anxiety.
- Daily selective serotonin reuptake inhibitors (SSRIs), such as paroxetine (most potent), delay ejaculation. Clomipramine (tricyclic antidepressant) also found to delay orgasm in men. Discontinuation of daily SSRIs often leads to recurrence of premature ejaculation.
- Sildenafil may be superior to antidepressants in delaying ejaculation.

DISPOSITION

- Premature ejaculation is frequently a chronic, lifelong problem.
- There is gradual improvement with age but frequently a chronic, lifelong problem with few spontaneous remissions.

REFERRAL

Behavioral sex therapy or psychotherapy may be helpful; refer to urologist if recurrent prostate infection is indicated.

PEARLS & CONSIDERATIONS

Various psychological risk factors are cited for premature ejaculation, including lack of sexual experience, infrequent sexual intercourse, fear, anxiety, social phobia, relationship problems, and a lack of sexual education.

EVIDENCE

Chronic use of SSRIs, particularly paroxetine, produces significant ejaculation delays, but discontinuation may lead to recurrence of premature ejaculation and SSRI-withdrawal symptoms. Tapering of SSRIs must occur gradually.[1,2]

Evidence-Based References

1. Waldinger MD et al: Relevance of methodological design for the interpretation of efficacy of drug treatment of premature ejaculation: a systematic review and meta-analysis, *Int J Impot Res* 16:369, 2004.
2. Monorsi AS: Medical therapy for premature ejaculation, *Lancet* 368:894, 2006.

SUGGESTED READINGS

Altof SE: Prevalence, characteristics, and implications of premature ejaculation/ rapid ejaculation, *J of Urology*, 175:842, 2006.

Wylie KR, Ralph D: Premature ejaculation: the current literature, *Curr Opin Urol* 15(6):393, 2005.

AUTHORS: **MITCHELL D. FELDMAN, M.D., M.PHIL.,** and **CINDY LAI, M.D.**

BASIC INFORMATION

DEFINITION

Injuries or wounds that occur as a result of contact with an electrical current.

ICD-9CM CODES
994.8 Electrical shock, nonfatal

EPIDEMIOLOGY & DEMOGRAPHICS

- Causes approximately 1000 deaths annually, with two thirds occurring in persons between ages 15 and 40 yr.
- Most electrical injuries in children occur at home (e.g., oral burns from electrical appliances).
- Most electrical injuries in adults are occupationally related. It ranks fifth as the cause of occupational fatalities.
- Accounts for 4% to 6.5% of all admissions to burn units.
- Lightning strikes kill on average 100 people per yr.
  - 8 of every 10 lightning strike victims are male, 75% of lightning deaths in the U.S. occur in the South and Midwest.
  - 25% of lightning deaths were work related.

PHYSICAL FINDINGS & CLINICAL PRESENTATION

- Cognitive changes: depending on the extent of injury, the patient may be unconscious, seizing, or confused and unable to present a history
- Extensive burns (>10% of the body surface)
  1. Located over the entry and exit sites
  2. Most common entry sites are the hands and skull
  3. Most common exit sites are the heels
  4. "Kissing burns" over the flexor creases
  5. Usually on the superficial partial thickness of the skin
  6. Oral burns are common in children; bleeding from the labial artery may present 7 to 10 days after the injury
- Asystole or ventricular fibrillation may be the initial presenting rhythm
- Fractures
- Compartment syndrome from severe muscle tissue damage
- Headaches
- Weakness and paresthesias
- Motor and sensory deficits
- Otologic injury, conductive loss secondary to tympanic membrane rupture or ossicular disruption
- Pneumothorax
- Stricture of the esophagus (delayed presentation)

ETIOLOGY

- Electricity causes tissue injury by converting electrical energy into heat; or by blunt trauma from being thrown from the electrical source or from continuous muscle contraction (tetany).
- The effects of electricity are determined by seven factors: type of current, amount of current, pathway of current, duration, area of contact, resistance of the body, and voltage.
- Tissue damage is greater with higher voltage, and longer the duration of contact.
- Direct current (DC) contact causes a single muscle contraction, throwing the patient away from the source. Alternating current (AC) contact precipitates a tetanic contraction, not allowing the patient to withdraw from the source and prolonging the duration of contact. AC contact is more ominous than DC contact.
- Electrical injuries are arbitrarily divided into high-voltage (>600 volts) and low-voltage (<600 volts) burns. Low-voltage burns involve almost exclusively either the hands or oral cavity. High-voltage injuries have a wide variety of systemic manifestations.
- The entry and exit path of the electrical current determines which tissues are affected.

DIAGNOSIS

WORKUP

Physical examination may not reveal the extent of damage that has occurred. Detailed testing to determine the extent of internal organ damage is indicated. However, in lightning injuries, male victims may suffer from scrotal (on the undersurface of the scrotum) and penile burns, which may often be overlooked. Hemorrhage behind the eardrum with or without perforation is not uncommon. An otoscopic exam is indicated in all victims struck by lightning.

LABORATORY TESTS

- CBC
- Electrolytes
- BUN/creatinine
- Arterial blood gases
- Myoglobin
- Creatinine kinase (CK) with isoenzyme fractionation
- Urinalysis including screening for myoglobinuria
- Liver function tests
- Type and cross-match
- EKG

IMAGING STUDIES

- X-ray: any suspicious area for bone fractures
- CT scan of the head and skull: in patients with major head injury
- Technetium pyrophosphate scanning may locate areas of myocardial necrosis

TREATMENT

NONPHARMACOLOGIC THERAPY

- At the scene of the injury: ensure the power source is turned off before approaching.
- Airway-Breathing-Cardiovascular assessments: respiratory arrest may be prolonged, but prognosis is excellent when breathing is supported.
- Cardiac monitoring.
- Oxygen.
- Tetanus prophylaxis.

ACUTE GENERAL Rx

- IV fluids to maintain urine output of at least 50 ml/hr (IV hydration should be reassessed with CNS expert in patients at risk of developing cerebral edema).
- Alkalinization of the urine (sodium bicarbonate 50 meq in 1 L of normal saline) in patients with or at risk of myoglobinuria.
- Furosemide 20 to 40 mg PO or IV and/or mannitol 12.5 g/kg/hr may be used to force diuresis.
- Seizures are treated in the standard fashion.
- Treat burns with sulfadiazine silver dressings.

CHRONIC Rx

- Hospitalization is indicated in patients with high-voltage injuries, extensive burns, central nervous system symptoms, myonecrosis (CK level >2 times normal, high serum myoglobin levels, or myoglobinuria), new cardiac arrhythmia or ECG changes, or any internal organ damage.
- Ophthalmology consultation at the follow-up to screen for cataract formation (occurs within 1 to 24 mo following a high-voltage electrical injury in 5% to 20% of patients).

DISPOSITION

- Patients with severe burns should be transferred to the regional burn center.
- Complications of electrical injuries include:
  1. Infection
  2. Renal failure from rhabdomyolysis
  3. Seizure disorder
  4. Fasciotomies
  5. Amputation
- Delayed neurologic damage may present as ascending paralysis, amoytrophic lateral sclerosis, or transverse myelitis, weeks to years after the injury.
- Vascular damage may also present in a delayed fashion.

REFERRAL

- Referrals to general surgery, burn, and/or critical care specialists in any patient that meets or may meet hospitalization criteria.
- Plastic surgery is recommended in children with oral burns.

PEARLS & CONSIDERATIONS

COMMENTS

- Lightning Strike and Electric Shock Survivors International is a support group that serves people from around the world who suffered electric injury (www.lightning-strike.org).
- Mobile phones are not at lightning-strike risk.
- Home safety education provided one to one in a clinical setting or at home, especially with the provision of safety equipment, is effective in increasing the range of safety practices.

SUGGESTED READINGS

Bailey B et al: Cardiac monitoring of high-risk patients after an electrical injury: a prospective multicentre study, *Emerg Med J* 24(5):348-352, 2007.

Edlich RF, Farinholt HM, Winters KL et al: Modern concepts of treatment and prevention of electrical burns, *J Long Term Eff Med Implants* 15(5):511-532, 2005.

Kendrick D et al: Home safety education and provision of safety equipment for injury prevention, *Cochrane Database Syst Rev* 1:CD005014, 2007.

Spies C, Trohman RG: Narrative review: electrocution and life-threatening electrical injuries, *Ann Intern Med* 145(7):531-537, 2006.

Zafren K et al: Lightning injuries: prevention and on-site treatment in mountains and remote areas. Official guidelines of the International Commission for Mountain Emergency Medicine and the Medical Commission of the International Mountaineering and Climbing Federation (ICAR and UIAA MEDCOM), *Resuscitation* 65(3):369-372, 2005.

AUTHOR: **ABDULBAKI ABDULRAHMAN, M.D.**

BASIC INFORMATION

DEFINITION

Electromechanical dissociation (EMD) is the absence of cardiac output in the presence of organized electrical activity.

SYNONYMS

Pulseless electrical activity (PEA)

ICD-9CM CODES
426.89 Electromechanical dissociation

EPIDEMIOLOGY & DEMOGRAPHICS

- Less frequent than ventricular tachycardia (VT)/ventricular fibrillation (VF), asystole. May account for 25% of cases in sudden cardiac death.
- Increasingly recognized as the cause of sudden cardiac death in patients with implantable cardioverter-defibrillators.

PHYSICAL FINDINGS & CLINICAL PRESENTATION

PRIMARY EMD:

- Organized electrical activity (not VT/VF)
- No detectable pulse

SECONDARY EMD:

Primary EMD and may also have:

- Bradycardia: drug overdose
- Tachycardia: hypovolemia, massive PE
- Decreased jugular venous pressure (JVP): hypovolemia
- Elevated JVP and no pulse with CPR: cardiac tamponade, massive PE, tension pneumothorax
- Absent unilateral breath sounds with mechanical ventilation and tracheal deviation: tension pneumothorax
- Cyanosis: hypoxia

ETIOLOGY

PRIMARY EMD: Myocardial excitation and contraction uncoupling secondary to advanced heart muscle disease

SECONDARY EMD: Because of changes in the loading conditions of the heart, ischemia, myocardial depressants

- Massive MI
- Massive PE
- Hypovolemia
- Cardiac tamponade
- Tension pneumothorax
- Hypothermia, hypoxia, acidosis
- Hyperkalemia/hypokalemia
- Hypomagnesemia
- Drug overdose: β-blockers, calcium channel blockers, digoxin, tricyclic antidepressants

DIAGNOSIS

DIFFERENTIAL DIAGNOSIS

- Pseudo-EMD
- Idioventricular rhythm
- Postdefibrillation idioventricular rhythm
- Ventricular escape rhythm
- Bradyasystolic rhythm

WORKUP

- Stabilizing patient and workup to establish etiology should proceed simultaneously
- History, physical examination, laboratory tests, imaging studies

LABORATORY TESTS

- CBC
- Potassium, magnesium
- Arterial blood gas
- ECG (Fig. 1-81):
  - Low voltage: tamponade
  - Right heart strain: PE, pneumothorax
  - Arrhythmias: MI, metabolic abnormalities, drug effects
  - ST changes, Q waves: MI

IMAGING STUDIES

- Chest x-ray: rule out pneumothorax
- Chest CT/pulmonary arteriogram: rule out PE
- Echocardiogram: rule out pseudo-EMD, tamponade, valve dysfunction, and atrial myxoma
- Abdominal x-ray: rule out rupture of abdominal aortic aneurysm

TREATMENT

Identifying and treating a reversible cause is critical.

NONPHARMACOLOGIC THERAPY

- Activate emergency medical service
- Begin CPR
- Intubate and ventilate
- Obtain IV access
- Fluid resuscitation
- Continuous cardiac monitor
- Confirm absence of blood flow with Doppler ultrasound, arterial line, or bedside echocardiogram

ACUTE GENERAL Rx

- Treat specific cause if known.
- Epinephrine 1 mg IV push, q3 to 5min or vasopressin 40U IV given once may be used to replace the first or second dose of epinephrine
- If bradycardic: atropine 1 mg IV q3 to 5min to a maximum of 3 mg.
- If preexisting hyperkalemia: sodium bicarbonate 1 mEq/kg.
- Normal saline (10 to 20 ml) should be given after the drug to improve distribution
- Alternate routes of medication delivery for epinephrine, vasopressin, and atropine. May take 2 min for medication to reach the heart via these routes:
  1. Intraosseous: safe and effective, use same dose
  2. Tracheal tube: least preferred as plasma concentrations are variable. Epinephrine and atropine given at 2 to 2.5 × the IV dose in 10 ml of sterile water

PROBABLY HELPFUL:

Sodium bicarbonate 1 mEq/kg if:

- Preexisting bicarbonate responsive acidosis
- Tricyclic antidepressant overdose
- Drug overdoses that respond to alkalization of urine

DISPOSITION

Of hospitalized patients who develop EMD, <15% survive to discharge. Survival rates much lower in patients with prehospital EMD.

REFERRAL

As needed for underlying condition

PEARLS & CONSIDERATIONS

- Some support the use of vasopressin instead of or in addition to epinephrine during resuscitation. Randomized trials show no benefit of vasopressin over epinephrine in survival to hospital discharge or improving neurological outcomes.
- Therapeutic hypothermia (32 to 34°C for 12 to 24hr) may improve neurological outcome in unconscious cardiac arrest survivors.
- Prognosis may be guided by median nerve somatosensory-evoked potentials (72 hr) or EEG (24 to 48 hr) after cardiac arrest.

SUGGESTED READINGS

Dager WE et al: Pharmacotherapy considerations in advanced cardiac life support, *Pharmacotherapy* 26(12):1703, 2006.

Guidelines 2000 for Cardiopulmonary Resuscitation and Emergency Cardiovascular Care, *Circulation* 102(suppl I):I136, 2000.

2005 International Consensus on Cardiopulmonary Resuscitation and Emergency Cardiovascular Care Science with Treatment Recommendations, Part 4: Advanced Life Support, *Circulation* 112(22 suppl):III-25, 2005.

Wenzel V et al: European Resuscitation Council Vasopressor during Cardiopulmonary Resuscitation Study Group: A comparison of vasopressin and epinephrine for out-of-hospital cardiopulmonary resuscitation, *N Engl J Med* 350:105, 2004.

AUTHOR: **SUDEEP K. AULAKH, M.D., F.R.C.P.C.**

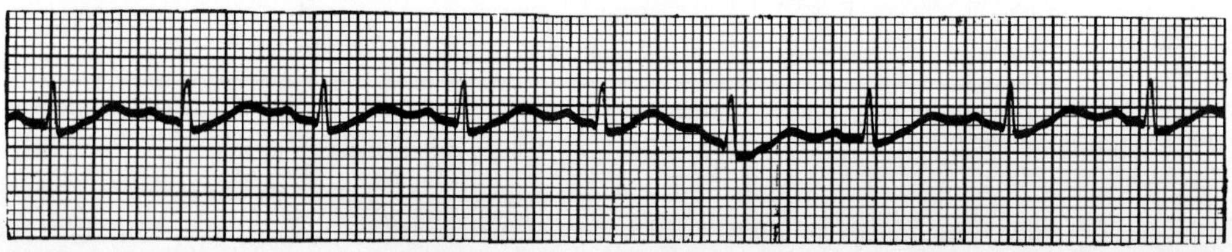

FIGURE 1-81 Sinus rhythm with electromechanical dissociation (EMD). Although the ECG showed sinus rhythm, the patient had no pulse or blood pressure. In this case the EMD was a result of depressed myocardial function after a cardiac arrest. (From Goldberg AL: *Clinical electrocardiography,* ed 5, St Louis, 1994, Mosby.)

BASIC INFORMATION

DEFINITION

Emergency contraception (EC) is a medical therapy women can use to prevent pregnancy soon after unprotected intercourse, sexual assault, or failure or improper use of a birth control method. EC reduces the risk of pregnancy when used up to 120 hours (5 days) after unprotected sex but is more effective if used earlier.

Options for emergency contraception:

- Plan B
  - Only FDA-approved product expressly designed for EC available in the United States.
  - Approved by the FDA in 2006 for sale to women and men age 18 and over without a prescription. Contains the progestin levonorgestrel.
- Combined oral contraceptives
  - Higher doses of available oral contraceptive pills containing ethinyl estradiol plus levonorgestrel or norgestrel can be used for EC (Table 1-10).
- Copper-bearing intrauterine device (IUD)
  - Emergency insertion of the copper-bearing IUD (Paraguard) can be used for EC.

MECHANISM: Current evidence indicates that the primary mechanism of Plan B is inhibition of ovulation and that Plan B is not effective after fertilization has occurred. Emergency insertion of the copper IUD may prevent fertilization or subsequent implantation.

EFFECTIVENESS: Plan B reduces the pregnancy rate by 89% after unprotected intercourse. Combined hormonal EC decreases the risk of pregnancy by about 75%.

SYNONYMS

Morning-after pill, postcoital contraception, Plan B

ICD-9CM CODES
V25.03 Emergency contraceptive counseling/Rx
V25.09 Family planning

EPIDEMIOLOGY & DEMOGRAPHICS

About 49% of all pregnancies and 80% of teen pregnancies in the U.S. are unintended. An estimated 1.7 million unintended pregnancies could be prevented annually if emergency contraception use were widespread.

LABORATORY TESTS

If there is doubt about whether a patient is already pregnant from intercourse that occurred more than a week ago, a pregnancy test may be helpful. However, there is no need for a pregnancy test before administering EC pills. Delays in administration of the medication will reduce its efficacy. The medications in EC pills will not harm an established pregnancy.

- A pregnancy test should be done prior to insertion of a copper IUD.

TREATMENT

ACUTE GENERAL Rx

- Administer EC as soon as possible after unprotected intercourse. EC reduces the risk of pregnancy when used up to 120 hours (5 days) after unprotected intercourse but is more effective if used earlier.
- Use of EC:
  - Plan B
    1. 2 tablets of 0.75-mg levonorgestrel.
    2. Both pills can be taken together as a single dose (1.5-mg levonorgestrel). A single dose is equally effective and causes no more side effects than two divided doses.
    3. Progestin-only EC pills are preferable to combined estrogen-progestin EC pills because of greater efficacy and lower incidence of nausea and vomiting.

NOTE: For women under age 18, a doctor's prescription is necessary to obtain plan B.

  - Combined oral contraceptive pills
    1. 2 doses, 12 hours apart, of 100 to 120 mcg ethinyl estradiol and 0.5 to 0.6 mg levonorgestrel (or 1.0 to 1.2 mg norgestrel) per dose.
    2. See Table 1-10 for dosing.
- Side effects:
  - Nausea occurs in 50% of women taking combined estrogen-progestin EC pills, vomiting in 20%. Plan B is associated with about half the incidence of nausea and vomiting. Side effects resolve within 1 to 2 days. Antinausea medication such as meclizine 25 mg orally is recommended 1 hour before taking combined EC pills.
- Contraindications:
  - Few contraindications to EC exist other than hypersensitivity to the product. EC will not affect an established pregnancy.
  - There are no other evidence-based medical contraindications to the use of EC pills, and very few adverse events have been reported. The benefits of EC in preventing pregnancy generally outweigh the theoretical risks for women who have contraindications to long-term use of combined hormonal contraception, such as thromboembolic disease, smoking over age 35, heart disease, or liver disease. Use of progestin-only EC may be preferable

TABLE 1-10 Oral Contraceptive Pills That Can Be Used for Emergency Contraception in the U.S.

Brand	Company	Pills per Dose	Ethinyl Estradiol per Dose (μg)	Levonorgestrel per Dose (mg)
Alesse	Wyeth	5 pink pills	100	0.50
Aviane	Barr	5 orange pills	100	0.50
Cryselle	Barr	4 white pills	120	0.60
Enpresse	Barr	4 orange pills	120	0.50
Lessina	Barr	5 pink pills	100	0.50
Levlen	Berlex	4 light-orange pills	120	0.60
Levlite	Berlex	5 pink pills	100	0.50
Levora	Watson	4 white pills	120	0.60
Lo/Ovral	Wyeth	4 white pills	120	0.60
Low-Ogestrel	Watson	4 white pills	120	0.60
Lutera	Watson	5 white pills	100	0.50
Nordette	Wyeth	4 light-orange pills	120	0.60
Ogestrel	Watson	2 white pills	100	0.50
Ovral	Wyeth	2 white pills	100	0.50
Portia	Barr	4 pink pills	120	0.60
Seasonale	Barr	4 pink pills	120	0.60
Seasonique	Barr	4 pink pills	120	0.60
Tri-Levlen	Berlex	4 yellow pills	120	0.50
Triphasil	Wyeth	4 yellow pills	120	0.50
Trivora	Watson	4 pink pills	120	0.50

Treatment schedule is 2 doses, 12 hours apart, as soon as possible within 120 hours after unprotected intercourse.

to use of combined estrogen-progestin EC for women with any of these conditions or who are breast-feeding.

- Alternative EC option: copper IUD.
  - Emergency insertion of the copper IUD is highly effective for EC up to 5 days after unprotected intercourse. This option may be preferable for women who desire effective long-term contraception and have no contraindications to IUD insertion. A pregnancy test should be done before IUD insertion.

CHRONIC Rx

Because EC pills are not as effective as other forms of contraception, they are not recommended as an ongoing method of contraception.

DISPOSITION

After using EC, menses will occur within 3 days of the expected onset date for most women. If a woman's next expected menses are delayed by more than a week, a pregnancy test should be done.

PEARLS & CONSIDERATIONS

COMMENTS

- EC is effective in preventing pregnancy up to 120 hours (5 days) after unprotected intercourse.
- A pregnancy test is not necessary before administering EC pills because the medicines in EC will not harm an existing pregnancy.
- Advanced prescription of EC at routine visits may increase timely utilization of EC and does not decrease use of more reliable means of contraception.

PREVENTION

- Patients should begin an effective method of birth control immediately after using EC. Hormonal contraceptives can be started the day after EC is administered. A backup method should be used for 7 days.
- Emergency contraception should be offered to all women after sexual assault.

PATIENT/FAMILY EDUCATION

- Emergency contraception website: http://Not-2-late.com
- Emergency contraception hotline: 1-888-NOT-2-LATE

SUGGESTED READINGS

Jackson RA et al: Advance supply of emergency contraception: effect on use and usual contraception—a randomized trial, *Obstet Gynecol* 102:8-16, 2003.

Gemzell-Danielsson K, Marions L: Mechanisms of action of mifepristone and levonorgestrel when used for emergency contraception, *Hum Reprod Update* 10:341-348, 2004.

Stewart F, Trussell J, Van Look P: Emergency contraception. In Hatcher R, Trussell J, Stewart F, Nelson A, Cates W, Guest F, Kowal D: *Contraceptive technology*, New York, 2004, Ardent Media, Inc., pp. 279-298.

AUTHORS: **JOANNA BROWN, M.D.,** and **MELISSA NOTHNAGLE, M.D.**

Empyema

BASIC INFORMATION

DEFINITION

An accumulation of pus in the pleural space, most often caused by bacterial infection.

SYNONYMS

Infected pleuritis
Infected pleural effusion
Purulent pleural effusion

ICD-9CM CODES
510.9 Empyema Lung

EPIDEMIOLOGY & DEMOGRAPHICS

- Empyema most commonly a complication of bacterial pneumonia, especially in association with pneumococcal or anaerobic infection
- Occur as a complication of thoracic surgery
- Penetrating chest trauma
- Bronchopleural fistulae resulting from malignancy or lung biopsy

PHYSICAL FINDINGS & CLINICAL PRESENTATION

- May be abrupt or chronic and insidious depending on the etiologic agent and host factors.
- Typically presents as progressive pleuritic chest pain, persistent fever, and other sustained signs and symptoms of infection.
- In anaerobic empyema, particularly that caused by the actinomycetes, the clinical picture is dominated by systemic symptoms and signs: weight loss, malaise, and low grade fever.
- A slowly enlarging chest wall mass.
- As a complication of thoracic trauma or surgery, empyema typically results from contamination of blood within the pleural space several days following the event.
- The physical findings of empyema are those of pleural effusion. Decreased breath sounds and dullness to percussion over the involved part of the thorax is typical. Systemic signs include fever, tachycardia, leukocytosis, and warmth and erythema over the involved area.

ETIOLOGY

Infection of the lung parenchyma spreading to pleural space caused by

- *Streptococcus pneumoniae*
- *Hemophilus influenzae*
- *Staphylococcus aureus*
- *Legionella species*
- *Mycobacterium tuberculosis*
- *Actinomyces spp.*
- A variety of oral anaerobic bacteria have been cultured in 36% to 37% of empyemas

DIAGNOSIS

DIFFERENTIAL DIAGNOSIS

- Uninfected parapneumonic effusion
- Congestive heart failure
- Malignancy involving the pleura
- Tuberculous pleurisy
- Collagen vascular disease (particularly rheumatoid lung and systemic lupus erythematosus)

LABORATORY TESTS

- Complete blood count; arterial blood gas.
- Blood cultures.
- Pleural fluid analysis in empyema has the characteristics of an exudate with a ratio of pleural fluid to serum protein >0.5 or pleural fluid to serum LDH >0.6. Characteristically, empyema fluid is grossly purulent with visible organisms on Gram stain with glucose <50 mg/dl and pH <7. These findings justify immediate drainage by chest tube or surgery because of the high risk of loculation and progressive systemic infection.

IMAGING STUDIES

- Chest roentgenogram
- Lateral decubitus view to establish the presence of free fluid in the pleural space
- Computed tomography to establish the presence of fluid loculation, underlying mass lesions, and other intrathoracic pathology

TREATMENT

NONPHARMACOLOGIC THERAPY

Prompt drainage by thoracostomy (chest tube) or open thoracotomy

ACUTE GENERAL Rx

- Maintenance of drainage until infection controlled.
- Antibiotics directed at suspected or proven bacterial or fungal pathogens.
- Thoracoscopy or instillation of thrombolytic agents (streptokinase or urokinase) may be considered in refractory, loculated empyema.

CHRONIC Rx

- If thorough drainage cannot be accomplished, open thoracotomy with pleural decortication may be required.
- Lung function should be monitored following completion of therapy.

DISPOSITION

Hospitalization with supplemental oxygen with ventilatory support if necessary

REFERRAL

Consultation by infectious diseases, pulmonary, or thoracic surgery specialists as needed.

PEARLS & CONSIDERATIONS

COMMENTS

- Empyema caused by actinomycetes may present with erosion through the chest wall and formation of a fistulous tract.
- Nosocomial infection caused by relatively resistant bacterial or fungal pathogens may result in empyema in patients with indwelling thoracostomy tubes.

SUGGESTED READINGS

Jaffe A, Cohen G: Thoracic empyema, *Arch Dis Child* 88(10):839, 2003.

Lardinois D et al: Delayed referral and gram-negative organisms increase the conversion thoracotomy rate in patients undergoing video-assisted thoracoscopic surgery for empyema, *Ann Thorac Surg* 79(6):1851, 2005.

Melloni G et al: Decortication for chronic parapneumonic empyema: results of a prospective study, *World J Surg* 28(5):488, 2004.

Schiza S, Siafakas NM: Clinical presentation and management of empyema, lung abscess and pleural effusion, *Curr Opin Pulm Med* 12(3):205, 2006.

AUTHORS: **GLENN G. FORT, M.D., M.P.H., DENNIS J. MIKOLICH, M.D.,** and **JOSEPH R. MASCI, M.D.**

BASIC INFORMATION

DEFINITION

Acute viral encephalitis is an acute febrile syndrome with evidence of meningeal involvement and of derangement of the function of the cerebrum, cerebellum, or brainstem.

SYNONYMS

Arboviral encephalitis
Brainstem encephalitis
Acute necrotizing encephalitis
Rasmussen encephalitis
Encephalitis lethargica

ICD-9CM CODES
049.9 Viral encephalitis, NOS

EPIDEMIOLOGY & DEMOGRAPHICS

INCIDENCE (IN U.S.): About 20,000 cases/yr are reported to the CDC.
PEAK INCIDENCE: Any age
PREVALENCE (IN U.S.): Unknown
PREDOMINANT SEX: Male = female
PREDOMINANT AGE: Any age
GENETICS: No specific genetic or congenital predisposition

ETIOLOGY

- Can be caused by a host of viruses, with herpes simplex the most common virus identified
- Arboviruses: agents causing Eastern equine encephalitis, Western equine encephalitis, St. Louis encephalitis, Venezuelan equine encephalitis, California virus encephalitis, Japanese B encephalitis, Murray Valley and West Nile encephalitis, Russian spring-summer encephalitis, as well as other lesser known agents
- Also implicated: rabies-causing agents, CMV, Epstein-Barr, varicella-zoster, echo virus, mumps, adenovirus, coxsackie, rubeola, and herpes viruses
- Meningoencephalitis: acute retroviral infection

PHYSICAL FINDINGS & CLINICAL PRESENTATION

- Initially, fever and evidence of meningeal irritation
- Headache and stiff neck
- Later, development of signs of cortical dysfunction: lethargy, coma, stupor, weakness, seizures, facial weakness, as well as brainstem findings
- Cerebellar findings: ataxia, nystagmus, hypotonia; myoclonus, cranial nerve palsies, and abnormal tendon reflexes
- Patients with rabies: hydrophobia, anxiety, facial numbness, psychosis, coma, or dysarthria
- Rarely, movement disorders, such as chorea, hemiballismus, or dystonia
- Recall of a prodromal viral-like illness (this finding is not at all uniform)

DIAGNOSIS

DIFFERENTIAL DIAGNOSIS

- Bacterial infections: brain abscess, toxic encephalopathies, TB
- Protozoal infections
- Behçet's disease
- Lupus encephalitis
- Sjögren's syndrome
- Multiple sclerosis
- Syphilis
- Cryptococcus
- Toxoplasmosis
- Brucellosis
- Leukemic or lymphomatous meningitis
- Other metastatic tumors
- Lyme disease
- Cat-scratch disease
- Vogt-Koyanagi-Harada syndrome
- Mollaret's meningitis

WORKUP

- Lumbar puncture to reveal pleocytosis, usually lymphocytic although neutrophils may be seen early on
- Usually, elevated CSF protein
- Normal or low CSF glucose
- In herpes simplex encephalitis: RBCs and xanthochromia
- EEG changes showing periodic high-voltage sharp waves in the temporal regions and slow wave complexes suggestive of herpes encephalitis
- CT scan and MRI to reveal edema and hemorrhage in the frontal and temporal lobes
- Arboviral infections suspected during outbreaks in specific areas
- Rising titers of neutralizing antibodies from the acute to the convalescent stage demonstrated but often not helpful in the acutely ill patient
- Polymerase chain reaction that amplifies DNA from the CSF for herpes simplex encephalitis
- Rarely, brain biopsy to assist in the diagnosis; viral culture of cerebral tissue obtained if biopsy done
- Classic herpetic skin lesions suggestive of herpes encephalitis
- In diagnosing arboviral encephalitis:
  1. Presence of antiviral IgM within the first few days of symptomatic disease; detected and quantified by ELISA
  2. Unusual to recover an arbovirus from the blood or CSF

LABORATORY TESTS

- Aside from the lumbar puncture, most other laboratory studies are nonspecific.
- Skin lesions and urine may be cultured for herpes simplex and CMV.

TREATMENT

ACUTE GENERAL Rx

- Supportive care, frequent evaluation, and neurologic examination
- Ventilatory assistance for patients who are moribund or at risk for aspiration
- Avoidance of infusion of hypotonic fluids to minimize the risk of hyponatremia
- For patients who develop seizures: anticonvulsant therapy and follow-up in a critical care setting
- For comatose patients:
  1. Aggressive care to avoid decubiti, contractures, and DVT
  2. Close attention to weights, input/output, and serum electrolytes
- Acyclovir 30 mg/kg/day IV for 14 days for herpes simplex encephalitis
- Short courses of corticosteroids to control brain edema and prevent herniation
- In patients with suspected rabies:
  1. Human rabies immune globulin (HRIG) should be given at a dose of 20 U/kg.
  2. Active immunization may be stimulated by recently developed rabies vaccine, which is grown on a human diploid cell line (HDCV) and has reduced the number of doses needed to five.
  3. If suspect animal is a dog or cat and can be found, observe closely for 10 days to detect rabid behavior; any significant illness in the animal should promptly initiate humane sacrifice of the animal with the brain submitted to local or state health departments for pathology and immunologic testing for rabies. Any wild animal suspected of rabies should be humanely sacrificed, if possible, and submitted for rabies testing immediately.
  4. If signs are seen, animal should be euthanized and its brain examined for signs of rabies.
- No specific pharmacologic therapy for most other viral pathogens

CHRONIC Rx

Some patients may develop permanent neurologic sequelae; these patients will benefit from intensive rehabilitation programs, including physical, occupational, and speech therapy.

DISPOSITION

- Patients with suspected encephalitis of any cause should generally be admitted for initial diagnostic workup and specific treatment (if available).
- Long-term management of patients with significant neurologic sequelae from encephalitis (e.g., memory de-

fects, depression, difficulty with organization of thoughts, movement disorders) may benefit from rehabilitation services, home care, or nursing home placement.

REFERRAL

- To a neurologist for initial workup and management
- To an infectious disease specialist for diagnostic and therapeutic plan
- To a rehabilitation service for long-term evaluation and convalescent services

PEARLS & CONSIDERATIONS

- West Nile virus encephalitis occurs primarily in elderly patients >65 years of age.
- Rabies may occur months after contact with the rabid animal, and the exposure (especially bat rabies) may have been seemingly insignificant and even inapparent.
- Experimental therapies are worthy of consideration for some forms of viral encephalitis (e.g., immune plasma, ribavirin, interferons), and expert consultation should be obtained early on for possible treatment interventions with promising experimental therapies.

SUGGESTED READINGS

Beckwith WH et al: Isolation of eastern equine encephalitis virus and West Nile virus from crows during increased arbovirus surveillance in Connecticut, 2000, *Am J Trop Med Hyg* 66(4):422, 2002.

De Tiege X et al : Postinfectious immune-mediated encephalitis after pediatric herpes simplex encephalitis, *Brain Dev* 27(4):304-307, 2005.

Frenkel LM: Challenges in the diagnosis and management of neonatal herpes simplex virus encephalitis, *Pediatrics* 115(3):795-797, 2005.

Kennedy PG: Viral encephalitis, *J Neurol* 252(3):268, 2005.

Roos KL: Fatal encephalitis due to rabies virus transmitted by organ transplantation, *Arch Neurol* 62(6):855-856, 2005.

Sellal F, Stoll-Keller F: Rabies: ancient yet contemporary cause of encephalitis, *Lancet* 365(9463):921-923, 2005.

Steiner I et al: Viral encephalitis: a review of diagnostic methods and guidelines for management, *Eur J Neurol* 12(5):331-343, 2005.

AUTHORS: **STEVEN M. OPAL, M.D.,** and **JOSEPH J. LIEBER, M.D.**

BASIC INFORMATION

DEFINITION

Encephalopathy is a clinical syndrome of global cognitive impairment that is characterized by impaired arousal, inattention, and disorientation.

SYNONYMS

Delirium, acute confusional state

ICD-9CM CODES
348.3 Encephalopathy, NOS
348.30 Encephalopathy, unspecified
348.31 Encephalopathy, metabolic
348.39 Encephalopathy, other
349.82 Encephalopathy, toxic

EPIDEMIOLOGY & DEMOGRAPHICS

POINT PREVALENCE: 1.1% of adults in the general population >55 years of age, 10% to 40% of hospitalized elderly, and 60% of nursing home patients >75 years of age; 100,000 to 200,000 cases annually with anoxic encephalopathy

RISK FACTORS: Age, cancer, AIDS, terminal illness, bone marrow transplant, surgery

PHYSICAL FINDINGS & CLINICAL PRESENTATION

- The essential feature of encephalopathy is the patient's inability to maintain a coherent stream of thought or action.
- The history may often suggest a waxing and waning of the level of arousal and general cognitive ability.
- Because toxins and metabolic disturbances are common causes of encephalopathy, the history should focus on exposure to toxins (including medications) and symptoms suggesting a concurrent illness such as a urinary tract infection or pneumonia.
- Common to all encephalopathies is a fluctuating level of arousal, poor attention, and disorientation.
- Some patients may appear agitated and others lethargic.
- Delusions (fixed false beliefs) and hallucinations are common.
- Asterixis (negative myoclonus) is extremely common.
- Other physical findings may vary depending on the underlying cause of encephalopathy: fever, ascites, jaundice, and tachycardia.

ETIOLOGY

- The final common pathway of all causes of encephalopathy is widespread cortical and subcortical neuronal dysfunction. The causes may be structural or functional.
- Many conditions are reversible and carry a good prognosis if treated in a timely manner.
- Organ failure (e.g., hepatic encephalopathy, hypoxia, hypercapnia, uremia).
- Infection—systemic (e.g., urinary tract, pneumonia) or involving the central nervous system (e.g., meningitis, encephalitis).
- Toxin ingestion or withdrawal (e.g., alcohol, medications, recreational drugs).
- Metabolic disturbances—hyperosmolar states, hypernatremia, hyponatremia, hyperglycemia, hypoglycemia, hypercalcemia, hypophosphatemia, acidosis, alkalosis, inborn errors of metabolism.
- Endocrinopathy—hyperthyroidism, hypothyroidism, Cushing's syndrome, adrenal insufficiency, pituitary failure.
- Neoplasm—tumors of the central nervous system, primary or metastatic. Also effect of distant tumors (e.g., paraneoplastic limbic encephalitis).
- Nutritional deficiency, mostly in alcoholics and chronically ill patients, such as vitamin B_{12} deficiency or folate deficiency (Wernicke's encephalopathy).
- Seizures—postictal state, nonconvulsive status epilepticus, complex partial seizures, absence seizures.
- Trauma—concussion, contusion, subdural hematoma, epidural hematoma, diffuse axonal injury.
- Vascular—both ischemic and hemorrhagic strokes, vasculitis, venous thrombosis.
- Postanoxic encephalopathy.
- Others—hypertensive encephalopathy, postoperative, sleep deprivation.

DIAGNOSIS

DIFFERENTIAL DIAGNOSIS

- Dementia—distinguished from encephalopathy by a history of slowly progressive cognitive decline over time (fluctuating cognitive function is rare except in diffuse Lewy body disease).
- Hypersomnia.
- Aphasia—distinguished from encephalopathy by virtue of it representing a specific disorder of language rather than a global disturbance of cognitive function.
- Depression.
- Psychosis—some overlap with encephalopathy as delusions and hallucinations may be common to both.
- Mania.
- Coma—a severe form of encephalopathy.
- Vegetative state—one potential outcome of coma; these patients appear awake (eyes are open) but there is no content to their consciousness.
- Akinetic mutism—these patients do not talk and do not move; there is little fluctuation in their state and there is no asterixis.
- Locked-in syndrome—may be distinguished from encephalopathy by the presence of fixed neurologic deficits (i.e., paralysis of all four limbs).

WORKUP

- EEG is helpful to confirm the presence of encephalopathy (diffuse slowing) and also to exclude nonconvulsive seizures.
- Chest x-ray to rule out pneumonia secondary to silent aspiration (common in elderly hospitalized patients).

LABORATORY TESTS

- General chemistry—electrolytes, glucose, creatinine, ammonia, blood urea nitrogen, transaminases, amylase, lipase
- Arterial blood gases
- Complete blood count
- Drug screen and alcohol level
- Lumbar puncture if meningitis, encephalitis, or subarachnoid hemorrhage with negative imaging are suspected
- HIV testing
- Endocrine testing—cortisol level, thyroid function test
- Urine analysis and microscopy

IMAGING STUDIES

- Computed tomography to rule out bleeding, hydrocephalus, tumors
- Magnetic resonance imaging with diffusion-weighted images for suspected encephalitis, tumors, and acute strokes
- Magnetic resonance angiography/venography for strokes, arterial dissection, venous thrombosis
- Conventional angiography for CNS vasculitis and aneurysms

TREATMENT

NONPHARMACOLOGIC THERAPY

The best approach is to treat the underlying toxic or metabolic disturbance. The encephalopathy itself is a symptom of these underlying problems. In general, it is best to avoid treating the symptom of encephalopathy with antipsychotics or sedatives.

GENERAL Rx

- Glucose if hypoglycemia
- Antibiotics in cases of infections (choice of an agent with good CNS penetration in cases of primary CNS infections)
- Insulin in hyperglycemic conditions (e.g., diabetic ketoacidosis, hyperosmolar nonketosis, and in sepsis)
- Lactulose in hepatic encephalopathy
- Folate replacement when deficiency suspected
- Anticonvulsants if seizures likely
- Librium or diazepam for delirium tremens (alcohol withdrawal)
- Assure hemodynamic stability (blood pressure and heart rate)

AUTHOR: **ACHRAF A. MAKKI, M.D., M.S.**

BASIC INFORMATION

DEFINITION

Encopresis is the voluntary or involuntary passage of stool into inappropriate places in children over the developmental age of 4 yr, with the absence of direct physiologic causes. Occurs at least once per month for at least 3 months.

SYNONYMS

Functional incontinence of stool

ICD-9CM CODES
787.6 Incontinence of feces
307.7 Encopresis

EPIDEMIOLOGY & DEMOGRAPHICS

PEAK INCIDENCE: 4 to 5 yr of age
PREVALANCE (IN U.S.): 1% to 1.5% of children ages 5 to 8.
PREDOMINANT SEX: Male > female (ratio of 4:1)
PREDOMINANT AGE: 4 to 9 yr of age
GENETICS: Factors that contribute to slow gut motility may predispose to encopresis

PHYSICAL FINDINGS & CLINICAL PRESENTATION

- Most children attain fecal continence by the age of 4. In "primary encopresis," continence is never fully established, whereas in "secondary encopresis" incontinence is preceded by a year or more of continence.
- In secondary encopresis, constipation is generally severe, causing an overflow incontinence in which soft or liquid stool flows around the retained feces, often several times per day.
- When constipation and overflow incontinence are causative, defecation is usually uncomfortable or painful, so patient avoids defecation with consequent stool retention.
- Stool is usually poorly formed and leakage is continuous (occurring during sleep and wakefulness).
- Encopresis resolves when the constipation is resolved.
- In primary encopresis, stool is more likely to be normal in character.
- Soiling is intermittent and usually in a prominent location.
- Coexisting oppositional-defiant or conduct disorders are frequent.

ETIOLOGY

- Children with encopresis exhibit abnormal anorectal dynamics.
- Primary encopresis may be related to developmental delay of sphincter control whereas secondary encopresis develops in the setting of constipation.
- Approximately 96% of children will have bowel movements between three times daily to once every other day. When bowel movements are less frequent, stool becomes drier and harder and much more uncomfortable to pass. Children may avoid the discomfort by avoiding elimination, but this only results in worsening constipation. Soiling results from liquid stool that leaks around the main stool mass.
- Constipation may begin gradually as a result of a slow decrease in elimination frequency or more acutely after an illness, dehydration, or prolonged bed rest.
- In encopresis without constipation and overflow incontinence, soiling is often intentional. This may occur in the setting of oppositional-defiant disorder or conduct disorder.
- Harsh or inconsistent toilet training and resultant anxiety may lead to retention of stool, constipation, and eventually encopresis.

DIAGNOSIS

DIFFERENTIAL DIAGNOSIS

- Hirschsprung's disease
- Endocrine disease (hypothyroidism)
- Cerebral palsy
- Myelomeningocele
- Pseudoobstruction
- Anorectal lesions (rectal stenosis)
- Malformations
- Trauma
- Rectal prolapse
- Hypothyroidism
- Medications

WORKUP

- History: pay particular attention to frequency of elimination, character of the stool, associated pain, and presence of enuresis (with which it is frequently associated).
- Evaluate child for other developmental or psychiatric problems.
- Physical examination: pay particular attention to the abdomen, anus, rectum, and saddle sensation.

LABORATORY TESTS

Consider thyroid function tests, electrolytes, calcium, urinalysis, and culture.

IMAGING STUDIES

- Abdominal imaging to determine extent of obstruction or megacolon
- Anorectal manometric studies to determine sphincter function if Hirschsprung's disease is suspected; if abnormal, follow up with a barium enema and rectal biopsy

TREATMENT

NONPHARMACOLOGIC THERAPY

- Behavioral and/or individual psychotherapy and family therapy.
- Biofeedback advocated by some to improve sphincter function.

ACUTE GENERAL Rx

- In secondary encopresis, disimpaction with hypertonic phosphate (30 ml/5 kg body weight) or isotonic saline enemas
- Resistant cases: repeated instillation of 200 to 600 ml of milk of magnesia enemas
- If child does not permit enemas: oral disimpaction with large doses of mineral oil or lactulose until stool mass is cleared

CHRONIC Rx

- Prevention of recurrence of constipation by increased dietary fiber and bulk agents and the use of laxatives (Senokot) and stool softeners (docusate sodium)
- In immediate postdisimpaction period (3 mo following acute treatment) laxatives needed because bowel tone remains low
- In primary encopresis, continue with nonpunitive toilet training and encourage regular toilet times (the latter is also helpful in secondary encopresis)

DISPOSITION

In most cases encopresis is self-limited and of relatively brief duration

REFERRAL

If patient is resistant to treatment, explore for complicating family factors, and/or encopresis.

PEARLS & CONSIDERATIONS

It is important to educate parents and children as to the nature of the problem and to defuse hostile or negative interactions between them.

EVIDENCE

Behavioral therapy

A systematic review found some evidence that behavioral intervention plus laxative therapy, rather than behavioral therapy or laxative therapy alone, improves continence in children with primary and secondary encopresis. There was no evidence that biofeedback adds any benefit to conventional management of encopresis and constipation in children.[1] Ⓐ

Evidence-Based Reference

1. Brazelli M, Griffiths P: Behavioural and cognitive interventions with or without other treatments for defaecation disorders in children, *Cochrane Database Syst Rev* 4:CD002240, 2001. Ⓐ

SUGGESTED READINGS

Klages T et al: Controlled study of encopresis and enuresis in children with a prepubertal and early adolescent bipolar-I disorder phenotype, *J Am Acad Child Adolesc Psychiatry* 44(10):1050, 2005.
Reid H, Bahar RJ: Treatment of encopresis and chronic constipation in young children: clinical results from interactive parent-child guidance, *Clin Pediatr* 45(2):157, 2006.

AUTHOR: **MITCHELL D. FELDMAN, M.D., M.PHIL.**

BASIC INFORMATION

DEFINITION

Infective endocarditis is an infection of the endocardial surface of the heart or mural endocardium.

ACUTE ENDOCARDITIS: Usually caused by *Staphylococcus aureus, Streptococcus pyogenes, Streptococcus pneumoniae,* and *Neisseria* organisms; classic clinical presentation of high fever, positive blood cultures, vascular and immunologic phenomenon

SUBACUTE ENDOCARDITIS: Usually caused by viridans streptococci in the presence of valvular pathology; less toxic, often indolent presentation with lower fevers, night sweats, fatigue

ENDOCARDITIS IN INJECTION DRUG USERS: Often involving *S. aureus* or *Pseudomonas aeruginosa* with variation that may be geographically influenced; tricuspid or multiple valvular involvement; high mortality rate of 50% to 60%

PROSTHETIC VALVE ENDOCARDITIS (EARLY): Usually caused by *S. epidermidis* within 2 mo of valve replacement; other organisms include *S. aureus,* gram-negative bacilli, diphtheroids, *Candida* organisms

PROSTHETIC VALVE ENDOCARDITIS (LATE): Typically develops >60 days after valvular replacement; involved organisms similar to early prosthetic valve endocarditis, including viridans streptococci, enterococci, and group D streptococci

NOSOCOMIAL ENDOCARDITIS: Secondary to intravenous catheters, TPN lines, pacemakers; coagulase-negative staphylococci, *S. aureus,* and streptococci most common

SYNONYMS

Bacterial endocarditis
Subacute bacterial endocarditis (SBE)
Endocarditis

ICD-9CM CODES
421.0 Infective endocarditis
996.61 Prosthetic valve endocarditis

EPIDEMIOLOGY & DEMOGRAPHICS

INCIDENCE (IN U.S.): 1.7 to 3.8 cases/100,000 persons/yr

PEAK INCIDENCE: Females: often <35 yr old; males: 45 to 65 yr old

NOSOCOMIAL ENDOCARDITIS: 14% to 28% of cases

PREVALENCE (IN U.S.): 0.3 to 3 cases/1000 hospital admissions

PREDOMINANT SEX: Male > female

PREDOMINANT AGE: 45 to 65 yr

PHYSICAL FINDINGS & CLINICAL PRESENTATION

- Fever may be variable in presentation; may be high, hectic, or absent.
- Fever, chills, fatigue, and rigors occur in 25% to 80% of patients.
- Heart murmur may be absent in right-sided endocarditis.
- Embolic phenomenon with peripheral manifestations is found in 50% of patients.
- Skin manifestations include petechiae, Osler nodes, splinter hemorrhages, Janeway lesions.
- Splenomegaly is more common with subacute course.

ETIOLOGY

Streptococcal and staphylococcal infections are the most common causes of infective endocarditis. Variation in incidence may occur that is influenced by the patient's risk for developing infection.

ACUTE ENDOCARDITIS:
- *S. aureus*
- *Streptococcus pneumoniae*
- Streptococcal species and groups A through G
- *Haemophilus influenzae*

SUBACUTE ENDOCARDITIS:
- Viridans streptococci (alpha-hemolytic)
- *S. bovis*
- Enterococci
- *S. aureus*

ENDOCARDITIS IN INJECTION DRUG USERS:
- *S. aureus*
- *P. aeruginosa*
- *Candida* species
- Enterococci

PROSTHETIC VALVE ENDOCARDITIS (EARLY):
- *S. epidermidis*
- *S. aureus*
- Gram-negative bacilli
- Group D streptococci

PROSTHETIC VALVE ENDOCARDITIS (LATE):
- *S. epidermidis*
- Viridans streptococci
- *S. aureus*
- Enterococci and group D streptococci

NOSOCOMIAL ENDOCARDITIS:
- Coagulase-negative *staphylococci*
- *S. aureus*
- Streptococci: viridans, group B, enterococcus

HACEK ORGANISMS:
- Fastidious gram-negative bacilli
- *Haemophilus parainfluenzae*
- *Haemophilus aphrophilus*
- *Actinobacillus actinomycetemcomitans*
- *Cardiobacterium hominis*
- *Eikenella corrodens*
- *Kingella kingae*

RISK FACTORS

- Poor dental hygiene
- Long-term hemodialysis
- Diabetes mellitus
- HIV infection
- Mitral valve prolapse

DIAGNOSIS

DIFFERENTIAL DIAGNOSIS

- Brain abscess
- FUO
- Pericarditis
- Meningitis
- Rheumatic fever
- Osteomyelitis
- Salmonella
- TB
- Bacteremia
- Pericarditis
- Glomerulonephritis

WORKUP

Physical examination to evaluate for the previous physical findings followed by laboratory testing (see "Laboratory Tests")

LABORATORY TESTS

- Blood cultures: three sets in first 24 hr
- More culturing if patient has received prior antibiotic
- CBC (anemia possibly present, subacute)
- WBC (leukocytosis is higher in acute endocarditis)
- ESR and C-reactive protein (elevated)
- Positive rheumatoid factor (subacute endocarditis)
- False-positive VDRL
- Proteinuria, hematuria, RBC casts
- Electrocardiogram: look for cardiac conduction abnormalities, injury pattern, or evidence of pericarditis—any such new findings are suggestive of myocardial abscess.

IMAGING STUDIES

- Echocardiogram: two-dimensional
- Transesophageal echocardiography (TEE): more sensitive in detecting vegetations if two dimensional is negative, especially helpful with prosthetic valves or in detecting perivalvular disease

TREATMENT

Initial IV antibiotic therapy (before culture results) is aimed at the most likely organism:

- In patients with prosthetic valves or patients with native valves who are allergic to penicillin: vancomycin (1 g IV every 12 hr for 4 wk) plus rifampin 600 mg by mouth daily and gentamicin (1mg/kg IV every 8 hr for 2 wk)—assuming normal renal function in adult patients.
- In IV drug users: nafcillin or oxacillin (2 g IV every 4 hr) plus gentamicin (1 mg/kg every 8 hr for 3 to 5 days until blood cultures are negative); if MRSA,

vancomycin (1 g IV every 12 hr for 4 wk) plus gentamicin (1 mg/kg every 8 hr for 3 to 5 days until blood cultures are negative).
- In native valve endocarditis with a penicillin-susceptible streptococcal isolate: combination of penicillin (18 to 24 million units/day IV for 4 wk) and gentamicin (1 mg/kg every 8 hr for 2 wk) assuming normal renal function. Extend the gentamicin therapy for 4 wk if a relatively penicillin-resistant strain of streptococcus is isolated (penicillin MIC >0.5 microgram/ml); a penicillase-resistant penicillin (oxacillin or nafcillin—2 g IV every 4 hr for 4 to 6 wk plus gentamicin 1mg/kg IV every 8 hr for 3 to 5 days) can be used if acute bacterial endocarditis is present or if *S. aureus* is suspected as one of the possible causative organisms; for Hacek organisms, treat with third-generation cephalosporin (ceftriaxone—2 g IV every 24 hr for 4 to 6 wk).
- Ceftriaxone: 2 g IV every 24 hr and an aminoglycoside (e.g., gentamicin 1 mg/kg IV every 8 hr for 2 wk) effective for *Streptococcus viridans* endocarditis.
- Daptomycin (6 mg/kg/day for 4 to 6 wk) has recently been approved for use in *S. aureus* bacteremia and right-sided endocarditis; may prove useful in MRSA infections.

Antibiotic therapy after identification of the organism should be guided by susceptibility testing—preferably by formal testing by MIC (minimum inhibitory testing).

DISPOSITION

- The patient may need outpatient IV antibiotic therapy, and arrangements need to be made to assure safe vascular access and continuity of care with outpatient IV therapy team.
- Long-term follow-up is essential after therapy has ended; relapse of endocarditis may occur.
- Prophylaxis with antibiotics will be needed before dental procedures as a previous episode of endocarditis increases the risk of recurrent endocarditis associated with transient bacteremia from dental procedures.

REFERRAL

- To an infectious disease specialist for an optimal antibiotic regimen
- To a cardiologist or a cardiac surgeon if evidence of heart failure, refractory infection, myocardial abscess, valve disruption, or major embolic events occur
- To a dentist or oral surgeon if dental work needs to be conducted with appropriate use of prophylactic antibiotics to prevent recurrent endocarditis

PEARLS & CONSIDERATIONS

COMMENTS

For endocarditis prophylaxis refer to Section V.

EVIDENCE

EBM

We are unable to cite evidence that meets our criteria for most therapies used in infective endocarditis.

A randomized controlled trial in patients with endocarditis due to penicillin-susceptible streptococci found monotherapy with ceftriaxone administered once daily for 4 weeks to be effective and safe.[1] (B)

Evidence-Based Reference

1. Sexton DJ et al: Endocarditis Treatment Consortium Group. Ceftriaxone once daily for four weeks compared with ceftriaxone plus gentamicin once daily for two weeks for treatment of endocarditis due to penicillin-susceptible streptococci, *Clin Infect Dis* 27:1470-1474, 1998. (B)

SUGGESTED READINGS

Cecchi E et al: Are the Duke criteria really useful for the early bedside diagnosis of infective endocarditis? Results of a prospective multicenter trial, *Ital Heart J* 6(1):41-48, 2005.

Cha R, Brown WJ, Rybak MJ: Bactericidal activities of daptomycin, quinupristin-dalfopristin, and linezolid against vancomycin-resistant *Staphylococcus aureus* in an in vitro pharmacodynamic model with simulated endocardial vegetations, *Antimicrob Agents Chemother* 47(12):3960-3963, 2003.

Fowler VG et al: Daptomycin versus standard therapy for bacteremia and endocarditis caused by *Staphylococcus aureus, N Engl J Med* 355(7):653, 2006.

McDonald JR et al: Enterococcal endocarditis: 107 cases from the international collaboration on endocarditis merged database, *Am J Med* 118(7):759, 2005.

Morris AJ et al: Gram stain, culture, and histopathological examination findings for heart valves removed because of infective endocarditis, *Clin Infect Dis* 36(6):697-704, 2003.

AUTHORS: **GLENN G. FORT, M.D., M.P.H.,** and **DENNIS J. MIKOLICH, M.D.**

BASIC INFORMATION

DEFINITION

Endometrial cancer is a malignant transformation of endometrial stroma and/or glands typified by irregular nuclear membranes, nuclear atypia, mitotic activity, loss of glandular pattern, irregular cell size (Fig. 1-82).

SYNONYMS

Uterine cancer (some forms)

ICD-9CM CODES
182 Malignant neoplasm of body of uterus

EPIDEMIOLOGY & DEMOGRAPHICS

INCIDENCE: 21.2 cases/100,000 persons; approximately 30,000 new cases annually

PREDOMINANCE: Median age at onset: 60 yr; only 5% occur in women <40 yr

RISK FACTORS: Obesity, diabetes, nulliparity, early menarche and late menopause, unopposed estrogen therapy, tamoxifen use, endometrial atypical hyperplasia

PHYSICAL FINDINGS & CLINICAL PRESENTATION

- Abnormal uterine bleeding or postmenopausal bleeding in 90%
- Pyometra or hematometra
- Abnormal Pap smear

ETIOLOGY

Endogenous or exogenous chronic unopposed estrogen stimulation of the endometrium

DIAGNOSIS

DIFFERENTIAL DIAGNOSIS

- Atypical hyperplasia
- Other genital tract malignancy
- Polyps
- Atrophic vaginitis
- Granuloma cell tumor
- Fibroid uterus

WORKUP

- Complete history and physical examination
- Endometrial biopsy or dilation and curettage
- Assessment of operative risk

LABORATORY TESTS

- CBC
- Chemistry profile including liver function tests
- Consider CA-125 level

IMAGING STUDIES

- Chest x-ray examination
- Possible CT scan, barium enema (BE), and/or pelvic ultrasound
- Endovaginal ultrasound in postmenopausal women with vaginal bleeding

TREATMENT

NONPHARMACOLOGIC THERAPY

- Surgery is the mainstay of treatment, with or without radiation, depending on tumor stage and grade.
- Surgery consists of pelvic washings, total abdominal hysterectomy and bilateral salpingo-oophorectomy, omental biopsy, and selective pelvic and periaortic lymphadenectomy, depending on stage and grade.
- Brachytherapy and/or teletherapy are added in an advanced stage.
- Chemotherapy (cisplatin, Adriamycin) or tamoxifen may also be used.

ACUTE GENERAL Rx

- A thorough workup should be completed before any therapy for endometrial cancer.
- Surgery is the treatment of choice.

CHRONIC Rx

- Physical and pelvic examination every 3 mo for 2 yr, then every 6 mo for 2 yr, annually thereafter
- Yearly Pap smear
- Hormone replacement (combination) a consideration in low-risk patients (stage I or early stage II)

DISPOSITION

The majority of cases present early, where the 5-yr survival is generally good:
Stage I 75% to 100%
Stage II 60%
Stage III 50%
Stage IV 20%
Some histologic types (clear cell, serous papillary) have poorer survival rates.

REFERRAL

A gynecologist may manage early-stage disease, otherwise refer to a gynecologic oncologist.

PEARLS & CONSIDERATIONS

COMMENTS

Estrogen replacement therapy (ERT) after surgery for endometrial cancer remains controversial. Recent data suggest that ERT does not increase endometrial cancer recurrence rates.

SUGGESTED READINGS

Amant et al: Endometrial cancer, *Lancet* 366 (9484):491, 2005.
Tabor A et al: Endometrial thickness as a test for endometrial cancer in women with postmenopausal vaginal bleeding, *Obstet Gynecol* 99:529, 2002.

AUTHORS: **GIL FARKASH, M.D.,** and **RUBEN ALVERO, M.D.**

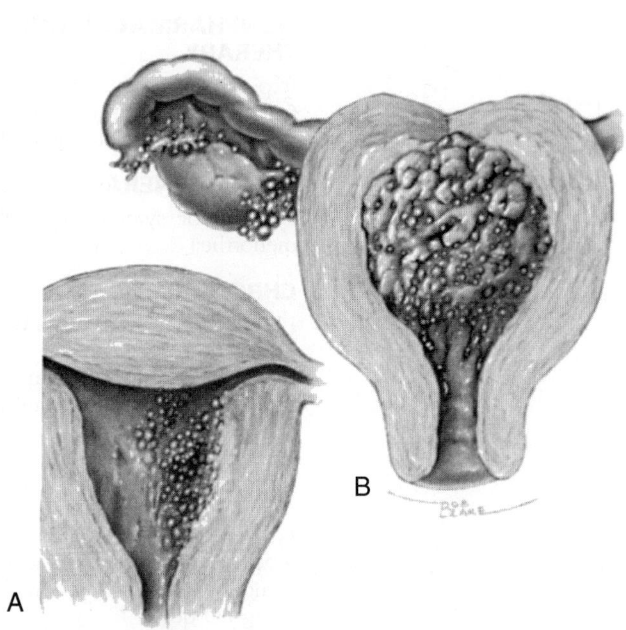

FIGURE 1-82 Carcinoma of the endometrium. **A,** Stage I. **B,** Stage III, myometrial invasion. (From Sabiston D: *Textbook of surgery,* ed 15, Philadelphia, 1997, WB Saunders.)

BASIC INFORMATION

DEFINITION

Endometriosis is defined as the presence of functioning endometrial glands and stroma outside the uterine cavity (Fig. 1-83).

ICD-9CM CODES
617.9 Endometriosis

EPIDEMIOLOGY & DEMOGRAPHICS

PREVALENCE:
- In asymptomatic women: 2% to 22%
- Women with dysmenorrhea: 40% to 60%
- Subfertile women: 20% to 30%
- Incidence peaks at about age 40

MOST COMMON AGE AT DIAGNOSIS: 25 to 29 yr

GENETICS:
- Multifactorial inheritance pattern
- 6.9% occurrence rate in first-degree female relatives

PHYSICAL FINDINGS & CLINICAL PRESENTATION

- Classic triad is dysmenorrhea, dyspareunia, and infertility.
- Presence of pelvic pain *not correlated* with the total area of endometriosis, type of lesion, or volume of disease, but it *is correlated* with the depth of infiltration.
- Other symptoms include: Abnormal bleeding (premenstrual spotting, menorrhagia), cyclic abdominal pain, intermittent constipation/diarrhea, dyschezia, dysuria, hematuria, urinary frequency.
- Rare manifestations: Catamenial hemothorax, bloody pleural effusion, massive ascites occurring during menses.
- Most severe discomfort is associated with lesions >1 cm in depth.
- Bimanual examination may reveal tender uterosacral ligaments, cul-de-sac nodularity, induration of the rectovaginal septum, fixed retroversion of the uterus, adnexal mass, and generalized or localized tenderness.

ETIOLOGY

- Reflux and direct implantation theory: retrograde menstruation with implantation of viable endometrial cells to surrounding pelvic structures
- Coelomic metaplasia theory: transformation of multipotential cells of the coelomic epithelium into endometrium-like cells
- Vascular dissemination theory: transport of endometrial cells to distant sites via the uterine vascular and lymphatic systems
- Autoimmune disease theory: disorder of immune surveillance allows growth of endometrial implants

DIAGNOSIS

DIFFERENTIAL DIAGNOSIS

- Ectopic pregnancy
- Acute appendicitis
- Chronic appendicitis
- PID
- Pelvic adhesions
- Hemorrhagic cyst
- Hernia
- Psychologic disorder
- Irritable bowel syndrome
- Uterine leiomyomata
- Adenomyosis
- Nerve entrapment syndrome
- Scoliosis
- Muscular/skeletal strain
- Interstitial cystitis

WORKUP

- Thorough history and physical examination, including inquiry about physical and emotional abuse
- Colonoscopy if rectal bleeding present
- Laparoscopy for definitive diagnosis
- Revised American Fertility Society (RAFS) scale to classify endometriosis (since 1985):
  Stage I minimal
  Stage II mild
  Stage III moderate
  Stage IV severe

LABORATORY TESTS

Cancer antigen 125 (CA125)
- Also elevated in ovarian epithelial neoplasm, myomas, adenomyosis, acute PID, ovarian cysts, pancreatitis, chronic liver disease, menstruation, and pregnancy
- CA 125 value >35 U/ml: positive predictive value of 0.58 and a negative predictive value of 0.96 for the presence of endometriosis

IMAGING STUDIES

- Ultrasound: for evaluating adnexal mass; cannot reliably distinguish endometriomas from other benign or malignant ovarian conditions
- MRI:
  1. Highly accurate in detecting endometriomas
  2. Limited sensitivity in detecting diffuse pelvic endometriosis

TREATMENT

NONPHARMACOLOGIC THERAPY

Expectant management (observation for 5 to 12 mo) for stage I or stage II endometriosis-associated infertility

ACUTE GENERAL Rx

NSAIDs for symptomatic relief of dysmenorrhea

CHRONIC Rx

PHARMACOLOGIC MANAGEMENT:
Estrogen-progesterone:
- State of "pseudopregnancy" created by continuous use of combination oral contraceptives for 6 to 12 mo
- Breakthrough bleeding treated by administering conjugated estrogens 1.25 mg/day for 2 wk

Progestins:
- Medroxyprogesterone acetate 10 to 30 mg PO qd and occasionally up to 100 mg PO qd
- Alternatively, 100 mg IM q2wk for four doses, followed by 200 mg IM monthly for 4 mo

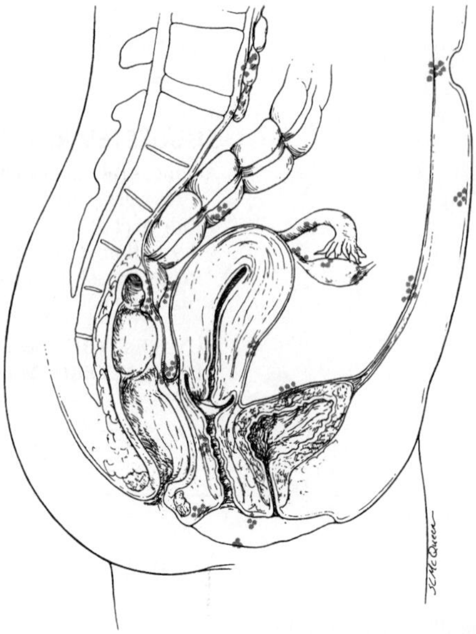

FIGURE 1-83 Common pelvic sites of endometriosis. (From Mishell D [ed]: *Comprehensive gynecology,* ed 3, St Louis, 1997, Mosby.)

- Breakthrough bleeding treated with ethinyl estradiol (20 μg/day) or conjugated estrogens (1.25 mg/day) for 1 to 2 wk
- Comparison with danazol: progestins cost less, have a more tolerable side-effect profile, and have comparable efficacy with regard to pain relief, so are often the first-line drug

Gonadotropin-releasing hormone (GnRH) agonists:

- Use usually limited to 6 mo
- Leuprolide acetate depot 3.75 mg IM monthly *or* 11.25 mg IM q3mo *or* nafarelin 200 μg nasal puffs bid *or* goserelin 3.6 mg SC monthly
- As effective as danazol for relief of pelvic pain
- Add-back therapy for protection against vasomotor symptoms and bone loss: norethindrone acetate 5 mg PO qd alone *or* in combination with conjugated estrogen 0.625 mg PO qd
- Add-back therapy allows GnRH agonist use to be extended to 1 yr

Alternative therapies for inhibition of estrogen action currently under investigation are:

- Aromatase inhibitors: Anastrozole, Letrozole
- SERM: Raloxifene
- Agents enhancing cell-mediated immunity are: Cytokines (interleukin-12 and interferon-α-2b)
- Immunomodulators (Loxaribine, Levamisole)
- Antiinflamatory: Pentoxifylline

SURGICAL MANAGEMENT:

Conservative:

- Directed at enhancing fertility or treating pain unresponsive to first line medical treatment
- Usually accomplished through laparoscopy
- Removal or destruction of endometriotic implants by excision, electrocautery, or laser
- Cystectomy for endometrioma
- LUNA (laparoscopic uterosacral nerve ablation) for midline pain such as dysmenorrheal or dyspareunia (evidence does not support its use)
- Unless pregnancy is desired, patient is usually started on GnRH agonist therapy immediately after surgery
- For those desiring pregnancy, surgery alone results in significant increase in fertility

Definitive:

- Directed at relieving endometriosis-associated pain
- Total abdominal hysterectomy with bilateral salpingo-oophorectomy and complete excision or ablation of endometriosis
- Thorough abdominal exploration to ensure removal of all disease
- Must be prepared to manage possible GI and urinary tract endometriosis
- 90% effective in pain relief
- Estrogen replacement therapy (ERT) to be considered in all women undergoing definitive surgical management; after ERT, recurrence rate of 0% to 5% in women with endometriosis confined to the pelvis but 18% in women with bowel involvement

MANAGEMENT OF ENDOMETRIOSIS-ASSOCIATED INFERTILITY:

Conservative surgery:

- Yields significantly increased pregnancy rate than does expectant management, in part because of correction of mechanical factors such as adhesions

Assisted reproductive technologies:

- Can be used to circumvent unknown mechanism of endometriosis-associated infertility
- Superovulation with clomiphene citrate or human menopausal gonadotropins; clomiphene citrate results in threefold pregnancy rate over either danazol or expectant management
- Further improvement with intrauterine insemination combined with superovulation
- In vitro fertilization if above mentioned unsuccessful

DISPOSITION

Tends to recur unless definitive surgery is performed and should be considered a chronic condition.

REFERRAL

To a reproductive endocrinologist for advanced surgical management or infertility management

PEARLS & CONSIDERATIONS

COMMENTS

Patient information can be obtained through the following organizations: Endometriosis Association, 8585 North 76th Place, Milwaukee, WI 53223, 414-355-2200 or 800-992-ENDO; Women's Reproductive Health Network, P.O. Box 30167, Portland, OR 97230-9067; phone: 503-667-7757.

EVIDENCE

EBM

The combined oral contraceptive and GnRH analogs are equally effective in reducing dyspareunia and nonmenstrual pain and relieve symptoms for up to 6 months after treatment. Both reduce dysmenorrhea.[1,2] Ⓐ

When used continuously following laparoscopy, the oral contraceptive is as effective as continuous low-dose cyproterone acetate in reducing painful symptoms.[3] Ⓐ

Treatment with medroxyprogesterone acetate for 6 months relieves symptoms of endometriosis and improves quality of life.[4] Ⓐ

Postoperatively, high-dose medroxyprogesterone is more effective than placebo in reducing pain due to moderate to severe disease.[5] Ⓐ

Medroxyprogesterone and danazol are no more effective than placebo in improving pregnancy outcomes in women with subfertility attributed to endometriosis.[6,7] Ⓐ

Postoperative leuprolide does not appear to improve long-term pain relief or fertility.[8] Ⓐ

Postoperative goserelin and nafarelin both reduce long-term pain and delay symptom recurrence.[9,10] Ⓐ

Nafarelin post laparotomy is not effective in improving pain due to endometriosis.[11] Ⓐ

Conflicting evidence exists with regard to the effectiveness of danazol, but most studies suggest that it is more effective than placebo in relieving painful symptoms.[12,13] Ⓐ

An RCT included in a systematic review found that laparoscopic ablation of endometrial deposits plus laparoscopic uterine nerve ablation significantly reduced pain in women with mild/moderate endometriosis vs. diagnostic laparoscopy alone. However, the reviewers comment that this was the only RCT they found meeting their criteria so conclusions need to be drawn with caution.[14] Ⓐ

It is not clear if the use of laparoscopic uterine nerve ablation has a role in the treatment of endometriosis.

Another RCT compared laparoscopic ablation of endometrial deposits plus laparoscopic uterine nerve ablation with laparoscopic deposit ablation alone. There was no significant difference in pain between the two groups at 6 to 9 months.[15] Ⓐ

A systematic review found one RCT comparing laparoscopic cystectomy vs. laparoscopic drainage and coagulation for ovarian endometrioma.

Symptom relief and fertility is improved more significantly following laparoscopic cystectomy than with endometrioma drainage.[16] Ⓐ

Evidence-Based References

1. Moore J, Kennedy S, Prentice A: Modern combined oral contraceptives for pain associated with endometriosis, *Cochrane Database Syst Rev* 4:1997. Ⓐ
2. Parazzini F et al: Estroprogestin vs. gonadotrophin agonists plus estroprogestin in the treatment of endometriosis-related pelvic pain: a randomized trial. Gruppo Italiano per lo Studio dell'Endometriosi, *Eur J Obstet Gynecol Reprod Biol* 88:11, 2000. Reviewed in: *Clin Evid* 11:2391, 2004. Ⓐ
3. Vercellini P et al: Cyproterone acetate versus a continuous monophasic oral contraceptive in the treatment of recurrent pelvic pain after conservative surgery for symptomatic endometriosis, *Fertil Steril* 77:52, 2002. Reviewed in *Clin Evid* 11:2391, 2004. Ⓐ
4. Bergqvist A, Theorell T: Changes in quality of life after hormonal treatment of endometriosis, *Acta Obstet Gynecol Scand* 80:628, 2001. Reviewed in: *Clin Evid* 11:2391, 2004. Ⓐ
5. Telimaa S, Ronnenberg L, Kauppila A: Placebo-controlled comparison of danazol and high-dose medroxyprogesterone acetate in the treatment of endometriosis after conservative surgery, *Gynecol Endocrinol* 1:363, 1987. Reviewed in: *Clin Evid* 11:2391, 2004. Ⓐ
6. Harrison RF, Barry-Kinsella C: Efficacy of medroxyprogesterone treatment in infertile women with endometriosis: a prospective, randomized, placebo-controlled study, *Fertil Steril* 74:24, 2000. Reviewed in: *Clin Evid* 11:2391, 2004. Ⓐ
7. Hughes E et al: Ovulation suppression for endometriosis, *Cochrane Database Syst Rev* 3,2003. Ⓐ
8. Busacca M et al: Post-operative GnRH analogue treatment after conservative surgery for symptomatic endometriosis stage III-IV: a randomized controlled trial, *Hum Reprod* 16:2399, 2001. Reviewed in: *Clin Evid* 11:2391, 2004. Ⓐ
9. Vercellini P et al: A gonadotrophin-releasing hormone agonist compared with expectant management after conservative surgery for symptomatic endometriosis, *Br J Obstet Gynaecol* 106:672, 1999. Reviewed in: *Clin Evid* 11:2391, 2004. Ⓐ
10. Hornstein MD et al: Use of nafarelin versus placebo after reductive laparoscopic surgery for endometriosis, *Fertil Steril* 68:860, 1997. Reviewed in: *Clin Evid* 11:2391, 2004. Ⓐ
11. Parazzini F et al: Postsurgical medical treatment of advanced endometriosis: results of a randomized clinical trial, *Am J Obstet Gynecol* 171:1205, 1994. Reviewed in: *Clin Evid* 11:2391, 2004. Ⓐ
12. Selak V et al: Danazol for pelvic pain associated with endometriosis, *Cochrane Database Syst Rev* 4,2001. Ⓐ
13. Bianchi S et al: Effects of 3 month therapy with danazol after laparoscopic surgery for stage III/IV: a randomized study, *Hum Reprod* 13:1335, 1999. Reviewed in: *Clin Evid* 11:2391, 2004. Ⓐ
14. Jacobson TZ et al: Laparoscopic surgery for pelvic pain associated with endometriosis, *Cochrane Database Syst Rev* 4,2001. Ⓐ
15. Proctor M et al: Surgical interruption of the pelvic nerve pathways for primary and secondary dysmenorrhoea, *Cochrane Database Syst Rev* 4,1999. Ⓐ
16. Beretta P et al: Randomised clinical trial of two laparoscopic treatments of endometriomas: cystectomy versus drainage and coagulation, *Fertil Steril* 709:1176, 1998. Reviewed in: *Clin Evid* 11:2391, 2004. Ⓐ

SUGGESTED READING

Winkel CA: Evaluation and management of women with endometriosis, *Obstetrics and gynecology,* 102(2):397, 2003.

AUTHORS: **WAN J. KIM, M.D.,** and **RUBEN ALVERO, M.D.**

BASIC INFORMATION

DEFINITION

Endometritis is defined as a uterine infection following delivery or abortion.

SYNONYMS

Endomyometritis
Metritis

ICD-9CM CODES
615.9 Endometritis

EPIDEMIOLOGY & DEMOGRAPHICS

- Overall rate of postpartum infection: estimated between 1% and 8%
- Most common genital tract infection following delivery
- Usually presents early in postpartum period; more commonly seen following C-section than vaginal delivery; also seen with an incomplete abortion (spontaneous abortion, legal abortion, or illegal abortion)
- More common in preterm deliveries
- Possible following any uterine manipulation in the presence of an undiagnosed cervicitis or vaginitis

PHYSICAL FINDINGS & CLINICAL PRESENTATION

- Postpartum oral temperature >37.8° C
- Localized uterine tenderness, purulent or foul lochia; physical examination revealing uterine or parametrial tenderness
- Nonspecific signs and symptoms such as malaise, abdominal pain, chills, and tachycardia

ETIOLOGY

Endometritis is usually associated with multiple organisms: group A or B streptococci, *Staphylococcus aureus* and *Bacteroides* species, *Neisseria gonorrhoeae, Chlamydia trachomatis,* enterococci, *Gardnerella vaginalis, E. coli,* and *Mycoplasma.*

DIAGNOSIS

DIFFERENTIAL DIAGNOSIS

Causes of postoperative or postprocedural infections

WORKUP

Diagnosis based on symptoms of fever, malaise, abdominal pain, uterine tenderness, and purulent, foul vaginal discharge

LABORATORY TESTS

CBC, blood cultures, and uterine culture

IMAGING STUDIES

Ultrasound may be useful if retained products are considered a possible source of infection.

TREATMENT

ACUTE GENERAL Rx

- In treating endometritis after a vaginal delivery, ampicillin 2 g IV q6h plus gentamicin loading dose IV or IM (2 mg/kg of body weight), followed by a maintenance dose (1.5 mg/kg of body weight) q8h are used.
- Regimen should be continued for at least 48 hr after substantial clinical improvement. If response is not adequate, check cultures and treat with appropriate antibiotics (Table 1-11).
- Endometritis following C-section should be treated with ampicillin 2 g IV q6h plus gentamicin loading dose IV or IM (2 mg/kg of body weight), followed by a maintenance dose (1.5 mg/kg of body weight) q8h and clindamycin 900 mg IV q8h. If *Chlamydia* is one of the etiologic agents, add doxycycline 100 mg PO bid for completion of a 14-day course of therapy (if breastfeeding, use erythromycin).

CHRONIC Rx

Watch for recurrent infection.

DISPOSITION

With appropriate antibiotic therapy, 95% to 98% cure rate

REFERRAL

For patients who do not respond within 48 to 72 hr of appropriate antibiotic therapy, obtain an infectious disease consult or gynecologic consultation.

EVIDENCE

Combined gentamicin and clindamycin is an appropriate treatment, and regimens with activity against penicillin-resistant anaerobic bacteria are better than those without.[1] Ⓐ

After clinical improvement of uncomplicated endometritis with intravenous therapy, oral therapy is unnecessary.[1] Ⓐ

Prophylactic antibiotics are effective in reducing endometritis in women undergoing cesarean section.

Prophylactic ampicillin and first-generation cephalosporins are equally effective in reducing postoperative endometritis following cesarean section and should be used as first line agents. The use of a more broad-spectrum agent or a multiple-dose regimen provides no additional clinical benefit.[2] Ⓐ

Antibiotics significantly reduce the risk of endometritis in women in preterm labor with intact membranes and in those with prelabor rupture of the membranes.

In the treatment of women in preterm labor with intact membranes, antibiotics, namely beta-lactams (alone or in combination with a macrolide), significantly reduce maternal chorioamnionitis and endometritis.[3] Ⓐ

The use of prophylactic antibiotics significantly reduces the risk of endometritis and chorioamnionitis in women with prelabor rupture of the membranes, at 36 weeks or beyond.[4] Ⓐ

Evidence-Based References

1. French LM, Smaill FM: Antibiotic regimens for endometritis after delivery. Reviewed in: Cochrane Library 4, Chichester, UK, 2004, John Wiley. Ⓐ
2. Hopkins L, Smaill F: Antibiotic prophylaxis regimens and drugs for cesarean section (Cochrane Review). Reviewed in: Cochrane Library 1, Chichester, UK, 2004, John Wiley.
3. King J, Flenady V: Prophylactic antibiotic for inhibiting preterm labour with intact membranes. Reviewed in: Cochrane Library 1, Chichester, UK, 2004, John Wiley. Ⓐ
4. Flenady V, King J: Antibiotics for prelabour rupture of membranes at or near term (Cochrane Review). Reviewed in: Cochrane Library 1, Chichester, UK, 2004, John Wiley.

AUTHORS: **GEORGE T. DANAKAS, M.D.,** and **RUBEN ALVERO, M.D.**

TABLE 1-11 Identified Causes of Poor Response to Antibiotic Therapy in Patients with Endometritis

Cause	Approximate Prevalence (%)
Infected mass, including abscess, hematoma, septic pelvic thrombophlebitis, pelvic cellulitis, retained placenta	40-50
Resistant organisms, commonly enterococci, in a patient receiving clindamycin-aminoglycoside or a cephalosporin	20
Additional cause, including catheter phlebitis, inadequate dose of antibiotics	10
No cause evident but response to empirical change in antibiotic therapy	20-30

From Gorbach SL: *Infectious diseases,* ed 2, Philadelphia, 1998, WB Saunders.

BASIC INFORMATION

DEFINITION

Enuresis refers to the voiding of urine into clothes or in bed that is usually involuntary in individuals who are expected to be continent (i.e., >5 yr of age). The diagnosis is made if voiding occurs at least twice a week for 3 mo. Primary enuresis refers to enuresis without a period of continence, whereas secondary enuresis occurs after a period of normal bladder control.

SYNONYMS

Urinary incontinence
Bed-wetting

ICD-9CM CODES
F98.0
DMS-IV Code 307.6

EPIDEMIOLOGY & DEMOGRAPHICS

PEAK INCIDENCE: Ages 5 to 10 yr
PREVALENCE (IN U.S.):
- Age 5: 7% of males and 3% of females
- Age 10: 3% of males and 2% of females
- Age 18: 1% of males

PREDOMINANT SEX: Twice as many males as females at all ages
PREDOMINANT AGE: By definition, enuresis does not begin before age 5, at which time the prevalence is highest, and decreases steadily thereafter at a rate of approximately 15% per year.
GENETICS:
- Approximately 75% of children with enuresis have a first-degree relative with enuresis.
- Almost twice as common in monozygotic than dizygotic twins.

PHYSICAL FINDINGS & CLINICAL PRESENTATION

Three enuresis subtypes are defined:
- Nocturnal only: usually occurs in first third of sleep, frequently during REM sleep; child may recall a dream with voiding
- Diurnal only: more frequent in girls and rarely after age 9 yr; voiding occurs in early afternoon on school days
- Combined nocturnal and diurnal enuresis; often called complex or complicated enuresis

ETIOLOGY

- Enuresis correlates with other maturational delays, particularly language, motor skills, and social development
- May be related to lax toilet training, stress, inability to concentrate urine, and altered smooth muscle physiology
- Diurnal enuresis associated with a higher rate of urinary tract infections

DIAGNOSIS

DIFFERENTIAL DIAGNOSIS

- May be associated with encopresis and sleep disorders such as sleep terrors; much less likely to be a primary psychological disorder.
- Organic causes of enuresis include diabetes mellitus, diabetes insipidus, bladder outlet obstruction, small bladder capacity, detrusor instability, urethral valves, meatal stenosis, cerebral palsy, spina bifida, pelvic mass, impacted stool, sedating medications, nocturnal seizures.

WORKUP

- History and physical examination to rule out anatomic abnormalities. Fluid intake and voiding diaries may be useful.
- Children frequently experience shame, so gentleness and care must be exercised when questioning or examining the child.

LABORATORY TESTS

- Urinalysis with specific gravity and urine culture if white cells or nitrites on analysis.
- Serum studies to rule out diabetes, electrolyte abnormalities, or renal dysfunction.

IMAGING STUDIES

- In complicated cases: sleep studies may be useful.
- If an anatomic abnormality suspected: renal ultrasound or intravenous pyelogram (IVP) possibly indicated, MRI of the spine if evidence of abnormalities of lower spine/perineum on exam.

TREATMENT

NONPHARMACOLOGIC THERAPY

Behavioral treatment:
- Alarm and pad technique—up to 80% cure rate, although 30% relapse
- Scheduled voiding to reduce the frequency of enuretic episodes
- Star charts to reward child for dry nights
- Punishment for enuresis is not effective

ACUTE GENERAL Rx

- Desmopressin (DDAVP) administered intranasally at bedtime significantly reduces the incidence of bed-wetting.
- Tricyclic antidepressants (imipramine)—efficacy supported by randomized control trials. Use with care in children.
- Serotonin reuptake inhibitors: lack of adequate trials is notable.
- Indomethacin suppositories may reduce normal prostaglandin inhibitory effects on antidiuretic hormone (ADH).

DISPOSITION

- After age 5 yr, the rate of spontaneous remissions is approximately 15% per year.
- Usually the disorder resolves by adolescence.
- Fewer than 1% will experience enuresis as adults.

REFERRAL

If coexisting psychiatric condition complicates the course of treatment

PEARLS & CONSIDERATIONS

Illness, hospitalization, family stressors may precipitate recurrent enuresis after a period of dryness

PATIENT/FAMILY EDUCATION

Bedwetting: Jasper to the Rescue! video available from Disney Educational Productions
(dep.disney.go.com/educational/index)

EVIDENCE

An enuresis alarm is an effective intervention for nocturnal enuresis in children.[1] Ⓐ

An alarm may be less effective initially than desmopressin, but an alarm appears to be more effective by the end of a treatment course and possibly in the long term. It appears to be more effective than tricyclic drugs both during treatment and afterwards.[1,2] Ⓑ

Relapse rates are reduced when overlearning (giving the child extra fluids at bedtime after he or she has become dry using the alarm) is added to the use of an alarm.[1] Ⓐ

Desmopressin significantly reduces the number of wet nights per week during treatment compared with placebo.[2] Ⓐ

However, there is some evidence that this reduction is not sustained after desmopressin therapy has been stopped.[2] Ⓑ

Most tricyclic drugs, including imipramine, are associated with a reduction of about one wet night per week during treatment, with about one fifth of children becoming dry while on treatment. However, these benefits may not be sustained after treatment has been stopped.[3] Ⓐ

Penalties for bed-wetting appear to be counterproductive.[1] Ⓐ

Evidence-Based References

1. Glazener CMA, Evans JHC, Peto RE: Alarm interventions for nocturnal enuresis in children. Reviewed in: Cochrane Library 1, Chichester, UK, 2004, John Wiley. ⒶⒷ
2. Glazener CMA, Evans JHC: Desmopressin for nocturnal enuresis in children. Reviewed in: Cochrane Library 1, Chichester, UK, 2004, John Wiley. ⒶⒷ
3. Glazener CMA, Evans JHC, Peto RE: Tricyclic and related drugs for nocturnal enuresis in children. Reviewed in: Cochrane Library 1, Chichester, UK, 2004, John Wiley. ⒶⒷ

SUGGESTED READINGS

Hjalmas K et al: Nocturnal enuresis: an international evidence based management strategy, *Urol* 171:2545, 2004.

Lyon C, Schnall J: What is the best treatment for nocturnal enuresis in children? *J Fam Pract* 54(10):905, 2005.

Makari J, Ruston HG: Nocturnal enuresis, *Am Fam Physician* 73(9):1611, 2006.

AUTHORS: **MITCHELL D. FELDMAN, M.D., M.PHIL.**, and **LAWRENCE HABER, M.D.**

BASIC INFORMATION

DEFINITION

Eosinophilic fasciitis is a rare inflammatory disease of the skin and subcutaneous tissue that is initially characterized by pain, swelling, and peripheral eosinophilia. This condition starts with symmetrical erythema, edema, and induration of an extremity or trunk and later may progress to sclerosis of the dermis and subcutaneous fascia leading to contractures.

SYNONYMS

Shulman's syndrome, diffuse fasciitis with eosinophilia

ICD-9CM CODES
728.89 Eosinophilic fasciitis

EPIDEMIOLOGY & DEMOGRAPHICS

- Males and females are affected equally.
- Most common in the fourth and fifth decades.

CLINICAL PRESENTATION

- Initial presentation consists of acute swelling and pain of the skin with or without erythema.
  - Extremities usually symmetrically involved.
  - Upper more commonly affected than lower extremities.
  - Face, fingers, and toes are spared.
  - Sunken veins may be seen when the extremity is elevated (Fig. 1-84). The groove sign marks the borders of different muscle groups.
  - Skin may appear deeply rippled (peau d'orange).
- Arthritis is found in 40% of cases in one series.
- Cranial and peripheral neuropathy (mononeuritis multiplex) may occur.
- Myalgia and weakness is common.
- Hematologic abnormalities are present in 10% of cases, including aplastic anemia, amegakaryocytic thrombocytopenia, myeloproliferative disorders, and hematological malignancies.
- Internal organs are generally not involved.
- Spontaneous resolution or improvement has been reported after 2 to 5 yr.

ETIOLOGY

The etiology is unclear. A defect in humoral immunity has been hypothesized to cause the disease.

DIAGNOSIS

DIFFERENTIAL DIAGNOSIS

- Systemic or localized sclerosis
- Systemic or localized scleroderma
- Scleroderma-like disorders
- Chemical-induced sclerosis
- Generalized lichen sclerosus et atrophicus
- Eosinophilia-myalgia syndrome
- Porphyria cutanea tarda
- Chronic Lyme borreliosis

WORKUP

- Physical examination to confirm characteristic distribution.
- Skin biopsy that penetrates to muscle is optimal for diagnosis:
  - Epidermis is usually normal.
  - Dermis may demonstrate mild inflammation with lymphocytes, histiocytes, plasma cells, and eosinophils with some fibrosis.
  - Moderate inflammation of subcutaneous tissue and sclerosis of fat septa.
  - Muscle demonstrates perivascular mixed inflammatory cell infiltrate.

LABORATORY TESTS

- Peripheral eosinophilia in up to 70%
- Elevated erythrocyte sedimentation rate (ESR) (29%)
- Hypergammaglobulinemia (35%)
- Creatine kinase is usually normal even in patients with myalgia
- Occasional thrombocytopenia, anemia

IMAGING STUDIES

MRI may be useful to detect the thickened fascia.

TREATMENT

ACUTE GENERAL Rx

- Although there are no controlled trials, corticosteroids (predonisone 1 mg/kg) are effective in most patients, but the duration and extent of symptom reduction are variable.
- Hydroxychloroquine is an alternative; may be as effective as steroids.
- In resistant cases, UVA photochemotherapy, cyclosporine, and antithymocyte globulin, methotrexate, D-penicillamine, and sulfasalasine have been successfully used.

CHRONIC Rx

Surgery is sometimes required to reduce contractures and maintain function.

DISPOSITION

- Prognosis is generally good with frequent spontaneous regression and response to steroids.
- Contractures are common.
- 10% may develop blood dyscrasias.

REFERRAL

To dermatology for biopsy to make definitive diagnosis. Functional impairment requires surgical evaluation.

PEARLS & CONSIDERATIONS

COMMENTS

- Eosinophilic fasciitis is a rare inflammatory disorder of unknown etiology with symmetric painful swelling and induration of the arms and legs with peripheral eosinophilia.
- Rapid onset, progression, and good response to systemic corticosteroids are characteristic of the disease.
- Prognosis is usually good.

SUGGESTED READINGS

Mosconi S et al: Eosinophilic fasciitis (Shulman syndrome), *Dermatology* 205(2):204, 2002.

Moulton SJ et al: Eosinophilic fasciitis: spectrum of MRI findings, *AJR Am J Roentgenol* 184(3):975, 2005.

AUTHOR: **ETSUKO AOKI, M.D., PH.D.**

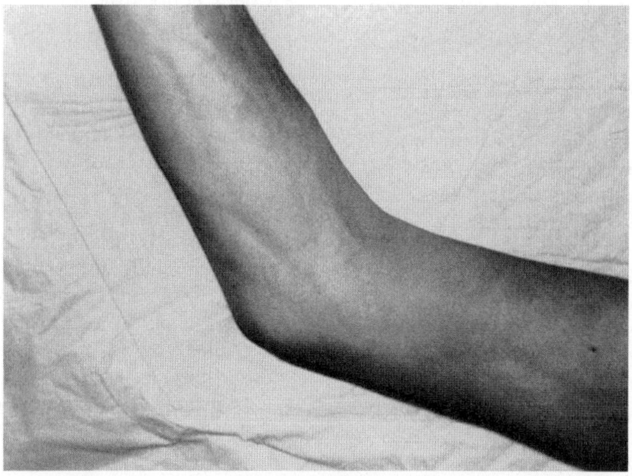

FIGURE 1-84 Eosinophilic fasciitis. This 29-year-old butcher had to stop working because of a generalized painful induration of his skin. Fingers were spared. As he raised his forearms, the collapsed veins appeared as grooves (the "groove sign"), which is pathognomonic of eosinophilic fasciitis. His condition subsided 4 years later, leaving joint contractures. (From Canoso J: *Rheumatology in primary care,* Philadelphia, 1997, WB Saunders.)

BASIC INFORMATION

DEFINITION

Eosinophilic pneumonias (EP) are a group of disorders characterized by pulmonary infiltrates, pulmonary parenchymal eosinophilia, and +/− peripheral blood eosinophilia. They manifest by different radiologic and clinical syndromes.

SYNONYMS

Simple pulmonary eosinophilia, chronic eosinophilic pneumonia, acute eosinophilic pneumonia, Churg-Strauss syndrome, idiopathic hypereosinophilic syndrome, allergic bronchopulmonary aspergillosis, parasite-induced, fungal-induced, and drug-induced pulmonary eosinophilia

ICD-9CM CODES
518.3 Eosinophilic pneumonia

EPIDEMIOLOGY & DEMOGRAPHICS

Varies depending on the specific cause

PHYSICAL FINDINGS & CLINICAL PRESENTATION

- Fever, cough, and shortness of breath
- Varies depending on the specific cause

ETIOLOGY

SIMPLE PULMONARY EOSINOPHILIA (LÖFFLER'S SYNDROME):
- Transient pulmonary infiltrates.
- Symptoms range from asymptomatic to dyspnea and dry cough.
- Usually idiopathic.
- May be secondary to parasitic infection or drugs (nitrofurantoin, penicillin).
- Remove the offending agent.
- If idiopathic and severe symptoms, then give glucocorticoid therapy.

IDIOPATHIC ACUTE EP:
- Absence of infection or other cause.
- Acute onset of fever, cough, dyspnea (<1 month).
- Bilateral diffuse infiltrates on CXR.
- Hypoxemia (P_aO_2 <60).
- Lung eosinophilia >25% on bronchoalveolar lavage (BAL).
- Steroids lead to rapid improvement.

IDIOPATHIC CHRONIC EP:
- Absence of infection or other cause.
- Productive cough, dyspnea, malaise, weight loss, night sweats, and fever (+/− hemoptysis/chest pain).
- Progressive pulmonary infiltrates.
- Blood eosinophilia not always present.
- Diagnose by BAL or lung biopsy.
- Spontaneous remission in 10% of cases.
- Treatment with glucocorticoids is rapidly effective.
- Relapses are common when glucocorticoids tapered.
- Prevalence of patients with asthma.

ALLERGIC BRONCHOPULMONARY ASPERGILLOSIS:
- Hypersensitivity reaction to *Aspergillus fungal spores.*
- Occurs most often in patients with asthma and atopy.
- Fever, flulike symptoms, myalgias, and lassitude.
- CXR: infiltrates (sometimes migratory) and atelectasis.
- Blood and sputum eosinophilia.
- Diagnosis by:
  1. *Aspergillus* isolation from multiple sputum samples
  2. Positive skin test to *Aspergillus*
  3. Elevated serum IgE
  4. *Aspergillus*-specific IgE and IgG
- Treatment: systemic corticosteroids.

TROPICAL PULMONARY EOSINOPHILIA:
- Onset of asthma, fever, paroxysmal cough and bronchospasm, marked blood eosinophilia.
- Basilar reticulonodular and alveolar infiltrates.
- High serum IgE levels.
- Presumed etiology: filariasis.

PULMONARY VASCULITIS (ALLERGIC GRANULOMATOSIS AND ANGIITIS):
- Vasculitis and necrotizing granulomatous inflammation that involves many organ systems.
- Blood eosinophilia and elevated IgE.

HYPEREOSINOPHILIC SYNDROME:
- A disease of persistently elevated eosinophils (>6 months) with no known cause.
- Cardiac problems are the prominent clinical feature with mural thrombi and endocardial/myocardial fibrosis.
- Hepatosplenomegaly is common.
- Fever, cough, weight loss, wheezing.
- Diagnosis of exclusion.
- Check echocardiogram.
- Treat with steroids if symptoms or cardiac abnormalities.

DRUG/TOXIN-INDUCED EP:
- Can have several different clinical presentations including simple pulmonary eosinophilia, chronic or acute.
- Symptoms resolve when offending drug is removed.
- Common drug/toxins cause: antibiotics, NSAIDs, amiodarone, bleomycin, captopril, gold salts, iodine, methotrexate, smoke, illicit drugs, radiation exposure.
- BAL is done to exclude infection or other lung disease.
- Lab evaluation is rarely diagnostic.

DIAGNOSIS

- Diagnosis varies depending on specific cause of pneumonia.
- Usually involves CXR, CT, peripheral eosinophil count, and BAL.

DIFFERENTIAL DIAGNOSIS

- Tuberculosis
- Brucellosis
- Fungal diseases
- Bronchogenic carcinoma
- Hodgkin's disease
- Immunoblastic lymphadenopathy
- Rheumatoid lung disease
- Sarcoidosis

WORKUP

Physical examination, laboratory tests, imaging, and bronchoscopy

LABORATORY TESTS

- WBC counts are often normal.
- Often blood eosinophilia.
- Elevated eosinophil count on BAL.

IMAGING STUDIES

CXR may show a variety of infiltrates depending on the cause of EP. CT demonstrates a more characteristic pattern and distribution of parenchymal opacities than CXR.

TREATMENT

- Varies depending on the cause.
- Remove offending agent or treat with appropriate antibiotic.
- Steroids may be helpful in many cases; doses and length of treatment depend on etiology of symptoms and response to treatment.
- Supportive respiratory care.

DISPOSITION

Prognosis is good if offending agent can be removed or an infectious etiology treated. Glucocorticoids have a good effect but relapse frequently recurs with tapering in the chronic idiopathic cases.

REFERRAL

To pulmonologist if a BAL is needed to establish the diagnosis.

PEARLS & CONSIDERATIONS

- History (including travel) and physical exam most important. Temporal association of eosinophilia and pulmonary abnormalities is an important diagnostic clue.

- Coccidiomycosis and Aspergillus can present as eosinophilic lung disease and are important to recognize because steroid therapy can produce progressive infection.
- Aspergillus from respiratory specimens does not always indicate true infection and may be colonization.
- Blood eosinophilia >1 × 10^9 eos/L or BAL >25% is helpful in narrowing diagnosis.
- Integrating the clinical, radiologic, and pathologic findings facilitates the initial and differential diagnoses of various eosinophilic lung diseases.

SUGGESTED READINGS

Alam M: Chronic eosinophilic pneumonia: a review, *South Med J* 100(1):49, 2007.

Allen J: Acute eosinophilic pneumonia, *Sem Resp Crit Care Med* 27(2):142, 2006.

Allen JN et al: The eosinophilic pneumonias, *Sem Resp Crit Care Med* 23(2):127, 2002.

Jeong YJ: Eosinophilic lung diseases: a clinical, radiologic and pathologic overview, *Radiographics* 27(3):617, 2007.

Leslie KO: Transbronchial biopsy interpretation in a patient with diffuse parenchymal lung disease, *Arch Pathol Lab Med* 131(3):407, 2007.

Marchand E: Idiopathic chronic eosinophilic pneumonia, *Sem Resp Crit Care Med* 27(2):134, 2006.

Mochimaru H et al: Clinicopathological differences between acute and chronic eosinophilic pneumonia, *Respirology* (10)1:76-85, 2005.

Solomon J: Drug, toxin, and radiation therapy-induced eosinophilic pneumonia, *Sem Resp Crit Care Med* 27(2):192, 2006.

AUTHOR: **CAROLYN J. O'CONNOR, M.D.**

BASIC INFORMATION

DEFINITION

Epicondylitis is an inflammation of the musculotendinous origin of the common extensors at the lateral elbow or the flexor pronator group at the medial elbow.

SYNONYMS

Tennis elbow (lateral epicondylitis)
Golfer's elbow (medial epicondylitis)

ICD-9CM CODES
726.31 Medial epicondylitis
726.32 Lateral epicondylitis
723.4 Radial nerve neuralgia

EPIDEMIOLOGY & DEMOGRAPHICS

PREVALENCE: 10% to 15% of regular (2 hr/wk) tennis players
PREVALENT AGE: 20 to 40 yr
The lateral side is involved 5 times more often than the medial.

PHYSICAL FINDINGS & CLINICAL PRESENTATION

- Local tenderness over affected epicondyle
- Reproduction of pain by resistance against wrist extension (lateral) (Fig. 1-85) or flexion (medial)

ETIOLOGY

- Unknown
- Overuse probably causing minor tendinous tears resulting in inflammation
- Posterior interosseous nerve syndrome: compression of this nerve has occasionally been cited as a possible etiology, especially in cases that have failed traditional medical and surgical treatment. In this disorder, the site of tenderness is 2 to 3 cm distal to the epicondyle

DIAGNOSIS

DIFFERENTIAL DIAGNOSIS

- Cervical radiculopathy
- Intraarticular elbow pathology (osteoarthritis, osteochondritis dissecans, loose body)
- Radial nerve compression
- Ulnar neuropathy
- Medial collateral ligament instability

IMAGING STUDIES

Traction spur or minor soft tissue calcification may be present on plain radiography. Other studies are not usually needed.

TREATMENT

- Rest, restricted activities
- Ice after exercise
- Stretching exercise program
- NSAIDs
- Local steroid/lidocaine injection (Table 1-12; Fig. 1-86)
- Counterforce brace
- Proper technique in sports activities
- Intermittent immobilization

DISPOSITION

Disorder is self-limited in most cases. Resolution of symptoms may take months to years.

REFERRAL

- If symptoms fail to respond to medical management
- For surgical consideration

PEARLS & CONSIDERATIONS

Concepts are changing in regard to the underlying pathology of epicondylitis and similar musculoskeletal conditions which were always thought to be inflammatory in nature. Many are now considered more degenerative as evidenced by tissue specimens that lack the cellular changes expected with inflammation.

EVIDENCE

The following evidence relates to lateral epicondylitis; it is not known whether these findings can be clinically applied to patients with medial epicondylitis.

Current evidence cannot support or refute the use of oral NSAIDs for lateral epicondylitis.[1]

Local corticosteroid injections are significantly more beneficial in the short term compared with oral NSAIDs, but this effect is not sustained.[1] Ⓐ

Evidence suggests that corticosteroid injections are effective and provide short-term benefits compared with placebo, local anesthetic injections, physical therapies, and orthoses, but these findings are limited by the small size and methodologic flaws of the relevant trials. More study is required to confirm these findings.[2–6] ⒶⒷ

Conflicting evidence exists regarding the role of extracorporeal shock wave therapy (ESWT) in the treatment of lateral elbow pain. A systematic review identified two randomized controlled trials (RCTs), the first finding that ESWT was significantly far more effective than placebo, and the second finding no difference between active and placebo treatment. Meta-analysis of these results failed to detect any significant benefits from ESWT. More research is required before the clinical role of shock wave therapy is understood.[7] Ⓑ

Evidence-Based References

1. Green S et al: Non-steroidal anti-inflammatory drugs (NSAIDs) for treating lateral elbow pain in adults. Reviewed in: Cochrane Library, 2, Chichester, UK, 2004, John Wiley. Ⓐ
2. Smidt N et al: Corticosteroid injections for lateral epicondylitis: a systematic review, *Pain* 96:23, 2002. Reviewed in: *Clin Evid* 11:1633, 2004. ⒶⒷ

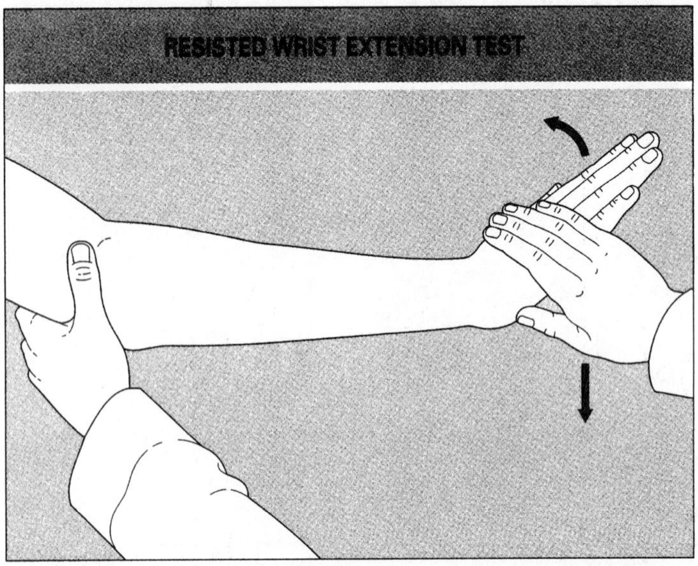

FIGURE 1-85 Resisted wrist extension to test for lateral epicondylitis. The examiner asks the patient to try to extend the wrist but prevents movement by fixing the wrist; this puts tension on the lateral epicondyle without moving the elbow and reproduces the pain of lateral epicondylitis. (From Klippel J, Dieppe P, Ferri F [eds]: *Primary care rheumatology,* London, 1999, Mosby.)

3. Newcomber K et al: Corticosteroid injection in early treatment of lateral epicondylitis, *Clin J Sport Med* 11:214, 2001. Reviewed in: *Clin Evid* 11:1633,2004. Ⓑ
4. Sems A et al: Extracorporeal shock wave therapy in the treatment of chronic tendinopathies, *J Am Acad Orthop Surg* 14:195, 2006.
5. Smidt N et al: Corticosteroid injections, physiotherapy, or a wait-and-see policy for lateral epicondylitis: a randomised controlled trial, *Lancet* 359:657, 2002. Reviewed in: *Clin Evid* 11:1633, 2004. Ⓐ
6. Struijs PAA et al: Orthotic devices for the treatment of tennis elbow (Cochrane Review). In: Cochrane Library, 2, Chichester, UK, 2004, John Wiley. Reviewed in: *Clin Evid* 11:1633, 2004. Ⓑ
7. Buchbinder R et al: Shock wave therapy for lateral elbow pain. Reviewed in: Cochrane Library, 2, Chichester, UK, 2004, John Wiley. Ⓑ

SUGGESTED READINGS

Ashe MC, McCauley T, Khan KM: Tendinopathies in the upper extremity: A paradigm shift, *J Hand Ther* 17(8):329, 2004.

Bunata RE et al: Anatomic factors related to the cause of tennis elbow, *J Bone Joint Surg* 89:1955, 2007.

Calfee RP et al: Management of lateral epicondylitis: current concepts, *J Am Acad Orthop Surg* 16:19, 2008.

Cole BJ, Schumacher HR: Injectable corticosteroids in modern practice, *J Am Acad Orthop Surg* 13:37, 2005.

David TS: Medial elbow pain in the throwing athlete, *Orthopedics* 26:94, 2003.

Haake M et al: Extracorporeal shock wave therapy in the treatment of lateral epicondylitis, *J Bone Joint Surg* 84(A):1982, 2002.

Nirschl RP, Ashman ES: Tennis elbow tendinosis (epicondylitis), *Instr Course Lect* 53:587, 2004.

Placzek R et al: Treatment of chronic radial epicondylitis with botulinum toxin A: a double-blind, placebo-controlled randomized multicenter study, *J Bone Joint Surg* 89A:255, 2007.

Rompe JD et al: Repetitive low-energy shock wave treatment for chronic lateral epicondylitis in tennis players, *Am J Sports Med* 32:734, 2004.

Sems A et al: Extracorporeal shock wave therapy in the treatment of chronic tendinopathies, *J Am Acad Orthop Surg* 14:195, 2006.

Smidt N et al: Corticosteroid injections, physiotherapy, or wait-and-see policy for lateral epicondylitis: a randomized controlled trial, *Lancet* 359:657, 2002.

AUTHOR: **LONNIE R. MERCIER, M.D.**

TABLE 1-12 Guidelines for Common Steroid Injections

Using 1 ml of the appropriate steroid, the volume is increased by the addition of local anesthetic. Injecting a "space" should not cause pain during the injection. If it does, the needle tip may be in the synovium, capsule, or fat pad, and the needle should be redirected or the shot may not be as effective. Injecting soft tissue should be performed slowly so as not to cause pain from the sudden volume pressure.

Site	Diagnosis	Needle Size (gauge, inches)	Anesthetic Volume (ml)
Subacromial bursa	Rotator cuff tendinitis	22, $1\frac{1}{2}$	4 to 5
Bicipital groove	Biceps tendinitis	22, $1\frac{1}{2}$	2 to 3
A-C joint	Arthritis	25, $1\frac{1}{2}$	1 to 2
Lat, med epicondyle	Epicondylitis	25, $\frac{5}{8}$	1.5
First extensor sheath	De Quervain's disease	25, $\frac{5}{8}$	1.5
Trochanteric bursa	Tendinitis	22, spinal	4 to 5
Knee joint	Arthritis	22, $1\frac{1}{2}$	5 to 10
Knee, soft tissue	Tendinitis	25, $1\frac{1}{2}$	3 to 4
Plantar fascia	Fasciitis	25, $1\frac{1}{2}$	1.0
Toe MPJ	Arthritis	25, $\frac{5}{8}$	1.5

From Mercier LR: *Practical orthopedics,* ed 5, St Louis, 2000, Mosby.

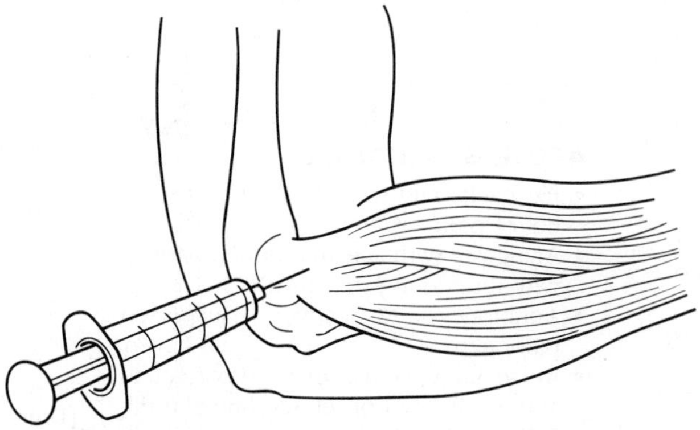

FIGURE 1-86 Soft-tissue injection for lateral epicondylitis. The patient is supine, and the elbow is flexed 90 degrees. A 25-gauge needle is used to inject the tender spot, which is usually about 1-cm distal to the bony epicondyle. (From Mercier L: *Practical orthopedics,* ed 5, St Louis, 2000, Mosby.)

BASIC INFORMATION

DEFINITION

Epididymitis is an inflammatory reaction of the epididymis caused by either an infectious agent or local trauma.

SYNONYMS

Nonspecific bacterial epididymitis
Sexually transmitted epididymitis

ICD-9CM CODES
604.90 Nonvenereal epididymitis
098.0 Gonococcal epididymitis

EPIDEMIOLOGY & DEMOGRAPHICS

INCIDENCE (IN U.S.): Cause of >600,000 visits to physicians per year
PEAK INCIDENCE: Sexually active years
PREDOMINANT SEX: Exclusive to males
PREDOMINANT AGE: All ages affected but usually in sexually active men or older males
CONGENITAL: Congenital urologic structural disorders possibly predisposing to infections

PHYSICAL FINDINGS & CLINICAL PRESENTATION

- Tender swelling of the scrotum with erythema, usually unilateral testicular pain and tenderness
- Dysuria and/or urethral discharge
- Fever and signs of systemic illness (less common)
- Pain and redness on scrotal examination
- Hydrocele or even epididymoorchitis, especially late
- Chronic draining scrotal sinuses with a "beadlike" enlargement of the vas deferens in tuberculous disease

ETIOLOGY

- In young, sexually active men, the most common infectious agents isolated are *N. gonorrhoeae* and *Chlamydia trachomatis*.
- In men >35 yr or with underlying urologic disease:
  1. Gram-negative aerobic rods are predominant.
  2. Similar organisms are found in men following invasive urologic procedures.
  3. Gram-positive cocci are rarely seen in these groups.
  4. Mycobacteria are also a cause of epididymitis.
- Young, prepubertal boys may present with epididymitis caused by coliform bacteria; almost always a complication of underlying urologic disease such as reflux.
- Recently, in AIDS patients, CMV and *Salmonella* epididymitis have been described. CMV may have a negative urine culture. Toxoplasmosis should also be considered as a cause of epididymitis in AIDS patients.

DIAGNOSIS

DIFFERENTIAL DIAGNOSIS

- Orchitis
- Testicular torsion, trauma, or tumor
- Epididymal cyst
- Hydrocele
- Varicocele
- Spermatocele
- Testicular torsion should be considered in all cases.

WORKUP

- Consideration of a full assessment of the urologic tract in patients with bacterial infection, especially if recurrent
- Imaging with sonogram or IVP (possibly procedures of choice)
- If discharge is present: cultures and Gram stain smear of urethral exudate
- In sexually active men: gonococcal cultures of the throat and rectum possibly of value
- If testicular torsion a consideration: radionuclear imaging
- Examination of first void uncentrifuged urine for leukocytes if the urethral Gram stain is negative. A culture and Gram-stained smear of this urine specimen should be obtained along with nucleic acid amplifications studies (ligase chain reaction [LCR]) from urine samples for gonorrhea and *Chlamydia spp.*

LABORATORY TESTS

- Urinalysis and urine culture if dysuria is present or if urinary tract infection is suspected
- VDRL in sexually active men
- PPD placed and chest x-ray viewed if TB suspected
- Rarely, biopsy to assure the diagnosis of tuberculous epididymitis
- HIV testing and counseling

TREATMENT

ACUTE GENERAL Rx

- Ice packs and scrotal elevation for relief of pain
- Analgesia with acetaminophen with or without codeine or NSAIDs
- Antibiotics to cover suspected pathogens
- In sexually active men, doxycycline 100 mg PO bid or tetracycline 500 mg PO qid for 10 days to cover both gonococci and chlamydia; ceftriaxone 250 mg IM is a single dose may be adequate for gonococci alone
- Best treatment for older men with gram-negative bacteriuria: ofloxacin 300 mg PO bid for 10 days or levofloxacin 500 mg PO qd for 10 days
- *Pseudomonas* covered by ciprofloxacin or cefepime (2 g IV q12h)
- Gentamicin in toxic-appearing patients (1 mg/kg IV q8h following a loading dose of 2 mg/kg): doses must be adjusted for renal function and these agents may be more toxic
- Vancomycin (1 g IV q12h) to cover suspected gram-positive infections
- Surgical aspiration of local abscesses or even open surgical drainage
- Diabetics: especially prone to develop more extensive scrotal infections, including Fournier's gangrene
- Reinforcement of compliance with antibiotics to avoid partial treatment

CHRONIC Rx

- Repair of underlying structural defects is considered especially if infections are severe or recur.
- Surgical repair of reflux in young boys should be undertaken promptly and at a young age when possible.
- Sex partners of patient should be referred for evaluation and treatment.

DISPOSITION

Usually self-limited

REFERRAL

- If abscess or chronic structural problems suspected
- If other diagnosis, such as testicular torsion, strongly considered

PEARLS & CONSIDERATIONS

- Recurrent epididymitis in sexually active men is usually related to failure to simultaneously treat sexual partners for STDs.
- Recurrent epididymitis in non-sexually active men is generally related to structural-anatomic defects in the genitourinary system or relapsing disease from inadequate initial treatment or antimicrobial resistance.
- Tuberculous epididymitis fails to respond to seemingly adequate antimicrobial therapy even without characteristic radiographic changes on chest films.

SUGGESTED READINGS

Abul F et al: The acute scrotum: a review of 40 cases, *Med Princ Pract* 14(3):177, 2005.
Chen MY et al: Trends in clinical encounters for pelvic inflammatory disease and epididymitis in a national sample of Australian general practices, *Int J STD AIDS* 17(6):384, 2006.
Drury NE et al: Management of acute epididymitis: are European guidelines being followed? *Eur Urol* 46(4):522, 2004.
Nickel JC et al: Prevalence, diagnosis, characterization, and treatment of prostatitis, interstitial cystitis, and epididymitis in outpatient urological practice: the Canadian PIE Study, *Urology* 66(5):935, 2005.

AUTHORS: **GLENN G. FORT, M.D., M.P.H., JOSEPH J. LIEBER, M.D.**, and **DENNIS J. MIKOLICH, M.D.**

BASIC INFORMATION

DEFINITION

Epiglottitis is a rapidly progressive cellulitis of the epiglottis and adjacent soft tissue structures with the potential to cause abrupt airway obstruction.

SYNONYMS

Supraglottitis
Cherry-red epiglottitis

ICD-9CM CODES
464.30 Epiglottitis

EPIDEMIOLOGY

INCIDENCE (IN U.S.): Highest in young children, 2 to 4 yr old
INCIDENCE (IN U.S.): Unknown
PEAK INCIDENCE: Peaks in young boys ages 2 to 4 yr, but it is reported in adults as well
PREDOMINANT SEX: Males

PHYSICAL FINDINGS & CLINICAL PRESENTATION

- Irritability, fever, dysphonia, and dysphagia
- Respiratory distress, with child tending to lean up and forward
- Often, drooling or oral secretions
- Often, presence of tachycardia and tachypnea
- On visualization, edematous and cherry-red epiglottis
- Often, no classic barking cough as seen in croup
- Possibly fulminant course (especially in children), leading to complete airway obstruction

ETIOLOGY

- In children, *Haemophilus influenzae* type b is usual.
- In adults, *H. influenzae* can be isolated from blood and/or epiglottis (about 26% of cases).
- Pneumococci, streptococci, and staphylococci are also implicated.
- Role of viruses in epiglottitis unclear.

DIAGNOSIS

DIFFERENTIAL DIAGNOSIS

- Croup
- Angioedema
- Retropharyngeal or peritonsillar abscess
- Diphtheria
- Foreign body aspiration
- Lingual tonsillitis

WORKUP

- Cultures of blood and urine
- Lateral neck radiograph to show an enlarged epiglottis, ballooning of the hypopharynx, and normal subglottic structures (Fig. 1-87)
  1. Radiographs are of only moderate sensitivity and specificity and take time to perform.
  2. Visualization of the epiglottis may be safer in adults than in children.
- Cultures of the epiglottis

LABORATORY TESTS

- CBC: may reveal a leukocytosis with a shift to the left
- Chest x-ray examination: may reveal evidence of pneumonia in close to 25% of cases
- Cultures of blood, urine, and the epiglottis, as noted previously

TREATMENT

ACUTE GENERAL Rx

- Maintenance of adequate airway is critical.
- Early placement of an endotracheal or nasotracheal tube in a child is advised.
- Closely follow the adult patient, if no signs of airway obstruction, and defer intubation.
- In children, visualization and intubation are best done in the most controlled environment.
- *H. influenzae* in children is less common thanks to the HIB vaccine.
- Use antibiotics such as ceftriaxone (80 to 100 mg/kg/day in two divided doses), cefotaxime (50 to 180 mg/kg/day in four divided doses), or ampicillin (200 mg/kg/day in four divided doses) with chloramphenicol (75 to 100 mg/kg/day in four divided doses).
- If possible, obtain cultures before initiating antibiotics.
- Treat adult patients with similar antibiotic regimens.
- If there is an unvaccinated child at home (or in a day care center) who is >4 yr and living with an index case, give close family contacts of the patient (including adults) rifampin 20 mg/kg/day for 4 days (up to 600 mg/day) for prophylaxis.
- Role of epinephrine or corticosteroids in the management of epiglottitis is not firmly established.

DISPOSITION

Invasive *Haemophilus influenzae* infections and epiglottitis are reportable illnesses; this may be particularly important in recognizing an outbreak in a day care center with unvaccinated children.

REFERRAL

- Close cooperation between the pediatrician or internist, anesthesiologist, and otorhinolaryngologist, especially when epiglottis is visualized and when the patient requires endotracheal intubation
- Best managed in a critical care setting or ICU

PEARLS & CONSIDERATIONS

The incidence of epiglottitis has diminished markedly since the introduction of the conjugate vaccine against *H. influenzae* serotype B into routine childhood immunization.

SUGGESTED READINGS

Hafidh MA et al: Acute epiglottitis in adults: a recent experience with 10 cases, *J Laryngol Otol* 120(4):310, 2006.

Wood N et al: Epiglottitis in Sydney before and after the introduction of vaccination against Haemophilus influenzae type b disease, *Intern Med J*, 35(9):530, 2005.

AUTHORS: **GLENN G. FORT, M.D., M.P.H., JOSEPH J. LIEBER, M.D.,** and **DENNIS J. MIKOLICH, M.D.**

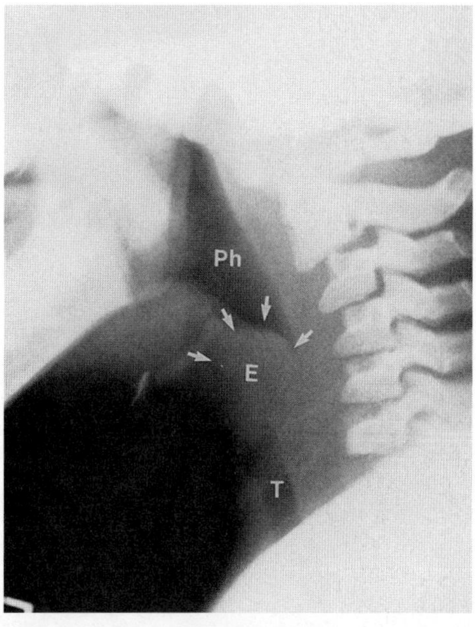

FIGURE 1-87 Epiglottitis. A lateral soft tissue view of the neck shows a ballooned pharynx *(Ph)* with swollen epiglottis *(E)* in the shape of a large thumbprint *(arrows)*. *T*, Trachea. (From Mettler FA [ed]: *Primary care radiology,* Philadelphia, 2000, WB Saunders.)

BASIC INFORMATION

DEFINITION

Episcleritis is an inflammation of the episclera, or thin layer of vascular elastic tissue between the sclera and conjunctiva.

ICD-9CM CODES
379.0 Scleritis and episcleritis

EPIDEMIOLOGY & DEMOGRAPHICS

INCIDENCE (IN U.S.): Relatively rare in an ophthalmologic practice
PEAK INCIDENCE: Most common in middle and old age
PREDOMINANT SEX: None
PREDOMINANT AGE: 43 yr

PHYSICAL FINDINGS & CLINIAL PRESENTATION

- Red, vascular injection of conjunctiva with engorged and enlarged blood vessels beneath the conjunctions (Fig. 1-88)
- Pain in area of inflammation which is usually localized

ETIOLOGY

Associated with collagen-vascular diseases, vasculitis, trauma, often nonspecific

DIAGNOSIS

DIFFERENTIAL DIAGNOSIS

- Acute glaucoma
- Conjunctivitis
- Scleritis
- Subconjunctival hemorrhage
- Congenital or lymphoid masses
- The differential diagnosis of "red eye" is described in Section II

WORKUP

Eye examination, general check-up for collagen vascular disease or other autoimmune diseases

LABORATORY TESTS

Studies for collagen-vascular disease (e.g., ANA, ESR, RF)

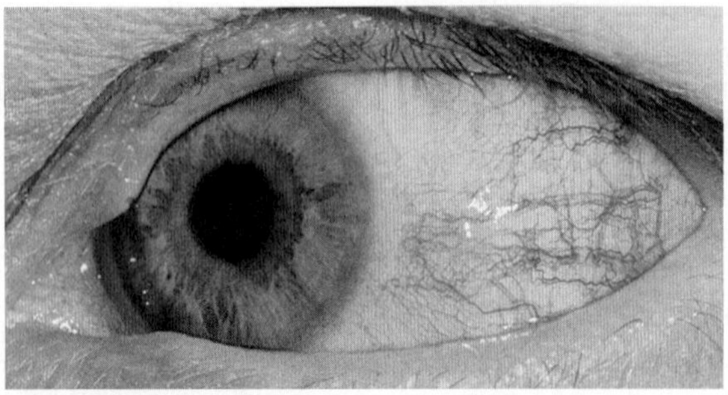

FIGURE 1-88 Nodular episcleritis in a patient with gout. (From Palay D [ed]: *Ophthalmology for the primary care physician,* St Louis, 1997, Mosby.)

TREATMENT

NONPHARMACOLOGIC THERAPY

Warm compresses

ACUTE GENERAL Rx

- Topical steroids, 1% prednisolone if no glaucoma; nonsteroidals if there is a tendency for glaucoma
- NSAIDs: treat underlying systemic disease

CHRONIC Rx

NSAIDs such as Voltaren or Acular qid

DISPOSITION

Close follow-up needed

REFERRAL

To ophthalmologist if patient unresponsive to treatment after a few days

PEARLS & CONSIDERATIONS

COMMENTS

- Often associated with collagen vascular disease
- Usually related to systemic disease

SUGGESTED READINGS

Jabs DA et al: Episcleritis and scleritis: clinical features and treatment results, *Am J Ophthalmol* 130(4):469, 2000.

Paresio CE, Meier FM: Systemic disorders associated with episcleritis and scleritis, *Curr Opin Ophthalmology* 12(6):471, 2002.

Shaw C et al: Rheumatoid arthritis and ocular involvement, *J Indian Med Assoc* 101(9)537, 2003.

AUTHOR: **MELVYN KOBY, M.D.**

BASIC INFORMATION

DEFINITION

Epistaxis is defined as bleeding from the nose or nasal hemorrhage and is classified as either anterior or posterior.

SYNONYMS

Nosebleed

ICD-9CM CODES
784.7 Epistaxis

EPIDEMIOLOGY & DEMOGRAPHICS

- Epistaxis accounts for 1 of 200 ED visits in the U.S.
- It increases in frequency after age 20 yr and reaches the highest levels among the elderly population.
- Over 80% of cases of epistaxis are anterior in origin (Little's area) and occur from Kiesselbach's plexus (Fig. 1-89).
- Only 5% of patients with epistaxis have posterior bleeds.

PHYSICAL FINDINGS & CLINICAL PRESENTATION

- Nosebleed
- Hypotension and hemodynamic instability with acute severe epistaxis

ETIOLOGY

- Approximately 90% of epistaxes are idiopathic.
- Common identifiable causes are:
  1. Cold, dry environment
  2. Trauma (nose picking, accidents, and physical altercations)
  3. Structural deformities (septal deviations/spurs, chronic perforations)
  4. Inflammatory (rhinosinusitis, nasal polyposis)
  5. Allergies
  6. Foreign bodies in the nasal cavity
  7. Tumors (juvenile angiofibroma)
  8. Irritants
  9. Hypertension
  10. Coagulopathy (hemophilia, von Willebrand's disease, thrombocytopenia)
  11. Osler-Weber-Rendu disease
  12. Renal failure
  13. Drugs: aspirin, NSAIDs, warfarin, alcohol, sildenafil, and tadalafil
  14. Blood vessel disorders (connective tissue disease, hereditary hemorrhagic telangiectasia)
  15. Pseudoaneurysm and aneurysm of the internal carotid artery might present as epistaxis

DIAGNOSIS

A good attempt should be made to directly visualize the source of bleeding to confirm the diagnosis and determine the best treatment.

DIFFERENTIAL DIAGNOSIS

Pseudoepistaxis must be ruled out. Common extranasal sites of bleeding that can simulate epistaxis include:

1. Pulmonary hemoptysis
2. Bleeding esophageal varices
3. Tumor bleeding from the pharynx, larynx, or trachea

WORKUP

The workup should include laboratory blood testing to exclude obvious causes. Type and cross in anticipation of transfusion if the bleeding is severe.

LABORATORY TESTS

- Hemoglobin and hematocrit
- Platelet count
- BUN/creatinine
- Coagulation studies (PT and PTT)
- Type and crossmatching of blood products

IMAGING STUDIES

X-ray studies are usually not helpful.

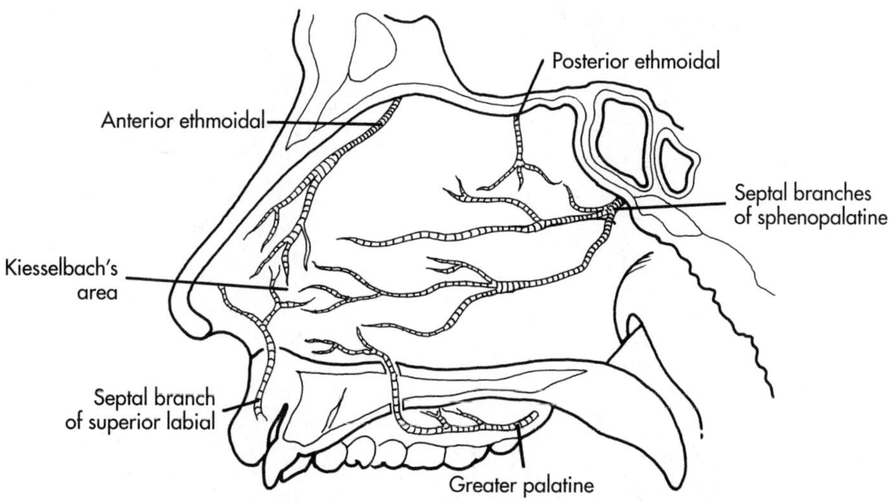

FIGURE 1-89 Kiesselbach's plexus on the anterior septum derives blood supply from the superior labial, descending palatine, and sphenopalatine arteries. (From Noble J: *Primary care medicine,* ed 3, St Louis, 2001, Mosby.)

TREATMENT

NONPHARMACOLOGIC THERAPY

- Digital compression or pinching of the lower soft cartilaginous part of the nose for 10 min is the method of choice
- Cotton or tissue plug
- The patient should be sitting and leaning forward, breathing through the mouth, allowing blood to flow out of the nostrils as opposed to bending backward, which would allow the blood to flow down the throat
- Application of cold compresses to the bridge of the nose to cause a vasoconstrictive effect; the patient may also suck on ice to achieve this effect

ACUTE GENERAL Rx

Anterior Epistaxis

- Local vasoconstriction is performed by moistening a cotton pledget with either:
  1. 4% lidocaine with 1:1000 epinephrine
  2. 4% lidocaine with 1% phenylephrine (Neo-Synephrine)
  3. 4% lidocaine with 0.05% oxymetazoline (Afrin)
  4. 4% cocaine or cocaine 25% in paraffin base ointment and inserting the pledget into the nasal cavity with bayonet forceps.
- Cauterization with silver nitrate or trichloroacetic acid is performed once hemostasis is achieved.
- Anterior nasal packing is needed when local measures are unsuccessful. Nasal packing is performed under local anesthesia, and is done by inserting Vaseline gauze strips in layers from the floor of the nasal cavity to the front entrance of the nasal orifice. Enough pressure is placed to tamponade the epistaxis (Fig. 1-90).
- Other commercially available nasal packing using sponge packs that expand when exposed to blood or moisture can be used for anterior epistaxis.

Posterior Epistaxis

- Posterior nasal packing
  1. Commercially available nasal sponge packing can be applied
  2. Rolled gauze technique (see Dai, Jurges, 2005)
- Foley catheter balloon insertion into the nasopharynx can be tried in patients with posterior epistaxis (for the proper technique, please refer to the reference).

CHRONIC Rx

- If acute treatment fails to stop the bleeding or the site of bleeding cannot be located, electrocautery, or endoscopic cauterization can be used.
- Electrocautery is performed after suitable anesthesia such as application of a topical anesthetic followed by local anesthetic injection. Only one side of the nasal septum should be cauterized at a time as perforation can result from bilateral cauterization.
- Arterial ligation or embolization has been used in refractory posterior epistaxis.
- For cases involving irritated or inflamed mucosa, a conservative regimen of triamcinolone 0.025%, nemdyn, nasalate, or equivalent cream should be applied once a week, combined with nightly application of a small quantity of petroleum jelly to the septum before bedtime.

DISPOSITION

- Most cases of anterior epistaxis from Kiesselbach's plexus can be stopped by nasal compression and local vasoconstriction or cauterization.
- Nasal packing with gauze or sponge can control 90% of anterior epistaxis.
- Anterior and posterior packs are removed in 2 to 3 days. Hospital admission should be considered in those patients who cannot be expected to return for prompt follow-up because prolonged packing increases the risk of pressure necrosis, toxic shock syndrome, sinus infections, and other complications.
- Although rare, epistaxis can lead to death by aspiration of blood, hemodynamic compromise from rapid excessive blood loss, or toxic shock syndrome.

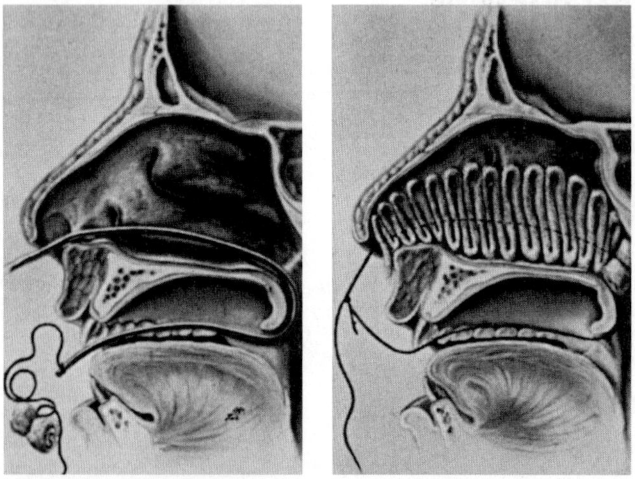

FIGURE 1-90 Packing of the nose for epistaxis with a postnasal pack and an anterior nose pack. (From Boies LR et al: *Fundamentals of otolaryngology: a textbook of ear, nose, and throat diseases*, ed 4, Philadelphia, 1964, WB Saunders.)

REFERRAL

- If epistaxis cannot be controlled, ENT specialist should be called for assistance.
- ENT specialist should be consulted in any patient with posterior epistaxis requiring posterior packing.

PEARLS & CONSIDERATIONS

COMMENTS

- Silver nitrate cauterization, if done on both sides of the nasal septum, can lead to septal perforation and should be discouraged.
- If anterior nasal packing is done, broad-spectrum antibiotics (e.g., amoxicillin-clavulanate 250 mg PO tid or trimethoprim-sulfamethoxazole 1 tab PO bid) are used until the anterior packs are removed.
- Complications of nasal packing include
  1. Aspiration
  2. Dislodged packing
  3. Infection
  4. Nasal trauma

SUGGESTED READINGS

Dai A, Jurges E: The problem with nose bleeds, *Emerg Med J* 22(8):596, 2005.

Leong SC et al: No frills management of epistaxis, *Emerg Med J* 22(7):470, 2005.

Pallin DJ et al: Epidemiology of epistaxis in U.S. emergency departments, 1992 to 2001, *Ann Emerg Med* 46(1):77, 2005.

Pope LE, Hobbs CG: Epistaxis: an update on current management, *Postgrad Med J* 81(955):309, 2005.

AUTHOR: **ABDULBAKI ABDULRAHMAN, M.D.**

BASIC INFORMATION

DEFINITION

Epstein-Barr virus infection refers to a disease caused by Epstein-Barr virus (EBV), a human herpesvirus.

SYNONYMS

Infectious mononucleosis (IM)

ICD-9CM CODES
075 Mononucleosis

EPIDEMIOLOGY & DEMOGRAPHICS

INCIDENCE (IN U.S.): 45 cases/100,000 persons/yr of infectious mononucleosis (IM)

PREDOMINANT SEX: Neither, although peak incidence occurs about 2 yr earlier in women

PREDOMINANT AGE:
- Clinical evidence of infectious mononucleosis: occurs most commonly at ages 15 to 24 yr.
- EBV infection: occurs earlier in life in lower socioeconomic groups.

PHYSICAL FINDINGS & CLINICAL PRESENTATION

- Most EBV infections either are asymptomatic or cause a nonspecific illness.
- Incubation period is 1 to 2 mo, possibly followed by a prodrome of anorexia, malaise, headache, and chills; after several days, clinical triad of pharyngitis, fever, and adenopathy may appear, accompanied by fatigue and malaise.
- Pharyngitis is usually the most severe symptom; exudates are common.
- Lymphadenopathy is most prominent in the cervical region but may be diffuse.
- Splenomegaly is possible, most commonly during the second week of illness.
- Rash is uncommon, but will occur in nearly all patients who receive ampicillin.
- Possible IM presentation: fever and adenopathy without pharyngitis.
- Although complications may be severe, they are also uncommon and tend to resolve completely.
- Involvement of the hematologic, pulmonary, cardiac, or nervous systems possible; splenic rupture is rare.
- IM is usually a self-limited illness, but symptoms of malaise and fatigue may last months before resolving.
- Besides IM, EBV is also related to lymphoproliferative syndromes in transplant recipients and in AIDS patients.
- Increasing evidence showing an association between EBV infection and both African Burkitt's lymphoma and nasopharyngeal carcinoma.

ETIOLOGY

- Ubiquitous virus
- Prevalence is higher in lower socioeconomic groups than in age-matched controls in more affluent groups
- Infection during childhood is much less likely to cause significant illness
- Frequency of IM in late adolescence is attributed to the onset of social contact between the sexes
- Close personal contact is usually necessary for transmission, although EBV is occasionally transmitted by blood transfusion; transfer via saliva while kissing may be responsible for many cases

DIAGNOSIS

DIFFERENTIAL DIAGNOSIS

- Heterophile-negative infectious mononucleosis caused by CMV
- Although clinical presentation similar, CMV more frequently follows transfusion
- Bacterial and viral causes of pharyngitis
- Toxoplasmosis
- Acute retroviral syndrome of HIV
- Lymphoma
- Lyme disease

WORKUP

Heterophile antibody and CBC

LABORATORY TESTS

- Increased WBC common, with a relative lymphocytosis and neutropenia
- Hallmark of IM: atypical lymphocytes (not pathognomonic)
- Mild thrombocytopenia
- Falling Hematocrit signals the possibility of splenic rupture or immune hemolytic anemia
- Elevated hepatocellular enzymes and cryoglobulins in most cases
- Heterophile antibody
  1. As measured by the Monospot test, may be positive at presentation or may appear later in the course of illness.
  2. Negative test is repeated if clinical suspicion is high.
  3. A positive test has been reported with primary HIV infection.
- Virus-specific antibodies possibly responding to IM: determination of these EBV-specific antibodies is rarely necessary to diagnose IM

IMAGING STUDIES

Chest x-ray examination
- May rarely show infiltrates
- Possible elevated left hemidiaphragm with splenic rupture

TREATMENT

NONPHARMACOLOGIC THERAPY

- Supportive
- Rest advocated by some; impact on outcome not clear
- Splenectomy if rupture occurs
- Transfusions for severe anemia or thrombocytopenia

ACUTE GENERAL Rx

- Pharmacologic therapy is not indicated in uncomplicated illness
- Use of steroids
  1. Suggested in patients who have severe thrombocytopenia or hemolytic anemia, or impending airway obstruction resulting from enlarged tonsils
  2. Prednisone 60 to 80 mg PO qd for 3 days, then tapered over 1 to 2 wk
- There is no role for antiviral agents such as acyclovir in the management of IM

CHRONIC Rx

An extremely rare, chronic form of IM with persistent fevers and other objective findings has been described and should be differentiated from chronic fatigue syndrome, which is not related to EBV.

DISPOSITION

Eventual resolution of all symptoms

REFERRAL

If more than mild illness

PEARLS & CONSIDERATIONS

COMMENTS

Avoidance of contact sports during the first month of illness, because splenic rupture can occur even in the absence of clinically detectable splenomegaly.

SUGGESTED READINGS

Bauer CC et al: Serum Epstein-Barr virus DNA load in primary Epstein-Barr virus infection, *J Med Virol* 75(1):54, 2005.

Crum NF: Epstein Barr virus hepatitis: case series and review, *South Med J* 99(5):544, 2006.

Ebell MH: Epstein-Barr virus: infectious mononucleosis, *Am Family Physician* 70:1279, 2004.

Kaygusuz I et al: The role of viruses in idiopathic peripheral facial palsy and cellular immune response, *Am J Otolaryngol* 25(6): 401, 2004.

Ozyar E et al: Prognostic role of Ebstein-Barr virus latent membrane protein-1 and interleukin-10 expression in patients with nasopharyngeal carcinoma, *Cancer Invest* 22(4):483, 2004.

Thorley-Lawson DA, Gross A: Persistence of the Epstein-Barr virus and the origins of associated lymphomas, *N Engl J Med* 350:1328, 2004.

Vernon SD et al: Preliminary evidence of mitochondrial dysfunction associated with post-infective fatigue after acute infection with Epstein Barr virus, *BMC Infect Dis* 6:15, 2006.

AUTHORS: **GLENN G. FORT, M.D., M.P.H., DENNIS J. MIKOLICH, M.D.,** and **MAURICE POLICAR, M.D.**

BASIC INFORMATION

DEFINITION

Erectile dysfunction (ED) is the persistent inability to achieve or sustain a penile erection of adequate rigidity to make intercourse possible or satisfactory.

SYNONYMS

Impotence
Male erectile disorder
Sexual dysfunction (a nonspecific term)

ICD-9CM CODES
F52.2 Male erectile disorder
(DSM-IV Code: 302.72 Male erectile disorder)

EPIDEMIOLOGY & DEMOGRAPHICS

PREVALENCE (IN U.S.):

- Increases with age.
- About 7% for men between 18 and 29 yr, 18% for men in their 50s, 25% for men in their 60s, 80% for men in their 80s.
- Likely underestimated because of social stigma but the number of patients presenting to their doctor with this complaint has increased considerably with greater availability and awareness of oral therapy.

PREDOMINANT SEX: By definition, only in males
PREDOMINANT AGE: Increases with age
PEAK INCIDENCE: Over age 70 yr

PHYSICAL FINDINGS & CLINICAL PRESENTATION

- Psychogenic impotence: inability to obtain erection, inability to obtain or maintain an adequate erection, or the loss of erection before completion of sexual intercourse; nocturnal penile tumescence usually normal
- Organic impotence: inability to obtain an erection or inability to obtain an adequate erection; nocturnal penile tumescence usually abnormal

ETIOLOGY

- Cover three issues with patients to uncover etiology: Is this an ongoing problem? What is the cause (psychogenic vs. organic)? Does the patient have a normal libido? Most cases are due to organic problem, related to neurologic, hormonal, or vascular abnormalities. If normal libido and exam normal, then unlikely testosterone deficiency and no need to check serum testosterone.
- Psychogenic erectile dysfunction resulting from mental stress, depression, widower syndrome, and performance anxiety. Characterized objectively by nocturnal and morning erections and otherwise negative test results.
- Vascular disease: Elicit history of hypertension (HTN), peripheral vascular disease, ischemic heart disease, diabetes, smoking. In approximately 40% of men >50 yr of age, the primary cause of ED is related to atherosclerotic disease.
- Diabetes mellitus (DM): neuropathy and vascular disease.
- Medications: Consider antihypertensives (especially thiazides and sympathetic blockers such as clonidine); antiandrogens (e.g., spironolactone, finasteride, ketoconazole); cimetidine; antidepressants (e.g., selective serotonin reuptake inhibitors [SSRIs]); and antipsychotics.
- Alcohol and nicotine.
- Recreational drugs, including cocaine, heroin, amphetamines, marijuana. These may increase libido but impair performance.
- Hormonal dysfunction such as testosterone deficiency (decreases libido and erection), hypothyroidism or hyperthyroidism, hyperprolactinemia, and adrenal insufficiency.
- Neurogenic causes including spinal cord lesions, cortical lesions, and peripheral neuropathies.
- Pelvic surgeries such as radical prostatectomy or cystectomy.

DIAGNOSIS

DIFFERENTIAL DIAGNOSIS

- A useful tool to diagnose and evaluate ED severity is the Sexual Health Inventory for Men.
- Psychogenic dysfunction distinguished from organic.
- Determine etiology of organic dysfunction.
- Erectile dysfunction possible in the setting of another psychiatric condition (e.g., depression or obsessive-compulsive disorder).

WORKUP

- Medical and social history (often including partner report) should address cardiac disease symptoms and risk factors (HTN, DM, hyperlipidemia, smoking and substance abuse), pelvic surgery, medications, and mental health.
- Report of spontaneous nocturnal or morning erections indicate intact neurologic reflexes and penile blood flow.
- Decreased libido may indicate endocrinologic or psychogenic cause.
- Physical examination to check blood pressure, femoral and peripheral pulses, femoral bruits; gynecomastia; neuronal damage (genital sensation, cremasteric reflex); direct penile damage (e.g., plaque formation such as Peyronie's disease); prostate exam; or testicular atrophy and other secondary sexual characteristics.

LABORATORY TESTS

- Only pursue serologic evaluation if suspect organic cause.
- Screen with fasting glucose in all men. Consider lipid panel, TSH, morning serum testosterone. If decreased testosterone, check prolactin, FSH, LH.

IMAGING STUDIES

Imaging studies rarely performed except in situations of pelvic trauma or surgery.

OTHER STUDIES

- Nocturnal penile tumescence testing very specific for distinguishing psychogenic vs. organic causes.
- Neurogenic etiologies examined by the cremasteric reflex (inner-thigh touch elicits scrotal contraction), the bulbocavernosus reflex, or the pudendal-evoked response.
- Intracorporeal injection of prostaglandin E1 to distinguish vascular and nonvascular etiologies (erection is achieved in patients with normal vascular systems). If no erection with direct injection of vasoactive substance, consider duplex ultrasound of penile vasculature.

TREATMENT

NONPHARMACOLOGIC THERAPY

- Various psychotherapeutic approaches: cognitive-behavioral therapy preferred because it is the most focused; success rates decrease with advancing age and duration of symptoms.
- Psychosexual therapy (sex therapy and couples therapy) is first line for psychogenic ED and for adjunctive therapy in ED due to any cause. Therapy is used to address social issues that contribute to impotence.
- Vacuum devices (70% to 90% effective) work for many men, but they are difficult to use and cumbersome.

ACUTE GENERAL Rx

- First-line treatment: In setting of sexual stimulation, three selective phosphodiesterase type 5 (PDE5) inhibitors prolong nitric-oxide induced vasodilation via increase of intracavernosal cyclic guanosine monophosphate levels. All three PDE5 inhibitors have similar efficacy and tolerability. Sildenafil (Viagra) 30 to 60 minutes before sexual activity, most commonly used as first-line therapy and lasts 4 hours. Vardenafil (Levitra) 30 to 60 minutes before sexual activity and lasts 4 hours. Must avoid food and excessive amounts of alcohol with sildenafil and vardenafil. Tadalafil (Cialis) with longer period of responsiveness (to 36 hr) gives it enhanced patient convenience. Patients can take tadalafil several hours prior to sexual activity, although about half of men respond by 30 minutes.

- With PDE5 inhibitors, avoid concomitant use of nitrates (absolute contraindication), alpha-adrenergic blockers, drugs that inhibit or induce cytochrome P450 CYP3A4, and drugs that prolong the QT interval. Caution in men who have had myocardial infarction in last 6 months, resting hypotension or uncontrolled hypertension, unstable angina, positive exercise stress test or poor exercise tolerance. Counsel on side effects of headache, flushing, dyspepsia, nasal congestion, changes in color perception, priapism (rare).
- Second-line treatment if PDE5 inhibitors fail: Intraurethral alprostadil (prostaglandin E1 [medicated urethral suppository (MUSE)]) applied into meatus of penis before intercourse; other more invasive intracavernosal injections of vasodilators (e.g., papaverine or prostaglandin E1 pellet). Consider combining intraurethral alprostadil with sildenafil.
- Second-line treatment alternative: Vacuum constriction pump. Draws blood into penile cavernosa. Variable satisfaction rate.

CHRONIC Rx

- Psychosexual therapy helpful as adjunctive treatment in all cases. Sexual therapists can also remotivate patients in whom PDE5 inhibitors initially failed.
- Psychogenic impotence: PDE5 inhibitors effective in patients with depression because tissues, nerves, hormones, and vasculature normal. Full psychologic evaluation recommended before starting treatment so underlying problem is addressed.
- For men failing other approaches: penile prosthesis.
- Testosterone therapy in elderly hypogonadal males. Must rule out prostate cancer prior to use.

DISPOSITION

- When erectile dysfunction is secondary to an organic cause, it does not remit unless the organic cause is corrected; therefore, it is usually a chronic condition.
- Psychogenic-acquired erectile dysfunction will remit spontaneously in 15% to 30% of cases.
- Lifelong erectile dysfunction is usually a chronic and unremitting condition.
- Situational erectile dysfunction may remit with changes in social environment, but it usually recurs.

REFERRAL

- If psychotherapy, sex therapy, or invasive organic treatment required.
- If PDE5 inhibitors fail, refer to urology.

PEARLS & CONSIDERATIONS

- Commonly evaluated and treated by primary care physician; refer to urologist if oral therapy fails or surgery is required.
- PDE5 inhibitors are treatment of choice for most causes of ED. Main contraindications include hypotension, nitrate use, decompensated cardiac disease, and alpha-adrenergic blockers.
- For optimal response, patients should be appropriately informed of proper use, precautions, and adverse effects of PDE5 inhibitors. Try 6 to 8 times at optimal doses before declaring PDE5 inhibitors a failure. Consider switching among the three PDE5 inhibitors if one fails.

EVIDENCE

EBM

Sildenafil is an effective treatment for impotence, regardless of etiology, including impotence associated with SSRIs that are being taken for depression[1] diabetes, spinal cord injury, and idiopathic.[2]

One third of patients may fail to respond to PDE5 inhibitors. If PDE5 inhibitors fail, consider reasons such as worsening atherosclerosis, hypogonadism, inadequate patient education or incorrect drug usage, tachyphylaxis, psychosocial issues.[3]

Intracavernosal alprostadil is an effective second-line treatment for erectile dysfunction regardless of its cause.[4]

Evidence-Based References

1. Nurnberg HG et al: Treatment of antidepressant-associated sexual dysfunction with sildenafil: a randomized controlled trial, *JAMA* 289:56, 2003. Reviewed in: *Clin Evid* 13:1120, 2005.
2. Fink HA et al: Sildenafil for male erectile dysfunction: a systematic review and meta-analysis, *Arch Intern Med* 162:1349, 2002. Reviewed in: *Clin Evid* 13:1120, 2005.
3. McMahon C.N., Smith CJ, Shabsigh R: Treating erectile dysfunction when PDE5 inhibitors fail, *BMJ* 332:589, 2006.
4. Urciuoli R et al: Prostaglandin E1 for treatment of erectile dysfunction, *Cochrane Database Syst Rev* 2, 2004.

SUGGESTED READINGS

Melnik T, Soares B, Nasselo A: Psychosocial interventions for erectile dysfunction, *Cochrane Database Syst Rev* 3:CD004825, 2007.

Mikhail N: Management of erectile dysfunction by the primary care physician, *Cleve Clin J Med* 72:293, 2005.

AUTHOR: **CINDY LAI, M.D.**

BASIC INFORMATION

DEFINITION

Erysipelas is a type of cellulitis caused by infection of the superficial layers of the skin and cutaneous lymphatics. Erysipelas is characterized by redness, induration, and a sharply demarcated, raised border.

SYNONYMS

St. Anthony's fire

ICD-9CM CODES
035 Erysipelas

EPIDEMIOLOGY & DEMOGRAPHICS

PREDOMINANT AGE: Occurs most often in the young or old
RISK FACTORS: Patients with impaired lymphatic or venous drainage (mastectomy, saphenous vein harvesting), and immunocompromised patients. Athlete's foot is a common portal of entry.
RECURRENCE RATE: Relatively common

PHYSICAL FINDINGS & CLINICAL PRESENTATION

- Distinctive red, warm, tender skin lesion with induration and a sharply defined, advancing, raised border is present (Fig. 1-91).
- Most common sites are lower extremities or face.
- Systemic signs of infection (fever) are often present.
- Vesicles or bullae may develop.
- After several days, lesions may appear ecchymotic.
- After 7 to 10 days desquamation of affected area may occur.

ETIOLOGY

- Usually group A β-hemolytic streptococci
- Less often group B, C, or G streptococci
- Rarely *Staphylococcus aureus*

COMPLICATIONS

- Abscess
- Necrotizing fasciitis
- Thrombophlebitis
- Gangrene
- Metastatic infection

DIAGNOSIS

DIFFERENTIAL DIAGNOSIS

- Other types of cellulitis
- Necrotizing fasciitis
- DVT
- Contact dermatitis
- Erythema migrans (Lyme disease)
- Insect bite
- Herpes zoster
- Erysipeloid
- Acute gout
- Pseudogout

WORKUP

History, physical examination, and laboratory evaluation

LABORATORY TESTS

Diagnosis is usually made by characteristic clinical setting and appearance.
- CBC and WBC often elevated
- Blood cultures positive in 5% of patients
- Gram stain and culture of any drainage from skin lesions
- Culture of aspirated fluid from leading edge of skin lesion has low yield

IMAGING STUDIES

- Duplex ultrasound for patients suspected of having DVT
- CT scan or MRI for patients with suspected necrotizing fasciitis

TREATMENT

NONPHARMACOLOGIC THERAPY

- Elevation of the affected limb
- Warm compresses

ACUTE GENERAL Rx

Typical erysipelas of extremity in nondiabetic patient:
- PO: penicillin V 250 mg to 500 mg qid
- IV: penicillin G (aqueous) 1 to 2 million units q6h

NOTE: Use erythromycin or cephalosporin in patients allergic to penicillin.
Facial erysipelas (include coverage for *Staphylococcus aureus*):
- PO dicloxacillin 500 mg q6h
- IV nafcillin or oxacillin 2 g q4h

DISPOSITION

Prognosis is good with antibiotic treatment, but recurrence is common.

REFERRAL

For surgical debridement for patients with necrotizing fasciitis or for drainage of abscess

PEARLS & CONSIDERATIONS

Consider early surgical referral when necrotizing fasciitis suspected. Consider skin biopsy when not responding to appropriate antibiotics.

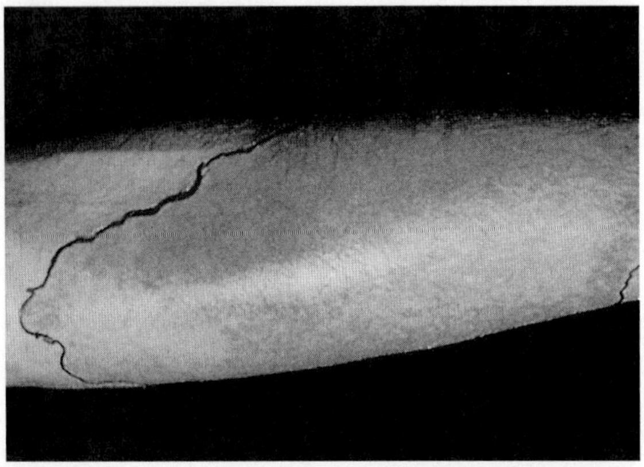

FIGURE 1-91 Erysipelas. Note well-demarcated erythematous plaque on arm. (From Goldstein B [ed]: *Practical dermatology,* ed 2, St Louis, 1997, Mosby. Courtesy Department of Dermatology, University of North Carolina at Chapel Hill.)

SUGGESTED READINGS

Falagas M et al: Narrative review: diseases that masquerade as infectious cellulites, *Ann Int Med* 142(1):47, 2005.

Guisto J, Meislin H: Soft tissue infections. In *Rosen's emergency medicine,* ed 6, Philadelphia, 2006, Mosby.

AUTHORS: **GAIL O'BRIEN, M.D.,** and **MARK J. FAGAN, M.D.**

BASIC INFORMATION

DEFINITION

Erythema multiforme is an inflammatory disease believed to be secondary to immune complex formation and subsequent deposition in the skin and mucous membranes. It is considered to be a hypersensitivity reaction to infection or drugs.

SYNONYMS

EM

ICD-9CM CODES
695.1 Erythema multiforme

EPIDEMIOLOGY & DEMOGRAPHICS

PREDOMINANT AGE: 20 to 40 yr
RISK FACTORS: Often associated with herpes simplex and other infectious agents, drugs, and connective tissue diseases

PHYSICAL FINDINGS & CLINICAL PRESENTATION

- Prodromal symptoms are mild or absent. Itching or burning at the site of eruption may occur.
- Symmetric skin lesions with a classic "target" appearance (caused by the centrifugal spread of red maculopapules to circumference of 1 to 3 cm with a purpuric, cyanotic, or vesicular center) are present (Fig. 1-92). The papules may enlarge into plaques measuring few centimeters in diameter with a dark or red central portion. Target lesions may not be apparent for several days.
- Lesions are most common in the back of the hands and feet and extensor aspect of the forearms and legs. Trunk involvement can occur in severe cases.
- Urticarial papules, vesicles, and bullae may also be present and generally indicate a more severe form of the disease.
- Individual lesions heal in 1 or 2 wk without scarring.
- Bullae and erosions may also be present in the oral cavity.

ETIOLOGY

- Immune complex formation and subsequent deposition in the cutaneous microvasculature may play a role in the pathogenesis of erythema multiforme.
- The majority of EM cases follow outbreaks of herpes simplex virus 1 and 2.
- Mycoplasma pneumoniae, fungal infections, medications, (bupropion, sulfonamides, penicillins, NSAIDs, barbiturates, phenothiazines, hydantoins)
- In >50% of patients, no specific cause is identified.

DIAGNOSIS

DIFFERENTIAL DIAGNOSIS

- Chronic urticaria
- Secondary syphilis
- Pityriasis rosea
- Contact dermatitis
- Pemphigus vulgaris
- Lichen planus
- Serum sickness
- Drug eruption
- Granuloma annulare
- Polymorphic light eruption
- Viral exanthem

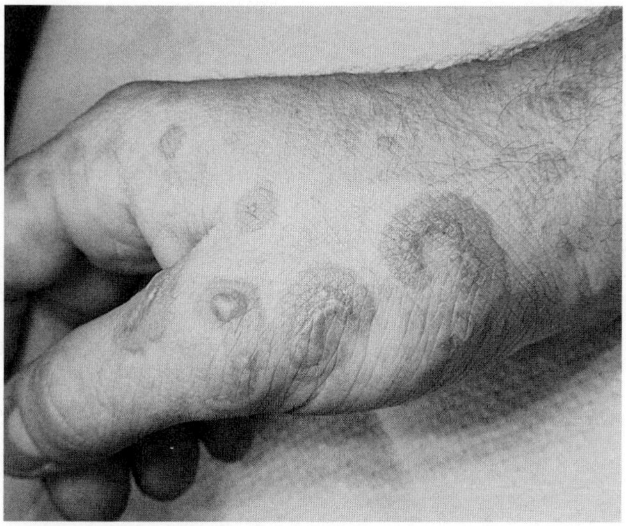

FIGURE 1-92 Iris and arcuate lesions of erythema multiforme. Note erythematous lesions with multiform configurations—target, arcuate, and vesicles. (From Noble J et al: *Textbook of primary care medicine,* ed 2, St Louis, 1995, Mosby.)

WORKUP

- Medical history with emphasis on drug ingestion
- Laboratory evaluation in patients with suspected collagen-vascular diseases
- Skin biopsy when diagnosis is unclear

LABORATORY TESTS

- CBC with differential
- ANA
- Serology for *Mycoplasma pneumoniae,* HSV-1, HSV-2
- Urinalysis

TREATMENT

NONPHARMACOLOGIC THERAPY

- Mild cases generally do not require treatment; lesions resolve spontaneously within 1 mo.
- Potential drug precipitants should be removed.

ACUTE GENERAL Rx

- Treatment of associated diseases (e.g., acyclovir for herpes simplex, erythromycin for *Mycoplasma* infection).
- Prednisone 40 to 80 mg/day for 1 to 3 wk may be tried in patients with many target lesions; however, the role of systemic steroids remains controversial.
- Levamisole, an immunomodulator, may be effective in treatment of patients with chronic or recurrent oral lesions (dose is 150 mg/day for 3 consecutive days used alone or in combination with prednisone).

DISPOSITION

The rash of EM generally evolves over a 2-wk period and resolves within 3 to 4 wk without scarring. A severe bullous form can occur (see "Stevens-Johnson Syndrome").

REFERRAL

Hospital admission in patients with Stevens-Johnson syndrome

PEARLS & CONSIDERATIONS

COMMENTS

The risk of recurrence of erythema multiforme exceeds 30%. Recurrent EM may be treated with valacyclovir 500 to 1000 mg/day, famcyclovir 125 to 250 mg/day, or acyclovir 400 mg bid. Dapsone, antimalarials, azathioprine, or cyclosporine use is reserved for cases resistant to antivirals.

SUGGESTED READING

Lamoreux M et al: Erythema multiforme, *Am Fam Phys* 74:1883, 2006.

AUTHOR: **FRED F. FERRI, M.D.**

BASIC INFORMATION

DEFINITION

Erythema nodosum is an acute, tender, erythematous, nodular skin eruption resulting from inflammation of subcutaneous fat, often associated with bruising. It is the most common form of panniculitis.

ICD-9CM CODES
695.2 Erythema nodosum
017.10 Erythema nodosum, tuberculous, NOS

EPIDEMIOLOGY & DEMOGRAPHICS

INCIDENCE: 2 to 3 cases/100,000 persons per yr
PREDOMINANT SEX: Female:male ratio of 3 to 4:1
PREDOMINANT AGE: 25 to 40 yr

PHYSICAL FINDINGS & CLINICAL PRESENTATION

- Acute onset of tender nodules typically located on shins (Fig. 1-93), occasionally seen on thighs and forearms.
- The nodules are usually ⅛ to 1 inch in diameter but can be as large as 4 inches; they begin as light red lesions, then become darker and often ecchymotic. The nodules heal within 8 wk without ulceration

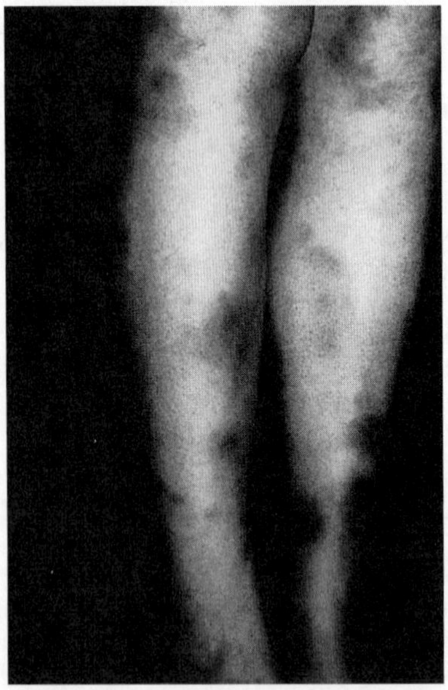

FIGURE 1-93 Erythema nodosum. (From Arndt KA et al: *Cutaneous medicine and surgery,* vol 1, Philadelphia, 1997, WB Saunders.)

- Associated findings:
  - Fever
  - Lymphadenopathy
  - Arthralgia
  - Signs of the underlying illness

ETIOLOGY

Cell-mediated hypersensitivity reaction seen more frequently in persons with human leukocyte antigen (HLA) B8. The lesion results from an exaggerated interaction between an antigen and cell-mediated immune mechanisms leading to granuloma formation. Up to 55% of cases of erythema nodosum are idiopathic.

Infections:
- Bacteria
  - Streptococcal pharyngitis (28% to 48%)
  - *Salmonella* enteritis
  - *Yersinia* enteritis
  - Psittacosis
  - *Chlamydia pneumoniae* infection
  - *Mycoplasma* pneumonia
  - Meningococcal infection
  - Gonorrhea
  - Syphilis
  - Lymphogranuloma venereum
  - Tularemia
  - Cat-scratch disease
  - Leprosy
  - Tuberculosis
- Fungi
  - Histoplasmosis
  - Coccidioidomycosis
  - Blastomycosis
  - *Trichophyton verrucosum*
- Viruses
  - Cytomegalovirus
  - Hepatitis B
  - Epstein-Barr virus
- Drugs (3% to 10%)
  - Sulfonamides
  - Penicillins
  - Oral contraceptives
  - Gold salts
  - Prazosin
  - Aspirin
  - Bromides
- Sarcoidosis (11% to 25%)
- Cancer, usually lymphoma
- Ankylosing spondylosis and reactive arthropathies (e.g., associated with inflammatory bowel disease)

DIAGNOSIS (Dx)

DIFFERENTIAL DIAGNOSIS

- Insect bites
- Posttraumatic ecchymoses
- Vasculitis
- Weber-Christian disease
- Fat necrosis associated with pancreatitis
- Necrobiosis lipoidica
- Scleroderma
- Lupus panniculitis
- Subcutaneous granuloma
- Alpha-1 antitrypsin deficiency

WORKUP

- Physical examination
- Diagnosis of underlying illness by history, physical examination, and laboratory tests as indicated

LABORATORY TESTS

- Erythrocyte sedimentation rate (ESR)
- Throat culture and antistreptolysin O titer
- PPD
- Others depending on index of suspicion (e.g., stool culture and evaluation for ova and parasites in patients with diarrhea and GI symptoms)
- Skin biopsy in doubtful cases:
  - Early lesion: inflammation and hemorrhage in subcutaneous tissue
  - Late lesion: giant cells and granulomata

IMAGING STUDIES

Chest x-ray to rule out sarcoidosis and TB

TREATMENT (Rx)

- The disease is self-limited and treatment is symptomatic. Erythema nodosum nodules develop in pretibial locations and resolve spontaneously over several weeks without scarring or ulceration.
- Treatment of underlying disorders.
- Avoidance of contact irritation of affected areas.
- NSAIDs for pain.
- Systemic steroids (prednisone 1mg/kg of body weight/day, tapered over several days) may be useful in severe cases if underlying risk of sepsis and malignancy have been excluded.

PROGNOSIS

Typical case:
- Pain for 2 wk
- Resolution within 8 wk

SUGGESTED READING

Schwartz RA, Nervi S: Erythema nodosum: a sign of systemic disease, *Am Fam Physician* 75: 695-700, 2007.

AUTHORS: **FRED F. FERRI, M.D.,** and **TOM J. WACHTEL, M.D.**

BASIC INFORMATION

DEFINITION

Esophageal tumors are defined as benign and malignant tumors arising from the esophagus. Approximately 15% of esophageal cancers arise in the cervical esophagus, 50% in the middle third of the esophagus, and 35% in the lower third. Eighty-five percent of esophageal tumors are squamous cell carcinoma (arising from squamous epithelium). Adenocarcinomas arise from columnar epithelium in the distal esophagus, which have become dysplastic secondary to chronic gastric reflux, Barrett's esophagus.

SYNONYMS

Neoplasm of the esophagus
Malignancy of the esophagus

ICD-9CM CODES
150.8 Esophageal cancer, NEC
150.9 Esophageal cancer, NOS
230.1 Carcinoma of esophagus, in situ

EPIDEMIOLOGY & DEMOGRAPHICS

Carcinomas of the esophageal epithelium, both squamous cell and adenocarcinoma, are by far the most common tumors of the esophagus. Benign neoplasms are much less common (leiomyoma, papilloma, and fibrovascular polyps).

PREVALENCE: Varies widely worldwide. It is the sixth leading cause of cancer death. Rates are highest in the Asian esophageal cancer belt, extending from the Caspian Sea to northern China, with certain high-incidence pockets in Finland, Ireland, SE Africa, and NW France. In the U.S., 14,550 new cases in 2006 and 13,000 deaths occur per year, making it the seventh leading cause of death by cancer among men.

AGE & SEX PREDOMINANCE: Esophageal cancer is more common among blacks than whites and has a high male:female ratio of 3:1. It usually develops in the seventh and eighth decades and is associated with lower socioeconomic status. The majority are diagnosed at an advanced stage (unresectable or metastatic disease).

GENETICS: Increasing evidence that genetics may play a role by incresing susceptibility to esophageal cancer.

CLINICAL PRESENTATION

Symptoms and signs:

- Dysphagia: initially occurs with solid foods and gradually progresses to include semisolids and liquids; latter signs usually indicate incurable disease with tumor involving more than 60% of the esophageal circumference. Occurs in 74%.
- Weight loss: usually of short duration. Weight loss >10% of body mass is an independent predictor of poor prognosis.
- Hoarseness: suggests recurrent laryngeal nerve involvement.
- Odynophagia: an unusual symptom.
- Cervical adenopathy: usually involving supraclavicular lymph nodes.
- Dry cough: suggests tracheal involvement.
- Aspiration pneumonia: caused by development of a fistula between the esophagus and trachea.
- Massive hemoptysis or hematemesis: results from the invasion of vascular structures.
- Advanced disease spreads to liver, lungs, and pleura.
- Hypercalcemia: associated with squamous cell carcinoma because of the secretion of a tumor peptide similar to the parathyroid hormone.

ETIOLOGY

Pathogenesis of esophageal cancers is due to chronic recurrent oxidative damage from any of the following etiologic agents, which cause inflammation, esophagitis, increased cell turnover, and ultimately, initiation of the carcinogenic process.

ETIOLOGIC AGENTS:

- Excess alcohol consumption: accounts for 80% to 90% of esophageal cancer in the U.S.; whiskey is associated with a higher incidence than wine or beer.
- Tobacco and alcohol use combined increases risk substantially.
- Obesity.
- Other ingested carcinogens:
  - Nitrates (converted to nitrites): South Asia, China
  - Smoked opiates: Northern Iran
  - Fungal toxins in pickled vegetables
- Mucosal damage:
  - Long-term exposure to extremely hot tea
  - Lye ingestion
- Radiation-induced strictures
- Chronic achalasia: incidence is 7×.
- Host susceptibility secondary to precancerous lesions:
  - Plummer-Vinson syndrome (Paterson-Kelly): glossitis with iron deficiency
  - Congenital hyperkeratosis and pitting of palms and soles
- Chronic GERD leading to Barrett's esophagus and adenocarcinoma (whites are affected more than blacks).
- Possible association with celiac sprue or dietary deficiencies of molybdenum, zinc, vitamin A.

DIAGNOSIS

DIFFERENTIAL DIAGNOSIS

- Achalasia
- Scleroderma of the esophagus
- Diffuse esophageal spasm
- Esophageal rings and webs

LABORATORY TESTS

Complete blood cell count, chemistries, liver enzymes

IMAGING STUDIES

- Double contrast esophagogram effectively identifies large esophageal lesions (Fig. 1-94).
  - In contrast to benign esophageal leiomyomata, which cause narrowing with preservation of normal mucosal pattern, esophageal carcinomas cause ragged ulcerating mucosal changes in association with deeper infiltration.
- Esophagoscopy is performed to visualize smaller tumors missed by esophagogram and obtain histopathologic confirmation. In conjunction, an endoscopic sonogram is often performed to determine the depth of tumor invasion.
  - Endoscopic inspection of the larynx, trachea, and bronchi may identify concomitant cancers of head, neck, and lung.
  - Endoscopic biopsies fail to recover malignant tissue one third of the time, thus cytologic examination of tumor brushings should be routinely performed.
  - Examination of the fundus of the stomach via retroflexion of the endoscope is also imperative.
- Chest and abdominal CT or integrated CT-PET scan should be performed to determine the extent of tumor spread to mediastinum, paraaortic lymph nodes, and liver.

TREATMENT

ACUTE GENERAL Rx

SURGICAL RESECTION:

- Surgical resection of squamous cell and adenocarcinoma of the lower third of the esophagus is indicated if there is no widespread metastasis. Usually stomach or colon is used for esophageal replacement.
- Endoscopic resections may replace radical surgical resections in early tumors with no lymph node involvement.

Complications of surgery:

- Anatomic fistula (usually with colon interposition, subphrenic abscesses).
- Respiratory complications.
- Cardiovascular complications are most common, including MI, CVA, and PE.

RADIATION THERAPY:

- Squamous cell carcinomas are more radiosensitive than adenocarcinoma, and radiation achieves good local control and is an excellent palliative modality for obstructive symptoms. Best used for upper esophageal tumors.
- About 40% of tumors cannot be destroyed even after 6000 rads.

- Palliative radiation therapy for bone metastasis is also effective.
- Preoperative radiotherapy:
  - No consistent evidence of effectiveness or that it improves survival in patients with potentially resectable esophageal tumors.

Complications of radiation therapy:

- Esophageal stricture, radiation-induced pulmonary fibrosis, transverse myelitis are the most feared complications.
- Radiation-induced cardiomyopathy and skin changes are rare.

COMBINATION CHEMOTHERAPY, RADIATION Rx, & SURGICAL Rx:

- Single-agent chemotherapy resulted in significant tumor regression in 15% to 25% of patients.
- Combination chemotherapy including cisplatin achieved significant tumor reduction in 30% to 60% of patients.
- Complications of chemotherapy include mucositis, GI toxicity, myelosuppression, nephrotoxicity; ototoxicity and neurotoxicity with cisplatin.
- Many centers are using preoperative chemoradiotherapy for patients with esophageal cancer.
- Chemoradiotherapy plus surgery significantly reduced the 3-year mortality rate compared with surgery alone in patients with resectable esophageal cancer.
- Most beneficial chemotherapy appeared to be a cisplatin, 5-fluorouracil-based combination.
- Conflicting evidence on the effects of cisplatin and 5-fluorouracil on survival time over surgery alone.
- Chemoradiotherapy is superior to radiotherapy alone for the primary treatment of esophageal carcinoma when a nonoperative approach is selected, but is associated with significant toxicity and perioperative mortality.

CHRONIC Rx

- Palliative procedures such as repeated endoscopic dilation, surgical placement of feeding tube, or polyvinyl prosthesis to bypass tumors have been used for unresectable patients.

DISPOSITION

- Overall 5-yr survival is 13%.
- Surgery: 5-yr survival rate is 48% in stages I and II, 20% in advanced stages.
- Radiation therapy: 5-yr survival rate is between 6% and 20%.
- Chemotherapy: Single-agent response rate 15% to 38%; combination response rate 80%.
- Combined modality: 18% response rate.
- Patients with stage IV disease receive palliative chemotherapy with a median survival of less than 1 year.

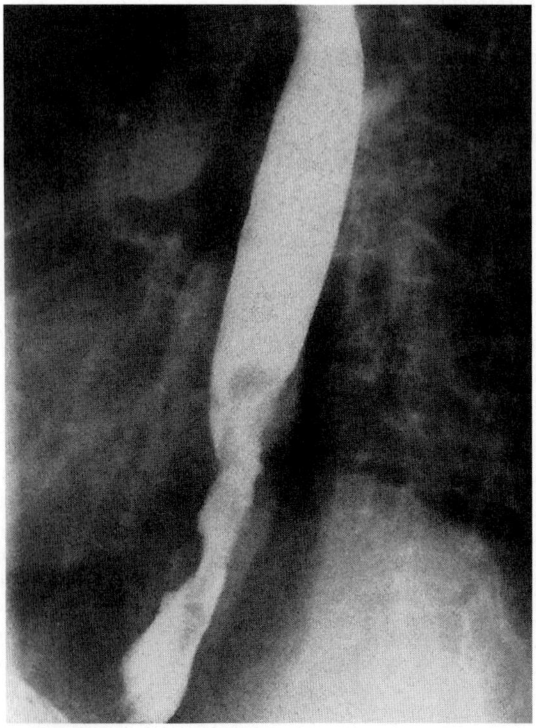

FIGURE 1-94 Barium swallow demonstrating the classic findings in cancer of the distal third of the espophagus. (From Nobel J [ed]: *Primary care medicine,* ed 2, St Louis, 1996, Mosby.)

REFERRAL

- Gastroenterologist or general surgeon for endoscopy for patients with chronic dysphagia, odynophagia, or unexplained weight loss
- Medical oncologist for evaluation of preoperative chemotherapy
- Radiation oncologist for palliative therapy if unresectable or obstruction
- Hospice referral if appropriate

PEARLS & CONSIDERATIONS

COMMENTS

>50% of patients with esophageal cancer are diagnosed when the disease is metastatic or unresectable.

PREVENTION

- A diet high in fruits and vegetables is associated with lower risk of esophageal cancer.
- Avoid excessive alcohol and tobacco use.
- Avoid ingested toxins known to cause esophageal cancers.
- Endoscopic evaluation of persons with chronic dysphagia, or GERD symptoms with regularly scheduled surveillance endoscopies if Barrett's esophagus is detected.

PATIENT/FAMILY EDUCATION

Provide education and support about the likely prognosis because most esophageal cancers are diagnosed at an advanced stage.

SUGGESTED READINGS

Arnott SJ et al: Preoperative radiotherapy for esophageal carcinoma, *Cochrane Database Syst Rev* 4:CD001799, 2005.

Chang JT, Katzka DA: Gastroesophageal reflux disease, Barrett esophagus, and esophageal adenocarcinoma, *Arch Intern Med* 164:1482, 2004.

Enzinger PC, Mayer RJ: Esophageal cancer, *N Engl J Med* 349:2241, 2003.

Walsh TN et al: A comparison of multimodal therapy and surgery for esophageal adenocarcinoma, *N Engl J Med* 335:462-467, 1996.

Wong R, Malthaner R: Combined chemotherapy and radiotherapy (without surgery) compared with radiotherapy alone in localized carcinoma of the esophagus, *Cochrane Database Syst Rev* 1:CD002092, 2006.

AUTHOR: **LYNN MCNICOLL, M.D., F.R.C.P.C.**

BASIC INFORMATION

DEFINITION

A predominantly postural and action tremor that is bilateral and tends to progress slowly over the years in the absence of other neurological abnormalities.

SYNONYMS

Benign essential tremor
Familial tremor

ICD-9CM CODES
333.1 Essential tremor

EPIDEMIOLOGY & DEMOGRAPHICS

PREDOMINANT AGE: About 415/100,000 in persons over 40

GENETICS: No gender or racial predominance

PHYSICAL FINDINGS & CLINICAL PRESENTATION

- Patients complain of tremor that is most bothersome when writing or holding something, such as a newspaper, or trying to drink from a cup. Worsens under emotional duress and drinking liquids.
- Tremor, 4 to 12 Hz, bilateral postural and action tremor of the upper extremities. May also affect the head, voice, trunk, and legs. Typically is the same amplitude throughout the action, such as bringing a cup to the mouth. No other neurologic abnormalities on examination, except for possibly some difficulty with tandem gait. Patients often note improvement with small amount of alcohol.

ETIOLOGY

Often an inherited disease, autosomal dominant; sporadic cases without a family history are frequently encountered

DIAGNOSIS

DIFFERENTIAL DIAGNOSIS

- Parkinson's disease—tremor is usually asymmetric, especially early on in the disease, and is predominantly a resting tremor. Patients with Parkinson's disease will also have increased tone, decreased facial expression, slowness of movement, and shuffling gait.
- Cerebellar tremor—an intention tremor that increases at the end of a goal-directed movement (such as finger to nose testing). Other associated neurologic abnormalities include ataxia, dysarthria, and difficulty with tandem gait.
- Drug-induced—there are many drugs that enhance normal, physiologic tremor. These include caffeine, nicotine, lithium, levothyroxine, β-adrenergic bronchodilators, valproate, and SSRIs.
- Wilson's Disease—wing-beating tremor that is most pronounced with shoulders abducted, elbows flexed, and fingers pointing towards each other. Usually there are other neurologic abnormalities including dysarthria, dystonia, and Keyser Fleischer rings on ophthalmologic examination.

WORKUP

- All imaging studies normal (MRI, CT) and are usually unnecessary unless there are other associated neurologic abnormalities
- Check TSH
- In patients younger than 40 yr with other neurologic abnormalities, send ceruloplasmin, serum Cu, 24-hr urine Cu to rule out Wilson's disease

TREATMENT

Do not need to treat essential tremor unless it is functionally impairing. Patients need to understand that treatments are only 40% to 70% effective.

NONPHARMACOLOGIC THERAPY

Reduction of stress. Minimize use of caffeine. Small quantities of alcohol at social functions tend to be beneficial.

ACUTE GENERAL Rx

Can take a dose of propranolol (20 to 40 mg) in preparation for specific event.

CHRONIC Rx

First-line agents

- Propranolol/Propranolol LA: Usual starting dose is 30 mg. The usual therapeutic dose is 160 to 320 mg. Although not contraindicated, they must be used with caution in those with asthma, depression, cardiac disease, and diabetes.
- Primidone: Usual starting dose is 12.5 to 25 mg qhs. Usual therapeutic dose is between 62.5 and 750 mg daily. Sedation and nausea when first begin medication are biggest side effects.

Other agents

- Gabapentin: 400 mg qhs, usual therapeutic dose is 1200 to 3600 mg
- Topiramate: 25 mg qhs, may titrate up to about 400 mg
- Alprazolam: 0.75 to 2.75 mg

For head tremor, propanolol may be more effective than others. Consideration should be given to referral for Botulinum toxin injections to treat head tremor. Not very useful for limb tremor.

The previously mentioned drugs can be tried in combination if monotherapy is ineffective.

SURGICAL Rx

Thalamic deep brain stimulation contralateral to side of tremor

DISPOSITION

Patients should be reassured that the condition is not associated with other neurologic disabilities; however, it can become quite functionally disabling over time.

REFERRAL

This is a condition that usually can be treated by the primary care physician; however, if patient fails first-line therapies then patient should be referred to specialists for other drug trials and possible surgical options.

PEARLS & CONSIDERATIONS

Essential tremor is the most common of all movement disorders.

EVIDENCE

A recent American Academy of Neurology Practice Parameter was released in June 2005.[1] They found that propranolol, propranolol LA, and primidone are effective in reducing limb tremor in essential tremor. Ⓐ Ⓑ The magnitude of effect of propranolol and primidone is roughly equivalent, and either can be tried as initial therapy. There is conflicting evidence for the use of gabapentin and limited evidence for the other drugs listed. Ⓑ Based on available studies, these agents are either "probably" or "possibly" effective in the treatment of limb tremor in essential tremor.

Evidence-Based Reference

1. Zesiewicz TA et al: Practice parameter: therapies for essential tremor. Report of the Quality Standards Subcommittee of the American Academy of Neurology, *Neurology* 64:2008, 2005.

SUGGESTED READINGS

Deuschel G, Volkmann J: Tremors: differential diagnosis, pathophysiology, and therapy. In Jankovic J, Tolosa E (eds): *Parkinson's disease and movement disorders*, ed 4, 2002, pp. 270-291.

Louis ED: Essential tremor, *N Engl J Med* 345(12):887, 2001.

Zesiewicz TA et al: Phenomenology and treatment of tremor disorders. In Hurtig H, Stern M (eds): *Neurologic clinics: movement disorders* 19:3, 2001, pp. 651-680.

AUTHOR: **CINDY ZADIKOFF, M.D.**

BASIC INFORMATION

DEFINITION

Factitious physical disorder is one in which an individual intentionally strives to create signs or symptoms of disease. The individual may create signs or symptoms by (1) lying, (2) simulating (e.g., putting drops of blood into a urine sample), or (3) actually creating disease (e.g., injecting bacteria or medications). The primary aim is to achieve the patient role, and the individual may seek invasive diagnostic testing, surgery, and treatment. Munchausen's syndrome is the most severe variant of factitious physical disorder and is exaggerated lying (pseudologia fantastica), sociopathy, geographic wandering from hospital to hospital, and a continuous life of patienthood.

SYNONYMS

Factitious disorder
Munchausen's syndrome (the most severe variant of factitious disorder)
Munchausen by proxy (factitious disorder created in another person, usually a child)
Deliberate disability
Hospital addiction syndrome
Artifactual illness
Peregrinating problem patients
Dermatitis artefacta
Surreptitious illness

ICD-9CM CODES
300.19 Factitious disorder

EPIDEMIOLOGY & DEMOGRAPHICS

INCIDENCE (IN U.S.): Unknown
PEAK INCIDENCE: 30s
PREVALENCE (IN U.S.): Unknown but considerable in specific illnesses. For example, 3.3% of patients with fever of unknown origin have a factitious disorder.
PREDOMINANT SEX: Male:female ratio of 2:1 for Munchausen's syndrome but 1:2 for individuals with non-Munchausen type of factitious physical disorder.
PREDOMINANT AGE: 30 to 40 yr
GENETICS: No genetic predisposition known.

PHYSICAL FINDINGS & CLINICAL PRESENTATION

- False complaints or self-inflicted injury or symptoms without clear secondary gain. The intentional aspect of the disorder is often evident, such as injecting bacteria to produce infection or taking medication to produce an abnormality.
- Presentation may be acute and dramatic but can be a chronic, recurring problem.
- Workup is usually negative for naturally occurring organic etiology.
- Clinical picture is atypical for the natural history of disease (e.g., an infection that fails to respond to multiple courses of appropriate antibiotics).

ETIOLOGY

- A history of significant childhood illness; physical or sexual abuse are thought to predispose.
- Personality disorders and psychodynamic factors often play a significant role.

DIAGNOSIS

The diagnosis can be made by (1) direct observation of fabrication, (2) the presence of signs or symptoms that contradict laboratory testing, (3) nonphysiologic response to treatment, (4) finding physical evidence of fabrication (e.g., syringes), and (5) recurrent patterns of illness exacerbation (e.g., just before discharge).

DIFFERENTIAL DIAGNOSIS

- Malingering: a clear secondary gain (e.g., financial gain or avoidance of unwanted duties) is present.
- Somatoform disorders or hypochondriasis: these disorders are produced unconsciously and are not intentionally produced.
- Self-injurious behavior is common in many other psychiatric conditions; in those conditions the patients confess the intentional self-harm and describe motivating factors; the main intent is the self-harm and not to attain the patient role as occurs in factitious disorder.
- May also present as Munchausen by proxy in which a mother (86% of time) or other caregiver induces illness in a child (52% between ages of 3 and 13 yr) for the purpose of obtaining medical attention or some other psychological need. Mothers often have a history of somatoform, factitious, or personality disorder themselves.

WORKUP

- Dictated by the presenting complaints.
- No specific tests for Munchausen's syndrome.
- Diagnosis may be made when the patient is caught in the act of lying or inducing an injury. The diagnosis often rests on organic workup failing to reveal a plausible natural organic disease. The failure of usual, or even extensive, treatment to ameliorate a condition is an important clue.

LABORATORY TESTS

- Laboratory testing often reveals inconsistencies.
- Other laboratory abnormalities may reflect the underlying factitious behavior (e.g., hypokalemia in an individual surreptitiously taking furosemide).

TREATMENT

NONPHARMACOLOGIC THERAPY

Two major approaches:

- Nonpunitive confrontation. Primary physician and psychiatrist conjointly meet with patient and say, "You must be in a lot of distress to be harming yourself as we believe you have been. We would like to help you deal with your distress more adaptively and get you into psychiatric treatment."
- Avoid overt confrontation with patient but provide him or her with a face-saving way to recover. For example, a therapeutic double bind would involve saying, "There are two possibilities here, one is that you have a medical problem that should respond to the next intervention we do, or two, you have a factitious disorder. The outcome will give us the answer."
- Munchausen's syndrome is the most severe variant and may be virtually impossible to treat except to avoid further invasive and iatrogenic disease.

ACUTE GENERAL Rx

Treatment of comorbid psychiatric disorders may be helpful. Treatment with antidepressants or psychotherapy may ameliorate the factitious behavior. Multidisciplinary staff meetings are useful to ventilate feelings and develop cohesive treatment plans.

DISPOSITION

- After being confronted with their behavior, patients may cease factitious behavior but more commonly seek other physicians or hospitals in the Munchausen variant. Other factitious disorder patients may enter psychotherapy, particularly when they have been given a face-saving approach with an avoidance of a humiliating confrontation.
- Extensive medical workups and exploratory surgery are frequent.

REFERRAL

Always obtain psychiatric referral. Risk management attorneys and hospital ethicists may contribute to challenging decision making in these patients.

PEARLS & CONSIDERATIONS

Think of factitious disorders whenever there is an unexplained medical course that continues to repeat despite appropriate treatment, particularly in patients associated with the health care field.

SUGGESTED READINGS

Eisendrath S, Young J: Factitious physical disorders. In Maj M et al (eds): *Somatoform disorders,* West Sussex, England, 2005, John Wiley and Sons, pp. 325-338.
Stone J, Carson A, Sharpe M: Functional symptoms in neurology: management, *J Neurol Neurosurg Psychiatry* 76(suppl 1):i13-i21, 2005.

AUTHOR: **STUART J. EISENDRATH, M.D.**

BASIC INFORMATION

DEFINITION

A fall is an "event which results in a person coming to rest inadvertently on the ground and other than a consequence of the following: loss of consciousness, sudden onset of paralysis, or epileptic seizure" (Kellogg International Work Group, *Danish Medical Bulletin,* 34, 1-24).

SYNONYMS

Syncope
Collapse

ICD-9CM CODES
Accidental fall (E880-E888.9)

EPIDEMIOLOGY & DEMOGRAPHICS

INCIDENCE:

- Falls are the leading cause of accidental death among older adults.
- The incidence of falls among community-dwelling older adults is 35% to 40%.
- The incidence of falls for nursing home and hospitalized older adults is three times the rate of community-dwelling older adults.
- Twenty to thirty percent of older adults, who fall, suffer significant injury leading to immobility and dependence.

PREDOMINANT SEX & AGE:

- Fall-related mortality is highest among older white men followed by white women, black men, and black women.
- The incidence rates of falls increase with advancing age.
- Older adults aged 85 years and over are 10 to 15 times more likely to have a fracture compared with those aged 60 to 65 years.

RISK FACTORS:

Three groups of risk factors for falls have been identified (Table 1-13):

1. Intrinsic factors inherent in the older adult who falls
2. Extrinsic factors circumstantial to the older adult who falls
3. Situational or the activity in which the older adult is engaged in when a fall occurs

CLINICAL PRESENTATION

- Older adults who fall may present with minor soft tissue injuries, such as lacerations or bruising, hip fracture or head trauma; however, most falls are not reported unless an injury has occurred.
- A detailed history of events and circumstances surrounding fall, risk factors, medications, chronic illnesses, and a review of systems for acute medical illnesses, cognitive status, and functional status should be obtained.
- Physical examination should focus on the identified risk factors and include:
  - Cardiovascular examination: heart rate and rhythm, orthostatics, carotid pulses
  - Neurologic examination: mental status, visual screen, lower extremity assessment of strength, tone, proprioception, sensation, reflexes and testing of cortical and cerebellar function
  - Gait and balance assessment: "Get up and go test"

ETIOLOGY

- Falls are a multifactorial syndrome resulting from the cumulative effects of impaired gait and balance, aging, polypharmacy, depression, cognitive impairment, acute medical illness, or environmental factors (Fig. 1-95).
- Most falls among community-dwelling older adults are due to environmental factors whereas falls among nursing home residents are a result of confusion, gait impairment, or postural hypotension.

DIAGNOSIS

DIFFERENTIAL DIAGNOSIS

Falls are often a nonspecific symptom of an acute illness (such as a UTI, acute anemia, or pneumonia) or an exacerbation of a chronic disease (CHF or COPD).

WORKUP

- Older adults presenting with a noninjurious fall need a detailed history and physical exam to identify acute medical illnesses and potential modifiable risk factors. Laboratory and neuroimaging studies may be necessary if the history and physical exam indicate a specific problem. ECG and Holter monitoring may be considered if cardiac arrhythmia is suspected.
- See Fig. 1-95

LABORATORY TESTS

CBC, chemistries, thyroid function, drug levels, and urinalysis depending on physical/historical findings

TABLE 1-13 Risk Factors for Falls in the Elderly

Intrinsic

Aging
Age-related decline in vestibular function might lead to increased sway, dizziness, and falls. Aging of the vision system may result in decreased visual acuity, inability to discriminate dark/light, and decreased spatial perception.

Cardiac
Cardiac arrhythmias, carotid sinus hypersensitivity

Neurologic
Parkinson's disease, normal pressure hydrocephalus (NPH), sensory neuropathy, dementia/impaired cognition, cervical myelopathy, senile gait disorder, prior stroke

Musculoskeletal
Lower extremity weakness, deconditioning, arthritis, foot abnormalities (such as bunions, calluses, or nail abnormalities)

Vascular
Vertebrobasilar insufficiency, postural hypotension, postprandial hypotension

Metabolic
Hypoglycemia, hypothyroidism, hyponatremia

Psychiatric
Depression

Extrinsic

Medications
Use of more than four medications may be associated with an increased risk of falls. Medications that may increase fall risk include benzodiazepines, sleeping medications, neuroleptics, antidepressants, anticonvulsants, class I antiarrythmics, and antihypertensives (Rao, 2005).

Environmental
Inadequate lighting, ill-fitting shoes, slippery floor surfaces, loose rugs, uneven steps

Situational

Tripping over obstacles, carrying heavy items, descending/ascending stairs, rapid turning, reaching overhead, climbing ladders

IMAGING STUDIES

- CT or MRI of the brain or cervical spine films in the presence of neurologic or gait impairment.
- Consider ECG, echocardiography, or Holter monitor if suspicious for structural cardiac abnormality or syncope.

TREATMENT (Rx)

NONPHARMACOLOGIC THERAPY

- Assisted devices such as a cane, walker to improve mobility
- Fall prevention equipment including bed alarms, low beds, and hip protectors
- Physical therapy evaluation for gait and balance training and home safety assessment
- Discontinuation of certain medications associated with falls
- Exercise program to improve strength and balance
- Evaluation of proper footwear, hard sole, and low heel height

ACUTE GENERAL Rx

Hospitalization may be necessary for treatment of hip fracture, subdural hematoma, lacerations, or trauma as well as the treatment of underlying cause of the fall such as infection, metabolic disturbances, cardiovascular or neurologic abnormality.

CHRONIC Rx

- Screen and treat for osteoporosis as low bone density increases the risk of hip or other fractures.
- Optimize treatment of chronic illnesses such as CHF, COPD, OA, Parkinson's disease, dementia and visual problems.

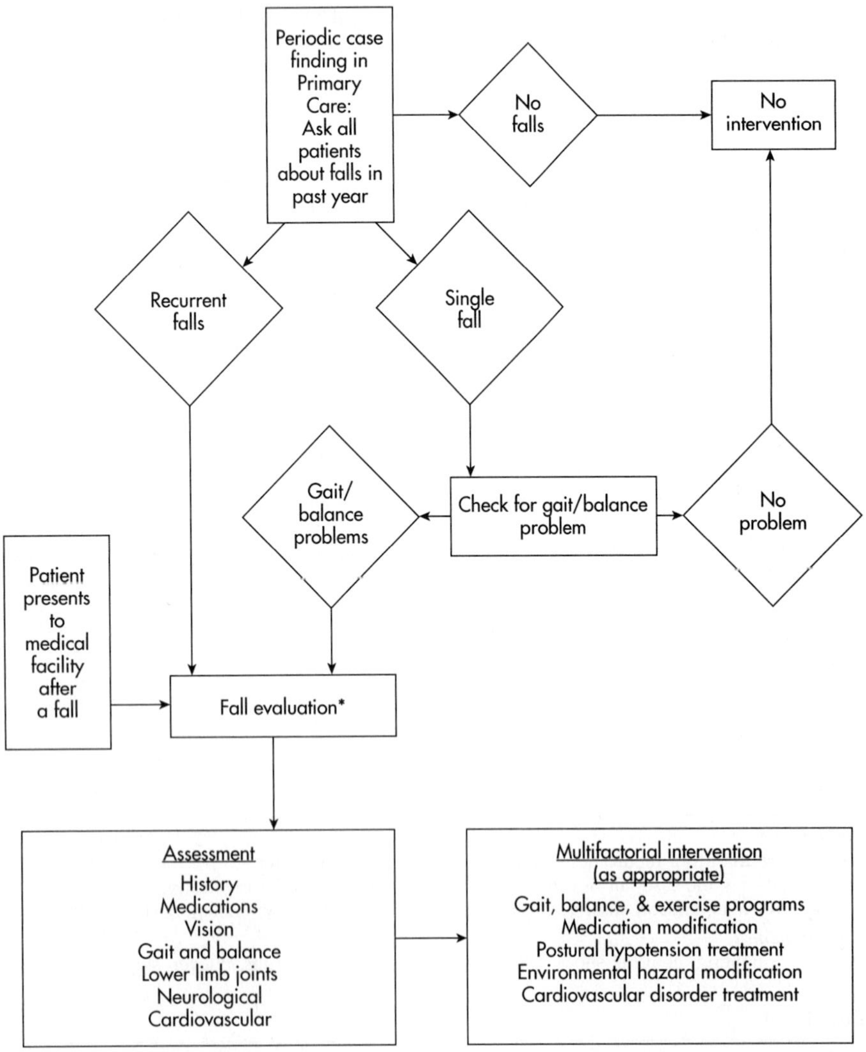

*See text for details

FIGURE 1-95 Guideline for the prevention of falls in older persons. Algorithm summarizing the assessment and management of falls. (From American Geriatrics Society, British Society, and American Academy of Orthopaedic Surgeons Panel on Falls Prevention.)

COMPLEMENTARY & ALTERNATIVE MEDICINE

Tai Chi has been shown to reduce the risk of falls in community-dwelling study participants.

DISPOSITION

Falls increase the older adult's risk of hospitalization, institutionalization, and mortality.

REFERRAL

- Referral may be appropriate to cardiologist, ophthalmologist, neurologist, or podiatrist depending on the presence of a specific condition.
- Consider referral to physical therapist for gait and balance training, evaluation for assisted device, or strengthening program.

PEARLS & CONSIDERATIONS (!)

COMMENTS

- Fear of falling may lead to restriction of activities, social isolation, and dependence.
- Older adults with four or more risk factors have a 78% chance of falling.

PREVENTION

The USPSTF does recommend counseling elderly patients about fall prevention during routine visits as well as arranging individualized multifactorial home interventions for high-risk elders (USPSTF Guidelines, 1996).

PATIENT/FAMILY EDUCATION

Counseling patient and family about reducing the risks of falling

SUGGESTED READINGS

American Geriatrics Society, British Geriatrics Society, and American Academy of Orthopedic Surgeons Panel on Falls Prevention: Guideline for the prevention of falls, *J Am Geriatr Soc* 49:664-672, 2001.

Centers for Disease Control and Prevention: http://www.cdc.gov/ncipc/factsheets/falls.htm

Rao S: Prevention of falls in older patients, *Am Fam Physician* 72:81-88, 2005.

Tinetti, M: Falls. *In* Cassel C et al (eds): *Geriatric medicine,* ed 3, New York, 1996, Springer-Verlag, pp. 528-534.

Tinetti ME: Preventing falls in the elderly, *N Engl J Med* 348:42-49, 2003.

U.S. Preventive Services Task Force: Guide to Clinical Preventive Services, 1996, Williams and Wilkins, Baltimore.

Wolf SL et al: Intense tai chi exercise training and fall occurrences in older, transitionally frail adults: a randomized, controlled trial, *J Am Geriatr Soc* 51:1693-16970, 2003.

AUTHORS: **SEAN H. UITERWYK, M.D.,** and **ALICIA J. CURTIN, PH.D., G.N.P.**

BASIC INFORMATION

DEFINITION

Acute fatty liver of pregnancy (AFLP) is characterized histologically by microvesicular fatty cytoplasmic infiltration of hepatocytes with minimal hepatocellular necrosis.

SYNONYMS

Acute fatty metamorphosis
Acute yellow atrophy

ICD-9CM CODES
646.7 Liver disorders in pregnancy

EPIDEMIOLOGY & DEMOGRAPHICS

INCIDENCE:
- Approximately 1 in 10,000 pregnancies
- Equal frequencies in all races and at all maternal ages

AVERAGE GESTATIONAL AGE: 37 wk (range 28 to 42 wk)

RISK FACTORS:
- Primiparity
- Multiple gestation
- Male fetus

GENETICS: Some with a familial deficiency of long-chain 3-hydroxyacyl-CoA dehydrogenase (LCHAD)

PHYSICAL FINDINGS & CLINICAL PRESENTATION

- Initial manifestations
  1. Nausea and vomiting (70%)
  2. Pain in RUQ or epigastrium (50% to 80%)
  3. Malaise and anorexia
- Jaundice often in 1 to 2 wk
- Late manifestations
  1. Fulminant hepatic failure
  2. Encephalopathy
  3. Renal failure
  4. Pancreatitis
  5. GI and uterine bleeding
  6. Disseminated intravascular coagulation
  7. Seizures
  8. Coma
- Liver
  1. Usually small
  2. Normal or enlarged in preeclampsia, eclampsia, HELLP (hemolysis, elevated liver enzymes, and low platelets) syndrome, and acute hepatitis
  3. Coexistent preeclampsia in up to 46% of patients

ETIOLOGY

- Postulated that inhibition of mitochondrial oxidation of fatty acids may lead to microvesicular fatty infiltration of liver
- Fatty metamorphosis of preeclamptic liver disease thought to be of different etiology

DIAGNOSIS

DIFFERENTIAL DIAGNOSIS

- Acute gastroenteritis
- Preeclampsia or eclampsia with liver involvement
- HELLP syndrome
- Acute viral hepatitis
- Fulminant hepatitis
- Drug-induced hepatitis caused by halothane, phenytoin, methyldopa, isoniazid, hydrochlorothiazide, or tetracycline
- Intrahepatic cholestasis of pregnancy
- Gallbladder disease
- Reye's syndrome
- Hemolytic-uremic syndrome
- Budd-Chiari syndrome
- SLE

WORKUP

- A clinical diagnosis is based predominantly on physical and laboratory findings.
- Most definitive diagnosis is through liver biopsy with oil red O staining and electron microscopy.
- Liver biopsy is reserved for atypical cases only and only after any existing coagulopathy corrected with FFP.

LABORATORY TESTS

Tests to determine the following:
- Hypoglycemia (often profound <60)
- Hyperammonemia
- Elevated aminotransferases (usually <500 U/ml)
- Thrombocytopenia
- Leucocytosis (WBC count >15,000)
- Hyperbilirubinemia (usually <10 mg/dl)
- Low albumin
- Hypofibrinogenemia (<300 mg/dl)
- DIC (in 75%)

IMAGING STUDIES

- Ultrasound: best used to rule out other diseases in the differential diagnosis such as gallbladder disease
- CT scan: plays minimal role because of a high false-negative rate

TREATMENT

NONPHARMACOLOGIC THERAPY

- Patient is admitted to intensive care unit for stabilization.
- Fetus is delivered; spontaneous resolution usually follows delivery.
- Mode of delivery is based on obstetric indications and clinical assessment of disease severity.

ACUTE GENERAL Rx

- Decrease in endogenous ammonia through dietary protein restriction; neomycin 6 to 12 g/day PO to decrease presence of ammonia-producing bacteria; magnesium citrate 30 to 50 ml PO or enema to evacuate nitrogenous wastes from colon
- Administration of intravenous fluids with glucose to keep glucose levels >60 mg/dl
- Coagulopathy corrected with FFP
- Avoidance of drugs metabolized by liver
- Aggressive avoidance and treatment for nosocomial infections; consideration of prophylactic antibiotics
- Monitor closely for development of complications like hepatic encephalopathy, pulmonary edema, DIC, and respiratory arrest

CHRONIC Rx

Orthotopic liver transplantation is the only treatment for irreversible liver failure.

DISPOSITION

- Before 1980, both maternal and fetal mortalities: approximately 85%
- After 1980, both maternal and fetal mortalities: below 20%
- Usually rapid return of liver function to normal after delivery
- Minimal risk of recurrence with future pregnancies

REFERRAL

- To tertiary health care facility as soon as diagnosis is suspected.
- Infants of mothers with AFLP should be evaluated for LCHAD deficiency.

SUGGESTED READINGS

Cunningham FG et al: Gastrointestinal disorders. In Cunningham FG et al (eds): *Williams' obstetrics,* ed 20, Stamford, Conn, 1997, Appleton & Lange.

Davidson KM: Acute fatty liver of pregnancy, *Postgrad Obstet Gynecol* 15:1, 1995.

Steingrub JS: Pregnancy-associated severe liver disfunction, *Crit Care Clin* 20(4):763, 2004.

Toro Ortiz JC et al: Acute fatty liver of pregnancy, *J Matern Fetal Neonatl Med* 12(4):277, 2003.

AUTHORS: **ARUNDATHI G. PRASAD, M.D.,** and **RUBEN ALVERO, M.D.**

BASIC INFORMATION

DEFINITION

Felty's syndrome (FS) is defined as the triad of rheumatoid arthritis (RA), splenomegaly, and neutropenia. The hallmark of FS is a persistent, idiopathic neutropenia, which is defined as a neutrophil count <2000/mm³. Splenomegaly is extremely variable in its extent and no longer required as an absolute diagnostic requirement. It is an extraarticular manifestation of seropositive RA in which recurrent local and systemic infections are the major source of morbidity and mortality.

ICD-9CM CODES
714.1 Felty's syndrome

EPIDEMIOLOGY & DEMOGRAPHICS

- FS occurs in less than 1% of patients with RA.
- 60% to 80% are women.
- Recognized in patients ages late 40s or early 50s who have had RA for 10 yr or more.
- Patients with FS are more likely to have a family history of RA and HLA-DRB1*0401.
- Rare in African Americans (low frequency of HLA-DRB1*0401).

CLINICAL PRESENTATION

- Rarely, splenomegaly and neutropenia are present before the arthritis.
- Articular involvement is usually more severe in patients with FS as compared with other patients with RA; however, one third may have relatively inactive synovitis with elevated erythrocyte sedimentation rate (ESR).
- Degree of splenomegaly varies and may be detectable only by imaging studies; degree of splenomegaly has no correlation with the degree of neutropenia.
- Patients with FS have a greater frequency of extraarticular manifestations (rheumatoid nodules, vasculitis, skin lesions, pleuropericarditis, etc.) than other patients with RA.
- Mild hepatomegaly is common (up to 68%).
- Patients with FS have a twentyfold increased frequency of infections as compared with other RA patients.

ETIOLOGY

The pathogenesis of FS is probably multifactorial and no clear explanation has been elucidated.

DIAGNOSIS

DIFFERENTIAL DIAGNOSIS

- Systemic lupus erythematosus
- Large granular lymphocytic leukemia
- Drug reaction
- Myeloproliferative disorders
- Lymphoma/reticuloendothelial malignancies
- Cirrhosis with portal hypertension
- Sarcoidosis
- Tuberculosis
- Amyloidosis
- HIV infection

LABORATORY TESTS

- There is no diagnostic test for FS.
- Complete blood count with differential to detect neutropenia, mild to moderate anemia, and mild to moderate thrombocytopenia.
- High ESR, C-reactive protein (CRP).
- Rheumatoid factor: positive in 98%, usually high titer.
- Antinuclear antibody (ANA): positive in 67%.
- Antihistone antibody: positive in 83%.
- Antineutrophil cytoplasmic antibodies (ANCA): positive in 77%.
- HLA-DRB1*0401: positive in 98%.
- Immunoglobulins: level may be higher than in RA patients.
- Complement: level may be lower than in RA patients.
- Bone marrow examination is often necessary to exclude other cause if neutropenia.

IMAGING STUDIES

Ultrasonography or CT scan may be useful in diagnosing splenomegaly.

TREATMENT

ACUTE GENERAL Rx

- Splenectomy
  - It was the principal treatment therapy for FS, but has now been replaced by drug therapy.
  - Usually reserved for patients with profound neutropenia (<1000/mm³) and severe recurrent infections.
  - Acutely reverses hematologic abnormalities.
  - 25% to 30% will have recurrent neutropenia, but the granulocyte count usually remains above the presplenectomy level.
  - Improvement in frequency of recurrent infection variable and not correlated with degree of hematologic improvement.
- Antirheumatic drugs: second-line drugs for rheumatological disorders may improve the neutropenia in FS.
  - Methotrexate: series of studies with small numbers of patients suggest the efficacy in FS. Follow-up durations are still short. Granulocyte count may begin to rise within several weeks in responders.
  - Gold salt injections: good hematologic response in 60%, partial response in 20%. The recovery of neutrophil count is usually slow.
  - Penicillamine, sulfasalazine: limited experience; not first choice for FS.
- Corticosteroids
  - Overwhelming infection is the main barrier to the use of corticosteroids.
  - Prednisone 30mg/day or more can elevate the neutrophil count, but this effect is often not sustained when the dose is reduced.
  - Pulse dosing is a potential alternative for short-term elevation of neutrophils.
- Others
  - Limited experience with cyclophosphamide, cyclosporine, azathioprine, leflunomide, anti-TNF-alpha antibody, and rituximab.
- Recombinant G-CSF
  - Improves neutrophil count but not arthritis and anemia of FS.
  - May be useful as adjunctive therapy during serious infection or in preparation for surgery.

DISPOSITION

- Poor prognosis with recurrent infections due to neutropenia.
- Articular involvement can be severe in FS.

REFERRAL

- To hematologist for treatment of neutropenia
- To rheumatologist for treatment of RA

PEARLS & CONSIDERATIONS

COMMENTS

- FS affects <1% of RA patients.
- Recurrent infections are the major cause of mortality.
- Neutropenia of FS can be effectively treated with disease-modifying antirheumatic drugs, the widest experience being with methotrexate.

SUGGESTED READINGS

Balint GP et al: Felty's syndrome, *Best Pract Res Clin Rheumatol* 18:631, 2004.

Bowman SJ: Hematological manifestations of rheumatoid arthritis, *Scand J Rheumatol* 31:251, 2002.

Burks EJ et al: Pathogenesis of neutropenia in large granular lymphocyte leukemia and Felty's syndrome, *Blood Rev* 20:245, 2006.

Capsoni F et al: Primary and secondary autoimmune neutropenia, *Arthritis Res Ther* 7:208, 2005.

Starkebaum G et al: Chronic neutropenia associated with autoimmune disease, *Semin Hematol* 39:121, 2002.

AUTHOR: **ETSUKO AOKI, M.D., PH.D.**

BASIC INFORMATION

DEFINITION

A femoral neck fracture occurs within the capsule of the hip joint between the base of the head and the intertrochanteric line.

SYNONYMS

Intracapsular fracture
Subcapital fracture

ICD-9CM CODES
820.8 Femoral neck fracture

EPIDEMIOLOGY & DEMOGRAPHICS

PREVALENCE: Lifetime risk in women approximately 16%
PREDOMINANT SEX: Female:male ratio of 3:1
PREDOMINANT AGE: 90% over age 60

PHYSICAL FINDINGS & CLINICAL PRESENTATION

- Hip or groin pain
- Affected limb usually shortened and externally rotated in displaced fractures
- Impacted fractures: possibly no deformity and only mild pain with hip motion
- Mild external bruising

ETIOLOGY

- Trauma
- Age-related bone weakness, usually caused by osteoporosis
- Increased risk of fractures in elderly (decline in muscle function, use of psychotropic medication, etc.)

DIAGNOSIS

DIFFERENTIAL DIAGNOSIS

- Osteoarthritis of hip
- Pathologic fracture
- Lumbar disc syndrome with radicular pain
- Insufficiency fracture of pelvis

WORKUP

Diagnosis usually obvious based on clinical and radiographic findings

IMAGING STUDIES

- Standard roentgenograms consisting of an AP of the pelvis and a cross-table lateral of the hip to confirm the diagnosis (Fig. 1-96)
- If initial roentgenograms negative and diagnosis of an occult femoral neck fracture suspected, hospital admission and further radiographic assessment with either bone scanning or MRI
- Bone scanning sensitive after 48 to 72 hr

TREATMENT

- Orthopedic consultation
- Surgery indicated in most cases, usually within 24 hr
- DVT prophylaxis

DISPOSITION

- Mortality rate within 1 yr in elderly patients is 25% to 30%.
- Dementia is a particularly poor prognostic sign.

REFERRAL

For surgical consideration when the diagnosis is made

PEARLS & CONSIDERATIONS

COMMENTS

- Complications: nonunion and avascular necrosis
- Intracapsular fractures: occasionally occur in nonambulatory patients
  1. Usually treated nonsurgically, especially in the patient with dementia and limited pain perception
  2. Early bed-to-chair mobilization and vigilant nursing care to avoid skin breakdown
  3. Fracture usually pain free in a short time even if solid bony healing does not occur
- As a result of the increasing life span of the female population, femoral neck fractures are becoming more common. The initial physical examination and roentgenographic studies may be completely negative. Groin pain, sometimes quite severe, may be the only early clue to the diagnosis
- The rate of hip fracture could be reduced by:
  1. Elimination of environmental hazards (poor lighting, loose rugs)
  2. Regular exercise for balance and strength
  3. Patient education about fall prevention
  4. Medication review to minimize side effects
  5. Prevention and treatment of osteoporosis

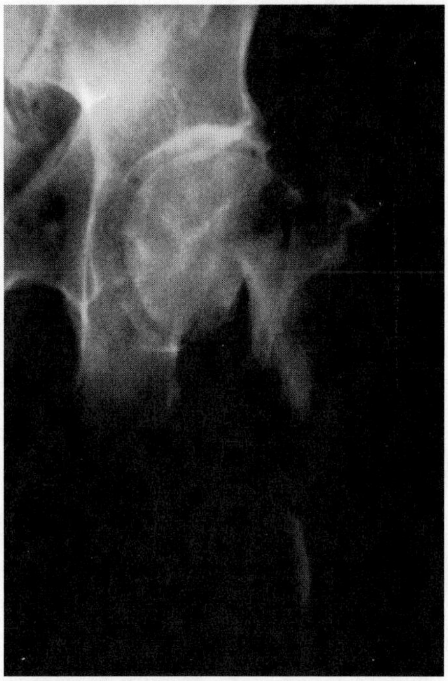

FIGURE 1-96 Femoral neck fracture. (From Scudieri G [ed]: *Sports medicine: principles of primary care,* St Louis, 1997, Mosby.)

SUGGESTED READINGS

Bettelli G et al: Relationship between mortality and proximal femur fractures in the elderly, *Orthopedics* 26:1045, 2003.

Bogoch ER et al: Effective initiation of osteoporosis diagnosis and treatment for patients with a fragility fracture in an orthopedic environment, *J Bone Joint Surg* 88A:25, 2006.

Feldstein AC et al: Older women with fractures: patients falling through the cracks of guideline recommended osteoporosis screening and treatment, *J Bone Joint Surg* 85A:2294, 2003.

Gardner MJ et al: Interventions to improve osteoporosis treatment following hip fracture, *J Bone Joint Surg* 87A:3, 2005.

Kaufman JD et al: Barriers and solutions to osteoporosis care in patients with a hip fracture, *J Bone Joint Surg* 85A:1837, 2003.

Lawrence VA et al: Medical complications and outcomes after hip fracture repair, *Ann Intern Med* 162:2053, 2003.

Logan K: Stress fractures in the adolescent athlete, *Pediatr Ann* 36:738, 2007.

Mirchandani S et al: The effects of weather and seasonality on hip fracture incidence in older adults, *Orthopedics* 28:149, 2005.

Parker MJ et al: Effectiveness of hip protectors for preventing hip fractures in elderly people, *BMJ* 332:571, 2006.

Radcliff TA et al: Patient risk factors, operative care, and outcomes among older community-dwelling male veterans with hip fracture, *J Bone Joint Surg* 90:34, 2008.

Schoofs MW et al: Thiazide diuretics and the risk for hip fractures, *Ann Intern Med* 139:476, 2003.

Tosi LL, Kyle RF: Fragility fractures: the fall and decline of bone health, *J Bone Joint Surg* 87A:1, 2005.

Van Helden S et al: Bone and fall-related fracture risks in women and men with a recent clinical fracture, *J Bone Joint Surg* 90:241, 2008.

AUTHOR: **LONNIE R. MERCIER, M.D.**

BASIC INFORMATION

DEFINITION

Fever of undetermined origin (FUO) was defined by Petersdorf and Beeson in 1961 as an illness characterized by temperatures >101° F on several occasions for >3 wk with no known cause despite extensive workup.

- Persistence for >2 wk separates an FUO from an insignificant viral illness.
- Traditionally, diagnosis made only after a 1-wk inpatient workup. In contemporary practice, much of the workup is performed as an outpatient.

SYNONYMS

Fever of unknown origin

ICD-9CM CODES
780.6 Pyrexia of undetermined origin

EPIDEMIOLOGY & DEMOGRAPHICS

- The incidence of undiagnosed FUO dropped to <10% in the 1950s but increased to approximately 30% in the 1990s.
- True FUOs are uncommon.

CLINICAL PRESENTATION

- Fever (101° F or more) >3 wk.

ETIOLOGY

(Most common etiologies italicized)

- Infection (16%)
  - *Abscess: abdominal, pelvic*
  - *Tuberculosis*
  - *HIV infection*
  - *Nosocomial* (febrile for 3 days in hospital): UTI, pneumonia, line-related bacteremia, *Clostridium difficile* diarrhea, or sinusitis
  - Bacterial endocarditis (especially caused by difficult-to-isolate organisms)
  - Biliary tract infection
  - Osteomyelitis, vertebral and mandibular
  - Less common infections: Q fever, leptospirosis, psittacosis, tularemia, secondary syphilis, gonococcemia, chronic meningococcemia, Whipple's disease, yersiniosis, and fungal infections
- Malignancy (7%): *lymphoma and leukemia,* renal cell carcinoma, hepatocellular carcinomas, and other tumors metastatic to liver
- Noninfectious inflammatory disease (22%)
  - Systemic lupus erythematosus
  - Juvenile rheumatoid arthritis (younger patients)
  - Temporal arteritis (elderly patients)
  - Other vasculitis: polyarteritis nodosa, Takayasu's arteritis, Wegener's granulomatosis, adult Still's disease
- Others (4%)
  - Drug-induced fever
  - Inflammatory bowel disease
  - Sarcoidosis
  - Granulomatous hepatitis
  - Deep venous thrombosis
  - Alcoholic hepatitis

DIAGNOSIS (Dx)

DIFFERENTIAL DIAGNOSIS

Factitious fever

WORKUP

- Accurate history and careful physical examination is essential.
- Laboratory tests and imaging dependent on historical clues, physical findings.
- When in doubt, perform another complete history and physical examination.

HISTORICAL CLUES

- Fever duration, tempo; inciting factors
- Rash, myalgia, weight loss, pain
- Sick contacts
- Past medical history: tuberculosis, HIV, malignancies, surgeries
- Medications
- Family history: tuberculosis, malignancies, familial Mediterranean fever
- Social history: daily routine, rural vs. urban, pets and animal contacts, arthropod bites, recent and remote travel, socioeconomic status, occupation, military service, sexual history

PHYSICAL FINDINGS

- HEENT: sinus tenderness, dental abscesses, funduscopic lesions
- Neck: adenopathy, palpable thyroid
- Lungs: auscultate for rales
- Heart: murmur
- Abdomen: organomegaly
- Rectal: prostate tenderness
- Pelvic: cervical motion tenderness, fundal or adnexal masses/pain; inguinal adenopathy
- Extremities: clubbing, splinter hemorrhages; tenderness/fluctuance at IV access site
- Musculoskeletal: joint effusions
- Skin: rashes, wounds

LABORATORY TESTS

- Most FUO workups will include
  - Blood cultures
  - CBC
  - Urinalysis
  - Transaminases
  - PPD testing
- Consider
  - HIV antibody testing
  - Lumbar puncture
  - Thyroid function testing
  - Stool culture and *C. difficile* assay
  - Bone marrow biopsy
  - Skin biopsy
  - ANA

May need to repeat tests at regular intervals until diagnosis is established.

IMAGING STUDIES

- Most workups eventually include
  - Chest x-ray
  - Abdominal CT scan
- Further imaging based on historical clues and physical findings

TREATMENT (Rx)

ACUTE GENERAL Rx

Antibiotics and other treatment indicated only after definitive or highly probable diagnosis is established, unless patient is severely ill or septic.

DISPOSITION

Diagnoses are found in majority of cases of FUO. In some cases, a diagnosis will not be made for years. At a 5-year follow-up, mortality among patients with undiagnosed FUO was only 3.2% in one study.

REFERRAL

To an infectious disease specialist, hematologist, or rheumatologist if no diagnosis after thoughtful workup

PEARLS & CONSIDERATIONS (!)

COMMENTS

Due to improvements in imaging and laboratory tests, fewer cases of FUO are attributed to infectious causes and more are diagnosed as secondary to tumors and collagen-vascular diseases.

SUGGESTED READINGS

Bleeker-Rovers CP et al: A prospective multicenter study on fever of unknown origin: the yield of a structured diagnostic approach, *Medicine (Baltimore)* 86:26, 2007.

Knockaert DC et al: Long-term follow-up of patients with undiagnosed fever of unknown origin, *Arch Intern Med* 156:6, 1996.

Mourad O et al: A comprehensive evidence-based approach to fever of unknown origin, *Arch Intern Med* 163:5, 2003.

Roth AR et al: Approach to the adult patient with fever of unknown origin, *Am Fam Physician* 68:2223, 2003.

AUTHOR: **ETSUKO AOKI, M.D., PH.D.**

BASIC INFORMATION

DEFINITION

Fibrocystic breast disease (FCD) is a "nondisease" that includes nonmalignant breast lesions such as microcystic and macrocystic changes, fibrosis, ductal or lobular hyperplasia, adenosis, apocrine metaplasia, fibroadenoma, papilloma, papillomatosis, and other changes. Atypical ductal or lobular hyperplasia is associated with a moderate increase in breast cancer risk.

SYNONYMS

Cystic changes
Chronic cystic mastitis
Mammary dysplasia

ICD-9CM CODES
610.0 Solitary cyst of the breast
610.1 Fibrocystic disease of the breast

EPIDEMIOLOGY & DEMOGRAPHICS

- Ubiquitous in premenopausal women after 20 yr of age
- Palpable nodular changes in the breast termed *FCD* clinically; such changes observable in more than half of adult women 20 to 50 yr of age

PHYSICAL FINDINGS & CLINICAL PRESENTATION

- Tender breasts
- Nodular areas
- Dominant mass
- Thickening
- Nipple discharge
- Can vary with menstrual cycle

ETIOLOGY

- Although frequently seen and diagnosed, mechanism of development not understood.
- Because found in majority of healthy breasts, regarded as nonpathologic process.
- With hormone replacement therapy, may be carried into menopausal age.

DIAGNOSIS

DIFFERENTIAL DIAGNOSIS

- If presenting as dominant mass or masses: exclude possible carcinoma.
- Carcinoma: detection is difficult with FCD, particularly among premenopausal women.
- If presenting with nipple discharge: differentiate from discharge of possible malignant origin.

WORKUP

- Exclude breast carcinoma if breast mass, thickening, discharge, and pain present.
- Perform biopsy of suspected area for histologic confirmation.

IMAGING STUDIES

Mammography and ultrasound studies required:

- For mammographic changes (suspicious densities, microcalcifications, architectural distortion): careful evaluation, including possibly biopsy to exclude breast cancer
- Ultrasound study: to establish cystic nature of clinical or mammographic mass lesion

TREATMENT

NONPHARMACOLOGIC THERAPY

- Not considered a "disease" and does not require treatment
- Surgical intervention diagnostic to eliminate possibility of breast cancer
- Periodic physician examination to follow patients with FCD who have pronounced nodular features
- Aspiration for palpable cysts (NOTE: Cysts often recur; repeat aspiration is not always required unless pain is a problem.)

ACUTE GENERAL Rx

Majority of women require no treatment.

CHRONIC Rx

For breast pain:

- Danocrine (Danazol): limited success reported
- Bromocriptine or tamoxifen: used less frequently
- Limited caffeine intake: not as successful in controlling pain or nodularity as originally suggested

DISPOSITION

- Careful evaluation to exclude suspicious changes for breast cancer, then reassurance and periodic reevaluation as required
- Regular self-examination, annual physician examination, and annual mammograms for women with atypical ductal or lobular hyperplasia

REFERRAL

- For further evaluation and/or biopsy if there are suspicious changes that may be associated with FCD (including changing of dominant mass or thickening, persistent or spontaneous discharge, suspicious mammographic changes or lesions)
- To alleviate anxiety associated with breast symptoms or changes

EVIDENCE

There is evidence that both danazol and tamoxifen are effective at relieving breast pain in benign breast conditions but their benefit needs to be balanced with their side effects.

A small randomized controlled trial (RCT) compared tamoxifen vs. placebo in premenopausal women with cyclical breast pain. Significantly more women in the tamoxifen group reported pain relief.[1] (A)

Another RCT compared tamoxifen vs. placebo for the treatment of mastalgia and found that the number of women who achieved complete recovery was increased in the tamoxifen group (90% with tamoxifen vs. 0% with placebo).[2] (A)

There is limited evidence that bromocriptine is effective in relieving breast pain. However, a high incidence of intolerable side effects is reported, which may outweigh any benefit.

One RCT found that bromocriptine significantly improved breast pain, tenderness, and heaviness compared with placebo in premenopausal women with diffuse fibrocystic breast changes. However, bromocriptine was associated with a significantly higher incidence of adverse effects. The high rate of withdrawal from this study means that the results should be interpreted with caution.[3] (B)

There is evidence that advice to eat a low-fat, high-carbohydrate diet leads to decreased self-reported breast tenderness.

A small RCT compared advice to follow a low-fat, high-carbohydrate diet vs. general dietary advice in women with severe cyclical mastalgia. There was a significant reduction in the severity of self-reported breast swelling and tenderness in patients in the low-fat, high-carbohydrate diet group after 6 months. However, there was no significant reduction in breast swelling, tenderness, or nodularity at physical examination.[4] (B)

Evidence-Based References

1. Fentiman IS et al: Double-blind controlled trial of tamoxifen therapy for mastalgia, *Lancet* 1:287, 1986. Reviewed in: *Clin Evid* 11:2334, 2004. (A)
2. Grio R et al: Clinical efficacy of tamoxifen in the treatment of premenstrual mastodynia, *Minerva Ginecol* 50:101, 1998. Reviewed in: *Clin Evid* 11:2334, 2004. (A)
3. Mansel RE, Dogliotti L: European multicentre trial of bromocriptine in cyclical mastalgia, *Lancet* 335:190, 1990. Reviewed in: *Clin Evid* 11:2334, 2004. (B)
4. Boyd NF et al: Effect of a low-fat high-carbohydrate diet on symptoms of cyclical mastopathy, *Lancet* 2:128, 1988. Reviewed in: *Clin Evid* 11:2334, 2004. (B)

AUTHORS: **TAKUMA NEMOTO, M.D.**, and **RUBEN ALVERO, M.D.**

BASIC INFORMATION

DEFINITION

Fibromyalgia is a poorly defined disorder characterized by multiple trigger points and referred pain.

SYNONYMS

Myofascial pain syndrome
Fibrositis
Psychogenic rheumatism
Nonarticular rheumatism
Fibromyalgia syndrome (FS)

ICD-9CM CODES
729.0 Rheumatism, unspecified and fibrositis
729.1 Myalgia and myositis, unspecified

EPIDEMIOLOGY & DEMOGRAPHICS

PREVALENCE: 1% to 2% of the general population
PREDOMINANT SEX: Female:male ratio of 9:1
PREDOMINANT AGE: 30 to 50 yr

PHYSICAL FINDINGS

Tender "nodules" and tender points (Fig. 1-97)

ETIOLOGY

- Unknown
- Pain magnification may play a role

DIAGNOSIS

DIFFERENTIAL DIAGNOSIS

- Polymyalgia rheumatica
- Referred discogenic spine pain
- Rheumatoid arthritis
- Localized tendinitis
- Connective tissue disease
- Osteoarthritis
- Thyroid disease
- Spondyloarthropathies

WORKUP

- Subsets of this disorder are often described:
  1. If symptoms develop in conjunction with other conditions (rheumatoid disease or acute stress)
  2. If findings are more regionally distributed, such as those in the neck following motor vehicle accidents
- The primary condition is often suggested by the following criteria from the American College of Rheumatology:
  1. History of widespread pain
  2. Pain in 11 of 18 selected tender spots on digital palpation (mainly in the spine, elbows, and knees)

LABORATORY TESTS

There are no abnormalities in fibromyalgia, but laboratory assessment may be required to rule out other conditions and may include:
- CBC, ESR, rheumatoid factor, ANA
- CPK, T_4

TREATMENT

ACUTE GENERAL Rx

- Self-management
- Explanation, reassurance
- Tricyclic antidepressants for sleep disturbance (amitriptyline 10 to 25 mg)
- Aerobic and stretching exercise, particularly swimming
- Mild analgesics; avoidance of chronic narcotic use
- Trigger point injections
- Physical therapy

DISPOSITION

- Prognosis is uncertain.
- Symptoms come and go for years in spite of an aggressive multifaceted approach to treatment.

REFERRAL

Consultation with rheumatology, psychiatry, and physical medicine may all be helpful.

PEARLS & CONSIDERATIONS

Some investigators consider myofacial pain syndrome to be a separate conditiion, perhaps with a better prognosis.

COMMENTS

- Before making this diagnosis, all other more likely disorders should be ruled out.
- The term "fibrositis" is often used, but no inflammation has ever been found.
- The number of trigger points needed to establish the diagnosis is debated.

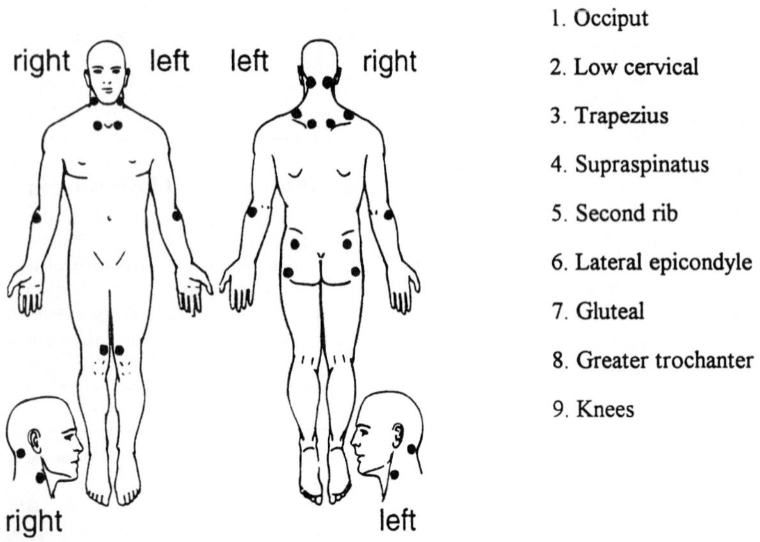

FIGURE 1-97 The sites of the 18 tender points of the 1990 ACR criteria for the classification of fibromyalgia. (From Conn R: *Current diagnosis,* ed 9, Philadelphia, 1997, WB Saunders.)

SUGGESTED READINGS

Bieber C et al: A shared decision-making communication training program for physicians treating fibromyalgia patients: effects of a randomized controlled trial, *J Psychom Res* 64:13, 2008.

Crofford LJ: Pharmaceutical treatment options for fibromyalgia, *Curr Rheumatol Rep* 6:274, 2004.

Freidberg F et al: Publication trends in chronic fatigue syndrome: comparisons with fibromyalgia and fatigue, *J Psychom Res* 63:143, 2007.

Goldenberg DL et al: Management of fibromyalgia syndrome, *JAMA* 292:2388, 2004.

Richards SCM, Scott DL: Prescribed exercise in people with fibromyalgia: parallel group randomized controlled trial, *BMJ* 325:185, 2002.

Robinson RL et al: Depression and fibromyalgia: treatment and cost when diagnosed separately or concurrently, *J Rheumatol* 31:1621, 2004.

Valkeinen H et al: Acute heavy-resistance exercise-induced pain and neuromuscular fatigue in elderly women with fibromyalgia and in healthy controls: effects of strength training, *Arthritis Rheum* 54:1334, 2006.

Van Middendorp H et al: Emotions and emotional approach and avoidance strategies in fibromyalgia, *J Psychom Res* 64:159, 2008.

Van Wilgen et al: Characteristics and healthcare costs of patients with fibromyalgia implemented in the primary care, *Disabil Rehabil* 29:1207, 2007.

Wahner-Roedler DL et al: Use of complementary and alternative medical therapies by patients referred to a fibromyalgia treatment program at a tertiary care center, *Mayo Clin Proc* 80:55, 2005.

AUTHOR: **LONNIE R. MERCIER, M.D.**

BASIC INFORMATION

DEFINITION

Fifth disease is a viral exanthem of childhood affecting primarily school-age children, which is caused by parvovirus B-19. Erythema infectiosum was the "fifth" in a series of described viral exanthems of childhood and is the most common clinical syndrome associated with parvovirus B-19.

SYNONYMS

Erythema infectiosum

ICD-9CM CODES
057.0 Fifth disease (eruptive)

EPIDEMIOLOGY & DEMOGRAPHICS

PEAK INCIDENCE: Late winter and spring, especially April and May
PREDOMINANT AGE: 5 to 18 yr old
GENETICS: Fifty to sixty percent of adults have demonstrated protective antibodies to parvovirus B-19

PHYSICAL FINDINGS & CLINICAL PRESENTATION

- Typical bright red nontender maxillary rash with circumoral pallor over cheeks, producing the classic "slapped cheek" appearance (Fig. 1-98)
- Reticular nonpruritic lacy, erythematous maculopapular rash over trunk and extremities lasting for up to several weeks after the acute episode. May be worsened by heat or sunlight
- Polyarthritis and arthralgias are commonly seen in older patients; less common in children. Arthritis involves small joints of extremities in symmetric fashion
- Mild fever seen in up to one third of patients

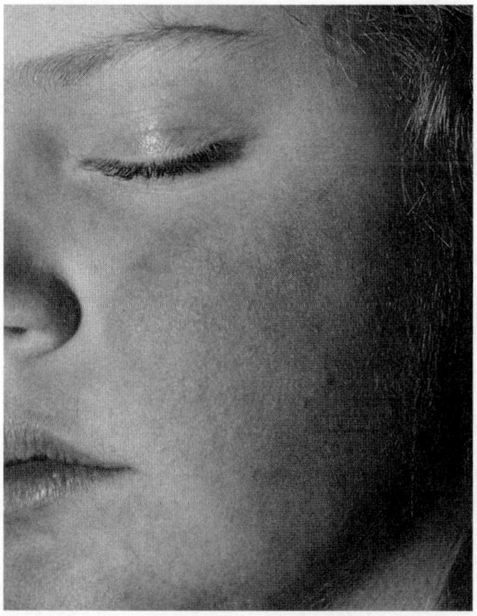

FIGURE 1-98 Fifth disease (erythema infectiosum). Facial erythema "slapped cheek." The red plaque covers the cheek and spares the nasolabial and the circumoral region. (From Habif TP: *Clinical dermatology: a color guide to diagnosis and therapy,* ed 3, St Louis, 1996, Mosby.)

ETIOLOGY

Syndrome caused by parvovirus B-19, a single-stranded DNA virus, which has been reclassified in a new genus "erythrovirus."

- It remains the only accepted member of this genus, although new variants have recently been described.
- Designation as "parvovirus" is still common in recent literature

DIAGNOSIS

DIFFERENTIAL DIAGNOSIS

- Juvenile rheumatoid arthritis (Still's disease)
- Rubella, measles (rubeola), and other childhood viral exanthems
- Mononucleosis
- Lyme disease
- Acute HIV infection
- Drug eruption

WORKUP

- Diagnosis made by typical clinical picture
- Parvovirus B-19 IgM antibody seen in 90% of patients with acute illness

LABORATORY TESTS

- CBC
  1. Transient aplastic crisis is a syndrome distinct from fifth disease, which may be seen in patients with chronic hematologic illness (described with sickle cell disease, spherocytosis, and other hemolytic processes) or AIDS, who are infected with parvovirus B-19.
     a. Usually self-limited and associated with prodrome of fever and malaise. Lasts for 1 to 2 wk followed by marrow recovery.
     b. Rash usually absent.
     c. These patients are highly infective.
- hCG in women of childbearing age.
  - Infection during early pregnancy may result in fetal death (10%) or severe anemia but is usually asymptomatic and not associated with congenital malformations.
- Antibody testing usually not necessary. IgM levels may be elevated early in the course of the illness.
- Lyme titers, monospot Ab.
- Testing for other viral diseases as indicated by clinical picture.
- Polymerase chain reaction (PCR) has been used for early, rapid diagnosis in immunocompromised patients.

TREATMENT

ACUTE GENERAL Rx

- Treatment is supportive only
- NSAIDs for arthralgias/arthritis
- Intravenous immunoglobulin and transfusion support may be used in patients with immunocompromised state with red cell aplasia
- Consider immunoglobulin treatment or prophylaxis in pregnancy

DISPOSITION & PROGNOSIS

- Self-limited illness lasting 1 to 2 wk
- Arthritis lasts for weeks. In some patients it may be chronic and develop into rheumatoid arthritis as adult
- Pregnant women should avoid contact with patients who have marrow suppression
- Patients with transient aplastic crisis or chronic parvovirus B-19 infection pose a risk for nosocomial spread and, when hospitalized, should be isolated with contact and respiratory precautions
- Children with fifth disease are not contagious and may attend school and day care
- Vaccine is under development

REFERRAL

- To hematologist for signs of marrow suppression
- To rheumatologist for signs of severe or erosive arthritis

PEARLS & CONSIDERATIONS

- Self-limited disease lasting 1-2 wk
- Symmetric arthritis involving small joints common in adults whereas facial rash is common in children
- Can cause aplastic anemia in patients with underlying hematologic disorder such as sickle cell disease, immunocompromised state, and posttransplantation

SUGGESTED READINGS

Katta, R: Parvovirus B19: a review, *Dermatol Clin* 20(2):333, 2002.
Sabella C, Goldfarls J: Parvovirus B19 infections, *Am Fam Physician* 60(5):1455, 1999.
Young NS: Parvovirus B19, *New Engl J Med* 350(6):586, 2004.

AUTHOR: **DOMINICK TAMMARO, M.D.**

BASIC INFORMATION

DEFINITION

Filariasis is a general term for an infection caused by subcutaneous nematodes (round-worms) of the genera *Wuchereria* and *Brugia,* found in the tropical and subtropical regions of the world. The disease is variably characterized by acute lymphatic inflammation or chronic lymphatic obstruction associated with intermittent fevers or recurrent episodes of dyspnea and bronchospasm.

SYNONYMS

Lymphatic filariasis
Elephantiasis

ICD-9CM CODES
125.0 Bancroftian
125.1 Brugian
125.9 Filariasis

EPIDEMIOLOGY & DEMOGRAPHICS

INCIDENCE (IN U.S.): Unknown
PEAK INCIDENCE: Unknown
PREDOMINANT SEX: Male
PREDOMINANT AGE: For both males and females, risk is greatest between the ages of 15 to 35 yr.

PHYSICAL FINDINGS & CLINICAL PRESENTATION

- Clinical manifestations result from acute lymphatic inflammation or chronic lymphatic obstruction.
- Many patients are asymptomatic despite the presence of microfilaremia.
- Episodes of lymphangitis and lymphadenitis are associated with fever, headache, and back pain.
- Acute funiculitis and epididymitis or orchitis may also be present; all usually resolve within days to weeks but tend to recur.
- Chronic infections may be associated with lymphedema, most commonly manifested by hydrocele.
- It is a progressive disease, leading to nonpitting edema and brawny changes that may involve a whole limb (Fig. 1-99).
- Elephantiasis occurs in about 10% of patients, with skin of the scrotum or leg becoming thickened and fissured; patient is thereafter plagued by recurrent ulceration and infection.
- Chyluria, a condition that develops when lymphatic vessels rupture into the urinary tract, may occur.

ETIOLOGY

Caused by one of three types of nematode parasites, all of which are transmitted to humans by *Culex spp.* mosquitoes.

- *W. bancrofti:* distributed in Africa, areas of Central and South America, the Pacific Islands, and the Caribbean Basin
- *B. malayi:* restricted to Southeast Asia
- *B. timori:* confined to the Indonesian archipelago

After bite of an infected mosquito:

- Filarial larvae move into lymphatic vessels and nodes, settling and maturing over 3 to 15 mo into adult male and female worms.
- After fertilization, the female nematode produces large numbers of larvae or microfilariae that enter into the blood stream via the lymphatics.
- Nocturnal periodicity, characteristic of *B. malayi,* is an increased presence of microfilariae in the circulation during the night.
- Microfilariae of *W. bancrofti* are maximal during late afternoon.
- Most microfilariae remain in the body as immature forms for 6 mo to 2 yr.
- Infected larvae are ingested by mosquitoes, then transmitted to humans where the microfilariae mature into new adult worms.

Acute and chronic inflammatory and granulomatous changes in the lymphatic channels:

- Result from complex interaction of adult worms and host's immune systems
- Eventually lead to fibrosis and obstruction
- Most likely to develop into obstructive lymphatic disease with recurrent exposure over many years

DIAGNOSIS

DIFFERENTIAL DIAGNOSIS

Elephantiasis is distinguished from other causes of chronic lymphedema, including Milroy's disease, postoperative scarring, and lymphedema of malignancy.

WORKUP

Diagnosis is suspected in individuals who have resided in endemic areas for at least 3 to 6 mo or more and complain of recurrent episodes of lymphangitis, lymphadenitis, scrotal edema, or thrombophlebitis, with or without fever.

LABORATORY TESTS

- Demonstration of microfilariae on a blood smear for definitive diagnosis
- For patients from southeastern Asia: blood sample drawn at night, especially between midnight and 2 A.M.
- Occasionally, microfilaremia in chylous urine or hydrocele fluid
- Prominent eosinophilia only during periods of acute lymphangitis or lymphadenitis
- Serologic tests for antibody, including enzyme-linked immunosorbent assay and indirect fluorescent antibody (often unable to distinguish among the various forms of filariasis or between acute and remote infection)
- Immunoassays (such as circulating filaria antigen [CFA]): more successful in antigen detection in patients who are

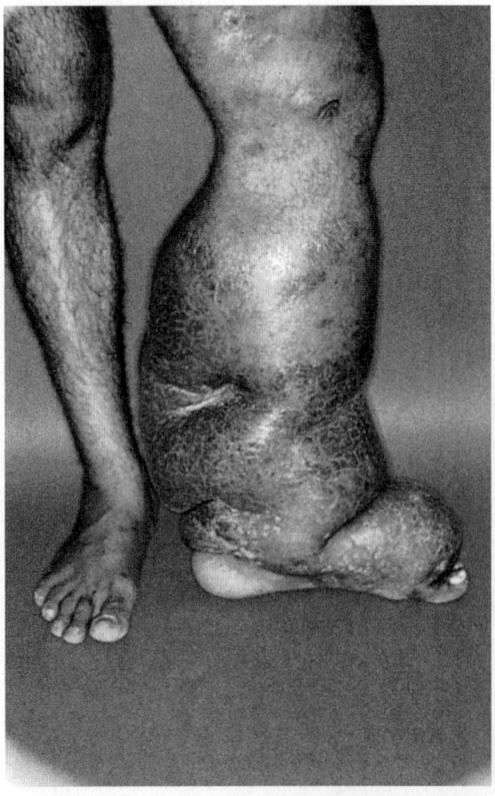

FIGURE 1-99 Filariasis that eventually leads to elephantiasis. Note massive swelling of the extremity. (From Goldstein B [ed]: *Practical dermatology,* ed 2, St Louis, 1997, Mosby.)

microfilaremic than in those who are amicrofilaremic

IMAGING STUDIES

- Chest x-ray examination: reticular nodular infiltrates (tropical pulmonary eosinophilia syndrome)
- In men proven to be microfilaremic, scrotal ultrasonography to aid in the detection of adult worms
- Compared with adults, children with FS have more sleep disturbances, fewer tender points, and a better prognosis

TREATMENT

Rx

NONPHARMACOLOGIC THERAPY

- Standard of care for elephantiasis:
  1. Elevation of the affected limb
  2. Use of elastic stockings
  3. Local foot care
- General wound care for chronic ulcers and prevention of secondary infection

ACUTE GENERAL Rx

- Diethylcarbamazine citrate (DEC) to reduce microfilaremia by 90%
  1. Effect on adult worms, especially those of the *Wuchereria* species, less certain
  2. Given in an oral dose of 6 mg/kg qd for 12 to 14 days
- Ivermectin alone or in combination with diethylcarbamazine citrate to decrease microfilaremia
- Both drugs are similar in efficacy and tolerability; advantage of ivermectin: administration in a single oral dose of 200 μg/kg
- World Health Organization (WHO) recommendation: DEC given as a single dose, alone or (preferably) in combination with ivermectin as treatment in endemic areas
- Antibacterial agents (a penicillin or cephalsporin) may be indicated to treat co-existing bacterial soft tissue infection (cellulitis or lymphangiitis), which frequently complicates filariasis of the lower extremities.

CHRONIC Rx

- Surgical drainage of hydroceles
- No satisfactory therapy for those patients with chyluria

DISPOSITION

Rarely fatal, but the psychologic impact of limb and scrotal deformities associated with elephantiasis is substantial.

REFERRAL

To a surgeon for management of hydrocele

PEARLS & CONSIDERATIONS

!

- Studies in endemic areas suggest that filarial-specific IgG1 is associated with amicrofilaremic states highest in children, regardless of sex.
- Levels of IgE and IgG4 increase with age and are associated with increased levels of microfilaremia.

COMMENTS

Individuals who intend to travel or reside in endemic areas should be advised to institute preventive measures such as the use of netting and insect repellents, especially at night.

SUGGESTED READINGS

Kerketta AS et al: A randomized clinical trial to compare the efficacy of three treatment regimens along with footcare in the morbidity management of filarial lymphoedema, *Trop Med Int Health* 10(7):698, 2005.

Malhotra I et al: Influence of maternal filariasis on childhood infection and immunity to Wuchereria bancrofti in Kenya, *Infect Immun* 71(9):5231, 2003.

Pal BK et al: Lymphatic filariasis: possible pathophysiological nexus with oxidative stress, *Trans R Soc Trop Med Hyg* 100(7):650, 2006.

Ramaiah KD et al: The prevalences of Wuchereria bancrofti antigenemia in communities given six rounds of treatment with diethylcarbamazine, ivermectin or placebo tablets, *Ann Trop Med Parasitol* 97(7):737, 2003.

Walther M, Muller R: Diagnosis of human filariases (except onchocerciasis), *Adv Parasitol* 53:149, 2003.

Watanabe K et al: Bancroftian filariasis in Nepal: a survey for circulating antigenemia of Wuchereria bancrofti and urinary IgG4 antibody in two rural areas of Nepal, *Acta Trop* 88(1):11, 2003.

AUTHORS: **GEORGE O. ALONSO, M.D., GLENN G. FORT, M.D., M.P.H.,** and **DENNIS J. MIKOLICH, M.D.**

BASIC INFORMATION

DEFINITION

Folliculitis is the inflammation of the hair follicle as a result of infection, physical injury, or chemical irritation.

SYNONYMS

Sycosis barbae

ICD-9CM CODES
704.8 Other specified diseases of hair and hair follicles

EPIDEMIOLOGY & DEMOGRAPHICS

PREVALENCE: Staphylococcal folliculitis is the most common form of infectious folliculitis; it occurs most commonly in persons with diabetes.

PREDOMINANT SEX: Sycosis barbae occurs most frequently in men who have commenced shaving.

PHYSICAL FINDINGS & CLINICAL PRESENTATION

- The lesions generally consist of painful yellow pustules surrounded by erythema; a central hair is present in the pustules.
- Patients with sycosis barbae may initially present with small follicular papules or pustules that increase in size with continued shaving; deep follicular pustules may occur surrounded by erythema and swelling; the upper lip is frequently involved (Fig. 1-100).
- "Hot tub" folliculitis occurs within 1 to 4 days following use of hot tub with poor chlorination, and it is characterized by pustules with surrounding erythema generally affecting torso, buttocks, and limbs.

ETIOLOGY

- *Staphylococcus* infection (e.g., sycosis barbae), *Pseudomonas aeruginosa* ("hot tub" folliculitis)
- Gram-negative folliculitis *(Klebsiella, Enterobacter, Proteus)* associated with antibiotic treatment of acne
- Chronic irritation of the hair follicle (use of cocoa butter or coconut oil, chronic irritation from workplace)
- Initial use of systemic corticosteroid therapy (steroid acne), eosinophilic folliculitis (AIDS patients), *Candida albicans* (immunocompromised patients)
- *Pityrosporum orbiculare*

DIAGNOSIS

DIFFERENTIAL DIAGNOSIS

- Pseudofolliculitis barbae (ingrown hairs)
- Acne vulgaris
- Dermatophyte fungal infections
- Keratosis biliaris
- Cutaneous candidiasis
- Superficial fungal infections
- Miliaris

WORKUP

Physical examination and medical history (e.g., use of hot tub: "hot tub" folliculitis; adolescent patients who have started shaving: sycosis barbae; use of occlusive topical steroid therapy: *Staphylococcus* folliculitis).

LABORATORY TESTS

Gram stain is useful to identify the infective organisms in infectious folliculitis and to differentiate infectious folliculitis from noninfectious.

TREATMENT

NONPHARMACOLOGIC THERAPY

- Prevention of chemical or mechanical skin irritation
- Glycemic control in diabetics
- Proper chlorination of hot tubs and spas
- Shaving with a clean razor

ACUTE GENERAL Rx

- Cleansing of the area with chlorhexidine and application of saline compresses to involved area
- Application of 2% mupirocin ointment (Bactroban) for bacterial folliculitis affecting a limited area (e.g., sycosis barbae)
- Treatment of severe cases of *Pseudomonas* folliculitis with ciprofloxacin
- Treatment of *S. aureus* folliculitis with dicloxacillin 250 mg qid for 10 days

CHRONIC Rx

- Chronic nasal or perineal *S. aureus* carriers with frequent folliculitis can be treated with rifampin 300 mg bid for 5 days.
- Mupirocin (Bactroban ointment 2%) applied to nares bid is also effective for nasal carriers.

DISPOSITION

- Most cases of bacterial folliculitis resolve completely with proper treatment.
- Steroid folliculitis responds to discontinuation of steroids.

PEARLS & CONSIDERATIONS

COMMENTS

Patients should be instructed in good personal hygiene and avoidance of sharing razors, towels, and washcloths.

AUTHOR: **FRED F. FERRI, M.D.**

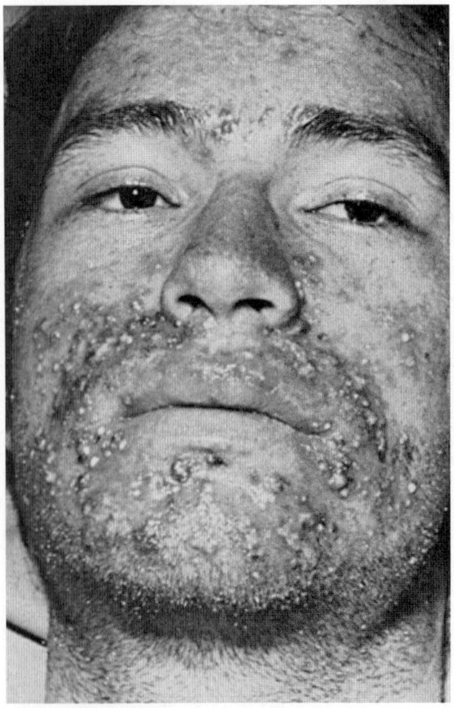

FIGURE 1-100 Folliculitis. Note the pustular eruption with small abscess formation in the hair-bearing areas of the face. General symptoms are usually absent. (From Mandell GL: *Mandell, Douglas, and Bennett's principles and practice of infectious diseases,* ed 6, New York, 2004, Churchill Livingstone.)

BASIC INFORMATION

DEFINITION

Food poisoning is an illness caused by ingestion of food contaminated by bacteria and/or bacterial toxins.

SYNONYMS

Enterotoxin-poisoning
Epidemic vomiting disease

ICD-9CM CODES
See specific illness.

EPIDEMIOLOGY & DEMOGRAPHICS

INCIDENCE (IN U.S.):
- Estimated range of 6 to 8 million cases/yr
- Majority of identifiable causes are bacterial

PEAK INCIDENCE: Varies with specific organism
- Summer: *Staphylococcus aureus, Salmonella, Shigella spp.*
- Summer and fall: *Clostridium botulinum, Vibrio parahaemolyticus*
- Spring and fall: *Campylobacter jejuni*
- Winter: *Clostridium perfringens, Yersinia enterocolitica*

PREDOMINANT AGE: Varies with specific agent

NEONATAL INFECTION: Rare but severe with *Shigella* and *Salmonella* spp.

PHYSICAL FINDINGS & CLINICAL PRESENTATION

- Any combination of GI symptoms and fever
- Specific organisms suspected on the basis of the incubation period and predominant symptoms, although a great deal of overlap exists
  1. Short incubation period (1 to 6 hr): involve the ingestion of preformed toxin; noninvasive
     a. *S. aureus:* nausea, profuse vomiting, and abdominal cramps common; diarrhea possible, but fever uncommon; usually resolves within 24 hr; foods implicated in outbreaks include meats, mayonnaise, and cream pastries
     b. *B. cereus:* two forms, a short incubation (emetic) form (characterized by vomiting and abdominal cramps in virtually all patients, diarrhea in one third of patients, fever uncommon) and a long incubation (diarrheal) form; illness usually mild, resolves within 12 hr; unrefrigerated rice most often implicated as vehicle
  2. Moderate incubation period (8 to 16 hr): involves the in vivo production of toxin; noninvasive
     a. *C. perfringens:* severe crampy abdominal pain and watery diarrhea common; fever and vomiting unlikely; symptoms usually resolving within 24 hr; outbreaks invariably related to cooked meat or poultry that is allowed to cool without refrigeration; most cases in the fall and winter months
     b. *B. cereus:* diarrheal (or long incubation) form most commonly beginning with diarrhea, abdominal cramps, and occasionally vomiting; fever uncommon; usually resolves within 24 hr; the responsible food is usually fried rice
  3. Long incubation period (>16 hr): some toxin-mediated, some invasive
     a. Toxin-producing organisms include:
        (1) *C. botulinum:* should be considered when a diarrheal illness coincides with or precedes paralysis; severity of illness related to the quantity of toxin ingested; characteristic cranial nerve palsies progressing to a descending paralysis; fever usually absent; usually associated with home-canned foods
        (2) Enterotoxigenic *E. coli* (ETEC): most common cause of travelers' diarrhea; after 1- to 2-day incubation period, abdominal cramps and copious diarrhea occur; vomiting and fever uncommon; usually resolves after 3 to 4 days; vehicle usually unbottled water or contaminated salad or ice
        (3) Enterohemorrhagic *E. coli* (EHEC): can cause severe abdominal cramps and watery diarrhea, which may eventually become bloody; bacteria (strain O157:H7) are noninvasive; no fever; illness may be complicated by hemolytic-uremic syndrome; associated with contaminated beef
        (4) *V. cholerae:* varies from a mild, self-limited illness to life-threatening cholera; diarrhea, nausea and vomiting, abdominal cramps, and muscle cramps; no fever; severe cases may progress to shock and death within hours of onset; survivors usually have resolution of symptoms in 1 wk; U.S. cases are either imported or result from ingestion of imported food
     b. Invasive organisms include:
        (1) *Salmonella:* associated most often with nontyphoidal strains; incubation period generally 12 to 48 hr; nausea, vomiting, diarrhea, and abdominal cramps typical; fever possible; outbreaks of gastroenteritis related to contaminated poultry, meat, and dairy products
        (2) *Shigella:* asymptomatic infection possible, but some with fever and watery diarrhea that may progress to bloody diarrhea and dysentery; with mild illness, usually self-limited, resolves in a few days; with severe illness, may develop complications; transmission usually from person to person but can occur via contaminated food or water
        (3) *C. jejuni:* the most common food-borne bacterial pathogen; incubation period is about 1 day, then a prodrome of fever, headache, and myalgias; intestinal phase marked by diarrhea associated with fever, malaise, and abdominal pain; diarrhea mild to profuse and bloody, usually resolves in about 7 days, but relapse is possible; associated with undercooked meats and poultry, unpasteurized dairy products, and drinking from freshwater streams
        (4) *Y. enterocolitica* and *Y. pseudotuberculosis:* infrequent causes of enteritis in U.S.; children affected more often than adults; fever, diarrhea, and abdominal pain lasting 1 to 3 wk; some with mesenteric adenitis that mimics acute appendicitis; contaminated food or water is usually responsible
        (5) *V. parahaemolyticus:* In U.S., most outbreaks in coastal states or on cruise ships during the summer months; incubation period usually <1 day, followed by explosive watery diarrhea in the majority of cases; nausea, vomiting, abdominal cramps, and

headache also common; fever less common; usually resolves by 1 wk; related to ingestion of seafood

(6) Enteroinvasive *E. coli* (EIEC): a rare cause of disease in the U.S.; high incidence of fever and bloody diarrhea; may resemble bacillary dysentery

(7) *V. vulnificus:* may cause serious, often fatal illness in persons with chronic liver disease; GI symptoms usually absent, but fever, chills, hypotension, and hemorrhagic skin lesions possible; patients with liver disease or at increased risk of developing liver disease should avoid eating raw oysters

ETIOLOGY

Classically categorized as either inflammatory (invasive) or noninflammatory:

- Noninflammatory: *B. cereus, S. aureus, C. botulinum, C. perfringens, V. cholerae,* enterotoxigenic *E. coli* (ETEC), and enterohemorrhagic *E. coli* (EHEC); toxin-producing organisms that are noninvasive; fecal leukocytes are not seen.
- Inflammatory: *Campylobacter,* enteroinvasive *E. coli* (EIEC), *Salmonella, Shigella, V. parahaemolyticus,* and *Yersinia;* cause disease by invasion of intestinal tissue; fecal leukocytes are seen.

DIAGNOSIS (Dx)

DIFFERENTIAL DIAGNOSIS

Gastroenteritis caused by viruses (Norwalk, Noro, or rotavirus), parasites *(Amoeba histolytica, Giardia lamblia),* or toxins (ciguatoxins, mushrooms, heavy metals)

LABORATORY TESTS

- Test stool for fecal leukocytes to help narrow the differential diagnosis:
  1. Send stool for culture and for ova and parasites.
  2. Send stool for *C. difficile* toxin in patients with current or recent antibiotic use.
  3. NOTE: Some pathogens are not identified on routine stool culture; laboratory should be advised if *Yersinia, C. botulinum, Vibrio,* or enterohemorrhagic *E. coli* (O157:H7) are suspected.
  4. Finding *B. cereus, C. perfringens,* or *E. coli* in stool is of little value, because these may be part of the normal bowel flora.
- If botulism suspected, send food, serum, and stool for toxin assay.
- Blood cultures are needed for all febrile patients.

TREATMENT (Rx)

NONPHARMACOLOGIC THERAPY

Adequate rehydration is the mainstay of therapy.

ACUTE GENERAL Rx

- Gastroenteritis caused by the following organisms requires no antimicrobial treatment: *B. cereus, S. aureus, C. perfringens, V. parahaemolyticus, Yersinia,* and enterohemorrhagic and enteroinvasive *E. coli.*
- The usual cause of traveler's diarrhea is enterotoxigenic *E. coli.* Although usually a self-limited illness, antibiotics can shorten the course.
  1. SMX/TMP one DS tab bid for 3 days
  2. Ciprofloxacin 500 mg PO bid for 3 days
- The mainstay of therapy for cholera is fluid replacement. Antibiotics should be given to decrease shedding and duration of illness.
  1. Doxycycline 100 mg PO bid for 3 days
  2. SMX/TMP one DS tab bid for 3 days
- Treatment is not indicated for *Salmonella* gastroenteritis. Patients who are at high risk of developing bacteremia may be treated for 48 to 72 hr (see "Salmonellosis").
- Although shigellosis tends to be a self-limited illness, antibiotics shorten the course of illness and may limit transmission of the illness (see "Shigellosis").
- Those with moderate or severe *Campylobacter* diarrhea may benefit from treatment.
  1. Erythromycin 500 mg PO qid for 5 days
  2. Ciprofloxacin 500 mg PO bid for 5 days
- *V. vulnificus* sepsis should be treated with:
  1. Doxycycline 100 mg IV bid for 2 wk
  2. Ceftazidime 2 g IV q8h for 2 wk
- For suspected botulism, antitoxin should be administered early (see "Botulism").

CHRONIC Rx

Patients with *Salmonella* infections may become carriers and may require treatment (see "Salmonellosis").

DISPOSITION

- Most infections are self-limited and do not require therapy.
- In immunocompromised host or patient with underlying disease, serious complications are possible.
- Postinfectious syndromes are important with some infections:
  1. Reiter's syndrome: *Salmonella, Shigella, Campylobacter, Yersinia spp.;* more common in genetically susceptible host (HLA-B27+)
  2. Guillain-Barré syndrome: *Campylobacter spp.*

REFERRAL

If more than a mild illness

PEARLS & CONSIDERATIONS (!)

COMMENTS

- Grossly underreported and undiagnosed
- All cases to be reported to the local health department

SUGGESTED READINGS

Allos BM et al: Surveillance for sporadic foodborne disease in the 21st century: the FoodNet perspective, *Clin Infect Dis* 38 (suppl 3)pS115, 2004.

Chiang YC et al: PCR primers for the detection of staphylococcal enterotoxins K, L, and M and survey of staphylococcal enterotoxin types in *Staphylococcus aureus* isolates from food poisoning cases in Taiwan, *J Food Prot* 69(5):1072, 2006.

Ikeda T et al: Mass outbreak of food poisoning disease caused by small amounts of staphylococcal enterotoxins A and H, *Appl Environ Microbiol* 71(5):2793, 2005.

Saito N et al: An outbreak of food poisoning caused by an enteropathogeic Escherichia coli O115:H19 in Miyagi Prefecture, *Jpn J Infect Dis* 58(3):189, 2005.

AUTHORS: **STEVEN M. OPAL, M.D.,** and **MAURICE POLICAR, M.D.**

BASIC INFORMATION

DEFINITION

Friedreich's ataxia is the most common neurodegenerative hereditary ataxic disorder, caused by degeneration of dorsal root ganglions, posterior columns, spinocerebellar and corticospinal tracts, and large sensory peripheral neurons.

ICD-9CM CODES
334.0 Friedreich's ataxia

EPIDEMIOLOGY & DEMOGRAPHICS

INCIDENCE (IN U.S.): Estimated at 1 in 30,000 Caucasians
PEAK INCIDENCE: 8 to 15 yr
PREVALENCE (IN U.S.): 2 to 4/100,000. Carrier rate 1:120 to 1:160. Lower prevalence in Asians and people of African descent.
PREDOMINANT SEX: Male = Female
GENETICS: Autosomal recessive; 96% of affected patients are homozygous, 4% compound heterozygous (two different mutations). Trinucleotide repeat expansion accounts for 98% of cases, whereas point mutations account for 2% of cases.

PHYSICAL FINDINGS & CLINICAL PRESENTATION

- Progressive gait ataxia; subsequently develop appendicular ataxia and dysarthria
- Loss of deep tendon reflexes, initially at the ankles, with extensor plantar responses
- Loss of vibration and joint position sense in the toes
- Pyramidal distribution weakness in the legs
- Progressive scoliosis, distal atrophy, and pes cavus
- Optic atrophy and hearing loss may develop
- Hypertrophic cardiomyopathy
- Insulin-requiring diabetes mellitus may occur in 10% of patients, with glucose intolerance occurring in an additional 10% to 20%

ETIOLOGY

- Genetic: GAA trinucleotide repeat expansion in the first intron of the Frataxin gene on chromosome 9q13.
- Frataxin deficiency leads to impaired mitochondrial iron homeostasis.

DIAGNOSIS

DIFFERENTIAL DIAGNOSIS

- Charcot-Marie-Tooth disease type 2
- Abetalipoproteinemia
- Severe vitamin E deficiency with malabsorption
- Early-onset cerebellar ataxia with retained reflexes
- Autosomal dominant cerebellar ataxia (spinocerebellar ataxia)

WORKUP

- Electrophysiologic evidence for a generalized axonal sensory neuropathy.
- Electrocardiogram (ECG) shows widespread T-wave inversion and evidence of left ventricular hypertrophy in most patients.
- Specific gene testing for the expanded GAA trinucleotide repeat.
- Sural nerve biopsy shows loss of large myelinated fibers (although not usually performed).

LABORATORY TESTS

- EMG/NCS
- ECG and echocardiogram
- Peripheral blood smear for acanthocytes
- Lipid profile
- Two-hour glucose tolerance test
- Vitamin E levels (if necessary)

IMAGING STUDIES

MRI of the spinal cord may demonstrate cervical cord atrophy with relatively normal brainstem and cerebellum (Fig. 1-101).

TREATMENT

NONPHARMACOLOGIC THERAPY

- Surgical correction of scoliosis and foot deformities in selected patients
- Prosthetic devices as required (e.g., ankle-foot orthosis for foot drop)
- Physical therapy
- Communication devices for patients with severe dysarthria

ACUTE GENERAL Rx

None established.

An antioxidant, idebenone (short-chain analogue of coenzyme Q10), administered orally at 5 to 10 mg/kg/day with or without vitamin E may improve outcomes in patients with cardiomyopathy without clinical deterioration. This treatment is experimental and research may be reviewed on www.idebenone.org.

Further research with various antioxidants and iron chelators is ongoing. A recently published open-labeled pilot study of antioxidants (coenzyme Q10, 400 mg/day and vitamin E, 2100U/day) suggested slowing in progression in generalized ataxia and kinetic function and significant improvement in cardiac function, with unaltered deterioration in posture, gait, and hand dexterity.

CHRONIC Rx

- Chronic management of congestive heart failure.
- Cardiac arrhythmias may warrant pacemaker implantation.

DISPOSITION

- Loss of ambulation typically occurs within 15 yr of symptom onset, and 95% are wheelchair bound by age 45 yr.
- Life expectancy is reduced, particularly if heart disease with or without diabetes mellitus is present. Mean survival from symptom onset is 36 years.

REFERRAL

- If uncertain about diagnosis
- For genetic counseling (recommended if available)

PEARLS & CONSIDERATIONS

Friedreich's ataxia should be considered in all preadolescent and adolescent children presenting with progressive ataxia. Early recognition of cardiac failure and arrhythmias and institution of appropriate therapy helps to prolong survival.

EVIDENCE

A small randomized controlled trial (RCT) of idebenone (a short-chain analogue of Coenzyme Q-10) shows modest benefit in terms of interventricular septal thickness and ventricular mass, but no effect on neurological outcome measures.[1]

A small RCT of L-carnitine compared to creatine and placebo showed no benefit in terms of neurological or cardiac outcome.[2]

Evidence-Based References

1. Mariotti C et al: Idebenone treatment in Friedreich patients: one-year-long randomized placebo-controlled trial, *Neurology* 60(10):1676, 2003.
2. Schols L et al: L-carnitine and creatine in Friedreich's ataxia: a randomized, placebo-controlled crossover trial, *J Neural Transm* 112(6):789, 2005.

SUGGESTED READING

Hart PE et al: Antioxidant treatment of patients with Friedreich ataxia: four-year follow-up, *Arch Neurol* 62:621-626, 2005.

AUTHOR: **EROBOGHENE UBOGU, M.D.**

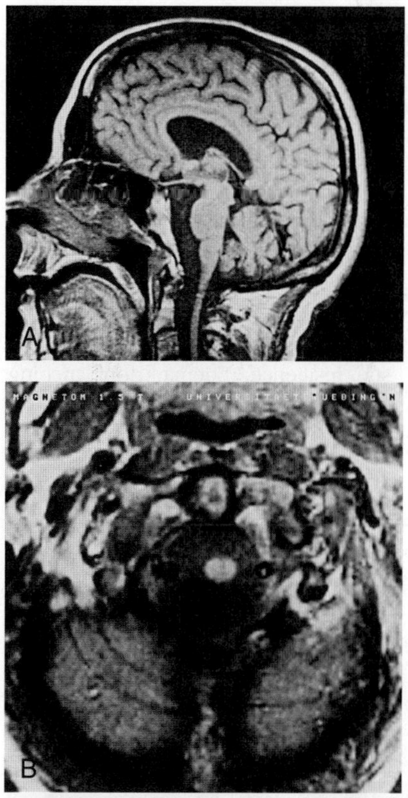

FIGURE 1-101 T1 MRI of the brain (midsagittal section) and spinal cord (axial slice at level of the dens) showing severe shrinkage of the cervical cord, but the cerebellum and brainstem are of normal size. (From Goetz CG: *Textbook of clinical neurology,* Philadelphia, 1999, WB Saunders.)

BASIC INFORMATION

DEFINITION

Frostbite represents tissue injury (or death) from freezing and vasoconstriction induced by severe environmental cold exposure.

SYNONYMS

Cold-induced tissue injury

ICD-9CM CODES

991.3 Frostbite

EPIDEMIOLOGY & DEMOGRAPHICS

- Environmental factors include wind chill factor, temperature, duration of exposure, altitude, and degree of wetness. Hands and feet account for 90% of injuries; earlobes, nose, and male genitalia are also more susceptible.
- Host factors include older age, psychiatric illness, neuroleptic and sedative drugs (especially alcohol), immobility, history of cold injuries, skin damage, malnutrition, tobacco use, peripheral neuropathy, hypothyroidism, hypoglycemia, hypoadrenalism, fatigue, and wearing constricting clothing/footwear.

PHYSICAL FINDINGS & CLINICAL PRESENTATION

- Frostbite may be classified into grades I to IV of injury severity or more practically, into *superficial* and *deep* groups.
- *Superficial* frostbite involves the skin and subcutaneous tissue. The frozen part is waxy, white, and firm but soft and resilient below the surface when gently depressed. After rewarming, the frostbitten area may appear mottled and swollen, and superficial blisters with clear or milky fluid may form within 6-24 hr (Fig.1-102). There is no ultimate tissue loss.
- *Deep* frostbite also involves muscles, nerves, tendons, or bones. The skin may be hard or wooden, without tissue resilience. Edema, nonblanching cyanosis, hemorrhagic blisters (after 3-7 days), tissue necrosis, and gangrene may develop. Affected tissue has a poor prognosis and debridement or amputation is generally required.
- Patients initially experience numbness, prickling, and itching. More severe injury can produce paresthesias and stiffness, with burning or throbbing pain upon thawing.

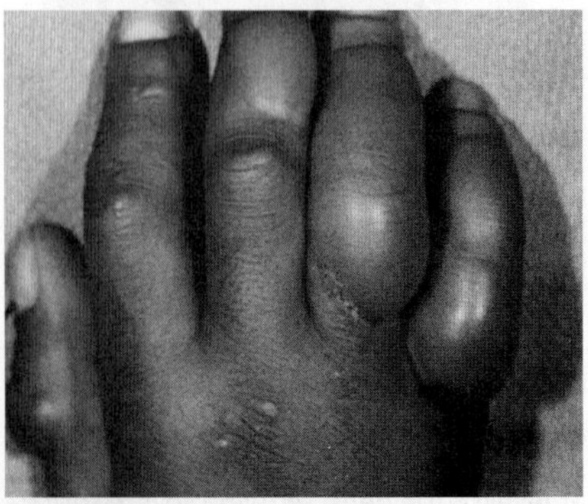

FIGURE 1-102 Large, clear frostbite blisters on the right hand. (From Rosen P [ed]: *Emergency medicine,* ed 4, St Louis, 1998, Mosby.)

ETIOLOGY

Two mechanisms of tissue injury:

1. Cellular death occurring at time of exposure from intracellular water crystallization and temperature-induced protein changes.
2. Vascular impairment from vasoconstriction, endothelial injury, and associated thrombosis as a result of tissue thawing and associated edema. Most frostbite injury occurs in this phase. Hemorrhage, necrosis, and gangrene may develop.

DIAGNOSIS

DIFFERENTIAL DIAGNOSIS

- Frostnip: transient tingling and numbness without associated permanent tissue damage
- Pernio (chilblains): self-limited, cold-induced vasculitis associated with purple plaques or nodules, often affecting dorsum of hands and feet; seen with prolonged cold exposure to above-freezing temperatures
- Cold immersion (trench) foot: caused by ischemic injury resulting from sustained severe vasoconstriction in appendages exposed to wet cold at temperatures above freezing

WORKUP

- Labwork is not indicated unless patient has systemic hypothermia.
- No reliable predictors of tissue viability. Technetium scintigraphy, MRI, and MRA are the most promising. (Some centers perform technetium scintigraphy or angiography within 24 hr and give thrombolytics to those with impaired blood flow.)

TREATMENT

NONPHARMACOLOGIC THERAPY

- Remove constricting/wet clothing. Gently insulate, splint, elevate affected area.
- Avoid thawing if any risk of refreezing.
- Never rub or massage the affected area. Avoid dry heat (e.g., fires/heaters) and exercising the affected area.
- If hypothermic (core body temperature <32° C), initiate active core rewarming (e.g., pleural and peritoneal irrigation, hemodialysis or cardiopulmonary bypass) and adjunctive treatment with warmed, humidified oxygen, heated IV saline (45° C) and warming blankets before thawing of frostbitten extremities.

ACUTE GENERAL Rx

- Rapid rewarming is the main objective.
- Immerse affected area in circulating warm water bath with a mild antibacterial agent (e.g., hexachlorophene or povidone-iodine) maintained at 40-42° C for 15-30 min. Repeat until capillary refill returns and tissue is supple and flushed. Active motion during rewarming is advisable, massage is not.
- IV narcotics for pain during thawing.
- Td prophylaxis and topical antibiotics if potentially contaminated skin wound.
- Streptococcal prophylaxis for 48-72 hr with IV penicillin for severe cases.
- Thrombolytic therapy followed by short-term anticoagulation appears to considerably improve reperfusion and reduce predicted digit amputations.
- Dextran, anticoagulants, vasodilators, hyperbaric oxygen, reserpine, and sympathectomy are of unproven benefit.

POST-THAW Rx

- Daily dressing changes with dry, sterile, noncompressive, and nonadherent dressings. Splint and elevate hands and feet to reduce edema and separate digits with cotton gauze. Avoid even slightest abrasion; preventing infection is highly important.
- Whirlpool hydrotherapy with warm water (38° C) and an antiseptic for 20-30 min bid to tid for several weeks.
- Debride broken clear vesicles and avoid disrupting intact blisters (especially hemorrhagic ones) unless they interfere with mobility.
- Topical aloe vera q6h and ibuprofen 400-600 mg TID for 1 wk may be beneficial as thromboxane inhibitors.
- Gentle, progressive physical therapy after edema resolves.
- Avoid all vasoconstrictors, including nicotine.

DISPOSITION

A majority of patients experience long-term residual symptoms including neuropathic pain, sensory deficits, hyperhidrosis, secondary Raynaud's disease, edema, hair or nail deformities, and (rarely) arthritis. Treatment with antiadrenergics or calcium-channel blockers and careful protection from further cold exposure is often helpful.

REFERRAL

- Hospitalize for hypothermia or deep frostbite. Burn unit best.
- Surgical decisions regarding amputation should be deferred until there is clear demarcation of viable tissue (1-3 mo) unless refractory pain, sepsis, or gangrene occurs.

SUGGESTED READINGS

Biem J et al: Out of the cold: management of hypothermia and frostbite, *CMAJ* 168(3):305, 2003.

Bruen KJ et al: Reduction of the incidence of amputation in frostbite injury with thrombolytic therapy, *Arch Surg* 142(6):546, 2007.

Jurkovich GJ: Environmental cold-induced injury, *Surg Clin N Am* 87(1), 247-267, 2007.

AUTHOR: **MICHAEL P. JOHNSON, M.D.**

BASIC INFORMATION

DEFINITION

Frozen shoulder is a condition unique to the shoulder and characterized by pain and restricted passive and active range of motion (Fig. 1-103).

SYNONYMS

Adhesive capsulitis
Periarthritis
Pericapsulitis
Check-rein shoulder

ICD-9CM CODES
726.0 Adhesive shoulder capsulitis

EPIDEMIOLOGY & DEMOGRAPHICS

PREDOMINANT SEX: Females > males
PREDOMINANT AGE: Over 40 yr

PHYSICAL FINDINGS & CLINICAL PRESENTATION

- Arm held protectively at the side with apprehension caused by pain
- Varying degrees of deltoid and spinatus atrophy
- Generalized shoulder tenderness
- Restricted active and passive shoulder motion of varying degrees

ETIOLOGY

- Unknown
- Fig. 1-103 illustrates the sequence of events terminating in frozen shoulder

DIAGNOSIS

DIFFERENTIAL DIAGNOSIS

- Secondary causes of shoulder stiffness (prolonged immobilization following trauma or surgery)
- Posterior shoulder dislocation
- Ruptured rotator cuff
- Glenohumeral osteoarthritis
- Rotator cuff inflammation
- Superior sulcus tumor
- Cervical disk disease
- Brachial neuritis

WORKUP

Laboratory and radiographic studies are generally normal.

TREATMENT

NONPHARMACOLOGIC THERAPY

Prevention is important. Shoulder motion should be maintained during those periods when the patient may be inactive as a result of illness or injury.

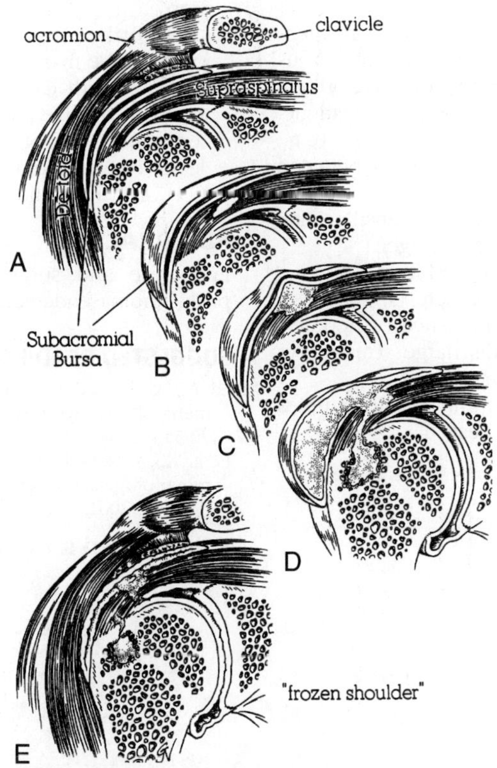

FIGURE 1-103 Sequence of events terminating in frozen shoulder. A, Normal structures of the shoulder. **B,** Supraspinatus tendonitis, sometimes calcific, in the "critical zone." **C,** Spread of inflammation to the tendon sheath and a bulge into the floor of the subacromial bursa. **D,** Rupture into the subacromial bursa and extension of the inflammatory process as an osteitis into the humeral head and greater tuberosity. **E,** Frozen shoulder with involvement of tendons, bursa, capsule, synovium, and muscle with fibrous contracture and markedly diminished volume of the shoulder joint space. (From Noble J [ed]: *Primary care medicine,* ed 2, St Louis, 1996, Mosby.)

ACUTE GENERAL Rx

- Moist heat, sedation, and analgesics as needed.
- A local steroid/lidocaine mixture injected into the subacromial space and joint (See Epicondylitis entry for guidelines to common steroid injections).
- Home exercise program. Should be performed on an hourly basis, if possible, at least in the early stages of treatment. PT may be needed.
- Manipulation of shoulder under anesthesia (rarely needed).

DISPOSITION

- The initial stage of pain followed by stiffness may last several months; recovery phase may also last several months; complete recovery is usually the case.
- Recurrence in the same shoulder is rare, although the opposite limb may develop the same symptoms.
- Some patients have mild residual loss of movement but without any significant functional impairment.

REFERRAL

Orthopedic consultation in patients with resistant disease

PEARLS & CONSIDERATIONS

COMMENTS

- "Capsulitis" with an inflammatory infiltrate is not consistently found pathologically.
- Frozen shoulder is increased in patients with diabetes, thyroid disease, and recent cardiopulmonary conditions.
- Some cases present with findings of reflex sympathetic dystrophy.

SUGGESTED READINGS

Berghs BM, Sole-Molins X, Bunker TD: Arthroscopic release of adhesive capsulitis, *J Shoulder Elbow Surg* 13:180, 2004.

Cheville AL, Tchou J: Barriers to rehabilitation following surgery for primary breast cancer, *J Surg Oncol* 95(5):409, 2007.

Cohen BL: Treatment of shoulder complaints, *Lancet* 363:492, 2004.

Hand GC et al: The pathology of frozen shoulder, *J Bone Joint Surg* 89(B):928, 2007.

Harrast MA, Rao AG: The stiff shoulder, *Phys Med Rehabil Clin N Am* 15(3):557, 2004.

Klauser A, Frauscher F: Treatment of shoulder complaints *Lancet* 363:491, 2004.

Placzek JD et al: Theory and technique of translational manipulation for adhesive capsulitis, *Am J Orthop* 33:173, 2004.

Tasto JP, Elias DW: Adhesive capsulitis, *Sports Med Arthrosc* 15:216, 2007.

Thomas SJ et al: Prevalence of symptoms and signs of shoulder problems in people with diabetes mellitus, *J Shoulder Elbow Surg* 16:748, 2007.

AUTHOR: **LONNIE R. MERCIER, M.D.**

BASIC INFORMATION

DEFINITION

Galactorrhea can be defined as inappropriate lactation (in absence of pregnancy and postpartum state) secondary to nonphysiologic augmentation of prolactin release.

ICD-9CM CODES
611.6 Galactorrhea

PHYSICAL FINDINGS AND CLINICAL PRESENTATION

- Milky discharge from nipples usually occurring bilaterally
- Evidence of chest wall irritation from ill-fitting clothing, herpes zoster, or atopic dermatitis may be present
- Visual field defects may be present with prolactinomas
- Evidence of acromegaly, Cushing's disease, or hypothyroidism when galactorrhea is secondary to these disorders

ETIOLOGY

- Medications (phenothiazines, metoclopramide, SSRIs, anxiolytics, buspirone, atenolol, valproic acid, conjugated estrogen and medroxyprogesterone, methyldopa, verapamil, H2 receptor blockers, octreotide, danazol, tricyclics, isoniazid, amphetamine, reserpine, opiates, sumatriptan, rimantadine, oral contraceptive formulations); after infancy, galactorrhea is usually medication-induced
- Breast stimulation (prolonged suckling), sexual intercourse
- Pituitary tumors (prolactinomas, craniopharyngiomas)
- Chest wall irritation from ill-fitting clothing, herpes zoster, atopic dermatitis, burns
- Hypothyroidism (elevated TSH increases TRH, which increases prolactin)
- Increased stress, major trauma
- Chronic renal failure (decreased prolactin clearance)
- Cushing's disease
- Herbs (e.g., fennel, red clover, anise, red raspberry, marshmallow)
- Cannabis
- Spinal cord surgery or injury, or tumors
- Severe GERD, esophagitis (stimulation of thoracic nerves via cervical and thoracic ganglia)
- Breast surgery
- Idiopathic
- Neonatal ("witch's milk" produced by 2% to 5% of neonates because of precipitous drop in maternal estrogen and progesterone postdelivery)
- Lymphomas, Hodgkin's disease, bronchogenic carcinoma, renal adenocarcinomas
- Sarcoidosis and other infiltrative disorders
- Tuberculosis affecting pituitary gland
- Pituitary stalk resection
- Multiple sclerosis
- Empty sella syndrome
- Acromegaly

DIAGNOSIS

DIFFERENTIAL DIAGNOSIS

- Intraductal papilloma
- Breast cancer
- Paget's disease of breast
- Breast abscess

WORKUP

- Complete history focusing on menstrual irregularity, infertility, previous pregnancies, duration of galactorrhea, medications, visual complaints, fatigue. Age of onset is also significant (e.g., prolactinoma most common between ages 20 to 35, neonatal galactorrhea is usually secondary to transplacental transfer of maternal estrogen)
- Physical examination: hirsutism, acne, obesity, visual field defects, goiter
- Breast exam for presence of nodules, evaluation of discharge (milky vs serosanguinous vs purulent)
- Laboratory testing and imaging studies (see "Laboratory Tests")

LABORATORY TESTS

- Prolactin level (elevated, usually >200 ng/ml in prolactinoma)
- Human chorionic gonadotropin level (positive in pregnancy)
- TSH, TRH (both elevated in hypothyroidism)
- BUN, creatinine (elevated in renal failure), glucose (elevated in Cushing's syndrome)
- Urinalysis (hematuria in renal cell carcinoma)
- Microscopic examination of nipple discharge (scant cellular material, numerous fat globules)

IMAGING STUDIES

- MRI of brain if prolactin level is elevated, amenorrhea is present or visual fields defects are detected on physical examination.
- High-resolution CT of brain with special coronal cuts through the pituitary region may be helpful in patients with contraindications to MRI; however, it may miss small lesions.

TREATMENT

- Discontinuation of potential offending agents.
- Avoidance of excessive breast stimulation.
- Galactorrhea resulting from prolactinoma can be managed medically, surgically, or with careful surveillance depending on size and growth of tumor, associated symptoms and prolactin level. Please refer to "Prolactinoma" in Section I for additional information.

REFERRAL

Endocrine and surgical consultation if prolactinoma is detected

SUGGESTED READINGS

Leung A, Pacaud D: Diagnosis and management of galactorrhea, *Am Fam Physician* 70:543, 2004.

Pena KS, Rosenfeld JA: Evaluation and treatment of galactorrhea, *Am Fam Physician* 63:1763, 2001.

AUTHOR: **FRED F. FERRI, M.D.**

BASIC INFORMATION

DEFINITION

Ganglia are cystic structures thought to derive from a tendon sheath or joint capsule.

SYNONYMS

Ganglion

ICD-9CM CODES
727.43 Ganglion

EPIDEMIOLOGY & DEMOGRAPHICS

- Ganglia are more common in women than men (3:1)
- Can occur at any age but usually occurs between second and fourth decades of life
- Most common soft tissue tumor of the hand and wrist

PHYSICAL FINDINGS & CLINICAL PRESENTATION

- Most ganglia occur on the dorsum of the wrist (50% to 70%) (Fig. 1-104).
- Volar wrist (18% to 20%) is the next most common site.
- Ganglia can also involve the proximal digital flexor tendons and the distal interphalangeal joints.
- Left and right hands are equally affected.
- Ganglia are usually solitary, firm, smooth, round, and fluctuant.
- Pain from mass effect or compression against nearby structure may be present (e.g., median nerve and radial nerve)
- Hand numbness may be present.
- Patient may experience hand muscle weakness.
- Ganglia usually develop over a period of months but may arise suddenly.

ETIOLOGY

Ganglia are thought to derive from synovial herniation or expansion from the joint capsule or tendon sheath.

DIAGNOSIS

Direct inspection and localization of the cyst often is enough to make the diagnosis of ganglia.

DIFFERENTIAL DIAGNOSIS

- Lipoma
- Fibroma
- Epidermoid inclusion cyst
- Osteochondroma
- Hemangioma
- Infection (tuberculosis, fungi, and secondary syphilis)
- Gout
- Rheumatoid nodule
- Radial artery aneurysm

WORKUP

The workup of ganglia usually consists of history, physical examination, and x-ray imaging.

LABORATORY TESTS

Blood tests are not specific in the diagnosis of ganglia.

IMAGING STUDIES

- X-ray of the hand and wrist is done to rule out other bone or joint abnormalities.
- Ultrasound studies are helpful in the diagnosis of ganglia, demonstrating smooth cystic walls that may be septated.
- CT scan can be done if the ultrasound is equivocal.
- MRI aids in differentiating malignant bone lesions from cystic structures.
- Arthrography may demonstrate a communication between the joint and ganglia (not commonly done).

TREATMENT

Treatment is indicated for pain, muscle weakness, and cosmetic purposes.

NONPHARMACOLOGIC THERAPY

- Attempts to rupture the cyst by sharp blows with a book or with finger compression.
- Aspiration, heat, and sclerotherapy have been tried but met with high recurrence rates (60%).

ACUTE GENERAL Rx

- Aspiration with a large-bore needle (18-gauge) followed by injection of 20 to 40 mg of triamcinolone acetonide can be tried.
- This may be repeated if the ganglia recurs (35% to 40%).

CHRONIC Rx

Total ganglionectomy is the surgical procedure of choice.

DISPOSITION

- Ganglia spontaneously resolve in approximately 40% to 50% of cases.
- Aspiration with steroid injection is successful in approximately 65% of cases.
- Surgery provides cure in 85% to 95% of the cases.
- Complications of ganglia include:
  1. Carpal tunnel syndrome with pain and muscle atrophy
  2. Radial nerve impingement
  3. Radial artery compression
- Complications of ganglion surgery include:
  1. Infection
  2. Recurrence (5% to 15%) usually secondary to inadequate excision
  3. Reflex sympathetic dystrophy
  4. Scar formation

REFERRAL

It is best to refer patients with symptomatic ganglia to a hand surgeon.

PEARLS & CONSIDERATIONS

- Dorsal ganglia usually originate from the scapholunate ligament.
- Volar ganglia typically originate between the tendons of the flexor carpi radialis and brachioradialis.

COMMENTS

Ganglia's synovial membrane maintains its secretory function. Aspiration of ganglia often demonstrates a viscous, mucinous clear fluid containing albumin, globulin, and hyaluronic acid.

SUGGESTED READINGS

Ho PC et al: Current treatment of ganglion of the wrist, *Hand Surg* 6(1):49, 2001.

Nahra ME, Bucchieri JS: Ganglion cysts and other tumor related cysts of the hand and wrist, *Hand Clin* 20(3):249, 2004.

Wang AA, Hutchinson DT: Longitudinal observation of pediatric hand and wrist ganglia, *J Hand Surg* 26(4):599, 2001.

AUTHOR: **PETER PETROPOULOS, M.D.**

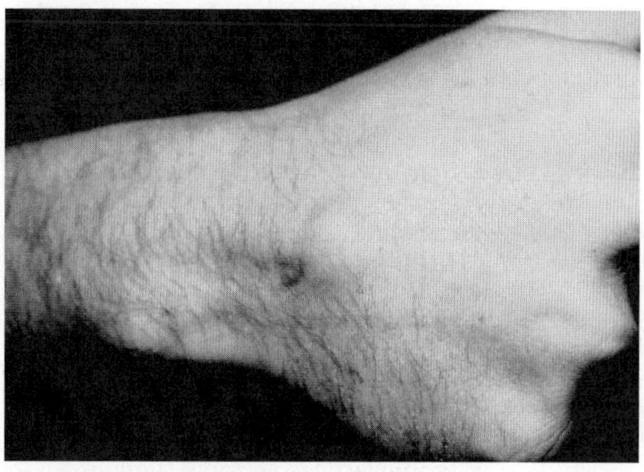

FIGURE 1-104 Round and firm ganglion cyst bulging from the dorsal aspect of the hand. (From Kelley WN: *Textbook of rheumatology,* ed 5, Philadelphia, 1997, WB Saunders.)

BASIC INFORMATION

DEFINITION

Gardner's syndrome is a variant of familial adenomatous polyposis (FAP), with prominent extraintestinal manifestations. It is an autosomal dominant condition characterized by:

- Adenomatous intestinal polyps
- Soft tissue tumors
- Osteomas

SYNONYMS

Familial adenomatous polyposis

ICD-9CM CODES
211.3 Gardner's syndrome

EPIDEMIOLOGY & DEMOGRAPHICS

- FAP is estimated to occur in 1 of 8000 to 14,000 live births.
- FAP accounts for <1% of all colorectal cancers.
- Individuals develop hundreds to thousands of colonic polyps.
- Polyps occur at a mean age of 16 yr.
- 100% lifetime risk for colorectal cancer, average age of diagnosis 35 to 40 yr.
- Gastric and duodenal polyps occur but have lower malignant potential.
- Increased risk for other cancers: about 15% develop desmoid tumors and 7% develop duodenal-ampullary cancer. Risk for nasopharyngeal angiofibroma, thyroid, childhood hepatoblastoma, adrenal, pancreatic, gastric, and CNS cancers also increased.

PHYSICAL FINDINGS & CLINICAL PRESENTATION

Phenotypic variability is seen in individuals and families with the same mutation. Soft tissue and bone abnormalities may precede intestinal disease.

- Congenital hypertrophy of the retinal pigment epithelium (CHRPE): benign fundus lesions, usually present at birth
- Dental abnormalities: supernumerary or unerupted teeth
- Soft tissue lesions: epidermal or sebaceous cysts, fibromas, lipomas, desmoid tumors (benign, locally aggressive, connective tissue tumors)
- Skull, mandible, long bone osteomas (benign bony growths)
- Anemia, abdominal mass, occult blood in stool, bowel obstruction

ETIOLOGY

- Caused by mutations of the tumor suppressor gene, adenomatous polyposis coli (APC) on chromosome 5q21; >700 disease causing mutations identified. The site of the mutation may explain the prominent extraintestinal lesions found in Gardner's syndrome.
- Spontaneous mutations are responsible for approximately 30% of FAP cases.

DIAGNOSIS

In individuals with a family history, >100 adenomatous polyps in the colon, CHRPE lesions, or genetic testing confirm diagnosis. In those without a family history, >100 adenomatous polyps in the colon suggest the diagnosis and genetic testing confirms it.

DIFFERENTIAL DIAGNOSIS

- Turcot's syndrome
- Attenuated familial adenomatous polyposis
- Peutz-Jeghers syndrome
- Juvenile polyposis syndrome
- MUTYH-associated polyposis
- Hereditary mixed polyposis syndrome
- Hyperplastic polyposis

WORKUP

History, physical examination, laboratory tests, imaging studies

DIAGNOSTIC SCREENING OPTIONS:

Genetic testing

- Should be offered to first-degree relatives of affected individuals (with an identified mutation) at 10 to 12 yr of age and clinically suspected individuals.
- Able to identify a mutation in about 80% of families. To ensure that the family has a detectable mutation, test an affected family member first.
- If positive in the affected individual, the test can differentiate with 100% accuracy affected and unaffected family members. If negative in the affected individual, screening family members will not be useful in determining disease status.
- If there is no known family history, screening the clinically suspected individual is reasonable. A positive test rules in FAP, but a negative test does not rule it out.
- May require multiple tests to identify the mutation.

NOTE: Genetic counseling should be performed and written informed consent obtained before genetic testing.

Sigmoidoscopy

- Individuals with a positive genetic test, untested at-risk family members, or patients from families with an unidentified APC mutation: annual flexible sigmoidoscopy from 12 to 25 yr, then decreasing frequency until 50 yr, at which point age-appropriate guidelines are followed
- Negative genetic test in patients from families with an identified mutation: standard risk screening

CHRPE

- Lesions occur in about 80% of families and are a reliable indicator of affected status in these families.

TREATMENT

- Prophylactic colectomy: timing determined by the number, size, and histology of polyps.
- Consider celecoxib therapy to reduce polyposis.
- Screening of remaining GI tract and screening for extraintestinal manifestations must continue after colectomy.
  - Annual physical exam: history, exam (palpation of thyroid), and blood tests.
  - Upper endoscopy to screen for gastric and duodenal/ampullary polyps: baseline at 25 yr and repeated every 1 to 5 yr based on findings.
  - Some recommend annual thyroid ultrasound.
  - Other possible cancer sites should be imaged if symptoms occur or if these cancers have occurred in relatives.
- Treat soft issue lesions and osteomas for symptoms or cosmetic concerns. Treat desmoid tumors if pose a risk to adjacent structures.

DISPOSITION

- There is a 100% chance of colorectal cancer in untreated individuals. Many other neoplasms occur at higher rates.
- Metastatic colorectal cancer is the leading cause of death (58%), followed by desmoid tumors (11%) and duodenal adenocarcinoma (8%).

REFERRAL

- Gastroenterologist
- Surgery
- Medical geneticist

PEARLS & CONSIDERATIONS

- Sulindac (nonselective NSAID) and celecoxib (cox-2 inhibitor) cause polyp regression in individuals with FAP. Celecoxib is FDA approved for this indication. Cancer risk remains; neither replaces colon resection for cancer prevention.
- Desmoid tumors frequently occur in the abdomen and are difficult to treat. Growth is stimulated by trauma (surgery) and estrogen.
- Screen children of affected parents yearly (from infancy to 7 yr) with alpha-fetoprotein level and liver ultrasound to rule out hepatoblastoma.
- High-risk cancer centers often provide genetic counseling and testing. Genetic counseling/testing sites can be found at GeneTests (www.genetests.org).

SUGGESTED READINGS

Galiatsatos P, Foulkes WD: Familial adenomatous polyposis, *Am J Gastroenterol* 101(2):385, 2006.

Giardiello FM, Brensinger JD, Petersen GM: American Gastroenterologic Association Practice Guidelines: AGA technical review on hereditary colorectal cancer and genetic testing, *Gastroenterology* 121(1):198, 2001.

AUTHOR: **SUDEEP K. AULAKH, M.D., F.R.C.P.C.**

BASIC INFORMATION

DEFINITION

Gastric cancer is an adenocarcinoma arising from the stomach.

SYNONYMS

Stomach cancer
Linitis plastica

ICD-9CM CODES
451 Malignant neoplasm of stomach

EPIDEMIOLOGY & DEMOGRAPHICS

- Annual incidence of gastric cancer in the U.S. is 7 cases/100,000 persons. The incidence is much higher in Japan, with rates as high as 80 cases/100,000 persons.
- Most gastric cancers arise in the antrum (35%).
- The incidence of distal stomach tumors has greatly declined whereas that of proximal tumors of the cardia and fundus is on the rise.
- Gastric cancer occurs most commonly in male patients >65 yr (70% of patients are >50 yr).
- Incidence of gastric cancer has been declining over the past 30 yr.
- Male:female ratio is 3:2.
- Familiar diffuse gastric cancer is a disease with autosomal dominant inheritance in which gastric cancer develops at a young age. Germ-line truncating mutations in the E-cadherin gene (CDH1) are found in these families.

PHYSICAL FINDINGS & CLINICAL PRESENTATION

- Medical history may reveal complaints of postprandial fullness with significant weight loss (70% to 80%), nausea/emesis (20% to 40%), dysphagia (20%), and dyspepsia, usually unrelieved by antacids; epigastric discomfort, usually lessened by fasting and exacerbated by food intake, is also common.
- Epigastric or abdominal mass (30% to 50%), epigastric pain.
- Skin pallor secondary to anemia.
- Hard, nodular liver: generally indicates metastatic disease to the liver.
- Hemoccult-positive stools.
- Ascites, lymphadenopathy, or pleural effusions: may indicate metastasis.

ETIOLOGY

Risk factors:

- Chronic *H. pylori* gastritis. Gastric cancer develops in persons infected with *H. pylori* but not in uninfected persons. Those with histologic findings of severe gastric atrophy, corpus-predominant gastritis, or intestinal metaplasia are at increased risk. Persons with *H. pylori* infection and duodenal ulcer are not at risk, whereas those with gastric ulcers, nonulcer dyspepsia, and gastric hyperplastic polyps are
- Tobacco abuse, alcohol consumption
- Food additives (nitrosamines), smoked foods, occupational exposure to heavy metals, rubber, asbestos
- Chronic atrophic gastritis with intestinal metaplasia, hypertrophic gastritis, and pernicious anemia

DIAGNOSIS

DIFFERENTIAL DIAGNOSIS

- Gastric lymphoma (5% of gastric malignancies)
- Hypertrophic gastritis
- Peptic ulcer
- Reflux esophagitis

WORKUP

Upper endoscopy with biopsy will confirm diagnosis. Endoscopic ultrasonography in combination with CT scannning and operative lymph node dissection can be used in staging of the tumor.

LABORATORY TESTS

- Microcytic anemia
- Hemoccult-positive stools
- Hypoalbuminemia
- Abnormal liver enzymes in patients with metastasis to the liver
- Mutation-specific predictive genetic testing by PCR amplification followed by restriction—enzyme digestion and DNA sequencing for truncating mutations in the E-cadherin gene (CDH1) is recommended in families of patients with familiar diffuse cancer because gastric cancer develops in three of every four carriers of a mutant CDH1 gene

IMAGING STUDIES

Abdominal CT scan to evaluate for metastasis (70% accurate for regional node metastases)

TREATMENT

ACUTE GENERAL Rx

- Gastrectomy with regional lymphadenectomy is performed in patients with curative potential (<30% of patients at time of diagnosis). In patients with operable gastric cancer, a perioperative regimen of epirubicin, cisplatin, and infused fluorouracil (ECF) decreases tumor size and stage and significantly improves progression-free and overall survival. Post-op adjuvant chemoradiatiotherapy using 5-fluorouracil and leucovorin is now the standard of care for resected patients able to tolerate such treatment. Postoperative chemotherapy and radiotherapy, compared with surgical resection alone, can extend the survival of patients with gastric cancer in those who are able to complete adjuvant therapy.
- When surgical cure is not possible, palliative resection may prolong duration and quality of life.
- Chemotherapy (FAM: 5-fluorouracil, Adriamycin, and mitomycin C) may provide some palliation; however, it generally does not prolong survival. Chemotherapy with docetaxel, cisplatin, and 5-fluorouracil can be used for chemotherapy-naive patients with metastatic or locally recurrent gastric cancer.

DISPOSITION

- 5-yr survival rate of gastric carcinoma is 12% overall.
- 5-yr survival for early gastric cancers (usually detected incidentally with endoscopy in populations where screening is recommended) is >35%.

PEARLS & CONSIDERATIONS

COMMENTS

- Gastrectomy patients will need vitamin B_{12} replacement. They are also at risk for dumping syndrome and should be advised to ingest frequent, small meals.
- Prophylactic gastrectomy should be considered in young asymptomatic carriers of germ-line truncating CDH1 mutations who belong to families with highly penetrant heredity diffuse gastric cancer.

EVIDENCE

Prospective and retrospective cohort studies have demonstrated that survival is dependent on complete tumor resection.[1]

Palliative gastrectomy improves survival.[2]

Lymphadenectomy, survival: RCTs have demonstrated no survival advantage from extended/regional lymph node resection (D-2, D-3 resection) vs. local lymph node resection (D-1 resection).[3]

Evidence-Based References

1. Boddie AW Jr et al: Palliative total gastrectomy and esophagogastrectomy: an evaluation. In: *Clin Evid* 4:266, 2000, London, BMJ Publishing Group.
2. Haugstvedt T: Benefits of resection in palliative surgery. Reviewed in: *Clin Evid* 4:266, 2000.
3. Dent DM, Madden MV, Price SK: Randomised comparison of R1 and R2 gastrectomy for gastric carcinoma. Reviewed in: *Clin Evid* 4:266, 2000, London, BMJ Publish ing Group.

SUGGESTED READING

Cunningham D et al: Perioperative chemotherapy versus surgery alone for respectable gastroesophageal cancer, *N Engl J Med* 355(1):11, 2006.

AUTHOR: **FRED F. FERRI, M.D.**

BASIC INFORMATION

DEFINITION

Histologically, gastritis refers to inflammation in the stomach. Endoscopically, gastritis refers to a number of abnormal features such as erythema, erosions, and subepithelial hemorrhages. Gastritis can also be subdivided into erosive, nonerosive, and specific types of gastritis with distinctive features both endoscopically and histologically.

SYNONYMS

Erosive gastritis
Hemorrhagic gastritis
Helicobacter pylori gastritis

ICD-9CM CODES
535.5 Gastritis (unless otherwise specified)
535.0 Gastritis, acute
535.3 Alcoholic gastritis
535.1 Atrophic (chronic) gastritis
535.4 Erosive gastritis
535.2 Hypertrophic gastritis

EPIDEMIOLOGY & DEMOGRAPHICS

- Erosive and hemorrhagic gastritis are most commonly seen in patients taking NSAIDs, alcoholics, and critically ill patients (usually on ventilator support).
- *H. pylori* infection with gastritis is believed to be present in 30% to 50% of the population; however, the majority are asymptomatic.
- The prevalence of *H. pylori* infection increases with age from <10% in Caucasians <40 yr old to >50% in patients >50 yr.

PHYSICAL FINDINGS & CLINICAL PRESENTATION

- Patients with gastritis generally present with nonspecific clinical signs and symptoms (e.g., epigastric pain, abdominal tenderness, bloating, anorexia, nausea [with or without vomiting]). Symptoms may be aggravated by eating.
- Epigastric tenderness in acute alcoholic gastritis (may be absent in chronic gastritis).
- Foul-smelling breath.
- Hematemesis ("coffee-ground" emesis).

ETIOLOGY

- Alcohol, NSAIDs, stress (critically ill patients usually on mechanical respiration), hepatic or renal failure, multiorgan failure
- Infection (bacterial, viral)
- Bile reflux, pancreatic enzyme reflux
- Gastric mucosal atrophy, portal hypertension gastropathy
- Irradiation

DIAGNOSIS

DIFFERENTIAL DIAGNOSIS

- Peptic ulcer disease
- GERD
- Nonulcer dyspepsia
- Gastric lymphoma or carcinoma
- Pancreatitis
- Gastroparesis

WORKUP

Diagnostic workup includes a comprehensive history and endoscopy with biopsy.

LABORATORY TESTS

- *H. pylori* testing via urea breath test, stool antigen test (*H. pylori* stool antigen), endoscopic biopsy, or specific antibody test is recommended:
  1. The urea breath test documents active infection (sensitivity and specificity >90%). Recently a new card test for ^{14}C urea has been developed providing a testing option in primary care settings. It uses a flat breath card that is read by a small analyzer.
  2. Stool antigen test is an enzymatic immunoassay (ELISA) that identifies *H. pylori* antigen in stool specimen through a polyclonal anti-*H. pylori* antibody. It is as accurate as the urea breath test for diagnosis of active infection and follow-up evaluation of patients treated for *H. pylori*. A negative result on the stool antigen test 8 wk after completion of therapy identifies patients in whom eradication of *H. pylori* was unsuccessful.
  3. Histologic evaluation of endoscopic biopsy samples is considered by many the gold standard for accurate diagnosis of *H. pylori* infection. However, detection of *H. pylori* depends on the site and number of biopsy samples, the method of staining, and experience of the pathologist.
  4. Serologic testing for antibodies to *H. pylori* is easy and inexpensive; however, the presence of antibodies demonstrates previous but not necessarily current infection. Antibodies to *H. pylori* can remain elevated for months to years after infection has cleared; therefore antibody levels must be interpreted in light of patient's symptoms and other test results (e.g., PUD seen on UGI series).
- Vitamin B_{12} level in patients with atrophic gastritis.
- Hct (low if significant bleeding has occurred).

TREATMENT

NONPHARMACOLOGIC THERAPY

- Avoidance of mucosal irritants such as alcohol and NSAIDs
- Lifestyle modifications with avoidance of tobacco and foods that trigger symptoms

ACUTE GENERAL Rx

Eradication of *H. pylori,* when present, can be accomplished with various regimens:

1. PPI bid *plus* amoxicillin 500 mg bid *plus* metronidazole 500 mg for 10 days.
2. PPI bid *plus* clarithromycin 500 mg bid *and* metronidazole 500 mg bid for 10 days. This regimen is useful in those with penicillin allergy.
3. A 1-day quadruple therapy may be as effective as a 7-day triple therapy regimen. The 1-day quadruple therapy regimen consists of two tablets of 262 mg bismouth subsalicylate qid, one 500 mg metronidazole tablet qid, 2 g of amoxicillin suspension qid, and two capsules of 30 mg of lansoprazole.
4. A 5-day treatment with three antibiotics (amoxicillin 1 g bid, clarithromycin 250 mg bid, and metronidazole 400 mg bid) plus either lansoprazole 30 mg bid or ranitidine 300 mg bid is an efficacious cost-saving option for patients older than 55 yr with no prior history of PUD.
5. A combination of levofloxacin 250 mg bid, amoxicillin 1000 mg bid, and a PPI bid for 10 to 14 days can be used as salvage therapy after unsuccessful attempts to eradicate *H. pylori* using other regimens.

- Prophylaxis and treatment of stress gastritis with sucralfate suspension 1 g orally q4 to 6h, H_2-receptor antagonists, or PPIs in patients on ventilator support
- Misoprostol (Cytotec) or PPIs in patients on chronic NSAIDs therapy

CHRONIC Rx

- Misoprostol 100 μg qid or Omeprazole 20 mg/qd in patients receiving chronic NSAIDs
- Avoidance of alcohol, tobacco, and prolonged NSAID use

DISPOSITION

- Undetectable stool antigen 4 wk after therapy accurately confirm cure of *H. pylori* infection in initially seropositive healthy subjects with reasonable sensitivity.
- Surveillance gastroscopy in patients with atrophic gastritis (increased risk of gastric cancer).

AUTHOR: **FRED F. FERRI, M.D.**

BASIC INFORMATION

DEFINITION

Gastroesophageal reflux disease (GERD) is a motility disorder characterized primarily by heartburn and caused by the reflux of gastric contents into the esophagus.

SYNONYMS

Peptic esophagitis
Reflux esophagitis
GERD

ICD-9CM CODES
530.81 Gastroesophageal reflux disease
530.1 Esophagitis
787.1 Heartburn

EPIDEMIOLOGY & DEMOGRAPHICS

GERD is one of the most prevalent GI disorders. Nearly 7% of persons in the United States experience heartburn daily, 20% experience it monthly, and 60% experience it intermittently. Incidence in pregnant women exceeds 80%. Nearly 20% of adults use antacids or OTC H_2-blockers at least once a week for relief of heartburn.

PHYSICAL FINDINGS & CLINICAL PRESENTATION

- Physical examination: generally unremarkable
- Clinical signs and symptoms: heartburn, dysphagia, sour taste, regurgitation of gastric contents into the mouth
- Chronic cough and bronchospasm
- Chest pain, laryngitis, early satiety, abdominal fullness, and bloating with belching
- Dental erosions in children

ETIOLOGY

- Incompetent LES
- Medications that lower LES pressure (calcium channel blockers, β-adrenergic blockers, theophylline, anticholinergics)
- Foods that lower LES pressure (chocolate, yellow onions, peppermint)
- Tobacco abuse, alcohol, coffee
- Pregnancy
- Gastric acid hypersecretion
- Hiatal hernia (controversial) present in >70% of patients with GERD; however, most patients with hiatal hernia are asymptomatic
- Obesity is associated with a statistically significant increase in the risk for GERD symptoms, erosive esophagitis, and esophageal carcinoma

DIAGNOSIS

DIFFERENTIAL DIAGNOSIS

- Peptic ulcer disease
- Unstable angina
- Esophagitis (from infections such as herpes, *Candida*), medication induced (doxycycline, potassium chloride)
- Esophageal spasm (nutcracker esophagus)
- Cancer of esophagus

WORKUP

- Aimed at eliminating the conditions noted in the differential diagnosis and documenting the type and extent of tissue damage.
- Upper GI endoscopy is useful to document the type and extent of tissue damage in GERD and to exclude potentially malignant conditions such as Barrett's esophagus. The American College of Gastroenterology recommends endoscopy to screen for Barrett's esophagus in patients who have chronic GERD symptoms. The data demonstrating the cost-effectiveness of endoscopic screening remain controversial.

LABORATORY TESTS

- 24-hr esophageal pH monitoring and Bernstein test are sensitive diagnostic tests; however, they are not very practical and generally not done. They are useful in patients with atypical manifestations of GERD, such as chest pain or chronic cough.
- Esophageal manometry is indicated in patients with refractory reflux in whom surgical therapy is planned.

IMAGING STUDIES

Upper GI series can identify ulcerations and strictures; however, it may miss mucosal abnormalities. It may be useful in patients unwilling to have endoscopy or with medical contraindications to the procedure. Only one third of patients with GERD have radiographic signs of esophagitis on UGI series.

TREATMENT

NONPHARMACOLOGIC THERAPY

- Lifestyle modifications with avoidance of foods (e.g., citrus- and tomato-based products) and drugs that exacerbate reflux (e.g., caffeine, β-blockers, calcium channel blockers, α-adrenergic agonists, theophylline)
- Avoidance of tobacco and alcohol use
- Elevation of head of bed (4 to 8 in) using blocks
- Avoidance of lying down directly after late or large evening meals
- Weight reduction, decreased fat intake
- Avoidance of clothing that is tight around the waist

GENERAL Rx

- Proton pump inhibitors (PPIs) (esomeprazole 40 mg qd, omeprazole 20 mg qd, lansoprazole 30 mg qd, rabeprazole 20 mg qd, or pantoprazole 40 mg qd) are safe, tolerated, and very effective in most patients.
- H_2-Blockers (nizatidine 300 mg qhs, famotidine 40 mg qhs, ranitidine 300 mg qhs, or cimetidine 800 mg qhs) can be used but are generally much less effective than PPIs.
- Antacids (may be useful for relief of mild symptoms; however, they are generally ineffective in severe cases of reflux).
- Prokinetic agents (metoclopramide) are indicated only when PPIs are not fully effective. They can be used in combination therapy; however, side effects limit their use.
- For refractory cases: surgery with Nissen fundoplication. Potential surgical candidates should have reflux esophagitis documented by EGD and normal esophageal motility as evaluated by manometry. Surgery generally consists of reduction of hiatal hernia when present and placement of a gastric wrap around the GE junction (fundoplication). Although laparoscopic fundoplication is now widely used, surgery should not be advised with the expectation that patients with GERD will no longer need to take antisecretory medications or that the procedure will prevent esophageal cancer among those with GERD and Barrett's esophagus.
- Endoscopic radiofrequency heating of the GE junction (Stretta procedure) is a newer treatment modality for GERD patients unresponsive to traditional therapy. Its mechanism of action remains unclear. Endoscopy gastroplasty (EndoCinch procedure) also aims at treating GERD. Initial results appear encouraging; however, long-term studies are needed before recommending these procedures.
- Lifestyle modification must be followed lifelong, because this is generally an irreversible condition.

DISPOSITION

- The majority of the patients respond well to therapy.
- Recurrence of reflux is common if treatment is discontinued.
- Postsurgical complications occur in nearly 20% of patients (dysphagia, gas, bloating, diarrhea, nausea). Long-term follow-up studies also reveal that within 3 to 5 yr, 52% of patients who had undergone antireflux surgery are taking antireflux medications again.

REFERRAL

- There is a strong and probably causal relation between symptomatic prolonged and untreated GERD, Barrett's esophagus, and esophageal adenocarcinoma. GI referral for upper endoscopy

is needed when there are concerns about associated PUD, Barrett's esophagus, or esophageal cancer.
- Patients with Barrett's esophagus should undergo surveillance endoscopy with mucosal biopsy every 2 yr or less because the risk of developing adenocarcinoma of esophagus is at least 30 times greater than that of the general population.
- Testing and treating for *Helicobactor pylori* in patients with GERD has not been shown to improve symptoms.
- All children with dental erosions should be evaluated for GERD.

EVIDENCE

EBM

Adults

H_2R antagonists are more effective than placebo but less effective than proton pump inhibitors (PPIs).

Antagonists vs. placebo are more likely to relieve heartburn in patients with endoscopy-negative reflux disease.[1] Ⓐ

Antagonists are less effective than PPIs in the empirical treatment of typical GERD symptoms, although the difference is not significant for heartburn remission.[1] Ⓐ

Antagonists are more effective than placebo but less effective than PPIs at reducing the risk of persistent esophagitis.[2] Ⓐ

Ranitidine is less effective at 6 months than PPIs at reducing relapse rate in people with healed esophagitis.[3] Ⓐ

Ranitidine is less effective than omeprazole at maintaining remission at 12 months in patients with healed esophagitis and no reflux symptoms.[4] Ⓐ

There is some evidence that esomeprazole may be more effective than other PPIs at promoting healing from esophagitis at 4 weeks. Otherwise there is little or no evidence to suggest that some PPIs are more effective than others.

A systematic review that compared various PPIs in people with reflux esophagitis found that esomeprazole was more effective than omeprazole at promoting healing at 4 weeks. There were no significant differences between lansoprazole and omeprazole, pantoprazole and omeprazole, or rabeprazole and omeprazole.[5] Ⓐ

Another systematic review and three RCTs also compared various PPIs with each other in people with reflux esophagitis. There were no significant differences in clinical benefit between other PPIs.[6] Ⓐ

Open surgery appears to be more effective than medical therapy in severe or complicated GERD in the short term; there may be no difference in the long term. There is no evidence to suggest a difference between open and laparoscopic fundoplication.

A systematic review of randomized controlled trials (RCTs) showed that open surgery vs. medical therapy in patients with severe or complicated GERD significantly reduced symptoms and produced endoscopic improvements in esophagitis.[7] Ⓐ

However, a 10-year follow-up of one of the RCTs in this review found no significant difference in endoscopic appearance between those who had been treated with open surgery and those who had received medical therapy.[8] Ⓐ

There appears to be no clear difference in efficacy between open and laparoscopic fundoplication.[9,10] Ⓐ

Evidence-Based References

1. van Pinxteren B et al: Short-term treatment with proton pump inhibitors, H2-receptor antagonists and prokinetics for gastro-oesophageal reflux disease-like symptoms and endoscopy negative reflux disease. Reviewed in: Cochrane Library, 3,2004, Chichester, UK, John Wiley. Ⓐ
2. Delaney B, Moayyedi P: Dyspepsia. In: Stevens A, Raftery J (Eds), *Health care needs assessment,* ed 4, 2002, NHS Executive. Reviewed in: *Clin Evid* 10:518, 2003. Ⓐ
3. Caro JJ, Salas M, Ward A: Healing and relapse rates in gastro-oesophageal reflux disease treated with the newer proton-pump inhibitors lansoprazole, rabeprazole and pantoprazole compared with omeprazole, ranitidine and placebo: evidence from randomized controlled trials, *Clin Ther* 23:998, 2001. Reviewed in: *Clin Evid* 10:518, 2003. Ⓐ
4. Festen HPM et al: Omeprazole versus high-dose ranitidine in mild gastro-oesophageal reflux disease: short- and long-term treatment, *Am J Gastroenterol* 94:931, 1999. Reviewed in: *Clin Evid* 10:518, 2003. Ⓐ
5. Edwards SJ, Lind T, Lundell L: Systematic review of proton pump inhibitors for the acute treatment of reflux oesophagitis, *Aliment Pharmacol Ther* 15:1729, 2001. Reviewed in: *Clin Evid* 10:518, 2003. Ⓐ
6. Moayyedi P, Delaney B, Forman D: Gastro-oesophageal reflux disease. Reviewed in: *Clin Evid* 10:518, 2003, London, BMJ Publishing Group. Ⓐ
7. Allgood PC, Bachmann M: Medical or surgical treatment for chronic gastro-oesophageal reflux? A systematic review of published evidence of effectiveness, *Eur J Surg* 166:713, 2000. Reviewed in: *Clin Evid* 10:518, 2003. Ⓐ
8. Spechler SJ et al: Long-term outcome of medical and surgical therapies for gastro-esophageal reflux disease, *JAMA* 285:2331, 2001. Reviewed in: *Clin Evid* 10:518, 2003. Ⓐ
9. Bias JE et al: Laparoscopic or conventional Nissen fundoplication for gastro-oesophageal reflux disease: randomized clinical trial, *Lancet* 355:170, 2000. Reviewed in: *Clin Evid* 10:518, 2003. Ⓐ
10. Heikkinen T-J et al: Comparison of laparoscopic and open Nissen fundoplication 2 years after operation, *Surg Endosc* 14:1019, 2000. Reviewed in: *Clin Evid* 10:518, 2003. Ⓐ

Children

Cimetidine has been found to be more effective than placebo for the treatment of children with GERD and esophagitis in a small randomized controlled trial (RCT).[1] Ⓐ

Another small RCT found that significantly more children achieved healing of esophagitis and symptomatic improvement when treated with nizatidine, compared with placebo.[2] Ⓐ

There is insufficient evidence for the use of metoclopramide in the treatment of GERD in children.[3] Ⓐ

A systematic review found that adults and children with asthma and GERD did not achieve an overall improvement in asthma following antireflux treatment. The patients were not specifically recruited on the basis of reflux-associated respiratory symptoms. Subgroups of patients may benefit, but it appears difficult to predict responders.[4] Ⓐ

Evidence-Based References

1. Cucchiara S et al: Cimetidine treatment of reflux esophagitis in children: an Italian multicenter study, *J Pediatr Gastroenterol Nutr* 8:150, 1989. Reviewed in: *Clin Evid* 11:414, 2004. Ⓐ
2. Simeone D et al: Treatment of childhood peptic esophagitis: a double-blind placebo-controlled trial of nizatidine, *J Pediatr Gastroenterol Nutr* 25:51, 1997. Ⓐ
3. Kumar Y, Sarvananthan R: Gastro-oesophageal reflux in children. Reviewed in: *Clin Evid* 11:414, 2004, London, BMJ Publishing Group. Ⓐ
4. Gibson PG, Henry RL, Coughlan JL: Gastro-oesophageal reflux treatment for asthma in adults and children, *Cochrane Database Syst Rev* 1,2003. Ⓐ

SUGGESTED READINGS

Hampel H et al: Meta-analysis: obesity and the risk for gastroesophageal reflux disease and its complications, *Ann Intern Med* 143(3):199, 2005.

Heidelbaugh JL et al: Management of gastroesophageal reflux disease, *Am Fam Physician* 68:1311, 2003.

Kabrilas PJ: Radiofrequency energy treatment of GERD, *Gastroenterology* 125:970, 2003.

Shaheen N, Ransohoff DF: Gastroesophageal reflux, Barret esophagus, and esophageal cancer, *JAMA* 287:1972, 2002.

AUTHOR: **FRED F. FERRI, M.D.**

BASIC INFORMATION

DEFINITION

Giant cell arteritis (GCA) is a segmental systemic granulomatous arteritis affecting medium- and large-sized arteries in individuals >50 years. Inflammation primarily targets extracranial blood vessels, and although the carotid system is usually affected, pathology in posterior cerebral artery has been reported.

SYNONYMS

Temporal arteritis
Cranial arteritis

ICD-9CM CODES
446.5 Temporal arteritis

EPIDEMIOLOGY & DEMOGRAPHICS

INCIDENCE: 17 to 23.3 new cases/100,000 persons >50 yr

PREVALENCE: 200 cases/100,000 persons; female-to-male predominance of two- to fourfold

PHYSICAL FINDINGS & CLINICAL PRESENTATION:

GCA can present with the following clinical manifestations:

- Headache, often associated with marked scalp tenderness
- Constitutional symptoms (fever, weight loss, anorexia, fatigue)
- Polymyalgia syndrome (aching and stiffness of the trunk and proximal muscle groups)
- Visual disturbances (transient or permanent monocular visual loss)
- Intermittent claudication of jaw and tongue on mastication

Important physical findings in GCA:

- Vascular examination: tenderness, decreased pulsation, and nodulation of temporal arteries; diminished or absent pulses in upper extremities

ETIOLOGY

Vasculitis of unknown etiology

DIAGNOSIS

Clinical history and vascular examination are cornerstones of diagnosis.

The presence of any three of the following five items allows the diagnosis of GCA with a sensitivity of 94% and a specificity of 91%:

- Age of onset >50 yr
- New-onset or new type of headache
- Temporal artery tenderness or decreased pulsation
- Westergren ESR >50 mm/hr
- Temporal artery biopsy with vasculitis and mononuclear cell infiltrate or granulomatous changes

DIFFERENTIAL DIAGNOSIS

- Other vasculitic syndromes
- Nonarteritic anterior ischemic optic neuropathy (AION)
- Primary amyloidosis
- TIA, stroke
- Infections
- Occult neoplasm, multiple myeloma

LABORATORY TESTS

- ESR >50 mm/hr; however, up to 22.5% patients with GCA have normal ESR before treatment.
- C-reactive protein is typically included in lab investigation; it has greater sensitivity than ESR.
- Mild to moderate normochromic normocytic anemia, elevated platelet count.

IMAGING STUDIES

- Reliability of color duplex ultrasonography of temporal artery is controversial as it is thought that it does not improve diagnostic accuracy over careful physical examination.
- Fluorescein angiogram of ophthalmic vessels may be warranted to differentiate between arteritic AION (i.e., GCA) and nonarteritic AION.

TREATMENT

ACUTE GENERAL Rx

- Intravenous methylprednisolone (500-1000 mg qd for 3 to 5 days) is indicated in those with significant clinical manifestations (e.g., visual loss).
- Oral prednisone (1 mg/kg/day) may be used under less urgent circumstances or following the initial period of treatment with intravenous methylprednisolone. High-dose oral regimen should be continued at least until symptoms resolve and ESR returns to normal. Prednisone treatment may last up to 2 yr and is tapered over several wk to mo.

DISPOSITION

If steroid therapy is initiated early, GCA has excellent prognosis; however, 20% of patients have permanent partial or complete loss of vision. Once there is visual loss, improvement is dismal: in one study, only 4% of eyes improved in both visual acuity and central visual field.

REFERRAL

- Surgical referral for biopsy of temporal artery
- Ophthalmology referral in patients with visual disturbances and following initiation of corticosteroid therapy
- Rheumatology referral for difficult cases

PEARLS & CONSIDERATIONS

The diagnostic utility of temporal artery biopsy is not compromised if performed within days of starting steroid therapy.

COMMENTS

- The relationship between polymyalgia rheumatica and GCA is unclear, but the two may frequently coexist.
- Clinical picture rather than ESR should be the prime yardstick for continuing prednisone therapy. A rising ESR in a clinically asymptomatic patient with normal hematocrit should raise suspicion for alternate explanations (e.g., infections, neoplasms).
- GCA is associated with a markedly increased risk for the development of aortic aneurysm, which is often a late complication and may cause death. Annual chest radiograph in chronic GCA patients has been suggested, as well as emergent chest CT or MRI for clinical suspicion.

EVIDENCE

The recommendation to perform temporal artery biopsy before beginning long-term corticosteroid therapy is based on consensus rather than evidence.

The recommendation that daily high-dose corticosteroid therapy should not be delayed pending confirmation of the diagnosis from temporal artery biopsy is similarly based on consensus rather than evidence.

Low-dose aspirin prophylaxis is proven to decrease visual loss and stroke in patients with GCA.

The efficacy of adding methotrexate or azathioprine to the steroid regimen for their steroid-sparing effect is unproven.

SUGGESTED READINGS

Gold R et al: Therapy of neurological disorders in systemic vasculitis, *Sem Neurol* 23(2):207, 2003.

Gonzalez-Gay MA: The diagnosis and management of patients with giant cell arteritis, *J Rheumatol* 32:1186, 2005.

Hoffman GS et al: A multicenter, randomized, double-blind, placebo-controlled trial of adjuvant methotrexate for giant-cell arteritis, *Arthritis Rheum* 46(5):1309, 2002.

Karassa FB et al: Meta-analysis: test performance of ultrasonography for giant cell arteritis, *Ann Intern Med* 142:359-369, 2005.

Nesher G et al: Low-dose aspirin and prevention of cranial ischemic complications in giant cell arteritis, *Arth & Rheum* 50(4):1332, 2004.

Norborg E, Norborg C: Giant cell arteritis: epidemiological clues to its pathogenesis and an update on its treatment, *Rheumatol* 42:413, 2003.

Salvarani C et al: Polymyalgia rheumatica and giant-cell arteritis, *N Engl J Med* 347(4):261, 2002.

Smetana GW, Shmerling RH: Does this patient have temporal arteritis? *JAMA* 287:92, 2002.

AUTHOR: **U. SHIVRAJ SOHUR, M.D., PH.D.**

BASIC INFORMATION

DEFINITION

Giardiasis is an intestinal and/or biliary tract infection caused by the protozoal parasite *Giardia lamblia*. The organism is a widespread zoonotic parasite and frequently contaminates fresh water sources worldwide.

SYNONYMS

Giardiasis
Giardia duodenalis
Giardia intestinalis

ICD-9CM CODES
007.1 Giardiasis

EPIDEMIOLOGY & DEMOGRAPHICS

INCIDENCE (IN U.S.):
- Exact incidence unknown
- Frequently occurs in outbreaks

PEAK INCIDENCE:
- Varies with risk factors, outbreaks
- All age groups affected

PREVALENCE (IN U.S.): 4%
PREDOMINANT SEX: Male = female
PREDOMINANT AGE:
- Preschool children, especially if in day care
- 20 to 40 yr of age, especially among sexually active homosexual men

GENETICS:
Familial Disposition: Patients with common variable immunodeficiency or X-linked agammaglobulinemia are at increased risk of infection.

PHYSICAL FINDINGS & CLINICAL PRESENTATION

- More than 70% with one or more intestinal symptoms (diarrhea, flatulence, cramps, bloating, nausea)
- Fever in <20%
- Chronic diarrhea, malabsorption, and weight loss
- GI bleeding is unusual
- Continuous or intermittent symptoms, lasting for weeks
- Of infected patients, 20% to 25% are asymptomatic

ETIOLOGY

Infection is acquired by ingestion of viable cysts of the organism, typically in contaminated water or by fecal-oral contact.

DIAGNOSIS

DIFFERENTIAL DIAGNOSIS

- Other agents of infective diarrhea (amebae, *Salmonella* sp., *Shigella* sp., *Staphylococcus aureus, Cryptosporidium,* etc.)
- Noninfectious causes of malabsorption

WORKUP

- Stool specimen (three specimens yield 90% sensitivity) or duodenal aspirate for microscopic examination to establish diagnosis and exclude other pathogens (Fig. 1-105)
- Immunoassays for *Giardia sp.* Antigens in stool samples are now routinely used in most clinical laboratories

LABORATORY TESTS

Serum albumin, vitamin B_{12} levels, and stool fat test to exclude malabsorption

IMAGING STUDIES

- Not necessary unless biliary obstruction is suspected
- In detection of organism, possible interference by barium in stool from radiographic studies

TREATMENT

NONPHARMACOLOGIC THERAPY

Avoidance of milk products to reduce symptoms of transient lactase deficiency that occur in many patients

ACUTE GENERAL Rx

Adults:
- Nitazoxanide 500 mg PO twice daily for 3 days
- Metronidazole 250 mg PO three times daily for 7 days (metronidazole avoided in pregnancy) *or* Tinidazole 2 mg PO once
- Paromomycin 25 to 30 mg/kg/day in three doses for 5 to 10 days

CHRONIC Rx

May require retreatment.

DISPOSITION

Reinfection is possible.

REFERRAL

For evaluation by gastroenterologist if malabsorption and persistent weight loss

PEARLS & CONSIDERATIONS

COMMENTS

Travelers to endemic areas (developing world, wilderness areas) should be cautioned to boil drinking water or use water purification tablets.

EVIDENCE

Randomized controlled trials (RCTs) have shown cure rates of 80%-90% at 7 to 14 days follow-up, after 5 to 7 days' treatment with metronidazole, in children with giardiasis.[1] B

An RCT comparing the efficacy and safety of furazolidone and metronidazole in liquid suspension found no significant differences between the treatments in children with giardiasis.[2] B

An RCT comparing the efficacy and safety of albendazole and metronidazole in suspension found no significant differences between the treatments in children with giardiasis.[3] B

Evidence-Based References

1. Ortiz JJ et al: Randomized clinical study of nitazoxanide compared to metronidazole in the treatment of symptomatic giardiasis in children from Northern Peru, *Aliment Pharmacol Ther* 15:1409, 2001. B
2. Quiros-Buelna E: Furazolidone and metronidazole for treatment of giardiasis in children, *Scand J Gastroenterol Suppl* 169:65, 1989. B
3. Misra PK et al: A comparative clinical trial of albendazole versus metronidazole in children with giardiasis, *Indian Pediatr* 32:779, 1995. B

SUGGESTED READINGS

Hlavsa MC et al: Giardiasis surveillance—United States, 1998-2002, *MMWR Surveill Summ* 54(1):9, 2005.
Lalle M et al: Genotyping of Giardia duodenalis from humans and dogs from Mexico using a beta-giardin nested polymerase chain reaction assay, *J Parasitol* 91(1):203, 2005.
Yakoob J et al: Giardiasis in patients with dyspeptic symptoms, *World J Gastroenterol* 11(42):6667, 2005.

AUTHORS: **GLENN G. FORT, M.D., M.P.H., JOSEPH R. MASCI, M.D.,** and **DENNIS J. MIKOLICH, M.D.**

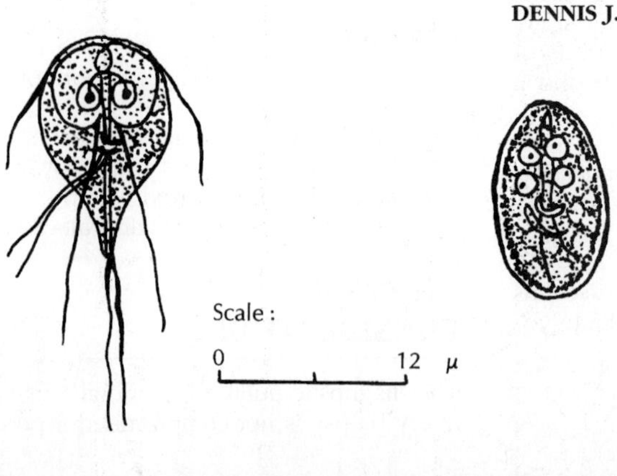

FIGURE 1-105 ***Giardia*** **organisms.** The trophozoite *(left)* is 12 to 15 μm long and has four pairs of flagella. This form is not commonly seen in stools. Cysts *(right)* are 9 to 19 μm long and may have two to four nuclei. (From Hoekelman R [ed]: *Primary pediatric care,* ed 3, St Louis, 1997, Mosby.)

BASIC INFORMATION

DEFINITION

Gilbert's disease is an autosomal dominant disease characterized by indirect hyperbilirubinemia caused by impaired glucuronyl transferase activity.

SYNONYMS

Gilbert's syndrome

ICD-9CM CODES
277.4 Gilbert's syndrome

EPIDEMIOLOGY & DEMOGRAPHICS

INCIDENCE (IN U.S.): Probable autosomal dominant disease affecting >5% of the U.S. population

PREDOMINANT SEX: Male:female ratio of 3:1

GENETICS: Most common hereditary hyperbilirubinemia (genotypic prevalence 12%)

PHYSICAL FINDINGS & CLINICAL PRESENTATION

- No abnormalities on physical examination other than mild jaundice when bilirubin exceeds 3 mg/dl.
- A family history of unconjugated hyperbilirubinemia may be present.

ETIOLOGY

- Decreased elimination of bilirubin in bile is caused by inadequate conjugation of bilirubin.
- Alcohol consumption and starvation diet can increase the bilirubin level.
- The pathogenesis of Gilbert's syndrome has been linked to a reduction in bilirubin UGT-1 gene (HUG-Brl) transcription resulting from a mutation in the promoter region.

DIAGNOSIS

DIFFERENTIAL DIAGNOSIS

- Hemolytic anemia
- Liver disease (chronic hepatitis, cirrhosis)
- Crigler-Najjar syndrome

WORKUP

- Most patients are diagnosed during or after adolescence, when isolated hyperbilirubinemia is detected as an incidental finding on routine biochemical testing
- Laboratory evaluation to exclude hemolysis and liver diseases as a cause of the elevated bilirubin level (Table 1-14)

LABORATORY TESTS

Elevated indirect (unconjugated) bilirubin (rarely exceeds 5 mg/dl)

TREATMENT

ACUTE GENERAL Rx

Treatment is generally unnecessary. Phenobarbital (if clinical jaundice is present) can rapidly decrease serum indirect bilirubin level.

DISPOSITION

Prognosis is excellent. Treatment is generally unnecessary.

REFERRAL

Referral is generally not necessary.

PEARLS & CONSIDERATIONS

COMMENTS

- Patients should be reassured about the benign nature of their condition.
- Fasting for 2 days or significant dehydration may raise the bilirubin level and result in the clinical recognition of jaundice.

AUTHOR: **FRED F. FERRI, M.D.**

TABLE 1-14 Characteristic Patterns of Liver Function Tests

Disorder	Bilirubin	Alkaline Phosphatase	AST	ALT	Prothrombin Time	Albumin
Gilbert's syndrome (abnormal bilirubin metabolism)	↑	NL	NL	NL	NL	NL
Bile duct obstruction (pancreatic cancer)	↑↑↑	↑↑↑	↑	↑	↑-↑↑	NL
Acute hepatocellular damage (toxic, viral hepatitis)	↑-↑↑↑	↑-↑↑	↑↑↑	↑↑↑	NL-↑↑↑	NL-↓↓
Cirrhosis	NL-↑	NL-↑	NL-↑	NL-↑	NL-↑↑	NL-↓↓

From Andreoli TE (ed): *Cecil essentials of medicine,* ed 6, Philadelphia, 2005, WB Saunders.
ALT, Alanine aminotransferase; *AST,* aspartate aminotransferase; *NL,* normal; ↑, increase; ↓, decrease (arrows indicate extent of change: ↑-↑↑↑, slight to large).

BASIC INFORMATION

DEFINITION

Inflammation of the gums covering the maxilla and mandible

SYNONYMS

None

ICD-9CM CODE
523.1

EPIDEMIOLOGY & DEMOGRAPHICS

Gingivitis generally occurs in adults.

PHYSICAL FINDINGS & CLINICAL PRESENTATION

- Inflammation is usually painless.
- Bleeding may occur with minor trauma such as brushing teeth.
- A bluish discoloration of the gums and halitosis are sometimes present.
- Subgingival plaque may be seen on close examination, and in time, there is detachment of soft tissue from the tooth surface.
- Long-standing infection may lead to destructive periodontal disease, which may involve teeth and bones.
- A dramatic form of gingivitis called *acute ulcerative necrotizing gingivitis* (ANUG or "trench mouth") can occur. This is manifested by acute, painful, inflammation of the gingivae, with bleeding, ulceration, and halitosis. At times this is accompanied by fever and lymphadenopathy.
- *Linear gingival erythema* ("HIV Gingivitis") presents as a brightly inflamed band of marginal gingiva. It may be painful, with easy bleeding and rapid destruction.
- Severe periodontitis can occur in patients with diabetes mellitus or HIV infection and in primary HIV infection (acute retroviral syndrome).
- Pregnancy may be associated with an acute form of gingivitis. Gingivae become inflamed and hypertrophic; this is likely due to hormonal shifts.

ETIOLOGY

- A variety of organisms may be found in the environment of plaque. Anaerobes play a predominant role in periodontal disease.
- Improper hygiene and poorly fitting dentures may contribute to development of gingivitis.
- Excessive use of tobacco and alcohol may predispose individuals to gingival disease.
- In patients with HIV infection, gram-negative anaerobes, enteric organisms, and yeast predominate.
- Appropriate oral hygiene, such as flossing and tooth brushing, can prevent the accumulation of bacterial plaque; once dense plaque is present, adequate hygiene becomes more difficult.

DIAGNOSIS

DIFFERENTIAL DIAGNOSIS

Gingival hyperplasia, which may be caused by long term use of phenytoin or nifedipine

WORKUP

Oral examination

LABORATORY TESTS

Elevated serum glucose in diabetics

IMAGING STUDIES

Radiographs of the teeth and facial bones may reveal extension of infection to these structures.

TREATMENT

NONPHARMACOLOGIC THERAPY

Removal of plaque, and at times, debridement of soft tissue

ACUTE GENERAL Rx

- Penicillin VK, 500 mg po qid for 1 to 2 wk *or*
- Clindamycin, 300 mg po qid for 1 to 2 wk
- For *linear gingival erythema,* chlorhexidene gluconate rinses and nystatin rinses or troches may be used

CHRONIC Rx

Extensive or recurrent infection may require periodic evaluation and debridement.

DISPOSITION

Continued inflammation can eventually lead to destruction of teeth and bone.

REFERRAL

Patients should be referred to a dentist or periodontist.

PEARLS & CONSIDERATIONS

COMMENTS

- Presence of periodontal disease is associated with an increased incidence of anaerobic pleuropulmonary infections.
- Existing data support the recommendation to change a toothbrush every 3 mo. Worn brushes seem to be less effective in plaque reduction.

EVIDENCE

Professional cleaning and scaling reaches subgingival areas not usually accessible to the patient through toothbrushing and flossing.[1]

Failure of the patient to remove plaque deposits regularly between visits will result in extension of plaque to subgingival crevices and accumulation of calculus.

Parameter on plaque-associated gingivitis. Chicago: American Academy of Periodontology, National Guideline Clearinghouse: patient education, including oral hygiene instruction; debridement of tooth surfaces to remove plaque and calculus; correction of restorations hindering oral hygiene; surgical correction of the gums where indicated; and outcomes assessment.[2]

Evidence-Based References

1. Axelsson P, Lindhe J: Effect of controlled oral hygiene procedures on caries and periodontal disease in adults: results after 6 years, *J Clin Periodontol* 8:239, 1981.
2. American Academy of Periodontology: Guidelines for periodontal therapy, *J Periodontol* 69:405, 1998.

SUGGESTED READINGS

Sharma NC et al: Antiplaque and antigingivitis effectiveness of a hexetidine mouthwash, *J Clin Periodontol* 30(7):590, 2003.

Rudiger SG et al: Dental biofilms at healthy and inflamed gingival margins, *J Clin Periodontol* 29(6):524, 2002.

AUTHORS: **GLENN G. FORT, M.D., M.P.H., DENNIS J. MIKOLICH, M.D.,** and **MAURICE POLICAR, M.D.**

BASIC INFORMATION

DEFINITION

Chronic open-angle glaucoma refers to optic nerve damage often associated with elevated intraocular pressure; it is a chronic, slowly progressive, usually bilateral disorder associated with visual loss, eye pain, and optic nerve damage. Now felt to be a primary disease of the optic nerve with high pressure a high risk factor for glaucoma.

SYNONYMS

Chronic simple glaucoma
Primary open-angle glaucoma (POAG)

ICD-9CM CODES
365.1 Open-angle glaucoma

EPIDEMIOLOGY & DEMOGRAPHICS

INCIDENCE (IN U.S.): Third most common cause of visual loss (75% to 95% of all glaucomas are open angle.)

PEAK INCIDENCE:
- Increases after 40 yr
- Because of rapid aging of the U.S. population, expect 3 million cases by year 2020.

PREVALENCE (IN U.S.):
- Overall prevalence in U.S. population >40 yr of age is estimated to be 1.86%, with 1.57 million white and 398,000 black patients affected.
- 150,000 patients suffer bilateral blindness.
- Disease occurs in 2% of people >40 yr old.
- Prevalence is higher in diabetics, with high myopia, and among older persons.
- More common in blacks (3× the age-adjusted prevalence than whites).

PREDOMINANT AGE:
- Persons >50 yr
- Can occur in 30s and 40s

GENETICS:
- Four to six times higher incidence in blacks than whites
- No clear-cut hereditary patterns but a strong hereditary tendency

PHYSICAL FINDINGS & CLINICAL PRESENTATION

- High intraocular pressures and large optic nerve cup (OHTS study—very important)
- Corneal edema causes vision loss and blurring
- Abnormal visual fields
- Open-angle gonioscopy
- Red eye
- Restricted vision and field

ETIOLOGY

- Uncertain hereditary tendency
- Topical steroids
- Trauma
- Inflammatory
- High-dose oral corticosteroids taken for prolonged periods

DIAGNOSIS

DIFFERENTIAL DIAGNOSIS

- Other optic neuropathies
- Secondary glaucoma from inflammation and steroid therapy
- Red eye differential
- Trauma
- Contact lens injury

WORKUP

- Intraocular pressure
- Slit lamp examination
- Visual fields
- Gonioscopy
- Nerve fiber analysis—GDx, etc.
- Corneal thickness—very important in prognosis

LABORATORY TESTS

Blood sugar

IMAGING STUDIES

- Optic nerve photography—stereo photographs
- Visual field testing
- GDx (laser scan of nerve fiber layer), OCT, HRT

TREATMENT

ACUTE GENERAL Rx

- β-Blockers (Timolol) qd to bid depending on individual response to drug
- Diamox 250 mg qid or 500 mg bid
- Hyperosmotic agents (mannitol) in acute treatment (IV)
- Prostaglandins very commonly used as first-line treatment
- Laser trabeculoplasty (SLT) as needed
- Pilocarpine qid

CHRONIC Rx

- At least biannual checks of intraocular pressure and adjustment of medication
- Poor control = frequent examinations; good control = drugs
- Trabeculectomy
- Filter valves

DISPOSITION

Must be followed by ophthalmologist

REFERRAL

Immediately to ophthalmologist

PEARLS & CONSIDERATIONS

COMMENTS

- Glaucoma is a serious blinding disease. Must be followed professionally by an ophthalmologist.
- Early diagnosis and treatment may minimize visual loss.
- Glaucoma is not solely caused by increased intraocular pressure, because approximately 20% of patients with glaucoma have normal intraocular pressure, but high pressure is definitely a risk factor to be considered. Potential sites of increased resistance to aqueous flow are described in Fig. 1-106.

EVIDENCE

One systematic review found that topical medical treatments significantly reduced intraocular pressure in patients with primary open-angle glaucoma after a minimum of 3 months of treatment. It is, however, not clear which types of medical treatments were used.[1] A

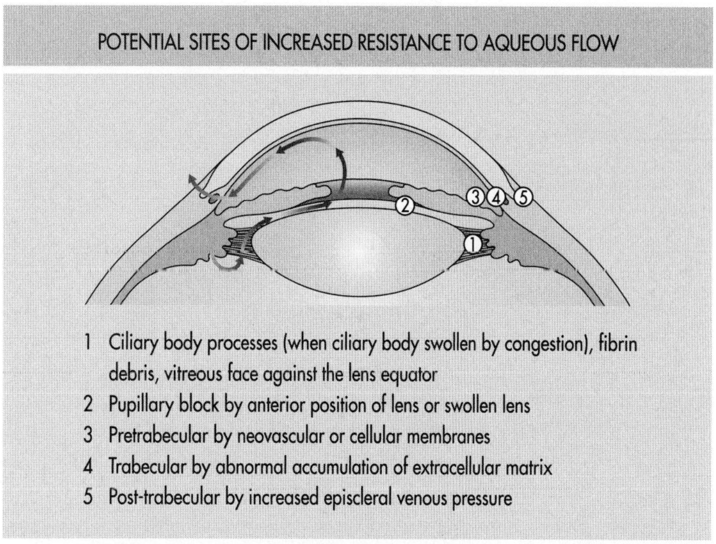

FIGURE 1-106 Potential sites of increased resistance to aqueous flow. (From Yanoff M, Duker JS: *Ophthalmology,* ed 2, St Louis, 2004, Mosby.)

One large randomized controlled trial (RCT) recruited 1636 participants with increased intraocular pressures but no other ophthalmologic changes aged between 40 and 80 years. Patients were randomized to observation or treatment groups. Treatment groups received commercially available topical ocular hypotensives. The study found that this treatment was effective in delaying or preventing the onset of primary open-angle glaucoma in patients after 5-year's follow-up compared with the observation group.[2] Ⓐ

RCTs have found that laser trabeculoplasty combined with medical treatment is more effective at decreasing intraocular pressures in patients with open-angle glaucoma than no initial treatment or medical treatment alone.[3,4] Ⓐ

There is some evidence to suggest that both surgical trabeculectomy and laser trabeculoplasty produce decreases in intraocular pressure, but the long-term differences between the efficacies of each treatment are less clear.[5,6] Ⓐ

There is evidence that there is no significant difference in visual acuity or intraocular pressure in the long term between Nd:YAG laser iridotomy and peripheral iridectomy for the treatment of acute angle-closure glaucoma.[7] Ⓐ

There is strong consensus for the efficacy of medical treatments that lower intraocular pressure in the treatment of acute angle-closure glaucoma. There is no apparent evidence available from any RCTs.[8]

An RCT of patients with normal-tension glaucoma showed that treatment to reduce the pressures by 30% significantly reduced the progression to visual field loss over 8 years compared with no treatment. The treatment consisted of drugs with or without surgical trabeculectomy.[9] Ⓐ

A Cochrane systematic review of the interventions for normal tension glaucoma was only able to find three studies that focused on patient relevant outcomes. In one study, the effect of intraocular pressure lowering on visual field outcome was only significant when data were corrected for cataract development. In two small studies, a calcium antagonist, brovincamine, produced a beneficial effect concerning visual field loss.[10] Ⓐ

Evidence-Based References

1. Rossetti L et al: Randomised clinical trials on medical treatment of glaucoma: are they appropriate to clinical practice? *Arch Ophthalmol* 111:96, 1993. Reviewed in: *Clin Evid* 9:729, 2003. Ⓐ
2. Kass M et al: The Ocular Hypertension Treatment Study: a randomized trial determines that topical ocular hypotensive medication delays or prevents the onset of primary open-angle glaucoma, *Arch Ophthalmol* 120:701, 2002. Ⓐ
3. Glaucoma Laser Research Group: The Glaucoma Laser Trial and Glaucoma Laser Trial follow-up study. 7. Results, *Am J Ophthalmol* 120:718, 1995. Reviewed in: *Clin Evid* 9:729, 2003. Ⓐ
4. Heijl A et al: Reduction of intraocular pressure and glaucoma progression: results from the Early Manifest Glaucoma Trial, *Arch Ophthalmol* 120:1268, 2002. Ⓐ
5. Migdal C et al: Long-term functional outcome after early surgery compared with laser and medicine in open angle glaucoma, *Ophthalmology* 101:1651, 1994. Reviewed in: *Clin Evid* 9:729, 2003. Ⓐ
6. The Advanced Glaucoma Intervention Study (AGIS): 4. Comparison of treatment outcomes with race. Seven year results, *Ophthalmology* 105:1146, 1998. Reviewed in: *Clin Evid* 9:729, 2003. Ⓐ
7. Fleck BW, Wright E, Fairley EA: A randomised prospective comparison of operative peripheral iridectomy and Nd:YAG laser iridotomy treatment of acute angle closure glaucoma: 3 year visual acuity and intraocular pressure control outcome, *Br J Ophthalmol* 81:884, 1997. Reviewed in: *Clin Evid* 9:729, 2003. Ⓐ
8. Shah R, Wormald R: Glaucoma. Reviewed in: *Clin Evid* 9:729, 2003, London, BMJ Publishing Group.
9. Collaborative Normal-Tension Glaucoma Study Group: Comparison of glaucomatous progression between untreated patients with normal-tension glaucoma and patients with therapeutically reduced intraocular pressure, *Am J Ophthalmol* 126:487, 1998. Reviewed in: *Clin Evid* 9:729, 2003. Ⓐ
10. Sycha T, Vass C, Findl O: Interventions for normal tension glaucoma, *Cochrane Database Syst Rev* 2,2004. Ⓐ

SUGGESTED READINGS

Gordon MO et al: Baseline factors that predict the onset of primary open-angle glaucoma, *Arch Ophthalmol* 120:714, 2002.

Heijl A et al: Reduction of intraocular pressure and glaucoma progression: Results from the early manifest glaucoma trial, *Arch Ophthalmol* 120:1268, 2002.

Higginbotham EJ et al: The Ocular Hypertension Treatment Study: topical medication delays or prevents primary open-angle glaucoma in African American individuals, *Arch Ophthalmol* 122(6):813, 2004.

Rezaie T et al: Adult-onset primary open-angle glaucoma caused by mutations in optineurin, Science 295:1077, 2002.

AUTHOR: **MELVYN KOBY, M.D.**

BASIC INFORMATION

DEFINITION

Primary angle-closure glaucoma (PACG) occurs when elevated intraocular pressure is associated with closure of the filtration angle or obstruction in the circulating pathway of the aqueous humor.

SYNONYMS

Acute glaucoma, angle-closure
Pupillary block glaucoma
Narrow-angle glaucoma

ICD-9CM CODES
365.2 Primary angle-closure glaucoma (PACG)

EPIDEMIOLOGY & DEMOGRAPHICS

INCIDENCE (IN U.S.):
- In 2% to 8% of all patients with glaucoma
- Higher incidence among those with hyperopia, small eyes, dense cataracts, shallow anterior chambers

PEAK INCIDENCE: Greater after 50 yr of age; high association with hypopia, cataracts, and eye trauma
PREDOMINANT SEX: Females > males
PREDOMINANT AGE: 50 to 60 yr
GENETICS: High family history

PHYSICAL FINDINGS & CLINICAL PRESENTATION

- Hazy cornea (Fig. 1-107)
- Narrow angle
- Red eyes
- Pain
- Injection of conjunctiva
- Shallow anterior chamber
- Thick cataract
- Old trauma
- Chronic eye infections

ETIOLOGY

- Narrow angles with acute closure—blockage of circulatory path of the aqueous humor causing increase in interior ocular pressure
- Secondary angle-closure glaucoma (SACG) resulting from neovascularization of iris, iris tumors, pharmacology, lens induced, iris scarring, trauma, chronic inflammation with scarring, malignant glaucoma with aqueous misdirection

DIAGNOSIS

DIFFERENTIAL DIAGNOSIS

- High pressure
- Optic nerve cupping
- Field loss
- Shallow chamber
- Open-angle glaucoma
- Conjunctivitis
- Corneal disease-keratitis
- Uveitis
- Scleritis
- Allergies
- Contact lens wearing with irritation

WORKUP

- Intraocular pressure
- Gonioscopy
- Slit lamp examination
- Visual field examination
- GDx examination (laser scan of nerve fiber layer), OCT
- Optic nerve evaluation
- Anterior chamber depth
- Cataract evaluation
- High hyperopia
- Dilatin provocative testing

LABORATORY TESTS

- Blood sugar and CBC (if diabetes or inflammatory disease is suspected)
- Visual field
- GDx nerve fiber analysis, OCT, HRT

IMAGING STUDIES

- Fundus photography
- Fluorescein angiography for neurovascular disease

TREATMENT

The goal of treatment is to acutely lower pressure on eye and keep it down.

NONPHARMACOLOGIC THERAPY

Laser iridotomy early in disease process

ACUTE GENERAL Rx

- IV mannitol
- Pilocarpine
- β-Blockers
- Diamox
- Laser iridotomy
- Anterior chamber paracentesis (as emergency treatment)

CHRONIC Rx

- Iridotomy
- Trabeculectomy
- Filter valves
- Other laser procedures

DISPOSITION

Refer to ophthalmologist immediately.

REFERRAL

This is an emergency—refer immediately to an ophthalmologist.

PEARLS & CONSIDERATIONS

COMMENTS

- Do not use antihistamines or vasodilators with narrow angle glaucoma.
- After iridotomy, the majority of patients will be totally cured and will need no further medication and have no visual loss.
- Lower socioeconomic status and higher levels of social deprivation are risk factors for delayed detection and probable worse outcomes in glaucoma.

EVIDENCE

One systematic review found that topical medical treatments significantly reduced intraocular pressure in patients with primary open-angle glaucoma after a minimum of 3 months of treatment. It is, however, not clear

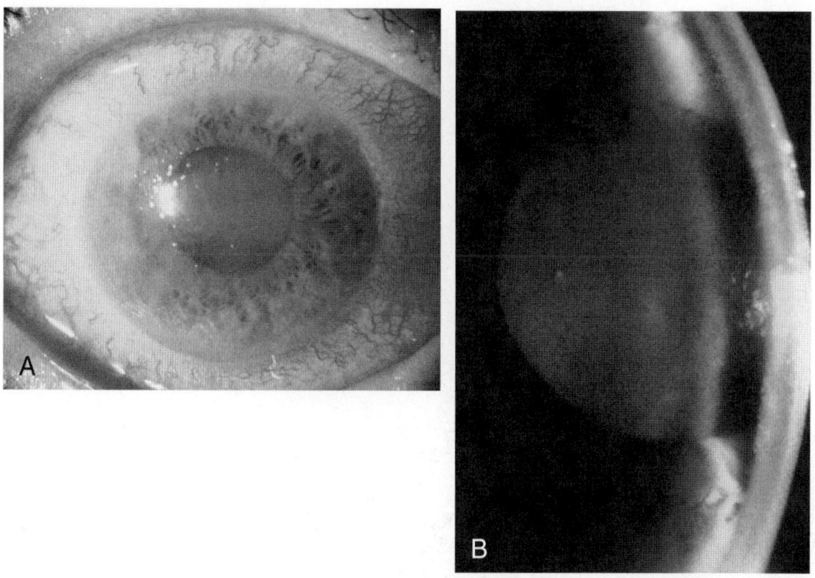

FIGURE 1-107 Acute angle-closure glaucoma. A, Acutely elevated pressure produces an inflamed eye with corneal edema (note fragmented light reflex) and a middilated pupil. B, Slit lamp examination shows a very shallow central anterior chamber (space between cornea and iris) and no peripheral chamber. (From Palay D [ed]: *Ophthalmology for the primary care physician,* St Louis, 1997, Mosby.)

which types of medical treatments were used.[1] Ⓐ

One large randomized controlled trial (RCT) recruited 1636 participants with increased intraocular pressures but no other ophthalmologic changes aged between 40 and 80 years. Patients were randomized to observation or treatment groups. Treatment groups received commercially available topical ocular hypotensives. The study found that this treatment was effective in delaying or preventing the onset of primary open-angle glaucoma in patients after 5-year's follow-up compared with the observation group.[2] Ⓐ

RCTs have found that laser trabeculoplasty combined with medical treatment is more effective at decreasing intraocular pressures in patients with open-angle glaucoma than no initial treatment or medical treatment alone.[3,4] Ⓐ

There is some evidence to suggest that both surgical trabeculectomy and laser trabeculoplasty produce decreases in intraocular pressure but the long-term differences between the efficacies of each treatment are less clear.[5,6] Ⓐ

There is evidence that there is no significant difference in visual acuity or intraocular pressure in the long term between Nd:YAG laser iridotomy and peripheral iridectomy for the treatment of acute angle-closure glaucoma.[7] Ⓐ

There is strong consensus for the efficacy of medical treatments that lower intraocular pressure in the treatment of acute angle-closure glaucoma. There is no apparent evidence available from any RCTs.[8]

An RCT of patients with normal-tension glaucoma showed that treatment to reduce the pressures by 30% significantly reduced the progression to visual field loss over 8 years compared with no treatment. The treatment consisted of drugs with or without surgical trabeculectomy.[9] Ⓐ

A Cochrane systematic review of the interventions for normal tension glaucoma was only able to find three studies that focused on patient relevant outcomes. In one study the effect of intraocular pressure lowering on visual field outcome was only significant when data were corrected for cataract development. In two small studies, a calcium antagonist, brovincamine, produced a beneficial effect concerning visual field loss.[10] Ⓐ

Evidence-Based References

1. Rossetti L et al: Randomised clinical trials on medical treatment of glaucoma; are they appropriate to clinical practice? *Arch Opthalmol* 111:96, 1993. Reviewed in: *Clin Evid* 9:729, 2003. Ⓐ
2. Kass M et al: The Ocular Hypertension Treatment Study: a randomized trial determines that topical ocular hypotensive medication delays or prevents the onset of primary open-angle glaucoma, *Arch Ophthalmol* 120:701, 2002. Ⓐ
3. Glaucoma Laser Research Group: The Glaucoma Laser Trial and Glaucoma Laser Trial follow-up study. 7. Results, *Am J Ophthalmol* 120:718, 1995. Reviewed in: *Clin Evid* 9:729, 2003. Ⓐ
4. Heijl A et al: Reduction of intraocular pressure and glaucoma progression: results from the Early Manifest Glaucoma Trial, *Arch Ophthalmol* 120:1268, 2002. Ⓐ
5. Migdal C et al: Long-term functional outcome after early surgery compared with laser and medicine in open angle glaucoma, *Ophthalmology* 101:1651, 1994. Reviewed in: *Clin Evid* 9:729, 2003. Ⓐ
6. The Advanced Glaucoma Intervention Study (AGIS): 4. Comparison of treatment outcomes with race. Seven year results, *Ophthalmology* 105:1146, 1998. Reviewed in: *Clin Evid* 9:729, 2003. Ⓐ
7. Fleck BW, Wright E, Fairley EA: A randomised prospective comparison of operative peripheral iridectomy and Nd:YAG laser iridotomy treatment of acute angle closure glaucoma: 3 year visual acuity and intraocular pressure control outcome, *Br J Ophthalmol* 81:884, 1997. Reviewed in: *Clin Evid* 9:729, 2003. Ⓐ
8. Shah R, Wormald R: Glaucoma. Reviewed in: *Clin Evid* 9:729, 2003, London, BMJ Publishing Group.
9. Collaborative Normal-Tension Glaucoma Study Group: Comparison of glaucomatous progression between untreated patients with normal-tension glaucoma and patients with therapeutically reduced intraocular pressure, *Am J Ophthalmol* 126:487, 1998. Reviewed in: *Clin Evid* 9:729, 2003. Ⓐ
10. Sycha T, Vass C, Findl O: Interventions for normal tension glaucoma, *Cochrane Database Syst Rev* 2:2004. Ⓐ

SUGGESTED READINGS

Foster PJ et al: Defining "occludable" angles in population surveys: drainage angle width, peripheral anterior synechiae, and glaucomatous optic neuropathy in East Asian people, *Br J Opthalmol* 88(4):486, 2004.

Fraser S et al: Deprivation and late presentation of glaucoma: case control study, *BMJ* 322:638, 2001.

Gazzard G et al: Intraocular pressure and visual field loss in primary angle closure and primary open angle glaucomas, *Br J Ophthalmol* 87(6):720, 2003.

Kapur SB: The lens and angle-closure glaucoma, *J Cataract Refract Surg* 27(2):176, 2001.

Lam DS et al: Angle-closure glaucoma, *Opthalmology* 109:1, 2002.

AUTHOR: **MELVYN KOBY, M.D.**

BASIC INFORMATION

DEFINITION

Complete separation or displacement of the humeral head from the glenoid surface. (Partial separation is termed *subluxation*.) Most often the cause is traumatic, and the humeral head dislocates anterior and inferior. This may cause a tear of the glenoid labrum (the Bankart lesion). Less commonly, the head dislocates posteriorly.

Rarely, multidirectional instability may be present in which dislocation or subluxation, often bilateral, may occur in multiple directions, usually the result of excessive joint laxity and generally without trauma.

ICD-9CM CODES
831.01 Anterior
831.02 Posterior
831.03 Inferior
718.31 Recurrent
718.81 Instability

PHYSICAL FINDINGS & CLINICAL PRESENTATION

Traumatic

- The arm is held in external rotation with anterior dislocation, internal rotation with posterior dislocation.
- Little movement is possible without pain.
- The acromion may appear more prominent and there is absence of the normal "fullness" beneath the acromion.
- The status of the axillary nerve must always be checked (sensation to the middeltoid should be assessed).
- The apprehension test may become positive if anterior instability persists (pain and apprehension that the shoulder will dislocate when the relaxed arm is manually placed in the "throwing position" of external rotation and abduction).
- Recurrent episodes of anterior dislocation may occur with minor movement such as putting on a coat or turning a light off at night.

Multidirectional

- Often difficult to diagnose, especially if only subluxation occurs
- Recurrent episodes of giving out, weakness, often bilateral without trauma
- Sulcus sign often positive (the arms are pulled downward with the patient standing; a sulcus [indentation] will form between the acromion and humeral head, indicating excessive inferior movement of the head)
- Other signs of generalized joint laxity may be present, such as joint hyperextensibility and the ability of the patient to touch the thumb against the flexor aspect of the forearm

ETIOLOGY

- Trauma
- Generalized joint laxity (multidirectional)
- Seizures (posterior dislocations)

DIAGNOSIS

DIFFERENTIAL DIAGNOSIS

- Rotator cuff rupture
- Frozen shoulder (posterior dislocation)
- Suprascapular nerve paralysis
- Anterior instability

IMAGING STUDIES

- Acute shoulder injury: True AP roentgenogram plus lateral view of the glenohumeral joint, either transaxillary or transcapular
- MRI: To determine soft tissue status, especially the presence of Bankart lesion or rotator cuff tear; may be indicated following a second episode of dislocation

TREATMENT

- Reduction of the acute dislocation by gentle straight traction in the relaxed patient followed by light immobilization
- Gentle limited range of motion exercises as pain subsides followed by strengthening exercises at 2 wk

DISPOSITION

- Recurrence of anterior dislocation is common in the young; this patient may have to avoid the arm position associated with dislocation (external rotation with abduction)
- Primary dislocations in patients over 40 yr are not generally complicated by recurrence, but may result in shoulder stiffness and may have associated rotator cuff injuries
- There is an almost 100% recurrence after the third dislocation

REFERRAL

Surgical reconstruction may be required in the recurrent dislocator

PEARLS & CONSIDERATIONS

COMMENTS

- It is important to know if there was an injury involved in the first episode and if a radiograph was taken to determine direction of the dislocation.
- Up to 50% of posterior dislocations are missed by the first examiner, usually the result of an inadequate lateral radiograph of the glenohumeral joint.
- "Voluntary" posterior dislocators should always be treated nonsurgically.
- Sports activities may be resumed when there is pain-free full flexibility and normal strength.
- Multidirectional instabilities are usually treated nonsurgically with strengthening exercises.

SUGGESTED READINGS

Caplan J et al: Multidirectional instability of the shoulder in elite female gymnasts, *Am J Orthop* 36:660, 2007.

Cicak N: Posterior dislocation of the shoulder, *J Bone Joint Surg Br* 86(3):324, 2004.

Matsen III FA et al: Principles for the evaluation and management of shoulder instability, *J Bone Joint Surg* 88A:648, 2006.

McFarland EG et al: The effect of variation in definition on the diagnosis of multidirectional instability of the shoulder, *J Bone Joint Surg* 85A:2138, 2003.

O'Connor DR et al: Painless reduction of acute anterior shoulder dislocations without anesthesia, *Orthopedics* 29:528, 2006.

Robinson CM, Dobson RJ: Anterior instability of the shoulder after trauma, *J Bone Joint Surg Br* 86(4):469, 2004.

Robinson CN, Kelly M, Wakefield AE: Redislocation of the shoulder during the first 6 weeks after a primary anterior dislocation: risk factor and results of treatment, *J Bone Joint Surg* 84:1552, 2002.

Sachs RA et al: Can the need for future surgery for acute traumatic anterior dislocation be predicted? *J Bone Joint Surg* 89A:1665, 2007.

Sugaya H, Moriishi J, et al: Glenoid rim morphology in recurrent anterior glenohumeral instability, *J Bone Joint Surg* 85:878, 2003.

te Slaa RL et al: The prognosis following acute primary glenohumeral dislocation, *J Bone Joint Surg Br* (86)1:58, 2004.

AUTHOR: **LONNIE R. MERCIER, M.D.**

BASIC INFORMATION

DEFINITION

Acute glomerulonephritis is an immunologically mediated inflammation primarily involving the glomerulus that can result in damage to the basement membrane, mesangium, or capillary endothelium. Table 1-15 summarizes primary renal diseases that present as acute glomerulonephritis.

SYNONYMS

Postinfectious glomerulonephritis
Acute nephritic syndrome

ICD-9CM CODES
583.9 Glomerulonephritis, acute

EPIDEMIOLOGY & DEMOGRAPHICS

- Over 50% of cases involve children <13 yr of age.
- Glomerulonephritis is the most common cause of chronic renal failure (25%).
- IgA nephropathy glomerulonephritis (Berger's disease) is the most common glomerulonephritis worldwide.

PHYSICAL FINDINGS & CLINICAL PRESENTATION

- Edema (peripheral, periorbital, or pulmonary)
- Joint pains, oral ulcers, malar rash (frequently seen with lupus nephritis)
- Dark urine
- Hypertension
- Findings of palpable purpura in patients with Henoch-Schönlein purpura
- Heart murmurs may indicate endocarditis
- Impetigo, skin pallor, tenderness in the abdomen and/or back, pharyngeal erythema may be present

ETIOLOGY

Acute glomerulonephritis may be due to primary renal disease or a systemic disease. A number of pathogenic processes (e.g., antibody deposition, cell-mediated immune mechanisms, complement activation, hemodynamic alterations) have been implicated in the pathogenesis of glomerular inflammation. Medical disorders generally associated with glomerulonephritis are:

- Post group A β-hemolytic *Streptococcus* infection (other infectious etiologies including endocarditis and visceral abscess)
- Collagen-vascular diseases (SLE)
- Vasculitis (Wegener's granulomatosis, polyarteritis nodosa)
- Idiopathic glomerulonephritis (membranoproliferative, idiopathic, crescentic, IgA nephropathy)
- Goodpasture's syndrome
- Other cryoglobulinemia (Henoch-Schönlein purpura)
- Drug-induced (gold, penicillamine)
- Table 1-15 is a summary of primary renal diseases that present as acute glomerulonephritis

DIAGNOSIS

DIFFERENTIAL DIAGNOSIS

- Cirrhosis with edema and ascites
- CHF
- Acute interstitial nephritis
- Severe hypertension
- Hemolytic-uremic syndrome
- SLE, diabetes mellitus, amyloidosis, preeclampsia, sclerodermal renal crisis

WORKUP

Initial evaluation of suspected glomerulonephritis consists of laboratory testing.

LABORATORY TESTS

- Urinalysis (hematuria [dysmorphic erythrocytes and red cell casts], proteinuria)
- Serum creatinine (to estimate GFR), BUN
- 24-hr urine for protein excretion and creatinine clearance (to document degree of renal dysfunction and amount of proteinuria). Proteinuria in acute glomerulonephritis typically ranges from 500 mg/day to 3 g/day but nephrotic-range proteinuria (>3.5 g/day) may be present
- Streptococcal tests (Streptozyme), antistreptolysin O (ASO) quantitative titer (highest in 3 to 5 wk); ASO titer, however, is not related to severity of renal disease, duration, or prognosis
- Additional useful tests depending on the history: Anti-DNA antibodies (rule out SLE), CH_{50} level (if elevated, obtain C_3, C_4 levels), triglycerides, cryoglobulins, hepatitis B and C serologies, ANCA (antineutrophil cytoplasmic antibody), c-ANCA (in suspected cases of Wegener's granulomatosis), p-ANCA found in pauciimmune (lack of immune deposits) idiopathic rapidly progressive glomerulonephritis with or without systemic vasculitis, anti-glomerular basement membrane (type alpha[3] IV collagen) antibodies
- Hct (decrease in glomerulonephritis), platelet count (thrombocytopenia in cases of lupus nephritis)
- Anti-GBM antibody (in Goodpasture's syndrome)
- Blood cultures are indicated in all febrile patients

IMAGING STUDIES

- Chest x-ray: pulmonary congestion, Wegener's granulomatosis, and Goodpasture's syndrome
- Renal ultrasound if GFR is depressed to evaluate renal size and determine extent of fibrosis. A kidney size of <9 cm is suggestive of extensive scarring and low likelihood of reversibility
- Echocardiogram in patients with new cardiac murmurs or positive blood cultures to rule out endocarditis and pericardial effusion
- Renal biopsy and light (Fig. 1-108), electron, and immunofluorescent microscopy to confirm diagnosis

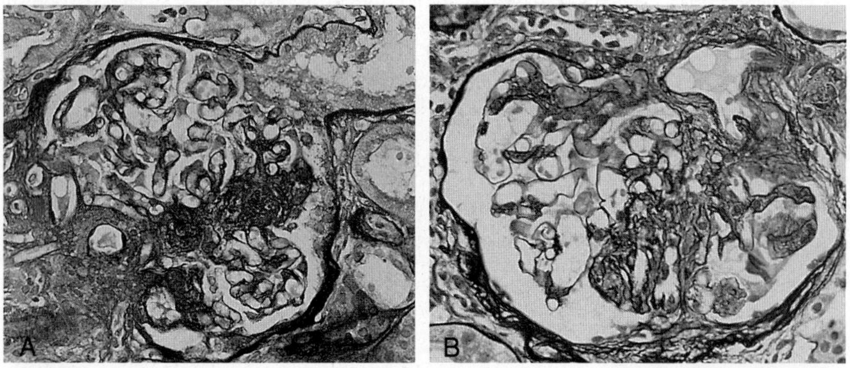

FIGURE 1-108 Light microscopic appearances in focal segmental glomerulosclerosis. Segmental scars with capsular adhesions in otherwise normal glomeruli. A, Periodic acid-Schiff, ×300; **B,** methenamine silver stain, x300. (Courtesy Dr. D. Davies. From Johnson RJ, Feehally J: *Comprehensive clinical nephrology,* ed 2, St Louis, 2000, Mosby.)

TABLE 1-15 **Summary of Primary Renal Diseases That Present as Acute Glomerulonephritis**

Diseases	Poststreptococcal Glomerulonephritis (PSGN)	IgA Nephropathy	Membranoproliferative Glomerulonephritis	Idiopathic Rapidly Progressive Glomerulonephritis (RPGN)
Clinical manifestations				
Age and sex	All ages, mean 7 yr, 2:1 male	15-35 yr, 2:1 male	15-30 yr, 6:1 male	Mean 58 yr, 2:1 male
Acute nephritic syndrome	90%	50%	90%	90%
Asymptomatic hematuria	Occasionally	50%	Rare	Rare
Nephrotic syndrome	10%-20%	Rare	Rare	10%-20%
Hypertension	70%	30%-50%	Rare	25%
Acute renal failure	50% (transient)	Very rare	50%	60%
Other	Latent period of 1-3 wk	Follows viral syndromes	Pulmonary hemorrhage; iron-deficiency anemia	None
Laboratory findings	↑ ASO titers (70%) Positive streptozyme (95%) ↓ C3-C9 Normal C1, C4	↑ Serum IgA (50%) IgA in dermal capillaries	Positive anti-GBM antibody	Positive ANCA
Immunogenetics	HLA-B12, D "EN" (9)*	HLA-Bw 35, DR4 (4)*	HLA-DR2 (16)*	None established
Renal pathology				
Light microscopy	Diffuse proliferation	Focal proliferation	Focal → diffuse proliferation with crescents	Crescentic GN
Immunofluorescence	Granular IgG, C3	Diffuse mesangial IgA	Linear IgG, C3	No immune deposits
Electron microscopy	Subepithelial humps	Mesangial deposits	No deposits	No deposits
Prognosis	95% resolve spontaneously 5% RPGN or slowly progressive	Slow progression in 25%-50%	75% stabilize or improve if treated early	75% stabilize or improve if treated early
Treatment	Supportive	None established	Plasma exchange, steroids, cyclophosphamide	Steroid pulse therapy

Modified from Goldman L, Ausiello D (eds): *Cecil textbook of medicine,* ed 22, Philadelphia, 2004, WB Saunders.
ANCA, Antineutrophil cytoplasm antibody; *GBM,* glomerular basement membrane; *GN,* glomerulonephritis; *Ig,* immunoglobulin.
*Relative risk.

- Kidney biopsy: generally reveals a granular pattern in poststreptococcal glomerulonephritis, linear pattern in Goodpasture's syndrome; absence of immune deposits suggests vasculitis; renal biopsy: although helpful to define the etiology of glomerulonephritis, is not usually essential. It is useful to determine the degree of inflammation and fibrosis. It is also especially important for patients with RPGN where prompt diagnosis and treatment is essential
- Immunofluorescence: generally reveals C_3; negative immunofluorescence suggests Wegener's granulomatosis, idiopathic crescentic glomerulonephritis, or polyarteritis nodosa
- Angiography or biopsy of other affected organs if systemic vasculitis is suspected

TREATMENT (Rx)

NONPHARMACOLOGIC THERAPY

- Avoidance of salt if edema or hypertension is present
- Low-protein intake (approximately 0.5 g/kg/day) in patients with renal failure
- Fluid restriction in patients with significant edema
- Avoidance of high-potassium foods

ACUTE GENERAL Rx

- Correction of electrolyte abnormalities (hypocalcemia, hyperkalemia) and acidosis (if present)
- Treatment of streptococcal infection with penicillin (or erythromycin in penicillin-allergic patients)
- Furosemide in patients with significant hypertension and/or edema; hydralazine or nifedipine in patients with hypertension
- Immunosuppressive treatment in patients with heavy proteinuria or rapidly decreasing glomerular filtration rate (high-dose steroids, cyclosporin A, cyclophosphamide); corticosteroids generally not useful in poststreptococcal glomerulonephritis
- Fish oil (n-3 fatty acids) 12 g/day: may prevent or slow down loss of renal function in patients with IgA nephropathy
- Plasma exchange therapy and immunosuppressive drugs (prednisone and cyclophosphamide): effective in Goodpasture's syndrome
- Short-term therapy with IV cyclophosphamide followed by maintenance therapy with mycophenolate mofetil or azathioprine is more efficacious and safer than long-term therapy with IV cyclophosphamide in patients with proliferative lupus nephritis

CHRONIC Rx

- Frequent monitoring of urinalysis, serum creatinine, and blood pressure in the initial 12 mo
- Monitoring for onset of hypertensive retinopathy, encephalopathy
- Aggressive treatment of infections, particularly streptococcal infections
- Dosage adjustment of all renally excreted medications

DISPOSITION

- Prognosis is generally related to histology with excellent prognosis in patients with minimal change glomerulonephritis and focal segmental proliferative glomerulonephritis; 25% to 30% of patients with mesangial IgA disease and membranous glomerulonephritis generally progress to chronic renal failure; >70% of patients with mesangial capillary glomerulonephritis will develop chronic renal failure.
- Generally prognosis is worse in patients with heavy proteinuria, severe hypertension, and significant elevations of creatinine.
- Recovery of renal function occurs within 8 to 12 wk in 95% of patients with poststreptococcal glomerulonephritis.

REFERRAL

- Nephrology consultation. The urgency for referral depends on the GFR. Urgent consultation is recommended if GFR is significantly abnormal, rapidly deteriorating, or if there are systemic symptoms
- Surgical referral for biopsy in selected cases

PEARLS & CONSIDERATIONS (!)

COMMENTS

- Anticoagulation to prevent DVT should be considered in patients with a low level of physical activity.
- Monitoring of lipids and aggressive treatment of hyperlipidemias is recommended.
- Close monitoring of side effects of immunosuppressive drugs and complications of corticosteroids is necessary.

SUGGESTED READINGS

Contreras G et al: Sequential therapies for proliferative lupus nephritis, *N Engl J Med* 350:971, 2004.

Hricik D et al: Glomerulonephritis, *N Engl J Med* 339:888, 1998.

Madaio MP, Harrington JT: The diagnosis of glomerular diseases, *Arch Intern Med* 161:25, 2001.

AUTHOR: **FRED F. FERRI, M.D.**

BASIC INFORMATION

DEFINITION

Glossitis is an inflammation of the tongue that can lead to loss of filiform papillae.

ICD-9CM CODES
529.0 Glossitis

EPIDEMIOLOGY & DEMOGRAPHICS

Glossitis is seen more frequently in patients of lower socioeconomic status, malnourished patients, alcoholics, smokers, elderly patients, immunocompromised patients, and patients with dentures.

PHYSICAL FINDINGS & CLINICAL PRESENTATION

- The appearance of the tongue is variable depending on the etiology of the glossitis. Loss of filiform papillae results in red, smooth-surfaced tongue (Fig. 1-109).
- The tongue may appear pale in patients with significant anemia.
- Pain and swelling of the tongue may be present when glossitis is associated with infections, trauma, or lichen planus.

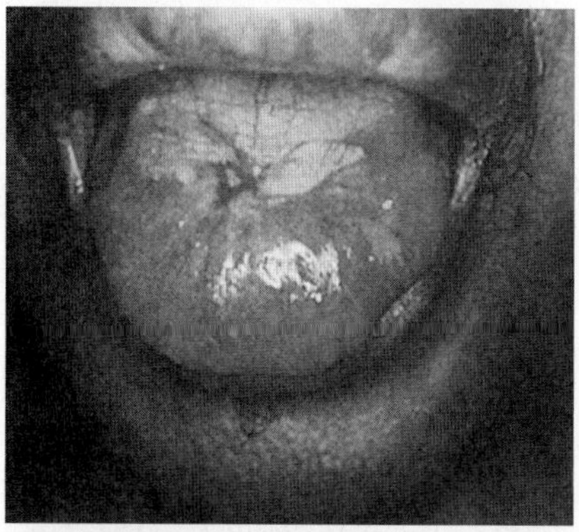

FIGURE 1-109 Glossitis. (From Seidel HM [ed]: *Mosby's guide to physical examination,* ed 4, St Louis, 1999, Mosby.)

- Ulcerations may be present in patients with herpetic glossitis, pemphigus, or streptococcal infection.
- Excessive use of mouthwash may result in a "hairy" appearance of the tongue.

ETIOLOGY

- Nutritional deficiencies (vitamin E, riboflavin, niacin, vitamin B_{12}, iron deficiency)
- Infections (viral, candidiasis, TB, syphilis)
- Trauma (generally caused by poorly fitting dentures)
- Irritation of the tongue secondary to toothpaste, medications, alcohol, tobacco, citrus
- Lichen planus, pemphigus vulgaris, erythema multiforme
- Neoplasms

DIAGNOSIS

DIFFERENTIAL DIAGNOSIS

- Infections
- Use of chemical irritants
- Neoplasms
- Skin disorders (e.g., Behçet's syndrome, erythema multiforme)

WORKUP

- Laboratory evaluation to exclude infectious processes, vitamin deficiencies, and systemic disorders
- Biopsy of lesion only when there is no response to treatment

LABORATORY TESTS

- CBC: Decreased Hgb and Hct, low MCV (iron deficiency anemia), elevated MCV (vitamin B_{12} deficiency)
- Vitamin B_{12} level
- 10% KOH scrapings in patients with white patches suspect for candidiasis

TREATMENT

NONPHARMACOLOGIC THERAPY

Avoidance of primary irritants such as hot foods, spices, tobacco, and alcohol

ACUTE GENERAL Rx

Treatment varies with the etiology of the glossitis.

- Malnutrition with avitaminosis: multivitamins
- Candidiasis: fluconazole 200 mg on day 1, then 100 mg/day for at least 2 wk or nystatin 400,000 U suspension qid for 10 days or 200,000 pastilles dissolved slowly in the mouth four to five times qd for 10 to 14 days
- Painful oral lesions: rinsing of the mouth with 2% lidocaine viscous, 1 to 2 tablespoons q4h prn; triamcinolone 0.1% applied to painful ulcers prn for symptomatic relief

CHRONIC Rx

- Lifestyle changes with elimination of tobacco, alcohol, and other primary irritants
- Dental evaluation for correction of ill-fitting dentures
- Correction of associated metabolic abnormalities such as hyperglycemia from diabetes mellitus

DISPOSITION

Most patients experience prompt improvement with identification and treatment of the cause of the glossitis.

REFERRAL

Surgical referral for biopsy of solitary lesions unresponsive to treatment to rule out neoplasm

PEARLS & CONSIDERATIONS

COMMENTS

If the primary cause of glossitis is not identified or cannot be corrected, enteric nutritional replacement therapy should be considered in malnourished patients.

AUTHOR: **FRED F. FERRI, M.D.**

BASIC INFORMATION

DEFINITION

Gonorrhea is a sexually transmitted bacterial infection with a predilection for columnar and transitional epithelial cells. It commonly manifests as urethritis, cervicitis, or salpingitis. Infection may be asymptomatic. It differs in males and females in course, severity, and ease of recognition.

SYNONYMS

Gonococcal urethritis
Gonococcal vulvovaginitis
Gonococcal cervicitis
Gonococcal bartholinitis
Clap; GC

ICD-9CM CODES
098 Gonococcal infections

EPIDEMIOLOGY & DEMOGRAPHICS

- The disease is common worldwide, affects both sexes, all ages, especially younger adults; highest incidence is in inner-city areas, with an estimated 3 million new cases annually.
- Asymptomatic anterior urethral carriage may occur in 12% to 50% of cases in men.
- Asymptomatic in 50% to 80% of cases in women. Most common dissemination by mucosal passage to fallopian tubes, resulting in PID in 10% to 15% of infected women. Hematogenous spread may result in septic arthritis and skin lesions. Conjunctivitis rarely occurs but may result in blindness if not rapidly treated. Infection can occur in both men and women in oropharynx and anorectally.
- 600,000 new infections/yr.

PHYSICAL FINDINGS & CLINICAL PRESENTATION

- Males: purulent discharge from anterior urethra with dysuria appearing 2 to 7 days after infecting exposure. May have rectal infection causing pruritus, tenesmus, and discharge or may be asymptomatic.
- Females: initial urethritis, cervicitis may occur a few days after exposure, frequently mild. In about 20% of cases, uterine invasion occurs after menstrual period with signs and symptoms of endometritis, salpingitis, or pelvic peritonitis. The patient may have purulent discharge, inflamed Skene's or Bartholin's glands.
- Classic presentation of acute gonococcal PID is fever, abdominal and adnexal tenderness, often absence of purulent discharge. Physical examination may be normal if asymptomatic.

ETIOLOGY

Neisseria gonorrhoeae is the gonococcus. Plasmids coding for β-lactamase render some strains resistant to penicillin or tetracycline (PPNG, TRNG). There is an increasing frequency of chromosomally mediated resistance to penicillin, tetracycline, and cefoxitin. In the Far East, high-level resistance to spectinomycin is endemic.

There are a rising number of cases of quinolone-resistant *N. gonorrhoeae* (QRNG) worldwide, with the expected number to rise in the U.S. from importation.

DIAGNOSIS

DIFFERENTIAL DIAGNOSIS

- Nongonococcal urethritis (NGU)
- Nongonococcal mucopurulent cervicitis
- *Chlamydia trachomatis*

WORKUP

- Diagnosis is dependent on bacteriologic investigation.
- Gram-negative intracellular diplococci are diagnostic in male urethral smears. There is a false-negative rate of 60% to 70% in female cervical or urethral smears. Culture is essential in women.

LABORATORY TESTS

- Gonorrhea culture on Thayer-Martin medium (Organism is fastidious, requires aerobic conditions with increased carbon dioxide atmosphere. Incubate ASAP.)
- Serologic testing for syphilis on all patients
- *Chlamydia* testing on all patients
- Offer of HIV counseling and testing

TREATMENT

ACUTE GENERAL Rx

Uncomplicated infections of the cervix, urethra, and rectum:
- Cefixime 400 mg PO × 1 dose *or*
- Ceftriaxone 125 mg IM × 1 dose *or*
- Ciprofloxacin 500 mg PO × 1 dose *or*
- Ofloxacin 400 mg PO × 1 dose *plus* azithromycin 1 g PO × 1 dose *or*
- Doxycycline 100 mg PO bid × 7 days
- Dual treatment with azithromax and doxycycline may prevent the development of antimicrobial resistant *N. gonorrhoeae.*

Alternatives: Spectinomycin 2 g IM × 1 dose

Quinolones:
- Gatifloxacin 400 mg PO × 1 dose
- Norfloxacin 800 mg PO × 1 dose
- Lomefloxacin 400 mg PO × 1 dose
- Not recommended for person <18 yr

Uncomplicated pharyngeal infection:
- Ceftriaxone 125 mg IM × 1 dose *or*
- Ciprofloxacin 500 mg PO × 1 dose *or*
- Ofloxacin 400 mg PO × 1 dose *plus* azithromycin 1 g PO × 1 dose *or*
- Doxycycline 100 mg PO bid × 7 days

Pregnancy: Patients should not be treated with quinolones or tetracyclines. They should be treated with one of the previous recommended or alternative cephalosporins.

DISPOSITION

- Pregnant patients require test of cure (as do those treated with regimens other than ceftriaxone/doxycycline); reculture 4 to 7 days after treatment.
- Treatment failure in nonpregnant patients is rare, and test of cure is not required. Rescreening in 1 to 2 mo detects treatment failures and reinfections.
- Sexual partners should all be identified, examined, cultured, and receive presumptive treatment.

REFERRAL

PID requiring hospitalization, disseminated gonococcal infection

PEARLS & CONSIDERATIONS

COMMENTS

This is a reportable disease.

EVIDENCE

Fluoroquinolones are no longer recommended as first line treatment for proven or suspected gonococcal infections in men who have sex with men or in those who provide a history suggesting acquisition of infection in an area with high prevalence of fluoroquinolone-resistant *N. gonorrhoeae* (QRNG); namely Asia, the Pacific Islands including Hawaii, California, and other areas such as England and Wales.[1]

In such cases, ceftriaxone 125 mg intramuscularly or cefixime 400 mg orally is recommended, with spectinomycin 2 g intramuscularly as an alternative. Spectinomycin may be used for urogenital and anorectal gonorrhea but is not sufficiently effective to treat pharyngeal gonorrhea.[1] C

Evidence-Based Reference

1. Centers for Disease Control and Prevention: Increases in fluoroquinolone-resistant *Neisseria gonorrhoeae* among men who have sex with men. United States, 2003, and Revised Recommendations for Gonorrhea Treatment, 2004, *MMWR Recomm Rep* 53(RR16):335, 2004.

AUTHORS: **MARIA A. CORIGLIANO, M.D.,** and **RUBEN ALVERO, M.D.**

BASIC INFORMATION

DEFINITION

Goodpasture's syndrome is characterized by idiopathic recurrence of alveolar hemorrhage and rapidly progressive glomerulonephritis. It can also be defined by the triad of glomerulonephritis, pulmonary hemorrhage, and antibody to basement membrane antigens.

ICD-9CM CODES
446.2 Goodpasture's syndrome

EPIDEMIOLOGY & DEMOGRAPHICS

- Goodpasture's syndrome affects predominantly young white male smokers.
- Male:female ratio is 6:1.
- Goodpasture's syndrome accounts for 5% of all cases of rapidly progressive glomerulonephritis.
- 80% of patients are HLA-BR2 positive.

PHYSICAL FINDINGS & CLINICAL PRESENTATION

- Dyspnea, cough, hemoptysis
- Skin pallor, fever, arthralgias (may be mild or absent at the time of initial presentation)

ETIOLOGY

Presence of glomerular basement membranes (GBM) antibody deposition in kidneys and lungs with subsequent pulmonary hemorrhage and glomerulonephritis.

DIAGNOSIS

DIFFERENTIAL DIAGNOSIS

- Wegener's granulomatosis
- SLE
- Systemic necrotizing vasculitis
- Idiopathic rapidly progressive glomerulonephritis
- Drug-induced renal pulmonary disease (e.g., penicillamine)

WORKUP

Laboratory evaluation, diagnostic imaging, immunofluorescence studies of renal biopsy

LABORATORY TESTS

- Presence of circulating serum anti-GBM antibodies
- Absence of circulating immunocomplexes, antineutrophils, cytoplasmic antibodies, and cryoglobulins
- Urinalysis revealing microscopic hematuria and proteinuria
- Elevated BUN and creatinine from rapidly progressive glomerulonephritis
- Immunofluorescence studies of renal biopsy material: linear deposits of anti-GBM antibody, often accompanied by C3 deposition
- Anemia from iron deficiency (secondary to blood loss and iron sequestration in the lungs)

IMAGING STUDIES

Chest x-ray: fluffy alveolar infiltrates, evidence of pulmonary hemorrhage (Fig. 1-110)

TREATMENT

ACUTE GENERAL Rx

- Plasma exchange therapy
- Immunosuppressive therapy with prednisone (1 mg/kg/day) and cyclophosphamide (2 mg/kg/day)
- Dialysis support in patients with renal failure

DISPOSITION

Life-threatening pulmonary hemorrhage and irreversible glomerular damage are the major causes of death.

REFERRAL

- Surgical referral for renal biopsy to guide the management
- Referral of patients with renal failure to dialysis center
- Consideration for renal transplantation in patients with end-stage renal failure

SUGGESTED READINGS

Levy JB et al: Long-term outcome of anti-glomerular basement membrane antibody disease treated with plasma exchange and immunosuppression, *Ann Intern Med* 134:1033, 2001.

Turner AN: Goodpasture's disease, *Nephrol Dial Transplant* 16:52, 2001.

AUTHOR: **FRED F. FERRI, M.D.**

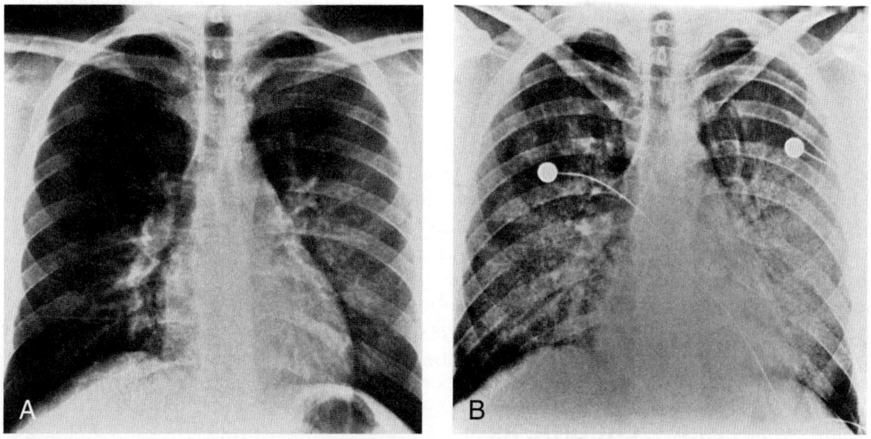

FIGURE 1-110 Goodpasture's syndrome. PA chest radiographs several days apart demonstrate consolidation in the left lung, **A,** which progressed to diffuse alveolar disease (consolidation), **B.** (From McLoud TC [ed]: *Thoracic radiology: the requisites,* St Louis, 1998, Mosby.)

BASIC INFORMATION

DEFINITION

Gout is a clinical disorder in which crystals of monosodium urate become deposited in tissue as a result of hyperuricemia. Gout and hyperuricemia can be classified as either primary or secondary if resulting from another disorder.

ICD-9CM CODES
274.9 Gout

EPIDEMIOLOGY & DEMOGRAPHICS

PREVALENCE: 3 cases/1000 persons
PREDOMINANT SEX: 95% males, rare in females before menopause
PREDOMINANT AGE: 30 to 50 yr

PHYSICAL FINDINGS & CLINICAL PRESENTATION

- Usually, initial attack in a single joint or an area of tenosynovium
- Mainly a disease of the lower extremities
- First site of involvement: classically, MP joint of the great toe
- Another common site of acute attack: extensor tenosynovium on the dorsum of the midfoot
- Severe pain and inflammation, which may be precipitated by exercise, dietary indiscretions, and physical or emotional stress
- Attacks following illness or surgery
- Presence of swelling, heat, redness, and other signs of inflammation (the physical findings simulating cellulitis)
- Exquisite soft tissue tenderness
- Fever, tachycardia, and other constitutional symptoms
- Eventually, deposits of urate crystals (tophi) in the subcutaneous tissue

ETIOLOGY

- Hyperuricemia and gout develop from excessive uric acid production, a decrease in the renal excretion of uric acid, or both.
- Primary gout results from an inborn error of metabolism and may be attributed to several biochemical defects.
- Secondary hyperuricemia may develop as a complication of acquired disorders (e.g., leukemia) or as a result of the use of certain drugs (e.g., diuretics).

DIAGNOSIS

DIFFERENTIAL DIAGNOSIS

- Pseudogout
- Rheumatoid arthritis
- Osteoarthritis
- Cellulitis
- Infectious arthritis

Section II describes the differential diagnosis of acute monoarticular and oligoarticular arthritis.

WORKUP

Hyperuricemia accompanying a typical history of monoarticular acute arthritis is usually sufficient to establish the diagnosis.

LABORATORY TESTS

- Mild leukocytosis
- Elevated ESR
- Hyperuricemia
- Synovial aspirate: usually cloudy and markedly inflammatory in nature; urate crystals in fluid: needle-shaped and birefringent under polarized light

IMAGING STUDIES

- Plain radiography to rule out other disorders
- No typical findings in early gouty arthritis but late disease possibly associated with characteristic punched-out lesions and joint destruction

TREATMENT

NONPHARMACOLOGIC THERAPY

- Modification of diet (avoidance of foods high in purines [e.g., anchovies, organ meat, liver, spinach, mushrooms, asparagus, oatmeal, cocoa, sweetbreads]) and lifestyle
- Treatment for obesity
- Moderation in alcohol intake, no more than two drinks per day
- Hypertension and its management requiring careful assessment and possibly nondiuretic drugs

ACUTE GENERAL Rx

- Quick-acting NSAIDs such as ibuprofen
- Colchicine (given PO or IV)
- Corticosteroids or ACTH for those who are intolerant of NSAIDs or colchicine
- Intraarticular cortisone when oral medication cannot be given
- General measures, such as rest, elevation, and analgesics as needed until acute pain subsides.
- Table 1-16 describes treatment options for gout

CHRONIC Rx

- Prevention is achieved through normalization of serum urate concentration.
- Uricosuric agents (e.g., probenecid) or xanthine oxidase inhibitors (allopurinol) are used in patients with recurrent attacks despite adequate dietary restrictions.
- A 24-hr urine collection is useful in deciding which antihyperuricemic agent is indicated. Allopurinol is generally used if the uric acid output is >900 mg/day on a regular diet. However, hyperuricemic therapy should not be started for at least 2 wk after the acute attack has resolved because it may prolong the acute attack and it can also precipitate new attacks by rapidly lowering the serum uric acid level.
- Urinary uric acid hypoexcretors (<700 mg/day) can be given probenecid (250 mg bid for 1 wk, then increased to 500 mg bid) to block absorption of uric acid. Probenecid should be started only after the acute attack of gout has completely subsided.
- Colchicine 0.6 mg bid is indicated for acute gout prophylaxis before starting hyperuricemic therapy. It is generally discontinued 6 to 8 wk after normalization of serum urate levels. Long-term colchicine therapy (0.6 mg qd or bid) may be necessary in patients with frequent gout attacks despite the use of uricosuric agents.
- Surgery usually limited to excision of large tophi and, occasionally, arthroplasty.

DISPOSITION

- Musculoskeletal complications are usually limited to joint disease.
- Surgical intervention may occasionally be indicated.
- Renal disease is the most frequent complication of gout after arthritis; most gouty patients develop renal disease as a result of parenchymal urate deposition but the involvement is only slowly progressive and often has no effect on life expectancy.
- Incidence of urolithiasis is increased, with 80% of calculi being uric acid stones.

REFERRAL

For orthopedic consultation when joint destruction has occurred

PEARLS & CONSIDERATIONS

COMMENTS

- No significant correlation between coronary artery disease and gout
- No indication to treat asymptomatic hyperuricemia
- Acute attacks of gout occasionally associated with normal levels of uric acid
- The main indication for prophylaxis is recurrent attacks of gouty joint inflammation, three or more per year

EVIDENCE

EBM

Acute

Limited evidence suggests nonsteroidal anti-inflammatory drugs may be effective in relieving pain in acute gout, but no one drug can be recommended over another. Systematic reviews and randomized controlled trials relating to the prevention of the recurrence of gout are lacking.

No systematic review has compared nonsteroidal anti-inflammatory drugs (NSAIDs) vs. placebo, or vs. each other, in the management of acute gout.[1]

Limited evidence suggests that colchicine is effective and provides more rapid pain relief during an acute episode of gout than placebo, although the gastrointestinal side effects are significant.[2] Ⓑ

We are unable to cite evidence that meets our criteria for any other treatment, or lifestyle intervention, used in the management or prevention of acute gout.

Evidence-Based References

1. Underwood M: Acute gout. Reviewed in: *Clin Evid* 11:1468, 2004.
2. Ahern MJ et al: Does colchicine work? The results of the first controlled study in acute gout, *Aust N Z J Med* 17:301, 1987. Reviewed in: *Clin Evid* 11:1468, 2004. Ⓑ

Chronic tophaceous

There is evidence that allopurinol reduces serum uric acid concentrations. However, the evidence showing a reduction in the likelihood of attacks of gout with this treatment is limited.[1]

Evidence-Based Reference

1. Allopurinol, oxipurinol, benzbromarone and probenecid for lowering uric acid, Bandolier, Knowledge Library. Accessed 10 August 2004.

SUGGESTED READINGS

Fitzgerald BT et al: Gout affecting the hand and wrist, *J Am Acad Orthop Surg* 15:625, 2007.

Fox R: Management of recurrent gout, *BMJ* 336:329, 2008.

Liote F, Ea HK: Recent developments in crystal-induced inflammation: pathogenesis and management, *Curr Rheumatol Rep* 9(3):243, 2007.

Riedel AA et al: Compliance with allopurinol therapy among managed care enrollees with gout: a retrospective analysis of administrative claims, *J Rheumatol* 31(8):1575, 2004.

Rosenthal AK: Crystal arthropathies and other unpopular rheumatic diseases, *Curr Opin Rheumatol* 16:262, 2004.

Schumacher HR et al: Outcome evaluations in gout, *J Rheumatol* 34(6):1381, 2007.

Velilla-Moliner J et al: Podagra, is it always gout? *Am J Emerg Med* 22(4):320, 2004.

Wallace KL et al: Increasing prevalence of gout and hyperuricemia over 10 years among older adults in a managed care population, *J Rheumatol* 31(8):1582, 2004.

AUTHOR: **LONNIE R. MERCIER, M.D.**

TABLE 1-16 **Treatment of Gout**

Acute Gout	Interval Gout	Long-Term Treatment
Therapeutic goal: Terminate acute inflammatory attack.	**Therapeutic goal:** Prevent recurrent attacks.	**Therapeutic goals:** Prevent attacks, resolve tophi, maintain serum urate at ≤6 mg/dl.
NSAIDs *(preferred):* Indomethacin, 50 mg qid, or ibuprofen, 800 mg tid (or other NSAIDs in full doses) *(lower dose in renal insufficiency; contraindicated with peptic ulcer disease).*	**Colchicine, oral:** 0.6-1.2 mg daily as prophylaxis against recurrent attacks.	**Colchicine, oral:** 0.6-1.2 mg daily for 1-2 wk before initiating hypouricemic therapy and for several months afterward to prevent recurrent attacks during initial period of hypouricemic therapy.
OR		
Colchicine, oral *(used infrequently):* 0.6-1.2 mg (1-2 tablets), then 0.6 mg (1 tablet) q1-2h until attack subsides or until nausea, diarrhea, or GI cramping develops. Maximum total dose, 4-6 mg. If ineffective in 48 hr, do not repeat.	**Hypouricemic agent:** Start only if indicated by frequent attacks, severe hyperuricemia, presence of tophi, urolithiasis, or urate overexcretion.	**Allopurinol:** Dose variable; usually 300 mg once daily, but up to 900 mg may be needed in occasional patient; dose should be reduced to 100 mg daily or every other day in patients with renal insufficiency.
		OR
Colchicine, IV *(only if oral medication is precluded):* 1-2 mg in 20 ml 0.9% saline infused slowly *(extravasation causes tissue necrosis);* dose may be repeated once in 6 hr. Few GI symptoms with IV use. Maximum total dose, 4 mg per attack. Monitor blood counts.	**Other:** Diet—moderate protein, low fat; avoid excessive alcohol. Treat hypertension if present. High fluid intake to promote uric acid excretion in a dilute urine (for uric acid overexcretors).	**Uricosuric agent** *(reduced efficacy if creatinine clearance <80 ml; ineffective if <30 ml):* Probenecid, 0.5-1 g bid, or sulfinpyrazone, 100 mg tid or qid; usually well tolerated, but may cause headache, GI upset, rash.
Steroids *(if NSAIDs or colchicines are contraindicated or if oral medication is precluded, e.g., postoperatively):* Triamcinolone acetonide, 60 mg IM, *or* ACTH, 40 U IM *or* 25 U by slow IV infusion, *or* prednisone, 20-40 mg daily. Intra-articular steroids may be used to treat a single inflamed joint: triamcinolone hexacetonide, 5-20 mg, or dexamethasone phosphate, 1-6 mg.		**Other:** Diet—moderate protein, low fat; avoid excessive alcohol. Treat hypertension if present. For uric acid overexcretors or when initiating uricosuric agent: high fluid intake, particularly at night, to promote uric acid excretion in a dilute urine. Acetazolamide, 250 mg at bedtime, may be used to keep urine pH >6.
Hypouricemic agents: Of no benefit for inflammatory attack and may initiate recurrent attack. Should not be started until attack has resolved, but *ongoing use should not be interrupted during an attack.*		

From Goldman L, Ausiello D (eds): *Cecil textbook of medicine,* ed 22, Philadelphia, 2004, WB Saunders.

ACTH, Adrenocorticotropic hormone; *bid,* twice daily; *GI,* gastrointestinal; *IM,* intramuscularly; *IV,* intravenously; *NSAIDs,* nonsteroidal anti-inflammatory drugs; *q1-2h,* every 1 to 2 hours; *qid,* four times daily; *tid,* three times daily.

BASIC INFORMATION

DEFINITION

A chronic, usually self-limited, inflammatory disorder of the dermis that classically presents as arciform to annular plaques located on the extremities.

SYNONYMS

Pseudorheumatoid nodule—subcutaneous granuloma annulare
GA

ICD-9CM CODES
695.89 Granuloma annulare

EPIDEMIOLOGY & DEMOGRAPHICS

- Most common in children and young adults; most cases of localized granuloma annulare are diagnosed in patients before 30 years of age
- Female predominance (2:1)
- Disseminated form associated with diabetes mellitus
- Recurrent in 40% of affected individuals
- A generalized form of GA can occur in up to 15% of patients

PHYSICAL FINDINGS & CLINICAL PRESENTATION

- The four main clinical variants of granuloma annulare are localized (75%), disseminated (>10 lesions), subcutaneous (occurring primarily in children 2 to 5 years of age), and perforating (rare form manifesting with 1- to 4-mm papules with a central crust).
- Localized granuloma annulare starts as a small ring of colored skin or pale erythematous papules.
- Lesions coalesce and evolve into annular plaques over several weeks.
- Plaques undergo central involution and increase in diameter over several months (0.5 to 5 cm) (Fig. 1-111).
- Most frequently found on the lateral and dorsal surfaces of the hands and feet.
- Most lesions resolve spontaneously after several months.
- The generalized form of GA is characterized by hundreds to thousands of small, flesh-colored papules in a symmetric distribution on the trunk and extremities.
- Deep dermal (subcutaneous GA) presents as a large, painless, skin-colored nodules that are frequently mistaken for rheumatoid nodules.

ETIOLOGY

Unknown, but may be related to vasculitis, trauma, monocyte activation, or delayed hypersensitivity.

DIAGNOSIS

DIFFERENTIAL DIAGNOSIS

- Tinea corporis
- Lichen planus
- Necrobiosis lipoidica diabeticorum
- Sarcoidosis
- Rheumatoid nodules
- Late secondary or tertiary syphilis
- Arcuate and annular plaques of mycosis fungoides
- Papular GA can simulate insect bites, secondary syphilis, xanthoma
- Annular elastolytic giant cell granuloma

WORKUP

- Diagnosis is based on clinical appearance and presentation.
- Biopsy when diagnosis is unclear

LABORATORY TESTS

There are no laboratory tests that will help confirm the diagnosis.

Biopsy shows focal degeneration of collagen and elastic fibers, mucin deposition, and perivascular and interstitial lymphohistiocytic infiltrate in the upper and mid dermis.

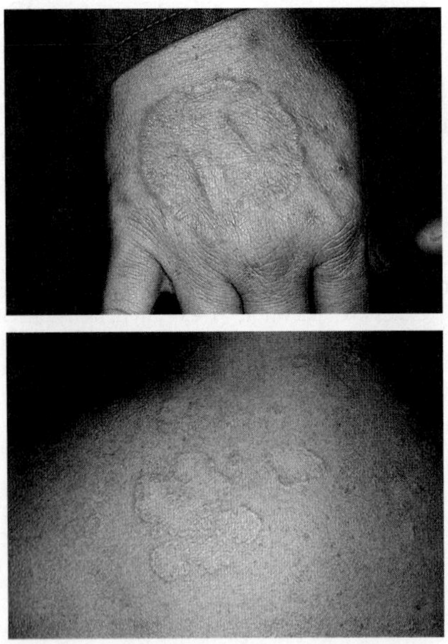

FIGURE 1-111 Granuloma annulare. (From Callen JP [ed]: *Color atlas of dermatology,* ed 2, Philadelphia, 2000, WB Saunders.)

TREATMENT

NONPHARMACOLOGIC THERAPY

Reassurance, given the self-limited and benign nature of GA

CHRONIC Rx

High potency topical corticalsteroids with or without occlusion and intralesional steroid injection into elevated border with triamcinolone 2.5 to 10 mg/ml are useful first-line local therapies.

- Cryosurgery, PUVA or UVA-1 therapy, and CO2 laser treatment can also be used.
- Systemic agents (e.g., niacinamide, hydroxychloroquine, chloroquine, cyclosporine, dapsone) are generally reserved for severe cases. Recent case reports indicate positive outcomes with tacrolimus and pimecrolimus and with the use of the tumor necrosis factor infliximab.

DISPOSITION

Most lesions will resolve spontaneously within 2 yr.

REFERRAL

Dermatology referral recommended for symptomatic, disseminated disease

PEARLS & CONSIDERATIONS

COMMENTS

GA has been described as a paraneoplastic granulomatous reaction to Hodgkin's disease, NHL, solid organ tumors, and mycosis fungoides.

SUGGESTED READING

Cyr PR: Diagnosis and management of granuloma annulare, *Am Fam Physician* 74:1729-1734, 2006.

AUTHOR: **JENNIFER R. SOUTHER, M.D.**

BASIC INFORMATION

DEFINITION

Granuloma inguinale is caused by a gram-negative bacterium, *Calymmatobacterium granulomatis,* that may be sexually transmitted, possibly by anal intercourse. It can also be spread through close, chronic nonsexual contact.

SYNONYMS

Donovanosis

ICD-9CM CODES
099.2 Granuloma inguinale

EPIDEMIOLOGY & DEMOGRAPHICS

INCIDENCE: Rare in the U.S. (<100 cases reported annually) and other developed countries

PREVALENCE: Endemic in Australia, India, Caribbean, and Africa. Incubation period is variable: 1 to 2 wk.

PREDOMINANT SEX: Can affect both males and females

PHYSICAL FINDINGS & CLINICAL PRESENTATION

- Indurated nodule is the primary lesion and is usually painless.
- Lesion erodes to granulomatous heaped ulcer (Fig. 1-112); progresses slowly.
- Pathogenic features are as follows:
  1. Large infected mononuclear cell containing many Donovan bodies
  2. Intracytoplasmic location

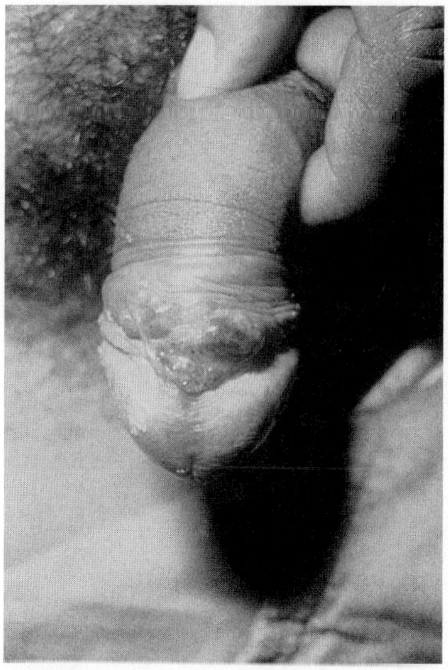

FIGURE 1-112 Involvement of the penis, with a beefy red, granulomatous ulceration in a patient with granuloma inguinale. (From Goldstein B [ed]: *Practical dermatology,* ed 2, St Louis, 1997, Mosby.)

ETIOLOGY

Calymmatobacterium granulomatis is a gram-negative bacillus that reproduces within PMNs, plasma cells, and histiocytes, causing the infected cells to rupture 20 to 30 organisms.

DIAGNOSIS

DIFFERENTIAL DIAGNOSIS

- Carcinoma
- Secondary syphilis: condylomata lata
- Amebiasis: necrotic ulceration
- Concurrent infections
- Lymphogranuloma venereum
- Chancroid
- Genital herpes

WORKUP

- Check for clinical manifestations.
  1. Lesions bleed easily.
  2. Lesions sharply defined and painless.
  3. Secondary infection may ensue.
  4. Inguinal involvement may cause pseudobuboes.
  5. Elephantiasis can result from obstruction of lymphatics.
  6. Suppuration and sinus formation are rare in female patients.
- Screen for other sexually transmitted diseases.
- Exclude other causes of lesions.
- Obtain stained, crushed prep from lesion.
- A clinical algorithm for evaluation of genital ulcer disease is described in Section III.

Section II describes the differential diagnosis of genital sores.

LABORATORY TESTS

Wright stain: observation of Donovan bodies (intracellular bacteria); organisms in vacuoles within macrophages

TREATMENT

ACUTE GENERAL Rx

Recommended regimens:
- Doxycycline 100 mg orally bid × 3 wk minimum

Alternative regimens:
- Ciprofloxacin 750 mg PO bid × 3 wk
- Erythromycin base 500 mg PO od × 3 wk
- Trimethoprim/sulfamethoxazole, one double-strength tablet orally bid × 3 wk minimum
- Azithromycin 1 g PO/wk × 3 wk
- All gentamicin 1 mg/kg IV q8h if no improvement within the first few days of therapy

CHRONIC Rx

If there is a poor initial response, extend treatment. Treatment of relapses is often necessary. Patients should be counseled to avoid risky sex practices and not resume having sex until infection is cleared.

DISPOSITION

Follow clinically until signs and symptoms have resolved, then routine annual or semiannual visits

REFERRAL

If response is poor, consider referral to infectious disease specialist.

PEARLS & CONSIDERATIONS

COMMENTS

- Sexual partners should be examined and offered therapy.
- Pregnant women should be treated with erythromycin regimen.
- Patient education material can be obtained from local and state health clinics and also from American College of Obstetricians and Gynecologists (ACOG).

SUGGESTED READING

Centers for Disease Control and Prevention: 2006 sexually transmitted diseases treatment guidelines, *MMWR Morb Mortal Wkly Rep* 55(RR-11), 2006.

AUTHORS: **GEORGE T. DANAKAS, M.D.,** and **RUBEN ALVERO, M.D.**

BASIC INFORMATION

DEFINITION

Graves' disease is a hypermetabolic state characterized by thyrotoxicosis, diffuse goiter, and infiltrative ophthalmopathy (edema and inflammation of the extraocular muscles and an increase in orbital connective tissue and fat); infiltrative dermopathy characterized by lymphocytic infiltration of the dermis, accumulation of glycosaminoglycans, and edema is occasionally present.

SYNONYMS

Thyrotoxicosis

ICD-9CM CODES
242.0 Toxic diffuse goiter

EPIDEMIOLOGY & DEMOGRAPHICS

INCIDENCE/PREVALENCE: Hyperthyroidism affects 2% of women and 0.2% of men in their lifetimes. More than 80% of these cases are caused by Graves' disease.
PREDOMINANT AGE: Most common before age 50 yr
GENETICS: Increased prevalence of HLA-B8 and HLA-DR3 in whites with Graves' disease. Concordance rate is 20% among monozygotic twins.

PHYSICAL FINDINGS & CLINICAL PRESENTATION

- Tachycardia, palpitations, tremor, hyperreflexia
- Goiter, exophthalmos (50% of patients), lid retraction, lid lag
- Nervousness, weight loss, heat intolerance, atrial fibrillation
- Increased sweating, brittle nails, clubbing of fingers
- Nervousness, weight loss, heat intolerance, and atrial fibrillation
- Localized dermopathy (1% to 2% of patients) is most frequent over the anterolateral aspects of the skin but can be found at other sites (especially after trauma)

ETIOLOGY

Autoimmune etiology: the activity of the thyroid gland is stimulated by the action of T cells, which induce specific B cells to synthesize antibodies against TSH receptors in the follicular cell membrane.

DIAGNOSIS

DIFFERENTIAL DIAGNOSIS

- Anxiety disorder
- Premenopausal state
- Thyroiditis
- Other causes of hyperthyroidism (e.g., toxic multinodular goiter, toxic adenoma)
- Other: metastatic neoplasm, diabetes mellitus, pheochromocytoma

WORKUP

The diagnostic workup includes a detailed medical history followed by laboratory and imaging studies. Patients often present with anxiety, heat intolerance, menstrual dysfunction, increased appetite, and weight loss. Elderly patients can have an atypical presentation (apathetic hyperparathyroidism). For additional information, refer to the topic "Hyperthyroidism."

LABORATORY TESTS

- Increased free thyroxine (T_4) and free triiodothyronine (T_3)
- Decreased TSH
- Presence of thyroid autoantibodies (useful in selected patients to differentiate Graves' disease from toxic nodular goiter)

IMAGING STUDIES

- 24-hr radioactive iodine uptake (RAIU): increased homogeneous uptake
- CT or MRI of the orbits is useful if there is uncertainty about the cause of ophthalmopathy

TREATMENT

NONPHARMACOLOGIC THERAPY

Patient education and discussion of therapeutic options

ACUTE GENERAL Rx

- Antithyroid drugs (ATDs) to inhibit thyroid hormone synthesis or peripheral conversion of T_4 to T_3
  1. Propylthiouracil (PTU) 50 to 100 mg q8h or methimazole (Tapazole) 10 to 20 mg q8h for 6 to 24 mo
  2. Side effects: skin rash (3% to 5%), arthralgias, myalgias, granulocytopenia (0.5%); rare side effects: aplastic anemia, hepatic necrosis (PTU), cholestatic jaundice (methimazole)
- Radioactive iodine (RAI)
  1. Treatment of choice for patients >21 yr of age and younger patients who have not achieved remission after 1 yr of ATD therapy
  2. Contraindicated during pregnancy and lactation
- Surgery: near-total thyroidectomy is rarely performed; indications: obstructing goiters despite RAI and ATD therapy, patients who refuse RAI and cannot be adequately managed with ATDs, and pregnant women inadequately managed with ATDs
- Adjunctive therapy: propranolol (20 to 40 mg q6h) to alleviate the β-adrenergic symptoms of hyperthyroidism (tachycardia, tremor); contraindicated in patients with CHF and bronchospasm
- Graves' ophthalmopathy: methylcellulose eye drops to protect against excessive dryness, sunglasses to decrease photophobia, systemic high-dose corticosteroids for severe exophthalmos; worsening of ophthalmopathy after RAI therapy often transient and can be prevented by the administration of prednisone

CHRONIC Rx

Patients undergoing treatment with ATDs should be seen every 1 to 3 mo until euthyroidism is achieved and every 3 to 4 mo while they are receiving ATDs.

DISPOSITION

- ATDs induce sustained remission in <60% of cases.
- The incidence of hypothyroidism post RAI is >50% within first year and 2%/yr thereafter.
- Complications of surgery include hypothyroidism (28% to 43% after 10 yr), hypoparathyroidism, and vocal cord paralysis (1%).
- Successful treatment of hyperthyroidism requires lifelong monitoring for the onset of hypothyroidism or the recurrence of thyrotoxicosis.
- RAI therapy is followed by the appearance or worsening of ophthalmopathy more often than is therapy with methimazole, particularly in patients who are cigarette smokers. It can be prevented with the administration of prednisone 0.5 mg/kg of body weight per day starting 2 to 3 days post RAI, continued for 1 mo, then tapered off over 2 mo.
- Mild to moderate ophthalmopathy often improves spontaneously. Severe cases can be treated with high-dose glucocorticoids, orbital irradiation, or both. Orbital decompression may be used in patients with optic neuropathy and exophthalmos (see "Hyperthyroidism").

SUGGESTED READING

Weetman AP: Graves' disease, *N Engl J Med* 343:1236, 2000.

AUTHOR: **FRED F. FERRI, M.D.**

BASIC INFORMATION

DEFINITION

Guillain-Barré syndrome (GBS) is an acute immune-mediated polyradiculoneuropathy (affects nerve roots and peripheral nerves), with predominant motor involvement. It is the most common cause of acute flaccid paralysis in the Western hemisphere and probably worldwide. By definition, maximal clinical weakness occurs within 4 wk of disease onset.

SYNONYMS

GBS consists of several clinical variants based on the pattern of clinical involvement and electrophysiologic findings. These include:

- Acute inflammatory demyelinating polyradiculoneuropathy (AIDP)—most common form in Europe and North America
- Acute motor axonal neuropathy (AMAN)—most prevalent form in China and Japan
- Acute motor and sensory axonal neuropathy (AMSAN)—has more severe sensory involvement and is associated with more severe clinical course and poorer prognosis
- Miller Fisher syndrome (MFS)—triad of ophthalmoplegia, ataxia, and areflexia
- Acute pandysautonomia—rapid onset of parasympathetic and sympathetic failure without motor or sensory involvement
- Regional variants such as pharyngeal-cervical-brachial and a pure ataxic form

ICD 9CM CODES
357.0 Guillain-Barré

EPIDEMIOLOGY & DEMOGRAPHICS

INCIDENCE: 0.6 to 1.9 cases/100,000 persons annually without geographic variation. Incidence increases with age.
PREDOMINANT SEX: There is a slight male preponderance (1.25:1).
PEAK INCIDENCE: A slight peak in incidence occurs between late adolescence and early adulthood.
PREDISPOSING FACTORS: Viral (HIV, CMV, EBV, influenza) and bacterial *(Campylobacter jejuni, Mycoplasma pneumonia)* infections; systemic illness (Hodgkin's lymphoma), immunizations

PHYSICAL FINDINGS & CLINICAL PRESENTATION

- Symmetric weakness, most commonly involving proximal muscles initially, subsequently involving both proximal and distal muscles
- Depressed or absent deep tendon reflexes in both arms and legs
- "Glove and stocking" pattern paresthesias/dysesthesia/anesthesia (often mild relative to severity of weakness)
- Pain, often paraspinal (caused by involvement of posterior nerve roots)
- Autonomic abnormalities (bradyarrhythmias or tachyarrhythmias, hypotension or hypertension)
- Respiratory insufficiency (caused by weakness of diaphragm and/or intercostal muscles
- Facial weakness
- Diplopia due to ophthalmoparesis
- Dysphagia due to pharyngeal weakness

ETIOLOGY

- Unknown
- Preceding infectious illness 1 to 4 wk before disease onset in approximately two thirds of patients
- Immune-mediated attack directed primarily against peripheral nerve myelin and/or Schwann cell antigens; secondary axonal loss may occur

DIAGNOSIS

DIFFERENTIAL DIAGNOSIS

- Toxic peripheral neuropathies: heavy metal poisoning (lead, thallium, arsenic), medications (vincristine, disulfiram), organophosphate poisoning, hexacarbon (glue sniffer's neuropathy)
- Nontoxic peripheral neuropathies: acute intermittent porphyria, vasculitic polyneuropathy, infectious (polio myelitis, diphtheria, Lyme disease, West Nile virus); tick paralysis
- Neuromuscular junction disorders: myasthenia gravis, botulism, snake envenomations
- Myopathies such as polymyositis, acute necrotizing myopathies caused by drugs
- Metabolic derangements such as hypermagnesemia, hypokalemia, hypophosphatemia
- Acute central nervous system disorders such as basilar artery thrombosis with brainstem infarction, brainstem encephalomyelitis, transverse myelitis, or spinal cord compression
- Hysterical paralysis or malingering

WORKUP

1. Exclude other causes based on clinical history, examination, and laboratory tests.
2. Lumbar puncture (may be normal in the first 1 to 2 wk of the illness).
    - Typical findings include elevated CSF protein with few mononuclear leukocytes (albuminocytologic dissociation) in 80% to 90% of patients. CSF pleocytosis is expected in cases associated with HIV seroconversion.
3. Electromyography/nerve conduction studies may be normal in the first 10-14 days of the disease. The earliest electrodiagnostic abnormalities are prolongation or absence of H-reflexes and reduced recruitment of motor units with normal morphology. EMG/NCS evidence of demyelination (prolonged distal latency, conduction velocity slowing, conduction block, temporal dispersion, and prolonged F-waves) in two or more motor nerves confirms diagnosis of AIDP in the appropriate clinical context.

LABORATORY TESTS

- CBC may reveal early leukocytosis with left shift. Electrolytes to exclude metabolic causes of weakness.
- Heavy metal testing, urine porphyria screen, creatine kinase, HIV titers, and neuroimaging of the brain and spinal cord if diagnosis uncertain. Nerve root enhancement may be seen on MRI of the lumbosacral spine.
- Antibodies against ganglioside GQ_{1b} may be present in up to 90% of patients with MFS. IgG antibodies against ganglioside GM_1 may be associated with AMAN. There are no antiganglioside antibodies commonly associated with AIDP.
- In equivocal cases (especially if peripheral nerve vasculitis is a concern), nerve biopsy may aid in confirming a diagnosis of GBS. Sensory nerve biopsy demonstrates segmental demyelination with infiltration of monocytes and T cells into the endoneurium. Axonal loss is commonly seen in sensory nerve biopsy specimens in GBS.

TREATMENT

NONPHARMACOLOGIC THERAPY

- Close monitoring of respiratory function (frequent measurements of vital capacity, negative inspiratory force, and pulmonary toilet), because respiratory failure is the most serious (and sometimes life-threatening) complication in GBS
- Frequent repositioning of immobile patients to minimize formation of pressure sores
- Prevention of thromboembolism with antithrombotic stockings and SC heparin (5000 U q12h) in nonambulatory patients
- Emotional support and social counseling

ACUTE GENERAL Rx

- Infusion of IV immunoglobulin (IVIg 0.4 g/kg/day for 5 days). Always check serum IgA levels before infusion to prevent anaphylaxis in deficient patients.
- Plasma exchange (PE): 200 to 250 ml/kg over five sessions every other day.
- IVIg and PE are equally effective. The selection of one or the other is determined by availability and risk of particular complications. For example, PE

should be avoided in patients with prominent autonomic dysfunction.
- There is no proven benefit from combining IVIg and PE.
- Mechanical ventilation may be needed if FVC is <12 to 15 ml/kg, vital capacity is rapidly decreasing or is <1000 ml, negative inspiratory force <−20 cm H_2O, PaO_2 is <70, or if the patient is having significant difficulty clearing secretions or is aspirating.

CHRONIC Rx

- Ventilatory support may be necessary in 10% to 20% of patients. Adequate fluid/electrolyte support and nutrition is necessary, especially in patients with dysautonomia or bulbar dysfunction.
- Aggressive nursing care is required to prevent decubiti, infections, fecal impactions, and pressure nerve palsies.
- Monitor and treat autonomic dysfunction (bradyarrhythmias or tachyarrhythmias, orthostatic hypotension, systemic hypertension, altered sweating).
- Treat back pain and dysesthesia with low-dose tricyclics, gabapentin, etc. Opiate narcotics can be used cautiously in the short term, but may compound dysautonomia.
- Stress ulcer prevention in patients receiving ventilator support.
- Discuss physical and occupational therapy rehabilitation, including supportive devices.

DISPOSITION

- Mortality is approximately 5% to 10%. Causes of death include cardiac arrest, pulmonary embolism, and fulminant infections.
- Full motor recovery occurs in approximately 60% of patients. There is mild residual weakness in 15%, moderately severe residual weakness in 10%, and 5% may remain in bed 1 year after the onset of symptoms.
- Predictors for poor recovery (inability to walk independently at 1 yr): age >60 yr, preceding diarrheal illness, recent CMV infection, fulminant or rapidly progressing course, ventilatory dependence, reduced motor amplitudes (<20% normal), or inexcitable nerves on NCS.
- Outcomes may also be influenced by complications of medical therapy.
- GBS is typically a monophasic illness. Recurrence may occur in <5% of patients following full recovery.

REFERRAL

- To ENT for tracheostomy if prolonged ventilatory support is required.
- To surgery for percutaneous endoscopic gastrostomy (PEG) if temporary nutritional support is required.

PEARLS & CONSIDERATIONS

- Guillain-Barré syndrome is the most common cause of acute flaccid paralysis.
- Close monitoring of ventilatory function with respiratory mechanics (FVC and NIF) is of paramount importance in all patients with suspected Guillain-Barré syndrome.

COMMENTS

Patient education information may be obtained from the Guillain-Barré Foundation International, Box 262, Wynnewood, PA 19096; phone: (610) 667-0131.

EVIDENCE

EBM

There is evidence from six randomized controlled trials (RCTs) that plasma exchange is of benefit to patients with GBS.[1] Ⓐ

There is evidence from six RCTs that IVIg is equally effective in the management of patients with GBS.[2] Ⓐ

The evidence does not support the combined use of IVIg and PE.[3]

The evidence does not support the use of steroids in the treatment of GBS.[4]

Evidence-Based References

1. Raphaël JC et al: Plasma exchange for Guillain-Barré syndrome, *Cochrane Database Syst Rev* 2:CD001798, 2002.
2. Hughes RAC et al: Intravenous immunoglobulin for Guillain-Barré syndrome, *Cochrane Database Syst Rev* 1:CD002063, 2006.
3. Hughes RAC et al: Corticosteroids for Guillain-Barré Syndrome, *Cochrane Database Syst Rev* 2:CD001446, 2006.
4. Hughes RAC, van der Meché FGA: Corticosteroids for Guillain-Barré syndrome, *Cochrane Database Syst Rev* 2:CD001446, 2006.

SUGGESTED READINGS

Bernsen RA et al: How Guillain-Barré patients experience their functioning after 1 year, *Acta Neurol Scand* 112:51, 2005.

Garssen MP et al: Physical training and fatigue, fitness, and quality of life in Guillain-Barré syndrome and CIDP, *Neurology* 63:2393, 2004.

Hughes RA et al: Guillain-Barré syndrome, *Lancet* 366(9497):1653, 2005.

Hughes RA et al: Multidisciplinary Consensus Group: supportive care for patients with Guillain-Barré syndrome, *Arch Neurol* 62:1194, 2005.

Hughes RA et al: Practice Parameter: report of the Quality Standards Subcommittee of the American Academy of Neurology, *Neurology* 61(6):746, 2003.

Kuwabara S: Guillain-Barré syndrome: epidemiology, pathophysiology and management, *Drugs* 64:597, 2004.

AUTHORS: **MICHAEL BENATAR, M.B.C.H.B., D.PHIL.,** and **EROBOGHENE UBOGU, M.D.**

BASIC INFORMATION

DEFINITION

Hand-foot-mouth (HFM) disease is a viral illness that is characterized by superficial lesions of the oral mucosa and of the skin of the extremities. HFM is transmitted primarily by the fecal-oral route and is highly contagious. Although children are predominantly affected, adults are also at risk. This disease is usually self-limited and benign.

SYNONYMS

Vesicular stomatitis with exanthem
Coxsackievirus infection

ICD-9CM CODES
074.0 Hand-foot-mouth disease

EPIDEMIOLOGY & DEMOGRAPHICS

- Children under the age of 5 yr are at the highest risk and have the most severe cases.
- HFM is usually found in children below the age of 10 yr.
- HFM is moderately contagious. Close contacts of affected children, including family members and health care workers, are the most commonly affected adults.
- Infection is spread from person to person by direct contact with nasal discharge or stool.
- A person is most contagious during the first wk of illness.
- Outbreaks tend to occur during the summer.
- Infection leads to immunity, but a second episode may occur after infection with a different agent.

PHYSICAL FINDINGS & CLINICAL PRESENTATION

Symptoms:
- After a 4- to 6-day incubation period, patients may complain of odynophagia, sore throat, malaise, and fever (38.3 to 40° C).
- One to 2 days later the characteristic oral lesions appear.
- In 75% of cases, skin lesions on the extremities accompany these oral manifestations.
- 11% of adults have cutaneous findings.
- Lesions appear over the course of 1 or 2 days.

Physical findings:
- Oral lesions, usually between five and ten, are commonly found on the tongue, buccal mucosa, gingivae, and hard palate.
- Oral lesions initially start as 1- to 3-mm erythematous macules and evolve into gray vesicles on an erythematous base.
- Vesicles are frequently broken by the time of presentation and appear as superficial gray ulcers with surrounding erythema.
- Skin lesions of the hands and feet start as linear erythematous papules (3 to 10 mm in diameter) that evolve into gray vesicles that may be mildly painful (Fig. 1-113). These vesicles are usually intact at presentation and remain so until they desquamate within 2 wk.
- Involvement of the buttocks and perineum is present in 31% of cases.
- In rare cases, encephalitis, meningitis, myocarditis, poliomyelitis-like paralysis, and pulmonary edema may develop. Sporadic acute paralysis has been reported with Enterovirus 71.
- Although information is limited, there is not clear evidence that pregnancy outcomes are affected.

ETIOLOGY

- Coxsackievirus group A, type 16, was the first and is the most common viral agent isolated.
- Coxsackieviruses A5, A7, A9, A10, B1, B2, B3, B5, and enterovirus 71 have also been implicated.

DIAGNOSIS

DIFFERENTIAL DIAGNOSIS

- Aphthous stomatitis
- Herpes simplex infection
- Herpangina
- Behçet's disease
- Erythema multiforme
- Pemphigus
- Gonorrhea
- Acute leukemia
- Lymphoma
- Allergic contact dermatitis

WORKUP

The diagnosis is usually made on the basis of history and characteristic physical examination.

LABORATORY TESTS

- Not indicated unless the diagnosis is in doubt
- Throat culture or stool specimen may be obtained for viral testing but may take from 2 to 4 wk for results

TREATMENT

ACUTE GENERAL Rx

- Palliative therapy is given for this usually self-limited disease.
- Limited data suggest acyclovir may have a role in treatment of certain cases.

DISPOSITION

Prognosis is excellent except in rare cases of CNS or cardiac involvement. Most are managed as outpatients.

REFERRAL

Not usually needed

PEARLS & CONSIDERATIONS

- Frequent hand washing, disinfection of contaminated surfaces, and washing of soiled articles of clothing can help reduce transmission.
- HFM has no relationship to hoof and mouth disease in cattle.

SUGGESTED READINGS

Chang LY et al: Transmission and clinical features of Enterovirus 71 infections in household contacts in Taiwan, *JAMA* 291(2):222, 2004.

Chang LY et al: Clinical features and risk of pulmonary edema after enterovirus related hand, foot, and mouth disease, *Lancet* 354(9191):1682, 1999.

Weir E: Foot-and-mouth disease in animals and humans, *Can Med Assoc J,* 164(9):1338, 2001.

AUTHORS: **JAMES J. NG, M.D.**, and **JENNIFER JEREMIAH, M.D.**

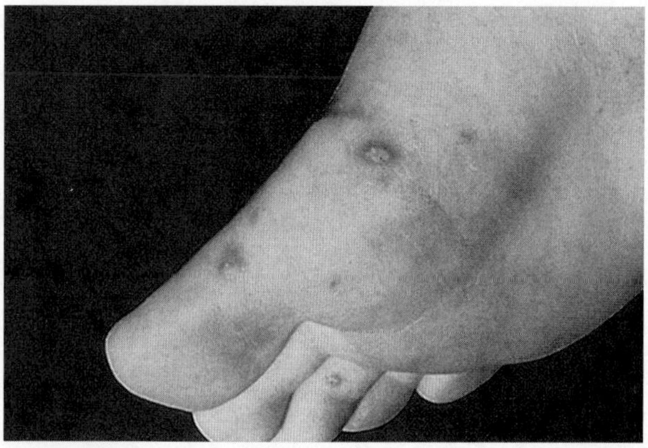

FIGURE 1-113 Hand-foot-mouth disease. Note oval lesions on an erythematous base. (From Goldstein B [ed]: *Practical dermatology,* ed 2, St Louis, 1997, Mosby.)

BASIC INFORMATION

DEFINITION

Hantavirus pulmonary syndrome (HPS) is a severe infectious cardiopulmonary illness usually caused by the Sin Nombre virus (SNV) whose main vector is the deer mouse.

SYNONYMS

Four Corners disease
Hantavirus cardiopulmonary syndrome

ICD-9CM CODES
079.81

EPIDEMIOLOGY & DEMOGRAPHICS

- First identified in the U.S. in 1993, hantavirus has been found throughout the Continental U.S. and the Americas.
- As of 2005, 396 cases have been identified in 31 states with a mortality rate of 37%.
- The peak incidence to date was in June and July 1993 in the Four Corners region of the U.S.
- HPS is more common in the spring and summer.
- HPS is more prevalent among males likely due to increased environmental exposure.
- Mean age is 38 years.
- HPS has not been found at the extremes of age.
- Risk factors include exposure to rodent populations, rural locales, occupations with increased exposure to rodents, and entering infrequently opened structures.

CLINICAL PRESENTATION

The most common symptoms are fever, headache, nausea, vomiting, cough, shortness of breath, and myalgia. It is not associated with rhinorrhea or nasal congestion.

The most common signs on physical exam include fever, hypoxemia, and tachypnea. Rash, mucosal bleeding, or peripheral edema are not found with HPS.

There are two phases of HPS, the prodromal phase and the cardiopulmonary phase.

The prodromal phase is characterized by:
- Fever, chills, headache, and myalgias especially in the legs and back
- Cough, nausea, vomiting, and general malaise
- Tachypnea, tachycardia, hypoxemia

The cardiopulmonary phase has the following characteristics:
- Cough and dyspnea
- Acute pulmonary edema
- Hypotension
- Decreased cardiac output

ETIOLOGY

- HPS is most often caused by the Sin Nombre virus.
- The main vector is the deer mouse.
- It is transmitted by inhalation of aerosolized feces, urine, or saliva from infected rodents.
- No cases of person-to-person transmission.

DIAGNOSIS

DIFFERENTIAL DIAGNOSIS

- ARDS
- Pneumonia
- CHF
- Pulmonary edema
- Acute bacterial endocarditis
- Gastroenteritis
- Plague
- Tularemia—"rabbit fever"
- Histoplasmosis
- Coccidioidomycosis
- Cardiogenic shock
- HIV/AIDS
- Myocardial infarction
- Goodpasture's syndrome—an autoimmune pulmonary disease

WORKUP

- CBC q8h.
  1. All patients manifest thrombocytopenia and its progression is the most consistent indicator heralding the cardiopulmonary phase of HPS.
  2. Differential usually reveals a left shift. WBC counts are an unreliable indicator of severity of infection.
- Lactate level greater than 4 mg/dl is associated with a high mortality rate.
- Rapid immunoblot strip assay (RIBA) for SNV antibodies.
- Diagnosis is confirmed by identification of IgM and IgG antibodies to SNV.

IMAGING STUDIES

Chest x-ray: pulmonary edema

TREATMENT

NONPHARMACOLOGIC THERAPY

- ICU admission in tertiary care center
- Mechanical ventilation with high PEEP and high FiO_2
- Pulmonary artery catheterization
- Extracorporeal membrane oxygenation (ECMO)

ACUTE GENERAL Rx

- Supportive measures
- Supplemental oxygen
- Intubation when indicated
- Fluid resuscitation
- Hemodynamic monitoring
- Initial broad-spectrum antibiotics
- Pressors
- No medication is effective against SNV.

DISPOSITION

- Patients that survive cardiopulmonary phase of HPS have rapid clinical improvement.
- There are no serious sequelae.

REFERRAL

University of New Mexico Hospital is the only facility with experience in ECMO for treatment of HPS and is only for hemodynamically unstable critically ill patients failing conventional therapies.

PEARLS & CONSIDERATIONS

COMMENTS

Although rare, HPS should be a consideration in those with acute respiratory illness and a history suggestive of HPS exposure. The combination of thrombocytopenia, left shift, circulating immunoblasts, and hemoconcentration is rare in other viral illnesses.

PREVENTION

Rodent control is the primary way to prevent hantavirus infection.

SUGGESTED READINGS

Graziano KL et al: Hantavirus pulmonary syndrome: a zebra worth knowing, *Am Fam Physician* 66(6):1015-1020, 2002.

Mertz GJ et al: Diagnosis and treatment of new world hantavirus infections, *Curr Opin Infect Dis* 19(5):437, 2006.

Mills JN et al: Hantavirus pulmonary syndrome—United States: updated recommendations for risk reduction, *MMWR Recomm Rep* 51(RR09):1-12, 2002.

National Center for Infectious Diseases, Special Pathogens Branch: All about hantaviruses, http://www.cdc.gov/ncidod/diseases/hanta/hps/noframes/generalinfoindex.htm Accessed Sept 2005.

AUTHOR: **CATHERINE SHAFTS, D.O.**

BASIC INFORMATION

DEFINITION

The term *cluster headache* refers to attacks of severe, strictly unilateral pain that is orbital, supraorbital, temporal, or in any combination of these sites, lasting 15 to 180 minutes, and occurring from once every other day to 8 times a day. The attacks are associated with one or more of the following, all of which are ipsilateral: conjunctival injection, lacrimation, nasal congestion, rhinorrhea, forehead and facial sweating, miosis, ptosis, eyelid edema. Most patients are restless or agitated during an attack.

SYNONYMS

Ciliary neuralgia
Erythro-melalgia of the head
Erythroprosopalgia of Bing
Horton's headache

ICD-9CM CODES
346.2 Variants of migraine

EPIDEMIOLOGY & DEMOGRAPHICS

INCIDENCE: Estimated to occur in 0.05% to 1% of the population
PREDOMINANT SEX: Occurs in males at least 5 times more commonly than in females
PREDOMINANT AGE: Peak age of onset between 20 and 40 yr
GENETICS: May be inherited (autosomal dominant) in about 5% of cases

PHYSICAL FINDINGS & CLINICAL PRESENTATION

- During attack: ipsilateral conjunctival injection, lacrimation, nasal congestion, rhinorrhea, facial sweating, Horner's syndrome.
- In contrast to migraine sufferers, patients are agitated and active during an attack.
- Permanent partial Horner's syndrome in 5% of patients; otherwise examination normal.

ETIOLOGY

Activation of the posterior hypothalamic grey matter resulting in trigeminal activation coupled with parasympathetic activation.

DIAGNOSIS

- Severe or very severe unilateral orbital, supraorbital and/or temporal pain lasting 15 to 180 minutes
- Frequency of every other day to 8 per day
- Headache is accompanied by at least one of the following (ipsilateral):
  1. conjunctival injection and/or lacrimation
  2. nasal congestion and/or rhinorrhea
  3. eyelid edema
  4. forehead and facial sweating
  5. miosis and/or ptosis
  6. restlessness or agitation

DIFFERENTIAL DIAGNOSIS

- Migraine
- Trigeminal neuralgia
- Temporal arteritis
- Postherpetic neuralgia
- Other trigeminal autonomic cephalagias
- Section II describes the differential diagnosis of headaches

WORKUP

Diagnosis is usually established by characteristic history.

IMAGING STUDIES

None, unless history or examination suggests focal neurological deficit

TREATMENT

NONPHARMACOLOGIC THERAPY

Avoidance of alcohol, histamine, nitroglycerine, or tobacco during clusters

ABORTIVE Rx

- Inhalation of 100% oxygen by face mask at 6 L/min for 15 min often aborts an attack.
- Triptans, cafergot, or dihydroergotamine may abort an attack or prevent one if given just before a predictable episode. Acute episode is typically resolved before oral analgesics become effective, although indomethacin and other NSAIDS may also be effective in prolonged attacks.

PROPHYLAXIS Rx

Various medications have been tried without great success, although good responses may be obtained in up to 50% of cases. Examples include:

- Verapamil: up to 480 mg/day as tolerated (the drug of choice)
- Lithium: 200 mg tid with frequent monitoring and adjustment to maintain therapeutic serum level of 0.4 to 1 mEq/L. Equally effective as verapamil, but more side effects
- Ergotamine tartrate: 3 to 4 mg/day during clusters
- Prednisone: 60 mg po qd × 1 wk followed by taper. Headaches can return during taper

DISPOSITION

Headache-free periods tend to increase with increasing age.

REFERRAL

Refractory cluster headaches

PEARLS & CONSIDERATIONS

COMMENTS

- Cluster headaches are divided into episodic (attacks lasting up to 1 yr with greater than 1 mo pain-free periods) and chronic (>1 yr without remission).
- Cluster headaches now classified as a trigeminal autonomic cephalalgia (TAC). Other TAC includes paroxysmal hemicrania and short-lasting unilateral neuralgiform headache attacks with conjunctival injection and tearing (SUNCT).

EVIDENCE

There is a randomized controlled trial (RCT) indicating that sumatriptan is an effective treatment for acute cluster headaches.[1]

There is evidence from a small RCT indicating that intranasal oxygen can provide significant pain relief from acute cluster headaches.[2]

There are two RCTs that suggest that verapamil is effective in episodic cluster headache prophylaxis.[3-4]

A small RCT showed oral prednisone was effective in treating cluster headaches.[5]

Evidence-Based References

1. Ekbom K et al: Treatment of acute cluster headache with sumatriptan, *N Engl J Med* 325:322, 1991.
2. Fogan L: Treatment of cluster headache, *Arch Neurol* 42:362, 1985.
3. Leone M et al: Verapamil in the prophylaxis of episodic cluster headache: a double-blind study versus placebo, *Neurology* 54:1382, 2000.
4. Bussone G et al: Double blind comparison of lithium and verapamil in cluster headache prophylaxis, *Headache* 30:411, 1990.
5. Jammes JL: The treatment of cluster headaches with prednisone, *Dis Nerv Syst* 36:375, 1975.

SUGGESTED READINGS

Headache Classification Committee of the International Headache Society: The International Classification of Headache Disorders, *Cephalgia* 24:s1, 2004.

May A: Cluster headache: pathogenesis, diagnosis, and management, *Lancet* 366:843, 2005.

AUTHOR: **CHUN LIM, M.D., PH.D.**

BASIC INFORMATION

DEFINITION

Migraine headaches are recurrent headaches that are preceded by a focal neurological symptom (migraine with aura), occur independently (migraine without aura), or have atypical presentations (migraine variants). Migraine with aura is characterized by visual or sensory symptoms that typically develop or march over a period of 5 to 20 min. In both migraine with and without aura, the headache is typically unilateral, pulsatile, and associated with nausea and vomiting, photophobia and phonophobia.

ICD-9CM CODES
346 Migraine

EPIDEMIOLOGY & DEMOGRAPHICS

INCIDENCE: Increases from infancy, peaks during the third decade of life then decreases

PREVALENCE (IN U.S.): Females: 18%; males: 6%

GENETICS:
- Familial predisposition, with over 50% of migraine sufferers having an affected family member
- Autosomal dominant transmission for some rare migraine variants (familial hemiplegic migraine, CADASIL)

PHYSICAL FINDINGS & CLINICAL PRESENTATION

- Normal between episodes
- Normal for migraine without aura. Focal motor or sensory abnormalities possible with migraine with aura or migraine variants
- Common aura types include scintillating scotomata, bright zigzags, homonymous visual disturbance such as paraethesias, speech disturbances, or hemiparesis (familial or sporadic hemiplegic migraine)

ETIOLOGY

A primary neuronal event resulting in a trigeminovascular reflex causing neurogenic inflammation. Serotonin, nitric oxide, and calcitonin-gene-related peptide also play a role but exact mechanism is unknown. Cortical spreading depression is responsible for the aura.

DIAGNOSIS

Migraine without aura
- 5 attacks fulfilling criteria
- Headache attacks lasting 4 to 72 hours
- Headache has at least two of the following characteristics:
  1. Unilateral location
  2. Pulsating quality
  3. Moderate or severe pain intensity
  4. Aggravation by or causing avoidance of routine physical activity
- During headache at least one of the following:
  1. Nausea and/or vomiting
  2. Photophobia and phonophobia

Migraine with aura
- At least two attacks
- Aura consisting of at least one of the following, but no motor weakness:
  1. Fully reversible visual symptoms including positive features and/or negative features.
  2. Fully reversible sensory symptoms including positive and/or negative features.
- At least two of the following:
  1. Homonymous visual symptoms and/or unilateral sensory symptoms.
  2. At least one aura symptom develops gradually over >5 minutes and/or different aura symptoms occur in succession over >5 minutes.
- A migraine occurring during or within 60 minutes of the aura.

DIFFERENTIAL DIAGNOSIS

- Subarachnoid hemorrhage
- Cluster headache
- Chronic daily headaches (drug rebound headaches)
- Tension headaches
- Tumor
- Section II describes the differential diagnosis of headaches

WORKUP

- Generally no additional investigation is needed with recurrent, typical attacks with usual age of onset, family history, and a normal physical examination.
- If there is an unusual presentation and/or unexpected findings on examination, investigation for other causes is required.

LABORATORY TESTS

Lumbar puncture for history of abrupt onset headaches and uncertain diagnosis of migraine

IMAGING STUDIES

- Imaging should be done in patients with headaches and an unexplained abnormal finding on the neurological examination.
- Imaging should be considered in patients with rapidly increasing headache frequency, history of dizziness or incoordination, headache causing wakening from sleep, or headaches worsening with Valsalva maneuver.

TREATMENT

Consider the use of a headache log/diary to identify triggers of headaches, to record efficacy of treatments, and to track history of the headaches.

NONPHARMACOLOGIC THERAPY

- Avoid any identifiable provoking factors: caffeine, tobacco, and alcohol may trigger attacks, as may dietary or other environmental precipitants (less common)
- Avoid stressors in life and minimize variations in daily routine with regular sleep, meals, and exercise
- Relaxation training and biofeedback

ACUTE ANALGESIC Rx

- Many oral agents are ineffective because of poor absorption secondary to migraine-induced gastric stasis. Nonoral route of administration should be selected in patients with severe nausea or vomiting
- Nonspecific treatment for pain.
- Acetaminophen, NSAIDS, combination analgesics, benzodiazepines, opioids, barbiturates

ACUTE ABORTIVE Rx

- Intravenous antiemetics (prochlorperazine, metoclopramide). Acute dystonic reactions and akathisia are rare side effects. Generally not used as monotherapy
- Ergotamine and ergotamine combinations (PO/PR), and dihydroergotamine (DHE 45) all have efficacy against migraines. DHE 45 usually administered in combination with an antiemetic drug (Table 1-17)
- Triptans (SC, PO, and intranasal) now considered drug of choice for abortive therapy. Meta-analysis suggests that 10 mg rizatriptan, 80 mg eletriptan, and 12.5 mg almotriptan are most effective
- Early administration improves effectiveness

PROPHYLAXIS Rx

- Prophylactic treatment is generally indicated when headaches occur more than once a week or when symptomatic treatments are contraindicated or not effective. They are most effective when initiated during headache-free period. All prophylaxis should be maintained for at least 3 mo before deeming the medication a failure.
- Well-established options for prophylactic treatment include β-blockers (propanolol, timolol), tricyclic antidepressants (amitriptyline), and the antiepileptic drugs valproic acid and topiramate.
- Less established options include Ca-channel blockers, SSRIs, and the antiepileptic drug gabapentin.

DISPOSITION

After age 30 yr, 40% of patients are migraine free.

REFERRAL

If uncertain about diagnosis or treatment not effective

PEARLS & CONSIDERATIONS

Avoid overuse of narcotics, barbiturates, caffeine, and benzodiazepines, as they are habit-forming and can result in drug-induced or rebound headaches.

EVIDENCE

Several randomized controlled trials (RCTs) have found that IV antiemetics are effective for acute treatment of migraine both as monotherapy or as adjunctive therapy.[1-2]

Many RCTs have reported on the efficacy and safety of DHE nasal spray for the treatment of moderate to severe migraine.[3]

Many RCTs show that triptans are an appropriate and effective treatment choice for use in patients with moderate-to-severe migraine who have no contraindications for its use.[4-6]

Many RCTs have shown that sodium valproate, topiramate, amitriptyline, and propanolol are the most effective medications in preventing migraine or reducing the frequency, severity, and duration of the attacks.[7-10]

Evidence-Based References

1. Tek DS et al: A prospective, double-blind study of metoclopramide hydrochloride for the control of migraine attacks, *Ann Emerg Med* 19:1083, 1990.
2. Coppola M et al: Randomized, placebo-controlled evaluation of prochlorperazine versus metroclopramide for emergency department treatment of migraine headache, *Ann Emerg Med* 24:541, 1995.
3. Ziegler D et al: Dihydroergotamine nasal spray for the acute treatment of migraine, *Neurology* 44:447, 1994.
4. Subcutaneous Sumatriptan International Study Group: Treatment of migraine attacks with sumatriptan, *N Engl J Med* 325:316, 1991.
5. Solomon GD et al: Clinical efficacy and tolerability of 2.5 mg zolmitriptan for the acute treatment of migraine. The 042 clinical trial study group, *Neurology* 49:1219, 1997.
6. Visser WH et al: Rizatriptan vs sumatriptan in the acute treatment of migraine. A placebo-controlled, dose-ranging study. Dutch/US rizatriptan study group, *Arch Neurol* 53:1132, 1996.
7. Hering R, Kuritzky A: Sodium valproate in the prophylactic treatment of migraine: a double-blind study versus placebo, *Cephalalgia* 12:81, 1992.
8. Couch JR, Hassanein RS: Amitriptyline in migraine prophylaxis, *Arch Neurol* 36:695, 1979.
9. Borgesen SE et al: Prophylactic treatment of migraine with propranolol. A clinical trial, *Acta Neurol Scand* 50:651, 1974.
10. Brandes JL et al: Topiramate for migraine prevention: a randomized controlled trial, *JAMA* 291:965, 2004.

SUGGESTED READINGS

Ferrari MD et al: Oral triptans (serotonin 5-HT1B/1D agonist) in acute migraine treatment: a meta-analysis of 53 trials, *Lancet* 358:1668, 2001.

Ferrari MD et al: Migraine—current understanding and treatment, *N Engl J Med* 346:257, 2002.

Silberstein SD: Practice parameter: evidence-based guidelines for migraine headache, *Neurology* 55:754, 2000.

AUTHOR: **CHUN LIM, M.D., PH.D.**

TABLE 1-17 Treatment for Acute Attacks of Migraine*

Drug	Route	Dose
Triptans (serotonin agonists)		
Sumatriptan	Subcutaneous	6 mg, repeat in 2 hr (max 2 doses/day)
Sumatriptan	Oral	25 mg, 50 mg, repeat in 2 hr (max 200 mg/day)
Sumatriptan	Nasal spray	5 mg and 20 mg, repeat in 2 hr (max 40 mg/day)
Zolmitriptan	Oral	1.25, 2.5 mg, 5 mg, repeat in 2 hr (max 10 mg/day)
Zolmitriptan	Nasal spray	5 mg, repeat in 2 hr (max 10 mg/day)
Zolmitriptan	Orally disintegrating tab	2.5, 5 mg, repeat in 2 hr (max 10 mg/day)
Naratriptan	Oral	1 mg, 2.5 mg, repeat in 4 hr (max 5 mg/day)
Rizatriptan	Oral	5 mg, 10 mg, repeat in 2 hr (max 30 mg/day)
Almotriptan	Oral	6.25 mg, 12.5 mg, may repeat in 2 hr (max 25 mg/day)
Eletriptan	Oral	20 mg, 40 mg, may repeat in 2 hr (max 80 mg/day)
Frovatriptan	Oral	2.5 mg, may repeat in 2 hr (max 7.5 mg/day)
Ergotamine preparations		
Ergotamine and caffeine	Oral	2 tablets, may repeat 1 tab q30 min; max 6/day
Ergotamine and caffeine	Rectal	1 suppository, repeat in 1 hr; max 2/day
Ergotaminel	Sublingual	1 tablet, repeat in 1 hr; max 2/day
Dihydroergotamine	Intramuscular Subcutaneous Intravenous Nasal spray	0.5-1.0 mg, repeat twice at 1-hr intervals (max 3 mg/attack)
Antiemetics		
Promethazine	Oral	50-125 mg
	Intramuscular	
Prochlorperazine	Oral	1-25 mg
	Rectal	2.5-25 mg (suppository)
	Intramuscular	5-10 mg
Chlorpromazine	Oral	10-25 mg
	Rectal	50-100 mg (suppository)
	Intravenous	Up to 35 mg
Trimetobenzamide	Oral	250 mg
	Rectal	200 mg
Metoclopramide	Oral	5-10 mg
	Intramuscular	10 mg
	Intravenous	5-10 mg
Dimenhydrinate	Oral	50 mg

Modified from Wiederholt WC: *Neurology for non-neurologists,* ed 4, Philadelphia, 2000, WB Saunders.

*For side effects and contraindications, consult the manufacturer's drug insert before prescribing any of these drugs.

BASIC INFORMATION

DEFINITION

Tension-type headaches (TTH) are recurrent headaches lasting 30 min to 7 days without nausea or vomiting and with at least two of the following characteristics: pressing or tightening quality (nonthrobbing), mild or moderate intensity, bilateral, and not aggravated by routine physical activity. The International Classification of Headache Disorders (ICHD-2) criteria include three subtypes: infrequent episodic TTH (<1 day/mo), frequent episodic TTH (1 to 14 days/mo), and chronic TTH (15 days/mo, perhaps without recognizable episodes).

SYNONYMS

Muscle contraction headache
Tension headache
Stress headache
Essential headache

ICD-9CM CODES
307.81 Tension headache

EPIDEMIOLOGY & DEMOGRAPHICS

INCIDENCE (IN U.S.): Most common type of headache; as high as 70% of all headaches presenting to primary care physician; first-degree relatives of probands confer increased risk

PEAK INCIDENCE: Occurs at all ages; may decrease with age

PREVALENCE (IN U.S.): Males: 63%/yr; females: 86%/yr

PREDOMINANT SEX: Females > males

PHYSICAL FINDINGS & CLINICAL PRESENTATION

Pressure or "bandlike" tightness all around the head, may be worse at the vertex. Cervical, paracervical and trapezius muscle spasm and/or tenderness on palpation may be present. Scalp tenderness or hypersensitivity to pain also occurs. Symptoms suggestive of migraine are usually not present (e.g., throbbing pain, nausea/vomiting, visual complaints, aura). Either one symptom of photo or phonophobia does not exclude the diagnosis of TTH.

ETIOLOGY

- Unclear; little data to support postulated muscle contraction component. More recently has been thought of as a multifactorial disorder with several possible concurrent pathophysiological mechanisms. Functional neuroimaging suggests gray matter decrease in regions known to be involved in pain processing.
- No recent data to support the longstanding belief that these headaches arise from stress or other psychologic factors. However, components of stress, sleep deprivation, hunger, and eyestrain may exacerbate symptoms.

DIAGNOSIS

DIFFERENTIAL DIAGNOSIS

- Migraine (would expect associated symptoms, see "Headache, Migraine")
- Cervical spine disease
- Intracranial mass (may present with focal neurologic signs, seizures, or headache awakening patient from sleep)
- Idiopathic intracranial hypertension (found more often in obese women of child-bearing age, may have papilledema, visual loss, or diplopia)
- Rebound headache from overuse of analgesics
- Secondary headache (e.g., temporomandibular joint syndrome, thyrotoxicosis, polycythemia, drug side-effects)
- Migraine and tension-type headache may often coexist and may be difficult to differentiate (suggest headache calendar)
- Section II describes the differential diagnosis of headaches

WORKUP

- Thorough history and physical examination for any new-onset headache
- Neuroimaging should be performed when unexplained neurologic findings are present on exam or in cases of atypical new-onset sudden and severe headaches.

LABORATORY TESTS

- No routine tests
- ESR in elderly patients suspected of having cranial arteritis

IMAGING STUDIES

CT scan and/or MRI may be used to exclude intracranial pathology. MRI is better for imaging the posterior fossa. Contrast should be used if mass lesion is suspected.

TREATMENT

NONPHARMACOLOGIC THERAPY

- Relaxation and cognitive behavioral therapy (especially in adolescents and children), Schultz-type autogenic training (relaxation technique based on passive concentration and body awareness of specific sensations), transcutaneous electrical nerve stimulation (TENS), heat
- Physical therapy including stretching exercises, massage, and ultrasound

ACUTE GENERAL Rx

Nonnarcotic analgesics with limited frequency to prevent drug-induced and/or rebound headache

CHRONIC Rx

- Tricyclic antidepressants (e.g., amitriptyline 10 to 150 mg hs) and SSRIs
- Avoid narcotics, limit NSAIDs, consider indomethacin; if related to cervical muscle spasm, may consider trial of muscle relaxants (e.g., Skelaxin 400 to 800 mg TID)

DISPOSITION

- May not respond fully to treatment
- Prognosis is fairly favorable for episodic forms; chronic forms, coexisting migraine, sleep difficulty, and not being married confer a less favorable prognosis

REFERRAL

If uncertain about diagnosis or unexplained focal neurologic findings on examination

PEARLS & CONSIDERATIONS

It is imperative to avoid overuse of caffeine- and barbiturate-containing medications because of the risk of rebound headaches

EVIDENCE

There is a paucity of high quality trials in the treatment of TTH. Various randomized controlled trials (RCT) have showed amitriptyline and cognitive therapy were more effective than placebo in various measures (e.g., headache-free days, symptom reduction). A small, double-blind cross-over trial of mirtazapine significantly reduced headache frequency. Systematic reviews have found that acupuncture is probably effective, although a small RCT did not show statistical benefit.

SUGGESTED READINGS

Bendtsen L, Jensen R: Mirtazapine is effective in the prophylactic treatment of chronic tension-type headache, *Neurology* 62:1706, 2004.

Bendtsen L, Jensen R: Tension-type headache: the most common, but also the most neglected, headache disorder, *Curr Opin Neurol* 19(3):305, 2006.

Bronfort G et al: Non-invasive physical treatments for chronic/recurrent headache, *Cochrane Database Syst Rev* 3, 2004.

Goadsby P: Headache (chronic tension-type), *BMJ* 12:1808, 2004.

Headache Classification Committee of the International Headache Society. The International Classification of Headache Disorders, *Cephalalgia* 24:1, 2004.

Holroyd KA et al: Management of chronic tension-type headache with tricyclic anti-depressant medication, stress management therapy, and their combination: a randomized controlled trial, *JAMA* 285(17):2208, 2001.

Jensen R: Pathophysiological mechanisms of tension-type headache: a review of epidemiological and experimental studies, *Cephalalgia* 19(6):602, 1999.

Lipton RB et al: Classification of primary headaches, *Neurology* 63:427, 2004.

May A: A review of diagnostic and functional imaging in headache, *J Headache Pain* 7(4):174, 2006. Epub ahead of print.

Russell MB: Genetics in primary headaches, *J Headache Pain* 8(3):190, 2007.

Silver N: Headache (chronic tension-type), *Am Fam Physician* 76:114, 2007.

Zsombok T et al: Effect of autogenic training on drug consumption in patients with primary headache: an 8-month follow-up study, *Headache* 43:251, 2003.

AUTHOR: **RICHARD S. ISAACSON, M.D.**

BASIC INFORMATION

DEFINITION

In complete heart block, there is complete blockage of all AV conduction. The atria and ventricles have separate, independent rhythms.

SYNONYMS

Third-degree AV block

ICD-9CM CODES
426.0 Complete heart block

EPIDEMIOLOGY & DEMOGRAPHICS

Over 100,000 permanent pacemakers are implanted worldwide each year for complete heart block.

PHYSICAL FINDINGS & CLINICAL PRESENTATION

Physical examination may be normal. Patients may present with the following clinical manifestations:

- Dizziness, palpitations
- Stokes-Adams syncopal attacks
- CHF
- Angina

ETIOLOGY

- Degenerative changes in His-Purkinje system
- Acute anterior wall MI
- Calcific aortic stenosis
- Cardiomyopathy
- Trauma
- Cardiovascular surgery
- Congenital

DIAGNOSIS

DIFFERENTIAL DIAGNOSIS

The differential diagnosis involves only the etiology. ECG will confirm diagnosis.

WORKUP

ECG:

- P waves constantly change their relationship to the QRS complexes (Fig. 1-114).
- Ventricular rate is usually <50 bpm (may be higher in congenital forms).
- Ventricular rate is generally lower than the atrial rate.
- QRS complex is wide.

TREATMENT

ACUTE GENERAL Rx

- Immediate pacemaker insertion unless the patient has congenital third-degree AV block and is completely asymptomatic
- Therapy of underlying etiology

CHRONIC Rx

Patients with permanent pacemakers need regular follow-up and pacemaker monitoring to ensure proper sensing.

DISPOSITION

Prognosis is favorable following insertion of pacemaker and related to the underlying etiology of complete AV block (e.g., MI, cardiomyopathy).

REFERRAL

Referral for implantation of permanent pacemaker

PEARLS & CONSIDERATIONS

COMMENTS

- Patients should be instructed on avoidance of activities that may damage the pacemaker (e.g., contact sports).
- Common environmental causes of pacemaker malformation are electrocautery, transthoracic defibrillation, MRI, extracorporeal shock wave lithotripsy, transcutaneous electrical nerve stimulation, therapeutic radiation, ECT, diathermy, radiofrequency ablation for treatment of tachyarrhythmias.

EVIDENCE

EBM

A systematic review analyzed 5 parallel and 26 crossover randomized controlled trials (RCTs) comparing dual-chamber pacing and single-chamber ventricular pacing for adult patients with atrioventricular block, sick sinus syndrome, or both. It found that there was a trend toward greater effectiveness with dual-chamber pacing compared with single-chamber ventricular pacing. None of the studies reported a significantly better outcome with single-chamber ventricular pacing.[1] Ⓐ

Evidence-Based Reference

1. Dretzke J et al: Dual chamber versus single chamber ventricular pacemakers for sick sinus syndrome and atrioventricular block. Reviewed in: Cochrane Library, 3, Chichester, UK, 2004, John Wiley. Ⓐ

SUGGESTED READING

Bayce M et al: Evolving indications for permanent pacemakers, *Ann Intern Med* 134:1130, 2001.

AUTHOR: **FRED F. FERRI, M.D.**

THIRD-DEGREE (COMPLETE) AV BLOCK

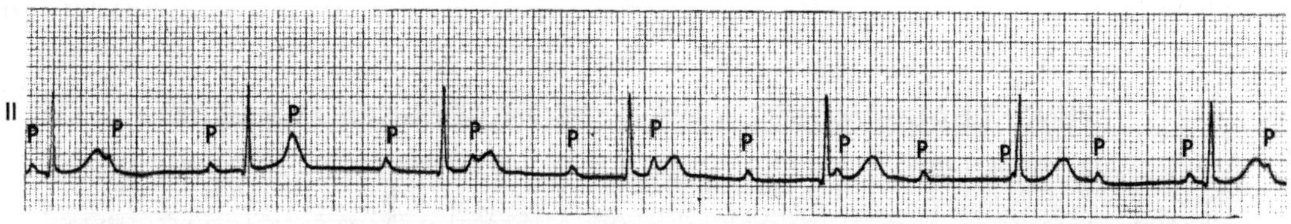

FIGURE 1-114 Third-degree complete AV heart block is characterized by independent atrial *(P)* and ventricular (QRS) activity. The atrial rate is always faster than the ventricular rate. The PR intervals are completely variable. Some P waves fall on the T wave, distorting its shape. Others may fall in the QRS complex and be "lost." Notice that the QRS complexes are of normal width, indicating that the ventricles are being paced from the AV junction. (From Goldberger AL [ed]: *Clinical electrocardiography,* ed 5, St Louis, 1994, Mosby.)

BASIC INFORMATION

DEFINITION

Second-degree heart block is the blockage of some (but not all) impulses from the atria to the ventricles. There are two types of second-degree AV block:

MOBITZ TYPE I (WENCKEBACH):

- There is a progressive prolongation of the PR interval before an impulse is completely blocked; the cycle repeats periodically.
- Cycle with dropped beat is less than two times the previous cycle.
- Site of block is usually AV node (proximal to the bundle of His).

MOBITZ TYPE II:

- There is a sudden interruption of AV conduction without prior prolongation of the PR interval.
- Site of block is infranodal.

SYNONYMS

Wenckebach block (Mobitz type I block)
Mobitz type II block

ICD-9CM CODES
426.13 Mobitz type I
426.12 Mobitz type II

EPIDEMIOLOGY & DEMOGRAPHICS

Mobitz type I block is more common and may occur in individuals with heightened vagal tone or secondary to some medications such as β-blockers or calcium channel blockers.

PHYSICAL FINDINGS & CLINICAL PRESENTATION

- Patients with Mobitz type I are usually asymptomatic.
- Sudden loss of consciousness without warning (Adams-Stokes attack) can occur in patients with Mobitz type II; however, it is much more common in patients with complete heart block.
- Irregular pulse with dropped beats is present (Mobitz type I).
- Irregular pulse with occasional dropped beats is present (Mobitz type II).

ETIOLOGY

MOBITZ TYPE I:

- Vagal stimulation
- Degenerative changes in the AV conduction system
- Ischemia at the AV nodes (particularly in inferior wall MI)
- Drugs (digitalis, quinidine, procainamide, adenosine, calcium channel blockers, β-blockers)
- Cardiomyopathies
- Aortic regurgitation
- Lyme carditis

MOBITZ TYPE II:

- Degenerative changes in the His-Purkinje system
- Acute anterior wall MI
- Calcific aortic stenosis

DIAGNOSIS

DIFFERENTIAL DIAGNOSIS

The ECG will distinguish between Mobitz type I and Mobitz type II block and other conduction abnormalities.

WORKUP

ECG, 24-hr Holter monitor (selected patients)

MOBITZ TYPE I (Fig. 1-115): ECG shows:

- Gradual prolongation of PR interval leading to a blocked beat
- Shortened PR interval after dropped beat

MOBITZ TYPE II: ECG shows:

- Fixed duration of PR interval
- Sudden appearance of blocked beats

TREATMENT

NONPHARMACOLOGIC THERAPY

Elimination of drugs that may induce AV block

ACUTE GENERAL Rx

MOBITZ TYPE I:

- Treatment generally is not necessary. This type of block is usually transient.
- If symptomatic (e.g., dizziness), atropine 1 mg (may repeat once after 5 min) may be tried to increase AV conduction; if no response, insert temporary pacemaker.
- If block is secondary to drugs (e.g., digitalis), discontinue the drug.
- If associated with anterior wall MI and wide QRS escape rhythm, consider insertion of temporary pacemaker.
- Significant AV block post-MI may be caused by adenosine produced by the ischemic myocardium. These arrhythmias (which may be resistant to conventional therapy such as atropine) may respond to theophylline (adenosine antagonist).

MOBITZ TYPE II:

Pacemaker insertion is needed, because this type of block is usually permanent and often progresses to complete AV block.

DISPOSITION

Prognosis is good with insertion of pacemaker in patients with Mobitz type II.

REFERRAL

Referral for pacemaker insertion (see "Acute General Rx")

PEARLS & CONSIDERATIONS

COMMENTS

Patients with Mobitz type I should be followed routinely for potential development of high-grade AV block.

SUGGESTED READING

Barold S, Hayes D: Second-degree atrioventricular block: a reappraisal, *Mayo Clin Proc* 76:44, 2001.

AUTHOR: **FRED F. FERRI, M.D.**

WENCKEBACH (MOBITZ TYPE I) SECOND-DEGREE AV BLOCK

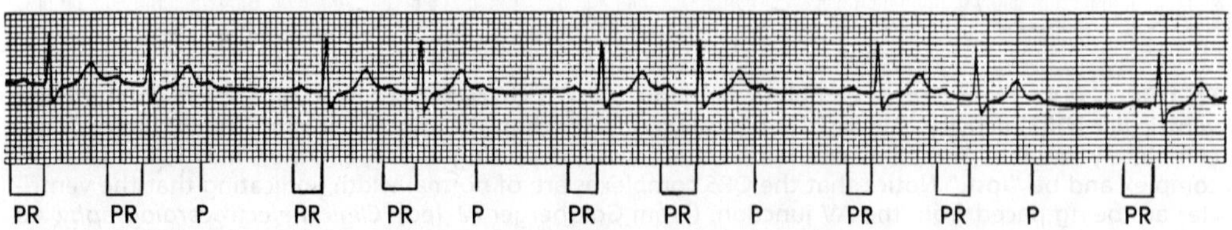

FIGURE 1-115 Wenckebach (Mobitz type I) second-degree AV block. Notice the progressive increase in PR intervals, with the third P wave in each sequence not followed by a QRS. Wenckebach block produces a characteristically syncopated rhythm with grouping of the QRS complexes (group beating). (From Goldberger AL [ed]: *Clinical electrocardiography,* ed 5, St Louis, 1994, Mosby.)

BASIC INFORMATION

DEFINITION

Heat exhaustion and heatstroke are part of a continuum of heat related illness, and unless factors leading to heat exhaustion are corrected swiftly, affected patients can progress to heatstroke

HEAT EXHAUSTION: An illness resulting from prolonged heavy activity in a hot environment with subsequent dehydration, electrolyte depletion, and rectal temperature >37.8° C but ≤40° C.

HEAT STROKE: A life-threatening heat illness characterized by extreme hyperthermia, dehydration, and neurologic manifestations (core temperature >40° C).

SYNONYMS

Heat illness
Hyperthermia

ICD-9CM CODES
992.0 Heat stroke
992.5 Heat exhaustion

EPIDEMIOLOGY & DEMOGRAPHICS

INCIDENCE (IN U.S.): Incidence of heat stroke is approximately 20 cases/100,000 population.

PREDOMINANT AGE: Heat exhaustion and stroke occur more frequently in elderly patients, especially those taking diuretics or medications that impair heat dissipation (e.g., phenothiazines, anticholinergics, antihistamines, β-blockers).

PHYSICAL FINDINGS & CLINICAL PRESENTATION

HEAT EXHAUSTION:

- Generalized malaise, weakness, headache, muscle and abdominal cramps, nausea, vomiting, hypotension, and tachycardia
- Rectal temperature is usually normal
- Sweating is usually present

HEAT STROKE:

- Neurologic manifestations (seizures, tremor, hemiplegia, coma, psychosis, and other bizarre behavior)
- Evidence of dehydration (poor skin turgor, sunken eyeballs)
- Tachycardia, hyperventilation
- Skin is hot, red, and flushed
- Sweating is often (not always) absent, particularly in elderly patients

ETIOLOGY

- Exogenous heat gain (increased ambient temperature)
- Increased heat production (exercise, infection, hyperthyroidism, drugs)
- Impaired heat dissipation (high humidity, heavy clothing, neonatal or elderly patients, drugs [phenothiazines, anticholinergics, antihistamines, butyrophenones, amphetamines, cocaine, alcohol, β-blockers])
- Diuretics, laxatives

DIAGNOSIS

DIFFERENTIAL DIAGNOSIS

- Infections (meningitis, encephalitis, sepsis)
- Head trauma
- Epilepsy
- Thyroid storm
- Acute cocaine intoxication
- Malignant hyperthermia
- Heat exhaustion can be differentiated from heat stroke by the following:
  1. Essentially intact mental function and lack of significant fever in heat exhaustion
  2. Mild or absent increases in CPK, AST, LDH, ALT in heat exhaustion

WORKUP

- Heat stroke: comprehensive history, physical examination, and laboratory evaluation
- Heat exhaustion: in most cases, laboratory tests are not necessary for diagnosis

LABORATORY TESTS

Laboratory abnormalities may include the following:

- Elevated BUN, creatinine, Hct
- Hyponatremia or hypernatremia, hyperkalemia or hypokalemia
- Elevated LDH, AST, ALT, CPK, bilirubin
- Lactic acidosis, respiratory alkalosis (secondary to hyperventilation)
- Myoglobinuria, hypofibrinogenemia, fibrinolysis, hypocalcemia

TREATMENT

- Treatment of **heat exhaustion** consists primarily of placing the patient in a cool, shaded area and providing rapid hydration and salt replacement.
  1. Fluid intake should be at least 2 L q4h in patients without history of CHF.
  2. Salt replacement can be accomplished by using one-quarter teaspoon of salt or two 10-grain salt tablets dissolved in 1 L of water.
  3. If IV fluid replacement is necessary, young athletes can be given normal saline IV (3 to 4 L over 6 to 8 hr); in elderly patients, consider using $D_5\frac{1}{2}$NS IV with rate titrated to cardiovascular status.
- Patients with **heat stroke** should undergo rapid cooling.
  1. Remove the patient's clothes and place the patient in a cool and well-ventilated room.
  2. If unconscious, position patient on his or her side and clear the airway. Protect airway and augment oxygenation (e.g., nasal O_2 at 4 L/min to keep oxygen saturation >90%).
  3. Monitor body temperature every 5 min. Measurement of the patient's core temperature with a rectal probe is recommended. The goal is to reduce the body temperature to 39° C (102.2° F) in 30 to 60 min.
  4. Spray the patient with a cool mist and use fans to enhance airflow over the body (rapid evaporation method).
  5. Immersion of the patient in ice water, stomach lavage with iced saline solution, intravenous administration of cooled fluids, and inhalation of cold air are advisable only when the means for rapid evaporation are not available. Immersion in tepid water (15° C, 59° F) is preferred over ice water immersion to minimize risk of shivering.
  6. Use of ice packs on axillae, neck, and groin is controversial because they increase peripheral vasoconstriction and may induce shivering.
  7. Antipyretics are ineffective because the hypothalamic set point during heat stroke is normal despite the increased body temperature.
  8. Intubate a comatose patient, insert a Foley catheter, and start nasal O_2. Continuous ECG monitoring is recommended.
  9. Insert at least two large-bore IV lines and begin IV hydration with NS or Ringer's lactate.
  10. Draw initial lab studies: electrolytes, CBC, BUN, creatinine, AST, ALT, CPK, LDH, glucose, INR, PTT, platelet count, Ca^{2+}, lactic acid, ABGs.
  11. Treat complications as follows:
      a. Hypotension: vigorous hydration with normal saline or Ringer's lactate.
      b. Convulsions: diazepam 5 to 10 mg IV (slowly).
      c. Shivering: chlorpromazine 10 to 50 mg IV.
      d. Acidosis: use bicarbonate judiciously (only in severe acidosis).
  12. Observe for evidence of rhabdomyolysis, hepatic, renal, or cardiac failure and treat accordingly.

DISPOSITION

Most patients recover completely within 48 hr. CNS injury is permanent in 20% of cases. Mortality can exceed 30% in patients with prolonged and severe hyperthermia.

SUGGESTED READING

Glazer JL: Management of heat stroke and exhaustion, *Am Fam Physician* 71:2133, 2005.

AUTHOR: **FRED F. FERRI, M.D.**

BASIC INFORMATION

DEFINITION

Infection of the human gastric mucosa with the organism *Helicobacter pylori,* a spiral-shaped gram-negative organism with unique features that allow it to survive in the hostile gastric environment.

SYNONYMS

The organism was previously known as *Campylobacter pylori.*

ICD-9CM CODES
041.86 *Helicobacter pylori (H. pylori)*

EPIDEMIOLOGY & DEMOGRAPHICS

H. pylori is the most common chronic bacterial infection in humans, with worldwide distribution, likely affecting 50% of the earth's population in all age groups, and probably 30% to 40% of the U.S. population. Infection is acquired at an earlier age and occurs more frequently in developing nations.

PHYSICAL FINDINGS & CLINICAL PRESENTATION

- *H. pylori* causes histologic gastritis in all affected individuals. However, the majority of cases are asymptomatic and unlikely to proceed to serious consequences.
- *H. pylori* is a causative agent in peptic ulcer disease (PUD), gastric adenocarcinoma, and gastric MALT (mucosa-associated lymphoid tissue) lymphoma, and may be a risk factor for iron deficiency anemia and chronic idiopathic thrombocytopenic purpura (ITP). Presenting signs and symptoms of these disorders may include abdominal pain, bloating, anorexia, and early satiety.
- Weight loss, dysphagia, protracted nausea or vomiting, anemia, melena, and palpable abdominal mass are "alarm signs and symptoms" and should prompt more immediate and aggressive workup.

ETIOLOGY

- Route of acquisition is unknown, but is presumed to be person to person, via oral-oral or fecal-oral exposure.
- The majority of cases are acquired in childhood. Socioeconomic status and living conditions in childhood affect risk of acquisition of infection. These factors include housing density, number of siblings, overcrowding, sharing a bed, and lack of running water.
- *H. pylori* does not invade gastroduodenal tissue, but disrupts the mucous layer, causing the underlying mucosa to be more vulnerable to acid peptic damage.
- It remains unclear what differentiates the subset of patients with *H. pylori* who go on to develop ulcers or cancer.

DIAGNOSIS

DIFFERENTIAL DIAGNOSIS

- Infection with *H. pylori* should be considered in the face of peptic ulcer disease, gastric cancer, gastritis, and gastric MALT lymphoma.
- Upper GI tract disease, including nonulcer dyspepsia, reflux esophagitis, biliary tract disease, gastroparesis, pancreatitis, and ischemic bowel, may be considered in the differential diagnosis of *H. pylori.*

WORKUP

- Workup is indicated in patients with active peptic ulcer disease, a past history of documented peptic ulcer, or with gastric MALT lymphoma. A test-and-treat strategy may be employed in patients under age 55 who have no alarm symptoms.
- The role of routine screening in high-risk population is not clear. However, there are numerous studies suggesting that *H. pylori* eradication is protective against progression of premalignant lesions. Consider a test-and-treat approach in asymptomatic first-degree relatives of gastric cancer patients.
- Routine identification and treatment of *H. pylori* in cases of non-ulcer dyspepsia, GERD, NSAID use, and of asymptomatic individuals in populations at high risk for gastric cancer is considered controversial although may be indicated in specific cases.
- Efficacy of testing is related to the individual patient's likelihood of *H. pylori* infection based on demographic risk factors. In the U.S. population, increased probability of infection exists in African Americans, Hispanics/Latinos, immigrants from developing nations, patients with poor socioeconomic status, Native Americans from Alaska, and persons older than 50.
- Routine screening for *H. pylori* in asymptomatic individuals is not indicated in low-risk patients.
- There is no evidence that *H. pylori* causes symptoms of nonulcer dyspepsia.

LABORATORY TESTS

- Testing may be invasive or noninvasive, depending on the need for endoscopy. There is no indication for endoscopy solely to diagnose *H. pylori.*
- Tests for *H. pylori* may be differentiated as active or passive tests. Active tests provide direct evidence that *H. pylori* infection is currently present and include urea breath testing and stool antigen testing. Passive testing, which includes all serologic testing for *H. pylori,* gives indirect evidence of its presence, by detecting the presence of antibodies to the organism. Serologic testing is limited by its inability to distinguish between current, active infection, and prior infection that has resolved.
- Where diagnostic endoscopy is indicated (for suspicion of or follow-up of PUD or gastric MALT), antral biopsy should be tested for urease activity, or for histologic exam, if false negative on urease testing is likely (see following section).
- In cases where biopsy is not indicated, urea breath testing or stool antigen testing are indicated to evaluate for active infection. The sensitivities and specificities of these two tests are similar, above 90%. Urea breath testing is slightly more expensive than stool antigen testing, but both costs are in a modest range. Choice can be made based on patient preference and availability.
- Tests that use urease as a marker (urea breath and stool antigen tests, and biopsy for urease activity) may result in false negatives in patients on antibiotics, bismuth, or antisecretory therapy as well as those with active ulcer bleeding. Patients should be off antibiotics for 4 weeks, and off protein pump inhibitors for 2 weeks, before urea breath or stool antigen testing.
- Serologic testing may be useful in cases where the pretest probability of infection is high or where it is impractical or contraindicated to stop antisecretory medication for the required duration. It cannot be used to document eradication of infection.

TREATMENT

ACUTE GENERAL Rx

- Test only those patients whom you intend to treat if positive (indications for workup discussed at length in previous "Workup" section). At this time, the value of eradicating *H. pylori* infection is proven in patients with peptic ulcer disease or gastric MALT lymphoma.
- The optimal antibiotic regimen has not been defined. In addition to efficacy, one must take into account side effects, cost, and ease of administration.
- The following regimens are effective in 85% of patients (see first "Suggested Reading" for specific dosages):
  - PPI twice daily, with twice-daily clarithromycin and amoxicillin.
  - In cases of PCN allergy, metronidazole may be substituted for amoxicillin. This may reduce effectiveness of treatment because metronidazole resistance has increased.

- PPI twice daily, combined with bismuth 4 times daily, as well as tetracycline and metronidazole 4 times daily.
- Current data support 2-week treatment regimens. Although there are encouraging data regarding the use of 1-week regimens, recommendation for optimal treatment duration has not yet been changed.
- Prior exposure to a macrolide or metronidazole, for any reason, is associated with increased resistance. A preferable regimen would include medications the patient has not been previously exposed to.
- Diarrhea and abdominal cramping are observed commonly with many of the regimens. Other side effects may include metallic taste with metronidazole or clarithromycin, neuropathy, seizures, and disulfiram-like reaction with metronidazole, diarrhea with amoxicillin, photosensitivity with tetracycline, and *Clostridium difficile* infection with any antibiotic exposure. Bismuth may cause black stool and constipation. Tetracycline is contraindicated in pregnant patients.
- 20% of patients may fail initial therapy. Optimal retreatment regimes are under investigation. Use either an alternative regimen with a different combination of medications, or quadruple therapy consisting of twice daily PPI and bismuth-based triple therapy. Levofloxacin-based triple therapy for persistent infections appears effective in international studies, but has not been evaluated in U.S. studies. It is important to reinforce compliance.

CHRONIC Rx

- Data do not yet support routinely testing for cure. Accepted indications for testing to prove eradication include *H. pylori* associated ulcers, MALT lymphoma, and early gastric cancer, as well as those with persistent dyspepsia despite a test-and-treat management strategy.
- Serology does not reliably revert to undetectable levels after treatment and should not be used to determine eradication.
- Active tests (urea breath test and stool antigen testing) are preferable. They are equally accurate in confirming eradication, and either may be used depending on availability and patient preference. To reduce the likelihood of false-negative results, testing should be performed 4 weeks after eradication therapy with PPI and antibiotics or 2 weeks after the cessation of PPI therapy.

DISPOSITION

Consider further evaluation in patients with recurrent symptoms after appropriate treatment.

REFERRAL

- Patients with gastric MALT lymphoma should be followed by a gastroenterologist and oncologist with expertise in the care of lymphoid neoplasms.
- Patients with dyspepsia who have tested positive for *H. pylori* and been treated, without resolution of symptoms, should be referred for endoscopy.
- Consider referral for biopsy for culture and sensitivity in patients who have failed two attempts at treatment.

PEARLS & CONSIDERATIONS

COMMENTS

- It is not clear if *H. pylori* eradication reduces the risk of gastric cancer.
- Outcomes in PUD and gastric MALT lymphoma are improved with treatment of associated *H. pylori* infection.
- Tests that provide direct evidence of active *H. pylori* infection (urea breath and stool antigen testing) are preferred, but may result in false negatives in patients on antibiotics, bismuth, or antisecretory testing.
- Serologic testing is unable to differentiate active from prior infection, but may be useful in the above situations, particularly in high-risk situations.
- Be aware of high-risk populations in low-prevalence settings, including immigrants from Mexico, South America, Southeast Asia, and Eastern Europe.

SUGGESTED READINGS

Chey W, Wong B: American College of Gastroenterology Guideline on the management of *Helicobacter pylori* infection, *Am J Gastroenterol* 102:1808-1825, 2007.

Malfertheiner P et al: Current concepts in the management of Helicobacter pylori infection: the Maastricht III Consensus Report, *Gut* 56:772-781, 2007.

AUTHOR: **MARGARET TRYFOROS, M.D.**

BASIC INFORMATION

DEFINITION

The HELLP syndrome is a serious variant of preeclampsia. HELLP is an acronym for *H*emolysis, *E*levated *L*iver function, and *L*ow *P*latelet count. It is the most frequently encountered microangiopathy of pregnancy. There are three classes of the syndrome based on the degree of maternal thrombocytopenia as a primary indicator of disease severity.

Class 1: platelets 50,000/mm^3

Class 2: platelets >50,000/mm^3 to 100,000/mm^3

Class 3: platelets >100,000/mm^3

ICD-9CM CODES

642.50 HELLP, episode of care

642.51 HELLP, delivered

642.52 HELLP, delivered with postpartum complications

642.53 HELLP, antepartum complications

642.54 HELLP, postpartum complications

EPIDEMIOLOGY & DEMOGRAPHICS

- Among women with severe preeclampsia, 6% will manifest with one abnormality suggestive of HELLP syndrome, 12% will develop two abnormalities, and approximately 10% will develop all three.
- The HELLP Syndrome, like preeclampsia, is rare before 20 wk gestation.
- One third of all cases occur postpartum; of these, only 80% were diagnosed with preeclampsia before delivery.

RISK FACTORS: Women older than 35 yr, Caucasian, multiparity

RECURRENCE RATE: 3% to 25%

PHYSICAL FINDINGS & CLINICAL PRESENTATION

- Definitive laboratory criteria remain to be validated prospectively.
- Most commonly used criteria include hemolysis defined by the presence of an abnormal peripheral smear with schistocytes, lactate dehydrogenase (LDH) >600 U/L, and total bilirubin >1.2 mg/dl; elevated liver enzymes as serum aspartate aminotransferase (AST) >70 U/L and LDH >600 U/L; low platelet count as less than 100,000/mm^3.
- Although many women with HELLP syndrome will be asymptomatic, 80% report right upper quadrant pain and 50% to 60% present with excessive weight gain and worsening edema.

ETIOLOGY

As with other microangiopathies, endothelial dysfunction, with resultant activation of the intravascular coagulation cascade, has been proposed as the central pathogenesis of HELLP syndrome.

DIAGNOSIS

DIFFERENTIAL DIAGNOSIS

- Appendicitis
- Gallbladder disease
- Peptic ulcer disease
- Enteritis
- Hepatitis
- Pyelonephritis
- Systemic lupus erythematosus
- Thrombotic thrombocytopenic purpura/hemolytic uremic syndrome
- Acute fatty liver of pregnancy

WORKUP

Because the HELLP syndrome is a disease entity based on laboratory values, initial assessment is detailed as follows.

LABORATORY TESTS

- Initial assessment of suspected HELLP syndrome should include a complete blood count (CBC) to evaluate platelets, urinalysis, serum creatinine, LDH, uric acid, indirect and total bilirubin levels, and AST/ALT.
- Tests of prothrombin time, partial thromboplastin time, fibrinogen and fibrin split products are reserved for those women with a platelet count well below 100,000/mm^3.

IMAGING STUDIES

There are none to aid in diagnosis.

TREATMENT

Treatment is dependent on gestational age of the fetus, severity of HELLP, and maternal status. Stabilization of the mother is the first priority.

ACUTE GENERAL Rx

- Assess gestational age thoroughly. Fetal status should be monitored with nonstress tests, contraction stress tests, and/or biophysical profile
- Maternal status should be evaluated by history, physical examination, and laboratory testing
- Magnesium sulfate is administered for seizure prophylaxis regardless of blood pressure
- Blood pressure control is achieved with agents such as hydralazine or labetalol
- Indwelling Foley catheter to monitor maternal volume status and urine output

CHRONIC Rx

- In those pregnancies 34 wk or class 1 HELLP syndrome, delivery, either vaginal or abdominal, within 24 hr is the goal.
- In the preterm fetus, corticosteroid therapy to enhance fetal lung maturation is indicated.
- Some reports have shown temporary amelioration of HELLP severity with the administration of high dose of steroids measured by increased urine output, improvement in platelet count and LFTs.
- Judicious use of blood products, especially in those requiring surgery.
- The patient requires intensive observation for 48 hr postpartum; laboratory levels should begin to improve during this time.

DISPOSITION

The natural history of this disorder is a rapidly deteriorating condition requiring close monitoring of maternal and fetal well-being.

REFERRAL

Preterm patients with the HELLP syndrome should be stabilized hemodynamically and transferred to a tertiary care center. Term patients can be treated at a local hospital depending on the availability of obstetric, neonatal, and blood banking services.

PEARLS & CONSIDERATIONS

Not all women with HELLP have hypertension or proteinuria.

SUGGESTED READINGS

Magann EF, Martin JN: Twelve steps to optimal management of HELLP syndrome, *Clin Obstet Gynecol* 42(3):532, 1999.

Norwitz ER, Hsu CD, Repke JT: Acute complications of preeclampsia, *Clin Obstet Gynecol* 45(2):308, 2002.

AUTHORS: **SONYA S. ABDEL-RAZEQ, M.D.,** and **RUBEN ALVERO, M.D.**

BASIC INFORMATION

DEFINITION

Hemochromatosis is an autosomal recessive disorder characterized by increased accumulation of iron in various organs (adrenals, liver, pancreas, heart, testes, kidneys, pituitary) and eventual dysfunction of these organs if not treated appropriately.

SYNONYMS

Bronze diabetes

ICD-9CM CODES
275.0 Hemochromatosis

EPIDEMIOLOGY & DEMOGRAPHICS

INCIDENCE: In whites, approximately 1 in 300 persons.

PREDOMINANT SEX AND AGE: Generally diagnosed in males in their fifth decade. Diagnosis in females is generally not made until 10 to 20 yr after menopause.

GENETICS: Most common genetic disorder in North European ancestry. Homozygosity for the C282Y mutation is now found in approximately 5 of every 1000 persons of European descent.

PHYSICAL FINDINGS & CLINICAL PRESENTATION

Examination may be normal; patient with advanced case may present with the following:

- Increased skin pigmentation
- Hepatomegaly, splenomegaly, hepatic tenderness, testicular atrophy
- Loss of body hair, peripheral edema, gynecomastia, ascites
- Amenorrhea (25% of females)
- Loss of libido (50% of males)
- Arthropathy
- Joint pain (44%)
- Fatigue (45%)

ETIOLOGY

Autosomal recessive disease linked to the region of the short arm of chromosome 6 encoding HLA-A*3; the gene HFE, which contains two missense mutations (C 282Y and H 63D), was recently identified.

DIAGNOSIS

DIFFERENTIAL DIAGNOSIS

- Hereditary anemias with defect of erythropoiesis
- Cirrhosis
- Repeated blood transfusions

WORKUP

Medical history, physical examination, and laboratory evaluation should be focused on affected organ systems (see Physical Findings). Liver biopsy is the gold standard for diagnosis; it reveals iron deposition in hepatocytes, bile ducts, and supporting tissues.

LABORATORY TESTS

- Transferrin saturation is the best screening test. Values >45% are an indication for further testing. When using transferring saturation to screen individuals <40 yr, a single test may not be sufficient and sequential measurements over a period of many years should be considered to detect hemochromatosis prior to onset of fibrosis or cirrhosis. Plasma ferritin is also a good indicator of total body iron stores but may be elevated in many other conditions (inflammation, malignancy). Some authors recommend measurement of both fasting transferrin saturation and serum ferritin level as initial tests for population-based screening to detect and treat hemochromatosis before iron loading occurs.
- Elevated AST, ALT, alkaline phosphatase.
- Hyperglycemia.
- Endocrine abnormalities (decreased testosterone, LH, FSH).
- Measurement of hepatic iron index (hepatic iron concentration [HIC] divided by age) in liver biopsy specimen can confirm diagnosis.
- Genetic testing (HFE genotyping for the C282Y and H63 D mutations) may be useful in selected patients with liver disease and suspected iron overload (e.g., patients with transferrin saturation >40%). Genetic testing should not be performed as part of initial routine evaluation for hereditary hemochromatosis. Once a patient has been identified, first-degree relatives of the index patient should also be screened. The HFE gene test is a PCR-based test usually performed on whole blood sample. Cost is approximately $150 to $200.

IMAGING STUDIES

CT scan or MRI of the liver is useful to exclude other etiologies and may in some cases show iron overload in the liver.

TREATMENT

NONPHARMACOLOGIC THERAPY

Weekly phlebotomies of one or two units of blood (each containing approximately 250 mg of iron) should be continued for several weeks until depletion of iron stores is achieved (ferritin level <50 μg/ml and transferring saturation <30%). Subsequent phlebotomies can be performed on a prn basis to maintain a transferrin saturation <50% and a ferritin level <100 μg/L.

ACUTE GENERAL Rx

Deferoxamine (iron chelating agent) is generally reserved for patients with severe hemochromatosis with diffuse organ involvement (e.g., liver disease, heart disease) and when phlebotomy is not possible. It is administered in a dose of 0.5 to 1 g IM qd or 20 mg SC over a 12- to 24-hr period with a constant infusion pump.

CHRONIC Rx

Phlebotomy on a prn basis depending on the Hct level; generally, Hct should not exceed 40%.

DISPOSITION

Prognosis is good if phlebotomy is started early (before onset of cirrhosis or diabetes mellitus); women can have the full phenotypic expression of the disease, including cirrhosis, and should also be aggressively treated.

REFERRAL

For liver biopsy if diagnosis is uncertain

PEARLS & CONSIDERATIONS

COMMENTS

- Patients with hemochromatosis and serum ferritin levels <1000 mcg/L are unlikely to have cirrhosis. Liver biopsy to screen for cirrhosis may be unnecessary in such patients.
- Cirrhotic patients must be periodically monitored (ultrasound or CT scan) because of their increased risk of hepatocellular carcinoma.
- HFE gene testing for C282Y mutation is a cost-effective method of screening relatives of patients with hereditary hemochromatosis. The American College of Gastroenterology recommends genotyping persons who have abnormal iron screening tests and first-degree relatives of those identified with C282Y homozygosity.
- Established cirrhosis, hypogonadism, destructive arthritis, and insulin-dependent diabetes mellitus secondary to hemochromatosis cannot be reversed with repeated phlebotomy but their progress can be slowed.

SUGGESTED READINGS

Allen KJ et al: Iron-overload related disease in HFE hereditary hemochromatosis, *N Engl J Med* 358:221-230, 2008.

Morrison ED et al: Serum ferritin level predicts advanced hepatic fibrosis among US patients with phenotypic hemochromatosis, *Ann Intern Med* 138:627, 2003.

Pietrangelo A: Hereditary hemochromatosis, a new look at an old disease, *N Engl J Med* 350:2383, 2004.

Whitlock EP et al: Screening for hereditary hemochromatosis: A systematic review for the US Preventive Services task force, *Ann Intern Med* 145:209, 2006.

AUTHOR: **FRED F. FERRI, M.D.**

BASIC INFORMATION

DEFINITION

Hemolytic-uremic syndrome (HUS) refers to an acute syndrome characterized by hemolytic anemia, thrombocytopenia, and severe renal failure.

SYNONYMS

HUS

ICD-9CM CODES
283.11 Hemolytic-uremic syndrome

EPIDEMIOLOGY & DEMOGRAPHICS

- HUS affects mainly children younger than 10 yr
- Incidence is 2.6 cases/100,000 in people younger than 5 yr
- Incidence is 0.97 cases/100,000 in people over the age of 18
- May be epidemic, most commonly occurring during the summer months
- Most common cause of acute renal failure in children
- In the United States 300 to 700 new cases occur each year

PHYSICAL FINDINGS & CLINICAL PRESENTATION

- HUS usually preceded by diarrhea in 90% of cases
- Bloody diarrhea (75%)
- Abdominal pain
- Vomiting
- Fever
- Irritability, lethargy, and seizures (10%)
- Hypertension
- Pallor
- Anuria or oliguria

ETIOLOGY

Pathologically, it is thought that thrombin generation (probably the result of accelerated thrombogenesis) and inhibition of fibrinolysis leads to renal arteriolar and capillary microthrombi preceding renal injury.
In children:

- *E. coli* serotype O157:H7 is the leading cause of HUS.
- The infection is acquired by eating undercooked red meat, especially hamburgers.

Other causes of HUS in children and adults are:

- Drugs (cyclosporine, mitomycin, tacrolimus, ticlopidine, clopidogrel, cisplatin, quinine, penicillin, penicillamine, oral contraceptives, and quinine used to treat muscle cramps)
- Infection (*Salmonella, Shigella, Yersinia,* Group A streptococci, *Clostridium difficile, Campylobacter,* coxsackievirus, rubella, influenza virus, Epstein-Barr virus)
- Toxins
- Pregnancy (usually postpartum) and oral contraceptives
- HIV-associated thrombotic microangiopathy
- Pneumococcal infection
- Persons with relative deficiency in von Willebrand factor cleaving protease are predisposed to nonenteric infection forms of HUS

DIAGNOSIS

The triad of thrombocytopenia, acute renal failure, and microangiopathic hemolytic anemia establishes the diagnosis of HUS.

DIFFERENTIAL DIAGNOSIS

- The differential is vast, including all causes of bloody and nonbloody diarrhea because the GI symptoms usually precede the triad of HUS
- Thrombotic thrombocytopenic purpura
- Disseminated intravascular coagulation
- Prosthetic valve hemolysis
- Malignant hypertension
- Vasculitis

WORKUP

The workup for suspected HUS patients includes blood tests and stool cultures.

LABORATORY TESTS

- CBC with hemoglobin <10 g/dl
- Peripheral smear shows the hallmark microangiopathic hemolytic anemia with schistocytes, burr cells, and helmet cells
- Thrombocytopenia (platelet counts usually <60,000/mm^3)
- Reticulocyte count is high
- LDH level is elevated
- Haptoglobin is low
- Indirect bilirubin is elevated
- BUN and creatinine are elevated
- Urinalysis reveals proteinuria, microscopic hematuria, and pyuria
- Stool cultures for *E. coli* O157:H7 are positive in over 90% of cases if obtained during the first week of illness. After the first week only one third are positive

IMAGING STUDIES

Imaging studies are not very helpful in the diagnosis of HUS.

TREATMENT

The treatment of HUS is primarily supportive.

NONPHARMACOLOGIC THERAPY

- Blood transfusions for severe anemia
- Antibiotics should be avoided and are not indicated for the treatment of *E. coli* O157:H7
- Correction of electrolyte abnormalities
- Fresh Frozen Plasma may benefit patients with non-enteric forms of HUS if they are deficient in VMF-CP (von Willebrand factor cleaving protease)

ACUTE GENERAL Rx

Hypertension control

CHRONIC Rx

For anuric or oliguric renal failure, dialysis may be required.

DISPOSITION

- Adults presenting with HUS have a worse prognosis than children do with HUS.
- Mortality rate is 5%.
- Morbidity includes:
  1. Proteinuria (31%)
  2. Renal insufficiency (31%)
  3. Hypertension (6%)

REFERRAL

- The local health department should be notified if the bacteria *E. coli* O157:H7 has been isolated; large food borne outbreaks have occurred with commercial beef products and asparagus.
- Consultation with hematology and nephrology specialist is recommended in patients with HUS.

PEARLS & CONSIDERATIONS

COMMENTS

- Hemolytic-uremic syndrome was first described by Gasser and colleagues in 1955.
- Children testing positive for the *E. coli* O157:H7 serotype should not return to school or day care facilities until two consecutive stools test negative for the microorganism.
- *E. coli* O157:H7 can be transmitted from person to person, therefore universal precautions and hand washing are recommended in preventing the spread of the infection.

SUGGESTED READINGS

Butani L: Hemolytic uremic syndrome associated with Clostridium difficile colitis, *Pediatr Nephrol* 19(12):1430, 2004.

Chandler WL et al: Prothrombotic coagulation abnormalities preceding the hemolytic-uremic syndrome, *N Engl J Med* 346:23, 2002.

George JN: ADAMTS13, thrombotic thrombocytopenic purpura, and hemolytic uremic syndrome, *Curr Hematol Rep* 4(3):167, 2005.

Zipfel PF, Skerka C: Complement dysfunction in hemolytic uremic syndrome, *Curr Opin Rheumatol* 18(5):548, 2006.

AUTHORS: **GLENN G. FORT, M.D., M.P.H.,** and **DENNIS J. MIKOLICH, M.D.**

BASIC INFORMATION

DEFINITION

Hemophilia is a hereditary bleeding disorder caused by low factor VIII coagulant activity (hemophilia A) or low levels of factor IX coagulant activity (hemophilia B).

SYNONYMS

Hemophilia A: Classic hemophilia, factor VIII deficiency hemophilia
Hemophilia B: Christmas disease, factor IX hemophilia

ICD-9CM CODES
286.0 Hemophilia A
286.1 Hemophilia B

EPIDEMIOLOGY & DEMOGRAPHICS

INCIDENCE/PREVALENCE (IN U.S.): Hemophilia A: 100 cases/1 million males, hemophilia B: 20 cases/1 million males. There are approximately 400,000 patients with severe hemophilia worldwide.

GENETIC: Both hemophilias have an X-linked recessive pattern of inheritance with only males affected.

PHYSICAL FINDINGS & CLINICAL PRESENTATION

- The clinical features of hemophilia A and B are generally indistinguishable from each other.
- Bleeding is most commonly seen in joints (knees, ankles, elbows) resulting in hot, swollen, painful joints and subsequent crippling joint deformity.
- Bleeding can also occur into the muscles and the GI tract.
- Compartment syndromes can occur from large hematomas.
- Hematuria may be present.

ETIOLOGY

- Hemophilia A: low factor VIII coagulant (VIII:C) activity; can be classified as mild if factor VIII:C levels are >5%, moderate: levels are 1% to 5%, severe: levels are <1%.
- Hemophilia B: low levels of factor IX coagulant activity.
- Both disorders are congenital.
- Spontaneous acquisition of factor VIII inhibitors (acquired hemophilia) is rare.

DIAGNOSIS

DIFFERENTIAL DIAGNOSIS

- Other clotting factor deficiencies
- Platelet function disorders
- Vitamin K deficiency

WORKUP

Patients with mild hemophilia bleed only in response to major trauma or surgery and may not be diagnosed until young adulthood. Diagnostic workup includes laboratory evaluation (see Laboratory Tests).

LABORATORY TESTS

- Partial thromboplastin time (PTT) is prolonged.
- Reduced factor VIII:C level distinguishes hemophilia A from other causes of prolonged PTT.
- Factor VIII antigen, PT, fibrinogen level, and bleeding time are normal.
- Factor IX coagulant activity levels are reduced in patients with hemophilia B.
- Coagulation factor activity measurement is useful to correlate with disease severity: normal range is 50 to 150 U/dl; 5 to 20 U/dl indicates mild disease, 2 to 5 U/dl indicates moderate disease, and <2 U/dl indicates severe disease with spontaneous bleeding episodes.

TREATMENT

NONPHARMACOLOGIC THERAPY

- Avoidance of contact sports
- Patient education regarding their disease; promotion of exercises such as swimming
- Avoidance of aspirin or other NSAIDs
- Orthopedic evaluation and physical therapy evaluation in patients with joint involvement
- Hepatitis vaccination

ACUTE GENERAL Rx

HEMOPHILIA A:

- Reversal and prevention of acute bleeding in hemophilia A and B are based on adequate replacement of deficient or missing factor protein.
- The choice of the product for replacement therapy is guided by availability, capacity, concerns, and cost. Recombinant factors cost 2 to 3 times as much as plasma-derived factors, and the limited capacity to produce recombinant factors often results in periods of shortage. In the U.S., 60% of patients with severe hemophilia use recombinant products.
- Factor VIII concentrates are effective in controlling spontaneous and traumatic hemorrhage in severe hemophilia. The new recombinant factor VIII is stable without added human serum albumin (decreased risk of transmission of infectious agents).
- Recombinant activated factor VII is useful to stop spontaneous hemorrhages and prevent excessive bleeding during surgery in 75% of patients with inhibitors. Recommended dose is 90 μg/mg of body weight every 2 to 3 hr for treatment of life-threatening hemorrhage. It is, however, very expensive ($1 per μg).
- Desmopressin acetate 0.3 μg/kg q24h (causes release of factor VIII:C) may be used in preparation for minor surgical procedures in mild hemophiliacs.
- Aminocaproic acid (EACA, Amicar) 4 g PO q4h can be given for persistent bleeding that is unresponsive to factor VIII concentrate or desmopressin.

HEMOPHILIA B:

- Infuse factor IX concentrates. It is important to remember that factor IX concentrates contain other proteins that may increase the risk of thrombosis with recurrent use. Therefore factor IX concentrates must be used only when clearly indicated.
- Daily administration of oral cyclophosphamide and prednisone without empirical factor VIII therapy is an effective and well-tolerated treatment for acquired hemophilia.

CHRONIC Rx

- The aim of chronic treatment is to prevent spontaneous bleeding and to prevent excessive bleeding during any surgical intervention.
- Prophylaxis with recombinant factor VIII can prevent joint damage and decrease the frequency of joint and other hemorrhages in young boys with severe hemophilia A. The estimated annual cost for treatment of one patient with recombinant factor VIII is $300,000.
- Implantation of genetically altered fibroblasts that produce factor VIII is safe and well tolerated. This form is feasible in patients with severe hemophilia. Hemophilia will likely be the first common, severe genetic disease to be cured by gene therapy.

DISPOSITION

- Despite the advent of virally safe blood products and blood treatment programs, nearly 70% of hemophiliacs are HIV seropositive. Survival is of normal expectancy in HIV-negative patients with mild disease.
- Intracranial bleeds are the second most common cause of death in hemophiliacs after AIDS. They are fatal in 30% of patients, occur in 10% of patients, and are generally secondary to trauma.

SUGGESTED READING

Manco-Johnson MJ et al: Prophylaxis versus episodic treatment to prevent joint disease in boys with severe hemophilia, *N Engl J Med* 357:535, 2007.

AUTHOR: **FRED F. FERRI, M.D.**

BASIC INFORMATION

DEFINITION

A hemorrhoid is a varicose dilation of a vein of the superior or inferior hemorrhoidal plexus, resulting from a persistent increase in venous pressure. External hemorrhoids are below the pectinate line (inferior plexus). Internal hemorrhoids are above the pectinate line (superior plexus) (Fig. 1-116).

SYNONYMS

Piles

ICD-9CM CODES
455.6 Hemorrhoids

EPIDEMIOLOGY & DEMOGRAPHICS

Potential for development of symptomatic hemorrhoids in all adults
PREVALENCE: Estimated 50% of the adult population in the U.S.
PREDOMINANT SEX: Males = females

PHYSICAL FINDINGS & CLINICAL PRESENTATION

- Painless bleeding with defecation; bleeding is bright red and staining on toilet paper
- Perianal irritation
- Mucofecal staining of underclothes
- Acute external hemorrhoids: painful, swollen, and often thrombosed
- Pain on sitting, standing, or defecating (thrombosed hemorrhoid)
- Prolapse
- Constipation

ETIOLOGY

- Low-fiber, high-fat diet
- Chronic constipation and straining with defecation
- High resting anal sphincter pressures
- Pregnancy
- Obesity
- Rectal surgery (i.e., episiotomy)
- Prolonged sitting
- Anal intercourse

DIAGNOSIS

DIFFERENTIAL DIAGNOSIS

- Fissure
- Abscess
- Anal fistula
- Condylomata acuminata
- Hypertrophied anal papillae
- Rectal prolapse
- Rectal polyp
- Neoplasm

WORKUP

- Inspection
- Digital rectal examination
- Anoscopy
- Sigmoidoscopy

TREATMENT

NONPHARMACOLOGIC THERAPY

- Avoidance of constipation and straining with defecation
- Avoidance of prolonged sitting on toilet
- High-fiber diet (20 to 30 g/day)
- Increased fluid intake (6 to 8 glasses of water per day)
- Cleaning with mild soap and water after defecation
- Warm soaks or ice to soothe
- Sitz baths

ACUTE GENERAL Rx

- Fiber supplements to provide bulk (psyllium extracts or mucilloids)
- Medicated compresses with witch hazel
- Topical hydrocortisone (1% to 3% cream or ointment)
- Topical anesthetic spray
- Glycerin suppositories
- Stool softeners
- Surgically remove during first 72 hr after onset

CHRONIC Rx

- Rubber-band ligation
- Injection sclerotherapy
- Photocoagulation
- Cryodestruction
- Hemorrhoidectomy
- Anal dilation
- Laser or cautery hemorrhoidectomy
- Observance for complications: thrombosis, bleeding, infection, anal stenosis or weakness

DISPOSITION

Should resolve, but there is a high rate of recurrence

REFERRAL

To colorectal or general surgeon for any hemorrhoid that does not respond to conservative therapy

PEARLS & CONSIDERATIONS

COMMENTS

- Patients need to understand the importance of a healthy diet, regular exercise, and rectal hygiene.
- Stress the importance of avoiding prolonged sitting and straining on the toilet.
- Stress the need not to defer the urge to defecate.

EVIDENCE

A meta-analysis of 16 randomized controlled trials (RCTs) of various treatments for hemorrhoids including manual dilation of the anus, rubber band ligation sclerotherapy, infrared photocoagulation, and hemorrhoidectomy found that hemorrhoidectomy was significantly more effective than manual dilation of the anus and rubber band ligation, although it was associated with significantly more pain in both cases.[1] B

The meta-analysis mentioned above also found that rubber band ligation was better than sclerotherapy in response to treatment for all hemorrhoids and patients were less likely to require further therapy than those treated with sclerotherapy or infrared coagulation. However, pain was greater after rubber band ligation than after sclerotherapy or infrared coagulation.[1] B

Evidence-Based Reference

1. MacRae HM, McLeod RS: Comparison of hemorrhoidal treatment modalities: a meta-analysis, *Dis Colon Rectum* 38:697, 1995. Reviewed in: DARE Document 123208, York, UK, Centre for Reviews and Dissemination. B

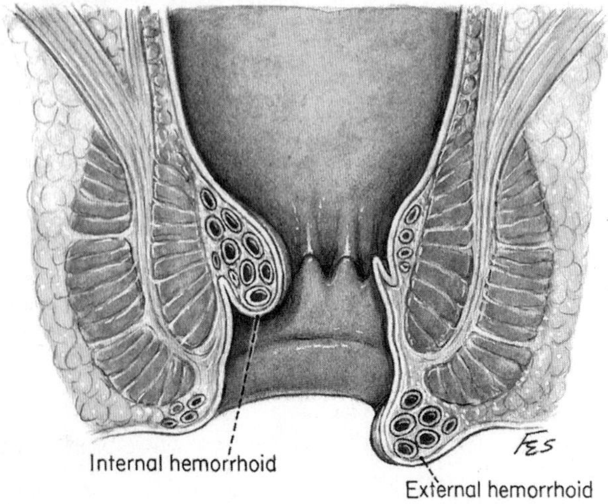

FIGURE 1-116 Anatomy of internal and external hemorrhoids. (From Noble J [ed]: *Textbook of primary care medicine,* ed 2, St Louis, 1996, Mosby.)

SUGGESTED READING

Zuber TJ: Hemorrhoidectomy for thrombosed external hemorrhoids, *Am Fam Physician* 65:1629, 2002.

AUTHORS: **MARIA A. CORIGLIANO, M.D.,** and **RUBEN ALVERO, M.D.**

BASIC INFORMATION

DEFINITION

Henoch-Schönlein purpura (HSP) is a systemic small-vessel immune-complex-mediated leukocytoclastic vasculitis characterized by a triad of palpable purpura, abdominal pain, and arthritis. It may also present with gastrointestinal bleeding, arthralgias, and renal involvement.

SYNONYMS

Anaphylactoid purpura
Allergic purpura

ICD-9CM CODES
287.0 Henoch-Schönlein purpura

EPIDEMIOLOGY & DEMOGRAPHICS

INCIDENCE: Annual incidence of 14 cases/100,000 population
PEAK INCIDENCE: Spring, although cases are seen throughout the year
PREVALENCE: Most common vasculitis seen in children and younger age groups
PREDOMINANT SEX: 2:1 male-to-female
PREDOMINANT AGE: Seen mostly from 4-15 yr, although can be seen in older adolescents and young adults

PHYSICAL FINDINGS & CLINICAL PRESENTATION

- Palpable purpura of dependent areas, especially lower extremities (Fig. 1-117), and areas subjected to pressure such as the beltline.
- Subcutaneous edema.
- Arthralgias and arthritis in 80%.
- GI symptoms are seen in approximately one third of patients. Common findings are nausea, vomiting, diarrhea, cramping, abdominal pain, hematochezia, and melena.
- Anecdotally may follow URI.
- Renal involvement is seen in up to 80% of older children, usually within the first month of illness. <5% progress to end-stage renal failure; major cause of morbidity.

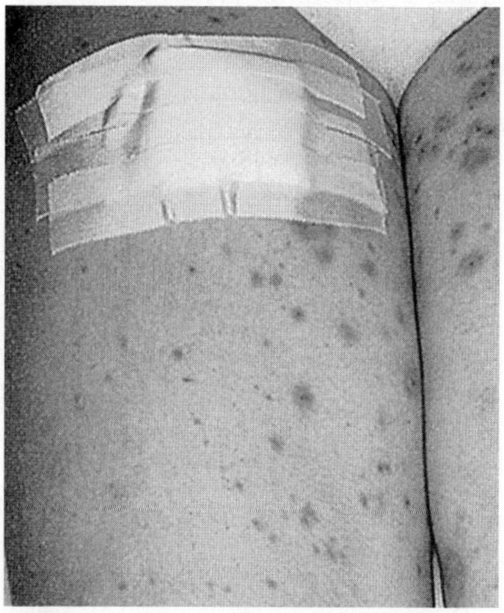

FIGURE 1-117 Henoch-Schönlein purpura on the lower extremities of a child. (Courtesy Medical College of Georgia, Division of Dermatology. From Goldstein B [ed]: *Practical dermatology,* ed 2, St Louis, 1997, Mosby.)

ETIOLOGY

- Presumptive etiology is exposure to a trigger Ag that causes Ab formation.
- Antigen-antibody (immune) complex deposition then occurs in arteriole and capillary walls of skin, renal mesangium, and GI tract. IgA deposition is most common.
- Antigen triggers postulated include drugs, foods, immunization, and upper respiratory and other viral illnesses. Group A Streptococcal infection is the most common precipitant in children, seen in up to one third of cases.
- Serologic and pathologic evidence suggests an association between Parvovirus B19 and HSP, which may explain observed cases of HSP that do not respond to corticosteroids or other immunosuppressive therapy.
- Case reports describing development of HSP following treatment with immunosuppressive agents such as etanercept have been published.

DIAGNOSIS

- Diagnosis is clinical.
- Skin manifestations are most common.
- Palpable purpura is seen in 70% of adult patients, whereas GI complaints are more common in children.
- Skin biopsy will show leukocytoclastic vasculitis.
- The presence of two of the following four American College of Rheumatology criteria yields a diagnostic sensitivity of 87.1% and specificity of 87.7%:
  - Palpable purpura unrelated to thrombocytopenia
  - Age <20 yr at onset of first symptoms
  - Bowel angina or ischemia
  - Granulocytic infiltration of arteriole or venule walls on biopsy

DIFFERENTIAL DIAGNOSIS

- Polyarteritis nodosa
- Meningococcemia
- Thrombocytopenic purpura

WORKUP

History, physical examination, laboratory testing, and skin biopsy

LABORATORY TESTS

- Electrolytes, BUN, and creatinine
- Urinalysis
- CBC
- Prothrombin time, fibrinogen, and fibrin degradation products
- Blood cultures

Laboratory abnormalities are not specific for HSP. Leukocytosis and eosinophilia may be seen. IgA levels are elevated in approximately 50% of patients. Glomerulonephritis may be present (microscopic hematuria, proteinuria, and RBC casts).

IMAGING STUDIES

Imaging studies are not useful in diagnosis of HSP. Arteriography or magnetic resonance angiography may be helpful in distinguishing from polyarteritis nodosa.

TREATMENT

- Prednisone 1 mg/kg po is given if renal or severe GI disease, although benefits are not clear.
- A recent double-blind randomized controlled trial found that early treatment with prednisone reduced abdominal pain and joint symptoms but did not prevent development of renal disease. It was effective in treatment of renal disease once established.
- Corticosteroids and azathioprine may be beneficial if rapidly progressive glomerulonephritis present. Pulse methylprednisolone therapy has also been proposed in patients with glomerulonephritis, mesenteric vasculitis, or pulmonary involvement.
- NSAIDs for arthritis and arthralgias.

NONPHARMACOLOGIC THERAPY

Supportive care with pain management, adequate hydration, and nutrition

DISPOSITION & PROGNOSIS

- Prognosis excellent with spontaneous recovery of most patients within 4 wk.
- End-stage renal disease occurs in 5% of patients. Chronic renal insufficiency is the most common long-term morbidity.
- GI complications (mesenteric infarction, perforation, and intussusception).
- Recurrences in up to one third of patients, especially within first 4 to 6 mo after initial episode, and most commonly in patients with renal involvement.

REFERRAL

To nephrologist or gastroenterologist

PEARLS & CONSIDERATIONS

- Most with spontaneous recovery within 4 wk of onset of symptoms.
- Organ systems involved are skin, joints, GI tract, and kidneys.
- Palpable purpura is more common in adults whereas GI symptoms are more common in children.
- End-stage renal disease occurs in only 5% of patients.
- Steroids and immunosuppressive agents may offer some benefit.

SUGGESTED READINGS

Ballinger S: Henoch-Schönlein purpura, *Curr Opin Rheumatol* 15:591, 2003.

Dedeoglu F: Vasculitis in children, *Pediatr Clin North Am* 52(2):547, 2005.

Dillon MJ: Henoch-Schönlein purpura (treatment and outcome), *Cleve Clin J Med* 69(Suppl 2):SII 121, 2002.

Ronkainen J et al: Early prednisone therapy in Henoch-Schönlein purpura: a randomized, double-blind, placebo controlled trial, *J Peds* 149(2):241, 2006.

AUTHOR: **DOMINICK TAMMARO, M.D.**

BASIC INFORMATION

DEFINITION

Hepatic encephalopathy (HE) is a neuropsychiatric syndrome occurring in patients with severe impairment of liver function and consequent accumulation of toxic products not metabolized by the liver.

SYNONYMS

Hepatic coma

ICD-9CM CODES
572.2 Hepatic encephalopathy

EPIDEMIOLOGY & DEMOGRAPHICS

INCIDENCE/PREVALENCE: Hepatic encephalopathy occurs in >50% of all cases of cirrhosis.

PHYSICAL FINDINGS & CLINICAL PRESENTATION

Hepatic encephalopathy can be classified in stages or grades 1 to 4:
- Grades 1 and 2: mild obtundation
- Grades 3 and 4: stupor to deep coma, with or without decerebrate posturing

The physical examination in hepatic encephalopathy varies with the stage and may reveal the following abnormalities:
- Skin: jaundice, palmar erythema, spider angiomata, ecchymosis, dilated superficial periumbilical veins (caput medusae) in patients with cirrhosis
- Eyes: scleral icterus, Kayser-Fleischer rings (Wilson's disease)
- Breath: fetor hepaticus
- Chest: gynecomastia in men with chronic liver disease
- Abdomen: ascites, small nodular liver (cirrhosis), tender hepatomegaly (congestive hepatomegaly)
- Rectal examination: hemorrhoids (portal hypertension), guaiac-positive stool (alcoholic gastritis, bleeding esophageal varices, PUD, bleeding hemorrhoids)
- Genitalia: testicular atrophy in males with chronic liver disease
- Extremities: pedal edema from hypoalbuminemia
- Neurologic: flapping tremor (asterixis), obtundation, coma with or without decerebrate posturing

ETIOLOGY

- Precipitating factors in patients with underlying cirrhosis (UGI bleeding, hypokalemia, hypomagnesemia, analgesic and sedative drugs, sepsis, alkalosis, increased dietary protein)
- Acute fulminant viral hepatitis
- Drugs and toxins (e.g., isoniazid, acetaminophen, diclofenac and other NSAIDs, statins, methyldopa, loratadine, PTU, lisinopril, labetalol, halothane, carbon tetrachloride, erythromycin, nitrofurantoin, troglitazone)
- Reye's syndrome
- Shock and/or sepsis
- Fatty liver of pregnancy
- Metastatic carcinoma, hepatocellular carcinoma
- Other: autoimmune hepatitis, ischemic venoocclusive disease, sclerosing cholangitis, heat stroke, amebic abscesses

DIAGNOSIS

DIFFERENTIAL DIAGNOSIS

- Delirium secondary to medications or illicit drugs
- CVA, subdural hematoma
- Meningitis, encephalitis
- Hypoglycemia
- Uremia
- Cerebral anoxia
- Hypercalcemia
- Metastatic neoplasm to brain
- Alcohol withdrawal syndrome

WORKUP

Exclude other etiologies with comprehensive history (obtained from patient, relatives, and others), physical examination, laboratory and imaging studies. A pertinent history should include exposure to hepatitis, ethanol intake, drug history, exposure to toxins, IV drug abuse, measles or influenza with aspirin use (Reye's syndrome), history of carcinoma (primary or metastatic).

LABORATORY TESTS

- ALT, AST, bilirubin, alkaline phosphatase glucose, calcium, electrolytes, BUN, creatinine, albumin
- CBC, platelet count, PT, PTT
- Serum and urine toxicology screen in suspected medication or illegal drug use
- Blood and urine cultures, urinalysis
- Venous ammonia level
- ABGs

IMAGING STUDIES

CT scan of head may be useful in selected patients to exclude other etiologies.

TREATMENT

NONPHARMACOLOGIC THERAPY

- Identification and treatment of precipitating factors
- Restriction of protein intake (30 to 40 g/day) to reduce toxic protein metabolites

ACUTE GENERAL Rx

REDUCTION OF COLONIC AMMONIA PRODUCTION:
- Lactulose 30 ml of 50% solution qid initially, dose is subsequently adjusted depending on clinical response. Ornithine aspartate 9 g tid is also effective. Lactulose may improve hepatic encephalopathy but may be less effective than antibiotics.
- Neomycin 1 g PO q4 to 6h or given as a 1% retention enema solution (1 g in 100 ml of isotonic saline solution); neomycin should be used with caution in patients with renal insufficiency; metronidazole 250 mg qid may be as effective as neomycin and is not nephrotoxic; however, long-term use can be associated with neurotoxicity. Rifaximin 1200 mg/day is a viable alternative to metronidazole.
- A combination of lactulose and neomycin can be used when either agent is ineffective alone.

TREATMENT OF CEREBRAL EDEMA: Cerebral edema is often present in patients with acute liver failure, and it accounts for nearly 50% of deaths. Monitoring intracranial pressure by epidural, intraparenchymal, or subdural transducers and treatment of cerebral edema with mannitol (100 to 200 ml of 20% solution [0.3 to 0.4 g/kg of body weight]) given by rapid IV infusion is helpful in selected patients (e.g., potential transplantation patients); dexamethasone and hyperventilation (useful in head injury) are of little value in treating cerebral edema from liver failure.

CHRONIC Rx

- Avoidance of any precipitating factors (e.g., high-protein diet, medications)
- Consideration of liver transplantation in selected patients with progressive or recurrent encephalopathy

DISPOSITION

Prognosis varies with the underlying etiology of the liver failure and the grade of encephalopathy (generally good for grades 1, 2; poor for grades 3, 4).

REFERRAL

The early stages of hepatic encephalopathy can be managed in the outpatient setting, whereas stages 3 or 4 require hospital admission.

PEARLS & CONSIDERATIONS

COMMENTS

Patients not responding to supportive therapy should be evaluated for liver transplantation.

AUTHOR: **FRED F. FERRI, M.D.**

BASIC INFORMATION

DEFINITION

Hepatitis A is generally an acute self-limiting infection of the liver by an enterically transmitted picorna virus, hepatitis A virus (HAV). Infection may range from asymptomatic to fulminant hepatitis.

SYNONYMS

Infectious hepatitis
Short incubation hepatitis
Type A hepatitis
HAV (hepatitis A virus)

ICD-9CM CODES
070.1 Hepatitis A

EPIDIMIOLOGY & DEMOGRAPHICS

INCIDENCE:
- It occurs worldwide, affecting 1.4 million people annually and accounting for 20% to 40% of cases of viral hepatitis in the U.S.
- The seroprevalence increases with age, ranging from 10% in individuals <5 yr to 74% in those >50 yr.
- In the U.S. average disease rate is approximately 15 cases/100,000 persons/yr.
- The incidence is relatively higher in some regions in the U.S., including Arizona, Alaska, California, Idaho, Nevada, New Mexico, Okalahoma, Oregon, South Dakota, and Washington.
- At-risk groups include:
  1. Residents and staff of group homes
  2. Children, employees of day care centers
  3. Persons who engage in oral-anal contact, regardless of sexual orientation
  4. Intravenous drug abusers
  5. Travel to endemic areas
  6. Areas of overcrowding, poor sanitation, inadequate sewage treatment

PREVALENCE:
- Approximately three fourths of U.S. population has serologic evidence of prior infection
- Anti-HAV prevalence has inverse relation to income and household size

PREDOMINANT SEX: None, except higher infection rates seen in homosexual males who engage in oral-anal contact.

PREDOMINANT AGE/PEAK INCIDENCE:
- In areas of high rates of hepatitis A, virtually all children are infected while younger than 10 yr, but disease is rare.
- In areas of moderate rates of hepatitis A, disease occurs in late childhood and young adults.
- In areas of low rates of hepatitis A, most cases occur in young adults.

INCUBATION PERIOD: Averages 30 days (15 to 50)

PHYSICAL FINDINGS & CLINICAL PRESENTATION

- Infection with HAV may have acute or subacute presentation, icteric or anicteric. Severity of illness seems to increase with age (90% of infection in children <5 yr may be subclinical)
- A preicteric, prodromal phase of approximately 1 to 14 days. 15% no apparent prodrome. Symptoms are usually abrupt in onset and may include anorexia, malaise, nausea, vomiting, fever, headache, abdominal pain
- Less common symptoms are chills, myalgias, arthralgias, upper respiratory symptoms, constipation, diarrhea, pruritis, urticaria
- Jaundice occurs in >70% of patients
- The icteric phase is preceded by dark urine
- Bilirubinuria is typically followed a few days later by clay-colored stools and icterus

PHYSICAL EXAMINATION

- Jaundice
- Hepatomegaly
- Splenomegaly
- Cervical lymphadenopathy
- Evanescent rash
- Petechiae
- Cardiac arrhythmias

COMPLICATIONS

- Cholestasis
- Fulminant hepatitis
- Arthritis
- Myocarditis
- Optic neuritis
- Transverse myelitis
- Thrombocytopenic purpura
- Aplastic anemia
- Red cell aplasia
- Henoch-Schonlein purpura
- IgA dominant glomerulonephritis

ETIOLOGY

- Caused by HAV, a 27 nm, nonenveloped, icosahedral, positive-stranded RNA virus.
- Transmission is fecal-oral route, from person to person. Transmission occurs with close contact or with food or water borne outbreaks with inadequately purified water or cooked foods. Recent outbreaks have involved green onions and tomatoes.
- Parenteral transmission is considered rare.
- Vertical transmission also reported.

DIAGNOSIS

DIFFERENTIAL DIAGNOSIS

- Other hepatitis virus (B, C, D, E)
- Infectious mononucleosis
- Cytomegalovirus infection
- Herpes simplex virus infection
- Leptospirosis
- Brucellosis
- Drug-induced liver disease
- Ischemic hepatitis
- Autoimmune hepatitis

WORKUP

- IgM antibody specific for HAV
- Liver function tests; ALT and AST elevations are sensitive for liver damage but not specific for HAV
- Elevated ESR
- CBC; may find mild lymphocytosis

LABORATORY TESTS

- Diagnosis confirmed by IgM anti HAV; it is detectable in almost all infected patients at presentation and remains positive for 3 to 6 mo
- A fourfold rise in titer of total antibody (IgM and IgG) to HAV confirms acute infection
- HAV detection in stool and body fluids by electron microscopy
- HAV RNA detection in stool, body fluids, serum, and liver tissue
- ALT and AST usually more than eight times normal in acute infection
- Bilirubin usually 5 to 15 times normal
- Alkaline phosphatase minimally elevated but higher level in cholestasis
- Albumin and prothrombin time are generally normal, if elevated may herald hepatic necrosis

IMAGING STUDIES

- Rarely useful
- Sonogram (fulminant hepatitis)

TREATMENT

- Usually self-limited
- Supportive care
- Those with fulminant hepatitis may require hospitalization and treatment of associated complications
- Activity as tolerated
- Advise to avoid alcohol and hepatotoxic drugs
- Patients with fulminant hepatitis should be assessed for liver transplantation

CHRONIC Rx

No chronic HAV and no chronic carrier state

DISPOSITION

Follow-up as outpatient

REFERRAL

- To a hepatologist if severe, fulminant hepatitis develops
- To a transplant surgeon if liver transplant becomes a consideration for fulminant hepatitis and liver failure

PEARLS & CONSIDERATIONS

- All cases of hepatitis A should be reported to the public heath authorities because food-borne or water-borne outbreaks may occur, and pubic health efforts (mass vaccination or immunoglobulin therapy) may avert secondary cases.
- Hepatitis A is a common illness in internationally traveled and developing countries. Pretravel vaccination is strongly recommended for travelers who are HAV susceptible.

PREVENTION

- Improvement in hygiene and sanitation
- Heating food
- Avoidance of water and foods from endemic area

PASSIVE IMMUNIZATION

- Immunoglobulin provides protection against HAV through passive transfer of antibody.
- Preexposure prophylaxis indicated for person traveling to endemic areas (IG 0.02 or 0.06 ml/kg given IM). The lower dose is effective for up to 3 months, and the higher dose is effective for up to 5 months.
- Postexposure prophylaxis (IG 0.02 ml/kg given IM) is indicated for persons with recent exposure (within 2 wk) to HAV and who have not been previously vaccinated. In high-risk patients vaccine may be administered with immunoglobulin.

ACTIVE IMMUNIZATION

- There are several inactivated and attenuated hepatitis vaccines; only the inactivated vaccines are currently available for use and they have been found to be safe and highly immunogenic: HAVRIX or VAQTA. These can be used in adults and children over the age of 12 months. A combined hepatitis A and hepatitis B vaccine called TWINRX is also available.
- Protective antibody levels were reached in 94% to 100% of adults 1 mo after the first dose, similar results have been found for children and adolescents.
- Theoretic analyses of antibody levels estimate duration of immunity to be 10 to 20 yr
- Vaccine should be considered for persons who are at risk: those traveling to or working in endemic areas, homosexual men, illegal drug users, persons with chronic liver disease, children in areas with high rates of hepatitis A infection

SUGGESTED READINGS

Fiore AE et al: Prevention of hepatitis A through active or passive immunization: recommendations of the Advisory Committee on Immunization Practices (ACIP), *MMWR Recomm Rep* 55(RR-7):1, 2006.

Jenson HB: The changing picture of hepatitis A in the United States, *Curr Opin Pediatr* 16(1):89, 2004.

Leach CT: Hepatitis A in the United States, *Pediatr Infect Dis J* 23(6):551, 2004.

Rezende G. et al: Viral and clinical factors associated with the fulminant course of hepatitis A infection, *Hepatology* 38:613, 2003.

Victor JC et al: Hepatitis A vaccine versus immuneglobulin for postexposure prophylaxis, *N Engl J Med* 357:1685-1694, 2007.

AUTHORS: **GLENN G. FORT, M.D., M.P.H., DENNIS J. MIKOLICH, M.D.,** and **VASANTHI ARUMUGAM, M.D.**

BASIC INFORMATION

DEFINITION

Hepatitis B is an acute infection of the liver parenchymal cells caused by the hepatitis B virus (HBV).

SYNONYMS

Serum hepatitis
Long incubation (30 to 180 days) Hepatitis

ICD-9CM CODES
070.3 Hepatitis B

EPIDEMIOLOGY & DEMOGRAPHICS

INCIDENCE (IN U.S.):

- Approximately 200,000 to 300,000 infections annually in U.S.
- Much higher incidence in Europe (approximately 1 million new cases annually) and in areas of high endemicity.
- In U.S., transmission is mainly horizontal (percutaneous and mucous membrane exposure to infectious blood and other body fluids, [e.g., sexual transmission, either homosexual or heterosexual]); also from needle sharing amongst drug abusers; occupational exposure to contaminated blood and blood products; persons receiving transfusions of blood and blood products; hemodialysis patients.

NOTE: Improved screening of blood and blood products has greatly reduced, although not eliminated, the risk of post-transfusion HBV infection.

- In areas of high endemicity, transmission is largely vertical (perinatal): HBV exists in the blood and body fluids. Perinatal transmission from HBsAg-positive mothers is as high as 90% unless immunoprophylaxis is given.

PEAK INCIDENCE: 30 to 45 yr of age, at rates of 5% to 20%

PREVALENCE (IN U.S.):

- North America, Western Europe, and Australia are areas of low prevalence, <2%.
- Africa, Asia, and the Western Pacific region are areas of high prevalence, ≥8%.
- Southern and Eastern Europe have intermediate rates, 2% to 7%.
- Chronically infected persons, those with positive HBsAg for >6 mo, represent the major source of infection.
- Up to 95% of infants and children <5 yr of age, who typically have subclinical acute infection, will become chronic HBV carriers.
- Adults are more likely to have clinically evident acute infection, but only 1% to 5% will develop chronic infection.
- Approximately 0.1% with acute infection will develop fulminant acute hepatitis resulting in death.

PREDOMINANT SEX:

- Predominant in males because of increased intravenous drug abuse, homosexuality
- Females more commonly terminate in chronic carrier state

PREDOMINANT AGE: 20 to 45 yr

GENETICS:

Neonatal infection:

- Rare in U.S.
- High (up to 90%) in areas of high endemicity (only 5% to 10% of perinatal infections occur in utero)

PHYSICAL FINDINGS & CLINICAL PRESENTATION (Fig. 1-118)

- Often nonspecific symptoms
- Profound malaise
- Many asymptomatic cases
- Prodrome:
  1. 15% to 20% serum sickness (urticaria, rash, arthralgia) during early HBsAg
  2. HBsAg-Ab complex disease (polyarteritis nodosa–arthritis, arteritis, glomerulonephritis)
- Hepatomegaly (87%) with RUQ tenderness
  1. Hepatic punch tenderness
  2. Splenomegaly: rare (10% to 15%)
- Jaundice, dark urine, with occasional pruritus
- Variable fever (when present, generally precedes jaundice and rapidly declines following onset of icteric phase)
- Spider angiomata: rare; resolves during recovery
- Rare polyarteritis nodosa, cryoglobulinemia

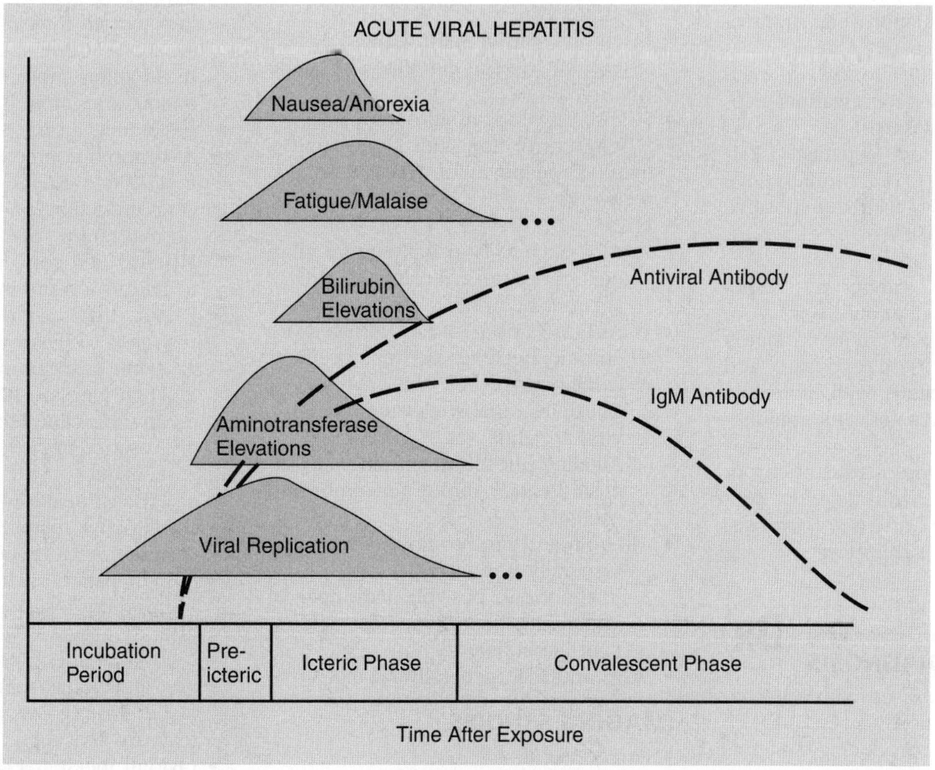

FIGURE 1-118 The typical course of acute viral hepatitis. (From Goldman L, Ausiello D [eds]: *Cecil textbook of medicine,* ed 22, Philadelphia, 2004, WB Saunders.)

ETIOLOGY

- Caused by hepatitis B virus (42-nm hepadnavirus with an outer surface coat [HBsAg], inner nucleocapsid core [HBcAg; HBeAg]; DNA polymerase; and partially double-stranded DNA genome)
- Transmission by parenteral route (needle use, tattooing, ear piercing, acupuncture, transfusion of blood and blood products, hemodialysis, sexual contact), perinatal transmission
- Infection may result from contact of infectious material with mucous membranes and open skin breaks (e.g., HBV is stable and can be transmitted from toothbrushes, utensils, razors, baby toys, various medical equipment [respirators, endoscopes])
- Oral intake of infectious material may result in infection through breaks in the oral mucosa
- Food or water virtually never found to be sources of HBV infection
- Infection occurring primarily in liver, where necrosis probably results from cytotoxic T-cell response, direct cytopathic effect of HBcAg (core antigen), high-level HBsAg (surface antigen) expression, or co-infection with delta (D) hepatitis virus (RNA delta core within HBsAg envelope)
- Recovery (>90%):
  1. Fulminant hepatitis occurring in <1% (especially if coinfected with hepatitis D); 80% fatal
  2. Unusual (5%) prolonged acute disease for 4 to 12 mo, with recovery
  3. Overall fatality increases with age and viral inoculation (e.g., transfusions)
- Chronic infection (1% to 2%):
  1. Persistent carrier state without hepatitis (HBsAg positive)
  2. Chronic persistent hepatitis (CPH) (clinically well), or chronic active hepatitis (CAH) (HBsAg positive and HBeAg positive)
  3. Cirrhosis
  4. Hepatocellular carcinoma (especially after neonatal infection)
  5. Chronic infection: more common following low-dose exposure and mild acute hepatitis, with earlier age of infection, in males, or if immunosuppressed
  6. One third to one quarter of chronically infected will develop progressive liver disease (cirrhosis, hepatocellular carcinoma)

DIAGNOSIS Dx

DIFFERENTIAL DIAGNOSIS

- Acute disease confused with other viral hepatitis infections (A, C, D, E)
- Any viral illness producing systemic disease and hepatitis (e.g., yellow fever, EBV, CMV, HIV, rubella, rubeola, coxsackie B, adenovirus, herpes simplex or zoster)
- Nonviral etiologies of hepatitis (e.g., leptospirosis, toxoplasmosis, alcoholic hepatitis, drug-induced [e.g., acetaminophen, INH], toxic hepatitis [carbon tetrachloride, benzene])

WORKUP

- Acute serum specimen for hepatitis B serology (HBsAg, HBsAb, HBcAb, HBeAg, HBeAb), HBDNA
- LFTs
- CBC
- Liver biopsy: rarely indicated for diagnosis of fulminant viral hepatitis, chronic hepatitis, cirrhosis, carcinoma

LABORATORY TESTS

- Diagnosis of acute HBV infection is best confirmed by IgM HBcAb in acute or early convalescent serum or by HBDNA.
  1. Generally, IgM present during onset of jaundice
  2. Coexisting HBsAg
- HBsAg and IgG-HBcAb during acute jaundice are strongly suggestive of remote HBV infection and another etiology for current illness.
- HBsAb alone is suggestive of immunization response.
- With recovery, HBeAg is rapidly replaced by HBeAb in 2 to 3 mo, and HBsAg is replaced by HBsAb in 5 to 6 mo.
- In chronic HBV hepatitis, HBsAg and HBeAg are persistent without corresponding Ab.
- In chronic carrier state, HBsAg is persistent, but HBeAg is replaced by HBe AB.
- HBcAb develops in all outcomes.
- HBeAg correlation with highest infectivity; appearance of HBeAb heralds recovery.
- LFTs:
  1. ALT and AST: usually more than eight times normal (often 1000 U/L) at onset of jaundice (minimal acute ALT/AST rises often followed by chronic hepatitis or hepatocellular carcinoma)
  2. Bilirubin: variably elevated in icteric viral hepatitis
  3. Alkaline phosphatase: minimally elevated (one to three times normal) acutely
- Albumin and prothrombin time:
  1. Generally normal
  2. If abnormal, possible harbinger of impending hepatic necrosis (fulminant hepatitis)
- WBC and ESR: generally normal

IMAGING STUDIES

- Rarely useful
- Sonogram to document rapid reduction in liver size during fulminant hepatitis or mass in hepatocellular carcinoma

TREATMENT Rx

NONPHARMACOLOGIC THERAPY

- Symptomatic treatment as necessary
- Activity as tolerated
- High-calorie diet preferred; often best tolerated in morning

ACUTE GENERAL Rx

- In most cases of acute HBV infection no treatment necessary; >90% of adults will spontaneously clear infection
- Hospitalization advisable for any patient in danger from dehydration caused by poor oral intake, whose PT is prolonged, who has rising bilirubin level >15 to 20 μg/dl, or who has any clinical evidence of hepatic failure
- IV therapy needed (rarely) for hydration during severe vomiting
- Avoid hepatically metabolized drugs
- No therapeutic measures are beneficial
- Steroids not shown helpful

CHRONIC Rx

The aim of therapy in chronic HBV infection is to eradicate the virus.

The two modalities of therapy available to achieve this goal have been: immune modulators (interferon alpha) and antiviral agents in the form of nucleoside analogues (e.g., lamivudine).

- Until recently, IFN-α given SQ either daily or thrice weekly for 16 to 24 weeks had been the mainstay of therapy. Its mechanism of action is to stimulate the immune system to attack HBV-infected hepatocytes, thus inhibiting viral protein synthesis. Currently, use of pegylated IFN-α offers more convenient administration and more sustained viral suppression as a once a week SQ injection.
- A 4-month course of treatment results in a 30% to 40% response with significant reduction of serum HBV DNA, normalization of ALT, and loss of HBeAg. Seroconversion from HBeAg to HBeAb occurs in 15% to 20%.
- Factors that increase the likelihood of response to IFN-α therapy include:
  1. Adult onset of infection
  2. High baseline ALT
  3. Low baseline HBV DNA
  4. Absence of cirrhosis
  5. Female
  6. HBeAg positive
- Infrequent relapse after successful completion of therapy.
- 80% of patients who lose HBeAg during therapy lose HBsAg in the decade after therapy.
- >50% of patients who do not seroconvert after initial therapy develop a delayed HBeAg seroconversion months to years after therapy.
- Overall incidence of cirrhosis and hepatocellular carcinoma is decreased in those treated with IFN-α.

- IFN-α is successful only in patients with an active immune response; therefore it is not effective in patients with HIV infection and organ transplant patients.
- Asians respond poorly to IFN-α.
- Treatment with IFN-α in general is also poorly tolerated: side effects include flulike symptoms, injection-site reactions, rash, weight loss, anxiety, depression, alopecia, thrombocytopenia, granulocytopenia, thyroid dysfunction.
- Nucleoside analogues block viral replication by inhibiting HBV polymerase.
- Lamivudine was the first nucleoside analogue approved for treatment of chronic HBV infection; it has been shown to rapidly reduce HBV replication and suppress HBV DNA to undetectable levels after a few weeks of treatment, and treatment for 1 yr is as effective as IFN-α with respect to loss of HBeAg seroconversion to HBeAb and loss of HBV DNA. Emergence of resistant HBV strains while on therapy has limited the use of lamivudine (YMDD variants [tyrosine-methionine-aspartate-aspartate]).
- Adefovir dipivoxil is a nucleotide reverse transcriptase inhibitor that also has antiviral activity against HBV. It is a prodrug that is converted to the active drug adefovir. It is highly active against HBV and may be useful as a first-line agent or as salvage therapy for patients who are refractory or intolerant to lamivudine. (Nephrotoxicity is a potential side effect, but emergence of resistant strains is less than with lamivudine.)
- Entecavir is the latest nucleoside agent approved for the treatment of hepatitis B, and it appears to be more effective and to present fewer concerns than lamivudine or adefovir regarding the emergence of resistant strains.
- Combination therapy with two or three nucleoside analogues or combination therapy with IFN-α currently under investigation.
- Liver transplantation (consider for fulminant hepatitis).

DISPOSITION

- Follow-up as outpatient
- Acute disease: usually <6 wk
- Rare fatalities (fulminant hepatitis)
- Possible chronic carrier state, cirrhosis, hepatocellular carcinoma

REFERRAL

To infectious disease specialist and gastroenterologist for consultation regarding fulminant hepatitis or prolonged cholestasis, for cases of uncertain etiology, or for treatment of chronic active hepatitis

PEARLS & CONSIDERATIONS

COMMENTS

- Virus and HBsAg in high titers in blood for 1 to 7 wk before jaundice and for a variable time thereafter.
- Transmission is possible during entire period of HBsAg (and especially during HBeAg) in serum.
- Universal precautions should be followed for all contacts with blood or secretions/excretions contaminated with blood.
- Preventing before exposure:
  1. Lifestyle changes
  2. Meticulous testing of blood supply (although some chronically infected, infectious donors are HBsAg negative)
  3. Sterilization via steam or hypochlorite
  4. Hepatitis B vaccine for high-risk groups given IM in deltoid to induce HBsAb (response should be confirmed) is protective (>90% effective)
  5. Recommendation for universal childhood immunization with doses at birth, 1 mo, and 6 mo
- Prevention after exposure:
  1. HBV hyperimmune globulin (HBIG) given immediately after needlestick, within 14 days of sexual exposure, or at birth, followed by HBV vaccination
  2. Standard immune globulin: nearly as effective as HBIG

Hepatitis B prophylaxis is described in Section V.

EVIDENCE

A meta-analysis of adults who were chronic carriers of hepatitis B virus and who were positive for HBsAg and HBeAg found that INF-α effectively terminated viral replication and eradicated the carrier state compared with control.[1] B

A systematic review found that loss of HBeAg and HBV DNA was significantly more frequent in patients receiving pretreatment corticosteroids before alpha-interferon therapy compared with those receiving INF-α treatment alone for chronic hepatitis B. Evidence for the effect of pretreatment with corticosteroids on clinical outcomes is lacking.[2] A

A randomized controlled trial (RCT) compared lamivudine with placebo in patients with chronic hepatitis B. Lamivudine was significantly more effective than placebo for the improvement of hepatic necroinflammatory activity.[3] B

Evidence-Based References

1. Wong DK et al: Effect of alpha-interferon treatment in patients with hepatitis B e antigen-positive chronic hepatitis B. A meta-analysis, *Ann Intern Med* 119:312, 1993. B
2. Mellerup MT et al: Sequential combination of glucocorticosteroids and alfa interferon versus alfa interferon alone for HBeAg-positive chronic hepatitis B, *Cochrane Database Syst Rev* 2, 2002. A
3. Lai CL et al: A one-year trial of lamivudine for chronic hepatitis B. Asia Hepatitis Lamivudine Study Group, *N Engl J Med* 339:61, 1998. B

SUGGESTED READINGS

Chang TT et al: A comparison of entecavir and lamivudine for HbeAg-positive chronic hepatitis B, *N Engl J Med* 354(10):1001, 2006.

Jonas MM et al: Clinical trial of lamivudine in children with chronic hepatitis B, *N Engl J Med* 346(22):1706, 2002.

Lai CL et al: Telbivudine versus lamivudine in patients with chronic hepatitis B, *N Engl J Med* 357:2576-2588, 2007.

Lok AS, McMahon BJ: Chronic hepatitis B (AASLD practice guidelines), *Hepatology* 45:507, 2007.

Van der Wielen M et al: Hepatitis A/B vaccination of adults over 40 years old: comparison of three vaccine regimens and effect of influencing factors, *Vaccine* 24(26):5509, 2006.

Westland CE et al: Activity of adefovir dipivoxil against all patterns of lamuvidine-resistant hepatitis B viruses in patients, *J Viral Hep* 12:67, 2005.

AUTHORS: **GLENN G. FORT, M.D., M.P.H., DENNIS J. MIKOLICH, M.D.,** and **JANE V. EASON, M.D.**

Section I DISEASES AND DISORDERS

BASIC INFORMATION

DEFINITION

Hepatitis C is an acute liver parenchymal infection caused by hepatitis C virus (HCV).

SYNONYMS

Transfusion-related non-A, non-B hepatitis (incubation period averages 6 wk, intermediate between hepatitis A and B)

ICD-9CM CODES
070.51 Other viral hepatitis

EPIDEMIOLOGY & DEMOGRAPHICS

Hepatitis C infection is the most common chronic blood-borne infection in the U.S.

INCIDENCE (IN U.S.):
- 150,000 new cases/yr (37,500, symptomatic; 93,000, later chronic liver disease; 30,700, cirrhosis)
- Approximately 9000 of these ultimately die of HCV infection; most common (40%) cause of nonalcoholic liver disease in U.S.

PREVALENCE (IN U.S.):
- Overall prevalence of anti-HCV antibody is 1.8% (an estimated 3.9 million persons nationwide)
- Highest prevalence in hemophiliacs transfused before 1987 and users of injection drugs, 72% to 90%
- Among low-risk groups, prevalence 0.6%

PREDOMINANT SEX: Slight male predominance

PREDOMINANT AGE: Highest prevalence in 30- to 49-yr age group (65%)

PEAK INCIDENCE:
- 20 to 39 yr of age
- African Americans and whites have similar incidence of acute disease; Hispanics have higher rates
- Prevalence substantially higher among non-Hispanic blacks than among non-Hispanic whites

GENETICS: Neonatal infection is rare; increased risk with maternal HIV-1 coinfection

PHYSICAL FINDINGS & CLINICAL PRESENTATION

- Symptoms usually develop 7 to 8 wk after infection (2 to 26 wk), but 70% to 80% of cases are subclinical.
- 10% to 20% report acute illness with jaundice and nonspecific symptoms (abdominal pain, anorexia, malaise).
- Fulminant hepatitis may rarely occur during this period.
- After acute infection, 15% to 25% have complete resolution (absence of HCV RNA in serum, normal ALT).
- Progression to chronic infection is common, 50% to 84%. 74% to 86% have persistent viremia; spontaneous clearance of viremia in chronic infection is rare. 60% to 70% of patients will have persistent or fluctuating ALT levels; 30% to 40% with chronic infection have normal ALT levels.
- 15% to 20% of those with chronic HCV will develop cirrhosis over a period of 20 to 30 yr; in most others, chronic infection leads to hepatitis and varying degrees of fibrosis.
- 0.4% to 2.5% of patients with chronic infection develop hepatocellular carcinoma.
- 25% of patients with chronic infection continue to have an asymptomatic course with normal LFTs and benign histology.
- In chronic HCV infection, extrahepatic sequelae include a variety of immunologic and lymphoproliferative disorders (e.g., cryoglobulinemia, membranoproliferative glomerulonephritis, and possibly Sjögren's syndrome, autoimmune thyroiditis, polyarteritis nodosa, aplastic anemia, lichen planus, porphyria cutanea tarda, B-cell lymphoma, others).

ETIOLOGY

- Caused by HCV (single-stranded RNA flavivirus).
- Most HCV transmission is parenteral.
- In the U.S., advances in screening of blood and blood products in 1990 and 1992 have made transfusion-related HCV infection rare (the risk is estimated to be 0.001% per unit transfused).
- Injecting-drug use accounts for most HCV transmission in the U.S. (60% of newly acquired cases, 20% to 50% of chronically infected persons).
- Occupational needlestick exposure from an HCV-positive source has a seroconversion rate of 1.8% (range 0% to 7%).
- Nosocomial transmission rates (from surgery and procedures such as colonoscopy, hemodialysis) are extremely low.
- Sexual transmission and maternal-fetal transmission are infrequent (estimated at 5%).
- No identifiable risk in 40% to 50% of community-acquired hepatitis C, but snorting of cocaine by shared use of straw or rolled-up paper has been identified as a risk factor due to microscopic bleeding of nasal mucosa.
- HCV infection may stimulate production of cytotoxic T lymphocytes and cytokines (inf-γ), which likely mediate hepatic necrosis.

DIAGNOSIS

DIFFERENTIAL DIAGNOSIS

- Other hepatitis viruses (A, B, D, E)
- Other viral illnesses producing systemic disease (e.g., yellow fever, EBV, CMV, HIV, rubella, rubeola, coxsackie B, adenovirus, HSV, HZV)
- Nonviral hepatitis (e.g., leptospirosis, toxoplasmosis, alcoholic hepatitis, drug-induced hepatitis [acetaminophen, INH], toxic hepatitis)

WORKUP

- Acute hepatitis C antibody (Table 1-18)
- LFTs; CBC

NOTE: ALT is an easy and inexpensive test to monitor infection and efficacy of therapy. However, ALT levels may fluctuate or even be normal in active or chronic infection and even with cirrhosis, and ALT may remain elevated even after clearance of viremia.

- Liver biopsy with histologic staging is the gold standard for assessing the degree of disease activity and the likelihood of disease progression, and also to help rule out other causes of liver disease

LABORATORY TESTS

Diagnosis is often by exclusion, because it takes 6 wk to 12 mo to develop anti-HCV antibody (70% positive by 6 wk, 90% positive by 6 mo).

Diagnostic tests include serologic assays for antibodies and molecular tests for viral particles.

1. Enzyme immunoassay is the test for anti-HCV antibody:
   - The current version can detect antibody within 4 to 10 wk after infection
   - False-negative rate in low-risk populations is 0.5% to 1%
   - False-negatives also in immune-compromised persons, HIV-1, renal failure, HCV-associated essential mixed cryoglobulinemia
   - False positives in autoimmune hepatitis, paraproteinemia, and persons with no risk factors
2. Recombinant immunoblot is used to confirm positive enzyme immunoassays:
   - Recommended only in low-risk settings
3. Qualitative and quantitative HCV RNA tests using PCR:
   - Lower limit of detection is <100 copies HCV RNA/ml
   - Used to confirm viremia and to assess response to treatment
   - Qualitative PCR useful in patients with negative enzyme immunoassay in whom infection is suspected
   - Quantitative tests use either branched-chain DNA or reverse transcription PCR; the latter is more sensitive
4. Viral genotyping can distinguish among genotypes 1, 2, 3, and 4, which is helpful in choosing therapy; most of these tests use PCR (NOTE: genotypes 1, 2, 3, and 4 predominate in the U.S. and Europe [1 is especially common in North America])

TABLE 1-18 Tests for Hepatitis C Virus Infection

Test/Type	Application	Comments
Hepatitis C Virus Antibody (anti-HCV)		
EIA	Indicates past or present infection but does not differentiate among acute, chronic, or resolved infection	Sensitivity ≥97%
Supplemental assay (i.e., RIBA)	All positive EIA results should be verified with a supplemental assay	EIA alone has low-positive predictive value in low-prevalence populations
HCV RNA		
*Qualitative Tests**†		
RT-PCR amplification of HCV RNA by in-house or commercial assays (e.g., Amplicor HCV)	Detect presence of circulating HCV RNA	Detects virus as early as 1-2 wk after exposure
	Monitor patients on antiviral therapy	Detection of HCV RNA during course of infection might be intermittent; a single negative RT-PCR is not conclusive
		False-positive and false-negative results might occur
*Quantitative Tests**†		
RT-PCR amplification of HCV RNA by in-house or commercial assays (e.g., Amplicor HCV monitor)	Determine concentration of HCV RNA	Less sensitive than qualitative RT-PCR
bDNA assays (e.g., Quantiplex HCV RNA assay)	Might be useful for assessing the likelihood of response to antiviral therapy	Should not be used to exclude the diagnosis of HCV infection or to determine treatment end point
*Genotype**†		
Several methodologies available (e.g., hybridization, sequencing)	Group isolates of HCV based on genetic differences, into 6 genotypes and >90 subtypes	Genotype 1 (subtypes 1a and 1b) most common in U.S. and associated with lower response to antiviral therapy
	With new therapies, length of treatment might vary based on genotype	
*Serotype**		
EIA based on immunoreactivity to synthetic peptides (e.g., Murex HCV Serotyping 1-6 assay)	No clinical utility	Cannot distinguish among subtypes
		Dual infections often observed

From *MMWR Morb Mortal Wkly Rep* 47(RR-19), 1998.
*Currently not U.S. Food and Drug Administration approved; lack standardization.
†Samples require special handling (e.g., serum must be separated within 2-4 hours of collection and stored frozen [−20° C or −70° C]; frozen samples should be shipped on dry ice).
bDNA, Branched-chain deoxyribonucleic acid; *EIA,* enzyme immunoassay; *HCV,* hepatitis C virus; *HCV RNA,* hepatitis C virus ribonucleic acid; *RIBA,* recombinant immunoblot assay; *RT-PCR,* reverse transcriptase polymerase chain reaction.

5. LFTs:
   - ALT and AST may be elevated to more than eight times normal in acute infection; in chronic infection ALT may be normal or fluctuate
   - Bilirubin may be 5 to 10 times normal
   - Albumin and prothrombin time generally normal; if abnormal, may be harbinger of impending hepatic necrosis
6. WBC and erythrocyte sedimentation rate (ESR) are generally normal

IMAGING STUDIES

Sonogram: rapid liver size reduction during fulminant hepatitis or mass in hepatocellular carcinoma

TREATMENT

Rx

NONPHARMACOLOGIC THERAPY

Activity and diet as tolerated

ACUTE GENERAL Rx

- Supportive care.
- Avoid hepatically metabolized drugs.
- Specific Rx for acute HCV infection.
- Recent studies demonstrate that *early* treatment with interferon-alpha-2b during acute HCV infection prevents chronic infection. The aim is to decrease viral load early in infection and allow the patient's immune system to control viral replication, thus preventing progression to chronic infection. The primary end point was sustained virologic response, with absence of HCV RNA in serum 24 wk after completion of therapy.
- Further investigations are in progress.

CHRONIC Rx

- Response to therapy is influenced by HCV genotype. Patients with genotype 1 and genotype 4 have sustained virologic response and cure rates much lower than patients with genotypes 2 and 3. Cure rates for genotypes 1 and 4 are about 45% to 50%, whereas cure rates for genotypes 2 and 3 are as high as 75% to 80%.
- Mainstay of therapy currently is with a pegylated interferon-alfa as a weekly subcutaneous injection and oral weight-based ribavirin. For genotypes 1 and 4, the therapy is for 48 wk. For genotypes 2 or 3, the length of therapy is 24 wk.
- Pegylated interferons are interferon-alpha with an attached polyethylene glycol (PEG) molecule. The PEG molecule confers a longer half-life and extended therapeutic activity compared with interferon-alfa and reduced dosing once a week. A third type of interferon, known as consensus interferon, is also available for treatment of hepatitis C, but it is not a long-acting form like the pegylated interferons.
- Two formulations of PEG interferon are available. Peginterferon alfa-2b (PEG INTRON) uses a weight-based

dosage in a once-a-week subcutaneous redipen injection. Peginterferon alfa-2a (Pegasys) uses a fixed dosage in a once-a-week premixed syringe, also subcutaneous.

- Both PEG interferon-alpha and ribavirin have numerous contraindications (absolute and relative) to use and may cause a variety of side effects. Interferon-alpha can cause flulike symptoms, thrombocytopenia, granulocytopenia, rash, alopecia, anorexia, psychiatric disturbances, others. Ribavirin can cause hemolysis, nausea, anemia, nasal congestion, pruritus. Ribavirin is contraindicated in pregnancy and patients should not get pregnant while on therapy and for 6 months after therapy
- In patients who fail to respond to interferon-alpha and ribavirin, <10% will respond to retreatment.
- Treatment trials have shown that pegylated interferon alone achieves higher hepatitis C-specific T-helper-1 response and clinical response rates than does interferon-alpha alone in patients with chronic hepatitis C without cirrhosis, and in patients with chronic hepatitis C with cirrhosis or bridging fibrosis.
- Liver transplantation:
  - Hepatitis C is the main indication for liver transplantation in the U.S.
  - It is the only option for patients with deteriorating HCV-related cirrhosis and for some patients with hepatocellular carcinoma.
  - Recurrent infection occurs in almost all patients with progressive fibrosis and cirrhosis; up to 20% progress to cirrhosis within 5 yr posttransplant.
- Coinfection with HIV:
  - These patients have a poor response to pegylated interferon-alpha and ribavirin if the immune system is depleted, with a low CD4 count as seen in the AIDS category. It is, however, important to treat patients co-infected with HIV and hepatitis C with HAART (highly active antiretroviral therapy). Many co-infected patients are stable from their HIV disease, but have significant morbidity and mortality from their hepatitis C.

DISPOSITION

- Follow-up as outpatient
- Monitor ALT levels as a clue for chronic disease
- Chronic carrier state, cirrhosis, hepatic carcinoma more common than with hepatitis A and B

REFERRAL

- To a hepatologist or infectious disease specialist for treatment for hepatitis C
- To an oncologist if hepatocellular carcinoma develops
- To a transplant surgeon for consideration of liver transplant if indicated

PEARLS & CONSIDERATIONS

- More rapid progression of disease in persons who drink alcohol regularly, persons of advanced age at time of infection, and those co-infected with other viruses (HIV, hepatitis B).
- No preventive vaccine available; post-exposure immune globulin provides minimal protection.
- Preventive measures include use of universal precautions, careful screening of blood and blood products, lifestyle changes.

EVIDENCE

A systematic review found that interferon-alpha is effective in improving biochemical outcomes (normalization of ALT) and achieving sustained virologic clearance in patients with transfusion-acquired acute hepatitis C. Limitations in current data meant that the effect on long-term outcomes could not be assessed.[1] Ⓐ

A systematic review of interferon-naive patients with chronic hepatitis C found that interferon was effective in improving viral clearance, liver histology, and liver biochemistries.

Although higher doses and prolonged duration of therapy were found to be more effective, they were associated with more adverse effects.[2] Ⓐ

Another systematic review of patients with chronic hepatitis C found that combination therapy with ribavirin and interferon-alpha was more effective than interferon-alpha alone. Combination therapy increased the number of patients (including interferon-naive patients, relapsers, and nonresponders) with a sustained virologic, biochemical, or histologic response. There was a significant increase in the risk of treatment discontinuation and adverse events with combination therapy.[3] Ⓐ

Evidence-Based References

1. Myers RP et al: Interferon for acute hepatitis C, *Cochrane Database Syst Rev* 4, 2001. Ⓐ
2. Myers RP et al: Interferon for interferon naive patients with chronic hepatitis C, *Cochrane Database Syst Rev* 2, 2002. Ⓐ
3. Kjaergard LL, Krogsgaard K, Gluud C: Ribavirin with or without alpha interferon for chronic hepatitis C, *Cochrane Database Syst Rev* 2, 2002. Ⓐ

SUGGESTED READINGS

Carrat F et al: Pegylated interferon alfa-2b vs standard interferon alfa-2b, plus ribavirin for chronic hepatitis C in HIV-infected patients: a randomized controlled trial, *JAMA* 292:2839, 2004.

Hadziyannis JJ et al: Peginterferon alpha-2a and ribavirin combination therapy in chronic hepatitis C, *Ann Intern Med* 140:346, 2004.

Pardo M et al: Effect of anti-viral therapy for occult hepatitis C virus infection, *Aliment Pharmacol Ther* 23(8):1153, 2006.

Sulkowski MS, Ray SC, Thomas DL: Needlestick transmission of hepatitis C, *JAMA* 287(18):2406, 2002.

Torriani FJ et al: Peginterferon alfa-2a plus ribavirin for chronic hepatitis C virus infection in HIV-infected patients, *N Engl J Med* 351:438, 2004.

AUTHORS: **GLENN G FORT, M.D., M.P.H., DENNIS J. MIKOLICH, M.D.,** and **JANE V. EASON, M.D.**

BASIC INFORMATION

DEFINITION

Autoimmune hepatitis is a chronic inflammatory condition of the liver, characterized by elevated serum globulin levels and the presence of circulating autoantibodies. Two types have been described:

- Type 1 or "classic" autoimmune hepatitis is the most predominant form in the U.S. and worldwide (80%) and patients are positive for antinuclear antibodies (ANA) and/or antismooth muscle antibodies (ASMA). Occurs across all age ranges and may be underdiagnosed in the elderly.
- Type 2 is rare in the U.S. and primarily affects young children. Type 2 is characterized by the presence of antibodies to liver/kidney microsomes (anti-LKM-1) or liver cytosol 1 (anti-LC-1).

SYNONYMS

Autoimmune chronic active hepatitis
Chronic active hepatitis
Lupoid hepatitis

ICD-9CM CODES
571.49 Chronic hepatitis

EPIDEMIOLOGY & DEMOGRAPHICS

Annual incidence (estimated): 1.9 cases/100,000
Point prevalence (estimated): 16.9/100,000
Type 1: all age groups; type 2: more common in teenagers and young adults
Female-to-male ratio is 3.6:1
Approximately 100,000-200,000 persons affected in the U.S
Accounts for 5.9% of liver transplants in U.S
Associated with HLA DR3 and HLA DR4

CLINICAL PRESENTATION

- Varies from asymptomatic elevations of liver enzymes, fulminant hepatitis to advanced cirrhosis.
- Symptoms may include fatigue, anorexia, nausea, abdominal pain, pruritus, and arthralgia.
- Jaundice.
- Hepatomegaly/splenomegaly.
- Autoimmune findings may include arthritis, xerostomia, keratoconjunctivitis, cutaneous vasculitis, and erythema nodosum.
- For patients presenting with advanced disease: ascites, edema, abnormal bleeding, jaundice.

ETIOLOGY

- Exact etiology unknown; liver histology demonstrates cell-mediated immune attack against hepatocytes.
- Presence of a variety of autoantibodies suggests an autoimmune mechanism.
- Strong genetic predisposition.
- Potential triggering agents such as virus (hepatitis A) or drugs (minocycline, atorvastatin).

DIAGNOSIS

DIFFERENTIAL DIAGNOSIS

- Acute viral hepatitis (A, B, C, D, E, cytomegalovirus, Epstein-Barr, herpes)
- Chronic viral hepatitis (B, C)
- Toxic hepatitis (alcohol, drugs)
- Primary biliary cirrhosis
- Primary sclerosing cholangitis
- Hemochromatosis
- Nonalcoholic steatohepatitis
- SLE
- Wilson's disease
- Alpha-1 antitrypsin deficiency

WORKUP

- History and physical examination with attention to the presence of autoimmune abnormalities such as thyroiditis, Graves' disease, ulcerative colitis, and rheumatoid arthritis
- LFTs and serum gamma globulins
- Tests for autoantibodies
- Liver biopsy for establishing diagnosis and disease severity

LABORATORY TESTS

- Aminotransferases generally elevated, may fluctuate.
- Bilirubin and alkaline phosphatase moderately elevated or normal.
- Elevation of gamma globulin and IgG.
- Circulating autoantibodies often present.
  1. Rheumatoid factor
  2. Antinuclear antibodies (ANA)
     a. Present in two thirds of patients.
     b. Typical pattern is homogeneous or speckled.
     c. Titer does not correlate with the stage, activity, or prognosis.
  3. Antismooth muscle antibodies (ASMA)
     a. Present in 87% of patients.
     b. Titer does not correlate with course or prognosis.
  4. Antibodies to liver/kidney microsomes (anti-LKM)
     a. Typically found in patients who are ANA-negative and ASMA-negative.
     b. Found in <1/25 of patients in U.S.
     c. Present in pediatric population and up to 20% of adults in Europe; also present in patients with drug-induced hepatitis.
  5. Autoantibodies against soluble liver antigen and liver-pancreas antigen (anti-SLA/LP)
     a. Present in 10% to 30% of patients.
     b. Associated with higher rate of relapse after corticosteroid therapy.
     c. Several studies suggest that patients with anti-SLA/LP have a more severe course.
- Hypoalbuminemia and prolonged prothrombin time with advanced disease.
- There is a well-described overlap syndrome with primary biliary cirrhosis (7%), primary sclerosing cholangitis (6%), and autoimmune cholangitis (11%).

IMAGING STUDIES

Ultrasound of liver and biliary tree to rule out obstruction or hepatic mass

TREATMENT

NONPHARMACOLOGIC THERAPY

- Avoid alcohol and hepatotoxic medications.
- Liver transplantation is an option for end-stage disease or fulminant hepatic failure.

PHARMACOLOGIC THERAPY

- Initial treatment:
  1. Prednisone 60 mg po/day or combination treatment with prednisone 30 mg po/day plus azathiaprine 50 mg po/day.
  2. Combination therapy allows for lower prednisone doses and less steroid side effects.
  3. Goal of therapy is remission (normalization of gammaglobulin and bilirubin, reduction of aminotransferases to <2 times the upper limit of normal).
- Indications for treatment:
  1. Serum aminotransferase >10 times the upper limit of normal
  2. Serum aminotransferase >5 times the upper limit of normal, with serum gammaglobulin level twice the upper limit of normal
  3. Young age
  4. Histologic features of bridging necrosis or multiacinar necrosis.
  5. Compensated cirrhosis:
     a. 3- to 6-mo treatment trial may be beneficial in patients with inflammation on liver biopsy.
     b. Fibrosis may improve during corticosteroid therapy and treatment may delay or obviate liver transplantation.
- Evaluation of treatment response:
  1. Goal is the absence of symptoms, resolution of LFT abnormalities, and histologic improvement.
  2. Patients who normalize their transaminase levels may continue to have ongoing active hepatitis involving inflammation and fibrosis. 5% to 10%

of patients with normal transaminase levels progress to cirrhosis.
3. Histologic improvement may lag behind clinical and laboratory improvement by as much as 6 mo.
4. Repeat liver biopsy should be considered after normalization of transaminase levels.
5. Complete normalization on biopsy is associated with 15% to 20% risk of relapse.
6. Persistent interface hepatitis is associated with 90% risk of relapse.

DISPOSITION

- Follow-up as outpatient.
- Long-term treatment may be necessary for sustained remission.
- 65% of patients achieve remission by 18 mo; 80% achieve remission by 3 yr.
- Approximately 10% of patients fail to improve with therapy.
- Patients who develop end-stage liver disease are candidates for liver transplantation. Recurrent disease may occur after liver transplantation.

REFERRAL

Patients who present with advanced cirrhosis or progress to end-stage liver disease are candidates for liver transplantation and should be referred to appropriate medical centers that provide liver transplantation services.

PEARLS & CONSIDERATIONS

COMMENTS

- A variety of autoimmune conditions can be seen in association with autoimmune hepatitis, including thyroiditis, Graves' disease, ulcerative colitis, rheumatoid arthritis, uveitis, pernicious anemia, Sjögren's syndrome, mixed connective tissue disease, CREST syndrome, and vitiligo.
- Variant forms of autoimmune hepatitis (overlap syndrome) have clinical and serologic findings of autoimmune hepatitis plus features of other forms of chronic liver disease such as primary biliary cirrhosis (PBC) or primary sclerosing cholangitis (PSC).

PREVENTION

None

PATIENT/FAMILY EDUCATION

- American Liver Foundation (ALF)
  Phone: 800-GO-LIVER (465-4837)
  E-mail: info@liverfoundation.org
  Internet: www.liverfoundation.org
- National Digestive Diseases Information clearinghouse
  http://digestive.niddk.nih.gov/ddiseases/pubs/autoimmunehep

SUGGESTED READINGS

Al-Khalidi JA, Czaja AJ: Current concepts in the diagnosis, pathogenesis, and treatment of autoimmune hepatitis, *Mayo Clin Proc* 76:1237, 2001.

Czaja AJ: Current concepts in autoimmune hepatitis, *Ann Hepatol* 4(1):6-24, 2005.

Czaja AJ, Freese AD: American Association for the Study of Liver Diseases guideline: diagnosis and treatment of autoimmune hepatitis, *Hepatology* 36:479, 2002.

Krawitt EL: Autoimmune hepatitis, *NEJM* 354:54, 2006.

AUTHORS: **KITTICHAI PROMRAT, M.D.**, and **CHRISTINE DUFFY, M.D.**

BASIC INFORMATION

DEFINITION

Hepatocellular carcinoma (HCC) is a malignant tumor of the hepatocytes.

SYNONYMS

Hepatoma

ICD-9CM CODES
155.0 Hepatocellular carcinoma

EPIDEMIOLOGY & DEMOGRAPHICS

Fifth most common cancer worldwide and third most common cause of cancer mortality. Incidence varies worldwide:

- Areas with high rates of hepatitis B and C (Asia, sub-Saharan Africa) have high rates of HCC.
- Males more affected than females with ratios between 2:1 and 4:1.
- Peak incidence: fifth and sixth decades in Western countries, earlier in areas with perinatal transmission of hepatitis B.
- Incidence rapidly growing in U.S. secondary to hepatitis C infection.
  - Incidence: increased more than twofold in the past 20 years; 3.3/100,000 per year between 1999 and 2001
  - Mean age of diagnosis ~ 65 years
- Risk factors:
  - Hepatitis B
  - Chronic hepatitis C
  - Cirrhosis due to causes other than viral hepatitis: alcoholic liver disease, nonalcoholic steatohepatitis, primary biliary cirrhosis, hemochromatosis, alpha-1-antitrypsin deficiency, and autoimmune hepatitis
  - Hepatotoxins: alcohol and aflatoxin B_1
  - Systemic diseases affecting the liver such as tyrosinemia
  - Obesity and diabetes mellitus

PHYSICAL FINDINGS & CLINICAL PRESENTATION

- One third of patients are asymptomatic. Abdominal pain may be initial presentation.
- Signs of underlying cirrhosis are often present.
- Previously compensated cirrhosis with new ascites, encephalopathy, jaundice, or bleeding.
- Paraneoplastic syndromes (hypoglycemia, erythrocytosis, hypercalcemia, severe diarrhea) may be present.

DIAGNOSIS

DIFFERENTIAL DIAGNOSIS

- Metastatic tumor to liver
- Benign liver tumors such as adenomas, focal nodular hyperplasia, and hemangiomas
- Focal fatty infiltration

WORKUP

- History with regard to risk factors
- Physical examination with attention to signs of chronic liver disease
- Laboratory evaluation and imaging studies

LABORATORY TESTS

- Liver function tests.
- Elevated alpha-fetoprotein (AFP) in 70% of patients (sensitivity 40% to 65%; specificity 80% to 94%).
- Paraneoplastic syndromes associated with HCC may cause hypercalcemia, hypoglycemia, and polycythemia.

IMAGING STUDIES

Ultrasound, CT scan, or MRI. Ultrasound is most commonly used as a screening test for HCC in high-risk patients. Multiphasic CT and MR scans are usually performed when there is a focal lesion on US or strong clinical suspicion of HCC.

BIOPSY

Percutaneous biopsy under ultrasound or CT scan usually is diagnostic. Tissue diagnosis is the gold standard. However, HCC can be reliably diagnosed when:

- Mass >2 cm that shows characteristic arterial vascularization that is seen on two imaging modalities *or*
- Single positive imaging method with AFP >200 μg/ml

SCREENING

Screening high-risk patients with US and AFP q6months may identify hepatocellular carcinoma at an early stage. Patients on transplant waiting lists should be screened for HCC because in the U.S. the development of HCC gives increased priority for liver transplantation. Screening at 6 to 12 mo intervals may be acceptable for healthy hepatitis B virus carriers without cirrhosis.

STAGING

According to the Barcelona-Clinic Liver Cancer (BCLC) staging classification, treatment is determined according to stage:

- Early stage: asymptomatic single tumor ≤5 cm or 3 nodules, each ≤3 cm (known as Milan criteria)
- Intermediate stage: patients with tumors that exceed early criteria but do not yet show cancer-related symptoms, vascular invasion, or metastases
- Advanced stage: patients with cancer-related symptoms
- End-stage: patients with advanced, symptomatic disease

TREATMENT

- Early stage: curative treatment (surgical resection or liver transplantation). Patients who have a single lesion can be offered surgical resection if they are noncirrhotic or have cirrhosis but still have well preserved liver function. Liver transplantation is an effective option for patients with HCC corresponding to the Milan criteria. Local ablation is safe and effective therapy for patients who cannot undergo resection, or as a bridge to transplantation.
- Intermediate stage: optimal therapeutic approach is controversial. Outcome may be improved with chemoembolization.
- Advanced stage: no curative treatment. In the absence of metastatic disease or portal invasion, chemoembolization is reasonable. Entry into clinical trials should be considered.
- End-stage: palliative care.
- For patients with unresectable HCC, chemoembolization using cisplatin or doxorubicin has been shown to improve 2-yr survival rates.

DISPOSITION

For unresectable tumors, prognosis is poor; 5-yr survival following surgical resection ranges from 30% to 50%.

REFERRAL

Referral to GI for treatment planning

PEARLS & CONSIDERATIONS

Prevention:

- Universal hepatitis B vaccination in children in endemic areas has been shown to decrease the incidence of HCC.
- Treatment of patients with chronic hepatitis B–associated cirrhosis with lamivudine reduces the incidence of HCC.
- For hepatitis C virus–associated HCC, postoperative treatment with interferon-alpha may decrease the rate of tumor recurrence.
- Eliminate aflatoxin from food.
- Decrease alcohol consumption.
- Identify and treat hemochromatosis.

SUGGESTED READINGS

Bruix J, Sherman M: Practice Guidelines Committee, American Association for the Study of Liver Diseases, *Hepatology*, 42(5):1208, 2005.

Cheng BQ et al: Chemoembolization combined with radio frequency abalation for patients with hepatocellular carcinoma larger than 3 cm: a randomized controlled trial, *JAMA* 299(14):1669-1677, 2008.

El-Serag H, Rudolph K: Hepatocellular carcinoma: epidemiology and molecular carcinogenesis, *Gastroenterology* 132(7):2557, 2007.

El-Serag HB et al: The continuing increase in the incidence of hepatocellular carcinoma in the United States: an update, *Ann Intern Med* 139:817, 2003.

Liaw YF et al: Lamivudine for patients with chronic hepatitis B and advanced liver disease, *N Engl J Med* 351:1521, 2004

Llovet JM, Bruix J: Systematic review of randomized trials for unresectable hepatocellular carcinoma: chemoembolization improves survival, *Hepatology* 37(2):429, 2003.

AUTHORS: **KITTICHAI PROMRAT, M.D.,** and **CHRISTINE DUFFY, M.D.**

BASIC INFORMATION

DEFINITION

Hepatorenal syndrome (HRS) is a condition of intense renal vasoconstriction resulting from loss of renal autoregulation occurring as a complication of severe liver disease. Criteria for hepatorenal syndrome are:

1. Serum creatinine concentration >1.5 mg/dl or 24 hr creatinine clearance <40 ml/min
2. Absence of shock, ongoing infection, and fluid loss, and no current treatment with nephrotoxic drugs
3. Absence of sustained improvement in renal function (decrease in serum creatinine to <1.5 mg/dl after discontinuation of diuretics and a trial of plasma expansion)
4. Absence of proteinuria (<500 mg/day) or hematuria (<50 RBC/high power field)
5. Absence of ultrasonographic evidence of obstructive uropathy or parenchymal renal disease
6. Urinary sodium concentration <10 mmol/L

There are two types of hepatorenal syndrome:

Type 1: progressive impairment in renal function as defined by a doubling of initial serum creatinine above 2.5 mg/dl in <2 wk

Type 2: stable or slowly progressive impairment of renal function not meeting the above criteria

SYNONYMS

Hepatic nephropathy
Oliguric renal failure of cirrhosis
HRS

ICD-9CM CODES
572.4 Hepatorenal syndrome

EPIDEMIOLOGY & DEMOGRAPHICS

The probability of HRS in patients with cirrhosis is 18% at 1 yr and 39% at 5 yr.

PHYSICAL FINDINGS & CLINICAL PRESENTATION

- Evidence of cirrhosis is usually present: jaundice, spider angiomas, splenomegaly, ascites, fetor hepaticus, pedal edema
- Hepatic encephalopathy: flapping tremor (asterixis), coma
- Tachycardia and bounding pulse
- Oliguria

ETIOLOGY

An exacerbation of end-stage liver disease, HRS may occur after significant reduction of effective blood volume (e.g., paracentesis, GI bleeding, diuretics) or in the absence of any precipitating factors.

DIAGNOSIS

DIFFERENTIAL DIAGNOSIS

- Prerenal azotemia: response to sustained plasma expansion is good (prompt diuresis with volume expansion).
- Acute tubular necrosis: urinary sodium >30, FENa >1.5%, urinary/plasma creatinine ratio <30, urine/plasma osmolality ratio = 1, urine sediment reveals casts and cellular debris, there is no significant response to sustained plasma expansion.

WORKUP

Patients with acute azotemia and oliguria in the setting of liver disease should undergo laboratory evaluation to differentiate HRS from acute tubular necrosis and volume challenge to differentiate HRS from prerenal azotemia if FENa <1%.

LABORATORY TESTS

- Obtain serum electrolytes, BUN, creatinine, osmolality, urinalysis, urinary sodium, urinary creatinine, urine osmolality.
- Calculate fractional excretion of sodium (FENa).
- In HRS: urinary sodium <10 mEq/L, FENa <1%, urinary plasma creatinine ratio >30, urinary-plasma osmolality ratio >1.5, urine sediment is unremarkable.

IMAGING STUDIES

Renal ultrasound may be indicated if renal obstruction is suspected.

TREATMENT

NONPHARMACOLOGIC THERAPY

Avoidance of precipitating factors

ACUTE GENERAL Rx

- Volume challenge (to increase mean arterial pressure) followed by large-volume paracentesis (to increase cardiac output and decrease renal venous pressure) may be useful to distinguish HRS from prerenal azotemia in patients with FENa <1%. In patients with prerenal azotemia, the increase in renal perfusion pressure and renal blood flow will result in prompt diuresis; the volume challenge can be accomplished by giving a solution of 100 g of albumin in 500 ml of isotonic saline.
- The only effective treatment of HRS is liver transplantation; ornipressin is used in some liver units to avoid further deterioration of renal function in patients awaiting liver transplantation. Generally dopamine and prostaglandins are ineffective in treating patients with hepatorenal syndrome.
- Vasopressin analogues may improve renal perfusion by reversing splanchnic vasodilation, which is the hallmark of HRS. Encouraging results were found in a recent study using continuous IV noradrenalin in combination with albumin and furosemide. In this study, reversal of HRS was achieved in 10 out of 12 patients.
- Treatment of hepatorenal syndrome with vasoconstrictors for 5 to 15 days in attempt to reduce serum creatinine to <1.5 mg/dl is as follows:
  1. Administration of one of the following drugs or drug combinations:
     a. Norepinephrine (0.5 to 3.0 mg/hr IV)
     b. Midodrine (7.5 mg PO tid, increased to 12.5 mg tid if needed) in combination with octretide (100 micrograms SC tid, increased to tid prn)
     c. Terlipressin (0.2 to 2.0 mg IV q 4 to 12 hr)
  2. Concomitant administration of albumin (1 g/kg IV on day 1, followed by 20 to 40 g daily)

DISPOSITION

Mortality rate exceeds 80%; liver transplantation is the only curative treatment.

REFERRAL

Referral for liver transplantation when indicated (see "Comments")

PEARLS & CONSIDERATIONS

COMMENTS

Liver transplantation may be indicated in otherwise healthy patients (age preferably <65 yr) with sclerosing cholangitis, chronic hepatitis with cirrhosis, or primary biliary cirrhosis; contraindications to liver transplantation are AIDS, most metastatic malignancies, active substance abuse, uncontrolled sepsis, uncontrolled cardiac or pulmonary disease.

SUGGESTED READINGS

Duvoux C et al: Effects of noradrenalin and albumin in patients with type 1 hepatorenal syndrome: a pilot study, *Hepatology* 36:374, 2002.

Gines P et al: Management of cirrhosis and ascites, *N Engl J Med* 350:1646, 2004.

AUTHOR: **FRED F. FERRI, M.D.**

BASIC INFORMATION

DEFINITION

Herpangina is a self-limited upper respiratory tract infection associated with a characteristic vesicular rash on the soft palate.

SYNONYMS

Vesicular stomatitis
Acute lymphonodular pharyngitis

ICD-9CM CODES
074.0 Herpangina

EPIDEMIOLOGY & DEMOGRAPHICS

INCIDENCE (IN U.S.): Unknown
PEAK INCIDENCE: Summer outbreaks common
PREVALENCE (IN U.S.): Unknown
PREDOMINANT SEX: Male = female
PREDOMINANT AGE: 3 to 10 yr

PHYSICAL FINDINGS & CLINICAL PRESENTATION

- Characterized by ulcerating lesions typically located on the soft palate (Fig. 1-119)
- Usually fewer than six lesions that evolve rapidly from a diffuse pharyngitis to erythematous macules and subsequently to vesicles that are moderately painful
- Fever, vomiting, and headache in the first few days of illness but subsiding spontaneously
- Pharyngeal lesions typical for several more days

ETIOLOGY

- Most caused by coxsackie A viruses (A2, A4, A5, A6, A10)
- Occasional cases caused by other enteroviruses (Echovirus and Enterovirus 71)

DIAGNOSIS

DIFFERENTIAL DIAGNOSIS

- Herpes simplex
- Bacterial pharyngitis
- Tonsillitis
- Aphthous stomatitis
- Hand-foot-mouth disease

WORKUP

Diagnosis is typically based on characteristic lesions on the soft palate.

LABORATORY TESTS

Viral and bacterial cultures of the pharynx to exclude herpes simplex infection and streptococcal pharyngitis if the diagnosis is in doubt

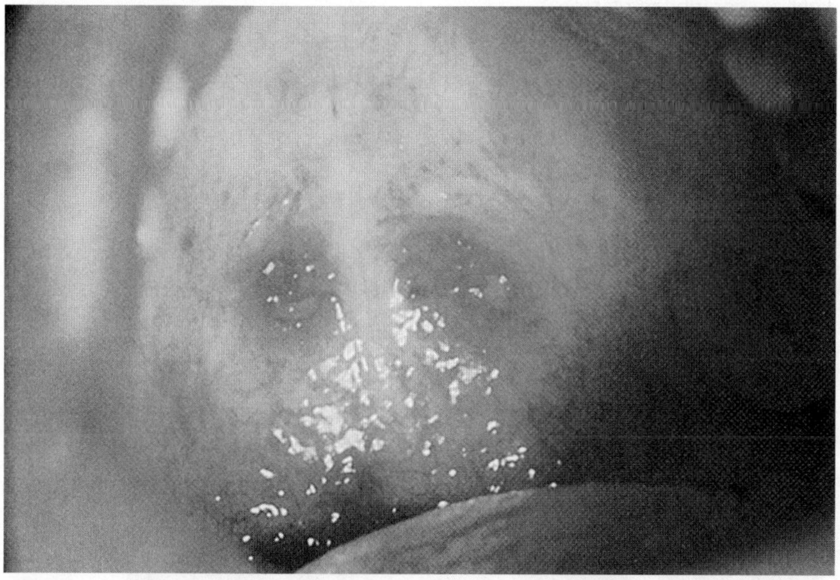

FIGURE 1-119 Herpangina with shallow ulcers in the roof of the mouth. (Courtesy Marshall Guill, M.D. From Goldstein B [ed]: *Practical dermatology,* ed 2, St Louis, 1997, Mosby.)

TREATMENT

- Symptomatic treatment for sore throat, saline gargles, analgesics, encourage oral fluids
- No antiviral therapy indicated; avoid antibacterial agents because they are ineffective, increase cost, might result in side effects, and promote antibiotic resistance

NONPHARMACOLOGIC THERAPY

Analgesic throat lozenges are helpful in some cases.

ACUTE GENERAL Rx

Antipyretics when indicated

CHRONIC Rx

Self-limited infection

DISPOSITION

- Generally, resolution of symptoms within 1 wk
- Persistence of fever or mouth lesions beyond 1 wk suggestive of an alternative diagnosis (see Differential Diagnosis)

REFERRAL

For consultation with otolaryngologist or infectious disease specialist if the diagnosis is in doubt

PEARLS & CONSIDERATIONS

COMMENTS

Household outbreaks may occur, especially during the summer months.

SUGGESTED READINGS

Chang LY et al: Outcome of enterovirus 71 infections with or without stage-based management: 1998 to 2002, *Pediatr Infect Dis J* 23(4):327, 2004.

Chang LY et al: Transmission and clinical features of enterovirus 71 infections in household contacts in Taiwan, *JAMA* 291(2):222, 2004.

Stone MS: Viral exanthems, *Dermatol Online J* 9(3):4, 2003.

Urashima M et al: Seasonal models of herpangina and hand-foot-mouth disease to simulate annual fluctuations in urban warming in Tokyo, *Jpn J Infect Dis* 56(2):48, 2003.

AUTHORS: **GLENN G. FORT, M.D., M.P.H., DENNIS J. MIKOLICH, M.D.,** and **JOSEPH R. MASCI, M.D.**

BASIC INFORMATION

DEFINITION

Herpes simplex is a viral infection caused by the herpes simplex virus (HSV). HSV-1 is associated primarily with oral infections, whereas HSV-2 causes mainly genital infections; however, each type can infect any site. Following the primary infection, the virus enters the nerve endings in the skin directly below the lesions and ascends to the dorsal root ganglia where it remains in a latent stage until it is reactivated.

SYNONYMS

Genital herpes
Herpes labialis
Herpes gladiatorum
Herpes digitalis

ICD-9CM CODES
054.10 Genital herpes
054.9 Herpes labialis

EPIDEMIOLOGY & DEMOGRAPHICS

- More than 85% of adults have serologic evidence of HSV-1 infection. The seroprevalence of adults with HSV-2 in the United States is 25%; however, only about 20% of these persons recall having symptoms of HSV infection.
- Most cases of eye or digital herpetic infections are caused by HSV-1.
- Frequency of recurrence of HSV-2 genital herpes is higher than HSV-1 oral labial infection.
- The frequency of recurrence is lowest for oral labial HSV-2 infections.
- The incidence of complications from herpes simplex (e.g., herpes encephalitis) is highest in immunocompromised hosts.

PHYSICAL FINDINGS & CLINICAL PRESENTATION

PRIMARY INFECTION:
- Symptoms occur from 3 to 7 days after contact (respiratory droplets, direct contact).
- Constitutional symptoms include low-grade fever, headache and myalgias, regional lymphadenopathy, and localized pain.
- Pain, burning, itching, and tingling last several hours.
- Grouped vesicles (Fig. 1-120) usually with surrounding erythema appear and generally ulcerate or crust within 48 hr.
- The vesicles are uniform in size (differentiating it from herpes zoster vesicles, which vary in size).
- During the acute eruption the patient is uncomfortable; involvement of lips and inside of mouth may make it unpleasant for the patient to eat; urinary retention may complicate involvement of the genital area.
- Lesions generally last from 2 to 6 wk and heal without scarring.

RECURRENT INFECTION:
- Generally caused by alteration in the immune system; fatigue, stress, menses, local skin trauma, and exposure to sunlight are contributing factors.
- The prodromal symptoms (fatigue, burning and tingling of the affected area) last 12 to 24 hr.
- A cluster of lesions generally evolve within 24 hr from a macule to a papule and then vesicles surrounded by erythema; the vesicles coalesce and subsequently rupture within 4 days, revealing erosions covered by crusts.
- The crusts are generally shed within 7 to 10 days, revealing a pink surface.
- The most frequent location of the lesions is on the vermilion border of the lips (HSV-1), the penile shaft or glans penis and the labia (HSV-2), buttocks (seen more frequently in women), fingertips (herpetic whitlow), and trunk (may be confused with herpes zoster).
- Rapid onset of diffuse cutaneous herpes simplex (eczema herpeticum) may occur in certain atopic infants and adults. It is a medical emergency, especially in young infants, and should be promptly treated with acyclovir.
- Herpes encephalitis, meningitis, and ocular herpes can occur in patients with immunocompromised status and occasionally in normal hosts.

ETIOLOGY

HSV-1 and HSV-2 are both DNA viruses.

DIAGNOSIS

DIFFERENTIAL DIAGNOSIS

- Impetigo
- Behçet's syndrome
- Coxsackie virus infection
- Syphilis
- Stevens-Johnson syndrome
- Herpangina
- Aphthous stomatitis
- Varicella
- Herpes zoster

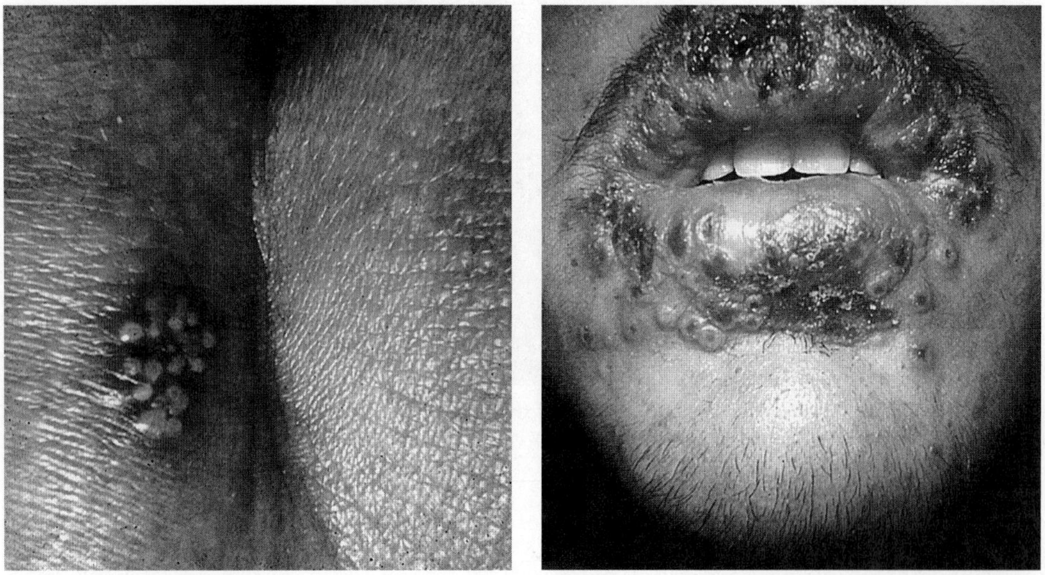

FIGURE 1-120 Herpes simplex. (From Scuderi G [ed]: *Sports medicine: principles of primary care,* St Louis, 1997, Mosby.)

WORKUP

Diagnosis is based on clinical presentation. Laboratory evaluation will confirm diagnosis.

LABORATORY TESTS

- Direct immunofluorescent antibody slide tests will provide a rapid diagnosis.
- Viral culture is the most definitive method for diagnosis; results are generally available in 1 or 2 days; the lesions should be sampled during the vesicular or early ulcerative stage; cervical samples should be taken from the endocervix with a swab.
- Tzanck smear is a readily available test; it will demonstrate multinucleated giant cells. However, it is not a very sensitive test.
- Pap smear will detect HSV-infected cells in cervical tissue from women without symptoms.
- Serologic tests for HSV: IgG and IgM serum antibodies. Antibodies to HSV occur in 50% to 90% of adults. Routine tests do not discriminate between antibodies that are HSV-1 and HSV-2; the presence of IgM or a fourfold or greater rise in IgG titers indicates a recent infection (convalescent sample should be drawn 2 to 3 wk after the acute specimen is drawn).

TREATMENT

Rx

NONPHARMACOLOGIC THERAPY

Application of topical cool compresses with Burow's solution for 15 min four to six times daily may be soothing in patients with extensive erosions on the vulva and penis (decrease edema and inflammation, debridement of crusts and purulent material).

ACUTE GENERAL Rx

- Acyclovir ointment or cream (Zovirax) applied using finger-cot or rubber glove q3 to 6h (6 times daily) for 7 days may be useful for the first clinical episode of genital herpes. Severe primary genital infections may be treated with IV acyclovir (5 mg/kg infused at a constant rate over 1 hr q8h for 7 days in patients with normal renal function) or oral acyclovir 200 mg 5 times daily for 10 days. Topical acyclovir 5% cream can also be used for herpes labialis; when started at the prodrome or papule stage, it decreases the duration of an episode by about one-half day.
- Valacyclovir caplets (Valtrex) can also be used for the initial episode of genital herpes (1 g bid for 10 days).
- Valacyclovir 2 g PO q12h for 1 day begun within the first symptoms of herpes labialis can modestly shorten its duration.
- Penciclovir 1% cream (Denavir) can be used for recurrent herpes labialis on the lips and face. It should be applied q2h while awake for 4 days. Treatment should be started at the earliest sign or symptom. Its use decreases healing time of orolabial herpes by about 1 day.
- Docosanol 10% cream (Abbreva), a long-chain saturated alcohol, inhibits fusion between the plasma membrane and the viral envelope, blocking viral entry and subsequent replication. It is available over the counter and, when applied at the first sign of recurrence of herpes labialis, may shorten the durations of the episode by about 12 hr.

CHRONIC Rx

- Recurrent episodes of genital herpes can be treated with acyclovir. A short course (800 mg tid for 2 days) is effective. Other treatment options include 800 mg PO bid for 3 to 5 days, generally started during the prodrome or within 2 days of onset of lesions; famciclovir (Famvir) is also useful for treatment of recurrent genital herpes (dose is 125 mg q12h for 5 days in patients with normal renal function) started at the first sign of symptoms, or valacyclovir (Valtrex) (dose is 500 mg q12h for 3 days in patients with normal renal function).
- Acyclovir-resistant mucocutaneous lesions in patients with HIV can be treated with foscarnet (40 to 60 mg/kg IV q8h in patients with normal renal function); HPMPC has also been reported to be effective in HSV infections resistant to acyclovir or foscarnet.
- Patients with 6 recurrences of genital herpes/year can be treated with valacyclovir 1 g qd, acyclovir 400 mg bid, or famciclovir 250 mg bid.

DISPOSITION

Most patients recover from the initial episode or recurrences without complications; immunocompromised hosts are at risk for complications (e.g., disseminated herpes simplex infection, herpes encephalitis).

REFERRAL

- Hospital admission in patients with herpes encephalitis, herpes meningitis, and in immunocompromised hosts with diffuse herpes simplex infection
- Ophthalmology referral in patients with suspected ocular herpes

PEARLS & CONSIDERATIONS

!

COMMENTS

- Provide patient education regarding transmission of HSV.
- Condom use offers significant protection against HSV-1 infection in susceptive women.
- Patients should be instructed on the use of condoms for sexual intercourse and on avoiding kissing or sexual intercourse until lesions are crusted.
- Patients should also avoid contact with immunocompromised hosts or neonates while lesions are present.
- Proper hand-washing techniques should be explained.
- Patients with herpes gladiatorum (cutaneous herpes in athletes involved in contact sports) should be excluded from participation in active sports until lesions have resolved.
- Many new HSV-2 infections are asymptomatic, but new symptoms may result from old infections.

EVIDENCE

EBM

There is limited evidence from randomized controlled trials (RCTs) that oral acyclovir may be effective as a preventive agent against recurrent herpes labialis.[1,2] Ⓐ

Regarding mother-to-baby transmission of herpes simplex during pregnancy and delivery, a systematic review recently concluded that prophylactic acyclovir starting at 36 weeks gestation reduces the risk of clinical herpes simplex virus recurrence at delivery, cesarean section rate for recurrent herpes, and viral shedding at delivery.[3] Ⓑ

Evidence-Based References

1. Spruance SL et al: Acyclovir prevents reactivation of herpes labialis in skiers, *JAMA* 260:1597, 1988. Reviewed in: *Clin Evid* 13:2105, 2005. Ⓐ
2. Raborn GW et al: Oral acyclovir in prevention of herpes labialis: a randomized, double-blind, placebo controlled trial, *Oral Surg Oral Med Oral Pathol Oral Radiol Endod* 85:55, 1998. Reviewed in: *Clin Evid* 10:1890, 2003. Ⓐ
3. Sheffield JS, Hollier LM, Hill JB: Acyclovir prophylaxis to prevent herpes simplex virus recurrence at delivery: a systematic review, *Obstet Gynecol* 102:1396, 2003. Ⓑ

SUGGESTED READING

Corey L et al: Once-daily valacyclovir to reduce the risk of transmission of genital herpes, *N Engl J Med* 350:11, 2004.

AUTHOR: **FRED F. FERRI, M.D.**

BASIC INFORMATION

DEFINITION

Herpes zoster is a disease caused by reactivation of the varicella-zoster virus. Following the primary infection (chickenpox) the virus becomes latent in the dorsal root ganglia and reemerges when there is a weakening of the immune system (secondary to disease or advanced age).

SYNONYMS

Shingles

ICD-9CM CODES
053.9 Herpes zoster

EPIDEMIOLOGY & DEMOGRAPHICS

- Herpes zoster occurs during lifetime in 10% to 20% of the population.
- There is an increased incidence in immunocompromised patients (AIDS, malignancy), the elderly, and children who acquired chickenpox when younger than 2 mo.

PHYSICAL FINDINGS & CLINICAL PRESENTATION

- Pain generally precedes skin manifestation by 3 to 5 days and is generally localized to the dermatome that will be affected by the skin lesions.
- Constitutional symptoms are often present (malaise, fever, headache).
- The initial rash consists of erythematous maculopapules generally affecting one dermatome (thoracic region in majority of cases); some patients (<50%) may have scattered vesicles outside of the affected dermatome.
- The initial maculopapules evolve into vesicles and pustules by the third or the fourth day.
- The vesicles have an erythematous base, are cloudy, and have various sizes (a distinguishing characteristic from herpes simplex in which the vesicles are of uniform size).
- The vesicles subsequently become umbilicated and then form crusts that generally fall off within 3 wk; scarring may occur.
- Pain during and after the rash is generally significant.
- Secondary bacterial infection with *Staphylococcus aureus* or *Streptococcus pyogenes* may occur.
- Regional lymphadenopathy may occur.
- Herpes zoster may involve the trigeminal nerve (most frequent cranial nerve involved); involvement of the geniculate ganglion can cause facial palsy and a painful ear, with the presence of vesicles on the pinna and external auditory canal (*Ramsay Hunt syndrome*).

ETIOLOGY

Reactivation of varicella virus (human herpes virus III)

DIAGNOSIS

DIFFERENTIAL DIAGNOSIS

- Rash: herpes simplex and other viral infections
- Pain from herpes zoster: may be confused with acute myocardial infarction, pulmonary embolism, pleuritis, pericarditis, renal colic

LABORATORY TESTS

Laboratory tests are generally not necessary (viral cultures and Tzanck smear will confirm diagnosis in patients with atypical presentation).

TREATMENT

NONPHARMACOLOGIC THERAPY

- Wet compresses (using Burow's solution or cool tap water) applied for 15 to 30 min 5 to 10 times a day are useful to break vesicles and remove serum and crust.
- Care must be taken to prevent any secondary bacterial infection.

ACUTE GENERAL Rx

- Gabapentin 300 to 1800 mg qd is effective in the treatment of pain and sleep interference associated with postherpetic neuralgia.
- Lidocaine patch 5% (Lidoderm) is also effective in relieving postherpetic neuralgia. Patches are applied to intact skin to cover the most painful area for up to 12 hr within a 24-hr period.
- Oral antiviral agents can decrease acute pain, inflammation, and vesicle formation when treatment is begun within 48 hr of onset of rash. Treatment options are:
    1. Acyclovir (Zovirax) 800 mg 5 times daily for 7 to 10 days
    2. Valacyclovir (Valtrex) 1000 mg tid for 7 days
    3. Famciclovir (Famvir) 500 mg tid for 7 days
- Immunocompromised patients should be treated with IV acyclovir 500 mg/m^2 or 10 mg/kg q8h in 1-hr infusions for 7 days, with close monitoring of renal function and adequate hydration; vidarabine (continuous 12-hr infusion of 10 mg/kg/day for 7 days) is also effective for treatment of disseminated herpes zoster in immunocompromised hosts.
- Patients with AIDS and transplant patients may develop acyclovir-resistant varicella-zoster; these patients can be treated with foscarnet (40 mg/kg IV q8h) continued for at least 10 days or until lesions are completely healed.
- Capsaicin cream (Zostrix) can be useful for treatment of postherpetic neuralgia. It is generally applied three to five times daily for several weeks after the crusts have fallen off.
- Sympathetic blocks (stellate ganglion or epidural) with 0.25% bupivacaine and rhizotomy are reserved for severe cases unresponsive to conservative treatment.
- Corticosteroids should be considered in older patients within 72 hours of clinical presentation or if new lesions are still appearing if there are no contraindications. Initial dose is prednisone 40 mg/day decreased by 5 mg/day until finished. When used there is a decrease in the use of analgesics and time to resumption of usual activities, but there is no effect on the incidence and duration of postherpetic neuralgia.

DISPOSITION

- The incidence of postherpetic neuralgia (defined as pain that persists more than 30 days after onset of rash) increases with age (30% by age 40 yr, >70% by age 70 yr); antivirals reduce the risk of postherpetic neuralgia.
- Incidence of disseminated herpes zoster is increased in immunocompromised hosts (e.g., 15% to 50% of patients with active Hodgkin's disease).
- Immunocompromised hosts are also more prone to neurologic complications (encephalitis, myelitis, cranial and peripheral nerve palsies, acute retinal necrosis). The mortality rate is 10% to 20% in immunocompromised hosts with disseminated zoster.
- Motor neuropathies occur in 5% of all cases of zoster; complete recovery occurs in >70% of patients.

REFERRAL

- Hospitalization for IV acyclovir in patients with disseminated herpes zoster
- Patients with herpes zoster ophthalmicus should be referred to an ophthalmologist

VACCINATION: Immunocompetent adults 60 years of age or older are appropriate candidates for a single dose of varicella zoster vaccine (VZV) whether or not they have had a previous episode of herpes zoster. Immunization with VZV (Zostavax) boosts waning immunity in older adults and reduces the severity and duration of pain caused by herpes zoster by 61%. Adults who are VZV seronegative (never had varicella) should be immunized against varicella with 2 doses of varicella vaccine (Varivax).

SUGGESTED READING

Kimberlin DW, Whitley RJ: Varicella-Zoster vaccine for the prevention of herpes zoster, *N Engl J Med* 356:1338, 2007.

AUTHOR: **FRED F. FERRI, M.D.**

BASIC INFORMATION

DEFINITION

A hiatal hernia is the herniation of a portion of the stomach into the thoracic cavity through the diaphragmatic esophageal hiatus.

SYNONYMS

Diaphragmatic hernias

ICD-9CM CODES
750.6 Hiatal hernia

EPIDEMIOLOGY & DEMOGRAPHICS

- Found in 50% of patients over the age of 50.
- Increases with age.
- More prevalent in Western countries than in Africa and Asia.
- Sliding hiatal hernias are more common in women than men (4:1).
- Associated with diverticulosis (25%), esophagitis (25%), duodenal ulcers (20%), and gallstones (18%).
- More than 90% of patients with endoscopic documentation of esophagitis have hiatal hernias.

PHYSICAL FINDINGS & CLINICAL PRESENTATION

Most patients are asymptomatic. If symptoms are present, it resembles those of gastroesophageal reflux disease (GERD).

- Heartburn
- Dysphagia
- Regurgitation of gastric contents
- Chest pain
- Postprandial fullness
- GI bleed
- Dyspnea
- Hoarseness
- Wheezing with bowel sounds heard over the left lung base

ETIOLOGY

- Imbalance between normal pulling forces of the esophagus through the diaphragmatic hiatus during swallowing and the supporting structures maintaining normal gastroesophageal (GE) junction positioning. The repetitive stretching and pulling of the GE junction causes widening of the hiatus, rupture of the phrenoesophageal ligament, and onset of the hernia.
- Hiatal hernias are classified as:
  1. Type I: Sliding (Fig. 1-121, *A*), axial, or concentric hiatal hernia (most common type, 99%). Only the GE junction protrudes into the thoracic cavity.
  2. Type II: Paraesophageal or rolling hernia (Fig. 1-121, *B*) (1%). The GE junction stays at the level of the diaphragm, but part of the stomach bulges into the thoracic cavity.
  3. Type III: Mixed (rare), a combination of type I and type II.
  4. Type IV: Large defect in hiatus that allows other intraabdominal organs to enter the hernia sac.

DIAGNOSIS

Imaging studies

DIFFERENTIAL DIAGNOSIS

- Peptic ulcer disease
- Unstable angina
- Esophagitis (caused by *Candida,* herpes, NSAIDs, etc.)
- Esophageal spasm
- Barrett's esophagus
- Schatzki's ring
- Achalasia
- Zenker's diverticulum
- Esophageal cancer

WORKUP

- Exclude conditions noted in the differential diagnosis and documenting the presence of a hiatal hernia. Upper endoscopy may also be needed to exclude abnormal metaplasia, dysplasia, or neoplasia.
- A clinical algorithm for evaluation of heartburn is described in Section III.

LABORATORY TESTS

- Blood tests are not specific.
- Esophageal manometry, although not commonly done, can be used in establishing a diagnosis (low sensitivity, but high specificity when compared with endoscopy).

IMAGING STUDIES

- Barium contrast upper gastrointestinal (UGI) series best defines the anatomic abnormality: demonstration that the gastric cardia is herniated 2 cm above the hiatus. UGI may reveal a tortuous esophagus (Fig. 1-122). If endoscopy is performed preoperatively, a barium swallow is generally not necessary.
- Upper GI endoscopy: documents the presence of a hiatal hernia and also excludes common associated findings of esophagitis and Barrett's esophagus (recommended at least once during the workup). Greater than 2 cm of gastric rugal fold seen above the margins of the diaphragmatic crura is diagnostic.
- Abdominal ultrasonography: simple, well tolerated; a transdiaphragmatic esophageal diameter of more than or equal to 18 mm is highly suggestive of the presence of a sliding hiatal hernia.

TREATMENT

NONPHARMACOLOGIC THERAPY

- Lifestyle modifications: avoidance of foods and drugs that decrease lower esophageal pressure (e.g. caffeine, chocolate, mint, calcium channel blockers, and anticholinergics)
- Weight loss
- Avoid large quantities of food with meals
- Sleep with the head of the bed elevated to 6 inches

ACUTE GENERAL Rx

- Antacids may be useful to relieve mild symptoms.
- H_2 antagonists (e.g., cimetidine 400 mg bid, ranitidine 150 mg bid, or famotidine 20 mg bid).
- If significant GERD is present with documented esophagitis, proton pump inhibitors (e.g., omeprazole 20 mg qd or lansoprazole 30 mg qd) are used. Refractory symptoms may require higher doses (e.g., bid dosing).
- Prokinetic agents (e.g., metoclopramide 10 mg taken 30 min before each meal) can be added to an H_2 antagonist or proton pump inhibitor.

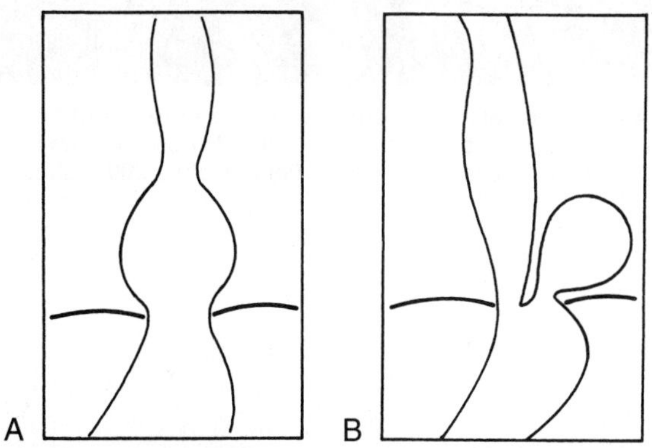

FIGURE 1-121 Types of esophageal hiatal hernia. **A,** Sliding hiatal hernia, the most common type. **B,** Paraesophageal hiatal hernia. (From Behrman RE: *Nelson textbook of pediatrics,* ed 17, Philadelphia, 2004, WB Saunders.)

CHRONIC Rx

- When indicated, surgery (laparoscopic or open) can be done in patients with refractory symptoms impairing quality of life, or causing intestinal (e.g., recurrent GI bleeds) or extraintestinal complications (e.g., aspiration pneumonia, asthma, or ear-nose-throat complications).
- Prophylactic surgery is a consideration in all paraesophageal hernias because they have a higher incidence of strangulation.

DISPOSITION

- More than 90% of patients having GERD symptoms respond well to medical therapy.
- Complications of hiatal hernias are similar to complications occurring in patients with GERD:
  1. Erosive esophagitis
  2. Ulcerative esophagitis
  3. Barrett's esophagus
  4. Peptic stricture
  5. GI hemorrhage
  6. Extraintestinal complications
  7. Lung collapse or heart failure (severe cases)

REFERRAL

Gastroenterologist: symptoms refractory to conventional therapy (H_2 antagonists, antacids, and proton pump inhibitors) or having complications mentioned above

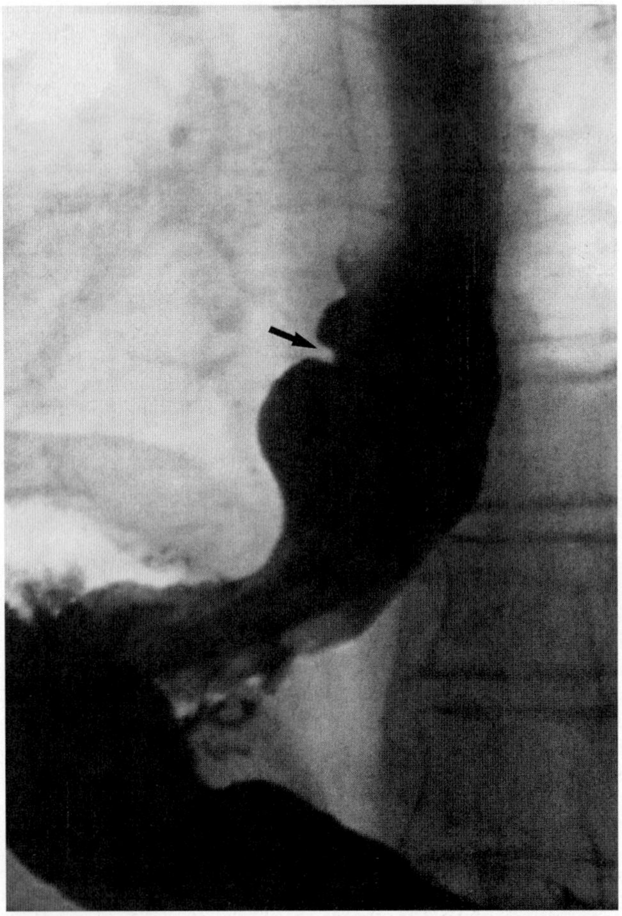

FIGURE 1-122 A sliding hiatal hernia confirmed by the presence of an incisural notch *(arrow)* on the greater curve aspect. (From Grainger RG, Allison DJ, Adam A, Dixon AK [eds]: *Grainger & Allison's diagnostic radiology,* ed 4, Philadelphia, 2001, Churchill Livingstone.)

PEARLS & CONSIDERATIONS

COMMENTS

- Gastric ulceration and erosions (Cameron's lesion) can occur in the hernia pouch and account for uncommon cause of upper GI bleeding.
- May cause iron deficiency anemia.
- Gastric volvulus or torsion can also occur and presents as dysphagia and postcibal pain.
- High incidence of esophagitis even after the eradication of *Helicobacter pylori.*
- The appearance of hiatal hernia may simulate left atrial mass by echocardiography.

SUGGESTED READINGS

Andujan JJ et al: Laparoscopic repair of large paraesophageal hernia is associated with low incidence of recurrence and reoperations, *Surg Endosc* 18(3):444, 2004.

Christensen J, Miftakhnr R: Hiatus hernia: a review of evidence for its origin in esophageal longitudinal muscle dysfunction, *Am J Med* 108(Suppl 4a):35, 2000.

Linke GR, Borovicka J, Schneider P et al: Is a barium swallow complementary to endoscopy essential in the preoperative assessment of laparoscopic antireflux and hiatal hernia surgery? *Surg Endosc.* Epub 2007 May 24.

Rosen M, Ponsky J: Laparoscopic repair of giant paraesophageal hernia: an update for internists, *Clev Clin J Med* 70(6):511, 2003.

Stylopoulos N, Rattner DW: Paraesophageal hernia: when to operate? *Adv Surg* 37:213, 2003.

AUTHOR: **ABDULBAKI ABDULRAHMAN, M.D.**

BASIC INFORMATION

DEFINITION

Hidradenitis suppurativa is a chronic, relapsing condition that occurs within the terminal follicular epithelium of the apocrine glands. Keritinous materials occlude the follicles causing secondary inflammation of the apocrine glands resulting in chronic infection and draining abscess that lead to scarring.

SYNONYMS

Suppurative hidradentis
Acne inversa
Verneuil's disease
Apocrinitis
Hidradenitis axillaris

ICD-9CM Codes
705.83

EPIDEMIOLOGY & DEMOGRAPHICS

- HS occurs more commonly in women in the U.S.
- It usually begins in the postpubertal age group, with an average age of onset of 23 yr.
- Its overall prevalence in the U.S. is approximately 1% to 2%.
- An increased frequency of this disease is seen in people of African American descent, though this has not been fully studied. The suspicion is that it is due to a greater density of apocrine glands.
- Predisposing factors thought to be involved are the following: hyperandrogenism, obesity, and familial predilection.
- HS has been associated with other endocrine disorders such as diabetes, Cushing's disease, and acromegaly.

PHYSICAL FINDINGS & CLINICAL PRESENTATION

The diagnosis is primarily clinical based on the development of typical lesions.
There are three key elements to typical lesions: typical lesions, characteristic distribution, and relapsing nature.

- Typical lesions can be as follows:
  - Painful and/or tender erythematous papules and nodules
  - Painful or tender abscesses and inflamed discharging papules or nodules
  - Dermal contractures and ropelike elevation of the skin
  - Comedones in the apocrine, gland-bearing skin
- Characteristic sites are:
  - Axilla (Fig. 1-123)
  - Inguinal perineal region
  - Areola of the breast
  - Submammary folds
- There is a strong tendency toward relapse and recurrence.
- Other characteristics of the disease are:
  - Poor response to conventional antibiotics
  - Often no pathogens from routine cultures of pus from boils
  - Personal or family history of acne or pilonidal cysts

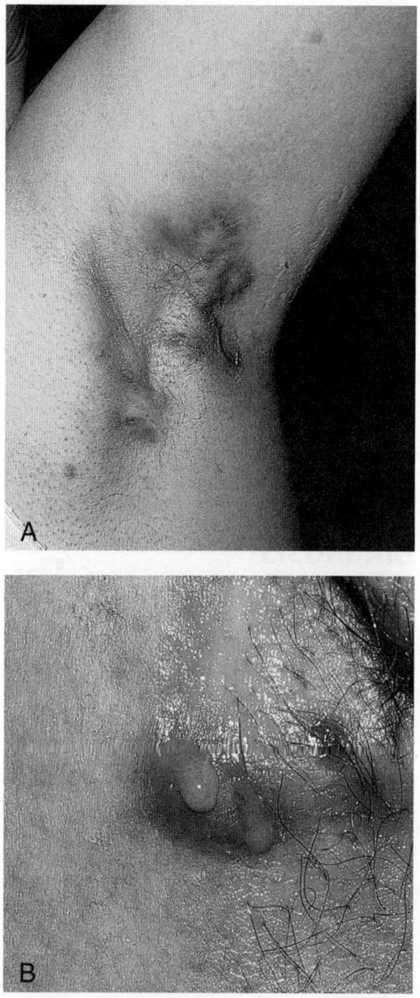

FIGURE 1-123 Hidradenitis suppurativa (HS). A, HS of the axilla. This is the classic appearance with inflammatory nodules and scarred areas. This condition is commonly misdiagnosed as a bacterial infection. **B,** HS of the axilla; a close-up view of the draining pus. When intact, the lesions represent sterile abscesses. Once open, they may become secondarily infected. (From White GM, Cox NH [eds]: *Diseases of the skin: a color atlas and text,* ed 2, St Louis, 2006, Mosby.)

ETIOLOGY

The exact cause of hidradentis suppurativa has not been determined, though a number of theories have been proposed:

1. Folliculitis is observed in almost all patients with HS, though whether or not this is causative has not been determined.
2. Local friction trauma could be a cause.
3. Infectious agents such as *Streptococcus, Staphylococcus,* and *E. coli* have been identified in cultures, but it is uncertain whether these are cause or result.
4. Low levels of estrogen are implicated, as are high levels of androgen.

DIAGNOSIS

DIFFERENTIAL DIAGNOSIS

- Follicular pyodermas such as folliculitis, furuncles, carbuncles, and pilonidal cysts
- Granuloma inguinale
- Perianal and vulvular manifestations of Crohn's disease
- Abscess
- Infection of a Bartholin's cyst
- Actinomycosis
- Lymphogranuloma venereum
- Infection of an epidermoid cyst
- Lymphadenitis
- Cat scratch disease
- Tularemia
- Erysipelas
- Ulcerative colitis

WORKUP

This is primarily a clinical diagnosis based on typical lesion (see "Physical Findings & Clinical Presentation").

LABORATORY TESTS

- Patients with acute lesions may have an elevated erythrocyte sedimentation rate or WBC. They also may have serum protein abnormalities on electrophoresis.
- Any pus should be sampled for bacterial culture and sensitivity.

AUTHOR: **CHRISTINE HARTLEY, M.D.**

BASIC INFORMATION

DEFINITION

The development of stiff, pigmented (terminal) facial and body hair in women as a result of excess androgen production.

SYNONYMS

Hypertrichosis
Acquired lanuginosa

ICD-9CM CODES
704.1 Hirsutism

EPIDEMIOLOGY & DEMOGRAPHICS

- Overall prevalence unknown, estimated 1% to 2% in women 18 to 38 years.
- Race and genetics should be considered as some distinct ethnic populations have minimal body hair and others have moderate to large amounts of body hair while serum androgen levels are similar.
- Social norms and culture also determine how much body hair is cosmetically acceptable.
- Incidence and presentation of hirsutism dependent on underlying cause of androgen excess (see "Differential Diagnosis").

CLINICAL PRESENTATION

- Timing of symptoms—abrupt onset, short duration, rapid progression, progressive worsening, more severe signs of virilization, or later age of onset suggest androgen-producing tumor, late-onset congenital adrenal hyperplasia, or Cushing's syndrome. Weight increases may produce increased androgen production.
- Menstrual history—menarche, cycle regularity and symptoms of ovulation, fertility, and contraception use. Anovulatory cycles are the most common underlying cause of androgen excess.
- Medication use history—some drugs cause hirsutism or produce androgenergic effects (donazol, phenytoin, androgenic progestins e.g., norgestrel, cyclosporin, minoxidil, metoclopramide, phenothiazines, methyldopa, diazoxide, penicillamine).
- Family history—known or suspected family history of hirsutism, congenital adrenal hyperplasia, insulin resistance, polycystic ovary syndrome (PCOS), infertility, obesity, menstrual irregularity.
- Physical exam—voice, body habitus, galactorrhea, abdominal and pelvic exam.
- Associated cutaneous manifestations—acne, acanthosis nigricans, striae, hair distribution, location and quantity, frontotemporal balding, muscle mass, clitoromegaly.

ETIOLOGY

- Presence of hirsutism indicates androgen excess. Total testosterone may be normal, but free testosterone is elevated.
- Anovulatory ovaries are usual source of excess androgens through thecal cell steroidogenesis and conversion of androstenedione to testosterone.
- Conditions that decrease hepatic production of sex hormone binding globulin (SHBG) decrease protein-bound testosterone and increase free testosterone fraction (e.g., low estrogen, high androgen, and hyperinsulinemic states).
- Late-onset, congenital adrenal hyperplasia enzyme deficiency (most commonly 21-hydroxylase deficiency) produces excess 17 alphahydroxyprogesterone (17-OHP) and overproduction of androstenedione.
- Rare ovarian tumors primarily derived from Sertoli-Leydig cells, granulosa theca cells, or hilus cells produce excess androgens.
- Rare adrenal tumors produce excess androgens.
- Rare pituitary or hypothalamic tumors produce excess prolactin and can lead to anovulation.

DIAGNOSIS

DIFFERENTIAL DIAGNOSIS

- Androgen-independent vellus hair—soft, unpigmented hair that covers entire body.
- Hypertrichosis—diffusely increased total body hair often an adverse response to a medication or systemic illness.
- PCOS 75%
- Idiopathic 5% to 15%
- Congenital adrenal hyperplasia 1% to 8%
- Insulin resistance syndrome 3% to 4%
- Drug induced <1%
- Ovarian tumor <1%
- Adrenal tumor <1%
- Hyperthecosis <1%
- Hyperprolactinemia <1%

WORKUP

Workup is directed to determine underlying cause of androgen excess. See specific conditions for more detailed workup of individual diagnoses.

LABORATORY TESTS

- Total serum testosterone or free testosterone—screen for testosterone secreting tumors. If markedly elevated may image adrenals and ovaries.
- DHEA-S (dehydroepiandrosterone sulfate)—screen for adrenal androgen production as almost entirely produced by adrenals.
- Prolactin—moderately elevated values should prompt imaging of pituitary-hypothalamic region.
- 17-OHP—screen for adrenal enzyme deficiencies.

Other laboratory test considerations if appropriate:

- FSH—rule out hypoestrogen state (perimenopausal).
- LH—typically elevated in PCOS with low or normal FSH.
- TSH—rule out hypothyroidism.
- 24-hr urinary free cortisol—rule out Cushing's syndrome and overproduction of cortisol.
- Overnight single-dose dexamethasone suppression test—rule out Cushing's syndrome and adrenal hyperfunction.
- FBS, 2-hr 75-g oral glucose tolerance test, fasting insulin levels—rule out insulin resistance syndrome.

IMAGING STUDIES

Imaging study considerations if appropriate:

- Abdominal CT/MRI—rule out adrenal tumor.
- Pituitary-hypothalamic region CT/MRI—rule out pituitary tumor.
- Pelvic ultrasound (high resolution, transvaginal)—rule out ovarian tumor.
- Laparoscopy/otomy—rule out small ovarian tumor in cases of elevated testosterone levels without radiologic evidence of adrenal or ovarian pathology.

TREATMENT

NONPHARMACOLOGIC THERAPY

- Weight reduction—can reduce androgen production, improve menstrual function, and slow hair growth in obese women.
- Cosmetic—temporary
  - Shaving—does not stimulate hair growth; lasts days.
  - Epilation—electronic plucking.
  - Bleaching.
  - Mechanical waxing/plucking.
  - Depilatories—chemically disrupts sulfide bonds of hair causing dissolution of hair shaft.
  - Pulsed laser—good for pigmented hair; lasts 3-6 months.
- Cosmetic—permanent
  - Electrolysis—destroys individual hair follicles.
  - Combined energies—bipolar radio frequency and pulsed light.

ACUTE GENERAL Rx

See "Pharmacologic Therapy."

CHRONIC Rx

See "Pharmacologic Therapy."

PHARMACOLOGIC THERAPY

- Temporary cosmetic treatment eflornithine topical 13.9% cream. Hair growth returns upon discontinuation of treatment. Slow response over 4 to 8 weeks. Applied directly to unwanted facial hair bid with at least 8 hrs spaced applications.
- Suppress ovarian steroidogenesis and LH through low-dose estrogen and low androgenic progestational agents. Slow response to treatment. Suppresses new hair growth. Established hair unaffected.
  - Low-dose OCPs e.g., norethindrone, desogestrel, norgestimate, cyproterone (not available in U.S.) Avoid norgestrel and levonorgestrel.
  - Medroxyprogesterone 150 mg IM q 3 months or 10 to 20 mg po daily.
- Spironolactone—when OCPs unacceptable or may be added for disappointing results after 6 months of OCP treatment.
  - Aldosterone-antagonist diuretic inhibits adrenal and ovarian biosynthesis of androgens. May get ovulation.
  - Slow response usually 6 months or more.
  - 200 mg po qD, then decrease to 25-50 mg qD maintenance.
  - May cause hyperkalemia.
  - Anovulatory, unopposed estrogen states require progestin management.
- Finasteride—antiandrogen, in hair follicle blocks 5 α–reductase conversion of testosterone to intranuclearly active dihydrotestosterone (DHT).
  - Use with reliable contraception because DHT necessary for normal male fetus urogenital development.
  - Not FDA approved for treatment of hirsutism.
  - 1-5 mg po qD.
- Flutamide—inhibits androgen uptake and receptor binding.
  - Not FDA approved for treatment of hirsutism, but used by some European endocrinologists.
  - Use with reliable contraception.
  - 250 mg po bid.
- GnRH agonists—inhibits gonadotropin and consequently ovarian androgen and estrogen secretion. May use in combination with low-dose estrogen/progestin or OCP to counter resulting estrogen deficiency.
- Dexamethasone—adrenal glucocorticoid suppression is reserved for diagnosis of adrenal enzyme deficiency.
- Metformin/troglitazone therapy reserved for insulin resistant states.
- Total abdominal hysterectomy/bilateral salpingo-oopherectomy reserved for recalcitrant hirsutism in older female with hyperthecosis and undesired fertility.

REFERRAL

To endocrinologist if difficulty in determining diagnosis, achieving therapeutic goals, or resistant to first line therapies.

PEARLS & CONSIDERATIONS

COMMENTS

- Hirsutism is both an endocrine and cosmetic problem for patients.
- Ovulation induction therapy is indicated in women desiring pregnancy.
- Evaluation of incidental adrenal mass is warranted.

SUGGESTED READINGS

Hunter M, Carek J: Evaluation and treatment of women with hirsutism, *Am Fam Physician* 67:2565-2572, 2003.

Speroff L, Glass RH, Kase NG (eds): Hirsutism. In *Clinical gynecologic endocrinology and infertility,* ed 6, Baltimore, 1999, Lippincott Williams & Wilkins, pp 529-556.

AUTHOR: **RICHARD LONG, M.D.**

BASIC INFORMATION

DEFINITION

Histiocytosis X, now known as Langerhans cell histiocytosis (LCH), is a rare disorder characterized by the abnormal proliferation of pathologic Langerhans cells. These dendritic cells form characteristic infiltrates with eosinophils, lymphocytes, and other histiocytes found in various organs.

SYNONYMS

Eosinophilic granuloma
Hand-Schüller-Christian disease
Letterer-Siwe disease
Langerhans cell histiocytosis
Langerhans cell granulomatosis

ICD-9CM CODES
277.8 Histiocytosis X

EPIDEMIOLOGY & DEMOGRAPHICS

- LCH is mainly a childhood disorder with a peak incidence from age 1 to 4 yr.
- In the pediatric population, it affects 2 to 5 per million population annually.
- LCH affects males more often than females, 2:1.
- Pulmonary LCH (a localized form more commonly found in adults) has an equal male:female incidence, if not female predominance, likely due to increased prevalence of smoking in women.
- Usually more common in Caucasians.
- Disseminated LCH usually occurs before 2 yr of age.

PHYSICAL FINDINGS & CLINICAL PRESENTATION

- Clinical presentation is variable, and ranges from:
  - A benign isolated bony lesion (eosinophilic granuloma), most often found in children younger than 15 yr of age.
  - Multiple bone lesions with soft tissue gingival and oral mucosal involvement (Hand-Schüller-Christian disease); generally occurs in children younger than10 yr of age.
  - An aggressive disseminated disease infiltrating organs and causing organ dysfunction (Letterer-Siwe disease). It is the rarest form of LCH, affecting mostly children younger than 2 yr.
- Bone lesions (80% to 100%).
  - May be isolated or multiple
  - Painful, often worse at night
  - Skull most often involved, followed by long bones; lesions rarely seen in small bones of hands and feet
  - Proptosis
  - Mastoiditis
  - Loose teeth
  - Gingival hypertrophy
- Skin is involved in >80% of patients with disseminated disease and in 30% of patients with less extensive disease.
  - Seborrhea-like scaling of scalp, petechial and purpuric lesions, ulcers, and bronzing of the skin may occur.
  - Common sites: scalp, neck, trunk, groin, and extremities.
- Lymphadenopathy (10%): cervical and inguinal.
- Pulmonary disease is very frequent in adults (usually as isolated disease), but can be seen in 23% to 50% of children as well. Lung involvement always occurs as part of the disseminated disease in children.
- Pulmonary involvement may manifest with cough, tachypnea, cyanosis, inspiratory crackles, pleural effusions, or pneumothorax. Diffuse emphysema associated with pulmonary fibrosis is the end stage of a mixed restrictive and obstructive pattern of disease.
- Liver involvement manifesting as hepatomegaly with or without jaundice (50% to 60%).
- Involvement of the biliary tree may be seen as biliary fibrosis or sclerosing cholangitis.
- Splenomegaly (5%).
- Central nervous system involvement occurs in 25% to 35% of patients, most often in those with disseminated disease. The most common cerebral site affected is the hypothalamic-neurohypophyseal region, where infiltration and destruction usually result in diabetes insipidus with insatiable thirst and urination. The second most common site of involvement is the cerebellum.
- Involvement of the thymus, parotid glands, and GI tract has been reported in rare cases.

ETIOLOGY

- The etiology of LCH is unknown, some degree of genetic predisposition has been proposed.
- Multiple theories have been proposed. Recent evidence suggests LCH as a monoclonal proliferative neoplastic disorder.
- In adults, pulmonary LCH appears to be primarily an immune-mediated reactive process and has been linked to cigarette smoking. Cigarette smoke had not been observed as a causative factor in other forms of LCH.

DIAGNOSIS

Tissue biopsy of organ lesions reveals pathological Langerhans cells characterized by the presence of multiple surface nucleoproteins including CD1a, the presence of which establishes definitively histological diagnosis of LCH. The infiltration by eosinophils forming pseudoabscesses is characteristic.

DIFFERENTIAL DIAGNOSIS

The differential diagnosis is extensive, including all causes of diabetes insipidus, lytic bone lesions, dermatitis, hepatomegaly, and lymphadenopathy.

WORKUP

Baseline evaluation should include bone scan, chest x-ray, skeletal x-ray, abdominal ultrasound, and routine laboratory to assess the extent of disease involvement. Depending on the results and symptoms, further diagnostic procedures may be necessary.

LABORATORY TESTS

- CBC is not specific, but may reveal cytopenias in patients with bone marrow involvement.
- Electrolytes, BUN, creatinine, urinalysis, and urine and serum osmolality are helpful in the diagnosis of diabetes insipidus during fluid deprivation testing.
- Liver function tests (LFTs) may be elevated in patients with liver involvement.
- Bronchoalveolar lavage may show increased numbers of CD1a-positive histiocytes or Langerhans cells in patients with pulmonary LCH.

IMAGING STUDIES

- X-ray studies of affected areas show lytic lesions with or without sclerotic margins.
- X-ray bone survey is done searching for other lesions.
- Bone scan complements the bone survey studies.
- Panoramic dental view of the mandible and maxilla for children with oral involvement.
- Chest x-ray can show interstitial reticulonodular infiltrates. This pattern typically progresses toward frank honeycombing fibrosis later in the course of the disease (Fig. 1-124).
- High-resolution CT scan of the chest confirms interstitial lung scarring, nodules, and cysts, and represents an excellent noninvasive means for diagnosis and follow-up of pulmonary LCH. Pulmonary cysts are bilateral and symmetric, showing slight upper-lobe predominance with relative sparing of the costophrenic angles.
- CT scans of the temporal bone searching for mastoid, and inner and middle ear involvement.
- Ultrasound of the abdomen may show hepatosplenomegaly.
- Conventional cholangiography or magnetic resonance cholangiopancreatography can confirm the presence of disease in patients suspected to have biliary involvement.

- MRI of the brain to visualize the hypothalamic-hypophyseal region in patients suspected of having diabetes insipidus.

TREATMENT

Rx

Treatment is still evolving and is based on organ involvement and the extent of disease.

ACUTE GENERAL Rx

Isolated bone lesions can be treated by:
- Curettage of affected site and implantation of allograft bone chips or polymethylmethacrylate
- Intralesional prednisone or prednisone and vinblastine
- Bisphosphonates
- NSAIDs
- Radiation therapy is useful only for bone lesions of the femoral vertebrae or femoral neck at risk of collapse

Single skin lesions are treated with:
- Topical steroid (e.g., triamcinolone acetonide) applied bid
- Nitrogen mustard in 20% solution
- Surgery
- Intralesional interferon
- Isotretinoin

Treatment of solitary lymph node involvement:
- Excision at the time of diagnosis
- Systemic oral prednisone

Treatment for multiple bone lesions, skull base lesions, or multisystem disease includes:
- Vinblastine 6 mg/m2 IV bolus qwk × 6 mo or etoposide 150 mg/m2 IV for 3 days q3wk for 6 mo plus oral prednisone for 6 mo

CHRONIC Rx

- For severe, high-risk, disseminated patients not responding within 6 weeks of initial treatment, salvage therapy, including high dose of the purine analog cladribine along with high-dose cytosine arabinoside followed by allogeneic blood stem cell transplantation, should be considered. Additionally, liver or lung transplantation might be the treatment of choice for terminal liver and lung failure patients.
- Diabetes insipidus is treated with DDAVP 0.1 to 0.8 mg PO or 1 spray bid to tid.
- Adults with isolated pulmonary LCH do not require aggressive treatment, and will benefit from smoking cessation.
- Empirical use of steroids, in either short pulses or longer exposures, has also been implicated in the treatment of pulmonary disease; however, data regarding effectiveness are still limited.
- Lung transplantation has been tried in both children and adults with advanced pulmonary disease and limited lung function, but failure rates are high because of local recurrence after transplantation.

DISPOSITION

- Patients with disease localized to only one organ system have a good prognosis and appear to need minimal, if any, treatment. For patients with isolated pulmonary LCH, the 5-yr survival rate is around 80%.
- Patients with disseminated disease have an increased risk for poor outcome, with a reported mortality rate of 10% to 20%, and 50% risk of life-impairing morbidity. A poor prognostic feature is the failure to respond to therapy in the first 6 wk.
- In patients with disseminated LCH and <2 yr of age, the mortality rate is 30%.

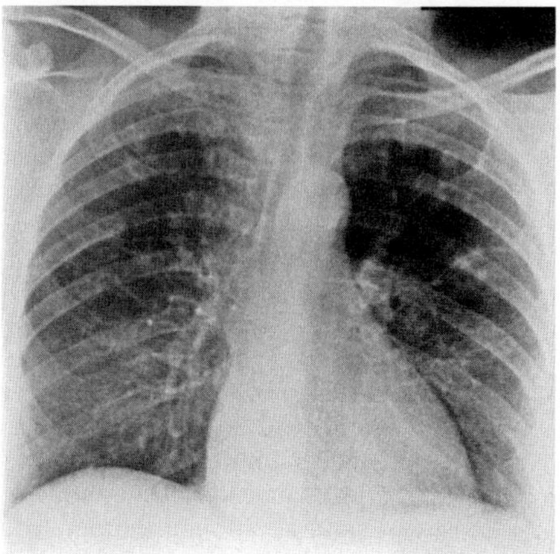

FIGURE 1-124 Langerhans cell histiocytosis (LCH; Histiocytosis X) There is a reticular nodular pattern in the upper lobes. The lung volumes are preserved. (From McLoud TC [ed]: *Thoracic radiology, the requisites,* St Louis, 1998, Mosby.)

REFERRAL

Multidisciplinary approach: pediatric oncologist, radiation oncologists, oral maxillary surgeons, ENT specialists, audiology, dermatology, endocrinology, and family counseling.

PEARLS & CONSIDERATIONS

!

COMMENTS

- The course of LCH is often unpredictable and varies from spontaneous resolution to rapid progression and death, or multiple recurrences and regressions with risk for permanent sequelae.
- The association of LCH with other malignancies (e.g., acute lymphocytic leukemia, acute nonlymphoblastic leukemia, and solid tumors) has been cited.

PREVENTION

Effective antismoking measures can prevent pulmonary LCH.

PATIENT/FAMILY EDUCATION

- Instruct patients to promptly report the development of hemoptysis. This symptom may indicate malignancy or superimposed bacterial/fungal infection, such as *Aspergillus* species infection.
- Educate about the likely etiologic role of cigarette smoking.

SUGGESTED READINGS

Dauriat G et al: Lung transplantation for pulmonary Langerhans' cell histiocytosis: a multicenter analysis, *Transplantation* 81:746, 2006.

Hoover KB et al: Langerhans cell histiocytosis, *Skeletal Radiol* 36(2):95-104, 2007. Epub 2006 Oct 7.

Schmidt S et al: Extra-osseous involvement of Langerhans' cell histiocytosis in children, *Pediatr Radiol* 34:313, 2004.

Stockschlaeder M, Sucker C: Adult Langerhans cell histiocytosis, *Eur J Haematol* 76(5):363368, 2006. Epub 2006 Mar 17.

AUTHOR: **RAMI ELTIBI, M.D.**

BASIC INFORMATION

DEFINITION

Histoplasmosis is caused by the fungus *Histoplasma capsulatum* and characterized by a primary pulmonary focus with occasional progression to chronic pulmonary histoplasmosis (CPH) or various forms of dissemination. Progressive disseminated histoplasmosis (PDH) may present with a diverse clinical spectrum, including adrenal necrosis, pulmonary and mediastinal fibrosis, and ulcerations of the oropharynx and GI tract. In those patients coinfected with the human immunodeficiency virus (HIV), it is a defining disease for acquired immunodeficiency syndrome (AIDS).

SYNONYMS

North American histoplasmosis
Ohio Valley fever
Vanderbilt disease

ICD-9CM CODES
115.90 Histoplasmosis
115.94 Histoplasmosis with endocarditis
115.91 Histoplasmosis with meningitis
115.93 Histoplasmosis with pericarditis
115.95 Histoplasmosis with pneumonia
115.92 Histoplasmosis with retinitis

EPIDEMIOLOGY & DEMOGRAPHICS

INCIDENCE (IN U.S.):
- Unknown for acute pulmonary disease
- For CPH, estimated at 1/100,000 cases in endemic areas
- For PDH in immunocompetent adults, estimated at 1/2000 cases of histoplasmosis

PREVALENCE: Unknown
PREDOMINANT SEX: Clinically evident disease is most common in males; male:female ratio of 4:1
PREDOMINANT AGE:
- CPH is most often seen in males >50 yr old with an associated history of COPD.
- Presumed ocular histoplasmosis syndrome (POHS) is seen between ages of 20 and 40 yr.

PEAK INCIDENCE: Unknown

PHYSICAL FINDINGS & CLINICAL PRESENTATION

- Conidia are deposited in alveoli then converted to yeast forms where they spread to regional lymph nodes and other organs, especially liver and spleen.
- 1 to 2 wk later, a granulomatous inflammatory response begins to contain the yeast in the form of discrete granulomas.
- Delayed-type hypersensitivity to *Histoplasma* antigens occurs 3 to 6 wk after exposure.
- Clinical disease manifests in various forms, depending on host cellular immunity and inoculum size:
  1. Acute primary pulmonary histoplasmosis
     a. Overwhelming number of patients are asymptomatic.
     b. Most clinically apparent infections manifest by complaints of fever, headache, malaise, pleuritic chest pain, nonproductive cough, and weight loss.
     c. Less than 10%, mainly women, complain of arthralgias, myalgias, and skin manifestations such as erythema multiforme or erythema nodosum.
     d. Acute pericarditis presents in smaller percentage of patients.
     e. Hepatosplenomegaly is most commonly observed in children.
     f. With particularly heavy exposure, there is severe dyspnea, marked hypoxemia, impending respiratory failure.
     g. Most patients are asymptomatic within 6 wk.
  2. CPH
     a. Presents insidiously with low-grade fever, malaise, weight loss, cough, sometimes with blood-streaked sputum or frank hemoptysis.
     b. Most patients with cavitary lesions present with associated COPD or chronic bronchitis, masking underlying fungal disease.
     c. Tends to worsen preexisting pulmonary disease and further contribute to eventual respiratory insufficiency.
  3. PDH
     a. In both acute and subacute forms, constitutional symptoms of fever, fatigue, malaise, and weight loss are common.
     b. Acute form (seen in infants and children) presents with respiratory symptoms, fever ≥101° F (38.3° C), generalized lymphadenopathy, marked hepatosplenomegaly, and fulminant course resembling septic shock associated with a high fatality rate.
     c. Subacute form is more common in adults and associated with lower temperatures, hepatosplenomegaly, oropharyngeal ulceration, focal organ involvement (including adrenal destruction, endocarditis, chronic meningitis, and intracerebral mass lesions).
     d. Course of subacute form is relentless, with untreated patient dying within 2 yr.
     e. Chronic PDH is found in adults and marked by gradual symptoms of weight loss, weakness, easy fatigability; low-grade fever when present; oropharyngeal ulcerations and hepatomegaly and/or splenomegaly in one third of patients.
     f. Less clinical evidence of focal organ involvement in chronic form than in subacute form.
     g. Natural history of chronic form protracted and intermittent, spanning months to years.
- Histoplasmoma
  1. A healed area of caseation necrosis surrounded by a fibrous capsule
  2. Usually asymptomatic
- Mediastinal fibrosis
  1. A rare consequence of a fibroblastic process that encases caseating mediastinal lymph nodes producing severe retraction, compression, and distortion of mediastinal structures
  2. Constriction of the bronchi resulting in bronchiectasis, also esophageal stenosis associated with dysphagia, and superior vena cava syndrome
- POHS
  1. Diagnosis characterized by distinct clinical features, including atrophic choroidal scars and maculopathy in patient with a history suggestive of exposure to the fungus (e.g., residence in an endemic area)
  2. Patient complains of distortion or loss of central vision without pain, redness, or photophobia
  3. Usually no evidence of infection except for a positive skin reaction to histoplasmin
- In patients with AIDS
  1. Possible presentation as overwhelming infection similar to acute PDH seen in children
  2. Constitutional symptoms: fever, weight loss, malaise, cough, dyspnea
  3. About 10% with cutaneous maculopapular, erythematous eruptions or purpuric lesions on face, trunk, and extremities
  4. Up to 20% with CNS involvement, manifesting as intracerebral mass lesions, chronic meningitis, or encephalopathy

ETIOLOGY

- *H. capsulatum* is a dimorphic fungus present in temperate zones and river valleys worldwide.
- In the U.S., it is highly endemic in southeastern, mid-Atlantic, and central states.
- Exists as mold at ambient temperature and favors soils enriched with bird or bat droppings.

DIAGNOSIS

DIFFERENTIAL DIAGNOSIS

- Acute pulmonary histoplasmosis
  1. *Mycobacterium tuberculosis*

2. Community-acquired pneumonias caused by *Mycoplasma* and *Chlamydia*
3. Other fungal diseases, such as *Blastomyces dermatitidis* and *Coccidioides immitis*

- Chronic cavitary pulmonary histoplasmosis: *M. tuberculosis*
- Histoplasmomas: true neoplasms

WORKUP

- Suspect diagnosis in patients who present with a history of residence or travel in an endemic area, especially if engaged in occupations (e.g., outside construction or street cleaning) or hobbies (e.g., cave exploring) that increase the likelihood of exposure to fungal spores.
- Suspect diagnosis in immunosuppressed patients with remote history of exposure, especially if associated with characteristic calcifications on chest x-ray examination.

LABORATORY TESTS

- Demonstration of organism on culture from body fluid or tissues to make definitive diagnosis
  1. Especially high yield in patients with AIDS
  2. Characteristic oval yeast cells in neutrophils with Giemsa stain from peripheral smear
  3. Preparations of infected tissue with Gomori's silver methenamine for revealing yeast forms, especially in areas of caseation necrosis
- Serologic tests, including complement-fixing (CF) antibodies and immunodiffusion assays
- Detection of *Histoplasma* antigen in urine: may be influenced by infections with *Blastomyces* and *Coccidioides*
- In PDH
  1. Pancytopenia
  2. Marked elevations in alkaline phosphatase and alanine aminotransferase (ALT) common
- In chronic meningitis (majority of cases)
  1. CSF pleocytosis with either lymphocytes or neutrophils predominating
  2. Elevated CSF protein levels
  3. Hypoglycorrhachia

IMAGING STUDIES

- Chest x-ray examination in acute pulmonary histoplasmosis
  1. Singular or multiple patchy infiltrates, especially in the lower lung fields
  2. Hilar or mediastinal lymphadenopathy with or without pneumonitis
  3. Diffuse nodular or confluent bilateral miliary infiltrates characteristic of heavier exposure
  4. Infrequent pleural effusions, except when associated with pericarditis
- Chest x-ray examination in histoplasmoma: coin lesion displaying central calcification, ranging from 1 to 4 cm in diameter, predominantly located in the subpleural regions
- Chest x-ray examination in CPH:
  1. Upper lobe disease frequently associated with cavities
  2. Preexisting calcifications in the hilum associated with peribronchial streaking extending to the parenchyma
- Chest x-ray examination in acute PDH: hilar adenopathy and/or diffuse nodular infiltrates
- CT scan of adrenals to reveal bilateral enlargement and low-attenuation centers

TREATMENT

Rx

NONPHARMACOLOGIC THERAPY

For life-threatening disease seen in acute disseminated disease or infection in patients with AIDS: supportive therapy with IV fluids

ACUTE GENERAL Rx

- No drug therapy is required for asymptomatic pulmonary disease.
- A course of therapy with ketoconazole 400 mg/day or itraconazole 200 mg/day PO for 3 to 6 wk may be beneficial in some patients with acute pulmonary distress. Avoid fluconazole because it is not as active.
- Same therapy appropriate for immunocompetent, mild to moderately symptomatic patients with CPH and subacute and chronic forms of PDH, but duration for 6 to 12 mo.
- Use amphotericin B 0.7 to 1 mg/kg IV for 6 to 12 mo in patients hypersensitive to or intolerant of azole therapy.
- Give amphotericin B for life-threatening disease or continued illness as a result of primary failure or relapse of adequate azole therapy. A lipid formulation of amphotericin b can be used to avoid nephrotoxicity.
  1. For acute pulmonary histoplasmosis associated with acute respiratory distress syndrome (ARDS), acute PDH, and histoplasma meningitis: dose of 0.7 to 1 mg/kg IV >4 hr
  2. End point of therapy for patient with complicated acute pulmonary disease: total dose of 500 mg
  3. End point for patient with acute PDH: total dose 35 mg/kg or 2.5 g total
  4. Prednisone 60 to 80 mg/day beneficial for severe fungal hypersensitivity complicating acute pulmonary disease
- Endocarditis: surgical treatment with excision of infected valve or graft combined with amphotericin for a total dose of 35 mg/kg or 2.5 g.
- For pericardial disease:
  1. Antifungal therapy: no apparent benefit
  2. Best managed with NSAIDs
- For POHS:
  1. Antifungal therapy: no apparent benefit
  2. May respond to laser therapy

CHRONIC Rx

In patients with AIDS: lifelong suppressive therapy with either itraconazole, given 200 mg PO qd, or IV amphotericin B at a dose of 50 mg once weekly; a triazole compound posaconazole (400 mg PO bid) may be useful in refractory cases, but clinical experience is limited at this point.

DISPOSITION

For those with chronic or progressive disease, especially if immunocompromised, prognosis is dependent on prompt recognition and timely administration of appropriate antifungal drugs.

REFERRAL

- To an infectious disease specialist in suspected cases of disseminated disease, especially if immunocompromised
- To a pulmonologist for patients with CPH form because progressive respiratory compromise
- To a thoracic surgeon for decompression procedures for progressive mediastinal fibrosis

PEARLS & CONSIDERATIONS

!

- *H. capsulatum,* variety *duboisii,* also known as African histoplasmosis, is restricted to Senegal, Nigeria, Zaire, and Uganda.
- Unlike *H. capsulatum,* pulmonary forms of *duboisii* are not seen, and the disease is limited to the skin, soft tissues, and bone.

COMMENTS

- Patients living in endemic areas, especially if immunocompromised, should take appropriate respiratory precautions when disposing of bird waste from rooftop or home aviaries.
- Appropriate respiratory precautions should also be taken when leisure traveling to areas that act as a natural haven for the fungus, such as bat caves.

SUGGESTED READINGS

Schestatsky P et al: Isolated central nervous system histoplasmosis in immunocompetent hosts: a series of 11 cases, *Scand J Infect Dis* 38(1):43, 2006.

Weinberg M et al: Severe histoplasmosis in travelers to Nicaragua, *Emerg Infect Dis* 9 (10):1322, 2003.

Wheat LJ, Kauffman CA: Histoplasmosis, *Infect Dis Clin North Am* 17(1):1, 2003.

AUTHORS: **GLENN G. FORT, M.D., M.P.H., DENNIS J. MIKOLICH, M.D.,** and **GEORGE O. ALONSO, M.D.**

BASIC INFORMATION

DEFINITION

Histrionic personality disorder is a cluster B personality disorder with a pervasive pattern of excessive emotionality and attention-seeking behavior that generally begins in early adulthood.

SYNONYMS

Hysterical personality disorder
Psycho-infantile personality disorder
Personality disorder (nonspecific)

ICD-9CM CODES
301.5 Histrionic personality disorder (ICD-9 and DSM IV Code)

EPIDEMIOLOGY & DEMOGRAPHICS

PREVALENCE (IN U.S.):

- Diagnosed more often in women.
- Prevalence: 2% to 3% for histrionic personality disorder; 10% to 13% for personality disorders (unspecified).

PREDOMINANT SEX: Predominant in women. Cultural factors may lead to more common diagnosis in women.

PREDOMINANT AGE: Generally begins in early childhood.

PHYSICAL FINDINGS & CLINICAL PRESENTATION

Features include five or more of the following:

1. Is uncomfortable in situations where he or she is not the center of attention.
2. Interaction with others is often characterized by inappropriate sexually seductive or provocative behavior.
3. Displays rapidly shifting and shallow expression of emotions.
4. Consistently uses physical appearance to draw attention to self.
5. Has a style of speech that is excessively impressionistic and lacking in detail.
6. Shows self-dramatization, theatricality, and exaggerated expression of emotion.
7. Is suggestible (i.e., easily influenced by others or circumstances).
8. Considers relationships to be more intimate than they actually are.

ETIOLOGY

- Unknown.
- As with other personality disorders, childhood events, psychosocial adversity, and genetics are contributory.

DIAGNOSIS

DIFFERENTIAL DIAGNOSIS

- Other personality disorders (e.g., borderline personality disorder, antisocial personality disorder, narcissistic personality disorder).
- Personality change secondary to general medical condition.
- Symptoms may develop in association with chronic substance abuse.

WORKUP

There is no formal test to establish diagnosis.

TREATMENT

NONPHARMACOLOGIC THERAPY

- Long-term individual psychotherapy is treatment of choice.
- Cognitive-behavioral or psychodynamically oriented outpatient individual psychotherapies are efficacious for some personality disorders, but the evidence is lacking for histrionic personality disorder.
- Persons with histrionic personality disorder may seek treatment (e.g., for cosmetic procedures) and exaggerate their symptoms and difficulties in functioning.
- Patients tend to be more emotionally needy and are often reluctant to terminate therapy.

ACUTE GENERAL Rx

- Small placebo-controlled trials suggest that patients with serious personality disorders (especially borderline PD) respond to optimal doses of selective serotonin reuptake inhibitors (SSRIs), with improvements in anger, impulsive, aggressive behavior, affective lability, and facilitation of psychotherapy.
- Care should be given when prescribing medications to someone who suffers from histrionic personality disorder because of the potential for using the medication to contribute to self-destructive or otherwise harmful behaviors.

DISPOSITION

- Therapy approaches should not be focused on the long-term personality change of the individual, but rather short-term alleviation of difficulties within the person's life.
- A "cure" is unlikely; the goal is to ameliorate symptoms.

REFERRAL

Referral to specialty mental health professionals is recommended.

PEARLS & CONSIDERATIONS

- Like most other personality disorders, people present for treatment only when stress or some other situational factor within their lives has made their ability to function and cope effectively impossible.
- Suicidality should be assessed on a regular basis and suicidal threats and self-mutilation should not be ignored or dismissed.

PATIENT/FAMILY EDUCATION

Group and family therapy approaches are generally not recommended, because the individual who suffers from this disorder often draws attention to himself or herself and exaggerates every action and reaction.

SUGGESTED READINGS

Gabbard GO: Mind, brain and personality disorders, *Am J Psychiatry* 162:4,2005.
Ritvo EV et al: Psychiatric conditions in cosmetic surgery patients, *Facial Plast Surg* 22(3):194, 2006.
Verheul R, Herbrink M: The efficacy of various modalities of psychotherapy for personality disorders: a systematic review of the evidence and clinical recommendations, *Int Rev Psychiatry* 19(1):25, 2007.

AUTHOR: **MITCHELL D. FELDMAN, M.D., M.PHIL.**

BASIC INFORMATION

DEFINITION

Hodgkin's disease is a malignant disorder of lymphoreticular origin, characterized histologically by the presence of multinucleated giant cells (Reed-Sternberg cells) usually originating from B lymphocytes in germinal centers of lymphoid tissue.

ICD-9CM CODES
201.9 Hodgkin's disease, unspecified
201.4 Hodgkin's disease, lymphocyte predominance
201.5 Hodgkin's disease, nodular sclerosis
201.6 Hodgkin's disease, mixed cellularity
201.7 Hodgkin's disease, lymphocyte depletion

EPIDEMIOLOGY & DEMOGRAPHICS

- There is a bimodal age distribution (15 to 34 yr and >50 yr).
- Concordance for Hodgkin's disease in identical twins suggests that a genetic susceptibility underlies Hodgkin's disease in young adulthood.
- The disease is more common in males (in childhood Hodgkin's disease, >80% occurs in males), in Caucasians, and in higher socioeconomic groups.
- Overall incidence of Hodgkin's disease in the U.S. is approximately 4:100,000. There are >7000 new cases of Hodgkin lymphoma diagnosed annually in the U.S.

PHYSICAL FINDINGS & CLINICAL PRESENTATION

- Palpable lymphadenopathy, generally painless
- Most common site of involvement: neck region
- See "Workup" for description of common symptoms

ETIOLOGY

Unknown; evidence implicating Epstein-Barr virus remains controversial.

DIAGNOSIS

DIFFERENTIAL DIAGNOSIS

- Non-Hodgkin's lymphoma
- Sarcoidosis
- Infections (e.g., CMV, Epstein-Barr virus, toxoplasma, HIV)
- Drug reaction

WORKUP

Symptomatic patients with Hodgkin's disease usually present with the following manifestations:

- Fever and night sweats: fever in a cyclical pattern (days or weeks of fever alternating with afebrile periods) is known as Pel-Epstein fever
- Weight loss, generalized malaise
- Persistent, nonproductive cough
- Pain associated with alcohol ingestion, often secondary to heavy eosinophil infiltration of the tumor sites
- Pruritus
- Others: superior vena cava syndrome and spinal cord compression (rare)

Diagnosis can be made with lymph node biopsy. There are four main *histologic subtypes,* based on the number of lymphocytes, Reed-Sternberg cells (Fig. 1-125), and the presence of fibrous tissue:

1. Lymphocyte predominance
2. Mixed cellularity
3. Nodular sclerosis
4. Lymphocyte depletion

Nodular sclerosis is the most common type and occurs mainly in young adulthood, whereas the mixed cellularity type is more prevalent after age 50 yr.

Staging for Hodgkin's disease follows the *Ann Arbor staging classification.*

Stage I: Involvement of a single lymph node region
Stage II: Two or more lymph node regions on the same side of the diaphragm
Stage III: Lymph node involvement on both sides of diaphragm, including spleen
Stage IV: Diffuse involvement of external sites
Suffix A: No systemic symptoms
Suffix B: Presence of fever, night sweats, or unexplained weight loss of 10% or more body weight over 6 mo
Suffix X: Indicates bulky disease >⅓ widening of mediastinum or >10 cm maximum dimension of nodal mass on a chest film

Proper staging requires the following:

- Detailed history (with documentation of "B symptoms" and physical examination)
- Surgical biopsy
- Laboratory evaluation (CBC, sedimentation rate, BUN, creatinine, alkaline phosphatase, LFTs, albumin, LDH, uric acid)
- Chest x-ray (PA and lateral)
- Bilateral bone marrow biopsy
- CT scan of the chest (when abnormal findings are noted on chest x-ray examination) and of the abdomen and pelvis to visualize the mesenteric, hepatic, portal, and splenic hilar nodes
- Positron emmision tomography (PET) scan
- Bipedal lymphangiography may be performed only in selected patients to define periaortic and iliac lymph node involvement
- Exploratory laparotomy and splenectomy (selected patients):
  1. Decision to perform staging laparotomy depends on the therapeutic plan; it is generally not indicated in patients who have a large mediastinal mass (these patients will generally be treated with combined chemotherapy and radiation). Staging laparotomy may also not be required in patients with clinical stage I or unlikely to have abdominal disease (e.g., females with supradiaphragmatic disease).
  2. Exploratory laparotomy and splenectomy may be used for patients with clinical stage I to IIA or IIB.
  3. It is useful in identifying patients who can be treated with irradiation alone with curative intent.
  4. Polyvalent pneumococcal vaccine should be given prophylactically to all patients before splenectomy (increased risk of sepsis from encapsulated organisms in splenectomized patients).

TREATMENT

ACUTE GENERAL Rx

The main therapeutic modalities are radiotherapy and chemotherapy; the indication for each vary with pathologic stage and other factors.

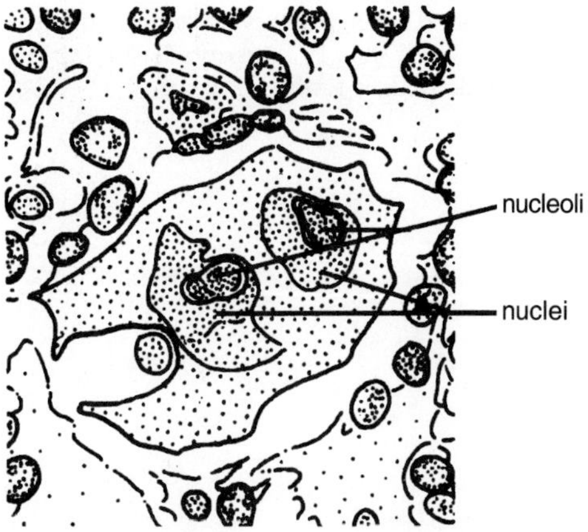

FIGURE 1-125 Hodgkin's disease. High-power photomicrograph demonstrates a binucleate Reed-Sternberg cell exhibiting prominent inclusion-like eosinophilic nucleoli giving it an "owl's eye" appearance. (From Skarin AT: *Atlas of diagnostic oncology,* ed 3, St Louis, 2003, Mosby.)

- Stage I and II: radiation therapy alone unless a large mediastinal mass is present (mediastinal to thoracic ratio ≥1.3); in the latter case, a combination of chemotherapy and radiation therapy is indicated.
- Stage IB or IIB: total nodal irradiation is often used, although chemotherapy is performed in many centers.
- Stage IIIA: treatment is controversial. It varies with the anatomic substage after splenectomy.
  1. III_1A and minimum splenic involvement: radiation therapy alone may be adequate.
  2. III_2 or III_1A with extensive splenic involvement: there is disagreement whether chemotherapy alone or a combination of chemotherapy and radiation therapy is the preferred treatment modality.
  3. IIIB and IVB: the treatment of choice is chemotherapy with or without adjuvant radiotherapy.

Various regimens can be used for combination of chemotherapy. Most oncologists prefer the combination of doxorubicin plus bleomycin plus vincristine plus dacarbazine (ABVD). Other commonly used regimens are MOPP, MOPP-ABV, MOPP-ABVD, MOPP-BAP.

- In patients with advanced Hodgkin's disease, increased-dose bleomycin, etoposide, doxorubicin, cyclophosphamide, vincristine, procarbazine, and prednisone (BEACOPP) offers better tumor control and overall survival than COPP-ABVD.

DISPOSITION

- The overall survival at 10 yr is approximately 60%.
- Cure rates as high as 75% to 80% are now possible with appropriate initial therapy.
- Poor prognostic features include presence of "B symptoms," advanced age, advanced stage at initial presentation, mixed-cellularity, and lymphocyte depletion histology.
- Chemotherapy significantly increases the risk of leukemia.
- The peak in risk of leukemia is seen approximately 5 yr after the initiation of chemotherapy.
- The risk of leukemia is greater for those who undergo splenectomy and for patients with advanced stages of Hodgkin's disease; the risk is unaffected by concomitant radiotherapy.
- Involved-field radiotherapy does not improve the outcome in patients with advanced-stage Hodgkin's lymphoma who have a complete remission after MOPP-ABV chemotherapy. Radiotherapy may benefit patients with a partial response after chemotherapy.
- Mediastinal irradiation increases the risk of subsequent death from heart disease caused by sclerosis of coronary artery secondary to irradiation. Risk increases with high mediastinal doses, minimal protective cardiac blocking, young age at irradiation, and increased duration of follow-up.
- Both chemotherapy and radiation therapy increase the risk of developing secondary solid tumors (e.g., carcinoma of the lung, breast, and stomach).

REFERRAL

- Surgical referral for lymph node biopsy
- Hematology/oncology referral

PEARLS & CONSIDERATIONS

COMMENTS

- Young male patients should consider sperm banking before the initiation of therapy.
- Chemotherapy plus involved-field radiotherapy should be the standard treatment for Hodgkin's disease with favorable prognostic features. In patients with unfavorable features, 4 courses of chemotherapy plus involved-field radiotherapy should be the standard of treatment.

EVIDENCE

For early stage Hodgkin's disease, experience and clinical trials over the last 50 years have shown the efficacy of radiotherapy alone. A retrospective study of 709 patients with early-stage disease and who were treated with primary radiation therapy revealed that 157 patients had relapsed at a median time of 2 years.[1]

Chemotherapy alone may prove to be equally as effective. The ultimate choice of therapy modality will then depend on differences in short-term and long-term toxic effects. The long-term effects (>15 years after completion of therapy) are not yet available for patients treated with chemotherapy alone.

For patients with early-stage, massive mediastinal disease, cure rates of 80% are achievable using combined modality treatments.[2]

For advanced-stage disease, chemotherapy alone or combined radiotherapy with chemotherapy for bulky disease is efficacious. A metaanalysis of >1700 patients treated on 14 different trials showed no improvement in overall 10-year survival for patients with advanced disease who received combined modality therapy vs. chemotherapy alone.[3]

In patients with advanced-stage disease with massive mediastinal involvement, relapse rates were lower in the group of patients treated with combined modalities than in the group treated with chemotherapy alone (20% vs. 50%).[4]

Evidence-Based References

1. Torrey PJ, Poen C, Hoppe RT: Detection of relapse in early-stage Hodgkin's disease: role of routine follow-up studies, *J Clin Oncol* 17:253, 1997.
2. Leopold KA et al: Stage IA-11B Hodgkin's disease: staging and treatment of patients with large mediastinal adenopathy, *J Clin Oncol* 7:1059, 1989.
3. Leoffler M et al: Meta-analysis of chemotherapy versus combined modality treatment trials in Hodgkin's disease, *J Clin Oncol* 16:818, 1998.
4. Longo DL et al: Treatment of advanced-stage mediastinal Hodgkin's disease: the case for combined modality treatment, *J Clin Oncol* 9:227, 1991.

SUGGESTED READINGS

Aleman B et al: Involved-field radiotherapy for advanced Hodgkin's lymphoma, *N Engl J Med* 348:2396, 2003.

Ansell S, Armitage JO: Management of Hodgkin Lymphoma, *Mayo Clin Proc* 81(3):419, 2006.

Diehl V et al: Standard and increased-dose BEACOPP chemotherapy compared with COPP-ABVD for advanced Hodgkin's disease, *N Engl J Med* 348:2386, 2003.

Ferme C et al: Chemotherapy plus involved-field radiation in early-stage Hodgkin's disease, *N Engl J Med* 357:1916-1927, 2007.

AUTHOR: **FRED F. FERRI, M.D.**

BASIC INFORMATION

DEFINITION

Hookworm is a parasitic infection of the intestine caused by helminths.

SYNONYMS

Ground itch
Ancylostoma duodenale infection
Necator americanus infection

ICD-9CM CODES
126.35 Hookworm

EPIDEMIOLOGY & DEMOGRAPHICS

INCIDENCE (IN U.S.):
- Varies greatly in different areas of the U.S.
- Most common in rural areas of southeastern U.S.
- Poor sanitation and increased rainfall increase likelihood

PREVALENCE (IN U.S.): Varies from 10% to 90% in regions where it is found
PREDOMINANT AGE: Schoolchildren

PHYSICAL FINDINGS & CLINICAL PRESENTATION

- Nonspecific abdominal complaints
- Because these organisms consume host RBCs, symptoms related to iron-deficiency anemia, depending on the amount of iron in the diet and the worm burden
- Fatigue, tachycardia, dyspnea, and high-output failure
- Hypoproteinemia and edema from loss of proteins into the intestinal tract
- Unusual for pulmonary manifestations to occur when the larvae migrate through the lungs
- Skin rash at sites of larval penetration in some individuals without prior exposure

ETIOLOGY

Two species can cause this disease: *N. americanus* and *A. duodenale*. *N. americanus* is the predominant cause of hookworm in the U.S. They are soil nematodes (Geohelminthic infections) that are acquired by skin contact (i.e., bare feet) with contaminated soils in moist, warm climate.
- Infection occurs via penetration of the skin by the larval form, with subsequent migration via the blood stream to the alveoli, up the respiratory tract, then into the GI tract
- *Ancylostoma spp* infection can also occur via the oral route through ingestion of contaminated water supplies
- Sharp mouth parts allow for attachment to intestinal mucosa
- *Ancylostoma spp* are more likely to cause iron deficiency anemia because they are larger and remove more blood daily from the bowel wall than the other hookworm species *N. americanus*

DIAGNOSIS

DIFFERENTIAL DIAGNOSIS

- Strongyloidiasis
- Ascariasis
- Other causes of iron deficiency anemia and malabsorption

WORKUP

Examine stool for hookworm eggs.

LABORATORY TESTS

CBC to show hypochromic, microcytic anemia; possible mild eosinophilia and hypoalbuminemia

IMAGING STUDIES

Chest x-ray examination: occasionally shows opacities

TREATMENT

NONPHARMACOLOGIC THERAPY

Prevention of disease by not walking barefoot and by improving sanitary conditions

ACUTE GENERAL Rx

- Albendazole 400 mg once by mouth has become preferred treatment
- Mebendazole 100 mg PO bid for 3 days is also effective
- Iron supplementation may be helpful in patients with iron deficiency

DISPOSITION

Easily treated

REFERRAL

If diagnosis uncertain

PEARLS & CONSIDERATIONS

COMMENTS

- Appropriate disposal of human wastes is important in controlling the disease in areas with a high prevalence of hookworm infestation.
- Wearing shoes will avoid contact with contaminated soils, and the provision of safe water and sanitation for disposing human excreta is important in control of hookworm.

SUGGESTED READINGS

Brooker S, Bethony J, Hotez PJ: Human hookworm infection in the 21st century, *Adv Parasitol* 58:197, 2004.

Brooker S et al: Epidemiologic, immunologic and practical considerations in developing and evaluating a human hookworm vaccine, *Expert Rev Vaccines* 4(1):35, 2005.

Hotez PJ et al: Hookworm infection, *N Engl J Med* 351(8):799, 2004.

Quinnell RJ, Bethony J, Pritchard DI: The immunoepidemiology of human hookworm infection, *Parasite Immunol* 26(11-12):443, 2004.

AUTHORS: **STEVEN M. OPAL, M.D.,** and **MAURICE POLICAR, M.D.**

BASIC INFORMATION

DEFINITION

A hordeolum is an acute inflammatory process affecting the eyelid and arising from the meibomian (posterior) or Zeis (anterior) glands. It is most often infectious and usually caused by *Staphylococcus aureus.*

SYNONYMS

Stye

ICD-9CM CODES
373.11 External hordeolum
373.12 Internal hordeolum

EPIDEMIOLOGY & DEMOGRAPHICS

INCIDENCE (IN U.S.): Unknown
PEAK INCIDENCE: May occur at any age
PREVALENCE (IN U.S.): Unknown
PREDOMINANT SEX: No gender predilection
PREDOMINANT AGE: May occur at any age
NEONATAL INFECTION: Rare in the neonatal period

PHYSICAL FINDINGS & CLINICAL PRESENTATION

- Abrupt onset with pain and erythema of the eyelid
- Localized, tender mass in the eyelid (Fig. 1-126)
- May be associated with blepharitis
- External hordeolum: points toward the skin surface of the lid and may spontaneously drain
- Internal hordeolum: can point toward the conjunctival side of the lid and may cause conjunctival inflammation

ETIOLOGY

- 75% to 95% of cases are caused by *S. aureus.*
- Occasional cases are caused by *Streptococcus pneumoniae,* other streptococci, gram-negative enteric organisms, or mixed bacterial flora.

DIAGNOSIS

DIFFERENTIAL DIAGNOSIS

- Eyelid abscess
- Chalazion
- Allergy or contact dermatitis with conjunctival edema
- Acute dacryocystitis
- Herpes simplex infection
- Cellulitis of the eyelid

LABORATORY TESTS

- Generally, none are necessary.
- If incision and drainage are performed, specimens should be sent for bacterial culture.

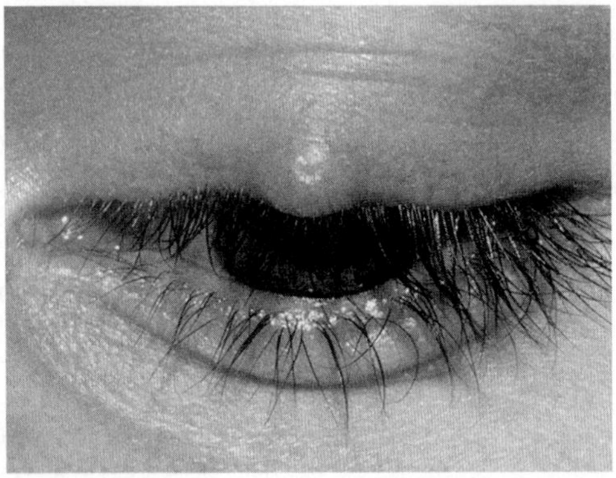

FIGURE 1-126 External stye. (From Palay D [ed]: *Ophthalmology for the primary care physician,* St Louis, 1997, Mosby.)

TREATMENT

NONPHARMACOLOGIC THERAPY

Usually responds to warm compresses

ACUTE GENERAL Rx

- Systemic antibiotics generally not necessary
- In refractory cases, an oral antistaphylococcal agent (e.g., dicloxacillin 500 mg PO qid) possibly helpful
- Topical erythromycin ophthalmic ointment applied to the lid margins two to four times daily until resolution
- Incision and drainage: rarely needed but should be considered for progressive infections

DISPOSITION

- Usually sporadic occurrence
- Possible relapse if resolution is not complete

REFERRAL

- For evaluation by an ophthalmologist if visual acuity or ocular movement is affected or if the diagnosis is in doubt
- For surgical drainage if necessary

PEARLS & CONSIDERATIONS

COMMENTS

Seborrheic dermatitis may coexist with hordeolum.

SUGGESTED READINGS

Hirunwiwatkul P, Wachirasereechai K: Effectiveness of combined antibiotic ophthalmic solution in the treatment of hordeolum after incision and curettage: a randomized, placebo-controlled trial: a pilot study, *J Med Assoc Thai* 88(5):647, 2005.

Kiratli HK, Akar Y: Multiple recurrent hordeola associated with selective IgM deficiency, *J AAPOS* 5(1):60, 2001.

Miller J: Acinetobacter as a causative agent in preseptal cellulitis, *Optometry* 76(3):176, 2005.

AUTHORS: **GLENN G. FORT, M.D., M.P.H., DENNIS J. MIKOLICH, M.D.,** and **JOSEPH R. MASCI, M.D.**

BASIC INFORMATION

DEFINITION

Horner's syndrome is the clinical triad of ipsilateral ptosis, miosis, and sometimes anhidrosis. Disruption of any of the three neurons in the oculosympathetic pathway (central, preganglionic, or postganglionic) can cause Horner's syndrome.

SYNONYMS

Oculosympathetic paresis
Raeder's paratrigeminal syndrome: Horner's syndrome of the postganglionic neuron associated with pain in the trigeminal nerve distribution

ICD-9CM CODES
337.9 Horner's syndrome

EPIDEMIOLOGY & DEMOGRAPHICS

Congenital or acquired

PHYSICAL FINDINGS & CLINICAL PRESENTATION

- Ptosis is usually mild. It results from loss of sympathetic tone to Müller's muscle, which contributes about 2 mm of upper eyelid elevation. Weakness of the corresponding muscle in the lower eyelid causes it to elevate slightly. This combination causes narrowing of the palpebral fissure. Levator function of the eyelid is preserved.
- Miosis results from loss of sympathetic pupillodilator activity of the iris (Fig. 1-127). The affected pupil reacts normally to bright light and accommodation. Anisocoria is greater in darkness.
  - Dilation lag: Horner's pupil dilates more slowly than the normal pupil when lights are dimmed (20 vs. 5 seconds) because it dilates passively due to relaxation of the iris sphincter.
- Presence of facial anhidrosis is variable and depends on the site of injury. It occurs with lesions affecting central or preganglionic neurons.
- Congenital Horner's syndrome may result in heterochromia. The affected eye has a lighter colored iris.
- Acute cases may also present with conjunctival injection due to the loss of sympathetic vasoconstriction.

ETIOLOGY

Lesions affecting any neuron in the oculosympathetic pathway. Central lesions are least common but usually due to pathology in hypothalamus, brainstem, or cervical spinal cord. Preganglionic lesions are often caused by disease involving the cervicothoracic spinal cord, lung apex, or anterior neck. Postganglionic lesions are usually seen with disease in superior cervical ganglion, internal carotid artery, or cavernous sinus or with vascular headaches. Location is often suggested by the presence of other findings. Vascular disease and neoplasms must be considered.

Mechanical:
- Syringomyelia
- Trauma
- Tumors: benign, malignant (thyroid, Pancoast, metastatic)
- Lymphadenopathy
- Neurofibromatosis
- Cervical rib
- Cervical spondylosis

Vascular (ischemia, hemorrhage or AVM):
- Brainstem lesion: commonly occlusion of the posterior inferior cerebellar artery but other arteries may be responsible (vertebral; superior, middle or inferior lateral medullary arteries; superior or anterior inferior cerebellar arteries)
- Carotid artery aneurysm or dissection. Can also be from injury to other major vessels (internal carotid artery, subclavian artery, ascending aorta)
- Cluster headache, migraine

Miscellaneous:
- Idiopathic
- Congenital
- Demyelination (multiple sclerosis)
- Infection (apical TB, herpes zoster, Lyme)
- Pneumothorax
- Iatrogenic (angiography, internal jugular/subclavian catheter, chest tube, surgery, epidural spinal anesthesia)
- Radiation

DIAGNOSIS

DIFFERENTIAL DIAGNOSIS

Causes of anisocoria (unequal pupils):
- Normal variant
- Mydriatic use
- Prosthetic eye
- Unilateral cataract
- Iritis

Causes of ptosis described in Section II.

WORKUP

History, physical examination, imaging

IMAGING STUDIES

Imaging the entire three neuron sympathetic pathway is usually warranted
- MRI head and neck: evaluate the central and cervical sympathetic pathway
- MR angiography (or ultrasound, CT angiography): assess the vessels in head and neck
- CT chest and neck: evaluate lung apex, perivertebral areas

TREATMENT

- Treatment depends on underlying cause.
- Ptosis can be surgically corrected or treated with medication (phenylephrine drops)

DISPOSITION

- Prognosis depends on underlying cause.
- Horner's syndrome is an uncommon presentation for malignancy.
- In one study, 40% of cases were idiopathic.

REFERRAL

- Ophthalmologist to confirm diagnosis and localize lesion. Topical cocaine test: failure of pupillary dilation after cocaine eye drops confirms presence of sympathetic denervation (drops dilate normal pupil but not Horner's pupil). Topical hydroxyamphetamine test: distinguishes central and preganglionic from postganglionic sympathetic lesions (drops dilate normal pupil but not postganglionic Horner's pupil).

PEARLS & CONSIDERATIONS

- May be the presentation of a life-threatening condition.
- Anisocoria greater in bright light is likely due to a defect in parasympathetic innervation, and anisocoria greater in dim light is likely due to a sympathetic defect.
- Normal variant anisocoria
  - Occurs in 20% of people
  - Usually <1 mm difference between pupils, more apparent in darkness
  - Pupils are round and display a normal, brisk constriction and dilation response to light

SUGGESTED READINGS

Murphy MA et al: Lyme disease associated with postganglionic Horner syndrome and Raeder paratrigeminal neuralgia, *J Neuro-ophthalmol* 27(2):123, 2007.

Walton KA, Buono LM: Horner syndrome, *Curr Opin Ophthalmol* 14(6):357, 2003.

AUTHOR: **SUDEEP K. AULAKH, M.D., F.R.C.P.C.**

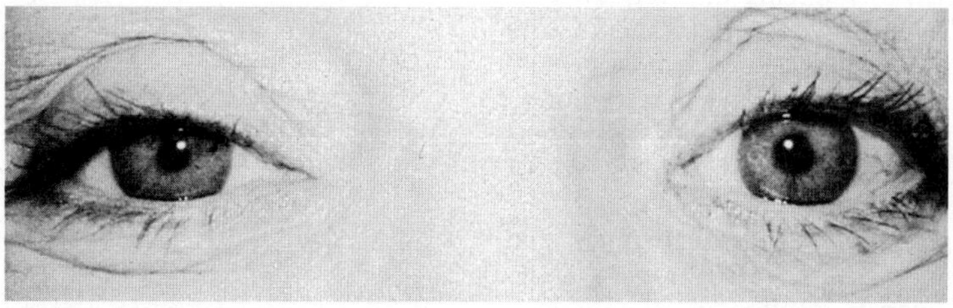

FIGURE 1-127 Horner's syndrome. The mild ptosis (1 to 2 mm) and the smaller pupil (in room light) can be seen on the affected right side. (From Palay D [ed]: *Ophthalmology for the primary care physician,* St Louis, 1997, Mosby.)

BASIC INFORMATION

DEFINITION

Sudden onset of intense warmth that begins in the neck or face or in the chest and progresses to the neck and face, often associated with profuse sweating, anxiety, and palpitations

ICD-9CM CODES
627.2 Hot flashes

EPIDEMIOLOGY & DEMOGRAPHICS

- Hot flashes affect 75% of postmenopausal women.
- Most hot flashes begin 1 to 2 yr before menopause and resolve after 2 yr.
- 15% of women report duration of hot flashes longer than 15 yr.

PHYSICAL FINDINGS & CLINICAL PRESENTATION

- Profuse sweating and red blotching of skin may be noted during the vasomotor event.
- Palpitations and hyperreflexia may be present during the hot flash.
- Hot flushes typically last 1 to 5 min.
- Each hot flush is associated with increase in temperature, increased pulse rate, and increased blood flow into the hands and face.
- Episodes of hot flush during sleep are common and are referred to as "night sweats."
- There is considerable variation in the frequency of hot flashes. One third of women report more than 10 flushes per day.

ETIOLOGY

- Dysfunction of central thermoregulatory centers caused by changes in estrogen level at the time of menopause
- Tamoxifen use
- Chemotherapy-induced ovarian failure
- Androgen ablation therapy for prostate carcinoma

DIAGNOSIS

DIFFERENTIAL DIAGNOSIS

- Carcinoid syndrome
- Anxiety disorder
- Idiopathic flushing
- Lymphoma (night sweats)
- Hyperthyroidism
- Hyperhydrosis

WORKUP

Evaluation of hot flashes is aimed at excluding conditions listed in the differential diagnosis

LABORATORY TESTS

- FSH, LH
- TSH

TREATMENT

NONPHARMACOLOGIC THERAPY

- Behavioral interventions such as relaxation training and paced respiration have been reported effective in reducing symptoms in some women.
- Avoidance of caffeine, alcohol, and tobacco, and spicy foods may be beneficial.

GENERAL Rx

- Estrogen replacement therapy reduces hot flashes by 80% to 90%. Estrogen therapy, however, is contraindicated in many women and others are fearful of its use. Potential risks and side effects should be considered before using estrogen in any patient. When using estrogen, it is best to use low-dose (e.g., Prempro [conjugated equine estrogen 0.45 mg or 0.3 mg plus medroxyprogesterone 1.5 mg]). Femring is an intravaginal ring that is changed every 3 mo and approved to treat vasomotor symptoms in women who have had a hysterectomy. It provides both local and systemic estrogen.
- Megestrol acetate, a progestational agent, is a safer alternative to estrogen in women with a history of breast or uterine cancer and in men receiving androgen ablation therapy for prostate cancer. Usual dose is 20 mg bid.
- The antidepressant venlaxefine has been reported to be 60% effective in reducing hot flashes and represents an alternative treatment modality in women unable or unwilling to use estrogens. Starting dose is 37.5 mg qd, increased as tolerated up to a maximum of 300 mg/day. Other antidepressants such as the SSRIs fluoxetine and paroxetine are also used by clinicians for hot flashes; however, they appear to be less effective than venlaxefine. A recent trial showed that paroxetine is an effective agent for diminishing hot flashes in men receiving androgen ablation therapy.
- The anticonvulsant gabapentin (300 to 1200 mg/day) represents another nonhormonal alternative in the treatment of hot flashes and can be used alone or in combination with venlafaxine.
- The antihypertensive clonidine is also effective in reducing the frequency of hot flashes. Adverse effects include dry mouth, sedation, and dizziness.
- Vitamin E (800 IU/day) may be effective in patients with mild symptoms that do not interfere with sleep or daily function.
- Soy protein (use of soy extracts that contain plant-derived estrogens [phytoestrogens]) is often used; however, clinical trials have not shown clear efficacy.
- Several classes of herbal remedies are available to patients and commonly used generally without significant benefit. Frequently used agents are *Cimicifuga racemosa* (black cohosh, snakeroot, bugbane), *angelica sinensis,* and evening primrose (evening star). Recent trials using the isopropanolic extract of black cohosh rootstock (Remefemin) did show some improvement in controlling menopausal symptoms.

EVIDENCE

The Agency for Healthcare Research and Quality (AHRQ) evidence report states that estrogen is the most consistently effective intervention for vasomotor symptoms. One trial showed no difference between combination testosterone and estrogen therapy alone for hot flashes. A few trials showed that tibolone (Livial) helped manage vasomotor symptoms but patients experienced more uterine bleeding, body pain, weight gain, and headaches compared to placebo.[1]

Evidence-Based Reference

1. Evidence, Report/Technology Assessment-Related Symptoms: http://www.ahrq.gov/clinic/epcsums/menosum.htm.

SUGGESTED READINGS

Loprinzi CL et al: Pilot evaluation of Gabapentin for treating hot flashes, *Mayo Clin Proc* 77:1159, 2002.

Loprinzi Cl et al: Pilot evaluation of paroxetine for treating hot flashes in men, *Mayo Clin Proc* 79(10):1247, 2004.

Nelson HD et al: Nonhormonal therapies for menopausal hot flashes, *JAMA* 295:2057, 2006.

Osmers R et al: Efficacy and safety of isopropanolic black cohosh extract for climacteric symptoms, *Obstet Gynecol* 105;1074, 2005.

Shanafelt TD et al: Pathophysiology and treatment of hot flashes, *Mayo Clin Proc* 77:1207, 2002.

Sikon A, Thacker HL: Treatment options for menopausal hot flashes, *Cleveland Clinic J Med* 71:578, 2004.

Women's Health Initiative Investigators: Risks and benefits of estrogen plus progestin in healthy postmenopausal women: principal results from the Women's Health initiative randomized controlled trial, *JAMA* 288:321, 2002.

AUTHOR: **FRED F. FERRI, M.D.**

BASIC INFORMATION

DEFINITION

Human granulocytic ehrlichiosis (HGE) is a zoonotic infection of granulocytes, caused by an *Ehrlichia* species closely related to *E. phagocytophila, E. equi,* and *E. ewingii,* with multisystem manifestations. The etiologic agent is now known as *Anaplasma phagocytophilum.*

SYNONYMS

Ehrlichia phagocytophila
Anaplasma phagocytophilum

ICD-9CM CODES

082-8 Other tick-borne rickettsiosis

EPIDEMIOLOGY & DEMOGRAPHICS

INCIDENCE (IN U.S.): Highest overall incidence in New York, New Jersey, Connecticut, Wisconsin, Minnesota, and northern California. >600 cases identified in the U.S. since 1990

PEAK INCIDENCE: Occurs throughout the year, with peak incidence between May and July and again in November

PREDOMINANT SEX: Males outnumber females by 2 to 1

PREDOMINANT AGE: Most severe disease 50 to 70 yr

PHYSICAL FINDINGS & CLINICAL PRESENTATION

- Most common initial symptoms
  1. Fever
  2. Chills, rigor
  3. Headache
  4. Myalgia
- Subsequent symptoms
  1. Anorexia, nausea
  2. Arthralgia
  3. Cough
  4. Confusion
  5. Abdominal pain
  6. Rash (erythematous to pustular) rare (<11%)
- Complications
  1. Hepatitis
  2. Interstitial pneumonitis
  3. Renal and respiratory failure
  4. Meningitis

ETIOLOGY

- Obligate intracellular gram-negative bacterium (family *Rickettsiaceae,* genus *Ehrlichia*), now renamed *Anaplasma phagocytophilum*
- Vector
  1. Almost certainly tick-borne, recently confirmed to be rarely transmitted by infected blood
  2. Transmitted by *Ixodes scapularis* in the northeastern and upper midwestern states and *Ixodes pacificus* in the Pacific western states
  3. Tick exposure reported in >90% of patients, with approximately 60% reporting tick bite
- Mammalian host: deer, horses, dogs, white-footed mice, cattle, sheep, goats, bison
- Host inflammatory and immune responses define final spectrum of disease beyond granulocytes, including hepatitis, interstitial pneumonitis, and nephritis with mild azotemia
- Between 6% and 21% of patients with HGE also have serologic evidence of other *Ixodes* spp. tick-borne diseases: Lyme disease or babesiosis
- Recovery is usual outcome; fatality rate of HGE is <1%

DIAGNOSIS

DIFFERENTIAL DIAGNOSIS

- Human monocytic ehrlichiosis (HME)
  1. Caused by *E. chaffeensis* (vector: tick *Amblyomma americanum*)
  2. Rash more common, sometimes petechial
  3. Morulae in monocytes
- Rocky Mountain spotted fever, Colorado tick fever, Q fever, relapsing fever
- Babesiosis
- Leptospirosis
- Lyme disease
- Tularemia
- Typhoid fever, paratyphoid fever
- Brucellosis
- Viral hepatitis
- Meningococcemia
- Infectious mononucleosis
- Hematologic malignancy

WORKUP

- Acute blood samples for Giemsa-stained smears
- CBC, Liver function, BUN/Cr
- Acute serum samples for serology
- Chest x-ray examination
- Bone marrow rarely needed

LABORATORY TESTS

- Giemsa-stained smear demonstrating morulae of the organism within granulocytes
- CBC progressive leukopenia and thrombocytopenia with nadir near day 7
- C reactive protein concentration is generally elevated
- LFT—increase in hepatic transaminases, lactate dehydrogenase, and alkaline phosphatase
- Elevated plasma creatinine concentration may be seen
- Serologic titer (IFA) >80 or fourfold increase in titer to *E. equi* antigen
- Polymerase chain reaction (PCR) to facilitate early diagnosis
- Culture on the first 7 days of illness; not readily available in most clinical laboratories

IMAGING STUDIES

- Chest x-ray examination to show interstitial pneumonitis (unusual)
- MRI of the brain

TREATMENT

ACUTE GENERAL Rx

- Immediate therapy to limit extent of acute illness and complication
- Doxycycline: 100 mg twice a day for 10 days is therapy of choice for adults and children >8 years (4 mg/kg/day in 2 divided doses)
- Rifampin: 300 mg twice a day for 7 to 10 days can be used in pregnancy and for children <8 years at 10 mg/kg twice per day

PROGNOSIS

Poor prognostic indicators include:

1. Advanced age
2. Concomitant chronic illness (such as diabetes mellitus, collagen-vascular disease)
3. Lack of diagnosis recognition
4. Delayed onset of specific antibiotic therapy

DISPOSITION

Repeat CBC every 2 to 4 wk until normal

REFERRAL

For consultation with infectious diseases specialist and hematologist in suspected cases

PEARLS & CONSIDERATIONS

COMMENTS

Duration of time tick must be attached to produce illness is at least 24 hr.

SUGGESTED READINGS

Bayard-McNeeley M et al: In vivo and in vitro studies on *Anaplasma phagocytophilum* infection of the myeloid cells of a patient with chronic myelogenous leukaemia and human granulocytic ehrlichiosis, *J Clin Pathol* 57(5):499, 2004.

Lotric-Furlan S et al: Concomitant tickborne encephalitis and human granulocytic ehrlichiosis, *Emerg Infect Dis* 11(3):485, 2005.

Moss WJ, Dumler JS: Simultaneous infection with Borrelia burgdorferi and human granulocytic ehrlichiosis, *Pediatr Infect Dis J* 22(1):91, 2003.

Singh-Behl D et al: Tick-borne infections, *Dermatol Clin* 21(2):237, 2003.

AUTHORS: **GLENN G. FORT, M.D., M.P.H., DENNIS J. MIKOLICH, M.D.,** and **VASANTHI ARUMUGAM, M.D.**

BASIC INFORMATION

DEFINITION

The human immunodeficiency virus, type 1 (HIV) causes a chronic infection that culminates, usually after several years, in acquired immunodeficiency syndrome (AIDS).

SYNONYMS

Acquired immunodeficiency syndrome (AIDS): when a patient with HIV infection meets specific diagnostic criteria (See "Acquired Immunodeficiency Syndrome" in Section I.)

ICD-9CM CODES
044.9 HIV, unspecified

EPIDEMIOLOGY & DEMOGRAPHICS

INCIDENCE (IN U.S.):
- No complete incidence data available.
- Greatest incidence is in metropolitan areas with population >500,000.

PEAK INCIDENCE: Age 30 to 35 yr
PREVALENCE (IN U.S.): Estimated at 1 to 2 million cases
PREDOMINANT SEX:
- Adults: most recently, estimated to be 74% males, 24% females, but is changing toward more women
- Children: male = female

PREDOMINANT AGE: 80% of cases occur between ages 20 and 40 yr
GENETICS:
Familial Disposition:
Although there is no proven genetic predisposition, individuals with deletions in the CCR5 gene are immune from infection with macrophage tropic virus (the predominant virus in sexual transmission).
Congenital Infection:
- 80% of childhood cases are caused by peripartum infection, which may occur in utero, during delivery, or after delivery via breastfeeding.
- No specific congenital abnormalities are associated with HIV infection, although risk of spontaneous abortion and low birth weight is greater.

Neonatal Infection:
- May occur during delivery or via breastfeeding
- Typically asymptomatic

PHYSICAL FINDINGS & CLINICAL PRESENTATION

- Signs and symptoms variable with stage of disease.
- In acute infection:
  1. May cause a self-limited mononucleosis-like illness characterized by fever, sore throat, lymphadenopathy, headache, and a rash resembling roseola
  2. In a minority of acute cases: frank aseptic meningitis, Bell's palsy, or peripheral neuropathy
- Later in the course of infection, after a prolonged asymptomatic phase: nonspecific symptoms of lymphadenopathy, weight loss, diarrhea, and skin changes including seborrheic dermatitis, localized herpes zoster, or fungal infection.
- Advanced disease: characterized by the infections and malignancies associated with acquired immunodeficiency syndrome (see specific disorders).
- Section II describes rheumatic syndromes in HIV infection.
- Some studies suggest that HIV infection in women is associated with lower levels of viral load at comparable degrees of immunosuppression when compared with men. Further, women may, on average, have higher CD4 lymphocyte counts at the time of AIDS diagnosis.
- Another special consideration in women infected with HIV is the high incidence of human papillomavirus (HPV) coinfection and the risk for cervical neoplasm that this presents. Even women with normal Pap smears should have this test repeated after 6 mo and annually thereafter.

ETIOLOGY

- RNA retrovirus (Fig. 1-128) HIV-1 was probably derived from transmission of a simian immunodeficiency virus (SIV) from chimpanzees in Central Africa; a related virus HIV-2 was derived from an SIV found in sooty mangebey monkeys from West Africa.
- HIV-1 is the predominant pathogenic retrovirus in human populations; HIV-2 has limited distribution (primarily in West Africa) and tends to be less rapidly immunosuppressive than HIV-1.
- Transmitted by sexual contact, shared needles, blood transfusion, or from mother to child during pregnancy, delivery, or breastfeeding.
- Primary target of infection: CD4 lymphocyte.
- Direct CNS involvement: manifested as encephalopathy, myelopathy, or neuropathy in advanced cases.
- Renal failure, rheumatologic disorders, thrombocytopenia, or cardiac abnormalities.

DIAGNOSIS

DIFFERENTIAL DIAGNOSIS

- Acute infection: mononucleosis or other respiratory viral infections
- Late symptoms: similar to those produced by other wasting illnesses such as neoplasms, TB, disseminated fungal infection, malabsorption, or depression
- HIV-related encephalopathy: confused with Alzheimer's disease or other causes of chronic dementia (cognitive impairment in HIV infection is described in Section II); myelopathy and neuropathy possibly resembling other demyelinating diseases such as multiple sclerosis

WORKUP

Diagnosis is established by voluntary testing for antibody to the virus; the CDC in the U.S. is now recommending that this test be done as a routine test in all hospital laboratories.

LABORATORY TESTS

HIV antibody detected by a two-step technique:
- ELISA as a sensitive screening test.
- Confirmation of positive ELISA tests with the more specific Western blot technique.

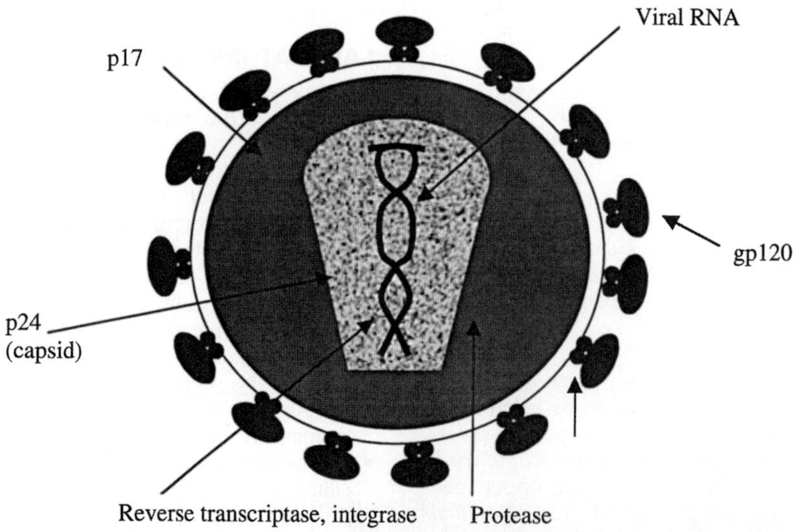

FIGURE 1-128 Locations of viral proteins and nucleic acids in the HIV-1 virion. (From Mandell GL [ed]: *Mandell, Douglas, and Bennett's principles and practice of infectious diseases,* ed 6, New York, 2005, Churchill Livingstone.)

- The CD4 count and HIV RNA PCR should be measured in all patients.
- The CD4 count is a marker of current immune status.
- The HIV RNA PCR (viral load) is predictive of disease progression.

Fig. 1-129 describes the immunologic response to HIV infection.

TREATMENT

Rx

NONPHARMACOLOGIC THERAPY

Maintenance of adequate nutrition

ACUTE GENERAL Rx

- Acute management of opportunistic infections and malignancies (See AIDS-associated disorders, "*Pneumocystis carinii* (now *P. jirovecii*) Pneumonia," "Cryptococcosis," "Tuberculosis," "Toxoplasmosis" elsewhere in this text.)
- Acute HIV syndrome:
  1. Treat with combination antiretroviral therapy, consisting of one or more (usually two) nucleoside agents (zidovudine [AZT], didanosine [DDI], zalcitabine [DDC], lamivudine [3TC], emtricitabine [FTC], abacavir, tenofovir) with a boostered (in combination with ritonavir) protease inhibitor (lopinavir, indinavir, saquinavir, nelfinavir, agenerase), or nonnucleoside reverse transcriptase inhibitors (nevirapine, delavirdine, efavirenz). Protease inhibitors, particularly lopinavir, are often administered in combination with low-dose ritonavir for enhanced drug levels. A new protease inhibitor, atazanavir, has been associated with a relatively low incidence of lipid abnormalities and insulin resistance than other protease inhibitors.
  2. Recommended doses of these drugs and specific combinations are currently being assessed.

CHRONIC Rx

- Naive chronically infected patients should be considered for therapy based on their current CD4 counts, likelihood for disease progression (viral loads), and ability to remain adherent with combination antiretroviral therapy. Please see current HIV treatment guidelines of the Department of Health and Human Services (http://www.aidsinfo.nih.gov/guidelines/).
  1. Patients with CD4 counts <200 cells/mm^3 should be treated regardless of viral load.
  2. Those with CD4 counts >350 cells/mm^3 should generally be observed without therapy; however, in cases of extremely elevated viral loads therapy should be considered.
  3. Patients should be treated when CD4 counts fall below 350 cells/mm^3 and before they reach 200 cells/mm^3. The precise starting point varies according to patient characteristics and viral parameters. It is currently recommended that treatment be initiated early if the CD4 count is <350 cells/mm^3 and if the viral load is >30,000 copies/ml or if the CD4 count is rapidly decreasing and viral load is >100,000 copies/ml. Compliant patients anxious to begin HAART should be started as the CD4 counts decline to less that 350 cells/mm^3.
  4. Antiretroviral therapy using combinations of nucleoside reverse transcriptase inhibitor (NRTI) agents: zidovudine (AZT), didanosine (DDI), zalcitabine (DDC), lamivudine (3TC), emtricitabine (FTC), stavudine (D4T), or abacavir; in addition to boosted (with ritonavir) protease inhibitors (PI) such as saquinavir, indinavir, nelfinavir, agenerase, ritonavir/lopinavir, or atazanavir; nonnucleoside reverse transcriptase inhibitors (NNRTI) such as nevirapine, delavirdine, or efavirenz; or the nucleotide agent tenofovir according to current recommendations based on clinical stage and viral load studies. The protease inhibitor ritonavir is often used, in low dose, in combination with other protease inhibitors to obtain more sustained drug levels. Adding a fourth drug to the three-drug regimen does not improve viral suppression or outcome and is not recommended. Treatment interruptions based upon CD4 responses appear harmful in recent comparative studies versus standard continous treatment protocols and should be avoided.
  5. Usual initial dosing regimen consists of two NRTIs and an NNRTI (or a PI). Standard regimens include:
     - Combivir (AZT and 3TC) one tablet by mouth twice a day and efavirenz 600 mg by mouth once daily
     - Combivir (AZT and 3TC) one tablet by mouth twice a day and ritonavir/lopinavir three tablets by mouth twice daily with food, or
     - Travuda (tenofovir plus Emtricitabine [FTC]) one tablet once daily and efavirenz 600 mg by mouth once daily

All these drugs have their own unique as well as class-specific side effects and require careful follow-up to achieve optimal antiviral effects. Compliance with the drug regimen and tolerance with common side effects are critically important to maintain drug efficacy. Antiviral response should be monitored by baseline HIV viral load and CD4 count and repeat measurement at 2 and 4 wk into treatment and the periodically (every 3 mo) to assure viral suppression.

- All patients should have genotypic resistance testing upon entry into medical care.
- Later antiretroviral regimen should be constructed based on past antiretroviral experience and the results of genotypic testing.
- Patients with CD4 lymphocyte count <200/mm^3 should be given preventive therapy for *Pneumocystis jirovecii* pneumonia (PJP) (see "*Pneumocystis jirovecii* [*P. carinii*] pneumonia").
- Evaluation of chronic diarrhea in patients with HIV is described in Section III, "HIV-Infected Patient, Acutely Ill."
- Criteria for discontinuing and restarting opportunistic prophylaxis for adults with HIV infection is described in Section I, "Acquired Immunodeficiency Syndrome."

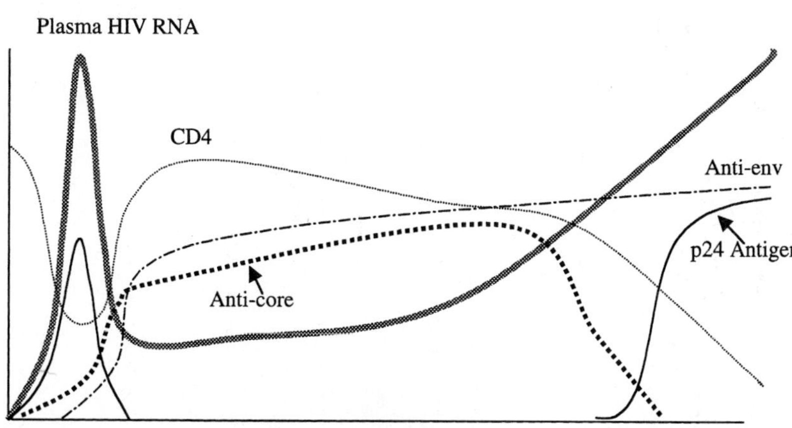

FIGURE 1-129 Course of human immunodeficiency virus infection. (From Mandell GL [ed]: *Mandell, Douglas, and Bennett's principles and practice of infectious diseases,* ed 6, New York, 2005, Churchill Livingstone.)

- HIV infection in a pregnant woman poses special challenges and considerations. Appropriate and timely antiretroviral therapy given to mother and newborn has been shown to dramatically reduce the risk of perinatal transmission of HIV. All pregnant women with newly diagnosed HIV infection should be offered antiretroviral therapy. Antiretroviral therapy should be initiated at the end of the first trimester, include zidovudine when possible, and continue through the baby's birth. The goal of therapy is to achieve an undetectable viral load. In women with viral loads persistently >1000 copies/ml despite appropriate ARV, cesarean section may further lower risk of transmission. Zidovudine (AZT) should also be given to the newborn for the first 6 wk of life, and mothers should completely avoid nursing. Efavirenz (Sustiva) should be avoided because of its potential teratogenic effects.

DISPOSITION

- Ongoing care consisting of frequent medical evaluations and T-lymphocyte subset analysis along with the plasma HIV load
- Long-term care focused on providing up-to-date antiretroviral therapy and prophylaxis of PJP and other opportunistic infections, as well as early detection of complications (See Section III.)

REFERRAL

To a physician knowledgeable and experienced in the management of HIV infection and its complications

PEARLS & CONSIDERATIONS

COMMENTS

- HIV chemoprophylaxis after occupational exposure is described in Section V.
- A recent analysis of the impact of the HAART era indicates that antiretroviral therapy has saved at least 3 million years of life since the introduction of HAART into medicine over 10 yr ago.

SUGGESTED READINGS

Bozzette SA: Routine screening for HIV infection—timely and cost-effective, *N Engl J Med* 352:620-621, 2005.

Danel C et al: CD4-guided antiretroviral treatment interruption strategy in HIV-infected adults in West Africa (Trivacan ANRS 1269 trial): A randomized trial, *Lancet* 367(9527):1981, 2006.

Gallant JE et al: Tenofir DF, emtricitabine, and efavirenz vs. zidovidine, lamivudine, and efaverenz for HIV, *N Engl J Med* 354(3):251, 2006.

Gulick RM et al: Three- vs four-drug antiretroviral regimens for the initial treatment of HIV-1 infection: a randomized controlled trial, *JAMA* 296(7):769, 2006.

Hammer SM et al: Treatment for adult HIV infection: 2006 recommendations of the International AIDS Society-USA panel, *JAMA* 296(7):827, 2006.

Kantor R et al: Evolution of resistance to drugs in HIV-1-infected patients failing antiretroviral therapy, *AIDS* 18(11):1503, 2004.

Klein MB et al: The impact of initial highly active antiretroviral therapy on future treatment sequences in HIV infection, *AIDS* 18(14):1895, 2004.

Walensky RP et al: The survival benefits of AIDS treatment in the United States, *J Infect Dis* 194(1):11, 2006.

AUTHORS: **STEVEN M. OPAL, M.D.,** and **JOSEPH R. MASCI, M.D.**

BASIC INFORMATION

DEFINITION

Huntington's chorea is an inherited neurodegenerative disorder characterized by involuntary movements, psychiatric disturbance, and cognitive decline.

SYNONYMS

Huntington's disease

ICD-9CM CODES
333.4 Huntington's chorea

EPIDEMIOLOGY & DEMOGRAPHICS

PEAK INCIDENCE: Late 30s and 40s, with onsets from age 2 to 70 yr
PREVALENCE (IN U.S.): 4.1 to 5.4 cases/100,000 persons
PREDOMINANT SEX: Female = male
PREDOMINANT AGE: Adulthood
GENETICS: Autosomal dominant

PHYSICAL FINDINGS & CLINICAL PRESENTATION

- Chorea (irregular rapid, flowing, nonstereotyped involuntary movements). When there is a writhing quality, it is referred to as choreoathetosis. Chorea is present early on and tends to decrease in end stages of disease.
- Dancelike, lurching gait, often caused by chorea.
- Westphal variant: cognitive dysfunction, bradykinesia, and rigidity. This variant is more commonly seen in juvenile onset Huntington's disease.
- Oculomotor abnormalities are common early on and include increased latency of response and insuppressible eye blinking.
- Psychiatric disorders (can be present early on): depression is commonly seen. Also, obsessive-compulsive behaviors and aggression associated with impaired impulse control.

ETIOLOGY

- Trinucleotide repeat disorder.
- The responsible gene is the Huntington gene located on chromosome 4. Its function is not known.

DIAGNOSIS

DIFFERENTIAL DIAGNOSIS

- Drug-induced chorea—dopamine, stimulants, anticonvulsants, antidepressants, and oral contraceptives have all been known to cause chorea.
- Sydenham's chorea—decreased incidence with decline of rheumatic fever.
- Benign hereditary chorea—autosomal dominant with onset in childhood. There is no progression of symptoms and no associated dementia or behavioral problems.
- Senile chorea—probably vascular in origin.
- Wilson's disease—autosomal recessive; tremor, dysarthria, and dystonia are more common presentations than chorea. 95% of patients with neurologic manifestations will have Keyser-Fleischer rings.
- Postinfectious.
- Systemic lupus erythematosus—can be the presenting feature of lupus. Rare.
- Chorea gravidarum—presents during first 4 to 5 mo of pregnancy and resolves after delivery.
- Paraneoplastic—seen most commonly in small cell lung cancer and lymphoma.

WORKUP

Onset of symptoms in an individual with an established family history requires no additional investigation.

LABORATORY TESTS

- Genetic testing.
- If normal, obtain CBC with smear, ESR, electrolytes, serum ceruloplasmin, 24-hr urinary copper excretion, TFTs, ANA, LFTs, HIV, and ASO titer. Consider paraneoplastic markers.

IMAGING STUDIES

CT scan or MRI scan will show atrophy most notably in the caudate and putamen. Cortex is involved to a lesser extent. A normal scan does not exclude the diagnosis.

TREATMENT

NONPHARMACOLOGIC THERAPY

- Supportive counseling
- Physical and occupational therapy
- Home health care
- Genetic counseling

CHRONIC Rx

- Chorea does not need to be treated unless disabling
- Chorea may be diminished by low doses of neuroleptics (e.g., haloperidol 1 to 10 mg/day)
- Amantadine (up to 300 to 400 mg divided tid)
- Tetrabenazine. This is a dopamine depletor that is not currently available in the United States. Side effects include parkinsonism and depression
- Depression with suicidal ideation is common; may improve with tricyclic or SSRI antidepressants

DISPOSITION

Relentless course of variable duration leading to progressive disability and death

REFERRAL

- Should refer to psychiatry and neurology for treatment of mood disorders and movement disorders
- Genetic counselors

PEARLS & CONSIDERATIONS

- Suicide rate is fivefold that of the general population.
- The number of repeats does correlate with age of onset but does not clearly correlate with disease severity. Interpretation of number of repeats is still difficult at this time and therefore it is debatable whether to disclose this information to patients.

EVIDENCE

Large placebo-controlled studies showing improved outcomes in patients with Huntington's disease are not available. Many drug trials have been undertaken but suffer either from small sample sizes, lack of blinding and placebo control, or negative results. However, amantadine,[1,2] tetrabenazine,[3,4] and fluphenazine[5] have fair (mediocre quality) evidence for symptomatic treatment of chorea when needed. Selective serotonin reuptake inhibitors are used most commonly for depression although there are small case reports and open label studies suggesting the use of risperidone and olanzapine,[6] especially if there is aggression or anxiety.

Evidence-Based References

1. Verhagen Metman L et al: Huntington's disease: a randomized, controlled trial using NMDA-antagonist amantadine, *Neurology* 59(5):694, 2002.
2. Heckmann JM et al: IV amantadine improves chorea in Huntington's disease: an acute randomized, controlled study, *Neurology* 10;63(3):597, 2004.
3. Swash M et al: Treatment of involuntary movement disorders with tetrabenazine, *J Neurol Neurosurg Psychiatry* 35:186, 1972.
4. Asher SW, Aminoff MJ: Tetrabenazine and movement disorders, *Neurology* 31:1051, 1981.
5. Terrence CF: Fluphenazine decanoate in the treatment of chorea: a double-blind study, *Curr Ther Res Clin Exp* 20:177, 1976.
6. Bonelli RM et al: Olanzapine for Huntington's disease: an open label study, *Clin Neuropharmacol* 25:263, 2002.

SUGGESTED READINGS

Biglan K, Shoulson I: Huntington's disease. In Jankovic J, Tolosa E (eds): *Parkinson's disease and movement disorders,* Philadelphia, 2002, Lippincott Williams & Wilkins.

Bonelli RM et al: Huntington's disease: present treatments and future therapeutic-modalities, *Intnl Clin Psychopharm* 19:51, 2004.

Higgins D: Chorea and its disorders, *Neuro Clin* 19(3):707, 2001.

AUTHOR: **CINDY ZADIKOFF M.D.**

BASIC INFORMATION

DEFINITION

A hydrocele is a fluid collection in a serous scrotal space usually between the layers of the tunica vaginalis (Figs. 1-130 and 1-131). A hydrocele that fills with fluid from the peritoneum is termed *communicating*. This is distinguished from a *noncommunicating* hydrocele by history of variation in size throughout the day and palpation of a thickened cord above the testicle on the affected side. A communicating hydrocele is basically a small inguinal hernia in which fluid, but not peritoneal structures, traverses the processus vaginalis.

ICD-9CM CODES
603.9 Hydrocele

PHYSICAL FINDINGS & CLINICAL PRESENTATION

Symptoms:
- Scrotal enlargement
- Scrotal heaviness or discomfort radiating to the inguinal area
- Back pain

Physical findings:
- Scrotal distention (testicle may be impossible to palpate)
- Transillumination

ETIOLOGY

Hydroceles may occur as a congenital abnormality where the processus vaginalis fails to close. In this case, an inguinal hernia is virtually always associated with the malformation. Congenital hydroceles are most common in infants and children. In adults, hydroceles are more frequently caused by infection, tumor, or trauma. Infection of the epididymis often results in the development of a secondary hydrocele. Tropical infections such as filariasis may produce hydroceles.

DIAGNOSIS

DIFFERENTIAL DIAGNOSIS

- Spermatocele
- Inguinoscrotal hernia
- Testicular tumor
- Varicocele
- Epididymitis

IMAGING STUDIES

Scrotal ultrasound (useful to rule out a testicular tumor as the cause of the hydrocele). The acute development of a hydrocele might be associated with the onset of epididymitis, testicular tumor, trauma, and torsion of a testicular appendage. An ultrasound of the scrotum may provide important diagnostic information.

TREATMENT

- No treatment if asymptomatic and testicle is thought to be normal.
- Surgical repair. Communicating hydroceles should be repaired in the same manner as an indirect hernia. The indications for repair of a noncommunicating hydrocele include failure to resolve and increase in size to one that is large and tense.

AUTHORS: **FRED F. FERRI, M.D.,** and **TOM J. WACHTEL, M.D.**

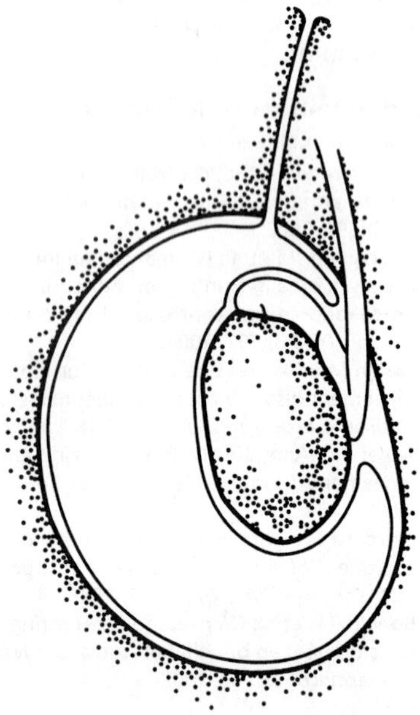

FIGURE 1-130 A hydrocele is a fluid collection in the serous space between the layers of the tunica vaginalis. The tunica vaginalis may or may not remain patent, allowing the hydrocele to communicate with the peritoneum.

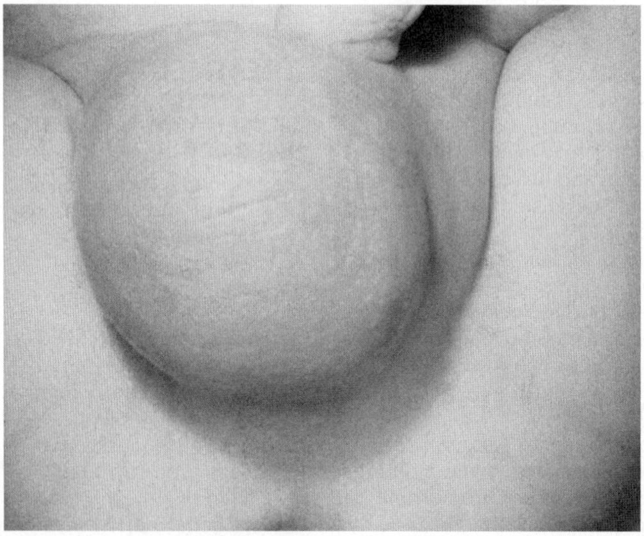

FIGURE 1-131 Newborn with large right hydrocele. (From Behrman RE: *Nelson textbook of pediatrics,* ed 16, Philadelphia, 2000, WB Saunders.)

BASIC INFORMATION

DEFINITION

Normal pressure hydrocephalus (NPH) is a syndrome of symptomatic hydrocephalus in the setting of normal CSF pressure. The classic clinical triad of NPH includes gait disturbance, cognitive decline, and incontinence.

SYNONYMS

Occult hydrocephalus
Extraventricular obstructive hydrocephalus
Chronic hydrocephalus

ICD-9CM CODES
331.3 Communicating hydrocephalus

EPIDEMIOLOGY & DEMOGRAPHICS

INCIDENCE: 1 per 100,0000; may account for 5% of dementia
PREDOMINANT SEX: Males = females
PREDOMINANT AGE: Fourth to sixth decades, but can occur at any age

PHYSICAL FINDINGS & CLINICAL PRESENTATION

- Gait difficulty: patients often have difficulty initiating ambulation, and the gait may be broad-based and shuffling, with the appearance that the feet are stuck to the floor (i.e., "magnetic gait" or "frontal gait disorder").
- Cognitive decline: mental slowing, forgetfulness and inattention without agnosia, aphasia, or other "cortical" disturbances.
- Incontinence: initially may have urinary urgency; later incontinence develops. Occasionally fecal incontinence also occurs.
- On physical examination, look for signs of disease that may mimic NPH.

ETIOLOGY

- Approximately 50% of cases are idiopathic; remaining cases are from secondary causes, including prior subarachnoid hemorrhage, meningitis, trauma, or intracranial surgery.
- Symptoms are presumed to result from stretching of sacral motor and limbic fibers that lie near the ventricles, as dilation occurs.

DIAGNOSIS

DIFFERENTIAL DIAGNOSIS

- Alzheimer's disease with extrapyramidal features
- Cognitive impairment in the setting of Parkinson's disease or parkinsonism-plus syndromes
- Diffuse Lewy body disease
- Frontotemporal dementia
- Cervical spondylosis with cord compromise in setting of degenerative dementia
- Multifactorial gait disorder
- Multi-infarct dementia

WORKUP

- Large-volume lumbar puncture
  1. Mental status testing and time to walk a prespecified distance (usually 25 feet) are measured, followed by removal of 40 to 50 ml of CSF.
  2. Retest of mental status and timed walking are done at 1 and 4 hr. Patients who have significant improvement in gait or mental status tend to have better surgical outcome; those with mild or negative response can have variable outcomes.
  3. Opening and closing pressure are measured; if pressure is elevated, alternative etiologies must be considered.
- Measurement of CSF outflow resistance by an infusion test, CSF pressure monitoring, or prolonged external lumbar drainage are sometimes used to help predict surgical outcome.

LABORATORY TESTS

CSF should be sent for routine fluid analyses to exclude other pathology.

IMAGING STUDIES

- CT scan or MRI can be used to document ventriculomegaly. The distinguishing feature of NPH is ventricular enlargement out of proportion to sulcal atrophy.
- MRI has advantages over CT, including better ability to visualize structures in the posterior fossa, visualize transependymal CSF flow, and to document extent of white matter lesions. On MRI, a flow void in the aqueduct and third ventricle ("jet sign") may be seen.
- Isotope cisternography and dynamic MRI studies have not been shown to be superior in predicting shunt outcome.

TREATMENT

There is no evidence that NPH can be effectively treated with medications.

NONPHARMACOLOGIC THERAPY

Response to ventriculoperitoneal shunting is variable. Some patients (30% of those with idiopathic NPH and 60% of patients with a known etiology) show significant improvement from shunting.

Factors that may predict positive outcome with surgery:
- NPH secondary to prior trauma, subarachnoid hemorrhage, or meningitis
- History of mild impairment in cognition <2 yr duration
- Onset of gait abnormality before cognitive decline
- Imaging demonstrates hydrocephalus without sulcal enlargement
- Transependymal CSF flow visualized on MRI
- Large-volume tap produces dramatic but temporary relief of symptoms

Factors that may predict negative outcome with surgery:
- Extensive white matter lesions or diffuse cerebral atrophy on MRI
- Moderate to severe cognitive impairment
- Onset of cognitive impairment before gait disorder
- History of alcohol abuse

ACUTE GENERAL Rx

Shunting in selected patients

DISPOSITION

Symptoms of NPH may progress over time. Prompt diagnosis may improve chance for treatment success.

REFERRAL

To neurologist for initial evaluation, including lumbar puncture, followed by neurosurgeon for shunting in appropriate patients

PEARLS & CONSIDERATIONS

Each of the cardinal symptoms of NPH is commonly seen in the elderly and occurs in multiple disease processes; therefore differential diagnosis should always be considered carefully.

CAUTION

Shunt complications, including subdural or intracerebral hematoma, may occur in 30% to 40% of patients.

SUGGESTED READINGS

Marmarou A et al: The value of supplemental prognostic tests for the preoperative assessment of idiopathic normal-pressure hydrocephalus, *Neurosurgery* 57(suppl 3):17-28, 2005.

Vanneste JA: Diagnosis and management of normal-pressure hydrocephalus, *J Neurol* 247(1):5, 2000.

AUTHOR: **TAMARA G. FONG, M.D., PH.D.**

BASIC INFORMATION

DEFINITION

Hydronephrosis is dilation of the renal pyelocalyceal system, most often as a result of impairment of urinary flow.

SYNONYMS

Hydroureter (dilation of ureter, often seen with hydronephrosis when obstruction is in lower urinary tract)
Urinary tract obstruction

ICD-9CM CODES
591 Acquired hydronephrosis
753.2 Congenital hydronephrosis

EPIDEMIOLOGY & DEMOGRAPHICS

Children usually have congenital malformations, whereas adults tend to have acquired defects as etiologies.

CLINICAL PRESENTATION

HISTORY:

- Pain is caused by distention of collecting system or renal capsule and is more related to the rate of onset than the degree of obstruction. It can vary in location from flank to lower abdomen to testes/labia. Pain in flank occurring only on micturition is highly suggestive of vesicoureteral reflux.
- Anuria can occur with total obstruction of urinary flow (bilateral hydronephrosis or unilateral if only one kidney is present).
- Polyuria or nocturia can occur with chronic (incomplete) obstruction because of deleterious effects on renal concentrating ability (nephrogenic diabetes insipidus).
- Urinary frequency, hesitancy, poor stream, and postvoid dribbling are all symptoms that can occur with obstruction at or below the bladder (e.g., prostatic hyperplasia).
- Chronic urinary infections can either result from chronic urinary obstruction (organisms favoring growth with stasis of urine) or lead to conditions (e.g., urine pH changes) that favor stone formation and subsequent obstruction.

PHYSICAL EXAMINATION:

- Hypertension can be caused by increased renin release in acute or subacute obstruction.
- Fever or CVA tenderness can suggest urinary tract infection.
- Palpate bladder to detect if distention present.
- Rectal examination to evaluate prostate for size and nodularity and also to check rectal sphincter tone.
- Pelvic examination to assess for vaginal anatomy, pelvic mass, or pelvic inflammatory disease (PID).
- Penile examination to rule out meatal stenosis or phimosis.
- Bladder catheterization to assess postvoid residual volume if urinary tract obstruction is considered. Should rule out postrenal obstruction in unexplained acute renal failure.

ETIOLOGY

MECHANICAL IMPAIRMENTS:

Congenital

- Ureteropelvic junction narrowing
- Ureterovesical junction narrowing
- Ureterocele
- Retrocaval ureter
- Bladder neck obstruction
- Urethral valve
- Urethral stricture
- Meatal stenosis

Acquired

- Intrinsic to urinary tract
  - Calculi
  - Inflammation
  - Trauma
  - Sloughed papillae
  - Ureteral tumor
  - Blood clots
  - Prostatic hypertrophy or cancer
  - Bladder cancer
  - Urethral stricture
  - Phimosis
- Extrinsic to urinary tract
  - Gravid uterus
  - Retroperitoneal fibrosis or tumor (e.g., lymphoma)
  - Aortic aneurysm
  - Uterine fibroids
  - Trauma (surgical or nonsurgical)
  - Pelvic inflammatory disease
  - Pelvic malignancies (e.g., prostate, colorectal, cervical, uterine, bladder)

FUNCTIONAL IMPAIRMENTS:

- Neurogenic bladder (often with adynamic ureter) can occur with spinal cord disease or diabetic neuropathy.
- Pharmacologic agents such as alpha-adrenergic antagonists and anticholinergic drugs can inhibit bladder emptying.
- Vesicoureteral reflux may occur.
- Pregnancy can cause hydroureter and hydronephrosis (right more often than left) as early as the second month. Hormonal effects on ureteral tone combine with mechanical factors.

DIAGNOSIS

DIFFERENTIAL DIAGNOSIS

- Urinary stones
- Neoplastic disease
- Prostatic hypertrophy
- Neurologic disease
- Urinary reflux
- Urinary tract infection
- Medication effects
- Trauma
- Congenital abnormality of urinary tract

LABORATORY TESTS

- Serum BUN and creatinine to assess for renal insufficiency (usually implies bilateral obstruction or unilateral obstruction of a solitary kidney).
- Electrolytes may reveal hypernatremia (if nephrogenic DI), hyperkalemia (from renal failure and effects on tubular function), or distal renal tubular acidosis.
- Urinalysis and examination of sediment may reveal WBCs, RBCs, or bacteria in the appropriate setting (e.g., infection, stones), but often the sediment is normal in obstructive renal disease.

IMAGING STUDIES

- Assess kidney and bladder size with ultrasound; contour of collecting system and ureters. Ultrasound is >90% sensitive and specific for hydronephrosis and is noninvasive, so it will not worsen preexisting renal insufficiency.
- Abdominal CT scan without IV contrast provides excellent localization of the site of obstruction.
- Once diagnosed, antegrade or retrograde ureterograms can further delineate with the point of obstruction.
- Voiding cystourethrogram is helpful in diagnosing vesicoureteral reflux and obstructions of the bladder neck or urethra.

TREATMENT

NONPHARMACOLOGIC THERAPY

- Urgent treatment is required if urinary tract obstruction is associated with urinary tract infection, acute renal failure, or uncontrollable pain.
- Conservative management of calculi with IV fluid, IV antibiotics (if evidence of infection), and aggressive analgesia may be enough to treat acute unilateral urinary tract obstruction depending on the size (90% of stones <5 mm will pass spontaneously).
- Urethral catheter is adequate to relieve most obstructions at or distal to the bladder, but occasionally a suprapubic catheter will be required (e.g., impassable urethral stricture or urethral injury). Neurogenic bladder may require intermittent clean catheterization if frequent voiding and pharmacologic treatments are ineffective.
- Nephrostomy tube can be placed percutaneously to facilitate urinary drainage.
- Extracorporeal shock wave lithotripsy (ESWL) is used to fragment large stones to facilitate spontaneous passage or subsequent extraction. (Note: ESWL is contraindicated in pregnancy.)

- Nephroscopy is performed for extraction of proximal stones under direct vision.
- Cystoscopy with ureteroscopy is used for removal of distal ureteral stones using a loop or basket with or without fragmentation by ultrasonic or laser lithotripsy.
- Ureteral stents can be used for extrinsic and some intrinsic ureteral obstructions.
- Urethral dilation or internal urethrotomy can be used for urethral strictures.
- Nephrectomy or ureteral diversion may be required in severe cases (e.g., malignancy).
- Ureterovesical reimplantation can be used for reflux disease.
- Transurethral retrograde prostatectomy (TURP) is used for severe obstruction from benign prostatic hypertrophy (BPH).
- IV fluid and electrolyte replacement is needed; the patient must be monitored closely during the postobstructive diuresis (usually lasting several days to a week).

ACUTE GENERAL Rx

Antibiotics if indicated

DISPOSITION

Aggressive treatment of infections and early relief of obstruction can usually prevent progressive loss of renal function; however, chronic bilateral obstruction (often from BPH) can lead to chronic renal failure.

REFERRAL

- Urologist consultation early for diagnostic or therapeutic procedures
- Oncologist if a neoplasm is diagnosed
- Gynecologist if pregnancy or female pelvic anatomy is involved

PEARLS & CONSIDERATIONS

COMMENTS

- Not a primary disorder: an underlying etiology should be sought.
- Treatment is relieving the obstruction, either directly or by addressing the underlying cause.

PREVENTION

May be achieved through prevention of an underlying potential etiology (e.g., medical or surgical management of BPH before obstruction occurring or medical treatment to avoid formation of renal stones)

SUGGESTED READINGS

Lameire N, Van Biesen W, Vanholder R: Acute renal failure, *Lancet* 365:417-430, 2005.

Mostbeck GH, Zontsich T, Turetschek K : Ultrasound of the kidney: obstruction and medical diseases, *Eur Radiol* 11(10):1878-1889, 2001.

AUTHORS: **SHEENAGH M. BODKIN, M.D.,** and **PAUL A. PIRRAGLIA, M.D., M.P.H.**

BASIC INFORMATION

DEFINITION

Hypercholesterolemia refers to a blood cholesterol measurement >200 mg/dl. A cholesterol level of 200 to 239 mg/dl is considered borderline high, and a level of >240 mg/dl is considered to be a high cholesterol measurement.

SYNONYMS

Hypercholesteremia
Hypercholesterinemia
Type II familial hyperlipoproteinemia

ICD-9CM CODES
272.0 Hypercholesterolemia

EPIDEMIOLOGY & DEMOGRAPHICS

- More than one-half of all U.S. adults have dyslipidemia; 50.4% of men and 50.9% of women.
- Only about 12% of people with high cholesterol are being treated.
- Elevated cholesterol requires drug therapy in about 60 million Americans.
- Incidence of heterozygous familial hypercholesterolemia: about 1:500.
- Incidence of homozygous familial hypercholesterolemia: about 1:1 million.
- Prevalence of hypercholesterolemia increases with increasing age.
- Familial hypercholesterolemia: autosomal dominant disorder.
- Familial combined hyperlipidemia: possibly an autosomal dominant disorder.
- Multifactorial predilection: apparent in majority of affected individuals.

PHYSICAL FINDINGS & CLINICAL PRESENTATION

- Most patients: no physical findings
- Possible findings particularly in the familial forms
  1. Tendon xanthomas
  2. Xanthelasma
  3. Arcus corneae
  4. Arterial bruits (young adulthood)

ETIOLOGY

Primary
1. Genetics
2. Obesity
3. Dietary intake

Secondary
1. Diabetes mellitus
2. Alcohol
3. Oral contraceptives
4. Hypothyroidism
5. Glucocorticoid use
6. Most diuretics
7. Nephrotic syndrome
8. Hepatoma
9. Extrahepatic biliary obstruction
10. Primary biliary cirrhosis

DIAGNOSIS

DIFFERENTIAL DIAGNOSIS

No real differential diagnosis; however, consider underlying secondary causes/ etiologies for the elevated cholesterol.

LABORATORY TESTS

PRIMARY PREVENTION WITHOUT ATHEROSCLEROSIS OR DIABETES MELLITUS:
1. Recommended to get a complete lipoprotein profile (total cholesterol, HDL, LDL, and triglycerides) on all adults 20 years and older.
2. Risk assessment to modify LDL goals: cigarette smoking, hypertension (BP >140/90 on medication), family history of premature CHD (first-degree relative with CHD in male <55 or female <65), age (male ≥45, female ≥55).
3. Evaluate for CHD equivalents, including atherosclerosis (peripheral arterial disease, aortic aneurism), diabetes, symptomatic carotid disease, or 10-year rise CHD >20%
4. LDL goal based on modifications:
   0 to 1 risk factors, LDL <160
   Multiple risk factors, LDL <130
   CHD or equivalents, LDL <100
5. Fasting lipid profile with LDL <130 and 0 to 1 risk factors: dietary guidance and repeat every 5 years.
6. Fasting lipid profile with LDL 130 to 159 mg/dl and less than two risk factors for CAD: diet and exercise modification, with repeat profile in 12 wk.
7. Fasting lipid profile with LDL >130 mg/dl and two or more risk factors for CAD: need diet and drug therapy.

SECONDARY PREVENTION WITH ATHEROSCLEROSIS OR DIABETES MELLITUS:
1. All patients: fasting lipid profile
2. If LDL <100 mg/dl: instruction on diet and exercise, and repeat annually
3. If LDL >100 mg/dl: drug therapy required

SECONDARY PREVENTION WITH ATHEROSCLEROSIS AND DIABETES MELLITUS:
1. Now classified as very high risk
2. Fasting lipid profile for all patients
3. If LDL >70, drug therapy required

METABOLIC SYNDROME:
1. A constellation of lipid and nonlipid risk factors of a metabolic origin
2. Diagnosed when three or more of the following present: abdominal obesity; triglycerides ≥150; HDL <40 in males, <50 in females; SBP >130; DBP >85; fasting glucose >110
3. Needs aggressive treatment with weight loss, increased physical activity, and pharmacologic therapy

TREATMENT

NONPHARMACOLOGIC THERAPY

- First line of treatment: dietary therapy (see "Hyperlipoproteinemia")
- Dietary modifications
  1. Low-cholesterol, low-fat diet (fat intake to 30% or less of the total caloric intake)
  2. Polyunsaturated fat up to 10% of total calories
  3. Monounsaturated fat up to 20% of total calories
  4. Saturated fats <7% of total calories
  5. No more than 200 mg/day of cholesterol
  6. Fiber 20 to 30 gm a day.
- Increased activity with aerobic exercise: encourage 20 to 30 min of aerobic exercise three to four times a week
- Smoking cessation encouraged
- Counseling on CAD risk factors

ACUTE GENERAL Rx

No acute treatment needed

CHRONIC Rx

- In primary prevention: needed for patients with LDL >130 mg/dl with two or more risk factors for CAD
- In secondary prevention: needed for patients with known CAD, vascular disease or diabetes mellitus, and LDL >70 mg/dl
- In primary prevention: considered in patients on dietary therapy with LDL >190 mg/dl with no risk factors, LDL >130 mg/dl with two or more risk factors, or HDL <30 mg/dl
- Medications that can be used (Table 1-19):
  1. Bile acid sequestrants (poorly tolerated)
  2. Niacin (poorly tolerated)
  3. HMG-CoA reductase inhibitors ("statins")
  4. Fibric acids
  5. Medication tailored to the patient's lipid profile, lifestyle, and the medication's side-effect profile
- Cholesterol absorption inhibitors (ezetimibe)
- Bile acid sequestrants to lower LDL
- Niacin to lower LDL and triglycerides and raise HDL
- HMG-CoA reductase inhibitors to lower LDL
- Fibric acids work to lower triglycerides more than LDL

DISPOSITION

- After initiation of therapy, repeat laboratory tests in 4 to 6 wk, with modifications as necessary.
- Once goal is achieved, lifelong medication and monitoring are needed at least three to four times a year.

- Dietary modification is needed to continue with drug therapy.
- Repeat review for additional CAD risk factors.

PEARLS & CONSIDERATIONS

COMMENTS

See "Hyperlipoproteinemia."

SUGGESTED READINGS

de Lemos JA et al: Early intensive vs a delayed conservative simvastatin strategy in patients with acute coronary syndromes: phase Z of the A to Z trial, *JAMA* 292:1307, 2004.

La Rosa JC et al: Intensive lipid lowering with atorvastatin in patients with stable coronary disease, *NEJM* 352:1425, 2005.

Mosca L et al: National study of physician awareness and adherence to cardiovascular disease prevention guidelines, *Circulation* 111:499, 2005.

National Cholesterol Education Program: Second Report on the Expert Panel on Detection, Evaluation, and Treatment of High Cholesterol in Adults (adult treatment panel IV), *JAMA* 285:2486, 2001.

Safeer R, Ugalat P: Cholesterol treatment guidelines update, *Am Fam Physician* 65:871, 2002.

AUTHORS: **BETH J. WUTZ, M.D.,** and **RUBEN ALVERO, M.D.**

TABLE 1-19 **Drugs Affecting Lipoprotein Metabolism**

Drug Class	Agents and Daily Doses	Lipid/Lipoprotein Effects		Side Effects	Contraindications
HMG-CoA reductase inhibitors (statins)	Lovastatin (20-80 mg) Pravastatin (20-80 mg) Simvastatin (20-80 mg) Fluvastatin (20-80 mg) Atorvastatin (10-80 mg) Rosuvastain (5-40 mg)	LDL HDL TG	↓18%-55% ↑5%-15% ↓7%-30%	Myopathy Increased liver enzymes	Absolute: • Active or chronic liver disease Relative: • Concomitant use of certain drugs*
Bile acid sequestrants	Cholestyramine (4-16 g) Colestipol (5-20 g) Colesevelam (2.6-3.8 g)	LDL HDL TG	↓1.5%-30% ↑3%-5% No change or increase	Gastrointestinal distress Constipation Decreased absorption of other drugs	Absolute: • Dysbetalipoproteinemia • TG >400 mg/dl Relative: • TG >200 mg/dl
Nicotinic acid	Immediate release (crystalline) nicotinic acid (1.5-3 g), extended-release nicotinic acid (Niaspan) 1-2 g, sustained release nicotinic acid (1-2 g)	LDL HDL TG	↓5%-25% ↑15%-35% ↓20%-50%	Flushing Hyperglycemia Hyperuricemia (or gout) Upper GI distress Hepatotoxicity	Absolute: • Chronic liver disease • Severe gout Relative: • Diabetes • Hyperuricemia • Peptic ulcer disease
Fibric acids	Gemfibrozil (600 mg bid) Fenofibrate (160 mg qd) Clofibrate (1000 mg bid)	LDL *(may be increased in patients with high TG)* HDL TG	↓5%-20% ↑10%-20% ↓20%-50%	Dyspepsia Gallstones Myopathy	Absolute: • Severe renal disease • Severe hepatic disease
Cholesterol absorption inhibitors	Ezetimibe (10 mg QD)	LDL HDL TG	↓18% ↑1% ↓7%-8%	Abdominal pain myalgias	• Severe renal disease • Severe hepatic disease

Modified from The National Cholestrol Education Program, *JAMA* 285:2486, 2001.
CoA, Coenzyme A; *GI,* gastrointestinal; *HDL,* high-density lipoprotein; *HMG,* 3-hydroxy-3 methylglutanyl; *LDL,* low-density lipoprotein; *TG,* triglyceride.
*Cyclosporine, macrolide antibiotics, various antifungal agents, and cytochrome P-450 inhibitors (fibrates and niacin should be used with appropriate caution).

BASIC INFORMATION

DEFINITION

A hypercoagulable state is an inherited or acquired condition associated with an increased risk of thrombosis.

SYNONYM

Thrombophilia

ICD-9CM CODES
289.8 Hypercoagulable syndrome
795.79 Antiphospholipid antibody syndrome

EPIDEMIOLOGY & DEMOGRAPHICS

See Table 1-20.

- Risk of thrombosis increases with age and with multiple risk factors.
- Most people with a genetic defect will not suffer thrombotic disease. When thrombosis occurs it is often associated with an acquired risk factor (surgery, pregnancy, oral contraceptive pill [OCP] use, etc.). Annual risk of thrombosis is <1%.
- About half of patients with unprovoked thrombosis have an identifiable inherited thrombophilia.
- Significant variations in the prevalence rates and thrombotic risks are reported in different studies. This may reflect geographic variation in the prevalence of genetic defects, the presence of other unmeasured coagulation defects, or different populations.

HISTORY

A hypercoagulable state is strongly suggested by:

- Spontaneous thrombosis: absence of other medical conditions associated with increased risk of thrombosis
- <50 yr of age at first episode of thrombosis
- Family history of thrombosis: first-degree relative with thrombosis at <50 yr
- Recurrent thrombotic events
- Thrombosis in unusual anatomic location (i.e., portal, hepatic, mesenteric, or cerebral vein)
- Thrombosis in pregnancy, postpartum, or associated with OCP use
- Warfarin-induced skin necrosis
- Adverse pregnancy outcomes may also be associated with thrombophilia: recurrent pregnancy loss, preeclampsia, placental abruption, intrauterine growth restriction

PHYSICAL FINDINGS & CLINICAL PRESENTATION

- Inherited thrombophilia is usually associated with venous thromboembolism (VTE), most commonly deep vein thrombosis (DVT)
- Some acquired thrombophilias are associated with arterial thrombosis
- Pregnancy complications
- Medical conditions associated with increased risk of thrombosis

ETIOLOGY

See Table 1-20.

- Often a multifactorial process with genetic, environmental, and acquired factors.
- Multiple genetic defects are not uncommon (1% to 2% prevalence in patients with idiopathic VTE); often strong synergistic effect when multiple risk factors are present.
- Among patients with inherited thrombophilia, thrombotic risk increases with use of OCP or hormone replacement therapy (HRT) and during pregnancy/postpartum.
- Adverse pregnancy outcomes may be caused by thrombosis of the uteroplacental circulation.

INHERITED:

Factor V Leiden (FVL) mutation:

- Autosomal dominant mutation with low penetrance.
- Causes activated protein C resistance (APCR); 90% of APCR is caused by FVL mutation.
- Most common genetic risk factor for venous thrombosis; accounts for thrombosis in 40% to 50% of inherited cases.
- OCP use in heterozygous carriers is associated with an eightfold increased risk of thrombosis compared with noncarriers and a thirty-fivefold increased risk of thrombosis compared with noncarriers not using OCP.
- Probably low risk of recurrent thrombotic events.
- May be associated with cardiovascular disease in select high-risk subgroups.

Prothrombin G20210A mutation:

- Autosomal dominant mutation with low penetrance.
- OCP use in heterozygous carriers is associated with a sixteenfold increased risk of thrombosis compared with noncarriers not using OCP.
- Probably low risk of recurrent thrombotic events.
- May be associated with cardiovascular disease in select high-risk subgroups and young patients with ischemic strokes.

Protein C, protein S, antithrombin (AT) deficiency:

- Autosomal dominant inheritance, many mutations identified for each of these conditions.
- Decreased level or abnormal function.
- First episode of thrombosis usually in young adults.
- Increased risk of recurrent thrombosis.

Protein C and protein S:

- Lifetime risk of thromboembolic event up to 50%.

TABLE 1-20 **Hypercoagulable Conditions**

	Prevalence in General Population (%)	Prevalence in Population with with Thrombosis (%)	Arterial (A)/ Venous (V) Events	Relative Risk of Thrombosis
FVL mutation	5% of whites Rare in nonwhites	12%-40%	V	Heterozygous: 3-7; homozygous: 80
Prothrombin G20210A mutation	3% of whites Rare in nonwhites	6%-18%	V	3
AT deficiency	0.02%	1%-3%	V	20-50
PC deficiency	0.2%-0.4%	3%-5%	V	7-15
PS deficiency	0.03%-0.1%	1%-5%	V	5-11
Antiphospholipid antibody syndrome	1%-2%	5%-21%	V + A	2-11
Hyperhomocysteinemia	5%-7%	10%	V + A	3
Elevated factor VIII level	11%	25%		5

AT, antithrombin; *FVL,* factor V Leiden; *PC,* protein C; *PS,* protein S.

- Homozygous condition very rare, usually associated with lethal thrombosis in infancy.
- Associated with warfarin-induced skin necrosis, which occurs secondary to depletion of vitamin K–dependent anticoagulant factors sooner than procoagulant factors in the first few days of therapy.

AT deficiency:
- Most thrombogenic of the identified inherited factors. Lifetime risk of thromboembolic event up to 70%.
- Homozygous condition very rare, probably not compatible with normal fetal development.
- Rarely, arterial thrombosis can occur.
- Recurrent thrombotic events reported in up to 60% of patients.
- Can cause heparin resistance.

Elevated factor VIII level:
- May be an important risk factor for thrombosis in African American population.
- Increased risk of recurrent thrombosis.
- Genetic etiology suspected but not yet identified.

Other possible causes: dysfibrinogenemias, elevated thrombin activatable fibrinolysis inhibitor, plasminogen deficiency, elevated factor IX and factor XI levels.

ACQUIRED:

Antiphospholipid antibody syndrome:
- Most common cause of acquired thrombophilia.
- Can present as arterial or venous thrombosis, recurrent pregnancy loss, and adverse pregnancy outcomes.
- Thromboembolic events occur in up to 30% of people. High risk of recurrent thrombosis (up to 70% reported).
- See "Antiphospholipid Antibody Syndrome" for more information.

Hyperhomocysteinemia:
- Can be inherited (most commonly an autosomal recessive mutation in methylene tetrahydrofolate reductase gene) but more often secondary to poor dietary intake. Deficiency of folate, vitamin B_6, or vitamin B_{12} accounts for two thirds of cases.
- May be associated with VTE, atherosclerotic disease (cardiovascular, cerebrovascular and peripheral vascular), and possibly adverse pregnancy outcomes.

Conditions associated with increased risk of thrombosis:
- Prior thrombosis
- Trauma
- Chronic medical illness: congestive heart failure, diabetes mellitus, obesity, nephrotic syndrome, inflammatory bowel disease, paroxysmal nocturnal hemoglobinuria, hemolytic-uremic syndrome/thrombotic thrombocytopenic purpura (HUS/TTP), disseminated intravascular coagulation (DIC), sickle cell anemia
- Pregnancy (sixfold increased risk of thrombosis compared with nonpregnant women), postpartum, OCP (threefold to fivefold increased risk of thrombosis with use, higher risk with third-generation OCP), HRT (twofold increased risk of thrombosis with use), tamoxifen, raloxifene
- Immobilization, travel
- Surgery (especially orthopedic), central venous catheters
- Hyperviscosity syndromes
- Myeloproliferative disorders
- Malignancy: disease or treatment related
- Heparin-induced thrombocytopenia and thrombosis
- Cigarette smoking
- IV drug use

DIAGNOSIS

Dx

WORKUP

- History (presence of conditions or use of medications predisposing to thrombosis, family history of thrombosis), physical examination, laboratory tests, imaging studies.

NOTE: Genetic counseling and written informed consent should be obtained prior to genetic testing.

- Varying recommendations on extent of workup. Little cost-effectiveness and outcomes data. Thrombophilia screening probably overutilized because results often do not impact therapy.
- It is not recommended that individuals with medical conditions associated with increased risk of thrombosis be screened for the inherited or acquired defects. A notable exception is made for thrombosis associated with pregnancy, postpartum, or OCP/HRT use.
- Some advocate for screening prior to OCP/HRT use and prior to pregnancy in women with a history of thrombosis and those with a first-degree relative with symptomatic inherited thrombophilia.
- Unprovoked venous thrombosis:
  - Screen individuals for APCR, prothrombin G20210A mutation, protein C, protein S, AT deficiency, hyperhomocysteinemia, and antiphospholipid antibody syndrome if any of the following are present: <50 yr of age at first episode of thrombosis, family history of thrombosis, recurrent thrombosis, thrombosis in unusual anatomic location, life-threatening thrombotic event, warfarin-induced skin necrosis, thrombosis in pregnancy/postpartum/with OCP use, or characteristic pregnancy complications.
  - Screen all Caucasians and all women on HRT for APCR, prothrombin G20210A mutation, hyperhomocysteinemia, and antiphospholipid antibody syndrome.
  - Screen all others for hyperhomocysteinemia and antiphospholipid antibody syndrome.
- Arterial thrombosis:
  - Screen for antiphospholipid antibody syndrome and hyperhomocysteinemia.

NOTE: Routine screening for factor VIII levels is not recommended by most experts.

TIMING OF WORKUP: Ideally >2 wk after discontinuation of anticoagulation (except for antiphospholipid antibodies because this will influence duration of anticoagulation).

NOTE: Acute thrombosis, anticoagulation, pregnancy, and many medical conditions can affect the results and must be considered in the timing and interpretation of the workup.

LABORATORY TESTS

- CBC with peripheral smear, electrolytes, renal and liver function tests, PT/PTT, PSA (in men >50 yr), urinalysis.

NOTE: Abnormal nongenetic tests should be repeated after 6 weeks to decrease false-positive diagnosis.

- APCR: APC-resistance assay (using factor V–deficient plasma) and if positive confirm with genetic test for FVL mutation; use genetic test in pregnancy and if lupus anticoagulant present.
- Prothrombin G20210A mutation: genetic test.
- AT deficiency: functional assay (AT-heparin cofactor assay).
- Protein C deficiency: functional assay (activity); may be falsely low in the presence of APCR, elevated factor VIII level, or lupus anticoagulant.
- Protein S deficiency: functional assay (activity) and immunologic assay (free and total level). Functional assay may be falsely low in the presence of APCR, elevated factor VIII level, or lupus anticoagulant.
- Antiphospholipid antibody syndrome: any of the following found on two occasions at least 12 wk apart: lupus anticoagulant or anticardiolipin antibody (IgG and IgM) or anti-B2-glycoprotein-1 antibody (IgG and IgM).
- Hyperhomocysteinemia: fasting plasma homocysteine level (if normal but suspicion is high, can proceed with methionine loading test and genotyping for methylene tetrahydrofolate reductase).
- Factor VIII level: functional assay.

IMAGING STUDIES

As appropriate to diagnose thrombosis and to rule out medical conditions associated with increased thrombotic risk.

TREATMENT

NONPHARMACOLOGIC THERAPY

OCP/HRT use and smoking should be avoided.

PROPHYLAXIS

- Symptomatic and asymptomatic carriers (identified by family screening) should receive prophylactic anticoagulation in high-risk situations.
- Patients with AT deficiency may benefit from antithrombin concentrates in the perioperative and postoperative periods.
- Though homocysteine levels can be lowered with folic acid, vitamin B_6, and vitamin B_{12} supplements, studies suggest that correcting mild/moderate hyperhomocysteinemia does not decrease risk of thrombosis and routine supplementation is not indicated.
- Pregnancy prophylaxis: timing and intensity of therapy is based on the patient's risk (genetic or acquired defect and clinical history).

ACUTE GENERAL Rx

- Initial therapy is the same as for individuals without thrombophilia (exceptions for protein C and AT deficiency)

Venous thrombosis:

- Unfractionated heparin or LMWH followed by warfarin. Continue heparin for at least 5 days and until international normalized ratio (INR) is therapeutic for 2 days, continue warfarin for 6 to 12 mo. Aim for INR of 2 to 3. The intensity of anticoagulation is not affected by the presence of thrombophilia.
- In pregnancy, full heparin anticoagulation during pregnancy and for at least 6 wk postpartum. Minimum duration of anticoagulation is 6 months.

Protein C deficiency:

- Warfarin-induced skin necrosis: FFP or protein C concentrates until full anticoagulation with heparin is achieved.
- After full heparin anticoagulation, begin gradual warfarin loading (2 mg qd for 3 days and increase by 2 to 3 mg qd until target INR is reached). Continue heparin for 5 to 7 days until warfarin-induced anticoagulation is achieved.

AT deficiency:

- AT concentrates may be used if difficulty achieving anticoagulation (heparin resistance), severe thrombosis, or recurrent thrombosis despite adequate anticoagulation.

Arterial thrombosis:

- Anticoagulation and surgical consult for definitive procedure.

Duration of therapy:

- Must consider risk and benefit, risk of major bleeding 2% to 3% per yr in general population on anticoagulation but as high as 7% to 9% per yr in the elderly. Long-term anticoagulation is usually not indicated given the low risk of recurrent thrombosis for most conditions and the bleeding risk associated with anticoagulation.

Indefinite anticoagulation considered if ≥2 spontaneous thromboses or spontaneous thrombosis associated with any of the following:

1. Life-threatening thrombosis
2. More than a single genetic defect
3. Presence of AT deficiency or antiphospholipid antibodies

DISPOSITION

Depends on underlying condition

REFERRAL

Hematology, maternal–fetal medicine, obstetric medicine

PEARLS & CONSIDERATIONS

- Consider screening family members: may be able to decrease risk with lifestyle modification and provide prophylaxis in high-risk situations.
- Previous episode of VTE is a major risk factor for recurrence regardless of the presence of thrombophilia. Risk is greatest in the first 2 yr after thrombosis. About 30% of all patients with unprovoked VTE have recurrence within 10 yr. Risk of recurrence may be assessed by evaluation of residual thrombosis by Doppler ultrasound and with D-dimer levels after completion of anticoagulation.
- Patients with pregnancy-related complications may benefit from prophylaxis with heparin and low-dose aspirin.
- Genetic risk factors for thrombosis in non-Caucasians remain largely unknown.
- Interpreting workup: many medical conditions cause acquired abnormalities.
  - Heparin therapy: antithrombin levels decrease by up to 30%, may affect testing of lupus anticoagulant and APC-resistance assay.
  - Warfarin therapy: protein C, protein S levels, and function decrease; antithrombin levels may increase.
  - Antithrombin decreases with acute thrombosis (<10 days), surgery, liver disease, DIC, nephrotic syndrome, chemotherapy, estrogen therapy (HRT, OCP).
  - Protein S levels decrease with acute thrombosis (<10 days), surgery, liver disease, DIC, nephrotic syndrome, HIV infection, chemotherapy, pregnancy (free and total levels may be reduced by 40% to 60%), estrogen therapy (HRT, OCP).
  - Protein C decreases with acute thrombosis (<10 days), surgery, liver disease, chemotherapy, severe infection, and DIC. Levels increase with age and hyperlipidemia.
  - APCR is increased with pregnancy, estrogen therapy (HRT, OCP), and certain cancers. Elevated factor VIII level and antiphospholipid antibodies can cause APCR.

SUGGESTED READINGS

Bauer KA: The thrombophilias: well-defined risk factors with uncertain therapeutic implications, *Ann Intern Med* 135:367, 2001.

Coppens M et al: Inherited thrombophilias, *Obstet Gynecol Clin N Am* 33:357, 2006.

Lim W et al: Inherited thrombophilia and pregnancy associated venous thromboembolism, *BMJ* 443:1318, 2007.

Marques MB, Triplett DA: When to suspect hypercoagulability and how to investigate it, *Ann Diagn Pathol* 5(3):177, 2001.

Simioni P et al: Inherited thrombophilia and venous thromboembolism, *Semin Thromb Hemost* 32:700, 2006.

Walker ID et al: Investigation and management of heritable thrombophilia, *Br J Haematol* 114:512, 2001.

AUTHOR: **SUDEEP K. AULAKH, M.D., F.R.C.P.C.**

BASIC INFORMATION

DEFINITION

Hyperemesis gravidarum is the persistent nausea and vomiting with onset in the first trimester of pregnancy, resulting in weight loss and fluid and electrolyte and acid-base imbalances.

ICD-9CM CODES
643.1 Hyperemesis gravidarum

EPIDEMIOLOGY & DEMOGRAPHICS

INCIDENCE: 0.5 to 10 cases/1000 pregnancies
GENETICS: No genetic disposition
RISK FACTORS:

- Multiple pregnancy
- Molar pregnancy
- Previous history of unsuccessful pregnancy
- Nulliparity
- Hyperemesis gravidarum in a prior pregnancy
- No correlation with race, socioeconomic status, or marital status

PEAK ONSET: 8 to 12 wk of gestation

PHYSICAL FINDINGS & CLINICAL PRESENTATION

- Weight loss
- Rapid heart rate
- Fall in blood pressure
- Dry mucous membranes
- Loss of skin elasticity
- Ketotic odor
- In severe cases, Wernicke's encephalopathy as a result of thiamine deficiency

ETIOLOGY

Specific etiology is unknown.

DIAGNOSIS

DIFFERENTIAL DIAGNOSIS

- Pancreatitis
- Cholecystitis
- Hepatitis
- Pyelonephritis

WORKUP

Hyperemesis gravidarum is a diagnosis of exclusion. A detailed history and physical examination along with laboratory tests to rule out other causes of vomiting in early pregnancy are indicated.

LABORATORY TESTS

- Urinalysis to document ketonuria and proteinuria
- Urine C&S to rule out pyelonephritis
- Serum electrolytes to rule out electrolyte and acid-base imbalance
- Serum concentration of aminotransferases and bilirubin to rule out hepatitis
- Serum amylase to rule out pancreatitis
- Free T_4 and TSH (Elevated T_4 with suppressed TSH levels present in up to 60% of patients with hyperemesis gravidarum. This biochemical hyperthyroidism usually spontaneously resolves after 18 wk.)

IMAGING STUDIES

- Pelvic ultrasound examination to rule out multiple gestation and molar pregnancy
- Ultrasound of the gallbladder to rule out cholecystitis

TREATMENT

NONPHARMACOLOGIC THERAPY

- Reassurance
- Psychologic support
- Avoidance of foods that trigger nausea
- Frequent small meals once oral intake has resumed
- Accupressure with the use of a wrist band
- Ginger has been studied as a promising herbal remedy, but data are relatively sparse

ACUTE GENERAL Rx

- NPO.
- Fluid and electrolyte replacement.
- Parenteral vitamin supplementation.
- Daily supplementation of thiamine 100 mg IM or IV to prevent Wernicke's encephalopathy.
- Pyridoxine (vitamin B_6) 30 mg daily may reduce nausea. It should not exceed 25 mg/day.
- Antiemetics, such as promethazine (Phenergan) or droperidol (Inapsine), have not been found to be associated with fetal malformations when given in early pregnancy. Promethazine given as a low-dose continuous infusion of 25 mg in each liter of IV fluid has been shown to be very effective in controlling nausea and vomiting.
- Restart oral intake gradually no less than 48 hr after vomiting has ceased.

CHRONIC Rx

If the previous acute therapy does not resolve vomiting and oral intake is not feasible, parenteral hyperalimentation may be necessary.

DISPOSITION

- Untreated hyperemesis gravidarum can result in maternal renal and hepatic damage or death from fluid and electrolyte imbalance.
- Hyperemesis gravidarum with severe weight loss has been associated with lower average birth weight and with CNS malformations in neonates.

REFERRAL

For parenteral hyperalimentation if required

PEARLS & CONSIDERATIONS

COMMENTS

Although the specific etiology of hyperemesis gravidarum is not known, psychogenic causes proposed in older literature have been largely discredited. "Behavioral therapies" for hyperemesis gravidarum are inappropriate.

SUGGESTED READING

Strong T: Alternative therapies of morning sickness, *Clin Obstet Gynecol* 44:653, 2001.

AUTHORS: **LAUREL WHITE, M.D.,** and **RUBEN ALVERO, M.D.**

BASIC INFORMATION

DEFINITION

Hypereosinophilic syndrome (HES) refers to a group of disorders of unknown cause characterized by sustained overproduction of eosinophils and organ dysfunction.

SYNONYMS

Idiopathic hypereosinophilic syndrome

ICD-9CM CODES
288.3 Hypereosinophilic syndrome

EPIDEMIOLOGY & DEMOGRAPHICS

PREDOMINANT SEX: Occurs in men more often than women (9:1)

PREDOMINANT AGE: Usually occurs between the ages of 20 and 50 yr

PHYSICAL FINDINGS & CLINICAL PRESENTATION

- Clinical presentation of HES may vary from an incidental finding of eosinophilia to sudden onset of cardiac or neurologic symptoms.
- *Cardiac manifestations* (58%) include dyspnea, orthopnea, signs and symptoms of congestive heart failure.
  1. Symptoms are the result of endocardial infiltration of eosinophils leading to tissue necrosis. Thrombosis of the damaged tissue ensues and ultimately results in scarring and fibrosis.
  2. The pathologic process may result in a restrictive cardiomyopathy, dilated cardiomyopathy, and valvular heart disease.
- *Neurologic manifestations* (54%) may be of three types:
  1. Thromboembolic (e.g., cardiac emboli or local vascular thrombosis)
  2. CNS dysfunction—confusion, loss of memory, ataxia, upper motor neuron signs, seizures, and behavior changes.
  3. Peripheral neuropathy may be symmetric or asymmetric, sensory or mixed sensory and motor deficits
- *Pulmonary manifestations* (40%) include a chronic persistent nonproductive cough, shortness of breath, and dyspnea on exertion.
- *Cutaneous manifestations* (56%) usually include urticaria, angioedema, or erythematous pruritic papules and nodules.
- *GI manifestations* (23%) include diarrhea but findings of gastritis, colitis, pancreatitis, and hepatitis can occur.
- *Ocular manifestations* (23%) are thought to be due to retinal microemboli.

ETIOLOGY

- The etiology of HES is unknown and is thought of as a composite of many diseases.
- In some cases, a fusion event generating an abnormal and oncogenic tyrosine kinase (FIP1L1-PDGF alpha kinase) appears to be causative.

DIAGNOSIS

Criteria for the diagnosis of idiopathic HES include:

- Persistent eosinophilia of >1500 eosinophils/mm^3 for more than 6 mo
- Exclusion of other conditions causing eosinophilia (e.g., parasites, allergies)
- Signs and symptoms of organ system dysfunction (e.g., heart, liver, lung)

DIFFERENTIAL DIAGNOSIS

The differential includes all causes of peripheral blood eosinophilia. Parasitic infections, coccidioidomycosis, cat-scratch disease, asthma, Churg-Strauss syndrome, allergic rhinitis, atopic dermatitis, drug reactions, aspergillosis, eosinophilic pneumonia, hypersensitivity pneumonitis, HIV, eosinophilic gastroenteritis, inflammatory bowel disease.

WORKUP

The workup of a patient who is suspected of having HES should exclude other causes mentioned in the Differential Diagnosis leading to peripheral eosinophilia.

LABORATORY TESTS

- CBC with total eosinophil count; often the total white cell count ranges from 10,000 to 30,000/mm^3 with eosinophilia of 30% to 70%
- Erythrocyte sedimentation rate (ESR)
- Electrolytes, BUN, and creatinine
- LFTs
- Urinalysis
- HIV assay
- Stools for ova and parasites × 3
- Serologic blood tests for parasitic infections (e.g., *Strongyloides*)
- Total IgE level
- Rheumatoid factor
- Bone marrow aspirate and biopsy
- Duodenal aspirate
- ECG

IMAGING STUDIES

- Chest x-ray may be clear or show infiltrates, effusions, or fibrotic scarring
- CT scan of chest, abdomen, and pelvis
- Echocardiogram can assess for ventricular function, valvular pathology including regurgitation and thrombi formation

TREATMENT

Treatment is usually not initiated unless there is evidence of organ involvement.

NONPHARMACOLOGIC THERAPY

In patients with hypereosinophilia without organ involvement, serial echocardiograms are recommended at 6-mo intervals.

ACUTE GENERAL Rx

- In patients with organ involvement, initial therapy is with prednisone 1 mg/kg/day or 60 mg/day in adults.
- Patient's symptoms and peripheral eosinophil counts are monitored.
- Doses may be tapered to alternate day prednisone use in patients whose eosinophil counts have been suppressed.

CHRONIC Rx

- Patients not responding to corticosteroids, hydroxyurea 1 to 2 g/day may be tried.
- In patients bearing the FIP1L1-PDGF alpha kinase fusion gene, a trial of a specific tyrosine kinase inhibitor (Gleevac) should be considered.
- Hydroxyurea is aimed at reducing the total WBC count to <10,000/mm^3.
- If the disease continues to progress, vincristine, etoposide, interferon-α, cyclosporine, and leukapheresis are alternative choices.
- Anticoagulation with warfarin and/or antiplatelet agents is often used in patients with HES.
- If all else fails, bone marrow transplantation may be considered.

DISPOSITION

- Before the use of cardiac imaging (echo) and cardiac surgeries (valve replacement), patients with HES had a poor prognosis with a mean survival of 9 mo and a 3-yr survival of 12%.
- Deaths usually result from congestive heart failure, endocarditis, and systemic emboli.
- There are now reports of 5-, 10-, and 15-yr survival rates.

REFERRAL

HES is a rare and complicated disorder requiring a multidisciplinary approach. Cardiology, neurology, pulmonary, ophthalmology, and hematology consultations should be requested in the appropriate clinical setting.

PEARLS & CONSIDERATIONS

COMMENTS

There is still much to be learned about HES. The etiology and exact mechanism of organ damage caused by eosinophils remains unknown.

SUGGESTED READINGS

Cools J et al: The FIP1L1-PDGFR alpha kinase in hypereosinophilic syndrome and chronic eosinophilic leukemia, *Curr Opin Hematol* 11(1):51, 2004.

Cools J et al: A tyrosine kinase created by fusion of the PDGFRA and FIP1L1 genes as a therapeutic target of imatinib in idiopathic hypereosinophilic syndrome, *N Engl J Med* 348(13):1201, 2003.

Katz HT, Haque SJ, Hsieh FH: Pediatric hypereosinophilic syndrome (HES) differs from adult HES, *J Pediatr* 146(1):134, 2005.

AUTHORS: **GLENN G. FORT, M.D., M.P.H.,** and **DENNIS J. MIKOLICH, M.D.**

BASIC INFORMATION

DEFINITION

Primary hyperlipoproteinemia refers to a group of genetic disorders of the lipid transport proteins in the blood, which manifests as abnormally elevated levels of cholesterol, triglycerides, or both in the serum of affected patients (Table 1-21).

SYNONYMS

Hyperlipidemia

ICD-9CM CODES
272.4 Hyperlipoproteinemia
272.3 Fredrickson type I
272.0 Fredrickson type IIa
272.2 Fredrickson type IIb, III
272.1 Fredrickson type IV
272.3 Fredrickson type V

EPIDEMIOLOGY & DEMOGRAPHICS

INCIDENCE:

- Variable depending on the genetic defect
- Spectrum spans the common familial hypercholesterolemia, with an incidence of 1:500, to the rare familial lipoprotein lipase deficiency

PREDOMINANT SEX: None

GENETICS:

- Familial lipoprotein lipase deficiency: autosomal recessive, resulting in an elevation in the plasma chylomicrons and triglycerides
- Familial apoprotein CII deficiency: autosomal recessive, resulting in increased serum chylomicrons, VLDL, and hypertriglyceridemia
- Familial type 3 hyperlipoproteinemia: single-gene defect requiring contributory factors to manifest
- Familial hypercholesterolemia: autosomal dominant defect of the LDL receptor resulting in an elevated serum cholesterol level and normal triglycerides
- Familial hypertriglyceridemia: common, autosomal dominant defect resulting in elevated VLDL and triglycerides
- Multiple lipoprotein–type hyperlipidemia: autosomal dominant, manifesting as isolated hypercholesterolemia, isolated hypertriglyceridemia, or hyperlipidemia
- Polygenic hypercholesterolemia: multifactorial
- Polygenic hyperalphalipoproteinemia: autosomal dominant or polygenic, causing an elevated HDL

PHYSICAL FINDINGS & CLINICAL PRESENTATION

- Familial lipoprotein lipase deficiency: recurrent bouts of abdominal pain in infancy, eruptive xanthomas, hepatomegaly, splenomegaly, lipemia retinalis
- Familial apoprotein CII deficiency: occasional eruptive xanthomas
- Familial type 3 hyperlipoproteinemia: after age 20 yr see xanthoma striata palmaris or tuberoeruptive xanthomas, xanthelasmas, arterial bruits at a young age, gangrene of the lower extremities at a young age
- Familial hypercholesterolemia: tendon xanthomas, arcus corneae, xanthelasma
- Familial hypertriglyceridemia: associated obesity; with exacerbations eruptive xanthomas can develop
- Multiple lipoprotein type hyperlipidemia: no discerning physical findings
- Polygenic hypercholesterolemia: no discerning physical findings
- Polygenic hyperalphalipoproteinemia: no discerning physical findings

ETIOLOGY

Genetic defects causing lipid abnormalities

DIAGNOSIS

DIFFERENTIAL DIAGNOSIS

Secondary causes of hyperlipoproteinemias:

- Diabetes mellitus
- Glycogen storage diseases
- Lipodystrophies
- Glucocorticoid use/excess
- Alcohol

TABLE 1-21 **Classification of Lipoprotein Disorders by Phenotypes, Genotypes, and Corresponding Clinical Manifestations**

	PLASMA LIPID LEVELS				
Phenotype	Cholesterol	Triglyceride	Genotype	Xanthomas	Other Clinical Manifestations
I	Normal or elevated	Elevated lipemia	Familial lipoprotein lipase deficiency, Apo C-II deficiency	Eruptive, tubero-eruptive	Recurrent abdominal pain, other gastrointestinal symptoms, hepatosplenomegaly
IIA	Normal	Elevated	FHC, familial combined hyperlipidemia—polygenic and sporadic hypercholesterolemia	Tendinous, xanthelasma, tuberous; planar (homozygous)	Premature CAD, arcus corneae, aortic stenosis (homozygous FHC), arthritic symptoms
IIB	Elevated	Elevated	Familial combined hyperlipidemia, FHC		
III	Elevated	Elevated	Familial dysbetalipoproteinemia	Planar (especially palmar), tuberous	Premature CAD and peripheral vascular disease, male > female, obesity, abnormal glucose tolerance, hyperuricemia, aggravated by hypothyroidism, good response to therapy
IV	Normal or elevated	Elevated	Familial hypertriglyceridemia, familial combined hyperlipidemia, sporadic hypertriglyceridemia	Usually none; rarely eruptive or tubero-eruptive	CAD and peripheral vascular disease, obesity, abnormal glucose tolerance, hyperuricemia, arthritic symptoms, gallbladder disease
V	Normal or elevated	Elevated	Homozygous FHC	Eruptive, tubero-eruptive	Recurrent abdominal pain, other gastrointestinal symptoms, hepatosplenomegaly, peripheral paresthesia

From Graber MA: *The family practice handbook,* ed 4, St Louis, 2001, Mosby.
CAD, Coronary artery disease; *FHC,* familial hypercholesterolemia.

- Oral contraceptives
- Renal disease
- Hepatic dysfunction

WORKUP

- Detailed family history for premature cardiac disease
- Recurrent pancreatitis
- Thorough physical examination

LABORATORY TESTS

- Lipoprotein analysis
- Lipoprotein electrophoresis
- Risk factor stratification for medications—see hypercholesterolemia

TREATMENT

NONPHARMACOLOGIC THERAPY

- Cornerstone of treatment: dietary therapy
  - TLC diet (therapeutic lifestyle changes): 7% total calories from saturated fat; up to 10% total calories from polyunsaturated fat; up to 20% total calories from monounsaturated fat
  - Fat 25% to 30% total calories
  - Fiber 20 to 30 gm/day
  - Cholesterol <200 mg/day
- Risk factor reduction includes smoking cessation, treatment of hypertension, exercise
- Familial lipoprotein lipase deficiency and familial apoprotein CII deficiency: fat-free diet
- Remainder of cases, except those with polygenic hyperalphalipoproteinemia: fat- and cholesterol-restricted diets

ACUTE GENERAL Rx

No acute treatment needed

CHRONIC Rx

- Familial lipoprotein lipase deficiency, polygenic hyperalphalipoproteinemia, or familial apoprotein CII deficiency: no chronic drug therapy
- Familial type 3 hyperlipoproteinemia: usually responds well to secondary causes being treated and diet therapy; if not, fibric acids may be tried
- Familial hypercholesterolemia: bile acid sequestrants, HMG-CoA reductase inhibitors, or niacin
- Familial hypertriglyceridemia: fibric acids
- Multiple lipoprotein type hyperlipidemia: drug therapy aimed at the predominant lipid abnormality noted
- Recent data suggest in patients with lipoprotein abnormalities that treatment goals should be based on non-HDLC rather than LDL-C

DISPOSITION

- Those with polygenic hyperalphalipoproteinemia: excellent prognosis for longevity
- Those with familial hypercholesterolemia, familial type 3 hypercholesterolemia, and multiple lipoprotein type hyperlipidemia: even with aggressive treatment, at high risk for accelerated atherosclerosis and CAD

PEARLS & CONSIDERATIONS

COMMENTS

Patient information is available through the American Heart Association.

See Tables 1-22 and 1-23 and Boxes 1-3 through 1-7.

SUGGESTED READINGS

Alawadhi M et al: Genetic lipoprotein disorders and coronary atherosclerosis, *Curr Atheroscler Rep* 7(3):196, 2005.

National Cholesterol Education Program: Second report on the Expert Panel on Detection, evaluation and treatment of high cholesterol in adults (adult treatment panel III), *JAMA* 285:2486, 2001.

Sveger T, Nordborg K: Apolipoprotein B as a marker of familial hyperlipoproteinemia, *J Atheroscler Thromb* 11(5):286, 2004.

AUTHORS: **BETH J. WUTZ, M.D.,** and **RUBEN ALVERO, M.D.**

TABLE 1-22 **LDL Cholesterol Goals and Cutpoints for Therapeutic Lifestyle Changes (TLC) and Drug Therapy in Different Risk Categories**

Risk Category	LDL Goal (mg/dl)	LDL Level at Which to Initiate Therapeutic Lifestyle Changes (mg/dl)	IDLD Level at Which to Consider Drug Therapy (mg/dl)
CHD or CHD risk equivalents (10-yr risk >20%)	<100	≥100	≥130 (100-129: drug optional)*
2+ Risk factors (10-yr risk ≤20%)	<130	≥130	10-yr risk 10%-20%: ≥130 10-yr risk <10%: ≥160
0-1 Risk factor†	<160	≥160	≥190 (160-189: LDL-lowering drug optional)

From National Cholesterol Education Program Expert Panel on Detection, Evaluation, and Treatment of High Blood Cholesterol in Adults (Adult Treatment Panel III), National Institutes of Health, *JAMA* 285:2486, 2001.
CHD, Coronary heart disease; *LDL,* low-density lipoprotein.
*Some authorities recommend use of LDL-lowering drugs in this category if an LDL cholesterol level of <100 mg/dl cannot be achieved by therapeutic lifestyle changes. Others prefer use of drugs that primarily modify triglycerides and HDL (e.g., nicotinic acid or fibrate). Clinical judgment also may call for deferring drug therapy in this subcategory.
†Almost all people with 0-1 risk factor have a 10-year risk <10%; thus 10-year risk assessment in people with 0-1 risk factor is not necessary.

TABLE 1-23 **Comparison of LDL Cholesterol and Non-HDL Cholesterol Goals for Three Risk Categories**

Risk Category	LDL Goal (mg/dl)	Non-HDL Goal (mg/dl)
CHD and CHD risk equivalent (10-yr risk for CHD >20%)	<70	<130
Multiple (2+) risk factors and 10-yr risk ≤20%	<130	<160
0-1 Risk factor	<160	<190

From National Cholesterol Education Program Expert Panel on Detection, Evaluation, and Treatment of High Blood Cholesterol in Adults (Adult Treatment Panel III), National Institutes of Health, *JAMA* 285:2486, 2001.
CHD, Coronary heart disease; *HDL,* high-density lipoprotein; *LDL,* low-density lipoprotein.

BOX 1-3 Nutrient Composition of the Therapeutic Lifestyle Changes (TLC) Diet

Nutrient	Recommended Intake
Saturated fat*	<7% of total calories
Polyunsaturated fat	Up to 10% of total calories
Monounsaturated fat	Up to 20% of total calories
Total fat	25%-35% of total calories
Carbohydrate†	50%-60% of total calories
Fiber	20-30 g/day
Protein	Approximately 15% of total calories
Cholesterol	<200 mg/day
Total calories‡	Balance energy intake and expenditure to maintain desirable body weight/prevent weight gain

From National Cholesterol Education Program Expert Panel on Detection, Evaluation, and Treatment of High Blood Cholesterol in Adults (Adult Treatment Panel III), National Institutes of Health, *JAMA* 285:2486, 2001.

*Trans fatty acids are another LDL-raising fat that should be kept at a low intake.

†Carbohydrates should be derived predominantly from foods rich in complex carbohydrates, including grains, especially whole grains, fruits, and vegetables.

‡Daily energy expenditure should include at least moderate physical activity (contributing approximately 200 kcal/day).

BOX 1-4 ATP III Classification of LDL, Total, and HDL Cholesterol (mg/dl)

LDL cholesterol	
<100	Optimal
100-129	Near or above optimal
130-159	Borderline high
160-189	High
≥190	Very high
Total cholesterol	
<200	Desirable
200-239	Borderline high
>240	High
HDL cholesterol	
<40	Low
>60	High

From National Cholesterol Education Program Expert Panel on Detection, Evaluation, and Treatment of High Blood Cholesterol in Adults (Adult Treatment Panel III), National Institutes of Health, *JAMA* 285:2486, 2001.

ATP, Adult treatment panel; *HDL,* high-density lipoprotein, *LDL,* low-density lipoprotein.

BOX 1-5 Major Risk Factors (Exclusive of LDL Cholesterol) That Modify LDL Goals*

Cigarette smoking
Hypertension (blood pressure ≥140/90 mm Hg or on antihypertensive medication)
Low HDL cholesterol (<40 mg/dl)†
Family history of premature CHD (CHD in male first-degree relative) (<55 yr; CHD in female first-degree relative <65 yr)
Age (men ≥45 yr; women ≥55 yr)

From National Cholesterol Education Program Expert Panel on Detection, Evaluation, and Treatment of High Blood Cholesterol in Adults (Adult Treatment Panel III), National Institutes of Health, *JAMA* 285:2486, 2001.

HDL, High-density lipoprotein; *LDL,* low-density lipoprotein.

*Diabetes is regarded as a coronary heart disese (CHD) risk equivalent.

†HDL cholesterol > 60 mg/dl counts as a "negative" risk factor; its presence removes 1 risk factor from the total count.

BOX 1-6 Interventions to Improve Adherence

Focus on the Patient
Simplify medication regimens
Provide explicit patient instruction and use good counseling techniques to teach the patient how to follow the prescribed treatment
Encourage the use of prompts to help patients remember treatment regimens
Use systems to reinforce adherence and maintain contact with the patient
Encourage the support of family and friends
Reinforce and reward adherence
Increase visits for patients unable to achieve treatment goal
Increase the convenience and access to care
Involve patients in their care through self-monitoring

Focus on the Physician and Medical Office
Teach physicians to implement lipid treatment guidelines
Use reminders to prompt physicians to attend to lipid management
Identify a patient advocate in the office to help deliver or prompt care
Use patients to prompt preventive care
Develop a standardized treatment plan to structure care
Use feedback from past performance to foster change in future care
Remind patients of appointments and follow up missed appointments

Focus on the Health Delivery System
Provide lipid management through a lipid clinic
Utilize case management by nurses
Deploy telemedicine
Utilize the collaborative care of pharmacists
Execute critical care pathways in hospitals

From National Cholesterol Education Program Expert Panel on Detection, Evaluation, and Treatment of High Blood Cholesterol in Adults (Adult Treatment Panel III), National Institutes of Health, *JAMA* 285:2486, 2001.

BOX 1-7 Clinical Identification of the Metabolic Syndrome

RISK FACTOR	DEFINING LEVEL
Abdominal obesity* (waist circumference)†	
Men	>102 cm (>40 in)
Women	>88 cm (>35 in)
Triglycerides	>150 mg/dl
High-density lipoprotein cholesterol	
Men	<40 mg/dl
Women	<50 mg/dl
Blood pressure	>130/>85 mm Hg
Fasting glucose	>110 mg/dl

From National Cholesterol Education Program Expert Panel on Detection, Evaluation, and Treatment of High Blood Cholesterol in Adults (Adult Treatment Panel III), National Institutes of Health, *JAMA* 285:2486, 2001.

*Overweight and obesity are associated with insulin resistance and the metabolic syndrome. However, the presence of abdominal obesity is more highly correlated with the metabolic risk factors than is an elevated body mass index (BMI). Therefore, the simple measure of waist circumference is recommended to identify the body weight component of the metabolic syndrome.

†Some male patients can develop multiple metabolic risk factors when the waist circumference is only marginally increased, for example, 94-102 cm (37-40 in). Such patients may have strong genetic contribution to insulin resistance, and they should benefit from changes in life habits, similarly to men with categorical increases in waist circumference.

BASIC INFORMATION

DEFINITION

Hyperosmolar hyperglycemic syndrome (HHS) is a state of extreme hyperglycemia, marked dehydration, serum hyperosmolarity, altered mental status, and absence of ketoacidosis.

SYNONYMS

HHS
Hyperosmolar coma
Nonketotic hyperosmolar syndrome
Hyperosmolar nonketotic state

ICD-9CM CODES
250.2 Hyperosmolar coma

PHYSICAL FINDINGS & CLINICAL PRESENTATION

- Evidence of extreme dehydration (poor skin turgor, sunken eyeballs, dry mucous membranes)
- Neurologic defects (reversible hemiplegia, focal seizures)
- Orthostatic hypotension, tachycardia
- Evidence of precipitating factors (pneumonia, infected skin ulcer)
- Coma (25% of patients), delirium

ETIOLOGY

- Infections, 20% to 25% (e.g., pneumonia, UTI, sepsis)
- New or previously unrecognized diabetes (30% to 50%)
- Reduction or omission of diabetic medication
- Stress (MI, CVA)
- Drugs: diuretics (dehydration), phenytoin, diazoxide (impaired insulin secretion), glucocorticoids, chemotherapeutic agents, calcium channel blockers, TPN, substance abuse (alcohol, cocaine)

DIAGNOSIS

DIFFERENTIAL DIAGNOSIS

- Diabetic ketoacidosis
- The differential diagnosis of coma is described in Section II

LABORATORY TESTS

- Hyperglycemia: serum glucose usually >600 mg/dl, serum/urine ketones absent or "small."
- Hyperosmolarity: serum osmolarity usually >320 mOsm/L.
- Serum sodium: may be low, normal, or high; if normal or high, the patient is severely dehydrated, because an elevated glucose draws fluid from intracellular space decreasing the serum sodium; the corrected sodium can be obtained by increasing the serum sodium concentration by 1.6 mEq/dl for every 100 mg/dl increase in the serum glucose level over normal.
- Serum potassium: may be low, normal, or high; regardless of the initial serum level, the total body deficit is approximately 5 to 15 mEq/kg.
- Serum bicarbonate: usually >15 mEq/L (average is 17 mEq/L).
- Arterial pH: usually >7.3; both serum bicarbonate and arterial pH may be lower if lactic acidosis is present.
- BUN: azotemia (prerenal) is usually present (BUN generally ranges from 60 to 90 mg/dl).
- Phosphorus: hypophosphatemia (average deficit is 70 to 140 mm).
- Calcium: hypocalcemia (average deficit is 50 to 100 mEq).
- Magnesium: hypomagnesemia (average deficit is 50 to 100 mEq).
- CBC with differential, urinalysis, blood and urine cultures should be performed to rule out infectious etiology.

IMAGING STUDIES

- Chest x-ray is useful to rule out infectious process. The initial chest x-ray may be negative if the patient has significant dehydration. Repeat chest x-ray examination after 24 hr of hydration if pulmonary infection is suspected.
- CT scan of head should be performed in patients with suspected CVA.

TREATMENT

NONPHARMACOLOGIC THERAPY

- Monitor mental status, vital signs, urine output qh until improved, then monitor q2 to 4h.
- Monitor electrolytes, renal function, and glucose level (see "Acute General Rx").

ACUTE GENERAL Rx

- Vigorous fluid replacement: the volume and rate of fluid replacement are determined by renal and cardiac function. Typically, infuse 1000 to 1500 ml/hr for the initial 1 to 2 L; then decrease the rate of infusion to 500 ml/hr and monitor urinary output, blood chemistries, and blood pressure; use 0.9% NS (isotonic solution) if the patient is hypotensive or serum osmolarity is <320 mOsm/L; otherwise use 0.45% NS solution. Slower infusion rate may be used initially in patients with compromised cardiovascular or renal status. When serum glucose reaches 300 mg/dl, change to 5% dextrose with 0.45% NS.
- Replace electrolytes and monitor serum levels frequently (e.g., serum sodium and potassium q2h for the first 12 hr). Serum KCl replacement in patients with normal renal function and adequate urinary output is started when the serum potassium level is <5.2 mEq/L (e.g., 10 mEq KCl/hr if potassium level is 4 to 5.2 mEq/L). Continuous ECG monitoring and hourly measurement of urinary output are recommended. In patients with severe hypokalemia (potassium <3.3 mEq/L), give 40 mEq of potassium/hr until potassium is >3.3 mEq/L.
- Correct hyperglycemia. The goal is for plasma glucose to decline by at least 50 to 100 mg/dl/hr.
  1. Vigorous IV hydration will decrease the serum glucose level in most patients by 80 mg/dl/hr; a regular insulin IV bolus (0.15 U/kg of body weight) is often not necessary. Insulin should not be administered until serum potassium is >3.3 mEq/L to prevent life-threatening hypokalemia.
  2. Low-dose insulin infusion at 0.1 U/kg/hr (e.g., 25 U of regular insulin in 250 ml of 0.9% saline solution at 20 ml/hr) until the serum glucose level approaches 300 mg/dl; then the patient is started on regular SC insulin with sliding scale coverage. If the plasma glucose does not decrease over 2 to 4 hr despite adequate fluid administration and urine output, consider doubling the hourly insulin dose.
  3. Glucose should be monitored q1-2h in the initial 12 hr.
- In the absence of renal failure, phosphate can be administered at a rate of 0.1 mmol/kg/hr (5 to 10 mmol/hr) to a maximum of 80 to 120 mmol in 24 hr. Magnesium replacement, in absence of renal failure, can be administered IM (0.05 to 0.10 ml/kg of 20% magnesium sulfate) or as IV infusion (4 to 8 ml of 20% magnesium sulfate [0.08 to 0.16 mEq/kg]). Repeat magnesium, phosphate, and calcium levels should be obtained after 12 to 24 hr.
- On day 2 begin/resume feeding if patient is able and glucose under control (<200 mg/dl). Begin/resume SC insulin. For patients with type 2 diabetes, a mixture of N+R insulin is preferred, timing the injection with a planned meal. Total daily dose (TDD) can be 0.5 units/kg. Insulin proportions are typically 60% in A.M., 40% in P.M.

  A.M. dose: TDD × 0.4 = A.M. NPH insulin
  TDD × 0.2 = A.M. Regular insulin
  P.M. dose: TDD × 0.2 = P.M. NPH insulin
  TDD × 0.2 = P.M. Regular insulin
- Individual patients may be appropriate for a trial of oral agents.

PEARLS & CONSIDERATIONS

COMMENTS

The typical patient presenting with hyperosmolar hyperglycemic syndrome is an elderly or bed-confined diabetic with impaired ability to communicate thirst who is evaluated after an interval of 1 to 2 wk of prolonged osmotic diuresis.

SUGGESTED READINGS

Inzucchi SE: Diabetes facts and guidelines, Yale Diabetes Center, 2007.

Stoner GD: Hyperosmolar hyperglycemic state, *Am Fam Physician* 71:1723, 2005.

AUTHOR: **FRED F. FERRI, M.D.**

BASIC INFORMATION

DEFINITION

Primary hyperparathyroidism is an endocrine disorder caused by the excessive secretion of parathyroid hormone (PTH) from the parathyroid glands.

ICD-9CM CODES
252.0 Primary hyperparathyroidism
253.9 Ectopic hyperparathyroidism
588.8 Secondary hyperparathyroidism in chronic renal disease

EPIDEMIOLOGY & DEMOGRAPHICS

INCIDENCE: 1 case/1000 men and 2 to 3 cases/1000 women
PREVALENCE: 1 case/1000 persons
PREDOMINANT SEX AND AGE:
- Primary hyperparathyroidism occurs most frequently in postmenopausal women; prevalence in this group may be as high as 3%. The condition is asymptomatic in >50% of patients
- Primary hyperparathyroidism is the most frequent cause of hypercalcemia in ambulatory patients whereas malignancy is the most frequent cause of hypercalcemia in hospitalized patients.

GENETICS: Hyperparathyroidism can occur in conjunction with multiple endocrine neoplasia (MEN) I or II.

PHYSICAL FINDINGS & CLINICAL PRESENTATION

Primary hyperparathyroidism can be classified as asymptomatic (75% to 80%) and symptomatic. Physical examination may be entirely normal. The presence of signs and symptoms varies with the rapidity of development and degree of hypercalcemia. The following abnormalities may be present:
- GI: constipation, anorexia, nausea, vomiting, pancreatitis, ulcers, abdominal pain
- CNS: confusion, anxiety, fatigue, obtundation, psychosis, lassitude, depression, coma
- GU: nephrolithiasis, renal insufficiency, polyuria, decreased urine-concentrating ability, nocturia, nephrocalcinosis
- Cardiovascular: hypertension, LVH, arrhythmia, prolonged QT interval, valvular calcification
- Musculoskeletal: myopathy, weakness, osteoporosis, pseudogout, bone pain, gout, cystic bone lesions, chondrocalcinosis
- Other: metastatic calcifications, band keratopathy (found in medial and lateral margin of the cornea), pruritus

ETIOLOGY

- A single adenoma is found in 80% of patients; 90% of the adenomas are found within one of the parathyroid glands, the other 10% are in ectopic sites (lateral neck, thyroid, mediastinum, retroesophagus).
- Parathyroid gland hyperplasia occurs in 20% of patients.
- Primary hyperthyroidism is associated with MEN I and II.

DIAGNOSIS

DIFFERENTIAL DIAGNOSIS

Other causes of hypercalcemia:
- Malignancy: neoplasms of breast, lung, kidney, ovary, pancreas; myeloma, lymphoma
- Granulomatous disorders (e.g., sarcoidosis)
- Paget's disease
- Vitamin D intoxication, milk-alkali syndrome
- Thiazide diuretics
- Other: familial hypocalciuric hypercalcemia, thyrotoxicosis, adrenal insufficiency, prolonged immobilization, vitamin A intoxication, recovery from acute renal failure, lithium administration, pheochromocytoma, disseminated SLE

WORKUP

- Persistent hypercalcemia and an elevated serum PTH confirm the diagnosis of primary hyperparathyroidism. Repeated measurements of serum calcium may be necessary because patients may not have persistently elevated serum calcium level. In malnourished patients, the serum calcium level needs to be corrected for low albumin levels by adding 0.8 mg/dl to the total serum calcium level for every 1.0 g/dl by which the serum albumin concentration is lower than 4 g/dl.
- The serum PTH level is the single best test for initial evaluation of confirmed hypercalcemia. The "intact" PTH (iPTH) is the best assay. The iPTH distinguishes primary hyperparathyroidism from hypercalcemia caused by malignancy when the serum calcium level is >12 mg/dl.
- A high level of urinary cyclic AMP is also suggestive of primary hyperparathyroidism.
- Parathyroid hormone–like protein (PLP) is increased in hypercalcemia associated with solid malignancies.
- ECG may reveal shortening of the QT interval secondary to hypercalcemia.

LABORATORY TESTS

- Elevated serum ionized calcium level, low serum phosphorus, and normal or elevated alkaline phosphatase
- Elevated urine calcium level (in contrast with very low urinary calcium levels seen in patients with familial hypocalciuric hypercalcemia)
- Possibly elevated serum chloride levels, decreased serum CO_2, hyperchloremic metabolic acidosis
- A serum albumin level should be obtained when measuring serum calcium and the calcium level should be adjusted (see previous) in hypoalbuminemic patients
- The differential diagnosis of hypercalcemia is described in Section II

IMAGING STUDIES

- A bone survey may show evidence of subperiosteal bone resorption suggesting PTH excess (Fig. 1-132). The classic bone disease of primary hyperparathyroidism is *osteitis fibrosa cystica.*
- Parathyroid localization with technetium-99m sestamibi has been shown to have a high sensitivity and specificity for single adenomas.
- Screen for osteopenia with measurement of bone mineral density in all postmenopausal women.

TREATMENT

NONPHARMACOLOGIC THERAPY

- Unless contraindicated, patients should maintain a high intake of fluids (3 to 5 L/day) and sodium chloride (>400 mEq/day) to increase renal calcium excretion. Calcium intake should be 1000 mg/day.
- Potential hypercalcemic agents (e.g., thiazide diuretics) should be discontinued.

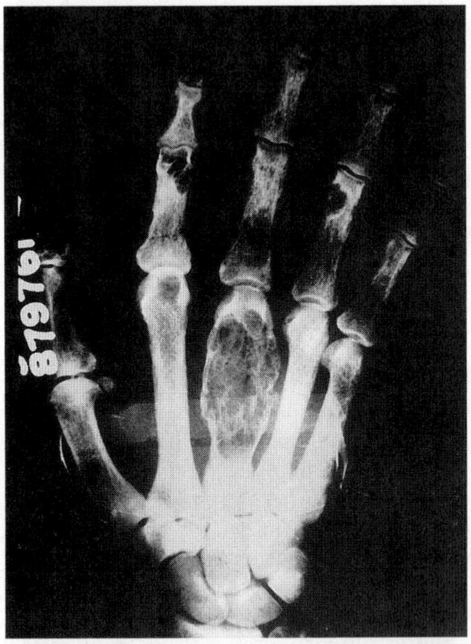

FIGURE 1-132 Radiograph of hand from a patient with severe primary hyperparathyroidism. Note the dramatic remodeling associated with the intense region of high bone turnover in the third metacarpal in addition to widespread evidence of subperiosteal, and trabecular resorption. (Courtesy Fuller Albright Collection, Masschusetts General Hospital. From Larsen PR, Kronenburg HM, Melmed S, Polonsky KS [eds]: *Williams textbook of endocrinology,* ed 10, Philadelphia, 2003, Saunders.)

- Surgery is the only effective treatment for primary hyperparathyroidism. It is generally indicated in all patients under age 50 and patients with complications from hyperthyroidism, such as nephrolithiasis and osteopenia. The conventional surgical approach is bilateral neck exploration under general anesthesia. Minimally invasive adenomectomy guided by preoperative technetium-99-m sestamibi scanning or ultrasound plus spiral CT is an alternative to conventional neck exploration. With the minimally invasive approach, the solitary adenoma is excised through a small unilateral incision with the patient under local cervical block anesthesia.
- Percutaneous ethanol injection into the parathyroid gland should be considered in selected patients who have undergone a subtotal parathyroidectomy for multigland disease and have recurrent hyperparathyroidism as a result of remnant gland. Percutaneous alcohol ablation of the parathyroid gland may also be a suitable treatment for patients who are unwilling or unable to undergo parathyroidectomy.
- Asymptomatic elderly patients can be followed conservatively with periodic monitoring of serum calcium level and review of symptoms. Serum creatinine and PTH levels should also be obtained at 6- to 12-mo intervals, bone density (cortical and trabecular) yearly. Criteria for medical monitoring of patients with asymptomatic primary hyperparathyroidism are as follows:
  1. Serum calcium level only mildly elevated
  2. Asymptomatic patient
  3. Normal bone status (no osteoporosis)
  4. Normal kidney function and no urolithiasis or nephrocalcinosis
  5. No previous episode of life-threatening hypercalcemia
- Nearly 25% of asymptomatic patients develop indications for surgery during observation.

ACUTE GENERAL Rx

Acute severe hypercalcemia (serum calcium >13 mg/dl) or symptomatic patients can be treated with the following:

- Vigorous IV hydration with NS followed by IV furosemide. Use NS with caution in patients with cardiac or renal insufficiency to avoid fluid overload.
- Biphosphonates are effective agents. Zoledronate (4 mg IV over a 15-min period in a solution of 50 ml of NS or D_5W) or pamidronate (60 to 90 mg IV infusion over a 2-hr period in a solution of 50 to 200 ml of saline or D_5W) are both very effective.
- Cinacalcet (Sensipar) is an oral calcimimetic agent that directly lowers PTH levels by increasing the Calcium-sensing receptor to extracellular calcium. The reduction in PTH is associated with a concomitant decrease in serum calcium levels. It is indicated in treatment of secondary hyperparathyroidism in patients with chronic kidney disease on dialysis and hypercalcemia in parathyroid carcinoma. Initial dose is 30 mg po qd.

PEARLS & CONSIDERATIONS

COMMENTS

- Patients should understand the importance of diet and exercise and be familiar with symptoms of disease progression.
- All patients with hyperparathyroidism should undergo further evaluation for the presence of MEN I or II.
- Decreased bone mineral density and nephrolithiasis are the major sequelae of untreated hyperparathyroidism.
- Treatment with alendronate or raloxifene should be considered in patients with hyperparathyroidism-induced osteoporosis.
- An experienced endocrine surgeon cures more than 95% of patients undergoing bilateral neck exploration and incurs <1% perioperative mortality.
- In pregnant women it is preferable to perform parathyroidectomy after the first trimester.

EVIDENCE

EBM

A systematic review concluded that the evidence base for less or minimally invasive parathyroidectomy techniques was inadequate for establishing their safety and efficacy.[1] (A)

A large cohort study, with 3213 patients, found patients treated surgically for primary hyperparathyroidism have a lower prevalence of fractures and gastric ulcers than patients treated conservatively.[2] (B)

A randomized controlled trial (RCT) of unilateral vs. bilateral neck exploration in cases of solitary parathyroid adenoma found the unilateral group had a lower incidence of biochemical and severe symptomatic hypocalcemia in the first 4 postoperative days.[3] (B)

Evidence-Based References

1. Scott NA et al: A systematic review of minimally invasive parathyroidectomy: update and re-appraisal. Australian Safety and Efficacy Register of New Interventional Procedures-Surgical (ASERNIP-S), ASERNIP-S Report No. 19, ed 2:105, 2001. Reviewed in: DARE Document 268021, York, UK, Centre for Reviews and Dissemination. (A)
2. Vestergaard P, Mosekilde L: Cohort study on effects of parathyroid surgery on multiple outcomes in primary hyperparathyroidism, *BMJ* 327:530, 2003. (B)
3. Bergenfelz A et al: Unilateral versus bilateral neck exploration for primary hyperparathyroidism: a prospective randomized controlled trial, *Ann Surg* 236:552, 2002. (B)

SUGGESTED READINGS

Farford B et al: Nonsurgical management of primary hyperparathyroidism, *Mayo Clin Proc* 82(3):351, 2007.

Monchik JM et al: Minimally invasive parathyroid surgery in 103 patients with local/regional anesthesia, without exclusion criteria, *Surgery* 131:502, 2002.

Taniegra ED: Hyperparathyroidism, *Am Fam Physician* 69:333, 2004.

Udelsman R: Six hundred fifty-six consecutive explorations for primary hyperparathyroidism, *Ann Surg* 235:665, 2002.

AUTHOR: **FRED F. FERRI, M.D.**

BASIC INFORMATION

DEFINITION

Hypersensitivity pneumonitis (HP) is a group of immunologically mediated pulmonary diseases provoked by recurrent exposure to various environmental agents.

SYNONYMS

Extrinsic allergic alveolitis (EAA)
Some specific examples:
- Bird fancier's lung
- Farmer's lung
- Chemical worker's lung
- Humidifier lung
- Hot tub lung
- Sauna taker's lung

ICD-9CM CODES
495.9 Pneumonitis, hypersensitivity

EPIDEMIOLOGY & DEMOGRAPHICS

- Prevalence and incidence of HP vary considerably.
- Depends on definition and methods to establish diagnosis, intensity of exposure, environmental conditions, and genetic risk factors that remain poorly understood.
- Greater than 300 causative agents have been identified and the number continues to grow.
- Causative agents have been established in residential and occupational exposures that include: birds, mold, humidifiers, organic and inorganic chemicals.
- Likely several genes are involved that cause an exaggerated lung response to offending agent. The major histocompatibility complex is the most studied thus far.
- A viral connection has been implicated that may enhance clinical exposure to an offending agent.

PHYSICAL FINDINGS & CLINICAL PRESENTATION

Vary depending on frequency and intensity of antigen exposure.
- *Acute:* fever, cough, and dyspnea 4 to 6 hr after an intense exposure, lasting 18 to 24 hr
- *Subacute:* insidious onset of productive cough, dyspnea on exertion, anorexia, and weight loss, usually from a heavy, sustained exposure
- *Chronic:* gradually progressive cough, dyspnea, malaise, and weight loss, usually from low-grade or recurrent exposure

Physical examination: cyanosis and "crepitant rales," possible fever

ETIOLOGY

- Numerous environmental agents, often encountered in occupational settings
- Common sources of antigens: "moldy" hay, silage, grain, or vegetables; bird droppings or feathers; low molecular weight chemicals (i.e., isocyanates), pharmaceutical products

DIAGNOSIS

- Accurate diagnosis is important for differentiating HP from other interstitial disorders because the prognosis and treatment may differ.
- No gold standard for diagnosis.
- The clinical syndrome is indistinguishable from an acute respiratory infection without a history of illness occurring within hours of exposure to an antigen.
- Need high index of suspicion.
- Detailed occupational and home exposure history.

DIFFERENTIAL DIAGNOSIS

Acute Stages:
Acute bronchopulmonary aspergillosis
Pulmonary embolism
Asthma
Aspiration pneumonia
Recurrent pneumonia
BOOP
Sarcoidosis
Churg-Strauss syndrome
Wegener's granulomatosis

Chronic Stages:
IPF
Bronchiectasis
Chronic bronchitis

WORKUP

There is no single radiologic, physiologic, or immunologic test specific for the diagnosis of HP. HP must be suspected in any patient presenting with cough, dyspnea, fever, and malaise. A thorough history focusing on potential exposures is essential.

Major criteria:
- History of symptoms compatible with HP that appear to worsen within hours after antigen exposure.
- Confirmation of exposure to the offending agent by history, investigation of the environment, serum precipitin test, or BAL antibody.
- Compatible changes on CXR or HRCT of the chest.
- BAL fluid lymphocytosis (if performed).
- Compatible histologic changes by lung bx (if performed).
- Positive natural challenge (reproduction of symptoms and laboratory abnormalities after exposure to the suspected environment) or by controlled inhalation challenge.

Minor criteria:
- Basilar crackles
- Decreased diffusion capacity
- Arterial hypoxemia (either at rest or with exercise)

LABORATORY TESTS

- Routine lab tests do not make the diagnosis, but typically the ESR, CRP, and leukocyte count are increased; elevated immunoglobulins IgG and IgM are nonspecific; RF and immune complexes are often positive; peripheral eosinophil count and serum IgE are generally normal.
- LDH is increased and tends to decrease with improvement.
- Pulmonary function tests: restrictive ventilatory patterns are typically seen. Decreased FEV1, decreased FVC, decreased TLC, decreased diffusing capacity, and decreased static compliance.
- ABG: mild hypoxemia (worsens with exercise).
- A-a gradient: slight increase.
- Serum precipitin test IgG antibody against offending antigen detected in serum. Sensitive but not specific for HP (asymptomatic patients may have IgG antibodies in serum).
- Skin testing: unclear if helpful. However, some feel it to be a safe, effective, and rapid procedure in the diagnosis and follow-up of patients with HP. Sensitivity is similar to that of the precipitin test but the specificity is higher.

IMAGING STUDIES

Chest x-ray: nonspecific; may be normal in early stage.
- *Acute/subacute:* bilateral interstitial and alveolar nodular infiltrates (Fig. 1-133) in a patchy or homogeneous distribution. Apices are often spared.
- *Chronic:* diffuse reticulonodular infiltrates and fibrosis. Honeycombing may develop.

High-resolution chest CT scan: no pathognomonic features but demonstrates airspace and interstitial patterns in the acute and subacute stage. The chronic stage reveals honeycombing and bronchiectasis.

TREATMENT

NONPHARMACOLOGIC THERAPY

Early recognition and avoidance of the causative antigen

ACUTE GENERAL Rx

- Glucocorticoids accelerate initial lung recovery but may have no effect long term (from a controlled study in

farmer's lung). There are no prospective, randomized, placebo-controlled trials for other types of HP or subacute and chronic stages.
- Prednisone 0.5 to 1mg/kg usually over 1 to 2 wk then tapered over 4 wk.

DISPOSITION/PROGNOSIS

Acute: 4 to 48 hr
- Clinical—fever, chills, cough, hypoxia, malaise
- HRCT—ground-glass infiltrates
- Immunopath—alveolitis, immune complex deposition
- Prognosis—good

Subacute: weeks to 4 mo
- Clinical—dyspnea, cough, episodic flares
- HRCT—micronodules, air trapping
- Immunopath—granulomas, bronchiolitis
- Prognosis—good

Chronic: 4 mo to years
- Clinical—dyspnea, cough, fatigue, weight loss
- HRCT—fibrosis (+/−), honeycombing, emphysema
- Immunopath—lymphocytic infiltration, fibrosis, neutrophil mediated air space destruction

REFERRAL

- Bronchoscopy: BAL provides useful supportive data in the diagnosis of HP. Usually reveals intense lymphocytosis (typically T cells >50%) of predominantly CD 8+ suppressor cells. In acute stages neutrophils predominate but as the disease progresses to chronic form the ratio of CD 4+ to CD 8+ cells increase. When fibrosis is present the number of neutrophils increase.
- Lung biopsy: the histopathologic features of HP are distinctive but not pathognomonic. Typically bronchiolitis and interstitial pneumonitis with granuloma formation is seen. Variable degrees of interstitial fibrosis are seen in the chronic form.
- Laboratory inhalation challenge: testing to prove a direct relationship between a suspected antigen and disease; extract of antigen is inhaled via a nebulizer.

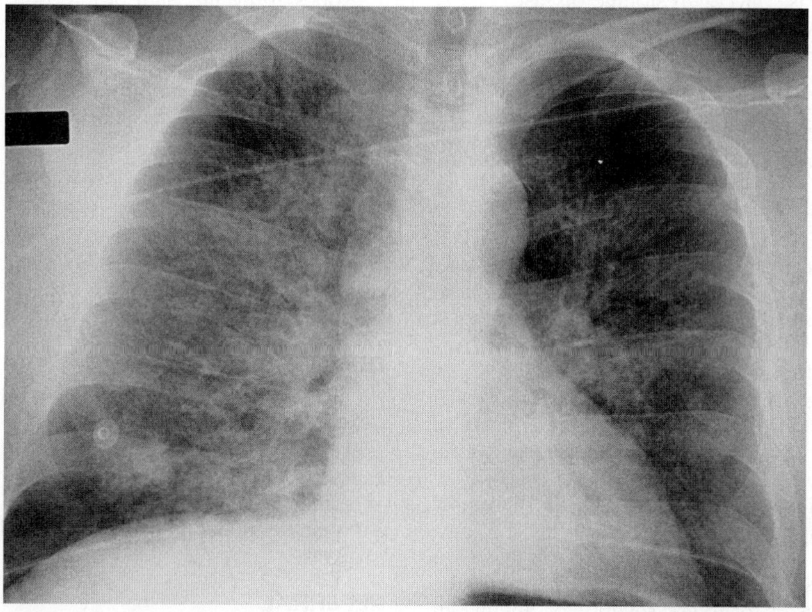

FIGURE 1-133 Chest radiograph of a patient with acute hypersensitivity pneumonitis. Bilateral interstitial infiltrates are evident, more on the right side than the left. Note the absence of pleural effusion, hilar adenopathy, and hyperinflation. (From Altman LV [ed]: *Allergy in primary care,* Philadelphia, 2000, WB Saunders.)

PEARLS & CONSIDERATIONS

A clinical prediction rule using six features has high specificity and sensitivity for the diagnosis of acute and subacute HP:
- Exposure to a known offending agent
- Positive specific precipitating AB
- Recurrent episodes of symptoms
- Inspiratory crackles
- Symptoms occurring 4 to 8 hr after exposure
- Weight loss

No diagnostic gold standards, requires combination of clinical, environmental, radiologic, physiologic, and pathologic findings that represent a diagnostic challenge.

HP occurs more frequently in smokers than nonsmokers (likely due to an immunosuppressive effect).

SUGGESTED READINGS

Churg A: Chronic hypersensitivity pneumonitis, *Am J Surg Path* 30(2):201, 2006.

Fink JN et al: Needs and opportunities for research in hypersensitivity pneumonitis, *Am J Respir Crit Care Med* 171:792-798, 2005.

Fraser et al: *Synopsis of diseases of the chest,* ed 2, Philadelphia, 1994, WB Saunders.

Lacasse Y et al: Clinical diagnosis of active hypersensitivity pneumonitis, *Am J Respir Crit Care Med* 168:952-958, 2003.

Morrell F, Roger A, Cruz MJ: Usefulness of specific skin tests in the diagnosis of hypersensitivity pneumonitis, *J Allergy Clin Immunol* 110(6):939, 2002.

Patel AM, Ryu JH, Reed CE: Hypersensitivity pneumonitis: current concepts and further questions, *J Allergy Clin Immunol* 108:661, 2001.

Schuyler M, Cormier Y: The diagnosis of hypersensitivity pneumonitis, *Chest* 111:534, 1997.

Selman M: Hypersensitivity pneumonitis: a multifaceted deceiving disorder, *Clin Chest Med* 25:3, 2004.

AUTHOR: **CAROLYN J. O'CONNOR, M.D.**

BASIC INFORMATION

DEFINITION

Hypersplenism is a syndrome characterized by splenomegaly, cytopenia (decrease of one or more peripheral cell lines), and compensatory hyperplastic bone marrow. The cytopenias are correctable with splenectomy.

ICD-9CM CODES
289.4 Hypersplenism

EPIDEMIOLOGY & DEMOGRAPHICS

Most often seen in patients with liver disease, hematologic malignancy, infection.

PHYSICAL FINDINGS & CLINICAL PRESENTATION

Symptoms depend on the size of the spleen, rate of growth, and underlying disease.

- History: early satiety, abdominal discomfort/fullness, left upper quadrant pleuritic pain (abscess, infarction), episodes of acute left upper quadrant pain (sequestration crisis), referred pain to left shoulder
- Physical examination: splenomegaly, presence of a rub in left upper quadrant (suggestive of a splenic infarct), stigmata of cytopenias

ETIOLOGY

The spleen is an important component of cellular and humoral immunity: antigen recognition, antibody production, clearance of antibody-coated particles, and bacteria from circulation. It is also responsible for the modification (removal of particles and parasites) and removal of old red blood cells from circulation. The spleen is a platelet reservoir, storing 30% of platelet mass. It can become the site of extramedullary hematopoiesis in certain disease states. The spleen's normal activities are augmented when it is enlarged.

- Splenomegaly increases the proportion of blood channeled through the red pulp (cords of Billroth), causing inappropriate splenic pooling of both normal and abnormal blood cells. The size of the spleen determines the amount of cell sequestration. Up to 90% of platelets may be pooled in an enlarged spleen.
- Splenomegaly leads to increased destruction of RBCs. Platelets and WBCs have about normal survival time even when sequestered and may be available if needed.
- Splenomegaly causes plasma volume expansion, exacerbating cytopenias by dilution.

DIAGNOSIS

DIFFERENTIAL DIAGNOSIS

Hypersplenism can be caused by splenomegaly of almost any cause.

- Splenic congestion: cirrhosis, CHF, portal, splenic or hepatic vein thrombosis
- Hematologic causes: hemolytic anemia, sickle cell anemia, thalassemia, spherocytosis, elliptocytosis, extramedullary hematopoiesis
- Infections: viral (hepatitis, infectious mononucleosis, CMV, HIV), bacterial (abscess, endocarditis, tuberculosis, salmonella, brucellosis, Lyme), parasitic (babesiosis, malaria, leishmaniasis, schistosomiasis, toxoplasmosis), fungal
- Malignancy: acute and chronic leukemia, lymphoma, polycythemia vera, myeloproliferative diseases, metastatic tumors
- Inflammatory diseases: rheumatic fever, Felty syndrome, SLE, sarcoid, serum sickness
- Infiltrative diseases: amyloidosis, Gaucher's disease, Niemann-Pick disease, glycogen storage disease
- Anatomic abnormalities: cyst, pseudocyst, hemangioma, hamartoma

WORKUP

History (including travel), physical examination, laboratory tests, imaging studies

LABORATORY TESTS

- CBC with differential: cytopenia, neutrophilia (infection)
- Peripheral smear: RBC and WBC morphology (abnormal cells may suggest infection, malignancy, bone marrow disease, rheumatologic disease), organisms (bacteria, malaria, babesiosis)
- Bone marrow biopsy: hyperplasia of cytopenic cell lines, hematologic, infiltrative disorders
- Tests to diagnose suspected cause of splenomegaly: LFT, hepatitis serology, HIV, RF, ANA, etc.
- Note: red cell mass (^{51}Cr assay) may be used to assess severity of anemia. If considering splenectomy secondary to severe anemia, RBC mass measurement will differentiate true anemia (decrease in red cells) from dilutional anemia (plasma volume expansion).

IMAGING STUDIES

- Ultrasound: splenic size, presence of cyst or abscess
- CT: estimate volume, obtain structural information: cyst, abscess, tumor, infarct
- MRI: most useful for assessing vascular lesions and infections
- Liver-spleen scan: assess anatomy and function; may suggest presence of portal hypertension
- Consider other studies as suggested by history and exam: CXR, echocardiogram, etc.

TREATMENT

ACUTE GENERAL Rx

- Treat underlying disease
- Splenectomy is considered if:
  1. Indicated for the management of the underlying cause
  2. Persistent symptomatic disease (severe cytopenia) not responding to therapy
  3. Necessary for diagnosis

Risks:

- Infections (especially encapsulated organisms): risk greatest in the first 2 yr after splenectomy. Mortality from sepsis is fiftyfold greater in asplenic patients. Attempts to decrease risk include:
  - Immunization with pneumococcal, meningococcal, and hemophilus vaccines 3 wk before splenectomy. Revaccination with pneumococcal every 10 yr.
  - Prophylactic antibiotics post splenectomy in highest risk patients.
  - Patient education regarding the importance of rapid initiation of antibiotics at the first sign of infection.
- Rapid increase in platelet count may cause thromboembolic complications.
- Possible increased risk of atherosclerotic heart disease.
- Splenectomy should not be performed if the spleen is the main site of hematopoiesis secondary to bone marrow failure (i.e., myelofibrosis).
- Other options include partial splenectomy, partial splenic embolization, portosystemic shunting (for congestive splenomegaly).

DISPOSITION

- Cytopenias are usually correctable with splenectomy, cell counts return to normal within a few weeks.
- Splenectomy may alleviate portal hypertension.
- Prognosis depends on the underlying disease.

REFERRAL

Hematology

PEARLS & CONSIDERATIONS

- Thrombocytopenia in hypersplenism is usually moderately severe ($>50 \times 10^9$/L) and asymptomatic; severe thrombocytopenia ($<20 \times 10^9$/L) suggests another diagnosis.
- Neutropenia of hypersplenism is rarely symptomatic.

SUGGESTED READING

Hoffman R et al: *Hematology basic principles and practice,* ed 4, Philadelphia, 2005, Elsevier Inc.

AUTHOR: **SUDEEP K. AULAKH, M.D., F.R.C.P.C.**

BASIC INFORMATION

DEFINITION

The Joint National Committee on Prevention, Detection, Evaluation, and Treatment of High Blood Pressure (JNC 7) classifies normal blood pressure in adults as <120 mm Hg systolic and <80 mm Hg diastolic. *Prehypertension* is defined as systolic pressure 120 to 139 mm Hg or diastolic pressure 80 to 89 mm Hg. *Stage 1 hypertension* is systolic BP 140 to 159 mm Hg or diastolic BP 90 to 99 mm HG. *Stage 2 hypertension* is systolic BP ≥160 mm Hg or diastolic BP ≥100 mm Hg.

SYNONYMS

Essential hypertension
Idiopathic hypertension
High blood pressure

ICD-9CM CODES
401.1 Essential hypertension
401.0 Malignant hypertension caused by renal artery stenosis
642 Hypertension complicating pregnancy
405.01 Malignant hypertension secondary to renal artery stenosis
437.2 Hypertensive encephalopathy

EPIDEMIOLOGY & DEMOGRAPHICS

INCIDENCE: 10% to 15% of adult population

PEAK INCIDENCE: Males and the elderly

PREVALENCE: 50 million individuals in the U.S. and approximately 1 billion individuals worldwide meet the criteria for diagnosis of hypertension.

PHYSICAL FINDINGS & CLINICAL PRESENTATION

Physical examination may be entirely within normal limits except for the presence of hypertension. A proper initial physical examination on a hypertensive patient should include the following:

- Measure height and weight.
- Evaluate skin for the presence of café-au-lait spots (neurofibromatosis), uremic appearance (CRF), striae (Cushing's syndrome).
- Perform careful funduscopic examination: check for papilledema, retinal exudates, hemorrhages, arterial narrowing, AV compression.
- Examine the neck for carotid bruits, distended neck veins, or enlarged thyroid gland.
- Perform extensive cardiopulmonary examination: check for loud aortic component of S_2, S_4, ventricular lift, murmurs, arrhythmias.
- Check abdomen for masses (pheochromocytoma, polycystic kidneys), presence of bruits over the renal artery (renal artery stenosis), dilation of the aorta.
- Obtain two or more BP measurements separated by 2 min with the patient either supine or seated and after standing for at least 2 min. Measure BP in both upper extremities (if values are discrepant, use the higher value).
- Examine arterial pulses (dilated or absent femoral pulses and BP greater in upper extremities than lower extremities suggest aortic coarctation).
- Note the presence of truncal obesity (Cushing's syndrome) and pedal edema (CHF, nephrosis).
- The clinical evaluation should help determine if the patient has primary or secondary (possibly reversible) hypertension, if there is target organ disease present, and if there are cardiovascular risk factors in addition to hypertension.

ETIOLOGY

- Essential (primary) hypertension (85%)
- Drug induced or drug related (5%)
- Renal hypertension (5%)
  1. Renal parenchymal disease (3%)
  2. Renovascular hypertension (<2%)
- Endocrine (4% to 5%)
  1. Oral contraceptives (4%)
  2. Primary aldosteronism (0.5%)
  3. Pheochromocytoma (0.2%)
  4. Cushing's syndrome and chronic steroid therapy (0.2%)
  5. Hyperparathyroidism or thyroid disease (0.2%)
- Coarctation of the aorta (0.2%)

DIAGNOSIS

WORKUP

Pertinent history:

- Age of onset of hypertension, previous antihypertensive therapy
- Family history of hypertension, stroke, cardiovascular disease
- Diet, salt intake, alcohol, drugs (e.g., oral contraceptives, NSAIDs, decongestants, steroids)
- Occupation, lifestyle, socioeconomic status, psychologic factors
- Other cardiovascular risk factors: hyperlipidemia, obesity, diabetes mellitus, carbohydrate intolerance
- Symptoms of secondary hypertension:
  1. Headache, palpitations, excessive perspiration (possible pheochromocytoma)
  2. Weakness, polyuria (consider hyperaldosteronism)
  3. Claudication of lower extremities (seen with coarctation of aorta)

An algorithm for investigation of suspected endocrine hypertension is described in Section III.

LABORATORY TESTS

- Urinalysis: for evidence of renal disease.
- BUN, creatinine: to rule out renal disease. High-serum creatinine is a predictor of cardiovascular risk in essential hypertension.
- Serum electrolyte levels: low potassium is suggestive of primary aldosteronism, diuretic use.
- Screening for coexisting diseases that may adversely affect prognosis:
  1. Fasting serum glucose
  2. Serum lipid panel, uric acid, calcium
  3. If pheochromocytoma is suspected: 24-hr urine for VMA and metanephrines

IMAGING STUDIES

- ECG: check for presence of left ventricular hypertrophy (LVH) with strain pattern.
- MRA of the renal arteries: in suspected renovascular hypertension (renal artery stenosis).

TREATMENT

NONPHARMACOLOGIC THERAPY

Lifestyle modifications:

- Lose weight if overweight.
- Limit alcohol intake to ≤1 oz of ethanol per day (<2 drinks/day) in men or ≤0.5 oz (<1 drink/day) in women.
- Exercise (aerobic) regularly (at least 30 min/day, most days).
- Reduce sodium intake to <100 mmol/day (<2.3 g of sodium/day).
- Maintain adequate dietary potassium (>3500 mg/day) intake.
- Stop smoking and reduce dietary saturated fat and cholesterol intake for overall cardiovascular health. Consume diet rich in fruits and vegetables.
- Alternative treatments such as vitamin C, coenzyme Q10, magnesium, and omega-3 fatty acids are often used but evidence for their effectiveness is lacking.

ACUTE GENERAL Rx

According to the Seventh Report of the Joint National Committee on Detection, Evaluation, and Treatment of High Blood Pressure:

- For patients with prehypertension and no other complications, recommend lifestyle modifications to prevent progression to sustained hypertension. For patients with prehypertension and diabetes or chronic kidney disease, aggressive pharmacologic treatment should be undertaken to reduce blood pressure to <130/80 mm Hg.
- Antihypertensive drug therapy should be initiated in patients with stage 1 hypertension. Diuretics are preferred for initial therapy unless there are compelling indications to use other agents for initial therapy.
- Compelling indications for individual drug classes:
  - CHF: ACE inhibitors, ARBs, beta blockers, diuretics, aldosterone antagonists

- ○ Post-MI: beta blockers, ACE inhibitors, aldosterone antagonists
- ○ High cardiovascular risk: beta blockers, ACE inhibitors, calcium channel blockers, diuretics
- ○ Diabetes: ACE inhibitors, ARBs, calcium channel blockers, beta blockers, diuretics
- ○ Chronic kidney disease: ACE inhibitors, ARBs
- ○ Recurrent stroke prevention: ACE inhibitors, diuretics
- Two-drug combination is necessary for most patients with stage 2 hypertension. Combination of diuretic with another agent is preferred unless there is compelling indications to use other agents.
- When selecting drugs, also consider the cost of the medication, metabolic and subjective side effects, and drug-drug interactions.
- The major advantages and limitations of each class of drugs are described as follows:
  1. Diuretics
     a. Advantages: inexpensive, once per day dosing. Useful in edema states, CHF, chronic renal disease, elderly patients (decreased incidence of hip fractures in elderly patients).
     b. Disadvantages: significant adverse metabolic effects, increased risk of cardiac arrhythmias, sexual dysfunction, possible adverse effects on lipids and glucose levels.
  2. Beta blockers
     a. Advantages: ideal in hypertensive patients with ischemic heart disease or post-MI. Favored in hyperkinetic, young patients (resting tachycardia, wide pulse pressure, hyperdynamic heart) and stable (Class II to III) CHF patients.
     b. Disadvantages: adverse effect on quality of life (increased incidence of fatigue, depression, impotence, bronchospasm, hypoglycemia, peripheral vascular disease, adverse effects on lipids, masking of signs and symptoms of hypoglycemia in diabetics).
  3. Calcium antagonists
     a. Advantages: helpful in hypertensive patients with ischemic heart disease. Generally favorable effect on quality of life; can be used in patients with bronchospastic disorders, renal disease, peripheral avascular disease, metabolic disorders, and salt sensitivity.
     b. Disadvantages: diltiazem and verapamil should be avoided in patients with CHF because of their chronotropic and inotropic effects; pedal edema may occur with nifedipine and amlodipine; constipation can be severe in elderly patients receiving verapamil.
  4. ACE inhibitors
     a. Advantages: well tolerated, favorable impact on quality of life; useful in hypertension complicated by CHF; helpful in prevention of diabetic renal disease; effective in decreasing LVH.
     b. Disadvantages: cough is a frequent side effect (5% to 20% of patients); hyperkalemia may occur in patients with diabetes or severe renal insufficiency; hypotension may occur in volume-depleted patients.
  5. Angiotensin II receptor blockers (ARB)
     a. Advantages: well tolerated, favorable impact on quality of life; useful in patients unable to tolerate ACE inhibitors because of persistent cough and in CHF and diabetic patients; single daily dose.
     b. Disadvantages: excessive cost; hypotension may occur in volume-depleted patients; contraindicated in pregnancy.
  6. Renin inhibitors: newest class of antihypertensives; Aliskiren (Tekturna)
     a. Advantages: generally well tolerated; once per day dosing; can be used alone or in combination with other antihypertensive agents.
     b. Disadvantages: contraindicated in pregnancy; should not be used in patients with impaired renal function; excessive cost.
  7. Alpha adrenergic blockers
     a. Advantages: no adverse effect on blood lipids or insulin sensitivity; helpful in BPH.
     b. Disadvantages: postural hypotension, sedation; syncope can be avoided by giving an initial low dose at bedtime.

TREATMENT OF RENOVASCULAR HYPERTENSION (RVH): The therapeutic approach varies with the cause of the RVH (refer to "Renal Artery Stenosis" for additional information).

1. Young patients with fibromuscular dysplasia can be treated with percutaneous transluminal renal angioplasty (PTRA).
2. Medical therapy is advisable in elderly patients with atheromatous renal vascular hypertension; useful agents are:
   a. Beta blockers: very effective in patients with elevated plasma renin.
   b. ACE inhibitors: very effective; however, should be avoided in patients. with bilateral renal artery stenosis or in patients with solitary kidney and renal stenosis.
   c. Diuretics: often used in combination with ACE inhibitors.
3. Surgical revascularization is generally reserved for atheromatous RVH in patients responding poorly to medical therapy (uncontrolled hypertension, deteriorating renal function).

HYPERTENSION DURING PREGNANCY:

1. Hypertension complicates 5% to 12% of all pregnancies.
2. The American Obstetrical Committee defines blood pressure of 130/80 mm Hg as the upper limit of normal at any time during pregnancy.
3. A rise of 30 mm Hg systolic or 15 mm Hg diastolic is also considered abnormal regardless of the absolute values obtained.
4. Chronic hypertension (occurring before pregnancy) must be distinguished from preeclampsia, because the risk to mother and fetus is much greater in the latter.
5. Treatment of chronic hypertension during pregnancy is as follows:
   a. Initial treatment with conservative measures (proper nutrition, limited physical activity).
   b. When drug therapy is necessary, initiation of one of the following agents—methyldopa, hydralazine, labetalol, or atenolol—is preferred.
   c. ACE inhibitors can cause fetal and neonatal complications; their use should be avoided in pregnancy.
   d. The safety of calcium channel blockers remains unclear.
   e. Diuretics should be used only if there is a specific reason for initiating and maintaining their use (e.g., hypertension associated with severe fluid overload or left ventricular dysfunction).

MALIGNANT HYPERTENSION, HYPERTENSIVE EMERGENCIES, AND HYPERTENSIVE URGENCIES:

- Definitions:
  1. Malignant hypertension is a potentially life-threatening situation that is secondary to elevated BP.
     a. The rate of BP rise is a critical factor.
     b. The clinical manifestations are grade IV hypertensive retinopathy (exudates, hemorrhages, and papilledema), cardiovascular or renal compromise, and encephalopathy.
     c. It requires immediate BP reduction (not necessarily into normal ranges) to prevent or limit target organ disease.
  2. Hypertensive emergencies are situations that require rapid (within 1 hr) lowering of BP to prevent end-organ damage.

3. Hypertensive urgencies are significant BP elevations that should be corrected within 24 hr of presentation.

- Therapy:

The choice of therapeutic agents in malignant hypertension varies with the cause.

1. Nitroprusside is the drug of choice in hypertensive encephalopathy, hypertension and intracranial bleeding, malignant hypertension, hypertension and heart failure, dissecting aortic aneurysm (used in combination with the propranolol); its onset of action is immediate.
2. Fenoldopam is a vasodilator agent useful for the short-term (up to 48 hr) management of severe hypertension when rapid but quickly reversible reduction of blood pressure is required.
3. The following are important points to remember when treating hypertensive emergencies:
   a. Introduce a plan for long-term therapy at the time of the initial emergency treatment.
   b. Agents that reduce arterial pressure can cause the kidney to retain sodium and water; therefore the judicious administration of diuretics should accompany their use.
   c. The initial goal of antihypertensive therapy is not to achieve a normal BP, but rather to gradually reduce the BP; cerebral hyperperfusion may occur if the mean BP is lowered >40% in the initial 24 hr.
4. Hypertensive urgencies can be effectively treated with oral clonidine 0.1 mg q20min (to a maximum of 0.8 mg); sedation is common.

PEARLS & CONSIDERATIONS

COMMENTS

- For patients with prehypertension, every 20/10 mm Hg increase in blood pressure doubles the risk of cardiovascular events.
- Most patients will require at least two medications for blood pressure control.
- Section III describes an algorithm for patients with "resistant" hypertension.

EVIDENCE (HYPERTENSION)

EBM

A systematic review found that treating systolic hypertension (>160 mm Hg) in people over 60 years of age reduced the total mortality rate and fatal and nonfatal cardiovascular events.[1] A

A systematic review found that in healthy elderly people (60 to 80 years of age), the treatment of hypertension with diuretics and beta blockers is clearly beneficial.[2] A

A randomized controlled trial (RCT) found that losartan and atenolol had similar efficacy in terms of blood pressure reduction in patients with essential hypertension and left ventricular hypertrophy. Cardiovascular events were significantly reduced in patients treated with losartan after 4 years.[3] A

Evidence from cohort, case-control, and randomized studies suggests that short-acting and intermediate-acting dihydropyridine calcium channel blockers may increase cardiovascular morbidity and mortality rates.[4] B

Lifestyle changes have been shown to effectively reduce blood pressure

A systematic review found that weight-reducing diets for overweight, hypertensive patients are effective in achieving modest weight reduction and are probably associated with modest reductions in blood pressure. Weight-reducing diets may allow a decrease in the required dose of antihypertensive medications. Two subsequent RCTs have confirmed these results.[5-7] A

Follow-up period

Follow-up every 6 months appears to be as effective as follow-up every 3 months. A randomized trial compared blood pressure control, satisfaction, and adherence to drug treatment in patients with treated hypertension followed up by their primary care physicians either every 3 months or every 6 months for 3 years. Mean blood pressure and control of hypertension was similar in the groups.[8] B

Evidence-Based References

1. Staessen JA et al: Risks of untreated and treated isolated systolic hypertension in the elderly: meta-analysis of outcome trials, *Lancet* 355:865-872, 2000. A
2. Mulrow C et al: Pharmacotherapy for hypertension in the elderly, *Cochrane Database Syst Rev* 2, 1998. A
3. Dahlof B et al: The LIFE Study Group. Cardiovascular morbidity and mortality in the Losartan Intervention for Endpoint reduction in hypertension study (LIFE): a randomised trial against atenolol, *Lancet* 359:995-1003, 2002. Reviewed in: *Clin Evid* 12:159-192, 2004. A
4. Cutler JA: Calcium channel blockers for hypertension—uncertainty continues, *N Engl J Med* 338:679-681, 1998. Reviewed in: *Clin Evid* 12:159-192, 2004. B
5. Mulrow CD et al: Dieting to reduce body weight for controlling hypertension in adults, *Cochrane Database Syst Rev* 4, 1998. Reviewed in: *Clin Evid* 12:159-192, 2004. A
6. Metz JA et al: A randomized trial of improved weight loss with a prepared meal plan in overweight and obese patients, *Arch Intern Med* 160:2150-2158, 2000. Reviewed in: *Clin Evid* 12:159-192, 2004. A
7. Stevens VJ et al: Long-term weight loss and changes in blood pressure: results of the Trials of Hypertension Prevention, phase II, *Ann Intern Med* 134:1-11, 2001. Reviewed in: *Clin Evid* 12:159-192, 2004. A
8. Birtwhistle RV et al: Randomised equivalence trial comparing three month and six month follow up of patients with hypertension by family practitioners, *BMJ* 328:204, 2004. B

EVIDENCE (HYPERTENSIVE DISORDERS IN PREGNANCY)

EBM

Methyldopa is recommended as first line therapy for the treatment of chronic hypertension in pregnancy. However, the evidence for this treatment does not reach our criteria for inclusion as evidence.

There is evidence for the use of hypertensive medication during pregnancy

A systematic review found that antihypertensive medication halved the risk of developing severe hypertension in women with mild-moderate hypertension during pregnancy. There was little evidence that antihypertensives reduced the risk of developing preeclampsia, and there was no clear effect on the risk of perinatal mortality, preterm birth, or small for gestational age babies.[1] A

Magnesium sulfate may be the best prophylactic anticonvulsant for women with severe preeclampsia. Magnesium sulfate is an effective treatment for eclampsia

Evidence-Based Reference

1. Abalos E et al: Antihypertensive drug therapy for mild to moderate hypertension during pregnancy. Reviewed in: Cochrane Library, 4, Chichester, UK, 2003, John Wiley. A

SUGGESTED READINGS

Moser M, Setaro JF: Resistant or difficult to control hypertension, *N Engl J Med* 355:385, 2006.

Seventh Report of the Joint National Committee on Prevention, Detection, Evaluation, and Treatment of High Blood Pressure, *JAMA* 289:2560, 2003.

Wexler R, Aukerman G: Nonpharmacologic strategies for managing hypertension, *Am Fam Physician* 73(11):1953, 2006.

AUTHOR: **FRED F. FERRI, M.D.**

BASIC INFORMATION

DEFINITION

Hyperthyroidism is a hypermetabolic state resulting from excess thyroid hormone.

SYNONYMS

Thyrotoxicosis

ICD-9CM CODES
242.9 Hyperthyroidism
242.0 Hyperthyroidism with goiter
242.2 Hyperthyroidism, multinodular
242.3 Hyperthyroidism, uninodular

EPIDEMIOLOGY & DEMOGRAPHICS

INCIDENCE/PREVALENCE:
- Hyperthyroidism affects 2% of women and 0.2% of men in their lifetime.
- Toxic multinodular goiter usually occurs in women >55 yr of age and is more common than Graves' disease in the elderly.

PHYSICAL FINDINGS & CLINICAL PRESENTATION

- Patients with hyperthyroidism generally present with the following clinical manifestations: tachycardia, tremor, hyperreflexia, anxiety, irritability, emotional lability, panic attacks, heat intolerance, sweating, increased appetite, diarrhea, weight loss, menstrual dysfunction (oligomenorrhea, amenorrhea); the presentation may be different in elderly patients (see third bullet).
- Patients with Graves' disease may present with exophthalmos, lid retraction (Fig. 1-134, *A*), lid lag (Graves' ophthalmopathy). The following signs and symptoms of ophthalmopathy may be present: blurring of vision, photophobia, increased lacrimation, double vision, deep orbital pressure. Clubbing of fingers associated with periosteal new bone formation in other skeletal areas (Graves' acropachy) and pretibial myxedema (Fig. 1-134, *B*) may also be noted.
- In the elderly the clinical signs of hyperthyroidism may be masked by manifestations of coexisting disease (e.g., new-onset atrial fibrillation, exacerbation of CHF).

ETIOLOGY

- Graves' disease (diffuse toxic goiter): 80% to 90% of all cases of hyperthyroidism
- Toxic multinodular goiter (Plummer's disease)
- Toxic adenoma
- Iatrogenic and factitious
- Transient hyperthyroidism (subacute thyroiditis, Hashimoto's thyroiditis)
- Rare causes: hypersecretion of TSH (e.g., pituitary neoplasms), struma ovarii, ingestion of large amount of iodine in a patient with preexisting thyroid hyperplasia or adenoma (Jod-Basedow phenomenon), hydatidiform mole, carcinoma of thyroid, amiodarone therapy

DIAGNOSIS

DIFFERENTIAL DIAGNOSIS

- Anxiety disorder
- Pheochromocytoma
- Metastatic neoplasm
- Diabetes mellitus
- Premenopausal state

WORKUP

Suspected hyperthyroidism requires laboratory confirmation and identification of its etiology, because treatment varies with its cause. A detailed medical history will often provide clues to the diagnosis and etiology of the hyperthyroidism.

LABORATORY TESTS

- Elevated free thyroxine (T_4)
- Elevated free triiodothyronine (T_3): generally not necessary for diagnosis
- Low TSH (unless hyperthyroidism is a result of the rare hypersecretion of TSH from a pituitary adenoma)
- Thyroid autoantibodies useful in selected cases to differentiate Graves' disease from toxic multinodular goiter (absent thyroid antibodies)

IMAGING STUDIES

- 24-hr radioactive iodine uptake (RAIU) is useful to distinguish hyperthyroidism from iatrogenic thyroid hor-

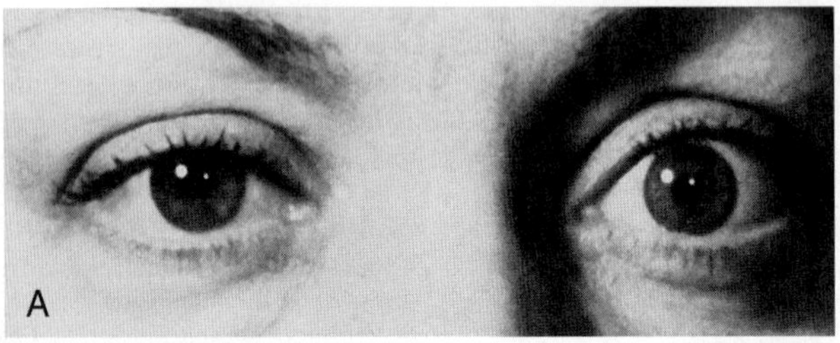

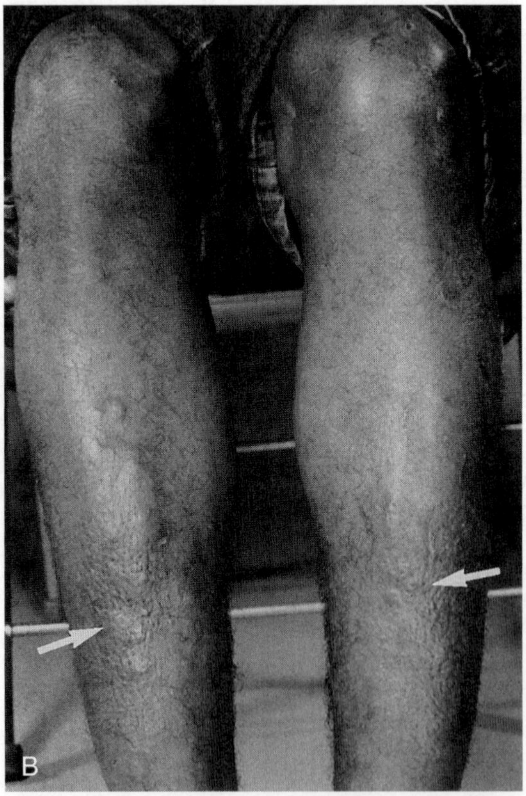

FIGURE 1-134 **A,** Unilateral (left) lid retraction in a patient with hyperthyroidism. **B,** Pretibial myxedema *(arrows)* in a patient with Graves' disease. (From Noble J [ed]: *Textbook of primary care medicine,* ed 2, St Louis, 1996, Mosby.)

mone synthesis (thyrotoxicosis factitia) and from thyroiditis.

- An overactive thyroid shows increased uptake, whereas a normal underactive thyroid (iatrogenic thyroid ingestion, painless or subacute thyroiditis) shows normal or decreased uptake.
- The RAIU results also vary with the etiology of the hyperthyroidism: Graves' disease: increased homogeneous uptake.

Multinodular goiter: increased heterogeneous uptake.

Hot nodule: single focus of increased uptake.

- RAIU is also generally performed before the therapeutic administration of radioactive iodine to determine the appropriate dose.

TREATMENT (Rx)

NONPHARMACOLOGIC THERAPY

Patient education regarding thyroid disease and discussion of the therapeutic options (medications, radioactive iodine, and thyroid surgery)

ACUTE GENERAL Rx

ANTITHYROID DRUGS (THIONAMIDES): Propylthiouracil (PTU) and methimazole (Tapazole) inhibit thyroid hormone synthesis by blocking production of thyroid peroxidase (PTU and methimazole) or inhibit peripheral conversion of T_4 to T_3 (PTU). PTU is preferred in pregnant women. CBC and differential count should be obtained prior to their use.

1. Dosage: PTU 50 to 100 mg PO q8h; methimazole 15 to 30 mg/day given as a single dose.
2. Antithyroid drugs can be used as the primary form of treatment or as adjunctive therapy before radioactive therapy or surgery or afterward if the hyperthyroidism recurs.
3. Side effects: skin rash (3% to 5% of patients), arthralgias, myalgias, granulocytopenia (0.5%). Rare side effects are aplastic anemia, hepatic necrosis from PTU, cholestatic jaundice from methimazole.
4. When antithyroid drugs are used as primary therapy, they are usually given for 6 to 18 mo; prolonged therapy may cause hypothyroidism. Monitor thyroid function every 2 mo for 6 mo, then less frequently.
5. The use of antithyroid drugs before radioactive iodine therapy is best reserved for patients in whom exacerbation of hyperthyroidism after radioactive iodine therapy is hazardous (e.g., elderly patients with coronary artery disease or significant coexisting morbidity). In these patients the antithyroid drug can be stopped 2 days before radioactive iodine therapy, resumed 2 days later, and continued for 4 to 6 wk.

RADIOACTIVE IODINE (RAI; ^{131}I):

1. RAI is the treatment of choice for patients >21 yr of age and younger patients who have not achieved remission after 1 yr of antithyroid drug therapy. Radioiodine is also used in hyperthyroidism caused by toxic adenoma or toxic multinodular goiter.
2. Contraindicated during pregnancy (can cause fetal hypothyroidism) and lactation. Pregnancy should be excluded in women of childbearing age before radioactive iodine is administered.
3. A single dose of radioactive iodine is effective in inducing euthyroid state in nearly 80% of patients.
4. There is a high incidence of postradioactive iodine hypothyroidism (>50% within first year and 2%/yr thereafter); therefore these patients should be frequently evaluated for the onset of hypothyroidism (see "Chronic Rx").

SURGICAL THERAPY (SUBTOTAL THYROIDECTOMY):

1. Indicated in obstructing goiters, in any patient who refuses radioactive iodine and cannot be adequately managed with antithyroid medications (e.g., patients with toxic adenoma or toxic multinodular goiter), and in pregnant patients who cannot be adequately managed with antithyroid medication or develop side effects to them.
2. Patients should be rendered euthyroid with antithyroid drugs before surgery.
3. Complications of surgery include hypothyroidism (28% to 43% after 10 yr), hypoparathyroidism, and vocal cord paralysis (1%).
4. Hyperthyroidism recurs after surgery in 10% to 15% of patients.

ADJUNCTIVE THERAPY: Propranolol alleviates the β-adrenergic symptoms of hyperthyroidism; initial dose is 20 to 40 mg PO q6h; dosage is gradually increased until symptoms are controlled; major contraindications to use of propranolol are CHF and bronchospasm. Diagnosis and treatment of thyrotoxic storm is also discussed in Section I.

CHRONIC Rx

- Patients undergoing treatment with antithyroid drugs should be seen every 1 to 3 mo until euthyroidism is achieved and every 3 to 4 mo while they remain on antithyroid therapy. After treatment is stopped, periodic monitoring of thyroid function tests with TSH every 3 mo for 1 yr, then every 6 mo for 1 yr, then annually is recommended.
- Orbital decompression surgery can be used to correct Graves' orbitopathy (Fig. 1-135).

DISPOSITION

Successful treatment of hyperthyroidism requires lifelong monitoring for the onset of hypothyroidism or the recurrence of thyrotoxicosis.

REFERRAL

- Endocrinology referral is recommended at the time of initial diagnosis and during treatment

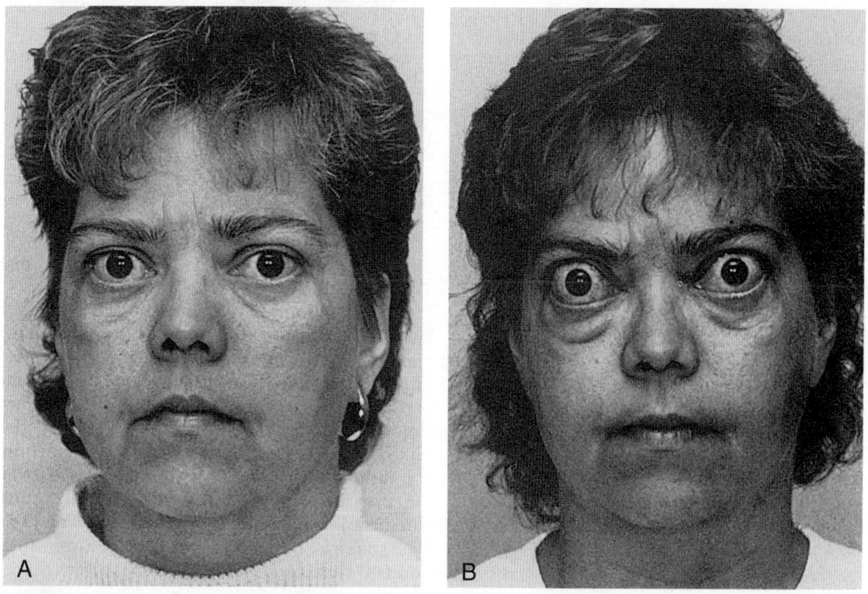

FIGURE 1-135 Characteristic signs of the Graves' orbitopathy. A, Subsequently corrected by orbital decompression surgery; **B,** note the thyroid stare, the asymmetry, the proptosis, and the periorbital edema prior to correction. (Courtesy Dr. Jack Rootman, University of British Columbia, Vancouver, Canada. From Larsen PR, Kronenburg HM, Melmed S, Polonsky KS [eds]: *Williams textbook of endocrinology,* ed 10, Philadelphia, 2003, Saunders.)

- Surgical referral in selected patients (see "Surgical Therapy")
- Hospitalization of all patients with thyroid storm

PEARLS & CONSIDERATIONS

COMMENTS

- Elderly hyperthyroid patients may have only subtle signs (weight loss, tachycardia, fine skin, brittle nails). This form is known as **apathetic hyperthyroidism** and manifests with lethargy rather than hyperkinetic activity. An enlarged thyroid gland may be absent. Coexisting medical disorders (most commonly cardiac disease) may also mask the symptoms. These patients often have unexplained CHF, worsening of angina, or new-onset atrial fibrillation resistant to treatment. See "Graves' Disease" in Section I for additional information on the diagnosis and treatment of Graves' disease.
- **Subclinical hyperthyroidism** is defined as a normal serum free thyroxine and free triiodothyronine levels with a thyroid-stimulating hormone level suppressed below the normal range and usually undetectable. These patients usually do not present with signs or symptoms of overt hyperthyroidism. Treatment options include observation or a therapeutic trial of low-dose antithyroid agents for 6 mo to attempt to induce remission.
- **Thyrotoxic periodic paralysis (TPP)** is a hyperthyroidism-related hypokalemia and muscle-weakening condition resulting from a sudden shift of potassium into cells. Many patients do not have other symptoms of hyperthyroidism. Typical presentation involves an Asian adult male with acute fatigue and muscle weakness initially presenting in the lower extremities. Physical exam reveals decreased DTRs, hypertension, and tachycardia. ECG often reveals U waves, high QRS voltage, and first degree AV block. Additional labs reveal normal, acid-base state, hypokalemia with low urinary potassium excretion (spot urinary potassium concentration <20 mEq/L due to potassium shift into cells), hypophosphatemia, hypophostaturia, and hypercalciuria. EMG during attacks show low-amplitude compound muscle action potential (CMAP) of the tested muscle. Therapy consists of cautious potassium supplementation (increased risk of rebound hyperkalemia). Use of non-selective beta blockers (e.g., propranolol) to counteract hyperadrenergic activity, which may be causing TPP, may also be useful.

EVIDENCE

Propylthiouracil and methimazole are both effective at inducing euthyroidism in Graves' disease, although single daily dose methimazole appears to be more effective than single daily dose propylthiouracil.[1] Ⓑ

Small trials have found that propranolol and diltiazem effectively lessen the adrenergic symptoms caused by hyperthyroidism.[2,3] Ⓑ

Thyroidectomy (either partial or total) is a successful treatment for hyperthyroidism.[4] Ⓑ

A systematic review of various regimen for medical treatment of Graves' hyperthyroidism found that a titration regimen was as effective as a block-replacement regimen and appeared to have fewer side effects. The evidence supported a 12- to 18-month duration for titration therapy. One trial found that a 6-month block-replacement regimen was as effective as a 12-month treatment. In general there was a high level of loss to follow-up in the trials reviewed.[5] Ⓑ

Evidence-Based References

1. Homsanit M et al: Efficacy of single daily dosage of methimazole vs. propylthiouracil in the induction of euthyroidism, *Clin Endocrinol (Oxf)* 54:385, 2001. Ⓑ
2. Henderson JM et al: Propranolol as an adjunct therapy for hyperthyroid tremor, *Eur Neurol* 37:182, 1997. Ⓑ
3. Kelestimur F, Aksu A: The effect of diltiazem on the manifestations of hyperthyroidism and thyroid function tests, *Exp Clin Endocrinol Diabetes* 104:38, 1996. Ⓑ
4. Palit TK, Miller CC 3rd, Miltenburg DM: The efficacy of thyroidectomy for Graves' disease: a meta-analysis, *J Surg Res* 90:161, 2000. Reviewed in: DARE Document 20001132, York, UK. Ⓑ
5. Abraham P et al: Antithyroid drug regimen for treating Graves' hyperthyroidism, *Cochrane Database Syst Rev* 2, 2004. Ⓑ

SUGGESTED READINGS

Cooper DS: Antithyroid drugs, *N Engl J Med* 352:905, 2005.

Reid JR, Wheeler SF: Hyperthyroidism, *Am Fam Physician* 72:623, 2005.

Shih HL: Thyrotoxic periodic paralysis, *Mayo Clin Proc* 80(10):99, 2005.

AUTHOR: **FRED F. FERRI, M.D.**

BASIC INFORMATION

DEFINITION

Hypertrophic osteoarthropathy (HOA) is a syndrome of clubbing of the digits, periostitis of long bones, and arthritis. HOA may be primary or secondary to other underlying disease processes.

SYNONYMS

- Primary hypertrophic osteoarthropathy
  1. Pachydermoperiostosis
  2. Idiopathic clubbing
  3. Touraine-Solente-Golé syndrome
- Secondary hypertrophic osteoarthropathy

ICD-9CM CODES

731.2 Hypertrophic osteoarthropathy

EPIDEMIOLOGY & DEMOGRAPHICS

- Primary HOA is a familial autosomal dominant disease affecting the age group between 1 and 20 years.
- Secondary HOA typically occurs in adults and is associated with other illnesses including:
  1. Pulmonary: Bronchogenic carcinoma, lung abscesses, bronchiectasis, cystic fibrosis, pulmonary fibrosis, mesothelioma, sarcoidosis
  2. Gastrointestinal: Esophageal carcinoma, colon cancer, inflammatory bowel disease (Crohn's disease, ulcerative colitis), hepatocellular carcinoma, liver cirrhosis, amebiasis
  3. Cardiac: Infective endocarditis, right-to-left cardiac shunts, aortic aneurysms
  4. Thymoma
  5. Lymphoma
  6. Connective tissue diseases
  7. Thyroid acropachy

PHYSICAL FINDINGS & CLINICAL PRESENTATION

- Primary HOA typically presents with the insidious onset of clubbing of the hands and feet and is described as "spadelike." Other signs and symptoms include:
  1. Joint pain and swelling
  2. Decreased use of the fingers and hands
  3. Facial changes, coarse facial skin grooves
  4. Thickening of the arms and legs
  5. Oily skin, diaphoresis, gynecomastia, and acne
- Secondary HOA patients may present with clinical symptoms before the underlying disorder can be detected. Signs and symptoms are similar to the above mentioned in addition to findings related to the underlying disease (e.g., bronchogenic carcinoma, infective endocarditis).

ETIOLOGY

Unknown; immunologic, endocrine, and vascular etiologies have been suggested.

DIAGNOSIS

DIFFERENTIAL DIAGNOSIS

- Other causes of periostitis include Paget's disease, Reiter's syndrome, psoriasis, syphilis, osteoarthritis, rheumatoid arthritis, and osteomyelitis.
- Hypertrophic osteoarthropathy with the classic finding of clubbing of the digits warrants an investigation into any associated illnesses.

WORKUP

Diagnosis is primarily clinical; x-rays and bone scans can help confirm the diagnosis

LABORATORY TESTS

- Routine lab studies such as CBC, electrolytes, and urine studies will typically be normal in primary and secondary HOA.
- ESR will be elevated in secondary HOA.
- LFTs may be abnormal in patients with secondary HOA from GI pathology.
- Alkaline phosphatase may be elevated secondary to periostitis of long bones.
- Analysis of the synovial fluid from joint effusions reveals a low WBC count with normal viscosity, color, and complement levels.

IMAGING STUDIES

- X-rays of the long bones show periosteal new bone formation.
- A chest x-ray should be obtained to rule out underlying lung cancer.
- Bone scan with technetium-99m reveals uptake along the long bones, phalanges, and periarticular joint spaces.

TREATMENT

ACUTE GENERAL Rx

- Treatment of primary HOA is symptomatic. Aspirin 325 mg PO q4 to 6 hr prn, salicylate 750 mg bid prn, ibuprofen 400 to 800 mg tid prn, naproxen 250 to 500 mg bid prn, indomethacin 25 to 50 mg qid prn will provide bone and joint pain relief.
- Treatment of secondary HOA is to eradicate the underlying disease (e.g., antibiotics for infective endocarditis, surgery for bronchogenic carcinoma).

CHRONIC Rx

In patients with secondary HOA refractory to NSAIDs and aspirin, vagotomy has been tried with some success. However, the definitive treatment is to treat the underlying disease.

DISPOSITION

- Patients with primary HOA will typically have symptoms of joint pains and swelling for the early part of their life. However, the disease becomes quiescent thereafter.
- Prognosis and disease course in patients with secondary HOA will depend on the underlying cause. The insidious development of clubbing suggests infectious process, whereas the rapid progression of clubbing may suggest underlying malignancy.

REFERRAL

Referral should be made to rheumatology when the diagnosis of HOA is suspected and the cause remains unclear.

PEARLS & CONSIDERATIONS

COMMENTS

HOA may be a marker for an underlying serious illness and a thorough investigation should be pursued. Infections and intrathoracic malignancies are the most common causes of secondary HOA.

SUGGESTED READINGS

Amital H et al: Hypertrophic pulmonary osteoarthropathy: control of pain and symptoms with pamidronate, *Clin Rheumatol* 23(4):330, 2004.

Viola JC, Jaffe S, Brent LH: Primary hypertrophic osteoarthropathy, *J Rheumatol* 27(6):1562, 2000.

AUTHOR: **MOHAMMAD HAJJIRI, M.D.**

BASIC INFORMATION

DEFINITION

Hypoaldosteronism is defined as an aldosterone deficiency or impaired aldosterone function.

ICD-9CM CODES
255.4 Hypoadrenalism

EPIDEMIOLOGY AND DEMOGRAPHICS

Selective hypoaldosteronism accounts for as many as 10% of cases of unexplained hyperkalemia.

PHYSICAL FINDINGS & CLINICAL PRESENTATION

- Physical examination may be entirely within normal limits.
- Hypertension may be present in some patients.
- Profound muscle weakness and cardiac arrhythmias may be present.

ETIOLOGY

- Hyporeninemic hypoaldosteronism (renin-angiotensin dependent): decreased aldosterone production secondary to decreased renin production; the typical patient has renal disease secondary to various factors (e.g., diabetes mellitus, interstitial nephritis, multiple myeloma).
- Hyperreninemic hypoaldosteronism (renin-angiotensin independent): renin production by the kidneys is intact; the defect is in aldosterone biosynthesis or in the action of angiotensin II. Common causes of this form of hypoaldosteronism are medications (ACE inhibitors, heparin), lead poisoning, aldosterone enzyme defects, and severe illness.

DIAGNOSIS

DIFFERENTIAL DIAGNOSIS

Pseudohypoaldosteronism: renal unresponsiveness to aldosterone. In this condition, both renin and aldosterone levels are elevated. Pseudohypoaldosteronism can be caused by medications (spironolactone), chronic interstitial nephritis, systemic disorders (SLE, amyloidosis), or primary mineralocorticoid resistance.

WORKUP

Measurement of plasma renin activity following 4 hr of upright posture can differentiate hyporeninemic from hyperreninemic causes. Renin levels in the normal or low range identify cases that are renin-angiotensin dependent, whereas high renin levels identify cases that are renin-angiotensin independent. The diagnosis and etiology of hypoaldosteronism can be confirmed with the renin-aldosterone stimulation test:

- Hyporeninemic hypoaldosteronism: low stimulated renin and aldosterone levels
- End-organ refractoriness to aldosterone action: high stimulated renin and aldosterone levels
- Adrenal gland abnormality: high stimulated renin and low aldosterone levels

LABORATORY TESTS

- Increased potassium, normal or decreased sodium
- Hyperchloremic metabolic acidosis (caused by the absence of hydrogen-secreting action of aldosterone)
- Increased BUN and creatinine (secondary to renal disease)
- Hyperglycemia (diabetes mellitus is common in these patients)

TREATMENT

NONPHARMACOLOGIC THERAPY

- Low-potassium diet with liberal sodium intake (at least 4 g of sodium chloride per day)
- Avoidance of ACE inhibitors and potassium-sparing diuretics

ACUTE GENERAL Rx

- Judicious use of fludrocortisone (0.05 to 0.1 mg PO qam) in patients with aldosterone deficiency associated with deficiency of adrenal glucocorticoid hormones
- Furosemide 20 to 40 mg qd to correct hyperkalemia of hyporeninemic hypoaldosteronism

DISPOSITION

Prognosis varies with the etiology of hypoaldosteronism and presence of associated disorders.

REFERRAL

Endocrinology referral for renin-aldosterone stimulation test

PEARLS & CONSIDERATIONS

COMMENTS

Treatment of pseudohypoaldosteronism is the same as for hypoaldosteronism; however, effect is limited because of impaired renal sensitivity.

AUTHOR: **FRED F. FERRI, M.D.**

BASIC INFORMATION

DEFINITION

According to DSM-IV, hypochondriasis is the preoccupation with the fear of having, or the idea that one has, a serious disease. The fear is usually based on a misinterpretation of bodily signs or symptoms and persists despite medical reassurance, although the belief does not have the intensity of a delusion. The preoccupation causes clinically significant distress or impairment in social, occupational, or other important areas of functioning and lasts for at least 6 months.

SYNONYMS

None

ICD-9CM CODES
300.7 Hypochondriasis

EPIDEMIOLOGY & DEMOGRAPHICS

PREVALENCE (IN GENERAL POPULATION): 1% to 5%, but it is thought to be higher in primary care outpatient settings where estimates range from 3% to 10%.

PREDOMINANT SEX: Occurs with equal frequency in men and women.

PREDOMINANT AGE: Onset can occur at any age, but incidence is most common between 20 and 30 yr of age.

GENETICS/RISK: No genetic component has been identified, and neither socioeconomic nor educational factors appear to predispose people to this disorder. j469Patients with hypochondriasis are more likely than the general population to have Axis I disorders, such as generalized anxiety, obsessive-compulsive disorder, and depression, as well as Axis II personality disorders.

PHYSICAL FINDINGS & CLINICAL PRESENTATION

- Patient presents with a complaint of a physical symptom or sign (e.g., dizziness, pain) and remains preoccupied with the concern, despite evidence to the contrary, that it represents a serious disease.
- Serious childhood illnesses common in past medical history.
- No specific physical examination findings.
- Degree of insight (i.e., recognition that the concern about serious illness is excessive or unreasonable) varies.

ETIOLOGY

Unknown etiology, but psychologic theories include disturbances of: (1) perception (i.e., amplification of normal somatic sensations); (2) cognition (i.e., tendency to attribute these sensations to a pathologic process); or (3) interpersonal relationships (i.e., learning and then reinforcement of the sick role); or (4) variant of another psychiatric condition such as depression.

DIAGNOSIS

DIFFERENTIAL DIAGNOSIS

- Underlying medical condition, such as multiple sclerosis, hypothyroidism, or systemic lupus erythematosus (SLE)
- Somatization disorder
- Body dysmorphic disorder (restricted to a circumscribed concern about appearance)
- Factitious disorder or malingering
- Generalized anxiety disorder with health concerns as one worry among many others
- Major depressive disorder with health concerns occurring only during depressive episodes
- Psychosis, as may occur with depression and schizophrenia

WORKUP

- History and physical examination, laboratory and imaging tests as directed by history, as appropriate, to exclude underlying medical condition.
- Symptom measures (e.g., Health Anxiety Inventory, Whiteley Index of Hypochondriasis) may be used for detection and monitoring of severity over time.
- Evaluation for other psychiatric disorders associated with hypochondriasis such as depression and anxiety.

TREATMENT

NONPHARMACOLOGIC THERAPY

- Reassurance and education, including linking the diagnosis to psychological stressors
- Brief and regularly scheduled appointments with the primary care physician
- Avoidance of laboratory tests, imaging studies, and diagnostic and surgical procedures unless clearly indicated
- Elimination of sources of secondary gain
- Limit on reading medical texts or websites
- Individual or group therapy, including problem-solving, focusing on understanding and coping with the disorder, or cognitive-behavioral, with techniques to alter or restructure hypochondriacal thinking
- Benign interventions (e.g., exercise, massage, vitamins)

CHRONIC Rx

- Pharmacologic treatment of comorbid psychiatric conditions, if present.
- Antidepressants may be helpful even in patients without features of depression—imipramine, fluoxetine, paroxetine, and fluvoxamine have all been studied in small, open-label trials.

DISPOSITION

Waxing and waning course over decades, with relapses often triggered by psychosocial stressors. Good prognostic features include acute onset, absence of secondary gain, lack of comorbid psychiatric disorder, and high socioeconomic status.

REFERRAL

Attempts can be made to refer patients to a psychiatrist; however, patients may resist referral given the belief that symptoms are due to an undiagnosed medical illness.

PEARLS & CONSIDERATIONS

- The onset of physical symptoms late in life is almost always the result of a medical disorder.
- Antidepressants and psychoeducational therapy may be helpful treatment modalities, although patients may be resistant to therapy not directed at the perceived illness.

SUGGESTED READINGS

Barsky AJ, Ahern DK: Cognitive behavior therapy for hypochondriasis: a randomized controlled trial, *JAMA* 291(12):1464, 2004.

Creed F, Barsky A: A systematic review of the epidemiology of somatisation disorder and hypochondriasis, *J Psychosom Res* 56(4):391, 2004.

Fink P et al: A new empirically established hypochondriasis diagnosis, *Am J Psychiatry* 161(9):1680, 2004.

Hiller W et al: Differentiating hypochondriasis from panic disorder, *J Anxiety Disord* 19(1):29, 2005.

AUTHOR: **LUCY KALANITHI, M.D.**

BASIC INFORMATION

DEFINITION

Hypopituitarism is the partial or complete loss of secretion of one or more pituitary hormones resulting from diseases of the hypothalamus or pituitary gland.

SYNONYMS

Panhypopituitarism
Pituitary insufficiency

ICD-9CM CODES
253.2 Panhypopituitarism

EPIDEMIOLOGY & DEMOGRAPHICS

- Pituitary tumors are the most common causes of hypopituitarism with an incidence of 0.2 to 2.8 cases per 100,000.
- Increased incidence of vascular or cerebrovascular disease in patients with panhypopituitarism.
- Predisposing factors for pituitary apoplexy (another cause of panhypopituitarism) include diabetes mellitus, anticoagulant therapy, head trauma, pituitary tumors, and radiation.
- Empty sella syndrome, a third cause of panhypopituitarism, can occur in both adults and children.

PHYSICAL FINDINGS & CLINICAL PRESENTATION

The onset of hypopituitarism is usually gradual, and symptoms are related to the lack of one or more hormones and/or mass effect if a pituitary tumor is the cause. Specific symptoms depend on the hormones involved, the severity of the deficiencies, and the patient's age at onset.

- Mass effect of a pituitary tumor can cause headaches and visual disturbances
- Corticotropin deficiency:
  1. Fatigue and weakness, no appetite, abdominal pain, nausea, and vomiting
  2. Hypotension, hair loss, and change in mental status
- Thyrotropin deficiency:
  1. Fatigue and weakness, weight gain, cold intolerance, and constipation
  2. Bradycardia, hung-up reflexes, pretibial edema, and hair loss
- Gonadotropin deficiency:
  1. Loss of libido, erectile dysfunction, amenorrhea, hot flashes, dyspareunia, infertility
  2. Gynecomastia with lack of hair growth and decreased muscle mass
- Growth hormone deficiency:
  1. Growth retardation in children
  2. Easy fatigue, hypoglycemia
  3. Decreased muscle mass and obesity
- Hyperprolactinemia
  1. Galactorrhea
  2. Hypogonadism
- Vasopressin deficiency:
  1. Polyuria, polydipsia and nocturia
  2. Hypotension and dehydration

ETIOLOGY

Hypopituitarism is the result of destruction of pituitary cells caused by:

- Pituitary tumors
  1. Macroadenomas >10 mm
  2. Microadenomas <10 mm
- Pituitary apoplexy caused by hemorrhage or infarction of the pituitary gland
- Pituitary radiation therapy
- Pituitary surgery
- Empty sella syndrome with enlargement of the sella turcica and flattening of the pituitary gland caused by extension of the subarachnoid space and filling of cerebrospinal fluid into the sella turcica
- Infiltrative disease including sarcoidosis, hemochromatosis, histiocytosis X, Wegener's granulomatosis, and lymphocytic hypophysitis
- Infection (tuberculosis, mycosis, and syphilis)
- Head trauma
- Internal carotid artery aneurysm

DIAGNOSIS

The diagnosis of hypopituitarism is suspected by clinical history and physical findings and is established by endocrine stimulation testing.

DIFFERENTIAL DIAGNOSIS

The differential diagnosis is as outlined under "Etiology." Other rare causes include postpartum necrosis (Sheehan's syndrome), hypopituitary tumors (e.g., craniopharyngiomas and meningioma), metastatic tumors (lung, colon, prostate, melanoma, plasmacytoma), and developmental abnormalities.

WORKUP

Includes basal determination of each anterior pituitary hormone followed by provocative stimulation tests and x-ray imaging

LABORATORY TESTS

- Corticotropin deficiency:
  1. Serum am cortisol level usually is low (<3 g/dl).
  2. Corticotropin stimulation test using 250 μg of corticotropin given IV and measuring serum cortisol before and 30 and 60 min after administration. A normal response is an increase in serum cortisol level >20 μg/dl.
  3. With pituitary disease, these tests may be indeterminate, and more dynamic testing such as an insulin-tolerance or metyrapone test may be necessary.
- Thyrotropin deficiency:
  1. TSH and free T_4 measurements
  2. Primary hypothyroidism shows elevated TSH with low free T_4. Secondary hypothyroidism shows normal or low TSH with low free T_4 and low T_3 resin uptake
- Gonadotropin deficiency:
  1. FSH, LH, estrogen, and testosterone measurements
  2. In men, hypogonadotropic hypogonadism is seen with low testosterone levels and normal or low FSH and LH levels
  3. In premenopausal women with amenorrhea, low estrogen with normal or low FSH and LH levels is typically seen
- Growth hormone deficiency:
  1. Insulin-induced hypoglycemia stimulation test using 0.1 to 0.15 unit/kg regular insulin given IV and measuring growth hormone 30, 60, and 120 min after administration. A normal response is a growth hormone level >10 μg/dl.
  2. Serum insulin-like growth factor I can also be measured after provocative testing.
- Hyperprolactinemia:
  1. Prolactin levels may be elevated in prolactin-secreting pituitary adenomas.
- Vasopressin deficiency:
  1. Urinalysis shows low specific gravity.
  2. Urine osmolality is low.
  3. Serum osmolality is high.
  4. Fluid deprivation test over 18 hr with inability to concentrate the urine.
  5. Serum vasopressin level is low.
  6. Electrolytes may show hyponatremia and exclude hyperglycemia.

IMAGING STUDIES

- When hypopituitarism has been established clinically and biochemically, imaging of the pituitary gland is necessary to identify the specific lesion.
- MRI is more sensitive than CT scan of the head in visualizing the pituitary fossa, sella turcica, optic chiasm, pituitary stalk, and cavernous sinuses. It is also more sensitive in detecting pituitary microadenomas.
- CT scan with coronal cuts through the sella turcica gives better images of bony structures.

TREATMENT

Hormone replacement therapy and either surgery, radiation, or medications in patients with pituitary tumors.

NONPHARMACOLOGIC THERAPY

- IV fluid resuscitation with normal saline to maintain hemodynamic stability may be needed in some circumstances

- Correction of electrolyte and metabolic abnormalities with potassium, bicarbonate, and oxygen therapy

ACUTE GENERAL Rx

Acute situations like adrenal crisis or myxedema coma can occur in untreated hypopituitarism and should be treated accordingly with IV corticosteroids (e.g., hydrocortisone 100 mg IV q6h for 24 hr) and levothyroxine (e.g., 5 to 8 μg/kg IV over 15 min, then 100 μg IV q24h).

CHRONIC Rx

Treatment is lifelong and requires the following hormone replacement therapy:

ACTH deficiency:

- Hydrocortisone 20 mg PO qam and 10 mg PO qpm or prednisone 5 mg PO qam and 2.5 mg PO qpm. Dexamethasone or prednisone are often preferred due to longer duration of action.

LH and FSH deficiency:

- In men, testosterone enanthate or propionate 200 to 300 mg IM q2 to 3 wk or transdermal testosterone scrotal patches can be tried.
- In women who are not interested in fertility, conjugated estrogen 0.3 to 1.25 mg/day and held the last 5 to 7 days of each month with the addition of medroxyprogesterone 10 mg/day given during days 15 to 25 of the normal menstrual cycle. In those who have secondary hypogonadism and wish to become pregnant, pulsatile GnRH may be of benefit.

TSH deficiency:

- Levothyroxine 0.05 to 0.15 mg/day.

GH deficiency:

- Growth hormone is not used in adults; however, can be given at 0.04 to 0.08 mg/kg/day subcutaneously in children.

ADH deficiency:

- Desmopressin (DDAVP) 10 to 20 μg via intranasal spray or 0.05 to 0.1 mg PO bid is used in patients with diabetes insipidus.

DISPOSITION

- Hormone replacement therapy is adjusted according to serum hormone blood monitoring.
- Hypopituitarism if untreated can lead to adrenal crisis, severe hyponatremia and hypothyroidism, metabolic abnormalities, and death.
- The prognosis for patients with hypopituitarism is excellent, and life expectancy can be normal in patients with eradication of the pituitary disease and adequate hormone replacement therapy that is closely monitored in long-term follow-up.

REFERRAL

Anyone suspected of having hypopituitarism should have an endocrine consultation. For patients with pituitary tumors, a radiation oncologist and neurosurgeon consultation should be consulted.

PEARLS & CONSIDERATIONS

- Hyperprolactinemia resulting in galactorrhea or hypogonadism may be associated with hypopituitarism in cases where the pituitary stalk is transected by tumor or trauma/surgery. In these cases, inhibitory dopaminergic effects on the prolactin-secreting cells of the anterior pituitary from neurons in the hypothalamus is disrupted.
- Thyroxine supplementation increases the rate of cortisol metabolism and can lead to adrenal crisis. It is therefore recommended to supplement corticosteroids first before administering thyroid hormone replacement therapy.
- All patients receiving glucocorticoid replacement therapy should wear proper identification stating the need for this therapy.
- Stress doses of corticosteroids are indicated before surgery or for any medical emergency (e.g., sepsis, acute myocardial infarction, etc.).

COMMENTS

- Mineralocorticoid replacement is not necessary in secondary adrenal insufficiency because the rennin-angiotensin-aldosterone system is unaffected by pituitary failure.
- Patients with adult acquired GH deficiency must meet at least two criteria before replacement therapy: a poor GH response to at least two standard stimuli and hypopituitarism due to pituitary or hypothalamic damage. The criteria are different in children in whom GH is required for normal growth.

EVIDENCE

Medical therapy should precede surgical therapy.

The order to replace treatment is cortisol, thyroxine, androgen/estrogen, and then in some cases, growth hormone.[1]

Transsphenoidal approach compared with the transcranial approach during surgery allowed for significantly more tumor to be removed, reduced hypothalamic dysfunction, and reduced visual complications.[2,3]

It is important to take account of the experience of the surgeon and maximize perioperative medical management to improve the safety of the pituitary surgery.[4]

The following features are poor prognostic indicators for pituitary surgery: large tumor size, infiltrating tumor, and very elevated levels of hypersecreted hormones.

There is a small but significant risk of surgical complications including nasal perforation and loss of vision with transsphenoidal surgery.

Evidence-Based References

1. Orrego et al: Pituitary disorders: drug treatment options, *Drugs* 59(1):93, 2000. Medline.
2. Czepko et al: Early results of treating pituitary adenomas by means of transcranial and trans-sphenoidal approach, *Przegl Lek* 56(10):638, 1999. Medline.
3. Woolons et al: Complications of trans-sphenoidal surgery: the Wellington experience, *Aust NZJ Surg* 70(6):405, 2000. Medline.
4. Giovenelli et al: Surgical therapy of pituitary adenoma, *Metab* 45(8):115, 1996. Medline.

SUGGESTED READINGS

American Association of Clinical Endocrinologists medical guidelines for clinical practice for growth hormone use in adults and children—2003 update, *Endocr Pract* 9:64, 2003.

American Association of Clinical Endocrinologists medical guidelines for clinical practice for the evaluation and treatment of hypogonadism in adult male patients—2002 update, *Endocr Pract* 8:439, 2002.

Hanberg A; Common disorders of the pituitary gland: hyposecretion versus hypersecretion, *J Infus Nurs* 28(1):36, 2005.

Sheehan JP et al: Stereotactic radiosurgery for pituitary adenomas: an intermediate review of its safety, efficacy, and role in the neurosurgical treatment armamentarium, *J Neurosurg* 102(4):678, 2005.

AUTHOR: **PURVA AGARWAL, M.D.**

BASIC INFORMATION

DEFINITION

Hypospadias is a developmental abnormality of the penis characterized by

- Abnormal ventral opening of the urethral meatus anywhere from the ventral aspect of the glans penis to the perineum
- Ventral curvature of the penis (chordee)
- Dorsal foreskin hood

ICD-9CM CODES
ICD-9CM: 752.61
Congenital Chordee: 752.63

EPIDEMIOLOGY & DEMOGRAPHICS

PREVALENCE: 1 in 250

GENETICS: Pertinent familial aspects of hypospadias include the finding of hypospadias in 6.8% of fathers of affected boys and in 14% of male siblings

- An 8.5-fold higher rate of hypospadias is reported in monozygotic twins suggesting that there is insufficient production of human chorionic gonadotropin by the single placenta

PHYSICAL FINDINGS & CLINICAL PRESENTATION

- Genetics: normal karyotypes are seen with glandular hypospadias; abnormal karyotypes are noted in more severe forms of hypospadias
- Cryptorchidism: 8% to 9% occurrence
- Inguinal hernia: 9% to 10% occurrence
- Hydrocele: 9% to 16% occurrence

PENILE CURVATURE (CHORDEE):
Three theories

- Abnormal development of the urethral plate
- Abnormal fibrotic mesenchymal tissue at the urethral meatus
- Corporal disproportion

ETIOLOGY

Multifactorial

- Endocrine factors
  1. Abnormal androgen production
  2. Limited androgen sensitivity in the target tissues
  3. Premature cessation of androgenic stimulation secondary to Leydig cell dysfunction
  4. Insufficient testosterone-dihydrotestosterone synthesis as a result of deficient 5-alpha reductase enzyme activity
- Arrested development

DIAGNOSIS

WORKUP

Made by observation and examination

LABORATORY TESTS

Intersex evaluation should be undertaken if there is associated cryptorchidism. The evaluation should include: ultrasound, genitographic studies, chromosomal, gonadal, biochemical, and molecular studies.

TREATMENT

ACUTE GENERAL Rx

DESIGNATION/CLASSIFICATION:
Anterior: 33%
Middle: 25%
Posterior: 41%

SPECIAL CONSIDERATION:

- The only reason for operating on any hypospadias patient is to correct deformities that interfere with the function of urination and procreation
- Other reasons for interventions: Cosmetic concerns
- The American Academy of Pediatrics recommends the best time for surgical intervention as 6 to 12 mo

HORMONAL MANIPULATION:

- Controversial
- hCG administration is given before repair of proximal hypospadias
- The effect of the hCG administration is decreased hypospadias and chordee severity in all patients, increased vascularity and thickness of the proximal corpus spongiosum
- Application of topical testosterone increased mean penile circumference and length without any lasting side effects
- Prepubertal exogenous testosterone does not adversely effect ultimate penile growth

CHRONIC Rx

SURGICAL PROCEDURES:

- Orthoplasty (correcting penile curvature)
- Urethroplasty
- Meatoplasty
- Glanuloplasty
- Skin coverage

There is no single universally acceptable applicable technique for hypospadias repair.

TYPES OF REPAIR:

- Anterior hypospadias: MAGPI, Thiersch-Duplay urethroplasty, glans approximation procedure (GAP), tubularized incised plate (TIP) urethroplasty, Mathieu perimeatal flap, Mustarde technique, megameatus intact prepuce (MIP), pyramid procedure
- Midlevel hypospadias: TIP, Mathieu, onlay island flap (OIF), King procedure
- Posterior hypospadias:
  1. One-stage repair: OIF, double onlay preputial flap, pedicled preputial flap, transverse preputial island flap (TPIF)
  2. Two-stage repair: Orthoplasty to correct chordee followed 6 mo later or longer by Thiersch-Duplay, bladder and/or buccal mucosal hypospadias repair

COMPLICATIONS OF REPAIR:
Hematoma, meatal stenosis, fistula, urethral stricture, urethral diverticulum, wound infection, impaired healing, balanitis xerotica obliterans, penile curvature

PEARLS & CONSIDERATIONS

- It must be kept in mind that apparent simple isolated hypospadias may be the only visible indication of an underlying abnormality.
- The dorsal hood of redundant foreskin is used in the repair of hypospadias, and the patient with hypospadias and a dorsal hood should not be circumcised.

SUGGESTED READINGS

American Academy of Pediatrics: Timing of elective surgery on the genitalia of male children with particular reference to the risks, benefits, and psychological effects of surgery and anesthesia, *Pediatrics* 97:590, 1996.

Belman AB: Hypospadias update, *Urology* 49:166, 1997.

Borer JG, Retik AB: Current trends in hypospadias repair, *Urol Clin North Am* 26:1:15, 1999.

Retik AB, Borer JG. In Walsh PC et al, eds: *Campbell's urology,* ed 8, Philadelphia, 2002, WB Saunders.

Zaontz MR, Packer MG: Abnormalities of the external genitalia. *Pediatr Clin North Am* 44:1267, 1997.

AUTHORS: **PHILIP J. ALIOTTA, M.D., M.S.H.A.,** and **RUBEN ALVERO, M.D.**

BASIC INFORMATION

DEFINITION

Hypothermia is a rectal temperature <35° C (95.8° F). *Accidental hypothermia* is unintentionally induced decrease in core temperature in absence of preoptic anterior hypothalamic conditions.

ICD-9CM CODES
991.6 Accidental hypothermia
780.9 Hypothermia not associated with low environmental temperature

EPIDEMIOLOGY & DEMOGRAPHICS

- Hypothermia occurs most frequently in the following groups: alcoholics, learning-impaired, patients with cardiovascular, cerebrovascular, or pituitary disorders, those using sedatives or tranquilizers, and elderly patients.
- Approximately 700 persons/yr in the U.S. die from hypothermia.

PHYSICAL FINDINGS & CLINICAL PRESENTATION

- The clinical presentation varies with the severity of hypothermia. Shivering may be absent if body temperature is <33.3° C (92° F) or in patients taking phenothiazines.
- Hypothermia may masquerade as CVA, ataxia, or slurred speech, or the patient may appear comatose or clinically dead.
- Physiologic stages of hypothermia:
  1. Mild hypothermia (32.2° to 35° C [90° to 95° F]): arrhythmias, ataxia
  2. Moderate hypothermia (28° to 32.2° C [82.4° to 90° F]):
     a. Progressive decrease of level of consciousness, pulse, cardiac output, and respiration
     b. Fibrillation, dysrhythmias (increased susceptibility to ventricular tachycardia)
     c. Elimination of shivering mechanism for thermogenesis
  3. Severe hypothermia (≤28° C [82.4° F]):
     a. Absence of reflexes or response to pain
     b. Decreased cerebral blood flow, decreased CO_2
     c. Increased risk of ventricular fibrillation or asystole

ETIOLOGY

Exposure to cold temperatures for a prolonged period. Contributing factors are listed below:

1. Drugs: ethanol, phenothiazines, sedative-hypnotics
2. Skin disorders: extensive burns, severe psoriasis, exfoliative dermatitis
3. Metabolic disorders: hypopituitarism, hypothyroidism, hypoadrenalism
4. Neurologic abnormalities: stroke, head trauma, acute spinal cord transaction, impaired shivering
5. Other: lack of acclimatization, aggressive fluid resuscitation, sepsis, heat stroke treatment

DIAGNOSIS

DIFFERENTIAL DIAGNOSIS

- CVA
- Myxedema coma
- Drug intoxication
- Hypoglycemia

LABORATORY TESTS

1. Metabolic and respiratory acidosis are usually present.
   a. When blood cools, the arterial pH increases, oxygen tension (Po_2) increases, and the Pco_2 falls:
      (1) pH ↑ 0.008 U/°F (or 0.015 U/°C), ↓ in temperature.
      (2) Pao_2 ↑ 3.3%/°F, ↓ in temperature.
      (3) $Paco_2$ ↓ 2.4%/°F, ↓ in temperature.
   b. Blood gas analyzers warm the blood to 37° C, increasing the partial pressure of dissolved gases, resulting in higher oxygen and carbon dioxide levels and a lower pH than the patient's actual values. Correction of ABGs for temperature is unnecessary as a guide to therapy. The use of uncorrected values also permits reference to the standard acid-base nomograms.
2. ↓ K^+ initially, then ↑ K^+ with increasing hypothermia; extreme hyperkalemia indicates a poor prognosis.
3. Hematocrit (Hct) ↑ (caused by hemoconcentration), ↓ leukocytes, ↓ platelets (caused by splenic sequestration).
4. Blood viscosity, ↑ clotting time

IMAGING STUDIES

- Chest x-ray: generally not helpful; may reveal evidence of aspiration (e.g., intoxicated patient with aspiration pneumonia).
- ECG: prolonged PR, QT, and QRS segments, depressed ST segments, inverted T waves, AV block, hypothermic J waves (Osborne waves) may appear at 25° to 30° C; characterized by notching of the junction of the QRS complex and ST segments (Fig. 1-136).

TREATMENT

NONPHARMACOLOGIC THERAPY

- Treatment of hypothermia varies with the following:
  1. Degree of hypothermia
  2. Existence of concomitant diseases (e.g., cardiovascular insufficiency)
  3. Patient's age and medical condition (e.g., elderly, debilitated patients vs. young, healthy patients)
- General measures:
  1. Secure an airway before warming all unconscious patients; precede endotracheal intubation with oxygenation (if possible) to minimize the risk of arrhythmias during the procedure.
  2. Peripheral vasoconstriction may impede placement of a peripheral intravenous catheter; consider femoral venous access as an alternative to the jugular or subclavian sites to avoid ventricular stimulation.
  3. A Foley catheter should be inserted, and urinary output should be monitored and maintained above 0.5 to 1 ml/kg/hr with intravascular volume replacement.

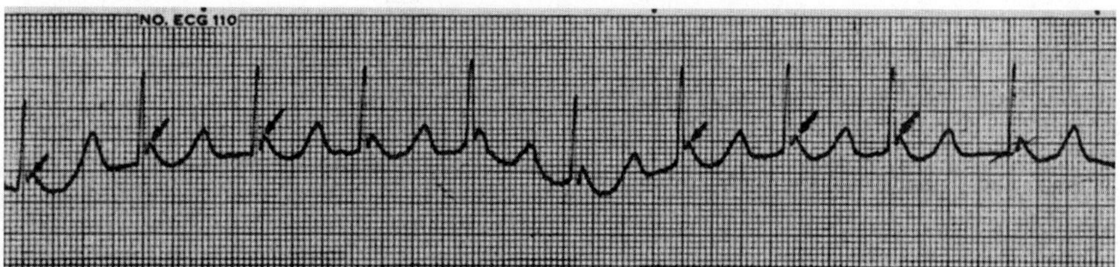

FIGURE 1-136 Osborne waves *(arrows)* in an 80-year-old man with core temperature of 86° F (30° C). These waves disappeared with rewarming. (From Morse CD, Rial WY: Emergency medicine. In Rakel RE [ed]: *Textbook of family practice,* ed 4, Philadelphia, 1990, WB Saunders.)

ACUTE GENERAL Rx

- Continuous ECG monitoring of patients is recommended; ventricular arrhythmias can be treated with bretylium; lidocaine is generally ineffective, and procainamide is associated with an increased incidence of ventricular fibrillation in hypothermic patients.
- Correct severe acidosis and electrolyte abnormalities.
- Hypothyroidism, if present, should be promptly treated (refer to "Myxedema Coma").
- If clinical evidence suggests adrenal insufficiency, administer IV methylprednisolone.
- In patients unresponsive to verbal or noxious stimuli or with altered mental status, 100 mg of thiamine, 0.4 mg of naloxone, and 1 ampule of 50% dextrose may be given.
- Warm (104° to 113° F [40° to 45° C]), humidified oxygen should also be given if it is available.
- Specific treatment:

1. Mild hypothermia (rectal temperature <32.3° C [90° F]): passive external rewarming is indicated. Place the patient in a warm room (temperature >21° C [69.8° F]), and cover with insulating material after gently removing wet clothing; recommended rewarming rates vary between 0.5° and 20° C/hr but should not exceed 0.55° C/hr in elderly persons.
2. Moderate to severe hypothermia:
   a. Active core rewarming
      (1) Delivery of heat via fluids: warm GI irrigation (with saline enemas and via NG tube); IV fluids (usually D_5NS without potassium) warmed to 104° to 107.6° F (40° to 42° C), peritoneal dialysis with dialysate heated to 40.5° to 42.5° C.
      (2) Inhalation of heated humidified oxygen (warmed to 40° C [104° F]) increases core temperature by 1° C (1.8° F) per hr and decreases evaporative heat loss via respiration.
   b. Active external rewarming: immersion in a bath of warm water (40° to 41° C); active external rewarming may produce shock because of excessive peripheral vasodilation. Ideal candidates are previously healthy, young patients with acute immersion hypothermia.
   c. Extracorporeal blood warming with cardiopulmonary bypass appears to be an efficacious rewarming technique in young, otherwise healthy persons.

EVIDENCE

EBM

Rewarming rates are controversial.

Evidence suggests aggressive rewarming is required to gain the best prognosis.

Evidence-Based Reference

Walpoth BH et al: Outcome of survivors of accidental deep hypothermia and circulatory arrest treated with extracorpeal blood warming, *N Engl J Med* 337:1500, 1997.

SUGGESTED READING

Mccullough L, Arora S: Diagnosis and treatment of hypothermia, *Am Fam Physician* 70:2325, 2004.

AUTHOR: **FRED F. FERRI, M.D.**

BASIC INFORMATION

DEFINITION

Hypothyroidism is a disorder caused by the inadequate secretion of thyroid hormone.

SYNONYMS

Myxedema

ICD-9CM CODES
244 Acquired hypothyroidism
243 Congenital hypothyroidism
244.1 Surgical hypothyroidism
244.3 Iatrogenic hypothyroidism
244.8 Pituitary hypothyroidism
246.1 Sporadic goitrous hypothyroidism

EPIDEMIOLOGY & DEMOGRAPHICS

INCIDENCE/PREVALENCE: 1.5% to 2% of women and 0.2% of men

PREDOMINANT AGE: Incidence of hypothyroidism increases with age; among persons older than 60 yr, 6% of women and 2.5% of men have laboratory evidence of hypothyroidism (TSH > twice normal).

PHYSICAL FINDINGS & CLINICAL PRESENTATION

- Hypothyroid patients generally present with the following signs and symptoms: fatigue, lethargy, weakness, constipation, weight gain, cold intolerance, muscle weakness, slow speech, slow cerebration with poor memory.
- Skin: dry, coarse, thick, cool, sallow (yellow color caused by carotenemia); nonpitting edema in skin of eyelids and hands (myxedema) secondary to infiltration of subcutaneous tissues by a hydrophilic mucopolysaccharide substance.
- Hair: brittle and coarse; loss of outer one third of eyebrows.
- Facies: dulled expression, thickened tongue, thick slow-moving lips.
- Thyroid gland: may or may not be palpable (depending on the cause of the hypothyroidism).
- Heart sounds: distant, possible pericardial effusion.
- Pulse: bradycardia.
- Neurologic: delayed relaxation phase of the DTRs, cerebellar ataxia, hearing impairment, poor memory, peripheral neuropathies with paresthesia.
- Musculoskeletal: carpal tunnel syndrome, muscular stiffness, weakness.

ETIOLOGY

PRIMARY HYPOTHYROIDISM (THYROID GLAND DYSFUNCTION): The cause of >90% of the cases of hypothyroidism

- Hashimoto's thyroiditis is the most common cause of hypothyroidism after 8 yr of age
- Idiopathic myxedema (nongoitrous form of Hashimoto's thyroiditis)
- Previous treatment of hyperthyroidism (radioiodine therapy, subtotal thyroidectomy)
- Subacute thyroiditis
- Radiation therapy to the neck (usually for malignant disease)
- Iodine deficiency or excess
- Drugs (lithium, PAS, sulfonamides, phenylbutazone, amiodarone, thiourea)
- Congenital (approximately 1 case per 4000 live births)
- Prolonged treatment with iodides

SECONDARY HYPOTHYROIDISM: Pituitary dysfunction, postpartum necrosis, neoplasm, infiltrative disease causing deficiency of TSH

TERTIARY HYPOTHYROIDISM: Hypothalamic disease (granuloma, neoplasm, or irradiation causing deficiency of TRH)

TISSUE RESISTANCE TO THYROID HORMONE: Rare

DIAGNOSIS

DIFFERENTIAL DIAGNOSIS

- Depression
- Dementia from other causes
- Systemic disorders (e.g., nephrotic syndrome, CHF, amyloidosis)

LABORATORY TESTS

- Increased TSH: TSH may be normal if patient has secondary or tertiary hypothyroidism, is receiving dopamine or corticosteroids, or the level is obtained following severe illness
- Decreased free T_4
- Other common laboratory abnormalities: hyperlipidemia, hyponatremia, and anemia
- Increased antimicrosomal and antithyroglobulin antibody titers: useful when autoimmune thyroiditis is suspected as the cause of the hypothyroidism

TREATMENT

NONPHARMACOLOGIC THERAPY

Patients should be educated regarding hypothyroidism and its possible complications. Patients should also be instructed about the need for lifelong treatment and monitoring of their thyroid abnormality.

ACUTE GENERAL Rx

Start replacement therapy with levothyroxine (L-thyroxine) 25 to 100 μg/day, depending on the patient's age and the severity of the disease. Physiologic combinations of L-thyroxine plus liothyronine do not offer any objective advantage over L-thyroxine alone. The levothyroxine dose may be increased every 6 to 8 wk, depending on the clinical response and serum TSH level. Elderly patients and patients with coronary artery disease should be started with 12.5 to 25 μg/day (higher doses may precipitate angina). The average maintenance dose of levothyroxine is 1.7 μg/kg/day (100 to 150 μg/day in adults). The elderly may require <1 μg/kg/day, whereas children generally require higher doses (up to 3 to 4 μg/kg/day). Pregnant patients also have increased requirements. Estrogen therapy may also increase the need for thyroxine. Women with hypothyroidism should increase their levothyroxine dose by approximately 30% as soon as pregnancy is confirmed. Close monitoring of serum thyrotropin levels and adjustment of levothyroxine dose is recommended throughout pregnancy.

CHRONIC Rx

- Periodic monitoring of TSH level is an essential part of treatment. Patients should be evaluated initially with office visit and TSH levels every 6 to 8 wk until the patient is clinically euthyroid and the TSH level is normalized. The frequency of subsequent visits and TSH measurement can then be decreased to every 6 to 12 mo. Pregnant patients should be checked every trimester.
- For monitoring therapy in patients with central hypothyroidism, measurement of serum free thyroxine (free T_4 level) is appropriate and should be maintained in the upper half of the normal range.

REFERRAL

Admission to the hospital ICU is recommended in all patients with myxedema coma. Additional information on the diagnosis and treatment of this life-threatening complication of hypothyroidism is available in the topic "Myxedema Coma" in Section I.

PEARLS & CONSIDERATIONS

COMMENTS

Subclinical hypothyroidism occurs in as many as 15% of elderly patients and is characterized by an elevated serum TSH and a normal free T_4 level. Treatment is individualized. Generally, replacement therapy is recommended for all patients with serum TSH >10 mU/L and with presence of goiter or thyroid autoantibodies.

SUGGESTED READING

Escobar-Morreale HF et al: Thyroid hormone replacement therapy in primary hypothyroidism: a randomized trial comparing L-Thyroxine plus liothyronine with L-thyronine alone, *Ann Intern Med* 142:412, 2005.

AUTHOR: **FRED F. FERRI, M.D.**

BASIC INFORMATION

DEFINITION

Idiopathic intracranial hypertension (IIH) is a syndrome of increased intracranial pressure without underlying hydrocephalus or mass lesion, and with normal cerebrospinal fluid analysis.

SYNONYMS

Pseudotumor cerebri
Benign intracranial hypertension

ICD-9CM CODES
348.2 Pseudotumor cerebri

EPIDEMIOLOGY & DEMOGRAPHICS

- 1 case/100,000 women
- 19 cases/100,000 women ages 20 to 44 and more than 20% of ideal body weight
- 0.3 to 1.5 cases/100,000 men
- Female:male ratio from 4.3:1 to 8:1
- More than 90% of IIH patients are obese
- Mean age at diagnosis is 30 years

PHYSICAL FINDINGS & CLINICAL PRESENTATION

Symptoms
- Headaches—generalized, throbbing, slowly progressive, worse with straining maneuvers, worse in the morning.
- Transient visual obscurations—described as a brief blurring of vision or scotomata. Lasting less than 30 sec. Frequently with Valsalva. May be monocular.
- Double vision—most often in the horizontal plane (due to pseudo-sixth nerve palsy).
- Pulsatile tinnitus—may be initial complaint.
- Photopsia—lights, sparkles in the eyes.
- Pain—mainly retro-orbital. Pain may also be located in the shoulders or neck. Could be present without a headache. May be associated with Lhermitte's sign.

Signs
- Papilledema—in virtually all cases. Bilateral, but may be asymmetric.
- Sixth nerve palsy—in approximately 10% to 20% of patients.
- Visual field defects—enlarged physiologic blind spot, constricted visual fields.
- Loss of vision—end result of longstanding and untreated IIH.

ETIOLOGY

IIH may be explained on the basis of decreased CSF absorption and increased intracerebral blood volume.
- Decreased CSF absorption due to increased venous sinus pressure—this hypothesis is supported by direct retrograde venography studies and would explain higher incidence of IIH in patients with CHF, hypertension, and obesity.
- Increase in cerebral blood volume—supported by magnetic resonance imaging and positron emission topography, as well as the presence of edema on microscopic evaluation.

DIAGNOSIS

DIFFERENTIAL DIAGNOSIS

- The symptoms and signs of IIH are essentially those of raised intracranial pressure (ICP), and the differential diagnosis includes any condition that may be associated with raised ICP. Here we consider only those disease processes in which elevated ICP occurs in the context of normal CSF analysis and normal MRI. (Of note, venous sinus thrombosis [VST] was placed on this list despite associated MRI findings. VST should be excluded in all individuals with suspected IIH.)
- Medications—vitamin A, steroids (both use and withdrawal), oral contraceptives
- Autoimmune disorders—systemic lupus erythematosus, Behçet's disease
- Vascular disease—venous sinus thrombosis
- Other conditions—hypertension, CHF, pregnancy, obesity, uremia, obstructive sleep apnea

LABORATORY TESTS

- Cerebrospinal fluid analysis
  1. Shows elevated opening pressure
  2. Shows normal protein, glucose, and cell count
- Hypercoagulability workup if suspicion for venous sinus thrombosis

IMAGING STUDIES

Magnetic resonance imaging of the brain to rule out underlying structural lesions
- "Empty sella sign" often associated with idiopathic intracranial hypertension but is not pathognomonic.

Cerebral venography to evaluate venous flow
- Magnetic resonance venography
- CT venography
- Conventional contrast venography

Computed tomography
- "Slitlike" ventricles

TREATMENT

NONPHARMACOLOGIC THERAPY

- Weight loss in obese patients
- Continuous positive airway pressure—if obstructive sleep apnea is suspected

ACUTE GENERAL Rx

- Acetazolamide 250 mg to 4 g per day—reduces CSF production by inhibition of carbonic anhydrase, occasionally causing anorexia and resultant weight loss. Should be avoided in pregnant women because of possible teratogenic risk.
- Furosemide 40 to 120 mg per day in divided doses—apparent mechanism of action is via reduced sodium transport, leading to decreased total CSF volume.
- Topiramate 100 to 400 mg per day—antiepileptic medication, recently reported to be effective in treatment of IIH. Weak carbonic anhydrase inhibitor associated with weight loss as one of its primary side effects. May cause word-finding difficulties and renal stone formation.
- Serial lumbar punctures—attempted in patients with severe headaches resistant to medical therapy. Goal is to reduce spinal fluid pressure allowing for immediate reduction in headache severity. This treatment should be reserved only for most resistant cases, and should be used as a conduit to future surgical intervention.
- IIH presents a special dilemma in pregnant women. Acetazolamide has been shown teratogenic in animals and caloric restriction is not advised in pregnancy. Symptomatic treatment of headache should be the mainstay of therapy. Recurrent lumbar punctures can be used to alleviate headache and delay the onset of visual loss.

CHRONIC Rx

Surgical intervention is indicated in cases of treatment failure and progressive visual loss.
- Optic nerve fenestration—preferred for patients with visual loss and easily controlled headaches. Proposed mechanism is decompression of the optic nerve. However, has been associated with significant failure rate.
- CSF shunting—neurosurgical procedure. Performed in patients with significant visual deterioration and difficult-to-control headaches. Provides rapid improvement in symptoms; however, reported to have significant rate of shunt malfunction requiring revision.

DISPOSITION

- Idiopathic intracranial hypertension is a self-limiting disease with occasional periods of relapses. Each episode may last from 1 to several years.
- All patients with IIH should undergo MR or CT venography to rule out the possibility of VST.
- The major complication of IIH is visual loss, and treatment should be directed toward reducing intracranial pressure to prevent visual loss.

REFERRAL

- Neuroophthalmologist for serial evaluation of visual fields and fundal photographs
- Nutritionist for weight loss
- General neurologist for the initial workup and eventual treatment of raised intracranial pressure

PEARLS & CONSIDERATIONS

COMMENTS

- Idiopathic intracranial hypertension is a diagnosis of exclusion.
- IIH is a disease of young obese women.
- Ongoing treatment is essential to avoid progressive visual loss, which is the most significant complication of this disorder.

PREVENTION

Maintenance of ideal body weight is one of the best preventative mechanisms for avoidance of IIH. However, it does occur in patients with normal body weight. In these cases, there are no known preventable risk factors.

PATIENT/FAMILY EDUCATION

Combination of weight loss and medical therapy is highly effective in treatment of IIH. Given that most patients with IIH are young and otherwise healthy, high success rates can be accomplished. Because IIH is a self-limiting condition, patients with IIH may expect to become both symptom- and medication-free after intracranial hypertension resolves.

EVIDENCE

EBM

Treatment of IIH includes a multitude of approaches, both acute and chronic in nature. While there have been studies looking specifically at the use of weight loss—acetazolamide therapy, optic nerve sheath fenestration, and ventriculo-peritoneal shunting—currently there are no randomized trials to show clear benefits of one treatment over the other. The majority of the studies are observational. It is clear that more research is needed in order to produce a definitive evidence-based approach to the treatment of IIH.

SUGGESTED READINGS

Acheson J: Idiopathic intracranial hypertension and visual function, *Br Med Bull* 79:233, 2007.

Binder D et al: Idiopathic intracranial hypertension, *Neurosurgery* 54:538, 2004.

Friedman D: Pseudotumor cerebri, *Neurol Clin* 22:99, 2004.

Friedman D, Jacobson D: Diagnostic criteria for idiopathic intracranial hypertension, *Neurology* 59:1492, 2002.

Friedman D, Jacobson D: Idiopathic intracranial hypertension, *J Neuroopthalmol* 24(2):138, 2004.

Goodwin J: Recent developments in idiopathic intracranial hypertension, *Semin Opthalmol* 18(4):181, 2003.

Lueck C, McIlwaine G: Interventions for idiopathic intracranial hypertension, *Cochrane Database Syst Rev* 3, 2005.

Mathews M, Sergott R, Savino P: Pseudotumor cerebri, *Curr Opin Ophthalmol* 14:364, 2003.

Miller N: Papilledema. In Miller N, Newman N (eds): *Clinical neuro-ophthalmology,* ed 5, Baltimore, 1998, Williams and Wilkins.

Salman MS, Kirkham FJ, MacGregor DL: Idiopathic "benign" intracranial hypertension: case series and review, *J Child Neurol* 16(7):465, 2001.

Wall M: Papilledema and idiopathic intracranial hypertension (pseudotumor cerebri). In Noseworthy J (ed): *Neurological therapeutics principles and practice,* London and New York, 2003, Martin Dunitz.

AUTHOR: **GENNA GEKHT, M.D.**

BASIC INFORMATION

DEFINITION

Specific form of chronic fibrosing interstitial pneumonia with histopathology characteristic of usual interstitial pneumonia (UIP). Disease characterized by progressive parenchymal scarring and loss of pulmonary function.

SYNONYMS

Cryptogenetic fibrosing alveolitis

ICD-9CM CODES
516.3 Idiopathic pulmonary fibrosis

EPIDEMIOLOGY & DEMOGRAPHICS

- Presents in fifth and sixth decades
- More common in men than women
- 3% appear to cluster in families, but no clear evidence for a genetic basis
- No distinct geographic distribution; no prediction by race or ethnicity
- Majority of patients with IPF are current or former smokers

PHYSICAL FINDINGS & CLINICAL PRESENTATION

- Most present with gradual onset (>6 months) of exertional dyspnea and nonproductive cough. Progressive dyspnea is usually the most prominent symptom.
- Tachypnea to compensate for stiff noncompliant lung.
- Fine bibasilar inspiratory crackles in >80% of patients, with progression upward as the disease advances.
- Clubbing in 25% to 50% of patients.
- Cyanosis, cor pumonale, right ventricular heave, peripheral edema may occur late in the disease course.
- Extrapulmonary involvement does not occur. Fever is rare and suggests alternative diagnosis.

ETIOLOGY

- Unknown.
- Numerous hypotheses, including environmental insults such as metal and wood dust, infectious causes, chronic aspiration, or exposure to certain drugs (antidepressants).
- New research suggests important role of aberrant tissue repair and fibrosis, and downplays the importance of generalized inflammation.

DIAGNOSIS

DIFFERENTIAL DIAGNOSIS

- Sarcoidosis
- Drug-induced lung diseases
- Connective tissue disease with similar clinical and pathologic presentations
- Other idiopathic interstitial pneumonias:
  - Desquamative interstitial pneumonia
  - Respiratory bronchitis interstitial lung disease
  - Acute interstitial pneumonia
  - Nonspecific interstitial pneumonia
  - Cryptogenic organizing pneumonia
  - Bronchiolitis obliterans organizing pneumonia
  - Occupational exposures (e.g., asbestos, silica) may cause pneumoconiosis that mimics IPF

WORKUP

- Almost all patients have abnormal CXR at presentation with bilateral reticular opacities most prominent in the periphery and lower lobes. Peripheral honeycombing may be seen.
- High-resolution CT scan shows patchy peripheral reticular abnormalities with intralobular linear opacities, irregular septal thickening, subpleural honeycombing, and ground glass appearance.
- Pulmonary function tests show restrictive impairment with reduced vital capacity and total lung capacity. Obstructive picture only seen in smokers with IPF. Reduced DLCO.
- Laboratory abnormalities (nondiagnostic): mild anemia; increases in ESR, LDH, CRP; low titer ANA seen in up to 30% of patients.
- Limited role for bronchioalveolar lavage either in diagnosis or monitoring IPF.
- Gold standard for diagnosis is lung biopsy (open thoracotomy or video-assisted thorascopy). Hallmark features: heterogeneous distribution of parenchymal fibrosis against background of mild inflammation (UIP).
- Transbronchial lung biopsies do not provide a large enough sample to make diagnosis.
- Lung biopsy is critical to distinguish IPF from diseases with better prognosis and treatment options, especially in patients with any atypical features.
- In absence of or contraindication to lung biopsy, the combination of the clinical and radiographic features are often enough to establish the diagnosis.

TREATMENT

- No proven treatment for IPF and little evidence to support the routine use of *any* specific therapy.
- Conventional treatment includes a trial of corticosteroids at 0.5 mg/kg × 4 wk, 0.25 mg/kg × 8 wk, then tapered down combined with azathioprine or cyclophosphamide for 3 to 6 mo; 10% to 30% of patients may respond.
- Treatment is continued for up to 24 months if the patient improves or is stable. Long-term treatment only with objective evidence of continued improvement or stabilization.
- Single lung transplantation is the only therapy shown to prolong survival in IPF. Posttransplant 5-year survival for IPF patients is about 40%.
- Treatment agents designed to target the fibrotic process include N-Acetylcysteine, pirfenidone, interferon-gamma 1b, coumadin, and etanercept. These are under investigation and show some initial promise.

DISPOSITION

- Spontaneous remissions do not occur.
- The course is progressive.
- No difference in clinical course, pathology, or prognosis in younger patients.
- Mean survival after the diagnosis of biopsy-confirmed IPF is 3 yr.
- 40% die of respiratory failure.
- The incidence of bronchiogenic carcinoma is increased.

REFERRAL

To pulmonologist for review of abnormal chest imaging and establishing diagnosis

PEARLS & CONSIDERATIONS

- The course is progressive with a high mortality rate.
- Critical to differentiate IPF from other interstitial lung diseases since prognosis and response to treatment differs.
- There is no proven treatment for IPF. A course of steroids combined with azathioprine or cyclophosphamide is often tried.
- Consider early referral for lung transplant.

SUGGESTED READINGS

American Thoracic Society: Idiopathic Pulmonary Fibrosis: Diagnosis and Treatment: International Consensus Statement, *Am J Respir Crit Care Med* 61:646, 2000.

Gross TJ, Hunninghake GW: Idiopathic pulmonary fibrosis, *N Engl J Med* 345(7):517, 2001.

Strieter RM: Pathogenesis and natural history of usual interstitial pneumonia, *Chest* 128 (5):526S, 2005.

Walter N et al: Current perspectives on the treatment of idiopathic pulmonary fibrosis, *Proc Am Thorac Soc* 3:3308, 2006.

AUTHORS: **MARA LINSCOTT, M.D.,** and **LYNN BOWLBY, M.D.**

BASIC INFORMATION

DEFINITION

IgA nephropathy is a proliferative glomerulonephritis associated with predominant deposition of IgA in the mesangium.

SYNONYMS

Berger's disease

ICD-9-CM CODES
583.81

EPIDEMIOLOGY & DEMOGRAPHICS

INCIDENCE: It is the most common type of glomerulonephropathy worldwide.

PREVALENCE: Prevalence rate is lower in the U.S. (10% to 15%) compared to Asian countries. Lower rates could be explained by conservative approach by nephrologists in the U.S. who are reluctant to do renal biopsy in asymptomatic patients with minimal renal abnormalities. In most reports, prevalence rates are expressed as a percentage of cases of primary glomerulonephritis or as a percentage of total series of renal biopsies.

PREDOMINANT SEX AND AGE: It is most prevalent in the second and third decade of life with a male:female ratio of 6:1 in the U.S.

GENETICS: Although it is considered to be a sporadic disease, genetic linkage to locus called IgAN1 on 6q22 and 6q23 has been shown.

RISK FACTORS: It has a higher association with Asians, Caucasians, and Native Americans and is rarely seen in African Americans.

PHYSICAL FINDINGS & CLINICAL PRESENTATION

- Two common presentations include (1) recurrent macroscopic hematuria often associated with upper respiratory infection or (2) persistent microscopic hematuria.
- Loin pain may be associated with macroscopic hematuria.
- Physical findings are usually unremarkable except hypertension seen in 20% to 30% of patients with chronic disease and edema in 5% of patients with nephrotic range proteinuria.
- Mild proteinuria is common.
- Rarely, IgA nephropathy could present as acute renal failure in 5% of patients and chronic renal failure in 10% to 20% of patients.

ETIOLOGY

- Most cases are idiopathic/primary.
- Secondary causes of IgA nephropathy include Henoch-Schönlein purpura, hepatitis B, alcoholic cirrhosis, celiac disease, inflammatory bowel disease, psoriasis, sarcoidosis, cystic fibrosis, cancer of lungs/larynx/pancreas, HIV infection, systemic lupus erythematosus (SLE), rheumatoid arthritis, diabetic nephropathy, Sjögren's syndrome, Reiter's syndrome, and so on.

DIAGNOSIS

DIFFERENTIAL DIAGNOSIS

- Henoch-Schönlein purpura
- Hereditary nephritis
- Thin glomerular basement membrane disease
- Lupus nephritis
- Poststreptococcal nephritis
- Above mentioned secondary causes associated with IgA nephropathy

WORKUP

- The diagnosis is suspected based on clinical history and laboratory data, but is confirmed by renal biopsy showing IgA deposits in the mesangium.
- Renal biopsy is restricted to patients with sustained proteinuria more than 1 gm/day or worsening renal function.

LABORATORY TESTS

- Urine analysis showing protein, RBC, WBC, and RBC casts.
- Serum creatinine may be elevated.
- 24-hour urine assay for quantifying proteinuria and to check creatinine clearance.
- Serum IgA is elevated in only 50% of patients. It has no clinical utility.

TREATMENT

Although initially considered to be a benign disease, IgA nephropathy is now recognized as a common cause of renal failure. Currently there is no cure for it.

NONPHARMACOLOGIC THERAPY

- Moderate dietary protein restriction
- Discourage smoking

ACUTE/CHRONIC GENERAL Rx

- Aggressive therapy for hypertension preferably with ACE inhibitors. Goal BP is less than 125/75 in presence of proteinuria over 1 gm/day.
- Patients with recurrent gross hematuria or isolated microscopic hematuria, no or minimal proteinuria (<1 gm/day), normotensives, and normal kidney function, should only be monitored every 6 to 12 months to assess disease progression.
- If bouts of recurrent macroscopic hematuria are associated with tonsillitis, tonsillectomy may benefit these patients.
- In patients with persistent proteinuria more than 1 gm/day with or without hypertension are treated with ACE inhibitors and/or ARB. Steroids are reserved for patients with persistent proteinuria greater than 1 gm/day in spite of ACE and/or ARB.
- Patients with nephrotic syndrome, preserved kidney function, and minimal change in disease are treated with steroids for 6 months.
- Patients with severe renal disease or crescentic, rapidly progressive glomerulonephritis in the absence of changes of chronic kidney disease in biopsy are treated with steroid and cyclophosphamide combination for the first 2 months, followed by steroids and azathioprine for 2 years for maintenance treatment.
- Patients with acute renal failure need renal biopsy to rule out acute tubular necrosis, which needs only supportive therapy, from crescentic IgA nephropathy, which needs aggressive medical management.
- Kidney transplantation is the treatment of choice for end-stage kidney disease. There is no difference in survival in living vs. cadaver donors. At present, kidneys with IgA deposits are not used for transplantation.
- Statins are indicated for all IgA nephropathy patients with dyslipidemia, hypertension, and other cardiovascular risks.
- Role of mycophenolate and plasmapheresis is controversial.

COMPLEMENTARY & ALTERNATIVE MEDICINE

Role of fish oil is controversial

DISPOSITION

- Complete remission occurs in less than 10% of patients.
- End-stage renal failure develops in 15% to 20% of patients within 10 years of onset and in 30% to 35% of patients within 20 years.

- Poor prognostic indicators include (1) male gender, (2) older age, (3) young age at the onset of the disease, (4) absence of episodes of recurrent macroscopic hematuria, (5) hypertension, (6) extent of renal insufficiency, (7) extent of proteinuria, (8) elevated serum uric acid, and (9) certain histological changes seen in renal biopsy such as crescents, glomerulosclerosis, and tubulointerstial fibrosis/atrophy.

REFERRAL

Patients with IgA nephropathy are commonly referred to nephrologists.

PEARLS & CONSIDERATIONS

COMMENTS

- IgA nephropathy seems to be a kidney-restricted form of Henoch-Schönlein purpura.
- IgA nephropathy is not an entirely benign condition, even when microhematuria is the only clinical presentation.

SUGGESTED READINGS

Appel et al: The IgA nephropathy treatment dilemma, *Kidney International* 69:1939-1944, 2006.

Barrett et al: Treatment of IgA nephropathy, *Kidney International* 69:1934-1938, 2006.

Barrett et al: IgA nephropathy, *J Am Soc Nephrol* 16:2088-2097, 2005.

Couser WG: Glomerulonephritis, *Lancet* 353(9163):1509-1515, 1999.

Dillon J: Treating IgA nephropathy, editorial, *J Am Soc Nephrol* 12:846-847, 2001.

Donadio JV, Grande JP: IgA nephropathy, *N Engl J Med* 347(10):738-748, 2002.

Floege et al: IgA nephropathy: recent developments, *J Am Soc Nephrol* 11:2395-2395, 2000.

Ibels LS, Gyory AZ: IgA nephropathy: analysis of the natural history, important factors in the progression of renal disease, and a review of the literature, *Medicine (Baltimore)* 73(2):79-102, 1994.

Schena FP: Immunoglobulin a nephropathy with mild renal lesions: a call in the forest for physicians and nephrologists, *Am J Med* 110(6):499-500, 2001.

Williams DG: IgA nephropathy, *BMJ* 308(6921):74-75, 1994.

AUTHOR: **HEMANT K. SATPATHY, M.D.**

BASIC INFORMATION

DEFINITION

Immune thrombocytopenic purpura (ITP) is an autoimmune disorder in which antibody-coated or immune complex-coated platelets are destroyed prematurely by the reticuloendothelial system resulting in peripheral thrombocytopenia.

ICD-9CM CODES
287.3 Idiopathic thrombocytopenic purpura (ITP)

EPIDEMIOLOGY & DEMOGRAPHICS

INCIDENCE: 100 cases/1 million persons/yr

PREVALENCE: 5 to 10 cases/100,000 persons

PREDOMINANT SEX: 72% of patients >10 yr old are female; in children, males = females

PREDOMINANT AGE: Children age 2 to 4 yr and young women (70% are <40 yr old)

PHYSICAL FINDINGS & CLINICAL PRESENTATION

The presentation of ITP is different in children and adults.

- Children generally present with sudden onset of bruising and petechiae from severe thrombocytopenia.
- In adults the presentation is insidious; a history of prolonged purpura may be present; many patients are diagnosed incidentally on the basis of automated laboratories that now routinely include platelet counts.
- The physical examination may be entirely normal.
- Patients with severe thrombocytopenia may have petechiae, purpura, epistaxis, or heme-positive stool from GI bleeding.
- Splenomegaly is unusual; its presence should alert to the possibility of other etiologies of thrombocytopenia.
- The presence of dysmorphic features (skeletal anomalies, auditory abnormalities) may indicate a congenital disorder as the etiology of the thrombocytopenia.

ETIOLOGY

Increased platelet destruction caused by autoantibodies to platelet-membrane antigens. Hundreds of medications can cause thrombocytopenia. Drugs commonly implicated are quinidine, heparin, antibiotics (linezolid, vancomycin, sulfonamides, rifampin), platelet inhibitors (tirofiban, abciximab, eptifibatide), cimetidine, NSAIDs, thiazide diuretics, antirheumatic agents (gold salts, penicillamine), acetaminophen, and chemotherapeutic agents (cyclosporine, fludarabine, oxaliplatin).

DIAGNOSIS

DIFFERENTIAL DIAGNOSIS

- Falsely low platelet count (resulting from EDTA-dependent or cold-dependent agglutinins)
- Viral infections (e.g., HIV, mononucleosis, rubella)
- Drug-induced (e.g., heparin, quinidine, sulfonamides)
- Hypersplenism resulting from liver disease
- Myelodysplastic and lymphoproliferative disorders
- Pregnancy, hypothyroidism
- SLE, TTP, hemolytic-uremic syndrome
- Congenital thrombocytopenias (e.g., Fanconi's syndrome, May-Hegglin anomaly, Bernard-Soulier syndrome)

LABORATORY TESTS

- CBC, platelet count, and peripheral smear: platelets are decreased but are normal in size or may appear larger than normal. RBCs and WBCs have a normal morphology.
- Additional tests may be ordered to exclude other etiologies of the thrombocytopenia when clinically indicated (e.g., HIV, ANA, TSH, liver enzymes, bone marrow examination).
- The direct assay for the measurement of platelet-bound antibodies has an estimated positive predictive value of 80% to 83%. A negative test cannot be used to rule out the diagnosis.

IMAGING STUDIES

CT scan of abdomen/pelvis in patients with splenomegaly to exclude other disorders causing thrombocytopenia

TREATMENT

NONPHARMACOLOGIC THERAPY

- Minimize activity to prevent injury or bruising (e.g., contact sports should be avoided).
- Stop any potentially offending drugs (see etiology). Avoid medications that increase the risk of bleeding (e.g., aspirin and other NSAIDs).

ACUTE GENERAL Rx

- Treatment varies with the platelet count, patient's age, and bleeding status.
- Observation and frequent monitoring of platelet count are needed in asymptomatic patients with platelet counts $>30{,}000/mm^3$.
- Methylprednisolone 30 mg/kg/day IV infused over a period of 20 to 30 min (max dose of 1 g/day for 2 or 3 days) plus IV immunoglobulin (1 g/kg/day for 2 or 3 days) and infusion of platelets should be given to patients with neurologic symptoms, internal bleeding, or those undergoing emergency surgery.
- Prednisone 1 to 2 mg/kg qd, continued until the platelet count is normalized then slowly tapered off, is indicated in adults with platelet counts $<20{,}000/mm^3$ and those who have counts $<50{,}000/mm^3$ and significant mucous membrane bleeding. Response rates range from 50% to 75%, and most responses occur within the first 3 wk. Oral dexamethasone at a dosage of 40 mg/day for 4 consecutive days has also been reported to induce a high response rate (85%).
- High-dose immunoglobulins (IgG 0.4 g/kg/day IV, infused on 3 to 5 consecutive days) or high-dose parenteral glucocorticoids (methylprednisolone 30 mg/kg/day) can be used in children with platelet count $<20{,}000/mm^3$ and significant bleeding or adults with severe thrombocytopenia or bleeding. However, responses are generally transient, lasting no longer than 4 wk.
- Splenectomy should be considered in adults with platelet count $<30{,}000/mm^3$ after 6 wk of medical treatment or after 6 mo if more than 10 to 20 mg of prednisone per day is required to maintain a platelet count $>30{,}000/mm^3$. In children, splenectomy is generally reserved for persistent thrombocytopenia (>1 yr) and clinically significant bleeding. Appropriate immunizations (pneumococcal vaccine in adults and children, *H. influenzae* vaccine, meningococcal vaccine in children) should be administered before splenectomy.
- Platelet transfusion is needed only in case of life-threatening hemorrhage.
- Use of Danazol, an attenuated androgen, and chemotherapy with cyclophosphamide, vincristine, and prednisone (CVP) has been partially effective in chronic ITP.
- Rituximab, a monoclonal antibody directed against the CD_{20} antigen, has been reported useful for patients with ITP who are resistant to conventional treatment, and it may help prevent serious or fatal bleeding. Encouraging results have also been shown in trials involving AMG 531, a thrombopoiesis-stimulating protein in patients with chronic ITP.
- The oral thrombopoietin-receptor agonist eltrombopag is effective in increasing platelet count in patients with chronic ITP.

DISPOSITION

- More than 80% of children have a complete remission within 8 weeks.
- In adults, the course of the disease is chronic and only 5% of adults have spontaneous remission.
- The principal cause of death from ITP is intracranial hemorrhage (1% of children, 5% of adults).

SUGGESTED READINGS

N Engl J Med 357:580, 2007.
N Engl J Med 355:1672, 2006.
N Engl J Med 357:2237-2247, 2007.

AUTHOR: **FRED F. FERRI, M.D.**

BASIC INFORMATION

DEFINITION

Impetigo is a superficial skin infection generally secondary to *Staphylococcus aureus* and/or *Streptococcus* spp.

Common presentations are bullous impetigo (generally secondary to staphylococcal disease) and nonbullous impetigo (secondary to streptococcal infection and possible staphylococcal infection); the bullous form is caused by an epidermolytic toxin produced at the site of infection.

SYNONYMS

Impetigo vulgaris
Pyoderma

ICD-9CM CODES
684 Impetigo

EPIDEMIOLOGY & DEMOGRAPHICS

- Bullous impetigo is most common in infants and children. The nonbullous form is most common in children ages 2 to 5 yr with poor hygiene in warm climates.
- The overall incidence of acute nephritis with impetigo varies between 2% and 5%.

PHYSICAL FINDINGS & CLINICAL PRESENTATION

- Nonbullous impetigo begins as a single red macule or papule that quickly becomes a vesicle. Rupture of the vesicle produces an erosion of which the contents dry to form honey-colored crusts. Multiple lesions with golden yellow crusts and weeping areas often found on the skin around the nose, mouth, and limbs (Fig. 1-137).
- Bullous impetigo is manifested by the presence of vesicles that enlarge rapidly to form bullae with contents that vary from clear to cloudy. There is subsequent collapse of the center of the bullae; the peripheral areas may retain fluid, and a honey-colored crust may appear in the center; as the lesions enlarge and become contiguous with the others, a scaling border replaces the fluid-filled rim; there is minimal erythema surrounding the lesions.
- Regional lymphadenopathy is most common with nonbullous impetigo.
- Constitutional symptoms are generally absent.

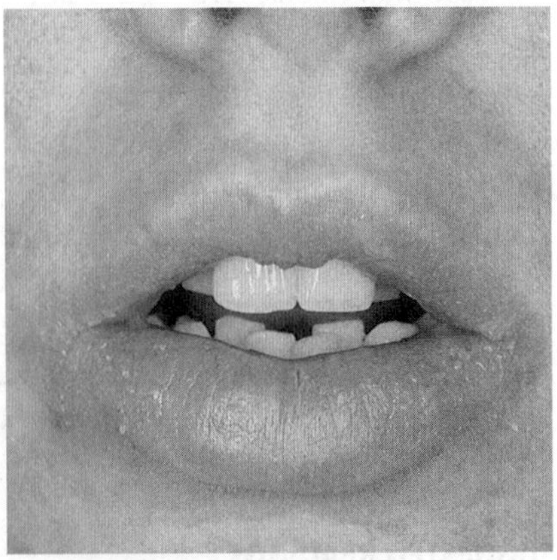

FIGURE 1-137 Impetigo. Serum and crust at the angle of the mouth is a common presentation for impetigo. (From Habif TB: *Clinical dermatology: a color guide to diagnosis and therapy,* ed 4, St Louis, 2000, Mosby.)

ETIOLOGY

- *S. aureus* coagulase positive is the dominant microorganism.
- *S. pyogenes* (group A β-hemolytic streptococci): M-T serotypes of this organism associated with acute nephritis are 2, 49, 55, 57, and 60.

DIAGNOSIS

DIFFERENTIAL DIAGNOSIS

- Atopic dermatitis
- Herpes simplex infection
- Ecthyma
- Folliculitis
- Eczema
- Insect bites
- Scabies
- Tinea corporis
- Pemphigus vulgaris and bullous pemphigoid
- Chickenpox

WORKUP

Diagnosis is clinical.

LABORATORY TESTS

- Generally not necessary
- Gram stain and C&S to confirm the diagnosis when the clinical presentation is unclear
- Sedimentation rate parallel to activity of the disease
- Increased anti-DNAse B and anti-hyaluronidase
- Urinalysis revealing hematuria with erythrocyte casts and proteinuria in patients with acute nephritis (most frequently occurring in children between 2 and 4 yr of age in the southern part of the U.S.)

TREATMENT

NONPHARMACOLOGIC THERAPY

Remove crusts by soaking with wet cloth compresses (crusts block the penetration of antibacterial creams).

GENERAL Rx

- Application of 2% mupirocin ointment (Bactroban) tid for 10 days or retapamulin 1% (Altabax) applied bid for 5 days to the affected area or until all lesions have cleared.
- Oral antibiotics are used in severe cases: commonly used agents are dicloxacillin 250 mg qid for 7 to 10 days, cephalexin 250 mg qid for 7 to 10 days, azithromycin 500 mg on day 1, 250 mg on days 2 through 5, amoxicillin/clavulanate 500 mg q8h.
- Impetigo can be prevented by prompt application of mupirocin or triple antibiotic ointment (bacitracin, Polysporin, and neomycin) to sites of skin trauma.
- Patients who are carriers of *S. aureus* in their nares should be treated with mupirocin ointment applied to their nares bid for 5 days.
- Fingernails should be kept short, and patients should be advised not to scratch any lesions to avoid spread of infection.

DISPOSITION

Most cases of impetigo resolve promptly with appropriate treatment. Both bullous and nonbullous forms of impetigo heal without scarring.

REFERRAL

Nephrology referral in patients with acute nephritis

PEARLS & CONSIDERATIONS

COMMENTS

- Patients should be instructed on use of antibacterial soaps and avoidance of sharing of towels and washcloths, because impetigo is extremely contagious.
- Children attending day care should be removed until 48 to 72 hr after initiation of antibiotic treatment.

EVIDENCE

A systematic review of interventions for impetigo found that topical antibiotics showed better cure rates than placebo, and topical mupirocin was superior to oral erythromycin. Topical and oral antibiotics did not show significantly different cure rates in general, nor did most oral antibiotics. Penicillin was inferior to erythromycin and cloxacillin, and there is little evidence that using disinfectant solutions improved impetigo. Erythromycin is the drug of choice in areas of low resistance because of high efficacy and relatively low cost.[1] Ⓐ

The same systematic review found oral antibiotic treatment caused more side effects than topical treatment.[1] Ⓐ

Evidence-Based Reference

1. Koning S et al: Interventions for impetigo. In The Cochrane Library, 3, Chichester, UK, 2004, John Wiley.

AUTHOR: **FRED F. FERRI, M.D.**

BASIC INFORMATION

DEFINITION

Inclusion body myositis (IBM) is an inflammatory myopathy with distinctive clinical and pathologic features.

ICD-9CM CODES
710.8 Other specified diffuse diseases of connective tissue

EPIDEMIOLOGY & DEMOGRAPHICS

INCIDENCE (IN U.S.): It is the third major form of idiopathic inflammatory myopathy (after polymyositis and dermatomyositis). It accounts for 15% to 28% of inflammatory myopathies in the U.S. and Canada.
PREVALENCE (IN U.S.): 4 to 9 cases/1,000,000 persons
PREDOMINANT SEX: Male > female (3:1); more common in white than black population
PREDOMINANT AGE: Older than 50 years of age; rare before the age of 30
PEAK INCIDENCE: Fifth decade
GENETICS:
- Two forms:
  1. Acquired sporadic: the majority of cases (discussed here)
  2. Familial: differs from the acquired form by the age of onset (early childhood), distribution of muscle weakness (spares quadriceps), and biopsy findings (lack of inflammation and less amyloid deposits). It is linked to chromosome 9 and can be expressed in an autosomal dominant or recessive fashion.
- HLA types: DR_1*0301, DR_3*0101 (or DR_3*0202) and DQ_1*0201

PHYSICAL FINDINGS & CLINICAL PRESENTATION

- Insidious onset (>6 yr from the onset of symptoms to diagnosis).
- Steadily progressive asymmetric and painless muscle weakness and atrophy of the finger or wrist flexors (commonly the flexor pollicis longus), knee extensor (quadriceps), and foot dorsiflexion. Over time weakness spreads to involve other muscles.
- A common complaint is difficulty with ambulation and frequent falls (due to buckling of knees caused by knee extensor weakness).
- Fatigue and reduced tolerance of exertion are common.
- Dysphagia (up to 60%).
- Weakness of the diaphragm resulting in subacute respiratory failure.
- Classic appearance is a scooped-out medial aspect of forearms and thin, atrophic quadriceps muscles.
- Facial and neck weakness can be seen.
- Early loss of patellar reflexes.
- Up to 15% of patients have other autoimmune diseases (systemic lupus erythematosus, Sjögren's syndrome, scleroderma, interstitial pneumonitis, psoriasis, and sarcoidosis), diabetes, and mild polyneuropathy.
- Cardiovascular abnormalities have been documented in some reports.
- There is no documented association with malignancies.
- Diagnostic criteria of either definite or possible IBM based on muscle biopsy, clinical features, and laboratory findings have been published.

ETIOLOGY

- Cell-mediated immune response: CD8 cytotoxic T-cell endomysial infiltration
- Of patients with sporadic form, 20% to 33% have a concomitant systemic or neurologic autoimmune disease
- Monoclonal gammopathies are found at higher frequency in these patients
- A strong association with a susceptibility gene in the central major histocompatibility (MHC) region (butyrophilin-like MHC class II–associated gene)
- Abundant proinflammatory and regulatory cytokines, chemokines, and chemokine receptors are upregulated
- Abnormal protein processing: accumulation of Alzheimer-type proteins (prion protein, beta amyloid protein, neuronal microtubule-associated protein, amyloid precursor protein, alpha-1 antichymotrypsin, phosphorylated tau, apolipoprotein E, ubiquitin, and presenilin) within the degenerating muscle fibers
- Deletion of mitochondrial DNA
- Nitric oxide induced oxidative stress
- Possible viral pathogenesis: filamentous inclusions resembling myxovirus nucleocapsids. Also seen in patients with chronic viral infection (HIV, HTLV-1, hepatitis C)

DIAGNOSIS

DIFFERENTIAL DIAGNOSIS

- Amyotrophic lateral sclerosis
- Polymyositis
- Polyneuropathy
- Oculopharyngeal dystrophy
- Emery-Dreifuss muscular dystrophy
- Vitamin E deficiency
- Chronic atrophic sarcoid myopathy
- Myasthenia gravis
- Acid maltase deficiency
- Chronic inflammatory demyelinating polyradiculoneuropathy

WORKUP

- Good history and physical exam demonstrating the characteristic pattern of weakness in a male who is older than 50.
- *Electromyography:* active myopathic changes (fibrillation potentials, positive sharp waves and short duration, low-amplitude, polyphasic motor unit action potentials). Mixed myopathic and neurogenic changes can also be seen.
- *Nerve conduction studies:* occasionally sensory nerve conduction studies are abnormal (if there is an associated neuropathy).
- *Muscle biopsy:* small angular atrophic and denervated fibers. CD8 cytotoxic T-cell endomysial infiltration. Intracytoplasmic rimmed vacuoles and cytoplasmic tubofilamentous inclusions on electromicrosopic examination of the affected muscle fiber.
- MRI has been used to visualize inflamed or atrophic muscles.

LABORATORY TESTS

- CPK (normal to increased 3 to 5 times normal)
- Thyroid function test to rule out thyroid disease
- Antinuclear antigen (ANA), rheumatoid factor (RF), double stranded DNA (ds-DNA), erythrocyte sedimentation rate (ESR), C-reactive protein (CRP), rapid plasma reagin (RPR), scl-70, anti-SS-A (Ro), and anti-SS-B (La) to rule out other autoimmune diseases
- Standard serum studies (hemogram and electrolytes)

TREATMENT

NONPHARMACOLOGIC THERAPY

- Exercise therapy: isotonic training program of the weak muscles
- Nutritional assessment if dysphagia is present
- Cricopharyngeal myotomy for dysphagia
- Braces/orthotics for weakness of tibialis anterior or quadriceps
- Routine follow-up visits

GENERAL Rx

- Resistant to treatment.
- Although there is no effective treatment, all available medical and nonmedical treatment should be discussed with the patient and considered.
- Corticosteroids, cyclophosphamide, chlorambucil, azathioprine, cyclosporine, methotrexate, anabolic steroid oxandrolone, and IVIG have been used but without evidence of benefit.
- IVIG might provide some benefit for patients with dysphagia (Cherin P et al.).
- IVIG in combination with prednisone results in reduction of endomysial inflammation but no clinical improvement (Dalakas, 2001).
- Beta interferon-1a at 30 and 60 mg IM/wk regimens did not result in significant improvement in muscle strength or muscle mass (Muscle Study Group, 2001 and 2004).

- Oxandrolone (a synthetic anabolic steroid) use resulted in muscle strength improvement but further studies are needed (Rutkow SB et al.).
- Several months' trial of prednisone (0.6 mg/kg) is recommended by some (Lotz et al., Alexandrescu et al.).
- Botulinum toxin A injection into the upper esophageal sphincter (Liu et al.).
- Patients should be given a trial of immunosuppressive therapy if a connective tissue disease coexists.

DISPOSITION

- The progression of the disease is very slow.
- The rate of decline in strength (based on handheld myometry or manual muscle testing) is 0.66%-1.4%/mo.
- The rate of functional decline from the onset of symptoms to use of a walker varies depending on the age of onset of symptoms (17 yr and 3.2 yr for age of onset 40 to 49 and 70 to 79, respectively).
- Periods of stabilization (3 to 6 mo) can be seen in 25% to 50% of patients.

REFERRAL

- Surgical evaluation for muscle biopsy
- A neurologist or a neuromuscular specialist
- Physical therapy

PEARLS & CONSIDERATIONS

COMMENTS

- Risk of falls should be assessed by a physical therapist.
- Quantitative measures of muscle strength (myometry) should be used to assess response to treatment and disease activity.

EVIDENCE

There is no strong evidence to support the benefit of corticosteroids in producing sustained or quantitatively demonstrated improvement. At best, short-term stabilization was noted.[1,2]

Azathioprine resulted in a slight improvement in some patients with IBM.[3]

Methotrexate might provide long term remission in some patients[3] and minor response in others.[3]

Cyclosporin might provide some stability or short-term benefit in selected patients.[4]

Total body irradiation, plasma exchange, IVIG, cyclophosphamide, and Chlorambucil did not show any significant benefit.

Evidence-Based References

1. Barohn RJ et al: Inclusion body myositis: explanation for poor response to immunosuppressive therapy, *Neurology* 45:1302-1304, 1995.
2. Dalakas MC et al: A controlled study of intravenous immunoglobulin combined with prednisone in the treatment of IBM, *Neurology* 56(3):323, 2001.
3. Love LA et al: A new approach to the classification of idiopathic inflammatory myopathy: myositis specific autoantibodies define useful homogenous patient groups, *Medicine (Baltimore)* 70:360, 1991.
4. Leff RL et al: The treatment of inclusion body myositis: a retrospective review and a randomised prospective trial of immunosuppressive therapy, *Medicine (Baltimore)* 72:225-235, 1993.

SUGGESTED READINGS

Alexandrescu DT et al: Steroid-responsive inclusion body myositis associated with endometrial cancer, *Clin Exp Rheumatol* 23(1):93-96, 2005.

Cherin P et al: Intravenous immunoglobulin for dysphagia of inclusion body myositis, *Neurology* 58:326, 2002.

Dalakas MC: Sporadic inclusion body myositis—diagnosis, pathogenesis and therapeutic strategies, *Nat Clin Pract Neurol* 2(8):437, 2006.

Katirji B et al: *Neuromuscular disorders in clinical practice,* Boston, 2002, Butterworth-Heinemann, pp 1169-1190.

Liu LW, Tarnopolsky M, Armstrong D: Injection of botulinum toxin A to the upper esophageal sphincter for oropharyngeal dysphagia in two patients with inclusion body myositis, *Can J Gastroenterol* 18(6):397-399, 2004.

Lotz BP et al: Inclusion body myositis: observation in 40 patients, *Brain* 112:727, 1989.

Muscle Study Group: Randomized pilot trial of betaINF1a (Avonex) in patients with inclusion body myositis, *Neurology* 57(9): 1566, 2001.

Muscle Study Group: Randomized pilot trial of high-dose beta INF-1a in patients with inclusion body myositis, *Neurology* 63(4):718, 2004.

Rutkove SB et al: A pilot randomized trial of oxandrolone in inclusion body myositis, *Neurology* 58:1081, 2002.

Sayers ME et al: Inclusion body myositis: analysis of 32 cases, *J Rheumatol* 19:1385, 1992.

Tawil R, Griggs RC: Inclusion body myositis, *Curr Opin Rheumatol* 14:653-657, 2002.

Toepfer M et al: Expression of chemokines in normal muscle and inflammatory myopathies, *Neurology* 50:A413, 1998.

AUTHOR: **MUSTAFA A. HAMMAD, M.D.**

BASIC INFORMATION

DEFINITION

Incontinence is the involuntary loss of urine.

ICD-9CM CODES
788.3 Incontinence
625.6 Stress incontinence
788.33 Mixed stress and urge incontinence
788.32 Male incontinence
788.39 Neurogenic incontinence
307.6 Nonorganic origin

EPIDEMIOLOGY & DEMOGRAPHICS

INCIDENCE/PREVALENCE: In the general population between the ages of 15 and 64 yr, 1.5% to 5% of men and 10% to 25% of women will suffer from incontinence. In the nursing home population, 50% of the population suffers some degree of incontinence. Nearly 20% of children through the midteenage years have episodes of urinary incontinence.

CLINICAL, PSYCHOLOGIC, & SOCIAL IMPACT

Less than 50% of the individuals with incontinence living in the community consult health care providers, preferring to "suffer silently," turning to "home remedies," commercially available absorbent materials, and supportive aids. As their condition worsens, they become depressed, sacrifice their independence, suffer from recurrent urinary tract infection and its sequelae, limit their social interaction, refrain from sexual intimacy, and become homebound. In terms of costs, for all ages living in the community, it is estimated that $7 billion is spent for incontinence annually.

MAJOR TYPES OF INCONTINENCE

TRANSIENT INCONTINENCE: Incontinence occurring as a result or reaction to an acute medical problem affecting the lower urinary tract. Many of these problems can be reversed with treatment of the underlying problem.

URGE INCONTINENCE: Involuntary loss of urine associated with an abrupt and strong desire to void. It is usually associated with involuntary detrusor contractions on urodynamic investigation. In *neurologically impaired patients,* the involuntary detrusor contraction is referred to as *detrusor hyperreflexia*. In *neurologically normal patients* the involuntary contraction is called *detrusor instability*.

STRESS INCONTINENCE: The involuntary loss of urine with physical activities that increase abdominal pressure in the absence of a detrusor contraction or an overdistended bladder. Classification of stress incontinence:

Type 0: Complaint of incontinence without demonstration of leakage

Type I: Incontinence in response to stress but little descent of the bladder neck and urethra

Type II: Incontinence in response to stress with >2 cm descent of the bladder neck and urethra

Type III: Bladder neck and urethra wide open without bladder contraction; intrinsic sphincter deficiency; and denervation of the urethra. The most common causes: urethral hypermobility and displacement of the bladder neck with exertion, intrinsic sphincter deficiency from failed antiincontinence surgery, prostatectomy, radiation, cord lesions, epispadias, or myelomeningocele

OVERFLOW INCONTINENCE: Loss of urine resulting from overdistention of the bladder with resultant "overflow" or "spilling" of the urine. Causes: hypotonic-to-atonic bladder resulting from drug effect, fecal impaction, or neurologic conditions such as diabetes, spinal cord injury, surgery, vitamin B_{12} deficiency. It is also caused by obstruction at the bladder neck and urethra. In this situation, prostatism, prostatic cancer, urethral stenosis, antiincontinence surgery, pelvic prolapse, and detrusor-sphincter dyssynergia cause the incontinence.

FUNCTIONAL INCONTINENCE: Involuntary loss of urine resulting from chronic impairments of physical and/or cognitive functioning. This is a diagnosis of exclusion. The condition can sometimes be improved or cured by improving the patient's functional status, treating comorbidities, changing medications, reducing environmental barriers, etc.

MIXED STRESS AND URGE INCONTINENCE

SENSORY URGENCY INCONTINENCE: Involuntary loss of urine as a result of decreased bladder compliance and increased intravesical pressures accompanied by severe urgency and bladder hypersensitivity without detrusor overactivity. This is seen with radiation cystitis, interstitial cystitis, eosinophilic cystitis, myelomeningocele, and radical pelvic surgery. Nephropathy can occur as a complication of this vesicoureteral reflux.

SPHINCTERIC INCONTINENCE:

Urethral Hypermobility: The basic abnormality is a weakness of pelvic floor support. Because of this weakness, during increases in abdominal pressure there is rotational descent of the vesical neck and proximal urethra. If the urethra opens concomitantly, stress urinary incontinence ensues. Urethral hypermobility is often present in women who are not incontinent. Its mere presence is not sufficient evidence to make the diagnosis of sphincteric abnormality unless incontinence is shown.

Intrinsic Sphincter Deficiency: There is an intrinsic malfunction of the sphincter itself. It is characterized by an open vesical neck at rest and a low leak point pressure (<65 cm water). Urethral hypermobility and intrinsic sphincter deficiency may coexist in the same patient. Causes of intrinsic sphincter deficiency are previous pelvic surgery, antiincontinence surgery, urethral diverticulectomy, radical hysterectomy, abdominoperineal resection of the rectum, urethrotomy, Y-V plasty of the vesical neck, myelodysplasia, anterior spinal artery syndrome, lumbo-sacral disease, aging, and hyperestrogenism.

DIAGNOSIS

HISTORY

- History of present illness, psychosocial factors, congenital disorders, access issues for the physically challenged, neurologic disorders, and disorders pertinent to the urologic tract
- Review of prescription and nonprescription medications
- Voiding diary to assess total voided volume, frequency of micturition, mean volume voided, largest single volume, diurnal distribution, nature and severity of incontinence

WORKUP

- Physical examination including general examination, gait of the patient (neuromuscular deficits), estrogen status, vaginal examination to include the periurethral region, evaluation for cystocele, rectocele, and enterocele
- Pelvic floor strength assessment
- Rectal examination to assess sphincter tone and bulbocavernosus reflex
- Neurologic examination
- Postvoid residual check using bladder scan or catheter

LABORATORY TESTS

Urinalysis, urine culture, urine cytology, BUN, and creatinine

IMAGING STUDIES

- KUB to assess bony skeleton
- IVP to rule out upper tract abnormalities, developmental anomalies, bladder configuration, and fistula
- Renal ultrasound if dye study is contraindicated

SPECIALIZED STUDIES

Simple cystometrogram, complex urodynamics including leak point pressures and uroflowmetry, endoscopic evaluation, and cystogram

TREATMENT

TRANSIENT INCONTINENCE

Treatment of underlying medical conditions and behavioral therapy to include habit training and timed voiding

URGE INCONTINENCE

Bladder relaxants (i.e., tolterodine [Detrol], oxybutynin [Ditropan], imipramine), trospium chloride, estrogen, biofeedback, Kegel exercises, and surgical removal of obstructing or other pathologic lesions

STRESS INCONTINENCE

Pelvic floor exercises, Kegel exercises, α-adrenergic agonists (i.e., ephedrine), estrogen, biofeedback

CYSTOURETHROPEXY: Marshall-Marchetti-Krantz procedure, Burch procedure, Raz procedure, Stamey-Raz procedure, Gittes procedure, in situ transvaginal sling, pubovaginal sling with autologous or cadaver graft, laparoscopic Burch procedure, laparoscopic sling, tension-free vaginal tape (TVT)

- For intrinsic sphincter deficiency: bulking agents (e.g., collagen), sling, and artificial sphincter

OVERFLOW INCONTINENCE

Surgical removal of any obstructing lesions, clean intermittent catheterization, and indwelling catheter

FUNCTIONAL INCONTINENCE

Behavioral training to include habit training and timed voiding, incontinence undergarments and pads, external collecting devices, and environmental manipulation

MIXED URGENCY AND STRESS INCONTINENCE

Use of measures recommended in the management of stress and urge incontinence

SENSORY URGENCY

Bladder relaxants (e.g., anticholinergics, muscle relaxants, and tricyclic antidepressants), behavior therapy to include habit training and timed voiding, cystoscopy and hydrodilation

SPHINCTERIC DEFICIENCY

Urethral bulking agents, sling procedure, artificial sphincter, mechanical clamp, and external collection devices

PEARLS & CONSIDERATIONS

COMMENTS

Other forms of incontinence:

NOCTURNAL ENURESIS: (ICD-9CM Code: 788.3) Can be caused by sphincter abnormalities and detrusor overactivity; can occur as idiopathic, neurogenic, and with outlet obstruction

POSTVOID DRIBBLE: (ICD-9CM Code: 599.2) A postsphincteric collection of urine that is seen with urethral diverticulum and can be idiopathic

EXTRAURETHRAL INCONTINENCE: Enterovesical (ICD-9CM Codes: 596.1 and 596.2), urethral (ICD-9CM Code: 599.1), also known as fistula

CONDITIONS THAT PREDISPOSE TO SURGICAL FAILURE: Advanced age, postmenopausal state, hysterectomy, prior failed incontinence surgery, concurrent detrusor instability, abnormal perineal electromyography, pelvic radiation

EVIDENCE

A systematic review found that approximately 50% of women treated with estrogen were cured or improved compared with approximately 25% on placebo. Combination estrogen/progestogen did not have the same cure or improvement rate. There was no evidence about long-term effects and the data were insufficient to address issues such as type of estrogen or mode of delivery.[1] Ⓐ

There is limited evidence to suggest that use of an adrenergic agonist is better than placebo in women with urinary incontinence. However, patients may suffer minor or rare but serious side effects such as cardiac arrhythmias and hypertension.[2] Ⓑ

A systematic review found that pelvic floor muscle training (PFMT) was more effective than no treatment or placebo for treating women with stress or mixed urinary incontinence. Methodologic problems with the trials included in this review limits the confidence that can be placed in these findings.[3] Ⓑ

A systematic review found limited evidence that weighted vaginal cones were more effective than no active treatment for the management of stress incontinence in women. Weighted cones may have similar efficacy to PFMT and electrostimulation. These conclusions are tentative.[4] Ⓑ

A systematic review and subsequent randomized controlled trials in women with stress incontinence have consistently found that pelvic floor electrical stimulation reduces the severity and frequency of incontinence episodes after 6 weeks compared with sham or no treatment.[5] Ⓐ

A systematic review found limited evidence suggesting that prompted voiding decreased incontinent episodes in elderly people in the short term. There was also suggestive but inconclusive evidence of short-term benefit when oxybutynin was combined with prompted voiding.[6] Ⓐ

A systematic review found limited evidence suggesting that bladder training may be helpful for the treatment of urge incontinence.[7] Ⓑ

A systematic review found that open retropubic colposuspension was the most effective treatment for stress incontinence in women. Urinary continence was achieved in approximately 85% to 90% of women in the first year after treatment, and approximately 70% at 5 years.[8] Ⓐ

A systematic review found that suburethral sling procedures have similar short-term cure rates to open abdominal retropubic suspension for women with stress or mixed urinary incontinence. This conclusion mainly reflects the preliminary results from one large trial on the tension-free vaginal tape (TVT) sling procedure.[9] Ⓐ

Evidence-Based References

1. Moehrer B, Hextall A, Jackson S: Oestrogens for urinary incontinence in women (Cochrane Review). Reviewed in: Cochrane Library, 1, Chichester, UK, 2004, John Wiley. Ⓐ
2. Alhasso A et al: Adrenergic drugs for urinary incontinence in adults (Cochrane Review). Reviewed in: Cochrane Library, 1, Chichester, UK, 2004, John Wiley. Ⓑ
3. Hay-Smith EJC et al: Pelvic floor muscle training for urinary incontinence in women (Cochrane Review). Reviewed in: Cochrane Library, 1, Chichester, UK, 2004, John Wiley. Ⓑ
4. Herbison P, Plevnik S, Mantle J: Weighted vaginal cones for urinary incontinence (Cochrane Review). Reviewed in: Cochrane Library, 1, Chichester, UK, 2004, John Wiley. Ⓑ
5. Bazian Ltd: Stress incontinence. Reviewed in: 10, 2003; web version only, London, BMJ Publishing Group. Ⓐ
6. Eustice S, Roe B, Paterson J: Prompted voiding for the management of urinary incontinence in adults (Cochrane Review). Reviewed in: Cochrane Library, 1, Chichester, UK, 2004, John Wiley. Ⓐ
7. Wallace SA et al: Bladder training for urinary incontinence in adults (Cochrane Review). Reviewed in: Cochrane Library, 1, Chichester, UK, 2004, John Wiley. Ⓑ
8. Lapitan MC, Cody DJ, Grant AM: Open retropubic colposuspension for urinary incontinence in women (Cochrane Review). Reviewed in: Cochrane Library, 1, Chichester, UK, 2004, John Wiley. Ⓐ
9. Bezzerra CA, Bruschini H, Cody DJ: Suburethral sling operations for urinary incontinence in women (Cochrane Review). Reviewed in: Cochrane Library, 1, Chichester, UK, 2004, John Wiley. Ⓐ

SUGGESTED READINGS

Holdroyd-Leduc JM et al: What type of urinary incontinence does this woman have? *JAMA* 299(12):1446-1456, 2008.

Rogers RG: Urinary stress incontinence in women, *N Engl J Med* 358:1029-1036, 2008.

Shamliyan TA et al: Systematic review: randomized controlled trials of nonsurgical treatment for urinary incontinence in women, *Ann Intern Med* 148:459-473, 2008.

AUTHORS: **PHILIP J. ALIOTTA, M.D., M.S.H.A.,** and **RUBEN ALVERO, M.D.**

BASIC INFORMATION

DEFINITION

Influenza is an acute febrile illness caused by infection with influenza type A or B virus.

SYNONYMS

Flu

ICD-9CM CODES
487.1 Influenza

EPIDEMIOLOGY & DEMOGRAPHICS

INCIDENCE (IN U.S.): Annual incidence of influenza-related deaths is approximately 20,000 deaths/yr
PEAK INCIDENCE: Winter outbreaks lasting 5 to 6 wk
PREDOMINANT SEX: Male = female
PREDOMINANT AGE: Attack rates are higher among children than adults, although children are less prone to develop pulmonary complications

PHYSICAL FINDINGS & CLINICAL PRESENTATION

- "Classic flu" is characterized by abrupt onset of fever, headache, myalgias, anorexia, and malaise after a 1- to 2-day incubation period.
- Clinical syndromes are similar to those produced by other respiratory viruses, including pharyngitis, common colds, tracheobronchitis, bronchiolitis, croup.
- Respiratory symptoms such as cough, sore throat, and nasal discharge are usually present at the onset of illness, but systemic symptoms predominate.
- Elderly patients may experience fever, weakness, and confusion without any respiratory complaints.
- Acute deterioration to status asthmaticus may occur in patients with asthma.
- Influenza pneumonia: rapidly progressive cough, dyspnea, and cyanosis may occur after typical flu onset. This may be caused by primary influenza pneumonia or secondary bacterial pneumonia (often pneumococcal or staphylococcal infection).

ETIOLOGY

- Variation in the surface antigens of the influenza virus, hemagglutinin (HA) and neuraminidase (NA), leading to infection with variants to which resistance is inadequate in the population at risk
- Transmitted by small-particle aerosols and deposited on the respiratory tract epithelium

DIAGNOSIS

DIFFERENTIAL DIAGNOSIS

- Respiratory syncytial virus, adenovirus, parainfluenza virus infection
- Secondary bacterial pneumonia or mixed bacterial-viral pneumonia

WORKUP

- Virus isolation from nasal or throat swab or sputum specimens is the most rapid diagnostic method in the setting of acute illness.
- Specimens are placed into virus transport medium and processed by a reference laboratory.
- For serologic diagnosis:
  1. Paired serum specimens, acute and convalescent, the latter obtained 10 to 20 days later
  2. Fourfold rises or falls in the titer of antibodies (various techniques) considered diagnostic of recent infection

LABORATORY TESTS

Septic syndrome presentation: CBC, ABG analysis, blood cultures

IMAGING STUDIES

- Chest x-ray examination to demonstrate findings of viral pneumonia: peribronchial and patchy interstitial infiltrates in multiple lobes with atelectasis
- Possible progression to diffuse interstitial pneumonitis

TREATMENT

NONPHARMACOLOGIC THERAPY

- Bed rest
- Hydration

ACUTE GENERAL Rx

- Supportive care: antipyretics—*Avoid use of aspirin in children because of the association with Reye's syndrome*
- Antibiotics if bacterial pneumonia is proven or suspected
- Amantadine (100 mg PO bid for children >10 yr and adults <65 yr; once daily in patients >65 yr) and rimantadine (same dose schedule as amantadine)
  1. Further dose adjustments needed with renal insufficiency
  2. Fewer CNS side effects with rimantadine
- Neuraminidase inhibitors block release of virions from infected cells, resulting in shortened duration of symptoms and decrease in complications; effective against both influenza A and B
  1. Zanamivir, administered via inhaler, 10 mg bid
  2. Oseltamivir, administered orally, 75 mg by mouth bid for 5 days
- Placebo-controlled studies have suggested that antiviral therapy with any of the above mentioned agents must be initiated within 1 to 2 days of the onset of symptoms and reduces the duration of illness by approximately 1 day
- Oseltamivir resistance has developed on therapy in individuals with avian flu (H5, N1) in Asia, and this is associated with poor outcome.

DISPOSITION

Patients are hospitalized if signs of pneumonia are present.

REFERRAL

Infectious disease and/or pulmonary consultation when influenza pneumonia is suspected

PEARLS & CONSIDERATIONS

COMMENTS

- Prevention of influenza in patients at high risk is an important goal of primary care.
- Vaccines reduce the risk of infection and the severity of illness.
  1. Antigenic composition of the vaccine is updated annually.
  2. Vaccination should be given at the start of the flu season (October) for the following groups:
     a. Adults ≥50 yr
     b. Adults and children with chronic cardiac or pulmonary disease, including asthma
     c. Adults and children with illness requiring frequent follow-up (e.g., hemoglobinopathies, diabetes mellitus)
     d. Children ages 6 to 59 mo and all those receiving long-term aspirin therapy
     e. Immunocompromised patients (including HIV-infected persons)
     f. Household contacts and caregivers of persons in the previous groups
     g. Health care workers, pregnant women
  3. Only contraindication to vaccination is hypersensitivity to hen's eggs.
  4. Special efforts should be made to vaccinate high-risk patients <65 yr, only 10% to 15% of whom are vaccinated each year.
- Chemoprophylaxis:
  1. Amantadine and rimantadine approved for prophylaxis against influenza A; they are ineffective against influenza B (NOTE: The avian flu strains [H5N1] are all intrinsically resistant to amantidine and rimantadine)
  2. Consider (after the current circulating strain of influenza has been shown to be sensitive):
     a. For high-risk patients in whom vaccination is contraindicated
     b. When the available vaccine is known not to include the circulating strain

c. To provide added protection to immunosuppressed patients likely to have a diminished response to vaccination
d. In the setting of an outbreak, when immediate protection of unvaccinated or recently vaccinated patients is desired
3. Give for 2 wk in the case of late vaccination and for the duration of the flu season in all other patients

EVIDENCE

EBM

There is evidence that amantadine and rimantadine are effective in the prevention of influenza and in reducing the duration of symptoms.

Amantadine has been shown, in adults, to prevent 25% of cases of influenza-like illness and 61% of cases of influenza A, as well as reducing duration of fever by 1 day.[1] Ⓐ

Rimantadine is comparably effective, although there are fewer trials and the results for prevention are not statistically significant.[1] Ⓐ

Both agents cause significant gastrointestinal adverse effects, but side effects of the central nervous system and study withdrawals have been significantly more common with amantadine than with rimantadine.[1] Ⓐ

There is evidence for the efficacy of neuraminidase inhibitors, such as zanamivir and oseltamivir, in reducing the duration of symptoms.

Neuraminidase inhibitors have been shown to reduce the duration of symptoms by 1 day in otherwise healthy adults with influenza infection. They are also effective for the prevention of influenza A and influenza B: they are 75% effective in preventing naturally occurring cases of clinically defined influenza and 60% effective in preventing cases of laboratory-confirmed influenza.[2] Ⓐ

Similarly, zanamivir (usually commenced within 48 hr of symptom onset) has been found by a systematic review to be significantly more effective than placebo in reducing the time to resolution of symptoms.[3] Ⓐ

However, a subsequent randomized controlled trial (RCT) found that although zanamivir reduced the time to alleviation of symptoms compared with placebo in healthy populations, the difference was not significant.[4] Ⓐ

Oseltamivir has been shown to be significantly more effective than placebo at reducing the time to alleviation of symptoms in otherwise healthy patients, but the difference is less clear in high-risk patients.[5] Ⓐ

No significant difference has been found between patients receiving oseltamivir and patients receiving placebo in terms of the need for antibiotics for complications of influenza.[5] Ⓐ

Evidence-Based References

1. Jefferson TO et al: Amantadine and rimantadine for preventing and treating influenza A in adults, *Cochrane Database Syst Rev* 3, 2004. Ⓐ
2. Jefferson T et al: Neuraminidase inhibitors for preventing and treating influenza in healthy adults, *Cochrane Database Syst Rev* 4, 1999. Ⓐ
3. Burls A et al: Zanamivir for the treatment of influenza in adults, West Midlands Development and Evaluation Service. Birmingham, 2000. Report for the National Institute for Clinical Excellence (NICE). Reviewed in: 12, 2004; web version only. Ⓐ
4. Puhakka T et al: Zanamivir: a significant reduction in viral load during treatment in military conscripts with influenza, *Scand J Infect Dis* 35:52, 2003. Reviewed in: *Clin Evid* 12, 2004; web version only. Ⓐ
5. Cooper NJ et al: Effectiveness of neuraminidase inhibitors in treatment and prevention of influenza A and B: systematic review and meta-analyses of randomised controlled trials, *BMJ* 326:1235, 2003. Reviewed in: *Clin Evid* 12, 2004; web version only. Ⓐ

SUGGESTED READINGS

Centers for Disease Control: Prevention and control of influenza, *MMWR* 55(RR-10):1, 2006.

De Jong M et al: Fatal outcome of human influenza A (H5N1) is associated with high viral load and hypercytokinemia, *Nature Med* 10:1038, 2006.

De Jong MD et al: Oseltamivir resistance during treatment of influenza A (H5N1) infection, *N Engl J Med* 353(25):2667, 2006.

WHO Global influenza program surveillance network: Evolution of H5N1 avian influenza viruses in Asia, *Emerg Infect Dis* 11:1515, 2005.

AUTHORS: **CLAUDIA L. DADE, M.D., GLENN G. FORT, M.D., M.P.H.,** and **DENNIS J. MIKOLICH, M.D.**

BASIC INFORMATION

DEFINITION

Avian influenza is a virus originating in birds that has the capacity to infect humans. The prior influenza pandemics of the twentieth century (from the devastating 1918 pandemic, in which between 40 million and 100 million people died, to the lesser pandemics of 1957 and 1968, with 1 million to 6 million deaths) were caused by highly virulent, efficiently transmitted influenzas that evolved from avian strains. The highly pathogenic avian influenza A (H5N1), which is capable of only incidentally infecting humans, but with a near 50% mortality rate, threatens to bring the next pandemic flu. It emerged in 1997 in Hong Kong, and by mid 2007 had infected more than 300 humans as it spread via migrating waterfowl from Asia to Europe and Africa.

SYNONYMS

Bird flu, pandemic flu

ICD-9-CM CODES
488

EPIDEMIOLOGY & DEMOGRAPHICS

Avian influenza A H5N1 is an influenza virus, related to those that bring our yearly flu, against which populations are routinely vaccinated. Influenza viruses are enveloped RNA viruses with segmented genomes and great antigenic diversity. They are categorized by their core proteins (A, B, C), species of origin (avian, swine), geographic site of isolation, serial number, and influenza subtypes based on the major antigenic surface glycoproteins, hemaglutinin (HA), and neuraminidase (NA).

Often human and avian viruses meet and resort in a pig respiratory system. Southeast Asia is often the birthplace of new flu strains because birds, pigs, and people live in close proximity. It is where avian influenza H5N1 emerged, first infecting domestic poultry, then wild birds that migrated across Eurasia. It is transmitted directly from birds to their keepers. Antigenic drift or shift may allow avian influenza A H5N1 to gain the ability to be easily transmissible from human to human, transforming it from a highly virulent influenza strain to a pandemic flu.

PREDOMINANT AGE: Children and young adults

RISK FACTORS: Poultry work, possibly swine work (in case of reassortment), travel to affected areas

PHYSICAL FINDINGS & CLINICAL PRESENTATION

- Symptoms include fever of at least 100.4° F (38° C) with leukopenia or lymphopenia, nearly always followed by viral pneumonia with escalating respiratory distress.
- Ventilatory support is often required within 48 hr of hospitalization for acute respiratory distress syndrome (ARDS).
- Symptom onset is 2 to 5 days after exposure, longer than with human influenza.
- Respiratory symptoms may also be accompanied by watery diarrhea and rarely encephalopathy.
- Complications include respiratory failure, renal dysfunction, cardiac compromise, pulmonary hemorrhage, pneumothorax, and multiorgan failure. A common cause of death is superinfection with bacterial pneumonias.

ETIOLOGY

H5N1 resists host antiviral cytokines, inducing excessive host proinflammatory responses. It may cause death by "cytokine storm" rather than by inherent pathogenecity. It attaches to sialic acid molecules via an alpha 2 to 3 galactose receptor (common in birds), also found in human alveoli, leading to heavy damage to lower lungs. It causes severe pulmonary injury with diffuse alveolar damage. In the bone marrow, there is a reactive histiocytosis with hemophagocytosis that may lead to pancytopenia.

DIAGNOSIS

DIFFERENTIAL DIAGNOSIS

- Atypical pneumonia, typical respiratory virus infections (e.g., influenza, RSV), SARS, upper respiratory infection with conjunctivitis (e.g., adenovirus).
- Clinical symptoms indistinguishable from other illnesses.

WORKUP

Comprehensive travel, occupational, and epidemiologic history

LABORATORY TESTS

- AST, ALT, BUN/Cr, CBC.
- Throat swab within 3 days of onset of symptoms to be sent for viral culture and PCR assay for avian influenza A H5N1 RNA with appropriate biosafety precautions. The throat swab is more effective than nasal swabs because avian flu preferentially infects the throat and lower respiratory tract. In the U.S., the FDA has approved the release of influenza H/A5 (Asian lineage) Virus Real-Time Reverse Transcription-PCR Primer and Probe Set for more than 140 labs in 50 states, which will return preliminary results in 4 hours.
- High-risk patients who must be tested include those with history of travel within 10 days of symptom onset to a country with documented H5N1 avian flu, as well as patients with radiographically confirmed pneumonia, ARDS, or severe respiratory illness without alternate etiology.
- Low-risk patients are those who have contact with domestic poultry, or contact with people who have traveled to a country with documented H5N1 avian flu, who have fever >38° C and cough/sore throat/shortness of breath.

IMAGING STUDIES

- Chest x-rays detect infiltrates a median of 7 days after onset of fever. They may be diffuse, multifocal/patchy infiltrates, or interstitial infiltrates, or segmental/lobular consolidation. Progression to respiratory failure is indicated by diffuse bilateral ground glass infiltrates
- Conduct ARDS imaging studies.

TREATMENT

Vaccines and antivirals are the usual means for preventing and treating flu, but there are limited supplies. It is difficult to manufacture avian influenza vaccines because the usual means of production using embryonated hens' eggs does not work; the bird flu kills the eggs. Alternative vaccine production methods are under experimentation.

NONPHARMACOLOGIC THERAPY

- N95 particulate masks should help prevent person-to-person transmission of H5N1. Surgical masks prevent only large-droplet transmission.
- In preparation for pandemic flu, increase worldwide surveillance and disease reporting. Kill infected birds. Increase the numbers of available ICU beds with mechanical ventilators and increase emergency capacity. Educate medical personnel and the public. Produce vaccines.
- In response, use influenza surveillance, social distancing (school closures), travel restrictions, quarantine, respirator masks, communications networking, and international teamwork to cordon off affected areas.

ACUTE GENERAL RX

- The neuraminidase inhibitor oseltamivir can reduce the severity and duration of symptoms if treatment is initiated in the first 48 hr after symptom onset.
  - Treatment: adults 75 mg po twice daily × 5 days
  - Postexposure prophylaxis: 75 mg po daily × 7 to 10 days
- H5N1 demonstrates amantadine and rimantadine resistance.

PEARLS & CONSIDERATIONS

The threat of pandemic has been called a "public health crisis" by the World Health Organization. Health care workers should stay abreast of developments, in terms of the epidemiology, preventive measures, and treatments.

PREVENTION

See "Nonpharmacologic Treatment"

PATIENT/FAMILY EDUCATION

The American Council on Science and Health's publication "Avian Influenza: What You Need to Know" is available at http://acsh.org/publications/pubid.1294/pub_detail.asp.

SUGGESTED READINGS

Arabi Y et al: The critically ill avian influenza A (H5N1) patient, *Crit Care Med* 35(5):1397, 2007.

Brundage JF: Interactions between influenza and bacterial respiratory pathogens: implications for pandemic preparedness, *Lancet Infect Dis* 6:303, 2006.

Cox MM: Vaccines in development against avian influenza, *Minerva Med* 98(2):145, 2007.

Juckett G: Avian influenza: preparing for a pandemic, *Am Fam Phys* 74(5): 783, 2006.

Stephenson I, Gust I, et al: Development of vaccines against influenza H5, *Lancet Infect Dis* 6: 458, 2006.

U.S. Centers for Disease Control: Avian influenza. Available at www.cdc.gov/flu/avian.

U.S. Government avian and pandemic flu information. Available at www.pandemicflu.gov.

WHO Rapid Advice Guidelines for pharmacological management of sporadic human infection with avian influenza A (H5N1) virus, *Lancet Infect Dis* 7(1):21, 2007.

Writing Committee of the Second World Health Organization: Consultation on clinical aspects of human infection with avian influenza A (H5N1) virus: update on avian influenza A (H5N1) virus infections in humans, *N Engl J Med* 358:261-273, 2008.

AUTHOR: **KOHAR JONES, M.D.**

BASIC INFORMATION

DEFINITION

Insomnia is a disturbance of initiating or maintaining sleep. Restless, nonrestorative sleep may also be described as insomnia. The disturbance may be purely subjective without daytime impairment or may be objectively measurable with daytime consequences of sleepiness and functional impairment.

SYNONYMS

Sleeplessness

Sleep disorder, sleep disturbance, dysomnia (Note: The terms *sleep disorder, sleep disturbance,* and *dysomnia* are generic and can refer to disorders of wakefulness [hypersomnia] or sleep-related behavior disorders [parasomnias]).

ICD-9CM CODES
780.52 Insomnia
780.51 Insomnia with sleep apnea
307.41 Insomnia, nonorganic origin
307.42 Insomnia, persistent (primary)
307.41 Insomnia, transient
307.49 Subjective complaint
DSM IV-TR Codes:
307.42 Primary insomnia
307.45 Circadian rhythm disorders
780.52 Insomnia due to a general medical condition
291.89 and 292.89 Substance-induced insomnia

EPIDEMIOLOGY & DEMOGRAPHICS

INCIDENCE (IN U.S.): 30% to 45% of adults experience insomnia per year.

PREVALENCE (IN U.S.): 1% to 15% of all adults develop persistent insomnia, 25% of older adults.

PREDOMINANT SEX: More common in women.

PREDOMINANT AGE: Transient insomnia can occur at any age, persistent insomnia is more common >60 yr.

GENETICS: Insomnia can run in families and may be genetically influenced. Sleep characteristics in monozygous twins are more similar than in dizygote twins. Some sleep disorders, such as circadian rhythm disorders and narcolepsy, have been traced to specific genes.

PHYSICAL FINDINGS & CLINICAL PRESENTATION

- Difficulty falling asleep, difficulty staying asleep, early morning awakening, restless or nonrestorative sleep, or difficulty sleeping at desired times.
- May have daytime sleepiness or fatigue.
- Symptoms may be acute and self-limited, chronic but intermittent, or chronic and frequent.

ETIOLOGY

- Transient insomnia:
  1. Stress
  2. Illness
  3. Travel (across time zones)
  4. Environmental disruptions (noise, heat, cold, poor bedding, unfamiliar surroundings, etc.)
- Persistent insomnia:
  1. Mood and anxiety disorders (depression, hypomania/mania, PTSD)
  2. Primary or psychophysiologic insomnia (with or without poor sleep hygiene)
  3. Sleep-related breathing disorders (e.g., obstructive apnea and hypopnea, increased upper airway resistance)
  4. Chronobiologic (also known as circadian rhythm) disorder (delayed sleep phase, advanced sleep phase, shift work, free-running rhythm secondary to blindness)
  5. Drug and alcohol abuse
  6. Restless legs syndrome and periodic leg movements
  7. Neurodegenerative (Alzheimer's disease, Parkinson's disease, etc.)
  8. Medical (pain, GERD, nocturia, orthopnea, medications, etc.)

DIAGNOSIS

DIFFERENTIAL DIAGNOSIS

Primary or psychophysiologic insomnia is diagnosed when other etiologies (see "Etiology") are ruled out. Primary insomnia may be related to counterproductive sleep hygiene, hyperarousal, or insufficient sleep drive.

WORKUP

- History (with bed partner interview, if possible)
- Sleep diary for 2 wk to document nightly sleep quality and daytime sleepiness or fatigue (sample sleep diary can be downloaded from the National Sleep Foundation website: www.sleepfoundation.org)
- Validated sleep-quality rating scale (optional)
  1. Pittsburgh Sleep Quality Index or Insomnia Severity Index
  2. Epworth Sleepiness Scale (see Daytime Sleepiness Test at www. sleepfoundation.org)

LABORATORY TESTS

- Evaluate for anemia, uremia (for restless legs), thyroid function (if other signs present).
- Polysomnography (in home or in sleep lab) for symptoms suggesting something other than primary insomnia: daytime sleepiness (obstructive sleep apnea, narcolepsy), nonrestorative sleep (periodic leg movements), or sleep behavior suggesting parasomnia (somnambulism, REM sleep behavior).

IMAGING STUDIES

- Not generally helpful for insomnia
- Brain CT or MRI for severe daytime sleepiness or acute onset

TREATMENT

NONPHARMACOLOGIC THERAPY

- Sleep hygiene measures (Box 1-8)
- Cognitive-behavioral therapy (CBT) can address anxiety and insomnia-perpetuating behaviors. CBT has been shown to reduce time to fall asleep and time awake during the night in placebo-controlled trials and can reduce reliance on sleep medications.
- The cognitive component of CBT involves education about sleep and insomnia to address concerns that might increase anxiety around sleeplessness. The behavioral component attempts to change habits that may perpetuate insomnia. The four components are *relaxation techniques; stimulus control* to address the conditioned cues that create arousal when attempting to sleep; *bed restriction* to sleep and sex and not tossing and turning, watching TV, reading, etc.; and improved *sleep hygiene* practices such as increased daytime exercise, avoiding heavy meals at night, and reduce or eliminate caffeine, nicotine, and alcohol intake.

BOX 1-8 Sleep Habits (Sleep Hygiene Measures) That May Improve Insomnia

1. Reduce caffeine, alcohol, or tobacco late in the day or evening.
2. Avoid heavy meals at night.
3. Increase daytime activity.
4. Increase daytime exposure to natural light.
5. Take warm bath as part of bedtime ritual.
6. Restrict bed to sleep and sex.
7. Get out of bed if not asleep after 30 minutes and return when drowsy.
8. Repeat above if awakened during the night.
9. Maintain regular sleep and wake times.
10. Go to bed with calm mind; resolve arguments or deal with problems earlier in day.

- Increased daytime activity improves sleep, especially in people (of any age) who were previously sedentary. Improvements are seen in total sleep duration, in sleep-onset latency, and in scores on a scale of global sleep quality.
- Insomnia secondary to circadian rhythm disturbances, as in shift workers, many blind individuals (lack of light-dark cycle to synchronize body-clock), adolescents and young adults with delayed sleep phase syndrome, and jet lag can be treated with chronobiological therapies such as bright light exposure, melatonin, or melatonin agonists. These therapies have to be given at specific times of the day or night, and referral to a sleep specialist may be necessary.

ACUTE GENERAL Rx

- Benzodiazepine sedative-hypnotics (e.g., temazepam 7.5 to 30 mg, triazolam 0.125 to 0.25 mg).
- In critical care: lorazepam 0.25 to 0.5 mg po, SL, or IV as needed for sleep. In patients with acute delirium, haloperidol 0.25 to 0.5 mg IV as needed up to 2 mg daily may be less likely to worsen confusion.
- Benzodiazepine receptor agonists zolpidem 5 to 10 mg and zaleplon 5 to 10 mg for sleep-onset insomnia, and zolpidem continuous release formulation 6.25 to 12.5 mg and eszopiclone 1 to 3 mg for maintenance insomnia.
- Melatonin agonist ramelteon 8 mg for sleep-onset insomnia when a mild agent without benzodiazepine side effects is desired.
- Avoid antihistamines except for occasional use.
- Optimize treatment of medical symptoms, especially pain.

CHRONIC Rx

- Controlled trials suggest that CBT is superior to medication for chronic insomnia. Long-term management of insomnia needs ongoing attention to sleep hygiene and other cognitive behavioral approaches for best results.
- Three sedative-hypnotics—zolpidem-continuous release, eszopiclone, and ramelteon—have been studied in 6-mo controlled trials and are FDA approved for chronic use.
- There is some evidence that benzodiazepines and benzodiazepine receptor agonists can be used for chronic insomnia on either intermittent or nightly use with moderate risk of tolerance and dependence but low risk of addiction.
- Sedating antidepressants (e.g., trazodone 25 to 150 mg, mirtazapine 7.5 to 30 mg, amitriptyline 25 to 50 mg) are in widespread use but there are limited data on safety and efficacy for insomnia. Amitriptyline should be avoided if possible in older adults.
- Sedating antipsychotics (e.g., quetiapine 25 to 200 mg, olanzapine 2.5 to 10 mg at night) for severe mood or psychotic disorders associated with insomnia.

COMPLEMENTARY & ALTERNATIVE MEDICINE

Melatonin is the only substance that has been studied in larger controlled trials. It may shorten sleep-onset latency in some individuals but not most. Valerian has been studied in small trials, but like melatonin, appears to be of minimal benefit for insomnia in most people.

DISPOSITION

- Transient insomnia: usually self-limited, but may require follow-up if stress-related or illness-related because of risk of depression or persistent insomnia.
- Persistent insomnia: patients have a chronic and recurrent disorder and will need periodic follow-up to reinforce good sleep hygiene measures and to reassess need for pharmacologic therapies. Increasingly, there is evidence that insomnia is associated with significant negative health effects over time.

REFERRAL

- Excessive daytime sleepiness not obviously due to insomnia (e.g., narcolepsy, sleep-related breathing disorder)
- Nighttime behavior suggestive of a parasomnia (e.g., somnambulism, REM behavior disorder)
- Severe insomnia not responsive to basic interventions

PEARLS & CONSIDERATIONS

COMMENTS

Treatment of insomnia should focus on reducing daytime sleepiness and improving daytime function, rather than trying to achieve the elusive goal of uninterrupted nighttime sleep.

PREVENTION

Not much is known about prevention of insomnia. Effective treatment of transient insomnia may reduce the risk of developing persistent insomnia.

PATIENT/FAMILY EDUCATION

The National Sleep Foundation (www.sleepfoundation.org) is a comprehensive resource for health care providers and patients.

EVIDENCE

EBM

The effects of CBT on reduced time to fall asleep are comparable to sleep medication, although may take several weeks to develop. CBT may be superior to pharmacotherapy for chronic insomnia.[1,2] Ⓐ

Regular, moderate-intensity exercise improves sleep in adults 60 years of age or older with primary insomnia. Improvements are seen in total sleep duration, in sleep-onset latency, and in scores on a scale of global sleep quality.[3] Ⓐ

Melatonin is effective in the prevention and reduction of jet lag, and occasional short-term use appears to be safe.[4] Ⓐ

A systematic review found inconsistent and contradictory evidence for the efficacy of valerian in the treatment of insomnia.[5] Ⓑ

Evidence-Based References

1. Jacobs GD et al: Cognitive behavior therapy and pharmacotherapy for insomnia: a randomized controlled trial and direct comparison, *Arch Int Med* 164(17):1888, 2004.
2. Silber MH: Chronic insomnia, *N Engl J Med* 353:803, 2005.
3. Montgomery P, Dennis J: Physical exercise for sleep problems in adults aged 60+, *Cochrane Database Syst Rev* 4, 2002. Ⓐ
4. Herxheimer A, Petrie KJ: Melatonin for the prevention and treatment of jet lag, *Cochrane Database Syst Rev* 2, 2002. Ⓐ
5. Stevinson C, Ernst E: Valerian for insomnia: a systematic review of randomized clinical trials, *Sleep Medicine* 1:91, 2000.

SUGGESTED READINGS

Carney PR, Berry RB, Geyer JD: *Clinical sleep disorders,* Philadelphia, 2005, Lippincott Williams & Wilkins, 2005.

Ramakrishnan K, Scheid DC: Treatment options for insomnia, *Am Fam Phys* 76(4):517, 2007.

AUTHORS: **MITCHELL D. FELDMAN, M.D., M.PHIL.,** and **CLIFFORD MILO SINGER, M.D.**

BASIC INFORMATION

DEFINITION

Insulinoma is a pancreatic insulin-secreting tumor that causes symptoms associated with hypoglycemia.

ICD-9CM CODES
M8151/0 Insulinoma

EPIDEMIOLOGY & DEMOGRAPHICS

INCIDENCE: 1 case/250,000 persons/yr. Ninety percent of insulinomas are benign.
PREDOMINANT SEX/AGE: Insulinomas occur in both sexes (approximately 60% in women) and at all ages. In the Mayo Clinic series, the median age at diagnosis was 50 yr in sporadic cases but 23 yr in patients with multiple endocrine neoplasia (MEN), type 1.

PHYSICAL FINDINGS & CLINICAL PRESENTATION

Symptoms occur typically in the morning before breakfast (i.e., fasting hypoglycemia as opposed to reactive hypoglycemia, which is not commonly associated with insulinoma)

Neuroglycopenic symptoms	**%**
Various combinations of diplopia, blurred vision, sweating, palpitations, or weakness	85
Confusion or abnormal behavior	80
Unconsciousness or amnesia	53
Grand mal seizures	12
Adrenergic symptoms	**%**
Sweating	43
Tremulousness	23
Hunger, nausea	12
Palpitations	10

ETIOLOGY, PATHOLOGY, PATHOPHYSIOLOGY

- Insulinomas are almost always solitary. Malignant insulinomas account for 5% of the total; they tend to be larger (6 cm). Metastases are usually to the liver (47%), regional lymph nodes (30%), or both.
- Insulinomas are evenly distributed in the head, body, and tail of the pancreas; ectopic insulinomas are rare (1% to 3%). Tumor size: 5% 0.5 cm or less, 34% 0.5 to 1 cm, 53% 1 to 5 cm, 8% >5 cm.
- Histologic classification includes insulinoma in 86% of patients, adenomatosis in 5% to 15%, nesidioblastosis in 4%, and hyperplasia in 1%. Adenomatosis consists of multiple macroadenomas or microadenomas and occurs especially in patients with MEN-1. Nesidioblastosis is also a diffuse lesion, in which islet cells form as buds on ductular structures.

DIAGNOSIS

DIFFERENTIAL DIAGNOSIS (OF FASTING HYPOGLYCEMIA)

HYPERINSULINISM:
- Insulinoma
- Nonpancreatic tumors
- Severe congestive heart failure
- Severe renal insufficiency in non-insulin-dependent diabetes

HEPATIC ENZYME DEFICIENCIES OR DECREASED HEPATIC GLUCOSE OUTPUT (PRIMARILY IN INFANTS, CHILDREN):
- Glycogen storage diseases
- Endocrine hypofunction
- Hypopituitarism
- Addison's disease
- Liver failure
- Alcohol abuse
- Malnutrition

EXOGENOUS AGENTS:
- Sulfonylureas, biguanides
- Insulin
- Other drugs (aspirin, pentamidine)

FUNCTIONAL FASTING HYPOGLYCEMIA: Autoantibodies to insulin receptor or insulin

LABORATORY TESTS

- An overnight fasting blood sugar level combined with a simultaneous plasma insulin, proinsulin, and/or C peptide level will establish the existence of fasting organic hypoglycemia in 60% of patients.
- If single overnight fasting glucose and insulin levels are nondiagnostic, a 72-hr fast is usually done with blood glucose and insulin levels determined at 2- to 4-hr intervals: 75% of patients with insulinoma develop symptoms and a blood sugar level of less than 40 mg/dl by 24 hr, 92% to 98% develop these by 48 hr, and virtually all patients develop them by 72 hr. The test is considered positive for insulinoma if the plasma insulin/glucose ratio is more than 0.3. If, at any point, the patient becomes symptomatic, plasma insulin and glucose values should be obtained and intravenous glucose should be administered.
- Plasma proinsulin, C-peptide, antibodies to insulin, and plasma sulfonylurea levels may be used to rule out factitious use of insulin or hypoglycemic agents or autoantibodies against the insulin receptor or insulin.
- See Section III, "Hypoglycemia," for a description of the diagnostic approach to patients with documented hypoglycemia and elevated insulin.

IMAGING STUDIES

- Abdominal CT scan or MRI detects half to two thirds of insulinomas (abdominal ultrasound is not effective). Should be done only after laboratory tests for insulinoma have confirmed the diagnosis
- Intraoperative ultrasound
- Arteriography
- Octreotide scan

TREATMENT

NONPHARMACOLOGIC THERAPY

- Enucleation of single insulinoma
- Partial pancreatectomy for multiple adenomas

ACUTE GENERAL Rx

- Carbohydrate administration
- Diazoxide directly inhibits insulin release and has an extrapancreatic, hyperglycemic effect that enhances glycogenolysis
- Lanreotide and octreotide (somatostatin analogs)
- Streptozotocin

REFERRAL

At some point in the workup the patient will probably be referred to an endocrinologist and then to a surgeon. A combination of fasting hypoglycemia and elevated insulin level is probably a good point at which to refer.

SUGGESTED READINGS

Axelrod L: Insulinoma: cost-effective care in patients with rare disease, *Ann Intern Med* 123:311, 1995.

Service FJ: Hypoglycemic disorders, *Endocrinol Metab Clin North Am* 28:467, 1999.

Service FJ et al: Functioning insulinoma—incidence, recurrence and long-term survival of patients, *Mayo Clin Proc* 66:711, 1991.

AUTHORS: **FRED F. FERRI, M.D.,** and **TOM J. WACHTEL, M.D.**

BASIC INFORMATION

DEFINITION

The International Continence Society defines interstitial cystitis (IC), otherwise known as painful bladder syndrome (PBS), as a clinical syndrome consisting of suprapubic pain related to bladder filling and accompanied by other symptoms such as increased daytime and nighttime frequency in the absence of proven infection or other obvious pathology.

SYNONYMS

Painful bladder syndrome
Tic douloureux of bladder

ICD-9-CM CODES
595.1

EPIDEMIOLOGY & DEMOGRAPHICS

INCIDENCE: 21 cases/100,000 women per yr, and 4 cases/100,000 men per yr

PREVALENCE:

- 197 per 100,000 women and 41 per 100,000 men in U.S.
- Because the disease is substantially underdiagnosed, it may actually affect 1 in 5 women and 1 in 20 men.
- More than 81% of women diagnosed with chronic pelvic pain (CPP) and up to 84% of men initially diagnosed with chronic prostatitis actually have IC.
- More than 90% of patients diagnosed with overactive bladder who do not respond to anticholinergics are subsequently diagnosed with IC.

PREDOMINANT SEX AND AGE:

- Caucasian women constitute 95% of patients with IC.
- Female:male ratio of 5 to 10:1.
- Most prevalent in fourth and fifth decades of life.

PHYSICAL FINDINGS & CLINICAL PRESENTATION

- Urinary urgency, frequency (>8 in daytime), nocturia (>2 at night), and suprapubic pain are the most common symptoms.
- Suprapubic pain is worse with bladder filling or urinating, and relieved after emptying.
- Dyspareunia.
- Symptoms lasting longer than 6 months.
- Intensity of symptoms waxes and wanes.
- Insidious onset and worsens to the final stage within 5 to 15 yr.
- Exercise, stress, sexual activity, ejaculation, certain foods with high potassium and acids (beer, spices, banana, tomatoes, chocolate, strawberries, artificial sweeteners, oranges, cranberries, caffeine, etc.), menstruation, prolonged sitting, activation of allergies, and so on exacerbates the symptoms.
- Often associated with irritable bowel syndrome, migraine, endometriosis, skin sensitivities, multiple drug allergies, other allergies, vulvodynia, fibromyalgia, chronic fatigue syndrome, systemic lupus erythematosus (SLE), mood disorders, and so on.
- Dysphoric mood.
- Lower abdominal tenderness.
- Tender prostate in digital rectal examination.
- Levator ani tenderness in female.
- Tenderness of anterior vaginal wall/bladder neck in female.

ETIOLOGY

Unknown

DIAGNOSIS

DIFFERENTIAL DIAGNOSIS

- Chronic pelvic pain
- Overactive bladder
- Recurrent UTI
- Endometriosis
- Pelvic adhesions
- Vulvar vestibulitis
- Vulvodynia
- Urethral pain syndrome
- Chronic nonbacterial prostatitis
- Frequent vaginitis
- Benign prostatic hyperplasia

WORKUP

- A clinical diagnosis should be a diagnosis of inclusion.
- There is no definite diagnostic test.
- Validated questionnaires such as Pelvic Pain and Urgency/Frequency scale (PUF), O'Leary-Sant symptoms and problem index, and Wisconsin IC scale. PUF is the most commonly used.
- Voiding diary shows low volume (<100 ml) and high frequency voiding pattern.
- National Institute of Diabetes and Diseases of the Kidney (NIDDK) diagnostic criteria misses 60% of IC patients and is not clinically used any more.
- Anesthetic Bladder Challenge (ABC): Here the symptoms dissipate on instillation of anesthetic cocktail into bladder.
- Cystoscopy and hydrodistension under general anesthesia may show terminal hematuria, glomerulation, Hunner's ulcers, and small bladder capacity of less than 350 ml.
- Bladder biopsy is not essential for diagnosis of IC.
- Parson's Potassium Sensitivity Test (PST).
- Urodynamics are unnecessary in diagnosis of IC.

LABORATORY TESTS

- Urine analysis and culture.
- Urine cytology should be performed if microscopic or gross hematuria is present, or with other risk factors such as smoking, age over 40 years, and other bladder cancer risk factors.
- Culture of sexually transmitted diseases if clinically indicated. Nonbacteriuric patients with pyuria should be screened for *Chlamydia*.
- Urine biomarkers (e.g., antiproliferative factor) are promising but not ready for clinical use.

IMAGING STUDIES

CT or ultrasound of abdomen and pelvis may be considered to rule out other pathology.

TREATMENT

- There is no consensus for optimal management.
- There is no cure for this disease.

NONPHARMACOLOGIC THERAPY

- Avoidance of activities associated with flare-up
- Avoidance of smoking
- Dietary restriction
- Physical therapy
- Exercise
- Behavioral therapy
- Bladder retraining
- Biofeedback
- Warm sitz bath, ice, heating pad
- Thiele massage (transrectal and transvaginal manual therapy of pelvic floor muscle) in presence of pelvic floor muscle tenderness and spasm
- Hydrodistension only gives temporary relief, so it is not commonly used anymore

ACUTE AND CHRONIC Rx

- A course of empiric antibiotics if not tried yet.
- Oral therapy is tried first.
- Pentosan polysulfate sodium (Elmiron) is the only FDA approved, most effective oral therapy.
- Most treatment takes 3 to 6 months before maximum benefit is seen.
- Adjunct oral therapy includes tricyclics (amitryptilin), antiallergy drugs (hydroxyzine, montelukast), neuroleptics (gabapentine, topiramate), analgesics (NSAIDS, opioid analgesics), and occasionally antimuscarinics.
- Oral therapies could be used in combination.
- Antihistaminics are preferred for patients with allergy history or those who show mast cells in bladder biopsy.
- Oral prednisone is used in presence of Hunner's ulcers.
- Other drugs rarely used for IC are cyclosporin A, IL-10, imatinib, methotrexate, suplatast, misoprostol, quercetin, and so on.
- Growth factor inhibitors, gene therapy, RDP 58, vitamin B_3 analogue (BXL 628) could be used in future.

- Intravesical treatment is used when oral medications fail, for acute flare-ups, or before the oral medications take full effect.
- Dimethyl sulfoxide (DMSO), heparin, lidocaine, hyaluronic acid, bacille Calmette-Guérin, capsaicin, resiniferatoxin (RTX), botulinum toxin A, chondroitin sulfate, steroids, elmiron, and so on are the drugs used for intravescical treatment.
- DMSO is the only FDA-approved intravesical treatment.
- DMSO is used less often these days because of its side effects, specifically garlic odor or taste on breath or skin that lasts 72 hours after treatment.
- Intravescical therapy typically involves mixture of heparin or elmiron with lidocaine and sodium bicarbonate.
- Silver nitrate and chloropactin have fallen out of favor.

SURGERY

- Major surgical intervention is not the mainstay of treatment.
- Patients whose condition is extreme and who are miserable may consider surgery if medications fail.
- Sacral neuromodulation (InterStim) is the current preferred surgical intervention.
- Laser ablation, fulguration, or resection is offered when Hunner's ulcers seen in cystoscopy.
- Augmentation cystoplasty is not recommended.
- Cystourethrectomy with urinary diversion is rarely done.

COMPLEMENTARY & ALTERNATIVE MEDICINE

- Transcutaneous electric nerve stimulation (TENS)
- Intravaginal electric nerve stimulation
- Acupuncture
- Urinary chelating agents such as Polycitra-K crystals, Urocit-K, and so on
- Prelief, an over-the-counter food additive
- Herbal remedies such as Algnot Plus, CystoProtek, Cysta-Q, aloe vera, and so on

DISPOSITION

- Close follow-up every month for 3 months and every 3 months thereafter.
- Voiding diary and symptom questionnaire are helpful to monitor response to treatment.

REFERRAL

- Urologist
- Pain specialist
- Physical therapist

PEARLS & CONSIDERATIONS

COMMENTS

- On average these patients see five physicians and endure irritating voiding symptoms for 5 yr before the disease is identified.
- Besides symptom questionnaire and urine analysis, all other diagnostic tests are optional.
- PST is well tolerated.
- Negative cystoscopy does not rule out IC.

PREVENTION

Early identification and timely intervention improves patient outcome.

PATIENT/FAMILY EDUCATION

- IC support groups
- Interstitial Cystitis Association
- Interstitial Cystitis Network

SUGGESTED READINGS

Chronic pelvic pain in women, *J Reproductive Medicine* 51(3):, 2006.
Dimitrakon J et al: Pharmacologic management of painful bladder syndrome/interstitial cystitis, *Arch Intern Med* 167(18):1922-1929, 2007.
Interstitial cystitis as a disease: a new paradigm emerges, *J Reproductive Medicine* 69(4):S1, 2007.

AUTHOR: **HEMANT K. SATPATHY, M.D.**

BASIC INFORMATION

DEFINITION

Diffuse interstitial lung disease (ILD) includes a large group of nonmalignant disorders, which are characterized by diffuse damage to the lung parenchyma via inflammation and fibrosis, and/or granulomatous reaction in interstitial or vascular areas.

SYNONYMS

Interstitial lung disease
ILD

ICD-9 CODES
136.3 Acute interstitial lung disease
515 Chronic interstitial lung disease

PREVALENCE: Varies with type of interstitial lung disease. The most common type of ILD is idiopathic interstitial fibrosis, with a prevalence of 20 cases/ 100,000 people in the general population, increasing with age to 175 cases/ 100,000 people aged 75 yr or older.

PREDOMINANT SEX & AGE: Some ILDs are more common in women, such as those resulting from connective tissues disorders. One exception is rheumatoid arthritis, which is more common in men. Lymphangiomyomatosis occurs exclusively in postmenopausal women. ILD caused by occupational exposures are more common in men. Generally, ILD occurs in people >50 yr.

RISK FACTORS: History of tobacco abuse; environmental exposures such as to silicone, asbestos or beryllium; reactions to drugs such as amiodarone, methotrexate, or bleomycin; history of connective tissue disease such as rheumatoid arthritis or systemic lupus erythematosus.

PHYSICAL FINDINGS & CLINICAL PRESENTATION

- Dyspnea
- Tachypnea
- Bibasilar end inspiratory dry crackles
- Pulmonary hypertension
- Cyanosis, clubbing

ETIOLOGY

- The hallmark of ILD is restriction caused by decreased lung compliance. The decreased compliance can be due to a number of factors depending on the type of ILD. Different types of interstitial lung disease are characterized by three distinct patterns in the alveolar walls:
  1. Inflammatory changes, which are early and potentially reversible
  2. Fibrotic changes
  3. Lung destruction
- Specific changes may be seen:
  - Granulomatous: accumulation of T lymphocytes, macrophages, and epithelioid cells into granulomas in lung parenchyma
  - Inflammation and fibrosis: injury to epithelium causes inflammation. If chronic, inflammation spreads to interstitium and vascular areas
  - Occupational exposure: pneumoconiosis, asbestosis, silicosis, organic dust
  - Drug induced
  - Connective tissue disorder: systemic lupus erythematosus, rheumatoid arthritis, dermatomyositis, interstitial pneumonitis

DIAGNOSIS

DIFFERENTIAL DIAGNOSIS

- Congestive heart failure
- Chronic renal failure

WORKUP

- Well-defined patterns in pulmonary function tests are usually consistent with restrictive defect (decreased FRC, RV, and TLC) owing to decreased lung compliance caused by alveolar wall thickening due to inflammation and fibrosis. Diffusing capacity is usually reduced also because of inflammation and thickening of alveolar walls, though nonspecific. FEV1/FVC is usually normal or increased because lung stiffness keeps small airways open, although some conditions (e.g., sarcoidosis) may reduce air flow.
- Bronchoscopy and BAL may help identify type of ILD. However, role in defining stage of disease and response to therapy is controversial.
- Biopsy is the most effective method for confirming diagnosis and assessing disease activity.

LABORATORY TESTS

- ABGs may be normal or show respiratory alkalosis.
- Antinuclear antibodies, anti-immunoglobulin antibodies (rheumatoid factors), LDH.
- Serum precipitins confirm exposure if hypersensitivity pneumonitis is suspected.
- Antineutrophil cytoplasmic antibodies or antibasement membrane antibodies if vasculitis is suspected.
- Elevation in angiotensin-converting enzyme level in sarcoidosis.
- ECG, echocardiogram to check for evidence of pulmonary hypertension.

IMAGING STUDIES

- Chest x-ray may be normal, but commonly shows a bibasilar reticular pattern.
- High-resolution CT superior to chest x-ray; also useful for determining potential biopsy sights.

TREATMENT

NONPHARMACOLOGIC THERAPY

Avoidance of tobacco and occupational exposures.

ACUTE GENERAL Rx

- Supplemental oxygen in patients with hypoxemia.
- Glucocorticoids are mainstay of therapy, but success rate is low. Common starting dose is prednisone 0.5 to 1 mg/kg once daily for 4 to 12 wk. Patients should be reevaluated after this initial course of treatment. If they are stable, steroids may be tapered. It not, the same course may be maintained for another 4 to 12 wk. If patient's condition continues to decline, may consider adding second agent (cyclophosphamide, azathioprine).

REFERRAL

- Surgical referral for biopsy
- Pulmonary referral for bronchoscopy or BAL

PEARLS & CONSIDERATIONS

SUGGESTED READINGS

Grippi MA: *Pulmonary science and medicine,* Philadelphia, 2001, J.B. Lippincott.
Kasper D A et al (eds): *Harrison's principles of internal medicine,* ed 16, 2005, McGraw-Hill Company.
Shah NR et al: A critical assessment of treatment options for idiopathic pulmonary fibrosis, *Sarcoidosis Vasc Diffuse Lung Dis* 22(3): 167, 2005.
Swigris JJ et al: Health-related quality of life in patients with idiopathic pulmonary fibrosis: a systematic review, *Thorax* 60:588, 2005.

AUTHORS: **GRACE SHIH, M.D.,** and **CINDY GLEIT, M.D.**

BASIC INFORMATION

DEFINITION

Interstitial nephritis falls into two broad categories: acute and chronic.

- Acute: defined as a decrease in renal function resulting from injury characterized histopathologically with edema and inflammation of the renal interstitium classically sparing the glomeruli and blood vessels. Most often induced by drugs.
- Chronic: represents a large and diverse group of disorders characterized by interstitial fibrosis with mononuclear leukocyte infiltration and tubular atrophy. It is a final common pathway of many chronic kidney diseases including chronic bacterial infections, obstruction, and high-grade vesicoureteral reflux. Histopathologically seen as atrophy and fibrosis of the renal interstitium.

SYNONYMS

Contracted kidney, cirrhosis of the kidney, granular kidney, gouty kidney, renal sclerosis, chronic productive nephritis without exudation

ICD-9CM CODES

583 Nephritis and nephropathy not specified as acute or chronic
583.0 With proliferative glomerular nephritis
583.1 With membranous glomerular nephritis
583.2 With membranoproliferative glomerular nephritis
583.4 With rapidly progressive glomerular nephritis
583.9 With unspecified pathological lesions in the kidney

EPIDEMIOLOGY & DEMOGRAPHICS

PEAK INCIDENCE: Median age at presentation is 65 yr.

PREVALENCE: 2% to 3% of all renal biopsies, in cases of acute renal failure, the incidence of acute interstitial nephritis is 7% to 15%.

PREDOMINANT SEX AND AGE: Older patients generally at higher risk given reduced glomerular filtration rates.

RISK FACTORS: Use of drugs known to cause acute interstitial nephritis, increases with age and decreasing glomerular filtration rate. Some autoimmune disorders are also risk factors.

PHYSICAL FINDINGS & CLINICAL PRESENTATION

Nonspecific but acutely can present with renal failure, oliguria, hematuria, malaise, mental status changes, rash, nausea, and vomiting. Chronically can be asymptomatic with elevations in BUN or creatinine or the appearance of abnormal urinary sediment.

ETIOLOGY

- Drug induced (71%): antibiotics (penicillins, cephalosporins sulfonamides) nonsteroidal anti-inflammatory drugs, diuretics, proton pump inhibitors, anticonvulsants
- Infection associated (15%):
  - Bacterial: *Corynebacterium diphtheriae,* legionella, staphylococci, streptococci, yersinia
  - Viral: cytomegalovirus, Epstein-Barr virus, hanta viruses, hepatitis C, herpes simplex virus, human immunodeficiency virus, mumps, polyoma virus
  - Other: mycobacterium, mycoplasma, rickettsia, syphilis, toxoplasmosis
- Cases associated with immune (systemic lupus erythematosus, Sjögren's, and Wegener's) or neoplastic disorders (5%)

DIAGNOSIS

DIFFERENTIAL DIAGNOSIS

Any other causes of acute renal failure including hypertensive nephrosclerosis, prerenal azotemia, obstructive nephropathy, interstitial nephritis, renal vascular disease, and various electrolyte abnormalities

WORKUP

Medical history with focus on recent infection illness or new medication in the presence of acute to chronic onset of kidney failure; evaluation for underlying infection or insult

LABORATORY TESTS

- Urinalysis, especially eosinophiluria, serum chemistry profile, complete blood count, liver function tests, 24-hour urine specimen collection, consider serum IgE levels.
- Renal biopsy indicated when diagnosis is unclear, removal of offending agent does not result in improvement and there are no contraindications to the procedure.

IMAGING STUDIES

Ultrasound; consider Gallium 67 scanning to discriminate acute tubular necrosis (ATN) from acute interstitial nephritis (AIN).

TREATMENT

NONPHARMACOLOGIC THERAPY

Largely supportive, removal of offending agent will resolve 60% of all cases.

ACUTE GENERAL Rx

- Correct fluid and electrolyte imbalances, maintain adequate hydration and urine output but avoid volume overload.
- Identify and treat infection as indicated.
- Remove offending drug, substitute as appropriate.
- Avoid medications that impair renal blood flow.
- If steroids are initiated, a reasonable choice is prednisone 1mg/kg/day for 2 to 3 wk.
- Consider treatment with cyclophosphamide (Cytoxan) if patients fail to respond to corticosteroids.

CHRONIC Rx

- Limit exposure to known nephrotoxic agents.
- Renally adjust medications as indicated by glomerular filtration rate.
- Tight control of blood pressure, diabetes and cholesterol to preserve kidney function as needed.

DISPOSITION

With acute interstitial nephritis 40% of patients will improve in time.

REFERRAL

Refer to nephrology with question in diagnosis, multiple comorbidities, with failure to respond to supportive care or initial therapies, or with decision to evaluate for biopsy.

PEARLS & CONSIDERATIONS

COMMENTS

Once known mainly as a complication of streptococcal infection, today acute interstitial nephritis is most often due to drugs; 88% of the time that drug has been started in the last 30 days. Significant fibrosis of the tubules seen in biopsy is the best predictor of transition to chronic interstitial nephritis. Corticosteroids cannot be recommended as empiric therapy because their efficacy has not been established, but may be indicated in specific cases.

PREVENTION

Use of known offending agents with care, especially in the elderly and those with known underlying kidney disease.

SUGGESTED READINGS

Clarkston MR et al: Acute interstitial nephritis: clinical features and response to cortical steroid therapy, *Nephol Dial Transplant* 19:2778-2283, 2004.

Councilman WT: Acute interstitial nephritis, *J Exp Med* 3:393-420, 1998.

Kodner, Kudrimoti: Diagnosis and management of acute interstitial nephritis, *AAFP* 12:2527-2534, 2003.

Michael R et al: Acute interstitial nephritis: clinical features response to cortical steroid therapy, *Nephrol Dial Transplant* 19:2778-2783, 2004.

Michel DM, Kelly CJ: Acute interstitial nephritis, *J Am Soc Nephrol* 9:506-515, 1998.

AUTHOR: **JOHN RAGSDALE, M.D.**

BASIC INFORMATION

DEFINITION

Irritable bowel syndrome (IBS) is a chronic functional disorder manifested by alteration in bowel habits and recurrent abdominal pain and bloating. IBS is a symptom complex influenced by a variety of physiologic determinants from gut to brain and back. The ROME III criteria for diagnosis of IBS is:

- Recurrent abdominal pain or discomfort at least 3 days per month in the past 3 months associated with two or more of the following:
  1. Pain is relieved or improved with defecation.
  2. Its onset is associated with a change in the frequency of bowel movement.
  3. Its onset is associated with a change in the form or appearance of the stool.
- The criteria must be fulfilled for at least the past 3 months with symptom onset at least 6 months before the diagnosis.

SYNONYMS

Irritable colon
Spastic colon
IBS

ICD-9CM CODES
564.1 Irritable bowel syndrome

EPIDEMIOLOGY & DEMOGRAPHICS

- IBS is the most common functional bowel disorder. It is estimated that 15 million people in the U.S. have IBS.
- IBS occurs in 20% of the population of industrialized countries and is responsible for >50% of GI referrals. Worldwide adult prevalence is 12%. Incidence increases during adolescence and peaks in third and fourth decades of life.
- Female:male ratio is 2:1.
- Nearly 50% of patients have psychiatric abnormalities, with anxiety disorders being most common.

PHYSICAL FINDINGS & CLINICAL PRESENTATION

- The clinical presentation of IBS consists of abdominal pain and abnormalities of defecation, which may include loose stools usually after meals and in the morning, alternating with episodes of constipation.
- Physical examination is generally normal.
- Nonspecific abdominal tenderness and distention may be present.

ETIOLOGY

- Unknown
- Associated pathophysiology includes altered GI motility, alteration in gut flora, and increased gut sensitivity
- Risk factors: anxiety, depression, personality disorders, history of childhood sexual abuse, and domestic abuse in women

DIAGNOSIS

DIFFERENTIAL DIAGNOSIS

- IBD
- Diverticulitis
- Colon malignancy
- Endometriosis
- PUD
- Biliary liver disease
- Chronic pancreatitis
- Constipation due to medications (opiates, calcium channel blockers, anticholinergics)
- Diarrhea due to medications (metformin, colchicine, proton pump inhibitors, antacids, antibiotics)
- Small bowel overgrowth
- Celiac disease
- Parasites
- Lymphoma of GI tract

WORKUP

Diagnostic workup is aimed primarily at excluding the conditions listed in the differential diagnoses. It is important to identify "red flags" of other diseases, such as weight loss, rectal bleeding, onset in patients >50 years of age, fever, nocturnal pain, family history of malignancy or IBD. Additional red flags include abnormal exam (e.g., mass, enlarged lymph nodes, stool positive for occult blood, muscle wasting) and abnormal labs (anemia, leukocytosis, abnormal chemistry).

Common clinical criteria for diagnosis of IBS are: more than 3 months of symptoms *including* abdominal pain that is relieved by a bowel movement, *or* pain accompanied by a change in bowel pattern, *and* abnormality in bowel movement 25% of the time, characterized by two of the following features:

- Abdominal distention
- Abnormal consistency
- Abnormal defecation (e.g., straining, sense of incomplete evacuation)
- Abnormal frequency
- Mucus with bowel movement

LABORATORY TESTS

- Blood work is generally normal. CBC and ESR are reasonable to evaluate for anemia. The presence of anemia should alert to the possibility of a colonic malignancy or IBD.
- Testing of stool for ova and parasites should be considered in patients with chronic diarrhea. Evaluation of stool for *Clostridium difficile* may be helpful in patients with predominant diarrhea symptoms who have recently taken antibiotics.

IMAGING STUDIES

Imaging studies (e.g., flat and upright abdominal radiograph, small bowel series, sonogram or CT of abdomen and pelvis) are normal and not necessary for diagnosis.

Lower endoscopy is generally normal except for the presence of some spasms.

TREATMENT

NONPHARMACOLOGIC THERAPY

- The patient should be encouraged to maintain an adequate fiber intake and to eliminate foods that aggravate symptoms. Avoidance of caffeine, dairy products, fatty foods, and dietary excesses is also helpful.
- Behavioral therapy is also recommended, particularly in younger patients because psychosocial stressors are important triggers of IBS. Reassurance and education about trigger avoidance and stress management are important.
- Importance of regular exercise and adequate fluid intake should be stressed.

GENERAL Rx

- The mainstay of treatment of IBS is a high-fiber diet. Fiber is helpful for relief of constipation but not for relief of pain. Because symptoms are chronic, the use of laxatives should generally be avoided.
- Fiber supplementation with psyllium 1 tablespoon bid or calcium polycarbophil (FiberCon) 2 tablets 1 to 4 times daily followed by 8 oz of water may be necessary in some patients.
- Patients should be instructed that there might be some increased bloating on initiation of fiber supplementation, which should resolve within 2 to 3 wk. It is important that patients take these fiber products on a regular basis and not only as needed. Fiber is not effective in patients with diarrhea-predominant IBS and may worsen symptoms in these patients.
- Antispasmodics–anticholinergics may be useful in refractory cases (e.g., dicyclomine [Bentyl] 10 to 20 mg up to 3 times daily).
- Patients who appear anxious can benefit from use of sedatives or SSRIs. Tricyclic antidepressants in low doses are also effective in some patients with IBS.
- Loperamide is effective for diarrhea. Alosetron (Lotronex), a serotonin type-3 receptor antagonist previously withdrawn because of severe constipation and ischemic colitis, has been reintroduced with limited availability. It is indicated only for women with severe chronic diarrhea-predominant IBS unresponsive to conventional therapy and not caused by anatomic or metabolic abnormality. Starting dose is 1 mg qd.
- Lubiprostone (Amitiza) is a chloride channel activator which stimulates chloride-rich intestinal fluid secretion and accelerates small intestine and

colonic transmit time. It may be effective in chronic constipation–predominant IBS unresponsive to conventional treatment. Usual dose is 24 mcg qd-bid with food. Side effects include headaches and nausea.

- Alterations in gut flora have been identified as potentially contributing to IBS (84% of IBS patients have an abnormal lactulose breath test suggesting small-intestinal bacterial overgrowth). Rifamixin, a gut selective antibiotic, has been used in recent trials to eradicate bacterial overgrowth (70% eradication rate). A dose of 400 mg tid for 10 days was reported effective in improving IBS symptoms up to 10 wk after discontinuation of therapy. Until additional evidence is available, use of rifamixin or other antibiotics in IBS should be reserved to patients with proven bacterial overgrowth.

DISPOSITION

Greater than 60% of patients respond successfully to treatment over the initial 12 mo; however, IBS is a chronic relapsing condition and requires prolonged therapy.

REFERRAL

GI referral is recommended in patients with rectal bleeding, fever, nocturnal diarrhea, anemia, weight loss, or onset of symptoms after age 40 yr. Consultation is also necessary if specialized diagnostic procedure such as endoscopy are necessary.

PEARLS & CONSIDERATIONS

COMMENTS

- Patients should be educated regarding maintenance of high-fiber diet and elimination of stressors, which can precipitate attacks of IBS. They should be reassured that their condition cannot lead to cancer.
- Recent drug efforts (alosetron, tegaserod) are aimed at serotonergic receptors in the gut because most of the serotonin in the body is found in the GI tract and is believed to be involved in the mediation of visceral sensation and motility.
- Cognitive-behavioral therapy (CBT) is effective in the treatment of patients with IBS and should be considered as part of the armamentarium against this disorder.

EVIDENCE

There is evidence that antidiarrheal agents are effective in the symptomatic management of IBS.

Patients with urgency and diarrhea can be successfully treated with loperamide at doses of 4-12 mg daily. Codeine is a reasonable alternative but more likely to cause unwanted sedation.[1] C

There is evidence from clinical trials that loperamide improves symptoms of IBS, most notably urgency and diarrhea.[2,3] B

Cholestyramine may be considered for patients with bile acid malabsorption.[1,4] C

There is limited evidence that dietary supplementation with fiber is of benefit in the management of IBS.

Increased dietary fiber (25 g/day), is recommended for simple constipation, although evidence for its effectiveness is limited.[4] C

Patients who fail to respond to, or are intolerant of, increased dietary fiber, may benefit from a fiber supplement.[1] C

There is evidence that smooth muscle relaxants are effective in the management of IBS.

Various antispasmodics can be given to reduce pain. Drugs with an anticholinergic action appear to be most effective.[1] C

A metaanalysis study of 26 randomized controlled trials (RCTs) that compared antispasmodics vs. placebo found a significant benefit for drug over placebo. Smooth muscle relaxants are consistently effective at reducing abdominal pain and improving symptoms of abdominal distension.[5] A

In particular, dicyclomine has been shown to improve patients' overall condition, decrease abdominal pain and tenderness, and improve bowel habits.[1,6] A B

There is evidence that antidepressants are effective in the treatment of IBS.

Antidepressants are recommended for moderate to severe pain symptoms and may be helpful for less severe symptoms.[4] C

A systematic review found that antidepressants, including amitriptyline, significantly improved symptoms in IBS.[7] A

It is not clear whether these effects are independent of the effects on psychologic symptoms.[8]

There is limited evidence for the use of drugs acting on the 5HT receptor in the treatment of constipation and diarrhea in patients with IBS.

A systematic review found that the $5HT_4$-agonist tegaserod was effective in improving bowel habit in patients with constipation-predominant IBS. However, individual symptoms of abdominal pain and discomfort were not significantly altered.[9] A

Another systematic review found that in patients with diarrhea-predominant IBS, the $5HT_3$-antagonist, alosetron, significantly improved symptoms compared with placebo. Alosetron was associated with an increased number of adverse effects.[10] B

There is limited evidence that psychologic interventions are of benefit in the management of IBS.

Cognitive behavioral treatment, dynamic psychotherapy, hypnosis, and stress management/relaxation seem to be effective in reducing pain and diarrhea (but not constipation), and also reduce anxiety and other psychologic symptoms.[4] C

One study found that hypnotherapy has been shown to be more effective than psychotherapy for the treatment of abdominal pain, abdominal distention, bowel habit, and general well-being in patients with IBS.[11] B

Evidence-Based References

1. Jones J et al: British Society of Gastroenterology for the management of irritable bowel syndrome, *Gut* 47(Suppl 2):ii1, 2000. C
2. Cann PA et al: Role of loperamide and placebo in management of irritable bowel syndrome (IBS), *Dig Dis Sci* 29:239, 1984. B
3. Efskind PS, Bernklev T, Vatn MH: A double-blind placebo controlled trial with loperamide in IBS, *Scand J Gastroenterol* 31:463, 1996. B
4. American Gastroenterological Association medical position statement, *Gastroenterology* 123:2105, 2002. C
5. Poynard T, Regimbeau C, Benhamou Y: Meta-analysis of smooth muscle relaxants in the treatment of irritable bowel syndrome, *Aliment Pharmacol Ther* 15:355, 2001. Reviewed in: 12:683, 2004. A
6. Page JG, Dirnberger GM: Treatment of the irritable bowel syndrome with Bentyl (dicyclomine hydrochloride), *J Clin Gastroenterol* 3:153, 1981. B
7. Jackson JL et al: Treatment of functional gastrointestinal disorders with antidepressant medications: a meta-analysis, *Am J Med* 108:65, 2000. Reviewed in: *Clin Evid* 12:683, 2004. A
8. Kennedy TM, Rubin G, Jones R: Irritable bowel syndrome, *Clin Evid* 12:683, 2004, London: BMJ Publishing Group.
9. Evans BW et al: Tegaserod for the treatment of irritable bowel syndrome, *Cochrane Database Syst Rev* 1, 2004. A
10. Cremonini F, Delgado-Aros S, Camilleri M: Efficacy ofalosetron in irritable bowel syndrome: a meta-analysis of randomized controlled trials, *Neurogastroenterol Motil* 15:79, 2003. Reviewed in: *Clin Evid* 12:683, 2004. B
11. Whorwell PJ, Prior A, Faragher EB: Controlled trial of hypnotherapy in treatment of severe refractory irritable-bowel syndrome, *Lancet* 2:1232, 1984. B

SUGGESTED READINGS

Drossman DA: The functional gastrointestinal disorders and the Rome III process, *Gastroenterology* 130:1377-1390, 2006.

Mayer EA: Irritable bowel syndrome, *N Engl J Med* 358:1692-1699, 2008.

Mertz HR: Irritable bowel syndrome, *N Engl J Med* 349:22, 2003.

Pimentel M et al: The effect of a nonabsorbed oral antibiotic (Rifaximin) on the symptoms of the irritable bowel syndrome, *Ann Intern Med* 145:557-563, 2006.

AUTHOR: **FRED F. FERRI, M.D.**

BASIC INFORMATION

DEFINITION

Jaundice is a yellowish discoloration of the sclera, skin, and mucous membranes caused by an excessive amount of bilirubin in the bloodstream. Clinically detectable jaundice in adults is a serum bilirubin of 2.5 to 3 mg/dl.

SYNONYMS

Icterus

ICD-9CM CODES
782.4 Jaundice
283.9 Hemolytic jaundice
576.8 Obstructive jaundice

EPIDEMIOLOGY & DEMOGRAPHICS

The major causes of jaundice by age and sex:
- Young adults—viral hepatitis
- Women over 30—choledocholithiasis
- Middle adulthood (both sexes)—drug induced and cirrhosis
- Middle-aged and older men—alcoholic liver disease, pancreatic cancer, hepatoma, primary hemochromatosis
- Women—primary biliary cirrhosis, chronic active hepatitis, choledocholithiasis, carcinoma of the gallbladder

CLINICAL PRESENTATION

Presentation can vary from asymptomatic to acute and life threatening. History and physical give important clues to the underlying condition.

KEY HISTORY:
- Duration of jaundice
- Previous episodes
- Pain
- Color of urine and stool
- Systemic symptoms (fever, chills)
- Alcohol use
- Medications
- Injection of illicit drugs
- Blood transfusions
- Hepatitis exposure (e.g., other jaundiced people)
- Shellfish ingestion
- Travel
- Occupation
- Anorexia/weight loss
- Prior abdominal/biliary surgery

KEY PHYSICAL: Vital signs, fever, signs of chronic liver disease (palmar erythema, spider angiomas, bruising, gynecomastia, testicular atrophy), size of liver, abdominal tenderness (and location), abdominal mass, splenomegaly, ascites, edema, weight loss, Kayser-Fleischer rings (Wilson's disease)

ETIOLOGY

Disruption in any of three phases of bilirubin metabolism can lead to jaundice.

PREHEPATIC PHASE: Bilirubin is produced from the metabolism of heme—80% from RBC catabolism, 20% from ineffective erythropoiesis and breakdown of muscle myoglobin and cytochromes—and transported to the liver for conjugation and excretion.

INTRAHEPATIC PHASE: Unconjugated (indirect) bilirubin, which is fat soluble but water insoluble, is conjugated within the hepatocyte to the water-soluble, conjugated (direct) bilirubin.

POSTHEPATIC PHASE: Conjugated bilirubin dissolves in the bile and travels through the biliary system to the gallbladder where it is stored, or passes into the duodenum through the ampulla of Vater. Some bilirubin is excreted in the stool and the rest is converted to urobilinogens by the gut flora and reabsorbed. Most of the urobilinogen is excreted by the kidney. A small amount is reabsorbed by the gut and reexcreted into the bile.

DIAGNOSIS

DIFFERENTIAL DIAGNOSIS

Prehepatic Causes:
- Unconjugated hyperbilirubinemia—excessive heme metabolism from hemolysis (e.g., sickle cell disease, spherocytosis, G6PD, immune hemolysis); ineffective erythropoiesis (e.g., thalassemia, folate, severe iron deficiency); or large hematoma reabsorption.

Intrahepatic Causes:
- Unconjugated hyperbilirubinemia—disorders of enzyme metabolism e.g., Gilbert's disease (common, benign), Crigler-Najjar (rare, severe); drugs e.g., rifampin, probenecid.
- Conjugated hyperbilirubinemia—intrahepatic cholestasis.
  1. Viruses: e.g., hepatitis A, B, and C; EB virus.
  2. Alcohol: alcoholic hepatitis, alcoholic cirrhosis.
  3. Autoimmune: e.g., primary biliary cirrhosis, primary sclerosing cholangitis.
  4. Drug induced: e.g., acetaminophen, penicillins, oral contraceptives, chlorpromazine (Thorazine), steroids (estrogenic or anabolic), some herbals.
  5. Hereditary metabolic: e.g., hemochromatosis, Wilson's disease, Dubin-Johnson and Rotor's syndromes, alpha-antitrypsin deficiency.
  6. Systemic disease: sarcoidosis, amyloidosis, glycogen storage diseases, celiac disease, TB, MAI.
  7. Other: sepsis, TPN, pregnancy, graft-versus-host disease, environmental toxins.

Posthepatic Causes:
- Conjugated hyperbilirubinemia—intrinsic or extrinsic obstruction of the biliary system
  1. Intrinsic blockage: gallstones, cholangitis, strictures, infection (e.g., CMV, cryptosporidium in AIDS patients, parasites, cholangiocarcinoma, gallbladder cancer).
  2. Extrinsic blockage: pancreatitis, pancreatic carcinoma, pancreatic pseudocyst.

Pseudojaundice—caused by an excessive ingestion of foods containing beta-carotene (carrots, melons, squash); does *not* result in hyperbilirubinemia or scleral icterus.

WORKUP

History and physical: as above are key to diagnosis.

LABORATORY TESTS

LABS:

First line tests:
- Serum total and direct bilirubin.
- Urinalysis.

If first line tests are normal, consider pseudojaundice.

If urine is positive for bilirubin and serum has elevated total and direct bilirubin (conjugated hyperbilirubinemia):
- Initial evaluation—liver function tests (AST, ALT, GGTP, AP), CBC, liver synthetic function (albumin, PT, PTT), pancreatic function (amylase, lipase).
- Additional tests—if diagnosis unclear.
  1. Screen for hepatitis A, B, and C—if still unclear then consider (2 to 6).
  2. Other viruses—EBV, CMV.
  3. Autoimmune disorders: antimitochondrial antibody, IgM (elevated in primary biliary cirrhosis); smooth muscle antibody, ANA, IgG (autoimmune chronic active hepatitis); antinuclear cytoplasmic antibody (primary sclerosing cholangitis).
  4. Ceruloplasmin (Wilson's disease).
  5. Alpha-1 antitrypsin deficiency (cirrhosis and emphysema).
  6. Ferritin, Fe saturation (elevated in hemochromatosis).

If urine is negative for bilirubin, increased t. bili and normal d. bili (unconjugated hyperbilirubinemia):
- Hemolysis? (CBC, smear for abnormal RBC types).
- Genetic syndrome? (e.g., Gilbert's).
- Hematoma?

Liver biopsy: essential in diagnosis of chronic hepatitis. Can be used for diagnosis of liver masses but carries a substantial risk.

IMAGING STUDIES

- Abdominal ultrasound—first line study. Most sensitive for biliary tract stones and extrahepatic biliary obstruction.

- Abdominal CT—more information on liver, pancreas, biliary system.
- Endoscopic retrograde cholangiopancreatography—best for lower duct obstruction.
- Percutaneous transhepatic cholangiography—best for hilar obstructions.
- Magnetic resonance cholangiopancreatography—noninvasive visualization of bile and pancreatic ducts. Becoming more available.

TREATMENT

Rx

NONPHARMACOLOGIC THERAPY

Depends on underlying cause of the jaundice, rapidity of onset, and clinical stability of the patient. Generally, obstructive causes require surgical treatment and nonobstructive medical treatment.

ACUTE GENERAL Rx

Acute, life-threatening illness such as acute cholecystitis or ascending cholangitis requires prompt diagnosis and emergent surgical or endoscopic intervention in conjunction with medical management.

CHRONIC Rx

Chronic causes may require such treatment as stopping certain medications; stopping alcohol; antihistamines for pruitis; cholestyramine to bind bilirubin and decrease pruritus; interferon for hepatitis B or C; penicillamine for Wilson's disease; phlebotomy for hemochromatosis; surgical resection for liver for pancreatic cancer; liver transplant for eligible patients with end-stage cirrhosis; N-acetylcysteine for acetaminophen overdose.

PEARLS & CONSIDERATIONS

!

COMMENTS

- The key to the management of the jaundiced adult is accurate diagnosis of the underlying cause.
- Prompt diagnosis and treatment of life-threatening illness is essential.
- Careful history and physical followed by selective lab and imaging studies will lead to accurate diagnosis.
- Collaboration with surgical and gastroenterology colleagues is helpful in complex patient care scenarios.

SUGGESTED READINGS

Beckingham IJ, Ryder SD: ABC of diseases of the liver, pancreas and biliary system: investigation of liver and biliary disease, *BMJ* 322:33-36, 2001.

Braunwald et al (eds): *Harrison's principles of internal medicine,* ed 15, New York, 2001, McGraw-Hill.

Roche SP, Kobos R: Jaundice in the adult patient, *Am Fam Physician* 69:299-304, 2004.

Ryder SD, Beckingham IJ: ABC of diseases of the liver, pancreas and biliary system: other causes of parenchymal liver disease, *BMJ* 322:290-292, 2001.

AUTHOR: **GOWRI ANANDARAJAH, M.D.**

BASIC INFORMATION

DEFINITION

Juvenile rheumatoid idiopathic arthritis is arthritis beginning before the age of 16 yr.

SYNONYMS

Still's disease
Juvenile chronic arthritis
Juvenile polyarthritis

ICD-9CM CODES
714.3 Juvenile chronic polyarthritis

EPIDEMIOLOGY & DEMOGRAPHICS

PREVALENCE (IN U.S.): 250,000 to 300,000 cases

PREDOMINANT SEX: Female:male ratio of 2:1

PREDOMINANT AGE: Two peak incidences, between ages of 1 and 3 yr and ages 8 and 12 yr.

PHYSICAL FINDINGS & CLINICAL PRESENTATION

Usually one of three types:

SYSTEMIC OR ACUTE FEBRILE JUVENILE RHEUMATOID ARTHRITIS (20% OF CASES):

- Characterized by extraarticular manifestations, especially spiking fevers and a typical rash that frequently appears in the evening and may be elicited by gently scratching the skin in susceptible areas (Koebner's phenomenon)
- Possible splenomegaly, generalized lymphadenopathy, pericarditis, and myocarditis
- Often, minimal articular findings overshadowed by systemic symptoms

PAUCIARTICULAR OR OLIGOARTICULAR FORM (50% OF CASES):

- Involves fewer than five joints
- Usually involves the larger joints, such as the knees, elbows, and ankles
- Systemic features often minimal, and only one to three joints usually involved
- Rarely causes impairment but chronic iridocyclitis develops in approximately 30% of cases with this form, and permanent loss of vision will develop in a high percentage of these patients (Fig. 1-138)
- Accelerated growth of the affected limb from chronic hyperemia possibly resulting in a temporary leg length discrepancy that is eventually equalized in most cases on control of the inflammation

POLYARTICULAR JUVENILE RHEUMATOID ARTHRITIS (30% OF CASES):

- Involves five or more joints
- Resembles the adult disease in its symmetric involvement of the small joints of the hands and feet (Fig. 1-139)
- Cervical spine involvement common and may produce marked loss of motion
- Early closure of the ossification centers of the mandible, often producing a markedly receding chin, a characteristic of this form
- Systemic manifestations similar to the febrile variety but not as dramatic

ETIOLOGY

Unknown. There is increasing evidence that the inflammation and destruction of bone and cartilage that occurs in many rheumatic diseases are the result of the activation, by some unknown mechanism, of proinflammatory cells that infiltrate the synovium. These cells, in turn, release various substances, such as cytokines and tumor necrosis factor (TNF) alpha, which subsequently cause the pathologic changes typical of this group of diseases. Many of the newer therapeutic agents are directed at the suppression of these final mediators of inflammation.

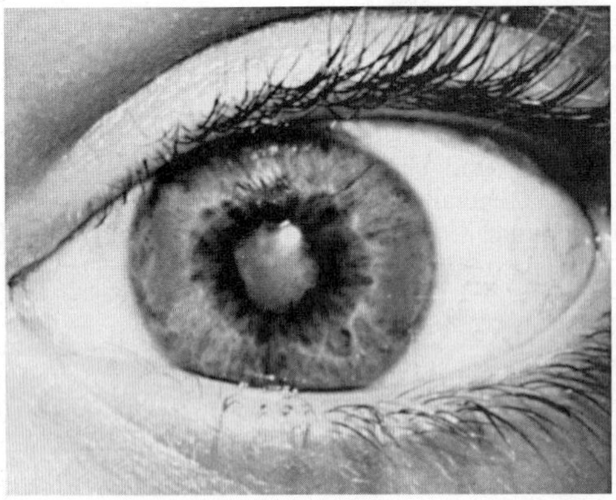

FIGURE 1-138 Chronic iridocyclitis of juvenile rheumatoid arthritis. Extensive posterior synechiae have resulted in a small, irregular pupil. There is a well-developed cataract and early band keratopathy at the medial and lateral margins of the cornea. (From Behrman RE [ed]: *Nelson textbook of pediatrics,* ed 17, Philadelphia, 2004, WB Saunders.)

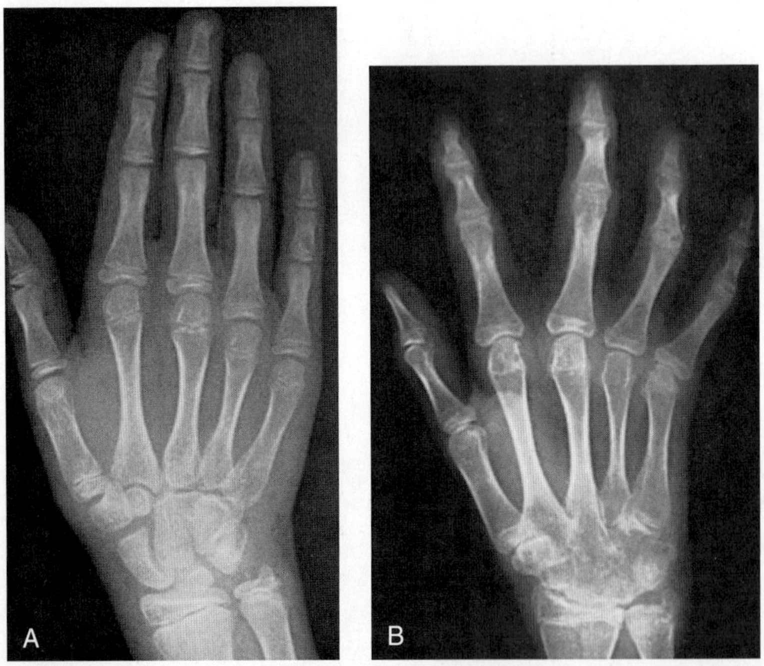

FIGURE 1-139 Progression of joint destruction in a girl with rheumatoid factor-positive juvenile rheumatoid arthritis despite doses of corticosteroids sufficient to suppress symptoms in the interval between A and B. **A,** Roentgenogram of the hand at onset. **B,** Roentgenogram 4 years later, showing a loss of articular cartilage and destruction changes in the distal and proximal interphalangeal and metacarpophalangeal joints and destruction and fusion of wrist bones. (From Behrman RE [ed]: *Nelson textbook of pediatrics,* ed 17, Philadelphia, 2004, WB Saunders.)

DIAGNOSIS

Dx

DIFFERENTIAL DIAGNOSIS

- Infectious causes of fever
- SLE
- Rheumatic fever
- Drug reaction
- Serum sickness
- "Viral arthritis"
- Lyme arthritis

WORKUP

Initial laboratory and imaging studies are often nonspecific in children with rheumatoid arthritis.

LABORATORY TESTS

- Increased ESR
- Low-grade anemia
- Very high peripheral WBC count
- Rheumatoid factor: rarely demonstrable in the serum of children
- Antinuclear antibodies: often found in children with ocular complications

IMAGING STUDIES

- Roentgenographic findings are similar to those in adult, with soft tissue swelling and osteoporosis early in the disease.
- Joint destruction is less frequent.
- Bony erosion and cyst formation may be present as a result of synovial hypertrophy.

TREATMENT

Rx

NONPHARMACOLOGIC THERAPY

Proper management requires close cooperation among primary physician, therapist, rheumatologist, and orthopedist.

- Rest
- Physical and occupational therapy
- Patient and family education
- Proper diet and weight maintenance

ACUTE GENERAL Rx

- NSAIDs
- DMARDs and biologic response modifiers (BMRs)
- Intraarticular steroids
- Systemic corticosteroids

DISPOSITION

- Complete remission occurs in the majority of patients and may occur at any age.
- 70% to 85% of children regain normal function.
- Mortality rate is 2%.
- Children with a protracted systemic phase of the disease are most at risk for developing serious intercurrent infection and potentially fatal amyloidosis.
- Myocarditis may develop in the systemic form.
- Blindness is the most serious complication of the pauciarticular form; joint deformity is the most serious problem of polyarticular disease.

REFERRAL

- Early rheumatology consultation
- For ophthalmology consultation when ocular involvement is suspected (frequent eye examinations, especially in oligoarticular form)
- For orthopedic consultation for corrective surgery

PEARLS & CONSIDERATIONS

!

COMMENTS

Patient information on juvenile idiopathic arthritis can be obtained from the National Arthritis Foundation, 1330 West Peachtree Street, Atlanta, GA 30309; 800-283-7800.

EVIDENCE

EBM

A randomized controlled trial (RCT) found that ibuprofen and aspirin had similar efficacy in treating juvenile idiopathic arthritis. There was no significant difference between the drugs in terms of response rates, or the amount of improvement in articular indexes of disease activity.[1] B

A systematic review found that methotrexate was associated with small to moderate positive effects on patient-centered disability outcomes. Methotrexate was more effective than placebo for increasing joint range of motion, decreasing the number of joints with pain and swelling, and improving assessment of disease activity.[2] A

An RCT found that sulfasalazine was significantly more effective than placebo for improving overall articular severity score, global assessments (by physicians, parents, and patients), and laboratory markers of inflammation in patients with juvenile idiopathic arthritis.[3] B

In a double-blind RCT significantly fewer etanercept-treated patients experienced a disease flare compared with patients who received placebo, and the median time to disease flare was much longer for those in the etanercept group.[4] B

Evidence-Based References

1. Giannini EH et al: Ibuprofen suspension in the treatment of juvenile rheumatoid arthritis. Pediatric Rheumatology Collaborative Study Group, *J Pediatr* 117:645, 1990. B
2. Takken T, Van der Net J, Helders, PJM: Methotrexate for treating juvenile idiopathic arthritis, *Cochrane Database Syst Rev* 3:CD003129, 2001. Reviewed in: *Cochrane Database Syst Rev* 4:CD003129, 2001. A
3. van Rossum MA et al: Sulfasalazine in the treatment of juvenile chronic arthritis: a randomized, double-blind, placebo-controlled, multicenter study. Dutch Juvenile Chronic Arthritis Study Group, *Arthritis Rheum* 41:808, 1998. B
4. Lovell DJ et al: Etanercept in children with polyarticular juvenile rheumatoid arthritis. Pediatric Rheumatology Collaborative Study Group, *N Engl J Med* 342:763, 2000. B

SUGGESTED READINGS

Dhillon S et al: Etenercept: a review of its use in the management of rheumatoid arthritis, *Drugs* 67(8):1211, 2007.

Edwards JC, Szczepanski L et al: Efficacy of β-cell-targeted therapy with rituximab in patients with rheumatoid arthritis, *N Engl J Med* 350:2572, 2004.

Feldman DE et al: Effects of adherence to treatment on short-term outcomes in children with juvenile idiopathic arthritis, *Arthritis Rheum* 57(6):905, 2007.

Glueck D, Gellman H: Management of the upper extremity in juvenile rheumatoid arthritis, *J Am Acad Orthop Surg* 13:254, 2005.

Hampton T: Trials reveal promising options for treating juvenile rheumatoid arthritis, *JAMA* 299:27, 2008.

Iesaka K et al: Orthopedic surgical management of hip and knee involvement in patients with juvenile rheumatoid arthritis, *Am J Orthop* 35:67, 2006.

Olsen NJ, Stein CM: New drugs for rheumatoid arthritis, *N Engl J Med* 350:2167, 2004.

Ravelli A, Martini A: Early predictors of outcome in juvenile idiopathic arthritis, *Clin Exp Rheumatol* 21:89, 2004.

Reiff AO: Developments in the treatment of juvenile arthritis, *Expert Opin Pharmacother* 5:1485, 2004.

Silverman E et al: Leflunomide of methotrexate for juvenile rheumatoid arthritis, *N Engl J Med* 352:1655, 2005.

Stinson JN et al: Asking the experts: exploring the self-management needs of adolescents with arthritis, *Arthritis Rheum* 59:65, 2008.

AUTHOR: **LONNIE R. MERCIER, M.D.**

BASIC INFORMATION

DEFINITION

Kaposi's sarcoma (KS) is a vascular neoplasm most frequently occurring in AIDS patients. It can be divided into the following four subsets:

1. *Classic Kaposi's sarcoma:* most frequently found in elderly Eastern European and Mediterranean males. It consists initially of violaceous macules and papules with subsequent development of plaques and red/purple nodules. Growth is slow, and most of the patients die of unrelated causes.
2. *Epidemic* or *AIDS-related Kaposi's sarcoma:* most frequently occurs in homosexual men. Lesions are generally multifocal and widespread. Lymphadenopathy may be associated.
3. *Endemic Kaposi's sarcoma:* usually affects African children and adults. An aggressive lymphadenopathic form affects African children in particular.
4. *Immunosuppression-associated,* or *transplantation-associated, Kaposi's sarcoma:* usually associated with chemotherapy.

SYNONYMS

KS

ICD-9CM CODES
173.9 Malignant neoplasm of the skin

EPIDEMIOLOGY & DEMOGRAPHICS

- AIDS-related KS affects >35% of AIDS cases.
- Highest incidence is in homosexual men.

PHYSICAL FINDINGS & CLINICAL PRESENTATION

- AIDS-related KS: multifocal and widespread red-purple or dark plaques and/or nodules on cutaneous or mucosal surfaces (Fig. 1-140).
- Generalized lymphadenopathy at the time of diagnosis is present in >50% of patients with AIDS-related KS; the initial lesions have a rust-colored appearance; subsequent progression to red or purple nodules or plaques occurs.
- Most frequently affected areas are the face, trunk, oral cavity, and upper and lower extremities.

ETIOLOGY

A herpesvirus (HHV-8, Kaposi's sarcoma-associated herpesvirus KSHV) has been isolated from patients with most forms of KS and is believed to be the causative agent. It can be transmitted sexually (homosexual, heterosexual activities) and by other forms of nonsexual contact such as maternal-infant transmission (common in African countries).

DIAGNOSIS

DIFFERENTIAL DIAGNOSIS

- Stasis dermatitis
- Pyogenic granuloma
- Capillary hemangiomas
- Granulation tissue
- Postinflammatory hyperpigmentation
- Cutaneous lymphoma
- Melanoma
- Dermatofibroma
- Hematoma
- Prurigo nodularis

The differential diagnosis of cutaneous lesions in patients with HIV infection is described in Section III.

WORKUP

Diagnosis can generally be made on clinical appearance; tissue biopsy will confirm diagnosis.

LABORATORY TESTS

HIV in patients suspected of AIDS

TREATMENT

NONPHARMACOLOGIC THERAPY

Observation is a reasonable option in patients with slowly progressive disease.

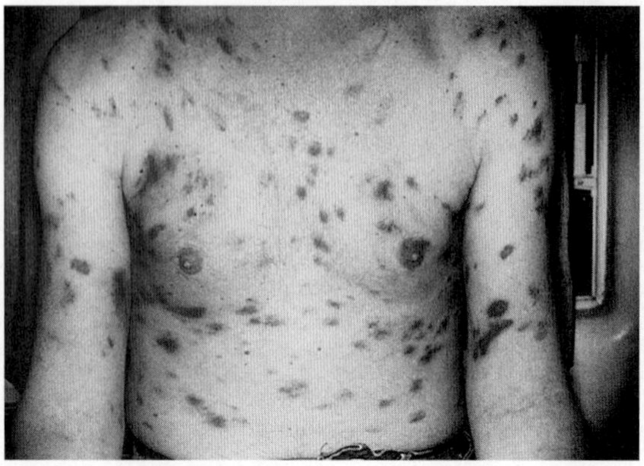

FIGURE 1-140 Kaposi's sarcoma. More advanced lesions. Note widespread hemorrhagic plaques and nodules. (From Noble J [ed]: *Textbook of primary care medicine,* ed 2, St Louis, 1995, Mosby.)

GENERAL Rx

- Excisional biopsy often provides adequate treatment for single lesions and resected recurrences in classic Kaposi's sarcoma.
- Liquid nitrogen cryotherapy can result in complete response in 80% of lesions.
- Interlesional chemotherapy with vinblastine is useful for nodular lesions >1 cm in diameter. Intralesional injection of interferon alfa-2b has also been reported as effective and well tolerated.
- Radiation therapy is effective in non-AIDS KS and for large tumor masses that interfere with normal function.
- Systemic therapy with interferon is also effective in AIDS-related KS and is often used in combination with AZT.
- Systemic chemotherapy (vinblastine, bleomycin, doxorubicin, and dacarbazine) can be used for rapidly progressive disease and for classic and African endemic KS.
- Sirolimus (rapamycin), an immunosuppressive drug, is effective in inhibiting the progression of dermal Kaposi's sarcoma in kidney transplant recipients.
- Oral etoposide is also effective and has less myelosuppression than vinblastine.
- Paclitaxel is also effective in patients with advanced KS and represents an excellent second-line therapy.

DISPOSITION

- Prognosis is poor in AIDS-related KS. Death is often a result of other AIDS-defining illnesses.
- Prognosis is better in African cutaneous KS and classic sarcoma (patients usually die of unrelated causes).

PEARLS & CONSIDERATIONS

COMMENTS

Immunosuppression-associated Kaposi's sarcoma usually regresses with the cessation, reduction, or modification of immunosuppression therapy in most patients. Similarly in HIV patients, Kaposi's sarcoma responds concurrently with the decrease in serum HIV RNA and increase in the CD4 count.

SUGGESTED READING

Stallone et al: Sirolimus for Kaposi's sarcoma in renal-transplant recipients, *N Eng J Med* 352:1317, 2005.

AUTHOR: **FRED F. FERRI, M.D.**

BASIC INFORMATION

DEFINITION

Kawasaki disease (also known as the mucocutaneous lymph node syndrome) is an acute, febrile, multisystem disease usually involving children, and is usually manifested by self-limited generalized vasculitis of unknown etiology.

SYNONYMS

Kawasaki syndrome
Mucocutaneous lymph node syndrome

ICD-9CM CODES
446.1 Kawasaki disease

EPIDEMIOLOGY & DEMOGRAPHICS

- Kawasaki disease is a leading cause of acquired heart disease in children.
- Commonly occurs under the age of 5 yr (80%). Peak age is 18 to 24 months.
- More prevalent in boys than in girls (1.5:1).
- The highest incidence is found in Japan (approximately 150 cases/100,000 children).
- Incidence of Kawasaki disease in the U.S. is 10 to 15 cases/100,000 children <5 yr of age.
- Children of Asian descent have the highest incidence of Kawasaki disease, compared to those of European and African descent.
- Approximately 4000 new cases are diagnosed each year in the U.S.
- In the U.S., Kawasaki disease has now surpassed acute rheumatic fever as the leading cause of acquired heart disease in children.

PHYSICAL FINDINGS & CLINICAL PRESENTATION

- Diagnosis of Kawasaki disease is based on characteristic clinical signs and symptoms and includes fever persisting for >5 days and the presence of at least four of the following five principal features:
  1. Predominantly unilateral cervical lymphadenopathy (>1.5 cm in diameter)
  2. Changes in extremities: (i) Acute: erythema and edema of hands and feet (Fig. 1-141, *A*); (ii) convalescent: membranous desquamation of fingertips
  3. Polymorphous exanthema (usually in truncal region)
  4. Bilateral, painless bulbar conjunctival injection without exudate
  5. Erythema and cracking of lips, strawberry tongue (Fig. 1-141, *B*), diffuse injection of the oral and pharyngeal mucosae
- The fever of Kawasaki disease is usually higher than 102.2°F (39°C) and often above 104.0°F (40°C); if untreated, it lasts for an average of 11 days.
- Coronary-artery aneurysms (>8 mm in diameter) develop in as many as 25% of untreated children and can lead, over time, to ischemic heart disease, myocardial infarction, congestive heart failure and occasionally, death.
- Children with Kawasaki disease who are less than 1 yr of age are more likely to develop the cardiac sequelae and are most likely to fail treatment.
- Patients with fever and fewer than four principal symptoms but evidence of coronary artery disease are diagnosed as having atypical Kawasaki disease.
- Mucous membrane changes involving the hands are the most common manifestation of Kawasaki disease (either typical or atypical).
- Cervical adenopathy is the most common physical manifestation in atypical Kawasaki disease.
- On rare occasions aneurysms of peripheral arteries (e.g., axillary) may be seen.
- Beau's lines (transverse grooves of the nails), diarrhea, dyspnea, arthralgia, and myalgia may also been seen.

ETIOLOGY

The cause of Kawasaki disease is not known, although evidence substantiates an infectious etiology precipitating an immune-mediated reaction.

DIAGNOSIS

There is no diagnostic test for this acute vasculitis. The illness begins with the abrupt onset of fever. Typically, the clinical signs appear over the course of several days. The clinical criteria (listed in "Physical Findings & Clinical Presentation") can be used to aid in the diagnosis of Kawasaki disease.

DIFFERENTIAL DIAGNOSIS

- Scarlet fever
- Stevens-Johnson syndrome
- Drug eruption
- Henoch-Schönlein purpura
- Toxic shock syndrome
- Measles
- Rocky Mountain spotted fever
- Infectious mononucleosis

WORKUP

Clinical findings in addition to laboratory and imaging studies are useful in searching for multiorgan system involvement and complications (e.g., cardiac, lung, liver).

LABORATORY TESTS

Clinical and laboratory findings observed in patients with this disease are frequently helpful in diagnosis. They include the following:

- CBC commonly shows a normochromic normocytic anemia, elevated platelet count, elevated white blood cell count with neutrophil predominance.
- Elevated liver function tests.
- Elevated erythrocyte sedimentation rate (often above 40 mm/hour and, not uncommonly, is elevated to levels of at least 100 mm/hour).
- Elevated C-reactive protein (levels of 3 mg/dl or more).
- Urinalysis may show sterile pyuria.

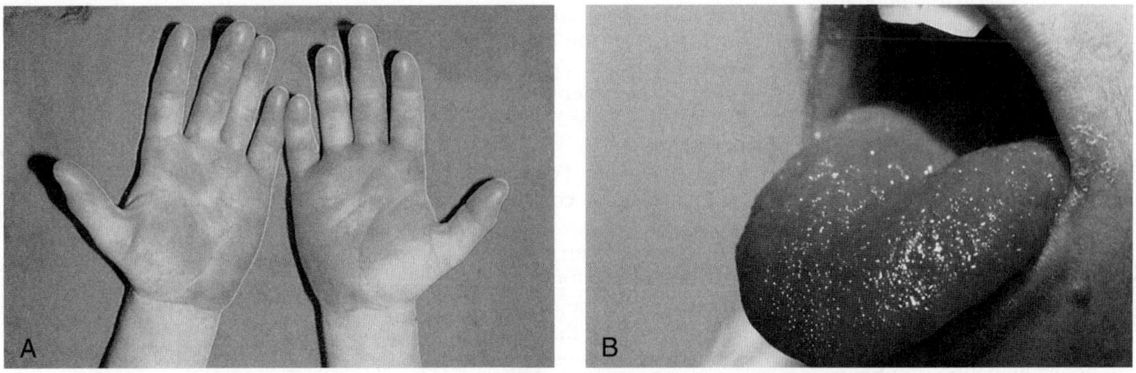

FIGURE 1-141 A, Erythema of the hands, to be followed by desquamation. **B,** Strawberry tongue in a patient with Kawasaki syndrome. (**A** Courtesy Department of Dermatology, University of North Carolina at Chapel Hill. In Goldstein B [ed]: *Practical dermatology,* ed 2, St Louis, 1997, Mosby. **B** Courtesy Marshall Guill, M.D. In Goldstein B [ed]: *Practical dermatology,* ed 2, St Louis, 1997, Mosby.)

IMAGING STUDIES

- Chest x-ray may reveal pulmonary infiltrates.
- Echocardiogram is very helpful and may show depressed left ventricular function with regional wall motion abnormalities, pericardial effusion (30%), and mitral valve regurgitation. The echocardiogram is also useful in the long-term follow-up of patients with Kawasaki disease.
- Coronary angiogram and MRI can be used to visualize the coronary arteries and for the presence of coronary artery aneurysms. Echocardiography may be able to visualize these aneurysms in infants.
- Intravascular ultrasound can assess for luminal irregularities of the coronary arteries.
- Exercise testing with myocardial perfusion studies can be done to assess for coronary blood flow and the presence of myocardial ischemia.
- ECG changes (arrhythmias, abnormal Q waves, prolonged PR and/or QT intervals, occasionally low voltage, or ST-T wave changes) can be seen. Chest x-ray abnormalities (cardiomegaly) may also be evident.

TREATMENT

Rx

Consists of treatment of the acute phase and long-term management of patients with Kawasaki disease. Treatment of Kawasaki disease in the acute phase is directed at reducing inflammation in the coronary artery wall and preventing coronary thrombosis, whereas long-term therapy in individuals who develop coronary aneurysms is aimed at preventing myocardial ischemia or infarction.

NONPHARMACOLOGIC THERAPY

- Oxygen in selected patients
- Salt restriction in patients with congestive heart failure

ACUTE GENERAL Rx

- Without treatment, coronary artery abnormalities develop in about 15% to 25% of patients with Kawasaki disease.
- Intravenous immunoglobulin (IVIG) 2 g/kg over 8 to 12 hr is the treatment of choice in children diagnosed with Kawasaki disease and ideally should be given within the first 10 days of the illness.
- Aspirin 80 to 100 mg/kg/day given in four divided doses until the patient is no longer febrile. Thereafter, aspirin 3 to 5 mg/kg/day is continued until lab studies (e.g., sedimentation rate) return to normal, generally within 6 to 8 wk.
- In patients that do not defervesce within 48 hr or have recrudescent fever after initial IVIG treatment, a second dose of IVIG 2 g/kg IV over 8 to 12 hr should be considered.
- Non steroidal anti-inflammatory drugs are not effective in the treatment of Kawasaki disease.
- The effect of corticosteroids on coronary artery aneurysms is unclear. Therefore, most experts recommend withholding steroids unless fever persists after at least two courses of IVIG.
- Other therapies, including pentoxifylline, infliximab (monoclonal antibody against tumor necrosis factor A), plasma exchange, abciximab (platelet glycoprotein IIb/IIIa receptor inhibitor), and cytotoxic agents (cyclophosphamide), have been used but there is limited data on their success.
- Acute management of patients with coronary artery abnormalities depends on the severity of the lesion.
- Most patients with large or giant coronary artery aneurysms (diameter >8 mm) are maintained on aspirin (or clopidogrel) and warfarin to prevent thrombosis within the aneurysm and myocardial infarction

CHRONIC Rx

Interventional and surgical procedures can be tried in children who have developed cardiac complications of Kawasaki disease:

- Percutaneous transluminal coronary angioplasty
- Coronary bypass graft surgery using the internal mammary artery or the gastroepiploic artery has met with greater patency success than saphenous vein grafts
- Cardiac transplantation is an option and is indicated in patients with:
  1. Severe left ventricular failure
  2. Malignant arrhythmias
  3. Multivessel coronary artery disease

DISPOSITION

- Mortality rate of children with Kawasaki disease is 0.5% to 2.8%, usually from coronary artery aneurysm, coronary thrombosis, and myocarditis.
- Death usually occurs in the third to fourth week of the illness.
- Before the use of IVIG, approximately 20% of all patients with Kawasaki disease developed coronary artery aneurysms.
- Treatment with IVIG has reduced the incidence of coronary aneurysms by 80%.
- IVIG has also been shown to improve left ventricular function during the acute stages of the disease.
- Risk factors for the development of coronary aneurysms or giant coronary aneurysms (>8 mm) are:
  1. Fever lasting >10 days
  2. Age <1 year
  3. Male
  4. Recurrence of fever
- 1% to 2% of patients have recurrences of Kawasaki disease.

REFERRAL

Multiple specialists may be consulted to assist in the diagnosis of Kawasaki disease, including dermatology, rheumatology, and infectious disease. Cardiology consultation is recommended in any patient with cardiac involvement and in the long-term follow-up of patients with Kawasaki disease.

PEARLS & CONSIDERATIONS

!

COMMENTS

- Kawasaki disease was first described by Dr. Tomasaku Kawasaki in 1967 and published in the *Journal of Allergology*.
- Kawasaki disease is not transmitted from person to person.
- The traditional means to diagnose Kawasaki disease include at least five days of fever plus at least four of five other findings common in the disease.
- Atypical or incomplete Kawasaki disease can be detected using clinical plus laboratory criteria along with typical findings on echocardiography.
- The mechanism of action of intravenous immunoglobulin therapy for Kawasaki disease remains unknown.

PREVENTION

- Without an etiologic agent for Kawasaki disease, primary prevention is not possible.
- Low-dose aspirin (3 to 5 mg/kg/day, given as a single dose) should be continued until 6 to 8 wk after disease onset if there are no coronary artery abnormalities or indefinitely if abnormalities are present.
- Thrombosis leading to myocardial infarction in a stenotic or aneurysmal coronary artery is the leading cause of death in these children and occurs most often in the first year after illness onset. Therefore, serial imaging and stress tests are necessary in patients with significant coronary artery abnormalities (via coronary angiography).

PATIENT/FAMILY EDUCATION

- The Kawasaki Disease Foundation, a nonprofit organization dedicated to Kawasaki Disease issues (http://www.kdfoundation.org).
- The American Heart Association has developed guidelines for the diagnosis of Kawasaki disease (http://www.americanheart.org).

EVIDENCE

EBM

Randomized, prospective clinical trials conducted in the U.S. in the 1980s established that intravenous immunoglobulin was an effective and safe therapy that reduced the rate of coronary-artery aneurysms detectable on echocardiography to 3% to 5%.[1,2] Ⓐ

Evidence-Based References

1. Newburger JW et al: Diagnosis, treatment, and long-term management of Kawasaki disease: a statement for health professionals from the Committee on Rheumatic Fever, Endocarditis, and Kawasaki Disease, Council on Cardiovascular Disease in the Young, American Heart Association, *Pediatrics* 114:1708-1733, 2004. (Published correction appears in *Pediatrics* 115:1118, 2005.)
2. Newburger JW et al: A single intravenous infusion of gamma globulin as compared with four infusions in the treatment of acute Kawasaki syndrome, *N Engl J Med* 324:1633-1639, 1991. (Abstract)

SUGGESTED READINGS

Burns JC et al: Kawasaki syndrome, *Lancet* 364:533-544, 2004.

Newburger JW, Fulton DR: Kawasaki disease, *Curr Opin Pediatr* 16(5):508, 2004.

Newburger JW et al: Diagnosis, treatment, and long-term management of Kawasaki disease: a statement for health professionals from the Committee on Rheumatic Fever, Endocarditis and Kawasaki Disease, Council on Cardiovascular Disease in the Young, American Heart Association, *Circulation* 110:2747-2771, 2004.

Royle J, Burgner D, Curtis N: The diagnosis and management of Kawasaki disease, *J Paediatr Child Health* 41(3):87, 2005.

AUTHOR: **PRANAV M. PATEL, M.D.**

BASIC INFORMATION

DEFINITION

Klinefelter's syndrome is a congenital disorder in which a 47,XXY chromosome complement is associated with hypogonadism and infertility.

SYNONYMS

47,XXY Hypogonadism

ICD-9CM CODES
758.7 Klinefelter's syndrome

EPIDEMIOLOGY & DEMOGRAPHICS

INCIDENCE: 1 in 500 men (most common sex chromosome disorder)

GENETICS: The most common mosaic complement is 46,XY/47,XXY. 47,XXY karyotype and occasional 48,XXYY; 48,XXXY; or 49,XXXXY have been reported. The manifestations vary in severity in patients. It is this sex chromosome mosaicism that is thought to account for the variable presentation. Fertility, although very rare, has been reported in men with Klinefelter's syndrome.

PHYSICAL FINDINGS & CLINICAL PRESENTATION

CLASSIC TRIAD: Small firm testes, azoospermia, and gynecomastia

Prepubertal: Small testes, gonadal volume <1.5 ml is a result of loss of germ cells before puberty.

Postpubertal: Gynecomastia (periductal fat growth) with small, firm testes. Exaggerated growth of the lower extremities results in a decreased crown-to-pubis:pubis-to-floor ratio (Fig. 1-142). There is diminished strength, diminished ability to grow a full beard or mustache, infertility. Decreased intellectual development and antisocial behavior are thought to occur with high frequency.

ETIOLOGY

- Several postulated mechanisms: nondisjunction during meiosis and mitosis and anaphase lag during mitosis or meiosis
- Reason: maternal age
  1. The incidence of Klinefelter's rises from 0.6% when the maternal age is 35 yr or less to 5.4% when the maternal age is in excess of 45 yr.
  2. It is of interest to note that the extra X chromosome has a paternal origin as often as a maternal origin.

DIAGNOSIS

- Markedly elevated FSH levels
- Total plasma testosterone are decreased in 50% to 60% of patients
- Free testosterone levels are decreased
- Plasma estradiol is increased stimulating the increase in levels of testosterone-binding globulin with resultant decrease in the testosterone-to-estradiol ratio, which is felt to be the cause of gynecomastia

LABORATORY TESTS

- Normal to low serum testosterone
- Elevated sex hormone binding globulin
- Increased sex hormone binding globin (acts to further suppress any available free testosterone)
- Normal to increased estradiol (a result of augmented peripheral conversion of testosterone to estradiol)
- Testis biopsy shows azoospermia, Leydig cell hyperplasia, hyalinization, and fibrosis of the seminiferous tubules. Mosaics may have focal areas of spermatogenesis, and, on rare occasions, a sperm may appear in the ejaculate. It is the extra X chromosome that is the pivotal factor controlling spermatogenesis as well as affecting neuronal function directly leading to the behavioral abnormalities related to decreased IQ
- Buccal smear: one sex chromatin body

PREPUBERTAL MALE: Gonadotropin levels are normal.

POSTPUBERTAL MALE: Gonadotropin levels are elevated even when the testosterone level is normal.

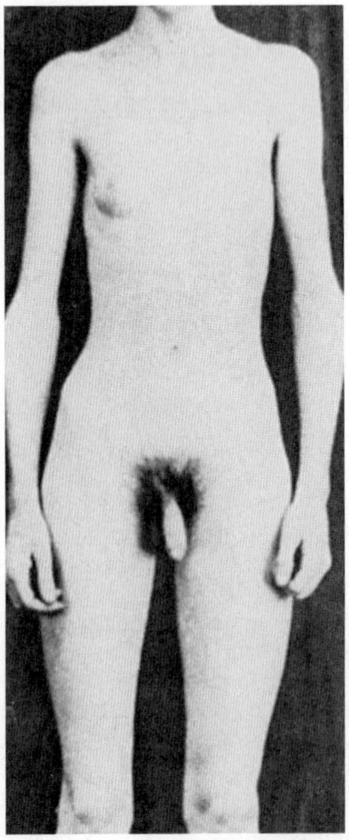

FIGURE 1-142 Klinefelter's syndrome. (From Harrison JH et al: *Campbell's urology,* ed 4, Philadelphia, 1979, WB Saunders.)

DISEASE ASSOCIATIONS:

Malignancies: Breast cancer (20 times greater than XY men and 20% the rate of occurrence in women), nonlymphocytic leukemia, lymphomas, marrow dysplastic syndromes, extragonadal germ cell neoplasms

Autoimmune Disorders: Chronic lymphocytic thyroiditis, Takayasu arteritis, taurodontism (enlarged molar teeth), mitral valve prolapse, varicose veins, asthma, bronchitis, osteoporosis, abnormal glucose tolerance testing, diabetes, varicose veins

TREATMENT

Revolves around three facets of Klinefelter's syndrome:

1. Hypogonadism: androgen replacement in the form of testosterone
2. Gynecomastia: cosmetic surgery
3. Psychosocial problems: androgen therapy and educational support
4. After extensive genetic counseling intracytoplasmic sperm insertion (ICSI) has been used to treat infertility with limited success in mosaic men

PEARLS & CONSIDERATIONS

COMMENTS

- Androgen therapy should not be used in the case of severe mental retardation.
- Also, rule out breast and prostate cancer before initiating or continuing androgen therapy.
- Furthermore, androgen therapy will not improve infertility; it may suppress any spermatogenesis that is taking place within the testes.
- Other causes of primary hypogonadism:
  1. Myotonic muscular dystrophy
  2. Sertoli-cell–only syndrome
  3. Kartagener's syndrome
  4. Anorchia
  5. Acquired hypogonadism
- A fifty-fold higher risk of breast cancer is reported in this population.

SUGGESTED READINGS

Manning MA, Hoyme HE: Diagnosis and management of the adolescent boy with Klinefelter syndrome, *Adolescent Medicine State of the Art Reviews* 13(2):367, 2002.

Palermo GD et al: Births after intracytoplasmic sperm insertion of sperm obtained by testicular extraction from men with non-mosaic Klinefelter's syndrome, *N Engl J Med* 338:588, 1998.

Smyth CM, Bremner WJ: Klinefelter syndrome, *Arch Intern Med* 158:1309, 1998.

AUTHORS: **PHILIP J. ALIOTTA, M.D., M.S.H.A.,** and **RUBEN ALVERO, M.D.**

BASIC INFORMATION

DEFINITION

Korsakoff's psychosis is a disorder of learning and memory, out of proportion to other cognitive functions, associated with thiamine deficiency. It is classically seen with chronic alcohol abuse and may follow the presentation of Wernicke's encephalopathy (see relevant entry).

SYNONYMS

Korsakoff's syndrome
Wernicke-Korsakoff syndrome
Alcoholic polyneuritic psychosis

ICD-9CM CODES
291.1 Alcohol amnestic syndrome

EPIDEMIOLOGY & DEMOGRAPHICS

- Formerly seen commonly in chronic alcohol users, but declining in recent years due to better nutrition and awareness by health professionals.
- Slightly more common in males.
- Age of onset evenly distributed between age 30 and 70.

PHYSICAL FINDINGS & CLINICAL PRESENTATION

- Impairment of ability to remember new material.
- Remote memory is relatively better preserved, but is commonly impaired on neuropsychologic testing.
- Confabulation (the fabrication of false memories to fill memory gaps) is common.

ETIOLOGY

Thiamine deficiency is the underlying cause. This is most commonly seen in alcoholics or other malnourished populations, although it may be iatrogenic from prolonged infusion of dextrose-containing fluids without thiamine repletion.

DIAGNOSIS

DIFFERENTIAL DIAGNOSIS

- Stroke, trauma, or tumor affecting the temporal lobes or hippocampus
- Cerebral anoxia
- Transient global amnesia
- Dementia of multiple causes

WORKUP

A high index of suspicion should be maintained in all alcoholics and other malnourished states.

LABORATORY TESTS

- CBC
- Serum chemistries
- Serum pyruvate is elevated
- Whole-blood or erythrocyte transketolase are decreased; rapid resolution to normal in 24 hr with thiamine repletion

IMAGING STUDIES

MRI may show T2 hyperintense diencephalic and mesencephalic lesions acutely, but there is no definitive radiologic study for diagnosis.

TREATMENT

NONPHARMACOLOGIC THERAPY

A supervised environment may be required. Alcohol cessation must be counseled.

ACUTE GENERAL Rx

- Thiamine 100 mg IV or IM should be given immediately.
- Avoid dextrose-containing fluids until thiamine repleted.
- Thiamine given acutely during Wernicke's phase (disorders of extraocular movements, confusion, and ataxia) may prevent the development of Korsakoff's psychosis.

CHRONIC Rx

- It is difficult to predict acutely the degree of recovery for an individual patient, although the vast majority will have lasting deficits. Decisions regarding long-term institutionalization should therefore be made cautiously.
- Chronic treatment with thiamine (typically 5 mg per day).

DISPOSITION

Patient often must live in assisted environment for the remainder of life.

REFERRAL

- A neurologist should assess the patient.
- Neuropsychologic testing may be helpful.

PEARLS & CONSIDERATIONS

COMMENTS

- This disease is probably underdiagnosed, and memory problems may persist, even in "recovered" patients.
- Replace thiamine in patients at risk, even if clinical symptoms are not evident.
- A preventable cause is prolonged dextrose-containing IV fluids without supplemental thiamine.

EVIDENCE

Thiamine has been established as the treatment of choice for more than 50 years. The evidence for its benefit is based on case reports and clinical experience. No randomized controlled trials (RCTs) are available to guide clinicians in the dosage, route, or duration of therapy in the acute presentation of the syndrome.

A recent RCT that looked at alcoholics without frank clinical evidence of Korsakoff's psychosis showed that those treated with the highest dose of thiamine showed neuropsychologic evidence of improvement in working memory, suggesting that even "asymptomatic" alcoholics may benefit from thiamine supplementation.[1,2]

At least one study suggests that the risk of developing Korsakoff's psychosis is far higher in alcoholic populations regardless of the severity of the underlying thiamine deficiency, suggesting that alcohol use is fundamental in its precipitation.[3]

Evidence-Based References

1. Ambrose ML et al: Thiamine treatment and working memory function of alcohol-dependent people: preliminary findings, *Alcohol Clin Exp Res* 25(1):112-116, 2001.
2. Day E et al: Thiamine for Wernicke-Korsakoff syndrome in people at risk from alcohol abuse, *Cochrane Database Syst Rev* 1:CD004033, 2004.
3. Homewood J, Bond NW: Thiamin deficiency and Korsakoff's syndrome: failure to find memory impairments following nonalcoholic Wernicke's encephalopathy, *Alcohol* 19(1):75-84, 1999.

SUGGESTED READINGS

Cook CC: Prevention and treatment of Wernicke-Korsakoff syndrome, *Alcohol Alcohol Suppl* 35(suppl):19, 2000.
Harper C: Thiamine (vitamin B1) deficiency and associated brain damage is still common throughout the world and prevention is simple and safe! *Eur J Neurol* 13(10):1078, 2006.
Martin PR et al: The role of thiamine deficiency in alcoholic brain disease, *Alcohol Res Health* 27(2):134, 2003.
Sechi G, Serra A: Wernicke's encephalopathy: new clinical settings and recent advances in diagnosis and management, *Lancet Neurol* 6(5):442, 2007.
Zubaran C, Fernandes JG, Rodnight R: Wernicke-Korsakoff syndrome, *Postgrad Med J* 78(855):27, 1997.

AUTHOR: **DANIEL MATTSON, M.D., M.SC. (MED.)**

BASIC INFORMATION

DEFINITION

Labyrinthitis is a peripheral vestibulopathy characterized by acute onset of vertigo usually associated with nausea and vomiting. It may or may not be associated with hearing loss. It may be either serous or purulent.

SYNONYMS

Acute labyrinthitis
Acute vestibular neuronopathy
Vestibular neuronitis
Viral neurolabyrinthitis

ICD-9CM CODES
386.12 Vestibular neuronitis (active and recurrent)
386.3 Labyrinthitis

EPIDEMIOLOGY & DEMOGRAPHICS

INCIDENCE (IN U.S.): Most common cause of prolonged spontaneous vertigo associated with nausea at any age.
PREDOMINANT AGE: Any

CLINICAL PRESENTATION

- Vertigo, nausea, and vomiting with onset over several hours.
- Symptoms usually peak within 24 hours, and then resolve gradually over several weeks.
- During the first day the patient usually has difficulty focusing the eyes because of spontaneous nystagmus.
- Usually has benign course, with complete recovery within 1 to 3 months, although older patients may have intractable dizziness that persists for many months.

PHYSICAL FINDINGS

- Nystagmus
- Nausea
- Vomiting
- Vertigo worsening with head movement
- Abnormal caloric ENG tests
- Possible hearing loss in the affected ear
- Normal otoscopic exam typically
- Otherwise normal neurologic exam, except may possibly have signs of vestibular loss, such as a positive head thrust test

ETIOLOGY

Often preceded 1 to 2 wk by a viral-like illness. It may be either bacterial or viral, and be either tympanogenic (i.e., due to spread of infection into the inner ear from the middle ear, antrum, or petrous apex), meningogenic, or hematogenic from encephalitis or brain abscess. The round window membrane is considered the most likely pathway of inflammatory mediators from the middle to the inner ear that subsequently give rise to labyrinthitis.

DIAGNOSIS

DIFFERENTIAL DIAGNOSIS

- Acute labyrinthine ischemia (vascular insufficiency)
- Other forms of labyrinthitis (bacterial and syphilitic)
- Labyrinthine fistula
- Benign positional vertigo
- Meniere's syndrome
- Cholesteatoma
- Drug induced
- Eighth nerve tumor
- Head trauma

WORKUP

- Otoscopic examination
- Neurologic examination, with close attention to cranial nerves
- Bedside test of vestibular function, i.e., head thrust or head heave test
- Audiogram if symptoms accompanied by hearing loss
- Caloric test if presentation is atypical

LABORATORY TESTS

- Routine laboratory tests are generally not helpful.
- If history of significant emesis, check electrolytes, BUN, and creatinine.

IMAGING STUDIES

Usually not necessary, but enhancement of bony labyrinth may be seen by MRI after injection of contrast material. Head CT with fine cuts through temporal bones if history of trauma or suspect cholesteatoma. MRI of the brain with and without contrast with fine cuts through the internal auditory canal if abnormal cranial nerve exam or suspect eighth nerve tumor.

TREATMENT

NONPHARMACOLOGIC THERAPY

Reassurance. Initial bed rest, then encourage increase in activity as tolerated.

ACUTE GENERAL Rx

- Phenergan or other antiemetics are effective.
- Vestibular suppressant: meclizine 12.5 to 25 mg qid often used. Scopolamine patch also effective.
- Methylprednisolone 100 mg per day for 3 days, with slow taper over 3 weeks.
- Valacyclovir has not been shown to be helpful.

CHRONIC Rx

Important to wean off vestibular suppressant therapy as soon as possible.

DISPOSITION

Usually does not require hospital admission unless patient is unable to tolerate oral intake of liquids.

REFERRAL

- If symptoms persist or neurologic abnormalities are present
- Vestibular rehabilitation

PEARLS & CONSIDERATIONS

COMMENTS

Labyrinthitis is a term that usually implies peripheral vestibulopathy associated with hearing loss. The term *vestibular neuronitis* is typically used when hearing is not affected. Despite this technical distinction, many physicians use both of these terms interchangeably.

SUGGESTED READINGS

Baloh RW et al: Neurotology, *Continuum, Lifelong Learning in Neurology* 2(2):37-53, 1996.

Cureoglu S et al: Round window membrane and labyrinthine pathological changes: an overview, *Acta Otolaryngol* 125(1):9-15, 2005.

Nuti D et al: Acute vestibular neuritis: prognosis based upon bedside clinical tests (thrusts and heaves), *Ann N Y Acad Sci* 1039:359-367, 2005.

Strupp M et al: Methylprednisolone, valacyclovir, or the combination for vestibular neuritis, *N Engl J Med* 351(4):322-323, 2004.

AUTHOR: **SHARON HARTMAN POLENSEK, M.D., PH.D.**

BASIC INFORMATION

DEFINITION

Lactose intolerance is the insufficient concentration of lactase enzyme, leading to fermentation of malabsorbed lactose by intestinal bacteria with subsequent production of intestinal gas and various organic acids.

SYNONYMS

Lactase deficiency
Milk intolerance

ICD-9CM CODES
271.3 Lactose intolerance

EPIDEMIOLOGY & DEMOGRAPHICS

Nearly 50 million people in the U.S. have partial or complete lactose intolerance. There are racial differences, with <25% of white adults being lactose intolerant, whereas >85% of Asian Americans and >60% of blacks have some form of lactose intolerance.

PHYSICAL FINDINGS & CLINICAL PRESENTATION

- Abdominal tenderness and cramping, bloating, flatulence
- Diarrhea
- Symptoms are directly related to the osmotic pressure of substrate in the colon and occur about 2 hr after ingestion of lactose
- Physical examination: may be entirely within normal limits

ETIOLOGY

- Congenital lactase deficiency: common in premature infants; rare in full-term infants and generally inherited as a chromosomal recessive trait
- Secondary lactose intolerance: usually a result of injury of the intestinal mucosa (Crohn's disease, viral gastroenteritis, AIDS enteropathy, cryptosporidiosis, Whipple's disease, sprue)

DIAGNOSIS

DIFFERENTIAL DIAGNOSIS

- IBD
- IBS
- Pancreatic insufficiency
- Nontropical and tropical sprue
- Cystic fibrosis
- Diverticular disease
- Bowel neoplasm
- Laxative abuse
- Celiac disease
- Parasitic disease (e.g., giardiasis)
- Viral or bacterial infections

WORKUP

- The diagnosis can usually be made on the basis of the history and improvement with dietary manipulation.
- Diagnostic workup may include confirming the diagnosis with hydrogen breath test and excluding other conditions listed in the differential diagnosis that may also coexist with lactase deficiency.

LABORATORY TESTS

- Lactose breath hydrogen test: A rise in breath hydrogen >20 ppm within 90 min of ingestion of 50 g of lactose is positive for lactase deficiency. This test is positive in 90% of patients with lactose malabsorption. Common causes of false-negative results are recent use of oral antibiotics or recent high colonic enema.
- The lactose tolerance test is an older and less accurate testing modality (20% rate of false positive and negative results). The patient is administered an oral dose of 1 to 1.5 gm of lactose/kg body weight. Serial measurement of blood glucose level on an hourly basis for 3 hr is then performed. The test is considered positive if the patient develops intestinal symptoms and the blood glucose level rises <20 mg/dl above the fasting baseline level.
- Diarrhea associated with lactase deficiency is osmotic in nature with an osmotic gap and a pH below 6.5.

IMAGING STUDIES

Imaging studies are generally not indicated. A small bowel series may be useful in patients with significant malabsorption.

TREATMENT

NONPHARMACOLOGIC THERAPY

A lactose-free diet generally results in prompt resolution of symptoms. Lactose is primarily found in dairy products but may be present as an ingredient or component of common foods and beverages. Possible sources of lactose are breads, candies, cold cuts, dessert mixes, cream soups, bologna, commercial sauces and gravies, chocolate, drink mixes, salad dressings, and medications. Labels should be read carefully to identify sources of lactose.

ACUTE GENERAL Rx

- Addition of lactase enzyme supplement (Lactaid tablets, Dairy Ease) before the ingestion of milk products may prevent symptoms in some patients. However, it is not effective for all lactose-intolerant patients.
- Lactose-intolerant patients must ensure adequate calcium intake. Calcium supplementation is recommended to prevent osteoporosis.

CHRONIC Rx

Patient education regarding foods high in lactose, such as milk, cottage cheese, or ice cream, is recommended.

DISPOSITION

Clinical improvement with restriction or elimination of milk products

REFERRAL

GI referral for endoscopic procedures if concomitant GI disorders are suspected

PEARLS & CONSIDERATIONS

COMMENTS

- There is great variability in signs and symptoms in patients with lactose intolerance depending on the degree of lactase deficiency.
- Most patients with lactose intolerance can ingest up to 12 oz of milk daily without symptoms.
- Nondairy synthetic drinks (e.g., Coffee-Mate) and use of rice milk are well tolerated.

SUGGESTED READING

Swagerty DL et al: Lactose intolerance, *Am Fam Physician* 65:1845, 2002.

AUTHOR: **FRED F. FERRI, M.D.**

BASIC INFORMATION

DEFINITION

Lambert-Eaton myasthenic syndrome (LEMS) is a disorder of neuromuscular transmission caused by antibodies directed against presynaptic voltage-gated P/Q calcium channels on motor and autonomic nerve terminals. There are two forms: paraneoplastic (most common) and nonparaneoplastic (autoimmune).

SYNONYMS

Eaton-Lambert syndrome

ICD-9CM CODES
199.1 Malignant neoplasm without specification of site, other

EPIDEMIOLOGY & DEMOGRAPHICS

INCIDENCE (IN U.S.): Uncertain; estimated at 5 cases/1 million persons per yr
PREVALENCE (IN U.S.): Uncertain; estimated at 1 per 100,000
PREDOMINANT SEX: Male:female ratio of 2:1
PEAK INCIDENCE: Sixth decade

PHYSICAL FINDINGS & CLINICAL PRESENTATION

- Weakness with diminished or absent muscle stretch reflexes
- Proximal lower extremity muscles most severely affected
- Ocular and bulbar muscles less commonly affected
- Transient improvement in strength and deep tendon reflexes following brief exercise
- Autonomic dysfunction common (dry eyes or dry mouth in 75%, sexual dysfunction, blurred vision, constipation, orthostasis, etc.)

ETIOLOGY

- Antibodies directed against presynaptic voltage-gated P/Q calcium channels are present in most patients. The reduction in calcium influx causes a reduction in acetylcholine release at motor and autonomic nerve terminals.
- Paraneoplastic forms, usually associated with small cell lung cancer (SCLC), are present in 50% to 70% of patients. About 1% to 3% of patients with SCLC develop LEMS.
- Autoimmune forms, usually in patients with other autoimmune diseases, occur in 10% to 30% of patients.

DIAGNOSIS

DIFFERENTIAL DIAGNOSIS

- Myasthenia gravis
- Polymyositis and other myopathies
- Polymyalgia rheumatica
- Botulism
- Guillain-Barré syndrome

Section II describes the differential diagnosis of muscle weakness.

WORKUP

Confirm diagnosis by characteristic electrodiagnostic (EMG/NCS) findings:
- Reduced motor amplitudes with normal sensory studies
- >10% decrement in motor amplitudes on slow (2 to 3 Hz) repetitive nerve stimulation
- >100% increment on fast RNS (20 to 30 Hz) or immediately after 10 seconds of intense muscle contraction (postexercise facilitation)

LABORATORY TESTS

Elevated P/Q calcium channel antibody titers

IMAGING STUDIES

Chest CT to screen for underlying SCLC. Since LEMS may precede diagnosis of SCLC by up to 5 yr, chest CT should be repeated every 6 to 12 mo for up to 5 yr.

TREATMENT

ACUTE GENERAL RX

Plasma exchange (200 to 250 ml/kg over 10 to 14 days) or IV immunoglobulins (2 g/kg over 2 to 5 days) often produce significant, temporary improvement.

CHRONIC Rx

- Anticholinesterase agents (pyridostigmine 30 to 60 mg q4 to 6h) may yield some improvement.
- Guanidine hydrochloride: start 5 to 10 mg/kg/day; up to 30 mg/kg/day in 3-day intervals.
- 3,4-diaminopyridine 10 to 20 mg PO qid (max 100 mg/day) may improve muscle strength and reduce autonomic symptoms in up to 85% of patients in uncontrolled series. (Available in Europe, but limited to research studies in the U.S.)
- Prednisone 1.0 to 1.5 mg/kg/day can be gradually tapered over months to minimal effective dose.
- Azathioprine can be given alone or in combination with prednisone. Give up to 2.5 mg/kg/day. If patient is intolerant of this, can administer cyclosporine up to 3 mg/kg/day instead.
- Manage symptoms of autonomic dysfunction (e.g., salt tablets, florinef, and/or midodrine for orthostatic hypotension).
- Treat underlying malignancy if present.

DISPOSITION

- Gradually progressive weakness leading to impaired mobility if untreated.
- Clinical remission may occur with chronic immunosuppressive therapy in 43% of cases.
- Possible substantial improvement with successful treatment of underlying malignancy.

REFERRAL

- To a neurologist (recommended) because of infrequency of this disease and risks associated with some treatments.
- Referral to specialist centers for 3,4-DAP therapy may be warranted in the U.S.
- Surgical referral for tumor debulking in paraneoplastic forms.

PEARLS & CONSIDERATIONS

COMMENTS

- Prominent autonomic symptoms (dry eyes, dry mouth, impotence, orthostasis) are often the clue to the diagnosis in the appropriate clinical context.
- Many drugs may worsen weakness and should be used only if absolutely necessary. These include succinylcholine, d-tubocurarine, quinine, quinidine, procainamide, aminoglycoside antibiotics, beta-blockers, and calcium channel blockers.

EVIDENCE

There is evidence from two randomized controlled trials (RCTs) that 3,4-diaminopyridine improves muscle strength in patients with LEMS.[1-3]

There is evidence from a single RCT that IV Ig leads to improved muscle strength in patients with LEMS.[3,4]

There is an absence of evidence regarding the efficacy of plasma exchange, steroids, and steroid-sparing agents such as azathioprine.

Evidence-Based References

1. McEvoy K et al: 3-4-Diaminopyridine in the treatment of Lambert-Eaton myasthenic syndrome, *New Engl J Med* 321:1567, 1989.
2. Sanders DB et al: A randomized trial of 3-4-diaminopyridine in Lambert-Eaton myasthenic syndrome, *Neurology* 54:603, 2000.
3. Maddison P, Newsom-Davis J: Treatment for Lambert-Eaton myasthenic syndrome, *Cochrane Database Syst Rev* 18:CD003279, 2005.
4. Bain P et al: Effects of intravenous immunoglobulin on muscle weakness and calcium-channel autoantibodies in the Lambert-Eaton myasthenic syndrome, *Neurology* 47:678, 1996.

SUGGESTED READINGS

Dropcho EJ: Remote neurologic manifestations of cancer, *Neurol Clin* 20:85, 2002.
Mareska M, Gutmann L: Lambert-Eaton myasthenic syndrome, *Semin Neurol* 24:149, 2004.
Sanders DB: The Lambert-Eaton myasthenic syndrome diagnosis and treatment, *Ann NY Acad Sci* 998:500, 2003.

AUTHORS: **MICHAEL BENATAR, M.B.CH.B., D.PHIL.,** and **EROBOGHENE UBOGU, M.D.**

BASIC INFORMATION

DEFINITION

Cancer of the larynx, including the vocal cords (glottis), supraglottis, and subglottis.

SYNONYMS

Laryngeal cancer
Head and neck cancer (subsite); other sites include oral cavity, pharynx, perinasal sinus, and salivary glands

ICD-9CM CODES
231.0 Carcinoma of larynx

EPIDEMIOLOGY & DEMOGRAPHICS

INCIDENCE: 12,000 new cases per year in the U.S.
PEAK INCIDENCE: Sixth decade
PREDOMINANT SEX: 80% male predominance (current, with past and projected increase in female rates as a result of changing smoking habits)

PHYSICAL FINDINGS & CLINICAL PRESENTATION

Glottis
- Early diagnosis possible because of voice change (hoarseness). Any voice change of more than 2 wk duration should prompt a laryngeal examination.
- Supraglottis
  1. No early symptom
  2. Cervical lymphadenopathy
  3. Neck pain or ear pain
  4. Discomfort during swallowing
  5. Odynophagia
  6. Later: hoarseness, dysphagia, airway obstruction
- Subglottis

Even more subtle than supraglottic lesion; the same signs occur, only later in the course

ETIOLOGY

- Smoking (cigarette, cigar, or pipe)
- Alcohol intake/abuse
- Diet and nutritional deficiencies
- Gastroesophageal reflux
- Voice abuse
- Chronic laryngitis
- Exposure to wood dust
- Asbestosis
- Exposure to radiation
- Possible role of human papilloma virus

DIAGNOSIS

DIFFERENTIAL DIAGNOSIS

- Laryngitis
- Allergic and nonallergic rhinosinusitis
- Gastroesophageal reflux
- Voice abuse leading to hoarseness
- Laryngeal papilloma
- Vocal cord paralysis secondary to a neurologic condition or secondary to entrapment of the recurrent laryngeal nerve caused by mediastinal compression
- Tracheomalacia

STAGING:

Supraglottic

T1 Tumor limited to one subsite with normal cord mobility
T2 Tumor invades mucosa of more than one subsite (e.g., base of tongue, vallecula, pyriform sinus) without fixation of larynx
T3 Tumor limited to larynx with vocal cord fixation or invasion of postcricoid area or preepiglottis
T4 Tumor invades thyroid cartilage or extends into soft tissue of the neck, thyroid, or esophagus

Glottic

T1 Tumor limited to vocal cord with normal mobility
T1a Tumor limited to one vocal cord
T1b Tumor involves both vocal cords
T2 Tumor extends to supra or subglottis or impairs cord mobility
T3 Tumor limited to larynx with cord fixation
T4 Tumor invades through cartilage or other tissues beyond larynx

Stage grouping

Stage I: T1, N0, M0
Stage II: T2, N0, M0
Stage III: T3, N0, M0
T1, T2, T3, N1, M0
Stage IV: T4, N0, N1, M0
Any T, N2, N3, M0
Any T, any N or M >0

WORKUP

- Laboratory: none
- Endoscopic laryngeal inspection
- After (and only after) diagnosis of the malignancy, imaging with CT or MRI should be undertaken to stage the disease

HISTOLOGIC CLASSIFICATION:

Epithelial cancers
- Squamous cell carcinoma in situ
- Superficially invasive cancer
- Verrucous carcinoma
- Pseudosarcoma
- Anaplastic cancer
- Transitional cell carcinoma
- Lymphoepithelial cancer
- Adenocarcinoma
- Neuroendocrine tumors, including small cell and carcinoid

Sarcomas
Metastatic malignancies

TREATMENT

ACUTE GENERAL Rx

- Early stage (T or T_2): two options
  1. Conservative surgery (partial laryngectomy) with neck dissection
  2. Primary radiation
- Intermediate stage: four options
  1. Primary radiation alone
  2. Supraglottic laryngectomy with neck dissection
  3. Supraglottic laryngectomy with postoperative radiation
  4. Chemotherapy with radiation
- Advanced stage

Chemotherapy and radiation with total laryngectomy reserved for treatment failure

Glottis
- Carcinoma in situ
  1. Microexcision
  2. Laser vaporization
  3. Radiation
- Early stage (T or T_2): two options
  1. Voice conservation surgery
  2. Radiation
- Intermediate stage (T_3)
  1. Combined radiation and chemotherapy (cisplatin and 5FU)
  2. Total laryngectomy for treatment failure
- Advanced stage (T_4)
  1. Combined radiation and chemotherapy
  2. Total laryngectomy and neck dissection followed by postoperative radiation in unfavorable lesion or treatment failure

Subglottis
Total laryngectomy and approximate neck surgery to excise the tumor, followed by radiation
Unresected cancers
- Induction chemotherapy and radiation followed by neck dissection in chemosensitive tumors, or by laryngectomy and neck dissection in chemoresistant tumors
- If hypopharyngeal involvement exists: laryngopharyngectomy, neck dissection, and postoperative radiation

DISPOSITION

Supraglottis 5-yr control
- T_1 95% to 100%
- T_2 80% to 90%
- T_3 65% to 85%
- T_4 40% to 55%

Glottis 5-yr control
- T_1 95% to 100%
- T_2 50% to 85%
- T_3 35% to 85%
- T_4 20% to 65%

EVIDENCE

EBM

Expert opinion supports the use of surgery in the management of laryngeal cancer.

Although there have been no definitive studies that compare the primary treatment options for oral cancer, there is a consensus that surgery is effective as a primary treatment of oral cancer.[1] C

Expert opinion supports the use of radiation therapy in the treatment of cancer of the head and neck, including laryngeal cancer.

Although there have been few definitive studies that compare the primary treatment options for laryngeal cancer, there is a consensus that radiation therapy is effective as a primary treatment of cancer of the larynx. It is also effective as an adjunctive treatment where surgical resection has been carried out as the primary treatment.[1] C

There is evidence that, in patients at high risk for local recurrence following surgical resection, the use of postoperative radiation therapy significantly improves treatment outcomes.

A nonrandomized study compared the effects of secondary surgery alone or with radiotherapy in patients with positive resection margins or evidence of extracapsular spread following primary radical neck resection. The study found that patients receiving the surgery/radiotherapy combination had significantly better rates of locoregional control and survival compared with those patients who were treated with further surgery alone.[2] B

There is evidence that delays in initiating radiation therapy, both as the primary treatment and as an adjunct to surgical resection, has a detrimental effect on locoregional control and survival.

A systematic review identified 12 case series that, retrospectively, assessed the relationship between delay in initiating radiation therapy and outcomes in patients with head and neck cancer.[3] A

In one study where radiation was the primary therapy the review found that patients in whom treatment was initiated more than 30 days after diagnosis had significantly higher rates of locoregional failure and significantly poorer 5-year survival than those patients treated within 30 days of diagnosis.[3] A

The same review also assessed the impact of timing of postoperative radiation therapy. It found that delays in initiating postoperative radiotherapy had a detrimental effect on locoregional control and survival. Patients treated with postoperative radiation therapy started 30 days after surgery had significantly poorer rates of locoregional control and 5-year survival compared with those patients where radiation therapy was started earlier.[3] A

There is limited evidence that patients with head and neck cancer who cease smoking during radiation therapy have better rates of response and survival than patients who continue to smoke.

One study evaluated the role of cigarette smoking during radiation therapy on the efficacy of treatment in 115 patients with head and neck cancer. The study found that the 53 patients who continued to smoke during treatment had significantly poorer response and 2-year survival compared with those patients who did not smoke or stopped before treatment.[4] B

There is limited evidence that the concomitant use of chemotherapy with surgery/radiation therapy is of benefit in the treatment of head and neck cancer.

A metaanalysis study of 69 trials comparing the impact on survival of chemotherapy added to locoregional treatment found that the use of concomitant chemotherapy had a small but significant overall benefit in survival.[5] A

Two recent randomized controlled trials (RCTs) each compared the use of concomitant cisplatin with postoperative radiotherapy vs. radiotherapy alone following surgical resection of mucosal squamous cell cancer of the head and neck. Both studies found that the use of cisplatin concurrent to postoperative radiotherapy significantly reduced the incidence of locoregional failure. Both RCTs, however, reported that the use of cisplatin was associated with a greater incidence of adverse effects.[6,7] B

One RCT also demonstrated that the concomitant use of cisplatin significantly improved 5-year survival rates compared with radiotherapy alone.[6] B

There is evidence that the combined use of chemotherapy with radiation therapy allows preservation of the larynx in patients with advanced carcinoma of the larynx.

A randomized controlled trial (RCT) compared induction chemotherapy (cisplatin plus fluorouracil) followed by radiation therapy vs. surgery followed by radiation therapy in 332 patients with stage III/IV laryngeal cancer. Patients initially assigned for nonsurgical treatment were evaluated during the initial treatment phase and those patients in whom there was no tumor response or who had locally recurrent cancers after chemotherapy and radiation therapy underwent salvage laryngectomy. This study reported that the 2-year survival was similar for both treatment groups (68%) and of the patients initially assigned for laryngeal preservation, by treatment with chemotherapy and radiation therapy, the larynx was preserved in 64% of cases.[8] B

A recent RCT compared induction chemotherapy (cisplatin plus fluorouracil) followed by radiation therapy vs. concomitant chemotherapy (cisplatin plus fluorouracil) plus radiation therapy vs. radiation therapy alone in 547 patients with stage III/IV laryngeal cancer, the surgical treatment for which would require total laryngectomy. In all patients who had either an inadequate response to chemotherapy or tumor recurrence following therapy, laryngectomy was performed. This study found that the use of concomitant chemotherapy (cisplatin plus fluorouracil) with radiation therapy resulted in significantly greater rates of locoregional control and laryngeal preservation than either induction chemotherapy followed by radiation therapy or radiation therapy alone. Survival rates were similar for all three regimens; 2 year (75%); 5 year (55%).[9] B

There is some evidence that the use of conventional analgesia is effective in the treatment of pain associated with cancer of the head and neck.

A systematic review found that morphine is effective in the management of moderate to severe cancer pain.[10] A

A systematic review found that single doses of NSAIDs are as equally effective as weak opioids in short-term symptomatic relief from cancer pain.[11] A

There is some evidence that pilocarpine is effective in the symptomatic management of xerostomia associated with radiation therapy for head and neck cancer.

A systematic review found that pilocarpine produced significant improvements in patient symptoms associated with postirradiation xerostomia.[12] B

There is some evidence that topical therapies are effective in the reduction and prevention of oral mucositis in patients undergoing treatment for cancer of the head and neck.

A systematic review found that, of a variety of topical measures, the use of ice chips was most effective in preventing or reducing the severity of mucositis.[13] A

A systematic review of patients undergoing radiation treatment, with or without chemotherapy, for squamous cancers of the head and neck found that there is some benefit from the use of prophylactic topical antibiotics in reducing the clinical severity of mucositis.[14] B

There is limited evidence that the use of retinoic acid is effective in preventing the development of a new second primary tumor of the aerodigestive tract.

A randomized controlled trial compared the use of the retinoid, 13-cis-retinoic acid, vs. placebo in 103 patients who were disease free after primary treatment of squamous cell carcinoma of the head and neck. Although no differences were observed in recurrence rates of the original tumor, the use of 13-cis-retinoic acid significantly reduced the incidence of new second primary tumors of the aerodigestive tract compared with placebo.[15] B

However, a recent large randomized controlled trial comparing the vitamin A analogue, retinyl palmitate, vs. placebo in the prevention of new second primaries in patients with head and neck cancer found no significant difference in the incidence of such tumors after 4 years' follow-up.[16] B

Another recent RCT involving 151 patients with primary head and neck cancer compared isotretinoin (at high or moderate doses) vs. placebo over a 3-year period. The study found that there were no significant differences in the incidence of new second primary carcinomas between the treatment groups.[17] B

Evidence-Based References

1. American Head and Neck Society: Los Angeles, CA. C
2. Huang DT et al: Postoperative radiotherapy in head and neck carcinoma with extracapsular lymph node extension and/or positive resection margins: a comparative study, *Int J Radiat Oncol Biol Phys* 23:737, 1992.
3. Huang J et al: Does delay in starting treatment affect the outcomes of radiotherapy? A systematic review, *J Clin Oncol* 21:555, 2003. A
4. Browman GP et al: Influence of cigarette smoking on the efficacy of radiation therapy in head and neck cancer, *N Engl J Med* 328:159, 1993. B
5. Pignon JP et al: Chemotherapy added to locoregional treatment for head and neck squamous-cell carcinoma: three meta-analyses of updated individual data, *Lancet* 355:949, 2000. A
6. Bernier J et al: Postoperative irradiation with or without concomitant chemotherapy for locally advanced head and neck cancer, *N Engl J Med* 350:1945, 2004. B
7. Cooper JS et al: Postoperative concurrent radiotherapy and chemotherapy in high-risk squamous-cell carcinoma of the head and neck, *N Engl J Med* 350:1937, 2004. B
8. The Department of Veterans Affairs Laryngeal Cancer Study Group: Induction chemotherapy plus radiation compared with surgery plus radiation in patients with advanced laryngeal cancer, *N Engl J Med* 324:1685, 1991. B
9. Forastiere AA et al: Concurrent chemotherapy and radiotherapy for organ preservation in advanced laryngeal cancer, *N Engl J Med* 349:2091, 2003. B
10. Wiffen PJ et al: Oral morphine for cancer pain, *Cochrane Database Syst Rev* 4, 2003. A
11. Eisenberg E et al: Efficacy and safety of nonsteroidal antiinflammatory drugs for cancer pain: a meta-analysis, *J Clin Oncol* 12:2756, 1994. Reviewed in: Bandolier: Knowledge Library. A
12. Hawthorne M, Sullivan K: Pilocarpine for radiation-induced xerostomia in head and neck cancer, *Int J Palliat Nurs* 6:228, 2000. Reviewed in: DARE Document 20005206, York, UK. B
13. Clarkson JE, Worthington HV, Eden OB: Interventions for preventing oral mucositis for patients with cancer receiving treatment, *Cochrane Database Syst Rev* 3, 2003. A
14. Sutherland SE, Browman GP: Prophylaxis of oral mucositis in irradiated head-and-neck cancer patients: a proposed classification scheme of interventions and meta-analysis of randomized controlled trials, *Int J Radiat Oncol Biol Phys* 49:917, 2001. B
15. Hong WK et al: Prevention of second primary tumors with isotretinoin in squamous-cell carcinoma of the head and neck, *N Engl J Med* 323:795, 1990. B
16. van Zandwijk N et al: EUROSCAN, a randomized trial of vitamin A and N-acetylcysteine in patients with head and neck cancer or lung cancer. For the European Organization for Research and Treatment of Cancer Head and Neck and Lung Cancer Cooperative Groups, *J Natl Cancer Inst* 92:977, 2000. B
17. Perry CF et al: Chemoprevention of head and neck cancer with retinoids: a negative result, *Arch Otolaryngol Head Neck Surg* 131:198, 2005. B

AUTHORS: **FRED F. FERRI, M.D.,** and **TOM J. WACHTEL, M.D.**

BASIC INFORMATION

DEFINITION

Laryngitis is an acute or chronic inflammation of the laryngeal mucous membranes.

SYNONYMS

Lower respiratory tract infection

ICD-9CM CODES
464.0 Acute laryngitis
476.0 Chronic laryngitis

EPIDEMIOLOGY & DEMOGRAPHICS

Common illness in both genders and all age groups, but the diagnosis is imprecise and therefore, statistics are not readily available with respect to incidence and prevalence.

PHYSICAL FINDINGS AND CLINICAL PRESENTATION

ACUTE LARYNGITIS:

- Clinical syndrome characterized by the onset of hoarseness, voice breaks, or episodes of aphonia. May also have accompanying sore throat, cough, nasal congestion, and rhinorrhea
- Usually associated with viral upper respiratory infection
- Larynx with diffuse erythema, edema, and vascular engorgement of the vocal folds, and occasionally mucosal ulceration
- In young children subglottis is often affected, resulting in airway narrowing with marked hoarseness, inspiratory stridor, dyspnea, and restlessness
- Respiratory compromise rare in adults

CHRONIC LARYNGITIS:

Characterized by hoarseness or dysphonia persisting for longer than 2 wk

ETIOLOGY

ACUTE LARYNGITIS:

- Most often caused by viruses so treatment consists of supportive measures as outlined in nonpharmacologic therapy section.
- Studies evaluating the use of antibiotics (erythromycin, penicillin) in acute laryngitis failed to show objective clinical benefit over placebo so they are not routinely recommended. Antibiotics and other antimicrobials may be indicated in cases where specific treatable pathogens are identified.
- Avoid decongestants secondary to their drying effect.
- Guaifenesin may be a useful adjunct as a mucolytic agent.
- In GERD-associated laryngitis use acid-suppressive therapy (H2 blockers, proton pump inhibitors) and nocturnal antireflux precautions.

CHRONIC LARYNGITIS:

- Results from any of the following: tuberculosis, usually through bronchogenic spread; leprosy, from nasopharyngeal or oropharyngeal spread; syphilis, in secondary and tertiary stages; rhinoscleroma, extending from the nose and nasopharynx; actinomycosis; histoplasmosis; blastomycosis; paracoccidiomycosis; coccidiosis; candidiasis; aspergillosis; sporotrichosis; rhinosporidiosis; parasitic infections including leishmaniasis and Clinostomum infection following raw freshwater fish ingestion
- Noninfectious causes of both acute and chronic laryngitis include malignancy, voice abuse (singers), gastroesophageal reflux disease, and chemical or environmental irritants such as cigarettes and allergens. Other causes of inflammatory or granulomatous lesions of the larynx include relapsing polychondritis, Wegener's granulomatosis, and sarcoidosis

DIAGNOSIS

DIFFERENTIAL DIAGNOSIS

Young children with signs of airway obstruction:

- Supraglottitis (epiglottitis)
- Laryngotracheobronchitis
- Tracheitis
- Foreign body aspiration

Adults with persistent hoarseness consider noninfectious causes of laryngitis as listed previously

WORKUP

- History and physical examination: diagnosis is usually apparent.
- Laryngoscopy for severe or persistent cases.
- Laryngeal cultures should be performed if etiology other than acute viral infection is suspected.
- Imaging not indicated unless evidence of airway compromise. Obtain plain radiographs of neck, anteroposterior and lateral views, to differentiate laryngitis from acute laryngotracheobronchitis or supraglottitis.

TREATMENT

NONPHARMACOLOGIC THERAPY

- Rest the voice.
- Use an air humidifier.
- Adequate hydration. Avoid alcohol and caffeine because of diuretic effect.

ACUTE GENERAL Rx

- Antibiotics and other antimicrobials: indicated only when a specific pathogen is isolated; commonly employed antibacterial agents are macrolides (clarithromycin 500 mg by mouth BID for 5 to 7 days or azithromycin 500 mg followed by 250 mg once daily for 4 to 5 days if the cause of laryngitis is found to be *Mycoplasma pneumoniae* or *Chlamydiophila pneumoniae* [the new name for what was formerly known as *Chlamydia pneumoniae*])
- Avoid decongestants secondary to their drying effect
- Guaifenesin may be a useful adjunct as a mucolytic agent
- In GERD-associated laryngitis use acid-suppressive therapy (H2 blockers, proton pump inhibitors) and nocturnal antireflux precautions

DISPOSITION

Uncomplicated laryngitis is usually benign, with gradual resolution of symptoms

REFERRAL

If symptoms persist for >2 wk, refer to otolaryngologist for laryngoscopy
Consider referral to gastroenterologist if GERD is suspected

PEARLS & CONSIDERATIONS

- Most cases of uncomplicated acute laryngitis are viral in origin, and bacterial agents should not be routinely administered.
- A recent Cochrane analysis found no evidence for the use of empiric antibiotics in adults with laryngitis.
- The most difficult clinical challenge is often convincing patients with acute laryngitis that they do not need and will not benefit from antibacterial agents.

SUGGESTED READINGS

Ebell MH: Antibiotics for acute laryngitis in adults, *Am Fam Phys* 72:76, 2005.

Mehanna HM et al: Fungal laryngitis in immunocompetent patients, *J Laryngol Otol* 118(5):379, 2004.

Reveiz L, Cardona AF, Ospina EG: Antibiotics for acute laryngitis in adults, *Cochrane Database Syst Rev* CD004783, 2005.

AUTHORS: **JANE V. EASON, M.D., MARILYN FABBRI, M.D., GLENN G. FORT, M.D., M.P.H.,** and **DENNIS J. MIKOLICH, M.D.**

BASIC INFORMATION

DEFINITION

Acute laryngotracheobronchitis is a viral infection of the upper and lower respiratory tract leading to erythema and edema of the tracheal walls and narrowing of the subglottic region.

SYNONYMS

Croup

ICD-9CM CODES
464.4 Croup

EPIDEMIOLOGY & DEMOGRAPHICS

- Croup is primarily a disease of children occurring between the ages of 1 and 6 yr.
- The peak incidence of croup is the second year of life (50 cases/1000 children).
- Most cases usually occur in the fall and represent parainfluenza type 1 viral infection.
- Winter outbreaks usually represent infection by influenza A and B viruses.
- Croup accounts for 10% to 15% of lower respiratory tract infections in young children.
- Boys are affected more often than girls.

PHYSICAL FINDINGS & CLINICAL PRESENTATION

- Most children with croup present with symptoms of an upper respiratory infection for several days
- Rhinorrhea
- Cough
- Low-grade fever
- Barking cough that usually occurs at night and wakes the child up
- Sore throat
- Stridor
- Apprehension
- Use of accessory muscles of respiration
- Tachypnea
- Tachycardia
- Wheezing

ETIOLOGY

- Parainfluenza viruses (types 1, 2, and 3) are the most common causes of croup in the U.S.
- Influenza A and B, although not a common cause of croup, does lead to more severe cases of the disease
- Adenovirus
- Respiratory syncytial virus
- *Mycoplasma pneumoniae* (rare)

DIAGNOSIS

The diagnosis of croup is usually based on the characteristic clinical presentation of a young child between the ages of 1 to 6 yr waking up with a barking cough ("seal's bark") and stridor.

DIFFERENTIAL DIAGNOSIS

- Spasmodic croup
- Epiglottitis
- Bacterial tracheitis
- Angioneurotic edema
- Diphtheria
- Peritonsillar abscess
- Retropharyngeal abscess
- Smoke inhalation
- Foreign body

WORKUP

- The workup of a child with croup is to differentiate viral laryngotracheobronchitis from noninfectious causes of stridor and epiglottitis caused by *H. influenzae*.
- The clinical presentation and plain films of the soft tissues of the neck assist in differentiating viral from nonviral and noninfectious causes.

LABORATORY TESTS

- Laboratory tests are not often used to make the diagnosis of viral tracheobronchitis.
- CBC, viral serology, and tissue cultures can be ordered and may detect the infecting agent in up to 65% of cases.
- Pulse oximetry and arterial blood gas determination for patients with tachypnea and respiratory distress.

IMAGING STUDIES

- Plain (AP and lateral) films of the soft tissues of the neck may show the classic radiographic finding of subglottic stenosis or "steeple" sign.
- CT scan of the soft tissues of the neck may be performed in the cases where the differential between croup, epiglottitis, and noninfectious is more difficult.
- Direct visualization via laryngoscopy may be useful in some situations under a controlled setting.

TREATMENT

Treatment of croup focuses on airway management.

NONPHARMACOLOGIC THERAPY

- Oxygen
- Cool mist
- Hot steam

ACUTE GENERAL Rx

- Use of 0.25 to 0.75 ml of 2.25% racemic epinephrine every 20 min is used in children with severe respiratory symptoms, rest stridor, and impending intubation.
- Corticosteroids (e.g., dexamethasone 0.6 mg/kg IV or PO, prednisone 2 mg/kg/day) have been shown to be effective.
- Budesonide, a nebulized corticosteroid given at 4 mg, has been shown to improve symptoms in patients with moderate to severe croup.

DISPOSITION

- Croup is usually benign and self-limited, resolving within 3 to 4 days.
- Complications include:
  1. Airway obstruction
  2. Otitis media
  3. Pneumonia
  4. Dehydration

REFERRAL

If intubation is needed (rarely), an emergency consultation with ENT and/or anesthesiology is recommended.

PEARLS & CONSIDERATIONS

COMMENTS

- Most patients with croup can be managed at home (e.g., patients without stridor and in no respiratory distress).
- Hospitalization and observation is required for children with moderate-to-severe croup (e.g., rest stridor, respiratory distress refractory to the above mentioned acute treatments).

EVIDENCE

Dexamethasone, budesonide, and inhaled epinephrine are effective in the management of croup in pediatric assessment units. Improvement in symptoms and reduction in hospital admissions have been noted in RCTs.[1,2] Ⓐ

Systemic dexamethasone and inhaled budesonide have similar efficacy in terms of symptom resolution rate and reattendance after discharge.[1] Ⓐ

Although humidification has been used for decades in the inpatient and outpatient treatment of croup, there is little evidence to support its use.

Evidence-Based References

1. Osmond M: Croup. Reviewed in: 6:268, London, 2001, BMJ Publishing Group. Ⓐ
2. Russell K et al: Glucocorticoids for croup (Cochrane Review). Reviewed in: 2, Chichester, UK, 2004, John Wiley. Ⓐ

SUGGESTED READINGS

Knutson D, Aring A: Viral croup, *Am Fam Physician* 69:535, 2004.

Reveiz L, Cardona AF, Ospina EG: Antibiotics for acute laryngitis in adults, *Cochrane Database Syst Rev* 1:CD004783, 2005.

Roe M, O'Donnell DR, Tasker RC: Acute laryngotracheobronchitis, *Paediatr Respir Rev* 4(3):267, 2003.

AUTHORS: **GLENN G. FORT, M.D., M.P.H.,** and **DENNIS J. MIKOLICH, M.D.**

BASIC INFORMATION

DEFINITION

Lead poisoning refers to multisystem abnormalities resulting from excessive lead exposure.

SYNONYMS

Plumbism

ICD-9CM CODES

984.0 Lead poisoning

EPIDEMIOLOGY & DEMOGRAPHICS

- Lead poisoning is most common in children ages 1 to 5 yr (17,000 cases/100,000 persons). The highest rates are among blacks, those with low income, and urban children.
- In 1991 the Centers for Disease Control and Prevention (CDC) lowered the definition of a safe blood lead level to <10 μg/dl of whole blood (a blood lead level of 25 μg/dl was considered acceptable before 1991).
- It is estimated that >15% of preschoolers in the U.S. have a blood lead level >15 μg/dl.

PHYSICAL FINDINGS & CLINICAL PRESENTATION

- Findings vary with the degree of toxicity. Examination may be normal in patients with mild toxicity.
- Myalgias, irritability, headache, and general fatigue may be present initially.
- Abdominal cramping, constipation, weight loss, tremor, paresthesias and peripheral neuritis, seizures, and coma may occur with severe toxicity.
- Motor neuropathy is common in children with lead poisoning; learning disorders are also frequent.

ETIOLOGY

Chronic repeated exposure to paint containing lead, plumbing, storage of batteries, pottery, lead soldering

DIAGNOSIS

DIFFERENTIAL DIAGNOSIS

- Polyneuropathies from other sources
- Anxiety disorder, attention deficit disorder
- Malabsorption, acute abdomen
- Iron deficiency anemia

WORKUP

Laboratory screening: all U.S. children should be considered to be at risk for lead poisoning and should be screened routinely starting at 1 yr of age for low-risk children and 6 mo of age for high-risk ones.

LABORATORY TESTS

- Venous blood lead level: normal level: <10 μg/dl; levels of 50 to 70 μg/dl: indicative of moderate toxicity; levels >70 μg/dl: associated with severe poisoning
- Mild anemia with basophilic stippling on peripheral smear
- Elevated zinc protoporphyrin levels or free erythrocyte protoporphyrin level
- An increased body burden of lead with previous high-level exposure in patients with occupational lead poisoning can be demonstrated by measuring the excretion of lead in urine after premedication with calcium EDTA or another chelating agent

IMAGING STUDIES

- Imaging studies are generally not necessary.
- A plain abdominal film can visualize lead particles in the gut.
- "Lead lines" may be noted on x-ray films of long bones.

TREATMENT

NONPHARMACOLOGIC THERAPY

- Provide adequate amounts of calcium, iron, zinc, and protein in patient's diet
- Family education on sources of lead exposure and potential adverse health effects

ACUTE GENERAL Rx

- For children with blood levels of 10 to 19 μg/dl the CDC recommends nonpharmacologic interventions (see "Nonpharmacologic Therapy").
- For children with blood levels between 20-44 μg/dl the CDC recommendations include case management by a qualified social worker, clinical management, environmental assessment, and lead hazard control. Chelation therapy should be considered in children with refractory blood lead levels.

Chelation therapy is indicated in children with blood lead levels 45 μg/dl:

- Succimer (DMSA) 10 mg/kg PO q8h for 5 days then q12h for 2 wk can be used in patients with levels between 45 and 70 μg/dl.
- Edetate calcium disodium (EDTA) and dimercaprol (BAL) are effective in patients with severe toxicity.
- Use of both EDTA and DMSA is indicated in children with blood levels >70 μg/dl.
- d-Penicillamine (Cuprimine) can also be used for lead poisoning, but it is not FDA approved for this condition.

CHRONIC Rx

- Reduce exposure, remove any potential lead sources.
- Correct iron deficiency and any other nutritional deficiencies.
- Recheck blood lead level 7 to 21 days after chelation therapy.

DISPOSITION

Patients with mild to moderate toxicity generally improve without any residual deficits. The presence of encephalopathy at diagnosis is a poor prognostic sign. Residual neurologic deficits may persist in these patients. Chelation therapy seems to slow the progression of renal insufficiency in patients with mildly elevated body lead burden.

REFERRAL

If exposure to lead is work related, it should be reported to the Office of the United States Occupational Safety and Health Administration (OSHA). Follow-up testing is mandatory in all patients following an abnormal screening blood lead level.

PEARLS & CONSIDERATIONS

COMMENTS

- Even blood lead concentrations <10 mcg/dl are inversely associated with children's IQ scores at 3 and 5 yr of age.
- Screening of household members of affected individuals is recommended.
- In children with blood lead levels ≤45 mg/dl, treatment with succimer does not improve scores on tests of cognition, behavior, or neuropsychological function.
- Lead toxicity may delay growth and pubertal development in girls.
- Low-level environmental lead exposure may accelerate progressive renal insufficiency in patients without diabetes who have chronic renal disease. Repeated chelation therapy may improve renal function and slow the progression of renal failure.

SUGGESTED READINGS

Canfield RL et al: Intellectual impairment in children with blood lead concentrations below 10 mcg/deciliter, *N Engl J Med* 348:1517, 2003.

Kemper AR et al: Follow-up testing among children with elevated screening blood lead levels, *JAMA* 293:2232, 2005.

Lin JL et al: Environmental lead exposure and progression of chronic renal diseases in patients without diabetes, *N Engl J Med* 348:277, 2003.

Selevan SG et al: Blood lead concentration and delayed puberty in girls, *N Engl J Med* 348:1527, 2003.

AUTHOR: **FRED F. FERRI, M.D.**

BASIC INFORMATION

DEFINITION

Legg-Calvé-Perthes disease is a self-limited disorder of unknown etiology caused by ischemia of the immature femoral head that leads to bone necrosis and variable amounts of collapse during the reparative process.

SYNONYMS

Coxa plana
Capital femoral osteochondrosis

ICD-9CM CODES
732.1 Perthes' disease

EPIDEMIOLOGY & DEMOGRAPHICS

PREVALENCE: 1 case/1300 children
PREDOMINANT SEX: Male:female ratio of 4:1
PREDOMINANT AGE: 3 to 10 yr

PHYSICAL FINDINGS & CLINICAL PRESENTATION

- Initial complaint: usually a mildly painful limp
- Pain referred down the inner aspect of the thigh to the knee
- Moderate restriction of motion resulting from hip synovitis (abduction and internal rotation are especially limited)
- Pain at the extremes of movement and tenderness over anterior hip joint

ETIOLOGY

Unknown

DIAGNOSIS

DIFFERENTIAL DIAGNOSIS

- Transient synovitis
- Low-grade septic arthritis
- JRA

WORKUP

Diagnosis is usually based on the physical findings and eventual radiographic findings.

IMAGING STUDIES

- Plain roentgenography to establish the diagnosis (Fig. 1-143)
- AP and frog-leg lateral radiographs
- Technetium bone scanning to assist in making the diagnosis in early cases

TREATMENT

ACUTE GENERAL Rx

- A brief period of bed rest (1 to 3 days) followed by bracing (except in mild cases)
- Bracing possibly required for 2 to 3 yr in small percent of patients

DISPOSITION

- Prognosis depends on age of patient and degree of involvement of the femoral head at onset.
- Young patients (under 6 yr) with minimal involvement do well.
- Older patients (over 8 yr) often do poorly.
- A few patients eventually develop degenerative arthritis.

REFERRAL

For orthopedic consultation when diagnosis is suspected

PEARLS & CONSIDERATIONS

Both the etiology and treatment of Perthes disease remain controversial. Treatment recommendations vary widely and continue to evolve.

COMMENTS

There is great uncertainty regarding treatment and its effect on outcome. It may be that bracing has no effect whatsoever on the end result.

SUGGESTED READINGS

Domzalski ME et al: The proximal femoral growth plate in Perthes disease, *Clin Orthop Relat Res* 458:150, 2007.

Frick SL: Evaluation of the child who has hip pain, *Orthop Clin North Am* 37:133, 2006.

Gough-Palmer A, McHugh K: Investigating hip pain in a well child, *BMJ* 334:1216, 2007.

Gregorzewski A et al: Treatment of the collapsed femoral head by containment in Legg-Calvé-Perthes disease, *J Pediatr Orthop* 23:15, 2003.

Herring JA, Kim HT, Browne R: Legg-Calvé-Perthes disease: Part I: Classification of radiographs with use of the modified lateral pillar and Stulberg classifications, *J Bone Joint Surg* 86A:2103, 2004.

Herring J, Kim HT, Browne R: Legg-Calvé-Perthes disease: Part II: Prospective multicenter study of the effect of treatment on outcome, *J Bone Joint Surg* 86A:2121, 2004.

Rosenfeld SB, Herring JA, Chao JC: Legg-Calvé-Perthes disease: a review of cases with onset before six years of age, *J Bone Joint Surg* 89:2712, 2007.

Scherl SA: Lower extremity problems in children, *Pediatr Rev* 25:52, 2004.

AUTHOR: **LONNIE R. MERCIER, M.D.**

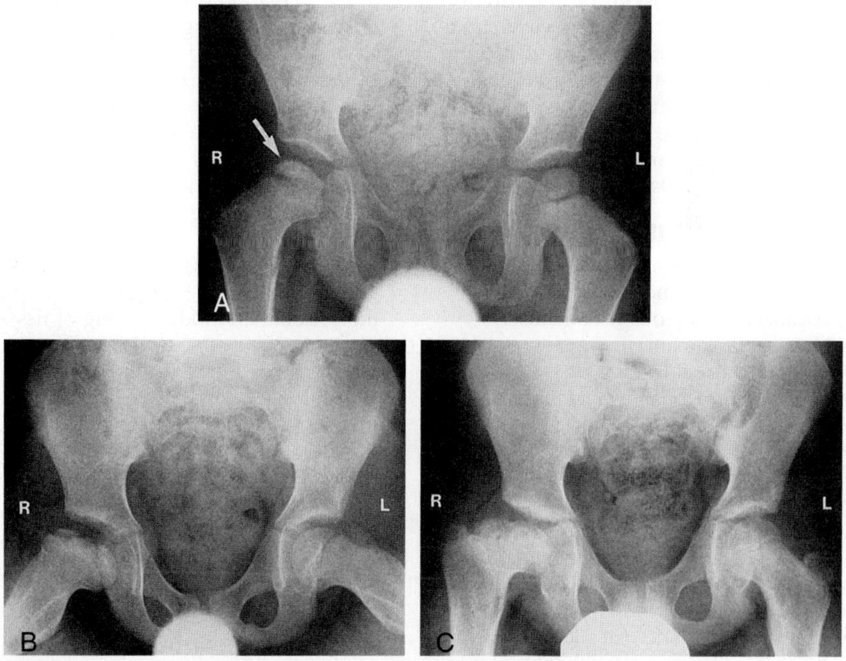

FIGURE 1-143 Legg-Calvé-Perthes disease. A, An anteroposterior view of the pelvis demonstrates fragmentation and sclerosis of the right femoral epiphysis *(arrow)* in this 6-year-old male. **B,** A follow-up film obtained 8 years later shows continuing deformity resulting from the osteonecrosis. The patient developed significant degenerative arthritis **(C)** by the age of 12 years. (From Mettler FA[ed]: *Primary care radiology,* Philadelphia, 2000, WB Saunders.)

BASIC INFORMATION

DEFINITION

Leishmaniasis is an infectious disease caused by a heterogeneous group of protozoan parasites belonging to the genus *Leishmania* and resulting in a variety of different clinical syndromes.

SYNONYMS

Kala azar
Old world leishmaniasis
New world leishmaniasis

ICD-9CM CODES
085.9 Leishmaniasis

EPIDEMIOLOGY & DEMOGRAPHICS

INCIDENCE: Approximately 400,000 new cases occur each year with almost 400 million people at risk for the disease.

- Can be classified geographically into new world versus old world disease
- Infection can be divided into cutaneous, mucocutaneous, visceral disease
- Incubation period: from 1 wk to many months for cutaneous and mucosal leishmaniasis; 2 to 6 mo (range is 10 days to years) for visceral leishmaniasis
- Mode of transmission: by the sandfly vector; can also be spread via shared needles, blood transfusions, vertically from the mother to fetus, or sexually
- Cutaneous leishmaniasis has been reported in United States military personnel in Iraq (more than 500 cases from 2002 to 2004)

PHYSICAL FINDINGS & CLINICAL PRESENTATION

Cutaneous syndrome

- Localized cutaneous leishmaniasis
- Mucosal leishmaniasis
- Leishmania recidivans
- Diffuse cutaneous leishmaniasis

Visceral syndrome

- Viscerotrophic leishmaniasis: fever, chronic fatigue, malaise, cough, intermittent diarrhea, and abdominal pain. Signs include adenopathy, hepatosplenomegaly, hyperpigmentation of skin, petechiae, jaundice, edema, and ascites
- Post–kala-azar dermal leishmaniasis: generalized cutaneous rash that is often papular or nodular; severe forms with desquamation of skin and mucosa

ETIOLOGY

- Old-world parasite: *Leishmania tropica, L. major, L. aethiopica, L. donovani, L. infantum*
- New-world parasite: *L. braziliensis* and *L. mexicana complex, L. chagasi, L.b. guyanensis, L.b. panamensis*

DIAGNOSIS

DIFFERENTIAL DIAGNOSIS

- Malaria
- African trypanosomiasis
- Brucellosis
- Enteric fever
- Bacterial endocarditis
- Generalized histoplasmosis
- Chronic myelocytic leukemia
- Hodgkin's disease and other lymphomas
- Sarcoidosis
- Hepatic cirrhosis
- Tuberculosis

WORKUP

- CBC
- LFTs
- Renal panel
- Serology
- Biopsy for histology and culture
- PCR

LABORATORY TESTS

- CBC: anemia, neutropenia, thrombocytopenia, and eosinophilia
- LFTs: hypergammaglobulinemia, hypoalbuminemia, and hyperbilirubinemia
- Elevated BUN and creatinine
- Specific diagnosis confirmed by intracellular amastigote in Giemsa-stained impression smears or sectioned tissue or culture performed in NMN (Novy, MacNeal, Nicolle) or Schneider's medium
- Serologic diagnosis: ELISA, direct agglutination tests, K39 ELISA, PCR, and monoclonal antibody staining of tissue smears
- Montenegro skin test

TREATMENT

- Nonspecific or supportive care
  1. Nutritional diet
  2. Antimicrobial agents for concurrent infections
  3. Blood transfusions
  4. Iron and vitamins
- Specific antileishmanial therapy
  1. Miltefosine (2.5 mg/kg/day orally in two divided doses for 28 days) now the treatment of choice for visceral disease
  2. Pentavalent antimonials: sodium stibogluconate and sodium antimony gluconate
  3. Lipid formations of Amphotericin B
  4. Fluconazole 200 mg po daily for 6 wks effective for cutaneous disease
  5. Pentamidine 2 to 4 mg/kg/day for 15 doses intravenously
  6. Other agents: allopurinol, ketoconazole, paromomycin (combined with other regimens)
  7. Immunotherapy: IFN-γ
  8. Local or tropical treatments and physical therapy, including thermal treatments
  9. Plastic surgery

DISPOSITION

Follow-up examination is important for the early detection and treatment relapse.

REFERRAL

To infectious disease experts for accurate diagnosis and management

PEARLS & CONSIDERATIONS

COMMENTS

- Prevention by reservoir control-destruction of animal reservoir hosts, mass treatment of human in kala-azar–prevalent areas
- Prevention by vector control: insecticide spraying in domestic and peridomestic areas
- Vaccines are in various stages of development and clinical trials. None are licensed or commercially available at this time

SUGGESTED READINGS

Jones J et al: Old world cutaneous leishmaniasis infection in children: a case series, *Arch Dis Child* 90(5):530, 2005.

Reithinger R et al: Social impact of leishmaniasis, Afghanistan, *Emerg Infect Dis* 11(4):634, 2005.

Sundar S et al: Low-dose liposomal amphotericin B in refractory Indian visceral leishmaniasis: a multicenter study, *Am J Trop Med Hyg* 66(2):143, 2002.

Sundar S et al: Oral miltefosine for Indian visceral leishmaniasis, *N Engl J Med* 347:1739, 2002.

AUTHORS: **GLENN G. FORT, M.D., M.P.H., DENNIS J. MIKOLICH, M.D.,** and **VASANTHI ARUMUGAM, M.D.**

BASIC INFORMATION

DEFINITION

Leprosy is a chronic granulomatous infection of humans that primarily affects the skin and peripheral nerves.

SYNONYMS

Hansen's disease

ICD-9CM CODES
030.9 Leprosy

EPIDEMIOLOGY & DEMOGRAPHICS

- The number of cases worldwide has fallen from more than 5 million cases in 1985 to less than 1 million cases in 1998.
- Nearly 75% of the cases of leprosy are found in India, Brazil, Bangladesh, Indonesia, and Myanmar.
- More than 85% of the cases diagnosed in the U.S. are found among immigrants.
- Worldwide incidence is 650,000 new cases per year.
- Annual incidence in the U.S. is 150 new cases per year.
- Leprosy is more common in men than women (2:1).
- Leprosy can occur at any age but usually is found in young children.

PHYSICAL FINDINGS & CLINICAL PRESENTATION

- A skin lesion: most common initial presentation
- Sensory loss
- Anhidrosis
- Neuritic pain
- Palpable peripheral nerves
- Nerve damage (most commonly affected nerves are ulnar, median, common peroneal, posterior tibial, radial cutaneous nerve of the wrist, facial, and posterior auricular)
- Muscle atrophy and weakness
- Foot drop
- Claw hand and claw toes
- Lagophthalmos, nasal septal perforation, collapse of bridge of nose (Fig. 1-144, *A*), loss of eyebrows resulting in "leonine" facies

Leprosy can present along a spectrum from simple cutaneous skin lesions with minimal sensory loss (Fig. 1-144, *B*) to severe extensive skin involvement, painful neuritis, muscle wasting and contractures, and multiple peripheral nerve damage.

ETIOLOGY

- Leprosy is caused by *Mycobacterium leprae,* an obligate intracellular acid-fast rod.
- The mode of transmission remains elusive. Spread in humans is thought to occur via the respiratory route or entry through broken skin in patients with multibacillary disease or extensive paucibacillary disease.
- Zoonotic transmission from armadillos has not been proven.
- The majority of people exposed to patients with leprosy do not develop the disease because of their natural immunity.
- Incubation period is 3 to 5 yr.

DIAGNOSIS

- The diagnosis of leprosy relies on a detailed history and physical examination and is established by the demonstration of acid-fast bacilli in skin smears or skin biopsies of the affected sites.
- Leprosy has been classified according to the WHO system into:
  1. Paucibacillary leprosy defined as fewer than five skin lesions with no bacilli on skin smear.
  2. Multibacillary leprosy defined as six or more skin lesions and may be skin-smear positive.
- Leprosy has also been classified more specifically according to the type of skin lesions, sensory and motor deficits, and biopsy into:
  1. Indeterminate leprosy
  2. Tuberculoid leprosy (paucibacillary [few organisms], intense inflamma-

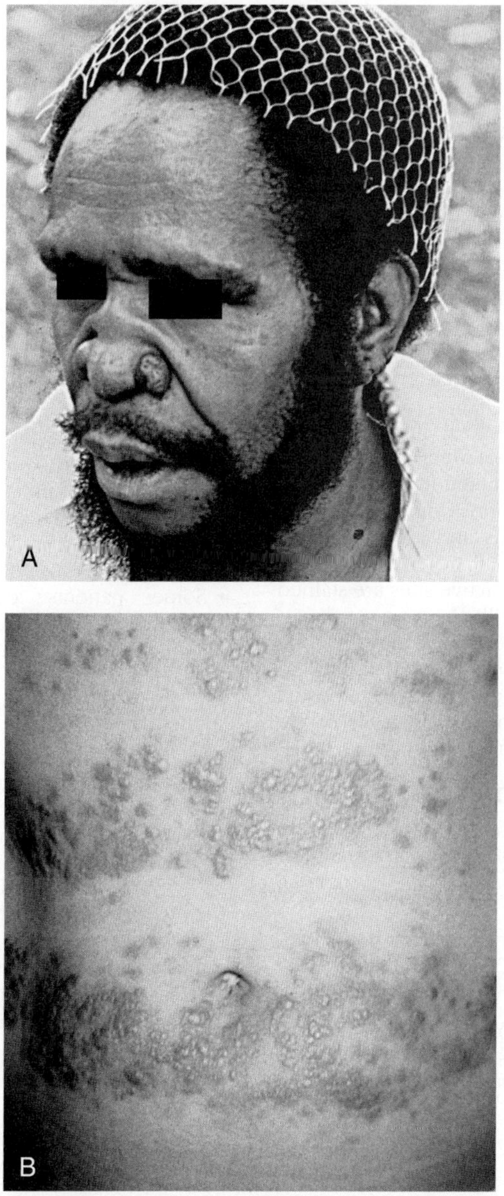

FIGURE 1-144 **A,** Advanced lepromatous leprosy with collapse of the nasal septum. **B,** Lepromatous leprosy characterized by extensive papule formation over abdomen. Minimal or no sensory loss is present in the affected areas. (**A** From Gorbach SL: *Infectious diseases,* ed 2, Philadelphia, 1998, WB Saunders; **B** from Mandell GL; *Mandell, Douglas, and Bennett's principles and practice of infectious diseases,* ed 5, New York, 2000, Churchill Livingstone.)

tory reaction; few, well-demarcated skin lesions)
3. Borderline tuberculoid leprosy
4. Borderline lepromatous leprosy
5. Lepromatous leprosy (multibacillary [numerous organisms], inadequate host response; diffuse, poorly organized skin lesions)

DIFFERENTIAL DIAGNOSIS

The differential diagnosis of leprosy includes: sarcoidosis, rheumatoid arthritis, systemic lupus erythematosus, lymphomatoid granulomatosis, carpal tunnel syndrome, cutaneous leishmaniasis, fungal infections and other causes of hypopigmented, hyperpigmented, and erythematous skin lesions.

WORKUP

Any patient who presents with skin lesions and a sensory or muscle deficit should have a workup for leprosy.

LABORATORY TESTS

- *Mycobacterium leprae* cannot be cultured on artificial media. The bacteria proliferate when injected into the footpads of mice or armadillos and can be used for drug-sensitivity testing.
- Serologic tests, including the antibody to phenolic glycolipid 1 (PGL-1), are available and used for diagnostic confirmation and research epidemiologic studies.
- Lepromin intradermal skin test is not diagnostic and not for commercial use.
- Skin smears are taken from active sites or most commonly from the earlobe, elbows, or knees and are stained for acid-fast bacilli.
- Skin biopsies of active sites are stained for acid-fast bacilli.
- Peripheral nerve biopsy can be done in patients with sensory loss and no skin lesions. Common nerves biopsied are the radial cutaneous nerve of the wrist and the sural nerve of the ankle.

IMAGING STUDIES

X-ray studies are usually of no benefit in the diagnosis or treatment of leprosy.

TREATMENT (Rx)

NONPHARMACOLOGIC THERAPY

- Physical therapy for patients with upper and lower extremity deformities
- Proper foot care and footwear to prevent ulcer formation

ACUTE GENERAL Rx

For paucibacillary leprosy:
- Dapsone 100 mg PO qd for 6 mo in an unsupervised setting is the treatment of choice.
- Rifampin 600 mg PO qd for 6 mo in a supervised setting is the recommendation by WHO.
- Ofloxacin 400 mg qd or minocycline 100 mg qd are other alternatives.

For multibacillary leprosy:
- Rifampin 600 mg PO qd and clofazimine 300 mg PO qd for 24 mo in a supervised setting. Rifampin can be given once monthly without loss of efficacy and at less cost.
- Rifampin 100 mg PO qd and clofazimine 50 mg PO qd for 24 mo in an unsupervised setting.
- Dapsone 100 mg PO qd is sometimes added as triple therapy in this group of patients.
- Clofazimine 50 mg daily is used with dapsone for better bacteriocidal effect.

CHRONIC Rx

- If relapse occurs, the patient is treated with the same medical regimen; drug resistance is low.
- If relapse is from paucibacillary to multibacillary, the medical regimen for multibacillary should be used for therapy.

DISPOSITION

- Relapse is <1% for multibacillary and just over 1% in paucibacillary cases.
- Patients are initially followed up monthly and when treatment is completed every 3 to 6 mo for the next 5 to 10 yr.
- Some patients develop reactions known as erythema nodosum leprosum and reversal reaction, usually during treatment.
  1. Erythema nodosum leprosum results in tender nodules and is treated with either prednisolone 40 to 60 mg qd until the reaction is controlled and tapered or thalidomide 300 to 400 mg qd and tapered to 100 mg qd with monthly attempts to wean down further.
  2. Reactive reaction results in the development of new skin lesions with swelling and erythema of existing lesions. Treatment is with either NSAIDs or prednisolone.

REFERRAL

- National Hansen's Disease Programs (NHDP) Center in Baton Rouge, Louisiana, and 15 outpatient clinics in the U.S. offer consultations and treatment. Telephone: 1-800-642-2477.
- Directly observed therapy (DOT), much like DOT for tuberculosis, is highly desirable and should be used if feasible, at least in the first 6 to 12 mo of therapy.
- Any suspected case of leprosy merits an infectious disease consultation. Consultation with orthopedic, podiatry, ophthalmology, physical therapy, plastic surgery, and psychology are all in order for any of the potential sequelae of the disease.

PEARLS & CONSIDERATIONS (!)

COMMENTS

- The risk of transmission is low in patients with leprosy, and therefore no infection control precautions of patients hospitalized is needed.
- Family members and close contacts need to be examined frequently for the development of lesions.
- Dapsone or rifampin prophylaxis is not recommended in the prevention of leprosy.
- BCG vaccination has a 50% efficacy in the prevention of leprosy and may be considered.

SUGGESTED READINGS

El-Darouti MA: Histopathological study of apparently normal skin of patients with leprosy, *Int J Dermatol* 45(3):292, 2006.

Moet FJ et al: Physical distance, genetic relationship, age, and leprosy classification are independent risk factors for leprosy in contacts of patients with leprosy, *J Infect Dis* 193(3):346, 2006.

Ohyama H et al: Polymorphism of the 5' flanking region of the IL-12 receptor beta2 gene partially determines the clinical types of leprosy through impaired transcriptional activity, *J Clin Pathol* 58(7):740, 2005.

Wilkinson RJ, Lockwood DN: Antigenic trigger for type 1 reaction in leprosy, *J Infect* 50(3):242, 2005.

AUTHORS: **GLENN G. FORT, M.D., M.P.H., DENNIS J. MIKOLICH, M.D.,** and **PETER PETROPOULOS, M.D.**

BASIC INFORMATION

DEFINITION

Leptospirosis is a zoonosis caused by the spirochete *Leptospira interrogans.*

SYNONYMS

Weil's disease

ICD-9CM CODES
100.9 Leptospirosis

EPIDEMIOLOGY & DEMOGRAPHICS

INCIDENCE (IN U.S.):

- 0.05 cases/100,000 persons
- Significant underestimation because of underreporting
- Hawaii consistently has the highest reported annual incidence rate in U.S.

PEAK INCIDENCE: Summer months, into the fall

PREDOMINANT SEX: Male (4:1)

PREDOMINANT AGE: Teenagers and young adults

GENETICS:

Neonatal Infection: Can occur

PHYSICAL FINDINGS & CLINICAL PRESENTATION

ANICTERIC FORM:

- Milder and more common presentation of disease
- A self-limited systemic illness with two stages:
  1. Septicemic stage: presents abruptly with fevers, headache, severe myalgias, rigors, prostration, and sometimes circulatory collapse; conjunctival suffusion is common; skin rash, pharyngitis, lymphadenopathy, hepatomegaly, splenomegaly.
  2. Immune stage: occurs a few days after first stage with similar symptoms; hallmark is aseptic meningitis.

ICTERIC LEPTOSPIROSIS (WEIL'S SYNDROME):

1. Denotes severe cases, with symptoms of hepatic, renal, and vascular dysfunction
2. Biphasic course: persistence of fever, jaundice, and azotemia
3. Complications: oliguria or anuria, hemorrhage, hypotension, vascular collapse

ETIOLOGY

Caused by a spirochete, *L. interrogans*

- Infects a variety of animals, including most mammals
- Specific serotypes associated with different hosts—*pomona* in livestock, *canicola* in dogs (Fig. 1-145), and *icterohaemorrhagiae* in rodents
- Exposure to animal urine or infected water method by which organism penetrates skin or mucous membranes

DIAGNOSIS

DIFFERENTIAL DIAGNOSIS

- Bacterial meningitis
- Viral hepatitis
- Influenza
- Legionnaire's disease

WORKUP

Culture of blood, CSF, and urine:

- Organism can be isolated from blood or CSF during first 10 days of illness.
- Urine should be cultured after first week and for up to 30 days after onset of illness.

LABORATORY TESTS

- Normal or elevated WBCs, at times with leukemoid reactions up to 70,000/mm^3
- Elevated transaminases or bilirubin
- Anemia, azotemia, hypoprothrombinemia in those with icteric illness
- Elevated CK in first phase
- Meningitis in both phases, but aseptic in second phase

IMAGING STUDIES

Chest radiographs to show interstitial nonlobar infiltrates

TREATMENT

NONPHARMACOLOGIC THERAPY

- Supportive
- Observation for dehydration, hypotension, renal failure, hemorrhage

ACUTE GENERAL Rx

- IV penicillin G 1 million U q4h
- Doxycycline 100 mg PO bid for 7 days
- Vitamin K administration if hypoprothrombinemia present
- Possible Jarisch-Herxheimer reaction when treated with penicillin

DISPOSITION

- In anicteric leptospirosis, antibiotics can decrease severity and duration of symptoms.
- Icteric leptospirosis, even with supportive therapy, may have a mortality as high as 10%.

REFERRAL

- If more than mild disease
- If no response to treatment

EVIDENCE

Penicillin and doxycycline may be effective in treating leptospirosis but evidence is insufficient to provide clear guidelines for practice.[1] Ⓐ

A randomized controlled trial (RCT) found that prophylactic doxycycline is no better than placebo in reducing infection rate but reduced the rate of clinical illness in those who become infected.[2] Ⓑ

An RCT found that ceftriaxone and penicillin G were equally effective for the treatment of severe leptospirosis.[3] Ⓑ

Evidence-Based References

1. Guidugli F, Castro AA, Atallah AN: Antibiotics for leptospirosis (Cochrane Review). Reviewed in: 2, Chichester, UK, 2004, John Wiley. Ⓐ
2. Sehgal SC et al: Randomized controlled trial of doxycycline prophylaxis against leptospirosis in an endemic area, *Int J Antimicrob Agents* 13:249, 2000. Ⓑ
3. Panaphut T et al: Ceftriaxone compared with sodium penicillin g for treatment of severe leptospirosis, *Clin Infect Dis* 36:1507, 2003. Ⓑ

SUGGESTED READINGS

Karande S et al: Acute aseptic meningitis as the only presenting feature of leptospirosis, *Pediatr Infect Dis J* 24(4):390, 2005.

Segura ER et al: Clinical spectrum of pulmonary involvement in leptospirosis in a region of endemicity, with quantification of leptospiral burden, *Clin Infect Dis* 40(3):343, 2005.

Suputtamongkol Y et al: An open, randomized, controlled trial of penicillin, doxycycline, and cefotaxime for patients with severe leptospirosis, *Clin Infect Dis* 39(10):1417, 2004.

AUTHORS: **STEVEN M. OPAL, M.D.,** and **MAURICE POLICAR, M.D.**

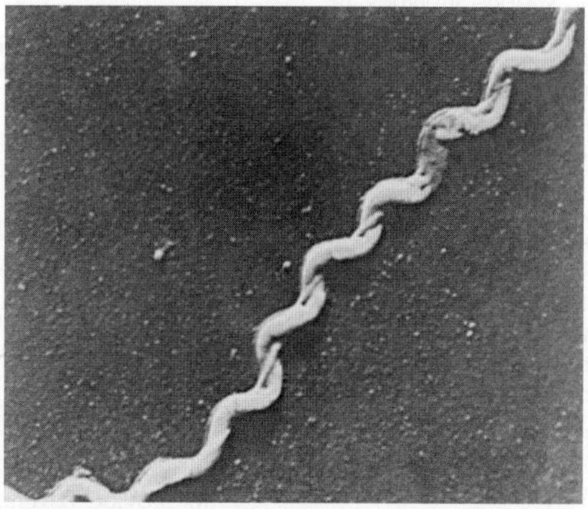

FIGURE 1-145 Electron micrograph of *Leptospira interrogans* (serovar *canicola*) showing the tightly coiled helicoids rod with the periplasmic axial filament. (Courtesy Armed Forces Institute of Pathology, AFIP No. 60-10941. In Gorbach SL: *Infectious diseases,* ed 2, Philadelphia, 1998, WB Saunders.)

BASIC INFORMATION

DEFINITION

Acute lymphoblastic leukemia (ALL) is characterized by uncontrolled proliferation of abnormal, immature lymphocytes and their progenitors, ultimately replacing normal bone marrow elements.

SYNONYMS

Lymphoid leukemia
ALL

ICD-9CM CODES
204.0 Acute lymphoblastic leukemia

EPIDEMIOLOGY & DEMOGRAPHICS

- ALL is primarily a disease of children (peak incidence at ages 2 to 10 yr).
- It is diagnosed in 3000 to 4000 persons in the U.S. each year; two thirds are children.

PHYSICAL FINDINGS & CLINICAL PRESENTATION

- Skin pallor, purpura, or easy bruising
- Lymphadenopathy or hepatosplenomegaly
- Fever, bone pain, oliguria, weakness, weight loss, mental status changes

ETIOLOGY

- Unknown; increased risk in patients with a previous use of antineoplastic agents (e.g., chemotherapy of NHL, Hodgkin's disease, ovarian cancer, myeloma)
- Environmental factors (e.g., ionizing radiation), toxins (e.g., benzene)

DIAGNOSIS

DIFFERENTIAL DIAGNOSIS

Acute myeloid leukemia (AML): the distinction between ALL and AML and the classification of the various subtypes are based on the following factors:

- Cell morphology
  1. Lymphoblasts: a high nucleus/cytoplasmic ratio; usually, cytoplasmic granules are not present.
  2. Myeloblasts: abundant cytoplasm; often, cytoplasmic granules (Auer rods) are present.
- Histochemical stains
  1. Peroxidase and Sudan black stains: negative in ALL; useful to distinguish nonlymphoid from lymphoid cells
  2. Chloroacetate esterase: a pink cytoplasmic reaction identifies granulocytes; useful to distinguish granulocytes from monocytes in patients with AML

Lymphoblastic lymphoma
Aplastic anemia
Infectious mononucleosis
Leukemoid reaction to infection
Multiple myeloma

WORKUP

- Laboratory evaluation
- Bone marrow examination (with biopsy, cytochemistry, immunophenotyping, and cytogenetics)
- Lumbar puncture and imaging studies

LABORATORY TESTS

- CBC reveals normochromic, normocytic anemia, thrombocytopenia.
- Peripheral smear will reveal lymphoblasts.
- Initial blood work should also include BUN, creatinine, serum electrolytes, uric acid, LDH.
- Special diagnostic tests include immunophenotyping, cytogenetics, and cytochemistry.
- The French, American, British (FAB) Cooperative Study Group has classified ALL into three groups (L1 to L3) based on cell size, cytoplasmic appearance, nucleus shape, and chromatin pattern; the most common form is the L2 type.
- Immunologic classification is on the basis of expression of surface antigens by blast cells: T lineage and B lineage.

IMAGING STUDIES

- Chest radiograph to evaluate for the presence of mediastinal mass
- CT scan or ultrasound of abdomen/pelvis to assess splenomegaly or leukemic infiltration of abdominal organs

TREATMENT

ACUTE GENERAL Rx

- Emergency treatment is indicated in patients with intracerebral leukostasis. It consists of one or more of the following:
  1. Cranial irradiation of the whole brain in one- or two-dose fractions
  2. Leukapheresis
  3. Oral hydroxyurea (requires 48 to 72 hr to significantly lower the circulating blast count)
- Urate nephropathy can be prevented by vigorous hydration and lowering uric acid level with allopurinol and urine alkalization with acetazolamide.
- Infections must be aggressively treated with broad-spectrum antibiotics.
  1. Any febrile or neutropenic patients must have cultures taken and be properly treated with IV antibiotics.
  2. If evidence of infection persists despite adequate treatment with antibiotics, amphotericin B may be added to provide coverage against fungal infections *(Candida, Aspergillus)*.
- Correct significant thrombocytopenia (platelet counts <20,000/mm^3) with platelet transfusion.
- Bleeding secondary to DIC is treated with heparin and replacement of clotting factors.
- Induction therapy is intensive chemotherapy to destroy a significant number of leukemic cells and achieve remission; it usually consists of a combination of vincristine (Oncovin), prednisone, and l-asparaginase (ELSPAR) in children or an anthracene in adults.
- Consolidation therapy consists of an aggressive course of chemotherapy with or without radiotherapy shortly after complete remission has been obtained. Its purpose is to prolong the remission period or cure. Commonly used agents are VM-26, VP-16, HiDAC.
- Meningeal prophylactic therapy with intrathecal methotrexate with or without cranial irradiation is indicated to prevent meningeal sequestration of leukemic cells.
- The goal of maintenance therapy is to maintain a state of remission. In patients with ALL, intermittent therapy is continued for at least 3 yr with a combination of methotrexate and 6-mercaptopurine (Purinethol).
- Bone marrow transplantation: patients should receive allograft in the first complete remission if they are between ages 20 and 50 yr and have matched a sibling donor.

DISPOSITION

- Prognosis is generally poorer in adult disease compared with childhood disease (40% adult cure rate versus 80% cure rate in children).
- Five-year leukemia-free survival is <40%.
- The different clinical outcomes associated with the various subtypes of ALL can be attributed primarily to drug sensitivity or resistance of leukemic blasts harboring specific genetic abnormalities. For example, cases of ALL expressing the TEL-AML1 fusion protein are very responsive to intensive chemotherapy with asparaginase, whereas the presence of Philadelphia chromosome (Ph$^+$), monosomy 5 and 7, and abnormalities of 11q23 are bad prognostic signs in ALL. Dasatinib (Sprycel) is a tyrosine kinase inhibitor that can be used as a second line in Philadelphia chromosome–positive ALL.

REFERRAL

Referral to hematologist is indicated in all cases of actue lymphoblastic leukemia.

SUGGESTED READING

Pui CH, Evans WE: Treatment of acute lymphoblastic leukemia, *N Engl J Med* 354:166, 2006.

AUTHOR: **FRED F. FERRI, M.D.**

BASIC INFORMATION

DEFINITION

Acute myelogenous leukemia (AML) is a disorder characterized by uncontrolled proliferation of primitive myeloid cells (blasts), ultimately replacing normal bone marrow elements frequently resulting in hematopoietic insufficiency (granulocytopenia, thrombocytopenia, or anemia) with or without leukocytosis.

SYNONYMS

Acute nonlymphoblastic leukemia (ANLL)
Acute nonlymphocytic leukemia
Acute myeloid leukemia (AML)

ICD-9CM CODES
205.0 Acute myelogenous leukemia

EPIDEMIOLOGY & DEMOGRAPHICS

- AML usually affects adults (most patients are 30 to 60 yr old; median age at presentation is 50 yr).
- Annual incidence is 2 to 4/100,000

PHYSICAL FINDINGS & CLINICAL PRESENTATION

Patients generally come to medical attention because of the effects of the cytopenias:

- Anemia manifests with weakness or fatigue.
- Thrombocytopenia can manifest with bleeding, petechiae, and ecchymosis.
- Neutropenia can result in infections and fever.
- Physical examination may reveal skin pallor, bruises, petechiae; abdominal examination may reveal hepatosplenomegaly; peripheral lymphadenopathy may also be present.
- Hyperleukocytosis can lead to symptoms of leukostasis, such as ocular and cerebrovascular dysfunction or bleeding.

ETIOLOGY

Risk factors are previous use of antineoplastic agents, chromosomal abnormalities, ionizing radiation, toxins, immunodeficiency states, and chronic myeloproliferative disorders.

DIAGNOSIS

DIFFERENTIAL DIAGNOSIS

- Acute lymphocytic leukemia
- Leukemoid reaction
- Myelodysplastic syndrome
- Infiltrative diseases of the bone marrow
- Epstein-Barr, other viral infection

LABORATORY TESTS

- CBC reveals anemia, thrombocytopenia. Peripheral WBC count varies from <5000/mm³ to >100,000/mm³.
- Additional laboratory findings may include elevated LDH and uric acid levels, decreased fibrinogen, and increased FDP secondary to DIC.
- Cytogenetic abnormalities are common (chromosome 8 is most frequently involved in AML).
- The distinction between ALL and AML and the classification of the various subtypes are based on the following factors:
  1. Cell morphology: myeloblasts reveal abundant cytoplasm; cytoplasmic granules are often present (Auer rods).
  2. Histochemical stains:
     a. Peroxidase and Sudan black stains are negative in ALL.
     b. Chloroacetate esterase: a pink cytoplasmic reaction identifies granulocytes; useful to distinguish granulocytes from monocytes in patients with AML.
- AML is diagnosed by the presence of at least 30% blast cells and positive peroxidase or Sudan black histochemical stain in the bone marrow aspirate.
- The French, American, British (FAB) Cooperative Study Group has classified AML into seven categories (M1 to M7) based on the type and percentage of immature cells.

IMAGING STUDIES

- Chest x-ray is useful to evaluate for the presence of mediastinal masses.
- CT scan of the abdomen may reveal hepatosplenomegaly or leukemic involvement of other organs.

TREATMENT

ACUTE GENERAL Rx

- Emergency treatment consisting of one or more of the following is indicated in patients with intracerebral leukostasis:
  1. Cranial irradiation
  2. Leukapheresis
  3. Oral hydroxyurea
- Urate nephropathy can be prevented by vigorous hydration and lowering uric acid level with allopurinol and urine alkalinization with acetazolamide.
- Infections must be aggressively treated with broad-spectrum antibiotics.
- Correct significant thrombocytopenia with platelet transfusions.
- Bleeding secondary to DIC is treated with heparin and replacement of clotting factors.
- Intensive induction chemotherapy to destroy a significant number of leukemic cells and achieve remission usually consists of cytarabine (Cytosar) and daunorubicin. Alltransretinoic acid is effective for the induction of remission of AML M3 subtype (acute promyelocytic leukemia).
- High-dose cytarabine (ARA-C) (HiDAC) can be used in patients with refractory or relapsed AML. It usually takes 28 to 32 days from the start of therapy to achieve remission. The duration of remission is variable; the median duration of remission in an adult with AML is 1 yr.
- Consolidation therapy consists of an aggressive course of chemotherapy with or without radiation shortly after complete remission has been obtained; its purpose is to prolong the remission period or cure. Complications of consolidation therapy are usually secondary to severe bone marrow suppression (anemia, thrombocytopenia, granulocytopenia).
- Goal of therapy is to maintain a state of remission. A postinduction course of high-dose cytarabine can provide equivalent disease-free survival and somewhat better overall survival than autologous marrow transplantation in adults.
- Autologous bone marrow transplantation is indicated in patients <55 yr without a sibling donor. Allogeneic bone marrow transplantation is generally available to <20% of patients; usually performed only in patients <40 yr of age because of higher incidence of GVHD with advancing age.

DISPOSITION

- Remission can be achieved in nearly 80% of patients <55 yr of age. Remission rates are highest in children.
- Cure for allogeneic bone marrow transplantation approaches 60%; cure rates with autologous transplantation are slightly lower.
- Favorable cytogenics are inv (16) (p13;q22) and t(8;21), t(15;17).

PEARLS & CONSIDERATIONS

COMMENTS

- The major complication of chemotherapy is profound marrow depression with pancytopenia lasting 3 to 4 wk. Treatment is aimed at RBC and platelet replacement and aggressive monitoring and treatment of suspected infections.
- Low doses of arsenic trioxide can induce complete remissions in patients with acute promyelocytic leukemia.

AUTHOR: **FRED F. FERRI, M.D.**

BASIC INFORMATION

DEFINITION

Chronic lymphocytic leukemia (CLL) is a lymphoproliferative disorder characterized by proliferation and accumulation of mature-appearing neoplastic lymphocytes.

SYNONYMS

CLL

ICD-9CM CODES
204.1 Leukemia, chronic lymphocytic

EPIDEMIOLOGY & DEMOGRAPHICS

- Most frequent form of leukemia in Western countries (10,000 new cases/yr in the U.S.)
- Generally occurs in middle-aged and elderly patients (median age of 65 yr)
- Male:female ratio of 2:1

PHYSICAL FINDINGS & CLINICAL PRESENTATION

- Lymphadenopathy, splenomegaly, and hepatomegaly in the majority of patients
- Variable clinical presentation according to stage of the disease
- Abnormal CBC: many cases are diagnosed on the basis of laboratory results obtained after routine physical examination
- Some patients come to medical attention because of weakness and fatigue (secondary to anemia) or lymphadenopathy

ETIOLOGY

CLL is a disease derived from antigen-experienced B lymphocytes that differ in the level of immunoglobulin V-gene mutations.

DIAGNOSIS

DIFFERENTIAL DIAGNOSIS

- Hairy cell leukemia
- Adult T cell lymphoma
- Prolymphocytic leukemia
- Viral infections
- Waldenström's macroglobulinemia

LABORATORY TESTS

- Proliferative lymphocytosis (≥15,000/dl) of well-differentiated lymphocytes is the hallmark of CLL.
- There is monotonous replacement of the bone marrow by small lymphocytes (marrow contains ≥30% of well-differentiated lymphocytes).
- Hypogammaglobulinemia and elevated LDH may be present at the time of diagnosis.
- Anemia or thrombocytopenia, if present, indicates poor prognosis.
- Trisomy-12 is the most common chromosomal abnormality, followed by 14 q+, 13 q, and 11 q; these all indicate a poor prognosis.
- New laboratory techniques (CD 38, fluorescence in situ hybridization [FISH]) can identify patients with early-stage CLL at higher risk of rapid disease progression. Staining of mononuclear cells by a 2-color (fluoresceinisothiocyanate/phycoerythrin) flow cytometric assay using antibodies to the chemokine receptors (CXCR1, CXCR2, etc.) can aid in staging and prognosis of patients. Increase in expression of chemokine receptors CXCR4 and CCR7 correlates with advanced Rai stage (stage IV). The presence of V-gene mutations, CD38+, or ZAP-70+ cells also has prognostic relevance. Patients with clones having few or no V-gene mutations or many CD38+ or ZAP-70+ B cells are associated with an aggressive, usually fatal course.
- The percentage of smudge cells (CLL cells ruptured during smear preparation) is associated with mutated IgVH gene status, a favorable prognostic factor. A high percentage of smudge cells on peripheral smear indicates a longer time to treatment (TTT) from initial diagnosis and better overall survival in patients with early stage CLL.

STAGING:

- Rai et al divided CLL into five clinical stages:

Stage 0—Characterized by lymphocytosis only (>15,000/mm³ on peripheral smear, bone marrow aspirate ≥40% lymphocytes). The coexistence of lymphocytosis and other factors increases the clinical stage.

Stage 1—Lymphadenopathy

Stage 2—Lymphadenopathy/hepatomegaly

Stage 3—Anemia (Hgb <11 g/mm³)

Stage 4—Thrombocytopenia (platelets <100,000/mm³)

- Another well-known staging system developed by Binet divides chronic lymphocytic leukemia into three stages:

Stage A—Hgb >10 g/dl, platelets >100,000/mm³, and fewer than three areas involved (the cervical, axillary, and inguinal lymph nodes [whether unilaterally or bilaterally]; the spleen; and the liver)

Stage B—Hgb >10 g/dl, platelets >100,000/mm³, and three or more areas involved

Stage C—Hgb <10 g/dl, low platelets (<100,000/mm³), or both (independent of the areas involved)

IMAGING STUDIES

CT scan of abdomen to evaluate for hepatomegaly and splenomegaly

TREATMENT

NONPHARMACOLOGIC THERAPY

- Treatment goals are relief of symptoms and prolongation of life.
- Observation is appropriate for patients in Rai stage 0 or Binet stage A.

ACUTE GENERAL Rx

- Symptomatic patients in Rai stage I and II or Binet stage B: chlorambucil; local irradiation for isolated symptomatic lymphadenopathy and lymph nodes that interfere with vital organs
- Fludarabine is an effective treatment for CLL that does not respond to initial treatment with chlorambucil. Recent reports indicate that when used as the initial treatment for CLL, fludarabine yields higher response rates and a longer duration of remission and progression-free survival than chlorambucil; overall survival, however, is not enhanced.
- Rai stages III and IV, Binet stage C: chlorambucil chemotherapy with or without prednisone
  1. Fludarabine, CAP (cyclophosphamide, Adriamycin, prednisone), or cyclophosphamide, doxorubicin, vincristine, and prednisone (mini-CHOP) can be used in patients who respond poorly to chlorambucil.
  2. Splenic irradiation can be used in selected patients with advanced disease.

CHRONIC Rx

Treatment of systemic complications:

- Hypogammaglobulinemia is frequent in CLL and is the chief cause of infections. Immune globulin (250 mg/kg IV every 4 wk) may prevent infections but has no effect on survival. Infections should be treated with broad-spectrum antibiotics. Patients should be monitored for opportunistic infections.
- Recombinant hematopoietic cofactors (e.g., granulocyte-macrophage colony–stimulating factor and granulocyte colony–stimulating factor) may be useful to overcome neutropenia related to treatment.
- Erythropoietin may be useful to treat anemia that is unresponsive to other measures.

DISPOSITION

The patient's prognosis is generally directly related to the clinical stage (e.g., the average survival in patients in Rai stage 0 or Binet stage A is >120 mo, whereas for RAI stage 4 or Binet stage C it is approximately 30 mo). Overall 5-yr survival is 60%. Measurement of ZAP-70 intracellular protein (where available) is also a useful indicator of prognosis.

SUGGESTED READINGS

Nowakowski GS et al: Using smudge cells on routine blood smears to predict clinical outcome in chronic lymphocytic leukemia: a universally available prognostic test. *Mayo Clin Proc* 82(4):449, 2007.

Yee K, O'Brien SM: Chronic lymphocytic leukemia: diagnosis and treatment, *Mayo Clin Proc* 81(8):1105, 2006.

AUTHOR: **FRED F. FERRI, M.D.**

BASIC INFORMATION

DEFINITION

Chronic myelogenous leukemia (CML) is a malignant clonal stem disease caused by an acquired somatic mutation that fuses, through chromosomal translocation, the ABL and BCR genes on chromosomes 9 and 22 and is characterized by abnormal proliferation and accumulation of immature granulocytes. CML manifests with a chronic phase (CP-CML) lasting months to years, followed by an advanced phase (AP-CML) characterized by poor response to therapy, worsening anemia, or decreased platelet count; the second phase then evolves into a terminal phase (acute transformation) that degenerates into acute leukemia (mostly myeloid and approximately 20% lymphoid subtype), characterized by elevated number of blast cells and numerous complications (e.g., sepsis, bleeding).

SYNONYMS

CML
Chronic granulocytic leukemia
Chronic myeloid leukemia

ICD-9CM CODES
201.1 Chronic myelogenous leukemia

EPIDEMIOLOGY & DEMOGRAPHICS

- CML usually affects elderly patients (median age at presentation is 65 yr) and accounts for 15% of adult leukemias
- Incidence is 1 to 2 cases per 100,000 people every year.

PHYSICAL FINDINGS & CLINICAL PRESENTATION

- The chronic phase usually reveals splenomegaly; hepatomegaly is not infrequent, but lymphadenopathy is very unusual and generally indicates the accelerated proliferative phase of the disease.
- Common complaints at the time of diagnosis are weakness or discomfort secondary to an enlarged spleen (abdominal discomfort or pain). Splenomegaly is present in up to 40% of patients at time of diagnosis.
- 40% of patients are asymptomatic and diagnosis is based solely on an abnormal blood count.

ETIOLOGY

Current evidence strongly implicates the chromosome translocation t (9;22) (q34;q11.2) as the cause of chronic granulocytic leukemia. This translocation is present in >95% of patients. The remaining patients have a complex or variant translocation involving additional chromosomes that have the same end result (fusion of the BCR [break point cluster region] gene on chromosome 22 to ABL [Ableson leukemia virus] gene on chromosome 9).

DIAGNOSIS

DIFFERENTIAL DIAGNOSIS

- Splenic lymphoma
- CLL
- Myelodysplastic syndrome

LABORATORY TESTS

- Elevated WBC count (generally >100,000/mm^3) with broad spectrum of granulocytic forms.
- Bone marrow demonstrates hypercellularity with granulocytic hyperplasia, increased ratio of myeloid cells to erythroid cells, and increased number of megakaryocytes. Blasts and promyelocytes constitute <10% of all cells.
- Philadelphia chromosome (which results from the reciprocal translocation between the long arms of chromosomes 9 and 22) is present in >95% of patients with CML; its presence (Ph^1) is a major prognostic factor because survival rate of patients with Philadelphia chromosome is approximately eight times better than that of those without it. Some believe that Ph$^+$ defines CML and that those who are Ph$^-$ have another disease.
- Leukocyte alkaline phosphatase (LAP) markedly decreased (used to distinguish CML from other myeloproliferative disorders).
- Anemia and thrombocytosis are often present.
- Additional laboratory results are elevated vitamin B_{12} levels (caused by increased transcobalamin 1 from granulocytes) and elevated blood histamine levels (because of increased basophils).

IMAGING STUDIES

Chest x-ray and CT scan of abdomen/pelvis

TREATMENT

ACUTE GENERAL Rx

Treatment with a potential to either cure CML or prolong survival should be used during the chronic phase of the disease because it is often futile when administered during the advanced phase. Imatinib mesylate (Gleevec), an oral tyrosine kinase inhibitor, is effective and indicated as first-line treatment for CML myeloid blast crisis, accelerated phase, or CML in its chronic phase. More than 75% of patients have major cytogenetic response (<35% Philadelphia chromosome-positive cells in the marrow) and more than 80% have progression-free survival after 24 mo. Complete hematologic response usually occurs in less than 1 mo.

- Symptomatic hyperleukocytosis (e.g., CNS symptoms) can be treated with leukapheresis and hydroxyurea; allopurinol should be started to prevent urate nephropathy following the rapid lysis of the leukemia cells.
- Allogeneic stem-cell transplantation (SCT) is the only curative treatment for CML in chronic phase unresponsive to imatinib. Generally only 20% of patients are candidates for SCT given the limitations of age or lack of HLA-matched related donors.
  1. It should be considered in "young" patients (increased survival in patients <55 yr) with compatible siblings.
  2. Early transplantation is also important for patient's survival.
- Nilotinib and dasatinib (Sprycel) are BCR-ABL tyrosine kinase inhibitors that are active in imatinib-resistant CML.
- Interferon-alfa is an acceptable alternative in the early chronic phase for patients who do not tolerate tyrosine kinase inhibitors.
- Transplantation of marrow from an HLA-matched, unrelated donor is also now recognized as safe and effective therapy for selected patients with chronic myelogenous leukemia.

SUGGESTED READINGS

Hehlmann R et al: Chronic myeloid leukemia, *Lancet* 370:342, 2007.

Kantarjian H et al: Nilotinib in imatinib-resistant CML and Philadelphia chromosome-positive ALL, *N Engl J Med* 354:2542, 2006.

Quintas-Cardam A, Cortes J: Chronic myeloid leukemia: diagnosis and treatment, *Mayo Clin Proc* 81(7):973, 2006.

Schiffer CA: BCR-ABL tyrosine kinase inhibitors for chronic myelogenous leukemia, *N Engl J Med* 357:258, 2007.

Talpaz M et al: Dasatinib in imatinib-resistant Philadelphia chromosome-positive leukemias, *N Engl J Med* 354:2531, 2006.

AUTHOR: **FRED F. FERRI, M.D.**

BASIC INFORMATION

DEFINITION

Hairy cell leukemia is a lymphoid neoplasm characterized by the proliferation of mature B cells with prominent cytoplasmic projections (hairs).

SYNONYMS

Leukemic reticuloendotheliosis

ICD-9CM CODES
202.4 Hairy cell leukemia

EPIDEMIOLOGY & DEMOGRAPHICS

PREVALENCE: Occurs predominantly in men between 40 and 60 yr of age. About 2% of leukemia cases are of the hairy cell type.
PREDOMINANT SEX: Male:female ratio of 4:1

PHYSICAL FINDINGS & CLINICAL PRESENTATION

- Usually, splenomegaly (present in >90% of cases) secondary to tumor cell infiltration
- Pallor, ecchymosis, and evidence of infection if the pancytopenia is severe
- Weakness, lethargy, and fatigue
- Infections (resulting from impaired resistance secondary to neutropenia) and easy bruising (secondary to thrombocytopenia) also common

ETIOLOGY

Neoplastic disease of the lymphoreticular system of unknown etiology

DIAGNOSIS

DIFFERENTIAL DIAGNOSIS

- Other forms of leukemia
- Lymphoma
- Viral syndrome

WORKUP

Comprehensive history, physical examination, and laboratory evaluation to confirm the diagnosis

LABORATORY TESTS

- Pancytopenia involving erythrocytes, neutrophils, and platelets is common; anemia is usually present and varies from minimal to severe.
- Hairy cells (Fig. 1-146) can account for 5% to 80% of cells in the peripheral blood. The cytoplasmic projections on the cells are redundant plasma membranes.
- Leukemic cells stain positively for tartrate-resistant acid phosphatase (TRAP) stain.
- Bone marrow may result in a "dry tap" (because of increased marrow reticulin).

TREATMENT

NONPHARMACOLOGIC THERAPY

Approximately 8% to 10% of patients are asymptomatic and have minimal splenomegaly and minor cytopenia. They are usually detected on routine laboratory evaluation and do not require initial therapy. They should, however, be frequently monitored for progression of their disease.

ACUTE GENERAL Rx

- Drugs of choice are the purine analogues 2-Chloro-2 deoxyadenosine (Cladribine) or 2-deoxycoformycin (DCF, Pentostatin). They induce complete remissions in up to 85% of patients and partial responses in 5% to 25%.
- 2-Chloro-2 deoxyadenosine (CdA) 0.14 mg/kg qd for 7 days has minimal toxicity and is able to induce complete durable responses with a single course of therapy.
- Interferon-α produces a partial remission in 30% to 70% of patients and complete remission, often of short duration, in 5% to 10% of patients.
- The anti-CD 22 recombinant immunotoxin BL 22 can induce complete remission in patients with hairy cell leukemia that is resistant to treatment with purine analogues.

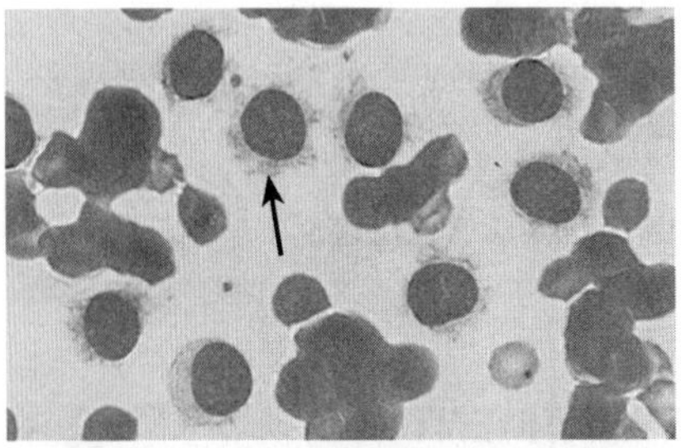

FIGURE 1-146 Hairy cell leukemia. Note the lymphocytes with hairlike cytoplasmic projections surrounding the nucleus. (From Rodak BF: *Diagnostic hematology,* Philadelphia, 1995, WB Saunders.)

CHRONIC Rx

Patients should be monitored with periodic examination and laboratory tests for progression of their disease.

DISPOSITION

Prognosis has become increasingly favorable with the newer agents. Approximately 90% of patients who are treated have a complete or partial response.

REFERRAL

Hematology consultation is recommended in all patients.

PEARLS & CONSIDERATIONS

COMMENTS

The diagnosis of hairy cell leukemia is occasionally missed and subsequently made by the histopathologist following removal of the spleen for diagnostic purposes.

EVIDENCE

We are unable to cite evidence that meets our criteria for some therapies, and there is only limited evidence for some other therapies. Initial therapies of choice are cladribine or pentostatin.

In a randomized controlled trial to compare pentostatin vs. interferon alpha-2a in previously untreated patients with hairy cell leukemia, 121 of 154 patients treated with pentostatin achieved confirmed complete or partial remission, compared with 60 of 159 who received interferon alpha-2a. Response rates were significantly higher and relapse-free survival was significantly longer with pentostatin than interferon.[1] Ⓑ

Evidence-Based Reference

1. Grever M et al: Randomized comparison of pentostatin versus interferon alpha in previously untreated patients with hairy cell leukemia: an intergroup study, *J Clin Oncol* 13:974, 1995.

SUGGESTED READING

Kreitman RJ et al: Efficacy of the anti-CD 22 recombinant immunotoxin BL 22 in chemotherapy resistant hairy-cell leukemia, *N Engl J Med* 345:241, 2001.

AUTHOR: **FRED F. FERRI, M.D.**

BASIC INFORMATION

DEFINITION

Oral hairy leukoplakia (OHL) is a painless, white, nonremovable, plaquelike lesion typically located on the lateral aspect of the tongue.

ICD-9CM CODES
528.6 Oral hairy leukoplakia

EPIDEMIOLOGY & DEMOGRAPHICS

INCIDENCE AND PREVALENCE: EBV seroprevalence occurs in high incidence in individuals who are HIV seropositive. However, OHL occurs in only 25% of these cases.

RISK FACTORS: OHL is usually found in human immunodeficiency virus (HIV) seropositive individuals (median CD4 count is 468/μl) but may also be identified in other immunocompromised patients such as transplant recipients (particularly renal) and patients taking steroids. Diagnosing OHL is an indication to institute a workup to evaluate and manage HIV disease.

PHYSICAL FINDINGS & CLINICAL PRESENTATION

- Varying morphology and appearance
- May be unilateral or bilateral
- White and can be small with fine vertical corrugations on the lateral margin of the tongue (Fig. 1-147)
- Irregular surface; may have prominent folds or projection, occasionally markedly resembling hairs
- May spread to cover the entire dorsal surface or spread onto the ventral surface of the tongue where they usually appear flat
- Rarely lesions manifest on the soft palate, buccal mucosa, and in the posterior oropharynx
- Usually asymptomatic, but some have mouth pain, soreness, or a burning sensation, impaired taste, or difficulty eating; others complain of its unsightly appearance
- OHL may progress to oral squamous cell carcinoma, which has a poor prognosis

ETIOLOGY

Epstein-Barr virus (EBV) is implicated in its etiology, and OHL is a result of replication EBV in the epithelium of keratinized cells. OHL differs from most EBV-related diseases in that infection is predominantly lytic rather than latent.

DIAGNOSIS

DIFFERENTIAL DIAGNOSIS

- *Candida albicans*
- Lichen planus
- Idiopathic leukoplakia
- White sponge nevus
- Dysplasia
- Squamous cell carcinoma

WORKUP

Requires physical examination and evaluation of HIV disease

LABORATORY TESTS

The *provisional* diagnosis is clinical and based on:

- Visual inspection
- Inability to scrape the lesion off the tongue with a blade
- Failure to respond to antifungal therapy

The *presumptive* diagnosis requires biopsy and histologic demonstration of:

- Epithelial hyperplasia with hairs
- Absence of inflammatory cell infiltrate

The *definitive* diagnosis requires:

- In situ hybridization of histologic or cytologic specimens revealing EBV DNA *or*
- Electron microscopy of specimens revealing herpes-like particles
- Measurement of the DNA content in cells of oral leukoplakia may be used to predict the risk of oral carcinoma

NOTE: Specimens obtained from lesions may demonstrate hyphae of *Candida albicans,* which may coexist and potentiate EBV-induced OHL.

TREATMENT

NONPHARMACOLOGIC THERAPY

OHL is usually asymptomatic and requires no specific therapy. It may resolve spontaneously and has no known premalignant potential.

ACUTE GENERAL Rx

- Highly active antiretroviral (HAART) therapy has considerably changed the frequency of oral lesions caused by opportunistic infections in HIV-seropositive individuals.
- Topical retinoids (0.1% vitamin A) may improve the appearance of OHL-affected oral surfaces through their dekeratinizing and immunomodulation effects; however, they are expensive and prolonged use may result in a burning sensation over the treated area.
- Topical podophyllin resin 25% solution has been reported to induce resolution.
- Surgical excision and cryotherapy may help, but the lesions may recur.
- High-dose acyclovir 800 mg 5× day, valacyclovir 1000 mg tid, famciclovir 500 mg tid, ganciclovir 1000 mg tid, or foscarnet 40 mg/kg IV tid will cause lesions to resolve but only temporarily.

PEARLS & CONSIDERATIONS

- Oral hairy leukoplakia is a nonmalignant lesion seen in patients with AIDS.
- Incidence has decreased significantly in the era of highly active antiretroviral therapy.

SUGGESTED READING

Sudbo J et al: DNA content as a prognostic marker in patients with oral leukoplakia, *N Engl J Med* 344:1270, 2001.

AUTHOR: **SAJEEV HANDA, M.D.**

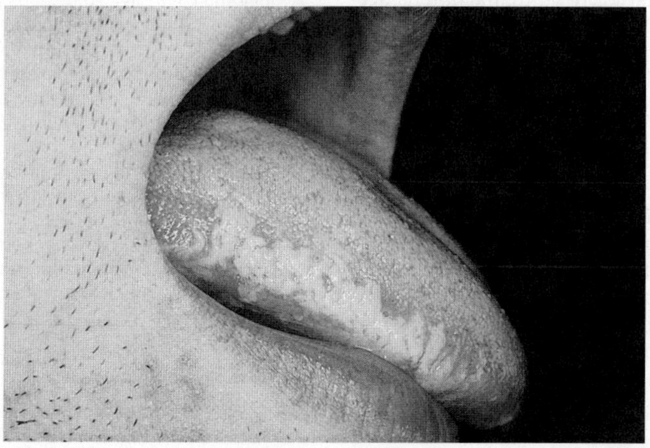

FIGURE 1-147 Oral hairy leukoplakia. Note white verrucoid plaques on the lateral border of the tongue. (From Noble J: *Primary care medicine,* ed 3, St Louis, 2001, Mosby.)

BASIC INFORMATION

DEFINITION

Lichen planus refers to a papular skin eruption characteristically found over the flexor surfaces of the extremities, genitalia, and mucous membranes.

SYNONYMS

Lichen
Lichen planus et atrophicus

ICD-9CM CODES
697.0 Lichen planus

EPIDEMIOLOGY & DEMOGRAPHICS

INCIDENCE: 1 in every 100 new patients seen in dermatology clinics in the U.S. is diagnosed with lichen planus
PREVALENCE: 440/100,000
PREDOMINANT SEX: Found equally between males and females (1:1)
PREDOMINANT AGE: Usually found in people between the ages of 30 to 60
PREDISPOSING FACTORS:
1. Associated with other autoimmune disorders (e.g., primary biliary cirrhosis, myasthenia gravis, ulcerative colitis, and diabetes)
2. Associated with hepatitis C infection
3. Drug-induced form affects any area of the body surface (e.g., beta-blocker, methyldopa, penicillamine, Quinidine, NSAIDS, ACE-I, sulfonylurea agents)

PHYSICAL FINDINGS & CLINICAL PRESENTATION

History
- Usually starts on an extremity and may remain localized or it can spread to involve other areas over a 1- to 4-mo time period.
- Pruritic

Physical findings
- Anatomic distribution:
  1. Flexor surface of wrists, forearms, shins, and upper thighs
  2. Neck and back area
  3. Nails
  4. Scalp (lichen planopilaris)
  5. Oral mucosa, buccal mucosa, tongue, gingiva, and lips
  6. Vulva, penis

Genital mucosa
- Lesion configuration:
  1. Linear
  2. Annular (more common)
  3. Reticular pattern noted on oral mucosa and genital area
- Lesion morphology:
  1. Papules (flat, smooth and shiny)—most common presentation
  2. Hypertrophic
  3. Follicular
  4. Vesicular
- Color:
  1. Dark red, bluish red, purplish-violaceous color is noted in cutaneous lichen planus
  2. Individual lesions characteristically have white lines visible (Wickham's striae)
  3. Oral and genital lichen planus have a reticular network of white lines that may be raised or annular in appearance
- Scalp lesions may result in alopecia.

ETIOLOGY

The cause of lichen planus is unknown.

DIAGNOSIS

- Clinical history and physical findings usually establish the diagnosis of lichen planus.
- Skin biopsy (deep shave or punch biopsy of the most developed lesion) can be done to confirm the diagnosis.

DIFFERENTIAL DIAGNOSIS

Drug eruption, psoriasis, Bowen's disease, leukoplakia, candidiasis, lupus rash, secondary syphilis, seborrheic dermatitis, chronic graft vs. host disease

WORKUP

If the diagnosis is questionable, a skin biopsy is performed.

LABORATORY TESTS

Laboratory tests are not specific for the diagnosis of lichen planus.

IMAGING STUDIES

Imaging studies are not helpful in diagnosing lichen planus.

TREATMENT

NONPHARMACOLOGIC THERAPY

- Avoid scratching.
- Use mild soaps and emollients after bathing to prevent dryness.

ACUTE GENERAL Rx

For cutaneous lichen planus
- Topical steroids (e.g., triamcinolone acetonide 0.1%, fluocinonide 0.05%, clobetasol propionate 0.05% cream or ointment) with occlusion used twice daily
- Acitretin 30 mg/day PO for 8 wk
- Systemic prednisone 30 to 60 mg/day as a starting dose and tapered to 15 to 20 mg/day maintenance for 6 wk
- Intradermal steroid triamcinolone acetonide 5 mg/ml can be tried for thick hyperkeratotic lesions
- Hydroxyzine 25 mg PO q6h can be used for pruritus

For oral lichen planus
- Topical steroid fluocinonide in an adhesive base used six times/day for 9 wk
- Topical calcineurin in steroid unresponsive cases
- Topical or systemic retinoids 0.1% retinoic acid in an adhesive base or gel
- Etretinate 75 mg/day for 2 mo

CHRONIC Rx

Refer to acute general treatment

DISPOSITION

- Spontaneous remissions of cutaneous lichen planus occur in over 65% of cases within the first year.
- Spontaneous remission of oral lichen planus usually occurs by 5 yr.
- Approximately 10% to 20% of patients will have recurrence.

REFERRAL

Dermatology

PEARLS & CONSIDERATIONS

COMMENTS

- Lichen planus can be remembered as purple, planar, pruritic, polygonal, papules, and plaques (Ps).
- Lesions can develop at the site of prior skin injury (Koebner's phenomenon).
- Although transformation to skin cancer has been seen in patients with lichen planus, it remains unclear if there is a true correlation.

EVIDENCE

There are small controlled trials on the use of oral acitretin vs. placebo in cutaneous lichen planus.[1]

There is a Cochrane review on interventions for treating oral lichen planus. This concludes that there is weak evidence for the superiority of any of the assessed interventions over placebo for palliation of symptomatic oral lichen planus.[2]

Trials have demonstrated the efficacy of topical tacrolimus in oral disease.[3,4]

Evidence-Based References

1. Laurberg G et al: Treatment of lichen planus with acitretin. A double blind placebo controlled study in 65 patients, *J Am Acad Dermatol* 24:434, 1991.
2. Kaliakatsou F et al: Management of recalcitrant ulcerative oral lichen planus with topical tacrolimus, *J Am Acad Dermatol* 46:35, 2002.
3. Dissemond J et al: Pimecrolimus in an adhesive ointment as a new treatment option for oral lichen planus. *Br J Dermatol* 150:782, 2004.
4. Swift JC et al: The effectiveness of 1% pimecrolimus cream in the treatment of oral erosive lichen planus. *J Periodontol* 76:627, 2005.

SUGGESTED READINGS

Chan ES, Thornhill M, Zakrzewska J: Interventions for treating oral lichen planus, *Cochrane Database Syst Rev* 2:CD001168, 2000.

Katta R: Lichen planus, *Am Fam Physician* 61(11):3319, 2000.

AUTHOR: **TANYA ALI, M.D.**

BASIC INFORMATION

DEFINITION

Chronic inflammatory condition of the skin usually affecting the vulva, perianal area, and groin

ICD-9CM CODES
701.0 Lichen sclerosus

EPIDEMIOLOGY & DEMOGRAPHICS

- Most common in postmenopausal women and men between ages 40 and 60 yr
- More common in females
- Can occur in children (usually prepubertal girls with involvement of the vulva and perineum)

PHYSICAL FINDINGS & CLINICAL PRESENTATION

- Erythema may be the only initial sign. A characteristic finding is the presence of ivory-white atrophic lesions on the involved area.
- Close inspection of the affected area will reveal the presence of white-to-brown follicular plugs on the surface (dells).
- When the genitals are involved, the white parchmentlike skin assumes an hourglass configuration around the introital and perianal area ("keyhole" distribution, Fig. 1-148). Inflammation, subepithelial hemorrhages, and chronic ulceration may develop.
- Dyspareunia, genital bleeding, and anal bleeding are common.

ETIOLOGY

Unknown. There may be an autoimmune association and a genetic familial component.

DIAGNOSIS

DIFFERENTIAL DIAGNOSIS

- Localized scleroderma (morphea)
- Cutaneous discoid lupus erythematosus
- Atrophic lichen planus
- Psoriasis

WORKUP

Diagnosis is based on close examination of the lesions for the presence of ivory-white atrophic lesions and typical location.

LABORATORY TESTS

Punch or deep shave biopsy can be used to confirm the diagnosis when in doubt.

TREATMENT

NONPHARMACOLOGIC THERAPY

Attention to hygiene and elimination of irritants or excessive bathing with harsh soaps

GENERAL Rx

- Application of clobetasol propionate 0.05% topically bid for up to 4 wk is usually effective. Repeat courses of corticosteroids may be necessary because of the chronic nature of this disorder. Continual application of topical steroids may lead to atrophy of the vulva.
- Use of topical testosterone (2%) has been found to be less effective than topical corticosteroids.
- Lubricants (e.g., Nutraplus cream) are useful to soothe dry tissues.
- Hydroxyzine 25 mg at hs is effective in decreasing nocturnal itching.
- Use of intralesional steroids, etretinate, and surgical management are usually reserved for refractory cases.

DISPOSITION

- The disease persists in approximately one third of patients.
- Most prepubertal girls improve spontaneously at menarche.
- Squamous cell carcinoma can develop within the lesions in 3% to 10% of older patients; therefore, periodic examination and biopsy of suspicious areas are indicated.

PEARLS & CONSIDERATIONS

COMMENTS

- Prepubertal lichen sclerosus may be confused with sexual abuse in prepubertal girls and may lead to false accusations and investigations.
- Lichen sclerosus of the vulva (kraurosis vulvae) usually occurs after menopause and is generally chronic. It can be painful and interfere with sexual activity.
- Lichen sclerosus of the penis (balanitis xerotica obliterans) is seen more commonly in uncircumcised males. It affects the glans and prepuce and may lead to stricture if it encroaches into the urinary meatus.

AUTHOR: **FRED F. FERRI, M.D.**

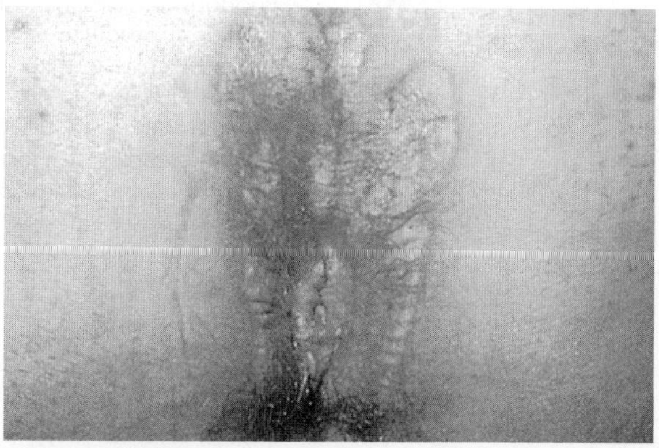

FIGURE 1-148 Lichen sclerosus. Perianal area is thinned and chalk white (keyhole distribution). (Courtesy Department of Dermatology, University of North Carolina at Chapel Hill. From Goldstein BG, Goldstein AO: *Practical dermatology,* ed 2, St Louis, 1997, Mosby.)

BASIC INFORMATION

DEFINITION

Listeriosis is a systemic infection caused by the gram-positive aerobic bacterium *Listeria monocytogenes.*

SYNONYMS

Listerial infection
Granulomatosis infantisepticum

ICD-9CM CODES
027.0 Listeriosis
771.2 Congenital listeriosis
771.2 Fetal listeriosis
665.4 Suspected fetal damage affecting management of pregnancy

EPIDEMIOLOGY & DEMOGRAPHICS

INCIDENCE (IN U.S.):

- Listeria meningitis: about 0.7 cases/100,000 persons (fourth most common cause of community-acquired bacterial meningitis in adults)
- Perinatal listeriosis: 8.6 cases/100,000 persons
- Nonperinatal listeriosis: 3 cases/1 million persons

PREDOMINANT SEX: Pregnant women are more susceptible to *Listeria* bacteremia, accounting for up to one third of reported cases.

PREDOMINANT AGE:

- Pregnant women
- Immunocompromised patients of any age
- Elderly patients are susceptible even in the absence of recognized immunocompromised states

GENETICS:

Congenital Infection:

- With transplacental transmission, syndrome termed *granulomatosis infantisepticum* in neonate
- Characterized by disseminated abscesses in multiple organs, skin lesions, conjunctivitis
- Mortality: 33% to 100%

Neonatal Infection:

- Infant becoming ill after 3 days of age; mother invariably asymptomatic
- Clinical picture of sepsis of unknown origin

PHYSICAL FINDINGS & CLINICAL PRESENTATION

- Infections in pregnancy
  1. More common in third trimester
  2. Usually present with fever and chills without localizing symptoms or signs of infection
- Meningoencephalitis
  1. More common in neonates and immunocompromised patients, but up to 30% of adults have no underlying condition
  2. In neonates: poor appetite with or without fever possibly the only presenting signs
  3. In adults: presentation often subacute, with low-grade fever and personality change as only signs
  4. Focal neurologic signs seen without demonstrable brain abscess on CT scan
- Cerebritis/rhombencephalitis:
  1. Headache and fever may be only presenting complaints
  2. Progressive cranial nerve palsies, hemiparesis, seizures, depressed level of consciousness, cerebellar signs, respiratory insufficiency may also be seen
- Focal infections
  1. Ocular infections (purulent conjunctivitis) and skin lesions (granulomatosis infantisepticum) as a result of inadvertent inoculation by laboratory and veterinary personnel
  2. Others: arthritis, prosthetic joint infections, peritonitis, osteomyelitis, organ abscesses, cholecystitis

ETIOLOGY

- Direct invasion of skin and eye has been documented, but mechanism of GI entry is unclear.
- Organism's intracellular life cycle explanatory of:
  1. Importance of cell-mediated immunity in host defense
  2. Increased infection in neonates, pregnant women, and immunocompromised hosts

DIAGNOSIS

DIFFERENTIAL DIAGNOSIS

- Meningitis caused by other bacteria, mycobacteria, or fungi
- CNS sarcoidosis
- Brain neoplasm or abscess
- Tuberculous and fungal (especially cryptococcal) meningitis
- Cerebral toxoplasmosis
- Lyme disease
- Sarcoidosis

WORKUP

Dictated by age, end-organ involvement, and immune status

LABORATORY TESTS

- Cultures of blood and other appropriate body fluids
- Variable CSF findings, but neutrophils usually predominate
- Organisms uncommonly seen on Gram stain and may be difficult to identify morphologically
- Monoclonal antibodies, polymerase chain reaction, and DNA probe techniques to detect *Listeria* in foods

IMAGING STUDIES

- If focal cerebral involvement suspected: CT scan or MRI
- MRI most sensitive for evaluation of brainstem and cerebellum

TREATMENT

Empiric therapy should be administered when diagnosis is suspected because overall mortality is 23%.

ACUTE GENERAL Rx

- Drugs of choice:
  1. IV ampicillin 8 to 12 g/day in divided doses
  2. IV penicillin 12 to 24 million U/day in divided doses
- Continuation of therapy for 2 wk
- Alternative (if penicillin allergic): trimethoprim/sulfamethoxazole or vancomycin
- Gentamicin added to provide synergy in meningitis or endocarditis

CHRONIC Rx

Relapses reported, especially in immunocompromised hosts, after 2 wk of therapy

DISPOSITION

Long-term follow-up of immunodeficiency state

REFERRAL

Infectious disease consultation for all patients

PEARLS & CONSIDERATIONS

COMMENTS

- Foodborne cases have been linked to various products: coleslaw, soft cheeses, unpasteurized milk and milk products, vegetables, undercooked chicken, hot dogs, luncheon meats, refrigerated smoked seafood, etc.
- Complete decontamination of food products is difficult because *Listeria* is resistant to pasteurization and refrigeration.

SUGGESTED READINGS

Gottlieb SL et al: Multistate outbreak of Listeriosis linked to turkey deli meat and subsequent changes in US regulatory policy, *Clin Infect Dis* 42(1):29, 2006.

Mylonakis E et al: Listeriosis during pregnancy: a case series and review of 222 cases, *Medicine* 81:260, 2002.

Pasche B et al: Sex-dependent susceptibility to *Listeria monocytogenes* infection is mediated by differential Interleukin-10 production, *Infect Immun* 73(9):5952, 2005.

Saunders BD et al: Molecular epidemiology and cluster analysis of human Listeriosis cases in three U.S. states, *J Food Prot* 69(7):1680, 2006.

Schlech WF et al: Does sporadic listeria gastroenteritis exist? A 2-year population-based survey in Nova Scotia, Canada, *Clin Infect Dis* 41(6):778, 2005.

AUTHORS: **GLENN G. FORT, M.D., M.P.H., DENNIS J. MIKOLICH, M.D.,** and **MAURICE POLICAR, M.D.**

BASIC INFORMATION

DEFINITION

Long QT syndrome is an electrocardiographic abnormality characterized by a corrected QT interval longer than 0.44 sec and associated with an increased risk of developing life-threatening ventricular arrhythmias.

SYNONYMS

QT interval prolongation

Congenital forms:

- Jervell and Lange-Nielsen syndrome (associated with deafness)
- Romano-Ward syndrome (associated with normal hearing)

Sporadic forms of long QT syndrome (nonfamilial)

ICD-9CM CODES

427.9 Unspecified cardiac dysrhythmia

EPIDEMIOLOGY & DEMOGRAPHICS

- Familial associated with deafness: autosomal recessive.
- Familial associated with normal hearing: autosomal dominant (the incidence is unknown). Although inheritance of long QT syndrome is autosomal dominant, female predominance has often been observed and has been attributed to an increased susceptibility to cardiac arrhythmias in women.

PHYSICAL FINDINGS & CLINICAL PRESENTATION

- Syncope caused by ventricular tachycardia
- Sudden death
- Abnormal ECG (prolonged QT) in asymptomatic relatives of known case. Bazett formula; QTc5QT/√RR. Calculated QTc should be <440 ms. If patient has atrial fibrillation, take the average of the longest and shortest QTc intervals.
- Routine (baseline) ECG finding.

ETIOLOGY

- Cardiac repolarization abnormality
- Congenital cause (chromosome 3 or chromosome 7 abnormality)
- Acquired causes:

Drugs (dofetilide, ibutilide, bepridil, quinidine, procainamide, sotalol, amiodarone, ranolazine, disopyramide, phenothiazines and antiemetic agents [droperidrol, domperidone], tricyclic antidepressants, quinolones, methadone, astemizole or cisapride given with ketoconazole or erythromycin, clarithromycin, and antimalarials), particularly among patients with asthma or those using potassium-lowering medications. Long QT syndrome is also common in patients receiving methadone.

Hypokalemia, hypomagnesemia

Liquid protein diet

CNS lesions

Mitral valve prolapse

DIAGNOSIS

DIFFERENTIAL DIAGNOSIS

See "Syncope."

Diagnostic criteria for the congenital long QT syndrome

ECG criteria	
Corrected QT >480 ms	3 points
Corrected QT 460 to 480 ms	2 points
Corrected QT 450 to 460 ms (males)	1 point
Torsades de pointe	2 points
T-wave alternans	1 point
Notched T wave in 3 leads	1 point
Bradycardia	0.5 points
History	
Syncope with stress	2 points
Syncope without stress	1 point
Congenital deafness	0.5 points
Definite family history of long QT	1 point
Unexplained cardiac death in first-degree relative under age 30	0.5 points

Total score ≥4: definite long QT syndrome

Total score 2 to 3: intermediate probability

Total score ≤1: low probability

WORKUP

In relatives of known patients with long QT syndrome or in young patients with syncope:

- Stress test may prolong the QT interval or cause T-wave alternans
- Valsalva maneuver: may prolong the QT interval or cause T-wave alternans
- Prolonged ECG monitoring with various stimulations aimed at increasing catecholamines (perform in a setting that can provide resuscitation)
- Epinephrine-induced prolongation of the 2T interval (Epinephrine infusion QT stress test)
- Genetic analysis

LQT1 locus of KCNQ1 potassium channel gene

LQT2 locus of KCNH2 potassium channel gene

LQT33 locus of SCN5A sodium channel gene

TREATMENT

- Asymptomatic sporadic forms with no complex ventricular arrhythmias: no treatment.
- Risk stratification.

High risk (<50% of cardiac event): QTc >500 ms and LQT1 and LQT2 or male with LQT3.

Moderate risk (30% to 50%): QTc >500 ms in female with LQT3 or L QTc <500 ms in male with LQT3 or in female with LQT2 or 3.

Low risk (<30%): QTc <500 ms and LQT1 and or male OQT2.

- General recommendations:

Avoid competitive sports.

β-blocker at maximum tolerated dose.

Cardiology referral is recommended for all cases. Pacemaker and implantable defibrillator recommended for survivors of cardiac arrest, for patients with syncope while receiving β-blockers, and for primary prevention in patients with characteristics that suggest high risk (these include LQT2, LQT3, and QTc interval >500 ms).

PROGNOSIS

The timing and frequency of syncope, QTc prolongation, and sex are predictive of risk for aborted cardiac arrest and sudden cardiac death during adolescence. Higher risk is present in those with one or two or more episodes of syncope in the last 10 years compared to those with no syncopal episodes, those with QTc ≥530 ms, and males between ages of 10 and 12 years.

SUGGESTED READINGS

Al-Khatib SM et al: What clinicians should know about the QT interval, *JAMA* 289:2120, 2003.

De Bruin ML, Hoes AW, Leufkens HGM: QTc-prolonging drugs and hospitalizations for cardiac arrhythmias, *Am J Cardiol* 91:59, 2003.

Ehret GB et al: Drug-induced long QT syndrome in injection drug users receiving methadone, *Arch Intern Med* 166:1280, 2006.

Hobbs et al: Risk of aborted cardiac arrest or sudden cardiac death during adolescence in the long QT syndrome, *JAMA* 296:1249, 2006.

Imboden M et al: Female predominance and transmission distortion in the long QT syndrome, *N Engl J Med* 355:2744, 2006.

Montanez Aetal: Prolonged QTc interval and risks of total and cardiovascular mortality and sudden death in the general population, *Arch Intern Med* 164:943, 2004.

Napolitano C et al: Genetic testing in the long QT syndrome, *JAMA* 294:2975, 2005.

Nemec J et al: Catecholamine-induced T-wave lability in congenital long qt syndrome, *Mayo Clin Proc* 78:40, 2003.

Priori SG et al: Risk stratification in the long-QT syndrome, *N Engl J Med* 348:1866, 2003.

Roden DM: Drug-induced prolongation of the QT interval, *N Engl J Med* 350:1013, 2004.

Roden DM: Long QT syndrome, *N Engl J Med* 358:169-176, 2008.

AUTHORS: **FRED F. FERRI, M.D.,** and **TOM J. WACHTEL, M.D.**

BASIC INFORMATION

DEFINITION

Lumbar disk syndromes are diseases resulting from disk disorder, either herniation or degenerative change (spondylosis). Massive disk protrusion may rarely lead to paralysis in the lower extremity, a condition termed *cauda equina syndrome*. Gradual narrowing of the spinal canal (lumbar stenosis), usually from spondylosis, may also cause lower extremity symptoms.

SYNONYMS

Lumbago
Sciatica

ICD-9CM CODES
722.10 Lumbar disk displacement
724.02 Lumbar stenosis
344.60 Cauda equina syndrome
721.3 Lumbar spondylosis

EPIDEMIOLOGY & DEMOGRAPHICS

PREVALENCE:
- Variable
- At least one episode in 80% of adults

PREDOMINANT SEX: Approximately equal

PREDOMINANT AGE:
- Herniation: 20 to 40 yr
- Stenosis: >40 to 50 yr
- Disk symptoms: rare <20 yr

PHYSICAL FINDINGS & CLINICAL PRESENTATION

- Overlapping clinical syndromes that may result:
  1. Mild herniation without nerve root compression
  2. Herniation with nerve root compression
  3. Cauda equina syndrome
  4. Chronic degenerative disease with or without leg symptoms
  5. Spinal stenosis
- Low back pain, often worsened by activity or coughing and sneezing
- Local lumbar or lumbosacral tenderness
- Paresthesias, usually unilateral
- Restricted low back motion
- Increased pain on bending toward affected side
- Weakness and reflex changes (L4-knee jerk and quadriceps, L5-extensor hallucis longus, S1-ankle jerk and toe walking)
- Sensory examination usually not helpful
- Lumbar stenosis that possibly produces symptoms (pseudoclaudication), which are often misinterpreted as being vascular (Pseudoclaudication usually recovers quickly with sitting or spine flexion. Vascular disease is unaffected by spine position and is typically associated with atrophic skin changes and diminished pulses.)
- Positive straight leg raising test if nerve root compression is present

ETIOLOGY

Unknown

DIAGNOSIS

DIFFERENTIAL DIAGNOSIS

- Soft-tissue strain/sprain
- Tumor
- Degenerative arthritis of hip
- Insufficiency fracture of hip or pelvis

Section II describes the differential diagnosis of common low back pain syndromes.

WORKUP

In most cases, the diagnosis can be established on a clinical basis alone.

IMAGING STUDIES

- Plain roentgenograms may be indicated within the first few weeks; they are usually normal in soft disk herniation, but with chronic degenerative disk disease, loss of height of the disk space and osteophyte formation can occur.
- Myelography, CT scanning, and MRI may be indicated in patients whose symptoms do not resolve or when other spinal pathology may be suspected.
- Electrodiagnostic studies may confirm the diagnosis or rule out peripheral nerve disorders.

TREATMENT

NONPHARMACOLOGIC THERAPY

- Short course (3 to 5 days) of bed rest for acute disk herniation with leg pain
- Physical therapy for modalities plus a careful gradual exercise program
- Lumbosacral corset brace during rehabilitation process in conjunction with exercise program
- Percutaneous electrical nerve stimulation (PENS) may be beneficial in selected patients with chronic back pain

ACUTE GENERAL Rx

- NSAIDs
- Muscle relaxants for sedative effect
- Analgesics
- Epidural steroid injection for leg symptoms in selected patients

DISPOSITION

- Almost all lumbar disk syndromes improve with time.
- Recurrent episodes usually respond to medical management.
- Recovery from the rare paralytic event is often incomplete.

REFERRAL

- For orthopedic or neurosurgical consultation for intractable pain or significant neurologic deficit
- Emergency referral for cauda equina syndrome

PEARLS & CONSIDERATIONS

Red flags suggesting a more serious condition as a cause of the back pain include:
1. Fever
2. History of malignancy
3. Pain at rest
4. Incontinence
5. Sudden worsening in level of pain
6. Weight loss
7. Significant motor loss, especially if associated with saddle anesthesia

COMMENTS

- Surgery is most consistently helpful when leg pain (not back pain) predominates.
- A clinical algorithm for evaluation of back pain is described in Section III.

SUGGESTED READINGS

Biyani A, Andersson GB: Low back pain: Pathophysiology and management, *J Am Acad Orthop Surg* 12:106, 2004.

Brodke DS, Ritter SM: Nonoperative management of low back pain and lumbar disc degeneration, *J Bone Joint Surg* 86A:1810, 2004.

Butterman GR: Treatment of lumbar disc herniation: epidural steroid injection compared with discectomy: a prospective, randomized study, *J Bone Joint Surg* 86A:670, 2004.

Cole BJ, Schumacher HR: Injectable corticosteroids in modern practice, *J Am Acad Orthop Surg* 13:37, 2005.

Dreyfuss P et al: Sacroiliac joint pain, *J Am Acad Orthop Surg* 12:255, 2004.

Haig AJ et al: Electromyographic and magnetic resonance imaging to predict lumbar stenosis, low back pain, and no back symptoms, *J Bone Joint Surg* 89A:358, 2007.

Katz JN: Lumbar disc disorders and low-back pain: socioeconomic factors and consequences, *J Bone Joint Surg* 88A(Suppl 2):21, 2006.

Lee DH, Claussen GC, Oh S: Clinical nerve conduction and needle electromyography studies, *J Am Acad Orthop Surg* 12:276, 2004.

Shen FH et al: Nonsurgical management of acute and chronic low back pain, *J Am Acad Orthop Surg* 14:477, 2006.

Thomas KC et al: Outcome evaluation of surgical and non surgical management of lumbar disc protrusion causing radiculopathy, *Spine* 32:1414, 2007.

Tribus CB: Degenerative lumbar scoliosis: evaluation and management, *J Am Acad Orthop Surg* 11:174, 2003.

Young IA et al: The use of lumbar epidural/transforaminal steroids for managing spinal disease, *J Am Acad Orthop Surg* 15:228, 2007.

AUTHOR: **LONNIE R. MERCIER, M.D.**

BASIC INFORMATION

DEFINITION

A primary lung neoplasm is a malignancy arising from lung tissue. The World Health Organization distinguishes 12 types of pulmonary neoplasms. Among them, the major types are *squamous cell carcinoma, adenocarcinoma, small cell carcinoma,* and *large cell carcinoma.* However, the crucial difference in the diagnosis of lung cancer is between small cell and non–small cell types, because the prognosis and therapeutic approach is different. Selective characteristics of lung carcinomas:

ADENOCARCINOMA: Represents 35%-40% of lung carcinomas; frequently located in mid lung and periphery; initial metastases are to lymphatics, frequently associated with peripheral scars

SQUAMOUS CELL (EPIDERMOID): 20% to 30% of lung cancers; central location; metastasis by local invasion; frequent cavitation and obstructive phenomena

SMALL CELL (OAT CELL): 20% of lung carcinomas; central location; metastasis through lymphatics; associated with lesion of the short arm of chromosome 3; high cavitation rate

LARGE CELL: 10% to 15% of lung carcinomas; frequently located in the periphery; metastasis to CNS and mediastinum; rapid growth rate with early metastasis

BRONCHOALVEOLAR: 5% of lung carcinomas; frequently located in the periphery; may be bilateral; initial metastasis through lymphatic, hematogenous, and local invasion; no correlation with cigarette smoking; cavitation rare

SYNONYMS

Lung cancer

ICD-9CM CODES
162.9 Malignant neoplasm of bronchus and lung, unspecified

EPIDEMIOLOGY & DEMOGRAPHICS

- Lung cancer is responsible for >30% of cancer deaths in males and >25% of cancer deaths in females. It has been the most common cancer in the world since 1985 and is the leading cause of cancer-related death.
- Tobacco smoking is implicated in 85% of cases; second-hand smoke is responsible for approximately 20% of cases.
- There are >180,000 new cases of lung cancer yearly in the U.S., most occurring >age 50 yr (<4% in patients <40 yr of age).
- Among women there has been a 600% increase in incidence of lung cancer during the past 80 years. The rates of death among women with lung cancer in the U.S. are the highest in the world.

PHYSICAL FINDINGS & CLINICAL PRESENTATION

- Weight loss, fatigue, fever, anorexia, dysphagia
- Cough, hemoptysis, dyspnea, wheezing
- Chest, shoulder, and bone pain
- Paraneoplastic syndromes:
  1. *Eaton-Lambert syndrome:* myopathy involving proximal muscle groups
  2. Endocrine manifestations: hypercalcemia, ectopic ACTH, SIADH
  3. Neurologic: subacute cerebellar degeneration, peripheral neuropathy, cortical degeneration
  4. Musculoskeletal: polymyositis, clubbing, hypertrophic pulmonary osteoarthropathy
  5. Hematologic or vascular: migratory thrombophlebitis, marantic thrombosis, anemia, thrombocytosis, or thrombocytopenia
  6. Cutaneous: acanthosis nigricans, dermatomyositis
- Pleural effusion (10% of patients), recurrent pneumonias (secondary to obstruction), localized wheezing
- *Superior vena cava syndrome:*
  1. Obstruction of venous return of the superior vena cava is most commonly caused by bronchogenic carcinoma or metastasis to paratracheal nodes.
  2. The patient usually complains of headache, nausea, dizziness, visual changes, syncope, and respiratory distress.
  3. Physical examination reveals distention of thoracic and neck veins, edema of face and upper extremities, facial plethora, and cyanosis.
- *Horner's syndrome:* constricted pupil, ptosis, facial anhidrosis caused by spinal cord damage between C8 and T1 secondary to a superior sulcus tumor (bronchogenic carcinoma of the extreme lung apex); a superior sulcus tumor associated with ipsilateral Horner's syndrome and shoulder pain is known as *"Pancoast" tumor.*

ETIOLOGY

- Tobacco abuse
- Environmental agents (e.g., radon) and industrial agents (e.g., ionizing radiation, asbestos, nickel, uranium, vinyl chloride, chromium, arsenic, coal dust)

DIAGNOSIS

DIFFERENTIAL DIAGNOSIS

- Pneumonia
- TB
- Metastatic carcinoma to the lung
- Lung abscess
- Granulomatous disease
- Carcinoid tumor
- Mycobacterial and fungal diseases
- Sarcoidosis
- Viral pneumonitis
- Benign lesions that simulate thoracic malignancy:
  1. Lobar atelectasis: pneumonia, TB, chronic inflammatory disease, allergic bronchopulmonary aspergillosis
  2. Multiple pulmonary nodules: septic emboli, Wegener's granulomatosis, sarcoidosis, rheumatoid nodules, fungal disease, multiple pulmonary AV fistulas
  3. Mediastinal adenopathy: sarcoidosis, lymphoma, primary TB, fungal disease, silicosis, pneumoconiosis, drug-induced (e.g., phenytoin, trimethadione)
  4. Pleural effusion: CHF, pneumonia with parapneumonic effusion, TB, viral pneumonitis, ascites, pancreatitis, collagen-vascular disease

WORKUP

Workup generally includes chest x-ray, CT scan of chest, PET scan, and tissue biopsy.

LABORATORY TESTS

Obtain tissue diagnosis. Various modalities are available:

- Biopsy of any suspicious lymph nodes (e.g., supraclavicular node)
- Flexible fiberoptic bronchoscopy: brush and biopsy specimens are obtained from any visualized endobronchial lesions
- Transbronchial needle aspiration: done via a special needle passed through the bronchoscope; this technique is useful to sample mediastinal masses or paratracheal lymph nodes
- Transthoracic fine-needle aspiration biopsy with fluoroscopic or CT scan guidance to evaluate peripheral pulmonary nodules
- Mediastinoscopy and anteromedial sternotomy in suspected tumor involvement of the mediastinum
- Pleural biopsy in patients with pleural effusion
- Thoracentesis of pleural effusion and cytologic evaluation of the obtained fluid: may confirm diagnosis

IMAGING STUDIES

- Chest x-ray: The radiographic presentation often varies with the cell type. Pleural effusion, lobar atelectasis, and mediastinal adenopathy can accompany any cell types.
- CT scan of chest: to evaluate mediastinal and pleural extension of suspected lung neoplasms.
- Positron emission tomography (PET) with 18F-fluorodeoxyglucose (18 FDG-PET), a metabolic marker of malignant tissue, is superior to CT scan in detecting mediastinal and distant metastases in non–small cell lung cancer. It is useful for preoperative staging of non–small cell lung cancer.

STAGING:

- Following confirmation of diagnosis, patients should undergo staging:
  1. The international staging system is the most widely accepted staging system for non–small cell lung cancer (NSLC). In this system, stage I (N0 [no lymph node involvement]), stage II (N1 [spread to ipsilateral bronchopulmonary or hilar lymph nodes]) include localized tumors for which surgical resection is the preferred treatment. Stage III is subdivided into IIIA (potentially resectable) and IIIB. The surgical management of stage IIIA disease (N2 [involvement of ipsilateral mediastinal nodes]) is controversial. Only 20% of N2 disease is considered minimal disease (involvement of only one node) and technically resectable. Stage IV indicates metastatic disease. The pathologic staging system uses a tumor/nodal involvement/metastasis system.
  2. In patients with small cell lung cancer, a more practical accepted staging system is the one developed by the Veterans Administration Lung Cancer Study Group (VALG). This system contains two stages:
     a. Limited stage: disease confined to the regional lymph nodes and to one hemithorax (excluding pleural surfaces)
     b. Extensive stage: disease spread beyond the confines of limited stage disease
  3. Pretreatment staging procedures for lung cancer patients, in addition to complete history and physical examination, generally include the following tests:
     a. Chest x-ray (PA and lateral), ECG.
     b. Laboratory evaluation: CBC, complete metabolic panel, ABGs, or pulse oximetry. The identification of molecular signatures of lung cancer to predict prognosis using data from microarray and/or RT-PCR analysis has been validated in recent trials. A five-gene signature (DUSP6, MMD, STAT1, ERBB3, and LCK) is closely associated with relapse-free and overall survival among patients with NSLC.
     c. Pulmonary function studies.
     d. CT scan of chest and PET scan: A recent Dutch trial revealed a 51% relative reduction in futile thoracotomies for patients with suspected non–small cell lung cancer who underwent preoperative assessment with PET with the tracer 18FDG-PET in addition to conventional workup.
     e. Mediastinoscopy or anterior mediastinotomy in patients being considered for possible curative lung resection.
     f. Biopsy of any accessible suspect lesions.
     g. CT scan of liver and brain; radionuclide scans of bone in all patients with small cell carcinoma of the lung and patients with non–small cell lung neoplasms suspected of involving these organs.
     h. Bone marrow aspiration and biopsy only in selected patients with small cell carcinoma of the lung. In the absence of an increased LDH or cytopenia, routine bone marrow examination is not recommended.

TREATMENT (Rx)

NONPHARMACOLOGIC THERAPY

- Nutritional support
- Avoidance of tobacco or other substances toxic to the lungs
- Supplemental O_2 prn

ACUTE GENERAL Rx

NON–SMALL CELL CARCINOMA:

- Surgical resection is the best hope for cure in patients with operable non–small cell lung cancer.
  1. Surgical resection is indicated in patients with limited disease (not involving mediastinal nodes, ribs, pleura, or distant sites). This represents approximately 15% to 30% of diagnosed cases.
  2. Preoperative evaluation includes review of cardiac status (e.g., recent MI, major arrhythmias) and evaluation of pulmonary function (to determine if the patient can tolerate any loss of lung tissue). Pneumonectomy is possible if the patient has a preoperative $FEV_1 \geq 2$ L or if the MVV is >50% of predicted capacity. Individuals with FEV_1 >1.5 L are suitable for lobectomy without further evaluation unless there is evidence of interstitial lung disease or undue dyspnea on exertion. In that case, DLCO should be measured. If the DLCO is <80% predicted normal, the individual is not clearly operable.
  3. Preoperative chemotherapy should be considered in patients with more advanced disease (stage IIIA) who are being considered for surgery, because it increases the median survival time in patients with non–small cell lung cancer compared with the use of surgery alone. Gene-expression profiles that predict the risk of recurrence in patients with early stage (IA) NSCLC have been identified. These patients are at high risk of recurrence and may also benefit from adjuvant chemotherapy.
  4. Postoperative adjuvant chemotherapy (chemotherapy given after surgical resection of an apparently localized tumor to eradicate occult metastases) with vinorelbine plus cisplatin significantly increases 5-year survival (69% vs. 54%) in patients with completely resected stage IB or stage II non–small cell lung cancer and good performance status.
- Treatment of unresectable non–small cell carcinoma of the lung:
  1. Radiotherapy can be used alone or in combination with chemotherapy; it is used primarily for treatment of CNS and skeletal metastases, superior vena cava syndrome, and obstructive atelectasis; although thoracic radiotherapy is generally considered standard therapy for stage 3 disease, it has limited effect on survival. Palliative radiotherapy should be delayed until symptoms occur since immediate therapy offers no advantage over delayed therapy and results in more adverse events from the radiotherapy.
  2. Chemotherapy: various combination regimens are available. Current drugs of choice are paclitaxel plus either carboplatin or cisplatin; cisplatin plus vinorelbine; gemcitabine plus cisplatin; carboplatin or cisplatin plus docetaxel. The overall results are disappointing, and none of the standard regimens for non–small cell lung cancer is clearly superior to the others. The addition of bevacizumab to paclitaxel plus carboplatin results in significant survival benefit but carries an increased risk of treatment-related death. Gefitinib (Iressa) and erlotinib (Tarceva) are oral inhibitors of epidermal growth factor receptor (EGFR) tyrosine kinase. Both agents are approved only for patients who have failed at least one prior chemotherapy regimen. Sensitivity of lung neoplasms to these agents is seen primarily in tumors with somatic mutations in the tyrosine kinase domain (more common in adenocarcinomas found in patients who never smoked and in Asian patients). Cost for one month of oral therapy exceeds $2,500.
  3. The addition of chemotherapy to radiotherapy improves survival in patients with locally advanced, unresectable non–small cell lung cancer. The absolute benefit is relatively small, however, and should be balanced against the increased toxicity associated with the addition of chemotherapy.

SMALL CELL LUNG CANCER:
- Limited stage disease: standard treatments include thoracic radiotherapy and chemotherapy (cisplatin and etoposide)
- Extensive stage disease: standard treatments include combination chemotherapy (cisplatin or carboplatin plus etoposide or combination of irinotecan and cisplatin)
- Prophylactic cranial irradiation for patients in complete remission to decrease the risk of CNS metastasis

DISPOSITION

- The 5-yr survival of patients with non–small cell carcinoma when the disease is resectable is approximately 30%.
- Median survival time in patients with limited stage disease and small cell lung cancer is 15 mo; in patients with extensive stage disease, it is 9 mo.
- Methylation of the promoter region of certain genes (P16, CDH13, APC, and RASSF1A) in a resected NSCLC specimen is associated with recurrence of the tumor.

PEARLS & CONSIDERATIONS

COMMENTS

CT screening for detection of lung cancer among persons with a heavy history of smoking increases the percentage of lung cancer cases that are diagnosed in stage 1. However, randomized trials to assess whether such screening reduces mortality have not shown a significant benefit for CT screening. Current data do not support screening for lung cancer with any method.

EVIDENCE

Non–small cell lung cancers

A systematic review of trials using modern cisplatin-containing regimens found a reduction in risk of death of between 13% and 27% when comparing radical radiotherapy with radical radiotherapy plus chemotherapy, surgery with surgery plus chemotherapy, and supportive care with supportive care plus chemotherapy.[1] A

In people with unresectable stage III non–small cell lung cancer (NSCLC), combining thoracic irradiation with chemotherapy improved survival compared with radiotherapy alone, but with unknown effects on quality of life.[2] A

A randomized controlled trial (RCT) to determine whether combination chemotherapy plus thoracic radiotherapy is superior to thoracic radiotherapy alone, in patients with completely resected stage II or IIIa NSCLC, found that radiotherapy and chemotherapy with cisplatin and etoposide did not decrease the risk of intrathoracic recurrence or prolong survival.[3] B

There is inconclusive evidence about the effects of preoperative chemotherapy in people with resectable stage III NSCLC.[2] B

One systematic review and five RCTs in people with advanced NSCLC found inconclusive evidence on the effects of first line single-agent vs. combined chemotherapy.[2] A

Five RCTs found insufficient evidence to compare first line platinum- vs. non-platinum-based chemotherapy in people with stage III or IV NSCLC.[2] B

Second line single-agent docetaxel has been found to significantly improve survival at 1 year compared each with best supportive care, vinorelbine, and ifosfamide.[4] B

A systematic review found a significant adverse effect of postoperative radiotherapy in the treatment of patients with completely resected stage I/II, N0-N1 NSCLC. However, there is no clear evidence of an adverse effect for stage II, N2 disease.[5] A

Small cell lung cancer

Two systematic reviews found that thoracic radiation plus chemotherapy compared with chemotherapy alone significantly increased 3-year survival in one review, and local control in the other review, in patients with limited-stage SCLC.[2] A

Early vs. late addition of thoracic radiotherapy to chemotherapy in patients with SCLC has produced mixed results, as was found for dose and fractionation.[2] B

RCTs compared oral etoposide with intravenous combination chemotherapy in patients with extensive-stage small cell lung cancer and found reduced survival at 1 year in two trials, and no significant difference in mortality at 3 years in another trial, although overall mortality was lower in the etoposide group.[2] B

RCTs also found that etoposide may reduce nausea, alopecia, and numbness in the short term compared with combination chemotherapy, but found no evidence that it offered better quality of life overall.[2] B

Prophylactic cranial irradiation has been found to significantly improve disease-free survival for patients with SCLC in complete remission.[7] A

Evidence-Based References

1. The Prophylactic Cranial Irradiation Overview Collaborative Group: Cranial irradiation for preventing brain metastases of small cell lung cancer in patients in complete remission, *Cochrane Database Syst Rev* 4, 2000. A
2. Neville A: Lung cancer. Reviewed in: 12:2167-2189, 2004, London, BMJ Publishing Group. AB
3. Keller SM et al: A randomized trial of postoperative adjuvant therapy in patients with completely resected stage II or stage IIIA non-small cell lung cancer, *N Engl J Med* 343:1217, 2000. B
4. Logan D et al: The role of single-agent docetaxel as second-line treatment for advanced non-small cell lung cancer, *Curr Oncol* 8:50, 2001. Reviewed in: *Clin Evid* 12:2167, 2004. B
5. PORT Meta-analysis Trialists Group: Postoperative radiotherapy for non-small cell lung cancer, *Cochrane Database Syst Rev* 1, 2003. A
6. Macbeth F et al: Palliative radiotherapy regimens for non-small cell lung cancer, *Cochrane Database Syst Rev* 4, 2001. A
7. The Prophylactic Cranial Irradiation Overview Collaborative Group: Cranial irradiation for preventing brain metastases of small cell lung cancer in patients in complete remission, *Cochrane Database Syst Rev* 4, 2000. A

SUGGESTED READINGS

Bach PB et al: Computed tomography screening and lung cancer outcomes, *JAMA* 297:953, 2007.

Brock MV et al: DNA methylation markers and early recurrence in stage I lung cancer, *N Engl J Med* 358:1118-1128, 2008.

Chen HY et al: A five-gene signature and clinical outcome in non-small cell lung cancer, *N Engl J Med* 356:11, 2007.

Sandler A et al: Paclitaxel-carboplatin alone or with bevacizumab for non–small-cell lung cancer, *N Engl J Med* 355:2542, 2006.

Shert DY et al: Small cell lung cancer, *Mayo Clin Proc* 83(3):355-367, 2008.

AUTHOR: **FRED F. FERRI, M.D.**

Section I DISEASES AND DISORDERS

BASIC INFORMATION

DEFINITION

Lyme disease is a multisystem inflammatory disorder caused by the transmission of a spirochete, *Borrelia burgdorferi*. Lyme disease is spread by the bite of infected *Ixodes* ticks, taking 36 to 48 hr for a tick to feed and transmit the infecting organism *B. burgdorferi* to the host.

SYNONYMS

Bannworth's syndrome (Europe)
Acrodermatitis chronica atrophicans

ICD-9CM CODES
088.8 Lyme disease

EPIDEMIOLOGY & DEMOGRAPHICS

INCIDENCE (IN U.S.): 4.4 cases/100,000 persons; 90% of cases in the U.S. are found in: Massachusetts, Connecticut, Rhode Island, New York, New Jersey, Pennsylvania, Minnesota, Wisconsin, and California.
PEAK INCIDENCE: May to November
PREDOMINANT SEX: Male = female
PREDOMINANT AGE: Median age of 28 yr

PHYSICAL FINDINGS & CLINICAL PRESENTATION

Lyme disease may present in the following stages:

- *Early localized:* early Lyme disease, erythema migrans (EM); skin rash, often at site of tick bite; possible fever, myalgias 3 to 32 days after tick bite
- *Early disseminated:* days to weeks later; multiorgan system involvement, including CNS, joints, cardiac; related to dissemination of spirochete
- *Late persistent:* months to years after tick exposure; affects central and peripheral nervous system, cardiac, joints

Common presenting signs and symptoms include:

- EM (Fig. 1-149).
- Lymphadenopathy, neck pains, pharyngeal erythema, myalgias, hepatosplenomegaly.
- Patients will complain of malaise, fatigue, lethargy, headache, fever/chills, neck pain, myalgias, back pain.

ETIOLOGY

B. burgdorferi transmitted from bite of an *Ixodes* tick.

DIAGNOSIS

Clinical presentation, exposure to ticks in endemic area, and diagnostic testing for antibody response to *B. burgdorferi*

DIFFERENTIAL DIAGNOSIS

- Chronic fatigue/fibromyalgia
- Acute viral illnesses
- Babesiosis
- Ehrlichiosis

WORKUP

- ELISA testing—Western blot IgM and IgG
- Immunofluorescent assay
- Early disease often difficult to diagnose serologically secondary to slow immune response
- Culturing of skin lesions (EM) and polymerase chain reaction (PCR) of skin biopsy and blood to give definitive diagnosis (available only in reference laboratories)

IMAGING STUDIES

- Echocardiogram if conduction abnormalities are present with cardiac involvement
- CT scan, MRI of head for CNS involvement

TREATMENT

- Early Lyme disease.
- Doxycycline 100 mg bid or amoxicillin 500 mg tid for 14 days (doxycycline should be avoided in children/pregnant females).
- Alternative treatments: cefuroxime axetil 500 mg bid for 14 to 21 days, azithromycin 500 mg po for 7 to 10 days but should not be used as a first-line agent.
- Early disseminated and late persistent infection: 30 days of treatment necessary; doxycycline and ceftriaxone appear equally effective for acute disseminated Lyme disease.
- Arthritis: 30 days of doxycycline or amoxicillin plus probenecid.
- Neurologic involvement requires parenteral antibiotics.
- Ceftriaxone 2 g/day for 21 to 28 days; alternative: cefotaxime 2 g q8h; alternative: penicillin G 5 million U qid.
- Cardiac involvement: IV ceftriaxone or penicillin plus cardiac monitoring.
- Prolonged treatment with IV or po antibiotic therapy for up to 90 days did not improve symptoms more than placebo.

DISPOSITION

The patient often needs careful follow-up and supportive care for the arthralgia-neuritis symptoms.

REFERRAL

- To a neurologist if significant neurologic complications (meningitis, myelitis, ophthalmoplegia, Bell's palsy)
- To a cardiologist if the patient develops evidence of cardiac conduction disturbances or pericarditis

PEARLS & CONSIDERATIONS

- The Lyme disease vaccine was taken off the U.S. market in 2002 because of concerns about possible side effects (arthralgia, arthritis) and its infrequent use.
- A physician diagnosis of classic erythema migrans in an endemic region of Lyme disease is sufficient to make a definitive diagnosis.
- In some patients with Lyme disease, nonspecific complaints such as headache, fatigue, and arthralgia may persist for months after appropriate (and ultimately successful) antibiotic treatment.
- A single dose of 200 mg doxycycline given within 72 hr of *Ixodes* tick bite can prevent development of Lyme disease.

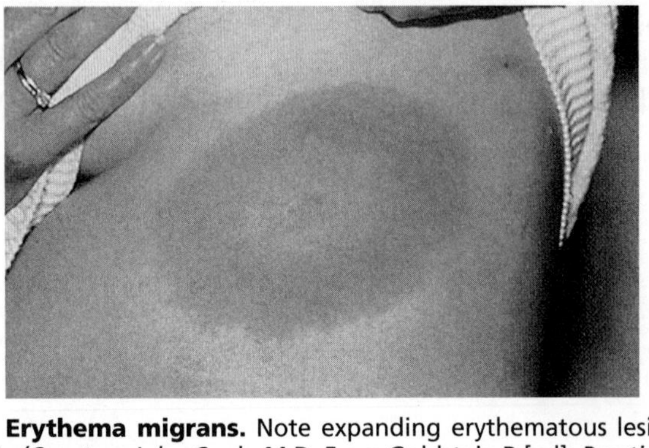

FIGURE 1-149 Erythema migrans. Note expanding erythematous lesion with central clearing on trunk. (Courtesy John Cook, M.D. From Goldstein B [ed]: *Practical dermatology,* ed 2, St Louis, 1997, Mosby.)

SUGGESTED READINGS

Nadelman RB et al: Prophylaxis with single dose doxycycline for the prevention of Lyme disease after an *Ixodes scapularis* tick bite, *N Engl J Med* 345:79, 2001.
Wormser GP et al: Duration of antibiotic therapy for early Lyme disease. A randomized, double-blind, placebo-controlled trial, *Ann Intern Med* 138:697, 2003.
Wormser GP et al: The clinical assessment, treatment, and prevention of Lyme disease, human granulocytic anaplasmosis, and babesiosis: clinical practice guidelines by the Infectious Diseases Society of America, *CID* 43:1089, 2006.

AUTHORS: **GLENN G. FORT, M.D., M.P.H., JOSEPH F. GRILLO, M.D.,** and **DENNIS J. MIKOLICH, M.D.**

BASIC INFORMATION

DEFINITION

Lymphangitis refers to the inflammation of lymphatic vessels.

SYNONYMS

Nodular lymphangitis
Sporotrichoid lymphangitis

ICD-9CM CODES
457.2 Lymphangitis

EPIDEMIOLOGY & DEMOGRAPHICS

INCIDENCE (IN U.S.): Several hundred cases/yr of sporotrichoid lymphangitis

PHYSICAL FINDINGS & CLINICAL PRESENTATION

ACUTE LYMPHANGITIS:
- Commonly associated with a bacterial cellulitis
- May or may not recognize site of skin trauma (i.e., laceration, puncture, ulcer)
- In hours to days, distal appearance of erythema, edema, and tenderness, with linear erythematous streaks extending proximally to regional lymph nodes
- Possible lymphadenitis and fever
- Predisposition to group A streptococcal infection of the skin in those with chronic lymphedema and superficial fungal infections (e.g., tinea pedis)

***SPOROTRICHOID* OR *NODULAR* LYMPHANGITIS:**
- Includes subcutaneous nodules that develop along the path of involved lymphatics
- Most commonly results from inoculation of the skin of the hand
- Usually preceded by well-defined episode of cutaneous inoculation or trauma
- Lesions apparent from one to several weeks after inoculation
- Initially, nodular or papular lesion; may ulcerate
- May have frank pus or a serosanguineous discharge
- Systemic complaints uncommon, but infection with certain microorganisms associated with fever, chills, myalgias, and headache

ETIOLOGY

- Acute lymphangitis: usually associated with *Streptococcus pyogenes* (group A streptococcus), but staphylococcal organisms are increasingly recognized as a cause of severe soft tissue infections such as lymphangitis, including community-acquired methicillin-resistant *S. aureus* (CA-MRSA)
- Nodular lymphangitis caused by one of several organisms
  1. *Sporothrix schenckii*
     a. Most common recognized cause in the U.S., usually in the Midwest
     b. Found in soil and plant debris
  2. *Nocardia brasiliensis:* found in soil
  3. *Mycobacterium marinum:* associated with trauma related to water (e.g., aquariums, swimming pools, fish)
  4. *Leishmania brasiliensis*
     a. Protozoal parasite transmitted to humans by sandflies, mostly to travelers in endemic areas
     b. Small endemic focus in Texas
  5. *Francisella tularensis*
     a. Most often in Midwestern states
     b. Associated with contact with infected mammals (e.g., rabbits) or tick bites

DIAGNOSIS

DIFFERENTIAL DIAGNOSIS

- Nodular lymphangitis
- Insect or snake bites
- Filariasis

WORKUP

- Acute lymphangitis: blood cultures
- Nodular lymphangitis: various stains and cultures of drainage or biopsy specimens of inoculation sites to make definitive diagnosis

LABORATORY TESTS

- WBCs possibly elevated with cellulitis
- Eosinophilia common with helminthic infections

TREATMENT

NONPHARMACOLOGIC THERAPY

Limb elevation

ACUTE GENERAL Rx

- Penicillin possibly sufficient, but 1 wk of dicloxacillin or cephalexin 500 mg PO qid commonly used to ensure antistaphylococcal coverage; if community-acquired MRSA (CA-MRSA) suspected, then oral Bactrin DS: one PO bid is the best oral agent and with vancomycin 1 g IV every 12 hr being reserved for patients requiring intravenous therapy.
- If allergic to penicillin:
  1. Clindamycin 300 mg PO qid for 7 days *or*
  2. Erythromycin 500 mg PO qid for 7 days
- Nodular lymphangitis: specific therapy directed at etiologic agent.
- For superficial fungal infections: treatment may prevent recurrence of acute lymphangitis.

DISPOSITION

- Acute lymphangitis: usually resolves with therapy
- Recurrent attacks: may lead to chronic lymphedema of limb, rarely resulting in elephantiasis nostras (nonfilarial elephantiasis)
- Nodular lymphangitis: usually responds to appropriate therapy

REFERRAL

- If acute lymphangitis is more than a mild disease or involves the face
- If nodular lymphangitis or filariasis is suspected

PEARLS & CONSIDERATIONS

COMMENTS

- Outside of the U.S., initial episodes of filariasis caused by *Brugia malayi* resemble acute lymphangitis.
- Chronic lymphedema or elephantiasis results from recurrent episodes.

SUGGESTED READINGS

Eijnden SV et al: Gloves and socks lymphangitis associated with acute parvovirus B19 infection, *Pediatr Dermatol* 20(2):184, 2003.

Kano Y, Inaoka M, Shiohara T: Superficial lymphangitis with interface dermatitis occurring shortly after a minor injury: possible involvement of a bacterial infection and contact allergens, *Dermatology* 203(3):217, 2001.

King MD et al: Emergence of community-acquired methicillin-resistant *Staphylococcus aureus* USA 300 clone as the predominant cause of skin and soft-tissue infections, *Ann Intern Med* 144(5):309, 2006.

Koehler JE, Duncan LM: A 56-year-old man with fever and axillary lymphadenopathy, *N Engl J Med* 355:1387, 2005.

AUTHORS: **GLENN G. FORT, M.D., M.P.H., DENNIS J. MIKOLICH, M.D.,** and **MAURICE POLICAR, M.D.**

BASIC INFORMATION

DEFINITION

Lymphedema refers to excessive accumulation of interstitial protein-rich fluid typically resulting from impaired regional lymphatic drainage.

SYNONYMS

Elephantiasis

ICD-9CM CODES
457.1 Lymphedema: acquired (chronic), praecox, secondary
457.1 Elephantiasis (nonfilarial)

EPIDEMIOLOGY & DEMOGRAPHICS

PRIMARY LYMPHEDEMA:

- Found in 1.1/100,000 people <20 yr old.
- Females outnumber males 3.5:1.
- Incidence peaks between ages 12 to 16 yr old.

SECONDARY LYMPHEDEMA: See specific etiology (e.g., filariasis, breast cancer, prostate cancer)

PHYSICAL FINDINGS & CLINICAL PRESENTATION

Edema:

- Painless and progressive
  1. Initially, the edema is pitting and smooth; however, with advanced cases, the edema becomes nonpitting (this depends on the extent of fibrosis that has occurred).
  2. Elevation of the leg resolves the swelling in the early stages but not in the advanced stages.
- More often unilateral but depending on the etiology can be bilateral
- Not always restricted to the lower extremities but may involve the genitals, face, or upper extremities (e.g., arm swelling after mastectomy)
- Stemmer's sign (squaring of the toes caused by edema in the digits)
- "Buffalo hump" appearance of the dorsum of the foot
- Loss of the ankle contour, giving a "tree trunk" appearance of the leg

Skin:

- Hard, thick, leathery skin secondary to fibrosis induced by chronic stasis
- Occasional drainage of lymph
- Infections (cellulitis, lymphangitis, onychomycosis)

ETIOLOGY

Lymphedema is caused by a reduction in lymphatic transport and is classified into primary and secondary forms.

Primary idiopathic lymphedema is thought to result from developmental abnormalities such as lymphatic hypoplasia and functional insufficiency or absence of lymphatic valves. Subclasses of this type of lymphedema include:

- Congenital lymphedema
  1. Detected at birth or recognized within first 2 yr of life
  2. Involving one or both extremities, usually the entire leg
  3. May be familial (Milroy's disease)
- Lymphedema praecox
  1. Onset in teenage years
  2. Usually unilateral; occurring in the teenage years
  3. Most common form of primary lymphedema (up to 94% of cases)
  4. More common in females (10:1), suggesting estrogen plays a role in pathogenesis
  5. May be familial (Meige's disease)
- Lymphedema tarda
  1. Usually occurs after the age of 30 yr
  2. Uncommon, accounting for less than 10% of cases of primary lymphedema

Secondary lymphedema develops after disruption or obstruction of the lymphatic system as a consequence of:

- Surgery for malignant tumors (e.g., breast, prostate, lymphoma)
- Edema of the arm after axillary lymph node dissection is the most common cause of lymphedema in the U.S.
- Incidence of lymphedema is ~14% in patients s/p mastectomy with adjuvant radiation treatment
- Inflammation (streptococci, filariasis)
- Filariasis is the most common cause of lymphedema in the world
- Trauma
- Radiation with lymph node removal

DIAGNOSIS

- Lymphedema is primarily a clinical diagnosis made on the basis of physical features that distinguish it from other causes of chronic edema of the extremities, such as the presence of cutaneous and subcutaneous fibrosis (peau d'orange) and the Stemmer sign.
- When physical examination is inconclusive, other available imaging tests can help make the diagnosis: isotopic lymphoscintigraphy, indirect and direct lymphography, lymphatic capillaroscopy, MRI, CT, or ultrasound.

DIFFERENTIAL DIAGNOSIS

Exclude other causes of edema (e.g., cirrhosis, nephrosis, CHF, myxedema, hypoalbuminemia, chronic venous stasis, reflex sympathetic dystrophy, obstruction from abdominal or pelvic malignancy).

WORKUP

A detailed history and physical examination should help exclude most of the differential diagnoses.

LABORATORY TESTS

- BUN, Cr, liver function tests, albumin, urine analysis, TFTs are obtained to exclude possible systemic causes of edema.
- Noninvasive venous studies help exclude venous insufficiency.
- Genetic testing may be practical in defining a specific hereditary syndrome with a discrete gene mutation such as lymphedema-distichiasis (FOXC2) and some forms of Milroy disease (VEGFR-3).

IMAGING STUDIES

- Lymphoscintigraphy:
  1. Diagnostic image of choice.
  2. Sensitivity and specificity of 100% in diagnosing lymphedema.
  3. It is currently considered the gold standard for diagnosis of lymphedema.
- CT scan: to exclude malignancy leading to obstruction
- Duplex ultrasound to rule out venous obstruction as a cause for edema
- Lymphangiography:
  1. Available but rarely used
  2. May be requested by surgeons considering repair or excision of tissue for lymphedema
  3. Difficult to perform; most information can be obtained from the nuclear lymphoscintigram

TREATMENT

NONPHARMACOLOGIC THERAPY

Complex decongestive therapy (CDT) is backed by longstanding experience as the primary treatment of choice for lymphedema in both children and adults. It involves a two-stage treatment program:

1. Reduce leg swelling and size:
   - Leg elevation
   - Limb massage
   - Pneumatic leg compression
2. Maintain edema-free state:
   - Elastic support stockings that are properly fitted according to compression pressure and length are essential to prevent edema from returning.
   - Compression pressures are graduated; most of the pressure is distal with less and less pressure from the stockings, moving proximally.
   - Compression pressures range from 20 to 30 mm Hg, 30 to 40 mm Hg, 40 to 50 mm Hg, and 50 to 60 mm Hg. Most prefer 40 to 50 mm Hg for lymphedema.
   - The length should cover the edematous site. Choices include below the knee, thigh-high, and pantyhose lengths.

ACUTE GENERAL Rx

- No drugs have been shown to be beneficial. Diuretics, in particular, should not be used because they may promote the development of volume depletion.
- Treat infections, such as lymphangitis (usually caused by group A streptococcus), with penicillin VK 250 mg qid for 10 days or erythromycin 250 mg qid in penicillin-allergic patients. If recurrent episodes of infection occur, many consider prophylaxis with penicillin VK 250 mg qid for 10 days at the beginning of each month. Clotrimazole 1% cream should be applied qd to dried fissured areas in between toes to prevent fungal infections.
- In secondary lymphedema, treating the underlying cause is indicated (e.g., prostate cancer, breast cancer). If the etiology is filariasis caused by the parasites *Wuchereria bancrofti* or *Brugia malayi,* treatment is diethylcarbamazine citrate (DEC) 5 mg/kg in divided doses for 3 wk.
- Mesotherapy (hyaluronidase), immunological therapy (autologous lymphocyte injection), and fluid restriction all have uncertain benefit in the treatment of lymphedema.
- In children with chylous reflux syndromes, a diet low in long-chain triglycerides and high in short and medium-chain triglycerides has been shown to be of benefit in treatment.

CHRONIC Rx

Surgery for chronic lymphedema should act as an adjunct to CDT or as an alternative if CDT has proven unsuccessful. Operative treatment is considered if:

- Continued increase in leg size despite medical treatment
- Impaired leg function
- Recurrent infections
- Emotional lability secondary to the cosmetic appearance

Surgical procedures are divided into two types:

- Those performed to improve lymph node drainage (e.g., anastomoses of the lymph system with the venous system)
- Those performed to excise the subcutaneous tissue (e.g., Charles' procedure, Thompson's procedure, and the modified Homans' procedure)
- Liposuction in combination with long-term decongestive therapy has been shown to be more effective in reducing edema than long-term decongestive therapy alone.

DISPOSITION

- Lymphedema is a slowly progressive disorder that can lead to significant disfigurement of the extremities or other body parts.
- The extent of fibrotic change to the skin of the affected limb increases with the chronicity of lymphatic stasis.
- In many patients, the maximum girth of the affected limb is reached within the first year after onset, unless complications like recurrent cellulitis supervene.
- Patients with lymphedema commonly manifest psychiatric comorbidities as a result of their disease, such as anxiety, depression, adjustment problems, and difficulty in vocational, domestic, or social domains.
- Chronic lymphedema can be complicated by cellulitis or, in rare cases, development of lymphagiosarcomata or other cutaneous malignancies.

REFERRAL

- If the diagnosis of lymphedema is unclear or in need of better definition for prognostic considerations, consultation with a clinical lymphologist or referral to a lymphohologic center if accessible is recommended.
- Consultation with vascular surgeons should be made if medical therapy for leg size reduction fails or if recurrent infections occur.

PEARLS & CONSIDERATIONS

- Lymphedema is a chronic, generally incurable ailment, and requires lifelong care and attention along with psychosocial support.
- It is important to remember that surgery is not a cure.
- Children and adolescents (along with parents and adults) should be encouraged to pursue a normal life, participating in school activities and sports (preferably noncontact, e.g., swimming).
- It should also be remembered that cases of lymphangiosarcomas have been associated, although rarely, with postmastectomy lymphedema.

COMMENTS

In the U.S., the leading cause of lymphedema of both upper and lower extremities is neoplastic disease and its related therapies. In a previously treated cancer patient with new or worsening edema, cancer recurrence leading to intrinsic or extrinsic lymphatic obstruction must be considered.

SUGGESTED READINGS

Caban ME: Trends in the evaluation of lymphedema, *Lymphology* 35(1):28, 2002.

International Society of Lymphology: The diagnosis and treatment of peripheral lymphedema: Consensus document of the International Society of Lymphology, *Lymphology* 36(2):84, 2003.

O'Brien JG, Chennubhotla SA, Chennubhotla RV: Treatment of edema, *Am Fam Physician* 71(11):2111, 2005.

Petrova TV et al: Defective valves and abnormal mural cell recruitment underlie lymphatic vascular failure in lymphedema distichiasis, *Nat Med* 10:974, 2004.

Rockson SG: Lymphedema, *Am J Med* 110:288, 2001.

AUTHOR: **TANYA ALI, M.D.**

BASIC INFORMATION

DEFINITION

Lymphogranuloma venereum (LGV) is a sexually transmitted, systemic disease caused by *Chlamydia trachomatis*.

SYNONYMS

Tropical bubo
Poradenitis inguinalis
LGV

ICD-9CM CODES
099.1 Lymphogranuloma venereum

EPIDEMIOLOGY & DEMOGRAPHICS

INCIDENCE (IN U.S.): Rare; 285 cases reported in 1993
PREVALENCE: Endemic in Africa, India, parts of Southeast Asia, South America, and the Caribbean
PREDOMINANT SEX: Male:female ratio is 5:1

PHYSICAL FINDINGS & CLINICAL PRESENTATION

Primary stage:
- Primary lesion caused by multiplication of organism at site of infection
- Papule, shallow ulcer
- Herpetiform lesion at site of inoculation (most common)
- Incubation period of 3 to 21 days
- Most common site of lesion in women: posterior wall, fourchette, or vulva
- Spontaneous healing, without scarring

Second stage:
- Inguinal syndrome: characteristic inguinal adenopathy
- Begins 1 to 4 wk after primary lesion
- Syndrome is the most frequent clinical sign of the disease
- Unilateral inguinal adenopathy in 70% of cases
- Symptoms: painful, extensive adenitis (bubo) and suppuration may occur with numerous sinus tracts
- "Groove sign" signaling femoral and inguinal node involvement (20%); most often seen in men
- Involvement of deep iliac and retroperitoneal lymph nodes in women may present as a pelvic mass

Third stage (anogenital syndrome):
- Subacute: proctocolitis
- Late: tissue destruction or scarring, sinuses, abscesses, fistulas, strictures of perineum, elephantiasis

ETIOLOGY

Chlamydia trachomatis is the causative agent. There are three serotypes: L1, L2, and L3.

DIAGNOSIS

DIFFERENTIAL DIAGNOSIS

- Inguinal adenitis, suppurative adenitis, retroperitoneal adenitis, proctitis, schistosomiasis
- Section II describes the differential diagnosis of genital sores.

WORKUP

- Clinical manifestation
- Screening for other STDs
- A clinical algorithm for evaluation of genital ulcer disease is described in Section III, "Genital Lesions."

LABORATORY TESTS

- Positive Frei test:
  1. Intradermal chlamydial antigen
  2. Nonspecific for all *Chlamydia*
  3. No longer available (historical significance only)
- Complement fixation test:
  1. Titer >1:64 in active infection
  2. Convalescent titers no difference
- Cell culture of *Chlamydia*—aspiration of fluctuant node yields highest rates of recovery
- CBC—mild leukocytosis with lymphocytosis or monocytosis
- Elevated sedimentation rate
- VDRL and HIV screening to rule out other STDs

IMAGING STUDIES

- Barium enema: may reveal elongated structure of LGV
- CT scan for retroperitoneal adenitis

TREATMENT

NONPHARMACOLOGIC THERAPY

- Avoid milk and milk products while taking medication.
- Practice sexual abstinence.
- Treat sexual partners.

ACUTE GENERAL Rx

- Doxycycline 100 mg PO bid × 21 days
- Erythromycin base 500 mg PO qid × 21 days
- Sulfisoxazole 500 mg PO qid × 21 days
- Surgical:
  1. Aspirate fluctuant nodes
  2. Incise and drain abscesses

CHRONIC Rx

- Longer course of therapy will be needed for chronic or relapsing cases, which may be caused by reinfection and/or inadequate treatment.
- A rectal stricture will require a colostomy.
- Surgery should be considered only after antibiotic treatment.

DISPOSITION

Good prognosis with early treatment, usually resulting in complete resolution of symptoms.

REFERRAL

Surgical consultation if patient develops obstruction, fistula, or rectal stricture. May need referral to plastic surgeon if patient has lymphatic obstruction.

PEARLS & CONSIDERATIONS

COMMENTS

- Pregnant and lactating women should be treated with erythromycin regimen.
- Congenital transmission does not occur, but infection may be acquired through an infected birth canal.
- Patient education materials may be obtained through local and state health clinics.

SUGGESTED READING

Centers for Disease Control and Prevention: 2006 sexually transmitted diseases treatment guidelines, *MMWR Morb Mortal Wkly Rep* 55(RR-11), 2006.

AUTHORS: **GEORGE T. DANAKAS, M.D.,** and **RUBEN ALVERO, M.D.**

BASIC INFORMATION

DEFINITION

Non-Hodgkin lymphoma is a heterogeneous group of malignancies of the lymphoreticular system.

SYNONYMS

NHL

ICD-9CM CODES
201.9 Lymphoma, non-Hodgkin

EPIDEMIOLOGY & DEMOGRAPHICS

INCIDENCE (IN U.S.): Sixth most common neoplasm (56,000 new cases/yr). Increasing incidence with age. In patients with HIV, non-Hodgkin lymphoma is the second most common tumor (after Kaposi sarcoma).

PREDOMINANT AGE: Median age at time of diagnosis is 50 yr

PHYSICAL FINDINGS & CLINICAL PRESENTATION

- Patients often present with asymptomatic lymphadenopathy.
- Approximately one third of NHL originates extranodally. Involvement of extranodal sites can result in unusual presentations (e.g., GI tract involvement can simulate PUD).
- NHL cases associated with HIV occur predominantly in the brain.
- Pruritus, fever, night sweats, weight loss are less common than in Hodgkin's disease.
- Hepatomegaly and splenomegaly may be present.

DIAGNOSIS

DIFFERENTIAL DIAGNOSIS

- Hodgkin's disease
- Viral infections
- Metastatic carcinoma
- A clinical algorithm for evaluation of lymphadenopathy is described in Section III
- The differential diagnosis of lymphadenopathy is described in Section II

WORKUP

Initial laboratory evaluation may reveal only mild anemia and elevated LDH and ESR. Proper staging of non-Hodgkin's lymphoma requires the following:

- A thorough history, physical examination, and adequate biopsy. Laparoscopic lymph node biopsy can be used on an outpatient basis for most patients with intra-abdominal lymphoma
- Routine laboratory evaluation (CBC, ESR, urinalysis, LDH, BUN, creatinine, serum calcium, uric acid, LFTs, serum protein electrophoresis)
- Chest x-ray examination (PA and lateral)
- Bone marrow evaluation (aspirate and full bone core biopsy)
- CT scan of abdomen and pelvis; CT scan of chest if chest x-ray films abnormal
- Bone scan (particularly in patients with histiocytic lymphoma)
- Depending on the histopathology, the results of the above studies and the planned therapy, some other tests may be performed (e.g., PET scan)
- β-2 Microglobulin levels should be obtained initially (prognostic value) and serially in patients with low-grade lymphomas (useful to monitor therapeutic response of the tumor)
- Serum interleukin levels have prognostic value in diffuse large cell lymphoma

CLASSIFICATION: The working formulation of non-Hodgkin lymphoma for clinical usage subdivides lymphomas into low grade, intermediate grade, high grade, and miscellaneous (Table 1-24).

STAGING: The Ann Arbor classification is used to stage non-Hodgkin lymphomas (see "Hodgkin's Disease" in Section I). Histopathology has greater therapeutic implications in NHL than in Hodgkin's disease.

TREATMENT

ACUTE GENERAL Rx

The therapeutic regimen varies with the histologic type and pathologic stage. Following are the commonly used therapeutic modalities:

LOW-GRADE NHL (E.G., NODULAR, POORLY DIFFERENTIATED):

1. Local radiotherapy for symptomatic obstructive adenopathy
2. Deferment of therapy and careful observation in asymptomatic patients
3. Single-agent chemotherapy with cyclophosphamide or chlorambucil and glucocorticoids
4. Combination chemotherapy alone or with radiotherapy: generally indicated only when the lymphoma becomes more invasive, with poor response to less aggressive treatment
5. Monoclonal antibodies directed against B-cell surface antigens can also be used to treat follicular lymphomas that are resistant to conventional therapy. The anti-CD20 monoclonal antibody rituximab is effective against low-grade NHL in patients who have not received previous treatment
6. The addition of rituximab to CHOP is generally well tolerated; however, additional studies may be necessary to clarify the role of CHOP plus rituximab in patients with indolent NHL
7. Ibritumomab tiuxetan (Zevalin), an immunoconjugate that combines the linker-chelator tiuxetan with the monoclonal antibody ibritumomab, can be used as part of a two-step regimen for treatment of patients with relapsed or refractory low-grade, follicular, or transformed B-cell NHL refractory to rituximab
8. New purine analogs (FLAMP, 2CDA) can be used in salvage treatment of refractory lymphomas. They all have activity in follicular lymphomas

INTERMEDIATE- AND HIGH-GRADE LYMPHOMAS (E.G., DIFFUSE HISTIOCYTIC LYMPHOMA):

Combination chemotherapy regimens (e.g., CHOP, PRO-MACE-CYTABOM, MACOP-B, M-BACOD). An anthracycline-containing regimen (such as CHOP) given in standard doses and schedule is generally best for treatment of older patients with advanced stage, aggressive-histology lymphoma who do not have significant comorbid illness.

1. High-dose sequential therapy is superior to standard-dose MACOP-B for patients with diffuse large-cell lymphoma of the B-cell type.
2. Dose-modified chemotherapy should be considered for most HIV-infected patients with lymphoma.
   - Three cycles of CHOP followed by involved-field radiotherapy may be superior to eight cycles of CHOP alone in patients with localized intermediate- and high-grade NHL.
   - High-dose chemotherapy with autologous stem-cell support has been reported to be superior to CHOP in adults with disseminated aggressive lymphoma.
   - The addition of rituximab against CD20 B-cell lymphoma to the CHOP regimen increases the complete response rate and prolongs event-free and overall survival in elderly patients with diffuse large B-cell lymphoma without a clinically significant increase in toxicity. Bexxar, a combination of the mononuclear antibody tositumomab and radiolabeled iodine-131 tositumomab can be used for a single treatment of relapsed follicular NHL in patients who are refractory to rituximab.
   - In patients under 61 yr of age, chemotherapy with 3 cycles of ACVBP (doxorubicin, cyclophosphamide, vindesine, bleomycin, and prednisone) followed by sequential consolidation has been reported to be superior to 3 cycles of CHOP plus radiotherapy for treatment of newly diagnosed aggressive lymphoma (diffuse mixed, diffuse large cell, or immunoblastic according to the working formulation).

- Granulocyte-colony stimulating factor (G-CSF): may be effective in reducing the risk of infection in patients with aggressive lymphoma undergoing chemotherapy.
- Radioimmunotherapy with (^{131}I) anti-B1 antibody therapy for NHL either by itself or in combination with other treatments represents a new modality in the armamentarium against lymphomas.
- Treatment with high-dose chemotherapy and autologous bone marrow transplant: as compared with conventional chemotherapy, increases event-free and overall survival in patients with chemotherapy-sensitive non-Hodgkin lymphoma in relapse.

DISPOSITION

- Patients with low-grade lymphoma, despite their long-term survival (6 to 10 yr average), are rarely cured, and the great majority (if not all) eventually die of the lymphoma, whereas patients with a high-grade lymphoma may achieve a cure with aggressive chemotherapy.
- Complete remission occurs in 35% to 50% of patients with intermediate- and high-grade lymphoma. Prognostic factors include the histiologic subtype, age of patient, and bulk of disease.
- Patients who present with AIDS-related non-Hodgkin lymphoma and a low CD4 cell count have a poor prognosis (median duration of survival is 15 to 34 mo).

SUGGESTED READINGS

Kaminski MS et al: ^{131}I-tositumomab therapy as initial treatment for follicular lymphoma, *N Engl J Med* 352:441, 2005.

Milpied N et al: Initial treatment of aggressive lymphoma with high-dose chemotherapy and autologous stem cell support, *N Engl J Med* 350:1287, 2004.

Reyes F et al: ACVBP versus CHOP plus radiotherapy for localized aggressive lymphoma, *N Engl J Med* 352:1197, 2005.

AUTHOR: **FRED F. FERRI, M.D.**

TABLE 1-24 Classification Systems for Grading Lymphomas

Kiel Classification	Working Formulation	Revised European-American Classification
Low-grade malignancy	Low grade	B-cell lymphomas
Lymphocytic, CLL	A. Malignant lymphoma, small lymphocytic	
Lymphocytic, other	Consistent with chronic lymphocytic leukemia	B-CLL/SLL
Lymphoplasmacytoid		Lymphoplasmacytoid lymphoma
Centrocytic	B. Malignant lymphoma, follicular, predominantly small cleaved cell	Follicle center lymphomas
Centroblastic/Centrocytic		Marginal zone lymphomas (MALT)
Follicular without sclerosis	Diffuse areas	Mantle cell lymphoma
Follicular with sclerosis	Sclerosis	
Follicular and diffuse, without sclerosis	C. Malignant lymphoma, follicular mixed, small cleaved and large cell	
Follicular and diffuse, with sclerosis	Diffuse areas	Diffuse large B-cell lymphoma
Diffuse	Sclerosis	Primary mediastinal large B-cell lymphoma
Low-grade malignant lymphoma, unclassified	Intermediate grade	Burkitt's lymphoma
High-grade malignancy	D. Malignant lymphoma, follicular	T-cell lymphomas
Centroblastic	Diffuse areas	
Lymphoblastic, Burkitt's type	E. Malignant lymphoma, diffuse small cleaved cell	
Lymphoblastic, convoluted cell type		T-CLL
Lymphoblastic, other (unclassified) immunoblastic		Mycosis fungoides/Sézary syndrome
High-grade malignant lymphoma, unclassified	F. Malignant lymphoma, diffuse mixed, small and large cell sclerosis	
Malignant lymphoma unclassified (unable to specify high grade or low grade)	G. Malignant lymphoma diffuse	Peripheral T-cell lymphoma, unspecified
Composite lymphoma	Large cell	Angioimmunoblastic T-cell lymphoma
	Cleaved cell	Angiocentric lymphoma
	Noncleaved cell	Intestinal T-cell lymphoma
	Sclerosis	Adult T-cell lymphoma/leukemia
	High grade	Anaplastic large cell lymphoma
	H. Malignant lymphoma large cell, immunoblastic	Precursor T-lymphoid lymphoma/leukemia
	Plasmacytoid	
	Clear cell	
	Polymorphous	
	Epithelioid cell component	
	I. Malignant lymphoma lymphoblastic	
	Convoluted cell	
	Nonconvoluted cell	
	J. Malignant lymphoma small noncleaved cell	
	Burkitt's	
	Follicular areas	

From Abeloff MD: *Clinical oncology,* ed 3, New York, 2004, Churchill Livingstone.
B-CLL, B-cell chronic lymphoid leukemia; *CLL,* chronic lymphocytic leukemia; *MALT,* mucosa-associated lymphoid tumor; *SLL,* lymphoid leukemia; *T-CLL,* T-cell CLL.

BASIC INFORMATION

DEFINITION

Lynch syndrome is a hereditary predisposition to malignancy of the colon that is explained by a germline mutation in a DNA mismatch repair gene.

SYNONYMS

Hereditary nonpolyposis colorectal cancer
Hereditary site-specific colon cancer

ICD-9-CM codes
1539 Lynch syndrome

EPIDEMIOLOGY & DEMOGRAPHICS

The lifetime risk for developing colon cancer in the U.S. is approximately 6%. Of these cases, 2% to 3% may be attributable to Lynch syndrome. The incidence of Lynch syndrome is estimated to be between 1:660 and 1:2000. The average age of diagnosis for Lynch syndrome is 48, although diagnosis can occur as early as the 20s or as late as the 70s.

RISK FACTORS: Family history of colon cancer or other hereditary nonpolyposis colorectal cancer (HNPCC)–related cancers such as endometrial (up to 43% of women with Lynch syndrome may develop endometrial cancer), biliary tract, ovarian, stomach, or pancreas

GENETICS: Autosomal dominant inheritance pattern

ETIOLOGY

Lynch syndrome is thought to be secondary to germline mutations in DNA mismatch repair genes. The predominant genes involved are *MSH2* and *MLH1,* which are tumor suppressor genes although other genes have documented involvement *(PMS1, PMS2, MSH6, MLH3).* Mutations in these genes prevent repair of DNA mismatches during DNA replication. This is most prevalent in regions of DNA called microsatellites causing DNA microsatellite instability and leading to an increased risk for malignancy, especially colon cancer.

PHYSICAL FINDINGS & CLINICAL PRESENTATION

- Changes in bowel habits (prolonged constipation)
- Melena
- Hematochezia
- Abdominal pain
- Unexplained weight loss
- Decreased appetite

DIAGNOSIS

DIFFERENTIAL DIAGNOSIS

- Familial adenomatosis polyposis
- Peutz-Jeghers syndrome
- Juvenile polyposis
- Nonhereditary colorectal cancer
- Gardner syndrome

WORKUP

If an individual presents with numerous adenomatous polyps or has multiple relatives with cancer at a young age, a family history complete with pedigree must be obtained. Clinical diagnosis of the Lynch syndrome can be made with the Amsterdam criteria or if these are not met, the Bethesda criteria, which are more sensitive (see following list).

- Amsterdam criteria (must meet all criteria):
  1. Colorectal carcinoma and/or endometrial carcinoma or transitional cell carcinoma of the ureter or carcinoma of the small bowel in at least three individuals in the family
  2. One of the patients is a first-degree family member of two other patients
  3. Involved patients occur in at least two successive generations
  4. At least one of the diagnoses was made before age 50
  5. The diagnoses are histologically confirmed
  6. Familial adenomatous polyposis is excluded
- Bethesda criteria (must meet all criteria):
  1. Colorectal cancer below age 50
  2. Multiple colorectal cancers or other HNPCC-related cancers such as biliary tract, endometrial, stomach, or ovary
  3. Colorectal cancer with microsatellite instability histology <60 years of age
  4. Colorectal cancer or HNPCC-related cancer in first-degree relative <50 years of age
  5. Colorectal cancer or HNPCC-related cancer in at least two first- or second-degree relatives, any age
- If criteria for the Lynch syndrome are not met, no further analysis is necessary (although a genetic syndrome cannot be definitively excluded and genetic referral may be warranted).

LABORATORY TESTS

- If a patient meets criteria for Lynch syndrome, immunohistochemistry can be performed for presence or absence of mismatch repair genes *MLH1, MSH2, MSH6* and *PMS2.*
- Microsatellite instability analysis should also be performed if criteria for Lynch syndrome are met.

TREATMENT

- If mutation has been identified in a family member, screening for this mutation can be performed via genetic testing. Informed consent after a thorough explanation has been provided to each individual must be obtained.
- Surveillance using colonoscopy can be performed in individuals who screen positive while those who screen negative can be discharged. The mismatch repair gene that is mutated guides screening.
- According to the Netherlands Surveillance Protocol, for example, individuals with mutations in *MLH1, MSH2* or *MSH6* should have colonoscopies every 1 to 2 yr starting at age 20 to 25; urine cytology every 1 to 2 yr starting at age 30 to 35; gastro copy every 1 to 2 yr starting at age 30 to 35; and, in females, ultrasound of endometrium and CA-125 every 1 to 2 yr starting at age 30 to 35.

REFERRALS

- To gastroenterology for surveillance colonoscopies
- To genetic counselor if patient satisfies Bethesda criteria
- To psychologist as necessary for psychologic support

PEARLS & CONSIDERATIONS

Prior to genetic testing being instituted, informed consent must be obtained because consequences of this testing include the necessity of lifelong screenings such as colonoscopies. Exclusion from life insurance must also be considered.

PATIENT/FAMILY EDUCATION

- For information on local genetic counselors, visit the National Society of Genetic Counselors' website at www.nsgc.org.
- For information on Lynch syndrome, visit www.mayoclinic.com/health/lynch-syndrome/DS00669.

SUGGESTED READINGS

Hampel H et al: Screening for the Lynch syndrome (hereditary non-polyposis colorectal cancer), *New Engl J Med,* 352:1851, 2005.

Hendriks YM et al: Management of Lynch syndrome (hereditary nonpolyposis colorectal carcinoma): guide for clinicians, *CA Cancer J Clin* 56:213, 2006.

Jass JR: Hereditary non-polyposis colorectal cancer: the rise and fall of a confusing term, *World J Gastroenterol* 12(31):4943, 2006.

AUTHORS: **PAUL GEORGE, M.D.,** and **JOANNE SILVIA, M.D.**

BASIC INFORMATION

DEFINITION

Macular degeneration refers to a group of diseases associated with loss of central vision and damage to the macula. Degenerative changes occur in the pigment, neural, and vascular layers of the macula. The dry macular degeneration is usually ischemic in etiology, and a wet macular degeneration is associated with leakage of fluid from blood vessels, usually referred to as age-related macular degeneration (ARMD).

ICD-9CM CODES
362.5 Degeneration of macula and posterior pole

EPIDEMIOLOGY & DEMOGRAPHICS

INCIDENCE (IN U.S.):
- Main cause of blindness in the U.S.
- Increases with age
- 1.75 million individuals in the U.S. currently affected; 3 million by year 2020

PEAK INCIDENCE:
- 75 to 80 yr old.
- Dramatic increases in incidence and prevalence with age until approximately 80% of people 75 yr or older have senile macular degeneration.

PREVALENCE (IN U.S.): Varies, but approximately 5% of people <50 yr old have some signs of macular degeneration.

PREDOMINANT SEX: Male = female (15% of white women >80 have severe ARMD)

PREDOMINANT AGE: >50 yr

GENETICS:
- Different syndrome: senile macular degeneration is age related.
- Several rare neurologic syndromes are associated with macular degeneration.

PHYSICAL FINDINGS & CLINICAL PRESENTATION

- Decreased central vision
- Macular hemorrhage, pigmentation, edema, atrophy
- The most common abnormality seen in age-related macular degeneration (AMD) is the presence of drusen, or yellowish deposits deep to the retina; this may be early in course of disease
- Choroidal neovascular membrane (CNVM) develops with rapid change in vision

ETIOLOGY

- Subretinal neovascular membrane early
- Pigmentary and vascular changes with exudate, edema, and scar tissue development
- Dry type atrophy of macular pigment epithelium

DIAGNOSIS

DIFFERENTIAL DIAGNOSIS

- Diabetic retinopathy (with neovascularization, can mimic CNVM)
- Hypertension
- Histoplasmosis (less common cause of CNVM)
- Trauma with scar

WORKUP

- Complete eye examination, including visual field and fluorescein angiography
- Optical coherence tomography (OCT)

LABORATORY TESTS

Evaluate for diabetes and other metabolic problems, as well as vascular diseases.

IMAGING STUDIES

- Optical coherence tomography (OCT)
- Fluorescein angiography

TREATMENT

NONPHARMACOLOGIC THERAPY

- Laser treatment to stop progression of disease—photodynamic treatment with verteporfin IV
- Laser (Argon)—for certain classic membranes (CNVM)
- A high dietary intake of antioxidants, vitamins C and E, and zinc has been reported to substantially reduce the risk of age-related macular degeneration in elderly persons

ACUTE GENERAL Rx

- Intravitral steroids, photodynamic treatment (PDT) with laser.
- Intravitreal administration of ranibizumab, a monoclonal antibody Fab that neutralizes all active forms of vascular endothelial growth factor A, is effective in preventing vision loss and improving mean visual acuity in patients with age-related macular degeneration. It has also been reported to be superior to photodynamic therapy with verteporfin in the treatment of predominantly classic neovascular age-related macular degeneration.
- Intravitreous injections of pegaptanib (Macugen), an antivascular endothelial growth factor, have been reported as effective therapy in slowing vision loss in neovascular age-related macular degeneration. Pegaptanib is administered once every 6 wk by intravitreous injection into one eye. Cost of each injection generally exceeds $1,000.

CHRONIC Rx

- Repeated laser treatments
- Antioxidants and zinc may slow down progression of ARMD

DISPOSITION

- Follow closely by ophthalmologist, retinal specialist.
- If vision deteriorates, refer urgently to an ophthalmologist.
- Avastin similar to Ranibizumab but not yet FDA approved for vitrial injection.

REFERRAL

- To ophthalmologist early in the course of the disease if the sight is to be saved
- Immediate referral if any change in vision

PEARLS & CONSIDERATIONS

COMMENTS

- Sildenafil has no significant effect on macular degeneration.
- The vision of only 1 out of 10 people can be saved, but the disease is so devastating that vigorous therapy should be attempted.
- Statins plus aspirin may slow down progression.
- Vitamins with zinc and antioxidants may slow down progression of ARMD.

EVIDENCE

A systematic review of two randomized controlled trials (RCTs) has found that photodynamic therapy is effective for the prevention of vision loss in patients with classic and occult choroidal neovascularization due to age-related macular degeneration (ARMD). It also found that photodynamic treatment with verteporfin significantly reduces the risk of moderate and severe visual loss compared with placebo at 24 months.[1] **A**

Laser photocoagulation has been compared with no treatment in four large RCTs. Laser photocoagulation significantly reduces the rate of severe vision loss, and contrast sensitivity is preserved in selected patients with exudative ARMD (those with well-demarcated lesions). Choroidal neovascularization recurs in 50% of patients within 2 years. Photocoagulation may initially reduce visual acuity. **A**

There is no evidence that antioxidant vitamins and minerals prevent or delay the onset of macular degeneration in people without the disease.[2] **A**

Evidence-Based References

1. Wormald R et al: Photodynamic therapy for neovascular age-related macular degeneration. Reviewed in: Cochrane Library, 3, Chichester, UK, 2004, John Wiley. **A**
2. Evans JR, Henshaw K: Antioxidant vitamin and mineral supplementation for preventing age-related macular degeneration. Reviewed in: Cochrane Library, 3, Chichester, UK, 2004, John Wiley. **A**

SUGGESTED READINGS

Brown DM et al: Ranibizumab versus verteporfin for neovascular age-related macular degeneration, *N Eng J Med* 355:1432, 2006.

De Jong P: Age-related macular degeneration, *N Engl J Med* 355:1474, 2006.

Rosenfeld P et al: Ranibizumab for neovascular age-related macular degeneration, *N Engl J Med* 355:1419, 2006.

Van Leeuwen R et al: Dietary intake of antioxidants and risk of age-related macular degeneration, *JAMA* 294:3101, 2005.

AUTHOR: **MELVYN KOBY, M.D.**

BASIC INFORMATION

DEFINITION

Malaria is a protozoan disease caused by the genus *Plasmodium* and transmitted by female *Anopheles spp.* mosquitoes. It is characterized by hectic fever and often presents with classic malarial paroxysm. Four species of genus plasmodium usually infect humans

- *P. falciparum*
- *P. vivax*
- *P. malariae*
- *P. ovale*

SYNONYMS

Periodic fever
Tertian malaria
Quartan malaria
Tropical splenomegaly

ICD-9CM CODES
084.6 Malaria

EPIDEMIOLOGY & DEMOGRAPHICS

Global:

- 300 to 500 million cases/yr
- 1 to 3 million deaths/yr
- 41% of the world's population lives in endemic area

U.S.:

- Between 1500 to 1800 cases reported by CDC in the last 5 yr
- 567 cases diagnosed as *P. falciparum*
- Most infections limited to
  1. Immigrant population
  2. Returned travelers or troops from endemic area
- Occasionally, transmission through exposure to infected blood product or shared intravenous needles by users of injection drugs
- Congenital transmission is possible
- Local mosquito borne transmission has been reported
- Competent mosquito vectors are present
  1. *A. albimanus* in eastern U.S.
  2. *A. freeborni* in western U.S.

Geographic distribution:

- *P. falciparum:* Sub-Saharan Africa, Papua New Guinea, Solomon Islands, Haiti, Indian subcontinent
- *P. vivax:* Central America, South America, North Africa, Middle East, Indian subcontinent
- *P. ovale:* West Africa
- *P. malariae:* worldwide

Parasite life cycle (Fig. 1-150):

- Human infection begins when a female anopheline mosquito bites (only female anopheline mosquito takes blood meal) and inoculates plasmodial sporozoites into bloodstream
- The sporozoites then travel to liver and invade to hepatocytes
- In the hepatocytes, the sporozoites mature to tissue schizont or become dormant hypnozoites
- The tissue schizont amplify the infection by producing large number of merozoites (10,000 to 30,000)
- Each merozoite is capable of invading an RBC and can establish the asexual cycle of replication in RBC
- Asexual cycles produce and release 24 to 32 merozoites at the end of 48- or 72-hr *(P. malariae)* cycle
- The hypnozoites are only found in relapsing malaria *P. vivax* or *P. ovale* and may remain dormant for up to 3 to 5 yr
- Eventually some intraerythrocytic parasites develop into gametocytes. Male and female gametocytes are taken up by a female anopheline mosquito with a blood meal where they fertilize in the mosquito gut to produce a diploid zygote that matures to an ookinete; haploid sporozoites are generated that migrate to the salivary gland of the mosquito to infect another human

PHYSICAL FINDINGS & CLINICAL PRESENTATION

- Fever is the hallmark of malaria, known as malarial paroxysm, initially daily until synchronization of infection after several weeks, when fever may occur every other day (tertian) in *P. vivax, P. ovale,* or *P. falciparum* malaria or every third day (quartan) in *P. malariae* malaria.
- Classic malarial paroxysm characterized by
  1. Cold stage: abrupt onset of cold feeling associated with rigors, shakes
  2. Hot stage: high fever (~40° C) associated with restlessness
  3. Sweating stage: patient defervesces
- Nonspecific symptoms are
  1. Headache
  2. Cough
  3. Myalgia
  4. Vomiting
  5. Diarrhea
  6. Jaundice

P. falciparum:

- Most pathogenic of the four species
- Rapidly progresses to high-level parasitemia
- Important cause of the fatal malaria
- Classic malarial paroxysm usually absent
- Incubation period after exposure is 12 days (range: 9 to 60 days)
- Cytoadherence and resetting of RBC play central role in pathogenesis
- The sequestration of RBC in vital organs leads to fatal complications

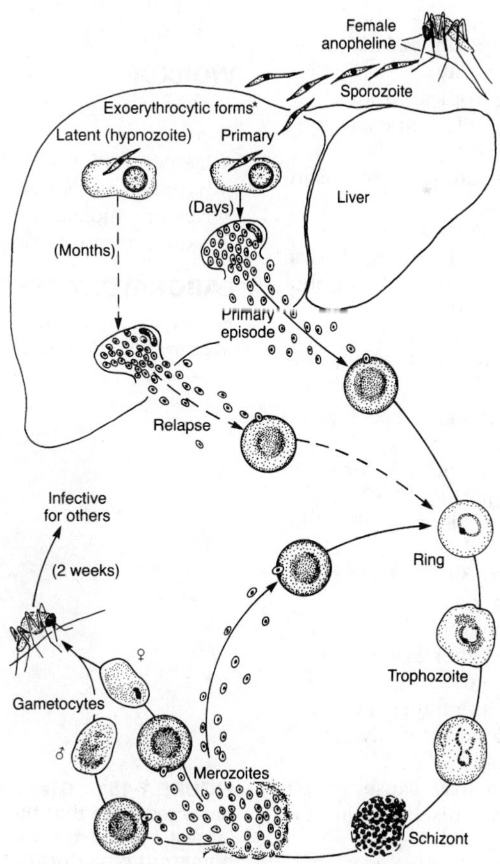

FIGURE 1-150 Life cycle of plasmodia in humans. *Exoerythrocytic forms are also called tissue schizonts. (From Gorbach SL: *Infectious diseases,* ed 2, Philadelphia, 1998, WB Saunders.)

- Cerebral malaria is a feared complication
- Invades erythrocytes of all ages
- Lacks hypnozoites (intrahepatic stage), does not relapse
- Blood smear usually shows ring form only
- Pigment color is black
- Banana-shaped gametocytes; if seen in blood, smear is diagnostic
- Chloroquine resistance widely present

P. vivax:
- Known as tertian malaria: fever occurs every other day
- Duffy blood-group antigen FYA- or FYB-related receptor needed for attachment to RBC
- FyFy phenotype (most West African) individuals are resistant to *P. vivax* malaria
- Incubation period after exposure is 14 days (range: 8 to 27 days)
- Hypnozoites may cause relapse of infection after years
- Infects mainly reticulocytes
- Irregularly shaped large rings and trophozoites, enlarged RBC, and Schüffner's dot are seen in peripheral blood smear (Fig. 1-151)
- Pigment color is yellow-brown
- *P. vivax* from Papua New Guinea have reduced sensitivity to chloroquine
- Primaquine needed to eradicate the hypnozoites

P. ovale:
- Also known as tertian malaria; fever occurs every other day
- Occurs mainly in tropical Africa
- Incubation period after exposure is 14 days (range: 8 to 27 days)
- Hypnozoites may cause relapse of infection
- Infects mainly reticulocytes
- Infected RBC seen as enlarged, oval shape containing large ring or trophozoites with Schüffner's dot
- Pigment color is dark brown
- Primaquine needed to eradicate the hypnozoites
- No chloroquine resistance encountered

P. malariae:
- Known as quartan malaria; fever occurs every third day
- Common cause of chronic malarial infection
- May persist 20 to 30 yr after leaving the endemic area
- Worldwide distribution
- Incubation period after exposure is 30 days (range: 16 to 60 days)
- Lacks hypnozoites (intrahepatic stage)
- May persist in blood for many years if treated inadequately
- Chronic infection may cause soluble immune-complex, resulting in nephritic syndrome
- Infects mainly mature RBC
- Band or rectangular forms of trophozoites are commonly seen in peripheral blood smear
- Pigment color is brown-black

Cerebral malaria:
- Feared complication of *P. falciparum* infection
- Mortality ~20%
- Pathogenesis is poorly understood
- Ischemia as a result of sequestration of parasites or cytokines induced by parasite toxin(s) is the key debate
- Seizure and altered mental status leading to coma are cardinal manifestation
- Hypoglycemia, lactic acidosis, and elevated circulating TNF-α may present
- CSF studies: no increase of WBC count or protein, raised lactate concentrate, and increased opening pressure, especially in children, may present

DIAGNOSIS (Dx)

DIFFERENTIAL DIAGNOSIS

- Typhoid fever
- Dengue fever
- Yellow fever
- Viral hepatitis
- Influenza
- Brucellosis
- UTI
- Leishmaniasis
- Trypanosomiasis
- Rickettsial diseases
- Leptospirosis

WORKUP

- Clinical diagnosis is notoriously inaccurate
- Demonstration of malarial parasites in blood smear is essential
- Newer molecular diagnostic techniques are promising

LABORATORY TESTS

- The thick and thin blood film is required to identify malarial parasites
- The thick smears are more sensitive and primarily used to detect the presence of parasites
- The thin smears are used for species differentiation and parasite density estimation
- Person suspected of having malaria but no parasite seen in blood smears should have blood smears repeated every 12 to 24 hr for 3 consecutive days

PREPARATION OF BLOOD SMEAR:
- Must be prepared from fresh blood obtained by pricking the fingers
- The thin smear is fixed in methanol before staining
- The thick smear is stained unfixed
- The smear should be stained with a 3% Giemsa solution (pH of 7.2) for 30 to 45 min
- The parasite density should be estimated by counting the percentage of RBC infected, not the number of parasites, under an oil immersion lens on thin film

COMMON ERRORS IN READING MALARIAL SMEARS:
- Platelets overlying an RBC
- Misreading artifacts as parasites
- Concern about missing a positive slide

MOLECULAR DIAGNOSIS OF MALARIA:
- Polymerase chain reaction (PCR)
  1. It is useful in accurate species diagnosis
  2. It can detect the low-level parasitemias
  3. Is expensive and time-consuming
  4. It needs technical expertise
- Quantitative buffy cost (QBC)
  1. This test detects nuclear material of parasites using acridine orange stain
  2. It is unable to speciate the parasites accurately
  3. It cannot quantitate parasitemias
- Para Sight F and Malaria PF Test
  1. This test uses a monoclonal antibody to detect *P. falciparum*-specific, histidine-rich protein (HRP)-2

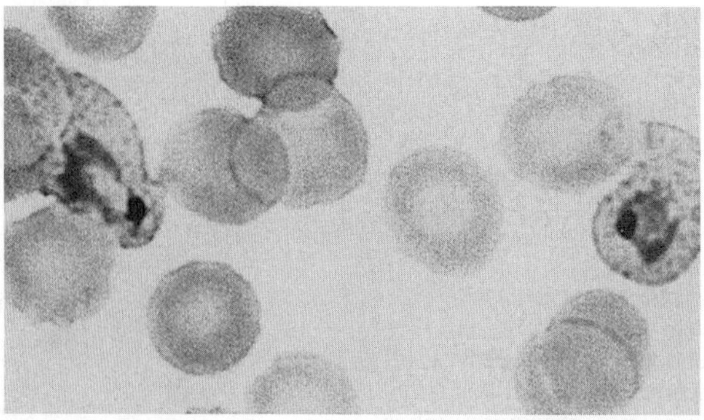

FIGURE 1-151 Giemsa-stained blood smear in *Plasmodium vivax* malaria. Asexual parasites. Note that the parasites are large and ameboid; the infected erythrocytes are the largest cells in the field (because they are reticulocytes), and the erythrocytes contain numerous pink dots (Schüffner's dots) (×2000). (From Klippel JH et al [eds]: *Internal medicine*, ed 5, St Louis, 1998, Mosby.)

2. It can detect *P. falciparum* only
3. Past infection may confuse diagnosis

- OptiMal test
  1. This test detects lactage dehydrogenase (LDH) of parasites
  2. It can differentiate *falciparum* from non-*falciparum* malaria

TREATMENT (Rx)

NONPHARMACOLOGIC THERAPY

ANTIMOSQUITO MEASURES:

1. Eradication of mosquito breeding places by chemical spray
2. Use of mosquito nets properly in the endemic areas
3. Use of protective clothing
4. Use of insect spray (permethrin), mosquito coils, or repellents (diethyltoluamide)

ACUTE GENERAL Rx

A definitive diagnosis of malaria is essential for specific antimalarial chemotherapy

NON-*FALCIPARUM* MALARIA:

- Chloroquine 600 mg base (1000 mg chloroquine phosphate) po loading dose, 6 hr later 300 mg base (500 mg salt), then 300 mg base (500 mg salt) daily for 2 days
- In the case of *P. vivax* and *P. ovale,* treatment with primaquine 15 mg daily for 14 days is needed to eradicate the exoerythrocytic forms, especially the hypnozoites responsible for relapses
- G6PD should be measured before primaquine is given
- Chloroquine-resistant *P. vivax* has been documented; in that case, quinine is given

***FALCIPARUM* MALARIA:**

- Chloroquine can be used cautiously for falciparum malaria acquired in chloroquine-sensitive areas (chloroquine is more rapidly effective than quinine)
- Mainstay of treatment is oral quinine sulfate 10 mg (salt)/kg (usually 650 mg) q8h for 3 to 7 days, followed by pyrimethamine with sulfadoxine (Fansider) 3 tablets (each tablets contains 500 mg sulfadoxine and 25 mg pyrimethamine) or doxycycline 200 mg loading dose, then 100 mg bid for 7 days to eradicate asexual forms of the parasite

ALTERNATIVES:

- Quinine followed by clindamycin 900 mg tid × 5 days, or
- Mefloquine 1250 mg as a single dose, or
- Halofantrine 500 mg q6h × 3 doses, repeat a week later, or
- Atovaquone 1000 mg daily × 3 days plus proguanil 400 mg daily × 3 days, or
- Atovaquone 1000 mg daily × 3 days plus doxycycline 100 mg bid × 3 days, or
- Artesunate 4 mg/kg daily × 3 days plus mefloquine 1250 mg single dose

NOTE: Parasitemia may paradoxically rise in the first 24 to 36 hr and is not an indication of treatment failure.

SEVERE *FALCIPARUM* MALARIA:

It is a medical emergency; intensive care is preferred

- Measurement of blood glucose, lactate, ABG is important
- Intravenous quinidine gluconate 10 mg salt/kg loading dose (maximum 600 mg) in NS infuse slowly over 1 to 2 hr, followed by continuous infusion of 0.02 mg/kg/min until patient can swallow
- Cardiac monitor needed for observation of QT interval
- Alternatively, artemether 3.2 mg/kg IM then 1.6 mg/kg daily × 3 days
- Plasmaparesis is an option for parasitemia >30% or in pregnant woman and in elderly with severe malaria

MULTIDRUG-RESISTANT MALARIA:

- Mefloquine 1250 mg as a single dose, or
- Halofantrine 500 mg every 6 hr for 3 doses, repeat same course after 1 wk
- Combination therapy usually preferred

DISPOSITION

RISK FACTORS FOR FATAL MALARIA:

- Failure to take chemoprophylaxis
- Delay in seeking medical care
- Misdiagnosis

COMPLICATIONS OF MALARIA:

- Anemia
- Acidosis
- Hypoglycemia
- Respiratory distress
- DIC
- Blackwater fever
- Renal failure
- Shock

REFERRAL

- To an infectious disease specialist or travel medicine expert for severe malaria complications
- To an intensive care specialist if severe cerebral malaria or other major organ failure develops

PEARLS & CONSIDERATIONS (!)

HOST RESPONSE:

- The specific immune response to malaria confers protection from high-level parasitemia and disease, but not from infection
- Asymptomatic parasitemia without illness (premunition) is common among adults in endemic area
- Immunity is specific for both the species and the strain of infecting malarial parasites
- Immunity to all strains is never achieved
- Normal spleen function is an important host factor because of immunologic as well as filtering functions of the spleen
- Both humoral and cellular immunity are necessary for protection
- Polyclonal increase in serum level of IgG, IgM, and IgA occur in immune individuals
- Antibody to antigenically variant protein PfEMP1 is important for protection in case of *P. falciparum* malaria
- Passively transferred IgG from immune individual has been shown protective
- Maternal antibody confers relative protection of infants from severe disease
- Genetic disorders (sickle cell disease, thalassemia, and G6PD deficiency) confer protection from death because parasites are unable to grow efficiently in low-oxygen tensions, thus preventing high-level parasitemias
- Individuals deficient of Duffy factor in RBC are resistant to infection by *P. vivax*
- Nonspecific defense mechanisms, cytokines (TNF-α, IL-1, 6, 8) also play an important role in protection; it causes fever (temperatures of 40° C damage mature parasites) and other pathologic effects

PREVENTION OF MALARIA:

Prophylaxis should be taken 1 wk before travel, continue weekly for the duration of stay and for 4 wk after leaving endemic area

NON-*FALCIPARUM* MALARIA:

Chloroquine 300 mg base (500 mg chloroquine phosphate) PO/wk

***FALCIPARUM* MALARIA:**

- Mefloquine 250 mg (228 mg base) PO/wk, or
- Doxycycline 100 mg PO/day, or
- Primaquine 0.5 mg base/kg/day, or
- Chloroquine (300 mg base) plus proguanil (200 mg) PO/day

SPECIAL CONSIDERATIONS:

- Long-term visitors or travelers
- Children <12 yr
- Immunocompromised host
- Pregnant women

VACCINATION:

- No effective and safe vaccine available yet
- A live, attenuated, whole sporozoite vaccine shown to work
- A synthetic peptide (SPf66) vaccine proved ineffective
- New DNA-based vaccines are in development

MALARIA INFORMATION:

CDC Travelers' Health Hotline (877) 394-8747; CDC Travelers' Health Fax (888) 232-3299

CDC Malaria Epidemiology (770) 488-7788; internet: http://www.cdc.gov

EVIDENCE

Evidence supporting the use of chloroquine in the treatment of malaria predated the widespread resistance of *P. falciparum* to chloroquine, now seen in Africa. Chloroquine is no longer recommended for malaria prophylaxis in this region, and its therapeutic use is limited to sensitive strains, in nonresistant areas only.[1] Ⓒ

There is evidence for the effectiveness of doxycycline in the prophylaxis of malaria, although the trials have not been conducted in Western tourists or business travelers. Doxycycline has been shown in randomized controlled trials (RCTs) to be effective in the prophylaxis of malaria. The RCTs have not been conducted in Western tourists or business travelers.[2,3] Ⓐ

There is evidence for the effectiveness of mefloquine in the prophylaxis of malaria, although adverse effects may limit its usefulness. Mefloquine has been found in a systematic review to be effective at preventing malaria in nonimmune adults. Five of the RCTs included in the review were field trials, mostly involving male soldiers.[4] Ⓐ Mefloquine has been shown to prevent episodes of malaria in one area of drug resistance.[4] Ⓐ

There is some evidence that atovaquone plus proguanil is effective in the prophylaxis of malaria. Atovaquone plus proguanil has been shown to be associated with a significant reduction in the proportion of people with malaria compared with placebo in an RCT that was conducted in Indonesian migrants with limited immunity who had moved to Papua.[5] Ⓐ

Atovaquone plus proguanil has been shown to be as effective as chloroquine plus proguanil in terms of the incidence of malaria in a group of travelers.[6] Ⓐ

There is evidence for the effectiveness of a number of lifestyle measures in the prophylaxis of malaria among those living in endemic areas. The use of bed nets and curtains treated with insecticide is associated with a reduction in childhood mortality and morbidity from malaria, and reduced the incidence of mild malarial episodes.[7] Ⓐ

The use of clothing or sheets treated with permethrin has been shown to reduce the incidence of malaria in endemic areas. Ⓐ

The indoor use of pyrethroid insecticide sprays has been shown to reduce the incidence of clinical malaria in endemic areas.[9] Ⓐ

Evidence-Based References

1. Centers for Disease Control and Prevention: Malaria: part 2, 2004. Ⓒ
2. Ohrt C et al: Mefloquine compared with doxycycline for the prophylaxis of malaria in Indonesian soldiers. A randomized, double-blind, placebo-controlled trial, *Ann Intern Med* 126:963, 1997. Reviewed in: *Clin Evid* 10:911, 2003. Ⓐ
3. Taylor WR et al: Malaria prophylaxis using azithromycin: a double-blind, placebo-controlled trial in Irian Jaya, Indonesia, *Clin Infect Dis* 28:74, 1999. Reviewed in: *Clin Evid* 10:911, 2003. Ⓐ
4. Croft AMJ, Garner P: Mefloquine for preventing malaria in non-immune adult travellers, *Cochrane Database Syst Rev* 4, 2000. Ⓐ
5. Ling J et al: Randomized, placebo-controlled trial of atovaquone/proguanil for the prevention of Plasmodium falciparum or Plasmodium vivax malaria among migrants to Papua, Indonesia, *Clin Infect Dis* 35:825, 2002. Reviewed in: *Clin Evid* 10:911, 2003. Ⓐ
6. Hogh B et al: Atovaquone/proguanil versus chloroquine/proguanil for malaria prophylaxis in non-immune travellers: a randomised, double-blind study, *Lancet* 356:1888, 2000. Reviewed in: *Clin Evid* 10:911, 2003. Ⓐ
7. Lengeler C: Insecticide-treated bed nets and curtains for preventing malaria, *Cochrane Database Syst Rev* 2, 2004. Ⓐ
8. Soto J et al: Efficacy of permethrin-impregnated uniforms in the prevention of malaria and lieshmaniasis in Colombian soldiers, *Clin Infect Dis* 21:599, 1995. Reviewed in: *Clin Evid* 10:911, 2003. Ⓐ
9. Misra SP et al: Spray versus treated nets using deltamethrin: a community randomized trial in India, *Trans R Soc Trop Med Hyg* 93:456, 1999. Reviewed in: *Clin Evid* 10:911, 2003. Ⓐ

SUGGESTED READINGS

Baird JK: Effectiveness of antimalarial drugs, *N Engl J Med* 352:1565, 2005.

Marx A et al: Meta-analysis: accuracy of rapid tests for malaria in travelers returning from endemic areas, *Ann Intern Med* 142:836, 2005.

Skarbinski J et al: Malaria surveillance—United States, 2004, *MMWR Surveill Summ* 55(4):23, 2006.

South East Asian Quinine Artesunate Malaria Trial (SEAQUAMAT) group: Artesunate versus quinine for treatment of severe falciparum malaria: a randomized trial, *Lancet* 366:7170725, 2005.

AUTHORS: **AMAR ASHRAF, M.D., GLENN G. FORT, M.D., M.P.H.,** and **DENNIS J. MIKOLICH, M.D.**

BASIC INFORMATION

DEFINITION

Malignant hyperthermia occurs when, in the setting of recently administered anesthetic agents, most commonly halogenated inhalation agents (halothane) or depolarizing muscle relaxants (succinylcholine), the patient quickly develops muscle rigidity and elevated temperature.

SYNONYMS

Malignant hyperthermia of anesthesia

ICD-9-CM CODES
995.86 Malignant hyperthermia

EPIDEMIOLOGY & DEMOGRAPHICS

INCIDENCE: Between 1/200 and 1/250,000

PREVALENCE: Difficult to determine because of great variations in both penetrance of gene and severity of illness.

PREDOMINANT SEX AND AGE: Any age and either sex may be affected.

PEAK INCIDENCE: Any age may be affected

RISK FACTORS: Known family history of malignant hyperthermia, or significant problems with general anesthesia.

GENETICS: Half of cases are autosomal dominant. Others unknown.

PHYSICAL FINDINGS & CLINICAL PRESENTATION

- Within minutes to hours after anesthetic is given, patient develops muscle rigidity (especially masseter spasm), hyperthermia (up to 45° C), tachycardia that may progress to other dysrhythmias, hypotension. Skin initially reddens but then becomes cyanotic and mottled. There is also increased carbon dioxide production.
- Rhabdomyolysis, acute renal failure, and disseminated intravascular coagulation may soon follow.

ETIOLOGY

- In contrast to fever, in which elevated core temperature is related to hypothalamus set point adjustment by cytokines, malignant hyperthermia results from overproduction of heat via skeletal muscle metabolism in the context of a normal hypothalamic set point.
- In genetically susceptible individuals, administration of anesthetic agents results in release of calcium from the sarcoplasmic reticulum of skeletal muscles causing muscle rigidity and hypermetabolism. This results in significant heat production, which overwhelms the body's normal ability to dissipate heat.

DIAGNOSIS

DIFFERENTIAL DIAGNOSIS

- Neuroleptic malignant syndrome
- Fever
- Heat stroke
- Thyrotoxicosis
- Pheochromocytoma
- Central nervous system infection or space occupying lesion
- MDMA (ecstasy), cocaine, alcohol withdrawal, or amphetamine use
- Serotonin syndrome
- Adverse reaction to monoamine oxidase inhibitor or anticholinergics drug
- Strychnine poisoning

WORKUP

Based upon history, it is usually easy to distinguish malignant hyperthermia from other causes of hyperthermia. A thorough history, especially including medications and any illicit substances, is important. Consider lumbar puncture to rule out infection.

LABORATORY TESTS

- If cause of hyperthermia is uncertain, a complete blood count, thyroid function studies, toxicology screen, and urine VMA may be useful.
- Once diagnosis is established, it is important to follow electrolytes (especially potassium, calcium, and phosphorus), creatinine, blood urea nitrogen, liver transaminases, as well as creatinine kinase.
- Prothrombin time and partial thromboplastin time should be followed to evaluate for disseminated intravascular coagulation.

IMAGING STUDIES

CT scan to assess for space occupying lesion if diagnosis is uncertain.

TREATMENT

The most important measures for treatment include stopping the anesthetic agents, starting dantrolene, physical cooling, and prevention of sequellae. Antipyretics are not useful because the hypothalamic set point is not altered by cytokines.

NONPHARMACOLOGIC THERAPY

- Cooling via ice bath, ice packs in groin and axillae, cool spray with fans, or cooling blankets. In severe instances, extracorporeal partial bypass or iced peritoneal lavage may be used. Stop cooling when core temperature reaches 38° C to prevent overcooling.
- Careful monitoring of cardiovascular and respiratory status with constant core temperature measurements.

ACUTE GENERAL Rx

- Dantrolene is the mainstay of treatment, starting with a bolus of 2.5mg/kg IV, which should be repeated every 5 minutes until symptoms abate or a maximum of 10-20mg/kg is reached. Then 24 hours of 10mg/kg/day IV should be given.
- Beta-blockers or lidocaine may be useful for dysrhythmias but verapamil should be avoided because its use with dantrolene has been shown to depress cardiac function.
- Sodium bicarbonate may be necessary to reverse acidosis.
- Aggressive hydration with forced diuresis and urine alkalinization should be instituted as treatment for rhabdomyolysis.

CHRONIC Rx

This is an acute illness.

COMPLEMENTARY AND ALTERNATIVE MEDICINE

None

DISPOSITION

Patient will likely need intensive monitoring, necessitating an intensive care unit bed.

REFERRAL

Anesthesia consultants will likely already be involved. Consider cardiac, renal, or hematologic consult if sequellae are significant.

PEARLS & CONSIDERATIONS

COMMENTS

Malignant hyperthermia is a life-threatening condition that requires prompt recognition of the signs and symptoms to minimize illness and prevent organ damage.

PREVENTION

- Careful family and personal history of significant adverse effects with general anesthesia are important tip-offs.
- Prophylactic dantrolene therapy is no longer recommended in susceptible individuals.

PATIENT/FAMILY EDUCATION

Because family history is so important in this illness, it is important for patients and families to be aware of a history of problems with general anesthesia.

SUGGESTED READINGS

Hadad E: Drug-induced hyperthermia and muscle rigidity: a practical approach, *Eur J Emerg Med* 10:2, 2003.

Krause T: Dantrolene: a review of its pharmacology, therapeutic use and new developments, *Anaesthesia* 59:346, 2004.

Litman R: Malignant hyperthermia, *JAMA* 293:23, 2005.

Simon H: Hyperthermia, *New Engl J Med* 329:7, 1993.

AUTHOR: **CRISTINA ANTONIO PACHECO, M.D.**

BASIC INFORMATION

DEFINITION

A Mallory-Weiss tear (MWT) is a longitudinal mucosal laceration in the region of the gastroesophageal junction.

SYNONYMS

Mallory-Weiss syndrome

ICD-9CM CODES
530.7 Gastroesophageal laceration-hemorrhage syndrome
530.82 Esophageal hemorrhage

EPIDEMIOLOGY & DEMOGRAPHICS

- Accounts for 5% to 15% of cases of upper GI bleeding
- Reported from early childhood to old age; the majority of patients are in their 40s to 60s
- More common in males
- Alcohol use is present in 30% to 60%

PHYSICAL FINDINGS & CLINICAL PRESENTATION

- Vomiting, retching, or vigorous coughing will often, but not always, precede hematemesis.
- Patients may be clinically stable or present with tachycardia, hypotension, melena, or hematochezia.
- Bleeding may be self-limited or severe.
- Tears may be seen in association with other upper GI tract lesions, including hiatus hernia (present in as many as 90% of patients), ulcers, and esophageal varices, particularly in alcoholics.

ETIOLOGY

- An acute increase in intraabdominal pressure is transmitted to the esophagus, resulting in mucosal laceration.
- Vomiting may be associated with alcohol use, ketoacidosis, ulcer disease, uremia, pancreatitis, cholecystitis, pregnancy, myocardial infarction, or the postoperative period.
- Tears may be iatrogenic, related to endoscopy (EGD), especially in struggling or retching patients, esophageal dilation, lower esophageal pneumatic disruption therapy for achalasia, transesophageal echocardiography, or in association with polyethylene glycol electrolyte colonic lavage preparation.

DIAGNOSIS

DIFFERENTIAL DIAGNOSIS

- Esophageal or gastric varices
- Esophagitis/esophageal ulcers (peptic or pill-induced)
- Gastric erosions
- Gastric or duodenal ulcer
- Dieulafoy lesion
- Arteriovenous malformations
- Neoplasms (usually gastric)
- Boerhaave's syndrome

WORKUP

EGD is the diagnostic method of choice.

LABORATORY TESTS

- Complete blood count, PT, PTT
- Lytes, BUN, creatinine, LFTs, pregnancy test, or others to evaluate for predisposing conditions

IMAGING STUDIES

Upper GI series usually not sensitive. Patients with concurrent chest pain, dyspnea, shock, or physical exam findings of crepitus or pleural effusion should have chest x-ray or CT to exclude Boerhaave's syndrome.

TREATMENT

NONPHARMACOLOGIC THERAPY

- Supportive care
- Aspirin, NSAIDs, and anticoagulants should be held

ACUTE GENERAL Rx

- Patients with active bleeding or hemodynamic instability require large-bore IVs, fluid resuscitation, and transfusion of blood products (red blood cells, FFP, and platelets) as appropriate
- NG decompression and antiemetics may be considered
- Endoscopic therapy for patients with active or ongoing hemorrhage. Therapeutic modalities include electrocoagulation, injection (e.g., 1:10,000 epinephrine, polidocanol), sclerotherapy (for bleeding associated with esophageal varices), band ligation, or endoscopic hemoclips (therapies may be used alone or in combination)
- Arterial embolization in patients with active bleeding who are poor surgical candidates
- Laparotomy, with gastrotomy and oversewing of the tear, is required in a small percentage of patients with uncontrolled bleeding

CHRONIC Rx

- Healing will usually occur without specific therapy.
- H_2-blockers or proton pump inhibitors may be given to help facilitate healing, but should not be used chronically unless appropriate indications are present.

DISPOSITION

- Prognosis is good, with spontaneous cessation of bleeding in upwards of 90% of patients. Endoscopic features can guide treatment.
- Delayed rebleeding is described in patients with high-risk stigmata (shock at initial presentation, spurting or oozing at initial endoscopy).
- Death has been reported in 3% to 12%; often with severe bleeding and underlying comorbid conditions, including coagulopathy, thrombocytopenia, alcohol use, and multisystem organ failure.

REFERRAL

- GI referral for endoscopy
- Surgical referral for bleeding unresponsive to endoscopic treatment, or in the setting of coexistent perforation

PEARLS & CONSIDERATIONS

Conditions predisposing to retching or vomiting should be identified and treated at presentation.

EVIDENCE

Endoscopic epinephrine treatment

- Endoscopic injection of epinephrine and polidocanol vs. placebo
    - Randomized controlled trial of 32 patients with MWT
    - Hemostasis obtained in all 32 patients
    - 2/32 patients (6.2%) had minor recurrent bleeding compared to 8/31 (25.8%) in the control group
    - No major episodes of rebleeding
- Endoscopic hemoclips vs. endoscopic injection of epinephrine
    - Prospective trial of 35 patients with MWT with spurting vessels or oozing
    - Randomized to either treatment
    - Primary hemostasis was achieved in 100% of patients in both groups
    - Each group had one patient who rebled, who was successfully retreated with the same modality. No second episodes of recurrent bleeding
    - No procedure-related complications
- Endoscopic band ligation vs. endoscopic injections of epinephrine
    - Prospective trial of 34 patients with actively bleeding MWT
    - Randomized to either treatment
    - Primary hemostasis achieved in all 17 (100%) of patients in band ligation group and 16 of 17 (94.1%) of patients in epinephrine injection group
    - No major complications or episodes of rebleeding in either group

SUGGESTED READINGS

Huang SP et al: Endoscopic hemoclip placement and epinephrine injection for Mallory-Weiss syndrome with active bleeding, *Gastrointest Endosc* 55:842, 2002.

Kortas DY et al: Mallory-Weiss tear: predisposing factors and predictors of a complicated course. *Am J Gastro* 96:2863, 2001.

Llach J et al: Endoscopic injection therapy in bleeding Mallory-Weiss syndrome: a randomized controlled trial, *Gastrointest Endosc* 54:679, 2001.

Park CH et al: A prospective, randomized trial of endoscopic band ligation vs. epinephrine injection for actively bleeding Mallory-Weiss syndrome, *Gastrointest Endosc* 60:22, 2004.

AUTHOR: **HARLAN G. RICH, M.D.**

BASIC INFORMATION

DEFINITION

Marfan's syndrome is an inherited disorder of connective tissue involving skeleton, cardiovascular system, eyes, lungs, and central nervous system.

ICD-9CM CODES
759.82 Marfan's syndrome

EPIDEMIOLOGY & DEMOGRAPHICS

PREVALENCE: 1 case/10,000 persons

- Both sexes are affected equally by this autosomal dominant syndrome.
- Approximately 30% of cases are a new mutation.

PHYSICAL FINDINGS & CLINICAL PRESENTATION

Diagnostic criteria for Marfan's syndrome (Fig. 1-152):

- Skeleton
  Joint hypermobility, tall stature, pectus excavatum, reduced thoracic kyphosis, scoliosis, arachnodactyly, dolichostenomelia, pectus carinatum, and erosion of the lumbosacral vertebrae from dural ectasia†
- Eye
  Myopia, retinal detachment, elongated globe, ectopia lentis†
- Cardiovascular
  Mitral valve prolapse, endocarditis, arrhythmia, dilated mitral annulus, mitral regurgitation, tricuspid valve prolapse, aortic regurgitation, aortic dissection,† dilation of the aortic root†
- Pulmonary
  Apical blebs, spontaneous pneumothorax
- Skin and integument
  Inguinal hernias, incisional hernias, striae atrophicae
- Central nervous system
  Attention deficit disorder, hyperactivity, verbal-performance discrepancy, dural ectasia, anterior pelvic meningocele.†

If the family history is positive for a close relative clearly affected by Marfan's syndrome, manifestations should be present in the skeleton and one of the other organ systems, and the diagnosis confirmed by linkage analysis or mutation detection.

If the family history is negative or unknown, the patient should have manifestations in the skeleton, the cardiovascular system, and one other system, and at least one of the manifestations indicated by †.

Manifestations are listed within each organ system in increasing specificity for Marfan's syndrome; although none is completely specific, those indicated by † are the most specific.

ETIOLOGY

Mutations in the gene that encodes fibrillin-1, the major constituent of microfibrils, which form the frame for elastic fibers. All the manifestations of Marfan's syndrome can be explained by the defective microfibrils.

DIAGNOSIS

DIFFERENTIAL DIAGNOSIS

Each of the clinical manifestations of the syndrome may have other causes; however, if the diagnostic criteria are met, the diagnosis is made.

WORKUP

- Echocardiography to establish:
  Mitral valve prolapse
  Mitral regurgitation
  Tricuspid valve prolapse
  Aortic regurgitation
  Dilation of the aortic root
- Chest x-ray
- Transesophageal echocardiography, chest CT scan, chest MRI, or aortography for suspected aortic dissection
- Chest x-ray for pulmonary apical bullae
- Ophthalmologic examination by ophthalmologist

TREATMENT

- Regular cardiac and aorta monitoring by physical examination and echocardiography
- Endocarditis prophylaxis
- Restriction of contact sports, weight lifting, and overexertion
- β-Blockers are commonly prescribed to slow the rate of aortic root dilation in children; recent trials, however, have shown that this approach is not effective
- Early use of angiotensin-converting enzyme inhibitors in young patients with Marfan syndrome and valvular regurgitation may lessen the need for mitral valve surgery
- Genetic counseling
- Monitor aorta during pregnancy (because of increased risk of dissection)

SUGGESTED READINGS

Selamet Tierney ES et al: Beta-blocker therapy does not alter the rate of aortic root dilation in pediatric patients with Marfan syndrome, *J Pediatr* 150:77, 2007.

Yetman AT et al: Comparison of outcome of the Marfan syndrome in patients diagnosed at age 6 years versus those diagnosed at age >6 years of age, *Am J Cardiol* 91:102, 2003.

AUTHORS: **FRED F. FERRI, M.D.**, and **TOM J. WACHTEL, M.D.**

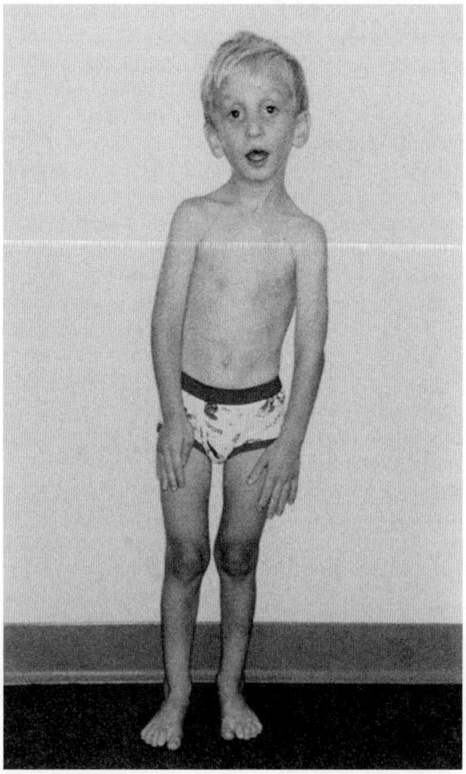

FIGURE 1-152 Marfan's syndrome. Note the elongated facies, droopy lids, apparent dolichostenomelia, and mild scoliosis. (From Behrman RE: *Nelson's textbook of pediatrics,* Philadelphia, 2004, WB Saunders.)

BASIC INFORMATION

DEFINITION

Mastitis is the inflammation of breast tissue either from irritation or infection resulting in subcutaneous cellulitis.

ICD-9CM CODES
611.0 Acute (infective, puerperal, nonpuerperal, diffuse, interstitial)
610.1 Chronic (cystic, fibrocystic)
610.4 Periductal/plasma cell
675.1 Postpartum/puerperal (purulent)
675.2 Postpartum/puerperal (nonpurulent)

EPIDEMIOLOGY & DEMOGRAPHICS

- When presenting in lactating mothers, mastitis typically occurs in the first 3 months postpartum (74% to 95% cases). When severe, mastitis can lead to a breast abscess (5% to 11%) or septicemia (TSS). Mastitis is a risk factor for vertical transmission of infections secondarily to changes in composition of milk and local immune response.
- In nonlactating women of childbearing age it often presents as granulomatous mastitis (GM).
- In older nonlactating women it is called periductal mastitis (PM) and is caused by inflamed milk ducts near the nipple.
- Mastitis can also occur in early infancy where breast hypertrophy due to maternal hormonal stimulation can lead to infection.
- Recurrent mastitis is typically secondary to incomplete or inappropriate antibiotic treatment.

PREVALENCE: 1% to 3% of women to as high as 1 in 3 lactating mothers; recurrence 4%

PREDOMINANT SEX: Females

RISK FACTORS:
- Mastitis in the past
- Cracked, fissured, or sore nipples
- Primiparity and improper nursing such that breast does not empty completely
- Milk stasis, engorgement
- Using antifungal nipple cream (presumably for nipple thrush) in the same week
- Employment outside home
- Tight clothing or bras
- Use of manual breast pump
- Stress/fatigue
- Diabetes
- Use of steroids
- Lumpectomy with radiation
- Breast implants

PHYSICAL FINDINGS & CLINICAL PRESENTATION

- Malaise and myalgia.
- Chills and fever above 38.3° C.
- Warmth, redness, tenderness in breast.
- Pain with nursing.
- Decreased milk output.
- Area of breast is hard, wedge-shaped, and swollen.
- Breast mass near nipple with retraction or discharge in periductal mastitis.
- Enlarged axillary lymph nodes or sinus tract formation in granulomatous mastitis.

ETIOLOGY

- Irritation.
- Blocked lactiferous duct and stasis of the duct leading to engorgement.
- Local adverse immune response to milk proteins.
- Infectious: *Staphylococcus aureus*, coagulase-negative staphylococci, Group A and B-hemolytic streptococci, *Escherichia coli* and *Bacteroides* species, increasing incidence of MRSA mastitis; rare instances with *Salmonella* spp., mycobacteria, candida, and Cryptococcus.
  - GM from inflammation with epithelioid histiocytes and multinucleated giant cells can be caused by etiologies like tuberculosis (TB), sarcoidosis, foreign body reaction, parasitic and mycotic infections, or idiopathic (IGM).
  - Mastitis in neonates is caused by infections with *Staphylococcus aureus* or gram-negative enteric bacteria.

DIAGNOSIS

DIFFERENTIAL DIAGNOSIS

- Plugged lactiferous ducts.
- Breast abscess.
- Inflammatory breast cancer.
- Mastitis as a symptom of hyperprolactinemia, galactorrhea.
- Other cancers—3% women diagnosed with breast cancer are lactating.
- GM can be a manifestation of systemic disease including sarcoidosis, Wegener granulomatosis, giant cell arteritis, or polyarteritis nodosa, TB, syphilis.

WORKUP

- History of signs and symptoms and clinical exam including thorough breast exam with assessment for axillary nodes and nipple discharge are sufficient to make diagnosis.
- Recurrent mastitis should include workup for underlying breast disease.

LABORATORY TESTS

- Simple mastitis requires no milk culture or studies.
- Obtain midstream sample of milk for culture for antibiotic sensitivities in refractory mastitis.
- CBC and blood cultures in toxic-appearing patients.
- Breast milk analysis reveals raised milk cell counts; increased sodium and protein levels; activation of milk leukocytes; increased factors such as TNF-alpha and IFN-gamma.
- Gram stain and culture indicated in early childhood mastitis.

IMAGING STUDIES

- Not necessary unless refractory mastitis.
- Consider ultrasound to evaluate for abscess or mammogram since cannot exclude carcinoma.
- In GM use of mammogram and ultrasound guided FNA are standard studies.

TREATMENT

NONPHARMACOLOGIC THERAPY

- Warm compresses.
- Continue frequent nursing and change feeding positions to completely empty breasts.
- Increase fluid intake and bedrest.
- Therapeutic ultrasound has been suggested for breast engorgement.
- In abscess formation, drainage is necessary followed by parenteral antibiotics.
- Surgery in severe periductal mastitis.

ACUTE GENERAL Rx

- Pain meds including anti-inflammatory and analgesics (e.g., Tylenol, Ibuprofen).
- Antimicrobials:
  - Dicloxacillin or Cloxacillin 500 mg po four times a day for 10 to 14 days.
  - If no response use Cephalexin or Augmentin or treat according to culture sensitivity.
  - PCN-allergic women can use erythromycin or clindamycin but sulfa drugs should be avoided if infant is under 1 month of age.
- Mastitis in early infancy should be treated with parenteral antibiotics based on results of Gram stain.

CHRONIC Rx

- Experimental vaccines (especially human staphylococcal vaccine) have shown protection against recurrent mastitis.
- Systemic corticosteroids or wide surgical resection in GM.
- New studies showing immunosuppressive therapy (methotrexate, azathioprine) as steroid-sparing agents in GM therapy.

COMPLEMENTARY & ALTERNATIVE MEDICINE

Complementary therapies (have not been assessed in prospective studies): belladonna, *Phytolacca*, *Chamomilla*, sulphur, and *Bellis perenis*

REFERRAL

Referral to a surgeon for severe periductal mastitis

PEARLS & CONSIDERATIONS

COMMENTS

- Antimicrobials are often not necessary for noninfective mastitis but 86% of women receive antibiotic treatment.
- In reassessing refractory mastitis the most important consideration is the possibility of cancer.
- Mastitis can be a manifestation of systemic disease.
- Delay in recognition and treatment may result in abscess formation or recurrent mastitis.
- Mastitis is a risk factor for vertical transmission of infections including increased transmission of retroviruses (especially HIV-1), CMV, measles, hepatitis B and C.
- Mastitis is the major cause of reduction in milk production.
- One quarter of breastfeeding mothers with one episode of mastitis will stop breastfeeding.
- GM mimics breast cancer both clinically and radiologically (more than 50% of reported cases are initially mistaken for carcinoma). This includes fine needle aspiration, which is sometimes interpreted as malignant.
- All infants with diagnosis of mastitis should receive parenteral antibiotics.

SUGGESTED READINGS

Asoglu O et al: Feasibility of surgical management in patients with granulomatous mastitis, *Breast J* 11:108-114, 2005.

Barbosa-Cesnik C, Schwartz K, Foxman B: Lactation mastitis, *JAMA* 289:1609-1612, 2003.

Foxman B et al: Lactation mastitis: occurrence and medical management among 946 breastfeeding women in the United States, *Am J Epidemiol* 55:103, 2002.

Mass S: Breast pain: engorgement, nipple pain and mastitis, *Clin Obstet Gynecol* 47(3):676-682, 2004.

Michie C, Lockie F, Lynn W: The challenge of mastitis, *Arch Dis Child* 88:818-821, 2003.

Pouchot J et al: Granulomatous mastitis: an uncommon cause of breast abscess, *Arch Int Med* 161:611-612, 2000.

Stricker T, Navratil F, Sennhauser F: Mastitis in early infancy, *Acta Paediatrica* 94:166-169, 2005.

AUTHOR: **AGNIESZKA K. BIALIKIEWICZ, M.D.**

BASIC INFORMATION

DEFINITION

- Pain in the breast.
- Mastodynia is synonymous with mastalgia.
- This condition is usually cyclical, but may be noncyclical or extramammary.

ICD-9CM CODES
611.71 Mastodynia

EPIDEMIOLOGY & DEMOGRAPHICS

- Mastodynia will affect up to 70% of women at some time in their reproductive lives.
- Severe cyclical mastodynia lasting more than 5 days/mo and of sufficient intensity to interfere with sexual, physical, social, and work-related activities is reported among 30% of premenopausal women.
- Underlying fear of breast cancer is the reason most of these women seek medical consultation.
- One tenth of women with mastodynia require pain-relieving therapy.

PHYSICAL FINDINGS & CLINICAL PRESENTATION

- Usually, the breasts are normal bilaterally
- Full, tender breasts
- Generalized breast nodularity without discrete lumps
- Chest wall tenderness: extramammary breast pain
- Distinguishing mammary from extramammary pain can be difficult
- With the patient lying on her side so that the breast tissue falls away from the chest wall, tenderness can then be reproduced by direct pressure over the offending site
- Cyclical mastodynia presents in the luteal phase of the menstrual cycle
- Women with cyclical mastodynia tend to have abdominal bloating, leg swelling, and other symptoms of premenstrual syndrome
- Noncyclical mastodynia, on the other hand, is unrelated to the menstrual cycle
- Extramammary breast pain simulates noncyclical mastodynia

ETIOLOGY

- Hormonal imbalance
- Abnormal lipid metabolism
- Premenstrual syndrome (20%)
- Fibrocystic breast disease
- Emotional abuse and anxiety
- Excessive caffeine intake
- Breast cancer (10%)
- Tietze syndrome (idiopathic costochondritis)

DIAGNOSIS

DIFFERENTIAL DIAGNOSIS

- See Etiology.
- The majority of women with mastodynia have no underlying abnormality.
- Breast fullness and tenderness associated with hormonal changes fluctuate with menstrual cycle.
- Similarly, the breast nodularity, which may or may not be the result of fibrocystic breast disease, also fluctuates with the menstrual cycle.
- Discrete breast lump needs full evaluation to rule out malignancy.
- Tietze syndrome is usually unilateral and may be associated with chest wall swelling.

WORKUP

- Complete history and thorough clinical examination.
- Pain analogue cards may be helpful in establishing the pattern of symptomatology. In patients >35 years of age, mammography should be performed as part of the baseline investigations.
- Most women presenting with severe mastodynia are <35. This group has a lower risk of subclinical breast cancer, and their breasts have increased density. In this younger group, radiologic investigations are of limited value, unless a discrete breast lump is palpated.

LABORATORY TESTS

Although hormonal imbalance and abnormal lipid metabolism have been implicated in the etiopathogenesis of mastodynia, there is no good evidence to support any consistent pattern of serum hormonal or lipid profile in women with mastodynia. These tests are therefore not recommended.

IMAGING STUDIES

- Mammography should be part of the baseline investigations if the woman is >35 yr.
- Ultrasound can be performed as needed; it is particularly helpful in the assessment of cystic breast lesions.
- In women <35 yr, imaging investigations are not helpful unless a lump has been palpated clinically.
- There are no radiologic features associated with mastodynia: rather, radiologic investigations are performed to exclude the rare presence of a subclinical carcinoma.

TREATMENT

NONPHARMACOLOGIC THERAPY

- 85% of the women with mastodynia can be reassured after full clinical evaluation
- The remaining 15% will require some form of therapy in addition to reassurance
- Firm, supportive brassiere designed for postpartum use; this is particularly helpful if mastodynia is associated with breast swelling
- Low-fat, high-carbohydrate diet
- Reduction of caffeine intake

ACUTE GENERAL Rx

- Evening primrose oil (EPO), which contains gamma-linolenic acid, has been shown to have some effectiveness and is an acceptable treatment for mastodynia.
- Topical NSAID preparations may confer some benefit and can be prescribed for these women.
- Hormonal therapy is the mainstay of treatment.
- Danazol is the only drug approved by the FDA for the treatment of mastodynia. Danazol is an antigonadotrophin with some androgenic and peripheral antiestrogenic effects. Its efficacy is well established with significant relief of mastodynia in 70% to 93% of cases.
- Widespread use of danazol is limited because of its adverse side effects. These include menstrual irregularities, depression, acne, hirsutism, and, in severe cases, voice deepening. Women taking danazol should be advised to use effective nonhormonal contraception because of its potential adverse effects on the fetus.
- The side effects of danazol can be significantly reduced by using a low dose (100 mg daily) and confining treatment to the fortnight preceding menstruation.
- Tamoxifen, a synthetic antiestrogen, has also been shown to be effective in the treatment of mastodynia. Although effective in relieving symptoms, its use is extremely limited because of side effects. When used, it should be at a low dosage of 10 mg/day, and duration should be limited to 6 mo at a time. In the U.S., this agent has no approval for use in women with mastodynia.
- Bromocriptine is a dopamine-receptor agonist whose primary action is inhibition of prolactin release. It has been used extensively in the treatment of severe cyclical mastodynia and is effective. Again, side effects such as headache and dizziness have limited its use.
- Lisuride maleate was recently found to be effective by one study.
- Other hormonal agents that have been reported to be effective in small studies cannot be recommended. They either have unacceptable side effect profiles or their efficacy is not established. These agents include gestrinone, GnRH analogues, progesterone, and hormone replacement therapy.

CHRONIC Rx

- Long-standing cases of mastodynia can be managed with intermittent low-dose danazol therapy to limit side effects. In between these courses of hormone, nonpharmacologic and non-hormonal therapy can be used.
- Severe, unremitting mastodynia that fails to respond to medical treatment may require mastectomy; this is rare.

DISPOSITION

- Cyclical mastodynia resolves spontaneously in 20% to 30% of women.
- Up to 60% of women may develop recurrent symptoms 2 yr after treatment.
- Noncyclical mastodynia responds poorly to treatment, but may resolve spontaneously in up to 50% of women.

REFERRAL

- Detection of a breast lump or any other findings suggestive of neoplasm should be fully investigated. In addition, an immediate referral should be arranged.
- Women with chronic, unremitting mastodynia that fails to respond to pharmacologic therapy should be referred for possible mastectomy; this is rare.

PEARLS & CONSIDERATIONS

COMMENTS

- There is no good evidence to support the use of vitamin B_6, diuretics, and vitamin E. Mastodynia may represent a presenting symptom of other more generalized disorder (e.g., premenstrual syndrome, psychologic disturbance).
- In these cases, treating mastodynia in isolation will not work; the underlying conditions must be appropriately addressed.

SUGGESTED READINGS

Colgrave S, Holcombe C, Salmon P: Psychological characteristics of women presenting with breast pain, *J Psychosom Res* 50:303, 2001.

Fentiman IS, Hamed H: Assessment of breast problems, *Int J Clin Pract* 55:458, 2001.

Kaleli S et al: Symptomatic treatment of premenstrual mastalgia in premenopausal women with lisuride maleate: a double-blind placebo-controlled randomized study, *Fertil Steril* 75:718, 2001.

Marchant DJ: Benign breast disease, *Obstet Gynecol Clin North Am* 29:1-20, 2002.

Norlock FE: Benign breast pain in women: a practical approach to evaluation and treatment, *J Am Med Womens Assoc* 57:85, 2002.

AUTHORS: **ALEXANDER OLAWAIYE, M.D.,** and **RUBEN ALVERO, M.D.**

Section I DISEASES AND DISORDERS

BASIC INFORMATION

DEFINITION

Mastoiditis is inflammation of the mastoid process and air cells, a complication of otitis media.

SYNONYMS

Mastoid abscess

ICD-9CM CODES
383.00 Mastoiditis, acute or subacute
383.1 Mastoiditis, chronic

EPIDEMIOLOGY & DEMOGRAPHICS

INCIDENCE (IN U.S.): Widespread use of broad-spectrum antibiotics has led to a marked decline in the incidence of acute mastoiditis

PEAK INCIDENCE: Early childhood

PREDOMINANT SEX: More common in males

PREDOMINANT AGE: 2 mo to 18 yr

PHYSICAL FINDINGS & CLINICAL PRESENTATION

- Acute mastoiditis is usually a complication of acute otitis media.
- Most common presenting symptom: pain and tenderness in the postauricular region.
- Other signs or symptoms include:
  1. Fever
  2. Postauricular erythema and edema
  3. Protrusion of the pinna inferiorly and anteriorly
  4. Tympanic membrane usually intact with signs of acute otitis media
- Complications of acute mastoiditis include:
  1. Subperiosteal abscess (most common complication)
  2. Hearing loss
  3. Facial nerve palsy
  4. Labyrinthitis
  5. Intracranial complications such as hydrocephalus, meningitis, encephalitis, intracranial abscess, and lateral sinus thrombosis
- Chronic mastoiditis is characterized by chronic otorrhea and chronic tympanic membrane perforation.

ETIOLOGY

- Continuity exists between the middle air space and the mastoid cavity.
- Initial hyperemia and edema of the mucosal lining of the air cells results in accumulation of purulent exudate.
- Dissolution of calcium from bony septae and osteoclastic activity in the inflamed periosteum lead to bone necrosis and coalescence of air cells.
- Most common bacterial isolates:
  1. *Streptococcus pneumoniae*
  2. *Streptococcus pyogenes*
  3. *Haemophilus influenzae*
  4. *Moraxella catarrhalis*
  5. *Staphylococcus aureus*
- Often, multiple organisms in chronic mastoiditis, with predominance of anaerobes and gram-negative bacteria.
- *Mycobacterium tuberculosis,* nontuberculous mycobacteria, *Aspergillus* and *Rhodococcus equi* have been reported in cases of mastoiditis in severely immunocompromised individuals.

DIAGNOSIS

DIFFERENTIAL DIAGNOSIS

- Children
  1. Rhabdomyosarcoma
  2. Histiocytosis X
  3. Leukemia
  4. Kawasaki syndrome
- Adults
  1. Fulminant otitis externa
  2. Histiocytosis X
  3. Metastatic disease

WORKUP

Thorough history and physical examination are important in establishing diagnosis.

LABORATORY TESTS

- Fluid for Gram stain and culture may be obtained by myringotomy.
- If there is a perforation in the tympanic membrane with drainage, cultures of this may be taken after carefully cleaning the external canal.

IMAGING STUDIES

- Plain x-rays of the mastoid region may demonstrate clouding or opacification in areas of pneumatization.
- CT scan can demonstrate early involvement of bone (mastoiditis with bone destruction).
- MRI is more sensitive than CT scan in evaluating soft tissue involvement and is useful in conjunction with CT scan to investigate other complications of mastoiditis.

TREATMENT

NONPHARMACOLOGIC THERAPY

Myringotomy, if the ear is not already draining

ACUTE GENERAL Rx

- Initiated with IV antibiotics directed against the common organisms *S. pneumoniae* and *H. influenzae*. If the disease in the mastoid has had a prolonged course, coverage for *Staphylococcus aureus* with gram-negative enteric bacilli may be considered for initial therapy until results of cultures become available.
- Continued until all signs of mastoiditis have resolved
- Directed against enteric gram-negative organisms and anaerobes in chronic mastoiditis
- Indications for mastoidectomy:
  1. Failure to improve after 72 hr of therapy
  2. Persistent fever
  3. Imminent or overt signs of intracranial complications
  4. Evidence of a subperiosteal abscess in the mastoid bone

DISPOSITION

Proceed with mastoidectomy when medical therapy fails.

REFERRAL

- To otorhinolaryngologist:
  1. If diagnosis in doubt
  2. If aural complications present
  3. To evaluate for surgical intervention
- To neurosurgeon if intratemporal or intracranial extension of infection suspected
  1. Aural complications: bone destruction, subperiosteal abscess, petrositis, facial paralysis, labyrinthitis
  2. Intracranial complications: extradural abscess, lateral sinus thrombophlebitis or thrombosis, subdural abscess, meningitis, brain abscess, otitic hydrocephalus

PEARLS & CONSIDERATIONS

Mastoiditis is particularly difficult to eradicate because the mastoid air cells are poorly vascularized and difficult to drain.

EVIDENCE

According to a retrospective case review of 13 patients with acute mastoiditis, eradication of microorganisms requires appropriate antibiotics based on the infecting microorganism's susceptibility. If there is no improvement despite the use of antibiotics, myringotomy or mastoidectomy may be necessary.[1]

Evidence-Based Reference

1. Lee E-S et al: Clinical experiences with acute mastoiditis—1988 through 1998, *Ear Nose Throat J* 79:884, 2000.

SUGGESTED READINGS

Migirov L, Eyal A, Kronenberg J: Intracranial complications following mastoidectomy, *Pediatr Neurosurg* 40(5):226, 2004.

Oestreicher-Kedem Y et al: Complications of mastoiditis in children at the onset of a new millenium, *Ann Otol Rhinol Laryngol* 114(2):147, 2005.

Taylor MF, Berkowitz RG: Indications for mastoidectomy in acute mastoiditis in children, *Ann Otol Rhinol Laryngol* 113(1):69, 2004.

AUTHORS: **JANE V. EASON, M.D., MARILYN FABBRI, M.D., GLENN G. FORT, M.D., M.P.H.,** and **DENNIS J. MIKOLICH, M.D.**

BASIC INFORMATION

DEFINITION

Measles is a childhood exanthem, caused by an RNA virus called *Morbillivirus,* belonging to the family *Paramyxoviridae.*

SYNONYMS

Rubeola

ICD-9CM CODES
055.9 Measles
055.0 Encephalitis
055.1 Pneumonia
V04.2 Vaccination

EPIDEMIOLOGY & DEMOGRAPHICS

- Before the introduction of an effective vaccine in 1963, measles was one of the most common childhood illnesses, and in developing countries, where it strikes mostly children under age 5 yr, it remains a leading cause of childhood mortality
- 30 million cases worldwide each year
- In developed countries, measles outbreaks occur occasionally in adolescents and young adults who have not been immunized (incidence 0 to 10/100,000 person-years)

PHYSICAL FINDINGS & CLINICAL PRESENTATION

- Incubation: 10 to 14 days (up to 3 wk in adults)
- Prodrome: 2 to 4 days; malaise, fever, rhinorrhea, conjunctivitis, cough
- Exanthem phase: 7 to 10 days
  The fever increases and peaks at 104° to 105° F together with the rash; it persists for 5 or 6 days. The patient's fever decreases over 24 hr.
  Rash: Erythematous maculopapular eruption begins behind the ears, progresses to forehead and neck (Fig. 1-153), then spreads to face, trunk, upper extremities, buttocks, and lower extremities in that order. After 3 days the rash fades in the same sequence by becoming copper brown and then desquamates.
  Enanthem: Koplik spots are white papules of 1 to 2 mm in diameter on an erythematous base. They first appear on the buccal mucosa opposite the lower molar 2 days before the rash and spread over 24 hours to involve most of the buccal and lower labial mucosa. They fade after 3 days.
  Other symptoms and signs: malaise, anorexia, vomiting, diarrhea, abdominal pain, pharyngitis, lymphadenopathy, and occasional splenomegaly.
- Atypical measles (in vaccinated persons)
  Incubation: 10 to 14 days
  Prodrome: 1 to 3 days; high fever and headache
  Rash: maculopapular, urticarial, or petechial rash that begins peripherally and progresses centrally
- Modified measles applies to patients who have received immune serum globulin and develop a milder illness
- Complications (30% of cases):
  Otitis media
  Laryngitis, tracheitis
  Pneumonia (accounts for 90% of measles deaths)
  Encephalitis with lethargy, irritability, and seizures; 60% recover completely, 25% have neurologic sequelae (mental retardation, hemiplegia, paraplegia, epilepsy, deafness), and 15% die
  Myocarditis, pericarditis, and hepatitis
  Complications more common in immunocompromised hosts and persons with AIDS

ETIOLOGY & PATHOGENESIS

- The measles virus is transmitted through the respiratory tract by airborne droplets.
- It initially infects the respiratory epithelium; the patient becomes viremic during the prodromal phase and the virus is disseminated to skin, respiratory tract, and other organs.
- Viral clearance is achieved via cellular immunity.

DIAGNOSIS

DIFFERENTIAL DIAGNOSIS

- Other viral infections by enteroviruses, adenoviruses, human parvovirus B-19, rubella
- Scarlet fever
- Allergic reaction
- Kawasaki disease

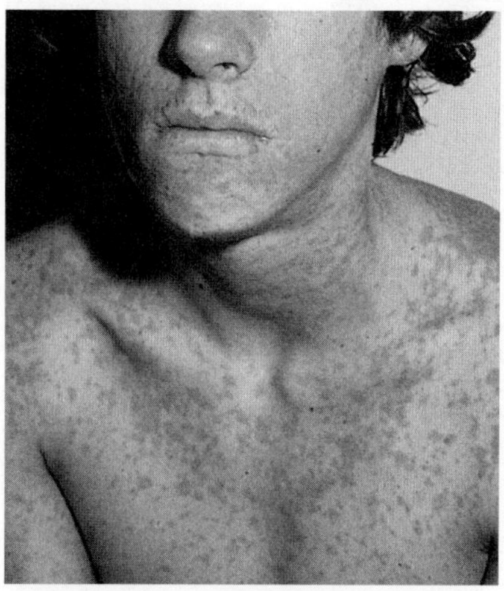

FIGURE 1-153 Rubeola. (From Zitelli BJ, Davis HW: *Atlas of pediatric physical diagnosis,* ed 5, St Louis, 2005, Mosby.)

WORKUP

Knowledge of outbreak, history and physical findings (Koplik spots are diagnostic), laboratory tests

LABORATORY TESTS

- CBC: leukopenia
- ELISA for measles antibodies, which appear shortly after the onset of the rash and peak 3 to 4 wk later
- CSF analysis in encephalitis may reveal a pleocytosis (lymphocytes) and an elevated protein

IMAGING STUDIES

Chest x-ray if pneumonia is suspected

TREATMENT

- Supportive
- Vitamin A
- Ribavirin for severe measles pneumonitis

PEARLS & CONSIDERATIONS

PREVENTION

- Passive immunization: Human immunoglobulin 0.25 ml/kg IM within 6 days of exposure. Double the dose for immunocompromised persons.
- Active immunization (see Section V).

EVIDENCE

Evidence for vaccination:

Monovalent measles and combined MMR vaccines are highly effective in preventing measles, with both vaccines having similar seroconversion rates at 6 wk.[1-3] Ⓐ

Evidence-Based References

1. Dezian Ltd: Measles. In: *Clin Evid* 11:436, London, 2004, BMJ Publishing Group. Ⓐ
2. Edees S, Pullan CR, Hull D: A randomised single blind trial of a combined mumps measles rubella vaccine to evaluate serological response and reactions in the UK population, *Public Health* 105:91, 1991. Reviewed in: *Clin Evid* 11:436, 2004. Ⓐ
3. Robertson CM et al: Serological evaluation of a measles, mumps and rubella vaccine, *Arch Dis Child* 63:612, 1988. Reviewed in: *Clin Evid* 11:436, 2004. Ⓐ

SUGGESTED READING

Mulholland EK: Measles in the United States, *N Engl J Med* 355:5, 2006.

AUTHORS: **FRED F. FERRI, M.D.,** and **TOM J. WACHTEL, M.D.**

BASIC INFORMATION

DEFINITION

Meckel diverticulum is an ileal diverticulum located 100 cm proximal to the cecum. It results from failure of the omphalomesenteric duct to obliterate completely (as it should by the eighth week of gestation).

SYNONYMS

MD

ICD-9CM CODES
751.0 Meckel diverticulum

EPIDEMIOLOGY & DEMOGRAPHICS

- Meckel diverticulum, based on autopsy studies and intraoperative evidence, occurs in 0.3% to 4% of the population and is the most prevalent congenital anomaly of the GI tract. Complications occur more frequently in males.
- Most patients who develop symptoms are younger than 10 yr.
- The lifetime risk of complications developing in a case of Meckel diverticulum is 4%.
- In adults, complications (small bowel obstruction [25% to 40%], diverticulitis [20%]) are usually due to factors other than heterotopic mucosa.
- Tumors have rarely been reported in symptomatic Meckel diverticulum, with carcinoid being the most common type.

PHYSICAL FINDINGS & CLINICAL PRESENTATION

- Painless lower GI bleeding (4%)
- Intestinal obstruction secondary to intussusception, volvulus, herniation, or entrapment of a loop of bowel through a defect in the diverticular mesentery (6%)
- Meckel's diverticulitis mimics acute appendicitis (5%)
- Rare primary tumor arising from diverticulum (carcinoid, sarcoma, leiomyoma, adenocarcinoma)
- Asymptomatic (80% to 95%)

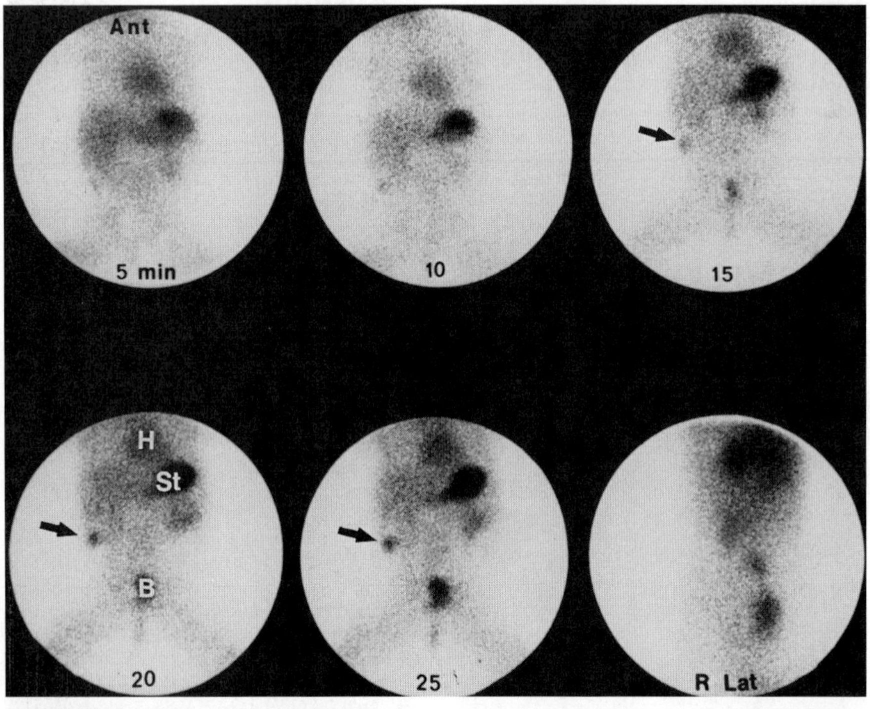

FIGURE 1-154 Meckel diverticulum. In this 2-year-old child who had unexplained rectal bleeding, a nuclear medicine study was performed using radioactive material that concentrates in gastric mucosa (technetium-99m pertechnetate). Sequential 5-minute images of the abdomen are obtained. On the 20-minute image, the heart *(H),* stomach *(St),* and bladder *(B)* are clearly seen, in addition to an ectopic focus of activity *(arrow)* representing a Meckel diverticulum. (From Mettler FA [ed]: *Primary care radiology,* Philadelphia, 2000, WB Saunders.)

ETIOLOGY & PATHOGENESIS

- As a remnant of the omphalomesenteric duct, Meckel diverticulum contains all layers of the intestinal wall and has its own mesentery and blood supply (branch of the superior mesenteric artery).
- The majority of complicated cases of Meckel diverticulum contain ectopic mucosa (75% gastric, 15% pancreatic). It causes ulceration and bleeding of ileal mucosa adjacent to the acidic ectopic gastric secretions. Alkaline secretions of ectopic pancreatic tissue can also cause ulcerations.

DIAGNOSIS

DIFFERENTIAL DIAGNOSIS

- Appendicitis
- Crohn's disease
- All causes of lower GI bleeding (polyp, colon cancer, AV malformation, diverticulosis, hemorrhoids)

WORKUP

- Diagnosis is often made intraoperatively when the preoperative diagnosis is appendicitis.
- Preoperative detection of symptomatic Meckel diverticulum requires a high index of suspicion.
- In the case of GI bleeding of unknown sources, a technetium scan will identify Meckel diverticulum (sensitivity: 85% in children, 62% in adults; specificity: 95% in children, 9% in adults) (Fig. 1-154).
- In patients with suspected small bowel obstruction, intussusception, or diverticulitis, a CT scan of the abdomen/pelvis is helpful.

TREATMENT

- Surgical resection in symptomatic patients.
- There is controversy regarding the need to remove an incidentally found diverticulum, with most surgeons arguing in favor of resection.

SUGGESTED READINGS

Feller A et al: Meckel diverticulum, *Arch Intern Med* 163:2093, 2003.

Martin JP et al: Meckel's diverticulum, *Am Fam Physician* 61:1037, 2000.

AUTHORS: **FRED F. FERRI, M.D.,** and **TOM J. WACHTEL, M.D.**

BASIC INFORMATION

DEFINITION

Meigs' syndrome is characterized by the presence of a benign solid ovarian tumor associated with ascites and right hydrothorax that disappear after tumor removal.

ICD-9CM CODES
620.2 Ovarian mass (unspecified)
220.0 Benign ovarian lesion
789.5 Ascites
511.9 Pleural effusion

EPIDEMIOLOGY & DEMOGRAPHICS

- Occurs in <1% of ovarian fibromas (associated with approximately 0.004% of ovarian tumors)
- Most frequently encountered during middle age (average age, approximately 48 yr)

PHYSICAL FINDINGS & CLINICAL PRESENTATION

- Asymptomatic pelvic mass on bimanual examination
- Intermittent pelvic pain (intermittent torsion)
- Acute pelvic tenderness
- Acute abdominal tenderness
- Abdominal pelvic mass
- Abdominal bloating
- Fluid wave
- Shifting dullness
- "Puddle sign"
- Hyperresonance or flatness to chest percussion, absence of tactile and vocal fremitus
- Absent or loud bronchial breath sounds, rales, mediastinal displacement, tracheal shift
- Weight loss and emaciation

ETIOLOGY

- Not specifically known
- Usually associated with "edematous" fibromas (or other benign ovarian solid tumor) in excess of 10 cm
- Plausible that large fibroma with narrow stalk has inadequate lymphatic drainage; when coupled with intermittent torsion, results in back flow transudation into the peritoneal cavity; accumulated peritoneal ascites then passes to the right pleural cavity via lymphatics (overloaded thoracic duct) or via abdominal pleural commutation (i.e., foramen of Bochdalek)

DIAGNOSIS

DIFFERENTIAL DIAGNOSIS

- Abdominal ovarian malignancy
- Various gynecologic disorders:
  1. Uterus; endometrial tumor, sarcoma, leiomyoma ("pseudo–Meigs' syndrome")
  2. Fallopian tube: hydrosalpinx, granulomatous salpingitis, fallopian tube malignancy
  3. Ovary: benign, serous, mucinous, endometrioid, clear cell, Brenner tumor, granulosa, stromal, dysgerminoma, fibroma, metastatic tumor
- Nongynecologic (GI tract or GU tract tumor or pathology) causes of pelvic mass
  1. Ascites
  2. Portal vein obstruction
  3. IVC obstruction
  4. Hypoproteinemia
  5. Thoracic duct obstruction
  6. TB
  7. Amyloidosis
  8. Pancreatitis
  9. Neoplasm
  10. Ovarian hyperstimulation
  11. Pleural effusion
  12. CHF
  13. Malignancy
  14. Collagen-vascular disease
  15. Pancreatitis
  16. Cirrhosis

WORKUP

- Clinical condition characterized by ovarian mass, ascites, and right-sided pleural effusion
- Ovarian malignancy and the other causes (see "Differential Diagnosis") of pelvic mass, ascites, and pleural effusion to be considered
- History of early satiety, weight loss with increased abdominal girth, bloating, intermittent abdominal pain, dyspnea, nonproductive cough

LABORATORY TESTS

- CBC to rule out inflammatory process
- Tumor markers (CA-125, hCG, AFP, CEA) to evaluate malignancy
- Chemical/LFT profile to evaluate metabolic or hepatic involvement

IMAGING STUDIES

- Pelvic sonography (color flow Doppler evaluation of adnexal mass) to evaluate pelvic pathology (CT scan or MRI if etiology indeterminate)
- Chest x-ray examination
- ABG if respiratory compromise

TREATMENT

NONPHARMACOLOGIC THERAPY

- Informed consent and proper preparation of patient for possible staging laparotomy (TAH-BSO, omentectomy, possible bowel resection, pelvic/periaortic lymphadenectomy)
- Bowel prep if considering pelvic malignancy

ACUTE GENERAL Rx

Depending on clinical presentation, size of pelvic mass, amount of ascites, and pleural effusion:

- If pelvic mass <10 cm, minimal ascites/pleural effusion: consider diagnostic open laparoscopy (possible exploratory laparotomy) and salpingo-oophorectomy with removal of ovarian fibroma (tumor).
- If pelvic mass >10 cm, moderate/large amount ascites/pleural effusion: consider pleurocentesis if respiratory compromise (cytology: AFB) and exploratory laparotomy with salpingo-oophorectomy and removal of ovarian fibroma (tumor).
- Treat pelvic malignancy, GI or GU tumor as indicated.

CHRONIC Rx

- Resolution of ascites and right-sided pleural effusion after removal of ovarian fibroma
- No long-term follow-up for benign ovarian fibroma

DISPOSITION

Excellent progress and complete survival are expected.

REFERRAL

To gynecologist or gynecologic oncologist for evaluation and treatment, especially if malignancy considered or encountered

SUGGESTED READINGS

Abramov Y et al: The role of inflammatory cytokines in Meigs' syndrome, *Obstet Gynecol* 99(5 Pt 2):917, 2002.

Buttin BM et al: Meigs' syndrome with an elevated CA 125 from benign Brenner tumors, *Obstet Gynecol* 98(5 Pt 2):980, 2001.

Meigs JV, Cass JW: Fibroma of the ovary with ascites and hydrothorax: with a report of seven cases, *Am J Obstet Gynecol* 33:249, 1937.

AUTHORS: **DENNIS M. WEPPNER, M.D.,** and **RUBEN ALVERO, M.D.**

BASIC INFORMATION

DEFINITION

Melanoma is a skin neoplasm arising from the malignant degeneration of melanocytes. It is classically subdivided in four types:

- Superficial spreading melanoma (70%) (Fig. 1-155, *A*)
- Nodular melanoma (15% to 20%) (Fig. 1-155, *B*)
- Lentigo maligna melanoma (5% to 10%)
- Acral lentiginous melanoma (7% to 10%)

SYNONYMS

Malignant melanoma

ICD-9CM CODES
172.9 Melanoma of the skin, site unspecified

EPIDEMIOLOGY & DEMOGRAPHICS

- Annual incidence of melanoma is 13 cases/100,000 persons.
- Melanoma has doubled to tripled in incidence over the past 25 years.
- Melanoma is the most common cancer among women 20 to 29 yr of age.
- Melanoma is much more common in whites (17.2/100,000 white men) than in blacks (1/100,000 black men).
- Lifetime risk of cutaneous melanoma for white Americans is 1/90.
- Melanoma is the leading cause of death from skin disease.
- Median age at diagnosis is 53 yr.
- Superficial spreading melanoma occurs most often in young adults on sun-exposed areas.
- Acral lentiginous melanoma is most often found in Asian Americans and African Americans and is not related to sun exposure.
- Death rate for white men with melanoma is 3/100,000.
- 8% to 10% of melanomas arise in people with a family history of the disease.

PHYSICAL FINDINGS & CLINICAL PRESENTATION

Variable depending on the subtype of melanoma:

- *Superficial spreading melanoma* is most often found on the lower legs, arms, and upper back. It may have a combination of many colors or may be uniformly brown or black.
- *Nodular melanoma* can be found anywhere on the body, but it most frequently occurs on the trunk on sun-exposed areas. It has a dark-brown or red-brown appearance, can be dome shaped or pedunculated; they are frequently misdiagnosed because they may resemble a blood blister or hemangioma and may also be amelanotic.
- *Lentigo maligna melanoma* is generally found in older adults in areas continually exposed to the sun and frequently arising from lentigo maligna (Hutchinson's freckle) or melanoma in situ. It might have a complex pattern and variable shape; color is more uniform than in superficial spreading melanoma.
- *Acral lentiginous melanoma* frequently occurs in soles, subungual mucous membranes, and palms (sole of the foot is the most prevalent site). Unlike other types of melanoma, it has a similar incidence in all ethnic groups.
- The warning signs that the lesion may be a melanoma can be summarized with the ABCD rules:

  A: Asymmetry (e.g., lesion is bisected and halves are not identical)

  B: Border irregularity (uneven, ragged border)

  C: Color variegation (presence of various shades of pigmentation)

  D: Diameter enlargement (>6 mm)

Recent data regarding small-diameter melanoma suggest that the ABCD criteria for gross inspection of pigmented skin lesions and early diagnosis of cutaneous melanoma should be expanded to ABCDE to include *Evolving* (i.e., lesions that have changed over time).

ETIOLOGY

- UV light is the most important cause of malignant melanoma.
- There is a modest increase in melanoma risk in patients with small nondysplastic nevi and a much greater risk in those with dysplastic lesions.
- The CDKN2A gene, residing at the 9p21 locus, is often deleted in people with familial melanoma.

DIAGNOSIS

DIFFERENTIAL DIAGNOSIS

- Dysplastic nevi
- Solar lentigo
- Vascular lesions
- Blue nevus
- Basal cell carcinoma
- Seborrheic keratosis

WORKUP

- Perform excisional biopsy with elliptical excision that includes 1 to 2 mm of normal skin surrounding the lesion and extends to the subcutaneous tissue; incisional punch biopsy is sometimes necessary in surgically sensitive areas (e.g., digits, nose).
- The sentinel lymph node dissection (SLND) should be considered in patients with intermediate (1 to 4 mm) melanomas or high-risk skin tumors to obtain information regarding a patient's subclinical lymph node status with minimal morbidity. It involves the use of radiologic lymphoscintigraphy to map lymphatic drainage from the site of the primary melanoma to the first "sentinel" lymph node in the region. When properly performed, if the sentinel node is negative, the remaining lymph nodes in the region will not have metastases in more than 98% of cases. The staging of intermediate thickness (1.2 to 3.5 mm) primary melanomas, according to the results of sentinel-node biopsy, provides important prognostic information and identifies patients with nodal metastases

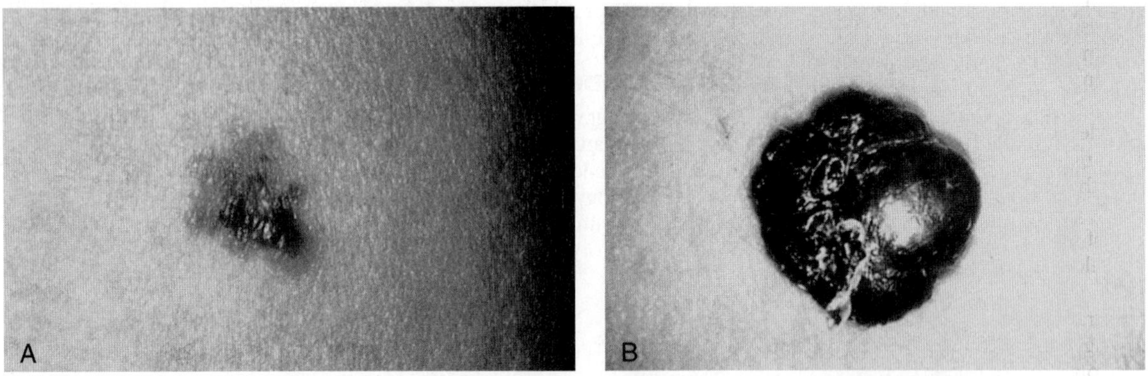

FIGURE 1-155 **A,** Superficial spreading melanoma. **B,** Nodular melanoma. (From Abeloff MD [ed]: *Clinical oncology,* ed 3, New York, 2004, Churchill Livingstone.)

whose survival can be prolonged by immediate lymphadenectomy.

- The staging system for melanoma adapted by the American Joint Committee on Cancer (AJCC) is as follows:

T*	Thickness of primary tumor
Tis	In situ
T1	≤1.0 mm
T2	1.01-2.0 mm
T3	2.01-4.0 mm
T4	>4.0 mm
N†	Number of positive lymph nodes
N0	0
N1	1
N2	2 or 3
N3	≥4 (or combination of in-transit metastases, satellite lesions, or an ulcerated primary lesion with any number of nodes)
M	Metastases
M0	0
M1	Distant subcutaneous or lymph node metastases
M2	Lung metastases
M3	All other visceral or any distant metastases or an elevated lactate dehydrogenase level not attributable to another cause
Clinical Stage	
0	(T0N0M0)
IA	(T1aN0M0)
IB	(T1bN0M0) (T2aN0M0)
IIA	(T2bN0M0) (T3aN0M0)
IIB	(T3bN0M0) (T4aN0M0)
IIC	(T4bN0M0)
IIIA	(T1-T4aN1bM0)
IIIB	(T1-T4aN2bM0)
IIIC	(AnyT,N2c,M0) (Any T, N3, M0)
IV	(Any T, Any N, >M1)

*a, Without ulceration; b, with ulceration
†a, Micrometastasis; b, macrometastases; c, in-transit metastases with metastatic lymph nodes

LABORATORY TESTS

The pathology report should indicate the following:

- Tumor thickness (Breslow microstage).
- Tumor depth (Clark level): The depth of invasion is the most important histologic prognostic parameter in evaluating the primary tumor.
- Mitotic rate: tabulated as mitosi per mm^2 in the dermal part of the tumor in which most mitoses are identified.
- Radial growth rates vs. vertical growth rate: Radial growth phase describes the growth of melanoma within the epidermis and along the dermal-epidermal junction.
- Tumor infiltrating lymphocytes: They have a strong predictive value in vertical growth phase melanomas and are defined as brisk, nonbrisk, and absent.
- Histologic regression: characterized by the absence of melanoma in the epidermis and dermis flanked on one or both sides by melanoma.
- Reverse transcriptase-polymerase chain reaction (RT-PCR) assay for tyrosine messenger RNA is a useful marker for the presence of melanoma cells. It is performed on sentinel lymph node biopsy and is useful for detection of submicroscopic metastases.

TREATMENT (Rx)

- Initial excision of the melanoma
- Reexcision of the involved area after histologic diagnosis:
  1. The margins of reexcision depend on the thickness of the tumor.
  2. Low-risk or intermediate-risk tumors require excision of 1 to 3 cm.
  3. Melanomas of moderate thickness (0.9 to 2.0 mm) can be excised safely with 2-cm margins.
  4. A 1-cm margin of excision for melanoma with a poor prognosis (as defined by a tumor thickness of at least 2 mm) is associated with a significantly greater risk of regional recurrence than is a 3-cm margin, but with a similar overall survival rate.
- Lymph node dissection: recommended in all patients with enlarged lymph nodes. Lymph node evaluation is important in patients with melanoma 1 mm in depth because it determines the overall prognosis and need for therapeutic lymph node dissection or adjuvant treatment.
  1. Elective lymph node dissection remains controversial.
  2. It is indicated with positive sentinel node. It may be considered in those with a primary melanoma that is between 1 and 4 mm thick (especially in patients <60 yr of age).
- Adjuvant therapy with interferon alfa-2b (intron A) in patients with metastatic melanoma is approved by the FDA for AJCC stages IIb and III melanoma; however, its statistical benefit remains unclear.
- Dacarbazine (DTIC) and interleukin 2 (IL-2) can be used in metastatic melanoma. Results are generally poor, with median survival in patients with distant metastatic melanoma approximately 6 mo.
- Recent attention has focused on combinations of dacarbazine and cisplatin with interleukin-2 and interferon alfa (biochemotherapy).
- Novel therapeutics involve cancer vaccines and use of granulocyte-macrophage colony-stimulating factor (GM-CSF) and angiogenesis inhibitors.
- Patients with a history of melanoma should be followed with skin examinations every 6 mo or sooner if patient detects any new lesions; the assessments usually consist of medical history, exam, labs, and chest x-ray.

DISPOSITION

- Prognosis varies with the stage of the melanoma. The 5-yr survival related to thickness is as follows: <0.76 mm, 99% survival; 0.6 to 1.49 mm, 85%; 1.5 to 2.49 mm, 84%; 2.5 to 3.9 mm, 70%; >4 mm, 44%.
- The 5-yr survival in patients with distant metastasis is <10%.
- Treatment of advanced disease consists (in addition to surgical excision and lymph node dissection) of chemotherapy, immunotherapy, and radiation therapy.

EVIDENCE (EBM)

Wide surgical margins have not been shown to improve survival rates.[1] (A)

Narrow margins are as effective in controlling local recurrence and reduce the need for skin grafting.[2] (A)

No significant survival benefit was noted for elective lymph node dissection (in patients with no clinical evidence of metastases) in four randomized controlled trials (RCTs). In a retrospective analysis, there was a trend toward benefit for elective dissection for certain patients.[2] (A)

Combination chemotherapy and dacarbazine have been compared with placebo in RCTs. No survival advantage was noted in patients receiving chemotherapy.[2] (A)

Increased disease-free and overall survival have been found in some trials with high-dose interferon alpha-2b, and there is evidence of increased time before relapse.[2] (A)

However, the evidence that any systemic treatments are superior to best available supportive care in metastatic malignant melanoma is inconsistent.[3] (A)

Evidence-Based References

1. Lens MB et al: Excision margins in the treatment of primary cutaneous melanoma: a systematic review of randomized controlled trials comparing narrow vs wide excision, *Arch Surg* 137:1101, 2002. (A)
2. Savage P, Crosby T, Mason M: Malignant melanoma: non-metastatic. Reviewed in: *Clin Evid* 10:1897, London, 2003, BMJ Publishing Group. (A)
3. Crosby T et al: Systemic treatments for metastatic cutaneous melanoma. Reviewed in: Cochrane Library, 1, Chichester, UK, 2004, John Wiley. (A)

SUGGESTED READINGS

Markovic S et al: Malignant melanoma in the 21st century, *Mayo Clin Proc* 82(3):364; 82(4):490, 2007.

Miller AJ, Mihm MC: Melanoma, *N Engl J Med* 355:51, 2006.

AUTHOR: **FRED F. FERRI, M.D.**

BASIC INFORMATION

DEFINITION

Meniere's disease is a syndrome characterized by recurrent vertigo with fluctuating hearing loss, tinnitus, and fullness in the ear.

SYNONYMS

Endolymphatic hydrops
Lermoyez's syndrome

ICD-9CM CODES
386.01 Meniere's disease, cochleovestibular (active)

EPIDEMIOLOGY & DEMOGRAPHICS

INCIDENCE (IN U.S.): 100 cases/100,000 persons
PREVALENCE (IN U.S.): 15 cases/100,000 persons
PREDOMINANT SEX: Male = female
PEAK INCIDENCE: 20 to 50 yr

PHYSICAL FINDINGS & CLINICAL PRESENTATION

- Hearing may be unilaterally decreased.
- Pallor, sweating, and nausea may occur during a severe attack.
- Usually the patient develops a sensation of fullness and pressure along with decreased hearing and tinnitus in a single ear.
- The patient typically experiences severe vertigo, which peaks within minutes, then slowly subsides over hours.
- May see spontaneous nystagmus on examination.
- Persistent sense of disequilibrium for days is typical after an acute episode
- May have vestibulopathy demonstrable with a positive head thrust test.

ETIOLOGY

- Unknown; viral and autoimmune etiologies have been suggested.
- Associated with endolymphatic hydrops.

DIAGNOSIS

Proposed criteria by the American Academy of Otolaryngology-Head and Neck Surgery (AAO-HNS) for diagnosis of Meniere's disease include the following four features, of which 1 and at least one of 2, 3, or 4 must be present:

1. Two spontaneous episodes of vertigo lasting 20 minutes or longer without loss of consciousness
2. Hearing loss that is usually, but not always, fluctuating
3. Tinnitus in the ear, which may fluctuate
4. Aural fullness in the ear, which may fluctuate

DIFFERENTIAL DIAGNOSIS

- Acoustic neuroma
- Migrainous vertigo
- Multiple sclerosis
- Autoimmune inner ear syndrome
- Otitis media
- Vertebrobasilar disease
- Labyrinthitis

WORKUP

- Electronystagmography may show peripheral vestibular deficit.
- Electrocochleography and glycerol test used by some otoneurologists and ENT specialists.

LABORATORY TESTS

Audiogram may show sensorineural hearing loss, with lower frequencies primarily affected.

IMAGING STUDIES

MRI to rule out acoustic neuroma, especially if cerebellar or CNS dysfunction is present

TREATMENT

ACUTE GENERAL Rx

- Prochlorperazine 5 to 10 mg po q6h or 25 mg po bid
- Promethazine 12.5 to 25 mg po q4 to 6h
- Diazepam 5 to 10 mg IV/po for acute attack
- Meclizine 25 mg q6h, during acute attack only
- Scopolamine patch

CHRONIC Rx

- Diuretics such as hydrochlorothiazide or acetazolamide, salt restriction (1 to 2 gm sodium/day), and avoidance of caffeine are traditional.
- For refractory cases, surgical interventions, such as transtympanic gentamycin injections or endolymphatic shunt placement. More recently, low-pressure micropulses to the inner ear using the Meniett device has been shown to be effective in some patients.

DISPOSITION

- Usually followed by an otoneurologist or ENT specialist.
- Usual course of disease consists of alternating attacks and remissions.
- Majority of patients can be managed medically. 10% to 30% of patients will undergo surgical intervention for persistent incapacitating vertigo.

REFERRAL

To an otolaryngologist for surgical intervention if attacks persist despite medical therapy

PEARLS & CONSIDERATIONS

COMMENTS

- Many variations of the classical clinical picture. The essential features for diagnosis are episodic vertigo and sensorineural hearing loss audiometrically documented on at least one occasion.
- In one third of patients both ears are eventually involved.
- Some evidence that Meniere's disease and migraines may be pathophysiologically linked.

EVIDENCE

Many management protocols have been published for the treatment of the symptoms of Meniere's disease with little evidence to support their efficacy.[1]

Seventeen out of 33 patients preferred dyazide to placebo in the only double-blind, crossover, placebo-controlled study of the effect of diuretic therapy on controlling symptoms of Meniere's disease.[2]

A small randomized double-blinded placebo-controlled trial found no statistically significant decrease in the number of vertigo spells in patients diagnosed with Meniere's disease treated with famciclovir.[3]

No randomized placebo-controlled trials have examined the effects of endolymphatic shunting procedures or vestibular neurectomy on controlling symptoms of Meniere's disease.

Vertigo control was achieved in 32 out of 37 patients receiving intratympanic injection of gentamycin for treatment of unilateral Meniere's disease in one study of a prospective case series.[4]

Results of a 2-year long-term unblinded follow-up after a prior randomized, placebo-controlled, multicenter clinical trial of the Meniett device for Meniere's disease found that use of the device was associated with a significant reduction in vertigo frequency in about two thirds of the participants, and this improvement was maintained long term.[5]

Evidence-Based References

1. Thorp MA et al: Does evidence-based medicine exist in the treatment of Ménière's disease? A critical review of the last decade of publications, *Clin Otolaryngol* 25:456-460, 2000.
2. van Deelen GW, Huizing EH: Use of a diuretic (dyazide) in the treatment of Ménière's disease. A double-blind cross-over placebo-controlled study, *ORL J Otorhinolaryngol Relat Spec* 48:287-292, 1986.

3. Derebery MJ, Fisher LM, Iqbal Z: Randomized double-blinded, placebo-controlled clinical trial of famciclovir for reduction of Meniere's disease symptoms, *Otolaryngol Head Neck Surg* 131(6):877-884, 2004.
4. Youssef TF, Poe DS: Intratympanic gentamycin injection for the treatment of Meniere's disease, *Am J Otol* 19(4):435, 1998.
5. Gates GA et al: Meniett clinical trial: long-term follow-up, *Arch Otolarygnol Head Neck Surg* 132(12):1311, 2006.

SUGGESTED READINGS

Committee on Hearing and Equilibrium of the AAO-HNS: Revised guidelines for the diagnosis and evaluation of therapy in Meniere's disease, *Otolaryngol Head Neck Surg* 113:181-185, 1995.

Gates GA: Meniere's disease review 2005, *J Am Acad Audiol,* 17(1):16, 2006.

Radtke A et al: Migraine and Meniere's disease: is there a link? *Neurology* 59(11): 1700-1704, 2002.

Thai-Von H, Bounaix MJ, Fraysse B: Meniere's disease: pathophysiology and treatment, *Drugs* 61(8):1089, 2001.

Weber PC, Adkins WY Jr: The differential diagnosis of Meniere's disease, *Otolaryngol Clin North Am* 30(6):977, 1997.

AUTHOR: **SHARON HARTMAN POLENSEK, M.D., PH.D.**

BASIC INFORMATION

DEFINITION

Meningiomas are generally slow-growing, intracranial tumors attached to the dura and arising from arachnoid cells of the arachnoid villi; most meningiomas (90%) are benign, with the remaining 10% being atypical or malignant.

ICD-9CM CODES
225.2 Cerebral meninges

EPIDEMIOLOGY & DEMOGRAPHICS

INCIDENCE (IN U.S.): 6 cases/100,000 persons per yr. Account for approximately 20% of primary intracranial tumors and are the second most common brain tumor in adults. Often underreported.

PEAK INCIDENCE: Males: sixth decade; females: seventh decade; rare in childhood.

PREDOMINANT SEX: Female:male ratio of almost 3:1 in the brain and up to 6:1 in the spinal cord; male > female in childhood and male = female among African Americans.

GENETICS: Approximately half of meningiomas have allelic losses involving chromosome 22q12. Allelic losses of chromosomes 1p, 6q, 9q, 10q, 14q, 17p, and 18q are seen in atypical meningiomas, suggesting that these loci may be important for progression.

ENVIRONMENTAL: Only known environmental risk factor is ionizing radiation.

PHYSICAL FINDINGS & CLINICAL PRESENTATION

- Neurologic symptoms vary with location and size; meningiomas can arise from the dura at any site, although most commonly occur over the cerebral convexities, often associated with the falx. Other common locations include the parasaggital regions, sphenoid wing, olfactory groove, and optic nerve sheath.
- May be asymptomatic and present incidentally on a neuroimaging study or at autopsy.
- Meningiomas may cause focal or generalized seizures, hemiparesis, headache, personality change/confusion, hearing loss, visual impairment, and obstructive hydrocephalus.
- Children are more likely to exhibit signs of increased intracranial pressure without further localizing features.

ETIOLOGY

- Mutations of the *NF2* gene on chromosome 22 are found in >50% of meningiomas. This gene is thought to act as a tumor suppressor gene; the protein product, merlin, is also involved in cytoskeletal organization.
- Mutations of the *DAL-1* gene, thought to be a meningioma susceptibility gene which is located on chromosome 18p, have been identified in a subset of the approximately 40% of sporadic meningiomas that have neither the *NF2* gene mutations nor allelic loss of chromosome 22q.
- Cranial radiation may be responsible for some cases following an appropriate latency period from 10 to 20 years. For example, survivors of Hiroshima have an increased incidence of meningiomas. More recent methods of delivering radiation with focused-beam techniques has limited exposure of areas outside the target, so are expected to be safer. Meningiomas that result from radiation are generally more aggressive.
- The link with steroid hormones and their receptors is suggested by the increase in growth rate and/or development of meningiomas during luteal phase of the menstrual cycle and during pregnancy, as well as in women who use postmenopausal hormones or in association with breast carcinomas.
- There is an increased incidence in individuals having suffered a head injury, though the relationship is not clearly understood.

DIAGNOSIS

DIFFERENTIAL DIAGNOSIS

- Other well-circumscribed intracranial tumors:
- Acoustic schwannoma (typically at the pontocerebellar junction)
- Ependymoma, lipoma, and metastases within the spinal cord
- Metastatic disease from lymphoma/adenocarcinoma, inflammatory disease, or infections such as tuberculosis

WORKUP

- Imaging studies with CT or MRI, followed by surgical removal with histologic confirmation.
- According to the World Health Organization (WHO) classification, there are nine benign histologic variants and four variants associated with increased recurrence and rates of metastasis. Ninety percent of meningiomas are classified as benign meningiomas or WHO grade I.
- Meningiomas may recur after surgical resection. In addition, some tumors show histologic progression to a higher grade. Features suggesting increased rate of recurrence include:
  - Allelic loss of chromosome 22 appears to happen early in the development of aggressive meningiomas
  - Loss of 14q, and later losses of other chromosomes such as 1p, 2p, 6q, and 9q, which are associated with histologic and clinical progression
  - Overexpression of p53 protein
  - Brain invasion, high rate of mitosis, and highly anaplastic features

IMAGING STUDIES

- Cranial CT scanning or MRI can detect and determine the extent of meningiomas (Fig. 1-156). CT can show hyperostosis and/or intratumoral calcifications. MRI is preferable to show the dural origin of the tumor in most cases, with the characteristic "dural tail."
- On nonenhanced scans, meningiomas typically are isodense to slightly hyperdense to brain and are homogeneous in appearance. Meningiomas show homogeneous enhancement; gadolinium can facilitate imaging of smaller additional lesions that are missed on unenhanced images (Fig 1-157).
- Indistinct margins, marked edema, mushroom-like projections from tumor, brain parenchymal infiltration, and heterogeneous enhancement are suggestive of more aggressive behavior.
- PET scan may help in predicting the aggressiveness of the tumor and the potential for recurrence.

TREATMENT

NONPHARMACOLOGIC THERAPY

Appropriate treatment options depend on location. The mainstay of treatment for meningiomas remains surgical removal if symptomatic. After total excision, recurrence rates of 0% to 20% have

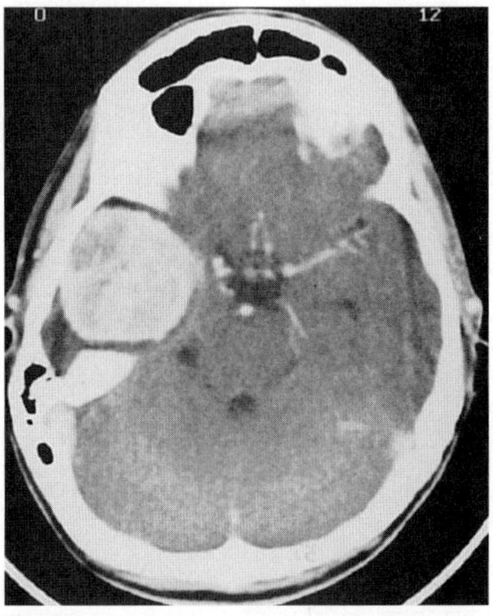

FIGURE 1-156 Contrast-enhanced CT scan demonstrates a large contrast-enhancing right sphenoid wing meningioma. (From Specht N [ed]: *Practical guide to diagnostic imaging,* St Louis, 1998, Mosby.)

been observed, whereas 20% to 50% of patients recur within 5 years of a subtotal resection.

ACUTE GENERAL Rx

- For lesions that cause significant mass effect, steroids are sometimes used to decrease brain edema.
- Anticonvulsants to control seizures. The use of prophylactic anticonvulsants is controversial without a clear history of seizures.

CHRONIC Rx

- Radiation therapy is the only validated form of adjuvant therapy and may be beneficial in patients with incomplete resections or inoperable tumors.
- Sterotactic radiosurgery can provide local control with more limited toxicity.
- Little information is available on the efficacy of traditional chemotherapy, and the evidence is largely anecdotal.
  - Regimens with some activity in malignant meningiomas include cyclophosphamide, Adriamycin and vincristine, dacarbazine and Adriamycin, or high-dose ifosfamide.
  - Hydroxyurea induces apoptosis and inhibits meningioma growth in culture.
  - Hormonal treatments, such as the progesterone and glucocorticoid receptor antagonist mifepristone (RU486), are currently under investigation based on the rationale that there is a link between progesterones and the development of meningiomas.

DISPOSITION

- Estimated surgical mortality is 7%. Significant morbidity and mortality can be observed in meningiomas with otherwise favorable pathology secondary to unfavorable location (e.g., skull base).
- Long-term outcome varies, based on pathology, tumor grade, location, and completeness of resection.
- Most incidentally discovered meningiomas remain asymptomatic and experience a slow rate of growth. Calcified tumors may be less likely to progress than noncalcified ones.

REFERRAL

Neurosurgical consultation for all cases

PEARLS & CONSIDERATIONS

- Many meningiomas are discovered incidentally; most are benign and remain asymptomatic.
- "Dural tail" is classic finding on neuroimaging studies.
- Individuals with neurofibromatosis type 2 are at high risk to develop meningiomas.

EVIDENCE

EBM

Postoperative radiotherapy greatly reduces the risk of recurrence and extends survival in patients with meningiomas who have undergone subtotal tumor resection.[1] Ⓑ

Evidence-Based Reference

1. Blomgren H: Brain tumors, *Acta Oncologica* suppl 7:16, 1996. Reviewed in: DARE Document 978123, York, UK, Centre for Reviews and Dissemination.

SUGGESTED READINGS

Drummond KJ et al: Meningiomas: updating basic science, management, and outcome, *Neurologist* 10(3):113, 2004.

Glantz MJ et al: Practice parameter: anticonvulsant prophylaxis in patients with newly diagnosed brain tumors. Report of the Quality Standards Subcommittee of the American Academy of Neurology, *Neurology* 54:1886, 2000.

Kleihues P et al: The WHO classification of tumors of the nervous system, *J Neuropathol Exp Neurol* 61(3):215, 2002.

Mason WP: Stabilization of disease progression by hydroxyurea in patients with recurrent or unresectable meningioma, *J Neurosurg* 97:341, 2002.

McMullen KP, Stieber VW: Meningioma: current treatment options and future directions, *Curr Treat Options Oncol* 5(6):499, 2004.

Perry A et al: Molecular pathogenesis of meningiomas, *J Neurooncol* 70(2):183, 2004.

Seizinger JP: Deletion mapping of a locus on human chromosome 22 involved in the oncogenesis of meningioma, *Proc Natl Acad Sci USA* 84:5419, 1987.

Whittle, IR et al: Meningiomas, *Lancet* 363:1535, 2004.

AUTHOR: **NICOLE J. ULLRICH, M.D., PH.D.**

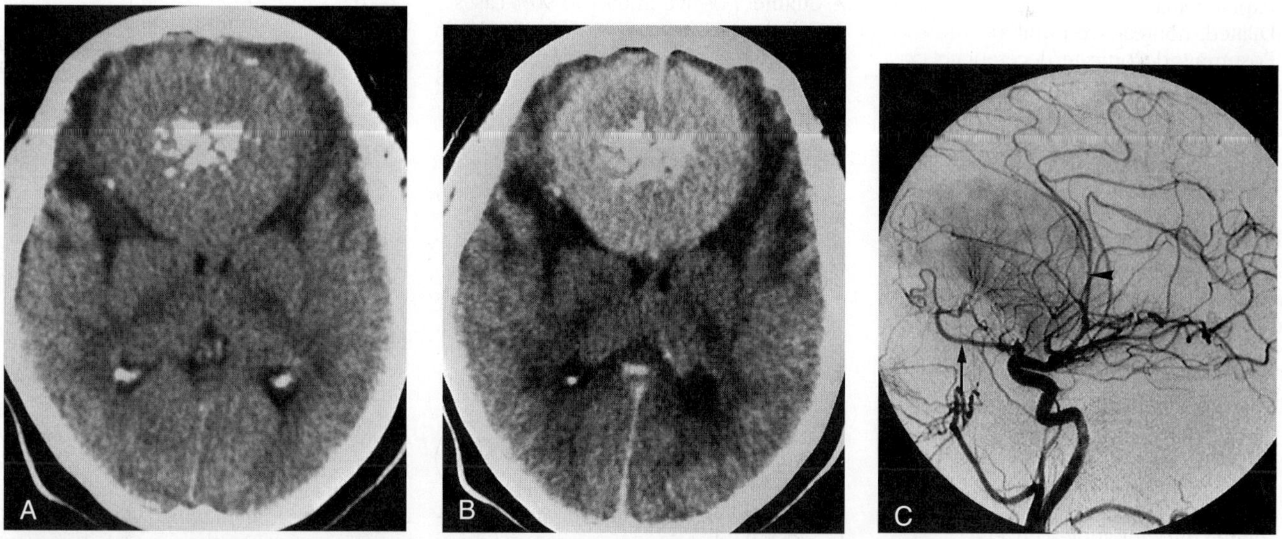

FIGURE 1-157 Subfrontal meningioma. CT before **(A)** and after **(B)** intravenous contrast medium, and lateral projection of common carotid arteriogram **(C)**. There is a large circumscribed mass in the anterior cranial fossa that is isodense to normal gray matter, contains foci or calcification centrally, and enhances homogenously. There is edema in the white matter of both frontal lobes and posterior displacement and splaying of the frontal horns of the lateral ventricles. On the arteriogram **(C)**, the mass is delineated by a tumor blush and there is posterior displacement of the anterior cerebral arteries *(arrowhead)* mirroring the mass effect seen on CT. The ophthalmic artery is enlarged as its ethmoidal branches supply the tumor *(arrow)*. (From Grainger RG et al [eds]: *Grainger & Allison's diagnostic radiology,* ed 4, Philadelphia, 2001, Churchill Livingstone.)

BASIC INFORMATION

DEFINITION

Bacterial meningitis is an inflammation of meninges with increased intracranial pressure, and pleocytosis or increased WBCs in CSF secondary to bacteria in the pia-subarachnoid space and ventricles, leading to neurologic sequelae and abnormalities.

SYNONYMS

Spinal meningitis

ICD-9CM CODES
320 Bacterial meningitis

EPIDEMIOLOGY & DEMOGRAPHICS

INCIDENCE (IN U.S.): 3 cases/100,000 persons
PREDOMINANT SEX: Male = female
PREDOMINANT AGE: All ages, neonate to geriatric

PHYSICAL FINDINGS & CLINICAL PRESENTATION

- Fever
- Headache
- Neck stiffness, nuchal rigidity, meningismus
- Altered mental state, lethargy
- Vomiting, nausea
- Photophobia
- Seizures
- Coma; lethargy, stupor
- Rash: petechial associated with meningococcal infection
- Myalgia
- Cranial nerve abnormality (unilateral)
- Papilledema
- Dilated, nonreactive pupil(s)
- Posturing: decorticate/decerebrate
- Physical examination findings of Kernig's sign and Brudzinski's sign in adults with meningitis are often not helpful in determining meningeal inflammation

ETIOLOGY

Neisseria meningitidis is now more common than *Haemophilus influenzae* as a cause of bacterial meningitis in children as well as adults. *H. influenzae* is the cause of >30% of cases of meningitis (usually in infants and children <6 yr of age). It is associated with sinusitis, otitis media.

- Neonates: group B streptococci, *Escherichia coli*, *Klebsiella* sp., *Listeria monocytogenes*
- Infants through adolescence:
  1. *N. meningitidis*
  2. *H. influenzae*
  3. *Streptococcus pneumoniae*
- Adults
  1. *N. meningitidis*
  2. *S. pneumoniae*
- Elderly
  1. *S. pneumoniae*
  2. *N. meningitidis*
  3. *L. monocytogenes*
  4. Gram-negative bacilli

DIAGNOSIS

Diagnostic approach is based on patient presentation and physical examination. Key elements to diagnosis are CSF evaluation and CT scan or MRI if the patient is in a coma or has focal neurologic deficits, pupillary abnormalities, or papilledema.

DIFFERENTIAL DIAGNOSIS

- Endocarditis, bacteremia
- Intracranial tumor
- Lyme disease
- Brain abscess
- Partially treated bacterial meningitis
- Medications
- SLE
- Seizures
- Acute mononucleosis
- Other infectious meningitides
- Neuroleptic malignant syndrome
- Subdural empyema
- Rocky Mountain spotted fever

WORKUP

CSF examination:

- Opening pressure >100 to 200 mm Hg
- WBC <5 to >100 mm^3
- Neutrophilic predominance: >80%
- Gram stain of CSF: positive in 60% to 90% patients
- CSF protein: >50 mg/dl
- CSF glucose: <40 mg/dl
- Culture: positive in 65% to 90% cases
- CSF bacterial antigen: 50% to 100% sensitivity
- E-test for susceptibility of pneumococcal isolates

LABORATORY TESTS

Blood culturing, WBC with differential, and CSF examination (see "Workup")

IMAGING STUDIES

- CT scan or MRI of head: necessary with increased intracranial pressure, coma, neurologic deficits
- Sinus CT: if sinusitis suspected

TREATMENT

Empiric therapy is necessary with IV antibiotic treatment if patient has purulent CSF fluid at time of lumbar puncture, is asplenic, or has signs of DIC/sepsis pending Gram stain and culture results. Therapy after Gram stain pending cultures is recommended for the following:

1. Neonates: ampicillin plus cefotaxime
2. Infants/children: ampicillin or third-generation cephalosporin (plus chloramphenicol if purulent or patient compromised)
3. Adults (18 to 50 yr): third-generation cephalosporin
4. Older adults (>50 yr): ampicillin plus third-generation cephalosporin

- Penicillin-resistant pneumococcus: because of an increasing incidence of this organism, empiric treatment with ceftriaxone or cefotaxime plus vancomycin (25 to 50 mg/kg/day) has been recommended.
- Table 1-25 describes common pathogens of bacterial meningitis and their empiric treatment based on age.
- Table 1-26 describes specific antibiotic treatments for known pathogens.
- Steroids: dexamethasone 0.15 mg/kg q6h for first 4 days of therapy should be used in adults with bacterial meningitis and mental status changes or acute neurologic phenomenon. Decreased mortality and neurologic sequelae are seen with adjunct therapy.
- Dexamethasone also benefits children with Hib or pneumococcal meningitis and should be given within the first 2 days of illness.

DISPOSITION

Bacterial meningitis is a reportable disease that needs to be reported to local health authorities.

REFERRAL

- To a neurologist if persistent neurologic sequelae develop after bacterial meningitis
- To an infectious disease consultant if a patient has recurrent bacterial meningitis. Such patients deserve a workup for an anatomic (CSF dural leak) or immunologic defect (complement defect, hyposplenism, immunoglobulin deficiency)

PEARLS & CONSIDERATIONS

COMMENTS

- Prevention of meningitis can be achieved through chemoprophylaxis of close contacts (household members and anyone exposed to oral secretions).
- Effective medications are rifampin 10 mg/kg PO bid for 2 days or ceftriaxone 250 mg IM single dose in patients over age 12; 125 mg IM if age 12 and under.
- Ciprofloxacin 500 mg for prevention of Neisseria meningitis can be given to patients over the age of 18 yr who cannot tolerate rifampin to eradicate pharyngeal colonization.
- Vaccines against serogroup A, C, Y, W-135 capsular polysaccharides are available for adults and children over the age of 2 yr; a protein-conjugate vaccine is now available.

EVIDENCE

EBM

A systematic review comparing third-generation cephalosporins vs. penicillin/ampicillin-chloramphenicol in patients with acute bacterial meningitis found that there were no significant differences between them apart from the third-generation cefalosporin group having a decreased risk of positive cerebrospinal fluid culture after 10 to 48 hr but also a significantly increased risk of diarrhea.[1] A

The studies included in the above review are not recent and concerns have been made that the results may not be applicable to routine clinical practice today.[1] A

A randomized controlled trial (RCT) concluded that chloramphenicol treatment of acute bacterial meningitis in children had the worst results compared with ampicillin, cefotaxime, or ceftriaxone. A 7-day course of ampicillin, cefotaxime, or ceftriaxone was considered sufficient in this trial, which included children suffering from Hib, meningococcal, or pneumococcal meningitis.[2] B

A prospective, randomized, double-blind trial found that dexamethasone

TABLE 1-25 Common Pathogens of Bacterial Meningitis and Their Empiric Treatment Based on Age

Age	Common Pathogens	Treatment*	Duration (days)
0-1 mo	Group B streptococcus *Listeria monocytogenes* *Escherichia coli*	Ampicillin + third-generation cephalosporin† or ampicillin + aminoglycoside	14-21 14-21 21
1-3 mo	*Streptococcus pneumoniae* Group B streptococcus, *E. coli, L. monocytogenes* *S. pneumoniae* *Neisseria meningitidis, Haemophilus influenzae*	Ampicillin + third-generation cephalosporin†	10-14 14-21 14-21 10-14 7-10
3 mo-18 yr	*H. influenzae, H. meningitidis, S. pneumoniae*	Third-generation cephalosporin† or meropenem or chloramphenicol	7-10 (*N. influenzae* and *N. meningitidis*) 10-14 *(S. pneumoniae)*
18-50 yr	*H. influenzae, N. meningitidis, S. pneumoniae*	Third-generation cephalosporin† or meropenem or ampicillin + chloramphenicol	Same as above
>50 yr	*S. pneumoniae, L. monocytogenes,* gram-negative bacilli	Ampicillin + third-generation cephalosporin† or ampicillin + fluoroquinolone‡ or meropenem	10-14 *(S. pneumoniae)* 14-21 *(L. monocytogenes)* 21 Gram-negative bacilli other than *H. influenzae*

From Rakel RE (ed): *Principles of family practice,* ed 6, Philadelphia, 2002, WB Saunders.
*Add vancomycin in areas where there is greater than 2% incidence of highly drug-resistant *S. pneumoniae.*
†Ceftriaxone or cefotaxime.
‡Ciprofloxacin or levofloxacin.

TABLE 1-26 Specific Antibiotic Treatments for Known Pathogens

Pathogen	Primary Therapy	Alternative*
Group B streptococcus	Penicillin G or ampicillin	Vancomycin or third-generation cephalosporin†
Streptococcus pneumoniae (MIC < 0.1)	Third-generation cephalosporin†	Meropenem, penicillin
S. pneumoniae (MIC > 0.1)	Vancomycin + third-generation cephalosporin*	Substitute rifampin for vancomycin; or meropenem; or vancomycin as monotherapy if highly allergic to other alternatives
Haemophilus influenzae (β-lactamase-negative)	Ampicillin	Third-generation cephalosporin† or chloramphenicol or aztreonam
H. influenzae (β-lactamase-positive)	Third-generation cephalosporin†	Chloramphenicol or aztreonam or fluoroquinolones‡
Listeria monocytogenes	Ampicillin + gentamicin	Trimethoprim-sulfamethoxazole
Neisseria meningitidis	Penicillin G or ampicillin	Third-generation cephalosporin†
Enterobacteriaceae	Third-generation cephalosporin† + aminoglycoside	Trimethoprim-sulfamethoxazole or aztreonam or fluoroquinolones or antipseudomonal penicillin (or ampicillin) + aminoglycoside
Pseudomonas aeruginosa	Ceftazidine + aminoglycoside	Aminoglycoside + aztreonam or aminoglycoside + antipseudomonal penicillin§
Staphylococcus aureus (methicillin-sensitive)	Antistaphylococcal penicillin¶ + rifampin	Vancomycin + rifampin or trimethoprim-sulfamethoxazole + rifampin
S. aureus (methicillin-resistant)	Vancomycin + rifampin	
Staphylococcus epidermidis	Vancomycin + rifampin	

From Rakel RE (ed): *Principles of family practice,* ed 6, Philadelphia, 2002, WB Saunders.
MIC, Minimum inhibitory concentration.
*If patient is highly allergic or intolerant of primary therapy.
†Ceftriaxone or cefotaxime.
‡Ciprofloxacin or levofloxacin.
§Piperacillin, mezlocillin, or ticarcillin.
¶Nafcillin, oxacillin, or methicillin.

treatment in adults with bacterial meningitis was associated with reduced mortality. It is therefore recommended that dexamethasone should be given to all adults with bacterial meningitis, and that it should be initiated with or before the first dose of antibiotics.[3] Ⓐ

A systematic review found that adjuvant corticosteroids reduced severe hearing loss in bacterial meningitis caused by *Haemophilus influenzae* as well as in meningitis caused by other bacteria.[4] Ⓐ

A meta-analysis of RCTs found that dexamethasone reduced the incidence of severe meningitis-related hearing loss in children with *H. influenzae* type b meningitis. In patients with pneumococcal meningitis, a reduction in the incidence of severe hearing loss was only found when dexamethasone was administered early.[5] Ⓑ

Evidence-Based References

1. Prasad K et al: Third generation cephalosporins versus conventional antibiotics for treating acute bacterial meningitis, *Cochrane Database Syst Rev* 2, 2004. Ⓐ
2. Peltota J, Anttila M, Renkonen OV: Randomized comparison of chloramphenicol, ampicillin, cefotaxime and ceftriaxone for childhood bacterial meningitis. Finnish Study Group, *Lancet* 1:1281, 1989. Ⓑ
3. de Gans J, van de Beek D, for the European Dexamethasone in Adulthood Bacterial Meningitis Study Investigators: Dexamethasone in adults with bacterial meningitis, *N Engl J Med* 347:1549, 2002. Discussed in: van de Beek D et al: Corticosteroids in acute bacterial meningitis, *Cochrane Database Syst Rev* 2, 2003. Ⓐ
4. van de Beek D et al: Corticosteroids in acute bacterial meningitis (Cochrane Review). Reviewed in: Cochrane Library, 1, Chichester, UK, 2004, John Wiley. Ⓐ
5. McIntyre PB et al: Dexamethasone as adjunctive therapy in bacterial meningitis. A meta-analysis of randomized clinical trials since 1988, *JAMA* 278:925, 1997. Ⓑ

SUGGESTED READINGS

Heyderman RS: Early management of suspected bacterial meningitis and meningococcal septicaemia in immunocompetent adults—second edition, *J Infect* 50(5):373, 2005.

Kutz JW et al: Clinical predictors for hearing loss in children with bacterial meningitis, *Arch Otolaryngol Head Neck Surg* 132(9): 941, 2006.

Sinner SW, Tunkel AR: Antimicrobial agents in the treatment of bacterial meningitis. *Infect Dis Clin North Am* 18(3):581, 2004.

van de Beek D et al: Clinical features and prognostic factors in adults with bacterial meningitis, *N Engl J Med* 351:1849, 2004.

Weisfelt M et al: Pneumococcal meningitis in adults: new approaches to management and prevention, Lancet Neurol 5(4):332, 2006.

AUTHORS: **STEVEN M. OPAL, M.D., GLENN G. FORT, M.D., M.P.H.,** and **DENNIS J. MIKOLICH, M.D.**

BASIC INFORMATION

DEFINITION

Viral meningitis is an acute aseptic meningitis usually with lymphocytic pleocytosis and negative CSF stains and cultures.

SYNONYMS

Aseptic meningitis

ICD-9CM CODES
047.8 Meningitis, aseptic

EPIDEMIOLOGY & DEMOGRAPHICS (Table 1-27)

INCIDENCE (IN U.S.): 11 cases/100,000 persons
PREDOMINANT SEX: Male = female
GENETICS: Those with abnormal humoral immunity and agammaglobulinemia have associated difficulty with viral clearance.

PHYSICAL FINDINGS & CLINICAL PRESENTATION

- Fever
- Headache
- Nuchal rigidity
- Photophobia
- Myalgias
- Vomiting
- Rash

ETIOLOGY

- Enterovirus
- Mumps virus
- Measles
- Arboviruses
- Herpes (simplex and zoster)
- HIV
- Lymphocytic choriomeningitis virus
- Adenovirus
- CMV
- Arthropod-borne viruses
- West Nile virus

DIAGNOSIS

The diagnostic approach is similar to bacterial meningitis (see "Bacterial Meningitis"); the foremost need is to rule out bacterial meningitis with CSF evaluation. Presentation may be similar to that of meningitis with bacterial involvement.

DIFFERENTIAL DIAGNOSIS

- Bacterial meningitis
- Meningitis secondary to Lyme disease, TB, syphilis, amebiasis, leptospirosis
- Rickettsial illnesses: Rocky Mountain spotted fever
- Migraine headache
- Medications
- SLE
- Acute mononucleosis/Epstein-Barr virus
- Seizures
- Carcinomatous meningitis

WORKUP

CSF examination:
- Usually shows pleocytosis
- Lymphocytic predominance (neutrophils in early stages)
- Opening pressure: 200 to 250 mm Hg
- WBC: 100 to 1000 mm^3
- Increased CSF protein
- Decreased or normal CSF glucose
- Negative Gram stain, cultures, CIE, latex agglutination
- Viral cultures or serologic testing may be diagnostic
- PCR for HSV, West Nile or enterovirus (which could shorten duration of antibiotic treatment and hospitalization if bacterial meningitis was suspected)

LABORATORY TESTS

CBC with differential, blood culturing, and CSF examination (see "Workup")

IMAGING STUDIES

CT scan or MRI: if cerebral edema, focal neurologic findings develop

TREATMENT

No specific antiviral therapy for most viruses. Treatment is supportive unless HSV is detected, which would be treated with IV acyclovir.

DISPOSITION

Viral meningitis is almost always an uncomplicated illness that will resolve; however, relapsing headache, myalgia, and weakness may occur for 2 to 3 wk after onset of symptoms.

PEARLS & CONSIDERATIONS

Enteroviruses are the most common cause of viral meningitis and are transmitted by fecal-oral and less commonly by the respiratory route.

SUGGESTED READINGS

Ellerin TB, Walsh SR, Hooper DC: Recurrent meningitis of unknown etiology, *Lancet* 363(9423):1772, 2004.

Shah SS et al: Early differentiation of Lyme from enteroviral meningitis, *Pediatr Infect Dis* 24(6):542, 2005.

AUTHORS: **STEVEN M. OPAL, M.D., GLENN G. FORT, M.D., M.P.H.,** and **DENNIS J. MIKOLICH, M.D.**

TABLE 1-27 **Epidemiology of Acute Viral Meningitis**

EPIDEMIOLOGIC FACTORS*

Season	Patient's Age (yr)	Patient's Sex	Risk Factor	Suggested Viral Agent
Summer-fall	Infant	—	Infected mother	Coxsackievirus B
	1-15	—	Swimming pools, closed communities	Enteroviruses
			Geographic area: California, southeastern United States	California serogroup virus
Winter	1-15	—	School exposure	Varicella virus, measles virus
		Male/female 3:1		Mumps virus
	16-21	—	College exposure	Measles virus
		Male/female 3:1		Mumps virus
		—		Epstein-Barr virus (mononucleosis)
	Any	—	Mice, rats, hamsters	Lymphocytic choriomeningitis virus
	Adults	—	Varicella-zoster	Varicella-zoster virus
Any	Any	—	Immunocompromise	Adenovirus
		—	Acquired immunodeficiency syndrome	Human immunodeficiency virus

From Gorbach SI: *Infectious diseases,* ed 2, Philadelphia, 1998, WB Saunders.
*Epidemiologic factors are suggestive but should not be used to exclude diagnoses in individual cases.

BASIC INFORMATION

DEFINITION

Meningomyelocele is the most common type of spina bifida and is characterized by herniation of the spinal cord, nerves, or both through a bony defect of the spine.

SYNONYMS

Myelomeningocele
Spina bifida cystica

ICD-9CM CODES
741.9 Spina bifida without mention of hydrocephalus
741.9 Meningomyelocele

EPIDEMIOLOGY & DEMOGRAPHICS

INCIDENCE (IN U.S.): 4.6/10,000 births
PREDOMINANT SEX: Male = female
PREDOMINANT INCIDENCE: Newborn
GENETICS: Environmental and genetic factors have a joint role.

ETIOLOGY

- Failure of neural tube to close completely at about 4 wk gestation
- Associated with maternal valproate use
- A small proportion of cases are associated with chromosomal or single-gene disorders

PHYSICAL FINDINGS & CLINICAL PRESENTATION

- Evident at birth—a sac protruding in the lumbar region (Fig. 1-158)
- Severity of neurologic deficits depends on the location of the lesion along the neuroaxis
- Motor dysfunction in the legs
- Lack of bladder or bowel control
- Often associated with Chiari II malformation and resulting obstructive hydrocephalus

DIAGNOSIS

- Prenatal diagnosis through ultrasound and MRI is being made more frequently.
- Coexisting hydrocephalus is detected by measurement of head size, ultrasonography, CT, or MRI.

DIFFERENTIAL DIAGNOSIS

- Teratoma
- Meningocele

WORKUP

- Evaluate for hydrocephalus.
- Evaluate for other congenital abnormalities, such as congenital heart disease, hydronephrosis, intestinal malformation, club foot, and skeletal deformities.

LABORATORY TESTS

Prenatal testing often reveals elevated alpha fetoprotein in amniotic fluid or maternal serum.

IMAGING STUDIES

- MRI of spine
- X-ray studies of skull exhibit craniolacuna, a honeycombed pattern associated with hydrocephalus
- CT or MRI of head may reveal hydrocephalus

TREATMENT

- Surgical closure of myelomeningocele is performed soon after birth
- Control of hydrocephalus (shunt)
- Management of urinary incontinence

ACUTE GENERAL Rx

- Immediate goal after delivery is to close defect and prevent infection; surgery usually performed within 24 hr of birth
- Shunt placement for obstructive hydrocephalus
- Treatment of seizures, if present

CHRONIC Rx

- Follow closely for development of hydrocephalus
- Bladder catheterization
- Avoid use of latex-containing products to prevent development of latex allergy

DISPOSITION

Followed by a team of specialists including neurosurgeons, urologists, orthopedists, and myelodysplasia nurses

PEARLS & CONSIDERATIONS

All mothers of children with neural tube defects should be instructed on nutritional supplementation with folate for future pregnancies.

COMMENTS

- Intrauterine repair of meningomyelocele decreases the incidence of hindbrain herniation and shunt-dependent hydrocephalus in infants, but increases the incidence of premature delivery.
- U.S. Public Health Service recommends 400 micrograms of folate intake per day for all women capable of becoming pregnant for primary prevention of neural tube defects.

SUGGESTED READINGS

Adzick NS, Walsh DS: Myelomeningocele: prenatal diagnosis, pathophysiology and management, *Semin Pediatr Surg* 12(3):168. 2003.
Mitchell LE: Epidemiology of neural tube defects, *Am J Med Genet C Semin Med Genet* 135(1):88, 2005.
Spina bifida and anencephaly before and after folic acid mandate—United States, 1995-1996 and 1999-2000, *MMWR Morb Mortal Wkly Rep* 53(17):362, 2004.

AUTHOR: **MAITREYI MAZUMDAR, M.D., M.P.H.**

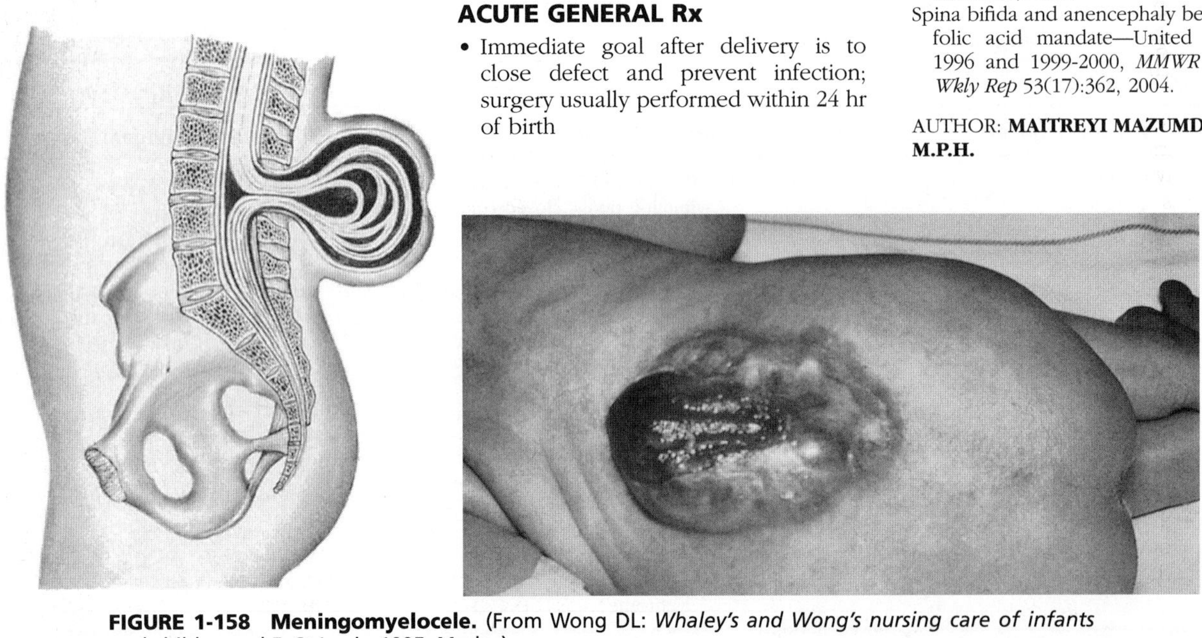

FIGURE 1-158 Meningomyelocele. (From Wong DL: *Whaley's and Wong's nursing care of infants and children,* ed 5, St Louis, 1995, Mosby.)

BASIC INFORMATION

DEFINITION

Menopause is the occurrence of no menstrual periods for 1 yr after age 40 yr or permanent cessation of ovulation following lost ovarian activity. It is a climacteric reproductive stage of life marked by waxing and waning estrogen levels followed by decreasing ovarian function. Premature ovarian failure and no menstrual periods may also occur because of depletion of ovarian follicles before the age of 40 yr.

SYNONYMS

Change of life
Climacteric ovarian failure

ICD-9CM CODES
627 Premenopausal menorrhagia
627.2 Menopausal or female climacteric states
627.4 States associated with artificial menopause
716.3 Climacteric arthritis

EPIDEMIOLOGY & DEMOGRAPHICS

- Average age of menopause in the U.S. is 51 yr.
- Age at which menopause occurs is genetically determined.
- Smokers experience menopause an average of 1.5 yr earlier than nonsmokers.
- More than one third of a woman's life will be spent after menopause.
- Onset of perimenopause is usually in a woman's mid- to late-40s.
- Approximately 4000 women each day begin menopause.

PHYSICAL FINDINGS & CLINICAL PRESENTATION

- Atrophic vaginitis, which can cause burning, itching, bleeding, dyspareunia
- Either complete cessation of menses or a period of irregular cycles and diminished or heavier bleeding
- Osteoporosis
- Psychologic dysfunction:
  1. Anxiety
  2. Depression
  3. Insomnia
  4. Nervousness
  5. Irritability
  6. Inability to concentrate
- Sexual changes, decreased libido, dyspareunia
- Urinary incontinence
- Vasomotor symptoms (hot flashes, flushes), night sweats, cardiovascular disease, coronary artery disease, atherosclerosis, headaches, tiredness, and lethargy

ETIOLOGY

- The most common etiology: physiologic, caused by depleted granulosa and theca cells that fail to react to endogenous gonadotropins, producing less estrogen; decreased negative feedback in the hypothalamic pituitary access, increased follicle-stimulating hormone (FSH), and increased luteinizing hormone (LH), which leads to stromal cells that continue to produce androgens as a result of the LH stimulation (Fig. 1-159)
- Surgical castration
- Family history of early menopause, cigarette smoking, blindness, abnormal chromosomal karyotype (Turner's syndrome, gonadal dysgenesis), precocious puberty, and left-handedness

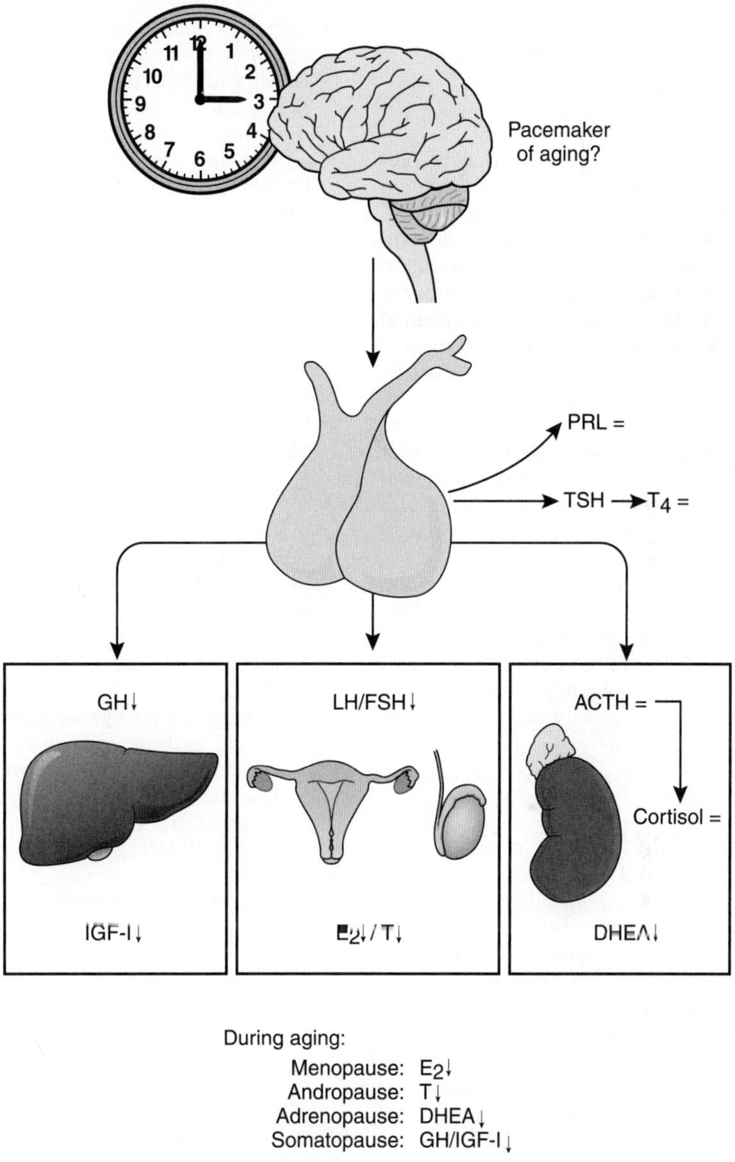

FIGURE 1-159 During aging, declines in the activities of a number of hormonal systems occur. *Left,* A decrease in growth hormone (GH) release by the pituitary gland causes a decrease in the production of insulin-like growth factor I (IGF-I) by the liver and other organs (somatopause). *Middle,* A decrease in release of gonadotropin luteinizing hormone (LH) and follicle-stimulating hormone (FSH) and decrease secretion at the gonadal level (from the ovaries, decreased estradiol [E2] from the testicle, decreased testosterone [T]) cause menopause and andropause, respectively. (Immediately after the initiation of menopause, serum LH and FSH levels increase sharply.) *Right,* The adrenocortical cells responsible for the production of dehydroepiandrosterone (DHEA) decrease in activity (adrenopause) without clinically evident changes in corticotrophin. A central pacemaker in the hypothalamus or higher brain areas (or both) is hypothesized, which together with changes in the peripheral organs (the ovaries, testicles, and adrenal cortex) regulates the aging process of these endocrine axes. PRL, Prolactin; T_4, thyroxine; TSH, thyrotropin. (From Larsen PR, Kronenburg HM, Melmed S, Polonsky KS [eds]: *Williams textbook of endocrinology,* ed 10, Philadelphia, 2003, Saunders.)

DIAGNOSIS (Dx)

DIFFERENTIAL DIAGNOSIS

- Asherman's syndrome
- Hypothalamic dysfunction
- Hypothyroidism
- Pituitary tumors
- Adrenal abnormalities
- Ovarian abnormalities
- Polycystic ovarian syndrome
- Pregnancy
- Ovarian neoplasm
- TB of the endometrium

WORKUP

- If the clinical picture is highly suggestive of menopause, estrogen can be prescribed. If all symptoms resolve, then diagnosis has essentially been made. Before estrogen is prescribed, a complete history and physical examination are needed. If a patient has estrogen-dependent malignancy, unexplained abnormal uterine bleeding, history of thrombophlebitis, or acute liver disease, estrogen therapy is contraindicated.
- Progesterone challenge test: progesterone 100 mg is given IM to induce withdrawal bleeding. If no withdrawal bleeding is obtained, it would be safe to assume that a hypoestrogenic state is present.
- Physical examination, height, weight, blood pressure, breast examination, and pelvic examination are needed.
- Assess risk for coronary artery disease, osteoporosis, cigarette smoking, personal history, history of breast cancer, liver disease, active coagulation disorder, or any unexplained vaginal bleeding.

LABORATORY TESTS

- FSH, LH, and estrogen levels: if the FSH is markedly elevated and the estrogen level is markedly depressed, constitutes laboratory diagnosis of ovarian failure; LH only if polycystic ovarian disease is to be ruled out in a younger patient
- TSH to rule out thyroid dysfunction and prolactin level if patient has symptoms of galactorrhea and if suspicion of pituitary adenoma exists
- A general chemistry profile to check for any systemic diseases
- Pap smear, endometrial biopsy, or D&C in patients who have had irregular periods or intermenstrual or postmenopausal bleeding
- Mammogram

IMAGING STUDIES

- CT scan or MRI of sella if pituitary tumor is suspected
- Bone density studies if high-risk condition for osteoporosis exists
- Pelvic ultrasound to check endometrial stripe

TREATMENT (Rx)

NONPHARMACOLOGIC THERAPY

- A balanced diet: low in fat, with total fat intake being <30% of calories; total calories sufficient to maintain body weight or to produce weight loss if that is needed
- Avoidance of smoking, excessive alcohol or caffeine intake
- Exercise: weight-bearing exercise for osteoporosis prevention
- Kegel exercises for strengthening the pelvic floor
- Adequate calcium intake: 1500 mg qd is necessary to maintain zero calcium balance in postmenopausal women
- Change in the ambient temperature (may ameliorate hot flashes and reduce night sweats)
- Vitamin E
- Avoidance of caffeine, alcohol, and spicy foods if they trigger hot flashes
- Vaginal lubricants to help with the dyspareunia secondary to vaginal dryness (e.g., Replens, K-Y Jelly, or Gyne-Moistrin cream)

ACUTE GENERAL Rx

Estrogen replacement in symptomatic patients can be done in a variety of forms, including oral estrogen and transdermal estrogen patch. The lowest effective dose should be prescribed.

- Examples of oral estrogen would include:
  1. Conjugated estrogens: start with 0.3 mg qd and increase up to 1.25 mg qd, depending on symptoms.
  2. Estradiol: start with 0.5 mg qd and increase to 2 mg qd.
  3. Esterified estrogens: start with 0.3 to 1.25 mg qd.
  4. Estropipate: start with 0.625 to 2.5 mg qd.
  5. Esterified estrogen/testosterone combination: give 1.25 mg and methyltestosterone 2.5 mg (Estratest) and esterified estrogen 0.625 mg and methyltestosterone 1.25 mg (Estratest HS). May improve sexual enjoyment and libido.
- If the patient has had a hysterectomy for benign disease, estrogen alone is sufficient. However, if she still has her uterus, progestin should be added for its protective effect against endometrial cancer. Progestins can be prescribed as continual daily dose or cyclic fashion. Most commonly prescribed progestins include medroxyprogesterone acetate 2.5 mg, 5 mg, 10 mg; Prometrieum 100 mg, 200 mg, 400 mg; Aygestin 5 mg. Continuous hormone replacement therapy is preferred, because after a period of time the patient should be amenorrheic. Patients should be counseled that they may experience some irregular spotting for the first 6 to 9 mo after starting the hormone replacement therapy. Cyclic therapy will cause withdrawal bleeding.
- Combination oral preparations Femhrt, Prefest, Prempro, Activella, Premphase.
- Transdermal patches can be either estradiol (Estraderm, Vivelle, Fempatch) 0.025 to 0.1 mg applied twice weekly or Climara 0.025 to 0.1 mg used once a week. With these preparations, progesterone should be used in a similar fashion. Combipatch—apply twice weekly (combination estrogen and progesterone)—or Climara Pro once/wk-patch.
- Vaginal creams can be used, and these should be reserved for local therapy of atrophic vaginitis. Systemic absorption does occur; however, blood levels are unpredictable. Usual dose 0.5 to 2 gm intravaginally daily cyclically 3 wk on 1 wk off. When symptoms improve, once to twice weekly is adequate maintenance.
- Vagifem estradiol vaginal tablets. Initial dosage: one Vagifem tablet, inserted vaginally, once daily for 2 wk. Maintenance dose: one Vagifem tablet, inserted vaginally, twice weekly.
- Femring vaginal ring delivering the equivalent of 0.5 mg/day inserted every 3 months or Estring 0.0075 mg/day.
- EstroGel 0.06% (estrodiol gel) One Pump (1.25 g/day) applied to one arm from wrist to shoulder.
- For women in whom estrogen is contraindicated or for those who do not wish to take estrogen, the following regimens can be used:
  1. Serotonin reuptake inhibitors
  2. Depo-Provera 150 mg IM every month (may be helpful in alleviating hot flashes)
  3. Clonidine 0.05 to 0.15 mg qd
  4. Bellergal-S (questionable efficacy)
- Tibolone significantly improves vasomotor symptoms, libido, and vaginal lubrication.

CHRONIC Rx

Hormone replacement therapy should be used only for the short term unless benefits outweigh the risks of long-term use.

DISPOSITION

If treated, the patient should have resolution of her symptoms and reduced incidence of osteoporosis. Lifelong medical supervision is necessary to monitor adequacy of treatment and prevention of complications. This should include annual Pap smears, pelvic examinations, breast examinations, mammography, and endometrial sampling of any type of abnormal bleeding. If untreated, the vasomotor symptoms will eventually disappear; however, this may take several years in a small percentage of women, and some women who are in their 80s have experienced hot flashes. Urogenital atrophy will continue to worsen. Osteoporosis and coronary artery disease risks will increase with every passing year. Women using ERT for >10 yr may have increased risk of developing ovarian cancer.

REFERRAL

Most menopausal women are managed by their gynecologist. However, this condition can be managed adequately by the patient's primary care physician who has an interest in treating menopausal women.

PEARLS & CONSIDERATIONS

COMMENTS

- Short-term risks of HRT include an 18-fold increased rise for cholecystitis, 3.5-fold risk of a thrombocardiac event in the first year, and probably increased risk of stroke and MI.
- Results of the WHI study found that for every 10,000 women taking HRT for 1 yr (10,000 person-yr), 7 more would have coronary events, 8 more strokes, 8 more pulmonary emboli, and 8 more with early breast cancer than would 10,000 women taking placebo. Benefits of HRT were 6 fewer cases of colorectal cancer and 5 fewer hip fractures per 10,000 women.
- HRT should not be initiated or continued for the primary or secondary prevention of CHD.
- ERT or HRT should only be prescribed for patients with sufficient menopausal symptoms that impact the patient's quality of life.

EVIDENCE

Benefits of hormonal therapy

A systematic review found that estrogen plus progesterone and estrogen alone significantly reduce the frequency and severity of hot flashes in postmenopausal women.[1] Ⓐ

Systematic reviews and randomized controlled trials (RCTs) have found that estrogen improves urogenital symptoms, depressed mood, and quality of life in menopausal women.[2-4] Ⓐ

RCTs have found that short-term treatment with progestogens is significantly more effective than placebo for treating vasomotor symptoms associated with menopause.[4] Ⓐ

Women receiving long-term combined HRT (conjugated estrogen plus medroxyprogesterone acetate) have a significantly reduced risk of colorectal cancer and hip fracture.[5] Ⓐ

Risks of hormonal therapy

The health risks of long-term HRT outweigh the benefits for the average healthy postmenopausal woman.[5] Ⓑ

Long-term combined HRT (conjugated estrogen plus medroxyprogesterone acetate) is associated with a significantly increased risk of coronary heart disease, stroke, and venous thromboembolism compared with placebo, in addition to a small increased risk of breast cancer.[5,6] Ⓐ

Long-term therapy with estrogen alone, in healthy postmenopausal women with prior history of a hysterectomy, is associated with an increased risk of stroke vs. placebo, and does not prevent coronary heart disease.[7] Ⓐ

The use of hormone therapy, either estrogen alone or combined therapy, is not recommended to prevent dementia or cognitive decline in women 65 years of age or older. Both regimens appear to be associated with an increased risk of developing probable dementia in women aged 65 and over.[8,9] Ⓐ

Unopposed estrogen therapy is associated with increased rates of endometrial hyperplasia and irregular bleeding. The addition of oral progestogens is associated with reduced rates of hyperplasia, and improves adherence to therapy.[10] Ⓐ

Another RCT comparing long-term HRT vs. placebo found an increased risk of ovarian cancer but no increase in risk of endometrial cancer.[11] Ⓑ

Unopposed estrogen and combined estrogen do not have an effect on body weight, but it is not known whether HRT helps prevent the body fat redistribution associated with menopause.[12]

Nonhormonal therapy

One RCT has found that clonidine significantly reduces vasomotor symptoms associated with menopause.[13] Ⓐ

There is limited and conflicting evidence from small RCTs for the use of phytoestrogens in the treatment of vasomotor symptoms.[4] Ⓐ

There is evidence for calcium supplementation having a limited effect on rate of bone loss.[14] Ⓐ

Evidence-Based References

1. MacLennan A, Lester S, Moore V: Oral oestrogen replacement therapy versus placebo for hot flushes. Reviewed in: Cochrane Library, 3, Chichester, UK, 2004, John Wiley. Ⓐ
2. Cardozo L et al: Meta-analysis of estrogen therapy in the management of urogenital atrophy in postmenopausal women: second report of the hormones and urogenital therapy committee, *Obstet Gynecol* 2:722, 1998. Reviewed in: 11:2459, 2004. Ⓐ
3. Zweifel JE, O'Brien WH: A meta-analysis of the effect of HRT upon depressed mood, *Psychoneuroendocrinology* 22:189, 1997. Reviewed in: *Clin Evid* 11:2459, 2004. Ⓐ
4. Morris E, Rymer J: Menopausal symptoms. Reviewed in: *Clin Evid* 11:2459, London, 2004, BMJ Publishing Group. Ⓐ
5. Manson JE et al: Women's Health Initiative Investigators. Estrogen plus progestin and the risk of coronary heart disease, *N Engl J Med* 349:523, 2003. Ⓐ
6. Collaborative Group on Hormonal Factors in Breast Cancer: Breast cancer and hormone replacement therapy: collaborative reanalysis of data from 51 epidemiological studies of 52,705 women with breast cancer and 108,411 women without breast cancer, *Lancet* 350:1047, 1997. Reviewed in: *Clin Evid* 11:2459, 2004. Ⓐ
7. Anderson GL et al: Women's Health Initiative Steering Committee, 2004. Effects of conjugated equine estrogen in postmenopausal women with hysterectomy. The Women's Health Initiative randomized controlled trial, *JAMA* 291:1701, 2004. Ⓐ

SUGGESTED READINGS

Gambrell RD: The Women's Health Initiative Reports: critical review of the findings, the female patient, *Menopause* 29.(11).23, 2004.

Lacey JV et al: Menopausal hormone replacement therapy and risk of ovarian cancer, *JAMA* 288:334, 2002.

NIH State of Sciences Panel: NIH State of Sciences Conference Statement: Management of menopause related symptoms, *Ann Int Med* 142:1003, 2005.

Speroff L: Efficacy and tolerability of a noval estradiol vaginal ring for relief of menopausal symptoms, *Obstet Gynecol* 102(4):823, 2003.

Writing Group for the Women's Health Initiative Investigators: Risks and benefits of estrogen plus progestin in healthy postmenopausal women, *JAMA* 288:321, 2002.

AUTHORS: **GEORGE T. DANAKAS, M.D.,** and **RUBEN ALVERO, M.D.**

BASIC INFORMATION

DEFINITION

Acute mesenteric lymphadenitis is a syndrome of acute right lower quadrant abdominal pain associated with mesenteric lymph node enlargement and a normal appendix.

ICD-9CM CODES
289.2 Mesenteric adenitis

EPIDEMIOLOGY & DEMOGRAPHICS

- Incidence unknown
- Affects mostly children (under age 18 yr) with no sex preference
- When *Yersinia* enterocolitis is the cause, boys are more frequently involved

PHYSICAL FINDINGS & CLINICAL PRESENTATION

- Abdominal pain of variable severity (mild ache to severe colic) beginning in upper abdomen or right lower quadrant, eventually localizes in right side but not in a precise location (unlike appendicitis)
- In *Yersinia* infection (Fig. 1-160) outbreaks, the symptoms include abdominal pain (84%), diarrhea (78%), fever (43%), anorexia (22%), nausea (13%), and vomiting (8%)
- Physical findings:
  Other lymphadenopathy (20% of cases)
  Right lower quadrant tenderness (site of maximum tenderness may vary from one examination to the next)
  Guarding (rare)
  Mild fever

ETIOLOGY & PATHOGENESIS

- Reactive hyperplasia of lymph nodes that drain the ileocecal region, similar to that seen in inflammatory or allergic conditions. One study reported that approximately two thirds of cases are secondary (reactive) and one third are primary (no demonstrable associated inflammatory process).
- *Yersinia enterocolitica, Yersinia pseudotuberculosis, Salmonella* species, *E. coli*, streptococci have been implicated with mesenteric adenitis.

DIAGNOSIS

Generally the diagnosis is made on exploration of the abdomen of a patient suspected of having acute appendicitis. On examination the appendix appears normal, and enlarged mesenteric lymph nodes are noted. Excision of an enlarged lymph node with culture and nodal histology may provide information regarding the etiology but is not routinely employed.

DIFFERENTIAL DIAGNOSIS

- Acute appendicitis (5% to 10% of patients admitted to hospitals with a diagnosis of appendicitis are discharged with a diagnosis of mesenteric adenitis)
- Crohn's disease

Section II describes the differential diagnosis of abdominal pain.

LABORATORY TESTS

- CBC may show leukocytosis
- Abdominal sonography and helical appendiceal CT scan may be useful
- Laparotomy if appendicitis is suspected

PROGNOSIS

Recurrent bouts are common; therefore if laparotomy is performed and a normal appendix is found, it should be removed.

SUGGESTED READINGS

Macari M et al: Mesenteric adenitis: CT diagnosis of primary versus secondary causes, incidence, and clinical significance on pediatric and adult patients, *Am J Roentgenol* 178:853, 2002.

Pearson RD, Guerrant RL: Enteric fever and other causes of abdominal symptoms with fever. In Mandell GL (ed): *Mandell, Douglas, and Bennett's principles and practice of infectious diseases,* ed 6, New York, 2005, Churchill Livingstone.

AUTHORS: **FRED F. FERRI, M.D.,** and **TOM J. WACHTEL, M.D.**

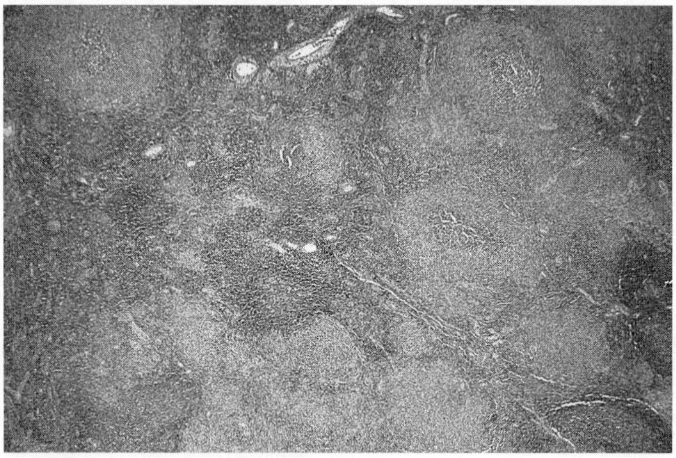

FIGURE 1-160 ***Yersinia* mesenteric lymphadenitis.** Multiple stellate granulomas with central necrosis replace a mesenteric lymph node. The inflammation extends into the surrounding perinodal fat. The preoperative diagnosis was acute suppurativa appendicitis, but the appendix was macroscopically and microscopically normal (H&E, ×5, *Yersinia pseudotuberloculosis* isolated from cultures). (From Silverberg SG, Delellis RA, Frable WJ, LiVolsi VA, Wick MR [eds]: *Silverberg's principles and practice of surgical pathology and cytopathology,* ed 4, Philadelphia, 2006, Churchill Livingstone.)

BASIC INFORMATION

DEFINITION

Acute mesenteric ischemia (AMI) is the sudden onset of intestinal hypoperfusion, caused by emboli, arterial or venous thrombosis, or by vasoconstriction resulting from low flow states.

ICD-9-CM CODES
557.1 Mesenteric vascular insufficiency

EPIDEMIOLOGY & DEMOGRAPHICS

INCIDENCE:
- AMI accounts for 0.1% of hospital admissions.
- The incidence appears to be increasing, probably due to increased awareness among clinicians, and the aging population.
- Increased use of ICUs, and more prolonged survival of sicker patients, has allowed mesenteric ischemia to occur more frequently as a complication of patients' initial illnesses.

PREDOMINANT SEX AND AGE:
- AMI caused by arterial embolism or thrombosis occurs in the elderly.
- Patients in whom the underlying mechanism is mesenteric venous thrombosis often are diagnosed at younger ages.

RISK FACTORS:
- These include advanced age, atherosclerosis, low cardiac output (especially atrial fibrillation), severe cardiac valvular disease, intraabdominal malignancy.
- In the subgroup of cases caused by venous thrombosis, risk factors include hypercoagulable states, portal hypertension, abdominal infection, blunt trauma, pancreatitis, and portal malignancy.
- Cases have been reported in patients younger than 50 years of age, with no identifiable risk factors, however.

GENETICS: No specific genetic predisposition, but may be related to the underlying factors such as cardiac disease, atherosclerosis, and hypercoagulable states.

PHYSICAL FINDINGS & CLINICAL PRESENTATION

- The classic presentation is in the patient with risk factors, exhibiting the rapid onset of severe periumbilical pain out of proportion to physical exam findings.
- Nausea and vomiting are commonly associated.
- Initial abdominal exam may be normal, with no rebound or guarding, or show minimal distension, or OB positive stool.
- Later in the course, the patient may present with gross distension, absence of bowel sounds, and peritoneal signs. In the elderly, mental status changes may be found.

ETIOLOGY

The pathophysiologic mechanisms that cause AMI include the following:
- Mesenteric arterial embolism: typically from the left atrium, left ventricle, or cardiac valves. The superior mesenteric artery is most commonly affected.
- Mesenteric arterial thrombosis: often in patients with prior progressive atherosclerotic stenoses, with superimposed abdominal trauma or infection.
- Mesenteric venous thrombosis (MVT): may occur in the setting of hypercoagulable states (acquired or inherited), blunt trauma, abdominal infection, portal hypertension, pancreatitis and portal malignancy.
- Nonocclusive mesenteric ischemia (NOMI): usually occurs in the setting of atherosclerotic vascular disease, often in a patient with an acute cardiovascular disease process, who is being treated with drugs that reduce intestinal perfusion. This may include patients with recent cardiac surgery, and dialysis patients. Cocaine use has also been a causative factor in a number of cases.

DIAGNOSIS

DIFFERENTIAL DIAGNOSIS

Initially include other causes of abdominal pain of acute onset including perforated peptic ulcer, early appendicitis. Ultimately include the varied causes of peritonitis.

WORKUP

- Success of treatment is related to the duration of symptoms prior to diagnosis.
- Consider early laparotomy for diagnosis in cases with a high index of suspicion, where angiography is not available.

LABORATORY TESTS

- Laboratory test results are nonspecific, especially early in the course. Later they can include leukocytosis, acidosis, and elevated hematocrit resulting from hemoconcentration. Most abnormalities occur after progression to bowel necrosis.
- When a hypercoagulable state is suspected, workup may include proteins C and S, antithrombin III, and factor V (Leiden). This will likely not affect the diagnosis of AMI but may help guide long-term therapy.

IMAGING STUDIES

- The gold standard is mesenteric angiography.
- With strong clinical suspicion, workup should proceed directly to angiography, without delay for CT scan or other testing.
- Plain films are normal 25% of the time in the early stages. Suggestive findings may include ileus, bowel wall thickening, or intramural gas. Intraluminal barium should not be used because it is rarely helpful in making a positive diagnosis, and will interfere with angiographic studies.
- Doppler ultrasound evaluation of intestinal blood flow is often limited by the presence of air-filled loops of bowel.
- CT scan findings also are commonly nonspecific, and more often found late in the course. Portal venous gas or intramural gas may be seen after the development of gangrene, but in many cases even at that advanced stage CT findings remain nonspecific.
- CT scanning has been found to be more useful in cases of mesenteric vein thrombosis causing AMI, with sensitivity approaching 90%. It has also been found useful in monitoring the progress of patients with superior mesenteric venous thrombosis who are treated nonsurgically.
- Magnetic resonance angiography (MRA) may prove to be useful, but data comparing this to angiography are needed.

TREATMENT

- The goal of treatment is to restore blood flow as rapidly as possible to ischemic bowel, prior to the occurrence of infarction.
- Treatment varies depending on etiology.

NONPHARMACOLOGIC THERAPY

- Signs of peritonitis mandate early laparotomy and resection of infarcted bowel.
- When workup is positive for major superior mesenteric artery (SMA) embolus, embolectomy is considered standard treatment, in the absence of peritoneal signs. Depending on the location and degree of occlusion of the embolus, surgical revascularization, intraarterial infusion of thrombolytics or vasodilators, or systemic anticoagulation may be considered.
- In cases of SMA thrombosis, emergency surgical revascularization is the treatment of choice.
- Angiography is needed to diagnose nonocclusive mesenteric ischemia

prior to infarct, and should be followed by intraarterial vasodilator infusion. This approach has been shown to significantly reduce mortality in this situation.
- In patients with mesenteric vein thrombosis, treatment is dependent on the presence or absence of peritoneal signs. Laparotomy and resection of infarcted bowel in more advanced cases, or if there are no peritoneal signs anticoagulant therapy, immediately with heparin, and ultimately with warfarin, may be adequate.

ACUTE GENERAL Rx

- Initial management should include hemodynamic monitoring and support, correction of acidosis, administration of broad-spectrum antibiotics, and gastric decompression via NG tube.
- Vasoconstricting agents should be avoided.
- Systemic anticoagulation may be started, although the timing of initiation is unclear.

CHRONIC Rx

In the subgroup of patients with mesenteric venous thrombosis, prevention of further thrombosis is indicated, although the optimal duration of anticoagulation is unclear.

DISPOSITION

- Prognosis is best in AMI resulting from mesenteric venous thrombosis and after surgical treatment for acute arterial embolism. It remains poor in cases of arterial thrombosis and nonocclusive ischemia.
- With delayed diagnosis, intestinal infarction, resulting in perforation or gangrenous bowel, sepsis, shock, and death is typical.

REFERRAL

Early surgical consultation should be considered, and should not be delayed if there are peritoneal signs, or if angiography is unavailable.

PEARLS & CONSIDERATIONS

COMMENTS

- The diagnosis of AMI should be considered in any patient with acute onset of abdominal pain out of proportion to physical findings, particularly in at-risk patients.
- Early diagnosis, before intestinal infarction occurs, is critical and correlates with improved survival rates.

PREVENTION

Prevention of the underlying factors, most notably atherosclerotic disease

SUGGESTED READINGS

Bingol H et al: Surgical therapy for acute superior mesenteric artery embolism, *Am J Surg* 188(1):68, 2004.

Brandt LJ et al: AGA technical review on intestinal ischemia, *Gastroenterology* 118:954, 2000.

Schoots IG et al: Systematic review of survival after acute mesenteric ischaemia according to disease aetiology, *Br J Surg* 91(1):17, 2004.

AUTHOR: **MARGARET TRYFOROS, M.D.**

BASIC INFORMATION

DEFINITION

Mesenteric venous thrombosis (MVT) is a thrombotic occlusion of the mesenteric venous system involving major trunks or smaller branches and leading to intestinal infarction in its acute form.

ICD-9CM CODES
557.0 Mesenteric venous thrombosis

EPIDEMIOLOGY & DEMOGRAPHICS

Between 5% and 15% of patients with acute mesenteric infarction have mesenteric venous thrombosis. MVT is slightly more common in men than women. The typical age of occurrence is 50 to 60 yr.

PHYSICAL FINDINGS & CLINICAL PRESENTATION

Acute MVT
- Symptoms: abdominal pain in 90% of patients, typically out of proportion to the physical findings. Nausea and vomiting occur in 50% and GI bleeding occurs in 50% (occult), 15% (gross).
- Physical findings:
  Early: abdominal tenderness, decreased bowel sounds, abdominal distention
  Later: guarding and rebound tenderness, fever, and septic shock

Subacute MVT
- Symptoms: nonspecific abdominal pain for weeks or months
- Physical findings: none

Chronic MVT
- Symptoms: upper GI hemorrhage from bleeding varices
- Physical findings: none other than signs of blood loss if significant

ETIOLOGY & PATHOGENESIS

Hypercoagulable states
- Peripheral deep venous thrombosis
- Neoplasms
- Antithrombin III, protein C, protein S deficiencies
- Lupus anticoagulant (antiphospholipid antibody)
- Oral contraceptive use, pregnancy
- Polycythemia vera
- Thrombocytosis
- Paroxysmal nocturnal hemoglobinuria

Portal hypertension
- Cirrhosis

Inflammation
- Pancreatitis
- Peritonitis (e.g., appendicitis, diverticulitis, perforated viscus)
- Inflammatory bowel disease
- Pelvic or intraabdominal abscess
- Intraabdominal cancer

Postoperative state or trauma
- Blunt abdominal trauma
- Postoperative states (abdominal surgery)

Thrombosis may begin in small mesenteric branches (e.g., in hypercoagulable states) and propagate to the major venous mesenteric trunks, or begin in large veins (e.g., in cirrhosis, intraabdominal cancer, surgery) and extend distally. If collateral drainage is inadequate, the intestine becomes congested, edematous, cyanotic, and hemorrhagic and eventually may infarct.

DIAGNOSIS

DIFFERENTIAL DIAGNOSIS

All other causes of abdominal pain (e.g., peritonitis, intestinal obstruction, pancreatitis, peptic ulcer disease, gastritis, inflammatory bowel disease, perforated viscus). Also to be considered in the differential diagnosis of GI hemorrhage

WORKUP

Laboratory tests and imaging studies

LABORATORY TESTS

- CBC: leukocytosis
- Electrolytes: metabolic acidosis (lactic) indicate bowel infarction
- Elevated amylase
- Tests for hypercoagulable status

IMAGING STUDIES

- Abdominal plain x-ray: ileus, ascites, bowel dilation, bowel wall thickening, loop separation, and thumbprinting
- Abdominal CT scan (diagnostic in 90%) bowel wall thickening, venous dilation, venous thrombus
- Arteriography if CT scan is not diagnostic

Occasionally the diagnosis is made by a laparotomy.

TREATMENT

- Anticoagulation or thrombolytic therapy
- Laparotomy if intestinal infarction is suspected

Short ischemic segment: resection
Long ischemic segment:
1. Nonviable: resection or close
2. Viable: intraarterial papaverine, and/or thrombectomy followed by "second look" intervention

- The treatment of chronic MVT is the same as for portal hypertension

PROGNOSIS

- Mortality of acute mesenteric venous thrombosis: 20% to 50%
- Recurrence rate: 15% to 25%

SUGGESTED READINGS

Brandt LJ, Smithline AE: Ischemic lesions of the bowel. In Feldman M, Scharsachmidt BF, Sleisenger MH (eds): *Gastrointestinal and liver disease,* ed 6, Philadelphia, 1998, WB Saunders.

Kumar S, Sarr MG, Kemeth PS: Mesenteric venous thrombosis, *N Engl J Med* 345:1683, 2002.

AUTHORS: **FRED F. FERRI, M.D.,** and **TOM J. WACHTEL, M.D.**

BASIC INFORMATION

DEFINITION

Malignant mesothelioma is a rare neoplastic lesion associated with asbestos exposure. There are three major histologic subtypes: epithelial (most common), sarcomatous, and mixed (epithelial/sarcomatous).

ICD-9CM CODES
199.1 Malignant mesothelioma, site NOS

EPIDEMIOLOGY & DEMOGRAPHICS

- Associated with asbestos exposure (all fiber types)
- Over 3000 new cases diagnosed in U.S. annually
- More common in men as a result of asbestos exposure in the workplace
- Right-sided involvement is more common
- Incidence of mesothelioma increases with age; median age at presentation is >60 yr
- There are currently more than 8 million persons in the U.S. who are at risk for mesothelioma because of prior asbestos exposure

PHYSICAL FINDINGS & CLINICAL PRESENTATION

- Dyspnea
- Nonpleuritic chest pain
- Fever, weight loss, sweats, fatigue, loss of appetite
- Dysphagia, superior vena cava syndrome, Horner's syndrome in advanced stages
- Auscultation may reveal unilateral loss of breath sounds
- Dullness on percussion may be present

ETIOLOGY

- Asbestos exposure
- Other reported potentially causal factors include prior radiation therapy and extravasated thorotrast, zeolite, and erionite fibers

DIAGNOSIS

DIFFERENTIAL DIAGNOSIS

Metastatic adenocarcinomas (from lung, breast, ovary, kidney, stomach, prostate)

WORKUP

- Staging evaluation includes complete history (including occupational history), physical examination, and testing to determine potential operability (CT, bone scan, PFTs)
- Thoracoscopy, pleuroscopy, and open lung biopsy are useful in obtaining adequate tissue samples for diagnosis
- Pulmonary function tests
- Staging: the UICC staging uses the TNM categories to organize mesothelioma in stages I to IV in a manner similar to that used for non–small cell lung cancer

LABORATORY TESTS

- Diagnostic thoracentesis is generally insufficient for diagnosis because pleural effusions may only reveal atypical mesothelial cells
- Immunohistochemistry is useful to distinguish adenocarcinoma from epithelial malignant mesothelioma (mesotheliomas are generally CEA negative and cytokeratin positive)
- Thrombocytosis and anemia may be found on initial lab evaluation
- Serum osteopontin levels (where available) can be used to distinguish persons with exposure to asbestos who do not have cancer from those with exposure to asbestos who have pleural mesothelioma

IMAGING STUDIES

- Chest radiographs may reveal pleural plaques or calcifications in the diaphragm
- CT scan of the chest/abdomen and bone scan are used to assess the extent of disease

TREATMENT

GENERAL Rx

- Operable patient (epithelial type, no positive nodes, confined to pleura, adequate PFTs): the two surgical techniques for therapeutic intervention are decortication (pleurectomy) and extrapleural pneumonectomy. Postoperative chemotherapy with cisplatin, doxorubicin, and cyclophosphamide and subsequent external beam radiation are used in some centers with limited success.
- Inoperable patient (disease too extensive, sarcomatous or mixed histology type, poor PFTs): supportive care plus/minus radiation therapy for symptoms or supportive care plus chemotherapy. Combined modality therapies (surgery, radiation therapy, chemotherapy, and biologics) have also been used to reduce both local and distant recurrences. The combination of pemetrexed (an antimetabolite that inhibits enzymes involved in folate metabolism) and cisplatin is used for chemotherapy of unresectable malignant pleural mesothelioma.
- Intrapleural instillation of cisplatin or biologics (e.g., interferons, interleukin-2) is generally limited to very early disease because it can only penetrate a very limited depth of the tumor and there is a propensity of the pleural space to become progressively obliterated with advancing disease.
- The role of radiation therapy in the treatment of mesotheliomas remains uncertain. It is often used for palliation of local pain despite lack of trials to prove its utility.
- Obliteration of the pleural space (pleurodesis) with instillation of tetracycline, bleomycin, or biologic substances such as *C. parvum* into the pleural cavity is often tried in attempting to treat recurrent symptomatic pleural effusions.

DISPOSITION

Median survival for patients undergoing pleurectomy ranges from 6.7 to 21 mo, for extrapleural pneumonectomy 4 to 21 mo. Survival is better for patients with epithelial form.

PEARLS & CONSIDERATIONS

COMMENTS

- Patients with early disease should be referred to treatment centers specializing in mesothelioma treatment before attempts are made to obliterate the pleural space with pleurodesis.
- An approach to the evaluation and treatment of mesothelioma is described in Section III.

SUGGESTED READINGS

Pass H et al: Asbestos exposure, pleural mesothelioma, and serum osteopontin levels, *N Engl J Med* 353:1564, 2005.

Robinson B, Lake R: Advances in malignant mesothelioma, *N Engl J Med* 353:1591, 2005.

AUTHOR: **FRED F. FERRI, M.D.**

BASIC INFORMATION

DEFINITION

Guidelines define the metabolic syndrome as the presence of any three of the following:

- Abdominal waist circumference >102 cm (40 inches) in men and >88 cm (35 inches) in women
- Serum hypertriglyceridemia ≥150 mg/dl (1.7 mmol/L) or drug treatment for elevated triglycerides
- Serum high-density lipoprotein (HDL) cholesterol <40 mg/dl (1 mmol/L) in men and <50 mg/dl (1.3 mmol/L) in women or drug treatment for low HDL
- Blood pressure ≥130/85 mm Hg or drug treatment for elevated blood pressure
- Fasting glucose ≥100 mg/dl (5.6 mmol/L) or drug treatment for elevated blood glucose

SYNONYMS

Syndrome X
Insulin resistance syndrome
Obesity dyslipidemia syndrome

ICD-9CM CODES
277.7 Metabolic syndrome

EPIDEMIOLOGY & DEMOGRAPHICS

- Affects 22% of U.S. adults.
- Prevalence increases with age affecting over 40% of individuals >60 yr.
- Greater prevalence in women compared with men (2:1).
- Weight or body mass index is a major risk factor. 5% of normal weight, 22% of overweight, and 60% of obese individuals have the metabolic syndrome.
- Up to 50% of the variation in the metabolic syndrome traits maybe accounted by genetic factors. Other risk factors include ethnic background such as Mexican American, low socioeconomic status, lack of physical activity, high carbohydrate diet, no alcohol intake, smoking, and postmenopausal status.

CLINICAL PRESENTATION

- Obesity, hypertension, dyslipidemia, and hyperglycemia as defined.
  - Blood pressure: ≥130/85 mm Hg
  - Waist circumference: >102 cm (40 inches) in men and >88 cm (35 inches) in women
  - Triglycerides: ≥150 mg/dl (1.7 mmol/L)
  - HDL: <40 mg/dl (1 mmol/L) in men and <50 mg/dl (1.3 mmol/L) in women
  - High fasting glucose: ≥100 mg/dl (5.6 mmol/L).
- Patients with the metabolic syndrome are at markedly increased risk for coronary artery disease and diabetes.
- Associated with several obesity-related disorders including fatty liver disease, polycystic ovary syndrome, and obstructive sleep apnea.
- Focus history on symptoms of diabetes and its complications, obesity and its complications, coronary artery disease (angina), and polycystic ovary syndrome.
- Complete physical examination including height, weight, waist circumference, and blood pressure.

ETIOLOGY

- Genetic predisposition and body fat distribution leads to development of the metabolic syndrome.
- Abdominal obesity is associated with insulin resistance and hyperinsulinemia.
- Elevations in inflammatory markers and cytokines (i.e., plasminogen activator inhibitor [PAI]-1, IL-6, and CRP) have been associated with insulin resistance.
- Insulin resistance results in ineffective glucose and fatty acid utilization leading to type 2 diabetes mellitus. Hyperinsulinemia and cytokines play an important role in development of abnormal lipid profile, hypertension, and vascular endothelial dysfunction, which can lead to the development of atherosclerotic cardiovascular disease (CVD).

DIAGNOSIS

DIFFERENTIAL DIAGNOSIS

- Other causes of weight gain or obesity (Cushing's syndrome, hypothyroidism, etc.)
- Other causes of hyperlipidemia (familial combined hyperlipidemia, hypothyroidism, etc.)
- Other causes of hypertension (Cushing's syndrome, hyperaldosteronism, etc.)
- Other forms of diabetes (type 1)

LABORATORY TESTS

- Fasting lipid profile (total cholesterol, LDL cholesterol, HDL cholesterol, and triglyceride)
- Fasting glucose

TREATMENT

NONPHARMACOLOGIC THERAPY

- Lifestyle modification:
  - Dietary modifications aimed at weight loss
  - Physical activity of moderate intensity: 30 minutes daily
  - Smoking cessation
- Consider bariatric surgery in the management of obesity:
  - BMI ≥40 kg/m^2 who have failed diet and exercise (with or without drug therapy).
  - Individuals with BMI >35 kg/m^2 and comorbidities (hypertension, impaired glucose tolerance, diabetes mellitus, dyslipidemia, sleep apnea) are also potential surgical candidates.

ACUTE GENERAL Rx

- Treat obesity (see "Obesity")
  - Pharmacologic treatment: consider sibutramine, orlistat, phentermine, diethylpropion, fluoxetine, and bupropion in individuals who have failed diet and exercise if BMI >30 kg/m2 or a BMI of 27 to 30 kg/m2 with comorbid conditions.
- Treat hypertension (see "Hypertension")
  - Systolic blood pressures >130/80: consider angiotensin converting-enzyme inhibitors, angiotensin II receptor blocker, or thiazide-type diuretics as first line.
- Treat hyperlipidemia
  - Serum LDL cholesterol of <100 mg/dL (2.6 mmol/L) is recommended for secondary prevention (i.e., CAD or CAD equivalent such as diabetes); however, recent studies suggest greater benefit with a more aggressive goal of <80 mg/dL (2.1 mmol/L). For primary prevention, an LDL goal <130 mg/dl (3.4 mmol/L) is recommended for individuals with greater than two coronary heart disease risk factors. HMG CoA reductase inhibitors (statins) commonly used as first line agents.
  - Patients with high triglycerides (>200 mg/dl) may benefit from the addition of a fibrate.
  - Must rule out hypothyroidism and normalize blood glucose.
- Treat diabetes
  - Goal fasting blood glucose <130 mg/dl.
  - Metformin as first line to improve insulin sensitivity.
- Treat cardiovascular risk factors
  - Consider aspirin.
  - Risk can be lowered with weight loss, exercise, smoking cessation, blood pressure control, diabetes management, and treatment of hyperlipidemia.

CHRONIC Rx

- Encourage lifestyle modification as above.
- Pharmacologic and surgical management to maintain therapeutic goals described above.

DISPOSITION

Weight loss can prevent disease progression. Appropriate treatment of obesity, hypertension, hyperlipidemia, and diabetes can improve morbidity and mortality.

REFERRAL

- To nutritionist for diet counseling
- To weight loss and exercise programs

- To endocrinologist if difficulty reaching therapeutic goals
- To bariatric surgeon if meet surgical criteria (as noted previously)

PEARLS & CONSIDERATIONS

PREVENTION

- Weight loss is essential to the prevention and treatment of metabolic syndrome.
- Recommend dietary modifications and physical activity of moderate intensity at least 30 minutes daily.
- Consider pharmacologic and surgical options in select individuals (as above).
- Recommend treatment of hypertension, hyperlipidemia, and diabetes.

PATIENT/FAMILY EDUCATION

- Weight Reduction Programs including Weight Watchers, Curves, etc.
- American Diabetes Association: www.diabetes.org
- Polycystic Ovarian Syndrome Association: www.pcosupport.org
- The Hormone Foundation: www.hormone.org

EVIDENCE

EBM

In the Diabetes Prevention Program, obese subjects with impaired fasting glucose or impaired glucose tolerance were randomly assigned to intensive lifestyle modifications (7% weight loss), metformin, or placebo. After an average follow-up of 3 years, 34% of individuals in the intensive lifestyle, 45% in the metformin, and 51% in the placebo group developed metabolic syndrome. Both lifestyle modification and metformin therapy reduced the incidence of metabolic syndrome in these high-risk individuals compared with placebo.[1]

Evidence-Based Reference

1. Orchard TJ et al: The effect of metformin and intensive lifestyle intervention on the metabolic syndrome: the Diabetes Prevention Program randomized trial, *Ann Intern Med* 142:611, 2005.

SUGGESTED READINGS

Genuth S et al: Follow-up report on the diagnosis of diabetes mellitus, *Diabetes Care* 26:3160, 2003.

Grundy SM et al: Diagnosis and management of the metabolic syndrome: an American Heart Association/National Heart, Lung, and Blood Institute Scientific Statement, *Circulation* 112:2735, 2005.

Grundy SM et al: Definition of metabolic syndrome: report of the National Heart, Lung, and Blood Institute/American Heart Association conference on scientific issues related to definition, *Circulation* 109:433, 2004.

Park YW et al: The metabolic syndrome: prevalence and associated risk factor findings in the US population from the Third National Health and Nutrition Examination Survey, 1988-1994, *Arch Intern Med* 163:427, 2003.

Pearson TA et al: AHA guidelines for primary prevention of cardiovascular disease and stroke: 2002 update: consensus panel guide to comprehensive risk reduction for adult patients without coronary or other atherosclerotic vascular diseases. American Heart Association Science Advisory and Coordinating Committee, *Circulation* 106:388, 2002.

AUTHOR: **GEETHA GOPALAKRISHNAN, M.D.**

BASIC INFORMATION

DEFINITION

Metatarsalgia refers to pain of the metatarsus, especially of the MTP articulation (Fig. 1-161). This is a nonspecific symptom usually involving the lesser toes.

ICD-9CM CODES
726.7 Metatarsalgia

PHYSICAL FINDINGS & CLINICAL PRESENTATION

- Pain beneath the metatarsal heads with ambulation
- Plantar callus formation beneath the metatarsal heads, usually involving one of the middle three toes
- Local tenderness
- Deformity
- Joint stiffness

ETIOLOGY

- Splayfoot
- Osteoarthritis, rheumatoid arthritis
- Freiberg's disease (avascular necrosis of second metatarsal head)
- Cavus foot (high arch)
- Bunion deformity
- Hallux rigidus
- MTP synovitis
- Morton's neuroma
- Often no obvious cause

DIAGNOSIS

DIFFERENTIAL DIAGNOSIS

See "Etiology."

WORKUP

Underlying cause should always be sought.

LABORATORY TESTS

Rheumatoid factor may be required to rule out rheumatoid synovitis.

IMAGING STUDIES

- Plain radiography to determine presence or absence of joint disease or deformity
- MRI may be able to detect neuroma

TREATMENT

NONPHARMACOLOGIC THERAPY

- Metatarsal bar or pad proximal to heads to redistribute weight
- Extra-depth shoe for contracture or deformity, if present
- Soft orthotic or well-padded liner to diffuse pressure around metatarsal heads
- Relief pads for plantar keratoses
- Soaks and pumice stone abrasion to decrease callus volume
- Rocker bottom shoe for resistant cases

CHRONIC Rx

- NSAIDs
- Intraarticular injection in selected cases with joint involvement

DISPOSITION

Prognosis is variable, depending on etiology.

REFERRAL

Failure to respond to medical management

SUGGESTED READINGS

Fuhrmann RA et al: Metatarsalgia: differential diagnosis and therapeutic algorithm, *Orthoade* 34(8):767, 2005.

Gorter K et al: Variation in diagnosis and management of common foot problems by GPs, *Fam Pract* 18(6):569, 2001.

Hassouna H, Singh D: Morton's metatarsalgia: pathogenesis, aetology and current management, *Acta Orthop Belg* 71(6):43, 2005.

Janisse DJ, Janisse E: Shoe modification and the use of orthotics in the treatment of foot and ankle pathology, *J Am Acad Orthop Surg* 16:152, 2008.

Jarboe NE, Quesada PM: The effects of cycling shoe stiffness on forefoot pressure, *Foot Ankle Int* 24:784, 2003.

Latinovic R et al: Incidence of common compression neuropathies in primary care, *J Neurol Neurosurg Psychiatry* 77(2):263, 2006.

Morscher E, Ulrich J, Dick W: Morton's intermetatarsal neuroma: morphology and histological substrate, *Foot Ankle Int* 21(7):558, 2000.

Sherry DD, Sapp LR: Enthesalgia in childhood, *J Rheumatol* 30:1335, 2003.

Waldecker U: Metatarsalgia in hallux valgus deformity: a pedographic analysis, *J Foot Ankle Surg* 41(5):300, 2002.

Yu JS, Tanner JR: Considerations in metatarsalgia and midfoot pain: an MR imaging perspective, *Semin Musculoskelet Radiol* 6(2):91, 2002.

AUTHOR: **LONNIE R. MERCIER, M.D.**

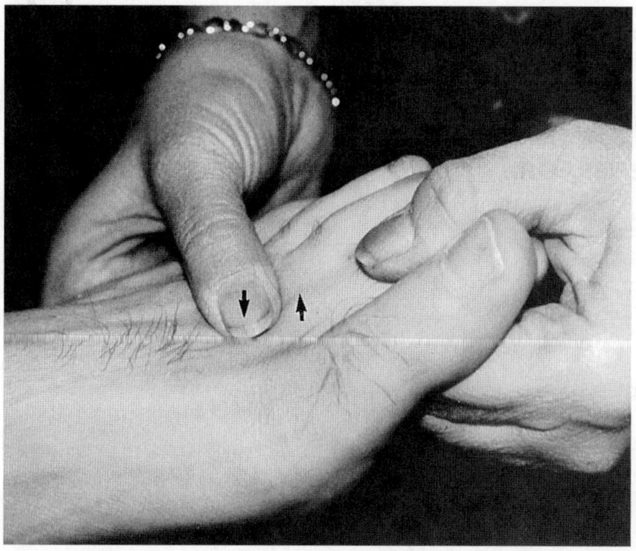

FIGURE 1-161 Vertical stress test for metatarsophalangeal stability. One of the examiner's hands stabilizes the metatarsal head while the other grasps the proximal phalanx. Examiner attempts to displace the proximal phalanx dorsally. A positive test result is the ability to displace dorsally while reproducing symptoms. (From Scuderi G [ed]: *Sports medicine: principles of primary care,* St Louis, 1997, Mosby.)

BASIC INFORMATION

DEFINITION

Milk-alkali syndrome is the consumption of large amounts of calcium and alkali resulting in the triad of hypercalcemia, metabolic alkalosis, and renal insufficiency.

SYNONYMS

Burnett's syndrome (acute form)
Cope's syndrome (subacute form)

ICD-9CM CODES
275.42 Milk-alkali syndrome

EPIDEMIOLOGY & DEMOGRAPHICS

In the early 20th century the milk-alkali syndrome was associated with an antacid regimen created by F.W. Sippy that included large amounts of calcium and bicarbonate. With the development of more effective and less toxic treatments, the syndrome virtually disappeared. Since the 1980s, however, there has been a small resurgence associated with use of calcium-containing products for the prevention of osteoporosis and the use of calcium bicarbonate rather than aluminum bicarbonate in patients with chronic renal failure. More recently, the milk-alkali syndrome was found to be the third leading cause of hypercalcemia (12%) in a review of hypercalcemia in hospitalized patients from 1990-1993.

PHYSICAL FINDINGS & CLINICAL PRESENTATION

- Asymptomatic hypercalcemia
  - Less than half of cases are made by an incidental finding of hypercalcemia and occasionally renal failure.
- Symptomatic hypercalcemia
  - Symptoms: nausea, vomiting, anorexia, fatigue, vague abdominal pain, nephrolithiasis- and pancreatitis-related pain and constipation. In more chronic cases, polyuria and polydipsia may be reported.
  - Physical exam and further testing: mental status changes such as anxiety, depression, and cognitive dysfunction, shortened QT interval.

ETIOLOGY

Overconsumption of supplemental calcium bicarbonate with reported ranges of 2.5 to 20 g/day particulary when associated with volume depletion, renal insufficiency, or use of hydrochlorothiazide or calcium-containing substances.

Betel nut chewing, a practice in Asia and the South Pacific, has been associated with a milk-alkali syndrome. Betel nuts are prepared with a compound that can be converted to calcium carbonate.

DIAGNOSIS

DIFFERENTIAL DIAGNOSIS

Hypercalcemia secondary to hyperparathyroidism or malignancy

LABORATORY TESTS

- Elevated plasma calcium (wide variation reported).
- Renal insufficiency.
- Elevated plasma bicarbonate and arterial pH, metabolic alkalosis.
- PTH, which is usually suppressed with milk-alkali syndrome, may be elevated, particularly if checked after treatment has begun.
- Phosphate level is variable.

TREATMENT

NONPHARMACOLOGIC THERAPY

Hemodialysis has been indicated for some patients with significant renal failure.

ACUTE GENERAL Rx

- Discontinuation of calcium bicarbonate supplements
- Aggressive hydration and furosemide if symptomatic hypercalcemia
- Monitor for rebound hypocalcemia as a result of elevation of PTH with treatment
- Patient education regarding appropriate calcium supplementation. Standard over-the-counter calcium supplements and some antacids contain calcium carbonate.

PROGNOSIS

Hypercalcemia and symptoms resolve with withdrawal of excess calcium supplementation and treatment of hypercalcemia. Patients initially presenting with renal failure may have residual renal insufficiency.

DISPOSITION

Treatment is determined by degree of hypercalcemia and symptomatology. Hospital admission is required for patients who require IV hydration and other intensive treatments for hypercalcemia.

REFERRAL

Differentiation from hyperparathyroidism can be difficult and may require the assistance of an endocrinologist. Referral to a nutritionist is generally not required as the excess calcium is from nutritional supplements rather than dietary factors.

PEARLS & CONSIDERATIONS

COMMENTS

Detailed history of dietary supplements and OTC medications can provide the most important clues. Many patients do not list dietary supplements as a medication.

SUGGESTED READINGS

Abreo K et al: The milk-alkali syndrome: a reversible form of acute renal failure, *Arch Intern Med* 153:1005, 1993.

Beall DP et al: Milk-alkali syndrome: a historical review and description of the modern version of the syndrome, *Am J Med Sci* 331(5):233, 2006.

Picolos MK et al: Milk-alkali syndrome is a major cause of hypercalcaemia among non–end-stage renal disease (non-ESRD) inpatients, *Clin Endocrinol* 63(5):566, 2005.

Sippy BW: Gastric and duodenal ulcer: medical cure by an efficient removal of gastric juice corrosion, *JAMA* 64:1625, 1915.

AUTHOR: **MICHELLE STOZEK ANVAR, M.D.**

BASIC INFORMATION

DEFINITION

Mitral regurgitation (MR) is retrograde blood flow through the left atrium secondary to an incompetent mitral valve. Eventually there is an increase in left atrial and pulmonary pressures, which may result in right ventricular failure.

SYNONYMS

Mitral insufficiency
MR

ICD-9CM CODES
424.0 Mitral regurgitation

EPIDEMIOLOGY & DEMOGRAPHICS

The incidence of MR has increased over the past 30 yr; however, this may be because of increasing availability of echocardiography rather than any real increases in this condition.

PHYSICAL FINDINGS & CLINICAL PRESENTATION

- Patients with MR generally present with the following symptoms:
  1. Fatigue, dyspnea, orthopnea, frank CHF
  2. Hemoptysis (caused by pulmonary hypertension)
  3. Possible systemic emboli in patients with left atrial mural thrombi associated with atrial fibrillation
- Hyperdynamic apex, often with palpable left ventricular lift and apical thrill
- Holosystolic murmur at apex with radiation to base or to left axilla; poor correlation between the intensity of the systolic murmur and the degree of regurgitation
- Apical early diastolic to middiastolic rumble (rare)

ETIOLOGY

- Papillary muscle dysfunction (as a result of ischemic heart disease)
- Ruptured chordae tendineae
- Infective endocarditis
- Calcified mitral valve annulus
- Left ventricular dilation
- Rheumatic valvulitis
- Primary or secondary mitral valve prolapse
- Hypertrophic cardiomyopathy
- Idiopathic myxomatous degeneration of the mitral valve
- Myxoma
- SLE
- Fenfluramine, dexfenfluramine, pergolide, cabergoline

DIAGNOSIS

DIFFERENTIAL DIAGNOSIS

- Hypertrophic cardiomyopathy
- Pulmonary regurgitation
- Tricuspid regurgitation
- VSD

WORKUP

Diagnostic workup consists of echocardiography, ECG, and chest x-ray.

IMAGING STUDIES

- Echocardiography: enlarged left atrium, hyperdynamic left ventricle (erratic motion of the leaflet is seen in patients with ruptured chordae tendineae); Doppler electrocardiography will show evidence of MR. The most important aspect of the echocardiographic examination is the quantification of left ventricular systolic performance.
- Chest x-ray study:
  1. Left atrial enlargement (usually more pronounced in mitral stenosis)
  2. Left ventricular enlargement
  3. Possible pulmonary congestion
- ECG:
  1. Left atrial enlargement
  2. Left ventricular hypertrophy
  3. Atrial fibrillation

TREATMENT

NONPHARMACOLOGIC THERAPY

Salt restriction

ACUTE GENERAL Rx

- Medical: Medical therapy is primarily directed toward treatment of complications (e.g., atrial fibrillation) and prevention of bacterial endocarditis.
  1. Consider digitalis for inotropic effect and to control ventricular response if atrial fibrillation with fast ventricular response is present
  2. Afterload reduction (to decrease the regurgitant fraction and to increase cardiac output): may be accomplished with nifedipine, hydralazine plus nitrates or ACE inhibitors
  3. Anticoagulants if atrial fibrillation occurs
- Surgery: Surgery is the only definitive treatment for MR. Transesophageal echocardiography allows accurate assessment of the feasibility of valve repair and is indicated before surgical intervention. The timing of surgical repair is controversial; generally surgery should be considered early in symptomatic patients despite optimal medical therapy and in patients with moderate to severe MR and minimal symptoms if there is echocardiographic evidence of rapidly progressive increase in left ventricular end-diastolic and end-systolic dimension (echocardiographic evidence of systolic failure includes end-systolic dimension >55 mm and fractional shortening <31%). Surgery is also indicated in asymptomatic patients with preserved ventricular function if there is a high likelihood of valve repair or if there is evidence of pulmonary hypertension or recent atrial fibrillation. Quantitative grading of mitral regurgitation is a powerful predictor of the clinical outcome of asymptomatic mitral regurgitation. Generally, patients with regurgitant orifices of ≥40 mm^2 should be considered for prompt surgery, whereas those with orifices between 20 and 39 mm^2 can be followed closely.

DISPOSITION

Prognosis is generally good unless there is significant impairment of left ventricle or significantly elevated pulmonary artery pressures. Most patients remain asymptomatic for many years (average interval from diagnosis to onset of symptoms is 16 yr).

REFERRAL

Surgical referral in selected patients (see "Acute General Rx"); emergency surgery may be necessary in patients with MR caused by ruptured chordae tendineae following MI.

PEARLS & CONSIDERATIONS

COMMENTS

Patients should be counseled regarding weight reduction (if obese), avoidance of tobacco, and maintenance of normal (nonstrenuous) activities.

SUGGESTED READINGS

Enriquez-Sarano M et al: Quantitative determinants of the outcome of asymptomatic mitral regurgitation, *N Engl J Med* 352:875, 2005.

Otto CM, Salerno CT: Timing of surgery in asymptomatic mitral regurgitation, *N Engl J Med* 3:352:928, 2005.

AUTHOR: **FRED F. FERRI, M.D.**

BASIC INFORMATION

DEFINITION

Mitral stenosis is a narrowing of the mitral valve orifice. The cross section of a normal orifice measures 4 to 6 cm^2. A murmur becomes audible when the valve orifice becomes smaller than 2 cm^2. When the orifice approaches 1 cm^2, the condition becomes critical, and symptoms become more evident.

SYNONYMS

MS

ICD-9CM CODES
394.0 Mitral stenosis

EPIDEMIOLOGY & DEMOGRAPHICS

- The occurrence of mitral valve stenosis has decreased worldwide over the past 30 yr (particularly in developed countries) as a result of declining incidence of rheumatic fever.
- The incidence of mitral stenosis is higher in women.

PHYSICAL FINDINGS & CLINICAL PRESENTATION

- Exertional dyspnea initially, followed by orthopnea and PND.
- Acute pulmonary edema (may develop after exertion).
- Systemic emboli (caused by stagnation of blood in the left atrium; may occur in patients with associated atrial fibrillation).
- Hemoptysis (may be present as a result of persistent pulmonary hypertension).
- Prominent jugular A waves are present in patients with normal sinus rhythm.
- Opening snap occurs in early diastole; a short (<0.07 second) A_2 to opening snap interval indicates severe mitral stenosis.
- Apical middiastolic or presystolic rumble that does not radiate is present.
- Accentuated S_1 (because of delayed and forceful closure of the valve) is present.
- If pulmonary hypertension is present, there may be an accentuated P_2 and/or a soft, early diastolic decrescendo murmur (Graham Steell murmur) caused by pulmonary regurgitation (it is best heard along the left sternal border and may be confused with aortic regurgitation).
- A palpable right ventricular heave may be present at the left sternal border.
- Patients with mitral stenosis usually have symptoms of left-sided heart failure: dyspnea on exertion, PND, orthopnea.
- Right ventricular dysfunction (in late stages) may be manifested by peripheral edema, enlarged and pulsatile liver, and ascites.

ETIOLOGY

- Progressive fibrosis, scarring, and calcification of the valve
- Rheumatic fever (still a common cause in underdeveloped countries); heart valves most frequently affected in rheumatic heart disease (in descending order of occurrence): mitral, aortic, tricuspid, and pulmonary
- Congenital defect (parachute valve)
- Rare causes: endomyocardial fibroelastosis, malignant carcinoid syndrome, SLE

DIAGNOSIS

DIFFERENTIAL DIAGNOSIS

- Left atrial myxoma
- Other valvular abnormalities (e.g., tricuspid stenosis, mitral regurgitation)
- Atrial septal defect

WORKUP

Physical examination and echocardiography

IMAGING STUDIES

- Echocardiography:
  1. The characteristic finding on echocardiogram is a markedly diminished E to F slope of the anterior mitral valve leaflet during diastole; there is also fusion of the commissures, resulting in anterior movement of the posterior mitral valve leaflet during diastole (calcification in the valve may also be noted).
     Two-dimensional echocardiogram can accurately establish valve area.
- Chest x-ray:
  1. Straightening of the left cardiac border caused by dilated left atrial appendage
  2. Left atrial enlargement on lateral chest x-ray (appearing as double density of PA chest x-ray)
  3. Prominence of pulmonary arteries
  4. Possible pulmonary congestion and edema (Kerley B lines)
- ECG:
  1. Right ventricular hypertrophy; right axis deviation caused by pulmonary hypertension
  2. Left atrial enlargement (broad notched P waves)
  3. Atrial fibrillation
- Cardiac catheterization to help establish the severity of mitral stenosis and diagnose associated valvular and coronary lesions. Findings on cardiac catheterization include:
  1. Normal left ventricular function
  2. Elevated left atrial and pulmonary pressures

TREATMENT

NONPHARMACOLOGIC THERAPY

Decrease level of activity in symptomatic patients.

ACUTE GENERAL Rx

- Medical:
  1. If the patient is in atrial fibrillation, control the rate response with diltiazem, digitalis, or esmolol. Although digitalis is the drug of choice for chronic heart rate control, IV diltiazem or esmolol may be acutely preferable when a rapid decrease in heart rate is required.
  2. If the patient has persistent atrial fibrillation (because of large left atrium), permanent anticoagulation is indicated to decrease the risk of serious thromboembolism.
  3. Treat CHF with diuretics and sodium restriction.
- Surgical: valve replacement is indicated when the valve orifice is <0.7 to 0.8 cm^2 or if symptoms persist despite optimal medical therapy; commissurotomy may be possible if the mitral valve is noncalcified and if there is pure mitral stenosis without significant subvalvular disease.
- Percutaneous transvenous mitral valvotomy (PTMV) is becoming the therapy of choice for many patients with mitral stenosis responding poorly to medical therapy, particularly those who are poor surgical candidates and whose valve is not heavily calcified; balloon valvotomy gives excellent mechanical relief, usually resulting in prolonged benefit.

DISPOSITION

- Prognosis is generally good except in patients with chronic pulmonary hypertension.
- Operative mortality rates for mitral valve replacement are 1% to 5% in most institutions.

AUTHOR: **FRED F. FERRI, M.D.**

BASIC INFORMATION

DEFINITION

Mitral valve prolapse (MVP) is the posterior bulging of interior and posterior leaflets in systole. Mitral valve prolapse syndrome refers to a constellation of MVP and associated symptoms (e.g., autonomic dysfunction, palpitations) or other physical abnormalities (e.g., pectus excavatum).

SYNONYMS

MVP
Mitral click murmur syndrome

ICD-9CM CODES
424.0 Mitral valve disorders
394.9 Other and unspecified mitral valve diseases

EPIDEMIOLOGY & DEMOGRAPHICS

- MVP can be found by 2D echocardiogram in 4% of the general population (females > males).
- Increased incidence is seen with autoimmune thyroid disorders, Ehlers-Danlos syndrome, Marfan's syndrome, pseudoxanthoma elasticum, pectus excavatum, anorexia nervosa, and bulimia.

PHYSICAL FINDINGS & CLINICAL PRESENTATION

- Usually, young female patient with narrow AP chest diameter, low body weight, low blood pressure
- Mid to late click, heard best at the apex
- Crescendo mid to late diastolic murmur
- Findings accentuated in the standing position
- Most patients with MVP are asymptomatic; symptoms (if present) consist primarily of chest pain and palpitations
- Neurologic abnormalities (e.g., TIA or stroke) are rare
- Patients may also complain of anxiety, fatigue, and dyspnea

ETIOLOGY

- Myxomatous degeneration of connective tissue of mitral valve
- Congenital deformity of mitral valve and supportive structures
- Secondary to other disorders (e.g., Ehlers-Danlos, pseudoxanthoma elasticum)

DIAGNOSIS

DIFFERENTIAL DIAGNOSIS

- Other valvular abnormalities
- Constrictive pericarditis
- Ventricular aneurysm

WORKUP

- Medical history and physical examination
- Workup consists primarily of echocardiography in patients with a systolic click or murmur on careful auscultation

IMAGING STUDIES

Echocardiography shows the anterior and posterior leaflets bulging posteriorly in systole.

TREATMENT

NONPHARMACOLOGIC THERAPY

Avoidance of stimulants (e.g., caffeine, nicotine) in patients with palpitations

ACUTE GENERAL Rx

The empiric use of antiarrhythmic drugs to prevent sudden death in patients with uncomplicated MVP is not advisable; β-blockers may be tried in symptomatic patients (e.g., palpitations, chest pain); they decrease the heart rate, thus decreasing the stretch on the prolapsing valve leaflets.

CHRONIC Rx

Monitoring for complications:

- Bacterial endocarditis (risk is three to eight times that of the general population)
- TIA or stroke secondary to embolic phenomena (from fibrin and platelet thrombi); risk in young patients: <0.05%/yr
- Cardiac arrhythmias (usually supraventricular)
- Sudden death (rare occurrence, most often caused by ventricular arrhythmias)
- Mitral regurgitation (most common complication of MVP)

DISPOSITION

The incidence of complications of MVP is very low (<1%/yr) and generally associated with an increase in mitral leaflet thickness to ≥5 mm; young patients (age <45) with absence of mitral systolic murmur or mitral regurgitation on Doppler echocardiography are at low risk for any complications.

REFERRAL

Surgical referral may be necessary in patients who develop symptomatic progressive mitral regurgitation.

PEARLS & CONSIDERATIONS

COMMENTS

- Recent studies suggest that the prevalence of MVP and its propensity to cause symptoms and serious complications have been overestimated in the past.
- Asymptomatic patients with MVP and mild or no mitral regurgitation can be evaluated clinically every 3 to 5 yr. High-risk patients should undergo a follow-up examination once a year.

SUGGESTED READINGS

Bouknight DP, O'Rourke RA: Current management of mitral valve prolapse, *Am Fam Physician* 61:3343, 2000.
Freed LA: Prevalence and clinical outcome of mitral valve prolapse, *N Engl J Med* 341:1, 1999.
Gilon D et al: Lack of evidence of an association between MVP and stroke in young patients, *N Engl J Med* 341:8, 1999.

AUTHOR: **FRED F. FERRI, M.D.**

BASIC INFORMATION

DEFINITION

The term *mixed connective tissue disease* (MCTD) describes a set of connective tissue symptoms that sometimes overlap with other known connective tissue diseases (SLE, progressive systemic sclerosis, polymyositis) but whose exact significance remains under debate. The disorder is sometimes referred to as an "overlap syndrome," but many prefer the term *undifferentiated connective tissue disease.*

ICD-9CM CODES
710.9 Diffuse connective tissue disease

EPIDEMIOLOGY & DEMOGRAPHICS

PREVALENCE: Approximately 10 to 15 cases/100,000 persons
PREDOMINANT SEX: Female:male ratio of 8:1
PREDOMINANT AGE: 4 to 80 yr

PHYSICAL FINDINGS & CLINICAL PRESENTATION

- Polyarthritis, polyarthralgia
- Raynaud's phenomenon, hand swelling, or sclerodactyly
- Esophageal hypomotility, myalgia, and muscle weakness
- Other: pericarditis, facial erythema, psychosis

ETIOLOGY

Autoimmune disorder

DIAGNOSIS

DIFFERENTIAL DIAGNOSIS

Other connective tissue disorders (SLE, progressive systemic sclerosis, polymyositis)

WORKUP

- Diagnosis is not well defined.
- Commonly used diagnostic tests are described in Laboratory Tests.

LABORATORY TESTS (Box 1-9)

- Rheumatoid factor is often present in low titers.
- If myositis is present, muscle enzyme (CPK) levels increase.
- Positive ANA is often present with a speckled pattern.
- ESR is elevated.
- Anti-RNP antibodies may be present.

TREATMENT

- Except for pulmonary and scleroderma-like symptoms, response to corticosteroids is excellent in most cases.
- Rheumatoid symptoms may respond to NSAIDs, but other cases may not even respond to gold or penicillamine.
- Immunosuppressive agents are used on occasion, but the best therapeutic options remain uncertain.

DISPOSITION

- Initially, this disorder was thought to be a mild variant of SLE, sometimes called "benign lupus," with excellent prognosis.
- Further studies suggested, however, that this was not always the case and serious renal, vascular, and neurologic complications were noted.
- Pulmonary involvement is a common clinical manifestation that may even lead to pulmonary hypertension and sometimes death.
- Whether MCTD is a separate entity continues under debate as concepts about the disorder evolve.
- Long-term outcomes remain uncertain.

REFERRAL

Rheumatology consultation for clarification and assistance in treatment

PEARLS & CONSIDERATIONS

COMMENTS

A clinical algorithm for evaluation of a positive ANA titer is described in Section III, "Antinuclear Antibody Testing."

SUGGESTED READINGS

Aringer M, Smolen JS: Mixed connective tissue disease: what is behind the curtain? *Best Pract Res Clin Rheumatol* 21:1037, 2007.

Bodolay E et al: Osteoporosis in mixed connective disease, *Clin Rheumatol* 22:213, 2003.

Chan AT, Wordsworth BP, McNally J: Overlap connective tissue disease, pulmonary fibrosis, and extensive soft tissue calcification, *Ann Rheum Dis* 62:690, 2003.

Keith MP et al: Anti-RNP immunity: implications for tissue injury and the pathogenesis of connective tissue disease, *Autoimmun Rev* 6(4):232, 2007.

Ling TC, Johnson BT: Esophageal investigations in connective tissue disease: which tests are most appropriate? *J Clin Gastroenterol* 32:33, 2001.

Lopez-Longo FJ et al: Does mixed connective tissue disease have a less favorable prognosis than systemic lupus erythematosis? *Arthritis Rheum* 44(suppl):119, 2001.

Lowe D, Kredich DW, Schanberg Durham LE: Thalidomide: an effective and safe agent for the treatment of pediatric mixed connective tissue disease, *Arthritis Rheum* 43(suppl): 117, 2000.

Tiddens HA et al: Juvenile-onset mixed connective tissue disease: longitudinal follow-up, *J Pediatr* 122(2):191, 2006.

AUTHOR: **LONNIE R. MERCIER, M.D.**

BOX 1-9 Guidelines for Diagnosing Mixed Connective Tissue Disease

General
Clinical features of a diffuse connective tissue disorder

Serologic
1. Positive ANA, speckled pattern, titer >1:1000
2. Antibodies to U1 RNP
3. Absence of antibodies to dsDNA, histones, Sm, Scl-70, and other specificities
4. Commonly: Hypergammaglobulinemia and positive rheumatoid factor

Clinical
1. Sequential evolution of overlap features over course of several years, including Raynaud's phenomenon, serositis, gastrointestinal dysmotility, myositis, arthritis, sclerodactyly, skin rashes, and an abnormal DLco on pulmonary function tests
2. Absence of truncal scleroderma, severe renal disease, and severe central nervous system involvement
3. A nail fold capillary pattern identical to that seen in systemic sclerosis (dropout and dilated vessels)

From Bennett RM: Mixed connective tissue disease and other overlap syndromes. In Kelley WN et al (eds): *Textbook of rheumatology,* ed 6, Philadelphia, 2005, WB Saunders.
ANA, Antinuclear antibodies; *dsDNA,* double-stranded DNA; *MCTD,* mixed connective tissue disease; *RNP,* ribonucleoprotein.

BASIC INFORMATION

DEFINITION

Viral infection characterized by discrete skin lesions with central umbilication (Fig. 1-162).

ICD-9CM CODES
078.0 Molluscum contagiosum

EPIDEMIOLOGY & DEMOGRAPHICS

- Molluscum contagiosum spreads by autoinoculation, scratching, or touching a lesion.
- It usually occurs in young children. It is also common in sexually active adults and patients with HIV infection.
- Incubation period varies between 4 and 8 wk.
- Spontaneous resolution in immunocompetent patients can occur after several months.

PHYSICAL FINDINGS & CLINICAL PRESENTATION

- The individual lesion appears initially as a flesh-colored, firm, smooth-surfaced papule with subsequent central umbilication. Lesions are frequently grouped. The size of each lesion generally varies from 2 to 6 mm in diameter.
- Typical distribution in children involves the face, extremities, and trunk. Mucous membranes are spared.
- Distribution in adults generally involves pubic and genital areas.
- Erythema and scaling at the periphery of the lesions may be present as a result of scratching or hypersensitivity reaction.
- Lesions are not present on the palms and soles.

ETIOLOGY

Viral infection of epithelial cells caused by a pox virus

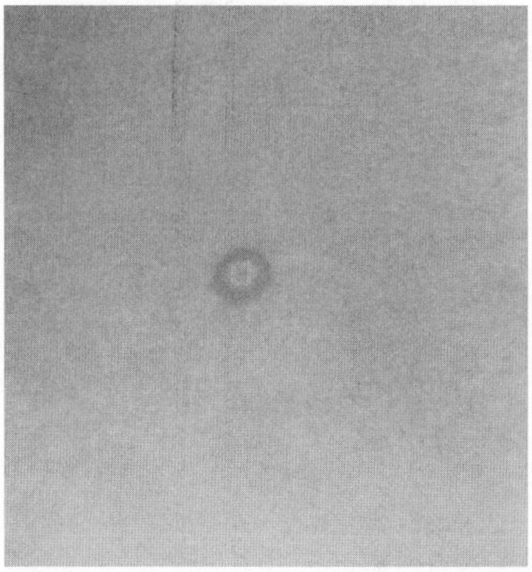

FIGURE 1-162 Molluscum contagiosum. (From Rakel RE: *Textbook of family practice, ed* 6, Philadelphia, 2002, WB Saunders.)

DIAGNOSIS

Diagnosis is usually established by the clinical appearance of the lesions (distribution and central umbilication). A magnifying lens can be used to observe the central umbilication. If necessary, the diagnosis can be confirmed by removing a typical lesion with a curette and examining the content on a slide after adding potassium hydroxide and gentle heating. Staining with toluidine blue will identify viral inclusions.

DIFFERENTIAL DIAGNOSIS

- Verruca plana (flat warts): no central umbilication, not dome shaped, irregular surface, can involve palms and soles
- Herpes simplex: lesions become rapidly umbilicated
- Varicella: blisters and vesicles are present
- Folliculitis: no central umbilication, presence of hair piercing the pustule or papule
- Cutaneous cryptococcosis in AIDS patients: budding yeasts will be present on cytologic examination of the lesions
- Basal cell carcinoma: multiple lesions are absent

WORKUP

Careful examination of the papules

LABORATORY TESTS

Generally not indicated in children. STD screening for other sexually transmitted diseases is recommended in all cases of genital molluscum contagiosum.

TREATMENT

GENERAL THERAPY

- Therapy is individualized depending on number of lesions, immune status, and patient's age and preference.
- Observation for spontaneous resolution is reasonable in patients with few, small, not irritated, and not-spreading lesions. Genital lesions should be treated in all sexually active patients.
- Liquid nitrogen cryotherapy
- Curettage following pretreatment of the area with combination prilocaine 2.5% with lidocaine 2.5% cream (EMLA) for anesthesia is useful for treatment of few lesions. Curettage should be avoided in cosmetically sensitive areas because scarring may develop.
- Treatments with liquid nitrogen therapy in combination with curettage are effective in older patients who do not object to some discomfort.
- Application of cantharidin 0.7% to individual lesions covered with clear tape will result in blistering over 24 hr and possible clearing without scarring. This medication should be avoided on facial lesions.
- Other treatment measures include use of imiquimod cream or tretinoin 0.025% gel or 0.1% cream at hs, daily use of salicylic acid (Occlusal) at hs, and use of laser therapy.
- Trichloroacetic acid peel generally repeated every 2 wk for several weeks is useful in immunocompromised patients with extensive lesions.

DISPOSITION

Most patients respond well to the therapeutic modalities listed previously. Spontaneous resolution can occur after 6 to 9 mo in some immunocompetent patients.

REFERRAL

To dermatology when diagnosis is in doubt or in patients with extensive lesions

PEARLS & CONSIDERATIONS

COMMENTS

Genital molluscum contagiosum in children may be indicative of sexual abuse.

EVIDENCE

A randomized controlled trial of males with molluscum contagiosum has found that treatment with 1% imiquimod analog in cream is significantly more effective than placebo, curing 82% of patients compared with 16% of patients cured with placebo.[1] B

A prospective clinical trial has evaluated the effectiveness of the 585 nm collagen remodeling pulsed dye laser in the treatment of cutaneous molluscum contagiosum and has found that 96.3% of the lesions healed after the first treatment and the remaining 3.7% healed after the second treatment (2 weeks later).[2] B

Evidence-Based References

1. Syed TA et al: Treatment of molluscum contagiosum in males with an analog of imiquimod 1% cream: a placebo-controlled double-blind study, *J Dermatol* 25:309, 1998. B
2. Michel JL: Treatment of molluscum contagiosum with 585nm collagen remodeling pulsed dye laser, *Eur J Dermatol* 14:103, 2004. B

AUTHOR: **FRED F. FERRI, M.D.**

BASIC INFORMATION

DEFINITION

Mononucleosis is a symptomatic infection caused by Epstein-Barr virus (EBV).

SYNONYMS

Infectious mononucleosis (IM)

ICD-9CM CODES
075 Infectious mononucleosis

EPIDEMIOLOGY & DEMOGRAPHICS

INCIDENCE IN U.S.: 45 cases/100,000 persons/yr
PREDOMINANT SEX: Incidence is the same, but occurs earlier in females.
PREDOMINANT AGE: Most common between the ages of 15 and 24 yr.

PHYSICAL FINDINGS & CLINICAL PRESENTATION

- Following an incubation period of 1 to 2 mo, a prodrome may occur, with fever, chills, malaise, and anorexia for several days. This is followed by the classic triad, which includes pharyngitis, fever, and adenopathy. Although fatigue and malaise may be prominent, pharyngitis is usually the most severe symptom. Exudates are common.
- Lymphadenopathy is most prominent in the cervical region but may be diffuse.
- Splenomegaly may occur, most commonly during the second week of illness.
- Rash is uncommon, but will occur in nearly all patients who receive ampicillin.
- At times, IM can present as fever and adenopathy without pharyngitis. Although complications may be severe, they are uncommon, and tend to resolve completely. Involvement of the hematologic, pulmonary, cardiac, or nervous system may occur; splenic rupture is rare. IM is usually a self-limited illness, but symptoms of malaise and fatigue may last months before resolving.

ETIOLOGY

The cause of IM is primary infection with EBV. Primary infection during childhood causes little or no symptoms. Infection during childhood is more common in lower socioeconomic groups. The frequency of IM in late adolescence is attributed to the onset of social contact between the sexes. Close personal contact is usually necessary for transmission, although EBV has occasionally been transmitted by blood transfusion. Transfer via saliva while kissing may be responsible for many cases.

DIAGNOSIS

DIFFERENTIAL DIAGNOSIS

- Heterophile-negative infectious mononucleosis caused by cytomegalovirus (CMV); although clinical presentation may be similar, CMV more frequently follows transfusion
- Bacterial and viral causes of pharyngitis
- Toxoplasmosis
- Acute retroviral syndrome of HIV, lymphoma

WORKUP

Heterophile antibody (monospot) and complete blood counts should be sent.

LABORATORY TESTS

- Increased WBC is common, with a relative lymphocytosis and neutropenia. Atypical lymphocytes are the hallmark of IM, but are not pathognomonic. Mild thrombocytopenia is common. A falling hematocrit may signal splenic rupture or severe immune-mediated hemolytic anemia. Elevated hepatocellular enzymes and cryoglobulins occur in most cases. Heterophile antibody, as measured by the Monospot test, may be positive at presentation, or may appear later in the course of illness. A negative test should be repeated if clinical suspicion is high. If this test remains negative for 8 wk, other causes of IM are likely. The monospot usually remains positive for 3 to 6 mo, but can last for 1 yr.
- A positive test has been reported with primary HIV infection.
- In addition to the heterophile antibody, virus-specific antibodies may result in response to IM. Determination of these EBV-specific antibodies is rarely necessary to diagnose IM, although early diagnosis in monospot negative cases may be made by isolating IgM to the viral capsid antigen (VCA), which is usually positive during the acute illness.

IMAGING STUDIES

Chest radiograph may rarely show infiltrates. An elevated left hemidiaphragm may occur in cases of splenic rupture.

TREATMENT

NONPHARMACOLOGIC THERAPY

- Supportive rest is advocated by some, but impact on outcome is not clear
- Splenectomy if rupture occurs. Transfusions for severe anemia or thrombocytopenia

ACUTE GENERAL Rx

- Pharmacologic therapy is not indicated in uncomplicated illness.
- The use of steroids is suggested in patients who have severe thrombocytopenia or hemolytic anemia, or impending airway obstruction as a result of enlarged tonsils. Prednisone, 60-80 mg PO qd for 3 days, then tapered over 1 to 2 wk. There is no role for antiviral agents such as acyclovir in the management of IM.

CHRONIC Rx

A rare, chronic form of IM with persistent organ infection and inflammation has been described. This should not be confused with chronic fatigue syndrome, which is unrelated to EBV.

DISPOSITION

Eventual resolution of all symptoms is the rule.

REFERRAL

More than mild illness

PEARLS & CONSIDERATIONS

COMMENTS

Contact sports should be avoided during the first month of illness, because splenic rupture can occur, even in the absence of clinically detectable splenomegaly.

SUGGESTED READINGS

Auwaerter PG: Infectious mononucleosis: return to play, *Clin Sports Med* 23:485, 2004.
Bauer CC et al: Serum Epstein-Barr virus DNA load in primary Epstein-Barr virus infection, *J Med Virol* 75(1):54, 2005.
Ebell MH: Epstein-Barr virus: infectious mononucleosis, *Am Family Physician* 70:1279, 2004.

AUTHORS: **GLENN G. FORT, M.D., M.P.H., DENNIS J. MIKOLICH, M.D.,** and **MAURICE POLICAR, M.D.**

BASIC INFORMATION

DEFINITION

Morton's neuroma refers to an inflammatory fibrosing process of the plantar digital nerve characterized by pain in the sole of the foot. Morton's neuroma is also described as an interdigital plantar neuropathy with or without plantar neuroma.

SYNONYMS

Morton's metatarsalgia
Morton's toe
Interdigital neuroma

ICD-9CM CODES
355.6 Morton's neuroma

EPIDEMIOLOGY & DEMOGRAPHICS

- Morton's neuroma most commonly involves the plantar digital nerve between the heads of the third and fourth metatarsals
- May also involve the second and third metatarsal and can involve both simultaneously
- Commonly occurs in people wearing tight-fitting shoes in toe region and high heels
- Morton's neuroma is usually unilateral
- Morton's neuroma is found more often in women than in men
- Can occur in both young and old

PHYSICAL FINDINGS & CLINICAL PRESENTATION

- Pain is usually located in a specific region, usually in the sole of the foot between the third and fourth metatarsal area and is unilateral in the majority of cases.
- Numbness may occur.
- Pain is exacerbated with exercise and relieved with rest and may radiate to the toes and to the ankle.
- Point tenderness is noted on examination, and palpation reveals fullness at the site of discomfort.
- An audible, painful click called *Murder's click* is noted in patients with Morton's neuroma after compressing and releasing the forefoot.
- Patients may have neuroma but silent lesions without symptoms.

ETIOLOGY

- Morton's neuroma is thought to be caused by nerve thickening from repeated injury.
- The typical finding is swelling of the plantar digital nerve that pathologically resembles other nerve entrapment syndromes (e.g., median nerve compression in carpal tunnel syndrome).

DIAGNOSIS

The diagnosis of Morton's neuroma is strictly made on clinical grounds alone as there are no laboratory tests or x-ray imaging studies that are specific for this disorder.

DIFFERENTIAL DIAGNOSIS

- Diabetic neuropathy
- Alcoholic neuropathy
- Nutritional neuropathy
- Toxic neuropathy
- Osteoarthritis
- Trauma (e.g., fracture)
- Gouty arthritis
- Rheumatoid arthritis

WORKUP

Exclude other causes as mentioned in the "Differential Diagnosis."

LABORATORY TESTS

- Laboratory studies are not specific for the diagnosis of Morton's neuroma
- CBC and ESR are usually normal
- Blood glucose
- B_{12} and folic acid level

IMAGING STUDIES

- X-ray imaging is primarily done to exclude other causes of foot pain (e.g., fractures, ostearthritis, gouty arthritis).
- MRI can detect and localize a neuroma but is rarely needed to make the diagnosis. An MRI can also be performed in patients with recurrent pain after surgical excision of a Morton's neuroma.
- Ultrasound imaging is also being used to locate Morton's neuroma but is rarely needed to make the diagnosis.

TREATMENT

NONPHARMACOLOGIC THERAPY

- Changing the type of footwear is the first line of treatment.
- Use open footwear and custom shoe inserts and avoid weight-bearing activities.
- Metatarsal pad with arch support is helpful.
- Participate in ultrasound therapy.

ACUTE GENERAL Rx

- If conservative measures are unsuccessful, injection of the intermetatarsal bursa with hydrocortisone may help
- Nonsteroidal anti-inflammatory agents (e.g., ibuprofen 400 to 800 mg PO tid or naproxen 250 to 500 mg bid)

CHRONIC Rx

- If nonpharmacologic and acute treatments do not give sufficient relief, surgical excision of the nerve has been successful in 95% of the cases.
- Surgery can be performed in the physician's office using local anesthesia.
- Numbness in the area where the nerve was excised is a common postoperative finding.

DISPOSITION

- Postoperative patients return to their normal activities by 3 to 6 wk.
- In cases where pain persists after surgery a "stump neuroma" may be present.
- Approximately 80% of patients who failed to have relief with the initial surgery did find relief with a second procedure.

REFERRAL

If surgery is being considered, a consultation with either a podiatrist or an orthopedic surgeon is indicated.

PEARLS & CONSIDERATIONS

COMMENTS

- Dr. Thomas G. Morton is given credit for describing this disorder in 1876.
- Morton's neuroma occurs just before the nerve bifurcates at the metatarsal area to innervate sides of two adjacent toes.
- A recent Cochrane analysis of treatment options for Morton's neuroma found insufficient evidence to support any treatment other than surgical excision for refractory cases.

SUGGESTED READINGS

Kay D, Bennett CL: Morton's neuroma, *Foot Ankle Clin* 8(1):49, 2003.

Sharp RJ et al: The role of MRI and ultrasound imaging in Morton's neuroma and the effect of size of lesion on symptoms, *J Bone Joint Surg Br* 85(7):999, 2003.

Thomson CE, Gibson JN, Martin D: Interventions for the treatment of Morton's neuroma, *Cochrane Database Syst Rev* 3:CD003118, 2004.

Weishaupt D et al: Morton neuroma: MR imaging in prone, supine, and upright weight-bearing body positions, *Radiology* 226(3):849, 2003.

AUTHORS: **GLENN G. FORT, M.D., M.P.H.,** and **DENNIS J. MIKOLICH, M.D.**

BASIC INFORMATION

DEFINITION

Patients with motion sickness suffer perspiration, nausea, vomiting, increased salivation, and generalized malaise in response to movement.

SYNONYMS

Physiologic vertigo

ICD-9CM CODES
994.6 Motion sickness

EPIDEMIOLOGY & DEMOGRAPHICS

INCIDENCE (IN U.S.): Common
PEAK INCIDENCE: Any age
PREVALENCE (IN U.S.): Common
PREDOMINANT SEX: Male = female
PREDOMINANT AGE: Any age
GENETICS: Not known to be genetic

PHYSICAL FINDINGS & CLINICAL PRESENTATION

- Vomiting
- Sweating
- Pallor

ETIOLOGY

- Motion (e.g., amusement rides, rides in automobiles or planes)
- Exacerbated by anxiety, fumes (e.g., industrial pollutants), visual stimuli

DIAGNOSIS

DIFFERENTIAL DIAGNOSIS

- Acute labyrinthitis
- Gastroenteritis
- Metabolic disorders
- Viral syndrome

WORKUP

None necessary in routine case

TREATMENT

NONPHARMACOLOGIC THERAPY

- Fixate on far object.
- Cease motion.
- Avoid reading.
- Avoid alcohol.

ACUTE GENERAL Rx

- Scopolamine patch (Transderm Scop) is most effective. It should be applied to hairless area behind ear every 3 days prn. It should be applied >4 hr before antiemetic effect is required.
- Over-the-counter oral preparations (e.g., Dramamine) are less effective.
- Meclizine (Antivert) 12.5 to 25 mg q6h may be effective.

CHRONIC Rx

- Rarely chronic
- Symptoms generally resolve completely with cessation of motion exposure

DISPOSITION

Follow-up is not needed.

REFERRAL

If another diagnosis is suspected (e.g., purulent ear, fever, cranial nerve abnormalities)

PEARLS & CONSIDERATIONS

COMMENTS

- Many patients with migraine report having severe motion sickness as a child.
- Improved ventilation, avoidance of large meals before travel, semirecumbent sitting, and avoidance of reading while in motion will minimize the risk of motion sickness.

EVIDENCE

A systematic review concluded that scopolamine was more effective than placebo in the prevention of motion sickness but no conclusions could be drawn from the comparative studies with other agents such as antihistamines and calcium channel antagonists.[1] Ⓐ

Limited evidence suggests that dimenhydrinate and cyclizine are equally effective in preventing motion sickness, but cyclizine is associated with less drowsiness and lower gastrointestinal symptom scores.[2] Ⓑ

Ginger may be effective in preventing seasickness, but evidence is still limited by the size of the trials.[3] Ⓑ

Evidence-Based References

1. Spinks AB et al: Scopolamine for preventing and treating motion sickness. Reviewed in: Cochrane Library, 3, Chichester, UK, 2004, John Wiley. Ⓐ
2. Weinstein SE, Stern RM: Comparison of Marezine and Dramamine in preventing symptoms of motion sickness, *Aviat Space Environ Med* 68:890, 1997. Ⓑ
3. Ernst E, Pittler MH: Efficacy of ginger for nausea and vomiting: a systematic review of randomized clinical trials, *Br J Anaesth* 84:367, 2000. Reviewed in: Does ginger prevent nausea and vomiting? Bandolier: Knowledge Library. Ⓑ

SUGGESTED READINGS

Koch KL: Illusory self-motion and motion sickness: a model for brain-gut interacting and nausea, *Dig Dis Sc* 48(8 Suppl):53S, 1999.

Yates BJ, Miller AD, Lacot JB: Physiological basis and pharmacology of motion sickness: an update, *Brain Res Bull* 45(5):395, 1998.

AUTHOR: **FRED F. FERRI, M.D.**

BASIC INFORMATION

DEFINITION

Mucormycosis is a fungal infection by *Zygomycetes* fungi, which include *Mucorales* spp. *(Mucor, Rhizopus, Absidia, Cunninghamella, Mortierella, Saksenaea, Syncephalastrum, Apophysomyces,* and *Thamnidium)* and *Entomophthorales* spp. *(Conidiobolus* and *Basidiobolus).*

ICD-9CM CODES
117.7 Mucormycosis

EPIDEMIOLOGY & DEMOGRAPHICS

- Infection by these ubiquitous organisms occurs in association with underlying conditions including diabetes mellitus, lymphoma, severe burns or trauma, prolonged postoperative course, multiple myeloma, hepatitis, cirrhosis, renal failure, steroid treatment, immunodeficiency states (e.g., AIDS), and use of contaminated Elastoplast bandages. Immunocompetent hosts may become infected in tropical climates.
- Most commonly the fungus gains entry to the body through the respiratory tract. The spores are deposited in the nasal turbinates and may be inhaled into the pulmonary alveoli. In cases of cutaneous mucormycosis, the spores are introduced directly into the skin lesion.

PHYSICAL FINDINGS & CLINICAL PRESENTATION

- Rhinocerebral-rhinoorbital-paranasal syndrome may present with fever, facial and orbital pain, headache, diplopia, loss of vision, facial or orbital cellulitis, facial anesthesia, cranial nerve dysfunction, black nasal discharge, epistaxis, and seizure. Physical findings in this situation include proptosis, chemosis, nasal, palatal or pharyngeal necrotic ulcerations, and retinal infarction. Thrombosis of the cavernous sinus or internal carotid artery may occur. This form of mucormycosis is found most commonly in diabetics, primarily in the presence of acidosis, and in patients with leukemia and neutropenia.
- Pulmonary mucormycosis can present with pneumonia, lung abscess, pulmonary infarction, pleurisy, pleural effusion, hemoptysis, chills, and fever. This form of mucormycosis is found most commonly in immunocompromised neutropenic hosts following chemotherapy for hematologic malignancies.
- Gastrointestinal zygomycosis presents with abdominal pain, diarrhea, GI hemorrhage, ulcers, peritonitis, and bowel infarction. This form of mucormycosis is found most commonly in patients with extreme malnutrition and is believed to arise from ingestion of the fungi.
- Cutaneous zygomycosis presents as nodular lesions (hematogenous seeding) or a wound infection. It involves primarily the epidermis and dermis following use of occlusive dressings that have not been properly sterilized.
- Cardiac mucormycosis is a form of endocarditis.
- Septic arthritis and osteomyelitis.
- Brain abscess occurs most often from extension of the fungus from the nose or paranasal sinuses through adjacent bones in severely debilitated patients.
- Disseminated zygomycosis (rare but uniformly fatal).
- Physical findings depend on the location of the infection.

ETIOLOGY & PATHOGENESIS

The cause of mucormycosis is infection by a fungus of the *Zygomycetes* class (see "Definition"). Normal host defenses include leukocytes and pulmonary macrophages. Quantitative (e.g., neutropenia) or qualitative (e.g., diabetes mellitus or steroid treatment) disruption in the host defenses predisposes the patient to infection.

DIAGNOSIS

The hallmark of mucormycosis is vascular invasion and tissue necrosis. Black eschars and discharges should be closely evaluated. Diagnosis depends on the demonstration of the organism in the tissue of a biopsy specimen.

DIFFERENTIAL DIAGNOSIS

- Infection of the sites described previously by other organisms (bacterial [including TB and leprosy], viral, fungal, or protozoan)
- Noninfectious tissue necrosis (e.g., neoplasia, vasculitis, degenerative) of the sites described previously

WORKUP

- Biopsy of infected tissue with direct light microscopy examination establishes the diagnosis within minutes of the biopsy in the case of nasopharyngeal infection. Typically the fungi appear as broad (10 to 20 micrometers in diameter) nonseptate hyphae with branches occurring at right angles.
- Bronchoalveolar lavage or bronchoscopy with biopsy for smear, culture, and histologic examination.
- X-rays and other imaging studies of symptomatic sites may be required before infection is suspected and tissue specimens are obtained.

TREATMENT

Aggressive correction of underlying disease (e.g., hyperglycemia, academia, high steroid doses, use of immunosuppressive drugs) should be undertaken.

Standard therapy for invasive mucormycosis is treatment with amphotericin B given IV at a daily dose of 1.0 to 1.5 mg/kg infused over 2 to 4 hr for a total of 1 to 4 g. Adverse reactions may be managed as follows:

- Fever, chills, headache, myalgias, nausea, and vomiting: premedicate with aspirin (650 mg po), acetaminophen (650 mg po), diphenhydramine (25 to 50 mg IV), hydrocortisone (25 to 100 mg IV), or meperidine (25 to 50 mg IV).
- Hypokalemia and hypomagnesemia are treated with potassium and magnesium replacement.
- Nephrotoxicity and renal tubular acidosis can be mitigated to some extent with 500 ml of normal saline infusion 30 min before and after each dose of amphotericin. Amphotericin dose reduction may also be necessary.
- Renal function and electrolytes should be monitored twice a week during the entire course of amphotericin.
- Lipid preparations of amphotericin B may be less toxic (i.e., amphotericin B lipid complex, amphotericin B colloidal dispersion, and liposomal amphotericin B).
- The role of flucytosine, rifampin, and tetracycline is controversial.
- Surgical debridement or radical resection.
- The role of colony-stimulating factors remains unclear, beyond that of increasing the neutrophil count in patients with neutropenia.

PROGNOSIS

- Sinus infection with no underlying disease: 75% survival.
- Sinus infection with diabetes: 60% survival.
- Sinus infection with renal disease: 25% survival.
- Surgery may increase survival by 5% to 20%.
- Early diagnosis improves survival as well as control of the underlying condition.

SUGGESTED READINGS

Larsen K et al: Unexpected expansive paranasal sinus mucormycosis, *J Otorhinolaryngol Relat Spec* 65:57-60, 2003.

Paydas S et al: Mucormycosis of the tongue in a patient with acute lymphoblastic leukemia: a possible relation with use of tongue depressor, *Am J Med* 114:618-620, 2003.

AUTHORS: **FRED F. FERRI, M.D.,** and **TOM J. WACHTEL, M.D.**

BASIC INFORMATION

DEFINITION

Multifocal atrial tachycardia is a supraventricular, moderately rapid arrhythmia (rate 100 to 140 bpm) with P waves having at least three or more different morphologies.

SYNONYMS

Chaotic atrial rhythm
The term *wandering pacemaker* is used for a similar arrhythmia associated with a normal or slow heart rate

ICD-9CM CODES
427.89 Multifocal atrial tachycardia

EPIDEMIOLOGY & DEMOGRAPHICS

Same as chronic lung disease (obstructive or restrictive), which the arrhythmia may complicate

PHYSICAL FINDINGS & CLINICAL PRESENTATION

Symptoms:
- Palpitation
- Lightheadedness
- Syncope
- Symptoms of the underlying pulmonary disease
- Physical findings associated with the underlying pulmonary disease

ETIOLOGY

- Exact mechanism unknown
- Associated abnormalities include hypoxia, hypercarbia, acidosis, electrolyte disturbances, digitalis toxicity

DIAGNOSIS

DIFFERENTIAL DIAGNOSIS

- Atrial fibrillation
- Atrial flutter
- Sinus tachycardia
- Paroxysmal atrial tachycardia
- Extrasystoles

WORKUP

- ECG (Fig. 1-163)
- Pulmonary function tests
- Electrolytes
- Arterial blood gases
- Digoxin level (if patient on digoxin)

TREATMENT

- Improve the pulmonary or metabolic dysfunction if possible
- Calcium blockers
- β-Blockers if not contraindicated by obstructive lung disease
- If the arrhythmia is asymptomatic, it can be left untreated

AUTHORS: **FRED F. FERRI, M.D.,** and **TOM J. WACHTEL, M.D.**

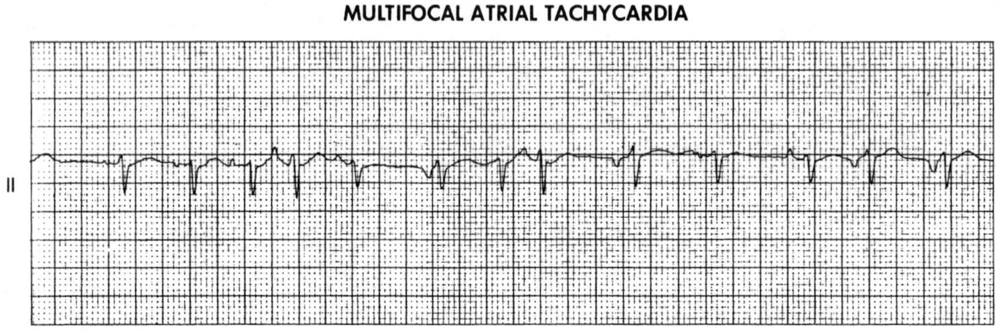

FIGURE 1-163 The P waves show variable shapes, variable PR intervals, or both. (From Goldberger AL: *Clinical electrocardiography,* ed 5, St Louis, 1994, Mosby.)

BASIC INFORMATION

DEFINITION

Multiple myeloma is a malignancy of plasma cells characterized by overproduction of intact monoclonal immunoglobulin or free monoclonal kappa or lambda chains. Diagnostic criteria require the following:

1. Presence of ≥10% plasma cells on examination of the bone marrow (or biopsy of a tissue with monoclonal plasma cells).
2. Monoclonal protein in the serum or urine. Occasional patients without detectable monoclonal protein are considered to have nonsecretory myeloma.
3. Evidence of end-organ damage (Calcium elevation, Renal insufficiency, Anemia, or Bone lesions [CRAB]).

ICD-9CM CODES
203.0 Multiple myeloma

EPIDEMIOLOGY & DEMOGRAPHICS

ANNUAL INCIDENCE: 4 cases/100,000 persons (blacks affected twice as frequently as whites); multiple myeloma accounts for 10% of all hematologic cancers.

PREDOMINANT AGE: Peak incidence in the seventh decade at a median age of 69 yr.

PHYSICAL FINDINGS & CLINICAL PRESENTATION:

The patient usually comes to medical attention because of one or more of the following:

- Bone pain (back, thorax) or pathologic fractures caused by osteolytic lesions
- Fatigue or weakness because of anemia secondary to bone marrow infiltration with plasma cells
- Recurrent infections as a result of impaired neutrophil function and deficiency of normal immunoglobulins
- Nausea and vomiting caused by constipation and uremia
- Delirium secondary to hypercalcemia
- Neurologic complications, such as spinal cord or nerve root compression, blurred vision from hyperviscosity
- Pallor and generalized weakness from anemia
- Purpura, epistaxis from thrombocytopenia
- Evidence of infections from impaired immune system
- Bone pain, weight loss
- Swelling on ribs, vertebrae, and other bones

DIAGNOSIS

DIFFERENTIAL DIAGNOSIS

- Metastatic carcinoma
- Lymphoma
- Bone neoplasms (e.g., sarcoma)
- Monoclonal gammopathy of undetermined significance (MGUS)
- Primary amyloidosis
- Chronic lymphocytic leukemia (CLL)

LABORATORY TESTS

- Normochromic, normocytic anemia; rouleaux formation on peripheral smear.
- Hypercalcemia is present in 15% of patients at diagnosis.
- Elevated BUN, creatinine, uric acid, and total protein.
- Proteinuria secondary to overproduction and secretion of free monoclonal kappa or lambda chains (Bence Jones protein).
- Tall homogeneous monoclonal spike (M spike) on protein immunoelectrophoresis (IEP) in approximately 75% of patients; decreased levels of normal immunoglobulins.
    1. The increased immunoglobulins are generally IgG (75%) or IgA (15%).
    2. Approximately 17% of patients have flat level of immunoglobulins but increased light chains in the urine by electrophoresis.
    3. A very small percentage (<2%) of patients have nonsecreting myeloma (no increase in immunoglobulins and no light chains in the urine) but have other evidence of the disease (e.g., positive bone marrow examination).
- Reduced ion gap resulting from the positive charge of the M proteins and the frequent presence of hyponatremia in myeloma patients.
- Hyponatremia, serum hyperviscosity (more common with production of IgA).
- Bone marrow examination: usually demonstrates nests or sheets of plasma cells, which comprise >30% of the bone marrow, and >10% are immature.
- Serum beta-2 microglobulin has little diagnostic value; it is useful for prognosis because levels >8 mg/L indicate high tumor mass and aggressive disease.
- Elevated serum levels of LDH at the time of diagnosis define a subgroup of myeloma patients with very poor prognosis.
- Increased interleukin-6 in serum during active stage of myeloma.
- The production of DKK1, an inhibitor of osteoblast differentiation, by myeloma cells is associated with the presence of lytic bone lesions in patients with multiple myeloma.
- Nearly all patients with myeloma present with abnormal chromosomes identified by fluorescence in situ hybridization (FISH). The Mayo Clinic Stratification of Myeloma, for purposes of therapy, identifies high-risk patients (~25% of patients at diagnosis) as those who have any of the following: FISH deletion 17p, FISH translocation 4;14, FISH translocation 14;16, cytogenetic deletion 13q, cytogenetic hypodiploidy, or plasma cell labeling index ≥3%.

IMAGING STUDIES

X-ray films of painful areas may demonstrate punched-out lytic lesions or osteoporosis. Bone scans are not useful, because lesions are not blastic.

TREATMENT

NONPHARMACOLOGIC THERAPY

Prevention of renal failure with adequate hydration and avoidance of nephrotoxic agents and dye contrast studies

ACUTE GENERAL Rx

- Newly diagnosed patients with good performance status are best treated with autologous stem cell transplantation. Allogenic transplantation is not recommended as routine therapy.
    1. Autologous transplantation is recommended for patients with stage II or III myeloma and good performance status.
    2. Induction therapy before stem-cell harvest is administered in four cycles. It includes dexamethasone alone or thalidomide-dexamethasone (thal-dex).
    3. High-dose chemotherapy (HDCT) with vincristine, melphalan, cyclophosphamide, and prednisone (VMCP) alternating with vincristine, carmustine, doxorubicin, and prednisone (BVAP) combined with bone marrow transplantation improves the response rate, event-free survival, and overall survival in patients with myeloma. Current HDCT regimen with autologous stem-cell support achieves complete response in approximately 20% to 30% of patients, with best results seen in good-risk patients, defined as young patients (<50 yr of age) with good performance status and a low tumor burden (beta-2 microglobulin ≤2.5 mg/L).
- Induction therapy in patients ineligible for transplantation (old age, coexisting conditions, poor physical conditions) includes the following chemotherapeutic agents:
    1. Thalidomide in combination with melphalan and prednisone.
    2. Melphalan and prednisone: the rates of response to this treatment range from 40% to 60%. Adding continuous low-dose interferon to standard melphalan-prednisone therapy does not improve response rate or survival; however, response duration and plateau phase dura-

tion are prolonged by maintenance therapy with interferon.
3. Vincristine, doxorubicin (Adriamycin), and dexamethasone (VAD) can be used in patients not responding or relapsing after treatment with melphalan and prednisone; methylprednisolone is substituted for dexamethasone (VAMP) in some centers.

- Therapy for relapsed and refractory myeloma:
  1. If the relapse occurs more than 6 mo after conventional therapy is stopped, the initial chemotherapy regimen can be reinstituted.
  2. Consider autologous stem-cell transplantation as salvage therapy in patients who had stem cell cryopreserved early in the course of the disease.
  3. Chemotherapy with vincristine, doxorubicin, and dexamethasone.
  4. Thalidomide, an agent with antiangiogenic properties, is also useful to induce responses in patients with multiple myeloma refractory to chemotherapy. Lenalidomide (CC-5013) is an active analogue of thalidomide developed to overcome the toxic effects of thalidomide.
  5. Bortezomib (Velcade) is a protease inhibitor that is cytotoxic for multiple myeloma. It is indicated for treatment of refractory multiple myeloma. It is superior to high-dose dexamethasone for treatment of patients who have had relapse. It is expensive, with an average course of treatment (five cycles) costing >$20,000.
- Approximately 15% of patients with newly diagnosed multiple myeloma are recognized incidentally and present without significant symptoms (smoldering myeloma). The rate of progression of smoldering myeloma to symptomatic disease is 10% per year for the initial 5 years, decreasing to 5% for the next 5 years, and decreasing further to 1.5% per year thereafter. Observation alone is reasonable in these patients because no survival advantage has been demonstrated by treating them.

CHRONIC Rx

- Promptly diagnose and treat infections. Common bacterial agents are *Streptococcus pneumoniae* and *Haemophilus influenzae*. Prophylactic therapy against *Pneumocystic carinii* with trimethoprim sulfamethoxazole must be considered in patients receiving chemotherapy and high-dose corticosteroid regimens. Vaccinate against *Streptococcus pneumoniae*, influenza, and *Haemophilus influenzae*.
- Control hypercalcemia with IV fluids and corticosteroids. Monthly infusions of the biphosphonate pamidronate provide significant protection against skeletal complications and improve the quality of life of patients with advanced multiple myeloma. Zoledronic acid (Zometa) at doses of 2 mg and 4 mg in patients with osteolytic lesions has been shown to be as effective as pamidronate in terms of reducing the need for radiation to bone, increasing bone mineral density, and decreasing bone resorption. It can be infused over 15 min for treatment of hypercalcemia of malignancy. Biphosphonates (pamidronate, zoledranate, and ibandronate) also appear to have an antitumor effect.
- Control pain with analgesics; radiation therapy to treat painful bone lesions or cord compression. Surgical stabilization of pathologic fractures. Consider vertebroplasty or kyphoplasty for selected vertebral lesions.
- Treat anemia with erythropoietin.
- Aggressive treatment of reversible causes of renal failure such as dehydration, hypercalcemia, and hyperuricemia.

DISPOSITION

- The median length of survival after diagnosis is 3 yr. Prognosis is better in asymptomatic patients with indolent or smoldering myeloma: median survival time is approximately 10 yr in persons with no lytic bone lesions and a serum myeloma protein concentration <3 g/dl. Adverse outcome is associated with increased levels of beta-2 microglobulin, low levels of serum albumin, circulating plasma cells, plasmablastic features in bone marrow, increased plasma cell labeling index, complete deletion of chromosome 13 or its long arm, t (4;14) or t (14;16) translocation, and increased density of bone marrow microvessels.
- As compared with a single autologus stem-cell transplantation, double transplantation (two successive autologus stem-cell transplantations) improves survival among patients with myeloma, especially those who do not have a very good partial response after undergoing one transplantation.
- Recent trials reveal that among patients with newly diagnosed myeloma, survival in recipients of a hematopoietic stem-cell autograft followed by a stem-cell allograft from an HLA-identical sibling is superior to that in recipients of tandem stem-cell autografts.

SUGGESTED READINGS

Attal M et al: Single versus double autologus stem-cell transplantation for multiple myeloma, *N Engl J Med* 349:2495, 2003.

Bruno B et al: A comparison of allografting with autografting for newly diagnosed myeloma, *N Engl J Med* 356:1110, 2007.

Dispenzieri A et al: Treatment of newly diagnosed multiple myeloma based on Mayo stratification of myeloma and risk-adapted therapy (mSMART): consensus statement, *Mayo Clin Proc* 82(3):323, 2007.

Facon T et al: Melphalan and prednisone plus thalidomide versus melphalan and prednisone alone or reduced-intensity autologous stem cell transplantation in elderly patients with multiple myeloma (IFM 99-06): a randomized trial, *Lancet* 370:1209-1218, 2007.

Imrie K et al: The role of high dose chemotherapy and stem-cell transplantation in patients with multiple myeloma: a practice guideline of the Cancer Care Ontario Practice Guidelines Initiative, *Ann Intern Med* 136:619, 2002.

International Myeloma Working Group: Criteria for the classification of monoclonal gammopathies, multiple myeloma, and related disorders: a report of the international Myeloma Working Group, *Br J Haematol* 121:749-757, 2003.

Kyle RA et al: Clinical course and prognosis of smoldering (asymptomatic) multiple myeloma, *N Engl J Med* 356:2582, 2007.

Kyle RA, Rajkumar SV: Multiple myeloma, *N Engl J Med* 351:1860-1873, 2004.

Rajkumar SV et al: Current therapy for multiple myeloma, *Mayo Clin Proc* 77:813, 2002.

Richardson PG et al: Bortezomib or high dose dexamethasone for relapsed multiple myeloma, *N Engl J Med* 352:2487-2498, 2005.

Tian E et al: The role of WNT-signaling antagonist DKK1 in the development of osteolytic lesions in multiple myeloma, *N Engl J Med* 349:2483, 2003.

AUTHOR: **FRED F. FERRI, M.D.**

BASIC INFORMATION

DEFINITION

Multiple sclerosis (MS) is a chronic autoimmune demyelinating disease of the central nervous system (CNS) characterized by clinical attacks (relapses) correlated with lesions separated in time and space. A relapse is the subacute onset of neurologic dysfunction that lasts for at least 24 hours. Subtypes include relapsing-remitting MS (RRMS) (relapses followed by complete or near complete recovery), secondary progressive MS (SPMS) (progression of disability with few or no relapses), and primary progressive MS (PPMS) (progression from onset). Rare MS variants include Balo's concentric sclerosis (alternating rings of myelination and demyelination), Marburg's disease (tumorlike lesion with significant edema), and Schilder's diffuse sclerosis (childhood onset with 1 to 2 large symmetric lesions). Neuromyelitis optica (NMO; Devic's disease) involves primarily the optic nerves and spinal cord, and is presently considered a separate disease.

SYNONYMS

MS
Disseminated sclerosis

ICD-9CM CODES
340 Multiple sclerosis

EPIDEMIOLOGY & DEMOGRAPHICS

PREVALENCE: Higher in northern latitudes and rare geographic clustering. Prevalence per 10^5 varies: 30 to 70 southern Europe, 100 to 200 Scandinavia, 40 to 177 U.S., 16 to 30 Middle Eastern Arabs, 30 to 38 Israeli Jews; <5 to 10 Asia, Central America, and most of Africa.

PREDOMINANT SEX/AGE: Female:male ratio is 1.5 to 2.4:1. Mean age (yr) of onset: overall 30, RRMS 28, SPMS 40, and PPMS 37.

SUBTYPES: 58% is RRMS (70% convert to SPMS after 25 yr), 27% SPMS, and 15% PPMS.

GENETICS: Frequency of MS in dizygotic twins and siblings is 3% to 5%; monozygotic twins 20% to 40%. Most common associations include HLA classes I and II (DRB1*1501, DQA1*0102, DQB1*0602).

PHYSICAL FINDINGS & CLINICAL PRESENTATION

- Common: fatigue, diplopia, vertigo, hemiparesis, paraparesis, monoparesis, numbness, paresthesias, ataxia, cognitive and urinary dysfunction
- Visual abnormalities: nystagmus, visual field defects, Marcus Gunn pupil (see topic "Optic Neuritis") and internuclear ophthalmoplegia—paresis of the adducting eye on conjugate lateral gaze with horizontal nystagmus of the abducting eye
- Upper motor neuron (UMN) signs: spasticity, increased deep tendon reflexes, extensor plantar response, clonus, and UMN pattern of weakness (shoulder abduction, elbow, hand and finger extension, hip and knee flexion, foot dorsiflexion)
- Sensory loss: pain/temp and/or vibration/position sense
- Ataxia: intention tremor, heel-to-shin ataxia, difficulty with tandem gait
- Bladder dysfunction: detrusor hyperreflexia (urge incontinence), flaccidity (neurogenic bladder), and dyssynergia (bladder contracts against a closed sphincter)
- Lhermitte's sign: flexion of the neck elicits an electrical sensation down the spine
- Uhthoff's phenomenon: exercise or heat-induced deterioration of function

ETIOLOGY

MS is thought to be caused by an interaction between multiple genes influencing the immune system and environmental factors, possibly including certain viruses, vitamin D, and sun exposure prior to adulthood.

DIAGNOSIS

- MS: primarily a clinical diagnosis based on a consistent clinical presentation with evidence of CNS demyelinating lesions disseminated in time and space not better explained by another disease.
- RRMS: a history of two relapses and confirmation on neurologic exam may be sufficient if *both* support the above definition. If there is only one lesion on exam or only one relapse, MRI or other paraclinical testing must be used (Table 1-28).
- PPMS: insidious progression of disability for ≥1 yr with two of three of the following:
  - Brain MRI: 9 T2 lesions in brain or ≥4 lesions plus positive delayed VEP
  - Spine MRI: ≥2 T2 lesions
  - Positive CSF: IgG index or oligoclonal bands (OCBs)

DIFFERENTIAL DIAGNOSIS

- Autoimmune: acute disseminated encephalomyelitis (ADEM), postvaccination encephalomyelitis
- Degenerative: subacute combined degeneration of the cord (B_{12} deficiency), inherited spastic paraparesis
- Infections: progressive multifocal leukoencephalopathy, Lyme, syphilis, HIV, HTLV-1, Whipple's, expand differential in immunocompromised patients
- Inflammatory: SLE, Sjögren's, Behçet's, vasculitis, sarcoidosis, celiac disease
- Inherited metabolic disorders: leukodystrophies
- Mitochondrial: Leber's hereditary optic neuropathy, mitochondrial encephalopathy lactic acidosis and stroke-like episodes (MELAS)
- Neoplasm: metastases, CNS lymphoma
- Vascular: subcortical infarcts, Binswanger's disease

WORKUP

- Lumbar puncture for all first relapses where the diagnosis of MS is not definite. Possible CSF abnormalities include increased protein and mononuclear WBCs (both usually only mild). An elevated CSF IgG Index and positive OCBs (send both with paired serum samples) are present in 70% and 90%, respectively, of clinically definite MS. False-positives occur with IgG Index in CNS infections and inflammation, but rarely with OCBs.

TABLE 1-28 Summary of McDonald's Criteria for Diagnosis of MS

Clinical Attacks	Clinical Lesions	Paraclinical Testing Needed
2	2	None
2	1	MRI dissemination in space *or* 2 lesions on MRI consistent with MS plus positive CSF
1	2	MRI dissemination in time
1	1	MRI dissemination in space *or* 2 MRI lesions consistent with MS plus positive CSF *and* MRI dissemination in time

CSF, Cerebrospinal fluid; *MRI,* magnetic resonance imaging; *MS,* multiple sclerosis.
1. Evidence of clinical lesions by physical exam or evoked potentials.
2. Positive CSF = positive oligoclonal bands (OCB) or elevated IgG index.
3. MRI dissemination in time = a new enhancing at least 3 mo or a new nonenhancing lesion (brain or spinal cord) at least 1 mo after the initial attack.
4. MRI dissemination in space = at least three of the following: (1) one enhancing lesion or nine T2 hyperintense lesions, (2) one infratentorial lesion, (3) one juxtacortical lesion, and (4) three periventricular lesions.
NOTE: One spinal cord lesion may count toward a T2 hyperintense lesion or be considered an infratentorial lesion.

- Serum: CBC, ESR, CRP, CHEM 7, LFTs, ANA, B12. Consider Lyme titer, ACE, other infectious and collagen vascular serologies, thyroid function tests, very-long-chain fatty acids, and arylsulfatase A. Also send NMO-IgG if suspected NMO.
- Consider evoked potentials (VEP, SSEP, BAER). Demyelination will slow conduction velocities.

IMAGING STUDIES

Head MRI with gadolinium is most sensitive (Fig. 1-164). MRI cervical spine can be helpful. MRI can assess acute and chronic lesions, and atrophy. A normal MRI, however, cannot exclude MS, especially in the first several years.

TREATMENT (Rx)

NONPHARMACOLOGIC THERAPY

Patient education regarding the disease, treatment options, and prognosis

ACUTE GENERAL Rx

Relapses: high-dose IV methylprednisolone (3 to 5 days of 1g MP/day; alternative dose is 15 mg/kg/day), often followed by a 7- to 10-day prednisone taper

CHRONIC Rx

- *Disease-modifying therapy* for RRMS includes: interferon beta-1a (IM Avonex, SC Rebif), interferon beta-1b (SC Betaseron), and glatiramer acetate (SC Copaxone). Interferons need CBC and LFT checks (month 1 followed by trimonthly), occasionally TSH. None needed with glatiramer acetate. Appropriate for PCP or neurologist to prescribe.
- Monoclonal antibody: refer to MS specialist. Natalizumab binds to an a4 subunit of leukocytes. It is a monthly infusion for RRMS associated with rare cases of progressive multifocal leukoencephalopathy (PML) when used in conjunction with other immunomodulatory medications.
- Cytotoxic: refer to MS specialist. Consider cyclophosphamide or mitoxantrone for frequent relapses with rapid disability progression and in early secondary progressive MS. Oral methotrexate or azathioprine is occasionally used.
- Spasticity: baclofen, tizanidine, diazepam, lorazepam, and intrathecal baclofen (oral medications not tolerated).
- Pain: carbamazepine, gabapentin, pregabalin, or amitriptyline.
- Spastic bladder: oxybutynin, tolterodine or propantheline. Prazosin for spastic sphincter.
- Fatigue: try amantadine 100 mg bid, modafinil (most effective for somnolence), or fluoxetine.
- Tremor: clonazepam, carbamazepine, or propanolol.

DISPOSITION

Most patients experience complete or near-complete recovery weeks to months after a relapse. The rate of disability progression over years is highly variable but often fastest in PPMS.

REFERRAL

- Initial neurology referral is highly recommended. Refer to MS specialist if poor response to therapy or MS variant.
- Consider referrals for PT, OT, social work, psychiatry, and urology.

PEARLS & CONSIDERATIONS (!)

Pseudorelapses may occur with heat, fever, or infections. Treat with antipyretic medication or cooling devices as appropriate.

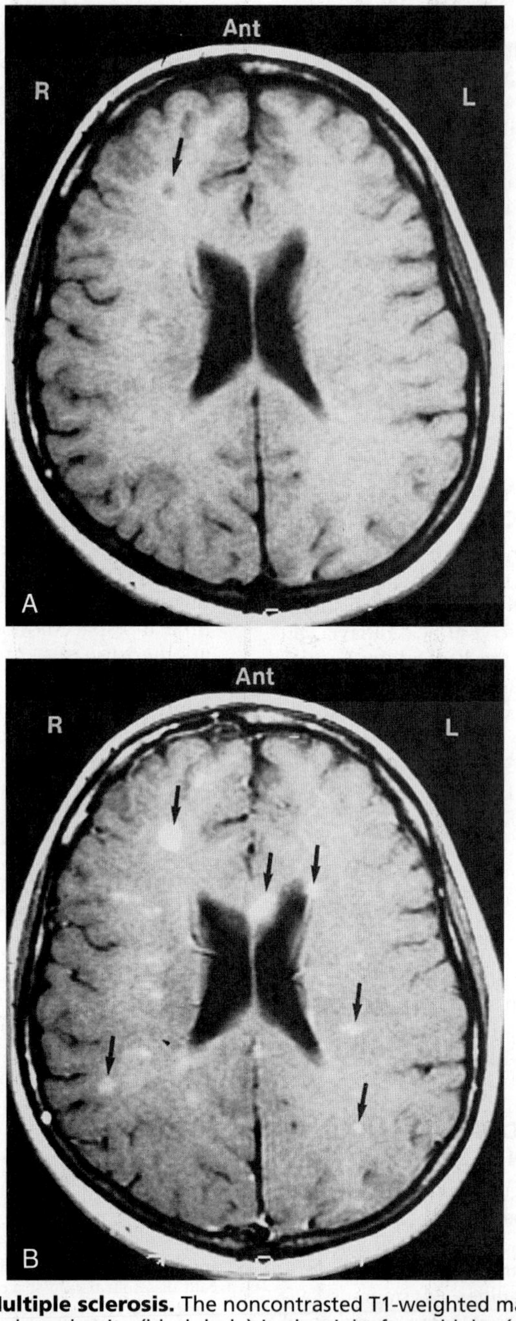

FIGURE 1-164 Multiple sclerosis. The noncontrasted T1-weighted magnetic resonance scan **(A)** shows one hypodensity (black hole) in the right frontal lobe *(arrow).* A gadolinium-enhanced scan **(B)** shows many enhancing lesions, only some of which are indicated *(arrows).* (From Mettler FA [ed]: *Primary care radiology,* Philadelphia, 2000, WB Saunders.)

EVIDENCE

EBM

Corticosteroids hasten recovery from acute relapses.

- A systematic review found that methylprednisolone significantly reduced the proportion of patients whose symptoms were worse or unimproved within 5 weeks of treatment. The long-term effect of such treatment, however, is uncertain.[1] **A**

Interferon-beta is effective in RRMS.

- Interferon beta-1a reduces the probability of conversion to definite multiple sclerosis if given to people with a first demyelinating event.[2,3] **B**
- There is a reduction in exacerbations (~30%) and disease progression over 2 years.[4] **A**
- Interferon beta-1b may slow progression in early SPMS.[5] **B**

Glatiramer acetate is effective in RRMS.

- Relapse rate has been shown to be reduced by 29% but without consistent evidence for reducing disability progression.[6-9] **B**

There is good evidence for limited use of natalizumab in RRMS.

- Reduces relapse rate by 68%, and disability progression by 42% over 2 years.[9] **A**
- Use with interferon beta-1a has rare risk of PML.[10] There is a theoretical risk of PML with natalizumab alone.

There is some evidence that cyclophosphamide and mitoxantrone are effective in select groups.[8]

Evidence-Based References

1. Filippini G et al: Corticosteroids or ACTH for acute exacerbations in multiple sclerosis, *Cochrane Database Syst Rev* 4, 2000.
2. Jacobs LD et al: Intramuscular interferon beta-1a therapy initiated during a first demyelinating event in multiple sclerosis, *N Engl J Med* 343:898, 2000.
3. Comi G et al: Effect of early interferon treatment on conversion to definite multiple sclerosis: a randomised study, *Lancet* 357:1576, 2001.
4. Rice GPA et al: Interferon in relapsing-remitting multiple sclerosis, *Cochrane Database Syst Rev* 4, 2001.
5. Kappos et al: Interferon beta-1b in secondary progressive MS: a combined analysis of the two trials, *Neurology* 63(10):1779, 2004.
6. Johnson et al: Copolymer 1 reduces relapse rate and improves disability in relapsing-remitting MS, *Neurology* 45:1268, 1995.
7. Munari L et al: Therapy with glatiramer acetate for multiple sclerosis, *Cochrane Database Syst Rev* 4, 2003.
8. Goodin DS et al: Disease modifying therapies in multiple sclerosis. Report of the Therapeutics and Technology Assessment Subcommittee of the American Academy of Neurology and the MS Council for Clinical Practice Guidelines, *Neurology* 58:169, 2002.
9. Polman CH et al: A randomized, placebo-controlled trial of natalizumab for relapsing multiple sclerosis, *N Engl J Med* 354(9):899, 2006.
10. Kleinschmidt-DeMasters BK, Tyler KL: Progressive multifocal leukoencephalopathy complicating treatment with natalizumab and interferon beta-1a for multiple sclerosis, *N Engl J Med* 353(4):369, 2005.

SUGGESTED READINGS

CHAMPS Study Group: MRI predictors of early conversion to clinically definite MS in the CHAMPS placebo group, *Neurology* 59:998, 2002.

Goodin et al: Disease-modifying therapies in multiple sclerosis, *Neurology* 58:169, 2002.

Polman et al: Diagnostic criteria for multiple sclerosis, *Ann Neurol* 58:840, 2005.

Weinshenker BG et al: The natural history of multiple sclerosis: a geographically based study, *Brain* 112:133, 1419, 1989.

AUTHOR: **ALEXANDRA DEGENHARDT, M.D.**

BASIC INFORMATION

DEFINITION

Mumps is an acute generalized viral infection that is usually characterized by nonsuppurative swelling and tenderness of one or both parotid glands. It is caused by mumps virus, a paramyxovirus and member of the paramyxoviridae family.

SYNONYMS

Viral parotitis
Parotitis

ICD-9CM CODES
072.9 Mumps

EPIDEMIOLOGY & DEMOGRAPHICS

INCIDENCE (IN U.S.):
- About 1600 infections/yr
- More than 150,000 cases/yr before licensure of mumps vaccine in 1967

PEAK INCIDENCE: Late winter and early spring months
PREDOMINANT SEX: Males = females
PREDOMINANT AGE: 75% of disease in teenage yr
GENETICS:
Congenital Infection:
- First-trimester infection is associated with excessive fetal deaths.
- Second- and third-trimester infection is not associated with increased fetal mortality.

Neonatal Infection:
- Uncommon
- Uncommon in infants <1 yr because of passive immunity conferred by placental transfer of maternal antibody

PHYSICAL FINDINGS & CLINICAL PRESENTATION

- Prodromal period:
  1. Low-grade fever
  2. Malaise
  3. Anorexia
  4. Headache
- Parotid swelling and tenderness are often first signs of infection.
  1. Progresses over 2 to 3 days, then opposite side may become involved
  2. Unilateral parotitis in 25% of cases
  3. Considerable pain with parotid swelling, causing trismus and difficulty with mastication and pronunciation
  4. Pain exacerbated by eating or drinking citrus and other acidic foods
  5. Possible fever with parotid swelling, ranging up to 40° C
  6. Parotid swelling usually resolving within 1 wk
- CNS involvement:
  1. May occur from 1 wk before to 2 wk after the onset of parotitis or even in its absence
  2. Meningitis
     a. Occurs in 1% to 10% of persons with mumps parotitis
     b. Occur three times more often in males than females
     c. Symptoms: headache, fever, nuchal rigidity, and vomiting
     d. Full recovery with no sequelae
  3. Encephalitis
     a. May develop early, as a result of direct viral invasion of neurons, or late, around the second week after onset of parotitis, and is a postinfectious demyelinating process
     b. Mumps accounted for only 0.5% of viral meningitis
     c. Symptoms: fever, alterations in the level of consciousness, possible seizures, paresis or paralysis, and aphasia. Fever can be quite high (40 to 41° C)
     d. Cerebellitis and hydrocephalus are serious complications of mumps encephalitis
     e. May result in permanent sequelae or death
  4. Other rare neurologic complications
     a. Cerebellar ataxia
     b. Transverse myelitis
     c. Gullain-Barré syndrome
     d. Facial palsy
- Epididymoorchitis:
  1. Most common extra salivary gland complication of mumps in adult men
  2. Occurs in 38% of postpubertal males who have mumps
  3. Most often unilateral but is bilateral in 30% of males who develop this complication
  4. May precede development of parotitis
  5. May be only manifestation of mumps
  6. Two thirds of cases develop during first week of parotitis
  7. One quarter of cases develop in second week
  8. Symptoms
     a. Severe pain, swelling, and tenderness of the testes and scrotal erythema
     b. Fever and chills
  9. Some degree of testicular atrophy in 50% of cases, months to years later
  10. Sterility from bilateral orchitis is rare
- Involvement of pancreas and ovaries:
  1. Abdominal pain
  2. Fever
  3. Vomiting
  4. Oophoritis
     a. Occurs in 5% of postpubertal women with mumps
     b. Symptoms include fever, nausea, vomiting, and lower abdominal pain
     c. May rarely result in decreased fertility and premature menopause
- Transient renal impairment:
  1. Common
  2. Manifest by hematuria and polyuria
- Joint involvement:
  1. Migratory polyarthritis is most frequent
  2. Infrequently affects adults with mumps
  3. Rarely in children
  4. Self-limited, with complete resolution
- Pancreatitis
  1. Uncommon as a severe illness
  2. Milder degree of upper abdominal discomfort
- Deafness:
  1. Most often unilateral, involving high frequencies; may rarely cause bilateral involvement
  2. Most patients recover
  3. Permanent unilateral deafness reported in 1 in 20,000 cases
  4. Labrynthitis and end lymphatic hydrops also reported
- Myocardial involvement:
  1. Uncommon
  2. Rarely causes progressive and culminant fatal myocarditis with dilated cardiomyopathy
  3. Refractory arrhythmia and congestive heart failure
  4. Coronary artery involvement
- Eye involvement:
  1. Corneal endothelitis following mumps parotitis

ETIOLOGY

- Virus is spread via direct contact, droplet nuclei, fomites, or oral or nasal secretions
- Patients are contagious from 48 hr before to 9 days after parotid swelling

DIAGNOSIS

DIFFERENTIAL DIAGNOSIS

- Other viruses that may cause acute parotitis:
  1. Parainfluenza types 1 and 3
  2. Coxsackie viruses
  3. Influenza A
  4. Cytomegalovirus
- Suppurative parotitis:
  1. Most often caused by *Staphylococcus aureus*
  2. May be differentiated from mumps
     a. Extreme indurations, tenderness and erythema overlying the gland
     b. Ability to express pus from Stensen's duct or massage of parotid
- Other conditions that may occur with parotid enlargement or swelling
  1. Sjögren's syndrome
  2. Leukemia
  3. Diabetes mellitus

4. Uremia
5. Malnutrition
6. Cirrhosis
- Drugs that cause parotid swelling:
  1. Phenothiazines
  2. Phenylbutazone
  3. Thiouracil
  4. Iodides
- Conditions that cause unilateral swelling:
  1. Tumors
  2. Cysts
  3. Stones causing obstruction
  4. Strictures causing obstruction

WORKUP

- Diagnosis based on history of exposure and physical finding of parotid tenderness with mild to moderate constitutional symptoms.
- Diagnosis is confirmed by a variety of serologic tests or isolation of the virus.

LABORATORY TESTS

- Diagnosis is confirmed by fourfold rise between acute and convalescent sera by CF, ELISA, or neutralization tests.
- Virus can be isolated from the saliva, usually from 2 to 3 days before to 4 to 5 days after the onset of parotitis.
- Virus can be isolated from CSF in patients with meningitis during the first 3 days of meningeal findings. More rapid confirmation of mumps in the CSF is IgM antibody capture Immunoassay and nested PCR assay.
- Virus can be detected in urine during the first 2 wk of infection.
- WBC
  1. May be normal or possible mild leucopenia with a relative lymphocytosis
  2. Leucocytosis with left shift with extra salivary gland involvement, such as meningitis, orchitis, or pancreatitis
- Serum amylase:
  1. Elevated in the presence of parotitis
  2. May remain elevated for 2 to 3 wk
  3. May be differentiated from mumps and parotids by isoenzyme analysis or serum pancreatic lipase
- Mumps meningitis:
  1. CSF WBCs from 10 to 2000 WBC/mm^3 with a predominance of lymphocytes
  2. In 20% to 25% of patients, predominance of polymorphonuclear cells
  3. CSF protein normal or mildly elevated
  4. CSF glucose low, <40mg/dl, in 6% to 30% of patients

TREATMENT

Rx

NONPHARMACOLOGIC THERAPY

- Supportive treatment
- Adequate hydration and nutrition

ACUTE GENERAL Rx

- Analgesics and antipyretics to relieve pain and fever
- Narcotic analgesics, along with bed rest, ice packs, and a testicular bridge, to relieve pain associated with mumps orchitis
- IV fluids for patients with frequent vomiting associated with mumps pancreatitis or meningitis

DISPOSITION

Most patients recover without incident.

REFERRAL

- To a neurologist if significant neurologic complications develop during or following mumps (myelitis, encephalitis, cranial nerve involvement, cerebellar ataxia, etc.)
- To a cardiologist if viral perimyocarditis develops
- To a urologist if orchitis develops

PEARLS & CONSIDERATIONS

!

COMMENTS

Prevention:
- Attenuated live mumps virus vaccine has been available since 1967.
  1. Usually given in combination with measles and rubella vaccines
  2. Should be given at 15 mo of age, and again at 5 to 12 yr
  3. Seroconversion in about 100% infants given the vaccine
  4. Contraindicated in pregnant women and immunocompromised patients
  5. Patients with asymptomatic HIV infection and patients with symptomatic HIV infection, in the absence of severe immunosuppression, can safely receive MMR vaccine
  6. Adverse events of vaccination include: local pain; indurations; thrombocytopenic purpura; Guillain-Barré syndrome; cerebellar ataxia
- Infected patients should be isolated until parotid swelling resolves.
- Because virus may be shed before the onset of parotid swelling, isolation possibly not of great value in limiting spread of infection.

EVIDENCE

EBM

The following statements concern the evidence for the MMR vaccine.

There are no randomized controlled trials comparing the clinical effects of combined measles, mumps, and rubella (MMR) vaccine vs. no vaccine or placebo.[1]

A large proportion of the literature on adverse events after immunization is based on passive reporting, which has major limitations (e.g., underreporting events or reporting events that are unassociated with the intervention).[1]

Existing evidence has failed to confirm an association between MMR vaccines and any autistic disorder, ulcerative colitis, Crohn's disease, or inflammatory bowel disease.[2-7] Ⓐ

Evidence-Based References

1. Bedford H et al: Measles: prevention. Reviewed in: 12:477, London, UK, 2004, BMJ Publishing Group.
2. Madsen KM et al: A population-based study of measles, mumps and rubella vaccination and autism, *New Engl J Med* 347:1477, 2002. Reviewed in: *Clin Evid* 12:477, 2004. Ⓐ
3. Institute of Medicine: *Immunization Safety Review: Measles-Mumps-Rubella Vaccine and Autism,* Washington, DC, 2001, National Academy Press. Reviewed in: *Clin Evid* 12:477, 2004. Ⓐ
4. Duclos P, Ward BJ: Measles vaccines: a review of adverse events, *Drug Saf* 6:435, 1998. Reviewed in: *Clin Evid* 12:477, 2004. Ⓐ
5. Morris DL, Montgomery SM, Thompson NP: Measles vaccination and inflammatory bowel disease: a National British Cohort study, *Am J Gastroenterol* 95:3507, 2000. Reviewed in: *Clin Evid* 12:477, 2004. Ⓐ
6. Patja A et al: Serious adverse events after measles-mumps-rubella vaccination during a fourteen-year prospective follow-up, *Pediatr Infect Dis J* 19:1127, 2000. Reviewed in: *Bandolier J* 84:2001. Ⓐ
7. Davis RL et al: Measles-mumps-rubella and other measles containing vaccines do not increase risk for inflammatory bowel disease: a case control study from the Vaccine Safety Datalink project, *Arch Pediatr Adolesc Med* 155:354, 2001. Reviewed in: *Clin Evid* 12:477, 2004. Ⓐ

SUGGESTED READINGS

Alp H et al: Acute hydrocephalus caused by mumps meningoencephalitis, *Pediatr Infect Dis J* 24(7):657, 2005.

Bloom S, Wharton M: Mumps outbreak among young adults in UK, *BMJ* 331(7508):363, 2005.

Centers for Disease Control and Prevention: Updated recommendations of the Advisory Committee on Immunization Practices (ACIP) for the control and elimination of mumps, *MMWR Morb Mortal Wkly Rep* 55(22):629, 2006.

Haas DM, Flowers CA, Congdon CL: Rubella, rubeola, and mumps in pregnant women: susceptibilities and strategies for testing and vaccinating, *Obstet Gynecol* 106(2):295, 2005.

Mackenzie DG, Hallam N, Stevenson J: Younger teenagers are also at risk of mumps outbreaks, *BMJ* 330(7506):1509, 2005.

AUTHORS: **VASANTHI ARUMUGAM, M.D., GLENN G. FORT, M.D., M.P.H.,** and **DENNIS J. MIKOLICH, M.D.**

BASIC INFORMATION

DEFINITION

Muscular dystrophy (MD) refers to a heterogeneous group of inherited disorders resulting in characteristic patterns of muscle weakness, some with cardiac involvement. Only disorders with childhood or adult onset will be considered here (i.e., excluding congenital myopathies).

ICD-9CM CODES
359 Muscular dystrophies and other myopathies
359.1 Hereditary progressive muscular dystrophy

EPIDEMIOLOGY & DEMOGRAPHICS

INCIDENCE:
- Most common childhood MD is Duchenne's muscular dystrophy with an incidence of 1/3500 male births
- Most common adult MD is myotonic dystrophy with an incidence as high as 1/8000

GENETICS:
- **Dystrophinopathies:** X-linked recessive defect in dystrophin gene resulting in either absence (Duchenne MD) or reduced/defective (Becker's MD) dystrophin.
- **Myotonic Dystrophy:** Autosomal dominant (AD) CTG trinucleotide repeat.
- **Limb-Girdle Muscular Dystrophy:** Autosomal recessive, also autosomal dominant forms with deficiency identified in multiple proteins (sarcoglycan, calpain, dysferlin, telethonin, lamin A/C, myotilin, and caveolin-3).
- **Emery-Dreifuss Muscular Dystrophy:** X-linked recessive defect in nuclear protein emerin or AR defect in inner nuclear lamina proteins lamin A/C.
- **Facioscapulohumeral Muscular Dystrophy:** AD; genetic mutation causes deletion of 3.3 kb repeat.
- **Oculopharyngeal Muscular Dystrophy:** AD GCG trinucleotide repeat resulting in deficient mRNA transfer from nucleus.

PHYSICAL FINDINGS & CLINICAL PRESENTATION

- **Dystrophinopathies:** Proximal arm and leg weakness with hypertrophic calf muscles, delayed motor milestones, cognitive impairment, cardiac involvement, progressive course resulting in respiratory complications and respiratory failure
  Duchenne's (DMD) onset 2 to 3 yr of age, typically wheelchair-bound by 12 yr
  Becker's (BMD) onset 5 to 15 yr of age, ambulatory beyond age 15
- **Myotonic Dystrophy:** Variable age of onset and severity manifesting as predominately distal weakness with long face, percussion and grip myotonia, temporalis and masseter wasting, ptosis, hypersomnolence, cognitive impairment, and cardiac conduction defects. May be associated with frontal balding, cataracts, impaired glucose tolerance, and male infertility.
- **Limb-Girdle Muscular Dystrophy:** Phenotypically and genetically heterogenous characterized by proximal hip and shoulder girdle weakness, some genotypes featuring cardiac involvement.
- **Emery-Dreifuss Muscular Dystrophy:** Early adulthood onset with predominately humeroperoneal weakness, early contractures, and cardiac dysfunction.
- **Facioscapulohumeral Muscular Dystrophy:** Onset typically in late childhood or adolescence with weakness mostly in face and shoulder girdle musculature and possible later, mild involvement of lower extremities.
- **Oculopharyngeal Muscular Dystrophy:** Symptom onset typically in mid-adult life with ptosis, dysphagia, dysarthria, and proximal muscle weakness.

DIAGNOSIS

DIFFERENTIAL DIAGNOSIS

Myasthenia gravis, inflammatory myopathy, metabolic myopathy, endocrine myopathy, toxic myopathy, mitochondrial myopathy

WORKUP

- Creatine kinase (CK)
- ECG, Holter monitor, echocardiography
- EMG
- Muscle biopsy with immunohistochemistry useful for diagnosis of dystrophinopathies and limb-girdle muscular dystrophy
- DNA analysis helpful if clinical suspicion is for myotonic, Emery-Drefuss, facioscapulohumeral, and oculopharyngeal muscular dystrophies
- Assessment of respiratory parameters, including forced vital capacity (FVC)

TREATMENT

NONPHARMACOLOGIC THERAPY

- Genetic counseling
- Physical, occupational, respiratory, speech therapy as symptoms dictate
- Screening for sleep-disordered breathing with overnight polysomnogram (PSG) if clinically indicated
- Pacemaker placement may be necessary if cardiac conduction defect present

ACUTE GENERAL Rx

Prednisone may modestly prolong ambulation in Duchenne MD.

CHRONIC Rx

Vigilance to avoid cardiac and respiratory complications, joint contractures

DISPOSITION

Variable course as severity of phenotype contingent upon both diagnosis and genotype.

REFERRAL

- Surgical referral for correction of scoliosis or contractures may be necessary
- Assessment and follow-up in a muscular dystrophy specialty clinic

PEARLS & CONSIDERATIONS

Formal evaluation recommended by anesthetist before any operation with general anesthesia in patients with dystrophinopathy

EVIDENCE

Clinical evidence supporting the use of corticosteroid therapy in Duchenne muscular dystrophy has been the subject of two recent reviews.[1,2] Prednisone at a dose of 0.75 mg/kg/day for boys aged 5 to 15 years has been shown to improve both muscle strength and function in this patient population for at least 18 months.[3,4] Timing the initiation of therapy and the exact duration of therapy has not been fully elucidated. Patients should be monitored for steroid-induced side effects and, if necessary, the steroid dose may be tapered to 0.3 mg/kg/day to minimize adverse effects with the recognition that clinical effect may be diminished.

Evidence-Based References

1. Moxley RT 3rd et al: Practice parameter: report of the Quality Standards Subcommittee of the American Academy of Neurology and the Practice Committee of the Child Neurology Society, *Neurology* 64:13, 2005. Ⓒ
2. Manzur AY et al: Glucocorticoid corticosteroids for Duchenne muscular dystrophy, *Cochrane Database Syst Rev* 2, 2004. Ⓐ
3. Griggs RC et al: Prednisone in Duchenne dystrophy. A randomized, controlled trial defining the time course and dose response. Clinical Investigation of Duchenne Dystrophy Group, *Arch Neurol* 48:383, 1991.
4. Griggs RC et al: Duchenne dystrophy: randomized, controlled trial of prednisone (18 months) and azathioprine (12 months), *Neurology* 43:520, 1993.

SUGGESTED READINGS

Emery AE: Muscular dystrophy into the new millennium, *Neuromuscul Disord* 12(4):843, 2002.

Emery AE: The muscular dystrophies, *Lancet* 359(9307):687, 2002.

Saperstein DS, Amato AA, Barohn RJ: Clinical and genetic aspects of distal myopathies, *Muscle Nerve* 24(11):1440, 2001.

AUTHOR: **TAYLOR HARRISON, M.D.**

BASIC INFORMATION

DEFINITION

Mushroom poisoning is intoxication resulting from ingestion of poisonous mushrooms.

ICD-9CM CODES
988.1 Mushroom poisoning

EPIDEMIOLOGY & DEMOGRAPHICS

- Five percent of all mushrooms are poisonous. Distinction between poisonous and edible mushrooms may be difficult even by experienced persons.
- Common poisonous species include *Amanita, Russula, Gyromitra,* and *Omphalotus*.

PHYSICAL FINDINGS & CLINICAL PRESENTATION (Table 1-29)

- *Russula* causes confusion, delirium, visual disturbance, tachycardia, and diarrhea within a few hours of ingestion. Prognosis: spontaneous recovery (mortality <1%).
- *Amanita* and *Gyromitra* intoxication begins with symptoms of gastroenteritis (nausea, vomiting, diarrhea, abdominal cramps) approximately 10 hr following ingestion. *Amanita* then goes on to cause cardiomyopathy and hepatic and renal failure. *Gyromitra* produces jaundice and seizures. Both mushrooms are associated with a 50% mortality rate.
- *Omphalotus* causes symptoms of gastroenteritis that subside spontaneously within 24 hr.

ETIOLOGY

- *Amanita* contains cytotoxic substances and isoxazoles that are gamma-aminobutyric acid neurotransmitter analogs.
- *Gyromitra* contains a pyridoxine antagonist that disrupts the GI mucosa and causes hemolysis.
- *Russula* contains a cholinergic substance.

DIAGNOSIS

DIFFERENTIAL DIAGNOSIS

- Food poisoning
- Overdose of prescription or illegal drug
- Other intoxications
- See topic on specific organ failure (e.g., renal or hepatic failure) for differential diagnosis of those conditions

WORKUP

- History
- Inspection and identification of suspected mushrooms
- Mushroom or gastric content analysis (by thin-layer chromatography or radioimmunoassay)

TREATMENT

- Gastric lavage
- Repeated administration of activated charcoal
- Supportive care as needed (may require respiratory assistance, hemodialysis, or emergency liver transplantation)

AUTHORS: **FRED F. FERRI, M.D.,** and **TOM J. WACHTEL, M.D.**

TABLE 1-29 **Mushroom Poisoning Syndromes**

Syndrome	Incubation Period (hr)	Species	Toxin
Confusion, restlessness, visual disturbances, lethargy	2	*Amanita muscaria* *Amanita pantherina*	Ibotenic acid, muscimol
Parasympathetic activity	2	*Inocybe* sp. *Clitocybe* sp.	Muscarine
Hallucinations	2	*Psilocybe* sp. *Panacolus* sp.	Psilocybin Psilocin
Disulfiram	2	*Coprinus atramentarius*	Disulfiram-like substances
Gastroenteritis	2	Many	Unknown
Hepatorenal failure	6-24	*Amanita phalloides* *Amanita virosa* *Amanita verna* *Galerina autumnalis* *Galerina marginata* *Galerina venenata*	Amatoxins Phallotoxins
Hepatic failure	6-24	*Gyromitra* sp.	Gyromitrin

From Gorbach SL: *Infectious diseases,* ed 2, Philadelphia, 1998, WB Saunders.

BASIC INFORMATION

DEFINITION

Myasthenia gravis (MG) is an autoimmune disorder of postsynaptic neuromuscular transmission classically directed against the nicotinic acetylcholine receptor (AChR) of the neuromuscular junction, resulting in a decrease in functional postsynaptic ACh receptors and consequent weakness.

ICD-9CM CODES
358.0 Myasthenia gravis

EPIDEMIOLOGY & DEMOGRAPHICS

INCIDENCE (IN U.S.): 2 to 5 cases/yr/1,000,000 persons
PEAK INCIDENCE: Female: second-third decade; male: sixth-seventh decade
PREVALENCE (IN U.S.): 1/20,000 persons
PREDOMINANT SEX: Female > male (3:2) in adults; female = male in elderly
GENETICS: Increased frequency of HLA-B8, DR3

PHYSICAL FINDINGS & CLINICAL PRESENTATION

- The hallmark of MG is fluctuating weakness worsened with exercise and improved with rest
- Generalized weakness involving proximal muscles, diaphragm, neck extensors in 85%
- Weakness confined to eyelids and extraocular muscles in about 15% of patients
- Bulbar symptoms of ptosis, diplopia, dysarthria, dysphagia common
- Normal reflexes, sensation, and coordination

ETIOLOGY

Antibody-mediated decrease in nicotinic acetylcholine receptors in the postsynaptic neuromuscular junction resulting in defective neuromuscular transmission and subsequent muscle weakness and fatigue

DIAGNOSIS

DIFFERENTIAL DIAGNOSIS

Lambert-Eaton myasthenic syndrome, botulism, medication-induced myasthenia, chronic progressive external ophthalmoplegia, congenital myasthenic syndromes, thyroid disease, basilar meningitis, intracranial mass lesion with cranial neuropathy, Miller-Fisher variant of Guillain-Barré Syndrome

WORKUP

Tensilon test: useful in MG patients with ocular symptoms.

Repetitive nerve stimulation (RNS): successive stimulation shows decrement of muscle action potential in clinically weak muscle, may be negative in up to 50%.

Single-fiber electromyography (SFEMG): highly sensitive, abnormal in up to 95% of myasthenics.

Serum AChR antibodies found in up to 80% of patients.

A subset of patients with seronegative MG may have muscle-specific tyrosine kinase (MuSK) antibodies.

ADDITIONAL TESTS

- Spirometry to document pulmonary function
- CT scan of anterior chest to rule out thymoma or residual thymic tissue
- TSH, free T_4: to rule out thyroid disease

TREATMENT

NONPHARMACOLOGIC THERAPY

- Patient education to facilitate recognition of worsening symptoms and impress need for medical evaluation at onset of clinical deterioration
- Avoidance of selected drugs known to provoke exacerbations of MG (β-blockers, aminoglycoside and quinolone antibiotics, class I antiarrhythmics)
- Prompt treatment of infections, diet modification, and speech evaluation with dysphagia

ACUTE GENERAL Rx

- Symptomatic treatment with acetylcholinesterase inhibitors:
  1. Pyridostigmine 30 to 60 mg PO q4 to 6h initially; onset of effects is 30 min, duration 4 hr
- Immunosuppressive treatment with corticosteroids, azathioprine, mycophenolate mofetil, cyclosporine for chronic disease-modifying therapy
  1. Prednisone initiated at 15 to 20 mg qd titrate by 5 mg increments to effect or dose of 1 mg/kg per day with improvement in 2 to 4 wk and maximal response by 3 to 6 mo
  2. Azathioprine initiated at 50 mg qd titrated to 2 to 3 mg/kg/day with clinical effect in 6 to 12 mo
  3. Mycophenolate mofetil initiated at 500 mg bid and titrated to 2 to 3 g per day, clinical effect in 2 wk to 2 mo
  4. Cyclosporine initiated at 5 mg/kg/day with clinical effect within 1 to 2 mo
- Plasmapheresis and intravenous immunoglobulin are possible short-term options for immunotherapy
- Mechanical ventilation is lifesaving in setting of a myasthenic crisis. Consider elective intubation if forced vital capacity <15 cc/kg, maximal expiratory pressure (<40 cm H_2O), or negative inspiratory pressure (<25 cm H_2O)

SURGICAL Rx

- In thymomatous MG, thymectomy is indicated in all patients.
- For nonthymomatous autoimmune MG: thymectomy is an option in patients less than 40 yr of age.

DISPOSITION

Course of disease is highly variable.

REFERRAL

Surgical referral for thymectomy in selected cases (see "Surgical Rx")

PEARLS & CONSIDERATIONS

Sustained upward or lateral gaze and arm abduction for 120 seconds may be necessary to elicit subtle signs on exam.

EVIDENCE

The use of corticosteroids in myasthenia gravis is supported more by clinical experience than by evidence from randomized controlled trials (RCTs).[1-3]

Azathioprine may afford a steroid-sparing effect and the frequency of clinical relapses may decrease in patients taking both medications.[4]

The use of plasmapheresis is supported by clinical experience although there are no RCTs that demonstrate its efficacy.

In patients with at least moderately severe disease and worsening weakness without severe dysphagia or respiratory failure, treatment with 2 g/kg intravenous immune globulin over 2 days has shown short-term improvement in strength (at 14 days) in one RCT.[5]

Evidence-Based References

1. Howard FM Jr et al: Alternate-day prednisone: preliminary report of a double-blind controlled study, *Ann N Y Acad Sci* 274:596, 1976.
2. Lindberg C, Andersen O, Lefvert AK: Treatment of myasthenia gravis with methylprednisolone pulse: a double blind study, *Acta Neurol Scand* 97:370, 1998.
3. Schneider-Gold C et al: Corticosteroids for myasthenia gravis, *Cochrane Database Syst Rev* 2, 2005. Ⓐ
4. Palace J, Newsom-Davis J, Lecky B: A randomized double-blind trial of prednisolone alone or with azathioprine in myasthenia gravis. Myasthenia Gravis Study Group, *Neurology* 50(6):1778, 1998.
5. Zinman L et al: IV immunoglobulin in patients with myasthenia gravis: a randomized controlled trial, *Neurology* 68(11):837, 2007.

SUGGESTED READING

Keesey JC: Clinical evaluation and management of myasthenia gravis, *Muscle Nerve* 29(4):484, 2004.

AUTHOR: **TAYLOR HARRISON, M.D.**

BASIC INFORMATION

DEFINITION

Mycosis fungoides refers to a T-cell lymphoproliferative disorder with characteristic cutaneous skin lesions and with the potential to disseminate into lymph nodes and viscera (Fig. 1-165).

SYNONYMS

Cutaneous T-cell lymphoma

ICD-9CM CODES
202.1 Mycosis fungoides

EPIDEMIOLOGY & DEMOGRAPHICS

- Incidence of mycosis fungoides is 4 cases per million persons.
- Approximately 1000 new cases are diagnosed annually in the U.S.
- More commonly affects males than females (2:1).
- Affects blacks > whites (2:1).
- Usually found in males 40 to 60 yr of age.

PHYSICAL FINDINGS & CLINICAL PRESENTATION

Mycosis fungoides characteristically progresses through three phases:

- A *premycotic phase* featuring scaly, erythematous patches that can last from months to years. During this stage the diagnosis can only be suspected, because the histopathologic features are not definitive for mycosis fungoides. Lesions are pruritic and can appear anywhere but are usually found in sun-shielded areas. Parapsoriasis en plaques, poikilodermatous parapsoriasis, parapsoriasis lichenoides, and variegata are skin lesions suspicious of representing premycotic cutaneous T-cell lymphoma.
- The *infiltrative plaque phase* features raised, indurated erythematous palpable plaques that are pruritic and may be associated with alopecia.
  - Stage IA disease is defined as a patch or plaque skin disease involving <10% of the skin surface area and with absence of blood involvement or with low blood tumor burden (<5% of atypical T-cells—Sézary cells—in the peripheral blood).
  - Stage IB disease is defined as a patch or plaque skin disease involving ≥10% of the skin surface area with absence of blood involvement or low blood tumor burden (<5% Sézary cells)
- The *tumor phase* is characterized by large, lumpy nodules arising from a premycotic patch, plaque, or unaffected skin and represents systemic infiltration and spreading. The tumors can be pruritic and large (>10 cm) and ulceration can occur.
  - Stage IIA and stage IIB diseases are defined by the presence of tumors with or without clinically abnormal peripheral lymph nodes with absence of blood involvement or low blood tumor burden. In approximately 5% of cases of mycosis fungoides, the presentation may be a diffuse, painful, pruritive erythroderma with Sézary cells in the peripheral blood (known as Sézary syndrome).
  - Stage III disease is defined by the presence of generalized erythroderma.
- Lymphadenopathy can occur during the plaque or tumor stages and may be regional or diffuse.
  - Stage IVA disease is defined by a lymph node biopsy showing large clusters of atypical cells, more than six cells, or showing total effacement by atypical cells.
- Infiltration of the liver, spleen, lungs, bone marrow, kidney, stomach, and brain can occur.
  - Stage IVB disease is defined by the presence of visceral involvement.

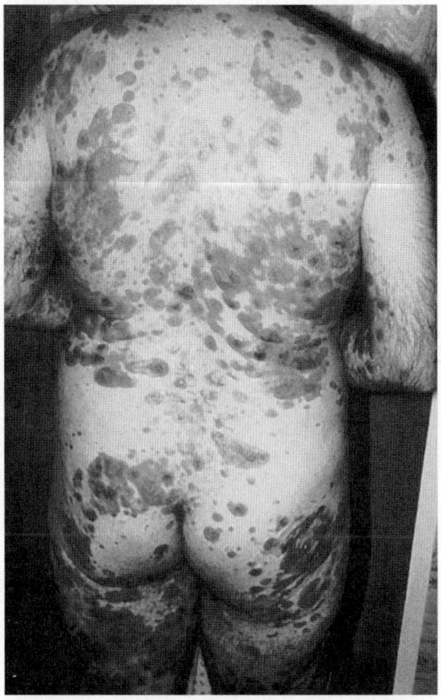

FIGURE 1-165 Cutaneous T-cell lymphoma (mycosis fungoides). Note patch, plaque, and tumor stages. (From Noble J [ed]: *Textbook of primary care medicine,* ed 2, St Louis, 1996, Mosby.)

ETIOLOGY

The specific cause of mycosis fungoides is not known. Infection with the retrovirus HTLV-1 has been suspected, given the association of individuals infected with HTLV-1 and those with T-cell leukemia. Other considerations listed but unsubstantiated include environmental toxins (e.g., tobacco, pesticides, herbicides, and solvents) and genetic predisposition.

DIAGNOSIS

The diagnosis of mycosis fungoides is established by skin biopsy. This may be difficult to differentiate from other skin lesions in the early phases of the disease (e.g., premycotic patch or early plaque lesions) and therefore the diagnosis can only be suspected.

DIFFERENTIAL DIAGNOSIS

- Contact dermatitis
- Atopic dermatitis
- Nummular dermatitis
- Parapsoriases
- Superficial fungal infections
- Drug eruptions
- Psoriasis
- Photodermatitis
- Alopecia mucinosa
- Lymphomatoid papulosis

WORKUP

Any patient who is suspected of having mycosis fungoides should have a staging workup done. Prognosis in patients with mycosis fungoides depends on the type of skin lesions and the extent of disease. The workup should focus on:

1. Complete physical exam
   - The type of skin lesion and the extent of skin involvement of the body (e.g., skin involvement is >10% or <10% of the skin surface)
   - Identification of palpable lymph node (especially those >1.5 cm in largest diameter)
   - Identification of organomegaly (e.g., lungs, liver)
2. Skin biopsy
   - Biopsy of the most indurated area
   - Immunophenotyping
   - Evaluation for clonality
3. Blood test
   - CBC with differential, liver function tests (LFTs), lactate dehydrogenase (LDH), chemistry
   - T-cell receptor gene rearrangement
   - Determination of Sézary cell count and/or flow cytometry
4. Radiologic tests
   - Depending on the stage of the disease, chest x-ray, ultrasound, CT scan of the chest, abdomen, and pelvis alone, with or without fluorodeoxyglucose positron emission tomography (FDG-PET) scan
5. Lymph node biopsy
   - Excisional biopsy
   - Biopsy of the largest lymph node

- If multiple nodes enlarged, order of preference is cervical, axillary, and inguinal areas
- Histopathology, flow cytometry, T-cell receptor gene rearrangement

TREATMENT

Rx

Treatment is guided according to the stage of disease.

NONPHARMACOLOGIC THERAPY

- For dry cracking skin, emollients (e.g., lanolin and petrolatum) are applied bid.
- Moisturizing lotion (e.g., ammonium lactate) applied bid.
- Topical antibiotics (e.g., bacitracin) are used on ulcerative tumors.

ACUTE GENERAL Rx

- Treatment of patients with stage IA limited patch or plaque phase include:
  - Topical nitrogen mustard 10 to 20 mg percent in water or ointment base applied to affected areas daily until cleared (usually 1 to 2 mo).
  - Psoralen ultraviolet light (PUVA) therapy where 0.6 mg/kg of 8-methoxypsoralen is ingested 1 to 2 hr before exposure of the skin to UV light (320 to 400 nm). This is done three times per week and tapered to 2 times per week until all the lesions have cleared. This is typically continued for 6 mo with a 90% complete remission rate.
- Treatment of patients with stage IB and IIA disease is similar to stage IA, with topical nitrogen mustard or PUVA.
  - Total skin electron beam therapy is considered in patients with thick plaques.
  - Interferon-alpha 5 million units SQ 3 times weekly can be considered in patients with stage IB or IIA disease.
  - Retinoids in combination with PUVA are used in refractory cases. Isotretinoin 1 mg/kg per day or acitretin 25 to 50 mg per day is the standard dosing.
- Treatment of patients with stage IIB disease with generalized tumor and plaque disease includes:
  - Total skin electron beam therapy in doses of 3000 to 3600 cGy given over 8 to 10 wk followed by adjuvant therapy with topical mustard can be used.

CHRONIC Rx

- In patients developing diffuse erythroderma, stage III disease (e.g., Sézary syndrome, extracorporeal photophoresis), 8-methoxypsoralen is ingested and peripheral blood is exposed to UVA through a membrane filter.
- Interferon and other systemic chemotherapeutic agents (e.g., methotrexate, cyclophosphamide, doxorubicin, vincristine, and prednisone) are considered in disseminated mycosis fungoides, stage IV disease.

DISPOSITION

- The median survival in patients with early patch or plaque phase disease and no extradermal involvement is 12 yr.
- The median survival of patients with skin involvement, lymph node involvement, but no visceral involvement, is approximately 5 yr.
- The median survival in patients with visceral involvement is 2.5 yr.

REFERRAL

Any patient with suspected mycosis fungoides should be referred to a dermatologist for definitive diagnosis and initial therapy. Oncology consultation is also indicated in patients with more advanced disease.

PEARLS & CONSIDERATIONS

!

A TNM staging classification of mycosis fungoides has been in use for guiding therapy since 1979. The International Society for Cutaneous Lymphomas (ISCL) and the Cutaneous Lymphoma Task Force of the European Organization of Research and Treatment of Cancer (EORTC) recommended revisions to the TNM classification and staging system of cutaneous T-cell lymphoma in 2007.

COMMENTS

Mycosis fungoides is thought to represent one class of the spectrum of cutaneous T-cell lymphomas.

SUGGESTED READINGS

Foss F: Mycosis fungoides and the Sézary syndrome, *Curr Opin Oncol* 16(5):421, 2004.

Girardi M, Heald PW, Wilson LD: The pathogenesis of mycosis fungoides, *N Engl J Med* 350(19):1978, 2004.

Lundin J, Osterborg A: Therapy for mycosis fungoides, *Curr Treat Options Oncol* 5(3):203, 2004.

Olsen E: Revisions to the staging and classification of mycosis fungoides and Sézary syndrome: a proposal of the International Society for Cutaneous Lymphomas (ISCL) and the Cutaneous Lymphoma Task Force of the European Organization of Research and Treatment of Cancer (EORTC), *Blood* 110(6):1713, 2007.

AUTHOR: **TANYA ALI, M.D.**

BASIC INFORMATION

DEFINITION

Myelodysplastic syndromes (MDS) are a group of acquired clonal disorders affecting the hemopoietic stem cells and characterized by cytopenias with hypercellular bone marrow and various morphologic abnormalities in the hemopoietic cell lines. MDS show abnormal (dysplastic) hemopoietic maturation. Marrow cellularity is increased, reflecting an effective hematopoiesis, but inadequate maturation results in peripheral cytopenias.

CLASSIFICATION

- Myelodysplasia encompasses several heterogenous syndromes. The French-American-British (FAB) classification of myelodysplastic syndromes is based on the proportion of immature blast cells in the blood and marrow and on the presence or absence of ringed sideroblasts or peripheral monocytosis. It includes the following: refractory anemia, refractory anemia with ringed sideroblasts, refractory anemia with excess blasts, chronic myelomonocytic leukemia, and refractory anemia with excess blasts in transformation.
- In 1999 the World Health Organization modified the FAB by incorporating newer morphologic insights and cytogenetic findings. It includes the following disease subtypes: refractory anemia, refractory anemia with ringed sideroblasts, refractory cytopenia with multilineage dysplasia, refractory cytopenia with multilineage dysplasia and ringed sideroblasts, refractory anemia with excessive blasts (1, 2), unclassified myelodysplastic syndrome, and myelodysplastic syndrome associated with isolated del(5q).

SYNONYMS

MDS
Preleukemia
Dysmyelopoietic syndrome

ICD-9CM CODES
238.7 Myelodysplastic syndrome

EPIDEMIOLOGY & DEMOGRAPHICS

INCIDENCE (IN U.S.): Approximately 82 cases/100,000 persons/yr. An estimated 7,000 to 12,000 new cases are diagnosed annually in the U.S.

PREDOMINANT AGE: More common in elderly patients, with a median age of >65 yr.

PHYSICAL FINDINGS & CLINICAL PRESENTATION:

- Splenomegaly, skin pallor, mucosal bleeding, ecchymosis may be present.
- Patients often present with fatigue.
- Fever, infection, and dyspnea are common.

ETIOLOGY

Unknown. However, exposure to radiation, chemotherapeutic agents, benzene, or other organic compounds is associated with myelodysplasia.

DIAGNOSIS

DIFFERENTIAL DIAGNOSIS

- Hereditary dysplasias (e.g., Fanconi's anemia, Diamond-Blackfan syndrome)
- Vitamin B_{12}/folate deficiency
- Exposure to toxins (drugs, alcohol, chemotherapy)
- Renal failure
- Irradiation
- Autoimmune disease
- Infections (TB, viral infections)
- Paroxysmal nocturnal hemoglobinuria

WORKUP

Diagnostic workup includes laboratory evaluation and bone marrow examination. Cytogenetic analysis by conventional metaphase karyotyping should be performed in patients with MDS.

TREATMENT

NONPHARMACOLOGIC THERAPY

RBC transfusions in patients with severe symptomatic anemia

ACUTE GENERAL Rx

- Results of chemotherapy are generally disappointing. Combination chemotherapy regimens (e.g., cytarabine plus doxorubicin) generally induce a complete response in only a minority of patients and the average duration of response is less than 1 yr.
- Azacitidine (Vidaza), a pyrimidine nucleoside analog of cytidine, has been shown to improve the quality of life for patients with myelodysplastic syndrome and probably prolong survival. Decitabine (Dacogen), another nucleoside analog, has also been FDA approved for patients with MDS.
- The role of myeloid growth factors (granulocyte colony–stimulating factor, granulocyte-macrophage colony–stimulating factor) and immunotherapy is undefined. In a recent trial, 34% of patients treated with antithymocyte globulin (40 mg/kg for 4 days) became transfusion independent. Response was also associated with a statistically significantly longer survival.
- Lenalidomide (Revlimid), a novel analogue of thalidomide, has demonstrated hematologic activity in patients with low-rise myelodysplastic syndrome who have no response to erythropoietin or who are unlikely to benefit from conventional therapy. Lenalidomide can also reduce transfusion requirements and reverse cytologic and cytogenetic abnormalities in patients who have myelodysplastic syndrome with the 5q31 deletion.
- Allogeneic stem-cell transplantation should be considered in patients <60 yr old because this is the established procedure with cure potential.

CHRONIC Rx

Monitor for infections, bleeding, and complications of anemia. Supportive measures include blood transfusions and erythropoietin for anemia, and antibiotics to treat opportunistic infections. Iron overload from frequent transfusions may require iron chelation therapy.

DISPOSITION

- Cure rates in young patients with allogeneic bone marrow transplantations approach 30% to 50%.
- The risk of transformation to acute myelogenous leukemia varies with the percentage of blasts in the bone marrow.
- Advanced age, male sex, and deletion of chromosomes 5 and 7 are associated with a poor prognosis.
- The 1997 International Prognostic Scoring System (IPSS) uses the following three elements for staging: (1) the proportion of myeloblasts in the patient's marrow, (2) the number of blood cell lineage deficits, and (3) the type of chromosomal abnormality present (e.g., poor risk includes abnormalities of chromosome 7; good risk includes clonal loss of the Y chromosome). According to the International Myelodysplastic Syndrome Risk Analysis Workshop, the most important variables in disease outcome are the specific cytogenetic abnormalities, the percentage of blasts in the bone marrow, and the number of hematopoietic lineages involved in the cytopenias.

REFERRAL

Hematology referral in all patients with MDS

PEARLS & CONSIDERATIONS

COMMENTS

- Patients with cytogenetic abnormalities associated with poor prognosis should be considered for aggressive treatment with high-dose chemotherapy and stem-cell transplantation.
- Nearly 50% of the deaths that result from myelodysplastic syndromes are the result of cytopenia associated with bone marrow failure.

SUGGESTED READINGS

List A et al: Lenalidomide in the myelodysplastic syndrome with chromosome 5q deletion, *N Engl J Med* 355:1456, 2006.

Steensma DP, Bennett JM: The myelodysplastic syndromes: diagnosis and treatment, *Mayo Clin Proc* 81(1)104, 2006.

AUTHOR: **FRED F. FERRI, M.D.**

BASIC INFORMATION

DEFINITION

Acute coronary syndromes are manifestations of ischemic heart disease and represent a broad clinical spectrum that includes non-ST segment elevation acute coronary syndrome (NSTEACS) (collectively unstable angina [UA]/non-ST elevation MI [NSTEMI]) and ST-elevation MI (STEMI).

1. Myocardial infarction is characterized by necrosis resulting from an insufficient supply of oxygenated blood to an area of the heart. According to the joint European Society of Cardiology/American College of Cardiology, either one of the following criteria for acute evolving or recent MI satisfies the diagnosis:
   a. Typical rise and gradual fall (troponin) or more rapid rise and fall (CK-MB) of biochemical markers of myocardial necrosis with at least one of the following:
      i. Ischemic symptoms
      ii. Development of pathologic Q waves on ECG
      iii. ECG changes indicative of ischemia (ST-segment elevation or depression)
      iv. Coronary artery intervention (e.g., coronary angioplasty)
   b. Pathologic findings of acute MI
2. ST elevation MI: area of ischemic necrosis that penetrates the entire thickness of the ventricular wall and results in ST-segment elevation.
3. Unstable angina: coronary arterial plaque rupture with fragmentation and distal arterial embolization resulting in myocardial necrosis. Usually occurs without ST elevation and is thus termed non-ST elevation MI.

SYNONYMS

MI
Myocardial infarction
Non-ST elevation MI
ST-elevation MI
Heart attack
Coronary thrombosis
Coronary occlusion

ICD-9CM CODES
410.9 Acute myocardial infarction, unspecified site

EPIDEMIOLOGY & DEMOGRAPHICS

INCIDENCE/PREVALENCE (IN U.S.):

- >500 cases/100,000 persons.
- >500,000 MIs in the U.S. yearly.
- More prominent in males between the ages of 40 and 65 yr; no predominant sex after age 65 yr.
- Women experience more lethal and severe first acute MIs than men, regardless of comorbidity, previous angina, or age.
- At least one fourth of all myocardial infections are clinically unrecognized.

PHYSICAL FINDINGS & CLINICAL PRESENTATION

Clinical presentation:

- Crushing substernal chest pain usually lasts longer than 30 min.
- Pain is unrelieved by rest or sublingual nitroglycerin or is rapidly recurring.
- Pain radiates to the left or right arm, neck, jaw, back, shoulders, or abdomen and is not pleuritic in character.
- Pain may be associated with dyspnea, diaphoresis, nausea, or vomiting.
- There is no pain in approximately 20% of infarctions (usually in diabetic or elderly patients).

Physical findings:

- Skin may be diaphoretic, with pallor (because of decreased oxygen).
- Rales may be present at the bases of lungs (indicative of CHF).
- Cardiac auscultation may reveal an apical systolic murmur caused by mitral regurgitation secondary to papillary muscle dysfunction; S_3 or S_4 may also be present.
- Physical examination may be completely normal.

ETIOLOGY

- Coronary atherosclerosis
- Coronary artery spasm
- Coronary embolism (caused by infective endocarditis, rheumatic heart disease, intracavitary thrombus)
- Periarteritis and other coronary artery inflammatory diseases
- Dissection into coronary arteries (aneurysmal or iatrogenic)
- Congenital abnormalities of coronary circulation
- MI with normal coronaries (MINC syndrome): more frequent in younger patients and cocaine addicts. The risk of acute MI is increased by a factor of 24 during the 60 min after the use of cocaine in persons who are otherwise at relatively low risk. Most patients with cocaine-related MI are young, nonwhite, male cigarette smokers without other risk factors for ASHD who have a history of repeated cocaine use. Blood and urine toxicology screen for cocaine is recommended in all young patients who present with acute MI.
- Hypercoagulable states, increased blood viscosity (polycythemia vera).

DIAGNOSIS

DIFFERENTIAL DIAGNOSIS

The various causes of myocardial ischemia are described in Section II along with the differential diagnosis of chest pain.

LABORATORY TESTS

- Cardiac troponin levels: cardiac-specific troponin T (cTnT) and cardiac-specific troponin I (cTnl) are generally indicative of myocardial injury. Increases in serum levels of cTnT and cTnI may occur relatively early after muscle damage (3 to 12 hr), peak within 24 hr, and may be present for several days after MI (up to 7 days for cTnI and up to 10 to 14 days for cTnT). Troponin T tests can be falsely positive in patients with renal failure. The threshold level of troponin T considered positive for MI is 0.1 ng/ml in patients with normal renal function or 0.5 ng/ml in patients with renal impairment. Although troponin is a sensitive biomarker to "rule out" NSTMI, it is less useful to "rule in" this event because many other diseases such as sepsis, hypovolemia, atrial fibrillation, CHF, pulmonary embolism, myocarditis, myocardial contusion, and renal failure can be associated with an increase in troponin level.
- Creatine kinase MB isoenzyme is a useful marker for MI. It is released in the circulation in amounts that correlate with the size of the infarct.
- Neither CK-MB nor troponin consistently appear in the blood within 6 hr after an ischemic event; therefore serial testing (e.g., on presentation and after 8 hr) is necessary to definitely rule out MI.
- ECG:
  1. In STEMI, there is development of:
     a. Inverted T waves, indicating an area of ischemia.
     b. Elevated ST segment, indicating an area of injury. Significant ST-segment elevation of ≥0.10 mV measured 0.02 sec after the J point is evident in two contiguous leads. The presence of this finding in leads V1-V6 indicates anterior or anterolateral MI, in leads I and aVL a lateral MI, and its presence in leads II, III, or aVF is diagnostic of inferior wall MI.
     c. Q waves (Fig. 1-166), indicating an area of infarction (usually develop over 12 to 36 hr).
  2. In NSTEMI:
     a. History and myocardial enzyme elevations are compatible with MI.
     b. ECG shows no ST-segment elevation and sometimes shows a small depression of the ST segment.

IMAGING STUDIES

- Chest radiography is useful to evaluate for pulmonary congestion and exclude other causes of chest pain.

- Echocardiography can evaluate wall motion abnormalities and identify mural thrombus or mitral regurgitation, which can occur acutely after MI.

RISK ASSESSMENT

Several risk assessment models are available. The TIMI risk score uses the seven following variables: age ≥65, at least three conventional risk factors for coronary artery disease, prior coronary stenosis ≥50%, ST-segment deviation on ECG at presentation, ≥2 anginal events in the preceding 24 hr, use of aspirin in the prior 7 days, and elevated serum cardiac markers.

TREATMENT Rx

NONPHARMACOLOGIC THERAPY

- Limit patient's activity: bed rest for the initial 12 to 24 hr; if the patient remains stable, gradually increase activity.
- Diet: NPO until stable, then no added salt and a low-cholesterol diet.
- Patient education to decrease the risk of subsequent cardiac events (proper diet, cessation of smoking, regular exercise) should be initiated when the patient is medically stable.

ACUTE GENERAL Rx

- Any patient with suspected acute MI should immediately receive the following:
  1. Antiplatelet therapy: aspirin, 160 to 325 mg po unless true aspirin allergy is suspected. If the first dose is chewed, a blood level is achieved more rapidly than if it is swallowed. Clopidogrel 75 mg qd may be substituted if true allergy is present or given in addition to aspirin. Clopidogrel pretreatment in patients with STEMI significantly reduces the incidence of cardiovascular death or ischemic complications both before and after PCI and without a significant increase in major or minor bleeding. For patients taking clopidogrel for whom CABG is planned, the drug should be withheld for at least 5 days unless the urgency of revascularization outweighs the risk of bleeding.
  2. Nitrates: they increase the supply of oxygen by reducing coronary vasospasm and decrease consumption of oxygen by reducing ventricular preload. Sublingual nitroglycerin (0.4 mg) can be administered immediately on suspicion of MI (unless systolic blood pressure is <90 mm Hg or ≤ to 30 mm Hg below baseline or heart rate is <50 bpm or >100 bpm); IV nitroglycerin can be subsequently used. Nitroglycerin should be used with great caution in patients with inferior wall MI; nitrate usage can result in hypotension because these patients are sensitive to change in preload. It should also be avoided in patients suspected of having right ventricular infarction (increased risk of preload reduction) and if a patient has used sildenafil (Viagra), or vardenafil (Levitra) within the previous 24 hr or tadalafil (Cialis) in the previous 48 hr.
  3. Adequate analgesia: morphine sulfate 2 to 4 mg IV initially with increments of 2 to 8 mg IV at 5 to 15 min intervals can be given for severe pain unrelieved by nitroglycerin. Hypotension secondary to morphine can be treated with careful IV hydration with saline solution. If sinus bradycardia accompanies hypotension, use atropine (0.5 to 1.0 mg IV q5min PRN to a total dose of 2.5 mg). Respiratory depression caused by morphine can be reversed with naloxone (Narcan) 0.8 mg.
  4. Nasal oxygen: administer at 2 to 4 L/min.
- Prompt myocardial reperfusion can be accomplished with percutaneous coronary intervention (PCI), fibrinolytic therapy, or coronary artery bypass graft (CABG) surgery. If readily available without delay, PCI is superior to thrombolytic therapy for treating patients with ST-segment elevation MI. It is effective and generally results in more favorable outcomes than thrombolytic therapy. When PCI is performed, use of heparin is recommended. In patients at high risk of bleeding from heparin, use of bivalirudin (Angiomax), a short-acting direct thrombin inhibitor, should be considered. Aspirin and clopidogrel should be started before PCI and continued for at least 3 to 6 mo afterwards (3 mo for sirolimus-coated stents and 6 mo for paclitaxel-coated stents) and up to 12 mo in patients who are not at high risk for bleeding. Addition of a GP IIb/IIIa inhibitor is also recommended, although it may not be necessary for low-risk patients pretreated with clopidogrel and aspirin. Coronary stents following PCI are useful to decrease ischemia, improve long-term patency, and lower the rate of restenosis of the infarct-related artery.

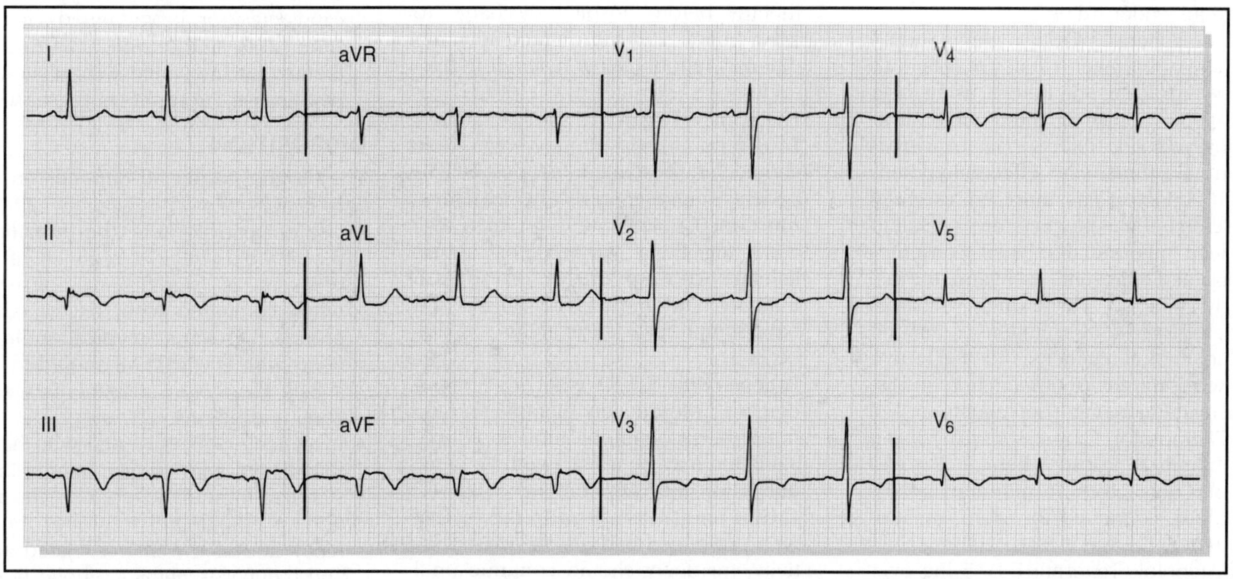

FIGURE 1-166 Evolving interoposterolateral infarction. Note the prominent Q waves in II, III, and aV_1, along with ST elevation and T wave inversion in these leads, as well as V_3 through V_6. ST depression in I, aV_1, V_1, and V_2 is consistent with a reciprocal change. Relatively tall R waves are also present in V_1 and V_2. (From Zipes DP, Libby P, Bonow RO, Braunwauld E [eds]: *Braunwald's heart disease,* ed 7, Philadelphia, 2005, Elsevier.)

- Thrombolytic therapy: if the duration of pain has been <6 hr and primary angioplasty is not readily available, recanalization of the occluded arteries should be attempted with thrombolytic agents, possibly in combination with glycoprotein IIb/IIIa inhibition. Because the effectiveness of thrombolytics is time dependent, ideally these agents should be administered either in the field or within 30 min of the patient's arrival in the emergency department. When tPA or rPA is used, heparin is given to increase the likelihood of patency in the infarct-related artery. In patients receiving fibrinolysis for ST-elevation myocardial infarction, treatment with enoxaparin is superior to treatment with unfractionated heparin for 48 hr but is associated with an increase in major bleeding episodes. In patients receiving streptokinase or APSAC, heparin is not indicated, because it does not offer any additional benefit and can result in increased bleeding complications. Tenecteplase and reteplase are comparable with accelerated infusion recombinant TPA in terms of efficacy and safety, but are more convenient because they are administered by bolus injection. Lanoplase and heparin bolus plus infusion is as effective as TPA with regard to mortality, but the rate of intracranial hemorrhage is significantly higher. Absolute contraindications to thrombolytic therapy include active internal bleeding, intracranial neoplasm or arteriovenous malformation, intracranial surgery in past 6 mo, stroke in past year, head trauma with loss of consciousness in past 6 mo, surgery in noncompressible location in past 6 wk, alteration in mental status, and infectious endocarditis.
- Beta-adrenergic blocking agents should generally be given to all patients with evolving acute MI. Before using beta blockers, some of the contraindications and side effects (i.e., exacerbation of asthma, CNS effects, hypotension, bradycardia) must be carefully assessed. Beta blockers are useful to reduce myocardial oxygen consumption and prevent tachyarrhythmias. Early IV beta blockage (in the initial 24 hr) followed by institution of an oral maintenance regimen is also effective in reducing recurrent infarction and ischemia. Frequently used agents are:
  1. Metoprolol (Lopressor): IV 5 mg q2min × 3 doses, then po 25 to 50 mg q6h, given 15 min after last IV dose, continued for 48 hr; maintenance dosage is 50 to 100 mg bid.
  2. Atenolol (Tenormin): IV 5 mg over 5 min, repeat in 10 min if initial dose is well tolerated, then start po dose 10 min after the last IV dose; po 50 mg qd, increasing to 100 mg as tolerated.
- ACE inhibitors reduce left ventricular dysfunction and dilation and slow the progression of CHF during and after acute MI. They should be initiated within hours of hospitalization, provided the patient does not have hypotension or a contraindication (bilateral renal stenosis, renal failure, or history of angioedema caused by previous treatment with ACE inhibitors). ARBs offer no advantage over ACEs and should be considered only in patients who have a contraindication to the use of ACEs or cannot tolerate them.
  1. Commonly used ACEs are ramipril 2.5 mg qd, captopril 12.5 mg po bid, enalapril 2.5 mg bid, or lisinopril 2.5 to 5 mg qd initially, with subsequent titration as needed. Ramipril is associated with lower mortality than most ACE inhibitors.
  2. ACE inhibitors may be stopped in patients without complications and no evidence of left ventricular dysfunction after 6 to 8 wk.
  3. ACE inhibitors should be continued indefinitely in patients with impaired left ventricular function (ejection fraction <40%) or clinical CHF.
- Glycoprotein IIb receptor inhibitors (tirofiban, eptifibatide), when administered with heparin and aspirin, further reduce the incidence of ischemic events in patients with NSTEMI. The use of IV glycoprotein IIb/IIIa inhibitors (e.g., abciximab) before and during PCI also reduces the risk of closure postangioplasty.
- Assess fasting lipid profile preferably with 24 hr of MI and initiate statin therapy before hospital discharge to keep LDL-C <70 mg/dl. Consider addition of fenofibrate or niacin if triglycerides are significantly elevated or HDL-C is very low.
- Long-term aldosterone blockade should be prescribed for post-STEMI patients without significant renal dysfunction (Cr ≤2.5 mg/dl in men and ≤2.0 mg/dl in women) or hyperkalemia who are already on an ACE inhibitor and have LVEF ≤0.40, and have symptomatic heart failure or diabetes.
- Patients with STEMI who are not undergoing reperfusion therapy and do not have a contraindication to anticoagulation may be treated with IV or SC unfractionated heparin or with SC LMWH for at least 48 hr. In the patient with prolonged bed rest or limited activity, treatment should continue until the patient is ambulatory.

CHRONIC Rx

Discharge medications in all patients with UA/NSTEMI (unless contraindicated) should include antiischemic medications (e.g., nitroglycerin, beta blocker), lipid-lowering agents, and aspirin (81-325 mg/day). Clopidogrel (Plavix) 75 mg/day can be given in addition to aspirin for up to 9 mo or in place of aspirin in those who cannot tolerate aspirin. If CABG is planned, clopidogrel should be withheld 5 to 7 days before the procedure.

The addition of ACE inhibitors is also recommended in all patients with diabetes, CHF, and in those with EF <40%.

Evaluation of post-MI patients.

- Submaximal (low level) treadmill test (can be done 1 to 3 wk after MI) in stable patients without any clinical evidence of significant left ventricular dysfunction or post-MI angina.
  1. Useful to assess the patient's functional capacity and formulate an at-home exercise program
  2. Helpful to determine the patient's prognosis
- Radionuclide angiography or two-dimensional echocardiography:
  1. To evaluate patient's left ventricular ejection fraction
  2. To evaluate ventricular size and segmental wall motion
  3. Echocardiography to rule out presence of mural thrombi in patients with anterior wall infarction; transesophageal echo is preferred if mural thrombosis is suspected
- A 24-hr Holter monitor study to evaluate patients who have demonstrated significant arrhythmias during their hospital stay; selected patients with complex ventricular ectopy may be candidates for programmed electrical stimulation studies and antiarrhythmic therapy or implanted defibrillator, depending on the results of these studies.

DISPOSITION

The prognosis after MI depends on multiple factors:

- Use of beta blockers: the mortality of patients on a regular regimen of beta blockers is significantly decreased when compared with that of control groups. Discharge medication in patients with UA/NSTEMI should include a beta blocker in all patients without contraindications.
- In patients ≤75 yr of age who have a STEMI and who receive aspirin and a standard fibrinolytic regimen, the addition of clopidogrel improves the patency rate of the infarct-related artery and reduces ischemic complications.
- Presence of arrhythmias, frequent ventricular ectopy (≥10/hr), or repetitive

forms of ventricular ectopic beats (couplets, triplets) indicates an increased risk (2 to 3 times greater) of sudden cardiac death. New bundle branch block, Mobitz II second-degree block, and third-degree heart block also adversely affect outcome.

- Size of infarct: the larger it is, the higher the post-MI mortality rate. Significant myocardial stunning with subsequent improvement of ventricular function occurs in most patients after anterior MI. A lower level of creatine kinase, an estimate of the extent of necrosis, is independently predictive of recovery of function.
- Site of infarct: inferior wall MI carries a better prognosis than anterior wall MI; however, patients with inferior wall MI and right ventricular involvement have a high risk for arrhythmic complications and cardiac shock.
- Ejection fraction after MI: the lower the left ventricular ejection fraction, the higher the mortality after MI. The risk of sudden death is highest in the first 30 days after MI among patients with left ventricular dysfunction, heart failure, or both.
- Presence of post-MI angina indicates a high mortality rate.
- Performance on low-level exercise test: the presence of ST segment changes during the test is a predictor of high mortality during the first year.
- Presence of pericarditis during the acute phase of MI increases mortality at 1 yr.
- Type A behavior (competitive drive, ambitiousness, hostility) is associated with a lower mortality rate after symptomatic MI.
- The Killip classification is an independent predictor of all-cause mortality in patients with non-ST elevation acute coronary syndromes.
- Self-reported moderate alcohol consumption in the year before acute MI is associated with reduced 1-yr mortality.
- Discharge medication in patients with UA/NSTEMI should include lipid-lowering agents in patients with hyperlipidemia unresponsive to exercise and dietary restrictions and is beneficial. Statins may also lower vascular inflammation and damage by mechanisms other than reduction of LDL cholesterol. Early initiation of statin treatment in patients with acute MI is associated with reduced 1-yr mortality.
- Additional poor prognostic factors include the following: cigarette smoking, history of hypertension or prior MI, presence of ST-segment depression in acute MI, increasing age, diabetes mellitus, and female sex (especially women >50 yr of age).
- Renal disease, even mild, as assessed by the estimated GFR, is a major risk factor for cardiovascular complications after MI.

PEARLS & CONSIDERATIONS

COMMENTS

Current guidelines recommend an early invasive strategy for patients who have acute coronary syndromes without ST-segment elevation and with an elevated cardiac troponin T level. However, a recent trial (ICTUS) comparing early invasive vs. selectively invasive management for acute coronary syndromes failed to show that, given optimized medical therapy, an early invasive strategy is superior to a selective invasive strategy in patients with acute coronary syndromes without ST-segment elevation and with an elevated cardiac troponin T level. All 1200 patients in this trial received aggressive medical therapy, including aspirin, clopidogrel, enoxaparin for 48 hr, abciximab during PCI, and intensive lipid-lowering therapy. The mortality rate was the same in the two groups (2.5%), myocardial infarction was significantly more frequent in the group assigned to early invasive management (15% vs. 10%), but rehospitalization rate was less frequent in that group (7.4% vs. 10.9%).

EVIDENCE

EBM

There is strong evidence supporting the rapid reestablishment of coronary artery flow in cases of myocardial infarction, with some evidence that primary percutaneous transluminal coronary angioplasty (PTCA) may be more beneficial than thrombolysis

There is good evidence for the short-term and long-term mortality benefits of thrombolysis. The benefits are greatest the earlier thrombolysis is given, and in patients with ST-segment elevation (especially with anterior infarction) or bundle branch block. It does, however, carry an increased risk of stroke.[1] A

Primary PCTA produces significantly better results than thrombolysis in the treatment of acute myocardial infarction as measured by separate and combined endpoints of death, reinfarction, and stroke. Benefit is present up to 18 months follow-up, is greatest in high-risk patients, and is present even if there is a short delay in transferring patients to a suitable facility. PCTA does, however, have a higher risk of major bleeding at 4 to 6 weeks than thrombolysis.[2-4] A B

There is strong evidence supporting the use of aspirin or thienopyridines (ticlopidine, clopidogrel) following myocardial infarction

There is evidence that treatment with aspirin significantly reduces the risk of death, reinfarction and stroke at 1 month following a myocardial infarct. A mortality benefit has been found to persist for at least 4 years. A loading dose of 160 mg to 325 mg has been shown to produce a prompt antiplatelet effect, and ongoing treatment with doses of 75 mg to 325 mg daily are similarly effective.[5-8] A

There is evidence that beta blockers reduce mortality when used in the treatment of MI, especially when given early

A systematic review found oral beta blockers given early after the onset of acute MI reduces the risk of death and major vascular events.[9] A

Benefit from beta blocker therapy has been shown in follow-up to 4 years after MI.[10] A

There is no evidence of benefit from calcium channel blockers in the treatment of patients with acute MI. This class of drug may increase mortality for some patients, notably those with congestive heart failure

Two systematic reviews found calcium channel blockers associated with nonsignificant increases in mortality of approximately 4% and 6%.[11,12] A B

ACE inhibitors are effective in reducing morbidity and mortality after an acute MI, though they also increase persistent hypotension and renal dysfunction

A systematic review of RCTs comparing ACE inhibitors vs. placebo, started within 14 days of a myocardial infarct, found ACE inhibitors significantly reduced the risk of death at 2 to 42 months follow-up.[13] A

There is good evidence for the benefit of HMG-CoA reductase inhibitors (statins) in the primary and secondary prevention of serious cardiovascular events including death, myocardial infarction, and stroke

Five systematic reviews found that, compared with placebo, 4 to 6 years of treatment with statins resulted in significantly lower rates of major coronary events and cardiovascular mortality, although there was no significant reduction in all-cause mortality or coronary heart disease mortality.[14] A

The American Heart Association and American College of Cardiology have reviewed the evidence regarding warfarin treatment post MI and have drawn the following conclusions:

The three options concerning anticoagulation post AMI are aspirin alone; aspirin plus moderate-intensity warfarin (INR 2.0 to 3.0); or high-intensity warfarin (INR 3.0 to 4.0). The aspirin alone regime is not as effective but is associated with less bleeding than the regimes including warfarin. It also should be noted that without tight monitoring, the high-intensity warfarin regime may result in unacceptable bleeding. An alternative approach is to use a combination of aspirin plus clopidogrel.[15] B

Although ACE inhibitors are the preferred agent, there is some evidence that may support the use of angiotensin-II receptor blockers in the treatment of myocardial infarction in those patients intolerant of ACE inhibitors.

A multicenter randomized controlled trial (RCT) compared losartan 50 mg daily with captopril 50 mg three times daily in patients over 50 years old with confirmed acute myocardial infarction and heart failure. It found a nonsignificant difference in total mortality in favor of captopril although losartan was better tolerated.[16] B

Another RCT compared the addition of valsartan alone vs. valsartan plus captopril vs. captopril alone to conventional therapy in patients 0.5 to 10 days after acute myocardial infarction. After follow-up for a median time of 24.7 months it was found that valsartan was as effective as captopril for those at high risk of cardiovascular events following acute MI but that the combination of the two drugs increased side effects without improving survival.[17] B

Evidence-Based References

1. French JK et al: Survival 12 years after randomization to streptokinase: the influence of thrombolysis in myocardial infarction flow at three to four weeks, *J Am Coll Cardiol* 34:62-69, 1999. Reviewed in: *Clin Evid* 12:20-50, 2004. A
2. Keeley EC, Boura JA, Grines CL: Primary angioplasty versus intravenous thrombolytic therapy for acute myocardial infarction: a quantitative review of 23 randomised trials, *Lancet* 361:13-20, 2003. Reviewed in: *Clin Evid* 12:20-50, 2004. A
3. Grines D et al. PCAT collaborators: Primary coronary angioplasty compared with intravenous thrombolytic therapy for acute myocardial infarction: six-month follow up and analysis of individual patient data from randomized trials, *Am Heart J* 145:47-57, 2003. B
4. Andersen HR et al: A comparison of coronary angioplasty with fibrinolytic therapy in acute myocardial infarction, *N Engl J Med* 349:733-742,2003. B
5. Second international study of infarct survival (ISIS-2) Collaborative group: Randomised trial of intravenous streptokinase, oral aspirin, both or neither among 17187 cases of suspected acute myocardial infarction, *Lancet* ii:349-ii360, 1988. Reviewed in: *Clin Evid* 12:20-50, 2004. A
6. Baigent BM, Collins R: ISIS-2: four year mortality of 17,187 patients after fibrinolytic and antiplatelet therapy in suspected acute myocardial infarction study, *Circulation* suppl 1:1-291, 1993. Reviewed in: *Clin Evid* 12:20-50, 2004. A
7. Yusuf S et al: Beta blockade during and after myocardial infarction: an overview of the randomized trials, *Prog Cardiovasc Dis* 27:355-371, 1985. Reviewed in: *Clin Evid* 12:20-50, 2004. A
8. Freemantle N et al: Beta blockade after myocardial infarction: systematic review and meta regression analysis, *BMJ* 318:1730-1737, 1999. Reviewed in: *Clin Evid* 12:20-50, 2004. A
9. Yusuf S, Furberg CD: Effects of calcium channel blockers on survival after myocardial infarction, *Cardiovasc Drugs Ther* 1:343-344, 1987. Reviewed in: *Clin Evid* 12:20-50, 2004. B
10. Teo KK, Yusuf S, Furberg CD: Effects of prophylactic antiarrhythmic drug therapy in acute myocardial infarction: an overview of results from randomized controlled trials, *JAMA* 270:1589-1595, 1993. Reviewed in: *Clin Evid* 12:20-50, 2004. A
11. Domanski MJ et al: Effect of angiotensin converting enzyme inhibition on sudden cardiac death in patients following acute myocardial infarction. A meta-analysis of randomized clinical trials, *J Am Coll Cardiol* 33:598-604, 1999. Reviewed in: *Clin Evid* 12:20-50, 2004. A
12. Foster C et al: Primary prevention. Reviewed in: Clinical Evidence 12:159-192, London, 2004, BMJ Publishing Group. A
13. Hirsh J et al: American Heart Association/American College of Cardiology Foundation guide to warfarin therapy, *Circulation* 107:1692-1711, 2003. C
14. Dickstein K, Kjekshus J, OPTIMAAL Steering Committee of the OPTIMAAL Study Group: Effects of losartan and captopril on mortality and morbidity in high-risk patients after acute myocardial infarction: the OPTIMAAL randomized trial, *Lancet* 360:752-760, 2002. B
15. Pfeffer MA et al: Valsartan, captopril, or both in myocardial infarction complicated by heart failure, left ventricular dysfunction, or both, *N Engl J Med* 349:1893-1906, 2003.

SUGGESTED READINGS

ACC/AHA task force on management of ST-elevation myocardial infarction (STEMI), *Circulation* 8/3/2004. Available at www.acc.org/clinical/guidelines/stemi/index.htm.

Antmam EM et al: Enoxaparin versus unfractionated heparin with fibrinolysis for ST-elevation myocardial infarction, *N Engl J Med* 354:1477, 2006.

Antman EM et al: The TIMI risk score for unstable angina/non-ST elevation MI: a method for prognostification and therapeutic decision making, *JAMA* 284:835-842, 2000.

Becker RC: Antithrombotic therapy after myocardial infarction, *N Engl J Med* 347:1019, 2002.

Cannon CP et al: Intensive versus moderate lipid lowering with statins after acute coronary syndromes, *N Eng L Med* 350:1495, 2004.

de Winter RJ et al: Early invasive versus selectively invasive management for acute coronary syndromes, *N Eng L Med* 353:1095-1104, 2005.

Gibbons RJ, Fuster V: Therapy for patients with acute coronary syndromes, new opportunities, *N Engl J Med* 354:1524, 2006.

Jeremias A, Gibson, M: Narrative review: alternative causes for elevated cardiac troponin levels when acute coronary syndromes are excluded, *Ann Intern Med* 142:786-791, 2005.

Meier MA et al: The new definition of myocardial infarction, *Arch Intern Med* 162:1585, 2002.

Newby LK et al: Early statin initiation and outcomes in patients with acute coronary syndromes, *JAMA* 287:3087, 2002.

Sabatine MS et al: Addition of clopidogrel to aspirin and fibrinolytic therapy for MI with ST-segment elevation, *N Engl J Med* 352:1179-1189, 2005.

Sabatine MS et al: Effect of clopidogrel pretreatment before percutaneous coronary intervention in patients with STEMI treated with fibrinolytics, *JAMA* 294:1224-1232, 2005.

AUTHOR: **FRED F. FERRI, M.D.**

BASIC INFORMATION

DEFINITION

Myocarditis is an inflammatory condition of the myocardium.

ICD-9CM CODES
429.0 Myocarditis, nonspecific
391.2 Myocarditis, rheumatic
422.91 Myocarditis, viral (except coxsackie)
074.23 Myocarditis, coxsackie
422.92 Myocarditis, bacterial

EPIDEMIOLOGY & DEMOGRAPHICS

- The incidence of focal myocarditis reported at autopsy is 1% to 7% in asymptomatic patients.
- Myocarditis is a major cause of sudden unexpected death (15% to 20% of cases) in adults <40 years of age.

PHYSICAL FINDINGS & CLINICAL PRESENTATION

- Persistent tachycardia out of proportion to fever
- Faint S_1, S_4 sound on auscultation
- Murmur of mitral regurgitation
- Pericardial friction rub if associated with pericarditis
- Signs of biventricular failure (hypotension, hepatomegaly, peripheral edema, distention of neck veins, S_3)
- Patients may present with a history of recent flulike syndrome (fever, arthralgias, malaise)

ETIOLOGY

- Infection
  1. Viral (coxsackie B virus, CMV, echovirus, polio virus, adenovirus, mumps, HIV, EBV)
  2. Bacterial *(Staphylococcus aureus, Clostridium perfringens,* diphtheria, and any severe bacterial infection)
  3. Mycoplasma
  4. Mycotic *(Candida, Mucor, Aspergillus)*
  5. Parasitic *(Trypanosoma cruzi, Trichinella, Echinococcus,* amoeba, *Toxoplasma)*
  6. *Rickettsia rickettsii*
  7. Spirochetal *(Borrelia burgdorferi*—Lyme carditis)
- Rheumatic fever
- Secondary to drugs (e.g., cocaine, emetine, doxorubicin, sulfonamides, isoniazid, methyldopa, amphotericin B, tetracycline, phenylbutazone, lithium, 5-FU, phenothiazines, interferon alfa, tricyclic antidepressants, cyclophosphamides)
- Toxins (carbon monoxide, ethanol, diphtheria toxin, lead, arsenicals)
- Collagen-vascular disease (SLE, scleroderma, sarcoidosis, Kawasaki syndrome)
- Sarcoidosis
- Radiation
- Postpartum

DIAGNOSIS

DIFFERENTIAL DIAGNOSIS

- Cardiomyopathy
- Acute myocardial infarction
- Valvulopathies

The differential diagnosis of chest pain is described in Section II

WORKUP

- Medical history: the clinical presentation of myocarditis is nonspecific and can consist of fatigue, palpitations, dyspnea, precordial discomfort, myalgias.
- Diagnostic workup includes chest x-ray examination, ECG, laboratory evaluation, echocardiogram, cardiac catheterization, and endomyocardial biopsy (selected patients).

LABORATORY TESTS

- Elevated cardiac troponin T (TnT) is suggestive of myocarditis in patients with clinically suspected myocarditis. A normal level does not rule out the diagnosis
- Increased CK (with elevated MB fraction, LDH), and AST secondary to myocardial necrosis
- Increased ESR (nonspecific but may be of value in following the progress of the disease and the response to therapy)
- Increased WBC (increased eosinophils if parasitic infection)
- Viral titers (acute and convalescent)
- Cold agglutinin titer, ASLO titer, blood cultures
- Lyme disease antibody titer

IMAGING STUDIES

- Chest x-ray: enlargement of cardiac silhouette
- ECG: sinus tachycardia with nonspecific ST-T wave changes; interventricular conduction defects and bundle branch block may be present
  1. Lyme disease and diphtheria cause all degrees of heart block.
  2. Changes of acute MI can occur with focal necrosis.
- Echocardiogram:
  1. Dilated and hypokinetic chambers
  2. Segmental wall motion abnormalities
- Cardiac catheterization and angiography:
  1. To rule out coronary artery disease and valvular disease.
  2. A right ventricular endomyocardial biopsy can confirm the diagnosis, although a negative biopsy result does not exclude myocarditis. Recent studies have shown that myocardial biopsy may be unnecessary, because immunosuppression therapy based on biopsy results is generally ineffective.

TREATMENT

NONPHARMACOLOGIC THERAPY

- Supportive care is the first line of therapy for patients with myocarditis.
- Restrict physical activity (to decrease cardiac work). Bed rest is advisable during viremia.

ACUTE GENERAL Rx

- Treat underlying cause (e.g., use specific antibiotics for bacterial infection).
- Treat CHF with diuretics, ACE inhibitors, and salt restriction. A β-blocker may be added once clinical stability has been achieved. Digoxin should be used with caution and only at low doses.
- If ventricular arrhythmias are present, treat with quinidine or procainamide.
- Provide anticoagulation to prevent thromboembolism.
- Use preload and afterload reducing agents for treating cardiac decompensation.
- Corticosteroid use is contraindicated in early infectious myocarditis; it may be justified in only selected patients with intractable CHF, severe systemic toxicity, and severe life-threatening arrhythmias.
- Immunosuppressive drugs (prednisone with cyclosporine or azathioprine) do not have any significant effect on the prognosis of myocarditis and should not be used in the routine treatment of patients with myocarditis. Immunosuppression may have a role in the treatment of myocarditis from systemic autoimmune disease (e.g., SLE, scleroderma) and in patients with idiopathic giant cell myocarditis.

DISPOSITION

Nearly 50% of patients with myocarditis will die within 5 yr of diagnosis. Prognosis is best for patients with "fulminant" lymphocytic myocarditis (severe hemodynamic compromise, rapid onset of symptoms, or high fever). These patients tend to have complete recovery with total resolution of myocarditis on repeat biopsy.

REFERRAL

Consider heart transplant if patient develops intractable CHF.

SUGGESTED READING

Wu LA et al: Current role of endomyocardial biopsy in the management of dilated cardiomyopathy and myocarditis, *Mayo Clin Proc* 76:1030, 2001.

AUTHOR: **FRED F. FERRI, M.D.**

BASIC INFORMATION

DEFINITION

Sudden, brief, involuntary jerks or contractions, either rhythmic or irregular, of single muscles or groups of muscles. It can occur at rest or in response to sensory stimulation (touch, auditory, visual) and can involve active muscle contraction (positive myoclonus) or inhibition of ongoing muscle activity (negative myoclonus). Myoclonus is not a disease entity, but rather a symptom that may result from a wide variety of disorders.

SYNONYMS

See "Definition."

ICD-9CM CODES
333.2 Myoclonus

EPIDEMIOLOGY & DEMOGRAPHICS

INCIDENCE: 1.3 cases/100,000 person-years. Incidence increases with age.
LIFETIME PREVALENCE: 8.6/100,000 persons

PHYSICAL FINDINGS & CLINICAL PRESENTATION

- Careful history of any precipitating or alleviating factors—sensory stimuli, startle, alcohol (may alleviate essential myoclonus).
- History of accompanying neurologic symptoms (seizures, cognitive decline, family history) provide an important clue to diagnoses like myoclonic epilepsies and essential myoclonus.
- Frequently normal physical examination.
- Myoclonic jerks may be seen on examination and persist during sleep.
- Spatial distribution of myoclonus (unilateral versus bilateral, focal versus generalized) may provide clues to the etiology.
- Try to determine whether myoclonus occurs spontaneously or with particular precipitants.
- Testing the patient with outstretched arms might reveal negative myoclonus (asterixis) in metabolic encephalopathy.

ETIOLOGY

Five major etiologic categories:
- Physiologic myoclonus—hiccups, hypnic jerks, anxiety induced, exercise induced, benign infantile.
- Essential myoclonus—autosomal dominant and sporadic varieties.
- Epileptic myoclonus—includes progressive degenerative disorders of the nervous system in which myoclonus may occur in association with dementia, ataxia, and multiple seizure types. Examples include myoclonic absence, infantile spasms, and Lennox-Gastaut syndrome.
- Symptomatic myoclonus in progressive myoclonic epilepsies—includes diseases where myoclonus is accompanied by other multisystem disturbances. Examples include mitochondrial and storage disease.
- Symptomatic myoclonus without prominent seizures—examples include posthypoxic (acute and chronic), posttraumatic, myoclonic dementias (e.g., Creutzfeldt-Jakob disease); basal ganglia disorders such as Parkinson's, Huntington's, and Wilson's disease; drug-induced myoclonus (many opioids at higher doses, when haloperidol or phenothiazines are administered concurrently); systemic metabolic disturbances such as uremia and liver failure; viral infections; and paraneoplastic conditions (opsoclonus-myoclonus in 2% to 3% of children with neuroblastoma).

DIAGNOSIS

DIFFERENTIAL DIAGNOSIS

- Tremor—usually rhythmic and oscillatory and significantly slower than myoclonus.
- Tics—often slower than myoclonus and are stereotyped and repetitive.
- Paroxysmal dyskinesias—episodic and sometimes triggered by voluntary movement.
- Dystonia—typically a sustained posture, but can sometimes have rapid clonic movements that mimic myoclonus.
- Psychogenic myoclonus—in patients with conversion disorder.

LABORATORY TESTS

- General chemistry (sodium, magnesium, carbon dioxide, creatinine, liver function test, renal function, toxicology screen)
- HIV testing
- Lumbar puncture (for suspected viral encephalopathies, or CJD)
- Genetic testing (if diagnosis of progressive myoclonic epilepsy is entertained)
- EEG (to determine whether myoclonus is epileptic or not)
- MRI (could rarely uncover a structural abnormality, e.g., cerebellar or brainstem mass, hypertrophy of inferior olive)

IMAGING STUDIES

MRI may show T1 hyperintensity in the putamen in hepatolenticular degeneration, or characteristic diffusion-weighted imaging abnormalities in CJD.

TREATMENT

NONPHARMACOLOGIC THERAPY

In cases where myoclonus is a consequence of an underlying metabolic abnormality, correction of the disturbance should be addressed.

ACUTE GENERAL Rx

Most commonly used are clonazepam and valproic acid (VPA).

CHRONIC Rx

- Posthypoxic myoclonus (Lance-Adams syndrome): clonazepam, VPA, levetiracetam.
- Progressive myoclonic epilepsy: piracetam (not FDA approved), VPA, clonazepam, zonisamide.
- Essential myoclonus: clonazepam; very responsive to small amounts of alcohol.
- Intractable hiccups: baclofen, amitriptyline, VPA.
- Palatal myoclonus: clonazepam, sumatriptan, botulinum toxin.
- Opiate-related myoclonus: discontinue the opiates and could use dantrolene, gabapentin.
- Positive myoclonus often responds to treatment, whereas therapy for negative myoclonus is extremely limited.

DISPOSITION

Prognosis depends on the underlying neurologic disorder responsible for the myoclonus.

REFERRAL

Neurologist with an interest in movement disorders.

PEARLS & CONSIDERATIONS

COMMENTS

Myoclonus should be regarded as the "tip of the iceberg" of an underlying disorder; it is a symptom rather than a disease.

SUGGESTED READINGS

Agarwal P et al: Myoclonus, *Curr Opin Neurol* 16:515, 2003.

Brashear A: Approach to the hyperkinetic patient. In Biller J (ed): *Practical neurology*, Philadelphia, 2002, Lippincott Williams and Wilkins.

Caviness JN, Brown P: Myoclonus: current concepts and recent advances, *Lancet Neurol* 3(10):598, 2004.

Fahn S et al: Definition and classification of myoclonus, *Adv Neurol* 143:1, 1986.

Frucht S: Myoclonus. In Noseworthy J (ed): *Neurological therapeutics, principle and practice,* London, 2003, Martin Dunitz.

Myoclonus Research Foundation: http://www.myoclonus.com.

NINDS Myoclonus fact sheet: http://www.ninds.nih.gov/health_and_medical/pubs/myoclonus_doc.htm.

AUTHOR: **ACHRAF A. MAKKI, M.D., M.S.**

BASIC INFORMATION

DEFINITION

Inflammatory myopathies are idiopathic diseases of muscle characterized clinically by muscle weakness and pathologically by inflammation and muscle fiber breakdown. The three most common are dermatomyositis, polymyositis, and inclusion body myositis. For details regarding inclusion body myositis, please see the separate section on this topic.

SYNONYMS

See "Definition."

ICD-9CM CODES
710.3 Dermatomyositis
710.4 Polymyositis

EPIDEMIOLOGY & DEMOGRAPHICS

Dermatomyositis (DM)
- Occurs in children and in adults.
- Incidence 1:100,000.
- Prevalence 1 to 10 cases/million in adults and 1 to 3.2 cases/million in children.
- More common in females than males (2:1).
- Average age at diagnosis is 40. The average age of onset in children is between 5 and 14 yr.
- Approximately 15% to 20% of patients with DM over the age of 50 have associated malignancies.

Polymyositis (PM)
- Incidence: 5 cases/1 million annually.
- Age >18 yr.

PHYSICAL FINDINGS & CLINICAL PRESENTATION

DM and PM:
- Most patients have a subacute onset, over weeks to months.
- Symmetric proximal muscle weakness involving the neck flexors, shoulder, and pelvic girdles.
- Difficulty getting up from a chair, climbing stairs, reaching for objects above head, or combing hair.
- Distal muscle and ocular involvement is uncommon.
- Sensation and reflexes are preserved.
- Dysphagia and dysphonia result from pharyngeal muscle involvement.
- Esophageal dysmotility often occurs in DM.
- Respiratory failure may be seen from associated pulmonary fibrosis, weakness of respiratory accessory muscles, or a combination of both.
- Cardiac conduction abnormalities can be seen with DM.
- Systemic autoimmune disease occurs frequently in PM, and rarely in DM.
- Skin findings in DM:
  1. Heliotrope rash on the upper eyelids (Fig. 1-167)
  2. Erythematous rash on the face (see Fig. 1-167)
  3. May also involve the back and shoulders (shawl sign), neck and chest (V-shape), knees and elbows
  4. Photosensitivity
  5. Gottron's papules (violaceous papules overlying dorsal interphalangeal or metacarpophalangeal areas, elbow or knee joints; Fig. 1-168)
  6. Nail cracking, thickening, and irregularity with periungual telangiectasia (see Fig. 1-168)
  7. Mechanic's hand: fissured, hyperpigmented, scaly, and hyperkeratotic; also associated with increased risk of interstitial lung disease

ETIOLOGY

- DM: complex, immune-mediated vasculitic microangiopathy
  1. Adaptive immune response via humorally mediated complement attack.
- PM: unknown
  1. Cell-mediated immune major histocompatibility-I (MHC-1) process directed against muscle fibers is likely, given biopsy features.
  2. A viral etiology has been proposed secondary to the presence of autoantibodies to histidyl transferase antibody, anti-Jo-1 antibody, and signal recognition particle.

DIAGNOSIS

- Characteristic pattern of muscle weakness for each type.
- EMG and nerve conduction studies should be consistent with myopathic features.
- Laboratory tests listed below.
- Biopsy is required for diagnosis and should confirm inflammation *before* treatment is started: myopathic features (variation in fiber size, fiber splitting, fatty replacement of muscle tissue, and increased endomysial connective tissue) should be seen in addition to the following:
  1. DM: perifascicular atrophy, MAC deposition along capillaries
  2. PM: endomysial infiltrates composed of CD8+ T cells and macrophages invading nonnecrotic muscle fibers that express MHC-I antigen.

DIFFERENTIAL DIAGNOSIS

- Muscular dystrophies
- Amyloid myoneuropathy
- Amyotrophic lateral sclerosis (ALS)
- Myasthenia gravis
- Lambert-Eaton myasthenic syndrome
- Drug-induced myopathies (e.g., quinidine, NSAIDs, penicillamine, HMG CoA-reductase inhibitors)
- Diabetic amyotrophy
- Guillain-Barré syndrome
- Hyperthyroidism or hypothyroidism
- Lichen planus
- Amyopathic DM (rash without weakness)
- SLE
- Contact atopic or seborrheic dermatitis
- Psoriasis

LABORATORY TESTS

- Creatine kinase is the most sensitive muscle enzyme test for muscle breakdown and can be elevated as much as 50 times above normal in DM and PM.
- Aldolase, AST, ALT, alkaline phosphatase, and LDH can be elevated.
- Anti-Jo-1 antibodies are seen in myositis with associated interstitial lung disease, but are not specific for either DM or PM.
- Electrolytes, TSH, Ca, and Mg should be requested to exclude other causes of weakness.
- ECG for cardiac involvement.

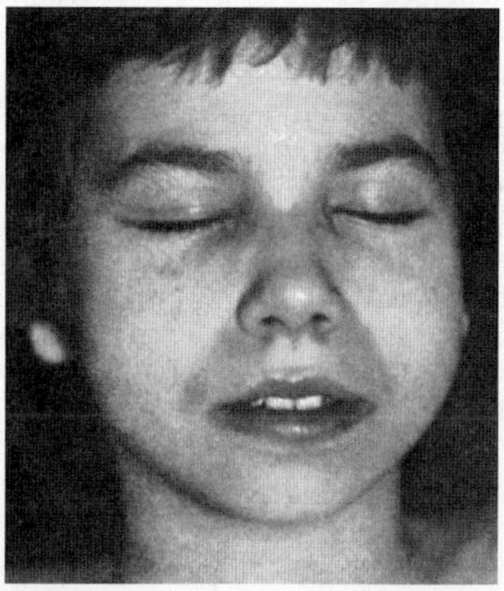

FIGURE 1-167 The facial rash of juvenile dermatomyositis. There is erythema over the bridge of the nose and malar areas, with violaceous (heliotropic) discoloration of the upper eyelids. (From Behrman RE: *Nelson textbook of pediatrics,* ed 17, Philadelphia, 2004, WB Saunders.)

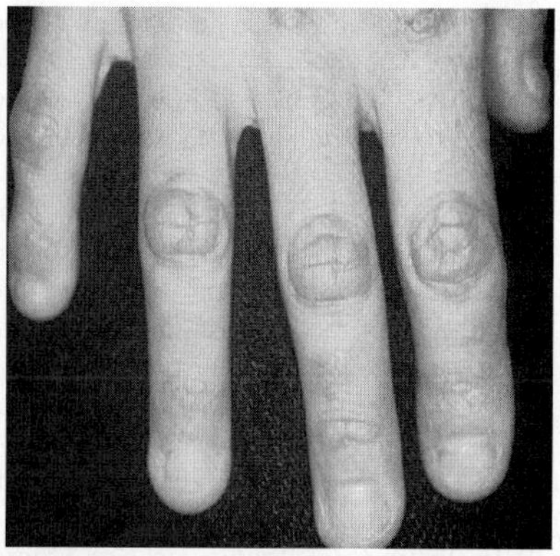

FIGURE 1-168 Dermatomyositis (Gottron's papules). Note erythematous papules over joints and periungual telangiectasias. (From Noble J [ed]: *Textbook of primary care medicine,* ed 2, St Louis, 1996, Mosby.)

IMAGING STUDIES

- Chest x-ray to rule out pulmonary involvement. If suspicious for pulmonary interstitial disease, a high-resolution CT scan of the chest may be helpful.
- Video fluoroscopy or barium swallow study to look for upper esophageal dysfunction in patients with dysphagia and DM.

TREATMENT

Rx

Goal: maintain strength, muscle function, and minimize disease/iatrogenic sequelae.

NONPHARMACOLOGIC THERAPY

- Sun-blocking agents with SPF 15 or greater for skin protection in patients with DM.
- Physical therapy is beneficial for gait training and increasing muscle tone and strength.
- Occupational therapy to assist with activities of daily living.
- Speech therapy for dysphagia and swallowing problems.

ACUTE GENERAL Rx

- Prednisone 1 to 2 mg/kg per day up to 100 mg/day. Continue dose until muscle strength improves or muscle enzymes have returned to normal for 4 wk. Begin taper by 10 mg/mo until 60 mg/day, then taper by 5 mg/mo. Consider every-other-day prednisone treatment at same dose (may decrease side effects).
- Use intravenous immunoglobulin or cyclophosphamide if patient fails to improve on prednisone, or muscle enzymes begin rising when tapering off prednisone. See "Chronic Rx" for specific dosage.
- Hydroxychloroquine can be used to treat the cutaneous lesions of DM.

CHRONIC Rx

- Chronic prednisone therapy may be needed for years, but other immunosuppressive agents should be added early to decrease long-term steroid side effects.
- Azathioprine 2 to 3 mg/kg per day tapered to 1 mg/kg per day once steroid is tapered to 15 mg/day. Reduce dosage monthly by 25-mg intervals. Maintenance dosage is 50 mg/day.
- Methotrexate 7.5 to 10 mg po/wk, increased by 2.5 mg/wk to total of 25 mg/wk; consider IM dosing if oral administration ineffective.
- IVIg 2g/kg total dose over 2 to 5 days can be used before azathioprine/methotrexate use. If initial improvement seen, repeat if relapse occurs.
- IV cyclophosphamide 1 g/M^2 monthly × 6 is preferred to oral dosing for refractory cases. However, oral dosing of cyclophosphamide is 1 to 3 mg/kg per day po or 2 to 4 mg/kg per day in conjunction with prednisone.
- Cyclosporin A: initial: 2.0 to 2.5 mg/kg bid; long-term maintenance is lowest effective dose.
- Mycophenolate mofetil 500 mg po bid, titrate to 1500 mg po bid over 1 to 2 mo.
- Hydroxychloroquine 200 mg po daily; monitor for visual changes.

DISPOSITION

- As treatment is initiated, the muscle enzymes should return to normal before symptoms improve.
- During exacerbations, enzymes may rise first before symptoms appear.
- Approximately 50% of the patients will go into remission and stop therapy within 5 yr. The remaining will have either active disease requiring ongoing treatment or inactive disease with permanent muscle atrophy and contractures.
- Poor prognostic indicators include delay in diagnosis, older age, recalcitrant disease, malignancy, interstitial pulmonary fibrosis, dysphagia, leukocytosis, fever, and anorexia.
- Infection, malignancy, cardiac and pulmonary dysfunction are the most common causes of death.
- With early treatment, 5- and 8-yr survival rates of 80% and 73%, respectively, have been reported.

REFERRAL

Neurology or rheumatology referral should be made to help establish the diagnosis and implement treatment.

PEARLS & CONSIDERATIONS

!

- Do *not* implement treatment before muscle biopsy.
- When assessing response to treatment, it is best to follow clinical muscle strength over muscle enzyme tests.
- The concern of malignancies (ovary, lung, breast, GI) associated with dermatomyositis is legitimate and merits screening in patients older than age 40 at time of diagnosis and every 2 to 3 yr thereafter.
- There does not appear to be any association between juvenile dermatomyositis and malignancy.
- Overlap syndrome refers to patients with dermatomyositis who also meet criteria for other connective tissue disorders (e.g., rheumatoid arthritis, scleroderma, SLE).
- If patient is taking steroids chronically, be sure to monitor for development of:
  1. Diabetes (oral glucose tolerance test)
  2. Osteopenia/osteoporosis (DEXA scan q6mo)
  3. Cataracts (yearly ophthalmologic appointment)
  4. Hypertension
  5. Psychiatric side effects including depression or psychosis
  6. Poor sleep
  7. Peptic ulcer disease (prescribe H2 antagonist or proton pump inhibitor)

EVIDENCE

EBM

Double-blind (DB), randomized (R), placebo-controlled (PC) trial of DM patients suggested intravenous immunoglobulin (IVIg) 2 gm/kg per month for 3 months was beneficial.[1]

DBRPC trial (PM patients) suggested trend toward benefit with 60 mg of prednisone per day plus azathioprine (2 mg/kg/day) for 3 months.[2]

DBRPC trial (DM, PM patients) suggested plasma exchange and leukapheresis offer no benefit.[3]

DBR trial (DM, PM patients) of prednisolone plus either methotrexate 15 mg weekly or azathioprine 2.5 mg/kg/daily showed equivalent efficacy; however, methotrexate was better tolerated.[4]

Randomized controlled trial (RCT) (DM, PM patients) suggested cyclosporin A 3.0 to 3.5 mg/kg/day vs. 7.5-15 mg weekly oral methotrexate showed no difference between groups.[5]

R, crossover, open label trial (DM, PM patients) of intramuscular methotrexate (50 mg/m2 every 6 hours for 4 doses every 2 weeks for 12 doses) vs. oral methotrexate plus azathioprine (up to 25 mg/week and 150 mg/day) for 6 months showed trend favoring combination therapy.[6]

Evidence-Based References

1. Dalakas MC et al: A controlled trial of high-dose intravenous immune globulin infusions as treatment for dermatomyositis, *N Engl J Med* 329(27):1993-2000, 1993.
2. Bunch TW et al: Azathioprine with prednisone for polymyositis, *Ann Int Med* 92(3):365-369, 1980.
3. Miller FW et al: Controlled trial of plasma exchange and leukapheresis in polymyositis and dermatomyositis, *N Engl J Med* 326(21):1380-1384, 1992.
4. Miller J et al: Randomised double blind controlled trial of methotrexate and steroids compared with azathioprine and steroids in the treatment of idiopathic inflammatory myopathy, *J Neurol Sci* 199(suppl 1):S53, 2002.
5. Vencovsky J et al: Cyclosporine A versus methotrexate in the treatment of polymyositis and dermatomyositis, *Scand J Rheumatol* 29(2):95-102, 2000.
6. Villalba L et al: Treatment of refractory myositis: a randomized crossover study of two new cytotoxic regimens, *Arthritis Rheum* 41(3):392-399, 1998.

AUTHOR: **GREGORY J. ESPER, M.D.**

BASIC INFORMATION

DEFINITION

Myotonia is a type of muscular dystrophy in which relaxation of a muscle after contraction is delayed or prolonged. The most common type of muscular dystrophy with myotonia is myotonic dystrophy, which is described below.

SYNONYMS

Myotonic dystrophy

ICD-9CM CODES
359.2 Myotonic disorders
728.85 Muscle spasm

EPIDEMIOLOGY & DEMOGRAPHICS

PREVALENCE: 3 to 5 cases/100,000 persons

- Genetic disorder inherited as an autosomal dominant illness
- Symptoms usually manifest during adolescence or early adulthood. Cases of infantile myotonic dystrophy have been described.

PHYSICAL FINDINGS & CLINICAL PRESENTATION

- Usual first complaint is distal extremity weakness sometimes associated with muscle stiffness, cramps, or difficulty relaxing the grasp.
- Weakness spreads to eventually involve all muscle groups. Flexor neck muscle weakness and masseter and temporal wasting are often prominent features, as is dysarthria.
- Percussion of a muscle produces a slow contraction followed by prolonged relaxation. The "myotonic reflex" is best tested by percussing the thenar muscles and observing a slow flexion followed by slow relaxation of the thumb.
- As the disease progresses, generalized weakness becomes more pronounced and myotonia becomes less evident.
- Extramuscular involvement:
  Mental retardation of variable severity (may be absent)
  Frontal baldness (Fig. 1-169)
  Cataracts
  Diabetes mellitus
  Hypogonadism
  Adrenal failure
  Cardiomyopathy
- Infantile myotonic dystrophy presents as neonatal extreme hypotonia with "shark mouth" deformity (upper lip forming an inverted V).

ETIOLOGY & PATHOGENESIS

Genetic disorder encoded on chromosome 19 leading to sustained firing of the muscle membrane, causing prolonged muscle contraction. Myotonic dystrophy 1 (the more common form) is caused by an expanded CTG repeat within the noncoding 3′ untranslated region of the myotonic dystrophy protein kinase *(DMPK)* gene. The less common form (myotonic dystrophy 2) is due to an expanded CCTG repeat in the first intron of the zinc finger protein 9 *(ZNF9)* gene.

DIAGNOSIS

DIFFERENTIAL DIAGNOSIS

- Myotonia congenita (Thomsen's disease)
  May be autosomal dominant or recessive (two distinct varieties)
  The disease is limited to muscles and causes hypertrophy and stiffness after rest. Muscle function normalizes with exercise. There is no weakness. Symptoms are exacerbated by exposure to cold.
- Paramyotonia congenita
  Autosomal dominant disease
  Weakness and stiffness of facial muscles and distal upper extremities, especially or exclusively on cold exposure
- Muscular dystrophies
- Inflammatory myopathies (polymyositis)
- Metabolic muscle diseases
- Myasthenic syndromes
- Motor neuron disease

WORKUP

- History and physical examination usually sufficient
- Muscle enzymes usually abnormal (CPK, aldolase, AST)
- EMG: typical myotonic "dive bomber" bursts
- Muscle biopsy: type I fiber atrophy, ring fibers, and increased central nucleation

TREATMENT

- Phenytoin
- Quinine
- Quinidine
- Procainamide
- Acetazolamide
- Genetic counseling
- Assistive devices, orthotics

DISPOSITION

In myotonic dystrophy, death is usually caused by the wasting of skeletal muscle and defects in cardiac function.

REFERRAL

To neurologist

SUGGESTED READINGS

Cooper TA: A reversal of misfortune for myotonic dystrophy, *N Engl J Med* 355:17, 2006.

Kanadia RN et al: Reversal of RNA missplicing and myotonia after muscleblind overexpression in a mouse poly (CUG) model for myotonic dystrophy, *Proc Natn Acad Sci USA* 103:11748, 2006.

AUTHORS: **FRED F. FERRI, M.D.,** and **TOM J. WACHTEL, M.D.**

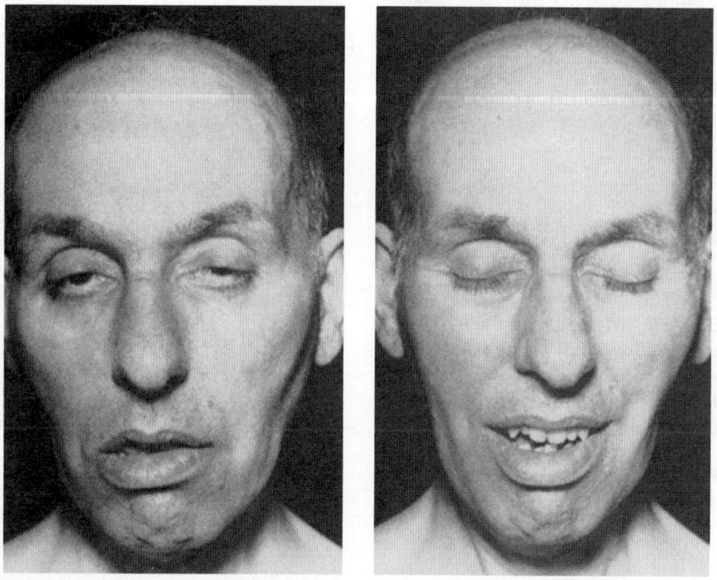

FIGURE 1-169 Myotonic dystrophy with typical myopathic facies, frontal balding, and sunken cheeks. (From Dubowitz V: *Muscle disorders in childhood,* London, 1995, WB Saunders.)

BASIC INFORMATION

DEFINITION

Myxedema coma is a life-threatening complication of hypothyroidism characterized by profound lethargy or coma and usually accompanied by hypothermia.

ICD-9CM CODES
244.8 Myxedema, pituitary
244.1 Myxedema, primary

PHYSICAL FINDINGS & CLINICAL PRESENTATION

- Profound lethargy or coma
- Hypothermia (rectal temperature <35° C [95° F]); often missed by using ordinary thermometers graduated only to 34.5° C or because the mercury is not shaken below 36° C
- Bradycardia, hypotension (secondary to circulatory collapse)
- Delayed relaxation phase of DTR, areflexia
- Myxedema facies (Fig. 1-170)
- Alopecia, macroglossia, ptosis, periorbital edema, nonpitting edema, doughy skin
- Bladder dystonia and distention

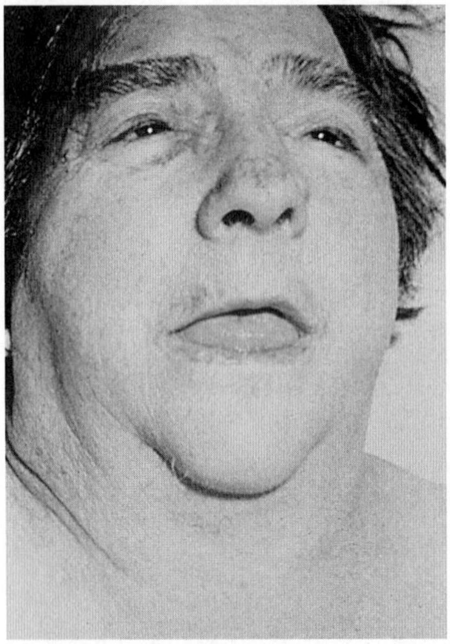

FIGURE 1-170 Myxedema facies. Note dull, puffy, yellowed skin; coarse, sparse hair; temporal loss of eyebrows; periorbital edema; prominent tongue. (Courtesy Paul W. Ladenson, M.D. The Johns Hopkins University and Hospital, Baltimore. In Seidel HM [ed]: *Mosby's guide to physical examination,* ed 5, St Louis, 2004, Mosby.)

ETIOLOGY

Decompensation of hypothyroidism secondary to:
- Sepsis
- Exposure to cold weather
- CNS depressants (sedatives, narcotics, antidepressants)
- Trauma, surgery

DIAGNOSIS

DIFFERENTIAL DIAGNOSIS

- Severe depression, primary psychosis
- Drug overdose
- CVA, liver failure, renal failure
- Hypoglycemia, CO_2 narcosis, encephalitis

WORKUP

Diagnosis of hypothyroidism and exclusion of contributing factors (e.g., sepsis, CVA) with laboratory and radiographic studies (see "Laboratory Tests")

LABORATORY TESTS

- Markedly increased TSH (if primary hypothyroidism), decreased serum free T_4
- CBC with differential, urine and blood cultures to rule out infectious process
- Electrolytes, BUN, creatinine, LFTs, calcium, glucose
- ABGs to rule out hypoxemia and carbon dioxide retention
- Cortisol level to rule out adrenal insufficiency
- Elevated CPK
- Hyperlipidemia

IMAGING STUDIES

- CT scan of head in suspected CVA
- Chest x-ray to rule out infectious process

TREATMENT

NONPHARMACOLOGIC THERAPY

- Prevent further heat loss; cover the patient but avoid external rewarming because it may produce vascular collapse.
- Support respiratory function; intubation and mechanical ventilation may be required.
- Monitor patients in the ICU.

ACUTE GENERAL Rx

- Give levothyroxine 5 to 8 μg/kg (300 to 500 μg) IV infused over 15 min, then 100 μg IV q24h.
- Glucocorticoids should also be administered until coexistent adrenal insufficiency can be ruled out. Hydrocortisone hemisuccinate 100 mg IV bolus is initially given, followed by 50 mg IV q12h or 25 mg IV q6h until initial plasma cortisol level is confirmed normal.
- IV hydration with D_5NS is used to correct hypotension and hypoglycemia (if present); avoid overhydration and possible water intoxication because clearance of free water is impaired in these patients.
- Rule out and treat precipitating factors (e.g., antibiotics in suspected sepsis).

CHRONIC Rx

Refer to "Hypothyroidism" in Section I.

DISPOSITION

Mortality rate in myxedema coma is 20% to 50%.

REFERRAL

Endocrinology consultation is appropriate in patients with myxedema coma.

PEARLS & CONSIDERATIONS

COMMENTS

If the diagnosis is suspected, initiate treatment immediately without waiting for confirming laboratory results.

SUGGESTED READING

Wall CR: Myxedema coma: diagnosis and treatment, *Am Fam Physician* 62:2485, 2000.

AUTHOR: **FRED F. FERRI, M.D.**

BASIC INFORMATION

DEFINITION

Narcissistic personality disorder (NPD) is characterized by a pattern of grandiosity, need for admiration, and lack of empathy that begins by early adulthood and causes significant distress or impairment in multiple domains of functioning. The individual must meet five or more of the following criteria:

1. Grandiose sense of self-importance. For example, the person may exaggerate achievements and talents or expect recognition as superior without commensurate achievements.
2. Preoccupied with fantasies of unlimited success, power, brilliance, beauty, or ideal love.
3. Views self as "special" and unique and should only associate with other special or highly regarded people and institutions.
4. Requires excessive admiration.
5. Sense of entitlement. For example, unreasonable expectations of especially favorable treatment or automatic compliance with his or her expectations.
6. Interpersonally exploitative.
7. Lacks empathy—unwilling to recognize or identify with the feelings or needs of others.
8. Often envious of others or believes others envious of him or her.
9. Shows arrogant or haughty behaviors.

SYNONYMS

None

ICD-9CM CODES
301.81

EPIDEMIOLOGY & DEMOGRAPHICS

PREVALENCE: Less than 1% of the general population. Estimates range from 2% to 16% in the clinical population.
PREDOMINANT SEX: More commonly diagnosed in males (up to 3:1).
PREDOMINANT AGE: 20s and 30s.

CLINICAL PRESENTATION

- Patients experience an underlying sense of inferiority and inadequacy.
- Often related to the failure of parents or parental surrogates to impart a sense of "self-worth."
- To avoid these beliefs and their associated painful affects, patients seek to convince self and others that they are special, the best, unusually talented.
- Astutely aware of status, pecking order.
- Vulnerability in self-esteem makes these patients exquisitely sensitive to "criticism," "defeat," or "perceived weakness," which in turn can lead to feeling humiliated, degraded, and empty.
- These patients react to perceived slights with either more intense grandiosity and admiration seeking or with disdain and rage. Either approach seeks to bolster their sense of self often by devaluing or criticizing the other person.
- Experiences of self-deflation lead to social withdrawal or depressed mood or to feigned humility that protects grandiosity.
- Interpersonal relationships typically shallow and limited.
- Though ambition and confidence may lead to high achievement, vocational functioning may be disrupted due to intolerance for criticism.

ETIOLOGY

- Limited knowledge about role of genetic loading and neurobiologic vulnerability.
- Prevailing hypotheses focus on impaired development of self as "worthy" due to insufficient affirmation and warmth from parents.

DIAGNOSIS

DIFFERENTIAL DIAGNOSIS

- Mania and hypomania.
- Dysthymia and major depressive episode.
- Substance-induced euphoria, especially cocaine abuse.
- Histrionic, borderline, antisocial, and paranoid personality disorders share common features and are often comorbid.
- Personality changes due to a general medical condition, including CNS processes in the frontal-temporal regions of the brain.

WORKUP

- History—collateral information essential to establishing presence of longstanding interpersonal pattern in multiple domains of the patient's life.
- Physical examination.
- Mental status examination.

LABORATORY TESTS

Those tests necessary to rule out medical causes of personality changes

IMAGING STUDIES

Those necessary to rule out medical causes of personality changes

TREATMENT

NONPHARMACOLOGIC THERAPY

- Cognitive behavioral therapy to help patients control rage, manage perceived criticism, and develop social skills
- Psychodynamic psychotherapy to help develop sense of self-worth

ACUTE GENERAL Rx

Benzodiazepines or low-dose antipsychotics to control rage

CHRONIC Rx

- SSRIs if comorbid depression
- Mood stabilizers if comorbid bipolar or to improve impulse control

DISPOSITION

- Severity is variable and course is chronic. The majority of patients obtain greater functioning in fifth decade and beyond when pessimism replaces grandiosity. Often lifelong difficulty maintaining intimate relationships.
- At increased risk for major depressive disorder and substance abuse or dependence (especially cocaine).

REFERRAL

If pharmacotherapy contemplated

PEARLS & CONSIDERATIONS

COMMENTS

- Illness threatens these patients' image of superiority.
- To defend against this threat, patients may minimize symptoms or deny presence of illness.
- Patients will commonly demand special treatment from senior and well-known physicians.
- Patients may devalue, criticize, or question the behavior or credentials of the treating physician.
- Management guidelines:
  1. Be respectful and nonconfrontational.
  2. Help patient use self-perceived talents in service of their treatment.
  3. Do not personalize patient's devaluation, but understand their criticalness as an attempt to manage their own intense insecurity.
  4. Appeal to the patient's narcissism. In other words, agree with the patient that they are "entitled" to appropriate care.

SUGGESTED READINGS

Grant BF et al: Prevalence, correlates, and disability of personality disorders in the United States: results from the national epidemiologic survey on alcohol and related conditions, *J Clin Psychiatry* 65(7):948-958, 2004.
Morana HC, Camara FP: International guidelines for the management of personality disorders, *Curr Opin Psychiatry* 19(5):539, 2006.
Ward RK: Assessment and management of personality disorders, *Am Fam Physician* 15;70(8):1505-1512, 2004.

AUTHOR: **JOHN Q. YOUNG, M.D., M.P.P.**

BASIC INFORMATION

DEFINITION

Narcolepsy is a chronic neurologic disorder characterized by excessive daytime sleepiness and a dysregulation of rapid eye movement (REM) sleep features. Symptoms associated with the dysregulation of REM sleep include cataplexy, sleep paralysis, and hallucinations during the transition between sleep and wakefulness.

SYNONYMS

Narcolepsy without cataplexy
Narcolepsy with cataplexy
Secondary narcolepsy
Narcolepsy-cataplexy syndrome
Gelineau syndrome

ICD-9CM CODES
347 Narcolepsy

EPIDEMIOLOGY & DEMOGRAPHICS

PREVALENCE: Approximately 1 in 2000 men and women in the U.S.
AGE OF ONSET: Two peaks, 14.7 and 35 yr (range 10 to 55 yr)
GENETICS:
- Associated with specific human leukocyte antigen (HLA) subtypes (i.e., DQB1*0602) in up to 98% of narcoleptics with cataplexy.
- There is a 20 to 40 times higher risk of developing narcolepsy if there is an affected family member.
- Monozygotic concordance rate is 17% to 36%, indicating incomplete penetrance with an environmental contribution to the disease process.

PHYSICAL FINDINGS & CLINICAL PRESENTATION

- Irresistible urges to sleep may occur during the day and lead to temporarily refreshing naps.
- Cataplexy occurs in 60% to 100% of narcoleptics and is reported as a partial or total loss of voluntary muscle control with preserved consciousness that is precipitated by a strong emotion. This is the most specific symptom associated with narcolepsy.
- Sleep paralysis, which occurs in 60% to 80% of narcoleptics, is a loss of muscle tone during the transition between sleep and wakefulness. It may be associated with frightening or vivid hallucinations and can be interrupted by sensory stimuli.
- Hypnagogic (wake to sleep) or hypnopompic (sleep to wake) hallucinations may occur in 60% to 80% of patients.
- Fragmented nighttime sleep is reported by 60% to 90% of narcoleptics and may be mistaken for insomnia or other intrinsic sleep disorder.

ETIOLOGY

Narcolepsy is a complex disorder with no clear etiology. Research suggests that a deficient hypocretin/orexin system in the hypothalamus may be associated with the development of narcolepsy. Human cerebrospinal fluid levels of hypocretin-1 are low to undetectable in narcolepsy with cataplexy but not in narcolepsy without cataplexy.

DIAGNOSIS

DIFFERENTIAL DIAGNOSIS

Excessive daytime somnolence:
- Sleep apnea
- Inadequate sleep time
- Insomnia
- Hypothyroidism
- Drugs and alcohol
- Seizures
- Sleep fragmentation (multiple causes)

Cataplexy:
- Seizures
- Periodic paralysis
- Cardiovascular insufficiency
- Psychogenic (multiple causes)

WORKUP

- Medical history should include questions regarding sleep apnea, seizures, dissociated REM sleep features, and a detailed family history. Questions concerning other hypothalamic dysfunction such as unexplained weight gain, depression, endocrinologic abnormalities, circadian dysrhythmias, and autonomic nervous system problems are also helpful.
- Overnight polysomnography followed by a multiple sleep latency test is the standard used for diagnosis. A clinical diagnosis of narcolepsy can be made with a clear history of cataplexy and excessive daytime somnolence. Without these features, the diagnosis depends upon the sleep laboratory testing.

LABORATORY TESTS

HLA subtyping and CSF hypocretin/orexin levels may be helpful in cases of suspected but unconfirmed narcolepsy; however, there is currently no clinical standard by which to interpret these results. Complicated cases should be referred to sleep specialists or institutions with active narcolepsy protocols for further workup and data collection.

TREATMENT

NONPHARMACOLOGIC THERAPY

Scheduled daily naps can be used for symptoms of excessive daytime somnolence and to combat irresistible sleep urges.

CHRONIC Rx

For excessive daytime somnolence:
1. Modafinil (Provigil) 200 to 600 mg PO qam, or divided bid
2. Methylphenidate (Ritalin) 5 to 15 mg PO bid-tid
3. Methylphenidate SR (Concerta) 18 to 54 mg PO qam, or divided bid
4. Dextroamphetamine (Dexedrine) 10 to 60 mg PO qd
5. Sodium Oxybate (Xyrem); contact the Xyrem Success Program for prescription information

For cataplexy and REM-related symptoms:
1. Fluoxetine (Prozac) 20 mg PO qd initially
2. Venlafaxine (Effexor) 25 mg PO qd initially
3. Sertraline (Zoloft) 25 mg PO qd initially
4. Clomipramine (Anafranil) 25 mg/day initially
5. Protriptyline (Vivactil) 5 mg tid initially
6. Imipramine (Tofranil) 25 to 50 mg/day initially
7. Desipramine (Norpramine) 10 mg bid initially
8. Sodium Oxybate (Xyrem); contact the Xyrem Success Program for prescription information

DISPOSITION

This is a chronic sleep disorder without periods of remission.

REFERRAL

Because this disorder is under intense investigation, patients should be referred to programs with sleep specialists who study, manage, and implement new therapies as they arise.

PEARLS & CONSIDERATIONS

Many narcoleptics report the onset of symptoms beginning in childhood to early adulthood. Often the symptoms of narcolepsy begin with excessive daytime sleepiness and progress with time to include REM-dysregulation (e.g., cataplexy, sleep paralysis, hypnagogic hallucinations). Patients with narcolepsy may have an increased incidence of rapid eye movement behavior disorder (RBD) and periodic limb movement disorder (PLMD).

COMMENTS

True narcolepsy is a relatively rare cause of excessive daytime sleepiness. Except for cataplexy, symptoms of REM dysregulation are not specific for narcolepsy. Sleep paralysis, hyponogogic hallucinations, and sleep onset REM may occur as a result of sleep deprivation.

EVIDENCE

EBM

There is evidence that pemoline, methylphenidate, dextroamphetamine, and modafinil are effective treatments of sleepiness in patients with narcolepsy.[1,2,4] Double-blind placebo-controlled trials demonstrate that Xyrem (sodium oxybate) is an effective treatment for symptoms of excessive daytime somnolence and cataplexy in narcoleptic patients.[3,4]

Evidence-Based References

1. American Sleep Disorders Association Standards of Practice. Practice parameters for the use of stimulants in the treatment of narcolepsy. Standards of the Practice Committee of the American Sleep Disorders Association. Adapted from *Sleep* 17:348, 1994.
2. Randomized trial of modafinil as a treatment for the excessive daytime somnolence of narcolepsy: US Modafinil in Narcolepsy Multicenter Study Group, *Neurology* 54(5):1166, 2000.
3. Xyrem International Study Group: Further evidence supporting the use of sodium oxybate for the treatment of cataplexy: a double-blind, placebo-controlled study in 228 patients, *Sleep Med* 6(5):415, 2005.
4. Black J, Houghton WC: Sodium oxybate improves excessive daytime sleepiness in narcolepsy, *Sleep* 29(9):939, 2006.

SUGGESTED READINGS

Baumann CR, Bassetti CL: Hypocretins (orexins) and sleep-wake disorders, *Lancet Neurol* (10):673, 2005.

Greenhill LL et al: Practice parameter for the use of stimulant medications in the treatment of children, adolescents, and adults, *J Am Acad Child Adolesc Psychiatry* 41(2 suppl):26S, 2002.

Littner et al: Practice parameters for clinical use of the multiple sleep latency test and the maintenance of wakefulness test, *Sleep* 28(1):113, 2005.

Mahmood M, Black J: Narcolepsy-cataplexy: how does recent understanding help in evaluation and treatment? *Curr Treat Options Neurol* 7(5):363, 2005.

Mignot E et al: The role of cerebrospinal fluid hypocretin measurement in the diagnosis of narcolepsy and other hypersomnias, *Arch Neurol* 59:1553, 2002.

Saletu M et al: EEG-tomographic studies with LORETA on vigilance differences between narcolepsy patients and controls and subsequent double-blind, placebo-controlled studies with modafinil, *J Neurol* 251(11):1354, 2004.

Scammell TE: The neurobiology, diagnosis, and treatment of narcolepsy, *Ann Neurol* 53:154, 2003.

Xyrem multicenter study group: A 12-month, open-label, multicenter extension trial of orally administered sodium oxybate for the treatment of narcolepsy, *Sleep* 26:31, 2003.

AUTHOR: **JEFFREY S. DURMER, M.D., PH.D.**

BASIC INFORMATION

DEFINITION

Malignant renal tumor derived from primitive metanephric blastome. Most tumors are unicentric, but some are multifocal in one or both kidneys. Associated anomalies may be present.

SYNONYM

Wilms' Tumor

ICD-9CM CODES
189.0 Nephroblastoma

EPIDEMIOLOGY & DEMOGRAPHICS

- Pediatric malignancy mean presentation is at 41.5 mo in boys and 46.9 mo in girls
- Slightly more frequent in girls
- Incidence rate is 7.9 cases/yr/million white children <15 yr (a little over 500 new cases/yr in the U.S.); the incidence is double in black children
- Associated syndromes:
  1. Cryptorchidism
  2. Hypospadias
  3. Hemihypertrophy with or without the Beckwith-Wiedemann syndrome, aniridia
  4. Denys-Drash syndrome (nephroblastoma, pseudohermaphrodism, glomerulonephritis)
  5. WAGR syndrome (Wilms' tumor, aniridia, genitourinary malformations, and mental retardation)
- Familial nephroblastoma occurs in 1.5% (with younger age at diagnosis and more frequent multifocal tumors)

PHYSICAL FINDINGS & CLINICAL PRESENTATION

- Wilms' tumor often is discovered when a parent notices a mass while bathing or dressing a child, most commonly a child who is about 3 yr old, or during a routine physical examination. The mass is unilateral, firm, and nontender and below the costal margin
- Abdominal swelling and/or pain
- Nausea
- Vomiting
- Constipation
- Loss of appetite
- Fever of unknown origin
- Night sweats
- Hematuria (less common than in adult renal malignancies)
- Malaise
- High blood pressure that is triggered when the tumor obstructs the renal artery
- Varicocele
- Signs of associated syndromes

ETIOLOGY & PATHOGENESIS

- Three cell types: blastomal, stromal, and epithelial may be present. Structural diversity is characteristic.
- Anaplasia is evidenced by the presence of gigantic polyploid nuclei. The term *focal anaplasia* is used to describe such findings when it is confined within the primary tumor in the kidney.
- Staging

Stage I: Tumor limited to the kidney whose capsule is intact. The tumor is completely excised.

Stage II: Tumor extends beyond the kidney but is completely excised. No peritoneal involvement.

Stage III: Residual tumor confined to the abdomen following surgery. No hematogenous metastases.

Stage IV: Hematogenous metastases present.

Stage V: Bilateral renal involvement at time of initial diagnosis.

DIAGNOSIS

DIFFERENTIAL DIAGNOSIS

- Other renal malignancies
  1. Hypernephroma
  2. Transitional cell carcinoma
  3. Lymphoma
  4. Clear cell sarcoma
  5. Rhabdoid tumor of the kidney
- Renal cyst
- Other intraabdominal or retroperitoneal tumors

LABORATORY TESTS

- CBC
- Transaminases (ALT, AST)
- Alkaline phosphatase
- BUN and creatinine
- Serum calcium
- Urinalysis

IMAGING STUDIES

- Renal ultrasound to confirm existence of a solid mass in a kidney
- Abdominal CT scan with contrast (Fig. 1-171)
- Chest x-ray or CT scan

TREATMENT

- Surgical resection and surgical staging
  1. Stages I and II: surgery followed by chemotherapy
  2. Stages III and IV: surgery followed by radiation and chemotherapy
- Chemotherapeutic agents used in the treatment of Wilms' tumor include vincristine, dactinomycin, and doxorubicin

PROGNOSIS

- Stage I: 95% survival
- Stage II: 91% survival
- Stage III: 91% survival
- Stage IV: 81% survival
- Prognosis is better for patients whose age is <2 yr

AUTHORS: **FRED F. FERRI, M.D.**, and **TOM J. WACHTEL, M.D.**

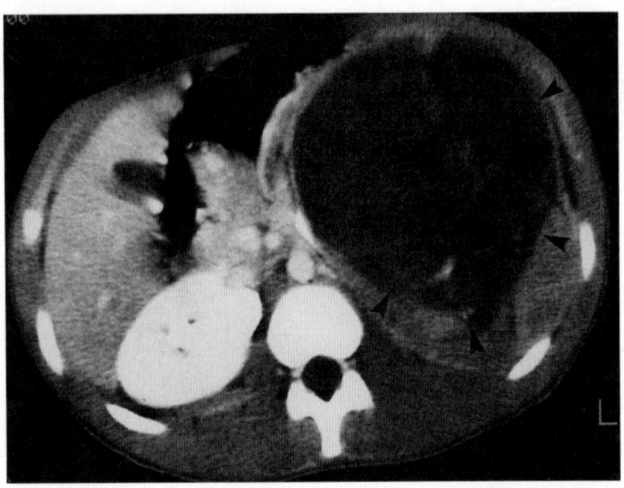

FIGURE 1-171 Transverse computed tomographic image of a Wilms' tumor shows a large intrarenal mass. (From Abeloff MD [ed]: *Clinical oncology,* ed 3, Philadelphia, 2004, Elsevier.)

BASIC INFORMATION

DEFINITION

Nephrotic syndrome is characterized by high urine protein excretion (>3.5g/1.73 m^3/24 hr), peripheral edema, and metabolic abnormalities (hypoalbuminemia, hypercholesterolemia).

ICD-9CM CODES
581.9 Nephrotic syndrome

EPIDEMIOLOGY & DEMOGRAPHICS

- Nephrotic syndrome occurs predominantly in children ages 2 to 6 yr (2 new cases/100,000 persons/yr) and in adults of all ages (3 to 4 new cases/100,000 persons/yr).
- Membranous glomerulonephritis is the most common cause of nephrotic syndrome.

PHYSICAL FINDINGS & CLINICAL PRESENTATION

- Peripheral edema
- Ascites, anasarca
- Hypertension
- Pleural effusion
- Typically patients present with severe peripheral edema, exertional dyspnea, and abdominal fullness secondary to ascites. There is a significant amount of weight gain in most patients

ETIOLOGY

- Idiopathic (may be secondary to the following glomerular diseases: minimal change disease [nil disease, lipoid nephrosis], focal segmental glomerular sclerosis, membranous nephropathy, membranoproliferative glomerular nephropathy)
- Associated with systemic diseases (diabetes mellitus, SLE, amyloidosis). Amyloidosis and dysproteinemias should be considered in patients older than 40 yr
- Majority of children with nephrotic syndrome have minimal change disease (this form also associated with allergy, nonsteroidals, and Hodgkin's disease)
- Focal glomerular disease: can be associated with HIV infection, heroin abuse. A more severe form of nephrotic syndrome associated with rapid progression to end-stage renal failure within months can also occur in HIV seropositive patients and is known as "collapsing glomerulopathy"
- Membranous nephropathy: can occur with Hodgkin's lymphoma, carcinomas, SLE, gold therapy
- Membranoproliferative glomerulonephropathy: often associated with upper respiratory infections

DIAGNOSIS

DIFFERENTIAL DIAGNOSIS

- Other edema states (CHF, cirrhosis)
- Primary renal disease (e.g., focal glomerulonephritis, membranoproliferative glomerulonephritis). Table 1-30 summarizes primary renal diseases that present as idiopathic nephrotic syndrome
- Carcinoma, infections
- Malignant hypertension
- Polyarteritis nodosa
- Serum sickness
- Toxemia of pregnancy

WORKUP

Diagnostic workup consists of family history and history of drug use or toxin exposure and laboratory evaluation. Renal biopsy is generally performed in individuals with persistent proteinuria in whom the etiology of the proteinuria is unclear.

LABORATORY TESTS

- Urinalysis reveals proteinuria. The presence of hematuria, cellular casts, and pyuria is suggestive of nephritic syndrome. Oval fat bodies (tubular epithelial cells with cholesterol esters) are also found in the urine in patients with nephrotic syndrome.
- 24-hr urine protein excretion is >3.5 g/1.73 m^3/24 hr.
- Abnormalities of blood chemistries include serum albumin <3 g/dl, decreased total protein, elevated serum cholesterol, glucose, azotemia.
- Additional tests in patients with nephrotic syndromes depending on the history and physical examination are ANA, serum and urine immunoelectrophoresis, C3, C4, CH-50, LDH, liver enzymes, alkaline phosphatase, hepatitis B and C screening, and HIV.

IMAGING STUDIES

- Ultrasound of kidneys
- Chest x-ray

TREATMENT

NONPHARMACOLOGIC THERAPY

- Bed rest as tolerated, avoidance of nephrotoxic drugs, low-fat diet, fluid restriction in hyponatremic patients; normal protein intake unless urinary protein loss exceeds 10 g/24 hr (some patients may require additional dietary protein to prevent negative nitrogen balance and significant protein malnutrition)
- Improved urinary protein excretion and serum lipid changes have been observed with a low-fat soy protein diet providing 0.7 g of protein/kg/day. However, because of increased risk of malnutrition, many nephrologists recommend normal protein intake
- Strict sodium restriction to help manage peripheral edema
- Close monitoring of patients for development of peripheral venous thrombosis and renal vein thrombosis because of hypercoagulable state secondary to loss of antithrombin III and other proteins involved in the clotting mechanism

ACUTE GENERAL Rx

- Furosemide is useful for severe edema.
- Use of ACE inhibitors to reduce proteinuria is generally indicated even in normotensive patients.
- Anticoagulant therapy should be administered as long as patients have nephrotic proteinuria, an albumin level <20 g/L, or both.

The mainstay of therapy is treatment of the underlying disorder:

- Minimal change disease generally responds to prednisone 1 mg/kg/day. Relapses can occur when steroids are discontinued. In these individuals, cyclophosphamide and chlorambucil may be useful.
- Focal and segmental glomerulosclerosis: steroid therapy is also recommended. However, response rate is approximately 35% to 40%, and most patients progress to end-stage renal disease within 3 yr.
- Membranous glomerulonephritis: prednisone 2 mg/kg/day may be useful in inducing remission. Cytotoxic agents can be added if there is poor response to prednisone.
- Membranoproliferative glomerulonephritis: most patients are treated with steroid therapy and antiplatelet drugs. Despite treatment, the majority of patients will progress to end-stage renal disease within 5 yr.

CHRONIC Rx

- Patients should be monitored for azotemia and should be aggressively treated for hypertension and hyperlipidemia. Furosemide is useful for severe edema. Anticoagulants may be necessary for thromboembolic events. Prophylactic anticoagulation should be considered in patients with membranous glomerulonephritis.
- Oral vitamin D is useful in the treatment of hypocalcemia (because of vitamin D loss).

REFERRAL

Nephrology consultation is recommended in all cases of nephrotic syndrome.

AUTHOR: **FRED F. FERRI, M.D.**

TABLE 1-30 Summary of Primary Renal Diseases That Present as Idiopathic Nephrotic Syndrome

	Minimal-Change Nephrotic Syndrome (MCNS)	Focal Segmental Sclerosis	Membranous Nephropathy	MEMBRANOPROLIFERATIVE GLOMERULONEPHRITIS (MPGN)	
				Type I	Type II
Frequency*					
Children	75%	10%	<5%	10%	10%
Adults	15%	15%	50%	10%	10%
Clinical Manifestations					
Age (yr)	2-6, some adults	2-10, some adults	40-50	5-15	5-15
Sex	2:1 male	1.3:1 male	2:1 male	Male-female	Male-female
Nephrotic syndrome	100%	90%	80%	60%	60%
Asymptomatic proteinuria	0	10%	20%	40%	40%
Hematuria	10%-20%	60%-80%	60%	80%	80%
Hypertension	10%	20% early	Infrequent	35%	35%
Rate of progression to renal failure	Does not progress	10 years	50% in 10-20 yr	10-20 yr	5-15 yr
Associated conditions	Allergy? Hodgkin's disease, usually none	None	Renal vein thrombosis, cancer, SLE, hepatitis B	None	Partial lipodystrophy
Laboratory Findings	Manifestations of nephrotic syndrome ↑ BUN in 15%-30%	Manifestations of nephrotic syndrome ↑ BUN in 20%-40%	Manifestations of nephrotic syndrome	Low C1, C4, C3–C9	Normal C1, C4, low C3–C9
Immunogenetics	HLA-B8, B12 (3.5)†	Not established	HLA-DRW3 (12–32)†	Not established	C3 nephritic factor Not established
Renal Pathology					
Light microscopy	Normal	Focal sclerotic lesions	Thickened GBM, spikes	Thickened GBM, proliferation	Lobulation
Immunofluorescence	Negative	IgM, C3 in lesions	Fine granular IgG, C3	Granular IgG, C3	C3 only
Electron microscopy	Foot process fusion	Foot process fusion	Subepithelial deposits	Mesangial and subendothelial deposits	Dense deposits
Response of Steroids	90%	15%-20%	May slow progression	Not established	Not established

Modified from Goldman L, Ausiello D (eds): *Cecil textbook of medicine,* ed 22, Philadelphia, 2004, WB Saunders.
*Approximate frequency as a cause of idiopathic nephrotic syndrome. About 10% of adult nephrotic syndrome is due to various diseases that usually present with acute glomerulonephritis.
†Relative risk.
↑, Elevated; *BUN,* blood urea nitrogen; *C,* complement; *GBM,* glomerular basement membrane; *hepatitis B,* hepatitis B virus; *HLA,* human leukocyte antigen; *Ig,* immunoglobulin; *SLE,* systemic lupus erythematosus.

BASIC INFORMATION

DEFINITION

Neuroblastomas are tumors of postganglionic sympathetic neurons that typically originate in the adrenal medulla or the paraspinal sites of the sympathetic nervous system ganglia. Often present at birth, but not diagnosed until later, when the child shows symptoms of the disease. Almost exclusively a disease of early childhood, with two thirds of cases presenting in children younger than 5 years.

ICD-9CM CODES
194.0 Neuroblastoma, unspecified site

EPIDEMIOLOGY & DEMOGRAPHICS

INCIDENCE (IN U.S.): 8% to 10% of all solid tumors of childhood; the third most common childhood cancer, after leukemia and brain tumors, and most common extracranial solid tumor; 1/10,000 children <15 yr

PREDOMINANT SEX: Male:female ratio of 1:1.3

PEAK AGE: Early childhood. Mean age of onset is 18 mo; 40% onset by 1 yr; 35% ages 1-2 yr, and 25% are older than 2 yr. In rare cases, neuroblastoma can be discovered by fetal ultrasound.

GENETICS: Chromosomal deletions found in nearly half of tumors, most commonly localized to chromosomes 1p, 11q, and 14q. Deletion of 1p36 (leading to amplification and overexpression of *N-myc*) associated with poor prognosis. A small subset of patients demonstrate autosomal dominant inheritance.

PHYSICAL FINDINGS & CLINICAL PRESENTATION

- Mass in abdomen, neck, or chest. Approximately two thirds of tumors arise in the abdomen; of these, two thirds arise in the adrenal glands. 70% to 80% of children have regional lymph node involvement or distant metastases at time of presentation.
- Neuroblastomas, because of the paraspinal location, can invade the spinal cord via the neural foramina, leading to back pain or signs of compression—paraplegia, stool/urine retention.
- Horner's syndrome: ptosis, miosis, anhidrosis.
- Thoracic: difficulty breathing, dysphagia, infections, chronic cough.
- High-risk patients typically present with symptoms related to the tumor size or from bony metastases, with pain or pancytopenia. Proptosis and periorbital ecchymosis are common in high-risk patients and typically arise from metastases to the retrobulbar region. Other constitutional symptoms are also frequently noted, including anorexia, weight loss, unexplained fever, multiple subcutaneous bluish nodules, and irritability.
- Paraneoplastic syndromes: opsoclonus-myoclonus syndrome appears to be caused by an immunologic mechanism, leading to myoclonic jerk of the extremities and chaotic eye movements in all directions. May be presenting symptom before tumor diagnosis; present in 1% to 3% of patients with neuroblastoma. Of all patients with opsoclonus-myoclonus, 20% to 50% have an underlying neuroblastoma. Pathology in patients who present with this syndrome often demonstrates more favorable biologic features. Adrenocorticotropic hormone (ACTH) treatment is thought to be effective, but many patients experience pervasive neurologic and cognitive deficits.
- Progressive cerebellar ataxia.
- Abnormal secretion of vasoactive intestinal peptide by the tumor, leading to distention of the abdomen and secretory diarrhea.

DIAGNOSIS

WORKUP

- Careful general physical examination
- Biopsy and resection of tumor when possible

LABORATORY TESTS

- Complete blood count, coagulation studies, erythrocyte sedimentation rate.
- 24-hour urine for catecholamines: homovanillic acid (HVA) and vanillylmandelic acid (VMA) are secreted by 90% to 95% of tumors.
- Nonspecific serum markers such as neuron-specific enolase, lactate dehydrogenase, and ferritin.
- Bone marrow biopsy and aspirate: karyotype, DNA index, *N-myc* copy number.
- Minimum diagnostic criteria includes one of the following: (1) unequivocal pathologic diagnosis made from tumor tissue or (2) combination of bone marrow aspirate with unequivocal tumor cells and increased levels of serum or urinary catecholamine metabolites, as described above.
- Genetic/biologic variables, including histology, aneuploidy of tumor DNA, and amplification of the *N-MYC* oncogene within tumor tissue are used to determine treatment.
  - Hyperdiploid DNA is associated with favorable prognosis, especially in infants.
  - *N-myc* amplification is associated with poor prognosis, regardless of patient age, likely owing to association with deletion of chromosome 1p and gain of chromosome 17q.
  - Other biologic factors have been studied but are not currently used in determining therapy; however, they may ultimately be useful as therapeutic targets or as prognostic factors in the future. These include the profile of GABAergic receptors, expression of neurotrophin receptors, level of telomerase RNA and serum ferritin and lactate dehydrogenase.
  - Neuroblastoma screening of infants was initiated in Japan using an assay for urinary catecholamine metabolites. A large population-based study in North America demonstrated that screening detects neuroblastoma with the most favorable characteristics, which would not otherwise be detected clinically likely due to spontaneous regression of these tumors. Current data do not support mass screening of infants.

IMAGING STUDIES

- Chest x-ray, abdominal x-ray, skeletal survey, abdominal ultrasound
- Renal/bladder ultrasound
- CT scan or MRI of the chest and abdomen to provide information about regional lymph nodes, vessel invasion, and distant metastases (Fig. 1-172)
- Body scan with ^{131}I-MIBG (meta-iodobenzylguanidine), which is taken up by neuroblasts and can demonstrate soft tissue and bony metastases.
- Bone scan with Tc-99 MDP to visualize lytic bone lesions and metastases

STAGING (INTERNATIONAL NEUROBLASTOMA STAGING SYSTEM)

I. Confined to single organ
IIA. Localized tumor with incomplete gross resection; lymph nodes negative
IIB. Localized tumor with incomplete gross resection; ipsilateral lymph nodes positive
III. Extension across midline, with or without lymph node involvement
IV. Distant metastases to lymph nodes, bone, bone marrow, liver, skin
IVs. Localized primary tumor with dissemination limited to skin, liver, or bone marrow; limited to infants <1 yr of age

DIFFERENTIAL DIAGNOSIS

- Other small, round, blue-cell childhood tumors, such as lymphoma, rhabdomyosarcoma, soft tissue sarcoma, and primitive neuroectodermal tumors (PNETs)
- Wilms' tumor
- Hepatoblastoma

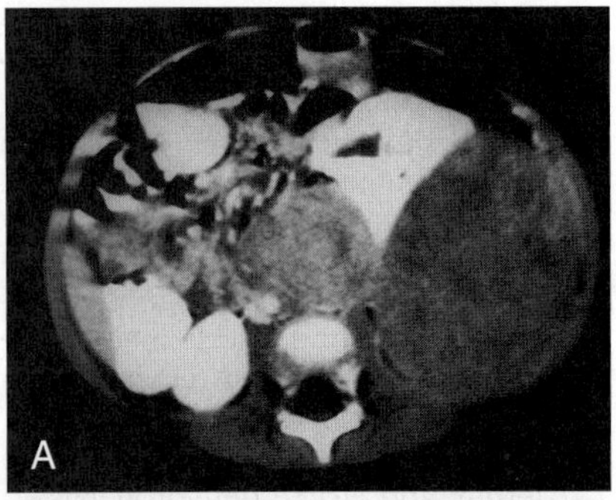

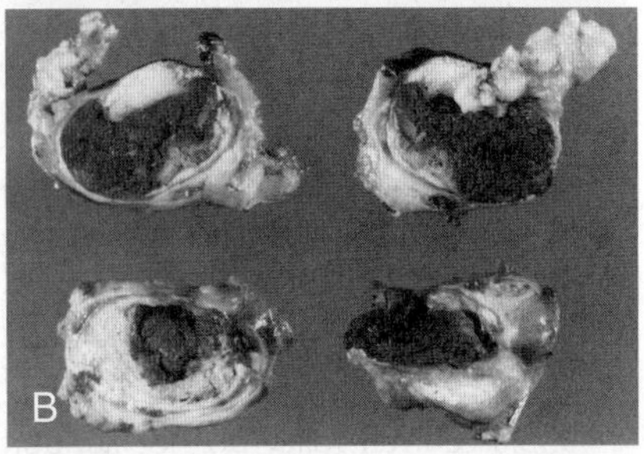

FIGURE 1-172 Computed tomographic scan **(A)** shows adrenal neuroblastoma at diagnosis. Serial sections through adrenal neuroblastoma **(B)** show tumor with large areas of diffuse hemorrhage and calcification. (From Abeloff MD [ed]: *Clinical oncology,* ed 3, Philadelphia, 2004, Elsevier.)

TREATMENT

Rx

- Assure patient that there is hope for recovery with aggressive treatment.
- Overall, treatment will be determined by several factors, including age at diagnosis, stage of disease, site of primary tumor and metastases, and tumor histology.
- Surgery, particularly for low-risk tumors.
- Radiation therapy is often reserved for unresectable tumors or tumors that are not responsive to chemotherapy and also with unfavorable biologic characteristics. Radiation therapy to the primary site is often recommended for high-risk patients even in the cases of complete resection.
- Multiagent chemotherapy is mainstay of treatment.
- Urgent treatment should be given for symptomatic spinal cord compression. Neurologic recovery is more likely with less severe and shorter duration of compromise and symptoms. For patients with low- or intermediate-risk neuroblastoma, immediate chemotherapy is recommended over surgery because of later concerns for scoliosis after laminectomy.
- Autologous bone marrow transplantation following aggressive chemotherapy for stage IV disease or in high-risk patients, based on age, presence of disseminated disease, or unfavorable markers. Radiation of residual tumor and original sites of metastases is often performed before, during, and after myeloablative therapy. After recovery, oral 13-*cis*-retinoic acid is used for 6 months and is thought to improve outcome.
- Novel therapies include immunotherapy using monoclonal antibodies and tumor-targeted vaccines with drugs that induce apoptosis or have antiangiogenic effect.
- ACTH treatment is thought to be effective for patients with opsoclonus/myoclonus syndrome.

DISPOSITION

- Overall survival is >40%. Children under the age of 1 yr have a cure rate as high as 90%.
- Approximately 70% of patients with neuroblastoma have metastases at diagnosis.
- Age, stage, and molecular abnormalities are important prognostic factors that are also used for risk-stratification and for determination of therapy. Children with localized disease and infants <1 year at diagnosis and favorable disease characteristics have better prognosis whereas poorer prognosis is noted in older children with stage IV disease (20% survival compared with >95% in stage I), age >1 year at diagnosis, increased number of *N-myc* copies, adrenal tumor, chronic 1p deletion.
- Children with neuroblastoma may be at risk for second malignancies, including renal cell carcinoma.

REFERRAL

Multidisciplinary oncology team with experience in treating cancers of childhood and adolescence.

PEARLS & CONSIDERATIONS

!

- Predominantly a tumor of early childhood that originates in the sites where the sympathetic nervous system tissue is present.
- Most common symptoms due to tumor mass or bone pain from metastases.
- Children can present with paraneoplastic neurologic symptoms including cerebellar ataxia and opsoclonus/myoclonus.

EVIDENCE

EBM

For patients with high-risk neuroblastoma, myoablative chemotherapy with hematopoetic stem-cell transplant is an effective treatment strategy. A large randomized controlled trial evaluated the role of conventional chemotherapy or myoablative therapy with stem-cell transplant. Event free survival was greater in those who received myoablative therapy plus hematopoietic cell transplantation (HCT) (34% vs. 22%).[1] Ⓐ

In most cases of stage IV, neuroblastoma is a favorable disease with minimal therapy achieving an excellent outcome. Infants <2 months of age may require more intensive treatment.[2] Ⓑ

Evidence-Based References

1. Matthay KK et al: Treatment of high-risk neuroblastoma with intensive chemotherapy, radiotherapy, autologous bone marrow transplantation, and 13-*cis*-retinoic acid: Children's Cancer Group, *N Engl J Med* 341:1165, 1999.
2. Nickerson HJ et al: Favorable biology and outcome of stage IV-S neuroblastoma with supportive care or minimal therapy: a Children's Cancer Group study, *J Clin Oncol* 18:477, 2000.

SUGGESTED READINGS

Marcus K et al: Primary tumor control in patients with stage 3/4 unfavorable neuroblastoma treated with tandem double autologous stem cell transplants, *J Pediatr Hematol Oncol* 25:934, 2003.

Maris JM: The biologic basis for neuroblastoma heterogeneity and risk stratification, *Curr Opin Pediatr* 17(1):7, 2005.

Pranzatelli MR et al: Screening for autoantibodies in children with opsoclonus-myoclonus-ataxia, *Pediatr Neurol* 27:384, 2002.

Riley RD et al: A systematic review of molecular and biological tumor markers in neuroblastoma, *Clin Cancer Res* 10(1 Pt 1):4, 2004.

Roberts SS et al: GABAergic system gene expression predicts clinical outcome in patients with neuroblastoma, *J Clin Oncol* 22(20):4127, 2004.

Rudnick E et al: Opsoclonus-myoclonus-ataxia syndrome in neuroblastoma: clinical outcome and antineuronal antibodies-a report from the Children's Cancer Group Study, *Med Pediatr Oncol* 36(6):612, 2001.

Schilling FH et al: Neuroblastoma screening at one year of age, *N Engl J Med* 346:1047, 2002.

Shimada H: International neuroblastoma pathology classification for prognostic evaluation of patients with peripheral neuroblastic tumors: a report from the Children's Cancer Group, *Cancer* 92:2451, 2001.

Woods WG et al: Screening of infants and mortality due to neuroblastoma, *N Engl J Med* 346:1041, 2002.

AUTHOR: **NICOLE J. ULLRICH, M.D., PH.D.**

BASIC INFORMATION

DEFINITION

Neurofibromatosis (NF) is an autosomal dominant disorder, affecting bone, nervous system, soft tissue, and skin. There are two major subtypes of neurofibromatosis disorders: NF type 1 (NF1) and NF type 2 (NF2).

SYNONYMS

NF1 is also called von Recklinghausen disease, peripheral NF

NF2 is also called bilateral acoustic neurofibromatosis, central NF

ICD-9CM CODES

237.71 Type 1, von Recklinghausen's

237.72 Type 2, acoustic

EPIDEMIOLOGY & DEMOGRAPHICS

- Incidence of NF1 (1 case/3000 persons), NF2 (1 case/33,000 persons).
- Prevalence of NF1 (1 case/5000 persons), NF2 (1 case/210,000 persons).
- NF1 and NF2 are autosomal dominant, with approximately 50% of cases having no family history.
- The two disorders affect approximately 100,000 people in the U.S.
- Equally affects males and females.
- NF1 may be associated with optic gliomas, astrocytomas, spinal neurofibromas, pheochromocytomas, and chronic myeloid leukemia.
- NF2 may be associated with meningiomas, spinal schwannomas, and cataracts.

PHYSICAL FINDINGS & CLINICAL PRESENTATION

- Common features of NF1 include:
  1. Café-au-lait macules (100% of children by age 2)
     a. Hyperpigmented skin lesions occurring anywhere on the body except the face, palms, and soles
     b. Appear early in life and increase in size and number during puberty
     c. Focal or diffuse
  2. Axillary and inguinal freckling (70%).
  3. Multiple neurofibromas (Fig. 1-173) can be soft or firm. Three subtypes:
     a. Cutaneous: circumscribed, not specific for NF1
     b. Subcutaneous: circumscribed, not specific for NF1
     c. Plexiform: noncircumscribed, thick and irregular, can cause disfigurement of supportive structures and specific for NF1
  4. Lisch nodule (small hamartoma of the iris) found in >90% of adult cases.
  5. Visual defects possibly related to optic gliomas (2% to 5%).
  6. Neurodevelopment problems (30% to 40%).
- Common features of NF2 include:
  1. Hearing loss and tinnitus related to bilateral acoustic neuromas (>90% of adults)
  2. Cataracts (81%)
  3. Headache
  4. Unsteady gait
  5. Cutaneous and subcutaneous neurofibromas, but less than NF1
  6. Café-au-lait macules (1%)

ETIOLOGY

- NF1 is caused by DNA mutations located on the long arm of chromosome 17 responsible for encoding the protein neurofibromin.
- NF2 is caused by DNA mutations located in the middle of the long arm of chromosome 22 responsible for encoding the protein merlin.
- Both proteins are speculated to act as tumor suppressors.

DIAGNOSIS

- NF1 is diagnosed if the person has two or more of the following features:
  1. Six or more café-au-lait macules >5 mm in prepubertal patients and >15 mm in postpubertal patients
  2. Two or more neurofibromas of any type or one plexiform neurofibroma
  3. Axillary or inguinal freckling
  4. Optic glioma
  5. Two or more Lisch nodules (iris hamartomas)
  6. Sphenoid wing dysplasia or cortical thinning of long bones, with or without pseudoarthrosis
  7. A first-degree relative (parent, sibling, or child) with NF1 based on the previous criteria
- NF2 is diagnosed if the person has either of the following two criteria:
  1. Bilateral eighth nerve masses seen by appropriate imaging studies (e.g., CT, MRI)
  2. A first-degree relative with NF2 and either a unilateral eighth nerve mass or two of the following: neurofibroma, meningioma, glioma, schwannoma, or juvenile posterior subcapsular lenticular opacity

DIFFERENTIAL DIAGNOSIS

- Abdominal neurofibromatosis
- Myxoid lipoma
- Nodular fasciitis
- Fibrous histiocytoma
- Segmental neurofibromatosis

WORKUP

The diagnosis of neurofibromatosis is usually self-evident. Workup is dictated by clinical symptoms in NF1 and usually includes MRI evaluation of the head and spine in NF2.

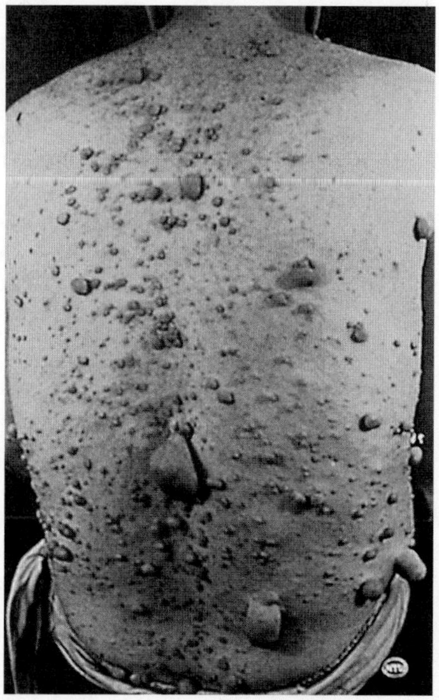

FIGURE 1-173 Nodules. Solid, large (>1 cm), deep-seated mass in dermal or subcutaneous tissues. These nodules are neurofibromas in a patient with neurofibromatosis. (From Goldman L, Ausiello D [eds]: *Cecil textbook of medicine,* ed 22, Philadelphia, 2004, WB Saunders.)

LABORATORY TESTS

- Genetic testing is possible in individuals who desire prenatal diagnosis for NF1. There is no single standard test and multiple tests are required. Results can only tell if an individual is affected but cannot predict the severity of the disease.
- In NF2, linkage analysis testing provides a >99% certainty the individual has NF2.

IMAGING STUDIES

- MRI with gadolinium is the imaging study of choice in both NF1 and NF2 patients. MRI increases detection of optic gliomas, tumors of the spine, acoustic neuromas, and "bright spots" thought to represent hamartomas.
- MRI of the spine is recommended in all patients diagnosed with NF2 to exclude intramedullary tumors.

OTHER TESTS

- Wood lamp examintation may be useful in patients with very pale skin for visualizing café-au-lait spots.
- Slit-lamp examination is recommended for children >6 years to confirm the presence of Lisch nodules and subcapsular opacity.

TREATMENT

Treatment is directed primarily at symptoms and complications of NF1 and NF2.

NONPHARMACOLOGIC THERAPY

- Counseling addressing prognosis, genetic, psychologic, and social issues
- Hearing testing and speech pathology evaluation

ACUTE GENERAL Rx

- Surgery is usually not done on skin tumors unless cosmetically requested or if suspicion of malignant transformation exists.
- Surgery may be indicated for spinal or cranial neurofibromas, gliomas, or meningiomas.
- Acoustic neuromas can be treated by surgical excision.

CHRONIC Rx

- Radiation may be indicated in NF1 patients with optic nerve gliomas.
- Stereotactic radiosurgery using gamma knife may be an alternative approach to surgery for acoustic neuromas.

DISPOSITION

- Prognosis varies according to the severity of involvement.
- There is no cure for neurofibromatosis.

REFERRAL

A multidisciplinary team of consultants is needed in patients with neurofibromatosis including neurosurgeon, otolaryngologist, dermatologist, neurologist, audiologist, speech pathologist, geneticist, and neuropsychologist.

PEARLS & CONSIDERATIONS

- Friedrich Daniel von Recklinghausen first reported his cases in 1882, although there had been similar accounts dating back to the 1600s.
- The first report in the literature of NF2 was by Wishart in 1822.

COMMENTS

For additional information refer to the National Neurofibromatosis Foundation (141 Fifth Avenue, Suite 7-S, New York, NY 10010, 800-323-7938) or Neurofibromatosis Inc. (PO Box 18246, Minneapolis, MN 55418, 301-918-4600).

SUGGESTED READINGS

Evans DG et al: Management of the patient and family with neurofibromatosis 2: a consensus conference statement, *Br J Neurosurg* 19(1):5, 2005.

Evans DG, Sainio M, Baser NE: Neurofibromatosis type 2, *J Med Genet* 37(12):897, 2000.

Kam JR et al: Neurofibromatosis, *eMedicine Journal,* last updated Jan 12, 2007. Accessed Aug 28, 2007. www.emedicine.com.

Korf BP: Diagnosis and management of neurofibronatosum type 1, *Curr Neurol Neurosci Rep* 1(2):162, 2001.

AUTHOR: **WEN-Y. WU-CHEN, M.D.**

BASIC INFORMATION

DEFINITION

Neuroleptic malignant syndrome (NMS) is a disorder characterized by hyperthermia, muscular rigidity, autonomic dysfunction, and depressed/fluctuating levels of arousal that evolve over 24 to 72 hr. This occurs as an idiosyncratic adverse reaction most commonly to dopamine-receptor antagonists (especially D2/4 receptor) or sudden withdrawal from a dopaminergic agent or agonist, such as antiparkinsonian medications.

SYNONYMS

None

ICD-9CM CODES
333.92 Neuroleptic malignant syndrome

EPIDEMIOLOGY & DEMOGRAPHICS

INCIDENCE (IN U.S.): 0.07% to 0.15% annual incidence in psychiatric population.
PREDOMINANT SEX: More than two thirds of patients are male.
PREDOMINANT AGE: Young and middle-aged adults
PREDISPOSING FACTORS:
- High-potency dopamine antagonists
- Long-acting depot preparations or multiple agents used
- Preexisting brain disease

PHYSICAL FINDINGS & CLINICAL PRESENTATION

- Muscle rigidity (hypertonia, cogwheeling, or "lead pipe" rigidity)
- Hyperthermia (38.6° to 42.3° C, usually <40° C)
- Autonomic symptoms: diaphoresis, sialorrhea, skin pallor, urinary incontinence
- Tachycardia, tachypnea
- Labile blood pressure (hypertension or postural hypotension)
- Agitation, catatonia, fluctuating consciousness, obtundation

ETIOLOGY

- Unknown. Impaired thermoregulation in hypothalamus and limbic cortex may occur as a result of central dopamine-blockade.
- Neuroleptic drugs have different potencies for inducing NMS:
  1. Typical neuroleptics: high potency—haloperidol; medium potency—chlorpromazine, fluphenazine; low potency—levomepromazine, loxapine
  2. Atypical neuroleptics: low potency—risperidone, olanzapine, clozapine, quetiapine

DIAGNOSIS

DIFFERENTIAL DIAGNOSIS

- Heatstroke, drug-induced states and overdose (ecstasy abuse, phencyclidine), thyrotoxicosis, pheochromocytoma, serotonin syndrome
- Malignant hyperthermia, catatonia, acute psychosis with agitation
- Central nervous system or systemic infections, including sepsis

WORKUP

Careful drug history

LABORATORY TESTS

- Elevated creatine phosphokinase (CPK) (sensitivity 0.71)
- Urinary myoglobin
- Leukocytosis, usually 10,000 to 40,000/mm³
- Electrolytes and renal function
- Blood gases
- Drug levels

TREATMENT

NONPHARMACOLOGIC THERAPY

- Stop all neuroleptic agents and reinstitute any recently discontinued dopaminergic agents.
- Respiratory support; nutritional support in cases with dysphagia or comatose.
- Careful fluid balance monitoring with adequate hydration (intravenous in severe cases).
- Active cooling (cooling blanket and antipyretics).
- Skilled nursing care to prevent decubitus ulcers in bed-confined patients.

ACUTE GENERAL Rx

- Intravenous benzodiazepines (e.g., diazepam 2 to 10 mg, with total daily dose of 10 to 60 mg) to relax muscles and control agitation.
- Bromocriptine, a dopamine receptor agonist, is the mainstay of therapy for patients with neuroleptic malignant syndrome. Initial doses of 2.5 to 10 mg are given IV q8h and are increased by 5 mg/day until clinical improvement is seen. The drug should be continued for at least 10 days after the syndrome has been controlled and then tapered slowly.
- Amantadine, a NMDA receptor antagonist with possible dopaminergic properties, administered orally at doses of 100 to 200 mg po bid, has been shown to reduce mortality in comparison to supportive therapy alone.
- Dantrolene therapy is also effective. Initially, patients can be given 0.25 mg/kg IV q6 to 12h, followed by a maintenance dose up to 3 mg/kg/day. After 2 to 3 days, patients may be given the drug orally (25 to 600 mg/day in divided doses). Oral dantrolene therapy (50 to 600 mg/day) may be continued for several days afterwards.
- Electroconvulsive therapy with neuromuscular blockage in pharmacologically refractory cases. Succinylcholine should not be used as it may cause hyperkalemia and cardiac arrhythmias in patients with rhabdomyolysis or dysautonomia.

CHRONIC Rx

- Respiratory care, nutritional support, and physical therapy may be required in more severe cases.
- Appropriate therapy would be required in patients with persistent neuropsychiatric sequelae of NMS (e.g., antidepressants for depression, cognitive behavioral therapy for cognitive deficits, rehabilitation for contractures).

DISPOSITION

- Mortality rate is currently 5% to 10% despite therapeutic measures. Serious sequelae may occur in a further 20%. Complete recovery occurs in >70% of patients. Causes of death include cardiac arrhythmias, myocardial infarction, renal failure secondary to rhabdomyolysis, seizures, pulmonary edema, and bronchopneumonia.
- Factors adversely affecting mortality are development of renal failure and core temperature >104°F (40°C).
- Late neuropsychiatric sequelae.
- Monitor closely for future complications of pharmacologic therapy.

REFERRAL

If patient's condition is critical, patient is preferably treated in a medical/neurologic ICU.

PEARLS & CONSIDERATIONS

COMMENTS

Early detection and diagnosis lead to a more favorable outcome. Treatment is a medical emergency.

EVIDENCE

There is no evidence from randomized controlled trials to guide therapy in neuroleptic malignant syndrome.

SUGGESTED READINGS

Adityanjee, Sajatovic M, Munshi KR: Neuropsychiatric sequelae of neuroleptic malignant syndrome, *Clin Neuropharmacol* 28:197-204, 2005.

Chandran GJ, Mikler JR, Keegan DL: Neuroleptic malignant syndrome: case report and discussion, *CMAJ* 169:439, 2003.

Kipps CM et al: Movement disorder emergencies, *Mov Disord* 20:322-334, 2005.

Sueman VL: Clinical management of neuroleptic malignant syndrome, *Psychiatr Q* 72(4):825, 2001.

Ty EB, Rothner AD: Neuroleptic malignant syndrome in children and adolescents, *J Child Neurol* 16(3):157, 2001.

AUTHORS: **EROBOGHENE E. UBOGU, M.D.,** and **MICHAEL BENATAR, M.B.CH.B., D.PHIL.**

BASIC INFORMATION

DEFINITION

Neuropathic pain is not a disease. It is a symptom, and at most, a syndrome. It may result from multiple illnesses, and it is not enough to define its presence without searching for its cause. It is defined as the sensation derived from the abnormal discharges of impaired or injured neural structures in either the peripheral or central nervous system. Descriptors include:

- Hyperalgesia: extreme sensitivity to painful stimuli, or reduced threshold to feel pain
- Hyperesthesia: abnormal acuteness of sensitivity to touch, pain, or other sensory stimuli
- Allodynia: a nonpainful stimulus is perceived as painful

ICD-9CM CODES
782.0 Numbness, paresthesias
729.1 Myositis/myalgia, not otherwise specified
729.2 Neuralgia, neuritis, or radiculitis, not otherwise specified

SYNONYMS

Neuralgia

EPIDEMIOLOGY & DEMOGRAPHICS

- Neuropathic pain affects at least 1.5% of the U.S. population.
- Demographics vary widely depending on etiology, for example:
  1. Postherpetic neuralgia: affects elderly, and pain seen in almost 100% of cases
  2. AIDS: 33% of patients affected
  3. Diabetes mellitus: 33% affected
  4. Fabry's disease: affects mostly children, pain in almost 90% of patients

PHYSICAL FINDINGS & CLINICAL PRESENATION

History: localize the disease with questions.

- Type of pain: burning, lancinating, shooting, sharp, hot or cold pain, pins and needles, broken glass, stinging, etc., can occur in any part of the body (e.g., V1 to V3 in trigeminal neuralgia).
- Identify if symptoms occur along a nerve distribution (i.e., superficial peroneal nerve) or plexus distribution (acute brachial neuritis or lumbosacral plexus in diabetic amyotrophy).
- Generalized small fiber neuropathy: dysesthesias without numbness common, but many etiologies (e.g., diabetes) cause both small and large fiber dysfunction.
- Large fiber neuropathy: coexisting numbness or weakness can be seen, usually worse distally than proximally.
- Nerve root: coexisting neck or low back pain that radiates along a specific dermatome; most common cause is structural compression.
- Spinal cord symptoms: coexisting spasticity, bowel or bladder involvement, sensory level.
- Past history of stroke in thalamic distribution.
- Family history suggests genetic cause.

Examination: see Table 1-31 and Section III, "Neuropathic Pain."

ETIOLOGY & LABORATORY EVALUATION (Table 1-32)

- Metabolic—diabetes mellitus; porphyria; Fabry's disease; thiamine deficiency, commonly seen in malnutrition and alcoholism; vitamin B_{12} deficiency
- Inflammatory—immune vasculitides (lupus, Sjögren's syndrome, polyarteritis nodosa, etc.), acute inflammatory demyelinating polyneuropathy (also classically presents with ascending weakness or numbness), chronic inflammatory demyelinating polyneuropathy, sarcoid, multiple sclerosis (common cause of trigeminal neuralgia), arachnoiditis
- Infiltrative—amyloidosis, paraproteinemias (e.g., MGUS)
- Infectious—postviral (brachial neuritis), HIV/AIDS, HSV, VZV, Lyme disease, leprosy (thickened nerves and skin lesions), syphilis
- Neoplastic and paraneoplastic—carcinomatous infiltration of nerve/nerve root, anti-Hu
- Drugs/toxins: determined by history—alcohol; chemotherapeutic agents: paclitaxel, vincristine; isoniazid; metronidazole; gold; thallium

DIAGNOSIS (Dx)

LABORATORY TESTS

- Hemoglobin A1c
- 2-hr glucose tolerance test
- Urine and stool protoporphyrins
- Vitamin B_1 level
- Vitamin B_{12} level; if normal, serum methylmalonic acid and homocysteine levels
- Serum ESR, ANA, SS-A and SS-B, c-ANCA, p-ANCA
- Serum ACE level (sarcoid)
- RPR or FTA-ABS
- HIV antibody
- SPEP, UPEP, immunofixation
- Hu antibody: may be positive without evidence of lung cancer, and it can be seen in both small cell and non–small cell lung cancer
- Lumbar puncture: oligoclonal bands, CSF/Serum IgG index, HSV, VZV, Lyme PCR, VDRL

TABLE 1-31 **Examination**

Exam Finding	Localization
Pinprick/temperature loss alone	Small fibers only
Pinprick/temperature loss + vibratory/proprioceptive loss	Small and large fibers
Sensory loss and motor dysfunction worse distally than proximal	Large fiber neuropathy
Sensory loss and motor dysfunction along single nerve distribution	Single nerve
Sensory loss and motor dysfunction along multiple single nerves	Multiple mononeuropathies (i.e., mononeuropathy multiplex)
Motor and sensory loss involving multiple nerves belonging to specific region of brachial or lumbar plexus	Plexopathy
Sensory loss along dermatome with multiple myotomal muscles affected	Nerve root lesion
Asymmetric sensory loss without weakness and pseudoathetosis	Dorsal root ganglion
Vibratory/proprioceptive loss without pinprick/temperature loss	Dorsal column dysfunction (from compressive lesion, B_{12} deficiency, or tabes dorsalis from neurosyphilis)
Sensory level with weakness below the level of lesion and long tract signs (spasticity/Babinski's sign)	Spinal cord lesion
Hemisensory hyperalgesia	Contralateral thalamus

ELECTROPHYSIOLOGY STUDIES

- Electrophysiology (electromyography with nerve conduction studies): normal in exclusively small fiber neuropathy, abnormal in large fiber neuropathy, normal in spinal cord disease
- Quantitative sensory testing: abnormal in small and large fiber neuropathy
- Evoked potentials (only if suspicion for spinal cord lesion)

PATHOLOGY STUDIES

- Nerve biopsy is helpful if there is evidence of large nerve fiber involvement: consider if vasculitis, sarcoid, or amyloid is in differential.
- Intraepidermal nerve fiber density (IENF): preferential diagnostic test for small fiber neuropathy when other studies are normal.
- Rectal mucosa biopsy: preferred study for amyloid deposition.

IMAGING STUDIES

MRI (with and without contrast)

- Of the brain to exclude thalamic pathology if symptoms and signs are consistent with thalamic lesion
- Of the spinal cord and nerve roots to exclude structural, inflammatory, neoplastic, or infectious causes
- Of the lumbar spine to evaluate for arachnoiditis

If MRI is not able to be performed, consider

- CT of the brain for thalamic pathology
- CT myelography of the spinal cord to evaluate for structural/neoplastic disease, but only if clinical signs of spinal or nerve root compromise are present

TREATMENT Rx

NONPHARMACOLOGIC THERAPY

- Counseling: should be initiated at the beginning of therapy to address psychologic issues exacerbating physiologic pain
- Physical therapy: especially in cases of chronic neck and low back pain

ACUTE GENERAL Rx

- Antidepressants:
  1. Tricyclic antidepressants: nortriptyline before amitriptyline (less anticholinergic side effects). Begin 10 mg po qd in elderly, but 25 mg po qd in adults. Can increase by 25 mg every week until usual maximal effective dose of 150 mg/day.

TABLE 1-32 **Clinical Presentation and Laboratory Findings**

Neuropathy Type	Predisposition	Examination Findings	EMG/NCS	Laboratory Analysis
Idiopathic small fiber PN	Age >50	Strength: normal Reflexes: normal Pos/Vib: normal Pain/Temp: decreased distally	Normal	Serum studies: normal Skin biopsy: abnormal Sudomotor studies: abnormal
Diabetic PN	Long-standing disease Family history	Strength normal to reduced, sensation reduced distally	Abnormal	Abnormal glucose tolerance High fasting glucose
Inherited PN	Family history	Pes cavus, hammer toes, reduced reflexes, sensation reduced distally	Abnormal	Genetic studies may be abnormal, other studies normal
Familial amyloid PN	Family history	Pain/temp loss Reduced reflexes Orthostasis	Abnormal if large fibers affected; also carpal tunnel syndrome	Transthyretin genetic study
Acquired amyloid PN	Monoclonal gammopathy	Pain/temp loss Reduced reflexes Orthostasis	Abnormal if large fibers affected; also carpal tunnel syndrome	SPEP, UPEP, immunofixation abnormal
Fabry's disease	Age <20 Renal failure Strokes	Normal; possible reduced pain/temp sensation	Normal	α-galactosidase levels in cultured fibroblasts
PN + mixed connective tissue disease	History of lupus, rheumatoid arthritis, Sjögren's syndrome	Reduced reflexes and distal sensation	Abnormal	ANA, RF, SS-A/SS-B, ANCA may be abnormal
Peripheral nerve vasculitis	Asymmetric disease	Multiple peripheral nerves involved	Abnormal	ANA, RF, SS-A/SS-B, ANCA, cryoglobulins may be abnormal
Paraneoplastic neuropathy	Lung cancer risk factors, chemical exposures	Asymmetric sensory loss, pseudoathetosis, relatively preserved strength	Abnormal	Anti-Hu
Sarcoidosis	Pulmonary sarcoid	Multiple mononeuropathies	Abnormal	Abnormal biopsy, elevated serum ACE, CXR abnormal
Arsenic	Pesticides, copper smelting	Reduced reflexes and distal sensation	Abnormal	Elevated arsenic in plasma, urine, and hair
HIV	Promiscuity, unprotected sex, IV drug abuse, blood transfusion	Variable, but most often reduced reflexes and distal sensation	Abnormal if large fibers involved	HIV antibody

Adapted from Mendell JR, Sahenk Z: Painful sensory neuropathy, *N Engl J Med* 348(13):1243, 2003.
ACE, Angiotensin-converting enzyme; *ANA,* antibody to nuclear antigens; *ANCA,* antineutrophil cytoplasmic antibodies; *CXR,* chest x-ray; *EMG,* electromyography; *HbA1C,* glycosylated hemoglobin; *HIV,* human immunodeficiency virus; *IV,* intravenous; *NCS,* nerve conduction studies; *PN,* polyneuropathy; *Pos,* position sensation; *RF,* rheumatoid factor; *SPEP,* serum protein electrophoresis; *SS-A,* Sjögren syndrome A; *SS-B,* Sjögren syndrome B; *Temp,* temperature sensation; *UPEP,* urine protein electrophoresis; *Vib,* vibration sensation.

2. Paroxetine: begin 10 mg po qd, increase by 10 mg/wk, max dose 60 mg po qd.
3. Duloxetine: begin 30 mg daily, increase to 60 to 120 mg daily, qd or bid.

- Antiepileptics:
  1. Gabapentin: begin 300 mg po qd, advance to 300 mg po tid by the end of the first week. Effective dose: higher than 1600 mg/day. Max dose: 1500 mg po tid.
  2. Carbamazepine: especially for trigeminal neuralgia. Begin 400 mg po bid, increase to tid if necessary. Side effects or drug levels should determine safe increase in dosing. Risk: aplastic anemia.
  3. Oxcarbazepine: better tolerated than carbamazepine. Initiate 150 mg po bid and increase gradually to 600 mg po bid if necessary.
  4. Lamotrigine: begin 25 mg po bid, increase slowly (by 100 mg biweekly) until maximum effective dose of 200 to 300 mg po bid. Risk: Stevens-Johnson syndrome.
  5. Pregabalin: begin 50 mg po tid, increase slowly to 100 to 200 mg po tid.
- Analgesics:
  1. Tramadol: 150 mg/day (50 mg tid), increase by 50 mg/wk, max 200 to 400 mg/day.
  2. Morphine (oral): 15 to 30 mg q8h, max 90 to 360 mg/day.
  3. Oxycodone: 20 mg q12h, increase by 10 mg/wk, max 40 to 160 mg/day.
  4. Fentanyl patch: 25 to 100 mcg transdermally q3 days.
- Topical anesthetics:
  1. 5% lidocaine patch, apply to area of pain, max three patches per 12 hr.
  2. Capsaicin is inconsistent in its ability to relieve pain and may exacerbate it. Use not recommended.

Procedural/Surgical: this option is considered mostly when the patient suffers from pain secondary to spinal cord or cauda equina injury. Studies are limited and benefit is not completely established. Procedures should be considered only when all other therapeutic modalities have failed. In addition, the patient should be cautioned that surgical procedures may not result in pain relief and may be associated with significant morbidity and even mortality.

- Dorsal root rhizotomy
- Nerve blocks
- Spinal cord stimulator

DISPOSITION

Prognosis is dependent on multiple factors including:

- Etiology of pain
- Initiation of multiple therapeutic modalities
- Acceptance by patient of therapeutic modalities
- Initial response to pain management

Most care is accomplished in the outpatient setting, except when surgery is required.

REFERRAL

- Pain clinic
- Psychiatry
- Psychology
- Physiatry
- Anesthesiology (nerve blocks)
- Neurosurgery if considering surgical management

PEARLS & CONSIDERATIONS

Factitious disorder and malingering, frequently manifested by pain complaints, are diagnoses of exclusion and require long-term follow-up and unequivocal proof before diagnosis is made.

EVIDENCE

Multiple placebo-controlled trials have been conducted to study the effects of various classes of medications on neuropathic pain resulting from a variety of diseases. Summarized below are the findings from rigorous analysis of available data reported in the four systematic reviews from the Cochrane Database; findings from additional studies are also listed.

Tricyclic antidepressants at varying doses are effective in reducing neuropathic pain induced by a variety of diseases, with a number needed to treat of two (CI 1.7 to 2.5).[1]

Selective serotonin reuptake inhibitors are potentially useful in treating pain, but should only be tried if tricyclic antidepressants are ineffective.[1]

Gabapentin at varying doses is effective in reducing neuropathic pain from postherpetic neuralgia, diabetic polyneuropathy, Guillain-Barré syndrome, and other diseases.[2]

Carbamazepine at varying doses is probably effective in reducing neuropathic pain from trigeminal neuralgia (NNT 1.8, 95% CI 1.4 to 2.8). NNT could not be calculated for diabetic polyneuropathy.[3]

Valproic acid is ineffective in controlling acute neuropathic pain. Phenytoin is effective in treating diabetic neuropathic pain. Gabapentin may not be superior to carbamazepine in the treatment of neuropathic pain.[4]

A randomized, placebo-controlled trial showed oxcarbazepine 300 to 1800 mg/day is effective in reducing pain from diabetic neuropathy as recorded on a visual analog scale (VAS).[5]

Oral pregabalin at fixed dosages of 300 and 600 mg/day, administered three times daily, was superior to placebo in relieving pain and improving pain-related sleep interference in three randomized, double-blind, multicenter studies in 724 patients with painful diabetic peripheral neuropathy.[6]

Lamotrigine was effective in alleviating HIV-associated neuropathic pain in a randomized, double-blind, placebo-controlled trial.[7]

Duloxetine 60 and 120 mg/day demonstrated greater improvement compared with placebo on the 24-hr Average Pain Score.[8]

Eight intermediate-term trials demonstrated opioid efficacy for neuropathic pain. Pain intensity after opioids was 14 units lower on a scale from 0 to 100 than after placebo (95% confidence interval [CI], −18 to −10; $P < .001$). Side effects were not life threatening.[9]

Evidence-Based References

1. Saarto T, Wiffen P: Antidepressants for neuropathic pain, *Cochrane Database Syst Rev* 3:CD005454, 2005.
2. Wiffen P et al: Gabapentin for acute and chronic pain, *Cochrane Database Syst Rev* 3:CD005452, 2005.
3. Wiffen P, McQuay H, Moore R: Carbamazepine for acute and chronic pain, *Cochrane Database Syst Rev* 3:CD005451, 2005.
4. Wiffen P et al: Anticonvulsant drugs for acute and chronic pain, *Cochrane Database Syst Rev* 3:CD001133, 2005.
5. Dogra S et al: Oxcarbazepine in painful diabetic neuropathy: a randomized, placebo-controlled study, *Eur J Pain* 9(5):543-554, 2005.
6. Frampton JE, Scott LJ: Pregabalin: in the treatment of painful diabetic peripheral neuropathy, *Drugs* 64(24):2813-2820; discussion 2821, 2004.
7. Simpson DM et al.; Lamotrigine HIV Neuropathy Study Team: Lamotrigine for HIV-associated painful sensory neuropathies: a placebo-controlled trial, *Neurology* 60(9):1508-1514, 2003.
8. Goldstein DJ et al: Duloxetine vs. placebo in patients with painful diabetic neuropathy, *Pain* 116(1-2):109-118, 2005.
9. Eisenberg E, McNicol ED, Carr DB: Efficacy and safety of opioid agonists in the treatment of neuropathic pain of nonmalignant origin: systematic review and meta-analysis of randomized controlled trials, *JAMA* 293(24):3043-3052, 2005.

SUGGESTED READING

Mendell JR, Sahenk Z: Painful sensory neuropathy, *N Engl J Med* 348(13):1243, 2003.

AUTHOR: **GREGORY ESPER, M.D.**

BASIC INFORMATION

DEFINITION

Any disorder affecting the peripheral nervous system, including nerve roots, plexuses, and individual peripheral nerves, that has a genetic basis of inheritance and has been or is capable of being transmitted along generations.

There are many different types of hereditary peripheral neuropathies, including Dejerine-Sottas disease, inherited metabolic neuropathies, hereditary sensory and autonomic neuropathies (HSANs), and hereditary motor neuropathies such as spinal muscular atrophy (SMA). Most disorders are diagnosed in infancy or childhood; as such, adult clinicians rarely see these patients. For this reason, this chapter discusses only the hereditary motor and sensory neuropathies that an adult clinician may encounter.

SYNONYMS

Charcot-Marie-Tooth (CMT) disease, a.k.a. hereditary motor-sensory neuropathy (HMSN)

Hereditary neuropathy with liability to pressure-sensitive palsies (HNPP)

ICD-9CM CODES
CMT: 356.1
HNPP: 689

EPIDEMIOLOGY & DEMOGRAPHICS

All CMT: approximately 30 per 100,000
- CMT type 1 (demyelinating pathophysiology): 1 in 2500
- CMT type 2 (axonal pathophysiology): 7 in 1000
- CMT type 4 and CMT-X: rare (either axonal or demyelinating pathophysiology)

HNPP: 2 to 5 per 100,000

PHYSICAL FINDINGS & CLINICAL PRESENATION

CMT: Highly variable
- Age at onset earlier for CMT-1 than CMT-2, but both may present from childhood to old age.
- Severely affected patients have severe distal weakness and muscle atrophy with hand (prominently affecting interossei) and foot deformities (pes cavus, high arched feet, hammer toes).
- Mildly affected patients may have only foot deformity (pes cavus) with little or no weakness/sensory loss.
- Legs can be affected greater than arms, and patients will complain of gait abnormalities (steppage), which cause them to trip and fall.
- Sensory complaints (paresthesias, numbness, dysesthesia) are uncommon despite physical findings of impaired sensation.
- Decreased or absent reflexes.
- Some patients may have postural tremor of the upper limbs.

HNPP (a.k.a. tomaculous neuropathy):
- Age at onset is commonly adolescence.
- Disorder is characterized by recurrent entrapment of peripheral nerves with accompanying signs and symptoms (paresthesias and/or weakness in anatomical distributions). Most common are:
  1. Median nerve at the wrist (carpal tunnel syndrome)
  2. Ulnar nerve at the elbow (cubital tunnel syndrome)
  3. Painless brachial plexopathies
  4. Lateral femoral cutaneous nerve (meralgia paresthetica)
  5. Peroneal nerve at the fibular head
- May be associated with a generalized polyneuropathy.

ETIOLOGY

CMT: more than 30 subgroups have been identified and have various chromosomal abnormalities.
- Most common mutation is PMP-22 duplication, giving rise to CMT 1A demyelinating phenotype.
- Other mutations include P0 (demyelinating) and neurofilament light chain mutations (demyelinating or axonal phenotype)—see the following.
- Updated information available at http://www.neuro.wustl.edu/neuromuscular.

HNPP: deletion of chromosome 17p11.2-12.

DIAGNOSIS

DIFFERENTIAL DIAGNOSIS

CMT: other genetic, metabolic, and multisystem disorders including:
- Spinocerebellar ataxias
- Friedreich's ataxia
- Leukodystrophies
- Refsum's disease (elevated serum phytanic acid)
- Distal spinal muscular atrophies and distal myopathies, which can present with pes cavus and other foot deformities
- Chronic inflammatory demyelinating polyneuropathy (CIDP)

HNPP:
- Hereditary neuralgic amyotrophy (HNA), which typically is painful rather than painless. In addition, in HNA, there is no evidence of generalized polyneuropathy.
- Multifocal motor neuropathy with conduction block (MMNCB)—autoimmune mediated and pure motor
- Neuropathy associated with renal failure
- Lead neuropathy
- Neuropathy relating to paraproteinemia (demyelinating pathophysiology)

EVALUATION

CMT
- History is very important (slow and gradual versus acute).
- Family history with *pedigree* is essential. Consider examination of multiple family members.
- Environmental history should be taken for possible heavy metal exposure.
- History of dysesthesias is uncommon and should prompt search for acquired neuropathy or other inherited neuropathies (e.g., Fabry's disease).

HNPP: genetic testing after identification of multiple entrapment neuropathies on EMG and nerve conduction studies

LABORATORY TESTS

- Neurophysiology: electromyography (EMG) and nerve conduction studies (NCSs) must be done first to determine type of pathophysiology: demyelinating or axonal. This will guide genetic testing.
- NCSs in CMT-1 will reveal demyelinating physiology characterized by very slow conduction velocities (around 15-30 m/s) with prolonged distal latencies. Inherited demyelinating disorders can be distinguished from acquired demyelinating disorders (e.g., chronic inflammatory demyelinating polyneuropathy or CIDP) by the presence of conduction block in the latter.
- In HNPP, diffusely prolonged distal latencies with superimposed entrapment neuropathies at common sites will be seen on NCSs.
- EMG will reveal reinnervation characterized by long-duration, large-amplitude, polyphasic motor unit potentials (MUPs) with decreased MUP recruitment.
- Genetic tests are available for some CMT subtypes:
  1. CMT-1A: chromosome 17p11 PMP-22 duplication
  2. CMT-1B: chromosome 1q22—P0 mutation
  3. CMT-2E: chromosome 8p21—neurofilament light chain (NF-L) point mutation
  4. CMT-X: connexin 32 mutations
  5. HNPP: chromosome 17p11 deletion—which includes the PMP-22 gene
- Serum heavy metals.
- SPEP, UPEP, immunofixation (for paraprotein).
- Anti-GM1 antibody (positive in ~50% of patients with MMNCB).
- Lumbar puncture may reveal elevated CSF protein in CIDP.
- Peripheral nerve biopsy:
  1. Demyelination with onion bulb pathology. Tomaculae, or focal thickening of myelin sheaths, seen in HNPP

2. Generally not indicated secondary to use of electrodiagnostic and DNA testing

IMAGING STUDIES

- Spine plain films: for evaluation of scoliosis.
- MRI: indicated if dissociative sensory loss (dorsal column dysfunction with intact spinothalamic tract function) or if upper motor neuron findings (spasticity, Babinski's sign, clonus, increased tendon reflexes) are present.
- Exclusion of involvement of brain or spinal cord compressive lesions causing arm or leg weakness.
- Some inherited peripheral demyelinating disorders (i.e., CMT-X) are associated with intracerebral white matter abnormalities on MRI.
- Exclusion of structural, infectious, or inflammatory nerve root pathology.

TREATMENT (Rx)

There is no known cure for any of these disorders. Management is supportive.

NONPHARMACOLOGIC THERAPY

- Physical therapy (PT) and occupational therapy (OT) to provide assistance with gait and coordination.
- PT and OT will also provide walking aids including ankle foot orthoses (AFO), canes, walkers, and possibly wheelchairs depending on the severity of the neuropathy.
- Wrist splints for superimposed carpal tunnel syndrome.
- Elbow pads (Heelbo Pads) to cushion the ulnar nerve at the elbow.
- Heel-cord strengthening.
- Stretching exercises.
- Analgesics for pain associated with foot deformity.
- Surgical correction of foot deformities by orthopedic surgeons if indicated.

Vincristine may worsen existing neuropathy. Therefore if patients develop cancer and need to receive chemotherapy, both they and covering physicians should be aware.

SURGICAL TREATMENT

- Patients with HNPP should probably not undergo surgical decompression of the median nerve at the wrist or the ulnar nerve at the elbow; these nerves are sensitive to manipulation. Poor results have been reported with ulnar nerve transposition.
- Anesthesiologists should be aware of HNPP diagnosis in patients undergoing surgery to prevent compression neuropathies from occurring during surgical procedures.

GENETIC COUNSELING

Must be routinely done for patient and family when diagnosis is established. Many aspects of the patient and family's life are affected including:

- Future progeny of patient and/or patient's parents or children
- Psychosocial aspects including social functioning, marriage, employment
- Financial needs
- Medical and life insurability

PROGNOSIS

- CMT—slowly progressive, and patients tend to continue walking until late in life. Life expectancy is normal. Patients with respiratory involvement (i.e., phrenic nerve involvement with diaphragm paresis) may have shorter life expectancy.
- HNPP—benign prognosis.

DISPOSITION

Outpatient care. Routine follow-up appointments should be done initially every 6 mo, and then every 1 to 2 yr.

REFERRAL

- Neurology and/or neuromuscular disease specialist
- Podiatry for recurrent foot problems, including appropriate arches

PEARLS & CONSIDERATIONS (!)

PATIENT/FAMILY EDUCATION

Patients can benefit from use of Muscular Dystrophy Association (MDA) resources.

SUGGESTED READINGS

Chance PF: Genetic evaluation of inherited motor/sensory neuropathy, *Suppl Clin Neurophysiol* 57:228, 2004.

Scott KR, Kothari MJ: Hereditary neuropathies, *Semin Neurol* 25(2):174, 2005.

Washington University Neuromuscular Disease Center: http://www.neuro.wustl.edu/neuromuscular.

AUTHOR: **GREGORY ESPER, M.D.**

BASIC INFORMATION

DEFINITION

Nocardiosis is an infection caused by aerobic actinomycetes found in soil and characterized by lung, soft tissue, or CNS involvement.

SYNONYMS

Mycetoma
Nocardia

ICD-9CM CODES
039 Actinomycotic infections
039.9 Nocardiosis NOS, of unspecified site

EPIDEMIOLOGY & DEMOGRAPHICS

- *Nocardia* species are found worldwide in the soil.
- Nocardiosis is found most commonly in patients who are immune compromised (e.g., receiving steroids, immunosuppressive therapy, lymphoma, leukemia, lung cancer, transplant patient, and other pulmonary infections).
- Other underlying conditions associated with nocardiosis are pemphigus vulgaris, Whipple's disease, Goodpasture's syndrome, Cushing's disease, cirrhosis, ulcerative colitis, and rheumatoid arthritis.
- Use of steroids is an independent risk factor for developing nocardiosis.
- Between 500 to 1000 new cases are diagnosed each year in the United States.
- Approximately 2% of patients with AIDS develop nocardiosis.
- Occurs more commonly in men than in women (2:1).
- Adults > children.

PHYSICAL FINDINGS & CLINICAL PRESENTATION

- Inhalation of *Nocardia* organisms is the most common mode of entry, and pneumonia is the most common presentation, with 75% manifesting with fever, chills, dyspnea, and a productive cough (Fig. 1-174).
  1. Presentation can be acute, subacute, or chronic.
  2. Nocardiosis should be suspected if soft tissue abscesses or CNS tumors or abscesses form in conjunction with the pulmonary infection.
  3. Pulmonary infection may spread into the pericardium, mediastinum, and superior vena cava.
- Cutaneous disease usually occurs via direct inoculation of the organism as a result of skin puncture by a thorn or splinter, surgery, IV catheter use, or animal scratches or bites manifesting in:
  1. Cellulitis
  2. Lymphocutaneous nodules appearing along lymphatic sites draining the infected puncture wound
  3. Mycetoma (Madura foot), a chronic deep nodular infection usually involving the hands or feet that can cause skin breakdown, fistula formation, and spread along the fascial planes to infect surrounding skin, subcutaneous tissue, and bone
- The CNS system is infected in approximately one third of all cases. Brain abscesses is the most common pathologic finding.
- Dissemination of nocardiosis may infect other tissues and organs including kidney, heart, skin, and bone.

ETIOLOGY

- The most common *Nocardia* species leading to infection in humans are:
  1. *N. asteroides* (causing more than 80% of the cases of pulmonary nocardiosis)
  2. *N. brasiliensis* (most common cause of mycetoma)
  3. *N. otitidiscaviarum*
- *N. asteroides* has two subgroups
  1. *N. farcinica*
  2. *N. nova*

DIAGNOSIS

Dx

The diagnosis of nocardiosis requires a high index of suspicion in the proper clinical setting and is confirmed by bacteriologic staining and growth of the organism in culture.

DIFFERENTIAL DIAGNOSIS

There are no pathognomonic findings separating nocardiosis pneumonia from other infectious etiologies of the lung. Diagnoses presenting in a similar manner and often confused for nocardiosis are:

1. Tuberculosis
2. Lung abscess
3. Lung tumor
4. Other causes of pneumonia
5. Actinomycosis
6. Mycosis
7. Cellulitis
8. Coccidioidomycosis
9. Histoplasmosis
10. Aspergillosis
11. Kaposi's sarcoma

WORKUP

All patients with suspected nocardiosis need laboratory identification of the microorganism by obtaining sputum in the case of pneumonia, cultures of the infected skin lesions in mycetoma or lymphocutaneous disease, or the sampling of any purulent material (e.g., brain abscess, lung abscess, and pleural effusion).

LABORATORY TESTS

- Blood tests are not very sensitive in the diagnosis of nocardiosis.
- Gram stain shows gram-positive beaded filaments with multiple branches (Fig. 1-175).
- Gomori methenamine silver staining may detect the organism.
- *Nocardia* species are acid-fast on a modified Ziehl-Neelsen stain.
- *Nocardia* are slow-growing organisms and colony growth in cultures may take up to 2 to 3 wk.

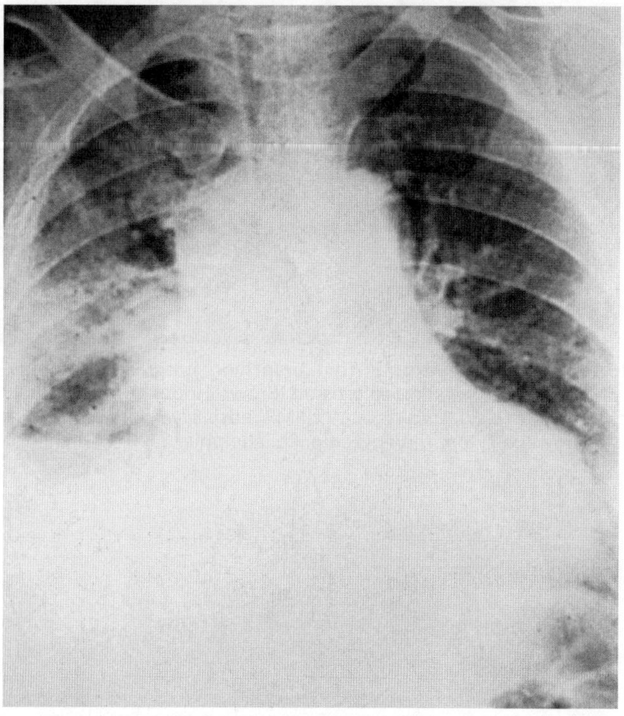

FIGURE 1-174 Right lower lobe *Nocardia* pneumonia in a renal transplant recipient. (From Gorbach SL: *Infectious diseases,* ed 2, Philadelphia, 1998, WB Saunders.)

IMAGING STUDIES

- Chest x-ray may demonstrate infiltrates, densities, nodules, cavitary masses, or multiple abscesses.
- CT scan of the brain is indicated in the appropriate clinical setting to exclude CNS brain abscesses.

TREATMENT

Rx

NONPHARMACOLOGIC THERAPY

- Supportive therapy with oxygen in patients with pneumonia
- Chest physiotherapy
- For any abscess formation, surgical drainage indicated (e.g., skin, lung, or brain)

ACUTE GENERAL Rx

- There are no prospective randomized trials to date highlighting the most effective treatment of nocardiosis. Nevertheless, sulfonamides are considered the treatment of choice. Sulfadiazine 6 to 10 g is given in 4 to 6 divided oral doses.
- For cutaneous infection Trimethoprim-sulfamethoxazole (TMX-SMX) (5 mg/kg/day divided in 2 doses)
- Severe infection—life-threatening pulmonary or disseminated disease, CNS disease, immunocompromised patients—two-drug therapy: TMP-SMX 15 mg/kg/day divided into 4 to 6 doses and amikacin 7.5 mg/kg/IV every 12 hours. In patients with CNS disease, ceftriaxone 2 g/IV daily is substituted for amikacin.
- Sulfonamide-resistant disease: any of the following two-drug regimen: amikacin plus one of the following: ampicillin/sulbactam, imipenem, meropenem, ceftriaxone, or cefotaxime.
- Alternative drug treatment includes:
  1. Imipenem
  2. Third-generation cephalosporin
  3. Minocycline 100 to 200 mg bid
  4. Extended spectrum fluoroquinolones (moxifloxacin)
  5. Linezolid (use of linezolid >4 wks is associated with hematologic toxicity)

CHRONIC Rx

- Although the optimal duration of therapy has not been determined, long-term therapy is generally recommended for all infections caused by *Nocardia.*
- Patients with cellulitis and lymphocutaneous syndrome are treated for 2 to 4 mo depending on whether there is bone involvement or not.
- Mycetomas are best treated with antibiotics for 6 to 12 mo but may require surgical drainage.
- Pulmonary and systemic nocardiosis excluding the CNS is treated for 6 to 12 mo.
- CNS involvement is treated with drainage and antibiotics for 12 mo.
- All immunosuppressed patients should receive 12 mo of antibiotic therapy.

DISPOSITION

- Patients with pulmonary nocardiosis have a mortality rate of 15% to 30%.
- CNS involvement carries a >40% mortality rate.
- Isolated skin lesions have a low mortality rate.

REFERRAL

Whenever the diagnosis of nocardiosis is suspected, consultation with infectious disease is indicated. Pulmonary evaluation and assistance may be needed in pulmonary nocardiosis. Neurosurgery consultation is indicated in patients with single or multiple brain abscesses.

PEARLS & CONSIDERATIONS

!

- Nocardiosis does not spread from animal to animal.
- Nocardiosis is not transmitted from person to person.
- Nocardiosis is distinguished by its ability to disseminate to any organ and its tendency to relapse despite appropriate antibiotic therapy.

COMMENTS

Tuberculosis and nocardiosis may coexist in the same patient.

SUGGESTED READINGS

Chapman S: Diagnosis and treatment of nocardiosis, *UpToDate,* 15.2, 2007. www.uptodateonline.com

Corti ME, Villafane-Fioti MF: Nocardiosis: a review, *Int J Infect Dis* 7(4):243, 2003.

Torres HA et al: Nocardiosis in cancer patients, *Medicine* 81(5):388, 2002.

AUTHOR: **TANYA ALI, M.D.**

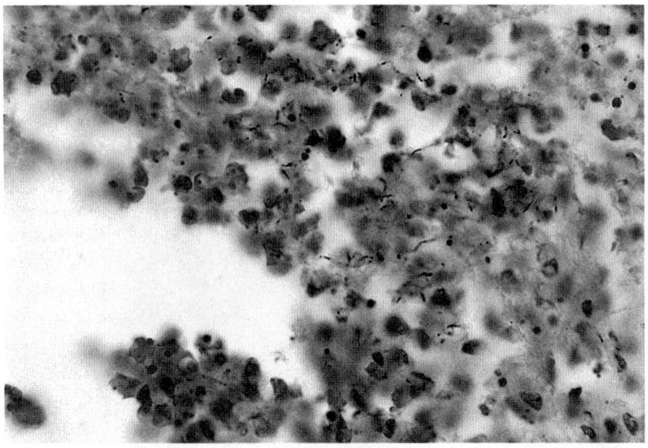

FIGURE 1-175 *Nocardia* pneumonia. Thin, branching, irregularly staining Gram-positive bacilli course through necrotic pulmonary tissue (Brown-Hopps Gram, ×1000). (From Silverberg SG, Delellis RA, Frable WJ, LiVolsi VA, Wick MR [eds]: *Silverberg's principles and practice of surgical pathology and cytopathology,* ed 4, Philadelphia, 2006, Churchill Livingstone.)

BASIC INFORMATION

DEFINITION

Spectrum of diseases based on histiopathologic findings and representing a morphologic rather than a clinical diagnosis. It is liver disease occurring in patients who do not abuse alcohol and manifesting histologically by mononuclear cells and/or polymorphonuclear cells, hepatocyte ballooning, and spotty necrosis.

SYNONYMS

- Nonalcoholic steatohepatitis (NASH)
- NAFLD
- Fatty liver hepatitis
- Diabetes hepatitis
- Alcohol-like liver disease
- Laënnec's disease

ICD-9CM CODES
571.8 Fatty liver

EPIDEMIOLOGY & DEMOGRAPHICS

- Nonalcoholic fatty liver disease (NAFLD) affects 10% to 24% of general population
- Increased prevalence in obese persons (57% to 74%), type 2 diabetes mellitus, and hyperlipidemia (primarily hypertriglyceridemia)
- Most common cause of abnormal liver test results in adults in the U.S. (accounts for up to 90% of cases of asymptomatic ALT elevations)
- 30 million obese adults have steatosis, 8.6 million may have steatohepatitis
- There is a 3:1 female-to-male predominance

PHYSICAL FINDINGS & CLINICAL PRESENTATION

- Most patients are asymptomatic
- Patients may report a sensation of fullness or discomfort on the right side of the upper abdomen
- Nonspecific complaints of fatigue or malaise may be reported
- Hepatomegaly is generally the only positive finding on physical examination
- Acanthosis nigricans may be found in children

ETIOLOGY

- Insulin resistance is the most reproducible factor in the development of nonalcoholic fatty liver disease
- Risk factors are obesity (especially truncal obesity), diabetes mellitus, hyperlipidemia

DIAGNOSIS

DIFFERENTIAL DIAGNOSIS

- Alcohol-induced liver disease (a daily alcohol intake of 20 g in females and 30 g in males [three 12-oz beers or 12 oz of wine] may be enough to cause alcohol-induced liver disease)
- Viral hepatitis
- Autoimmune hepatitis
- Toxin or drug-induced liver disease

WORKUP

Diagnosis is usually suspected on the basis of hepatomegaly, asymptomatic elevations of transaminases, or "fatty liver" on sonogram of abdomen in obese patients with little or no alcohol use. Liver biopsy will confirm diagnosis and provide prognostic information. It should be considered in patients with suspected advanced liver fibrosis (presence of obesity or type 2 diabetes, AST/ALT ratio 1, age 45 yr).

LABORATORY TESTS

- Elevated ALT, AST: AST/ALT ratio is usually <1, but can increase as fibrosis advances
- Negative serology for infectious hepatitis; generally normal GGTP, and serum alkaline phosphatase
- Hyperlipidemia (primarily hypertriglyceridemia) may be present
- Elevated glucose levels may be present
- Prolonged prothrombin time, hypoalbuminuria, and elevated bilirubin may be present in advanced stages
- Elevated serum ferritin and increased transferrin saturation may be found in up to 10% of patients; however, hepatic iron index and hepatic iron level are normal
- Liver biopsy may show a wide spectrum of liver damage, ranging from simple steatosis to advanced fibrosis and cirrhosis

IMAGING STUDIES

- Ultrasound generally reveals diffuse increase in echogenicity as compared with that of the kidneys; CT scan reveals diffuse low-density hepatic parenchyma.
- Occasionally patients may have focal rather than diffuse steatosis, which may be misinterpreted as a liver mass on ultrasound or CT; use of MRI in these cases will identify focal fatty infiltration.

TREATMENT

NONPHARMACOLOGIC THERAPY

- Weight reduction of 55% to 10% in all obese patients (500 g per week in children and 1600 g per week in adults is preferred)
- Increase physical activity

GENERAL Rx

- No medications have been proved to directly improve liver damage from nonalcoholic fatty liver disease.
- Medications to control hyperlipidemia (e.g., fenofibrates for elevated triglycerides) and hyperglycemia (e.g., metformin) can lead to improvement in abnormal liver test results.
- In a recent trial of pioglitazone therapy in NASH it was associated with several favorable histologic and metabolic outcomes.

DISPOSITION

- Patients with pure steatosis on liver biopsy generally have a relatively benign course.
- The presence of steatohepatitis or advanced fibrosis on liver biopsy is associated with a worse prognosis.

REFERRAL

Liver transplantation should be considered in patients with decompensated, end-stage disease; however, in these patients there may be a recurrence of nonalcoholic fatty liver disease post-transplantation.

PEARLS & CONSIDERATIONS

COMMENTS

- Nonalcoholic fatty liver disease is closely associated with metabolic disorders, even in nonobese, nondiabetic subjects. It can be considered an early predictor of metabolic disorders, particularly in the normal-weight population. The presence of metabolic syndrome is a strong predictor of nonalcoholic fatty liver disease.
- A diagnosis of nonalcoholic fatty liver disease is contingent on the following factors:
  1. Alcohol consumption in amounts less than those considered hepatotoxic
  2. Absence of serologic evidence of other hepatic diseases or disorders
  3. Liver biopsy showing predominant macrovesicular steatosis or steatohepatitis

SUGGESTED READINGS

Angulo P: Nonalcoholic fatty liver disease, *N Engl J Med* 346:1221, 2002.

Bayard M et al: Nonalcoholic fatty liver disease, *Am Fam Physician* 73:1961, 2006.

Belfort R et al: A placebo-controlled trial of pioglitazone in subjects with nonalcoholic steatohepatitis, *N Engl J Med* 355:2297, 2006.

Clark JM: Nonalcoholic fatty liver disease, *JAMA* 289:3000, 2003.

Ekstedt M et al: Long-term follow-up of patients with NAFLD and elevated liver enzymes, *Hepatology* 44:865, 2006.

Hamaguchi M et al: The metabolic syndrome as a predictor of nonalcoholic fatty liver disease, *Ann Intern Med* 143:722, 2005.

Kim HJ et al: Metabolic significance of nonalcoholic fatty liver disease in nonobese, nondiabetic adults, *Arch Intern Med* 164:2169, 2004.

AUTHOR: **FRED F. FERRI, M.D.**

BASIC INFORMATION

DEFINITION

Nosocomial infections (NI) are infections acquired as a result of hospitalization, generally after 48 to 72 hr of admission.

SYNONYMS

Hospital-acquired infections

EPIDEMIOLOGY & DEMOGRAPHICS

INCIDENCE (IN U.S.):

- Develop in at least 5% of hospitalized patients
- In 2002 these nosocomial infections accounted for more than 98,000 deaths

In 2002 the annual cost of nosocomial infections was estimated as >$5 to 10 billion to health care in the U.S.

PREVALENCE (IN U.S.): 2 to 4 million cases/yr

PREDOMINANT SEX:

- Overall, approximately equal
- Elderly women: predominantly nosocomial urinary tract infections

PREDOMINANT AGE: Elderly patients (>60 yr old) at highest risk

RISK FACTORS: Patients with the following conditions may develop NI at any age.

1. ICU
2. Intubation
3. Chronic lung disease
4. Renal disease
5. Comatose
6. Chronic urethral or vascular catheterization
7. Malnutrition
8. Postoperative state

PEAK INCIDENCE: Varies widely with infection site

PHYSICAL FINDINGS & CLINICAL PRESENTATION

Vary with specific NI

ETIOLOGY

- Bacteria
- Fungi
- Viruses

SOURCES AND MODES OF TRANSMISSION:

1. Patient's own flora
   a. Comprises resistant organisms acquired during hospitalization
   b. Frequently maintained thereafter by persistent GI colonization
2. Unwashed hands of staff
   a. Physicians
   b. Nurses
3. Invasion of protective defenses (intact skin, respiratory cilia, urinary sphincters, and mucosa)
   a. IV lines
   b. Catheters
   c. Respiratory equipment
   d. Surgical wounds
   e. Scopes and other imaging devices
4. Failure to provide adequate negative pressure, high-volume air flow chambers for respiratory isolation of patients with TB
5. Failure to rapidly identify and provide appropriate care (with isolation or precautions) for patients with communicable diseases
6. Inanimate environment
7. Food
8. Fomites

RISKS AMPLIFIED:

1. Use of broad-spectrum antibiotics
   a. Select highly resistant bacteria
   b. Establish highly resistant bacteria as endemic flora in microenvironments within the hospital
2. Highly vulnerable patients with specific risk factors
   a. Immunosuppression (as a result of therapy, transplantation, AIDS)
   b. Old age
   c. Postsurgery
   d. Prolonged surgery
   e. Chronic lung disease
   f. Ventilator dependence
   g. Antacid therapy
   h. Vascular lines
   i. Hyperalimentation
   j. ICU stay
   k. Recent antibiotic therapy
3. Clustering of seriously ill patients
   a. Often with wounds or drainage of contaminated materials
   b. Intensifying probability of cross-infection

HANDWASHING BETWEEN ALL PATIENT CONTACTS: Single most important method of decreasing NI

1. Regular soap and water for at least 15 seconds
2. Chlorhexidine for methicillin-resistant *Staphylococcus aureus* (MRSA) and other resistant Gram-positive organisms
3. Iodophor for resistant Gram-negative organisms
4. Purpose
   a. Degrease hand surfaces
   b. Wash away oils and associated bacteria
5. Procedure
   a. Lukewarm water
   b. Must include all surfaces
   c. Special attention to areas between fingers and to the dirtier dominant hand (most people reflexively wash their cleaner, nondominant hand more vigorously)
6. The widespread availability of alcohol-based hand hygiene solutions throughout hospital settings has been shown to improve hand-washing frequency (less drying to hands, faster, and no need for wash basin and towels for drying) and to significantly reduce nosocomial infections in hospitals that have adopted this hand-washing technique. It is now recommended in essentially all routine health care settings

VANCOMYCIN-RESISTANT *ENTEROCOCCUS FAECIUM* (VREF):

1. The percentage of nosocomial infections caused by VREF increased more than twentyfold between 1989 and 1993, rising from 0% to 3% to 7% to 9%. By 2005, VREF, vancomycin-resistant *E. faecalis,* and other vancomycin-resistant species of enterococci had become common and endemic nosocomial pathogens accounting for 15% to 40% of all enterococci isolated in the hospital setting.
2. A high percentage of VREF isolated, 80% are also ampicillin resistant.
3. Factors predisposing to VREF colonization or infection include percentage of hospital days receiving antimicrobial therapy, use of IV, underlying disease, immunosuppression, and abdominal surgery.
4. Evidence suggests that vehicle is the hands of medical personnel.
5. Control measures
   a. Aggressive isolation of colonized and infected patients
   b. Restraint in using broad-spectrum antibiotics

CLOSTRIDIUM DIFFICILE:

1. Causes diarrhea as a result of pseudomembranous colitis
2. May be transmitted among hospitalized patients
3. Warrants stool (contact) precautions
4. Alcohol-based hand gels may not eliminate spores of this organism

SURVEILLANCE:

1. Crucial for early identification of infections
   a. Enabling immediate intervention
   b. Education
2. Prospective, concurrent, total hospital surveillance
   a. Provides most complete data
   b. Feasible with sophisticated computerized data collection and analysis
3. Daily plotting of all infections on comprehensive wall maps
   a. Including all beds on all wards
   b. Enhances early recognition of microclusters of infections by body site and by organism
   c. Facilitates proper early control of potential outbreaks

DIAGNOSIS

MOST COMMON NOSOCOMIAL INFECTIONS:

- Urinary tract infections (40% to 45%)
- Surgical wound and other soft tissue infections (25% to 30%)
- Pneumonia (15% to 20%)
- Bacteremia (5% to 12%)

NOSOCOMIAL URINARY TRACT INFECTIONS:

- General associations:
  1. Foley catheters
  2. Inappropriate catheter care (including opening catheter junctions)

3. Female sex
4. Absence of systemic antibiotics
- Physical findings:
1. Fever
2. Dysuria
3. Leukocytosis
4. Pyuria
5. Flank or costovertebral angle tenderness
- Usual organisms:
1. *E. coli*
2. *Klebsiella*
3. *Enterobacter*
4. *Pseudomonas*
5. *Enterococcus*
- Sepsis in 1% to 3% of nosocomial UTIs
- Prevention:
1. Meticulous technique during insertion and daily perineal care
2. Never open the catheter-collection tubing junction
3. Obtain all specimens using sterile syringe
4. Substitute intermittent catheterization for Foley catheters

NOSOCOMIAL BACTEREMIAS:
- General associations:
1. IV lines
2. Arterial lines
3. CVP lines
4. Phlebitis
5. Hyperalimentation
- Fever possibly only presenting sign
- Exit site of all vascular lines carefully evaluated for:
1. Erythema
2. Induration
3. Tenderness
4. Purulent drainage
- Usual organism for device-associated bacteremia
1. *S. aureus* (including MRSA)
2. *Staphylococcus epidermidis* for long-term IV lines
3. *Enterobacter*
4. *Klebsiella*
5. *Candida* spp.
6. *Pseudomonas aeruginosa* may come from a water source or reflect cutaneous bacteria
- Phlebitis in 1.3 million patients yearly
- Approximately 10,000 annual deaths from IV sepsis
- Prevention:
1. Meticulous sterile technique during IV insertion
2. Emphasis should be placed on attention to detail, including handwashing, adherence to guidelines for catheter insertion and maintenance, appropriate use of antiseptic solutions such as chlorhexidine or iodine to prepare the skin around the catheter insertion site, and use of sterile technique for central catheter insertion
3. Modified catheter may reduce risk for endoluminal colonization and catheter-related sepsis in subclavian lines
4. Decrease use of routine IVs (patients would rather drink)

NOSOCOMIAL PNEUMONIAS:
- More common in ICUs
- General associations:
1. Aspiration
2. Intubation
3. Altered consciousness
4. Old age
5. Chronic lung disease
6. Postsurgery
7. Antacids
- Signs of pneumonia common among patients on general wards:
1. Cough
2. Sputum
3. Fever
4. Leukocytosis
5. New infiltrate on chest x-ray examination
- Signs more subtle in ICUs, because many patients have purulent sputum because of chronic intubation
1. Change in sputum character or volume
2. Small changes on chest x-ray examination
- Usual organisms:
1. *Klebsiella*
2. *Acinetobacter*
3. *Enterobacter*
4. *Pseudomonas aeruginosa*
5. *S. aureus* (including MRSA)
- Less common organisms:
1. *Stenotrophomonas* spp.
2. *Legionella, Flavobacterium*
3. Respiratory syncytial virus (infants)
4. Adenovirus
- 1% of hospitalized patients affected
- Mortality rate high (40%)
- Prevention:
1. Meticulous sterile technique during suctioning and handling airway
2. Do not routinely change ventilator breathing circuits and components more frequently than q48h
3. Drain respirator tubing without allowing fluid to return to respirator
4. Handwashing routinely to prevent colonization of patients and transfer of organisms among patients

NOSOCOMIAL SOFT TISSUE INFECTIONS:
- Associations:
1. Decubitus ulcers
2. Surgical wound classification (contaminated or dirty-infected)
3. Abdominal surgery
4. Presence of drain
5. Preoperative length of stay
6. Duration of surgery >2 hr
7. Surgeon
8. Presence of other infection
- Physical findings:
1. Decubitus ulcer with fluctuance at margin or under firm eschar
2. Erythema extending >2 cm beyond margin of surgical wound
3. Tenderness
4. Induration
5. Erythema
6. Fluctuance
7. Purulent drainage
8. Dehiscence of sutures
- Usual organisms:
1. *S. aureus* (including MRSA)
2. *Enterococcus*
3. *Enterobacter*
4. *Acinetobacter*
5. *E. coli*
- Prevention:
1. Careful skin care and frequent, proper positioning of patient to prevent decubitus ulcer
2. Meticulous sterile surgical technique
3. Handwashing to decrease colonization when handling postoperative wound
4. Limit prophylactic antibiotics to 24 hr perioperatively
5. Double-wrap contaminated dressings (hold in gloved hand and evert gloves over dressings) before disposal

LABORATORY TESTS

- Appropriate to specific NI and specific patient's condition
- Cultures generally indicated for proper confirmation of responsible pathogens
1. Urine
2. Blood
3. Sputum
4. Soft tissue infection
- Molecular analysis of nosocomial epidemics
1. Plasmid fingerprinting
2. Restriction endonuclease digestion (plasmid and genomic DNA)
3. Peptide analysis by SDS-PAGE
4. Immunoblotting
5. Ribosomal (rRNA) typing
6. DNA probes
7. Multilocus enzyme electrophoresis
8. Restriction fragment length polymorphism (RFLP)
9. Polymerase chain reaction (PCR)
10. Provide confirmation of point-source or common strains and corroboration of hypotheses reached utilizing classic epidemiology

IMAGING STUDIES

Rarely needed for diagnosis of NI

TREATMENT

Rx

ACUTE GENERAL Rx

- Appropriate to etiologic organism:
1. Antibiotic
2. Antifungal
3. Antiviral
- Specific therapy determined after careful consideration of resident flora

within the microenvironment in which the patient was hospitalized
1. Empiric therapy
   a. Frequently difficult to fashion accurately
   b. Often undesirable, unless the patient's clinical condition requires urgent treatment
2. Consultation for expert advice regarding antibiotic selection in view of known epidemiologic risks within the hospital
   a. Nosocomial infection control nurses
   b. Hospital epidemiologist

- Avoid unnecessary treatment for organisms that are colonizing but not infecting patients
- Prevention of spread of communicable diseases often requiring Isolation or Precautions
  1. Classic Schema (Strict, Respiratory Isolation and Contact [Skin and Wound] Precautions) being replaced by more streamlined Revised Guidelines (Airborne, Droplet, Contact Isolation Precautions)
  2. Less careful response to some diseases (e.g., hemorrhagic fevers) inadvertently induced by removal of strict isolation category
  3. Universal/Standard Precautions and Body Substance Isolation continue within a new Standard Isolation Precautions Guideline
- Universal Precautions used for all patients during all contacts with blood, body fluids, or secretions
  1. Gloves
  2. Goggles
  3. Impermeable gowns if aerosol or splash is likely
- Consider aggressive isolation to restrict spread of resistant organisms and their plasmids
  1. MRSA
  2. VREF
  3. Highly resistant Gram-negative organisms, including ESBL (extended sprectrum β-lactamases) Gram-negative rods

DISPOSITION

The infection control service and/or hospital epidemiologist should be notified when infectious complications occur in hospital setting; most, but not all, nosocomial infections are potentially avoidable, and every effort should be taken to minimize the risk of infections associated with health care.

REFERRAL

- To nosocomial infection control nurses
- To hospital epidemiologist

PEARLS & CONSIDERATIONS

COMMENTS

- Sharps and splash injuries to staff relatively are rare, but nearly all are preventable.
  1. Nurses incur most injuries.
  2. Usual causes:
     a. Needle sticks
     b. Scalpel and surgical needle injuries
     c. Blood splashes
  3. Prevention:
     a. Never recap needles
     b. Needle disposal only in rigid, impermeable plastic containers
     c. Clearly announce instrument passes in operating room or during procedures and use passing trays
     d. Use needleless systems for vascular access and connectors whenever possible to limit health care workers' use of sharp medical devices
     e. Gloves, masks, and goggles if aerosol or splash is likely
     f. Never leave needles or other sharp items in beds
     g. Never dispose of sharp items in regular trash bags
  4. Infection control staff should be consulted immediately after exposure to determine need for prophylaxis for hepatitis B or HIV.
  5. All staff should be immune to hepatitis B (natural or vaccine).
- Fungi previously considered to be contaminants now risks for patients with cancer and organ transplantation
  1. *Candida* spp.
     a. *C. guilliermondii*
     b. *C. krusei*
     c. *C. parapsilosis*
     d. *C. tropicalis*
  2. *Aspergillus* spp.
  3. *Curvularia* spp.
  4. *Bipolaris* spp.
  5. *Exserohilum* spp.
  6. *Alternaria* spp.
  7. *Fusarium* spp.
  8. *Scopulariopsis* spp.
  9. *Pseudallescheria boydii*
  10. *Trichosporon beigelii*
  11. *Malassezia furfur*
  12. *Hansenula* spp.
  13. *Microsporum canis*
- Focused, committed efforts by the entire health care staff continuously directed toward prevention
  1. Each NI addressed as an opportunity to improve the organization and delivery of care
  2. Essential that individual staff members understand that small risks applied to large populations result in a large number of total events (i.e., NI)

SUGGESTED READINGS

Brossette SE et al: A laboratory-based, hospital-wider, electronic marker for nosocomial infection: the future of infection control surveillance? *Am J Clin Pathol* 125(1):34, 2006.

Eriksen HM, Iversen BG, Aavitsland P: Prevalence of nosocomial infections and use of antibiotics in long-term care facilities in Norway, 2002 and 2003, *J Hosp Infect* 57(4):316, 2004.

Gastmeier P: Nosocomial infection surveillance and control policies, *Curr Opin Infect Dis* 17(4):295, 2004.

Merle V et al: Knowledge and opinions of surgical patients regarding nosocomial infections, *J Hosp Infect* 60(2):169, 2005.

Won SP et al: Handwashing program for the prevention of nosocomial infections in a neonatal intensive care unit, *Infect Control Hosp Epidemiol* 25(9):742, 2004.

AUTHORS: **GLENN G. FORT, M.D., M.P.H., DENNIS J. MIKOLICH, M.D.,** and **ZEENA LOBO, M.D.**

BASIC INFORMATION

DEFINITION

Obesity refers to having an excess amount of body fat in relation to lean body mass, or a body mass index (BMI) of ≥30 kg/m². Overweight is defined as BMI of 25 to 29.9 kg/m². These conditions result from a problem of imbalance between energy intake and expenditure.

SYNONYMS

Overweight

ICD-9CM CODES
278.0 Obesity

EPIDEMIOLOGY & DEMOGRAPHICS

- The Behavioral Risk Factor Surveillance System (BRFSS) of the Centers for Disease Control and Prevention (CDC) has suggested that during the past 20 years there has been a dramatic increase in obesity in the U.S.
- In 1990, four states in the U.S. had obesity prevalence rates of 15% to 19%, and no states had rates of 20% or more. By 2005, all but four states had obesity prevalence rates of 20% or more.
- The prevalence of obesity has increased from 23% to 31% over the recent past in the U.S, and 66% of adults are overweight.
- Approximately 33% of all U.S. women and 28% of all U.S. men are obese.
- The prevalence of overweight and obesity increases with advancing age until the sixth decade, after which it begins to decline.
- The Third National Health and Nutrition Examination Survey (NHANES III) estimated that 13.7% of children and 11.5% of adolescents are overweight.
- The present costs of obesity in the U.S. population are estimated to run at 5% to 8% of total health care spending, which equates to $92.6 to $99.2 billion annually.
- For persons with a BMI of ≥30 kg/m², all-cause mortality is increased by 50% to 100% above that of persons with BMI in the range of 20 to 25 kg/m².
- Obese individuals are at increased risk of morbidity/mortality from type 2 diabetes, hypertension, coronary artery disease (CAD), cancer (particularly colon, prostate, and breast cancer), sleep apnea, degenerative joint disease, thromboembolic disorders, digestive tract diseases (gallstones), and dermatologic disorders.
- The effects of obesity on health outcome appear to be reversible with weight loss.

PHYSICAL FINDINGS & CLINICAL PRESENTATION

- Physical examination should assess the degree and distribution of body fat and signs of secondary causes of obesity.
- Increased waist circumference is apparent. Excess abdominal fat is clinically defined as a waist circumference >40 inches (>102 cm) in men and >35 inches (>88 cm) in women.
- Symptoms associated with hypertension, CAD, and diabetes (e.g., polyuria, polydipsia, retinopathy, and neuropathy) may be present.
- Joint pain and swelling are associated with degenerative joint disease and obesity.

ETIOLOGY

- The cause of obesity is multifactorial, involving social, nutritional, physiological, psychological, environmental, and genetic factors.
- Environmental factors such as a sedentary lifestyle and the chronic ingestion of excess calories can cause obesity in some cases.
- Most human obesity may be related to genetic factors. It is thought that obesity may be polygenic. Genetic studies with adopted children have demonstrated that they have similar BMIs to their biologic parents, but not to their adoptive parents. Twin studies also demonstrate a genetic influence on BMI.
- Current data also suggest that obesity may spread in social networks in a quantifiable and discernable pattern that depends on the nature of social ties. Moreover, social distance appears to be more important than geographic distance within these networks.

DIAGNOSIS

- BMI will help to establish the diagnosis of obesity. BMI is a measure of an adult's weight in relationship to his or her weight: more specifically, the adult's weight in kilograms divided by the square of his or her height.
- BMI values can categorize patients into three classes of obesity:

Class I (mild)	BMI = 30.0 to 34.9 kg/m²
Class II (moderate)	BMI = 35.0 to 39.9 kg/m²
Class III (severe)	BMI ≥ 40 kg/m²

- Although BMI is commonly used to define obesity, it is not a very accurate indicator of body fat composition in children, who are undergoing rapid changes in height, or in bodybuilders or athletes who have large amounts of muscle tissue.
- Measure waist circumference because the health risks of overweight and obesity are independently associated with excess abdominal fat.

DIFFERENTIAL DIAGNOSIS

It is important to rule out specific causative medical disorders in obese patients. Metabolic syndrome, hypothalamic disorders, hypothyroidism, Cushing's syndrome, insulinoma, depression, diabetes mellitus, drugs (corticosteroids, antidepressants, antipsychotics, antihistamine agents, antihypertensive agents, and HIV protease inhibitors) can cause obesity.

WORKUP

History should be obtained regarding weight change, family history of obesity, social circles, and eating and exercise behavior. Assessment for eating disorders and depression should be made. Attention should be directed to the use of nutritional supplements, over-the-counter medications, hormones, diuretics, and laxatives. The workup of an obese patient typically requires laboratory work to assess for risks and complications as well as to rule out underlying causative medical conditions.

LABORATORY TESTS

- Obese patients should be assessed for medical consequences of their obesity by screening for metabolic syndrome (measure high density lipoprotein [HDL], triglycerides, blood pressure, fasting glucose, and waist circumference).
- In the proper clinical setting, thyroid function studies, dexamethasone suppression testing, A.M. cortisol level, and insulin level with C-peptide measurements will exclude hypothyroidism, Cushing's syndrome, and insulinoma as underlying causes of obesity.

IMAGING STUDIES

- Several methods are available for determining or calculating total body fat but offer no significant advantage over the BMI. These include measurement of total body water, total body potassium, bioelectrical impedance, and dual-energy x-ray absorptiometry.
- Buoyancy testing is an accurate method for determining total body fat composition.

TREATMENT

- The National Heart, Lung, and Blood Institute (NHLBI) has developed guidelines for selecting treatment strategies for overweight and obese patients based on BMI and comorbidities. They recommend a combination

of dietary management, physical activity management, and behavior therapy for any patient with a BMI ≥30 and for those with a BMI between 25 and 29.9 with comorbidities. Pharmacotherapy should be considered for patients with a BMI between 27 and 29.9 with comorbidities and for any patient with a BMI ≥30.
- Surgery is indicated for patients with a BMI between 35 and 39.9 with comorbidities and for any patient with a BMI ≥40.

NONPHARMACOLOGIC THERAPY

- The major principle of dietary management for weight loss is calorie reduction.
- The NHLBI guidelines recommend an initial diet to produce a calorie deficit of 500-1000 kcal/day. This has been shown to reduce total body weight by an average of 8% over 3 to 12 months.
- These guidelines recommend the use of a food diary to focus on dietary substitutes.
- Thirty minutes of moderate intensity activity on 5 or more days of the week results in health benefits for obese individuals. Today several studies also indicate that 60 to 80 minutes of moderate to vigorous physical activity can be more beneficial.
- Behavioral therapy is also necessary.

ACUTE GENERAL Rx

- According to the NHLBI *Guidelines on the Identification, Evaluation, and Treatment of Overweight and Obesity in Adults* and the U.S. Food and Drug Administration (FDA), pharmacotherapy is indicated for:
  - Obese patients with a BMI ≥30 *or*
  - Overweight patients with a BMI of ≥27 and concomitant obesity related risk factors or diseases, such as hypertension, diabetes, or dyslipidemia
- There are three general classes of medications currently approved by the FDA for treating obesity:
  1. Sympathomimetic medications approved for long-term use
  2. Gastrointestinal (GI) lipase inhibitors
  3. Sympathomimetic medications approved for short-term use
- Sibutramine (Meridia) acts as a serotonin norepinephrine reuptake inhibitor (SNRI) and suppresses appetite primarily by increasing satiation.
- Orlistat (Xenical) blocks the digestion and absorption of ingested dietary fat. It is a reversible inhibitor of pancreatic, gastric, and carboxylester lipases and phospholipase A2, which are required for the hydrolysis of dietary fat in the gastrointestinal tract.
- Phentermine is an amphetamine derivative that increases the amount of norepinephrine (NE) in the neuronal cleft, resulting in appetite suppression. Similar drugs include diethylpropion, benzphetamine, and phendimetrazine.
- In 1997 both dexfenfluramine and fenfluramine were withdrawn from the market secondary to side effects of valvular heart lesions and pulmonary hypertension.
- Other medications in clinical trials include bupropion (Wellbutrin), topiramate (Topamax), and metformin (Glucophage).

CHRONIC Rx

- According to the NHLBI guidelines surgical intervention is an option for selected patients with clinically severe obesity (a BMI ≥ 40 or a BMI ≥ 35 with co-morbid conditions), when patients are at high risk for obesity-associated morbidity or mortality and when less invasive methods of weight loss have failed.
- Bariatric surgery for weight loss falls into one of two categories:
  1. Restrictive surgeries that limit the amount of food the stomach can hold and slow the rate of gastric emptying. These include vertical banded gastroplasty and laparoscopic adjustable silicone gastric banding.
  2. Restrictive malabsorptive bypass procedures combine the elements of gastric restriction and selective malabsorption. These include Roux-en-Y gastric bypass and biliopancreatic diversion.

DISPOSITION

- Obesity increases the risk of developing hypertension, hyperlipidemia, type 2 diabetes, coronary artery disease, cerebrovascular disease, degenerative joint disease, digestive tract disease, sleep apnea, and endometrial, breast, prostate, and colon cancers.
- Obesity accelerates the progression of coronary atherosclerosis.
- All-cause mortality is increased in obese patients as increased body fat corresponds to increased health risks.

REFERRAL

Obesity is commonly seen in the primary care setting. If pharmacologic therapy is considered, consultation with physicians specializing in obesity and experienced with the use of the drug is recommended. In addition, consultation with nutritionists and behavioral therapists is also helpful. A consultation with general surgery is indicated in patients being considered for surgical intervention.

PEARLS & CONSIDERATIONS

COMMENTS

- The National Heart, Lung, and Blood Institute (NHLBI) of the National Institutes of Health (NIH) launched the Obesity Education Initiative (OEI) in January 1991. The overall purpose of the initiative is to help reduce the prevalence of overweight along with the prevalence of physical inactivity in order to reduce the risk of coronary heart disease (CHD) and overall morbidity and mortality from CHD.
- The American Medical Association produced, with support from the Robert Wood Johnson Foundation, and developed, in collaboration with the U.S. Department of Health and Human Services, a primer for the assessment and management of adult obesity. The primer consists of 10 booklets that offer practical recommendations for addressing adult obesity in the primary care setting.

PREVENTION

- Prevention of overweight and obesity involves both increasing physical activity and dietary modification to reduce caloric intake.
- Clinicians can help guide patients to develop personalized eating plans and help them to recognize the contributions of fat, concentrated carbohydrates, and large portion sizes.
- Clinicians must work with patients to modify other risk factors such as tobacco use, high glycemic intake, and elevated blood pressure in order to prevent the long-term chronic disease sequelae of obesity.
- Regular screening of body weight and BMI measurements at routine office visits can help to identify early weight gain.

PATIENT/FAMILY EDUCATION

Information can be obtained on the American Obesity Association website (http://www.obesity.org) and the American Medical Association website (http://www.ama-assn.org).

EVIDENCE

EBM

The prevalence of obesity has increased from 23% to 31% over the last 20 years in the United States, and 66% of adults are overweight.[1,2] Ⓐ

Proposed explanations for the obesity epidemic include societal changes that promote both inactivity and food consumption, [3] as well as genetic factors.[4,5] Ⓑ

Network phenomena appear to be relevant to the biologic and behavioral trait of obesity, and obesity appears to spread through social ties.[6] Ⓐ

Health care professionals should be concerned about overweight and obesity because of the well-established relations between excess body weight and such medical conditions as type 2 diabetes, hypertension, and osteoarthritis.[7] Ⓐ

Evidence-based guidelines issued by the National Institutes of Health call for weight loss both in obese persons and in overweight persons with two or more risk factors for obesity-related diseases.[8] Ⓐ

In regard to pharmacologic therapy, there is evidence that Orlistat is modestly effective in promoting weight loss in obese people.[9,10] Ⓑ

There is evidence that sibutramine is modestly effective at promoting weight loss in obese people, and doses of 10 to 20 mg daily results in greater weight loss than placebo after 8 weeks and after 6 months.[11] Ⓑ

A systematic review found evidence that gastric surgery results in good weight loss in very obese patients in whom all other remedies have failed, with surgical patients losing 23 to 28 kg more weight on average than nonsurgical patients after 2 years. One study with 8 years' follow-up found that surgical patients had lost an average of 21 kg, whereas nonsurgical patients had gained weight.[12] Ⓑ

Evidence-Based References

1. Chang VW, Lauderdale DS: Income disparities in body mass index and obesity in the United States, 1971-2002, *Arch Intern Med* 165:2122-2128, 2005.
2. Hedley AA et al: Prevalence of overweight and obesity among US children, adolescents, and adults, 1999-2002, *JAMA* 291:2847-2850, 2004.
3. Hill JO et al: Environmental contributions to the obesity epidemic, *Science* 280:1371-1374, 1998.
4. Stunkard AJ et al: An adoption study of human obesity, *N Engl J Med* 314:193-198, 1986.
5. Stunkard AJ et al: The body-mass index of twins who have been reared apart, *N Engl J Med* 322:1483-1487, 1990.
6. Christakis NA, Fowler, JH: The spread of obesity over a large social network over 32 years, *N Engl J Med* 357:370-379, 2007.
7. National Task Force on the Prevention and Treatment of Obesity: Overweight, obesity, and health risk, *Arch Intern Med* 160:898-904, 2000.
8. Clinical guidelines on the identification, evaluation, and treatment of overweight and obesity in adults—the evidence report, *Obes Res* 6(Suppl 2):51S-209S, 1998.
9. O'Meara S et al: A rapid and systematic review of the clinical effectiveness and cost-effectiveness of orlistat in the management of obesity, *Health Technol Assess* 5:1, 2001. Reviewed in: *Clin Evid* 10:676, 2004.
10. Hill JO et al: Orlistat, a lipase inhibitor, for weight maintenance after conventional dieting: a 1-year study, *Am J Clin Nutr* 69:1108, 1999. Reviewed in: *Clin Evid* 10:676, 2004.
11. University of York, NHS Centre for Reviews and Dissemination: A systematic review of the clinical effectiveness of sibutramine and orlistat in the management of obesity, York, UK, 2000, NHS Centre for Reviews and Dissemination. Reviewed in: *Clin Evid* 10:676, 2004.
12. Colquitt J et al: Surgery for morbid obesity (Cochrane Review). Reviewed in: Cochrane Library 1, Chichester, UK, 2004, John Wiley.

SUGGESTED READINGS

Chang VW, Lauderdale DS: Income disparities in body mass index and obesity in the United States, 1971-2002, *Arch Intern Med* 165:2122-2128, 2005.

Li Z et al: Meta-analysis: pharmacologic treatment of obesity, *Ann Intern Med* 142:532, 2005.

Maggard MA et al: Meta-analysis: surgical treatment of obesity, *Ann Intern Med* 142:547, 2005.

Ogden, CL, Carroll, MD, Curtin, LR, et al: Prevalence of overweight and obesity in the United States, 1999-2004, *JAMA* 295:1549, 2006.

Snow V et al: Pharmacologic and surgical management of obesity in primary care: a clinical practice guideline from the American College of Physicians, *Ann Intern Med* 142:525, 2005.

Speakman JR: Obesity: the integrated roles of environment and genetics, *J Nutr* 134:2090S, 2004.

AUTHOR: **PRANAV M. PATEL, M.D.**

BASIC INFORMATION

DEFINITION

Obsessive-compulsive disorder (OCD) involves recurrent obsessions (intrusive and inappropriate thoughts, impulses, or images) and/or compulsions (behaviors or mental acts performed in response to obsessions or rigid application of rules) that consume >1 hr/day or cause marked impairment or distress. The symptoms are perceived as excessive and unreasonable.

SYNONYMS

Compulsive hoarding, washing, list-making

Intrusive thoughts with ritualized and repetitive behaviors

ICD-9CM CODES
F42.8 Obsessive-compulsive disorder (DSM-IV 300.3)

EPIDEMIOLOGY & DEMOGRAPHICS

PEAK INCIDENCE: Mean age at onset is 19.6 yr.

LIFETIME PREVALENCE (IN U.S.): 2.5% of adults

PREDOMINANT SEX: Approximately equal distribution between sexes.

PREDOMINANT AGE:
- Modal age of onset for females is between 20 and 29 yr.
- Modal age of onset for males is between 6 and 15 yr.

DISEASE COURSE:
- Condition is chronic with waxing and waning.
- Symptoms typically worsen with stress.
- 15% show progressive deterioration while 5% show an episodic course with little impairment between episodes.

GENETICS:
- There is no clear genetic pattern.
- Rate of concordance is higher in monozygotic (33%) vs. dizygotic (7%) twins.
- Rate of disorder is also higher in first-degree relatives of individuals with OCD and Tourette's disorder than the general population.

PHYSICAL FINDINGS & CLINICAL PRESENTATION

- Persistent and recurrent intrusive and ego-dystonic obsessive ideas, thoughts, impulses, or images that are perceived as alien and beyond one's control.
- Frequent experiencing of obsessions related to contamination (e.g., when using the telephone), excessive doubt (e.g., was the door locked?), organization (the need for a particular order), violent impulses (e.g., to yell obscenities in church), or intrusive sexual imagery.
- Obsessions possibly leading to compulsive behaviors meant to temporarily ameliorate the anxiety caused by obsessions (e.g., repeated hand washing, checking, rearranging), or mental tasks (e.g., counting, repeating phrases).
- Obsessions and compulsions almost always accompanied with high anxiety and subjective distress. Both are seen as excessive and unreasonable.

ETIOLOGY

- Strong evidence of neurobiological etiology.
- OCD may have onset after infectious illness of CNS (e.g., Von Economo's encephalitis, Sydenham's chorea).
- OCD may follow head trauma or other premorbid neurological conditions including birth hypoxia and Tourette's syndrome.
- Serotonergic pathways believed important in some ritualistic instinctual behaviors, with dysfunction of these pathways possibly giving rise to OCD.

DIAGNOSIS

DIFFERENTIAL DIAGNOSIS

- Obsessive-compulsive personality disorder (OCPD) is a maladaptive personality style defined by excessive rigidity, need for order/control, preoccupation with details, and excessive perfectionism. Unlike OCD, OCPD is ego syntonic.
- Other psychiatric disorders in which obsessive or intrusive thoughts occur (e.g., body dysmorphic disorder, phobias, posttraumatic stress disorder).
- Other conditions in which compulsive or impulse control behaviors are seen (e.g., trichotillomania, gambling, paraphilias).
- Major depression, hypochondriasis, and several anxiety disorders with predominant obsessions or compulsions; however, in these disorders the thoughts are not anxiety provoking or are extremes of normal concern.
- Delusions or psychosis, which may be mistaken for obsessive thoughts; unlike OCD, these individuals do not believe their obsessions are unreal and may likely meet criteria for another psychotic spectrum disorder that fully accounts for the obsessions (e.g., schizophrenia).

WORKUP

- Careful history leading to diagnosis
- Neurologic examination to rule out concomitant Tourette's or other tic disorder
- In adolescents and children: psychological testing to reveal learning disabilities

LABORATORY TESTS

No specific tests are indicated.

IMAGING STUDIES

No specific studies are indicated.

TREATMENT

NONPHARMACOLOGIC THERAPY

- Average delay between symptom onset and treatment is 17 yr.
- Initiation of treatment will help about 50% of patients achieve partial remission within the first 6 mo.
- Cognitive-behavioral therapy (especially exposure with response prevention) is successful in up to 70% of patients but nearly 25% drop out of treatment due to the initial anxiety the exposures create. Best results are found for contamination obsessions and washing compulsions.

ACUTE GENERAL Rx

PRN clonazapam may be helpful in patients with extreme anxiety or those with a history of seizure disorder.

CHRONIC Rx

- Antidepressants with serotonergic reuptake blockade, including fluoxetine, clomipramine, fluvoxamine, paroxetine, sertraline, venlafaxine, escitalopram, and citalopram; optimal dosages are typically at the high end of the prescription range.
- No response in only 15% of patients.
- Indefinite treatment.
- It is unclear if combination cognitive-behavioral therapy and pharmacotherapy yields superior outcomes.
- Patients with comorbid psychosis and/or tic disorders may benefit from the addition of a neuroleptic.
- Surgical interventions (e.g., cingulotomy) are available for the most extreme, refractory cases.

DISPOSITION

- Course is chronic with waxing and waning. Symptoms tend to worsen with stress.
- Most mild to moderate cases can be managed on a regular outpatient basis. Treatment should typically start with SSRI monotherapy with regular follow-up to assess treatment response and side effect management. Dose should be increased to maximum tolerated.
- Patient and family education may help improve medical adherence and support.

REFERRAL

- If distinction from other psychiatric conditions, particularly delusional disorder, is not clear

- If patient refractory to drug treatment and/or requests cognitive-behavioral therapy

PEARLS & CONSIDERATIONS

Patients with OCD typically have insight regarding the irrationality of their obsessions and compulsions but lack the ability to control them. This may cause intense shame and avoidance of medical care unless patient education and support are provided.

EVIDENCE

Selective serotonin reuptake inhibitors (SSRIs) have been found to be more effective than placebo at reducing symptoms of obsessive-compulsive disorder (OCD).[1,2] Ⓐ

Systematic reviews have also found clomipramine to be more effective than SSRIs (paroxetine, fluoxetine, fluvoxamine, sertraline) in the management of OCD in children and adolescents, and more effective than desipramine, imipramine, or nortriptyline. All of the SSRIs were equally effective.[1,3] Ⓐ

A randomized controlled trial compared fluvoxamine vs. clomipramine and found no significant difference in symptom severity after 10 wk. Fluvoxamine was better tolerated.[4]

A randomized controlled trial found that there was no significant difference in symptoms between treatment with venlafaxine and clomipramine at 12 wk. This trial may have been underpowered.[5] Ⓑ

Both behavioral therapy and cognitive therapy have been found to be significantly more effective than relaxation therapy for the reduction of symptoms in patients with obsessive-compulsive disorder.[6] Ⓐ

It is unclear if the addition of fluvoxamine to behavioral or cognitive therapy produces superior outcomes.[7,8]

Evidence-Based References

1. Math SB, Janardhan Reddy YC. Issues in the pharmacological treatment of obsessive-compulsive disorder, *Int J Clin Pract* 61:1188, 2007. Ⓐ
2. Ackerman DL, Greenland S: Multivariate meta-analysis of controlled drug studies for obsessive-compulsive disorder, *J Clin Psychopharmacol* 22:309, 2002. Reviewed in: *Clin Evid* 10:1172, 2003. Ⓐ
3. Geller DA et al: Which SSRI? A meta-analysis of pharmacotherapy trials in pediatric obsessive-compulsive disorder, *Am J Psychiatry* 160:1919, 2003. Ⓐ
4. Mundo E et al: Fluvoxamine in obsessive-compulsive disorder: similar efficacy but superior tolerability in comparison with clomipramine, *Hum Psychopharmacol* 16:461, 2001. Reviewed in: *Clin Evid* 13:1297, 2005.
5. Albert U et al: Venlafaxine versus clomipramine in the treatment of obsessive-compulsive disorder: A preliminary single-blind, 12-week, controlled study, *J Clin Psychiatry* 63:1004, 2002. Ⓑ
6. Abramowitz JS: Effectiveness of psychological and pharmacological treatments for obsessive compulsive disorder: a quantitative review, *J Consult Clin Psychol* 65:44, 1997. Reviewed in: *Clin Evid* 9:1073, 2003. Ⓐ
7. van Balkom AJ et al: Cognitive and behavioral therapies alone versus in combination with fluvoxamine in the treatment of obsessive compulsive disorder, *J Nerv Ment Dis* 186:492, 1998. Reviewed in: *Clin Evid* 13:1297, 2005.
8. Hohagen F et al: Combination of behaviour therapy with fluvoxamine in comparison with behaviour therapy and placebo: results of a multicentre study, *Br J Psychiatry* 35(suppl):718, 1998. Reviewed in: *Clin Evid* 13:1297, 2005.

SUGGESTED READINGS

Eddy MF, Walbroehl GS: Recognition and treatment of obsessive-compulsive disorder, *Am Fam Physician* 57:1623, 1998.

Fineberg NA, Gale TM: Evidence-based pharmacotherapy of obsessive-compulsive disorder, *Int J Neuropsychopharmacol* 8(1):107, 2005.

Schruers K et al: Obsessive-compulsive disorder: a critical review of therapeutic perspectives, *Acta Psychiatr Scand* 111(4):261, 2005.

AUTHORS: **JASON M. SATTERFIELD, PH.D.,** and **MITCHELL D. FELDMAN, M.D., M.PHIL.**

BASIC INFORMATION

DEFINITION

The term *ocular foreign body* refers to a foreign body on the surface of the corneal epithelium.

ICD-9CM CODES
930 Foreign body in external eye

EPIDEMIOLOGY & DEMOGRAPHICS

INCIDENCE (IN U.S.): Universal, with a predominance in active people
PEAK INCIDENCE: Childhood through active adult years
PREDOMINANT SEX: Perhaps slightly more common in men
PREDOMINANT AGE: Childhood through active adult years

PHYSICAL FINDINGS & CLINICAL PRESENTATION

Pain is most common symptom
Most common foreign bodies:
- Grinding (Fig. 1-176)
- Drilling
- Auto mechanics
- Working beneath cars
- Airborne particles blown by fans and so forth

DIAGNOSIS

DIFFERENTIAL DIAGNOSIS

- History of corneal foreign body seen
- Hemorrhage, loss of vision
- Distorted anterior chamber, soft eye
- Corneal abrasion
- Corneal ulceration or laceration
- Glaucoma
- Herpes ulcers
- Infection
- Other keratitis
- Intraocular foreign body

WORKUP

- Fluorescein stain, slit lamp examination if no foreign body is found
- Ultrasound exam
- Plain x-ray

LABORATORY TESTS

Intraocular pressure to make certain that eye has not been penetrated

IMAGING STUDIES

Occasionally, MRI of the orbits to identify foreign bodies not found by other means. Do not do MRI if suspect metallic foreign body. Plain x-ray and ultrasound are sufficient.

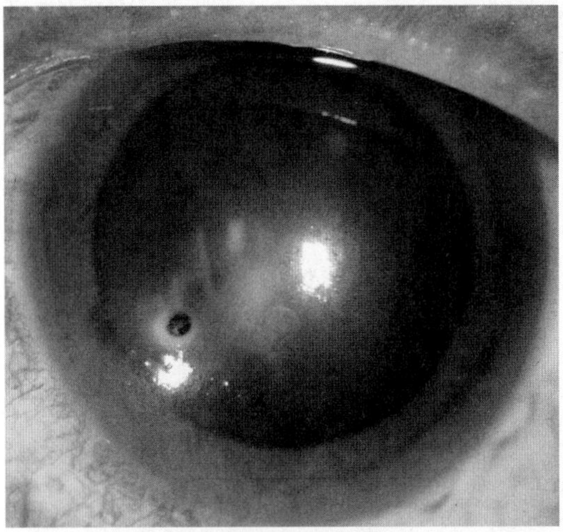

FIGURE 1-176 A small, iron foreign body may be seen on external examination. (Courtesy Department of Dermatology, University of North Carolina at Chapel Hill. In Goldstein GB, Goldstein AO: *Practical dermatology,* ed 2, St Louis, 1997, Mosby.)

TREATMENT

NONPHARMACOLOGIC THERAPY

- Remove foreign body
- Treat infection
- Repair eye if ruptured
- Treat corneal abrasion or injury

ACUTE GENERAL Rx

- Saline irrigation
- Removal of foreign body with moist cotton-tipped applicator after instillation of topical anesthetic drops
- Use Burr or more aggressive treatment if needed
- Cycloplegics, antibiotics, and pressure dressing after removal of foreign body
- Repair corneal laceration or damaged eye

DISPOSITION

If symptoms persist 24 hr after examination, refer to an ophthalmologist.

REFERRAL

To ophthalmology within 24 hr if patient not completely comfortable

PEARLS & CONSIDERATIONS

COMMENTS

- Make sure foreign body is not intraocular inside eye.
- Alkaline or acidic chemical foreign bodies can be dangerous, and pH test must be performed if either of these is suspected (for all chemical foreign bodies).

SUGGESTED READING

Ta CN, Bowman RW: Hyphema caused by a metallic intraocular foreign body during magnetic resonance imaging, *Am J Ophthalmol* 129(4):533, 2000.

AUTHOR: **MELVYN KOBY, M.D.**

BASIC INFORMATION

DEFINITION

Onychomycosis is defined as a persistent fungal infection affecting the toenails and fingernails.

SYNONYMS

Tinea unguium
Ringworm of the nails

ICD-9CM CODES
110.1 Onychomycosis

EPIDEMIOLOGY & DEMOGRAPHICS

- Onychomycosis is most commonly found in people between the ages of 40 to 60 yr.
- Onychomycosis rarely occurs before puberty.
- Incidence: 20 to 100 cases/1000 population.
- Toenail infection is 4 to 6 times more common than fingernail infections.
- Onychomycosis affects men more often than women.
- Occurs more frequently in patients with diabetes, peripheral vascular disease, and any conditions resulting in the suppression of the immune system.
- Occlusive footwear, physical exercise followed by communal showering, and incompletely drying the feet predisposes the individual to developing onychomycosis.

PHYSICAL FINDINGS & CLINICAL PRESENTATION

- Onychomycosis causes nails to become thick, brittle, hard, distorted, and discolored (yellow to brown color). Eventually, the nail may loosen, separate from the nail bed, and fall off.
- Onychomycosis is frequently associated with tinea pedis (athlete's foot).

ETIOLOGY

- The most common causes of onychomycosis are dermatophyte, yeast, and nondermatophyte molds.
- The dermatophyte *Trichophyton rubrum* accounts for 80% of all nail infections caused by fungus.
- *Trichophyton interdigitale* and *Trichophyton mentagrophytes* are other fungi causing onychomycosis.
- The yeast *Candida albicans* is responsible for 5% of the cases of onychomycosis.
- Nondermatophyte molds *Scopulariopsis brevicaulis* and *Aspergillus niger,* although rare, can also cause onychomycosis.

- Onychomycosis is classified according to the clinical pattern of nail bed involvement. The main types are:
  1. Distal and lateral subungual onychomycosis (DLSO)
  2. Superficial onychomycosis
  3. Proximal subungual onychomycosis
  4. Endonyx onychomycosis
  5. Total dystrophic onychomycosis

DIAGNOSIS

The diagnosis of onychomycosis is based on the clinical nail findings and confirmed by direct microscopy and culture.

DIFFERENTIAL DIAGNOSIS

- Psoriasis
- Contact dermatitis
- Lichen planus
- Subungual keratosis
- Paronychia
- Infection (e.g., *Pseudomonas*)
- Trauma
- Peripheral vascular disease
- Yellow nail syndrome

WORKUP

The workup of suspected onychomycosis is directed at confirming the diagnosis of onychomycosis by visualizing hyphae under the microscope or by culturing the organism.

LABORATORY TESTS

- Blood tests are not specific in the diagnosis of onychomycosis
- KOH prep
- Fungal cultures on Sabouraud medium

IMAGING STUDIES

- Imaging studies are not very specific in making the diagnosis of onychomycosis.
- If an infection is present and osteomyelitis is a consideration, an x-ray of the specific area and a bone scan may help establish the diagnosis.

TREATMENT

NONPHARMACOLOGIC THERAPY

- Surgical removal of the nail plate is a treatment option; however, the relapse rate is high.
- Prevention of reinfection by wearing properly fitted shoes, avoiding public showers, and keeping feet and nails clean and dry.

ACUTE GENERAL Rx

- Topical antifungal creams are used for early superficial nail infections.
  1. Miconazole 2% cream applied over the nail plate bid
  2. Clotrimazole 1% cream bid
- Oral agents.
  1. *Itraconazole*
     a. For toenails: 200 mg qd × 3 mo
     b. For fingernails: 200 mg PO bid × 7 days, followed by 3 wk of no medicine, for two pulses
  2. *Terbinafine*
     a. For toenails: 250 mg/day for 3 mo
     b. For fingernails: 250 mg/day for 6 wk
  3. *Fluconazole*
     a. For toenails: 150 to 300 mg once weekly, until infection clears
     b. For fingernails: 150 to 300 mg once weekly until infection clears
- All oral agents used for onychomycosis require periodic monitoring of liver function blood tests. Patients should be advised to watch for symptoms of drug-induced hepatitis (anorexia, fatigue, nausea, right upper quadrant pain) while taking these oral antifungal agents. They should stop their medication and contact their physician immediately if symptoms occur.
- Itraconazole is contraindicated in patients taking cisapride, astemizole, triazolam, midazolam, and terfenadine. Statins should be discontinued during itraconazole therapy. Itraconazole requires gastric acidity for absorption; patients should be advised not to take oral antacids, H2 blockers, or proton pump inhibitors while taking itraconazole.
- Fluconazole is contraindicated in patients taking cisapride and terfenadine.
- Oral antifungal agents should not be initiated during pregnancy.
- Ciclopirox, a topical nail lacquer antifungal agent, is FDA approved for treatment of mild to moderate disease not involving the lunula.

DISPOSITION

- Spontaneous remission of onychomycosis is rare.
- A disease-free toenail is reported to occur in approximately 25% to 50% of patients treated with the oral antifungal agents mentioned previously.

REFERRAL

- Podiatry consultation is indicated in diabetic patients for proper instruction in foot care, footwear, and nail debridement or surgical removal of the toenail.
- Dermatology consultation is indicated in patients refractory to treatment or if another diagnosis is considered (e.g., psoriasis).

PEARLS & CONSIDERATIONS

COMMENTS

- The growth of fungus on an infected nail typically begins at the end of the nail and spreads under the nail plate to infect the nail bed as well.

- Carefully consider the informational insert regarding drug-drug interactions and contraindications before initiating oral antifungal agents.

EVIDENCE

EBM

A systematic review found insufficient evidence to draw conclusions on the efficacy of topical antifungals for the treatment of nail infections.[1] Ⓐ

Terbinafine is more effective than griseofulvin for the treatment of patients with dermatophyte onychomycosis.[2,3] Ⓑ

Continuous terbinafine was found to be more effective than intermittent itraconazole in patients with fungal toenail infections in one randomized controlled trial (RCT).[4] Ⓑ

Continuous terbinafine was also found to be more effective than continuous itraconazole for fungal toenail infections, in the pooled results of two RCTs included in a systematic review.[5] Ⓑ

Evidence-Based References

1. Crawford F et al: Topical treatments for fungal infections of the skin and nails of the foot (Cochrane Review), 4, Chichester, UK, 2003, John Wiley. Ⓐ
2. Haneke E et al: Short-duration treatment of fingernail dermatophytosis: a randomized, double-blind study with terbinafine and griseofulvin. LAGOS III Study Group, *J Am Acad Dermatol* 32:72, 1995. Ⓑ
3. Faergemann J et al: Double-blind, parallel-group comparison of terbinafine and griseofulvin in the treatment of toenail onychomycosis, *J Am Acad Dermatol* 32:750, 1995. Ⓑ
4. Evans EG, Sigurgeirsson B: Double blind, randomised study of continuous terbinafine compared with intermittent itraconazole in treatment of toenail onychomycosis. The LION Study Group, *BMJ* 318:1031, 1999. Ⓑ
5. Crawford F et al: Oral treatments for toenail onychomycosis, *Arch Dermatol* 138:811, 2002. Ⓑ

SUGGESTED READINGS

Baran R, Kaoukhov A: Topical antifungal drugs for the treatment of onychomycosis: an overview of current strategies for monotherapy and combination therapy, *J Eur Acad Dermatol Venereol* 19(1):21, 2005.

Gupta AK et al: The use of terbinafine in the treatment of onychomycosis in adults and special populations: a review of the evidence, *J Drugs Dermatol* 4(3):302, 2005.

Kulac M et al: Venous insufficiency in patients with toenail onychomycosis, *J Ultrasound Med* 24(8):1085, 2005.

Romano C, Gianni C, Difonzo EM: Retrospective study of onychomycosis in Italy: 1985-2000, *Mycoses* 48(1):42, 2005.

Sigurgeirsson B, Steingrimsson O: Risk factors associated with onychomycosis, *J Eur Acad Dermatol Venereol* 18(1):48, 2004.

AUTHORS: **GLENN G. FORT, M.D., M.P.H.,** and **DENNIS J. MIKOLICH, M.D.**

BASIC INFORMATION

DEFINITION

- Opiate addiction is defined as a cluster of cognitive, behavioral, and physiological symptoms in which the individual continues use of opiates despite significant opiate-induced problems. Opiate dependence is a chronic, relapsing disorder characterized by repeated self-administration that usually results in opiate tolerance, withdrawal, and compulsive drug use. Dependence may occur with or without the physiological symptoms of tolerance and withdrawal.
- There are four stages of addiction:
  - Stage I, acute drug effects: rewarding effects of drug result from neurobiological changes in response to the acute drug use. Duration varies from hours to days.
  - Stage II, transformation to addiction: associated with changes in neuronal function that accumulate with repeated administration and diminish over days or weeks after discontinuation of drug use.
  - Stage III, relapse after extended periods of abstinence: precipitated by an incubation of cue-induced craving (people, places, and things as triggers) and priming (relapse precipitated by drug exposure).
  - Stage IV, end-stage addiction: vulnerability to relapse endures for years and results from prolonged changes at the cellular level.
- Pseudoaddiction: undertreatment of pain resulting in "opiate-seeking" behaviors such as "doctor shopping" and multiple emergency room visits. These behaviors disappear with adequate treatment of pain.

SYNONYMS

Opioid addiction
Opiate abuse
Narcotic addiction
Narcotic abuse

ICD-9-CM CODES
304.7X/304.8X Opioid dependence

EPIDEMIOLOGY & DEMOGRAPHICS

INCIDENCE: There are 980,000 opiate addicts in the U.S.; less than one third are in treatment.

PREVALENCE:

- Approximately 6 million persons age 12 yr and older used psychotherapeutic drugs for nonmedical purposes in 2004, which represents 2.5% of the population. Most of them reported abusing opiate pain relievers.
- In 2004, 2.4 million persons age 12 yr or older initiated nonmedical use of prescription pain relievers, surpassing for the first time those who initiated abuse of marijuana (2.1 million).
- Opiate addiction is becoming an adolescent disease. Among twelfth-graders, in 2005, 9.5% reported past year nonmedical use of oxycodone (Vicodin) and 5.5% reported past year nonmedical use of oxycodone slow-release tablets (Oxycontin).
- The percentage of eighth-, tenth-, and twelfth-graders who have used heroin has more than doubled since the late 1990s. This increase has largely been attributed to decreased price and increased purity in the last decade.

PREDOMINANT SEX: Males abuse opiates more commonly than females, with a male:female ratio of 3:1 for heroin and 1.5:1 for prescription opiates.

PEAK INCIDENCE: The majority of new abusers of opiates are less than 26 yr old.

RISK FACTORS:

- Family history
- Prior history of addiction
- Psychiatric disorders

GENETICS:

- Genetic epidemiologic studies suggest a high degree of heritable vulnerability for opiate dependence.
- Gene polymorphism for dopamine receptor/transporters, opioid receptors, serotonin receptors/transporters, proenkephlin, and catachol-o-methytrasferase (COMT) all appear to be associated with vulnerability to opiate dependence. Future interventions for opiate dependence may include medications identified through genetic research.

PHYSICAL FINDINGS & CLINICAL PRESENTATION

- Physical exam is often noncontributory.
- Small-sized pupils may be the only observable sign of use because only mild tolerance develops for miosis.
- Scars or tracks from chronic intravenous (IV) use may be visible in the veins of the arms, hands, ankles, neck, and breasts.
- Inflamed nasal mucosa or respiratory wheezing may be apparent in patients who are snorting heroin or Oxycontin.
- Patients in withdrawal may have more dramatic findings such as tachycardia, hypertension, fever, piloerection (goose flesh), mydriasis, lacrimation, central nervous system (CNS) arousal, irritability, and repeated yawning. In patients presenting with sympathetic overactivity and panic attacks, use of CNS stimulants, such as amphetamines or cocaine, should also be ruled out.
- Although gastrointestinal symptoms of nausea, vomiting, and abdominal pain are common in opiate withdrawal, other causes such as gastroenteritis, pancreatitis, peptic ulcer disease, and intestinal obstruction need to be ruled out.
- The history may provide relevant information in making the diagnosis. Significant findings may include:
  - A long history of opiate self-administration typically via the IV or intranasal route but sometimes through smoking as well.
  - Polysubstance use. Intoxication by drugs other than narcotics (e.g., benzodiazepines, barbiturates) should be ruled out in unconscious patients.
  - A high incidence of non–opiate related psychiatric disorders (>80%).
  - History of problems at work, school, or relationships associated with drug use.
  - History of legal problems associated with drug use such as arrest for possession, robberies, or prostitution.
  - History of interpersonal violence (perpetrator or victim).
  - History of physical problems such as skin infections, phlebitis, endocarditis, liver diseases due to acetaminophen toxicity (Vicodin/Percocet), and viral hepatitis. Hepatitis C is the most prevalent blood-borne pathogen. It is present in approximately 90% of opiate-dependant people and is often spread by sharing IV drug "works" or snorting devices. There is also a higher incidence of HIV infection.

ETIOLOGY

Opiate dependence is a biopsychosocial disorder. Pharmacologic, social, genetic, and psychodynamic factors interact to influence abusive behaviors. Pharmacologic factors are especially prominent in opiate addiction because these drugs are strong reinforcing agents owing to their euphoric effects and their ability to reduce anxiety and increase self-esteem and the patient's subjective feelings of improved ability to cope with daily challenges.

DIAGNOSIS

DIFFERENTIAL DIAGNOSIS

- Psychiatric disorders (e.g., anxiety, depression, bipolar disorder).
- Acute medical illness (e.g., hypoglycemia, seizure disorder, sepsis, renal or hepatic insufficiency) may mimic opiate withdrawal symptoms.

WORKUP

- The history is the most important part of the workup.
- Observation of opiate withdrawal is indicative of opiate addiction.
- Observation of purposeful behaviors such as complaints and manipulations directed at getting more drugs and anxiety during withdrawal is suggestive of opiate addiction.
- Screen blood and urine for opiate metabolites.
- Screen for communicable diseases: HIV, hepatitis B and hepatitis C, tuberculosis.
- Screen for endocarditis in patients with newly diagnosed murmurs.

LABORATORY TESTS

- Urine and serum toxicology screen
- CBC
- Chemistries (ALT, AST, serum creatinine): elevated liver function tests (LFTs) may be secondary to viral hepatitis or acetaminophen toxicity
- Hepatitis screen: if hepatitis C antibody–positive, follow up with hepatitis C PCR (viral load) even in patients with normal LFTs
- HIV
- PPD

IMAGING STUDIES

Generally not helpful in routine diagnosis and treatment. Consider echocardiography in patients with heart murmurs and liver sonography or CT scan in patients with elevated LFTs or positive for hepatitis C or B (increased risk of hepatocellular carcinoma).

TREATMENT

Rx

NONPHARMACOLOGIC THERAPY

- Brief counseling interventions during a visit with their primary care physician or OB/GYN have proven efficacious in motivating patients for treatment.
- Therapeutic communities (residential).
- 12-step or other self-help groups (e.g., Alcoholics Anonymous, Narcotics Anonymous).
- Relapse prevention (counseling).

ACUTE Rx

- Medical withdrawal (not overdosed).
- Short (30 days) or long-term (30 to 180 days) protocols.
- Buprenorphine (opioid partial agonist) or methadone (opioid agonist) is initiated in tapering doses.
- Clonidine 0.1 mg bid-tid can be used to minimize autonomic symptoms (sweating) and craving.
- NSAIDs for body/muscle aches.
- The anticholinergic dicyclomine (Bentyl) can be used to minimize GI hyperactivity.
- Nonbenzodiazepine hypnotics, low-dose atypical antipsychotics (e.g., Quetiapine [Seroquel]), or low-dose tricyclics are effective for promoting adequate sleep.

CHRONIC Rx

Opioid antagonist treatment:

- Naltrexone: does not stabilize neuronal circuitry like partial or full opioid agonists and generally results in poor outcomes, much like Antabuse for alcohol.
- Opioid partial agonist therapy: buprenorphine.
- Opioid agonist therapy: methadone.

NOTE: Buprenorphine and methadone are both metabolized by the cytochrome P450 3a4 and 2d6 I isoenzyme pathways. Prescribers should be aware of multiple possible drug interactions.

PATIENT SELECTION FOR BUPRENORPHINE OR METHADONE

- Appropriate patients for buprenorphine office-based treatment:
  - Patients interested (highly motivated) for treatment
  - Have no major contraindications (see following)
  - Can be expected to be reasonably compliant with treatment
  - Understand the benefits and risks of buprenorphine treatment
  - Willing to follow safety precautions
- Less likely to be appropriate for office-based treatment:
  - Have comorbid dependence on benzodiazepines or other CNS depressants (including ETOH)
  - Have significant untreated psychiatric comorbidities
  - Have active or chronic suicidal or homicidal ideation or attempts
  - Have multiple previous treatments with frequent relapses
  - Have poor response to previous treatment with buprenorphine
  - Have significant medical complications (e.g., hepatic insufficiency, bacterial endocarditis, active TB)
- Methadone maintenance: narcotic treatment program (clinic setting) indications
- Evidence of opiate addiction >1yr
- Two failed previous treatment attempts
- Patients not appropriate for office-based treatment
- Eligible without active "use" if prior methadone maintenance patient within previous 2 months
- Pregnancy

DISPOSITION

- Opiate addiction is a chronic relapsing disease.
- High rate of relapse after "detox."
- Relapse potential after medically supervised withdrawal from methadone:
  - 90% after 1 yr stable in treatment
  - 80% after 3 yr stable in treatment
  - 70% after 5 yr stable in treatment

REFERRAL

Refer to addiction medicine specialist or narcotic treatment program when the neurobiological disease of opiate addiction is identified.

PEARLS & CONSIDERATIONS

!

COMMENTS

- Methadone maintenance is the gold standard for the pregnant opiate-addicted patient regardless of the duration of the addiction or prior treatment attempts. Detoxification is contraindicated during pregnancy.
- Breastfeeding is encouraged in mothers on methadone maintenance (MOMS). The American Academy of Pediatrics statement regarding "Transfer of Drugs and Other Chemicals into Human Milk" has placed methadone into the "usually compatible with breastfeeding" group, based on the assumption that maternal urines are monitored to detect use of illicit drugs. The U.S. Department of Health and Human Services also recommends that mothers on methadone be encouraged to breastfeed.
- When a physician identifies a patient as a "drug seeker," it is imperative that the physician avoids abruptly stopping the opiate prescription because this will often result in the patient buying the drugs illegally. These patients should be counseled and referred for treatment.
- Patients on methadone or buprenorphine who have pain resulting from an acute injury will need pain medication in addition to their daily dose of methadone or buprenorphine. They will require higher than usual doses of pain medications because of opiate receptor "blockade" secondary to their methadone or buprenorphine use.
- Opiate-dependant patients have a lower pain threshold resulting from hyperalgesia caused by the long-term use of opiates.

PREVENTION

Education is the hallmark of prevention.

- School drug prevention education programs.
- Educate children about their family medical history including diseases of addiction.
- Address childhood psychiatric disorders to prevent self-medicating.

PATIENT/FAMILY EDUCATION

- Stigma of addictions and treatment often interferes with good treatment.
- Family needs to be educated so they can support the patient's efforts.
- Encourage family meeting with addiction specialist, counselor.
- Recommend support groups for family members.

SUGGESTED READINGS

Daniel A: Acute pain management for patients receiving methadone or buprenorphine therapy, *Ann Int Med* 144:127, 2006.

Kalinas PW, Volkow ND: The neural basis of addiction: a pathology of motivation and choice, *Am J Psych* 162:1403, 2005.

Minkoff K: Best practices: developing standards of care for individuals with co-occurring psychiatric and substance abuse disorders, *Psych Serv* 52:597, 2001.

Olsen Y, Alford D: Chronic pain management in patients with substance use disorders, *Johns Hopkins Advanced Studies in Medicine* 6:110, 2006.

Puredes A, Zweban J: The hepatitis C epidemic: shall we remain silent? *J Addict Dis* 1:1, 2001.

Wilford B: *Principles of addiction medicine,* ed 3, Chevy Chase, MD, 2003, American Society of Addiction Medicine.

AUTHOR: **STEVEN PELIGIAN, D.O.**

BASIC INFORMATION

DEFINITION

Optic atrophy refers to the degeneration of the axons of the optic nerve.
It is a symptom rather than a disease.

SYNONYMS

Unilateral/Bilateral optic atrophy

ICD-9CM CODES
377.10 Atrophy, optic nerve

EPIDEMIOLOGY & DEMOGRAPHICS

PEAK INCIDENCE: Varies depending on etiology
PREDOMINANT SEX: Unilateral optic atrophy in women is most commonly MS; may also occur after head injury (more commonly in men)
PREDOMINANT AGE: 21 to 40 yr

PHYSICAL FINDINGS & CLINICAL PRESENTATION

- Asymmetry of disc color is often first subtle finding
- Temporal part of optic disc is pale initially (Fig. 1-177); later the entire disc becomes pale/white
- Optic disc pallor occurs 4 to 6 wk after optic nerve injury
- Unilateral lesion produces a relative afferent pupillary defect (RAPD): swing flashlight eye to eye; abnormal pupil dilates to direct light
- Decreased visual acuity, blurred vision, visual field deficits (e.g., central scotoma), abnormal color vision (e.g., red desaturation)

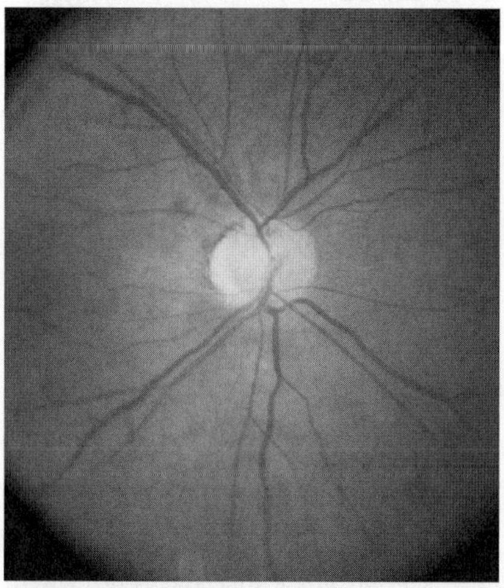

FIGURE 1-177 Optic atrophy. Patient's right eye shows atrophy. (Courtesy John W. Payne, M.D., The Wilmer Ophthalmological Institute, The Johns Hopkins University and Hospital, Baltimore. From Seidel HM [ed]: *Mosby's guide to physical examination,* ed 4, St Louis, 1999, Mosby.)

ETIOLOGY

- Optic neuritis—multiple sclerosis, sarcoidosis, infections (syphilis, CMV, HIV, Lyme, TB, bartonella, West Nile)
- Vascular—ischemic optic neuropathy, central retinal artery occlusion, temporal arteritis
- Compression—glaucoma, pituitary tumor, meningioma, thyroid eye disease, pseudotumor cerebri
- Hereditary—Leber's hereditary optic neuropathy
- Nutritional, toxic and metabolic—Amiodarone, Isoniazid, B_{12} deficiency, tobacco-alcohol
- Trauma

DIAGNOSIS

DIFFERENTIAL DIAGNOSIS

- Nutritional, toxic, and hereditary causes are usually bilateral.
- Unilateral optic atrophy in a young person is more commonly MS.
- Postviral atrophy may be seen in childhood.

WORKUP

- Depends on suspected etiology/clinical presentation. History including age of onset, risk factors, acuity of onset of symptoms, trauma, presence of pain, family history, toxic/nutritional factors, and other associated neurologic findings should be considered. When accompanied by other systemic signs and symptoms, a metabolic disorder should be considered.
- Visual field testing may help identify etiology (e.g., centrocecal field defects may occur with nutritional/toxic causes), but specificity is low.
- To differentiate between optic nerve vs. macular disease an Amsler chart and/or visual evoked responses may be helpful.
- If high clinical suspicion for MS, consider MRI of brain with contrast and LP with oligoclonal bands.
- Measure intraocular pressure (glaucoma).
- If pseudotumor cerebri is suspected, suggest LP; if bartenellosis (catscratch disease) is suspected, check bartonella titers.

LABORATORY TESTS

- Depends on suspected etiology: none for trauma, tumor, MS
- Serum B_{12}
- Autoimmune diseases: ESR, ANA, ACE

IMAGING STUDIES

- MRI brain with contrast, need fat suppression and special (thin) cuts through orbits to identify compressive lesions in all patients with unexplained optic atrophy; especially important in patients with positive predictive factors for abnormal imaging (e.g., young age, progression, bilateral findings)
- If sarcoid is suspected, order chest x-ray

TREATMENT

ACUTE GENERAL Rx

Treat the underlying cause—discontinue identifiable toxins, B_{12} replacement, neurosurgical intervention if tumor found; consider IV steroids if there is evidence for active demyelinating disease.

CHRONIC Rx

The optic nerve does not regenerate although symptoms often improve.

DISPOSITION

- Visual loss occurs over weeks to months
- Usually follow-up by neurologist or ophthalmologist

REFERRAL

If tumor or demyelinating lesions are found or if etiology is unknown

PEARLS & CONSIDERATIONS

COMMENTS

- An experienced clinician should be able to identify pale optic discs and a relative afferent pupillary defect.
- Pupillary dilation with mydriatic agents (e.g., Pilocarpine) may be necessary for a better funduscopic examination.
- Patient education material can be obtained from the National Eye Institute, Department of Health and Human Services, 9000 Rockville Pike, Bethesda, MD 20892.

EVIDENCE

Optic atrophy is a syndrome with multiple potential etiologies, rather than a single disorder, and there are no randomized, controlled clinical trials for the diagnosis or treatment of this syndrome.

SUGGESTED READINGS

Huizing M et al: Optic atrophies in metabolic disorders, *Mol Genet Metab* 86:51, 2005.

Lee AG et al: The diagnostic yield of the evaluation for isolated unexplained optic atrophy, *Ophthalmol* 112(5):757, 2005.

Newman NJ: Hereditary optic neuropathies: from the mitochondria to the optic nerve, *Am J Ophthalmol* 140(3):517, 2005.

Van Stavern GP, Newman NJ: Optic neuropathies. An overview, *Ophthalmol Clin North Am* 14(1):61, 2001.

AUTHOR: **RICHARD S. ISAACSON, M.D.**

BASIC INFORMATION

DEFINITION

Optic neuritis is an inflammation of the optic nerve resulting in a reduction of visual function.

SYNONYMS

Optic papillitis
Retrobulbar neuritis

ICD-9CM CODES
377.3 Optic neuritis

EPIDEMIOLOGY & DEMOGRAPHICS

INCIDENCE (IN U.S.): 1 to 5/100,000 person years; rates vary according to incidence of multiple sclerosis (MS).

PEAK INCIDENCE: 20 to 49 yr, mean 30.

PREVALENCE (IN U.S.): Common in multiple sclerosis.

PREDOMINANT SEX: Female 1.8:1 male.

GENETICS: MS more common in patients with certain HLA blood types. See "Multiple Sclerosis."

PHYSICAL FINDINGS & CLINICAL PRESENTATION

- Visual loss develops over hours or days, most often accompanied by pain and tenderness with movement of affected eye.
- Marcus Gunn pupil (RAPD = relative afferent pupillary defect): direct and consensual responses are normal. However, when swinging the flashlight from eye to eye, the affected eye's pupil dilates transiently to direct light.
- Decreased visual acuity.
- Unilateral visual field abnormalities—often a central scotoma.
- Color desaturation—red most affected.
- Normal orbit and fundus; occasionally there is disc edema acutely (Fig. 1-178), uveitis, or periphlebitis.
- May have movement or light-induced phosphenes (flashes of light lasting 1 to 2 sec) or Uhtoff's phenomenon (see "Multiple Sclerosis").
- After several months the optic disc may atrophy and develop pallor.

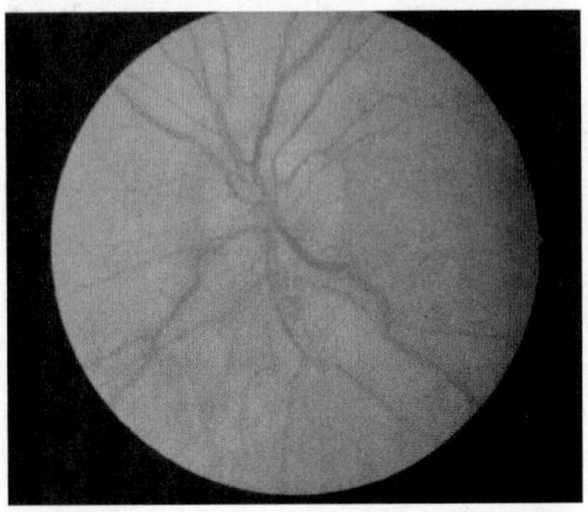

FIGURE 1-178 A case of optic neuritis. The optic disc edema seen here is often not present. Note the otherwise normal fundus. (Courtesy of J. Barton, M.D., Beth Israel Deaconess Medical Center, Boston.)

ETIOLOGY

An inflammatory response associated with an infection, autoimmune disease (such as multiple sclerosis), or rarely a mitochondrial disorder.

DIAGNOSIS

The classic triad includes loss of vision, pain, and dyschromatopsia. Alternate ocular pathology, infection, and CNS mass lesions should be excluded. 30% of cases are bilateral.

DIFFERENTIAL DIAGNOSIS

- Inflammatory: multiple sclerosis, neuromyelitis optica, sarcoidosis, SLE, Sjögren's, Behçet's, postinfectious, postvaccination
- Infectious: syphilis, TB, Lyme, *Bartonella*, HIV, CMV, herpes, orbital infection
- Ischemic: giant cell arteritis, anterior and posterior ischemic optic neuropathies, diabetic papillopathy, branch or central retinal artery or vein occlusion (sudden onset loss of vision)
- Mitochondrial: Leber's hereditary optic neuropathy
- Mass lesion: pituitary tumor, aneurysm, meningioma, glioma, metastases, sinus mucocele
- Ocular: optic drusen, retinal detachment, vitreous hemorrhage, uveitis, posterior scleritis, neuroretinitis, maculopathies and retinopathies
- Toxic: B_{12} deficiency, tobacco-ethanol amblyopia, methanol or ethambutol intoxication (painless, slowly progressive, and mostly bilateral)
- Other: acute papilledema, retinal migraine, factitious visual loss

WORKUP

The neurologic examination should otherwise be normal. Recommend dilated ophthalmoscopy.

LABORATORY TESTS

- Recommend: CBC, ANA, ESR, CRP.
- Consider: HIV Ab, Lyme titer, ACE, RPR, LHON mtDNA mutations.

IMAGING STUDIES

MRI of the brain and orbits (thin section fat-suppressed T2-weighted) with gadolinium to rule out compressive and infiltrative etiologies and to assess the risk of MS.

TREATMENT

NONPHARMACOLOGIC THERAPY

Assure patient that in most cases there is nearly complete recovery of vision.

ACUTE GENERAL Rx

Treat if the visual loss is moderate to severe or if there is an abnormal MRI (higher risk of MS). Methylprednisolone 250 mg IV every 6 hr for 3 days followed by an oral prednisone taper over 11 days.

CHRONIC Rx

None, unless at high risk to develop MS. See "Multiple Sclerosis."

DISPOSITION

Recovery over several months. In the ONTT (see below), 90% had 20/40 or better at 1 yr and 3% had 20/200 or worse. Of initial 20/200 or worse, only 5% remained in that group at 6 mo.

REFERRAL

- To neurologist if patient has other neurologic signs or an abnormal brain MRI.
- Urgent if proptosis, ophthalmoplegia, or brain MRI demonstrates a mass lesion.
- To ophthalmologist when atypical features, sudden onset, slowly progressive, other ocular pathology; if vision worsens or does not improve after several weeks; if severe or persistent pain; or if vision deteriorates as steroids are tapered.

PEARLS & CONSIDERATIONS

- Bilateral ON with poor recovery suggests possible Leber's hereditary optic neuropathy or toxic optic neuropathies.
- Consider pituitary apoplexy with severe headache or diplopia.

EVIDENCE

IV methylprednisolone hastens recovery with slight improvement in visual function tests at 6 mo. Oral prednisone may increase the risk of recurrent ON.[1]

Evidence-Based Reference

1. Beck RW et al: A randomized, controlled trial of corticosteroids in the treatment of acute optic neuritis. The Optic Neuritis Study Group, *N Engl J Med* 326(9):581, 1992.

SUGGESTED READINGS

Beck R et al: High and low risk profiles for the development of MS within 10 years after optic neuritis, *Arch Ophthalmol* 121(7):944, 2003.

Beck R et al: Visual function more than 10 years after optic neuritis, *Am J Ophthalmol* 137:77, 2004.

AUTHOR: **ALEXANDRA DEGENHARDT, M.D.**

BASIC INFORMATION

DEFINITION

Orchitis is an inflammatory process (usually infectious) involving the testicles. Infection may be viral or bacterial and can be associated with infection of other male sex organs (prostate, epididymis, bladder) or lower urogenital tract or sexually transmitted diseases often via hematogenous spread. Common causes are:

- Viral: Mumps—20% postpubertal; coxsackie B virus
- Bacterial: Pyogenic via spread from involving epididymis; bacteria include *Escherichia coli, Klebsiella pneumoniae, P. aeruginosa, Staphylococcus, Streptococcus* or *Rickettsia, Brucella spp.*
- Other:
  Viral-HIV associated, CMV
  Fungi
  1. Cryptococcosis
  2. Histoplasmosis
  3. *Candida*
  4. Blastomycosis

Mycobacterium tuberculosis and *M. leprae*

Parasitic causes: toxoplasmosis, filiariasis, schistosomiasis

SYNONYMS

Epididymiorchitis
Testicular infection
Testicular inflammation

ICD-9CM CODES
0.72 Mumps
098.13 Acute gonococcal orchitis
095.8 Syphilitic orchitis
016.50 Tuberculous orchitis, unspecified

EPIDEMIOLOGY & DEMOGRAPHICS

PREDOMINANT SEX: Male

PREDOMINANT ORGANISM: The leading cause of viral orchitis is mumps. The mumps virus rarely causes orchitis in prepubertal males but involves one or both testicles in nearly 30% of postpubertal males.

PHYSICAL FINDINGS & CLINICAL PRESENTATION

- Testicular pain, unilateral or bilateral swelling
- May have associated epididymitis, prostatitis, fever, scrotal edema, erythema cellulitis
- Inguinal lymphadenopathy
- Acute hydrocele (bacterial)
- Rare development—abscess formation, pyocele of scrotum, testicular infarction
- Spermatic cord tenderness may be present

DIAGNOSIS

Clinical presentation as described previously with possible history of acute viral illness or concomitant epididymitis.

DIFFERENTIAL DIAGNOSIS

- Epididymoorchitis—gonococcal
- Autoimmune disease
- Vasculitis
- Epididymyosis
- Mumps—with or without parotitis
- Neoplasm
- Hematoma
- Spermatic cord torsion

LABORATORY TESTS

- CBC with differential
- Urinalysis
- Viral titer—mumps
- Urine culture
- Ultrasound of testicle to rule out abscess

IMAGING STUDIES

Ultrasound if abscess suspected

TREATMENT

- Dependent on etiology
- Viral (mumps)—observation; bed rest, ice packs, analgesics, and a scrotal sling for support may provide some relief of discomfort that accompanies mumps orchitis
- Bacterial—empiric antibiotic treatment with parenteral antibiotic treatment until pathogen identified: ceftriaxone (250 mg IM × 1) plus doxycycline (100 mg PO bid × 10 days), ofloxacin (300 mg PO bid × 10 days), ciprofloxacin (500 mg PO bid or 400 mg IV bid)
- Surgery for abscess, pyogenic process

DISPOSITION

Follow up for evidence of recurrence, hypogonadism, and infertility may be needed with bilateral orchitis

REFERRAL

To a urologist if surgical drainage is needed
To an endocrinologist if hypogonadism develops
To a fertility specialist if infertility develops

PEARLS & CONSIDERATIONS

Consider tuberculous orchitis if symptoms fail to respond to standard antibacterial therapy, even in the absence of chest radiographic evidence of pulmonary tuberculosis

SUGGESTED READINGS

Niizuma T et al: Elevated serum C-reactive protein in mumps orchitis, *Pediatr Infect Dis J* 23(10):971, 2004.
Rajagopal AS: Pseudomonas orchitis in puberty, *Int J STD AIDS* 15(10):707, 2004.

AUTHORS: **GLENN G. FORT, M.D., M.P.H.,** and **DENNIS J. MIKOLICH, M.D.**

BASIC INFORMATION

DEFINITION

Orthostatic hypotension (OH) is defined as the presence of at least one of the following: a decrease in systolic blood pressure by greater than or equal to 20 mm Hg or a decrease in diastolic blood pressure by greater than or equal to 10 mm Hg within 5 minutes of standing.

SYNONYMS

Postural hypotension

ICD-9CM CODES
458.0 Orthostatic hypotension

EPIDEMIOLOGY & DEMOGRAPHICS

- The incidence of OH is increased in the elderly, most likely due to an impaired baroreceptor response to postural changes in these patients.
- OH may cause up to 30% of all syncopal events in the elderly.

CLINICAL PRESENTATION

- Symptoms include dizziness, lightheadedness, syncope, visual and auditory disturbances, weakness, diaphoresis, pallor, gastrointestinal upset, and urinary dysfunction.
- Associated with increased autonomic activity during meals (from increased splanchnic blood flow), exercise, and hot weather.
- Supine and nocturnal *hyper*tension in patients with OH may be secondary to underlying autonomic dysfunction.

ETIOLOGY

- The assumption of an upright posture results in a lower arterial pressure and decreased carotid baroreceptor activity. The consequent increase in sympathetic tone at the expense of parasympathetic tone causes arterial and venous constriction as well as positive inotropic and chronotropic effects, thereby limiting the fall in blood pressure in the upright position.
- When OH is caused by central or peripheral autonomic dysfunction, this baroreceptor reflex is impaired, and thus decreased blood pressure cannot be counteracted by the aforementioned compensatory mechanisms.

DIAGNOSIS

DIFFERENTIAL DIAGNOSIS

Common:
- Medications: antihypertensives, antidepressants (tricyclics), antipsychotics (phenothiazines), alcohol, narcotics, barbiturates, insulin, nitrates
- Reduced intravascular volume (hemorrhage, dehydration, hyperglycemia, hypoalbuminemia)
- Postprandial effect (especially in the elderly)
- Vasovagal syncope
- Deconditioning
- Peripheral autonomic dysfunction (diabetes mellitus, Guillain-Barré syndrome)

Uncommon:
- Central autonomic dysfunction (Shy-Drager syndrome)
- Postganglionic autonomic dysfunction: impaired norepinephrine release
- Autoimmune autonomic dysfunction: nAChR autoantibodies
- Paraneoplastic autonomic dysfunction: anti-Hu antibodies (in small cell lung cancer)
- POTS (postural tachycardia syndrome): usually occurs in young women; an abnormally large increase in heart rate is observed in the upright position due to increased venous pooling from autonomic dysfunction of the lower extremities, but blood pressure is not affected due to an excess of plasma norepinephrine.
- Impaired cardiac output
- Cerebrovascular accident
- Adrenal insufficiency
- Deconditioning
- Carotid sinus hypersensitivity
- Anxiety, panic attacks
- Seizures
- Idiopathic

WORKUP

- Measure supine blood pressure, stand for 5 minutes, then measure upright blood pressure.
- Thorough neurologic exam.
- Rule out treatable causes (e.g., medications, volume depletion).

LABORATORY TESTS

- Hemoglobin and hematocrit.
- Serum erythropoietin level if anemia is suspected.
- Consider when treatable causes of OH have been ruled out:
  - Blood pressure and heart rate monitoring using the tilt table test.
  - Plasma norepinephrine measurements (to distinguish postganglionic from preganglionic autonomic dysfunction).
  - Other methods use the Valsalva maneuver or measure sweating as indirect means of evaluating the autonomic nervous system.

IMAGING STUDIES

None

TREATMENT

NONPHARMACOLOGIC THERAPY

- High-salt diet (e.g., bouillon cubes)
- Liberal fluid intake
- Raising the head of the bed at night
- Compression stockings to waist (to include splanchnic circulation)
- Multiple low-carbohydrate meals to avoid postprandial orthostatic hypotension
- Patient education (leg crossing, prolonged sitting before first standing in the morning)

ACUTE GENERAL Rx

- Correction of volume status
- Discontinuation of medications that may cause OH

CHRONIC Rx

- Fludrocortisone: 0.1 mg/d (may combine with an alpha-1 agonist to lower the dose of each)
- Midodrine (alpha-1 agonist): 10 mg three times a day
- Erythropoietin (if anemic)
- Caffeine

OTHER TREATMENTS

- Pyridostigmine (enhances renal sodium reabsorption): 0.2 to 0.6 mg/d (not FDA approved for this indication)
- Octreotide: 300 to 600 mg/d (not FDA approved for this indication)
- Indomethacin (prostaglandin inhibitor)
- DdAVP (experimental)

PEARLS & CONSIDERATIONS

COMMENTS

- Orthostatic hypotension is diagnosed by observing changes in blood pressure, but not by observing changes in heart rate.
- Volume depletion should cause an increased heart rate upon standing, but the heart rate may not change upon standing in patients with autonomic dysfunction.
- Pharmacotherapy with mineralocorticoids may require concomitant potassium replenishment and monitoring for hypertension.
- Suspect OH when a patient has preexisting supine *hyper*tension.
- Suspect POTS in young women with a marked increase in heart rate but no change in blood pressure upon standing.

SUGGESTED READINGS

Jacob G et al: The neuropathic postural tachycardia syndrome, *N Engl J Med* 343:1008, 2000.

Kaufman H et al: Mechanisms and causes of orthostatic and postprandial hypotension. In Kasper et al (eds): *Harrison's principles of internal medicine,* ed 16, New York, NY, 2005, McGraw Hill, pp 2430-2434.

Shannon J et al: Orthostatic intolerance and tachycardia associated with norepinephrine transporter deficiency, *N Engl J Med* 342:541, 2000.

AUTHOR: **TIMOTHY W. FARRELL, M.D.**

BASIC INFORMATION

DEFINITION

Osgood-Schlatter disease is a painful swelling of the tibial tuberosity that occurs in adolescence.

ICD-9CM CODES
732.4 Osgood-Schlatter disease

EPIDEMIOLOGY & DEMOGRAPHICS

PREVALENCE: 4 cases/100 adolescents
PREDOMINANT SEX: Male:female ratio of 3:1
PREDOMINANT AGE: 11 to 15 yr (bilateral in 20%)

PHYSICAL FINDINGS & CLINICAL PRESENTATION

- Pain at the tibial tubercle that is aggravated by activity, especially stairwalking and squatting
- Tender swelling and enlargement of the tibial tubercle
- Increased pain with knee extension against resistance

ETIOLOGY

- Unknown
- May be traumatically induced inflammation

DIAGNOSIS

DIFFERENTIAL DIAGNOSIS

- Referred hip pain (any child with hip pain should have a thorough clinical hip examination)
- Patellar tendinitis

WORKUP

In most cases, the diagnosis is obvious on a clinical basis.

IMAGING STUDIES

- Lateral roentgenogram of the upper portion of the tibia with the leg slightly internally rotated may reveal variable degrees of separation and fragmentation of the upper tibial epiphysis (Fig. 1-179).
- Occasionally, fragmented area fails to unite to the tibia and persists into adulthood.

TREATMENT

ACUTE GENERAL Rx

- Ice, especially after exercise
- NSAIDs
- Gentle hamstring and quadriceps stretching exercises
- Abstinence from physical activity
- Temporary immobilization in a knee splint for 2 to 4 wk in resistant cases

DISPOSITION

- Prognosis for complete restoration of function and relief from pain is excellent.
- Condition usually heals when the epiphysis closes.
- Complications are rare.
- Symptoms in the adult:
  1. Although unusual, prominence of the tibial tubercle is usually permanent
  2. May be more susceptible to local irritation, especially when kneeling
  3. Rarely, nonunion of the epiphyseal fragment, but it is usually asymptomatic
  4. Surgery rarely required

REFERRAL

For orthopedic consultation when diagnosis is uncertain or when symptoms persist.

PEARLS & CONSIDERATIONS

COMMENTS

Larsen-Johansson disease is a similar disorder that can develop where either the quadriceps or patellar tendon inserts into the patella. Treatment and prognosis are the same as with Osgood-Schlatter disease.

SUGGESTED READINGS

Bloom OJ, Mackler L, Barbee J: What is the best treatment for Osgood-Schlatter disease? *J Fam Pract* 53(2):153, 2004.

Cohen DA, Hinton RY: Bilateral tibial tubercle avulsion fractures associated with Osgood-Schlatter's disease, *Am J Orthop* 37:92, 2008.

Duri ZA, Patel DV, Aichroth PM: The immature athlete, *Clin Sports Med* 21(3):461, 2002.

Frank JB et al: Lower extremity injuries in the skeletally immature athlete, *J Am Acad Orthop Surg* 15(6):356, 2007.

Gholve PA et al: Osgood Schlatter syndrome, *Curr Opin Pediatr* 19(1):44, 2007.

Hirano A et al: Magnetic resonance imaging of Osgood-Schlatter disease: the course of the disease, *Skeletal Radiol* 31(6):334, 2002.

Ross MD, Villard D: Disability levels of college-aged men with history of Osgood-Schlatter disease, *J Strength Cond Res* 17(4)659, 2003.

AUTHOR: **LONNIE R. MERCIER, M.D.**

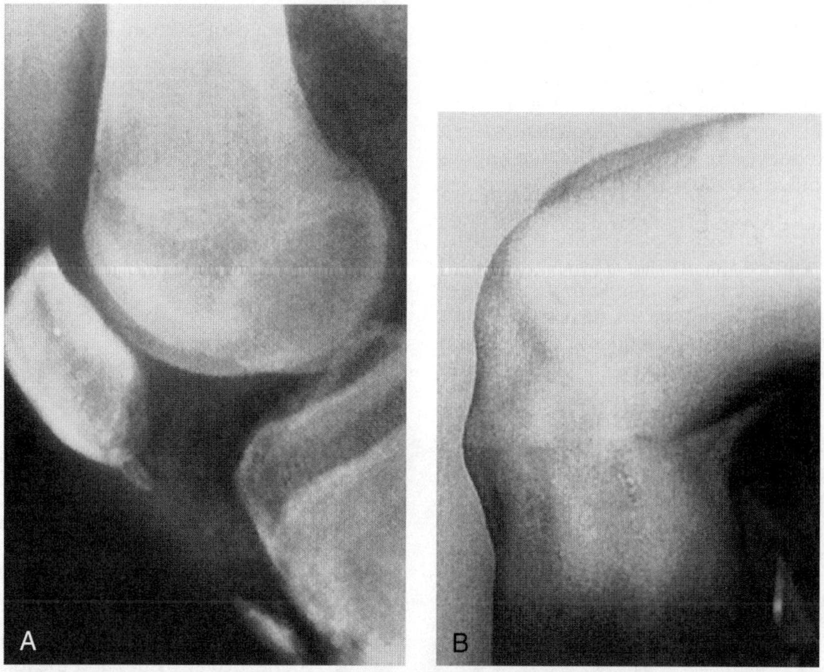

FIGURE 1-179 **A,** Radiograph of Osgood-Schlatter disease demonstrating thickening of patella tendon, fragmentation of the tibial tubercle, and soft tissue swelling. **B,** Clinical picture of bony prominence anteriorly at the tibial tubercle. (From Scuderi G [ed]: *Sports medicine: principles of primary care,* St Louis, 1997, Mosby.)

BASIC INFORMATION

DEFINITION

Osteoarthritis is a joint condition in which degeneration and loss of articular cartilage occur, leading to pain and deformity. Two forms are usually recognized: primary (idiopathic) and secondary. The primary form may be localized or generalized.

SYNONYMS

Degenerative joint disease
Osteoarthrosis
Arthrosis

ICD-9CM CODES
715.0 Osteoarthrosis and allied disorders

EPIDEMIOLOGY & DEMOGRAPHICS

PREVALENCE: 2% to 6% of general population
PREDOMINANT SEX: Female = male
PREDOMINANT AGE: >50 yr

PHYSICAL FINDINGS & CLINICAL PRESENTATION

- Similar symptoms in most forms: stiffness, pain, and crepitus
- Joint tenderness, swelling
- Decreased range of motion
- Crepitus with motion
- Bony hypertrophy
- Pain with range of motion
- DIP joint involvement possibly leading to development of nodular swellings called Heberden's nodes (Fig. 1-180)
- PIP joint involvement possibly leading to development of nodular swellings called Bouchard's nodes

ETIOLOGY

Primary osteoarthritis is of unknown cause. Secondary osteoarthritis may result from a number of disorders including trauma, metabolic conditions, and other forms of arthritis.

DIAGNOSIS

DIFFERENTIAL DIAGNOSIS

- Bursitis, tendinitis
- Radicular spine pain
- Inflammatory arthritides
- Infectious arthritis

WORKUP

- No diagnostic test exists for degenerative joint disease.
- Laboratory evaluation is normal.
- Rheumatoid factor, ESR, CBC, and ANA tests may be required if inflammatory component is present.
- Synovial fluid examination is generally normal.

IMAGING STUDIES

- When knee is involved with pain, x-rays should always be taken with the patient standing
- Roentgenographic evaluation reveals:
  1. Joint space narrowing
  2. Subchondral sclerosis
  3. New bone formation in the form of osteophytes

TREATMENT

- Rest, restricted use or weight bearing, and heat
- Walking aids such as a cane (often helpful for weight-bearing joints)
- Suitable footwear
- Gentle range of motion and strengthening exercise
- Local creams and liniments to provide a counterirritant effect
- Education, reassurance

ACUTE GENERAL Rx

- Mild analgesics for joint pain
- NSAIDs if inflammation is present
- Occasional local corticosteroid injections
- Mild antidepressants, especially at night, if depression is present
- Viscosupplementation (injection of hyaluronic acid products into the degenerative joint) is of uncertain benefit
- Nutritional supplements (glucosamine and chondroitin) are unproven

DISPOSITION

Progression is not always inevitable, and the prognosis is variable depending on the site and extent of the disease.

REFERRAL

Surgical consultation for patients not responding to medical management

PEARLS & CONSIDERATIONS

COMMENTS

Surgical intervention is generally helpful in degenerative joint disease. Arthroplasty, arthrodesis, and realignment osteotomy are the most common procedures performed. Arthroscopic debridement (of the knee) appears to be of questionable value.

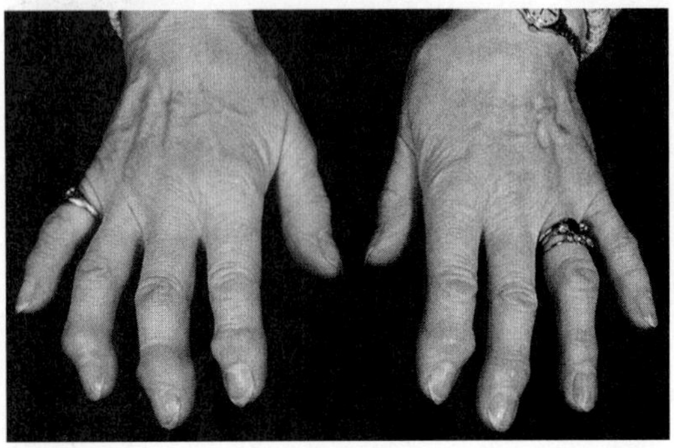

FIGURE 1-180 Osteoarthritis of the distal interphalangeal (DIP) joints. This patient has the typical clinical findings of advanced osteoarthritis of the DIP joints, including large, firm swellings (Heberden's nodes), some of which are tender and red because of associated inflammation of the periarticular tissues and the joint. (From Klippel J, Dieppe P, Ferri F [eds]: *Primary care rheumatology,* London, 1999, Mosby.)

EVIDENCE

Evidence for pharmacologic therapy

There is some evidence for the effectiveness of acetaminophen compared with placebo in the treatment of pain caused by osteoarthritis, although NSAIDs may be slightly more effective.[1-3] (A)

Two systematic reviews found that NSAIDs were effective at reducing short-term pain from osteoarthritis vs. placebo, the first in the hip and the second in the knee.[4,5] (A)

There is limited evidence for the efficacy of intraarticular corticosteroid injections in the short-term treatment of osteoarthritic knee pain.[6,7] (B)

There is good evidence for the effectiveness of joint replacement as a treatment in osteoarthritis.[8-11] (A) (B)

Evidence-Based References

1. Towheed TE et al: Acetaminophen for osteoarthritis, *Cochrane Database Syst Rev* 1, 2003. (A)
2. Zhang W, Jones A, Doherty M: Does paracetamol (acetaminophen) reduce the pain of osteoarthritis? A meta-analysis of randomised controlled trials, *Ann Rheum Dis* 63:901, 2004. Reviewed in: *Bandolier J* 127:2004. (B)
3. Wegman A et al: Nonsteroidal anti-inflammatory drugs or acetaminophen for osteoarthritis of hip or knee? A systematic review of evidence and guidelines, *J Rheumatol* 31:344, 2004. Reviewed in: Paracetamol for osteoarthritis, *Bandolier J* 127:2004. (B)

4. Towheed T et al: Analgesia and non-aspirin, non-steroidal anti-inflammatory drugs for osteoarthritis of the hip, *Cochrane Database Syst Rev* 4, 1997 (Cochrane Review). Reviewed in *Clin Evid* 11:1560, 2004. Ⓐ
5. Watson MC et al: Non-aspirin, non-steroidal anti-inflammatory drugs for treating osteoarthritis of the knee, *Cochrane Database Syst Rev* 1, 1997. Ⓐ
6. Godwin M, Dawes M: Intra-articular steroid injections for painful knees: systematic review with meta-analysis, *Can Fam Physician* 50:241, 2004. Ⓑ
7. Arroll B, Goodyear-Smith F: Corticosteroid injections for osteoarthritis of the knee: meta-analysis, *BMJ* 328:869, 2004. Ⓑ
8. Callahan CM et al: Patient outcomes following tricompartmental total knee replacement. A meta-analysis, *JAMA* 271:1349, 1994. Reviewed in: *Clin Evid* 11:1560, 2004. Ⓐ
9. Callahan CM et al: Patient outcomes following unicompartmental or bicompartmental knee arthroplasty. A meta-analysis, *J Arthroplasty* 10:141, 1994. Reviewed in: *Clin Evid* 11:1560, 2004. Ⓐ
10. Kiebzak GM et al: SF-36 general health status survey to determine patient satisfaction at short-term follow up after total hip and knee arthroplasty, *J South Orthop Assoc* 6:169, 1997. Reviewed in: *Clin Evid* 11:1560, 2004. Ⓑ
11. Hawker G et al: Health-related quality of life after knee replacement, *J Bone Joint Surg Am* 80:163-173, 1998. Reviewed in: *Clin Evid* 11:1560-1588, 2004. Ⓑ

SUGGESTED READINGS

Callahan JJ et al: Results of Charnley total hip arthroplasty at a minimum of thirty years, *J Bone Joint Surg* 86A:690, 2004.

Felson DT: Hyaluronate sodium injections for osteoarthritis: hope, hype and hard truths, *Arch Intern Med* 162:245, 2002.

Hartofilakidis G, Karachalios T: Idiopathic osteoarthritis of the hip: incidence, classification and natural history of 272 cases, *Orthopedics* 26:161, 2003.

Hinton R et al: Osteoarthritis: diagnosis and therapeutic considerations, *Am Fam Physician* 65:841, 2002.

Hunt SA, Jazrawi LM, Sherman OH: Arthroscopic management of osteoarthritis of the knee, *J Am Orthop Surg* 10:356, 2002.

Kelly MA et al: Osteoarthritis and beyond: a consensus on the past, present and future of hyaluronans in orthopedics, *Orthopedics* 26:1064, 2003.

Leopold S et al: Corticosteroid compared with hyaluronic acid injections for the treatment of osteoarthritis of the knee, *J Bone Joint Surg* 85:1197, 2003.

Lo HG: Intra-articular hyaluronic acid in treatment of knee osteoarthritis, *JAMA* 290:3115, 2003.

Moseley JB et al: A controlled trial of arthroscopic surgery for osteoarthritis of the knee, *N Engl J Med* 347:81, 2002.

O'Connor MI: Sex differences in osteoarthritis of the hip and knee, *J Am Acad Orthop Surg* 15(suppl 1):S22, 2007.

Ottaviani RA et al: Inflammatory and immunological responses to hyaluronan preparations: study of a murine biocompatibility model, *J Bone Joint Surg* 89A:148, 2007

Pollo FE, Jackson RW: Knee bracing for unicompartmental osteoarthritis, *J Am Acad Orthop Surg* 14:5, 2006.

Ramsey DK et al: A mechanical theory for the effectiveness of bracing for medial compartment osteoarthritis of the knee, *J Bone Joint Surg* 89:2398, 2007.

Salk RS et al: Sodium hyaluronate in the treatment of osteoarthritis of the ankle: a controlled, randomized double-blind study, *J Bone Joint Surg* 88A:295, 2006.

Saltzman CL et al: Impact of comorbidities on the measurement of health in patients with ankle osteoarthritis, *J Bone Joint Surg* 88A:2366, 2006.

Scott WN, Clarke HD: Early knee arthritis: the role of arthroscopy, *Orthopedics* 26:943, 2003.

Wai EK, Kreder HJ, Williams JI: Arthroscopic debridement of the knee for osteoarthritis in patients fifty years of age or older, *J Bone Joint Surg* 84(A):17, 2002.

Wang C et al: Therapeutic effects of hyaluronic acid in osteoarthritis of the knee, *J Bone Joint Surg* 86A:538, 2004.

Wegman A et al: Nonsteroidal antiinflammatory drugs or acetominophen for osteoarthritis of the hip or knee? A systematic review of evidence and guidelines, *J Rheumatol* 31:344, 2004.

AUTHOR: **LONNIE R. MERCIER, M.D.**

BASIC INFORMATION

DEFINITION

Osteochondritis dissecans is a disorder in which a portion of cartilage and underlying subchondral bone separates from a joint surface and may even become detached.

SYNONYMS

Osteochondrosis
Talar dome fracture: commonly used in describing the lesion of the talus
Panners disease (capitellum)

ICD-9CM CODES
732.7 Osteochondritis dissecans

EPIDEMIOLOGY & DEMOGRAPHICS

PREVALENCE: 0.3 cases/1000 persons
PREDOMINANT SEX: Male:female ratio of 3:1
PREDOMINANT AGE: Onset at 10 to 30 yr
The most common joint affected is the knee, with the lateral surface of the medial femoral condyle the most frequent area involved. The capitellum of the humerus, dome of the talus, shoulder, and hip may also be affected.

PHYSICAL FINDINGS & CLINICAL PRESENTATION

- Pain, stiffness, and swelling
- Intermittent locking if the fragment becomes detached
- Occasionally palpable loose body
- Tenderness at the site of the lesion
- When the knee is involved, positive Wilson's sign (pain with knee extension and internal rotation)
- Some asymptomatic cases

ETIOLOGY

Unknown

DIAGNOSIS

DIFFERENTIAL DIAGNOSIS

- Acute fracture
- Neoplasm

IMAGING STUDIES

- Plain roentgenography to confirm the diagnosis (Fig. 1-181)
- "Tunnel view" helpful in knee cases
- Typical finding: radiolucent, semilunar line outlining the oval fragment of bone (but findings variable, depending on the amount of healing and stability)
- MRI or bone scanning usually not necessary in establishing diagnosis but helpful in determining prognosis and management, especially with regards to the stability of the lesion

TREATMENT

ACUTE GENERAL Rx

- Observation every 4 to 6 mo for patients in whom the lesion is asymptomatic
- Symptomatic patients who are skeletally immature:
  1. Observation with an initial period of non–weight bearing for 6 to 8 wk (in knee cases)
  2. When symptoms subside, gradual resumption of activities

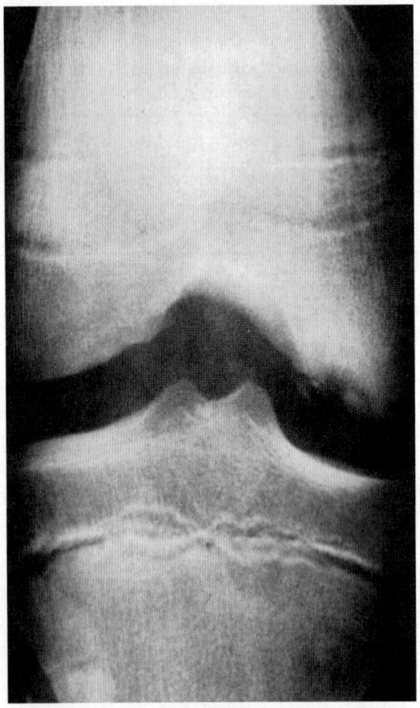

FIGURE 1-181 Osteochondritis dissecans of the knee. The "tunnel" view is often helpful in visualizing the defect. This fragment may become detached and form a loose body. This area should not be confused with the normal irregularity of the distal femoral epiphysis in young children.

DISPOSITION

- Juvenile cases with open epiphyses have a favorable prognosis.
- Cases developing after skeletal maturity are more likely to develop osteoarthritis.
- Large fragments, especially those in weight-bearing areas, have a more unfavorable prognosis, especially if they involve the lateral femoral condyle.
- Loose body formation and degenerative joint disease are more common when condition develops after age 20 yr.

REFERRAL

For orthopedic consultation:
- For most adults with unstable lesions
- If a loose body is present
- If symptomatic care has failed

PEARLS & CONSIDERATIONS

COMMENTS

- Although inflammation is suggested by the name, it has not been shown to be of significance in this disorder. *Osteochondral lesion* or *osteochondrosis dissecans* may be more appropriate terms to describe these disorders.
- Repetitive trauma with ischemic necrosis is the most likely cause.
- The condition is often bilateral, especially in the knee, which could suggest the possibility of an endocrine or genetic basis.
- This condition should always be considered in the patient whose "sprained ankle" does not improve over the usual course of treatment.

SUGGESTED READINGS

Bramer JA et al: Increased external tibial torsion and osteochondritis dissecans of the knee, *Clin Orthop* 422:175, 2004.
Crawford DC, Safran MR: Osteochondritis dissecans of the knee, *J Am Acad Orthop Surg* 14:90, 2006.
Frank JB et al: Lower extremity injuries in the skeletally immature athlete, *J Am Acad Orthop Surg* 15:356, 2007.
Hanna SA et al: Bicondylar osteochondritis dissecans in the knee: a report of two cases, *J Bone Joint Surg* 90:232, 2008.
Kobaynsh, K, Burton KJ et al: Lateral compression injuries in the pediatric elbow. Panner's disease and osteochondritis dissecans of the capitellum, *J Am Acad Orthop Surg* 12:246, 2004.
Peh WC: Osteochondritis dissecans, *Am J Orthop* 33(1):46, 2004.
Perumal V et al: Juvenile osteochondritis dissecans of the talus, *J Pediatr Orthop* 27:821, 2007.
Takahara M et al: Classification, treatment and outcome of osteochondritis dissecans of the humeral capitellum, *J Bone Joint Surg* 89A:1205, 2007.

AUTHOR: **LONNIE R. MERCIER, M.D.**

BASIC INFORMATION

DEFINITION

Osteomyelitis is an acute or chronic infection of the bone secondary to the hematogenous or contiguous source of infection or direct traumatic inoculation, which is usually bacterial.

SYNONYMS

Bone infection

ICD-9CM CODES
730.1 Chronic osteomyelitis
730.2 Acute or subacute osteomyelitis

EPIDEMIOLOGY & DEMOGRAPHICS

PREDOMINANT SEX: Male > female
PREDOMINANT AGE: All ages

PHYSICAL FINDINGS & CLINICAL PRESENTATION

HEMATOGENOUS OSTEOMYELITIS: Usually occurs in tibia/fibula (children).

- Localized inflammation: often secondary to trauma with accompanying hematoma or cellulitis
- Abrupt fever
- Lethargy
- Irritability
- Pain in involved bone

VERTEBRAL OSTEOMYELITIS: Usually hematogenous.

- Fever: 50%
- Localized pain/tenderness
- Neurologic defects: motor/sensory

CONTIGUOUS OSTEOMYELITIS: Direct inoculation.

- Associated with trauma, fractures, surgical fixation
- Chronic infection of skin/soft tissue
- Fever, drainage from surgical site

CHRONIC OSTEOMYELITIS:

- Bone pain
- Sinus tract drainage, nonhealing ulcer
- Chronic low-grade fever
- Chronic localized pain

ETIOLOGY

- *Staphylococcus aureus*
- *S. aureus* (methicillin-resistant)
- *Pseudomonas aeruginosa*
- Enterobacteriaceae
- *Streptococcus pyogenes*
- *Enterococcus*
- Mycobacteria
- Fungi
- Coagulase-negative staphylococci
- *Salmonella* (in sickle cell disease)

DIAGNOSIS

DIFFERENTIAL DIAGNOSIS

- Gaucher's disease
- Bone infarction
- Charcot's joint
- Fracture

WORKUP

- ESR, C-reactive protein
- Blood culturing
- Bone culture
- Pathologic evaluation of bone biopsy for acute/chronic changes consistent with necrosis or acute inflammation

IMAGING STUDIES

- Bone x-ray examination
- Triple-phase bone scan (Fig. 1-182)
- Gallium scan
- Indium scan
- CT or MRI (most accurate imaging study)

TREATMENT

Surgical debridement in biopsy-positive cases will guide direction for antibiotic therapy. This will vary with type of osteomyelitis. Duration of therapy is usually 6 wk for acute osteomyelitis; chronic osteomyelitis may need a longer course of medication.

- *S. aureus:* cefazolin IV, nafcillin IV, vancomycin IV (in patient allergic to penicillin)
- *S. aureus* (methicillin resistant): vancomycin IV, linezolid, daptomycin, or tigecycline
- *Streptococcus* spp.: cefazolin or ceftriaxone
- *P. aeruginosa:* piperacillin plus aminoglycoside or cefepime plus aminoglycoside
- Enterobacteriaceae: ceftriaxone or fluoroquinolone
- Hyperbaric oxygen therapy: may be useful in chronic osteomyelitis
- Surgical debridement of all devitalized bone and tissue
- Immobilization of affected bone (plaster, traction) if bone is unstable

DISPOSITION

Acute hematogenous osteomyelitis usually resolves without recurrence or long-term complications, but contiguous focus osteomyelitis, bone infections from open fractures, or osteomyelitis frequently recur.

REFERRAL

- To an orthopedic surgeon if chronic osteomyelitis with need for bone debridement, bone grafting, or stabilization of infected tissue adjacent to a bone fracture
- To an infectious disease specialist for appropriate treatment for difficult-to-treat or recalcitrant infections
- To an hyberbaric oxygen chamber service for nonhealing, chronic osteomyelitis

PEARLS & CONSIDERATIONS

Chronic osteomyelitis is one of the most challenging infections to treat; the high failure rate is a consequence of poor vascular supply, nondistensible bone tissue, and limited penetration of bone tissue

EVIDENCE

The use of antibiotics had a protective effect against early infection in open fractures compared with no antibiotics or placebo.[1] (A)

We are unable to cite evidence for the other therapies used in osteomyelitis.

Evidence-Based Reference

1. Gosselin RA, Roberts I, Gillespie WJ: Antibiotics for preventing infection in open limb fractures, *Cochrane Database Syst Rev* 3, 2003. (A)

SUGGESTED READINGS

Joosten U et al: Effectiveness of hydroxyapatite-vancomycin bone cement in the treatment of Staphylococcus aureus induced chronic osteomyelitis, *Biomaterials* 26(25):5251, 2005.

Schinabeck MK, Johnson JL: Osteomyelitis in diabetic foot ulcers. Prompt diagnosis can avert amputation, *Postgrad Med* 118(1):11, 2005.

Yin LY et al: Comparative evaluation of tigecycline and vancomycin, with and without rifampicin, in the treatment of methicillin-resistant Staphylococcus aureus experimental osteomyelitis in a rabbit model, *J Antimicrob Chemother* 55(6):995, 2005.

AUTHORS: **GLENN G. FORT, M.D., M.P.H.,** and **DENNIS J. MIKOLICH, M.D.**

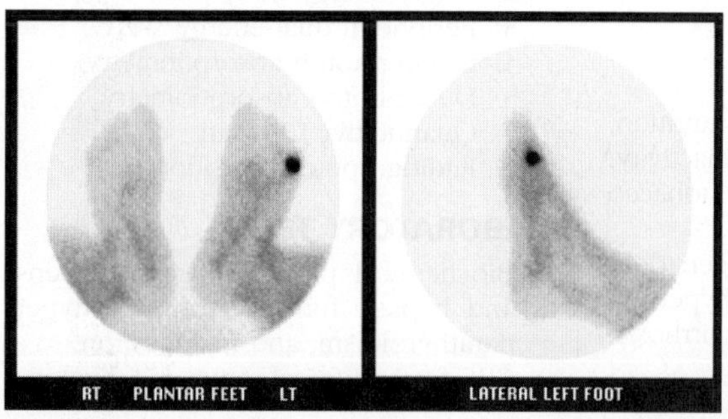

FIGURE 1-182 Osteomyelitis. Intense accumulation of Tc-99m WBC in proximal phalanx of fifth digit of left foot at 4 hours after injection. (From Specht N [ed]: *Practical guide to diagnostic imaging,* St Louis, 1998, Mosby.)

BASIC INFORMATION

DEFINITION

Osteoporosis is characterized by a progressive decrease in bone mass that results in increased bone fragility and a higher fracture risk. The various types are as follows:

PRIMARY OSTEOPOROSIS: 80% of women and 60% of men with osteoporosis

- Idiopathic osteoporosis: unknown pathogenesis; may occur in children and young adults
- Type I osteoporosis: may occur in postmenopausal women (age range: 51 to 75 yr); characterized by accelerated and disproportionate trabecular bone loss and associated with vertebral body and distal forearm fractures (estrogen withdrawal effect)
- Type II osteoporosis (involutional): occurs in both men and women >70 yr of age; characterized by both trabecular and cortical bone loss, and associated with fractures of the proximal humerus and tibia, femoral neck, and pelvis

SECONDARY OSTEOPOROSIS: 20% of women and 40% of men with osteoporosis; osteoporosis that exists as a common feature of another disease process, heritable disorder of connective tissue, or drug side effect (see "Differential Diagnosis")

ICD-9CM CODES
733.0 Osteoporosis

EPIDEMIOLOGY & DEMOGRAPHICS

PREVALENCE (IN U.S.):

- Approximately 25 million men and women
- Twice as common in women
- Results in 1.5 million fractures annually (70% women)
- Osteoporosis-related fractures in 50% women and 20% men >65 yr
- Results: institutionalization, mortality, and costs in excess of $10 billion annually

RISK FACTORS:

- Age: each decade after 40 yr associated with a fivefold increase risk
- Genetics:
  1. Ethnicity (white/Asian > black > Polynesian)
  2. Gender (female > male)
  3. Family history
- Environmental factors: poor nutrition, calcium deficiency, physical inactivity, medication (steroids/heparin), tobacco use, ETOH, traumatic injury
- Chronic disease states: estrogen deficiency, androgen deficiency, hyperthyroidism, hypercortisolism, cirrhosis, gastrectomy

PHYSICAL FINDINGS & CLINICAL PRESENTATION

- Most commonly silent with no signs and symptoms
- Insidious and progressive development of dorsal kyphosis (dowager's hump), loss of height, and skeletal pain typically associated with fracture, other physical findings related to other conditions with associated increased risk for osteoporosis (see "Risk Factors")

ETIOLOGY

- Primary osteoporosis; multifactorial resulting from a combination of factors including nutrition, peak bone mass, genetics, level of physical activity, age of menopause (spontaneous vs. surgical), and estrogen status
- Secondary osteoporosis: associated decrease in bone mass resulting from an identified cause, including endocrinopathies—hypogonadism, hyperthyroidism, hyperparathyroidism, Cushing's syndrome, hyperprolactinemia, acromegaly, diabetes mellitus, gastrointestinal disease, malabsorption, primary biliary cirrhosis, gastrectomy, malnutrition (including anorexia nervosa)

DIAGNOSIS

DIFFERENTIAL DIAGNOSIS

- Malignancy (multiple myeloma, lymphoma, leukemia, metastatic carcinoma)
- Primary hyperparathyroidism
- Osteomalacia
- Paget's disease
- Osteogenesis imperfecta: types I, III, and IV (see also "Epidemiology and Demographics" and "Etiology")

WORKUP

- History and physical examination (20% of women with type I osteoporosis have associated secondary cause), with appropriate evaluation for identified risk factors and secondary causes
- Diagnosis of osteoporosis made by bone mineral density (BMD) determination (BMD should ideally evaluate the hip, spine, and wrist):
  1. Dual-energy x-ray absorptiometry (DEXA)
  2. Single-energy x-ray
  3. Peripheral dual-energy x-ray
  4. Single-photon absorptiometry
  5. Dual-photon absorptiometry
  6. Quantitative CT scan
  7. Radiographic absorptiometry

LABORATORY TESTS

- Biochemical profile to evaluate renal and hepatic function, primary hyperparathyroidism, and malnutrition
- CBC for nutritional status and myeloma
- TSH to rule out the presence of hyperthyroidism
- Consideration of 24-hr urine collection for calcium (excess skeletal loss, vitamin D malabsorption/deficiency), creatinine, sodium, and free cortisol (to detect occult Cushing's disease); no need to measure calcitropic hormones (PTH, calcitriol, calcitonin) unless specifically indicated
- Biochemical markers of bone remodeling; may be useful to predict rate of bone loss and/or follow therapy response; specific biochemical markers followed (e.g., 3-mo interval) to document normalization as a response to therapy
  1. High turnover osteoporosis: high levels of resorption markers (lysyl pyridinoline [LP], deoxy lysyl pyridinoline [DPD], n-telopeptide of collagen cross-links [NTX], C-telopeptide of collagen cross-links [PICP]) and formation markers (osteocalcin [OCN], bone-specific alkaline phosphatase [BSAP], carboxy-terminal extension peptide of type I procollagen [PICP]); accelerated bone loss responding best to antiresorptive therapy
  2. Low-normal turnover osteoporosis: normal or low levels of the markers of resorption and formation (see "high turnover osteoporosis" above); no accelerated bone loss; responds best to drugs that enhance bone formation

IMAGING STUDIES

- BMD determination (see "Workup") should be performed on all women with determined risk factors and/or associated secondary causes; accepted screening criteria are currently being investigated.
  1. Normal: BMD <1 SD of the young adult reference mean
  2. Osteopenia: BMD <1 to 2.5 SD below the young adult reference mean
  3. Osteoporosis: BMD >2.5 SD below the young adult reference mean
- For patient undergoing treatment: annual BMD to follow response to therapy
- X-ray examination of appropriate part of skeleton to evaluate clinical osteoporotic fracture only (Fig. 1-183)

TREATMENT

NONPHARMACOLOGIC THERAPY

Prevention:

- Identification and minimization of risk factors
- Appropriate diagnosis and treatment of secondary causes

- Behavioral modification: proper nutrition (dietary calcium >800 mg/day, vitamin D 400 to 800 U/day), physical activity, fracture prevention strategies

ACUTE GENERAL Rx

- Vitamin D supplement: 400 U/day
- Calcium supplement: 1000 to 1500 mg/day
- Estrogen (conjugated equine estrogen or equivalent): 0.3 to 0.625 mg/day
- Progestin: continuous (e.g., 2.5 mg medroxyprogesterone acetate/day or equivalent) or cyclic (e.g., 10 mg medroxyprogesterone acetate days 16 to 25 each month or equivalent) coadministered in nonhysterectomized women
- Ibandronate (Boniva) 150 mg once monthly, swallow whole with 8 oz water on empty stomach, with no oral intake for at least 60 min. Do not lie down for 60 min after dose
- Alendronate (10 mg/day) or risedronate (5 mg/day) on awakening with 8 oz water on empty stomach with no oral intake for at least 30 min
- Alendronate (Fosamax): 70 mg once weekly on awakening, with 8 oz water on empty stomach, with no oral intake for at least 30 min. Use 70 mg dose for treatment of postmenopausal osteoporosis and a 35-mg tablet for the prevention of osteoporosis in postmenopausal women
- Synthetic salmon calcitonin (Miacalcin): 100 U/day SC or 200 U/day intranasally
- Raloxifene (Evista): 60 mg qd
- Risedronate (Actonel): 35 mg once weekly on awakening with 8 oz water or empty stomach with no oral intake for at least 30 min. Do not lie down for 30 min after dose
- Teriparatide (Forteo) is a recombinant human parathyroid hormone used for postmenopausal women with osteoporosis who are at high risk for fracture. It is also used in men with primary or hypogonadal osteoporosis who are at high risk of fracture. It is administered via injection 20 mcg qd SQ into thigh or abdominal wall. Use for >2 yr not recommended
- Other FDA-approved drugs (without osteoporosis indication) used to treat osteoporosis:
  1. Calcitriol
  2. Etidronate
  3. Thiazide
- Combination estrogen/alendronate or estrogen-progestin/alendronate may be considered in individualized patients on HRT with identified osteoporosis
- BMD baseline obtained before onset of therapy and at 1 yr; decrease of 2% or greater results in dosage adjustment or medication change
- Baseline biochemical markers of remodeling baseline considered; identified high turnover osteoporosis patients rescreened at 3 mo to document marker return to normal

CHRONIC Rx

- Lifelong disorder requiring lifelong attention to behavior modification issues (nutrition, physical activity, fracture prevention strategies) and compliance with pharmacologic intervention
- Continuing need to eliminate high-risk factors where possible and to diagnose and optimally manage secondary causes of osteoporosis

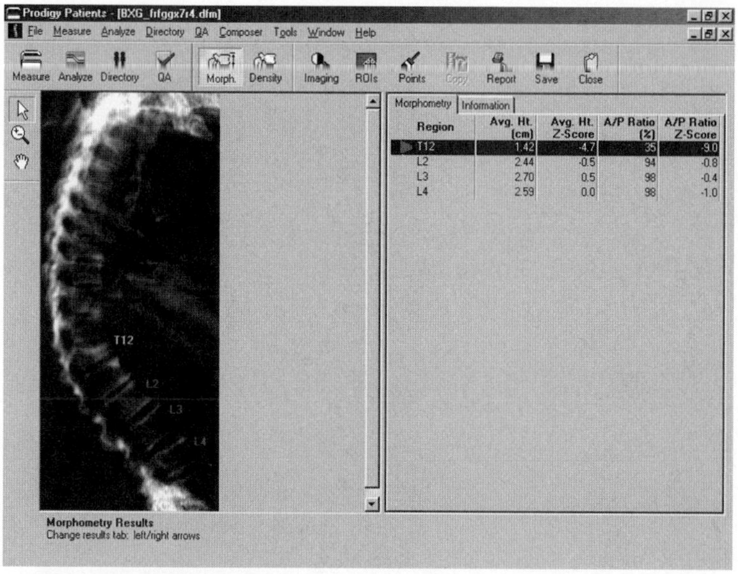

FIGURE 1-183 Vertebral fracture assessment from a dual x-ray absorptiometry image of the spine. Use of dual energy images facilitates the visualization of the lumbar and thoracic spine in a single image. In this example, a fracture has been identified at T12. (From Hochberg MC, Silman AJ, Smolen JS, Weinblatt ME, Weisman MH [eds]: *Rheumatology,* ed 3, St Louis, 2003, Mosby.)

DISPOSITION

Goal for diagnosis and treatment: identification of women at risk, initiation of preventive measures for all women lifelong, institution of treatment modalities that will result in a decrease in fracture risk, and reduction of morbidity, mortality, and unnecessary institutionalization, thereby improving quality of independent life and productivity.

REFERRAL

- To reproductive endocrinologist, endocrinologist, gynecologist, or rheumatologist if unfamiliar with diagnosis and management of osteoporosis
- If multidisciplinary management is required, to other specialties depending on presence of acute fracture and/or secondary associated disorders

EVIDENCE

EBM

In patients taking corticosteroids, calcium and vitamin D therapy are effective at preventing bone loss. In postmenopausal women, calcium and vitamin D appear to reduce the risk of hip fractures and other nonvertebral fractures after 18 months; the effect of either treatment alone is less clear.

Calcium supplementation alone has a small positive effect on bone mineral density (BMD) in postmenopausal women. It probably also reduces the incidence of vertebral fractures.[1] (A)

Vitamin D with or without calcium supplementation appeared to decrease vertebral fractures in one meta-analysis and may also decrease nonvertebral fractures. No conclusions can be drawn about the relative effects of standard vitamin D and hydroxylated vitamin D.[2] (A)

However, another review of 14 randomized controlled trials (RCTs), has concluded that there is still uncertainty about the efficacy of treatment with vitamin D or its analogs in the prevention of fractures in elderly men and in women with involutional or postmenopausal osteoporosis.[3] (A)

Two further RCTs examining the effects of vitamin D_3 alone vs. placebo have produced conflicting results.[4] (A)

Hormone replacement therapy (HRT) improves BMD and probably reduces the incidence of fracture in postmenopausal women. However, the overall health risks from HRT in this population appear to exceed the possible benefits.

HRT has been shown to have a consistent, favorable, and large effect on BMD at all sites, with a nonsignificant trend toward a reduced incidence of vertebral and nonvertebral fractures.[5] (A)

Two recent large RCTs have concluded that the risks of HRT for indications such as the prevention of osteoporosis outweigh the benefits.[6] Ⓐ

Risedronate substantially reduces the risk of both vertebral and nonvertebral fracture after the menopause.[7] Ⓐ

Evidence suggests that alendronate increases BMD in men with osteoporosis.

Calcitriol can reduce the rate of new vertebral deformity at 1 year in postmenopausal women.

Two small RCTs included in a systematic review found a decrease in development of new vertebral deformity with women taking calcitriol vs. control.[3] Ⓑ

The evidence concerning exercise as a means of decreasing the rate of fractures due to falls is not clear.

Two systematic reviews have studied the effect of exercise on fall reduction and subsequent fracture. They have produced conflicting results that have been difficult to analyze due to the differences in methods used and types of exercise studied.[8] Ⓐ

The use of hip protectors may be associated with a reduction of hip fractures in the frail and elderly but the evidence is inconsistent.

One systematic review analyzing only the results from cluster randomized studies indicates that, for those living in institutional care, the incidence of hip fracture can be reduced by the provision of hip protectors. There may however, be difficulties due to discomfort and practicality of use.[9] Ⓐ

However, three RCTs found no significant difference in hip fracture occurrence in the groups using hip protectors vs. control, and one RCT only found a decrease in hip fracture rate of borderline significance in the hip protector group.[10,11] Ⓐ

A multifactorial interventional approach including nursing home staff education, exercise, walking aid provision, environmental manipulation, drug regime reviews, and the use of hip protectors significantly decreases the rate of hip fractures.

Evidence-Based References

1. Shea B et al: The Osteoporosis Methodology Group, and the Osteoporosis Research Advisory Group. Calcium supplementation on bone loss in postmenopausal women.
2. Papadimitropoulos E et al: The Osteo porosis Methodology Group and the Osteoporosis Research Advisory Group. Meta-analyses of therapies for postmenopausal osteoporosis. VIII: Meta-analysis of the efficacy of vitamin D treatment in preventing osteoporosis in postmenopausal women, *Endocr Rev* 23:560, 2002. Reviewed in: 11:1450, 2004. Ⓐ
3. Gillespie WJ et al: Vitamin D and vitamin D analogues for preventing fractures associated with involutional and postmenopausal osteoporosis. Reviewed in: Cochrane Library, 3, Chichester, UK, 2004, John Wiley. Ⓐ
4. Trivedi DP, Doll R, Khaw KT: Effect of four monthly oral vitamin D3 (cholecalciferol) supplementation on fractures and mortality in men and women living in the community: randomised double blind controlled trial, *BMJ* 326:469, 2003. 11:1450, 2004. Ⓐ
5. Wells G et al: The Osteoporosis Methodology Group and The Osteoporosis Research Advisory Group: Meta-analyses of therapies for postmenopausal osteoporosis. V. Meta-analysis of the efficacy of hormone replacement therapy in treating and preventing osteoporosis in postmenopausal women, *Endocr Rev* 23:529, 2002. Ⓑ
6. Writing Group for the Women's Health Initiative Investigators: Risks and benefits of estrogen plus progestin in healthy postmenopausal women: principal results from the Women's Health Initiative randomized controlled trial, *JAMA* 288:321, 2002. 11:1450, 2004. Ⓐ
7. Cranney A et al: Risedronate for the prevention and treatment of postmenopausal osteoporosis, *Cochrane Database Syst Rev* 4, 2003. Ⓐ
8. Gillespie LD et al: Interventions for preventing falls in elderly people, *Cochrane Database Syst Rev* 4, 2003. Ⓐ
9. Parker MJ, Gillespie LD, Gillespie WJ: Hip protectors for preventing hip fractures in the elderly, *Cochrane Database Syst Rev* 3, 2004. Ⓐ
10. van Schoor NM et al: Prevention of hip fractures by external hip protectors: a randomised controlled trial, *JAMA* 289:1957, 2003. 11:1450, 2004. Ⓐ
11. Meyer G et al: Effect on hip fractures of increased use of hip protectors in nursing homes: cluster randomised controlled trial, *BMJ* 326:76, 2003. 11:1450. Ⓐ

SUGGESTED READINGS

Bone HG et al: Ten years' experience with alendronate for osteoporosis in postmenopausal women, *N Engl J Med* 350:12, 2004.

Raisz LG: Screening for osteoporosis, *N Engl J Med* 353:164, 2005.

Rosen CJ: Postmenopausal osteoporosis, *N Engl J Med* 353:595, 2005.

AUTHORS: **DENNIS M. WEPPNER, M.D.,** and **RUBEN ALVERO, M.D.**

BASIC INFORMATION

DEFINITION

Otitis externa is a term encompassing a variety of conditions causing inflammation and/or infection of the external auditory canal (and/or auricle and tympanic membrane). There are six subgroups of otitis externa:

- Acute localized otitis externa (furunculosis)
- Acute diffuse bacterial otitis externa (swimmer's ear)
- Chronic otitis externa
- Eczematous otitis externa
- Fungal otitis externa (otomycosis)
- Invasive or necrotizing (malignant) otitis externa (Fig. 1-184.)

SYNONYMS

See "Definition."

ICD-9CM CODES
38.10 Otitis externa

EPIDEMIOLOGY & DEMOGRAPHICS

INCIDENCE (IN U.S.)

- Among the most common disorders
- Affects 3% to 10% of patients seeking otologic care

PREVALENCE (IN U.S.)

- Diffuse otitis externa (swimmer's ear) is most often seen in swimmers and in hot, humid climates, conditions that lead to water retention in the ear canal.
- Necrotizing otitis externa is more common in elderly, diabetics, immunocompromised patients.

PREDOMINANT SEX: None

PREDOMINANT AGE:

- Occurs at all ages
- Necrotizing otitis externa: typically occurs in elderly: mean age >65 yr

PHYSICAL FINDINGS & CLINICAL PRESENTATION

The two most common symptoms are otalgia, ranging from pruritus to severe pain exacerbated by motion (e.g., chewing), and otorrhea. Patients may also experience aural fullness and hearing loss secondary to swelling with occlusion of the canal. More intense symptoms may occur with bacterial otitis externa, with or without fever, and lymphadenopathy (anterior to tragus). There are also findings unique to the various forms of the infection:

- Acute localized otitis externa (furunculosis):
  1. Occurs from infected hair follicles, usually in the outer third of the ear canal, forming pustules and furuncles
  2. Furuncles are superficial and pointing or deep and diffuse
- Impetigo:
  1. In contrast to furunculosis, this is a superficial spreading infection of the ear canal that may also involve the concha and the auricle
  2. Begins as a small blister that ruptures, releasing straw-colored fluid that dries as a golden crust
- Erysipelas:
  1. Caused by group A streptococcus
  2. May involve the concha and canal
  3. May involve the dermis and deeper tissues
  4. Area of cellulitis, often with severe pain
  5. Fever chills, malaise
  6. Regional adenopathy
- Eczematous otitis externa:
  1. Stems from a variety of dermatologic problems that can involve the external auditory canal
  2. Severe itching, erythema, scaling, crusting, and fissuring possible
- Acute diffuse otitis externa (swimmer's ear):
  1. Begins with itching and a feeling of pressure and fullness in the ear that becomes increasingly tender and painful
  2. Mild erythema and edema of the external auditory canal, which may cause narrowing and occlusion of the canal, leading to hearing loss
  3. Minimal serous secretions, which may become profuse and purulent
  4. Tympanic membrane may appear dull and infected
  5. Usually absence of systemic symptoms such as fever, chills
- Otomycosis:
  1. Chronic superficial infection of the ear canal and tympanic membrane
  2. In primary fungal infection, major symptom is intense itching
  3. In secondary infection (fungal infection superimposed on bacterial infection), major symptom is pain
  4. Fungal growth of variety of colors
- Chronic otitis externa:
  1. Dry and atrophic canal
  2. Typically, lack of cerumen
  3. Itching, often severe, and mild discomfort rather than pain
  4. Occasionally, mucopurulent discharge
  5. With time, thickening of the walls of the canal, causing narrowing of the lumen
- Necrotizing otitis externa (also known as malignant otitis externa). Typically seen in older patients with diabetes or in patients who are immunocompromised.
  1. Redness, swelling, and tenderness of the ear canal
  2. Classic finding of granulation tissue on the floor of the canal and the bone-cartilage junction
  3. Small ulceration of necrotic soft tissue at bone-cartilage junction
  4. Most common complaints: pain (often severe) and otorrhea
  5. Lessening of purulent drainage as infection advances
  6. Facial nerve palsy often the first and only cranial nerve defect
  7. Possible involvement of other cranial nerves

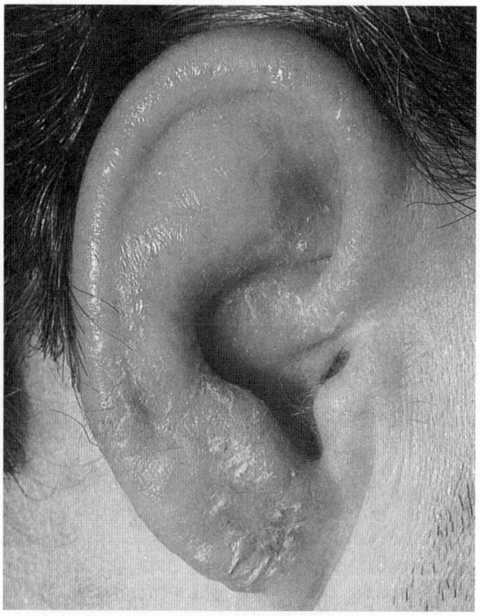

FIGURE 1-184 Malignant external otitis. Severe infection of the ear has occurred after months of chronic inflammation of the pinna. (From Habif TP: *Clinical dermatology: a color guide to diagnosis and therapy,* ed 3, St Louis, 1996, Mosby.)

ETIOLOGY

- Acute localized otitis externa: *Staphylococcus aureus*
- Impetigo:
  1. *S. aureus*
  2. *Streptococcus pyogenes*
- Erysipelas: *S. pyogenes*

- Eczematous otitis externa:
  1. Seborrheic dermatitis
  2. Atopic dermatitis
  3. Psoriasis
  4. Neurodermatitis
  5. Lupus erythematosus
- Acute diffuse otitis externa:
  1. Swimming
  2. Hot, humid climates
  3. Tightly fitting hearing aids
  4. Use of ear plugs
  5. *Pseudomonas aeruginosa*
  6. *S. aureus*
- Otomycosis:
  1. Prolonged use of topical antibiotics and steroid preparations
  2. *Aspergillus* (80% to 90%)
  3. *Candida*
- Chronic otitis externa: persistent low-grade infection and inflammation
- Necrotizing otitis externa (NOE):
  1. Complication of persistent otitis externa
  2. Extends through Santorini's fissures, small apertures at the bone-cartilage junction of the canal, into the mastoid and along the base of the skull
  3. *P. aeruginosa*

DIAGNOSIS (Dx)

DIFFERENTIAL DIAGNOSIS

- Acute otitis media
- Bullous myringitis
- Mastoiditis
- Foreign bodies
- Neoplasms

WORKUP

Thorough history and physical examination

LABORATORY TESTS

- Cultures from the canal are usually not necessary unless the patient is refractory to treatment.
- Leukocyte count normal or mildly elevated.
- ESR is often quite elevated in malignant otitis externa.

IMAGING STUDIES

- CT scan is the best technique for defining bone involvement and extent of disease in malignant otitis externa.
- MRI is slightly more sensitive in evaluation of soft tissue changes.
- Gallium scans are more specific than bone scans in diagnosing NOE.
- Follow-up scans are helpful in determining efficacy of treatment.

NOTE: Expert opinion supports history and physical examination as the best means of diagnosis. Persistent pain that is constant and severe should raise the question of NOE (particularly in elderly, diabetics, and immunocompromised).

TREATMENT (Rx)

NONPHARMACOLOGIC THERAPY

- Cleansing and debridement of the ear canal with cotton swabs and hydrogen peroxide or other antiseptic solution allows for a more thorough examination of the ear.
- If the canal lumen is edematous and too narrow to allow adequate cleansing, a cotton wick or gauze strip inserted into the canal serves as a conduit for topical medications to be drawn into the canal. Usually remove wick after 2 days.
- Local heat is useful in treating deep furunculosis.
- Incision and drainage is indicated in treatment of superficial pointing furunculosis.

ACUTE GENERAL Rx

Topical medications:

- An acidifying agent, such as 2% acetic acid, inhibits growth of bacteria and fungi
- Topical antibiotics (in the form of otic or ophthalmic solutions) or antifungals, often in combination with an acidifying agent and a steroid preparation
- The following are some of the available preparations:
  1. Neomycin otic solutions and suspensions:
     a. with polymyxin-B-hydrocortisone (Corticosporin)
     b. with hydrocortisone-thonzonium (Coly-Mycin S)
  2. Polymyxin-B-hydrocortisone (Otobiotic)
  3. Quinolone otic solutions:
     a. Ofloxacin 0.3% solution (Floxin Otic)
     b. Ciprofloxacin 0.3% with hydrocortisone (Cipro HC)
  4. Quinolone ophthalmic solutions:
     a. Ofloxacin 0.3% (Ocuflox)
     b. Ciprofloxacin 0.3% (Ciloxan)
  5. Aminoglycoside ophthalmic solutions:
     a. Gentamicin sulfate 0.3% (Garamycin)
     b. Tobramycin sulfate 0.3% (Tobrex)
     c. Tobramycin 0.3% and dexamethasone 0.1% (TobraDex)
  6. Chloramphenicol 0.5% otic solution or 0.25% ophthalmic solution (Chloromycetin)
  7. Gentian violet (methylrosaniline chloride 1%, 2%)
  8. Antifungals:
     a. Amphotericin B 3% (Fungizone lotion)
     b. Clotrimazole 1% solution (Lotrimin)
     c. Tolnaftate 1% (Tinactin)
- Topical preparations should be applied qid (bid for quinolones, antifungals), generally for 3 days after cessation of symptoms (average 10 to 14 days total)

Systemic antibiotics:

- Reserved for severe cases, most often infections with *P. aeruginosa* or *S. aureus*
- Treatment usually for 10 days with ciprofloxacin 750 mg q12h or ofloxacin 400 mg q12h, or with antistaphylococcal agent (e.g., dicloxacillin or cephalexin 500 mg q6h)

Treatment for NOE:

- Requires prolonged therapy up to 3 mo. Whether to use oral parenteral therapy is based on clinical judgment
- Oral quinolones, ciprofloxacin 750 mg q12h or ofloxacin 400 mg q12h may be appropriate initial therapy or used to shorten the course of IV therapy
- Intravenous antipseudomonals with or without aminoglycosides are also appropriate
- Local debridement

Pain control:

- May require NSAIDs or opioids
- Topical corticosteroids to reduce swelling and inflammation

CHRONIC Rx

- Patients prone to recurrent infections should try to identify and avoid precipitants to infection.
- Swimmers should try tight-fitting ear plugs or tight-fitting bathing caps, and remove all excess water from the ears after swimming.
- Treat underlying systemic diseases and dermatologic conditions that predispose to infection.

DISPOSITION

Inadequate treatment of otitis externa may lead to NOE and mastoiditis.

REFERRAL

To an otolaryngologist:

- NOE
- Treatment failure
- Severe pain

PEARLS & CONSIDERATIONS (!)

Otitis externa varies in severity from a mild irritation of the external acoustic canal (swimmer's ear) that resolves spontaneously by simply removing the offending agent (stay out of fresh water or wear ear plugs) to a life-threatening infection with the risk of intracranial extension, gram-negative bacterial meningitis, and severe neurologic impairment with multiple cranial neuropathy. Don't miss severe malignant otitis externa in patients who are diabetic or immunocompromised.

EVIDENCE

EBM

Topical methylprednisolone-neomycin drops are an effective treatment of acute and chronic diffuse otitis externa.[1] Ⓐ

Treatment with drops containing acetic acid alone results in a significantly lower cure rate and higher recurrence of symptoms of acute otitis media compared with treatment with corticosteroid and acetic acid or steroid and antibiotic drops.[2] Ⓑ

In the treatment of acute diffuse otitis externa, no clinical benefit is derived from the addition of an oral antibiotic to a regimen of topical triamcinolone-neomycin-gramicidin ointment.[3] Ⓐ

Evidence has not found topical quinolone preparations to be superior to other topical antiinfectives in the treatment of acute otitis externa.[4,5] Ⓐ

In the treatment of moderate to severe acute or chronic diffuse otitis externa, topical treatment with triamcinolone-neomycin undecenoate is associated with a higher resolution rate than hydrocortisone-neomycin sulfate-polymyxin B treatment.[6] Ⓐ

Limited evidence suggests that topical preparations of neomycin-dexamethasone-acetic acid may be associated with an improved clinical outcome compared with agents not containing acetic acid.[7,8] Ⓐ

Evidence-Based References

1. Cannon SJ, Grunwaldt E: Treatment of otitis externa with a topical steroid-antibiotic combination, *Eye Ear Nose Throat Mon* 46:1296-1302, 1967. Reviewed by *Clin Evid* 11:677, 2004. Ⓐ
2. van Balen FA et al: Clinical efficacy of three common treatments in acute otitis externa in primary care: randomised controlled trial, *BMJ* 327:1201, 2003. Ⓑ
3. Yelland MJ: The efficacy of co-trimoxazole in the treatment of otitis externa in general practice, *Med J Aust* 158:697-699, 1999. Reviewed in: *Clin Evid* 11:677, 2004. Ⓐ
4. Pistorius B et al: Prospective, randomized, comparative trial of ciprofloxacin otic drops, with or without hydrocortisone, vs polymyxin B-neomycin-hydrocortisone otic suspension in the treatment of acute diffuse otitis externa, *Infect Dis Clin Pract* 8:387, 1999. Reviewed in: *Clin Evid* 11:677, 2004. Ⓐ
5. Jones RN, Milazzo J, Seidlin M: Ofloxacin otic solution for treatment of otitis externa in children and adults, *Arch Otolaryngol Head Neck Surg* 123:1193, 1997. Reviewed in: *Clin Evid* 11:677, 2004. Ⓐ
6. Worgan D: Treatment of otitis externa. Report of a clinical trial, *Practitioner* 202:817-820, 1969. Reviewed in: *Clin Evid* 11:677, 2004. Ⓐ
7. Smith RB, Moodie J: A general practice study to compare the efficacy and tolerability of a spray ("Otomize") versus a standard drop formulation ("Sofradex") in the treatment of patients with otitis externa, *Curr Med Res Opin* 12:12, 1990. Reviewed in: *Clin Evid* 11:677, 2004. Ⓐ
8. Smith RB, Moodie J: Comparative efficacy and tolerability of two antibacterial/anti-inflammatory formulations ('Otomize' spray and 'Otosporin' drops) in the treatment of otitis externa in general practice, *Curr Res Med Opin* 11:661, 1990. Reviewed in: *Clin Evid* 11:677, 2004. Ⓐ

SUGGESTED READINGS

Block SL: Otitis externa: providing relief while avoiding complications, *J Fam Pract* 54(8):669, 2005.

Cantrell HF et al: Declining susceptibility to neomycin and polymyxin B of pathogens recovered in otitis externa clinical trials, *South Med J* 97(5):465, 2004.

Hajioff D: Otitis externa, *Clin Evid* (12):755, 2004.

McCoy SI, Zell ER, Besser RE: Antimicrobial prescribing for otitis externa in children, *Pediatr Infect Dis J* 23(2):181, 2004.

Rutka J: Acute otitis externa: treatment perspectives, *Ear Nose Throat J* 83(9 Suppl 4):20, 2004.

AUTHORS: **GLENN G. FORT, M.D., M.P.H., DENNIS J. MIKOLICH, M.D.,** and **JANE V. EASON, M.D.**

BASIC INFORMATION

DEFINITION

Otitis media is the presence of fluid in the middle ear accompanied by signs and symptoms of infection.

SYNONYMS

Acute suppurative otitis media
Purulent otitis media

ICD-9CM CODES
382.9 Acute or chronic otitis media
382.10 381.00 Otitis media with effusion

EPIDEMIOLOGY & DEMOGRAPHICS

INCIDENCE (IN U.S.):
- Affects patients of all ages, but is largely a disease of infants and young children
- Occurs once in about 75% of all children
- Occurs three or more times in one third of all children by 3 yr of age
- The diagnosis of acute otitis media increased from 9.9 million in 1975 to 25.5 million in 1990
- From 1975 to 1990, office visits for acute otitis media increased threefold for children <2 yr, doubled for children ages 2 to 5, and almost doubled for children ages 6 to 10 yr

PEAK INCIDENCE:
- Between 6 and 36 mo
- Second peak between ages 4 and 6 yr
- Fall, winter, early spring

PREDOMINANT SEX: Males

PREDOMINANT AGE:
- 47% to 60% of all children have their first episode of OM during their first year of life, 60% to 70% by their fourth birthday
- Incidence of infection declines with age; seen infrequently in adults

GENETICS:

Familial Disposition:
- Native Americans
- Eskimos
- Australian aborigines
- Those with a strong family history

Congenital Infection: High incidence in children born with cleft palates and other craniofacial abnormalities

PHYSICAL FINDINGS & CLINICAL PRESENTATION

- Fluid in the middle ear along with signs and symptoms of local inflammation (Figs. 1-185 and 1-186).
  1. Erythema with diminished light reflex
- Erythema of the tympanic membrane without other abnormalities is not a diagnostic criterion for acute otitis media because it may occur with any inflammation of the upper respiratory tract, crying, or nose blowing.
- As infection progresses, middle ear exudation occurs (exudative phase); the exudate rapidly changes from serous to purulent (suppurative phase).
  1. Retraction and poor motility of the tympanic membrane, which then becomes bulging and convex
- At any time during the suppurative phase the tympanic membrane may rupture, releasing the middle ear contents.
- Symptoms:
  1. Otalgia, ranging from slight discomfort to severe, spreading to the temporal region
  2. Ear stuffiness and hearing loss may precede or follow otalgia
  3. Otorrhea
  4. Vertigo, nystagmus, tinnitus, fever, lethargy, irritability, nausea, vomiting, anorexia
- After an episode of acute otitis media:
  1. Persistence of effusion for weeks or months (called secretory, serous, or nonsuppurative otitis media)
  2. Fever and otalgia usually absent
  3. Hearing loss possible (10 to 50 dB, with predominant involvement of the low frequencies)

ETIOLOGY

- Most common etiologic factor is an upper respiratory tract infection (often viral), which causes inflammation and obstruction of the eustachian tube. Bacterial colonization of the nasopharynx in conjunction with eustachian tube dysfunction leads to infection.
- May occasionally develop as a result of hematogenous spread or via direct invasion from the nasopharynx.
- Most common bacterial pathogens:
  1. *Streptococcus pneumoniae* causes 40% to 50% of cases and is the least likely of the major pathogens to resolve without treatment
  2. *Haemophilus influenzae* causes 20% to 30% of cases
  3. *Moraxella catarrhalis* causes 10% to 15% of cases
  4. Of increasing importance, infection caused by penicillin-nonsusceptible *S. pneumoniae* (MIC >0.1 μg/ml), ranging from 8% to 34%. About 50% of PNSSP isolates are penicillin-intermediate (MIC-0.1 to 2.0 μg/ml)
- Viral pathogens:
  1. Respiratory syncytial virus
  2. Rhinovirus

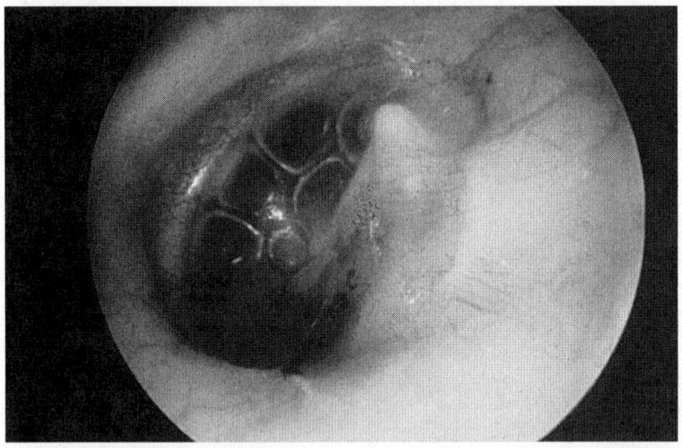

FIGURE 1-185 Otitis media with effusion of left ear. Retracted eardrum, prominent short process of malleus, and air bubbles seen anteriorly through the tympanic membrane. (From Behrman RE: *Nelson textbook of pediatrics,* ed 16, Philadelphia, 1996, WB Saunders.)

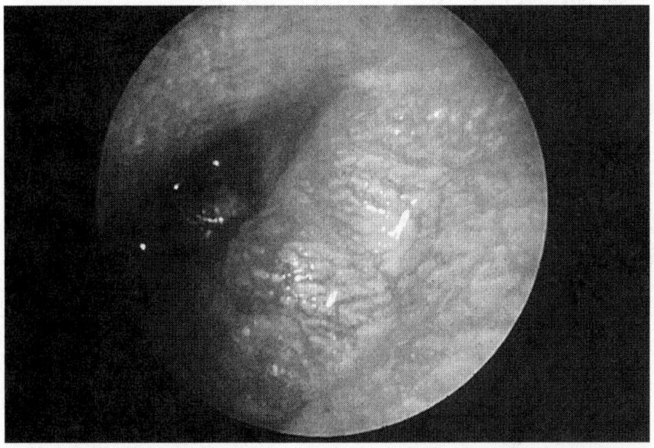

FIGURE 1-186 Acute left otitis media. (From Behrman RE: *Nelson textbook of pediatrics,* ed 16, Philadelphia, 1996, WB Saunders.)

3. Adenovirus
4. Influenza
- Others:
1. *Mycoplasma pneumoniae*
2. *Chlamydia trachomatis*

DIAGNOSIS

Dx

DIFFERENTIAL DIAGNOSIS

- Otitis externa
- Referred pain
1. Mouth
2. Nasopharynx
3. Tonsils
4. Other parts of the upper respiratory tract
- Section II describes the differential diagnosis of earache

WORKUP

Thorough otoscopic examination; adequate visualization of the tympanic membrane requires removal of cerumen and debris.

- Tympanometry
1. Measures compliance of the tympanic membrane and middle ear pressure
2. Detects the presence of fluid
- Acoustic reflectometry
1. Measures sound waves reflected from the middle ear
2. Useful in infants >3 mo
3. Increased reflected sound correlated with the presence of effusion

LABORATORY TESTS

- Tympanocentesis
1. Not necessary in most cases as the microbiology of middle ear effusions has been shown to be quite consistent
2. May be indicated in:
   a. Highly toxic patients
   b. Patients who fail to respond to treatment in 48 to 72 hr
   c. Immunocompromised patients
- Cultures of the nasopharynx: sensitive but not specific
- Blood counts: usually show a leukocytosis with polymorphonuclear elevation
- Plain mastoid radiographs: generally not indicated; will reveal haziness in the periantral cells that may extend to entire mastoid
- CT or MRI may be indicated if serious complications suspected (meningitis, brain abscess)

TREATMENT

Rx

ACUTE GENERAL Rx

Hydration, avoidance of irritants (e.g., tobacco smoke), nasal systemic decongestants, cool mist humidifier

Antimicrobials:

NOTE: Most uncomplicated cases of acute otitis media resolve spontaneously, without complications. Studies have demonstrated limited therapeutic benefit from antibiotic therapy. However, when opting to employ antibiotic therapy:

- Amoxicillin remains the drug of choice for first-line treatment of uncomplicated acute otitis media, despite increasing prevalence of drug-resistant *S. pneumoniae.*
- Treatment failure is defined by lack of clinical improvement of signs or symptoms after 3 days of therapy.
- With treatment failure, in the absence of an identified etiologic pathogen, therapy should be redirected to cover.
1. Drug-resistant *S. pneumoniae*
2. β-lactamase–producing strains of *H. influenzae* and *M. catarrhalis*
- Agents fulfilling these criteria include amoxicillin/clavulanate, second-generation cephalosporins (e.g., cefuroxime axetil, cefaclor); ceftriaxone (given IM). Cefaclor, cefixime, loracarbef and ceftibuten are active against *H. influenzae* and *M. catarrhalis,* but less active against pneumococci, especially drug resistant strains, than the agents listed previously.
- TMP/SMX and macrolides have been used as first- and second-line agents, but pneumococcal resistance to these agents is rising (up to 25% resistance to TMP/SMX, and up to 10% resistance to erythromycin).
- Cross-resistance between these drugs and the β-lactams exist; therefore patients who are treatment failures on amoxicillin are more likely to have infections resistant to TMP/SMX and macrolides.
- Newer fluoroquinolones (grepafloxacin, levofloxacin, moxifloxacin) have enhanced activity against pneumococci as compared with older agents (ciprofloxacin, ofloxacin).
- Treatment should be modified according to cultures and sensitivities.
- Generally treatment course is 10 to 14 days.
- Follow up approximately 4 wk after discontinuation of therapy to verify resolution of all symptoms, return to normal otoscopic findings, and restoration of normal hearing.

NOTE: Effusions may persist for 2 to 6 wk or longer in many cases of adequately treated otitis media.

SURGICAL Rx

- No evidence to support the routine of myringotomy, but in severe cases it provides prompt pain relief and accelerates resolution of infection.
- Purulent secretions retained in the middle ear lead to increased pressure that may lead to spread of infection to contiguous areas. Myringotomy to decompress the middle ear is necessary to avoid complications.
- Complications include mastoiditis, facial nerve paralysis, labyrinthitis, meningitis, brain abscess.
- Other procedures used for drainage of the middle ear include insertion of a ventilation tube and/or simple mastoidectomy.

CHRONIC Rx

- Myringotomy and tympanostomy tube placement for persistent middle ear effusion unresponsive to medical therapy for ≥3 mo if bilateral or ≥6 mo if unilateral.
- Adenoidectomy, with or without tonsillectomy, often advocated for treatment of recurrent otitis media, although indications for this procedure are controversial.
- Chronic complications include tympanic membrane perforations, cholesteatoma, tympanosclerosis, ossicular necrosis, toxic or suppurative labyrinthitis, and intracranial suppuration.

DISPOSITION

Patients can be treated at home as outpatients with the rare exception of patients with evidence of local suppurative complications (e.g., meningitis, acute mastoiditis, brain abscess, cavernous sinus, or lateral vein thrombosis).

REFERRAL

- To otorhinolaryngologist if:
1. Medical treatment failure
2. Diagnosis uncertain: adults with ≥1 episode of otitis media should be referred for ENT evaluation to rule out underlying process (e.g., malignancy)
3. Any of the above mentioned acute and chronic complications

PEARLS & CONSIDERATIONS

!

COMMENTS

Prevention:

- Multiple component conjugate vaccines hold promise for decreasing recurrent episodes of acute otitis media
- Breast-feeding, bottle-feeding infants in an upright position
- Avoidance of irritants (e.g., tobacco smoke)

EVIDENCE

EBM

Antibiotics appear to have a modest role in the management of acute otitis media.

In acute otitis media in children, a short course of an appropriate antibiotic is modestly effective.[1-4] Ⓐ

There is no evidence that the choice of a particular antibiotic influences the outcome, and extending antimicrobial coverage to include beta-lactamase-producing organisms did not significantly increase the rates of primary control or resolution of middle ear effusion.[1] Ⓐ

However, in children younger than 2 years with acute otitis media, antibiotic therapy may not be effective.[5] Ⓐ

Immediate use of antibiotics vs. delayed use reduces the duration of earache, the number of disturbed nights, the number of days of crying, and the consumption of acetaminophen. However, it does not reduce the mean daily pain score, the number of episodes of pain each day, or the number of days of absence from school.[6] Ⓐ

There is conflicting evidence about the effects of antibiotics in otitis media with effusion.

A systematic review found that antibiotics vs. placebo or vs. no treatment significantly increased resolution of effusion at follow-up for up to 1 month.[7] Ⓐ

However, another systematic review failed to find a significant effect on cure rate of effusion with antibiotics vs. placebo.[8] Ⓐ

In chronic otitis media with suppuration, oral antibiotics seem to be associated with resolution of otorrhea but are less effective than topical antibiotics.

A systematic review of randomized trials of any method of management for patients with eardrum perforation and persistent otorrhea concluded that treatment with antibiotics or antiseptics accompanied by aural toilet was more effective in resolving otorrhea than no treatment or aural toilet alone.[9] Ⓐ

However, the review concluded that long-term outcomes, such as prevention of recurrence, closure of tympanic perforation, and hearing improvement, need to be further evaluated.[9] Ⓐ

Trials included in this review compared topical vs. systemic antibiotics and found that systemic treatment was less effective.[10,11] Ⓐ

There is some evidence supporting the effectiveness of tympanostomy tubes in the management of otitis media with effusion.

The insertion of tympanostomy tubes in children with otitis media with effusion has been found to result in hearing improvement.[12] Ⓐ

There is conflicting evidence about the efficacy of adenoidectomy in the treatment of otitis media with effusion.

Adenoidectomy has been shown to give little additional benefit over tympanostomy tubes alone in terms of hearing gain.[12] Ⓐ

However, a subsequent randomized controlled trial of adenotonsillectomy or adenoidectomy vs. neither procedure found that there was a statistically significant benefit in combining adenoidectomy with tympanostomy tubes in terms of reduced duration of otitis media with effusion.[13] Ⓐ

Analgesia may be effective in reducing earache but not other outcomes.

A randomized controlled trial in children with acute otitis media, receiving antibiotic treatment with cefaclor for 7 days, compared the effect of three times daily ibuprofen or paracetamol vs. placebo (for 48 hr). It found that paracetamol vs. placebo significantly reduced earache. No difference was found between paracetamol and ibuprofen, and none between ibuprofen or paracetamol and placebo for other outcomes.[14] Ⓐ

Evidence-Based References

1. Rosenfeld RM et al: Clinical efficacy of antimicrobial drugs for acute otitis media: metaanalysis of 5400 children from thirty-three randomized trials, *J Pediatr* 124:355, 1994. Reviewed in: *Clin Evid* 11:314, 2004. Ⓐ
2. Marcy M et al: Management of acute otitis media. Evidence Report/Technology Assessment No.15. AHRQ Publication No 01-E010. Rockville, MD: Agency for Healthcare Research and Quality, May 2001. Reviewed in: *Clin Evid* 11:314, 2004. Ⓐ
3. Glasziou PP et al: Antibiotics for acute otitis media in children. Reviewed in: Cochrane Library, 2, Chichester, UK, 2004, John Wiley. Ⓐ
4. Kozyrskyj AL et al: Short course antibiotics for acute otitis media. Reviewed in: Cochrane Library, 2, Chichester, UK, 2004, John Wiley. Ⓐ
5. Damoiseaux RA et al: Antibiotic treatment of acute otitis media in children under two years of age: evidence based? *Br J Gen Pract* 48:1861, 1998. Reviewed in: *Clin Evid* 11:314, 2004. Ⓐ
6. Little P et al: Pragmatic randomised controlled trial of two prescribing strategies for childhood acute otitis media, *BMJ* 322:336, 2001. Reviewed in: *Clin Evid* 11:314, 2004. Ⓐ
7. Stool SE et al: Otitis media with effusion in young children: clinical practice guideline number 12. AHPCR Publication 94-0622, Rockville, MD, Agency of Health Care Policy and Research, Public Health Service, United States Department of Health and Human Services, July 1994. Reviewed in: *Clin Evid* 11:684, 2004. Ⓐ
8. Cantekin EI, McGuire TW: Antibiotics are not effective for otitis media with effusion: reanalysis of meta-analysis, *Otorhinolaryngol Nova* 8:214, 1998. Reviewed in: *Clin Evid* 11:684, 2004. Ⓐ
9. Acuin J, Smith A, Mackenzie I: Interventions for chronic suppurative otitis media. Reviewed in: Cochrane Library, 2, Chichester, UK, 2004, John Wiley. Ⓐ
10. Browning G et al: Controlled trial of medical treatment of active chronic otitis media, *BMJ* 287:1024, 1983. Reviewed in: *Clin Evid* 11:645, 2004. Ⓐ
11. Yuen P et al: Ofloxacin eardrop treatment for active chronic suppurative otitis media: prospective randomized study, *Am J Otol* 15:670, 1994. Reviewed in: *Clin Evid* 11:645, 2004. Ⓐ
12. University of York. Centre for Reviews and Dissemination: The treatment of persistent glue ear in children, *Effective Health Care* 1(4):1992. Reviewed in: *Clin Evid* 11:684, 2004. Ⓐ
13. Maw R, Bawden R: Spontaneous resolution of severe chronic glue ear in children and the effect of adenoidectomy, tonsillectomy, and insertion of ventilation tubes, *BMJ* 306:756, 1993. Reviewed in: *Clin Evid* 11:684, 2004. Ⓐ
14. Bertin L et al: A randomized double blind multicentre controlled trial of ibuprofen versus acetaminophen and placebo for symptoms of acute otitis media in children, *Fundam Clin Pharmacol* 10:387, 1996. Reviewed in: *Clin Evid* 11:314, 2004. Ⓐ

SUGGESTED READINGS

American Academy of Pediatrics/American Academy of Family Physicians: Diagnosis and management of acute otitis media, *Pediatrics* 113(5):1451, 2004.

Brook I, Gober AE: Antimicrobial resistance in the nasopharyngeal flora of children with acute otitis media and otitis media recurring after amoxicillin therapy, *J Med Microbiol* 54(Pt1):83, 2005.

Damoiseaux RA et al: Long-term prognosis of acute otitis media in infancy: determinants of recurrent acute otitis media and persistent middle ear effusion, *Fam Pract* 23(1):40, 2006.

Kenna MA: Otitis media and the new guidelines, *J Otolaryngol* 34 (suppl 1):S24, 2005.

Plasschaert AL et al: Trends in doctor consultations, antibiotic prescription, and specialist referrals for otitis media in children: 1995-2003, *Pediatrics* 117(6):1879, 2006.

Rovers MM et al: Otitis media, *Lancet* 363(9407):465, 2004.

AUTHORS: **GLENN G. FORT, M.D., M.P.H., DENNIS J. MIKOLICH, M.D., JANE V. EASON, M.D.,** and **JOSEPH R. MASCI, M.D.**

BASIC INFORMATION

DEFINITION

Otosclerosis is a conductive hearing loss secondary to fixation of the stapes resulting in gradual hearing loss. About 15% of cases affect only one ear.

ICD-9CM CODES
387.9 Otosclerosis

EPIDEMIOLOGY & DEMOGRAPHICS

INCIDENCE (IN U.S.): Most common cause of hearing loss in young adults
PEAK INCIDENCE: Middle age
PREVALENCE (IN U.S.): 5 cases/1000 persons
PREDOMINANT SEX: Male:female ratio of 2:1
PREDOMINANT AGE: Symptoms start between 15 and 30 yr, with slowly progressive hearing loss.
GENETICS: One half of cases are dominantly inherited.

PHYSICAL FINDINGS & CLINICAL PRESENTATION

- Tympanic membrane is normal in most cases (tested with tuning fork).
- Bone conduction is greater than air conduction.
- Weber test localizes to affected ear.

ETIOLOGY

- A disease where vascular type of spongy bone is laid down
- Unknown

DIAGNOSIS

DIFFERENTIAL DIAGNOSIS

- Hearing loss from any cause: cochlear otosclerosis, polyps, granulomas, tumors, osteogenesis imperfecta, chronic ear infections, trauma.
- A clinical algorithm for evaluation of hearing loss is described in Section III.
- Table 1-33 describes common types of conductive and sensorineural hearing loss.

WORKUP

Audiometry

LABORATORY TESTS

None, unless infection suspected

IMAGING STUDIES

MRI or CT with specific cuts through inner ear (Fig. 1-187)

TREATMENT

NONPHARMACOLOGIC THERAPY

Hearing aid only of temporary use

CHRONIC Rx

Progresses to deafness without surgical intervention

DISPOSITION

Referral to ENT specialist

REFERRAL

To ENT specialist for surgery if moderate hearing loss suspected

PEARLS & CONSIDERATIONS

COMMENTS

A full ENT evaluation in a young or middle-aged person with hearing loss is mandatory unless cause is obvious (such as trauma or repeated infection).

SUGGESTED READING

Chole RA, McKenna M: Pathophysiology of otosclerosis, *Otol Neurotol* 22(2):249, 2001.

AUTHOR: **FRED F. FERRI, M.D.**

TABLE 1-33 Common Types of Conductive and Sensorineural Hearing Loss

Conductive Hearing Loss	Sensorineural Hearing Loss
Otitis media with effusion	Presbycusis (hearing loss with aging)
TM perforation	Ototoxicity
Tympanosclerosis	Meniere's disease
Retracted TM (eustachian tube dysfunction)	Idiopathic loss
Ossicular problems	Noise-induced loss
Otosclerosis	Perilymphatic fistula
Foreign body in ear canal	Hereditary (congenital) loss
Cerumen impaction	Multiple sclerosis
Tumor of the ear canal or middle ear	Diabetes
Cholesteatoma	Syphilis
	Acoustic neuroma

From Rakel RE (ed): *Principles of family practice,* ed 6, Philadelphia, 2002, WB Saunders.
TM, Tympanic membrane.

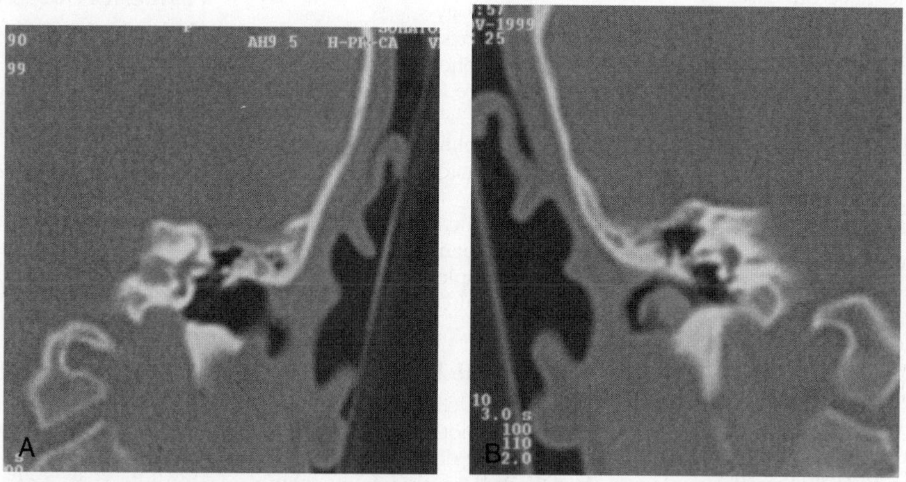

FIGURE 1-187 A patient with conductive hearing loss. By comparing the normal **(A)** and abnormal **(B)** sides on CT scan, the narrowing of the oval window can be clearly appreciated. This results in fixation of the stapes footplate and conductive hearing loss. (From Grainger RG, Allison DJ, Adam A, Dixon AK [eds]: *Grainger & Allison's diagnostic radiology,* ed 4, Philadelphia, 2001, Churchill Livingstone.)

BASIC INFORMATION

DEFINITION

Ovarian tumors can be benign, requiring operative intervention but not recurring or metastasizing; malignant, recurring, metastasizing, and having decreased survival; or borderline, having a small risk of recurrence or metastases but generally having a good prognosis.

SYNONYMS

Epithelial ovarian cancer
Germ cell tumor
Sex cord stromal tumor
Ovarian tumor of low malignant potential

ICD-9CM CODES
183.0 Malignant neoplasm of ovary

EPIDEMIOLOGY & DEMOGRAPHICS

INCIDENCE: 12.9 to 15.1 cases/100,000 persons; approximately 25,000 new cases annually

PREVALENCE: Median age of 61 yr, peaks at age 75 to 79 yr (54/100,000)

GENETICS: Familial susceptibility has been shown with the BRCA1 gene located on 17q12 to 21. This correlates with breast-ovarian cancer syndrome.

RISK FACTORS: Low parity, delayed childbearing, use of talc on the perineum (unlikely), high-fat diet, fertility drugs (unlikely), Lynch II syndrome (nonpolyposis colon cancer, endometrial cancer, breast cancer, and ovarian cancer clusters in first- and second-degree relatives), breast-ovarian familial cancer syndrome, site-specific familial ovarian cancer (NOTE: Use of oral contraceptives appears to have a protective effect.)

PHYSICAL FINDINGS & CLINICAL PRESENTATION

- 60% present with advanced disease
- Abdominal fullness, early satiety, dyspepsia
- Pelvic pain, back pain, constipation
- Pelvic or abdominal mass
- Lymphadenopathy (inguinal)
- Sister Mary Joseph nodule (umbilical mass)

ETIOLOGY

- Can be inherited as site-specific familial ovarian cancer (two or more first-degree relatives have ovarian cancer)
- Breast-ovarian cancer syndrome (clusters of breast and ovarian cancer among first- and second-degree relatives)
- Lynch syndrome
- No family history and unknown etiology in the majority of ovarian cancer cases

DIAGNOSIS (Dx)

DIFFERENTIAL DIAGNOSIS

- Primary peritoneal cancer mesothelioma
- Benign ovarian tumor
- Functional ovarian cyst
- Endometriosis
- Ovarian torsion
- Pelvic kidney
- Pedunculated uterine fibroid
- Primary cancer from breast, GI tract, or other pelvic organ metastasized to the ovary

WORKUP

- Definitive diagnosis made at laparotomy
- Careful physical and history including family history
- Exclusion of nongynecologic etiologies
- Observation of small, cystic masses in premenopausal women for regression for 2 mo

LABORATORY TESTS

- CBC
- Chemistry profile
- CA-125 or lysophosphatidic acid level
- Consider: hCG, Inhibin, AFP, neuron-specific enolase (NSE), and LDH in patients at risk for germ cell tumors

IMAGING STUDIES

- Ultrasound
- Chest x-ray examination
- Mammogram
- CT scan to help evaluate extent of disease
- Other studies (BE, MRI, IVP, etc.) as clinically indicated

TREATMENT (Rx)

NONPHARMACOLOGIC THERAPY

Virtually all cases of ovarian cancer involve surgical exploration. This includes:

- Abdominal cytology
- Total abdominal hysterectomy and bilateral salpingo-oophorectomy (except in early stages where fertility is an issue)
- Omentectomy
- Diaphragm sampling
- Selective lymphadenectomy (pelvis and paraaortic)
- Primary cytoreduction with a goal of residual tumor diameter <2 cm
- Bowel surgery, splenectomy if needed to obtain optimal (<2 cm) cytoreduction

ACUTE GENERAL Rx

- Optimal cytoreduction is generally followed by chemotherapy (except in some early-stage disease).
- Cisplatin-based combination chemotherapy is used for stage II or greater, 6 mo treatment. As compared with intravenous paclitaxel plus cisplatin, IV paclitaxel plus intraperitoneal cisplatin and paclitaxel improves survival in patients with optimally debulked stage III ovarian cancer.
- Chemotherapy regimens continue to change as research continues.
- Consider second-look surgery when chemotherapy is complete.

CHRONIC Rx

- If CA-125 have recurrent disease
- Physical and pelvic examinations every 3 mo for 2 yr, every 4 mo during third year, then every 6 mo
- CA-125 every visit
- Yearly Pap smear

DISPOSITION

- Overall 5-yr survival rates remain low because of the preponderance of late-stage disease:
  Stage I and II 80% to 100%
  Stage III 15% to 20%
  Stage IV 5%
- Younger patients (<50 yr) in all stages have a considerably better 5-yr survival than older patients (40% vs. 15%).

EVIDENCE (EBM)

A systematic review found some evidence in favor of platinum-based therapy compared with non-platinum-based therapy, and there is some evidence for combination regimens compared with platinum alone. However, the evidence is not conclusive.[1] Ⓐ

Women with advanced ovarian cancer who had responded to platinum-paclitaxel combination therapy were found to have significantly longer progression-free survival with 12 further cycles of single-agent paclitaxel than with 3 further cycles. There was no difference between treatment groups in terms of overall survival.[2] Ⓑ

Evidence-Based References

1. Advanced Ovarian Cancer Trialists Group: Chemotherapy for advanced ovarian cancer. Reviewed in: Cochrane Library, 3, Chichester, UK, 2004, John Wiley. Ⓐ
2. Markman M et al: Southwest Oncology Group. Gynecologic Oncology Group: Phase III randomized trial of 12 versus 3 months of maintenance paclitaxel in patients with advanced ovarian cancer after complete response to platinum and paclitaxel-based chemotherapy: a Southwest Oncology Group and Gynecologic Oncology Group, *J Clin Oncol* 21:2460, 2003. Ⓑ

SUGGESTED READINGS

Armstrong D et al: Intraperitoneal cisplatin and paclitaxel in ovarian cancer, *N Engl J Med* 354:34, 2006.

Yawn BP et al: Ovarian cancer: the neglected diagnosis, *Mayo Clinic Proc* 79(10):1277, 2004.

AUTHORS: **GIL FARKASH, M.D.**, and **RUBEN ALVERO, M.D.**

BASIC INFORMATION

DEFINITION

Benign ovarian neoplasms are often clinically indistinguishable from their malignant counterparts. Therefore all persistent adnexal masses must be considered malignant until proven otherwise. Nonneoplastic tumors are as follows:

- Germinal inclusion cyst
- Follicle cyst
- Corpus luteum cyst
- Pregnancy luteoma
- Theca lutein cysts
- Sclerocystic ovaries
- Endometrioma

Neoplastic tumors that are derived from coelomic epithelium are as follows:

- Cystic tumors: serous cystoma, mucinous cystoma, mixed forms
- Tumors with stromal overgrowth: fibroma, adenofibroma, Brenner tumor

Tumors derived from germ cells are dermoids (benign cystic teratomas).

ICD-9CM CODES
220 Benign neoplasm of ovary

EPIDEMIOLOGY & DEMOGRAPHICS

- Reproductive years:
  1. Most common benign ovarian neoplasms: serous cystadenoma and benign cystic teratoma
  2. Most common adnexal mass: functional cyst
- Risk of malignancy increases after age 40 yr.
- Infants: adnexal masses are usually follicular cysts secondary to maternal hormone stimulation that regress during first few months of life.
- Childhood:
  1. Adnexal masses are rare.
  2. 8% are malignant.
  3. Almost always dysgerminomas or teratomas (germ cell origin).
  4. Frequency of malignancy is inversely correlated with age.
- Adolescence:
  1. Most common adnexal mass is a functional cyst.
  2. Most common neoplastic ovarian tumor is a benign cystic teratoma.
  3. Solid/cystic adnexal tumors are rare and almost always dysgerminomas or malignant teratomas.

PHYSICAL FINDINGS & CLINICAL PRESENTATION

- Usually asymptomatic
- Pelvic pain/pressure
- Dyspareunia
- Abdominal pain ranging from mild to severe peritoneal irritation
- Increasing abdominal girth/distention
- Adnexal mass of pelvic examination
- Children: abdominal/rectal mass

ETIOLOGY

- Physiologic
- Endometriosis
- Unknown

DIAGNOSIS

DIFFERENTIAL DIAGNOSIS

- Ovarian torsion
- Malignancy: ovary, fallopian tube, colon
- Uterine fibroid
- Diverticular abscess/diverticulitis
- Appendiceal abscess/appendicitis (especially in children)
- Tuboovarian abscess
- Paraovarian cyst
- Distended bladder
- Pelvic kidney
- Ectopic pregnancy
- Retroperitoneal cyst/neoplasm

WORKUP

- Complete history and physical examination
- Pelvic examination/rectovaginal examination to reveal firm, irregular, mobile mass
- Laparoscopy/laparotomy to establish diagnosis

LABORATORY TESTS

- Pregnancy test
- Serum tumor markers:
  1. Cancer antigen 125 (CA 125)
  2. α-Fetoprotein (AFP) (endodermal sinus tumor, immature teratoma)
  3. β-Human chorionic gonadotropin (hCG)
  4. Lactic dehydrogenase (LDH) (dysgerminoma)

IMAGING STUDIES

Ultrasound:

- May differentiate adnexal mass from other pelvic masses
- Features that increase risk of malignancy include solid component, papillae, multiple septations/solitary thick septa, ascites, matted bowel, bilaterality, irregular borders
- CT scan with contrast or IVP
- Colonoscopy/barium enema, if symptomatic

TREATMENT

NONPHARMACOLOGIC THERAPY

Repeat pelvic examination for premenopausal women in 4 to 6 wk.

ACUTE GENERAL Rx

Indications for surgery:

- Postmenopausal or premenarcheal palpable adnexal mass
- Adnexal mass with suspicious ultrasound features
- Premenopausal woman with persistent cyst >5 cm
- Any adnexal mass >10 cm
- Suspected torsion or rupture

CHRONIC Rx

- Depends on diagnosis
- Possible suppression of formation of new cysts by oral contraceptives

DISPOSITION

Depends on diagnosis

REFERRAL

- If malignancy suspected
- If surgery required

SUGGESTED READINGS

Dayal M, Barnhart KT: Noncontraceptive benefits and therapeutic uses of the oral contraceptive pill, *Semin Reprod Med* 19(4):295, 2001.

Doret M, Raudrant D: Functional ovarian cysts and the need to remove them, *Euro J Obstet Gynecol Reprod Biol* 100(1):1, 2001.

Kurjak A, Kupesic S, Simunic V: Ultrasonic assessment of the peri- and postmenopausal ovary, *Maturitas* 41(4):245, 2002.

AUTHORS: **GEORGE T. DANAKAS, M.D.,** and **RUBEN ALVERO, M.D.**

Section I DISEASES AND DISORDERS

BASIC INFORMATION

DEFINITION

Paget's disease of the bone is a nonmetabolic disease of bone characterized by repeated episodes of osteolysis and excessive attempts at repair that results in a weakened bone of increased mass. Monostotic (solitary lesion) and polyostotic (numerous lesions) disease are both described.

SYNONYMS

Osteitis deformans

ICD-9CM CODES
731.0 Paget's disease (osteitis deformans)

EPIDEMIOLOGY & DEMOGRAPHICS

PREVALENCE: Localized lesions in 3% of patients >50 yr
PREDOMINANT SEX: Male:female ratio of 2:1
PREDOMINANT AGE: Rare before 40 yr

PHYSICAL FINDINGS & CLINICAL PRESENTATION

- Many lesions are asymptomatic.
- Onset is variable.
- Symptoms result mainly from the effects of complications:
  1. Skeletal pain, especially hip and pelvis
  2. Bowing of long bones, sometimes leading to pathologic fracture
  3. Increased heat of extremity (resulting from increased vascularity)
  4. Skull enlargement and spinal involvement caused by characteristic bone enlargement, which can produce neurologic complications (vision and hearing loss, radicular pain, and cord compression)
  5. Thoracic kyphoscoliosis
  6. Secondary osteoarthritis, especially of hip
  7. Heart failure as a result of chest and spine deformity and blood shunting

ETIOLOGY

Unknown

DIAGNOSIS

DIFFERENTIAL DIAGNOSIS

- Fibrous dysplasia
- Skeletal neoplasm (primary or metastatic)
- Osteomyelitis
- Hyperparathyroidism
- Vertebral hemangioma

LABORATORY TESTS

- Increased serum alkaline phosphatase (SAP)
- Normal serum calcium and phosphorus levels
- Increased urinary excretion of pyridinoline cross-links, although test is expensive and not usually required in routine cases
- Other: bone biopsy only in uncertain cases or if sarcomatous degeneration is suspected

IMAGING STUDIES

- Appropriate radiographs reflect the characteristic radiolucency and opacity (Fig. 1-188).
- Bone scanning usually reflects the activity and extent of the disease.

TREATMENT

NONPHARMACOLOGIC THERAPY

- Counseling regarding home environment to prevent falls
- Cane for balance and weight-bearing pain

ACUTE GENERAL Rx

- Calcitonin
- Biphosphonates
- NSAIDs for pain relief
- General indications for treatment
  1. All symptomatic patients
  2. Asymptomatic patients with high level of metabolic activity or those at risk for deformity
  3. Preoperative, if surgery involves pagetic site

DISPOSITION

- Many monostotic lesions probably remain asymptomatic.
- Progression of the disease is common.
- Malignant degeneration occurs in <1% of patients and should be considered when there is a sudden increase in pain.
- Sarcomatous change carries a grave prognosis.

REFERRAL

- For dental evaluation if there is involvement of the mandible or maxilla
- For ENT evaluation if there is hearing loss
- For ophthalmologic evaluation if there is impaired vision
- For orthopedic consultation for assessment of pain in bone or joint

PEARLS & CONSIDERATIONS

COMMENTS

Surgical intervention is often required for neurologic complications or joint symptoms

- Often associated with profuse blood loss
- Elective cases: benefit from preoperative treatment to suppress bone activity and vascularity

SUGGESTED READINGS

Bone HG: Nonmalignant complications of Paget's disease, *J Bone Mineral Res* 21(suppl 2):64, 2006.

Haddaway MJ et al: Effect of age and gender on the number and distribution of sites in Paget's disease of bone, *Br J Radiol* 80:532, 2007.

Keating GM, Scott LJ: Zoledronic acid: a review of its use in the treatment of Paget's disease of bone, *Drugs* 67:793, 2007.

Kotocvicz MA: Paget's disease of bone: Diagnosis and indications for treatment, *Aust Fam Physician* 33(3):127, 2004.

Langston AL et al: Clinical determinants of quality of life in Paget's disease of bone, *Calcif Tissue Int* 80(1):1, 2007.

Langston AL, Ralston SH: Management of Paget's disease of bone, *Rheumatology* 43(8):955, 2004.

Lin JT, Lane JM: Bisphosphonates, *J Am Acad Orthop Surg* 11:1, 2003.

AUTHOR: **LONNIE R. MERCIER, M.D.**

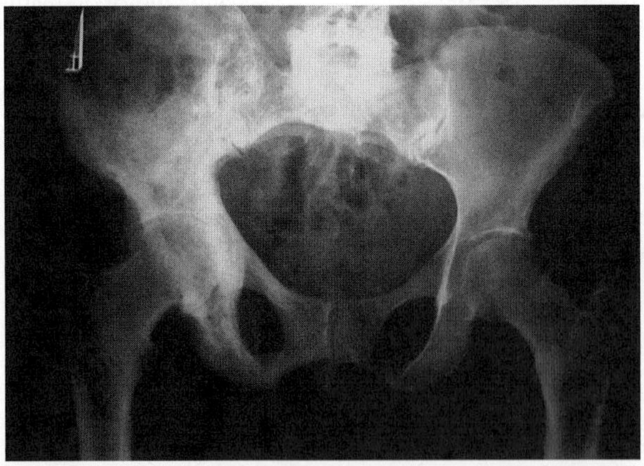

FIGURE 1-188 Frontal radiograph of the pelvis shows marked prominence to the trabeculae in the right ilium, ischium, and pubic bones with small lytic areas identified compatible with the later stages of Paget's disease. (From Specht N [ed]: *Practical guide to diagnostic imaging,* St Louis, 1998, Mosby.)

BASIC INFORMATION

DEFINITION

Paget's disease of the breast is a malignant disease that presents itself as a scaly, sore, eroding, bleeding ulcer of the nipple. Microscopically, typical large clear cells (Paget's cells) with pale and abundant cytoplasm and hyperchromatic nuclei with prominent nucleoli are found in the epidermal layer. Paget's disease is more often associated with primary invasive or in situ carcinoma of the breast.

ICD-9CM CODES
174.0 Malignant neoplasm of female breast, nipple, and areola

EPIDEMIOLOGY & DEMOGRAPHICS

- Not common
- Found in 1 in 100 to 200 breast cancer patients

PHYSICAL FINDINGS & CLINICAL PRESENTATION

- Variable
- Itching or burning nipple and/or reported lump
- Very minimal scaly lesion that may bleed when scales are lifted
- Typical ulcer located on nipple with serous fluid weeping or small amount of bleeding coming from it (Fig. 1-189)
- Palpable carcinoma in the breast of some patients

ETIOLOGY

- Exact origin unknown
- Possibly migration of either in situ or invasive carcinoma cells in breast to nipple skin to produce Paget's disease

DIAGNOSIS

DIFFERENTIAL DIAGNOSIS

- Chronic dermatitis
- Florid papillomatosis of the nipple or nipple adenoma
- Eczema

WORKUP

- Clinically apparent
- Careful breast examination with diagnosis in mind
- Palpable mass or mammographic lesions in 60% to 70% of patients
- A clinical algorithm for the evaluation of nipple discharge is described in Section III, "Breast, Nipple Discharge Evaluation"

LABORATORY TESTS

Biopsy of nipple lesion

IMAGING STUDIES

Mammograms to search for possible primary carcinoma

TREATMENT

NONPHARMACOLOGIC THERAPY

- Fewer patients:
  1. Paget's disease of nipple only finding when mammographically negative breast
  2. Consideration of wide excision of nipple with or without radiation
- Other patients: additional invasive or in situ carcinoma recognized
- Either modified mastectomy or breast conservation treatment
- Presence of underlying in situ or invasive carcinoma in mastectomy specimen of majority of patients

ACUTE GENERAL Rx

Systemic adjuvant therapy, depending on extent of invasive carcinoma found

DISPOSITION

- Parallel prognosis to that of breast cancer patient without Paget's disease
- Regular follow up as in other invasive or in situ carcinoma patients

REFERRAL

At outset, all suspicious nipple lesions should be referred for evaluation and treatment.

SUGGESTED READINGS

Sakoratias GH et al: Paget's disease of the breast, *Canc Treat Rev* 27(1):9, 2001.

Sakoratias GH et al: Paget's disease of the breast: a clinical perspective, *Langenbecks Arch Surg* 386(6):444, 2001.

AUTHORS: **TAKUMA NEMOTO, M.D.,** and **RUBEN ALVERO, M.D.**

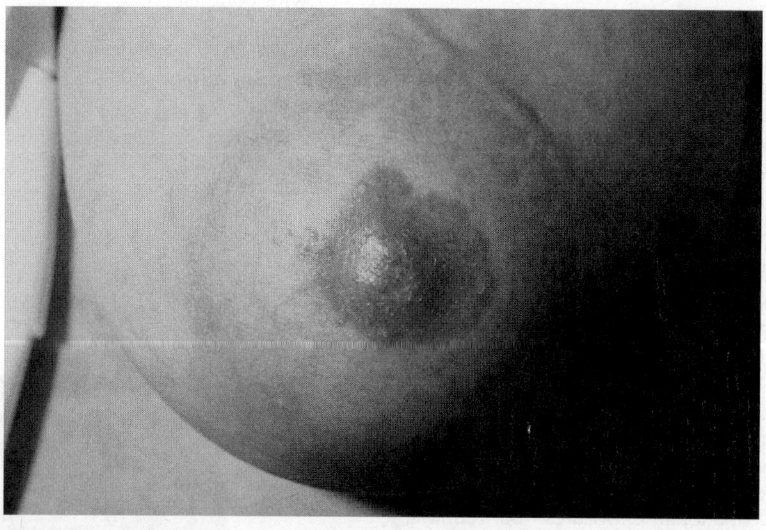

FIGURE 1-189 Paget's disease of the breast. The lesion has insidiously spread for 1 year to infiltrate the areola and surrounding skin. (From Habif TP: *Clinical dermatology: a color guide to diagnosis and therapy,* ed 3, St Louis, 1996, Mosby.)

BASIC INFORMATION

DEFINITION

Pancreatic cancer is an adenocarcinoma derived from the epithelium of the pancreatic duct.

ICD-9CM CODES
157.9 Pancreatic cancer
157.0 (head)
157.1 (body)
157.2 (tail)
157.3 (duct)
230.9 (in situ)

EPIDEMIOLOGY & DEMOGRAPHICS

INCIDENCE: 1 case/10,000 persons/yr. In the U.S. there are over 30,000 patients diagnosed with pancreatic cancer and over 30,000 deaths yearly.

PREDOMINANT SEX: Male:female ratio of 2:1

PREDOMINANT AGE: Seventh and eighth decades of life

PHYSICAL FINDINGS & CLINICAL PRESENTATION

Presenting symptoms:
- Jaundice
- Abdominal pain
- Weight loss
- Anorexia/change in taste
- Nausea
- Uncommonly: depression, GI bleeding, acute pancreatitis, back pain

Physical findings:
- Icterus
- Cachexia
- Excoriations from scratching pruritic skin

ETIOLOGY

Unknown, but several conditions have been associated with pancreatic cancer:
- Smoking
- Alcoholism
- Gallstones
- Diabetes mellitus
- Chronic pancreatitis
- Diet rich in animal fat
- Occupational exposures: oil refining, paper manufacturing, chemical industry

DIAGNOSIS

DIFFERENTIAL DIAGNOSIS

- Common duct cholelithiasis
- Cholangiocarcinoma
- Common duct stricture
- Sclerosing cholangitis
- Primary biliary cirrhosis
- Drug-induced cholestasis (e.g., phenothiazines)
- Chronic hepatitis
- Sarcoidosis
- Other pancreatic tumors (islet cell tumor, cystadenocarcinoma, epidermoid carcinoma, sarcomas, lymphomas)

WORKUP

Routine laboratory tests	% abnormal
Alkaline phosphatase	80
Bilirubin	55
Total protein	15
Amylase	15
Hematocrit	60

IMAGING STUDIES

There is no evidence-based consensus on the optimal preoperative imaging assessment of patients with suspected pancreatic cancer. Helical CT is often the initial study. Multidetector CT and endoscopic ultrasonography represent newer modalities. Compared with multidetector CT, endoscopic ultrasonography is superior for tumor detection and staging but similar for nodal staging and respectability of preoperatively suspected, non-metastatic pancreatic cancer.

Noninvasive imaging	% abnormal
Abdominal ultrasonography	60
Abdominal CT scan (Fig. 1-190) (without or with contrast [IV or oral])	90
Abdominal MRI scan	90
Invasive imaging	
Endoscopic retrograde cholangiopancreatography (ERCP)	90
CT scan or ultrasonography-guided needle aspiration cytology	90-95

STAGING FOR PANCREATIC CANCER

PRIMARY TUMOR (T):
TX Primary tumor cannot be assessed
T0 No evidence of primary tumor
T1 Tumor <2 cm
T2 Tumor >2 cm, confined to the pancreas
T3 Tumor extends locally beyond the pancreas
T4 Tumor involves celiac or superior mesenteric arteries

LYMPH NODES (N):
NX Regional lymph nodes cannot be assessed
N0 No regional lymph node metastasis
N1 Regional lymph node metastasis

DISTANT METASTASES (M):
MX Presence of distant metastasis cannot be assessed
M0 No distant metastasis
M1 Distant metastasis

STAGING GROUP:
IA T1, N0, M0
IB T2, N0, M0
IIA T3, N0, M0
IIB T1-3, N1, M0
III T4, N0-1, M0
IV T1-4, N0-1, M1

TREATMENT

- Surgery

Curative pancreatectomy (Whipple's procedure) appropriate for only 10% to 20% of patients whose lesion is <5 cm, solitary, and without metastases. Surgical mortality is 5%. Adjuvant chemotherapy may improve postoperative survival.

Palliative surgery (for biliary decompression/diversion)

Palliative therapeutic endoscopic retrograde cholangiopancreatography (ERCP) using stents

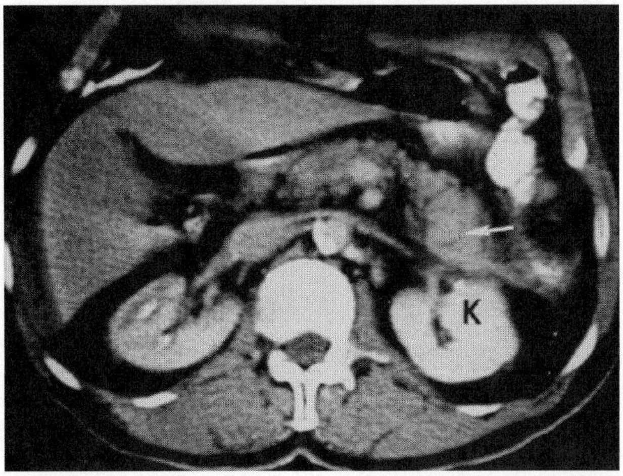

FIGURE 1-190 CT scan of a patient with adenocarcinoma of the body and tail of the pancreas. The tumor *(arrow)* is seen anterior and adjacent to the left kidney *(K)*. At operation, the tumor was invading Gerota's fascia. (From Sabiston D: *Textbook of surgery,* ed 17, Philadelphia, 2005, WB Saunders.)

- Chemotherapy

The best combination chemotherapy using streptozotocin, mitomycin C, and 5-FU provides only a 19-wk median survival.

- Radiation

External beam radiation for palliation of pain.

- Combined chemotherapy and radiation provides a median survival of 11 mo
- Celiac plexus block by an experienced anesthesiologist provides pain relief in 80% to 90% of cases

DISPOSITION

- Adjunct chemotherapy has a significant survival benefit in patients with resected pancreatic cancer.
- Recent trials have shown that adjuvant postoperative chemotherapy with gemcitabine significantly delays the development of recurrent disease after complete resection of pancreatic cancer.

PEARLS & CONSIDERATIONS

COMMENTS

- The U.S. Preventive Services Task Force (USPSTF) recommends against routine screening for pancreatic cancer in asymptomatic adults using abdominal palpation, ultrasonography, or serologic markers. The USPSTF found no evidence that screening for pancreatic cancer is effective in reducing mortality. There is potential for significant harm because of the low prevalence of pancreatic cancer, limited accuracy of available screening tests, invasive nature of diagnostic tests, and poor outcome of treatment. As a result, the USPSTF concluded that the harms of screening for pancreatic cancer exceed any potential benefits.
- Recent trials indicate that pancreatic cancer may have a distinct microRNA (miRNA) expression pattern that may differentiate it from normal pancreas and chronic pancreatitis. Current research is aimed at using miRNA expression patterns to distinguish between long- and short-term survivors.

EVIDENCE

EBM

Surgical treatment

In people with resectable pancreatic cancer, both Whipple's procedure and pylorus-preserving surgery appear to have similar efficacy in terms of quality of life and 5-year survival. However, the trials supporting this finding may have lacked power to detect any clinically significant differences.[1-3] Ⓑ

Adjuvant therapy following surgical resection

A retrospective analysis has shown that following radical surgery, treatment with adjuvant external beam radiation therapy (EBRT) is associated with a significant survival benefit vs. surgery alone. Patients managed with surgery, intraoperative radiation therapy, and EBRT have the best median survival time.[4] Ⓑ

Fluorouracil-based chemotherapy significantly improves short-term median survival following surgical resection, compared with no adjuvant treatment. Five-year survival, however, is the same for both groups.[5,6] Ⓐ Ⓑ

Following surgical resection, combined chemoradiotherapy (with fluorouracil-based chemotherapy), significantly improves survival compared with no chemoradiotherapy. It is not apparent whether these findings are due to chemotherapy or concomitant radiotherapy.[7] Ⓑ

Evidence-Based References

1. Wenger F et al: Gastrointestinal quality of life after duodenopancreatectomy in pancreatic carcinoma. Preliminary results of a prospective randomized study: pancreatoduodenectomy or pylorus-preserving pancreatoduodenectomy, *Chirurg Gastroenterol* 70:1454, 1999. Reviewed in: *Clin Evid* 10:549, 2003. Ⓑ
2. Paquet K-J: Comparison of Whipple's pancreaticoduodenectomy with the pylorus-preserving pancreaticoduodenectomy—a prospectively controlled, randomized long-term trial, *Chirurg Gastroenterol* 14:54, 1998. Reviewed in: *Clin Evid* 10:549, 2003. Ⓑ
3. Seiler C et al: Randomized prospective trial of pylorus-preserving vs. Classic duodenopancreatectomy (Whipple procedure): initial clinical results, *J Gastrointest Surg* 4:443, 2000. Reviewed in: *Clin Evid* 10:549, 2003. Ⓑ
4. Dobelbower RR et al: Adjuvant radiation therapy for pancreatic cancer: a 15 year experience, *Int J Radiat Oncol Biol Phys* 39:31, 1997. Ⓑ
5. Bakkevold KE et al: Adjuvant combination chemotherapy (AMF) following radical resection of carcinoma of the pancreas and papilla of Vater—results of a controlled, prospective, randomised multicentre study, *Eur J Cancer* 29A:698, 1993. Reviewed in: *Clin Evid* 10:549, 2003. Ⓑ
6. Takada T et al: Is postoperative adjuvant chemotherapy useful for gallbladder carcinoma? A Phase III multicenter prospective randomized controlled trial in patients with resected pancreaticobiliary carcinoma, *Cancer* 95:1685, 2002. Ⓐ
7. Neoptolemos JP et al: Adjuvant chemoradiotherapy and chemotherapy in resectable pancreatic cancer: a randomised controlled trial, *Lancet* 358:1576, 2001. Reviewed in: *Clin Evid* 10:549, 2003. Ⓑ

SUGGESTED READINGS

Abbruzzese JL: Adjuvant therapy for surgically resected pancreatic adenocarcinoma, *JAMA* 299:1066, 2008.

Bloomston M et al: MicroRNA expression patterns to differentiate pancreatic adenocarcinoma from normal pancreas and chronic pancreatitis, *JAMA* 297:1901, 2007.

DeWitt J et al: Comparison of endoscopic ultrasonography and multidetector computed tomography for detecting and staging pancreatic cancer, *Ann Intern Med* 141:753, 2004.

Freelove R, Walling AD: Pancreatic cancer: Diagnosis and management, *Am Fam Physician* 73:485, 2006.

Michaud DS et al: Physical activity, obesity, height, and the risk of pancreatic cancer, *JAMA* 286:821, 2001.

Neoptolemos JP et al: A randomized trial of chemotherapy and radiochemotherapy after resection of pancreatic cancer, *N Engl J Med* 350:1200, 2004.

Oettle H et al: Adjuvant chemotherapy with gemcitabine vs observation in patients undergoing curative-intent resection of pancreatic cancer, *JAMA* 297:267, 2007.

U.S. Preventive Task Force: Screening for pancreatic cancer: a brief evidence update for the USPTS. Agency for Healthcare Research and Quality, 2005: http://ahrq.gov/clinic/uspstf/uspspanc.htm.

AUTHORS: **FRED F. FERRI, M.D.**, and **TOM J. WACHTEL, M.D.**

BASIC INFORMATION

DEFINITION

- Acute pancreatitis is an inflammatory process of the pancreas with intrapancreatic activation of enzymes that may also involve peripancreatic tissue and/or remote organ systems.
- Severe acute pancreatitis (SAP) is diagnosed by the presence of any of the following four criteria:
  1. Organ failure with one or more of the following: shock (systolic BP <90 mmHg), pulmonary insufficiency (PaO2 ≤60 mmHg), renal failure (serum creatinine >2 mg/dl after rehydration), and GI bleeding (>500 ml/24 hr)
  2. Local complications such as necrosis, pseudocyst, or abscess
  3. At least three of Ranson's criteria (see below) or
  4. At least eight of the Acute Physiology and Chronic Health Evaluation II (APACHE II) criteria

ICD-9CM CODES
577.0 Acute pancreatitis

EPIDEMIOLOGY & DEMOGRAPHICS

- Acute pancreatitis is most often secondary to biliary tract disease and alcohol.
- Incidence in urban areas is twice that of rural areas (20 cases/100,000 persons in urban areas).
- 20% of patients have necrotizing pancreatitis; the remainder have interstitial, or endematous pancreatitis.
- Acute pancreatitis accounts for >220,000 hospital admissions in the U.S. each year.

PHYSICAL FINDINGS & CLINICAL PRESENTATION

- Epigastric tenderness and guarding; pain usually developing suddenly, reaching peak intensity within 10 to 30 min, severe and lasting several hours without relief
- Hypoactive bowel sounds (secondary to ileus)
- Tachycardia, shock (secondary to decreased intravascular volume)
- Confusion (secondary to metabolic disturbances)
- Fever
- Tachycardia, decreased breath sounds (atelectasis, pleural effusions, ARDS)
- Jaundice (secondary to obstruction or compression of biliary tract)
- Ascites (secondary to tear in pancreatic duct, leaking pseudocyst)
- Palpable abdominal mass (pseudocyst, phlegmon, abscess, carcinoma)
- Evidence of hypocalcemia (Chvostek's sign, Trousseau's sign)
- Evidence of intraabdominal bleeding (hemorrhagic pancreatitis):
  1. Gray-bluish discoloration around the umbilicus (Cullen's sign)
  2. Bluish discoloration involving the flanks (Grey Turner's sign)
- Tender subcutaneous nodules (caused by subcutaneous fat necrosis)

ETIOLOGY

- In >90% of cases: biliary tract disease (calculi or sludge) or alcohol
- Drugs (e.g., thiazides, furosemide, corticosteroids, tetracycline, estrogens, valproic acid, metronidazole, azathioprine, methyldopa, pentamidine, ethacrynic acid, procainamide, sulindac, nitrofurantoin, ACE inhibitors, danazol, cimetidine, piroxicam, gold, ranitidine, sulfasalazine, isoniazid, acetaminophen, cisplatin, opiates, erythromycin)
- Abdominal trauma
- Surgery
- ERCP
- Infections (predominantly viral infections)
- Peptic ulcer (penetrating duodenal ulcer)
- Pancreas divisum (congenital failure to fuse of dorsal or ventral pancreas)
- Idiopathic
- Pregnancy
- Vascular (vasculitis, ischemic)
- Hypolipoproteinemia (types I, IV, and V)
- Hypercalcemia
- Pancreatic carcinoma (primary or metastatic)
- Renal failure
- Hereditary pancreatitis
- Occupational exposure to chemicals: methanol, cobalt, zinc, mercuric chloride, creosol, lead, organophosphates, chlorinated naphthalenes
- Others: scorpion bite, obstruction at ampulla region (neoplasm, duodenal diverticula, Crohn's disease), hypotensive shock, autoimmune pancreatitis

DIAGNOSIS

DIFFERENTIAL DIAGNOSIS

- PUD
- Acute cholangitis, biliary colic
- High intestinal obstruction
- Early acute appendicitis
- Mesenteric vascular obstruction
- DKA
- Pneumonia (basilar)
- Myocardial infarction (inferior wall)
- Renal colic
- Ruptured or dissecting aortic aneurysm
- Mesenteric ischemia

LABORATORY TESTS

Pancreatic enzymes

- Amylase is increased, usually elevated in the initial 3 to 5 days of acute pancreatitis. Isoamylase determinations (separation of pancreatic cell isoenzyme components of amylase) are useful in excluding occasional cases of salivary hyperamylasemia. The use of isoamylase rather than total serum amylase reduces the risk of erroneously diagnosing pancreatitis and is preferred by some as initial biochemical test in patients suspected of having acute pancreatitis.
- Urinary amylase determinations are useful to diagnose acute pancreatitis in patients with lipemic serum, to rule out elevated serum amylase secondary to macroamylasemia, and to diagnose acute pancreatitis in patients whose serum amylase is normal.
- Serum lipase levels are elevated in acute pancreatitis; the elevation is less transient than serum amylase; concomitant evaluation of serum amylase and lipase increases diagnostic accuracy of acute pancreatitis. An elevated lipase/amylase ratio is suggestive of alcoholic pancreatitis.
- Elevated serum trypsin levels are diagnostic of pancreatitis (in absence of renal failure); measurement is made by radioimmunoassay. Although not routinely available, the serum trypsin level is the most accurate laboratory indicator for pancreatitis.
- Rapid measurement of urinary trypsinogen-2 (if available) is useful in the ER as a screening test for acute pancreatitis in patients with abdominal pain; a negative dipstick test for urinary trypsinogen-2 rules out acute pancreatitis with a high degree of probability, whereas a positive test indicates need for further evaluation.

Additional tests:

- CBC: reveals leukocytosis; Hct may be initially increased secondary to hemoconcentration; decreased Hct may indicate hemorrhage or hemolysis.
- BUN is increased secondary to dehydration.
- Elevation of serum glucose in previously normal patient correlates with the degree of pancreatic malfunction and may be related to increased release of glycogen, catecholamines, and glucocorticoid release and decreased insulin release.
- Liver profile: AST and LDH are increased secondary to tissue necrosis; bilirubin and alkaline phosphatase may be increased secondary to common bile duct obstruction. A threefold or greater rise in serum ALT concentrations is an excellent indicator (95% probability) of biliary pancreatitis.
- Serum calcium is decreased secondary to saponification, precipitation, and decreased PTH response.
- ABGs: Pao_2 may be decreased secondary to ARDS, pleural effusion(s); pH

may be decreased secondary to lactic acidosis, respiratory acidosis, and renal insufficiency.

- Serum electrolytes: potassium may be increased secondary to acidosis or renal insufficiency, sodium may be increased secondary to dehydration.

IMAGING STUDIES

- Abdominal plain film is useful initially to distinguish other conditions that may mimic pancreatitis (perforated viscus); it may reveal localized ileus (sentinel loop), pancreatic calcifications (chronic pancreatitis), blurring of left psoas shadow, dilation of transverse colon, calcified gallstones.
- Chest x-ray may reveal elevation of one or both diaphragms, pleural effusions, basilar infiltrates, platelike atelectasis.
- Abdominal ultrasonography is useful in detecting gallstones (sensitivity of 60% to 70% for detecting stones associated with pancreatitis). It is also useful for detecting pancreatic pseudocysts; its major limitation is the presence of distended bowel loops overlying the pancreas.
- CT scan is superior to ultrasonography in identifying pancreatitis and defining its extent, and it also plays a role in diagnosing pseudocysts (they appear as a well-defined area surrounded by a high-density capsule); GI fistulation or infection of a pseudocyst can also be identified by the presence of gas within the pseudocyst. Sequential contrast enhanced CT is useful for detection of pancreatic necrosis (Fig. 1-191). The severity of pancreatitis can also be graded by CT scan. (A = normal pancreas, B = enlarged pancreas [1 point], C = pancreatic and/or peripancreatic inflammation [2 points], D = single peripancreatic collection [3 points], E = at least 2 peripancreatic collections and/or retroperitoneal air [4 points]. Percentage of pancreatic necrosis <30% [2 points], 30% to 50% [4 points], >50% [6 points]. The CT severity index is calculated by adding grade points to points assigned for percentage of necrosis.)
- Magnetic resonance cholangiopancreatography (MRCP) is also a useful diagnostic modality if a surgical procedure is not anticipated.
- ERCP should not be performed during the acute stage of disease unless it is necessary to remove an impacted stone in the ampulla of Vater; patients with severe or worsening pancreatitis but without obstructive jaundice (biliary obstruction) do not benefit from early ERCP and papillotomy.

TREATMENT Rx

NONPHARMACOLOGIC THERAPY

- Bowel rest with avoidance of PO liquids or solids during the acute illness
- Avoidance of alcohol and any drugs associated with pancreatitis

ACUTE GENERAL Rx

General measures:

- Maintain adequate intravascular volume with vigorous IV hydration.
- Patient should remain NPO until clinically improved, stable, and hungry. Enteral feedings are preferred over total parenteral nutrition (TPN). Parenteral nutrition may be necessary in patients who do not tolerate enteral feeding or in whom an adequate infusion rate cannot be reached within 2 to 4 days.
- Nasogastric suction is useful only in severe pancreatitis to decompress the abdomen in patients with ileus.
- Control pain: IV morphine or fentanyl
- Correct metabolic abnormalities (e.g., replace calcium and magnesium as necessary).

Specific measures:

- Pancreatic or peripancreatic infection develops in 40% to 70% of patients with pancreatic necrosis. However, IV antibiotics should not be used prophylactically for all cases of pancreatitis; their use is justified if the patient has evidence of septicemia, pancreatic abscess, or pancreatitis secondary to biliary calculi. Their use should generally be limited to 5 to 7 days to prevent development of fungal superinfection. Appropriate empiric antibiotic therapy should cover:
  1. *B. fragilis* and other anaerobes (cefotetan, cefoxitin, metronidazole, or clindamycin plus aminoglycoside)
  2. *Enterococcus* (ampicillin)
- Surgical therapy has a limited role in acute pancreatitis; it is indicated in the following:
  1. Gallstone-induced pancreatitis: cholecystectomy when acute pancreatitis subsides
  2. Perforated peptic ulcer
  3. Excision or drainage of necrotic or infected foci. Necrosectomy (debridement) with placement of wide-bore drains for continuous postoperative irrigation is the preferred surgical procedure. Surgery is not indicated for patients with sterile necrosis unless there is clinical deterioration despite intensive medical care
- Identification and treatment of complications:
  1. Pseudocyst: round or spheroid collection of fluid, tissue, pancreatic enzymes, and blood.
     a. Diagnosed by CT scan or sonography
     b. Treatment: CT scan or ultrasound-guided percutaneous drainage (with a pigtail catheter left in place for continuous drainage) can be used, but the recurrence rate is high; the conservative approach is to reevaluate the pseudocyst (with CT scan or sonography) after 6 to 7 wk and surgically drain it if the pseudocyst has not decreased in size. Generally pseudocysts <5 cm in diameter are reabsorbed without intervention whereas those >5 cm require surgical intervention after the wall has matured.
  2. Phlegmon: represents pancreatic edema. It can be diagnosed by CT scan or sonography. Treatment is

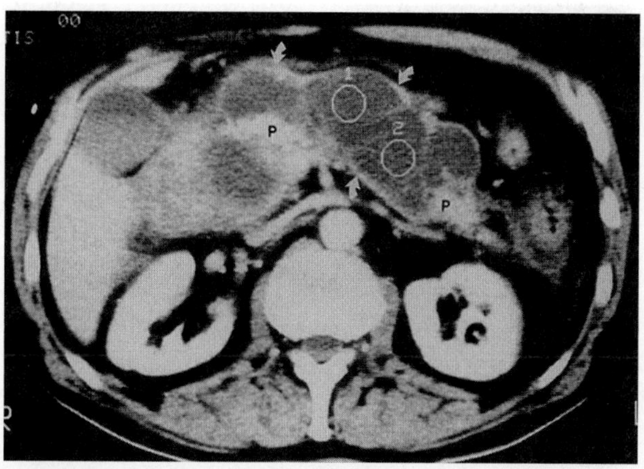

FIGURE 1-191 Acute necrotizing pancreatitis. Dynamic CT shows enlargement of the pancreas, a thin rim of contrast-enhancement *(arrows),* and lack of enhancement of the pancreatic parenchyma indicating almost complete gland necrosis (cursors 1 and 2 measure soft tissue density: 25 to 30 Hounsfield units). Small islands of normally enhancing parenchyma are seen *(P).* Patient died despite surgery. (From Grainger RG, Allison DJ, Adam A, Dixon AK [eds]: *Grainger & Allison's diagnostic radiology,* ed 4, Philadelphia, 2001, Churchill Livingstone.)

supportive measures, because it usually resolves spontaneously.

3. Pancreatic abscess: diagnosed by CT scan (presence of bubbles in the retroperitoneum); Gram staining and cultures of fluid obtained from guided percutaneous aspiration (GPA) usually identify bacterial organism. Therapy is surgical (or catheter) drainage and IV antibiotics (imipenem-cilastin [Primaxin] is the drug of choice).
4. Pancreatic ascites: usually caused by leaking of pseudocyst or tear in pancreatic duct. Paracentesis reveals very high amylase and lipase levels in the pancreatic fluid; ERCP may demonstrate the lesion. Treatment is surgical correction if exudative ascites from severe pancreatitis does not resolve spontaneously.
5. GI bleeding: caused by alcoholic gastritis, bleeding varices, stress ulceration, or DIC.
6. Renal failure: caused by hypovolemia resulting in oliguria or anuria, cortical or tubular necrosis (shock, DIC), or thrombosis of renal artery or vein.
7. Hypoxia: caused by ARDS, pleural effusion, or atelectasis.

DISPOSITION

Prognosis varies with the severity of pancreatitis; overall mortality in acute pancreatitis is 5% to 10%; poor prognostic signs according to the Ranson criteria are as follows:

- Age >55 yr
- Fluid sequestration >6000 ml
- Laboratory abnormalities on admission: WBC >16,000, blood glucose >200 ml/dl, serum LDH >350 IU/L, AST >250 IU/L
- Laboratory abnormalities during the initial 48 hr: decreased Hct >10% with hydration or Hct <30%, BUN rise >5 mg/dl, serum calcium <8 mg/dl, arterial Po_2 <60 mm Hg, and base deficit >4 mEq/L

REFERRAL

- Hospitalization is indicated in moderate/severe cases of pancreatitis.
- Surgical consultation is needed in suspected gallstone pancreatitis, perforated peptic ulcer, or presence of necrotic or infected foci.

EVIDENCE

EBM

We are unable to cite evidence that meets our criteria for many of the supportive therapies for pancreatitis.

A systematic review concluded that available data were insufficient to draw firm conclusions about the effectiveness and safety of enteral nutrition vs. total parenteral nutrition in patients with acute pancreatitis; however, the authors did note there is a trend toward reductions in the adverse outcomes of acute pancreatitis after administration of enteral nutrition.[1] Ⓑ

A more recent systematic review found six relevant trials comparing enteral vs. parenteral nutrition in pancreatitis and concluded enteral nutrition was associated with a significantly lower incidence of infections, reduced pancreatitis-related surgical interventions, and a shorter hospital stay. However, there were no significant differences in mortality rates or noninfectious complication rates.[2] Ⓐ

There is evidence supporting prophylactic antibiotics in patients with severe acute pancreatitis and proven pancreatic necrosis.

A systematic review found strong evidence for the use of prophylaxis with broad-spectrum antibiotics active against enteric organisms (such as impinem with cilastatin, cefuroxime, or ofloxacin with metronidazole) in the treatment of patients with severe acute pancreatitis and pancreatic necrosis proven by intravenous contrast-enhanced computed tomography.[3] Ⓐ

In predicted severe gallstone-associated acute pancreatitis there is evidence that early endoscopic retrograde cholangiopancreatography (ERCP) results in a reduction in complications.

A systematic review found that early ERCP +/− endoscopic sphincterotomy resulted in reduced odds of complications in patients that are predicted a severe attack of gallstone-associated pancreatitis. However, this benefit was not found in patients predicted a mild attack.[4] Ⓐ

Evidence-Based References

1. Al-Omran M, Groof A, Wilke D: Enteral versus parenteral nutrition for acute pancreatitis, *Cochrane Database Syst Rev* 1, 2003. Ⓑ
2. Marik PE, Zaloga GP: Meta-analysis of parenteral nutrition versus enteral nutrition in patients with acute pancreatitis, *BMJ* 328:1407, 2004.
3. Villatoro E, Larvin M, Bassi C: Antibiotic therapy for prophylaxis against infection of pancreatic necrosis in acute pancreatitis, *Cochrane Database Syst Rev* 4, 2003. Ⓐ
4. Ayub K, Imada R, Slavin J: Endoscopic retrograde cholangiopancreatography in gallstone-associated acute pancreatitis, *Cochrane Database Syst Rev* 3, 2004. Ⓐ

SUGGESTED READINGS

Balthazar EJ: Acute pancreatitis: assessment of severity with clinical and CT evaluation, *Radiology* 223:603, 2002.

Finkelberg D et al: Autoimmune pancreatitis, *N Engl J Med* 355:2670, 2006.

Knaus WA et al: APACHE II: a severity of disease classification system, *Crit Care Med* 13:818, 1984.

Swaroop VS et al: Severe acute pancreatitis, *JAMA* 291:2865, 2004.

Vitale GC: Early management of acute gallstone pancreatitis, *Ann Surg* 245:18, 2007.

Whitcomb DC: Acute pancreatitis, *N Engl J Med* 354:2142, 2006.

AUTHOR: **FRED F. FERRI, M.D.**

BASIC INFORMATION

DEFINITION

Chronic pancreatitis is a recurrent or persistent inflammatory process of the pancreas characterized by chronic pain and by pancreatic exocrine and/or endocrine insufficiency.

ICD-9CM CODES
577.1 Chronic pancreatitis

EPIDEMIOLOGY & DEMOGRAPHICS

- Chronic pancreatitis occurs in approximately 5 to 10/100,000 persons in industrialized countries.
- Male:female ratio is 5:1.

PHYSICAL FINDINGS & CLINICAL PRESENTATION

- Persistent or recurrent epigastric and left upper quadrant pain, may radiate to the back
- Tenderness over the pancreas, muscle guarding
- Significant weight loss
- Bulky, foul-smelling stools, greasy in appearance
- Epigastric mass (10% of patients)
- Jaundice (5% to 10% of patients)

ETIOLOGY

- Chronic alcoholism.
- Obstruction (ampullary stenosis, tumor, trauma, pancreas divisum, annular pancreas).
- Hereditary pancreatitis.
- Severe malnutrition.
- Idiopathic.
- Untreated hyperparathyroidism (hypercalcemia).
- Mutations of the cystic fibrosis transmembrane conductance regulator (CFTR) gene and the TF genotype.
- Autoimmune pancreatitis (5% of chronic pancreatitis cases): presents clinically with jaundice (63% of patients) and abdominal pain (35%). CT may reveal diffusely enlarged pancreas, enhanced peripheral rim of hypoattenuation 'halo,' and low-attenuation mass in head of pancreas. Labs reveal elevated serum IgG4, elevated serum Ig or gamma globulin level, presence of antilactoferrin antibody (ALA), anticarbonic anhydrase (ACA) II level, anti-smooth-muscle antibody (ASMA), or antinuclear antibody (ANA).
- Sclerosing pancreatitis: a form of chronic pancreatitis characterized by infrequent attacks of abdominal pain, irregular narrowing of the pancreatic duct, and swelling of the pancreatic parenchyma; these patients have high levels of serum immunoglobins (IgG4). Chronic sclerosing pancreatitis is also known as autoimmune pancreatitis.

DIAGNOSIS

DIFFERENTIAL DIAGNOSIS

- Pancreatic cancer
- PUD
- Cholelithiasis with biliary obstruction
- Malabsorption from other etiologies
- Recurrent acute pancreatitis

WORKUP

Medical history with focus on alcohol use, laboratory tests, diagnostic imaging

LABORATORY TESTS

- Serum amylase and lipase may be elevated (normal amylase levels, however, do not exclude the diagnosis).
- Hyperglycemia, glycosuria, hyperbilirubinemia, and elevated serum alkaline phosphatase may also be present.
- 72-hr fecal fat determination (rarely performed) reveals excess fecal fat.
- Bentiromide test or secretin stimulation test can confirm pancreatic insufficiency.
- Elevated levels of serum IgG4 are found in sclerosing pancreatitis and autoimmune pancreatitis.
- Elevated serum Ig or gamma globulin level, presence of ALA, ACA II level, ASMA, or ANA in autoimmune pancreatitis.

IMAGING STUDIES

- Plain abdominal radiographs may reveal pancreatic calcifications (95% specific for chronic pancreatitis).
- Ultrasound of abdomen may reveal duct dilation, pseudocyst, calcification, and presence of ascites.
- CT scan of abdomen is useful for the detection of calcifications, to evaluate for ductal dilation, and for ruling out pancreatic cancer.
- ERCP can be used to evaluate for the presence of dilated ducts, strictures, pseudocysts, and intraductal stones.
- Use of fine needle aspiration (FNA) and endoscopic ultrasound (EUS) are newer diagnostic modalities.

TREATMENT

NONPHARMACOLOGIC THERAPY

- Avoidance of alcohol
- Frequent, small-volume, low-fat meals

ACUTE GENERAL Rx

- Avoidance of narcotics if possible (simple analgesics or NSAIDs can be used)
- Treatment of steatorrhea with pancreatic supplements (e.g., Pancrease, Creon, Pancrelipase titrated prn based on the amount of steatorrhea and patient's weight loss)
- Octreotide 200 μg SC tid may be useful for pain secondary to idiopathic chronic pancreatitis
- Treatment of complications (e.g., type 1 DM)
- Glucocorticoid therapy in patients with autoimmune pancreatitis and sclerosing pancreatitis can induce clinical remission and significantly decrease serum concentrations of IgG4, immune complexes, and the IgG4 subclass of immune complexes

CHRONIC Rx

- Surgical intervention may be necessary to eliminate biliary tract disease and improve flow of bile into the duodenum by eliminating obstruction of pancreatic duct.
- ERCP with endoscopic sphincterectomy and stone extraction is useful in selected patients.
- Transduodenal sphincteroplasty or pancreaticojejunostomy in selected patients. Surgery should also be considered in patients with intractable pain.

DISPOSITION

- Long-term survival is poor (50% of patients die within 10 yr from chronic pancreatitis or malignancy).
- Prognosis is best in patients with recurrent acute pancreatitis resulting from cholelithiasis, hyperparathyroidism, or stenosis of the sphincter of Oddi.

REFERRAL

GI referral for ERCP, surgical referral in selected patients (see "Chronic Rx").

SUGGESTED READINGS

Finkelberg DL et al: Autoimmune pancreatitis, *N Engl J Med* 355:2670, 2006.

Hamano H et al: High serum IgG4 concentrations in patients with sclerosing pancreatitis, *N Engl J Med* 344:732, 2001.

Hollerbach S et al: Endoscopic ultrasonography and fine needle aspiration cytology for diagnosis of chronic pancreatitis, *Endoscopy* 33:824, 2001.

Nair R et al: Chronic pancreatitis, *Am Fam Physician* 76:1679-1688, 2007.

AUTHOR: **FRED F. FERRI, M.D.**

BASIC INFORMATION

DEFINITION

A panic attack is a relatively brief, sudden episode of intense fear or apprehension, often associated with a sense of impending doom and various uncomfortable and disquieting physical symptoms. Panic attacks may be uncued ("out of the blue") or cued (i.e., triggered by a particular object or situation). Panic attacks may be present in a variety of different anxiety-related disorders (e.g., phobias, social anxiety, obsessive-compulsive disorder). Panic disorder is diagnosed after two uncued panic attacks have occurred followed by at least 1 month (or more) of significant concern about future attacks, worry about their implications, or a major change in behavior related to these attacks. Agoraphobia is anxiety about, and avoidance of, places or situations in which the ability to escape is limited or embarrassing or in which help might not be available in the event of having a panic attack.

SYNONYMS

Anxiety attacks
Fear attacks
Ataque de nervios

ICD-9CM CODES
F41.0 Panic disorder without agoraphobia (DSM-IV: 300.01)
F40.01 Panic disorder with agoraphobia (DSM-IV 300.21)

EPIDEMIOLOGY & DEMOGRAPHICS

INCIDENCE (IN U.S.): 1% 1-mo incidence of panic attacks.

PREVALENCE (IN U.S.):
- 15% to 20% lifetime prevalence of one or more panic attacks.
- Panic disorder much more uncommon, with a lifetime prevalence of 1.5% to 3.5%; chronicity of condition reflected by a similar 1-yr prevalence rate of 1% to 2%.
- Agoraphobia relatively rare; 0.3% to 1% lifetime prevalence; 30% to 50% of patients diagnosed with panic disorder also have agoraphobia.

PEAK INCIDENCE:
- Chronic condition with a waxing and waning course.
- Bimodal incidence peaks noted, with the first peak between ages 15 and 24 and second peak between ages 35 and 44.

PREDOMINANT SEX:
- Women more commonly affected (>85% of clinical population).
- Panic disorder twice as common in women.
- Panic disorder with agoraphobia three times as common in women.

PREDOMINANT AGE:
- Age of onset is typically late adolescence to mid-30s. Onset earlier in males (24 yr) than females (28 yr).
- Onset after age 45 yr rare and should raise suspicion of different etiology.

GENETICS:
- Risk of developing panic disorder in first-degree relatives of individuals with panic disorder four to seven times that of general population.
- Findings in twin studies: about 60% of contributing factors to panic are genetic.

PHYSICAL FINDINGS & CLINICAL PRESENTATION

Panic disorder
- Present either with a panic attack or with fear and anxiety related to anticipation of a future panic attack or its implications.
- Typical presentation: unexpected, untriggered periods of intense anxiety and fear with associated physiologic changes (e.g., palpitations, sweating, tremulousness, shortness of breath, chest pain, GI distress, faintness, derealization, paresthesia). Panic attacks are often described as "the most terrifying" episode an individual has experienced.
- Emergency or physician visits often occasioned by physical symptoms such as chest pain, dizziness, or difficulty breathing.

Agoraphobia
- Rare complaints to physician. May manifest in missed office visits or tardiness. Patients may request home visits or telephone care.
- Activities usually self-limited by avoiding public situations where the patient might experience a panic attack and would be unable to exit readily, such as the following:
  1. Crowded public areas (stores, public transportation, flying, church)
  2. Individual interactions (hairdresser, neighborhood meetings)
  3. Driving (especially if alone, over bridges, or isolated roads)
- On exposure to or anticipation of exposure to such situations, significant anxiety occurs. Anxiety may generate somatic symptoms that trigger a full-blown panic attack, further reinforcing avoidance of such situations.

ETIOLOGY

Hypotheses (Note: There are sufficient data to support each model. Models are not mutually exclusive.)
1. Central dyscontrol of autonomic arousal (typically localized to the locus ceruleus); similar symptoms may be chemically induced with yohimbine, caffeine, or cholecystokinin (CKK).
2. Cognitive overreaction (i.e., "catastrophic misinterpretation") to relatively mild or benign physiologic cues that then triggers a genuine autonomic cascade and further misinterpretations.
3. Dysfunction of a central suffocation alarm mechanism; some signs of compensated respiratory alkalosis. Can be experimentally induced with sodium lactate or carbon dioxide.

DIAGNOSIS

DIFFERENTIAL DIAGNOSIS

Medical conditions
- Endocrinopathies
  1. Hyperthyroidism
  2. Hyperparathyroidism
  3. Pheochromocytoma
  4. Carcinoid tumor
- Cardiac and respiratory diseases
  1. Arrhythmias
  2. Myocardial infarction
  3. Chronic obstructive pulmonary disease (COPD)
  4. Asthma
- Metabolic
  1. Hypoglycemia
  2. Electrolyte imbalances
  3. Porphyria
- Seizure disorders
- Psychiatric disorders (Note: Panic attacks are common in a variety of psychiatric disorders. Panic disorder could be conceptualized as a phobia of the somatic sensations or situations that have become paired with panic attacks.)
  1. Phobias (e.g., specific phobia or social phobia)
  2. Obsessive-compulsive disorder (cued by exposure to the object of the obsession)
  3. Posttraumatic stress disorder (cued by recall of a stressor)
- Therapeutic (theophylline, steroids) and recreational (cocaine, amphetamine, caffeine, diet pills) drugs and drug withdrawal (alcohol, barbiturates, benzodiazepines)

WORKUP

- Emergency presentation: cardiac, respiratory, or neurologic symptoms
- History and physical examination to rule out a concomitant medical or substance-related condition

NOTE: Panic disorder and agoraphobia are not diagnoses of exclusion, but exclusion of other conditions is usually required.

LABORATORY TESTS

- Thyroid profile
- Electrolyte measures, including calcium
- Toxicology screen
- ECG
- Acute cases: possible monitoring and cardiac enzymes to rule out arrhythmia or ischemia

IMAGING STUDIES

- For temporal lobe dysfunction (e.g., temporal lesions or as ictal or interictal manifestation of temporal lobe seizures): brain CT scan or MRI or an EEG in some patients
- Holter monitor to rule out occult or episodic arrhythmias
- Chest x-ray examination, ABG, or pulmonary function tests if respiratory compromise suspected

TREATMENT

Rx

NONPHARMACOLOGIC THERAPY

Cognitive-behavioral therapy (CBT) generally very effective with strongest results for cognitive restructuring (i.e., challenging catastrophic misinterpretations of somatic symptoms) and interoceptive exposures (i.e., recreation and management of feared somatic sensations). CBT effect sizes are equal to or larger than for pharmacotherapy, attrition rates are lower, and relapse rates are lower.

ACUTE GENERAL Rx

- Benzodiazepines, particularly alprazolam: very effective in acute setting.
- Low-dose alprazolam for patients with rare panic attacks and asymptomatic interattack periods (0.25 to 0.5 mg po or sublingually prn).
- Start patient on selective serotonin reuptake inhibitor (SSRI) or similar agent and taper patient off of benzodiazepine by wk 2 to 3.

CHRONIC Rx

- Preferred pharmacologic agents: antidepressants with a significant serotonin reuptake inhibitory action. Generally start at low dose and titrate upward. Minimum treatment duration is 6-8 mo but many patients need to take medications indefinitely.
  1. SSRIs; paroxetine (10 to 60 mg/day), sertraline (50 to 200 mg/day), citalopram (20 to 60 mg/day), escitalopram (5 to 30 mg/day), and fluoxetine (5 to 60 mg/day)
  2. Imipramine (100 to 300 mg/day)
  3. Venlafaxine (75 to 225 mg/day)
- Combination CBT plus SSRI has shown good long-term effects but is not notably better than CBT alone. Combination CBT plus benzodiazepine does not provide any added benefit and may undermine CBT (interoceptive exposures are less effective if patient is on benzodiazepine).

DISPOSITION

- Typical course chronic but with significant waxing and waning (common to have long periods of remission).
- Presence of agoraphobia associated with a more chronic course.
- Findings with long-term follow-up studies: 6 to 10 yr after treatment some 30% in remission, 40% to 50% improved with residual symptoms, and the remainder either unchanged or worse.

REFERRAL

Referral needed if:

- Patients do not respond to a serotonin reuptake inhibitor.
- Cognitive-behavioral therapy is the preferred treatment.

PEARLS & CONSIDERATIONS

!

- Patient and family education is an important first step in the management of panic disorder. Education provides more adaptive explanations for the benign somatic sensations paired with panic.
- Resumption of avoided activities or situations is a positive prognostic sign and may promote further therapeutic gains.

EVIDENCE

EBM

A systematic review found that SSRIs (paroxetine, fluvoxamine, zimelidine, clomipramine) were significantly better than placebo at alleviating panic. They were also significantly superior to both imipramine and alprazolam. Imipramine and alprazolam were both superior to placebo.[1] Ⓐ

Imipramine may be effective as maintenance therapy in the management of agoraphobia, and can protect against relapse.[2] Ⓐ

Alprazolam can reduce the number of panic attacks in patients with agoraphobia, and there is evidence that some other benzodiazepines are as effective as alprazolam.[2-4] Ⓐ Ⓑ

Because benzodiazepines have been associated with a wide range of adverse effects, both during and after treatment, the benefit of these drugs must be balanced against their potential harm.[5]

A randomized controlled trial (RCT) included in a systematic review compared five interventions in people with panic disorder and agoraphobia: CBT; fixed dose fluvoxamine 150 mg; fluvoxamine 150 mg plus CBT; pharmacological placebo; and pharmacological placebo plus CBT. At day 84 and at 6 months follow-up, the trial found that CBT increased the proportion of people with statistically and clinically significant improvement on all measures of panic symptoms compared with placebo.[6,7] Ⓐ

Evidence-Based References

1. Boyer W: Serotonin uptake inhibitors are superior to imipramine and alprazolam in alleviating panic attacks: a meta-analysis, *Int Clin Psychopharmacol* 10:45, 1995.
2. Curtis GC et al: Maintenance drug therapy of panic disorder, *J Psychiatr Res* 27:127, 1993. Reviewed in: *Clin Evid* 12:1474, 2004. Ⓐ
3. Charney DS, Woods SW: Benzodiazepine treatment of panic disorder: a comparison of alprazolam and lorazepam, *J Clin Psychiatry* 50:418, 1989. Ⓑ
4. Noyes R et al: Diazepam versus alprazolam for the treatment of panic disorder, *J Clin Psychiatry* 57:349, 1996. Ⓑ
5. Kumar S, Oakley-Browne M: Panic disorder, *Clin Evid* 15:1438-1452, 2006.
6. Sharp DM et al: Fluvoxamine, placebo, and cognitive behaviour therapy used alone and in combination in the treatment of panic disorder and agoraphobia, *J Anxiety Disord* 10:219, 1996.
7. Oei TPS et al: The efficacy and cognitive processes of cognitive behaviour therapy in the treatment of panic disorder with agoraphobia, *Behav Cogn Psychotherapy* 27:63, 1999.

SUGGESTED READINGS

Ham P et al: Treatment of panic disorder, *Am Fam Physician* 71:733, 2005.

Katon WJ: Clinical practice: panic disorder, *N Engl J Med* 354(22):2360, 2006.

Roy-Byrne PP et al: Understanding and treating panic disorder in the primary care setting, *J Clin Psychiatry* 66(suppl 4):16, 2005.

AUTHORS: **JASON M. SATTERFIELD, PH.D.,** and **MITCHELL D. FELDMAN, M.D., M.PHIL.**

BASIC INFORMATION

DEFINITION

Paranoid personality disorder (PPD) is characterized by a pattern of pervasive distrust and suspiciousness of others that leads the person to assign malevolence to the motives of others. PPD begins by early adulthood and causes significant distress or impairment in multiple domains of functioning. Individuals must meet four or more of the following criteria:

1. Suspect, without justification, that others are exploiting, harming, or deceiving them.
2. Preoccupied with unwarranted doubts about the loyalty or trustworthiness of friends or associates.
3. Reluctant to confide in others because of unjustified fear that the information will be used against them in a malicious fashion.
4. Infer demeaning or threatening statements from benign remarks or events.
5. Bear grudges for extended periods. For example, PPD patients are unforgiving of perceived or real insults and slights.
6. Perceive attacks on their character that are not apparent to others. Quick to react angrily or to counterattack.
7. Recurrent suspicions, without justification, regarding fidelity of spouse or partner.

SYNONYMS

None

ICD-9CM CODES
301.0

EPIDEMIOLOGY & DEMOGRAPHICS

PREVALENCE: 0.5% to 4.4% in the general population, 10% to 30% in inpatient psychiatric settings, and 2% to 10% in outpatient mental health clinics.

PREDOMINANT SEX: More commonly diagnosed in males in clinical samples.

GENETICS: Increased prevalence of PPD in relatives of probands with schizophrenia and delusional disorder, paranoid type.

CLINICAL PRESENTATION

- Signs of PPD in childhood include solitariness, poor peer relationships, social anxiety, underachievement in school, hypersensitivity, peculiar thoughts and language, and idiosyncratic fantasies.
- As children, these patients may have appeared "odd" or "eccentric" and attracted teasing.
- Their excessive suspiciousness often leads to either overt argumentativeness and recurrent complaining or quiet, hostile aloofness.
- These patients maintain interpersonal distance and may refuse to answer personal questions saying the information is "nobody's business."
- Misinterpret benign actions by others as malicious assaults. PPD patients may, for example, interpret an honest mistake as a deliberate attempt to harm, a casual humorous remark as a serious character attack, a compliment as a veiled criticism, and an offer of help as a judgment of failure.
- Close relationships are impaired by hypervigilance for threats and associated guardedness. May appear as "cold." Suspiciousness can lead to pathologic jealousy where they gather circumstantial evidence to support contention of betrayal.
- To protect themselves from the perceived malice of others, these patients often maintain a high degree control of relationships and interactions, constantly questioning the whereabouts, intentions, or actions of the other.
- Often rigid and critical of others but have great difficulty accepting criticism themselves.
- Given their lack of trust of others, PPD patients have an excessive need for self-sufficiency and autonomy.
- Quick to counterattack and may be litigious.
- May join "cults" or groups who share their paranoid belief system.
- In response to stress, may experience very brief psychotic episodes (minutes to hours).

ETIOLOGY

- At this point, limited knowledge about role of genetic loading and neurobiologic vulnerability.
- However, increased prevalence in families of probands with schizophrenia and delusional disorder, paranoid type, suggests possible genetic role.

DIAGNOSIS

DIFFERENTIAL DIAGNOSIS

- Schizophrenia, paranoid type, delusional disorder, paranoid type, and mood disorder with psychotic symptoms: require presence of persistent positive psychotic symptoms such as delusions and hallucinations. To give an additional diagnosis of PPD, the personality disorder must be present before the onset of psychotic symptoms and must persist when the psychotic symptoms are in remission.
- Substance-induced paranoia, especially in the context of cocaine or methamphetamine abuse or dependence.
- Personality changes due to a general medical condition that affects the central nervous system.
- Paranoid traits associated with a sensory disability. For example, hearing impairment.
- Increased risk for major depressive disorder, obsessive-compulsive disorder, agoraphobia, and substance abuse or dependence.
- The most common co-occurring personality disorders are schizotypal, schizoid, narcissistic, avoidant, and borderline:
  1. Schizotypal personality disorder includes magical thinking and unusual perceptual experiences.
  2. Schizoid and borderline personality disorders do not have prominent paranoid ideation.
  3. Avoidant personality disorder includes fear of embarrassment.
  4. Narcissistic personality disorder includes the fear that hidden "flaws" or "inferiority" may be revealed.

WORKUP

- History—collateral information essential to establishing presence of longstanding interpersonal pattern in multiple domains of the patient's life
- Physical examination
- Mental status examination

LABORATORY TESTS

Those necessary to rule out medical causes of personality changes

IMAGING STUDIES

Those necessary to rule out medical causes of personality changes

TREATMENT

NONPHARMACOLOGIC THERAPY

- No randomized trials assessing treatment.
- Cognitive behavioral therapy to help patients control rage, manage perceived criticism, and develop social skills.
- Psychodynamic psychotherapy to help patient develop capacity to trust.

ACUTE GENERAL Rx

Benzodiazepines or low-dose antipsychotics to control hostility and paranoia

CHRONIC Rx

- Low-dose antipsychotic medication. Increase dose in small increments to minimize risk of side effects.
- SSRIs if comorbid depression, obsessive-compulsive disorder, or agoraphobia.
- Substance abuse treatment if comorbid dependence.

COMPLEMENTARY & ALTERNATIVE MEDICINE

No evidence of efficacy in PPD.

DISPOSITION

- Severity is variable and course is chronic. Often lifelong difficulty maintaining intimate relationships.
- At increased risk for major depressive disorder, obsessive-compulsive disorder, agoraphobia, and substance abuse or dependence.
- In some cases, PPD a prepsychotic antecedent of delusional disorder, paranoid type.

REFERRAL

- If pharmacotherapy or psychotherapy contemplated
- If patient's social or occupational functioning impaired

PEARLS & CONSIDERATIONS

COMMENTS

- Illness exacerbates these patients' sense of vulnerability.
- Communicating personal information to the physician challenges the guarded, self-protective approach to others and will often heighten PPD patients' fear that the physician will harm them.
- The encounter with the physician intensifies hypervigilance. As a result, innocuous or even overtly helpful behaviors by the physician may be perceived as threatening.
- With the perceived threat, these patients will often confront and challenge the physician on their motives and their rationale for diagnosis and treatment. Conflict and argument are not uncommon.
- Thus, establishing an alliance with the patient can be challenging.
- Faced with such a patient, physicians may understandably react defensively to unfounded suspicion or distance and not respond to the patient's concerns. Both responses increase the patient's anxiety and paranoia.
- Management guidelines:
  1. Convey intent "to do no harm."
  2. Address the patient's fears and concerns, no matter how irrational, in a clear, direct, and detailed manner.
  3. Remember that behind the patient's hostility lie fears that are real to him or her.
  4. Maintain a professional and neutral stance.
  5. Responding with too much warmth and friendliness will intensify paranoia.
  6. Give patient detailed and factual information about treatment plan.
  7. Give patient as much control as possible, including maximum participation at each decision node.
  8. Do not personalize patient's hostility and suspicion, but understand their distrust as an attempt to manage their own intense fear.
  9. Validate patient's concerns about the diagnosis or treatment plan.

SUGGESTED READINGS

Gomez-Benyto M et al: Posttraumatic stress disorder in primary care with special reference to personality disorder comorbidity, *Br J Gen Pract* 56(526):349, 2006.

Shea MT et al: Associations in the course of personality disorders and Axis I disorders over time, *J Abnorm Psychol* 113(4):499-508, 2004.

Ward RK: Assessment and management of personality disorders, *Am Fam Physician* 70(8):1505-1512, 2004.

AUTHOR: **JOHN Q. YOUNG, M.D., M.P.P.**

BASIC INFORMATION

DEFINITION

Idiopathic Parkinson's disease (PD) is a progressive neurodegenerative disorder characterized clinically by rigidity, tremor, and bradykinesia.

SYNONYMS

Paralysis agitans

ICD-9CM CODES
332.0 Idiopathic Parkinson's disease, primary
332.1 Parkinson's disease, secondary

EPIDEMIOLOGY & DEMOGRAPHICS

PREVALENCE:

- Affects over 1 million people in North America.
- In age group <40 yr, <5/100,000 are affected.In those >70 yr, 700/100,000 are affected.
- Highest incidence in whites; lowest incidence in Asians and black Africans.

PHYSICAL FINDINGS & CLINICAL PRESENTATION

- Tremor—typically a resting tremor with a frequency of 4 to 6 Hz that is often first noted in the hand as a pill-rolling tremor (thumb and forefinger). Can also involve the leg and lip. Tremor improves with purposeful movement. Usually starts asymmetrically (Fig. 1-192).
- Rigidity—increased muscle tone that persists throughout the range of passive movement of a joint. This, too, is usually asymmetric in onset.
- Akinesia/Bradykinesia—slowness in initiating movement.
- Masked facies—face seems expressionless, "poker face." Decreased blink, often there is excess drooling.
- Gait disturbance—difficulty initiating the first step; small shuffling steps that increase in speed (festinating gait). Steps become progressively faster and shorter while the trunk inclines further forward. Decreased arm swing.
- Stooped posture.
- Other complaints and findings early on include micrographia (handwriting becomes smaller) and hypophonia (voice becomes softer).
- Postural instability—tested by "pull test." Ask patient to stand in place with back to examiner. Examiner pulls patient back by the shoulders, and proper response would be to take no steps back or very few steps back without falling. Retropulsion is a positive test as is falling straight back. This is not usually severe early on. If falls occur and postural reflexes are greatly impaired early on, then consider other disorders.

ETIOLOGY

- Unknown.
- Most cases are sporadic, with age being the most common risk factor, although there is probably a combination of both environmental and genetic factors contributing to disease expression. There are rare familial forms with at least five different genes identified. The most well known is the parkin gene, which is a significant cause of early-onset autosomal recessive Parkinson's disease and isolated juvenile-onset Parkinson's disease (at or before age 20).

DIAGNOSIS

A presumptive clinical diagnosis can be made based on a comprehensive history and physical examination. The combination of asymmetric signs, resting tremor, and good response to levodopa best differentiates idiopathic Parkinson's disease from other causes of parkinsonism (see "Differential Diagnosis").

DIFFERENTIAL DIAGNOSIS

- Multiple system atrophy—distinguishing features include autonomic dysfunction, (including urinary incontinence, orthostatic hypotension, and erectile dysfunction), parkinsonism, cerebellar signs, and normal cognition.
- Diffuse Lewy body disease—parkinsonism with concomitant dementia. Patients often have early hallucinations and fluctuations in level of alertness and mental status.
- Corticobasal degeneration—often begins asymmetrically with apraxia, cortical sensory loss in one limb, and sometimes alien limb phenomenon.
- Progressive supranuclear palsy—tends to have axial rigidity greater than appendicular (limb) rigidity. These patients have early and severe postural instability. Hallmark is supranuclear gaze palsy that usually involves vertical gaze before horizontal.
- Essential tremor—bilateral postural and action tremor.
- Secondary (acquired) parkinsonism:
  1. Postinfectious parkinsonism—von Economo's encephalitis.
  2. Parkinson's pugilistica—after repeated head trauma.
  3. Iatrogenic—any of the neuroleptics and antipsychotics. The high potency D_2-blocker neuroleptics are most likely to cause parkinsonism. Quetiapine is an atypical antipsychotic with a lower risk of causing parkinsonism. Clozaril does not cause parkinsonism.
  4. Toxins (e.g., MPTP, manganese, carbon monoxide).

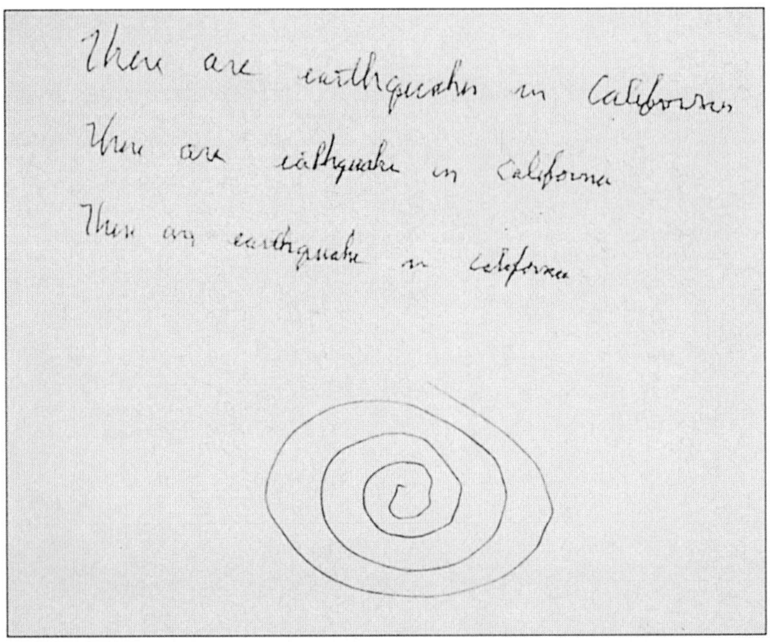

FIGURE 1-192 Handwriting sample of a patient with mild Parkinson's disease. The handwriting is slower and smaller, and the Archimedes spiral tends to be cramped and less open. Notice the progressive shortening of the length of the sentence as it is repeatedly written. If a tremor is present, it can usually be seen in the handwriting. Bradykinesia manifests in many other ways: decreased blinking and loss of facial expression (masked facies), decreased automatic swallowing leading to drooling, loss of arm swing while walking, and soft voice (hypophonia). During walking, some patients take faster and faster steps as the step size becomes smaller (festination). (From Rosenberg RN: *Atlas of clinical neurology,* Boston, 1998, Butterworth-Heinemann.)

5. Vascular parkinsonism (basal ganglia infarcts, multiinfarcts, Binswanger's).

WORKUP

Identification of clinical signs and symptoms associated with Parkinson's disease (see "Physical Findings") and elimination of conditions that may mimic it with a comprehensive history and physical examination

IMAGING STUDIES

CT scan has almost no role in investigations. MRI of the head may sometimes distinguish between idiopathic Parkinson's disease and other conditions that present with signs of parkinsonism (see "Differential Diagnosis").

TREATMENT

Rx

NONPHARMACOLOGIC THERAPY

- Physical therapy, patient education and reassurance, treatment of associated conditions (e.g., depression)
- Avoidance of drugs that can induce or worsen parkinsonism: neuroleptics (especially high potency), certain antiemetics (prochlorperazine, trimethobenzamide), metoclopramide, nonselective MAO inhibitors (may induce hypertensive crisis), reserpine, methyldopa

TREATMENT APPROACH WHEN INITIATING THERAPY

- Therapy should be initiated when disease starts to impact patient's quality of life.
- Goal of therapy is symptomatic and not curative.
- If symptoms very mild, can consider MAO-B inhibitor or amantadine.
- Once decision is made to start dopaminergic therapy, either agonists or levodopa can be used as first line. Decision is based on relative impact of improving motor disability (L-dopa) compared with lessening of motor complications (dopamine agonist). In general, consider use of dopamine agonist in young patients as first-line therapy. In patients >70 years of age, levodopa is the drug of choice.
- Motor complications do develop during the course of the disease and likely reflect the combination of disease progression together with the side effects of dopaminergic medications.

CHRONIC Rx

- Levodopa therapy
  1. Cornerstone of symptomatic therapy. Should be used with a peripheral dopa decarboxylase inhibitor (carbidopa) to minimize side effects (nausea, lightheadedness, postural hypotension). The combination of the two drugs is marketed under the trade name Sinemet.
  2. Usual starting dose is 25/100 mg (carbidopa/levodopa) tid 1 hr before meals.
  3. Controlled-release preparations (Sinemet CR) are available, but they do not delay onset of motor fluctuations (wearing off or dyskinesias) and have similar efficacy to immediate-release preparations. Higher doses are required because of decreased bioavailability. In general, use should be deferred to a neurologist.
  4. Stalevo (combination Sinemet and entacapone, a COMT inhibitor). Useful for patients with motor fluctuations (wearing off). There is no evidence for its use in patients without fluctuations, so it currently has no role in the early treatment of PD.
- Dopamine receptor agonists (Ropinirole, Pramipexole, Bromocriptine, and Rotigotine) are not as potent as levodopa, but they are often used as initial treatment in younger patients to attempt to delay the onset of complications (dyskinesias, motor fluctuations). These medications are more expensive than levodopa. In general they cause more side effects such as nausea, vomiting, light-headedness, peripheral edema, confusion, and somnolence than levodopa. They can also cause a dopamine dysregulation syndrome, which includes compulsive behaviors such as pathologic gambling and hypersexuality. All patients on these drugs should be asked about the presence of these symptoms. Nothing suggests that one agonist is better than another.
  1. Ropinirole (Requip): initial dose of 0.25 mg tid.
  2. Pramipexole (Mirapex): initial dose of 0.125 mg tid.
  3. Bromocriptine (Parlodel): initial dose, 1.25 mg qhs.
  4. Rotigotine (Neupro): transdermal patch initial dose of 2 mg qd.
- MAO B inhibitors can be used early as initial therapy in those with very mild disease or as adjunctive therapy. It is still unknown whether these drugs have neuroprotective effects or only mild symptomatic benefits.
  1. Selegiline: usual dose, 5 mg bid with breakfast and lunch. It can be useful in treating the fatigue that is commonly associated with PD. Concurrent use of stimulants and sympathomimetics should be avoided.
  2. Rasagaline: a newer MAO B inhibitor. Usual dose 1 to 2 mg/day.
- Amantadine (Symmetrel) can be used alone early in the disease. It is especially useful in the treatment of dyskinesias. Dosage is 100 mg tid (titrate q week from 100 mg qd). Must adjust for elderly and renal impairment. Most notable side effect, especially in elderly, is confusion and livedo reticularis.
- Anticholinergic agents are helpful in treating the tremor and drooling in patients with Parkinson's disease and can be used alone or in combination with levodopa; potential side effects include constipation, urinary retention, memory impairment, and hallucinations. They should be avoided in the elderly. In general, role is limited to young patients with tremor and no (or minimal) other associated signs/symptoms of PD.
  1. Trihexyphenidyl (Artane): initial dose, 1 mg tid po
  2. Benztropine (Cogentin): usual dose, 0.5 to 1 mg qd or bid
- Surgical options
  1. Pallidal (globus pallidus interna) and subthalamic deep brain stimulation are currently the surgical options of choice; thalamic DBS may be useful for refractory tremor.
  2. Surgery is limited to patients with disabling, medically refractory problems, and patients must still have a good response to L-dopa to undergo surgery. DBS results in decreased dyskinesias, fluctuations, rigidity, and tremor.

DISPOSITION

Parkinson's disease usually follows a slowly progressive course leading to disability over the course of several years. However, every patient will progress individually and patients should be reassured that this diagnosis does not, by definition, result in being either wheelchair or bed bound.

REFERRAL

- Neurology consultation is recommended on initial diagnosis of Parkinson's disease.
- Participation in outpatient physical therapy program is recommended for patients with moderate to advanced disease. The most useful speech therapy method available is the Lee Silverman technique, which focuses on projection.

PEARLS & CONSIDERATIONS

!

- Asymmetry of symptoms at onset is very useful in distinguishing PD from other causes of parkinsonism.
- Although resting tremor is a common presenting symptom, up to one fourth of patients with idiopathic PD do not have classic resting tremor.

COMMENTS

Additional patient information on Parkinson's disease can be obtained from the Internet at www.parkinson.org and from the National Parkinson Foundation, Inc., 1501 Ninth Avenue NW, Miami, FL 33136; phone: (800) 327-4545.

EVIDENCE

EBM

An American Academy of Neurology Practice Parameter on the initiation of treatment of Parkinson's disease was released in October 2002.[1] Controversy still exists as to whether treatment should be initiated with dopamine agonists or levodopa. Evidence shows that either can be used and the choice depends on the relative impact of improving motor disability (better with levodopa) compared with the lessening of motor complications (better with dopamine agonists). Ⓐ

There is little convincing evidence that one dopamine agonist is better than another with respect to control of parkinsonian symptoms.[2-5]

There are no large randomized controlled trials regarding the use of levodopa; however, experts agree that it is the most potent symptomatic treatment for PD.

Evidence from randomized controlled trials (RCTs) shows that selegiline delays the need for levodopa in early Parkinson's disease; however, there is no convincing evidence for either the neuroprotective benefit of or increased mortality with selegiline.[6] Ⓐ

Evidence from two RCTs suggests that there is no significant difference in motor complications or disease control at 5 years between modified-release and immediate-release levodopa in patients with early Parkinson's disease.[7,8] Ⓐ

A systematic review of double-blind crossover trials found that anticholinergics used in de novo or advanced Parkinson's disease are superior to placebo in at least one outcome measure, although reporting of methods and results was incomplete and outcome measures were often heterogenous.[9] Ⓑ

A systematic review of the efficacy of amantadine in the treatment of dyskinesias found insufficient data due to poor design of studies to comment on its utility; however, subsequent studies and clinical experience suggest that it is an effective drug in the treatment of dyskinesias.[10] Ⓐ

Evidence-Based References

1. Miyasaki JM et al: Practice parameter: initiation of treatment for Parkinson's disease: an evidence-based review, *Report of the Quality Standards Subcommittee of the American Academy of Neurology* 58:11, 2002.
2. Suchowersky O et al: Practice parameter: neuroprotective strategies and alternative therapies for Parkinson disease (an evidence-based review), *Neurology* 66:976, 2006.
3. Suchowersky O et al: Practice parameter: diagnosis and prognosis of new onset Parkinson disease (an evidence-based review), *Neurology* 66:968, 2006
4. Clarke CE, Deane KHO: Ropinirole versus bromocriptine for levodopa-induced complications in Parkinson's disease, Cochrane Movement Disorders Group, *Cochrane Database Syst Rev* 3, 2005.
5. Clarke JA: Pramipexole versus bromocriptine for levodopa-induced complications in Parkinson's disease, Cochrane Movement Disorders Group, *Cochrane Database Syst Rev* 3, 2005.
6. Macleod AD et al: Monoamine oxidase B inhibitors for early Parkinson's disease, Cochrane Movement Disorders Group, *Cochrane Database Syst Rev* 3, 2005.
7. Dupont E et al: Sustained-release Madopar HBS compared with standard Madopar in the long-term treatment of de novo Parkinsonian patients, *Acta Neurol Scand* 93:14, 1996. Reviewed in: *Clin Evid* 11:1736, 2004.
8. Block G et al: Comparison of immediate release and controlled release carbidopa/levodopa in Parkinson's disease, *Eur Neurol* 37:23, 1997. Reviewed in: *Clin Evid* 11:1736, 2004.
9. Katzenschlager R et al: Anticholinergics for symptomatic management of Parkinson's disease, Cochrane Movement Disorders Group, *Cochrane Database Syst Rev* 3, 2005.
10. Crosby NJ, Deane KHO, Clarke CE: Amantadine for dyskinesia in Parkinson's disease, Cochrane Movement Disorders Group, *Cochrane Database Syst Rev* 3, 2005.

SUGGESTED READINGS

Goetz C et al: Evidence-based medical review update: pharmacological and surgical treatments of Parkinson's disease: 2001 to 2004, *Mov Disord* 20:523, 2005.

Samii A et al: Parkinson's disease, *Lancet* 363(9423):1783, 2004.

Tetrud J et al: Treatment challenges in early stage Parkinson's disease, *Neurol Clin* 22:S19, 2004.

AUTHOR: **CINDY ZADIKOFF, M.D.**

BASIC INFORMATION

DEFINITION

Paronychia is a localized superficial infection or abscess of the lateral and proximal nail fold. Paronychia may be acute or chronic.

SYNONYMS

Nail bed infection
Nail bed abscess

ICD-9CM CODES
681.9 Paronychia

EPIDEMIOLOGY & DEMOGRAPHICS

- Acute paronychia affects males and females equally.
- Chronic paronychia more common in females than males (9:1).
- Acute paronychia most often occurs in children.
- Chronic paronychia usually presents in the fifth or sixth decade of life.
- Paronychia is the most common infection of the hand.

PHYSICAL FINDINGS & CLINICAL PRESENTATION

- Acute paronychia usually presents with the sudden onset of redness, swelling, and pain with abscess or cellulitis formation in the nail fold. Fluid with purulence is often present.
- Chronic paronychia is insidious, presenting with mild swelling and erythema of the nail folds.
- Acute paronychia usually involves only one finger.
- Chronic paronychia may involve more than one finger.
- Acute paronychia usually involves the thumb.
- Chronic paronychia commonly involves the middle finger.

ETIOLOGY

- Any disruption of the seal between the proximal nail fold and the nail plate can cause paronychial infections.
- Acute paronychia is almost always bacterial in origin (e.g., *Staphylococcus aureus* [most common], *Streptococcus pyogenes, Enterococcus faecalis, Proteus* and *Pseudomonas* species, and anaerobes).
- Chronic paronychia is commonly caused by *Candida albicans* (70%) with bacterial organisms accounting for the remaining 30%.
- Trauma, nail biting, hangnails, diabetes, and chronic exposure to water are common predisposing features of paronychia.

DIAGNOSIS

The diagnosis of paronychia is self-evident on physical examination.

DIFFERENTIAL DIAGNOSIS

- Herpetic whitlow
- Pyogenic granuloma
- Viral warts
- Ganglions
- Squamous cell carcinoma

WORKUP

A workup is usually not pursued unless there is treatment failure.

LABORATORY TESTS

- Gram stain and culture any purulent drainage.
- KOH mount may show pseudohyphae.

IMAGING STUDIES

X-ray the digit if concerned about osteomyelitis.

TREATMENT

NONPHARMACOLOGIC THERAPY

- For acute paronychia without purulent drainage, warm soaks tid or qid are helpful. If pus is present, surgical drainage is required.
- For chronic paronychia, avoid chronic immersion in water or exposure to moisture.

ACUTE GENERAL Rx

- First-generation cephalosporin (e.g., cephalexin 250 to 500 mg qid) or penicillinase-resistant penicillin (e.g., dicloxacillin 250 to 500 mg qid) are usually the antibiotics of choice for acute paronychia.
- Alternative antibiotic choices include clindamycin and amoxicillin-clavulanate potassium
- Surgical drainage is indicated if purulent discharge is noted.
- A No. 11 blade scalpel is used to lift the lateral perionychium and proximal eponychium off the nail, facilitating drainage.
- If the pus is located beneath the nail, the lateral edge of the nail can be lifted off the nail bed and excised.

CHRONIC Rx

- If no fungal organism is found, tincture of iodine (2 drops bid) helps keep the nail and skin dry.
- Chronic paronychia caused by *Candida albicans* is treated with topical antifungal agents (e.g., miconazole or ketoconazole applied tid).
- Unresponsive cases may be treated with itraconazole or fluconazole but should be done in consultation with dermatology and/or infectious disease.
- Surgery may be needed in refractory cases.

DISPOSITION

- Most acute paronychias with appropriate treatment resolve within 7 to 10 days.
- Osteomyelitis is a potential complication of paronychia.
- Untreated chronic paronychia leads to thickening and discoloration with eventual nail loss.

REFERRAL

Chronic paronychia refractory to topical medical therapy is best referred to dermatology and/or infectious disease. A hand surgeon is consulted if abscess drainage or surgery is being considered.

PEARLS & CONSIDERATIONS

COMMENTS

The GI tract, including the mouth and bowel, or the GU tract in women, are the usual sources of *Candida albicans* in chronic paronychia.

SUGGESTED READINGS

Daniel CR et al: Managing simple chronic paronychia and onycholysis with ciclopirox 0.77% and an irritant-avoidance regimen, *Cutis* 73(1):81, 2004.
Griffiths G et al: Paronychia or an abscess: early diagnosis, *Hosp Med* 65(11):696, 2004.

AUTHORS: **GLENN G. FORT, M.D., M.P.H.,** and **DENNIS J. MIKOLICH, M.D.**

BASIC INFORMATION

DEFINITION

Paroxysmal atrial tachycardia (PAT) is a group of arrhythmias that generally originate as reentrant rhythm from the AV node and are characterized by sudden onset and abrupt termination.

SYNONYMS

PAT
SVT
Supraventricular tachycardia

ICD-9CM CODES
427.0 Paroxysmal atrial tachycardia

PHYSICAL FINDINGS & CLINICAL PRESENTATION

- Patient is usually asymptomatic.
- Patient may be aware of "fast" heartbeat.
- Persistent tachycardia may precipitate CHF or hypotension during acute MI.

ETIOLOGY

- Preexcitation syndromes (Wolff-Parkinson-White [WPW] syndrome)
- Atrial septal defect
- Acute MI

DIAGNOSIS

WORKUP

ECG:

- Absolutely regular rhythm at rate of 150 to 220 bpm is present.
- P waves may or may not be seen (the presence of P waves depends on the relationship of atrial to ventricular depolarization).
- Wide QRS complex (>0.12 sec) with initial slurring (delta wave) during sinus rhythm and short PR (≤0.12 sec) is characteristic of WPW syndrome; this syndrome is a result of an accessory AV pathway (bundle of Kent) that preexcites the ventricular muscle earlier than would be expected if the impulse reached the ventricles by way of normal conduction system; arrhythmias associated with WPW are narrow-complex SVT, atrial fibrillation, and ventricular fibrillation; digoxin and verapamil use should be avoided because they can lead to arrhythmia acceleration through the accessory pathway. Radiofrequency catheter ablation of accessory pathways (performed in conjunction with diagnostic electrophysiology testing) is a safe and effective treatment of patients with WPW syndrome.

TREATMENT

NONPHARMACOLOGIC THERAPY

- Valsalva maneuver in the supine position is the most effective way to terminate SVT; carotid sinus massage (after excluding occlusive carotid disease) is also commonly used to elicit vagal efferent impulses.
- Synchronized DC shock is used if patient shows signs of cardiogenic shock, angina, or CHF.

ACUTE GENERAL Rx

- Adenosine (Adenocard), an endogenous nucleoside, is useful for treatment of paroxysmal SVT, particularly that associated with WPW; it is considered by many the first choice of therapy for treatment of almost all episodes of SVT unresponsive to vagal maneuvers; the dose is 6 mg given as a rapid IV bolus; tachycardia is usually terminated within a few seconds; if necessary, may repeat with 12 mg IV bolus. Contraindications are second- or third-degree AV block, sick sinus syndrome (SSS), atrial fibrillation, and ventricular tachycardia. Adenosine may cause bronchospasm in asthmatics. Patients receiving theophylline (a competitive antagonist of adenosine receptors) are usually refractory to treatment. Dipyridamole enhances the effect of adenosine; therefore patients receiving dipyridamole should be started at lower doses.
- Verapamil 5 to 10 mg IV is given over 5 min; if no effect, may repeat in 30 min.
  1. Verapamil should be used cautiously in patients with SVT associated with hypotension.
  2. Slow injection of calcium chloride (10 ml of a 10% solution given over 5 to 8 min before verapamil administration) decreases the hypotensive effect without compromising its antiarrhythmic effect.
- Repeat carotid massage after IV verapamil if SVT persists.
- Metoprolol (IV 5 mg/2 min up to 15 mg) or esmolol (500 μg/kg IV bolus, then 50 μg/kg/min) may be effective in the treatment of SVT.
- IV digitalization (0.75 to 1 mg slow IV loading) if other agents are not effective
  1. Repeat carotid massage 30 min later; if not successful, give additional 0.25 mg IV digoxin and repeat carotid sinus massage 1 hr later.
  2. Digoxin should be avoided in patients with WPW syndrome and narrow QRS tachycardia (increased risk of atrial fibrillation during AV reentrant tachycardia).

DISPOSITION

Most patients respond well with resolution of the paroxysmal atrial tachycardia with treatment (see "Acute General Rx").

REFERRAL

Radiofrequency ablation is the procedure of choice in patients with accessory pathways and recurrent symptomatic episodes.

PEARLS & CONSIDERATIONS

COMMENTS

Accessory pathways occur in 0.1% to 0.3% of the general population.

SUGGESTED READING

Marine JE: Catheter ablation therapy for supraventricular arrhythmias, *JAMA* 298(3):2768-2778, 2007.

AUTHOR: **FRED F. FERRI, M.D.**

BASIC INFORMATION

DEFINITION

Paroxysmal cold hemoglobinuria (PCH) is a rare disease characterized by episodic massive intravascular hemolysis after exposure to cold temperatures. Hemolysis may occur in an idiopathic form in adults or, more commonly, after a viral infection in children. It was first described in patients with secondary or tertiary syphilis.

SYNONYMS

PCH
Donath-Landsteiner hemoglobinuria

ICD-9CM CODES
283.2 Hemoglobinuria caused by hemolysis from external causes

EPIDEMIOLOGY & DEMOGRAPHICS

- No race or sex predilection
- Accounts for up to 5% of adult cases of autoimmune hemolytic anemia
- Accounts for nearly 30% of childhood cases of autoimmune hemolytic anemia

PHYSICAL FINDINGS & CLINICAL PRESENTATION

- Following cold exposure, red to brown urination begins within minutes to hours.
- Associated symptoms include back, leg, and abdominal pain.
- Headaches, nausea, vomiting, and diarrhea are common.
- May be associated with Raynaud's phenomenon.
- Associated with cold urticaria.
- Transient splenomegaly and jaundice may occur.
- Symptoms and gross hemoglobinuria usually resolve within hours.
- Symptoms thought to be mediated by smooth muscle dysfunction secondary to nitric oxide toxicity associated with hemoglobinemia.

ETIOLOGY & PATHOGENESIS

- Polyclonal IgG (Donath-Landsteiner antibody) binds to P antigen on RBC membrane when blood is exposed to cold temperatures. As blood warms to body temperature, complement-mediated hemolysis ensues.
- In children, the appearance of the antibody usually follows the onset of a viral respiratory illness by 7-10 days. Symptoms may persist for several weeks.
- PCH has been associated with multiple infectious pathogens, including syphilis, H. influenza, EBV, CMV, influenza A, varicella, measles, mumps, and adenovirus.

DIAGNOSIS

DIFFERENTIAL DIAGNOSIS

- Cold agglutinin disease associated with hemoglobinuria, paroxysmal nocturnal hemoglobinuria, rhabdomyolysis.
- Other causes of acute massive intravascular hemolysis.

LABORATORY TESTS

- The presence of IgG that reacts with the red blood cell at reduced temperatures but not at body temperature. In the Donath-Landsteiner test, a patient's serum is incubated with donated RBCs and complement at 4° C then warmed to 37° C. Lysis is observed in a positive test.
- A more sensitive test involves using radiolabelled monoclonal antiIgG. This is incubated at 4° C with the patient's serum and donor RBCs. The degree of radioactivity on the separated RBCs will be elevated in PCH as compared with a control run at 37° C.
- Elevated bilirubin and LDH.
- Abnormal RBC forms such as poikilocytosis, spherocytosis, and anisocytosis.
- Erythrophagocytosis by neutrophils and monocytes may be seen.

TREATMENT

NONPHARMACOLOGIC THERAPY

The mainstay of treatment is the avoidance of exposure to cold.

ACUTE GENERAL Rx

- In children in particular, transfusion may be necessary as the anemia may become life threatening and hemolysis may be ongoing for several weeks.
- Testing and treatment for syphilis if present.
- Steroids generally are not found to be helpful.
- Splenectomy is not indicated.

DISPOSITION

- Postinfectious varieties are self-limited.
- Adult idiopathic form is generally manageable by avoidance of environmental exposure.

REFERRAL

To hematologist to aid in diagnosis

PEARLS & CONSIDERATIONS

- PCH is associated with brown or red discoloration of urine after cold exposure in adults or after a viral infection in children.
- PCH can be associated with viral or bacterial infections, including syphilis, H. influenza, EBV, CMV, influenza A, varicella, measles, mumps, and adenovirus.
- PCH can cause life-threatening hemolysis in children.

SUGGESTED READINGS

Packman CH: Cryopathic hemolytic syndromes. In Beutler et al (eds): *Williams hematology,* ed 6, New York, 2001, McGraw Hill.

Thomas AT: Autoimmune hemolytic anemias. In Lee et al (eds): *Wintrobes' clinical hematology,* Philadelphia, 1999, Lippincott Williams & Wilkins.

AUTHOR: **MICHAEL MAHER, M.D.**

BASIC INFORMATION

DEFINITION

Paroxysmal nocturnal hemoglobinuria (PNH) is a rare disease characterized by episodes of intravascular hemolysis and hemoglobinuria usually occurring at night. Thrombocytopenia, leukopenia, and recurrent venous thrombosis are also associated with PNH.

SYNONYMS

PNH

ICD-9CM CODES
283.2 Paroxysmal nocturnal hemoglobinuria

EPIDEMIOLOGY & DEMOGRAPHICS

- Affects patients of any age (reported spectrum 6 to 82 yr) but most common in patients aged 30 to 50 yr
- Affects both sexes (slight female predominance) and all races

PHYSICAL FINDINGS & CLINICAL PRESENTATION

Initial manifestations
- Anemia symptoms (35%)
- Hemoglobinuria (25%)
- Bleeding (20%)
- Aplastic anemia (15%)
- GI symptoms (10%)
- Hemolytic anemia (10%)
- Iron deficiency anemia (5%)
- Venous thrombosis (5%)
- Infections (5%)
- Neurologic symptoms

Hemoglobinuria
- Typically the first morning void reveals dark urine with progressive clearing during the day. The cause for the circadian rhythm is unknown.

Hemolysis
- In addition to the circadian hemolysis and resulting hemoglobinuria, episodes of hemolytic exacerbations can accompany infections, menstruation, transfusion, surgery, iron therapy, and vaccinations. Symptoms of severe hemolysis include chest, back, or abdominal pain, headache, fever, malaise, and fatigue.

Aplastic anemia
- Aplastic anemia may be the presenting manifestation of PNH (therefore PNH must be in the differential diagnosis of aplastic anemia) or may develop as a later complication of PNH.

Thrombosis
- Lower extremity DVT
- Subclavian thrombosis
- Portal or mesenteric vein thrombosis
- Hepatic vein thrombosis (Budd-Chiari syndrome)
- Cerebrovascular thromboses

Renal failure
- Acute renal failure associated with massive hemoglobinuria (acute tubular necrosis)
- Progressive renal failure associated with thrombosis within renal small veins

Dysphagia

Infections (associated with leukopenia or steroid treatment)

Physical findings include:
- Pallor (anemia)
- Jaundice (hemolysis)
- Splenomegaly
- Unilateral extremity swelling (DVT)
- Ascites (Budd-Chiari syndrome)

ETIOLOGY & PATHOGENESIS

- Complement-mediated hemolysis; the erythrocytes are abnormally sensitive to acidified serum.
- Patients have two populations of RBCs, some sensitive to hemolysis (PNH III cells) and others not (PNH I cells) in variable proportions (10% to 75% PNH III cells). About 20% PNH III are required for hemoglobinuria to be detectable.
- The RBC defects in PNH are in the membrane proteins as follows:
  Decay-accelerating factor deficiency
  Membrane inhibitor of reactive lysis deficiency
  C-8 binding protein deficiency
- These protein deficiencies are the result of an acquired mutation located in the X chromosome, which regulates glycosylphosphatidylinositol (GPI). GPI anchors the abovementioned proteins in the RBC membrane; GPI-deficient RBCs proliferate as an abnormal clone. Because women are affected at least as frequently as men are, the mutation must be expressed as dominant gene. The mechanism whereby the mutant stem cells can dominate hematopoiesis in PNH is unknown.
- The pathophysiology of the relationship of PNH and aplastic anemia is unknown.

DIAGNOSIS

Clinical situations:
- Intravascular hemolysis
- Hemoglobinuria
- Pancytopenia associated with hemolysis
- Iron deficiency associated with hemolysis
- Recurrent venous thrombosis
- Recurrent episodes of abdominal pain, headache, or back pain associated with hemolysis

DIFFERENTIAL DIAGNOSIS

- See "Hemolytic Anemia" in Section I.
- See "Aplastic Anemia" in Section I.
- See "Anemia" algorithm in Section III.

LABORATORY TESTS

- CBC: anemia, leukopenia, thrombocytopenia
- Reticulocytosis
- RBC smear: spherocytes
- Negative Coombs' test
- Low leukocyte alkaline phosphatase
- Elevated LDH
- Low serum haptoglobin
- Low serum iron saturation, low ferritin
- Elevated urine hemoglobin
- Elevated urine urobilinogen
- Elevated urine hemosiderin
- Positive Ham test (acidified serum RBC lysis)
- Normoblastic hyperplasia on bone marrow aspirate or biopsy
- Identification of GPI-anchored protein deficiency on hematopoietic cells using monoclonal antibodies or flow cytometry
- Cytogenetic studies are not diagnostic

TREATMENT

- Androgenic steroids
- Prednisone (15 to 40 mg qod)
- Eculizumab, a humanized antibody that inhibits the activation of terminal complement components, is an effective therapy for PNH; it reduces intravascular hemolysis, hemoglobinuria, and need for transfusion in patients with PNH
- Iron replacement
- Transfusions
- Treatment and prevention of thrombosis (heparin, coumadin)
- Avoidance of oral contraceptives
- Bone marrow transplantation

REFERRAL

To hematologist

PROGNOSIS

- 50% survival to 10 to 15 yr
- 25% survival to 25 yr
- If thrombosis at presentation, only 40% survival to 4 yr
- 1% incidence of leukemia
- 5% incidence of myelodysplastic syndrome

SUGGESTED READINGS

Brodsky RA: Narrative review: paroxysmal nocturnal hemoglobinuria: the physiology of complement-related hemolytic anemia, *Ann Intern Med* 148:587-595, 2008.

Hillmen P et al: The complement inhibitor eculizumab in paroxysmal nocturnal hemoglobinuria, *N Engl J Med* 355:1233, 2006.

AUTHORS: **FRED F. FERRI, M.D.,** and **TOM J. WACHTEL, M.D.**

BASIC INFORMATION

DEFINITION

Medication errors represent failure of intended prescription, dispensation, or administration of desired drug therapy. Medication errors may result in inappropriate medication use or an adverse drug event (ADE) (i.e., direct harm or injury to the patient).

SYNONYMS

Dosing errors or mistakes. Medication errors are not synonymous with ADEs because not all cause harm (a requirement of ADEs).

ICD-9CM CODES
Not applicable

EPIDEMIOLOGY & DEMOGRAPHICS

INCIDENCE:

- 15% of pediatric outpatient prescriptions are either underdosed (7%) or overdosed (8%).
- Nearly 6% of medication orders for a hospitalized child contain an error. 1% of medication orders for a child will result in a potential ADE (i.e., an error that would have caused harm but was intercepted before reaching the patient). Less than 1% of medication orders for a child will contain an error that ultimately results in harm or injury.

PEAK INCIDENCE: Among outpatient prescriptions, medication errors occur more frequently in children younger than 4 years of age compared with older children (20% vs. 13%)

PREVALENCE: Not applicable

PREDOMINANT SEX AND AGE: Children younger than 4 years of age

GENETICS: Not applicable

RISK FACTORS:

- Patient age younger than 4 years, particularly with prescriptions for asthma and allergy medications or antibiotics
- Off-label (non-FDA approved) medication use
- Prescriptions for analgesics (most commonly written for potential overdose)
- Lack of computerized prescriber order entry (CPOE), standardized order sets, or alert systems
- Prescriptions for antiseizure medications (most commonly written for potential underdose)
- Infants or children with multiple health care needs or those in intensive care

PHYSICAL FINDINGS & CLINICAL PRESENTATION

- Signs and symptoms of toxicity specific to the current drug regimen
- Lack of clinical efficacy of the current drug regimen

ETIOLOGY

Common sources of pediatric medication errors include:

- Prescribing errors: lack of knowledge of medication; lack of recognition of the impact growth and development may have on the pharmacokinetics of a specific drug; use of medical abbreviations within the prescription or medication order
- Calculation errors: mg/kg/*dose* vs. mg/kg/*day* dosing recommendations; "tenfold" decimal mistakes such as the use of trailing zeros (1 vs. 1.0) and naked decimals (0.1 vs. 1); patient weight in pounds vs. kilograms
- Administration errors: incomplete education provided to patient or caregiver; lack of appropriate drug administration tools such as graduated oral syringes, medication spoons, and so on; deviation from the "five rights," (i.e., the *right* drug at the *right* dose for the *right* patient by the *right* route at the *right* time)
- Dispensing errors: inappropriate formulation recommended, prescribed, or dispensed; use of adult formulations for children

DIAGNOSIS

DIFFERENTIAL DIAGNOSIS

- Iatrogenic adverse drug reaction (unpreventable ADEs)
- Patient nonadherence (may be considered a medication error if appropriate instructions and/or education are not provided to the patient or caregiver)

WORKUP

Alert from CPOE systems, deviation from standardized order set, or detection upon review of prescription or medication order by pharmacist or nurse:

- Immediately discontinue medication order or prescription
- Determine if suspected error has reached the patient
- Assess harm to patient and intervene if necessary (if ADE has occurred)
- Determine source of error if possible
- Resume correct drug therapy with appropriate monitoring of efficacy and toxicity
- Report error to institution or facility for tracking and quality improvement purposes
- Report sentinel events (an adverse event that led to death, serious physical or psychologic injury, or the risk of such injury) to the Joint Commission

LABORATORY TESTS

Supratherapeutic or subtherapeutic serum drug concentrations (if applicable)

TREATMENT

Management of a medication error resulting in harm to the patient may include acute treatment of a toxic ADE or long-term management of a suboptimally treated condition. It should always include the workup described above.

ACUTE GENERAL Rx

If the medication error has reached the patient and resulted in an ADE, immediate intervention may be required. Disclosure to the patient or caregiver of an error resulting in harm to the patient is necessary.

CHRONIC Rx

Long-term management of injury or harm resulting from a medication error may be necessary.

DISPOSITION

- Prescribers may need to reestablish trust with the patient or caregiver following an error that resulted in harm to ensure optimal care in the future.
- The reporting of medication errors should be nonpunitive in nature and intent on individual education and correction of health-systems-related flaws.

REFERRAL

Consultation with a pharmacist trained in pediatric pharmacotherapy may improve individual drug therapy and ensure age-specific drug dosing. Interpreters may be necessary to ensure drug information is accurately relayed to non-English-speaking patients or caregivers.

PEARLS & CONSIDERATIONS

COMMENTS

- 20% of ADEs occurring in hospitalized children are preventable
- Medication errors must be reported for health-systems-related flaws to be identified and corrected.
- Careful attention must always be focused on the impact growth and development has on the pharmacokinetic characteristics of drugs used in children. From birth through adolescence, the absorption, distribution, metabolism, and elimination of a particular drug must not be assumed constant, and age-specific dosing recommendations should be used. A child's dose should not exceed that of an adult. Equations that calculate proportionate doses based on body weight or body surface area do not take into consideration these age-related changes.

PREVENTION

- Health systems management: Double-checking of calculations and verification of medication orders by pharmacists and nurses will reduce preventable ADEs. Eliminate the use of medical abbreviations within medication orders and prescriptions. The use of CPOE, standardized order sets, and electronic prescription filing can provide a prompt at the time of prescribing or ordering and will reduce medication errors resulting from illegible handwriting.
- Communication: Open lines of communication between the prescriber, nurse, and pharmacist will help ensure medication errors do not occur. Drug information must be presented and reinforced at a level and in a language understandable to patients or caregivers.
- Education: Health care professionals must remain knowledgeable of current standards of care, as well as new drug therapy options.
- Review of drug therapy: Reassessment of prescriptions for accurate age-appropriate dosing and the indication for drug therapy, monitoring of efficacy and toxicity, and reconfirming a patient or caregiver's understanding of the drug regimen will limit medication errors and potential harm in chronic medication use.

PATIENT/FAMILY EDUCATION

- Caregivers should always remind a child's doctor of any drug allergies or side effects the child has had in the past.
- A list of all the medicines a child uses should be kept and shared all the doctors the child sees. Remember to include over-the-counter medicine like cough medicine and analgesics.
- Caregivers should ask a child's doctor or pharmacist as many questions as needed so that they understand how to correctly use the child's medicine.

Evidence-Based References

Cowley E et al: Medication errors in children: a descriptive summary of medication error reports submitted to the United States Pharmacopeia, *Cur Ther Res Clin Exp* 62:627, 2001.

Kaushal R et al: Medication errors and adverse drug events in pediatric inpatients, *JAMA* 285:2114, 2001.

SUGGESTED READINGS

Kozer E, Berkovitch M, Koren G: Medication errors in children, *Pediatr Clin N Am* 53:1155, 2006.

Sharek PJ, Classen D: The incidence of adverse events and medical error in pediatrics, *Pediatr Clin N Am* 53:1067, 2006.

Stucky ER: Prevention of medication errors in the pediatric inpatient setting, *Pediatrics* 112:431, 2003.

AUTHOR: **BRIAN J. COWLES, PHARM.D.**

BASIC INFORMATION

DEFINITION

Pediculosis is lice infestation. Humans can be infested with three kinds of lice: *Pediculus capitis* (head louse [Fig. 1-193]), *Pediculus corporis* (body louse), and *Phthirus pubis* (pubic, or crab, louse). Lice feed on human blood and deposit their eggs (nits) on the hair shafts (head lice and pubic lice) and along the seams of clothing (body lice). Nits generally hatch within 7 to 10 days. Lice are obligate human parasites and cannot survive away from their hosts for longer than 7 to 10 days.

SYNONYMS

Lice

ICD-9CM CODES
132.9 Pediculosis

EPIDEMIOLOGY & DEMOGRAPHICS

- There are 6 million to 12 million cases of head lice in the U.S. yearly.
- Lice infestation of the scalp is most common in children (girls > boys).
- Infestation of the eyelashes is most frequently seen in children and may indicate sexual abuse.
- The chance of acquiring pubic lice from one sexual exposure with an infested partner is >90% (most contagious STD known).
- Body lice is most common in conditions of poor hygiene.

PHYSICAL FINDINGS & CLINICAL PRESENTATION

- Pruritus with excoriation may be caused by hypersensitivity reaction, inflammation from saliva, and fecal material from the lice.
- Nits can be identified by examining hair shafts.
- The presence of nits on clothes is indicative of body lice.
- Lymphadenopathy may be present (cervical adenopathy with head lice, inguinal lymphadenopathy with pubic lice).
- Head lice is most frequently found in the back of the head and neck, behind the ears.
- Scratching can result in pustules and crusting.
- Pubic lice may affect the hair around the anus.

ETIOLOGY

Lice are transmitted by close personal contact or use of contaminated objects (e.g., combs, clothing, bed linen, hats).

DIAGNOSIS

DIFFERENTIAL DIAGNOSIS

- Seborrheic dermatitis
- Scabies
- Eczema
- Other: pilar casts, trichonodosis (knotted hair), monilethrix

WORKUP

Diagnosis is made by seeing the lice or their nits. Combing hair with a fine-toothed comb is recommended because visual inspection of the hair and scalp may miss more than 50% of infestations.

LABORATORY TESTS

Wood's light examination is useful to screen a large number of children: live nits fluoresce, empty nits have a gray fluorescence, nits with unborn louse reveal white fluorescence.

TREATMENT

NONPHARMACOLOGIC THERAPY

- Patients with body lice should discard infested clothes and improve their hygiene.
- Combing out nits is a widely recommended but unproven adjunctive therapy.
- Personal items such as combs and brushes should be soaked in hot water for 15 to 30 min.
- Close contacts and household members should also be examined for the presence of lice.

ACUTE GENERAL Rx

The following products are available for treatment of lice:

- Permethrin: available over the counter (1% permethrin [Nix]) or by prescription (5% permethrin [Elimite]); should be applied to the hair and scalp and rinsed out after 10 min. A repeat application is generally not necessary in patients with head lice. It can be applied to clean, dry hair and left on overnight (8 to 14 hours) under a shower cap.
- Lindane 1% (Kwell), pyrethrin S (Rid): available as shampoos or lotions; they are applied to the affected area and washed off in 5 min; treatment should be repeated in 7 to 10 days to destroy hatching nits. Resistance to this medication is increasing. Lindane is potentially neurotoxic and should be avoided in infants and children weighing <50 kg.
- Malathion (Ovide) or organophosphate is effective in head lice. It is available by prescription. Use should be avoided in children ≤2 yr. It is not commonly used due to its objectionable odor, fear of flammability, and prolonged application time (8 to 12 hours).
- Eyelash infestation can be treated with the application of petroleum jelly rubbed into the eyelashes three times a day for 5 to 7 days. The application of baby shampoo to the eyelashes and brows three or four times a day for 5 days is also effective. The use of fluorescein drops applied to the lids and eyelashes is also toxic to lice.
- In patients who have previously failed treatment or in whom resistance with 1% permethrin cream rinse occurs, a 10-day course of trimethoprim-sulfamethoxazole (TMP-SMX) 8 mg/kg/day of trimethoprim in divided doses is an effective treatment for head lice infestation especially for eyelash infestations with *phthirus pubis.*
- Ivermectin (Mectizan), an antiparasitic drug, given in a single oral dose of 200 μg/kg is effective for head lice resistant to other treatments (currently not FDA approved for pediculosis).

PEARLS & CONSIDERATIONS

COMMENTS

- Patients with pubic lice should notify their sexual contacts. Sex partners within the last month should be treated.
- Parents of patients should also be educated that head lice infestation (unlike body lice) does not indicate poor hygiene.

SUGGESTED READINGS

Flinders DC, DeSchweinitz P: Pediculosis and scabies, *Am Fam Physician* 69:341, 2004.
Roberts RJ: Head lice, *N Engl J Med* 346:1645, 2002.

AUTHOR: **FRED F. FERRI, M.D.**

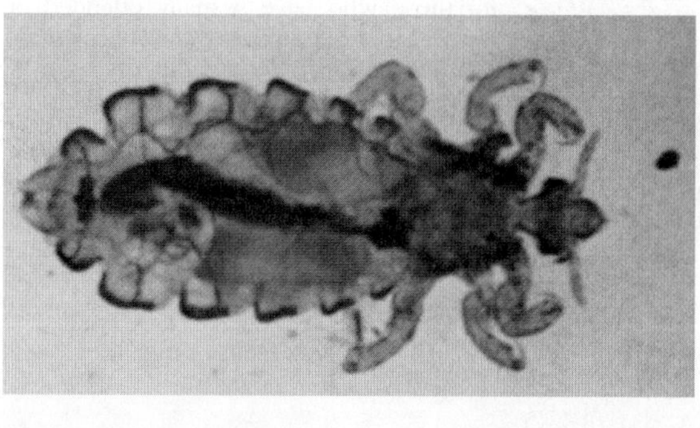

FIGURE 1-193 *Pediculus humanus* var. *capitis* (head louse). (From Mandell GL [ed]: *Mandell, Douglas, and Bennett's principles and practice of infectious diseases,* ed 6, New York, 2005, Churchill Livingstone.)

BASIC INFORMATION

DEFINITION

Pedophilia is a sexual disorder that involves recurrent, intense, distressing sexual urges and/or fantasies involving prepubescent children. A person must be at least 16 yr of age and at least 5 yr older than the child affected. The behavior may range from looking, to fondling, masturbation, and various degrees of penetration and coercion.

SYNONYMS

Pedophilia erotica
Acts referred to as child sexual abuse or child molestation

ICD-9CM CODES
302.2 Pedophilia

EPIDEMIOLOGY & DEMOGRAPHICS

PEAK INCIDENCE: Onset in adolescence

PREVALENCE (IN U.S.): 12% of men and 17% of women report being sexually touched by an older person when they were children.

PREDOMINANT SEX:

- Majority of perpetrators are men: 75% attracted to females exclusively; 25% attracted to males exclusively
- Girls sexually abused 3 times more often than boys; children from the lowest-income families 18 times more likely to be sexually abused.

PREDOMINANT AGE: 1 of every 7 sexual assaults of juveniles occurs in children younger than 6 yr and one third are younger than 12 yr.

GENETICS: None identified.

PHYSICAL FINDINGS & CLINICAL PRESENTATION

- Often shy, passive, and with social and interpersonal difficulties
- Frequently, has experienced early abuse himself/herself
- May occasionally seek help before any sexual acts with children
- "Belief" among some of those who molest children that their behavior is good for or welcomed by the child

ETIOLOGY

- Personal experience with early molestation may be important, though only a minority of molested children develop pedophilia.
- Influence of personality factors is cited by some experts (i.e., inadequate attachment style rooted in a dysfunctional family).
- Neurodevelopmental perturbations increase the risk of pedophilia in males.

DIAGNOSIS

DIFFERENTIAL DIAGNOSIS

- Psychosis: may present with unusual ideas or statements that may rarely be confused with pedophilia.
- Incest: not necessarily based in pedophilia, but may instead reflect a dysfunctional family unit.
- Paraphilic sexual behavior in the setting of another condition such as mental retardation, brain injury, or drug intoxication.

WORKUP

- History is essential for diagnosis; however, most pedophiles are less than forthcoming even to direct questions by a physician.
- Children who have been sexually abused may display depression and aggressive behaviors, have an increased frequency of anxiety disorders, and have problems with age-appropriate sex roles and sexual functioning.
- Collateral information should be obtained from family members, suspected victims, or legal and social organizations; but even experienced interviewers may be unable to diagnose pedophilia consistently.

LABORATORY TESTS

Hormone profile is sometimes recommended.

IMAGING STUDIES

Useful only if pedophilic behavior is believed to be a consequence of CNS damage

TREATMENT

NONPHARMACOLOGIC THERAPY

- Usually obtain treatment under legal coercion after child molestation charge.
- Behavioral approaches are centered on aversion conditioning in which an aversive stimulus is paired with the pedophilic fantasy.
- Outpatient group therapy sometimes combined with the administration of antiandrogenic medications.
- For incestuous adult-child relationships not based in pedophilia, intensive family systems investigation and therapy are needed.
- Pedophilia is considered a chronic disorder. Therefore, treatment should focus on achieving long-term behavioral change in the community.
- Treat comorbid conditions, such as alcoholism and affective illness.

ACUTE GENERAL Rx & CHRONIC Rx

- Brief periods of inpatient hospitalization may be required as a precaution during periods of heightened stress.
- Chemical castration with antiandrogen compounds; they are generally believed to be safe, effective, and reversible.
- Medroxyprogesterone acetate (Provera) can be administered PO (60 mg/day) or in a depot IM form (200 to 400 mg IM once weekly).
- Testosterone-lowering medications. Although these drugs suppress the intensity of libidinal drive, they generally allow erectile function.
- Serotonin reuptake inhibitors to suppress sexual drive.

DISPOSITION

Untreated, child molesters are highly likely to be repeat offenders.

REFERRAL

Refer to specialty mental health.

PEARLS & CONSIDERATIONS

Physicians should be aware of reporting requirements in their jurisdiction.

EVIDENCE

A systematic review studied randomized, controlled trials of psychological treatments for children who had been sexually abused. It found that cognitive–behavioral therapy, particularly for young children, had the strongest evidence for improving psychological symptoms.[1] (B)

Evidence-Based Reference

1. Ramchandani P, Jones DP: Treating psychological symptoms in sexually abused children: from research findings to service provision, *Br J Psychiatry* 183:484, 2003. (B)

SUGGESTED READINGS

Blanchard R et al: IQ, handedness, and pedophilia in adult male patients stratified by referral source, *Sex Abuse* 19(3):285, 2007.
Fagan PJ et al: Pedophilia, *JAMA* 288(19):2458, 2002.
Kenworthy T et al: Psychological interventions for those who have sexually offended or are at risk of offending, *Cochrane Database Syst Rev* 3:CD004858, 2004. Review.
Schober JM et al: Leuprolide acetate is a familiar drug that may modify sex-offender behaviour: the urologist's role, *BJU Int* 97(4):684, 2006.

AUTHOR: **MITCHELL D. FELDMAN, M.D., M.PHIL.**

BASIC INFORMATION

DEFINITION

Pelvic inflammatory disease (PID) is a spectrum of inflammatory disorders of the upper genital tract including a combination of any of the following:

- Endometritis, salpingitis, tuboovarian abscess, or pelvic peritonitis
- Resulting from an ascending lower genital tract infection
- Not related to obstetric or surgical intervention

SYNONYMS

Adnexitis
Pyosalpinx
Salpingitis
Tuboovarian abscess

ICD-9CM CODES
614.9 Unspecified inflammatory disease of female pelvic organs and tissue

EPIDEMIOLOGY & DEMOGRAPHICS

INCIDENCE/PREVALENCE:

- Estimated 600,000 to 1 million cases annually (U.S.)
- Diagnosed in 2% to 5% of women seen in STD clinics
- Most common cause of female infertility and ectopic pregnancy

RISK FACTORS:

- Adolescent sexually active females <20 yr of age (1:8)
- Previous episode of gonococcal PID
- Multiple sexual partners
- Vaginal douching

PHYSICAL FINDINGS & CLINICAL PRESENTATION

- Lower abdominal pain
- Abnormal vaginal discharge
- Abnormal uterine bleeding
- Dysuria
- Dyspareunia
- Nausea and vomiting (suggestive of peritonitis)
- Fever
- Right upper quadrant tenderness (perihepatitis): 5% of PID cases
- Cervical motion tenderness and adnexal tenderness
- Adnexal mass

ETIOLOGY

- *Chlamydia trachomatis*
- *Neisseria gonorrhoeae*
- Polymicrobial infection—*Bacteroides fragilis, Escherichia coli, Gardnerella vaginalis, Haemophilus influenzae, Mycoplasma hominis, U. urealyticum*
- *Mycobacterium tuberculosis* (an important cause in developing countries)
- Cytomegalovirus (CMV)

DIAGNOSIS

DIFFERENTIAL DIAGNOSIS

- Ectopic pregnancy
- Appendicitis
- Ruptured ovarian cyst
- Endometriosis
- Urinary tract infection (cystitis or pyelonephritis)
- Renal calculus
- Adnexal torsion
- Proctocolitis

WORKUP

DIAGNOSTIC CONSIDERATIONS:

- Clinical diagnosis is difficult and imprecise. A clinical algorithm for the evaluation of pelvic pain is described in Section III, "Pelvic Pain, Reproductive-Age Woman"; evaluation of vaginal discharge is described in Section III, "Vaginal Discharge."
- Clinical diagnosis of symptomatic PID has a positive predictive value of 65% to 90% when compared with laparoscopy as the standard.
- No single historical, physical, or laboratory finding is both sensitive and specific for the diagnosis of PID.

2002 CDC DIAGNOSTIC CRITERIA FOR PID:

- Empiric treatment is based on the presence of all of the following minimum criteria:
  1. Uterine tenderness
  2. Adnexal tenderness
  3. Cervical motion tenderness
- Additional criteria to increase the specificity of the diagnosis of PID in women with severe clinical signs:
  1. Oral temperature >38.3° C (101° F)
  2. Abnormal cervical or vaginal discharge
  3. Elevated ESR
  4. Elevated C-reactive protein
  5. Laboratory documentation of cervical infection with *N. gonorrhoeae* or *C. trachomatis*
- Definitive criteria for diagnosing PID, which are warranted in selected cases:
  1. Laparoscopic abnormalities consistent with PID
  2. Histopathologic evidence of endometritis on biopsy
  3. Transvaginal sonography or other imaging techniques showing thickened fluid-filled tubes with or without free pelvic fluid or tuboovarian complex

LABORATORY TESTS

- Leukocytosis
- Elevated acute phase reactants: ESR >15 mm/hr, C-reactive protein
- Gram stain of endocervical exudate: >30 PMNs per high-power field correlates with chlamydial or gonococcal infection
- Endocervical cultures for *N. gonorrhoeae* and *C. trachomatis*
- Fallopian tube aspirate or peritoneal exudate culture if laparoscopy performed
- hCG to rule out ectopic pregnancy

IMAGING STUDIES

- Transvaginal ultrasound to look for adnexal mass has sensitivity for PID of 81%, specificity 78%, accuracy 80%.
- MRI has sensitivity for PID of 95%, specificity 89%, accuracy 93%. It is useful not only for establishing the diagnosis of PID, but also for detecting other processes responsible for the symptoms. Disadvantages are its higher cost and unavailability in certain areas.

TREATMENT

NONPHARMACOLOGIC THERAPY

- Most patients are treated as outpatients.
- Criteria for hospitalization (CDC, 2006) as follows:
  1. Surgical emergencies such as appendicitis cannot be excluded
  2. Tuboovarian abscess
  3. Pregnant patient
  4. Patient is immunodeficient
  5. Severe illness, nausea, or vomiting precluding outpatient management
  6. Patient unable to follow or tolerate outpatient regimen
  7. No clinical response to outpatient therapy

ACUTE GENERAL Rx

REGIMENS FOR TREATMENT OF PID RECOMMENDED BY THE CDC, 2006:

- Outpatient treatment: Regimen A:
  1. Ofloxacin 400 mg PO bid × 14 days or Levofloxacin 500 mg PO × 14 days with or without metronidazole 500 mg PO bid × 14 days
- Outpatient treatment: Regimen B:
  1. Cefoxitin 2 g IM plus probenecid 1 g PO single dose plus doxycycline 100 mg PO bid × 14 days with or without metronidazole 500 mg PO bid × 14 days *or*
  2. Ceftriaxone 250 mg IM once single dose plus doxycycline 100 mg PO bid × 14 days with or without metronidazole 500 mg PO bid × 14 days

- Inpatient treatment: Regimen A:
  1. Cefoxitin 2 g IV q6h or cefotetan 2 g IV q12h plus doxycycline 100 mg IV or PO q12h
  2. Continuation of regimen for at least 24 hr after substantial clinical improvement, after which doxycycline 100 mg PO bid is continued for a total of 14 days
- Inpatient treatment: Regimen B:
  1. Clindamycin 900 mg IV q8h plus gentamicin loading dose IV or IM (2 mg/kg of body weight), followed by a maintenance dose (1.5 mg/kg) q8h
  2. Continuation of regimen for at least 24 hr after substantial clinical improvement, followed by doxycycline 100 mg PO bid or clindamycin 450 mg PO qid to complete a total of 14 days of thcrapy
- Alternative parental regimens:
  1. Ofloxacin 400 mg IV q12h or
  2. Levofloxacin 500 mg IV once daily with or without Metronidazole 500 mg IV q8h or
  3. Ampicillin/sulbactam 3 gm IV q6h plus doxycycline 100 mg PO or IV q12h

CHRONIC Rx

Hospitalized patients receiving IV therapy:

1. Significant clinical improvement is characterized by defervescence, decreased abdominal tenderness, and decreased uterine, adnexal, and cervical motion tenderness within 3 to 5 days.
2. If no clinical improvement occurs, further diagnostic workup is necessary, including possible surgical intervention.

DISPOSITION

- Long-term sequelae of PID: recurrent PID, chronic pelvic pain, ectopic pregnancy, infertility, Fitz-Hugh–Curtis syndrome (Fig. 1-194)
- Risk of tubal infertility related to episodes of PID: first episode, 8%; second episode, 20%; third episode, 40%
- Essential to evaluate and treat male sex partners

REFERRAL

If there is no clinical improvement with outpatient therapy observed within 72 hr, patient should be hospitalized and gynecology consult requested.

PEARLS & CONSIDERATIONS

COMMENTS

Maintain a low threshold for the diagnosis of PID

EVIDENCE

EBM

One randomized, controlled trial compared inpatient with outpatient care, with various intramuscular and oral antibiotics, and found no significant difference for recurrence, chronic pelvic pain, infertility, or ectopic pregnancy at 35 mo.[1] Ⓐ

Evidence-Based Reference

1. Ness RB et al: Effectiveness of inpatient and outpatient treatment strategies for women with pelvic inflammatory disease: results from the Pelvic Inflammatory Disease Evaluation and Clinical Health (PEACH) randomized trial, *Am J Obstet Gynecol* 186:929, 2002. Reviewed in: *Clin Evid* 11:2121, 2004. Ⓐ

SUGGESTED READING

Centers for Disease Control and Prevention: 2006 sexually transmitted diseases treatment guidelines, *MMWR Morb Mortal Wkly Rep* 55(RR-11):1, 2006.

AUTHORS: **GEORGE T. DANAKAS, M.D.,** and **RUBEN ALVERO, M.D.**

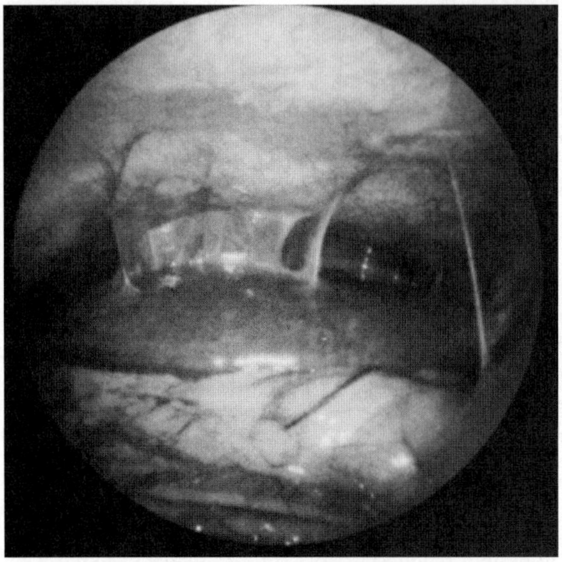

FIGURE 1-194 "Violin string" adhesions are visualized in this patient with Fitz-Hugh-Curtis syndrome. (From Copeland LJ: *Textbook of gynecology,* ed 2, Philadelphia, 2000, WB Saunders.)

BASIC INFORMATION

DEFINITION

- Pemphigus refers to a group of rare, potentially fatal, chronic, autoimmune blistering diseases of the skin and mucous membranes.
- Pemphigus has four main subtypes:
    1. Pemphigus vulgaris (PV) (Fig. 1-195)
        - Pemphigus vegetans, a rare clinical variant of PV
    2. Pemphigus foliaceus (PF)
        - Pemphigus erythematosus, a variant of PF
    3. Paraneoplastic pemphigus
    4. IgA pemphigus
- Pemphigus vulgaris is the most common form of pemphigus and refers to an intraepidermal autoimmune mucocutaneous blistering disorder characterized by the formation of a flaccid blister.

SYNONYMS

Pemphigus

ICD-9CM CODES

694.4 Pemphigus

EPIDEMIOLOGY & DEMOGRAPHICS

- Incidence is 1 case/100,000 persons
- More common in Ashkenazi Jews
- Typically occurs in the fourth and fifth decades of life
- Males = females
- Can occur in the young

PHYSICAL FINDINGS & CLINICAL PRESENTATION

- History
    1. Multiple oropharyngeal mucosal lesions typically occur first; these are followed by a generalized bullous eruption involving the skin within several weeks or months.
    2. Lesions are fragile and rupture easily, leaving painful denuded crusted erosions, which may be the only presenting symptom.
    3. Pain associated with oral mucosal blistering often results in dysphagia and hoarseness in voice.
    4. Usually not pruritic.
- Physical findings
    1. Anatomic distribution
        a. Oral mucosa
        b. Can also involve the pharynx, larynx, vagina, penis, anus, and conjunctival mucosa
        c. Generalized cutaneous involvement (Figs. 1-196 and 1-197)
    2. Lesion configuration
        a. All stratified squamous epithelium can become involved

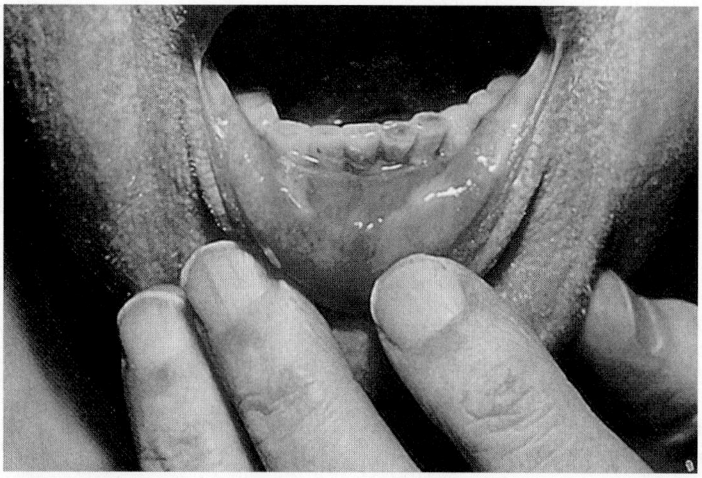

FIGURE 1-195 Pemphigus vulgaris with oral lesions and no intact bullae. (Courtesy Department of Dermatology, University of North Carolina at Chapel Hill. In Goldstein BG, Goldstein AO: *Practical dermatology,* ed 2, St Louis, 1997, Mosby.)

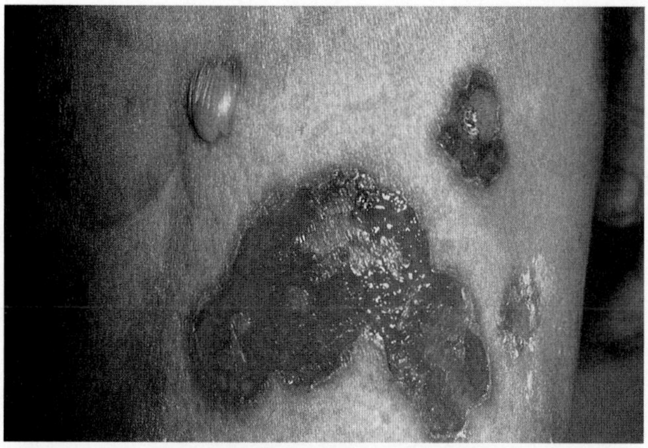

FIGURE 1-196 Pemphigus vulgaris: extensive erosions and blisters are present on the shin. (Courtesy R. A. Marsden, MD, St. George's Hospital, London, UK. From McKee PH, Calonje E, Granter SR [eds]: *Pathology of the skin with clinical correlations,* ed 3, St Louis, 2005, Mosby.)

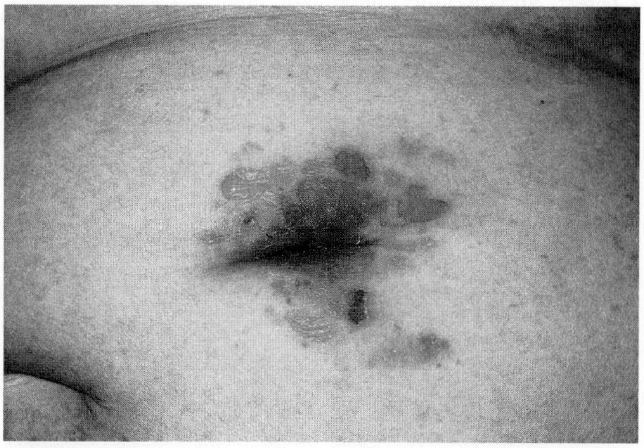

FIGURE 1-197 Pemphigus vulgaris: umbilical lesions showing intact blisters as well as raw erosions. (Courtesy R. A. Marsden, MD, St. George's Hospital, London, UK. From McKee PH, Calonje E, Granter SR [eds]: *Pathology of the skin with clinical correlations,* ed 3, St Louis, 2005, Mosby.)

3. Lesion morphology
   a. Flaccid bullae
   b. Denuded crusting and erosion commonly occurs
4. Nikolsky sign: nonspecific but clinically sensitive sign in which clinician applies sliding pressure to skin, causing separation of superficial epidermal layer of skin from basal layer

ETIOLOGY

Autoimmune disease caused by autoantibodies binding to antigens within the epithelial layer of the skin.

DIAGNOSIS (Dx)

The diagnosis of pemphigus vulgaris should be suspected in patients with oral lesion and flaccid bullae on the skin.

DIFFERENTIAL DIAGNOSIS

- Bullous pemphigoid (Table 1-34)
- Cicatricial pemphigoid
- Behçet's syndrome
- Erythema multiforme
- Systemic lupus erythematosus
- Aphthous stomatitis
- Dermatitis herpetiformis
- Drug eruptions

WORKUP

Specific laboratory tests, and histology and immunofluorescence testing of skin biopsies to establish the diagnosis.

LABORATORY TESTS

- Autoantibodies can be detected in the serum by indirect immunofluorescence assays.
- Skin biopsy reveals intraepidermal bulla formation, also called acantholysis (loss of cell adhesion between the epidermal cells).
- Direct and indirect immunofluorescence studies of the lesion show deposits of IgG and C3 in the epidermal layers of the skin.

IMAGING STUDIES

X-ray imaging is not useful in the diagnosis of pemphigus vulgaris.

TREATMENT (Rx)

NONPHARMACOLOGIC THERAPY

- Use mild soaps.
- Soak lesions with Burow's solution.
- Soft diet and viscous lidocaine can be used in patients with oral lesions.

ACUTE GENERAL Rx

- For mild cases, topical or intralesional steroids, triamcinolone acetonide 5 to 10 mg/ml, can be used for individual lesions. Topicals used for prevention of secondary infections on skin lesions include gentamicin and tetracycline.
- Systemic corticosteroids are cornerstone of therapy and critical to eliminating the inflammatory component of PV. They are very effective and work rapidly, but are associated with significant complications such as secondary infections, hypertension, osteoporosis, aseptic necrosis, and Cushing's syndrome.
- For more severe cases of PV, systemic corticosteroids are indicated at high dosages: Prednisone 1 mg/kg/day, titrating the dose to a clinical response. The drug is tapered as the condition is improved. The duration of treatment is variable; however, one should expect long-term management. Initial treatment duration and dosing changes usually occur at 6-8 wk.

CHRONIC Rx

- Adjuvant therapy such as immunosuppressants, anti-inflammatories, chemotherapeutic agents, and biologicals (e.g., Rituximab) are tried in patients as a steroid-sparing mechanism:
  1. Azathioprine 50 to 100 mg/day; treatment duration and dosing is determined by clinical response
  2. Cyclophosphamide 1 to 3 mg/kg/day
  3. Dapsone 25 to 100 mg/day
  4. Others: low-dose methotrexate, cyclosporine, mycophenolate, hydroxychlorine rituximab (monoclonal antibody)

DISPOSITION

- Before the use of corticosteroids, approximately 75% of patients die of pemphigus.
- Combined corticosteroids and adjuvant therapy has decreased mortality rates to <10%.
- Patients usually die from sepsis or complications from therapy.

REFERRAL

A dermatology consult is recommended for any patient with PV.

PEARLS & CONSIDERATIONS (!)

COMMENTS

PV, unlike bullous pemphigoid, rarely occurs in the elderly population.

It is important to diagnose PV early in its course for prompt treatment.

SUGGESTED READINGS

Bickle K, Roark TR, Hsu S: Autoimmune bullous dermatoses: a review, *Am Fam Physician* 65(9):1861, 2002.

Dick SE, Werth V: Pemphigus: a treatment update, *Autoimmunity* 39(7):591-599, 2006.

Yeh SW, Sami N, Ahmed RA: Treatment of pemphigus vulgaris: current and emerging options, *Am J Clin Dermatol* 6(5):327, 2005.

AUTHOR: **RAMI ELTIBI, M.D.**

TABLE 1-34 Differentiation of Pemphigus Vulgaris and Bullous Pemphigoid

Characteristics	Pemphigus Vulgaris	Bullous Pemphigoid
Age	>50 years	≥60 years
Site	Oral mucosa, face, chest, groin	Flexural areas, groin, axilla, less often oral
Findings	Flaccid bullae, intraepidermal blisters, IgG autoantibodies	Intact bullae, subepidermal blisters, IgG and complement autoantibodies
Treatment	Prednisone 40-60 mg/day, immunosuppressant agents; often chronically steroid-dependent	Prednisone 1 mg/kg/day or higher initially; taper over months to years
Prognosis	>90% respond; steroid side effects significant	>90% respond; remissions and recurrences common

BASIC INFORMATION

DEFINITION

Peptic ulcer disease (PUD) is an ulceration in the stomach or duodenum resulting from an imbalance between mucosal protective factors and various mucosal damaging mechanisms (see "Etiology").

SYNONYMS

PUD
Duodenal ulcer (DU)
Gastric ulcer (GU)

ICD-9CM CODES
536.8 Peptic ulcer disease
531.3 Peptic ulcer, stomach, acute
531.7 Peptic ulcer, stomach, chronic
532.3 Peptic ulcer, duodenum, acute
532.7 Peptic ulcer, duodenum, chronic

EPIDEMIOLOGY & DEMOGRAPHICS

- Incidence: 250,000 to 500,000 (200,000 to 400,000 DU; 50,000 to 100,000 GU) annually; duodenal ulcer:gastric ulcer ratio is 4:1.
- Anatomic location: >90% of DUs occur in the first portion of the duodenum; GU occurs most frequently in the lesser curvature near the incisura angularis.

PHYSICAL FINDINGS & CLINICAL PRESENTATION

- Physical examination is often unremarkable.
- Patient may have epigastric tenderness, tachycardia, pallor, hypotension (from acute or chronic blood loss), nausea and vomiting (if pyloric channel is obstructed), boardlike abdomen and rebound tenderness (if perforated), and hematemesis or melena (with a bleeding ulcer).

ETIOLOGY

Often multifactorial; the following are common mucosal damaging factors:

- *Helicobacter pylori* infection. *H. pylori* is the major cause of peptic ulcer disease. It is found in more than 70% of patients with duodenal ulcers and gastric ulcers in the U.S. Rates are much higher (>90%) in other parts of the world. Eradication of *H. pylori* markedly reduces peptic ulcer recurrence.
- Medications (NSAIDs, glucocorticoids)
- Incompetent pylorus or LES
- Bile acids
- Impaired proximal duodenal bicarbonate secretion
- Decreased blood flow to gastric mucosa
- Acid secreted by parietal cells and pepsin secreted as pepsinogen by chief cells
- Cigarette smoking
- Alcohol

DIAGNOSIS

DIFFERENTIAL DIAGNOSIS

- GERD
- Cholelithiasis syndrome
- Pancreatitis
- Gastritis
- Nonulcer dyspepsia
- Neoplasm (gastric carcinoma, lymphoma, pancreatic carcinoma)
- Angina pectoris, MI, pericarditis
- Dissecting aneurysm
- Other: high small bowel obstruction, pneumonia, subphrenic abscess, early appendicitis

WORKUP

- Comprehensive history and physical examination to exclude other diagnoses. Diagnostic modalities include endoscopy or UGI series. Endoscopy is invasive and more expensive; however, it is preferred for the following reasons:
  1. Highest accuracy (approximately 90% to 95%)
  2. Useful to identify superficial or very small ulcerations
  3. Essential to diagnose gastric ulcers (1% to 4% of gastric ulcers diagnosed as benign by UGI series are eventually diagnosed as gastric carcinoma)
  4. Additional advantages over UGI series include:
- Biopsy of suspicious looking ulcers
- Electrocautery of bleeding ulcers
- Measurement of gastric pH in suspected gastrinoma (e.g., patient with multiple ulcers)
- Diagnosis of esophagitis, gastritis, duodenitis
- Endoscopic biopsy for *H. pylori*

LABORATORY TESTS

- Routine laboratory evaluation is usually unremarkable.
- Anemia may be present in patients with significant GI bleeding.
- *H. pylori* testing via endoscopic biopsy, urea breath test, stool antigen test (*H. pylori* stool antigen), or specific antibody test is recommended:
  1. Serologic testing for antibodies to *H. pylori* is easy and inexpensive; however, the presence of antibodies demonstrates previous but not necessarily current infection. Antibodies to *H. pylori* can remain elevated for months to years after infection has cleared; therefore antibody levels must be interpreted in light of patient's symptoms and other test results (e.g., PUD seen on UGI series).
  2. The urea breath test documents active infection (sensitivity and specificity >90%). The patient ingests a small amount of urea labeled with carbon 13 (^{13}C) or carbon 14. If urease is present (produced by the organism), the urea is hydrolyzed and the patient exhales labeled carbon dioxide that is then collected and measured. This test is more expensive and not as readily available. Use of proton pump inhibitors (PPI) within 2 wk of the urea breath test may interfere with test results. Recently a new card test for ^{14}C urea has been developed providing a testing option in primary care settings. It uses a flat breath card that is read by a small analyzer.
  3. Histologic evaluation of endoscopic biopsy samples is considered by many the gold standard for accurate diagnosis of *H. pylori* infection. However, detection of *H. pylori* depends on the site and number of biopsy samples, the method of staining, and experience of the pathologist.
  4. Stool antigen test is an enzymatic immunoassay (ELISA) that identifies *H. pylori* antigen in stool specimen through a polyclonal anti-*H. pylori* antibody. It is as accurate as the urea breath test for diagnosis of active infection and follow-up evaluation of patients treated for *H. pylori*. A negative result on the stool antigen test 8 wk after completion of therapy identifies patients in whom eradication of *H. pylori* was unsuccessful.
- Additional laboratory evaluation is indicated only in specific cases (e.g., amylase level in suspected pancreatitis, serum gastrin level in suspected Zollinger-Ellison [ZE] syndrome).

IMAGING STUDIES

Conventional UGI barium studies identify approximately 70% to 80% of PUD; accuracy can be increased to approximately 90% by using double contrast.

TREATMENT

NONPHARMACOLOGIC THERAPY

- Stop smoking; smoking increases the risk of PUD, decreases the healing rate, and increases the frequency of recurrence.
- Avoid NSAIDs and alcohol.
- Special diets have been proved *unrelated* to ulcer development and healing; however, avoid foods that cause symptoms.

ACUTE GENERAL Rx

Eradication of *H. pylori*, when present, can be accomplished with various regimens:

1. PPI (e.g., omeprazole 20 mg bid or lansoprazole 30 mg bid, esomeprazole 40 mg qd) *plus* clarithromycin

500 mg bid *and* amoxicillin 1000 mg bid for 10 days. This regimen achieves an eradication rate of 80%-90% and can be used first line for patients not allergic to penicillin.
2. PPI bid *plus* amoxicillin 500 mg bid *plus* metronidazole 500 mg for 10 days.
3. PPI bid *plus* clarithromycin 500 mg bid *and* metronidazole 500 mg bid for 10 days. This regimen is useful in those with penicillin allergy.
4. A 1-day quadruple therapy may be as effective as a 7-day triple therapy regimen. The 1-day quadruple therapy regimen consists of two tablets of 262 mg bismouth subsalicylate qid, one 500-mg metronidazole tablet qid, 2 g of amoxicillin suspension qid, and two capsules of 30 mg of lansoprazole.
5. Bismouth compound qid *plus* tetracycline 500 mg qid *and* metronidazole 500 mg qid for 14 days.
6. A combination of levofloxacin 250 mg bid, amoxicillin 1000 mg bid, and a PPI bid for 10 to 14 days can be used as salvage therapy after unsuccessful attempts to eradicate *H. pylori* using other regimens.

PUD patients testing negative for *H. pylori* should be treated with antisecretory agents:

- Histamine-2 receptor antagonists (H_2RAs): cimetidine, ranitidine, famotidine, and nizatidine are all effective; they are usually given in split dose or at nighttime.
- Proton pump inhibitors (PPIs): can also induce rapid healing; they are usually given 30 min before meals.

Antacids and sucralfate are also effective agents for the treatment and prevention of PUD.

CHRONIC Rx

Maintenance therapy in duodenal ulcer patients is indicated in the following situations:

- Persistent smokers
- Recurrent ulcerations
- Chronic treatment with NSAIDs, glucocorticoids
- Elderly or debilitated patients
- Aggressive or complicated ulcer disease (e.g., perforation, hemorrhage)
- Asymptomatic bleeders

Misoprostol therapy (100 μg qid with food, increased to 200 μg qid if well tolerated) is useful for the prevention of NSAID-induced gastric ulcers in all patients on long-term NSAID therapy; it is contraindicated in women of childbearing age because of its abortifacient properties. Proton pump inhibitors are also effective at healing ulcers and maintaining remission in patients on long-term NSAIDs.

DISPOSITION

- The recurrence rate for untreated PUD is approximately 60% (>70% in smokers). Treatment decreases the recurrence rate by nearly 30%.
- Patients with recurrent ulcers should be retreated for an additional 8 wk and then placed on maintenance therapy with H_2RAs, PPIs, sucralfate, or antacids.
- An ulcer is considered refractory to treatment if healing is not evident after 8 wk for duodenal ulcers and 12 wk for gastric ulcers. In these patients maximum acid inhibition (e.g., Esomeprazole 40 mg bid) is preferred over continued therapy with standard antiulcer therapy.
- Eradication of *H. pylori* (when present) is indicated in all patients. A negative stool antigen test for *H. pylori* 6 wk after treatment accurately confirms cure of *H. pylori* infection with reasonable sensitivity in initially seropositive healthy subjects.
- Screening for Zollinger-Ellison (Z-E) syndrome should also be considered in patients with multiple recurrent ulcers; in patients with ZE, the serum gastrin level is >1000 pg/ml and the basal acid output is usually >15 mEq/hr.
- Surgery for refractory ulcers is now only rarely performed; it consists of highly selective vagotomy for duodenal ulcers or ulcer removal with antrectomy or hemigastrectomy without vagotomy for gastric ulcers.

REFERRAL

- GI referral for patients requiring endoscopy
- Surgical referral for patients with nonhealing ulcers despite appropriate medical therapy

PEARLS & CONSIDERATIONS

COMMENTS

- Patients with gastric ulcers should have repeat endoscopy after 4 to 6 wk of therapy to document healing and test exfoliative cytology for gastric carcinoma.
- After endoscopic treatment of bleeding peptic ulcers, bleeding recurs in up to 20% of patients. PPI administration intravenously by continuous infusion substantially reduces the risk of recurrent bleeding.

EVIDENCE

EBM

Treatment of peptic ulcers

Treatment of acute peptic ulcer bleeding with proton pump inhibitors significantly reduces rebleeding and surgical intervention rates compared with control (placebo or H_2 receptor antagonist), but there is no evidence of an effect on mortality.[1] Ⓐ

A systematic review has found; in patients with duodenal ulcers, eradication therapy is superior to ulcer-healing drug (UHD) and no treatment; in patients with gastric ulcers, no significant difference has been detected between eradication therapy and UHD; and that eradication therapy is superior to no treatment in preventing ulcer recurrence for both.[2] Ⓐ

A second systematic review has found that triple regimens are more effective than antisecretory therapy alone in healing duodenal ulcers. The review also found that *H. pylori* eradication regimens are significantly more effective than antisecretory therapy in reducing gastric and duodenal ulcer recurrence rates at 1 year.[3] Ⓐ

H. pylori eradication therapy has been shown in an RCT to be as effective as proton pump inhibitors in healing NSAID-related peptic ulcers.[4] Ⓐ

Prevention of peptic ulcers

In patients with no history of peptic ulceration, both proton pump inhibitor therapy alone and eradication therapy are effective in preventing NSAID associated ulcers.[5,6] Ⓐ

Evidence-Based References

1. Leontiadis GI et al: Proton pump inhibitor treatment for acute peptic ulcer bleeding. Reviewed in: Cochrane Library, 3, Chichester, UK, 2004, John Wiley. Ⓐ
2. Ford A et al: Eradication therapy for peptic ulcer disease in Helicobacter pylori positive patients. Reviewed in: Cochrane Library, 3, Chichester, UK, 2004, John Wiley. Ⓐ
3. Penston JG: Review article: clinical aspects of *Helicobacter pylori* eradication therapy in peptic ulcer disease, *Aliment Pharmacol Ther* 10:469-486, 1996. Reviewed in: *Clin Evid* 12:2004. Ⓐ
4. Chan FKL et al: Does eradication of *Helicobacter pylori* impair healing of nonsteroidal anti-inflammatory drug associated bleeding peptic ulcers? A prospective randomized study, *Aliment Pharmacol Ther* 12:1201-1205, 1998. Reviewed in: *Clin Evid* 12:2004. Ⓐ
5. Chan FKL et al: Randomised trial of eradication of *Helicobacter pylori* before nonsteroidal anti-inflammatory drug therapy to prevent peptic ulcers, *Lancet* 350:975-979, 1997. Reviewed in: *Clin Evid* 12:2004. Ⓐ
6. Labenz J et al: Primary prevention of diclofenac associated ulcers and dyspepsia by omeprazole or triple therapy in *Helicobacter pylori* positive patients: a randomised, double blind, placebo controlled, clinical trial, *Gut* 51:329-335, 2002. Reviewed in: *Clin Evid* 12:2004. Ⓐ

SUGGESTED READING

Lara LF et al: One day quadruple therapy compared with 7-day triple therapy for helicobacter pylori infection, *Arch Intern Med* 163:2079, 2003.

AUTHOR: **FRED F. FERRI, M.D.**

BASIC INFORMATION

DEFINITION

Pericarditis is the inflammation (or infiltration) of the pericardium associated with a wide variety of causes (see "Etiology").

ICD-9CM CODES
420.91 Pericarditis

EPIDEMIOLOGY & DEMOGRAPHICS

- The incidence of acute pericarditis is 2% to 6%.
- Increased incidence in males and in adults compared with children.
- Most common cause (>40%) of constrictive pericarditis is idiopathic.
- The use of thrombolytic agents has greatly reduced the incidence of both early postinfarction pericarditis and Dressler's syndrome.

PHYSICAL FINDINGS & CLINICAL PRESENTATION

- Severe constant pain that localizes over the anterior chest and may radiate to arms and back; it can be differentiated from myocardial ischemia, because the pain intensifies with inspiration and is relieved by sitting up and leaning forward (the pain of myocardial ischemia is not pleuritic).
- Pericardial friction rub is best heard with patient upright and leaning forward and by pressing the stethoscope firmly against the chest. It is often confused with the pleural rub. The pericardial friction rub corresponds temporally to movement of the heart within the pericardial sac. Typically the rub is a high-pitched scratchy or squeaky sound heard best at the left sternal border at end expiration. It consists classically of three short, scratchy sounds:
  1. Systolic component
  2. Diastolic component
  3. Late diastolic component (associated with atrial contraction)

However, in reality, the rub is reported to be triphasic in about half the patients, biphasic in a third, and monophasic in the remainder.

- Cardiac tamponade may be occurring if the following are observed:
  1. Tachycardia
  2. Low blood pressure and pulse pressure
  3. Distended neck veins
  4. Paradoxical pulse (pulsus paradoxus)

ETIOLOGY

- Idiopathic (possibly postviral). In 9 of 10 patients with acute pericarditis, the cause is either viral or unknown (idiopathic).
- Infectious (viral, bacterial [1% to 2%], tuberculous [4%], fungal, amebic, toxoplasmosis)
- Collagen-vascular disease (SLE, rheumatoid arthritis, scleroderma, vasculitis, dermatomyositis): 3% to 5 % of cases
- Drug-induced lupus syndrome (procainamide, hydralazine, phenytoin, isoniazid, rifampin, doxorubicin, mesalamine)
- Acute MI (transmural myocardial infarction)
- Trauma or posttraumatic
- After MI (Dressler's syndrome)
- After pericardiotomy
- After mediastinal radiation (e.g., patients with Hodgkin's disease)
- Uremia
- Sarcoidosis
- Neoplasm (primary or metastatic): 7% of cases
- Leakage of aortic aneurysm in pericardial sac
- Familial Mediterranean fever
- Rheumatic fever
- Leukemic infiltration
- Other: anticoagulants, amyloidosis, ITP

DIAGNOSIS

DIFFERENTIAL DIAGNOSIS

- Angina pectoris
- Pulmonary infarction
- Dissecting aneurysm
- GI abnormalities (e.g., hiatal hernia, esophageal rupture)
- Pneumothorax
- Hepatitis
- Cholecystitis
- Pneumonia with pleurisy

WORKUP

ECG, laboratory tests, and echocardiogram

LABORATORY TESTS

Generally lab tests are not clinically helpful and the clinical presentation should guide the ordering of any. The following tests may be useful in absence of an obvious cause:

- CBC with differential
- Viral titers (acute and convalescent)
- ESR (not specific but may be of value in following the course of the disease and the response to therapy)
- ANA, rheumatoid factor
- PPD, ASLO titers
- BUN, creatinine
- Blood cultures
- Cardiac isoenzymes (usually normal, but mild elevations of CK-MB may occur because of associated epicarditis). Plasma troponins are elevated in 35%-50% of patients with pericarditis.
- Pericardiocentesis is indicated in patients with pericardial tamponade and in those with known or suspected purulent or neoplastic pericarditis. The fluid should be analyzed for RBC and WBC counts, cytology, glucose, LDH, protein, pH, triglyceride level and cultured. PCR assays or elevated levels of adenosine deaminase activity (>30 U/L) are useful when suspecting tuberculous pericarditis.
- Pericardial biopsy may be helpful in recurrent tamponade.

IMAGING STUDIES

- Echocardiogram to detect and determine amount of pericardial effusion; absence of effusion does not rule out the diagnosis of pericarditis. Divergence of right and left ventricular systolic pressures is present in cardiac tamponade and constrictive pericarditis.
- ECG: varies with the evolutionary stage of pericarditis
  1. Acute phase: PR segment depression and diffuse ST-segment elevations (particularly evident in the precordial leads), which can be distinguished from acute MI by:
     a. Absence of reciprocal ST-segment depression in oppositely oriented leads (reciprocal ST-segment depression may be seen in aV_R and VI)
     b. Elevated ST segments concave upward
     c. Absence of Q waves
  2. Intermediate phase: return of ST segment to baseline, and T wave inversion in leads previously showing ST-segment elevation (Fig. 1-198)
  3. Late phase: resolution of the T wave changes
- Chest radiography: done primarily to rule out abnormalities of the mediastinum or lung fields that may be responsible for the pericarditis
  1. Cardiac silhouette appears enlarged if more than 250 ml of fluid has accumulated.
  2. Calcifications around the heart may be seen with constrictive pericarditis.

TREATMENT

NONPHARMACOLOGIC THERAPY

- Limitation of activity until the pain abates
- Patient education regarding potential complications (e.g., cardiac tamponade, constrictive pericarditis)

ACUTE GENERAL Rx

- Anti-inflammatory therapy (NSAIDs, [e.g., ibuprofen 800 mg tid, naproxen 500 mg bid]). Aspirin is preferred in patients with recent MI.
- Colchicine 0.6 mg bid may be used as an alternative in patients intolerant to

NSAIDs and corticosteroids or can be used in combination with NSAIDs.
- Prednisone 1.5 mg/kg of body weight qd for up to 4 wk may be added in patients with severe forms of acute pericarditis and suspected connective tissue disease.
- Consider ventricular rate control with verapamil or diltiazem because of the propensity for atrial fibrillation in these patients.
- Close observation of patients for signs of cardiac tamponade.
- Avoidance of anticoagulants (increased risk of hemopericardium).

TREATMENT OF UNDERLYING CAUSE:
1. Bacterial pericarditis: systemic antibiotics and surgical drainage of pericardium
2. Collagen vascular disease and idiopathic: NSAIDs, prednisone
3. Uremic: dialysis

POTENTIAL COMPLICATIONS FROM PERICARDITIS:
1. **Pericardial effusion:** the time required for pericardial effusion to develop is of critical importance; if the rate of accumulation is slow, the pericardium can gradually stretch and accommodate a large effusion (up to 1000 ml), whereas rapid accumulation can cause tamponade with as little as 200 ml of fluid.
2. **Chronic constrictive pericarditis:**
   a. Physical examination reveals jugular venous distention, Kussmaul's sign (increase in jugular venous distention during inspiration as a result of increased venous pulse), pericardial knock (early diastolic filling sound heard 0.06 to 0.1 sec after S_2), clear lungs, tender hepatomegaly, pedal edema, ascites.
   b. Chest x-ray: clear lung fields, normal or slightly enlarged heart, pericardial calcification.
   c. ECG: low-voltage QRS complex.
   d. Echocardiography: may show pericardial thickening or may be normal.
   e. Cardiac catheterization.
   f. Therapy: surgical stripping or removal of both layers of the constricting pericardium.
3. **Cardiac tamponade:** occurs in 15% of patients with idiopathic pericarditis but in nearly 60% of those with neoplastic, tuberculous, or purulent pericarditis.
   a. Signs and symptoms: dyspnea, orthopnea, interscapular pain.
   b. Physical examination: distended neck veins, distant heart sounds, decreased apical impulse, diaphoresis, tachypnea, tachycardia, Ewart's sign (an area of dullness at the angle of the left scapula caused by compression of the lungs by the pericardial effusion), pulsus paradoxus (decrease in systolic blood pressure >10 mm Hg during inspiration), hypotension, narrowed pulse pressure. Of all the clinical signs, a pulsus paradoxus >10 mm Hg in patients with pericardial effusion helps distinguish those with cardiac tamponade from those without.
   c. Chest x-ray: cardiomegaly (water bottle configuration of the cardiac silhouette may be seen) with clear lungs; the chest x-ray film may be normal when acute tamponade occurs rapidly in the absence of prior pericardial effusion.
   d. ECG reveals decreased amplitude of the QRS complex, variation of the R wave amplitude from beat to beat (electrical alternans). This results from the heart's oscillating in the pericardial sac from beat to beat and frequently occurs with neoplastic effusions.
   e. Echocardiography: detects effusions as small as 30 ml; a paradoxical wall motion may also be seen.
   f. Cardiac catheterization: equalization of pressures within chambers of the heart, elevation of right atrial pressure with a prominent x but no significant y descent.
   g. MRI can also be used to diagnose pericardial effusions.
   h. Therapy for pericardial tamponade consists of immediate pericardiocentesis preferably by needle paracentesis with the use of echocardiography, fluoroscopy, or CT; in patients with recurrent effusions (e.g., neoplasms), placement of a percutaneous drainage catheter or pericardial window draining in the pleural cavity may be necessary.
4. **Effusive-constrictive pericarditis:**
   a. Uncommon pericardial syndrome characterized by concomitant tamponade caused by tense pericardial effusion and constriction caused by the visceral pericardium.
   b. Extensive epicardiectomy is the procedure of choice in patients requiring surgery.

PERICARDITIS, EVOLVING PATTERN

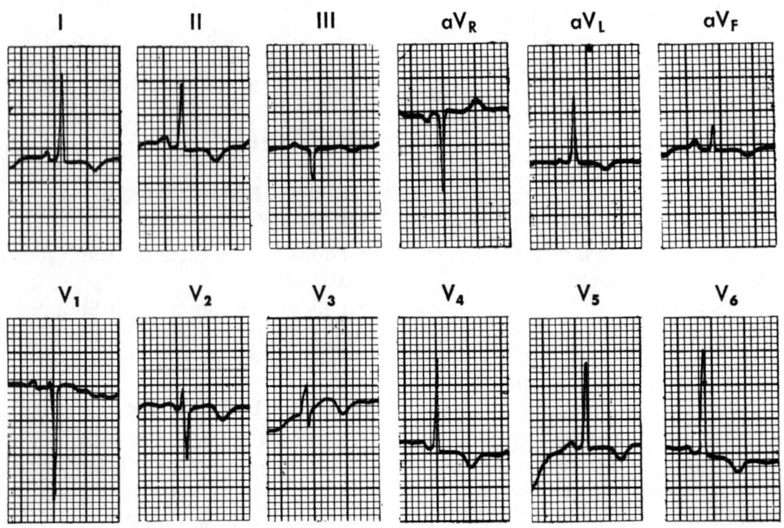

FIGURE 1-198 Notice the diffuse T wave inversions in leads I, II, III, aV_L, aV_F, and V_2 to V_6. (From Goldberg AL [ed]: *Clinical electrocardiography,* ed 5, St Louis, 1994, Mosby.)

DISPOSITION

- Complete resolution of pain and other signs and symptoms during the initial 3 wk of therapy.
- Recurrence in 10% to 15% of patients within the initial 12 mo.
- Recurrent pericarditis in 28% of patients.
- Recurrence of large effusion after pericardiocentesis is common in patients with idiopathic chronic pericardial effusion. Pericardiectomy should be considered in these patients.
- Most cases of pericarditis can be treated in the outpatient setting. Indications for hospitalization are fever >38°C, immunosuppressed state, history of trauma, subacute onset, oral anticoagulant therapy, presence of myocarditis, large pericardial effusion, or tamponade.

SUGGESTED READINGS

Lange RA, Hillis LD: Acute pericarditis, *N Engl J Med* 351:2195-2202, 2005.
Roy C et al: Does this patient with pericardial effusion have cardiac tamponade? *JAMA* 297:1810, 2007.
Tingle LE et al: Acute pericarditis, *Am Fam Physician* 76:1509-1514, 2007.

AUTHOR: **FRED F. FERRI, M.D.**

BASIC INFORMATION

DEFINITION

Peripheral arterial disease (PAD) refers to stenotic, occlusive, and aneurysmal diseases of the aorta and its branch arteries, exclusive of the coronary arteries. This chapter deals specifically with the arteries of the lower extremities.

SYNONYMS

Peripheral vascular disease (PVD), arteriosclerosis obliterans, atherosclerotic occlusive disease, atherosclerosis of the extremities, peripheral arterial stenosis, vaso-occlusive disease of the legs, chronic critical limb ischemia

ICD-9CM CODES
443.9 Peripheral vascular disease

EPIDEMIOLOGY & DEMOGRAPHICS

- The likelihood of developing PAD increases after age 40 yr. As a result it is an increasingly prevalent problem given the aging populations in most Western countries.
- The 1999-2000 National Health and Nutrition Examination Survey (NHANES) found the incidence of PAD to be approximately 14.5% in patients aged 70 yr or older.
- Other studies have shown a prevalence of up to 29% in patients aged 50-69 yr with a history of diabetes and smoking.
- PAD is a common manifestation of atherosclerosis and its prevalence increases with age and the presence of cardiovascular risk factors.
- Cigarette smoking and diabetes mellitus are the strongest risk factors.
- Greater than 80% of patients with PAD are current or former smokers.
- PAD affects men and women equally.
- African Americans and Hispanics with diabetes have a higher prevalence of PAD than whites.
- Cardiovascular disease is the major cause of death in patients with intermittent claudication.
- Patients with newly diagnosed PAD are 6 times more likely to die within the next 10 years when compared with patients without PAD.
- Risk factors associated with PAD are similar to coronary artery disease including tobacco use, diabetes, hyperlipidemia, hypertension, and advanced age.
- Other potential risk factors include elevated levels of C-reactive protein, fibrinogen, homocysteine, apolipoprotein A, and plasma viscosity.
- An inverse relationship has been suggested between PAD and alcohol consumption.
- In 2006 American College of Cardiology/American Heart Association (ACC/AHA) suggested that the following individuals would be at risk from lower extremity PAD:
    - Age <50 yr, with diabetes and one other atherosclerosis risk factor (smoking, dyslipidemia, hypertension, or hyperhomocysteinemia)
    - Age 50-69 yr and history of smoking or diabetes
    - Age ≥70 yr
    - Leg symptoms with exertion (suggestive of claudication) or ischemic rest pain
    - Abnormal lower extremity pulse examination
    - Known atherosclerotic coronary, carotid, or renal artery disease

PHYSICAL FINDINGS & CLINICAL PRESENTATION

Nearly 50% of the patients with PAD experience no symptoms, making PAD an underdiagnosed and undertreated condition. Approximately one third of patients with PAD present with intermittent claudication described as an aching or cramping leg pain brought on by exertion and relieved with rest, and can progress with time. However, relying on the classic history of claudication alone will miss the majority of patients with PAD.

A person with PAD may have various symptoms, including the following:

- Painful cramping in buttocks, hip, or leg that occurs while walking but goes away while resting
- Diminished pedal pulses
- Bruits heard over the distal aorta, iliac, or femoral arteries
- Changes in skin color, especially on feet (rubor with prolonged capillary refill on dependency or delayed pallor)
- Cool skin temperature
- Trophic changes of hair loss and muscle atrophy
- Nonhealing ulcers, necrotic tissue, and gangrene
- Weakness, numbness, or a feeling of heaviness in legs
- Aching or burning in toes and feet during rest and especially while lying flat, which may be a sign of ischemia and more serious PAD

ETIOLOGY

The primary cause of PAD is atherosclerosis: atherosclerotic lesions lead to stenosis of peripheral vessels and inability to supply oxygenated blood to meet the demand of limb muscles.

DIAGNOSIS

DIFFERENTIAL DIAGNOSIS

- Spinal stenosis
- Musculoskeletal disorder
- Lumbar spinal stenosis or nerve root compression (neurogenic or pseudoclaudication)
- Peripheral neuropathy
- Reflex sympathetic dystrophy
- Raynaud's disease
- Compartment syndrome

WORKUP

The initial history is very important and should concentrate on symptoms of claudication, walking impairment, ischemic rest pain and nonhealing wounds involving the lower extremities for individuals with risk factors for atherosclerosis who are age 50 yr or older. If individuals are 70 yr or older, then this should be a routine part of their review of systems.

Workup for PAD should also involve other arterial trees, and would include the following:

- Measurement of blood pressure in both arms and notation of any asymmetry.
- Palpation and recording of carotid pulses, upstroke, amplitude, and presence of bruits.
- Auscultation and palpation of abdomen for bruits, aortic pulsation, and diameter.
- Palpation of brachial, radial, ulnar, femoral, popliteal, dorsalis pedis, and posterior tibial pulses. Pulse intensity should be recorded as follows: 0, absent; 1, diminished; 2, normal; 3, bounding.
- Auscultation of femoral arteries for the presence of bruits.
- Feet should be inspected for color, temperature, and integrity of the skin
- Findings suggestive of severe PAD—hair loss, trophic skin changes, and hypertrophic nails—should be sought and recorded.
- In patients with symptoms of intermittent claudication, the ankle-brachial index (ABI) should be measured after exercise (especially if the resting study is normal).
- Individuals with asymptomatic lower extremity PAD should be identified by examination and/or measurement of the ABI so that therapeutic interventions known to diminish their risk of myocardial infarction, stroke, and death may be offered.

The ankle-brachial index (ABI) is calculated by dividing the highest ankle systolic pressure using either the dorsalis pedis or posterior tibial artery by the highest systolic pressure from either arm.

- A diagnosis of PAD is based on the presence of limb symptoms or a low ABI
- The severity of PAD is based on the ABI at rest and during treadmill exercise (1 to 2 mph, 5 min, or symptom limited). It is classified as follows:
    - Mild: ABI at rest 0.71 to 0.90 or ABI during exercise 0.50 to 0.90

- Moderate: ABI at rest 0.41 to 0.70 or ABI during exercise 0.20 to 0.50
- Severe: ABI at rest <0.40 or ABI during exercise <0.20

LABORATORY TESTS

Lipid profile, hemoglobin A1C, homocysteine levels, fibrinogen

IMAGING STUDIES

- The diagnosis of PAD can be confirmed by measuring the ABI or toe-brachial index (determined according to the return of pulsatile flow on deflation of a small blood pressure cuff on the great or second toe with a plethysmographic device).
- Rest or exercise pulse volume recordings (PVR) and segmental limb pressures are also useful. PVR measures volume of limb flow per pulse in different segments of the limb (e.g., thigh, calf, ankle, metatarsal, and toes). They help to assess the location and severity of the lesion.
- MRA can be used as a noninvasive approach to visualize the aorta and peripheral lower extremity arteries. A major advantage of MRA is that it does not require contrast agents.
- Contrast CT may be used, but alternative modalities should be used in patients with renal failure.
- Angiography remains the gold standard for visualizing the arterial anatomy before revascularization.

TREATMENT

Rx

NONPHARMACOLOGIC THERAPY

The mainstays of treatment for PAD include risk-factor modification, exercise, antiplatelet therapy, additional pharmacologic therapy (if symptoms warrant), and revascularization (endovascular or surgical).

Aggressive management of risk factors for PAD includes:

- Smoking-cessation programs, diet counseling, and weight-loss programs.
- Smoking goal: complete cessation and no exposure to environmental tobacco smoke.
- Physical activity: 30 to 60 min/day at about 2 miles/hr to near maximal pain every day for 6 months, and resistance training, is encouraged in patients with PAD.
- Weight management: goal BMI 18.5 to 24.9 kg/m^2. Waist circumference: men <40 inches, women <35 inches.
- Management of hypertension with goal <140/90 or <130/80 if the patient has diabetes or chronic renal disease.
- Tight glycemic control (A1C <7%) in diabetic patients with PAD results in prevention of microvascular complications.
- Control of dyslipidemia with goal for LDL-C of <100 mg/dl or <70 in very high risk patients. Alternatively, reduction of LDL-C levels by 50% in patients with high baseline LDL if levels <70 could not be achieved. If triglycerides are >200 mg/dl, non-HDL-C should be lowered to <130 mg/dl.

ACUTE GENERAL Rx

Most individuals will respond fairly well to risk factor modification and exercise. If symptoms become so severe then endovascular or surgical therapy is performed for symptom relief.

CHRONIC Rx

- Aspirin 75 to 325 mg daily is recommended for secondary prevention.
- The thienopyridines (ticlopidine and clopidogrel) may be considered as alternatives to aspirin, particularly in patients who cannot tolerate aspirin.
- Pentoxyphylline (Trental, Pentoxil) 400 mg tid provides a small benefit in walking distance when compared with placebo
- Cilostazol (Pletal) 100 mg bid has been shown to increase the distance by up to 50% in symptomatic patients with infrainguinal PAD. It should not be given to patients with congestive heart failure and an ejection fraction <40%. Cilostazol may be used in patients with aspirin and/or clopidogrel.

The ACC/AHA have suggested the following guidelines for revascularization therapy:

- Revascularization (surgery or percutaneous transluminal angioplasty [PTA]) is indicated for relief in patients with claudication that limits their lifestyle and that has proved to be unresponsive to exercise and pharmacologic therapy or if there is a very favorable risk-benefit ratio (e.g., focal aortoiliac occlusive disease).
- Endovascular intervention is recommended for TransAtlantic Inter-Society Consensus type A iliac and femoropopliteal arterial lesions.
- Endovascular therapy is preferred when possible in patients who are 50 yr of age or younger, because they have a higher risk of graft failure after surgical therapy than do older patients.
- Endovascular intervention is not indicated if there is no significant pressure gradient across a stenosis even after augmentation of flow with vasodilators.
- Endovascular intervention is not indicated as prophylactic therapy in an asymptomatic patient with lower extremity PAD.
- Primary stent placement is not recommended in the femoral, popliteal, or tibial arteries.
- Surgical intervention is not indicated to prevent progression to limb-threatening ischemia in patients with intermittent claudication.
- Surgical interventions are indicated for individuals with claudication symptoms who have lifestyle-limiting disability, who are unresponsive to exercise or pharmacotherapy, and who have a reasonable chance of symptomatic improvement. Prior to any surgical therapy, patients should have a preoperative cardiovascular risk evaluation.

DISPOSITION

Risk factors for atherosclerosis should be assessed, and appropriate modification instituted. Focus should be placed on smoking cessation, dietary adjustment, and pharmacotherapy for dyslipidemia, hyperglycemia, and hypertension. All patients with PAD should receive aspirin therapy (75 to 325 mg/day) unless contraindicated for some other medical reason. Revascularization is performed if the symptoms of PAD do not improve with conservative therapy.

REFERRAL

Consultation with vascular medicine, vascular surgery, or other physicians with expertise in PAD is recommended in patients with rest pain, functional disability from pain, ABI <0.50 at rest, or any physical signs of limb ischemia or gangrene.

PEARLS & CONSIDERATIONS

!

COMMENTS

- Although the prevalence of PAD in Europe and North America is estimated at approximately 27 million people, PAD remains underdiagnosed and undertreated.
- Studies of the natural history of claudication show the relative safety of initial conservative treatment of PAD in absence of critical limb ischemia.
- When PAD limits a patient's ability to walk and exercise, percutaneous revascularization can be considered. Data reveal excellent outcomes with angioplasty and stenting in selected patients. Outcomes will likely be better as peripheral interventional technology and skills improve.

PREVENTION

Cardiovascular disease is the major cause of death in patients with intermittent claudication. Therefore, the treatment of claudication is directed not only at improving walking distance but also at reducing cardiovascular risk.

BASIC INFORMATION

DEFINITION

Spontaneous bacterial peritonitis (SBP) is an inflammatory reaction of the peritoneum secondary to the presence of bacteria or other microorganisms. More specifically, SBP is defined as an ascitic fluid infection without an evident intra-abdominal surgically treatable source occurring primarily in patients with advanced cirrhosis of the liver.

SYNONYMS

Primary peritonitis
SBP

ICD-9CM CODES
567.2 Peritonitis

EPIDEMIOLOGY & DEMOGRAPHICS

PREDOMINANT SEX: Male > female

PHYSICAL FINDINGS & CLINICAL PRESENTATION

- Acute fever with accompanying abdominal pain/ascites, nausea, vomiting, diarrhea
- In cirrhotic patients, presentation may be subtle when low-grade temperature (100° F) with or without abdominal abnormalities
- In patients with ascites, a heightened degree of awareness is necessary for detection
- Jaundice and encephalopathy
- Deterioration of mental status and/or renal function

ETIOLOGY

- *Escherichia coli*
- *Klebsiella pneumoniae*
- *Streptococcus pneumoniae*
- *Streptococcus* and *Enterococcus* spp.
- *Staphylococcus aureus*
- Anaerobic pathogens: *Bacteroides, Clostridium* organisms
- Other: fungal, mycobacterial, viral

DIAGNOSIS

The diagnosis of SBP is established by a positive ascitic fluid bacterial culture and an elevated ascitic fluid absolute polymorphonuclear leukocyte (PMN) count (≥250 cells/mm³).

DIFFERENTIAL DIAGNOSIS

- Appendicitis (in children)
- Perforated peptic ulcer
- Secondary peritonitis
- Peritoneal abscess
- Splenic, hepatic, or pancreatic abscess
- Cholecystitis
- Cholangitis

WORKUP

Paracentesis and ascitic fluid analysis (see "Laboratory Tests") will confirm diagnosis.

LABORATORY TESTS

Ascitic fluid analysis reveals the following:
- Polymorphonuclear (PMN) cell count: >250/mm³
- Presence of bacteria on Gram stain
- pH: <7.31
- Lactic acid: >32 mg/dl
- Protein: <1 g/dl
- Glucose: >50 mg/dl
- LDH: <225 mU/ml
- Positive culture of peritoneal fluid
- Measurement of the serum-ascites albumin gradient: The serum-ascites albumin gradient indirectly measures portal pressure. The albumin concentration of ascitic fluid and serum must be obtained on the same day. The ascitic fluid value is subtracted from the serum value to obtain the gradient. If the difference (not a ratio) is >1.1 g/dl, the patient has portal hypertension, with 97% accuracy. If the difference is <1.1 g/dl, portal hypertension is not present. The vast majority of patients with SBP have portal hypertension secondary to cirrhosis

IMAGING STUDIES

- Abdominal ultrasound: if there is clinical difficulty in performing paracentesis
- CT scan: to rule out secondary peritonitis (if indicated) and to exclude abscess, mass

TREATMENT

ACUTE GENERAL Rx

Cefotaxime 1 to 2 g IV q8h or ceftriaxone 2 g IV q24h in patients with normal renal function; duration of treatment is generally 7 to 10 days. Oral quinolone therapy (ofloxacin 400 to 800 mg/day) or ciprofloxacin may be an acceptable alternative in selected patients.

PROPHYLAXIS

Give double-strength trimethoprim/sulfamethoxazole qd 5 days/wk or ciprofloxacin 750 mg/wk PO. Both have been shown to decrease occurrence of SBP in patients with cirrhosis.

DISPOSITION

- If possible, the initial management of SBP should be undertaken in the hospital setting—this permits careful follow-up for treatment-related complications, management of underlying portal hypertension, and work up for concomitant diseases
- Once the diagnosis is confirmed and the patient is stabilized, oral antibiotic therapy can be continued in an outpatient setting, if careful follow-up of the patient is assured

REFERRAL

- To a gastroenterologist for management of ascites and prevention of recurrent SBP
- To an infectious disease specialist for management of difficult-to-treat infections, antibiotic-resistant bacterial infections, or antibiotic drug intolerance

PEARLS & CONSIDERATIONS

COMMENTS

- Renal failure is a major cause of morbidity in cirrhotic patients with SBP. The use of IV albumin (1.5 g/kg at the time of diagnosis and 1 g/kg on day 3) may lower the rate of renal failure and mortality in patients with SBP.
- The criteria for the diagnosis of SBP require that abdominal paracentesis be performed and ascitic fluid be analyzed before a diagnosis of SBP can be made.
- Culturing ascitic fluid as if it were blood (with bedside inoculation of ascitic fluid into blood culture bottles) has been shown to significantly increase the culture-positivity of the ascitic fluid.
- Laparotomy may be life threatening in end-stage cirrhosis.
- Positive blood cultures in an individual with ascites require exclusion of a peritoneal source by paracentesis.

SUGGESTED READINGS

Cholongitas E et al: Spontaneous bacterial peritonitis in cirrhotic patients: Is prophylactic propranolol therapy beneficial? *J Gastroenterol Hepatol* 21(3):581, 2006.

Gonzalez-Suarez B et al: Pharmacologic treatment of portal hypertension in the prevention of community-acquired spontaneous bacterial peritonitis, *Eur J Gastroenterol Hepatol* 18(1):49, 2006.

Parsi MA, Atreja A, Zein NN: Spontaneous bacterial peritonitis: recent data on incidence and treatment, *Cleve Clin J Med* 71(7):569, 2004.

Runyon BA: Early events in spontaneous bacterial peritonitis, *Gut* 53(6):782, 2004.

Shaw E et al: Clinical features and outcome of spontaneous bacterial peritonitis in HIV-infected cirrhotic patients: a case control study, *Eur J Clin Microbiol Infect Dis* 25(5):291, 2006.

Sorrentino P et al: Clinical presentation and prevalence of spontaneous bacterial peritonitis in patients with cryptogenic cirrhosis and features of metabolic syndrome, *Can J Gastroenterol* 18(6):381, 2004.

Tuncer I et al: Oral ciprofloxacin versus intravenous cefotaxime and ceftriaxone in the treatment of spontaneous bacterial peritonitis, *Hepatogastroenterology* 50(53):1426, 2003.

AUTHORS: **GLENN G. FORT, M.D., M.P.H.,** and **DENNIS J. MIKOLICH, M.D.**

BASIC INFORMATION

DEFINITION

Peritonsillar abscess is an acute infection located between the capsule of the palatine tonsil and the superior constrictor muscle of the pharynx.

SYNONYMS

Quinsy

ICD-9CM CODES
475.0 Peritonsillar abscess

EPIDEMIOLOGY & DEMOGRAPHICS

INCIDENCE: 30:100,000 per year in the U.S.
FREQUENCY: There is a bimodal frequency during the year with highest occurrence between November to December and April to May.
SEX: Male = Female
Age: Common during adolescence and 20s. Young children may be affected if immunocompromised.

CLINICAL PRESENTATION

- Sore throat, which may be severe
- Dysphagia and odynophagia
- Otalgia
- Foul-smelling breath
- Facial swelling
- Drooling
- Headache
- Fever
- Trismus
- Hoarseness
- Tender submandibular and anterior cervical lymph nodes
- Tonsillar hypertrophy
- Contralateral deflection of the uvula
- Stridor

ETIOLOGY

- Peritonsillar abscess is a complication of tonsillitis.
- Group A beta-hemolytic Streptococcus is the most common bacterial cause, accounting for 15% to 30% of cases in children and 5% to 10% of cases in adults.
- Less common aerobic causes are *Staphylococcus aureus, Haemophilus influenzae, Neisseria* species.
- The most common anaerobic organism is *Fusobacterium.*

DIAGNOSIS (Dx)

DIFFERENTIAL DIAGNOSIS

- Tonsillitis
- Infectious mononucleosis
- Peritonsillar cellulitis
- Retropharyngeal abscess
- Epiglottitis
- Dental abscess
- Lymphoma

WORKUP

Thorough history and physical exam

LABORATORY TESTS

- Rapid strep antigen detecting testing and throat swab culture and sensitivity
- Aspiration of the abscess for culture and sensitivity

IMAGING STUDIES

Ultrasound vs. CT scan can be considered to help differentiate mass vs. abscess, but the gold standard still remains a culture of the abscess.

TREATMENT (Rx)

NONPHARMACOLOGIC THERAPY

- Surgical drainage of the abscess by needle aspiration or by incision and drainage
- Possible subsequent surgery for tonsillectomy

ACUTE GENERAL Rx

Appropriate selection of antibiotic guided by culture and sensitivity of the organism. After performing aspiration or drainage, appropriate antibiotic therapy, possibly including penicillin, clindamycin, cephalosporins, or metronidazole, must be started.

CHRONIC Rx

- Tonsillectomy usually occurs 3 to 6 months after diagnosis of abscess or recurrent tonsillitis.
- Though rare, in adults and children with peritonsillar abscess and a history of recurrent pharyngitis or previous peritonsillar abscess, the specialist may proceed with removal of the tonsils directly after placing the patient on intravenous antibiotics. This is known as a quinsy or hot tonsillectomy.

REFERRAL

Emergently consider hospitalization or consultation with an otolaryngologist if the patient's airway has the potential to become obstructed or if stridor is appreciated.

PEARLS & CONSIDERATIONS (!)

COMMENTS

- Any person who has had a peritonsillar abscess is at risk for a recurrence, both immediately (within 4 days) and long term (2 to 3 years).
- Most recurrences occur shortly after the initial presentation, suggesting continued infection rather than recurrence.
- Regardless of treatment modality, the overall recurrence rate is from 6% to 36%.

PREVENTION

- Strongly encourage completion of the full course of antibiotic treatment for acute pharyngitis (10 to 14 days) to prevent incomplete treatment of infection leading to abscess formation.
- Tonsillectomy is recommended in the event of recurrent peritonsillar abscess or tonsillitis in both children and adults.

SUGGESTED READING

Steyer TE: Peritonsillar abscess: diagnosis and treatment, *Am Fam Physician* 65:93-96, 2002.

AUTHOR: **CHRISTINE HEALY, D.O.**

BASIC INFORMATION

DEFINITION

Pertussis is a prolonged bacterial infection of the upper respiratory tract characterized by paroxysms of an intense cough.

SYNONYMS

Whooping cough

ICD-9CM CODES
033.9 Pertussis

EPIDEMIOLOGY

INCIDENCE (IN U.S.): Approximately 5000 new cases/yr (Fig. 1-199)

PEAK INCIDENCE:
- Childhood
- Usually affects children <1 yr of age

PREDOMINANT AGE:
- 50% in children <1 yr of age
- 20% in children >15 yr of age

PHYSICAL FINDINGS & CLINICAL PRESENTATION

- Usually begins with a 1- to 2-wk prodrome that resembles a common cold
- Following this initial phase, increased production of mucus is noted
- Increased mucus production is followed by an intense, paroxysmal cough, ending with gasps and an inspiratory whoop
- In some children, cyanosis and anoxia are noted
- When prolonged, frank exhaustion and even apnea occur
- Pertussis is characterized by the finding of intense cough with a marked lymphocytosis; post-tussive gagging and vomiting is characteristic of pertussis

ETIOLOGY

Gram-negative rod, *Bordetella pertussis,* which adheres to human cilia

DIAGNOSIS

DIFFERENTIAL DIAGNOSIS

- Croup
- Epiglottitis
- Foreign body aspiration
- Bacterial pneumonia

WORKUP

- Blood cultures
- Chest x-ray examination
- Culture of bacteria, usually from nasopharynx
- Immunofluorescent staining of nasopharyngeal secretions
- ELISA for detection of antibody to pertussis

LABORATORY TESTS

CBC, which usually demonstrates marked lymphocytosis:
1. Up to 18,000 WBCs
2. 70% to 80% lymphocytes

IMAGING STUDIES

Chest x-ray examination is of value if secondary bacterial pneumonia is suspected.

TREATMENT

ACUTE GENERAL Rx

- Intensive supportive care:
  1. Adequate hydration
  2. Control of secretions
  3. Maintenance of airway
- Antibiotics are indicated even though their ability to alter the course of the disease is controversial.
  1. Erythromycin 50 mg/kg/day for 14 days. Recent literature reports indicate that a 7-day treatment regimen may be as effective as a 14-day course of erythromycin
  2. Although unproved, dexamethasone 1 mg/kg/day in 4 doses for severe, life-threatening paroxysms
  3. Ceftriaxone 75 mg/kg/day in 2 doses for broad coverage of secondary bacterial pneumonias
- Vaccination is successful in preventing the disease: universal vaccination is advised for all children <7 yr of age.
- Erythromycin is recommended for all close contacts in the household: TMP/SMX in two oral doses per day for those intolerant to erythromycin.

DISPOSITION

Close attention to accepted vaccination schedules is the best prevention.

REFERRAL

To intensive care setting for life-threatening infections:
1. Pulmonologist
2. Infectious disease specialist

PEARLS & CONSIDERATIONS

The diagnosis of pertussis in a young child is easily recognized, but in adults pertussis can be a very subtle diagnosis and is often missed. The tip-off is often a persistent, hacking, and productive cough with minor or no fever in a previously healthy person that lasts greater than 2 wk.

EVIDENCE

Multicomponent acellular pertussis vaccines are effective and have fewer systemic and local adverse effects than whole cell pertussis vaccines.[1] Ⓐ

Evidence-Based Reference

1. Tinnion ON, Hanlon M: Acellular vaccines for preventing whooping cough in children. In: Cochrane Library 3, Chichester, UK, 2004, John Wiley.

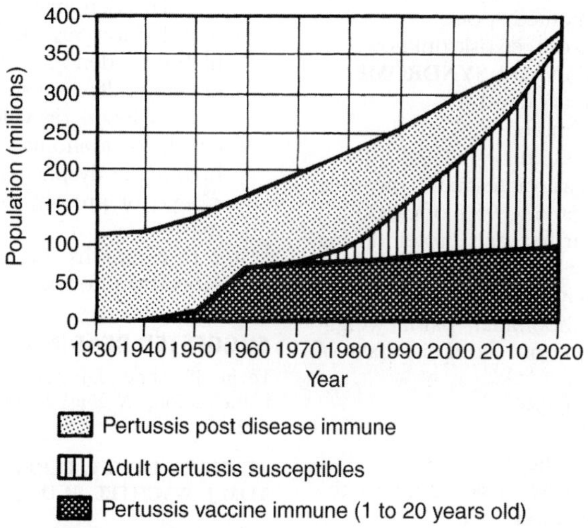

FIGURE 1-199 Projected pertussis epidemiology in the United States through the year 2020 with continued use of present-day whole-cell pertussis vaccines. (Modified from Bass JW, Stephenson SR: *Pediatr Infect Dis J 6:141,* 1987.)

SUGGESTED READINGS

Bisgard KM et al: Pertussis vaccine effectiveness among children 6 to 59 months of age in the United States, 1998-2001, *Pediatrics* 116(2):285, 2005.

Byrne S, Slack AT: Analysis of *Bordetella pertussis* pertactin and pertussis toxin types from Queensland, Australia, 1999-2003, *BMC Infect Dis* 6:53, 2006.

Cherry JD: The epidemiology of pertussis: a comparison of the epidemiology of the disease pertussis with the epidemiology of *Bordetella pertussis* infection, *Pediatrics* 115(5):1422, 2005.

Heininger U, Cherry JD: Pertussis immunization in adolescents and adults—*Bordetella pertussis* epidemiology should guide vaccination recommendations, *Expert Opin Biol Ther* 6(7):685, 2006.

Hewlett EL, Edwards KM: Pertussis—not just for kids, *N Engl J Med* 352:1215, 2005.

AUTHORS: **GLENN G. FORT, M.D., M.P.H., JOSEPH J. LIEBER, M.D.,** and **DENNIS J. MIKOLICH, M.D.**

BASIC INFORMATION

DEFINITION

- A hamartomatous polyp is a benign intestinal growth that may contain all components of the intestinal mucosa. In gastrointestinal polyposis, multiple such polyps coexist within the intestinal tract, and associated manifestations are usually also present.
- Juvenile polyps are benign polyps composed of cystic dilatations of glandular structures within the fibroblastic stroma of the lamina propria. They may cause bleeding or intussusception.
- Commonly recognized syndromes are Peutz-Jeghers syndrome, juvenile polyposis syndrome, Cowden's disease, Bannagan-Ruvalcaba-Riley syndrome, and Cronkhite-Canada syndrome. Other lesser known inherited hamartomatous polyposis syndromes are hereditary mixed polyposis syndrome, intestinal ganglioneuromatosis and neurofibromatosis (variant of von Recklinghausen's syndrome), Devon family syndrome, basal cell nevus syndrome, and tuberous sclerosis (may involve GI tract).

ICD-9CM CODES
759.6 (Peutz-Jeghers syndrome)
211.3 (Cronkhite-Canada syndrome)

EPIDEMIOLOGY

- Colonic adenomas, the precursors of nearly all colorectal cancers, are found in nearly 40% of patients by 60 yr of age.
- 25% of men and 155 of women who undergo colonoscopy are found to have one or more adenomas.
- Detection of any adenoma in patients younger than 60 yr of age confers an increased risk of colorectal cancer (by a factor of 2.6) in their first-degree relatives.

PHYSICAL FINDINGS & CLINICAL PRESENTATION

PEUTZ-JEGHERS SYNDROME:

- Transmission: autosomal dominant with incomplete penetrance
- Disease expression
  - Stomach, small and large intestinal hamartomas with bands of smooth muscle in the lamina propria
  - Pigmented lesions around mouth (lips and buccal mucosa), nose, hands, feet, genital, and perineal areas
  - Ovarian tumors
  - Sertoli cell testicular tumors
  - Airway polyps
  - Pancreatic cancer
  - Breast cancer
  - Urinary tract polyps
- Cumulative lifetime cancer risk
  - Colon cancer: 39%
  - Stomach cancer: 29%
  - Small intestine cancer: 13%
  - Pancreatic cancer: 36%
  - Breast cancer: 54%
  - Ovarian cancer: 10%
  - Sertoli cell tumor: 9%
  - Overall cancer risk: 93%
- Clinical manifestation
  - Gastrointestinal, small bowel obstruction, intussusception, GI bleeding
  - See chapters on relevant malignancies for their signs and symptoms

JUVENILE POLYPOSIS SYNDROME:

- Transmission: autosomal dominant
- Disease expression
  - Solitary juvenile polyps numbering 10 or more in the rectum or throughout the gastrointestinal tract; the polyps are smooth and covered with normal epithelium
  - Various congenital abnormalities coexist in 20%
- Cumulative cancer risk is increased (may be as high as 50%)
- Clinical manifestation
  - Intestinal obstruction
  - Intussusception
  - GI bleeding

COWDEN'S DISEASE:

- Transmission: autosomal dominant, rare
- Disease expression
  - Juvenile intestinal polyposis
  - Orocutaneous hamartomas
  - Fibrocystic breast disease and breast cancer
  - Goiter and thyroid cancer
  - Facial tricholemmomas (papules) in 83%
- Cumulative cancer risk
  - GI: same as general population
  - Thyroid: 3% to 10%
  - Breast: 25% to 50%

BANNAGAN-RUVALCABA-RILEY SYNDROME:

- Transmission: autosomal dominant, rare
- Disease expression
  - Juvenile intestinal polyposis
  - Macrocephaly
  - Developmental delay
  - Penile pigmented spots
  - Cumulative cancer risk unknown

CRONKHITE-CANADA SYNDROME:

- Transmission: acquired
- Age of onset: midlife
- Disease expression
  - Diffuse gastrointestinal juvenile polyposis (50% to 95% of cases)
  - Chronic diarrhea and protein-losing enteropathy (the entire intestinal mucosa may be inflamed), which leads to abdominal pain, weight loss, and various complications of malnutrition
  - Dystrophic nails
  - Alopecia
  - Hyperpigmentation
- Cumulative cancer risk: same as the average population

DIAGNOSIS

Diagnosis is suggested in many cases by family history and confirmed by colonoscopy and physical findings described previously.

TREATMENT

GENERAL Rx

Peutz-Jeghers syndrome:
- Colonoscopies with polypectomies
- Screening for breast cancer, testicular cancer, possibly ovarian cancer

Juvenile polyposis syndrome:
- Colonoscopies with polypectomies if few colon polyps
- Total colectomy if numerous polyps
- Esophagogastroscopies and polypectomies

Cowden's disease: Rigorous breast cancer screening or prophylactic simple bilateral mastectomy with reconstruction.

Cronkhite-Canada syndrome: Progressive malabsorption syndrome is the hallmark of this syndrome, and no specific treatment exists for it. Enteral or parenteral feeding is the cornerstone of management and can result in remission.

DISPOSITION

- The screening of first-degree relatives of patients with colonic adenomas detected before 60 yr of age is controversial. Some recommend beginning colonoscopic screening at 40 yr of age or 10 yr younger than the age at diagnosis of the youngest person in the family with an adenoma.
- Recommended interval between colonoscopies from the U.S. Consensus Guidelines for Colonoscopic Surveillance after Polypectomy are as follows:
  - 10 yr for small, rectal hyperplastic polyps
  - 5-10 yr for 1 to 2 low-risk adenomas (tubular adenomas <1 cm)
  - 3 yr for low-risk adenomas or any high-risk adenoma (large [≥1 cm] or histologically advanced adenomas [tubulovillous or villous adenomas or villous adenomas and those with high-grade dysplasia)]
  - <3 yr for presence of >10 adenomas
  - 2 to 6 months for inadequately removed adenomas

SUGGESTED READING

Levine JS, Ahnen DJ: Adenomatous polyps of the colon, *N Engl J Med* 355:2551-2557, 2006.

AUTHORS: **FRED F. FERRI, M.D.,** and **TOM J. WACHTEL, M.D.**

BASIC INFORMATION

DEFINITION

Peyronie's disease is an abnormal curvature and shortening of the penis during an erection. This is caused by scarring of the tunica albuginea of the corpora cavernosa.

SYNONYMS

Plastic induration of the penis
Penile fibromatosis

ICD-9CM CODES
607.89 Peyronie's disease

EPIDEMIOLOGY & DEMOGRAPHICS

- Peyronie's disease occurs in approximately 1% of men (7:700).
- It is commonly seen between the ages of 45 to 60.
- A genetic predisposition has been suggested.
- There are no incidence and prevalence data available in the literature.

PHYSICAL FINDINGS & CLINICAL PRESENTATION

- Painful erections
- Tenderness over the scar tissue area
- Erectile dysfunction
- Curvature of the erected penis interfering with penetration
- Dupuytren's contracture is a commonly associated finding in patients with Peyronie's disease

ETIOLOGY

- Specific cause is unknown. It is thought that scar tissue forms on either the dorsal or ventral midline surface of the penile shaft. The scar restricts expansion at the involved site, causing the penis to bend or curve in one direction.
- The precipitating factor appears to be trauma either from repetitive microvascular injury caused by vigorous sexual intercourse, accidents, or from prior surgeries (e.g., transurethral or radical prostatectomy, cystoscopy).

DIAGNOSIS

Diagnosis is made based on the clinical finding.

DIFFERENTIAL DIAGNOSIS

- The history differentiates congenital from acquired curvatures of the penis.
- Other causes of erectile dysfunction must be excluded including metabolic, diabetic, thyroid, and renal causes, in addition to hypogonadism and hyperprolactinemia.

WORKUP

History and physical examination alone will usually establish the diagnosis of Peyronie's disease.

LABORATORY TESTS

There are no specific blood tests to diagnose Peyronie's disease. Electrolytes, BUN, creatinine, glucose, thyroid function tests (TSH, T_3U, T_4), testosterone, and prolactin levels are blood tests to exclude other medical causes of erectile dysfunction.

IMAGING STUDIES

Imaging studies are not specific.

TREATMENT

NONPHARMACOLOGIC THERAPY

A conservative approach of reassurance and observation is taken at first because the disease process may be self-limiting.

ACUTE GENERAL Rx

Although not substantiated by direct randomized controlled clinical trials, the following treatment modalities have been tried:

- Vitamin E 400 mg bid.
- Paraaminobenzoic acid 12 g/day.
- Colchicine 0.6 mg bid for 2 to 3 wk.
- Fexofenadine 60 mg bid for 3 mo.
- Steroid injection into the scar tissue.
- Collagenase injection into the scar tissue.
- Radiation to the scar tissue area.
- Extracorporeal shockwave therapy (ESWT): Current evidence on the safety, but not the efficacy, of ESWT appears adequate. From comparative studies, the main benefits of ESWT were the alleviation of pain and reduction of angulation of the penis. In one comparative study, 10 in 20 patients receiving ESWT experienced a decrease in the curvature of at least 30%. Case series evidence also suggested some improvement of sexual performance.
- Other medications that can be helpful include: verapamil, tamoxifen, and interferon.

CHRONIC Rx

In patients who have progressed to intractable pain with erection or erectile dysfunction, surgical treatment with excision of the plaque and skin grafting may be indicated.

DISPOSITION

Peyronie's disease evolves slowly and in some cases can resolve on its own. Waiting for 1 yr before proceeding with surgical attempts is recommended.

REFERRAL

A urologic consultation is recommended in patients with progressive symptoms and erectile dysfunction.

PEARLS & CONSIDERATIONS

COMMENTS

- Peyronie's disease is not commonly seen in younger patients because they are able to sustain intracorporeal pressures high enough to stretch the scar tissue, preventing it from deforming the penis during erection.
- Trauma from buckling of the erected penis is thought to be the precipitant cause of scar formation and Peyronie's disease. It is found more often in men who are sexually very active and vigorous, having sexual intercourse daily or almost daily.
- Sexual positions with the women being on top or thrusting the penis into the anterior vaginal wall is thought to increase the chances of developing Peyronie's disease.

SUGGESTED READINGS

Ralph DJ, Minhas S: The management of Peyronie's disease, *BJU Int* 93(2):208, 2004.

Smith CJ, McMahon C, Shabsigh R: Peyronie's disease: the epidemiology, aetiology and clinical evaluation of deformity, *BJU Int* 95(6):729, 2005.

AUTHOR: **MOHAMMED HAJJIRI, M.D.**

BASIC INFORMATION

DEFINITION

Pharyngitis/tonsillitis is inflammation of the pharynx or tonsils.

SYNONYMS

Sore throat

ICD-9CM CODES
462 Pharyngitis

EPIDEMIOLOGY & DEMOGRAPHICS

PEAK INCIDENCE: Late winter/early spring (group A streptococcal infections)
PREDOMINANT SEX: Female = male
PREDOMINANT AGE:
- All ages affected
- Streptococcal pharyngitis most common among school-age children

GENETICS:
Neonatal Infection: Pharyngitis below the age of 3 yr is almost always of viral etiology.

PHYSICAL FINDINGS & CLINICAL PRESENTATION

- Pharynx:
  1. May appear normal to severely erythematous
  2. Tonsillar hypertrophy and exudates commonly seen but do not indicate etiology
- Viral infection:
  1. Rhinorrhea
  2. Conjunctivitis
  3. Cough
- Bacterial infection, especially group A streptococci:
  1. High fever
  2. Systemic signs of infection
- Herpes simplex or enterovirus infection: vesicles
- Streptococcal infection:
  1. Rare complications:
     a. Scarlet fever
     b. Rheumatic fever
     c. Acute glomerulonephritis
  2. Extension of infection: tonsillar, parapharyngeal, or retropharyngeal abscess presenting with severe pain, high fever, trismus

ETIOLOGY

- Viruses:
  1. Respiratory syncytial virus
  2. Influenza A and B
  3. Epstein-Barr virus
  4. Adenovirus
  5. Herpes simplex
- Bacteria:
  1. *Streptococcus pyogenes*
  2. *Neisseria gonorrhoeae*
  3. *Arcanobacterium haemolyticum*
- Other organisms:
  1. *Mycoplasma pneumoniae*
  2. *Chlamydophila pneumoniae*

DIAGNOSIS

DIFFERENTIAL DIAGNOSIS

- Sore throat associated with granulocytopenia, thyroiditis
- Tonsillar hypertrophy associated with lymphoma
- Section II describes the differential diagnosis of sore throat.

WORKUP

- Throat swab for culture to exclude *S. pyogenes, N. gonorrhoeae* (requires specific transport medium)
- Rapid streptococcal antigen test (culture should be performed if rapid test negative)
- Monospot

LABORATORY TESTS

- CBC with differential
  1. May help support diagnosis of bacterial infection
  2. Streptococcal infection suggested by leukocytosis >15,000/mm^3
- Viral cultures, serologic studies rarely needed

IMAGING STUDIES

Seldom indicated

TREATMENT

NONPHARMACOLOGIC THERAPY

- Fluids
- Salt water gargles

ACUTE GENERAL Rx

- Aspirin (acetaminophen culture)
- If streptococcal infection proven or suspected:
  1. Penicillin V 500 mg PO bid for 10 days or benzathine penicillin 1.2 million U IM once (adults)
  2. Erythromycin 500 mg PO bid or 250 mg qid for 10 days if penicillin allergic
- If gonococcal infection proven or suspected: ceftriaxone 125 mg IM once

CHRONIC Rx

- Recurrent streptococcal infections are common and may represent reinfection from other household.
- There is no conclusive evidence from randomized clinical trials that tonsillectomy is superior to antibiotic therapy for recurrent tonsillitis in adults.

Tonsillopharyngitis is generally managed as in an outpatient setting with follow-up arranged in a week or two. Admission to the hospital is indicated for local suppurative complications (peritonsillar abscess, lateral pharyngeal or posterior pharyngeal abscess, impending airway closure, or inability to swallow food, medications, or water).

REFERRAL

- To otolaryngologist:
  1. If peritonsillar or other abscess is suspected
  2. If tonsillar hypertrophy persists
- To infectious diseases expert if unusual pathogen is suspected

PEARLS & CONSIDERATIONS

COMMENTS

Antibiotic therapy should be avoided unless bacterial etiology is suspected or proven, especially in adults.

EVIDENCE

Pharyngitis
A systematic review found that antibiotics confer relative benefits in the treatment of sore throat, shortening the duration of symptoms by a mean of 1 day about halfway through the illness (the time of maximal effect), and by about 16 hours overall, and preventing nonsuppurative complications of beta-hemolytic streptococcal pharyngitis. However, the absolute benefits are modest in modern Western societies given the rarity of suppurative and nonsuppurative complications.[1] Ⓐ

In children with tonsillopharyngitis, bacteriologic and clinical cure are significantly more likely following treatment with an oral cephalosporin compared with an oral penicillin.[2] Ⓑ

Another systematic review found that NSAIDs and acetaminophen are more effective than placebo for the treatment of sore throat.[3] Ⓐ

Flurbiprofen lozenges significantly improve short-term symptoms of a sore throat compared with placebo.[4] Ⓐ

Tonsillitis
A systematic review found a lack of evidence from randomized controlled trials (RCTs) demonstrating the efficacy of tonsillectomy in the management of tonsillitis.[5]

A subsequent RCT compared surgery (tonsillectomy or adenotonsillectomy) vs. medical treatment in children with recurrent, moderately severe throat infections. Although surgical treatment significantly reduced the frequency of throat infections over a 3-year follow-up period, there was also a low rate of infections in the medical treatment group. The authors concluded that the modest benefit associated with surgery did not justify the risks in these children.[5] Ⓐ

A systematic review assessed the benefits of antibiotics in the treatment of "sore throat." It found that about 90% of treated and untreated patients were symptom free by 1 week. Concerning throat swabs, it found that if the swab was positive, antibiotics were more effective than if it was negative. Overall antibiotics resulted in modest benefits vs. placebo in the reduction of suppurative and nonsuppurative complications. However, the reviewers comment that in Western society protection against these complications could only be achieved by treating many who would have no benefit. Antibiotics were also found to decrease the length of illness but only by about 16 hours overall.[6] Ⓐ

Evidence-Based References

1. Del Mar CB, Glasziou PP, Spinks AB: Antibiotics for sore throat, *Cochrane Database Syst Rev* 2, 2004. Ⓐ
2. Casey JR, Pichichero ME: Meta-analysis of cephalosporin versus penicillin treatment of group A streptococcal tonsillopharyngitis in children, *Pediatrics* 113:866, 2004. Ⓑ
3. Thomas M, Del Mar C, Glaziou P: How effective are treatments other than antibiotics for acute sore throat? *Br J Gen Pract* 50:817, 2000. Reviewed in: *Clin Evid* 11:1956, 2004. Ⓐ
4. Schachtel, BP et al: Demonstration of a dose response of flurbiprofen lozenges with the sore throat pain model, *Clin Pharmacol Ther* 71:375, 2002. Reviewed in: *Clin Evid* 11:1956, 2004. Ⓐ
5. Paradise JL et al: Tonsillectomy and adenotonsillectomy for recurrent throat infection in moderately affected children, *Pediatrics* 110:7, 2002. Reviewed in: *Clin Evid* 13:663, 2005. Ⓐ
6. Del Mar CB, Glasziou PP, Spinks AB: Antibiotics for sore throat (Cochrane Review). Reviewed in: Cochrane Library, 1, Chichester, UK, 2004, John Wiley. Ⓐ

SUGGESTED READINGS

Brook I, Gober AE: Treatment of non-streptococcal tonsillitis with metronidazole, *Int J Pediatr Otorhinolaryngol* 69(1):65, 2005.

Chen Y et al: Pharyngotonsillitis due to Arcanobacterium haemolyticum in northern Israel, *Isr Med Assoc J* 7(4):241, 2005.

Frohna JG: Effectiveness of adenotonsillectomy in children with mild symptoms of throat infections or adenotonsillar hypertrophy: open, randomised controlled trial, *J Pediatr* 146(3):435, 2005.

Hersh EV: Comparison of 5 days of ER clarithromycin versus 10 days of penicillin V for the treatment of streptococcal pharyngitis/tonsillitis, *Curr Med Res Opin* 20(4):451, 2004.

Tewfik TL, Al Garni M: Tonsillopharyngitis: clinical highlights, *J Otolaryngol* 34 Suppl 1:S45, 2005.

AUTHORS: **GLENN G. FORT, M.D., M.P.H., JOSEPH R. MASCI, M.D.,** and **DENNIS J. MIKOLICH, M.D.**

BASIC INFORMATION

DEFINITION

Pheochromocytomas are catecholamine-producing tumors that originate from chromaffin cells of the adrenergic system. They generally secrete both norepinephrine and epinephrine, but norepinephrine is usually the predominant amine.

SYNONYMS

Paraganglioma

ICD-9CM CODES
194.0 Pheochromocytoma

EPIDEMIOLOGY & DEMOGRAPHICS

- Incidence: 0.05% of population; peak incidence in 30s and 40s.
- "Rough" rule of 10: 10% are extra-adrenal, 10% are malignant, 10% are familial, 10% occur in children, 10% involve both adrenals, 10% are multiple (other than bilateral adrenal).
- Approximately 25% of patients with apparently sporadic pheochromocytoma may be carriers of mutations.
- Pheochromocytoma is a feature of two disorders with autosomal dominant pattern of inheritance:
  1. Multiple endocrine neoplasia II
  2. Von Hippel-Lindau disease: angioma of the retina, hemangioblastoma of the CNS, renal cell carcinoma, pancreatic cysts, and epididymal cystoadenoma
- Pheochromocytomas occur in 5% of patients with neurofibromatosis type 1.

PHYSICAL FINDINGS & CLINICAL PRESENTATION

- Hypertension: can be sustained (55%) or paroxysmal (45%).
- Headache (80%): usually paroxysmal in nature and described as "pounding" and severe.
- Palpitations (70%): can be present with or without tachycardia.
- Hyperhidrosis (60%): most evident during paroxysmal attacks of hypertension.
- Physical examination may be entirely normal if done in a symptom-free interval; during a paroxysm the patient may demonstrate marked increase in both systolic and diastolic pressure, profuse sweating, visual disturbances (caused by hypertensive retinopathy), dilated pupils (secondary to catecholamine excess), paresthesias in the lower extremities (caused by severe vasoconstriction), tremor, tachycardia.

ETIOLOGY

- Catecholamine-producing tumors that are usually located in the adrenal medulla.
- Specific mutations of the RET protooncogene cause familial predisposition to pheochromocytoma in MEN II.
- Mutations in the von Hippel-Lindau tumor suppressor gene (VHL gene) cause familial disposition to pheochromocytoma in von Hippel-Lindau disease.
- Recently identified genes for succinate dehydrogenase subunit D (SDHD) and succinate dehydrogenase subunit B (SDHB) predispose carriers to pheochromocytoma and globus tumors.

DIAGNOSIS

DIFFERENTIAL DIAGNOSIS

- Anxiety disorder
- Thyrotoxicosis
- Amphetamine or cocaine abuse
- Carcinoid
- Essential hypertension

WORKUP

Laboratory evaluation and imaging studies to locate the neoplasm.

LABORATORY TESTS

- Plasma-free metanephrines are the best test for excluding or confirming pheochromocytoma and should be the test of first choice for diagnosis of the tumor. Plasma concentrations of normetanephrines >2.5 pmol/ml or metanephrine levels >1.4 pmol/ml indicate a pheochromocytoma with 100% specificity.
- 24-hr urine collection for metanephrines (100% sensitive) will also show increased metanephrines; the accuracy of the 24-hr urinary levels for metanephrines can be improved by indexing urinary metanephrine levels by urine creatinine levels.
- The clonidine suppression test is useful for distinguishing between high levels of plasma norepinephrine caused by release from sympathetic nerves and those caused by release from a pheochromocytoma. A decrease <50% in plasma norepinephrine levels after clonidine administration is normal, whereas persistent elevations are indicative of pheochromocytoma.

IMAGING STUDIES

- Abdominal CT scan (88% sensitivity) is useful in locating pheochromocytomas >0.5 inch in diameter (90% to 95% accurate).
- MRI: pheochromocytomas demonstrate a distinctive MRI appearance (100% sensitivity); MRI may become the diagnostic imaging modality of choice.
- Scintigraphy with ^{131}I-MIBG (100% sensitivity): this norepinephrine analog localizes in adrenergic tissue; it is particularly useful in locating extraadrenal pheochromocytomas.
- 6 [^{18}F] Fluorodopamine positron emission tomography is reserved for cases in which clinical symptoms and signs suggest pheochromocytoma and results of biochemical tests are positive but conventional imaging studies cannot locate the tumor. An alternative approach is to use vena caval sampling for plasma catecholamines and metanephrines.

TREATMENT

GENERAL Rx

Laparoscopic removal of the tumor (surgical resection for both benign and malignant disease):

1. Preoperative stabilization with combination of phenoxybenzamine, β-blocker, metyrosine, and liberal fluid and salt intake starting 10 to 14 days before surgery.
2. Hypertensive crisis preoperatively and intraoperatively can be controlled with phentolamine (Regitine) 2 to 5 mg IV q1 to 2h prn or nitroprusside used in combination with β-adrenergic blockers.

PEARLS & CONSIDERATIONS

COMMENTS

- Obtaining a detailed family history is important because 10% of pheochromocytomas are familial.
- Screening for pheochromocytoma should be considered in patients with any of the following:
  1. Malignant hypertension
  2. Poor response to antihypertensive therapy
  3. Paradoxical hypertensive response
  4. Hypertension during induction of anesthesia, parturition, surgery, or thyrotropin-releasing hormone testing
  5. Hypertension associated with imipramine or desipramine
  6. Neurofibromatosis (increased incidence of pheochromocytoma)
- All patients with pheochromocytoma should be screened for MEN-II and von Hippel-Lindau disease with pentagastrin test, serum PTH, ophthalmoscopy, MRI of the brain, CT scan of the kidneys and pancreas, and ultrasonography of the testes.
- In patients with pheochromocytoma, routine analysis for mutations of RET, VHL, SDHD, and SDHB is indicated to identify pheochromocytoma-associated syndromes.

AUTHOR: **FRED F. FERRI, M.D.**

BASIC INFORMATION

DEFINITION

Phobic anxiety disorders have at their core an extreme anxiety that is elicited by a specific object or situation that is usually perceived as more threatening than it really is and that often leads to avoidance behavior. The provoking stimuli may be social or performance situations (social phobia) or any other stimulus (specific phobia of objects, e.g., animals, natural environments, blood, or situational). Additionally, a person may experience intense anxiety about being in a place or situation from which they will not be able to escape in the event of a panic attack (agoraphobia in conjunction with or independent of panic disorder).

SYNONYMS

Simple phobia (obsolete name for specific phobia)
Phobias named according to the inducing stimulus, for example, arachnophobia (fear of spiders), claustrophobia (fear of tight spaces)
Social anxiety disorder

ICD-9CM CODES
F40.2 Specific phobia (DSM-IV: 300.29)
F40.1 Social phobia (DSM-IV: 300.23) Agoraphobia (DSM-IV: 300.21 [with panic disorder], 300.22 [without panic disorder])

EPIDEMIOLOGY & DEMOGRAPHICS

PEAK INCIDENCE: Specific phobias: often lifelong condition, but phobias with onset in childhood (e.g., animal phobias) tend to remit spontaneously.

PREVALENCE (IN U.S.):
- Specific phobias affect 5% to 10% of the general population.
- Social phobias affect about 13%.
- Agoraphobias without panic disorder affect 3% to 7% of the general population.

PREDOMINANT SEX AND AGE:
- Females with specific phobias outnumber males, though rates vary according to the phobia.
- More women are affected with social phobia; however, men are more likely to seek treatment.
- Agoraphobia also affects more women than men.
- Childhood onset for most specific phobias.
- Situational phobias have two peaks—the first in childhood and the second in the mid-20s.
- Fears are generally stable.
- Roots of social phobia may be in childhood, with described shyness or social inhibition, but onset usually in the midteens or into late adulthood; disorder is generally lifelong.

GENETICS: Both specific phobias and social phobias are more common in first-degree relatives than the general population.

PHYSICAL FINDINGS & CLINICAL PRESENTATION

- Specific phobias: frequently occur with other anxiety disorders, particularly panic and agoraphobias.
- When approaching the phobic object the patient experiences extreme anxiety often accompanied by autonomic symptoms such as tachycardia, tremor, and diaphoresis. In addition, depersonalization may occur. In blood phobias, however, these symptoms are often followed by a parasympathetic response consisting of hypotension and in some instances vasovagal syncope.
- Social phobias are distinguished from specific phobias in that what is feared is humiliation or embarrassment rather than the thing itself.

ETIOLOGY

Unknown

DIAGNOSIS

DIFFERENTIAL DIAGNOSIS

- Body dysmorphic disorder (BDD): similar to social phobia but in BDD the fear arises from the patient's belief that they are misshapen in some way.
- Panic attacks (with or without agoraphobia): anxiety symptoms seen in specific phobia may resemble panic attacks, but the stimulus in specific phobias or social phobias is clear, whereas panic attacks are unexpected.
- Generalized anxiety disorder: may be difficult to distinguish from social phobia, but in social phobia the cognitive focus is fear of embarrassment or humiliation, whereas in generalized anxiety disorder the focus is more internal on the subjective sensations of discomfort.
- Avoidant personality disorder is often comorbid with social phobia.
- Psychotic disorders: fear of being in public arises from delusions.

WORKUP

- History: usually diagnostic. Should elicit information about other medical disorders, medications, any history of physical or emotional abuse and substance abuse.
- Social phobia is a chronic condition. Individuals with social phobia often underachieve, drop out of school, avoid seeking work as a result of anxiety about interviews, refrain from dating and remain with family of origin, and are less likely to marry.
- Physical examination: to confirm absence of cardiovascular abnormalities (e.g., a chronic sinus arrhythmia).

LABORATORY TESTS

No specific laboratory tests are indicated.

IMAGING STUDIES

No specific imaging studies are recommended.

TREATMENT

NONPHARMACOLOGIC THERAPY

- Cognitive-behavioral therapy (CBT) and other psychotherapeutic approaches found to be effective in controlled trials.
- Behavioral treatment involves relaxation training, usually paired with visualization and progressive desensitization.
- Success rates are higher when the phobia is not complicated by other anxiety disorders.
- Social phobia is more problematic to treat because the psychological difficulties are more pervasive, but cognitive-behavioral therapy and other psychotherapies are quite effective.

ACUTE GENERAL Rx

- Benzodiazepines provide rapid relief of anxiety associated with exposure to fearful stimuli.
- Alprazolam or lorazepam: both administered sublingually to increase rate of absorption.
- Beta-blockers (e.g., propanolol) have been used to decrease autonomic hyperarousal and tremor associated with performance situations (e.g., before a public speech).

CHRONIC Rx

- If the phobic stimulus is rarely encountered, benzodiazepines as needed may be appropriate long-term treatment.
- Selective serotonin reuptake inhibitors (SSRIs), particularly paroxetine and sertraline, are effective in reducing symptoms and improving function for persons with social phobia.

COMPLEMENTARY & ALTERNATIVE MEDICINE

There is no definitive evidence for complementary and alternative medicine in treatment of phobic disorders. Several studies of supplements (e.g., valerian, St. John's wort, passiflora) have been done without statistically significant outcomes.

DISPOSITION

Usually present for life without treatment. Treatment may effectively reduce symptoms but not eliminate the fear.

REFERRAL

Recommended to confirm diagnosis and to evaluate for psychotherapy.

PEARLS & CONSIDERATIONS

Persons with social phobia usually have low self-esteem and fear of evaluation from others; they avoid or are fearful of any situation in which others may assess or evaluate them directly or indirectly. Concurrent anxiety disorders are common. Patients with social phobias may have comorbid substance abuse issues.

EVIDENCE

SSRIs

There is evidence that SSRIs are effective in the management of social phobia.

A systematic review identified 36 randomized controlled trials (RCTs) that compared antidepressants with placebo in the treatment of social phobia. The review found that in 26 of the studies short-term treatment with antidepressant therapy of all classes produced significant response compared with placebo.[1] Ⓐ

The review found that the response was significantly greater with SSRIs than other classes of antidepressant.[1] Ⓐ

Two subsequent RCTs compared paroxetine with placebo over 12 weeks in adults with social phobia. Both studies found that paroxetine significantly improved patient response over the period of treatment.[2,3] Ⓐ

Another RCT found that sertraline produced significantly greater improvements in clinical outcome, over a 20-week period, compared to placebo in adults with generalized social phobia.[4] Ⓐ

One RCT compared fluvoxamine with placebo over an 8-week period in children diagnosed with social phobia, separation anxiety disorder, or generalized anxiety disorder. The study found that fluvaxamine was superior to placebo in reducing anxiety symptoms with significant benefit at the end of the treatment.[5] Ⓐ

Cognitive-Behavioral Therapy (CBT)

There is evidence that CBT is of benefit in the management of social phobia.

An RCT compared phenelzine (a monoamine oxidase inhibitor [MAOI]) or cognitive-behavioral group therapy with placebo/attention placebo procedure over a 12-week period in adults with social phobia. At 12 weeks both CBT and phenelzine were equally effective in significantly improving patient responses compared to placebo.[6] Ⓐ

Exposure Therapy

There is evidence that exposure therapy is effective in the treatment of social phobia.

An RCT involving 375 adults suffering from social phobia compared sertraline with placebo with or without exposure therapy for 24 weeks. At the end of the trial all patients receiving active treatment showed an improved response compared to placebo, with the greatest response being seen in those patients receiving sertraline alone. Patients were followed up for a further 28 weeks at which point those patients receiving exposure therapy showed continued improvement whereas there was some deterioration in those patients receiving sertraline. The study suggests that better long-term outcome may be achieved with exposure therapy.[7] Ⓐ

Evidence-Based References

1. Stein DJ et al: Pharmacotherapy for social anxiety disorder, *Cochrane Database Syst Rev* 4, 2000. Ⓐ
2. Baldwin D et al: Paroxetine in social phobia/social anxiety disorder. Randomised, double-blind, placebo-controlled study, *Br J Psychiatry* 175:120, 1999. Reviewed in: *Evidence Based Mental Health* 3:41, 2000. Ⓐ
3. Stein MB et al: Paroxetine treatment of generalised social phobia (social anxiety disorder): a randomized controlled trial, *JAMA* 280:708, 1998. Reviewed in: *Evidence Based Mental Health* 2:53, 1999. Ⓐ
4. Van Ameringen MA et al: Sertraline treatment of generalized social phobia: a 20-week, double-blind, placebo-controlled study, *Am J Psychiatry* 158:275, 2001. Reviewed in: *Evidence Based Mental Health* 4:91, 2001. Ⓐ
5. The Research Unit on Pediatric Psychopharmacology Anxiety Study Group: Fluvoxamine for the treatment of anxiety disorders in children and adolescents, *N Engl J Med* 344:1279, 2001. Reviewed in: *Evidence Based Mental Health* 4:116, 2001. Ⓐ
6. Heimberg RG et al: Cognitive behavioural group therapy vs phenelzine therapy for social phobia: 12 week outcome, *Arch Gen Psychiatry* 55:1131, 1998. Reviewed in: *Evidence Based Mental Health* 2:80,1999. Ⓐ
7. Haug TT et al: Exposure therapy and sertraline in social phobia: 1-year follow up of a randomised control trial, *Br J Psychiatry* 182:312, 2003. Reviewed in: *Evidence Based Mental Health* 6:90, 2003. Ⓐ

SUGGESTED READINGS

Anxiety Disorders Association of America: http://www.adaa.org

Kripke C: Is pharmacotherapy useful in social phobia? *Am Fam Physician* 71(9):1700, 2005.

Schneir FR: Clinical practice: social anxiety disorder, *N Engl J Med* 355(10):1029, 2006.

AUTHORS: **MITCHELL D. FELDMAN, M.D., M.PHIL.,** and **AMANDA A. WULFSTAT, M.D.**

BASIC INFORMATION

DEFINITION

From Latin: *pilus* = hair and *nidus* = nest. A *pilonidal sinus* is a short tract that extends from the skin surface, is most commonly found in the intergluteal fold sacrococcygeal region, additionally described in the interdigital area, umbilicus, chest wall, and scalp. It most likely represents a distended hair follicle. An *acute pilonidal abscess,* which consists of pus and a wall of edematous fat, results from rupture of an infected follicle into fat. A *chronic pilonidal abscess* results when an infected follicle ruptures directly into surrounding tissues; the wall of a chronic pilonidal abscess consists of fibrous tissue. A *pilonidal cyst* develops from a chronic abscess of long duration as a thin and flat lining of epithelium grows into the cavity from the skin surface.

SYNONYMS

Jeep disease

ICD-9CM CODES
685.1 Pilonidal cyst

EPIDEMIOLOGY & DEMOGRAPHICS

INCIDENCE: 26 cases/100,000 persons
PREDOMINANT SEX: Male > female (2.2:1)
AVERAGE AGE OF PRESENTATION: 21 yr
RISK FACTORS:
- Male sex
- Caucasian race
- Family predisposition
- Obesity
- Sedentary lifestyle
- Occupation requiring prolonged sitting
- Local hirsutism
- Poor hygiene
- Increased sweat activity

PHYSICAL FINDINGS & CLINICAL PRESENTATION

- May manifest as asymptomatic pits or pores in the natal cleft
- Tenderness after physical activity or prolonged sitting
- Acute pilonidal abscess in 20% of patients with pilonidal disease
- Presents as a hot, tender, fluctuant swelling just lateral to the midline over the sacrum that may exude pus through the midline pit
- Chronic pilonidal abscess in 80% of patients with pilonidal disease
- Acute suppuration, tenderness, swelling, and heat
- Infrequently, systemic reaction: occasionally fever, leukocytosis, and malaise

ETIOLOGY

- Currently, thought to be acquired rather than congenital.
- Drilling of hair shed from the perineum or the head into sebaceous or hair follicles in the natal cleft.
- Drilling is facilitated by the friction of the natal cleft.
- Subsequent infection by skin organisms leads to pilonidal abscess.

DIAGNOSIS

DIFFERENTIAL DIAGNOSIS

- Perianal abscess arising from the posterior midline crypt
- Hidradenitis suppurativa
- Carbuncle
- Furuncle
- Osteomyelitis
- Anal fistula
- Coccygeal sinus

WORKUP

- Diagnosis is based on history and physical examination.
- Midline pits present behind the anus overlying the sacrum and coccyx.
- Broken hairs are often seen extruding from the midline pits.
- Insert probe in pilonidal sinus in path away from the anus.
- Complicated anal fistula may be angulating posteriorly before passing into a retrorectal abscess, but thorough examination of the anal cavity usually discloses point of origin.

LABORATORY TESTS

CBC

IMAGING STUDIES

CT scan in advanced recurrent cases

TREATMENT

NONPHARMACOLOGIC THERAPY

Prevention of exacerbations:
1. Local hygiene
2. Avoidance of prolonged sitting position
3. Weight reduction

ACUTE GENERAL Rx

- Procedure of choice for first-episode acute abscess: simple incision and drainage in an outpatient setting
- Cure rate of 76% after 18 mo
- Antibiotics: generally not indicated unless the patient has a medical condition such as rheumatic heart disease or is immunosuppressed

CHRONIC Rx

Elective treatment of pilonidal disease:
1. Minimal surgery
   a. Remove hair from midline pits and shave buttocks.
   b. May use a fine wire brush with local anesthesia to clear the pits and any lateral openings of granulation tissue and hair.
   c. Keep area clean.
2. Fistulotomy and curettage
   a. Used when minimal surgery does not control episodes of suppuration
   b. Pass probe to outline the pilonidal sinus and open tract surgically
   c. Curette granulation tissue at the base of the sinus and excise edges of the skin
   d. Keep open granulating wound meticulously clean and allow to heal
   e. If complete healing does not take place, use a skin graft or advancement flap to close the defect
3. Marsupialization
   a. This is the treatment of choice for chronic pilonidal disease.
   b. Wide excision of the pilonidal area is performed, including all affected skin and subcutaneous tissues down to the presacral fascia.
   c. Wound is left open, allowed to marsupialize, or closed as a primary procedure.
   d. Give antibiotics for 24 hr (particularly those directed against *Staphylococcus* and *Bacteroides* spp).
4. Other procedures
   a. Excision and closure
   b. Excision and skin grafting
   c. Bascom procedure (follicle removal & lateral drainage)
   d. Flaps: Z-plasty, V-Y advancement flap, rhomboid flap, gluteus maximus myocutaneous flap

DISPOSITION

- Recurrence rate for excision (most definitive procedure): 1% to 6%
- Incidence of squamous cell carcinoma in a chronic, recurrent pilonidal sinus is rare <1%

REFERRAL

- Emergency room for incision and drainage for an acute abscess
- To a surgeon for elective treatment or management of chronic or recurrent disease

PEARLS & CONSIDERATIONS

COMMENTS

Because of significant associated morbidity, the elective surgical procedures outlined are performed only after the potential risks vs. benefits are carefully weighed.

SUGGESTED READINGS

Church JM: Pilonidal cyst: cause and treatment, *Dis Colon Rectum* 43(8):1146, 2000.
Hull TL, Wu J: Pilonidal disease, *Surg Clin North Am* 82(6):1169, 2002.

AUTHORS: **ARUNDATHI G. PRASAD, M.D.,** and **RUBEN ALVERO, M.D.**

BASIC INFORMATION

DEFINITION

Pinworms are a noninvasive infestation of the intestinal tract by *Enterobius vermicularis,* a helminth of the nematode family.

SYNONYMS

Enterobiasis

ICD-9CM CODES
127.4 Enterobiasis

EPIDEMIOLOGY & DEMOGRAPHICS

- Most common intestinal nematode with approximately 30,000 cases/yr in the U.S.
- Worldwide distribution, but most common in temperate climates.
- The prevalence of pinworm infection is lowest in infants and reaches highest infection rate in school-age children (5 to 14 yr old).
- Eggs are infective within 6 hr of oviposition and may remain so for 20 days.
- Clusters are found in families, institutionalized persons, and homosexual men.

PHYSICAL FINDINGS & CLINICAL PRESENTATION

- Most infested persons are asymptomatic.
- Perianal itching is the most common reported symptom, with scratching leading to excoriation and sometimes secondary infection.
- Rarely insomnia, irritability, anorexia, and weight loss are described.
- Granulomas have been described in various organs resulting from worms wandering outside the intestines and dying there.

ETIOLOGY & PATHOGENESIS

- *E. vermicularis* is highly prevalent throughout the world, particularly in countries of the temperate zone. Humans are the only host for this worm. Infestation is by fecal-oral route; ingested eggs hatch in the stomach and the larvae migrate to the colon where they mature. Gravid female worms containing an average of 10,000 ova migrate to the perianal skin at night, lay their eggs there, and die. The eggs embryonate within 6 hr and cause itching; scratching causes egg deposition under fingernails, from which they can contaminate food or lead to autoreinfection.
- *E. vermicularis* may be transmitted between sexual partners, especially those engaging in oral-anal sex.

DIAGNOSIS

DIFFERENTIAL DIAGNOSIS

- Perianal itching related to poor hygiene
- Hemorrhoidal disease and anal fissures
- Perineal yeast/fungal infections
- Section II describes the causes of pruritus ani

WORKUP

Identification of adult worms or eggs. *E. vermicularis* ova are ovoid but flattened on one side and measure approximately 56 × 27 micrometers (Fig. 1-200). The eggs can be identified on transparent tape placed on the perianal skin upon awakening (NOTE: Five consecutive negative tests rule out the diagnosis.). A single examination detects 50% of infections, three examinations detect 90%, and five examinations detect 99%.

TREATMENT

- Single dose of mebendazole (100 mg) with a repeat dose given after 2 wk.
- Single dose of albendazole (400 mg) with a second dose given 2 wk later is also highly effective.
- Pyrantel pamoate (11mg/kg up to 1 g) can prevent against *Enterobius vermicularis.* It is available as a suspension and has minimal toxicity (mild transient GI symptoms, headache, drowsiness). A repeat dose after 2 wk is recommended because of the frequency of reinfection and autoinfection.
- Other infected family members, classmates, or residents of long-term care facilities should be treated at the same time as the index case.

SUGGESTED READING

Lohiya GS et al: Epidemiology and control of enterobiasis in a developmental center, *West J Med* 172:305-308, 2000.

AUTHORS: **FRED F. FERRI, M.D.,** and **TOM J. WACHTEL, M.D.**

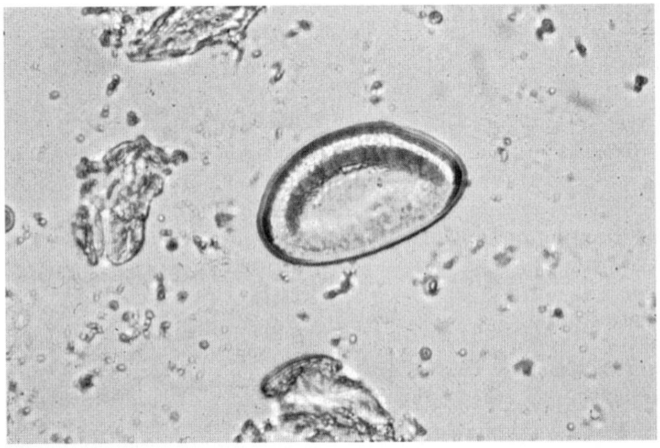

FIGURE 1-200 *Enterobius vermicularis* embryonated egg. Note larva inside (40 × 10 μm). (From Gorbach SL, Bartlett JG, Blacklow NR (eds): *Infectious diseases,* ed 2, Philadelphia, 1998, WB Saunders.)

BASIC INFORMATION

DEFINITION

Pituitary adenoma is a benign neoplasm of the anterior lobe of the pituitary that causes symptoms, either by excess secretion of hormones or by a local mass effect as the tumor impinges on other, nearby structures (e.g., optic chiasm, hypothalamus, pituitary stalk). Pituitary adenomas are classified by their size, function, and features that characterize their appearance. Microadenomas are <10 mm in size, and macroadenomas are >10 mm in size.

- *Acromegaly* is the disease state characterized by a pituitary adenoma that secretes growth hormone (GH).
- A *prolactinoma* secretes prolactin (PRL).
- *Cushing's disease* is a disease state in which there is hypersecretion of adrenocorticotropic hormone (ACTH).
- *Thyrotropin-secreting pituitary adenomas* secrete primarily thyroid-stimulating hormone (TSH).
- *Nonsecretory pituitary adenomas* are those in which the neoplasm is a space-occupying lesion whose secretory products do not cause a specific disease state.

ICD-9CM CODES
253 Pituitary adenoma
253.0 Acromegaly
253.1 Prolactinoma

EPIDEMIOLOGY & DEMOGRAPHICS

CLASSIFICATION (BY HORMONE SECRETED):
- PRL only 35%
- No hormone 30%
- GH only 20%
- PRL and GH 7%
- ACTH 7%
- LF/FSH/TSH 1%

PREVALENCE/INCIDENCE:
Pituitary adenomas: Up to 10% to 15% of all intracranial neoplasms; 3% to 27% autopsy series
Prolactinomas: Up to 20% in women with unexplained primary or secondary amenorrhea
Growth hormone–secreting pituitary adenoma: 50 to 60 cases/1,000,000 persons
Thyrotropin-secreting pituitary adenoma: 2.8% of pituitary adenomas with a slight female:male predominance of 1.7:1
Corticotropin-secreting pituitary adenomas: Female:male predominance of 8:1

PHYSICAL FINDINGS & CLINICAL PRESENTATION

PROLACTINOMAS:
- Females:
  1. Galactorrhea
  2. Amenorrhea
  3. Oligomenorrhea with anovulation
  4. Infertility
  5. Estrogen deficiency leading to hirsutism
  6. Decreased vaginal lubrication
  7. Osteopenia
- Males:
  1. Large tumors more common secondary to delayed diagnosis
  2. Possible impotence or decreased libido or hypogonadism
  3. Galactorrhea rare because males lack the estrogen-dependent breast growth and differentiation

GROWTH HORMONE–SECRETING PITUITARY ADENOMA: Acromegaly
- Coarse facial features
- Oily skin
- Prognathism
- Carpal tunnel syndrome
- Osteoarthritis
- History of increased hat, glove, or shoe size
- Decreased exercise capacity
- Visual field deficits
- Diabetes mellitus

CORTICOTROPIN-SECRETING PITUITARY ADENOMA: Cushing's disease
- Usually present when the tumor is small (1 to 2 mm)
- 50% of the tumors <5 mm
- Other symptoms:
  1. Truncal obesity
  2. Round facies (moon face)
  3. Dorsocervical fat accumulation (buffalo hump)
  4. Hirsutism
  5. Acne
  6. Menstrual disorders
  7. Hypertension
  8. Striae
  9. Bruising
  10. Thin skin
  11. Hyperglycemia

THYROTROPIN-SECRETING PITUITARY ADENOMA:
- In males, larger, more invasive, and more rapidly growing tumors that present later in life
- Other symptoms: thyrotoxicosis, goiter, visual impairment

NONSECRETORY PITUITARY ADENOMAS (ENDOCRINE INACTIVE PITUITARY ADENOMA):
- Usually large at the time of diagnosis
- Symptoms:
  1. Bitemporal hemianopsia secondary to compression of the optic chiasm
  2. Hypopituitarism secondary to compression of the pituitary gland
  3. Hypogonadism in men and in premenopausal women
  4. Cranial nerve deficits, secondary to extension into the cavernous sinus
  5. Hydrocephalus, secondary to extension into the third ventricle, compressing the foramen of Monro
  6. Diabetes insipidus, secondary to compression of the hypothalamus or pituitary stalk (a rare complication)

ETIOLOGY

Benign neoplasms of epithelial origin

DIAGNOSIS

DIFFERENTIAL DIAGNOSIS

PROLACTINOMA:
- Pregnancy
- Postpartum puerperium
- Primary hypothyroidism
- Breast disease
- Breast stimulation
- Drug ingestion (especially phenothiazines, antidepressants, haloperidol, methyldopa, reserpine, opiates, amphetamines, and cimetidine)
- Chronic renal failure
- Liver disease
- Polycystic ovarian disease
- Chest wall disorders
- Spinal cord lesions
- Previous cranial irradiation

ACROMEGALY: Ectopic production of growth hormone–releasing hormone from a carcinoid or other neuroendocrine tumor

CUSHING'S DISEASE:
- Diseases that cause ectopic sources of ACTH overproduction (including small cell carcinoma of the lung, bronchial carcinoid, intestinal carcinoid, pancreatic islet cell tumor, medullary thyroid carcinoma, or pheochromocytoma)
- Adrenal adenomas, adrenal carcinoma
- Nelson's syndrome

THYROTROPIN-SECRETNG PITUITARY ADENOMAS: Primary hypothyroidism

NONSECRETORY PITUITARY ADENOMA: Nonneoplastic mass lesions of various etiologies (e.g., infectious, granulomatous)

WORKUP (See Section III, "Pituitary Tumor")

PROLACTINOMA: First step: measurement of basal PRL levels
- Elevated PRL levels are correlated with tumor size.
- Levels >200 ng/ml are diagnostic, with levels of 100 to 200 ng/ml being equivocal.
- Basal PRL levels between 20 and 100 suggest a microprolactinoma, as well as other conditions such as drug ingestion.
- Basal level <20 is normal.

ACROMEGALY:
- First screening test is the measurement of the serum IGF-I level, postprandial serum GH, TRH stimulation test.
- Follow with an oral glucose tolerance test.

- Failure to suppress serum GH to <2 ng/ml with an oral load of 100 g glucose is considered conclusive.
- A GHRH level >300 ng/ml is indicative of an ectopic source of GH.

CUSHING'S DISEASE:
- Normal or slightly elevated corticotropin levels ranging from 20 to 200 pg/ml; normal is 10 to 50 pg/ml.
- Levels <10 pg/ml usually indicate an autonomously secreting adrenal tumor.
- Levels >200 pg/ml suggest an ectopic corticotropin-secreting neoplasm.
- Cushing's disease is confirmed by demonstration of low-dose dexamethasone, which shows presence of abnormal cortisol suppressibility.
- 24-hr urine collection should demonstrate an increased level of cortisol excretion.

THYROTROPIN-SECRETING PITUITARY ADENOMA:
- Highly sensitive thyrotropin assays, which evaluate the presence of thyrotoxicosis, are one way to detect a thyrotropin-secreting tumor.
- Free alpha subunit is secreted by >80% of tumors with the ratio of the alpha subunit to thyrotropin <1.
- With central resistance to thyroid hormone, ratio is <1 and the sella is normal.
- Laboratory tests show elevated serum levels of both T_3 and T_4.

NONSECRETORY PITUITARY ADENOMA:
- Visual field testing
- Assessment of the pituitary and organ function to determine if there is hypopituitarism or hypersecretion of hormones (even if the effects of hypersecretion are subclinical)
- TRH to provoke secretion of FSH, LH, and LH-beta-subunit; will not elicit response in normal persons
- Exclusion of Klinefelter's syndrome in patient with long-standing primary hypogonadism, elevated gonadotropin levels, and enlargement of the sella

IMAGING STUDIES

- Study of choice: MRI of the pituitary and hypothalamus
  1. When evaluating Cushing's disease, small size at the onset of symptoms noted
- MRI, in this case, only 60% sensitive at best and may yield false-positive results
- CT scan only when MRI is unavailable or is otherwise contraindicated

TREATMENT (Rx)

NONPHARMACOLOGIC THERAPY

SURGERY:
- Selective transsphenoidal resection of the adenoma is the treatment of choice for acromegaly, Cushing's disease, and thyrotropin-secreting pituitary adenomas, which all tend to be microadenomas at the time of onset of symptoms.
- Macroadenomas, such as the nonsecretory pituitary adenoma, may also be surgically removed, but risk of recurrence is greater with these tumors, and adjunctive therapy such as irradiation may also be necessary.
- Radiotherapy is reserved for patients who have failed surgical treatment and who still experience the symptoms of their adenoma.
- Bilateral adrenalectomy has been done in patients with Cushing's disease on failure of other therapies; complications requiring lifelong hormone replacement or Nelson's syndrome may occur.

RADIOTHERAPY:
- Generally reserved for patients who have failed surgical treatment
- Used with varying degrees of success in all of the different pituitary adenomas

ACUTE GENERAL Rx

PROLACTINOMA:
- Bromocriptine, a dopamine analog, is generally given orally in divided doses of 1.5 to 10 mg.
- Side effects include orthostatic hypotension, nausea, and dizziness; avoided by beginning with low-dose therapy.
- Other compounds under investigation include pergolide mesylate, a long-acting ergot derivative with dopaminergic properties, as well as other nonergot derivatives.

ACROMEGALY:
- Octreotide, a somatostatin analog, 100 μg SC, is the medical therapy of choice but is limited by side effects such as biliary sludge and gallstones, nausea, cramps, steatorrhea, and its parenteral administration.
- Bromocriptine 10 to 20 mg po tid-qid is less effective than octreotide, but has the advantage of oral administration.

CUSHING'S DISEASE:
- Ketoconazole, which inhibits the cytochrome P-450 enzymes involved in steroid biosynthesis, is effective in managing mild to moderate disease in daily oral dosages of 600 to 1200 mg.
- Metyrapone and aminoglutethimide can be used to control hypersecretion of cortisol but are generally used when preparing a patient for surgery or while waiting for a response to radiotherapy.

THYROTROPIN-SECRETING PITUITARY ADENOMA:
- Ablative therapy with either radioactive iodide or surgery is indicated.
- Treatment directed to the thyroid alone may accelerate growth of the pituitary adenoma.
- Octreotide has been shown to be effective in doses similar to those used for acromegaly.

NONSECRETORY PITUITARY ADENOMA:
- There is no role for medical therapy at this time.
- Surgery and radiotherapy are indicated.

CHRONIC Rx

For all pituitary adenomas:
- Careful follow-up is important. Patients undergoing transsphenoidal microsurgical resection should be seen in 4 to 6 wk to ensure that the adenoma has been completely removed and that the endocrine hypersecretion is resolved.
- If there is good clinical response, patient should be monitored yearly for recurrence and to follow the level of the hypersecreted hormone.
- Patients who have undergone irradiation should have close follow-up with backup medical therapy because response to radiotherapy may be delayed; incidence of hypopituitarism also increases with time.

SUGGESTED READINGS

Davis AK, Farrell WE, Clayton RN: Pituitary tumors, *Reproduction* 121(3):363, 2001.

Kovacs K, Horvath E, Vidal S: Classification of pituitary adenomas, *J Neurooncol* 54(2): 121, 2001.

AUTHORS: **BETH J. WUTZ, M.D.,** and **RUBEN ALVEERO, M.D.**

BASIC INFORMATION

DEFINITION

Pityriasis is a common self-limiting skin eruption of unknown etiology.

ICD-9CM CODES
696.3 Pityriasis rosea

EPIDEMIOLOGY & DEMOGRAPHICS

- Most cases of pityriasis rosea occur between ages 10 and 35 yr; mean age is 23 yr.
- The incidence of disease is highest in the fall and spring.
- Female:male ratio is 1.5:1.

PHYSICAL FINDINGS & CLINICAL PRESENTATION

- Initial lesion (herald patch) precedes the eruption by approximately 1 to 2 wk; typically measures 3 to 6 cm; it is round to oval in appearance and most frequently located on the trunk.
- Eruptive phase follows within 2 wk and peaks after 7 to 14 days.
- Lesions are most frequently located in the lower abdominal area. They have a salmon-pink appearance in whites and a hyperpigmented appearance in blacks.
- Most lesions are 4 to 5 mm in diameter; center has a "cigarette paper" appearance; border has a characteristic ring of scale (collarette).
- Lesions occur in a symmetric distribution and follow the cleavage lines of the trunk (Christmas tree pattern [Fig. 1-201]).
- The number of lesions varies from a few to hundreds.
- Most patients are asymptomatic; pruritus is the most common symptom.
- History of recent fatigue, headache, sore throat, and low-grade fever is present in approximately 25% of cases.

ETIOLOGY

Unknown, possibly viral (picornavirus)

DIAGNOSIS

DIFFERENTIAL DIAGNOSIS

- Tinea corporis (can be ruled out by potassium hydroxide examination)
- Secondary syphilis (absence of herald patch, positive serologic test for syphilis)
- Psoriasis
- Nummular eczema
- Drug eruption: medications that may cause rashes similar to pityriasis rosea include clonidine, captopril, interferon, bismuth, barbiturates, gold, hepatitis B vaccine, and imatinib mesylate
- Viral exanthem
- Eczema
- Lichen planus
- Tinea versicolor (the lesions are more brown and the borders are not as ovoid)

WORKUP

Presence of herald lesion and characteristic rash are diagnostic. Skin biopsy is generally reserved for atypical cases.

LABORATORY TESTS

Generally not necessary; serologic test for syphilis if clinically indicated

TREATMENT

NONPHARMACOLOGIC THERAPY

The disease is self-limited and generally does not require any therapeutic intervention.

ACUTE GENERAL Rx

- Use calamine lotion or oral antihistamines in patients with significant pruritus.
- Use prednisone tapered over 2 wk in patients with severe pruritus.
- Direct sun exposure or use of ultraviolet light within the first week of eruption is beneficial in decreasing the severity of disease.

DISPOSITION

- Spontaneous complete resolution of the rash within 4 to 8 wk
- Recurrence rare (<2% of cases)

PEARLS & CONSIDERATIONS

COMMENTS

Reassure patient that the disease is not contagious and its course is benign.

SUGGESTED READING

Stulberg D, Wolfrey J: Pityriasis rosea, *Am Fam Physician,* 69:87, 2004.

AUTHOR: **FRED F. FERRI, M.D.**

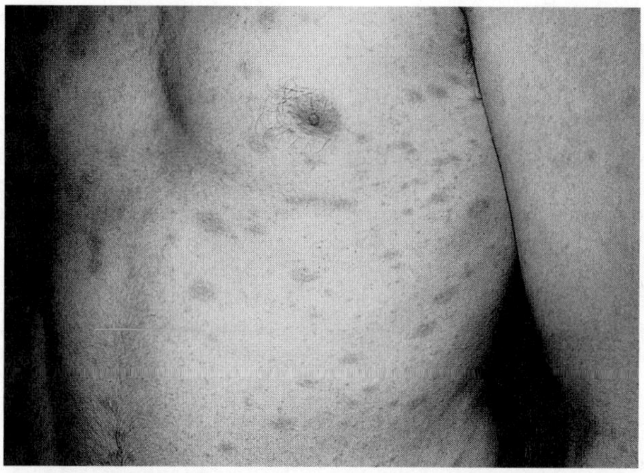

FIGURE 1-201 Scale (pityriasis rosea). Shows example of how unique scaling (collarette of fine scale within several lesions), distribution and shape of lesions (oval lesions with long axis paralleling natural skin cleavage lines), and color (salmon-pink) help in diagnosing skin disease. (From Noble J [ed]: *Textbook of primary care medicine,* ed 3, St Louis, 2001, Mosby.)

BASIC INFORMATION

DEFINITION

Placenta previa is the implantation of the placenta over the internal os. Four degrees of this abnormality have been defined:

- Total placenta previa: the internal os is covered completely.
- Partial placenta previa: the internal os is partially covered.
- Marginal placenta previa: the edge of the placenta is at the margin of the internal os.
- Low-lying placenta: the placenta is implanted in the lower uterine segment, and although its edge does not reach the internal os, it is in close proximity to it.

See Fig. 1-202.

ICD-9CM CODES
641.1 Placenta previa

EPIDEMIOLOGY & DEMOGRAPHICS INCIDENCE

INCIDENCE: 0.26% to 0.7% of pregnancies

RISK FACTORS:

- Previous cesarean delivery (after one such delivery, the risk is 1% to 4%; after four or more cesarean deliveries, the risk approaches 10%).
- Multiparity has also been associated with placenta previa.

PHYSICAL FINDINGS & CLINICAL PRESENTATION

The classic presentation of placenta previa is painless vaginal bleeding, usually in the second or third trimester. Uterine contractions may or may not be present. On physical examination, the uterus is soft and pain-free. The fetus is often in breech, transverse lie, or high. Fetal distress is usually not present.

ETIOLOGY

Uncertain

DIAGNOSIS

DIFFERENTIAL DIAGNOSIS

- Placenta accreta
- Placenta percreta
- Placenta increta
- Vasa previa
- Abruptio placentae
- Vaginal or cervical trauma
- Labor
- Local malignancy

WORKUP

- Do *not* perform a digital vaginal examination.
- The diagnosis of placenta previa can seldom be firmly established by physical examination alone. A speculum examination in a hospital setting to exclude any local bleeding may be performed.
- This diagnosis should not be dismissed until thorough evaluation, including sonography, has completely excluded its presence.

LABORATORY TESTS

- A complete blood count (CBC) can be used to monitor hemoglobin and hematocrit
- A Kleihauer-Betke preparation of maternal blood in all Rh-negative women and Rh-immune globulin when indicated

IMAGING STUDIES

- The simplest, most precise, and safest method of placental localization is transabdominal sonography with confirmatory imaging by transvaginal ultrasonography. Transperineal sonography has also proven effective in detection.
- Magnetic resonance imaging has also been effective in detecting placenta previa, although sonography remains the preferred method.

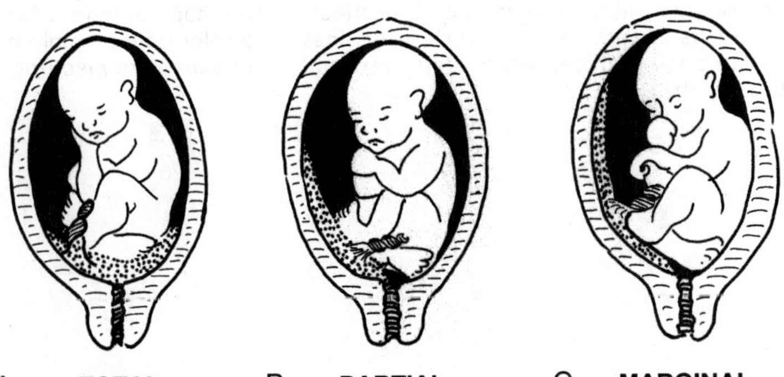

FIGURE 1-202 Various types of placenta previa. **A,** The cervical os is completely covered by placenta. **B,** The cervical os is partially covered by placenta. **C,** The placenta extends to the edge of the cervical os. (From Rakel RE: *Textbook of family practice,* ed 6, Philadelphia, 2002, WB Saunders.)

TREATMENT

NONPHARMACOLOGIC THERAPY

- In preterm pregnancies with no active bleeding, close observation and expectant management are indicated. In those with active bleeding, conservative management, including blood transfusions for severe bleeds, is appropriate. The woman should stay in the hospital for at least 48 hr after the bleeding has stopped.
- Bedrest, preferably in a hospital setting, should be prescribed.

ACUTE GENERAL Rx

- Initial assessment for signs of maternal hemodynamic compromise or hemorrhagic shock; large-bore intravenous access with crystalloid fluid resuscitation
- Assess fetal status and gestational age using sonogram and continuous fetal heart rate monitoring
- Cross-matched blood should be made available during bleeding episodes; if the hemorrhage is severe, cesarean delivery is indicated despite fetal immaturity
- Tocolytic therapy may be considered in those women in preterm labor, as well as the administration of corticosteroids to enhance fetal lung maturity

CHRONIC Rx

- Cesarean delivery is necessary in nearly all cases of placenta previa.
- Uncontrollable hemorrhage after placental removal should be anticipated secondary to the poorly contractile nature of the lower uterine segment. The need for hysterectomy to control bleeding should be discussed with the patient before delivery, if possible.

DISPOSITION

Because of the unpredictable nature of placenta previa, not all women with placenta previa can be treated expectantly.

REFERRAL

Affected women and their families should be aware of all signs and symptoms that would necessitate immediate transport to the hospital. The possibility of hysterectomy should also be discussed early during pregnancy.

SUGGESTED READING

Faiz AS, Ananth CV: Etiology and risk factors for placenta previa: an overview and meta-analysis of observational studies, *J Matern Fetal Neonatal Med* 13(3):175, 2003.

AUTHORS: **SONYA S. ABDEL-RAZEQ, M.D.,** and **RUBEN ALVERO, M.D.**

BASIC INFORMATION

DEFINITION

Plantar fasciitis is a common, painful inflammation or degeneration of the plantar fascia, a tissue that extends from the calcaneus to the proximal phalanges of each toe.

SYNONYMS

Painful heel syndrome
Painful heel spur

ICD-9CM CODES
728.71 Plantar fasciitis
726.73 Calcaneal spur

EPIDEMIOLOGY & DEMOGRAPHICS

PREDOMINANT SEX: Males = females
PREDOMINANT AGE: Middle age
Bilateral in 10% to 20% of cases

PHYSICAL FINDINGS & CLINICAL PRESENTATION

- Pain is characteristically worse on arising and after periods of rest; "warming up" often lessens the pain
- Local tenderness at site involvement, usually the medial tubercle of the calcaneus, sometimes in the midfascia
- Pain sometimes elicited by passive dorsiflexion of toes and ankle, which stretches the plantar fascia
- A tight heel cord may be present

ETIOLOGY

- Uncertain.
- Inflammation, microscopic tears, and/or degeneration.
- The role of the calcaneal traction osteophyte (spur) is unclear. The rate of plantar fascial pain appears unrelated to the occurrence or presence of a calcaneal osteophyte.
- May be associated with tight heel cord.

DIAGNOSIS

DIFFERENTIAL DIAGNOSIS

- Other regional tendonitis
- Stress fracture
- Tarsal tunnel syndrome
- Tumor, infection

IMAGING STUDIES

Traction osteophyte or minor soft tissue calcification may be present on plain radiography. Other studies are usually not required.

TREATMENT

- Sensible activity restriction
- Gentle stretching exercises
- NSAIDS
- Local steroid/lidocaine injections (Fig. 1-203)
- Heel lift
- Night brace, daytime cast brace

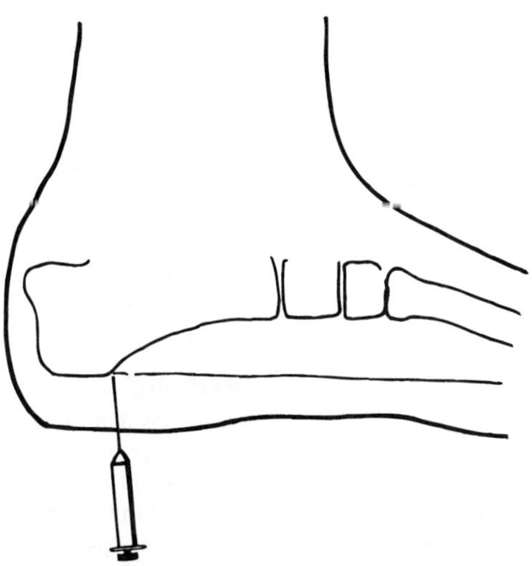

FIGURE 1-203 Injection site for plantar fasciitis. Injection should be through the sole into the area of maximum tenderness. A 25- or 27-gauge needle should be used and the medication injected slowly as some pain may occur. The total volume should be no greater than 1.5 ml. (From Mercier L: *Practical orthopedics,* ed 5, St Louis, 2002, Mosby.)

DISPOSITION

Disorder is usually self-limited, although full recovery may take 1 to 2 yr.

REFERRAL

- If symptoms fail to respond to medical management
- For surgical consideration (plantar fascia release, excision of osteophyte)

PEARLS & CONSIDERATIONS

Fasciitis may be a misnomer. Inflammation is usually not present on pathologic evaluation of tissue samples in most cases. Tendinosis may be a more proper term. Involvement of the plantar fascia and/or heel cord insertion in the spondyloarthropathies (enthesitis, enthesopathy) is a common association.

COMMENTS

- Various cushions and heel cups are generally ineffective because stretching, not heel strikes, is probably cause of disorder.
- Surgical intervention is rarely necessary.
- Shock wave therapy is of unproven benefit.

SUGGESTED READINGS

Aldridge J: Diagnosing heel pain in adults, *Am Fam Physician* 70:332, 2004.
Bachbinder R: Plantar fasciitis, *N Engl J Med* 350:2159, 2004.
Cosca DD, Navazio F: Common problems in endurance athletes, *Am Fam Physician* 76:237, 2007.
DiGiovanni BF et al: Tissue specific plantar fascia stretching exercises enhances outcomes in patients with chronic heel pain, *J Bone Joint Surg* 85:1270, 2003.
Flanigan RM et al: The influence of foot position on stretching of the plantar fascia, *Foot Ankle Int* 28(7):815, 2007.
Fredericson M, Misra AK: Epidemiology and aetiology of marathon running injuries, *Sports Med* 37:437, 2007.
Furia JP: The safety and efficacy of high energy extracorporeal shock wave therapy in active, moderately active and sedentary patients with chronic plantar fasciitis, *Orthopedics* 28:685, 2005.
Khoury V et al: Ultrasound of ankle and foot: overuse and sports injuries, *Semin Musculoskeletal Radiol* 11:149, 2007.
Riddle DL et al: Risk factors for plantar fasciitis: a matched case-control study, *J Bone Joint Surg* 85:872, 2003.

AUTHOR: **LONNIE R. MERCIER, M.D.**

BASIC INFORMATION

DEFINITION

Aspiration pneumonia is a lung infection caused by bacterial organisms aspirated from nasopharyngeal space.

ICD-9CM CODES
507.0 Aspiration pneumonia

EPIDEMIOLOGY & DEMOGRAPHICS

INCIDENCE (IN U.S.):
- Few reliable data
- 20% to 35% of all pneumonias
- 5% to 15% of all community acquired pneumonias

PEAK INCIDENCE: Elderly patients in hospitals or nursing homes
PREVALENCE (IN U.S.): Unreliable data
PREDOMINANT SEX: Equal
PREDOMINANT AGE: Elderly

PHYSICAL FINDINGS & CLINICAL PRESENTATION

- Shortness of breath, tachypnea, cough, sputum, fever after vomiting, or difficulty swallowing
- Rales, rhonchi, often diffusely throughout lung

ETIOLOGY

Complex interaction of etiologies, ranging from chemical (often acid) pneumonitis following aspiration of sterile gastric contents (generally not requiring antibiotic treatment) to bacterial aspiration

COMMUNITY-ACQUIRED ASPIRATION PNEUMONIA:
- Generally results from predominantly anaerobic mouth bacteria (anaerobic and microaerophilic streptococci, fusobacteria, gram-positive anaerobic non–spore-forming rods), *Bacteroides* species *(melaninogenicus, intermedius, oralis, ureolyticus), Haemophilus influenzae,* and *Streptococcus pneumoniae*
- Rarely caused by *Bacteroides fragilis* (of uncertain validity in published studies) or *Eikenella corrodens*
- High-risk groups: elderly, alcoholics, IV drug users, patients who are obtunded, those with esophageal disorders, seizures, poor dentition, stroke victims, or recent dental manipulations

HOSPITAL-ACQUIRED ASPIRATION PNEUMONIA:
- Often occurs among elderly patients and others with diminished gag reflex; those with nasogastric tubes, intestinal obstruction, or ventilator support; and especially those exposed to contaminated nebulizers or unsterile suctioning
- High-risk groups: seriously ill hospitalized patients (especially patients with coma, acidosis, alcoholism, uremia, diabetes mellitus, nasogastric intubation, or recent antimicrobial therapy, who are frequently colonized with aerobic gram-negative rods); patients undergoing anesthesia; those with strokes, dementia, swallowing disorders; the elderly; and those receiving antacids or H_2 blockers (but not sucralfate)
- Hypoxic patients receiving concentrated O_2 have diminished ciliary activity, encouraging aspiration
- Causative organisms:
  1. Anaerobes listed previously, although in many studies gram-negative aerobes (60%) and gram-positive aerobes (20%) predominate
  2. *E. coli, P. aeruginosa, S. aureus, Klebsiella, Enterobacter, Serratia,* and *Proteus* spp. *H. influenzae, S. pneumoniae, Legionella,* and *Acinetobacter* spp. (sporadic pneumonias) in two thirds of cases
  3. Fungi, including *Candida albicans,* in fewer than 1%

DIAGNOSIS

DIFFERENTIAL DIAGNOSIS

- Other necrotizing or cavitary pneumonias (especially tuberculosis, gram-negative pneumonias)
- See "Pulmonary Tuberculosis"

WORKUP

- Chest x-ray examination
- CBC, blood cultures
- Sputum Gram stain and culture
- Consideration of tracheal aspirate

LABORATORY TESTS

- CBC: leukocytosis often present
- Sputum Gram stain
  1. Often useful when carefully prepared immediately after obtaining suctioned or expectorated specimen, examined by experienced observer.
  2. Only specimens with multiple WBCs and rare or absent epithelial cells should be examined.
  3. Unlike nonaspiration pneumonias (e.g., pneumococcal), multiple organisms may be present.
  4. Long, slender rods suggest anaerobes.
  5. Sputum from pneumonia caused by acid aspiration may be devoid of organisms.
  6. Cultures should be interpreted in light of morphology of visualized organisms.

IMAGING STUDIES

- Chest x-ray examination often reveals bilateral, diffuse, patchy infiltrates, and posterior segment upper lobes.
- Aspiration pneumonias of several days' or longer duration may reveal necrosis (especially community-acquired anaerobic pneumonias) and even cavitation with air-fluid levels, indicating lung abscess.

TREATMENT

NONPHARMACOLOGIC THERAPY

- Airway management to prevent repeated aspiration
- Ventilatory support if necessary

ACUTE GENERAL Rx

Acute aspiration of acidic gastric contents without bacteria may not require antibiotic therapy; consult infectious diseases or pulmonary expert.

COMMUNITY-ACQUIRED ANAEROBIC ASPIRATION PNEUMONIA: Levofloxacin 500 mg qd or ceftriaxone 1 to 2 g/day

NURSING HOME ASPIRATIONS: Levofloxacin 500 mg qd or piperacillin-tazobactam 3.375 g q6h or ceftazidime 2 g q8h

HOSPITAL-ACQUIRED ASPIRATION PNEUMONIA:
- Piperacillin-tazobactam 3.375 g IV q6h, or clindamycin 450 to 900 mg IV q8h, or cefoxitin 2 g IV q8h.
- Knowledge of resident flora in the microenvironment of the aspiration within the hospital is crucial to intelligent antibiotic selection; consult infection control nurses or hospital epidemiologist.
- Confirmed *Pseudomonas* pneumonia should be treated with antipseudomonal β-lactam agent plus an aminoglycoside until antimicrobial sensitivities confirm that less toxic agents may replace aminoglycoside.
- Do not use metronidazole alone for anaerobes.

DISPOSITION

Repeat chest x-ray examination in 6 to 8 wk.

REFERRAL

For consultation with infectious disease and/or pulmonary experts for patients with respiratory distress, hypoxia, ventilatory support, pneumonia in more than one lobe, necrosis or cavitation on x-ray examination, or not responding to antibiotic therapy within 2 to 3 days

SUGGESTED READING

Marik PE: Aspiration pneumonitis and aspiration pneumonia, *N Engl J Med* 344:665, 2001.

AUTHORS: **BETH J. WUTZ, M.D.,** and **RUBEN ALVERO, M.D.**

BASIC INFORMATION

DEFINITION

Bacterial pneumonia is an infection involving the lung parenchyma

ICD-9CM CODES
486.0 Pneumonia, acute
507.0 Pneumonia, aspiration
482.9 Pneumonia, bacterial
481 Pneumonia, pneumococcal
482.1 Pneumonia, *Pseudomonas*
482.4 Pneumonia, staphylococcal
482.0 Pneumonia, *Klebsiella*
482.2 Pneumonia, *Haemophilus influenzae*

EPIDEMIOLOGY & DEMOGRAPHICS

- Incidence of community-acquired pneumonia is 1/100 persons.
- Incidence of nosocomial pneumonia is 8 cases/1000 persons/yr.
- Primary care physicians see an average of 10 cases of pneumonia annually.
- Hospitalization rate for pneumonia is 15% to 20%.
- Most cases of pneumonia occur in the winter and in elderly patients.

PHYSICAL FINDINGS & CLINICAL PRESENTATION

- Fever, tachypnea, chills, tachycardia, cough
- Presentation varies with the cause of pneumonia, the patient's age, and the clinical situation:
  1. Patients with streptococcal pneumonia usually present with high fever, shaking chills, pleuritic chest pain, cough, and copious production of purulent sputum.
  2. *Mycoplasma pneumoniae:* insidious onset; headache; dry, paroxysmal cough, worse at night; myalgias; malaise; sore throat; extrapulmonary manifestations (e.g., erythema multiforme, aseptic meningitis, urticaria, erythema nodosum) may be present.
  3. *Chlamydia pneumoniae:* persistent, non-productive cough; low-grade fever; headache; sore throat.
  4. *Legionella pneumophila:* fever, mild cough, mental status change, myalgias, diarrhea, respiratory failure.
  5. Elderly or immunocompromised hosts with pneumonia may initially present with only minimal symptoms (e.g., low-grade fever, confusion); respiratory and nonrespiratory symptoms are less commonly reported by older patients with pneumonia.
  6. Generally, auscultation of patients with pneumonia reveals crackles and diminished breath sounds.
  7. Percussion dullness is present if the patient has pleural effusion.

ETIOLOGY

- *Streptococcus pneumoniae*
- *Haemophilus influenzae*
- *Legionella pneumophila* (1% to 5% of adult pneumonias)
- *Klebsiella, Pseudomonas, E. coli*
- *Staphylococcus aureus*
- Atypical organisms such as *Mycoplasma pneumoniae, Chlamydia pneumoniae,* and *Legionella pneumophila* are implicated in up to 40% of cases of community-acquired pneumonia
- Pneumococcal infection is responsible for 50% to 75% of community-acquired pneumonias, whereas gram-negative organisms cause >80% of nosocomial pneumonias
- Predisposing factors are:
  1. COPD: *H. influenzae, S. pneumoniae, Legionella*
  2. Seizures: aspiration pneumonia
  3. Compromised hosts: *Legionella,* gram-negative organisms
  4. Alcoholism: *Klebsiella, S. pneumoniae, H. influenzae*
  5. HIV: *S. pneumoniae*
  6. IV drug addicts with right-sided bacterial endocarditis: *S. aureus*
  7. Older patient with comorbid diseases: *Chlamydia pneumoniae*

DIAGNOSIS

DIFFERENTIAL DIAGNOSIS

- Exacerbation of chronic bronchitis
- Pulmonary embolism or infarction
- Lung neoplasm
- Bronchiolitis
- Sarcoidosis
- Hypersensitivity pneumonitis
- Pulmonary edema
- Drug-induced lung injury
- Viral pneumonias
- Fungal pneumonias
- Parasitic pneumonias
- Atypical pneumonia
- Tuberculosis

WORKUP

Laboratory evaluation and chest x-ray examination

LABORATORY TESTS

- CBC with differential. WBC count is elevated, usually with left shift
- Blood cultures (hospitalized patients only): positive in approximately 20% of cases of pneumococcal pneumonia
- Pulse oximetry or ABGs: hypoxemia with partial pressure of oxygen <60 mm Hg while the patient is breathing room air is a standard criterion for hospital admission
- Direct immunofluorescent examination of sputum when suspecting *Legionella* (e.g., direct fluorescent antibody [DFA] stain is a highly specific and rapid test for detecting legionellae in clinical specimen)
- Serologic testing for HIV in selected patients

IMAGING STUDIES

Chest x-ray: findings vary with the stage and type of pneumonia and the hydration of the patient (Fig. 1-204).

- Classically, pneumococcal pneumonia presents with a segmental lobe infiltrate.
- Diffuse infiltrates on chest x-ray can be seen with *L. pneumophila, M. pneumoniae,* viral pneumonias, *P. carinii,* miliary TB, aspiration, aspergillosis.
- An initial chest x-ray is also useful to rule out the presence of any complications (pneumothorax, empyema, abscesses).

TREATMENT

NONPHARMACOLOGIC THERAPY

- Avoidance of tobacco use
- Oxygen to maintain partial oxygen pressure in arterial blood >60 mm Hg
- IV hydration, correction of dehydration
- Assisted ventilation in patients with significant respiratory failure

ACUTE GENERAL Rx

- Initial antibiotic therapy should be based on clinical, radiographic, and laboratory evaluation.
- Macrolides (azithromycin or clarithromycin) or levofloxacin is recommended for empirical out-patient treatment of community-acquired pneumonia; cefotaxime or a beta-lactam/beta-lactamase inhibitor can be added in patients with more severe presentation who insist on out-patient therapy. Duration of treatment ranges from 7 to 14 days.
- In the hospital setting, patients admitted to the general ward can be treated empirically with a second- or third-generation cephalosporin (ceftriaxone, ceftizoxime, cefotaxime, or cefuroxime) plus a macrolide (azithromycin or clarithromycin) or doxycycline. An antipseudomonal quinolone (levofloxacin or moxifloxacin) may be substituted in place of the macrolide or doxycycline.
- Empiric therapy in ICU patients: IV beta-lactam (ceftriaxone, cefotaxime, ampicillin-sulbactam) plus an IV quinolone (levofloxacin, moxifloxacin) or IV azithromycin.
- In hospitalized patients at risk for *P. aeruginosa* infection, empirical treatment should consist of an antipseudomonal beta-lactam (cefepime or piperacillin-tazobactam) *plus* an aminoglycoside *plus* an antipseudomonal quinolone or macrolide.
- In patients with suspected MRSA, use vancomycin or linezolid.

CHRONIC Rx

Parapneumonic effusion-empyema can be managed with chest tube placement for drainage. Instillation of fibrinolytic agents (streptokinase, urokinase) via the chest tube may be necessary in resistant cases.

DISPOSITION

- Most patients respond well to antibiotic therapy.
- Indications for hospital admission are:
  1. Hypoxemia (oxygen saturation <90% while patient is breathing room air)
  2. Hemodynamic instability
  3. Inability to tolerate medications
  4. Active co-existing condition requiring hospitalization

PEARLS & CONSIDERATIONS

COMMENTS

- Use of gastric acid suppressive therapy (H2 receptor antagonists, PPIs) is associated with an increased risk of community-acquired pneumonia.
- Causes of slowly resolving or nonresolving pneumonia:
  - Difficult to treat infections: viral pneumonia, *Legionella,* pneumococci, or staphylococci with impaired host response, TB, fungi
  - Neoplasm: lung, lymphoma, metastasis
  - CHF
  - Pulmonary embolism
  - Immunologic or idiopathic: Wegener's granulomatosis, pulmonary eosinophilic syndromes, SLE
  - Drug toxicity (e.g., amiodarone)

SUGGESTED READINGS

Carratala J et al: Outpatient care compared with hospitalization for community-acquired pneumonia, *Ann Intern Med* 142:165, 2005.

Davidson R et al: Resistance to levofloxacin and failure of treatment of pneumococcal pneumonia, *N Engl J Med* 346:747, 2002.

Halm EA, Teirstein AS: Management of community-acquired pneumonia, *N Engl J Med* 347:2039, 2002.

Laheij RJ et al: Risk of community-acquired pneumonia and use of gastric acid suppressive drugs, *JAMA* 292:1955, 2004.

Thibodeau K, Viera AJ: Atypical pathogens and challenges in community-acquired pneumonia, *Am Fam Physician* 69:1699, 2004.

AUTHOR: **FRED F. FERRI, M.D.**

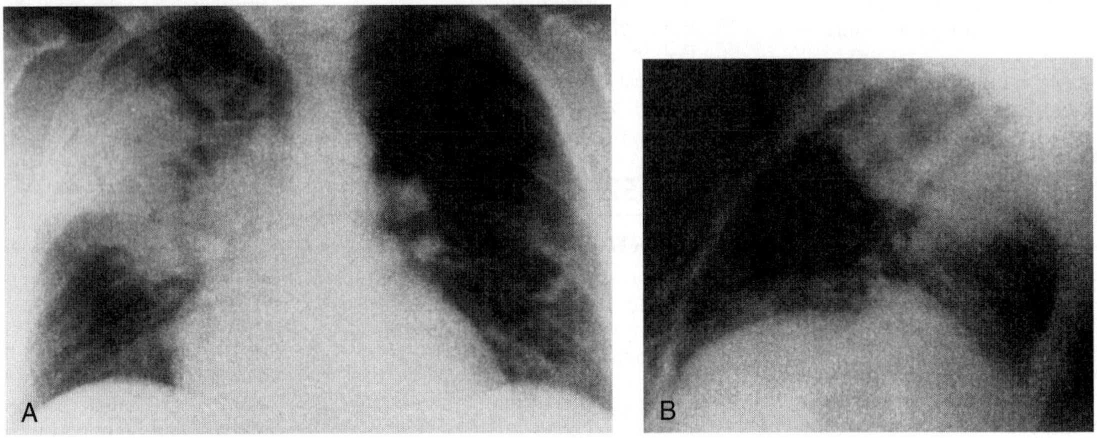

FIGURE 1-204 **A,** PA and, **B,** lateral chest radiographs reveal right upper lobe pneumonia and patchy left lower lobe infiltrate. A variety of organisms can produce this pattern, including *S. pneumoniae* and *H. influenzae.* (From Marx J [ed]: *Rosen's emergency medicine,* ed 5, St Louis, 2003, Mosby.)

BASIC INFORMATION

DEFINITION

Mycoplasma pneumonia is an infection of the lung parenchyma caused by *Mycoplasma pneumoniae*.

SYNONYMS

Primary atypical pneumonia
Eaton's pneumonia
Walking pneumonia

ICD-9CM CODES
483 *Mycoplasma* pneumonia

EPIDEMIOLOGY & DEMOGRAPHICS

INCIDENCE (IN U.S.):
- Hard to determine incidence precisely because of difficulty in making the diagnosis, but it is a frequent cause of community-acquired pneumonia.
- Probably many cases resolve without coming to medical attention.
- Incidence is estimated at 1 case/1000 persons/yr.
- Incidence is estimated to at least triple every (approximately) 5 yr during epidemics.

PEAK INCIDENCE:
- Some increased incidence in fall to early winter
- Seems more prevalent in temperate climates

PREVALENCE (IN U.S.):
- Estimated to be present in 1 of 5 patients hospitalized for pneumonia (generally a self-limited disease, so its true prevalence is unknown)
- Estimated to cause 7% of all pneumonias and about half in those aged 5 to 20 yr

PREDOMINANT SEX: Equal distribution

PREDOMINANT AGE:
- Most commonly affected: school-age children and young adults (ages 5 to 20 yr)
- Occurs in older adults as well, especially with household exposure to a young child
- More severe infections in affected elderly patients

GENETICS:

Familial Disposition:
- None known
- May be more severe in patients with sickle cell anemia

Neonatal Infection: Severe respiratory distress, sometimes requiring intubation, attributed to this disease in infants.

PHYSICAL FINDINGS & CLINICAL PRESENTATION

- Nonexudative pharyngitis (common)
- Headache, otalgia common
- Fever may be mild or no fever at all may be seen with *Mycoplasma* pneumonia
- Rhonchi or rales, without evidence of consolidation (common) in lower lung zones
- Associated with bullous myringitis (nonspecific finding; perhaps no more frequently than in other pneumonias)
- Skin rashes in up to one fourth of patients
  1. Morbilliform
  2. Urticaria
  3. Erythema nodosum (unusual)
  4. Erythema multiforme (unusual)
  5. Stevens-Johnson syndrome (rare)
- Muscle tenderness (<50% of the patients)
- On examination (and confirmed with testing):
  1. Mononeuritis or polyneuritis
  2. Transverse myelitis
  3. Cranial nerve palsies
  4. Meningoencephalitis
- Lymphadenopathy and splenomegaly
- Conjunctivitis

ETIOLOGY

Infection is spread by droplet infection from respiratory tract secretions.

DIAGNOSIS

DIFFERENTIAL DIAGNOSIS

- *Chlamydia* (now known as *Chlamydophila*) *pneumoniae*
- *C. psittaci*
- *Legionella* spp.
- *Coxiella burnetii*
- Several viral agents
- Q fever
- *Streptococcus pneumoniae*
- Pulmonary embolism/infarction

WORKUP

- Chest x-ray examination
- Thorough history and physical examination
- Laboratory tests
- Evaluation guided by symptoms and findings

LABORATORY TESTS

- WBC:
  1. WBC count >10,000/mm^3 in about a quarter of patients
  2. Differential count nonspecific
  3. Leukopenia rare
- Cold agglutinins:
  1. Detected in about half of the patients
  2. Also may be found in:
     a. Lymphoproliferative diseases
     b. Influenza
     c. Mononucleosis
     d. Adenovirus infections
     e. Occasionally, Legionnaires' disease
  3. Titers typically >1:64
     a. May be detectable with bedside testing
     b. Appear between days 5 and 10 of the illness (so may be demonstrable when patient is first examined) and disappear within about 1 mo
- Complement fixation testing or other immunoassays specific for mycoplasm antigens of paired sera (fourfold rise) in patients with pneumonia and a compatible history:
  1. Considered diagnostic in the appropriate clinical setting
- Culture of the organism from specimens
  1. Only truly specific test for infection
  2. Technically difficult and done reliably by few laboratories
  3. May require weeks to get results
- Sputum
  1. Often no sputum produced for laboratory testing
  2. When present, gram-stained specimens show PMNs without organisms
- Infection occasionally complicated by pancreatitis or glomerulitis
- Disseminated intravascular coagulation is a rare complication
- Electrocardiographic evidence of pericarditis or myocarditis may be present

IMAGING STUDIES

- Predilection for lower lobe involvement (upper lobes involved in less than a fourth), with radiographic abnormalities frequently out of proportion to those on physical examination (Fig. 1-205)
- Small pleural effusions in about 30% of patients
- Large effusions: rare
- Infiltrates: patchy, unilateral, and with a segmental distribution, although multilobar involvement may be seen
- Evidence of hilar adenopathy on chest films in 20% to 25%
- Rare cases reported:
  1. Associated lung abscess
  2. Residual pneumatoceles
  3. Lobar collapse
  4. Hyperlucent lung syndrome

TREATMENT

ACUTE GENERAL Rx

- Therapy (10 to 14 days) with erythromycin (500 mg qid), azithromycin (500 mg initially, then 250 mg daily for 4 days), or clarithromycin (500 mg bid) is preferred to tetracycline, especially in young children or women of childbearing age. Respiratory fluoroquinolones such as levaquin or moxifloxacin are alternative agents for treatment but should not be used in young children.
- Therapy shortens the duration and severity of symptoms and may hasten radiographic clearing, but the disease is self-limiting.

CHRONIC Rx

- Effective antimicrobial therapy does not eliminate the organism from the respiratory secretions, which may be positive for weeks.
- Serum antibody response does not necessarily provide lifelong immunity.
- Chronic symptoms do not occur, although clinical relapses may occur 7 to 10 days following the initial response and may be associated with new areas of infiltration.

DISPOSITION

- Clinical improvement is almost universal within 10 days.
- Infiltrates generally clear within 5 to 8 wk.
- Rare deaths are likely attributable to underlying medical diseases.
- Person-to-person spread can be minimized by avoiding open coughing, especially in enclosed areas.

REFERRAL

- Not responding to treatment
- Severe infection
- Severe extrapulmonary manifestations
- Multilobe involvement accompanied by respiratory embarrassment (very rare)

PEARLS & CONSIDERATIONS

COMMENTS

X-ray resolution complete by 8 wk in about 90% of patients.

EVIDENCE

Much of the data on treatment of atypical pneumonia have been taken from studies on patients with community-acquired pneumonia, which include a large number of patients with atypical pneumonia.[1]

Oral antibiotic therapy results in a 90% rate of clinical cure or improvement in outpatients with community-acquired pneumonia.[2] Ⓐ

Little evidence exists suggesting superior clinical efficacy of one oral antibiotic over another. Oral azithromycin may be more effective than other macrolides, penicillins, and cephalosporins in the treatment of community-acquired pneumonia, but further study is required in this area to confirm this finding. Beta-lactam agents are ineffective against *M. pneumoniae*.[1,3] Ⓐ Ⓑ

In hospitalized and nonhospitalized patients with community-acquired pneumonia, clinical outcome at 5 to 7 days is significantly better when treated with levofloxacin (oral or intravenous) compared with intravenous ceftriaxone or oral cefuroxime axetil.[4] Ⓑ

Monotherapy with levofloxacin is as effective as combination therapy with intravenous azithromycin plus ceftriaxone in patients hospitalized with community-acquired pneumonia.[5] Ⓑ

Evidence-Based References

1. Loeb M: Community acquired pneumonia. 10:1724, 2003, London, BMJ Publishing Group.
2. Pomilla PV, Brown RB: Outpatient treatment of community-acquired pneumonia in adults, *Arch Intern Med* 154:1793, 1994. Reviewed in: *Clin Evid* 10:1724, 2003. Ⓐ
3. Contopoulos-Ioannidis DG et al: Meta-analysis of randomized controlled trials on the comparative efficacy and safety of azithromycin against other antibiotics for lower respiratory tract infections, *J Antimicrob Chemother* 48:691, 2001. Ⓑ
4. File TM et al: A multicenter, randomized study comparing the efficacy and safety of intravenous and/or oral levofloxacin versus ceftriaxone and/or cefuroxime axetil in treatment of adults with community-acquired pneumonia, *Antimocrob Agents Chemother* 41:1965, 1997. Reviewed in: *Clin Evid* 10:1724, 2003. Ⓑ
5. Frank E et al: A multicenter, open-label, randomized comparison of levofloxacin and azithromycin plus ceftriaxone in hospitalized adults with moderate to severe community-acquired pneumonia, *Clin Ther* 24:1292, 2002. Reviewed in: *Clin Evid* 10:1724, 2003. Ⓑ

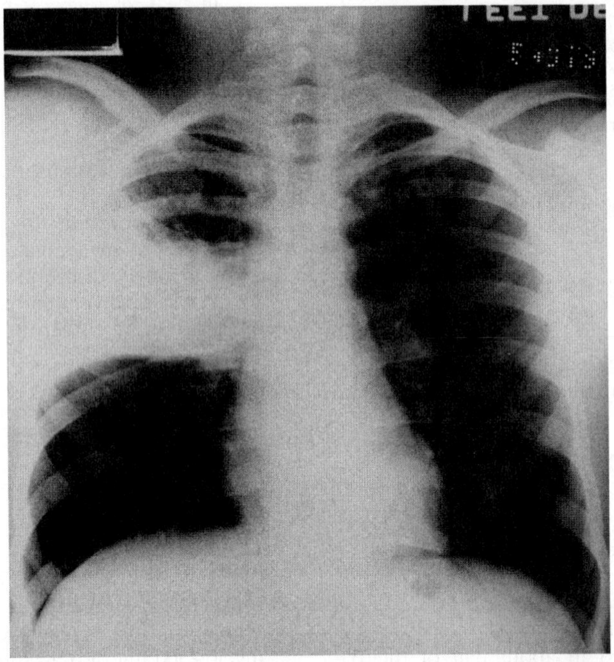

FIGURE 1-205 Localized airspace opacification secondary to *Mycoplasma pneumoniae.* (From Specht N [ed]: *Practical guide to diagnostic imaging,* St Louis, 1998, Mosby.)

SUGGESTED READINGS

La Scola B et al: *Mycoplasma pneumoniae:* a rarely diagnosed agent in ventilator-acquired pneumonia, *J Hosp Infect* 59(1):74, 2005.

Meloni F et al: Acute *Chlamydia pneumoniae* and *Mycoplasma pneumoniae* infections in community-acquired pneumonia and exacerbations of COPD or asthma: therapeutic considerations, *J Chemother* 16(1):70, 2004.

Michelow IC et al: Diagnostic utility and clinical significance of naso- and oropharyngeal samples used in a PCR assay to diagnose *Mycoplasma pneumoniae* infection in children with community-acquired pneumonia, *J Clin Microbiol* 42(7):3339, 2004.

Waites KG, Talkington DF: *Mycoplasma pneumoniae* and its role as a human pathogen, *Clin Microbiol Rev* 17(4):697, 2004.

AUTHORS: **GLENN G. FORT, M.D., M.P.H., DENNIS J. MIKOLICH, M.D.,** and **HARVEY M. SHANIES, M.D., PH.D.**

BASIC INFORMATION

DEFINITION

Pneumocystis jirovecii pneumonia is a serious respiratory infection caused by the fungal or protozoal organism *P. jirovecii* (formerly known as *P. carinii*).

SYNONYMS

PCP
PJP

ICD-9CM CODES
136.3 *Pneumocystis jirovecii (P. carinii)* pneumonia

EPIDEMIOLOGY & DEMOGRAPHICS

INCIDENCE (IN U.S.):
- Seen primarily in the setting of acquired immunodeficiency syndrome (AIDS)
- Approximately 11 cases/100 patient-years among HIV-infected patients with CD4 lymphocyte counts $<100/mm^3$
- Also seen in other immunocompromised patients with severe cell-mediated immune deficiency (congenital T cell deficiency, acute leukemia, lymphoma, bone marrow or organ transplant deficiency)

PEAK INCIDENCE: 20 to 40 yr (parallel to AIDS epidemic)

PREDOMINANT SEX: Equal incidence when corrected for HIV status

PREDOMINANT AGE:
- <2 yr
- 20 to 40 yr

GENETICS:

Neonatal Infection:
- Most frequent opportunistic infection among HIV-infected children, occurring in approximately 30%
- Neonatal occurrence unusual

PHYSICAL FINDINGS & CLINICAL PRESENTATION

- Fever, cough, shortness of breath present in almost all cases
- Lungs frequently clear to auscultation, although rales occasionally present
- Cyanosis and pronounced tachypnea in severe cases
- Hemoptysis unusual
- Spontaneous pneumothorax

ETIOLOGY

- *P. jirovecii* (formerly *P. carinii*) recently reclassified as a fungal organism
- Reactivation of dormant infection
- Extrapulmonary involvement rare

DIAGNOSIS

DIFFERENTIAL DIAGNOSIS

- Other opportunistic respiratory infections:
  1. Tuberculosis
  2. Histoplasmosis
  3. Cryptococcosis
- Nonopportunistic infections:
  1. Bacterial pneumonia
  2. Viral pneumonia
  3. Mycoplasmal pneumonia
  4. Legionellosis
- Occurs virtually exclusively in the setting of profound depression of cellular immunity

WORKUP

- Chest x-ray examination.
- ABG.
- Sputum examination for cysts of PCP (PJP) and to exclude other pathogens.
- Bronchoscopy with bronchoalveolar lavage or lung biopsy for diagnosis if sputum examination is negative or equivocal. Stains such as Gomori methenamine silver stain or toluidine blue O are used to identify the organism.

LABORATORY TESTS

- ABG monitoring
- Elevated lactate dehydrogenase (LDH) in majority of cases
- HIV antibody test if cause of underlying immune deficiency state is unclear

IMAGING STUDIES

Diffuse uptake on gallium scanning of the lungs is suggestive but not diagnostic.

TREATMENT

NONPHARMACOLOGIC THERAPY

- Supplemental oxygen
- Ventilatory support if needed
- Prompt thoracotomy if pneumothorax develops

ACUTE GENERAL Rx

For confirmed or suspected PCP:
- Trimethoprim-sulfamethoxazole (15 to 20 mg/kg trimethoprim and 75 to 100 mg/kg sulfamethoxazole qd) PO or IV per day divided and given in q6 to 8h
- Pentamidine (4 mg/kg IV qd)
- Either regimen with prednisone (40 mg PO bid):
  1. If arterial oxygen pressure <70 mm Hg
  2. If arterial-alveolar oxygen pressure difference >35 mm Hg
  3. Dose tapered to 20 mg bid after 5 days and 20 mg qd after 10 days
- Therapy continued for 3 wk
- Alternative therapies available for patients unable to tolerate conventional therapy:
  1. Dapsone/trimethoprim
  2. Clindamycin/primaquine
  3. Atovaquone

CHRONIC Rx

- After completion of therapy, lifelong prophylaxis should be maintained with trimethoprim-sulfamethoxazole (one single-strength tablet PO qd or double-strength three times weekly).
- Patients intolerant of this therapy should be treated with dapsone (50 mg PO qd) plus pyrimethamine (50 mg PO weekly) plus leucovorin (25 mg PO weekly).
- Inhaled pentamidine (300 mg monthly by standardized nebulizer) is less effective and is reserved for patients intolerant to other forms of prophylaxis.
- Same approach taken to all HIV-infected patients with CD4 lymphocyte counts <200 to $250/mm^3$ or <20% of the total lymphocyte count because of their high risk of PCP.

DISPOSITION

After completion of therapy, long-term ambulatory follow-up is mandatory to provide secondary prevention of PCP (see "Chronic Rx") and management of the underlying immunodeficiency syndrome.

REFERRAL

- To pulmonologist for bronchoscopy if diagnosis cannot be confirmed by sputum examination
- To an infectious disease specialist if severe or difficult to manage

PEARLS & CONSIDERATIONS

COMMENTS

All patients, especially those with severe infection or intolerant of conventional therapy, should be followed by a physician experienced in the management of PCP and, if appropriate, in the long-term management of HIV infection or other underlying disease.

Severe and life-threatening hypoglycemia may occur after one or two wk after start of intravenous pentamidine. Monitor closely and advise the patient of symptoms of hypoglycemia.

SUGGESTED READINGS

Briel M et al: Adjunctive corticosteroids for *Pneumocystis jiroveci* pneumonia in patients with HIV infection: a meta-analysis of randomized controlled trials, *BMC Infect Dis* 5:101, 2005.

Kazanjian PH et al: Increase in prevalence of *Pneumocystis carinii* mutations in patients with AIDS and *P carinii* pneumonia, in the United States and China, *J Infect Dis* 189(9):1684, 2004.

Torres HA et al: Influence of type of cancer and hematopoietic stem cell transplantation on clinical presentation of *Pneumocystis jiroveci* pneumonia in cancer patients, *Eur J Clin Microbiol Infect Dis* 25(6):382, 2006.

AUTHORS: **GLENN G. FORT, M.D., M.P.H., DENNIS J. MIKOLICH, M.D.,** and **JOSEPH R. MASCI, M.D.**

BASIC INFORMATION

DEFINITION

Viral pneumonia is infection of the pulmonary parenchyma caused by any of a large number of viral agents. The most important viruses are discussed in the following sections.

SYNONYMS

Nonbacterial pneumonia
Atypical pneumonia

ICD-9CM CODES
480.9 Viral pneumonia

EPIDEMIOLOGY & DEMOGRAPHICS

INCIDENCE (IN U.S.):
- Influenza virus:
  1. 10% to 20% of population in temperate zones infected during 1- to 2-mo epidemics occurring yearly during winter months.
  2. Up to 50% infected during pandemics.
  3. Pneumonia develops in small percentage of infected persons.
- Incidence of other important viral pneumonias is not known precisely.

PEAK INCIDENCE:
Influenza:
- Winter months for influenza A
- Year round for influenza B
- Peak of pneumonia seen weeks into the outbreak of infection

RSV and Parainfluenza virus: Winter and spring
Adenovirus: Endemic (military)
Varicella: Spring in temperate zones
Measles: Year round
CMV: Year round

PREVALENCE (IN U.S.):
- Often related to immune status of the population or presence of an epidemic
- Normal hosts (estimates):
  1. 86% of cases of pneumonia resulting in hospitalization in American adults
  2. 16% of pediatric pneumonias managed as outpatients
  3. 49% of hospitalized infants with pneumonia
- Important problem in hosts with impaired immunity

PREDOMINANT SEX:
- None generally
- Male sex may predispose to more severe respiratory disease in respiratory syncytial virus (RSV) infection

PREDOMINANT AGE:
Influenza:
- Overall incidence greatest at age 5 yr
- Falls with increasing age
- The most serious sequelae in those with chronic medical illnesses, especially cardiopulmonary disease
- Hospitalizations greatest in infants and adults >64 yr of age

RSV and Parainfluenza virus:
- Young children (as the major cause of pneumonia)
- Occurs throughout life

Adenoviruses:
- Young children
- Adults, primarily military recruits

Varicella:
- About 16% of adults (not infected in childhood) who contract chickenpox
- Acute varicella during pregnancy more likely to be complicated by severe pneumonia
- 90% of reported varicella pneumonia cases are in adults (highest incidence 20 to 60 yr old)

Measles:
- Young adults and older children who received a single vaccination (5% failure rate)
- Measles during pregnancy more likely to be complicated by pneumonia
- Underlying cardiopulmonary diseases and immunosuppression predispose to serious pneumonia complicating measles
- Before availability of measles vaccine, 90% of pneumonias in those <10 yr
- Currently more than a third of U.S. patients >14 yr old
- 3% to 50% of measles cases are complicated by pneumonia

CMV:
- Neonatal through adult
- Immunosuppression is key predisposing factor

GENETICS:
Familial Disposition:
- Close contact, not genetics, is important in acquisition
- Congenital anomalies and immunosuppression worsen course of RSV pneumonia

Congenital Infection:
- CMV is the most common intrauterine infection in the U.S.
- Pneumonia occurs occasionally in infants with symptomatic congenital infection.

Neonatal Infection:
- Severe RSV pneumonia
- Adenovirus pneumonia
  1. 5% to 20% fatality rate
  2. Can lead to residual restrictive or obstructive functional abnormalities
- "Varicella neonatorum"
  1. Disseminated visceral disease including pneumonia
  2. May develop in neonates whose mothers develop peripartum chickenpox
- CMV pneumonia
  1. Generally fatal
  2. Associated with severe cerebral damage in this population

PHYSICAL FINDINGS & CLINICAL PRESENTATION

INFLUENZA:
- Fever
- Uncomfortable or lethargic appearance
- Prominent dry cough (rarely hemoptysis)
- Flushed integument and erythematous mucous membranes
- Rales or rhonchi

RSV AND PARAINFLUENZA:
- Fever
- Tachypnea
- Prolonged expiration
- Wheezes and rales

ADENOVIRUSES:
- Hoarseness
- Pharyngitis
- Tachypnea
- Cervical adenitis

MEASLES:
- Conjunctivitis
- Rhinorrhea
- Koplik's spots
- Exanthem
- Pneumonitis
  1. May occur as a complication in 3% to 4% of adolescents and young adults
  2. Coincident with rash
  3. May also develop following apparent recovery from measles
- Fever
- Dry cough

VARICELLA:
- Fever
- Maculopapular or vesicular rash
  1. Becomes encrusted
  2. Pneumonia typical 1 to 6 days after rash appears
  3. Pneumonia accompanied by cough, and occasionally hemoptysis
- Few auscultatory abnormalities noted on examination of the lungs

CMV:
- Fever
- Paroxysmal cough
- Occasional hemoptysis
- Diffuse adenopathy when pneumonia occurs after transfusion

ETIOLOGY

Viral infection can lead to pneumonia in both immunocompetent and immunocompromised hosts.

DIAGNOSIS

DIFFERENTIAL DIAGNOSIS

- Bacterial pneumonia, which frequently complicates (i.e., can follow or be simultaneous with) viral (especially influenza) pneumonia
- Other causes of atypical pneumonia:
  1. *Mycoplasma*
  2. *Chlamydia*
  3. *Coxiella*
  4. Legionnaires' disease

- ARDS
- Physical findings and associated hypoxemia confused with pulmonary emboli

WORKUP

- Information about the prevalent strain of influenza virus can be obtained from local health departments or from the Centers for Disease Control and Prevention.
- Viral diagnostic tests are usually not necessary once an outbreak has been defined.
- Influenza and other viruses can be cultured from respiratory secretions during the initial few days of the illness (special media and techniques necessary).
- Paired sera antibody titers are also useful.
- Monoclonal antibody tests are available for influenza and other respiratory viruses.
- Measles and adenovirus pneumonia are usually diagnosed clinically.
- Polymerase chain reaction may be able to rapidly detect and identify viral nucleic acid.
- Open lung biopsy is required for definite diagnosis of CMV pneumonia.

LABORATORY TESTS

- Sputum Gram stain (usually produced in scanty amounts) typically shows few polymorphonuclear leukocytes and few bacteria.
- WBC count may vary from leukopenic to modest elevation, usually without a leftward shift.
- Disseminated intravascular coagulation has occasionally complicated adenovirus type 7 pneumonia.
- Multinucleated giant cells on Tzanck preparation of an unroofed vesicular lesion are useful in diagnosing varicella in a patient with an infiltrate (also found in herpes simplex).
- Severe immunosuppression is associated with symptomatic CMV pneumonia (usually reactivation of latent infection, or in previously seronegative recipients from the donor).
- Hypoxemia may be profound.
- Cultures may be helpful in identifying superinfecting bacterial pathogens.
- When they occur, parapneumonic pleural effusions are exudative.

IMAGING STUDIES

- Chest x-ray examination may demonstrate a spectrum of findings from ill-defined, patchy, or generalized interstitial infiltrates, which can be associated with ARDS.
- A localized dense alveolar infiltrate suggests a superimposed bacterial pneumonia.
- Small calcified nodules may develop as a radiographic residual of varicella pneumonia (Fig. 1-206).

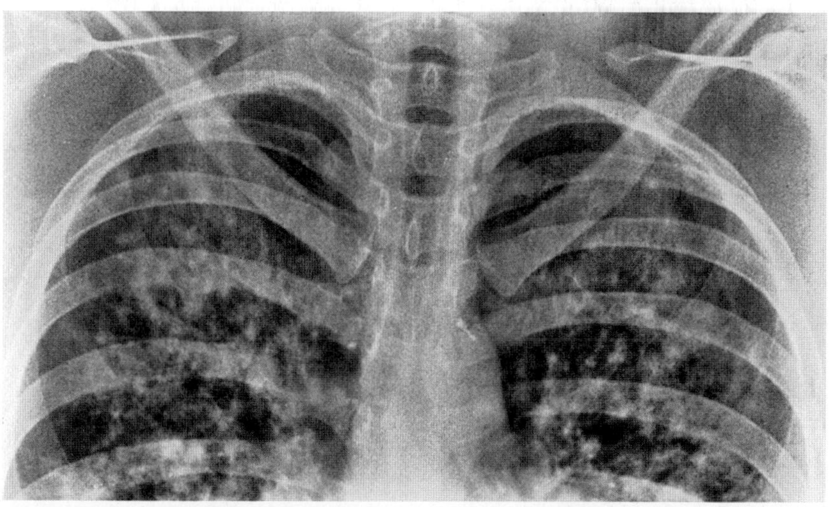

FIGURE 1-206 Chickenpox—varicella pneumonia. Coned-down view of the upper lobes shows multiple ill-defined nodules in both upper lobes. (From McLoud TC: *Thoracic radiology: the requisites,* St Louis, 1998, Mosby.)

TREATMENT (Rx)

NONPHARMACOLOGIC THERAPY

GENERAL:

- Measures to diminish person-to-person transmission
- Modified bed rest
- Maintenance of adequate hydration
- Possible ventilatory support for severe pneumonia or ARDS

INFLUENZA:

- Yearly prophylactic strain-specific influenza vaccination (only subvirion vaccine should be used in children <13 yr) can be given to prevent infection.
- Live, attenuated influenza vaccines administered by nose drops as effective as injected inactivated viral vaccines.

RSV:

- Isolation techniques are important in limiting spread of RSV infections.
- Immunoglobulins with a high RSV-neutralizing antibody titer are beneficial in treatment.

ADENOVIRUSES:

- Intestinal inoculation of respiratory adenoviruses has been used to successfully immunize military recruits.
- Although they produce no disease in recipients, the viruses may be shed chronically and may infect others at a later date.
- These vaccines are not available for civilian populations.

VARICELLA:

- Live, attenuated varicella vaccine has been successfully used in clinical trials.
- Varicella-zoster immune globulin should be administered within 4 days of exposure to prevent or modify the disease in susceptible persons.
- Nonimmunized persons exposed to varicella are potentially infectious between 10 and 21 days after exposure.

MEASLES:

- Effective measles vaccine is available:
  1. The vaccine should be administered at 15 mo.
  2. A second dose should be administered at the time of school entry.
- Live, attenuated vaccine or γ-globulin can prevent measles in unvaccinated persons if administered early following exposure.
- Vitamin A given PO for 2 days reduces morbidity and mortality from measles in exposed children.
- SARS = associated coronaviruses:
  1. No vaccine currently available.
  2. Supportive care: ribavirin ineffective, use of steroids or interferon alpha of unclear value.

ACUTE GENERAL Rx

GENERAL: Administer appropriate antibiotics for bacterial superinfections.

INFLUENZA:

- Amantadine and rimantadine for influenza A (not active against influenza B). Early use can speed recovery from small airways dysfunction, but whether it influences the development or course of pneumonia is uncertain.
- The neuraminidase inhibitors oseltamivir and zanamivir are effective if given in the first 48 hours of symptoms of influenza; their efficacy in established influenza pneumonia is unclear.
- Aerosolized ribavirin or amantadine may have a role in severe influenza pneumonia but have not been approved for this indication.

RSV AND PARAINFLUENZA:

- Ribavirin aerosol is effective for severe RSV pneumonia.
- There is no approved antiviral therapy for parainfluenza virus pneumonia.

ADENOVIRUSES: No effective agent; some case reports of cidofovir use but unproved.

VARICELLA:

- Varicella pneumonia can be treated with IV acyclovir.
- Adults who develop chickenpox should be considered for acyclovir treatment, which may prevent the development of pneumonia.

MEASLES: No effective antimeasles agent.

CMV:

- Acyclovir can prevent CMV infection in renal transplant recipients.
- Ganciclovir and foscarnet, with or without CMV hyperimmune globulin, show promise in the treatment of serious CMV infection, including pneumonia, in compromised hosts.

DISPOSITION

- Supportive therapy is useful.
- Deaths are possible during acute illness.
- Residual functional abnormalities may be persistent, develop into, or predispose to chronic respiratory diseases in later life.
- Morbidity and mortality following most viral pneumonias are increased by bacterial superinfection.

REFERRAL

- Uncertainty about the diagnosis in a compromised host
- Symptoms or findings progressive
- Severe respiratory compromise, diffuse infiltrates, or the development of ARDS

PEARLS & CONSIDERATIONS

COMMENTS

- Influenza spreads by close contact and by small droplets transmitted by cough.
- RSV is effectively transmitted by fomites and by direct contact (little by aerosol).
- Varicella is transmitted by direct contact or by aerosol.
- Of the three major forms of parainfluenza viruses (types 1 to 3), type 3 is the most common cause of viral pneumonia; types 1 and 2 primarily cause laryngotracheitis.
- Recent evidence indicates that a newly discovered virus known as metapneumovirus is a common cause of upper respiratory infections worldwide; this virus can cause pneumonia.

EVIDENCE

Although there is evidence that many antiviral agents reduce the duration of influenza, there is no evidence that these drugs are effective in preventing pneumonia.[1]

A systematic review found limited evidence on the efficacy of ribavirin in the management of hospitalized infants with respiratory syncytial virus infection of the lower respiratory tract. Mortality rate and respiratory deterioration were not significantly reduced with ribavirin compared with placebo. Cumulative results from three small trials showed that ribavirin reduced the duration of mechanical ventilator support and may reduce the duration of hospitalization.[2] (A)

Evidence-Based References

1. Hansen L: Influenza. 10:867, London, 2003, BMJ Publishing Group.
2. Ventre K, Randolph AG: Ribavirin for respiratory syncytial virus infection of the lower respiratory tract in infants and young children, *Cochrane Database Syst Rev* 4, 2004. (A)

SUGGESTED READINGS

Cheng VC et al: Medical treatment of viral pneumonia including SARS in immunocompetent adults, *J Infect* 49(4):262, 2004.

Falsey AR, Walsh EE: Viral pneumonia in older adults, *Clin Infect Dis* 42(4):518, 2006.

Hohenthal U et al: Measurement of complement receptor 1 on neutrophils in bacterial and viral pneumonia, *BMC Infect Dis* 6:11, 2006.

Michelow IC et al: Epidemiology and clinical characteristics of community-acquired pneumonia in hospitalized children, *Pediatrics* 113(4):701, 2004.

Moreno L et al: Development and validation of a clinical prediction rule to distinguish bacterial from viral pneumonia in children, *Pediatr Pulmonol* 41(4):331, 2006.

Tsolia MN et al: Etiology of community-acquired pneumonia in hospitalized school-age children: evidence for high prevalence of viral infections, *Clin Infect Dis* 39(5):681, 2004.

Werno AM et al: Human metapneumovirus in children with bronchiolitis or pneumonia in New Zealand, *J Paediatr Child Health* 40(9–10):549, 2004.

AUTHORS: **STEVEN M. OPAL, M.D., HARVEY M. SHANIES, M.D., PH.D.,** and **JOSEPH R. MASCI, M.D.**

BASIC INFORMATION

DEFINITION

A spontaneous pneumothorax (SP) is defined as the accumulation of air into the pleural space, collapsing the lung (Fig. 1-207). This can be primary SP (i.e., without any obvious underlying lung disease) or secondary SP (i.e., with underlying lung disease).

SYNONYMS

Primary spontaneous pneumothorax
Secondary spontaneous pneumothorax

ICD-9CM CODES
512.0 Spontaneous tension pneumothorax
512.8 Other spontaneous pneumothorax

EPIDEMIOLOGY & DEMOGRAPHICS

- Approximately 20,000 new cases of SP occur each year in the U.S.
- SP is more common in men than women (6:1).
- Incidence of primary SP is 7.4 cases/100,000 in men and 1.2 cases/100,000 in women.
- Incidence of secondary SP is 6.3 cases/100,000 in men and 2.0 cases/100,000 in women.
- SP is commonly seen in tall, thin young men 20 to 40 yr of age.
- Tobacco increases the risk of SP.

PHYSICAL FINDINGS & CLINICAL PRESENTATION

- Sudden onset of pleuritic chest pain (90%), which often becomes dull after a few hours
- Dyspnea (80%), which often resolves within 24 hr, despite persistence of pneumothorax
- Cough (10%)
- Asymptomatic (5%), may take up to 7 days to come to medical attention
- Tachycardia
- Diminished breath sounds
- Decreased tactile fremitus
- Hyperresonance

ETIOLOGY

- In primary SP, rupture of small blebs, usually located near the apex of the upper lobes, is a common cause. The check-valve mechanism is uncommon in this case; therefore, tension pneumothorax rarely occurs.
- In secondary SP, chronic obstructive pulmonary disease (COPD) is the most common cause, but it can also be associated with pneumonia, bronchogenic carcinoma, mesothelioma, sarcoidosis, tuberculosis, cystic fibrosis, and many other lung diseases.

DIAGNOSIS

Established by the chest x-ray

DIFFERENTIAL DIAGNOSIS

- Pleurisy
- Pulmonary embolism
- Myocardial infarction
- Pericarditis
- Asthma
- Pneumonia

WORKUP

Includes arterial blood gases, chest x-ray, and in some cases, CT scan of the chest

LABORATORY TESTS

ABGs may show hypoxemia and hypocapnia secondary to hyperventilation.

IMAGING STUDIES

- Spontaneous pneumothorax is usually confirmed by upright chest x-ray. X-ray findings include:
  - Identification of white visceral pleural line with absence of vessel markings peripheral to this line helps differentiation from mimicking conditions like an overlying skin fold.
  - The increased sensitivity of expiratory films in detecting pneumothorax has never been demonstrated in studies. The left lateral decubitus position is the most sensitive, and the supine position the least sensitive.
  - As little as 50 ml of air can be detected on upright film and a lateral width of 1 cm corresponds to 10% pneumothorax.
  - Tension pneumothorax should be suspected with contralateral tracheal and mediastinal deviation and ipsilateral flattening, or inversion of the diaphragm.
- CT scan can be done in suspected but difficult-to-visualize pneumothoraces, or to differentiate from large subpleural bullae.

TREATMENT

NONPHARMACOLOGIC THERAPY

- 100% oxygen administration reduces the partial pressure of nitrogen in pleural capillaries and consequently quadruples the rate of pneumothorax absorption.
- Observation alone is acceptable in the asymptomatic patient with <15% pneumothorax, once a repeat chest x-ray demonstrates stability of the condition; but it requires close outpatient monitoring.

ACUTE GENERAL Rx

- Aspiration is used only in a stable pneumothorax and can be done using a thoracentesis catheter, introduced in the second intercostal space midclavicular line attached to a three-way stopcock and a large syringe. Air is aspirated until resistance, excess cough by the patient, or >2.5 L is taken out. Repeat films are done immediately after aspiration and again in 24 hr. If the lungs fails to expand after 4 L, surgical exploration should be considered
- If there is improvement, but not complete resolution of pneumothorax after the aspiration, the catheter can be attached to a Heimlich (one-way) valve to allow for outpatient management of this condition.
- Chest tube insertion has been recommended for patients with primary SP who failed observation and simple aspiration and for all patients with secondary SP.
- There is no firm conclusion on the optimal treatment (simple aspiration vs. chest tube insertion) for a first episode of primary SP. Studies suggest that shorter hospital stay can be achieved with the aspiration technique, but there is a potential risk of lung laceration.
- Air leak for 3 days after tube thoracostomy insertion suggests the presence of bronchopleural fistula. Most will resolve with conservative measures only, including continued observation; increase the suction applied to pleural space to 35 cm H_2O or reposition of the tube.
- The absence of visible leak does not guarantee the leak has resolved because air might bubble out intermittently. Therefore, chest tube should be clamped for 24 hr prior to removal.
- Thoracoscopy or video-assisted thoracoscopy (VAT) is indicated in patients who have persistent air leak for seven days. Application of Heimlich valve to chest tube or intrabronchial bronchoscopic instillation of fibrin glue to occlude fistula should be considered in poor surgical candidates.

PREVENTION

- Multiple techniques have been utilized to prevent recurrence, including pleural pleurectomy, laser abrasion of parietal pleural, intrapleural instillation of sclerosing agents, and pleural abrasion with dry gauze. The overall recurrence rates are estimated at less than 5%.
- The current technique of choice is VAT, but its timing in the prevention of primary SP recurrence remains controversial. Most recommend definitive

management after the first recurrence. However, high-risk occupations such as divers or pilots should be considered for surgery after first pneumothorax. Similarly, complex conditions such as patients with persistent bronchopleural fistula should also be considered for early surgical intervention.

- The recurrence rates for the instillation of sclerosing agents (minocycline 5 mg/kg in 50 ml of normal saline or doxycycline 500 mg in 50 ml of normal saline) are higher than VATS. Therefore, this should be reserved for patients who are poor surgical candidates.
- Talc has also been used as a sclerosing agent, however there are case reports of acute respiratory distress syndrome (ARDS) and pleural calcification occurring after usage.
- Open thoracotomy is done in patients who fail VATS or where VATS is not available.

DISPOSITION

- Approximately 25% of patients with primary SP will have recurrence within 2 yr.
- Smoking cessation should be advised.
- The rates of recurrence after the second and third episode of SP are 60% and 80%, respectively, with the majority of recurrences occurring on the same side as the first pneumothorax.
- Death from primary SP is uncommon. In patients with secondary SP and COPD, mortality ranges from 1% to 16%.

REFERRAL

A pulmonary specialist and general surgeon consultation is recommended.

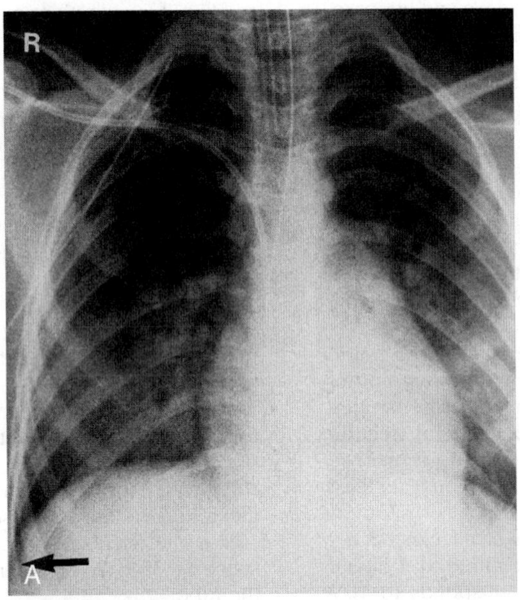

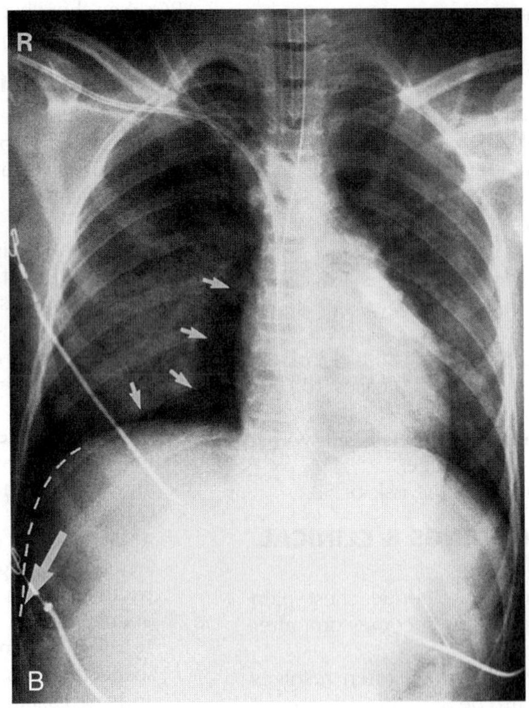

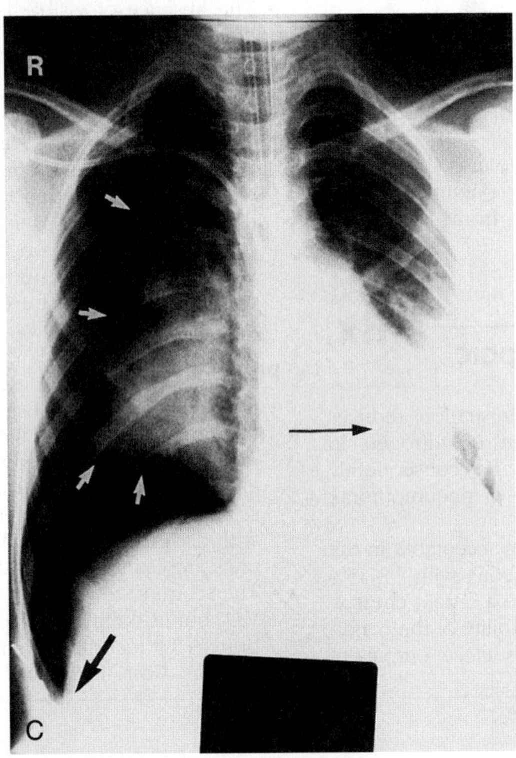

FIGURE 1-207 Deep sulcus sign of pneumothorax. On posterior-anterior (PA) chest radiograph **(A)** the costophrenic angle is normally acute *(arrow)*. In a supine patient, a pneumothorax will often be anterior, medical, and basilar. On a subsequent supine film **(B)** the dark area along the right cardiac border and lung base angle became much deeper and more acute than normal *(large arrow)*. These findings were not recognized, and as a result, the same patient developed a tension pneumothorax **(C)** with an extremely deep costophrenic angle *(large black arrow)* and almost completely collapsed right lung *(small white arrows)* and shift of the mediastinum to the left. (From Mettler FA [ed]: *Primary care radiology,* Philadelphia, 2000, WB Saunders.)

PEARLS & CONSIDERATIONS

The rate of pleural air absorption is about 1.25% of the volume of the hemithorax per day. Hence, the time interval for complete resolution of pneumothorax with observation can be estimated.

COMMENTS

Patients with AIDS and *Pneumocystis carinii* infection have a high incidence of SP. Treatment typically requires chest tube placement and either thoracoscopy or open thoracotomy.

SUGGESTED READINGS

Baumann MH et al: Pneumothorax, *Respirology* 9(2):137, 2004.

Baumann MH et al: Management of spontaneous pneumothorax: an American College of Chest Physicians Delphi consensus statement, *Chest* 119(2):590, 2001.

Chen F et al: Position of a chest tube at video-assisted thoracoscopic surgery for spontaneous pneumothorax, *Respiration.* Epub 2005 Sept 29.

Deavanand A et al: Simple aspiration versus chest tube insertion in the management of primary spontaneous pneumothorax: a systematic review, *Respir Med* 98(7):579, 2004.

Morimoto T et al: Effects of timing of thoracoscopic surgery for primary spontaneous pneumothorax on prognosis and cost, *Am J Surg* 187(6):767, 2004.

Noppen M et al: Music: a new cause of primary spontaneous pneumothorax, *Thorax* 59(8):722, 2004.

Wakai A: Spontaneous pneumothorax, *Clin Evid* 13:1884, 2005.

AUTHORS: **BRIAN CASSERLY, M.D.,** and **GAURAV CHOUDHARY, M.D.**

BASIC INFORMATION

DEFINITION

Poliomyelitis is a symptomatic infection caused by poliovirus, which (on rare occasions) may result in paralysis.

SYNONYMS

Polio
Infantile paralysis

ICD-9CM CODES
045.9 Poliomyelitis

EPIDEMIOLOGY & DEMOGRAPHICS

INCIDENCE (IN U.S.):
- Approximately 8 cases/yr.
- All cases in the U.S. and Western Hemisphere are now vaccine associated (because of oral polio vaccine [OPV]).

PREDOMINANT AGE: Almost always infants or young children

GENETICS:
Neonatal Infection: Most cases occur in otherwise healthy infants who receive OPV, or their contacts.

PHYSICAL FINDINGS & CLINICAL PRESENTATION

- Exposure of a nonimmune host to poliovirus usually results in asymptomatic infection.
- A small percentage of individuals may have one of three presentations:
  1. Abortive poliomyelitis: a flulike illness
     a. Fever
     b. Malaise
     c. Headache
     d. Sore throat
  2. Nonparalytic poliomyelitis: an aseptic meningitis that correlates with invasion of the CNS
     a. Headache
     b. Neck stiffness
     c. Change in mental status
  3. Paralytic poliomyelitis
     a. Most commonly affects the lumbar or bulbar regions
     b. Following paralysis, a period of variable degrees of recovery, the majority of which occurs in 2 to 6 mo
     c. Paralysis from involvement of motor neurons in the spinal cord
     d. Flaccid paralysis without sensory defects
     e. Postpolio syndrome late sequela, which may occur many years after the acute illness
     f. Functional deterioration of muscle groups that had recovered from initial paralysis thought to result from failure of reinnervation, which initially was able to restore function to weakened or paralyzed areas

ETIOLOGY

- Virus of genus *Enterovirus* (3 serotypes of polio virus [types 1 to 3])
- Classic endemic and epidemic disease caused by wild-type poliovirus
- All cases in the U.S. currently caused by a live, attenuated virus in the OPV
  1. Extremely rare complication that occurs in vaccine recipients or their contacts
  2. Paralysis from lower motor neuron damage caused by viral infection

DIAGNOSIS

DIFFERENTIAL DIAGNOSIS

- Guillain-Barré syndrome
- CVA
- Botulism food poisoning
- Spinal cord compression
- Other enteroviruses:
  1. Aseptic meningitis
  2. Paralysis (rare)

WORKUP

- Isolation of virus:
  1. Stool or a rectal swab
  2. Throat swabs
  3. Rarely CSF
- Paired sera for antibody titer determinations

LABORATORY TESTS

CSF:
- Aseptic meningitis
- Elevated WBCs
- Elevated protein
- Normal glucose

IMAGING STUDIES

MRI may show involvement of anterior horn of the spinal cord.

TREATMENT

NONPHARMACOLOGIC THERAPY

- Maintenance of respiration and hydration
- Early mobilization and exercise once fever subsides

ACUTE GENERAL Rx

- Aimed at reduction of pain and muscle spasm
- No agent to alter the course of disease

CHRONIC Rx

Physical therapy

DISPOSITION

- In the abortive and nonparalytic forms, complete recovery
- Paralytic disease:
  1. Variable degrees of recovery
  2. 80% usually in the first 6 mo following illness

REFERRAL

Always refer to an infectious disease consultant. Cases should be reported to public health agencies.

PEARLS & CONSIDERATIONS

COMMENTS

- Risk of disease in recipients of OPV is approximately 1 in 2.5 million.
- Use of inactivated polio vaccine (IPV) is not associated with disease:
  1. Does not confer local (mucosal) immunity
  2. Will not immunize nonvaccinated contacts
  3. Requires boosters
  4. Is given by injection
- To decrease the incidence of vaccine-associated polio, the routine childhood vaccination schedule has been changed. A recent recommendation for use of a sequential IPV-OPV schedule has again been modified. Exclusive use of IPV is now recommended. OPV use is limited to unvaccinated persons with plans for imminent (<4 wk) travel to polio-endemic areas.

SUGGESTED READINGS

Alexander LN et al: Vaccine policy changes and epidemiology of poliomyelitis in the United States, *JAMA* 292(14):1696, 2004.
Howard RS: Poliomyelitis and the postpolio syndrome, *BMJ* 330(7503):1314, 2005.
Progress towards poliomyelitis eradication in India, January 2004 to May 2005, *Wkly Epidemiol Rec* 80(27):235, 2005.
Wiysonge CS et al: Eradication of poliomyelitis, *Lancet* 366(9492):1163, 2005.

AUTHORS: **STEVEN M. OPAL, M.D.,** and **MAURICE POLICAR, M.D.**

BASIC INFORMATION

DEFINITION

Polyarteritis nodosa is a vasculitic syndrome involving medium-size to small arteries, characterized histologically by necrotizing inflammation of the arterial media and inflammatory cell infiltration.

SYNONYMS

Periarteritis nodosa
PAN
Necrotizing arteritis

ICD-9CM CODES
446.0 Polyarteritis nodosa

EPIDEMIOLOGY & DEMOGRAPHICS

INCIDENCE: 1:100,000 annually. Increased incidence in patients with hepatitis B surface antigen, hepatitis C virus.
PREDOMINANT SEX: Male:female ratio is 2:1.

PHYSICAL FINDINGS & CLINICAL PRESENTATION

- Typical presentation is subacute, with the onset of constitutional symptoms over weeks to months
- Weight loss, nausea, vomiting
- Testicular pain or tenderness
- Myalgias, weakness, or leg tenderness
- Neuropathy (mononeuritis multiplex), foot drop
- Livedo reticularis, ulceration of digits, abdominal pain after meals, hematemesis, hematochezia, hypertension, asymmetric polyarthritis (tending to involve large joints of lower extremities); true synovitis occurs only in a minority of patients
- Fever may be present (polyarteritis nodosa is often a cause of fever of unknown origin) and can range from intermittent, low-grade fevers to high fevers with chills
- Tachycardia is common and often striking

ETIOLOGY

- Unknown
- Hepatitis B virus-associated PAN appears to be an immune complex-mediated disease

DIAGNOSIS

DIFFERENTIAL DIAGNOSIS

Cryoglobulinemia, SLE, infections (e.g., SBE, trichinosis, *Rickettsia*), lymphoma

WORKUP

- Laboratory evaluation, arteriography, and biopsy of small or medium-size arteries can confirm diagnosis. Clinical manifestations are variable and depend on the arteries involved and the organs affected (e.g., kidney involvement occurs in >80% of cases).
- The presence of any three of the following ten items allows the diagnosis of polyarteritis nodosa with a sensitivity of 82% and a specificity of 86%:
  1. Weight loss >4 kg
  2. Livedo reticularis
  3. Testicular pain or tenderness
  4. Myalgias, weakness, or leg tenderness
  5. Neuropathy
  6. Diastolic blood pressure >90 mm Hg
  7. Elevated BUN or creatinine
  8. Positive test for hepatitis B virus
  9. Arteriography revealing small or large aneurysms and focal constrictions between dilated segments
  10. Biopsy of small or medium-size artery containing WBC

LABORATORY TESTS

- Elevated BUN or creatinine, positive test for hepatitis B virus or hepatitis C
- Elevated ESR and C-reactive protein, anemia, elevated platelets, eosinophilia, proteinuria, hematuria
- Biopsy of small or medium-size artery of symptomatic sites (muscle, nerve) is >90% specific. Biopsy of the gastrocnemius muscle and sural nerve are commonly performed
- Assays for ANA and RF are negative; however, low, nonspecific titers may be detected

IMAGING STUDIES

Arteriography can be done in patients with negative biopsies or if there are no symptomatic sites. Visceral angiography will reveal aneurysmal dilation of the renal, mesenteric, or hepatic arteries.

TREATMENT

NONPHARMACOLOGIC THERAPY

Low-sodium diet in hypertensive patients

ACUTE GENERAL Rx

Prednisone 1 to 2 mg/kg/day; cyclophosphamide in refractory cases

CHRONIC Rx

Monitoring for infections and potential complications such as thrombosis, infarction, or organ necrosis

DISPOSITION

The 5-yr survival is <20% in untreated patients. Treatment with corticosteroids increases survival to approximately 50%. Usage of both corticosteroids and immunosuppressive drugs may increase 5-yr survival >80%. Poor prognostic signs are severe renal or GI involvement.

REFERRAL

Surgical referral for biopsy

EVIDENCE

Treatment with prednisone plus plasma exchange was compared with prednisone, plasma exchange, and cyclophosphamide in patients with polyarteritis nodosa and Churg-Strauss angiitis in a small randomized controlled trial. The two groups had comparable survival but the patients who had received cyclophosphamide had fewer relapses.[1] B

Because polyarteritis nodosa is such a rare disease, few definitive studies have been performed that compare treatment options. Therefore, in the absence of such evidence, clinical experience and longitudinal studies will provide the basis for treatment.

Evidence-Based Reference

1. Guillevin L et al: Long-term follow-up after treatment of polyarteritis nodosa and Churg-Strauss angiitis with comparison of steroids, plasma exchange and cyclophosphamide to steroids and plasma exchange: a prospective randomized trial of 71 patients. The Cooperative Study Group for Polyarteritis Nodosa, *J Rheumatol* 18:567, 1991. B

SUGGESTED READING

Stone JH: Polyarteritis nodosa, *JAMA* 288:1632, 2002.

AUTHOR: **FRED F. FERRI, M.D.**

BASIC INFORMATION

DEFINITION

Polycystic kidney disease refers to a systemic hereditary disorder characterized by the formation of cysts in the cortex and medulla of both kidneys (Figs. 1-208 and 1-209).

SYNONYMS

Autosomal dominant polycystic kidney disease (ADPKD)

ICD-9CM CODES
753.1 Polycystic kidney, unspecified type
753.13 Polycystic kidney, autosomal dominant

EPIDEMIOLOGY & DEMOGRAPHICS

- Occurs in between 1:400 and 1:1000 people
- Incidence: 6000 new cases per year
- Approximately 500,000 people with ADPKD in the U.S.
- Found in all ages
- Accounts for 10% of end-stage renal disease
- Associated with liver cysts (50% to 70%), pancreatic cysts (10%), splenic cysts (5%), and CNS arachnoid cysts (5%), and cerebral aneurysms (20%)
- Increased incidence of diverticular disease and mitral valve prolapse

PHYSICAL FINDINGS & CLINICAL PRESENTATION

- Usually presents in the third to fourth decade of life
- Pain (abdominal, flank, or back)
- Palpable flank mass
- Hypertension
- Headache
- Nocturia
- Hematuria
- Nephrolithiasis (20%)
- Urinary tract infection

ETIOLOGY

- Approximately 90% of cases are inherited as an autosomal dominant trait.
- Spontaneous mutations occur in 10% of cases.
- The abnormal gene in the majority of cases has been located to the short arm of chromosome 16. In the minority of cases the defect is located on chromosome 4.
- All cysts develop from preexisting renal tubules segments and only a small portion of the nephrons (1%) undergoes cystic formation.

DIAGNOSIS

A person is considered to have polycystic kidney disease if three or more cysts are noted in both kidneys and there is a positive family member with ADPKD.

DIFFERENTIAL DIAGNOSIS

- Simple cysts
- Autosomal recessive polycystic kidney disease in children
- Tuberous sclerosis
- von Hippel Lindau syndrome
- Acquired cystic kidney disease

WORKUP

The workup to establish the diagnosis of ADPKD includes a detailed family history and either an ultrasound or a CT scan of the abdomen to visualize bilateral renal cysts.

- Complications of ADPKD should be excluded and they are:
  - End-stage renal failure
  - Infected cysts and urinary tract infections
  - Pyelonephritis
  - Nephrolithiasis
  - Electrolyte abnormalities
  - Cerebral aneurysm rupture
  - Intractable pain from enlarging cysts
  - Hypertension

LABORATORY TESTS

- Hemoglobin and hematocrit is elevated because of increased secretion of erythropoietin from functioning renal cysts. This also explains the relatively mild severity of anemia found in patients with ADPKD and severe renal insufficiency.
- Electrolyte abnormalities commonly seen in any patients with renal insufficiency may be present.
- BUN and creatinine can be elevated.
- Urinalysis can show microscopic hematuria, WBC casts in pyelonephritis, or proteinuria (seldom >1 g/24 hr).
- Increased erythropoietin level.
- Patients with a strong positive family history of ADPKD and no cysts detected by imaging studies can undergo genetic linkage analysis.

IMAGING STUDIES

- Abdominal renal ultrasound is the easiest and more cost-efficient test for renal cysts. Renal ultrasound can detect cysts from 1 to 1.5 cm.
- Abdominal CT scan is more sensitive than ultrasound and can detect cysts as small as 0.5 cm.
- Both studies can detect associated hepatic, splenic, and pancreatic cysts.
- MRI is more sensitive than ultrasound and may help in distinguishing renal cell carcinomas from simple cysts.

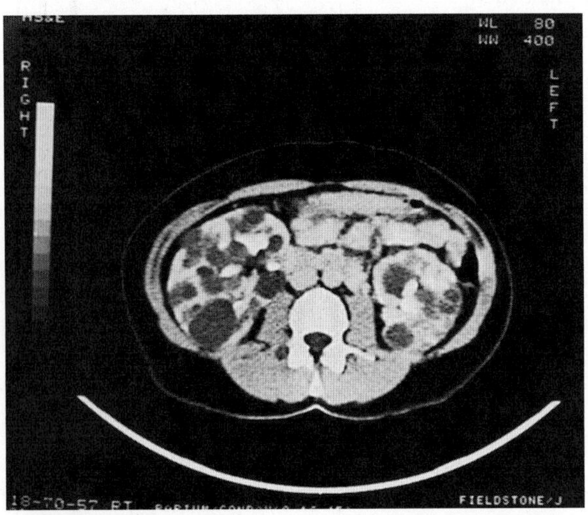

FIGURE 1-208 Tomogram of autosomal dominant polycystic kidney disease. Kidney cysts. (From Stein JH [ed]: *Internal medicine,* ed 5, St Louis, 1998, Mosby.)

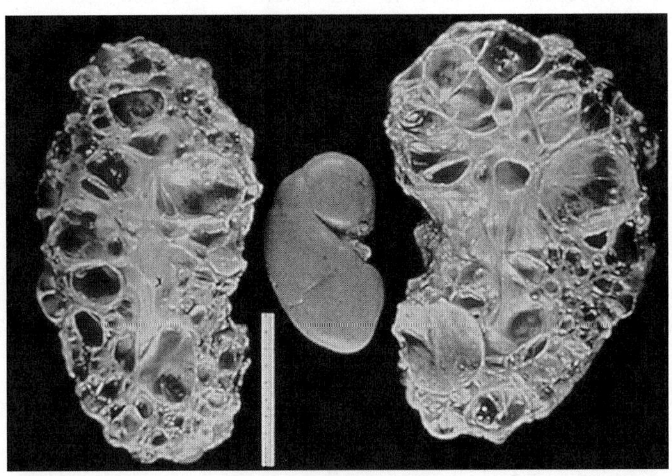

FIGURE 1-209 Markedly enlarged polycystic kidneys from a patient with ADPKD in comparison to a normal kidney in the middle. (From Johnson RJ, Feehally J: *Comprehensive clinical nephrology,* ed 2, St Louis, 2000, Mosby.)

TREATMENT

Rx

NONPHARMACOLOGIC THERAPY

- Associated nephrolithiasis can be treated in a similar manner with either IV or PO hydration. If stones remain lodged, lithotripsy or percutaneous nephrostolithotomy can also be done.
- Hypertension treatment is initiated with salt restriction, weight loss, and daily exercise.
- Avoidance of physical contact sports is advised.

ACUTE GENERAL Rx

- Kidney infections should be treated with antibiotics known to penetrate the cyst (e.g., trimethoprim-sulfamethoxazole 1 tablet PO bid or ciprofloxacin 250 mg PO bid).
- Angiotensin-converting enzyme inhibitors (e.g., captopril 25 mg bid or tid, lisinopril 10 mg PO qd, fosinopril 10 mg PO qd, or enalapril 10 mg qd) are effective in the treatment of hypertension associated with ADPKD.
- Calcium channel blockers (e.g., nifedipine 30 to 90 mg PO qd, amlodipine 5 to 10 mg PO qd, or felodipine 5 to 10 mg PO qd) can be used with or without ACE inhibitors in the treatment of hypertension.
- Alpha-blockers and diuretics can be added as adjunctive therapy for hypertension.
- Blood pressure <130/85 mm Hg is the goal for patients with renal disease. If there is >1 g of urinary protein per 24 hr, the target blood pressure is <125/75 mm Hg.

CHRONIC Rx

- Dialysis for end-stage renal failure
- Nephrectomy
- Renal transplantation
- Cystic decompression in patients with intractable pain caused by enlarging cysts

DISPOSITION

- Approximately half the patients with ADPKD will progress to renal failure.
- Gross hematuria is usually self-limited.

REFERRAL

Nephrology consultation should be made in patients with renal insufficiency, difficult-to-control hypertension, recurrent infections, or renal stones. Urology can also be consulted in patients with nephrolithiasis, recurrent episodes of gross hematuria, or consideration for nephrectomy before transplantation.

PEARLS & CONSIDERATIONS

!

- Cardiac disease is the most common cause of death followed by infections and neurologic events.
- A cyst is considered to be present if it measures >2 mm in diameter.
- A positive family history of ADPKD is found in approximately 60% of the cases. Renal ultrasound performed on patient's parents reveals ADPKD in about 30% of the cases.
- Up to 25% of patients may not have cysts present before the age of 30.

COMMENTS

Routine screening patients with ADPKD for cerebral aneurysms is not recommended unless there is a positive family history of cerebral aneurysms.

EVIDENCE

EBM

For low-protein diet in chronic renal failure: It appears that reducing protein intake in patients with chronic renal failure reduces the occurrence of renal death by about 40% as compared with higher or unrestricted protein intake. The optimum level of protein intake cannot be confirmed from available studies.[1]

For use of angiotensin-converting enzyme inhibitors: Enalapril slows the rate of progression to end-stage renal failure in patients with chronic renal failure without diabetes, but these studies did not provide specific data regarding autosomal-dominant polycystic kidney disease.

For method of continuous ambulatory peritoneal dialysis (CAPD): double-bag system should be the preferred exchange system in CAPD. Significantly fewer patients suffered peritonitis, and number of patient months on CAPD per episode of peritonitis was consistently greater with double bag system compared with standard system.[2]

Evidence-Based References

1. Fouque D et al: Low protein diets for chronic renal failure in non-diabetic adults (Cochrane review). Reviewed in: Cochrane Library 3, Oxford, 2001, Update Software.
2. Daly C et al: Double bag or Y set versus standard transfer systems for continuous ambulatory peritoneal dialysis in end stage renal disease (Cochrane review). Reviewed in: Cochrane Library 3, Oxford, 2001, Update Software.

SUGGESTED READINGS

Chapman AB: Autosomal dominant polycystic kidney disease: time for a change? *J Am Soc Nephrol* 18(5):1399, 2007.

Pei Y: Diagnostic approach in autosomal dominant polycystic kidney disease, *Clin J Am Soc Nephrol* 1(5):1108, 2006.

Torres VE, Harris PC, Pirson Y: Autosomal dominant polycystic kidney disease, *Lancet* 369(9569):1287, 2007.

AUTHOR: **PURVA AGARWAL, M.D.**

BASIC INFORMATION

DEFINITION

Polycystic ovary syndrome (PCOS) in its complete form associates polycystic ovaries, amenorrhea, hirsutism, and obesity.

SYNONYMS

Stein-Leventhal syndrome
PCOS

ICD-9CM CODES

256.4 Polycystic ovary syndrome

EPIDEMIOLOGY & DEMOGRAPHICS

PREVALENCE: 3% of adolescent and adult women.

- Symptoms usually begin around the time of menarche, and the diagnosis is often made during adolescence or young adulthood.
- Increased risk of endometrial and ovarian cancers.

PHYSICAL FINDINGS & CLINICAL PRESENTATION

- Oligomenorrhea or amenorrhea
- Dysfunctional uterine bleeding
- Infertility
- Hirsutism
- Acne
- Obesity (40% only)
- Insulin resistance (type 2 diabetes mellitus)

ETIOLOGY & PATHOGENESIS

Elevated serum LH concentrations and an increased serum LH:FSH ratio result either from an increased GnRH hypothalamic secretion or less likely from a primary pituitary abnormality. This results in dysregulation of androgen secretion and increased intraovarian androgen, the effect of which in the ovary is follicular atresia, maturation arrest, polycystic ovaries, and anovulation. Hyperinsulinemia is a contributing factor to ovarian hyperandrogenism, independent of LH excess. A role for insulin growth factor (IGF) receptors has been postulated for the association of PCOS and diabetes.

DIAGNOSIS

Clinical:

- PCOS is the most common cause of chronic anovulation with estrogen present. A positive progesterone withdrawal test establishes the presence of estrogen. Medroxyprogesterone (Provera) 10 mg qd is administered for 5 days and bleeding occurs if estrogen is present.
- The presence of oligomenorrhea, hirsutism, obesity, and documentation of polycystic ovaries establishes the diagnosis.

DIFFERENTIAL DIAGNOSIS

Causes of amenorrhea:

- Primary (unusual in PCOS)

Genetic disorder (Turner's syndrome)
Anatomic abnormality (e.g., imperforate hymen)

- Secondary

Pregnancy
Functional (cause unknown, anorexia nervosa, stress, excessive exercise, hyperthyroidism, less commonly hypothyroidism, adrenal dysfunction, pituitary dysfunction, severe systemic illness, drugs such as oral contraceptives, estrogens, or dopamine agonists)
Abnormalities of the genital tract (uterine tumor, endometrial scarring, ovarian tumor)

LABORATORY TESTS

Fasting blood glucose to rule out diabetes
Elevated LH/FSH ratio >2.5
Prolactin level elevation in 25%
Elevated androgens (testosterone, DHEA-S)

IMAGING STUDIES

Pelvic ultrasound (or CT scan) reveals the presence of twofold to fivefold ovarian enlargement with a thickened tunica albuginea, thecal hyperplasia, and 20 or more subcapsular follicles from 1 to 15 mm in diameter (Fig. 1-210).

TREATMENT

The goal is to interrupt the self-perpetuating abnormal hormone cycle:

- Reduction of ovarian androgen secretion by laparoscopic ovarian wedge resection
- Reduction of ovarian androgen secretion by using oral contraceptives or LHRH analogs
- Weight reduction for all obese women with PCOS
- FSH stimulation with clomiphene HMG, or pulsatile LHRH
- Urofollitropin (pure FSH) administration
- Glitazones (e.g., rosiglitazone, pioglitazone) may improve ovulation and hirsutism in the polycystic ovary syndrome

Choice of treatment:

- The management of hirsutism without risking pregnancy includes oral contraceptives, glucocorticoids, LHRH analogs, or spironolactone (an antiandrogen)
- Pregnancy can be achieved with clomiphene (alone or with glucocorticoids, hCG, or bromocriptine), HMG, urofollitropin, pulsatile LHRH, or ovarian wedge resection.

(Metformin may induce ovulation.)

EVIDENCE

Oral contraceptives containing desogestrel or norgestrel significantly improve acne and hirsutism.[1] Ⓑ

Spironolactone, 100 mg for 6 mo, results in significant, subjective improvement in hair growth and decrease in hair scores, compared with placebo.[2] Ⓐ

Evidence-Based References

1. Shaw JC: Antiandrogen and hormonal treatment of acne, *Dermatol Clin* 14:803, 1996. Ⓑ
2. Farquhar C et al: Spironolactone versus placebo or in combination with steroids for hirsutism and/or acne, *Cochrane Database Syst Rev* 4, 2003 (Cochrane Review). Ⓐ

SUGGESTED READING

Ehrmann DA: Polycystic ovary syndrome, *N Engl J Med* 352:1223, 2005.

AUTHORS: **FRED F. FERRI, M.D.,** and **TOM J. WACHTEL, M.D.**

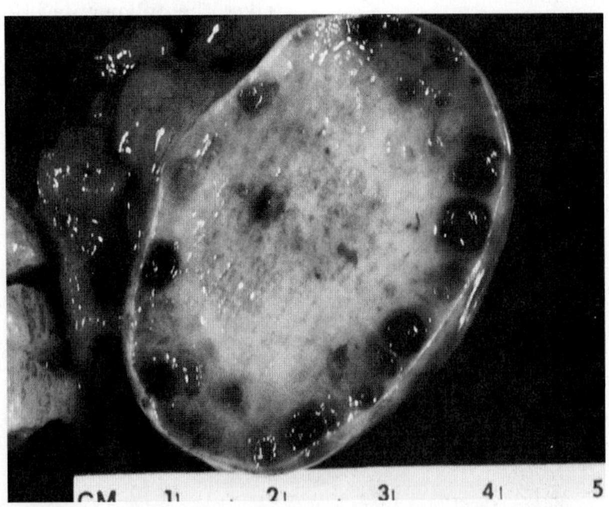

FIGURE 1-210 Sagittal section of a polycystic ovary illustrating large number of follicular cysts and thickened stroma. (From Mishell DR: *Comprehensive gynecology,* ed 3, St Louis, 1997, Mosby.)

BASIC INFORMATION

DEFINITION

Polycythemia vera is a chronic myeloproliferative disorder characterized mainly by erythrocytosis (increase in RBC mass).

SYNONYMS Primary polycythemia, vaquez disease

ICD-9CM CODES
238.4 Polycythemia vera

EPIDEMIOLOGY & DEMOGRAPHICS

INCIDENCE/PREVALENCE: 0.5 cases/100,000 persons; mean age at onset is 60 yr; men are more affected than women.

PHYSICAL FINDINGS & CLINICAL PRESENTATION

The patient generally comes to medical attention because of symptoms associated with increased blood volume and viscosity or impaired platelet function:

- Impaired cerebral circulation resulting in headache, vertigo, blurred vision, dizziness, TIA, CVA
- Fatigue, poor exercise tolerance
- Pruritus, particularly following bathing (caused by overproduction of histamine)
- Bleeding: epistaxis, UGI bleeding (increased incidence of PUD)
- Abdominal discomfort secondary to splenomegaly; hepatomegaly may be present
- Hyperuricemia may result in nephrolithiasis and gouty arthritis

The physical examination may reveal:
Facial plethora, congestion of oral mucosa, ruddy complexion
Enlargement and tortuosity of retinal veins
Splenomegaly (found in >75% of patients)

DIAGNOSIS

DIFFERENTIAL DIAGNOSIS

SMOKING:

- Polycythemia is secondary to increased carboxyhemoglobin, resulting in left shift in the Hgb dissociation curve.
- Laboratory evaluation shows increased Hct, RBC mass, erythropoietin level, and carboxyhemoglobin.
- Splenomegaly is not present on physical examination.

HYPOXEMIA (SECONDARY POLYCYTHEMIA): Living for prolonged periods at high altitudes, pulmonary fibrosis, congenital cardiac lesions with right-to-left shunts

- Laboratory evaluation shows decreased arterial oxygen saturation and elevated erythropoietin level.
- Splenomegaly is not present on physical examination.

ERYTHROPOIETIN-PRODUCING STATES: Renal cell carcinoma, hepatoma, cerebral hemangioma, uterine fibroids, polycystic kidneys

- The erythropoietin level is elevated in these patients; the arterial oxygen saturation is normal.
- Splenomegaly may be present with metastatic neoplasms.

STRESS POLYCYTHEMIA (GAISBÖCK'S SYNDROME, RELATIVE POLYCYTHEMIA):

- Laboratory evaluation demonstrates normal RBC mass, arterial oxygen saturation, and erythropoietin level; plasma volume is decreased.
- Splenomegaly is not present on physical examination.

HEMOGLOBINOPATHIES ASSOCIATED WITH HIGH OXYGEN AFFINITY: An abnormal oxyhemoglobin-dissociation curve (P50) is present.

WORKUP

Recent developments in molecular biology have identified a single, acquired point mutation in the Janus kinase 2 (JAK2) gene in the majority of patients with polycythemia vera and other pH-negative myeloproliferative disorders. The JAK2 mutation is found in .95% of patients with polycythemia vera and can be used for diagnostic purposes. Testing for the JAK2 V617F mutation with PCR assay is now available. In patients with high hematocrit (.52% in men or .48% in women) and in the absence of coexisting secondary erythrocytosis, the presence of the JAK2 mutation is sufficient for the diagnosis of polycythemia vera.

The diagnosis of polycythemia vera, using standards from the classic Polycythemia Vera Study Group, generally requires the following three major criteria or the first two major criteria plus two minor criteria:

- Major criteria
  1. Increased RBC mass (>36 ml/kg in men, >32 ml/kg in women)
  2. Normal arterial oxygen saturation (>92%)
  3. Splenomegaly
- Minor criteria
  1. Thrombocytosis (>400,000/mm^3)
  2. Leukocytosis (>12,000/mm^3)
  3. Elevated leukocyte alkaline phosphatase (>100)
  4. Elevated serum vitamin B_{12} (>900 pg/ml) or vitamin B_{12} binding protein (>2200 pg/ml)

Serum erythropoietin level is the best initial test for the diagnosis of polycythemia vera. A low serum erythropoietin level is highly suggestive of polycythemia vera. A normal level does not exclude the diagnosis. If the erythropoietin level is elevated, obtain abdominal and pelvic CT to rule out renal cercal carcinoma and other causes of polycythemia.

In patients with elevated erythropoietin level, evaluate for secondary erythrocytosis:

- Measure RBC mass by isotope dilution using ^{51}Cr-labeled autologous RBCs (expensive test); a high value eliminates stress polycythemia.
- Measure arterial saturation; a normal value eliminates polycythemia secondary to smoking.
- The diagnosis of hemoglobinopathy with high affinity is ruled out by a normal oxyhemoglobin dissociation curve.
- A diagnostic algorithm for polycythemia is described in Section III.

LABORATORY TESTS

- Elevated RBC count (>6 million/mm^3), elevated Hgb (>18 g/dl in men, >16 g/dl in women), elevated Hct (>54% in men, >49% in women)
- Increased WBC (often with basophilia); thrombocytosis in the majority of patients
- Elevated leukocyte alkaline phosphatase, serum vitamin B_{12}, and uric acid levels
- Low serum erythropoietin level
- Bone marrow aspiration revealing RBC hyperplasia and absent iron stores

TREATMENT

NONPHARMACOLOGIC THERAPY

Phlebotomy to keep Hct <45% in men and <42% in women is the mainstay of therapy.

ACUTE GENERAL Rx

- Hydroxyurea can be used in conjunction with phlebotomy to decrease the incidence of thrombotic events.
- Interferon α-2b is also effective in controlling RBC values without significant side effects.
- Myelosuppressive therapy with chlorambucil is effective but not routinely used because of its leukemogenic potential.

CHRONIC Rx

- Patient education regarding need for lifelong monitoring and treatment
- Adjunctive therapy: treatment of pruritus with antihistamines, control of significant hyperuricemia with allopurinol, reduction of gastric hyperacidity with antacids of H_2 blockers, low-dose aspirin to treat vasomotor symptoms in patients without bleeding diathesis. Low-dose aspirin can safely prevent thrombotic complications in patients with P. vera.

DISPOSITION

- The median survival time without treatment is 6 to 18 mo following diagnosis; phlebotomy extends the average survival time to 12 yr.
- Prognosis is worse in patients >60 yr of age and those who have a history of thrombosis.

SUGGESTED READINGS

Campbell PJ, Green AR: The myeloproliferative disorders, *N Engl J Med* 355:2452, 2006.
Stuart BJ, Vieira AJ: Polycythemia vera, *Am Fam Physician* 69:2139, 2004.

AUTHOR: **FRED F. FERRI, M.D.**

BASIC INFORMATION

DEFINITION

Polymyalgia rheumatica is a disorder of unknown cause affecting older patients. It is characterized by shoulder and hip stiffness and an elevated erythrocyte sedimentation rate (ESR).

SYNONYMS

Anarthritic rheumatoid syndrome

ICD-9CM CODES
725.0 Polymyalgia rheumatica

EPIDEMIOLOGY & DEMOGRAPHICS

PREVALENCE: 1 case/135 persons >50 yr of age
PREDOMINANT SEX: Female:male ratio of 2:1
PREDOMINANT AGE: Rare under age 50 yr; average age at onset: 70 yr

PHYSICAL FINDINGS & CLINICAL PRESENTATION

- Symptoms are frequently of sudden onset but are often present for months before the diagnosis is made.
- Neck, shoulder, low back, and thigh pain are common complaints.
- Morning stiffness lasting 2 to 3 hr is typical, and patients often have difficulty getting out of bed.
- Malaise, weight loss, depression, and a low-grade fever are common constitutional symptoms and may suggest systemic inflammation.
- Physical findings are usually limited. Synovitis may be present in peripheral joints and may also be responsible for the proximal girdle symptoms in spite of the fact that they appear to be "muscular" in nature.
- Mild soft tissue tenderness may be present.
- Distal extremity manifestations (knee, wrist, metacarpophalangeal joints) may occur in 25% to 45% of patients.
- The temporal arteries should be carefully examined because of the strong relation of polymyalgia rheumatica with temporal or giant cell arteritis.

ETIOLOGY

Unknown

DIAGNOSIS

DIFFERENTIAL DIAGNOSIS (Table 1-35)

- Rheumatoid arthritis: rheumatoid factor is negative in polymyalgia.
- Polymyositis: enzyme studies are negative in polymyalgia.
- Fibromyalgia.

WORKUP

The diagnosis of polymyalgia rheumatica is suggested by the following findings:

- Pain and stiffness of pectoral and pelvic musculature
- Patient >50 yr old
- Morning stiffness >1 hr
- Normal motor strength
- Symptoms for at least 4 to 6 wk
- Elevated ESR (>45)
- Rapid clinical response to low-dose corticosteroid therapy

LABORATORY TESTS

- CBC, ESR, and rheumatoid factor should be performed.
- Mild anemia may be present.

TREATMENT

ACUTE GENERAL Rx

- Prednisone 10 to 20 mg/day is given. The response is often so dramatic that it can be used to confirm the diagnosis. Improvement is usually noted within 24 to 48 hr. Generally, if the initial prednisone dose is 20 mg/day, reduce by 2.5 mg every wk to 10 mg/day, then by 1 mg/day every month if tolerated.
- Steroids are gradually tapered over the next few weeks as soon as symptoms permit, but small doses (5 mg/day) may be needed for 2 yr.
- NSAIDs may be tried in mild cases.
- Physical therapy is usually unnecessary.

PEARLS & CONSIDERATIONS

COMMENTS

The prognosis is generally favorable. Relapse occasionally occurs in several years, but again responds well to prednisone.

SUGGESTED READINGS

Bird HA: Criteria for polymyalgia rheumatica: tale without end, *J Rheumatol* 35:188, 2008.
Cimmino MA, Macchioni P et al: Pulse steroid treatment of polymyalgia rheumatica, *Clin Exp Rheumatol* 22(3):381, 2004.
Clough JD: Polymyalgia rheumatica: not well understood, but important to consider, *Cleve Clin J Med* 71(6):446, 2004.
Dasgupta B et al: Management guidelines and outcome measures in polymyalgia rheumatica (PMR), *Clin Exp Rheumatol* 25(suppl 47):130, 2007.
Hennell S et al: Evidence-based management for polymyalgia rheumatica for rheumatology practitioners, nurses and physiotherapists, *Musculoskeletal Care* 5(2):65, 2007.
Hutchings A et al: Clinical outcomes, quality of life and diagnostic uncertainty in the first year of polymyalgia rheumatica, *Arthritis Rheum* 57(5):803, 2007.
Mandell BF: Polymyalgia rheumatica: clinical presentation is key to diagnosis and treatment, *Cleve Clin J Med* 71(6):489, 2004.
Salvarani C et al: Polymyalgia rheumatica and giant-cell arteritis, *N Engl J Med* 347:261, 2002.

AUTHOR: **LONNIE R. MERCIER, M.D.**

TABLE 1-35 **Differential Features in Polymyalgia Rheumatica and Similar Disorders**

Signs/Symptoms	Polymyalgia Rheumatica	Giant Cell Arteritis	Rheumatoid Arthritis	Dermatomyositis	Fibromyalgia
Morning stiffness >30 min	+	±	+*	±	Variable
Headache and/or scalp tenderness	0	+	0	0	Variable
Pain with active joint movement	+	0	+*	0	Inconstant
Tender joints	±	0	+*	0	Tender spots
Swollen joints	±	±	+	0	0
Muscle weakness	±†	0	+*	+	0
Normochromic anemia	+	+	+	0	0
Elevated erythrocyte sedimentation rate	+	+	+	±	0
Elevated serum creatine kinase	0	0	0	+	0
Serum rheumatoid factor	0	0	70%	0	0
Distinct electromyographic abnormality	0	0	0	+	0
Response to nonsteroidal anti-inflammatory drug	±	0	+	0	0

From Goldman L, Ausiello D, (eds): *Cecil textbook of medicine,* ed 22, Philadelphia, 2004, WB Saunders.
0, Absent; +, present; ±, present in minority of cases.
*Associated with affected joints
†Pain inhibits movement. Disuse atrophy may occur.

BASIC INFORMATION

DEFINITION

Polypharmacy is the concomitant use of more drugs than are clinically necessary. Older definitions have emphasized specific numbers of medications, commonly more than four or five drugs per day. The primary issue is that the drugs are inappropriate and increase the risk of medication errors, adverse drug reactions, drug interactions, hospitalizations, and/or cost without a clear benefit to the patient.

SYNONYMS

Inappropriate prescribing

ICD-9CM CODES
Not applicable

EPIDEMIOLOGY & DEMOGRAPHICS

PEAK INCIDENCE: Estimates vary, but incidence appears to increase between 70 and 84 yr of age.

PREVALENCE: Approximately one in five Americans receives potentially inappropriate drug therapy although prevalence may be substantially higher in different clinical settings.

PREDOMINANT SEX AND AGE:
- Older adults
- Women (evidence supporting this is controversial)

RISK FACTORS:
- Multiple chronic diseases
- Frequent hospitalizations
- Multiple providers
- Multiple pharmacies

PHYSICAL FINDINGS & CLINICAL PRESENTATION

- Presence of one or more drugs without a clearly defined purpose or indication
- Presence of therapeutic duplication such as multiple proton pump inhibitors (PPIs)
- Presence of prescriptions for both generic and brand name version of the same drug
- Unexpected response to drug therapy ranging from lack of efficacy to exaggerated responses
- Failure to use appropriate drugs (aspirin, calcium, etc.) in patients who would clearly benefit
- Expanding list of new medications for a patient late in life or at the end of life

ETIOLOGY

- Inadequate communication between physicians, pharmacists, patients, and their families
- Lack of coordination of medical care
- Extensive use of self-care with over-the-counter (OTC) drugs by patients
- Prescribing cascade (not recognizing new problem as a drug side effect and prescribing a second drug)

DIAGNOSIS

DIFFERENTIAL DIAGNOSIS

Misuse, overuse, or underuse of drug therapy

WORKUP

- Obtain thorough medication history including prescription and OTC drugs, and dietary supplements.
- Visually verify all medication bottles for actual ingredients.
- Although presence of many drugs does not necessarily identify inappropriate prescribing, the likelihood of at least one or more problem drugs being present increases if at least seven drugs are prescribed.
- Use standard tools to evaluate drug regimen:
  - Beers criteria drugs to recognize potentially dangerous or ineffective drugs [1]
    - Some of these drugs include propoxyphene, pentazocine, meperidine, indomethacin, ketoralac, amitriptyline and imipramine (in antidepressant dosages), long-acting benzodiazepines, muscle relaxants and antispasmodic agents, short-acting dipyridamole, ticlopidine, disopyramide, chlorpropamide, drugs with strong anticholinergic properties.
  - Medication Appropriateness Index evaluates key elements of appropriate prescribing [2-4]
    - Is there an indication for the drug?
    - Is the medication effective for the condition?
    - Are the directions correct?
    - Are the directions practical?
    - Are there clinically significant drug-drug interactions?
    - Are there clinically significant drug-disease interactions?
    - Is there unnecessary duplication with other drugs?
    - Is the duration of therapy appropriate?
    - Is this drug the least expensive alternative compared with others of equal utility?
  - Assessment of Underutilization of Medication instrument asks whether or not there is a needed drug that has been omitted from a patient's regimen [5]

TREATMENT

The most important consideration in "treating" polypharmacy is to establish which conditions have the greatest priority for drug treatment, especially from the patient's perspective.

NONPHARMACOLOGIC THERAPY

As drugs are identified that could be discontinued, ask the patient about his or her interest in nondrug therapies.

ACUTE GENERAL Rx

If acute drug-related problems are identified, establish priorities for safely withdrawing or tapering the offending drugs (as appropriate for the specific agents).

CHRONIC Rx

- A key issue is whether or not the individual is likely to receive a benefit from a specific medication, especially if multiple co-morbid conditions exist and/or life expectancy is limited.
- Also, consideration should be given to the likely incremental benefit from each drug added to a complex drug regimen. For example, what would be the benefit to individuals in their 80s from the addition of spironolactone to a regimen consisting of lisiniopril, candesartan, and carvedilol for heart failure?

DISPOSITION

Safe discontinuation of inappropriate medications from a drug regimen may take at least several months depending on the specific drugs.

REFERRAL

Referral to a clinical pharmacist for a comprehensive drug regimen review and potentially to a geriatrician especially for frail older adults.

PEARLS & CONSIDERATIONS

COMMENTS

The prevention and/or identification of polypharmacy should focus on the "appropriateness" of the medications for the *individual* person and not necessarily on the number of medications. The decision regarding what is appropriate for an individual should first consider the patient's own priorities and expected risk and benefit to that individual before focusing on clinical practice guidelines, which may or may not be applicable to a specific patient.

PREVENTION

- Polypharmacy is prevented by considering whether or not a drug is needed for a new symptom and whether or not a new symptom is actually an unrecognized adverse drug reaction.
- The use of technology such as electronic health records, in which the complete medication history is up-

dated on a regular basis, and personal digital assistants at the point of care to identify adverse drug reactions, drug interactions, and appropriate dosage, may help to prevent polypharmacy.

- OTC drugs and dietary supplements such as vitamins and herbs should always be identified when taking a medication history as more prescription drugs are becoming OTC. In addition, manufacturers are making slight changes to common brand names in order to introduce new OTC products. However, the actual ingredients have been completely altered.
- Certain points in the continuum of care should be recognized for their high risk of polypharmacy and inappropriate prescribing. Discharge from the hospital to home (or to a nursing home) is a common time when medications are inappropriately added to drug regimens resulting in patients taking two PPIs, two angiotensin-converting enzyme inhibitors, two beta-blockers, etc. This duplication occurs when the home medication was not on the hospital formulary.
- Consistent use of generic drug names can decrease the risk of polypharmacy. Duplicate prescriptions for the same drug (furosemide and Lasix) commonly occur.
- Perform a complete review of medications for the appropriateness of their continued use at least every 6 months (for older adults), after discharge from the hospital, and whenever new drugs are added.

PATIENT/FAMILY EDUCATION

- Keep an up-to-date list of all drugs taken on a regular or as needed basis. The list should include all prescription and OTC drugs including eye drops, inhalers, and skin creams. Dietary supplements such as vitamins should also be on the list.
- Patients should ask their physician or pharmacist to review all of their drugs at least once a year.
- After any discharge from a hospital, patients should compare newly prescribed drugs to their existing drugs. They should ask which drugs should be continued and which should be stopped.

Evidence-Based References

1. Fick DM et al: Updating the Beers criteria for potentially inappropriate medication use in older adults: results of a US consensus panel of experts, *Arch Intern Med* 163:2716, 2003.
2. Hajjar ER et al: Unnecessary drug use in frail older people at hospital discharge, *J Am Geriatr Soc* 53:1518, 2005.
3. Hanlon JT et al: A method for assessing drug therapy appropriateness, *J Clin Epidemiol* 45:1045, 1992.
4. Samsa GP et al: A summated score for the medication appropriateness index: development and assessment of clinimetric properties including content validity, *J Clin Epidemiol* 47:891, 1994.
5. Lipton HL et al: Undermedication among geriatric outpatients: results of a randomized controlled trial, *Ann Rev Gerontol Ger* 12:95, 1992.

SUGGESTED READINGS

Holmes HM et al: Reconsidering medication appropriateness for patients late in life, *Arch Intern Med* 166:605, 2006.

Steinman MA et al: Polypharmacy and prescribing quality in older people, *J Am Geriatr Soc* 54:1516, 2006.

Tinetti ME, Fried T: The end of the disease era, *Am J Med* 116:179, 2004.

AUTHOR: **ANNE L. HUME, PHARM.D.**

BASIC INFORMATION

DEFINITION

Clinically significant portal hypertension is defined as a portal vein pressure >10 mm Hg, most commonly due to liver disease.

SYNONYMS

None

ICD-9CM CODES
572.3 Portal hypertension

EPIDEMIOLOGY & DEMOGRAPHICS

- Incidence of portal hypertension is not known.
- Cirrhosis is the most common cause of portal hypertension in the U.S.
- More than 90% of patients with cirrhosis develop portal hypertension.
- Alcoholic and viral liver diseases are the most common causes of cirrhosis and portal hypertension in the U.S.
- Schistosomiasis is the main cause of portal hypertension outside of the U.S.
- Esophageal varices may appear when portal vein pressures rise above 10 mm Hg.
- Variceal hemorrhage is the most serious complication of portal hypertension and may occur when portal pressures rise above 12 mm Hg.

PHYSICAL FINDINGS & CLINICAL PRESENTATION

- Jaundice
- Ascites (Figs. 1-211 and 1-212)
- Spider angiomata
- Testicular atrophy
- Gynecomastia
- Palmar erythema
- Dupuytren's contracture
- Asterixis (with advanced liver failure)
- Irritability, encephalopathy
- Splenomegaly
- Dilated veins in the anterior abdominal wall
- Venous pattern on the flanks
- Caput medusae (tortuous collateral veins around the umbilicus)
- Hemorrhoids
- Hematemesis
- Melena
- Pruritus

ETIOLOGY

- Pathophysiologically caused by:
  1. Conditions resulting in an increased resistance to flow
     a. Prehepatic (e.g., portal vein thrombosis, splenic vein thrombosis, congenital stenosis)
     b. Hepatic (e.g., cirrhosis, alcoholic liver disease, primary biliary cirrhosis, schistosomiasis)
     c. Posthepatic (e.g., Budd-Chiari syndrome, constrictive pericarditis, inferior vena cava obstruction, cor pulmonale, tricuspid regurgitation)
  2. Conditions leading to increase in portal blood flow
     a. Splanchnic arterial vasodilation accompanying portal hypertension, mediated by local release of nitric oxide
     b. Arterial-portal venous fistulae

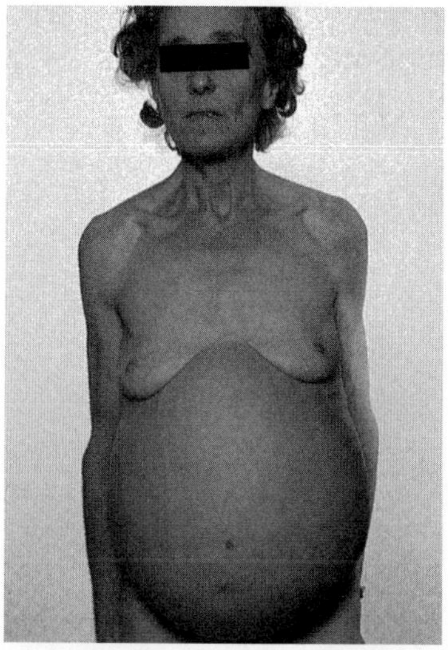

FIGURE 1-211 Ascites secondary to portal hypertension. Note the dilated collateral vein running up the right side of the abdomen. (From Forbes A, Misiewicz JJ, Crompton CC, Levine M et al [eds]: *Atlas of clinical gastroenterology,* ed 3, Oxford, 2005, Mosby.)

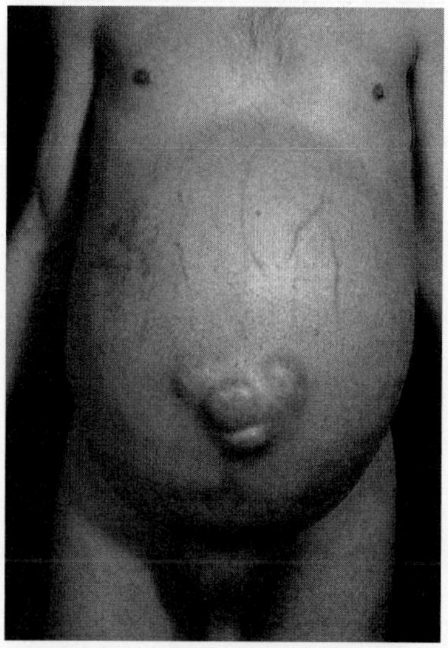

FIGURE 1-212 Ascites in a patient with alcoholic cirrhosis showing distended abdomen; dilated superficial collateral veins; hemorrhagic scratch marks due to pruritus and coagulopathy; umbilical varices; plaster in left iliac fossa indicating diagnostic paracentesis. (From Forbes A, Misiewicz JJ, Crompton CC, Levine M et al [eds]: *Atlas of clinical gastroenterology,* ed 3, Oxford, 2005, Mosby.)

DIAGNOSIS

- The diagnosis of portal hypertension is made on clinical grounds after a comprehensive history and physical examination.
- Noninvasive and invasive procedures serve to confirm diagnosis and determine the severity of portal hypertension.

DIFFERENTIAL DIAGNOSIS

- Ascites due to infection, neoplasm, or other inflammatory processes
- Obesity
- Abdominal organomegaly

WORKUP

The workup of portal hypertension includes blood tests and noninvasive imaging studies to determine if the cause of portal hypertension is prehepatic, hepatic, or posthepatic in origin. Ascitic fluid analysis is a key part of the diagnosis.

LABORATORY TESTS

- CBC w/platelet count
- LFTs w/serum albumin
- PT/PTT
- Hepatitis B surface antigen and antibody
- Hepatitis C antibody
- In selected cases: iron, TIBC, and ferritin; ANA, anti-smooth muscle antibodies (ASMA), antimitochondrial antibody (AMA), ceruloplasmin, alpha-1 antitrypsin
- Ascitic fluid analysis: a serum-ascites albumin gradient (SAAG) ≥1.1 mg/dl suggests portal hypertension. PMNs ≥250 cells/ml, positive Gram stain or culture suggest complicating spontaneous bacterial peritonitis (SBP).

IMAGING STUDIES

- Duplex-Doppler ultrasound is effective in screening for portal hypertension.
- Less commonly, CT/MRI scanning or liver-spleen nuclear medicine scanning can be used if the results from ultrasound are equivocal.
- Upper endoscopy is the most reliable test documenting the presence of esophageal varices.

TREATMENT

The treatment of portal hypertension is complex and involves measures to reduce portal hypertension directly, minimize volume overload, correct underlying disorders, and prevent complications (most notably SBP and variceal bleeding).

NONPHARMACOLOGIC THERAPY

Dietary sodium restriction to generally 2000 mg per day forms the basis of therapy to limit fluid overload.

ACUTE GENERAL Rx

- For tense ascites, large volume paracentesis (LVP) is generally recommended. The use of albumin infusion (8 to 10 grams per liter of ascites fluid removed) during LVP >5 liters has been shown to reduce the incidence of postparacentesis circulatory dysfunction, although its use remains somewhat controversial.
- Intravenous diuretics, typically furosemide and spironolactone, are used to achieve natriuresis and net negative fluid balance. Renal function and serum electrolytes are monitored frequently, with transition to an oral regimen for chronic therapy.
- SBP is treated with intravenous antibiotics directed against enteric bacteria.
- Acute variceal hemorrhage is treated with crystalloid and blood product resuscitation, intravenous octreotide, terlipressin/vasopressin or somatostatin, and urgent upper endoscopy, often with sclerotherapy or band ligation. Patients with acute variceal hemorrhage should receive antibiotic prophylaxis against SBP.
- For patients failing the above measures, a transjugular intrahepatic portosystemic shunt (TIPS) or surgical shunt placement may be considered.

CHRONIC Rx

- Dietary sodium restriction in combination with diuretics: the typical ratio of furosemide 40 mg to spironolactone 100 mg retains normal serum potassium levels in most patients.
- Nonselective beta blockers (propranolol and nadolol) in dosages sufficient to reduce the resting heart rate by 25% have been shown to be effective in primary prophylaxis for first-time variceal bleeding and for preventing recurrent variceal bleeding. Dosages are usually given bid and decreased if heart rate falls <55 beats/min or systolic BP <90 mm Hg. The addition of a long-acting nitrate (e.g., isosorbide-5-mononitrate) has been shown to improve portal hemodynamics. A prospective trial of beta blockers to prevent the formation of varices was negative.
- Serial LVP may be needed in "diuretic resistant" patients.
- Patients with prior SBP merit lifelong antibiotics for secondary prevention.
- Abstinence from alcohol or treatment for hepatitis B or hepatitis C. Vaccination for hepatitis A and B as appropriate.
- Hepatic transplantation is an option in selected patients.

DISPOSITION

- The most common complication associated with portal hypertension is variceal bleeding. The risk of bleeding from varices is approximately 15% at 1 yr.
- Development of the hepatorenal syndrome (HRS) is associated with high near-term mortality. In particular, HRS may complicate SBP, which emphasizes the importance of making the dx of SBP and instituting appropriate prophylaxis.

REFERRAL

Consultation with a gastroenterologist is recommended in all patients with portal hypertension in order to screen for esophageal varices.

PEARLS & CONSIDERATIONS

Splanchnic arterial vasodilation is increasingly recognized as an important component of the pathophysiology of portal hypertension and ascites. There may be vasodilation in other capillary beds as well: of note, pulmonary arteriolar vasodilation can create a significant shunt fraction and resultant hypoxemia in the absence of chest x-ray or CT chest evidence of parenchymal disease. The diagnosis is suspected when otherwise unexplained hypoxia arises in a patient with cirrhosis, along with platypnea (dyspnea worse when sitting upright) and orthodeoxia (desaturation with upright posture). The diagnosis is confirmed by echocardiography with agitated saline, in which there is delayed appearance of bubbles in the left heart after injection into a peripheral vein.

COMMENTS

Portal hypertension and its complications carry significant morbidity and mortality. Emphasize ethanol abstinence, provide vaccinations and prophylactic therapy where indicated, and consider early referral to a specialist for assistance with management and consideration for hepatic transplantation.

SUGGESTED READINGS

Blei AT: Portal hypertension and its complications, *Curr Opin Gastroenterol* 23(3):275, 2007.

De Francis R: Evolving consensus in portal hypertension. Report of the Baveno IV consensus workshop on methodology of diagnosis and therapy in portal hypertension, *J Hepatol* 43(1):167-176, 2005.

Gines P et al: Current concepts: management of cirrhosis and ascites, *N Engl J Med* 350:1646, 2004.

Runyon B: Practice Guidelines Committee, American Association for the Study of Liver Diseases (AASLD): Management of adult patients with ascites due to cirrhosis, *Hepatology* 39:841, 2004.

AUTHOR: **MEL ANDERSON, M.D.**

BASIC INFORMATION

DEFINITION

Portal vein thrombosis is thrombotic occlusion of the portal vein.

SYNONYMS

Pylethrombosis

ICD-9CM CODES
452 Portal vein thrombosis
572.1 Septic portal vein thrombosis

EPIDEMIOLOGY & DEMOGRAPHICS

Occurs with equal frequency in children (peak age: 6 yr) and adults (peak age: 40 yr)

PHYSICAL FINDINGS & CLINICAL PRESENTATION

Upper GI hemorrhage (hematemesis and/or melena) caused by esophageal varices. If abdominal pain is present, mesenteric venous thrombosis should be suspected (see "Mesenteric Venous Thrombosis" in Section I).

ETIOLOGY AND PATHOPHYSIOLOGY

In children: umbilical sepsis (pathophysiology unknown)
In adults:

1. Hypercoagulable states
   - Antiphospholipid syndrome
   - Neoplasm (common cause)
   - Paroxysmal nocturnal hemoglobinuria
   - Myeloproliferative diseases
   - Oral contraceptives
   - Polycythemia vera
   - Pregnancy
   - Protein S or C deficiency
   - Sickle cell disease
   - Thrombocytosis
2. Inflammatory diseases
   - Crohn's disease
   - Pancreatitis
   - Ulcerative colitis
3. Complications of medical intervention
   - Ambulatory dialysis
   - Chemoembolization
   - Liver transplantation
   - Partial hepatectomy
   - Sclerotherapy
   - Splenectomy
   - Transjugular intrahepatic portosystemic shunt
4. Infections
   - Appendicitis
   - Diverticulitis
   - Cholecystitis
5. Miscellaneous
   - Cirrhosis (common cause)
   - Bladder cancer

Pathophysiology: portal vein thrombosis results in portal hypertension leading to esophageal and gastrointestinal varices. The liver sustained by the hepatic artery maintains normal function.

DIAGNOSIS

DIFFERENTIAL DIAGNOSIS

Causes of upper GI hemorrhage are covered in Section II.

WORKUP

- Esophagogastroscopy shows esophageal varices.
- Abdominal ultrasound (Fig. 1-213) or MRI may show the portal vein thrombosis.

TREATMENT

- Variceal sclerotherapy or banding
- Surgical mesocaval or splenorenal shunt

REFERRAL

To gastroenterologist, surgeon, or both

AUTHORS: **FRED F. FERRI, M.D.,** and **TOM J. WACHTEL, M.D.**

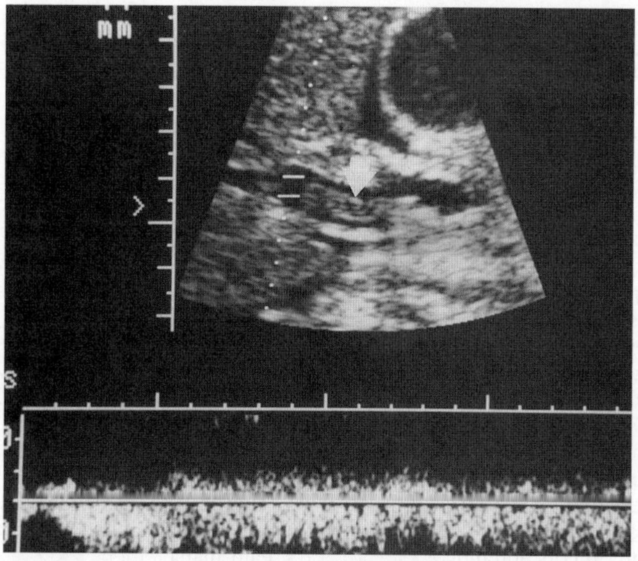

FIGURE 1-213 Thrombus in portal vein evident on pulsed Doppler ultrasonography. An echogenic thrombus *(arrow)* is within the lumen of the portal vein. Doppler tracing indicates flow within portal vein. (From Sabiston D: *Textbook of surgery,* ed 17, Philadelphia, 2005, WB Saunders.)

BASIC INFORMATION

DEFINITION

Postconcussive syndrome (PCS) refers to persistent neurologic symptoms (listed in "Physical Findings & Clinical Presentation") that result from minor head injury or concussion. Concussion is an acute trauma-induced alteration of mental function lasting fewer than 24 hr, with or without preceding loss of consciousness.

SYNONYMS

Posttraumatic nervous instability or brain injury

ICD-9CM CODES
310.2 Postconcussive syndrome

EPIDEMIOLOGY & DEMOGRAPHICS

- Incidence is approximately 27 cases/ 100,000 persons.
- More often seen in men than in women.
- Usually seen in the young, ages 20 to 30 yr.

PHYSICAL FINDINGS & CLINICAL PRESENTATION

- Usually present without focal neurologic deficits on examination.
- Symptoms start within a few days after the head injury, and usually persist after 3 months.
- Can be divided into early and late or persistent (>6 months).
- 15% of patients will have persistent symptoms 1 yr later.
- Symptoms include (at least three of the following to meet ICD-10 criteria):
  - Headache (usually of frontooccipital location and of migraine or tension type)
  - Fatigue
  - Dizziness and/or vertigo
  - Impaired memory
  - Difficulty in concentrating
  - Insomnia
  - Irritability
  - Lowered tolerance of stress, emotion, or alcohol
- Other associated symptoms: neck pain, paresthesias, interference with social role functioning.

ETIOLOGY

- Caused by traumatic brain injury from falls, motor vehicle accidents, contact sports, etc.
- Postmortem findings reveal diffuse axonal injury as the primary pathologic finding along with small petechial hemorrhages and local edema.
- Diffuse axon injury is thought to lead to altered neurotransmitters and possibly to clinical manifestations.

DIAGNOSIS

A careful history, a nonfocal neurologic examination, and a normal neurologic testing will usually establish the diagnosis.

DIFFERENTIAL DIAGNOSIS

- Headache (dissection of the vertebral artery, occipital neuralgia)
- Epidural hematoma
- Subdural hematoma
- Skull fracture
- Cervical spine disk disease
- Whiplash
- Cerebrovascular accident
- Depression
- Anxiety

WORKUP

To exclude other causes of neurologic symptoms following traumatic brain injury:
- EEG is normal.
- Evoked potentials are normal.
- Neuropsychologic testing is useful as it reveals difficulties in concentration, memory, language, and executive function.

LABORATORY TESTS

Blood tests are not specific.

IMAGING STUDIES

- CT scan of the head is normal.
- MRI of the head is often normal, but may show irregular brain contours, or old cerebral contusions.

TREATMENT

Must be recognized as a physiologic and psychologic problem and treated accordingly.

GENERAL Rx

- Supportive care may include the use of nonnarcotic analgesics and antiemetics.
- Pain management.
- Depression can be treated with SSRIs, but may not respond as well when compared with patients without PCS who have depression.
- Some patients may be admitted for severe symptoms; most can be managed as an outpatient.

NONPHARMACOLOGIC THERAPY

- Early psychological intervention and cognitive rehabilitation are key for full recovery.
- Physical and occupational therapy.
- Avoidance of alcohol, narcotics, and sleep deprivation.
- Explanation of symptoms and expectations, combined with early follow-up with reassurance may hasten resolution of symptoms.

DISPOSITION

- Most patients improve after mild traumatic brain injury without any residual deficits within 3 months.
- Predictors for the development of persistent PCS include:
  - Female
  - Ongoing litigation
  - Low socioeconomic status
  - Prior headaches
  - Prior traumatic brain injury
  - Prior psychiatry illnesses

REFERRAL

Early consultations with psychologists, psychiatrists, neurologists, and rehabilitation specialists in an outpatient setting would be beneficial.

PEARLS & CONSIDERATIONS

- PCS syndrome starts within a few days after the injury.
- Recognizing depression and treating pain symptoms early in the course may help prevent the development of persistent PCS (>1 yr).
- The severity of the trauma determines the severity of axonal injury.
- The severity of the brain injury can be determined by the initial Glasgow coma scale, the length of unconsciousness, and the duration of amnesia.

COMMENTS

- Attempts to determine how much of a role psychologic and/or neurologic factors play in the PCS are important, but very difficult.
- No medication at hospital discharge has been proven to change the natural course of the disease.

SUGGESTED READINGS

Legome E, Wu T: Postconcussive syndrome, *eMedicine Journal,* last updated Sept 6, 2006. Accessed Aug 29, 2007. www.emedicine.com.

McAllister TW, Arciniegas D: Evaluation and treatment of postconcussive symptoms, *NeuroRehabilitation* 17(4):265, 2002.

Wood RL: Post concussional syndrome: all in the minds eye! *J Neurol Neurosurg Psychiatry,* 78:552, 2007.

AUTHOR: **WEN Y. WU-CHEN, M.D.**

BASIC INFORMATION

DEFINITION

Postpoliomyelitis syndrome (PPS) is a lower motor neuron disease characterized by late-onset chronic progressive weakness, muscle cramps, joint pain, and fatigue (focal muscles or generalized) occurring several years after recovering from an acute poliomyelitis infection.

SYNONYMS

Progressive postpoliomyelitis muscular atrophy

ICD-9CM CODES
138 Late effects of acute poliomyelitis

EPIDEMIOLOGY & DEMOGRAPHICS

INCIDENCE (IN U.S.): 250,000 to 640,000 people survived acute poliomyelitis from the 1940 and 1950 epidemics; of those, 28.5% to 64% will develop PPS.

PEAK INCIDENCE: Occurs 8 to 71 yr (mean 36 yr) from the time of the acute poliomyelitis infection.

RISK FACTORS:
- Severe acute poliomyelitis infection
- Older age of onset of the acute infection
- Less recovery and greater physical activity during the intervening years
- Longer interval since the acute illness
- Recent weight gain
- Muscle and joint pain

PHYSICAL FINDINGS & CLINICAL PRESENTATION

- Polio "wall": generalized fatigue occurring with minimal activity
- A slow progressive asymmetric, proximal, distal or patchy weakness and atrophy, involving predominately previously affected muscles by the acute infection
- Focal muscle fatigue (decreased endurance)
- Muscle tenderness on palpation, pain (aches and soreness), fasciculations, cramps, arthralgia, and joint deformities
- Bulbar muscle dysfunction (dysphasia, dysarthria, aphonia, and less commonly facial weakness)
- Cold intolerance and vasomotor instability
- Respiratory dysfunction
- Sleep apnea and sleep disturbances
- Diagnostic criteria (set by the PostPolio Task Force in 1997):
    - A confirmed episode of acute poliomyelitis infection with residual motor neuron loss documented by a typical history, neurologic examination, or electromyographic studies
    - Neurologic and functional stability after recovery from the acute episode for several decades (median 25 yr)
    - Insidious onset (can be acute) of new muscle weakness, atrophy, or fatigue (focal muscle fatigability or generalized)
    - Exclusion of other conditions that can present like PPS

ETIOLOGY

- Controversial.
- *The overuse of a weak muscle (most widely held hypothesis):* many years of muscle overuse causes excessive metabolic stress on the remaining motor neurons that already have branched out to innervate denervated muscle fibers from the acute infection. This results in the gradual degeneration of those nerve terminals (and eventually the motor neurons) that are supplying the denervated muscles.
- *Vulnerability of the anterior horns:* due to an earlier acute infection or preexistent since birth.
- *A scar tissue forming in the anterior horn:* forms "a locus resistentiae minoris" (an area of little resistance) or "a latent inflammatory focus" that could produce new symptoms at any time.
- *Chronic persistent polio virus infection.*
- *Persistent immune-mediated mechanism:* supported by the presence of oligoclonal bands in the CSF and lymphocytic infiltration of muscles and spinal cord of some patients.

DIAGNOSIS

DIFFERENTIAL DIAGNOSIS

- Amyotrophic lateral sclerosis
- Cervical and lumbosacral radiculopathy
- Adult spinal muscular atrophy
- Diabetic amyotrophy
- Multifocal motor neuropathy with conduction block
- Chronic inflammatory demyelinating polyneuropathy
- Entrapment neuropathies
- Inflammatory and metabolic myopathies
- Vasculitis
- Connective tissue disease associated myopathies

WORKUP

- A good history and physical examination demonstrating the characteristic pattern of weakness in an individual who has a history of a documented acute poliomyelitis illness.
- *Electromyography:* ongoing denervation and chronic reinnervation. Fibrillation potentials and fasciculations may be present in symptomatic muscles. Single fiber EMG may show increased jitter and blocking. However, those findings cannot separate PPS from asymptomatic patients with previous poliomyelitis.
- *Nerve conduction studies:* decreased compound muscle action potential amplitudes with normal distal latencies and conduction velocities. Sensory nerve action potentials are normal.
- *Muscle biopsy:* fiber type grouping (remote denervation), isolated angular atrophic fibers (recent localized denervation), and neural cell adhesion molecule (N-CAM)-positive myofibers (denervation).
- *Lumbar puncture:* CSF might show a nonspecific protein elevation and oligoclonal bands.
- *Imaging studies (MRI, CT, x-ray):* to rule out spine disease, such as spondylosis, spinal stenosis, or radiculopathy.
- *Pulmonary function test:* to assess respiratory muscle strength.
- *Sleep study:* if there is a suggestion of obstructive sleep apnea.
- *Swallow evaluation:* using dynamic imaging.
- *Cardiac evaluation:* check for conduction abnormalities.

LABORATORY TESTS

- Creatine kinase (CPK) (mildly elevated in many patients).
- Thyroid function test to rule out thyroid disease causing myopathy.
- Antinuclear antigen (ANA), rheumatoid factor (RF), double-stranded DNA (ds-DNA), erythrocyte sedimentation rate (ESR), C-reactive protein (CRP), scl-70, anti-Ro and anti-La to rule out other autoimmune diseases.
- Heavy metal screening should be considered.
- Standard serum studies (complete blood count and electrolytes).

TREATMENT

NONPHARMACOLOGIC THERAPY

- Treatment is supportive and focused on reducing physical exhaustion.
- Generalized fatigue:
    - Energy conservation (pacing of physical activities, frequent rest periods and daytime naps), weight loss, and assistive devices (orthoses, canes, intermittent use of wheelchairs)
- New weakness: nonfatiguing aerobic exercise and isometric or isokinetic exercise (short intervals, frequent rest, and should be performed on alternate days). A physical therapist should be involved.
- Respiratory insufficiency: nighttime noninvasive positive-pressure ventilation. Some patients might require tracheostomy and permanent ventilation.
- Dysphagia: speech therapist to teach proper food and swallowing techniques.

- Musculoskeletal pain (joint or muscle pain) and joint instability: pacing activities, lifestyle changes, decrease mechanical stress, bracing and wheelchairs. Heat and massage might be used. Anti-inflammatory medications, antidepressant pain medications, lamotrigine can provide some relief.
- Pneumonia and influenza vaccines should be given.
- Smoking cessation.
- Avoid certain medications: beta blockers, benzodiazepines, neuromuscular blockers, tetracycline, aminoglycosides, phenytoin, lithium, phenothiazines, and barbiturates.
- Cardiac conditioning using aerobic or general conditioning exercise with lower-limb cycle or arm ergometers significantly improves cardiorespiratory.
- Social support for psychosocial difficulties.

GENERAL Rx

- Weakness and fatigue
  - Anticholinesterases (pyridostigmine): an open trial reported improvement of fatigue with pyridostigmine (Trojan & Cashman). Preliminary data from a double-blinded, placebo-controlled crossover trial suggested subjective improvement of fatigue and strength in the upper extremities with the same drug (Seizert et al).
  - Amantadine, amitriptyline, bromocriptine, fluoxetine, and pemoline might be considered.
- Postpolio tinnitus
  - Botulinum toxin A (Scolozzi et al)
- Depression
  - SRRIs

DISPOSITION

Slow progression with an average decline in strength of about 1% to 2% per year

REFERRAL

- Surgical evaluation for muscle biopsy
- A neurologist or a neuromuscular specialist for neurophysiologic testing
- Physical and occupational therapists

PEARLS & CONSIDERATIONS

COMMENTS

- Risk of falls should be assessed by a physical therapist.
- Interdisciplinary approach should be used in the management of those patients, including primary care physician, physiatrist, neurologist, pulmonologist, psychiatrist, physical, occupational, and respiratory therapists, nurse, and social worker.

EVIDENCE

EBM

Pyridostigmine provided improvement of fatigue[1] and subjective improvement of fatigue and strength in the upper extremities.[2]

Moderate intensity strength training exercise is safe and effective in postpolio patients.[3]

Evidence-Based References

1. Trojan DA, Cashman NR: An open trial of pyridostigmine in post-poliomyelitis syndrome, *Can J Neurol Sci* 22(3):223-237, 1995.
2. Seizert BP, Speier JL, Canine JK: Pyridostigmine effect on strength, endurance, and fatigue in post-polio patients, *Arch Phys Med Rehabil* 75:1049, 1994 (abstract).
3. Chan KM et al: Randomized controlled trial of strength training in post-polio patients, *Muscle Nerve* 27(3):332 338, 2003.

SUGGESTED READINGS

Katirji B et al: *Neuromuscular disorders in clinical practice,* Boston, 2002, Butterworth-Heinemann, pp 403-415.

Nollet F, de Visser M: Postpolio syndrome, *Arch Neurol* 61(7):1142-1144, 2004.

Scolozzi P et al: Successful treatment of a postpolio tinnitus with type A botulinum toxin, *Laryngoscope* 115(7):1288-1290, 2005.

Trojan DA, Cashman NR: Post-poliomyelitis syndrome, *Muscle Nerve* 31(1):6-19, 2005.

AUTHOR: **MUSTAFA A. HAMMAD, M.D.**

BASIC INFORMATION

DEFINITION

Posttraumatic stress disorder (PTSD) is a disorder that arises when an individual has witnessed or experienced a potentially fatal or serious injury, during which he or she felt helpless or horrified. The individual continues to experience the event in the form of flashbacks (reliving the trauma), intrusive recollections, dreams, or physiologic reactivity. These responses are associated with persistent hyperarousal (e.g., hypervigilance, exaggerated startle response, sleep disturbance, irritability, and difficulty concentrating) and avoidance (both physically and cognitively) of stimuli associated with the traumatic event.

SYNONYMS

Soldier's heart
Effort syndrome
Shell shock
Irritable heart
Traumatic necrosis
Survivor syndrome
Concentration camp syndrome
Gross stress reaction (DSM-I, published in 1952)

ICD-9CM CODES

308.3 Posttraumatic stress syndrome, acute
309.81 Posttraumatic stress syndrome, chronic

EPIDEMIOLOGY & DEMOGRAPHICS

INCIDENCE: PTSD cannot be diagnosed until at least 1 month after the traumatic event.

PREVALENCE (IN U.S.):

- PTSD is one of the most common psychiatric disorders, with an estimated lifetime prevalence of 7.8% to 12.3%.
- Prevalence estimates among high-risk populations (e.g., combat veterans or victims of violent crimes) range up to 58%.
- PTSD is associated with high rates of depression, anxiety disorders, and substance use. Overall, about 80% of persons with PTSD also have a comorbid psychiatric disorder.

PREDOMINANT SEX: Twice as many women as men are affected, with prevalence rates of 10% to 14% of women and 5% to 6% of men; more than 50% of cases in women are related to sexual assault.

PREDOMINANT AGE: No predisposing age factors have been identified.

GENETICS: Twin studies have demonstrated the important role of genetic vulnerability in the development of PTSD related to combat. There are no comparable studies for civilian trauma.

PHYSICAL FINDINGS & CLINICAL PRESENTATION

- Reexperiencing of traumatic events in the form of dreams, flashbacks, and intrusive memories is required in the diagnostic criteria.
- Depersonalization, detachment, emotional numbing and dissociation, with avoidance of physical or cognitive reminders of the event.
- Hyperarousal, hypervigilance and exaggerated startle response, irritability, anxiety, and difficulty concentrating.
- The symptoms may be disabling.

ETIOLOGY

- By definition, the patient must have been exposed to a traumatic event that involved actual or threatened death or serious injury. Events that involve interpersonal violence are more likely to give rise to PTSD than are events such as motor vehicle accidents and natural disasters.
- The severity of the physical injury is a weaker predictor of the likelihood of developing PTSD than the psychologic distress; the duration of the stress is the most important factor.
- Symptoms are mediated, in part, by the autonomic nervous system and the hypothalamic-pituitary-adrenal (HPA) system. Studies have proposed mechanisms including an excessive release of norepinephrine and an exaggerated negative feedback inhibition of the HPA axis by glucocorticoids and enhanced postsynaptic alpha-1 response in the central nervous system (CNS) to norepinephrine.

DIAGNOSIS

DIFFERENTIAL DIAGNOSIS

- Adjustment disorders are distinguished from PTSD in that the precipitating stress is less catastrophic and the psychologic reaction less specific.
- Acute stress reaction typically lasts <48 hr; acute stress disorder begins during or shortly after the precipitating event (within 4 wk) and must last at least 48 hr.
- Borderline personality disorder and dissociative identity disorder.
- Patients with major depression should be screened for PTSD because up to 30% of primary care patients with depression also have PTSD.

WORKUP

- After a traumatic event, the presence of the following symptoms for greater than one month: at least one reexperiencing symptom, at least three avoidance/numbing symptoms, and at least one hypervigilance symptom meet DSM-IV criteria for diagnosis of PTSD.
  - Symptoms 1 to 3 months = acute PTSD
  - Symptoms >3 months = chronic PTSD
  - Development of symptoms years after the event = delayed-onset PTSD
- There are numerous self-report questionnaires and structured diagnostic instruments; mainly useful in research settings.
- Laboratory and imaging not sufficiently validated or replicated to be clinically useful, although other medical conditions can be ruled out with studies including a TSH, CBC, urine toxicology, and glucose.

TREATMENT

NONPHARMACOLOGIC THERAPY

- In most cases, treatment of PTSD should be multidimensional, consisting of patient education and support, cognitive-behavioral therapy (CBT), and psychopharmacotherapy. Alcohol or drug abuse cessation programs if indicated.
- CBT is the nonpharmacologic treatment of choice. Prolonged exposure (PE), a type of CBT that includes education on stress response, breathing training, and prolonged mental recounting of the event to decrease the emotional response, was found to be more effective than standard CBT in female veterans.
- Group therapy is often helpful for many PTSD victims, particularly combat veterans.

ACUTE GENERAL Rx

- Symptomatic and generally aimed at alleviating distress.
- Benzodiazepines for reducing anxiety symptoms.
- Sedating antidepressants to treat initial insomnia and prazosin to suppress trauma nightmares.

CHRONIC Rx

- SSRIs are the pharmacologic treatment of choice for PTSD. Paroxetine and fluoxetine are the best studied.
- Other antidepressants (TCAs and MAOs) are also helpful in reducing symptoms associated with PTSD.
- Preliminary data suggests that memantine may be useful in the treatment of cognitive and psychiatric components.

COMPLEMENTARY & ALTERNATIVE APPROACHES

- Acupuncture was shown to be as effective at CBT in decreasing symptoms of PTSD.

- Eye movement desensitization reprocessing (EMDR); results from controlled trials have shown mixed results.
- β-adrenergic antagonists and clonidine may be helpful for treating aggression and other psychophysiologic arousal symptoms.

DISPOSITION

- Recovery rates are highest in the first 12 mo after onset of symptoms.
- Average duration of symptoms is 36 mo for those who undergo treatment and 64 mo for those never treated.
- Up to half of patients experience chronic symptoms.
- Predictors of chronic course:
  - Premorbid psychiatric function
  - Acute response to stress (e.g., individuals who experience an acute stress disorder immediately after the trauma do better in the long term)

REFERRAL

Because early intervention improves outcome, refer to psychiatry as soon as diagnosis made.

PEARLS & CONSIDERATIONS

A personal or family history of psychiatric disorder, a prior history of traumatic experiences, and a history of childhood behavioral problems are associated with an increased risk of developing PTSD.

EVIDENCE

A systematic review concludes that psychologic intervention improves both immediate and long-term outcomes compared with supportive counseling.[1] Ⓐ

CBT, specifically PE, improves symptoms of posttraumatic stress disorder compared with supportive counseling, relaxation therapy, and minimal attention.[1-3] Ⓐ

EMDR and acupuncture are significantly more effective than no treatment in reducing symptoms of posttraumatic stress disorder. They have not, however, been shown to be any more effective than cognitive-behavioral therapy or exposure techniques.[4,5] Ⓐ Ⓑ

Despite there being no direct comparative studies of pharmacotherapeutic and psychotherapeutic interventions in posttraumatic stress disorder, drug therapy can be effective and should be considered as part of the overall management.[6]

One systematic review analyzed nine randomized controlled trials (RCTs) assessing the use of antidepressants, including sertraline, fluoxetine, and paroxetine, in PTSD. Despite methodologic limitations and trial inconsistencies, the majority showed that drug treatment was more effective than placebo.[7]

Trials to date have been unable to suggest any predictors of response to treatment because the subjects studied have been so diverse with regard to the trauma experienced, duration of trauma, and comorbidity.[6] Ⓐ

Evidence-Based References

1. Sherman JJ: Effects of psychotherapeutic treatments for PTSD: a meta-analysis of controlled clinical trials, *J Trauma Stress* 11:413, 1998. Ⓐ
2. Marks I et al: Treatment of posttraumatic stress disorder by exposure and/or cognitive restructuring: a controlled study, *Arch Gen Psychiatry* 55:317, 1998. Reviewed in: *Clin Evid* 11:1343, 2004. Ⓐ
3. Resick A et al: A comparison of cognitive-processing therapy with prolonged exposure and a waiting condition for the treatment of chronic posttraumatic stress disorder in female rape victims, *J Consult Clin Psychol* 70:867, 2002. Reviewed in: *Clin Evid* 11:1343, 2004. Ⓐ
4. Davidson PR, Parker KC: Eye movement desensitisation and reprocessing (EMDR): a meta-analysis, *J Consult Clin Psychol* 69:305, 2001. Reviewed in: *Clin Evid* 11:1343, 2004. Ⓐ
5. Lee C et al: Treatment of PTSD: stress inoculation training with prolonged exposure compared to EMDR, *J Clin Psychol* 58:1071, 2002. Reviewed in: *Clin Evid* 11:1343, 2004. Ⓐ
6. Stein DJ et al: Pharmacotherapy for posttraumatic stress disorder (PTSD). Reviewed in: Cochrane Library 3, Chichester, UK, 2004, John Wiley. Ⓐ
7. Stein DJ et al: Pharmacotherapy for post traumatic stress disorder (PTSD), *Cochrane Database of Syst Rev* 4, Chichester, UK, 2000, John Wiley.

SUGGESTED READINGS

Bisson JI: Post-traumatic stress disorder, *BMJ* 334:789-793, 2007.

De Bellis MD, Van Dillen T: Childhood posttraumatic stress disorder: an overview, *Child Adolesc Psychiatr Clin N Am* 14(4):745, 2005.

Grubaugh AL et al: Subthreshold PTSD in primary care: prevalence, psychiatric disorders, healthcare use, and functional status, *J Nerv Ment Dis* 193(10):658, 2005.

Schoenfeld FB et al: Current concepts in pharmacotherapy for posttraumatic stress disorder, *Psychiatr Serv* 55(5):519, 2004.

Vieweg WV et al: Posttraumatic stress disorder: clinical features, pathophysiology, and treatment, *Am J Med* 119(5):383, 2006.

AUTHORS: **MITCHELL D. FELDMAN, M.D., M.PHIL.,** and **NICOLE SIROTIN, M.D.**

BASIC INFORMATION

DEFINITION

Precocious puberty is defined as sexual development occurring before 8 yr of age in females and 9 yr of age in males.

SYNONYMS

Pubertas praecox

ICD-9CM CODES
259.1 Precocious puberty

EPIDEMIOLOGY & DEMOGRAPHICS

INCIDENCE: Estimated to be between 1:5000 and 1:10,000.

PREDOMINANT SEX: Females > males for the idiopathic variant; for other causes, dependent on the underlying etiology.

GENETICS: The genetics for some of the etiologies of precocious puberty are known.

PHYSICAL FINDINGS & CLINICAL PRESENTATION

- In females: breast development, pubic hair development, accelerated growth, and menarche
- In males: increase in testicular volume and penile length, pubic hair development, accelerated growth, muscular development, acne, change in voice, and penile erections

ETIOLOGY

- Idiopathic or true: diagnosis of exclusion
- CNS pathology: tumors, hydrocephalus, ventricular cysts, benign lesions
- Severe hypothyroidism
- Posttraumatic head injury
- Genetic disorders: neurofibromatosis, tuberous sclerosis, McCune-Albright syndrome, congenital adrenal hyperplasia
- Gonadal tumors
- Nongonadal tumors: hepatoblastoma
- Exposure to exogenous sex steroids

DIAGNOSIS

DIFFERENTIAL DIAGNOSIS

- Most common diagnoses to consider: premature thelarche and premature adrenarche
- Gonadotropin hormone–releasing hormone (GnRH)–dependent precocious puberty: idiopathic, CNS tumors, hypothalamic hamartomas, neurofibromatosis, tuberous sclerosis, hydrocephalus, post acute head injury, ventricular cysts, post CNS infection
- GnRH-independent precocious puberty: congenital adrenal hyperplasia, adrenocortical tumors (males), McCune-Albright syndrome (females), gonadal tumors, ectopic hCG-secreting tumors (chorioblastoma, hepatoblastoma), exposure to exogenous sex steroids, severe hypothyroidism

WORKUP

Thorough history and physical examination are essential to determine if the patient has true precocious puberty. Particular attention should be paid to growth, development, order of appearance of the secondary sexual characteristics, pubertal development in family members, medications, neurologic symptoms, Tanner staging, abdominal and neurologic examination. Section III, Puberty, Precocious describes a clinical approach to precocious puberty.

LABORATORY TESTS

- GnRH testing will help determine if dependent or independent cause
- Sex hormone studies: LH, FSH, hCG, testosterone (males), estrogen (females)
- T_4, TSH

IMAGING STUDIES

- CT scan or MRI of the brain to evaluate for CNS pathology
- Consideration of pelvic ultrasound in female patients to evaluate for cysts/tumors
- Abdominal imaging with CT scan if intraabdominal pathology suspected

TREATMENT

NONPHARMACOLOGIC THERAPY

- Good communication with the parents is essential to care.
- Psychologic support for the child may be needed with regard to self-image and problems with peer acceptance.

ACUTE GENERAL Rx

There is no acute therapy for precocious puberty.

CHRONIC Rx

Therapy depends on the etiology of precocious puberty:

- For true precocious puberty and some CNS lesions, the treatment of choice is leuprolide 0.25 to 0.3 mg/kg with a 7.5 mg minimum IM every 4 wk.
- For other CNS lesions and extragonadal tumors, therapy is dependent on the type of lesion, location of the lesion, and the overall prognosis of the underlying problem.
- For severe hypothyroidism, treatment with thyroid hormone will result in regression of the sexual development. The child will subsequently undergo appropriate pubertal development later in life.
- For familial male gonadotropin-independent precocious puberty, ketoconazole can be used at doses of 600 mg/day divided tid, or a combination of testolactone and spironolactone can be used.

DISPOSITION

- For true precocious puberty and some CNS lesions, long-term outcome is usually very good. When drug therapy is instituted, it is continued until a time when further pubertal development is appropriate. It is then discontinued, allowing the child to progress through puberty.
- For other cases, long-term outcomes are dependent on the prognosis of the underlying cause.

REFERRAL

- Initial workup can be instituted by the primary care provider.
- Referral to an endocrinologist is indicated for most children because they will need long-term management, monitoring, and treatment.

SUGGESTED READING

Root AW: Precocious puberty, *Pediatr Rev* 21(1):10, 2000.

AUTHORS: **BETH J. WUTZ, M.D.**, and **RUBEN ALVERO, M.D.**

BASIC INFORMATION

DEFINITION

Preeclampsia involves a triad of hypertension, proteinuria, and edema that develops after the twentieth week of gestation. Mild preeclampsia is defined as a blood pressure of <140/90 mm Hg. Severe preeclampsia is associated with a blood pressure >160/110 mm Hg, proteinuria >5 g in a 24-hr urine collection, oliguria (<400 ml/24 hr), cerebral or visual disturbances, epigastric pain, pulmonary edema, thrombocytopenia, hepatic dysfunction, or severe intrauterine growth retardation.

SYNONYMS

Pregnancy-induced hypertension
Toxemia of pregnancy

ICD-9CM CODES
642.6 Preeclampsia

EPIDEMIOLOGY & DEMOGRAPHICS

INCIDENCE: 10% to 14% in primigravidas, 5.7% to 7.3% in multigravidas
RISK FACTORS: Increased incidence and severity with multiple gestations, renal or collagen-vascular diseases. Extremes of reproductive age, <20 or >35 yr of age, obesity, African Americans, thrombophilia, previous preeclampsia.
GENETICS: Positive correlation with maternal and paternal family history.

PHYSICAL FINDINGS & CLINICAL PRESENTATION

- Generalized swelling or nondependent edema, possibly manifested by rapid weight gain (>4 lb/wk) even in the absence of edema
- Auscultation of pulmonary rales
- Right upper quadrant pain (HELLP syndrome or subcapsular liver hematoma)
- Hyperreflexia or clonus
- Vaginal bleeding (placental abruption)
- Acute or chronic fetal compromise manifested by intrauterine growth restriction or fetal tachycardia with late decelerations, respectively
- Wide range of symptoms attributable to multiorgan system dysfunction, involving hepatic, hematologic, renal, pulmonary, and CNS
- Possibility of severe disease despite "normal" blood pressure readings, so a high index of suspicion must be maintained in high-risk situations

ETIOLOGY

- Exact etiology or toxic substance is unknown
- Theories
  1. Imbalance between thromboxane A_2 (vasoconstrictor and platelet aggregator) and prostacyclin (vasodilator)
  2. Abnormal trophoblastic invasion of spiral arteries
  3. Increased sensitivity to angiotensin II by the muscular walls of the arteries
  4. Excess circulating soluble fms-like tyrosine kinase 1 (SFlT-1), which binds placental growth factor (PlGF) and vascular endothelial growth factor (VEGF), may have a pathogenic role

DIAGNOSIS

DIFFERENTIAL DIAGNOSIS

- Acute fatty liver of pregnancy
- Appendicitis
- Diabetic ketoacidosis
- Gallbladder disease
- Gastroenteritis
- Glomerulonephritis
- Hemolytic-uremic syndrome
- Hepatic encephalopathy
- Hyperemesis gravidarum
- Idiopathic thrombocytopenia
- Thrombotic thrombocytopenic purpura
- Nephrolithiasis
- Pyelonephritis
- PUD
- SLE
- Viral hepatitis

WORKUP

- Two blood pressure measurements in lateral recumbent position 6 hr apart, with an absolute pressure >140/90 mm Hg or an increase of 30 mm Hg systolic or 15 mm Hg diastolic from baseline, an increase in the mean arterial pressure (MAP) of 20 mm Hg, or an absolute MAP >105 mm Hg
- Evaluation for proteinuria as defined by >0.1 g/L on urine dipstick or >300 mg protein on a 24-hr urine collection
- Evaluation of fetal status for evidence of intrauterine growth restriction, oligohydramnios, alteration in umbilical or uterine artery Doppler flow, or acute compromise, such as abruption
- Because of the insidious nature of the disease with potential for multiple organ involvement, complete evaluation for preeclampsia in any pregnant patient presenting with CNS derangement or GI complaints after 20 wk of gestation
- Evaluation for associated conditions such as disseminated intravascular coagulation, hepatic dysfunction, or subcapsular hematoma

LABORATORY TESTS

- High-risk patients: baseline assessment of renal function (24-hr urine collection for protein and creatinine clearance), platelets, BUN, creatinine, LFTs, and uric acid should be obtained at the first prenatal visit.
- CBC (Hgb, HCT, platelets) may show signs of volume contraction or HELLP syndrome.
- LFTs (AST, ALT, LDH) are useful in evaluation for HELLP syndrome or to exclude important differentials.
- Hyperuricemia or increased creatinine may indicate decreasing renal function.
- PT, PTT, and fibrinogen should be checked to rule out disseminated intravascular coagulation.
- Peripheral smear may demonstrate microangiopathic hemolytic anemia.
- Complement levels can be used to differentiate from an acute exacerbation of a collagen-vascular disease.
- Increased levels of SFlT-1 and reduced levels of PlGF predict subsequent development of preeclampsia.

IMAGING STUDIES

- CT scan of head if atypical presentation of eclampsia, possibility of intracerebral bleed, or prolonged postictal state
- Sonogram of fetus to evaluate for IUGR, amniotic fluid, placenta
- Sonogram of maternal liver if suspect subcapsular hematoma

TREATMENT

NONPHARMACOLOGIC THERAPY

Bed rest in left lateral decubitus position

ACUTE GENERAL Rx

Delivery is the treatment of choice and the only cure for the disease. This must be taken in the context of the gestational age of the fetus, severity of the preeclampsia, and the likelihood of a successful induction and reliability of patient.

- Administer magnesium sulfate 6 g IV loading dose, with 2 to 3 g maintenance or phenytoin at 10 to 15 mg/kg loading dose, then 200 mg IV q8h starting 12 hr after loading dose.
- Hydralazine 10 mg IV, labetalol hydrochloride 20 to 40 mg IV, nifedipine 20 mg SL can be used for acute blood pressure control.
- Continuous fetal monitoring is needed.
- Epidural is anesthesia of choice for pain management in labor or C-section.
- All patients undergoing induction of labor should receive antiseizure medications regardless of severity of disease.

CHRONIC Rx

- Mild preeclampsia <37 wk: close observation for worsening maternal or fetal condition, with delivery at >37 wk with favorable cervix or at 40 wk regardless of cervical status.
- Severe preeclampsia: delivery in the presence of maternal or fetal compromise, labor, or >34 wk; at 28 to 34 wk

consider steroids with close monitoring, and at <24 wk consider termination of pregnancy.
- Methyldopa is drug of choice for chronic blood pressure control during pregnancy.

DISPOSITION

Preeclampsia is a progressive and unpredictable disease process; a course of expectancy should be managed with caution. Up to 20% of patients who have seizures are normotensive.

REFERRAL

Obstetric management is indicated because of the insidious nature of the disease, with transfer of all cases <34 wk to a facility with a level three nursery.

PEARLS & CONSIDERATIONS

COMMENTS

- Low-dose aspirin 81 mg qd and calcium supplementation 1500 mg qd can be considered in high-risk patients to decrease the risk of recurrence.
- Begin after first trimester.

EVIDENCE

EBM

There is evidence for the use of hypertensive medication during pregnancy.

A systematic review found that antihypertensive medication halved the risk of developing severe hypertension in women with mild-moderate hypertension during pregnancy. There was little evidence that antihypertensives reduced the risk of developing preeclampsia, and there was no clear effect on the risk of perinatal mortality, preterm birth, or small for gestational age babies.[1] Ⓐ

A systematic review compared different antihypertensives (hydralazine, labetalol, nifedipine, diazoxide, and katanserin) for the treatment of severe high blood pressure in pregnancy. There was no clear evidence that any one drug was more effective than another for blood pressure control.[2] Ⓐ

Beta blockers were found to decrease the risk of severe hypertension and to have comparable efficacy and safety to methyldopa.

A systematic review found that oral beta blockers decrease the risk of severe hypertension and the need for additional antihypertensives in pregnant women with mild-moderate hypertension. There was no evidence that there was any additional substantial benefit to be gained for mother or baby.[3] Ⓐ

Magnesium sulfate may be the best prophylactic anticonvulsant for women with severe preeclampsia.

A metaanalysis of five randomized controlled trials (RCTs) comparing magnesium sulfate with placebo found that prophylactic magnesium sulfate halved the risk of eclampsia, and reduced maternal mortality (although the latter results did not reach statistical significance). There was no significant difference for rate of stillbirth or perinatal death.[4] Ⓐ

A systematic review found that magnesium sulfate was superior to phenytoin for the prevention of eclampsia (although magnesium sulfate was associated with a higher risk of cesarean section).[5] Ⓐ

A large RCT of preeclamptic peripartum women found that the rate of eclampsia was halved in those treated with magnesium sulfate vs. placebo. The investigators concluded that magnesium sulfate probably reduces maternal death.[6] Ⓑ

Magnesium sulfate is an effective treatment for eclampsia.

Systematic reviews found that magnesium sulfate was more effective than "lytic cocktail" (usually a combination of chlorpromazine, promethazine, and pethidine), phenytoin, and diazepam in preventing further seizures in women with eclampsia. Magnesium sulfate was associated with a reduction in maternal deaths, but this result did not reach statistical significance.[7-9] Ⓐ

There is insufficient evidence to assess the effects of hospital admission, bed rest, or day care compared with outpatient care.

Systematic reviews compared hospital admission vs. outpatient clinic assessment, bed rest in hospital vs. normal ambulation in hospital, and antenatal day care units vs. hospital admission in women who develop hypertension during pregnancy, but the trials were too small for any reliable conclusions to be drawn.[4]

Evidence-Based References

1. Abalos E et al: Antihypertensive drug therapy for mild to moderate hypertension during pregnancy. Reviewed in: Cochrane Library 4, Chichester, UK, 2003, John Wiley. Ⓐ
2. Duley L, Henderson-Smart DJ: Drugs for treatment of very high blood pressure during pregnancy. Reviewed in: Cochrane Library 4, Chichester, UK, 2003, John Wiley. Ⓐ
3. Magee LA, Duley L: Oral beta-blockers for mild to moderate hypertension during pregnancy. Reviewed in: Cochrane Library 4, Chichester, UK, 2003, John Wiley. Ⓐ
4. Duley L: Preeclampsia and hypertension. 10:1683, London, 2003, BMJ Publishing Group. Ⓐ
5. Duley L, Gulmezoglu AM, Henderson-Smart DJ: Magnesium sulphate and other anticonvulsants for women with preeclampsia. Reviewed in: Cochrane Library 4, Chichester, UK, 2003, John Wiley. Ⓐ
6. Duley L et al: Do women with preeclampsia, and their babies, benefit from magnesium sulphate? The Magpie Trial: a randomised placebo-controlled trial, *Lancet* 359:1877, 2002. Ⓑ
7. Duley L, Gulmezoglu AM: Magnesium sulphate versus lytic cocktail for eclampsia. Reviewed in: Cochrane Library 4, Chichester, UK, 2003, John Wiley. Ⓐ
8. Duley L, Henderson-Smart D: Magnesium sulphate versus phenytoin for eclampsia. Reviewed in: Cochrane Library 4, Chichester, UK, 2003, John Wiley. Ⓐ
9. Duley L, Henderson-Smart D: Magnesium sulphate versus diazepam for eclampsia. Reviewed in: Cochrane Library 4, Chichester, UK, 2003, John Wiley. Ⓐ

SUGGESTED READINGS

Lain KY, Roberts JM: Contemporary concepts of the pathogenesis and management of preeclampsia, *JAMA* 287:3183, 2002.

Levine RJ et al: Circulating angiogonic factors and risk of preeclampsia, *N Enl J Med* 350:672, 2004.

AUTHORS: **SCOTT J. ZUCCALA, D.O.,** and **RUBEN ALVERO, M.D.**

BASIC INFORMATION

DEFINITION

The Diagnostic and Statistical Manual of Mental Disorders, 4th edition, classifies premenstrual dysphoric disorder (PMDD) as a "depressive disorder not otherwise specified" and requires as criteria for definition the presence of five or more of the following symptoms in most menstrual cycles for the past year.

- The symptoms should be present most of the time during the last week of the luteal phase, with remission beginning within a few days after the onset of the follicular phase, and absent during the week after menses, with at least one of the symptoms being either 1, 2, 3, or 4:
  1. Marked depressed mood, feeling of hopelessness, or self-deprecating thoughts
  2. Marked anxiety, tension, feeling of being "keyed up" or "on edge"
  3. Marked affective lability (e.g., feeling suddenly sad or tearful or increased sensitivity to rejection)
  4. Persistent and marked anger or irritability or increased interpersonal conflicts
  5. Decreased interest in usual activities (e.g., work, school, friends, hobbies)
  6. Subjective sense of difficulty in concentrating
  7. Lethargy, easy fatigability, or marked lack of energy
  8. Marked change in appetite, overeating, or specific food cravings
  9. Hypersomnia or insomnia
  10. A subjective sense of being overwhelmed or out of control
  11. Other physical symptoms, such as breast tenderness or swelling, headaches, joint or muscle pain, a sensation of "bloating," or weight gain
- The disturbance markedly interferes with work or school or with usual social activities and relationships with others (e.g., avoidance of social activities, decreased production and efficiency at work or school).
- The disturbance is not merely an exacerbation of the symptoms of another disorder, such as major depressive disorder, panic disorder, dysthymic disorder, or a personality disorder (although it may be superimposed on any of these disorders).
- The first three criteria must be confirmed by prospective daily ratings during at least two consecutive symptomatic cycles (diagnosis may be made provisionally before such confirmation).

NOTE: In menstruating women, the luteal phase corresponds to the period between ovulation and the onset of menses, and the follicular phase begins with menses. In nonmenstruating women (e.g., women who have had a hysterectomy), determination of the timing of the luteal and follicular phases may require measurement of circulating reproductive hormones.

ICD-9CM CODES
625.4 Premenstrual dysphoric syndrome

EPIDEMIOLOGY & DEMOGRAPHICS

- PMDD affects 3% to 10% of women of reproductive age.
- Genetic factors play a significant role (increased incidence in monozygotic twins and in women whose mothers had PMDD).
- 30% to 76% of women with PMDD have a lifetime history of depression.

PHYSICAL FINDINGS & CLINICAL PRESENTATION

- Physical examination may be completely normal.
- Depressed mood, tachycardia, sweating from comorbid disorders (e.g., panic disorder, major depression) may be present.
- Symptoms occur during the last half of the menstrual cycle (the luteal phase) and are absent from the first day of menstruation until ovulation (follicular phase).

ETIOLOGY

Unknown. Serotonin deficiency and altered sensitivity in serotoninergic system in response to phasic hormone fluctuations in the menstrual cycle are believed to play a role.

DIAGNOSIS

DIFFERENTIAL DIAGNOSIS

- Premenstrual syndrome
- Dysthymic syndrome
- Personality disorder
- Panic disorder
- Major depressive disorder
- Hyperthyroidism
- Polycystic ovarian syndrome
- Drug or alcohol abuse
- Irritable bowel syndrome
- Endometriosis

WORKUP

- Diagnosis is based on obtaining a detailed history and ruling out the presence of physical or psychiatric disorders. No objective diagnostic tests exist.
- The diagnosis should be confirmed using a symptom checklist prospectively for two consecutive menstrual cycles. Commonly used diagnostic instruments include the Calendar of Premenstrual Experiences and the Premenstrual Syndrome Diary.

LABORATORY TESTS

- None are usually necessary.
- A serum TSH to exclude thyroid problems, CBC to rule out anemia, and a chemistry profile to assess electrolytes may be ordered if diagnosis is unclear.

TREATMENT

NONPHARMACOLOGIC THERAPY

- Reduction in intake of caffeine, refined sugars, or sodium may be helpful in some patients.
- Increased aerobic exercise, smoking cessation, alcohol restriction, and regular sleep are often beneficial.
- Stress reduction and management will decrease severity of symptoms.

GENERAL Rx

- Selective serotonin reuptake inhibitors (SSRIs) are first-line agents for the treatment of PMDD. Commonly used agents and initial doses are fluoxetine 10 mg qd, sertraline 50 mg qd, paroxetine 10 mg qd, and citalopram 20 mg qd. Many patients will require titration to significantly higher doses to achieve therapeutic benefit. These medications can be administered continuously during the menstrual cycle or only when the patients experience symptoms. Luteal-phase or intermittent administration involves initiating medication at the time of ovulation and stopping it at the beginning of menses.
- Second-line agents are benzodiazepines (alprazolam 0.25 mg tid prn) and the tricyclic antidepressant (clomipramine 25 mg qd as starting dose).
- Hormonal intervention with monthly IM injections of leuprolide has been reported effective in some patients; however, it should be reserved only for patients unresponsive to first- and second-line agents.
- Nutritional supplementation (vitamin B_6 up to 100 mg/day, vitamin E up to 600 IU/day, calcium carbonate up to 1200 mg/day, and magnesium up to 500 mg/day) are also commonly used and effective in symptom reduction in some patients.
- Ovariectomy may be considered in severe refractory cases.

AUTHOR: **FRED F. FERRI, M.D.**

BASIC INFORMATION

DEFINITION

Premenstrual syndrome (PMS) is a cyclic recurrence during the luteal phase of the menstrual cycle of somatic, affective, and behavioral disturbances that are of sufficient severity to affect interpersonal relationships adversely or interfere with normal activities.

SYNONYMS

PMS
PMDD

ICD-9CM CODES
625.4 Premenstrual tension syndromes

EPIDEMIOLOGY & DEMOGRAPHICS

- PMS is thought to be extremely prevalent, intermittently affecting approximately one third of all premenopausal women.
- Severe cases occur in approximately 2% to 10% of women with PMS.
- Those seeking treatment for PMS are usually in their 30s or 40s.
- The natural history of PMS has not been clearly elucidated.

PHYSICAL FINDINGS & CLINICAL PRESENTATION

- Diverse and potentially disabling symptoms
- Associated with >150 psychologic, physical, and behavioral symptoms
- Most frequent reason for seeking treatment: emotional symptoms
- Most common emotional symptoms: depression, irritability, anxiety, labile moods, anger, crying easily, sadness, overly sensitive, nervous tension
- Most common physical complaints: headache, bloating, cramps, breast tenderness, migraines, fatigue, weight gain, aches and pains, palpitations
- Most common behavior symptom: food cravings
- Other behavioral symptoms: increased appetite, increased alcohol intake, decreased motivation, decreased efficiency, avoidance of activities, staying home, sleep changes, libido changes, forgetfulness, decreased concentration

ETIOLOGY

- Etiology remains obscure.
- Because of multifactorial-multiorgan nature of PMS, a single etiologic cause is unlikely.

DIAGNOSIS

DIFFERENTIAL DIAGNOSIS

- A diagnosis of exclusion, so other medical or psychologic disorders should be ruled out
- Most common disorders: depression or anxiety, thyroid disease
- Section II describes the differential diagnosis of menstrual pain

WORKUP

- History
- Physical examination
- Laboratory studies to rule out alternative diagnosis
- If no alternative diagnosis confirms diagnosis of PMS, basal body temperature charting is used to determine if the patient is ovulating:
  1. If she is not ovulating, it is not PMS.
  2. If she is ovulating, symptoms should be charted for at least two cycles to determine if the symptoms occur in the luteal phase.
  3. If symptoms are not occurring in the luteal phase, it is not PMS, and further investigation is needed.
     a. If symptoms occur in the follicular phase, patient has premenstrual exacerbation of another condition.
     b. If symptoms do not occur in the follicular phase, diagnosis of PMS is confirmed.

LABORATORY TESTS

- None available to specifically confirm the diagnosis of PMS
- Thyroid function tests to rule out thyroid disease

TREATMENT

NONPHARMACOLOGIC THERAPY

- Individualization of the treatment plan to maximize therapeutic response
- Psychosocial intervention:
  1. Education
  2. Stress management
  3. Environmental changes
  4. Adequate rest and sleep
  5. Regular exercise
- Nutritional recommendations:
  1. Regularly eaten, well-balanced meals
  2. Adequate amounts of protein, fiber, and complex carbohydrates; low fat
  3. Avoidance of foods that are high in salt and simple sugars; may promote water retention, weight gain, and physical discomfort
  4. Avoidance of caffeine-containing beverages; stimulant effects of caffeine may worsen tension, irritability, and insomnia
  5. Avoidance of alcohol and illicit drugs; may worsen emotional lability
  6. Calcium supplementation (1000 mg/day for women 19 to 50 yr, 1300 mg/day for girls 14 to 18 yr) to reduce the physical and emotional symptoms
  7. Magnesium (360 mg/day) to reduce water retention and the negative effect associated with PMS
  8. Pyridoxine (vitamin B_6) 50 mg bid to improve depression, fatigue, irritability and natural diuretic ability; neurotoxicity observed at higher dosages

ACUTE GENERAL Rx

SUPPRESSION OF OVULATION:

- Oral contraceptives—one pill per day
- Progestin-only oral contraceptive—one pill per day
- Oral micronized progesterone—100 mg qam and 200 mg qpm on days 17 through 28 of menstrual cycle
- Progestin suppository—200 to 400 mg bid on days 17 through 28 of menstrual cycle
- Oral contraceptive containing arosperenone/ethinyl estradiol—very effective in decreasing physical symptoms
- Medroxyprogesterone—150 mg IM every 3 mo
- Levonorgestrel implants—surgical insertion every 5 yr
- Transdermal estradiol—one or two 100-μg patches every 3 days
- Danazol—100 to 200 mg/day (ovulation not suppressed at this dose)
- Gonadotropin-releasing hormone (GnRH) agonists—daily by intranasal spray or monthly by depot injection

SUPPRESSION OF PHYSICAL SYMPTOMS:

- Spironolactone—25 to 50 mg bid on days 14 through 28 of menstrual cycle
- Mefenamic acid
  1. For fluid retention: 250 mg tid on days 24 through 28 of cycle
  2. For pain: 500 mg tid on days 19 through 28 of cycle
- Bromocriptine—5 mg/day on days 10 through 26 of cycle
- Danazol—200 mg/day on days 19 through 28 of cycle
- Naproxen—550 mg bid on days 17 through 28 of cycle; Naprosyn—500 mg bid on days 17 through 28 of cycle

SUPPRESSION OF PSYCHOLOGIC SYMPTOMS:

- Nortriptyline—50 to 125 mg/day
- Fluoxetine—20 mg/day or 90 mg weekly (this medication has indications for premenstrual dysphoric disorder)
- Buspirone—10 mg bid or tid on days 16 through 28 of cycle, then taper drug
- Alprazolam—25 mg tid on days 16 through 28 of cycle, then taper drug
- Clonidine—0.1 mg bid
- Naltrexone—0.25 mg/day on days 9 through 18 of cycle
- Atenolol—50 mg/day
- Paroxetine—20 mg/day

- Sertraline (Zoloft)—50 to 100 mg/day
- Nefazodone (Serzone)—Initial dosage 100 mg bid; after 1 wk increase to 150 mg bid
- Propranolol—20 to 40 mg bid
- Verapamil—100 to 320 mg qd

CHRONIC Rx

- Therapy is largely trial and error, with the goal of providing effective treatment with the safest and most simple therapy.
- For severe intractable PMS: hysterectomy with bilateral oophorectomy; give trial of GnRH therapy or danazol before surgery.
- Estrogen replacement therapy recommended postoperatively to reduce the risk of osteoporosis, heart disease, and genitourinary atrophy.

DISPOSITION

Improved symptoms in 90% of women over time.

REFERRAL

- For counseling with a psychologist or psychiatrist if underlying psychiatric disorder is discovered (cognitive behavioral therapy)
- To a gynecologist if surgical therapy is contemplated

EVIDENCE

EBM

A systematic review showed inconsistent results for the benefit of magnesium supplements.[1] Ⓑ

The same systematic review found calcium to be more effective than placebo in reducing overall premenstrual syndrome symptoms. However, the reviewers concluded that the evidence was not compelling, due to methodologic limitations of the trial.[1] Ⓑ

The aforementioned systematic review also included trials using herbal medicine, homeopathy, dietary supplementation, relaxation, massage, reflexology, chiropractice, and biofeedback. The authors concluded that on the basis of the current evidence, no complementary or alternative therapy could be recommended as a treatment for premenstrual syndrome.[1] Ⓑ

There is a small but significant improvement in symptoms with progesterone treatment, but the clinical significance of this is uncertain, and the preferred route and timing of delivery remains unclear.[2] Ⓑ

Three randomized controlled trials (RCTs) have found that spironolactone is effective in improving irritability, breast tenderness, and bloating, and one trial failed to find it superior to placebo.[3-6] Ⓑ

Treatments for which there is good evidence often have significant side effects or potential harms.

GnRH analogs are effective in reducing premenstrual symptoms. Evidence suggests that the use of add-back estrogen and progesterone therapy is less effective than the use of GnRH analogs alone, but more effective than placebo, but the addition of tibolone to GnRH analogs provides no benefit.[7-9] Ⓐ Ⓑ

Alprazolam in daily doses of 0.75 mg and above are significantly more effective than placebo in reducing premenstrual symptoms. There is a risk of significant side effects with long-term use.[10] Ⓑ

There is good evidence to support the use of selective serotonin reuptake inhibitors in the management of severe premenstrual syndrome.

A systematic review has confirmed that selective serotonin reuptake inhibitors are significantly better at relieving premenstrual symptoms than placebo in women with severe premenstrual syndrome. However their long-term use in this chronic condition has not been extensively studied as yet.[11] Ⓐ

Evidence-Based References

1. Stevinson C, Ernst E: Complementary/alternative therapies for premenstrual syndrome: a systematic review of randomized controlled trials, *Am J Obstet Gynecol* 185:227, 2001. Reviewed in: *Clin Evid* 11:2507, 2004. Ⓑ
2. Wyatt K et al: Efficacy of progesterone and progestogens in management of premenstrual syndrome: systematic review, *BMJ* 323:776, 2001. Reviewed in: *Clin Evid* 11:2507, 2004. Ⓑ
3. Hellberg D, Claesson B, Nilsson S: Premenstrual tension: a placebo-controlled efficacy study with spironolactone and medroxyprogesterone acetate, *Int J Gynecol Obstet* 34:243, 1991. Reviewed in: *Clin Evid* 11:2507, 2004. Ⓐ
4. Vellacott ID et al: A double-blind, placebo-controlled evaluation of spironolactone in the premenstrual syndrome, *Curr Med Res Opin* 10:450, 1987. Reviewed in: *Clin Evid* 11:2507, 2004. Ⓐ
5. Wang M et al: Treatment of premenstrual syndrome by spironolactone: a double-blind, placebo-controlled study, *Acta Obstet Gynecol Scand* 74:803, 1995. Reviewed in: *Clin Evid* 11:2507, 2004. Ⓐ
6. Burnet RB et al: Premenstrual syndrome and spironolactone, *Aust NZ J Obstet Gynaecol* 31:366, 1991. Reviewed in: *Clin Evid* 11:2507, 2004. Ⓐ
7. Mortola JF, Girton L, Fischer U: Successful treatment of severe premenstrual syndrome by combined use of gonadotrophin-releasing hormone agonist and estrogen/progestin, *J Clin Endocrinol Metab* 72:252A, 1991. Reviewed in: *Clin Evid* 11:2507, 2004. Ⓑ
8. Mezrow G et al: Depot leuprolide acetate with estrogen and progestin add-back for long-term treatment of premenstrual syndrome, *Fertil Steril* 62:932, 1994. Reviewed in: *Clin Evid* 11:2507, 2004. Ⓑ
9. Wyatt K: Premenstrual syndrome. Reviewed in: *Clin Evid* 11:2507, 2004. Ⓐ
10. Di Carlo C et al: Use of leuprolide acetate plus tibolone in the treatment of severe premenstrual syndrome, *Fertil Steril* 75:380, 2001. Reviewed in: *Clin Evid* 11:2507, 2004. Ⓐ
11. Wyatt KM, Dimmock PW, O'Brien PMS: Selective serotonin reuptake inhibitors for premenstrual syndrome. Reviewed in: Cochrane Library 3, Oxford, 2004, Update Software. Ⓐ

SUGGESTED READINGS

Brown C: A new monophasic oral contraceptive containing drospirenone: effect on premenstrual symptoms, *J Reprod Med* 47(1):14, 2002.

Miner C, Brown E: Weekly luteal-phase dosing with enteric-coated fluoxetine 90 mg in premenstrual dysphoric disorder: a randomized, double blind, placebo-controlled clinical trial, *Clin Therapeut* 24(3):417, 2002.

Pearlstein T: Selective serotonin reuptake inhibitors for premenstrual dysphoric disorder: the emerging gold standard? *Drugs* 62(13):1869, 2002.

Wyatt K: Premenstrual syndrome, *Clin Evid* 7:338, 2002.

AUTHORS: **GEORGE T. DANAKAS, M.D.**, and **RUBEN ALVERO, M.D.**

BASIC INFORMATION

DEFINITION

Priapism is the persistent, usually painful, erection associated or unassociated with sexual stimulation. There are two major forms: low-flow (venoocclusive) priapism and high-flow priapism (associated with increased arterial inflow without increased venous outflow resistance).

ICD-9CM CODES
607.3 Priapism

EPIDEMIOLOGY & DEMOGRAPHICS

- Peak incidence is seen from ages 5 to 10 and 20 to 50 yr.
- In the younger group, priapism is often associated with sickle cell disease or neoplasm. In the older group it is often caused by pharmacologic agents.
- Low-flow (venoocclusive priapism [type I]) is much more common than high-flow (type II).

PHYSICAL FINDINGS & CLINICAL PRESENTATION

- In idiopathic priapism the initial erection is associated with prolonged sexual excitement. Previous transient episodes are frequently reported. The erection involves the corpora cavernosa alone. Detumescence does not occur spontaneously.
- In secondary priapism, sexual excitement need not be involved. Otherwise the clinical picture is the same as in idiopathic priapism.
- Table 1-36 compares normal erection and priapism.

ETIOLOGY

Idiopathic: prolonged sexual arousal
Secondary or associated causes:
- Sickle cell disease
- Diabetes
- Leukemia (especially chronic myelogenous leukemia)
- Solid tumor (malignant) penile infiltration
- Spinal cord injury
- Peineal or penile trauma

Iatrogenic
- TPN, which includes a fat emulsion
- Hyperosmolar IV contrast
- Spinal or general anesthesia
- Anticoagulant therapy
- Phenothiazines
- Trazodone
- Intracorporeal injection therapy for impotence
- Phosphodiesterase type 5 inhibitors (e.g., sildenafil [Viagra], tadalafil [Cialis], vardenafil [Levitra])

PATHOPHYSIOLOGY

- Low-flow priapism: prolonged erection leads to edema of the cavernosal trabeculae, resulting in a sequence of statis, thrombosis, venous occlusion, fibrosis, scarring, and possibly impotence.
- High-flow priapism: cavernosal artery rupture leading to an arteriocavernous fistula.

DIAGNOSIS

WORKUP

None if the associated underlying causes are known to be present. Otherwise they should be ruled out. Low-flow priapism can be distinguished from high-flow priapism by obtaining a corporeal blood gas value. A PO2 <30 mm Hg, PCO2 >60 mm Hg, and a pH <7.25 are consistent with low-flow priapism. High-flow priapism can be confirmed by a perineal Doppler ultrasound or arteriography (useful to identify arterial-lacunar fistula).

TREATMENT

Goal: achieve detumescence with preservation of potency.

1. Medical therapies:
   - Ice packs
   - Ice water enemas
   - Hot water enemas
   - Pressure dressing
   - Sedatives
   - Analgesics
   - Antispasmodic/anticholinergic drugs
   - Estrogens
   - Anticoagulants
   - Procaine
   - Amyl nitrite
   - Local or general anesthesia
   - Ketamine (1 mg/lb)
2. In the patient with sickle cell disease: intravenous hydration, alkalinization, transfusion or exchange-transfusion, oxygen.
3. Corporeal irrigation with normal saline may be used for low-flow priapism. The midshaft of the penis can be injected with a small-gauge butterfly needle and irrigated with 10 to 20 ml of normal saline, followed by an intracorporeal injection of an alpha-adrenergic agonist every 5 min until detumescence. Commonly used intracavernous vasoconstrictor agents are epinephrine (10 to 20 micrograms), phenylephrine (250 to 500 micrograms), and ephedrine (50 to 100 mg). It is mandatory to monitor the patient's blood pressure and pulse when using alpha-adrenergic agonists.
4. Surgery:
   - Cavernospongiosum shunt
   - Glans-cavernosum shunt
   - Cavernosaphenous shunt
   - In the less common situation of high-flow priapism (diagnosed by the finding of bright red arterial blood on aspiration), arterial embolization or surgical ligation is recommended.

PROGNOSIS

Impotence is associated with the duration of priapism, with 36 hr being an important threshold.

REFERRAL

To urologist

AUTHORS: **FRED F. FERRI, M.D.,** and **TOM J. WACHTEL, M.D.**

TABLE 1-36 Comparison of Normal Erection and Priapism

Factor	Normal Erection	Priapism
Portion of penis involved	Corpora cavernosa and corpus spongiosum and glans	Corpora cavernosa
Cause	Vasodilatation of penile arteries	Obstruction of venous outflow Disturbance of neuroarterial mechanism (imbalance between it and adrenergic activity) Increased viscosity
Sexual desire	Present	Absent
Pain	Absent	Present
Duration	Minutes to hours	Hours to days

From Nseyo UO (ed): *Urology for primary care physicians,* Philadelphia, 1999, WB Saunders.

BASIC INFORMATION

DEFINITION

Progressive supranuclear palsy (PSP) is a progressive degenerative disease of the central nervous system particularly affecting the brainstem and basal ganglia with core features of supranuclear ophthalmoplegia, rigidity, postural instability, and cognitive decline.

SYNONYMS

Steele-Richardson-Olszewski syndrome
Progressive supranuclear ophthalmoplegia

ICD-9CM CODES
333.0 Other degenerative diseases of the basal ganglia

EPIDEMIOLOGY & DEMOGRAPHICS

- Peak incidence is between ages 50 to 70.
- Onset is nearly always after age 40.
- Age-adjusted prevalence is 1.3 to 6.4 cases per 100,000.
- There is no gender predilection.

PHYSICAL FINDINGS & CLINICAL PRESENTATION

- Common early symptoms include slowness (bradykinesia) and stiffness, as well as falls.
- Differences from PD become more pronounced with progression. Tremor is present in only 5% to 10% of patients.
- Hallmark on examination is supranuclear gaze palsy; impaired voluntary conjugate eye movements, primarily on attempted up-and-down gaze.
- Predominantly axial rigidity leading to typical neck extension. This plus low blink rate and facial muscle contraction gives a characteristic appearance of "sustained surprise" (Fig. 1-214).
- Limb rigidity is typically proximal in contrast to the distal rigidity seen in idiopathic PD.
- Gait is slow and stiff, with marked postural instability leading to unheralded, often backward falls.

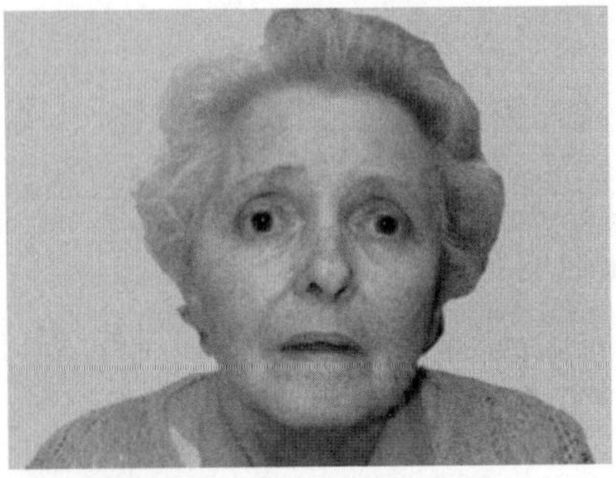

FIGURE 1-214 A patient with PSP, with staring expression, frontalis overactivity, and retrocolitis. She is wearing a neck sling for a fractured wrist sustained in a fall. (From Burn D, Lees A: Progressive supranuclear palsy: where are we now? *Lancet Neurol* 1:359, 2002.)

- Cognitive impairment is frequent and consists of mental slowness, irritability, and social withdrawal.

ETIOLOGY

Pathogenesis is believed to be related to accumulation of hyperphosphorylated tau protein in neurons and glia in basal ganglia and brainstem nuclei. In this regard, PSP is thought to be pathophysiologically related to frontotemporal dementia and corticobasal degeneration.

DIAGNOSIS

DIFFERENTIAL DIAGNOSIS

- Parkinson's disease—differs from PSP in which early falls are prominent, tremor is unusual, and there is very little response to levodopa.
- Cortical basal ganglionic degeneration—differentiated from PSP by presence of cortical sensory signs and asymmetrical limb apraxia.
- Multiple systems atrophy—differs from PSP by the presence of prominent autonomic symptoms and/or cerebellar signs.
- Dementia with Lewy bodies (DLB)—in PSP visual hallucinations typically only occur if provoked by dopaminergic therapy, whereas in DLB there are prominent visual hallucinations that may be spontaneous or provoked.

WORKUP

- Diagnosis is largely clinical. National Institute of Neurologic Disorders and Stroke (NINDS) provides inclusion and exclusion criteria. Mandatory exclusion criteria include:
  1. Recent history of encephalitis
  2. Cortical sensory deficits
  3. Hallucinations or delusions unrelated to dopaminergic therapy
  4. Cortical dementia of Alzheimer type
- There are no diagnostic laboratory tests at present.

LABORATORY TESTS

If there is a question of recent encephalitis, spinal fluid analysis may be indicated.

IMAGING STUDIES

- If atypical features such as unilateral symptoms or signs are present, brain MRI may be helpful in ruling out structural lesions.
- Conventional neuroimaging is often unable to differentiate PSP from the major differential diagnoses; however, use of volumetric measures of midbrain atrophy are gaining acceptance as a way to improve teh specificity of conventional MRI.
- Functional neuroimaging such as PET and SPECT show promise, but are not yet routinely indicated or available.

TREATMENT

NONPHARMACOLOGIC THERAPY

- Physical, occupational, and speech/swallowing therapies can be helpful for both patients and caregivers.
- Patients with significant dysphagia may require a feeding gastrostomy.

ACUTE GENERAL Rx

None available.

CHRONIC Rx

- Levodopa may be mildly helpful with rigidity and bradykinesia early in the disease course, but typically loses effectiveness quickly. Dopamine receptor agonists are not typically effective.
- Cholinesterase inhibitors have not been shown to help with the cognitive impairment.

DISPOSITION

Median survival after diagnosis is <10 yr.

REFERRAL

Referral to a general neurologist or movement disorders center is appropriate.

PEARLS & CONSIDERATIONS

COMMENTS

- Unheralded, often backward falling is one of the most common initial presentations.
- Poor downgaze is an especially helpful examination finding because upgaze palsy is common in normal aging.
- Poor or unsustained response to levodopa therapy suggests a diagnosis other than idiopathic Parkinson's disease.

PATIENT/FAMILY EDUCATION

Comprehensive movement disorders website with disease information as well as links to support and discussion groups: http://www.wemove.org

SUGGESTED READINGS

Burn D, Lees A: Progressive supranuclear palsy: where are we now? *Lancet Neurol* 1:359, 2002.

Kertesz A: Pick complex: an integrative approach to frontotemporal dementia: primary progressive aphasia, corticobasal degeneration, and progressive supranuclear palsy, *Neurologist* 9(6):311, 2003.

Oba H et al: New and reliable MRI diagnosis for progressive supranuclear palsy, *Neurology* 64:2050, 2005.

Pastor P, Tolosa E: Progressive supranuclear palsy: clinical and genetic aspects, *Curr Opin Neurol* 15:429, 2002.

AUTHOR: **DAVID P. WILLIAMS, M.D.**

BASIC INFORMATION

DEFINITION

Prolactinomas are monoclonal tumors that secrete prolactin.

ICD-9CM CODES

253.1 Forbes-Albright syndrome

EPIDEMIOLOGY & DEMOGRAPHICS

INCIDENCE: Most common pituitary tumor; nearly 30% of all pituitary adenomas secrete enough prolactin to cause hyperprolactinemia.

PREDOMINANT SEX: Microadenomas are more common in women; macroadenomas are more frequent in men.

PHYSICAL FINDINGS & CLINICAL PRESENTATION

MEN: Decreased facial and body hair, small testicles; may also have decreased libido, impotence, and delayed puberty (caused by decreased testosterone secondary to inhibition of gonadotropin secretion).

WOMEN: Physical examination may be normal; history may reveal amenorrhea, galactorrhea, oligomenorrhea, and anovulation.

BOTH SEXES: Visual field defects and headache may occur depending on size of tumor and its expansion.

ETIOLOGY

Prolactin-secreting pituitary adenomas: microadenomas (<10 mm diameter) or macroadenomas (>10 mm diameter)

DIAGNOSIS

DIFFERENTIAL DIAGNOSIS

Hyperprolactinemia may be caused by the following:

- Drugs: phenothiazines, methyldopa, reserpine, MAO inhibitors, androgens, progesterone, cimetidine, tricyclic antidepressants, haloperidol, meprobamate, chlordiazepoxide, estrogens, narcotics, metoclopramide, verapamil, amoxapine, cocaine, oral contraceptives
- Hepatic cirrhosis, renal failure, primary hypothyroidism
- Ectopic prolactin-secreting tumors (hypernephroma, bronchogenic carcinoma)
- Infiltrating diseases of the pituitary (sarcoidosis, histiocytosis)
- Head trauma, chest wall injury, spinal cord injury
- Polycystic ovary disease, pregnancy, nipple stimulation
- Idiopathic hyperprolactinemia, stress, exercise

WORKUP

- The diagnosis of prolactinoma is established by demonstration of an elevated serum prolactin level (after exclusion of other causes of hyperprolactinemia) and radiographic evidence of a pituitary adenoma.
  1. Normal mean prolactin levels are 8 ng/ml in women and 5 ng/ml in men.
  2. Levels >300 ng/ml are virtually diagnostic of prolactinomas.
  3. Prolactin levels can vary with time of day, stress, sleep cycle, and meals. More accurate measurements can be obtained 2 to 3 hr after awakening, preprandially, and when patient is not distressed.
  4. Serial measurements are recommended in patients with mild prolactin elevations.
- TRH stimulation test may be useful in equivocal cases. The normal response is an increase in serum prolactin levels by 100% within 1 hr of TRH infusion; failure to demonstrate an increase in prolactin level is suggestive of pituitary lesion.
- All patients with prolactinomas should undergo visual field testing. Serial evaluation is recommended, particularly during pregnancy in patients with macroadenomas.

IMAGING STUDIES

- MRI with gadolinium enhancement (Fig. 1-215) is the procedure of choice in the radiographic evaluation of pituitary disease.
- In absence of MRI, a radiographic diagnosis is best accomplished with a high-resolution CT scanner and special coronal cuts through the pituitary region.

TREATMENT

NONPHARMACOLOGIC THERAPY

Pregnancy and breast-feeding should be avoided, because they can encourage tumor growth.

ACUTE GENERAL Rx

- Management of prolactinomas depends on their size and encroachment on the optic chiasm and other vital structures, the presence or absence of gonadal dysfunction, and the patient's desires with respect to fertility.
- Medical therapy is preferred when fertility is an important consideration.
  1. Bromocriptine (Parlodel): Initial dose is 0.625 at hs for the first week. After 1 wk, add AM dose of 1.25 mg. Gradually increase dose by 1.25 mg/wk until dose of 5 to 10 mg/day is achieved; Bromocriptine decreases size of the tumor and generally lowers the prolactin level into the normal range when the initial serum prolactin is <500 ng/ml. Side effects of bromocriptine are nausea, constipation, dizziness, and nasal stuffiness. Bromocriptine appears to be safe during pregnancy.
  2. Cabergoline (Dostinex) is a longer-acting dopamine agonist that is more expensive but may be more effective and better tolerated than bromocriptine; initial dose is 0.25 mg twice weekly.
- Transsphenoidal resection: option in an infertile patient who cannot tolerate bromocriptine or cabergoline or when medical therapy is ineffective. The success rate depends on the location of the tumor (entirely intrasellar), experience of the neurosurgeon, and size of the tumor (<10 mm in diameter); the recurrence rate may reach 80% within 5 yr. Possible complications of transsphenoidal surgery include transient diabetes insipidus, hypopituitarism, CSF rhinorrhea, and infections (meningitis, wound infection).
- Pituitary irradiation is useful as adjunctive therapy of macroadenomas (>10 mm in diameter) and in patients with persistent hypersecretion following surgery. Potential complications include cranial nerve damage, radionecrosis, and cognitive abnormalities.
- Stereotactic radiosurgery (gamma knife) has become popular as a modality in the treatment of prolactinomas. A high dose of ionizing radiation is delivered to the tumor through multiple ports. Its advantage is minimal irradiation to surrounding tissues. Proximity of the tumor to the optic chiasm limits this therapeutic modality.

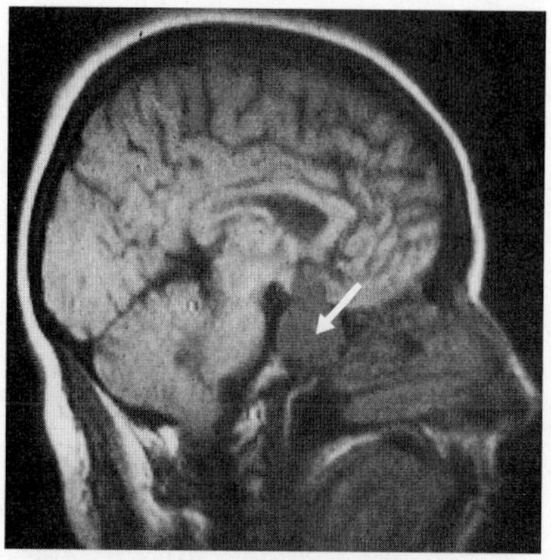

FIGURE 1-215 T1 Sagittal MRI depicting a large pituitary prolactinoma *(arrow)* in a 13-year-old girl presenting with headaches and galactorrhea. (From Grainger RG, Allison DJ, Adam A, Dixon AK [eds]: *Grainger & Allison's diagnostic radiology,* ed 4, Philadelphia, 2001, Churchill Livingstone.)

CHRONIC Rx

- Patients on medical therapy require periodic measurement of prolactin levels. An attempt to reduce the dose of bromocriptine or cabergoline can be made after the prolactin level has been normal for 2 yr. An MRI scan of the pituitary should be obtained to rule out tumor enlargement within 6 mo of initiation of tapering regimen.
- Evaluation and monitoring of pituitary function are recommended following transsphenoidal surgery.

DISPOSITION

- Transsphenoidal surgery will result in a cure in nearly 50% to 75% of patients with microadenomas and 10% to 20% of patients with macroadenomas.
- Nearly 20% of microprolactinomas resolve during long-term dopamine agonist treatment.

PEARLS & CONSIDERATIONS

COMMENTS

Patients must be monitored for several years after surgery, because up to 50% of microadenomas and nearly 90% of macroadenomas can recur.

EVIDENCE

Evidence for the treatment of prolactinoma is limited. High-quality trials for the main therapies mentioned in this medifile are lacking, although some small or nonrandomized trials exist. One retrospective study of 46 men with prolactinomas found that treatment with dopamine agonists (bromocriptine/carbegoline) normalized serum prolactin levels in approximately 80% of patients.[1] (B)

Treatment with dopamine agonists resulted in similar biochemical remission rates in men with microprolactinomas and macroprolactinomas.[1] (B)

The same study found that patients with macroadenomas treated with dopamine agonists required additional hormone replacement therapy. No patients with microadenomas required additional hormonal therapy.[1] (B)

One metaanalysis study of 271 patients with macroprolactinoma found that treatment with dopamine agonists (chiefly bromocriptine) produced useful tumor shrinkage in 79% of patients.[2] (B)

A study evaluated the outcome of cabergoline treatment in 52 male patients with prolactinomas. It found that after 24 months of treatment with carbegoline, serum prolactin levels had normalized in 75% of patients and no patients had galactorrhea. Restoration of normal ACTH, growth hormone, and testosterone levels was achieved in approximately 60% of patients.[3] (A)

A randomized controlled trial (RCT) compared the use of carbegoline vs. bromocriptine in the treatment of amenorrhea in 479 females with hyperprolactinema, 282 of whom had prolactinomas. It found that carbegoline produced significantly greater stable normal prolactin levels compared with bromocriptine. Restoration of normal ovulation was significantly better with carbegoline.[4] (B)

Withdrawal of carbegoline therapy in patients with prolactinomas, after normalization of prolactin levels and clinical evidence of tumor shrinkage, can be undertaken. However, such patients must be carefully monitored for at least 36 months to assess possible tumor recurrence.[5] (B)

Evidence-Based References

1. Pinzone JJ et al: Primary medical therapy of micro- and macroprolactinomas in men, *J Clin Endocrinol Metab* 86:1838, 2001. (B)
2. Bevan JS et al: Dopamine agonists and pituitary tumor shrinkage, *Endocr Rev* 13:220, 1992. (B)
3. Colao A et al: Outcome of cabergoline treatment in men with prolactinoma: effects of a 24-month treatment on prolactin levels, tumor mass, recovery of pituitary function, and semen analysis, *J Clin Endocrinol Metab* 89:1704, 2004. (A)
4. Webster J et al: A comparison of cabergoline and bromocriptine in the treatment of hyperprolactinemic amenorrhea. Cabergoline Comparative Study Group, *N Engl J Med* 331:904, 1994. (B)
5. Colao A et al: Withdrawal of long-term cabergoline therapy for tumoral and nontumoral hyperprolactinemia, *N Engl J Med* 349:2023, 2003. (B)

SUGGESTED READINGS

Leung A, Pacaud D: Diagnosis and management of galactorrhea, *Am Fam Physician* 70:543, 2004.

Schlechte JA: Prolactinoma, *N Engl J Med* 349:2035, 2003.

AUTHOR: **FRED F. FERRI, M.D.**

BASIC INFORMATION

DEFINITION

A form of compression neuropathy of the median nerve in the proximal forearm caused primarily by the pronator teres muscle. Occasionally, only the anterior interosseus motor branch is affected, sometimes causing a very specific separate clinical presentation.

SYNONYMS

Kiloh-Nevin syndrome (anterior interosseus syndrome)

ICD-9CM CODES
354.1 Median nerve entrapment
354.9 Mononeuritis of upper limb

EPIDEMIOLOGY & DEMOGRAPHICS

PREDOMINANT SEX:
Males = females

INCIDENCE:
Rare (≤1% median nerve entrapment disorders). Most common in dominant arm

PHYSICAL FINDINGS & CLINICAL PRESENTATION

- Forearm discomfort and fatigue, often resulting from repetitive pronation
- Insidious onset
- Nocturnal paresthesias are not typical
- Vague numbness in hand, primarily in thumb and index finger, may be present
- Tenderness and enlargement of the pronator teres may be present
- Tinel's sign may be positive at the site of compression
- Although there are no reliable provocative tests, painful paresthesias may occasionally be elicited with forced pronation of the forearm against resistance
- Motor impairment is rare

Anterior interosseus nerve syndrome:
- Forearm pain and weakness
- Patient may be unable to form a circle when trying to pinch the index finger and thumb because of inability to flex distal phalanges of thumb and index finger
- Sensation to the hand is not affected

ETIOLOGY

- Localized anatomic compression
- Trauma
- Traumatic cut down or phlebotomy

DIAGNOSIS

DIFFERENTIAL DIAGNOSIS

- Carpal tunnel syndrome
- Cervical disc syndrome with radiculopathy
- Tendon rupture
- Tendinitis

WORKUP

- Electrodiagnostic studies may be helpful; they are indicated if symptoms persist longer than 4 to 6 wk or if motor weakness is suspected
- Plain radiography to rule out bony abnormalities causing compression

TREATMENT

- Rest, bracing of forearm, sling
- Stretching exercises, physical therapy
- NSAIDs

DISPOSITION

Patients whose symptoms are mainly subjective often respond to nonsurgical management. Motor deficits may not be reversible in spite of surgery.

REFERRAL

Surgical referral in cases of failed medical management or when motor weakness is present

PEARLS & CONSIDERATIONS

COMMENTS

Prognosis for recovery is good. When indicated, surgical intervention is most effective if the diagnosis can be firmly established by objective testing.

SUGGESTED READINGS

Bridgeman C et al: Clinical and electrophysiological presentation of pronator syndrome, *Electromyogr Clin Neurophysiol* 47(2):89, 2007.

Cain EL et al: Elbow injuries in throwing athletes: a current concepts review, *Am J Sports Med* 31(4):621, 2003.

Rehak DC: Pronator syndrome, *Clin Sports Med* 20(3):531, 2001.

Sellards R, Kuebrich C: The elbow: diagnosis and treatment of common injuries, *Prim Care* 32(1):1, 2005.

AUTHOR: **LONNIE R. MERCIER, M.D.**

BASIC INFORMATION

DEFINITION AND CLASSIFICATION

Prostate cancer is a neoplasm involving the prostate; various classifications have been developed to evaluate malignancy potential and prognosis:

- The degree of malignancy varies with the stage

Stage A: Confined to the prostate, no nodule palpable
Stage B: Palpable nodule confined to the gland
Stage C: Local extension
Stage D: Regional lymph nodes or distant metastases

- In the Gleason classification, two histologic patterns are independently assigned numbers 1 to 5 (best to least differentiated). These numbers are added to give a total tumor score between 2 and 10. Prognosis is best for highly differentiated tumors (e.g., Gleason score 2 to 4) as compared with most poorly differentiated tumors (Gleason score 7 to 10).
- Another commonly used classification is the Tumor-Node-Metastasis (TNM) classification of prostate cancer.

ICD-9CM CODES
185 Malignant neoplasm of prostate

EPIDEMIOLOGY & DEMOGRAPHICS

- Prostate cancer has surpassed lung cancer as the most common non-skin cancer in men.
- More than 100,000 cases are diagnosed yearly, and nearly 30,000 males die from prostate cancer each year (second leading cause of death from cancer in U.S. men).
- Incidence of prostate cancer increases with age: uncommon <50 yr; 80% of new cases are diagnosed in patients ≥65 yr.
- Average age at time of diagnosis is 72 yr.
- Blacks in the U.S. have the highest incidence of prostate cancer in the world (1 in every 9 males).
- Incidence is low in Asians.
- Approximately 9% of all prostate cancers may be familial.
- Mortality rates of prostate cancer have declined substantially in the past 15 yr from 34% in 1990 to <20% currently.

PHYSICAL FINDINGS & CLINICAL PRESENTATION

- Generally silent disease until it reaches advanced stages.
- Bone pain and pathologic fractures may be initial symptoms of prostate cancer.
- Local growth can cause symptoms of outflow obstruction.
- Digital rectal examination (DRE) may reveal an area of increased firmness; 10% of patients will have a negative DRE.
- Prostate may be hard, fixed, with extension of tumor to the seminal vesicles in advanced stages.

DIAGNOSIS

DIFFERENTIAL DIAGNOSIS

- Benign prostatic hypertrophy
- Prostatitis
- Prostate stones

LABORATORY TESTS

- Measurement of PSA is controversial in early diagnosis of prostate cancer. Normal PSA is found in >20% of patients with prostate cancer, whereas only 20% of men with PSA levels between 4 ng/ml and 10 ng/ml have prostate cancer. The American Cancer Society recommends offering the PSA test and digital rectal examination yearly to men 50 yr or older who have a life expectancy of at least 10 yr. Earlier testing, starting at age 45, is recommended for men at high risk (e.g., blacks, men with family history of prostate cancer). An isolated elevation in PSA level should be confirmed several weeks later before proceeding with further testing, including prostate biopsy.
- Free PSA: the use of serum-free PSA for prostate screening has been proposed by some urologists as a means to decrease unwarranted biopsies without missing a significant number of prostate cancers. This approach is based on the higher free PSA in men with benign prostatic hyperplasia and the higher protein-bound PSA levels in men with prostate cancer. For example, in men with total PSA levels of 4 to 10 ng/ml, the cancer probability is 0.25, but if the percentage of free PSA is ≤17%, the probability of cancer increases to 0.45.
- PSA velocity: the rate of increase of serum PSA (PSA velocity) can aid in the diagnosis of prostate cancer. A yearly PSA velocity >0.75 ng/ml increases the likelihood of later malignancy when total PSA is still within normal range. Proper interpretation of PSA velocity requires at least three PSA measurements over an 18-month period because most PSA variations are physiologic.
- Age-adjusted PSA: there is evidence that the current threshold of 4.0 ng/ml is inadequate for younger men, because in a recent study 22% of men with PSA levels between 2.6 and 4.0 were found to have prostate cancer. The concept of age-related cutoffs remains controversial. Lowering the upper limit of normal for PSA would improve sensitivity but decrease specificity.
- Prostatic acid phosphatase (PAP) can be used for evaluation of nonlocalized disease.
- Transrectal biopsy and fine-needle aspiration of prostate can confirm the diagnosis. Indications for biopsy include an abnormal PSA level, an abnormal digital rectal exam (DRE), or a previous biopsy specimen that showed prostatic intraepithelial neoplasia (PIN) or prostatic atypia. The number of cores taken is patient specific, typically including a minimum of 10 cores. Prostate volume negatively affects cancer detection rate (23% in glands >50 cm^3, 38% in glands <50 cm^3).

IMAGING STUDIES

- Bone scan is useful to evaluate bone metastasis (present or eventually develops in almost 80% of patients). However, according to the American Urological Association (AUA), the routine use of bone scanning is not required for staging of prostate cancer in asymptomatic men with clinically localized cancer if the PSA level is ≤20 ng/ml.
- CT scan, MRI, and transrectal ultrasonography may be useful in selected patients to assess extent of prostate cancer. High-resolution MRI with magnetic nanoparticles has been used for the detection of small and otherwise undetectable lymph-node metastases in patients with prostate cancer. However, according to the AUA, transrectal ultrasonography adds little to the combination of PSA and digital rectal examination. Similarly, CT and MRI imaging are generally not indicated for cancer staging in men with clinically localized cancer and PSA <25 ng/ml. With regard to pelvic lymph node dissection in staging, the AUA states that it may not be required in patients with PSA levels <10 ng/ml and when PSA level is <20 ng/ml and the Gleason score is <6.

TREATMENT

NONPHARMACOLOGIC THERAPY

Watchful waiting is reasonable in selected patients with early-stage (T-IA) and projected life expectancy <10 yr or in patients with focal and moderately differentiated carcinoma.

ACUTE GENERAL Rx

- Therapeutic approach varies with the following:
  1. Stage of the tumor
  2. Patient's life expectancy

3. General medical condition
4. Patient's treatment preference (e.g., patient may be opposed to orchiectomy)

- The optimal treatment of clinically localized prostate cancer is unclear.
  1. Radical prostatectomy is generally performed in patients with localized prostate cancer and life expectancy >10 yr. Radical prostatectomy reduces disease-specific mortality, overall mortality, and the risks of metastasis and local progression. The absolute reduction in the risk of death after 10 yr is small, but the reductions in the risks of metastasis and local tumor progression are substantial. Postoperative complications of radical prostatectomy include urinary incontinence (10%-20% depending on degree of neurovascular bundle and urethral preservation, patient age, and correct mucosal apposition) and erectile dysfunction (percentage exceeds 50% and varies with patient age, preoperative erectile dysfunction, stage of tumor at time of surgery, and preservation of neurovascular bundle). Lower complication rates occur in hospitals that perform a large number of prostatectomies. Fewer men will have postsurgical erectile dysfunction after unilateral or bilateral nerve-sparing surgery.
  2. Radiation therapy (external beam irradiation or brachytherapy with implantation of radioactive pellets [iodine-125 or palladium-103 seeds] into the prostate gland) represents an alternative in patients with localized prostate cancer, especially poor surgical candidates or patients with a high-grade malignancy. The efficacy of brachytherapy is comparable to external radiation. In patients receiving external beam radiation, a total dose of 79.2 Gy (high dose) as compared with a total dose of 70.2 Gy (conventional dose) has been reported to lower the risk of recurrence without increased risk of morbidity and mortality. Patients with localized prostate cancer and high risk for extraprostatic disease and disease recurrence (e.g., Gleason score ≥7 with multiple positive biopsy cores and clinical stage T1b-T2b) may benefit (increased overall survival) with the addition of 6 mo of androgen suppression therapy to radiation therapy.
  3. Watchful waiting is reasonable in patients who are too old or too ill to survive longer than 10 yr. If the cancer progresses to the point where it becomes symptomatic, palliation can be attempted with several methods. Conservative management is also reasonable for patients with Gleason 2 to 4 cancer because these patients do not have a shortened life expectancy, and treatment is associated with long-term side effects.
- Patients with advanced disease and projected life expectancy <10 yr are candidates for radiation therapy and hormonal therapy (DES, LHRH analogs, antiandrogens, bilateral orchiectomy).
- Recommended treatment of patients with regional metastatic prostate cancer with projected life expectancy ≥10 yr includes radiation therapy, hormonal therapy.
- Androgen-deprivation therapy (ADT) with a gonadotropin-releasing hormone agonist is the mainstay of treatment for metastatic prostate cancer. Adverse effects of ADT include decreased libido, impotence, hot flashes, osteopenia with increased fracture risk, metabolic alterations, and changes in mood and cognition. Adjuvant treatment with GnRH agonists (goserelin leuprolide, or triptorelin) plus antiandrogens (flutamide, bicalutamide, or nilutamide), when started simultaneously with external irradiation, improves local control and survival in patients with locally advanced prostate cancer. Pamidronate inhibits osteoclast-mediated bone resorption and prevents bone loss in the hip and lumbar spine in men receiving treatment for prostate cancer with a GnRH. Abarelix (Plenaxis) is an injectable GnRH agonist useful to suppress testosterone in patients with prostate cancer who are not good candidates for LHRH agonists and refuse surgical castration. Assessment of bone density and treatment with once-weekly oral alendronate can prevent and improve the bone loss that occurs in men receiving ADT for prostate cancer.
- Docetaxel plus prednisone or doxacetel plus estramustine can be used in metastatic hormone-refractory prostate cancer.

CHRONIC Rx

- Patients should be monitored at 3- to 6-mo intervals with clinical examination, and PSA for the first year, then every 6 mo for the second year, then yearly if stable. For patients who have undergone radical prostatectomy, a rising PSA level suggests evidence of residual or recurrent prostate cancer. Salvage radiotherapy may potentially cure patients with disease recurrence after radical prostatectomy.
- Chest x-ray and bone scan should be performed yearly or sooner if patient develops symptoms.

DISPOSITION

- Prognosis varies with the stage of the disease (see "Definition") and the Gleason classification (see "Definition"). For patients between 65 and 69 yr of age at diagnosis and a Gleason score of 2 to 4, the probability of dying from prostate cancer 15 yr after diagnosis is 0.06 and that of dying from other causes is 0.56. If the Gleason score is 7 to 10, the probability of dying from prostate cancer increases up to 0.72 and from other causes varies from 0.25 to 0.36.
- The ploidy of the tumor also has prognostic value: prognosis is better with diploid tumor cells, worse with aneuploid tumor cells.
- For grade 1 tumors, the extended 10-yr, disease-specific survival is similar for patients with prostatectomy (94%), radiotherapy (90%), and conservative management (93%); survival rate is better with surgery than with radiotherapy or conservative management in patients with grade 2 or 3 localized prostate cancer.
- Expression of the gene *EZH2* has been identified as an important factor in the determination of the aggressiveness of prostate cancer. A recent study revealed that expression of the *EZH2* gene may be a better predictor of clinical failure than Gleason score, tumor stage, or surgical margin status. Testing for *EZH2* protein in prostate cancer tissue may be useful to determine prognosis and direct treatment.
- Preoperative PSA level and PSA velocity have prognostic significance. Men whose PSA level increases by >2.0 μg/ml during the year before the diagnosis of cancer may have a relatively high risk of death from prostate cancer despite undergoing radical prostatectomy.
- Extraprostatic disease is detected at radical prostatectomy in 38% to 52% of patients and is associated with a risk of disease recurrence, progression, and death. In these patients, adjuvant radiotherapy results in significantly reduced risk of PSA relapse and disease recurrence; however, the improvements in metastases-free survival and overall survival are not statistically significant.

EVIDENCE

EBM

Any benefits of radical prostatectomy need to be balanced with potential harms

A systematic review including two randomized controlled trials (RCTs) comparing radical prostatectomy with watchful waiting in men with localized disease was unable to show any difference in death rates from any cause. However, the larger trial found a significant reduction in death rates at 6 years due to prostate cancer with surgery vs. watchful waiting. Twenty to seventy percent reported sexual dysfunction and 15% to 50% reported urinary difficulties after radical prostatectomy.[1] Ⓐ

More evidence should result from the completion of the U.S. Prostatectomy Intervention Versus Observation Trial (PIVOT), which started in 1994 and is scheduled for 12 to 15 years.

One RCT comparing radical prostatectomy vs. external beam radiation for men with either localized or locally advanced disease found that radical prostatectomy significantly increased prostate cancer specific survival rates vs. external beam radiation after 5 years.[1] Ⓐ

Another RCT comparing radical prostatectomy vs. external beam radiation therapy in men with clinically localized prostate cancer found that prostatectomy was associated with a lower risk of metastatic disease.[2] Ⓐ

The outcome of watchful waiting varies widely according to the stage at presentation and the degree of differentiation of the tumor

Two large prospective clinical cohort studies found that watchful waiting was associated with a 15-year disease-specific survival rate of 80% in men with clinically localized disease. This ranged from 95% for well-differentiated tumors to 30% for poorly differentiated tumors.[3,4] Ⓐ

Androgen deprivation therapy is effective in prolonging survival among men with prostate cancer outside the capsule

A systematic review found that early androgen deprivation improved overall 5-year survival compared with deferred treatment in patients with locally advanced prostate cancer who were receiving external beam radiation therapy.[5] Ⓐ

An RCT compared immediate androgen deprivation vs. delayed androgen deprivation in men with node-positive disease following radical prostatectomy. There was a significant improvement in survival and a reduction in recurrence in the immediate-treatment group.[6] Ⓐ

An RCT compared immediate androgen deprivation (at time of diagnosis) vs. delayed androgen deprivation (at time of disease progression) in men with stage C or D prostate cancer. Disease-related mortality was significantly reduced in patients with stage C disease receiving immediate treatment, and the risk of major complications was also reduced.[7] Ⓐ

Inconclusive evidence from systematic reviews suggests that combined androgen blockade (androgen deprivation plus nonsteroidal antiandrogen) improves survival in patients with metastatic prostate cancer compared with androgen deprivation alone.[8] Ⓐ

An RCT found no significant difference between orchiectomy, radiotherapy, and both treatments in combination for overall survival or need for further treatment of local disease progression in patients with locally advanced prostate cancer.[9] Ⓐ

The evidence for different forms of androgen deprivation for metastatic prostate cancer has produced similar overall survival rates

A systematic review compared different forms of androgen deprivation (diethylstilbestrol, orchiectomy, and GnRH agonists) in men with metastatic prostate cancer. There were no significant differences between the therapies in terms of overall progression-free survival, time to progression, or overall survival.[10] Ⓐ

Patients with symptomatic metastatic prostate cancer (androgen independent) may benefit from chemotherapy

RCTs have shown that some men have reduced pain and prolonged palliation with chemotherapy, but there is no evidence of improved survival.[8] Ⓐ

Evidence-Based References

1. Harris RP et al: Screening for prostate cancer. Systematic Evidence Review no. 16. Rockville, MD, 2001, Agency for Healthcare Research and Quality. Reviewed in: *Clin Evid* 13:1128, 2005. Ⓐ
2. Paulson DF et al. and the Uro-Oncology Research Group: Radical surgery versus radiotherapy for adenocarcinoma of the prostate, *J Urol* 128:502-504, 1982. Reviewed in: *Clin Evid* 11:1169-1185, 2004. Ⓐ
3. Albertsen PC et al: Competing risk analysis of men aged 55 to 74 years at diagnosis managed conservatively for clinically localized prostate cancer, *JAMA* 280:975-980, 1998. Reviewed in: *Clin Evid* 11:1169-1185, 2004. Ⓐ
4. Lu-Yao GL, Yao S: Population-based study of long-term survival in patients with clinically localized prostate cancer, *Lancet* 349:906-910, 1997. Reviewed in: *Clin Evid* 11:1169-1185, 2004. Ⓐ
5. Agency for Health Care Policy and Research: Relative effectiveness and cost-effectiveness of methods of androgen suppression in the treatment of advanced prostatic cancer: summary. Rockville, MD: Agency for Health Care Policy and Research, 1999. Reviewed in: *Clin Evid* 11:1169-1185, 2004. Ⓐ
6. Messing EM et al: Immediate hormonal therapy compared with observation after radical prostatectomy and pelvic lymphadenectomy in men with node-positive prostate cancer, *N Engl J Med* 341:1781-1789, 1999. Reviewed in: *Clin Evid* 11:1169-1185, 2004. Ⓐ
7. Medical Research Council Prostate Cancer Working Party Investigators Group: Immediate versus deferred treatment for advanced prostatic cancer: initial results of the Medical Research Council Trial, *Br J Urol* 79:235-246, 1997. Reviewed in: *Clin Evid* 11:1169-1185, 2004. Ⓐ
8. Michaelson MD, Smith MR, Talcott JA: Prostate cancer (metastatic). Reviewed in: *Clin Evid* 11:1158-1168, London, 2004, BMJ Publishing Group. Ⓐ
9. Fellows GJ et al: Treatment of advanced localised prostatic cancer by orchiectomy, radiotherapy, or combined treatment, *Br J Urol* 70:304-309, 1992. Reviewed in: *Clin Evid* 11:1169-1185, 2004. Ⓐ
10. Seidenfeld J et al: Single-therapy androgen suppression in men with advanced prostate cancer: a systematic review and meta-analysis, *Ann Intern Med* 132:566-577, 2000. Reviewed in: *Clin Evid* 11:1158-1168, 2004. Ⓐ

SUGGESTED READINGS

Bill-Axelson A et al: Radical prostatectomy versus watchful waiting for early prostate cancer, *N Engl J Med* 352:1977-1984, 2005.

Freenspan S et al: Effect of once-weekly oral alendronate on bone loss in men receiving androgen deprivation therapy for prostate cancer, *Ann Intern Med* 146:416, 2007.

Hoffman RM et al: Health outcomes in older men with localized prostate cancer: results from the prostate cancer outcomes study, *Am J Med* 119:418, 2006.

Petrylak DP et al: Docetaxel and estramustine compared with mitoxantrone and prednisone for advanced prostate cancer, *N Engl J Med* 351:1513-1520, 2005.

Routh JC, Leibovich BC: Adenocarcinoma of the prostate: epidemiological trends, screening, diagnosis, and surgical management of localized disease, *Mayo Clin Proc* 80(7):899-907, 2005.

Sanda MG et al: Quality of life and satisfaction with outcome among prostate cancer survivors, *N Engl J Med* 358:1250-1261, 2008.

Sharifi N et al: Androgen deprivation therapy for prostate cancer, *JAMA* 294:238-244, 2005.

Tannock IF et al: Docetaxel plus prednisone or mitoxantrone plus prednisone for advanced prostate cancer, *N Engl J Med* 351:1502-1512, 2005.

Thompson IM et al: Adjuvant radiotherapy for pathologically advanced prostate cancer, *JAMA* 296:2329, 2006.

Walczak J, Carducci M: Prostate cancer: a practical approach to current management of recurrent disease, *Mayo Clin Proc* 82(2):243, 2007.

Walsh PC et al: Localized prostate cancer, *N Engl J Med* 357:26, 2007.

Wilt TS et al: Systematic review: comparative effectiveness and harms of treatments for clinically localized prostate cancer, *Ann Intern Med* 148:435-448, 2008.

AUTHOR: **FRED F. FERRI, M.D.**

BASIC INFORMATION

DEFINITION

Benign prostatic hyperplasia is the benign growth of the prostate, generally originating in the periureteral and transition zones, with subsequent obstructive and irritative voiding symptoms.

SYNONYMS

BPH
Prostatic hypertrophy

ICD-9CM CODES
600 Benign prostatic hyperplasia

EPIDEMIOLOGY & DEMOGRAPHICS

- 80% of men have evidence of benign prostatic hypertrophy by age 80 yr.
- Medical and surgical intervention for problems caused by BPH is required in >20% of males by age 75 yr.
- Transurethral resection of the prostate (TURP) is the tenth most common operative procedure (>400,000/yr in U.S.).
- 10% to 30% of men with BPH have occult prostate cancer.

PHYSICAL FINDINGS & CLINICAL PRESENTATION

- Digital rectal examination (DRE) reveals enlargement of the prostate.
- Focal enlargement may be indicative of malignancy.
- There is poor correlation between size of prostate and symptoms (BPH may be asymptomatic if it does not encroach on the urethral lumen).
- Most patients with BPH complain of difficulty in initiating urination (hesitancy), decrease in caliber and force of stream, incomplete emptying of bladder often resulting in double voiding (need to urinate again a few minutes after voiding), postvoid "dribbling," and nocturia.

ETIOLOGY

Multifactorial; a functioning testicle is necessary for development of BPH (as evidenced by the absence in males who were castrated before puberty).

DIAGNOSIS

DIFFERENTIAL DIAGNOSIS

- Prostatitis
- Prostate cancer
- Strictures (urethral)
- Medication interfering with the muscle fibers in the prostate and also with bladder function

WORKUP

Symptom assessment (use of American Urological Association [AUA] Symptom Index for BPH [Table 1-37]), laboratory tests, and imaging studies

LABORATORY TESTS

- Prostate specific antigen (PSA): protease secreted by epithelial cells of the prostate; elevated in 30% to 50% of patients with BPH. Testing for PSA increases detection rate for prostate cancer and tends to detect cancer at an earlier stage. However, the PSA test does not discriminate well between patients with symptomatic BPH and those with prostate cancer, particularly if the cancers are pathologically localized and curable. The test may also trigger additional evaluation, including ultrasound biopsy of the prostate. Asymptomatic men with PSA levels <2 ng/ml do not need annual testing. According to the AUA, PSA testing and digital rectal examination should be offered to any asymptomatic man older than 50 yr of age with a life expectancy of 10 yr. PSA testing can also

TABLE 1-37 International Prostate Symptom Score (I-PSS)

SCORE							
Symptom	**Not At All**	**Less Than 1 Time in 5**	**Less Than Half the Time**	**About Half the Time**	**More Than Half the Time**	**Almost Always**	**Total Score**
Incomplete emptying: Over the past month, how often have you had a sensation of not emptying your bladder completely after you finished urinating?	0	1	2	3	4	5	
Frequency: Over the past month, how often have you had to urinate again <2 hr after you finished urinating?	0	1	2	3	4	5	
Intermittency: Over the past month, how often have you found you stopped and started again several times when you urinated?	0	1	2	3	4	5	
Urgency: Over the past month, how often have you found it difficult to postpone urination?	0	1	2	3	4	5	
Weak stream: Over the past month, how often have you had a weak urinary stream?	0	1	2	3	4	5	
Straining: Over the past month, how often have you had to push or strain to begin urination?	0	1	2	3	4	5	
	None	**1 Time**	**2 Times**	**3 Times**	**4 Times**	**5 or More Times**	
Nocturia: Over the past month, how many times did you most typically get up to urinate from the time you went to bed at night until the time you got up in the morning?	0	1	2	3	4	5	
Total I-PSS score =							

be offered at an earlier age in men at higher risk of prostatic cancer (e.g., first-degree relatives with prostate cancer; black men)
- Measurement of "free" PSA is useful to assess the probability of prostate cancer in patients with normal digital rectal examination and total PSA between 4 and 10 ng/ml. In these patients the global risk of prostate cancer is 25%; however, if the free PSA is >25%, the risk of prostate cancer decreases to 8%, whereas if the free PSA is <10%, the risk of cancer increases to 56%. Free PSA is also useful to evaluate the aggressiveness of prostate cancer. A low free PSA percentage generally indicates a high-grade cancer, whereas a high free PSA percentage is generally associated with a slower growing tumor
- Urinalysis, urine C&S to rule out infection (if suspected)
- BUN and creatinine to rule out postrenal insufficiency

IMAGING STUDIES

- Transrectal ultrasound may be indicated in patients with palpable nodules or significant elevation of PSA. It is also useful to estimate prostate size. BPH may also be evident in suprapubic ultrasound and MRI (Fig. 1-216).
- Uroflowmetry may be used to determine relative impact of obstruction on urine flow. Urethral pressure profile is useful to predict prostatic hypertrophy within the urethral lumen.
- Pressure flow studies, although invasive, are particularly helpful in patients whose history and/or examination suggest primary bladder dysfunction as a cause of symptoms of prostatism. They are also useful in patients for whom a distinction between prostatic obstruction and impaired detrusor contractility may affect the choice of therapy. However, pressure flow studies may not be useful in the workup of the usual patient with symptoms of prostatism.
- Postvoid residual urine measurement has not been proved useful in predicting the need for or response to treatment; may be useful in monitoring the course of the disease in patients who elect nonsurgical treatment.
- Urethral cystoscopy is an option during later evaluation if invasive treatment is being planned.

TREATMENT (Rx)

NONPHARMACOLOGIC THERAPY

- Avoidance of caffeine or any other foods that may exacerbate symptoms
- Avoidance of medications that may exacerbate symptoms (e.g., most cold and allergy remedies)

GENERAL Rx

- Asymptomatic patients with prostate enlargement caused by BPH generally do not require treatment. Patients with mild to moderate symptoms are candidates for pharmacologic treatment (see below). For those patients who have specific complications from BPH, prostate surgery is usually the most appropriate form of treatment. However, surgery may result in significant complications (e.g., incontinence, infection).
- TURP is the most commonly used surgical procedure for BPH. Transurethral incision of the prostate (TUIP), a procedure almost equivalent in efficacy, is limited to patients whose estimated resection tissue weight would be 30 g or less. TUIP can be performed in an ambulatory setting or during a 1-day hospitalization. Open prostatectomy is typically performed on patients with very large prostates.
- Laser therapy for BPH is a less invasive alternative to TURP; however, recent studies indicate that at least in the initial 7 mo after surgery, TURP is moderately more effective than laser therapy in relieving symptoms of BPH.
- Surgery need not be treatment of last resort for most patients; that is, patients need not undergo other treatments for BPH before they can have surgery. However, recommending surgery on the grounds that a patient's surgical risk will "only increase with age" is generally inappropriate.
- Balloon dilation of the prostatic urethra is less effective than surgery for relieving symptoms but is associated with fewer complications. It is a reasonable treatment option for patients with smaller prostates and no middle lobe enlargement.
- The dietary supplement saw palmetto is effective in relieving BPH symptoms in patients with mild obstruction.
- α-Blockers (e.g., tamsulosin [Flomax], alfuzosin [Uroxatral], doxazosin, prazosin, and terazosin) relax smooth muscle of the bladder neck and prostate and can increase peak urinary flow rate. They have no effect on the size of the prostate. α-1 blockers are useful in symptomatic patients to relieve symptoms of obstruction by causing relaxation of smooth muscle tone in the prostatic capsule and urethra and bladder neck.
- Hormonal manipulation with finasteride (Proscar), a 5-α-reductase inhibitor that blocks conversion of testosterone to dihydrotestosterone, can reduce the size of the prostate. Usual dose is 5 mg qd. Treatment requires 6 mo or more for maximal effect.
- Dutasteride (Avodart) is also a 5-α-reductase inhibitor useful to decrease prostate size and improve urinary flow. In addition to inhibiting the isoform of 5-α-reductase located in the prostate, the medication also inhibits a second isoform and reduces DHT formation in the skin and liver. Usual dose is 0.5 mg qd.
- Saw palmetto is commonly used for relief of symptoms of BPH. Recent trials using 160 mg of saw palmetto bid did not improve symptoms of BPH. This contrasts with the positive findings of many previous studies. Trials with higher dose-ranging protocols are currently in progress.

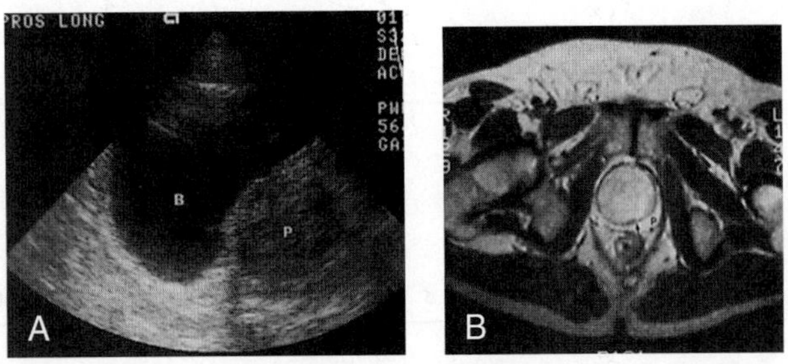

FIGURE 1-216 Benign prostatic nodular hyperplasia. A, US (suprapubic abdominal approach) and **B,** T2-weighted MRI. On US the prostate *(P)* demonstrates uniform low-level acoustic reflectivity, while on the MRI the adenomatous enlargement of the prostate and the peripheral zone *(P)* can be distinguished. The two are separated by a low-intensity surgical pseudocapsule *(arrow)*. (From Grainger RG, Allison DJ, Adam A, Dixon AK [eds]: *Grainger & Allison's diagnostic radiology,* ed 4, Philadelphia, 2001, Churchill Livingstone.)

CHRONIC Rx

- Avoid medications and foods that exacerbate symptoms.
- Symptomatic improvement occurs in >70% of patients with proper treatment.

DISPOSITION

With appropriate therapy, symptoms improve or stabilize in >70% of patients with BPH.

REFERRAL

Urology referral for patients with severe or intolerable symptoms and for any patient suspected of having prostate cancer (10% to 30% of men with BPH).

PEARLS & CONSIDERATIONS

COMMENTS

- Emerging technologies for treating BPH include lasers, coils, stents, thermal therapy, and hyperthermia. Laser prostatectomy appears promising; however, long-term effectiveness has not yet been demonstrated.
- The increase in the use of pharmacologic management has resulted in more than 30% reduction in the total number of transurethral resections of the prostate.

EVIDENCE

Alpha blockers are effective in the management of BPH and may be more effective than 5-α-reductase inhibitors (finasteride).

Three systematic reviews of randomized controlled trials (RCTs) found that alpha blockers are more effective than placebo in relieving symptoms of BPH.[1-3] Ⓐ

One of the reviews noted there was comparable efficacy among the alpha blockers on the basis of three trials, which included tamsulosin vs. alfuzosin, alfuzosin vs. prazosin, and tamsulosin vs. terazosin.[2] Ⓐ

Two RCTs compared finasteride with an alpha blocker and with both treatments combined. The trials found that the alpha blocker was associated with a greater reduction in symptoms than finasteride and that addition of finasteride to alpha-blocking therapy conferred no additional benefit. Neither trial selected patients on the basis of prostate size.[4,5] Ⓐ

There is evidence for the efficacy of 5-α-reductase inhibitors (finasteride and dutasteride) in the management of BPH, and they may be most useful for men with large prostates.

A systematic review found that finasteride was significantly more effective than placebo at reducing symptom scores.[3] Ⓐ

A nonsystematic review also found that treatment with finasteride was significantly more effective than placebo at reducing symptom scores and that the benefit over placebo was greatest in men with larger prostates (40 g or more).[6] Ⓐ

Another nonsystematic review (a meta-analysis) found that finasteride vs. placebo reduced the 2-year risk of acute urinary retention and of progression to prostatectomy.[7] Ⓐ

A large RCT compared finasteride with placebo in men with symptomatic BPH. After 4 years, finasteride vs. placebo significantly reduced symptoms, the risk of acute urinary retention (AUR), or the need for prostatectomy. The risk reduction was greatest in men with a higher baseline level of prostate-specific antigen (reflecting larger prostates). Further follow-up at 6 years found the decrease in the incidence of AUR- or BPH-related surgery was sustained in those that had continued on finasteride.[8,9] ⒶⒷ

A good-quality RCT with mean follow-up of 4.5 years, in men with moderate to severe symptoms and an average prostate volume of 31 ml, found the risk of overall clinical progression was significantly reduced by both doxazosin alone (39% risk reduction) and finasteride alone (34% risk reduction), and that combination therapy (doxazosin and finasteride together) produced a significantly better risk reduction (66%) than either drug used alone. The particular risks of acute retention and the need for invasive therapy were significantly reduced by combination therapy and finasteride alone, but not by doxazosin alone.[10] Ⓑ

Daily dutasteride (a dual inhibitor of the 5-α-reductase isoenzymes types 1 and 2) was compared with placebo in men with benign prostatic hyperplasia. At 24 months, treatment with dutasteride was associated with a significant reduction in serum dihydrotestosterone, prostate volume, and symptoms, and a significant increase in maximum urinary flow rates. The risk of acute urinary retention and the need for surgical intervention was also reduced compared with placebo.[11] Ⓑ

There is limited evidence that TURP is more effective than watchful waiting for improving symptoms and reducing complications. There is no evidence for any significant difference in outcome between TURP and TUIP. TURP is more effective than transurethral needle ablation (TUNA) but is associated with more adverse effects.

TURP has been found to be associated with more symptomatic improvement and lower rates of treatment failure than watchful waiting.[12,13] Ⓐ

There is little clear evidence that TURP is more effective than laser therapy or electrical vaporization.[14] Ⓐ

A systematic review found no significant difference between TURP and TUIP in terms of symptom scores at 1 year. The review found little good evidence for longer-term results.[15] Ⓐ

TURP was found to be associated with more symptomatic improvement than TUNA. However, TURP was also associated with increased incidence of retrograde ejaculation and bleeding.[16] Ⓐ

Transurethral microwave therapy (TUMT) is more effective than sham treatment or terazosin for the treatment of BPH.

Three RCTs comparing TUMT with sham treatment found that TUMT improved symptoms more than sham treatment.[17-19] Ⓐ

Transurethral microwave therapy (TUMT) has been shown to produce significantly more symptomatic improvement than terazosin at both 6 and 18 months.[20,21] Ⓐ

Symptoms of BPH may be effectively treated with saw palmetto.

A systematic review found that saw palmetto provides mild to moderate improvement in urinary symptoms and flow measures compared with placebo and has efficacy comparable with that of finasteride.[22] Ⓐ

Symptoms and flow measures have been improved in BPH with the use of beta-sitosterols.

A systematic review assessing the use of nonglucosidic beta-sitosterols for the treatment of mild to moderate BPH showed that urinary symptoms and flow measures were improved, although the long-term effectiveness and safety of beta-sitosterols are not known.[23] Ⓐ

Pygeum africanum may be a useful treatment option for men with lower urinary symptoms consistent with BPH.

A systematic review showed that compared with placebo, *Pygeum africanum* provided a moderately large improvement in overall symptoms, although the trials were small in size, of short duration, and different methods of reporting outcomes were used.[24] Ⓐ

Evidence-Based References

1. Wilt TJ, MacDonald R, Rutks I: Tamsulosin for benign prostatic hyperplasia, *Cochrane Database Syst Rev* 4, 2002. Ⓐ
2. Djavan B, Marberger M: A meta-analysis on the efficacy and tolerability of alpha-1 adrenoceptor antagonists in patients with lower urinary tract symptoms suggestive of benign prostatic obstruction, *Eur Urol* 36:1, 1999. Reviewed in *Clin Evid* 11:1119, 2004. Ⓐ
3. Clifford GM, Farmer RD: Medical therapy for benign prostatic hyperplasia: a review of the literature, *Eur Urol* 38:2, 2000. Reviewed in: *Clin Evid* 11:1119, 2004. Ⓐ

4. Lepor H, Williford WO, Barry MJ: The efficacy of terazosin, finasteride, or both in benign prostatic hyperplasia. Veterans Affairs Cooperative Studies Benign Prostatic Hyperplasia Study Group, *N Engl J Med* 335:533, 1996. Reviewed in: *Clin Evid* 11:1119, 2004. Ⓐ
5. Debruyne FMJ et al: Sustained-release alfuzosin, finasteride and the combination of both in the treatment of benign prostatic hyperplasia, *Eur Urol* 34:169, 1998. Reviewed in: *Clin Evid* 11:1119, 2004. Ⓐ
6. Boyle P, Gould AL, Roehrborn CG: Prostate volume predicts outcome of treatment of benign prostatic hyperplasia with finasteride: meta-analysis of randomized clinical trials, *Urology* 48:398, 1996. Reviewed in: *Clin Evid* 11:1119, 2004. Ⓐ
7. Andersen JT et al: Finasteride significantly reduces acute urinary retention and need for surgery in patients with symptomatic benign prostatic hyperplasia, *Urology* 49:839, 1997. Reviewed in: *Clin Evid* 11:1119, 2004. Ⓐ
8. McConnell J et al: The effect of finasteride on the risk of acute urinary retention and the need for surgical treatment among men with benign prostatic hyperplasia, *N Engl J Med* 338:557, 1998. Reviewed in: *Clin Evid* 11:1119, 2004. Ⓐ
9. Roehrborn CG et al: Proscar Long-Term Efficacy and Safety Study Group. Sustained decrease in incidence of acute urinary retention and surgery with finasteride for 6 years in men with benign prostatic hyperplasia, *J Urol* 171:1194, 2004. Ⓑ
10. McConnell JD et al: Medical Therapy of Prostatic Symptoms (MTOPS) Research Group. The long-term effect of doxazosin, finasteride, and combination therapy on the clinical progression of benign prostatic hyperplasia, *N Engl J Med* 349:2387, 2003. Reviewed in: Bandolier, Knowledge Library. Ⓐ
11. Roehrborn CP et al: Efficacy and safety of a dual inhibitor of 5 alpha reductase types 1 and 2 (dutasteride) in men with benign prostatic hyperplasia, *Urology* 60:434, 2002. Ⓑ
12. Wasson JH et al: A comparison of transurethral surgery (TURP) with watchful waiting for moderate symptoms of benign prostatic hyperplasia. The Veterans Affairs Cooperative Study Group on Transurethral Resection of the Prostate, *N Engl J Med* 332:75, 1995. Reviewed in: *Clin Evid* 11:1119, 2004. Ⓐ
13. Donovan JL et al: A randomized trial comparing transurethral resection of the prostate, laser therapy and conservative treatment of men with symptoms associated with benign prostatic enlargement: the ClasP study, *J Urol* 164:65, 2000. Reviewed in: *Clin Evid* 11:1119, 2004. Ⓐ
14. Webber R: Benign prostatic hyperplasia, *Clin Evid* 11:1119, 2004. Ⓐ
15. Yang Q et al: Transurethral incision compared with transurethral resection of the prostate for bladder outlet obstruction: a systematic review and meta-analysis of randomized controlled trials, *J Urol* 165:1526, 2001. Reviewed in: *Clin Evid* 11:1119, 2004. Ⓐ
16. Bruskewitz R et al: A prospective, randomized 1-year clinical trial comparing transurethral needle ablation to transurethral resection of the prostate for the treatment of symptomatic benign prostatic hyperplasia, *J Urol* 159:1588, 1998. Reviewed in: *Clin Evid* 11:1119, 2004. Ⓐ
17. Roehrborn CG et al: Microwave thermotherapy for benign prostatic hyperplasia with the Dornier Urowave: results of a randomized, double blind, multicenter, sham-controlled trial, *Urology* 51:19, 1998. Reviewed in: *Clin Evid* 11:1119, 2004. Ⓐ
18. Larson T et al: A high-efficiency microwave thermoablation system for the treatment of benign prostatic hyperplasia: results of a randomized, sham-controlled, prospective, double-blind, multicenter clinical trial, *Urology* 51:731, 1998. Reviewed in: *Clin Evid* 11:1119, 2004. Ⓐ
19. de la Rosette J et al: Transurethral microwave thermotherapy (TUMT) in benign prostatic hyperplasia: placebo versus TUMT, *Urology* 44:58, 1994. Reviewed in: *Clin Evid* 11:1119, 2004. Ⓐ
20. Djavan B et al: Prospective randomized comparison of high energy transurethral microwave thermotherapy versus alpha blocker treatment of patients with benign prostatic hyperplasia, *J Urol* 161:139, 1999. Reviewed in: *Clin Evid* 11:1119, 2004. Ⓐ
21. Djavan B et al: Targeted transurethral microwave thermotherapy versus alpha-blockade in benign prostatic hyperplasia: outcomes at 18 months, *Urology* 57:66, 2001. Reviewed in: *Clin Evid* 11:1119, 2004. Ⓐ
22. Wilt T, Ishani A, MacDonald R: Serenoa repens for benign prostatic hyperplasia, *Cochrane Database Syst Rev* 3:2002. Ⓐ
23. Wilt T et al: Beta-sitosterols for benign prostatic hyperplasia, *Cochrane Database Syst Rev* 3, 1999. Ⓐ
24. Wilt T et al: Pygeum africanum for benign prostatic hyperplasia, *Cochrane Database Syst Rev* 1, 1998. Ⓐ

SUGGESTED READINGS

AUA Practice Guidelines Committee: AUA guideline on management of benign prostatic hyperplasia, *J Urol* 170:2003.
Bent S et al: Saw palmetto for benign prostatic hyperplasia, *N Engl J Med* 354:557, 2006.
Lepor H: Insights into the natural history and treatment of benign prostatic hyperplasia, *J Urol* 175:815, 2006.

AUTHOR: **FRED F. FERRI, M.D.**

BASIC INFORMATION

DEFINITION

Prostatitis refers to inflammation of the prostate gland. There are four major categories:

- Acute bacterial prostatitis (type I)
- Chronic bacterial prostatitis (type II)
- Chronic prostatitis/pelvic pain syndrome (CP/CPPS) (type III): subdivided in type IIIA (inflammatory) and IIIB (noninflammatory)
- Asymptomatic inflammatory prostatitis (type IV)

ICD-9CM CODES
601.0 Prostatitis (acute)
601.1 Prostatitis (chronic)
099.54 Prostatitis (chlamydial)

EPIDEMIOLOGY & DEMOGRAPHICS

- 50% of men experience symptoms of prostatitis in their lifetime.
- Acute bacterial prostatitis is uncommon.
- The prevalence of chronic bacterial prostatitis is 5% to 10%.
- Chronic prostatitis/pelvic pain syndrome (CP/CPPS) is the most common of the clinically defined prostatitis syndromes, with the prevalence of the syndrome ranging from 9% to 12% among men.

PHYSICAL FINDINGS & CLINICAL PRESENTATION

ACUTE BACTERIAL PROSTATITIS:

- Sudden or rapidly progressive onset of:
  1. Dysuria
  2. Frequency
  3. Urgency
  4. Nocturia
  5. Perineal pain that may radiate to the back, the rectum, or the penis
- Hematuria or a purulent urethral discharge may occur.
- Occasionally urinary retention complicates the course.
- Fever, chills, and signs of sepsis can also be part of the clinical picture.
- On rectal examination the prostate is typically tender.

CHRONIC BACTERIAL PROSTATITIS:

- Characterized by positive culture of expressed prostatic secretions. May cause symptoms such as suprapubic, low back, or perineal pain, mild urgency, frequency, and dysuria with urination, and may be associated with recurrent urinary tract infections.
- May be asymptomatic when the infection is confined to the prostate.
- May present as an increase in severity of baseline symptoms of benign prostatic hypertrophy.
- When cystitis is also present, urinary frequency, urgency, and burning may be reported.
- Hematuria may be a presenting complaint.
- In elderly men, new onset of urinary incontinence may be noted.

CHRONIC PROSTATITIS/CHRONIC PAIN SYNDROME:

- Presents similarly with pain in the pelvic region lasting more than 3 mo. Symptoms also can include pain in the suprapubic region, low back, penis, testes, or scrotum.
- The symptoms can be of variable severity and may include lower urinary tract symptoms, sexual dysfunction, and reduced quality of life.

ETIOLOGY

ACUTE BACTERIAL PROSTATITIS:

- Acute usually gram-negative infection of the prostate gland.
  1. Generally associated with cystitis
  2. Resulting from the ascent of bacteria in the urethra
- Occasionally the route of infection is hematogenous or a lymphatogenous spread of rectal bacteria.
- The condition is seen in young or middle-aged men.

CHRONIC BACTERIAL PROSTATITIS:

- Often asymptomatic.
- Exacerbation of symptoms of benign prostatic hypertrophy caused by the same mechanism as in acute bacterial prostatitis.

CHRONIC PROSTATITIS/CHRONIC PAIN SYNDROME:

- Type IIIA: refers to symptoms of prostatic inflammation associated with the presence of WBCs in prostatic secretions with no identifiable bacterial organism.
- Chlamydia infection may be etiologically implicated in some cases.
- Type IIIB: refers to symptoms of prostatic inflammation with no or few WBCs in the prostatic secretion.
- Its cause is unknown. Spasm in the bladder neck or urethra may be responsible for the symptoms.

DIAGNOSIS

DIFFERENTIAL DIAGNOSIS

- Benign prostatic hypertrophy with lower urinary tract symptoms
- Prostate cancer
- Also see differential diagnosis of hematuria

WORKUP

- Rectal examination:
  1. Tender prostate most suggestive of acute bacterial prostatitis.
  2. Enlarged prostate common in chronic bacterial prostatitis.
  3. Normal prostate is consistent with chronic bacterial prostatitis and chronic prostatitis/chronic pain syndrome.
- Expression of prostatic secretions (EPS) by prostate massage is contraindicated in acute bacterial prostatitis but is appropriate in the other three situations.

LABORATORY TESTS

- Urinalysis.
- Urine culture and sensitivity.
- Bacterial localization studies can be performed but are cumbersome and impractical in most clinical settings.
- Cell count and culture of expressed prostatic secretions.
- The yield of a urine culture may be increased if the specimen is obtained after a prostatic massage.
- PSA is not used to diagnose prostatitis and is not recommended unless a nodule is present on digital examination. A rapid rise over baseline should raise the possibility of prostatitis even in the absence of symptoms. In such cases, a follow-up PSA after treatment of prostatitis is appropriate.
- CBC and blood cultures if fever, chills, or signs of sepsis exist.
- If hematuria is present, a workup to rule out a urologic malignancy should be considered if the hematuria does not clear after treatment of prostatitis.

TREATMENT

ACUTE BACTERIAL PROSTATITIS

Culture-guided antibiotic therapy for 4 wk (beginning with a few days of intravenous antibiotics if the infection is serious or if the patient is bacteremic)

CHRONIC BACTERIAL PROSTATITIS

- Trimethoprim-sulfamethoxazole is first line choice for 4 wk if the organism is sensitive.
- Second line choice for treatment failure or organisms resistant to TMP-SMX is with a quinolone.
- Patient with refractory infection or with multiple relapses may be offered long-term suppressive therapy.

CHRONIC PROSTATITIS/ CHRONIC PAIN SYNDROME

- No specific treatment. A brief course of NSAIDs may be tried until urine localization cultures are completed.
- Antibiotics are not effective and should be avoided in patients who are afebrile and have normal urinalysis results.
- A trial of treatment with an alpha-adrenergic blocker (terazosin, doxazosin, or tamsulosin) may be considered, but recent trials failed to show a significant reduction in symptoms.
- Contributing factors (e.g., stress, neuromuscular factors) should be addressed.
- Any underlying bladder pathology should be ruled out by cystoscopy and treated if identified.

AUTHORS: **FRED F. FERRI, M.D.,** and **TOM J. WACHTEL, M.D.**

BASIC INFORMATION

DEFINITION

Pruritus ani refers to an intense chronic itching of the anus and perianal skin.

ICD-9CM CODES
698.0 Pruritus ani

EPIDEMIOLOGY & DEMOGRAPHICS

- Any age can be affected.
- Occurs in 1% to 5% of the population.
- Male to female predominance of 4:1.

PHYSICAL FINDINGS & CLINICAL PRESENTATION

- Anal itching
- Anal fissures
- Hemorrhoids
- Excoriations
- Pinworms
- Fecal incontinence

ETIOLOGY

ANORECTAL DISEASES AND FECAL CONTAMINATION:
- Diarrhea
- Anal incontinence
- Hemorrhoids
- Fissures
- Fistulae
- Rectal prolapse
- Malignancy: Bowen's disease, epidermoid cancer, perianal Paget's disease

INFECTIONS:
- Fungal: candidiasis, dermatophytes
- Parasitic: pinworms, scabies
- Bacterial: *Staphylococcus aureus,* erythrasma
- Lymphogranuloma venereum
- Granuloma inguinale
- Chancroid
- Molluscum contagiosa
- Trichomoniasis
- Venereal: herpes, gonococcal syphilis, human papillomavirus

LOCAL IRRITANTS:
- Moisture, obesity, excessive perspiration
- Soaps, hygiene products
- Toilet paper: perfumed, dyed
- Underwear: irritating fabrics, detergents
- Anal creams, suppositories
- Dietary: coffee, beer, acidic foods
- Drugs: mineral oil, ascorbic acid, hydrocortisone sodium succinate, quinine, colchicine

DERMATOLOGIC DISEASES:
- Psoriasis
- Atopic dermatitis
- Seborrheic dermatitis

Section II also describes the various causes of pruritus ani.

DIAGNOSIS (Dx)

DIFFERENTIAL DIAGNOSIS

- Allergies
- Anxiety
- Dermatologic conditions
- Infections
- Parasites
- Diabetes mellitus
- Chronic liver disease
- Neoplasia
- Proctalgia fugax

WORKUP

- Detailed history regarding bowel habits, hygiene, use of perfumed products, and medical history
- Inspection of perianal area
- Possible biopsy to exclude neoplasia
- Microscopic inspection of scrapings
- Colposcopy of perineum

LABORATORY TESTS

- Chemistry profile
- Urinalysis
- Cultures
- Stool for ova and parasites
- Tape test
- Glucose tolerance test, if necessary

TREATMENT (Rx)

NONPHARMACOLOGIC THERAPY

- Avoidance of tight, nonporous clothing and underclothing
- Discontinuation or curtailment of coffee, beer, citrus fruits, tomatoes, chocolate, and tea
- Cleansing of anal area after bowel movements with a premoistened pad or tissue and avoidance of perfumes and dyes present in toilet paper and soaps
- Avoidance of excessive perspiration
- Aggressive management of fecal leakage or incontinence to avoid soiling of perianal skin

ACUTE GENERAL Rx

- Minimization of frequent loose stools with antidiarrheals and fiber agents if appropriate
- Use of a 1% hydrocortisone cream sparingly bid during the acute phase of pruritus ani but not for >2 wk to avoid atrophy
- Treatment of predisposing factors, such as parasites, diabetes, liver disease, hemorrhoids, and other infections

CHRONIC Rx

- Possible complications: excoriation and secondary bacterial infection; must be treated aggressively
- Long-standing, intractable pruritus ani: good response to intracutaneous injections of methylene blue and other agents, steroid injection

DISPOSITION

- Usually good results with total resolution of symptoms
- In some, persistent and recurrent symptoms

REFERRAL

To colorectal specialist if conservative measures fail

SUGGESTED READING

Heard S: Puritus ani, *Aust Fam Physician* 33(7):511, 2004.

AUTHORS: **MARIA A. CORIGLIANO, M.D.,** and **RUBEN ALVERO, M.D.**

BASIC INFORMATION

DEFINITION

Pruritus vulvae refers to intense itching of the female external genitalia.

SYNONYMS

Vulvodynia

ICD-9CM CODES
698.1 Pruritus of genital organs

EPIDEMIOLOGY & DEMOGRAPHICS

- A female disorder that can affect women at any age
- Young girls: infection is usually causative
- Postmenopausal women: frequently affected because of hypoestrogenic state

PHYSICAL FINDINGS & CLINICAL PRESENTATION

Constant intense itching or burning of the vulva

ETIOLOGY

- About 50% are caused by monilial infection or trichomoniasis.
- Other infectious causes are herpes simplex, condylomata acuminata, and molluscum contagiosum.
- Other causes:
  1. Infestations with scabies, pediculosis pubis, and pinworms
  2. Dermatoses such as hypertrophic dystrophy, lichen sclerosus, lichen planus, and psoriasis
  3. Neoplasms such as Bowen's disease, Paget's disease, and squamous cell carcinoma
  4. Allergic or chemical dermatitis caused by dyes in clothing or toilet paper, detergents, contraceptive gels, vaginal medications, douches, or soaps
  5. Vulvar or vaginal atrophy
- Severe pruritus is probably caused by degeneration and inflammation of terminal nerve fibers.
- Most intense itching occurs with hyperplastic lesions.
- Children (75%) nonspecific pruritus, lichen sclerosus, bacterial infections, yeast infection, and pinworm infestation.

DIAGNOSIS

DIFFERENTIAL DIAGNOSIS

- Vulvitis
- Vaginitis
- Lichen sclerosus
- Squamous cell hyperplasia
- Pinworms
- Vulvar cancer
- Syringoma of the vulva

WORKUP

- Inspection of vulva, vagina, and perianal area looking for infection, fissures, ulcerations, induration, or thick plaques
- Must rule out trichomoniasis, candidiasis, bacterial vaginosis, allergy, vitamin deficiencies, diabetes

LABORATORY TESTS

- Wet prep of saline and KOH of vaginal discharge
- Tape test to look for pinworms
- Vaginal cultures
- Biopsy when needed

TREATMENT

NONPHARMACOLOGIC THERAPY

- Keep vulva clean and dry.
- Wear white cotton panties.
- Avoid perfumes and body creams over vulvar area because they can cause irritation.
- Reduce stress.
- Apply wet dressings with aluminum acetate (Burow's) solution frequently.
- Avoid coffee and caffeine-containing beverages, chocolate, tomatoes.
- Sitz baths may be helpful.

ACUTE GENERAL Rx

Need to treat underlying problem:

- Yeast infection: any of the vaginal creams or Diflucan 150-mg one-time dose
- Trichomoniasis or *Gardnerella vaginalis:* Flagyl 500 mg or 375 mg PO bid for 7 days
- Urinary tract infection: treatment of specific organism
- Estrogen replacement therapy if atrophy is the cause of pruritus
- Pinworms: mebendazole (Vermox) 100 mg one tablet at diagnosis and repeated in 1 to 2 wk; also treat other members in family >2 yr of age
- Squamous cell hyperplasia: local application of corticosteroids
  1. One of the high- or medium-potency corticosteroids (0.025% or 0.01% fluocinolone acetonide or 0.01% triamcinolone acetonide) can be used to relieve itching.
  2. Rub into vulva bid or tid for 4 to 6 wk.
  3. Once itching is controlled, fluorinated steroid can be discontinued and patient can be switched to hydrocortisone preparation.
- Lichen sclerosus: topical 2% testosterone in petrolatum massaged into the vulvar tissue bid or tid; Temovate (clobetasol propionate gel 0.05%) cream tid × 5 days is very effective
- Treatment with immune response modifiers

CHRONIC Rx

- If not relieved by topical measures: intradermal injection of triamcinolone (10 mg/ml diluted 2:1 saline) 0.1 ml of the suspension injected at 1-cm intervals and tissue gently massaged
- If symptoms still uncontrollable: SC injection of absolute alcohol 0.1 ml at 1-cm intervals

DISPOSITION

Usually controlled with conservative measures and topical steroids

REFERRAL

To a gynecologist for further workup if conservative measures do not give relief

SUGGESTED READINGS

Boardman LA et al: Recurrent vulvar itching, *Obstet Gynecol* 105(6):1451, 2005.

Welch B et al: Vulval itch, *Aust Fam Physcian* 33(7):505, 2004.

AUTHORS: **MARIA A. CORIGLIANO, M.D.,** and **RUBEN ALVERO, M.D.**

BASIC INFORMATION

DEFINITION

Pseudogout is one of the clinical patterns associated with a crystal-induced synovitis resulting from the deposition of calcium pyrophosphate dehydrate (CPPD) crystals in joint hyaline and fibrocartilage. The cartilage deposition is termed *chondrocalcinosis.*

SYNONYMS

Calcium pyrophosphate dehydrate crystal deposition disease (CPDD)
Chondrocalcinosis
Pyrophosphate arthropathy

ICD-9CM CODES
275.4 Chondrocalcinosis

EPIDEMIOLOGY & DEMOGRAPHICS

PREVALENCE:
- Uncertain
- Probably similar to gout (3/1000 persons)
- Chondrocalcinosis is present in >20% of all people at age 80 yr, but most are asymptomatic

PREDOMINANT SEX: Female:male ratio of approximately 1.5:1

PREDOMINANT AGE: 60 to 70 yr at onset

PHYSICAL FINDINGS & CLINICAL PRESENTATION

- Symptoms are similar to those of gouty arthritis with acute attacks and chronic arthritis
- Knee joint is most commonly affected
- Swelling, stiffness, and increased heat in affected joint

ETIOLOGY

- Unknown
- Often associated with various medical conditions, including hyperparathyroidism and amyloidosis

DIAGNOSIS

DIFFERENTIAL DIAGNOSIS

- Gouty arthritis
- Rheumatoid arthritis
- Osteoarthritis
- Neuropathic joint

Section II describes the differential diagnosis of acute monoarticular and oligoarticular arthritis and crystal-induced arthritides. An algorithm for evaluation of arthralgia is described in Section III, "Arthralgia Limited to One or Few Joints."

WORKUP

- Variable clinical presentation
- Diagnosis dependent on the identification of CPPD crystals
- The American Rheumatism Association revised diagnostic criteria for CPPD crystal deposition disease (pseudogout) are often used:

1. Criteria
   - I. Demonstration of CPPD crystals (obtained by biopsy, necroscopy, or aspirated synovial fluid) by definitive means (e.g., characteristic "fingerprint" by x-ray diffraction powder pattern or by chemical analysis)
   - II. (a) Identification of monoclinic and/or triclinic crystals showing either no or only a weakly positive birefringence by compensated polarized light microscopy
     (b) Presence of typical calcifications in roentgenograms
   - III. (a) Acute arthritis, especially of knees or other large joints, with or without concomitant hyperuricemia
     (b) Chronic arthritis, especially of knees, hips, wrists, carpus, elbow, shoulder, and metacarpophalangeal joints, especially if accompanied by acute exacerbations; the following features are helpful in differentiating chronic arthritis from osteoarthritis:
       1. Uncommon site—for example, wrist, MCP, elbow, shoulder
       2. Appearance of lesion radiologically—for example, radiocarpal or patellofemoral joint space narrowing, especially if isolated (patella "wrapped around" the femur)
       3. Subchondral cyst formation
       4. Severity of degeneration—progressive, with subchondral bony collapse (microfractures), and fragmentation, with formation of intraarticular radiodense bodies
       5. Osteophyte formation—variable and inconstant
       6. Tendon calcifications, especially Achilles, triceps, obturators
2. Categories

Definite—Criteria I or II (a) plus (b) must be fulfilled.
Probable—Criteria II(a) or II(b) must be fulfilled.
Possible—Criteria III(a) or (b) should alert the clinician to the possibility of underlying CPPD deposition.

LABORATORY TESTS

Crystal analysis of the synovial fluid aspirate to reveal rhomboid calcium pyrophosphate crystals

IMAGING STUDIES

Plain radiographs to reveal the following:
- Stippled calcification in bands running parallel to the subchondral bone margins
- Crystal deposition in menisci, synovium, and ligament tissue; triangular wrist cartilage and symphysis pubis are often affected

TREATMENT

NONPHARMACOLOGIC THERAPY

General measures such as heat, rest, and elevation as needed

ACUTE GENERAL Rx

- NSAIDs (as for gout)
- Colchicine
- Aspiration/steroid injection

DISPOSITION

Structural joint damage may occasionally occur, requiring arthroplasty in rare cases.

REFERRAL

For orthopedic consultation for destructive joint changes

PEARLS & CONSIDERATIONS

COMMENTS

As with gout, acute attacks may be triggered by various surgical or medical events.

SUGGESTED READINGS

Liote F, Ea HK: Recent developments in crystal-induced inflammation pathogenesis and management, *Curr Rheumatol Rep* 9(3):243, 2007.

McGonagle D et al: Successful treatment of resistant pseudogout with anakinra, *Arthritis Rheum* 58:631, 2008.

Mader B: Calcium pyrophosphate dihydrate deposition disease of the wrist, *Clin Rheumatol* 23(1):95, 2004.

Rosenthal AK: Crystal arthropathies and other unpopular rheumatic diseases, *Curr Opin Rheumatol* 16(3):262, 2004.

Wise CM: Crystal-associated arthritis in the elderly, *Rheum Dis Clin North Am* 33(1):33, 2007.

AUTHOR: **LONNIE R. MERCIER, M.D.**

BASIC INFORMATION

DEFINITION

Pseudomembranous colitis is the occurrence of diarrhea and bowel inflammation associated with antibiotic use.

SYNONYMS

Antibiotic-induced colitis

ICD-9CM CODES
008.45 *Clostridium difficile,* pseudomembranous colitis

EPIDEMIOLOGY & DEMOGRAPHICS

- Cephalosporins are the most frequent offending agent in pseudomembranous colitis because of their high rates of use.
- The antibiotic with the highest incidence is clindamycin (10% incidence of pseudomembranous colitis with its use).
- *Clostridium difficile* is responsible for approximately 3 million cases of diarrhea and colitis in the U.S. every year.

PHYSICAL FINDINGS & CLINICAL PRESENTATION

- Abdominal tenderness (generalized or lower abdominal)
- Fever
- In patients with prolonged diarrhea, poor skin turgor, dry mucous membranes, and other signs of dehydration may be present

ETIOLOGY

Risk factors for *C. difficile* (the major identifiable agent of antibiotic-induced diarrhea and colitis):

- Administration of antibiotics: can occur with any antibiotic, but occurs most frequently with clindamycin, ampicillin, and cephalosporins
- Prolonged hospitalization
- Advanced age
- Abdominal surgery
- Hospitalized, tube-fed patients are at risk for *C. difficile*–associated diarrhea. Clinicians should consider testing for *C. difficile* in tube-fed patients with diarrhea unrelated to the feeding solution

DIAGNOSIS

The clinical signs of pseudomembranous colitis generally include diarrhea, fever, and abdominal cramps following use of antibiotics.

DIFFERENTIAL DIAGNOSIS

- GI bacterial infections (e.g., *Salmonella, Shigella, Campylobacter, Yersinia*)
- Enteric parasites (e.g., *Cryptosporidium, Entamoeba histolytica*)
- IBD
- Celiac sprue
- Irritable bowel syndrome
- Ischemic colitis
- Antibiotic intolerance

WORKUP

- All patients with diarrhea accompanied by current or recent antibiotic use should be tested for *C. difficile* (see "Laboratory Tests").
- Sigmoidoscopy (without cleansing enema) may be necessary when the clinical and laboratory diagnosis is inconclusive and the diarrhea persists.
- In antibiotic-induced pseudomembranous colitis, the sigmoidoscopy often reveals raised white-yellow exudative plaques adherent to the colonic mucosa (Fig. 1-217).

LABORATORY TESTS

- *C. difficile* toxin can be detected by cytotoxin tissue-culture assay (gold standard for identifying *C. difficile* toxin in stool specimen). This test is difficult to perform and results are not available for 24-48 hr. A more useful test enzyme-linked immunoabsorbent assay (ELISA) for *C. difficile* toxins A and B. The latter is used most widely in the clinical setting. It has a sensitivity of 85% and a specificity of 100%.
- Fecal leukocytes (assessed by microscopy or lactoferrin assay) are generally present in stool samples.
- CBC usually reveals leukocytosis. A sudden increase in WBC to $>30,000/mm^3$ may be indicative of fulminant colitis.

IMAGING STUDIES

Abdominal film (flat plate and upright) is useful in patients presenting with abdominal pain or evidence of obstruction on physical examination.

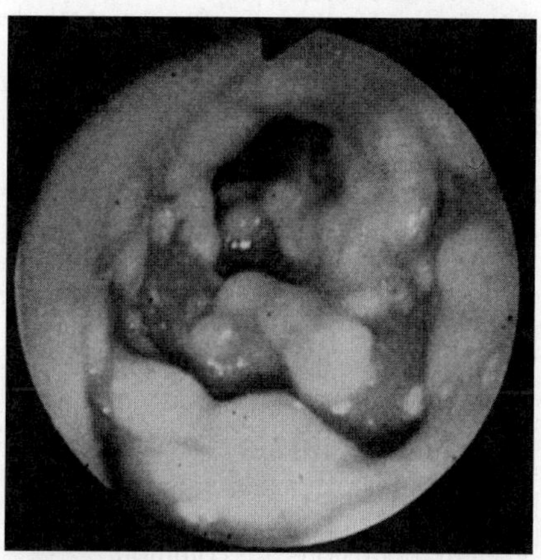

FIGURE 1-217 Pseudomembranous plaques seen with colonoscopy in a patient with *C. difficile*–associated PMC. (From Gorbach SL: *Infectious diseases,* ed 2, Philadelphia, 1998, WB Saunders.)

TREATMENT

NONPHARMACOLOGIC THERAPY

- Discontinue offending antibiotic
- Fluid hydration and correct electrolyte abnormalities

ACUTE GENERAL Rx

- Metronidazole 500 mg PO qid for 10 to 14 days.
- Vancomycin 125 mg PO qid for 10 to 14 days in cases resistant to metronidazole. However, vancomycin may be considered as first-line therapy in hospitalized patients who are seriously ill.
- Cholestyramine 4 g PO qid for 10 days in addition to metronidazole to control severe diarrhea (avoid use with vancomycin).
- When parenteral therapy is necessary (e.g., patient with paralytic ileus), IV metronidazole 500 mg qid can be used. It can also be supplemented with vancomycin 500 mg via NG tube with intermittant clamping or retention enema.

CHRONIC Rx

Judicious future use of antibiotics to prevent recurrences (e.g., avoid prolonged antibiotic therapy)

DISPOSITION

Most patients recover completely with appropriate therapy. Fever resolves within 48 hr and diarrhea within 4 to 5 days. Overall mortality is 1% to 2.5% but exceeds 10% in untreated patients.

REFERRAL

Hospital admission and IV hydration in severe cases

PEARLS & CONSIDERATIONS

COMMENTS

Possible complications of pseudomembranous colitis include dehydration, bowel perforation, toxic megacolon, electrolyte imbalance, and reactive arthritis.

SUGGESTED READINGS

Bartlett JG: Antibiotic-associated diarrhea, *N Engl J Med* 346:334, 2002.

Hurley BW, Nguyen CC: The spectrum of pseudomembranous enterocolitis and antibiotic-associated diarrhea, *Arch Intern Med* 162:2177, 2002.

Schroeder MS: *Clostridium difficile*-associated diarrhea, *Am Fam Physician* 71:921, 2005.

AUTHOR: **FRED F. FERRI, M.D.**

BASIC INFORMATION

DEFINITION

Psittacosis is a systemic infection caused by *Chlamydophila psittaci* (formerly known as *Chlamydia psittaci*).

SYNONYMS

Ornithosis
Parrot pneumonia

ICD-9CM CODES
073.9 Psittacosis

EPIDEMIOLOGY & DEMOGRAPHICS

INCIDENCE (IN U.S.):
- 21 cases reported in 2005
- True incidence possibly higher because infections may be subclinical
- Highest incidence among pet owners and people working in contact with birds

PEAK INCIDENCE: 30 to 60 yr of age
PREVALENCE (IN U.S.):
- Low among humans
- Organism carried in 5% to 8% of birds

PREDOMINANT SEX: Equal sex distribution
PREDOMINANT AGE: More common in adults

PHYSICAL FINDINGS & CLINICAL PRESENTATION

- Incubation period of 5 to 15 days
- Subclinical infection
- Onset abrupt or insidious
- Most common symptoms:
  1. Fever
  2. Myalgias
  3. Chills
  4. Cough
- Most common clinical syndrome: atypical pneumonia with fever, headache, dry cough, and a chest x-ray more dramatically abnormal than the physical examination
- Ranges from mild disease to respiratory failure and death, although this is extremely unusual
- Other clinical presentations:
  1. Mononucleosis-like syndrome
  2. Typhoidal form
- Most frequent physical findings:
  1. Fever
  2. Pharyngeal erythema
  3. Rales
  4. Hepatomegaly
- Less common findings:
  1. Somnolence
  2. Confusion
  3. Relative bradycardia
  4. Pleural rub
  5. Adenopathy
  6. Splenomegaly
  7. Horder's spots (pink blanching maculopapular rash)
- Besides the lungs, other specific end-organ involvement:
  1. Pericarditis
  2. Myocarditis
  3. Endocarditis
  4. Hepatitis
  5. Joints
  6. Kidneys (glomerulonephritis)
  7. CNS

ETIOLOGY

- *Chlamydophila* (formerly *Chlamydia*) *psittaci* is an obligate intracellular bacterium.
- Infection is usually spread by the respiratory route from infected birds.
- There is a history of exposure to birds in 85% of patients.
- Strains from turkeys and psittacine birds are most virulent for humans.
- Cows, goats, and sheep are occasionally implicated.

DIAGNOSIS

DIFFERENTIAL DIAGNOSIS

- *Legionella*
- *Mycoplasma*
- *Chlamydophila pneumoniae* (TWAR)
- Viral respiratory infections
- Typhoid fever
- Viral hepatitis
- Aseptic meningitis
- Mononucleosis

WORKUP

- CBC, renal and liver function tests
- Chlamydophila serology
- Chest x-ray examination
- Special immunostaining of respiratory secretions

LABORATORY TESTS

- WBC count is normal or slightly elevated.
- Mild liver function abnormalities are common (50%).
- Blood cultures are almost always negative.
- Studies on respiratory secretions:
  1. Direct immunofluorescent antibody (DFA) of respiratory secretions with monoclonal antibodies to chlamydial antigens
  2. Chlamydophila LPS (lipopolysaccharide) antigen by enzyme immunoassay (EIA)
  3. Polymerase chain reaction (PCR)
- Serologic studies:
  1. Complement-fixing antibodies
  2. Microimmunofluorescence
  3. Possible false-negative results and cross-reaction with other chlamydial species with both techniques

IMAGING STUDIES

- Chest x-ray examination is abnormal in 50% to 90% with a variety of patterns.
- Pleural effusions are common.

TREATMENT

NONPHARMACOLOGIC THERAPY

Oxygen supplementation as needed

ACUTE GENERAL Rx

- Tetracycline (500 mg PO qid) *or*
- Doxycycline (100 mg PO bid) *or*
- Erythromycin (500 mg PO qid): less effective

CHRONIC Rx

In the rare cases of endocarditis, combination of heart valve replacement and prolonged antibiotic course may be the treatment of choice.

DISPOSITION

- Mortality low (0.7%)
- Poor prognostic factors:
  1. Advanced age
  2. Leukopenia
  3. Severe hypoxemia
  4. Renal failure
  5. Confusion
  6. Multilobe pulmonary involvement
- Possible reinfection

REFERRAL

- To infectious disease expert:
  1. Complicated atypical pneumonia or other end-organ involvement
  2. Suspicion of an outbreak
- To pulmonologist for diagnostic bronchoscopy

PEARLS & CONSIDERATIONS

COMMENTS

- Hospitalized patients do not require specific isolation precautions.
- Any confirmed or suspected case of psittacosis should be reported to public health authorities.
- Recent evidence indicates that *C. psittaci* may be associated with induction of a rare form of lymphoma found in the ocular adnexa; case reports have described regression of ocular lymphoma with antibiotic treatment for *C. psittaci*.

SUGGESTED READINGS

Cunha BA: The atypical pneumonias: clinical diagnosis and importance, *Clin Microbiol Infect* 3:12, 2006.

Ferreri AJ et al: Regression of ocular adnexal lymphoma after *Chlamydia psittaci*-eradicating antibiotic therapy, *J Clin Oncol* 23(22):5067, 2005.

Ferreri AJ et al: Evidence for an association between *Chlamydia psittaci* and ocular adnexal lymphomas, *J Natl Cancer Inst* 96(8):586, 2004.

Smith KA et al: Compendium of measures to control *Chlamydophila psittaci* (formerly *Chlamydia psittaci*) infection among humans (psittacosis) and pet birds, 2005, *J Am Vet Med Assoc* 226(4):532, 2005.

Vargas RL et al: Is there an association between ocular adnexal lymphoma and infection with *Chlamydia psittaci?* The University of Rochester experience, *Leuk Res* 30(5)547, 2006.

AUTHORS: **GLENN G. FORT, M.D., M.P.H., MICHELE HALPERN, M.D.,** and **DENNIS J. MIKOLICH, M.D.**

BASIC INFORMATION

DEFINITION

Psoriasis is a chronic skin disorder characterized by excessive proliferation of keratinocytes, resulting in the formation of thickened scaly plaques, itching, and inflammatory changes of the epidermis and dermis. The various forms of psoriasis include guttate, pustular, and arthritis variants.

ICD-9CM CODES
696.0 Psoriasis, arthritis, arthropathic
696.1 Psoriasis, any type except arthropathic

EPIDEMIOLOGY & DEMOGRAPHICS

- Psoriasis affects 1% to 3% of the world's population. Most patients have limited psoriasis involving <5% of their body surface.
- There is a strong association between psoriasis and HLA B13, B17, and B27 (pustular psoriasis).
- Peak age of onset is bimodal (adolescents and at 60 yr of age).
- Men and women are equally affected.

PHYSICAL FINDINGS & CLINICAL PRESENTATION

- The primary psoriatic lesion is an erythematous papule topped by a loosely adherent scale. Scraping the scale results in several bleeding points (Auspitz sign).
- Chronic plaque psoriasis generally manifests with symmetric, sharply demarcated, erythromatous, silver-scaled patches affecting primarily the intergluteal folds, elbows, scalp, fingernails, toenails, and knees (Fig. 1-218, *A*). This form accounts for 80% of psoriasis cases.
- Psoriasis can also develop at the site of any physical trauma (sunburn, scratching). This is known as Koebner's phenomenon.
- Nail involvement is common (pitting of the nail plate), resulting in hyperkeratosis, onychodystrophy with onycholysis (Fig. 1-218, *B*).
- Pruritus is variable. Soreness and bleeding may occur.
- Joint involvement can result in sacroiliitis and spondylitis.
- Guttate psoriasis is generally preceded by streptococcal pharyngitis and manifests with multiple droplike lesions on the extremities and the trunk (Fig. 1-218, *C*).
- Adverse effect on psychologic and social functioning, with affected persons often feeling stigmatized.

ETIOLOGY

- Unknown, but there is a strong genetic component and high heritability.
- Familial clustering (genetic transmission with a dominant mode with variable penetrants).
- One third of persons affected have a positive family history.
- Within the past decade, several putative loci for genetic susceptibility to psoriasis have been reported. One locus (psoriasis susceptibility 1 [PSORS1] locus) in the major-histocompatibility-complex (MHC) region on chromosome 6 is considered the most important susceptibility locus.

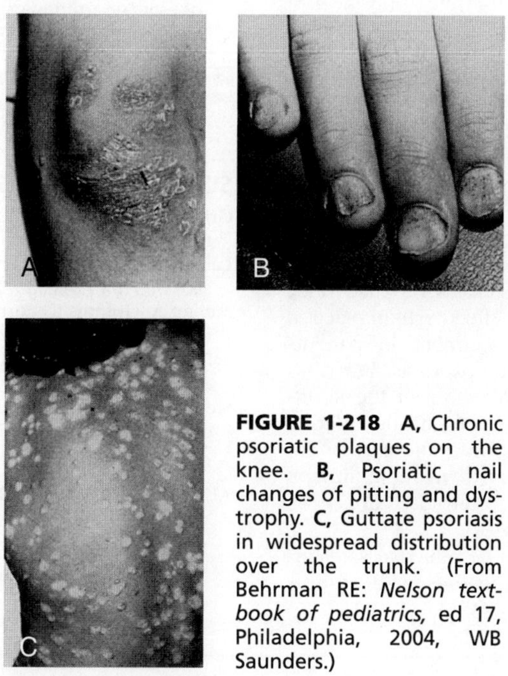

FIGURE 1-218 **A,** Chronic psoriatic plaques on the knee. **B,** Psoriatic nail changes of pitting and dystrophy. **C,** Guttate psoriasis in widespread distribution over the trunk. (From Behrman RE: *Nelson textbook of pediatrics,* ed 17, Philadelphia, 2004, WB Saunders.)

DIAGNOSIS

DIFFERENTIAL DIAGNOSIS

- Contact dermatitis
- Atopic dermatitis
- Stasis dermatitis
- Tinea
- Nummular dermatitis
- Candidiasis
- Mycosis fungoides
- Cutaneous SLE
- Secondary and tertiary syphilis
- Drug eruption

WORKUP

- Diagnosis is clinical.
- Skin biopsy is rarely necessary.

LABORATORY TESTS

Generally not necessary for diagnosis

TREATMENT

NONPHARMACOLOGIC THERAPY

- Sunbathing generally leads to improvement.
- Eliminate triggering factors (e.g., stress, certain medications [e.g., lithium, β-blockers, antimalarials]).
- Patients with psoriasis benefit from a daily bath in warm water followed by application of a cream or ointment moisturizer. Regular use or an emollient moisturizer limits evaporation of water from the skin and allows the stratum corneum to rehydrate itself.

GENERAL Rx

Therapeutic options vary according to the extent of disease. Approximately 70% to 80% of all patients can be treated adequately with use of topical therapy.

- Patients with limited disease (<20% of the body) can be treated with the following:
  1. Topical steroids: disadvantages are brief remissions, expense, and decreased effect with continued use. Salicylic acid can be compounded by pharmacist in concentrations of 2% to 10% and used in combination with a corticosteroid to decrease amount of scale.
  2. Calcipotriene (Dovonex): a vitamin D analogue, is effective for moderate plaque psoriasis; adults should comb the hair, apply solution to the lesions, and rub it in, avoiding uninvolved skin; disadvantages are its cost and potential burning and skin irritation. It should not be used concurrently with salicylic acid because calcipotriene is inactivated by the acidic nature of salicylic acid. Taclonex ointment is a combination of calcipotriene and the high potency corticosteroid betamethasone dipropionate. It is well tolerated and

more effective than either agent used alone but also much more expensive.
3. Tar products (Estar, LCD, psoriGel) can be used overnight and are most effective when combined with UVB light (Goeckerman regimen).
4. Anthralin (Drithocreme): useful for chronic plaques, can result in purple/brown staining; best used with UVB light.
5. Retinoids such as tazarotene 0.05%, 0.1% cream or gel, are effective in thinning plaques but are expensive and can produce irritation.
6. Other useful measures include tape or occlusive dressing, UVB and lubricating agents, interlesional steroids.

- Therapeutic options for persons with generalized disease (affecting >20% of the body) and for those with inadequate response to topical agents:
  1. UVB light exposure three times a week: This therapy does not require administration of a systemic drug (unlike PUVA), but to be effective, it requires removal of scale with keratolytic agents and emollients.
  2. Oral PUVA (psoralen plus ultraviolet A) administered two to three times weekly is effective for generalized disease. It is often considered in patients for whom narrowband UVB therapy is ineffective. However, many PUVA treatments are required, necessitating frequent office visits, and it may be associated with phototoxicity, such as erythema and blistering, and increased risk of skin cancer.
- Systemic treatments include methotrexate 25 mg every week for severe psoriasis. Etretinate (Tegison) (a synthetic retinoid) is most effective for palmar-plantar pustular psoriasis. Dose is 0.5 to 1 mg/kg/day. It can cause liver enzyme and lipid abnormalities and is teratogenic.
- Cyclosporine is also effective in severe psoriasis; however, relapses are common.
- Chronic plaque psoriasis may be treated with alefacept, a recombinant protein that selectively targets T lymphocytes. Treatment with alefacept for 12 wk (0.025, 0.075, or 0.150 mg/kg of body weight IV weekly) may result in significant improvement. Some patients also experience a sustained clinical response after the cessation of treatment. This medication is very expensive (a 12-wk course costs >$8,000). Treatment with etanercept, a tumor necrosis factor (TNF) antagonist, for 24 wk can also lead to a reduction in severity of plaque psoriasis. Efalizumab, a humanized monoclonal antibody that inhibits the activation of T cells, has also been reported to produce significant improvement in plaque psoriasis over a 24-wk treatment period. Adalimumab—a fully human, anti-TNF-alpha monoclonal antibody—has been reported effective for joint and skin manifestations of psoriasis.

DISPOSITION

The course of psoriasis is chronic, and the disease may be refractory to treatment.

REFERRAL

- Dermatology referral is recommended in all patients with generalized disease.
- Hospital admission may be necessary for severe diffuse or poorly responsive psoriasis. The Goeckerman regimen combines daily application of tar with UVB exposure and can result in prolonged remissions.

PEARLS & CONSIDERATIONS

COMMENTS

Psoriasis is more emotionally than physically disabling for most patients. Counseling may be indicated, particularly when it affects younger patients.

EVIDENCE

Topical therapies

Anthralin improves chronic plaque psoriasis more effectively than placebo.[1] Ⓐ

Calcipotriene is more effective than placebo, and has been found to have similar or better efficacy than other medications used for chronic plaque psoriasis (including tar, topical, and anthralin short-contact treatment).[1] Ⓐ

Combination therapy with calcipotriene and topical corticosteroids leads to better clearance and maintenance in patients with chronic plaque psoriasis.[1] Ⓐ

Mid- to high-potency topical corticosteroids have been shown to produce temporary improvement in psoriatic lesions.[1] Ⓐ

Topical corticosteroids (applied once a week) are more effective than placebo as maintenance treatment in patients with chronic plaque psoriasis.[2] Ⓐ

Tazarotene is effective in the short-term management of chronic plaque psoriasis. The response rate may be increased when used in combination with topical corticosteroids.[1] Ⓐ

Systemic therapies

Cyclosporine may be effective as clearance therapy in patients with chronic plaque psoriasis.[3] Ⓐ

A systematic review found limited evidence from randomized controlled trials (RCTs) that oral retinoids improved symptoms of chronic plaque psoriasis. Combination therapy with oral retinoids plus UVB was more effective than UVB alone for the treatment of chronic plaque psoriasis. Oral retinoids plus topical corticosteroids were also more effective than either treatment alone.[3] Ⓐ

RCTs have found monotherapy with subcutaneous etanercept to be more effective than placebo in patients with plaque psoriasis when treated for up to 24 weeks, with a positive association between strength and duration of therapy also being noted.[4-6] Ⓑ

Subcutaneous efalizumab has been shown to significantly improve clinical response in patients with psoriasis, with improvement in response over placebo reaching significance as early as week 4.[7] Ⓑ

Evidence-Based References

1. Naldi L, Rzany B: Chronic plaque psoriasis. Reviewed in: *Clin Evid* 12:2275, 2004 Ⓐ
2. Katz HI et al: Intermittent corticosteroid treatment of psoriasis: a double-blind multicenter trial of augmented betamethasone dipropionate ointment in a pulse dose treatment regimen, *Dermatologica* 183:269, 1991. Reviewed in: *Clin Evid* 12:2275, 2004. Ⓐ
3. Griffiths GE et al: A systematic review of treatments for severe psoriasis, *Health Technol Assess* 4:1, 2000. Reviewed in: *Clin Evid* 12:2275, 2004. Ⓐ
4. Gottlieb AB et al: A randomized trial of etanercept as monotherapy for psoriasis, *Arch Dermatol* 139:1627, 2003. Ⓑ
5. Leonardi CL et al: Etanercept as monotherapy in patients with psoriasis, *N Engl J Med* 349:2014, 2003. Ⓑ
6. Mease PJ et al: Etanercept in the treatment of psoriatic arthritis and psoriasis: a randomised trial, *Lancet* 356:385, 2000. Reviewed in *Clin Evid* 12:2275, 2004. Ⓑ
7. Lebwohl M et al: A novel targeted T-cell modulator, efalizumab, for plaque psoriasis, *N Engl J Med* 349:2004, 2003. Ⓑ

SUGGESTED READINGS

Griffiths C, Barker J: Pathogenesis and clinical features of psoriasis, *Lancet* 370:263, 2007.

Luba KM, Stulberg DL: Chronic plaque psoriasis, *Am Fam Physician* 73:636, 2006.

Menter A, Griffiths C: Current and future management of psoriasis, *Lancet* 370:272, 2007.

Schon MP, Boehncke WH: Psoriasis, *N Engl J Med* 353:1899, 2005.

Stern RS: Psoralen and ultraviolet A light therapy for psoriasis, *N Engl J Med* 357:682, 2007.

AUTHOR: **FRED F. FERRI, M.D.**

BASIC INFORMATION

DEFINITION

A state in which external reality is distorted by delusions and/or hallucinations (where a delusion is a fixed false belief, and a hallucination is a false auditory, visual, olfactory, tactile, or taste perception).

SYNONYMS

Psychosis is a key finding in many mental illnesses, such as brief psychotic disorder, delusional disorder, schizoaffective disorder, schizophrenia, schizophreniform disorder, or shared psychotic disorder.

EPIDEMIOLOGY & DEMOGRAPHICS

One year prevalence: 4.5 per 1000. The demographics of psychosis depend on the underlying disorder.

PHYSICAL FINDINGS & CLINICAL PRESENTATION

History
- Past medical history of any of the etiologies
- Use of possible offending medications
- Use of illicit substances
- Impaired function
- ICU stay >5 days

Physical examination
- If associated with a mood disorder, delusions/hallucinations are usually consistent with mood (e.g., auditory hallucinations in a depressed patient may tell the patient what a terrible person he is).
- Altered, disorganized thought pattern, which is usually reflected in disorganized speech (including word salad, thought blocking, rhyming, clang).
- Lack insight into problems.
- Behavior is odd or unpredictable; patient may clearly be responding to internal stimuli.
- Signs of Parkinson's disease, dementia.

ETIOLOGY

- Pathophysiologically, an interaction among:
  1. Dopaminergic overactivity (particularly in the mesolimbic, nigrostriatal, and mesocortical systems)
  2. Environmental, social/childhood factors
  3. Genetic predisposition
- Underlying mental disorder: schizophrenia, major depression, brief psychotic disorder, delusional disorder, schizoaffective disorder, schizophreniform disorder, shared psychotic disorder
- Underlying personality disorder: borderline, paranoid, schizoid, schizotypal
- Underlying medical condition: HIV/AIDS, Parkinson's, Huntington's, leprosy, malaria, sarcoidosis, SLE, prion disease, hypoglycemia, postpartum state, cerebrovascular event, temporal lobe epilepsy, brain neoplasm
- Medications: systemic steroids, anticonvulsants, anti-parkinsonian medications, some chemotherapy, scopolamine
- Underlying dementia: Alzheimer's, Lewy body dementia
- Illicit drugs (usually with chronic use; can be with intoxication or withdrawal): LSD, PCP, cocaine, GHB (withdrawal), alcohol, amphetamines, marijuana
- Traumatic brain injury
- ICU stay: hypoxia, decreased cardiac output, infection, medications, sleep deprivation, alteration of diurnal cycle, sensory deprivation/overload, pain
- Emotional stress

DIAGNOSIS

WORKUP

Any workup would be to better assess etiology and would depend on the clinical situation.

LABORATORY TESTS

Consider checking chemistry panel (calcium), complete blood count, liver function tests, cortisol, HIV, RPR, TSH, toxicology screen, LP.

IMAGING STUDIES

Consider CXR (sarcoid), EEG, head CT/MRI.

TREATMENT

NONPHARMACOLOGIC THERAPY

- Cognitive behavioral therapy.
- Social/behavioral skills training.
- Training for self-management of disease.
- Aforementioned strategies favored over psychoanalytic techniques given the relative inability for abstract thought and lack of insight in psychotic patients.
- Family intervention, including education and strategies to reduce emotional expression.
- Counseling for substance abuse.

ACUTE GENERAL Rx

- Antipsychotics; low doses should control first episode. Use with caution in elderly patients because adverse effects limit effectiveness.
- Benzodiazepines if agitation is severe.
- Discontinue offending medication if present.

CHRONIC Rx

Antipsychotics, second-generation antipsychotics may reduce incidence of tardive dyskinesia, but may increase incidence of metabolic disorders compared to first-generation antipsychotics.

DISPOSITION

Prognosis varies according to etiology of psychosis. In general, the more severe and longer the psychotic episode, the worse the prognosis.

REFERRAL

Patient should be admitted for acute stabilization if actively psychotic to prevent harm to self and others, as well as to ensure administration of medications.

PEARLS & CONSIDERATIONS

- Delusions and/or hallucinations are hallmarks of psychosis.
- Rule out medical or drug causes of psychosis.
- Antipsychotics are the mainstay of acute and chronic treatment.
- Consider alternatives to antipsychotics in elderly patients.

SUGGESTED READINGS

Byrne P: Managing the acute psychotic episode, *BMJ* 334(7595):686, 2007.

Petersen L et al: A randomised multicentre trial of integrated versus standard treatment for patients with a first episode of psychotic illness, *BMJ* 17;331(7517):602, 2005.

Schneider LS et al: Effectiveness of atypical antipsychotic drugs in patients with Alzheimer's disease, *N Engl J Med* 355(15):1525, 2006.

Wang PS et al: Risk of death in elderly users of conventional vs. atypical antipsychotic medications, *N Engl J Med* 353(22):2335, 2005.

AUTHOR: **MICHAEL K. ONG, M.D., PH.D.**

BASIC INFORMATION

DEFINITION

Pubertal delay refers to delayed development and maturation of the reproductive system. The diagnostic criterion is a delay of more than 2 to 3 standard deviations from the mean age of pubertal onset. See Figure 3-238 in Section III.

ICD-9CM CODES
259.0 Delay in sexual development and puberty, not elsewhere classified

EPIDEMIOLOGY & DEMOGRAPHICS

PREVALENCE: 2.5% of healthy adolescents have a diagnosis of pubertal delay using the statistical diagnostic criteria
GENETICS: Constitutional delay of puberty often runs in families. Pubertal delay occurs with some congenital syndromes, such as Prader-Willi syndrome and Noonan syndrome, and in patients with enzyme defects in sex steroid synthesis, as well as others.

PHYSICAL FINDINGS & CLINICAL PRESENTATION

Puberty is clinically delayed for girls if there is no evidence of breast development by 13 yr of age, absence of menarche by age 16 yr, or absence of menarche within 5 yr of pubertal onset. Puberty is clinically delayed for boys if there is no evidence of testicular enlargement by 14 yr of age, or >5 yr between start and completion of growth of genitalia.

ETIOLOGY

Puberty begins with increased pulsatile secretion of gonadotropin-releasing hormone (GnRH) from the hypothalamus, increased pituitary responsiveness to GnRH, secretion of gonadotropins, gonadal maturation, and increasing production of sex steroids. Increased concentration of sex steroids induces the development of secondary sexual characteristics, acceleration of growth, and fertility. Numerous causes can lead to pubertal delay including chronic disease, normal variation, abnormal chromosomes, or other factors.

DIAGNOSIS

DIFFERENTIAL DIAGNOSIS

Normal or low serum gonadotropins
- Constitutional delay
- Hypothalamic dysfunction
  - Malnutrition or eating disorder
  - Strenuous exercise
  - Chronic illness
  - Severe obesity
  - Central nervous system tumors
- Hypopituitarism
  - Panhypopituitarism
  - Isolated gonadotropin deficiency
  - Kallman syndrome (associated with anosmia)
  - Growth hormone deficiency
- Hypothyroidism
- Hyperprolactinemia
  - Pituitary adenoma
  - Drug-associated (cannabis, cocaine)

Increased serum gonadotropins
- Turner syndrome (gonadal dysgenesis)
- Klinefelter syndrome
- Bilateral gonadal failure
  - Primary testicular failure
  - Anorchia
  - Premature ovarian failure
  - Resistant ovary syndrome
  - Irradiation, cytotoxic therapy
  - Trauma
  - Infections (e.g., mumps, orchitis)

Other conditions
- Anatomic abnormalities
- Prader-Willi syndrome
- Noonan syndrome
- Androgen resistance
- Steroidogenic enzyme defects

WORKUP

- Given the extensive differential diagnosis for pubertal delay, a systematic and focused approach is necessary. A careful history, including family history and social history, can identify eating and exercise habits, chronic illnesses, and parental history of pubertal delay.
- Growth measurement should include height and weight, a growth chart to assess rate of growth, and calculation of the sex-adjusted midparental height that represents the statistically most probable adult height for the child.
  - For boys add 2.5 inches (or 6.5 cm) from the mean of the parents' heights. For girls, subtract 2.5 inches (or 6.5 cm) from the mean of the parents' height.
  - Physical exam can reveal signs of sexual maturation, stigmata of congenital syndromes, nutritional status. Include neurologic exam (visual fields, ophthalmologic), thyroid, chest, heart, abdomen, Tanner staging.

LABORATORY TESTS

- Serum gonadotropin levels (LH/FSH) distinguish disorders of congenital or acquired gonadal failure from other causes. By bone age 10 to 12 yr gonadal failure produces elevated levels of serum gonadotropins. If levels are low or normal constitutional delay is the most frequent diagnosis.
- Chromosomal analysis if there is a suspicion of gonadal dysgenesis or Klinefelter syndrome.
- Screening studies include CBC, erythrocyte sedimentation rate, serum prolactin, serum TSH.
- Endocrinologist may do further studies including: GH testing, GnRH stimulation testing, hCG stimulation with testosterone levels.

IMAGING STUDIES

Consider bone age (left hand and wrist film), which is delayed in constitutional delay and GnRH deficiency; CT or MRI of head to evaluate for tumors of pituitary or hypothalamus and absence of olfactory bulb and tract, which occurs in Kallman syndrome (absence of GnRH); and pelvic ultrasound.

TREATMENT

- Treat underlying cause if it is identified.
- Constitutional delay can be managed with reassurance that the delay will have no effect on final adult height or development. Short-term hormonal therapy can be used to hasten puberty if the delay is causing severe psychosocial difficulties. Monthly testosterone injections are used for boys who have begun pubertal development while oral oxandrolone is used for boys who have not yet begun puberty. Potential side effects include premature epiphyseal closure and hepatic peliosis. Treatment is discontinued when endogenous hormone production has begun.
- Gonadotropin deficiency or hypogonadism requires lifelong sex steroid replacement.
- Psychosocial evaluation, support, and treatment as needed.

REFERRAL

Pediatric endocrinology

PEARLS & CONSIDERATIONS

COMMENTS

- Constitutional delay is the most common cause of pubertal delay and is often associated with a positive family history in parents and/or siblings, but other causes, such as Turner syndrome and systemic disorders, should be excluded.
- No studies reliably distinguish constitutional delay from gonadotropin deficiency.

PATIENT/FAMILY EDUCATION

- The Magic Foundation, a support group for patients and their families (http://www.magicfoundation.org)
- The American Academy of Family Physicians (http://www.aafp.org)
- American Academy of Pediatrics (http://www.aap.org)

Evidence-Based References

Blondell RD, Foster MB, Kamlesh CD: Disorders of puberty, *Am Fam Physician.* Available at http://www.aafp.org/afp/990700ap/209.html. Accessed online July 2, 2007.
Master-Hunter T, Heiman D: Amenorrhea: evaluation and treatment, *Am Fam Physician* 73:1376-1382, 2006.
Rosen D, Foster C: Delayed puberty, *Pediatr Rev* 27:9, 2001.
Sedlmeyer IL, Palmort MR: Delayed puberty: analysis of a large case series from an academic center, *J Clin Endocrinol Metab* 87:1613-1620, 2002.

SUGGESTED READING

Rosen D, Foster C: Delayed puberty, *Pediatr Rev* 27:9, 2001.

AUTHOR: **NIRALI BORA, M.D.**

BASIC INFORMATION

DEFINITION

Cardiogenic pulmonary edema is a life-threatening condition caused by severe left ventricular decompensation.

SYNONYMS

Cardiogenic pulmonary edema

ICD-9CM CODES
428.1 Acute pulmonary edema with heart disease

PHYSICAL FINDINGS & CLINICAL PRESENTATION

- Dyspnea with rapid, shallow breathing
- Diaphoresis, perioral and peripheral cyanosis
- Pink, frothy sputum
- Moist, bilateral pulmonary rales
- Increased pulmonary second sound, S_3 gallop (in association with tachycardia)
- Bulging neck veins

ETIOLOGY

Increased pulmonary capillary pressure secondary to:
- Acute myocardial infarction
- Exacerbation of CHF
- Valvular regurgitation (e.g., mitral regurgitation)
- Ventricular septal defect
- Severe myocardial ischemia
- Mitral stenosis
- Other: cardiac tamponade, endocarditis, myocarditis, arrhythmias, cardiomyopathy, hypertensive crisis

DIAGNOSIS

DIFFERENTIAL DIAGNOSIS

- Noncardiogenic pulmonary edema
- Pulmonary embolism
- Exacerbation of asthma
- Exacerbation of COPD
- Sarcoidosis
- Pulmonary fibrosis
- Viral pneumonitis and other pulmonary infections

LABORATORY TESTS

- ABGs: respiratory and metabolic acidosis, decreased Pao_2, increased Pco_2, low pH. (NOTE: The patient may initially show respiratory alkalosis secondary to hyperventilation in attempts to maintain Pao_2.)
- Measurement of plasma BNP (elevated).

IMAGING STUDIES

- Chest x-ray examination:
  1. Pulmonary congestion with Kerley B lines; fluffy perihilar infiltrates in the early stages; bilateral interstitial alveolar infiltrates
  2. Pleural effusions
- Echocardiogram:
  1. Useful to evaluate valvular abnormalities, diastolic vs. systolic dysfunction
  2. Can aid in differentiation of cardiogenic vs. noncardiogenic pulmonary edema
  3. Can also estimate pulmonary capillary wedge pressure and rule out presence of myxoma or atrial thrombus
- Right heart catheterization (selected patients): cardiac pressures and cardiogenic pulmonary edema reveal increased PADP and PCWP ≥25 mm Hg

TREATMENT

ACUTE GENERAL Rx

All the following steps can be performed concomitantly:
- 100% oxygen by face mask. Both CPAP and BiPAP systems can improve oxygenation and lower carbon dioxide tensions. Check ABGs; if marked hypoxemia or severe respiratory acidosis, intubate the patient and place on a ventilator. Positive end-expiratory pressure (PEEP) increases functional capacity and improves oxygenation.
- Furosemide: 1 mg/kg IV bolus (typically 40 to 100 mg) to rapidly establish diuresis and decrease venous return through its venodilator action; may double the dose in 30 min if no effect.
- Vasodilator therapy:
  1. Nitrates: particularly useful if the patient has concomitant chest pain.
     a. Nitroglycerin: 150 to 600 μg SL or nitroglycerin spray (Nitrolingual) may be given immediately on arrival and repeated multiple times if the patient remains symptomatic and blood pressure remains stable.
     b. 2% nitroglycerin ointment: 1 to 3 inches out of the tube applied continuously; absorption may be erratic.
     c. IV nitroglycerin: 100 mg in 500 ml of D_5W solution; start at 6 μg/min (2 ml/hr).
  2. Nitroprusside: useful for afterload reduction in hypertensive patients with decreased cardiac index (CI).
     a. Increases the CI and decreases left ventricular filling pressure.
     b. Vasodilator and diuretic therapy should be tailored to achieve PCWP ≤18 mm Hg, RAP ≤8 mm Hg, systolic blood pressure >90 mm Hg, SVR >1200 dynes/sec/cm^{-5}. The use of nitroprusside in patients with acute MI is controversial because it may intensify ischemia by decreasing the blood flow to the ischemic left ventricular myocardium.
  3. Nesiritide (Natrecor): dosage is 2 mcg/kg IV bolus, then 0.01 mcg/kg/min. Use of nesiritide should be reserved for patients who present to the hospital with acutely decompensated heart failure and dyspnea at rest, in whom standard combination therapy with diuretics and nitroglycerin has been inadequate. It should not be substituted for diuretics, used for intermittent outpatient infusion, or used repetitively.
  4. Morphine: 2 to 4 mg IV/SC/IM, may repeat q15 min prn. It decreases venous return, anxiety, and systemic vascular resistance (naloxone should be available at bedside to reverse the effects of morphine if respiratory depression occurs). Morphine may induce hypotension in volume-depleted patients.
  5. Afterload reduction with ACE inhibitors. Captopril 25 mg PO tablet can be used for SL administration (placing a drop or two of water on the tablet and placing it under the tongue helps dissolve it), onset of action is <10 min, peak effect can be reached in 30 min. ACE inhibitors can also be given IV (e.g., enalaprilat 1 mg IV given q2h prn).
  6. Dobutamine: parenteral inotropic agent of choice in severe cases of cardiogenic pulmonary edema. It can be administered at a dosage of 2.5 to 10 μg/kg/min IV. IV phosphodiesterase inhibitors (amrinone, milrinone) may be useful in refractory cases.

SUGGESTED READING

Ware LB, Matthay MA: Acute pulmonary edema, *N Engl J Med* 353:2788, 2005.

AUTHOR: **FRED F. FERRI, M.D.**

BASIC INFORMATION

DEFINITION

Pulmonary embolism (PE) refers to the lodging of a thrombus or other embolic material from a distant site in the pulmonary circulation.

SYNONYMS

Pulmonary thromboembolism
PE

ICD-9CM CODES
415.1 Pulmonary embolism and infarction

EPIDEMIOLOGY & DEMOGRAPHICS

- 650,000 cases of PE occur in the U.S. each year; 50,000 result in death (increased incidence in women and with advanced age).
- More than 90% of pulmonary emboli originate in the deep venous system of the lower extremities.
- Pulmonary thromboembolism is associated with >200,000 hospitalizations each year in the U.S.
- 8% to 10% of victims of PE die within the first hour.

PHYSICAL FINDINGS & CLINICAL PRESENTATION

- Most common symptom: dyspnea
- Chest pain: may be nonpleuritic or pleuritic (infarction)
- Syncope (massive PE)
- Fever, diaphoresis, apprehension
- Hemoptysis, cough
- Evidence of DVT may be present (e.g., swelling and tenderness of extremities)
- Cardiac examination: may reveal tachycardia, increased pulmonic component of S_2, murmur of tricuspid insufficiency, right ventricular heave, right-sided S_3
- Pulmonary examination: may demonstrate rales, localized wheezing, friction rub
- Most common physical finding: tachypnea

ETIOLOGY

- Thrombus, fat, or other foreign material
- Risk factors for PE:
  1. Prolonged immobilization
  2. Postoperative state
  3. Trauma to lower extremities
  4. Estrogen-containing birth control pills
  5. Prior history of DVT or PE
  6. CHF
  7. Pregnancy and early puerperium
  8. Visceral cancer (lung, pancreas, alimentary and genitourinary tracts)
  9. Trauma, burns
  10. Advanced age
  11. Obesity
  12. Hematologic disease (e.g., antithrombin III deficiency, protein C deficiency, protein S deficiency, lupus anticoagulant, polycythemia vera, dysfibrinogenemia, paroxysmal nocturnal hemoglobinuria, factor V Leiden mutation, G20210A prothrombin mutation)
  13. COPD, diabetes mellitus
  14. Prolonged air travel

DIAGNOSIS

DIFFERENTIAL DIAGNOSIS

- Myocardial infarction
- Pericarditis
- Pneumonia
- Pneumothorax
- Chest wall pain
- GI abnormalities (e.g., peptic ulcer, esophageal rupture, gastritis)
- CHF
- Pleuritis
- Anxiety disorder with hyperventilation
- Pericardial tamponade
- Dissection of aorta
- Asthma

WORKUP

- Clinical assessment alone is insufficient to diagnose or rule out PE. It is also important to remember that no single noninvasive test has both high sensitivity and high specificity for PE. Consequently, in addition to clinical assessment, most patients will require several noninvasive tests or pulmonary angiography to diagnose PE. The Wells prediction rules (Box 1-10) can be used to estimate the probability of pulmonary embolism.
- Spiral CT of chest or lung scan may be diagnostic. Pulmonary angiogram (when indicated) will confirm the diagnosis.
- Serial compressive duplex ultrasonography of lower extremities can be used in patients with "low-probability" lung scan and high clinical suspicion (see "Imaging Studies"). It is useful if positive, negative results do not exclude pulmonary embolism.
- A diagnostic approach to pulmonary embolism is described in Section III.

LABORATORY TESTS

- ABGs generally reveal decreased Pao_2 and $Paco_2$ and increased pH; normal results do not rule out PE.
- Alveolar-arteriolar (A-a) oxygen gradient, a measure of the difference in oxygen concentration between alveoli and arterial blood, is a more sensitive indicator of the alteration in oxygenation than Pao_2; it can easily be calculated using the information from ABGs; a normal A-a gradient among patients without history of PE or DVT makes the diagnosis of PE unlikely.
- Plasma D-dimer measurement: D-dimer assays by ELISA detect the presence of plasmin-mediated degradation products of fibrin that contain cross-linked D fragments in the whole blood or plasma. A normal plasma D-dimer level is useful to exclude pulmonary embolism in patients with a nondiagnostic lung scan and a low pretest probability of PE. However, it cannot be used to "rule in" the diagnosis because it increases with many other disorders (e.g., metastatic cancer, trauma, sepsis, postoperative state). Plasma D-dimer can also be used in conjunction with lower-extremity compression ultrasonography in patients with indeterminate V/Q and spiral CT scans. Absence of DVT and presence of a normal D-dimer level in these settings generally rules out clinically significant pulmonary embolism.
- Elevated cardiac troponin levels also occur in patients with pulmonary embolism because of right ventricular dilation and myocardial injury; therefore, PE should be considered in the differential diagnosis of all patients presenting with chest pain or dyspnea and elevated cardiac troponin levels.
- ECG is abnormal in 85% of patients with acute PE. Frequent abnormalities are sinus tachycardia; nonspecific ST-segment or T wave changes; S-I, Q-III, T-III pattern (10% of patients); S-I, S-II, S-III pattern; T wave inversion in V_1 to V_6; acute RBBB; new-onset atrial fibrillation; ST segment depression in lead II; right ventricular strain.

IMAGING STUDIES

- Chest x-ray may be normal; suggestive findings include elevated diaphragm, pleural effusion, dilation of pulmonary artery, infiltrate or consolidation, abrupt vessel cut-off, or atelectasis. A wedge-shaped consolidation in the middle and lower lobes is suggestive of a pulmonary infarction and is known as "Hampton's hump."
- Lung scan (in patient with normal chest x-ray examination):
  1. A normal lung scan rules out PE.
  2. A ventilation-perfusion mismatch is suggestive of PE, and a lung scan interpretation of high probability is confirmatory.
  3. If the clinical suspicion of PE is high and the lung scan is interpreted as low probability, moderate probability, or indeterminate, a pulmonary arteriogram is diagnostic; a positive arteriogram confirms diagnosis; a positive compressive duplex ultrasonography for DVT obviates the need for an arteriogram, because treatment with IV anticoagulants is indicated in these patients; the overall sensitivity of compres-

sive ultrasonography for DVT in patients with PE is 29%, specificity 97%; adding ultrasonography in patients with a nondiagnostic lung scan prevents 9% of angiographies; however, this improvement in efficacy is achieved at the cost of unnecessary anticoagulant therapy in 26% of patients who have false-positive ultrasonography results.

- Spiral CT is an excellent modality for diagnosing PE. It may be used in place of the lung scan and is favored in patients with baseline lung abnormalities on initial chest x-ray. It has the added advantage of detecting other pulmonary pathology that can mimic pulmonary embolism. Newer generation CT scanners (4-slice multidetector-row CT) are highly accurate in diagnosing PE, and when coupled with d-dimer testing, may eliminate the need for additional testing.
- Angiography: pulmonary angiography is the gold standard; however, it is invasive, expensive, and not readily available in some clinical settings. False-positive pulmonary angiograms may result from mediastinal disorders such as radiation fibrosis and tumors. CT angiography is an accurate, noninvasive tool in the diagnosis of PE at the main, lobar, and segmental pulmonary artery levels. A major advantage of CT angiography over standard pulmonary angiography is its ability to diagnose intrathoracic disease other than PE that may account for the patient's clinical picture. It is also less invasive, less costly, and more widely available. Its major shortcoming is its poor sensitivity for subsegmental emboli. Gadolinium-enhanced magnetic resonance angiography of the pulmonary arteries has a moderate sensitivity and high specificity for the diagnosis of PE; MRA is best reserved for selected patients when CT scan and/or lung scan are inconclusive and the risk of pulmonary angiography is high.

TREATMENT (Rx)

NONPHARMACOLOGIC THERAPY

Correction of risk factors (see "Etiology") to prevent future PE

ACUTE GENERAL Rx

- Unfractionated heparin by continuous infusion for at least 5 days or low-molecular-weight heparin (LMWH); many experts recommend a larger initial IV heparin bolus (15,000 to 20,000 U) to block platelet aggregation and thrombi and subsequent release of vasoconstrictive substances.
- Thrombolytic agents (urokinase, tPA, streptokinase): provide rapid resolution of clots; thrombolytic agents are the treatment of choice in patients with massive PE who are hemodynamically unstable and with no contraindication to their use. The use of thrombolytic agents in the treatment of hemodynamically stable patients with acute submassive pulmonary embolism remains controversial. Use of the thrombolytic agents alteplase (100 mg IV over a 2-hr period) in normotensive patients with moderate or severe right ventricular dysfunction identified by echocardiography has been advocated by some physicians. Use of alteplase in conjunction with heparin has been shown to improve the clinical course of stable patients who have acute submassive PE without internal bleeding. Additional studies are needed to confirm these findings before recommending routine use of this therapeutic approach.
- Long-term treatment is generally carried out with warfarin therapy started on day 1 or 2 and given in a dose to maintain the INR at 2 to 3. Preliminary trials reveal that idraparinux, a long-acting inhibitor of activated factor X, given once weekly SC as a fixed dose for 3 or 6 months has efficacy similar to that of heparin plus a vitamin K antagonist in the treatment of DVT and causes less bleeding. However, in patients with PE, idraparinux was less efficacious than standard therapy.
- If thrombolytics and anticoagulants are contraindicated (e.g., GI bleeding, recent CNS surgery, recent trauma) or if the patient continues to have recurrent PE despite anticoagulation therapy, vena caval interruption is indicated by transvenous placement of a Greenfield vena caval filter.
- Acute pulmonary artery embolectomy may be indicated in a patient with massive pulmonary emboli and refractory hypotension.

CHRONIC Rx

Elimination of risk factors (see "Etiology") and monitoring of warfarin dose with INR on a routine basis

DISPOSITION

- Mortality can be reduced to <10% by rapid and effective treatment.
- Mortality from recurrent pulmonary emboli is 8% with effective treatment and >30% in patients with untreated pulmonary emboli.

BOX 1-10 Probability Assessment Methods for Pulmonary Embolism

Wells et al* have developed the following clinical prediction rules to determine the probability of PE, assigning a score to each finding:

a. Clinical signs/symptoms of DVT (minimum of leg swelling and pain with palpation of the deep veins of the legs (score = 3.0)
b. No alternate diagnosis likely or more likely than PE (score = 3.0)
c. Heart rate > 100/min (score = 1.5)
d. Immobilization or surgery in last 4 wk (score = 1.5)
e. Previous history of DVT or PE (score = 1.5)
f. Hemoptysis (score = 1.0)
g. Cancer actively treated within last 6 months (score = 1.0)

Probability of PE is high if total score is >6; moderate if 2-6; and low if <2.

Le Gal et al† have developed another clinical prediction rule that does not require subjective diagnostic judgments or tests. The score consists of eight variables:

a. Age > 65 yr (1 point)
b. Previous DVT or PE (3 points)
c. Surgery or fracture within 1 month (2 points)
d. Active malignant condition (2 points)
e. Unilateral lower limb pain (3 points)
f. Hemoptysis (2 points)
g. Heart rate of 75-94 beats/min (3 points)
h. Heart rate ≥ 95 beats/min (5 points)
i. Pain on lower deep venous palpation and unilateral edema (4 points)

Probability of PE = 8% (low probability) in patients with 0-3 points; 28% (intermediate probability) with 4-10 points; 74 % (high probability) with ≥11 points.

*Wells PS et al: Use of a clinical model for safe management of patients with suspected PE, *Ann Intern Med* 129:997, 1998.
†Le Gal et al: Prediction of pulmonary embolism in the emergency department: the revised Geneva score, *Ann Intern Med* 144:165-171, 2006.
DVT, Deep vein thrombosis; *PE,* pulmonary embolism.

PEARLS & CONSIDERATIONS

COMMENTS

- In hemodynamically stable patients with pulmonary embolism, initial treatment with once-daily SC administration of the synthetic antithrombotic agent fondaparinux without monitoring has been reported to be at least as safe and as effective as adjusted-dose IV unfractionated heparin. Several other trials have also demonstrated that fixed-dose low molecular weight heparin to be as effective and safe as dose-adjusted IV unfractionated heparin for the initial treatment of nonmassive PE.
- The duration of oral anticoagulant treatment is 6 mo in patients with reversible risk factors and indefinitely in patients with persistence of risk factors that caused the initial PE.
- See Box 1-10.

SUGGESTED READINGS

Agnelli G et al: Extended oral anticoagulant therapy after a first episode of pulmonary embolism, *Ann Intern Med* 139:19, 2003.

Fedullo PF, Tapson VF: The evaluation of suspected pulmonary embolism, *N Engl J Med* 349:1247, 2003.

Perrier A et al: Multidector-row computed tomography in suspected pulmonary embolism, *N Engl J Med* 352:1760, 2005.

Qaseem A et al: Current diagnosis of venous thromboembolism in primary care: a clinical practice guideline from the American Academy of Family Physicians and the American College of Physicians, *Ann Intern Med* 146:454, 2007.

Quinlan DJ et al: Low-molecular weight heparin compared with IV unfractionated heparin for treatment of pulmonary embolism, *Ann Intern Med* 140:175, 2004.

The van Gogh Investigators: Idraparinux versus standard therapy for venous thromboembolic disease, *N Engl J Med* 357:1094, 2007.

AUTHOR: **FRED F. FERRI, M.D.**

BASIC INFORMATION

DEFINITION

Pulmonary hypertension (PH) is abnormally elevated pressure in the arterial side of the pulmonary circulation, usually defined as mean pulmonary artery pressure (PAP) >25 mm Hg at rest or greater than 30 mm Hg with exercise. Sustained elevation in PAP due to increased pulmonary venous pressure, hypoxic pulmonary vasoconstriction, or increased flow is often referred to as secondary pulmonary hypertension.

SYNONYMS

Primary pulmonary hypertension (PPH)
Secondary pulmonary hypertension

ICD-9CM CODES
416.0 Primary pulmonary hypertension
416.8 Secondary pulmonary hypertension

EPIDEMIOLOGY & DEMOGRAPHICS

- Primary pulmonary hypertension (PPH) is rare, occurring in 1 to 2 cases per 1 million people per year, with an overall prevalence estimated at 1300 per million.
- PPH is more common in women than men (1.7:1), usually presenting in the third to fourth decade of life.
- Secondary pulmonary hypertension is more common than PPH.
- Secondary pulmonary hypertension is the common pathophysiologic mechanism leading to cor pulmonale in patients with underlying pulmonary disease (e.g., chronic obstructive pulmonary disease [COPD], pulmonary embolism).

PHYSICAL FINDINGS & CLINICAL PRESENTATION

Primary pulmonary hypertension:
- PPH is insidious and may go undetected for years.
- Exertional dyspnea is the most common presenting symptom (60%).
- Fatigue and weakness.
- Syncope, classically exertion related or after a warm shower with peripheral vasodilation.
- Chest pain.
- Hoarse voice due to compression of recurrent laryngeal nerve by an enlarged pulmonary artery (Ortner's syndrome).
- Loud P2 component of the second heart sound and paradoxical splitting of second heart sound.
- Right-sided S4.
- Jugular venous distension.
- Abdominal distention/ascites.
- Prominent parasternal (right ventricular [RV]) impulse.
- Holosystolic tricuspid regurgitation murmur heard best along the left fourth parasternal line that increases in intensity with inspiration.
- Peripheral edema.

Secondary pulmonary hypertension:
- Similar to PPH, but caused by an underlying cause (e.g., left-sided congestive heart failure, mitral stenosis, COPD).

ETIOLOGY

- The etiology of PPH is unknown. Most cases are sporadic, but there is a 6% to 12% familial incidence.
- PPH is associated with several known risk factors: portal hypertension and liver cirrhosis, appetite-suppressant drugs (fenfluramine), and HIV disease.
- Several genetic abnormalities have been associated with the familial form of PPH, many of which are mutations in the genes that code for members of the TGF-β family of receptors (BMPR-II, ALK-1) on chromosome 2q33.
- Familial PPH is an autosomal dominant disease with variable penetrance, affecting only about 10% to 20% of carriers.
- Several factors play a role in the pathogenesis of PPH, including a genetic predisposition, endothelial cell dysfunction, abnormalities in vasomotor control, thrombotic obliteration of the vascular lumen, and vascular remodeling through cell proliferation and matrix production.
- New WHO classification of pulmonary hypertension (based on common clinical features):

  Pulmonary arterial hypertension
  - Primary: familial and sporadic
  - Related to: collagen vascular diseases, congenital systemic to pulmonary shunts, HIV, portal hypertension, drugs and toxins

  Pulmonary venous hypertension
  - Left-sided atrial, ventricular, or valvular heart disease
  - Fibrosing mediastinitis, adenopathy, and tumors

  Pulmonary veno-occlusive disease

  PH associated with disorders of the respiratory system or hypoxemia
  - COPD, interstitial lung disease, sleep disordered breathing, alveolar hypoventilation syndromes, chronic exposure to high altitude, neonatal lung disease, alveolar capillary dysplasia

  PH due to chronic thrombotic and or embolic disease
  - Pulmonary embolus (thrombus, tumor, parasites, foreign material)

  Miscellaneous: schistosomiasis, sarcoidosis, other

DIAGNOSIS

- PH is a hemodynamic diagnosis involving the detection of elevated pressure in the pulmonary arteries, and characterization of this abnormality to determine its etiology.
- Right-sided heart catheterization must be performed in all patients suspected of having PH to establish the diagnosis and document pulmonary hemodynamics.
- Primary pulmonary hypertension is a diagnosis of exclusion.

DIFFERENTIAL DIAGNOSIS

The differential diagnosis is as listed under "Etiology."

WORKUP

- Screening for the presence of PH using Doppler echocardiography is warranted in individuals with a known predisposing genetic mutation or first-degree relative with idiopathic PPH, scleroderma, congenital heart disease with left-to-right shunt, or portal hypertension undergoing evaluation for orthotopic liver transplantation.
- The workup of a patient suspected of having PPH includes a detailed evaluation of the heart and lungs. Blood tests, chest x-ray, pulmonary function tests, CT scan of the chest, radionuclide studies of the heart and lungs, echocardiogram, electrocardiograms, pulmonary angiogram, and right- and left-sided heart catheterization are all required to exclude secondary causes of pulmonary hypertension.
- Once the diagnosis has been made, functional assessment should be done to determine disease prognosis and potential therapeutic options.
- Determining the degree of functional impairment, as assessed by the WHO classification system and the 6-minute-walk test (6MWT), is a useful way to monitor disease progression and assess response to treatment.

LABORATORY TESTS

- CBC is usually normal in PPH, but may show secondary polycythemia.
- ABGs show low PO_2 and oxygen saturation.
- Pulmonary function tests (PFTs) are done to exclude obstructive or restrictive lung disease.
- Overnight oximetry and sleep study to rule out sleep apnea/hypopnea.
- ECG may show evidence of both right atrial enlargement (tall P wave >2.5 mV in leads II, III, aVF) and right ventricular enlargement (right axis deviation > 100 and R wave > S wave in lead V1).

- Other blood tests: ANA titer to screen for underlying connective tissue disease, HIV serology, liver function tests, and antiphospholipid antibodies.
- Assessment of exercise capacity is a key part of the evaluation of PH. The 6MWT is most commonly used. It has been shown to determine prognosis and identify those patients who require treatment, and allows noninvasive monitoring of response to treatment.

IMAGING STUDIES

- Chest x-ray shows enlargement of the main and hilar pulmonary arteries with rapid tapering of the distal vessels, described as peripheral oligemia (Fig. 1-219). Right ventricular enlargement may be evident on lateral films.
- Lung perfusion scan (V/Q scan) is the test of choice in excluding chronic pulmonary embolism.
- Transthoracic Doppler echocardiogram including M-mode, 2D mode, pulse, continuous, and color Doppler assesses ventricular function, excludes significant valvular pathology, and visualizes abnormal shunting of blood between heart chambers if present. It also provides an estimate of the pulmonary artery systolic pressure that has been shown to correlate well (0.57 to 0.93) with pressures measured by right-sided heart catheterization.
- Pulmonary angiogram is done in patients with inconclusive V/Q scans.
- Cardiac catheterization is performed to directly measure PAPs, assess pulmonary vasodilator response, and detect any shunting of blood.

TREATMENT (Rx)

NONPHARMACOLOGIC THERAPY

- Oxygen therapy to improve alveolar oxygen flow in both primary and secondary pulmonary hypertension.
- Avoidance of vigorous exercise and pregnancy.

ACUTE GENERAL Rx

- PPH
  1. Diuretics (e.g., furosemide 40 to 80 mg qd) improve dyspnea and peripheral edema.
  2. Digoxin 0.25 mg qd has been used in patients with PPH, although no benefit has been demonstrated unless patients have atrial fibrillation or left ventricular dysfunction.
  3. Right-sided heart catheterization to establish diagnosis and evaluation for treatment with vasodilators.
  4. Short-acting vasodilators to test for vasodilator response including: IV adenosine, epoprostenol, or inhaled nitric oxide.
- Secondary pulmonary hypertension treatment is aimed at the underlying cause.

CHRONIC Rx

- Vasodilator trials showing at least 10 mm Hg drop in mean PAP and mean PAP ≤40, while maintaining cardiac output, may benefit from treatment with calcium channel blockers (diltiazem, amlodipine, or nifedipine). Verapamil is not recommended due to its negative inotropic effects. All patients should be reassessed in 6 to 8 wk to demonstrate continued benefit from calcium channel blocker.
- Nonresponders are eligible for selective pulmonary vasodilators.
- Warfarin therapy with goal INR 1.5 to 2.0 is recommended for all patients with PPH and although not proven may be indicated in secondary PH.
- Prostanoids (epoprostenol, treprostinil, and iloprost) act as potent vasodilators of pulmonary arteries, and inhibitors of platelet aggregation.
  - Epoprostenol: IV formulation with very short half-life. Requires long-term IV access with associated risks of infection and thrombosis. Rapid tachyphylaxis, thus, dose escalation is seen. Common side effects include jaw pain, abdominal cramping, and diarrhea. Limited evidence exists for use in secondary PH patients.
  - Treprostinil: IV and SQ formulation with longer half-life. Main disadvantage is pain at SQ pump site (no long-term evidence for IV formulation).
  - Iloprost: aerosolized formulation with short half-life requiring 6 to 8 treatments/day.
- Endothelin receptor antagonists: (bosentan, ambrisentan, and sitaxsentan).
  - Bosentan (nonselective endothelin A and B receptor blocker): only oral pulmonary vasodilator, requires monthly liver function tests (LFT), often response delay by weeks. Thus, it is not an ideal starting therapy for WHO class IV patients.
  - Sitaxsentan and ambrisentan (selective endothelin A receptor blockers): both with limited long-term evidence.

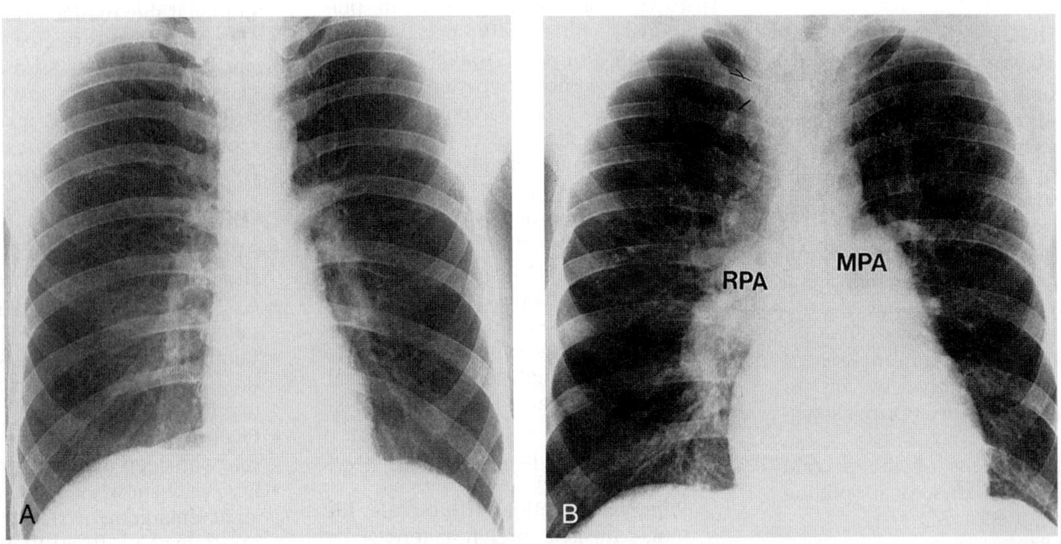

FIGURE 1-219 Progressive pulmonary arterial hypertension. This patient initially presented with a relatively normal chest radiograph **(A)**. However, several years later **(B)** there is increasing heart size and marked dilation of the main pulmonary artery (MPA) and right pulmonary artery (RPA). Rapid tapering of the arteries as they proceed peripherally is suggestive of pulmonary hypertension and is sometimes referred to as pruning. (From Mettler FA [ed]: *Primary care radiology,* Philadelphia, 2000, WB Saunders.)

- Phosphodiesterase inhibitors: (sildenafil and tadalafil).
- Combination therapies: limited evidence at this point.
- Lung transplantation and heart-lung transplantation are other options in patients with end-stage class IV disease. Atrial septostomy may be performed as a bridge to transplant. The defect can be closed at the time of transplantation.
- Atrial septostomy is recommended for individuals with a room air SaO_2 >90% who suffer from severe right-sided heart failure (with refractory ascites) despite maximal diuretic therapy, or who have signs of impaired systemic blood flow (such as syncope) due to reduced left heart filling.
- Lung transplant recipients with PPH had survival rates of 73% at 1 yr, 55% at 3 yr, and 45% at 5 yr.

DISPOSITION

- The 6MWT is predictive of survival in patients with idiopathic PPH. Desaturation >10% during the test increases mortality risk 2.9 times over a median follow-up of 26 mo.
- The actual 6-minute-walk distance on chronic epoprostenol treatment is more predictive of survival than the change in 6-minute-walk distance before and after treatment.
- WHO class II and III patients with PPH have a mean survival of 3.5 yr.
- WHO class IV patients have a mean survival of 6 mo.

REFERRAL

If the diagnosis of PPH is suspected, a consultation with a pulmonary specialist is recommended. Secondary causes of pulmonary hypertension may require disease specific consultations.

PEARLS & CONSIDERATIONS

- The exertional dyspnea of PH is typically described by patients as being relentlessly progressive over several months to a year, often out of proportion to, or in the absence of, underlying heart or lung disease.
- Chest x-ray may reveal evidence of interstitial fluid within the lungs in cases of secondary pulmonary hypertension. PPH is not associated with infiltrates on chest x-ray.

COMMENTS

- Right ventricular systolic pressure (RVSP) as estimated by echocardiography is not a very good indicator of the presence of PH because RVSP increases with age and body mass index (BMI). Athletically conditioned men also have a higher resting RVSP. Thus, these measurements can be misleading.
- Abrupt development of pulmonary edema during acute vasodilator testing suggests pulmonary veno-occlusive disease or pulmonary capillary hemangiomatosis and is a contraindication to chronic vasodilator treatment.

EVIDENCE

EBM

Medical Therapy

Many of the therapies used in the treatment of pulmonary hypertension considered important and effective are not supported by randomized controlled trials (RCTs). The evidence for the use of calcium channel antagonists is mainly derived from expert opinion. Recommendations include the following.

Calcium Channel Antagonists

In the absence of right-sided heart failure, patients who demonstrate a favorable acute response to vasodilator should be considered candidates for a trial of therapy with an oral calcium channel antagonist.[1] C

In patients with PAH, calcium channel antagonists should not be used empirically in the absence of demonstrated acute vasoreactivity.[1] C

Epoprostenol: A recently updated systematic review identified nine RCTs involving 1175 participants that evaluated the use of prostacyclin/prostacyclin analogues in the treatment of pulmonary hypertension. These studies showed a consistent, significant improvement in exercise capacity, cardiopulmonary hemodynamics, and New York Heart Association (NYHA) function with epoprostenol, compared with placebo. The review concluded that the use of prostacyclin, in addition to conventional therapy, can result in some short-term benefit in exercise capacity and cardiopulmonary hemodynamics. In addition, subgroup analysis suggested that such benefits were greater in those patients with primary pulmonary hypertension.[2] A

Treprostinil: A recently updated systematic review identified nine RCTs involving 1175 participants that evaluated the use of prostacyclin or prostacyclin analogues in the treatment of pulmonary hypertension. Cardiopulmonary hemodynamics and symptom scores favored the treprostinil group and there was a significant improvement in exercise capacity reported in the larger study. However, treatment with treprostinil was associated with a number of withdrawals due to adverse effects.[2] A

Iloprost: A recently updated systematic review identified nine RCTs involving 1175 participants that evaluated the use of prostacyclin or prostacyclin analogues in the treatment of pulmonary hypertension. Use of inhaled iloprost was associated with a significant increase in exercise capacity, and improved hemodynamic and symptom scores compared with placebo.[2] A

Sildenafil: There is a lack of clinical trials evaluating the role of sildenafil in the long-term management of PH. Early reports from clinical studies show promising results and, as such, the use of sildenafil is supported by expert opinion. In patients with PAH who have failed or are not candidates for other available therapy, treatment with sildenafil should be considered.[1] C

Bosentan: A systematic review identified three RCTs, involving 423 patients that compared short-term (12 to 16 weeks) use of endothelin antagonists (bosentan or sitaxsentan) vs. placebo in the management of pulmonary hypertension. The review found that the use of endothelin antagonists improved exercise capacity, Borg dyspnea scores, and cardiopulmonary hemodynamic values compared with placebo. The reviewers concluded that, in the short term, endothelin antagonists may benefit patients with pulmonary hypertension.[3] A

Anticoagulation

The evidence for the use of anticoagulants is mainly derived from expert opinion. Patients with idiopathic pulmonary hypertension (IPAH) should receive anticoagulation with warfarin; for patients with PAH associated with other underlying processes, anticoagulation should be considered.[1] C

Surgical Treatment

Recommendations are based, in part, upon expert opinion from clinicians with experience in the surgical management of pulmonary hypertension. Recommendations for lung transplant/heart-lung transplant (LT/HLT) include:

- Patients with pulmonary hypertension with NYHA functional class III/IV symptoms should be referred to a transplant center for evaluation and listing for LT or HLT.[4] C
- Listed patients whose prognosis remains poor despite medical therapy should undergo LT or HLT.[4] C
- In patients undergoing transplantation, the procedure of choice is bilateral LT.[4] C

- In adults with simple congenital heart lesions, bilateral LT with repair of the cardiac defect is the procedure of choice.[4] C
- In adults with complex congenital defects, HLT is the procedure of choice.[4] C

Supplemental Oxygen Therapy

Recommendation regarding the use of oxygen in patients with pulmonary hypertension are supported by expert opinion. In patients with PAH, supplemental oxygen should be used as necessary to maintain oxygen saturations >90% at all times.[1] C

Evidence-Based References

1. Badesch DB et al; American College of Chest Physicians: Medical therapy for pulmonary arterial hypertension: ACCP evidence-based clinical practice guidelines, *Chest* 126(suppl 1):35S-62S, 2004. C
2. Paramothyan NS et al: Prostacyclin for pulmonary hypertension in adults, *Cochrane Database Syst Rev* 2, 2005. A
3. Liu C, Chen J: Endothelin receptor antagonists for pulmonary arterial hypertension, *Cochrane Database Syst Rev* 4, 2004. A
4. Doyle RL et al; American College of Chest Physicians: Surgical treatments/interventions for pulmonary arterial hypertension: ACCP evidence-based clinical practice guidelines, *Chest* 126(suppl 1):63S-71S, 2004. C

SUGGESTED READINGS

Barst RJ et al: Diagnosis and differential assessment of pulmonary arterial hypertension, *J Am Coll Cardiol* 43:40S, 2004.

Lee SH, Rubin LJ: Current treatment strategies for pulmonary arterial hypertension, *J Intern Med* 258(3):199, 2005.

McLaughlin VV et al: Prognosis of pulmonary arterial hypertension: ACCP evidence-based clinical practice guidelines, *Chest* 126:(suppl 1)S78, 2004.

Rubin LJ, Badesch DB: Evaluation and management of the patient with pulmonary arterial hypertension, *Ann Intern Med* 143:282, 2005.

AUTHORS: **JEFFREY MAZER, M.D.,** and **GAURAV CHOUDHARY, M.D.**

BASIC INFORMATION

DEFINITION

Pyelonephritis is an infection, usually bacterial in origin, of the upper urinary tract.

SYNONYMS

Acute pyelonephritis
Pyonephrosis
Renal carbuncle
Lobar nephronia
Acute bacterial nephritis

ICD-9CM CODES
590.81 Pyelonephritis
599.0 Urinary tract infection
595.9 Cystitis

EPIDEMIOLOGY & DEMOGRAPHICS

INCIDENCE (IN U.S.): Extremely common

PREDOMINANT SEX: Female

PREDOMINANT AGE:

- Sexually active years in women
- Usually >50 yr of age in men

GENETICS:

Congenital Infection: Congenital urologic structural disorders may predispose to infections at an early age.

PHYSICAL FINDINGS & CLINICAL PRESENTATION

- Fever, rigors, chills
- Flank pain
- Dysuria
- Polyuria
- Hematuria
- Toxic feeling and appearance
- Nausea and vomiting
- Headache
- Diarrhea
- Physical examination notable
  1. Costovertebral angle tenderness
  2. Exquisite flank pain

ETIOLOGY

- Gram-negative bacilli such as *E. coli* and *Klebsiella* spp. in more than 95% of cases
- Other, more unusual gram-negative organisms, especially if instrumentation of the urinary system has occurred
- Resistant gram-negative organisms or even fungi in hospitalized patients with indwelling catheters
- Gram-positive organisms such as enterococci
- *Staphylococcus aureus:* presence in urine indicates hematogenous origin
- Viruses: rarely, but these are usually limited to the lower tract

DIAGNOSIS

DIFFERENTIAL DIAGNOSIS

- Nephrolithiasis
- Appendicitis
- Ovarian cyst torsion or rupture
- Acute glomerulonephritis
- PID
- Endometritis
- Other causes of acute abdomen
- Perinephric abscess
- Hydronephrosis

WORKUP

- No workup usually indicated in sexually active women
- Poorly responding infections, especially with azotemia and frank bacteremia
  1. Renal sonogram or CT scan to assess for underlying urologic pathology such as hydronephrosis
- Urologic imaging studies in all young men and boys
- Prostate assessment in older men

LABORATORY TESTS

- CBC with differential
- Renal panel
- Blood cultures
- Gram stain of urine, urinalysis and urine cultures
- Urgent renal sonography if obstruction or closed space infection suspected
- CT scans may better define the extent of collections of pus
- Helical CT scans excellent to detect calculi

TREATMENT

ACUTE GENERAL Rx

- Hospitalization for:
  1. Toxic patients
  2. Complicated infections
  3. Diabetes
  4. Suspected bacteremia
- Keep patients well hydrated.
- IV fluids are indicated for those unable to take adequate amounts of liquids.
- Give antipyretics such as acetaminophen when necessary.
- Antibiotic therapy should be initiated after cultures are obtained and guided by the results of culture and sensitivity testing.
  1. Oral TMP-SMX DS (bid for 10 days) or ciprofloxacin (500 mg orally bid for 10 days): adequate for stable patients who can tolerate oral medications with sensitive pathogens
  2. TMP-SMX or ciprofloxacin IV for more toxic patients
  3. Ceftazidime 1 g IV q6 to 8h
  4. Aminoglycosides such as gentamicin (2 mg/kg IV load followed by 1 mg/kg IV q8h adjusted for renal function) added but nephrotoxic especially in diabetics with azotemia
  5. Vancomycin 1 g IV q12h or linezlid to cover gram-positive cocci such as enterococci or staphylococci
  6. Ampicillin 1 to 2 g IV q4 to 6h to cover enterococci with an aminoglycoside for synergy
  7. Oral ampicillin or amoxicillin: no longer adequate for therapy of gram-negative infections because of resistance
- Prompt drainage with nephrostomy tube placement for obstruction.
- Surgical drainage of large collections of pus to control infection.
- Diabetic patients, as well as those with indwelling catheters, are especially prone to complicated infections and abscess formation.

CHRONIC Rx

- Repair underlying structural problems, especially when renal function is compromised.
  1. Reflux
  2. Obstruction
  3. Nephrolithiasis should be considered
- Patients with diabetes mellitus and indwelling urinary catheters are at particular risk of severe and complicated infections.
- When possible, remove catheters.

DISPOSITION

Most patients with uncomplicated pyelonephritis are now treated as outpatients or in short hospitalizations. Indications to admit a patient with pyelonephritis include: pregnancy, suspected urinary obstruction, suspected renal abscess or perinephric abscess, bacterial sepsis, diabetic or other immunocompromised patients, recurrent or refractory pyelonephritis, or infection with an unusual or antibiotic resistant microorganism.

REFERRAL

- To a surgeon for correction of underlying urologic problems (e.g., reflux and hydronephrosis)
- To a pediatrician for detection of reflux to avoid recurrent UTI and loss of renal function
- To an internist for aggressive metabolic and urologic evaluation for patients with nephrolithiasis

PEARLS & CONSIDERATIONS

Pyelonephritis is a systemic illness and may be a source of bacteremia and sepsis, especially if accompanied by urinary obstruction. Workup for abscess, obstruction, papillary necrosis, and other local complications of pyelonephritis should be initiated if the patient is septic, fails to respond to antibiotic therapy after 72 hr of treatment, or if infection is accompanied by worsening renal function.

EVIDENCE

In children with acute pyelonephritis:

Oral cefixime for 14 days, or short courses of intravenous (IV) therapy (ceftriaxone) followed by oral therapy, are as effective as longer duration IV therapy regimens.[1] Ⓐ

Aminoglycosides are just as effective given as a single daily dose as given three times daily.[1] Ⓐ

In adults with acute pyelonephritis:

Evidence suggests that oral levofloxacin, ciprofloxacin, and lomefloxacin are equally effective in treating acute, uncomplicated pyelonephritis.[2] Ⓐ

A single dose of IV tobramycin does not enhance the efficacy of a 10-day course of oral ciprofloxacin in hospitalized women with acute, uncomplicated pyelonephritis.[3] Ⓐ

Existing evidence does not allow for a comparison of efficacies of intravenous antibiotic regimens.[4]

In pregnant patients:

Antibiotic treatment of asymptomatic bacteriuria is effective in reducing the risk of pyelonephritis in pregnancy and preterm delivery, but the optimal duration of antibiotic treatment has yet to be established.[5,6] Ⓑ

There is insufficient evidence to recommend any specific treatment regimen for symptomatic urinary tract infections during pregnancy.[7] Ⓐ

Evidence-Based References

1. Bloomfield P, Hodson EM, Craig JC: Antibiotics for acute pyelonephritis in children. Reviewed in: Cochrane Library 2, Chichester, UK, 2004, John Wiley. Ⓐ
2. Richard GA et al: Levofloxacin versus ciprofloxacin versus lomefloxacin in acute pyelonephritis, *Urology* 52:51-55, 1998. Reviewed in: *Clin Evid*11:2527, 2004. Ⓐ
3. Le Conte P et al: Acute pyelonephritis. Randomized multicentre double-blind study comparing ciprofloxacin with combined ciprofloxacin and tobramycin, *Presse Med* 30:11, 2001. Reviewed in: *Clin Evid* 11:2527, 2004. Ⓐ
4. Wechsler A: Pyelonephritis in non-pregnant women. Reviewed in: *Clin Evid* 11:2527, London, 2004, BMJ Publishing Group.
5. Smaill F: Antibiotics for asymptomatic bacteriuria in pregnancy. Reviewed in: Cochrane Library 2, Chichester, UK, 2004, John Wiley. Ⓐ
6. Villar J et al: Duration of treatment for asymptomatic bacteriuria during pregnancy. Reviewed in: Cochrane Library 2, Chichester, UK, 2004, John Wiley. Ⓑ
7. Vazquez JC, Villar J: Treatments for symptomatic urinary tract infections during pregnancy. Reviewed in: Cochrane Library 2, Chichester, UK, 2004, John Wiley. Ⓐ

SUGGESTED READINGS

Bloomfield P, Hodson EM, Craig JC: Antibiotics for acute pyelonephritis in children, *Cochrane Database Syst Rev* 1:CD003772, 2005.

Hill JB et al: Acute pyelonephritis in pregnancy, *Obstet Gynecol* 105(1):18, 2005.

Pitukkijronnakorn S, Chittacharoen A, Herabutya Y: Maternal and perinatal outcomes in pregnancy with acute pyelonephritis, *Int J Gynaecol Obstet* 89(3): 286, 2005.

Scholes D et al: Risk factors associated with acute pyelonephritis in healthy women, *Ann Intern Med* 142(1):20, 2005.

Taskinen S, Ronnholm K: Post-pyelonephritic renal scars are not associated with vesicoureteral reflux in children, *J Urol* 173(4):1345, 2005.

AUTHORS: **GLENN G. FORT, M.D., M.P.H., JOSEPH J. LIEBER, M.D.,** and **DENNIS J. MIKOLICH, M.D.**

BASIC INFORMATION

DEFINITION

Pyogenic granuloma is a benign vascular lesion of the skin and mucus membranes. They are a result of capillary proliferation generally secondary to trauma.

SYNONYMS

Granuloma pyogenicum
Tumor of pregnancy
Eruptive hemangioma
Lobular capillary hemangioma
Granulation tissue-type hemangioma

ICD-9CM CODES
686.1 Pyogenic granuloma

EPIDEMIOLOGY & DEMOGRAPHICS

- Common in children and young adults.
- Equally prevalent in males and females and show no racial or familial predisposition.
- Caused by trauma or surgery.
- Gingival lesions occur more frequently during pregnancy.

PHYSICAL FINDINGS & CLINICAL PRESENTATION

- Small (<1 cm), yellow-to-red, dome-shaped lesions (Fig 1-220)
- May have surrounding scale at base
- Most commonly found on the head, neck, and extremities
- Often found on the gingiva during pregnancy (called *epulis*)
- Extremely friable, can easily ulcerate, and may bleed profusely with minor trauma

ETIOLOGY

Trauma causing focal capillary growth. These lesions are neither infectious in etiology nor granulomatous in histology.

DIAGNOSIS

DIFFERENTIAL DIAGNOSIS

Amelanotic melanoma
Bacillary angiomatosis
Glomus tumor
Hemangioma
Irritated nevus
Wart
Kaposi's sarcoma

WORKUP

Diagnosis is based on clinical history and appearance. Generally begins with trauma followed by the development of an erythematous papule. The lesion tends to bleed easily and develops over several days to weeks.

LABORATORY TESTS

Pathologic examination should be performed after excision to rule out melanoma.

TREATMENT

ACUTE GENERAL Rx

- Excision: using 1% lidocaine for anesthesia, shave or curette at base and border. Follow with electrocauterization or cryotherapy.
- Pulsed-dye laser is also a safe and effective treatment modality.
- Pregnancy epulis generally resolve spontaneously following childbirth.

REFERRAL

Dermatology referral recommended if lesion recurs or multiple satellite lesions occur after excision.

PEARLS & CONSIDERATIONS

COMMENTS

- Removal of entire lesion is essential because lesions may recur at the site of residual tissue.
- Patients and parents should be alerted to the possibility of recurrence after removal
- Multiple satellite lesions occasionally develop near a primary pyogenic granuloma, usually after destruction of that lesion.

AUTHOR: **JENNIFER R. SOUTHER, M.D.**

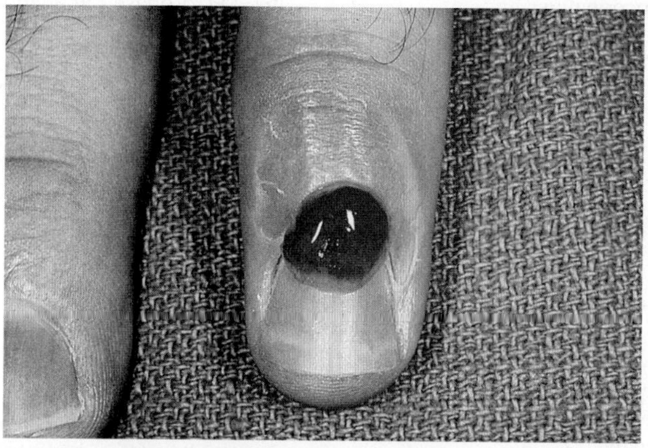

FIGURE 1-220 Pyogenic granuloma. Often the lesions have a collar or moat. (From Callen JP [ed]: *Color atlas of dermatology,* ed 2, Philadelphia, 2000, WB Saunders.)

BASIC INFORMATION

DEFINITION

Q fever is a systemic febrile illness caused by *Coxiella burnetii* that may be acute or chronic.

SYNONYMS

C. burnetii infection

ICD-9CM CODES
083.0 Q fever

EPIDEMIOLOGY & DEMOGRAPHICS

- *C. burnetii* is found worldwide.
- Common animal reservoirs are cattle, sheep, and goats.
- Most cases are found in individuals who have direct contact with infected animals (e.g., farmers, veterinarians) or who are exposed to contaminated animal urine, feces, milk, or placental tissues.
- Q fever is seen more in men than in women (3:1).

PHYSICAL FINDINGS & CLINICAL PRESENTATION

Acute Q fever presentation:
- Fever
- Pneumonia
- Hepatitis
- Meningoencephalitis

Chronic Q fever presentation:
- Endocarditis

Most common clinical symptoms:
- Chills
- Sweats
- Nausea
- Vomiting
- Cough, nonproductive
- Headache
- Fatigue

Most frequent physical findings:
- Fever
- Inspiratory rales
- Purpuric rash
- Hepatomegaly
- Splenomegaly

ETIOLOGY

- Q fever is caused by the rickettsial organism *C. burnetii.*
- *C. burnetii* is a gram-negative coccobacillus that is transmitted from arthropods to animals to humans.
- The disease is acquired most often via inhalation of aerosols. In the lungs, it proliferates in macrophases and then gains access to the blood, producing a transient bacteria. Thereafter it can invade many organs, but most commonly invades the lungs and liver.
- There is an incubation period between 3 to 30 days before systemic symptoms manifest.

DIAGNOSIS

DIFFERENTIAL DIAGNOSIS

Q fever can have various presentations and must be in the differential diagnosis of fever, hepatitis, pneumonia, endocarditis, and meningitis.

WORKUP

- CBC, ESR, and LFTs
- Urinalysis
- Serology
- Chest x-ray

LABORATORY TESTS

In acute Q fever:
- CBC and white blood cell count is usually normal.
- Thrombocytopenia can occur (25%).
- Elevation of hepatic transaminases (two to three times the abnormal range) may be seen.
- Complement fixation (CF) shows a fourfold rise in titer between acute and convalescent samples.

In chronic Q fever (almost always endocarditis):
- ESR is elevated
- Anemia is present
- Microscopic hematuria
- Blood cultures are almost always negative
- Complement fixation (CF) titer of >1:200 to phase I antigen is diagnostic

IMAGING STUDIES

- Chest x-ray examination is abnormal, showing segmental lobe consolidation
- Pleural effusions (35%)

TREATMENT

NONPHARMACOLOGIC THERAPY

Oxygen as needed in patients with pneumonia

ACUTE GENERAL Rx

- Acute Q fever can be treated with doxycycline (100 mg bid) for 14 to 21 days *or*
- Erythromycin (500 mg qid) for 14 days *or*
- Ofloxacin 200 mg PO q8h for 14 to 21 days
- Hydroxychloroquine plus doxycycline for endocarditis associated with Q fever
- Fluoroquinolones are recommended for suspected meningoencephalitis

CHRONIC Rx

- Chronic Q fever is treated with a combination of two antibiotics, doxycycline 100 mg bid and rifampin 300 mg qd *or*
- Doxycycline 100 mg bid and Ofloxacin 200 mg po q8h *or*
- Doxycycline 100 mg bid and hydroxychloroquine 200 mg PO tid
- Duration of treatment: 2 to 3 yr

DISPOSITION

- Patients with acute Q fever respond well with antibiotics, with rare deaths reported.
- Mortality rate in chronic Q fever endocarditis is high (24%). Most patients will need valve replacement surgery.

REFERRAL

Referral to an infectious disease expert is recommended in any cases of suspected acute or chronic Q fever.

PEARLS & CONSIDERATIONS

COMMENTS

- No vaccines are available.
- Infected patients do not require specific isolation precautions.
- Q fever derived its name in 1935 from Derrick, who was suspicious of a new disease during a series of acute febrile illnesses in abattoir workers of Queensland, Australia, justifying the name of Q fever (for query).

SUGGESTED READINGS

Healy B et al: The value of follow-up after acute Q fever infection, *J Infect* 52(4):e109, 2006.

McQuiston JH et al: National surveillance and the epidemiology of human Q-fever in the United States, 1978-2004, *Am J Trop Med Hyg* 75(1): 2006.

Milazzo A et al: Q fever vaccine uptake in South Australian meat processors prior to the introduction of the National Q Fever Management Program, *Commun Dis Intell* 29(4):400, 2005.

Oren I et al: An outbreak of Q fever in an urban area in Israel, *Eur J Clin Microbiol Infect Dis* 24(5):338, 2005.

Raoult D, Marrie T, Mege J: Natural history and pathophysiology of Q fever, *Lancet Infect Dis* 5(4):219, 2005.

Rolain JM, Raoult D: Molecular detection of *Coxiella burnetii* in blood and sera during Q fever, *QJM* 98(8):615, 2005.

Wagner-Wiening C et al: Serological diagnosis and follow-up of asymptomatic and acute Q fever infections, *Int J Med Microbiol* 40:294, 2006.

AUTHORS: **GLENN G. FORT, M.D., M.P.H.,** and **DENNIS J. MIKOLICH, M.D.**

BASIC INFORMATION

DEFINITION

Rabies is a fatal illness caused by the rabies virus and transmitted to humans by the bite of an infected animal.

SYNONYMS

Hydrophobia

ICD-9CM CODES
071 Rabies

EPIDEMIOLOGY & DEMOGRAPHICS

INCIDENCE (IN U.S.): Approximately 2 cases/yr
PREDOMINANT SEX: Men (70% of cases)
PREDOMINANT AGE: <16 yr and >55 yr

PHYSICAL FINDINGS & CLINICAL PRESENTATION

- Incubation period of 10 to 90 days
  1. Shorter with bites of the face
  2. Longer if extremities involved
- Prodrome
  1. Fever
  2. Headache
  3. Malaise
  4. Pain or anesthesia at exposure site
  5. Sore throat
  6. GI symptoms
  7. Psychiatric symptoms
- Acute neurologic period, with objective evidence of CNS involvement
  1. Extreme hyperactivity and bizarre behavior alternating with periods of relative calm
  2. Hallucinations, disorientation
  3. Seizures
  4. Paralysis
  5. Fear, pain, and spasm of the pharynx and larynx caused by drinking
  6. Coma, death

ETIOLOGY

- Rabies virus
- Cases in U.S. are associated with:
  1. Bats
  2. Raccoons
  3. Foxes
  4. Skunks
- In 8 of the 32 cases occurring in the U.S. since 1980, there was a history of exposure to bats without a clinically evident bite or scratch.
- Imported cases are usually associated with dogs.
- Unusual acquisition:
  1. Via organ transplantation
  2. Via aerosol transmission in laboratory workers and spelunkers

DIAGNOSIS

DIFFERENTIAL DIAGNOSIS

- Delirium tremens
- Tetanus
- Hysteria
- Psychiatric disorders
- Other viral encephalitides
- Guillain-Barré syndrome
- Poliomyelitis

WORKUP

- Rabies antibody
  1. Serum
  2. CSF
- Viral isolation
  1. Saliva
  2. CSF
  3. Serum
- Rabies fluorescent antibody: skin biopsy from the hair-covered area of the neck
- Characteristic eosinophilic inclusions (Negri bodies) in infected neurons

TREATMENT

NONPHARMACOLOGIC THERAPY

- Isolation of the patient to prevent transmission to others
- Supportive therapy

ACUTE GENERAL Rx

- No known beneficial therapy. A recent report describes a 15-year-old girl who survived rabies and had been treated with a combination of ketamine, midazolam, ribavirin, and amamtadine. This therapy is worth trying despite the fact this is a single case report.
- Emphasis is placed on prophylaxis of potentially exposed individuals following an exposure:
  1. Thorough wound cleansing and irrigation of the wound as soon as possible
  2. Active and passive immunization most effective when used within 72 hr of exposure
- Vaccinations:
  1. Human diploid cell vaccine (HDCV) or rhesus monkey diploid cell vaccine (RVA), 1 ml IM (deltoid) on days 0, 3, 7, 14, and 28
  2. Human rabies hyperimmune globulin (RIG) 20 IU/kg, to persons not previously vaccinated. If anatomically feasible, the full dose should be infiltrated into the wound; any remaining volume should be given IM at a site separate from vaccine administration
- Preexposure prophylaxis using HDCV or RVA (1 ml IM days 0, 7, and 21 or 28) in individuals at high risk for acquisition:
  1. Veterinarians
  2. Laboratory workers working with rabies virus
  3. Spelunkers
  4. Visitors to endemic areas

DISPOSITION

Virtually always fatal

REFERRAL

- To infectious disease consultant
- To local health authorities

PEARLS & CONSIDERATIONS

COMMENTS

- Most cases in the U.S. are caused by:
  1. Bat bites, often after minimal contact and inapparent exposure to infected bat saliva
  2. Dog bites occurring outside the U.S.
- Rare cases can be transmitted by mucous membrane contact of aerosolized virus (caves, laboratory acquired cases).

EVIDENCE

Studies conducted in the U.S. by the CDC have documented that a regimen of one dose of RIG and five doses of HDCV over a 28-day period was safe and induced an excellent antibody response in all recipients.[1]

Rabies vaccines induce an active immune response with neutralizing antibodies. This antibody response requires 7 to 10 days to develop and usually persists for 2 years or longer.[2]

RIG provides a rapid, passive, short-lived immunity (half-life of approximately 21 days).[1]

Evidence-Based References

1. CDC: Human rabies prevention—United States, 1999: recommendations of the Advisory Committee on Immunization Practices (ACIP), *MMWR Recomm Rep* 48:RR-1, 1999.
2. Dreesen DW et al: Two-year comparative trial on the immunogenicity and adverse effects of purified chick embryo cell rabies vaccine for pre-exposure immunization, *Vaccine* 7:397, 1989.

SUGGESTED READINGS

Hemachudha T, Wilde H: Survival after treatment of rabies, *N Engl J Med* 353(10):1068, 2005.

Rupprecht CE, Gibbons RV: Prophylaxis against rabies, *N Engl J Med* 351:2626, 2004.

Srinivasan A et al: Transmission of rabies virus from an organ donor to four transplant recipients, *N Engl J Med* 352:1103, 2005.

AUTHORS: **GLENN G. FORT, M.D., M.P.H., DENNIS J. MIKOLICH, M.D.,** and **MAURICE POLICAR, M.D.**

BASIC INFORMATION

DEFINITION

Exposure to ionizing radiation has the potential for radiation injury. Radionuclides present a danger to humans through the particles emitted during radioactive decay. These particles can damage cellular structures and may result in mutation, cancer, or cell death. Radiation injury can occur from external irradiation, external contamination with radioactive materials, and internal contamination by inhalation, ingestion, or transdermal absorption with incorporation of radiologic materials into the body's cells and tissues. These three types of exposure can occur in combination and can be associated with thermal burns and traumatic injuries.

PRINCIPLES OF RADIOACTIVITY, ADDITIONAL DEFINITIONS:

Particles of radiation

- Photons: massless particles that travel at the speed of light and produce electromagnetic radiation. Their wavelength determines their energy; the longer the wavelength the lower the energy. In order of increasing energy, they are called ultraviolet, visible light, infrared, microwave, gamma, and x-rays. X-rays consist of a spectrum of wavelengths whereas gamma rays have a fixed wavelength specific to the radioactive material that produces them. X-rays and gamma rays are highly penetrating.
- Beta particles are electrons. They may be emitted during decay of a radionuclide (atom) that disintegrates. Positrons (positively charged electrons) may also be produced during radioactive decay. Beta particles are less penetrating than x-rays and gamma rays, but can still pass through several centimeters of human tissue. Nonetheless, their main toxic effect is through inhalation.
- Alpha particles are helium nuclei (2 protons and 2 neutrons) stripped of their electrons. They are stopped by clothing; therefore, they need to be "incorporated" to cause health problems.
- Neutrons are released during nuclear fission, not during natural radionuclide decay. They can cause a stable atom to become radioactive by collision (e.g., during nuclear fallout).
- Cosmic rays are streams of electrons, protons, and alpha particles that come from outer space. Most of their energy is dissipated by the earth's atmosphere.
- Ionizing radiation describes any radiation with sufficient energy to break up an atom or molecule with which it collides. This is the mechanism of radiation toxicity.
- Nonionizing radiation has insufficient energy to break up atoms; nonetheless sufficient energy in the form of heat may be produced to cause localized tissue damage.
- Radioactive decay: process of transformation of unstable nuclei into more stable ones via the emissions of various particles. Decay is described by half-life, which is a characteristic of every radioisotope.
- Radiation units of measure:
  1. Roentgen: amount of radiation to which an object is exposed.
  2. Rad (radiation absorbed dose) and Gray (Gy, the same concept in the international system): amount of radiation absorbed by tissue (1 Gy = 100 Rad).
  3. Rem (roentgen equivalent man) and Sievert (Sv, the same concept in the International System): a measure that standardizes the amount of cel lular damage produced by different types of radiation. One Rem (or 0.01 Sv) is the dose of radiation that produces damage equivalent to one Rad of x-ray.

IRRADIATION, CONTAMINATION, AND INCORPORATION:

- Irradiation: exposure to ionizing radiation
- Contamination: an object or person covered with a radioactive substance
- Incorporation: exposure to a radionuclide by inhalation, ingestion, intravenous infusion, or percutaneously

STOCHASTIC EFFECTS OF IONIZING RADIATION:

Any dose of ionizing radiation can alter DNA, causing mutations or carcinogenic changes that may take years to be expressed. There is no dose threshold, and the effect is cumulative. The stochastic effects of radiation are mostly a concern with small but prolonged exposure to radiation.

DETERMINISTIC EFFECTS OF IONIZING RADIATION:

The dose of radiation is sufficient to kill cells; the higher the dose, the greater the number of killed cells and the greater the impact on an organ system. The deterministic effects of radiation are the consequence of a large whole-body exposure.

SYNONYMS

Acute radiation syndrome
Radiation sickness

ICD-9CM CODE
990 Radiation exposure

PHYSICAL FINDINGS & CLINICAL PRESENTATION

ACUTE RADIATION SYNDROME:

Follows a large whole-body exposure of 2 Sv or more (500 times the average annual exposure) or greater than 1 Gy delivered at a relatively high dose rate. The mean lethal dose of radiation required to kill 50% of humans at 60 days (LD 50/60) of whole body radiation is between 3.25 and 4 Gy in persons managed without supportive care and 6 to 7 Gy when antibiotics and transfusion support are provided.

Sequence of events: four stages:

- Stage 1 (prodromal phase): usually occurs in the first 48 hr but may develop up to 6 days after exposure.
- Stage 2 (latent phase): short period characterized by improvement of symptoms, as the person appears to have recovered. Unfortunately this effect is transient, lasting for several days to a month.
- Stage 3 (manifest illness phase): third to fifth week following exposure. This stage is characterized by intense immunosuppression and is the most difficult to manage. If the person survives this stage, recovery is likely. Signs and symptoms consist of abdominal pain, diarrhea, hair loss, bleeding, infection. During this stage, several subsyndromes may coexist, overlap, or occur in sequence.
  1. Cerebrovascular syndrome: fever, hypotension, ataxia, apathy, lethargy, and seizures. These symptoms may be observed in those receiving more than 20 to 30 Gy of radiation. The prodromal phase is characterized by disorientation, confusion, and prostration. The physical exam may show papilledema, ataxia, decreased or absent DTRs, and corneal reflexes.
  2. Cutaneous syndrome: due from thermal or radiation burns and characterized by loss of epidermis, local edema, and increased risk for a compartmental syndrome.
  3. GI syndrome: radiation induces loss of intestinal crypts and breakdown of mucosal barrier. These changes result in abdominal pain, anorexia, nausea, vomiting, diarrhea, and dehydration, and predispose patients to superinfection and sepsis.
  4. Hematopoietic syndrome: lymphopenia is common and occurs before the onset of other cytopenias; pancytopenia with bleeding diathesis and sepsis often follow. A predictable decline in lymphocytes occurs after irradiation. A potentially lethal exposure is characterized by a 50% decline in absolute lymphocyte count within the first 24 hr after exposure, followed by a further, more severe decline within 48 hr. The onset of cytopenias varies, depending on the dose and dose rate. Granulocyte counts may transiently increase before decreas-

ing in patients with exposure to less than 5 Gy. This transient increase before decline is known as an "abortive rise" and may indicate a survivable exposure.

- Stage 4: recovery, lasting weeks to months.

DIAGNOSIS

DOSE ESTIMATION AND PROGNOSIS:

Because radiation is often mixed and because body parts may be exposed to different amounts of radiation, the dose received is difficult to estimate in the field. Therefore, it is usually the acute radiation syndrome itself that allows prognosis. At a dose received under 3 Sv a lymphocyte count >1200/mm^3 at 48 hr confers a favorable prognosis; if the count is <1200/mm^3, a fatal dose is possible and more aggressive medical management is warranted. A drop in the number of granulocytes or platelets also portends a severe exposure. Patients exposed to less than 2 Sv will survive with no or minimal care. Patients exposed to 2 to 5 Sv are likely to survive with medical care. A dose of 5 to 20 Sv is survivable. A dose above 20 Sv is supralethal, and the patient will die within 24 to 48 hr from CNS or CV syndrome. At the Chernobyl nuclear reactor accident, mortality was 33% among those receiving 4 to 6 Sv and 95% among those receiving 6 to 16 Sv. When expressed in Gy units:

- Exposure <1 Gy: almost certain survival
- Exposure 1 to 2 Gy: 90% survival
- Exposure 2 to 3.5 Gy: probable survival
- Exposure 3.5 to 5.5 Gy: 50% survival
- Exposure 5.5 to 10 Gy: probable death
- Exposure >10 Gy: certain death

CARCINOGENESIS:

Leukemia, breast cancer, lung cancer, and thyroid cancer incidence increase following exposure to ionizing exposure. This is a stochastic effect that can occur with or without a history of acute radiation syndrome.

ETIOLOGY

SOURCE OF RADIATION:

- Natural
  1. Radon (domestic and mining industry)
  2. Cosmic
  3. Terrestrial
  4. Ingested (from food)
- Industrial
  1. X-ray diagnosis
  2. Nuclear medicine
  3. Consumer products
  4. Occupational (e.g., nuclear energy)
  5. Weapons

TREATMENT

- Decontamination
  1. Perform at site of exposure unless there is ongoing radiation.
  2. Remove all clothing (and treat those as radioactive waste). Providers should use strict isolation precautions including donning of gown, mask, cap, double gloves, and shoe covers when evaluating and treating contaminated patients.
  3. Wash patient with soap and water. Dispose of the used water as radioactive waste.
  4. Scrub any open wound.
  5. Depending on the situation, the regional emergency response system should be called for additional measures such as evacuation.
- Management of the acute radiation syndrome
  1. Establish IV access.
  2. Manage the airway if needed.
  3. Manage burns.
  4. Identify and treat other injuries.
  5. Provide analgesia.
  6. Give antiemetics (e.g., ondansetron).
  7. Manage bleeding and transfuse if necessary.
  8. Diagnose and treat sepsis. Administration of antibiotics reduces mortality. In nonneutropenic patients, antibiotic therapy should be directed toward foci of infection and the most likely pathogens. Fluoroquinolones are useful for prophylaxis in neutropenic patients.
  9. Consider colony-stimulating factors. In any adult with a whole body or significant partial body exposure >3 Gy, treatment with CSFs should be rapidly initiated (e.g., G-CSF or filgrastim, 5 mcg/kg of body weight per day). CSF may be withdrawn when the absolute neutrophil count reaches a level greater than 1.0 × 10 9 after recovery from the nadir.
  10. Consider stem-cell transplantation in people with exposure dose of 7 to 10 Gy who do not have significant burns or other major organ toxicity and who have an appropriate donor.
  11. Provide counseling: 75% of individuals exposed to nuclear weapon denotations exhibit some form of psychologic symptoms, ranging from insomnia to difficulty concentrating and social withdrawal.

PEARLS & CONSIDERATIONS

COMMENTS

Individual biodosimetry is essential for predicting the clinical severity, treatment, and survivability of exposed individuals. The three most useful elements for calculating the exposure dose are time to onset of vomiting, lymphocyte depletion kinetics, and the presence of chromosome dicentrics.

A radiation casualty management software program (biologic assessment tool) is available at the Armed Forces' Radiobiology Research Institute website (www.afrri.usuhs.mil).

Monitoring of lymphocyte count requires obtaining a CBC with leukocyte differential immediately after exposure, three times/day for next 3 days, then twice/day for the following 6 days. CBC with differential should then be obtained weekly until a nadir in neutrophil count is defined.

The chromosome-aberration cytogenetic bioassay should be obtained from a qualified radiation cytogenetic biodosimetry laboratory.

SUGGESTED READINGS

Rella J: Radiation. In Goldfrank LR et al (eds): *Toxicologic emergencies,* ed 7, New York, 2002, McGraw-Hill.

Turai I et al: Medical response to radiation incidents and radionuclear threats, *BMJ* 4:247, 2004.

Waselenko JK et al: Medical management of the acute radiation syndrome, *Ann Intern Med* 140:1037, 2004.

AUTHORS: **FRED F. FERRI, M.D.,** and **TOM J. WACHTEL, M.D.**

BASIC INFORMATION

DEFINITION

Ramsay Hunt syndrome is a localized herpes zoster infection involving the seventh nerve and geniculate ganglia, resulting in hearing loss, vertigo, and facial nerve palsy.

SYNONYMS

Herpes zoster oticus
Geniculate herpes
Herpetic geniculate ganglionitis

ICD-9CM CODES
053.11 Ramsay Hunt syndrome

EPIDEMIOLOGY & DEMOGRAPHICS

PREDOMINANT SEX: Equal sex distribution

PREDOMINANT AGE:
- Increasingly common with advancing age
- Rare in childhood

PHYSICAL FINDINGS & CLINICAL PRESENTATION

- Characteristic vesicles:
  1. On pinna
  2. In external auditory canal
  3. In distribution of the facial nerve and, occasionally, adjacent cranial nerves
- Facial paralysis on the involved side

ETIOLOGY

Reactivation of dormant infection with varicella-zoster virus following primary varicella

DIAGNOSIS

- Usually made by recognition of the clinical features detailed previously
- Viral culture and/or microscopic examination of specimens taken from active vesicles

DIFFERENTIAL DIAGNOSIS

- Herpes simplex
- External otitis
- Impetigo
- Enteroviral infection
- Bell's palsy of other etiologies
- Acoustic neuroma (before appearance of skin lesions)
- The differential diagnosis of headache and facial pain is described in Section II

WORKUP

If the diagnosis is in doubt, confirmation of varicella-zoster virus infection should be sought.

LABORATORY TESTS

- Viral culture of specimens of vesicular fluid and scrapings of the vesicle base
- Tzanck preparation, which may reveal multinucleated giant cells
- Direct immunofluorescent staining of scrapings

IMAGING STUDIES

MRI may demonstrate enhancement of the facial and vestibulocochlear nerves before appearance of vesicles.

TREATMENT

ACUTE GENERAL Rx

- Prednisone (40 mg PO for 2 days; 30 mg for 7 days; followed by tapering course) is recommended by some authors.
- Acyclovir (800 mg PO 5 times qd for 10 days), famciclovir (500 mg tid for 7 days), or valacyclovir (1 g every 8 hr for 7 days) may hasten healing.
- Analgesics should be used as indicated.

CHRONIC Rx

- Amitriptyline is effective in some cases of postherpetic pain.
- Other agents for postherpetic pain include gabapentin (Neurontin) and pregabalin (Lyrica).
- Narcotic analgesics may occasionally be necessary.

DISPOSITION

Recurrences are unusual.

REFERRAL

To otolaryngologist: patients with persistent facial paralysis for potential surgical decompression of the facial nerve

PEARLS & CONSIDERATIONS

COMMENTS

Immunodeficiency states, particularly infection with the human immunodeficiency virus (HIV), should be considered in:
- Younger patients
- Severe cases
- Patients with a history of specific risk behavior

SUGGESTED READINGS

Diaz GA, Rakita RM, Koelle DM: A case of Ramsay Hunt-like syndrome caused by herpes simplex virus type 2, *Clin Infect Dis* 40(10):1545, 2005.

Kinishi M et al: Acyclovir improves recovery rate of facial nerve palsy in Ramsay Hunt syndrome, *Auris Nasus Larynx* 28(3):223, 2001.

Verm AM, Scott IU, Davis JL: Necrotizing herpetic retinopathy associated with Ramsay Hunt syndrome, *Arch Ophthalmol* 120(7): 989, 2002.

AUTHORS: **GLENN G. FORT, M.D., M.P.H., DENNIS J. MIKOLICH, M.D.,** and **JOSEPH R. MASCI, M.D.**

BASIC INFORMATION

DEFINITION

Raynaud's phenomenon (RP) is a vasospastic disorder that produces an exaggerated response to cold temperatures and/or emotional stress resulting in transient digital ischemia. It is manifested as a triphasic discoloration of the fingers and toes (a result of pallor, cyanosis, and rubor).

SYNONYMS

Primary Raynaud's phenomenon or Raynaud's disease
Secondary Raynaud's phenomenon

ICD-9CM CODES
443.0 Raynaud's syndrome, Raynaud's disease, Raynaud's phenomenon (secondary)
785.4 If gangrene present

EPIDEMIOLOGY & DEMOGRAPHICS

- RP is classified clinically into primary or secondary forms and affects approximately 3% of the general population.
- Primary RP usually occurs between the ages of 15 and 25 yr. It is more likely to effect women than men, and appears to be more common in colder climates.
- Secondary RP tends to begin after 35 to 40 yr of age.
- Secondary RP occurs in more than 90% of patients with scleroderma, and in about 30% of patients with systemic lupus erythematosus and with Sjögren's syndrome.
- There is also some suggestion that secondary RP may be associated with drugs (nicotine, caffeine, ergotamine, vinyl chloride) or trauma to the hands from vibrating tools such as jack hammers.

PHYSICAL FINDINGS & CLINICAL PRESENTATION

- The classic manifestation is the triphasic color response to cold exposure, which may or may not be accompanied by pain (Fig. 1-221):
  1. Pallor of the digit resulting from vasospasm.
  2. Blue discoloration (cyanosis) secondary to desaturated venous blood.
  3. Red (rubor) with or without pain and paresthesia when vasospasm resolves and blood returns to the digit.
- Initial pallor is typically necessary for the diagnosis to be made.
- The triphasic color changes can sometimes be induced in the office by placing the hand in an ice bath.
- Color changes are well delineated, symmetric, and usually bilateral involving the fingers and toes. The index, middle, and ring fingers are commonly involved.
- Fingertips are most often involved, but feet, ears, and nose can be affected.
- Duration of attacks can range from seconds to hours.
- Chronic skin changes resulting from repeated attacks may include skin thickening and brittle nails. Ulcerations and, rarely, gangrene may occur.
- Physical exam should also include examination for symptoms associated with autoimmune disease, such as fever, rash, arthritis, dry eyes, dry mouth, myalgias, or cardiopulmonary abnormalities.

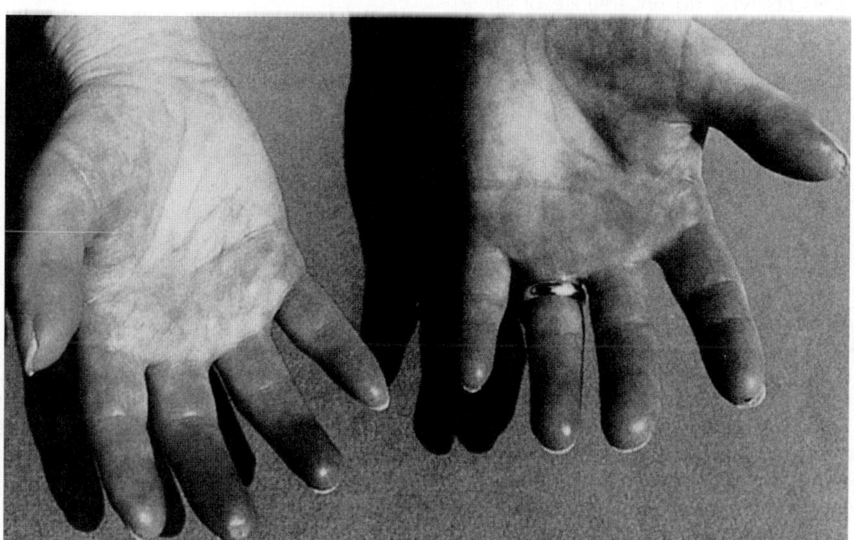

FIGURE 1-221 Raynaud's phenomenon. Sharply demarcated cyanosis of the fingers with proximal venular congestion (livedo reticularis) is seen. (From Klippel J, Dieppe P, Ferri F [eds]: *Primary care rheumatology,* London, 1999, Mosby.)

ETIOLOGY

- Primary RP can also be called idiopathic Raynaud's phenomenon, primary Raynaud's syndrome, or Raynaud's disease. It occurs in the absence of any associated disease.
- With primary RP, the possibility that another first-degree family member is affected is reported as approximately 25%.
- Secondary RP is associated with an underlying pathologic condition or disease and may include the following:
  1. CREST syndrome (calcinosis, RP, esophageal dysmotility, sclerodactyly, and telangiectasia)
  2. Scleroderma
  3. Mixed connective tissue disease, polymyositis, and dermatomyositis
  4. Systemic lupus erythematosus
  5. Rheumatoid arthritis
  6. Thromboangiitis obliterans (Buerger's disease)
  7. Drug induced (beta-blockers, ergotamine, methysergide, vinblastine, bleomycin, oral contraceptives, nicotine, caffeine, vinyl chloride)
  8. Hematological disorders (polycythemia, cryoglobulinemia, cold agglutinins, paraproteinemia)
  9. Carpal tunnel syndrome
  10. Use of tools that vibrate
  11. Endocrine disorders (hypothyroidism, carcinoid syndrome)

DIAGNOSIS

The suggested criteria for primary RP are:
- Symmetric attacks.
- Absence of tissue necrosis, ulceration, or gangrene.
- Absence of a secondary cause on the basis of a patient's history and general physical examination.
- Normal nail-fold capillaries.
- Negative test for antinuclear antibody.
- Normal erythrocyte sedimentation rate (ESR).

Secondary RP is suggested by the following findings:
- Onset of symptoms after the age of 30 years.
- Episodes that are painful, asymmetric, or associated with ischemic skin lesions.
- Clinical features suggestive of a connective-tissue disease.
- Specific autoantibody tests and ESR are elevated.
- Evidence of microvascular disease on microscopy of nail-fold capillaries.

DIFFERENTIAL DIAGNOSIS

- Neurogenic thoracic outlet syndrome or carpal tunnel syndrome

- Frostbite or cold weather injury
- Medication reaction (ergotamine, chemotherapeutic agents)
- Atherosclerosis, thromboembolic disease
- Buerger's disease, embolic disease
- Acrocyanosis
- Livedo reticularis
- Injury from repetitive motion

WORKUP

- Once the diagnosis of RP is established, differentiating primary from secondary is helpful in treatment and prognosis.
- Patients who are younger when their symptoms occur; have a normal history and physical examination and normal nail-fold capillaries; and have no history of digital ischemic lesions can be considered as having primary RP. These patients can be monitored clinically without any further testing.
- If a secondary cause of RP is suspected, appropriate lab testing is recommended (see "Laboratory Testing"). Secondary RP will reveal abnormal nail-fold microscopy.

LABORATORY TESTS

- Complete blood count, serum electrolytes, blood urea nitrogen (BUN), creatinine, ESR, antinuclear antibodies (ANA), VDRL antibody test, rheumatoid factor (RF), and urinalysis should be included in the initial evaluation.
- If the history, physical examination, and initial laboratory tests suggest a possible secondary cause, specific serologic testing (e.g., anticentromere antibodies, anti-Scl 70, cryoglobulins, complement testing, and protein electrophoresis) may be indicated.
- Noninvasive vascular testing includes finger systolic blood pressures, segmental blood pressure measurements, cold recovery time (measure vasoconstrictor and vasodilator responses of finger to cold), finger tip thermography, and laser Doppler with thermal challenge (measure relative change in skin blood flow with ambient warming).

IMAGING STUDIES

- The diagnosis of RP should not be made on the basis of laboratory tests and imaging studies should not replace a good history and physical exam.
- Duplex ultrasound can image the palmar arch and digital arteries for patency.
- Magnetic resonance angiography (MRA) is useful imaging larger arteries.
- Contrast angiography is the gold standard for arterial imaging.
- Nail-fold capillary microscopy can differentiate primary from secondary RP.

TREATMENT (Rx)

NONPHARMACOLOGIC THERAPY

- Avoid drugs that may precipitate RP (see "Etiology").
- Avoid cold exposure. Use warm gloves, hats, and garments during the winter months or before going into cold environments (e.g., air-conditioned rooms). Sudden shifts in temperature are more likely to precipitate RP.
- Avoid stressful situations, and use relaxation techniques in preventing RP attacks.

ACUTE GENERAL Rx

- Typically, patients with RP respond well to nonpharmacologic measures.
- Medications are indicated in the treatment of RP if there are signs of critical ischemia or if the quality of life of the patient is affected to the degree that activities of normal living are no longer possible, and preventative techniques do not work.

CHRONIC Rx

- Calcium channel blockers are the most effective treatment for RP.
- Calcium channel blockers differ in their peripheral vasodilator properties. Nifedipine, amlodipine, felodipine, nisoldipine, and isradipine appear more effective than diltiazem and verapamil in the treatment of RP.
- Nifedipine is most often prescribed at a dose of 10 to 20 mg 30 min before going outside. If symptoms occur with long duration, nifedipine XL 30 to 180 mg PO qd is effective.
- Patients who do not tolerate or fail to respond to calcium channel blocker therapy can try other vasodilator drugs alone or in combination. Options include nitroglycerin, nitroprusside, hydralazine, papaverine, minoxidil, niacin, and topical nitrates.
- Agents that indirectly cause vasodilation (selective serotonin reuptake inhibitors, ACE inhibitors, phosphodiesterase inhibitors) may be useful, but there is no convincing evidence that they are better than calcium channel blockers alone.
- Sympatholytic agents (reserpine, guanethidine) may be helpful for acute treatment, but their effect tends to decrease with time, and they often have intolerable side effects.
- Alpha receptor blockers such as prazosin or doxazosin counteract the actions of norepinephrine, which will constrict blood vessels.
- The prostaglandins, including inhaled iloprost, intravenous epoprostenol, and alprostadil, may be promising in severe RP. However, additional experience and controlled studies are needed to substantiate this claim.
- Phosphodiesterase inhibitors (such as cilostazol [Pletal], pentoxifylline [Trental], and sildenafil [Viagra], and angiotensin II receptor antagonists (such as losartan [Cozaar]) have also been used with some limited success.
- Anticoagulation with aspirin and heparin can be considered during the acute phase of an ischemic event. Aspirin (81 mg/day) therapy can be considered in all patients with secondary RP with a history of ischemic ulcers or thrombotic events; however, caution should be exercised because aspirin can theoretically worsen vasospasm via inhibition of prostacyclin. Long-term anticoagulation with heparin or warfarin is not recommended unless there is evidence of a hypercoagulable disorder.
- Bypass surgery can be performed for severe RP associated with reconstructible arterial occlusive disease.
- Sympathectomy is available for unreconstructable occlusive disease or pure vasospastic disease refractory to medical treatment.

DISPOSITION

The prognosis of patients with RP depends on the etiology.

- Primary RP is fairly benign, usually remaining stable and controlled with nonpharmacologic medical treatment.
- Patients with secondary RP, specifically those with scleroderma, CREST syndrome, and thromboangiitis obliterans, may develop severe ischemic digits with ulceration, gangrene, and autoamputation.

REFERRAL

- Rheumatology consult is indicated if secondary collagen vascular disease is diagnosed.
- Vascular surgery consult is indicated if ulcers, gangrene, or threatened digit loss is noted.

PEARLS & CONSIDERATIONS (!)

- Most patients with RP can be managed by a primary care provider.
- It is important to differentiate primary from secondary forms. Secondary forms may become manifest as far out as 10 yr from the diagnosis of RP. It is important to take immediate action during an attack and patients' are encouraged to:
  1. Keep warm
  2. Not smoke
  3. Avoid aggravating medications
  4. Control stress

5. Exercise
6. Follow up with a physician

EVIDENCE

EBM

A meta-analysis of calcium channel blockers in systemic sclerosis concluded that there is moderate evidence for the efficacy of nifedipine in reducing the frequency and severity of attacks of Raynaud's in this group.[1] A Other medical therapies have been shown to be beneficial in some trials, but the evidence so far is limited:

A crossover randomized controlled trial (RCT) comparing prazosin 1 mg twice daily vs. placebo in 24 people (14 with the primary disease) found that prazosin significantly reduced the mean number and duration of attacks vs. placebo but not the severity of attacks.[2] A

Topical nitrates have been shown to reduce severity and frequency of attacks but side effects are not unusual.[3] B

The synthetic prostacyclin analog iloprost was found to reduce the frequency and severity of Raynaud's attacks significantly and also to prevent and heal digital ulcers.[4] There is evidence for the successful use of surgical sympathectomy to reduce symptoms and avoid amputation.[5-7] B

Evidence-Based References

1. Thompson AE et al: Calcium-channel blockers for Raynaud's phenomenon in systemic sclerosis, *Arthritis Rheum* 44:1841, 2001.
2. Wollersheim H et al: Double-blind, placebo-controlled study of prazosin in Raynaud's phenomenon, *Clin Pharmacol Ther* 40:219, 1986. Reviewed in: *Clin Evid* 11:1603, 2004.
3. Teh LS et al: Sustained-release transdermal glyceral trinitrate patches as treatment for primary and secondary Raynaud's phenomenon, *Br J Rheumatol* 34:636, 1995.
4. Pope J et al: Iloprost and cisaprost for Raynaud's phenomenon in progressive systemic sclerosis. Reviewed in: Cochrane Library 2, Chichester, UK, 2004, John Wiley.
5. McCall TE et al: The use of digital artery sympathectomy as a salvage procedure for severe ischaemia of Raynaud's disease and phenomenon, *J Hand Surg [Am]* 24:173, 1999.
6. Tomaino MM et al: Surgery for ischemic pain and Raynaud's phenomenon in scleroderma: description of treatment protocol and evaluation of results, *Microsurgery* 21:75, 2001.
7. Tham S et al: Limited microsurgical arteriolysis for complications of digital vasospasm, *J Hand Surg [Br]* 22:359, 1997.

SUGGESTED READINGS

Cook JP et al: Mechanisms of Raynaud's disease, *Vasc Med* 10:297-307, 2005.

Thompson AE, Pope JE: Calcium channel blockers for primary Raynaud's phenomenon: a meta-analysis, *Rheumatology* (Oxford) 44:145, 2005.

Wigley FM: Raynaud's phenomenon, *N Engl J Med* 347:1001-1008, 2002.

AUTHOR: **PRANAV M. PATEL, M.D.**

BASIC INFORMATION

DEFINITION

Reflex sympathetic dystrophy (RSD) or complex regional pain syndrome (CRPS) type 1 is a pain disorder characterized by constant and intense limb pain associated with vasomotor and sudomotor abnormalities that occurs without a definable nerve lesion. RSD or CRPS type 1 should be distinguished from CRPS type 2, which refers to pain disorders where a definable nerve lesion exists.

SYNONYMS

CRPS type 1
Causalgia (or CRPS type 2)
Shoulder-hand syndrome
Sudeck's atrophy
Posttraumatic pain syndrome

ICD-9CM CODES
337.20 Dystrophy sympathetic (posttraumatic) (reflex)

EPIDEMIOLOGY & DEMOGRAPHICS

- First described by Mitchell et al during the American Civil War.
- The incidence and prevalence is not known.
- Usually initiated by trauma, mostly after orthopedic procedures, especially those on the extremities
- Can occur in adults or children.
- Often associated with psychiatric and emotional lability, anxiety, and depression.

PHYSICAL FINDINGS & CLINICAL PRESENTATION

RSD is divided into three stages:

- Acute stage (occurring within hours to days after the injury)
  1. Burning or aching pain occurring over the injured extremity
  2. Hyperalgesia (exquisitely sensitive to touch)
  3. Edema
  4. Dysthermia
  5. Increased hair and nail growth
- Dystrophic stage (3 to 6 mo after the injury)
  1. Burning pain radiating both distal and proximally from the site of injury
  2. Brawny edema
  3. Hyperhidrosis
  4. Hypothermia and cyanosis
  5. Muscle tremors and spasms
  6. Increased muscle tone and reflexes
- Atrophic stage (6 mo after injury)
  1. Spread of pain proximally
  2. Cold, pale cyanotic skin
  3. Trophic skin changes with subcutaneous atrophy
  4. Fixed joints
  5. Contractures

ETIOLOGY

- The cause is unknown. It is thought to represent dysfunction of the sympathetic nervous system.
- Any injury can precipitate RSD including:
  1. Crush blunt trauma, burns, frostbite
  2. Surgery
  3. Parkinson's disease
  4. Cerebrovascular accident
  5. Myocardial infarction
  6. Osteoarthritis, cervical and lumbar disk disease
  7. Carpal tunnel and tarsal tunnel syndrome
  8. Diabetes
  9. Hyperthyroidism
  10. Isoniazid therapy

DIAGNOSIS

The diagnosis is primarily clinical, based on the patient's history and physical presentation.

DIFFERENTIAL DIAGNOSIS

The differential diagnosis includes all the causes mentioned under "Etiology."

WORKUP

- No workup is needed because there are no specific diagnostic tests establishing the diagnosis.
- Electrophysiologic testing is useful to identify patients with type 2 CRPS.

LABORATORY TESTS

Blood tests are not specific.

IMAGING STUDIES

- No imaging studies are diagnostic. Three-phase bone imaging may be helpful.
- Autonomic testing, although not commonly done, has been proposed.
  1. Measuring resting sweat output
  2. Measuring resting skin temperature
  3. Quantitative sudomotor axon reflex test
- X-ray studies of the affected limb may show osteoporosis from disuse.

TREATMENT

Treatment is aimed at relieving the pain and improving disuse atrophy with physical therapy.

NONPHARMACOLOGIC THERAPY

- Physical therapy
- Transcutaneous nerve stimulation

ACUTE GENERAL Rx

- The following has been tried for neuropathic pain relief:
  1. Amitriptyline 10 mg to 150 mg qd
  2. Phenytoin 300 mg qd
  3. Carbamazepine 100 mg bid
  4. Calcium channel blockers, nifedipine extended release 30 to 60 mg qd
  5. Prednisone 60 to 80 mg qd × 2 wk and then tapered over 1 to 2 wk to a maintenance dose of 5 mg qd for 2 to 3 mo
  6. Vitamin C 500 mg daily for 50 days after wrist fracture can decrease the occurrence of CRPS
  7. Gabapentin 300 mg daily up to 3 times a day
- Regional nerve block that provides a perioperative sympathectomy may be advantageous for patients with a history of CRPS who require orthopedic surgery.
- Because CRPS type 2 is the result of a definable nerve lesion, using a surgical technique that minimizes the risk of nerve damage is important.

CHRONIC Rx

- Stellate ganglion and lumbar sympathetic blocks can be tried
- Intravenous alpha-adrenergic blockade with phentolamine may predict response to subsequent sympatholytic treatment.
- Surgical sympathectomy.

DISPOSITION

Spontaneous remission can occur after several weeks to months.

REFERRAL

RSD is a very difficult diagnosis to make and referral to either rheumatology, neurology, orthopedic, or psychiatry is recommended.

PEARLS & CONSIDERATIONS

COMMENTS

- RSD is a common clinical entity without clear definition, pathophysiologic features, or treatment.
- Pain is the most disabling symptom for most patients and is usually out of proportion to the extent of the injury.

SUGGESTED READINGS

Baron R: Reflex sympathetic dystrophy and causalgia, *Suppl Clin Neurophysiol* 57:24, 2004.

Dowd GSE et al: Complex regional pain syndrome with special emphasis on the knee, *J Bone Joint Surg* 89-B(3):285-290, 2007.

Low AK et al: Pediatric complex regional pain syndrome, *J Pediatr Orthop* 27(5):567-572, 2007.

Reuben SS, Buvanendran A: Preventing the development of chronic pain after orthopaedic surgery with preventive multimodal analgesic techniques, *J Bone Joint Surg [Am]* 89(6):1343-1358, 2007.

Teasdall RD et al: Complex regional pain syndrome (reflex sympathetic dystrophy), *Clin Sports Med* 23(1):145, 2004.

AUTHOR: **JORGE WILLAFUERTE, M.D.**

BASIC INFORMATION

DEFINITION

Reiter's syndrome is one of the seronegative spondyloarthropathies, so called because serum rheumatoid factor is not present in these forms of inflammatory arthritis. There is an international consensus that the term *reactive arthritis* should replace the name Reiter's syndrome to describe this constellation of signs and symptoms. Unfortunately, the original name is still associated with the syndrome. Reiter's syndrome is an asymmetric polyarthritis that affects mainly the lower extremities and is associated with one or more of the following:

- Urethritis
- Cervicitis
- Dysentery
- Inflammatory eye disease
- Mucocutaneous lesions

SYNONYMS

Reiter's disease
Reactive arthritis
Seronegative spondyloarthropathy

ICD-9CM CODES
099.3 Reiter's syndrome

EPIDEMIOLOGY & DEMOGRAPHICS

INCIDENCE (IN U.S.): 0.0035% annually of men <50 yr
PEAK INCIDENCE: Most common in the third decade
PREDOMINANT SEX: Male
PREDOMINANT AGE: 20 to 40 yr
GENETICS:
Familial Disposition: Strongly associated with HLA-B27 (63% to 96%)

PHYSICAL FINDINGS & CLINICAL PRESENTATION

- Polyarthritis
  1. Affecting the knee and ankle
  2. Commonly asymmetric
- Heel pain and Achilles tendinitis, especially at the insertion of the Achilles tendon
- Plantar fasciitis
- Large effusions
- Dactylitis or "sausage toe"
- Urethritis
- Uveitis or conjunctivitis; uveitis can progress to blindness without treatment
- Keratoderma blennorrhagicum, circinate balinitis
  1. Hyperkeratotic lesions on soles of the feet, toes, penis, hands
  2. Closely resembles psoriasis
- Aortic regurgitation similar to that seen in ankylosing spondylitis

ETIOLOGY

- Epidemic Reiter's syndrome following outbreaks of dysentery has been well described.
- Genetically susceptible HLA-B27 individuals are at risk for developing Reiter's syndrome following infection with certain pathogens:
  1. *Salmonella*
  2. *Shigella*
  3. *Yersinia enterocolitica*
  4. *Chlamydia trachomatis*
  5. Molecular mimicry mechanism suspected
- Symptom complex indistinguishable from Reiter's syndrome has been described in association with HIV infection.

DIAGNOSIS

DIFFERENTIAL DIAGNOSIS

- Ankylosing spondylitis
- Psoriatic arthritis
- Rheumatoid arthritis
- Gonococcal arthritis-tenosynovitis
- Rheumatic fever

WORKUP

- X-ray examination of affected joints
- Synovial fluid examination and culture
- Careful examination of eyes and skin
- Cultures for gonococcus (urethral, cervical, stool)

LABORATORY TESTS

- Elevated but nonspecific ESR
- No specific laboratory tests to diagnose Reiter's syndrome

IMAGING STUDIES

Plain radiographs:

- Juxtaarticular osteopenia of affected joints
- Erosions and joint space narrowing in more advanced disease
- Periostitis and reactive new bone formation at the insertions of the Achilles tendon and the plantar fascia
- Sacroiliitis:
  1. Unilateral or bilateral
  2. Indistinguishable from ankylosing spondylitis
- Vertebral bridging osteophytes

TREATMENT

NONPHARMACOLOGIC THERAPY

Physical therapy to maintain range of motion of the back and other joints

ACUTE GENERAL Rx

Flares treated with NSAIDs such as indomethacin (25 to 50 mg PO tid)

- Enteric or urethral infection should be treated with appropriate antibiotic coverage.
- Uveitis should be treated with steroid eye drops in consultation with an ophthalmologist.
- Achilles tendinitis and plantar fasciitis should be treated with injections of methylprednisolone (40 to 80 mg).
- Sulfasalazine (2 to 3 g PO tid) may be effective.
- Careful monitoring for the following is essential:
  1. GI toxicity
  2. Hypersensitivity
  3. Bone marrow suppression
- Persistent and uncontrolled disease should be managed with cytotoxic drugs (methotrexate, azathioprine) in consultation with a rheumatologist.

CHRONIC Rx

Chronic disease is best managed by a team approach with the collaboration of a rheumatologist or other experienced physician and physical therapist.

DISPOSITION

- Recurrences are frequent, even with treatment.
- Long-term sequelae:
  1. Persistent polyarthritis
  2. Chronic back pain
  3. Heel pain
  4. Progressive iridocyclitis
  5. Aortic regurgitation

REFERRAL

- To ophthalmologist if uveitis is suspected
- To rheumatologist if arthritis and tendinitis fail to improve rapidly after a course of NSAIDs

PEARLS & CONSIDERATIONS

COMMENTS

- Infection with HIV is associated with particularly severe cases of Reiter's syndrome.
- HIV testing is recommended, especially if risk factors such as unprotected sexual activity or IV drug use are identified.

SUGGESTED READINGS

Eapen BR: A new insight into the pathogenesis of Reiter's syndrome using bioinformatics tools, *Int J Dermatol* 42(3):242, 2003.

Klecker RJ, Weissman BN: Imaging features of psoriatic arthritis and Reiter's syndrome, *Semin Musculoskelet Radiol* 7(2):115, 2003.

Neumann S et al: Reiter's syndrome as a manifestation of an immune reconstitution syndrome in an HIV-infected patient: successful treatment with doxycycline, *Clin Infect Dis* 36(12):1628, 2003.

Schneider JM, Matthews JH, Graham BS: Reiter's syndrome, *Cutis* 71(3):198, 2003.

AUTHORS: **GLENN G. FORT, M.D., M.P.H., DENNIS J. MIKOLICH, M.D.,** and **DEBORAH L. SHAPIRO, M.D.**

BASIC INFORMATION

DEFINITION

Renal artery stenosis is the narrowing or occlusion of a renal artery, which can occur acutely (thrombosis or embolism) and cause renal infarction or progressively (e.g., atheroma or fibromuscular dysphasia) and cause renovascular hypertension and/or lead to ischemic nephropathy. In addition, renal atheroembolism caused by showers of cholesterol microemboli can lead to progressive renal failure if sustained or recurrent.

SYNONYMS

Acute:
Renal artery thrombosis
Renal artery embolism
Chronic:
Renovascular hypertension

ICD-9CM CODES
593.81 Renal artery occlusion
440.1 Renal artery stenosis
405.01 Renovascular hypertension, secondary
447.9 Renal artery hyperplasia

EPIDEMIOLOGY & DEMOGRAPHICS

- In acute renal artery occlusion, the epidemiology depends on the underlying cause (see below).
- Renovascular hypertension:

Prevalence of 0.2% to 5% of all hypertensive patients.

The prevalence is higher in patients with severe hypertension, reaching 43% of white patients and 7% of black patients with malignant hypertension.

- Approximately 1 in 6 patients with end-stage renal disease has ischemic nephropathy, and survival of patients with end-stage renal disease associated with ischemic nephropathy is half that of patients with end-stage renal disease from other causes.
- The demographics of atheromatous renal artery stenosis mirrors the pattern seen in other arteriosclerotic conditions (coronary artery disease, cerebrovascular disease, peripheral vascular disease) and is influenced by the usual risk factors (smoking, family history, diabetes, hyperlipidemia). For example, the prevalence of renal artery stenosis among hypertensive patients undergoing coronary catheterization is high (47%), with 19% having a stenosis of 50% or more. Fibromuscular dysplasia is most likely to be seen in young adult women. Takayasu's arteritis can involve the renal arteries and is also seen in young to middle-aged women.

PHYSICAL FINDINGS & CLINICAL PRESENTATION

Acute renal artery occlusion

- Flank or abdominal pain
- Fever
- Nausea or vomiting
- Leukocytosis
- Hematuria (microscopic or gross)
- Elevated AST, LDH, and alkaline phosphatase
- Oliguric renal failure if occlusion is bilateral; normal or near normal renal function in unilateral occlusion

Cholesterol emboli

- Multisystem manifestations resembling vasculitis (visual disturbance, painful distal extremities, abdominal pain, signs of organ or limb ischemia). Laboratory findings include eosinophiluria, proteinuria, renal failure, elevated ESR.

Progressive renal artery stenosis

- Hypertension in a young, white woman without a family history of such (fibromuscular dysplasia)
- Hypertension in a middle-aged man with other evidence of atheromatous disease
- Abdominal bruit (40% of cases)
- Renal failure
- Hypertensive retinopathy
- Pulmonary edema in a hypertensive patient
- Hypokalemia
- Renal failure following the administration of an angiotensin-converting enzyme inhibitor (if bilateral renal artery stenosis)

ETIOLOGY & PATHOGENESIS

Etiology of renal artery thrombosis

- Atherosclerosis
- Fibromuscular dysphasia
- Arteritis
- Aneurysm
- Arteriography
- Syphilis
- Hypercoagulable state
- Complication of renal transplantation (role of cyclosporine)

Etiology of renal artery embolism (cardiac conditions [90%])

- Myocardial infarction
- Atrial fibrillation
- Cardiomyopathy
- Endocarditis
- Paradoxical emboli from DVT in patient with cardiac septal defect
- Atheromatous plaques (cholesterol emboli)

PATHOGENESIS: Renal hypoperfusion or ischemia produces an increase in plasma renin that stimulates the conversion of angiotensin I to angiotensin II, causing vasoconstriction and aldosterone secretion, sodium retention, and potassium wasting. Hypertension results and can be self-sustaining after some time, even in the case of unilateral renal artery stenosis because of hypertensive damage to the other kidney.

DIAGNOSIS (Dx)

LABORATORY TESTS

- Creatinine
- Potassium level
- Urinalysis
- Peripheral plasma renin activity
- Captopril test (stimulation of excessive renin secretion)

IMAGING STUDIES

- Magnetic resonance angiography
- Renal scan (70% sensitivity and 79% specificity)
- Captopril renal scan (85% sensitivity and 90% specificity)
- Intravenous digital substraction angiography (88% sensitivity and 90% specificity) is the reference standard for anatomic diagnosis of renal artery stenosis
- Section III describes an algorithm for the diagnosis of renal artery stenosis

TREATMENT (Rx)

Acute renal artery thrombosis or embolism

- Thrombolytic therapy
- Anticoagulation
- Revascularization (surgery)
- Blood pressure control

Cholesterol emboli

- No treatment

Renal artery stenosis

- Blood pressure control (role of ACE inhibitors and angiotensin receptor blockers is controversial, but neither should be continued if renal function worsens)
- Angioplasty or revascularization should be reserved for patients whose blood pressure control with medication is difficult and for patients with progressive renal failure

NATURAL HISTORY

- Renal artery stenosis caused by fibromuscular dysplasia does not progress.
- Renal artery stenosis associated with atherosclerosis is progressive. Of patients with >60% stenosis, 5% progress to total occlusion in 1 yr and 11% progress in 2 yr.

SUGGESTED READINGS

Boudewijn G et al: Accuracy of computed tomographic angiography and magnetic resonance angiography for diagnosing renal artery stenosis, *Ann Intern Med* 141:674, 2004.

Slovut DP, Olin JW: Fibromuscular dysplasia, *N Engl J Med* 350:1862, 2004.

AUTHORS: **FRED F. FERRI, M.D.,** and **TOM J. WACHTEL, M.D.**

BASIC INFORMATION

DEFINITION

Renal cell adenocarcinoma (RCA) is a primary adenocarcinoma originating in the renal parenchyma from the malignant transformation of proximal renal tubular epithelial cells.

SYNONYMS

Hypernephroma
Clear cell carcinoma of the kidney
Grawitz tumor

ICD-9CM CODES
189.0 Adenocarcinoma of kidney
189.1 (Renal pelvis)

EPIDEMIOLOGY & DEMOGRAPHICS

INCIDENCE: Approximately 1:10,000 persons/yr (3% of all adult malignancies). In the U.S., renal cancer is the 7th leading malignant condition among men and 12th among women. Two percent of cases of renal cancer are associated with inherited syndromes.

PREDOMINANT SEX: Male:female ratio of 2:1.

PREDOMINANT AGE: Peak in age 50 to 70 yr.

PHYSICAL FINDINGS & CLINICAL PRESENTATION

The classic presentation of renal cell adenocarcinoma includes teh triad of flank pain, hematuria, and a palpable abdominal mass. This represents an unusual presentation nowadays. Presenting findings in RCA patients:

Hematuria	50% to 60%
Elevated erythrocyte sedimentation rate	50% to 60%
Abdominal mass	25% to 45%
Anemia	20% to 40%
Flank pain	35% to 40%
Hypertension	20% to 40%
Weight loss	30% to 35%
Fever	5% to 15%
Hepatic dysfunction	10% to 15%
Classic triad (hematuria, abdominal mass, flank pain)	5% to 10%
Hypercalcemia	3% to 6%
Erythrocytosis	3% to 4%
Varicocele	2% to 3%

ETIOLOGY

Hereditary forms
- Familial renal carcinoma
- Renal carcinoma associated with von Hippel-Lindau disease
- Hereditary papillary renal cell carcinoma

Risk factors
- Cigarette smoking
- Obesity
- Use of diuretics
- Phenacetin-containing analgesics
- Asbestos exposure
- Gasoline and other petroleum products
- Lead
- Cadmium
- Thorotrast
- Role of the VHL gene located on chromosome 3

DIAGNOSIS

DIFFERENTIAL DIAGNOSIS

- Transitional cell carcinomas of the renal pelvis (8% of all renal cancers)
- Wilms' tumor
- Other rare primary renal carcinomas and sarcomas
- Renal cysts
- All causes of hematuria (see Section II)
- Retroperitoneal tumors

WORKUP

- Laboratory tests and imaging studies
- Section III, "Renal Mass," describes the patients evaluation.

LABORATORY TESTS

- CBC: anemia or erythrocytosis
- Elevated sedimentation rate
- Nonmetastatic hepatic dysfunction with elevated alkaline phosphatase, prolonged prothrombin time, and hypoalbuminemia
- Hypercalcemia (secondary to parathyroid related protein)
- Other: elevated ferritin, elevated insulin and glucagon levels, elevated alpha-fetoprotein, and elevated beta-human chorionic gonadotropin

IMAGING STUDIES

Nearly 50% of renal cancers are now detected because a renal mass is incidentally detected on radiographic evaluation.
- Renal ultrasound
- Abdominal CT scan with contrast (Fig. 1-222)
- MRI
- Renal arteriogram
- Intravenous pyelography (IVP)

STAGING

See Table 1-38.

COMMON SITES OF METASTASES

Lung	50% to 60%
Bone	30% to 40%
Regional nodes	15% to 30%
Main renal vein	15% to 20%
Perirenal fat	10% to 20%
Adrenal (ipsilateral)	10% to 15%
Vena cava	10% to 15%
Brain	10% to 15%
Adjacent organs (colon, pancreas)	10%
Kidney (contralateral)	2%

TREATMENT

- Surgery
  Surgical nephrectomy is the only effective management for stages I, II, and some stage III tumors.
  Various forms of partial nephrectomy may be available for patients with bilateral cancers or with a solitary kidney.
  The role of nephrectomy in patients with metastatic renal cell carcinoma is controversial and should probably be reserved for patients who have a solitary metastasis amenable to surgical resection.
- Angioinfarction (for palliation)
- Radiotherapy (for palliation)
- Chemotherapy (only 5% response rate)
- Hormonal therapy (high-dose progesterone may achieve a 15% to 20% response rate)
- Immunotherapy (interleukin-2 may achieve a 15% to 30% response rate; alpha, beta, and gamma interferons are somewhat less effective; for example, interferon alfa-2b increased post-nephrectomy median survival by 30% in one recent trial)

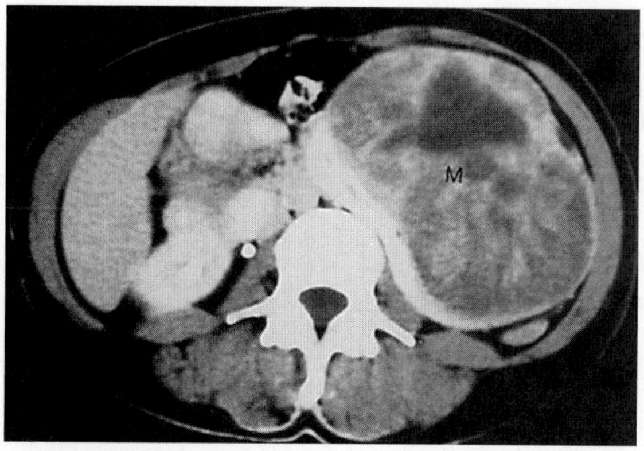

FIGURE 1-222 Large renal cell carcioma. Large mass *(M)* containing areas of high enhancement, low enhancement, and necrosis. (From Stein JH [ed]: *Internal medicine,* ed 5, St Louis, 1998, Mosby.)

- Antivascular endothelial growth factor antibody Bevacizumab slows disease progression in metastatic renal cancer.
- Sunitinib and sorafenib are oral tyrosine kinase inhibitors useful for therapy of advanced renal cell carcinoma (as first-line therapy) or in patients failing or intolerant to cytokine therapy.
- Recent trials with temsirolimus, a specific inhibitor of the mammalian target of rapamycin kinase, have shown promising results. Compared with interferon-alpha, temsirolimus improved overall survival among patients with metastatic renal cell carcinoma and a poor prognosis. The addition of temsirolimus to interferon did not improve survival.

PROGNOSIS

Prognosis of surgically treated patients

TNM stage	5-year survival (%)
I	95
II	88
III (renal vein or vena cava)	50 to 60
III (nodal involvement)	15 to 25
IV	5 to 20

REFERRAL

To urologist

EVIDENCE

EBM

Generally, surgery is the gold standard for treatment of RCC and has high cure rates and long-term survival rates, especially in stage I and II disease, and sometimes in stage III disease.

Those patients with stage IV metastatic disease are usually amenable to palliative surgery.

Evidence-Based Reference

Coppin C et al: Immunotherapy for advanced renal cell cancer, *Cochrane Database Syst Rev* 3:CD001425, 2000.

SUGGESTED READINGS

Cohen HT, McGovern FJ: Renal cell carcinoma, *N Engl J Med* 353:2477, 2005.

Curti BD: Renal cell carcinoma, *JAMA* 292:97, 2004.

Flanigan RC et al: Nephrectomy followed by interferon alfa-2b compared with interferon alfa-2b alone for metastatic renal-cell cancer, *N Engl J Med* 345:1655, 2002.

Hudes G et al: Temsirolimus, interferon alfa, or both for advanced renal-cell carcinoma, *N Engl J Med* 356:2271, 2007.

Motzer RJ et al: Sunitinib in patients with metastatic renal cell carcinoma, *JAMA* 295:2516, 2006.

Motzer RJ et al: Sunitinib versus interferon alfa in metastatic renal-cell carcinoma, *N Engl J Med* 356:115, 2007.

Yang CJ: A randomized trial of Bevacizumab, an anti-vascular endothelial growth factor antibody, for metastatic renal cancer, *N Engl J Med* 349:427, 2003.

AUTHORS: **FRED F. FERRI, M.D.,** and **TOM J. WACHTEL, M.D.**

TABLE 1-38 Comparison of Conventional and TNM Staging Classification of RCC

Robson Stage	T	N	M
I: Tumor confined by capsule	T_1 (tumor 2.5 cm or less) T_2 (tumor >2.5 cm, limited to kidney)		
II: Tumor extension to perirenal fat or ipsilateral adrenal but confined by Gerota's fascia	T_3a (tumor invades adrenal gland or perinephric fat but not beyond Gerota's fascia)		
IIIa: Renal vein or inferior vena caval involvement	T_3b (renal vein or caval involvement below diaphragm) T_3c (caval involvement above diaphragm)	N_0 (nodes negative)	M_0 (no distant metastases)
IIIb: Lymphatic involvement	$T_{1\text{-}4}$	N_1 (single lymph node 2 cm or less) N_2 (single node between 2 and 5 cm, or multiple nodes <5 cm) N3 (single or multiple nodes >5 cm)	
IIIc: Combination of IIIa and IIIb	$T_{3,\,4}$		
IVa: Spread to contiguous organs except ipsilateral adrenal	T_4 (tumor extends beyond Gerota's fascia)		
IVb: Distant metastases	$T_{1\text{-}4}$		M_1 (distant metastases)

RCC, Renal cell carcinoma.

BASIC INFORMATION

DEFINITION

Acute renal failure (ARF) is the rapid impairment in renal function resulting in retention of products in the blood that are normally excreted by the kidneys.

SYNONYMS

ARF

ICD-9CM CODES
584.9 Acute renal failure, unspecified

EPIDEMIOLOGY & DEMOGRAPHICS

- ARF requiring dialysis develops in 5/100,000 persons annually.
- >10% of ICU patients develop ARF.
- >40% of hospital ARF is iatrogenic.
- The most common cause of ARF in hospitalized patients is intrinsic renal failure caused by acute tubular necrosis (ATN).
- Acute renal failure occurs in 20% of patients with moderate sepsis and over 50% of patients with septic shock and positive blood cultures.

PHYSICAL FINDINGS & CLINICAL PRESENTATION

- The physical examination should focus on volume status. The physical findings noted below vary with the duration and rapidity of onset of renal failure
- Peripheral edema
- Skin pallor, ecchymoses
- Oliguria (however, patients can have nonoliguric renal failure), anuria
- Delirium, lethargy, myoclonus, seizures
- Back pain, fasciculations, muscle cramps
- Tachypnea, tachycardia
- Weakness, anorexia, generalized malaise, nausea

ETIOLOGY

- Prerenal: inadequate perfusion caused by hypovolemia, CHF, cirrhosis, sepsis. Sixty percent of community-acquired cases of ARF are due to prerenal conditions.
- Postrenal: outlet obstruction from prostatic enlargement, ureteral obstruction (stones), bilateral renal vein occlusion. Postrenal causes account for 5% to 15% of community-acquired ARF.
- Intrinsic renal: glomerulonephritis, acute tubular necrosis, drug toxicity, contrast nephropathy.
- Causes of acute renal failure are described in Section II.

DIAGNOSIS

DIFFERENTIAL DIAGNOSIS

Refer to "Etiology."

LABORATORY TESTS

- Elevated serum creatinine: the rate of rise of creatinine is approximately 1 mg/dl/day in complete renal failure.
- Elevated BUN: BUN/creatinine ratio is >20:1 in prerenal azotemia, postrenal azotemia, and acute glomerulonephritis; it is <20:1 in acute interstitial nephritis and acute tubular necrosis (Table 1-39).
- Electrolytes (potassium, phosphate) are elevated; bicarbonate level and calcium are decreased.
- CBC may reveal anemia because of decreased erythropoietin production, hemoconcentration, or hemolysis.
- Urinalysis may reveal the presence of hematuria (GN), proteinuria (nephrotic syndrome), casts (e.g., granular casts in ATN, RBC casts in acute GN, WBC casts in acute interstitial nephritis), eosinophiluria (acute interstitial nephritis).
- Urinary sodium and urinary creatinine should also be obtained to calculate the fractional excretion of sodium (FE_{Na}) (FE_{Na} = urine sodium/plasma sodium × plasma creatinine/urine creatinine × 100). The fractional excretion of sodium is <1 in prerenal failure, >1 in intrinsic renal failure in patients with urine output <400 ml/day.
- Urinary osmolarity is 250 to 300 mOsm/kg in ATN, <400 mOsm/kg in postrenal azotemia, and >500 mOsm/kg in prerenal azotemia and acute glomerulonephritis (Table 1-40).
- Additional useful studies are blood cultures for patients suspected of sepsis, LFTs, immunoglobulins, and protein electrophoresis in patients suspected of myeloma, creatinine kinase in patients with suspected rhabdomyolysis.
- Renal biopsy may be indicated in patients with intrinsic renal failure when considering specific therapy; major uses of renal biopsy are differential diagnosis of nephrotic syndrome, separation of lupus vasculitis from other vasculitis and lupus membranous from idiopathic membranous, confirmation of hereditary nephropathies on the basis of the ultrastructure, diagnosis of rapidly progressing glomerulonephritis, separation of allergic interstitial nephritis from ATN, separation of primary glomerulonephritis syndromes. The biopsy may be performed percutaneously or by open method. The percutaneous approach is favored and generally yields adequate tissue in >90% of cases. Open biopsy is generally reserved for uncooperative patients, those with solitary

TABLE 1-39 Serum and Radiographic Abnormalities in Renal Failure

	Prerenal	Postrenal (Acute)	Intrinsic Renal (Acute)	Intrinsic Renal (Chronic)
BUN	↑10:1 > Cr	↑ 20-40/day	↑ 20-40/day	Stable, ↑ varies with protein intake
Serum creatinine	N/moderate ↑	↑ 2-4/day	↑ 2-4/day	Stable ↑ (production equals excretion)
Serum potassium	N/moderate ↑	↑ varies with urinary volume	↑↑ (particularly when patient is oliguric) ↑↑↑ with rhabdomyolysis	Normal until end stage, unless tubular dysfunction (type 4 RTA)
Serum phosphorus	N/moderate ↑	Moderate ↑ ↑↑ with rhabdomyolysis	↑ Poor correlation with duration of renal disease	Becomes significantly elevated when serum creatinine level surpasses 3 mg/dl
Serum calcium	N	N/↓ with PO_4^{-3} retention	↓ (poor correlation with duration of renal failure)	Usually ↓
Renal size				
By ultrasound	N/↑	↑ and dilated calyces	N/↑	↓ and with ↑ echogenicity
FE_{Na}*	<1	<1 → 1	>1	>1

From Kiss B: Renal failure. In Ferri FF (ed): *Practical guide to the care of the medical patient,* ed 6, St Louis, 2004, Mosby.
↑, Increase; ↓, decrease; ↑↑, large increase, *Cr,* creatinine; *N,* normal; *Na,* sodium; *P,* plasma; *RTA,* renal tubular acidosis; *U,* urine.
*$FE_{Na} = U_{Na}/P_{Na}U_{Cr}/P_{cr} \times 100$.

kidney, and patients at risk for uncontrolled bleeding.

IMAGING STUDIES

- Chest x-ray is useful to evaluate for CHF and for pulmonary renal syndromes (Goodpasture's syndrome, Wegener's granulomatosis).
- Ultrasound of kidneys is used to evaluate for kidney size (useful to distinguish ARF from CRF), to evaluate for the presence of obstruction, and to evaluate renal vascular status (with Doppler evaluation).

TREATMENT Rx

NONPHARMACOLOGIC THERAPY

- Stop all nephrotoxic medications
- Dietary modification to supply adequate calories while minimizing accumulation of toxins; appropriate control of fluid balance. Physicians should recommend a nutrition program with an energy prescription of 120 to 150 KJ/kg/day and restriction of potassium (60 mEq/day), sodium (90 mEq/day), and phosphorus (800 mg/day). Ideal protein supplementation ranges from 0.6 to 1.4 g/kg depending on whether dialysis is required
- Daily weight
- Modifications of dosage of renally excreted drugs

ACUTE GENERAL Rx

Treatment is variable with etiology of ARF:

- Prerenal: IV volume expansion in hypovolemic patients.
- Intrinsic renal: discontinuation of any potential toxins and treatment of condition causing the renal failure.
  1. Low-dose dopamine is at times used to influence renal dysfunction and may offer transient improvement in renal physiology; however, there is lack of evidence that it offers significant clinical benefits to patients with or at risk for acute renal failure.
  2. Fenoldopam, a dopamine alpha-1 receptor agonist currently approved for inpatient management of severe hypertension has been reported beneficial in patients who are at risk for renal failure related to reduced renal blood flow.
  3. Although furosemide is used frequently to convert oliguric to nonoliguric renal failure in patients with early acute renal failure, it has no effect on mortality, dialysis requirement, and proportion of patients with persistent oliguria. Its use in high dose is also associated with increased risk of tinnitus and temporary deafness.
- Postrenal: removal of obstruction.

CHRONIC Rx

- Monitoring of renal function and electrolytes.
- Prevention of further insults to the kidneys with proper hydration, especially before contrast studies, and avoidance of nephrotoxic agents. Hydration with sodium bicarbonate (addition of 154 ml of 1000 mEq/l sodium bicarbonate to 846 mL of 5% dextrose in water) before contrast exposure is more effective than hydration with sodium chloride for prophylaxis of contrast-induced renal failure. After appropriate clinical evaluation and measurement of blood pressure, patients should receive an initial IV bolus of 3 ml/kg/hr for 1 hr immediately before radiocontrast injection and the same fluid at a rate of 1 ml/kg/hr during the contrast exposure and for 6 hr after the procedure.
- Refer to topic on chronic renal failure for indications for initiation of dialysis. Daily hemodialysis is superior to every-other-day hemodialysis in patients with acute tubular necrosis and ARF.

DISPOSITION

- General indications for initiation of dialysis are:
  1. Florid symptoms of uremia (encephalopathy, pericarditis)
  2. Severe volume overload
  3. Severe acid-base imbalance
  4. Significant derangement in electrolyte concentrations (e.g., hyperkalemia, hyponatremia)
- Renal function recovery (ability to discontinue dialysis) varies from 50% to 75% in survivors of ARF.
- Overall mortality rate in ARF is nearly 50%, varying from 60% in patients with ATN to 35% in patients with prerenal or postrenal ARF.
- The combination of acute renal failure and sepsis is associated with a 70% mortality rate.

SUGGESTED READINGS

Abuelo G: Normotensive ischemic acute renal failure, *N Engl J Med* 357:797, 2007.

AUTHOR: **FRED F. FERRI, M.D.**

TABLE 1-40 **Urinary Abnormalities in Renal Failure**

	Prerenal	Postrenal (Acute)	Intrinsic Renal (Acute)	Intrinsic Renal (Chronic)
Urinary volume	↓	Absent-to-wide fluctuation	Oliguric or nonoliguric	1000 ml + until end stage
Urinary creatinine	↑ (U/P Cr ±40)	↓ (U/P Cr ±20)	↓ (U/P Cr <20)	↓ (U/P Cr <20)
Osmolarity	↑ (±400 mOsm/kg)	(<350 mOsm/kg)	(<350 mOsm/kg)	(<350 mOsm/kg)
Degree of proteinuria	Minimum	Absent	Varies with cause of renal failure: Modest with ATN; Nephrotic range common with acute glomerulopathies, usually <2 g/24 hr with interstitial disease*	Varies with cause of renal disease (from 1-2 g/day to nephrotic range)
Urinary sediment	Negative, or occasional hyaline cast	Negative or hematuria with stones or papillary necrosis; Pyuria with infectious prostatic disease	ATN: muddy brown; Interstitial nephritis: lymphocytes, eosinophils (in stained preparations), and WBC casts; RPGN: RBC casts; Nephrosis: oval fat bodies	Broad casts with variable renal "residual" acute findings

From Kiss B: Renal failure. In Ferri FF (ed): *Practical guide to the care of the medical patient,* ed 6, St Louis, 2004, Mosby.

↑, Increased; ↓, decreased; *ATN,* acute tubular necrosis; clearance = $\frac{\text{urinary concentration} \times \text{urinary volume}}{\text{plasma concentration}}$; *Cr,* creatinine; *RBC,* red blood cell; *RPGN,* rapidly progressive glomerulonephritis; *U/P,* urine/plasma; *WBC,* white blood cell.

BASIC INFORMATION

DEFINITION

Chronic renal failure (CRF) is a progressive decrease in renal function (CFR <60 ml/min for >3 mo) with subsequent accumulation of waste products in the blood, electrolyte abnormalities, and anemia.

SYNONYMS

CRF
Chronic kidney disease
CKD
End-stage renal disease

ICD-9CM CODES
585 Chronic renal failure

EPIDEMIOLOGY & DEMOGRAPHICS

- The prevalence of patients with chronic kidney disease in the U.S. is approximately 11%.
- The number of patients with ESRD is increasing at the rate of 7% to 9%/yr in the U.S. Each year 2/10,000 persons develop end-stage CRF.
- In the U.S., >250,000/yr receive dialysis treatment for ESRD.

PHYSICAL FINDINGS & CLINICAL PRESENTATION

- Skin pallor, ecchymoses
- Edema
- Hypertension
- Emotional lability and depression
- The clinical presentation varies with the degree of renal failure and its underlying etiology. Common symptoms are generalized fatigue, nausea, anorexia, pruritus, insomnia, taste disturbances

ETIOLOGY

- Diabetes (37%), hypertension (30%), chronic glomerulonephritis (12%)
- Polycystic kidney disease
- Tubular interstitial nephritis (e.g., drug hypersensitivity, analgesic nephropathy), obstructive nephropathies (e.g., nephrolithiasis, prostatic disease)
- Vascular diseases (renal artery stenosis, hypertensive nephrosclerosis)

DIAGNOSIS

- CRF is primarily distinguished from ARF by the duration (progression over several months).
- Sonographic evaluation of the kidneys reveals smaller kidneys with increased echogenicity in CRF.

WORKUP

- Laboratory evaluation and imaging studies should be aimed at identifying reversible causes of acute decrements in GFR (e.g., volume depletion, urinary tract obstruction, CHF) superimposed on chronic renal disease
- Kidney biopsy: generally not performed in patients with small kidneys or with advanced disease
- The glomerular filtration rate is the best overall indicator of kidney function. It can be estimated using prediction equations that take into account the serum creatinine level and some or all of specific variables (body size, age, sex, race). GFR calculators are available on the National Kidney Foundation website (http://www.kidney.org/kls/professionals/gfr_calculator.cfm)

LABORATORY TESTS

- Elevated BUN, creatinine, creatinine clearance.
- Urinalysis: may reveal proteinuria, RBC casts.
- Serum chemistry: elevated BUN and creatinine, hyperkalemia, hyperuricemia, hypocalcemia, hyperphosphatemia, hyperglycemia, decreased bicarbonate.
- Measure urinary protein excretion. The finding of a ratio of protein to creatinine of >1000 mg/g suggests the presence of glomerular disease.
- Special studies: serum and urine immunoelectrophoresis (in suspected multiple myeloma), ANA (in suspected SLE).
- Cystatin C is a cysteine proteinase inhibitor produced by all nucleated cells, freely filtered at the glomerulus but not secreted by tubular cells. Given these characteristics, it may be superior to creatinine concentration both in kidney disease and as a marker of acute kidney injury. It is a better index of kidney function in elderly patients and a better predictor of outcomes than creatinine. The association of cystatin C is stronger than the association of measured GFR with all-cause and CVD mortality in patients with advanced chronic kidney disease.

IMAGING STUDIES

Ultrasound of kidneys to measure kidney size and to rule out obstruction

TREATMENT

NONPHARMACOLOGIC THERAPY

- Provide adequate nutrition and calories (147 to 168 kJ/kg/day in energy intake, chiefly from carbohydrate and polyunsaturated fats). Referral to a dietician for nutritional therapy for patients with GFR <50 ml/1.73 m² is recommended and is now a covered service by Medicare.
- Restrict sodium (approximately 100 mmol/day), potassium (≤60 mmol/day), and phosphate (<800 mg/day).
- Adjust drug doses to correct for prolonged half-lives.
- Restrict fluid if significant edema is present.
- Protein restriction (≤0.8 g/kg/day) may slow deterioration of renal function; however, recent studies have not confirmed this benefit. There is insufficient evidence to recommend or advise against routine restriction of protein intake.
- Resistance exercise training can preserve lean body mass, nutritional status, and muscle function in patients with moderate chronic kidney disease.
- Avoid radiocontrast agents. Hydration with sodium bicarbonate before contrast exposure is more effective than hydration with sodium chloride for prophylaxis of contrast-induced renal failure.
- Smoking cessation.
- Initiate hemodialysis or peritoneal dialysis (see "Acute General Rx").
- Prompt referral to nephrologist is essential. Late evaluation of patients with chronic renal disease is associated with greater burden and severity of comorbid disease and shorter survival.
- Kidney transplantation in selected patients.

GENERAL Rx

- ACE inhibitors and ARBs are useful in reducing proteinuria and slowing the progression of chronic renal disease, especially in hypertensive diabetic patients. A systolic blood pressure between 110 and 129 mm Hg may be beneficial in patients with urine protein excretion >1.0 g/day. Systolic BP <110 mm Hg may be associated with a higher risk for kidney disease progression.
- Initiation of dialysis
  1. Urgent indications: uremic pericarditis, neuropathy, neuromuscular abnormalities, CHF, hyperkalemia, seizures.
  2. Judgmental indications: creatinine clearance 10 to 15 ml/min; progressive anorexia, weight loss, reversal of sleep pattern, pruritus, uncontrolled fluid gain with hypertension and signs of CHF.
- Erythropoiesis-stimulating agents epoetin alpha (Epogen, Procrit) and darbepoetin alpha (Aranesp) can be used to reduce the need for transfusions in patients with anemia. Anemia should not be fully corrected in patients with chronic kidney disease. Maintaining a target hemoglobin of 11 to 12 g/dl or Hct 30% to 33% is satisfactory.
- Diuretics for significant fluid overload (loop diuretics are preferred).

- Correction of hypertension to at least 130/85 mm Hg with ACE inhibitors (avoid in patients with significant hyperkalemia), ARBs, and/or nondihydropyridene calcium channel blockers (verapamil, diltiazem) can be used in patients intolerant to ACE inhibitors or when other agents are needed to control blood pressure.
- Correction of electrolyte abnormalities (e.g., calcium chloride, glucose, sodium polystyrene sulfonate for hyperkalemia), sodium bicarbonate in patients with severe metabolic acidosis.
- Lipid-lowering agents in patients with dyslipidemia, target LDL cholesterol is <100 mg/dl.
- Control of renal osteodystrophy with calcium supplementation and vitamin D. Starting dose of calcium carbonate is 0.5 g with each meal, increased until the serum phosphorus concentration is normalized (most patients require 5 to 10 g/day). Calcitriol 0.125 to 0.25 μg/day PO is effective in increasing serum calcium concentration. Paricalcitol, a new vitamin-D analogue has been reported as more effective than calcitriol in lessening the elevations in serum calcium and phosphorus levels.
- Sevelamer (Renagel) is a useful phosphate binder to reduce serum phosphate levels.

DISPOSITION

- Prognosis is influenced by comorbidity of multisystem diseases. Late referral of patients to a nephrologist is associated with higher mortality, morbidity, and costs. Despite recommendations for early referral, up to 64% of patients with CRF are still referred late.
- Apolipoprotein E (APOE) variation predicts chronic kidney disease progression, independent of diabetes, race, lipid, and nonlipid factors. The e2 allele moderately increases risk of kidney disease progression, whereas allele e4 decreases the risk.
- Kidney transplantation in selected patients improves survival. The 2-yr kidney graft survival rate for living related donor transplantations is >80%, whereas the 2-yr graft survival rate for cadaveric donor transplantation is approximately 70%.

EVIDENCE

EBM

In recent years, several comprehensive clinical trials conducted in the U.S. and in Europe have provided reasonably strong evidence for the following factors affecting progression of renal disease and treatments altering the rate of progression to end-stage disease:

ACE inhibitors slow the rate of progression of type 1 diabetic nephropathy.[1]

ACE inhibitors slow the rate of progression of nondiabetic proteinuric nephropathies.[2]

Blood pressure control and magnitude of proteinuria influences rate of progression of renal disease (but no good evidence for protein-restricted diet).[3]

Validity of spot urine albumin:creatinine ratio as predictor of progression.[4]

Evidence-Based References

1. Lewis EJ et al: The effect of angiotensin converting enzyme inhibition on diabetic nephropathy, *N Engl J Med* 329:359, 1993.
2. Ruggenenti P et al: Renoprotective properties of ACE inhibition in non-diabetic nephropathies with non-nephrotic proteinuria, *Lancet* 354:359, 1999.
3. Peterson JC et al. for the Modification of Diet in Renal Disease (MDRD) Study Group: Blood pressure control, proteinuria and the progression of renal disease, *Ann Int Med* 123:754, 1995.
4. Ruggenenti P et al: Cross sectional longitudinal study of spot morning urine protein:creatinine ratio, 24 hour protein excretion rate, glomerular filtration rate, and end stage renal failure in chronic renal disease in patients without diabetes, *BMJ* 316:504, 1998.

SUGGESTED READINGS

Herget-Rosenthal S et al: Early detection of acute renal failure by serum cystain C, *Kidney Int* 66:1115, 2004.

Hsu CC et al: Apolipoprotein E and progression of chronic kidney disease, *JAMA* 293:2892, 2005.

Jafar TH et al: Progression of chronic kidney disease: the role of blood pressure control, proteinuria, and angiotensin-converting enzyme inhibition, *Ann Intern Med* 139:244, 2003.

Johnson CA et al: Clinical practice guidelines for chronic kidney disease in adults, *Am Fam Physician* 70:869, 2004.

Kinchen KS et al: The timing of specialist evaluation in chronic kidney disease and mortality, *Ann Intern Med* 137:479, 2003.

Levey AS: Nondiabetic kidney disease, *N Engl J Med* 347:1505, 2002.

Lewey AS et al: National Kidney Foundation practice guidelines for chronic kidney disease: evaluation, classification, and stratification, *Ann Intern Med* 139:137, 2003.

Lewinsky NG: Specialist evaluation in chronic kidney disease: too little too late, *Ann Intern Med* 137:542, 2002.

Menon V et al: Cystatin C as a risk factor for outcomes in chronic kidney disease, *Ann Intern Med* 147:19, 2007.

Merten GJ et al: Prevention of contrast-induced nephropathy with sodium bicarbonate, *JAMA* 291:2328, 2004.

Remuzzi G et al: Chronic renal diseases: renoprotective benefits of renin-angiotensin system inhibition, *Ann Intern Med* 136:604, 2002.

Singh AK et al: Correction of anemia with epoetin alfa in chronic kidney disease, *N Engl J Med* 355:2085, 2006.

Snively C, Gutierrez C: Chronic kidney disease: prevention and treatment of common complications, *Am Fam Physician* 70:1921, 2004.

Sprangers B et al: Late referral of patients with chronic kidney disease: no time to waste, *Mayo Clin Proc* 81:1487, 2006.

Yu HT: Progression of chronic renal failure, *Arch Intern Med* 163:1417, 2003.

AUTHOR: **FRED F. FERRI, M.D.**

BASIC INFORMATION

DEFINITION

Renal tubular acidosis (RTA) is a disorder characterized by inability to excrete H^+ or inadequate generation of new HCO_3^-. There are four types of renal tubular acidosis:

- Type I (classic, distal RTA): abnormality in distal hydrogen secretion resulting in hypokalemic hyperchloremic metabolic acidosis.
- Type II (proximal RTA): decreased proximal bicarbonate reabsorption resulting in hypokalemic hyperchloremic metabolic acidosis.
- Type III (RTA of glomerular insufficiency): normokalemic hyperchloremic metabolic acidosis as a result of impaired ability to generate sufficient NH_3 in the setting of decreased glomerular filtration rate (<30 ml/min). This type of RTA is described in older textbooks and is considered by many not to be a distinct entity.
- Type IV (hyporeninemic hypoaldosteronemic RTA): aldosterone deficiency or antagonism resulting in decreased distal acidification and decreased distal sodium reabsorption with subsequent hyperkalemic hyperchloremic acidosis.

SYNONYMS

RTA

ICD-9CM CODES
588.8 Renal tubular acidosis

EPIDEMIOLOGY & DEMOGRAPHICS

RTA type IV affects mostly adults, whereas RTA type I and II are more frequent in children.

PHYSICAL FINDINGS & CLINICAL PRESENTATION

- Examination may be normal.
- Poor skin turgor may be present from dehydration.
- Muscle weakness and muscle aches from hypokalemia may occur.
- Low back pain and bone pain may be present in patients with abnormalities of calcium metabolism (RTA II).
- There is failure to thrive in children (RTA II).

ETIOLOGY

- Type I RTA: autoimmune disorders, primary biliary cirrhosis and other liver diseases, medications (amphotericin, nonsteroidals), SLE, Sjögren's syndrome, genetic disorders (Ehlers-Danlos syndrome, Marfan syndrome, hereditary elliptocytosis), toxins (toluene), disorders with nephrocalcinosis (hyperparathyroidism, vitamin D intoxication, idiopathic hypercalciuria), tubulointerstitial disease (obstructive uropathy, renal transplantation)
- Type II RTA: Fanconi's syndrome, primary hyperparathyroidism, multiple myeloma, medications (acetazolamide)
- Type IV RTA: diabetes mellitus, sickle cell disease, Addison's disease, urinary obstruction

DIAGNOSIS

DIFFERENTIAL DIAGNOSIS

- Diarrhea with significant bicarbonate loss
- Other causes of metabolic acidosis
- Respiratory acidosis

WORKUP

Detection of hyperchloremic metabolic acidosis with ABGs and serum electrolytes and evaluation of potential causes (see "Etiology")

LABORATORY TESTS

- ABGs reveal metabolic acidosis; serum potassium is low in RTA types I and II, normal in type III, and high in type IV.
- Minimal urine pH is >5.5 in RTA type I, <5.5 in types II, III, and IV.
- Urinary anion gap is 0 or positive in all types of RTA.
- Additional useful studies include serum calcium level and urine calcium.
- Anion gap is normal.
- PTH measurement is useful in patients suspected of primary hyperparathyroidism (may be associated with type II RTA).

IMAGING STUDIES

- Plain abdominal radiography is useful to evaluate for nephrocalcinosis
- Renal sonogram can be used to evaluate renal size or presence of stones
- IVP in patients with nephrocalcinosis or nephrolithiasis

TREATMENT

ACUTE GENERAL Rx

- Type I and type II are treated with oral sodium bicarbonate (1 to 2 mEq/kg/day in RTA 1, 2 to 4 mEq/kg/day in RTA type II) titrated to correct acidosis.
- Potassium supplementation is needed in hypokalemic patients.
- Type IV RTA can be treated with furosemide to lower elevated potassium levels and sodium bicarbonate to correct significant acidosis. Fludrocortisone 100 to 300 μg/day can be used to correct mineralocorticoid deficiency.

CHRONIC Rx

- Frequent monitoring of potassium levels in type IV RTA
- Monitoring for bone disease in RTA type II
- Monitoring for nephrocalcinosis and nephrolithiasis in RTA type I

DISPOSITION

- Prognosis varies with the presence of associated conditions (see "Etiology").
- Untreated distal RTA may result in hypercalcemia, hyperphosphaturia, nephrolithiasis, and nephrocalcinosis.

PEARLS & CONSIDERATIONS

COMMENTS

Patient education material can be obtained from the National Kidney and Urologic Diseases Information Clearinghouse, Box NKUDIC, Bethesda, MD 20893.

AUTHOR: **FRED F. FERRI, M.D.**

BASIC INFORMATION

DEFINITION

Renal vein thrombosis is the thrombotic occlusion of one or both renal veins.

ICD-9CM CODES
453.3 Renal vein thrombosis

EPIDEMIOLOGY & DEMOGRAPHICS

- Incidence unknown, probably an underdiagnosed condition
- May occur at any age with no gender preference
- Epidemiology tied to the underlying cause

PHYSICAL FINDINGS & CLINICAL PRESENTATION

Acute bilateral renal vein thrombosis
- Back and bilateral flank pain
- Acute renal failure

Acute unilateral renal vein thrombosis
- Flank pain
- Decline in renal function
- Hematuria
- Increase in the amount of proteinuria if associated with nephrotic syndrome

Chronic unilateral renal vein thrombosis
- May be silent
- Pulmonary emboli and hemolysis
- Back pain
- DVT in lower extremities
- Edema
- Glycosuria
- Hyperchloremic acidosis
- Left varicocele (if the left renal vein is thrombosed)
- Dilated abdominal veins

ETIOLOGY & PATHOGENESIS

- Extrinsic compression by a tumor or retroperitoneal mass
- Invasion of the renal vein or inferior vena cava by tumor (almost always renal cell cancer)
- Trauma
- Hypercoagulable states
- Dehydration
- Glomerulopathies (membranous glomerulonephritis, crescenting glomerulonephritis, SLE, amyloidosis) especially in the presence of nephrotic syndrome when the serum albumin is lower than 2 g/dl
- NOTE: For unknown reasons, diabetic nephropathy is not commonly associated with renal vein thrombosis even if the nephrotic syndrome is present

A controversy has existed as to whether the renal vein thrombosis association with nephrotic syndrome is a complication of nephrotic syndrome or whether renal vein thrombosis occurring in the setting of increased renal vein pressure (e.g., with congestive heart failure, constrictive pericarditis, or extrinsic compression) can independently cause proteinuria. Current evidence is that renal vein thrombosis does not cause nephrotic syndrome.

DIAGNOSIS

DIFFERENTIAL DIAGNOSIS

The diagnosis of renal vein thrombosis does not include any differential consideration. The differential diagnosis is that of proteinuria. Renal vein thrombosis should be considered if proteinuria worsens or if renal function worsens in a patient with glomerulonephritis. Renal vein thrombosis should also be considered in patients with pulmonary emboli and no lower-extremity DVT.

WORKUP

Clinical suspicion (see "Differential Diagnosis") and imaging studies

IMAGING STUDIES

- Abdominal ultrasound
- Abdominal MRI or CT with contrast (Fig. 1-223)
- Renal arteriography (delayed films during venous phase)
- Selective renal vein venography (inferior venacavogram images should be obtained before advancing the catheter in the vena cava because clots, if present, could be dislodged)
- Renal biopsy may be indicated if evidence of nephritis is present (e.g., active urinary sediment)

TREATMENT

- Anticoagulation in acute renal vein thrombosis to prevent pulmonary emboli and in attempt to improve renal function and decrease proteinuria
- Thrombolytic therapy or surgical thrombectomy has also been reported to be effective
- The value of anticoagulation in chronic renal vein thrombosis is dubious except in nephrotic patients with membranous glomerulonephritis with profound hypoalbuminemia where prolonged prophylactic anticoagulation may be of benefit even if renal vein thrombosis has not been documented

PROGNOSIS

Probable worsening of the underlying glomerulonephritis by acute renal vein thrombosis; the effect of chronic renal vein thrombosis is unclear.

AUTHORS: **FRED F. FERRI, M.D.**, and **TOM J. WACHTEL, M.D.**

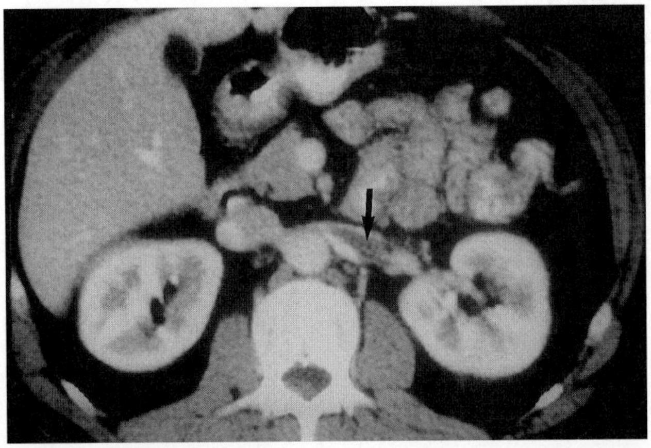

FIGURE 1-223 Renal vein thrombus in a patient with nephritic syndrome. Contrast medium enhanced CT at the level of the renal vein shows thrombus in the left renal vein *(arrow)*. (From Grainger RG, Allison DJ, Adam A, Dixon AK [eds]: *Grainger & Allison's diagnostic radiology,* ed 4, Philadelphia, 2001, Churchill Livingstone.)

BASIC INFORMATION

DEFINITION

Respiratory syncytial virus (RSV) is an RNA virus that tends to form syncytia in tissue culture. RSV causes repeated acute respiratory tract infections in people of all ages. It is the leading cause of severe lower respiratory tract infections in infants and young children, whereas it usually manifests as upper respiratory tract infections or tracheobronchitis in older children and adults.

ICD-9-CM CODES
079.6

EPIDEMIOLOGY & DEMOGRAPHICS

INCIDENCE: 64 million infections worldwide annually, resulting in 160,000 deaths; RSV is associated with 120,000 U.S. pediatric hospitalizations annually.
PREVALENCE: Nearly all patients are infected by age 2, with reinfections occurring throughout life.
PREDOMINANT SEX AND AGE: None generally, but male sex may predispose to more severe respiratory disease in RSV infection. Occurs at all ages, but is more likely to be severe in infants, young children, and the elderly
PEAK INCIDENCE: In nontropical areas of the northern hemisphere, seasonal outbreaks usually occur November to April, with a peak in January or February; in nontropical areas of the southern hemisphere, May to September, with a peak in May, June, or July. In the tropics, seasonal outbreaks usually occur during the rainy season.
RISK FACTORS: For children, risk factors include inpatient hospitalization and attending daycare or school. Severe disease is seen primarily in infants and young children (especially those born before 35 weeks gestation), the elderly, and patients with cardiac, pulmonary, or immune system dysfunction.
GENETICS: Severe disease is associated with polymorphisms in genes *IL-4* (and its receptor), *IL-8, IL-10,* and *CCR5* (UTD).

PHYSICAL FINDINGS & CLINICAL PRESENTATION

Physical findings include fever, tachypnea, prolonged expiration, wheezes and "rales," cough, rhinorrhea coryza, conjunctivitis, and otitis media. Clinical presentation can include pneumonia and bronchiolitis.

ETIOLOGY

Humans are the only known reservoir. Transmission is by large respiratory droplets via close contact or contaminated surfaces, where the virus can survive for several hours. The CDC recommends handwashing, gowns, and gloves to prevent nosocomial infection, which is especially common on pediatric wards. However, the CDC does not recommend excluding children with respiratory illnesses who are well enough to attend school or daycare because RSV is often spread during early stages of illness.

DIAGNOSIS

DIFFERENTIAL DIAGNOSIS

Infants: influenza, parainfluenza, and adenovirus
Elderly: influenza (UTD)
Immunocompromised: parainfluenza (UTD)

WORKUP

- History with a focus on upper and lower respiratory symptoms, fever, and (in infants) apnea
- Focused physical exam including temperature and pulse oximetry, as well as lung and head, eyes, ears, nose, and throat (HEENT) exam

LABORATORY TESTS

- Analysis of respiratory secretions (especially nasal washings) for virus isolation (the standard for definitive diagnosis), viral antigens (most labs use this rapid assay), or viral RNA.
- Other tests include serum antibodies, but this is of dubious usefulness; in infants it is confounded by maternal antibodies and in other patients antibodies are almost universally present due to repeated infections.

IMAGING STUDIES

Chest x-ray for suspected pneumonia or bronchiolitis

TREATMENT

NONPHARMACOLOGIC THERAPY

Isolation techniques are important in limiting spread of RSV infections.

ACUTE GENERAL Rx

- Mild disease: symptomatic treatment.
- Immunoglobulins with a high RSV-neutralizing antibody titer are beneficial in treatment.
- Severe disease may require oxygen therapy, mechanical ventilation, bronchodilators, and corticosteroids.
- Ribavarin aerosol is effective for severe RSV pneumonia.

REFERRAL

To pulmonology for severe disease

PEARLS & CONSIDERATIONS

PREVENTION

- For infants and children with chronic lung disease and those who are premature or otherwise at high risk for RSV complications, preventive treatment may include RSV prophylaxis immune globulin (IG) IV 750 mg/kg and/or RSV IG monoclonal antibody (Synagis) 15 mg/kg IM.
- The American Academy of Pediatrics recommendations state that there are three types of infants who are most likely to benefit from preventive treatment: those being treated for heart failure; those with moderate to severe pulmonary hypertension; or those with cyanotic heart disease.

PATIENT/FAMILY EDUCATION

Stress the importance of handwashing.

SUGGESTED READINGS

American Academy of Pediatrics, Committee on Infectious Diseases and Committee on Fetus and Newborn: Policy statement: revised indications for the use of palivizumab and respiratory syncytial virus immune globulin intravenous for the prevention of respiratory syncytial virus infections, *Pediatrics* 112:1442, 2003.
Centers for Disease Control: www.cdc.gov.
Meissner HC et al: Revised indications for the use of palivizumab and respiratory syncytial virus immune globulin intravenous for the prevention of respiratory syncytial virus infections, *Pediatrics* 112:1447, 2003.
World Health Organization: www.who.int.

AUTHOR: **STEVEN BUSSELEN, M.D.**

BASIC INFORMATION

DEFINITION

Restless legs syndrome is a sensory-motor disorder with four cardinal features: (1) an uncomfortable sensation or urge to move the legs, (2) discomfort worse in the evening or night, (3) discomfort worse at rest, and (4) discomfort better with movement of the affected limb(s). There are two forms of RLS: primary (familial) and secondary (acquired). Most RLS sufferers (>85%) have periodic leg movements in sleep (PLMS), which also may disrupt sleep.

SYNONYMS

Restless limb syndrome
Growing pains
Night kicking
Night walker syndrome

ICD-9CM CODES
333.99 Restless legs syndrome

EPIDEMIOLOGY & DEMOGRAPHICS

PREVALENCE: 8% to 12% depending on population and severity of symptoms
DEMOGRAPHICS: Age 2 and up (youngest case: 8 wk of age)

- Age <18: 2%; 18-29: 3%; 30-79: 10%; ≥80: 20%.
- Prevalence increases with age.
- Symptoms may worsen with age and may spread to the arms.
- Primary RLS follows an autosomal-dominant or pseudodominant mode of inheritance, shows genetic anticipation, and follows a female:male ratio of 3:2.

PHYSICAL FINDINGS & CLINICAL PRESENTATION

- Sensory complaints usually affecting one or both lower extremities during rest:
  1. "Worms" or "bugs" under the skin
  2. Sense of pressure under the skin
  3. Throbbing muscular ache or pain
  4. "Growing pains"
  5. Irresistible urge to move the symptomatic limb(s)
- Many other words used by patients to describe the leg symptoms: creeping, burning, searing, tugging, pulling, drawing, like water flowing, restless, and very often "indescribable."
- Temporary symptomatic relief or improvement with leg movement, rubbing, pressure, walking, or added warmth (bath or heating pad).
- Sleep disruption resulting from leg discomfort, PLMS, and urges to move or walk.
- Leg movements during sleep almost always occur and may be reported by a spouse or parent as kicking or constant movement during the night. These movements are stereotypic, and rhythmic ankle/leg shaking lasting <5 sec can cause arousals during sleep.
- Physical examination is normal in primary RLS, but may reveal subtle neuropathy, radiculopathy, or myelopathy in secondary RLS.
- Excessive daytime somnolence, insomnia, and occasional leg symptoms during the day while sedentary are common complaints.

ETIOLOGY

- The most likely mechanism is related to dopaminergic dysregulation at the level of the spinal cord or higher in the central nervous system.
- Genome wide studies of patients with RLS and PLMS (periodic limb movements of sleep) reveal associations on chromosomes 2, 6, and 15.
- Primary RLS (50% to 60%) may be related to iron deficiency.
- Secondary RLS associated with anemia, iron deficiency, pregnancy, renal failure, repetitive blood donation, neuropathy, radiculopathy, myelopathy, and rheumatologic conditions.
- Symptoms may be precipitated by medications (SSRIs and TCAs), caffeine, alcohol, and sleep deprivation.

DIAGNOSIS

DIFFERENTIAL DIAGNOSIS

- Periodic limb movement disorder (PLMD): repetitive limb movements (lower extremities > upper extremities) occurring during sleep; no sensory complaints or urges to move the limbs for comfort during periods of rest; associated with arousals in sleep and excessive daytime sleepiness; patient is typically unaware, but bed partner may report restlessness or kicking during sleep.
- Peripheral neuropathy, radiculopathy, myelopathy, or other CNS injury (i.e., stroke)
- Anxiety and mood disorders
- Narcolepsy
- REM behavior disorder
- Parasomnias (i.e., sleepwalking, confusional arousals, head-banging)
- Obstructive sleep apnea
- Iron deficiency
- Neuroleptic-induced akathisia
- Dyskinesias while awake
- Nocturnal leg cramps with or without peripheral arterial disease

WORKUP

- History is typically diagnostic, with sensitivity and specificity both >90%.
- Family history of RLS, growing pains, or "night walking."
- Polysomnography with arm and leg leads.
- Ambulatory recording of leg activity over several nights with sleep logs.
- Serum iron studies including TIBC, ferritin, and CBC.
- Serum B_{12}, folate, and magnesium.
- EMG for neuropathy, radiculopathy, or myelopathy, if suspected.
- Central nervous system MRI for myelopathy or stroke, if suspected.

TREATMENT

NONPHARMACOLOGIC THERAPY

- Avoid RLS triggers, which include sleep deprivation, alcohol, caffeine, many antidepressants (most often SSRIs and TCAs), antinausea medications, antihistamines antipsychotics, and calcium channel blockers.
- Maintain a regular sleep schedule and good sleep hygiene (e.g., use the bed only for sleep, no alerting or light-related activities before bed, avoid daytime cues such as clocks).

CHRONIC Rx

- Dopaminergic meds are first line (may divide dose bid or tid as needed):
  1. Requip (ropinirole): start 0.25 mg; avg dose 2 mg; max 12 mg/day
  2. Mirapex (pramipexole): start 0.125 mg; avg dose 0.375 mg; max 5 mg/day
  3. Permax (pergolide): start 0.05 mg; avg dose 0.5 mg; max 3 mg/day
  4. Sinemet (levodopa/carbidopa): start 25/100; max 3 to 4 doses
  5. Sinemet CR (continuous release): start 25/100; max 50/200
- Antiepileptics:
  1. Neurontin (gabapentin): start 300 mg; max 3600 mg/day
  2. Carbatrol (carbamazepine): start 200 mg; max 1200 mg/day
  3. Keppra (levetiracetam): start 250 mg; max 2000 mg/day
  4. Topamax (topiramate): start 25 mg; max 200 mg/day
- Opiates:
  1. Ultram (tramadol): start 25 mg; max 400 mg/day
  2. Dilaudid (hydromorphone): start 2 mg; max 24 mg/day
  3. Darvon (propoxyphene HCl): start 65 mg; max 195 mg/day
  4. Oxycontin (oxycodone-XR): start 10 mg; max 30 mg/day
  5. Roxicodone (oxycodone): start 5 mg; max 120 mg/day
- Opiate/analgesic combinations:
  1. Vicodin/Lortab (hydrocodone/acetaminophen): start 5/500 mg; max 6 doses/day
  2. Percocet (oxycodone/acetaminophen): start 10/325 mg; max 8 doses/day

BASIC INFORMATION

DEFINITION

In a retinal hemorrhage, blood accumulates in the retinal and subretinal areas as a result of multiple causes.

SYNONYMS

Pseudoxanthoma elasticum
Coats' disease
Retinal trauma
High-altitude retinopathy

ICD-9CM CODES
362.81 Retinal hemorrhage

EPIDEMIOLOGY & DEMOGRAPHICS

INCIDENCE (IN U.S.): Busy ophthalmologist sees one or two cases a month.

PEAK INCIDENCE:

- Children—associated primarily with trauma and hematologic disorders (must consider shaken baby syndrome)
- Associated with trauma, diabetes, vascular disease, macular degeneration, altitude changes (mountain climbing)

PREDOMINANT AGE: Degenerative disease in older patients

PHYSICAL FINDINGS & CLINICAL PRESENTATION

- Hemorrhage within the retina or subretinal area (Fig. 1-225)
- Evidence of retinal tears, tumors, and inflammation, macular degeneration, drugs, diabetes

ETIOLOGY

- Diabetes
- Hypertension
- Trauma
- Inflammation
- Tumors
- Subretinal neovascularization
- Associated with diabetes and aging
- Rapid changes in altitude (mountain climbing or scuba diving)

DIAGNOSIS

DIFFERENTIAL DIAGNOSIS

- Evaluate patients for local and systemic diseases.
- Trauma in children or adults.
- Either venous or arterial occlusion may cause retinal hemorrhage, and such occlusion is associated with atherosclerotic or heart disease, so look for these.
- Rule out malignant melanoma, trauma, hypertensive cardiovascular disease.

Section II describes the differential diagnosis of acute painless loss of vision.

WORKUP

Complete general physical examination, evaluate for trauma

Look for systemic diseases and medication etiologies.

LABORATORY TESTS

- Minimum: CBC, sedimentation rate, and complete blood chemistries
- Fluorescein
- Angiography
- Visual field testing

IMAGING STUDIES

- Usually not necessary
- Trauma—skull x-rays or head CT
- Ultrasound
- Fluorescein angiography

TREATMENT

NONPHARMACOLOGIC THERAPY

- Laser or treatment of underlying disorder
- Treat medical problems (ARMD, etc.)

ACUTE GENERAL Rx

- Laser is often indicated.
- Steroids may be indicated, with macular degeneration (intravitrial injection).
- Treat underlying disease.
- Repair damage if from trauma.

CHRONIC Rx

- Laser if hemorrhage is recurrent
- Vitamin therapy—high in zinc and antioxidants

DISPOSITION

Consider this an emergency.

REFERRAL

- Immediate referral to an ophthalmologist
- An emergency, with early treatment significantly affecting outcome

PEARLS & CONSIDERATIONS

COMMENTS

- Vision may return substantially
- Complete recovery dependent on amount of scar tissue formed.
- Chronic situations have poor prognosis.

SUGGESTED READINGS

Duncan BB et al: Hypertensive retinopathy and incident coronary heart disease in high risk men, *Br J Ophth* 86(9):1002, 2002.

Gardner HB: Retinal hemorrhages in children, *Ophthalmology* 110(9):1863, 2003.

Lauritzen DB, Weiter JJ: Management of subretinal hemorrhage, *Int Ophthalmol Clin* 42(3):87, 2002.

Schloff S et al: Retinal findings in children with intracranial hemorrhage, *Ophthalmology* 109(8):1472, 2002.

AUTHOR: **MELVYN KOBY, M.D.**

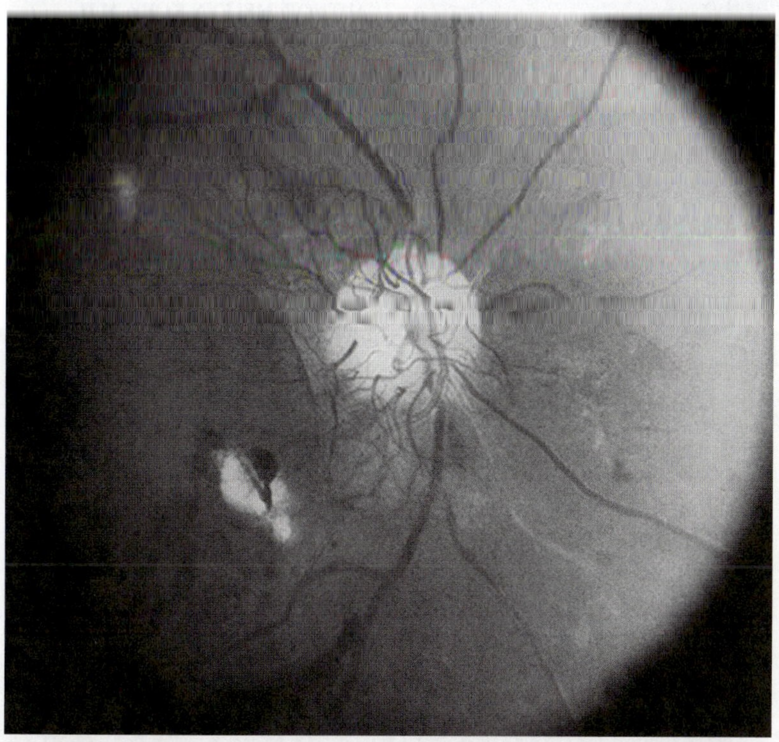

FIGURE 1-225 Fronds of neovascularization on the disc are present in this right eye. Temporally, two cotton-wool spots have adjacent intraretinal hemorrhage and preretinal hemorrhage. Native retinal arteries are narrowed and show evidence of sclerosis. (From Palay D [ed]: *Ophthalmology for the primary care physician,* St Louis, 1997, Mosby.)

BASIC INFORMATION

DEFINITION

Retinitis pigmentosa is a generalized retinal pigment degeneration associated with a variety of inheritance patterns resulting in decreased vision. A simple recessive pattern is most severe. It may be associated with some rare neurologic syndromes.

ICD-9CM CODES
362.74 Retinitis pigmentosa, pigmentary retinal dystrophy

EPIDEMIOLOGY & DEMOGRAPHICS

PEAK INCIDENCE:
- Recessive incidence: in the 20s
- Dominant form: in the 40s

PREVALENCE (IN U.S.): 1 in 4000 people
PREDOMINANT SEX: Depends on inheritance
PREDOMINANT AGE: 60 yr
GENETICS:
- 19% dominant
- 19% recessive
- 8% X-linked
- 46% not known to be genetically related (mutations)
- 8% undetermined cause

PHYSICAL FINDINGS & CLINICAL PRESENTATION

- Deposition of retinal pigment in midperiphery and centrally in the retina with a pale optic nerve and narrowing of blood vessels (Fig. 1-226)

- Old inflammatory scars
- Old hemorrhage
- Diabetes
- Toxic retinopathies (phenothiazines, chloroquine)

WORKUP

- Electrophysiologic studies
- Dark adaptation studies
- Visual fields

LABORATORY TESTS

- Usually not necessary
- VDRL, glucose (selected patients)

IMAGING STUDIES

- Usually not necessary
- Rate of decline of vision for different groups cannot be accurately determined; decline rates are fastest with patients with mutations

TREATMENT

CHRONIC Rx

- No proven effective therapy
- Sometimes vitamin E or vitamin A may be helpful

DISPOSITION

Disease may be either mild or severe, but if the patient is expected to progress to total blindness, counseling and early education are important.

REFERRAL

To ophthalmologist to confirm diagnosis

PEARLS & CONSIDERATIONS

COMMENTS

- The spiderweb-like appearance of macular degeneration should not be confused with the extra pigments sometimes seen in dark-skinned individuals.
- Patient education material can be obtained from the Retinitis Pigmentosa Foundation Fighting Blindness, 1401 Mt. Royal Avenue, 4th Floor, Baltimore, MD 21217.
- Research in fetal retinal pigment transplantation and computer chip implantation are ongoing.

EVIDENCE

Vitamin A

had typical retinitis pigmentosa showed a modest but positive slowing of visual loss. Visual loss slowed to a decline of 8.3% per year compared with 10% per year in controls.[1]

Acetazolamide

Treating those with cystoid macular edema: initial dose 250 mg daily increased to 500 mg daily if no effect apparent.

Some studies showed that it may be of benefit (as measured by improved visual acuity or decreased cystoid macular edema on fluorescein angiogram).[2]

A trial of several weeks is given.

Docosahexaenoic acid

Trials currently underway.

Evidence-Based References

1. Berson EL et al: A randomized trial of vitamin A and vitamin E supplementation for retinitis pigmentosa, *Arch Opthalmol* 111:761, 1993.
2. Steinmertz RL, Fitzke FW, Bird ZC: Treatment of cystoid macular edema with acetazolamide in a patient with serpiginous choroidopathy, *Retina* 11:412, 1991.

SUGGESTED READINGS

Chow AY et al: The artificial silicon retina microchip for the treatment of vision loss from retinitis pigmentosa, *Arch Ophthalmol* 122(4):460, 2004.
Radtke ND et al: Vision change after sheet transplant of fetal retina with retinal pigment epithelium to a patient with retinitis pigmentosa, *Arch Ophthalmol* 122(8):1159, 2004.

AUTHOR: MELVYN KOBY, M.D.

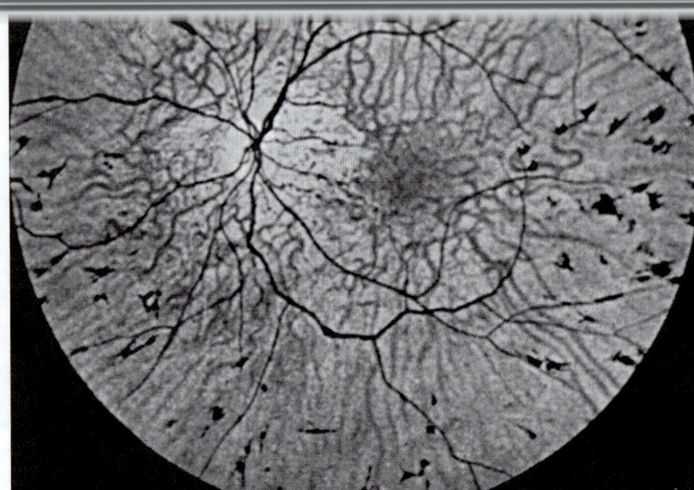

FIGURE 1-226 Retinitis pigmentosa. (From Behrman RE [ed]: *Nelson textbook of pediatrics,* Philadelphia, 2005, WB Saunders.)

BASIC INFORMATION

DEFINITION

Retropharyngeal abscess is a soft tissue infection of the throat involving retropharyngeal space. The anatomic boundaries of the retropharyngeal space are the middle layer of the deep cervical fascia (abutting the posterior oesophageal wall) anteriorly and the deep layer of the deep cervical fascia posteriorly (Fig. 1-229). These two fasciae fuse inferiorly at the level between the first and second thoracic vertebra.

ICD-9CM CODES
478.79

EPIDEMIOLOGY & DEMOGRAPHICS

PREDOMINANT SEX AND AGE: Retropharyngeal abscess occurs most commonly in children between the ages of 2 and 4 yr, analogous to suppurative cervical adenitis. This represents the peak age group for numerous viral upper respiratory tract infections (URI) and their attendant complications, acute otitis media and sinusitis. Retropharyngeal space infection is less common in older children and adults because the lymph nodes atrophy by the age of 3 or 4 yr.

PHYSICAL FINDINGS & CLINICAL PRESENTATION

- The onset of a retropharyngeal infection may be insidious, with little more than fever, irritability, drooling, a muffled voice (dysphonia), or possibly nuchal rigidity.
- The acute symptoms relate to pressure and inflammation produced by the abscess on either the airway or the upper digestive tract and pharynx. The patient may have intense dysphagia, drooling, and odynophagia, or there may be some element of respiratory distress from edema and inflammation of the airway (stridor, tachypnea, or both).
- Unwillingness to move the neck because of discomfort is often a prominent presenting feature and should lead to consideration of retropharyngeal abscess if the child is febrile and irritable.
- Usually extension of the neck is affected more than flexion. This causes the patient to hold his or her neck stiffly or to present with torticollis.
- Trismus is unusual.
- On physical examination it may be possible to appreciate midline or unilateral swelling of the posterior pharyngeal wall. The mass may be fluctuant to the examining finger, and care must be taken to avoid rupture of the abscess into the upper airway.

Complications are numerous and could be fatal; these include airway obstruction, septicemia, thrombosis of the internal jugular vein, carotid artery rupture, and acute necrotizing mediastinitis. Aspiration with resultant pneumonia may complicate retropharyngeal abscess if rupture of the abscess occurs and empties into the airway. Infection can spread from one space in the neck to another.

The most dreaded complication is jugular vein suppurative thrombophlebitis (Lemierre's syndrome), in which the vessels of the carotid sheath become infected, leading to bacteremia and metastatic spread of infection to the lungs, brain, and mediastinum.

ETIOLOGY

- The retropharyngeal space is comprised of two chains of lymph nodes that drain the nasopharynx, adenoids, posterior paranasal sinuses, middle ear, and eustachian tube. Accordingly, suppurative infections in these areas may provide the seeds for infection for retropharyngeal abscess.
- The predominant bacterial species are *Streptococcus pyogenes* (group A *Streptococcus*), *Staphylococcus aureus,* and respiratory anaerobes (including *Fusobacteria, Prevotella,* and *Veillonella* species). *Haemophilus* species are also occasionally found.
- In young children, infection usually reaches this space by lymphatic spread from a septic focus in the pharynx or sinuses.
- In adults, infection may reach the retropharyngeal space from either local or distant sites. Penetrating trauma (e.g., from chicken bones or following instrumentation) is the usual source of local spread. More distant sources of infection include odontogenic sepsis and peritonsillar abscess (now a rare cause).

DIAGNOSIS

DIFFERENTIAL DIAGNOSIS

- Cervical osteomyelitis
- Pott's disease
- Meningitis
- Calcific tendonitis of the long muscle of the neck

IMAGING STUDIES

- A lateral neck film may be helpful in delineating the presence of a retropharyngeal abscess and may demonstrate cervical lordosis; the retropharyngeal space is considered widened and pathologic if it is greater than 7 mm at C2 or 14 mm at C6 (Fig. 1-230).

There must be attention to technical issues when performing the study, especially in children. The film should be a perfect lateral, and the child must

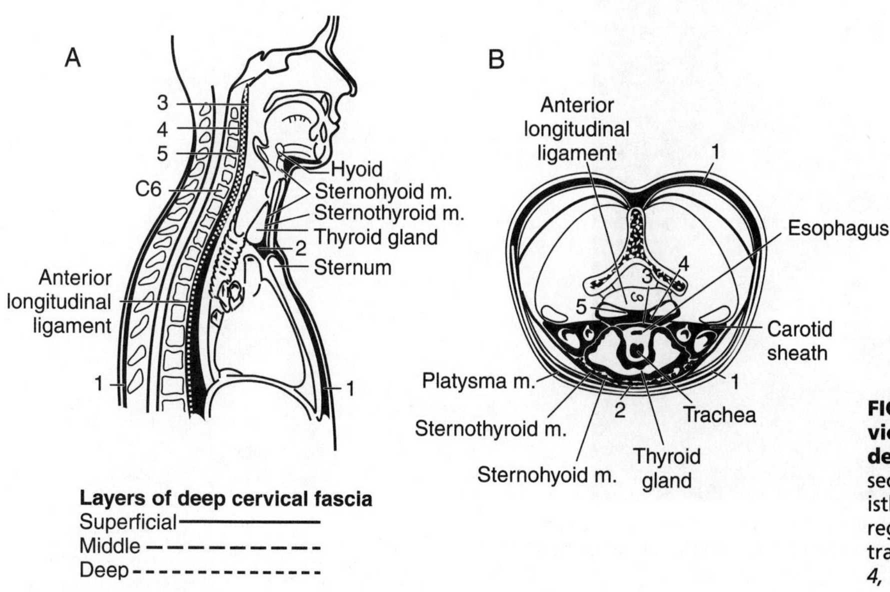

FIGURE 1-229 Relationship of various cervical fascial spaces to the superficial and deep layers of the cervical fascia. A, Cross section of the neck at the level of the thyroid isthmus. **B,** Coronal section in the suprahyoid region of the neck. *1,* Superficial space; *2,* pretracheal space; *3,* retropharyngeal space; *4,* "danger" space; *5,* prevertebral space.

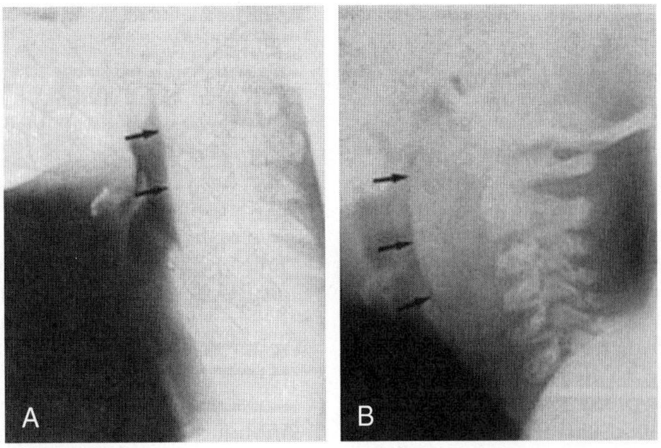

FIGURE 1-230 Lateral radiographs of the neck show **(A)** normal lateral cervical view and **(B)** expansion of the prevertebral soft tissues by a retropharyngeal abscess.

keep the neck in extension during inspiration to avoid a false thickening of the retropharyngeal space. Crying, particularly in infants, may also cause false thickening of the retropharyngeal space.

- A computed tomographic (CT) scan of the neck is the best tool to identify abscesses in the retropharyngeal area, but it is not a perfect tool. Both the sensitivity and specificity of the CT scan in predicting the presence of drainable purulent material are quite variable from study to study, ranging between 68% and 100%.

  The CT provides more information than the plain radiograph because it can generally differentiate between retropharyngeal cellulitis and retropharyngeal abscess and can demonstrate extension of the retropharyngeal abscess to contiguous spaces in the neck. Findings on CT that are common to both cellulitis and abscess are a low-density core, soft-tissue swelling, obliterated fat planes, and mass effect. The best differential finding on CT scan is "complete rim enhancement," which is indicative of abscess (Fig. 1-231). The abscess may be seen as a mass impinging on the posterior pharyngeal wall.
- MRI of the neck is more sensitive than CT and probably technetium scanning is helpful in detecting bone involvement. T2-weighted images may identify and localize areas of pus for drainage or aspiration. Gadolinium enhancement is important to accurately define the soft tissue component. Finally, MRI is useful for imaging vascular lesions, such as jugular thrombophlebitis.

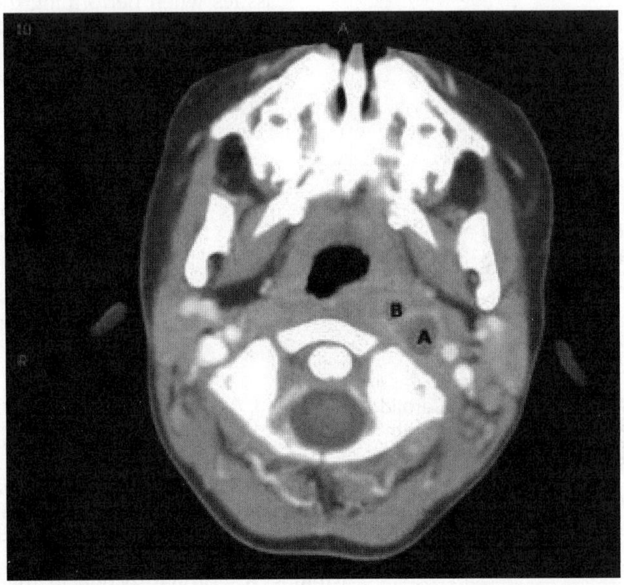

FIGURE 1-231 CT scan of a retropharyngeal abscess **(A, B)** demonstrates a low-density core, soft tissue swelling, obliterated fat planes, mass effect, and rim enhancement.

TREATMENT

Rx

ACUTE GENERAL Rx/CHRONIC Rx

- High-dose penicillin (2 to 4 million units IV q4h) plus metronidazole (500 mg IV q8h) or ampicillin-sulbactam (50 mg/kg/dose IV q6h) or clindamycin (13 mg/kg/dose IV q8h) are effective antimicrobial selections. Parenteral treatment is maintained until the patient is afebrile and clinically improved. Antibiotics should be adjusted as culture data become available, and oral therapy is continued to complete at least a 14-day course.
- Surgical intervention has historically played a prominent role in the management of retropharyngeal abscess in conjunction with antibiotic therapy. Drainage is indicated when there is a large hypodense area or when a patient has failed to respond to parenteral therapy alone.
- When the CT does not demonstrate a large hypodense area, a trial of antibiotic therapy without drainage is appropriate. Some investigators also support a trial of IV antibiotic therapy alone when small abscesses are identified by CT scans, as long as there is no compromise of the airway.

PEARLS & CONSIDERATIONS

!

PREVENTION

The complications of deep neck infection in any space are numerous and potentially fatal. Early diagnosis, with prompt and appropriate management, is key to avoiding these complications.

AUTHOR: **RUBY SATPATHY, M.D.**

BASIC INFORMATION

DEFINITION

Reye's syndrome is a postinfectious triad consisting of encephalopathy, fatty liver degeneration, and transaminase elevation.

ICD-9CM CODES
331.81 Reye's syndrome

EPIDEMIOLOGY & DEMOGRAPHICS

- During the 1970s, 300 to 600 cases were being reported yearly in the U.S
- Since the mid-1980s, following the understanding that aspirin is associated with Reye's syndrome, the yearly count has fallen to <20 cases
- Seasonal relation with influenza and varicella outbreaks
- Age: rare in persons over age 18 yr; peak age (in the U.S.) is 6 to 8 yr
- Case fatality rate: 25% to 50%

PHYSICAL FINDINGS & CLINICAL PRESENTATION

Shortly following recovery from a viral infection (flu or chicken pox) an afebrile child begins to vomit intractably. Hepatomegaly is often present. The vomiting can lead to dehydration. Occasionally, symptoms of hypoglycemia are present. After 2 days, symptoms of encephalopathy dominate the clinical picture (lethargy, confusion, stupor, coma, seizures, decorticate or decerebrate posture) (Table 1-41).

ETIOLOGY

- Temporal association with influenza and varicella infection
- Epidemiologic association with aspirin or other salicylate use to treat the viral infection
- Possible association with aflatoxin and pesticides
- Pathology

Liver: no inflammation; the striking finding is panlobular microvesicular hepatocyte infiltration on light microscopy and mitochondrial injury on electron microscopy.

Brain: no inflammation; there are cerebral edema and anoxic degeneration.

- Pathogenesis: not fully understood but mitochondrial dysfunction is clearly at the center stage

DIAGNOSIS

DIFFERENTIAL DIAGNOSIS

- Inborn errors of metabolism
  Carnitine deficiency
  Ornithine transcarbamylase deficiency
  Others
- Salicylate or amiodarone intoxication
- Jamaican vomiting sickness
- Hepatic encephalopathy of any cause

WORKUP

According to the CDC's case definition, the following conditions must be met for consideration as a Reye's syndrome case:

- Acute noninflammatory encephalopathy documented by:

Alteration in the level of consciousness and, if available, a record of cerebrospinal fluid containing ≤8 leukocytes per mm³ *or*

Histologic specimen demonstrating cerebral edema without perivascular or meningeal inflammation

- Hepatopathy documented either by a liver biopsy or autopsy considered to be diagnostic of Reye's syndrome or by a threefold or greater rise in the levels of serum aspartate aminotransferase, serum alanine aminotransferase, or serum ammonia *and*
- No more reasonable explanation for the cerebral and hepatic abnormalities

LABORATORY TESTS

- Elevated transaminase (ALT and AST)
- Elevated ammonia level
- Occasional elevation of CPK, LDH, and bilirubin and prolongation of prothrombin time
- Occasional hypoglycemia (in patients under the age of 4 yr)
- Cerebrospinal fluid is normal or contains <8 WBCs/ml
- Rarely a liver biopsy is indicated (in infants or in recurrent cases)

TREATMENT

- Supportive
- Mannitol, glycerol, or hyperventilation for cerebral edema if present
- Interferon alfa (experimental)
- Prevention
  Influenza vaccine
  Varicella vaccine
  Avoidance of aspirin in children, especially during influenza and varicella outbreaks

AUTHORS: **FRED F. FERRI, M.D.,** and **TOM J. WACHTEL, M.D.**

TABLE 1-41 Clinical Staging of Reye's Syndrome

Grade	Symptoms at Time of Admission
I	Usually quiet, **lethargic** and sleepy, vomiting, laboratory evidence of liver dysfunction
II	Deep lethargy, **confusion,** delirium, combative, hyperventilation, hyperreflexic
III	Obtunded, **light coma,** seizures, decorticate rigidity, intact pupillary light reaction
IV	Seizures, deepening coma, **decerebrate rigidity,** loss of oculocephalic reflexes, fixed pupils
V	Coma, loss of deep tendon reflexes, respiratory arrest, fixed dilated pupils, **flaccidity/decerebrate** intermittent isoelectric electroencephalogram

From Behrman RE: *Nelson textbook of pediatrics,* ed 17, Philadelphia, 2005, WB Saunders.

BASIC INFORMATION

DEFINITION

Rh incompatibility occurs when an absence of the D antigen on maternal RBCs and its presence on fetal RBCs causes risk of Rh isoimmunization.

ICD-9CM CODES
656.1 Rh incompatibility

EPIDEMIOLOGY & DEMOGRAPHICS

INCIDENCE:

- The absence of the D antigen (Rh^- blood type) occurs in 15% of whites, 8% of blacks, and virtually no Asians or Native Americans. If the father's blood type is not known, the chance that an Rh^- pregnant woman is bearing an Rh^+ fetus is about 60%.
- Of those pregnancies complicated by Rh incompatibility, the risk of maternal isoimmunization to the D antigen is about 8% for each ABO compatible pregnancy *if no prophylaxis is given*.
- Maternal-fetal ABO incompatibility is somewhat protective against Rh isoimmunization.

GENETICS: Five major loci determine Rh status: C, D, E, c, e. The presence of the D antigen results in an Rh^+ individual. Its absence results in an Rh^- individual. Of Rh^+ fathers, 45% are homozygotes, 55% are heterozygotes. For homozygous Rh^+ fathers, the probability of an Rh^+ offspring is 100%. The probability for heterozygotes is about 50%.

RISK FACTORS FOR ISOIMMUNIZATION:

- Antepartum: fetal-to-maternal transfusion
- Intrapartum: fetal-to-maternal transfusion, spontaneous abortion, ectopic pregnancy, abruptio placentae, abdominal trauma, chorionic villus sampling, amniocentesis, percutaneous umbilical blood sampling (PUBS), external cephalic version, manual removal of the placenta, therapeutic abortion, autologous blood product administration

ETIOLOGY

The initial response to D antigen exposure is production of IgM (MW 900,000) that does not cross the placenta. With a repeated exposure, IgG (MW 160,000) is produced. IgG can cross the placenta and enter the fetal circulation, producing hemolysis in the fetus. This may produce erythroblastosis fetalis or hemolytic disease in the newborn, resulting in antepartum or neonatal death or neurologic damage to the fetus because of hyperbilirubinemia and kernicterus.

DIAGNOSIS

LABORATORY TESTS

ABO and Rh blood type and an antibody screen as part of the initial prenatal profile

- If antibody screen negative:
  1. Repeat antibody screen at 28 wk gestation.
  2. Obtain neonatal blood type after delivery.
  3. If Rh incompatibility is confirmed by the neonatal blood type, a Kleihauer-Betke or rosette test should be performed to determine the amount of fetomaternal transfusion in the following high-risk circumstances: abruptio placentae, placenta previa, cesarean delivery, intrauterine manipulation, manual removal of the placenta.
- If anti-D antibody screen is positive:
  1. Maternal indirect Coombs' test is needed to determine antibody titer.
  2. Determine paternal Rh status and zygosity.
  3. If father is heterozygous, PUBS or amniotic fluid is needed to determine fetal Rh status.

IMAGING STUDIES

Ultrasound evaluation can diagnose hydrops fetalis, but it cannot predict it.

TREATMENT

PREVENTION OF D ISOIMMUNIZATION

- Give 50 μg of D immunoglobulin: after spontaneous or induced abortion or ectopic pregnancy <13 wk gestation.
- Give 300 μg of D immunoglobulin (protects against 30 ml of fetal blood):
  1. After spontaneous or induced abortion >13 wk gestation, amniocentesis, CVS, PUBS, external cephalic version or other intrauterine manipulation.
  2. As antepartum prophylaxis at 28 wk gestation. Maternal anti-D prophylaxis does not cause hemolysis in the fetus or newborn.
  3. At delivery if the neonate is D- or Du-positive.
  4. If Kleihauer-Betke or rosette test confirms >30 ml of fetal red blood in maternal circulation, additional D immunoglobulin is indicated. Confirm adequacy of therapy by a maternal indirect Coombs' test 48 to 72 hr after Rh immune globulin is given.

MANAGEMENT OF D ISOIMMUNIZED PREGNANCIES

- Serial amniocentesis for assessment of OD_{450} after 25 wk gestation with interpretation of the Delta OD_{450} according to criteria established by Liley
- PUBS if ultrasonographic evidence of hydrops, rising zone II Delta OD_{450} values on amniocentesis, maternal history of a severely affected child
- Intrauterine exchange transfusion if severe anemia is documented remote from term
- Initiation of steroids for lung maturation at 28 wk in severely affected pregnancies with delivery at lung maturity
- Delivery as soon as lung maturation is achieved in mild to moderately affected pregnancies

DISPOSITION

Survival of nonhydropic infants is 90%. Of infants with hydrops, 82% survive.

REFERRAL

Refer all Rh isoimmunized pregnancies to a tertiary care center before 18 to 20 wk gestation.

SUGGESTED READING

Maayan-Metzger A et al: Maternal anti-D prophylaxis during pregnancy does not cause neonatal hemolysis, *Arch Dis Child* 84:60, 2001.

AUTHORS: **LAUREL M. WHITE, M.D.,** and **RUBEN ALVERO, M.D.**

BASIC INFORMATION

DEFINITION

Rhabdomyolysis is the dissolution or disintegration of muscle, which causes membrane lysis and leakage of muscle constituents, resulting in the excretion of myoglobin in the urine. Renal damage can occur as a result of tubular obstruction by myoglobin as well as hypovolemia.

ICD-9CM CODES
728.89 Rhabdomyolysis

EPIDEMIOLOGY & DEMOGRAPHICS

PREDOMINANT AGE: Rare in children

PHYSICAL FINDINGS & CLINICAL PRESENTATION

- Variable muscle tenderness
- Weakness
- Muscular rigidity
- Fever
- Altered consciousness
- Muscle swelling
- Malaise
- Dark urine

ETIOLOGY

- Exertion (exercise-induced)
- Electrical injury
- Drug-induced (statins, combination of statins with fibrates, amphetamines, haloperidol)
- Compartment syndrome
- Multiple trauma
- Malignant hyperthermia
- Limb ischemia
- Reperfusion after revascularization procedures for ischemia
- Extensive surgical (spinal) dissection, bariatric surgery
- Tourniquet ischemia
- Prolonged static positioning during surgery
- Infectious and inflammatory myositis
- Metabolic myopathies
- Hypovolemia and urinary acidification are important precipitating causes in the development of acute renal failure
- Sickle cell trait is a predisposing condition.

DIAGNOSIS

DIFFERENTIAL DIAGNOSIS

Section III, "Creatine Kinase Elevation," describes a clinical algorithm for the evaluation of CPK elevation.

LABORATORY TESTS

- Screening for myoglobinuria with a simple urine dipstick test using orthotoluidine or benzidine
- BUN, creatinine
- Increased CPK (Fig. 1-232)
- Hyperkalemia
- Hypocalcemia
- Hyperphosphatemia
  - Increased urinary myoglobin
- Pigmented granular casts
- Hyperuricemia

TREATMENT

ACUTE GENERAL Rx

- Early, aggressive high-volume IV fluid replacement with mannitol, to induce diuresis to prevent acute renal failure
- Treatment of electrolyte imbalances
- Alkalinization of urine is controversial but appears helpful in research models

DISPOSITION

The condition is easily treatable, but early diagnosis and management are necessary to avoid renal failure, which occurs in 30% of cases.

REFERRAL

Renal consultation in difficult cases

PEARLS & CONSIDERATIONS

COMMENTS

A clinical algorithm for the evaluation of muscle cramps and aches is described in Fig. 3-187.

EVIDENCE

There is overwhelming support in the literature for the efficacy of early volume expansion in volume-depleted patients.

Prevention of acute renal failure (ARF) is imperative with liberal use of intravenous fluids.

Myoglobin precipitation is prevented with this treatment.

Myoglobinuria usually resolves in 3 to 4 days.

Evidence-Based References

Better OS, Stein JH: Early management of shock and prophylaxis of acute renal failure in traumatic rhabdomyolysis, *N Engl J Med* 322:825, 1990.

Zager R: Rhabdomyolysis and myohemoglobinuric acute renal failure, *Kidney Int* 49:314, 1996.

SUGGESTED READINGS

Alsheikh-Ali AA et al: Effect of the magnitude of lipid lowering on risk of elevated liver enzymes, rhabdomyolysis, and cancer: insights from large randomized statin trials, *J Am Coll Cardiol* 50(5):409, 2007.

Ahn SC: Neuromuscular complications of statins, *Phys Med Rehabil Clin N Am* 19:47, 2008.

Brown CV et al: Preventing renal failure in patients with rhabdomyolisis: do bicarbonate and mannitol make a difference? *J Trauma* 56(6):1191, 2004.

Ettinger JE et al: Rhabdomyolysis: diagnosis and treatment in bariatric surgery, *Obes Surg* 17(4):525, 2007.

Finsterer J et al: Severe rhabdomyolysis after excessive bodybuilding, *J Sports Med Phys Fitness* 47:502, 2007.

Gunal AI et al: Early and vigorous fluid resuscitation prevents acute renal failure in the crush victims of catastrophic earthquakes, *J Am Soc Nephrol* 15(7):1862, 2004.

AUTHOR: **LONNIE R. MERCIER, M.D.**

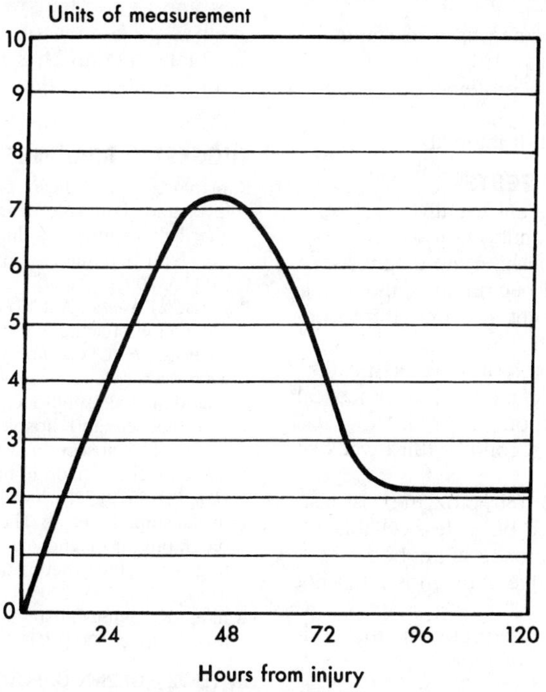

FIGURE 1-232 Typical CK elimination curve. (From Rosen P [ed]: *Emergency medicine*, ed 4, St Louis, 1998, Mosby.)

BASIC INFORMATION

DEFINITION

Rheumatic fever is a multisystem inflammatory disease that occurs in the genetically susceptible host after a pharyngeal infection with group A streptococci.

SYNONYMS

Acute rheumatic fever
Rheumatic carditis

ICD-9CM CODES
390; 716.9 Rheumatic fever

EPIDEMIOLOGY & DEMOGRAPHICS

INCIDENCE (IN U.S.):
- 0.1% to 3% in patients with untreated streptococcal pharyngitis
- Higher incidence of streptococcal pharyngitis with:
  1. Crowding
  2. Poverty
  3. Young age

PEAK INCIDENCE: School-age children

PREDOMINANT AGE:
- Age 5 to 15 yr for first attack
- Possible relapses later

GENETICS:
Familial Disposition: Predisposition to the disease is likely to be genetically determined.

PHYSICAL FINDINGS & CLINICAL PRESENTATION

- Acute streptococcal pharyngitis, which may be subclinical and not reported by the patient
- After latent period of 1 to 5 wk (average, 19 days), acute rheumatic attack
- Patient is febrile, with a migratory polyarthritis of knees, ankles, wrists, elbows; typically severe for 1 wk, remits by 3 to 4 wk
- Carditis
  1. New heart murmur
     a. Mitral regurgitation
     b. Aortic insufficiency
     c. Diastolic mitral murmur
  2. Cardiomegaly
  3. CHF
  4. Pericardial friction rub or effusion
- Rarely, pancarditis is severe and fatal.
- Subcutaneous nodules can be palpated over extensor tendon surfaces or bony prominences, such as the skull.
- Chorea (Sydenham's chorea) is characterized by rapid involuntary movements affecting all muscles.
  1. Muscular weakness
  2. Emotional lability
  3. Rarely seen after adolescence and almost never in adult males
- Erythema marginatum
  1. Evanescent, pink, well-demarcated spreading to trunk and proximal extremities
  2. Not specific
- Arthralgias (joint pain without swelling)
- Abdominal pain

ETIOLOGY

- Group A streptococci not recovered from tissue lesions.
- It does not occur in the absence of a streptococcal antibody response.
- Immunologic cross-reactivity between certain streptococcal antigens and human tissue antigens suggests an autoimmune etiology.
- Both initial attacks and recurrences can be completely prevented by prompt treatment of streptococcal pharyngitis with penicillin.

DIAGNOSIS

DIFFERENTIAL DIAGNOSIS

- Rheumatoid arthritis
- Juvenile rheumatoid arthritis (Still's disease)
- Bacterial endocarditis
- Systemic lupus
- Viral infections
- Serum sickness

WORKUP

- "Jones Criteria (revised) for Guidance in the Diagnosis of Rheumatic Fever" published by the American Heart Association

One major and two minor criteria if supported by evidence of an antecedent group A streptococcal infection
- Major criteria
  1. Carditis
  2. Migratory arthritis
  3. Chorea
  4. Erythema marginatum
  5. Subcutaneous nodules
- Minor criteria
  1. Previous rheumatic fever or rheumatic heart disease
  2. Fever
  3. Arthralgia
  4. Increased acute-phase reactants
     a. ESR
     b. C-reactive protein
     c. Leukocytosis
  5. Prolonged P-R interval

LABORATORY TESTS

- Throat cultures are usually negative.
- Streptococcal antibody tests are more useful in establishing the diagnosis.
  1. Peak at the beginning of the attack
  2. Can document a recent streptococcal infection
- ASO (antistreptolysin O) titers peak:
  1. 4 to 5 wk after a streptococcal throat infection
  2. During the second or third week of illness
- Anti-DNase B (Streptozyme) is also commonly used but is less reliable.
- High-titer streptococcal antibodies:
  1. Are supportive of diagnosis, but not proof
  2. Should be interpreted in the context of clinical criteria

IMAGING STUDIES

- Chest x-ray to assess heart size
- Echocardiogram:
  1. To evaluate murmurs
  2. To rule out pericardial effusion

TREATMENT

ACUTE GENERAL Rx

- Course of penicillin to eradicate throat carriage of group A streptococci
- Arthralgia or arthritis without carditis: aspirin 40 mg/lb/day for 2 wk, followed by 20 mg/lb/day for 4 to 6 wk
- Carditis and heart failure:
  1. Prednisone 40 to 60 mg/day
  2. IV corticosteroids, such as methylprednisolone, 10 to 40 mg/day for severe carditis

CHRONIC Rx

Secondary prevention (prevention of recurrences):
- Monthly treatment with benzathine penicillin 1.2 million U IM
- Erythromycin in patients with penicillin allergy

DISPOSITION

- Damage of heart valves because of fibrosis
  1. Late sequela of recurrent attacks
  2. Frequent cause of valvular heart disease in developing countries
- May progress to heart failure

REFERRAL

To cardiologist for management of severe carditis

EVIDENCE

Practical application of bed rest and aspirin for symptom relief, as well as prevention of recurrence with antibiotic therapy, has resulted in dramatic declines in adult rheumatic heart disease.

SUGGESTED READINGS

Kaplan EL: Pathogenesis of acute rheumatic fever and rheumatic heart disease: evasive after half a century of clinical, epidemiological, and laboratory investigation, *Heart* 91(1):3, 2005.

Robertson KA et al: Antibiotics for the primary prevention of acute rheumatic fever: a meta-analysis, *BMC Cardiovasc Disord* 5(1):11, 2005.

Sharland M et al: Antibiotic prescribing in general practice and hospital admissions for peritonsillar abscess, mastoiditis, and rheumatic fever in children: time trend analysis, *BMJ* 331(7512):328, 2005.

Vijayalakshmi IB et al: The role of echocardiography in diagnosing carditis in the setting of acute rheumatic fever, *Cardiol Young* 15(6):583, 2005.

Walker K, Wilmshurst J: Acute rheumatic fever, *Lancet* 366(9494):1354, 2005.

AUTHORS: **GLENN G. FORT, M.D., M.P.H., DENNIS J. MIKOLICH, M.D.,** and **DEBORAH L. SHAPIRO, M.D.**

BASIC INFORMATION

DEFINITION

Rheumatoid arthritis (RA) is a systemic disorder characterized by chronic joint inflammation that most commonly affects peripheral joints. This process results in the development of pannus, a destructive tissue that damages cartilage.

ICD-9CM CODES
714.0 Rheumatoid arthritis

EPIDEMIOLOGY & DEMOGRAPHICS

PREVALENCE: 5 cases/1000 adults
PREDOMINANT SEX:
- Female:male ratio of 3:1
- After age 50 yr, sex difference less marked

PREDOMINANT AGE: 35 to 45 yr

PHYSICAL FINDINGS & CLINICAL PRESENTATION

- Usually gradual onset; common prodromal symptoms of weakness, fatigue, and anorexia
- Initial presentation: multiple symmetric joint involvement, most often in the hands and feet, usually MCP, MTP, and PIP joints (Fig. 1-233)
- Joint effusions, tenderness, and restricted motion usually present early in the disease
- Eventual characteristic deformities: subluxations, dislocations, and joint contractures
- Extraarticular findings:
  1. Tendon sheaths and bursae frequently affected by chronic inflammation
  2. Possible tendon rupture
  3. Rheumatoid nodules over bony prominences such as the elbow and shaft of the ulna
  4. Splenomegaly, pericarditis, and vasculitis
  5. Findings of carpal tunnel syndrome resulting from flexor tenosynovitis

ETIOLOGY

Unknown. There is increasing evidence that the inflammation and destruction of bone and cartilage that occurs in many rheumatic diseases are the result of the activation by some unknown mechanism of proinflammatory cells that infiltrate the synovium. These cells, in turn, release various substances, such as cytokines and tumor necrosis factor (TNF) alpha, which subsequently cause the pathologic changes typical of this group of diseases. Many of the newer therapeutic agents are directed at the suppression of these final mediators of inflammation.

DIAGNOSIS

DIFFERENTIAL DIAGNOSIS

- SLE
- Seronegative spondyloarthropathies
- Polymyalgia rheumatica
- Acute rheumatic fever
- Scleroderma

According to the American College of Rheumatology, RA exists when four of seven criteria are present, with criteria 1 to 4 being present for at least 6 wk.

1. Morning stiffness over 1 hr
2. Arthritis in three or more joints with swelling
3. Arthritis of hand joints with swelling
4. Symmetric arthritis
5. Rheumatoid nodules
6. Roentgenographic changes typical of RA
7. Positive serum rheumatoid factor

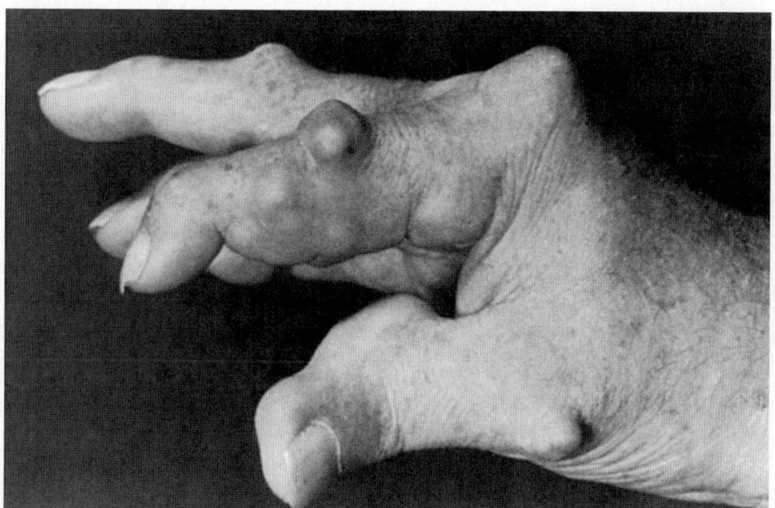

FIGURE 1-233 Rheumatoid arthritis. Hand of a 60-year-old man with seropositive rheumatoid arthritis. There are fixed deformities and gross rheumatoid nodules. (From Canoso JJ: *Rheumatology in primary care,* Philadelphia, 1997, WB Saunders.)

LABORATORY TESTS

- Increase in rheumatoid factor in 80% of cases (rheumatoid factor also present in the normal population)
- Possible mild anemia
- Usually, elevated acute phase reactants (ESR, C-reactive protein)
- Possible mild leukocytosis
- Usually, turbid joint fluid, which forms a poor mucin clot; elevated cell count, with an increase in polymorphonuclear leukocytes

IMAGING STUDIES

Plain radiography
- Usually reveals soft-tissue swelling and osteoporosis early (Fig. 1-234)
- Eventually, joint space narrowing, erosion, and deformity visible as a result of continued inflammation and cartilage destruction

TREATMENT

NONPHARMACOLOGIC THERAPY

Proper management requires close cooperation among primary physician, therapist, rheumatologist, and orthopedist.
- Patient education is important.
- Rest with proper exercise and splinting can prevent or correct joint deformities.
- Maintain proper diet and control obesity.

CHRONIC Rx

- NSAIDs: commonly used as the initial treatment to relieve inflammation (drug of choice for most patients: aspirin, but other NSAIDs also effective)
- Disease-modifying drugs (DMARDs): are traditionally begun when NSAIDs are not effective; current recommendations favor early aggressive treatment with DMARDs, seeking to minimize long-term joint damage. Commonly used agents are methotrexate, cyclosporine, hydroxychloroquine, sulfasalazine, leflunomide, and infliximab. Most of these are associated with potential toxicity and require close monitoring. They are also usually slow-acting drugs that require more than 8 wk to become effective (Table 1-42)
- Oral prednisone
- Intrasynovial steroid injections
- Etanercept (Enbrel), a tumor necrosis factor α-blocker, is indicated in moderately to severely active RA in patients who respond inadequately to DMARDs. The combination of etanercept and methotrexate has been reported to be effective and promising in the treatment of RA

DISPOSITION

- Remissions and exacerbations are common, but condition is chronically progressive in the majority of cases.
- Joint degeneration and deformity often lead to disability.
- Early diagnosis and treatment are important and can improve quality of life.

REFERRAL

Early referral to rheumatologist

Orthopedic consultation for corrective surgery

PEARLS & CONSIDERATIONS

- RA often develops acutely in the postpartum patient, a common time for the onset of autoimmune diseases.
- Because of the poor outcomes associated with previous treatment protocols, a much more aggressive approach, often using IV therapies, is presently advocated by many rheumatologists.

EVIDENCE

EBM

Combinations of certain DMARDs may be more effective than using individual drugs alone. However, the balance of benefits and harms varies for different combinations.[1] Ⓐ

Low-dose methotrexate is significantly more effective than placebo for the short-term treatment of patients with rheumatoid arthritis.[2] Ⓐ

The addition of subcutaneous adalimumab to long-term treatment with methotrexate in patients with active rheumatoid arthritis produces significant improvement in disease activity.[3] Ⓑ

Hydroxychloroquine significantly reduces disease activity and joint inflammation compared with placebo. It also has a low toxicity profile.[4] Ⓐ

Sulfasalazine is significantly more effective than placebo for the treatment of tender and swollen joints and for decreasing pain and erythrocyte sedimentation rate in rheumatoid arthritis.[5,6] Ⓐ

Leflunomide appears to improve all clinical outcomes and delay radiologic progression of rheumatoid arthritis at both 6 and 12 months.[7] Ⓐ

Etanercept and infliximab have been shown to be effective than placebo in improving symptoms and in reducing long-term disease and joint inflammation, although there are significant questions about their long-term safety.[1] Ⓐ

Minocycline is more effective than placebo at improving control of disease activity in rheumatoid arthritis.[1] Ⓐ

Evidence-Based References

1. Emery P, Suarez-Almazor M: Rheumatoid arthritis. 11, web version only, London, 2003, BMJ Publishing Group. Ⓐ
2. Suarez-Almazor ME et al: Methotrexate for treating rheumatoid arthritis. Reviewed in: Cochrane Library 2, Chichester, UK, 2004, John Wiley. Ⓐ
3. Weinblatt ME, Keystone EC, Furst DE: Adalimumab, a fully human anti-tumor necrosis factor alpha monoclonal antibody, for the treatment of rheumatoid arthritis in patients taking concomitant methotrexate: the ARMADA trial, *Arthritis Rheum* 48:35, 2003. Ⓑ
4. Suarez-Almazor ME et al: Antimalarials for treating rheumatoid arthritis. Reviewed in: Cochrane Library 2, Chichester, UK, 2004, John Wiley. Ⓐ
5. Suarez-Almazor ME et al: Sulfasalazine for treating rheumatoid arthritis. Reviewed in: Cochrane Library 2, Chichester, UK, 2004, John Wiley. Ⓐ
6. Weinblatt ME et al: Sulfasalazine treatment for rheumatoid arthritis: a metaanalysis of 15 randomized trials, *J Rheumatol* 26:2:2123-, 1999. Reviewed in: *Clin Evid* 11, 2003, web version only. Ⓐ
7. Osiri M et al: Leflunomide for treating rheumatoid arthritis. Reviewed in: Cochrane Library 2, Chichester, UK, 2004, John Wiley. Ⓐ

SUGGESTED READINGS

Chen AL, Joseph TN, Zuckerman JD: Rheumatoid arthritis of the shoulder, *J Am Acad Orthop Surg* 11:12, 2003.

Edwards JC, Szczepanski L et al: Efficacy of β-cell-targeted therapy with ritaximab in patients with rheumatoid arthritis, *N Engl J Med* 350:2572, 2004.

Gardner GC, Kadel MJ: Ordering and interpreting rheumatologic laboratory tests, *J Am Acad Orthop Surg* 11:60, 2003.

Heiberg MS et al: The comparative one-year performance of anti-tumor necrosis factor alpha drugs in patients with rheumatoid arthritis, psoriatic arthritis and ankylosing spondylitis: results from a longitudinal, observational, multicenter study, *Arthritis Rheum* 59:234, 2008.

Olsen NJ, Stein CM: New drugs for rheumatoid arthritis, *N Engl J Med* 350:2167, 2004.

Maini SR: Infliximab treatment of rheumatoid arthritis, *Rheum Dis Clin North Am* 30:329, 2004.

Papp SR et al: The rheumatoid wrist, *J Am Acad Orthop Surg* 14:65, 2006.

Smith AM et al: Rotator cuff repair in patients with rheumatoid arthritis, *J Bone Joint Surg* 87A:1782, 2005.

Sokka T: Quantitative assessment of rheumatoid arthritis in standard clinical care: turning clinical care into clinical science, *Best Pract Res Clin Rheumatol* 21(4):653, 2007.

AUTHOR: **LONNIE R. MERCIER, M.D.**

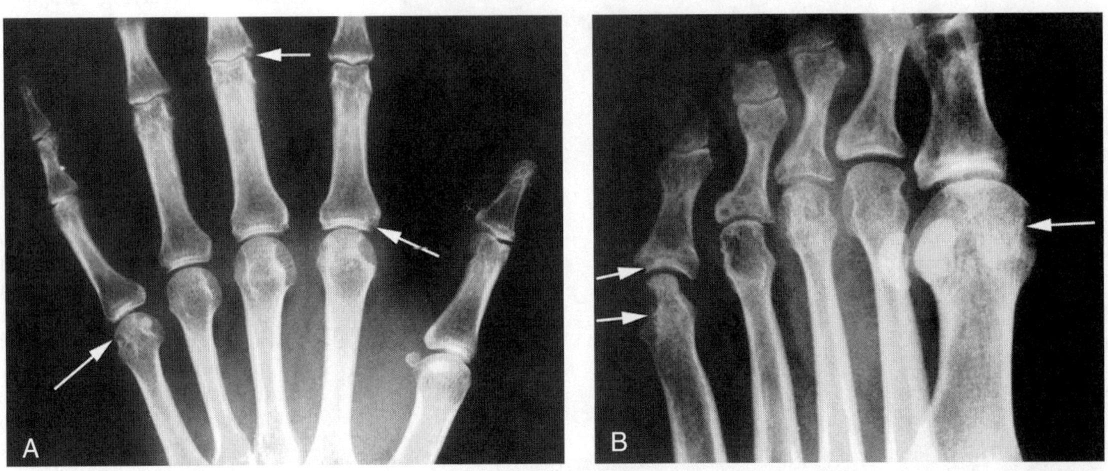

FIGURE 1-234 Rheumatoid arthritis. A, Periarticular osteopenia and marginal erosions in MCPs and a PIP *(arrows)*. **B,** In the same patient, marginal erosions at metatarsal heads. (From Canoso JJ [ed]: *Rheumatology in primary care,* Philadelphia, 1997, WB Saunders.)

TABLE 1-42 Selected Disease-Modifying Antirheumatic Drugs

Type/Generic (Trade) Name	Recommended Dosages	Toxic Effects	Recommended Monitoring
Gold compounds (Myochrysine)	IM: 10 mg followed by 25 mg 1 wk later, then 25-50 mg wkly until there is toxicity, major clinical improvement, or cumulative dose = 1 g. If effective, interval between doses is increased.	Pruritus, dermatitis (frequent—⅓ of pts), stomatitis, nephrotoxicity, blood dyscrasias, "nitritoid" reaction: flushing, weakness, nausea, dizziness 30 min after injection.	CBC, platelet count before every other injection. Urinalysis before each dose.
Aurothioglucose (Solganal)	IM: 10 mg; 2nd and 3rd doses 25 mg, 4th and subsequent 50 mg. Interval between doses: 1 wk. If improvement, no toxicity→decrease dose to 25 mg or increase interval between doses.	Dermatitis, stomatitis, nephrotoxicity, blood dyscrasias.	CBC, platelet count every 2 wk. Urinalysis before each dose.
Auranofin (Ridaura)	Oral: 3 mg bid or 6 mg qd. May increase to 3 mg tid after 6 months.	Loose stools, diarrhea (up to 50%), dermatitis.	Baseline CBC, platelet count, U/A, renal, liver function, at onset then CBC with platelet count, U/A 9 months.
Antimalarial Hydroxychloroquine (Plaquenil)	Oral: 400-600 mg qd with meals then 200-400 mg qd.	Retinopathy, dermatitis, muscle weakness, hypoactive DTRs, CNS.	Ophthalmologic examination every 3 months (visual acuity, slitlamp, funduscopic, visual field tests), neuromuscular examination.
Penicillamine (Cuprimine, Depen)	Oral: 125-250 mg qd, then increasing at monthly intervals doses to max 750-1000 mg by 125-250 mg.	Pruritus, rash/mouth ulcers, bone marrow depression, proteinuria, hematuria, hypogeusia, myesthenia, myositis, GI distress, pulmonary toxicity, teratogenic.	CBC every 2 weeks until dose stable, then every month. U/A weekly until dose stable, then every month. HCG as needed.
Methotrexate (Rheumatrex)	Oral: 7.5-15 mg weekly.	Pulmonary toxicity, ulcerative stomatitis, leukopenia, thrombocytopenia, GI distress, malaise, fatigue, chills, fever, CNS, elevated LFTs/liver disease, lymphoma, infection.	CBC with platelet count, LFTs weekly × 6 wk then monthly LFTs, U/A periodically, HCG as needed.
Azathioprine (Imuran)	Oral: 50-100 mg qd, increase at 4-wk intervals by 0.5 mg/kg/d up to 2.5 mg/kg/d	Leukopenia, thrombocytopenia, GI, neoplastic if previous Rx with alkylating agents.	CBC with platelet count, wkly × 1 mo, 2×/mo. × 2 mo, then monthly, HCG as needed.
Sulfasalazine (Azulfidine)	Oral: 500 mg daily then increase up to 3 g daily.	GI, skin rash, pruritus, blood dyscrasias, oligospermia.	CBC, U/A q 2 wk × 3 mo, then monthly × 9 mo, then every 6 mo.
Alkylating agents Cyclophosphamide (Cytoxan)	Oral: 50-100 mg daily up to 2.5 mg/kg/d.	Leukopenia, thrombocytopenia, hematuria, GI, alopecia, rash, bladder cancer, non-Hodgkin's lymphoma, infection.	CBC with platelet count, regularly. HCG as needed.
Chlorambucil (Leukeran)	Oral: 0.1-0.2 mg/kg/d.	Bone marrow suppression, GI, CNS, infection.	CBC with platelet count every wk. WBCs 3-4 days after each CBC during 1st 3-6 wk at therapy. HCG as needed.
Cyclosporine (Sandimmune)	Oral 2.5-5 mg/kg/d.	Nephrotoxicity, tremor, hirsutism, hypertension, gum hyperplasia.	Renal function, liver function.
Pyrimidine, synthesis inhibitors Leflunomide (Arava)	Loading dose: 100 mg/d for 3 days. Maintenance therapy: 20 mg/d; if not tolerated, 10 mg/d.	Hepatotoxicity, carcinogenesis. Immunosuppression, long half-life.	LFTs every month, drug levels after discontinuation (after 1 month therapy, remains in blood for 2 years without use of cholestyramine).

From Rakel RE (ed): *Principles of family practice,* ed 6, Philadelphia, 2002, WB Saunders.
bid, Twice a day; *CBC,* complete blood count; *CNS,* central nervous system; *DTR,* deep tendon reflex; *GI,* gastrointestinal; *HCG,* human chorionic gonadotropin; *IM,* intramuscular; *LFT,* liver function test; *qd,* every day; *tid,* three times a day; *U/A,* urinalysis; *WBC,* white blood cell count.

BASIC INFORMATION

DEFINITION

Rickets is a systemic disease of infancy and childhood in which mineralization of growing bone is deficient as a result of abnormal calcium, phosphorus, or vitamin D metabolism. *Osteomalacia* is the same condition in the adult. *Renal osteodystrophy* is a term used to describe a similar condition in patients with chronic kidney disease. Certain forms of the disorder may respond only to high doses of vitamin D and are referred to as vitamin D–resistant rickets (VDRR).

ICD-9CM CODES
268.0 Active rickets
275.3 Vitamin D–resistant rickets
588.0 Renal rickets (renal osteodystrophy)
268.2 Osteomalacia

PHYSICAL FINDINGS & CLINICAL PRESENTATION

The child with classic rickets usually develops a number of specific abnormalities:
- Softening of the skull bones (craniotabes) early in the disorder
- Enlargement of the ribs at the costochondral junctions, producing the "rachitic rosary"
- Limb deformities and epiphyseal swelling (Fig. 1-235)
- Height below normal range
- Irritability and easy fatigability
- Pigeon breast deformity and an indentation of the lower ribcage at the insertion of the diaphragm, sometimes referred to as Harrison's groove; possible decrease in thoracic volume, resulting in diminished pulmonary ventilation

Physical findings in the adult with osteomalacia are more subtle:
- Possible malaise and bone pain
- Many patients presumed to have osteoporosis but may also have osteomalacia

ETIOLOGY

- Deficiency states
  1. True classic VDDR is rare in Western society.
  2. Absorption of vitamin D, however, may be blocked in several GI disorders.
  3. Similar disorders may also prevent absorption of calcium and phosphorus, but in the absence of these other diseases, deficiencies of calcium and phosphorus are also rare.
- Acquired or inherited renal tubular abnormalities that cause resorptive defects and result in rickets and osteomalacia; syndromes include classical VDRR (probably the most common form of rickets seen in general practice)
- Chronic renal failure:
  1. Can produce renal rickets or renal osteodystrophy
  2. Results in the retention of phosphate

DIAGNOSIS

DIFFERENTIAL DIAGNOSIS

- Osteoporosis
- Hyperparathyroidism
- Hyperthyroidism

LABORATORY TESTS

- Requires a high degree of interest because many of the conditions are so similar that only a complicated laboratory evaluation may establish the diagnosis
- BUN, creatinine, alkaline phosphatase, calcium, and phosphorus levels in any patient suspected of having metabolic bone disease

IMAGING STUDIES

- In rickets:
  1. Characteristic radiographic changes in the ends of growing long bones caused by the lack of calcification of the cartilage matrix
  2. Widening and irregularity of the epiphyseal plate
- Radiographs in the adult with osteomalacia:
  1. More subtle and often confused with osteoporosis
  2. Possible pseudofractures (Looser's zones) where major arteries cross bone
  3. Insufficiency compression deformities in the vertebral bodies

TREATMENT

REFERRAL

- Because of the complex nature of many of these disorders, a qualified endocrinologist and nephrologist should be consulted for treatment.
- The need for orthopedic intervention is rare.
- Surgical care is indicated for slipped capital femoral epiphysis, which is fairly common in renal rickets.
- Deformity may require bracing.

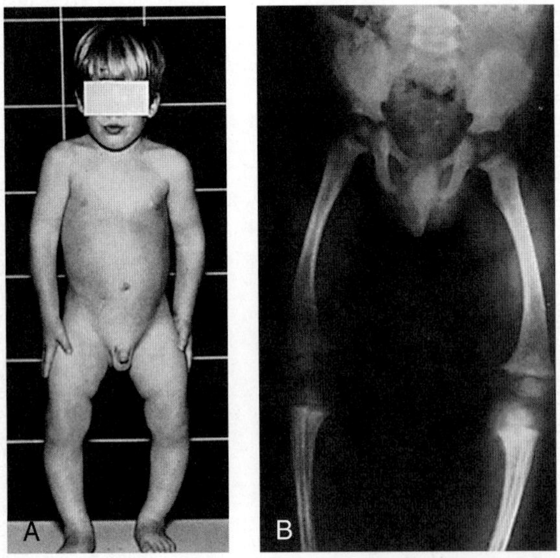

FIGURE 1-235 A, Clinical and, B, radiographic appearance of a young boy with X-linked hypophosphatemic rickets. Note the striking bowing of the legs, apparent in both femora and tibiae, with flaring of the ends of the bones at the knee. (Courtesy Dr. Sara B. Arnaud. From Bikle DB: Osteomalacia and rickets. In Wyngaarden JB, Smith LH Jr, Bennett JB [eds]: *Cecil textbook of medicine,* ed 19, Philadelphia, 1992, WB Saunders.)

SUGGESTED READINGS

Abrams SA: Nutritional rickets: an old disease returns, *Nutr Rev* 60(4):111, 2002.
Allgrove J: Is nutritional rickets returning? *Arch Dis Child* 89(8):699, 2004.
Ashraf S, Mughal MZ: The prevalence of rickets among non-Caucasian children, *Arch Dis Child* 87(3):263, 2002.
Eliot MM: The control of rickets, *Am J Public Health* 94(8):1321, 2004.
Fulop M, Mackay M: Renal tubular acidosis, Sjogren Syndrome and bone disease, *Arch Intern Med* 164(8):905, 2004.
Goodman SB et al: The effects of medications on bone, *J Am Acad Orthop Surg* 15(8):450, 2007.
Joiner TA et al: Primary care pediatrician knowledge of nutritional rickets, *J Natl Med Assoc* 94(11):971, 2002.
Tejwani NC et al: Renal osteodystrophy, *J Am Acad Orthop Surg* 14:303, 2006.
Ward LM et al: Vitamin D-deficiency rickets among children in Canada, *CMAJ* 177(2): 161, 2007

AUTHOR: **LONNIE R. MERCIER, M.D.**

BASIC INFORMATION

DEFINITION

Rocky Mountain spotted fever (RMSF) is a life-threatening, tick-borne febrile illness caused by infection with *Rickettsia rickettsii*. The infection occurs when *R. rickettsii* in the salivary glands of a vector tick is transmitted into the dermis, spreading and replicating in the cytoplasm of endothelial cells and eliciting widespread vasculitis and end-organ damage.

ICD-9CM CODES
082.0 Rocky Mountain spotted fever

EPIDEMIOLOGY & DEMOGRAPHICS

INCIDENCE: 0.18 to 0.32 cases/100,000 person-years

PREVALENCE: Most prevalent in the Southeast, followed by the South Central states, but seen anywhere. It has recently been reported in eastern Arizona, with common brown dog ticks (*Rhipicephalus sanguineus*) implicated as a vector of *R. rickettsii.*

PREDOMINANT SEX: Affects both genders equally

PREDOMINANT AGE: Occurs at any age, but more likely in children aged 5 to 14 yr

PHYSICAL FINDINGS & CLINICAL PRESENTATION

- Incubation: 3 to 12 days
- First symptoms: fever, headache, malaise, and myalgias

Common history, signs, or symptoms	**%**
Tick bite	65
Fever	100
Rash	90
Rash on palms and soles	80
Headache	90
Myalgia	75
Nausea or vomiting	60
Abdominal pain	40
Conjunctivitis	30
Edema	20
Pneumonitis	15
Any severe neurologic complication (including stupor, delirium, seizures, ataxia, papilledema, focal neurologic deficits, and coma)	30

Rash:
- Appears during first 3 days in 50%; by day 5, 80% have it. No rash in 10%.
- Initial appearance: blanching erythematous macules on wrists and ankles that then spread to trunk, palms, and soles.
- Lesions may evolve into papules and eventually become nonblanching (petechiae or palpable purpura).

Gastrointestinal symptoms:
- Nausea, vomiting, and abdominal pain are common
- Occasionally may mimic an "acute abdomen" (e.g., appendicitis, cholecystitis)
- Mild hepatitis

Cardiopulmonary involvement:
- Interstitial pneumonitis
- Myocarditis

Renal problems:
- Prerenal azotemia
- Interstitial nephritis
- Glomerulonephritis

Neurologic involvement:
- Encephalitis (confusion, lethargy, delirium)
- Ataxia
- Convulsion
- Cranial nerve palsy
- Speech impediment
- Hemiparesis or paraparesis
- Spasticity

Fulminant Rocky Mountain spotted fever
- Early, widespread vascular necrosis leading to multisystem illness and death

ETIOLOGY & PATHOGENESIS

- Infectious agent: *R. rickettsii* (an intracellular bacterium).
- Vector: dog tick and wood tick (vertical transmission exists in ticks, but horizontal transmission involving rodents represents an important reservoir for the agent). In the United States *R. rickettsii* is transmitted mainly by the American dog tick *(Dermacentor variabilis)* and the Rocky Mountain wood tick *(D. andersoni).*
- Pathogenesis: the spread of *R. rickettsii* is hematogenous with attachment to the vascular endothelium, causing a vasculitis. The manifestations of this illness are caused by increased vascular permeability.

DIAGNOSIS

DIFFERENTIAL DIAGNOSIS

Influenza A, enteroviral infection, typhoid fever, leptospirosis, infectious mononucleosis, viral hepatitis, sepsis, ehrlichiosis, gastroenteritis, acute abdomen, bronchitis, pneumonia, meningococcemia, disseminated gonococcal infection, secondary syphilis, bacterial endocarditis, toxic shock syndrome, scarlet fever, rheumatic fever, measles, rubella, typhus, rickettsialpox, Lyme disease, drug hypersensitivity reactions, idiopathic thrombocytopenic purpura, thrombotic thrombocytopenic purpura, Kawasaki disease, immune complex vasculitis, connective tissue disorders

WORKUP

Consider RMSF in any patient with an acute febrile illness with headache and myalgia, especially with an associated history of tick exposure. Absence of rash does not rule out the diagnosis.

LABORATORY TESTS

Routine tests	**%**
White cell count	
<10,000/mm^3	72
>10% bands	69
Platelet count	
<150,000/mm^3	52
<99,000/mm^3	32
Serum sodium value <132 mEq/L	56
Aspartate aminotransferase ≥2× normal	62
Alanine aminotransferase ≥2× normal	39
Bilirubin value >1.4 mg/dl	30
Cerebrospinal fluid	
Opening pressure ≥250 mm H_2O	14
Glucose value ≤50 mg/dl	8
Protein value ≥50 mg/dl	35
White cell count ≥5/mm^3	38
Mononuclear cell predominance	46
Polymorphonuclear cell predominance	50

Etiologic tests
- Antibody titers to *R. rickettsii* (by indirect fluorescent antibody test). The diagnosis of RMSF requires a fourfold increase 2 wk apart and thus is not helpful in the care of the patients despite a sensitivity and specificity of near 100%.
- The only test that can provide a timely diagnosis is the immunohistologic demonstration of *R. rickettsii* in skin biopsy specimens.

TREATMENT

- Oral or intravenous doxycycline, 200 mg/day in two divided doses
- Oral tetracycline, 25 to 50 mg/kg/day in four divided doses
- Chloramphenicol, 50 to 75 mg/kg/day in four divided doses; therapy continued for at least 2 days after defervescence

PROGNOSIS

Fatality rate: 1% to 4% (five times greater if treatment is initiated after day 5 of illness, which is more likely in absence of rash and during seasonal nonpeak tick activity). Long-term sequelae seen in patients who recover from severe RMSF: paraparesis, hearing loss; peripheral neuropathy; bladder and bowel incontinence; cerebellar, vestibular, and motor dysfunction; language disorders; limb amputation; and scrotal pain after cutaneous necrosis.

SUGGESTED READINGS

Demma LJ et al: Rocky Mountain spotted fever from an unexpected tick vector in Arizona, *N Engl J Med* 353:587, 2005.

Masters EJ: Rocky Mountain spotted fever, *Arch Intern Med* 163:769, 2003.

AUTHORS: **FRED F. FERRI, M.D.,** and **TOM J. WACHTEL, M.D.**

BASIC INFORMATION

DEFINITION

Rosacea is a chronic skin disorder characterized by papules and pustules affecting the face and often associated with flushing and erythema.

SYNONYMS

Acne rosacea

ICD-9CM CODES
695.3 Rosacea

EPIDEMIOLOGY & DEMOGRAPHICS

- Rosacea occurs in 1 in 20 Americans
- Onset often between age 30 and 50 yr
- More common in people of Celtic origin; however, this disease may be overlooked in nonwhites because skin pigmentation results in atypical presentation
- Female:male ratio of 3:1

PHYSICAL FINDINGS & CLINICAL PRESENTATION

- Facial erythema, presence of papules, pustules, and telangiectasia.
- Excessive facial warmth and redness is the predominant presenting complaint.
- Itching is generally absent.
- Comedones are absent (unlike acne).
- Women are more likely to show symptoms on the chin and cheeks, whereas in men the nose is commonly involved.
- Ocular findings (mild dryness and irritation with blepharitis, conjunctival injection, burning, stinging, tearing, eyelid inflammation, swelling, and redness) are present in 50% of patients.

CLASSIFICATION:

Rosacea can be classified in 4 major subtypes:

1. Erythematotelengiectatic: erythema in central part of face, telengiectasia, flushing
2. Papulopustular: presence of dome-shaped erythematous papules and small postules, in addition to facial erythema, flushing, and telengiectasia
3. Phymatous: presence of thickened skin with prominent pores that may affect the nose (rhinophyma), chin (gnathophyma), forehead (metophyma), eyelids (blepharophyma), and ears (otophyma)
4. Ocular: conjunctival injection, sensation of foreign body in the eye, telengiectasia and erythema of lid margins, scaling.

ETIOLOGY

- Unknown.
- Hot drinks, alcohol, and sun exposure may accentuate the erythema by causing vasodilation of the skin.
- Flare-ups may also result from reactions to medications (e.g., simvastatin, ACE inhibitors, vasodilators, fluorinated corticosteroids), stress, extreme heat or cold, spicy drinks, menstruation.

DIAGNOSIS

DIFFERENTIAL DIAGNOSIS

- Drug eruption
- Acne vulgaris
- Contact dermatitis
- SLE
- Carcinoid flush
- Idiopathic facial flushing
- Seborrheic dermatitis
- Facial sarcoidosis
- Photodermatitis
- Mastocytosis

WORKUP

Diagnosis is based on clinical findings. Distinguishing features between acne and rosacea are the presence of telengiectasia and deep diffuse erythema and absence of comedones in rosacea.

TREATMENT

NONPHARMACOLOGIC THERAPY

- Avoid alcohol, excessive sun exposure, and hot drinks of any type.
- Use of mild, nondrying soap is recommended; local skin irritants should be avoided.
- Reassure patient that rosacea is completely unrelated to poor hygiene.

GENERAL Rx

- Several classes of drugs are used in treatment of rosacea, including the metronidazole family, the tetracycline family, and azelic acid.
- Topical therapy with metronidazole aqueous gel (MetroGel) applied bid is effective as initial therapy for mild cases or following the use of oral antibiotics. A new 1% formulation of metronidazole (Noritate) applied qd may improve patient compliance. Azelaic cream (20% or gel 15%), clindamycin lotion (Cleocin), sulfacetamide, or erythromycin 2% solution may also be effective.
- Systemic antibiotics: tetracycline 250 mg qid until symptoms diminish, then taper off; doxycycline 100 mg bid is also effective.
- Minocycline 50 to 100 mg qd should be used only in resistant cases, because this medication is expensive.
- Oral metronidazole (200 mg qd-bid) for 4 to 6 wk is also effective.
- Isotretinoin (Accutane) 0.5 to 1 mg/kg/day in two divided doses for 15 to 20 wk can be used for refractory papular and pustular rosacea; use of retinoids may, however, worsen erythema and telangiectasis.
- Laser treatment is an option for progressive telangiectasias or rhinophyma.
- Erythema and flushing may respond to low dose clonidine (0.05 mg bid).
- Another topical treatment modality for pustular and papular forms of rosacea is the use of azelaic acid (Finacea, Azelex). Azelex is available in a 20% cream base, Finacea as a 15% gel. Azelaic acid is as least as effective as topical metronidazole but may be more irritating.

DISPOSITION

- Rosacea is often resistant to initial treatment and recurrent. Periods of remission and relapse are common.
- The progression of rosacea is variable. Typical stages include:
  1. Facial flushing
  2. Erythema and/or edema and ocular symptoms
  3. Papules and pustules
  4. Rhinophyma

PEARLS & CONSIDERATIONS

COMMENTS

- The course of the disease is typically chronic, with remissions and relapses.
- Patients with resistant cases may have *Demodex folliculorum* mite infestation or tinea infection (diagnosis can be confirmed with potassium hydroxide examination); the role of *D. folliculorum* in rosacea is unclear. These mites can sometimes be found in large numbers in the lesions; however, their numbers do not generally decline with treatment.
- Rosacea can result in emotional and social stigmas, especially because many people associate rosacea and rhinophyma with alcohol abuse.
- Early consultation with an ophthalmologist is recommended in patients with suspected ocular involvement.

SUGGESTED READING

Powell FC: Rosacea, *N Engl J Med* 352:793, 2005.

AUTHOR: **FRED F. FERRI, M.D.**

BASIC INFORMATION

DEFINITION

Roseola is a benign viral illness found in infants and characterized by high fevers, followed by a rash.

SYNONYMS

Exanthem subitum
Sixth disease
Roseola infantum

ICD-9CM CODES
057.8 Roseola

EPIDEMIOLOGY & DEMOGRAPHICS

- Nearly one third of all infants develop roseola before the age of 2 yr.
- More than 90% of children older than 2 yr of age are seropositive for the virus causing roseola.
- Roseola is spread from person to person. It is not known how it is spread, but it must be very efficiently spread and presumably via the respiratory tract.
- There is no predilection for gender or time of year.

PHYSICAL FINDINGS & CLINICAL PRESENTATION

- Typically the child develops a high fever, usually up to 104° F (40° C) that lasts for 3 to 5 days
- Fever may be associated with a runny nose, irritability, and fatigue
- A rash appears within 48 hr of defervescence, mainly on the face, neck, trunk, arms, and legs
- The rash is a faint pink maculopapular rash that blanches when palpated
- The rash usually fades away within 48 hr
- Anorexia
- Seizures
- Cervical adenopathy

ETIOLOGY

- Roseola is caused by human herpesvirus-6 (HHV-6).
- The incubation period is between 5 and 15 days.

DIAGNOSIS

The diagnosis of roseola is usually made by the clinical presentation as stated previously.

DIFFERENTIAL DIAGNOSIS

- Measles
- Rubella
- Fifth disease
- Drug eruption
- Mononucleosis
- All causes of fever (e.g., otitis media, pneumonia, and urinary tract infection)
- Meningitis

WORKUP

- If unsure of the diagnosis of roseola in a febrile infant, a fever workup is done to rule out other infectious causes.
- The decision to proceed with a fever workup is a clinical judgment call.

LABORATORY TESTS

- CBC with differential, erythrocyte sedimentation rate (ESR), blood cultures as indicated
- Urinalysis and urine cultures
- Stool cultures if diarrhea is present
- Lumbar puncture if needed to rule out meningitis
- Commercial assays can be used to detect HHV-6–specific immunoglobulin G (IgG) antibody responses but IgM assays are not always reliable for acute infection

IMAGING STUDIES

Chest x-ray to rule out pneumonia

TREATMENT

NONPHARMACOLOGIC THERAPY

- Supportive care
- Maintain hydration by drinking clear fluids: water, fruit juice, lemonade, and so forth
- Sponge bathe with lukewarm water if febrile

ACUTE GENERAL Rx

- Acetaminophen 10-15 mg/kg per dose at 4-hr intervals for fever
- Ibuprofen 5-10 mg/kg per dose at 6-hr intervals (maximal dose 600 mg)

CHRONIC Rx

Roseola is a viral disease that is short lasting; chronic treatment is usually not an issue.

DISPOSITION

- Roseola is generally a benign, self-limited disease that usually lasts approximately 1 wk.
- Complications, although rare, can occur and include:
  1. Febrile seizures
  2. Meningitis
  3. Encephalitis
  4. Pneumonitis
  5. Hepatitis

REFERRAL

Subspecialty consultation is made with the appropriate discipline if any of the above mentioned complications occur (e.g., neurology for seizures).

PEARLS & CONSIDERATIONS

COMMENTS

- A child with fever and rash should be excluded from daycare.
- Human herpesvirus 6 is named accordingly because it is the sixth herpesvirus discovered after herpes simplex 1 (HSV-1), HSV-2, cytomegalovirus (CMV), Epstein-Barr virus (EBV), and varicella-zoster virus (VZV).
- Roseola is called sixth disease because it represents the sixth childhood "exanthem"; the other five are measles, scarlet fever, rubella, Dukes disease, and erythema infectiosum.

SUGGESTED READINGS

Caserta MT, Mock DJ, Dewhurst S: Human herpesvirus 6, *Clin Infect Dis* 33(6):829, 2001.
Ward KN: The natural history and laboratory diagnosis of human herpesviruses-6 and -7 infections in the immunocompetent, *J Clin Virol* 32(3):183, 2005.
Zerr DM et al: A population-based study of primary human herpesvirus 6 infection, *N Engl J Med* 352(8):768, 2005.

AUTHORS: **GLENN G. FORT, M.D., M.P.H.,** and **DENNIS J. MIKOLICH, M.D.**

BASIC INFORMATION

DEFINITION

Rotator cuff syndrome refers to a spectrum of afflictions involving the tendons of the rotator cuff (primarily the supraspinatus), ranging from simple strains and tendinitis to complete, massive rupture with cuff-tear arthropathy.

SYNONYMS

Impingement syndrome
Painful arc syndrome
Internal derangement of the subacromial joint
Supraspinatus syndrome
Bursitis of shoulder

ICD-9CM CODES
726.10 Rotator cuff syndrome
727.61 Rotator cuff rupture

EPIDEMIOLOGY & DEMOGRAPHICS

PREVALENCE: 5% to 10% of the general population
PREDOMINANT SEX: More common in males than females
PREDOMINANT AGE: Uncommon under 20 yr of age

PHYSICAL FINDINGS & CLINICAL PRESENTATION

- Pain, often at night
- Rotator cuff tenderness
- Referred pain down deltoid, especially with abduction between 70 and 120 degrees ("the painful arc") (Fig. 1-236)
- Weakness in abduction or forward flexion
- Increased pain with overhead activities
- Atrophy in long-standing cases of complete tear
- Positive "drop-arm" test (weakness of abduction against downward pressure at 90 degrees)

ETIOLOGY

- Microtrauma from repetitive use
- Abnormally shaped acromion
- Shoulder instability
- Worsening of process by the overhead throwing motion
- Microcirculatory changes at the musculotendinous junction

DIAGNOSIS

DIFFERENTIAL DIAGNOSIS

- Shoulder instability
- Degenerative arthritis
- Cervical radiculopathy
- Avascular necrosis
- Suprascapular nerve entrapment

WORKUP

- In chronic tendinitis, clinical findings similar to those seen in partial rupture
- Even with complete rupture, may have full, active range of motion in shoulder

IMAGING STUDIES

- Plain radiography
- Ultrasonography may be useful but only in diagnosing moderately large tears
- MRI to evaluate full- or partial-thickness tears, chronic tendinitis, and other causes of shoulder pain
- Since MRI, arthrography is rarely used

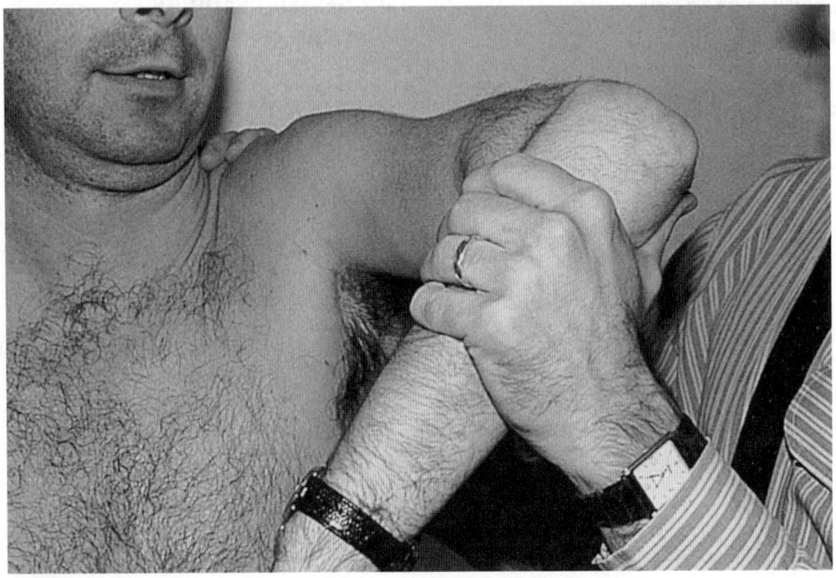

FIGURE 1-236 Rotator cuff lesions are often accompanied by painful impingement of the upwardly subluxating humerus onto the acromion. Evidence for this as a cause of pain is elicited by impingement tests, for example, by forced, passive, internal rotation, and abduction of the shoulder, as shown here. (From Klippel J, Dieppe P, Ferri F [eds]: *Primary care rheumatology,* London, 1999, Mosby.)

TREATMENT

ACUTE GENERAL Rx

- Rest to avoid overhead activity
- Ice or heat for comfort
- Carefully supervised program of stretching and strengthening
- Medication: NSAIDs, subacromial corticosteroid injection (once or twice at 2-wk intervals)

DISPOSITION

- All forms are likely to respond to nonsurgical management.
- Even many complete rotator cuff tears have minimal pain and little loss of function.

REFERRAL

For orthopedic consultation in cases that fail to respond to medical management or in which rotator cuff tear is suspected

PEARLS & CONSIDERATIONS

COMMENTS

- There is considerable disagreement regarding the likelihood of recovery once a significant rotator cuff rupture has developed.
- Indications for surgery vary among surgeons.
- Injection is contraindicated in the presence of local infection.
- As with other similar musculoskeletal disorders, the underlying pathology involved may be more degenerative (tendinopathy, tendinosis) than inflammatory.
- Once a separation ("tear") develops, there is no way to predict whether it will ever become worse or not.

SUGGESTED READINGS

Cohen BL: Treatment of shoulder complaints, *Lancet* 363:492, 2004.
Ebell MH: Diagnosing rotator cuff tears, *Am Fam Phys* 71:1587, 2005.
Koester MC et al: The efficacy of subacromial corticosteroid injection in the treatment of rotator cuff disease: a systematic review, *J Am Acad Orthop Surg* 15:3, 2007.
Mcfarland EG et al: Clinical evaluation of impingement: what to do and what works, *J Bone Joint Surg* 88A:432, 2006.
Tashjian RZ et al: Effect of medical comorbidity on self-assessed pain, function, and general health status after rotator cuff repair, *J Bone Joint Surg* 88A:536, 2006.
Teefey SA et al: Detection and quantification of rotator cuff tears, *J Bone Joint Surg* 86A:708, 2004.
Wolff AB et al: Partial-thickness rotator cuff tears, *J Am Acad Orthop Surg* 14:715, 2006.
Zing PO et al: Clinical and structural outcomes of nonoperative management of massive rotator cuff tears, *J Bone Joint Surg* 89A:1928, 2008.

AUTHOR: **LONNIE R. MERCIER, M.D.**

BASIC INFORMATION

DEFINITION

Rubella is a mild illness caused by the rubella virus that can cause severe congenital problems via in vitro transmission to the fetus when a pregnant woman becomes infected.

SYNONYMS

German measles

ICD-9CM CODES
056.9 Rubella
771.0 (Congenital)
V04.3 (Vaccination)

EPIDEMIOLOGY & DEMOGRAPHICS

- Before vaccination (i.e., before 1969): 28 reported cases per 100,000 person-years, 8 of which were in persons over age 15 yr

  Four cases of congenital rubella syndrome per 100,000 live births
- After mass vaccination (i.e., after 1980) most cases have occurred in unimmunized people, with fewer than 1 case/100,000 person-years (acquired and congenital).
- Currently, 10% to 20% of childbearing-age women are susceptible.
- The highest risk of developing long-term complications of congenital infection exists during the first trimester of gestation; both risk of congenital infection and long-term complications drop during the second trimester, and although the risk of congenital infection increases during the third trimester, there is no risk of long-term complication at that point.

PHYSICAL FINDINGS & CLINICAL PRESENTATION

Acquired infection
- Incubation: 14 to 21 days
- Prodrome: 1 to 5 days; low-grade fever, headache, malaise, anorexia, mild conjunctivitis, coryza, pharyngitis, cough, and cervical, suboccipital, and postauricular lymphadenopathy
- Rash: 1 to 5 days

Enanthema: palatal macules

Exanthema (rash): blotchy eruption beginning on face and neck and then spreading to trunk and limbs
- Occasional splenomegaly and hepatitis (during rash)
- Complications: arthritis (15%, mostly in adult women), thrombocytopenia, myocarditis, optic neuritis, encephalitis (all less than 0.1%)

Congenital infection
- Deafness: 85%
- Intrauterine growth retardation: 70%
- Cataracts: 35%
- Retinopathy: 35%
- Patent ductus arteriosus: 30%
- Pulmonary artery hypoplasia: 25%
- In utero death: 20%
- Mental retardation: 10% to 20%
- Meningoencephalitis: 10% to 20%
- Behavior disorder: 10% to 20%
- Hepatosplenomegaly: 10% to 20%
- Bone radiolucencies: 10% to 20%
- Diabetes mellitus (type 1): 10% to 20% by age 35 yr
- Other congenital heart defects: 2% to 5%

ETIOLOGY & PATHOGENESIS

Acquired infection
- Viral portal of entry is upper respiratory tract.
- Viral replication occurs in lymph nodes, then hematogenous dissemination occurs to many organs, including placenta if present.
- Immune complexes may be cause of rash and arthritis.

Congenital infection
- Fetus is infected via placenta during maternal acquired infection.
- Cellular damage in the fetus results from cytolysis of fetal cells, mostly via a fetal vasculitis or from an immune-mediated inflammation and damage.

DIAGNOSIS

DIFFERENTIAL DIAGNOSIS

Acquired rubella syndrome
- Other viral infections by enteroviruses, adenoviruses, human parvovirus B-19, measles
- Scarlet fever
- Allergic reaction
- Kawasaki disease

Congenital rubella syndrome
- Congenital syphilis, toxoplasmosis, herpes simplex, cytomegalovirus, and enterovirus can cause a similar set of problems.

WORKUP

Acquired infection
- Serologic test (hemagglutination inhibition, neutralization tests, complement fixation tests, passive agglutination, enzyme immunoassay [EIA], enzyme-linked immunosorbent assay [ELISA])
- IgM antibodies (by EIA) are detected early: second to fourth week
- IgG antibodies (by ELISA) can be measured as acute phase (7 days after rash onset) and convalescent phase (14 days later)

Congenital infection
- Viral culture (from nasopharynx)
- Serologic studies: IgM antirubella virus detection by EIA is the method of choice (after the newborn is 5 mo old)

IMMUNIZATION

Four existing vaccines provide persisting immunity in 92% of vaccinees. Indications:
- All children 12 mo or older (as part of the measles-mumps-rubella vaccine)
- Postpubertal women

Vaccinate if not known to be immunized (advise not to become pregnant within 3 mo of vaccination)

Premarital serologic screening for rubella immunity

Prenatal or antepartum serologic screening for rubella

Vaccinate susceptible women postpartum

Serologic screening for female workers likely to be exposed to rubella (e.g., teachers, child care employees, health care workers)

Contraindications
- Pregnancy
- Recent receipt of immune globulin or blood transfusion (2 wk before to 3 mo after)
- Immunodeficiency (except AIDS)

Adverse reaction
- Fever, rash, or lymphadenopathy: 5% to 15%
- Arthralgias: 0.5% in children; 25% in adult women
- Transient peripheral neuropathy (rare)

TREATMENT

- No known effective antiviral therapy
- Management of specific congenital problems as appropriate

SUGGESTED READINGS

Madsen KM et al: A population-based study of measles, mumps, and rubella vaccination and autism, *New Eng J Med* 347(19)1477, 2002.

U.S. Department of Health: Control and prevention of rubella: evaluation and management of suspected outbreaks, rubella in pregnant women, and surveillance for congenital rubella syndrome, *MMWR* 50(RR-12):1, 2001.

AUTHORS: **FRED F. FERRI, M.D.,** and **TOM J. WACHTEL, M.D.**

BASIC INFORMATION

DEFINITION

Salivary gland neoplasms are benign or malignant tumors of a salivary gland (parotid, submandibular, or sublingual).

SYNONYMS

These tumors are often named according to their histologic type (see "Diagnosis").

ICD-9CM CODES
142.9 Salivary gland neoplasm
142.0 (Parotid)
142.1 (Submandibular)
142.2 (Sublingual)

EPIDEMIOLOGY & DEMOGRAPHICS

INCIDENCE: 1 to 2 cases/100,000 person-years (1% of all head and neck tumors)

DISTRIBUTION:
- Parotid gland 85% (80% are benign)
- Submandibular gland 10% (55% are benign)
- Sublingual and minor glands 5% (35% are benign)

PHYSICAL FINDINGS & CLINICAL PRESENTATION

- Parotid gland:
  1. Painless swelling overlying the masseter muscle (under the temporomandibular joint)
  2. Pain
  3. Facial nerve palsy
  4. Cervical lymph nodes
  5. Mass in oral cavity
- Submandibular gland: swelling under anterior portion of the mandible
- Sublingual gland: intraoral swelling under the tongue, medial to the mandible

DIAGNOSIS

PATHOLOGY

History

BENIGN TUMORS:
- Mixed tumor (usually parotid)
- Adenolymphoma (Warthin's tumor)
- Pleomorphic adenoma
- Capillary hemangioma, lymphangioma (in children)
- Intraductal papilloma
- Other (e.g., myoepithelioma, canalicular adenoma, basal cell adenoma)

MALIGNANT TUMORS:
- Mucoepidermoid carcinoma (most common malignant tumor of the parotid gland)
- Adenoid cystic carcinoma
- Adenocarcinoma
- Malignant mixed tumor
- Squamous cell carcinoma
- Other

Stage (TNM)

T_0 No evidence of primary tumor
T_1 Tumor <2 cm
T_2 Tumor 2 to 4 cm
T_3 Tumor 4 to 6 cm
T_4 Tumor >6 cm

All subdivided into
- Without local extension
- With local extension

N_0 No lymph node metastasis
N_1 Single ipsilateral node <3 cm
N_2 Ipsilateral, contralateral, or bilateral node <6 cm
N_3 Any node >6 cm
M_0 No distant metastasis
M_1 Distant metastasis

Stage I T_{1a} or ${}_{2a}N_0M_0$
Stage II $T_{1b,2b,3a}$ N_0M_0
Stage III $T_{3b,4a}$ N_0M_0 or any T except ${}_{4b}N_1M_0$
Stage IV T_{4b} any N any M or any T $N_{2,3}M_0$ or any T, any N_1M_1

WORKUP

- Fine-needle aspiration. The sensitivity, specificity, and accuracy of parotid gland aspirates is approximately 92%, 100%, and 98%, respectively
- Imaging by CT scan or MRI
- Open biopsy (rarely indicated)

TREATMENT

Malignant tumors:
- Surgery is the mainstay of treatment; gland resection and neck dissection if lymph nodes are involved.
- A lateral lobectomy with preservation of facial nerve should be considered for tumors confined to the superficial lobe of the parotid gland. Gross tumor should not be left in situ, but if the facial nerve is able to be preserved by "peeling" tumor off the nerve, it should be attempted, followed by radiation therapy for microscopic disease.
- Postoperative radiation is indicated for high-grade malignancies demonstrating extraglandular disease, perineural invasion, direct invasion of surrounding tissues, or regional metastases.
- Chemotherapy.

Benign tumors: surgery for tumor resection

PROGNOSIS OF MALIGNANT TUMORS

Five-year survival rates:
- Mucoepidermoid carcinoma: 75% to 95%
- Adenoid cystic carcinoma: 40% to 80%
- Adenocarcinoma: 20% to 75%
- Malignant mixed tumor: 35% to 75%
- Squamous cell carcinoma: 25% to 60%

PEARLS & CONSIDERATIONS

COMMENTS

Salivary gland neoplasms most often present as slow-growing, well-circumscribed masses. Pain, rapid growth, nerve weakness, fixation to skin or underlying muscle, and paresthesias usually are indicative of malignancy.

SUGGESTED READING

Stewart CJ et al: Fine needle aspiration cytology of salivary gland: a review of 341 cases, *Diagn Cytopathol* 22:139, 2000.

AUTHORS: **FRED F. FERRI, M.D.,** and **TOM J. WACHTEL, M.D.**

BASIC INFORMATION

DEFINITION

Salmonellosis is an infection caused by one of several serotypes of *Salmonella.*

SYNONYMS

Typhoid fever
Paratyphoid fever
Enteric fever

ICD-9CM CODES
003.0 Salmonellosis

EPIDEMIOLOGY & DEMOGRAPHICS

INCIDENCE (IN U.S.):

- Estimated 1 million cases/yr of nontyphoidal salmonellosis
- Approximately 500 cases of *Salmonella typhi* infection reported each year
- Largest outbreak: 200,000 persons who ingested contaminated milk

PEAK INCIDENCE: Summer and fall

PREDOMINANT AGE:

- <20 yr old
- >70 yr old
- Highest rates of infection in infants, especially neonates

GENETICS:

Neonatal Infection: Highly susceptible to infection with nontyphoidal Salmonella

PHYSICAL FINDINGS & CLINICAL PRESENTATION

- Infections
  1. Localized to GI tract (gastroenteritis)
  2. Systemic (typhoid fever)
  3. Localized outside of GI tract
- Gastroenteritis
  1. Incubation period: 12 to 48 hr
  2. Nausea, vomiting
  3. Diarrhea, abdominal cramps
  4. Fever
  5. Bacteremia: Occurs mostly in the immunocompromised host or those with underlying conditions, including HIV infection
  6. Self-limited illness lasting 3 or 4 days
  7. Colonization of GI tract persistent for months, especially in those treated with antibiotics
- Typhoid fever
  1. Incubation period of few days to several weeks
  2. Prolonged fever, often with a stepwise-increasing temperature pattern
  3. Myalgias
  4. Headache, cough, sore throat
  5. Malaise, anorexia
  6. Abdominal pain
  7. Hepatosplenomegaly
  8. Diarrhea or constipation early in the course of illness
  9. Rose spots (faint, maculopapular, blanching lesions) sometimes seen on chest or abdomen
- Untreated disease
  1. Fever lasting 1 to 2 mo
  2. Main complication: GI bleeding caused by perforation from ulceration of Peyer's patches in the ileum (Fig. 1-237)
  3. Rare complications:
     a. Mental status changes
     b. Shock
  4. Relapse rate of approximately 10%
- Infections outside GI tract
  1. Can occur in virtually any location
  2. Usually occur in patients with underlying diseases
  3. Endocarditis, endovascular infections are caused by seeding of atherosclerotic plaques or aneurysms
  4. Hepatic or splenic abscesses in patients with underlying disease in these organs
  5. Urinary tract infections in patients with renal TB or schistosomiasis
  6. Salmonellae are a frequent cause of gram-negative meningitis in neonates
  7. Osteomyelitis in children with hemoglobinopathies (particularly sickle cell disease)

ETIOLOGY

- More than 2000 serotypes of *Salmonella* exist, but only a few cause disease in humans.
- Some found only in humans are the cause of enteric fever.
  1. *S. typhi*
  2. *S. paratyphi*
- Some responsible for gastroenteritis and frequently isolated from raw meat and poultry and uncooked or undercooked eggs.
  1. *S. typhimurium*
  2. *S. enteritidis*
- *S. cholerae-suis* is a prototype organism that causes extraintestinal nontyphoidal disease.
- Transmission generally via ingestion of contaminated food or drink.
- Outbreaks of gastroenteritis related to contaminated poultry, meat, and dairy products.
- Typhoid fever is a systemic illness caused by serotypes exclusive to humans.
  1. Acquisition by ingestion of food or water contaminated by other humans

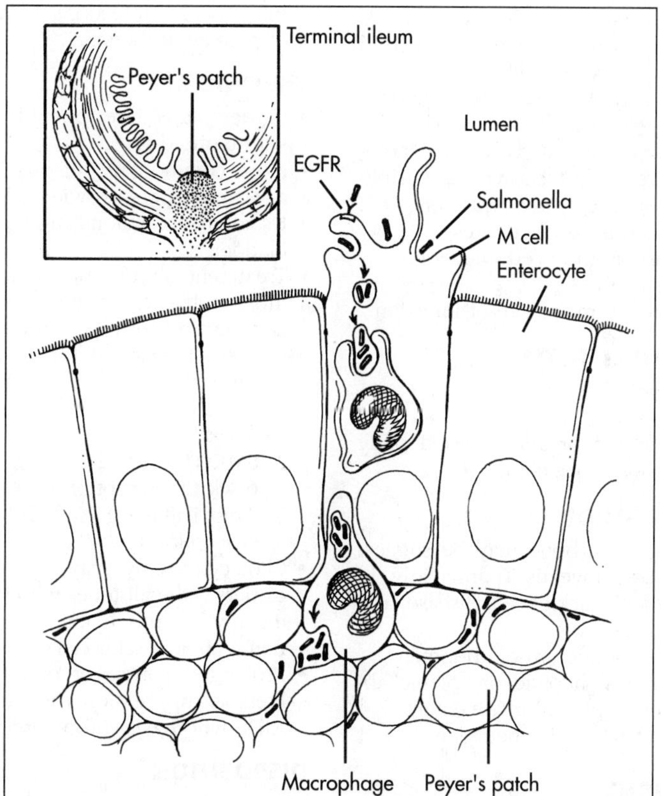

FIGURE 1-237 *Salmonella typhi* invade M cells through membrane ruffling and EGF receptor-dependent pathways. Macrophages originating from Peyer's patch take up *S. typhi* in close association with M cells. *S. typhi* replicate in Peyer's patches and then enter the lymphatic system, leading to bacteremia. Replication in Peyer's patches causes hypertrophy followed by necrosis, which can cause intestinal perforation. (From Stein JH [ed]: *Internal medicine,* ed 5, St Louis, 1998, Mosby.)

2. Most cases in the U.S. are:
   a. Acquired during foreign travel
   b. Acquired by ingestion of food prepared by chronic carriers, many of whom have acquired the organism outside of the U.S.

DIAGNOSIS (Dx)

DIFFERENTIAL DIAGNOSIS

- Other causes of prolonged fever:
  1. Malaria
  2. TB
  3. Brucellosis
  4. Amebic liver abscess
- Other causes of gastroenteritis:
  1. Bacterial: *Shigella, Yersinia, Campylobacter spp.*
  2. Viral: Norwalk virus, rotavirus
  3. Parasitic: *Entamoeba histolytica, Giardia lamblia*
  4. Toxic: enterotoxigenic *E. coli, Clostridium difficile*

WORKUP

- Typhoid fever
  1. Cultures of blood, stool, urine; repeat if initially negative.
  2. Blood cultures are more likely to be positive early in the course of illness.
  3. Stool and urine cultures are more commonly positive in the second and third week of illness.
  4. Highest yield with bone marrow biopsy cultures: 90% positive
  5. Serology using Widal's test is helpful in retrospect, showing a fourfold increase in convalescent titers.
- Gastroenteritis: stool cultures
- Extraintestinal localized infection:
  1. Blood cultures
  2. Cultures from the site of infection

LABORATORY TESTS

- Neutropenia is common
- Transaminitis is possible
- Culture to grow organism: blood, body fluids, biopsy specimens

IMAGING STUDIES

- Radiographs of bone may be suggestive of osteomyelitis (particularly in patients with sickle cell disease and bone infarctions).
- CT scan or sonogram of abdomen:
  1. May reveal hepatic or splenic abscesses or pleural involvement
  2. May reveal aortic aneurysm

TREATMENT (Rx)

NONPHARMACOLOGIC THERAPY

Adequate hydration and electrolyte replacement in persons with diarrhea

ACUTE GENERAL Rx

- Typhoid fever:
  1. Ciprofloxacin 500 mg PO bid or 400 mg IV bid for 14 days
  2. Ceftriaxone 2 g IV qd for 14 days
  3. If sensitive, may switch therapy to TMP/SMX 1 to 2 DS tabs PO bid or amoxicillin 2 g PO q8h to complete 14 days
  4. Dexamethasone 3 mg IV initially, followed by 1 mg IV q6h for eight doses for patients with shock or mental status changes
- Gastroenteritis:
  1. Usually not indicated for gastroenteritis alone because this illness usually self-limited
  2. May prolong the carrier state
  3. Prophylactic treatment for patients who are at high risk of developing complications from bacteremia
     a. Neonates
     b. Patients with hemoglobinopathies
     c. Patients with atherosclerosis
     d. Patients with aneurysms
     e. Patients with prosthetic devices
     f. Immunocompromised patients
  4. Treatment can be oral or parenteral, with the same regimens used for typhoid, but only for 48 to 72 hr
- Intravascular infections require 6 wk of parenteral therapy.

CHRONIC Rx

- Carrier states are possible in those with typhoid fever.
- More common in persons >60 yr of age and in persons with gallstones.
- Usual site of colonization is the gallbladder.
- Treatment should be considered for those with persistently positive stool cultures and for food handlers.
- Suggested regimens for eradication of carrier state:
  1. Ciprofloxacin 500 mg PO bid for 4 wk
  2. SMX/TMP 1 to 2 DS tabs PO bid for 6 wk (if susceptible)
  3. Amoxicillin 2 g PO q8h for 6 wk (if susceptible)
- Cholecystectomy may be required in carriers with gallstones who fail medical therapy but this is rarely indicated for non-typhoidal salmonellosis currently.
- Prolonged course of oral therapy or lifetime suppression for patients with AIDS who have chronic infection

DISPOSITION

- Typhoid fever
  1. Treated patients usually respond to therapy; small percentage of chronic carriers.
  2. Untreated patients may have serious complications.
- Gastroenteritis
  1. Usually self-limited
  2. May be recurrent or persistent in AIDS patients

REFERRAL

- If gastroenteritis is persistent or recurrent
- If there is evidence of extraintestinal infection, typhoid fever, or chronic carriers

PEARLS & CONSIDERATIONS (!)

COMMENTS

- Quinolones should not be used in children or pregnant women.
- Infections should be reported to local health departments.
- Recent outbreaks in the U.S. have been traced back to raw tomatoes, peanut butter, and frozen pot pies.

EVIDENCE (EBM)

Antibiotic therapy has not been shown to have any positive clinical effect in healthy children and adults with mild diarrhea caused by *Salmonella* spp.[1] Ⓐ

Oral rehydration fluids are as effective as intravenous rehydration fluids in children with mild or moderate dehydration caused by gastroenteritis.[2,3] Ⓐ

Oral rehydration fluid has been shown to be associated with significant reductions in the duration of diarrhea and with increased weight gain at discharge compared with intravenous rehydration fluid, in a randomized controlled trial conducted in a developing country.[4] Ⓐ

Evidence-Based References

1. Sirinavin S, Garner P: Antibiotics for treating salmonella gut infections, *Cochrane Database Syst Rev* 1, 1999. Ⓐ
2. Gavin N, Merrick N, Davidson B: Efficacy of glucose-based oral rehydration therapy, *Pediatrics* 98:45, 1996. Reviewed in: *Clin Evid* 10:86, 2003. Ⓐ
3. Singh M et al: Controlled trial of oral versus intravenous rehydration in the management of acute gastroenteritis, *Indian J Med Res* 75:691, 1982. Reviewed in: *Clin Evid* 9:367, 2003. Ⓐ
4. Sharifi J et al: Oral versus intravenous rehydration therapy in severe gastroenteritis, *Arch Dis Child* 60:856, 1985. Reviewed in: *Clin Evid* 9:367, 2003. Ⓐ

SUGGESTED READINGS

CDC: Salmonellosis associated with pet turtles—Wisconsin and Wyoming, 2004, *MMWR Morb Mortal Wkly Rep* 54(9):223, 2005.

Delaloye J et al: Nosocomial nontyphoidal salmonellosis after antineoplastic chemotherapy reactivation of asymptomatic colonization? *Eur J Clin Microbiol Infect Dis* 23(10):751, 2004.

Wells EV et al: Reptile-associated salmonellosis in pre-school aged children in Michigan, January 2001-June 2003, *Clin Infect Dis* 39(5):687, 2004.

AUTHORS: **GLENN G. FORT, M.D., M.P.H.,** and **MAURICE POLICAR, M.D.**

BASIC INFORMATION

DEFINITION

Sarcoidosis is a chronic systemic granulomatous disease characterized histologically by the presence of nonspecific, noncaseating granulomas.

SYNONYMS

Boeck's sarcoid

ICD-9CM CODES
135.0 Sarcoidosis

EPIDEMIOLOGY & DEMOGRAPHICS

INCIDENCE (IN U.S.)
10.9/100,000 whites, 35.5/100,000 blacks
- Presents most commonly in the winter and early spring

PREDOMINANT SEX:
Increased incidence in females

PREDOMINANT AGE:
20 to 40 yr old

PHYSICAL FINDINGS & CLINICAL PRESENTATION

- Clinical manifestations often vary with the stage of the disease and degree of organ involvement; patients may be asymptomatic, but a chest x-ray may demonstrate findings consistent with sarcoidosis (see "Imaging Studies"). Nearly 50% of patients with sarcoidosis are diagnosed by incidental findings on chest x-ray.
- Frequent manifestations:
  1. Pulmonary manifestations: dry, nonproductive cough, dyspnea, chest discomfort
  2. Constitutional symptoms: fatigue, weight loss, anorexia, malaise
  3. Visual disturbances: blurred vision, ocular discomfort, conjunctivitis, iritis, uveitis
  4. Dermatologic manifestations: erythema nodosum, macules, papules, subcutaneous nodules, hyperpigmentation, lupus pernio
  5. Myocardial disturbances: arrhythmias, cardiomyopathy
  6. Splenomegaly, hepatomegaly
  7. Rheumatologic manifestations: arthralgias have been reported in up to 40% of patients
  8. Neurologic and other manifestations: cranial nerve palsies, diabetes insipidus, meningeal involvement, parotid enlargement, hypothalamic and pituitary lesions, peripheral adenopathy

ETIOLOGY

Unknown. Multiple lines of evidence suggest that sarcoidosis may result from the interaction of multiple genes with environmental exposures or infection.

DIAGNOSIS

DIFFERENTIAL DIAGNOSIS

- TB
- Lymphoma
- Hodgkin's disease
- Metastases
- Pneumoconioses
- Enlarged pulmonary arteries
- Infectious mononucleosis
- Lymphangitic carcinomatosis
- Idiopathic hemosiderosis
- Alveolar cell carcinoma
- Pulmonary eosinophilia
- Hypersensitivity pneumonitis
- Fibrosing alveolitis
- Collagen disorders
- Parasitic infection

Section II describes the differential diagnosis of granulomatous lung disease and a classification of granulomatous disorders.

WORKUP

- Workup is aimed at excluding critical organ involvement, determining extent and severity of disease, and excluding other disease. A complete neurologic and ophthalmologic exam is mandatory. A complete occupational and environmental exposure history is recommended.
- Initial lab evaluation should include CBC, serum chemistries (ALT, AST, lytes, BUN, creatinine, serum calcium), urinalysis, and tuberculin test.
- Chest x-ray and ECG should also be obtained in all patients with sarcoidosis.
- Pulmonary function testing; spirometry, diffusion capacity of carbon monoxide-single breath.
- Biopsy should be done on accessible tissues suspected of sarcoid involvement (conjunctiva, skin, lymph nodes); bronchoscopy with transbronchial biopsy is the procedure of choice in patients without any readily accessible site.

LABORATORY TESTS

Laboratory abnormalities:
- Hypergammaglobulinemia, anemia, leukopenia
- LFT abnormalities
- Hypercalcemia, hypercalciuria (secondary to increased GI absorption, abnormal vitamin D metabolism, and increased calcitriol production by sarcoid granuloma)
- Cutaneous anergy to *Trichophyton, Candida,* mumps, and tuberculin
- Angiotensin-converting enzyme (ACE): elevated in approximately 60% of patients with sarcoidosis; nonspecific and generally not useful in following the course of the disease

IMAGING STUDIES

- Chest x-ray (Fig. 1-238): adenopathy of the hilar and paratracheal nodes is a frequent finding; parenchymal changes may also be present, depending on the stage of the disease (stage 0, normal x-ray; stage I, bilateral hilar adenopathy; stage II, stage I plus pulmonary infiltrate; stage III, pulmonary infiltrate without adenopathy); stage IV, advanced fibrosis with evidence of honey-combing, hilar retraction, bullae, cysts, and emphysema.
- PFTs (spirometry and diffusing capacity of the lung for carbon dioxide): may be normal or may reveal a restrictive pattern and/or obstructive pattern.
- Gallium-67 scan: will localize in areas of granulomatous infiltrates; however, it is not specific. The "panda" sign (localization in the lacrimal and salivary glands, giving a "panda" appearance to the face) is suggestive of sarcoidosis.

TREATMENT

GENERAL Rx

- Corticosteroids (Table 1-43) remain the mainstay of therapy when treatment is required (e.g., prednisone 40 mg qd for 8 to 12 wk with gradual tapering of the dose to 10 mg qod over 8 to 12 mo); corticosteroids should be considered in patients with severe symptoms (e.g., dyspnea, chest pain), hypercalcemia, ocular, CNS, or cardiac involvement, and progressive pulmonary disease. Patients with interstitial lung disease benefit from oral steroid therapy for 6 to 24 mo.
- Patients with progressive disease refractory to corticosteroids may be treated with methotrexate 7.5 to 15 mg once/week or azathioprine.
- Hydroxychloroquine is effective for chronic disfiguring skin lesions.
- NSAIDs are useful for musculoskeletal symptoms and erythema nodosum.
- Pulmonary rehabilitation in patients with significant respiratory insufficiency.

DISPOSITION

- The majority of patients with sarcoidosis have spontaneous remission within 2 yr and do not require treatment. Their course can be followed by periodic clinical evaluation, chest x-ray, and PFTs.
- Blacks have increased rates of pulmonary involvement, a worse long-term prognosis, and more frequent relapses.
- Adverse prognostic factors in sarcoidosis include age of onset >40 yr, cardiac involvement, neurosarcoidosis, progressive pulmonary fibrosis, chronic hypercalcemia, chronic uveitis, involvement of nasal mucosa, nephrocalcinosis, and presence of cystic bone lesions and lupus pernio.

REFERRAL

Ophthalmologic examination is indicated in all patients with suspected sarcoidosis, because ocular findings (iridocyclitis, uveitis, conjunctivitis, and keratopathy) are found in >25% of documented cases.

PEARLS & CONSIDERATIONS

COMMENTS

Approximately 15% to 20% of patients with lung involvement advance to irreversible lung impairment (bronchiectasis, cavitation, progressive fibrosis, pneumothorax, and respiratory failure). Death from pulmonary failure occurs in 5% to 7% of patients with sarcoidosis.

EVIDENCE

EBM

Oral corticosteroids improve chest x-ray findings over 6 to 24 months, and they improve global scores (a combination of symptoms, chest x-ray changes, and lung function) in patients with stages II and III pulmonary sarcoidosis, but not in patients with stage I disease. A systematic review found little evidence of an improvement in lung function, and there were insufficient data on the effects of corticosteroids on long-term disease progression.[1] Ⓐ

Evidence-Based Reference

1. Paramothayan NS, Jones PW: Corticosteroids for pulmonary sarcoidosis (Cochrane Review), 1, Chichester, UK, 2004, John Wiley. ⒶⒷ

SUGGESTED READINGS

Judson MA: The management of sarcoidosis by the primary care physician, *Am J Med* 120:403, 2007.

Fannuzzi MC et al: Sarcoidosis, *N Engl J Med* 357:2153-2165, 2007.

AUTHOR: **FRED F. FERRI, M.D.**

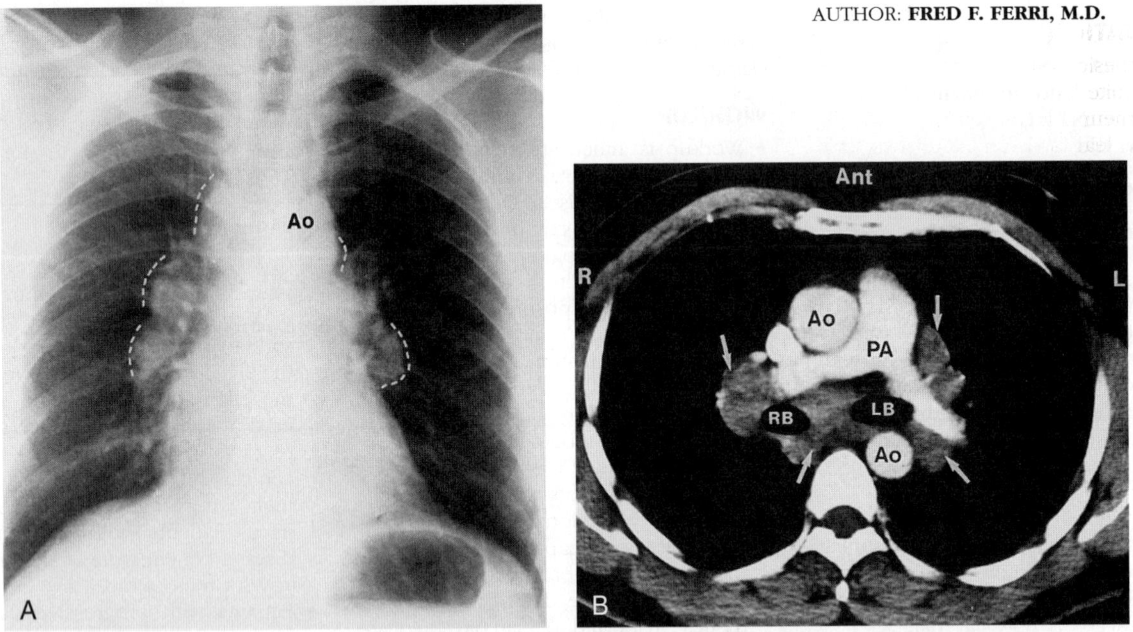

FIGURE 1-238 Sarcoid. Marked lymphadenopathy *(dotted lines)* is seen in the region of both hila in the right paratracheal region **(A)**. The transverse contrast-enhanced CT scan of the upper chest **(B)** clearly shows the ascending and descending aorta *(Ao)* as well as the pulmonary artery *(PA)* and superior vena cava. The right and left mainstem bronchus area is also seen. The *arrows* indicate the extensive lymphadenopathy. *LB,* Left bronchus; *RB,* right bronchus. (From Mettler FA [ed]: *Primary care radiology,* Philadelphia, 2000, WB Saunders.)

TABLE 1-43 Indications for Use of Corticosteroids in Sarcoidosis

Disorder	Treatment
Iridocyclitis	Corticosteroid eyedrops Local subjunctival deposit of cortisone
Posterior uveitis	Oral prednisone
Pulmonary involvement	Steroids rarely recommended for stage I; usually employed if infiltrate remains static or worsens over 3-mo period or the patient is symptomatic
Upper airway obstruction	Rare indication for intravenous steroids
Lupus pernio	Oral prednisone shrinks the disfiguring lesions
Hypercalcemia	Responds well to corticosteroids
Cardiac involvement	Corticosteroids usually recommended if patient has arrhythmias or conduction disturbances
CNS involvement	Response is best in patients with acute symptoms
Lacrimal/salivary gland involvement	Corticosteroids recommended for disordered function, not gland swelling
Bone cysts	Corticosteroids recommended if symptomatic

From Andreoli TE (ed): *Cecil essentials of medicine,* ed 5, Philadelphia, 2001, WB Saunders.
CNS, Central nervous system.

BASIC INFORMATION

DEFINITION

Scabies is a contagious disease caused by the mite *Sarcoptes scabiei.*

ICD-9CM CODES
133.0 Scabies

EPIDEMIOLOGY & DEMOGRAPHICS

- Scabies is generally acquired by sleeping with or in the bedding of infested individuals.
- It is generally associated with poor living conditions and is also common in hospitals and nursing homes.

PHYSICAL FINDINGS & CLINICAL PRESENTATION

- Primary lesions are caused when the female mite burrows within the stratum corneum, laying eggs within the tract she leaves behind; burrows (linear or serpiginous tracts) end with a minute papule or vesicle.
- Primary lesions are most commonly found in the web spaces of the hands, wrists, buttocks, scrotum, penis, breasts, axillae, and knees.
- Secondary lesions result from scratching or infection.
- Intense pruritus, especially nocturnal, is common; it is caused by an acquired sensitivity to the mite or fecal pellets and is usually noted 1 to 4 wk after the primary infestation.
- Examination of the skin may reveal burrows, tiny vesicles, excoriations, inflammatory papules.
- Widespread and crusted lesions (Norwegian or crusted scabies) may be seen in elderly and immunocompromised patients.

ETIOLOGY

Human scabies is caused by the mite *S. scabiei,* var. *hominis* (Fig. 1-239).

DIAGNOSIS

DIFFERENTIAL DIAGNOSIS

- Pediculosis
- Atopic dermatitis
- Flea bites
- Seborrheic dermatitis
- Dermatitis herpetiformis
- Contact dermatitis
- Nummular eczema
- Syphilis
- Other insect infestation

WORKUP

Diagnosis is made on the clinical presentation and on the demonstration of mites, eggs, or mite feces.

LABORATORY TESTS

- Microscopic demonstration of the organism, feces, or eggs: a drop of mineral oil may be placed over the suspected lesion before removal; the scrapings are transferred directly to a glass slide; a drop of potassium hydroxide is added and a cover slip is applied.
- Skin biopsy is rarely necessary to make the diagnosis.

TREATMENT

NONPHARMACOLOGIC THERAPY

Clothing, underwear, and towels used in the 48 hr before treatment must be laundered.

ACUTE GENERAL Rx

- Following a warm bath or shower, Lindane (Kwell, Scabene) lotion should be applied to all skin surfaces below the neck (can be applied to the face if area is infested); it should be washed off 8 to 12 hr after application. Repeat application 1 wk later is usually sufficient to eradicate infestation.
- Pruritus generally abates 24 to 48 hr after treatment, but it can last up to 2 wk; oral antihistamines are effective in decreasing postscabietic pruritus.
- Topical corticosteroid creams may hasten the resolution of secondary eczematous dermatitis.
- If the patient is a resident of an extended care facility, it is important to educate the patients, staff, family, and frequent visitors about scabies and the need to have full cooperation in treatment. Scabicide should be applied to all patients, staff, and frequent visitors, whether symptomatic or not; symptomatic family members of staff and visitors should also receive treatment.
- Permethrin 5% cream (Elimite) is also effective with usually one treatment; it should be massaged into the skin from head to soles of feet; remove 8-14 hr later by washing. If living mites are present after 14 days, treat again.
- A single dose (150 to 200 mg/kg in 6-mg tablets) of ivermectin, an antihelminthic agent, is as effective as topical lindane for the treatment of scabies. It is the best treatment for generalized crusted scabies.

DISPOSITION

Refractory cases usually are seen with immunocompromised hosts or patients with underlying skin diseases.

PEARLS & CONSIDERATIONS

COMMENTS

- Lindane is potentially neurotoxic and should not be used for infants and pregnant women (permethrin is safe and effective in these situations).
- Sexual partners should be notified and treated.

EVIDENCE

EBM

A systematic review concludes that, on balance, permethrin should be used as the treatment of choice. However, this recommendation is based on information from small trials, together with professional opinion and traditional reviews.[1] Ⓐ

All the commonly used treatments are effective, and in general, there is little evidence to suggest that any one is superior.[1,2] Ⓐ

Evidence-Based References

1. Walker GJA, Johnstone PW: Interventions for treating scabies. In: Cochrane Library 1, Chichester, UK, 2004, John Wiley. Ⓐ
2. Walker G, Johnstone P: Scabies. 10:1910, London, 2003, BMJ Publishing Group. Ⓐ

AUTHOR: **FRED F. FERRI, M.D.**

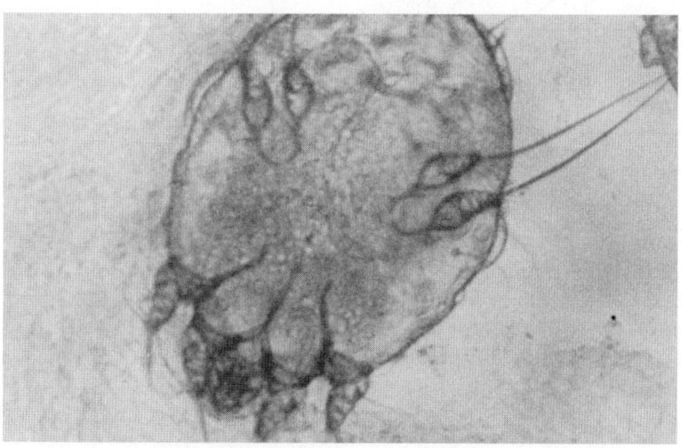

FIGURE 1-239 Scabies organism in a wet mount preparation. (From Mandell GL: *Mandell, Douglas, and Bennett's principles and practice of infectious diseases,* ed 5, New York, 2000, Churchill Livingstone.)

BASIC INFORMATION

DEFINITION

Scarlet fever is a rash involving skin and tongue and complicating a streptococcal group A pharyngitis.

SYNONYMS

Scarlatina
SF

ICD-9CM CODES
034.1 Scarlet fever

EPIDEMIOLOGY & DEMOGRAPHICS

- Same as streptococcal pharyngitis; namely, children aged 5 to 15 yr. May also complicate impetigo.
- Most common in cooler climates during the late fall, winter, and early spring.
- Most cases follow tonsillitis or pharyngitis; however, it has also been reported following wounds ("surgical scarlet fever"), burns, and pelvic or puerperal infections.

PHYSICAL FINDINGS & CLINICAL PRESENTATION

- Diffuse erythema, beginning on face and spreading to neck, back, chest, rest of trunk, and extremities. Most intense on inner aspects of arms and thighs.
- Erythema blanches, but nonblanching petechiae may be present or produced by a tourniquet.
- Strawberry or raspberry tongue.
- Rash lasts about 1 wk and then desquamates.
- Febrile illness with headache, malaise, anorexia, and pharyngitis begins after a 2- to 4-day incubation period.
- Scarlatinal rash begins 1 or 2 days after the onset of pharyngitis (Fig. 1-240).

ETIOLOGY

Caused by group A beta-hemolytic *Streptococcus* infection, which produces one of three erythrogenic toxins (NOTE: Some streptococcal species have the ability to cause both scarlet fever and rheumatic fever).

DIAGNOSIS

DIFFERENTIAL DIAGNOSIS

- Viral exanthems (covered in Section II)
- Kawasaki disease
- Toxic shock syndrome
- Drug rashes

See differential diagnosis of "Pharyngitis" in Section I.

WORKUP

- Identification of group A *Streptococcus* by throat culture
- SLO antibody titers

TREATMENT

- Penicillin 250 mg po qid for 10 days or erythromycin 250 mg po qid for 10 days in penicillin-allergic patients. A clinical response can be expected in 24 to 48 hr.
- Benzathine penicillin 1 to 2 million U IM once; may be used for a patient who cannot swallow pills.

COMPLICATIONS (RARE)

- Peritonsillar abscess
- Mastoiditis
- Otitis media
- Pneumonia
- Sepsis and distant foci of infection
- Acute rheumatic fever
- Inability to swallow liquids or upper airway obstruction requires hospitalization.

Note: Failure to respond to penicillin should raise doubt about the diagnosis because *Streptococcus* may be carried in the pharynx without causing infection.

PEARLS & CONSIDERATIONS

COMMENTS

Patients with antibodies against the toxin are spared the rash but still develop other symptoms of the infection (e.g., sore throat).

AUTHORS: **FRED F. FERRI, M.D.,** and **TOM J. WACHTEL, M.D.**

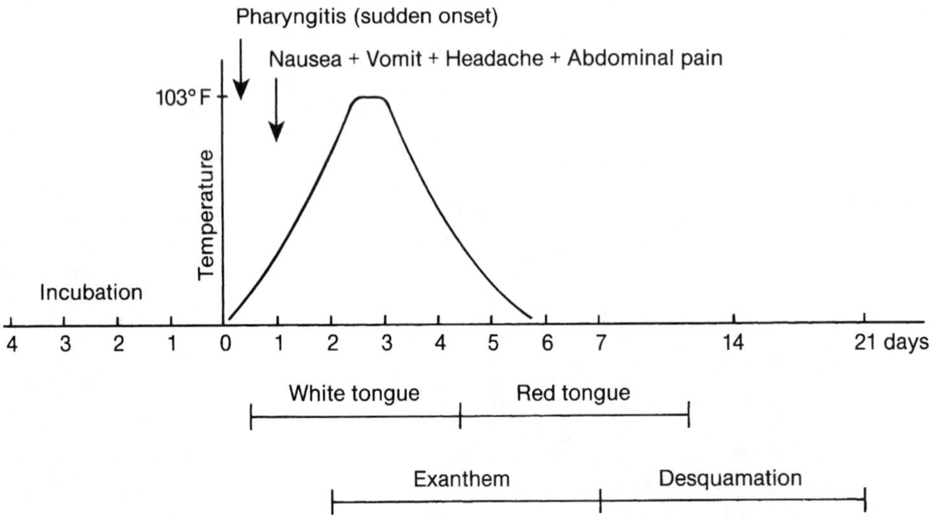

FIGURE 1-240 Scarlet fever. Evolution of signs and symptoms. (From Habif TP: *Clinical dermatology: a color guide to diagnosis and therapy,* ed 3, St Louis, 1996, Mosby.)

BASIC INFORMATION

DEFINITION

Schistosomiasis is caused by infection with parasite blood flukes known as schistosomes.

SYNONYMS

Bilharziasis
Urinary schistosomiasis
Hepatosplenic schistosomiasis
Swimmers itch
Katayama fever

ICD-9CM CODES
120.9 Schistosomiasis

EPIDEMIOLOGY & DEMOGRAPHICS

INCIDENCE:
- More than 200 million people worldwide and more than 200,000 deaths annually. In U.S., estimated to exceed 400,000 persons.
- Geographic distribution of schistosomiasis is confined to an area between 36° north and 34° south latitude, where fresh water temperatures average 25 to 30° C.

PREVALENCE:
The greatest cercarial exposure usually occurs in boys aged 5 to 10 yr

DISTRIBUTION:
- *S. mansoni* in tropical and subtropical areas of sub-Saharan Africa, the Middle East, South America, and the Caribbean
- *S. haematobium* in North Africa, sub-Saharan Africa, the Middle East, and India
- *S. japonicum* in Asia, particularly in China, the Philippines, Thailand, and Indonesia
- *S. intercalatum* in central and west Africa
- *S. mekongi* in Cambodia

ETIOLOGY & PATHOGENESIS

- Human infections are caused by *S. mansoni, S. haematobium, S. japonicum, S. mekongi,* and *S. intercalatum.*
- Acquisition of disease via contact with fresh water containing infectious free-living cercarial larvae.
- In U.S., most cases are acquired during foreign travel.
- Human disease is primarily associated with the host's granulomatous response to eggs retained in the tissue.

PHYSICAL FINDINGS & CLINICAL PRESENTATION

ACUTE SYMPTOMS:
- Swimmers itch
- Katayama fever

CHRONIC SYMPTOMS:
- Intestinal schistosomiasis
  1. Abdominal pain
  2. Bloody diarrhea
  3. Iron deficiency anemia
  4. Intestinal polyp
  5. Bowel ulcer and strictures
- Hepatic schistosomiasis
  1. Hepatomegaly
  2. Splenomegaly
  3. Portal hypertension
  4. Esophageal varices
- Urinary schistosomiasis
  1. Hematuria
  2. Dysuria
  3. Urinary frequency
  4. Fibrosis of bladder and ureters
  5. Squamous cell ca of bladder
  6. Proteinuria
  7. Nephrotic syndrome

COMPLICATIONS:
- Neurologic complication
  1. Granuloma of spinal cord or brain
  2. Transverse myelitis
  3. Epilepsy or focal neurologic deficit
- Pulmonary complication
  1. Granulomatous pulmonary endarteritis
  2. Pulmonary hypertension
  3. Cor pulmonale
- Other complications include tubal obstruction and infertility
- Recurrent bacteremia and recurrent UTI

DIAGNOSIS

DIFFERENTIAL DIAGNOSIS

- Amebiasis
- Bacillary dysentery
- Bowel polyp
- Prostatic disease
- Genitourinary tract cancer
- Bacterial infections of the urinary tract

WORKUP

- Microscopy in urine or stool
- Tissue biopsy
- Serology
- CBC
- LFT
- US of abdomen
- CT scan of abdomen

LABORATORY TESTS

- CBC shows eosinophilia, anemia, thrombocytopenia
- LFT with mild increase in alkaline phosphatase and GGT
- Microscopy: stool and urine
- Serology: ELISA for detecting both schistosomal antibodies and antigen
- Rectal biopsy or bladder mucosal biopsy

IMAGING STUDIES

- X-ray of abdomen shows "fetal head" calcification.
- Sonography also documents a thickened bladder wall, hydronephrosis and hydroureter, and bladder polyps or calcification. It also demonstrates the thickened fibrosed portal tracts.
- Esophagoscopy documents esophageal varices.
- Liver biopsy may also demonstrate granuloma and clay pipestem fibrosis.

TREATMENT

- Praziquantel 40 mg/kg of body weight orally in one or two doses
- Oxamniquine 15 mg/kg orally once or 20 mg/kg orally daily for 3 days for recalcitrant infections
- Metrifonate 7.5 to 10 mg/kg of body weight given orally in three doses at 2-wk intervals

DISPOSITION

Treated patients usually respond to therapy. Definitive cure has occurred only when there is total disappearance of viable eggs from the excreta for a total of 6 mo after treatment.

REFERRAL

- To an infectious disease specialist knowledgeable in parasitology and geographic medicine for treatment and follow-up
- To a gastroenterologist for sclerotherapy of bleeding esophageal varices, if needed in advanced hepatosplenic schistosomiasis
- To a urologist for management and follow-up of urinary complications of *S. haematobium* infection of the genitor-urinary tract

PEARLS & CONSIDERATIONS

COMMENTS

Prevention:
- Chemotherapy
  1. Mass
  2. Targeted population
- Snail control
  1. Mollusciciding
  2. Environmental modification
  3. Biologic control
- Reduction of water contact and contamination
  1. Provision of domestic water supplies
  2. Provision for sanitary disposal of excreta
- Vaccination
- Improved living standards

SUGGESTED READINGS

Steinmann P et al: Schistosomiasis and water resources development: systematic review, meta-analysis, and estimates of people at risk, *Lancet Infect Dis* 6(7):411, 2006.

Swai B et al: Female genital schistosomiasis as an evidence of a neglected cause for reproductive ill-health: a retrospective histopathological study from Tanzania, *BMC Infect Dis* 6:134, 2006.

Vennervald BJ et al: Morbidity in schistosomiasis: an update, *Curr Opin Infect Dis* 17(5): 439, 2004.

AUTHORS: **VASANTHI ARUMUGAM, M.D., GLENN G. FORT, M.D., M.P.H.,** and **DENNIS J. MIKOLICH, M.D.**

BASIC INFORMATION

DEFINITION

Schizophrenia is a disorder that causes significant distortions in thinking, perception, speech, and behavior. Characteristics include psychosis, apathy and social withdrawal, and cognitive impairment, which result in significant social impairment.

SYNONYMS

Dementia praecox

ICD-9CM CODES
295.9 Schizophrenia

EPIDEMIOLOGY & DEMOGRAPHICS

PREVALENCE: 0.5%, incidence 0.2 per 1000. Lifetime prevalence risk is 0.4%.

PEAK INCIDENCE: Ages 16 to 30

PREDOMINANT SEX: Males have a more severe illness with earlier onset; however, distribution is probably equal.

PREDOMINANT AGE:

- Age at onset of psychotic symptoms is in the early 20s for males and late 20s for females.
- Age of onset of the negative symptoms is usually earlier (midteenage years).

GENETICS:

- Accounts for 70% of risk, remaining 30% is biologic or psychosocial.
- First-degree relatives of schizophrenics have 10 times greater chance of becoming schizophrenic than the general population.
- Discordant rates among identical twins are higher than expected with simple inheritance pattern.
- Associations with several chromosomes have been described, but none have been replicated.
- Evidence exists that triplet nucleotide repeat expansion (such as seen with Huntington's disease) may play a role in inheritance of the disease.

PHYSICAL FINDINGS & CLINICAL PRESENTATION

- Best defined as a dementing illness beginning in early life and progressing slowly throughout the lifetime.
- Initial "negative" symptoms of adolescence—cognitive decline, social withdrawal and awkwardness, loss of motivation and pleasure, and loss of emotional expressiveness—begin after a period of normal development.
- In early adulthood, positive symptoms of psychosis and thought disturbance occur; psychotic symptoms then wax and wane throughout life; treatment ameliorates positive symptoms but generally does little for negative ones.
- It is also accompanied by cognitive impairment, including problems in attention and concentration, psychomotor speed, learning and memory, and executive functions (e.g., abstract thinking, problem solving).
- Social and occupational dysfunction can be profound.

ETIOLOGY

- Basic distinction of whether this is a degenerative or a developmental condition is not settled.
- Frequent findings include enlargement of ventricular system and loss of brain volume and cortical gray matter.
- Major hypothesis: generation of the mesocortical pathways produce the hypofrontality and negative symptoms, along with a compensatory hyperactivation of the mesolimbic pathways, which produce the positive symptoms of psychosis.

DIAGNOSIS

DIFFERENTIAL DIAGNOSIS

- Schizophrenia is diagnosed when an individual has experienced at least 1 month of hallucinations, delusions, thought disorder, catatonia, or negative symptoms (avolition, anhedonia, social isolation, affective flattening).
- Any medical condition, medicine, or substance of abuse that can affect brain homeostasis and cause psychosis: distinguished from schizophrenia by their relatively brief course and the alteration in mental status that could suggest an underlying delirium.
- Other neurologic conditions (e.g., Huntington's) that have psychosis as the initial presentation.
- Other psychiatric disorders: source of greatest confusion.
- Mood disorders with psychosis: indistinguishable from schizophrenia cross-sectionally, but have a longitudinal course that includes full recovery.
- Delusional disorder: has nonbizarre delusions and lacks the thought disturbance, hallucinations, and negative symptoms of schizophrenia.
- Autism in the adult: has an early age at onset and lacks significant hallucinations or delusions.

WORKUP

- History and physical examination to aid in determining if psychosis is secondary or primary
- Neurologic examination to uncover soft neurologic signs (clumsy, cortical thumb, loss of fine motor movements) common in schizophrenia

LABORATORY TESTS

- No laboratory tests are specific for schizophrenia.
- Laboratory examinations (chemistry profile, blood count, sedimentation rate, toxicology screen, and urinalysis) are geared toward excluding a primary medical condition.

IMAGING STUDIES

- CT scan or MRI of brain during initial workup; repeated if the course of the illness varies from expected
- Sometimes EEG to reveal slowing when psychosis is secondary to an encephalopathy
- Chest x-ray examination during initial workup to rule out a primary medical condition

TREATMENT

NONPHARMACOLOGIC THERAPY

- Significant social support is required by most schizophrenic patients; available support services are grossly inadequate, and schizophrenia patients constitute nearly one third of all homeless individuals. They usually require help with basic social, occupational, and interactive skills.
- For schizophrenic patients who continue to live with their families, family stress can precipitate relapse and rehospitalization; family interventions can reduce morbidity.
- Cognitive behavioral therapy can reduce severity of both psychotic and negative symptoms.
- Illness management training for patients can increase medication adherence and reduce distress due to symptoms.
- Integrated treatment of assertive community treatment, family involvement programs, and social skills training reduces severity of both psychotic and negative symptoms, reduces comorbid substance misuse, reduces hospital days, increases adherence to treatment, and increases satisfaction with treatment.

ACUTE GENERAL Rx

- Acute psychosis is usually adequately controlled by antipsychotic agents.
- Mainstay of therapy is the second-generation antipsychotics (risperidone, olanzapine, quetiapine, ziprasidone, aripiprazole, and clozapine). Traditional neuroleptic (e.g., haloperidol, perphenazine, fluphenazine, chlorpromazine) use is decreasing in part because of their propensity to cause a parkinsonian state and eventual tardive dyskinesia (rate of tardive dyskinesia 15% to 30%). Antiparkinsonian drugs (benztropine, amantadine) are

used to ameliorate the parkinsonism. Risperidone has been shown to be superior to haloperidol in preventing acute psychotic relapse.
- Sedatives (benzodiazepines, and to a lesser degree, barbiturates) can be used transiently if there is an agitated state.

CHRONIC Rx

- Relapse prevention is a major goal of treatment. Noncompliance is common and leads to high relapse rates. Antipsychotic agents usually must be continued at the same doses that controlled psychosis. For noncompliant patients, depot preparations that are given biweekly or monthly can be used.
- Most patients frequently switch between antipsychotics; fewer patients discontinue olanzapine compared to other second-generation antipsychotics for all causes, lack of efficacy, or by patient choice.
- Neurocognitive improvement associated with antipsychotic treatment in patients with schizophrenia is small and does not differ between first-generation and second-generation antipsychotics.
- Antiparkinsonian agents may also need to be continued chronically.
- Tardive dyskinesia (choreoathetoid movements of the muscles of tongue, face, and occasionally other muscle groups) can occur in as many as 30% of patients with long-term use of the neuroleptics.
- The negative symptoms of schizophrenia can resemble depression. In addition, depressive disorders may occur in schizophrenic patients. Antidepressant treatment of the negative symptoms is usually without effect. However, antidepressants can improve the symptoms of a discrete comorbid depressive episode.
- Mood stabilizers, such as lithium, valproate, or carbamazepine, are of little use unless there is a comorbid impulse control disorder.
- Substance abuse is a major problem in more than one third of schizophrenics. Unfortunately, these patients do poorly in traditional substance abuse treatment programs. Specialized "dual diagnosis" programs with highly structured aftercare are required.
- Specific antipsychotics have been associated with weight gain (olanzapine and clozapine) and QT prolongation. Hyperlipidemia and diabetes mellitus are associated with second-generation antipsychotics, and hyperprolactinemia is associated with first-generation antipsychotics. Clozapine is associated with agranulocytosis.

DISPOSITION

- The positive symptoms of as many as 20% to 30% of schizophrenic patients do not respond to available treatments. A much higher fraction relapse as a result of poor compliance.
- The negative symptoms are responsible for the 50% to 70% of cases in which deterioration in occupational and social function continues.
- Approximately 10% of patients will complete suicide.
- Course of illness most strongly predicted by level of social development attained at onset of psychosis.

REFERRAL

- If hospitalization is required
- If patient is noncompliant
- If patient is resistant to treatment

PEARLS & CONSIDERATIONS

- Rule out delirium due to medical condition, medicine, or substance abuse before diagnosing psychotic behavior as schizophrenia.
- All antipsychotics have high discontinuation rates in chronic schizophrenia treatment. Olanzapine and clozapine may be more effective than other antipsychotics for chronic treatment but have significant side effects.
- Significant social support is required by most patients with schizophrenia, and nonpharmacologic therapy should be used in conjunction with pharmacotherapy.

EVIDENCE

Typical antipsychotic drugs

Typical antipsychotic drugs, such as chlorpromazine and haloperidol, are effective in the management of schizophrenia, although they have high rates of adverse effects, which may limit their acceptability.[1,2] (A)

Atypical antipsychotic drugs

Atypical antipsychotic drugs, such as clozapine, olanzapine, and risperidone, are in general at least as effective as the typical agents and tend to have fewer extrapyramidal side effects, which may improve acceptability.[3] (A)

Cognitive behavioral therapy (CBT)

CBT plus standard care has significant beneficial effects on discharge from hospital, as well on improvement in mental state at 13 to 26 weeks compared with standard care alone; the effects on mental state are not apparent by 52 weeks.[4] (A)

Family therapy

Multiple session family interventions are effective in reducing relapse rates at 12 months compared with single session, psychoeducational intervention and usual care practices.[5] (A)

Social skills training

Social skills training reduces relapse rates at 24 months, but not at 12 months, compared with standard or psychoeducational care.[6] (A)

Evidence-Based References

1. Adams CE et al: Chlorpromazine versus placebo for schizophrenia, *Cochrane Database Syst Rev* 2, 2007.
2. Joy CB, Adams CE, Lawrie SM: Haloperidol versus placebo for schizophrenia, *Cochrane Database Syst Rev* 2, 2001. (A)
3. Leucht S et al: Relapse prevention in schizophrenia with new generation antipsychotics: a systematic review, and exploratory meta-analysis of randomized, controlled trials, *Am J Psychiatry* 160:1209-1222, 2003. Reviewed in: *Evid Based Ment Health* 7, 2004.
4. Jones C et al: Cognitive behaviour therapy for schizophrenia, *Cochrane Database Syst Rev* 4, 2004. (A)
5. Pilling S et al: Psychological treatments in schizophrenia: I. Meta-analysis of family interventions and cognitive behaviour therapy, *Psychol Med* 32:763, 2002. Reviewed in: *Clin Evid* 12:1500, 2004. (A)
6. Pilling S et al: Psychological treatments in schizophrenia: II. Meta-analysis of randomised controlled trials of social skills training and cognitive remediation, *Psychol Med* 32:783, 2002. Reviewed in: *Clin Evid* 12:1500, 2004. (A)

SUGGESTED READINGS

Lieberman JA et al: Effectiveness of antipsychotic drugs in patients with chronic schizophrenia, *N Engl J Med* 353:1209, 2005.

Mueser KT, McGurk SR: Schizophrenia, *Lancet* 363:2063, 2004.

Petersen L et al: A randomised multicentre trial of integrated versus standard treatment for patients with a first episode of psychotic illness, *BMJ* 331:602, 2005.

Picchioni MM, Murray RM: Schizophrenia, *BMJ* 335:91, 2007.

AUTHOR: **MICHAEL K. ONG, M.D., PH.D.**

BASIC INFORMATION

DEFINITION

Scleritis is inflammation of the sclera.

SYNONYMS

Anterior scleritis
Diffuse nodular, necrotizing scleritis
Scleromalacia perforans
Scleral melt syndrome

ICD-9CM CODES
379.0 Scleritis and episcleritis

EPIDEMIOLOGY & DEMOGRAPHICS

PEAK INCIDENCE: Increases with increasing age
INCIDENCE (IN U.S.): Busy ophthalmologist may see 1 or 2 cases a year
PREVALENCE (IN U.S.): Relatively rare
PREDOMINANT SEX: 61% women
PREDOMINANT AGE: 52 yr

PHYSICAL FINDINGS & CLINICAL PRESENTATION

- Deep, boring eye pain
- Photophobia
- Tearing
- Conjunctival injection (Fig. 1-241)
- Thinning of the sclera
- 44% of patients have associated medical conditions: 7% infections, 37% rheumatic disease. Most common infection is Herpes zoster. Most common rheumatic problem is rheumatoid arthritis. 4% have systemic vasculitis. Most patients with systemic disease are diagnosed before development of scleritis

ETIOLOGY

- Inflammatory
- Allergic
- Toxic

DIAGNOSIS

DIFFERENTIAL DIAGNOSIS

- Most common causes are rheumatoid arthritis and other collagen-vascular disease.
- Occasionally, there are allergic, infectious, or traumatic causes.
- Conjunctivitis, iritis, and episcleritis should be considered in the differential diagnosis.

WORKUP

- Fluorescein angiography
- Eye examination
- Visual field examination
- Workup for autoimmune disease
- Workup for vasculitis
- Collagen vascular workup

LABORATORY TESTS

- RF, ANA, ESR may be useful
- For underlying etiology

IMAGING STUDIES

Usually not necessary; CT scan of orbit may be useful in selected patients for collagen vascular disease or vasculitis

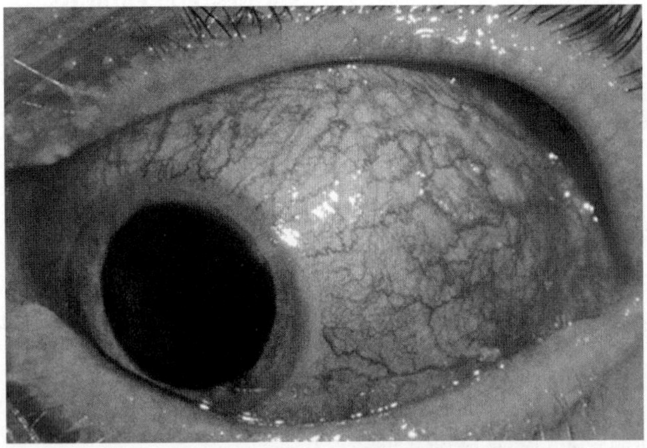

FIGURE 1-241 In diffuse anterior scleritis, widespread injection of the conjunctival and deep episcleral vessels occurs. (From Palay D [ed]: *Ophthalmology for the primary care physician,* St Louis, 1997, Mosby.)

TREATMENT

NONPHARMACOLOGIC THERAPY

- Bandage lenses
- Surgery if thinning of the sclera is severe to prevent eye rupture

ACUTE GENERAL Rx

Immunotherapy (with steroids and Imuran, etc.):
- Steroids (topical, periocular, and systemic)
- Cycloplegic drops
- NSAIDs (topical and systemic); systemic more effective than topical
- Other immunosuppressive drugs

CHRONIC Rx

- Systemic steroids can be given for the underlying disease.
- Local steroids may be helpful.
- Control underlying disease.

DISPOSITION

Urgent referral to ophthalmologist

REFERRAL

If not referred to an ophthalmologist early, patients may develop uveitis and other complications.

PEARLS & CONSIDERATIONS

COMMENTS

An ominous diagnosis because these patients often have other severe underlying debilitating disease processes.

SUGGESTED READINGS

Akpek EK et al: Evaluation of patients with scleritis for systemic disease, *Ophthalmology* 111(3):501, 2004.
Paresio CG et al: Systemic disorders associated with episcleritis and scleritis, *Curr Opin Ophthalmal* 12(6):471, 2001.
Sainz de la Maza M et al: Ocular characteristics and disease associations in scleritis: associated peripheral keatopathy, *Arch Ophth* 120(1):15, 2002.
Thorne JE et al: Severe scleritis and urticarial lesions, *Am J Ophthalmol* 134(6):932, 2002.

AUTHOR: **MELVYN KOBY, M.D.**

BASIC INFORMATION

DEFINITION

Scleroderma is a connective tissue disorder characterized by thickening and fibrosis of the skin and variably severe involvement of diverse internal organs.

SYNONYMS

Systemic sclerosis; morphea applies to localized scleroderma affecting only the skin. Scleredema is a disease of the skin distinct from scleroderma.

ICD-9CM CODES
710.1 (Morphea: 701.0)

EPIDEMIOLOGY & DEMOGRAPHICS

INCIDENCE: 4 to 12 cases/million persons per year, but many mild cases go unrecognized

PREDOMINANT SEX: Female:male ratio of 4:1

PREDOMINANT AGE: 30 to 50 yr

DISTRIBUTION: Worldwide

PHYSICAL FINDINGS & CLINICAL PRESENTATION

PHYSICAL FINDINGS:

Skin
- Begins on hands, then face; skin is shiny, taut, sometimes red with loss of creases and hair
- Later skin tightening may limit movement
- Pigmentary changes occur
- Skin atrophy occurs in late stages

Musculoskeletal
- Symmetric inflammatory arthritis
- Myopathy

GI involvement
- Esophageal dysmotility with heartburn, dysphagia, odynophagia
- Delayed gastric emptying
- Small bowel dysmotility with abdominal cramps and diarrhea
- Colon dysmotility with constipation
- Primary biliary cirrhosis (see “Cirrhosis, Primary Biliary” in Section I)

Pulmonary manifestations
- Pulmonary fibrosis with symptoms of dyspnea and nonproductive cough and fine inspiratory crackles on examination
- Pulmonary hypertension

Cardiac involvement
- Myocardial fibrosis leading to congestive heart failure

Renal involvement
- Malignant hypertension
- Rapidly progressive renal failure

Other organ involvement
- Hypothyroidism
- Erectile dysfunction
- Sjögren’s syndrome
- Entrapment neuropathies

CREST syndrome
- Calcinosis, Raynaud’s syndrome, esophageal dysmotility, sclerodactyly, telangiectasias (in CREST scleroderma is limited to distal extremities)

CLINICAL PRESENTATION:
- Raynaud’s phenomenon: initial complaint in 70% (NOTE: The prevalence of Raynaud’s is 5% to 10% of the general population; most do not progress to scleroderma)
- Finger or hand swelling, sometimes associated with carpal tunnel syndrome
- Arthralgias/arthritis
- Internal organ involvement

ETIOLOGY

Etiology is unknown. Stimulatory autoantibodies against platelet-derived growth factor (PDGF) appear to be a specific hallmark of scleroderma. Their biologic activity on fibroblasts suggests that they have a causal role in the pathogenesis of the disease. In scleroderma, unifying features exist in spite of heterogenous patterns of organ involvement and disease progression:
- Extracellular connective tissue activation
- Frequent immunologic abnormalities
- Inflammation
- Vasoconstriction

DIAGNOSIS

DIFFERENTIAL DIAGNOSIS

Dermatologic
- Mycosis fungoides
- Amyloidosis
- Porphyria cutanea tarda
- Eosinophilic fasciitis
- Reflex sympathetic dystrophy

Systemic
- Idiopathic pulmonary fibrosis
- Primary pulmonary hypertension
- Primary biliary cirrhosis
- Cardiomyopathies
- GI dysmotility problems
- SLE and overlap syndromes

WORKUP

Laboratory tests and imaging studies

LABORATORY TESTS

- Antinuclear antibodies (homogeneous, speckled, or nucleolar patterns)
- Negative antibody to native DNA
- Negative anti-Sm antibody
- Anti-nRNP positive in 20%
- Rheumatoid factor positive in 30%
- Anticentromere antibodies in fewer than 10% with systemic illness and in 50% to 95% with limited scleroderma (i.e., good prognosis if positive)
- Positive extractable nuclear antibody to SCL 70 in 30%
- Routine biochemistry tests may indicate specific organ involvement (e.g., liver, kidney, muscle)

IMAGING AND OTHER STUDIES

Arthritis: joint x-rays

GI
- Barium swallow
- Cine esophagography
- Endoscopy
- Esophageal manometry

Pulmonary
- Chest x-ray
- PFTs
- Chest CT scan
- Bronchoscopy with biopsy
- Gallium lung scan
- Bronchoalveolar lavage

Heart
- ECG
- Ambulatory (Holter) ECG monitoring
- Echocardiography
- Cardiac catheterization

Kidney: renal biopsy

Skin: skin biopsy

TREATMENT

D-penicillamine; recombinant human relaxin; supportive therapies used.

Raynaud’s syndrome:
- Calcium channel blockers
- Peripheral α_1-adrenergic blockers

Arthralgias: NSAIDs

Skin: moisturizing agents

Esophageal reflux
- H_2-receptor blockers
- Proton pump inhibitors

Pulmonary hypertension and fibrosis
- Oxygen
- Lung transplant
- Cyclophosphamide chemotherapy in symptomatic scleroderma-related interstitial lung disease

Renal involvement
- Angiotensin-converting enzyme inhibitors
- Dialysis
- Renal transplantation

REFERRAL

To rheumatologist

SUGGESTED READINGS

Baron: SS et al: Stimulatory autoantibodies to the PDGF receptor in systemic sclerosis, *N Engl J Med* 354:2667, 2006.

Pope JE et al: A randomized, controlled trial of methotrexate versus placebo in early diffuse scleroderma, *Arthritis Rheum* 44(6):1351, 2001.

Seibold JR, Koan JH, Simms R, et al: Recombinant human relaxin in the treatment of scleroderma, *Ann Intern Med* 132:871, 2000.

Tashkin DP et al: Cyclophosphamide versus placebo in scleroderma lung disease, *N Engl J Med* 354:2655, 2006.

Thompson AE et al: Calcium-channel blockers for Raynaud’s phenomenon in systemic sclerosis, *Arthritis Rheum* 44(8):1841, 2001.

AUTHORS: **FRED F. FERRI, M.D.,** and **TOM J. WACHTEL, M.D.**

BASIC INFORMATION

DEFINITION

Scoliosis is a lateral curvature of the spine in the upright position, usually 10 degrees or greater. Scoliosis may be classified as either structural (fixed, nonflexible) or nonstructural (flexible, correctable).

ICD-9CM CODES
737.30 Idiopathic scoliosis
737.39 Paralytic scoliosis
754.2 Congenital scoliosis
724.3 Sciatic scoliosis
737.43 Associated with neurofibromatosis

EPIDEMIOLOGY & DEMOGRAPHICS (IDIOPATHIC FORM)

PREDOMINANT SEX: Females > males (7:1)
PREVALENCE: 4 cases/1000 persons
PREDOMINANT AGE:
- Onset is variable.
- Most curves are found in adolescents (age 11 yr and over).

PHYSICAL FINDINGS & CLINICAL PRESENTATION

- Record patient age (in years plus months) and height.
- Perform neurologic examination to rule out neuromuscular disease.
- Inspect the shoulders and iliac crests to determine if they are level.
- Palpate the spinous processes to determine their alignment.
- Have the patient bend forward symmetrically at the waist with the arms hanging free (Adams' position); observe from the back or front to detect abnormal spine rotation (Fig. 1-242).

ETIOLOGY

- 90% unknown, usually referred to as idiopathic (genetic)
- Congenital spine deformity
- Neuromuscular disease
- Leg length inequality
- Local inflammation or infection
- Acute pain (disc disease)
- Chronic degenerative disc disease with asymmetric disc narrowing

Curves of an idiopathic nature or those accompanying congenital deformity or neuromuscular disease are those associated with structural changes. The nonstructural types (leg length discrepancy, inflammation, or acute pain) disappear when the offending disorder is corrected.

DIAGNOSIS

WORKUP

- Curvatures associated with congenital spine abnormalities, neuromuscular disease, and the other less common forms of scoliosis can usually be identified by history or associated radiographic or physical findings.
- Section III, "Scoliosis," describes an approach to scoliosis screening.

IMAGING STUDIES

- Diagnosis of idiopathic scoliosis is confirmed by a standing roentgenogram of the spine.
- Severity of the curve is measured in degrees, usually by the Cobb method.
- MRI is usually not indicated unless there is: (1) pain, (2) a neurologic deficit, or (3) a left thoracic curve (which is often associated with an underlying spinal disorder).

TREATMENT

ACUTE GENERAL Rx

- Treatment or correction of cause if curve is nonstructural
- Early detection is key in treating genetic curve
- Regular observation for curves <20 degrees
- Bracing for idiopathic curves of 20 to 40 degrees to prevent progression
- Surgery for idiopathic curves >40 to 50 degrees in immature patient

DISPOSITION

- The larger the curve at detection, the greater the chance of progression.
- Progression is more common in young children who are beginning their growth spurt.
- Curves in females are more likely to progress.
- Curves <20 degrees will improve spontaneously more than 50% of the time.
- Failure to diagnose and treat these curves may allow progressive deformity, pain, and cardiopulmonary compromise to develop.
- Spinal deformities >50 degrees in adults may progress and eventually become painful.
- There is no difference in the rate of back pain in the general population and patients with adolescent idiopathic scoliosis.

REFERRAL

For orthopedic consultation if structural curve is present

PEARLS & CONSIDERATIONS

COMMENTS

- Congenital scoliosis has a high incidence of cardiac and urinary tract abnormalities.
- Bracing is not intended to completely straighten the idiopathic curve. It may improve the curvature but is mainly used to stabilize and prevent progression.

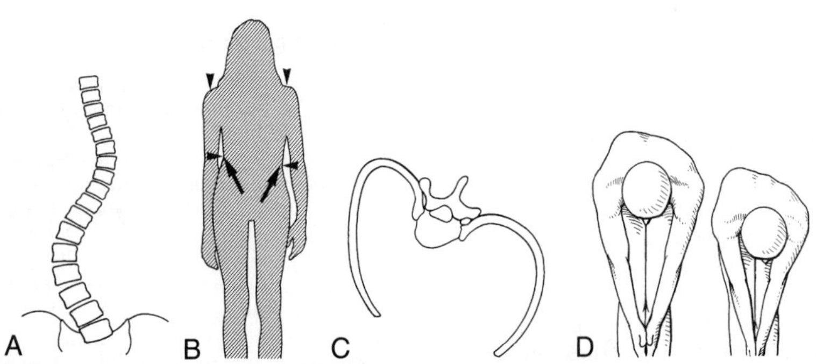

FIGURE 1-242 Structural changes in idiopathic scoliosis. A, As curvature increases, alterations in body configuration develop in both the primary and compensatory curve regions. **B,** Asymmetry of shoulder height, waistline, and the elbow-to-flank distance are common findings. **C,** Vertebral rotation and associated posterior displacement of the ribs on the convex side of the curve are responsible for the characteristic deformity of the chest wall in scoliosis patients. **D,** In the school screening examination for scoliosis, the patient bends forward at the waist. Rib asymmetry of even a small degree is obvious. (From Scoles PV: Spinal deformity in childhood and adolescence. In Behrman RE, Vaughn VC III [eds]: *Nelson textbook of pediatrics,* ed 5, Philadelphia, 1989, WB Saunders.)

SUGGESTED READINGS

Davids JR, Chamberlin E, Blackhurst DW: Indications for magnetic resonance imaging in presumed adolescent idiopathic scoliosis, *J Bone Joint Surg* 86A:2187, 2004.
Fernandes P, Weinstein SL: Natural history of early onset scoliosis, *J Bone Joint Surg* 89A (suppl 1):21, 2007.
Gillingham BL et al: Early onset idiopathic scoliosis, *J Am Acad Orthop Surg* 14:101, 2006.
Lenke LG, Dobbs MB: Management of juvenile idiopathic scoliosis, *J Bone Joint Surg* 89A(suppl 1):55, 2007.
McCarthy JJ et al: Scoliosis in the child with cerebral palsy, *J Am Acad Orthop Surg* 14:367, 2006.
Richards BS, Vitale MG: Screening for idiopathic scoliosis in adolescents, *J Bone Joint Surg* 90A:195, 2008.
Sanders JO et al: Predicting scoliosis progression from skeletal maturity: a simplified classification during adolescence, *J Bone Joint Surg Am* 90:540, 2008.
Ugwonali OF et al: Effect of bracing on the quality of life of adolescents with idiopathic scoliosis, *Spine J* 4:254, 2004.

AUTHOR: **LONNIE R. MERCIER, M.D.**

BASIC INFORMATION

DEFINITION

Recurrent depressive episodes during autumn and winter alternating with nondepressive episodes during spring and summer. Patients with the disorder have experienced two episodes of major depression in the last 2 yr that demonstrate temporal seasonal relationships and there have been no nonseasonal episodes over this time period.

SYNONYMS

Seasonal depression
Winter depression
Wintertime blues

ICD-9CM CODES
296.30 Seasonal affective disorder

EPIDEMIOLOGY & DEMOGRAPHICS

- Climate, genetic vulnerability, and social-cultural factors all play a role. The risk of seasonal mood swings is clearly associated with northern latitudes. The prevalence of seasonal affective disorder (SAD) is estimated to be 0.5% to 1.5% in northern European populations, and 10% to 20% of these populations report milder, recurrent episodes consistent with subsyndromal SAD.
- As with other depressive disorders, women are affected disproportionate to men.

PHYSICAL FINDINGS & CLINICAL PRESENTATION

- The symptoms of SAD are similar to those of other depressive episodes, but tend to include those features associated with an atypical major depression, including low energy, irritability, weight gain, and overeating.
- The average duration of symptoms is 5 mo, generally commencing in November.

ETIOLOGY

- Explanations for SAD tend to focus on biologic models. The shorter photoperiod and decrease in sunlight exposure experienced by people living in temperate and higher latitudes during the winter is hypothesized to be the main trigger for SAD.
- Several neurotransmitters have been implicated in SAD, including dopamine, serotonin, and norepinephrine. Current research is focused on the role of serotonin in the mediation of seasonal affective changes.

DIAGNOSIS

Diagnostic workup similar to that for major depression but with focus on the seasonal nature of the symptoms.

DIFFERENTIAL DIAGNOSIS

- Depressive disorders
- Bipolar affective disorder
- Evaluate for substance use (especially alcohol)
- Medical illness or medications that may contribute to depression (e.g., endocrine or neurologic disorders)

WORKUP

- As with major depression, consider medical etiologies and rule out as indicated by the presenting signs and symptoms.
- Structured Interview Guide for the Hamilton Depression Rating Scale-Seasonal Affective Disorders Version (SIGH-SAD) used in research settings.

LABORATORY TESTS

As directed by presenting complaints

IMAGING STUDIES

Generally not indicated

TREATMENT

NONPHARMACOLOGIC THERAPY

- Phototherapy is based on the principle that the presentation of artificial light at a similar strength to natural sunlight will prevent the biologic changes that mediate SAD during the winter.
- There have been at least 20 randomized trials comparing light treatment with placebo in the treatment of SAD. Some of these trials have found a benefit; others have been unable to demonstrate a benefit over placebo.
- Phototherapy for SAD tends to use 2500 to 10,000 lux delivered via a commercial light box or a portable head-mounted unit. Phototherapy is recommended to commence within 2 wk of the start of symptoms and to continue through the winter months. Patients are instructed to sit approximately 18 inches away from the light box for 30 min up to several hours once or twice per day for a minimum of 1 wk.
- One study suggests that cognitive-behavioral therapy plus light therapy may improve short-term remission rates over light therapy alone.

ACUTE GENERAL Rx

None necessary unless patient is suicidal.

CHRONIC Rx

There is some evidence from randomized trials to support the use of selective serotonin reuptake inhibitors (SSRIs) in the treatment of SAD.

DISPOSITION

Psychiatric referral may be helpful to confirm diagnosis. Recommended for high-risk and suicidal patients.

REFERRAL

For active suicidal ideation, psychosis, symptoms suggestive of bipolar disorder

PEARLS & CONSIDERATIONS

Patients with SAD may present with a complaint of overeating, particularly food high in carbohydrates.

EVIDENCE

Light Therapy (Phototherapy)
A small randomized controlled trial compared light-box treatment with dawn simulation in patients with winter depression. Improvement in symptoms was noted in both groups, but there was significantly greater improvement in the light-box group. The majority of patients in both treatment groups maintained improvement at 9-week follow-up.[1] Ⓑ

SSRIs
A randomized controlled trial compared fluoxetine with placebo over 5 weeks in patients with SAD. The rate of clinical response (>50% reduction in depression score between baseline and study termination) was greater in the fluoxetine group.[2] Ⓑ

Evidence-Based References

1. Lingjaerde O et al: Dawn simulation vs. lightbox treatment in winter depression: a comparative study, *Acta Psychiatr Scand* 98:73, 1998. Ⓑ
2. Lam RW et al: Multicenter, placebo-controlled study of fluoxetine in seasonal affective disorder, *Am J Psychiatry* 152:1765, 1995. Ⓑ

SUGGESTED READINGS

Glickman G et al: Light therapy for seasonal affective disorder with blue narrow-band light-emitting diodes (LEDs), *Biol Psychiatry* 59(6):502, 2006.

Lam RW et al: The Can-SAD study: a randomized controlled trial of the effectiveness of light therapy and fluoxetine in patients with winter seasonal affective disorder, *Am J Psychiatry* 163(5):805, 2006.

Rohan KJ et al: A randomized controlled trial of cognitive-behavioral therapy, light therapy, and their combination for seasonal affective disorder, *J Consult Clin Psychol* 75(3):489, 2007.

AUTHOR: **MITCHELL D. FELDMAN, M.D., M.PHIL.**

BASIC INFORMATION

DEFINITION

Absence seizures are a common type of generalized onset seizure characterized by brief episodes of loss of awareness (typically 10 to 15 seconds) followed by abrupt return to full consciousness. They are associated with a classic EEG pattern of 3 Hz generalized spike and slow wave discharges.

SYNONYMS

Petit mal seizures (obsolete)
Childhood absence epilepsy

ICD-9CM CODES
345.0 Generalized nonconvulsive epilepsy

EPIDEMIOLOGY & DEMOGRAPHICS

INCIDENCE (IN U.S.): 11 cases/100,000 persons from ages 3 to 10 yr, rare after age 14 yr
PEAK INCIDENCE: 6 to 7 yr
PREVALENCE (IN U.S.): Accounts for 2% to 15% of the cases of childhood epilepsy
PREDOMINANT AGE: 4 to 8 yr but can persist into adulthood
GENETICS: Clear genetic predisposition; undetermined mode of inheritance

PHYSICAL FINDINGS & CLINICAL PRESENTATION

- Findings are normal between seizures in children with typical absence epilepsy.
- During the seizure, patients typically appear awake but have sudden behavioral arrest typically lasting less than 30 seconds followed by immediate resumption of activity.
- There may be associated automatisms and therefore can be mistaken for complex partial seizures.
- Tonic-clonic seizures can occur in approximately 40% of patients.

ETIOLOGY

- Idiopathic with a presumed genetic cause
- Absence seizures are most commonly seen in childhood absence epilepsy with onset between age 4 and 8 but can also be seen with other idiopathic generalized epilepsy syndromes such as juvenile absence epilepsy or juvenile myoclonic epilepsy where onset is later, generalized tonic-clonic seizures are more common, and seizures are less likely to spontaneously resolve with age.

DIAGNOSIS

DIFFERENTIAL DIAGNOSIS

- Complex partial seizures
- Daydreaming
- Psychogenic unresponsiveness

WORKUP

- EEG is the most powerful tool for identification of this seizure type.
- In the vast majority of untreated individuals, vigorous hyperventilation for 3-5 min will provoke a typical absence seizure.

IMAGING STUDIES

None needed for typical presentation

TREATMENT

NONPHARMACOLOGIC THERAPY

Avoid sleep deprivation and hyperventilation.

ACUTE GENERAL Rx

Not indicated for individual typical seizures

CHRONIC Rx

- Drug of choice is ethosuximide or valproate.
- Ethosuximide does not suppress tonic-clonic seizures. Thus, valproate is the drug of choice for patients with absence and tonic clonic seizures.
- In patients with child-bearing potential, valproate should be used with caution due to the high risk of teratogenicity.
- The initial dose of ethosuximide in children is 10 to 15 mg/kg/day with maintenance dose of 15 to 40 mg/kg/day divided into a bid or tid dosing schedule. Can result in gastrointestinal side-effects so may be best to take with meals.
- Common pediatric doses for valproate are 15 to 60 mg/kg/day (bid-qid). Can result in hepatotoxity and blood dyscrasias.
- Lamotrigine has been shown to be effective, but is not FDA approved for the treatment of absence seizures.
- Because most patients will have spontaneous resolution of their seizures, one can consider withdrawing anticonvulsant therapy when the patient has been seizure-free for at least 2 yr and EEG is normal.

DISPOSITION

- Favorable prognosis in typical childhood absence epilepsy without other seizure types
- Excellent response to medication
- Subsidence of seizures with advancing age in 70% to 90% of patients

REFERRAL

If uncertain about diagnosis or treatment

PEARLS & CONSIDERATIONS

COMMENTS

- Absence seizures may be mistakenly diagnosed as complex partial seizures based on clinical descriptions. The EEG is essential for making this distinction.
- Administering other anticonvulsants (particularly carbamazepine or phenytoin) to patients with typical absence epilepsy may exacerbate seizures.
- Patient education information can be obtained from the Epilepsy Foundation, 4351 Garden City Drive, Landover, MD 20785; phone: (800) 332-1000, web address: www.epilepsyfoundation.org.

EVIDENCE

A systematic review assessing the efficacy of valproate, ethosuximide, and lamotrigine in the treatment of absence seizures in children and adolescents found insufficient evidence to guide clinical practice due to the poor methodological quality of the included trials.[1]

A more recent review found lamotrigine to be effective for newly diagnosed absence seizures in children.[2]

Evidence-Based References

1. Posner EB, Mohamed K, Marson AG: Ethosuximide, sodium valproate or lamotrigine for absence seizures in children and adolescents, *Cochrane Database Syst Rev* 3, 2003.
2. French JA et al: Efficacy and tolerability of the new antiepileptic drugs I: treatment of new onset epilepsy, *Neurology* 62:1252, 2004.

SUGGESTED READINGS

Bourgeois BF: Chronic management of seizures in the syndromes of idiopathic generalized epilepsy, *Epilepsia* 44(2):27, 2003.
Mattson RH: Overview: idiopathic generalized epilepsies, *Epilepsia* 44(2):2, 2003.
Panayiotopoulos CP: Treatment of typical absence seizures and related epileptic syndromes, *Paediatr Drugs* 3(5):379, 2001.

AUTHORS: **JOHN E. CROOM, M.D., PH.D.,** and **SUZETTE LAROCHE, M.D.**

BASIC INFORMATION

DEFINITION
A febrile seizure is a seizure in infancy or childhood, usually occurring between 6 mo and 5 yr of age, associated with fever but without evidence of intracranial infection or defined cause.

SYNONYMS
Benign febrile seizure
Febrile convulsions

ICD-9CM CODES
780.3 Convulsions

EPIDEMIOLOGY & DEMOGRAPHICS
INCIDENCE (IN U.S.): Not reported
PREVALENCE (IN U.S.): 2% to 4% in children <5 yr of age
PREDOMINANT SEX: Male = female
PREDOMINANT AGE: 18 to 24 mo of age
GENETICS:
- Family history increases risk two- to threefold.
- Susceptibility genes have been identified, some with autosomal dominant inheritance pattern, others have complex inheritance.

PHYSICAL FINDINGS & CLINICAL PRESENTATION
- Typically occurs early in the course of an illness when temperature is rising.
- Most commonly associated with a viral upper respiratory or gastrointestinal infection.
- Febrile seizures can be either simple or complex.
- Simple febrile seizures are single events lacking focality and lasting less than 15 min. The children are neurologically normal and there are no persistent deficits following the seizure.
- Features of complex febrile seizures include: duration longer than 15 min, focal seizures, seizure recurrence within 24 hr, or abnormal neurologic examination. Children with complex febrile seizures are at greater risk of developing subsequent epilepsy.
- Physical and neurologic examination and developmental history are usually normal especially with simple febrile seizures.
- Rarely associated with a familial epilepsy syndrome called generalized epilepsy with febrile seizure plus (GEFS+) which includes other types of generalized onset seizures.

ETIOLOGY
Unknown

DIAGNOSIS

DIFFERENTIAL DIAGNOSIS
- Epilepsy
- Meningitis
- Encephalitis

WORKUP
- In children with simple febrile seizures, no further evaluation is usually required.
- In children with complex febrile seizures, more aggressive investigation is required.

LABORATORY TESTS
- Lumbar puncture is indicated in all children under 6 mo of age, in children with complex febrile seizures, or if signs or symptoms of meningitis are present.
- Complex febrile seizures may warrant EEG, toxicology screening, assessment of electrolytes, and so forth, depending on history and examination findings.

IMAGING STUDIES
- Not needed in simple febrile seizures
- Complex febrile seizures warrant head imaging studies

TREATMENT

NONPHARMACOLOGIC THERAPY
- Avoid excessive clothing.
- Encourage fluids.
- Apply tepid sponge bath to control fever.

ACUTE GENERAL Rx
- Antipyretics.
- For prolonged seizures, can use parenteral or rectal diazepam or lorazepam (parenteral only).
- Febrile status epilepticus should be treated as a medical emergency (see "Status Epilepticus" in Section I).

CHRONIC Rx
- Prophylactic treatment with anticonvulsants is not indicated in children with typical simple febrile seizures.
- Phenobarbital and valproate have each been shown to prevent recurrence of febrile seizures, but no drug has been shown to alter the subsequent risk of developing afebrile seizures or epilepsy. Due to the high rate of associated adverse drug effects and the generally benign nature of simple febrile seizures, neither drug is indicated for chronic prophylactic therapy.
- May consider anticonvulsant use in children with complex febrile seizures, but risks and benefits must be considered.

DISPOSITION
- Approximately one third of patients will experience additional febrile seizures. Less than 6% of patients will suffer three or more febrile seizures.
- Independent predictors of febrile seizure recurrence include: (1) young age at onset (particularly less than 1 yr of age), (2) history of first degree-relatives with febrile seizures, (3) low degree of fever while in the emergency room, and (4) brief interval between fever onset and seizure presentation.
- Risk of subsequent epilepsy is estimated at 1% to 2.5%. Risk of developing subsequent epilepsy is highest in children with complex febrile seizures and can be up to 13% to 50%.
- Available data: there is no risk reduction with prophylactic anticonvulsants.

REFERRAL
If uncertain about diagnosis or with atypical presentation

PEARLS & CONSIDERATIONS

COMMENTS
Febrile seizures typically occur early in the course of a fever. Often the febrile seizure occurs before the fever is noticed by the patient's caregivers, and the patient is only found to have a fever after the seizure has occurred.

CAUTION
A child who presents with a seizure after having been febrile for more than a day should be considered to have encephalitis until proven otherwise, and should undergo a workup for meningoencephalitis, including lumbar puncture.

EVIDENCE

EBM

Randomized controlled trials have found that in children with febrile seizures diazepam given during febrile illnesses, daily phenobarbital, and daily valproate are each effective at reducing the risk of recurrent febrile seizures. However, phenobarbital was not found to be effective at reducing the incidence of subsequent afebrile seizures or epilepsy in children with febrile seizures.[1-7] Data are lacking for other antiepileptic drugs.

Evidence-Based References

1. *N Engl J Med* 329:79-84, 1993.
2. *J Pediatr* 97:16-21, 1980.
3. *Lancet* 2:600-604, 1981.
4. *Neuropediatrics* 15:37-42, 1984.
5. *Arch Dis Child* 55:171-174, 1980.
6. *Pediatrics* 59:378-385, 1977.
7. *Acta Paediatr Scand* 78:291-295, 1989.

SUGGESTED READINGS

Baumann RJ: Prevention and management of febrile seizures, *Paediatr Drugs* 3(8):585, 2001.
Knudsen FU: Febrile seizures: treatment and prognosis, *Epilepsia* 41(1):2, 2000.
Shinnar S, Glauser TA: Febrile seizures, *J Child Neurol* 17(suppl 1):S44, 2002.
Waruiru C, Appleton R: Febrile seizures: an update, *Arch Dis Child* 89(8):751-756, 2004.

AUTHORS: **JOHN E. CROOM, M.D., PH.D.,** and **SUZETTE LAROCHE, M.D.**

BASIC INFORMATION

DEFINITION

Generalized onset seizures consist of paroxysmal hypersynchronous neuronal activity originating in both hemispheres simultaneously. Patients with generalized onset seizures are classified as having either idiopathic/primary generalized epilepsy or symptomatic generalized epilepsy based on seizure type, age of onset, neurological exam and EEG findings (Table 1-44).

SYNONYMS Grand mal seizure (obsolete), drop attacks

ICD-9-CM CODES
345.1 Generalized convulsive epilepsy

EPIDEMIOLOGY & DEMOGRAPHICS

INCIDENCE (IN U.S.): 10/100,000 persons/yr highest rates in childhood
PREVALENCE (IN U.S.): Approximately 6.5 cases/1000 persons for all types of epilepsy
GENETICS: Genetic predisposition

PHYSICAL FINDINGS & CLINICAL PRESENTATION

- Patients with idiopathic/primary generalized epilepsy have normal neurological exam between seizures.
- Lennox-Gastaut syndrome is the most common type of symptomatic generalized epilepsy; it is characterized by childhood onset, cognitive dysfunction, and the presence of multiple seizure types.
- Generalized onset seizure types include:
  - Tonic-clonic: Tonic stiffening then clonic movements of the extremities for 1 to 2 minutes, followed by postictal confusion
  - Tonic: Spasms of the trunk with flexion of the upper extremities, usually less than 1 minute duration
  - Clonic: Repetitive, rhythmic motor movements of the extremities
  - Atonic (drop attacks): Sudden loss of muscle tone and consciousness accompanied by falling
  - Myoclonic: Brief muscle jerk without loss of consciousness
  - Absence: Behavioral arrest and loss of awareness commonly accompanied by eye blinking lasting up to 30 seconds

ETIOLOGY

- Idiopathic epilepsies have no known underlying cause although a genetic predisposition has been established in many syndromes.
- Symptomatic generalized epilepsies can be caused by a variety of causes including perinatal injury, metabolic disorders, congenital brain malformations, and some genetic disorders including tuberous sclerosis.

DIAGNOSIS

DIFFERENTIAL DIAGNOSIS

- Syncope
- Sleep disorder
- Psychogenic or behavioral phenomena

WORKUP

EEG is extremely useful in distinguishing generalized onset seizures from focal onset seizures when history alone is unclear.

LABORATORY TESTS

- New onset seizures: Glucose, electrolytes and urine toxicology screen to exclude a provoked etiology
- Recurrent seizures: Antiepileptic drug levels

IMAGING STUDIES

MRI or CT aids in excluding a focal cause for seizures if diagnosis is not clear by history and EEG alone.

TREATMENT

NONPHARMACOLOGIC THERAPY

Medically refractory patients
- Vagus nerve stimulation.
- Corpus callosotomy can be performed as a palliative surgery in symptomatic generalized epilepsies.

ACUTE GENERAL Rx

- Individual seizures lasting <5 min require no acute pharmacologic intervention.
- Status epilepticus requiring urgent intervention is common in symptomatic generalized epilepsies.

CHRONIC Rx

- Therapeutic choices are more limited than for treatment of partial onset seizures and, in fact, some antiepileptic drugs, such as carbamazepine, may worsen myoclonic or absence seizures.
- Valproate, lamotrigine, topiramate, and levetiracetam are indicated as first-line antiepileptic drugs for the treatment of generalized onset seizures.

DISPOSITION

- Idiopathic generalized epilepsies may remit in childhood or can be easily controlled with medication in most cases.
- Symptomatic generalized epilepsies are usually difficult to control and require polytherapy.

REFERRAL

Refer to neurologist or epilepsy specialist if diagnosis is uncertain or patient fails to respond to therapy. Female patients considering pregnancy should also have evaluation and management by a specialist.

PEARLS & CONSIDERATIONS

COMMENTS

Generalized onset generalized tonic-clonic seizures can be impossible to differentiate from partial onset generalized tonic-clonic seizures by history and/or visual inspection alone.

EVIDENCE

Lamotrigine and topiramate have been found to be effective for the treatment of seizures associated with symptomatic generalized epilepsy such as Lennox-Gastaut.[1]

Topiramate and more recently lamotrigine and levetiracetam have been found to be effective for treatment of generalized tonic-clonic seizures seen in primary generalized epilepsy.[1-4]

Evidence-Based References

1. *Neurology* 62:1261-1273, 2004.
2. *Neurology* 65:1737-1743, 2005.
3. *Pediatrics* 118:371-378, 2006.
4. *Neurology* 69:1751-1760, 2007.

SUGGESTED READINGS

Neurologic Clinics 19:251, 2001.
J Child Neurol 17(suppl 1):S70, 2002.

AUTHOR: **SUZETTE M. LAROCHE, M.D.**

TABLE 1-44 **Classification of Generalized Onset Seizures**

	Idiopathic/Primary Epilepsy	Symptomatic Epilepsy
Examples of syndromes	Childhood absence, juvenile absence, juvenile myoclonic	Lennox-Gastaut, progressive myoclonic epilepsy
Major seizure types	GTC, myoclonic, absence	GTC, tonic, atonic, clonic, atypical absence
MRI	Normal	Normal or diffuse or focal abnormalities
EEG	Generalized epileptiform discharges, background normal	Generalized epileptiform discharges, background slow
Exam	Normal	Cognitive dysfunction in most patients
Prognosis	Good, may remit after childhood (varies by syndrome)	Poor

GTC, Generalized tonic-clonic.

BASIC INFORMATION

DEFINITION

In partial onset seizures, abnormal electrical activity originates in a focal region or lobe of the brain but may spread rapidly to the entire brain. There are three types of partial onset seizures: simple partial (consciousness preserved), complex partial (consciousness impaired), and secondary generalized tonic-clonic seizures.

SYNONYMS

Focal epilepsy
Localization-related seizures

ICD-9CM CODES
345.4 Partial epilepsy, with impairment of consciousness
345.5 Partial epilepsy, without impairment of consciousness

EPIDEMIOLOGY & DEMOGRAPHICS

INCIDENCE (IN U.S.): 20 cases/100,000 persons through age 65 yr, then rises sharply
PREVALENCE (IN U.S.): 6.5 cases/1000 persons for all types of epilepsy
RISK FACTORS: History of congenital abnormalities, febrile seizures, central nervous system (CNS) infection, head trauma, stroke, or family history of epilepsy
GENETICS: Predominantly acquired

PHYSICAL FINDINGS & CLINICAL PRESENTATION

- Clinical presentation is varied and depends on the site of origin of the abnormal electrical discharges.
- Symptoms of simple partial seizures can include focal motor or sensory symptoms; language disturbance; olfactory, visual, or auditory hallucinations; visceral sensation, fear, or panic.
- With complex partial seizures, there is a loss or reduction of awareness. This may be preceded by an aura (simple partial seizure). There may be associated automatisms or alterations in behavior.
- Secondarily generalized tonic-clonic seizures may be preceded by symptoms of a simple or complex partial seizure or may present with tonic followed by clonic activity from the onset.
- Post-ictal confusion and/or fatigue is common after complex partial seizures as well as secondarily generalized tonic-clonic seizures.
- Benign partial epilepsy of childhood is also known as *rolandic epilepsy*. This epilepsy syndrome is a common type of partial motor epilepsy in childhood, most often affecting males between age 5 and 8. The seizures typically occur during sleep, with the child often awakening with one side of the face twitching. An EEG may reveal centrotemporal (Fig. 1-243) or midtemporal spike discharges. Neurologic studies

A

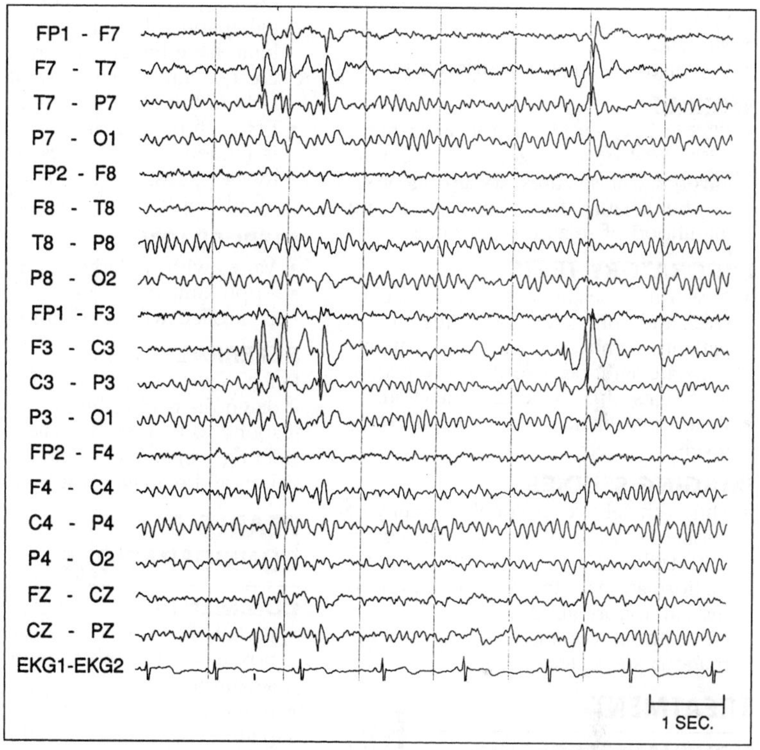

B

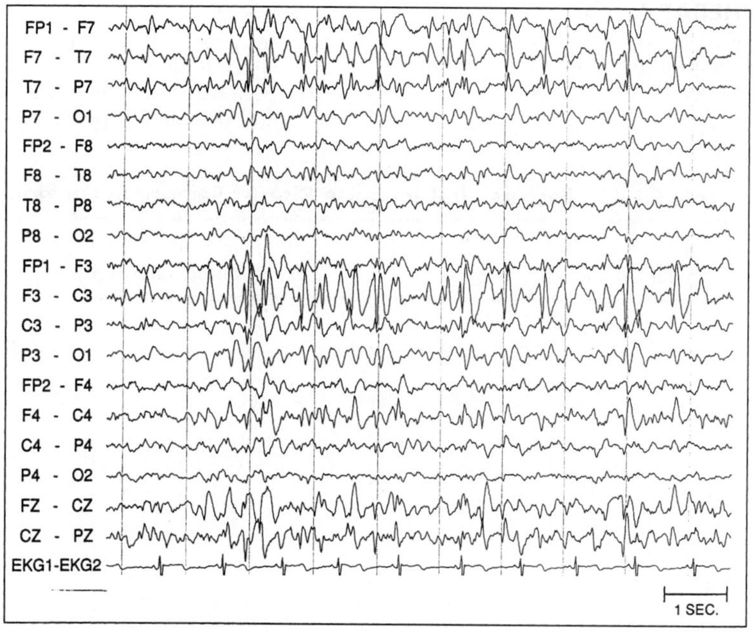

FIGURE 1-243 Benign rolandic epilepsy. Electroencephalograms (EEGs) from a 9-year-old boy with a history of nocturnal generalized tonic-clonic seizures that responded well to antiepileptic drugs. **A,** EEG from the awake background with several sharp waves in the left centrotemporal region. This distribution is typical for benign rolandic epilepsy, but it is not diagnostic for rolandic epilepsy, because other entities such as structural lesions can present with similar spiking. If the clinical history is appropriate, however, the best clinical correlation of these waveforms would be rolandic epilepsy. **B,** There is significant activation of the EEG spiking in sleep. The discharges are often quite continuous. The patients are usually asymptomatic at this time. This fascinating disorder may have a genetic component, and is almost always resolved by the age of 16. If seizures occur they can include simple partial motor seizures of the lower face and generalized tonic-clonic seizures. (From Rosenberg RN: *Atlas of clinical neurology,* Boston, 1998, Butterworth-Heinemann.)

usually do not reveal any abnormalities to correlate with the EEG abnormality. Most seizure episodes remit when the child is around 10 to 12 years of age and almost always by age 16.

ETIOLOGY

- Partial onset seizures may be caused by underlying disorders including stroke, tumor, infection, trauma, or vascular malformations.
- In 65% of patients, there is no cause identified (cryptogenic).

DIAGNOSIS

Dx

DIFFERENTIAL DIAGNOSIS

- Transient ischemic attack (TIA)
- Syncope
- Migraine
- Psychiatric (conversion disorder)

WORKUP

- EEG is a powerful tool for differentiating partial onset seizures from generalized onset seizures, localizing onset of the seizure focus and predicting likelihood of seizure recurrence.

LABORATORY TESTS

- New onset seizures: Glucose, electrolytes, and urine toxicology screen for all patients; lumbar puncture for patients who are HIV positive and any patient with signs of possible CNS infection.
- Recurrent seizures: Antiepileptic drug levels.

IMAGING STUDIES

- MRI with seizure protocol: modality of choice because of its high sensitivity for stroke, tumor, abscess, vascular malformations, and subtle developmental abnormalities.
- CT without contrast if acute hemorrhage is suspected.

TREATMENT

Rx

NONPHARMACOLOGIC THERAPY

Medically refractory patients

- Surgical resection of the seizure focus
- Vagus nerve stimulation

ACUTE GENERAL Rx

- Individual seizures lasting <5 min require no acute pharmacologic intervention.
- See "Status Epilepticus" for management of recurrent or prolonged seizures.

CHRONIC Rx

- Treatment is indicated if there is a significant risk of recurrence (Table 1-45) or the patient has experienced more than one unprovoked seizure.
- Phenytoin, carbamazepine, and valproate are traditional therapeutic agents but are limited by drug interactions and side effects.
- Newer agents such as lamotrigine, topiramate, oxcarbazepine, zonisamide, gabapentin, levetiracetam, and pregabalin have fewer drug interactions and are generally better tolerated, particularly in the elderly population.
- For each patient, anticonvulsant choice is influenced by factors such as effectiveness, cost, adverse effects, and ease of administration.

DISPOSITION

- Varies with underlying etiology.
- Approximately 70% of patients are controlled with medications.

REFERRAL

Refer to neurologist or epilepsy specialist if diagnosis is uncertain or patient fails to respond to therapy. Female patients considering pregnancy should also have evaluation and management by a specialist.

PEARLS & CONSIDERATIONS

!

COMMENTS

- Partial onset is the most underdiagnosed, yet the most common, type of seizure in adults.
- Initial EEG is normal in up to 50% of patients with epilepsy; thus diagnosis is primarily based on history.
- Partial onset generalized tonic-clonic seizures and generalized onset generalized tonic-clonic seizures can be impossible to differentiate by history and/or visual inspection alone.

PATIENT/FAMILY EDUCATION

Information is available from the Epilepsy Foundation of America, 4351 Garden City Drive, Landover, MD 20785; phone: (800) 332-1000; website: www.epilepsyfoundation.org.

EVIDENCE

EBM

Phenobarbital, phenytoin, primidone, carbamazepine and valproate have been found to be equally efficacious in the treatment of partial onset seizures.[1,2]

Lamotrigine, topiramate, gabapentin, oxcarbazepine, zonisamide, levetiracetam, and tiagabine have each been found to be effective as adjunctive treatment for refractory, partial onset seizures.[3] Ⓐ

Lamotrigine, topiramate, and oxcarbazepine have been found to be as effective as monotherapy in refractory or new onset epilepsy.[4] Ⓐ

Gabapentin has been found to be effective as monotherapy in new onset epilepsy.[4] Ⓐ

In a large, multicenter study of seizures in the elderly population, both lamotrigine and gabapentin were found to be better tolerated than carbamazepine, but there was no significant difference in efficacy.[5]

Evidence-Based References

1. *N Engl J Med* 313:145, 1985.
2. *N Engl J Med* 327:765, 1992.
3. *Neurology* 62:1261, 2004.
4. *Neurology* 62:1252, 2004.
5. *Neurology* 64:1868, 2005.

SUGGESTED READINGS

American College of Emergency Physicians (ACEP) Clinical Policies Committee and the Clinical Policies Subcommittee on Seizures: Clinical policy: critical issues in the evaluation of adult patients presenting to an emergency department with seizures, *Ann Emer Med* 43:605, 2004.

Browne TR, Holmes GL: Epilepsy, *N Engl J Med* 344:1145, 2001.

Chang BS, Lowenstein DH: Mechanisms of disease: epilepsy, *N Engl J Med* 349:1257, 2003.

AUTHOR: **SUZETTE M. LAROCHE, M.D.**

TABLE 1-45 **Factors That Increase Risk of Seizure Recurrence**

Epileptiform activity on EEG	Abnormal neurological exam
Structural brain lesions	Family history of epilepsy

BASIC INFORMATION

DEFINITION

Septicemia is a systemic illness caused by generalized bacterial or fungal infection and characterized by evidence of infection, fever or hypothermia, hypotension, and evidence of end-organ compromise.

SYNONYMS

Sepsis
Sepsis syndrome
Severe sepsis
Systemic inflammatory response syndrome
Septic shock

ICD-9CM CODES
038.9 Sepsis
038.40 Sepsis, gram-negative bacteremia
038.1 Sepsis, *Staphylococcus*

EPIDEMIOLOGY & DEMOGRAPHICS

INCIDENCE (IN U.S.):
- Exact incidence is unknown
- Approximately 750,000 cases of severe sepsis occur among hospitalized patients each year in the U.S.
- Complicates a minority of bacteremia cases and may occur in the absence of documented bacteremia

PREDOMINANT SEX: Males slightly more commonly affected than females
PREDOMINANT AGE:
- Neonatal period
- Patients >65 yr of age account for 60% of all cases of severe sepsis

GENETICS:
Familial Disposition: A great variety of congenital immunodeficiency states and other inherited disorders may predispose to septicemia.
Neonatal Infection: Incidence is high in neonatal period.

PHYSICAL FINDINGS & CLINICAL PRESENTATION

- Fever or hypothermia
- Hypotension
- Tachycardia
- Tachypnea
- Altered mental status
- Bleeding diathesis
- Skin rashes
- Symptoms that reflect primary site of infection: urinary tract, GI tract, CNS, respiratory tract

ETIOLOGY

- Disseminated infection with a great variety of bacteria:
  A. Gram-negative bacteria
    1. *E. coli*
    2. *Klebsiella* spp.
    3. *Pseudomonas aeruginosa*
    4. *Proteus* spp.
    5. *Neisseria meningitidis*
  B. Gram-positive bacteria
    1. *Staphylococcus aureus*
    2. *Streptococcus* spp.
    3. *Enterococcus* spp.
- Less common infections:
  1. Fungal
  2. Viral
  3. Rickettsial
  4. Parasitic
- Activation of coagulation, inflammatory cytokines, complement, and kinin cascades with release of a variety of vasoactive endogenous mediators
- Predisposing host factors:
  1. General medical condition
  2. Age
  3. Immunosuppressive therapy
  4. Recent surgery
  5. Granulocytopenia
  6. Hyposplenism
  7. Diabetes
  8. Instrumentation

DIAGNOSIS

DIFFERENTIAL DIAGNOSIS

- Cardiogenic shock
- Acute pancreatitis
- Pulmonary embolism
- Systemic vasculitis
- Toxic ingestion
- Exposure-induced hypothermia
- Fulminant hepatic failure
- Collagen-vascular diseases

WORKUP

- Evaluation should focus on identifying a specific pathogen and localizing the site of primary infection.
- Hemodynamic, metabolic, coagulation disorders should be carefully characterized.
- Intensive monitoring, including the use of central venous or Swan-Ganz catheters, may be necessary.

LABORATORY TESTS

- Cultures of blood and examination and culture of sputum, urine, wound drainage, stool, CSF
- CBC with differential, coagulation profile
- Routine chemistries, LFTs
- ABGs, lactic acid level; Procalcitonin might be useful as a general marker of infection/sepsis
- Urinalysis

IMAGING STUDIES

- Chest x-ray examination
- Other radiographic and radioisotope procedures according to suspected site of primary infection

TREATMENT

NONPHARMACOLOGIC THERAPY

- Tissue oxygenation: mixed venous oxygen saturation maintained >70% if possible; early mechanical ventilation
- Focal infection drained, if possible

ACUTE GENERAL Rx

- Blood pressure support, rapid intravenous fluid resuscitation and vasopressors, if needed, with the goal of reestablishing a mean arterial blood pressure >65 mmHg; reduction in blood lactate and mixed venous oxygen saturation >70% within 6 hr of recognition of septic shock is associated with improved survival
  1. IV hydration; crystalloids are as effective as colloids as resuscitation fluids
  2. Therapy with pressors (e.g., dopamine, norepinephrine, vasopressin) if mean blood pressure of 70 to 75 mm Hg cannot be maintained by hydration alone
- Correction of acidosis by improving the tissue perfusion, not by giving bicarbonate
  1. Mechanical ventilation
- Antibiotics
  1. Directed at the most likely sources of infection
  2. Should generally provide broad coverage of gram-positive and gram-negative bacteria (or fungi if clinically indicated)
  3. Typical regimens:
     a. For hospital-acquired sepsis (pending culture results): vancomycin plus cefepime, imipenem, aztreonam, quinolones, or an aminoglycoside. Monotherapy with appropriate agents appears to be as effective as combination therapy in immunocompetent hosts.
     b. For community-acquired infection in the absence of granulocytopenia: above or single-drug therapy with third-generation cephalosporin.
     c. For infection in the granulocytopenic host: above or dual gram-negative coverage (e.g., cephalosporin and aminoglycoside).
  4. Biological treatment Drotrecogin alfa (Xigris), a genetically engineered form of activated protein C, is approved for use in patients with severe sepsis with multiorgan dysfunction (or APACHE II score >24); when combined with conventional therapy, there may be a reduction in mortality.

5. The role of corticosteroids in the acute management of septicemia has long been debated. Although most well-constructed clinical trials have demonstrated no benefit, recent data suggest that patients with relative adrenal insufficiency may benefit from low-dose therapy with hydrocortisone (50 mg IV q6h) and fludrocortisone (50 microgram daily PO) given together for 7 days. Recent data suggest that physiologic doses of corticosteroids with subsequent tapering may improve survival in some patients without proven adrenal insufficiency.

CHRONIC Rx

- Adjust antibiotic therapy on the basis of culture results.
- In general, continue therapy for a minimum of 2 wk.

DISPOSITION

All patients with suspected septicemia should be hospitalized and given access to intensive monitoring and nursing care.

REFERRAL

- To infectious diseases expert
- To physician experienced in critical care

PEARLS & CONSIDERATIONS

COMMENTS

Mortality rises quickly if antibiotic therapy is not instituted promptly and metabolic derangements are not treated aggressively.

EVIDENCE

EBM

A systematic review of 15 trials found corticosteroids did not change 28-day all-cause mortality or hospital mortality in patients with severe sepsis and septic shock. However, there was some evidence of reduction in intensive care unit mortality and an increase in the proportion of shock reversal by days 7 and 28.[1] Ⓐ

A randomized controlled trial (RCT) compared low-dose corticosteroids (hydrocortisone and fludrocortisone) vs. placebo in patients with septic shock and relative adrenal insufficiency. There was a significantly lower risk of death over 28 days in the treatment group.[2] Ⓑ

Early goal-directed therapy provides significant benefits in patients with septic shock. An RCT compared early goal-directed therapy (in which cardiac output was adjusted to balance oxygen delivery with oxygen demand) vs. standard therapy during the first 6 hr of ER admission in patients with septic shock. In-hospital mortality was significantly lower in the patients who received early goal-directed therapy, and during the period from 7 to 72 hr, these patients had more rapid hemodynamic and oxygenization improvement than standard care.[3] Ⓑ

Evidence-Based References

1. Annane D et al: Corticosteroids for treating severe sepsis and septic shock, *Cochrane Database Syst Rev* 1, 2004. Ⓐ
2. Annane D et al: Effect of treatment with low doses of hydrocortisone and fludrocortisone on mortality in patients with septic shock, *JAMA* 288:862, 2002. Ⓑ
3. Rivers E et al: Early goal-directed therapy in the treatment of severe sepsis and septic shock, *N Engl J Med* 345:1368, 2001. Ⓑ

SUGGESTED READINGS

Calandra T, Cohen J: The international sepsis forum consensus conference on definitions of infection in the intensive care unit, *Crit Care Med* 33(7):1538, 2005.

Hackman DG et al: Statins and sepsis in patients with cardiovascular disease: a population-based cohort analysis, *Lancet* 367(9508):413, 2006.

Johnson SB et al: Gene expression profiles differentiate between sterile SIRS and early sepsis, *Ann Surg* 245(4):611, 2007.

Uzzan B et al: Procalcitonin as a diagnostic test for sepsis in critically ill patients and after surgery and trauma: a systemic review and meta-analysis, *Crit Care Med* 34(7): 1996, 2006.

AUTHORS: **GLENN G. FORT, M.D., M.P.H., STEVEN M. OPAL, M.D.,** and **JOSEPH R. MASCI, M.D.**

BASIC INFORMATION

DEFINITION

Serotonin syndrome (SS) refers to a group of symptoms resulting from increased activity of serotonin (5-hydroxytryptamine) in the central nervous system. Serotonin syndrome is a drug-induced disorder that is characterized by a change in mental status and alteration in neuromuscular activity and autonomic function.

SYNONYMS

SS

ICD-9CM CODES
333.99 Syndrome serotonin

EPIDEMIOLOGY & DEMOGRAPHICS

- The incidence of serotonin syndrome is not known.
- Serotonin syndrome is seen in all age groups, from neonates to elderly.
- Serotonin syndrome commonly occurs in patients receiving two or more serotonergic drugs.
- Concomitant use of a selective serotonin reuptake inhibitor (SSRI) with a monoamine oxidase inhibitor (MAOI) poses the greatest risk of developing SS.
- Combination of SSRIs with other serotonergic drugs (e.g., tryptophan) or drugs with serotonin properties (e.g., lithium, meperidine) can also lead to SS.

PHYSICAL FINDINGS & CLINICAL PRESENTATION

- Findings of clonus with hyperreflexia in the setting of recent (<5 wk) use of serotonergic agents strongly suggests the diagnosis of serotonin syndrome.
- Symptoms can manifest within minutes to hours after starting a new psychopharmacologic treatment or after administering a second serotonergic drug.
- Clonus (inducible, spontaneous, and ocular) is the key finding in establishing a diagnosis of serotonin syndrome.
- Other pertinent findings include:
  - Confusion, agitation, hypomania
  - Fever >38° C (100° F), tachycardia, and tachypnea
  - Nausea, vomiting, abdominal pain, and diaphoresis
  - Diarrhea, tremors, shivering, and seizures
  - Hyperreflexia and muscle rigidity

ETIOLOGY

- Hyperstimulation of the brainstem and spinal cord serotonin receptors because of blocking reuptake of serotonin and catecholamines leading to the neuromuscular and autonomic symptoms.
- Psychopharmacologic drugs—in particular, fluoxetine and sertraline coadministered with MAOI (e.g., tranylcypromine and phenelzine)—have been cited in the literature as a common cause of SS.

DIAGNOSIS

- The diagnosis of SS is made on clinical grounds. There are no specific laboratory tests for SS. A high index of suspicion along with a detailed medication history is the mainstay of diagnosis.
- Diagnostic criteria: most accurate is Hunter Serotonin Toxicity Criteria (sensitivity 84%, specificity 97%).
- To fulfill Hunter criteria a patient must have consumed a serotonergic drug and should have one of the following:
  1. Spontaneous clonus
  2. Inducible clonus plus agitation or diaphoresis
  3. Ocular clonus plus agitation or diaphoresis
  4. Tremor and hyperreflexia
  5. Temperature above 38° C (100° F) plus clonus or inducible clonus

DIFFERENTIAL DIAGNOSIS

- Neuroleptic malignant syndrome (NMS), substance abuse (e.g., cocaine, amphetamines), thyroid storm, infection, alcohol and opioid withdrawal.
- Classic features in differentiation of NMS vs. SS are that SS develops over 24 hr, involves neuromuscular hyperactivity, and begins to resolve within 24 hr with appropriate therapy, whereas NMS develops gradually over days to weeks, involves sluggish neuromuscular response, and resolves over an average period of 1 week to 10 days.

WORKUP

- Because SS is a clinical diagnosis, there is no laboratory test that confirms the diagnosis and serum serotonin concentration does not correlate with clinical picture. Other causes are described in "Differential Diagnosis." Thus, all patients should have blood tests and diagnostic imaging studies to rule out infectious, toxic, and metabolic etiologies.
- Additional laboratory tests are performed to exclude complicating features of SS (e.g., renal failure secondary to rhabdomyolysis).

LABORATORY TESTS

- CBC with differential to rule out sepsis
- Electrolytes, BUN, and creatinine to rule out acidosis and renal failure
- Blood and urine toxicology screen
- Thyroid function tests
- Creatine-phosphokinase (CPK) with isoenzymes
- Urine and blood cultures
- ECG because ventricular rhythm disturbance is a potentially fatal complication

IMAGING STUDIES

Imaging studies are not very specific in the diagnosis of SS and are only ordered to exclude other causes with similar clinical presentations as SS.

TREATMENT

Once a diagnosis of SS is established, appropriate consultation with a medical toxicologist, clinical pharmacologist, and/or poison control center should be sought.

Management includes:

- Discontinue use of all potential precipitating drugs
- Provide supportive management
- Control agitation
- Administer serotonin antagonists
- Control autonomic instability
- Control hyperthermia
- Reassess the need to resume the use of the serotonergic agent once the symptoms have resolved

NONPHARMACOLOGIC THERAPY

- Discontinuation of the drug is the mainstay of therapy.
- Treatment is supportive: maintaining oxygenation and blood pressure and monitoring respiratory status. Hypotensive patients may require both intravenous fluids and vasopressor therapy.
- Patients who are severely hyperthermic with temperatures greater than 41° C (106° F) should be given intravenous sedation, paralyzed, and intubated. Cooling blankets can be used for patients with mild-moderate hyperthermia. There is no role of acetaminophen here.
- Mechanical intubation is recommended for patients unable to protect their airways as a result of mental status changes or seizures.

ACUTE GENERAL Rx

- Serotonin antagonists
  1. Cyproheptadine 4-mg tablet or 2 mg/5 ml syrup is given in 4- to 8-mg doses q1 to 4h (up to 32 mg for adults, 12 mg in children) until a therapeutic response is achieved.
  2. Atypical antipsychotic agents with serotonin antagonist properties (e.g., olanzapine 10 mg SL) have been tried with some success.
  3. Chlorpromazine 50 to 100 mg IM may be considered in severe cases.
- Benzodiazepines
  1. Lorazepam 1 to 2 mg IV q30 min has been used effectively in treating agitation, muscle rigidity, myoclonus, and seizure complications.
  2. Diazepam is an alternative choice.

3. Blood pressure management with short-acting agents such as esmolol and nitroprusside.

CHRONIC Rx

For patients not requiring hospital admission, cyproheptadine and lorazepam can be given in an oral dose on a prn basis with close follow-up.

DISPOSITION

- Serotonin syndrome is a potentially life-threatening condition if not recognized early.
- Prompt diagnosis and withdrawal of the medication results in improvement of symptoms within 24 hr.
- Seizures, rhabdomyolysis, hyperthermia, ventricular arrhythmia, respiratory arrest, and coma are all complicating features of SS.

REFERRAL

All cases of SS secondary to psychotropic medications should be referred to a psychiatrist.

PREVENTION

Modify prescription practices by avoiding multidrug regimens.

PEARLS & CONSIDERATIONS

The combined use of SSRIs and MAOIs is contraindicated.

COMMENTS

- The use of SSRIs and other serotonergic agents is not an absolute contraindication; however, prompt withdrawal of the medication is recommended if any symptoms suggesting SS occur.
- Serotonin syndrome is usually found in patients being treated for depression, bipolar disorders, obsessive-compulsive disorder, attention-deficit disorder, and Parkinson's disease.

SUGGESTED READINGS

Boyer EW, Shannon M: The serotonin syndrome, *N Engl J Med* 352:1112-1120, 2005.

Dunkley EJ et al: The Hunter Serotonin Toxicity Criteria: simple and accurate diagnostic decision rules for serotonin toxicity, *QJM* 96:635, 2003.

AUTHOR: **PURVA AGARWAL, M.D.**

BASIC INFORMATION

DEFINITION

Severe acute respiratory syndrome (SARS) is a respiratory illness caused by a coronavirus called SARS-associated coronavirus (SARS-CoV).

CLINICAL CRITERIA:

A. Asymptomatic or mild respiratory illness

B. Moderate respiratory illness

1. Temperature of >100.4° F (>38° C),* and
2. One or more clinical findings of respiratory illness (e.g., cough, shortness of breath, difficulty breathing, or hypoxia)

C. Severe respiratory illness

1. Temperature of >100.4° F (>38° C)*, and
2. One or more clinical findings of respiratory illness (e.g., cough, shortness of breath, difficulty breathing, or hypoxia), and
   a. Radiographic evidence of pneumonia, or
   b. Respiratory distress syndrome, or
   c. Autopsy findings consistent with pneumonia or respiratory distress syndrome without an identifiable cause

EPIDEMIOLOGIC CRITERIA:

- Travel (including transit in an airport) within 10 days of onset of symptoms to an area with current or previously documented or suspected community transmission of SARS, or
- Close contact† within 10 days of onset of symptoms with a person known or suspected to have SARS
- The Chinese horseshoe bat, which is a healthy carrier of SARS, has been identified as the reservoir of the virus in nature. The spread of the virus was facilitated by people eating bats or using bat feces in traditional medicine for asthma, kidney ailments, and general malaise

Laboratory criteria

- Confirmed
  1. Detection of antibody to SARS-associated coronavirus (SARS-CoV) in a serum sample, or
  2. Detection of SARS-CoV RNA by RT-PCR confirmed by a second PCR assay, by using a second aliquot of the specimen and a different set of PCR primers, or
  3. Isolation of SARS-CoV
- Negative
  1. Absence of antibody to SARS-CoV in a convalescent-phase serum sample obtained >28 days after symptom onset‡
- Undetermined
  1. Laboratory testing either not performed or incomplete

Case classification§

- Probable case: meets the clinical criteria for severe respiratory illness of unknown etiology and epidemiologic criteria for exposure; laboratory criteria confirmed or undetermined.
- Suspect case: meets the clinical criteria for moderate respiratory illness of unknown etiology, and epidemiologic criteria for exposure; laboratory criteria confirmed or undetermined.

Exclusion criteria

A case may be excluded as a suspect or probable SARS case if:

- An alternative diagnosis can fully explain the illness.||
- The case has a convalescent-phase serum sample (i.e., obtained >28 days after symptom onset) that is negative for antibody to SARS-CoV.‡
- The case was reported on the basis of contact with an index case that was subsequently excluded as a case of SARS, provided other possible epidemiologic exposure criteria are not present.

SYNONYMS

SARS

ICD-9CM CODES
Not available

EPIDEMIOLOGY & DEMOGRAPHICS

- The disease was first recognized in Asia in February 2003, and over the next several months spread to more than 2 dozen countries in North and South America, Europe, and Asia affecting more than 8000 patients and resulting in more than 750 deaths. In July 2003, cases were no longer being reported, and SARS outbreaks worldwide were considered contained.
- Most reported cases of SARS in the United States were exposed through foreign travel to countries with community transmission of SARS, with only limited secondary spread to close contacts such as family members and health care workers.
- Incubation period is 2 to 10 days.
- Evidence of airborne transmission of the SARS virus and laboratory-acquired SARS has now been documented.

PHYSICAL FINDINGS & CLINICAL PRESENTATION

- Early manifestations: fever, myalgias and headache. Fever is often high and associated with chills or rigors. Fever may be absent in elderly patients.

*A measured documented temperature of >100.4° F (>38° C) is preferred. However, clinical judgment should be used when evaluating patients for whom a measured temperature of >100.4° F (>38° C) has not been documented. Factors that might be considered include patient self-report of fever, use of antipyretics, presence of immunocompromising conditions or therapies, lack of access to health care, or inability to obtain a measured temperature. Reporting authorities should consider these factors when classifying patients who do not strictly meet the clinical criteria for this case definition.

†Close contact is defined as having cared for or lived with a person known to have SARS or having a high likelihood of direct contact with respiratory secretions and/or body fluids of a patient known to have SARS. Examples of close contact include kissing or embracing, sharing eating or drinking utensils, close conversation (<3 ft), physical examination, and any other direct physical contact between persons. Close contact does not include activities such as walking by a person or sitting across a waiting room or office for a brief period.

‡The WHO has specified that the surveillance period for China should begin on November 1; the first recognized cases in Hong Kong, Singapore, and Hanoi (Vietnam) had onset in February 2003. The date for Toronto is linked to the occurrence of a laboratory confirmed case of SARS in a U.S. resident who had traveled to Toronto; the date for Taiwan is linked to CDC's issuance of travel recommendations.

§The last date for illness onset is 10 days (i.e., one incubation period) after removal of a CDC travel alert. The case patient's travel should have occurred on or before the last date the travel alert was in place.

Assays for the laboratory diagnosis of SARS-CoV infection include enzyme-linked immunosorbent assay, indirect fluorescent-antibody assay, and reverse transcription polymerase chain reaction (RT-PCR) assays of appropriately collected clinical specimens (Source: CDC. Guidelines for collection of specimens from potential cases of SARS. Available at http://www.cdc.gov/ncidod/sars/specimen_collection_sars2.htm). Absence of SARS-CoV antibody from serum obtained <28 days after illness onset,‡ a negative PCR test, or a negative viral culture does not exclude SARS-CoV infection and is not considered a definitive laboratory result. In these instances, a convalescent serum sample obtained >28 days after illness is needed to determine infection with SARS-CoV.‡ All SARS diagnostic assays are under evaluation.

‡Does not apply to serum samples collected before July 11, 2003. Testing results from serum samples collected before July 11, 2003, and between 22 and 28 days after symptom onset are acceptable and will not require collection of an additional sample >28 days after symptom onset.

§Asymptomatic SARS-CoV infection or clinical manifestations other than respiratory illness might be identified as more is learned about SARS-CoV infection.

||Factors that may be considered in assigning alternate diagnoses include the strength of the epidemiologic exposure criteria for SARS, the specificity of the diagnostic test, and the compatibility of the clinical presentation and course of illness for the alternative diagnosis.

- Dry nonproductive cough occurs within 2 to 4 days of onset of fever.
- Diarrhea may occur in up to 25% of cases.
- Dyspnea and hypoxemia follow the cough and may require intubation in nearly 20% of patients.
- A biphasic course of illness may occur with initial improvement followed by subsequent deterioration in some patients.

ETIOLOGY

SARS-associated coronavirus

DIAGNOSIS (Dx)

DIFFERENTIAL DIAGNOSIS

- Legionella pneumonia
- Influenza A and B
- Respiratory syncytial virus
- Acute respiratory distress syndrome (ARDS)

WORKUP

- Initial diagnostic testing for suspected SARS patients should include chest radiograph, pulse oximetry, blood cultures, sputum Gram's stain and culture, and testing for viral respiratory pathogens, notably influenza A and B and respiratory syncytial virus. A specimen for Legionella and pneumococcal urinary antigen testing should also be considered.

LABORATORY TESTS

When to test for SARS:

- In the absence of documented SARS transmission, diagnostic testing for SARS-associated coronavirus (SARS-CoV) should *not* be considered unless the clinician and health department have a high index of suspicion for SARS (e.g., a hospitalized pneumonia patient has a possible SARS exposure during travel and no other explanation for their pneumonia).
- Respiratory specimens should be collected as soon as possible in the course of the illness. The likelihood of recovering most viruses diminishes markedly >72 hours after symptom onset.
- Three types of specimens may be collected for viral or bacterial isolation and PCR. These include (1) nasopharyngeal wash/aspirates, (2) nasopharyngeal swabs, or (3) oropharyngeal swabs. Nasopharyngeal aspirates are the specimen of choice for detection of respiratory viruses and are the preferred collection method among children aged <2 yr.
- Laboratory testing on initial evaluation should also include CBC with differential, platelet count, liver enzymes, LDH, and CPK. Common laboratory abnormalities in SARS include thrombocytopenia, lymphopenia, elevated LDH, and elevated CPK, ALT, AST.

IMAGING STUDIES

- Chest x-ray: patchy focal infiltrates or consolidation with peripheral distribution.
- Chest x-ray may be normal in up to 25% of patients.
- Pleural effusions generally are not present.

TREATMENT (Rx)

NONPHARMACOLOGIC THERAPY

- Supportive care.
- Nearly 25% of cases will require ventilator assistance.
- Nutritional support.

ACUTE GENERAL Rx

- There is no specific treatment currently available for SARS.
- Broad-spectrum antibiotics (quinolone or macrolide) are generally started pending laboratory testing.
- Use of corticosteroids (methylprednisolone 40 mg bid or doses up to 2 mg/kg/day) is controversial but may be beneficial in patients with significant hypoxemia and progressive pulmonary infiltrates.
- In a preliminary, uncontrolled study of patients with SARS, use of interferon alfacon-1 plus corticosteroids was beneficial.

DISPOSITION

- Case fatality rate is 3% to 12%.
- Mortality rate is higher in elderly and immunocompromised patients and lower in pediatric age group.

REFERRAL

- Infectious disease consultation and pulmonary consultation is recommended in all cases.
- Notification of state Department of Health is mandatory.

PEARLS & CONSIDERATIONS (!)

COMMENTS

- Persons who may have been exposed to SARS should be vigilant for fever (i.e., measure temperature twice daily) and respiratory symptoms over the 10 days after exposure. During this time, in the absence of both fever and respiratory symptoms, persons who may have been exposed to SARS patients need not limit their activities outside the home and should not be excluded from work, school, out-of-home child care, church, or other public areas.
- Exposed persons should notify their health care provider immediately if fever or respiratory symptoms develop.
- Symptomatic persons exposed to SARS should follow the following infection control precautions:
    1. If fever or respiratory symptoms develop, the person should limit interactions outside the home and not go to work, school, out-of-home child care, church, or other public areas. In addition, the person should use infection control precautions in the home to minimize the risk for transmission, and continue to measure temperature twice daily.
    2. If symptoms improve or resolve within 72 hr after first symptom onset, the person may be allowed, after consultation with local public health authorities, to return to work, school, out-of-home child care, church, or other public areas, and infection control precautions can be discontinued.
    3. For persons who meet or progress to meet the case definition for suspected SARS (e.g., develop fever and respiratory symptoms), infection control precautions should be continued until 10 days after the resolution of fever, provided respiratory symptoms are absent or improving.
    4. If the illness does not progress to meet the case definition, but the individual has persistent fever or unresolving respiratory symptoms, infection control precautions should be continued for an additional 72 hr, at the end of which time a clinical evaluation should be performed. If the illness progresses to meet the case definition, infection control precautions should be continued as described earlier. If case definition criteria are not met, infection control precautions can be discontinued after consultation with local public health authorities and the evaluating clinician.
- Persons who meet or progress to meet the case definition for suspected SARS (e.g., develop fever and respiratory symptoms) or whose illness does not meet the case definition, but who have persistent fever or unresolving respiratory symptoms over the 72 hr after onset of symptoms should be tested for SARS coronavirus infection.

SUGGESTED READINGS

Lim PL et al: Laboratory-acquired SARS, *N Engl J Med* 350:1740, 2004.

Poutanen SM et al: Identification of severe acute respiratory syndrome in Canada, *N Engl J Med* 348:20, 2004.

Yu, IT et al: Evidence of airborne transmission of SARS virus, *N Engl J Med* 350:1731, 2004.

AUTHOR: **FRED F. FERRI, M.D.**

BASIC INFORMATION

DEFINITION

Any disorder that interferes with female sexuality and causes marked distress to that person.

Generally categorized into four types:

1. Disorders of desire
2. Disorders of arousal
3. Orgasmic disorders
4. Sexual pain disorders (includes dyspareunia, vaginismus, vulvodynia)

SYNONYMS

Female sexual dysfunction (FSD)

ICD-9CM CODES
302.70 Decreased libido
302.72 Disorders of arousal
302.73 Orgasmic disorders
625.x Sexual pain disorders

EPIDEMIOLOGY & DEMOGRAPHICS

According to the National Health and Social Life Survey (1999), approximately 20% to 50% of women report some form of sexual dysfunction in their lifetime. One third of women report a decrease in sexual interest and one fourth report inability to achieve orgasm.

PHYSICAL FINDINGS & CLINICAL PRESENTATION

- History:
  - Important to obtain the patient's definition of dysfunction including onset, duration, determination if dysfunction is situational vs. global, and if more than one dysfunction exists and the interrelationship of these dysfunctions
  - Related medical and gynecologic conditions
  - Psychosocial factors including sexual abuse, sexual orientation, depression/anxiety
  - Current medications
- Physical examination: external genitalia, vaginal vault, uterus/adenexa, rectovaginal, as well as other body systems (as indicated)

ETIOLOGY

- Chronic medical conditions (diabetes, coronary vascular disease, arthritis, urinary incontinence)
- Medication induced (e.g., antihypertensives, SSRIs)
- Gynecologic conditions (cystitis, posthysterectomy), gynecologic cancers, breast cancer (both femininity/self-image issues and/or postchemotherapy), postpregnancy, postmenopausal
- Psychosocial (religion, taboos, identity conflicts, guilt, relationship problems, abuse/rape, life stressors)

DIAGNOSIS

DIFFERENTIAL DIAGNOSIS

- Depression
- Psychosocial stressors
- Medical disease

LABORATORY TESTS

- Cervical cultures and vaginal swabs for infectious disease, pap smear
- Appropriate laboratory tests if comorbid or chronic disease is suspected

IMAGING STUDIES

Appropriate imaging studies if comorbid or chronic disease is suspected

TREATMENT

NONPHARMACOLOGIC THERAPY

- Education
- Activities to enhance stimulation and eliminate routine
- Distraction techniques
- Noncoital behavior
- Position changes (e.g., female astride)
- Lubricants (non-petroleum based)

ACUTE GENERAL Rx

NSAIDs before intercourse for sexual pain disorders

CHRONIC Rx

- Treat underlying medical, gynecologic, or psychologic condition.
- Reduce comorbidities.
- Medication induced: decrease dose or change medication.
- Postmenopausal women/hypoestrogenism: ERT +/− progesterone.
- Testosterone therapy (controversial).
- Sildenafil (controversial).
- Behavioral therapy.

REFERRAL

- Gynecologic referral for conditions that may be amenable to surgical therapy
- Psychologic conditions (e.g., depression, abuse) that may benefit from counseling for psychotherapy
- Social services referrals for active abuse issues

PEARLS & CONSIDERATIONS

COMMENTS

Identify the earliest cause in the chain and treat first.

PATIENT/FAMILY EDUCATION

When appropriate, involve patient's partner or significant other in treatment.

SUGGESTED READINGS

Basson R et al: Report of the International Consensus Development Conference on Female Sexual Dysfunction: definitions and classifications, *J Urology* 163(3): 888-893, 2000.

Laumann EO et al: Sexual dysfunction in the United States: prevalence and predictors, *JAMA* 281:537-544, 1999.

Phillips NA: Female sexual dysfunction: evaluation and treatment, *Am Fam Physician* 62(1):127-136, 2000.

AUTHOR: **ANNGENE A. GIUSTOZZI, M.D., M.P.H.**

BASIC INFORMATION

DEFINITION

Sheehan's syndrome is a state of hypopituitarism resulting from an infarct of the pituitary secondary to postpartum hemorrhage or shock, causing partial or complete loss of the anterior pituitary hormones (i.e., ACTH, FSH, LH, GH, PRL, TSH) and their target organ functions.

ICD-9CM CODES
253.2 Sheehan's syndrome

EPIDEMIOLOGY & DEMOGRAPHICS

INCIDENCE: 1 case/10,000 deliveries (perhaps more rare in the U.S.)
PREDOMINANT SEX: Affects only females
RISK FACTORS:
- Hypovolemic shock
- Type I (insulin-dependent) diabetes mellitus (secondary to microvascular disease)
- Sickle cell anemia (secondary to occlusion of the small vessels in the pituitary)

ONSET OF SYMPTOMS: Average delay of 5 to 7 yr between onset of symptoms and diagnosis of disease.

PHYSICAL FINDINGS & CLINICAL PRESENTATION

- Failure of lactation
- Infertility
- Failure to resume menses after delivery
- Failure to regrow shaved pubic or axillary hair
- Skin depigmentation (including areola)
- Rapid breast involution
- Superinvolution of the uterus
- Hypothyroidism
- Adrenal cortical insufficiency
- Diabetes insipidus (rare)

ETIOLOGY

- Compromise of the blood supply to the low-pressure pituitary sinusoidal system may occur with postpartum hemorrhage or shock, resulting in pituitary infarct and/or necrosis.
- It is hypothesized that locally released factors may mediate vascular spasm of the pituitary blood supply.
- Severity of postpartum hemorrhage does not always correlate with the presence of Sheehan's syndrome.

DIAGNOSIS

DIFFERENTIAL DIAGNOSIS

- Chronic infections
- HIV
- Sarcoidosis
- Amyloidosis
- Rheumatoid disease
- Hemochromatosis
- Metastatic carcinoma
- Lymphocytic hypophysitis

WORKUP

- Target gland deficiency should be investigated by measuring levels of ACTH, FSH, LH, TSH (which may be normal or low), and T_4. Cortisol and estradiol (which may be low) should also be measured.
- Provocative testing of pituitary hormone reserves (e.g., metyrapone test, insulin tolerance test, and cosyntropin test): normal, subnormal, or delayed responses may suggest the presence of islands of pituitary cells that no longer have the support of the hypothalamic-portal circulation.
- Measurement of IGF-I to screen for GH deficiency: subnormal levels suggest decreased GH.
- Impaired prolactin response to TRH or dopamine antagonist stimulation is frequently found.
- During pregnancy, adjustments must be made in interpreting both hormone levels and responses to various stimuli because of normal physiologic changes.

IMAGING STUDIES

- Study of choice: MRI of the pituitary
  1. Sella turcica partially or totally empty
  2. Rules out mass lesion
- CT scan of the pituitary when MRI is unavailable or contraindicated

TREATMENT

ACUTE GENERAL Rx

- Acute form can be lethal, presenting with hypotension, tachycardia, failure to lactate, and hypoglycemia.
- A high degree of suspicion is required with any woman who has undergone postpartum hemorrhage and shock.
- Intravenous corticosteroids and fluid replacement should be given initially.
- Diagnosis is confirmed with a full endocrinologic workup as noted previously.
- Thyroid hormone is replaced as l-thyroxin in doses of 0.1 to 0.2 mg qd.

CHRONIC Rx

- With late-onset disease (symptoms of general hypopituitarism, such as oligomenorrhea or amenorrhea, vaginal atrophic changes, and loss of libido): a full endocrinologic workup and replacement of the appropriate hormones are needed.
- With symptoms of adrenal insufficiency: corticosteroids should be given.
  1. A maintenance dose of cortisone acetate or prednisone may be given.
  2. Because adrenal production of cortisol is not entirely dependent on ACTH, replacement of mineralocorticoids is rarely necessary.
  3. Stress doses of glucocorticoids should be administered during surgery or during labor and delivery.

DISPOSITION

Patients who receive early diagnosis and adequate hormonal replacement may expect favorable outcomes, including subsequent pregnancy.

REFERRAL

Patients should have yearly examinations by endocrinologist.

SUGGESTED READING

Kovacs K: Sheehan's syndrome, *Lancet* 361(9356):520, 2003.

AUTHORS: **BETH J. WUTZ, M.D.**, and **RUBEN ALVERO, M.D.**

BASIC INFORMATION

DEFINITION

Shigellosis is an inflammatory disease of the bowel caused by one of several species of *Shigella*. It is the most common cause of bacillary dysentery in the U.S.

SYNONYMS

Bacillary dysentery

ICD-9CM CODES
004.9 Shigellosis

EPIDEMIOLOGY & DEMOGRAPHICS

INCIDENCE (IN U.S.): Approximately 15,000 cases/yr
PREDOMINANT SEX: Male homosexuals at increased risk
PREDOMINANT AGE: Young children
PEAK INCIDENCE: Summer
GENETICS:
Neonatal Infection: Rare but severe

PHYSICAL FINDINGS & CLINICAL PRESENTATION

- Possibly asymptomatic, but incubation period can range from 1 to 7 days with an average of 3 days
- Mild illness that is usually self-limited, resolving in a few days
- Fever
- Watery diarrhea
- Bloody diarrhea
- Dysentery (abdominal cramps, tenesmus, and numerous, small-volume stools with blood, mucus, and pus)
- Descending intestinal tract illness, reflecting infection of small bowel first and then the colon
- Severe disease is more common in children and elderly and outside of U.S.
- Complications of severe illness:
  1. Seizures
  2. Megacolon
  3. Intestinal perforation
  4. Death
- Extraintestinal manifestations are rare
- Bacteremia is more common in children; in adults it has been described in patients with AIDS, the elderly, and diabetics
- Hemolytic-uremic syndrome (HUS): usually occurs as the initial illness seems to be resolving
- Reactive arthritis, sometimes as part of Reiter's syndrome

ETIOLOGY

- *Shigella*
  1. *S. flexneri*
  2. *S. dysenteriae*
  3. *S. sonnei*
  4. *S. boydii*
- *S. sonnei* is the most commonly isolated species in the U.S., and it usually causes a mild watery diarrhea.
- Direct person-to-person transmission is thought to be the most common route. Outbreaks among men who have sex with men have occurred because of direct or indirect oral-anal contact.
- Contaminated food or water may transmit disease.
- A recent outbreak occurred at a community wading pool frequented by toddlers.

DIAGNOSIS

DIFFERENTIAL DIAGNOSIS

- May mimic any bacterial or viral gastroenteritis
- Dysentery also caused by *Entamoeba histolytica*
- Bloody diarrhea may resemble disease caused by enterotoxigenic *E. coli*

LABORATORY TESTS

- Total WBCs may be low, normal, or high. Leukemoid reactions can occur in children.
- Stool should be cultured from fresh samples, because the yield is increased by processing the specimen soon after passage. The best yield is from the mucoid part of the stool.
- Serology is available but rarely useful.
- Polymerase chain reaction may be diagnostic.
- Fecal leukocyte preparation may show WBCs.

IMAGING STUDIES

Abdominal radiographs may suggest megacolon or perforation in rare, severe cases.

TREATMENT

NONPHARMACOLOGIC THERAPY

- Adequate hydration
- Electrolyte replacement

ACUTE GENERAL Rx

Antibiotics:
- To shorten course of illness.
- To limit transmission of illness.
- For children: IV ceftriaxone (50 mg/kg/day) for severe disease. For oral therapy, can use SMX/TMP or ampicillin for 5 days for susceptible strains. Azithromycin can be used for 5 days when susceptibilities still not known or in areas of high resistance (12 mg/kg for the first day, then 6 mg/kg/day for 4 days).
- For adults: Pending susceptibilities, ciprofloxacin 500 mg PO bid for 5 days should be used. If susceptible, can also use SMX/TMP one DS PO bid for 5 days. Azithromycin is a second alternative.

DISPOSITION

- Most disease is self-limited.
- Severe illness may be fatal.

REFERRAL

For severe illness or complications

PEARLS & CONSIDERATIONS

COMMENTS

- *Shigella* is one cause of "gay bowel syndrome."
- Illness is worsened by agents that decrease intestinal motility.
- Food handlers, child-care providers, and health care workers should have a negative stool culture documented following treatment.

SUGGESTED READINGS

Ashkenazi S: Shigella infections in children: new insights, *Semin Pediatr Infect Dis* 15(4):246, 2004.

Ekdahl K, Andersson Y: The epidemiology of travel-associated shigellosis—regional risks, seasonality and serogroups, *J Infect* 51(3): 222, 2005.

Taylor DN et al: Rifaximin, a nonabsorbed oral antibiotic, prevents shigellosis after experimental challenge, *Clin Infect Dis* 42(9):1283, 2006.

AUTHORS: **GLENN G. FORT, M.D., M.P.H., DENNIS J. MIKOLICH, M.D.,** and **MAURICE POLICAR, M.D.**

BASIC INFORMATION

DEFINITION

Short bowel syndrome is a malabsorption syndrome that results from extensive small intestinal resection.

SYNONYMS

Short bowel

ICD-9CM CODES
579.3 (postsurgical malabsorption)

EPIDEMIOLOGY & DEMOGRAPHICS

- Parallels Crohn's disease (see "Crohn's Disease" in Section I), which is the most common cause of the syndrome in adults
- In children, two thirds of short bowels are related to congenital abnormalities (intestinal atresia, gastroschisis, volvulus, aganglionosis) and one third are related to necrotizing enterocolitis
- Prevalence: 10,000 to 20,000 cases are estimated to exist in the U.S.

PHYSICAL FINDINGS & CLINICAL PRESENTATION

- Diarrhea and steatorrhea
- Weight loss
- Anemia related to iron or vitamin B_{12} absorption
- Bleeding diathesis related to vitamin K malabsorption
- Osteoporosis/osteomalacia related to vitamin D and calcium malabsorption
- Hyponatremia, hypokalemia
- Hypovolemia
- Other macronutrient or micronutrient deficiency states

ETIOLOGY

- Extensive bowel resection for treatment of the conditions mentioned previously (see "Epidemiology").
- Pathogenesis (Fig. 1-244).

The human intestine is 3 to 8 m in length. Removal of up to one half of the small intestine produces no disruption in nutrient absorption, and most patients can maintain nutritional balance on oral feeding if they have more than 100 cm (3 ft) of jejunum. Similarly, 100 cm of intact jejunum can maintain a normal water, sodium, and potassium balance under normal circumstances. The presence of an intact colon can compensate for some small intestine loss.

Site-specific functions:
- Calcium, magnesium, phosphorus, iron, and vitamins are absorbed in the duodenum and proximal jejunum.
- Vitamin B_{12} and bile acids are absorbed in the ileum. The resection of more than 60 cm of ileum results in vitamin B_{12} malabsorption. The loss of more than 100 cm results in fat malabsorption (from the loss of bile acids).
- The loss of gastrointestinal endocrine hormones can affect intestinal motility.
- Intestinal bacterial overgrowth may also occur, especially if the ileocecal valve is lost.

DIAGNOSIS

Presence of macronutrient and/or micronutrient loss in a patient with a known history of bowel resection

DIFFERENTIAL DIAGNOSIS

Because the history of significant bowel resection is typically known, there is no differential diagnosis. If that history is not known, all causes of weight loss, malabsorption, and diarrhea must be considered (see respective chapters).

TREATMENT

Extensive small bowel resection with colectomy (<100 cm of jejunum)
- Rx: long-term parenteral nutrition (TPN). Some patients can switch to oral intake after 1 to 2 yr of TPN. In jejunostomy patients, excessive fluid loss can be reduced with H_2 blockers, proton pump inhibitors, or octreotide. Micronutrients are supplemented.

Extensive small bowel resection with partial colectomy (usually patients with Crohn's disease)
- Rx: oral intake alone is possible in all patients with >100 cm of jejunum. In addition to vitamin B_{12} deficiency, these patients often have diarrhea. Consider lactose malabsorption and bacterial overgrowth treated, respectively, with lactose restriction and antibiotics (tetracycline 250 mg tid or metronidazole 500 mg tid for 2 wk). Nonspecific antidiarrheal agents may also be indicated (e.g., Imodium or codeine). The patient must be monitored for micronutrient losses.

COMPLICATIONS

- Oxalate kidney stones
- Cholesterol gallstones
- D-Lactic acidosis

PROGNOSIS

Directly dependent on the extent of the bowel resection and in the case of Crohn's disease by the underlying illness

AUTHORS: **FRED F. FERRI, M.D.,** and **TOM J. WACHTEL, M.D.**

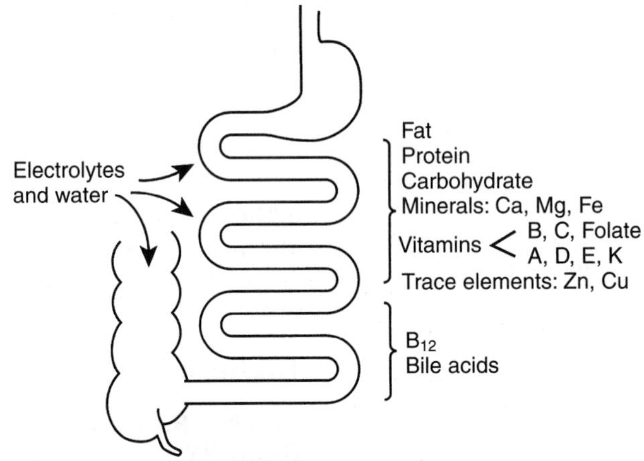

FIGURE 1-244 Specific areas of absorption of constituents of diet and secretions in the gastrointestinal tract. Macronutrients and micronutrients are predominantly absorbed in the proximal jejunum. Bile acids and vitamin B_{12} are only absorbed in the ileum. Electrolytes and water are absorbed in both the small and the large intestine. (From Feldman M, Scharschmidt BF, Sleisenger MH [eds]: *Sleisenger and Fordtran's gastrointestinal and liver disease: pathophysiology, diagnosis, and management,* ed 6, Philadelphia, 1998, WB Saunders.)

BASIC INFORMATION

DEFINITION

Sialadenitis is an inflammation of the salivary glands.

ICD-9CM CODES
527.2 Sialadenitis

EPIDEMIOLOGY & DEMOGRAPHICS

Parotid or submandibular glands are most frequently affected (Fig. 1-245).

PHYSICAL FINDINGS & CLINICAL PRESENTATION

- Pain and swelling of the affected salivary gland
- Increased pain with meals
- Erythema, tenderness at the duct opening
- Purulent discharge from duct orifice
- Induration and pitting of the skin with involvement of the masseteric and submandibular spatial planes in severe cases

ETIOLOGY

- Ductal obstruction is generally secondary to a mucus plug caused by stasis of saliva with increased viscosity with subsequent stasis and infection.
- Most frequent infecting organisms are *Staphylococcus aureus, Pseudomonas, Enterobacter, Klebsiella, Enterococcus, Proteus,* and *Candida* spp.
- Sjögren's syndrome, trauma, radiation therapy, chemotherapy, dehydration, and chronic illness are predisposing factors.

DIAGNOSIS

DIFFERENTIAL DIAGNOSIS

- Salivary gland neoplasm
- Ductal stricture
- Sialolithiasis
- Decreased salivary secretion secondary to medications (e.g., amitriptyline, diphenhydramine, anticholinergics)

WORKUP

- Generally not necessary
- Ultrasound or CT scan in patients not responding to medical treatment (see "Imaging Studies")

LABORATORY TESTS

- Generally not indicated
- CBC with differential to possibly reveal leukocytosis with left shift

IMAGING STUDIES

- Ultrasound or CT scan may be needed in patients not responding to medical therapy.
- Sialography should not be performed during the acute phase.

TREATMENT

NONPHARMACOLOGIC THERAPY

- Massage of the gland: may express pus and relieve some of the pressure
- Rehydration
- Warm compresses
- Oral cavity irrigations

ACUTE GENERAL Rx

- Amoxicillin-clavulanate 500 to 875 mg or cefuroxime 250 to 500 mg bid should be given for 10 days. Clindamycin is an alternative choice in patients allergic to penicillin.
- IV antibiotics (e.g., cefoxitin, nafcillin) can be given in severe cases.

DISPOSITION

Complete recovery unless the patient has underlying obstruction (e.g., ductal stricture, tumor, or stone)

REFERRAL

- To ENT for nonresolving cases despite appropriate antibiotic therapy
- For salivary gland incision and drainage, which may be necessary in resistant cases

PEARLS & CONSIDERATIONS

COMMENTS

Prevention of dehydration will decrease the risk of sialadenitis.

AUTHOR: **FRED F. FERRI, M.D.**

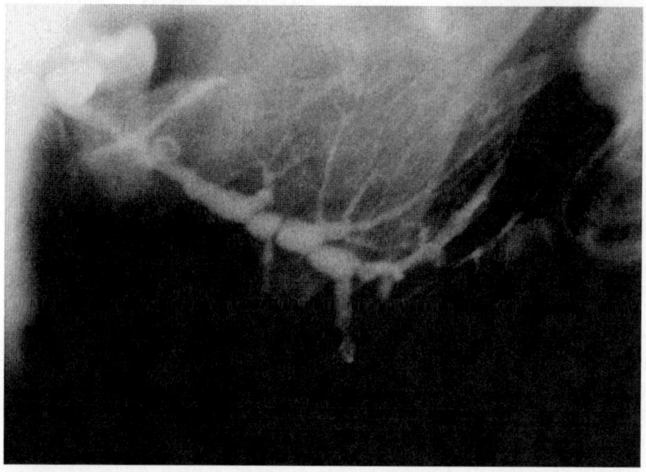

FIGURE 1-245 Sialogram of patient with chronic sialadenitis showing sausage link–like patterns and massive duct dilation. (From Blitzer CE, Lawson W, Reino A: Sialadenitis. In Johnson JT, Yu VL [eds]: *Infectious diseases and antimicrobial therapy of the ears, nose, and throat,* Philadelphia, 1997, WB Saunders.)

BASIC INFORMATION

DEFINITION

Sialolithiasis is the existence of hardened intraluminal deposits in the ductal system of a salivary gland.

SYNONYMS

Salivary gland stone
Salivary calculus

ICD-9CM CODES
527.5 Sialolithiasis

EPIDEMIOLOGY & DEMOGRAPHICS

Affects patients mostly in their fifth to eighth decade and occurs most commonly in the submandibular gland (80%); only 14% are located in a parotid gland.

PHYSICAL FINDINGS & CLINICAL PRESENTATION

- Symptoms: colicky postprandial pain and swelling of a salivary gland. Tends to have a remitting/relapsing course.
- Signs: swelling and tenderness of a salivary gland. The stone may be felt by palpation of the floor of the mouth (Fig. 1-246).

ETIOLOGY

- The cause is unknown. Contributing factors include saliva stagnation, sialadenitis (inflammation of a salivary gland), ductal inflammation or injury.
- Salivary calculus composition is mainly calcium phosphate and carbonate, often combined with small proportions of magnesium, zinc, ammonium salts, and organic materials/debris.

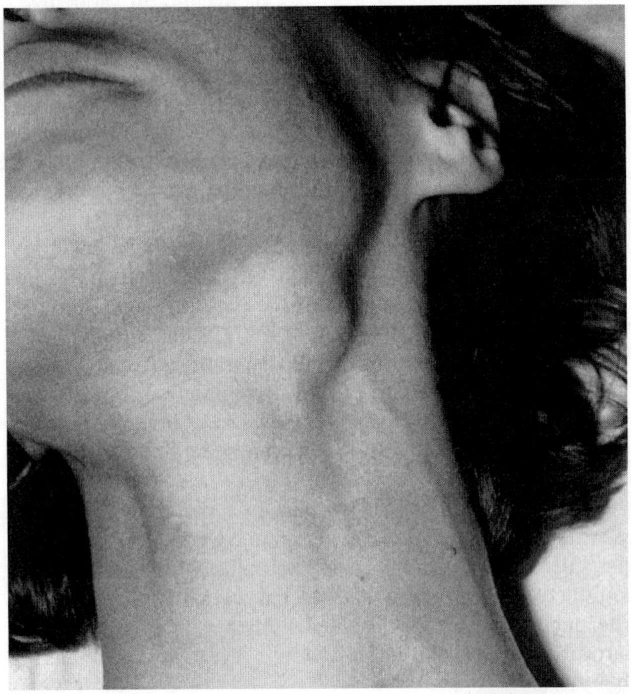

FIGURE 1-246 Patient with large calculus and obstruction of the left submandibular gland. (From Blitzer CE, Lawson W, Reino A: Sialadenitis. In Johnson JT, Yu VL [eds]: *Infectious diseases and antimicrobial therapy of the ears, nose, and throat,* Philadelphia, 1997, WB Saunders.)

DIAGNOSIS

DIFFERENTIAL DIAGNOSIS

- Lymphadenitis
- Salivary gland tumor
- Salivary gland bacterial *(Staphylococcus* or *Streptococcus),* viral (mumps), or fungal infection (sialadenitis)
- Noninfectious salivary gland inflammation (e.g., Sjögren's syndrome, sarcoidosis, lymphoma)
- Salivary duct stricture
- Dental abscess

IMAGING STUDIES

- Plain x-ray
- Sialography

TREATMENT

- Warm soaks to area
- Antibiotics if associated bacterial sialadenitis is present
- Bland diet—avoid citrus fruit and spices
- Manual stone extraction sometimes associated with incisional enlargement of the ductal orifice
- Surgical salivary gland removal for retained hilar calculi

REFERRAL

To otorhinolaryngologist

AUTHORS: **FRED F. FERRI, M.D.,** and **TOM J. WACHTEL, M.D.**

BASIC INFORMATION

DEFINITION

Sick sinus syndrome is a group of cardiac rhythm disturbances characterized by abnormalities of the sinus node including (1) sinus bradycardia, (2) sinus arrest or exit block, (3) combinations of sinoatrial or atrioventricular conduction defects, and (4) supraventricular tachyarrhythmias. These abnormalities may coexist in a single patient so that a patient may have episodes of bradycardia and episodes of tachycardia.

SYNONYMS

Bradycardia-tachycardia syndrome

ICD-9CM CODES
427.81 Sick sinus syndrome

EPIDEMIOLOGY & DEMOGRAPHICS

- In children: associated with congenital heart disease
- In adults: typically associated with ischemic heart disease but may occur in the presence of a normal heart

PHYSICAL FINDINGS & CLINICAL PRESENTATION

- Lightheadedness, dizziness, syncope, palpitation
- Arterial embolization (e.g., stroke) associated with atrial fibrillation
- Physical examination may be normal or reveal abnormalities (e.g., heart murmurs or gallop sounds) associated with the underlying heart disease

ETIOLOGY

- Fibrosis or fatty infiltration involving the sinus node, atrioventricular node, the His bundle, or its branches
- In addition, inflammatory or degenerative changes of the nerves and ganglia surrounding the sinus nodes and other sclerodegenerative changes may be found.

DIAGNOSIS

DIFFERENTIAL DIAGNOSIS

- Bradycardia: atrioventricular block
- Tachycardia: atrial fibrillation
- Atrial flutter
- Paroxysmal atrial tachycardia
- Sinus tachycardia
- Syncope (see "Syncope" in Section I)

WORKUP

- ECG
- Ambulatory cardiac rhythm monitoring
- 24-hour ambulatory ECG (Holter) (Fig. 1-247)
- Event recorder
- Electrophysiologic testing including sinus nodal recovery time and sino-atrial conduction time

TREATMENT

- Permanent pacemaker placement if symptoms are present
- The drug treatment of the tachycardia (e.g., with digitalis or calcium channel blockers) may worsen or bring out the bradycardia and become the reason for pacemaker requirement

REFERRAL

To cardiologist

AUTHORS: **FRED F. FERRI, M.D.**, and **TOM J. WACHTEL, M.D.**

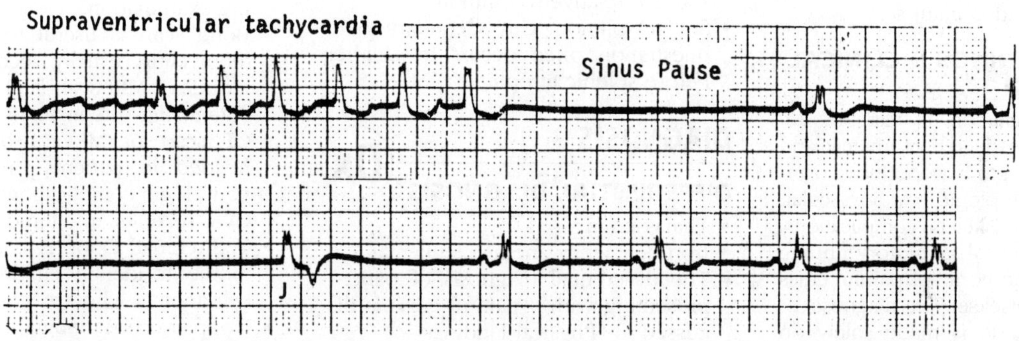

FIGURE 1-247 Brady-tachy (sick sinus) syndrome. This rhythm strip shows a narrow-complex tachycardia (probably atrial flutter) followed by a sinus pause, an AV junctional escape beat *(J)*, and then sinus rhythm. (From Goldberger AL: *Clinical electrocardiography,* ed 5, St Louis, 1994, Mosby.)

BASIC INFORMATION

DEFINITION

Sickle cell disease is a hemoglobinopathy characterized by the production of hemoglobin S caused by substitution of the amino acid valine for glutamic acid in the sixth position of the γ-globin chain. When exposed to lower oxygen tension, RBCs assume a sickle shape resulting in stasis of RBCs in capillaries. Painful crises are caused by ischemic tissue injury resulting from obstruction of blood flow produced by sickled erythrocytes.

SYNONYMS

Sickle cell anemia
Hemoglobin S disease

ICD-9CM CODES
286.60 Sickle cell anemia

EPIDEMIOLOGY & DEMOGRAPHICS

- Sickle cell hemoglobin S is transmitted by an autosomal recessive gene. It is found mostly in blacks (1 in 400 black Americans).
- Sickle cell trait occurs in nearly 10% of black Americans.
- There is no predominant sex.

PHYSICAL FINDINGS & CLINICAL PRESENTATION

- Physical examination is variable depending on the degree of anemia and presence of acute vasoocclusive syndromes or neurologic, cardiovascular, GU, and musculoskeletal complications.
- There is no clinical laboratory finding that is pathognomonic of painful crisis of sickle cell disease. The diagnosis of a painful episode is made solely on the basis of the medical therapy and physical examination.
- Bones are the most common site of pain. Dactylitis, or hand-foot syndrome (acute, painful swelling of the hands and feet), is the first manifestation of sickle cell disease in many infants. Irritability and refusal to walk are other common symptoms. After infancy, musculoskeletal pain can be symmetric, asymmetric, or migratory, and it may or may not be associated with swelling, low-grade fever, redness, or warmth.
- In both children and adults, sickle vasoocclusive episodes are difficult to distinguish from osteomyelitis, septic arthritis, synovitis, rheumatic fever, or gout.
- When abdominal or visceral pain is present, care should be taken to exclude sequestration syndromes (spleen, liver) or the possibility of an acute condition such as appendicitis, pancreatitis, cholecystitis, urinary tract infection, PID, or malignancy.
- Pneumonia develops during the course of 20% of painful events and can present as chest and abdominal pain. In adults chest pain may be a result of vasoocclusion in the ribs and often precedes a pulmonary event. The lower back is also a frequent site of painful crisis in adults.
- The "acute chest syndrome" manifests with chest pain, fever, wheezing, tachypnea, and cough. Chest x-ray reveals pulmonary infiltrates. Common causes include infection (mycoplasma, chlamydia, viruses), infarction, and fat embolism.
- Musculoskeletal and skin abnormalities seen in sickle cell anemia include leg ulcers (particularly on the malleoli) and limb-girdle deformities caused by avascular necrosis of the femoral and humeral heads.
- Endocrine abnormalities include delayed sexual maturation and late physical maturation, especially evident in boys.
- Neurologic abnormalities on examination may include seizures and altered mental status.
- Infections, particularly involving *Salmonella, Mycoplasma,* and *Streptococcus,* are relatively common.
- Severe splenomegaly secondary to sequestration often occurs in children before splenic atrophy.

DIAGNOSIS

DIFFERENTIAL DIAGNOSIS

- Thalassemia
- Iron deficiency anemia, leukemia
- The differential diagnosis of patients presenting with a painful crisis is discussed in "Physical Findings"

WORKUP

- Screening of all newborns regardless of racial background is recommended. Screening can be performed with sodium metabisulfite reduction test (Sickledex test).
- Hemoglobin electrophoresis will also confirm the diagnosis and is useful to identify hemoglobin variants such as fetal hemoglobin and hemoglobin A2.

LABORATORY TESTS

- Anemia (resulting from chronic hemolysis), reticulocytosis, leukocytosis, and thrombocytosis are common.
- Elevations of bilirubin and LDH are also common.
- Peripheral blood smear may reveal sickle cells, target cells, poikilocytosis, and hypochromia (Fig. 1-248).
- Elevated BUN and creatinine may be present in patients with progressive renal insufficiency.
- Urinalysis may reveal hematuria and proteinuria.

IMAGING STUDIES

- Chest x-ray is useful in patients presenting with "chest syndrome." Cardiomegaly may be present on chest x-ray examination.
- Bone scan is useful to rule out osteomyelitis (usually secondary to salmonella). MRI scan is also effective in diagnosing osteomyelitis.
- CT scan or MRI of brain is often needed in patients presenting with neurologic complications such as TIA, CVA, seizures, or altered mental status.
- Transcranial Doppler is a useful commodity to identify children with sickle cell anemia who are at risk for stroke.
- Doppler echocardiography can be used to diagnose pulmonary hypertension.

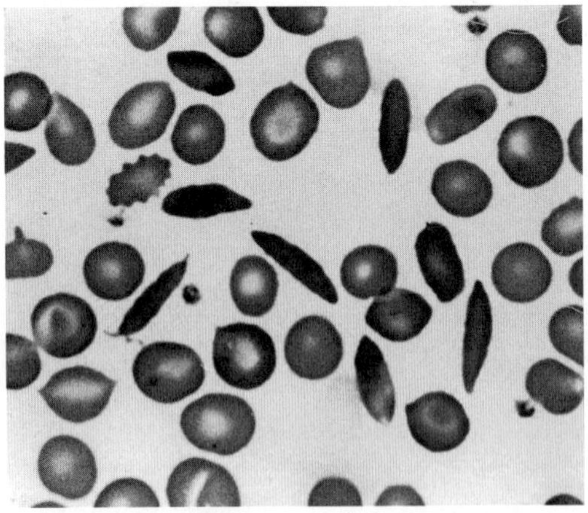

FIGURE 1-248 Photomicrograph of peripheral blood smear, sickle cells, typical of sickle cell anemia. (From Andreoli TE [ed]: *Cecil essential of medicine,* ed 4, Philadelphia, 1997, WB Saunders.)

TREATMENT

Rx

NONPHARMACOLOGIC THERAPY

- Patients should be instructed to avoid conditions that may precipitate sickling crisis, such as hypoxia, infections, acidosis, and dehydration.
- Maintain adequate hydration (PO or IV).
- Correct hypoxia.

ACUTE GENERAL Rx

- Aggressively diagnose and treat suspected infections (*Salmonella* osteomyelitis and pneumococcal infections occur more often in patients with sickle cell anemia because of splenic infarcts and atrophy). Combination therapy with a cephalosporin and erythromycin plus incentive spirometry and bronchodilators are useful in patients with acute chest syndrome.
- Provide pain relief during the vasoocclusive crisis. Medications should be administered on a fixed time schedule with a dosing interval that does not extend beyond the duration of the desired pharmacologic effect.
  1. Meperidine is contraindicated in patients with renal dysfunction or CNS disease because its metabolite, normeperidine (which is excreted by the kidneys) can cause seizures.
  2. Narcotics (e.g., morphine 0.1 mg/kg IV q3 to 4h or 0.3 mg/kg PO q4h) should be given on a fixed schedule (not prn for pain), with rescue dosing for breakthrough pain as needed.
  3. Except when contraindications exist, concomitant use of NSAIDs should be standard treatment.
  4. Nurses should be instructed not to give narcotics if the patient is heavily sedated or respirations are depressed.
  5. When the patient shows signs of improvement, narcotic drugs should be tapered gradually to prevent withdrawal syndrome. It is advisable to observe the patient on oral pain relief medications for 12 to 24 hr before discharge from the hospital.
  6. Analgesic medications should be used in combination with psychologic, behavioral, and physical modalities in the management of sickle cell disease.
- Aggressively diagnose and treat any potential complications (e.g., septic necrosis of the femoral head, priapism, bony infarcts, and acute "chest syndrome").
- Avoid "routine" transfusions but consider early transfusions for patients at high risk for complications. Indications for transfusion: aplastic crises, severe hemolytic crises (particularly during third trimester of pregnancy), acute chest syndrome, and high risk of stroke.
- Hydroxyurea (500 to 750 mg/day) increases hemoglobin F levels and reduces the incidence of vasoocclusive complications. It is generally well tolerated. Side effects consist primarily of mild reversible neutropenia.
- Replace folic acid (1 mg PO qd).

CHRONIC Rx

- Guidelines for prompt management of fever, infections, pain, and specific complications should be reviewed.
- Genetic counseling is recommended in all cases.
- Avoid unnecessary transfusions. Exchange transfusions may be necessary for patients with acute neurologic signs, in aplastic crisis, or undergoing surgery.
- Allogeneic stem cell transplantation can be curative in young patients with symptomatic sickle cell disease; however, the death rate from the procedure is nearly 10%, the marrow recipients are likely to be infertile, and there is an undefined risk of chemotherapy-induced malignancy.
- Penicillin V 125 mg PO bid should be administered by age 2 mo and increased to 250 mg bid by age 3. Penicillin prophylaxis can be discontinued after age 5 except in children who have had splenectomy.

REFERRAL

- Hospitalization is generally recommended for most crises and complications.
- Psychosocial counseling and support structures should be developed.

PEARLS & CONSIDERATIONS

!

COMMENTS

- Pain in adults with sickle cell disease is the rule rather than the exception and needs to be treated appropriately.
- Patients and their families should receive genetic counseling and should be made aware of the difference between sickle cell trait and sickle cell disease.
- Regular immunizations and pneumococcal vaccination are recommended. The prophylactic administration of penicillin soon after birth and the timely administration of pneumococcal and *H. influenzae* type b vaccines have resulted in a significant decline in the incidence of these infections. The heptavalent conjugated pneumococcal vaccine (Prevan) should be administered from 2 mo of age. The 23-valent unconjugated pneumococcal vaccine is given from age 2 and can be boosted once 3 yr later. Influenza vaccination can be given after 6 mo of age.
- Patients should be instructed on a well-balanced diet and appropriate folic acid supplementation.
- The presence of dactylitis, Hb 7, or leukocytosis in the absence of infection during the first 2 yr of life, indicates a higher risk of severe sickle cell disease later in life.
- Among patients with sickle cell disease, the acute chest syndrome is commonly precipitated by fat embolism and infection, especially community-acquired pneumonia. Among older patients and those with neurologic symptoms, the syndrome often progresses to respiratory failure.
- Poloxamer 188, a nonionic surfactant with hemorrheologic and antithrombotic properties, has been reported to produce a significant but relatively small decrease in the duration of painful episodes and an increase in the proportion of patients who achieved resolution of the symptoms. A more significant effect was observed in patients who received concomitant hydroxyurea.
- Pulmonary hypertension is a complication of chronic hemolysis and is associated with a high risk of death. It can be detected by Doppler echocardiography in over 30% of adult patients with sickle cell disease. Cardiac catheterization will confirm the diagnosis. It is resistant to hydroxyurea therapy.

EVIDENCE

EBM

There is some evidence for the effectiveness of specific analgesics or analgesic regimens in relieving the pain of a sickle cell crisis.

Oral controlled-release morphine has been shown to be as effective as intravenous morphine, after a loading dose of intravenous morphine, in children and adolescents.[1] Ⓐ

There is some evidence for the effectiveness of parenteral ketorolac, but the trials are generally small, some show conflicting results, and overall the evidence is insufficient.[2]

There is some evidence for the effectiveness of prophylactic penicillin in preventing pneumococcal infection in children with sickle cell disease.

Prophylactic penicillin significantly reduces the risk of pneumococcal infection, although the ideal age for safely withdrawing penicillin has not been established.[3] Ⓐ

There is evidence for the effectiveness of conjugate pneumococcal vaccines in preventing pneumococcal infection in people with sickle cell disease.

Conjugate pneumococcal vaccines are immunogenic and should be used in people with sickle cell disease.[4] Ⓐ

There is evidence for the effectiveness of hydroxyurea in the management of sickle cell disease in those with severe disease.

Hydroxyurea reduces the crisis rate, the use of transfusions, and the rate of life-threatening complications (in particular, the acute sickle chest syndrome).[5] Ⓐ

Available data refer to severely affected adults with sickle cell disease; further studies are needed to elucidate the role of hydroxyurea in other groups of sickle cell patients.[5]

There is some evidence for the use of blood transfusions for some indications in patients with sickle cell disease.

Aggressive preoperative blood transfusion is no more effective than a more conservative regimen, and the more conservative regimen is associated with fewer transfusion-related adverse events.[6] Ⓐ

However, further research is needed to identify the optimal regimen for different types of surgery and to address the question of whether preoperative transfusion is needed in all situations.[6]

There is insufficient evidence to draw firm conclusions about the prophylactic use of blood transfusion for pregnant women with sickle cell disease. Comparison of routine blood transfusion with a policy of selective transfusion shows that selective transfusion reduces the number of transfusions required, but at the expense of more frequent crises.[7] Ⓐ

There is evidence that long-term blood transfusion regimens prevent stroke in high-risk patients with sickle cell disease, but the benefits must be carefully weighed against the risks.[8] Ⓐ

Evidence-Based References

1. Jacobson SJ et al: Randomised trial of oral morphine for painful episodes of sickle-cell disease in children, *Lancet* 350:1358, 1997. Reviewed in: *Clin Evid* 10:21, 2003. Ⓐ
2. Meremikwu MM: Sickle cell disease. Reviewed in: *Clin Evid* 10:21, London, 2003, BMJ Publishing Group.
3. Riddington C, Owusu-Ofori S: Prophylactic antibiotics for preventing pneumococcal infection in children with sickle cell disease, *Cochrane Database Syst Rev* 3, 2002. Ⓐ
4. Davies EG et al: Pneumococcal vaccines for sickle cell disease, *Cochrane Database Syst Rev* 1, 2004. Ⓐ
5. Davies S, Olujohungbe A, Jones AP: Hydroxyurea for sickle cell disease, *Cochrane Database Syst Rev* 4, 2002. Ⓐ
6. Riddington C, Williamson L: Preoperative blood transfusions for sickle cell disease, *Cochrane Database Syst Rev* 3, 2001. Ⓐ
7. Mahomed K: Prophylactic versus selective blood transfusion for sickle cell anaemia during pregnancy, *Cochrane Database Syst Rev* 2, 1996. Ⓐ
8. Riddington C, Wang W: Blood transfusion for preventing stroke in people with sickle cell disease, *Cochrane Database Syst Rev* 1, 2002. Ⓐ

SUGGESTED READINGS

Gladwin MT et al: Pulmonary hypertension as a risk factor for death in patients with sickle cell disease, *N Engl J Med* 350:886, 2004.

Mehta S et al: Opportunities to improve outcomes in sickle cell disease, *Am Fam Physician* 74:303, 2006.

Orringer E et al: Purified poloxamer 188 for treatment of acute vaso-occlusive crisis of sickle cell disease, *JAMA* 286:2099, 2001.

Platt OS: Hydroxyurea for the treatment of sickle cell anemia, *N Engl J Med* 358:1362-1369, 2008.

Smith WR et al: Daily assessment of pain in adults with sickle cell disease, *Ann Intern Med* 148:94-101, 2008.

Vichinski EP et al: Causes and outcomes of the acute chest syndrome in sickle cell disease, *N Engl J Med* 342:1855, 2000.

Wethers DL: Sickle cell disease in childhood, *Am Fam Physician* 62:1013, 2000.

AUTHOR: **FRED F. FERRI, M.D.**

BASIC INFORMATION

DEFINITION

Silicosis is a lung disease attributable to the inhalation of silica (silicon dioxide) in crystalline form (quartz) or in cristobalite or tridymite forms.

SYNONYMS

Pneumoconiosis caused by silica

ICD-9CM CODES
502 Silicosis, occupational
503 Pneumoconiosis caused by other inorganic dust

EPIDEMIOLOGY & DEMOGRAPHICS

- Occupational disease affecting men and women involved in gathering, milling, processing, or using silica-containing rock or sand
- An estimated 1 million Americans are exposed

PHYSICAL FINDINGS & CLINICAL PRESENTATION

- Dyspnea
- Cough
- Wheezing
- Abnormal chest x-ray in an asymptomatic person

ETIOLOGY

- Silica particles are ingested by alveolar macrophages, which in turn release oxidants causing cell injury and cell death, attract fibroblasts, and activate lymphocytes, increasing immunoglobulins in the alveolar space.
- Hyperplasia of alveolar epithelial cells occurs.
- Collagen accumulates in the interstitium.
- Neutrophils also accumulate and secrete proteolytic enzymes, which leads to tissue destruction and emphysema.
- Silica dust may be carcinogenic (not proven).
- Exposure to silicosis predisposes to tuberculosis.
- Some patients develop rheumatoid silicotic pulmonary nodules and may have arthritic symptoms of rheumatoid arthritis (Caplan's syndrome). Scleroderma has also been associated with silicosis.

DIAGNOSIS

DIFFERENTIAL DIAGNOSIS

- Other pneumoconiosis, berylliosis, hard metal disease, asbestosis
- Sarcoidosis
- Tuberculosis
- Interstitial lung disease
- Hypersensitivity pneumonitis
- Lung cancer
- Langerhans' cell granulomatosis (histiocytosis X)
- Granulomatous pulmonary vasculitis

WORKUP

- History of occupational exposure
- Chest x-ray (Fig. 1-249)

Chronic silicosis

- Characteristic finding: small, rounded lung parenchymal opacities
- Hilar lymphadenopathy with "eggshell" calcifications
- Pleural plaques (uncommon)

Accelerated silicosis (progressive massive fibrosis)

- Large parenchymal lesions resulting from coalesced small nodules

Acute silicosis

- Ground-glass appearance of the lung fields
- Chest CT scan
- Pulmonary function tests

Combination of obstructive and restrictive changes with or without reduction in diffusing capacity

- Bronchoscopy with lung biopsy in uncertain cases

COURSE

CHRONIC SILICOSIS:

- May not progress with absence of further exposure
- Accelerated silicosis: progressive respiratory failure and cor pulmonale

ACUTE SILICOSIS: Fatal course from respiratory failure over several months to a few years

TREATMENT

- Prevention (industrial hygiene)
- Treatment of associated tuberculosis if present
- Supportive measures (oxygen, bronchodilators)
- Lung transplant

AUTHORS: **FRED F. FERRI, M.D.,** and **TOM J. WACHTEL, M.D.**

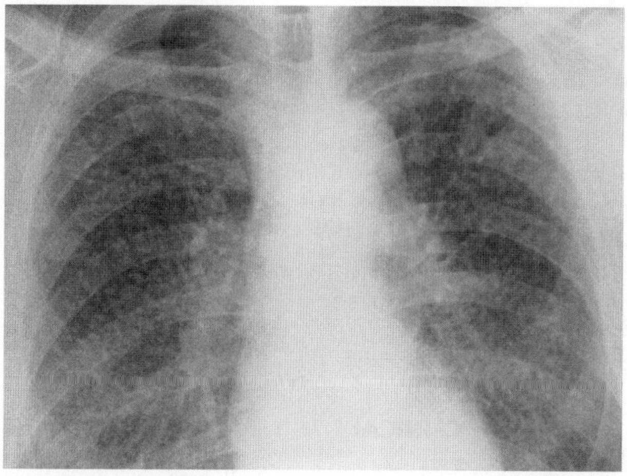

FIGURE 1-249 Simple silicosis. There are multiple small (2- to 4-mm) nodules distributed throughout the lungs, with an upper lobe predominance. (From McLoud TC: *Thoracic radiology: the requisites,* St Louis, 1998, Mosby.)

BASIC INFORMATION

DEFINITION

Sinusitis is inflammation of the mucous membranes lining one or more of the paranasal sinuses. The various presentations are:

- Acute sinusitis: infection lasting <30 days, with complete resolution of symptoms.
- Subacute infection: lasts from 30 to 90 days, with complete resolution of symptoms.
- Recurrent acute infection: episodes of acute infection lasting <30 days, with resolution of symptoms, which recur at intervals at least 10 days apart.
- Chronic sinusitis: inflammation lasting >90 days, with persistent upper respiratory symptoms.
- Acute bacterial sinusitis superimposed on chronic sinusitis: new symptoms that occur in patients with residual symptoms from prior infection(s). With treatment, the new symptoms resolve but the residual ones do not.

SYNONYMS

Rhinosinusitis: Sinusitis is almost always accompanied by inflammation of the nasal mucosa; thus it is now the preferred term.

ICD-9CM CODES
473.9 Sinusitis (accessory) (nasal) (hyperplastic) (nonpurulent) (purulent) (chronic)
461.9 Acute sinusitis

EPIDEMIOLOGY & DEMOGRAPHICS

INCIDENCE (IN U.S.): Seems to correlate with the incidence of upper respiratory tract infections

PEAK INCIDENCE: Fall, winter, spring: September through March

PHYSICAL FINDINGS & CLINICAL PRESENTATION

- Patients often give a history of a recent upper respiratory illness with some improvement, then a relapse
- Mucopurulent secretions in the nasal passage
  1. Purulent nasal and postnasal discharge lasting >7 to 10 days
  2. Facial tightness, pressure, or pain
  3. Nasal obstruction
  4. Headache
  5. Decreased sense of smell
  6. Purulent pharyngeal secretions, brought up with cough, often worse at night
- Erythema, swelling, and tenderness over the infected sinus in a small proportion of patients
  1. Diagnosis cannot be excluded by the absence of such findings.
  2. These findings are not common, and do not correlate with number of positive sinus aspirates.
- Intermittent low-grade fever in about half of adults with acute bacterial sinusitis
- Toothache is a common complaint when the maxillary sinus is involved
- Periorbital cellulitis and excessive tearing with ethmoid sinusitis
  1. Orbital extension of infection: chemosis, proptosis, impaired extraocular movements
- Characteristics of acute sinusitis in children with upper respiratory tract infections:
  1. Persistence of symptoms
  2. Cough
  3. Bad breath
- Symptoms of chronic sinusitis (may or may not be present)
  1. Nasal or postnasal discharge
  2. Fever
  3. Facial pain or pressure
  4. Headache
- Nosocomial sinusitis is typically seen in patients with nasogastric tubes or nasotracheal intubation.

ETIOLOGY

- Each of the four paranasal sinuses is connected to the nasal cavity by narrow tubes (ostia), 1- to 3-mm diameter; these drain directly into the nose through the turbinates. The sinuses are lined with a ciliated mucous membrane (mucoperiosteum).
- Acute viral infection
  1. Infection with the common cold or influenza
  2. Mucosal edema and sinus inflammation
  3. Decreased drainage of thick secretions/obstruction of the sinus ostia
  4. Subsequent entrapment of bacteria
     a. Multiplication of bacteria
     b. Secondary bacterial infection
- Other predisposing factors
  1. Tumors
  2. Polyps
  3. Foreign bodies
  4. Congenital choanal atresia
  5. Other entities that cause obstruction of sinus drainage
  6. Allergies
  7. Asthma
- Dental infections lead to maxillary sinusitis.
- Viruses recovered alone or in combination with bacteria (in 16% of cases):
  1. Rhinovirus
  2. Coronavirus
  3. Adenovirus
  4. Parainfluenza virus
  5. Respiratory syncytial virus
- The principal bacterial pathogens in sinusitis are *Streptococcus pneumoniae*, nontypeable *Haemophilus influenzae*, and *Moraxella catarrhalis*.
- In the remainder of cases find *Streptococcus pyogenes, Staphylococcus aureus*, α-hemolytic streptococci, and mixed anaerobic infections *(Peptostreptococcus, Fusobacterium, Bacteroides, Prevotella spp.)*.
- Infection is polymicrobial in about one third of cases.
- Anaerobic infections seen more often in cases of chronic sinusitis and in cases associated with dental infection; anaerobes are unlikely pathogens in sinusitis in children.
- Fungal pathogens are isolated with increasing frequency in immunocompromised patients but remain uncommon pathogens in the paranasal sinuses. Fungal pathogens include: *Phaeohyphomycoses, Aspergillus, Pseudallescheria, Sporothrix*, and *Zygomycetes spp.*
- Nosocomial infections: occur in patients with nasogastric tubes, nasotracheal intubation, cystic fibrosis, immunocompromised.
  1. *S. aureus* (including MRSA)
  2. *Pseudomonas aeruginosa*
  3. *Klebsiella pneumoniae*
  4. *Enterobacter spp.*
  5. *Proteus mirabilis*
- Organisms typically isolated in chronic sinusitis:
  1. *S. aureus*
  2. *S. pneumoniae*
  3. *H. influenzae*
  4. *P. aeruginosa*
  5. Anaerobes

DIAGNOSIS

DIFFERENTIAL DIAGNOSIS

- Temporomandibular joint disease
- Migraine headache
- Cluster headache
- Dental infection
- Trigeminal neuralgia

WORKUP

- In the normal healthy host the paranasal sinuses should be sterile. Although the contiguous structures are colonized with bacteria and likely contaminate the sinuses, the mucociliary lining functions to remove these bacteria.
- Gold standard for diagnosis: recovery of bacteria in high density ($\geq 10^4$ colony-forming units/ml) from a paranasal sinus, in the setting of a patient with history of upper respiratory infection and symptoms persisting 7 to 10 days. Sinus aspiration is the best method for obtaining cultures; however, it must be performed by an otorhinolaryngologist and is not practical for the primary care practitioner. Therefore most diagnoses are based

on the clinical history and presentation, possibly supported by radiologic evaluations.

1. Standard four-view sinus radiographs
   a. Complete opacification and air-fluid levels are most specific findings (average 85% and 80%, respectively)
   b. Mucosal thickening has low specificity (40% to 50%)
   c. Absence of all three of the previous findings has estimated sensitivity of 90%
   d. Overall, standard radiographs are of limited use in diagnosis, although negative films are strong evidence against the diagnosis
2. CT scans:
   a. Much more sensitive than plain radiographs in detecting acute changes and disease in the sinuses
   b. Recommended for patients requiring surgical intervention, including sinus aspiration; it is a useful adjunct to guide therapy
3. Transillumination:
   a. Used for diagnosis of frontal and maxillary sinusitis
   b. Place transilluminator in the mouth or against cheek to assess maxillary sinuses, under medial aspect of the supraorbital ridge to assess frontal sinuses
   c. Absence of light transmission indicates that sinus is filled with fluid
   d. Dullness (decreased light transmission) is less helpful in diagnosing infection
4. Endoscopy:
   a. Used to visualize secretions coming from the ostia of infected sinuses
   b. Culture collection via endoscopy often contaminated by nasal flora; not nearly as good as sinus puncture
5. Sinus puncture:
   a. Gold standard for collecting sinus cultures
   b. Generally reserved for treatment failures, suspected intracranial extension, and nosocomial sinusitis

TREATMENT

Rx

NONPHARMACOLOGIC THERAPY

To help promote sinus drainage:

- Air humidification with vaporizers (for steam) or humidifiers (for a cool mist)
- Application of hot, wet towel over the face
- Sipping hot beverages
- Hydration

ACUTE GENERAL Rx

- Sinus drainage:
  1. Nasal vasoconstrictors, such as phenylephrine nose drops, 0.25% or 0.5%
  2. Topical decongestants should not be used for more than a few days because of the risk of rebound congestion
  3. Systemic decongestants
  4. Nasal or systemic corticosteroids, such as nasal beclomethasone, short course oral prednisone
  5. Nasal irrigation, with hypertonic or normal saline (saline may act as a mild vasoconstrictor of nasal blood flow)
  6. Use of antihistamines has no proven benefit, and the drying effect on the mucous membranes may cause crusting, which blocks the ostia, thus interfering with sinus drainage
- Analgesics, antipyretics

Antimicrobial therapy:

- Most cases of acute sinusitis have a viral etiology and will resolve within 2 wk without antibiotics.
- Current treatment recommendations favor symptomatic treatment for those with mild symptoms.
- Antibiotics should be reserved for those with moderate to severe symptoms who meet the criteria for diagnosis of sinusitis.
- Antibiotic therapy is usually empiric, targeting the common pathogens:
  1. First-line antibiotics include amoxicillin, erythromycin, TMP/SMX.
  2. Second-line antibiotics include the newer macrolides: clarithromycin, azithromycin, amoxicillin/clavulanate, cefuroxime axetil, cefprozil, cefaclor, loracarbef, ciprofloxacin, levofloxacin, moxifloxacin, clindamycin, metronidazole, others.
  3. For patients with uncomplicated acute sinusitis, the less expensive first-line agents appear to be as effective as the costlier second-line agents.
- Hospitalization and IV antibiotics may be required for more severe infection and those with suspected intracranial complications. Broader-spectrum antibiotic coverage may be indicated in severe cases, to cover for MRSA, *Pseudomonas,* and fungal pathogens.

Duration of therapy generally 10 to 14 days, although some have success with much shorter regimens

Surgery:

- Surgical drainage indicated
  1. If intracranial or orbital complications suspected
  2. Many cases of frontal and sphenoid sinusitis
  3. Chronic sinusitis recalcitrant to medical therapy
- Surgical debridement imperative in the treatment of fungal sinusitis

Complications:

- Untreated, sinusitis may lead to a number of serious, life-threatening complications.
- Intracranial complications include meningitis, brain abscess, epidural and subdural empyema.
- Intracranial sequelae are more common with frontal and ethmoid infections.
- Extracranial complications include orbital cellulitis, blindness, orbital abscess, osteomyelitis.
- Extracranial sequelae are more commonly seen with ethmoid sinusitis.

CHRONIC Rx

- Broad-spectrum antibiotics that cover both aerobes and anaerobes
- Duration of therapy not clearly established: range 3 to 6 wk
- Adjunctive therapy: one or more of the various options listed previously
- Surgical intervention may be necessary in nonresponders

DISPOSITION

Appropriate diagnosis and treatment necessary to avoid the various sequelae that can occur without proper therapy

REFERRAL

- To infectious disease specialist if failure to respond to initial therapy
- To otorhinolaryngologist for:
  1. Failure to respond to therapy
  2. Fungal infection suspected
  3. Intracranial or orbital complications suspected

PEARLS & CONSIDERATIONS

- Recurrent sinusitis is usually related to anatomic defects, poor drainage, or immunocompromised states; such patients deserve a thorough workup by an ENT specialist and/or an infectious disease specialist.
- Nosocomial sinusitis from obstruction by nasotracheal or nasogastric tubes is not uncommon and can be difficult to recognize in patients in the critical care units.

EVIDENCE

EBM

Antibiotics are effective in radiologically or bacteriologically confirmed sinusitis, although the benefits are modest.

There is limited evidence that antibiotics (including amoxicillin, cephalosporins, and macrolides) for 7 to 10 days are effective in the treatment of radiologically or bacteriologically confirmed acute maxillary sinusitis. Nevertheless, the moderate benefits of antibiotic treatment should be weighed against the potential for adverse effects.[1] Ⓐ

However, one randomized controlled trial of amoxicillin vs. placebo for 10 days did not find any difference between treatments in patients with clinically diagnosed sinusitis.[2] Ⓐ

A systematic review of RCTs that compared antibiotics vs. placebo or standard therapy in children with rhinosinusitis found that antibiotics, including amoxicillin, trimethoprim-sulfamethoxazole, and erythromycin, for 10 days reduces the probability of persistent symptoms. Erythromycin may be associated with more clinical failures than amoxicillin and trimethoprim-sulfamethoxazole. Again, the benefits are modest and the risk of side effects should be borne in mind.[3] Ⓐ

We are unable to cite evidence for other therapies that meets our criteria.

Evidence-Based References

1. Williams JW Jr. et al: Antibiotics for acute maxillary sinusitis, *Cochrane Database Syst Rev* 3, 2002. Reviewed in: *Clin Evid* 11:710-717, 2004. Ⓐ
2. De Sutter AI et al: Does amoxicillin improve outcomes in patients with purulent rhinorrhea? A pragmatic randomized double-blind controlled trial in family practice, *J Fam Pract* 51:317, 2002. Reviewed in: *Clin Evid* 11:710, 2004. Ⓐ
3. Morris P, Leach A: Antibiotics for persistent nasal discharge (rhinosinusitis) in children (Cochrane Review). 2, Chichester, UK, 2004, John Wiley. Ⓐ

SUGGESTED READINGS

Brook I: Microbiology of acute and chronic maxillary sinusitis associated with an odontogenic origin, *Laryngoscope* 115(5):823,. 2005.

Gerencer RZ: Successful outpatient treatment of sinusitis exacerbations caused by community-acquired methicillin-resistant *Staphylococcus aureus, Otolaryngol Head Neck Surg* 132(6):828, 2005.

Lindback M: Acute sinusitis: guide to selection of antibacterial therapy, *Drugs* 64(8):805, 2004.

Llki A, Ulger N, Inanli S: Microbiology of sinusitis and the predictive value of throat culture for the aetiology of sinusitis, *Clin Microbiol Infect* 11(5):407, 2005.

Oxford LE, McClay J: Complications of acute sinusitis in children, *Otolaryngol Head Neck Surg* 133(1):32, 2005.

Stein M, Caplan ES: Nosocomial sinusitis: a unique subset of sinusitis, *Curr Opin Infect Dis* 18(2):147, 2005.

Taxy JB: Paranasal funal sinusitis: contributions of histopathology to diagnosis: a report of 60 cases and literature review, *Am J Surg Pathol* 30(6):713, 2006.

AUTHORS: **GLENN G. FORT, M.D., M.P.H., DENNIS J. MIKOLICH, M.D.,** and **JANE V. EASON, M.D.**

BASIC INFORMATION

DEFINITION

Sjögren's syndrome (SS) is an autoimmune disorder characterized by lymphocytic and plasma cell infiltration and destruction of salivary and lacrimal glands with subsequent diminished lacrimal and salivary gland secretions.

- *Primary:* dry mouth (xerostomia) and dry eyes (xerophthalmia) develop as isolated entities.
- *Secondary:* associated with other disorders.

SYNONYMS

SS
Sicca syndrome

ICD-9CM CODES
710.2 Sjögren's syndrome

EPIDEMIOLOGY & DEMOGRAPHICS

INCIDENCE/PREVALENCE: 1 case/2500 persons; secondary SS is just as common and can affect up to one third of SLE patients and nearly 20% of RA patients.
PREDOMINANT SEX: Female > male
PREDOMINANT AGE: Peak incidence is in the sixth decade.

PHYSICAL FINDINGS & CLINICAL PRESENTATION

- Dry mouth with dry lips (cheilosis), erythema of tongue (Fig. 1-250), and other mucosal surfaces, carious teeth
- Dry eyes (conjunctival injection, decreased luster, and irregularity of the corneal light reflex)
- Possible salivary gland enlargement and dysfunction with subsequent difficulty in chewing and swallowing food and in speaking without frequent water intake
- Purpura (nonthrombocytopenic, hyperglobulinemic, vasculitic) may be present
- Evidence of associated conditions (e.g., RA or other connective disease, lymphoma, hypothyroidism, COPD, trigeminal neuropathy, chronic liver disease, polymyopathy)

ETIOLOGY

Autoimmune disorder

DIAGNOSIS

DIFFERENTIAL DIAGNOSIS

- Medication-related dryness (e.g., anticholinergics)
- Age-related exocrine gland dysfunction
- Mouth breathing
- Anxiety
- Other: sarcoidosis, primary salivary hypofunction, radiation injury, amyloidosis

WORKUP

Workup involves occular and oral examination and laboratory and radiographic testing to demonstrate the following criteria for diagnosis of primary and secondary Sjögren's syndrome:

PRIMARY:

- Symptoms and objective signs of ocular dryness:
  1. Schirmer's test: <8 mm wetting per 5 min
  2. Positive rose bengal or fluorescein staining of cornea and conjunctiva to demonstrate keratoconjunctivitis sicca
- Symptoms and objective signs of dry mouth:
  1. Decreased parotid flow using Lashley cups or other methods
  2. Abnormal biopsy result of minor salivary gland (focus score >2 based on average of four assessable lobules)
- Evidence of systemic autoimmune disorder:
  1. Elevated titer of rheumatoid factor >1:320
  2. Elevated titer of ANA >1:320
  3. Presence of anti-SS A (Ro) or anti-SS B (La) antibodies

SECONDARY:

- Characteristic signs and symptoms of SS (described in "Physical Findings")
- Clinical features sufficient to allow a diagnosis of RA, SLE, polymyositis, or scleroderma

LABORATORY TESTS

- Positive ANA (>60% of patients) with autoantibodies anti-SS A and anti-SS B may be present.
- Additional laboratory abnormalities may include elevated ESR, anemia (normochromic, normocytic), abnormal liver function studies, elevated serum β_2 microglobulin levels, rheumatoid factor.
- A definite diagnosis SS can be made with a salivary gland biopsy.

TREATMENT

NONPHARMACOLOGIC THERAPY

- Adequate fluid replacement. Ameliorate skin dryness by gently blotting dry after bathing, leaving a small amount of moisture, and then applying a moisturizer.
- Proper oral hygiene to reduce the incidence of caries

GENERAL Rx

- Use artificial tears frequently.
- Pilocarpine 5 mg PO qid is useful to improve dryness. A cyclosporine 0.05% ophthalmic emulsion (Restasis) may also be useful for dry eyes. Recommended dose is one drop bid in both eyes.
- Cevimeline (Evoxac), a cholinergic agent with muscarinic agonist activity, 30 mg PO tid is effective for the treatment of dry mouth in patients with Sjögren's syndrome.
- Interferon alfa, 150 IU tid for 12 wk has been shown to significantly improve stimulated whole saliva output and decrease complaints of xerostomia
- Periodic dental and ophthalmology evaluations to screen for complications

PEARLS & CONSIDERATIONS

COMMENTS

Unusual presentations of SS may occur in association with polymyalgia rheumatica, chronic fatigue syndrome, FUO, and inflammatory myositis.

SUGGESTED READING

Kassan SS, Moutsopoulos HM: Clinical manifestations and early diagnosis of Sjogren syndrome, *Arch Intern Med* 164:1275, 2004.

AUTHOR: **FRED F. FERRI, M.D.**

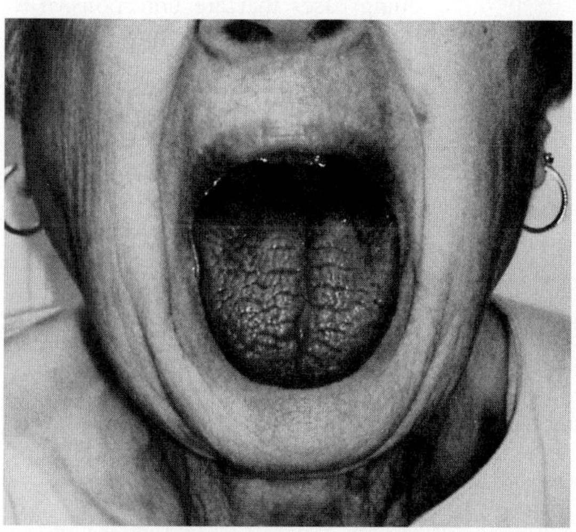

FIGURE 1-250 "Crocodile tongue" in a patient, with Sjögren's syndrome. (From Noble J: *Primary care medicine,* ed 3, St Louis, 2001, Mosby.)

BASIC INFORMATION

DEFINITION

The American Academy of Sleep Disorders defines obstructive sleep apnea as "characterized by repetitive episodes of upper airway obstruction that occur during sleep, usually associated with a reduction in blood oxygen saturation."

SYNONYMS

Sleep apnea syndrome
Obstructive sleep apnea-hypopnea syndrome
Complex sleep apnea syndrome

ICD-9CM CODES
780.57 Obstructive sleep apnea syndrome

EPIDEMIOLOGY & DEMOGRAPHICS

Obstructive sleep apnea (OSA) occurs most frequently in 40- to 65-year-old men (4%) and women (2%). The prevalence is higher in obese and hypertensive individuals. Pediatric OSA most frequently occurs in preschool-aged children (2%) and is associated with hypertrophy of the tonsils and adenoids, but can be similar to adult apnea in obese children.

PHYSICAL FINDINGS & CLINICAL PRESENTATION

- Systemic hypertension, type II diabetes, stroke, or heart failure
- History of snoring, witnessed apneas, frequent arousals and/or nocturnal urination, and excessive daytime somnolence.
- Obesity with body mass index >27 kg/m², neck circumference >43 cm (17 in.) in men.
- Working memory impairment, inability to concentrate, short-temperedness, inattention, and hyperactivity in children.
- Examination of oropharynx may reveal erythema caused by snoring and lateral narrowing secondary to large tonsils, pendulous uvula, excessive soft tissue, prominent tongue, and retrognathia.
- Patient's bed partner may report loud snoring, episodic choking sounds, disrupted sleep with repetitive arousals, thrashing movements of extremities during sleep.
- Decreased libido, mood swings, and depression.

ETIOLOGY

Narrowing of upper airway secondary to:
- Obesity
- Macroglossia
- Tonsillar and adenoid hypertrophy
- Micrognathia
- Muscular weakness
- Use of alcohol or sedatives at bedtime

Upper airway muscular weakness secondary to:
- Neuromuscular disorders
- Metabolic disorders
- Primary CNS disorder (e.g., stroke, Down's syndrome)
- Proposed genetic predisposition

DIAGNOSIS

DIFFERENTIAL DIAGNOSIS

- Excessive daytime somnolence
- Inadequate sleep time
- Pulmonary disease
- Heart disease
- Parkinsonism
- Narcolepsy
- Hypothyroidism
- Anemia
- Sleep fragmentation
- Sleep-related asthma
- Sleep-related GERD
- Periodic limb movement disorder
- Restless legs syndrome
- Parasomnias
- Psychophysiologic insomnia
- Panic disorder

WORKUP

- Medical history should include questions about snoring, witnessed apneas, sleep fragmentation, and excessive daytime sleepiness. Additional history concerning morning headaches, alcohol intake, weight gain, and mood/personality changes also may help implicate apnea.
- Sleep apnea can be confirmed by overnight polysomnography (PSG) (gold standard). Testing is performed during the patient's habitual sleep hours and ideally includes all stages of sleep and body positions. Patients with sleep apnea have more than five apneic/hypopneic episodes per hour (termed apnea hypopnea index, or AHI) with desaturations of at least 3% by oximetry or coincidental arousals. Overnight oximetry tests can suggest the presence of sleep apnea but are not sufficient to rule out sleep apnea.
- Portable monitors that measure respiratory flow are available but they lack the EEG, EMG, and technical observations necessary to diagnose sleep apnea with reliable accuracy. The use of such devices is usually related to limited availability of polysomnography or adjustment of OSA therapy.

LABORATORY TESTS

- TSH level is indicated in suspected hypothyroidism.
- CBC (with iron studies) is indicated for detecting anemia.
- Pulmonary function tests are indicated for detecting related pulmonary disorders.
- ECG is indicated for detecting related heart disease.

IMAGING STUDIES

Radiography of soft tissues in the neck in patients with suspected anatomic abnormalities

TREATMENT

NONPHARMACOLOGIC THERAPY

- Weight loss in overweight patients including bariatric surgery.
- Avoidance of sedating medications and alcohol.
- Sleep hygiene training.
- Elimination of the supine sleeping position.
- For mild to moderate obstructive sleep apnea in select patient populations (e.g., retrognathia) an oral appliance (constructed by a qualified dentist) may be useful to push the mandible forward.
- Uvulopalatopharyngoplasty (UPPP, both standard and laser-assisted [LAUP]) in patients with significant obstruction of retropalatal airway can treat snoring but is not an accepted therapy for OSA.
- Nasal septoplasty in patients with nasoseptal deformity may reduce snoring but is not an accepted therapy for OSA.
- Adenotonsillectomy in children is often curative if indicated by an overnight PSG.

ACUTE GENERAL Rx

- Nighttime treatment with continuous positive airway pressure (CPAP) provides immediate resolution of sleep apnea. Symptoms of excessive daytime somnolence may linger and necessitate further investigation or medical therapy.
- Complex apnea (a combination of obstructive and central apnea) may necessitate therapy with bilevel PAP or require a period of adaptation with repeated nocturnal respiratory measures to demonstrate efficacy.
- Tracheostomy: reserved for life-threatening cases that are unresponsive to other treatments.
- Nasal steroids in allergy or sinusitis patients.

CHRONIC Rx

- CPAP therapy
- Weight loss

COMPLEMENTARY & ALTERNATIVE MEDICINE

Treatment with low-dose mirtazapine may reduce the AHI in patients with mild OSA.

DISPOSITION

- Most patients improve with weight loss, CPAP, or oral appliance therapy.

- Complex apnea syndrome may result in Cheyne-Stokes respiratory patterns that can complicate CPAP therapy.
- Overall success rate for UPPP is about 40% for snoring; much less effective for apnea.
- Weight loss over time may reduce the need for CPAP pressure or obviate its use entirely.

REFERRAL

- Sleep physician for proper study type(s) or complex symptoms
- Dental referral for patients unresponsive to weight loss and CPAP
- Consider surgical evaluation in select patients (i.e., need for mandibular/maxilla advancement)

PEARLS & CONSIDERATIONS

- In a primary care setting, patients with high risk of sleep apnea are those who meet two of the following three criteria: (1) snoring, (2) persistent daytime sleepiness or drowsiness while driving, (3) obesity or hypertension.
- Children with OSA may have symptoms of excessive daytime somnolence, hyperactivity, insomnia, inattention, declining academic performance, growth retardation, and a history of recurrent ear or throat infections.
- Some patients with sleep apnea experience nocturnal dysrhythmias (bradycardia, paroxysmal tachyarrhythmias). In cardiac patients, trials using atrial overdrive pacing have demonstrated a reduction in the number of episodes of sleep apnea without reduction in the total sleep time.
- The use of vagal nerve stimulators (VNS) in epilepsy patients has been associated with an increase in apneas and hypopneas. VNS-related respiratory events may be reduced by altering VNS stimulation parameters or by initiating CPAP.

EVIDENCE

The following therapies have been evaluated with varying levels of clinical evidence:

Randomized controlled trials (RCTs) demonstrate that nasal CPAP is an effective treatment of moderate to severe obstructive sleep apnea-hypopnea syndrome[1,2] and is more effective than placebo in improving sleepiness and several quality of life and depression measures in people with obstructive sleep apnea.[3] Treatment of OSA with CPAP shows a significant improvement in left ventricular ejection fraction and daytime systolic blood pressure in people with heart failure compared with those without CPAP.[4] CPAP therapy provides secondary ischemic stroke prevention in patients with moderately severe apnea.[5]

RCTs demonstrate that mandibular advancement devices (oral appliances) are effective in treating moderate to severe OSA[6,7] and show significant improvement in measures of daytime sleepiness and sleep disordered breathing when compared with no treatment in moderately severe OSA.[8] CPAP is significantly more effective than oral appliances in improving the AHI and minimum oxygen saturation during sleep,[3] as well as functional outcomes and quality of life measures.[9]

In patients with mild obstructive sleep apnea-hypopnea syndrome, an oral mandibular advancement appliance is significantly more effective in improving AHI at 12 months and at 4-year follow-up compared with uvulopalatopharyngoplasty. Both interventions are equivalent in terms of daytime sleepiness and quality of life measures. Patients treated with uvulopalatopharyngoplasty, however, have better contentment scores.[10-12]

A systematic review failed to find randomized controlled trials demonstrating the efficacy of surgical treatments for obstructive sleep apnea.[13] Variability in experimental design as well as limited sample sizes and a lack of common outcomes measures further limits the comparison of studies related to surgical treatments.[14]

Evidence-Based References

1. Montserrat JM et al: Effectiveness of CPAP treatment in daytime function in sleep apnea syndrome: a randomized controlled study with an optimized placebo, *Am J Respir Crit Care Med* 164:608-613, 2001.
2. Faccenda JF et al: Randomized placebo-controlled trial of continuous positive airway pressure on blood pressure in the sleep apnea-hypopnea syndrome, *Am J Respir Crit Care Med* 163:344-348, 2001. Reviewed in: *Clin Evid* 11:2249-2265, 2004.
3. White J, Cates C, Wright J: Continuous positive airways pressure for obstructive sleep apnoea, *Cochrane Database Syst Rev* 4, 2001.
4. Kaneko Y et al: Cardiovascular effects of continuous positive airway pressure in patients with heart failure and obstructive sleep apnea, *N Engl J Med* 348:1233-1241, 2003.
5. Martinez-Garcia MA et al: Continuous positive airway pressure treatment prevents new vascular events after ischemic stroke, *Chest* 128(4):2123, 2005.
6. Hans MG et al: Comparison of two dental devices for treatment of obstructive sleep apnea syndrome (OSAS), *Am J Orthod Dentofac Orthop* 111:562-570, 1997. Reviewed in: *Clin Evid* 11:2249-2265, 2004.
7. Mehta A et al: A randomized controlled study of a mandibular advancement splint for obstructive sleep apnea, *Am J Respir Crit Care Med* 163:1457-1461, 2001. Reviewed in: *Clin Evid* 11:2249-2265, 2004.
8. Bloch KE et al: A randomized, controlled crossover trial of two oral appliances for sleep apnea treatment, *Am J Respir Crit Care Med* 162:246-251, 2000. Reviewed in: *Clin Evid* 11:2249-2265, 2004.
9. Engleman HM et al: Randomized crossover trial of two treatments for sleep apnoea/hypopnea syndrome: continuous positive airway pressure and mandibular repositioning splint, *Am J Respir Crit Care Med* 166:855-859, 2002. Reviewed in: *Clin Evid* 11:2249-2265, 2004.
10. Wilhelmsson B et al: A prospective randomized study of a dental appliance compared with uvulopalatopharyngoplasty in the treatment of obstructive sleep apnoea, *Acta Otolaryngol* 119:503-509, 1999. Reviewed in: *Clin Evid* 11:2249-2265, 2004.
11. Walker-Engstrom ML et al: Quality of life assessment of treatment with dental appliance or UPPP in patients with mild to moderate obstructive sleep apnoea. A prospective randomized 1-year follow-up study, *J Sleep Res* 9:303-308, 2000. Reviewed in: *Clin Evid* 11:2249-2265, 2004.
12. Walker-Engstrom ML et al: 4-year follow-up of treatment with dental appliance or uvulopalatopharyngoplasty in patients with obstructive sleep apnea: a randomized study, *Chest* 121:739-746, 2002.
13. Bridgman SA, Dunn KM, Ducharme F: Surgery for obstructive sleep apnoea, *Cochrane Database Syst Rev* 1:1998.
14. Sundaram S et al: Surgery for obstructive sleep apnea, *Cochrane Database Syst Rev* 4:CD001004, 2005.

SUGGESTED READINGS

American Academy of Pediatrics: Clinical practice guideline: diagnosis and management of childhood obstructive sleep apnea syndrome, *Pediatrics* 109:704, 2002.

American Academy of Sleep Medicine: *International classification of sleep disorders: diagnostic and coding manual,* ed 2, Westchester, IL, 2005, Author.

Beebe DW: Neurobehavioral effects of obstructive sleep apnea: an overview and heuristic model, *Curr Opin Pulm Med* 11(6):494-500, 2005.

Chervin RD et al: Inattention, hyperactivity and symptoms of sleep-disordered breathing, *Pediatrics* 109:449, 2002.

Flemons WW: Obstructive sleep apnea, *N Engl J Med* 347:498, 2002.

Garrigue A et al: Benefit of atrial pacing in sleep apnea syndrome, *N Engl J Med* 346:404, 2002.

Guilleminault C, Lee JH, Chan A: Pediatric obstructive sleep apnea syndrome, *Arch Pediatr Adolesc Med* 159(8):775-785, 2005. Review.

Marzec M et al: Effects of vagal nerve stimulation on sleep-related breathing in epilepsy patients, *Epilepsia* 44:930, 2003.

Qureshi A, Lee-Chiong TL: Medical treatment of obstructive sleep apnea, *Semin Respir Crit Care Med* 26(1):96-108, 2005. Review.

Sharabi Y, Rabin K, Grossman E: Sleep apnea-induced hypertension: mechanisms of vascular changes, *Expert Rev Cardiovasc Ther* 3(5):937-940, 2005.

AUTHOR: **JEFFREY S. DURMER, M.D., PH.D.**

BASIC INFORMATION

DEFINITION

Smallpox infection is due to the variola virus, a DNA virus member of the genus *Orthopoxvirus*. It is a human virus with no known nonhuman reservoir of disease. Natural infection occurs following implantation of the virus on the oropharyngeal or respiratory mucosa.

ICD-9CM CODES
050.9 Smallpox NOS
V01.3 Smallpox exposure
050.0 Smallpox, hemorrhagic (pustular)
050.1 Variola minor (alastrim)
050.0 Variola major

EPIDEMIOLOGY & DEMOGRAPHICS

- Smallpox infection was eliminated from the world in 1977. The last cases of smallpox, from laboratory exposure, occurred in 1978. The threat of bioterrorism has brought on renewed interest in smallpox virus.
- Routine vaccination against smallpox ended in 1972.
- Smallpox is spread from one person to another by infected saliva droplets that expose a susceptible person who has face-to-face contact with the ill person.
- Persons with smallpox are most infectious during the first wk of illness, when the largest amount of virus is present in saliva; however, some risk of transmission lasts until all scabs have fallen off.
- The incubation period is about 12 days (range: 7 to 17 days) following exposure.
- Contaminated clothing or bed linen could also spread the virus. Special precautions need to be taken to ensure that all bedding and clothing of patients are cleaned appropriately with bleach and hot water. Disinfectants such as bleach and quaternary ammonia can be used for cleaning contaminated surfaces.

PHYSICAL FINDINGS & CLINICAL PRESENTATION

- Initial symptoms include high fever, fatigue, and headaches and back aches. A characteristic rash, most prominent on the face, arms, and legs, follows in 2 to 3 days (Fig. 1-251).
- The rash starts with flat red lesions that evolve at the same rate. The rash follows a centrifugal pattern.
- Lesions are firm to the touch, domed, or umbilicated. They become pus-filled and begin to crust early in the second wk.
- Scabs develop and then separate and fall off after about 3 to 4 wk. Depigmentation persists at the base of the skin lesions for 3 to 6 mo after illness. Scarring is usually most extensive on the face.
- Associated with the rash may be fever, headache, generalized malaise, vomiting, and colicky abdominal pain.
- Variola major may produce a rapidly fatal toxemia in some patients.
- Complications of smallpox include dehydration, pneumonia, blepharitis, conjunctivitis, and corneal ulcerations.

ETIOLOGY

Smallpox is caused by the variola virus. There are at least two strains of the virus, the most virulent known as *variola major* and a less virulent strain known as *variola minor* (elastrim).

DIAGNOSIS

DIFFERENTIAL DIAGNOSIS

- Rash from other viral illnesses (e.g., hemorrhagic chicken pox, measles, coxsackievirus)
- Abdominal pain may mimic appendicitis
- Meningococcemia
- Insect bites
- Impetigo
- Dermatitis herpetiformis
- Pemphigus
- Papular urticaria

WORKUP & LABORATORY TESTS

- Laboratory examination requires high-containment (BL-4) facilities.
- Electron microscopy of vesicular scrapings can be used to distinguish poxvirus particles from varicella-zoster virus or herpes simplex. To obtain vesicular or pustular fluid it may be necessary to open lesions with the blunt edge of a scalpel. A cotton swab may be used to harvest the fluid.
- In absence of electron microscopy, light microscopy can be used to visualize variola viral particles (Guarnieri bodies) following Giemsa staining.
- Polymerase chain reaction (PCR) techniques and restriction fragment-length polymorphisms can rapidly identify variola.

IMAGING STUDIES

Chest x-ray in patients with suspected pneumonia

TREATMENT

NONPHARMACOLOGIC THERAPY

- Supportive therapy
- IV hydration in severe cases
- A suspect case of smallpox should be placed in strict respiratory and contact isolation

ACUTE GENERAL Rx

- There is no proven treatment for smallpox. Vaccination administered within 3 to 4 days may prevent or significantly ameliorate subsequent illness. Vaccinia immune globulin can be used for treatment of vaccine complications and for administration with vaccine to those for whom vaccine is otherwise contraindicated.
- Patients can benefit from supportive therapy (e.g., IV fluids, acetaminophen for pain or fever).
- Antibiotics are indicated only if secondary bacterial infections occur. Penicillase-resistant antimicrobial agents should be used if smallpox lesions are secondarily infected.
- Topical idoxuridine should be considered for corneal lesions.

DISPOSITION

- Mortality for variola major is 20% to 50%. Variola minor has a mortality rate of 1%.

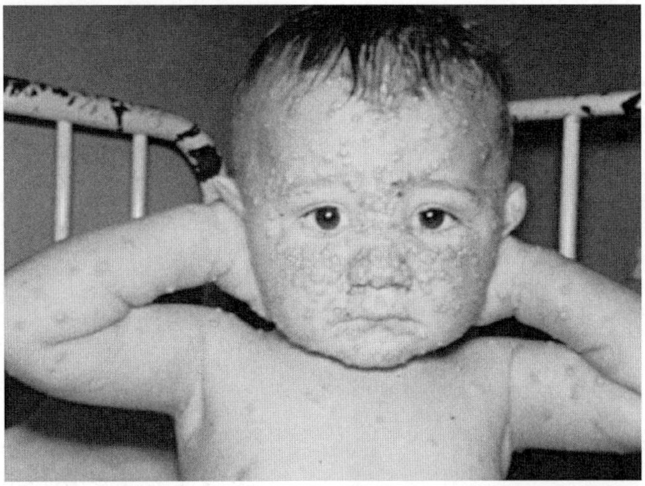

FIGURE 1-251 Appearance of the rash of smallpox on day 6 to 7. All of the lesions are in the same stage of development. (From Gorbach SL: *Infectious diseases,* ed 2, Philadelphia, 1998, WB Saunders.)

- After severe smallpox, pitted lesions (most commonly on the face) are seen in up to 80% of survivors.
- Panophthalmitis and blindness from viral keratitis or secondary eye infection occur in 1% of patients.
- Arthritis caused by viral infection of the metaphysis of growing bones occurs in 2% of children.

REFERRAL

ID consultation and notification of local health authorities is mandatory in all cases of smallpox.

PEARLS & CONSIDERATIONS

- The smallpox virus is fragile and in the event of an aerosol release of smallpox, all viruses will be inactivated or dissipated within 1 to 2 days. Buildings exposed to the initial aerosol release of the virus do not need to be decontaminated. By the time the first cases are identified, typically 2 wk after release, the virus in the building will be gone. Infected patients, however, will be capable of spreading the virus and possibly contaminating surfaces while they are sick. Standard hospital-grade disinfectants such as quaternary ammonias are effective in killing the virus on surfaces and should be used for disinfecting hospitalized patients' rooms or other contaminated surfaces. In the hospital setting, patients' linens should be autoclaved or washed in hot water with bleach added. Infectious waste should be placed in biohazard bags and autoclaved before incineration.
- Symptomatic patients with suspected or confirmed smallpox are capable of spreading the virus. Patients should be placed in medical isolation to avoid spread of the virus. In addition, people who have come into close contact with smallpox patients should be vaccinated immediately and closely watched for symptoms of smallpox.

COMMENTS

- In people exposed to smallpox, the vaccine can lessen the severity of or even prevent illness if given within 4 days of exposure.
- Vaccine against smallpox contains another live virus called vaccinia. The vaccine does not contain smallpox virus. Smallpox vaccination produces a skin lesion that is infectious. Vaccine virus in the skin lesion can be transferred to others if the skin lesion is touched directly or if the bandage is handled casually with ungloved hands. The vaccination site is infectious until the scab falls off, approximately 21 days after vaccination.
- Primary vaccination confers full immunity to smallpox in more than 95% of persons for up to 10 yr.

SUGGESTED READINGS

Breman JG, Henderson DA: Diagnosis and management of smallpox, *N Engl J Med* 346:1300, 2002.

Frey SE et al: Clinical responses to undiluted and diluted smallpox vaccine, *N Engl J Med* 346:1265, 2002.

Henderson DA et al: Smallpox as a biological weapon, *JAMA* 281:2127, 1999. www.bt.cdc.gov/Agent/Smallpox/SmallpoxGen.asp

AUTHOR: **FRED F. FERRI, M.D.**

BASIC INFORMATION

DEFINITION

Somatization disorder refers to a pattern of recurring multiple somatic complaints that begin before the age of 30 yr and persist over several years. Patients complain of multiple sites of pain (a minimum of four), GI symptoms (a minimum of two), a sexual or reproductive symptom, and a pseudoneurologic symptom. These cannot be explained by a medical condition or are in excess to expected disability from a coexisting medical condition.

SYNONYMS

Briquet's syndrome
Nonorganic physical symptoms
Medically unexplained symptoms
Functional somatic symptoms

ICD-9CM CODES
300.81 Somatization disorder

EPIDEMIOLOGY & DEMOGRAPHICS

PREVALENCE (IN U.S.): Lifetime rates of 0.25% to 2% in women, <0.2% in men
PEAK INCIDENCE: Typically before age 25 yr
PREDOMINANT SEX: Women are more commonly affected in the U.S. by 10:1 ratio
PREDOMINANT AGE: Onset occurs before age 30 yr and usually in adolescence.
GENETICS: In males, there is a high risk of associated substance abuse or antisocial personality disorder.

PHYSICAL FINDINGS & CLINICAL PRESENTATION

- Onset is characteristically in the teens; course is marked by frequent, unexplained, and frequently disabling pain and physical complaints.
- Patient frequently undergoes multiple procedures and seeks treatment from multiple physicians. Symptom focus rotates periodically with new physicians sought for new complaints.
- Patient often has a comorbid psychiatric disorder, most commonly generalized anxiety, panic disorder, or depression.

ETIOLOGY

- Believed to be the physical expression of psychologic distress; there appears to be a biological predisposition.
- May be more common in individuals without sufficient verbal or intellectual capacity to communicate psychologic distress, individuals with alexithymia (inability to describe emotional states), or individuals from cultural backgrounds that consider emotional distress as an undesirable quality.
- Some aspects of somatization behavior possibly learned from somatizing parents.

DIAGNOSIS

DIFFERENTIAL DIAGNOSIS

- Undifferentiated somatoform disorder (ICD-10 F45.1, DMS-IV 300.81): one or more physical complaints that cannot be explained by a medical condition are present for at least 6 mo (NOTE: Somatization disorder is more severe and less common).
- Conversion disorder: there is an alteration or loss of voluntary motor or sensory function without demonstrable physical cause and related to a psychologic stress or a conflict (NOTE: With multiple complaints, the diagnosis of conversion is not made).
- Pain disorder: distinguished from somatization disorder by the latter featuring multiple nonpain symptoms.
- Factitious disorder (e.g., Munchausen's syndrome) and malingering: the psychologic basis of the complaints in somatization disorder is not conscious as in factitious disorder where the goal is to be in the patient role and malingering, in which symptoms are also produced consciously for some secondary gain.

WORKUP

- Rule out a general medical condition.
- If somatization is suspected on the basis of a history of repeated, multiple, unexplained complaints, restraint in ordering tests is recommended.

LABORATORY TESTS

No specific laboratory tests are required.

IMAGING STUDIES

No specific imaging studies are required.

TREATMENT

NONPHARMACOLOGIC THERAPY

- Legitimize patient's complaints.
- Minimize diagnostic investigation and symptomatic treatment. Only do invasive testing or procedures when there are clear-cut signs, not just symptom reports.
- Set attainable treatment goals. Patients may benefit from realizing that even though they cannot be cured, that they will be cared for. This may help reassure them that they will continue to have a relationship with the physician.
- Treat coexisting psychiatric conditions such as depression and anxiety.

ACUTE GENERAL Rx

- At each visit do a brief physical examination focusing on the area of complaint.
- Gently praise increased functioning rather than focusing on symptoms.
- Explore recent life events and ask how the patient is handling these.
- Convey empathy with the patient's suffering and psychosocial difficulties.
- No specific pharmacologic therapy has been clearly proven effective, although a number of agents including gabapentin and St. John's wort have been useful in some studies.

CHRONIC Rx

- Provide one primary care practitioner to manage care.
- Avoid confronting the patient regarding the psychological origin of symptoms.
- Ensure follow-up visits at regular (e.g., 2- to 4-wk intervals that are not symptom-contingent; i.e., maintain the regularity even if the symptoms improve).
- Avoid invasive or expensive diagnostic procedures unless there are clear signs of new illness, not just symptoms.
- Diagnose and treat mood or anxiety disorders.
- Cognitive behavior therapy groups have been helpful for patients with unexplained somatic symptoms and can dramatically improve functioning.

DISPOSITION

A chronic condition with frequent exacerbations

REFERRAL

If the patient is open to discussing psychological issues a referral for psychotherapy can be made.

PEARLS & CONSIDERATIONS

Patients with somatization disorder respond best to establishing a regular, working relationship with a primary care provider. Avoiding confrontations about the origins of symptoms, investigating symptoms when related to actual signs of disease, and gently investigating concurrent stressors will help avoid most of the common problems with this population.

SUGGESTED READINGS

Allen LA et al: Cognitive-behavioral therapy for somatization disorder: a randomized controlled trial, *Arch Intern Med* 166(14):1512, 2006.
Barsky AJ et al: Distinctive patterns of medical care utilization in patients who somatize, *Med Care* 44(9):803, 2006.
Mai F: Somatization disorder: a practical review, *Can J Psychiatry* 49(10):652, 2004.

AUTHOR: **STUART J. EISENDRATH, M.D.**

BASIC INFORMATION

DEFINITION

Spinal cord compression is the neurologic loss of spine function. Lesions may be complete or incomplete and develop gradually or acutely. Incomplete lesions often present as distinct syndromes, as follows:

- Central cord syndrome
- Anterior cord syndrome
- Brown-Séquard syndrome
- Conus medullaris syndrome
- Cauda equina syndrome

ICD-9CM CODES
344.89 Brown-Séquard syndrome
344.60 Cauda equina syndrome
336.8 Conus medullaris syndrome
Other lesions listed by site

PHYSICAL FINDINGS & CLINICAL PRESENTATION

Clinical features reflect the amount of spinal cord involvement:

- Motor loss and sensory abnormalities
- Babinski testing usually positive
- Clonus
- Gradual compression, often manifested by progressive difficulty walking, clonus with weight bearing, and involuntary spasm; development of sensory symptoms; bladder dysfunction (late)
- Central cord syndrome: results in a variable quadriparesis with the upper extremities more severely involved than the lower extremities; some sensory sparing
- Anterior cord syndrome: results in motor, pain, and temperature loss below the lesion
- Brown-Séquard syndrome:
  1. Spinal cord syndrome caused by injury to either half of the spinal cord and resulting in the loss of motor function, position, vibration, and light touch on the affected side
  2. Pain and temperature sense loss on the opposite side
- Conus medullaris syndrome: results in variable motor loss in the lower extremities with loss of bowel and bladder function
- Cauda equina syndrome: typical low back pain, weakness in both lower extremities, saddle anesthesia, and loss of voluntary bladder and bowel control

ETIOLOGY

- Trauma
- Tumor
- Infection
- Inflammatory processes
- Degenerative disk conditions with spinal stenosis
- Acute disk herniation
- Cystic abnormalities

DIAGNOSIS

DIFFERENTIAL DIAGNOSIS

- See "Etiology."
- Section II describes the differential diagnosis of paraplegia.

WORKUP

- Spinal cord compression: requires an immediate referral for radiographic and neurologic assessment
- Laboratory results usually unremarkable unless infectious or inflammatory causes suspected

IMAGING STUDIES

- Depend on the suspected etiology
- MRI usually required

TREATMENT

Urgent surgical decompression is usually indicated as soon as the etiology is established.

DISPOSITION

Important indicators regarding prognosis (Leventhal):

- The greater the distal motor and sensory sparing, the greater the expected recovery.
- When a plateau of recovery is reached, no further improvement is expected.
- The quicker the recovery, the greater the recovery

REFERRAL

Immediate referral for radiographic and neurologic evaluation and treatment in all suspected cases of spinal cord compression

SUGGESTED READINGS

Baines MJ: Spinal cord compression—a personal and palliative care perspective, *Clin Oncol (R Coll Radiol)* 14(2):135, 2002.

Banerjee R, Stanley J, Palumbo M: Spinal Epidural Hematoma induced by leukemia, *Orthopedics* 27:864, 2004.

Benjamin R: Neurologic complications of prostate cancer, *Am Fam Physician* 65(9):1834, 2002.

Buchner M, Schiltenwolf M: Cauda equina syndrome caused by intervertebral lumbar disc prolapse: mid-term results of 22 patients and literature review, *Orthopedics* 25:727, 2002.

Carlson GD et al: Sustained spinal cord compression. Part I: time-dependent effect on long-term pathophysiology, *J Bone Joint Surg* 85:86, 2003.

Carlson GD et al: Sustained spinal cord compression. Part II: effect of methylprednisolone on regional blood flow and recovery of somatosensory evoked potentials, *J Bone Joint Surg* 85:95, 2003.

Casey AT et al: Rheumatoid arthritis of the cervical spine: current techniques for management, *Orthop Clin North Am* 33(2):291, 2002.

Jagas M et al: Vertebroplasty with methacrylate bone cement and radiotherapy in the treatment of spinal metastases with epidural spinal cord compression, *Ortop Traumatol Rehabil* 7(5):491, 2005.

Kadanka Z et al: Approaches to spondylotic cervical myelopathy: conservative versus surgical in a 3-year follow-up study, *Spine* 27(20):2205, 2002.

Malcolm GP: Surgical disorders of the cervical spine: presentation and management of common disorders, *J Neurosurg Psychiatry* 73(Suppl 1):134, 2002.

Matsunaga S et al: Trauma-induced myelopathy in patients with ossification of the posterior longitudinal ligament, *J Neurosurg* 97(2 Suppl):172, 2002.

Mohanty SP, Venkatram N: Does neurological recovery in thoracolumbar and lumbar burst fractures depend on the extent of canal compromise? *Spinal Cord* 40(6):295, 2002.

Rades D et al: Do bladder cancer patients with metastatic spinal cord compression benefit from radiotherapy alone? *Urology* 69(6): 1081, 2007.

Shimomura T et al: Prognostic factors for deterioration of patients with cervical spondylotic myelopathy after nonsurgical treatment, *Spine* 32:2474, 2007.

Sorar M et al: Cervical compression myelopathy: is fusion the main prognostic indicator? *J Neurosurg Spine* 6(6)531, 2007.

Tang HJ et al: Spinal epidural abscess—experience with 46 patients and evaluation of prognostic factors, *J Infect* 45(2):76, 2002.

Venkitaraman R et al: Outcome of early detection and radiotherapy for occult spinal cord compression, *Radiother Oncol* 85:469, 2007.

AUTHOR: **LONNIE R. MERCIER, M.D.**

BASIC INFORMATION

DEFINITION

A spinal epidural abscess (SEA) is a focal suppurative infection occurring in the spinal epidural space.

ICD-9CM CODES
324.1 Spinal epidural abscess

EPIDEMIOLOGY & DEMOGRAPHICS

INCIDENCE (IN U.S.):
- 2 to 25 cases/100,000 hospitalized patients/yr
- May be increasing over the past 3 decades

PREDOMINANT AGE:
- Median age of onset approximately 50 yr (35 yr in intravenous drug users)
- Peak incidence in seventh and eighth decades of life

PHYSICAL FINDINGS & CLINICAL PRESENTATION

The presentation of SEA can be nonspecific.
- Fever, malaise, and back pain are the most consistent early symptoms.
- Pain is often focal. It may initially be mild but can progress to become severe.
- As the disease progresses, root pain can occur, followed by motor weakness, sensory changes, bladder and bowel dysfunction, and paralysis.
- Physical findings may be limited to fever or spinal tenderness.
- The evolution to neurologic deficits can occur as quickly as a few hours, or over weeks to months.
- Once paralysis occurs, it may quickly become irreversible without the appropriate intervention.

ETIOLOGY

- Pyogenic bacteria account for the majority of cases in the U.S. Immigrants from tuberculosis-endemic areas may present with tuberculous SEAs. Fungi and parasites can also cause this condition. The most common causative organism is *Staphylococcus aureus*. Most posterior EAs thought to originate from distant focus (e.g., skin and soft tissue infections), while anterior EAs commonly associated with diskitis or vertebral osteomyelitis. No source found in approximately one third of cases.
- Associated predisposing conditions include diabetes mellitus, alcoholism, cancer, AIDS, and chronic renal failure, or following epidural anesthesia, spinal surgery or trauma, or intravenous drug use. No predisposing condition is found in approximately 20% of patients.
- Damage to the spinal cord can be caused by direct compression of the spinal cord, vascular compromise, bacterial toxins, and inflammation.

DIAGNOSIS

DIFFERENTIAL DIAGNOSIS

- Herniated disc
- Vertebral osteomyelitis and diskitis
- Metastic tumors
- Meningitis

LABORATORY TESTS

- WBC may be normal or elevated.
- ESR usually elevated over 30 mm/hr.
- Blood cultures are positive in approximately 60% of patients with SEA.
- CSF cultures positive in 19%, but lumbar puncture unnecessary, and may be contraindicated.
- Once imaging is done, CT-guided aspiration or open biopsy should be done to determine causative organism. Abscess content culture positive in 90%.

IMAGING STUDIES

- MRI with gadolinium is the imaging modality of choice; CT scan with contrast may show the abscess but is less sensitive than MRI.
- CT with myelography is more sensitive for cord compression.

TREATMENT

NONPHARMACOLOGIC THERAPY

- Surgical decompression is the mainstay of treatment. Decompression within the first 24 hr has been related to an improved prognosis.
- Nonsurgical treatment is effective in some patients, but failure rate may be excessive. This approach should not be considered but should only be attempted in the absence of signs of compressive myelopathy and with very careful follow-up.

ACUTE GENERAL Rx

- In addition to surgery, antibiotics directed at the most likely organism should be initiated.
- If the organism is unknown, broad coverage against staphylococci, streptococci and gram-negative bacilli should be initiated. The regimen can be adjusted according to culture results. Therapy should continue for at least 4 to 6 wk.

CHRONIC Rx

Neurologic deficits may remain despite aggressive treatment.

DISPOSITION

Irreversible paralysis and death can occur in up to 25% of patients.

REFERRAL

All cases should be referred to a neurosurgeon and an infectious diseases specialist.

PEARLS & CONSIDERATIONS

It is critically important to recognize this process early; the prognosis is generally excellent if treatment is initiated while symptoms are localized and before evidence of myelopathy develops.

SUGGESTED READINGS

Curry WT et al: Spinal epidural abscess: clinical presentation, management, and outcome, *Surg Neurol* 63(4):364, 2005.

Moriya M et al: Successful management of cervical spinal epidural abscess without surgery, *Intern Med* 44(10):1110, 2005.

Savage K, Holtom PD, Zalavras CG: Spinal epidural abscess: early clinical outcome in patients treated medically, *Clin Orthop Relat Res* 439:56, 2005.

Torgovnick J, Sethi N, Wyss J: Spinal epidural abscess: clinical presentation, management and outcome, *Surg Neurol* 63:364, 2005.

AUTHORS: **GLENN G. FORT, M.D., M.P.H., DENNIS J. MIKOLICH, M.D.,** and **MAURICE POLICAR, M.D.**

BASIC INFORMATION

DEFINITION

Spinal stenosis is the pathologic condition caused by the compressing or narrowing of the spinal canal, nerve root canal, or intervertebral foramina at the lumbar region.

SYNONYMS

Central spinal stenosis
Lateral spinal stenosis
Spondylosis

ICD-9CM CODES
724.02 Spinal stenosis lumbar, lumbosacral

EPIDEMIOLOGY & DEMOGRAPHICS

More common between 50 and 60 yr of age

PHYSICAL FINDINGS & CLINICAL PRESENTATION

- Symptoms caused by direct mechanical compression or indirect vascular compression of the nerve roots or the cauda equina
- Neurogenic claudication: leg, buttock, or back pain precipitated by walking and relieved by sitting
- Pain may radiate down to ankles and is associated with numbness, tingling, and weakness
- Taking a flexed posture reduces symptoms because it increases the available space in the lumbar spinal canal
- Decreased lumbar extension
- Normal peripheral pulses
- Positive Romberg's sign (decreased proprioception)
- Wide-based gait
- Reduced knee and ankle reflex
- Urine incontinence

ETIOLOGY

Spinal stenosis may be primary or secondary

- Primary stenosis (congenital or developmental narrowing)
  1. Idiopathic
  2. Achondroplasia
  3. Morquio-Ullrich syndrome
- Secondary stenosis (acquired)
  1. Degenerative (hypertrophy of the articular processes, disk degeneration, ligamentum flavum hypertrophy, spondylolisthesis)
  2. Fracture/trauma
  3. Postoperative (postlaminectomy)
  4. Paget's disease
  5. Ankylosing spondylitis
  6. Tumors
  7. Acromegaly

DIAGNOSIS

DIFFERENTIAL DIAGNOSIS

- Osteoarthritis of the knee or hip
- Acute cauda equina syndrome, due to compression by epidural abscess or tumors
- Pain and weakness caused by multiple myeloma or osteomyelitis
- Intermittent claudication-peripheral vascular disease
- Peripheral neuropathy such as that caused by a herniated nucleus pulposus
- Scoliosis or spondylolisthesis
- Rheumatoid diseases: ankylosing spondylitis, Reiter's syndrome, fibromyalgia

WORKUP

History, physical examination, and specific imaging studies

IMAGING STUDIES

- Lumbar spine film sensitivity 66%, specificity 93%.
- Ultrasound of the spinal canal has also been used.
- CT scan of the lumbosacral spine: sensitivity (75% to 85%), specificity (80%).
- MRI of the lumbosacral spine: sensitivity (80% to 90%), specificity (95%).
- Myelogram: sensitivity (77%), specificity (72%). Absolute stenosis is defined as the anterior-posterior (AP) diameter of the spinal canal <10 mm. Relative stenosis: 10 to 12 mm AP diameter.
- Electromyography (EMG) and nerve conduction velocity (NCV) are additional studies particularly useful in differentiating peripheral neuropathy from lumbar spinal stenosis.

TREATMENT

NONPHARMACOLOGIC THERAPY

- Physiotherapy
- Lumbar corsets
- Back exercises
- Abdominal muscle strengthening
- Aquatic exercises

ACUTE GENERAL Rx

- Surgery is indicated in patients with significant compression of nerve roots as determined by MRI or CT and incapacitating symptoms limiting activities of daily living or bladder and bowel incontinence.
- Surgical procedures include decompressive laminectomy, arthrodesis, hemilaminectomy, and medial facetectomy.
- Lumbar interspinous process decompression using X-STOP device: a titanium oval spacer placed between the two adjacent spinous processes of the affected level; provides an unloading distractive force to the stenotic middle column part of the motion segment

CHRONIC Rx

Conservative therapy with NSAIDs (ibuprofen 800 mg PO tid, naproxen 500 mg PO bid) may be tried for symptomatic relief in addition to acetaminophen 1 g PO qid.

Epidural steroid injections may provide temporary relief.

DISPOSITION

- Approximately 20% of patients having surgery require repeat surgery within 10 yr. Nearly one third of these patients continue to experience pain.
- The natural history of spinal stenosis is one of slow progression. Although not very common, cord compression with resultant bowel and bladder incontinence and paresis can occur.
- Operative treatment is more effective in reducing pain and disability than nonoperative treatment.

REFERRAL

- Patients who have spinal stenosis should be referred to an orthopedic surgeon specializing in back surgery or to a neurosurgeon.
- Pain clinic referrals should be made if surgery is contraindicated or if the patient does not want surgery.

PEARLS & CONSIDERATIONS

COMMENTS

- Approximately one third of patients have coexisting peripheral vascular disease.
- The severity of cauda equina constriction is directly related to the walking ability and the pain intensity in the legs and back.
- Spinal stenosis is also a cause of chronic low back pain in the young.

SUGGESTED READINGS

de Graaf I et al: Diagnosis of lumbar spinal stenosis: a systematic review of the accuracy of diagnostic tests, *Spine* 31(10):1168-1176, 2006.

Malmivaara A et al (for the Finnish Lumbar Spinal Research Group): Surgical or nonoperative treatment for lumbar spinal stenosis? A randomized controlled trial, *Spine* 32(1): 1-8, 2007.

AUTHOR: **JORGE A. VILLAFUERTE, M.D.**

BASIC INFORMATION

DEFINITION

A heterogenous group of autosomal dominantly inherited diseases with core features of progressive ataxia and spasticity. Current nomenclature (e.g., SCA1, SCA6) is based on genotyping of mutations.

SYNONYMS

Autosomal dominant spinocerebellar ataxia (ADCA)

- Machado-Joseph disease (MJD) is a subset, the most common type (SCA3).

ICD-9CM CODES
334.2 Primary cerebellar degeneration

EPIDEMIOLOGY & DEMOGRAPHICS

Epidemiology has not been well studied outside of isolated geographic regions. A conservative estimate of prevalence is 3 cases per 100,000 people. The most common subtypes worldwide are SCA3 (30% to 50%) and SCA1, SCA2, SCA6, SCA7, SCA8.

PHYSICAL FINDINGS & CLINICAL PRESENTATION

A. Chronic, slowly progressive ataxia is the hallmark of all of these diseases. Ataxia refers to incoordination or clumsiness of movements. Cerebellar ataxia is defined as lack of accuracy or coordination that is not due to weakness, alteration in tone, sensory loss, or the presence of involuntary movements.

B. Most often the SCAs present in adulthood (see later). Many of the diseases show the phenomenon of genetic anticipation, in that successive generations (within a family) will be affected at earlier ages.

C. Within a family, there can be significant phenotypic variability.

D. Although the nomenclature of these diseases is moving toward that based on genotyping, an older clinical classification still provides a useful framework (note that because of phenotypic variability within a genotype, some mutations can fit into more than one of the clinical groups):

1. Autosomal dominant cerebellar ataxia (ADCA) type I:
   a. Progressive cerebellar ataxia variably associated with other extracerebellar neurologic features, such as ophthalmoplegia, neuropathy, optic atrophy, pyramidal or extrapyramidal signs, or sleep disorders.
   b. The largest clinical subtype.
   c. Symptoms typically appear in third or fourth decades, but range from first to seventh.
   d. Gait is usually affected first, followed by arms, speech.
   e. Genetically heterogenous, includes most patients with SCA1, SCA2, SCA3, SCA4, SCA8, SCA10, SCA12.
2. ADCA type II:
   a. Progressive cerebellar ataxia invariably associated with pigmentary retinopathy. Other neurologic features may also be present, the most common of which is supranuclear ophthalmoplegia.
   b. Symptoms typically appear in third or fourth decades, but range from first to seventh.
   c. Onset may occur with either ataxia or vision loss.
   d. Early retinal changes subtle and only visible with indirect ophthalmoscopy.
   e. Genetically homogenous, most patients have SCA7.
3. ADCA type III:
   a. Progressive cerebellar ataxia without prominent visual or extracerebellar neurologic symptoms.
   b. Symptoms typically appear in third or fourth decades, but range from first to seventh.
   c. Genetically heterogenous, includes most patients with SCA5, SCA6, SCA11, SCA15, SCA16.

ETIOLOGY

Many of the currently identified mutations in the SCA genes are expansion of exonic CAG repeats. As in other diseases of this type (Huntington's chorea), the severity/age of onset of the disease is proportional to the number of CAG repeats in an individual's gene.

DIAGNOSIS

DIFFERENTIAL DIAGNOSIS

- Friedrich's ataxia (FA)—differs from the SCAs in that inheritance is autosomal recessive, that it almost always begins in childhood or adolescence, and that it is associated with early lower-limb areflexia.
- Sensory ataxias—differ from the SCAs in that the primary defect is not one of cerebellar function but of sensory inputs into the cerebellum. Can be the result of peripheral neuropathies or spinal cord disease that involves the posterior columns.
- Posterior fossa mass lesions.
- Acquired vitamin E deficiency—differs from SCAs in that patients almost always have clinically evident disorder of fat malabsorption.
- Chronic toxin exposure (alcohol, phenytoin, organic mercury).
- Multiple sclerosis, other CNS inflammatory diseases—differ from SCAs in that ataxia, when present, usually presents acutely to subacutely.
- Antigliadin antibodies—present in most patients with gluten enteropathy (celiac sprue); however, they can also be found in some ataxia patients without clinically evident celiac disease (this association remains controversial).
- Paraneoplastic cerebellar degeneration—differs from SCAs in that the ataxia progresses relatively rapidly.
- Creutzfeldt-Jakob disease—differs from the SCAs in that the ataxia progresses relatively rapidly, and is accompanied by dementia and myoclonus.
- Wilson's disease—differs from the SCAs in that there is often accompanying parkinsonism, psychiatric manifestations, and hepatic dysfunction.
- Superficial siderosis—differs from the SCAs in that it also often produces sensorineural hearing loss, anosmia, dementia, and bladder disturbance.
- Mitochondrial encephalomyopathies.
- Multiple systems atrophy—differs from the SCAs in that age of onset is usually later and that parkinsonism, long-tract signs, or orthostatic hypotension are often present.

LABORATORY TESTS

- Genetic testing:
  1. Available commercially for many of the SCAs. Given the number of available tests and significant expense for each, referral to a specialist is probably prudent before testing.
  2. In patients with a positive family history, this is an appropriate first step.
  3. In patients without a positive family history, testing for acquired/potentially reversible causes should be done first.
  4. There are significant ethical issues involved when testing presymptomatic individuals at risk within a family. Genetic and psychologic counseling is appropriate for these patients before testing is performed.
- Anti-Purkinje cell antibodies (anti-Yo, less commonly anti-Hu)—present in approximately half of patients with paraneoplastic cerebellar degeneration.
- Antigliadin antibodies (serum and spinal fluid).
- Serum vitamin E levels.
- If Wilson's disease is a consideration: serum transaminases and ceruloplasmin, 24-hr urine copper, ophthalmologic evaluation for Kayser-Fleischer rings.
- If Creutzfeldt-Jakob disease is a consideration: MRI, EEG, spinal fluid analysis for 14-3-3 protein.
- Testing for organic mercury poisoning is beyond the scope of this article but

note that urinary mercury testing will not detect it.

IMAGING STUDIES

- MRI of the brain with and without contrast is the preferred imaging modality, mostly as a means of eliminating other differential diagnoses.
- Cerebellar atrophy, with or without brainstem atrophy is the typical picture seen in the SCAs. This finding on MRI is not terribly sensitive or specific for the SCAs, however.

TREATMENT

Rx

NONPHARMACOLOGIC

Physical, occupational, and speech therapies to help patients adapt to progressive disability

ACUTE GENERAL Rx

None available.

CHRONIC Rx

There are currently no disease-modifying treatments available. Symptomatic treatment of specific symptoms can be of benefit (e.g., treatment of spasticity with antispasticity agents, treatment of parkinsonism and/or restless leg syndrome with dopaminergic agents).

DISPOSITION

Variable life expectancies, roughly inversely related to age of onset.

REFERRAL

Referral to a general neurologist or movement disorders center is appropriate.

PEARLS & CONSIDERATIONS

!

COMMENTS

- In symptomatic patients with a family history of dominantly inherited ataxia, the diagnostic process is relatively straightforward. Genetic testing, directed toward likely mutations by phenotype and ethnic origin, should be the first step.
- In patients with subacute to chronic onset of cerebellar ataxia without a clear family history, the initial step in diagnosis should be brain MRI to look for structural lesions. If negative, or only showing atrophy, one should proceed with serologic/spinal fluid evaluation.

PREVENTION

None available.

PATIENT/FAMILY EDUCATION

Patient educational materials as well as contact information for support groups and advocacy available at the website for the National Ataxia Foundation: http://www.ataxia.org.

SUGGESTED READINGS

Koeppen A: The pathogenosis of spinocerebellar ataxia, *Cerebellum* 4:62, 2005.

Paulson H: Dominantly inherited ataxias: lessons learned from Machado-Joseph disease/spinocerebellar ataxia type 3, *Semin Neurol* 27:133, 2007.

Schols L et al: Autosomal dominant cerebellar ataxias: clinical features, genetics, and pathogenesis, *Lancet Neurol* 3:291, 2004.

Wood N, Harding A: Cerebellar and spinocerebellar disorders. In Bradley W et al (eds): *Neurology in Clinical Practice,* ed 3, Boston, 2000, Butterworth-Heinemann.

AUTHOR: **DAVID P. WILLIAMS, M.D.**

BASIC INFORMATION

DEFINITION

Spontaneous miscarriage is fetal loss before wk 20 of pregnancy, calculated from the patient's last menstrual period or the delivery of a fetus weighing <500 g. *Early loss* is before menstrual wk 12, while *late loss* refers to losses from 12 to 20 wk.

Miscarriage can also be classified as *incomplete* (partial passage of fetal tissue through partially dilated cervix), *complete* (spontaneous passage of all fetal tissue), *threatened* (uterine bleeding without cervical dilation or passage of tissue), *inevitable* (bleeding with cervical dilation without passage of fetal tissue), or *missed abortion* (intrauterine fetal demise without passage of tissue).

Recurrent miscarriage involves three or more spontaneous pregnancy losses before wk 20.

ICD-9CM CODES
634.0 Spontaneous abortion

SYNONYMS

Abortion

EPIDEMIOLOGY & DEMOGRAPHICS

INCIDENCE: 15% to 20% of clinically recognized pregnancies, with 80% of miscarriages occurring in the first trimester

GENETICS:

- Distribution of abnormal karyotypes: autosomal trisomy (50%), monosomy 45,X (20%), triploidy (15%), tetraploidy (10%), structural chromosomal abnormalities (5%).
- With two or more spontaneous miscarriages, a karyotype should be performed to evaluate for balanced translocation, which has 80% risk for abortion, and, if the pregnancy is carried to term, has 3% to 5% risk for unbalanced karyotype.

RISK FACTORS: Prior pregnancy history (risk after live birth = 5%, prior pregnancy aborted = 20% subsequent risk) is the most significant risk factor. Vaginal bleeding, especially >3 days, carries with it a 15% to 20% chance of miscarriage.

PHYSICAL FINDINGS & CLINICAL PRESENTATION

- Profuse bleeding and cramping has a higher association with miscarriage than bleeding without cramping, which is more consistent with a threatened miscarriage.
- Cervical dilation with history or finding of fetal tissue at cervical os may be present.
- In cases of missed abortion, uterine size may be smaller than menstrual dating, in contrast to molar gestation, where size may be greater than dates.

ETIOLOGY

- In a general overview the etiology can be classified in terms of maternal (environmental) and fetal (genetic) factors, with the majority of miscarriages being related to genetic or chromosomal causes
- Causes: uterine anomalies (unicornuate uterus risk = 50%, bicornuate or septate uterus risk = 25% to 30%), incompetent cervix (iatrogenic or congenital, associated with 20% of midtrimester losses), diethylstilbestrol exposure in utero (T-shaped uterus), submucous leiomyomas, intrauterine adhesions or synechiae, luteal phase or progesterone deficiency, autoimmune disease such as anticardiolipin antibodies, uncontrolled diabetes mellitus, HLA associations between mother and father, infections such as TB, *Chlamydia, Ureaplasma,* smoking and alcohol use, irradiation, and environmental toxins

DIAGNOSIS

DIFFERENTIAL DIAGNOSIS

- Normal pregnancy
- Hydatidiform molar gestation
- Ectopic pregnancy
- Dysfunctional uterine bleeding
- Pathologic endometrial or cervical lesions

WORKUP

- All patients with bleeding in the first trimester should have an evaluation for possible ectopic pregnancy.
- If there are three early, prior pregnancy losses, a workup and treatment for recurrent miscarriage should begin before next conception. If there is a strong history for second-trimester loss, consideration for cerclage should be given, especially if the history is consistent with incompetent cervix (e.g., painless cervical dilation).

LABORATORY TESTS

- Type and antibody screen is used to evaluate for the need for Rh immune globulin.
- During the preconception period, Hgb A1C, anticardiolipin antibody, lupus anticoagulant, factor V, Leiden, MTHFR, Antithrombin III, Prothrombin gene 2210A, karyotyping, endometrial biopsy with progesterone level, and cervical cultures or serum antibodies can be checked for suspected disease processes.
- Progesterone level <5 mg/dl indicates nonviable gestation vs. >25 mg/dl, which suggests a good prognosis.

IMAGING STUDIES

Transabdominal or transvaginal sonogram (preferably) can be used in combination with menstrual dating and serum quantitative hCG to document pregnancy location, fetal heart presence, gestational sac size, and adnexal pathology.

TREATMENT

NONPHARMACOLOGIC THERAPY

Depending on the patient's clinical status, desire to continue the pregnancy, and certainty of the diagnosis, expectant management can be considered. In pregnancies <6 wk or >14 wk, complete expulsion of fetal tissue usually occurs and surgical intervention such as dilation and curettage (D&C) can be avoided.

ACUTE GENERAL Rx

- *Incomplete miscarriage* between 6 and 14 wk can be associated with large amounts of blood loss, and thus these patients should undergo D&C.
- In cases of *missed abortion,* if fetal demise has occurred >6 wk before or gestational age is >14 wk, there is an increased risk of hypofibrinogenemia with disseminated intravascular coagulation, and thus D&C should be performed early in the disease course. Can consider use of misoprostol (Cytotec) 200 mg po q6h × 4 doses.
- *Threatened abortions* may be managed expectantly, watching for signs of cervical dilation or sonographic evidence of missed abortion.
- If surgical intervention is required, preoperative use of 40 U of oxytocin (Pitocin) in 1000 ml lactated Ringer's solution may be used to decrease the amount of bleeding and shorten the operative time.
- Postoperatively all patients undergoing a D&C should receive antibiotics (doxycycline 100 mg bid for 7 days), methylergonovine (Methergine) 0.2 mg q6h for four doses, and Motrin or NSAIDs prn for pain.
- In all cases of first- or second-trimester bleeding in Rh-negative patients, Rh immune globulin 300 μg should be given to prevent Rh sensitization.

REFERRAL

Refer to OB/GYN.

PEARLS & CONSIDERATIONS

"Spontaneous pregnancy loss" has been recommended to avoid the term "abortion" and acknowledge the emotional aspects of losing a pregnancy.

SUGGESTED READING

Griebel CP et al: Management of spontaneous abortion, *Am Fam Physician* 72:1243, 2005.

AUTHORS: **SCOTT J. ZUCCALA, D.O.,** and **RUBEN ALVERO, M.D.**

BASIC INFORMATION

DEFINITION

Sporotrichosis is a granulomatous disease caused by *Sporothrix schenckii.*

SYNONYMS

Lymphocutaneous sporotrichosis
Cutaneous sporotrichosis
Pulmonary sporotrichosis

ICD-9CM CODES
117.1 Sporotrichosis

EPIDEMIOLOGY & DEMOGRAPHICS

PREDOMINANT SEX: The most common form, lymphocutaneous sporotrichosis, occurs equally in both sexes. Males predominate in both pulmonary and osteoarticular sporotrichosis.

PREDOMINANT AGE: Generally, lymphocutaneous sporotrichosis occurs in persons 35 yr of age or younger, and pulmonary sporotrichosis occurs in persons between the ages of 30 to 60 yr.

GENETICS:

Neonatal Infection: At least one case of transmission from the cheek lesion of the mother to the skin of the infant has been reported.

PHYSICAL FINDINGS & CLINICAL PRESENTATION

- Cutaneous disease
  1. Arises at the site of inoculation
  2. Initial lesion usually located on the distal part of an extremity, although any area may be affected, including the face
  3. Variable incubation period of approximately 3 wk once introduced into the skin
  4. Granulomatous reaction provoked
  5. Lesion becomes papulonodular, erythematous, elastic, variable in size
  6. Subsequently, nodule becomes fluctuant, undergoes central necrosis, breaks down, discharges mucoid pus from which fungus may be isolated
  7. Indolent ulcer with raised erythematous or violaceous borders
  8. Secondary lesions:
     a. Develop along superficial lymphatic channels
     b. Evolve in the same manner as the primary lesion, with subsequent inflammation, induration, and suppuration
- Fixed, or plaque form
  1. Erythematous verrucous, ulcerated, or crusted lesions
  2. Does not spread locally
  3. Does not involve lymphatic vessels
  4. Rarely undergoes spontaneous resolution
  5. More often persists for years without systemic symptoms and within a setting of normal laboratory examinations
- Osteoarticular involvement
  1. Most common extracutaneous form
  2. Usually presents as monoarticular arthritis
  3. Left untreated, may progress to:
     a. Synovitis
     b. Osteitis
     c. Periostitis
     d. All involving elbows, knees, wrists, and ankles
  4. Joint inflamed
     a. Associated with an effusion
     b. Painful on motion
- Early pulmonary disease
  1. Usually associated with a paucity of clinical findings
     a. Low-grade fever
     b. Cough
     c. Fatigue
     d. Malaise
     e. Weight loss
  2. Untreated
     a. Cavitary pulmonary disease
     b. Frank pulmonary dysfunction
  3. Meningitis uncommon
     a. Except perhaps in the immunocompromised patient
     b. Presents with few signs or symptoms of neurologic involvement
  4. Few reported cases
     a. Infection of the ocular adnexa
     b. Endophthalmitis without antecedent trauma
     c. Infection of the testes and epididymis

ETIOLOGY

- *Sporothrix schenckii*
  1. Global in distribution
  2. Often isolated from soil, plants, and plant products
  3. Majority of case reports from tropical and subtropical regions of the Americas
- Occupational or recreational exposure
  1. Hay
  2. Straw
  3. Sphagnum moss
  4. Timber
  5. Thorny plants (e.g., roses and barberry bushes)
- Animal contact
  1. Armadillos
  2. Cats
  3. Squirrels
- Human-to-human transmission
- Tattooing

DIAGNOSIS

DIFFERENTIAL DIAGNOSIS

- Fixed, or plaque, sporotrichosis
  1. Bacterial pyoderma
  2. Foreign body granuloma
  3. Tularemia
  4. Anthrax
  5. Other mycoses: blastomycosis, chromoblastomycosis
- Lymphocutaneous sporotrichosis
  1. *Nocardia brasiliensis*
  2. *Leishmania braziliensis*
  3. Atypical mycobacterial disease: *M. marinum, M. kansasii*
- Pulmonary sporotrichosis
  1. Pulmonary TB
  2. Histoplasmosis
  3. Coccidioidomycosis
- Osteoarticular sporotrichosis
  1. Pigmented villonodular synovitis
  2. Gout
  3. Rheumatoid arthritis
  4. Infection with *M. tuberculosis*
  5. Atypical mycobacteria: *M. marinum, M. kansasii, M. avium-intracellulare*
- Meningitis
  1. Histoplasmosis
  2. Cryptococcosis
  3. TB

WORKUP

- The diagnosis should be considered in individuals who are occupationally exposed to soil, decaying plant matter, and thorny plants (gardeners, horticulturists, farmers) who present with chronic nonhealing ulcers or lesions with or without associated arthritis or pulmonary symptoms.
- Diagnosis is made by culture:
  1. Pus
  2. Joint fluid
  3. Sputum
  4. Blood
  5. Skin biopsy
- Isolation of the fungus from any site is considered diagnostic of infection.
- Saprophytic colonization of the respiratory tract has been described.
- A positive blood culture may indicate infection in an immunocompromised host.
- Increasingly sensitive laboratory culturing systems may detect the fungus in the normal host.
- Biopsy specimens are diagnostic if characteristic cigar-shaped, round, oval, or budding yeast forms are seen.
- Despite special staining, the yeast may remain difficult to detect unless multiple sections are examined.
- No standard method of serologic testing is available.
- Previously described techniques have been hampered by the presence of antibody in the absence of infection.

LABORATORY TESTS

- CBCs and serum chemistries are generally normal.
- Elevated ESR is seen with extracutaneous disease.

- CSF analysis in meningeal disease reveals:
  1. Lymphocytic pleocytosis
  2. Elevated protein
  3. Hypoglycorrhachia
- Nested PCR assay represents a future clinical modality to rapidly detect *Sporothrix schenckii*.

IMAGING STUDIES

- Chest x-ray examination: unilateral or bilateral upper lobe cavitary or noncavitary lesions
- Radiographic findings of affected joints:
  1. Loss of articular cartilage
  2. Periosteal reaction
  3. Periarticular osteopenia
  4. Cystic changes

TREATMENT

Rx

NONPHARMACOLOGIC THERAPY

Local heat and prevention of bacterial superinfection in cutaneous or plaque form

ACUTE GENERAL Rx

CUTANEOUS AND LYMPHOCUTANEOUS SPOROTRICHOSIS:

- Itraconazole at doses of 100 to 200 mg/day is the drug of choice and should be given for 3 to 6 mo.
- Use saturated solution of potassium iodide (SSKI) 5 to 10 drops PO tid or 1.5 ml PO tid, gradually increasing to 40 to 50 drops PO tid or 3 ml PO tid after meals.
- Maximum tolerated dose should be continued until cutaneous lesions have resolved, approximately 6 to 12 wk.
- Adjunctive therapy with heat is useful and occasionally curative.
- Side effects:
  1. Nausea
  2. Anorexia
  3. Diarrhea
  4. Parotid or lacrimal gland hypertrophy
  5. Acneiform rash

DEEP-SEATED MYCOSES (E.G., OSTEOARTICULAR, NONCAVITARY PULMONARY DISEASE):

- Itraconazole
  1. Appropriate initial chemotherapy
  2. Probably as effective as amphotericin B
  3. Less toxic than amphotericin B
  4. Better tolerated than ketoconazole
  5. 100 to 200 mg bid for 1 to 2 yr with continued lifelong suppressive therapy in selected patients
  6. Absence of relapses from 40 to 68 mo has been documented when at least 200 mg/day administered for 24 mo
  7. Insufficient data for use in disseminated disease (e.g., fungemia and meningitis)
- Parenteral amphotericin B, total course of 2 to 2.5 g or more, results in cure in approximately two thirds of cases
  1. Relapses are common.
  2. Amphotericin B–resistant isolates of *Sporothrix schenckii* have been reported.
  3. Remains the drug of choice for severely ill patients with disseminated disease.
  4. In cavitary pulmonary disease, given perioperatively as an adjunct to surgical resection.
  5. In meningitis, amphotericin B may be used alone or in combination with 5-fluorocytosine.
- Fluconazole
  1. Less effective than itraconazole
  2. Requires daily doses of 400 mg/day for lymphocutaneous disease and 800 mg/day for visceral or osteoarticular disease

CHRONIC Rx

For lymphocutaneous and visceral disease, therapy with itraconazole 200 mg/day for periods of 24 mo or greater; newer agents such as voriconazole and posaconazole might be useful in refractory to standard therapy but existing data for these new agents is very limited at present.

DISPOSITION

- Prognosis for cutaneous disease is good.
- Prognosis is less satisfactory for extracutaneous disease, especially if associated with abnormal immunologic states or other underlying systemic diseases.

REFERRAL

To surgeon; with an established diagnosis of pulmonary sporotrichosis, cavitary lesions require resection of involved tissue

PEARLS & CONSIDERATIONS

!

COMMENTS

- In patients with underlying immunosuppression (e.g., hematologic malignancy or infection with HIV), progression of the initial infection may develop into multifocal extracutaneous sporotrichosis.
- In this subset of patients, dissemination of cutaneous lesions is accompanied by hematogenous spread to lungs, bone, mucous membranes, CNS.
- Osteoarticular and pulmonary manifestations predominate with the development of polyarticular arthritis and osteolytic bone lesions.
- In the absence of therapy, the infection is ultimately fatal.
- Patients with underlying immunosuppressive states should be carefully evaluated even when presenting with single cutaneous lesions.
- Diagnostic modalities should include:
  1. Radiographic examination of chest
  2. Technetium pyrophosphate bone scan
  3. Culture of synovial fluid, blood, skin lesion(s)
- In patients with AIDS, itraconazole appears to be the drug of choice, although meningitis and pulmonary disease may warrant the use of amphotericin B.
- In patients with AIDS, lifetime suppressive therapy with itraconazole should follow initial therapy given the potential for relapse and dissemination.

SUGGESTED READINGS

Bernardes-Engermann AR et al: Development of an enzyme-linked immunosorbent assay for the serodiagnosis of several clinical forms of sporotrichosis, *Med Mycol* 43(6):487, 2005.

Da Rosa AC et al: Epidemiology of sporotrichosis; a study of 304 cases in Brazil, *J Am Acad Dermatol* 52(3 Pt 1):451, 2005.

Neyra E et al: Epidemiology of human sporotrichosis investigated by amplified fragment length polymorphism, *J Clin Microbiol* 43(3):1348, 2005.

Schubach AO, Schubach TM, Barros MB: Epidemic cat-transmitted sporotrichosis, *N Engl J Med* 353(11):1185, 2005.

AUTHORS: **GEORGE O. ALONSO, M.D., GLENN G. FORT, M.D., M.P.H.,** and **DENNIS J. MIKOLICH, M.D.**

BASIC INFORMATION

DEFINITION

Squamous cell carcinoma (SCC) is a malignant tumor of the skin arising in the epithelium.

SYNONYMS

SCC
Skin cancer

ICD-9CM CODES
173.9 Skin neoplasm, site unspecified

EPIDEMIOLOGY & DEMOGRAPHICS

- SCC is the second most common cutaneous malignancy, comprising 20% of all cases of nonmelanoma skin cancer.
- Incidence is highest in lower latitudes (e.g., southern U.S., Australia).
- Male:female ratio of 2:1.
- Incidence increases with age and sun exposure.
- Average age at diagnosis is 66 yr.

PHYSICAL FINDINGS & CLINICAL PRESENTATION

- SCC commonly affects scalp, neck region, back of hands, superior surface of the pinna, and the lip.
- The lesion may have a scaly, erythematous macule or plaque.
- Telangiectasia, central ulceration may also be present (Fig. 1-252).
- Most SCC present as exophytic lesions that grow over a period of months.

ETIOLOGY

Risk factors include UVB radiation and immunosuppression (renal transplant recipients have a threefold increased risk).

DIAGNOSIS

DIFFERENTIAL DIAGNOSIS

- Keratoacanthomas
- Actinic keratosis
- Amelanotic melanoma
- Basal cell carcinoma
- Benign tumors
- Healing traumatic wounds
- Spindle cell tumors
- Warts

WORKUP

Diagnosis is made with full-thickness skin biopsy (incisional or excisional).

TREATMENT

ACUTE GENERAL Rx

- Electrodesiccation and curettage for small SCCs (<2 cm in diameter), superficial tumors and lesions located in extremity and trunk.
- Tumors thinner than 4 mm can be managed by simple local removal.
- Lesions between 4 and 8 mm thick or those with deep dermal invasion should be excised.
- Tumors penetrating the dermis can be treated with several modalities, including excision and Mohs' surgery, radiation therapy, and chemotherapy.
- Metastatic SCC can be treated with cryotherapy and combination of chemotherapy using 13-*cis*-retinoic acid and interferon α-2A.

DISPOSITION

- Survival is related to size, location, degree of differentiation, immunologic status of the patient, depth of invasion, and presence of metastases. Risk factors for metastasis include lesions on the lip or ear, increasing lesion depth, and poor cell differentiation.
- Patients whose tumors penetrate through the dermis or exceed 8 mm in thickness are at risk of tumor recurrence.
- The most common metastatic locations are regional lymph nodes, liver, and lung.
- Tumors on the scalp, forehead, ears, nose, and lips also carry a higher risk.
- SCCs originating in the lip and pinna metastasize in 10% to 20% of cases.
- Five-year survival for metastatic squamous cell carcinoma is 34%.

REFERRAL

Oncology referral for metastatic SCC

PEARLS & CONSIDERATIONS

COMMENTS

SCC arising in areas of prior radiation, thermal injury, and areas of chronic ulcers or chronic draining sinuses are more aggressive and have a higher frequency of metastases than those originating in actinic damaged skin.

EVIDENCE

There is insufficient evidence for the use of radiation therapy after surgery to prevent recurrence of squamous cell carcinoma.[1] Ⓐ

A 40% reduction in incidence of squamous cell carcinoma was found with daily application of sunscreen to head, neck, arms, and hands compared with discretionary application in a 4.5-year randomized controlled trial.[2] Ⓐ

Evidence-Based References

1. Green A, Marks R: Squamous cell carcinoma of the skin (non-metastatic). In: *Clin Evid* 13:2142, 2005. Ⓐ
2. Green A et al: Daily sunscreen application and betacarotene supplementation in prevention of basal cell and squamous cell carcinomas of the skin: a randomised controlled trial, *Lancet* 354:723, 1999. Reviewed in: *Clin Evid* 11:2203, 2004. Ⓐ

SUGGESTED READING

Stulberg DL et al: Diagnosis and treatment of basal cell and squamous cell carcinomas, *Am Fam Physician* 70:1481, 2004.

AUTHOR: **FRED F. FERRI, M.D.**

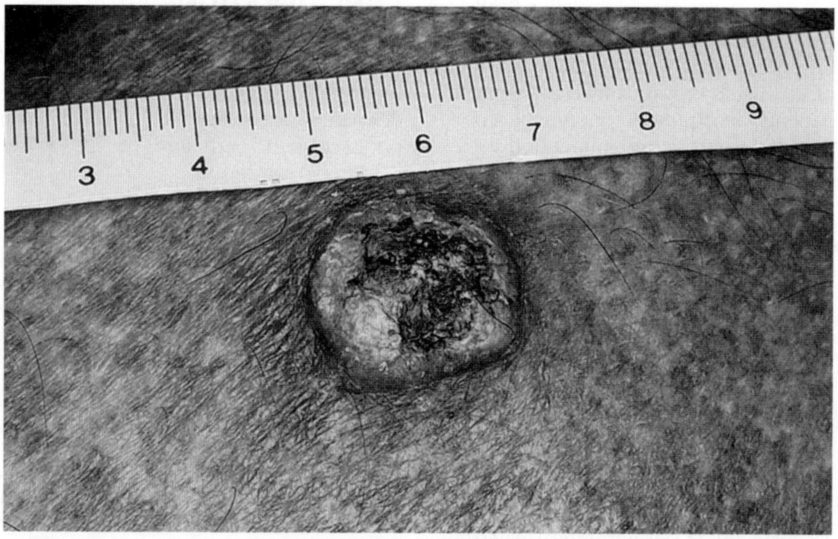

FIGURE 1-252 Squamous cell carcinoma. Nodular hyperkeratotic lesion with central erosion. (From Noble J et al: *Textbook of primary care medicine,* ed 3, St Louis, 2001, Mosby.)

BASIC INFORMATION

DEFINITION

Stasis dermatitis refers to an inflammatory skin disease of the lower extremities, commonly seen in patients with chronic venous insufficiency. (Fig. 1-253)

SYNONYMS Chronic venous insufficiency

ICD-9CM CODES
459.81 Stasis dermatitis

EPIDEMIOLOGY & DEMOGRAPHICS

- Stasis dermatitis occurs more frequently in the elderly
- Rarely seen before the age of 50 yr
- Estimated to occur in up to 6% to 7% of the patients >50 yr
- Occurs in woman more often than men, perhaps related to lower extremity venous impairment aggravated through pregnancy

PHYSICAL FINDINGS & CLINICAL PRESENTATION

- Insidious onset
- Pruritus
- Chronic edema usually described as "brawny" edema as stasis dermatitis pathologically is associated with dermal fibrosis
- Erythema
- Scaly
- Eczematous patches
- Commonly located over the medial malleolus
- Progressive pigment changes can occur as a result of extravasation of red blood cells and hemosiderin deposition within the cutaneous tissue.
- Secondary infections can occur

ETIOLOGY

- Stasis dermatitis is thought to occur as a direct result from any insult or injury of the lower extremity venous system leading to venous insufficiency including:
  1. Deep vein thrombosis
  2. Trauma
  3. Pregnancy
  4. Vein stripping
  5. Vein harvesting in patients requiring coronary artery bypass grafting (CABG)
- Venous insufficiency subsequently results in venous hypertension, causing skin inflammation and the aforementioned physical findings and clinical presentation.

DIAGNOSIS

The diagnosis of stasis dermatitis is primarily made by a detailed history and physical examination.

DIFFERENTIAL DIAGNOSIS

- Contact dermatitis
- Atopic dermatitis
- Cellulitis
- Tinea dermatophyte infection
- Pretibial myxedema
- Nummular eczema
- Lichen simplex chronicus
- Xerosis
- Asteatotic eczema
- Deep vein thrombosis

WORKUP Directed at excluding potential life-threatening causes (e.g., deep vein thrombosis) and complications (e.g., cellulites and sepsis).

LABORATORY TESTS Generally not very helpful unless a secondary infection is present.

IMAGING STUDIES

- X-rays, CT scans, and MRIs are generally not very helpful.
- Doppler studies are indicated in any patient suspected of having a deep vein thrombosis.

TREATMENT

NONPHARMACOLOGIC THERAPY

- Leg elevation above heart level for 30 min 3 to 4 times a day (avoid in arterial occlusive diseases).
- Compression stocking with a gradient of at least 30 to 40 mm Hg. In obese patients, intermittent pneumatic compression pump is recommended.
- For weeping skin lesions, wet to dry dressing changes are helpful.

ACUTE GENERAL Rx

- The mainstay of treatment of stasis dermatitis is to control leg edema and prevent venous stasis ulcers from developing.
- In patients with acute stasis dermatitis, a compression (Unna) boot can be applied.
- Topical corticosteroid creams or ointments (e.g., triamcinolone 0.1% bid) are used frequently to help reduce inflammation and itching.
- Secondary infections should be treated with appropriate antibiotics. Most secondary infections are the result of *Staphylococcus* or *Streptococcus* organisms.
- Diuretics for controlling edema.
- Aspirin (300 to 325 mg) promotes healing of chronic venous ulcers.

CHRONIC Rx

- Patients with chronic stasis dermatitis can be treated with topical emollients (e.g., white petrolatum, lanolin, Eucerin).
- Topical dressings (e.g., DuoDerm) are effective in the treatment of chronic venous stasis ulcers.
- Surgical therapy:
  - Venous stripping
  - Superficial and deep perforator vein ligation
  - Endovenous stenting

REFERRAL

- Dermatology
- Vascular surgery
- Indications for referral:
  - Nonhealing ulcers
  - Uncertainty in the diagnosis
  - Associated arterial insufficiency
  - Persistent stasis dermatitis
  - Suspected contact dermatitis
  - Consideration of superficial venous surgery

PEARLS & CONSIDERATIONS

COMMENTS

Inflammatory skin changes from stasis dermatitis are thought to result from poor oxygen perfusion to the lower-extremity skin tissue.

SUGGESTED READINGS

Felty CL, Rooke TW: Compression therapy for chronic venous insufficiency, *Semin Vasc Surg* 18(1):36, 2005.

Mussa FF: Iliac vein stenting for chronic venous insufficiency, *Tex Heart Inst J* 34(1):60, 2007.

Pascarella L, Schonbein GW, Bergan JJ: Microcirculation and venous ulcers: a review, *Ann Vasc Surg* 19(6):921, 2005.

Yuwono HS: Diagnosis and treatment in the management of chronic venous insufficiency, *Clin Hemorheol Microcirc* 23(2-4):233, 2000.

AUTHOR: **PURVA AGARWAL, M.D.**

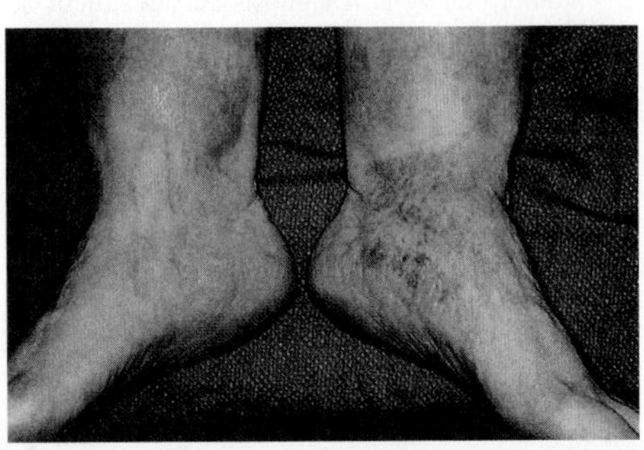

FIGURE 1-253 Moderate stasis dermatitis with hyperpigmentation and bilateral venous insufficiency. (Courtesy Department of Dermatology, University of North Carolina at Chapel Hill. From Goldstein BG, Goldstein AO: *Practical dermatology,* ed 2, St Louis, 1997, Mosby.)

BASIC INFORMATION

DEFINITION

The term *status epilepticus* refers to continuous seizure activity lasting at least 5 min, or two or more discrete seizures between which there is incomplete recovery of consciousness.

SYNONYMS

Generalized convulsive status epilepticus
Nonconvulsive status epilepticus
Complex partial status epilepticus
Absence status epilepticus

ICD-9CM CODES
345.3 Grand mal status

EPIDEMIOLOGY & DEMOGRAPHICS

INCIDENCE (IN U.S.): 100,000 to 152,000 cases per year
PREDOMINANT SEX: Male = female

PHYSICAL FINDINGS & CLINICAL PRESENTATION

- In convulsive status epilepticus, patients are unresponsive and have obvious tonic, clonic, or tonic-clonic movements of the extremities.
- Presentation of patients in nonconvulsive status epilepticus varies from complete unresponsiveness with little or no observable motor activity to confusion with or without repetitive behaviors or automatisms.

ETIOLOGY

- Preexisting epilepsy with break-through seizures or low anticonvulsant drug levels
- Central nervous system (CNS) infection or tumor
- Drug/alcohol toxicity or withdrawal
- Metabolic disturbance
- Hypoxia
- Head trauma
- Stroke

DIAGNOSIS

DIFFERENTIAL DIAGNOSIS

- Coma
- Encephalopathy
- Psychogenic unresponsiveness

WORKUP

Because convulsive status epilepticus is an emergency with substantial morbidity and mortality, treatment must be early and aggressive, not postponed until an etiology is determined.

LABORATORY TESTS

- While treatment is being initiated: glucose, electrolytes, BUN, ABG, drug levels, CBC, UA, toxicology screen.
- Lumbar puncture in patients with fever or other signs/symptoms suspicious of CNS infection and all patients who are HIV positive.

IMAGING STUDIES

CT or MRI of the brain is recommended as soon as possible after seizures have been controlled.

TREATMENT

NONPHARMACOLOGIC THERAPY

- Give oxygen by nasal cannula or non-rebreathing mask.
- Maintain blood pressure, monitor ECG.
- Obtain IV access.
- Endotracheal intubation for refractory status epilepticus or signs of respiratory distress.

ACUTE GENERAL Rx

- 0 to 5 minutes: Thiamine 100 mg IV and glucose 50 mg D_{50} by IV push (2 ml/kg D_{25} in children) unless hyperglycemic.
- 5 to 10 minutes: Lorazepam 2 mg/min IV up to 0.1 mg/kg.
- >10 minutes: Fosphenytoin 20 mg/kg, Fosphenytoin equivalents (PE) IV up to 150 mg/min (if not available, use phenytoin 20 mg/kg IV at up to 50 mg/min). Can be followed by an additional 5 to 10 mg/kg PE IV if seizures persist.
- >45 minutes (refractory status epilepticus): Load phenobarbital 20 mg/kg IV *or* induce general anesthesia with midazolam, propofol, or pentobarbital by continuous intravenous drip.
- An electroencephalogram (EEG) should be obtained to evaluate for nonconvulsive status epilepticus in any patient who does not regain consciousness within 1 to 2 hr of cessation of convulsive activity and for all patients requiring general anesthesia for seizure control.

CHRONIC Rx

Chronic treatment with anticonvulsants should be considered for all patients presenting with status epilepticus, particularly if there is significant risk of recurrence (e.g., known epilepsy, brain lesion, epileptiform EEG abnormalities).

DISPOSITION

- Favorable if status is treated promptly and there is no underlying acute symptomatic cause such as an underlying CNS lesion.
- Overall mortality is 22%, but higher in the elderly (38%) and substantially lower in children (2.5%). Difference in mortality is mainly because status epilepticus in the elderly is more often the result of an acute symptomatic cause.

REFERRAL

All patients with refractory status epilepticus should be evaluated by a neurologist or epilepsy specialist.

PEARLS & CONSIDERATIONS

COMMENTS

- Because of varied clinical presentations of status epilepticus, there is no clinical basis for being certain that seizures have stopped unless the patient regains full consciousness.
- EEG provides the only definitive information about seizure cessation.
- All patients being treated with continuous IV infusion of anesthetic agents should have continuous EEG monitoring to assess treatment response.

EVIDENCE

In the Veterans Affairs cooperative randomized controlled trial, status epilepticus was terminated within 20 min in 64.9% of patients treated with lorazepam (0.1 mg/kg), 58.2% treated with phenobarbital (15 mg/kg), 55.8% treated with diazepam (0.15 mg/kg) and phenytoin (18 mg/kg), and 43.6% treated with phenytoin alone.[1]

The San Francisco Emergency Medical Services Study, a randomized controlled trial, found that prehospital administration of intravenous benzodiazepines safely and effectively terminated convulsive status epilepticus in up to 60% of patients.[2] Ⓐ

A meta-analysis comparing treatments for refractory status epilepticus found no difference in mortality between midazolam, pentobarbital, and propofol.[3]

A retrospective review of all EEGs recorded in an academic hospital on comatose patients with no overt signs of seizure activity found nonconvulsive status epilepticus in 8% of patients.[4]

In a study of EEGs performed following cessation of convulsive status epilepticus, discrete electrographic seizures were found in 48% and nonconvulsive status epilepticus was found in 14%.[5]

Evidence-Based References

1. *N Engl J Med* 339:792, 1998.
2. *N Engl J Med* 345:631, 2001.
3. *Epilepsia* 43:146, 2002.
4. *Neurology* 54:340, 2000.
5. *Epilepsia* 39:833, 1998.

SUGGESTED READINGS

Gaitanis JN, Drislane FW: Status epilepticus: a review of different syndromes, their current evaluation, and treatment, *Neurologist* 9(2):61, 2003.
Manno EM: New management strategies in the treatment of status epilepticus, *Mayo Clin Proc* 78(4):508, 2003.

AUTHORS: **JOHN E. CROOM, M.D., PH.D.,** and **SUZETTE LAROCHE, M.D.**

BASIC INFORMATION

DEFINITION

Stevens-Johnson syndrome (SJS) is a severe vesiculobullous form of erythema multiforme affecting skin, mouth, eyes, and genitalia.

SYNONYMS

SJS
Herpes iris
Febrile mucocutaneous syndrome

ICD-9CM CODES
695.1 Stevens-Johnson syndrome

EPIDEMIOLOGY & DEMOGRAPHICS

- SJS affects predominantly children and young adults.
- Male:female ratio of 2:1.

PHYSICAL FINDINGS & CLINICAL PRESENTATION

- The cutaneous eruption is generally preceded by vague, nonspecific symptoms of low-grade fever and fatigue occurring 1 to 14 days before the skin lesions. Cough is often present. Fever may be high during the active stages.
- Bullae generally occur on the conjunctiva, mucous membranes of the mouth, nares, and genital regions.
- Corneal ulcerations may result in blindness.
- Ulcerative stomatitis results in hemorrhagic crusting.
- Flat, atypical target lesions or purpuric maculae may be distributed on the trunk or be widespread (Fig. 1-254).
- The pain from oral lesions may compromise fluid intake and result in dehydration.
- Thick, mucopurulent sputum and oral lesions may interfere with breathing.

ETIOLOGY

- Drugs (e.g., phenytoin, penicillins, phenobarbital, sulfonamides) are the most common cause.
- Upper respiratory tract infections (e.g., *Mycoplasma pneumoniae*) and herpes simplex viral infections have also been implicated in SJS.

DIAGNOSIS

DIFFERENTIAL DIAGNOSIS

- Toxic erythema (drugs or infection)
- Pemphigus
- Pemphigoid
- Urticaria
- Hemorrhagic fevers
- Serum sickness
- *Staphylococcus* scalded-skin syndrome
- Behçet's syndrome

WORKUP

- Diagnosis is generally based on clinical presentation and characteristic appearance of the lesions.
- Skin biopsy is generally reserved for when classic lesions are absent and diagnosis is uncertain.

LABORATORY TESTS

CBC with differential, cultures in cases of suspected infection

IMAGING STUDIES

Chest x-ray may show patchy changes in patients with pulmonary involvement.

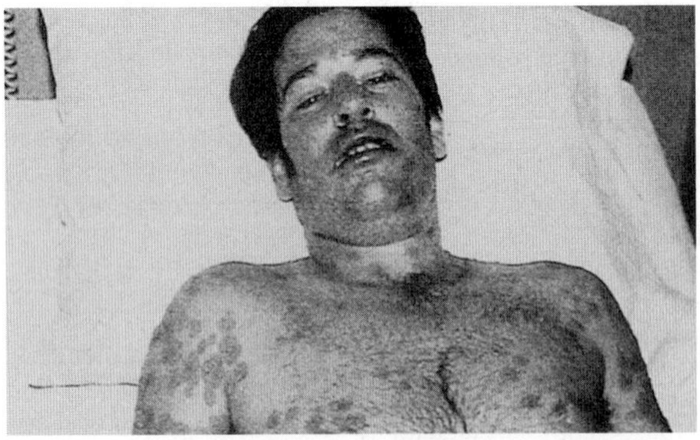

FIGURE 1-254 Stevens-Johnson syndrome. (From Stein JH: *Internal medicine,* ed 5, St Louis, 1998, Mosby.)

TREATMENT

NONPHARMACOLOGIC THERAPY

- Withdrawal of any potential drug precipitants
- Careful skin nursing to prevent secondary infection

ACUTE GENERAL Rx

- Treatment of associated conditions, (e.g., acyclovir for herpes simplex virus infection, erythromycin for mycoplasma infection)
- Antihistamines for pruritus
- Treatment of the cutaneous blisters with cool, wet Burow's compresses
- Relief of oral symptoms by frequent rinsing with lidocaine (Xylocaine Viscous)
- Liquid or soft diet with plenty of fluids to ensure proper hydration
- Treatment of secondary infections with antibiotics
- Corticosteroids: use remains controversial; when used, prednisone 20 to 30 mg bid until new lesions no longer appear, then rapidly tapered
- Topical steroids: may use to treat papules and plaques; however, should not be applied to eroded areas
- Vitamin A: may be used for lacrimal hyposecretion

DISPOSITION

- Prognosis varies with severity of disease. It is generally good in patients with limited disease; however, mortality may approach 10% in patients with extensive involvement.
- Oral lesions may continue for several months.
- Scarring and corneal abnormalities may occur in 20% of patients.

REFERRAL

- Hospital admission in a unit used for burn care is recommended in severe cases.
- Urethral involvement may necessitate catheterization.
- Ocular involvement should be monitored by an ophthalmologist.

PEARLS & CONSIDERATIONS

COMMENTS

Risk of recurrence of SJS is 30% to 40%.

AUTHOR: **FRED F. FERRI, M.D.**

BASIC INFORMATION

DEFINITION

Stomatitis is inflammation involving the oral mucous membranes.

SYNONYMS

Heterogeneous grouping of unrelated illnesses, each with their own designation(s)

ICD-9CM CODES
528.0 Stomatitis
054.2 (herpetic)
528.2 (aphthous)
112.0 (monilial)

PHYSICAL FINDINGS & CLINICAL PRESENTATION

WHITE LESIONS: Candidiasis (thrush)
Caused by yeast infection *(Candida albicans)*

Examination: white, curdlike material that when wiped off leaves a raw bleeding surface

Epidemiology: seen in the very young and the very old, those with immunodeficiency (AIDS, cancer), persons with diabetes, and patients treated with antibacterial agents

Other

- Leukoedema: filmy opalescent-appearing mucosa, which can be reverted to normal appearance by stretching. This condition is benign.
- White sponge nevus: thick, white corrugated folds involving the buccal mucosa. Appears in childhood as an autosomal dominant trait. Benign condition.
- Darier's disease (keratosis follicularis): white papules on the gingivae, alveolar mucosa, and dorsal tongue. Skin lesions also present (erythematous papules). Inherited as an autosomal dominant trait.
- Chemical injury: white sloughing mucosa.
- Nicotine stomatitis: whitened palate with red papules.
- Lichen planus: linear, reticular, slightly raised striae on buccal mucosa. Skin is involved by pruritic violaceous papules on forearms and inner thighs.
- Discoid lupus erythematosus: lesion resembles lichen planus.
- Leukoplakia: white lesions that cannot be scraped off; 20% are premalignant epithelial dysplasia or squamous cell carcinoma.
- Hairy leukoplakia: shaggy white surface that cannot be wiped off; seen in HIV infection, caused by EBV.

RED LESIONS:

- Candidiasis may present with red instead of the more frequent white lesion (see "White Lesions"). Median rhomboid glossitis is a chronic variant.
- Benign migratory glossitis (geographic tongue): area of atrophic depapillated mucosa surrounded by a keratotic border. Benign lesion, no treatment required.
- Hemangiomas.
- Histoplasmosis: ill-defined irregular patch with a granulomatous surface, sometimes ulcerated.
- Allergy.
- Anemia: atrophic reddened glossal mucosa seen with pernicious anemia.
- Erythroplakia: red patch usually caused by epithelial dysplasia or squamous cell carcinoma.
- Burning tongue (glossopyrosis): normal examination; sometimes associated with denture trauma, anemia, diabetes, vitamin B_{12} deficiency, psychogenic problems.

DARK LESIONS (BROWN, BLUE, BLACK):

- Coated tongue: accumulation of keratin; harmless condition that can be treated by scraping
- Melanotic lesions: freckles, lentigines, lentigo, melanoma, Peutz-Jeghers syndrome, Addison's disease
- Varices
- Kaposi's sarcoma: red or purple macules that enlarge to form tumors; seen in patients with AIDS

RAISED LESIONS:

- Papilloma
- Verruca vulgaris
- Condyloma acuminatum
- Fibroma
- Epulis
- Pyogenic granuloma
- Mucocele
- Retention cyst

BLISTERS:

- Primary herpetic gingivostomatitis

Caused by herpes simplex virus type 1 or less frequently type 2
Course: day 1: malaise, fever, headache, sore throat, cervical lymph-adenopathy; days 2 and 3: appearance of vesicles that develop into painful ulcers of 2 to 4 mm in diameter; duration of up to 2 wk

Recurrent intraoral herpes: rare, recurrences typically involve only the keratinized epithelium (lips)

- Pemphigus and pemphigoid
- Hand-foot-mouth disease: caused by coxsackievirus group A
- Erythema multiforme
- Herpangina: caused by echovirus
- Traumatic ulcer
- Primary syphilis
- Perlèche (or angular cheilitis)
- Recurrent aphthous stomatitis (canker sores)
- Behçet's syndrome (aphthous ulcers, uveitis, genital ulcerations, arthritis, and aseptic meningitis)
- Reiter's syndrome (conjunctivitis, urethritis, and arthritis with occasional oral ulcerations)
- Unknown cause

Course: solitary or multiple painful ulcers may develop simultaneously and heal over 10 to 14 days. The size of the lesions and the frequency of recurrences are variable.

DIAGNOSIS

WORKUP

WHITE LESIONS: Candidiasis (thrush) diagnosis: ovoid yeast and hyphae seen in scrapings treated with KOH culture

BLISTERS:

- Exfoliative cytology
- Viral culture
- Immunofluorescence for herpes antigen

TREATMENT

WHITE LESIONS: Candidiasis (thrush) treatment:

- Topical with nystatin or clotrimazole
- Systemic with ketoconazole or fluconazole

BLISTERS:

- Supportive
- Consider acyclovir

RECURRENT INTRAORAL HERPES: Topical corticosteroids or systemic steroids for severe cases

SUGGESTED READINGS

Amir J et al: Treatment of herpes simplex gingivostomatitis with acyclovir in children: a randomized double blind placebo controlled study, *BMJ* 314:1800, 1997.

Khandwala A et al: 5% amlexanox oral paste, a new treatment for recurrent minor aphthous ulcers. Clinical demonstration of acceleration of healing and resolution of pain, *Oral Surg Oral Med Oral Pathol* 83:222, 1997.

AUTHORS: **FRED F. FERRI, M.D.,** and **TOM J. WACHTEL, M.D.**

BASIC INFORMATION

DEFINITION

Strabismus is a condition of the eyes in which the visual axes of the eyes are not straight in the primary position or in which the eyes do not follow each other in the different positions of gaze.

SYNONYMS

Esotropia
Exotropia
Restrictive eye movement

ICD-9CM CODES
378.9 Strabismus

EPIDEMIOLOGY & DEMOGRAPHICS

INCIDENCE (IN U.S.): 2% of all children
PEAK INCIDENCE: Childhood
PREDOMINANT SEX: None
PREDOMINANT AGE: Birth to 5 yr of age
GENETICS: None known

PHYSICAL FINDINGS & CLINICAL PRESENTATION

- Conjugate gaze loss in both eyes with the eyes focusing independently (Fig. 1-255)
- Amblyopia

ETIOLOGY

- Many cases are congenital.
- Accomodative cases occur later with focusing.
- Rarely, there is neurologic disease or severe refractive errors.
- Hereditary common, with hyperopia (far-sightedness) most common.

DIAGNOSIS

DIFFERENTIAL DIAGNOSIS

- Measuring eye position and movement
- Vision testing
- Refractive errors
- CNS tumors
- Orbital tumors
- Brain and CNS dysfunction

WORKUP

- Eye examination
- Visual field
- MRI to rule out tumors when develops later with no apparent cause

LABORATORY TESTS

Generally not needed

IMAGING STUDIES

Necessary only if other neurologic findings are found

TREATMENT

NONPHARMACOLOGIC THERAPY

- Glasses
- Patching—best between 3 to 7 yr old; vision most improved by 3 to 6 mo
- Prisms
- Atropine—same as patching most of time although patching may give better results in resistant cases

CHRONIC Rx

- Glasses
- Alternate eye patching
- Surgery
- Prisms

DISPOSITION

- The earlier the condition is treated, the more likely it is that the child will have normal vision in both eyes.
- After age 7 yr, visual loss is usually permanent from amblyopia.

REFERRAL

- Early for full rehabilitation of eye cosmetically and functionally
- To an ophthalmologist for management (usually)

EVIDENCE

A systematic review of randomized controlled trials of surgical and nonsurgical treatments for intermittent distance exotropia found that the literature consists mainly of retrospective case reviews, which are difficult to compare and analyze because of large variations in definition, intervention criteria, and outcome measures. The reviewers noted, however, that there seems to be general agreement that nonsurgical treatment is most appropriate in small-angle deviations or as a supplement to surgery. They found studies that supported early surgical intervention and others that supported late surgical intervention, and so were unable to draw conclusions about the optimal timing of surgical intervention. They also noted that recent work suggests that bilateral surgery may be the most effective surgical procedure.[1]

A systematic review of the literature concerning the surgical treatment of strabismus in adults identified one randomized controlled trial, which found that surgical treatment was significantly more effective than chemodenervation with botulinum toxin A.[2] Ⓐ

Evidence-Based References

1. Richardson S, Gnanaraj L: Interventions for intermittent distance exotropia, *Cochrane Database Syst Rev* 2, 2003.
2. Mills MD et al: Strabismus surgery for adults. A report by the American Academy of Ophthalmology, *Ophthalmology* 111:1255, 2004. Ⓐ

SUGGESTED READING

Donahue SP: Pediatric strabismus, *N Engl J Med* 356:1040, 2007.

AUTHOR: **MELVYN KOBY, M.D.**

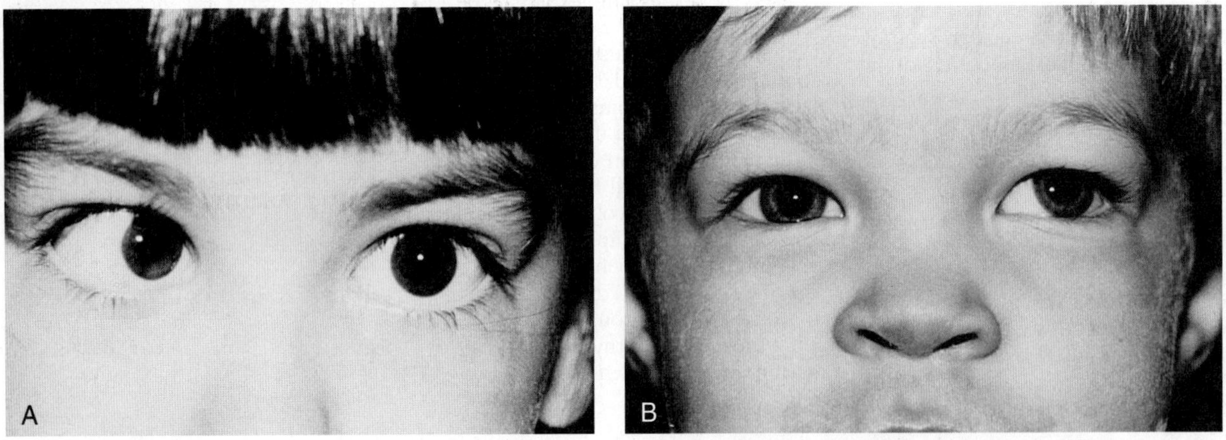

FIGURE 1-255 **A,** Note the nasal deviation of the right eye with the corneal light reflection temporally displaced on the right eye and centered in the left pupil, indicating an esotropia. **B,** Divergent strabismus of the left eye, defining an exotropia. (From Hodkelman [ed]: *Primary pediatric care,* ed 3, St Louis, 1997, Mosby.)

BASIC INFORMATION

DEFINITION

Stroke describes acute brain injury caused by decreased blood supply or hemorrhage.

SYNONYMS

Cerebrovascular accident (CVA)

ICD-9CM CODES
436 Acute stroke

EPIDEMIOLOGY & DEMOGRAPHICS

INCIDENCE (IN U.S.):

- Occurs in 5 to 10/100,000 persons <40 yr of age
- Occurs in 10 to 20/100,000 persons >65 yr of age

PEAK INCIDENCE: 80 to 84 yr

PREVALENCE (IN U.S.): Estimated at 5.8 million persons

PREDOMINANT SEX: Incidence is 30% higher in males

PHYSICAL FINDINGS & CLINICAL PRESENTATION

Motor and/or sensory and/or cognitive deficits, depending on distribution and extent of involved vascular territory. More common manifestations include contralateral motor weakness or sensory loss, as well as language difficulties (aphasia; predominantly left-sided lesions) and visuospatial/neglect phenomena (predominantly right-sided lesions). Onset is usually sudden; however, this depends on specific etiology.

ETIOLOGY

- 70% to 80% are caused by ischemic infarcts; 20% to 30% are hemorrhagic.
- 80% of ischemic infarcts are from occlusion of large or small vessels caused by atherosclerotic vascular disease (due to hypertension, hyperlipidemia, diabetes, tobacco abuse), 15% are caused by cardiac embolism, 5% are from other causes, including hypercoagulable states and vasculitis.
- Small vessel occlusion is most often caused by lipohyalinosis precipitated by chronic hypertension.
- Risk factors for ischemic stroke are described in Box 1-11.

DIAGNOSIS

DIFFERENTIAL DIAGNOSIS

- TIA (transient ischemic attack), defined as focal neurologic deficits (brain or retina) lasting <24 hr [usually lasting <60 min])
- Migraine, seizure, mass lesion

WORKUP

- Thorough history and physical examination, including detailed neurologic and cardiovascular evaluation to identify vascular territory and likely etiology (Table 1-46). Infectious, toxic, and metabolic causes should be excluded because each may cause clinical deterioration of old stroke symptoms.
- Cardiac: mandatory ECG, telemetry; serial cardiac enzymes, transthoracic and/or transesophageal echocardiography, Holter monitor, should be seriously considered especially in setting of suspected embolic etiology. Carotid Doppler should be performed in cases of embolic stroke to anterior or middle cerebral artery territory.

LABORATORY TESTS

- STAT (acute stroke): CBC, platelets, PT (INR), PTT, BUN, creatinine, glucose, electrolytes, urinalysis
- Additional tests, depending on suspected etiology (in younger patients; e.g., coagulopathies)

IMAGING STUDIES

- CT scan without contrast to distinguish hemorrhage from infarct (Figs. 1-256 and 1-257)
- An MRI is superior to CT in identifying abnormalities in the posterior fossa and, in particular, lacunar (small vessel) infarcts. Diffusion weighted imaging (DWI) is best to determine hyperacute ischemia (positive within minutes of symptom onset). MRA is recommended to help identify vascular pathology (e.g., extent of intracranial atherosclerosis or vascular distribution of ischemia)
- In select cases (e.g., hemorrhagic stroke), conventional angiography may identify aneurysms or other vascular malformations

TREATMENT

NONPHARMACOLOGIC THERAPY

- To prevent pulmonary emboli, above-the-knee elastic stockings, pneumatic

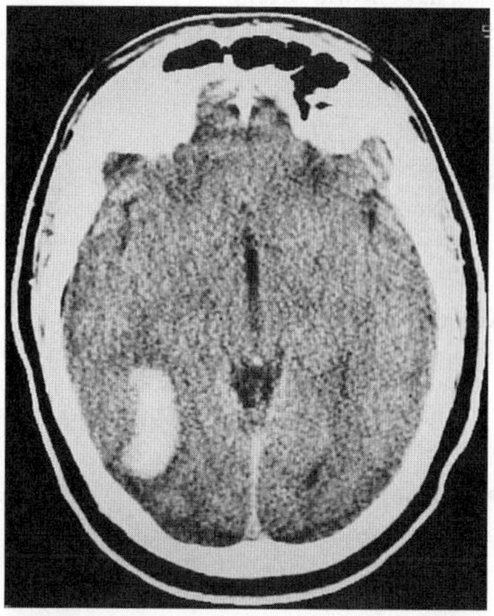

FIGURE 1-256 Intracerebral hemorrhage. Noncontrast CT scan demonstrates an intracerebral hemorrhage in the right occipital lobe. (From Specht N [ed]: *Practical guide to diagnostic imaging,* St Louis, 1998, Mosby.)

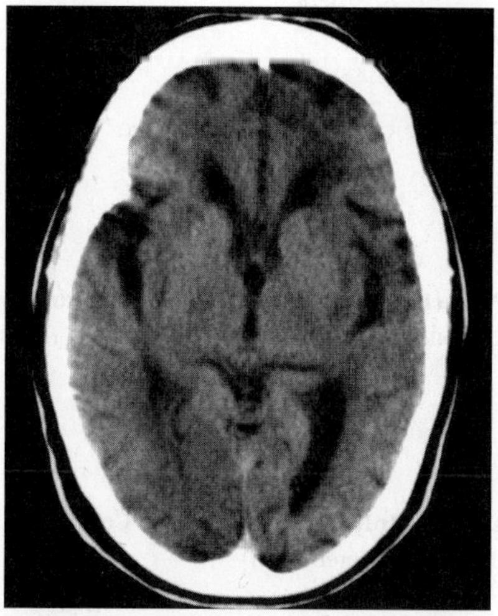

FIGURE 1-257 Occipital lobe infarct (posterior cerebral artery territory). Note the large right occipital hypodensity with mass effect caused by infarction and subsequent edema. (From Cwinn AA, Grahovac SZ [eds]: *Emergency CT scans of the head: a practical atlas,* St Louis, 1998, Mosby.)

BOX 1-11 Risk Factors for Ischemic Stroke

Nonmodifiable:
Age, gender, race, sociocultural
Family history of premature vascular disease

Modifiable:
Diabetes, hypertension, hyperlipidemia
Smoking (prior smoker 1.3 × risk, current smoker 2.1 × risk)
Alcohol (1-2 drinks/day decreases risk × 0.75 vs. no alcohol; >2 drinks/day increases risk)
Waist circumference
Atrial fibrillation
History of transient ischemic attack (TIA)
History of congestive heart failure (left ventricular [LV] ejection fraction <25%)
Drugs (sympathomimetics, oral contraceptive pill, cocaine)

Modified from Andreoli TE (ed): *Cecil essentials of medicine,* ed 5, Philadelphia, 2001, WB Saunders.

boots, or SQ Heparin if nonhemorrhagic etiology and patient is immobile in bed
- Carotid endarterectomy (CEA) is recommended in patients with carotid territory stroke associated with 70% to 99% ipsilateral carotid stenosis, performed by an experienced surgeon who has demonstrated low morbidity and mortality
- Modification of risk factors (e.g., smoking cessation, exercise, diet)

ACUTE GENERAL Rx

- Box 1-12 describes initial considerations for patients with stroke.
- Judicious control of blood pressure; patients with chronic hypertension may extend the area of infarction if the blood pressure is lowered into the "normal" range. Adequate hydration and bed rest (e.g., head of bed down in pressure dependent ischemia vs. head of bed up if patient is aspiration risk). Tight glycemic control is also recommended (e.g., sliding scale insulin).
- Patients presenting <3 hr after onset of nonhemorrhagic stroke: thrombolytic therapy is standard of care.

ACUTE SPECIFIC Rx

- Depends on several factors, including etiology, vascular territory involved, risk factors, and elapsed time from symptom onset to arrival at hospital.

TABLE 1-46 Neurologic Signs Associated with Stroke by Location

Artery Affected	Neurologic Signs
Internal Carotid Artery	
(Supplies the cerebral hemispheres and diencephalon by the ophthalmic and ipsilateral hemisphere arteries)	Occasional unilateral (ipsilateral) blindness Severe contralateral hemiplegia, hemianesthesia, and hemianopia Profound aphasia if left hemisphere involved
Middle Cerebral Artery	
(Supplies structures of higher cerebral processes of communication; language interpretation; perception and interpretation of space, sensation, form, and voluntary movement)	Alterations in communication, cognition, mobility, and sensation Homonymous hemianopia Contralateral hemiplegia or hemiparesis
Anterior Cerebral Artery	
(Supplies medial surfaces and upper convexities of frontal and parietal lobes and medial surface of hemisphere, which includes motor and somesthetic cortex serving the legs)	Emotional lability Confusion, amnesia, personality changes Urinary incontinence Impaired mobility, with weakness greater in lower extremities than in upper
Posterior Cerebral Artery	
(Supplies medial and inferior temporal lobes, medial occipital lobe, thalamus, posterior hypothalamus, and visual receptive area)	Homonymous hemianopia Hemianesthesia Cortical blindness Memory deficits
Vertebral or Basilar Arteries	
(Supply the brainstem and cerebellum) Incomplete occlusion	Drop attacks (rare) Unilateral and bilateral weakness of extremities Diplopia, homonymous hemianopia Nausea, vertigo, tinnitus, and syncope Dysphagia Dysarthria Sometimes confusion and drowsiness
Anterior portion of pons	"Locked-in" syndrome—no movement except eyelids; sensation and consciousness preserved
Complete occlusion or hemorrhage	Coma Miotic pupils Decerebrate rigidity Respiratory and circulatory abnormalities Death
Posterior Inferior Cerebellar Artery and/or Vertebral Artery	
(Supplies the lateral and posterior portion of the medulla)	Wallenberg syndrome Dysphagia, dysphonia Ipsilateral anesthesia of face and cornea for pain and temperature (touch preserved) Ipsilateral Horner syndrome Contralateral loss of pain and temperature sensation in trunk and extremities Ipsilateral decompensation of movement (cerebellar signs)
Anterior Inferior and Superior Cerebellar Arteries	
(Supply the cerebellum)	Difficulty in articulation, swallowing, gross movements of limbs; nystagmus (cerebellar signs)
Anterior Spinal Artery	
(Supplies the anterior spinal cord)	Flaccid paralysis, below level of lesion Loss of pain, touch, temperature sensation (proprioception preserved, sensory level)
Posterior Spinal Artery	
(Supplies the posterior spinal cord)	Sensory loss, particularly proprioception, vibration, touch, and pressure (movement preserved)

Adapted from Seidel HM (ed): *Mosby's guide to physical examination,* ed 4, St Louis, 1999, Mosby.

- Box 1-13 describes criteria for thrombolytic therapy in patients with thromboembolic stroke.
- If atrial fibrillation and/or a cardiac mural thrombus is found on echocardiography, heparin may be considered.
- If a subarachnoid or intracerebral hemorrhage is found on CT, MR angiography and/or cerebral angiography may be indicated to identify aneurysm. If no aneurysm is found and clot is expanding, neurosurgical evacuation of clot may be attempted, but outcomes are generally poor.
- In select cases of patients presenting >3 hr but <8 hr, a neurointerventionalist may be able to offer either direct injection of a clot-busting agent (e.g., intraarterial tPA) or direct clot extraction (e.g., Merci Retrieval System). However, this remains investigational.

CHRONIC Rx

- Antiplatelet therapy (aspirin, dipyridamole/aspirin [Aggrenox], clopidogrel [Plavix], or ticlopidine) reduces the risk of subsequent stroke.
- In patients with first TIA/stroke on no prior antiplatelet agent, aspirin (325 mg vs. 81 mg each day) is usually chosen initially. Evidence suggests that if a TIA occurs while on aspirin, the patient should be switched to dipyridamole/aspirin.
- Warfarin is usually reserved for patients with cardioembolic stroke as well as for patients with atrial fibrillation.
- Evidence supports BP <120/80 mm Hg, glucose control to near-normoglycemic levels in diabetics (HbA1C <7%), and LDL cholesterol <100 mg/dl (comorbid CHD/symptomatic atherosclerotic disease) or <70 mg/dl (very high risk with multiple risk factors).
- Recurrent stroke rates are lowered by the combination of an ace inhibitor (ACEI) and thiazide-type diuretic.
- ACEI and angiotensin receptor blockers are recommended for patients with comorbid diabetes.
- In patients with recent stroke or TIA and without history of coronary heart disease, atorvastatin 80 mg/day reduced the risk of stroke and cardiovascular events.
- Combination therapy with antiplatelets, statins, and ACEI has been shown in one retrospective study to reduce stroke severity, shorten length of hospitalization, and improve functional status upon discharge; further prospective study is warranted.

DISPOSITION

Prognosis depends on severity of deficits, etiology, and other concurrent medical/surgical illness. A polymodality physical medicine and rehabilitative approach is an integral part of poststroke recovery. This includes physical, occupational, and speech therapy individualized based on deficits.

REFERRAL

- Neurology/neurosurgical referral depending on etiology and resources available.
- Vascular surgery if patient is candidate for CEA. If not a surgical candidate and endovascular treatment is available, refer to interventional neuroradiologist for carotid stenting.

PEARLS & CONSIDERATIONS

- Evidence supports CEA for severe (70% to 99%) symptomatic stenosis.
- Evidence supports that patent foramen ovale (PFO) is *not* associated with increased risk of subsequent stroke or death among medically treated patients with cryptogenic stroke. However, having both PFO and atrial septal abnormalities possibly increases the risk of subsequent stroke (but not death) in medically treated patients <55.

EVIDENCE

EBM

Thrombolysis, given soon after the onset of acute ischemic stroke, reduces the overall risk of death and long-term dependency.[1]

BOX 1-12 Initial Considerations for Patients with Strokes

Initial care
- Stabilize the patient, secure the airway, and provide adequate oxygenation
- Assess level of consciousness, language, visual fields, eye movements, and pupillary movements
- Obtain history and perform physical examination
- Perform CT of head without contrast: consider MRI with DWI in select cases
- Obtain CBC with platelets and differential, electrolytes, creatinine, BUN, glucose, PT/PTT, arterial blood gas, or oxygen saturation
- Consider a toxicology screen
- Consider special coagulation studies such as antiphospholipid antibodies, factor V Leiden assay, protein C and protein S, antithrombin III, ANA, fibrinogen, RPR, homocysteine, serum protein electrophoresis

Consider acute intervention with t-PA if symptoms for less than 3 hr

Consider the following with admission orders
- Transthoracic echocardiogram (consider transesophageal echocardiogram if transthoracic echocardiogram is equivocal or there is a high suspicion of cardiogenic thromboembolism)
- Carotid duplex ultrasonography
- Telemetry
- Supplemental oxygen and appropriate oxygen saturation monitoring
- Antiplatelet therapy
- Fluid restriction if infarct is large, to reduce cerebral edema
- Close monitoring of intake and output
- Regular determinations of blood glucose levels to avoid hyperglycemia
- NPO if there are concerns about the pharyngeal reflex pending swallowing evaluation
- Elevate the head of the bed 20-30 degrees to reduce cerebral edema
- Bed rest for the first 24 hr with fall precautions, then advance as appropriate
- Vital signs and neurologic checks every 2 hr times four until stable
- Prophylaxis for DVT if immobile (elastic stockings at a minimum)
- Speech therapy consultation to evaluate swallowing
- Neurology, physical therapy, occupational therapy, nutrition, and social services consultations

From Rakel RE (ed): *Principles of family practice,* ed 6, Philadelphia, 2002, WB Saunders.

ANA, Antinuclear antibodies; *BUN,* blood urea nitrogen; *CBC,* complete blood count; *CT,* computed tomography; *DVT,* deep vein thrombosis; *DWI,* diffusion weighted imaging; *MRI,* magnetic resonance imaging; *NPO,* nothing by mouth; *PT/PTT,* prothrombin time/partial thromboplastin time; *RPR,* rapid plasma reagin; *t-PA,* tissue plasminogen activator.

Aspirin, given within 48 hours of acute ischemic stroke, reduces mortality and dependency at 6 months, and increases the likelihood of complete recovery.[2]

Heparins and oral anticoagulants provide *no* net short- or long-term benefits, due to the increased risk of death, symptomatic intracranial hemorrhage, and recurrent stroke during treatment. Evidence does not support their routine use in acute ischemic stroke.[3]

Patients are significantly more likely to be alive, independent, and living at home 1 year after a stroke if they have received specialized stroke rehabilitation (specialist unit/organized stroke team) vs. nonstroke unit.[4]

In patients with and without cardiovascular disease, statins alone (not associated with multifactorial interventions or other cholesterol-lowering agents) reduce the relative risk of stroke by 24% over 4 years, when the mean total cholesterol is reduced by 21%. Additionally, they produce a definite and substantial reduction in ischemic stroke, irrespective of the patient's age, sex, or blood lipid levels.[5]

Anticoagulation is beneficial for patients in atrial fibrillation at high risk of stroke, providing there are no contraindications. Antiplatelet agents are less effective than warfarin but may be used if there are contraindications to warfarin or the risk of stroke is low.[6]

Fish consumption confers relative risk reduction compared to no consumption.[7]

One RCT demonstrated a moderate decrease in homocysteine level but no effect on vascular outcomes over 2 years in patients treated with folic acid and vitamins B_6 and B_{12}.[8]

Evidence-Based References

1. *Cochrane Library* 3:CD000213, 2003.
2. *Lancet* 349:1641, 1997.
3. *Cochrane Library* 3:CD000024, 2004.
4. *Stroke* 34:101, 2003.
5. *JAMA* 278:313, 1997.
6. *Clin Evid* 11:257, 2004.
7. *Am J Prev Med* 29:347, 2005.
8. *JAMA* 291:565, 2004.

SUGGESTED READINGS

Adams HP et al: Guidelines for the early management of adults with ischemic stroke, *Circulation* 115:478, 2007.

Amarenco P et al: High-dose atorvastatin after stroke or transient ischemic attack, *N Engl J Med* 355:549, 2006.

Diener HC et al: Aspirin and clopidogrel compared with clopidogrel alone after recent ischaemic stroke or transient ischaemic attack in high-risk patients (MATCH): randomised, double-blind, placebo-controlled trial, *Lancet* 364(9431):331, 2004.

Endovascular versus surgical treatment in patients with carotid stenosis in the Carotid and Vertebral Artery Transluminal Angioplasty Study (CAVATAS): a randomised trial, *Lancet* 357(9270):1729, 2001.

Goldstein LB et al: Primary prevention of ischemic stroke, *Stroke* 37:1583, 2006.

International Stroke Trial Collaborative Group: The International Stroke Trial (IST): a randomized trial of aspirin, heparin, both or neither among 19,435 patients with acute ischemic stroke, *Lancet* 349:1569, 1997.

Kumar S et al: Antiplatelets, ACE inhibitors, and statins combination reduces stroke severity and tissue at risk, *Neurology* 66(8):1153, 2006.

Sacco R et al: Guidelines for prevention of stroke in patients with ischemic stroke or transient ischemic attack, *Stroke* 37:577, 2006.

AUTHOR: **RICHARD S. ISAACSON, M.D.**

BOX 1-13 Criteria for Tissue Plasminogen Activator (Alteplase [Activase]) Use in Patients with Thromboembolic Stroke

Criteria for considering t-PA as a treatment option
- Age ≥18 yr
- Noncontrast CT without evidence of hemorrhage
- Time since onset of symptoms clearly <3 hr before t-PA administration would begin

Criteria for excluding t-PA as a treatment option

Historical and clinical findings
- Clinical presentation suggests subarachnoid hemorrhage, even if CT is normal
  - Sudden, severe headache, often with loss of consciousness at onset
  - Vomiting common
- Active internal bleeding, increased risk of bleeding, or known bleeding diathesis, including:
  - Recent use of warfarin with a prolonged international normalized ratio (INR)—some would add current use of warfarin regardless of INR
  - Use of heparin within 48 hr with a prolonged aPTT
  - Platelet count <100,000/mm3
  - History of intracranial hemorrhage
  - Known arteriovenous malformation or aneurysm
  - GI or GU bleeding within the past 21 days
  - Arterial puncture within the past 7 days
- Recent lumbar puncture
- Stroke, intracranial surgery, or head trauma within the previous 3 mo
- Major surgery or serious trauma within the preceding 14 days
- Persistent systolic blood pressure >185 mm Hg or diastolic blood pressure >110 mm Hg
- Seizure at stroke onset
- Rapidly improving neurologic signs
- Isolated, mild neurologic deficits
- Acute myocardial infarction
- Post–myocardial infarction pericarditis
- Blood glucose >50 mg/dl or <400 mg/dl
- Patient pregnant or lactating

CT findings
- Evidence of intracranial hemorrhage
- Hypodensity or effacement of the sulci in 1/3 of the territory of the middle cerebral artery

From Rakel RE (ed): *Principles of family practice,* ed 6, Philadelphia, 2002, WB Saunders.

aPTT, Activated partial thromboplastin time; *CT,* computed tomography; *GI,* gastrointestinal; *GU,* genitourinary; *t-PA,* tissue plasminogen activator.

BASIC INFORMATION

DEFINITION

Sturge-Weber syndrome (SWS) is a sporadic congenital disorder characterized by a dermal capillary malformation (port-wine stain) occurring in association with vascular malformations of the leptomeninges and the eye.

Sturge first described a patient with epilepsy, a facial capillary malformation, and buphthalmos in 1879. Parkes Weber better characterized the pattern and distribution of the characteristic intracranial calcifications. The complete syndrome generally includes the triad of facial dermal capillary malformation (port-wine stain), ipsilateral central nervous system (CNS) vascular malformation (leptomeningeal angiomatosis), and vascular malformation of the choroid of the eye associated with glaucoma. Partial forms have been reported.

SYNONYMS

Sturge (-Weber) (-Dimitri) disease or syndrome

Encephalocutaneous angiomatosis

ICD-9CM CODES

759.6

EPIDEMIOLOGY & DEMOGRAPHICS

GENETICS: SWS is not a heritable disorder. Thus, recurrence is unlikely.

PHYSICAL FINDINGS & CLINICAL PRESENTATION

SWS is characterized by a facial angioma (port-wine stain) and an associated leptomeningeal angioma. These vascular malformations are associated with specific ocular and neurologic abnormalities.

Cutaneous manifestations

- Cutaneous port-wine stain is the most common type of vascular malformation, occurring in 0.3% of newborns (Fig. 1-258, *A*). However, only a small proportion of children with port-wine stains have SWS.
- In SWS, the port-wine stain typically is present on the forehead and upper eyelid, primarily in the distribution of the first or second division of the trigeminal nerve. Extension of the skin lesion to both sides of the face and the trunk and extremities is common.
- The distribution of the cutaneous angioma influences the risk of an associated leptomeningeal angioma. Leptomeningeal angioma occurs in approximately 90% of cases when the port-wine stain involves both the upper and lower eyelids, compared to 10% when only one eyelid is affected.
- The skin lesion usually is obvious at birth. However, its appearance changes with age and its size increases as the patient grows. In the newborn, the lesion is flat and usually light pink in color. It typically darkens with age to a deep red, port-wine appearance and vascular ectasias develop (Fig. 1-258, *B*). The vascular ectasias produce nodularity and superficial blebbing, which lead to overgrowth of the underlying soft tissues and sometimes the bone.
- It may extend to mucosal surfaces with concomitant gingival hypertrophy, which may be even further accentuated in patients being treated with phenytoin for seizures. Some patients exhibit accelerated eruption of teeth

Leptomeningeal angioma

- Leptomeningeal angioma occurs in 10% to 20% of cases when a typical facial lesion is present. The intracerebral lesion usually occurs on the same side as the port-wine stain. Leptomeningeal angiomatosis seldom occurs without an accompanying facial angioma.
- The parietal and occipital areas are affected most commonly, although any portion of the cerebrum can be involved.
- The pathologic appearance of the leptomeninges includes thickening and discoloration caused by the increased vascularity. The angiomatous tissue typically fills the subarachnoid space in the sulci, and large tortuous venous structures drain superficially or into the deep venous system. The underlying parenchyma may be atrophic and contain multiple calcific granular deposits. The intraparenchymal calcification may result from chronic tissue hypoxia caused by venous stasis.

Ocular manifestations

- Ocular features of SWS include glaucoma and vascular malformations of the conjunctiva, episclera, choroid, and retina.
- The predominant ocular abnormality is glaucoma (increased intraocular pressure), which occurs in 30% to 70% of affected patients. The risk of glaucoma is highest in the first decade. Congenital glaucoma is seen in approximately one half of patients with SWS and presents in newborns with enlargement of the globe *(buphthalmos)*. Occasional patients develop glaucoma as adults. Thus, continued vigilance is needed, even in patients with initially normal intraocular pressure.
- Angioma of the choroid occurs in 30% to 40% of patients with SWS and can lead to increased intraocular pressure. These lesions may be diffuse or localized within the retina.
- Episcleral and conjunctival lesions include anomalous vessels or true angiomata. These may be caused by increased venous pressure in the eye.
- Weber originally noted heterochromia of the iris. The more deeply pigmented iris usually is ipsilateral to the facial angioma. The pigmentation is caused by aggregated melanocytic hamartomata on the anterior surface of the iris.

Neurologic features

- The neurologic features of SWS are progressive and include seizures, focal neurologic deficits, and mental retardation. These disorders occur with variable severity. A small proportion of patients have no neurologic abnormalities.
- The reasons for neurologic progression are uncertain. A possible mechanism is hypoxic-ischemic injury to tissue adjacent to the leptomeningeal angioma. Other proposed mechanisms are venous occlusion and increased venous pressure.

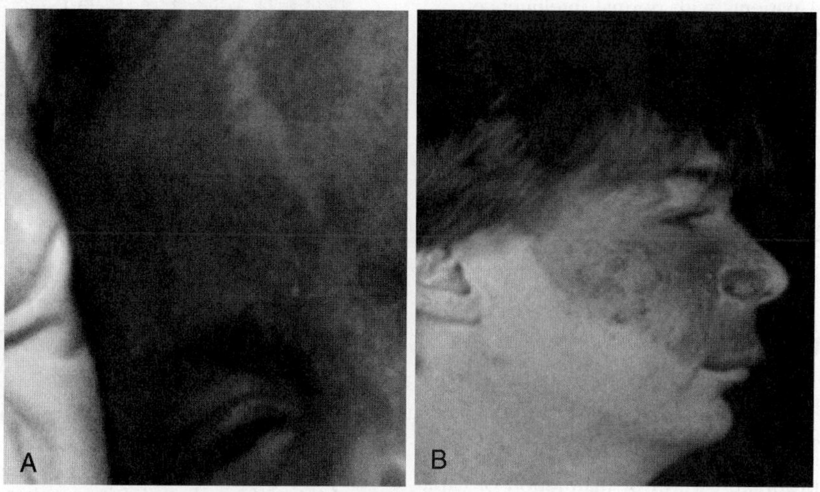

FIGURE 1-258 Port-wine stain at different stages.

- Seizures:
  1. Seizures occur in 80 percent of patients with SWS and are more common with bilateral than unilateral port-wine stains. Seizures may develop at any age, although they usually start in early childhood.
  2. Seizures are often the first symptom to appear. Initially, seizures are typically focal but often become generalized tonic-clonic. Less often, infantile spasms or myoclonic or atonic seizures are seen. The occurrence of seizures, the age at onset, and the response to treatment affect prognosis. Onset before 1 yr of age and poor response to anticonvulsant therapy are associated with a greater likelihood of cognitive impairment.
- Hemiparesis: Hemiparesis often develops acutely in conjunction with the onset of seizures. The deficit occurs contralateral to the facial and intracranial lesions. The affected extremity usually does not grow at a normal rate, resulting in hemiatrophy. Some affected children have progressive loss of motor function or have a series of stroke-like events.
- Mental retardation: Children with SWS typically develop normally for several months after birth, then manifest developmental delay. However, impairment can be obvious soon after birth, especially in infants with extensive brain involvement. Cognitive function is poorest in patients with bilateral intracerebral lesions. In one report, only 8% of patients with bilateral leptomeningeal angiomata were intellectually normal.
- Behavior problems: Behavior problems are more common in SWS patients than in their unaffected siblings. Higher risk for psychological problems is associated with poorer cognitive function and frequent seizures. However, behavior problems can occur in patients with normal intelligence.
- Other deficits: Many patients have visual field defects, typically homonymous hemianopia. This is due to the involvement of the leptomeningeal angioma with one or both occipital lobes or optic tracts. Hydrocephalus also may occur. This disorder is thought to result from increased venous pressure caused by thrombosis of the deep venous channels or extensive arteriovenous anastomoses.

ETIOLOGY

The etiology of SWS is unknown. One hypothesis suggests that the capillary angiomata result from somatic mutations in fetal ectodermal tissues that cause inappropriate control or maturation of capillary blood vessel formation.

DIAGNOSIS Dx

DIFFERENTIAL DIAGNOSIS

- Klippel-Trenaunay-Weber syndrome (extensive capillary angiomata associated with dysplastic veins involve the limbs and trunk, often with hypertrophy of the affected extremity)
- Von Hippel-Lindau disease (associated with capillary retinal angiomata in contrast to cavernous angiomata seen in SWS)

WORKUP

SWS should be suspected in all patients with facial capillary malformations involving the trigeminal dermatome. At-risk infants should undergo careful physical examination to determine the extent of the malformation.

IMAGING STUDIES

- Most children with facial port-wine stains without an intracranial lesion would be expected to develop normally. Therefore, performing neuroimaging studies is helpful to provide prognostic information.
- Plain radiographs of the skull may detect intracranial calcifications, revealing the classic "tram-line" appearance, but calcifications are often not present before 2 yr of age. Newer radiographic techniques have made plain films obsolete.
- The preferred technique is magnetic resonance imaging (MRI) with gadolinium contrast, which demonstrates the presence of the leptomeningeal angioma and the extent of involvement with brain structures (Fig. 1-259).
- If MRI is not readily available, cranial computed tomography reliably identifies brain calcification and provides some anatomic information.
- In some cases, leptomeningeal involvement may not be detected by neuroimaging during infancy and becomes apparent later. There is no absolute way to exclude intracerebral lesions during the first year after birth.

TREATMENT Rx

No specific treatment exists for SWS. The cutaneous, ocular, and neurologic manifestations are treated with mixed success.

ACUTE GENERAL Rx/CHRONIC Rx

Port-wine stain

- Port-wine stains can be treated by selective photothermolysis using a pulsed dye laser. Treatment can be further optimized for individual patients so that blanching of the lesion can be accomplished in the fewest possible sessions.
- The response of facial port-wine stains to laser treatment depends upon the location and size of the lesion and the patient's age. The greatest decrease in size occurs in the smallest lesions and in the youngest children (<1 yr of age). The greater success in the youngest patients may reflect treatment before the development of ectasias.
- Complications of laser therapy include scarring and transient hyperpigmentation. Retinal injury can occur if the eyes are not shielded properly.

Glaucoma

- The development of new medications has improved the medical management of glaucoma in SWS. However, topical treatment often is ineffective in normalizing intraocular pressure. In these cases, the surgical treatment depends upon the etiology of the glaucoma.

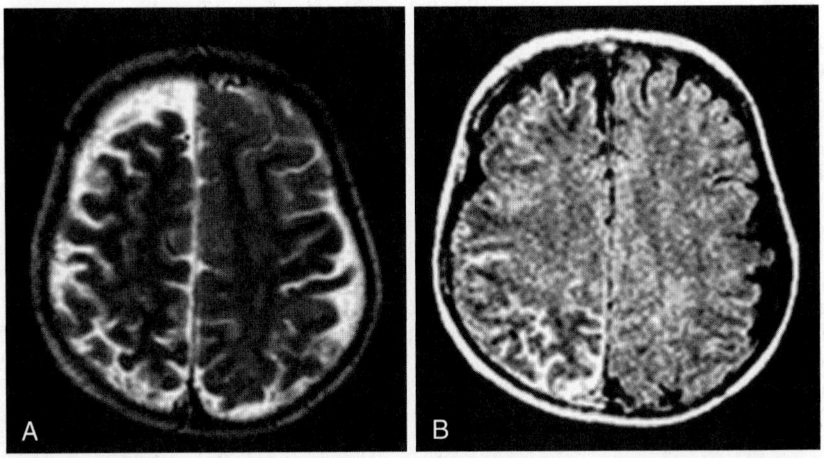

FIGURE 1-259 Axial magnetic resonance image (MRI) of child with Sturge-Weber Syndrome demonstrating atrophy of the left hemisphere and contrast enhancement of the surface of the left hemisphere particularly prominent over the occipital lobe.

Seizures

- Management of seizures in SWS often is difficult. The success of controlling seizures with anticonvulsant medication is variable and unpredictable. Carbamazepine is the recommended antiepileptic of choice. In refractory cases, hemispherectomy or more limited surgical resection of epileptogenic tissue may be beneficial, although risks often outweigh benefits.

REFERRAL

- Initial ophthalmologic evaluation should be performed in the neonatal period because of the risk of congenital glaucoma.
- If the first complete ophthalmologic evaluation is normal, it should be repeated frequently (some authors have suggested quarterly evaluations) for the first 2 yr of life.
- If the examination results remain normal, the vision should be reevaluated at least annually throughout the patient's lifetime.
- Periodic evaluation by a pediatric neurologist is an essential component of the management of SWS.

PEARLS & CONSIDERATIONS

COMMENTS

- The prognosis for SWS depends upon the extent of the leptomeningeal angioma and its effect on the perfusion of the cerebral cortex, as well as the severity of ocular involvement.
- Prognosis also is affected by the age of onset of seizures and whether they can be controlled.
- Neurologic function may deteriorate with age. As a result, approximately one half of affected adults are impaired, including those who initially were normal.

PATIENT/FAMILY EDUCATION

- The Sturge-Weber Foundation is an active support group for patients and families (http://www.sturge-weber.com).

SUGGESTED READINGS

Garzon MC et al: Vascular malformations; Part II: associated syndromes, *J Am Acad Dermatol,* 56(4):541-564, 2007.

Nathan N, Thaller SR: Sturge-Weber syndrome and associated congenital vascular disorders: a review, *J Cranifac Surg,* 17(4):724-728, 2006.

AUTHOR: **RUBY SATPATHY, M.D.**

BASIC INFORMATION

DEFINITION

Subarachnoid hemorrhage (SAH) is the presence of active bleeding into the subarachnoid space usually secondary to a spontaneous ruptured aneurysm or after head trauma.

SYNONYMS

SAH, subarachnoid bleed

ICD-9CM CODES
430 Subarachnoid hemorrhage

EPIDEMIOLOGY & DEMOGRAPHICS

INCIDENCE (IN U.S.): 6 to 28 cases/100,000 persons/yr
PEAK INCIDENCE: 50 to 60 yr
PREDOMINANT SEX: Males > females in persons <40 yr of age; then female:male ratio of 3:2 in persons >40 yr old
PREDOMINANT AGE: >50 yr
GENETICS:

- First-degree relatives have a 4% to 9% risk of intracranial aneurysms (as compared with about 2% in the general population) and these may tend to rupture at a younger age and at a smaller size than sporadic ones. Recommendations on screening unaffected family members depend on the number of relatives with aneurysms. There may also be a familial predisposition to multiple aneurysms.
- Increased incidence in some inherited systemic diseases (e.g., autosomal dominant polycystic kidney disease and connective tissue diseases such as Ehlers-Danlos syndrome).
- No single gene has yet been identified for intracranial aneurysm formation or rupture.

PHYSICAL FINDINGS & CLINICAL PRESENTATION

- Patients typically present with sudden onset of a severe headache with maximal intensity at onset. Additional findings may include nuchal rigidity, nausea, and vomiting.
- Transient loss of consciousness occurs in 45% of patients.
- Focal neurologic deficits may be present.
- Funduscopic examination may reveal subhyaloid hemorrhage.

ETIOLOGY

- Key distinction is aneurysmal (nontraumatic etiology in >60% of cases, most commonly after rupture of saccular "berry" aneurysms) vs. nonaneurysmal (traumatic) SAH
- Others: Arteriovenous malformation (AVM), angioma, fusiform or mycotic aneurysm, dissecting and tumor-related aneurysms

DIAGNOSIS

DIFFERENTIAL DIAGNOSIS

- Intraparenchymal hemorrhage
- Subarachnoid extension of an extracranial arterial dissection or intracerebral hemorrhage
- Meningoencephalitis (e.g., hemorrhagic meningoencephalitis caused by HSV)
- Headache associated with sexual activity (e.g., coital/postcoital headache; usually acute onset of severe headache around time of orgasm)

WORKUP

- CT scan without contrast is initial test of choice, with a sensitivity of 90% or higher in the first 12 to 24 hr. If CT is negative and there is a high clinical suspicion for SAH, lumbar puncture must be considered as there is an approximately 7% (or 1 in 14) chance of having a SAH. Spinal fluid is considered positive if there is xanthochromia and if there is a constant amount of red cells in each LP tube. LP performed <12 hr after onset of headache may be falsely negative for xanthochromia.
- If CT scan is unavailable, transfer patient immediately.
- ECG (nonspecific ST-and T-wave changes, "cerebral T-waves").

LABORATORY TESTS

PT, PTT, platelet count at a minimum for clotting abnormality

IMAGING STUDIES

CT scan (Fig. 1-260) followed by cerebral angiography if hemorrhage is confirmed. May also use Transcranial Doppler (TCD) as a baseline to more adequately assess for vasospasm later

TREATMENT

NONPHARMACOLOGIC THERAPY

- Intubation as necessary
- Bed rest, isotonic fluids
- Neurosurgical or interventional neuroradiologic referral mandatory if aneurysm or arteriovenous malformation demonstrated by angiography; also, invasive ICP monitoring and/or ventriculostomy may be required on an emergent basis (e.g., deteriorating level of consciousness and/or development of hydrocephalus); elevated ICP is associated with a worse patient outcome, particularly if ICP does not respond to treatment

ACUTE GENERAL Rx

- Short-acting analgesics (e.g., morphine 1 to 4 mg IV) and sedation (e.g., midazolam 1 to 5 mg IV); avoid oversedation and watch neurologic examination closely
- Seizure prophylaxis controversial (consider phenytoin 15 to 20 mg/kg IV load, 100 mg TID maintenance)
- Vasospasm prophylaxis (nimodipine 60 mg PO q4h)
- BP control (e.g., labetalol 10 to 40 mg IV q30min); lower BP for unprotected aneurysms vs. higher BP if protected (post-coiling/clipping)
- Stool softeners
- Hypertonic saline (HS) solutions have been used in various concentrations (e.g., 7.5%, 10%, 23.5%) to treat elevated ICP and augment cerebral blood flow (CBF); in one study, HS 23.5% bolus (2 ml/kg IV x 1) exerted an early CBF-augmenting effect which lasted for up to 7.5 hr; despite this evidence, there are limited studies in this area and the exact recommended doses have yet to be determined; neurosurgical consultation is mandatory for persistently elevated ICP management
- Vasospasm occurs in 20% to 30% of patients and peaks at about 1 wk; monitor closely for this. Consider TCD monitoring in high-risk patients. "Triple H" therapy for prevention of vasospasm includes hemodilution, hypertension (consider pressors), and hypervolemia. Goals of Triple H include a hematocrit of 30%, central venous pressure of 8 to 12 mm Hg, and enough artificially induced hypertension to prevent or reverse new neurologic deficits

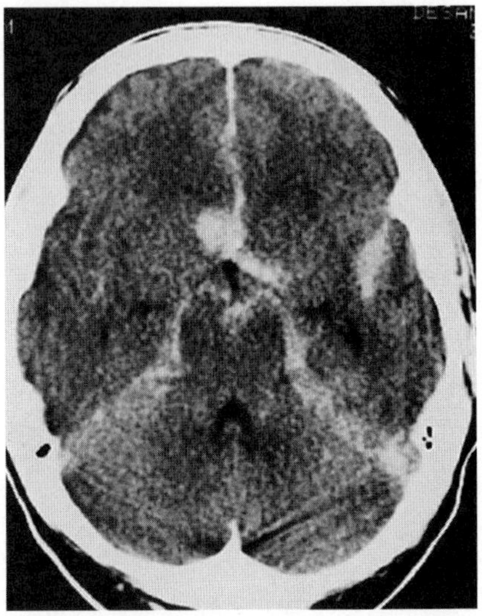

FIGURE 1-260 Noncontrast CT demonstrates diffuse subarachnoid hemorrhage. The rounded area of hyperdensity anterior to the suprasellar cistern represents an aneurysm of the anterior communicating artery. (From Specht N [ed]: *Practical guide to diagnostic imaging,* St Louis, 1998, Mosby.)

- Patients with any persistent new neurologic deficit who do not respond to medical treatment should have urgent catheter angiography to confirm the presence of vasospasm, followed by intraarterial papaverine and/or balloon angioplasty in those cases
- While a systematic review of randomized trials suggested a positive effect of antiplatelet therapy after aneurysmal SAH, a randomized controlled trial concluded that aspirin did not reduce the risk of delayed ischemic neurological deficit

CHRONIC Rx

It is unclear whether the increased risk for recurrent aneurysms justifies continued screening. A review of 752 cases found the cumulative incidence of recurrent SAH was 3.2% (22 times higher than expected in comparable populations). Risk factors for recurrence were smoking, age, and multiple aneurysms at the time of the initial SAH. The issue requires further study.

DISPOSITION

Approximately 35% early mortality, 45% at 1 mo

REFERRAL

Transfer as soon as possible to a facility with neurosurgical care.

PEARLS & CONSIDERATIONS

COMMENTS

About 20% of patients experience warning signs within 3 mo before aneurysm rupture, including moderate or severe headache ("sentinel headache"), dizziness, nausea and vomiting, transient motor or sensory deficits, loss of consciousness, or visual disturbances.

EVIDENCE

Oral nimodipine (60 mg every 4 hours) significantly reduces the proportion of patients with poor outcome and ischemic neurologic deficits after aneurysmal SAH.

Limited evidence suggests that the timing of surgery is not a critical factor in determining outcome following an SAH, although results from one trial suggest that patients who undergo early surgery (day 0-3) tend to fare best.

Antifibrinolytic therapy does not improve clinical outcome following SAH, as the benefit gained from a reduction of rebleeding is offset by an increase in poor outcome caused by cerebral ischemia.

A randomized trial comparing neurosurgical clipping vs. endovascular coiling in 2143 patients with ruptured intracranial aneurysms showed the outcome in terms of survival free of disability at 1 year is significantly better with endovascular coiling. The data also suggested that the long-term risks of further bleeding from the treated aneurysm are low with either therapy, although somewhat more frequent with endovascular coiling.

A prospective pilot study of 19 patients confirmed the safety and feasibility of continuous high-dose intravenous magnesium sulfate (MgSO4) for the prevention of cerebral vasospasm and ischemic cerebral injury. A randomized, double-blind, placebo-controlled trial with MgSO4 (64 mmol/day IV) is currently under way. A randomized trial of intravenous magnesium vs. nimodipine showed comparable results between groups.

A randomized trial of mild intraoperative hypothermia during surgery for intracranial aneurysm did not improve neurologic outcomes.

There is no evidence of a beneficial or adverse effect of corticosteroids, and we are unable to cite evidence that meets our criteria for the other treatments for SAH.

SUGGESTED READINGS

Beck J et al: Sentinel headache and the risk of rebleeding after aneurysmal subarachnoid hemorrhage, *Stroke* 37(11):2733, 2006. Epub Sept 28, 2006.

Bederson JB et al: Recommendations for the management of patients with unruptured intracranial aneurysms: a statement for healthcare professionals from the Stroke Council of the American Heart Association, *Circulation* 102(18):2300, 2000.

Brisman JL et al: Cerebral aneurysms, *N Engl J Med* 355:928, 2006.

Dorhout Mees S et al: Calcium antagonists for aneurysmal subarachnoid haemorrhage, *Cochrane Library* 3:CD000277, 2007.

Edlow JA: Diagnosis of subarachnoid hemorrhage, *Neurocri Care* 2(2):99, 2005.

Edlow JA, Caplan LR: Avoiding pitfalls in the diagnosis of subarachnoid hemorrhage, *N Engl J Med* 342:29, 2000.

Edlow JA, Wyer PC: How good is a negative cranial computed tomographic scan result in excluding subarachnoid hemorrhage? *Ann Emerg Med* 36:507, 2000.

Feigin V et al: Corticosteroids for aneurysmal subarachnoid haemorrhage and primary intracerebral haemorrhage, *Cochrane Database Syst Rev* 20;(3):CD004583, 2005.

Heuer GG et al: Relationship between intracranial pressure and other clinical variables in patients with aneurysmal subarachnoid hemorrhage, *J Neurosurg* 101(3):408, 2004.

Krischek B, Inoue I: The genetics of intracranial aneurysms, *J Hum Genet* 51:587, 2006.

Molyneux A et al: International Subarachnoid Aneurysm Trial (ISAT) of neurosurgical clipping versus endovascular coiling in 2143 patients with ruptured intracranial aneurysms: a randomised trial, *Lancet* 26;360(9342):1267, 2002.

Morgenstern LB et al: Worst headache and subarachnoid hemorrhage: prospective modern computed tomography and spinal fluid analysis, *Ann Emerg Med* 32:297, 1998.

Morris PG et al: Anxiety and depression after spontaneous subarachnoid hemorrhage, *Neurosurgery* 54(1):47, discussion 52, 2004.

Pickard JD et al: Effect of oral nimodipine on cerebral infarction and outcome after subarachnoid haemorrhage: British aneurysm nimodipine trial, *BMJ* 298:636, 1989.

Qureshi AI, Suarez JI: Use of hypertonic saline solutions in treatment of cerebral edema and intracranial hypertension, *Crit Care Med* 28(9):3301, 2000.

Raaymakers TW, and the MARS Study Group: Aneurysms in relatives of patients with subarachnoid hemorrhage. Frequency and risk factors, *Neurology* 53:982, 1999.

Roos YB et al: Antifibrinolytic therapy for aneurysmal subarachnoid haemorrhage, *Cochrane Library* 1:2004.

Schmid-Elsaesser R et al: Intravenous magnesium versus nimodipine in the treatment of patients with aneurismal subarachnoid hemorrhage: a randomized study, *Neurosurg* 58:1054, 2006.

Suarez JI: Editorial comment: salting the brain to improve CBF in SAH patients, *Stroke* 34:1396, 2003.

Todd MM: Mild intraoperative hypothermia during surgery for intracranial aneurysm, *N Engl J Med* 352:135, 2005.

Treggiari, MM et al: Systematic review of the prevention of delayed ischemic neurological deficits with hypertension, hypervolemia, and hemodilution therapy following subarachnoid hemorrhage, *J Neurosurg* 98:978, 2003.

Tseng MY et al: Effect of hypertonic saline on cerebral blood flow in poor-grade patients with subarachnoid hemorrhage, *Stroke* 34:1389, 2003.

Van den Bergh WB et al: Randomized controlled trial of acetylsalicylic acid in aneurysmal subarachnoid hemorrhage: the MASH study, *Stroke* 37:2326, 2006.

Wermer MJ et al: Incidence of recurrent subarachnoid hemorrhage after clipping for ruptured intracranial aneurysms, *Stroke* 36:2394, 2005.

Whitfield PC, Kirkpatrick PJ: Timing of surgery for aneurysmal subarachnoid haemorrhage, *Cochrane Library* 1:2004.

Yahia AM et al: The safety and feasibility of continuous intravenous magnesium sulfate for prevention of cerebral vasospasm in aneurysmal subarachnoid hemorrhage, *Neurocrit Care* 3(1):16, 2005.

AUTHOR: **RICHARD S. ISAACSON, M.D.**

Subclavian Steal Syndrome

BASIC INFORMATION

DEFINITION

Subclavian steal syndrome is an occlusion or severe stenosis of the proximal subclavian artery leading to decreased antegrade flow or retrograde flow in the ipsilateral vertebral artery and neurologic symptoms referable to the posterior circulation.

SYNONYMS

Proximal subclavian (or innominate) artery stenosis or occlusion

ICD-9CM CODES
435.2 Subclavian steal syndrome

EPIDEMIOLOGY & DEMOGRAPHICS

- Similar to that of other manifestations of atherosclerosis (coronary artery disease, cerebrovascular disease, or peripheral vascular disease)
- Affects middle-aged persons (men somewhat younger than women on average) with arteriosclerotic risk factors including family history, smoking, diabetes mellitus, hyperlipidemia, hypertension, sedentary lifestyle

PHYSICAL FINDINGS & CLINICAL PRESENTATION

Symptoms:
- Many patients are asymptomatic.
- Upper extremity ischemic symptoms: fatigue, exercise-related aching, coolness, numbness of the involved upper extremity.
- Neurologic symptoms are reported by 25% of patients with known unilateral subclavian steal. These include brief spells of:
  1. Vertigo
  2. Diplopia
  3. Decreased vision
  4. Oscillopsia
  5. Gait unsteadiness

  These spells are only occasionally provoked by exercising the ischemic upper extremity (classic subclavian steal). Left subclavian steal is more common than right, but the latter is more serious.
- Posterior circulation stroke related to subclavian steal is rare.
- Innominate artery stenosis can cause decreased right carotid artery flow and cerebrovascular symptoms of the anterior cerebral circulation, but this is uncommon.

Physical findings:
- Delayed and smaller volume pulse (wrist or antecubital) in the affected upper extremity
- Lower blood pressure in the affected upper extremity
- Supraclavicular bruit

NOTE: Inflating a blood pressure cuff will increase the bruit if it originates from a vertebral artery stenosis and decrease the bruit if it originates from a subclavian artery stenosis.

ETIOLOGY & PATHOGENESIS

Etiology:
- Atherosclerosis
- Arteritis (Takayasu's disease and temporal arteritis)
- Embolism to the subclavian or innominate artery
- Cervical rib
- Chronic use of a crutch
- Occupational (baseball pitchers and cricket bowlers)

Pathogenesis: The vertebral artery originates from the subclavian artery. For subclavian steal to occur, the occlusion must be proximal to the takeoff of the vertebral artery. On the right side, only a small distance separates the bifurcation of the innominate artery and the takeoff of the vertebral artery, explaining why the condition occurs less commonly on the right side. Occlusion of the innominate artery must affect right carotid artery flow.

DIAGNOSIS

- See "History," "Physical Findings," and "Imaging Studies."
- The carotid arteries should be evaluated at least noninvasively in all cases.

DIFFERENTIAL DIAGNOSIS

- Posterior circulation TIA (and stroke)
- Upper extremity ischemia
  1. Distal subclavian artery stenosis/occlusion
  2. Raynaud's syndrome
  3. Thoracic outlet syndrome

WORKUP

- Noninvasive upper extremity arterial flow studies
- Doppler sonography of the vertebral, subclavian, and innominate arteries
- Arteriography

TREATMENT

- In most patients the disease is benign and requires no treatment other than atherosclerosis risk factor modification and aspirin. Symptoms tend to improve over time as collateral circulation develops.
- Vascular surgical reconstruction requires a thoracotomy; it may be indicated in innominate artery stenosis or when upper extremity ischemia is incapacitating.

AUTHORS: **FRED F. FERRI, M.D.,** and **TOM J. WACHTEL, M.D.**

BASIC INFORMATION

DEFINITION

A subdural hematoma is bleeding into the subdural space, caused by rupture of bridging veins between the brain and venous sinuses.

ICD-9CM CODES
432.1 Subdural hematoma

SYNONYMS

Acute subdural hematoma
Chronic subdural hematoma
Subdural hemorrhage

EPIDEMIOLOGY & DEMOGRAPHICS

Nearly all cases are caused by trauma, although the trauma may be quite trivial. Patients are commonly at the extremes of age. Coagulation abnormalities, especially use of anticoagulation in the elderly, is a significant risk factor.

PHYSICAL FINDINGS & CLINICAL PRESENTATION

- Vague headache, often worse in morning than evening.
- Some apathy, confusion, and clouding of consciousness is common, although frank coma may complicate late cases. Chronic subdural hematomas may cause a dementia picture.
- Neurologic symptoms may be transient, simulating TIA.
- Almost any sign of cortical dysfunction may occur, including hemiparesis, sensory deficits, or language abnormalities, depending on which part of the cortex is compressed by the hematoma.
- New-onset seizures should raise the index of suspicion.

ETIOLOGY

Traumatic rupture of cortical bridging veins, especially where stretched by underlying cerebral atrophy

DIAGNOSIS

DIFFERENTIAL DIAGNOSIS

- Epidural hematoma
- Subarachnoid hemorrhage
- Mass lesion (e.g., tumor)
- Ischemic stroke
- Intraparenchymal hemorrhage

WORKUP

- CT scan is sensitive for diagnosis and should be performed in a timely fashion (Fig. 1-261).
- Hematocrit, platelet count, PTT, and PT/INR should be routinely checked.

TREATMENT

NONPHARMACOLOGIC THERAPY

Small subdural hematomas may be left untreated and the patient observed, but if there is an underlying cause, such as anticoagulation, this should be rapidly corrected to prevent further accumulation of blood.

ACUTE GENERAL Rx

- Neurosurgical drainage of blood from subdural space via burr hole is the definitive procedure, although it is common for the hematoma to reaccumulate.
- There is an increased risk of seizures, which should be treated appropriately if they arise.

DISPOSITION

Admit to hospital, may require ICU admission. Neurosurgical evacuation may be required.

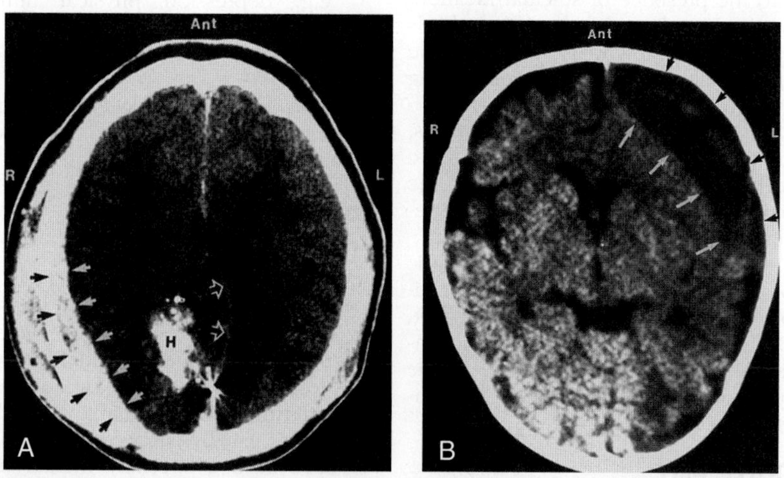

FIGURE 1-261 Subdural hematomas. A noncontrasted computed tomography scan of an acute subdural hematoma **(A)** shows a crescentic area of increased density in the right posterior parietal region between the brain and the skull *(black and white arrows)*. An area of intraparenchymal hemorrhage *(H)* is also seen; a chronic subdural hematoma for a different patient is shown in **(B)**. There is an area of decreased density in the left frontoparietal region *(arrows)* effacing the sulci, compressing the anterior horn of the left lateral ventricle, and shifting the midline somewhat to the right. (From Mettler FA [ed]: *Primary care radiology,* Philadelphia, 2000, WB Saunders.)

REFERRALS

Neurology, neurosurgery, critical care

PEARLS & CONSIDERATIONS

- The very young and very old are particularly susceptible to subdural hematomas.
- Relatively minor trauma may cause a subdural hematoma.
- Caution should be taken in interpreting CT findings in the subacute stage, where blood appears as isodense to brain, and therefore the distance from the cortical sulci to the skull needs to be evaluated.

EVIDENCE

EBM

There are no RCTs to guide the selection of treatment in SDH. In particular, no defined criteria for selecting patients who would benefit from surgical evacuation exist. Advanced age and severity of underlying cerebral lesions were negatively correlated with outcome in a large retrospective study of patients who received surgical intervention.[1,2]

Review of the literature does not show a clear benefit for prophylactic antiepileptic medications in SDH.[3]

Use of factor IX complex vs. FFP for reversal of warfarin-induced bleeding was associated with improved speed of anticoagulation reversal by factor IX complex in an RCT. No studies, however, establish that rapid reversal improves outcome.[4]

A recent retrospective analysis suggested no difference in outcome between craniotomy vs. decompressive craniectomy in acute traumatic SDH, but found advanced age and evidence of herniation independently correlated with poor outcome.[5]

Evidence-Based References

1. *Neurosurg Rev* 20(4):239-244, 1997.
2. *Clin Neurol Neurosurg* 107(3):223-229, 2005.
3. *Cochrane Database Syst Rev* 3:CD004893, 2005.
4. *Neurosurgery* 45(5):1113-1118; discussion 1118-1119, 1999.
5. *J Clin Neurosci* 13(7):718, 2006. Epub 2006.

SUGGESTED READINGS

Adhiyaman V et al: Chronic subdural haematoma in the elderly, *Postgrad Med J* 78(916):71-75, 2002.

Chen JC, Levy ML: Causes, epidemiology, and risk factors of chronic subdural hematoma, *Neurosurg Clin N Am* 11(3):399, 2000.

Voelker JL: Nonoperative treatment of chronic subdural hematoma, *Neurosurg Clin N Am* 11(3):507, 2000.

AUTHOR: **DANIEL MATTSON, M.D., M.SC.(MED.)**

BASIC INFORMATION

DEFINITION

Suicide refers to successful and unsuccessful attempts to kill oneself. Suicide ideation is defined as the presence of passive or active thoughts about a premature end of life.

SYNONYMS

Self-murder

ICD-9CM CODES
Categorized by method (e.g., poisoning)

EPIDEMIOLOGY & DEMOGRAPHICS

INCIDENCE (IN U.S.):

- Suicide is among the top 10 leading causes of death and the seventh leading cause of years of potential life lost in the U.S.
- Suicide ideation is present in 7% to 10% of primary care patients.
- Overall rate in U.S. is 11 cases/100,000 persons.
- Rate in men is 18.7 cases/100,000 persons.
- Rate in women is 4.4 cases/100,000 persons.

PEAK INCIDENCE: >65 yr of age for completed suicide

PREDOMINANT AGE:

- Increases with age (13.1 cases/100,000 persons aged 15 to 24 yr, 16.9 cases/100,000 persons aged 65 to 74 yr, and 23.5 cases/100,000 persons aged 75 to 84 yr)
- Third leading cause of death in ages 15 to 24 in U.S.

GENETICS:

- Biologic factors may increase the risk of suicide directly (e.g., by increasing impulsivity) or indirectly (e.g., by predisposing to a mental illness).
- Family history of suicide is associated with suicidal behavior.
- Pediatric trials suggest that selective serotonin reuptake inhibitors (SSRIs) are associated with slight increased risk of suicidal behavior.

PHYSICAL FINDINGS & CLINICAL PRESENTATION

Methods used in attempted (unsuccessful) suicides differ from those used in completed suicides.

- Overdose used in >70% of attempted suicides.
- About 60% of completed suicides are accomplished with firearms. Hanging is the second most common method for completed suicides.
- Several risk factors for completed suicide include psychiatric illness such as depression or anxiety, middle age or advanced age, white race, male gender, a recent divorce or separation, comorbid substance abuse (particularly when intoxicated), previous history of suicide attempts, fatal plan (e.g., firearms or hanging), history of violence, and family history of suicide. Concurrent chronic physical illness increases the risk for suicide greatly (e.g., the risk for suicide among AIDS or renal dialysis patients is nearly 30 times that of the general population).

ETIOLOGY

- Individuals with a mental disorder or substance abuse are responsible for >90% of all suicides.
- The concurrence of more than one condition (e.g., depression and alcohol abuse) greatly increases the risk of suicide.
- Hopelessness is a strong predictor of suicide potential.
- Same-gender sexual orientation has been shown to exert an independent influence on suicide attempts.

DIAGNOSIS

DIFFERENTIAL DIAGNOSIS

- Some disorders are associated with self-injurious behavior that is not suicidal. Borderline personality disorder, for example, manifests with self-mutilation without active suicidal intent. Eating disorders are harmful and may be fatal, but death is rarely the goal.
- Some suicidal behavior is intended as a "call for help." In these situations individuals usually design the suicide so that they will be discovered before significant damage has been done.

WORKUP

- The physician must directly inquire into the presence of suicidal ideation. Approximately one half to two thirds of individuals who commit suicide visit physicians within 1 mo of taking their lives.
- Explicit suicidal intent, hopelessness, and a well-formulated plan indicate high risk. Clinicians can use the mnemonic SAL: Is the method Specific? Is it Available? Is it Lethal?
- The concurrence of multiple psychiatric problems, substance abuse, and multiple physical problems increases the risk.
- Covert suicidal ideation occurs in patients primarily with multiple vague physical complaints, depression, anxiety, or substance abuse.

TREATMENT

NONPHARMACOLOGIC THERAPY

- Major immediate intervention: placement of the patient in a safe environment (usually hospitalization in a psychiatric unit or a medical unit with continuous observation)
- Long-term: psychotherapy aimed at factors that underlie the decision to pursue suicide or at the risk factors contributing to suicidal behavior
- Substance abuse treatment (e.g., AA, NA) when substance abuse is present

ACUTE GENERAL Rx

- Benzodiazepines are useful in reducing the extreme anxiety and dysphoria in a suicidal patient; however, these agents are depressive and should be used only when patient is in a safe environment.
- Antipsychotics can be used if psychosis is present (e.g., voices telling patient to hurt self).
- Mood stabilizers and antidepressants should be started in the acute setting but may have up to a 2-wk latency period.

CHRONIC Rx

- Therapy should be aimed at the underlying condition (e.g., antidepressants for depression, anxiolytics or antidepressants for anxiety, ongoing substance abuse treatment for substance abuse history, or psychotherapy for chronic low self-esteem, hopelessness).
- In elderly, loneliness and medical disability are major reasons for suicide and therefore major targets for intervention.

DISPOSITION

- Prior suicide attempt is the best predictor for completed suicides (i.e., patients who attempt suicide once are at high risk for completing suicide in the future).
- Conditions associated with suicide (e.g., depression, physical ailments) are usually chronic and recurring.

REFERRAL

Patients with active suicidal ideation and intent should be referred to specialty mental health.

PEARLS & CONSIDERATIONS

- Past suicidal behavior is strongly associated with an increased risk for subsequent suicidal behavior.
- Most people who die by suicide are suffering from a treatable mental disorder, usually depression, but few have seen a specialty mental health provider.
- Although many patients are reluctant to seek and actively engage in mental health treatment, up to 75% of those who complete suicide have seen a pri-

mary care provider in the prior 30 days.

PREVENTION

The U.S. Preventive Services Task Force has produced the following document:

Gaynes BN et al: Screening for suicide risk in adults: a summary of the evidence for the U.S. Preventive Services Task Force, *Ann Intern Med* 140:822, 2004.

EVIDENCE

EBM

Cognitive-behavioral therapy (CBT)

There is limited evidence from randomized studies that CBT is of benefit in reducing further suicide attempts in patients who have previously attempted suicide.

A randomized controlled trial (RCT) compared CBT vs. enhanced usual care over 18 months in 120 adults who had recently attempted suicide. This study found that treatment with CBT resulted in significantly lower reattempt rate compared with usual care (24% vs. 41%) and had significantly reduced rate of self-reported depression.[1] B

Electroconvulsive therapy (ECT)

The use of ECT in the short-term management of suicidality is supported by expert opinion.

Recommendations from the American Psychiatric Association are that, because ECT is associated with a rapid and robust antidepressant response and a rapid diminution in associated suicidal thoughts, ECT may be recommended as a treatment for severe episodes of major depression that are accompanied by suicidal thoughts or behaviors.[2] C

Further recommendations are that, because there is no evidence of a long-term reduction of suicide risk with ECT, continuation or maintenance treatment with pharmacotherapy or with ECT is recommended after an acute ECT course.[2] C

Interpersonal therapy

A systematic review of 13 RCTs analyzed the efficacy of interpersonal therapy in the treatment of depressive spectrum disorders using a metaanalytic approach. Four metaanalyses were performed, showing that interpersonal therapy was superior to placebo, similar to treatment with medication alone (and efficacy did not increase when combined with medication), and superior to CBT.[3] A

Recommendations from the American Psychiatric Association are that, in patients with suicidality, psychotherapies such as interpersonal psychotherapy and CBT may be considered appropriate treatments for suicidal behavior, especially in the context of depression.[2] C

Evidence-Based References

1. Brown GK et al: Cognitive therapy for the prevention of suicide attempts: a randomized controlled trial, *JAMA* 294:563-570, 2005. B
2. American Psychiatric Association: *Practice guideline for the assessment and treatment of patients with suicidal behaviors,* Arlington, VA, 2003, American Psychiatric Association. C
3. de Mello MF et al: A systematic review of research findings on the efficacy of interpersonal therapy for depressive disorders, *Eur Arch Psychiatry Clin Neurosci* 255:75-82, 2005. B

SUGGESTED READINGS

Feldman MD et al: Let's not talk about it: suicide inquiry in primary care, *Ann Fam Med* 5(5):412-418, 2007.

Mann JJ et al: Suicide prevention strategies: a systematic review, *JAMA* 294(16):2064, 2005.

AUTHOR: **MITCHELL D. FELDMAN, M.D., M.PHIL.**

BASIC INFORMATION

DEFINITION

Superior vena cava syndrome is a set of symptoms that results when a mediastinal mass compresses the superior vena cava (SVC) or the veins that drain into it.

ICD-9CM CODES
453.2 Vena cava thrombosis

EPIDEMIOLOGY & DEMOGRAPHICS

- The superior vena cava syndrome occurs in 15,000 persons in the U.S. every year.
- Mirrors lung cancer (especially small cell carcinoma) and lymphoma: see "Lung Neoplasm" and "Lymphoma" in Section I.

PHYSICAL FINDINGS & CLINICAL PRESENTATION

The pathophysiology of the syndrome involves the increased pressure in the venous system draining into the superior vena cava, producing edema of the head, neck, and upper extremities. Symptoms develop over a period of 2 weeks in one third of patients.

Symptoms:
- Shortness of breath
- Chest pain
- Cough
- Dysphagia, hoarseness, stridor
- Headache
- Syncope
- Visual trouble

Signs:
- Chest wall vein distention (Fig. 1-262)
- Neck vein distention
- Facial edema
- Upper extremity swelling
- Cyanosis

ETIOLOGY

- Lung cancer (80% of all cases, of which half are small cell lung cancer)
- Lymphoma (15%)
- Thymoma
- Tuberculosis
- Goiter
- Aortic aneurysm (arteriosclerotic or syphilitic)
- SVC thrombosis
  1. Primary: associated with a central venous catheter
  2. Secondary: as a complication of SVC syndrome associated with one of the abovementioned causes
- Inflammatory process, fibrosing mediastinitis

DIAGNOSIS

CT of the chest wth contrast is the most useful diagnostic study. MRI is usually adequate to establish the diagnosis of superior vena cava obstruction and to assist in the differential diagnosis of probable cause.

DIFFERENTIAL DIAGNOSIS

The syndrome is characteristic enough to exclude other diagnoses. The differential diagnosis concerns the underlying etiologies listed previously.

WORKUP

- Chest x-ray
- Chest CT with contrast or MRI (in patient who cannot tolerate contrast medium)
- Venography: warranted only when an intervention (e.g., stent or surgery) is planned
- Percutaneous needle biopsy (usually the initial diagnostic modality used to establish a histologic diagnosis)
- Bronchoscopy
- Mediastinoscopy
- Thoracotomy

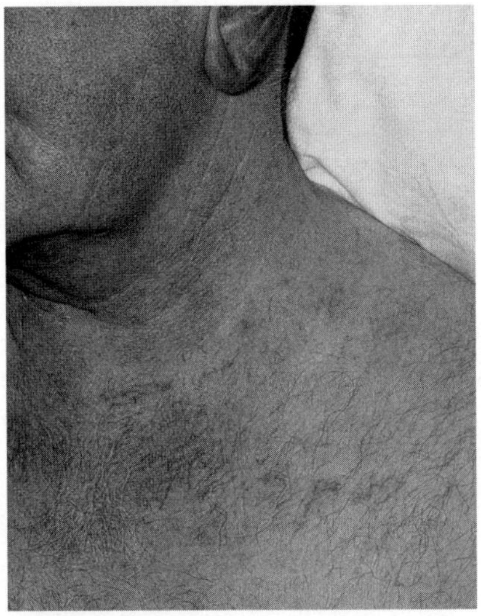

FIGURE 1-262 Superior vena cava obstruction causing dilated veins and plethora of the upper trunk and neck in a patient with bronchial carcinoma. Patients with superior vena cava obstruction are occasionally referred to dermatologists with suspected contact allergy (eyelid swelling) or angioedema (facial or hand swelling). (From White GM, Cox NH [eds]: *Diseases of the skin, a color atlas and text,* ed 2, St. Louis, 2006, Mosby.)

TREATMENT

Although invasive procedures such as mediastinoscopy or thoracotomy are associated with higher than usual risk of bleeding, a tissue diagnosis is usually needed before commencing therapy.

Management is guided by the severity of the symptoms and the underlying etiology.

Emergency empiric radiation is indicated in critical situations such as respiratory failure or central nervous system signs associated with increased intracranial pressure.

- Treatment of the underlying malignancy:
  1. Radiotherapy: the majority of tumors causing the SVC syndrome are sensitive to radiotherapy
  2. Systemic/chemotherapy
- Anticoagulant or fibrinolytic therapy in patients who do not respond to cancer treatment within a week or if an obstructing thrombus has been documented.
- Loop diuretics are often used, but their effect is limited.
- Upright positioning and fluid restriction until collateral channels develop and allow for clinical regression are useful modalities for SVC syndrome secondary to benign disease.
- Steroids (dexamethasone 4 mg q6h) may be useful in reducing the tumor burden in lymphoma and thymoma.
- Percutaneous self-expandable stents that can be placed under local anesthesia with radiologic manipulation are useful in the treatment of SVC syndrome to bypass the obstruction, especially in cases associated with malignant tumors.
- Surgical bypass grafting is infrequently used to treat the superior vena cava syndrome.

REFERRAL

To a thoracic surgeon, pulmonary specialist, or oncologist

AUTHORS: **FRED F. FERRI, M.D.,** and **TOM J. WACHTEL, M.D.**

BASIC INFORMATION

DEFINITION

Syncope is the transient loss of consciousness that results from an acute global reduction in cerebral blood flow. Syncope should be distinguished from other causes of transient loss of consciousness.

ICD-9CM CODES
720.2 Syncope

EPIDEMIOLOGY & DEMOGRAPHICS

- Syncope accounts for 3% to 5% of emergency room visits.
- 30% of the adult population will experience at least one syncopal episode during their lifetime.
- Incidence of syncope is highest in elderly men and young women.

PHYSICAL FINDINGS & CLINICAL PRESENTATION

- Blood pressure: if low, consider orthostatic hypotension; if unequal in both arms (difference >20 mm Hg), consider subclavian steal or dissecting aneurysm. (NOTE: Blood pressure and heart rate should be recorded in the supine and standing positions.) If there is drop in BP but no change in HR, the patient may be on a beta blocker or may have an autonomic neuropathy.
- Pulse: if patient has tachycardia, bradycardia, or irregular rhythm, consider arrhythmia.
- Heart: if there are murmurs present suggestive of AS or IHSS, consider syncope secondary to left ventricular outflow obstruction; if there are JVD and distal heart sounds, consider cardiac tamponade.
- Carotid sinus pressure: can be diagnostic if it reproduces symptoms and other causes are excluded; a pause >3 sec or a systolic BP drop >50 mm Hg without symptoms or <30 mm Hg with symptoms when sinus pressure is applied separately on each side for <5 sec is considered abnormal. This test should be avoided in patients with carotid bruits or cerebrovascular disease; ECG monitoring, IV access, and bedside atropine should be available when carotid sinus pressure is applied.

ETIOLOGY

- Neurally mediated syncope
  1. Psychophysiologic (emotional upset, panic disorders, hysteria)
  2. Visceral reflex (micturition, defecation, food ingestion, coughing, ventricular contraction; glossopharyngeal neuralgia)
  3. Carotid sinus pressure
  4. Reduction of venous return caused by Valsalva maneuver
- Orthostatic hypotension
  1. Hypovolemia
  2. Vasodilator medications
  3. Autonomic neuropathy (diabetes, amyloid, Parkinson's disease, multisystem atrophy)
  4. Pheochromocytoma
  5. Carcinoid syndrome
- Cardiac
  1. Reduced cardiac output
     a. Left ventricular outflow obstruction (aortic stenosis, hypertrophic cardiomyopathy)
     b. Obstruction to pulmonary flow (pulmonary embolism, pulmonic stenosis, primary pulmonary hypertension)
     c. MI with pump failure
     d. Cardiac tamponade
     e. Mitral stenosis
     f. Reduction of venous return (atrial myxoma, valve thrombus)
     g. β-blockers
  2. Arrhythmias or asystole
     a. Extreme tachycardia (>160 to 180 bpm)
     b. Severe bradycardia (<30 to 40 bpm)
     c. Sick sinus syndrome
     d. AV block (second- or third-degree)
     e. Ventricular tachycardia or fibrillation
     f. Long QT syndrome
     g. Pacemaker malfunction
     h. Psychotropic medications and beta blockers

DIAGNOSIS

DIFFERENTIAL DIAGNOSIS

1. Seizure (see "Workup")
2. Vertebrobasilar TIA usually manifests as diplopia, vertigo, ataxia but not loss of consciousness. Isolated episodes of transient loss of consciousness (TLOC) without accompanying neurologic symptoms are very unlikely to be a TIA
3. Recreational drugs/alcohol
4. Functional causes, such as stress and somatoform disorders
5. Sleep disorders, such as sleep attacks and narcolepsy, are also in the differential for TLOC
6. Head trauma

WORKUP

The history is crucial to diagnosing the cause of syncope and may suggest a diagnosis that can be evaluated with directed testing. History is also important to determine other etiologies for TLOC, such as seizure.

- Sudden loss of consciousness: consider cardiac arrhythmias.
- Gradual loss of consciousness: consider orthostatic hypotension, vasodepressor syncope, hypoglycemia.
- History of aura before loss of consciousness (LOC) or prolonged confusion (>1 min), amnesia or lethargy after LOC suggests seizure rather than syncope.
- Patient's activity at the time of syncope:
  1. Micturition, coughing, defecation: consider syncope secondary to decreased venous return.
  2. Turning head or while shaving: consider carotid sinus syndrome.
  3. Physical exertion in a patient with murmur: consider aortic stenosis.
  4. Arm exercise: consider subclavian steal syndrome.
  5. Assuming an upright position: consider orthostatic hypotension.
- Associated events:
  1. Chest pain: consider MI, pulmonary embolism.
  2. Palpitations: consider arrhythmias.
  3. Incontinence (urine or fecal) and tongue biting are associated with seizure or syncope.
  4. Brief, transient shaking after LOC may represent myoclonus from global cerebral hypoperfusion and not seizures. However, sustained tonic/clonic muscle action is more suggestive of seizure.
  5. Focal neurologic symptoms or signs point to a neurologic event such as a seizure with residual deficits (e.g., Todd's paralysis) or cerebral ischemic injury.
  6. Psychologic stress: syncope may be vasovagal.
- Review current medications, particularly antihypertensive and psychotropic drugs.

LABORATORY TESTS

Routine blood tests rarely yield diagnostically useful information and should be done only if they are specifically suggested by the results of the history and physical examination. The following are commonly ordered tests.

- Pregnancy test should be considered in women of childbearing age
- CBC to rule out anemia, infection
- Electrolytes, BUN, creatinine, magnesium, calcium to rule out electrolyte abnormalities and evaluate fluid status
- Serum glucose level
- Cardiac isoenzymes should be obtained if the patient gives a history of chest pain before the syncopal episode
- ABGs to rule out pulmonary embolus, hyperventilation (when suspected)
- Evaluate drug and alcohol levels when suspecting toxicity

IMAGING STUDIES

- Echocardiogram is useful to rule out major pathology such as AS, IHSS, atrial myxoma, and left ventricular dysfunction.

- If seizure is suspected, CT scan and/or MRI of the head and EEG may be useful.
- If head trauma or neurologic signs on examination, CT or MRI may be helpful.
- If pulmonary embolism is suspected, ventilation-perfusion scan should be done.
- If arrhythmias are suspected, a 24-hr Holter monitor and admission to a telemetry unit is appropriate. Generally, Holter monitoring is rarely useful, revealing a cause for syncope in <3% of cases. Loop recorders that can be activated after syncopal episode to retrieve information about the cardiac rhythm during the preceding 4 min add considerable diagnostic yield in patients with unexplained syncope.
- Implantable cardiac monitors that function as permanent loop recorders or implantable cardioverter-defibrillators, which are placed subcutaneously in the pectoral region with the patient under local anesthesia, may be useful in patients with cardiac syncope.
- Electrophysiologic studies may be indicated in patients with structural heart disease and/or recurrent syncope.
- ECG to rule out arrhythmias; may be diagnostic in 5% to 10% of patients.

TILT-TABLE TESTING

- Useful to support a diagnosis of neurally mediated syncope or orthostatic hypotension. Head-up tilt-table (HUT) testing should be performed after ruling out structural cardiac abnormalities of the heart (e.g., valvular stenosis, left ventricular dysfunction, hypertrophied cardiomyopathy by echocardiography). Patients older than age 50 should also have stress testing before tilt-table testing. Positive results would preclude tilt-table testing.
- Indicated in patients with recurrent episodes of unexplained syncope as well as for patients in high-risk occupations (e.g., pilots, bus drivers) (Fig. 1-263).
- It is performed by keeping the patient in an upright posture on a tilt table with footboard support. The angle of the tilt table varies from 60 to 80 degrees. The duration of upright posture during tilt-table testing varies from 25 to 45 min. Provocative measures such as intravenous isoproterenol or sublingual nitroglycerine may be used during tilt-table test.
- The hallmark of neurally mediated syncope is severe hypotension associated with a paradoxical bradycardia triggered by a specific stimulus. The diagnosis of orthostatic hypotension is made by observance of a drop in systolic blood pressure of 20 mm Hg or a drop in diastolic blood pressure of 10 mm Hg within 3 min of upright tilt table testing. A number of patients may have delayed orthostatic hypotension, with falls in blood pressure beyond 30 min.

PSYCHIATRIC EVALUATION

- May be indicated in young patients without heart disease who have frequently recurring transient loss of consciousness and other somatic symptoms.
- Generalized anxiety disorder, pain disorder, and major depression predispose patients to neurally mediated reactions and may result in syncope.

TREATMENT (Rx)

GENERAL THERAPY

- Teach patients to recognize and avoid triggering factors leading to syncope. Advise patients to assume a recumbent position to maintain cerebral perfusion when they develop premonitory symptoms.
- Ensure proper hydration; consider TED stockings and salt tablets.
- Eliminate medications that may induce hypotension.

PHARMACOLOGIC Rx

- Pharmacologic approaches include beta-adrenergic receptor blockers (if not contraindicated) as first-line therapy. Other agents that are used include selective serotonin reuptake inhibitors (SSRIs), methylxanthines, anticholinergic agents, and alpha agonists. A progressive approach to pharmacologic therapy is advisable.
- Syncope caused by orthostatic hypotension is treated with volume replacement in patients with intravascular volume depletion. Also consider midodrine to promote venous return via adrenergic-mediated vasoconstriction and fludrocortisone for its mineralocorticoid effects to increase intravascular volume.

NONPHARMACOLOGIC RX

- Permanent dual-chamber pacemaker with algorithm for rapid pacing at detection of sudden rate drop may help those patients who have recurrent refractory symptomatic neurocardiogenic syncope associated with bradycardia documented spontaneously or at the time of HUT testing.
- Other nonpharmacologic and more definitive therapies vary with the underlying etiology of syncope (e.g., pacemaker in patients with syncope secondary to complete heart block; cardiac defibrillator in patients with ventricular tachyarrhythmias; radiofrequency ablation for supraventricular tachyarrhythmias; surgery for stenotic valvular heart disease).
- Varies with the underlying etiology of syncope (e.g., pacemaker in patients with syncope secondary to complete heart block).
- Syncope caused by orthostatic hypotension is treated with volume replacement in patients with intravascular volume depletion. Also consider midodrine to promote venous return via adrenergic-mediated vasoconstriction and Florinef for its mineralocorticoid effects to increase intravascular volume.

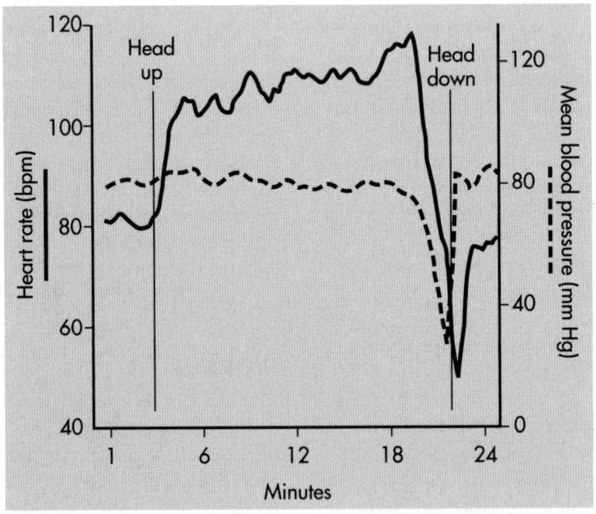

FIGURE 1-263 Head-up tilt test performed on an 18-year-old woman with a history of syncope associated with pain, preceded by a prodrome of dizziness, graying vision, and diaphoresis. A similar prodrome preceded syncope during the test. Note the precipitous, nearly simultaneous, decline of heart rate and blood pressure after an initial rise in heart rate. Vital signs returned to normal rapidly after the head was lowered. (Courtesy Robert F. Sprung, University of Utah. In Goldman L, Ausiello D [eds]: *Cecil textbook of medicine*, ed 22, Philadelphia, 2004, WB Saunders.)

DISPOSITION

Prognosis varies with the age of the patient and the etiology of the syncope. Generally:

- Benign prognosis (very low 1-yr morbidity) in patients:
  1. Age <30 yr and having noncardiac syncope
  2. Age <70 yr and having vasovagal/psychogenic syncope or syncope of unknown cause
- Poor prognosis (high mortality and morbidity) in patients with cardiac syncope
- Patients with the following risk factors have a higher 1-yr mortality: abnormal ECG, history of ventricular arrhythmia, history of CHF

REFERRAL

Hospital admission in elderly patients without prior history of syncope or unknown etiology of their syncope and in any patients suspected of having cardiac syncope.

PEARLS & CONSIDERATIONS

COMMENTS

- Section III, "Syncope," describes an algorithmic approach to the patient.
- The etiology of syncope is identified in <50% of cases during the initial evaluation.
- A thorough history and physical examination are the most productive means of establishing a diagnosis in patients with syncope.

EVIDENCE

Evidence-based treatment depends upon the cause of syncope and is discussed in other areas of the text.

SUGGESTED READINGS

Brignole M et al: Guidelines on management (diagnosis and treatment) of syncope—update 2004, *Europace* 6:467, 2004.

Fenton AM et al: Vasovagal syncope, *Ann Intern Med* 133:722, 2000.

Kapoor WN: Syncope, *N Engl J Med* 343:1856, 2000.

Menozzi C et al: Mechanism of syncope in patients with heart disease and negative electrophysiologic test, *Circulation* 105:2741, 2002.

AUTHORS: **SEAN I. SAVITZ, M.D.,** and **BHARAT K. KANTHARIA, M.D.**

BASIC INFORMATION

DEFINITION

Syndrome of inappropriate antidiuresis (SIAD) is a syndrome characterized by excessive secretion of antidiuretic hormone (ADH) in absence of normal osmotic or physiologic stimuli (increased serum osmolarity, decreased plasma volume, hypotension).

SYNONYMS

SIAD
SIADH
Syndrome of inappropriate antidiuretic hormone secretion
Inappropriate secretion of antidiuretic hormone

ICD-9CM CODES
276.9 Inappropriate secretion of antidiuretic hormone

EPIDEMIOLOGY & DEMOGRAPHICS

Nearly 50% of hyponatremia detected in the hospital setting is caused by SIAD.

PHYSICAL FINDINGS & CLINICAL PRESENTATION

- The patient is generally normovolemic or slightly hypervolemic; edema is absent.
- Delirium, lethargy, and seizures may be present if the hyponatremia is severe or of rapid onset.
- Manifestations of the underlying disease may be evident (e.g., fever from an infectious process or headaches and visual field defects from an intracranial mass).
- Diminished reflexes and extensor plantar responses may occur with severe hyponatremia.

ETIOLOGY

- Neoplasm: lung, duodenum, pancreas, brain, thymus, bladder, prostate, mesothelioma, lymphoma, Ewing's sarcoma
- Pulmonary disorders: pneumonia, TB, bronchiectasis, emphysema, cystic fibrosis, status asthmaticus
- Intracranial pathology: trauma, neoplasms, infections (meningitis, encephalitis, brain abscess), hemorrhage, hydrocephalus
- Postoperative period: surgical stress, ventilators with positive pressure, anesthetic agents
- Drugs: chlorpropamide, thiazide diuretics, vasopressin, desmopressin, oxytocin, chemotherapeutic agents (vincristine, vinblastine, cyclophosphamide), carbamazepine, phenothiazines, MAO inhibitors, tricyclic antidepressants, narcotics, nicotine, clofibrate, haloperidol, SSRIs, NSAIDs, arginine vasopressin analogues (desmopressin, oxytocin, vasopressin)
- Other: multiple sclerosis, acute intermittent porphyria, Guillain-Barré syndrome, myxedema, psychosis, delirium tremens, ACTH deficiency (hypopituitarism)

DIAGNOSIS

DIFFERENTIAL DIAGNOSIS

- Hyponatremia associated with hypervolemia (congestive heart failure, cirrhosis, nephrotic syndrome)
- Factitious hyponatremia (hyperglycemia, abnormal proteins, hyperlipidemia)
- Hyponatremia associated with hypovolemia (e.g., burns, GI fluid loss)

WORKUP

- Demonstration through laboratory evaluation (see "Laboratory Tests") of excessive secretion of ADH in absence of appropriate osmotic or physiologic stimuli (abnormal result on test of water load, elevated plasma arginine vasopressin levels despite the presence of hypotonicity and clinical euvolemia)
- Demonstration of normal thyroid, adrenal, and cardiac function
- No recent or concurrent use of diuretics
- Failure to correct hyponatremia after 0.9% saline infusion
- Correction of hyponatremia through fluid restriction

LABORATORY TESTS

- Hyponatremia
- Decreased effective osmolality (<275 mOsm/kg of water)
- Urine osmolality >100 mOsm/kg of water during hypotonicity
- Urinary osmolarity > serum osmolarity
- Urinary sodium usually >40 mEq/L with normal dietary salt intake
- Normal BUN, creatinine (indicative of normal renal function and absence of dehydration), normal TSH
- Decreased uric acid

IMAGING STUDIES

Chest x-ray to rule out neoplasm or infectious process

TREATMENT

NONPHARMACOLOGIC THERAPY

Fluid restriction to 500 to 800 ml/day with close monitoring of levels of urinary and plasma electrolytes. Adequate intake of dietary protein and salt should be encouraged.

ACUTE GENERAL Rx

- In emergency situations (seizures, coma) SIAD can be treated with combination of:
  1. Hypertonic saline solution (slow infusion of 250 ml of 3% NaCl). Infuse 3% saline (513 mmol/L) at a rate of 1 to 2 ml/kg of body weight per hour to increase the serum sodium level by 1 to 2 mmol/L/hr.
  2. Furosemide, 20 to 40 mg IV. This combination increases the serum sodium by causing diuresis of urine that is more dilute than plasma and prevents extracellular fluid volume expansion.
- The rapidity of correction varies depending on the degree of hyponatremia and if the hyponatremia is acute or chronic; generally the serum sodium should be corrected only halfway to normal in the initial 24 hr. A prudent approach is to increase serum sodium by <0.5 mEq/L/hr and limit the total increase to 8 to 12 mmol/L during the first 24 hr.
- Close monitoring of the rate of correction (every 2 to 3 hr) is recommended to avoid overcorrection. In patients with hyponatremia of chronic duration, correction of serum sodium level by >12 mmol/L over a period of 24 hr increases the risk of osmotic demyelination.
- Conivaptan (Vaprisol) is an intravenous (20 to 40 mg/day) vasopressin receptor antagonist useful in selected hospitalized patients with moderate-to-severe hyponatremia. Potential problems associated with its use are infusion-site reactions (50% of patients) and risk of osmotic demyelination if serum sodium levels are corrected too rapidly. Oral vasopressin-receptor antagonists (tolvaptan, lixivaptan, satavaptan) are pending FDA approval.

CHRONIC Rx

- Depending on the underlying etiology, fluid restriction may be needed indefinitely. Monthly monitoring of electrolytes is recommended in patients with chronic SIAD.
- Demeclocycline (Declomycin) 300 to 600 mg PO bid reduces urinary osmolality and increases serum sodium levels. It may be useful in patients with chronic SIAD (e.g., secondary to neoplasm) but use with caution in patients with hepatic disease; its side effects include nephrogenic diabetes insipidus (DI) and photosensitivity. This medication is also very expensive.
- Successful treatment of chronic nephrogenic SIAD with urea to induce osmotic diuresis has been reported in children and adults. However, oral in-

take of urea (30 g/day) is generally poorly tolerated

DISPOSITION

- Prognosis varies depending on the cause. Generally, prognosis is benign when SIAD is caused by an infectious process.
- Morbidity and mortality are high (>40%) when serum sodium concentration is <110 mEq/L.

REFERRAL

Hospital admission depending on severity of symptoms and degree of hyponatremia

PEARLS & CONSIDERATIONS

COMMENTS

- Use of hypertonic (3%) saline is contraindicated in patients with CHF, nephrotic syndrome, or cirrhosis.
- Too rapid correction of hyponatremia can cause demyelination and permanent central nervous system damage.

SUGGESTED READING

Ellison DH, Berl T: The syndrome of inappropriate antidiuresis, *N Engl J Med* 356:2064-2072, 2007.

AUTHOR: **FRED F. FERRI, M.D.**

BASIC INFORMATION

DEFINITION

Syphilis is a sexually transmitted treponemal disease, acute and chronic, characterized by primary skin lesion, secondary eruption involving skin and mucous membranes, long periods of latency, and late lesions of skin, bone, viscera, CNS, and cardiovascular system.

SYNONYMS

Lues

ICD-9CM CODES
097.9 Syphilis, acquired unspecified

EPIDEMIOLOGY & DEMOGRAPHICS

- Widespread, primarily involving ages 20 to 35 yr. Racial differences in incidence are related to social factors. Usually more prevalent in urban areas. Estimated annual incidence of 90,000 cases in the U.S. Increase in incidence in the late 1980s to 1990s, likely related to illicit drug use and prostitution. Increase occurred primarily in lower socioeconomic groups.
- Communicability is indefinite and variable. Communicable during primary, secondary, and latent mucocutaneous lesions in up to first 4 yr of latency. Most probable congenital transmission occurs in early maternal syphilis. Adequate penicillin treatment ends infectivity within 24 to 48 hr.

PHYSICAL FINDINGS & CLINICAL PRESENTATION

PRIMARY SYPHILIS: Characteristic lesion is a painless chancre on genitalia, mouth, or anus; atypical primary lesions may occur. Usually appears 3 wk after exposure and may spontaneously involute.

SECONDARY SYPHILIS:

- Localized or diffuse mucocutaneous lesions and generalized lymphadenopathy. Common to have constitutional symptoms, flulike symptoms. May begin about 4 to 6 wk after appearance of primary lesion. Manifestations may resolve in 1 wk to 12 mo.
- 60% to 80% of patients have maculopapular lesions on their palms and soles.
- Condylomata lata intertriginous papules form at areas of friction and moisture, such as the vulva.
- 21% to 58% have mucocutaneous or mucosal lesions (pharyngitis, tonsillitis, "mucous patch" lesion on oral and genital mucosa).

EARLY LATENT (<1 YR): Generally asymptomatic

LATE LATENT (>1 YR):

- Characterized by gummas (nodular, ulcerative lesions) that can involve the skin, mucous membranes, skeletal system, and viscera.
- Manifestations of cardiovascular syphilis include aortitis, aneurysm, or aortic regurgitation.
- Neurosyphilis may be asymptomatic or symptomatic. Tabes dorsalis, meningovascular syphilis, general paralysis, or insanity may occur. Iritis, choroidoretinitis, and leukoplakia may also occur.

ETIOLOGY

- *Treponema pallidum,* a spirochete
- Spread by sexual intercourse or by intrauterine transfer

DIAGNOSIS

DIFFERENTIAL DIAGNOSIS

- Other genitoulcerative diseases such as herpes, chancroid (see Section II)
- See Section III for a clinical algorithm for the evaluation of genital ulcer disease

WORKUP

Confirmation is primarily through laboratory diagnosis.

LABORATORY TESTS

- Dark-field microscopy of fluid from lesion to look for treponeme
- Serologic testing, both nontreponemal (VDRL, RPR) and treponemal (FTA, MHA)
- Lumbar puncture for CSF VDRL in patients with evidence of latent syphilis

TREATMENT

ACUTE GENERAL Rx

- Early (primary, secondary, early latent): penicillin G benzathine 2.4 million U IM × 1 or doxycycline 100 mg PO bid × 14 days
- Late (late latent, cardiovascular, gumma): penicillin G benzathine 2.4 million U IM qwk × 3 wk or doxycycline 100 mg PO bid × 4 wk
- Neurosyphilis: aqueous crystalline penicillin G 18 to 24 million U/day, administered as 3 to 4 million U IV q4h × 10 to 14 days or procaine penicillin 2.4 million U IM/day plus probenecid 500 mg PO qid, both for 10 to 14 days
- Congenital syphilis: aqueous crystalline penicillin G 50,000 U/kg/dose IV q12h × first 7 days of life and q8h after that for total of 10 days or procaine penicillin G 50,000 U/kg/dose IM/day × 10 days
- Penicillin-allergic patients with primary or secondary syphilis: doxycycline 100 mg PO bid × 14 days, or tetracycline 500 mg PO qid × 14 days, or ceftriaxone 1 g IM or IV × 8 to 10 days, or azithromycin 2 g PO stat (preliminary data only)
- Latent syphilis in penicillin-allergic patient: doxycycline 100 mg PO bid or tetracycline 500 mg qid for 28 days
- Tetracyclines are contraindicated in pregnancy. If pregnant and penicillin allergic, must be desensitized

DISPOSITION

- Repeat quantitative nontreponemal tests at 3, 6, and 12 mo. Pregnancy requires monthly tests until delivery.
- If a fourfold increase in titer occurs, if initial high titer fails to drop by fourfold within a year, or persistent signs, retreatment may be indicated. Use treatment regimen for late syphilis.
- Pregnant women without a fourfold drop in titer in a 3-mo period need to be retreated.
- Cases should be reported to local or state health department for referral, follow-up, and partner notification.

REFERRAL

- Pregnant and possible congenital syphilis
- Pregnant and allergic to penicillin, with need to be desensitized
- Late latent syphilis with serious CNS, cardiovascular, or other organ system compromise

PEARLS & CONSIDERATIONS

COMMENTS

- Jarisch-Herxheimer reaction (fever, myalgia, tachycardia, hypotension) may occur within 24 hr of treatment.
- One third of untreated patients develop CNS and/or cardiovascular sequelae.
- Up to 80% of those treated during late stages remain seropositive indefinitely.
- Treponemal tests remain positive even after adequate therapy.

SUGGESTED READINGS

Centers for Disease Control and Prevention: 2006 sexually transmitted diseases treatment guidelines, *MMWR Morb Mortal Wkly Rep* 55(RR-11), 2006.

Golden MR, Marra CM, Holmes KK: Update on syphilis: resurgence of an old problem, *JAMA* 290(11):1510, 2003.

AUTHORS: **MARIA A. CORIGLIANO, M.D.,** and **RUBEN ALVERO, M.D.**

BASIC INFORMATION

DEFINITION

Syringomyelia is a disease of the spine characterized by the formation of fluid-filled cavities within the spinal cord, sometimes extending into the brainstem.

ICD-9CM CODES
336.0 Syringomyelia

PHYSICAL FINDINGS & CLINICAL PRESENTATION

- Onset is usually insidious, with symptoms often not beginning until the third or fourth decade.
- Cervical spine is the most commonly affected area.
  1. Intrinsic hand atrophy, weakness, and anesthetic sensory loss may develop.
  2. The latter may lead to unnoticed burns or other injuries in the hand.
  3. Loss of pain and temperature sensation may occur, but tactile sense in the upper extremity is preserved.
  4. Sharp testing elicits no pain, but patient often perceives the sharpness of the object.
  5. A Charcot joint in the shoulder or elbow may develop.
- Reflexes are absent in the upper extremity.
- Spasticity and hyperreflexia are present in the lower extremity.
- Scoliosis is common.
- Nystagmus and Horner's syndrome may also occur.
- Trophic skin changes eventually develop in many cases.

ETIOLOGY

- Cause is unknown, but condition is thought to result from obstruction of the outlet of the fourth ventricle, often associated with a Chiari I malformation, which causes fluid to be diverted down the central cord.
- Often a history of birth injury exists.
- Syringes later in life may be the result of trauma or an intramedullary tumor.

DIAGNOSIS

DIFFERENTIAL DIAGNOSIS

- ALS
- MS
- Spinal cord tumor
- Tabes dorsalis
- Progressive spinal muscular atrophy

WORKUP

- Plain radiographs usually reveal widening of the bony canal in the region of involvement.
- Bony anomalies are often present at the base of the skull and at the C1-C2 spinal segments.
- Myelography, MRI (Fig. 1-264), and other imaging studies are recommended.

TREATMENT

Drainage and operative repair of any bony anomalies are undertaken, often with decompression laminectomy of C1 and C2.

DISPOSITION

- Condition is slowly progressive in most cases, but course may be quite variable, ranging from death in a few months to slow incapacitation over several years: progression may halt at any time.
- Surgical intervention often stops progression but frequently does not lead to improvement in neurologic findings.

REFERRAL

For neurosurgical consultation when diagnosis is suspected

EVIDENCE

Ergun et al. reviewed their surgical results in 18 patients with syringomyelia-Chiari complex who underwent foramen magnum decompression and syringosubarachnoid shunting. Sixteen patients improved and there was no change in two patients.

Lorenzo et al. prospectively evaluated 20 patients with syringomyelia-Chiari I complex who underwent surgery. After an average follow-up of 2.4 years, 8 patients were improved and 11 stabilized.

Rauzzino and Oakes reviewed several studies on patients with syringomyelia and Chiari II malformations treated surgically, all showing positive results with favorable outcomes.

Evidence-Based References

1. Lindsay KW, Bone I: *Neurology and Neurosurgery Illustrated,* ed 3, New York, 1997, Churchill Livingstone, pp 387-388.
2. Ergun R et al: Surgical management of syringomyelia-Chiari complex, *Eur Spine J* 9(6):553, 2000.
3. Di Lorenzo N et al: "Conservative" craniocervical decompression in the treatment of syringomyelia-Chiari I complex. A prospective study of 20 adult cases, *Spine* 20:2479, 1995.
4. Rauzzino M, Oakes WJ: Chiari II malformation and syringomyelia, *Neurosurg Clin N Am* 6:293, 1995.

SUGGESTED READINGS

Chu WC et al: A detailed morphologic and functional magnetic resonance imaging study of the craniocervical junction in adolescent idiopathic scoliosis, *Spine* 32(15): 1667, 2007.

Kimura R et al: Syringomyelia caused be cervical spondylosis, *Acta Neurochir* 146:175, 2004.

Klekamp J: The pathophysiology of syringomyelia: historical overview and current concepts, *Acta Neurochir* 144(7):649, 2002.

Mallucci C, Brodbelt A: The enigma of syringomyelia, *Br J Neurosurg* 21:423, 2007.

Riente L, Frigelli S, Delle SA: Neuropathic shoulder arthropathy associated with syringomyelia and Arnold-Chiari malformation (type I), *J Rheumatol* 29(3):638, 2002.

Wang R et al: Atypical syringomyelia without cavity in a patient with Chiari malformation and hydrocephalus, *Spine* 32(16):467, 2007.

AUTHOR: **LONNIE R. MERCIER, M.D.**

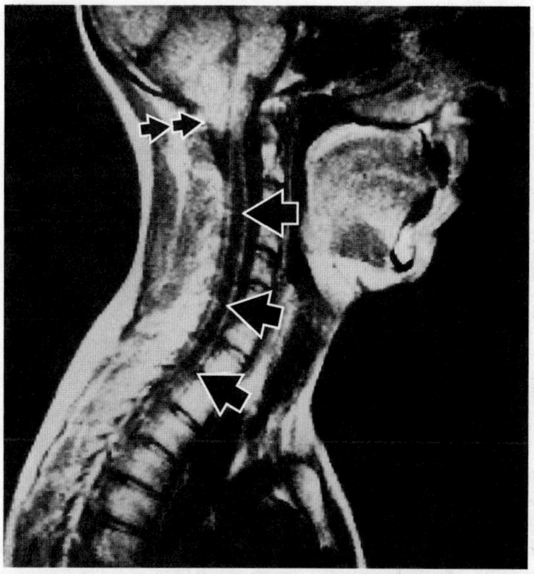

FIGURE 1-264 Midsagittal magnetic resonance image of Arnold-Chiari malformation *(small black arrows)* and syringomyelia *(three large black arrows)* in a 31-year-old man. Note the cerebellar tonsils extending below the posterior rim of the foramen magnum *(dark structure immediately above the black arrow).* The syrinx extends from the medulla well into the thoracic cord. (From Andreoli TE [ed]: *Cecil essentials of medicine,* ed 4, Philadelphia, 1997, WB Saunders.)

BASIC INFORMATION

DEFINITION

Systemic lupus erythematosus (SLE) is a chronic multisystemic disease characterized by production of autoantibodies and protean clinical manifestations.

SYNONYMS

SLE

ICD-9CM CODES
710.0 Systemic lupus erythematosus

EPIDEMIOLOGY & DEMOGRAPHICS

PREVALENCE: 20 cases/100,000 persons
PREDOMINANT SEX: Female:male ratio of 7:1
PREDOMINANT AGE: 20-45 yr (childbearing years)

PHYSICAL FINDINGS & CLINICAL PRESENTATION

- Skin: erythematous rash over the malar eminences (Fig. 1-265), generally with sparing of the nasolabial folds (butterfly rash); alopecia; raised erythematous patches with subsequent edematous plaques and adherent scales (discoid lupus); leg, nasal, or oropharyngeal ulcerations; livedo reticularis; pallor (from anemia); petechiae (from thrombocytopenia)
- Joints: tenderness, swelling, or effusion, generally involving peripheral joints
- Cardiac: pericardial rub (in patients with pericarditis), heart murmurs (if endocarditis or valvular thickening or dysfunction)
- Other: fever, conjunctivitis, dry eyes, dry mouth (sicca syndrome), oral ulcers, abdominal tenderness, decreased breath sounds (pleural effusions)

ETIOLOGY

Unknown. Autoantibodies are typically present many years before the diagnosis of SLE. A haplotype of STAT4 is associated with increased risk for both rheumatoid arthritis and SLE, suggesting a shared pathway for these illnesses.

DIAGNOSIS

DIFFERENTIAL DIAGNOSIS

- Other connective tissue disorders (e.g., RA, MCTD, progressive systemic sclerosis)
- Metastatic neoplasm
- Infection

WORKUP

The diagnosis of SLE can be made by demonstrating the presence of any four or more of the following criteria of the American Rheumatism Association:

1. Butterfly rash
2. Discoid rash
3. Photosensitivity (particularly leg ulcerations)
4. Oral ulcers
5. Arthritis
6. Serositis (pleuritis, pericarditis)
7. Renal disorder (persistent proteinuria >0.5 g/day or 3+ if quantitation not performed, cellular casts)
8. Neurologic disorder (seizures, psychosis [in absence of offending drugs or metabolic derangement])
9. Hematologic disorder:
   a. Hemolytic anemia with reticulocytosis
   b. Leukopenia (<4000/mm^3 total on two or more occasions)
   c. Lymphopenia (<1500/mm^3 on two or more occasions)
   d. Thrombocytopenia (<100,000/mm^3 in the absence of offending drugs)
10. Immunologic disorder:
    a. Positive SLE cell preparation
    b. Anti-DNA (presence of antibody to native DNA in abnormal titer)
    c. Anti-Sm (presence of antibody to Smith nuclear antigen)
    d. False-positive STS known to be positive for at least 6 mo and confirmed by negative TPI or FTA tests
11. ANA: an abnormal titer of ANA by immunofluorescence or equivalent assay at any time in the absence of drugs known to be associated with "drug-induced lupus" syndrome

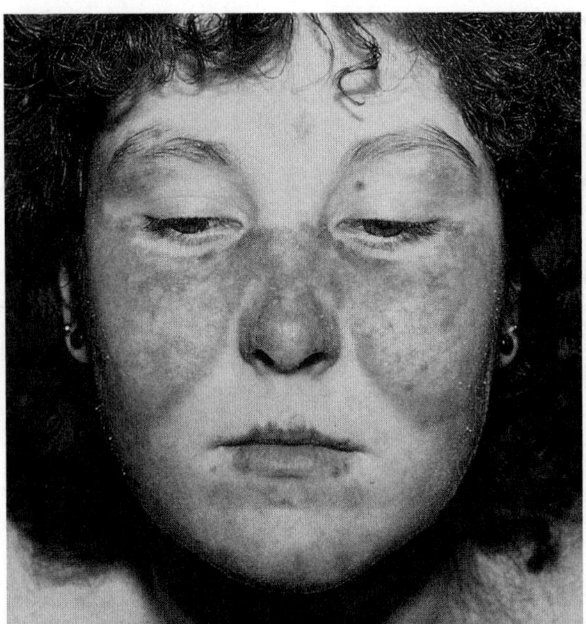

FIGURE 1-265 Acute cutaneous LE (systemic LE). The classic butterfly rash occurs in 10% to 50% of patients with acute LE. (From Habif TP: *Clinical dermatology: a color guide to diagnosis and therapy,* ed 3, St Louis, 1996, Mosby.)

LABORATORY TESTS

Suggested initial laboratory evaluation of suspected SLE:

- Immunologic evaluation: ANA, anti-DNA antibody, anti-Sm antibody
- Other laboratory tests: CBC with differential, platelet count (Coombs' test if anemia detected), urinalysis (24-hr urine collection for protein if proteinuria is detected), PTT and anticardiolipin antibodies in patients with thrombotic events, BUN, creatinine to evaluate renal function

IMAGING STUDIES

- Chest x-ray for evaluation of pulmonary involvement (e.g., pleural effusions, pulmonary infiltrates)
- Echocardiogram to screen for significant valvular heart disease (present in 18% of patients with SLE); echocardiography can identify a subset of lesions (valvular thickening and dysfunction) other than verrucous (Libman-Sacks) endocarditis that are prone to hemodynamic deterioration

TREATMENT

NONPHARMACOLOGIC THERAPY

Patients with photosensitivity should avoid sunlight and use high-factor sunscreen.

GENERAL Rx

- Joint pain and mild serositis are generally well controlled with NSAIDs; antimalarials are also effective (e.g., hydroxychloroquine [Plaquenil]).

- Cutaneous manifestations are treated with the following:
  1. Topical corticosteroids; intradermal corticosteroids are helpful for individual discoid lesions, especially in the scalp
  2. Antimalarials (e.g., hydroxychloroquine [Plaquenil] and quinacrine)
  3. Sunscreens that block ultraviolet (UV) A and UVB radiation
  4. Immunosuppressive drugs (methotrexate or azathioprine) are used as steroid-sparing drugs
- Renal disease (lupus nephritis)
  1. The use of high-pulsed doses of cyclophosphamide given at monthly intervals is more effective in preserving renal function than is treatment with glucocorticoids alone. The present standard of care with monthly high-dose IV cyclophosphamide has been challenged on several fronts. Alternative ways of administering cyclophosphamide in much lower doses for shorter periods have emerged. The combination of methylprednisolone and cyclophosphamide is superior to bolus therapy with methylprednisolone or cyclophosphamide alone in patients with lupus nephritis. For patients with proliferative lupus nephritis, short-term therapy with IV cyclophosphamide followed by maintenance therapy with mycophenolate mofetil or azathioprine appears to be more efficacious and safer than long-term therapy with IV cyclophosphamide. In the treatment of severe proliferative lupus nephritis, mycophenolate mofetil represents an excellent alternative to cyclophosphamide.
  2. The use of plasmapheresis in combination with immunosuppressive agents (to prevent the rebound phenomenon of antibody levels after plasmapheresis) is generally reserved for rapidly progressive renal failure or life-threatening systemic vasculitis.
- CNS involvement: treatment generally consists of corticosteroid therapy; however, its efficacy is uncertain, and it is generally reserved for organic brain syndrome. Anticonvulsants and antipsychotics are also indicated in selected cases; headaches are treated symptomatically.
- Hemolytic anemia: treatment of Coombs'-positive hemolytic anemia consists of high doses of corticosteroids; nonhemolytic anemia (secondary to chronic disease) does not require specific therapy.
- Thrombocytopenia
  1. Initial treatment consists of corticosteroids.
  2. In patients with poor response to steroids, encouraging results have been reported with the use of danazol, vincristine, and immunoglobulins. Combination chemotherapy with cyclophosphamide and prednisone combined with vincristine, vincristine and procarbazine, or etoposide may be useful in patients with severe refractory idiopathic thrombocytopenic purpura.
  3. Splenectomy generally does not cure the thrombocytopenia of SLE, but it may be necessary as an adjunct in managing selected cases.
- Infections are common because of compromised immune function secondary to SLE and the use of corticosteroid, cytotoxic, and antimetabolite drugs; pneumococcal bacteremia is associated with high mortality rate.
- Close monitoring for exacerbation of the disease and for potential side effects from medications (corticosteroids, cytotoxic agents) with frequent laboratory evaluation and office visits is necessary in all patients with SLE.
- Valvular heart disease is present in 18% of patients with SLE. The prevalence of infective endocarditis is approximately 1% (similar to the prevalence after prosthetic valve surgery, but greater than that following rheumatic valvulitis). Valvular heart disease in patients with SLE frequently changes over time (e.g., vegetations can appear unexpectedly for the first time, resolve, or change in size or appearance). These frequent changes are temporarily unrelated to other clinical features of SLE and can be associated with substantial morbidity and mortality.
- Newer treatment modalities include the use of rituximab (a chimeric human-murine monoclonal antibody directed against CD20 on B cells and their precursors) to induce substantial remissions in patients previously unresponsive to conventional agents. Intravenous immunoglobulins are also increasingly being used in the treatment of patients with resistant lupus.

DISPOSITION

- Most patients with lupus experience remissions and exacerbations.
- The leading cause of death in SLE is infection (one third of all deaths); active nephritis causes approximately 18% of deaths, and CNS disease causes 7% of deaths; the survival rate is 75% over the first 10 yr. Blacks and Hispanics generally have a worse prognosis.
- Symptomatic pericarditis occurs in one fourth of patients with SLE at some point during the course of the disease. Asymptomatic involvement is estimated to be more than 60% based on autopsy reports.
- Renal histologic studies and evaluation of renal function are useful in determining disease activity and predicting disease outcome (e.g., serum creatinine levels >3 mg/dl or evidence of diffuse proliferative involvement on renal biopsy are poor prognostic factors).
- Atherosclerosis occurs prematurely in patients with SLE and is independent of traditional risk factors for cardiovascular disease.
- Antiphospholipid syndrome with thrombotic manifestations is a major predictor of irreversible organ damage and death in patients with SLE.

REFERRAL

- Rheumatology consultation in all patients with SLE
- Hematology consultation in patients with significant hematologic abnormalities (e.g., severe hemolytic anemia or thrombocytopenia)
- Nephrology consultation in patients with significant renal involvement

EVIDENCE

EBM

We are unable to cite evidence that meets our criteria for many treatments for SLE.

Another systematic review found that, in patients with proliferative lupus nephritis, cyclophosphamide plus corticosteroids reduced the risk of doubling serum creatinine compared with corticosteroids alone, although there was no impact on mortality, and the risk of ovarian failure was increased in the cyclophosphamide group. The reviewers concluded that cyclophosphamide combined with corticosteroids is the best option for preserving renal function, and that the smallest effective dose and the shortest duration of treatment should be used.[1] (A)

This same systematic review found that azathioprine plus corticosteroids reduced the risk of death from any cause compared with corticosteroids alone, but it had no impact on renal outcomes.[1] (A)

Evidence-Based Reference

1. Flanc RS et al: Treatment for lupus nephritis. Reviewed in: Cochrane Library 3:2004, Chichester, UK, John Wiley. (A)

SUGGESTED READINGS

D'Cruz DP et al: Systemic lupus erythematosus, *Lancet* 369:587, 2007.
Fine DM: Pharmacologic therapy of lupus nephritis, *JAMA* 293:3053, 2005.
Remmers EF et al: STAT4 and the risk of rheumatoid arthritis and systemic lupus erythematosus, *N Engl J Med* 357:977, 2007.

AUTHOR: **FRED F. FERRI, M.D.**

BASIC INFORMATION

DEFINITION

Tabes dorsalis is a form of tertiary neurosyphilis affecting the dorsal columns of the spinal cord and peripheral nerves, characterized by paroxysmal pain, particularly in the abdomen and legs; sensory ataxia; normal strength; autonomic dysfunction, and Argyll-Robertson pupils.

SYNONYMS

Posterior spinal sclerosis
Tabetic neurosyphilis
Syphilitic myeloneuropathy

ICD-9CM CODES
094.0 Tabes dorsalis, ataxia, locomotor

EPIDEMIOLOGY & DEMOGRAPHICS

INCIDENCE (IN U.S.): Rare, but increasing with HIV/AIDS

PEAK INCIDENCE: 15 to 20 yr after initial infection

PREVALENCE (IN U.S.): Rare; more common with HIV/AIDS epidemic. 10% of untreated cases of syphilis develop neurosyphilis, of which 2% to 5% may develop tabes dorsalis.

PREDOMINANT SEX: Male

PHYSICAL FINDINGS & CLINICAL PRESENTATION

- Argyll-Robertson pupil in 50% (pupil reacts poorly to light but well to accommodation)
- Loss of position and vibration at ankles (wide-based gait; inability to walk in the dark: sensory ataxia)
- Loss of deep pain sensation, resulting in deep foot ulcers
- Degenerative joint disease, especially in knees caused by severe neuropathy (Charcot joints)
- Normal strength with areflexia in the legs
- Lightning pains in the legs
- Severe intermittent visceral pains, such as gastrointestinal, laryngeal (visceral crises)
- Autonomic dysfunction (urinary and fecal incontinence)

ETIOLOGY

Infectious *(Treponema pallidum)*

DIAGNOSIS

DIFFERENTIAL DIAGNOSIS

- Vitamin B_{12} deficiency (subacute combined degeneration of the spinal cord)
- Vitamin E deficiency
- Chronic nitrous oxide abuse
- Spinal cord neoplasm (involving conus medullaris)
- Lyme disease

WORKUP

Thorough neurologic history and examination

LABORATORY TESTS

- Lumbar puncture for elevated VDRL and FTA-ABS titers. False-positive CSF VDRL titers may occur with traumatic tap. CSF mononuclear pleocytosis (>5 white cells/microL) with increased protein support the diagnosis.
- Serum venereal disease research laboratory test (VDRL). This may be normal in 25% to 30% of patients. Serum microhemagglutination-Treponema Pallidum (MHA-TP) or Fluorescent Treponemal Antigen-Antibody test (FTA-ABS) is necessary if clinical suspicion high.
- False-positive serum VDRL may occur in Lyme disease, nonvenereal treponematoses, genital herpes simplex, pregnancy, SLE, alcoholic cirrhosis, scleroderma, and mixed connective tissue disease.

IMAGING STUDIES

Not necessary if diagnosis confirmed

TREATMENT

ACUTE GENERAL Rx

- Procaine penicillin 2 to 4 million U IM qd, along with probenecid 500 mg PO qid, for 14 days, or aqueous penicillin G 3 to 4 million U IV q4h for 10 to 14 days.
- If penicillin allergic, doxycycline 200 mg PO bid for 4 wk.
- Many of the symptoms—degenerative neuropathic joint disease, lightning pains—persist after treatment.

CHRONIC Rx

- Physical therapy
- Analgesics, carbamazepine, gabapentin, or steroids may help "lightning" pain
- Supportive care (wheelchair, toileting issues, etc.)

DISPOSITION

Close follow-up required. Repeat lumbar puncture every 6 mo until CSF pleocytosis normalizes. If pleocytosis does not normalize in 6 mo or CSF is still abnormal in 2 yr, repeat treatment.

Further indication for retreatment: if there is a fourfold increase in titers or a failure of titers >1:32 to decrease at least fourfold by 12 to 24 mo.

REFERRAL

Joint replacement in moderate cases

PEARLS & CONSIDERATIONS

COMMENTS

Diagnosis should be considered in all patients with a progressive neuropsychiatric disorder with signs of spinal cord dysfunction and peripheral neuropathy.

EVIDENCE

There is no evidence from randomized controlled trials to guide treatment of tabes dorsalis.

SUGGESTED READINGS

Centers for Disease Control and Prevention: 2002 sexually transmitted diseases treatment guidelines, *MMWR Morb Mortal Wkly Rep* 51(RR-6), 2002.

Conde-Sendin MA et al: Current clinical spectrum of neurosyphilis in immunocompetent patients, *Eur Neurol* 52:29, 2004.

Timmermans M, Carr J: Neurosyphilis in the modern era, *J Neurol Neurosurg Psychiatry* 75:1727, 2004.

AUTHOR: **EROBOGHENE E. UBOGU, M.D.**

BASIC INFORMATION

DEFINITION

Takayasu's arteritis refers to a chronic systemic granulomatous vasculitis primarily affecting large arteries (aorta and its branches).

SYNONYMS

Pulseless disease
Aortitis syndrome
Aortic arch arteritis

ICD-9CM CODES
446.7 Takayasu disease or syndrome

EPIDEMIOLOGY & DEMOGRAPHICS

- Most cases have been reported from Japan, China, India, and Mexico
- Exact incidence and prevalence is not known
- Incidence in the U.S. 2.6/1 million
- Females > males 9:1
- Seen predominantly in patients <30 yr old

PHYSICAL FINDINGS & CLINICAL PRESENTATION

Takayasu's arteritis most frequently involves the aortic arch and its branches and can manifest as:

- Arm claudication, weakness, and numbness
- Amaurosis fugax, diplopia, headache, and postural dizziness
- Systemic symptoms
  1. Low-grade fever
  2. Malaise
  3. Weight loss
  4. Fatigue
  5. Arthralgia and myalgia
- Vascular bruits of the carotid artery, subclavian artery, and aorta
- Discrepancy of blood pressures between the upper extremities
- Absent pulses
- Hypertension
- Retinopathy
- Aortic insufficiency murmur

ETIOLOGY

- The cause of Takayasu's arteritis is unknown. A delayed hypersensitivity to mycobacteria and spirochetes is a theory but remains to be substantiated.
- Infiltration of inflammatory cells into the vasa vasorum and media of large elastic arteries leads to thickening and narrowing or obliteration as well as aneurysmal dilation.

DIAGNOSIS

Criteria have been established for the diagnosis of Takayasu's arteritis by the American College of Rheumatology in 1990 and include:

- Age of disease <40 yr
- Claudication of extremities
- Decreased brachial artery pulse
- Systolic BP difference >10 mm Hg between left and right arms
- Bruit over subclavian arteries or aorta
- Abnormal arteriogram
- Takayasu's arteritis is diagnosed if at least three of the six criteria are present, giving a sensitivity of 90% and a specificity of 98%

DIFFERENTIAL DIAGNOSIS

Other causes of inflammatory aortitis must be excluded:

- Giant cell arteritis
- Syphilis
- Tuberculosis
- SLE
- Rheumatoid arthritis
- Buerger's disease
- Behçet's disease
- Cogan's syndrome
- Kawasaki disease
- Spondyloarthropathies

WORKUP

Any young patient with findings of absence pulses and loud bruits merits a workup for Takayasu's arteritis. The workup generally includes blood testing to look for signs of inflammation and imaging studies with the angiogram being the diagnostic gold standard.

LABORATORY TESTS

- CBC may reveal an elevated WBC count
- ESR is elevated in active disease

IMAGING STUDIES

- Ultrasound: Carotid, thoracic, and abdominal ultrasound are useful adjunctive imaging studies in diagnosing occlusive disease resulting from Takayasu's arteritis (Fig. 1-266).
- Doppler and noninvasive upper and lower extremity studies are helpful in assessing blood flow and absent pulses.
- CT scan is used to assess the thickness of the aorta.
- Angiogram can show narrowing of the aorta and/or branches of the aorta, aneurysm formation, and poststenotic

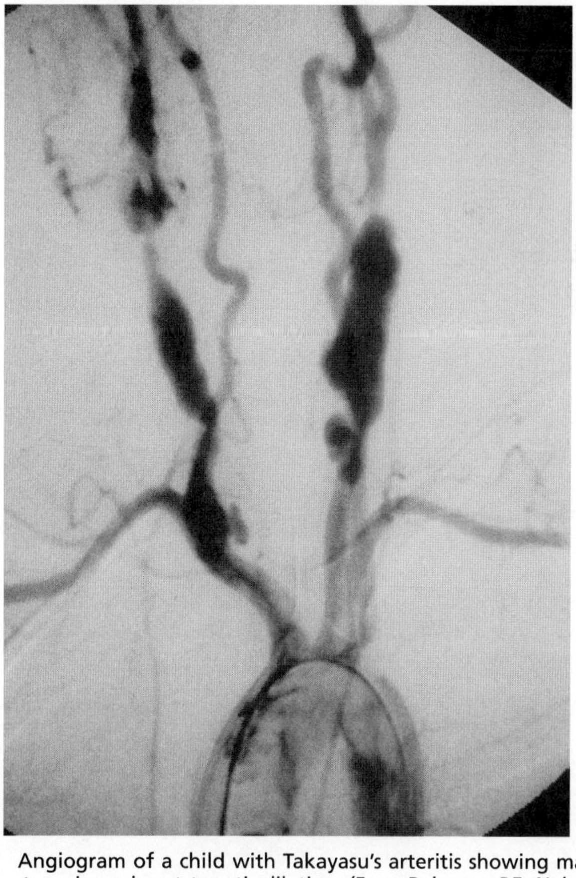

FIGURE 1-266 Angiogram of a child with Takayasu's arteritis showing massive bilateral carotid dilation, stenosis, and poststenotic dilation. (From Behrman RE: *Nelson textbook of pediatrics,* ed 16, Philadelphia, 2000, WB Saunders.)

dilation. Angiographic findings are classified as four types:

1. Type I: Lesions involve only the aortic arch and its branches.
2. Type II: Lesions only involving the abdominal aorta and its branches.
3. Type III: Lesions involving the aorta above and below the diaphragm.
4. Type IV: Lesions involving the pulmonary artery.

TREATMENT

ACUTE GENERAL Rx

- Corticosteroids are the treatment of choice. Prednisone 40 to 60 mg PO qd or 1 mg/kg/day is used for 3 mo.
- Patients are monitored for symptoms and by following the ESR. If symptoms have resolved and the ESR is normal, attempts to taper prednisone are made.

CHRONIC Rx

- Patients who cannot be tapered off the corticosteroids or who have relapse of the disease are given methotrexate 0.15 to 0.35 mg/kg or approximately 15 mg/wk.
- Cyclophosphamide 1 to 2 mg/kg/day can be given with glucocorticoids as adjunctive therapy in relapse or treatment-resistant patients.

DISPOSITION

- Treatment improves symptoms within days with relief of ischemic claudication, return of pulses on examination, and reversal of lumen narrowing on angiograms. However, some patients may continue to have progression of arterial lesions despite therapy.
- With the addition of a second agent in patients with treatment resistance or relapse, 50% remission has been seen.
- Mortality results are mixed, showing high rates in reports from Asia and lower rates in studies done in the U.S. (2%).
- Death can occur suddenly from ruptured aneurysm, myocardial infarction, and stroke.

REFERRAL

Whenever the diagnosis of vasculitis is suspected, a rheumatology consult is appropriate. Vascular surgery and cardiology consultations are recommended for any evidence of carotid, peripheral, and coronary artery disease or if a large abdominal aneurysm is found.

PEARLS & CONSIDERATIONS

With long term corticosteroid use, consider measures to protect against bone loss. Bisphosphonates have been studied prospectively with corticosteroid use in this fashion; remember to ensure adequate dietary calcium and vitamin D intake as well.

COMMENTS

The long-term prognosis of treated patients with Takayasu's disease is good, with >90% of patients surviving more than 15 yr.

SUGGESTED READINGS

Arend WP et al: American College of Rheumatology 1990 criteria for the classification of Takayasu's arteritis, *Arthr Rheum* 33:1129, 1990.

Hahn-Kover K, Folzenlogen D: Diagnosis of Takayasu arteritis, *J Clin Rheumatol* 11(3):170, 2005.

Mwipatayi B et al: Takayasu arteritis: clinical features and management: report of 272 cases, *ANZ J Surg* 75(3):110, 2005.

Seko Y: Giant cell and Takayasu arteritis, *Curr Opin Rheumatol* 19(1)39, 2007.

Weyend CM, Goronzy JJ: Mechanisms of disease: medium and large vessel vasculitis, *N Engl J Med* 349:160, 2003.

AUTHOR: **MEL ANDERSON, M.D.**

BASIC INFORMATION

DEFINITION

Four species of adult tapeworm may infect humans as the definitive host: *Taenia saginata* (beef tapeworm), *Taenia solium* (pork tapeworm), *Diphyllobothrium latum* (fish tapeworm), and *Hymenolepis nana*. In addition, *T. solium* may infect humans in its larval form (cysticercosis), and several animal tapeworms (see "Echinococcosis" in Section I) may cause infection in an analogous manner.

SYNONYMS

Cysticercosis (larval infection by *T. solium*)

ICD-9CM CODES
123.9 Tapeworm infestation

EPIDEMIOLOGY & DEMOGRAPHICS

INCIDENCE (IN U.S.):
- Diagnosed primarily in immigrants
- Varies widely by country of origin and dietary practices

PREVALENCE (IN U.S.):
- *T. saginata:* <0.1%
- *D. latum:* <0.05%
- *T. solium:* <0.1%
- *H. nana:* sporadic, often in setting of outbreak

PREDOMINANT SEX: Equal sex distribution

PREDOMINANT AGE:
- *T. saginata, T. solium, D. latum:* 20 to 39 yr of age
- *H. nana* in setting of institution outbreaks: children

PHYSICAL FINDINGS & CLINICAL PRESENTATION

- Adult worms
  1. Attach to bowel mucosa
  2. Feed and grow
  3. Cause minimal or no symptoms or sequelae
- Cysticercosis
  1. Mass lesions of brain (neurocysticercosis), soft tissue, viscera
  2. Neurocysticercosis may cause seizures, hydrocephalus
- Prolonged infection with *D. latum*
  1. Vitamin B_{12} deficiency
  2. Megaloblastic anemia

ETIOLOGY

TAPEWORM:
- Adult worm resides in small or large bowel; proglottids and eggs passed in stool.
- Eggs are ingested by the animal intermediate host.
- Eggs hatch into larvae.
- Larvae disseminate largely in skeletal muscle, brain, viscera.
- Humans eat infected beef *(T. saginata),* infected pork *(T. solium),* or infected fish *(D. latum).*
- Larvae mature into adults within the GI lumen.
- *H. nana* infection is acquired by ingesting eggs in human or rodent feces.

CYSTICERCOSIS:
- Humans ingest eggs of *T. solium* in food contaminated with human feces that contain the eggs.
- Eggs hatch into larvae in gut.
- Larvae disseminate widely through tissues (particularly soft tissue and CNS) forming cystic lesions containing either viable or nonviable larvae.

DIAGNOSIS

DIFFERENTIAL DIAGNOSIS

Section II describes the differential diagnosis of intestinal helminths.

WORKUP

- Stool examination for eggs or proglottids (tapeworm)
- Cerebral CT scan (neurocysticercosis)
- Serum antibody (neurocysticercosis)

IMAGING STUDIES

- Tapeworm: incidental finding on upper GI series
- Neurocysticercosis:
  1. Cerebral cysts are readily demonstrated by CT scan or MRI.
  2. Calcified lesions are an incidental finding.

TREATMENT

ACUTE GENERAL Rx

- All patients with intestinal tapeworm infections should be treated with a single oral dose of praziquantel.
  1. *T. solium:* 5 mg/kg
  2. *T. saginata:* 20 mg/kg
  3. *D. latum:* 10 mg/kg
  4. *H. nana:* 25 mg/kg
- An alternative therapy to praziquantel for tapeworm infections is niclosamide, 2 gm by mouth once or 500 mg by mouth daily for 3 days.
- Therapy that may be considered for symptomatic cysticercosis:
  1. May regress spontaneously
  2. Surgery
  3. Albendazole 15 mg/kg PO qd in three doses for 28 days
  4. Praziquantel 50 mg/kg PO qd in three doses for 15 days
- Therapy contraindicated with:
  1. Ocular infections
  2. Cerebral infections in which local inflammation caused by destruction of the parasite may cause significant damage

CHRONIC Rx

- Retreatment if required
- Avoidance of undercooked pork, meat, or fish
- Cysticercosis: proper hand washing, proper disposal of human waste

DISPOSITION

- Neurologic follow-up for patients with neurocysticercosis
- Ophthalmologic follow-up for patients with ocular involvement

REFERRAL

Patients treated for neurocysticercosis should be evaluated by a physician experienced in managing this infection, if possible.

PEARLS & CONSIDERATIONS

COMMENTS

T. solium is the most dangerous of the tapeworms because of the potential for cysticercosis by means of autoinfection.

SUGGESTED READINGS

Buyuk Y et al : Non-ruptured hydatid cyst can lead to death by spread of cyst content into bloodstream: an autopsy case, *Eur J Gastroenterol Hepatol* 17(6):671, 2005.

DeGiorgio C, Pietsch-Escueta S, Tsang V: Sero-prevalence of *Taenia solium* cysticercosis and *Taenia solium* taeniasis in California, USA, *Acta Neurol Scand* 111(2):84, 2005.

Flisser A et al: Short report: evaluation of a self-detection tool for tapeworm carriers for use in public health, *Am J Trop Med Hyg* 72(5):510, 2005.

Infanger M et al: Surgical and medical management of rare echinococcosis of the extremities. Pre- and postoperative long-term chemotherapy, *Scand J Infect Dis* 37(11): 954, 2005.

Liu YM et al: Acute pancreatitis cause by tapeworm in the biliary tract, *AM J Trop Med Hyg* 73(2):377, 2005.

AUTHORS: **GLENN G. FORT, M.D., M.P.H., DENNIS J. MIKOLICH, M.D.,** and **JOSEPH R. MASCI, M.D.**

BASIC INFORMATION

DEFINITION

Tardive dyskinesia (TD) is a syndrome of involuntary movements associated with the long-term use of antipsychotic medication, particularly dopamine-blocking neuroleptics. Patients usually exhibit rapid, repetitive, stereotypic movements mostly involving the oral, lingual, trunk, and limb areas.

SYNONYMS

Tardive syndrome
Tardive dystonia

ICD-9CM CODES
333.82 Tardive dyskinesia

EPIDEMIOLOGY & DEMOGRAPHICS

- The disorder is caused by dopamine-blocking neuroleptics (e.g., haloperidol).
- Incidence is declining with the use of newer generation antipsychotics.
- At least 20% of patients treated with standard neuroleptic drugs are affected with TD, and approximately 5% are expected to develop TD with each year of neuroleptic treatment.
- The risk is greatest in the early years of exposure and in elderly patients.

PHYSICAL FINDINGS & CLINICAL PRESENTATION

- Typically appears with the reduction or withdrawal of the antipsychotics.
- TD is characterized by:
  - Primarily involves the tongue, lips, and jaw. A combination of tongue twisting and protrusion, lip smacking and puckering, and chewing movements in a repetitive and stereotypic fashion is often observed.
  - Slow, writhing movements of the arms and legs.
  - The involuntary mouth movements in TD may be voluntarily suppressed by patients. They are also suppressed by voluntary actions such as putting food in the mouth or talking.

ETIOLOGY

TD is generally thought to result from chronic exposure to dopamine receptor blocking agents—drugs primarily used to treat psychosis. TD has not been reported with dopamine depleters (e.g., reserpine) and is seldom reported with atypical antipsychotic drugs. Some drugs for nausea (e.g., metoclopramide and prochlorperazine) and depression (e.g., amoxapine, fluoxetine, and paroxetine) can also cause TD. Recent evidence suggests that TD may result from antipsychotic-induced damage to striatal cholinergic neurons.

DIAGNOSIS

DIFFERENTIAL DIAGNOSIS

- Huntington's chorea
- Excessive treatment with L-dopa
- Tourette's syndrome
- Wilson's disease
- Sydenham's chorea

WORKUP

Diagnosis of exclusion with emphasis on complete neuropsychiatric history (including medication history) and examination.

IMAGING STUDIES

Brain imaging normal in TD.

TREATMENT

ACUTE GENERAL Rx

- Treatment predicated on prevention-limiting the indications for neuroleptics and using the lowest effective dose and withdrawing them when feasible.
- Use atypical antipsychotics if possible. Clozapine, risperidone, and olanzapine have lower reported rates of TD in long-term studies.

CHRONIC Rx

- Clozapine has best evidence for improvement of symptoms in TD. Risperidone, olanzapine, and amisulpride also have been shown to benefit.
- Piracetam, an antioxidant and neuronal enhancer, was effective in reducing symptoms of TD in randomized clinical trial with short-term follow-up.
- Benzodiazepines, vitamin E, vitamin B_6, donepezil, clonazepam, and melatonin may be helpful, but controlled trial evidence is weak.

DISPOSITION

Potentially irreversible, long-term adverse effect of treatment with first-generation antipsychotic medications.

REFERRAL

Movement disorder specialist if symptoms are severe.

PEARLS & CONSIDERATIONS

- Neuroleptics should be resumed to treat TD in the absence of active psychosis only as a last resort for persistent, disabling, and treatment-resistant TD.
- Worsening in overall psychopathology in schizophrenia is longitudinally associated with the emergence of TD.

SUGGESTED READINGS

Bhoopathi PS et al: Benzodiazepines for neuroleptic-induced tardive dyskinesia, *Cochrane Database Syst Rev* 3:CD000205, 2006.

Libov I et al: Efficacy of piracetam in the treatment of tardive dyskinesia in schizophrenic patients: a randomized, double-blind, placebo-controlled crossover study, *J Clin Psychiatry* 68(7):1031-1037, 2007.

Margolese HC et al: Tardive dyskinesia in the era of typical and atypical antipsychotics. Part 2: Incidence and management strategies in patients with schizophrenia, *Can J Psychiatry* 50(11):703, 2005.

Rosenheck RA: Evaluating the cost-effectiveness of reduced tardive dyskinesia with second-generation antipsychotics, *Br J Psychiatry* 191:238-245, 2007.

Skidmore F, Reich SG: Tardive dystonia, *Curr Treat Options Neurol* 7(3):231, 2005.

AUTHORS: **MITCHELL D. FELDMAN, M.D., M.PHIL.,** and **SHALINI PATEL, M.D.**

BASIC INFORMATION

DEFINITION

Tarsal tunnel syndrome is a rare entrapment neuropathy that develops as a result of compression of the posterior tibial nerve in the tunnel formed by the flexor retinaculum behind the medial malleolus of the ankle (Fig. 1-267). This retinaculum arises from the medial malleolus and inserts into the medial aspect of the calcaneus.

ICD-9CM CODES
355.5 Tarsal tunnel syndrome

SYNONYMS

None

EPIDEMIOLOGY & DEMOGRAPHICS

PREVALENCE: Unknown
PREDOMINANT SEX: Female = male

PHYSICAL FINDINGS & CLINICAL PRESENTATION

- Symptoms are often vague in contrast to other compression neuropathies such as carpal tunnel syndrome.
- Neuritic symptoms along the course of the posterior tibial nerve in the sole and heel.
- The Valleix phenomenon (proximal radiation of the pain) may occur.
- Swelling over tarsal tunnel.
- Possible positive Tinel's sign.
- Possible reproduction of symptoms with sustained eversion of hindfoot or digital compression of tunnel.
- Sensory loss and motor changes unusual.

ETIOLOGY

Space-occupying lesions (ganglia, varicosities, lipomas, synovial hypertrophy) or local tendonitis
Possibly traction on nerve

DIAGNOSIS

DIFFERENTIAL DIAGNOSIS

- Plantar fasciitis
- Peripheral neuropathy
- Proximal radiculopathy
- Local tendinitis
- Peripheral vascular disease
- Morton's neuroma

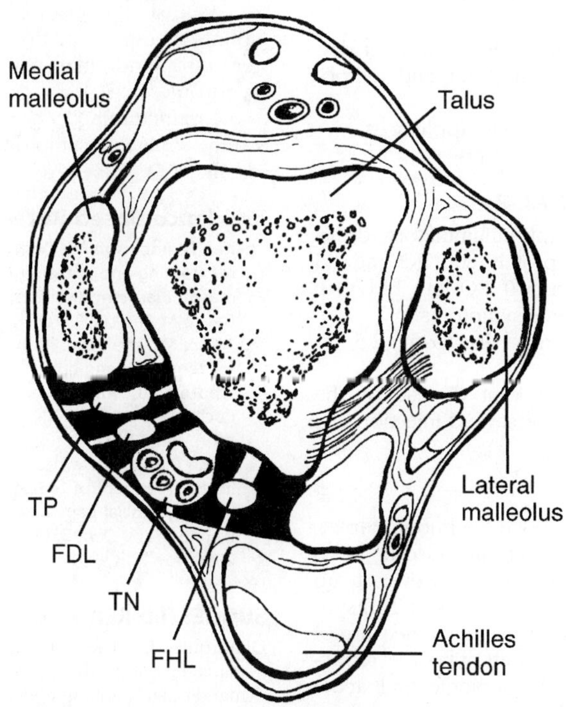

FIGURE 1-267 Anatomy of tarsal tunnel syndrome. Transverse view of ankle. *FDL,* Flexor digitorum longus; *FHL,* flexor hallucis longus tendon; *TN,* tibial nerve (single contour), posterior tibial artery, veins; *TP,* tibialis posterior tendon. Tendons and neurovascular elements are included into individual fibrous septa that connect periosteum with the deep fascia. (From Canoso J: *Rheumatology in primary care,* Philadelphia, 1997, WB Saunders.)

ELECTRICAL STUDIES

Electrodiagnostic testing is often inconclusive. Delayed sensory conduction or increased motor latency may be seen.

TREATMENT

- NSAIDs
- Immobilization for 4 to 6 wk with ankle orthosis or fracture cast boot
- Medial heel wedge or orthotic to minimize heel eversion
- Local steroid injection into tunnel (avoiding the posterior tibial nerve) if symptoms persist

DISPOSITION

Many patients are successfully treated conservatively.

REFERRAL

For surgical decompression if needed. Results of surgery are mixed unless an obvious compressive lesion is found.

PEARLS & CONSIDERATIONS

The disorder is controversial and there are many unanswered questions regarding its diagnosis and incidence.
The condition may be difficult to differentiate from plantar fasciitis and the two conditions may occur together.

SUGGESTED READINGS

Aldridge T: Diagnosing heel pain in adults, *Am Fam Physician* 70:332, 2004.
Bracilovic A et al: Effect of foot and ankle position on tarsal tunnel compartment volume, *Foot Ankle Int* 27:431, 2006.
Campbell SE: MRI of sports injuries of the ankle, *Clin Sports Med* 25(4):727, 2007.
Gorter K et al: Variation in diagnosis and management of common foot problems by GPs, *Fam Pract* 18(6):569, 2001.
Labib SA et al: Heel pain triad (HPT): the combination of plantar fasciitis, posterior tibial tendon dysfunction and tarsal tunnel syndrome, *Foot Ankle Int* 23(3):212, 2002.
Mizel MS et al: Evaluation and treatment of chronic ankle pain, *Instr Course Lect* 53:311, 2004.
Mondelli M, Morana P, Padua L: An electrophysiological severity scale in tarsal tunnel syndrome, *Acta Neurol Scand* 109:284, 2004.
Pecina M: Diagnostic tests for tarsal tunnel syndrome, *J Bone Joint Surg Am* 84-A(9):1714, 2002.
Pessis E et al: Nerve and vascular entrapment in athletes, *J Radiol* 88:156, 2007.

AUTHOR: **LONNIE R. MERCIER, M.D.**

BASIC INFORMATION

DEFINITION

Temporomandibular joint (TMJ) syndrome refers to a group of disorders leading to symptoms of the temporomandibular joint.

SYNONYMS

Temporomandibular dysfunction
Painful temporomandibular joint

ICD-9CM CODES
524.60 Temporomandibular joint pain-dysfunction syndrome

EPIDEMIOLOGY & DEMOGRAPHICS

- 15% of the population have TMJ disorders
- Females > males 4:1
- Occurs between the second and fourth decades of life
- Usually unilateral, affecting either side with equal frequency

PHYSICAL FINDINGS & CLINICAL PRESENTATION

- Otalgia
- Odontalgia
- Headaches (frontal, temporal, retro-orbital)
- Tinnitus
- Dizziness
- Clicking or popping sounds with movement of the TMJ
- Joint locking
- Tender to palpation
- Limited range of motion of the TMJ

ETIOLOGY

- Multifactorial, encompassing local anatomic anomalies to familiar disease processes that can involve the TMJ.
- Myofascial pain-dysfunction syndrome: the most common cause of TMJ syndrome and results from teeth grinding and clenching the jaw (bruxism)
- Internal TMJ derangement: abnormal connection of the articular disk to the mandibular condyle
- Degenerative joint disease
- Rheumatoid arthritis
- Gouty arthritis
- Pseudogout
- Ankylosing spondylitis
- Trauma
- Prior surgery (orthodontic, intraarticular steroid injection)
- Tumors

DIAGNOSIS

DIFFERENTIAL DIAGNOSIS

Can be made based on history and physical examination in most cases. Includes the list as mentioned previously under Etiology. Myofascial pain-dysfunction syndrome, internal TMJ derangement, and degenerative joint disease represent >90% of all causes of TMJ syndrome.

WORKUP

Radiographic imaging evaluation is helpful to exclude anatomic or systemic causes of disease.

LABORATORY TESTS

Laboratory examination is not very helpful.

IMAGING STUDIES

- Plain x-rays: The most common x-rays are the panoramic, transorbital, and transpharyngeal views in both opened and closed positions.
- Arthrography is helpful in looking for meniscus involvement.
- CT scan is very accurate in diagnosing meniscal and osseous derangements of the TMJ.
- MRI can better visualize soft tissue inflammation, if present.

TREATMENT

NONPHARMACOLOGIC THERAPY

- Soft diet to rest the muscles of mastication
- Heat 15 to 20 min 4 to 6 times per day
- Massage of the masseter and temporalis muscles
- Formed splints or bite appliances
- Range-of-motion exercises

ACUTE GENERAL Rx

- Nonsteroidal anti-inflammatory drugs (NSAIDs): ibuprofen 800 PO mg tid prn, naproxen 500 PO mg bid prn, titrated to relieve symptoms
- Muscle relaxants: diazepam 2.5 to 5 mg PO tid prn
- In degenerative joint disease of the TMJ, intraarticular steroid injection can be tried

CHRONIC Rx

- Most of the above mentioned treatment is used for myofascial pain-dysfunction syndrome; however, it can be applied to other causes of TMJ syndrome. Surgery is usually a measure of last resort in patients who are refractory to nonpharmacologic and acute general treatment.
- Surgical procedures include:
  1. Meniscoplasty
  2. Meniscectomy
  3. Subcondylar osteotomy
  4. TMJ reconstruction

DISPOSITION

The course depends on the underlying etiology; however, a lengthy course with exacerbations of symptoms can be expected.

REFERRAL

All patients with TMJ syndrome refractory to conservative nonpharmacologic and acute therapy should be referred to a periodontist, oral maxillofacial surgeon, or ENT surgeon.

PEARLS & CONSIDERATIONS

Patients with rheumatoid arthritis involving the TMJ usually will have bilateral involvement.

COMMENTS

Frequently, emotional stress initiates the myofascial pain-dysfunction, which accounts for 85% of all cases of TMJ syndrome.

EVIDENCE

A systematic review of occlusal adjustment in the management of temporomandibular disorders (TMD) found no difference between occlusal adjustment and control groups (reassurance or no treatment) in terms of symptom-based outcomes.[1] Ⓐ

There is insufficient evidence for or against the use of stabilization splint therapy for the treatment of temporomandibular pain dysfunction syndrome.[2]

Acupuncture had a positive influence on the signs and symptoms of TMJ syndrome.[3] Ⓐ

Evidence-Based References

1. Koh H, Robinson PG: Occlusal adjustment for treating and preventing temporomandibular joint disorders, *Cochrane Database Syst Rev* 1:2003 (Cochrane Review). Ⓐ
2. Al-Ani MZ et al: Stabilisation splint therapy for temporomandibular pain dysfunction syndrome (Cochrane Review). Reviewed in: Cochrane Library 2:2004, Chichester, UK, John Wiley. Ⓐ
3. Smith P et al: The efficacy of acupuncture in the treatment of temporomandibular joint myofascial pain: a randomised controlled trial, *J Dent* 35(3):259, 2007. Epub 2006 Nov 13. Ⓐ

SUGGESTED READINGS

Dimitroulis G: The role of surgery in the management of disorders of the temporomandibular joint: a critical review of the literature. Part 1 and Part 2, *Int J Oral Maxillofac Surg* 34(2):107, 2005; 34(3):231, 2005.

Herb K et al: Temporomandibular joint pain and dysfunction, *Curr Pain Headache Rep* 10(6):408, 2006.

Sommer OJ et al: Cross-sectional and functional imaging of the temporomandibular joint: radiology, pathology, and basic biomechanics of the jaw, *Radiographics* 23(6):e14, 2003.

AUTHOR: **WEN-CHIH WU, M.D.**

BASIC INFORMATION

DEFINITION

Testicular neoplasms are primary cancers originating in a testis.

SYNONYMS

Testis tumor
Testicular cancer

ICD-9CM CODES
186.9 Testicular neoplasm
M906/3 (seminoma)
M9101/3 (embryonal carcinoma or teratoma)
M9100/3 (choriocarcinoma)

EPIDEMIOLOGY & DEMOGRAPHICS

INCIDENCE: 2 to 3 cases/100,000 men/yr
PREVALENCE: 1% to 2% of all cancers in males
PREDOMINANT AGE: Can occur in any age but most common in young adults; average age for embryonal cell carcinoma: 30 yr; average age for seminoma: 36 yr

PHYSICAL FINDINGS & CLINICAL PRESENTATION

- Any mass within the testicle should be considered cancer until proven otherwise. It may be found by the patient who brings it to the attention of a physician or it may be found by a physician on a routine examination.
- Symptoms other than scrotal or testicular swelling are typically absent unless the cancer has metastasized. Occasionally a patient may complain of scrotal fullness or heaviness.
- Testicular palpation should be performed with two hands. Transillumination may distinguish a solid mass (e.g., cancer) and a fluid-filled lesion (e.g., hydrocele or spermatocele). The mass is nontender, indeed less sensitive than a normal testicle.

ETIOLOGY & PATHOLOGY

- Cryptorchidism (undescended testes) even if corrected by orchiopexy; however, treatment of undescended testis before puberty decreases the risk of testicular cancer.
- Pathology.

Cell type	Frequency %
Seminoma	42
Embryonal cell carcinoma	26
Teratocarcinoma	26
Teratoma	5
Choriocarcinoma	1

Other rare types:
  Yolk sac carcinoma
  Mixed germ cell tumors
  Carcinoid tumor
  Sertoli cell tumors
  Leydig cell tumors
  Lymphoma
  Metastatic cancer to the testes

- TNM staging system for testicular cancer

T_0 No apparent primary
T_1 Testis only (excludes rete testis)
T_2 Beyond the tunica albuginea
T_3 Rete testis or epididymal involvement
T_4 Spermatic cord
  1. Spermatic cord
  2. Scrotum
N_0 No nodal involvement
N_1 Ipsilateral regional nodal involvement
N_2 Contralateral or bilateral abdominal or groin nodes
N_3 Palpable abdominal nodes or fixed groin nodes
N_4 Juxtaregional nodes
M_0 No distant metastases
M_1 Distant metastases present

The clinical stages consist of stage A, with tumor confined to the testis and cord structures; stage B, with tumor confined to the retroperitoneal lymph nodes; and stage C, with tumor involving the abdominal viscera or disease above the diaphragm.

DIAGNOSIS

DIFFERENTIAL DIAGNOSIS

- Spermatocele
- Varicocele
- Hydrocele
- Epididymitis
- Epidermoid cyst of the testicle
- Epididymis tumors

WORKUP

Physical examination, laboratory tests, and imaging studies (Section III, "Testicular Mass")

LABORATORY TESTS

- Serum human chorionic gonadotropin (hCG)
- Serum alpha-fetoprotein (AFP)

One or both of these tumor markers will be elevated in 70% of cases of testicular cancer.

- Testicular biopsy is contraindicated.

IMAGING STUDIES

- Ultrasound
- CT scan or MRI of pelvis and abdomen
- Chest x-ray

TREATMENT

- Surgical exploration of the testicle through an inguinal incision with a noncrushing clamp placed on the cord before direct testicular examination. If a mass is confined within the body of the testicle, an orchiectomy is performed
- Retroperitoneal lymph node dissection for clinical stage A and low stage B (lymph nodes under 6 cm in greatest diameter) provides cure in 70%
- Chemotherapy: cisplatin, vinblastine, and bleomycin
  1. Not indicated in clinical stage A
  2. Controversial in low stage B
  3. Cornerstone of treatment in high stage B or stage C
- Radiation therapy for stage A and low stage B seminoma provides cure in 85%
- Posttreatment surveillance for testicular cancer survivors (annually)
  1. General maintenance
  2. Fertility assessment
  3. Sexuality status
  4. Skin examination (increased risk of dysplastic nevi)
  5. Testicular examination (3% to 4% risk of second testicular cancer)
  6. Serum tumor markers (hCG, AFP)
  7. Chest x-ray (for late relapse)
  8. Complications of cisplatin: hypertension, hyperlipidemia, renal failure, hypomagnesemia, hearing loss, tinnitus, peripheral neuropathy, and infertility

EVIDENCE

A randomized trial of paraaortic (PA) vs. PA plus ipsilateral iliac lymph node radiation for stage I testicular seminoma found low recurrence rates for either treatment and reduced hematologic, gastrointestinal, and gonadal toxicity with adjuvant radiotherapy confined to the PA nodes.[1] (B)

Evidence-Based Reference

1. Fossa SD et al: Optimal planning target volume for stage I testicular seminoma: a Medical Research Council randomized trial Medical Research Council Testicular Tumor Working Group, *J Clin Oncol* 17:1146, 1999. (B)

SUGGESTED READINGS

Feldman DR et al: Medical treatment of advanced testicular cancer, *JAMA* 299(6):672-684, 2008.
Petterson A et al: Age at surgery for undescended testis and risk of testicular cancer, *N Engl J Med* 356:1835, 2007.
Shaw J: Diagnosis and treatment of testicular cancer, *Am Fam Physician* 77(4):469-474, 2008.

AUTHORS: **FRED F. FERRI, M.D.,** and **TOM J. WACHTEL, M.D.**

BASIC INFORMATION

DEFINITION

Testicular torsion is a twisting of the spermatic cord leading to cessation of testicular blood flow, ischemia, and infarction if left untreated.

SYNONYMS

Spermatic cord torsion

ICD-9CM CODES
608.2 Testicular torsion

EPIDEMIOLOGY & DEMOGRAPHICS

INCIDENCE: Affects 1:4000 males younger than 25 years

PREDOMINANT AGE: Two thirds of all cases occur between the ages of 12 and 18 yr, but may occur at any age, including antenatally.

PHYSICAL FINDINGS & CLINICAL PRESENTATION

- Typical sequence is sudden onset of hemiscrotal pain, then swelling, nausea, and vomiting without fever or urinary symptoms.
- Physical examination may reveal a tender firm testis, high-riding testis, horizontal lie of testis, absent cremasteric reflex, and no pain with elevation of testis. Absence of the cremasteric reflex (stroking or pinching the medial thigh normally causes contraction of the cremaster muscle and elevation of the testis) is the most sensitive physical finding.
- Painless testicular swelling occurs in 10%.
- One out of three patients reports previous episodes of spontaneously remitting scrotal pain.
- In the neonate, testicular torsion should be presumed in patients with a painless, discolored hemiscrotal swelling.
- In rare cases, torsion may involve an undescended testicle. In such situations an empty hemiscrotum is palpated together with a tender lump in the inguinal area.

ETIOLOGY

- There are two types of testicular torsion: extravaginal caused by nonadherence of the tunica vaginalis to the dartos layer and intravaginal due to malrotation of the spermatic cord with the tunica vaginalis. Intravaginal torsion accounts for 90% of cases.
- Torsion usually occurs in the absence of any precipitating events. Trauma accounts for <10% of cases.

DIAGNOSIS

Diagnosis is made mainly by clinical suspicion. Color Doppler ultrasound evaluation or a nuclear testicular scan (Fig. 1-268) may help with the diagnosis. Ultrasonography will show absent or decreased blood flow; scintigraphy reveals decreased perfusion on symptomatic side.

DIFFERENTIAL DIAGNOSIS (See also Section II)

- Torsion of the testicular appendages (appendix testis)
- Testicular tumor
- Epididymitis
- Incarcerated inguinoscrotal hernia
- Orchitis
- Spermatocele
- Hydrocele, varicocele

WORKUP

The diagnosis is usually based on history and physical examination.

IMAGING STUDIES

- Radionuclide scrotal scanning (technetium-99m): cold testicle
- Doppler ultrasonic stethoscope (Doppler flowmetry)

TREATMENT

Surgical derotation of the spermatic cord followed by bilateral testicular fixation with nonabsorbable sutures. If the affected testis is nonviable, orchiectomy of the affected testis and orchiopexy of the contralateral side are performed. Attempts at manual detorsion should not delay surgical consultation.

PROGNOSIS

- The degree of ischemia depends on the duration of torsion and the degree of rotation of the spermatic cord.
- There is an 80% testicular salvage rate if detorsion occurs within 12 hr of onset.
- After 24 hr, irreversible testicular infarction is expected.
- Because the contralateral testes can be affected (immunologic process), when treatment is delayed and return of blood flow does not occur after detorsion, some recommend orchiectomy of the infarcted testicle.

REFERRAL

To urologist

COMMENTS

- Manual detorsion by external rotation of the testis toward the thigh can be attempted for adolescent intravaginal torsion if an operating facility is not readily available.
- Extravaginal torsion is diagnosed in the newborn. Intravaginal torsion can occur at any age but is usually diagnosed in males ages 12 to 18 yr.

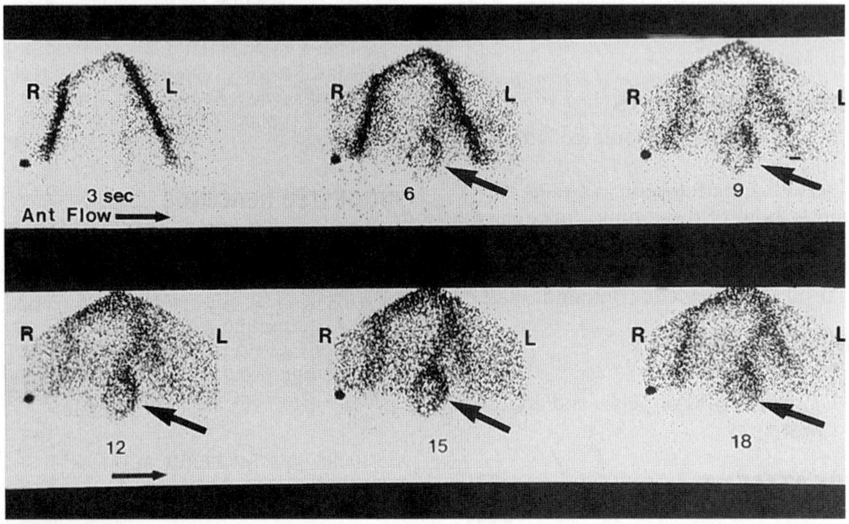

FIGURE 1-268 Testicular torsion. Evaluation of blood flow to the testicle has been done by giving an intravenous bolus of radioactive material. The right and left iliac vessels are clearly identified, and sequential images are obtained every 3 sec. Here, increased flow is seen to the rim of the left testicle *(arrows),* and there is no blood flow centrally. This is the appearance of a testicular torsion in which the torsion has been present for more than approximately 24 hr. (From Mettler FA [ed]: *Primary care radiology,* Philadelphia, 2000, WB Saunders.)

SUGGESTED READING

Ringdahl E, Teague L: Testicular torsion, *Am Fam Physician* 74:1739, 2006.

AUTHORS: **FRED F. FERRI, M.D.,** and **TOM J. WACHTEL, M.D.**

BASIC INFORMATION

DEFINITION

Tetanus is a life-threatening illness manifested by muscle rigidity and spasms; it is caused by a neurotoxin (tetanospasmin) produced by *Clostridium tetani.*

SYNONYMS

Lockjaw
Generalized tetanus
Neonatal tetanus
Cephalic tetanus
Localized tetanus

ICD-9CM CODES
037 Tetanus

EPIDEMIOLOGY & DEMOGRAPHICS

INCIDENCE (IN U.S.): 48 to 64 cases reported annually since 1986
PREDOMINANT AGE: >60 yr of age
GENETICS:
Neonatal Infection:
- Rare in U.S.
- Among the leading causes of neonatal mortality in many parts of the world (caused by infection of the umbilical cord stump)

PHYSICAL FINDINGS & CLINICAL PRESENTATION

- Trismus ("lockjaw")
- Risus sardonicus (peculiar grin), characteristic grimace that results from contraction of the facial muscles
- Generalized muscle spasms causing severe pain and, at times, respiratory compromise and death
- Rigid abdominal muscles, flexed arms, and extended legs
- Autonomic dysfunction several days after onset of illness
- Leading cause of death: fluctuations in heart rate and blood pressure
- Usually, absence of fever
- Localized tetanus
  1. Rigidity of muscles near the injury
  2. Weakness as a result of lower motor neuron injury
  3. May be self-limited and resolve spontaneously
  4. More often progresses to generalized tetanus
  5. Cephalic tetanus:
     a. May occur with head injuries or chronic otitis with localized ear or mastoid infection with *C. tetani*
     b. Can manifest as cranial nerve dysfunction

ETIOLOGY

- *C. tetani* is a gram-positive, spore-forming bacillus that resides primarily in the soil.
- Majority of cases are caused by punctures and lacerations.
- Toxin is elaborated from organisms in a contaminated wound.
- Local symptoms are caused by inhibition of neurotransmitter at presynaptic sites.
  1. Over the next 2 to 14 days, the toxin travels up the neurons to the CNS, where it acts on inhibitory neurons to prevent neurotransmitter release.
  2. Unopposed motor activity results in tonic contractions of muscles.

DIAGNOSIS

DIFFERENTIAL DIAGNOSIS

- Strychnine poisoning
- Dystonic reaction caused by neuroleptic agents
- Local infection (dental or masseter muscle) causing trismus
- Severe hypocalcemia
- Hysteria

WORKUP

- Positive wound culture is not helpful in diagnosis.
- Isolation of organism is possible in patients without the illness.

LABORATORY TESTS

- Usually, normal blood counts and chemistries
- Toxicology of serum and urine to rule out strychnine poisoning

TREATMENT

NONPHARMACOLOGIC THERAPY

- Monitoring in a hospital ICU: keep surroundings dark and quiet
- Intubation or tracheostomy for severe laryngospasm
- Debridement of wound

ACUTE GENERAL Rx

- Human tetanus immunoglobulin (HTIg) 500 U via IM injection
- Tetanus toxoid (Td) 0.5 ml by IM injection at a different site
- Metronidazole 500 mg IV q6h, or penicillin G 1 million U IV q4h for 10 days
- IV diazepam to control muscle spasms
- Neuromuscular blockade if necessary

CHRONIC Rx

- Supportive care
- Possible mechanical ventilation
- Minimal external stimuli
- Control of heart rate and blood pressure:
  1. Labetalol for sympathetic hyperactivity
  2. Pacemaker for sustained bradycardia
- Physical therapy once spasms subside

DISPOSITION

Full recovery over weeks to months if complications can be avoided

REFERRAL

- To emergency department
- To infectious disease specialist

PEARLS & CONSIDERATIONS

COMMENTS

- Illness is preventable.
- Boosters of Td should be given every 10 yr to maintain immune status.
- Passive as well as active immunization (HTIg + Td) should be given for patients with tetanus-prone wounds who have not been adequately immunized in the previous 5 yr.
- A recent U.S. study showed that only 72% of people >6 yr had protective levels of antibody.

EVIDENCE

Limited evidence suggests that diazepam is an effective treatment for the muscular spasms and rigidity of tetanus, in children. Survival rates are higher when children are treated with diazepam alone, compared with a combination of phenobarbitone and chlorpromazine. Those receiving diazepam experience a significantly milder clinical course and shorter duration of hospitalization.[1] Ⓑ

Limited evidence suggests that in the treatment of moderate tetanus, metronidazole is associated with a significantly lower mortality rate, shorter hospital stay, and an improved response to treatment compared with procaine penicillin.[1] Ⓑ

A substantial proportion of adults in the U.S. do not have antibody levels that are protective against diphtheria and tetanus, with rates of immunity substantially reducing after 20 years of age.[2] Ⓑ

Evidence-Based References

1. Okoromah CN, Lesi FEA: Diazepam for treating tetanus, *Cochrane Database Syst Rev* 1, 2004. Ⓑ
2. McQuillan GM et al: Serologic immunity to diphtheria and tetanus in the United States, *Ann Intern Med* 136:660, 2002. Ⓑ

SUGGESTED READINGS

Demicheli V et al: Vaccines for women to prevent neonatal tetanus, *Cochrane Database Syst Rev* 4:CD002959, 2005.

Rao KN et al: Structural analysis of the catalytic domain of tetanus neurotoxin, *Toxicon* 45(7):929, 2005.

Rhee P et al: Tetanus and trauma: a review and recommendations, *J Trauma* 58(5):1082, 2005.

Talan DA et al: Tetanus immunity and physician compliance with tetanus prophylaxis practices among emergency department patients presenting with wounds, *Ann Emerg Med* 43(3):305, 2004.

AUTHORS: **GLENN G. FORT, M.D., M.P.H., DENNIS J. MIKOLICH, M.D.,** and **MAURICE POLICAR, M.D.**

BASIC INFORMATION

DEFINITION

Tetralogy of Fallot (TOF) is a congenital heart deformity consisting of the following four features:
- Ventricular septal defect (VSD)
- Infundibular stenosis leading to obstruction to the right ventricular (RV) outflow tract
- Overriding aorta
- Right ventricular hypertrophy (RVH)

See Fig. 1-269.

ICD-9CM CODES
745.2 Tetralogy of Fallot

EPIDEMIOLOGY & DEMOGRAPHICS

- TOF is the most common cyanotic congenital heart malformation diagnosed after age 1 yr.
- TOF accounts for nearly 10% of all congenital heart disease.
- TOF occurs in approximately 3000 newborns/yr.

PHYSICAL FINDINGS & CLINICAL PRESENTATION

- Of the four major features of TOF, infundibular stenosis leading to RV outflow tract obstruction and VSD are the primary defects leading to:
  1. Right-to-left shunting and hypoxemia
  2. Altered RV hemodynamics
  3. Decreased pulmonary blood flow
- The aforementioned pathophysiologic concepts subsequently result in common manifestations of TOF, including:
  1. Cyanosis secondary to shunting of deoxygenated blood from the RV through the VSD into the left ventricle, thus bypassing the lungs
  2. Dyspnea on exertion
  3. Clubbing
  4. Child assuming a squatting position after exercise increasing systemic vascular resistance, thereby decreasing right-to-left shunting
  5. Low birth weight and growth rate
  6. Palpable RV impulse
  7. Systolic thrill along the left sternal border
  8. Single second heart sound, inaudible P2 component
  9. Systolic ejection murmur resulting from RV outflow tract obstruction

ETIOLOGY

Unknown

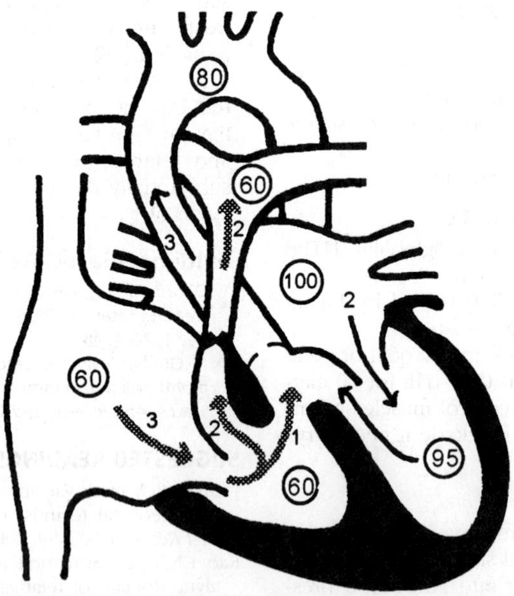

FIGURE 1-269 Physiology of tetralogy of Fallot (TOF). The circled numbers represent oxygen saturations. The numbers next to the arrows represent volumes of blood flow (in L/min/m²). The atrial (mixed venous) oxygen saturation is decreased secondary to the systemic hypoxemia. Three liters per minute per square meter of desaturated blood enter the right atrium and traverse the tricuspid valve. Two liters flow through the right ventricular outflow tract into the lungs, whereas 1 L shunts right to left through the ventricular septal defect (VSD) into the ascending aorta. Thus, the pulmonary blood flow is two-thirds normal (Qp:Qs of 0.7:1). Blood returning to the left atrium is fully saturated. Only 2 L of blood flows across the mitral valve. The oxygen saturation in the left ventricle may be slightly decreased owing to right-to-left shunting across the VSD. Two liters of saturated left ventricular blood, mixing with 1 L of desaturated right ventricular blood, are ejected into the ascending aorta. The aortic saturation is decreased, and the cardiac output is normal. (From Behrman RE: *Nelson textbook of pediatrics,* ed 16, Philadelphia, 2000, WB Saunders.)

DIAGNOSIS

The diagnosis of TOF is suspected in any neonate, infant, or child presenting with cyanosis and a heart murmur.

DIFFERENTIAL DIAGNOSIS

- Asthma
- Isolated VSD
- Pulmonary atresia
- Patent ductus arteriosus
- Aortic stenosis
- Pneumothorax

WORKUP

- Detailed history and physical examination
- Echocardiography, chest x-ray, ECG, and routine laboratory tests.

LABORATORY TESTS

- CBC with polycythemia resulting from long-standing cyanosis
- Arterial blood gases (ABGs) with hypoxemia, normal pH, and pCO_2
- Pulse oximetry
- ECG commonly demonstrating RVH and/or right atrial enlargement

IMAGING STUDIES

- Chest x-ray revealing boot-shaped heart commonly described as "coeur en sabot"; prominent RV with decreased pulmonary vascularity.
- Echocardiography demonstrating VSD with a stenotic RV outflow tract and an overriding aorta.
- Cardiac catheterization and angiography aid in the determination of the severity of right-to-left shunting, localization of the VSD, and anatomic assessment of the RV outflow tract, pulmonary artery, and coronary artery anatomy.
- Cardiac MRI: used for localization of the VSD and anatomic assessment of the RV outflow tract, as well as assessment of RV function, quantification of pulmonary regurgitation, and detection of RV myocardial fibrosis. Magnetic resonance angiography (MRA) can be an alternative noninvasive method to cardiac catheterization in the evaluation of pulmonary vascular anatomy.
- 64-slice spiral CT can also be used for the diagnosis and is extremely important for the planning of the repair procedure. Its use may be limited by the risks associated with radiation exposure in children.

TREATMENT

NONPHARMACOLOGIC THERAPY

- Oxygen.

- Knee-chest position in hypoxemic spells helps reduce venous return and increase systemic vascular resistance, thus decreases right-to-left shunting.

ACUTE Rx

Acute treatment of any infant or child with TOF who is cyanotic with respiratory distress is aimed at increasing systemic vascular resistance and decreasing right-to-left shunting (e.g., phenylephrine 0.1 to 0.5 μg/kg/min IV). Intravenous beta-blockers (e.g., propranolol 0.15 to 0.25 mg/kg slow IV push) are used to decrease RV outflow tract contractility, and subcutaneous morphine can be used to decrease venous return.

CHRONIC Rx

- Palliative repair includes procedures increasing pulmonary blood flow, thus reducing right-to-left shunting. Examples of palliative procedures include the Blalock-Taussig shunt, in which a shunt is made between the subclavian artery and the pulmonary artery; the Waterston shunt, which attaches the ascending aorta to the right pulmonary artery; and the Potts shunt, which attaches the descending aorta to the left pulmonary artery.
- Complete surgical repair has good success and involves closing the VSD with a Dacron patch and relieving the RV outflow tract obstruction. It is recommended for nearly every patient with TOF.

DISPOSITION

- Almost all TOF patients have either palliative or complete surgical repair before reaching adulthood.
- Less than 3% of patients with TOF reach 40 yr of age without having surgery.
- Survival after complete operative repair for TOF is excellent provided the RV outflow tract obstruction has been relieved and the VSD has been closed. Most adults lead unrestricted lives and are asymptomatic.
- 85% of patients who have operative repair of TOF survive >36 yr.
- Early and late postoperative complications can occur and generally manifest in arrhythmias from atrial and ventricular tachycardias, and diminished exercise tolerance from RV failure.
- A prolonged QRS duration in the preoperative ECG predicts an increased risk of postoperative supraventricular and ventricular arrhythmias. Prolongation of QRS beyond 180 ms identifies patients at increased risk of ventricular tachycardia after surgery.
- Ventricular arrhythmias can lead to sudden cardiac death in 8.3% of surgically repaired patients by age 35.
- Reduced exercise capacity is usually secondary to chronic pulmonary regurgitation or residual RV outflow tract obstruction. The precise indications and timing for undergoing pulmonary valve replacement after TOF repair are under research. An RV end-diastolic volume index of 150 ml/m^2 is a practical cutoff value for pulmonic valve replacement.
- TEI index (a measurement of myocardial performance) by echocardiography, increased serum brain natriuretic peptide (BNP) levels, and a decreased peak O_2 consumption on exercise testing help to identify significant pulmonic valve lesions before they are clinically symptomatic.
- Women with repaired TOF should be assessed by a cardiologist before considering pregnancy to determine if pulmonic valve replacement is needed first.
- Selected patients with normal RV pressures and function, without evidence of residual shunt, and without atrial or ventricular tachyarrhythmias are eligible to participate in competitive sports.

REFERRAL

- Infants and children with cyanotic heart disease should be referred to a pediatric cardiologist for further diagnostic evaluation. On diagnosing TOF, patients should be referred to centers experienced in palliative and complete surgical repair.
- Adult patients with repaired TOF should be co-managed with cardiology.

PEARLS & CONSIDERATIONS

- TOF was first described by the French physician Etienne Fallot in 1888.
- The first palliative surgical treatment for TOF was performed by Dr. Alfred Blalock at Johns Hopkins University in 1945 (Taussig-Blalock shunt).
- The first surgical repair for TOF was performed by Dr. C. Walton Lillehei at the University of Minnesota in 1954.

COMMENTS

- The severity of right ventricular outflow tract obstruction is the primary determinant of clinical symptoms and outcome.
- Coexisting cardiac abnormalities occur in nearly 40% of patients with TOF, including patent ductus arteriosus, atrial septal defect, multiple VSDs, absence of a pulmonary artery, complete AV septal defects, and anomalous coronary arteries.
- TOF requires bacterial endocarditis prophylaxis before any dental work or nonsterile surgical procedures, such as surgery on the bowel or bladder.
- Screening of patients with TOF for 22q11 deletions is helpful to detect concomitant immune deficiency syndromes.
- Long-term follow-up of children with surgically corrected TOF is warranted. Even hemodynamically stable, they are at risk for neurodevelopment delay at school age.

SUGGESTED READINGS

Dave HH et al: Early insertion of a pulmonary valve for chronic regurgitation helps restoration of ventricular dimensions, *Ann Thorac Surg* 80(5):1615-1620, 2005.

Graham TP Jr et al: Task Force 2: congenital heart disease, *J Am Coll Cardiol* 45(8):1326-1333, 2005.

Shinebourne E et al: Tetralogy of Fallot: from fetus to adult, *Heart* 92(9):1353-1359, 2006.

Warnes CA: The adult with congenital heart disease: born to be bad? *J Am Coll Cardiol* 46(1):1-8, 2005.

AUTHORS: **ABDULBAKI ABDULRAHMAN, M.D.,** and **WEN-CHIH WU, M.D.**

BASIC INFORMATION

DEFINITION

Thalassemias are a heterogeneous group of disorders of hemoglobin synthesis that have in common a deficient synthesis of one or more of the polypeptide chains of the normal human hemoglobin, resulting in a quantitative abnormality of the hemoglobin thus produced. There are no qualitative changes such as those encountered in the hemoglobinopathies (e.g., sickle cell disease).

SYNONYMS

Mediterranean anemia
Cooley's anemia

ICD-9CM CODES
282.4 Thalassemia

EPIDEMIOLOGY & DEMOGRAPHICS

- Thalassemia is among the most common genetic disorders worldwide. 4.83% of the world's population carry globin variants, including 1.67% of the population who are heterozygous for alpha-thalassemia and beta-thalassemia.
- The highest concentration of alpha-thalassemia is found in Southeast Asia and the African west coast. For example, in Thailand the prevalence is 5% to 10%. It is also common among blacks, with a prevalence of approximately 5%.
- The worldwide prevalence of beta-thalassemia is approximately 3%; in certain regions of Italy and Greece the prevalence reaches 15% to 30%. This high prevalence can be found in Americans of Italian or Greek descent.
- The distribution of thalassemia in Europe and Africa parallels that of malaria, suggesting that thalassemic persons are more resistant to the parasite, thus permitting evolutionary survival advantage.

CLASSIFICATION

BETA THALASSEMIA:
- Beta (+) thalassemia (suboptimal beta-globin synthesis)
- Beta (o) thalassemia (total absence of beta-globin synthesis)
- Delta-beta thalassemia (total absence of both delta-globin and beta-globin synthesis)
- Lepore hemoglobin (synthesis of small amounts of fused delta-beta-globin and total absence of delta- and beta-globin)
- Hereditary persistence of fetal hemoglobin (HPHF) (increased hemoglobin F synthesis and reduced or absence of delta- and beta-globin)

ALPHA THALASSEMIA:
- Silent carrier (three alpha-globin genes present)
- Alpha thalassemia trait (two alpha-globin genes present)
- Hemoglobin H disease (one alpha-globin gene present)
- Hydrops fetalis (no alpha-globin gene)
- Hemoglobin constant sprint (elongated alpha-globin chain)

THALASSEMIC HEMOGLOBINOPATHIES: Hb Terre Haute, Hb Quong Sze, HbE, Hb Knossos

PHYSICAL FINDINGS & CLINICAL PRESENTATION

BETA THALASSEMIA:
- Heterozygous beta thalassemia (thalassemia minor): no or mild anemia, microcytosis and hypochromia, mild hemolysis manifested by slight reticulocytosis and splenomegaly
- Homozygous beta thalassemia (thalassemia major): intense hemolytic anemia; transfusion dependency; bone deformities (skull and long bones); hepatomegaly; splenomegaly; iron overload leading to cardiomyopathy, diabetes mellitus, and hypogonadism; growth retardation; pigment gallstones; susceptibility to infection
- Thalassemia intermedia caused by combination of beta and alpha thalassemia or beta thalassemia and Hb Lepore: resembles thalassemia major but is milder

ALPHA THALASSEMIA:
- Silent carrier: no symptoms.
- Alpha thalassemia trait: microcytosis only.
- Hemoglobin H disease: moderately severe hemolysis with microcytosis and splenomegaly.
- The loss of all four alpha-globin genes is incompatible with life (stillbirth of hydropic fetus). Note: Pregnancies with hydrops fetalis are associated with a high incidence of toxemia.

ETIOLOGY

- Beta thalassemia: it is caused by more than 200 point mutations and, rarely, by deletions. The reduction of beta-globin synthesis results in redundant alpha-globin chains (Heinz bodies), which are cytotoxic and cause intramedullary hemolysis and ineffective erythropoiesis. Fetal hemoglobin may be increased.
- Alpha thalassemia: several mutations can result in insufficient amounts of alpha globin available for combination with non–alpha globins.

DIAGNOSIS

LABORATORY TESTS

BETA THALASSEMIA:
- Microcytosis (MCV: 55 to 80 FL)
- Normal RDW (RBC distribution width)
- Smear: nucleated RBCs, anisocytosis, poikilocytosis, polychromatophilia, Pappenheimer and Howell-Jolly bodies
- Hemoglobin electrophoresis: absent or reduced hemoglobin A, increased fetal hemoglobin, variable increase in the amount of hemoglobin A_2
- Markers of hemolysis: elevated indirect bilirubin and LDH, decreased haptoglobin

ALPHA THALASSEMIA:
- Microcytosis in the absence of iron deficiency.
- Hemoglobin electrophoresis is normal, except for the presence of hemoglobin H in hemoglobin H disease.

TREATMENT

- Thalassemia minor: no treatment but avoid iron administration for incorrect diagnosis of iron deficiency.
- Beta thalassemia major (and hemoglobin H disease):
  1. Transfusion as required together with chelation of iron with desferrioxamine (by intravenous or subcutaneous administration, 8 to 12 hr nightly, 5 to 6 days a week at a dose of 2 to 6 g/day using a portable infusion pump).
  2. Splenectomy for hypersplenism if present.
  3. Bone marrow transplantation. Although hematopoietic stem-cell transplantation is the only curative approach for thalassemia, it has been limited by the high cost and scarcity of HLA-matched donors. Before transplantation it is necessary to administer myeloablative regimens to eradicate the endogenous thalassemic bone marrow. Commonly used agents are hydroxyurea, azathioprine, fludarabine, busulfan, and cyclophosphamide.
  4. Hydroxyurea may increase the level of hemoglobin F.

PEARLS & CONSIDERATIONS

- Polymerase chain reaction (PCR) can be used to detect point mutations or deletions in chorionic-villous samples, enabling first-trimester, DNA-based testing for thalassemia.
- Preimplantation genetic diagnosis can be extended to HLA typing on embryonic biopsies allowing the selection of an embryo that is not affected by thalassemia and that may also serve as a stem-cell donor for a previously affected child within the same family.

SUGGESTED READING

Round D, Rachmilewitz E: Beta thalassemia, *N Engl J Med* 353:1135-1146, 2005.

AUTHORS: **FRED F. FERRI, M.D.,** and **TOM J. WACHTEL, M.D.**

BASIC INFORMATION

DEFINITION

Thoracic outlet syndrome is the term used to describe a condition producing upper extremity symptoms thought to result from neurovascular compression at the thoracic outlet. Three types are described based on the point of compression: (1) cervical rib and scalenus syndrome, in which abnormal scalene muscles or the presence of a cervical rib may cause compression; (2) costoclavicular syndrome, in which compression may occur under the clavicle; and (3) hyperabduction syndrome, in which compression may occur in the subcoracoid area.

ICD-9CM CODES
353.0 Thoracic outlet syndrome

EPIDEMIOLOGY & DEMOGRAPHICS

PREVALENCE: Varies from source to source; presence of cervical ribs in 0.5% to 1% of population (50% bilateral), but most are asymptomatic

PREDOMINANT SEX: Female > male (3.5:1)

PREDOMINANT AGE: Rare under 20 yr of age

PHYSICAL FINDINGS & CLINICAL PRESENTATION

- Symptoms and signs are related to the degree of involvement of each of the various structures at the level of the first rib.
- True venous or arterial involvement is not common.
- Diagnosis is most often used in the consideration of neural pain affecting the arm, which would suggest involvement of the brachial plexus.
  1. *Arterial compression:* pallor, paresthesias, diminished pulses, coolness, digital gangrene, and a supraclavicular bruit or mass
  2. *Venous compression:* edema and pain; thrombosis causing superficial venous dilation about the shoulder
  3. *"True" neural compression:* lower trunk (C8, T1) findings with intrinsic weakness and diminished sensation to the finger and small fingers and ulnar aspect of the forearm
  4. Possible supraclavicular tenderness
  5. Provocative tests (Adson's, Wright's): may reproduce pain but are of disputed usefulness

ETIOLOGY

- Congenital cervical rib or fibrous extension of cervical rib (Fig. 1-270)
- Abnormal scalene muscle insertion
- Drooping of shoulder girdle resulting from generalized hypotonia or trauma
- Narrowed costoclavicular interval as a result of downward and backward pressure on shoulder (sometimes seen in individuals who carry heavy backpacks)
- Acute venous thrombosis with exercise (effort thrombosis)
- Bony abnormalities of first rib
- Abnormal fibromuscular bands
- Malunion of clavicle fracture

DIAGNOSIS

DIFFERENTIAL DIAGNOSIS

- Carpal tunnel syndrome
- Cervical radiculopathy
- Brachial neuritis
- Ulnar nerve compression
- Reflex sympathetic dystrophy
- Superior sulcus tumor

WORKUP

Except for venous or arterial pathology, no ancillary diagnostic tests are reliable for diagnostic confirmation.

IMAGING STUDIES

- Arteriography or venography when vascular pathology is strongly suspected clinically
- Cervical spine radiographs to rule out cervical disk disease
- Chest film to rule out lung tumor
- EMG, NCV studies to rule out carpal tunnel syndrome, cervical radiculopathy

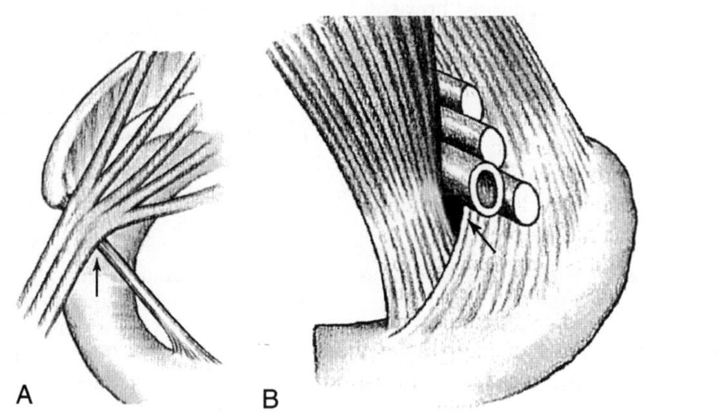

FIGURE 1-270 **A,** Compression caused by a cervical rib *(arrow).* **B,** Abnormal scalene muscle insertions that may cause compression at the cervicobrachial region *(arrow).* (From Mercier LR: *Practical orthopedics,* ed 5, St Louis, 2000, Mosby.)

TREATMENT

ACUTE GENERAL Rx

- Sling for pain relief
- Physical therapy modalities plus shoulder girdle–strengthening exercises
- Postural reeducation
- NSAIDs

DISPOSITION

- Surgery: generally successful for vascular disorders
- Nonsurgical treatment: often successful for patients with pain as the primary symptom

REFERRAL

For vascular surgery consultation when venous or arterial impairment is present

PEARLS & CONSIDERATIONS

COMMENTS

- True thoracic outlet syndrome is probably an uncommon condition.
- Diagnosis is often used to describe a wide variety of clinical symptoms.
- Considerable disagreement exists regarding the frequency of this disorder.

EVIDENCE

Home exercise treatment program provides relief to patients with thoracic outlet syndrome symptoms.

Evidence-Based Reference

1. Lindgren KA: Conservative treatment of thoracic outlet syndrome: a 2-year follow-up, *Arch Phys Med Rehab* 78:373, 1997.

SUGGESTED READINGS

Kaymak B, Ozcakar L: Complex regional pain syndrome in thoracic outlet syndrome, *Br J Sports Med* 38:364, 2004.

Malas FU et al: Etiologic factors in thoracic outlet syndrome, *Orthopedics* 30(6):425, 2007.

Monica JT et al: Thoracic outlet syndrome with subclavian artery thrombosis undetectable by magnetic resonance angiography, *J Bone Joint Surg* 89:1589, 2007.

Sanders RJ et al: Diagnosis of thoracic outlet syndrome, *J Vasc Surg* 46:601, 2007.

Urschel HC, Kourlis H: Thoracic outlet syndrome: a 50-year experience at Baylor University Medical Center, *Proc (Bayl Univ Med Cent)* 20(2):125, 2007.

Wehbe MA, Leinberry CF: Current trends in treatment of thoracic outlet syndrome, *Hand Clin* 20:119, 2004.

AUTHOR: **LONNIE R. MERCIER, M.D.**

Section I DISEASES AND DISORDERS

BASIC INFORMATION

DEFINITION

Thromboangiitis obliterans (TAO), or Buerger's disease, is a nonatherosclerotic inflammatory disease that commonly affects the small- and medium-sized arteries, veins, and nerves of the upper and lower extremities.

SYNONYMS

Buerger's disease
Presenile gangrene

ICD-9CM CODES
443.1 Thromboangiitis obliterans (Buerger's disease)

EPIDEMIOLOGY & DEMOGRAPHICS

- TAO is most prevalent in the Middle East, Far East, and Asia, where the prevalence can be as high as 45% to 63%.
- In the U.S., the prevalence has been estimated at 12.6 to 20 cases/100,000 persons.
- A genetic predisposition has been proposed based on the higher incidence in Israel among Jews of Ashkenazi ancestry with peripheral artery disease.
- The symptoms almost always begin before the age of 40 yr, and almost all the patients affected are smokers.
- TAO was initially thought to affect almost exclusively men. It still predominantly affects young men; however, more recently there has been an increase in the prevalence of TAO in women. This increase may be a result of an increase in smoking among women.
- Death from TAO is rare.

PHYSICAL FINDINGS & CLINICAL PRESENTATION

- TAO generally begins with hand or foot ischemia due to involvement of the distal small arteries and veins of the limbs.
- In 70% to 80% of cases, rest pain and diminished sensation from ischemic neuropathy is seen. Sometimes this can lead to ischemic ulcerations of the toes or feet before diagnosis of TAO is made.
- Rest pain generally occurs on the forefoot, causing continuous pain and, therefore, patients may sleep with their legs dangling downward.
- Ischemia of the upper limbs is clinically evident in 40% to 50% of patients, but may be detected in 63% of patients by the Allen's test.
- There is evidence of prolonged capillary refill with dependent rubor, and migratory thrombophlebitis.
- Systemic involvement, intestinal involvement, and central nervous system involvement are rare.

ETIOLOGY

- Unknown.
- Exposure to tobacco is essential for initiation and progression of the disease (a small number of cases have been reported to be attributed to the use of chewing tobacco).
- Studies have suggested the presence of impaired endothelium-dependent vasorelaxation in the peripheral vasculature in patients with TAO.
- There is no evidence to suggest that hypercoagulability abnormalities play a role in the disease mechanism.
- There is no overwhelming evidence to suggest a predominantly genetic or immunologic etiology for TAO.

DIAGNOSIS

DIFFERENTIAL DIAGNOSIS

- Limb ischemia resulting from emboli or atherosclerotic occlusive disease
- Antiphospholipid antibody syndrome
- Autoimmune disorders
- Acrocyanosis
- Carpal tunnel syndrome
- CREST (calcinosis cutis, Raynaud's phenomenon, esophageal motility disorder, sclerodactyly, and telangiectasia) syndrome
- Systemic lupus erythematosus
- Diabetes mellitus
- Repetitive vibratory equipment use
- Hypothenar hammer syndrome
- Raynaud's phenomenon
- Ergotamine intoxication
- Polyarteritis nodosa
- Cannabis arteritis
- Peripheral neuropathy

WORKUP

The diagnosis of TAO is rendered difficult by the lack of specific clinical, radiological, and biological features in the disease. Point scoring systems are available to aid with the diagnosis; however, at this time no criteria is validated or accepted internationally. The diagnosis is therefore made by trying to eliminate differential diagnoses and to search for other signs of the disease:

1. Peripheral vascular disease occurring predominantly in men before the age of 40 yr
2. Typically, affects the arms and the legs and not just the lower extremities as arteriosclerosis does
3. Found solely in tobacco smokers, with improvement in those who abstain
4. Associated with migratory thrombophlebitis
5. No other atherosclerotic risk factors (e.g., diabetes, cholesterol, or hypertension)

- Angiographic criteria (see "Imaging Studies")
- TAO is an inflammatory disease; however, in contrast to all of the major arteritis, fibrinoid necrosis of the arterial wall is *not* observed and the vascular wall is preserved. This feature distinguishes TAO from other types of systemic vasculitis and from arteriosclerosis, in which there is usually disruption of the internal elastic lamina and the media.

LABORATORY TESTS

TAO can not be diagnosed on the basis of a specific laboratory test. The primary goal of a laboratory workup in patients thought to have the disease is to exclude other disease processes in the differential diagnosis.

IMAGING STUDIES

- Noninvasive vascular studies help differentiate proximal occlusive disease characteristic of arteriosclerosis from distal disease typical of TAO.
- Echocardiography should be performed in patients thought to have TAO in order to exclude a proximal source of emboli as the cause of distal vessel occlusion.
- Angiography findings in TAO include:
  - Involvement of distal small- and medium-size vessels
  - Occlusions are segmental, multiple, smooth, and tapered
  - Collateral circulation gives a "tree root" or "spider leg" appearance
  - Both upper and lower extremities are involved

TREATMENT

NONPHARMACOLOGIC THERAPY

Abstaining from smoking is the only way to stop the progression of the disease. Medical and surgical treatments will prove to be futile if the patient continues to smoke. Exacerbation of ischemic ulcers is directly related to tobacco use.

ACUTE GENERAL Rx

- The goal of medical treatment is to provide relief of ischemic pain and healing of ischemic ulcers. If the patient does not completely abstain from tobacco, medical measures will not be helpful.
- Treatment with intravenous iloprost (a prostaglandin analogue) has been shown to be effective in improving symptoms and reducing the amputation rate among patients with TAO.

- Epidural anesthesia and hyperbaric oxygen have a vasodilator effect and have been shown to aid in pain relief from ischemic ulcers.

CHRONIC Rx

- Surgical bypass procedures and sympathectomy, as with medical treatment, will not be efficacious unless the patient stops smoking.
- Surgical bypass may be difficult because the occlusions of TAO are distal.
- Sympathectomy leads to increased blood flow by decreasing the vasoconstriction of distal vessels and also has been shown to aid in the healing and relief of pain from ischemic ulcers.
- Debridement must be done on necrotic ulcers if needed.
- Amputation is frequently required for gangrenous digits.
- There is limited data on experimental gene transfer to induce therapeutic angiogenesis in TAO.

DISPOSITION

The course of TAO can be dramatically changed by the cessation of tobacco smoking. If a patient continues to smoke, recurrent exacerbation of ischemic ulcers, necrosis, and gangrene leading to small digit amputations are inevitable.

REFERRAL

Smoking cessation counseling, rheumatology consultation, and vascular surgery consultation are recommended in any young smoker with claudication and ischemic ulcers, especially if both the upper and lower extremities are involved.

PEARLS & CONSIDERATIONS

COMMENTS

Smoking cessation is mandatory. In individuals who quit smoking, prognosis is markedly improved.

PATIENT/FAMILY EDUCATION

Patients with TAO must be warned about tobacco use and secondhand smoke.
Information for patients:

- Vascular Disease Foundation (http://www.vdf.org)
- Mayo Foundation for Medical Education and Research (http://www.mayoclinic.com)

EVIDENCE

The discontinuation of tobacco use is the only definitive therapy for TAO.[1] Ⓐ

Prostacyclin analogues may help patients with critical limb ischemia seen in TAO.[2] Ⓑ

Recent experimental genetic and cell-based therapeutic approaches have been proposed to help in the treatment of TAO; however, further study is required.[3,4] Ⓒ

Evidence-Based References

1. Olin JW et al: Thromboangiitis obliterans (Buerger's disease), *N Engl J Med* 343:864-869, 2000.
2. Fiessinger JN et al: Trial of iloprost versus aspirin treatment for critical limb ischemia of thromboangiitis obliterans: the TAO study, *Lancet* 335:555-557, 1990.
3. Kim DI et al: Angiogenesis facilitated by autologous whole bone marrow stem cell transplantation for Buerger's disease, *Stem Cells* 24:1194-1200, 2006.
4. Kim SW et al: Successful stem cell therapy using umbilical cord blood derived multipotent stem cells for Buerger's disease and ischemic limb disease animal model, *Stem Cells* 24:1620-1626, 2006.

SUGGESTED READINGS

Puéchal X et al: Thromboangiitis obliterans or Buerger's disease: challenges for the rheumatologist, *Rheumatology* 46(2):192-199, 2007.

AUTHOR: **PRANAV M. PATEL, M.D.**

BASIC INFORMATION

DEFINITION

Superficial thrombophlebitis is inflammatory thrombosis in subcutaneous veins. Superficial suppurative thrombophlebitis is an inflammation of the vein wall due to the presence of microorganisms occurring as a complication of either dermal infection or use of an indwelling intravenous catheter.

SYNONYMS

Phlebitis
Superficial suppurative thrombophlebitis

ICD-9CM CODES
451.0 Thrombophlebitis, superficial

EPIDEMIOLOGY & DEMOGRAPHICS

- 20% of superficial thrombophlebitis cases are associated with occult DVT.
- Catheter-related thrombophlebitis incidence is 100:100,000. The disease occurs more frequently when plastic catheters are inserted in the lower extremities. The mean duration of preceding venous cannulation is 4.8 days and the latent interval from removal of the catheter to development of symptoms ranges from 2 to 10 days.

PHYSICAL FINDINGS & CLINICAL PRESENTATION

- Subcutaneous vein is palpable, tender; tender cord is present with erythema and edema of the overlying skin and subcutaneous tissue.
- Induration, redness, and tenderness are localized along the course of the vein. This linear appearance rather than circular appearance is useful to distinguish thrombophlebitis from other conditions (cellulitis, erythema nodosum).
- There is no significant swelling of the limb (superficial thrombophlebitis generally does not produce swelling of the limb).
- Low-grade fever may be present. High fever and chills are suggestive of septic phlebitis.
- Superficial suppurative thrombophlebitis may be difficult to identify because local findings of inflammation may be absent. Fever is present in >70% of cases but rigors are rare. Local findings (warmth, erythema, tenderness, swelling, lymphangitis) are present in only one third of patients.

ETIOLOGY

- Trauma to preexisting varices.
- Intravenous cannulation of veins (most common cause).
- Abdominal cancer (e.g., carcinoma of pancreas).
- Infection: *Staphylococcus aureus* was the most common pathogen, found in 65% to 78% of the cases of superficial suppurative thrombophlebitis before 1970; now most cases are due to *Enterobacteriaceae*, especially *Klebsiella-Enterobacter* spp. These agents are acquired nosocomially and are often resistant to multiple antibiotics. Infection with fungi or gram-negative aerobic bacilli is often seen in patients who are receiving broad-spectrum antibiotics at the time of the superficial suppurative phlebitis.
- Hypercoagulable state.
- DVT.

DIAGNOSIS

DIFFERENTIAL DIAGNOSIS

- Lymphangitis
- Cellulitis
- Erythema nodosum
- Panniculitis
- Kaposi's sarcoma

WORKUP

Laboratory evaluation to exclude infectious etiology and imaging studies to rule out DVT in suspected cases

LABORATORY TESTS

- CBC with differential, blood cultures, culture of IV catheter tip (when secondary to intravenous cannulation). Bacteremia occurs in 80%-90% of the cases of superficial suppurative thrombophlebitis.
- Culture of the catheter may be misleading because even though bacteria are isolated in 60% of the cases, a positive culture does not correlate with inflammation.
- Exploratory venotomy may be necessary in suspected superficial suppurative thrombophlebitis.

IMAGING STUDIES

- Serial ultrasound or venography in patients with suspected DVT
- CT scan of abdomen in patients with suspected malignancy (Trousseau's syndrome: recurrent migratory thrombophlebitis)

TREATMENT

NONPHARMACOLOGIC THERAPY

- Warm, moist compresses.
- It is not necessary to restrict activity; however, if there is extensive thrombophlebitis, bed rest with the leg elevated will limit the thrombosis and improve symptoms.

ACUTE GENERAL Rx

- NSAIDs to relieve symptoms
- Treatment of septic thrombophlebitis with antibiotics with adequate coverage of *Enterobacteriaceae* and *Staphylococcus*. Initial empirical treatment with a semisynthetic penicillin (IV Nafcillin 2 g q4 to 6h plus either an aminoglycoside [gentamicin 1 mk/kg IV q8h] or a third-generation cephalosporin [cefotaxime] or a quinolone [ciprofloxacin]).
- Ligation and division of the superficial vein at the junction to avoid propagation of the clot in the deep venous system when the thrombophlebitis progresses toward the junction of the involved superficial vein with deep veins.
- The role of antifungal therapy for superficial suppurative thrombophlebitis due to *C. albicans* is controversial. Most of these infections can be cured by vein excision. Because of the propensity of these infections for hematogenous spread, a 10- to 14-day course of amphotericin B or fluconazole is advisable.

DISPOSITION

Clinical improvement within 7 to 10 days

REFERRAL

Surgical referral in selected cases (see "Acute General Rx")

PEARLS & CONSIDERATIONS

COMMENTS

- Patients with positive cultures should be evaluated and treated for endocarditis.
- Suppurative thrombophlebitis is a particular problem in burned patients, for whom it represents a common cause of death due to infection.
- Septic thrombophlebitis is more common in IV drug addicts.

SUGGESTED READING

Gillespie P et al: Cannula related suppurative thrombophlebitis in the burned patient, *Burns* 26:200-204, 2000.

AUTHOR: **FRED F. FERRI, M.D.**

BASIC INFORMATION

DEFINITION

Thrombotic thrombocytopenic purpura (TTP) is a rare disorder characterized by thrombocytopenia (often accompanied by purpura) and microangiopathic hemolytic anemia; neurologic impairment, renal dysfunction, and fever may also be present.

SYNONYMS

TTP

ICD-9CM CODES
446.6 Thrombotic thrombocytopenic purpura

EPIDEMIOLOGY & DEMOGRAPHICS

- TTP primarily affects females between 10 and 50 yr of age.
- Frequency is 3.7 cases/yr/1 million persons.

PHYSICAL FINDINGS & CLINICAL PRESENTATION

- Purpura (secondary to thrombocytopenia)
- Jaundice, pallor (secondary to hemolysis)
- Mucosal bleeding
- Fever
- Fluctuating levels of consciousness (secondary to thrombotic occlusion of the cerebral vessels)

ETIOLOGY

- The exact cause of TTP remains unknown. Recent studies reveal that there is platelet aggregation as a result of abnormalities in circulating von Willebrand factor caused by endothelial injury.
- Many drugs, including clopidogrel, penicillin, antineoplastic agents, oral contraceptives, quinine, and ticlopidine, have been associated with TTP. Other precipitating causes include infectious agents, pregnancy, malignancies, allogenic bone marrow transplantation, and neurologic disorders.

DIAGNOSIS

DIFFERENTIAL DIAGNOSIS

- DIC
- Malignant hypertension
- Vasculitis
- Eclampsia or preeclampsia
- Hemolytic-uremic syndrome (typically encountered in children, often following a viral infection)
- Gastroenteritis as a result of a serotoxin-producing serotype of *Escherichia coli*
- Medications: clopidogrel, ticlopidine, penicillin, antineoplastic chemotherapeutic agents, oral contraceptives

WORKUP

- A comprehensive history, physical examination, and laboratory evaluation usually confirms the diagnosis.
- The disease often begins as a flulike illness ultimately followed by clinical and laboratory abnormalities.
- An algorithm for the diagnosis of TTP is described in Section III.

LABORATORY TESTS

- Severe anemia and thrombocytopenia
- Elevated BUN and creatinine
- Evidence of hemolysis: elevated reticulocyte count, indirect bilirubin, LDH, decreased haptoglobin
- Urinalysis: hematuria (red cells and red cell casts in urine sediment) and proteinuria
- Peripheral smear: severely fragmented RBCs (schistocytes)
- No laboratory evidence of DIC (normal FDP, fibrinogen)

TREATMENT

ACUTE GENERAL Rx

- Discontinue potential offending agents.
- The America Association of Blood Banks, the American Society for Apheresis, and the British Committee for Standards in Haematology recommend daily plasma exchange with replacement of 1.0 to 1.5 times the predicted plasma volume of the patient as standard therapy for TTP. The British guidelines recommend that plasma exchange therapy be continued for a minimum of 2 days after the platelet count returns to normal (>150,000 per cubic millimeter).
- Corticosteroids (prednisone 1 to 2 mg/kg/day) may be effective alone in patients with mild disease or may be administered concomitantly with plasmapheresis plus plasma exchange with FFP.
- Vincristine has been used in patients refractory to plasmapheresis.
- Use of antiplatelet agents (ASA, dipyridamole) is controversial.
- Platelet transfusions are contraindicated except in severely thrombocytopenic patients with documented bleeding.
- Splenectomy is performed in refractory cases.

CHRONIC Rx

- Relapsing TTP may be treated with plasma exchange.
- Remission of chronic TTP that is unresponsive to conventional therapy has been reported after treatment with cyclophosphamide and the monoclonal antibody rituximab.
- Splenectomy done while the patients are in remission has been used in some centers to decrease the frequency of relapse in TTP.

DISPOSITION

- Survival of patients with TTP currently exceeds 80% with plasma exchange therapy.
- Relapse occurs in 20% to 40% of patients who have TTP in remission.

REFERRAL

Surgical referral for splenectomy in selected patients (see "Acute General Rx" and "Chronic Rx")

PEARLS & CONSIDERATIONS

COMMENTS

Thrombotic microangiopathy can also be associated with administration of cyclosporine and mitomycin C, and with HIV infection.

EVIDENCE

Plasma exchange vs. plasma infusion with fresh frozen plasma is associated with a significantly higher response rate (increase in platelet count) and lower mortality rate in patients receiving treatment with aspirin and dypridamole for TTP.[1] B

There is no significant difference in outcome between plasma exchange with fresh frozen plasma vs. exchange with cryoprecipitate-poor plasma as initial treatment for patients with TTP.[2] B

Evidence-Based References

1. Rock GA et al: Comparison of plasma exchange with plasma infusion in the treatment of thrombotic thrombocytopenic purpura. Canadian Apheresis Study Group, *N Engl J Med* 325:393, 1991. B
2. Zeigler ZR et al: Cryoprecipitate poor plasma does not improve early response in primary adult thrombotic thrombocytopenic purpura (TTP), *J Clin Apheresis* 16:19, 2001. B

SUGGESTED READING

George JN: Thrombotic thrombocytopenic purpura, *N Engl J Med* 354:1927, 2006.

AUTHOR: **FRED F. FERRI, M.D.**

BASIC INFORMATION

DEFINITION

Thyroid carcinoma is a primary neoplasm of the thyroid. There are four major types of thyroid carcinoma: papillary, follicular, anaplastic, and medullary.

SYNONYMS

Papillary carcinoma of thyroid
Follicular carcinoma of thyroid
Anaplastic carcinoma of thyroid
Medullary carcinoma of thyroid

ICD-9CM CODES
193 Malignant neoplasm of thyroid

EPIDEMIOLOGY & DEMOGRAPHICS

- Thyroid cancer is the most common endocrine cancer, with an annual incidence of 14,000 new cases in the U.S. and about 1100 deaths.
- Female:male ratio of 3:1.
- Most common type (50% to 60%) is papillary carcinoma.
- Median age at diagnosis: 45 to 50 yr.

PHYSICAL FINDINGS & CLINICAL PRESENTATION

- Presence of thyroid nodule
- Hoarseness and cervical lymphadenopathy
- Painless swelling in the region of the thyroid

ETIOLOGY

- Risk factors: prior neck irradiation
- Multiple endocrine neoplasia II (medullary carcinoma)

DIAGNOSIS

DIFFERENTIAL DIAGNOSIS

- Multinodular goiter
- Lymphocytic thyroiditis
- Ectopic thyroid

WORKUP

The workup of thyroid carcinoma includes laboratory evaluation and diagnostic imaging. However, diagnosis is confirmed with fine-needle aspiration (FNA) or surgical biopsy. The characteristics of thyroid carcinoma vary with the type:

- Papillary carcinoma
  1. Most frequently occurs in women during second or third decades
  2. Histologically, psammoma bodies (calcific bodies present in papillary projections) are pathognomonic; they are found in 35% to 45% of papillary thyroid carcinomas
  3. Majority are not papillary lesions but mixed papillary follicular carcinomas
  4. Spread is via lymphatics and by local invasion
- Follicular carcinoma
  1. More aggressive than papillary carcinoma
  2. Incidence increases with age
  3. Tends to metastasize hematogenously to bone, producing pathologic fractures
  4. Tends to concentrate iodine (useful for radiation therapy)
- Anaplastic carcinoma
  1. Very aggressive neoplasm
  2. Two major histologic types: small cell (less aggressive, 5-yr survival approximately 20%) and giant cell (death usually within 6 mo of diagnosis)
- Medullary carcinoma
  1. Unifocal lesion: found sporadically in elderly patients
  2. Bilateral lesions: associated with pheochromocytoma and hyperparathyroidism; this combination is known as MEN-II and is inherited as an autosomal dominant disorder

LABORATORY TESTS

- Thyroid function studies are generally normal. TSH, T_4, and serum thyroglobulin levels should be obtained before thyroidectomy in patients with confirmed thyroid carcinoma
- Increased plasma calcitonin assay in patients with medullary carcinoma (tumors produce thyrocalcitonin)

IMAGING STUDIES

- Thyroid scanning with iodine-123 or technetium-99m can identify hypofunctioning (cold) nodules, which are more likely to be malignant. However, warm nodules can also be malignant.
- Thyroid ultrasound can detect solitary solid nodules that have a high risk of malignancy. However, a negative ultrasound does not exclude diagnosis of thyroid carcinoma.
- FNA biopsy is the best method to assess a thyroid nodule (refer to "Thyroid Nodule" in Section I).

TREATMENT

ACUTE GENERAL Rx

- Papillary carcinoma
  1. Total thyroidectomy is indicated if the patient has:
     a. Extrapyramidal extension of carcinoma
     b. Papillary carcinoma limited to thyroid but a positive history of irradiation to the neck
     c. Lesion >2 cm
  2. Lobectomy with isthmectomy may be considered in patients with intrathyroid papillary carcinoma <2 cm and no history of neck or head irradiation; most follow surgery with suppressive therapy with thyroid hormone because these tumors are TSH responsive. The accepted practice is to suppress serum TSH concentrations to <0.1 μU/ml.
  3. Radiotherapy with iodine-131 (after total thyroidectomy), followed by thyroid suppression therapy with triiodothyronine, can be used in metastatic papillary carcinoma.
- Follicular carcinoma
  1. Total thyroidectomy followed by TSH suppression as noted previously
  2. Radiotherapy with iodine-131 followed by thyroid suppression therapy with triiodothyronine is useful in patients with metastasis
- Anaplastic carcinoma
  1. At diagnosis, this neoplasm is rarely operable; palliative surgery is indicated for extremely large tumor compressing the trachea.
  2. Management is usually restricted to radiation therapy or chemotherapy (combination of doxorubicin, cisplatin, and other antineoplastic agents); these measures rarely provide significant palliation.
- Medullary carcinoma
  1. Thyroidectomy should be performed.
  2. Patients and their families should be screened for pheochromocytoma and hyperparathyroidism.

DISPOSITION

Prognosis varies with the type of thyroid carcinoma: 5-yr survival approaches 80% for follicular carcinoma and is approximately 5% with anaplastic carcinoma.

PEARLS & CONSIDERATIONS

COMMENTS

Family members of patients with medullary carcinoma should be screened; DNA analysis for the detection of mutations in the RET gene structure permits the identification of MEN IIA gene carriers.

AUTHOR: **FRED F. FERRI, M.D.**

BASIC INFORMATION

DEFINITION

A thyroid nodule is an abnormality found on physical examination of the thyroid gland; nodules can be benign (70%) or malignant.

ICD-9CM CODES
241.0 Nodule, thyroid

EPIDEMIOLOGY & DEMOGRAPHICS

- Palpable thyroid nodules occur in 4% to 7% of the population.
- Thyroid nodules can be found in 50% of autopsies; however, only 1 in 10 is palpable.
- Malignancy is present in 5% to 30% of palpable nodules.
- Incidence of thyroid nodules increases after 45 yr of age. They are found more frequently in women.
- History of prior head and neck irradiation increases the risk of thyroid cancer.
- Increased likelihood that nodule is malignant: nodule increasing in size or >2 cm, regional lymphadenopathy, fixation to adjacent tissues, age <40 yr, symptoms of local invasion (dysphagia, hoarseness, neck pain, male sex, family history of thyroid cancer or polyposis [Gardner syndrome]), rapid growth during levothyroxine therapy.

PHYSICAL FINDINGS & CLINICAL PRESENTATION

- Palpable, firm, and nontender nodule in the thyroid area should prompt suspicion of carcinoma. Signs of metastasis are regional lymphadenopathy, inspiratory stridor.
- Signs and symptoms of thyrotoxicosis can be found in functioning nodules.

ETIOLOGY

- History of prior head and neck irradiation
- Family history of pheochromocytoma, carcinoma of the thyroid, and hyperparathyroidism (medullary carcinoma of the thyroid is a component of MEN-II)

DIAGNOSIS

DIFFERENTIAL DIAGNOSIS

- Thyroid carcinoma
- Multinodular goiter
- Thyroglossal duct cyst
- Epidermoid cyst
- Laryngocele
- Nonthyroid neck neoplasm
- Branchial cleft cyst

WORKUP

- Fine-needle aspiration (FNA) biopsy is the best diagnostic study; the accuracy can be >90%, but it is directly related to the level of experience of the physician and the cytopathologist interpreting the aspirate.
- FNA biopsy is less reliable with thyroid cystic lesions; surgical excision should be considered for most thyroid cysts not abolished by aspiration.
- A diagnostic approach to thyroid nodule is described in Section III.

LABORATORY TESTS

- TSH, T_4, and serum thyroglobulin levels should be obtained before thyroidectomy in patients with confirmed thyroid carcinoma on FNA biopsy.
- Serum calcitonin at random or after pentagastrin stimulation is useful when suspecting medullary carcinoma of the thyroid and in anyone with a family history of medullary thyroid carcinoma.
- Serum thyroid autoantibodies (see "Thyroiditis" in Section I) are useful when suspecting thyroiditis.

IMAGING STUDIES

- Thyroid ultrasound is done in some patients to evaluate the size of the thyroid and the number, composition (solid vs. cystic), and dimensions of the thyroid nodule; solid thyroid nodules have a higher incidence of malignancy, but cystic nodules can also be malignant.
- The introduction of high-resolution ultrasonography has made it possible to detect many nonpalpable nodules (incidentalomas) in the thyroid (found at autopsy in 30% to 60% of cadavers). Most of these lesions are benign. For most patients with nonpalpable nodules that are incidentally detected by thyroid imaging, simple follow-up neck palpation is sufficient.
- Thyroid scan can be performed with technetium-99m pertechnetate, iodine-123, or iodine-131. Iodine isotopes are preferred because 35% to 8% of nodules that appear functioning on pertechnetate scanning may appear nonfunctioning on radioiodine scanning. A thyroid scan:
  1. Classifies nodules as hyperfunctioning (hot), normally functioning (warm), or nonfunctioning (cold); cold nodules have a higher incidence of malignancy.
  2. Scan has difficulty evaluating nodules near the thyroid isthmus or at the periphery of the gland.
  3. Normal tissue over a nonfunctioning nodule might mask the nodule as "warm" or normally functioning.
- Both thyroid scan and ultrasound provide information about the risk of malignant neoplasia based on the characteristics of the thyroid nodule, but their value in the initial evaluation of a thyroid nodule is limited because neither provides a definite tissue diagnosis.

TREATMENT

GENERAL Rx

- Evaluation of results of FNA
  1. Normal cells: may repeat biopsy during present evaluation or reevaluate patient after 3 to 6 mo of suppressive therapy (l-thyroxine, prescribed in doses to suppress the TSH level to 0.1 to 0.5)
     a. Failure to regress indicates increased likelihood of malignancy.
     b. Reliance on repeat needle biopsy is preferable to routine surgery for nodules not responding to thyroxine.
  2. Malignant cells: surgery
  3. Hypercellularity: thyroid scan
     a. Hot nodule: ^{131}I therapy if the patient is hyperthyroid
     b. Warm or cold nodule: surgery (rule out follicular adenoma vs. carcinoma)

DISPOSITION

Variable with results of FNA biopsy

REFERRAL

Surgical referral for FNA biopsy

PEARLS & CONSIDERATIONS

COMMENTS

- Most solid, benign nodules grow, therefore an increase in nodule volume alone is not a reliable predictor of malignancy.
- Surgery is indicated in hard or fixed nodule, presence of dysphagia or hoarseness, and rapidly growing solid masses regardless of "benign" results on FNA.
- Suppressive therapy of malignant thyroid nodules postoperatively with thyroxine is indicated. The use of suppressive therapy for benign solitary nodules is controversial.
- The preferred approach when repeated FNA fails to yield an adequate specimen remains a challenge. Immunohistochemical markers (galectin-3, human bone marrow endothelial cell [HBME-1]) have shown promise in preliminary studies. Routine calcitonin measurement for early detection of medullary carcinoma remains controversial due to the low frequency of this cancer and the high cost associated with case detection.

SUGGESTED READINGS

Castro MR, Gharib H: Continuing controversies in the management of thyroid nodules, *Ann Intern Med* 142:926, 2005.

Shetty SK et al: Significance of incidental thyroid lesions detected on CT: correlation among CT, sonography, and pathology, *Am J Roentgenol* 187:1349, 2006.

AUTHOR: **FRED F. FERRI, M.D.**

BASIC INFORMATION

DEFINITION

Thyroiditis is an inflammatory disease of the thyroid. It is a multifaceted disease with varying etiology, different clinical characteristics (depending on the stage), and distinct histopathology. Thyroiditis can be subdivided into three common types (Hashimoto's, painful, painless) and two rare forms (suppurative, Riedel's). To add to the confusion, there are various synonyms for each form, and there is no internationally accepted classification of autoimmune thyroid disease.

SYNONYMS

Hashimoto's thyroiditis: *chronic lymphocytic thyroiditis, chronic autoimmune thyroiditis, lymphadenoid goiter*
Painful subacute thyroiditis: subacute thyroiditis, *giant cell thyroiditis, de Quervain's thyroiditis, subacute granulomatous thyroiditis, pseudogranulomatous thyroiditis*
Painless postpartum thyroiditis: *subacute lymphocytic thyroiditis, postpartum thyroiditis*
Painless sporadic thyroiditis: *silent sporadic thyroiditis, subacute lymphocytic thyroiditis*
Suppurative thyroiditis: *acute suppurative thyroiditis, bacterial thyroiditis microbial inflammatory thyroiditis, pyogenic thyroiditis*
Riedel's thyroiditis: *fibrous thyroiditis*

ICD-9CM CODES
245.2 Hashimoto's thyroiditis
245.1 Subacute thyroiditis
245.9 Silent thyroiditis
245.0 Suppurative thyroiditis
245.3 Riedel's thyroiditis

PHYSICAL FINDINGS & CLINICAL PRESENTATION

- Hashimoto's: patients may have signs of hyperthyroidism (tachycardia, diaphoresis, palpitations, weight loss) or hypothyroidism (fatigue, weight gain, delayed reflexes) depending on the stage of the disease. Usually there is diffuse, firm enlargement of the thyroid gland; thyroid gland may also be of normal size (atrophic form with clinically manifested hypothyroidism).
- Painful subacute: exquisitely tender, enlarged thyroid, fever; signs of hyperthyroidism are initially present; signs of hypothyroidism can subsequently develop.
- Painless thyroiditis: clinical features are similar to subacute thyroiditis except for the absence of tenderness of the thyroid gland.
- Suppurative: patient is febrile with severe neck pain, focal tenderness of the involved portion of the thyroid, erythema of the overlying skin.
- Riedel's: slowly enlarging hard mass in the anterior neck; often mistaken for thyroid cancer; signs of hypothyroidism occur in advanced stages.

ETIOLOGY

- Hashimoto's: autoimmune disorder that begins with the activation of CD4 (helper) T-lymphocytes specific for thyroid antigens. The etiologic factor for the activation of these cells is unknown.
- Painful subacute: possibly postviral; usually follows a respiratory illness; it is not considered to be a form of autoimmune thyroiditis.
- Painless thyroiditis: it frequently occurs postpartum.
- Suppurative: infectious etiology, generally bacterial, although fungi and parasites have also been implicated; it often occurs in immunocompromised hosts or following a penetrating neck injury.
- Riedel's: fibrous infiltration of the thyroid; etiology is unknown.
- Drug induced: lithium, interferon alfa, amiodarone, interleukin-2.

DIAGNOSIS

DIFFERENTIAL DIAGNOSIS

- The hyperthyroid phase of Hashimoto's, subacute, or silent thyroiditis can be mistaken for Graves' disease.
- Riedel's thyroiditis can be mistaken for carcinoma of the thyroid.
- Painful subacute thyroiditis can be mistaken for infections of the oropharynx and trachea or for suppurative thyroiditis.
- Factitious hyperthyroidism can mimic silent thyroiditis.

WORKUP

- The diagnostic workup includes laboratory and radiologic evaluation to rule out other conditions that may mimic thyroiditis (see "Differential Diagnosis") and to differentiate the various forms of thyroiditis.
- The patient's medical history may be helpful in differentiating the various types of thyroiditis (e.g., presentation following childbirth is suggestive of silent [postpartum, painless] thyroiditis; occurrence following a viral respiratory infection suggests subacute thyroiditis; history of penetrating injury to the neck indicates suppurative thyroiditis).

LABORATORY TESTS

- TSH, free T_4: may be normal, or indicative of hypo- or hyperthyroidism depending on the stage of the thyroiditis.
- WBC with differential: increased WBC with "shift to the left" occurs with subacute and suppurative thyroiditis.
- Antimicrosomal antibodies: detected in >90% of patients with Hashimoto's thyroiditis and 50% to 80% of patients with silent thyroiditis.
- Serum thyroglobulin levels are elevated in patients with subacute and silent thyroiditis; this test is nonspecific but may be useful in monitoring the course of subacute thyroiditis and distinguishing silent thyroiditis from factitious hyperthyroidism (low or absent serum thyroglobulin level).

IMAGING STUDIES

24-hr radioactive iodine uptake (RAIU) is useful to distinguish Graves' disease (increased RAIU) from thyroiditis (normal or low RAIU).

TREATMENT

ACUTE GENERAL Rx

- Treat hypothyroid phase with levothyroxine 25 to 50 μg/day initially and monitor serum TSH initially every 6 to 8 wk.
- Control symptoms of hyperthyroidism with β-blockers (e.g., propranolol 20 to 40 mg PO q6h).
- Control pain in patients with subacute thyroiditis with NSAIDs. Prednisone 20 to 40 mg qd may be used if NSAIDs are insufficient, but it should be gradually tapered off over several weeks.
- Use IV antibiotics and drain abscess (if present) in patients with suppurative thyroiditis.

DISPOSITION

- Hashimoto's thyroiditis: long-term prognosis is favorable; most patients recover their thyroid function.
- Painful subacute thyroiditis: permanent hypothyroidism occurs in 10% of patients.
- Painless thyroiditis: 6% of patients have permanent hypothyroidism.
- Suppurative thyroiditis: there is usually full recovery following treatment.
- Riedel's thyroiditis: hypothyroidism occurs when fibrous infiltration involves the entire thyroid.

REFERRAL

Surgical referral in patients with compression of adjacent neck structures and in some patients with suppurative thyroiditis

SUGGESTED READINGS

Bindra A, Braunstein GD: Thyroiditis, *Am Fam Physician* 73:1769, 2006.
Pearce EN et al: Thyroiditis, *N Engl J Med* 348:2646, 2003.

AUTHOR: **FRED F. FERRI, M.D.**

BASIC INFORMATION

DEFINITION

Thyrotoxic storm is the abrupt and severe exacerbation of thyrotoxicosis.

ICD-9CM CODES
242.9 Thyrotoxic storm
242.0 With goiter
242.2 Multinodular
242.3 Adenomatous
242.8 Thyrotoxicosis factitia

PHYSICAL FINDINGS & CLINICAL PRESENTATION

- Goiter
- Tremor, tachycardia, fever
- Warm, moist skin
- Lid lag, lid retraction, proptosis
- Altered mental status (psychosis, coma, seizures)
- Other: evidence of precipitating factors (infection, trauma)

ETIOLOGY

- Major stress (e.g., infection, MI, DKA) in an undiagnosed hyperthyroid patient
- Inadequate therapy in a hyperthyroid patient

DIAGNOSIS

The clinical presentation is variable. The patient may present with the following signs and symptoms:

- Fever
- Marked anxiety and agitation, psychosis
- Hyperhidrosis, heat intolerance
- Marked weakness and muscle wasting
- Tachyarrhythmias, palpitations
- Diarrhea, nausea, vomiting
- Elderly patients may have a combination of tachycardia, CHF, and mental status changes

DIFFERENTIAL DIAGNOSIS

- Psychiatric disorders
- Alcohol or other drug withdrawal
- Pheochromocytoma
- Metastatic neoplasm

WORKUP

- Laboratory evaluation to confirm hyperthyroidism (elevated free T_4, decreased TSH)
- Evaluation for precipitating factors (e.g., ECG and cardiac enzymes in suspected MI, blood and urine cultures to rule out sepsis)
- Elimination of disorders noted in the differential diagnosis (e.g., psychiatric history, evidence of drug and alcohol abuse)

LABORATORY TESTS

- Free T_4, TSH
- CBC with differential
- Blood and urine cultures
- Glucose
- Liver enzymes
- BUN, creatinine
- Serum calcium
- CPK

IMAGING STUDIES

Chest x-ray to exclude infectious process, neoplasm, CHF in suspected cases

TREATMENT

NONPHARMACOLOGIC THERAPY

- Nutritional care: replace fluid deficit aggressively (daily fluid requirement may reach 6 L); use solutions containing glucose and add multivitamins to the hydrating solution.
- Monitor for fluid overload and CHF in the elderly and in those with underlying cardiovascular or renal disease.
- Treat significant hyperthermia with cooling blankets.

ACUTE GENERAL Rx

- Inhibition of thyroid hormone synthesis
  1. Administer propylthiouracil (PTU) 300 to 600 mg initially (PO or via NG tube), then 150 to 300 mg q6h.
  2. If the patient is allergic to PTU, use methimazole (Tapazole) 80 to 100 mg PO or PR followed by 30 mg PR q8h.
- Inhibition of stored thyroid hormone
  1. Iodide can be administered as sodium iodine 250 mg IV q6h, potassium iodide (SSKI) 5 gtt PO q8h, or Lugol's solution, 10 gtt q8h. It is important to administer PTU or methimazole 1 hr *before* the iodide to prevent the oxidation of iodide to iodine and its incorporation in the synthesis of additional thyroid hormone.
  2. Corticosteroids: dexamethasone 2 mg IV q6h or hydrocortisone 100 mg IV q6h for approximately 48 hr is useful to inhibit thyroid hormone release, impair peripheral conversion of T_3 from T_4, and provide additional adrenocortical hormone to correct deficiency (if present).
- Suppression of peripheral effects of thyroid hormone
  1. β-Adrenergic blockers: Administer propranolol 80 to 120 mg PO q4 to 6h. Propranolol may also be given IV 1 mg/min for 2 to 10 min under continuous ECG and blood pressure monitoring. β-Adrenergic blockers must be used with caution in patients with severe CHF or bronchospasm. Cardioselective β-blockers (e.g., esmolol or metoprolol) may be more appropriate for patients with bronchospasm, but these patients must be closely monitored for exacerbation of bronchospasm because these agents lose their cardioselectivity at high doses.
- Control of fever with acetaminophen 325 to 650 mg q4h; avoidance of aspirin because it displaces thyroid hormone from its binding protein
- Consider digitalization of patients with CHF and atrial fibrillation (these patients may require higher than usual digoxin doses)
- Treatment of any precipitating factors (e.g., antibiotics if infection is strongly suspected)

DISPOSITION

Patients with thyrotoxic crisis should be treated and appropriately monitored in the ICU.

REFERRAL

Endocrinology referral is appropriate in patients with thyrotoxic crisis.

PEARLS & CONSIDERATIONS

COMMENTS

If the diagnosis is strongly suspected, therapy should be started immediately without waiting for laboratory confirmation.

AUTHOR: **FRED F. FERRI, M.D.**

BASIC INFORMATION

DEFINITION

Tinea capitis is a dermatophyte infection of the scalp.

SYNONYMS

Ringworm of the scalp, ringworm of the head, gray patch tinea capitis, black dot tinea capitis, tinea tonsurans, superficial mycosis, dermatophytosis, kerion

ICD-9CM CODES

110.0 Tinea capitis

EPIDEMIOLOGY & DEMOGRAPHICS

Tinea capitis is the most common dermatophytosis of childhood, primarily affecting children between 3 and 7 yr of age. About 3% to 8% of American children are affected, and 34% of household contacts are asymptomatic carriers. African American children are particularly susceptible. Adult and geriatric populations are less frequently affected, possibly because of the fungistatic effect of the sebum found in older persons. In urban populations, large family size, low socioeconomic status, and crowded living conditions may contribute to an increased incidence of tinea capitis. The predominant etiologic agent of tinea capitis in the U.S. and in Western Europe has changed from *Microsporum audouinii* to *Trichophyton tonsurans* in the past 50 years.

PHYSICAL FINDINGS & CLINICAL PRESENTATION

- Triad of scalp scaling, alopecia, and cervical adenopathy.
- Primary lesions including plaques, papules, pustules, or nodules on the scalp (usually occipital region).
- Secondary lesions include scales, alopecia (usually reversible), erythema, exudates, and edema.
- Two distinctly different forms:
  - Gray patch: Lesions are scaly and well demarcated. The hairs within the patch break off a few millimeters above the scalp. One or several lesions may be present; sometimes the lesions join to form larger ones.
  - Black dot: Early lesions with erythema and scaling patch are easily overlooked until areas of alopecia develop. Hairs within the patches break at the surface of the scalp, leaving behind a pattern of swollen black dots.
- Scalp pruritus may be present.
- Fever, pain, and lymphadenopathy (commonly postcervical) with inflammatory lesions.
- Kerion: inflamed, exudative, pustular, boggy, tender nodules exhibiting marked edema, and hair loss seen in severe tinea capitis. Caused by immune response to the fungus. May lead to some scarring.
- Favus: production of scutula (hair matted together with dermatophyte hyphae and keratin debris), characterized by yellow cup-shaped crusts around hair shafts. A fetid odor may be present.

ETIOLOGY

Most commonly caused by the *Trichophyton* (80% of the cases in the U.S.) or *Microsporum* genera. Most common causative species for black dot tinea capitis is *T. tonsurans* and for gray patch tinea capitis are *M. andouinii* and *M. canis.* Transmission occurs via infected persons or asymptomatic carriers, fallen infected hairs, animal vectors, and fomites. *M. audouinii* is commonly spread by dogs and cats. Infectious fungal particles may remain viable for many months.

DIAGNOSIS

DIFFERENTIAL DIAGNOSIS

Alopecia areata, impetigo, pediculosis, trichotillomania, traction alopecia, folliculitis, pseudopelade, seborrhea/atopic dermatitis, psoriasis, carbuncles, pyoderma, lichen ruber planus, lupus erythematosus

WORKUP

- KOH testing of hair shaft extracted from the lesion, not the scale, because the *T. tonsurans* spores attach to or reside inside hair shafts and will rarely be found in the scales.
- Wood's ultraviolet light fluoresces blue-green on hair shafts for *Microsporum* infections but will fail to identify *T. tonsurans.*
- Fungal culture of hairs and scales on fungal medium such as Sabouraud's agar may be used to confirm the diagnosis, especially if uncertain.
- Histology of biopsies with fungal staining in cases where mycology tests are negative because of treatment initiation.

TREATMENT

- Griseofulvin—gold standard FDA-approved treatment with excellent long-term safety profile. Micronized and ultramicronized preparations are absorbed better, and side effects are infrequent, especially when administered with fatty meals. Periodic monitoring of hematologic, liver, and renal function may be indicated, especially in prolonged treatment over 8 weeks.
  - Children: higher doses of 20 to 25 mg/kg/d orally (to a maximum of 0.5 to 1.0 gram per day) now recommended for at least 6 to 8 weeks (until hair regrowth occurs or 2 weeks beyond cure to prevent relapse).
  - Adults: 250 mg orally bid or 500 mg qd (or tid for a few cases of black dot type) for 4 to 12 weeks.
- New alternative treatments: oral terbinafine, itraconazole, or fluconazole are comparable in efficacy and safety to griseofulvin, with shorter treatment and better patient compliance. Monitoring of CBC, liver function tests, and renal function may be indicated.
- The adjuvant use of antifungal shampoos is recommended for all patients and household contacts. Shampoo like selenium sulfide 2.5% used for 5 minutes or ketoconazole shampoo used 2 to 3 times/week can help prevent infection or eradicate asymptomatic carrier state by inhibiting fungal growth.
- Severe inflammatory kerion can be managed with additional prednisone 1 mg/kg/day and erythromycin.

PEARLS & CONSIDERATIONS

COMMENTS

- Confirming the diagnosis of tinea capitis with a laboratory specimen is important because misdiagnosis will result in delay or improper treatment.
- Patients and their families should look for sources of infections and disinfect contaminated objects such as combs, brushes, towels, and headgear. Avoid sharing personal hygiene utensils.
- Culture of hairs and scalp dander facilitates carrier identification and prevention.
- Pets that are infected or asymptomatic carriers should be treated.
- Recommend follow-up visit every 2 to 4 weeks using Wood's light, microscopic study, and fungal culture. A mycologically documented cure is the goal of treatment.

SUGGESTED READINGS

Elewski BE: Tinea capitis: a current perspective, *J Am Acad Dermatol* 41:1-20, 2000.

Gilbert DN et al: *The Sanford Guide to Antimicrobial Therapy 2005,* Hyde Park, VT, 2005, Antimicrobial Therapy.

Goldstein AO et al: Mycotic infections: effective management of conditions involving the skin, hair, and nails, *Geriatrics* 55(5):40-52, 2000.

Mohrenschlager M et al: Pediatric tinea capitis: recognition and management, *Am J Clin Dermatol* 6(4):203-213, 2005.

Roberts BJ, Friedlander SF: Tinea capitis: a treatment update, *Pediatr Ann* 34(3):191-200, 2005.

Seebacher C et al: Tinea capitis: ringworm of the scalp, *Mycoses* 50(3):218-226, 2007.

Shy R: Tinea corporis and tinea capitis, *Pediatr Rev* 28(5):164-174, 2007.

Strober BE: Tinea capitis, *Dermatol Online J* 7(1):12, 2000.

Trovato MJ et al: Tinea capitis: current concepts in clinical practice, *Cutis* 77(2):93-99, 2006.

AUTHOR: **MARIE ELIZABETH WONG, M.D.**

BASIC INFORMATION

DEFINITION

Tinea corporis is a dermatophyte fungal infection caused by the genera *Trichophyton* or *Microsporum*.

SYNONYMS

Ringworm
Body ringworm
Tinea circinata

ICD-9CM CODES
110.5 Tinea corporis

EPIDEMIOLOGY & DEMOGRAPHICS

- The disease is more common in warm climates.
- There is no predominant age or sex.

PHYSICAL FINDINGS & CLINICAL PRESENTATION

- Typically appears as single or multiple annular lesions with an advancing scaly border; the margin is slightly raised, reddened, and may be pustular.
- The central area becomes hypopigmented and less scaly as the active border progresses outward (Fig. 1-271).
- The trunk and legs are primarily involved.
- Pruritus is variable.
- It is important to remember that recent topical corticosteroid use can significantly alter the appearance of the lesions.

ETIOLOGY

Trichophyton rubrum is the most common pathogen.

DIAGNOSIS

DIFFERENTIAL DIAGNOSIS

- Pityriasis rosea
- Erythema multiforme
- Psoriasis
- SLE
- Syphilis
- Nummular eczema
- Eczema
- Granuloma annulare
- Lyme disease
- Tinea versicolor
- Contact dermatitis

WORKUP

Diagnosis is usually made on clinical grounds. It can be confirmed by direct visualization under the microscope of a small fragment of the scale using wet mount preparation and potassium hydroxide solution; dermatophytes appear as translucent branching filaments (hyphae) with lines of separation appearing at irregular intervals.

LABORATORY TESTS

- Microscopic examination of hyphae
- Mycotic culture is usually not necessary
- Biopsy is indicated only when the diagnosis is uncertain and the patient has failed to respond to treatment

TREATMENT

NONPHARMACOLOGIC THERAPY

Affected areas should be kept clean and dry.

ACUTE GENERAL Rx

- Various creams are effective; the application area should include normal skin about 2 cm beyond the affected area:
  1. Miconazole 2% cream (Monistat-Derm) applied bid for 2 wk
  2. Clotrimazole 1% cream (Mycelex) applied and gently massaged into the affected areas and surrounding areas bid for up to 4 wk
  3. Naftifine 1% cream (Naftin) applied qd
  4. Econazole 1% (Spectazole) applied qd
- Systemic therapy is reserved for severe cases and is usually given up to 4 wk; commonly used agents:
  1. Ketoconazole (Nizoral), 200 mg qd
  2. Fluconazole (Diflucan), 200 mg qd
  3. Terbinafine (Lamisil), 250 mg qd

DISPOSITION

Majority of cases resolve without sequelae within 3 to 4 wk of therapy.

REFERRAL

Dermatology referral in patients with persistent or recurrent infections

SUGGESTED READINGS

Friedlander SF et al: Terbinafine in the treatment of trichophytin tinea capitis, *Pediatrics* 109:602, 2002.
Hainer BL: Dermatophyte infections, *Am Fam Physician* 67:101, 2003.
Weinstein A, Berman B: Topical treatment of common superficial tinea infections, *Am Fam Physician* 65:2095, 2002.

AUTHOR: **FRED F. FERRI, M.D.**

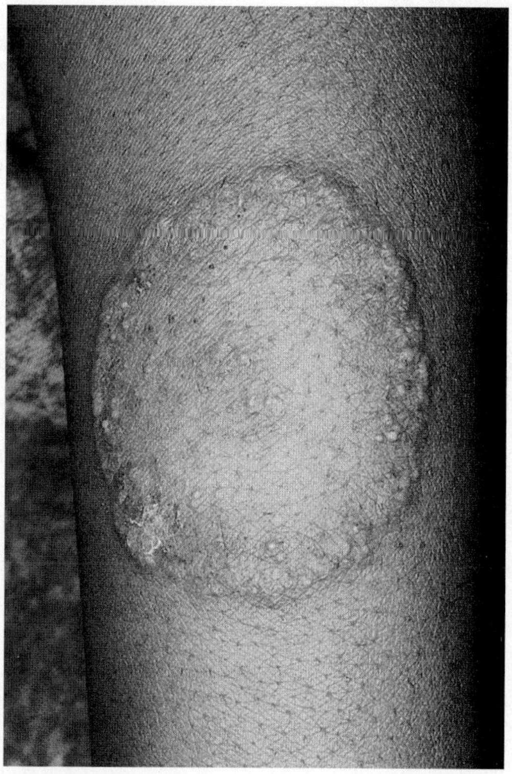

FIGURE 1-271 Annular lesion (tinea corporis). Note raised erythematous scaling border and central clearing. (From Noble J et al: *Textbook of primary care medicine,* ed 3, St Louis, 2001, Mosby.)

BASIC INFORMATION

DEFINITION

Tinea cruris is a dermatophyte infection of the groin.

SYNONYMS

Jock itch
Ringworm

ICD-9CM CODES
110.3 Tinea cruris

EPIDEMIOLOGY & DEMOGRAPHICS

- Most common during the summer
- Men are affected more frequently than women

PHYSICAL FINDINGS & CLINICAL PRESENTATION

- Erythematous plaques have a half-moon shape and a scaling border.
- The acute inflammation tends to move down the inner thigh and usually spares the scrotum; in severe cases the fungus may spread onto the buttocks.
- Itching may be severe.
- Red papules and pustules may be present.
- An important diagnostic sign is the advancing well-defined border with a tendency toward central clearing (Fig. 1-272).

ETIOLOGY

- Dermatophytes of the genera *Trichophyton, Epidermophyton,* and *Microsporum. T. rubrum* and *E. floccosum* are the most common causes.
- Transmission from direct contact (e.g., infected persons, animals). The patient's feet should be evaluated as a source of infection because tinea cruris is often associated with tinea pedis.

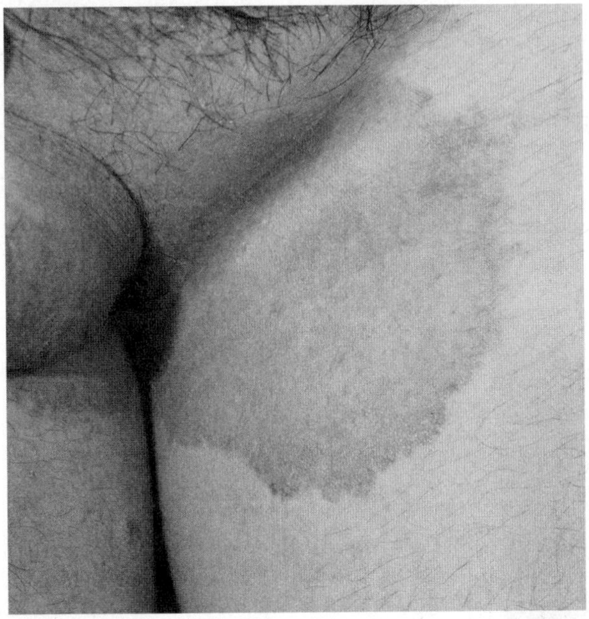

FIGURE 1-272 Tinea cruris. A halfmoon-shaped plaque has a well-defined, scaling border. (From Habif TB: *Clinical dermatology: a color guide to diagnosis and therapy,* ed 3, St Louis, 1996, Mosby.)

DIAGNOSIS

DIFFERENTIAL DIAGNOSIS

- Intertrigo
- Psoriasis
- Seborrheic dermatitis
- Erythrasma
- Candidiasis
- Tinea versicolor

WORKUP

Diagnosis is based on clinical presentation and demonstration of hyphae microscopically using potassium hydroxide.

LABORATORY TESTS

- Microscopic examination
- Cultures are generally not necessary

TREATMENT

NONPHARMACOLOGIC THERAPY

- Keep infected area clean and dry.
- Use of boxer shorts is preferred to regular underwear.

ACUTE GENERAL Rx

- Drying powders (e.g., Miconazole nitrate [Zeasorb AF]) may be useful in patients with excessive perspiration.
- Various topical antifungal agents are available: miconazole (Lotrimin), terbinafine (Lamisil), sulconazole nitrate (Exelderm), betamethasone dipropionate/clotrimazole (Lotrisone).
- Oral antifungal therapy is generally reserved for cases unresponsive to topical agents. Effective medications are itraconazole (Sporonax) 100 mg/day for 2 to 4 wk, ketoconazole (Nizoral) 200 mg qd, fluconazole (Diflucan) 200 mg qd, and terbinafine (Lamisil) 250 mg qd.

DISPOSITION

Most cases respond promptly to therapy with complete resolution within 2 to 3 wk.

SUGGESTED READING

Hainer BL: Dermatophyte infections, *Am Fam Physician* 67:101, 2003.

AUTHOR: **FRED F. FERRI, M.D.**

BASIC INFORMATION

DEFINITION

Tinea pedis is a dermatophyte infection of the feet.

SYNONYMS

Athlete's foot

ICD-CM CODES
110.4 Tinea pedis

EPIDEMIOLOGY & DEMOGRAPHICS

- Most common dermatophyte infection
- Increased incidence in hot humid weather. Occlusive footwear is a contributing factor
- Occurrence is rare before adolescence
- More common in adult males

PHYSICAL FINDINGS & CLINICAL PRESENTATION

- Typical presentation is variable and ranges from erythematous scaling plaques (Fig. 1-273) and isolated blisters to interdigital maceration.
- The infection usually starts in the interdigital spaces of the foot. Most infections are found in the toe webs or in the soles.
- Fourth or fifth toes are most commonly involved.
- Pruritus is common and is most intense following removal of shoes and socks.
- Infection with *tinea rubrum* often manifests with a moccasin distribution affecting the soles and lateral feet.

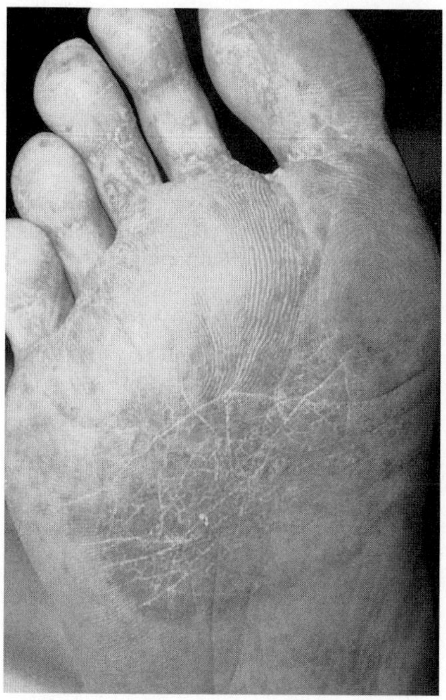

FIGURE 1-273 Tinea pedis. (From Goldstein BG, Goldstein AO: *Practical dermatology,* ed 2, St Louis, 1997, Mosby.)

ETIOLOGY

Dermatophyte infection caused by *T. rubrum, T. mentagrophytes,* or less commonly *E. floccosum*

DIAGNOSIS

DIFFERENTIAL DIAGNOSIS

- Contact dermatitis
- Toe web infection
- Eczema
- Psoriasis
- Keratolysis exfoliativa
- Juvenile plantar dermatosis

WORKUP

- Diagnosis is usually made by clinical observation.
- Laboratory testing, when performed, generally consists of a simple potassium hydroxide (KOH) preparation with mycologic examination under a light microscope to confirm the presence of dermatophytes.

LABORATORY TESTS

- Microscopic examination of a scale or the roof of a blister with 10% KOH under low or medium power will reveal hyphae.
- Mycologic culture is rarely indicated in the diagnosis of tinea pedis.
- Biopsy is reserved for when the diagnosis remains in question after testing or failure to respond to treatment.

TREATMENT

NONPHARMACOLOGIC THERAPY

- Keep infected area clean and dry. Aerate feet by using sandals when possible.
- Use 100% cotton socks rather than nylon socks to reduce moisture.
- Areas likely to become infected should be dried completely before being covered with clothes.

ACUTE GENERAL Rx

- Butenafine Hcl 1% (Mentax) cream applied bid for 1 wk or qd for 4 wk is effective in interdigital tinea pedis.
- Ciclopirox 0.77 % (Loprox) cream applied bid for 4 wk is also effective.
- Clotrimazole 1% (Lotrimin AF) cream is an OTC treatment. It should be applied to affected and surrounding area bid for up to 4 wk.
- Naftifine (Naftin) 1 % cream applied qd or gel applied bid for 4 wk also produces a significantly high cure rate.
- When using topical preparations, the application area should include normal skin about 2 cm beyond the affected area.
- Areas of maceration can be treated with Burow's solution soaks for 10 to 20 min bid followed by foot elevation.
- Oral agents (fluconazole 150 mg once/wk for 4 wk) can be used in combination with topical agents in resistant cases.

PEARLS & CONSIDERATIONS

Combination therapy of antifungal and corticosteroid (clotrimazole/betamethasone [Lotrisone]) should only be used when the diagnosis of fungal infection is confirmed and inflammation is a significant issue.

EVIDENCE

A systematic review found that topical allylamines are significantly more effective than placebo for the treatment of fungal infections of the foot. Allylamines were found to be slightly more effective than azoles, although they are more expensive.[1] Ⓐ

Terbinafine cream has been shown to be more effective than placebo for the treatment of interdigital tinea pedis.[2] Ⓐ

Terbinafine cream and butenafine cream have been shown to be more effective than placebo for the treatment of moccasin-type tinea pedis. There was no significant difference in cure rates between the treatment groups in this randomized controlled trial (RCT).[3] Ⓐ

A systematic review compared various oral antifungals for treatment of tinea pedis. Terbinafine and itraconazole were found to be more effective than placebo in two RCTs. There was no difference in efficacy between fluconazole and itraconazole; terbinafine was found to be more effective than griseofulvin.[4] Ⓐ

Evidence-Based References

1. Crawford F et al: Topical treatments for fungal infections of the skin and nails of the foot, *Cochrane Database Syst Rev* 3:1999. Ⓐ
2. Korting HC et al. for the LAS-INT-06 Study Group: One week terbinafine 1% cream (Lamisil) once daily is effective in the treatment of interdigital tinea pedis: a vehicle controlled study, *Med Mycology* 39:335, 2000. Reviewed in: *Clin Evid* 13:2060, 2005. Ⓐ
3. Syed TA et al: Butenafine 1% versus terbenafine 1% in cream for the treatment of tinea pedis. A placebo controlled double-blind comparative study, *Clin Drug Invest* 19:393, 2000. Reviewed in: *Clin Evid* 11:2128, 2004. Ⓐ
4. Bell-Syer SEM et al: Oral treatments for fungal infections of the skin of the foot (Cochrane Review). Reviewed in: Cochrane Library 1:2004, Chichester, UK, John Wiley. Ⓐ

SUGGESTED READING

Weinstein A, Berman B: Topical treatment of common superficial tinea infections, *Am Fam Physician* 65:2095, 2002.

AUTHOR: **FRED F. FERRI, M.D.**

BASIC INFORMATION

DEFINITION

Tinea versicolor is a fungal infection of the skin caused by the yeast *Pityrosporum orbiculare (Malassezia furfur)*.

SYNONYMS

Pityriasis versicolor

ICD-9CM CODES
111.0 Tinea versicolor

EPIDEMIOLOGY & DEMOGRAPHICS

- Increased incidence in adolescence and young adulthood
- More common during the summer (hypopigmented lesions are more evident when the skin is tanned)

PHYSICAL FINDINGS & CLINICAL PRESENTATION

- Most lesions begin as multiple small, circular macules of various colors.
- The macules may be darker or lighter than the surrounding normal skin and will scale with scraping.
- Most frequent site of distribution is trunk.
- Facial lesions are more common in children (forehead is most common facial site).
- Eruption is generally of insidious onset and asymptomatic.
- Lesions may be hyperpigmented in blacks.
- Lesions may be inconspicuous in fair-complexioned individuals, especially during the winter.
- Most patients become aware of the eruption when the involved areas do not tan (Fig. 1-274).

ETIOLOGY

The infection is caused by the lipophilic yeast *P. orbiculare* (round form) and *P. ovale* (oval form); these organisms are normal inhabitants of the skin flora; factors that favor their proliferation are pregnancy, malnutrition, immunosuppression, oral contraceptives, and excess heat and humidity.

DIAGNOSIS

DIFFERENTIAL DIAGNOSIS

- Vitiligo
- Pityriasis alba
- Secondary syphilis
- Pityriasis rosea
- Seborrheic dermatitis

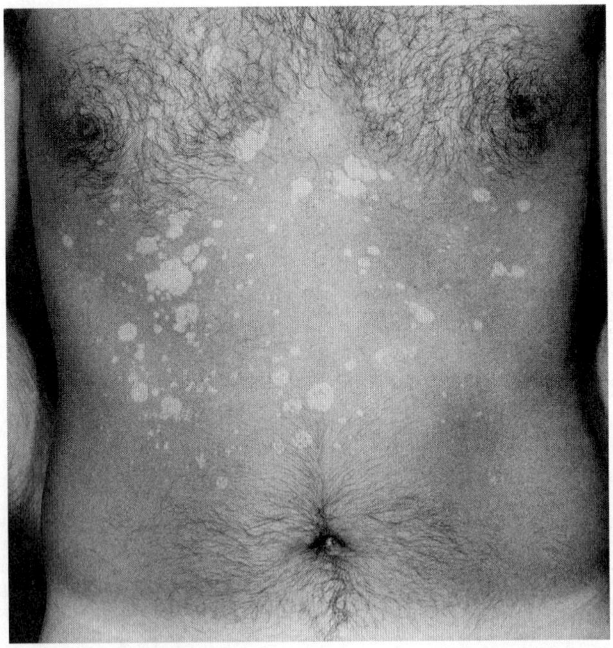

FIGURE 1-274 The classic presentation of tinea versicolor with white, oval, or circular patches on tan skin. (From Habif TB: *Clinical dermatology: a color guide to diagnosis and therapy,* ed 3, St Louis, 1996, Mosby.)

WORKUP

Diagnosis is based on clinical appearance; identification of hyphae and budding spores (spaghetti and meatballs appearance) with microscopy confirms diagnosis.

LABORATORY TESTS

Microscopic examination using potassium hydroxide confirms diagnosis when in doubt.

TREATMENT

NONPHARMACOLOGIC THERAPY

Sunlight accelerates repigmentation of hypopigmented areas.

ACUTE GENERAL Rx

- Topical treatment: selenium sulfide 2.5% suspension (Selsun or Exsel) applied daily for 10 min for 7 consecutive days results in a cure rate of 80% to 90%.
- Antifungal topical agents (e.g., miconazole, ciclopirox, clotrimazole) are also effective but generally expensive.
- Oral treatment is generally reserved for resistant cases. Effective agents are ketoconazole (Nizoral) 200 mg qd for 5 days, or single 400-mg dose (cure rate >80%), fluconazole (Diflucan) 400 mg given as a single dose (cure rate >70% at 3 wk after treatment), or itraconazole 200 mg/day for 5 days.

DISPOSITION

The prognosis is good, with death of the fungus usually occurring within 3 to 4 wk of treatment; however, recurrence is common.

PEARLS & CONSIDERATIONS

COMMENTS

Patients should be informed that the hypopigmented areas will not disappear immediately after treatment and that several months may be necessary for the hypopigmented areas to regain their pigmentation.

AUTHOR: **FRED F. FERRI, M.D.**

BASIC INFORMATION

DEFINITION

Tinnitus is an unwanted auditory perception of internal origin, usually localized and rarely heard by others. It usually involves a high-pitched sound with a buzzing or ringing quality.

SYNONYM

Ringing in the ear(s)

ICD-9CM CODES
388.30 Tinnitus

EPIDEMIOLOGY & DEMOGRAPHICS

Tinnitus increases with age. The most recent prevalence statistics from the National Center for Health Statistics (1999) indicate that tinnitus affects approximately 18% of the population. The American Tinnitus Association reports that 50 million Americans have tinnitus. It is slightly more common in men, frequently associated with hearing impairment, and more common in Caucasians than African Americans. The prevalence is double in the southern states compared to the northern states. It is most prevalent at ages 40 to 70 yr.

PHYSICAL FINDINGS & CLINICAL PRESENTATION

- Patient complaints are of sounds in ears: determine onset, localization, pitch, loudness, duration, and nature: can be pulsatile, or described as ringing, buzzing, cricketlike, hissing, humming, or whistling.
- Objective tinnitus is pulsatile, with bursts of sound energy coinciding with the pulse.

ETIOLOGY

- Mechanism poorly understood; central in origin, it may originate at any point along the auditory pathway. Theories include injured cochlear hair cells, spontaneous activity in auditory nerve fibers, hyperactivity in the auditory nuclei in the brainstem, or a reduction in suppressive activity of the central auditory cortex.
- Medications implicated in tinnitus: aspirin, NSAIDs, aminoglycosides, chloramphenicol, erythromycin, tetracycline, vancomycin, bleomycin, cisplatin, mechlorethamine, vincristine, bumetanide, ethacrynic acid, furosemide, chloroquine, heavy metals, heterocyclic antidepressants, quinine.
- Classified as either objective or subjective.
  - Subjective causes: (1) otologic: hearing loss, Meniere's disease, acoustic neuroma, cerumen impaction; (2) ototoxic medications; (3) neurologic: multiple sclerosis, head injury; (4) metabolic: thyroid disorder, hyperlipidemia, vitamin B12 deficiency; (5) psychogenic: depression, anxiety, fibromyalgia; and (6) infectious: otitis media, Lyme disease, meningitis, syphllis
  - Objective causes: (1) vascular: arterial bruit, venous hum, AV malformation, vascular tumors; (2) neurologic: palatomyoclonus, idiopathic stapedial muscle spasm; and (3) patulous (lax) Eustachian tube

DIAGNOSIS

DIFFERENTIAL DIAGNOSIS

Subjective vs. objective tinnitus

WORKUP

- History of exposure to ototoxic substances or disease processes that predispose to tinnitus
- Association with depression: screen for depression

LABORATORY TESTS

- Audiometry, tympanometry, pitch masking
- Evaluate for metabolic abnormalities: thyroid disease, hyperlipidemia, anemia, B12 deficiency, zinc deficiency, CBC, complete blood chemistry
- Electronystagmograph: Meniere's disease

IMAGING STUDIES

- MRI/CT: Consider brain imaging to rule out multiple sclerosis, acoustic neuroma, brainstem tumor
- MRI/MRA for pulsatile tinnitus

TREATMENT

NONPHARMACOLOGIC THERAPY

Unknown effectiveness: psychotherapy, biofeedback, acupuncture, tinnitus-masking devices

ACUTE GENERAL Rx

- No FDA-approved medications: possibly beneficial are tricyclic antidepressants (one randomized controlled trial [RCT])
- Benzodiazapines possibly effective
- Lidocaine not found to be effective

CHRONIC Rx

Tinnitus retraining therapy: education, support, counseling and feedback device, multidisciplinary team. Duration of therapy is >1 yr; success rates of 80%, but no RCTs have been done.

COMPLEMENTARY & ALTERNATIVE MEDICINE

- Possibly effective: acupuncture, relaxation therapy, hypnosis (based on systemic reviews)
- *Ginkgo biloba* not found to be effective (based on one systemic review, one RCT)

DISPOSITION

Evaluate for all treatable causes, careful history to raise awareness of pulsatile tinnitus; determine subjective vs. objective

REFERRAL

ENT, neurology

PEARLS & CONSIDERATIONS

COMMENTS

- Up to 18% of population may have tinnitus, with 0.5% severely effected; be aware of high prevalence.
- Be aware of concurrent depression; screen and treat for it. Treat all treatable underlying causes.

PREVENTION

Avoid ototoxic drugs and loud, chronic noise exposure.

PATIENT/FAMILY EDUCATION

- American Tinnitus Association: 800-634-8978, www.ata.org
- American Academy of Audiology: 800-AAA-2336, www.audiology.org
- Hear USA: www.hearusa.org
- Counsel families and patients that tinnitus may be irreversible and that they should be aware of the condition's effect on their lives.

EVIDENCE

Patients with difficulty sleeping as a result of tinnitus reported a significant overall improvement with melatonin in a crossover randomized controlled trial. Patients with bilateral tinnitus had significantly more improvement with melatonin than patients with unilateral tinnitus.[1] Ⓐ

There is little evidence to support the use of *Ginkgo biloba* in the treatment of tinnitus.[2]

There is insufficient evidence about the effects of masking to comment on whether it is effective in the treatment of tinnitus.[2]

Evidence-Based References

1. Rosenberg SI et al: Effect of melatonin on tinnitus, *Laryngoscope* 108:305, 1998. Ⓐ
2. Waddell A: Tinnitus. Reviewed in: *Clin Evid* 12:798, London, 2004, BMJ Publishing Group.

SUGGESTED READINGS

Crummer RW: Diagnostic approach to tinnitus, *Am Fam Physician* 69(1):120, 2004.

Waddell A: Tinnitus: clinical evidence concise, *Am Fam Physician* 69(3):591, 2004.

Lockwood A: Tinnitus, *Neurology Clinics* 23:893, 2005.

Lockwood A: Tinnitus, *N Engl J Med* 347(12): 904, 2002.

AUTHOR: **JUDITH NUDELMAN, M.D.**

BASIC INFORMATION

DEFINITION

Torticollis is a contraction or contracture of the muscles of the neck that causes the head to be tilted to one side. It is usually accompanied by rotation of the chin to the opposite side with flexion (Fig 1-275). Usually it is a symptom of some underlying disorder. This term is often used incorrectly in cases when the torticollis may simply be positional.

SYNONYMS

Twisted neck
"Wry neck"

ICD-9CM CODES
723.5 Spastic (intermittent) torticollis
754.1 Congenital muscular (sternocleidomastoid)
300.11 Hysterical
714.0 Rheumatoid
333.83 Spasmodic

PHYSICAL FINDINGS & CLINICAL PRESENTATION

- Congenital muscular torticollis:
  1. Palpable soft tissue "mass" in the sternocleidomastoid shortly after birth
  2. Mass gradually subsides, leaving a shortened, contracted sternocleidomastoid muscle
  3. Head characteristically tilted toward the side of the mass and rotated in the opposite direction
  4. Facial asymmetry and other secondary changes persisting into adulthood
- Spasmodic torticollis:
  1. "Spasms" in the cervical musculature; may be bilateral and uncontrollable
  2. Head often tilted toward the affected side
- Findings in other cases depend on etiology.

ETIOLOGY

Torticollis has been attributed to more than 50 different causes:

- Localized fibrous shortening of unknown cause involving the sternocleidomastoid, leading to the condition termed *congenital muscular torticollis*
- Spasmodic torticollis: of uncertain etiology, possibly a variant of dystonia musculorum deformans
- Infection, specifically pharyngitis, tonsillitis, retropharyngeal abscess
- Miscellaneous rare causes: congenital musculoskeletal deformities, trauma, inflammation from rheumatoid arthritis, vestibular disturbances, posterior fossa tumor, syringomyelia, neuritis of spinal accessory nerve, and drug reactions

DIAGNOSIS

DIFFERENTIAL DIAGNOSIS

- Usually involves separating each disorder from the others
- Acquired positional disorders (e.g., ocular disturbances, acute disk herniation)

WORKUP

- Workup is dependent on the clinical situation.
- Laboratory studies are usually not helpful unless infection or rheumatoid disease is suspected.
- Section II describes a differential diagnosis for the evaluation and therapy of neck pain.
- Any child with a gradually increasing torticollis should have a complete eye examination.

IMAGING STUDIES

- Plain radiographs in cases of trauma or to rule out congenital abnormalities
- MRI in appropriate cases
- Electrodiagnostic studies: only rarely indicated to rule out neurologic causes

TREATMENT

- Congenital muscular torticollis: gentle stretching exercises carried out by the parent
- Spasmodic torticollis: physical therapy, psychotherapy, cervical braces, biofeedback, and pain control
- Other forms: treated according to etiology

DISPOSITION

- Most patients with congenital muscular torticollis respond well to conservative treatment.
- Spasmodic torticollis is often resistant to normal conservative treatment.
- Prognosis of other forms of torticollis is dependent on etiology.

REFERRAL

- Torticollis often requires a multidisciplinary approach unless the etiology is obvious.
- Children usually do not require any specific studies; however, an orthopedic consultation is recommended.
- Fixed deformity in the child; may need orthopedic referral for surgical release.

SUGGESTED READINGS

Crowner BE: Cervical dystonia: disease profile and clinical management, *Phys Ther* 87:1511, 2007.
Ferreira JJ et al: The management of cervical dystonia, *Expert Opin Pharmacother* 8(2):129, 2007.
Hosalkar HS et al: Congenital osseous anomalies of the upper cervical spine, *J Bone Joint Surg* 90A:337, 2008.
Papadimitriou NG et al: Acute torticollis after isolated stress fracture of the first rib in a child, *J Bone Joint Surg* 87A:2537, 2005.
Parikh SN, Crawford AH, Choudhary S: Magnetic resonance imaging in the evaluation of infantile torticollis, *Orthopedics* 27:509, 2004.
Slawek J et al: Factors affecting the health-related quality of life of patients with cervical dystonia and the impact of botulinum toxin type A injections, *Funct Neurol* 22(2):95, 2007.

AUTHOR: **LONNIE R. MERCIER, M.D.**

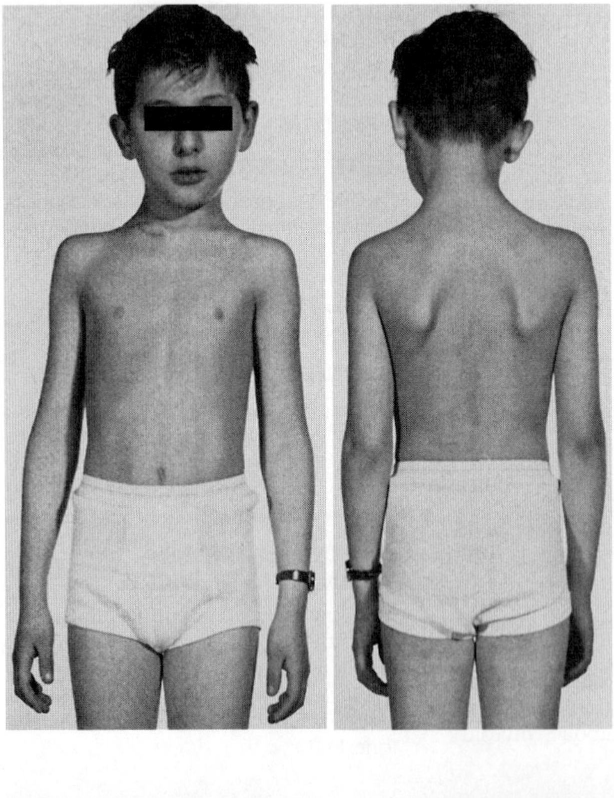

FIGURE 1-275 Torticollis. In this child, the right sternocleidomastoid muscle is contracted. (From Brinker MR, Miller MD: *Fundamentals of orthopaedics,* Philadelphia, 1999, WB Saunders.)

BASIC INFORMATION

DEFINITION

Tics are sudden, brief, intermittent involuntary or semivoluntary movements (motor tics) or sounds (phonic or vocal tics) that mimic fragments of normal behavior.

Tourette's syndrome (TS) is an inherited neuropsychiatric disorder characterized by multiple motor and vocal tics that change during the course of the illness. Onset is before age 18.

SYNONYMS

Gilles de la Tourette syndrome

ICD-9CM CODES
307.23 Gilles de la Tourette disorder

EPIDEMIOLOGY & DEMOGRAPHICS

PREVALENCE (IN U.S.): Unknown. Estimates range from 0.7% to 5%.

PREDOMINANT SEX: Male:female ratio of 3:1

PREDOMINANT AGE: Typical age of onset is between 2 to 15 yr. Mean is 5 to 7 yr.

PHYSICAL FINDINGS & CLINICAL PRESENTATION

- Neurologic examination is normal.
- Vocal tics (clearing of throat, repetitive short phrases, e.g., "You bet," swearing [coprolalia]).
- Motor tics can be simple (e.g., blinking, grimacing, head jerking) or complex (e.g., gesturing). Tics wax, wane, and change over time. Often they can be suppressed for short periods. Commonly they are preceded by an urge to perform the tic.
- Often TS is associated with a variety of behavioral symptoms, most commonly ADHD and OCD.

ETIOLOGY

There is a large genetic contribution to TS. There is a strong family history of OCD or TS in patients with tics, and twin studies provide evidence for importance of genetic factors. However, although multiple candidate genes have been identified no simple mutation has been found thus far. Dopamine is thought to be one of the major neurotransmitters involved.

DIAGNOSIS

DIFFERENTIAL DIAGNOSIS

- Sydenham's chorea—occurs after infection with group A streptococcus.
- PANDAS—pediatric autoimmune neurolopsychiatric disorder associated with streptococcal infection.
- Sporadic tic disorders—these tend to be motor or vocal but not both.
- Head trauma.
- Drug intoxication—there are many drugs that are known to induce or exacerbate tic disorder, including methylphenidate, amphetamines, pemoline, anticholinergics, and antihistamines.
- Postinfectious encephalitis.
- Inherited disorders—these include Huntington's disease, Hallervorden Spatz, and neuroacanthocytosis. All these should have other abnormalities on neurologic examination.

WORKUP

Clinical observation and history to confirm diagnosis

LABORATORY TESTS

No definitive laboratory tests.

IMAGING STUDIES

CT scan and MRI of brain are normal and unnecessary in the absence of abnormal neurologic examination.

TREATMENT

NONPHARMACOLOGIC THERAPY

Multidisciplinary: parents, teachers, psychologists, school nurses

ACUTE GENERAL Rx

Dopamine-blocking agents may be used to reduce severity of tics acutely (e.g., haloperidol 0.25 mg po qhs initially).

CHRONIC Rx

Tics only require treatment when they interfere with psychosocial, educational, and occupational functioning of a person.

TICS

- Clonidine—many choose this as a first line agent because of fewer long-term side effects. Start at 0.05 mg and slowly titrate to about 0.45 mg daily (needs tid/qid dosing). May also help with symptoms of ADHD.
- Guanfacine (Tenex), another alpha agonist similar to clonidine but can be administered once daily. Typical starting dose is 0.5 mg titrating to 1 to 3 mg qd.
- Tetrabenazine—dopamine-depleting agent that is not currently available in the U.S. Avoids many of the typical side effects of the neuroleptics.
- Atypical antipsychotics such as ziprasidone (Geodon), risperidone (Risperdal), and olanzapine (Zyprexa). These have fewer side effects than typical neuroleptics.
- Dopamine-blocking agents—neuroleptics (Pimozide, Haldol, Prolixin). These should be avoided until other options have been exhausted.
- Dopamine agonists—recent small, open label studies have found that ropinirole and pramipexole in low doses may be effective in reducing tic severity.

ADHD

Stimulants (dextroamphetamine, methylphenidate) are useful for symptoms of ADHD but may exacerbate tics.

OCD

SSRIs, such as fluoxetine, are the most effective.

DISPOSITION

- In the later teen years, intensity and frequency of tics diminish.
- One third of patients will achieve significant remission although complete, lifelong remission is rare.
- One third will have mild, persistent, but "unimpairing" tics.

REFERRAL

To neurologist to confirm initial diagnosis

PEARLS & CONSIDERATIONS

Tics do not need treatment unless they interfere with an individual's ability to function.

COMMENTS

Patient education may be obtained from the Tourette's Syndrome Association (TSA), 4240 Bell Blvd., Bayside, NY 11361-2864; phone: (800) 237-0717, (718) 224-2999; www.tsa-usa.org.

EVIDENCE

Evidence for specific therapies is limited. A recent double-blind, placebo-controlled study confirmed that methylphenidate (as compared with clonidine) does not actually cause a worsening of tics.[1]

Evidence-Based Reference

1. *Neurology* 58:527-536, 2002.

SUGGESTED READINGS

Jankovic J: Tourette's syndrome, *N Engl J Med* 345:1184, 2001.

Jankovic J: Tics and Tourette's syndrome. *In* Jankovic J, Tolosa E (eds): *Parkinson's Disease and Movement Disorders,* Philadelphia, 2002, Lippincott Williams & Wilkins.

Kurlan R: Future and alternative therapies in Tourette syndrome, *Adv Neurol* 99:248, 2006.

Pringsheim T: Tics, *Curr Opin Neurol* 16:523-527, 2003.

Sandor P: Pharmacological management of tics in patients with TS, *J Psychosom Res* 55:41-48, 2003.

AUTHOR: **CINDY ZADIKOFF, M.D.**

BASIC INFORMATION

DEFINITION

Toxic shock syndrome is an acute febrile illness resulting in multiple organ system dysfunction caused most commonly by a bacterial exotoxin. Disease characteristics also include hypotension, vomiting, myalgia, watery diarrhea, vascular collapse, and an erythematous sunburnlike cutaneous rash that desquamates during recovery.

ICD-9CM CODES
040.89 Toxic shock syndrome

EPIDEMIOLOGY & DEMOGRAPHICS

- Case reported incidence peak: 14 cases/100,000 menstruating women/yr in 1980; has since fallen to 1 case/100,000 persons
- Occurs most commonly between ages 10 and 30 yr in healthy, young menstruating white females
- Case fatality ratio of 3%

PHYSICAL FINDINGS & CLINICAL PRESENTATION

- Fever (≥38.9° C)
- Diffuse macular erythrodermatous rash that desquamates 1 to 2 wk after disease onset in survivors
- Orthostatic hypotension
- GI symptoms: vomiting, diarrhea, abdominal tenderness
- Constitutional symptoms: myalgia, headache, photophobia, rigors, altered sensorium, conjunctivitis, arthralgia
- Respiratory symptoms: dysphagia, pharyngeal hyperemia, strawberry tongue
- Genitourinary symptoms: vaginal discharge, vaginal hyperemia, adnexal tenderness
- End-organ failure
- Severe hypotension and acute renal failure
- Hepatic failure
- Cardiovascular symptoms: DIC, pulmonary edema, ARDS, endomyocarditis, heart block

ETIOLOGY

- Menstrually associated TSS: 45% of cases associated with tampons, diaphragm, or vaginal sponge use
- Nonmenstruating associated TSS: 55% of cases associated with puerperal sepsis, post–cesarean section endometritis, mastitis, wound or skin infection, insect bite, pelvic inflammatory disease, and postoperative fever
- Causative agent: *S. aureus* infection of a susceptible individual (10% of population lacking sufficient levels of antitoxin antibodies), which liberates the disease mediator TSST-1 (exotoxin)
- Other causative agents: coagulase-negative streptococci producing enterotoxins B or C, and exotoxin A producing group A β-hemolytic streptococci

DIAGNOSIS

DIFFERENTIAL DIAGNOSIS

- Staphylococcal food poisoning
- Septic shock
- Mucocutaneous lymph node syndrome
- Scarlet fever
- Rocky Mountain spotted fever
- Meningococcemia
- Toxic epidermal necrolysis
- Kawasaki's syndrome
- Leptospirosis
- Legionnaires' disease
- Hemolytic-uremic syndrome
- Stevens-Johnson syndrome
- Scalded skin syndrome
- Erythema multiforme
- Acute rheumatic fever

WORKUP

Broad-spectrum syndrome with multiorgan system involvement and variable but acute clinical presentation, including the following:

1. Fever ≥38.1° C
2. Classic desquamating (1 to 2 wk) rash
3. Hypotension/orthostatic SBP 90 or less
4. Syncope
5. Negative throat/CSF cultures
6. Negative serologic test for Rocky Mountain spotted fever, rubeola, and leptospirosis
7. Clinical involvement of three or more of the following:
   a. Cardiopulmonary: ARDS, pulmonary edema, endomyocarditis, second- or third-degree AV block
   b. CNS: altered sensorium without focal neurologic findings
   c. Hematologic: thrombocytopenia (PLT <100 k)
   d. Liver: elevated LFT results
   e. Renal: >5/HPF, negative urine cultures, azotemia, and increased creatinine double normal
   f. Mucous membrane involvement: vagina, oropharynx, conjunctiva
   g. Musculoskeletal: myalgia, CPK twice normal
   h. GI: vomiting, diarrhea

LABORATORY TESTS

- Pan culture (cervix/vagina, throat, nasal passages, urine, blood, CSF, wound) for *Staphylococcus, Streptococcus,* or other pathogenic organisms
- Electrolytes to detect hypokalemia, hyponatremia
- CBC with differential and clotting profile for anemia (normocytic/normochromic), thrombocytopenia, leukocytosis, coagulopathy, and bacteremia
- Chemistry profile to detect decreased protein, increased AST, increased ALT, hypocalcemia, elevated BUN/creatinine, hypophosphatemia, increased LDH, increased CPK
- Urinalysis to detect WBC (>5/HPF), proteinemia, microhematuria
- ABGs to assess respiratory function and acid-base status
- Serologic tests considered for Rocky Mountain spotted fever, rubeola, and leptospirosis

IMAGING STUDIES

- Chest x-ray examination to evaluate pulmonary edema
- ECG to evaluate arrhythmia
- Sonography/CT scan/MRI considered if pelvic abscess or TOA suspected

TREATMENT

NONPHARMACOLOGIC THERAPY

- For optimal outcome: high index of suspicion and early and aggressive supportive management in an ICU setting
- Aggressive fluid resuscitation (maintenance of circulating volume, CO, SBP)
- Thorough search for a localized infection or nidus: incision and drainage, debridement, removal of tampon or vaginal sponge
- Central hemodynamic monitoring, Swan-Ganz catheter and arterial line for surveillance of hemodynamic status and response to therapy
- Foley catheter to monitor hourly urine output
- Possible MAST trousers as temporary measure
- Acute ventilator management if severe respiratory compromise
- Renal dialysis for severe renal impairment
- Surgical intervention for indicated conditions (i.e., ruptured TOA, wound abscess, mastitis)

ACUTE GENERAL Rx

- Isotonic crystalloid (normal saline solution) for volume replacement following "7-3" rule
- Electrolyte replacement (K^+, Ca^+)
- PRBC/coagulation factor replacement/FFP to treat anemia or D&C
- Vasopressor therapy for hypotension refractory to fluid volume replacement (i.e., dopamine beginning at 2 to 5 μg/kg/min)
- Naloxone infusion (i.e., 0.5 mg/kg/hr) to improve SBP by blocking endogenous endorphin effects
- Parenteral antibiotic therapy; β-lactamase resistant antibiotic (methicillin, nafcillin, or oxacillin) initiated early

- Broad-spectrum antibiotic added if concurrent sepsis suspected
- Tetracycline added if considering Rocky Mountain spotted fever

CHRONIC Rx

- Severely ill patient: may require prolonged hospitalization and supportive management with gradual recovery and/or sequelae from severe end-organ involvement (ARDS or renal failure requiring dialysis)
- Majority of patients: complete recovery
- Early late-onset complications (within 2 wk):
  1. Skin desquamation
  2. Impaired digit sensation
  3. Denuded tongue
  4. Vocal cord paralysis
  5. ATN
  6. ARDS
- Late-onset complications (after 8 wk):
  1. Nail splitting/loss
  2. Alopecia
  3. CNS sequelae
  4. Renal impairment
  5. Cardiac dysfunction
- Recurrent TSS:
  1. More common in menstrually related cases
  2. Less common in patient treated with β-lactamase–resistant antistaphylococcal antibiotics
  3. Patients with history of TSS: if suspect signs and symptoms occur, should have high index of suspicion and low threshold for evaluation and treatment

PREVENTION

- Avoidance of tampons or use of low-absorbency tampons only (<4 hr in situ) and alternate with napkins
- Education for patients concerning signs and symptoms of TSS
- Avoidance of tampons for patients with history of TSS

DISPOSITION

- Complete recovery for most patients
- Long-term management of early- and late-onset complications for minority of patients

REFERRAL

- For multidisciplinary management, involving primary physician, gynecologist, internist, infectious disease specialist, and other supportive care specialists
- To tertiary level hospital

PEARLS & CONSIDERATIONS

COMMENTS

Patient information available from American College of Gynecologists and Obstetricians.

EVIDENCE

In patients with bacterial sepsis or septic shock, treatment with polyclonal intravenous immunoglobulin (IVIG) has been shown to significantly reduce both overall and sepsis-related mortality, but larger multicenter trials are needed to support these findings.[1,2] Ⓐ

Existing evidence has not determined whether any particular vasopressor agent has superiority in the management of septic shock.[3] Ⓑ

Treatment with a long course of low-dose corticosteroids has been shown to significantly reduce 28-day all-cause mortality, and intensive care unit and hospital mortality in patients with severe sepsis or septic shock, compared with control groups.[4] Ⓐ

A randomized controlled trial has found that early goal-directed therapy, commenced in the emergency department before admission to the intensive care unit, provides significant benefits with respect to outcome (including in-hospital mortality) in patients with severe sepsis and septic shock.[5] Ⓑ

Evidence-Based References

1. Alejandria MM et al: Intravenous immunoglobulin for treating sepsis and septic shock, *Cochrane Database Syst Rev* 1, 2002 (Cochrane Review).
2. Darenberg J et al: Intravenous immunoglobulin G therapy in streptococcal toxic shock syndrome: a European randomized, double-blind, placebo-controlled trial, *Clin Infect Dis* 37:333, 2003. Ⓑ
3. Müllner M et al: Vasopressors for shock, *Cochrane Database Syst Rev* 2, 2004 (Cochrane Review).
4. Annane D et al: Corticosteroids for treating severe sepsis and septic shock, *Cochrane Database Syst Rev* 1, 2004 (Cochrane Review).
5. Rivers E et al; Early Goal-Directed Therapy Collaborative Group: Early goal-directed therapy in the treatment of severe sepsis and septic shock, *N Engl J Med* 345:1368, 2001. Ⓑ

SUGGESTED READINGS

Issa NC et al: Staphylococcal toxic shock syndrome: suspicion and prevention are keys to control, *Postgrad Med* 110(4):55, 2001.

Miche CA, Shah V: Managing toxic shock syndrome. *Nursing Times* 99(5):26, 2003.

AUTHORS: **DENNIS M. WEPPNER, M.D.,** and **RUBEN ALVERO, M.D.**

BASIC INFORMATION

DEFINITION

Toxoplasmosis is an infection caused by the protozoal parasite *Toxoplasma gondii.*

ICD-9CM CODES
130.9 Toxoplasmosis

EPIDEMIOLOGY & DEMOGRAPHICS

INCIDENCE (IN U.S.):
- 3% to 70% of healthy adults
- Increases with age
- Increases with certain activities
  1. Slaughterhouse workers
  2. Cat owners
- Increases with certain geographic locations: high prevalence of cats

PEAK INCIDENCE: Temperate climates
PREDOMINANT SEX: Equal gender distribution
PREDOMINANT AGE:
- Infancy (congenital infection)
- Prevalence increases with age

GENETICS:
Congenital Infection:
- Incidence and severity vary with the trimester of gestation during which the mother acquired infection.
  1. 10% to 25% (first trimester)
  2. 30% to 54% (second trimester)
  3. 60% to 65% (third trimester)
- Congenital infection occurring in the first trimester is the most severe.
- 89% to 100% of infections in the third trimester are asymptomatic.
- Risk to the fetus is not correlated with symptoms in the mother.

PHYSICAL FINDINGS & CLINICAL PRESENTATION

- Acquired (immunocompetent host)
  1. 80% to 90% asymptomatic
  2. Adenopathy (usually cervical)
  3. Fever
  4. Myalgias
  5. Malaise
  6. Sore throat
  7. Maculopapular rash
  8. Hepatosplenomegaly
  9. Chorioretinitis rare
- Acquired (in patients with AIDS)
  1. 89% of symptomatic cases
     a. Encephalitis
     b. Intracerebral mass lesions
  2. Pneumonitis
  3. Chorioretinitis
  4. Other end organ
- Acquired (immunocompromised patients)
  1. Encephalitis
  2. Myocarditis (especially in heart transplant patients)
  3. Pneumonitis
- Ocular infection in the immunocompetent host
  1. Congenital infection
  2. Blurred vision
  3. Photophobia
  4. Pain
  5. Loss of central vision if macula involved
  6. Focal necrotizing retinitis
  7. Typically presents in second or third decade
- Congenital
  1. Results from acute infection acquired by the mother within 6 to 8 wk before conception or during gestation
  2. Usually, asymptomatic mother
  3. No sign of disease
  4. Chorioretinitis
  5. Blindness
  6. Epilepsy
  7. Psychomotor or mental retardation
  8. Intracranial calcifications
  9. Hydrocephalus
  10. Microcephaly
  11. Encephalitis
  12. Anemia
  13. Thrombocytopenia
  14. Hepatosplenomegaly
  15. Lymphadenopathy
  16. Jaundice
  17. Rash
  18. Pneumonitis
  19. Most infected infants are asymptomatic at birth

ETIOLOGY

- *Toxoplasma gondii*
  1. Ubiquitous intracellular protozoan
  2. Present worldwide
  3. Cat is definitive host
- Human infection
  1. Ingestion of oocysts shed by cats
  2. Ingestion of meat containing tissue cysts
  3. Vertical transmission

DIAGNOSIS

DIFFERENTIAL DIAGNOSIS

- Lymphadenopathy
  1. Infectious mononucleosis
  2. CMV mononucleosis
  3. Cat-scratch disease
  4. Sarcoidosis
  5. Tuberculosis
  6. Lymphoma
  7. Metastatic cancer
- Cerebral mass lesions in immunocompromised host
  1. Lymphoma
  2. Tuberculosis
  3. Bacterial abscess
- Pneumonitis in immunocompromised host
  1. *Pneumocystis jirovecii (carinii)* pneumonia
  2. Tuberculosis
  3. Fungal infection
- Chorioretinitis
  1. Syphilis
  2. Tuberculosis
  3. Histoplasmosis (competent host)
  4. CMV
  5. Syphilis
  6. Herpes simplex
  7. Fungal infection
  8. Tuberculosis (AIDS patient)
- Myocarditis
  1. Organ rejection in heart transplant recipients
- Congenital infection
  1. Rubella
  2. CMV
  3. Herpes simplex
  4. Syphilis
  5. Listeriosis
  6. Erythroblastosis fetalis
  7. Sepsis

WORKUP

- Acute infection, immunocompetent host
  1. CBC
  2. *Toxoplasma* serology (IgG, IgM) in serial blood specimens 3 wk apart
  3. Lymph node biopsy if diagnosis uncertain
- Immunocompromised host
  1. CNS symptoms
     a. Cerebral CT scan or MRI if CNS symptoms present
     b. Spinal tap, if safe
     c. Brain biopsy if no response to empiric therapy
  2. Ocular symptoms
     a. Funduscopic examination
     b. Serologic studies
     c. Rarely, vitreous tap
  3. Pulmonary symptoms
     a. Chest x-ray examination
     b. Bronchoalveolar lavage
     c. Transbronchial or open lung biopsy
  4. Myocarditis
     a. Cardiac enzymes
     b. Electrocardiogram
     c. Endomyocardial biopsy for definitive diagnosis
- Toxoplasmosis in pregnancy
  1. Initial maternal screening with IgM and IgG
     a. If negative, mother at risk of acute infection and should be retested monthly
     b. If both IgG and IgM positive, obtain IgA and IgE ELISA, AC/HS test
     c. IgA and IgE ELISA, AC/HS test elevated in acute infection
     d. Ig high for 1 yr or more
     e. IgG repeated 3 to 4 wk later to determine if titer is stable
  2. Acute maternal infection not excluded or documented
     a. Fetal blood sampling (for culture, Ig, IgA, IgE)
     b. Amniotic fluid PCR

3. Fetal ultrasound every other week if maternal infection documented
- Congenital toxoplasmosis
  1. Placental histology
  2. Specific IgM or IgA in infant's blood

LABORATORY TESTS

- Antibody studies
  1. More than one test necessary to establish diagnosis of acute toxoplasmosis
  2. IgM antibody
     a. Appears 5 days into infection
     b. Peaks at 2 wk
     c. Falls to low level or disappears within 2 mo
     d. May persist at low levels for 1 yr or more
  3. Antibody not measurable
     a. Ocular toxoplasmosis
     b. Reactivation
     c. Immunocompromised hosts
  4. IgA ELISA, IgE ELISA, and IgE ASAGA
     a. More sensitive tests
     b. Disappear more rapidly than Ig, establishing diagnosis of acute infection
  5. IgG antibody
     a. Appears 1 to 2 wk after infection
     b. Peaks at 6 to 8 wk
     c. Gradually declines over months to years

IMAGING STUDIES

- Chest x-ray examination if pulmonary involvement suspected
- Cerebral CT scan or MRI if encephalitis suspected

TREATMENT

Rx

NONPHARMACOLOGIC THERAPY

- Selected cases of ocular infection
  1. Photocoagulation
  2. Vitrectomy
  3. Lentectomy
- Selected cases of congenital cerebral infection
  1. Ventricular shunting

ACUTE GENERAL Rx

- Acute infection, immunocompetent host
  1. No treatment, unless severe and persistent symptoms or vital organ damage
- Acute infection, immunocompromised host, non-AIDS
  1. Treat even if asymptomatic
  2. Duration
     a. Until 4 to 6 wk after resolution of all signs and symptoms
     b. Usually 6 mo or longer
- Reactivated infection, immunocompromised host, non-AIDS
  1. Treat if symptomatic
- Acute or reactivated infection, AIDS
  1. Treat in all cases
  2. Induction course
     a. 3 to 6 wk
     b. Maintenance therapy continued for life; consider discontinuation of suppressive therapy if the patient has a good response to highly active antiretroviral therapy and if the CD4 count remains >200 cell/mm³ for more than 3 mo
  3. Empiric therapy
     a. AIDS with positive IgG
     b. Multiple ring-enhancing lesions on cerebral CT scan or MRI
     c. Response seen by day 7 in 71% and day 14 in 91%
- Ocular infection
  1. Treat in all cases
  2. Therapy continued for 1 mo or longer if needed
  3. Response seen in 70% within 10 days
  4. Retreat as needed
  5. Steroids may be indicated
  6. Surgical treatment in selected cases
- Treatment regimens
  1. Pyrimethamine 100 to 200 mg loading dose once PO, then 25 mg PO qd (50 to 75 mg in AIDS) *plus*
  2. Leucovorin 10 to 20 mg PO qd *plus*
  3. Sulfadiazine 1 to 1.5 g PO q6h

Other treatment options (if sulfa-hypersensitivity or allergy is present): pyrimethamine 50 to 75 mg/day orally with leucovorin 10 to 20 mg/day po and either (1) clindamycin 600 mg iv or po q6h, or (2) clarithromycin 1 gm po bid, or (3) dapsone 100 mg/day po, or (4) atovaquone 750 mg po q6h.

- Acute infection in pregnancy
  1. Treat immediately
  2. Risk of fetal infection reduced by 60% with treatment
     a. First trimester
        i. Spiramycin 3 g PO qd in two to four divided doses
        ii. Sulfadiazine 4 g PO qd in four divided doses
     b. Second and third trimester
        i. Sulfadiazine as above *plus*
        ii. Pyrimethamine 25 mg PO qd *plus*
        iii. Leucovorin 5 to 15 mg PO qd
        iv. Spiramycin as above
- Congenital infection
  1. Sulfadiazine 50 mg/kg PO bid *plus*
  2. Pyrimethamine 2 mg/kg PO for 2 days, then 1 mg/kg PO, three times weekly *plus*
  3. Leucovorin 5 to 20 mg PO three times weekly
  4. Minimum duration of treatment: 12 mo

CHRONIC Rx

- Maintenance therapy in AIDS patients because of the high risk (80%) of relapse
  1. Pyrimethamine 25 mg PO qd
  2. Sulfadiazine 500 mg PO qid
  3. Leucovorin 10 to 20 mg PO qd

DISPOSITION

- Prognosis
  1. Excellent in the immunocompetent host
  2. Good in ocular infection (although relapses are common)
- Treatment of acute infection in pregnancy
  1. Reduces incidence and severity of congenital toxoplasmosis
- Treatment of congenital infection
  1. Improvement in intellectual function
  2. Regression of retinal lesions
- AIDS
  1. 70% to 95% response to therapy

REFERRAL

- To infectious disease expert:
  1. Immunocompromised hosts
  2. Pregnant women
  3. Difficulty in making a diagnosis or deciding on treatment
- To pediatric infectious disease expert:
  1. Congenital infection
- To obstetrician:
  1. Pregnant seronegative mother
  2. Acute seroconversion
- To ophthalmologist:
  1. Congenital infection
  2. Any case of ocular infection

PEARLS & CONSIDERATIONS

COMMENTS

- Prevention of toxoplasmosis is most important in seronegative pregnant women and immunocompromised hosts.
- Patient instructions:
  1. Cook meat to 66° C.
  2. Cook eggs.
  3. Do not drink unpasteurized milk.
  4. Wash hands thoroughly after handling raw meat.
  5. Wash kitchen surfaces that come in contact with raw meat.
  6. Wash fruits and vegetables.
  7. Avoid contact with materials potentially contaminated with cat feces.

EVIDENCE

EBM

Treatment of toxoplasmosis in pregnancy

Two systematic reviews in women with acute toxoplasmosis in pregnancy found little evidence to suggest a benefit for mother or baby from treatment with current antiparasitics compared with no treatment.[1,2] Ⓑ

However, a long-term multicenter observational study concluded that even though prenatal antibiotic therapy for toxoplasmosis infection during pregnancy had no impact on the fetomaternal transmission rate, it did reduce the rate of sequelae among the infected infants. Also, starting treatment early resulted in significantly fewer severely affected children.[3] Ⓑ

Treatment and prophylaxis of toxoplasmic encephalitis in HIV-infected patients

A European multicenter trial found no difference in efficacy during acute treatment between pyrimethamine plus sulfadiazine or pyrimethamine plus clindamycin.[4] Ⓑ This trial also found that during maintenance therapy the relapse rate was twice as high among patients in the group receiving pyrimethamine plus clindamycin.[4] Ⓑ A small, randomized controlled trial (RCT) found that trimethoprim-sulfamethoxazole was as effective and better tolerated than pyrimethamine-sulfadiazine.[5] Ⓑ

A trial of patients in the early stages of HIV infection in sub-Saharan Africa found that there was no significant difference between trimethoprim-sulfamethoxazole vs. placebo terms of preventing toxoplasmosis.[6] Ⓐ A systematic review found no significant difference between trimethoprim-sulfamethoxazole vs. dapsone (alone or in combination with pyrimethamine) in the prevention of toxoplasmosis in HIV-infected patients.[7] Ⓐ

An RCT found that, in patients who were able to tolerate it, dapsone/pyrimethamine was a more effective prophylactic treatment for toxoplasmic encephalitis in HIV-infected people vs. aerosolized pentamidine. However, 30% of patients were unable to tolerate dapsone/pyrimethamine.[8] Ⓑ We were unable to cite any evidence that meets our criteria concerning the newer agents azithromycin and atovaquone.

Evidence-Based References

1. Wallon M et al: Congenital toxoplasmosis: systematic review of evidence of efficacy of treatment in pregnancy, *BMJ* 318:1511, 1999. Reviewed in: *Clin Evid* 12:1058, 2004. Ⓑ
2. Peyron F et al: Treatments for toxoplasmosis in pregnancy, *Cochrane Database Syst Rev* 3, 1999.
3. Foulon W et al: Treatment of toxoplasmosis during pregnancy: a multicenter study of impact on fetal transmission and children's sequelae at age 1 year, *Am J Obstet Gynecol* 180:410, 1999. Ⓑ
4. Katlama C et al: Pyrimethamine-clindamycin vs. pyrimethamine-sulfadiazine as acute and long-term therapy for toxoplasmic encephalitis in patients with AIDS, *Clin Infect Dis* 22:268, 1996. Ⓑ
5. Torre D et al: Randomized trial of trimethoprim-sulfamethoxazole versus pyrimethamine-sulfadiazine for therapy of toxoplasmic encephalitis in patients with AIDS, *Antimicrob Agents Chemother* 42(6):1346, 1998. Ⓑ
6. Anglaret X et al: Early chemoprophylaxis with trimethroprim-sulphamethoxazole for HIV-1-infected adults in Abidjan, Cote d'Ivoire: a randomized trial, *Lancet* 353:1463, 1999. Reviewed in: *Clin Evid* 12:1004, 2004. Ⓐ
7. Bucher HC et al: Meta-analysis of prophylactic treatments against *Pneumocystis carinii* pneumonia and toxoplasma encephalitis in HIV-infected patients, *J Acquir Immune Defic Syndr Hum Retrovirol* 15:104, 1997. Reviewed in: *Clin Evid* 12:1004, 2004. Ⓐ
8. Opravil M et al: Once-weekly administration of dapsone/pyrimethamine vs. aerosolized pentamidine as combined prophylaxis for *Pneumocystis carinii* pneumonia and toxoplasmic encephalitis in human immunodeficiency virus-infected patients, *Clin Infect Dis* 20:531, 1995. Ⓑ

SUGGESTED READINGS

Boyer KM et al: Risk factors for Toxoplasma gondii infection in mothers of infants with congenital toxoplasmosis: implications for prenatal management and screening, *Am J Obstet Gynecol* 192(2):564, 2005.

Campbell AL et al: First case of toxoplasmosis following small bowel transplantation and systematic review of tissue-invasive toxoplasmosis following noncardiac solid organ transplantation, *Transplantation* 81(3):408, 2006.

Fricker-Hidalgo H et al: Disseminated toxoplasmosis with pulmonary involvement after heart transplantation, *Transpl Infect Dis* 7(1):38, 2005.

Kravetz JD, Federman DG: Prevention of toxoplasmosis in pregnancy: knowledge of risk factors, *Infect Dis Obstet Gynecol* 13(3):161, 2005.

Kravetz JD, Federman DG: Toxoplasmosis in pregnancy, *Am J Med* 118:212, 2005.

Montoya JG, Rosso F: Diagnosis and management of toxoplasmosis, *Clin Perinatol* 32(3):705, 2005.

Soheilian M et al: Prospective randomized trial of trimethoprim/sulfamethoxazole versus pyrimethamine and sulfadiazine in the treatment of ocular toxoplasmosis, *Ophthalmology* 112(11):1876, 2005.

AUTHORS: **GLENN G. FORT, M.D., M.P.H., MICHELE HALPERN, M.D.,** and **DENNIS J. MIKOLICH, M.D.**

BASIC INFORMATION

DEFINITION

Bacterial tracheitis is an acute infectious disease affecting the trachea and large conducting airways. Tracheal inflammation may be caused by a large number of inhaled stimuli, but bacterial infection is a life-threatening illness associated with purulent secretions and subglottic edema.

SYNONYMS

Bacterial tracheobronchitis
Pseudomembranous croup
Membranous laryngotracheobronchitis

ICD-9CM CODES
464.10 Tracheitis

EPIDEMIOLOGY & DEMOGRAPHICS

INCIDENCE (IN U.S.):

- Uncommon
- May be the most common cause of acute upper airway obstruction requiring admission to pediatric ICUs

PEAK INCIDENCE: Three fourths of cases reported in winter

PREDOMINANT SEX: Boys > girls in one series

PREDOMINANT AGE:

- 1 mo to 8 yr
- Almost all <13 yr (most <3 yr)

GENETICS: Down syndrome is a possible predisposing factor.

Congenital Infection: Some cases found in those with anatomic abnormalities of the upper airways.

PHYSICAL FINDINGS & CLINICAL PRESENTATION

- Croupy or "brassy" cough
- Inspiratory stridor (frequent)
- Wheezing (unusual)
- Fever (often >102° F)
- Thick, purulent secretions expectorated
  1. Minority of patients expectorate "ricelike" pellets.
  2. Most patients are unable to mobilize secretions.
     a. Become inspissated
     b. Form pseudomembranes

ETIOLOGY

- *Staphylococcus aureus*
- *Haemophilus influenzae*
- β-Hemolytic streptococcal infection
- Secondary to viral infections of the respiratory tract
  1. Primary influenza
  2. RSV
  3. Parainfluenza
- Many cases follow measles
  1. Especially when accompanied by chest radiographic infiltrates
  2. Sometimes fatal outcome
  3. Associated with prolonged endotracheal intubation

DIAGNOSIS

DIFFERENTIAL DIAGNOSIS

- Viral croup
- Epiglottitis
- Diphtheria
- Necrotizing herpes simplex infection in the elderly
- CMV in immunocompromised patients
- Invasive aspergillosis in immunocompromised patients

WORKUP

Direct laryngoscopy

1. Typical secretions
   a. May form pseudomembranes
   b. Airway obstruction
2. Normal epiglottis rules out epiglottitis
3. Possible subglottic edema

LABORATORY TESTS

- WBC is sometimes elevated.
- On differential, left shift is almost universal.
- Gram stain and culture of tracheal secretions confirm diagnosis.
- Blood cultures are positive in a minority.

IMAGING STUDIES

- Lateral x-ray examination of neck
  1. Normal epiglottis
  2. Vague density or a "dripping candle" appearance of tracheal mucosa
     a. Secretions
     b. Pseudomembranes
- Chest radiograms
  1. Not diagnostic
  2. Should not be performed on patients in acute respiratory distress, because severe or fatal upper airway obstruction can develop suddenly
- Pneumonic infiltrates frequent
- Atelectasis: unusual but can lead to lobar collapse

TREATMENT

NONPHARMACOLOGIC THERAPY

- Aggressive maintenance of a patent airway
  1. Laryngoscopy or bronchoscopy used diagnostically and therapeutically to strip away pseudomembranes
  2. Voluminous and tenacious secretions suctioned from the underlying friable mucosa
     a. May extend from between the vocal cords to the main carina
     b. Larger channels of rigid instruments for more effective suctioning
- Prevention of complete large airway obstruction
  1. Nasotracheal intubation
  2. Humidification of inspired gas
  3. Frequent saline instillation and suctioning
  4. Intubation with general anesthesia, performed in the operating room, is preferred by some
- Ventilatory support necessary with initial management in ICU

ACUTE GENERAL Rx

- Antibiotic therapy: start immediately, generally continued for 1 to 2 wk
- Initial therapy directed against *H. influenzae* and *S. aureus* (e.g., cefotaxime and vancomycin)
- Oral therapy is usually sufficient after 5 or 6 days of IV administration

DISPOSITION

- Most patients are extubated in 5 to 6 days after initiating antibiotic therapy.
- Anoxic encephalopathy is reported in 7% of survivors.

REFERRAL

Suspected diagnosis

PEARLS & CONSIDERATIONS

COMMENTS

- Infants are at increased risk of airway obstruction because of the small airway dimension.
- Presence of pneumonia and a staphylococcal etiology are thought to worsen prognosis.
- Reported complications: toxic shock syndrome, persistent postextubation stridor, pneumothorax, and volutrauma

SUGGESTED READINGS

Gaugler C et al: Neonatal necrotizing tracheobronchitis: three case reports, *J Perinatol* 24(4):259, 2004.

Kinebuchi S et al: Tracheo-bronchitis associated with Crohn's disease improved on inhaled corticotherapy, *Intern Med* 43(9):829, 2004.

Salamone FN et al: Bacterial tracheitis reexamined: is there a less severe manifestation? *Otolaryngol Head Neck Surg* 131(6):871, 2004.

AUTHORS: **GLENN G. FORT, M.D., M.P.H., JOSEPH R. MASCI, M.D.,** and **HARVEY M. SHANIES, M.D., PH.D.**

BASIC INFORMATION

DEFINITION

Hemolytic transfusion reaction is an acute intravascular hemolysis caused by mismatches in the ABO system. It is caused by complement-fixing Ig and IgG antibodies to group A and B RBCs. Hemolytic transfusion reactions can also be caused by minor antigen systems; however, they are usually less severe. In delayed serologic transfusion reactions, hemolysis with hemoglobinemia is unusual; in these delayed reactions the only manifestations may be the development of a newly positive Coombs' test and fever.

ICD-9CM CODES
999.8 Other transfusion reaction

EPIDEMIOLOGY & DEMOGRAPHICS

Acute intravascular hemolysis occurs in <1 in 50,000 transfusions.

PHYSICAL FINDINGS & CLINICAL PRESENTATION (Table 1-47)

- Hypotension
- Pain at the infusion site
- Fever, tachycardia, chest or back pain, dyspnea
- Often, severe reactions occur in surgical patients under anesthesia who are unable to give any warning signs

ETIOLOGY

Most fatal hemolytic reactions are caused by clerical errors and mislabeled specimens.

DIAGNOSIS

DIFFERENTIAL DIAGNOSIS

- Bacterial contamination of blood
- Hemoglobinopathies

WORKUP

The transfusion must be stopped immediately. The blood bank must be notified, and the donor transfusion bag must be returned to the blood bank along with a freshly drawn posttransfusion specimen.

LABORATORY TESTS

- Positive Coombs' test, elevated BUN, creatinine, and bilirubin
- Hemoglobinuria (wine-colored urine), hemoglobinemia (pink plasma)
- Decreased Hct, decreased serum haptoglobin

TREATMENT

NONPHARMACOLOGIC THERAPY

- Stop transfusion immediately. Test anticoagulated blood from the recipient for the presence of free Hgb in the plasma.
- Monitor vital signs.

ACUTE GENERAL Rx

- Vigorous IV hydration to maintain urine flow at >100 ml/hr until hypotension is corrected and hemoglobinuria clears. IV furosemide may be necessary to maintain adequate renal flow.
- The addition of mannitol may prevent renal damage (controversial).
- Monitor for the presence of DIC.
- Use of IV steroids is controversial.

DISPOSITION

Mortality exceeds 50% in severe transfusion reactions.

PEARLS & CONSIDERATIONS

COMMENTS

Hemolysis caused by minor antigen systems is generally less severe and may be delayed 5 to 10 days after transfusion.

AUTHOR: **FRED F. FERRI, M.D.**

TABLE 1-47 Signs and Symptoms of Acute Adverse Reactions to Blood Transfusion

Reaction	Fever	Chills/ Rigors	Nausea/ Vomiting	Chest Discomfort/ Pain	Facial Flushing	Wheezing/ Dyspnea	Back/ Lumbar Pain	Discomfort at Infusion Site	Hypotension
Acute hemolytic	X	X	X	X	X	X	X	X	X
Febrile nonhemolytic	X	X		X	X				
Nonimmune hemolysis									
Acute lung injury	X			X		X			X
Allergic									
Massive transfusion complications									
Anaphylaxis	X	X	X	X	X	X	X	X	X
Passive cytokine infusion	X	X	X						
Hypervolemia						X			
Bacterial sepsis	X	X	X				X	X	X
Air embolus				X		X			

From Goldman L, Bennett JC (eds): *Cecil textbook of medicine,* ed 22, Philadelphia, 2004, WB Saunders.

BASIC INFORMATION

DEFINITION

Transient ischemic attack (TIA) refers to a transient neurologic dysfunction caused by focal brain or retinal ischemia with symptoms lasting less than 60 min and followed by a full recovery of function. Acute brain ischemia is a medical emergency requiring prompt neurologic evaluation and potential intervention.

SYNONYMS

TIA

ICD-9CM CODES
435.9 Unspecified transient cerebral ischemia

EPIDEMIOLOGY & DEMOGRAPHICS

INCIDENCE (IN U.S.): 49 cases/100,000 persons/yr
PEAK INCIDENCE: >60 yr
PREDOMINANT SEX: Males > females

PHYSICAL FINDINGS & CLINICAL PRESENTATION

- During an episode, neurologic abnormalities are confined to discrete vascular territory.
- Typical carotid territory symptoms are ipsilateral monocular visual disturbance, contralateral homonymous hemianopsia, contralateral hemimotor or sensory dysfunction, and language dysfunction (dominant hemisphere) alone or in combination.
- Typical vertebrobasilar territory symptoms are binocular visual disturbance, vertigo, diplopia, dysphagia, dysarthria, and motor or sensory dysfunction involving the ipsilateral face and contralateral body.

ETIOLOGY

- Cardioembolic
- Large vessel atherothrombotic disease
- Lacunar disease
- Hypoperfusion with fixed arterial stenosis
- Hypercoagulable states

DIAGNOSIS

DIFFERENTIAL DIAGNOSIS

- Hypoglycemia
- Seizures
- Migraine
- Subdural hemorrhage
- Mass lesions
- Vestibular disease
- Section II describes the differential diagnosis of neurologic deficits, focal and multifocal.

WORKUP

- Thorough history and physical examination
- Ancillary investigations including neuroimaging aimed at identifying the etiology quickly

LABORATORY TESTS

- CBC with platelets
- PT (INR) and PTT
- Glucose
- Lipid profile
- ESR (if clinical suspicion for infectious or inflammatory process)
- Urinalysis
- Chest x-ray
- ECG and consider cycling cardiac enzymes
- Other tests as dictated by suspected etiology

IMAGING STUDIES

- Head CT scan to exclude hemorrhage including a subdural hemorrhage
- MRI and MRA. (In several studies, MRI with diffusion-weighted imaging has identified early ischemic brain injury in up to 50% of patients with TIA, and in such cases the patient has had a stroke). MRA of the brain and neck can identify large vessel intracranial and extracranial stenoses, arteriovenous malformations, and aneurysms
- Carotid Doppler studies identify carotid stenosis; neck ultrasound can also visualize stenoses of the vertebrobasilar arteries
- Echocardiography if cardiac source is suspected
- Telemetry for hospitalized patients for at least 24 hr. May consider 24-hr Holter if patient is being discharged
- CT angiogram or supraaortic vessel MRA if considering carotid endarterectomy or carotid stent. Four-vessel angiogram if Doppler ultrasound does not agree with MRA/CTA.

TREATMENT

NONPHARMACOLOGIC THERAPY

- Carotid endarterectomy for carotid territory TIA associated with an ipsilateral stenosis of 70% to 99%: should be done by a surgeon who is experienced with and performs this procedure frequently. The procedure should be performed as soon as the patient is fit for surgery, preferably within 2 weeks of TIA. Carotid stenting is also being performed in patients who are not surgical candidates. Trials are comparing stenting versus surgery for carotid disease.
- Modification of risk factors including smoking cessation.

ACUTE GENERAL Rx

- Depends on etiology.
- If the time of the onset of symptoms is clear, and there are significant deficits on neurologic examination, and brain hemorrhage has been ruled out, then the patient may be a candidate for thrombolytic therapy, and it is advisable to discuss the case with a neurologist or a specialist in cerebrovascular disease.
- Acute anticoagulation: no data supporting benefits in the acute setting. Heparin is considered for new-onset atrial fibrillation and atherothrombotic carotid disease causing recurrent transient neurologic symptoms especially in the setting before carotid endarterectomy or carotid stenting. Also considered for basilar artery thrombosis given concern for progression to brainstem stroke with high morbidity and mortality.
- Section III, "Transient Ischemic Attacks," describes a treatment algorithm.

CHRONIC Rx

- For cardioembolic TIA, long-term anticoagulation is considered. Stroke patients with atrial fibrillation or demonstrated cardiac thrombi have been shown to benefit from long-term warfarin therapy. Target INR of 2.5 is recommended.
- For noncardioembolic TIA, first line of treatment has traditionally been aspirin. No significant benefit of high-dose aspirin (up to 1500 mg/day) has been conclusively found over lower doses (75 mg to 325 mg/day). A baby aspirin (81 mg/day) is therefore appropriate.
- Aspirin/dipyridamole extended-release capsules (Aggrenox, 1 capsule po bid) is now recommended as a first-line therapy for noncardioembolic TIA. In a study of patients with TIA or stroke, aspirin/dipyridamole reduced subsequent cerebrovascular events to a greater extent than either drug alone. Clopidrogel is equally effective to aspirin in secondary prevention but the combination of aspirin and clopidrogel for patients with TIA or stroke causes more life threatening bleeding than clopidrogel alone. Recommend Aggrenox or oral anticoagulation for patients who continue to have TIAs while on aspirin (aspirin failures), but there are no data to support this recommendation.
- In patients with cerebrovascular disease, HMG-CoA reductase inhibitors (statins) have been shown to provide significant protection against subsequent vascular events such as MI and stroke even for LDLs <100. Consider starting a statin agent unless LDL is <70.

DISPOSITION

- Studies indicate a significant 90-day risk for stroke in patients with a TIA. The risk varies depending on comorbidities, age, and specific neurologic deficits. The 7-point ABCD2 score predicts the risk of ischemic stroke and has been validated on a large number of patients.
- One-year and 3-yr survival rates are 98% and 94%, respectively.

REFERRAL

Recommend referring all patients with TIA for an urgent neurologic evaluation and management. TIA patients should be evaluated with the same urgency as stroke.

PEARLS & CONSIDERATIONS

CAVEAT

Urgently evaluate all patients who present with symptoms suggestive of acute brain ischemia. Do not wait for symptoms to resolve to distinguish TIA versus stroke, as patients who present with acute neurologic deficits within three hours of symptom onset may be eligible for t-PA.

EVIDENCE

Prolonged antiplatelet therapy significantly reduces the risk of serious vascular events in patients with a prior stroke or TIA.[1]

A systematic review, which compared dipyridamole plus aspirin with aspirin alone, in patients presenting after TIA or stroke has found no clear difference in vascular deaths, but has found that the combination is associated with fewer vascular events.[2]

There is no benefit from oral anticoagulation following a TIA in the absence of atrial fibrillation.[3]

Warfarin has been shown to be superior to antiplatelet agents in the prevention of stroke in patients with atrial fibrillation. Antiplatelet agents may be used if there are contraindications to warfarin or the risk of ischemic stroke is low.[4]

In people with atrial fibrillation at a high risk of stroke (but no history of previous stroke or TIA), adjusted-dose warfarin significantly reduces the combined rate of ischemic stroke or systemic embolism, and reduces the rate of disabling or fatal stroke compared with low, fixed-dose warfarin plus aspirin.[5]

Carotid endarterectomy has been shown to reduce the risk of major stroke or death in patients with symptomatic severe or moderate carotid stenosis. Patients with mild stenosis did not benefit from surgery.[6,7]

RCTs comparing carotid angioplasty plus stenting vs. endarterectomy, in patients with symptomatic carotid stenosis, have produced conflicting results, are limited by trial design, and are ongoing. The Stenting and Angioplasty with Protection in Patients at High Risk for Endarterectomy (SAPPHIRE) study reported improved outcomes in patients at high risk for surgery who were treated with carotid stenting.[8]

In patients with a history of previous stroke or TIA, antihypertensive treatment is associated with a significantly reduced risk of stroke and major cardiovascular events compared with placebo, no treatment, or usual medical care.[9]

Simvastatin 40 mg daily for 5 years has significantly reduced mean total cholesterol by 24%, and has significantly reduced stroke, major vascular events, and deaths vs. placebo, in people with coronary heart disease, other occlusive vascular disease, or diabetes, with or without a history of cerebrovascular disease.[10] In patients with stroke or TIA, simvistatin 80 mg reduces the risk of stroke and coronary events.[11]

Statin therapy has reduced the relative risk of a major vascular event, irrespective of a patient's medical history or pretreatment cholesterol or triglyceride level.[10]

Evidence-Based References

1. Antithrombotic Trialists' Collaboration: Collaborative meta-analysis of randomised trials of antiplatelet therapy for prevention of death, myocardial infarction, and stroke in high risk patients, *BMJ* 324:71, 2002. Corrections: *BMJ* 324:141, 2002. Reviewed in: *Clin Evid* 11:257, 2004.
2. De Schryver EL, Algra A, van Gijn J: Dipyridamole for preventing stroke and other vascular events in patients with vascular disease, *Cochrane Database Syst Rev* 1:CD001820, 2002.
3. Sandercock P et al: Anticoagulants for preventing recurrence following presumed non-cardioembolic ischaemic stroke or transient ischaemic attack, *Cochrane Database Syst Rev* 4, 2002.
4. Freestone B et al: Stroke prevention. Reviewed in: *Clin Evid* 11:257, 2004, London, BMJ Publishing Group.
5. Stroke Prevention in Atrial Fibrillation Investigators: Adjusted-dose warfarin versus low-intensity, fixed-dose warfarin plus aspirin for high-risk patients with atrial fibrillation III randomized clinical trial, *Lancet* 348:633, 1996. Reviewed in: *Clin Evid* 11:257, 2004.
6. Rothwell PM et al: Analysis of pooled data from the randomised controlled trials of endarterectomy for symptomatic carotid stenosis, *Lancet* 361:107, 2003.
7. Cina CS, Clase CM, Haynes RB: Carotid endarterectomy for symptomatic carotid stenosis, *Cochrane Database Syst Rev* 3, 1999.
8. Yadav JS et al: Protected carotid-artery stenting versus endarterectomy in high-risk patients, *N Engl J Med* 351:1493, 2004.
9. The INDANA Project Collaborators: Effect of antihypertensive treatment in patients having already suffered from stroke, *Stroke* 28:2557, 1997. Reviewed in: *Clin Evid* 11:257, 2004.
10. Heart Protection Study Collaborative Group: MRC/BHF Heart Protection Study of cholesterol lowering with simvastatin in 20,536 high-risk individuals: a randomised placebo-controlled trial, *Lancet* 360:7, 2002. Reviewed in: *Clin Evid* 11:257, 2004.
11. Stroke Prevention by Aggressive Reduction in Cholesterol Levels (SPARCL) investigators: High-dose atorvastatin after stroke or TIA, *N Engl J Med* 355:549, 2006.

SUGGESTED READINGS

Albers GW: A review of published TIA treatment recommendations, *Neurology* 62:S26, 2004.

Albers GW et al: Antithrombotic and thrombolytic therapy for ischemic stroke, *Chest* 126:483S, 2004.

Albers GW et al: Transient ischemic attack—proposal for a new definition, *N Engl J Med* 347:1713, 2002.

Algra A et al: Oral anticoagulants versus antiplatelet therapy for preventing further vascular events after transient ischemic attack or minor stroke of presumed arterial origin, *Stroke* 34:234, 2003.

Chaturvedi S et al: Carotid endarterectomy—an evidence-based review: report of the Therapeutics and Technology Assessment Subcommittee of the American Academy of Neurology, *Neurology* 65:794, 2005.

Diener HC et al: Aspirin and clopidrogrel compared with clopidogrel alone after recent ischemic stroke or transient ischaemic attack in high risk patients (MATCH): randomized, double-blind, placebo-controlled trial, *Lancet* 364:331, 2004.

Heart Protection Study Collaborative Group: MRC/BHF heart protection study of cholesterol lowering with simvastatin in 20,536 high-risk individuals: a randomized placebo-controlled trial, *Lancet* 360:7, 2002.

Johnston SC: Clinical practice. Transient ischemic attack, *N Engl J Med* 347:1687, 2002.

Johnston SC et al: National Stroke Association guidelines for the management of transient ischemic attacks, *Annals of Neurology* 60:301, 2006.

Johnston SC et al: Validation and refinement of scores to predict very early stroke risk after transient ischaemic attack, *Lancet* 369:283, 2007.

AUTHOR: **SEAN I. SAVITZ, M.D.**

BASIC INFORMATION

DEFINITION

Trichinosis is an infection by one of various species of *Trichinella.*

SYNONYMS

Trichinella spiralis muscle infection

ICD-9CM CODES
124 Trichinosis

EPIDEMIOLOGY & DEMOGRAPHICS

INCIDENCE (IN U.S.): <100 cases/yr
GENETICS:
Congenital Infection:
- Abrupt delivery of stillbirths in infected pregnant women
- Vertical infection of the fetus

PHYSICAL FINDINGS & CLINICAL PRESENTATION

- Symptoms
  1. May vary widely depending on the time from ingestion of contaminated meat and on worm burden
  2. Most persons asymptomatic
- Enteral phase
  1. Correlates with penetration of ingested larvae into the intestinal mucosa
  2. May last from 2 to 6 wk
  3. Mild, transient diarrhea and nausea
  4. Abdominal pain
  5. Diarrhea or constipation
  6. Vomiting
  7. Malaise
  8. Low-grade fevers
- Migratory or parenteral phase
  1. In the intestine, maturation and mating
  2. Newborn larvae
     a. Penetrate into lymphatic and blood vessels
     b. Migrate to muscles where they penetrate into muscle cells, enlarge, coil, and develop a cyst wall
  3. Patients may present with
     a. Fever
     b. Myalgias
     c. Periorbital or facial edema
     d. Headache
     e. Skin rash
     f. Other symptoms caused by the penetration of tissues by the newborn migrating larvae
  4. Peak in symptoms 2 to 3 wk after infection, then slowly subside
- Severe complications
  1. Brain damage by granulomatous inflammation or occlusion of arteries
  2. Cardiac involvement
  3. Can lead to death

ETIOLOGY

- The nematode responsible for this illness is an obligate intracellular parasite belonging to the genus *Trichinella.*
- It is one of the most ubiquitous parasites in the world and may be found in virtually all warm-blooded animals.
- Infection in humans occurs by the ingestion of contaminated animal meat that is raw or partially cooked and contains viable cysts.
- Most cases are now related to the consumption of poorly processed pork or wild game (bear, wild boar, cougar, and walrus).

DIAGNOSIS

DIFFERENTIAL DIAGNOSIS

- Different presentations have different differential diagnoses.
- Early illness may resemble gastroenteritis.
- Later symptoms may be confused with:
  1. Measles
  2. Dermatomyositis
  3. Glomerulonephritis
- The differential diagnosis of nematode tissue infections is described in Section II.

WORKUP

- Antibody assay of serum is usually positive by approximately 2 wk after infection.
- Muscle biopsy is used to detect the larva in muscle tissue if diagnosis unclear; best done by placing the tissue between two slides.

LABORATORY TESTS

- CBC: leukocytosis with prominent eosinophilia
- ESR: usually normal
- Elevation of muscle enzymes common (i.e., CPK, aldolase)

IMAGING STUDIES

Soft-tissue radiographs may show calcified cyst walls.

TREATMENT

NONPHARMACOLOGIC THERAPY

Bed rest for myalgias

ACUTE GENERAL Rx

- Albendazole 400 mg po for 1 to 2 wk.
- Salicylates to decrease muscle discomfort.
- Steroids in critically ill patients.
- Mebendazole 200 mg po TID for 3 days, followed by mebendazole 400 mg po TID is an alternative to albendazole.

DISPOSITION

- Most symptoms subside over time.
- Reports of long-term sequelae:
  1. Myalgias
  2. Headaches
- Occasionally, death occurs.

REFERRAL

Diagnosis uncertain

PEARLS & CONSIDERATIONS

COMMENTS

- Prevention by thorough cooking of meats
- Inadequate to smoke, cure, or dry meats
- Freezing at specified temperatures kills *T. spiralis* larvae in pork
- *T. nativa* is a freeze-resistant species that remains viable after freezing, even for months or years—has been associated with infection from ingestion of bear meat

SUGGESTED READINGS

Astudillo LM, Arlet PM: Images in clinical medicine. The chemosis of trichinosis, *N Engl J Med* 351(5):487, 2004.

Awada A, Kojan S: Neurological disorders and travel, *Int J Antimicrob Agents* 21(2):189, 2003.

Centers for Disease Control and Prevention (CDC): Trichinellosis associated with bear meat—New York and Tennessee, *MMWR* 53(27):606, 2004.

Moller LN et al: Outbreak of trichinellosis associated with consumption of game meat in West Greenland, *Vet Parasitol* 132(1-2):131, 2005.

Piergili-Fioretti D et al: Re-evaluation of patients involved in a trichinellosis outbreak caused by *Trichinella britovi* 15 years after infection, *Vet Parasitol* 132(1-2):119, 2005.

Wu Z et al: Tumor necrosis factor receptor-mediated apoptosis in *Trichinella spiralis*-infected muscle cells, *Parasitology* 131(Pt 3):373, 2005.

AUTHORS: **GLENN G. FORT, M.D., M.P.H., DENNIS J. MIKOLICH, M.D.,** and **MAURICE POLICAR, M.D.**

BASIC INFORMATION

DEFINITION

Tricuspid regurgitation (TR) refers to an abnormal flow of blood from the right ventricle to the right atrium during systole (Fig. 1-276).

SYNONYMS

Tricuspid insufficiency

ICD-9CM CODES
397.0 Disease of the tricuspid valve
424.2 Tricuspid valve disorders, specified as nonrheumatic

EPIDEMIOLOGY & DEMOGRAPHICS

- In the adult population, TR is usually functional rather than structural.
- In adolescents and young adults, most cases of TR are caused by congenital cardiac abnormalities.
- In patients with rheumatic heart disease, TR rarely occurs alone and is usually associated with mitral or aortic valve disease.
- A small degree (trace to mild) of TR is present in approximately 70% of normal adults. On echocardiography, this "normal" degree of regurgitation is localized to a small region adjacent to valve closure, often does not extend throughout systole, and has a low signal strength.

PHYSICAL FINDINGS & CLINICAL PRESENTATION

- Isolated TR can cause nonspecific symptoms, such as exercise intolerance.
- Signs and symptoms in the presence of TR are usually caused by the underlying etiology.
- Signs and symptoms may be caused by accompanying right-sided heart failure (e.g., jugular venous distention, peripheral edema, ascites, hepatomegaly, right-sided S3).
- Holosystolic murmur, heard best along the left sternal border in the fourth intercostal space. The murmur becomes louder during inspiration (Carvallo's sign) and during maneuvers that increase venous return.
- Prominent V waves in the jugular venous waveform (see Fig. 1-276).
- Pulsatile liver.

ETIOLOGY

- Functional TR refers to conditions leading to dilation of the tricuspid annulus or right ventricle, including the following:
  1. Any cause of pulmonary hypertension (e.g., COPD, pulmonary embolism, restrictive lung disease, collagen vascular disease, and primary pulmonary hypertension)
  2. Left-sided heart failure leading to right-sided heart failure
  3. Dilated cardiomyopathy
  4. Right ventricular infarction
- Structural TR refers to conditions directly affecting the tricuspid valve apparatus, including the following:
  1. Rheumatic fever
  2. Congenital (e.g., Ebstein's anomaly, tricuspid atresia)
  3. Endocarditis—bacterial (particularly related to intravenous drug use) or marantic (e.g., systemic lupus erythematosus or rheumatoid arthritis)
  4. Tricuspid valve prolapse
  5. Carcinoid syndrome
  6. Marfan's syndrome
  7. Iatrogenic damage to the valve (e.g., pacemaker or implantable cardiac defibrillator insertion, endocardial biopsy)
  8. External trauma (deceleration injury)
  9. Right atrial myxoma
  10. Collagen-vascular disease
  11. Radiation injury

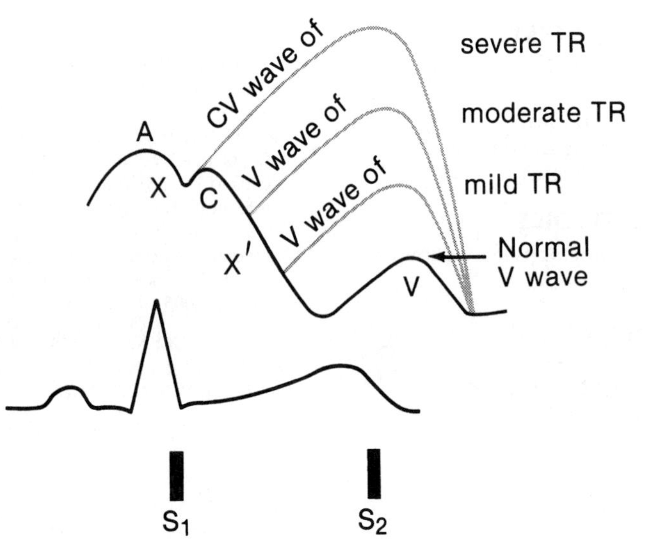

FIGURE 1-276 The jugular venous pulse in tricuspid regurgitation (TR). The jugular venous pulse wave normally drops during ventricular systole. As TR becomes more severe, the CV wave becomes more obvious during ventricular systole. (From Conn R: *Current diagnosis,* ed 9, Philadelphia, 1997, WB Saunders.)

DIAGNOSIS

The diagnosis of TR is made by clinical history, physical examination, and adjunctive studies including ECG, chest x-ray, echocardiography, and right-sided heart catheterization in selected cases.

DIFFERENTIAL DIAGNOSIS

Based on heart auscultation, the diagnosis of TR may be confused with other causes of systolic murmurs such as mitral regurgitation, aortic stenosis, pulmonary stenosis, ventricular septal defect, and hypertrophic cardiomyopathy.

WORKUP

Any patient suspected of having significant TR should undergo the following:
1. Chest x-ray
2. Electrocardiogram
3. Echocardiogram (confirmatory)
4. Right-sided heart cardiac catheterization (in selected cases)

LABORATORY TESTS

Electrocardiogram may show evidence of:
1. Right atrial enlargement (e.g., P-wave amplitude in leads II, III, aVF >2.5 mV)
2. Right ventricular enlargement/hypertrophy (e.g., R wave > S wave in lead V_1)
3. Right axis deviation >100 degrees
4. Atrial fibrillation

IMAGING STUDIES

- Chest x-ray may show:
  1. Evidence of COPD (e.g., flattened diaphragms, barrel chest, dilated pulmonary arteries, and increased retrosternal air space) or restrictive lung disease
  2. Enlarged right atrium
  3. Enlarged right ventricle
- Echocardiogram (Fig. 1-277) will:
  1. Detect TR
  2. Estimate the severity of TR
  3. Estimate the pulmonary artery pressure
  4. Exclude vegetation, mass or prolapse
  5. Assess left and right ventricular function
- Right-sided heart catheterization shows:

1. Elevated right atrial and right ventricular end-diastolic pressures
2. Large V waves

TREATMENT

Rx

Treatment of TR is usually directed at the underlying cause.

NONPHARMACOLOGIC THERAPY

Oxygen therapy is beneficial in patients with functional TR secondary to underlying pulmonary hypertension provoked by alveolar hypoxia.

ACUTE GENERAL Rx

- Functional TR caused by left-sided heart failure is treated in the standard way with preload reduction, afterload reduction, or inotropic therapy (see "Heart Failure").
- Reversal of pulmonary hypertension with vasodilators or pulmonary thromboendarterectomy has been shown to reverse functional TR.
- Structural TR treatment depends on the underlying cause of heart disease.

CHRONIC Rx

- Tricuspid valve repair is beneficial for severe TR in patients with mitral valve (MV) disease requiring MV surgery but carries a high morbidity/mortality. In rheumatic valvular disease, the 30-day morbidity/mortality rate may be as high as 15% to 20%.
- Tricuspid annuloplasty may be considered in mild and moderate TR in patients undergoing MV surgery when there is suspicion that their TR will progress despite MV surgery (e.g., pulmonary hypertension, tricuspid annular dilatation, or myxomatous involvement of the tricuspid valve).
- Tricuspid valve replacement or annuloplasty is reasonable in a symptomatic patient with severe TR and diseased or abnormal tricuspid valve leaflets not amenable to annuloplasty or repair.

DISPOSITION

- Regardless of the etiology, greater than mild degree of TR is associated with decreased survival.
- Isolated TR should not pose a significant problem during pregnancy, although greater care may be necessary to protect against diuretic-induced hypoperfusion.
- Isolated TR with normal right ventricular function does not preclude involvement in competitive sports.

REFERRAL

For patients with significant symptomatic TR, a cardiology consultation is recommended.

PEARLS & CONSIDERATIONS

!

TR caused by tricuspid valve prolapse is often associated with concurrent mitral valve prolapse.

COMMENTS

Antibiotic prophylaxis for dental, GI, or GU procedures is *no* longer recommended in patients with only structural tricuspid valve abnormalities.

SUGGESTED READINGS

Bonow RO et al: ACC/AHA 2006 guidelines for the management of patients with valvular heart disease: a report of the American College of Cardiology/American Heart Association Task Force on Practice Guidelines (Writing Committee to Develop Guidelines for the Management of Patients With Valvular Heart Disease), *Circulation* 48(3):598-675, 2006.

Raman SV et al: Tricuspid valve disease: tricuspid valve complex perspective, *Curr Prob Cardiol* 27(3):103-142, 2002.

Trichon BH, O'Connor CM: Secondary mitral and tricuspid regurgitation accompanying left ventricular systolic function: is it important, and how is it treated? *Am Heart J* 144(3):373-376, 2002.

AUTHORS: **BRIAN CASSERLY, M.D.**, and **GAURAV CHOUDHARY, M.D.**

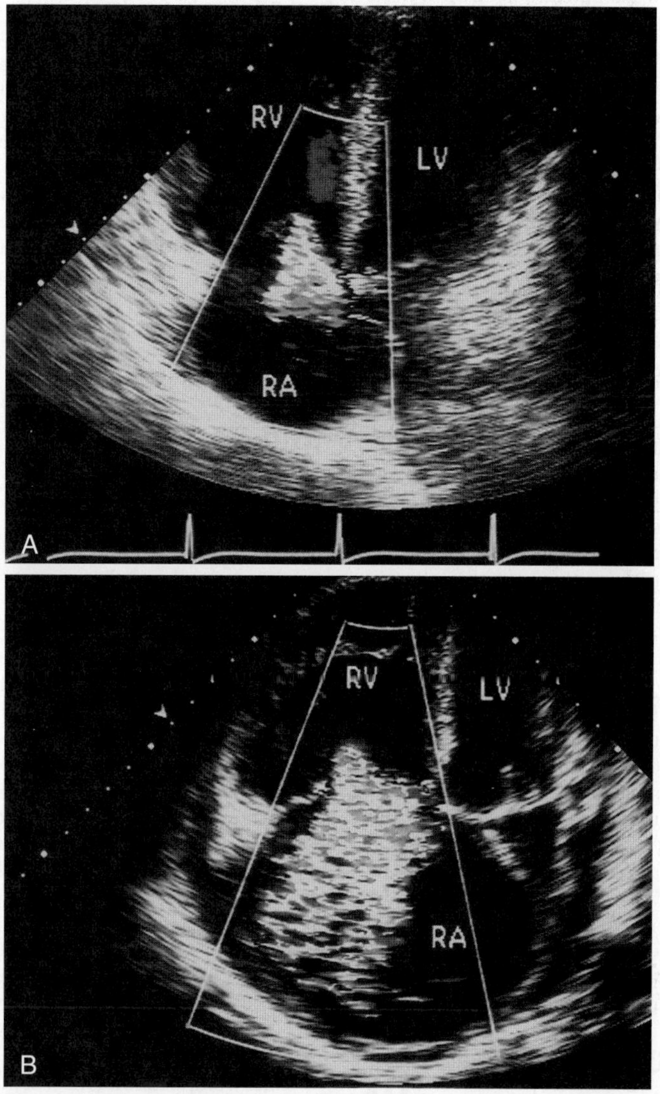

FIGURE 1-277 Two-dimensional echocardiograms with color flow imaging of patients with tricuspid regurgitation. A, Echocardiogram of a patient with severe tricuspid insufficiency. **B,** Echocardiogram of a patient with severe tricuspid regurgitation. *LV,* Left ventricle; *RA,* right atrium; *RV,* right ventricle. (From Zipes DP, Libby P, Bonow RO, Braunwauld E [eds]: *Braunwauld's heart disease,* ed 7, Philadelphia, 2005, Elsevier.)

BASIC INFORMATION

DEFINITION

Tricuspid stenosis (TS) is an uncommon valvular pathology caused by narrowing of the tricuspid valve orifice resulting in the restriction of right atrial emptying. TS is most often rheumatic in origin.

SYNONYMS

Tricuspid valve stenosis
TS

ICD-9CM CODES
397.0 Disease of the tricuspid valve

EPIDEMIOLOGY & DEMOGRAPHICS

- Most commonly a result of rheumatic heart disease and almost always occurs with associated mitral or aortic valve disease.
- Antibiotic therapy has made rheumatic heart disease and TS a rarity in the U.S.
- Present at autopsy in 15% of patients with rheumatic heart disease, but clinically significant in only 5%.

PHYSICAL FINDINGS & CLINICAL PRESENTATION

- Symptoms of right heart failure: fatigue, right upper quadrant abdominal pain (because of hepatic congestion), ascites, hepatomegaly, and peripheral edema.
- Jugular venous distention with a prominent "a" wave is noted along with a palpable hepatic pulsation.
- Right atrial pulsation may be palpated to the right of the sternum and a diastolic thrill that increases with inspiration may be felt over the left sternal edge.
- An opening snap and a diastolic murmur are best heard along the left sternal border of the fourth intercostal space and are augmented by inspiration.

ETIOLOGY

- Rheumatic heart disease results in scarring of the valve leaflets, shortening of the chordae tendineae, and fusion of the commissures, leading to immobility of the valve leaflets and narrowing of the tricuspid valve orifice.
- Other causes are congenital, infectious (e.g., endocarditis), metabolic or enzymatic (carcinoid syndrome, Whipple's disease, Fabry's disease), and systemic (e.g., lupus endocarditis).

DIAGNOSIS

DIFFERENTIAL DIAGNOSIS

- Congenital tricuspid atresia
- Right heart diastolic dysfunction: endomyocardial fibrosis, constrictive pericarditis
- Extrinsic compression of the right venticle: severe pectum excavatum, massive ascites, pleural effusion, pericardial effusion, or tumor
- Obstruction of right atrial emptying: right atrial myxoma, metastatic tumor (e.g., lymphoma), right atrial thrombi, tricuspid valve vegetation

WORKUP

- Echocardiography is the diagnostic test of choice
- Chest x-ray examination
- ECG: atrial arrhythmias, enlarged right atrium
- Right-heart catheterization in patients for whom echocardiography cannot make a definitive diagnosis

IMAGING STUDIES

- Echocardiography reveals thickening and shortening of the tricuspid valve leaflets, with restriction of movement of the leaflets and leaflet tips. Evidence of right atrial enlargement is present in most cases.
- Doppler echocardiography or cardiac catheterization demonstrates a reduced tricuspid valve area (severe: <1 cm^2) and a diastolic pressure gradient across the tricuspid valve (normal gradient <1 mm Hg).
- Chest x-ray may reveal an enlarged right atrium and reduced pulmonary blood volume.

TREATMENT

NONPHARMACOLOGIC THERAPY

Salt and fluid restrictions are essential to decrease peripheral edema.

ACUTE GENERAL Rx

- Diuretics to manage volume overload
- Rate-controlling AV nodal blockers and anticoagulation, especially in patients with atrial fibrillation

CHRONIC Rx

- Symptoms of systemic venous hypertension and congestion can be controlled with diuretics and ACE inhibitors or angiotensin receptor antagonists.
- Balloon valvotomy or dilation of the stenosed tricuspid valve has been described in both rheumatic and congenital TS with some success and low morbidity, but experience is limited and complications may occur (e.g., advanced heart block, significant tricuspid regurgitation).
- Surgery for TS is usually recommended when the tricuspid valve area falls below 2 cm^2 with a mean diastolic gradient across the tricuspid valve of >5 mm Hg.
- Isolated tricuspid valve replacement surgery almost never occurs and is typically performed in the setting of concomitant mitral or aortic valve surgery.
- Surgical procedures for TS include commissurotomy and tricuspid valve replacement.

DISPOSITION

The natural course of severe TS is not well known.

REFERRAL

TS may be difficult to diagnose and therefore consultation with a cardiology specialist is recommended.

PEARLS & CONSIDERATIONS

- Rheumatic heart disease accounts for over 90% of stenotic tricuspid valves.
- Rheumatic TS almost always occurs in association with mitral valve disease and sometimes aortic valve disease.
- Most cases present with tricuspid regurgitation or a combination of regurgitation and stenosis.

COMMENTS

- Tricuspid valve replacement carries a 30-day operative morbidity/mortality of 15% to 20%, in addition to a high risk of right heart thrombus formation. Therefore, surgical procedures are reserved for patients who are not candidates for balloon dilation techniques.
- Unlike mitral stenosis patients, TS patients typically do not complain of dyspnea, orthopnea, or paroxysmal nocturnal dyspnea.

SUGGESTED READINGS

AHA/ACC guidelines for the management of patients with valvular heart disease, *J Am Coll Cardiol* 48:e1, 2006.

Block PC, Bonhoeffer P: Percutaneous approaches to valvular heart disease, *Curr Cardiol Rep* 7(2):108, 2005.

Mehra MR et al: Difficult cases in heart failure: isolated tricuspid stenosis and heart failure: a focus on carcinoid heart disease, *Congest Heart Fail* 9(5):294, 2003.

Raman SV et al: Tricuspid valve disease: tricuspid valve complex perspective, *Curr Prob Cardiol* 27(3):103, 2002.

AUTHORS: **CRAIG McMACKIN, M.D.,** and **WEN-CHIH WU, M.D.**

BASIC INFORMATION

DEFINITION

Tricyclic antidepressants (TCAs) are secondary or tertiary amines that have variable abilities to inhibit reuptake of neurotransmitters (norepinephrine, dopamine, and serotonin) and to be anticholinergic, antihistaminic, and sedating. These properties are important to consider when prescribing these agents and when managing an intentional or accidental overdose.

SYNONYMS

Tricyclic antidepressant intoxication or poisoning
TCA OD

ICD-9CM CODES
969.0

EPIDEMIOLOGY & DEMOGRAPHICS

- TCAs are the most common cause of death resulting from prescription drug overdose in the U.S.
- Available TCAs: amitriptyline, imipramine, desipramine, nortriptyline, doxepin, amoxapine, clomipramine, protriptyline, and others.

PHYSICAL FINDINGS & CLINICAL PRESENTATION

Cardiovascular
- Intraventricular conduction delay (QRS prolongation)
- Sinus tachycardia
- Atrioventricular block
- Prolongation of the QT interval
- Ventricular tachycardia
- Wide complex tachycardia without P waves
- Refractory hypotension (the most common cause of death from TCA OD)
- Late arrhythmias or sudden death (in addition to the previous, which occur during the first 24 to 48 hr: late problems can occur up to 5 days after the OD)

Central nervous system
- Coma
- Delirium
- Myoclonus
- Seizures

Other
- Hyperthermia
- Ileus
- Urinary retention
- Pulmonary complications (e.g., aspiration pneumonitis)
- Life-threatening overdose exists with the ingestion of more than 1 g of TCA. Among patients who reach a hospital, most deaths occur within the first 24 hr; lack of initial symptoms can be deceptive

ETIOLOGY & PATHOGENESIS

Mechanisms of tricyclic antidepressant cardiovascular toxicity (Table 1-48)
CNS toxicity
- Cholinergic blockade is believed to cause hyperthermia, ileus, urinary retention, pupillary dilation, delirium, and coma.
- The mechanism of myoclonus and seizures is not fully understood.

DIAGNOSIS

DIFFERENTIAL DIAGNOSIS

Cardiotoxicity from TCA can be confused with intoxication by drugs that cause QRS prolongation. These include class Ia antiarrhythmic agents (disopyramide, procainamide, quinidine), class Ic antiarrhythmic agents (encainide, flecainide, propafenone), cocaine, propranolol, quinine, chloroquine, neuroleptics, propoxyphene, and digoxin. Other causes of QRS prolongation include hyperkalemia, ischemic heart disease, cardiomyopathy, and cardiac conduction system dysfunction.

WORKUP

- Clinical presentation
- Knowledge of the overdose
- Serum drug levels (TCA concentration >1 μg/ml is life threatening and TCA concentration >3 μg/ml is often fatal)
- Baseline CBC, prothrombin time, BUN, creatinine, and electrolytes

TREATMENT

ACUTE GENERAL Rx

Initial measures
- Hospitalization with cardiac monitoring as well as monitoring of vital signs and temperature
- Initiate intravenous access
- Administer activated charcoal with sorbitol
- Large-bore tube gastric lavage is of unproven benefit
- Ipecac is contraindicated
- 12-Lead ECG
- If no evidence of cardiotoxicity has been noted during the first 6 hr of observation, further monitoring is not necessary; if there is evidence of cardiotoxicity, monitoring should continue for 24 hr after all signs of toxicity have resolved

Treatment of specific complications of TCA toxicity: see Table 1-49.
When the patient is medically stable, psychiatric evaluation should be obtained.

SUGGESTED READING

Glauser J: Tricyclic antidepressant poisoning, *Cleve Clin J Med* 67:704, 2000.

AUTHORS: **FRED F. FERRI, M.D.**, and **TOM J. WACHTEL, M.D.**

TABLE 1-48 **Mechanism of Tricyclic Antidepressant Cardiovascular Toxicity**

Toxic Effect	Mechanism
Conduction Delays, Arrhythmias	
QRS prolongation atrioventricular block	Cardiac sodium channel → slowed depolarization in atrioventricular node, His-Purkinje fibers, and ventricular myocardium
Sinus tachycardia	Cholinergic blockade, inhibition of norepinephrine reuptake
Ventricular tachycardia	
Monomorphic	Cardiac sodium channel inhibition → reentry
Torsades de pointes	Cardiac potassium channel inhibition → prolonged repolarization
Ventricular bradycardia	Impaired cardiac automaticity
Hypotension	
Vasodilation	Vascular a-adrenergic receptor blockade
Decreased cardiac contractility	Cardiac sodium channel inhibition → impaired excitation-contraction coupling

TABLE 1-49 **Treatment of Complications of Tricyclic Antidepressant Toxicity**

Toxic Effect	Treatment
Cardiovascular	
QRS prolongation	Hypertonic $NaHCO_3$ if QRS prolongation is marked or progressing; not clear if treatment is needed in the absence of hypotension or arrhythmias
Hypotension	Intravascular volume expansion, $NaHCO_3$ Vasopressors (norepinephrine) or inotropic agents (dopamine) Correct hyperthermia, acidosis, seizures Consider mechanical support
Ventricular tachycardia	$NaHCO_3$, lidocaine, overdrive, pacing Correct hypotension, hypothermia, acidosis, seizures
Torsades de pointes	Overdrive, pacing
Ventricular bradycardia	Chronotropic agent (epinephrine), pacemaker
Sinus tachycardia	Treatment rarely needed
Atrioventricular block type II second or third degree	Pacemaker
Hypertension	Rapidly titratable antihypertensive agent (nitroprusside)
Central Nervous System	
Delirium	Restraints, benzodiazepine Neuromuscular blockade for hyperthermia, acidosis
Seizures	Benzodiazepine Neuromuscular blockade for hyperthermia, acidosis
Coma	Intubation, ventilation if needed
Other	
Hyperthermia	Control seizures, agitation Cooling measures
Acidosis	$NaHCO_3$ Correct hypotension, hypoventilation

BASIC INFORMATION

DEFINITION

Trigeminal neuralgia is a syndrome characterized by recurrent excruciating paroxysms of lancinating pain in the distribution of one or more divisions of the trigeminal (fifth) nerve.

SYNONYMS

Tic douloureux

ICD-9CM CODES
350.1 Trigeminal neuralgia

EPIDEMIOLOGY & DEMOGRAPHICS

INCIDENCE (IN U.S.): 3 to 5/100,000
PREVALENCE (IN U.S.): 155/1 million persons
PREDOMINANT SEX: Slight predominance of females to males
PEAK INCIDENCE: Median age 67 years
GENETICS: Uncommonly familial and possibly caused by underlying genetic etiology (see "Etiology" under "Rare causes")

PHYSICAL FINDINGS & CLINICAL PRESENTATION

- Each attack lasts only seconds but may cluster.
- Often, attacks are brought on by mild stimulation of trigger zones, located in the affected division of the fifth nerve. These triggers include light touching, eating, drinking, shaving, and draught of air.

ETIOLOGY

- It is thought that 80% to 90% of cases are due to compression of the trigeminal nerve root at the cerebellopontine angle by an aberrant loop of artery or vein, and rarely a saccular aneurysm or arteriovenous malformation
- Compressive lesions such as schwannomas, epidermoid cysts and meningiomas, also typically at the cerebellopontine angle
- Bony compression of the fifth nerve (e.g., from an osteoma or deformity resulting from osteogenesis imperfecta)
- Primary demyelinating disorders: multiple sclerosis (2% to 4% of patients) and rarely Charcot-Marie-Tooth disease. In multiple sclerosis, usually there is a plaque of demyelination at the root entry zone of the fifth nerve in the pons
- Rare causes: (a) infiltrative disorders such as carcinomatous or amyloid deposits in the fifth nerve root, nerve proper, or ganglion; (b) familial occurrence has been reported in Charcot-Marie-Tooth disease

DIAGNOSIS

DIFFERENTIAL DIAGNOSIS

- Dental pathology
- The differential diagnosis of headache and facial pain is described in Section II.

WORKUP

MRI scans (CT scan with thin posterior fossa cuts if MRI not available) for all patients to exclude mass lesions or evidence of central demyelination as in multiple sclerosis

TREATMENT

NONPHARMACOLOGIC THERAPY

- In refractory cases, surgical options, including percutaneous radiofrequency gangliolysis and microvascular decompression. Motor cortex stimulation has provided hopeful results; however, this is a new approach, and evidence is largely based on case reports at this stage.
- Gamma-knife radiosurgery is an increasingly popular alternative to conventional surgery for trigeminal neuralgia.

ACUTE GENERAL Rx

None, episodes are too brief

CHRONIC Rx

- Carbamazepine is the treatment of choice, providing relief to at least 75% of patients. Begin with 100 mg bid and increase gradually as tolerated using a tid regimen.
- If carbamazepine is not tolerated or effective, use gabapentin, 400 mg PO tid. Doses as high as 3600 mg/day are easily tolerated. Topiramate (Topamax) 25 mg qhs gradually titrated up to 100 mg bid is also effective. Other drugs in practice include oxcarbazepine and baclofen.

DISPOSITION

Spontaneous remissions occur after months to years.

REFERRAL

If uncertain about diagnosis or if surgical treatment is necessary

PEARLS & CONSIDERATIONS

Even in patients with multiple sclerosis, a vascular compression may be the source of symptoms and thus may benefit from intervention such as surgery.

COMMENTS

Because prolonged remission may occur, drug tapering at yearly intervals is recommended.

EVIDENCE

Carbamazepine is the first-line drug for trigeminal neuralgia, with high quality evidence from multiple crossover RCTs. In summary, all other medical (and nonmedical) modalities are based on anecdotal evidence (see Zakrzewska and Chesire reviews). Although pimozide was shown to be of benefit in carbamazapine failures in an RCT, its use remains limited in practice due to cardiac side effects.

SUGGESTED READINGS

Chesire WP: Trigeminal neuralgia: diagnosis and treatment, *Curr Neurol and Neurosci Rep* 5:79, 2005.

Elias WJ and Burchiel KJ: Trigeminal neuralgia and other neuropathic pain syndromes of the head and face, *Curr Pain Headache Rep* 6(2):115, 2002.

Kitt CA et al. Trigeminal neuralgia: opportunities for research and treatment, *Pain* 85: 3, 2000

Loeser JD: Tic douloureux, *Pain Res Manag* 6(3):156, 2001.

Love S, Coakham HB: Trigeminal neuralgia: pathology and pathogenesis, *Brain* 124(Pt 12):2347, 2001.

Maesawa S et al: Clinical outcomes after stereotactic radiosurgery for idiopathic trigeminal neuralgia, *J Neurosurg* 94:16, 2001.

Zakrzewska JM, Lopez BC: Trigeminal neuralgia, *Clin Evid* 14(1-2), 2005.

AUTHOR: **U. SHIVRAJ SOHUR, M.D., PH.D.**

BASIC INFORMATION

DEFINITION

"Trigger finger," or digital stenosing tenosynovitis, refers to an inflammatory process of the digital flexor tendon sheath.

SYNONYMS

Digital stenosing tenosynovitis

ICD-9CM CODES
727.03 Trigger finger (acquired)

EPIDEMIOLOGY & DEMOGRAPHICS

- Trigger finger can be found in all age groups but is commonly found in patients older than 45 yr
- More frequently affects females (4:1)
- Occupational risk groups: meat cutters, seamstress, tailors, and dentists
- In adults, the middle finger is most often affected (Fig. 1-278)
- In children, the thumb is most often affected

PHYSICAL FINDINGS & CLINICAL PRESENTATION

- Hand pain
- Painful triggering or snapping with flexion and extension of the affected digit
- Locking or loss of active digital extension is the most common symptom
- The digit is usually fixed in flexion (trapped or incarcerated)
- Usually affects one digit
- If more digits are involved, a systemic cause is most likely present (e.g., diabetes, rheumatoid arthritis)
- A palpable tender nodule is noted at the MCP joint of the affected digit
- Pain over the flexor tendon with resisted flexion
- Pain with passive stretching

ETIOLOGY

Trigger finger is described as being primary or secondary:
- Primary (idiopathic)
- Secondary
  1. Diabetes
  2. Rheumatoid arthritis
  3. Hypothyroidism
  4. Histiocytosis
  5. Amyloidosis
  6. Gout

DIAGNOSIS

Clinical history and physical examination

DIFFERENTIAL DIAGNOSIS

- Dupuytren's contracture
- De Quervain's tenosynovitis
- Acute digital tenosynovitis
- Proliferative tenosynovitis
- Carpal tunnel syndrome
- Flexion tendon rupture
- Trauma

WORKUP

Pursued if a secondary cause is suspected.

LABORATORY TESTS

- CBC with differential
- Electrolytes, BUN, and creatinine
- Blood glucose
- Thyroid function tests
- Uric acid
- Rheumatoid factor

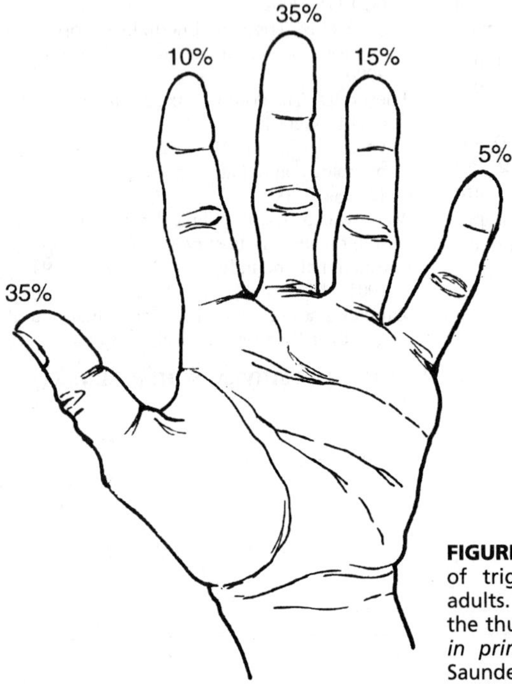

FIGURE 1-278 Trigger finger. Frequency of trigger finger according to digit in adults. In children, virtually all cases occur in the thumb. (From Canoso J: *Rheumatology in primary care,* Philadelphia, 1997, WB Saunders.)

IMAGING STUDIES

X-ray studies are not very helpful unless a secondary cause has affected other organs (e.g., rheumatoid lung).

TREATMENT

NONPHARMACOLOGIC THERAPY

Splinting can be tried early in the course but has not been very successful.

ACUTE GENERAL Rx

- In idiopathic trigger finger, steroid injection with 15 to 20 mg depomethylprenisolone acetate in 1 ml 1% Xylocaine has been used with success.
- Triamcinolone 10 mg with 1 ml of 1% Xylocaine is an alternative steroid choice to be used in patients who do not respond to the first injection.
- If symptoms do not resolve in 3 wk, a repeat injection can be tried.

CHRONIC Rx

- Surgical release is indicated in patients with refractory symptoms (e.g., locked digits) despite nonpharmacologic and acute treatment.
- Surgery is also indicated in patients with recurrent symptoms despite steroid injection.

DISPOSITION

- Following steroid injection, symptoms usually resolve in 3 to 5 days, and locking resolves in 60% of the cases in 2 to 3 wk.
- If symptoms recur, a repeat steroid injection improves the symptoms in >80% of patients.
- Diabetic patients do not have the same success rate with steroid injections as the primary group.

REFERRAL

If steroid injection therapy is considered, a rheumatology consult is requested.

PEARLS & CONSIDERATIONS

COMMENTS

If more than one digit is involved, a workup for a secondary systemic cause is in order.

SUGGESTED READINGS

Akhtar S et al: Management and referral for trigger finger/thumb, *BMJ* 331(7507):30, 2005.
Ryzewicz M, Wolf J: Trigger digits: principles, management and complications, *J Hand Surg* 31(1):135, 2006.
Saldana MJ: Trigger digits: diagnosis and treatment, *J Am Acad Orthop Surg* 9(4):246, 2001.

AUTHOR: **PETER PETROPOULOS, M.D.**

BASIC INFORMATION

DEFINITION

Trochanteric bursitis is a presumed inflammation or irritation of the gluteus maximus bursa or the bursa separating the greater trochanter from the gluteus medius and gluteus minimus (Fig. 1-279).

SYNONYMS

Greater trochanteric pain syndrome

ICD-9CM CODES
726.5 Bursitis trochanteric area

EPIDEMIOLOGY & DEMOGRAPHICS

- Trochanteric bursitis is commonly associated with other conditions:
  1. Osteoarthritis of the hip
  2. Lumbar spinal degenerative joint disease
  3. Rheumatoid arthritis
- Incidence peaks between the fourth and sixth decades of life but can occur at any age group
- Occurs in females > males (4:1)

PHYSICAL FINDINGS & CLINICAL PRESENTATION

- Hip pain is the most common complaint. The pain is chronic, intermittent, and located over the lateral thigh.
- Numbness can be present.
- Pain is precipitated with prolonged lying or standing on the affected side.
- Walking, climbing, and running exacerbate the pain.
- Point tenderness over the greater trochanter is noted.
- Pain is reproduced with resisted hip abduction.

ETIOLOGY

- The specific cause of trochanteric bursitis is not known although repetitive high-intensity use of the hip joint, trauma, infection (tuberculosis and bacterial), and crystal deposition can precipitate the disease.
- Trochanteric bursitis can occur when other conditions such as osteoarthritis of the knee and hip and bunions of the feet cause changes in the patient's gait, placing varus stress on the hip joint.

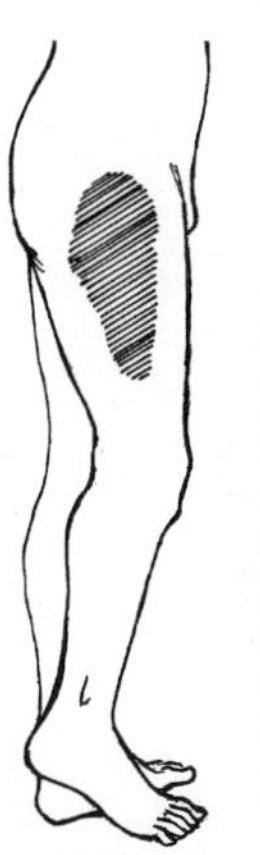

FIGURE 1-279 Typical location of pain in trochanteric bursitis syndrome. This is also a frequent pain radiation site for lumbar spine lesion, various nerve compression syndromes, and hip disease, particularly in osteonecrosis of the femoral head. (From Canoso J: *Rhematology in primary care,* Philadelphia, 1997, WB Saunders.)

DIAGNOSIS

A detailed physical examination and clinical presentation usually make the diagnosis of trochanteric bursitis. Laboratory tests and x-ray images are helpful adjunctive studies used to exclude other conditions either associated with or mimicking trochanteric bursitis.

DIFFERENTIAL DIAGNOSIS

- Osteoarthritis of the hip
- Osteonecrosis of the hip
- Stress fracture of the hip
- Osteoarthritis of the lumbar spine
- Fibromyalgia
- Iliopsoas bursitis
- Trochanteric tendonitis
- Gout
- Pseudogout
- Trauma
- Neuropathy
- Tuberculosis of the greater trochanter
- Metastatic bone disease

WORKUP

A workup is indicated if suspected associated conditions exist; otherwise treatment can be started on clinical grounds alone.

LABORATORY TESTS

CBC with differential may show elevated white count if infection is present.
ESR is elevated in an inflammatory process.

IMAGING STUDIES

- Plain x-rays of the hip are not very helpful in diagnosing trochanteric bursitis. Sometimes calcifications may be seen around the greater trochanter.
- Bone scan can be done but is usually not necessary.
- CT and MRI may show bursitis but are usually not warranted because it will not alter treatment.

TREATMENT

NONPHARMACOLOGIC THERAPY

- Heat 15 to 20 min 4 to 6 times per day
- Ultrasound therapy
- Rest
- Partial weight bearing
- Physical therapy to strengthen back, hip, and knee muscles

ACUTE GENERAL Rx

- NSAIDs, ibuprofen 800 mg PO tid, or naproxen 500 mg PO bid is used for pain relief.
- Acetaminophen 500-mg tablet, 1 to 2 tablets PO q6h prn can be used with NSAIDs or alternating with NSAIDs.
- Corticosteroid injection (30 to 40 mg depomethylprednisolone acetate mixed with 3 ml 1% Xylocaine).

CHRONIC Rx

Although rarely done, surgical removal of the bursa is possible for patients with refractory symptoms or infection.

DISPOSITION

- Most patients respond to NSAIDs and/or nonpharmacologic therapy.
- If steroid injection is used, approximately 70% of patients respond after the first injection and more than 90% respond to two injections.
- 25% of patients receiving steroid injection may develop a relapse.

REFERRAL

A rheumatology or orthopedics referral is made if steroid injection therapy is needed or if the etiology is thought to be infectious.

PEARLS & CONSIDERATIONS

Patients with trochanteric bursitis will commonly complain of "hip" pain. The physical examination readily distinguishes true hip pain from trochanteric bursitis.

COMMENTS

- The absence of pain with flexion and extension differentiates trochanteric bursitis from degenerative joint disease of the hip.
- Localization of pain over the lateral thigh differentiates trochanteric bursitis from pain caused by meralgia paresthetica located over the anterolateral thigh and pain from osteoarthritis located over the inner thigh groin area.

SUGGESTED READINGS

Adkins SB, Figler RA: Hip pain in athletes, *Am Fam Physician* 61(7):2109, 2000.

Canoso JJ: Hip pain. In Canoso JJ, Kersey R (eds): *Rheumatology in primary care.* Philadelphia, 1997, WB Saunders.

Cardone DA, Tallia AF: Diagnostic and therapeutic injection of the hip and knee, *Am Fam Physician* 67:2147, 2003.

Segal NA et al, Multicenter Osteoarthritis Study Group: Greater trochanteric pain syndrome: epidemiology and associated factors, *Arch Phys Med Rehabil* 88(8):988, 2007.

AUTHOR: **MEL ANDERSON, M.D.**

BASIC INFORMATION

DEFINITION

Tropical sprue is a malabsorption syndrome occurring primarily in tropical regions, including Puerto Rico, India, and Southeast Asia.

SYNONYMS

Postinfectious tropical malabsorption
"Tropical enteropathy" refers to a subclinical form of tropical sprue.

ICD-9CM CODES
579.1 Tropical sprue

EPIDEMIOLOGY & DEMOGRAPHICS

- Tropical sprue is endemic in tropical regions, Venezuela, Colombia, the Middle East, the Far East, the Caribbean [Puerto Rico, Haiti, Dominican Republic, Cuba], and India.
- The disease affects mainly adults although it has been reported in all age groups.

PHYSICAL FINDINGS & CLINICAL PRESENTATION

- The classic clinical features of tropical sprue are nonspecific and simply reflect the symptom of malabsorption. Onset is generally not insidious and most patients can pinpoint when their disorder began.
- Diffuse, nonspecific abdominal tenderness and distention. Abdominal pain is crampy in nature.
- Low-grade fever.
- Glossitis, cheilosis, hyperkeratosis, hyperpigmentation.
- Diarrhea, often with mucus and foul-smelling stools due to fat malabsorption.
- Nausea, which leads to decreased appetite and decreased oral intake.
- Lactose intolerance often develops early in the course of tropical sprue.

ETIOLOGY

- Unknown. There is a strong presumption that it is caused by an enteric infection, perhaps in individuals predisposed by some nutritional deficiency.
- Associated with overgrowth of predominantly coliform bacteria in the small intestine.

DIAGNOSIS

The clinical features of tropical sprue include anorexia, diarrhea, weight loss, abdominal pain, and steatorrhea; these symptoms can develop in expatriates even several months after immigrating to temperate regions.

DIFFERENTIAL DIAGNOSIS

- Celiac disease
- Parasitic infestation
- Inflammatory bowel disease
- Other causes of malabsorption (e.g., Whipple's disease)
- Lymphoma
- Pancreatic tumor
- Intestinal TB
- Microsporidia-associated HIV enteropathy

WORKUP

Diagnostic workup includes a comprehensive history (especially travel history), physical examination, laboratory evidence of malabsorption (see "Laboratory Tests"), and jejunal biopsy; the biopsy results are nonspecific, with blunting, atrophy, and even disappearance of the villi and subepithelial lymphocytic infiltration. Partial villus atrophy distinguishes tropical sprue histologically from celiac sprue, which reveals flattened mucosa.

LABORATORY TESTS

- Megaloblastic anemia (>50% of cases)
- Vitamin B_{12} deficiency, folate deficiency
- Abnormal D-xylose absorption (72-hour fecal fat determination or serum carotene concentration)
- Stool examination to exclude *Giardia*

IMAGING STUDIES

GI series with small bowel follow-through may reveal coarsening of the jejunal folds.

TREATMENT

NONPHARMACOLOGIC THERAPY

Monitoring of weight and calorie intake

ACUTE GENERAL Rx

- Folic acid therapy (5 mg bid for 2 wk followed by a maintenance dose of 1 mg tid) will improve anemia and malabsorption in more than two thirds of patients.
- Tetracycline 250 mg qid for 4 to 6 wk in individuals who have returned to temperate zones, up to 6 mo in patients in endemic areas; ampicillin 500 mg bid for at least 4 wk in patients intolerant to tetracycline.
- Correction of vitamin B_{12} deficiency: vitamin B_{12} 1000 μg IM weekly for 4 wk, then monthly for 3 to 6 mo.
- Correction of other nutritional deficiencies (e.g., calcium, iron).

DISPOSITION

Complete recovery with appropriate therapy

REFERRAL

GI referral for jejunal biopsy

PEARLS & CONSIDERATIONS

COMMENTS

- Tropical sprue should be considered in any patient who presents with chronic diarrhea, weight loss, and malabsorption, especially if there is significant travel and exposure history.
- Important factors in the medical history in addition to travel history are use of medications that may predispose to a small bowel overgrowth, HIV exposure (increased risk of chronic diarrhea), and any surgical procedure that may predispose to blind loop syndrome.
- Most of the functional changes in tropical sprue may be related to small bowel mucosal damage; however, there is also dysfunctional hormonal regulation of the gut (increased enteroglucagon, motilin levels, decreased postprandial insulin and gastric inhibitory peptide) and decreased ability of the colon to absorb water.
- Even with prolonged therapy, relapses can occur; however, some may be reexposure to an infecting organism rather than relapsing disease.

AUTHOR: **FRED F. FERRI, M.D.**

BASIC INFORMATION

DEFINITION

Miliary tuberculosis (TB) is an infection of disseminated hematogenous disease, caused by the bacterium *Mycobacterium tuberculosis,* and is often characterized as resembling millet seeds on examination. Extrapulmonary disease may occur in virtually every organ site.

SYNONYMS

Disseminated TB

ICD-9CM CODES
018.94 Miliary tuberculosis

EPIDEMIOLOGY & DEMOGRAPHICS

INCIDENCE (IN U.S.): >38% of AIDS patients with TB have disseminated disease, often with concurrent pulmonary and extrapulmonary active sites. (See "Pulmonary Tuberculosis" in Section I.)

PEAK INCIDENCE: HIV-positive patients, regardless of age

PREVALENCE (IN U.S.):
- Undetermined
- Highest prevalence
  1. AIDS patients
  2. Minorities
  3. Children
  4. Foreign-born persons
  5. Elderly

PREDOMINANT SEX:
- No specific predilection
- Male predominance in AIDS, shelters, and prisons reflected in disproportionate male TB incidence

PREDOMINANT AGE: Predominantly among 24- to 45-yr-olds

PHYSICAL FINDINGS & CLINICAL PRESENTATION

- See also "Etiology"
- Common symptoms
  1. High intermittent fever
  2. Night sweats
  3. Weight loss
- Symptoms referable to individual organ systems may predominate
  1. Meninges
  2. Pericardium
  3. Liver
  4. Kidney
  5. Bone
  6. GI tract
  7. Lymph nodes
  8. Serous spaces
     a. Pleural
     b. Pericardial
     c. Peritoneal
     d. Joint
  9. Skin
  10. Lung: cough, shortness of breath
- Adrenal insufficiency possible caused by infection of adrenal gland
- Pancytopenia
  1. With fever and weight loss *or*
  2. Without other localizing symptoms or signs *or*
  3. With only splenomegaly
- TB hepatitis
  1. Tender liver
  2. Obstructive enzymes (alkaline phosphatase) elevated out of proportion to minimal hepatocellular enzymes (SGOT, SGPT) and bilirubin
- TB meningitis
  1. Gradual-onset headache
  2. Minimal meningeal signs
  3. Malaise
  4. Low-grade fever (may be absent)
  5. Sudden stupor or coma
  6. Cranial nerve VI palsy
- TB pericarditis
  1. Effusions resembling TB pleurisy
  2. Cardiac tamponade
- Skeletal TB
  1. Large joint arthritis (with effusions resembling TB pericarditis)
  2. Bone lesions (especially ribs)
  3. Pott's disease
     a. TB spondylitis, especially of lower thoracic spine
     b. Paraspinous TB abscess
     c. Possible psoas abscess
     d. Frequent cord compression (often relieved by steroids)
- Genitourinary TB
  1. Renal TB
     a. Papillary necrosis
     b. Destruction of renal pelvis
     c. Strictures of upper third of ureters
     d. Hematuria
     e. Pyuria with misleading bacterial cultures
     f. Preserved renal function
  2. TB orchitis or epididymitis
     a. Scrotal mass
     b. Draining abscess
  3. Chronic prostatic TB
- Gastrointestinal TB
  1. Diarrhea
  2. Pain
  3. Obstruction
  4. Bleeding
  5. Especially common with AIDS
  6. Bowel lesions
     a. Circumferential ulcers
     b. Short strictures
     c. Calcified granulomas
     d. TB mesenteric caseous adenitis
     e. Abscess, but rare fistula formation
     f. Often difficult to distinguish from granulomatous bowel disease (Crohn's disease)
- TB peritonitis
  1. Fluid resembles TB pleurisy
  2. PPD often negative
  3. Tender abdomen
  4. Doughy peritoneal consistency, often with ascites
  5. Peritoneal biopsy indicated for diagnosis
- TB lymphadenitis (scrofula)
  1. May involve all node groups
  2. Common adenopathies
     a. Cervical
     b. Supraclavicular
     c. Axillary
     d. Retroperitoneal
  3. Biopsy generally needed for diagnosis
  4. Surgical resection of nodes may be necessary
  5. Especially common with AIDS
- Cutaneous TB
  1. Skin infection from autoinoculation or dissemination
  2. Nodules or abscesses
  3. Tuberculids (possibly allergic reactions)
  4. Erythema nodosum
- Miscellaneous presentations
  1. TB laryngitis
  2. TB otitis
  3. Ocular TB
     a. Choroidal tubercles
     b. Iritis
     c. Uveitis
     d. Episcleritis
  4. Adrenal TB
  5. Breast TB

ETIOLOGY

- See also "Pulmonary Tuberculosis" in Section I
- *Mycobacterium tuberculosis* (Mtb), a slow growing, aerobic, non–spore-forming, nonmotile bacillus
- Humans are the only reservoir for Mtb
- Pathogenesis:
  1. AFB (Mtb) are ingested by macrophages in alveoli, then transported to regional lymph nodes where spread is contained.
  2. Some AFB reach the bloodstream and disseminate widely.
  3. Immediate active disseminated disease may ensue or a latent period may develop.
  4. During latent period, T-cell immune mechanisms contain infection in granulomas until later reactivation occurs as a result of immunosuppression or other undefined factors in conjunction with reactivated pulmonary TB or alone.
- Miliary TB may occur as a consequence of the following:
  1. Primary infection: inability to contain primary infection leads to a hematogenous spread and progressive disseminated disease.
  2. In late chronic TB and in those with advanced age or poor immunity, a continuous seeding of the blood may develop and lead to disseminated disease.

DIAGNOSIS

DIFFERENTIAL DIAGNOSIS

- Widespread sites of possible dissemination associated with myriad differential diagnostic possibilities
- Lymphoma
- Typhoid fever
- Brucellosis
- Other tumors
- Collagen-vascular disease

WORKUP

- Prompt evaluation is essential
- Sputum for AFB stain and culture
- Chest x-ray examination
- PPD
- Fluid analysis and culture wherever available
  1. Sputum
  2. Blood: particularly helpful in patients with AIDS
  3. Urine
  4. CSF
  5. Pleural
  6. Pericardial
  7. Peritoneal
  8. Gastric aspirates
- Biopsy of any involved tissue is advisable to make immediate diagnosis
  1. Transbronchial biopsy preferred and easily accessible
  2. Bone marrow
  3. Lymph node
  4. Scrotal mass if present
  5. Any other involved site
  6. Positive granuloma or AFB on biopsy specimen is diagnostic
- Imaging studies as needed

LABORATORY TESTS

- Culture and fluid analysis as described previously
- Smear-negative sputum often is positive weeks later on culture
- CBC is usually normal
- ESR is usually elevated

IMAGING STUDIES

- Chest x-ray examination (may or may not be positive) (See "Pulmonary Tuberculosis" in Section I)
- CT scan or MRI of brain
  1. Tuberculoma
  2. Basilar arachnoiditis
- Barium studies of bowel

TREATMENT

NONPHARMACOLOGIC THERAPY

- Bed rest during acute phase of treatment
- High-calorie, high-protein diet to reverse malnutrition and enhance immune response to TB
- Isolation in negative-pressure rooms with high-volume air replacement and circulation (with health care provider wearing proper protective 0.5- to 1-micron filter respirators)
  1. Until three consecutive sputum AFB smears are negative, if pulmonary disease coexists
  2. Isolation not required for closed-space TB infections

ACUTE GENERAL Rx

- See "Pulmonary Tuberculosis" in Section I.
- Therapy should be initiated immediately. Do not wait for definitive diagnosis.
- More rapid response to chemotherapy by disseminated TB foci than cavitary pulmonary TB.
- Treatment for 6 mo with INH plus rifampin plus PZA.
  1. Treatment for 12 mo often required for bone and renal TB.
  2. Prolonged treatment often required for CNS and pericardial.
  3. Prolonged treatment often required for all disseminated TB in infants.
- Compliance (rigid adherence to treatment regimen) is the chief determinant of success.
  1. Supervised DOT is recommended for all patients.
  2. Supervised DOT is mandatory for unreliable patients.
- Steroids are often helpful additions in fulminant miliary disease with the hypoxemia and DIC.

CHRONIC Rx

- Generally not indicated beyond treatment described previously
- Prolonged treatment supervised by ID expert required in a few complicated infections caused by resistant organisms

DISPOSITION

- Monthly follow-up by physician experienced in TB treatment
- Confirm sensitivity testing, and alter treatment appropriately (see "Pulmonary Tuberculosis" in Section I)

REFERRAL

- To infectious disease expert for:
  1. HIV-positive patient
  2. Patient with suspected drug-resistant TB
  3. Patients previously treated for TB
  4. Patients whose fever has not decreased and sputum (if positive) has not converted to negative in 2 to 4 wk
  5. Patients with overwhelming pulmonary or extrapulmonary tuberculosis
- To pulmonary, orthopedic, or GI physicians for examinations or biopsy

PEARLS & CONSIDERATIONS

COMMENTS

- All contacts (especially close household contacts and infants) should be properly tested for PPD conversions >3 mo following exposure.
- Those with positive PPD should be evaluated for active TB and properly treated or given prophylaxis.

EVIDENCE

A systematic review compared various treatment regimens in patients with newly diagnosed, active pulmonary tuberculosis. Treatment for <6 months was associated with higher relapse rates.[1] Ⓐ Two randomized controlled trials (RCTs) found no difference in relapse rates when 6-month treatment regimens were compared with longer (8- to 9-month) regimens in patients with newly diagnosed pulmonary tuberculosis. The regimens included different combinations of isoniazid, rifampin, ethambutol, streptomycin, and pyrazinamide for initial and continuation treatment.[2,3] Ⓐ

A systematic review identified one RCT, which compared treatment regimens of daily vs. three-times-weekly over 6 months in patients with pulmonary tuberculosis. There was no significant difference in cure rates between the groups at 1 month after completion of the treatment. A clinically important difference between the dosing regimens could not be ruled out.[4] Ⓑ

A systematic review found insufficient evidence from RCTs demonstrating the efficacy of direct observation of tablet swallowing in the treatment of tuberculosis in low-, middle-, and high-income country settings. There was no significant difference between direct observation and self-treatment for cure or treatment completion.[5] Ⓐ However, the most recent American guidelines recommend this form of therapy, based on three key references.[6-9] Ⓑ Ⓒ

A systematic review of RCTs studied the effectiveness of tuberculosis preventive therapy in reducing the risk of active tuberculosis and death in persons infected with HIV. Preventive therapy (with any anti-TB regimen) was associated with a significantly lower incidence of active tuberculosis compared with placebo, but all-cause mortality rates were similar in both groups. Those with a positive tuberculin skin test were more likely to benefit from treatment than those with a negative test.[10] Ⓐ

Limited evidence from this review suggested that the protective effect of therapy may have declined over the short to medium term. No one regimen was found to be superior; however, short-course multidrug regimens were much more likely to be discontinued due to adverse effects, compared with INH monotherapy.[10] Ⓐ

A systematic review found that isoniazid is effective for the prevention of active tuberculosis in HIV-negative patients who are at increased risk of developing the infection.[11] Ⓐ

Evidence-Based References

1. Gelband H: Regimens of less than six months for treating tuberculosis, *Cochrane Database Syst Rev* 4, 1999 (Cochrane Review). Ⓐ
2. East and Central African/British Medical Research Council Fifth Collaborative Study: Controlled clinical trial of 4 short-course regimens of chemotherapy (three 6-month and one 8-month) for pulmonary tuberculosis, *Tubercle* 64:153, 1983. Reviewed in: *Clin Evid* 12:1194, 2004. Ⓐ
3. British Thoracic Society: A controlled trial of 6 months' chemotherapy in pulmonary tuberculosis, final report: results during the 36 months after the end of chemotherapy and beyond, *Br J Dis Chest* 78:330, 1984. Reviewed in: *Clin Evid* 9:901, 2003. Ⓐ
4. Mwandumba HC, Squire SB: Fully intermittent dosing with drugs for treating tuberculosis in adults (Cochrane Review). Reviewed in: Cochrane Library 1, Chichester, UK, 2004, John Wiley. Ⓑ
5. Volmink J, Garner P: Directly observed therapy for treating tuberculosis (Cochrane Review). Reviewed in: Cochrane Library 1, Chichester, UK, 2004, John Wiley. Ⓐ
6. The Infectious Diseases Society of America, the American Thoracic Society, the Centers for Disease Control and Prevention: Treatment of tuberculosis, *MMWR Recomm Rep* 52(RR-11):1, 2003. Ⓒ
7. Chaulk CP: Eleven years of community-based directly observed therapy for tuberculosis, *JAMA* 274;945, 1995. Ⓑ
8. Chaulk CP: Directly observed therapy for treatment completion of tuberculosis: concensus statement of the Public Health Tuberculosis Guidelines Panel, *JAMA* 279:943, 1998. Ⓒ
9. Weis SE et al: The effect of directly observed therapy on the rates of drug resistance and relapse in tuberculosis, *N Engl J Med* 330:1179, 1994. Ⓑ
10. Woldehanna S, Volmink J: Treatment of latent tuberculosis infection in HIV infected persons (Cochrane Review). Reviewed in: Cochrane Library 1, Chichester, UK, 2004, John Wiley. Ⓐ
11. Smieja MJ et al: Isoniazid for preventing tuberculosis in non-HIV infected persons (Cochrane Review). Reviewed in: Cochrane Library 1, Chichester, UK, 2004, John Wiley. Ⓐ

SUGGESTED READINGS

American Thoracic Society, CDC and the Infectious Disease Society of America: Controlling tuberculosis in the United States, *MMWR* 54(RR-12):1, 2005.

Golden MP, Vikram HR: Extrapulmonary tuberculosis: an overview, *Am Fam Physician* 72(9):1761, 2005.

Maher D et al: Tuberculosis deaths in countries with high HIV prevalence: what is their use as an indicator in tuberculosis programme monitoring and epidemiological surveillance? *Int J Tuberc Lung Dis* 9(2):123, 2005.

Matsushima T: Miliary tuberculosis or disseminated tuberculosis, *Intern Med* 44(7):687, 2005.

Miyoshi I et al: Miliary tuberculosis not affecting the lungs but complicated by acute respiratory distress syndrome, *Intern Med* 44(6):622, 2005.

Sharma SK et al: Miliary tuberculosis: new insights into an old disease, *Lancet Infect Dis* 5(7):415, 2005.

Torgersen J et al: Molecular epidemiology of pleural and other extrapulmonary tuberculosis: a Maryland state review, *Clin Infect Dis* 42(10):1375, 2006.

AUTHORS: **GEORGE O. ALONSO, M.D., GLENN G. FORT, M.D., M.P.H.,** and **DENNIS J. MIKOLICH, M.D.**

BASIC INFORMATION

DEFINITION

Pulmonary tuberculosis (TB) is an infection of the lung and, occasionally, surrounding structures, caused by the bacterium *Mycobacterium tuberculosis*.

SYNONYMS

TB

ICD-9CM CODES
011.9 Pulmonary tuberculosis

EPIDEMIOLOGY & DEMOGRAPHICS

INCIDENCE (IN U.S.):
- Approximately 7 cases/100,000 persons—lowest in reported history
- >90% of new cases each year from reactivated prior infections
- 9% newly infected
- Only 10% of patients with PPD conversions (higher [8%/yr] in HIV-positive patients) will develop TB, most within 1 to 2 yr
- Two thirds of all new cases in racial and ethnic minorities
- 80% of new cases in children in racial and ethnic minorities
- Occurs most frequently in geographic areas and among populations with highest AIDS prevalence
  1. Urban blacks and Hispanics between 25 and 45 yr old
  2. Poor, crowded urban communities
- Nearly 36% of new cases from new immigrants

PEAK INCIDENCE:
- Infancy
- Teenage years
- Pregnancy
- Elderly
- HIV-positive patients, regardless of age, at highest risk

PREVALENCE (IN U.S.):
- Estimated 10 million people infected
- Varies widely among population groups

PREDOMINANT SEX:
- No specific predilection
- Male predominance in AIDS, shelters, and prisons reflected in disproportionate male incidence

PREDOMINANT AGE:
- 24 to 45 yr old
- Childhood cases common among minorities
- Nursing home outbreaks among elderly

GENETICS:
- Populations with widespread low native resistance have been intensely infected when initially exposed to TB.
- Following elimination of those with least native resistance, incidence and prevalence of TB tend to decline.

PHYSICAL FINDINGS & CLINICAL PRESENTATION

- See "Etiology"
- Primary pulmonary TB infection generally asymptomatic
- Reactivation pulmonary TB
  1. Fever
  2. Night sweats
  3. Cough
  4. Hemoptysis
  5. Scanty nonpurulent sputum
  6. Weight loss
- Progressive primary pulmonary TB disease: same as reactivation pulmonary TB
- TB pleurisy
  1. Pleuritic chest pain
  2. Fever
  3. Shortness of breath
- Rare massive, suffocating, fatal hemoptysis secondary to erosion of pulmonary artery within a cavity (Rassmussen's aneurysm)
- Chest examination
  1. Not specific
  2. Usually underestimates extent of disease
  3. Rales accentuated following a cough (posttussive rales)

ETIOLOGY

- *Mycobacterium tuberculosis* (Mtb), a slow-growing, aerobic, non–spore-forming, nonmotile bacillus, with a lipid-rich cell wall
  1. Lacks pigment
  2. Produces niacin
  3. Reduces nitrate
  4. Produces heat-labile catalase
  5. Mtb staining, acid-fast and acid-alcohol fast by Ziehl-Neelsen method, appearing as red, slightly bent, beaded rods 2 to 4 microns long (acid-fast bacilli [AFB]), against a blue background
  6. Polymerase chain reaction (PCR) to detect <10 organisms/ml in sputum (compared with the requisite 10,000 organisms/ml for AFB smear detection)
  7. Culture
     a. Growth on solid media (Löwenstein-Jensen; Middlebrook 7H11) in 2 to 6 wk
     b. Growth in liquid media (BACTEC, using a radioactive carbon source for early growth detection) often in 9 to 16 days
     c. Enhanced in a 5% to 10% carbon dioxide atmosphere
  8. DNA fingerprinting (based on restriction fragment length polymorphism [RFLP])
     a. Facilitates immediate identification of Mtb strains in early growing cultures
     b. False-negatives possible if growth suboptimal
  9. Humans are the only reservoir for Mtb
  10. Transmission
      a. Facilitated by close exposure to high-velocity cough (unprotected by proper mask or respirators) from patient with AFB-positive sputum and cavitary lesions, producing aerosolized droplets containing AFB, which are inhaled directly into alveoli
      b. Occurs within prisons, nursing homes, and hospitals
- Pathogenesis
  1. AFB (Mtb) ingested by macrophages in alveoli, then transported to regional lymph nodes where spread is contained
  2. Some AFB may reach bloodstream and disseminate widely
  3. Primary TB (asymptomatic, minimal pneumonitis in lower or midlung fields, with hilar lymphadenopathy) essentially an intracellular infection, with multiplication of organisms continuing for 2 to 12 wk after primary exposure, until cell-mediated hypersensitivity (detected by positive skin test reaction to tuberculin purified protein derivative [PPD]) matures, with subsequent containment of infection
  4. Local and disseminated AFB thus contained by T-cell–mediated immune responses
     a. Recruitment of monocytes
     b. Transformation of lymphocytes with secretion of lymphokines
     c. Activation of macrophages and histiocytes
     d. Organization into granulomas, where organisms may survive within macrophages (Langhans' giant cells), but within which multiplication essentially ceases (95%) and from which spread is prohibited
  5. Progressive primary pulmonary disease
     a. May immediately follow the asymptomatic phase
     b. Necrotizing pulmonary infiltrates
     c. Tuberculous bronchopneumonia
     d. Endobronchial TB
     e. Interstitial TB
     f. Widespread miliary lung lesions
  6. Postprimary TB pleurisy with pleural effusion
     a. Develops after early primary infection, although often before conversion to positive PPD
     b. Results from pleural seeding from a peripheral lung lesion or rupture of lymph node into pleural space
     c. May produce a large (sometimes hemorrhagic) exudative effusion (with polymorphonuclear cells

early, rapidly replaced by lymphocytes), frequently without pulmonary infiltrates
    d. Generally resolves without treatment
    e. Portends a high risk of subsequent clinical disease, and therefore must be diagnosed and treated early (pleural biopsy and culture) to prevent future catastrophic TB illness
    f. May result in disseminated extrapulmonary infection
7. Reactivation pulmonary TB
    a. Occurs months to years following primary TB
    b. Preferentially involves the apical posterior segments of the upper lobes and superior segments of the lower lobes
    c. Associated with necrosis and cavitation of involved lung, hemoptysis, chronic fever, night sweats, weight loss
    d. Spread within lung occurs via cough and inhalation
8. Reinfection TB
    a. May mimic reactivation TB
    b. Ruptured caseous foci and cavities, which may produce endobronchial spread
9. Mtb in both progressive primary and reactivation pulmonary TB
    a. Intracellular (macrophage) lesions (undergoing slow multiplication)
    b. Closed caseous lesions (undergoing slow multiplication)
    c. Extracellular, open cavities (undergoing rapid multiplication)
    d. INH and rifampin are cidal in all three sites
    e. PZA especially active within acidic macrophage environment
    f. Extrapulmonary reactivation disease also possible
10. Rapid local progression and dissemination in infants with devastating illness before PPD conversion occurs
11. Most symptoms (fever, weight loss, anorexia) and tissue destruction (caseous necrosis) from cytokines and cell-mediated immune responses
12. Mtb has no important endotoxins or exotoxins
13. Granuloma formation related to tumor necrosis factor (TNF) secreted by activated macrophages

DIAGNOSIS (Dx)

DIFFERENTIAL DIAGNOSIS

- Necrotizing pneumonia (anaerobic, gram-negative)
- Histoplasmosis
- Coccidioidomycosis
- Melioidosis
- Interstitial lung diseases (rarely)
- Cancer
- Sarcoidosis
- Silicosis
- Paragonimiasis
- Rare pneumonias
    1. *Rhodococcus equi* (cavitation)
    2. *Bacillus cereus* (50% hemoptysis)
    3. *Eikenella corrodens* (cavitation)

WORKUP

- Sputum for AFB stains
- Chest x-ray examination
- PPD
    1. Recent conversion from negative to positive within 3 mo of exposure is highly suggestive of recent infection.
    2. Single positive PPD is not helpful diagnostically.
    3. Negative PPD never rules out acute TB.
    4. Be certain that positive PPD does not reflect "booster phenomenon" (prior positive PPD may become negative after several years and return to positive only after second repeated PPD; repeat second PPD within 1 wk), which thus may mimic skin test conversion.
    5. Positive PPD reaction is determined as follows:
        a. Induration after 72 hr of intradermal injection of 0.1 ml of 5 TU-PPD
        b. 5-mm induration if HIV-positive (or other severe immunosuppressed state affecting cellular immune function), close contact of active TB, fibrotic chest lesions
        c. 10-mm induration if in high–medical risk groups (immunosuppressive disease or therapy, renal failure, gastrectomy, silicosis, diabetes), foreign-born high-risk group (Southeast Asia, Latin America, Africa, India), low socioeconomic groups, IV drug addict, prisoner, health care worker
        d. 15-mm induration if low risk
    6. Anergy antigen testing (using mumps, *Candida,* tetanus toxoid) may identify patients who are truly anergic to PPD and these antigens, but results are often confusing. Not recommended.
    7. Patients with TB may be selectively anergic only to PPD.
    8. Positive PPD indicates prior infection but does not itself confirm active disease.
- A new diagnostic test for latent tuberculosis infection, known as the quantaferon test (QFT-G), is now available. This is a blood test that measures interferon response to specific *M. tuberculosis* antigens. The test is FDA approved and is available in some large TB centers and state health departments. It may assist in distinguishing true positive reactions, from individuals with latent tuberculosis, from PPD reactions related to: non-tuberculous mycobacteria; prior BCG vaccination; or difficult-to-interpret skin test results from persons with dermatologic conditions or immediate allergic reactions to PPD. The diagnostic utility of the test as a replacement or supplement to the standard PPD is not yet fully determined.

LABORATORY TESTS

- Sputum for AFB stains and culture
    1. Induced sputum if patient not coughing productively
- Sputum from bronchoscopy if high suspicion of TB with negative expectorated induced sputum for AFB
    1. Positive AFB smear is essential before or shortly after treatment to ensure subsequent growth for definitive diagnosis and sensitivity testing
    2. Consider lung biopsy if sputum negative, especially if infiltrates are predominantly interstitial
- AFB stain-negative sputum may grow Mtb subsequently
- Gastric aspirates reliable, especially in HIV-negative patients
- CBC
    1. Variable values
        a. WBCs: low, normal, or elevated (including leukemoid reaction: >50,000)
        b. Normocytic, normochromic anemia often
    2. Rarely helpful diagnostically
- ESR usually elevated
- Thoracentesis
    1. Exudative effusion
        a. Elevated protein
        b. Decreased glucose
        c. Elevated WBCs (polymorphonuclear leukocytes early, replaced later by lymphocytes)
        d. May be hemorrhagic
    2. Pleural fluid usually AFB-negative
    3. Pleural biopsy often diagnostic—may need to be repeated for diagnosis
    4. Culture pleural biopsy tissue for AFB
- Bone marrow biopsy is often diagnostic in difficult-to-diagnose cases, especially miliary tuberculosis

IMAGING STUDIES

- Chest x-ray examination
    1. Primary infection reflected by calcified peripheral lung nodule with calcified hilar lymph node
    2. Reactivation pulmonary TB
        a. Necrosis
        b. Cavitation (especially on apical lordotic views)
        c. Fibrosis and hilar retraction
        d. Bronchopneumonia
        e. Interstitial infiltrates

f. Miliary pattern
g. Many of previous may also accompany progressive primary TB
3. TB pleurisy
a. Pleural effusion, often rapidly accumulating and massive
4. TB activity not established by single chest x-ray examination
5. Serial chest x-ray examinations are excellent indicators of progression or regression

TREATMENT

Rx

NONPHARMACOLOGIC THERAPY

- Bed rest during acute phase of treatment
- High-calorie, high-protein diet to reverse malnutrition and enhance immune response to TB
- Isolation in negative-pressure rooms with high-volume air replacement and circulation, with health care provider wearing proper protective 0.5- to 1-micron filter respirators, until three consecutive sputum AFB smears are negative

ACUTE GENERAL Rx

- Compliance (rigid adherence to treatment regimen) chief determinant of success.
  1. Supervised directly observed therapy (DOT) recommended for all patients and mandatory for unreliable patients
- Preferred adult regimen: DOT.
  1. Isoniazid (INH) 15 mg/kg (max 900 mg) + rifampin 600 mg + ethambutol (EMB) 30 mg/kg (max 2500 mg) + pyrazinamide (PZA) (2 g [<50 kg]; 2.5 g [51 to 74 kg]; 3 g [>75 kg]) thrice weekly for 6 mo
  2. Alternative, more complicated DOT regimens
- Rifapentine, a rifampin derivative with a much longer serum half-life, was shown to be as effective when administered weekly (with weekly isoniazid) as conventional regimens for drug-sensitive pulmonary tuberculosis in non-HIV-infected patients.
- Short-course daily therapy: adult.
  1. HIV-negative patient: 6 mo total therapy (2 mo INH 300 mg + rifampin 600 mg + EMB 15 mg/kg [max 2500 mg]) + PZA (1.5 g [<50 kg]; 2 g [51 to 74 kg]; 2.5 g [>75 kg]) daily and until smear negative and sensitivity confirmed; then INH + rifampin daily × 4 mo
  2. HIV-positive patient: 9 mo total therapy (2 mo INH + rifampin + EMB + PZA daily until smear negative and sensitivity confirmed; then INH + rifampin qd × 7 mo)
  3. Continue treatment at least 3 mo following conversion to negative cultures
- Drug resistance (often multiple drug resistance [MDRTB]) increased by:
  1. Prior treatment
  2. Acquisition of TB in developing countries
  3. Homelessness
  4. AIDS
  5. Prisoners
  6. IV drug addicts
  7. Known contact with MDRTB
- Never add single drug to failing regimen.
- Never treat TB with fewer than two to three drugs or two to three new additional drugs.
- Monitor for clinical toxicity (especially hepatitis).
  1. Patient and physician awareness that anorexia, nausea, RUQ pain, and unexplained malaise require immediate cessation of treatment
  2. Evaluation of LFTs
     a. Minimal SGOT/SGPT elevations without symptoms generally transient and not clinically significant
- Preventive treatment for PPD conversion only (infection without disease).
  1. Must be certain that chest x-ray examination is negative and patient has no symptoms of TB
  2. INH 300 mg daily for 9 to 12 mo; at least 12 mo if HIV-positive
  3. Most important groups:
     a. HIV-positive and other severely immunocompromised patients
     b. Close contact of active TB
     c. Recent converter
     d. Old TB on chest x-ray examination
     e. IV drug addict
     f. Medical risk factor
     g. High-risk foreign country
     h. Homeless
- Infants generally given prophylaxis immediately if recent contact of active TB (even if infant PPD negative), then retested with PPD in 3 mo (continuing INH if PPD becomes positive and stopping INH if PPD remains negative).
- Chronic, stable PPD (several years) given INH prophylaxis generally only if patient is <35 yr old.
  1. INH toxicity may outweigh benefit
  2. Individualize decision
- Preventive therapy for suspected INH-resistant organisms is unclear.

CHRONIC Rx

- Generally not indicated beyond treatment described previously
- Prolonged treatment, supervised by infectious disease expert, in a few very complicated infections caused by resistant organisms

DISPOSITION

- Monthly follow up by physician experienced in TB treatment
- Confirm sensitivity testing and alter treatment appropriately
- Frequent sputum samples until culture is negative
- Confirm chest x-ray regression at 2 to 3 mo

REFERRAL

- To infectious disease expert for:
  1. HIV-positive patient
  2. Patient with suspected drug-resistant TB
  3. Patients previously treated for TB
  4. Patients whose fever has not decreased and sputum has not converted to negative in 2 to 4 wk
  5. Patients with overwhelming pulmonary or extrapulmonary tuberculosis
- To pulmonologist for bronchoscopy or pleural biopsy

PEARLS & CONSIDERATIONS

!

COMMENTS

- All contacts (especially close household contacts and infants) should be properly tested for PPD conversions during 3 mo following exposure.
- Those with positive PPD should be evaluated for active TB and properly treated or given prophylaxis.

EVIDENCE

EBM

A systematic review compared various treatment regimens in patients with newly diagnosed, active pulmonary tuberculosis. Treatment for <6 months was associated with higher relapse rates.[1] Ⓐ

Two randomized controlled trials (RCTs) found no difference in relapse rates when 6-month treatment regimens were compared with longer (8- to 9-month) regimens in patients with newly diagnosed pulmonary tuberculosis. The regimens included different combinations of isoniazid, rifampin, ethambutol, streptomycin, and pyrazinamide for initial and continuation treatment.[2,3] Ⓐ

A systematic review identified one RCT, which compared treatment regimens of daily vs. three-times-weekly over 6 months in patients with pulmonary tuberculosis. There was no significant difference in cure rates between the groups at 1 month after completion of the treatment. A clinically important difference between the dosing regimens could not be ruled out.[4] Ⓑ

A systematic review found insufficient evidence from RCTs demonstrating the efficacy of direct observation of tablet swallowing in the treatment of tuberculosis in low-, middle-, and high-income country settings. There was no significant difference between direct observation and self-treatment for cure or treatment completion.[5] Ⓐ However, the most recent American guidelines recommend this form of therapy, based on three key references.[6-9] Ⓑ Ⓒ

A systematic review of RCTs studied the effectiveness of tuberculosis preventive therapy in reducing the risk of active tuberculosis and death in persons infected with HIV. Preventive therapy (with any anti-TB regimen) was associated with a significantly lower incidence of active tuberculosis compared with placebo, but all-cause mortality rates were similar in both groups. Those with a positive tuberculin skin test were more likely to benefit from treatment than those with a negative test.[10] Ⓐ

Limited evidence from this review suggested that the protective effect of therapy may have declined over the short to medium term. No one regimen was found to be superior; however, short-course multidrug regimens were much more likely to be discontinued due to adverse effects, compared with INH monotherapy.[10] Ⓐ

A systematic review found that isoniazid is effective for the prevention of active tuberculosis in HIV-negative patients who are at increased risk of developing the infection.[11] Ⓐ

Evidence-Based References

1. Gelband H: Regimens of less than six months for treating tuberculosis, *Cochrane Database Syst Rev* 4, 1999 (Cochrane Review). Ⓐ
2 East and Central African/British Medical Research Council Fifth Collaborative Study: Controlled clinical trial of 4 short-course regimens of chemotherapy (three 6-month and one 8-month) for pulmonary tuberculosis, *Tubercle* 64:153, 1983. Reviewed in: *Clin Evid* 12:1194, 2004. Ⓐ
3. British Thoracic Society: A controlled trial of 6 months' chemotherapy in pulmonary tuberculosis, final report: results during the 36 months after the end of chemotherapy and beyond, *Br J Dis Chest* 78:330, 1984. Reviewed in: *Clin Evid* 9:901, 2003. Ⓐ
4. Mwandumba HC, Squire SB: Fully intermittent dosing with drugs for treating tuberculosis in adults (Cochrane Review). Reviewed in: Cochrane Library 1, Chichester, UK, 2004, John Wiley. Ⓑ
5. Volmink J, Garner P: Directly observed therapy for treating tuberculosis (Cochrane Review). Reviewed in: Cochrane Library 1, Chichester, UK, 2004, John Wiley. Ⓐ
6. The Infectious Diseases Society of America, the American Thoracic Society, the Centers for Disease Control and Prevention: Treatment of tuberculosis, *MMWR Recomm Rep* 52(RR-11):1, 2003. Ⓒ
7. Chaulk CP: Eleven years of community-based directly observed therapy for tuberculosis, *JAMA* 274;945, 1995. Ⓑ
8. Chaulk CP: Directly observed therapy for treatment completion of tuberculosis: concensus statement of the Public Health Tuberculosis Guidelines Panel, *JAMA* 279:943, 1998. Ⓒ
9. Weis SE et al: The effect of directly observed therapy on the rates of drug resistance and relapse in tuberculosis, *N Engl J Med* 330:1179, 1994. Ⓑ
10. Woldehanna S, Volmink J: Treatment of latent tuberculosis infection in HIV infected persons (Cochrane Review). Reviewed in: Cochrane Library 1, Chichester, UK, 2004, John Wiley. Ⓐ
11. Smieja MJ et al: Isoniazid for preventing tuberculosis in non-HIV infected persons (Cochrane Review). Reviewed in: Cochrane Library 1, Chichester, UK, 2004, John Wiley. Ⓐ

SUGGESTED READINGS

Aderaye G et al: The relationship between disease pattern and disease burden by chest radiography, *M. tuberculosis* load, and HIV status in patients with pulmonary tuberculosis in Addis Ababa, *Infection* 32(6):333, 2004.

American Thoracic Society, CDC, and the Infectious Disease Society of America: Controlling tuberculosis in the United States, *MMWR* 54(RR-12):1, 2005.

Ismail Y: Pulmonary tuberculosis—a review of clinical features and diagnosis in 232 cases, *Med J Malaysia* 59(1):56, 2004.

Rubin EJ: Toward a new therapy for tuberculosis, *N Engl J Med* 352:933, 2005.

van Lettow M et al: Micronutrient malnutrition and wasting in adults with pulmonary tuberculosis with and without HIV co-infection in Malawi, *BMC Infect Dis* 4(1):61, 2004.

Wei CJ et al: Computed tomaography features of acute pulmonary tuberculosis, *Am J Emerg Med* 22(3):171, 2004.

AUTHORS: **GEORGE O. ALONSO, M.D., GLENN G. FORT, M.D., M.P.H.,** and **DENNIS J. MIKOLICH, M.D.**

BASIC INFORMATION

DEFINITION

Tuberous sclerosis (TS) is an inherited neurocutaneous disorder that is characterized by pleomorphic features involving many organ systems, including multiple benign neoplasms (hamartomas) of the brain, kidney, and skin.

ICD-9CM CODES
759.5

EPIDEMIOLOGY & DEMOGRAPHICS

INCIDENCE: TS has an estimated incidence of 1 case per 6000 live births. Thus, it is the second most common neurocutaneous syndrome after neurofibromatosis.

PREVALENCE: The disorder affects about 1 in 10,000 persons in the general population.

PREDOMINANT SEX AND AGE: TS has no predilection for gender or race.

GENETICS:

- TS is an autosomal dominant disorder with almost complete penetrance but a wide range of clinical severity. However, only one third of cases are familial. The apparently nonfamilial cases can represent either spontaneous mutations or mosaicism.
- Genetic research has identified two TS genes. One is located on chromosome 9 (*TSC1* gene) and the other on chromosome 16 (*TSC2* gene). About 68% of cases occur as a result of new gene mutations. Because of the genetic transmission and new mutations, antenatal diagnosis is difficult.

PHYSICAL FINDINGS & CLINICAL PRESENTATION

- Dermatologic manifestations may be the only clues the family physician has to the diagnosis of the disorder, which is also marked by childhood seizures and mental retardation (Figs. 1-280 through 1-282).
- The diagnostic criteria for TS were recently revised at a consensus conference. Major and minor features are listed in Table 1-50.
- The classic diagnostic triad of seizures, mental retardation, and facial angiofibromas (Vogt's triad) occurs in fewer than 50% of patients with TS.
- All of the clinical features of TS may not be apparent in the first year of life. Thus, a child is often initially diagnosed with possible or probable TS and the diagnosis of definite TS is made after additional features are identified.
- Dermatologic manifestations: A careful skin examination of patients at risk for TS continues to be the easiest and most accessible method of establishing the diagnosis (Table 1-51).
- Neurologic manifestations: These are the leading cause of morbidity and mortality in patients with TS. Brain hamartomas in the form of cortical tubers, subependymal nodules, and subependymal giant cell astrocytomas are often responsible for intractable seizures, most commonly as infantile spasms. Approximately 90% to 96% of TS patients suffer from seizures. Approximately 85% of patients have their first epileptic episode in the first 2 years of life. Behavioral and cognitive dysfunction, including autism and mental retardation, can be seen in 40% to 50% of patients.
- Renal and pulmonary manifestations: They are strongly associated with TS. Angiomyolipoma is the most common renal lesion found in TS patients. Clinically evident pulmonary involvement in TS patients is relatively rare, with an estimated incidence of 1% to 6%. The most common lesion is lymphangiomyomatosis (LAM), a progressive cystic lung disease with progressive dyspnea and spontaneous pneumothorax in a childbearing woman.
- Cardiovascular manifestations: These are often the earliest diagnostic findings in patients with TS. Rhabdomyoma is the most common primary cardiac tumour in infants and children. Its incidence in TS patients ranges between 47% and 60%. In fact, 80% to 95% of patients with cardiac rhabdomyomas have TS.

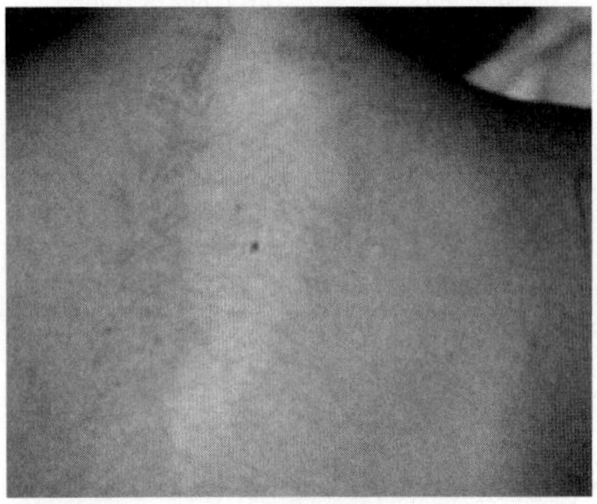

FIGURE 1-280 Hypomelanotic macules ("ash left" spots).

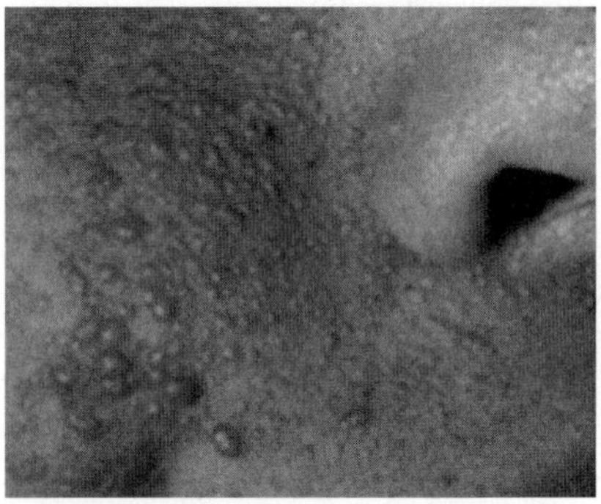

FIGURE 1-281 Facial angiofibromas.

TABLE 1-50 Revised Diagnostic Criteria for Tuberous Sclerosis Complex (TSC)

Major features

1. Facial angiofibromas or forehead plaque
2. Nontraumatic ungual or periungual fibroma
3. Hypomelanotic macule (3 or more)
4. Shagreen patch (connective tissue nevus)
5. Multiple retinal nodular hamartomas
6. Cortical tuber
7. Subependymal nodule
8. Subependymal giant cell astrocytoma
9. Cardiac rhabdomyoma, single or multiple
10. Lymphangiomyomatosis
11. Renal angiomyolipoma

Minor features

1. Multiple, randomly distributed pits in dental enamel
2. Hamartomatous rectal polyps
3. Bone cysts
4. Cerebral white matter radial migration lines
5. Gingival fibromas
6. Nonrenal hamartomas
7. Retinal achromic patch
8. "Confetti" skin lesions
9. Multiple renal cysts

Definite TSC: Either two major features or one major feature plus two minor features. Probable TSC: One major plus one minor feature. Possible TSC: Either one major feature or two or more minor features.

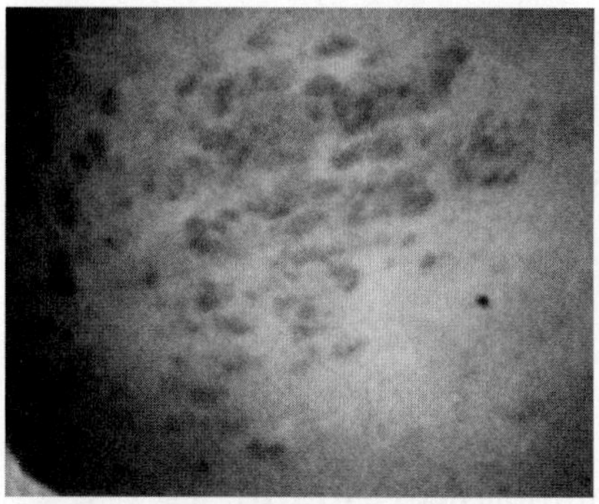

FIGURE 1-282 Shagreen patches.

- The most common ocular findings in TS are retinal hamartomas, appearing in 40% to 50% of patients.

ETIOLOGY

TS is an autosomal dominant disorder.

DIAGNOSIS

Dx

DIFFERENTIAL DIAGNOSIS

Cutaneous manifestations:

- Nevus anemicus
- Nevus depigmentosus (nevus achromicus)
- Vitiligo

WORKUP

- The dermatologic manifestations of TS are helpful in diagnosing this disorder. When TS has been inherited in the autosomal dominant form, dermatologic signs are almost universally present in one of the patient's parents.
- No specific prenatal laboratory test is available.
- Early recognition of TS is vital because prompt implementation of the recommended diagnostic evaluation (neuroimaging studies, electroencephalogram, electrocardiography, renal ultrasonography, and chest computed tomography) may prevent serious clinical consequences.

LABORATORY TESTS

Molecular genetic testing: In recent years, molecular genetic testing for TS has become clinically available. Such testing identifies mutations in the *TSC1* and *TSC2* genes by one of several methods, most commonly polymerase chain reaction (PCR) amplification of individual exons, followed by DNA sequencing on DNA obtained from a patient's blood sample.

DNA testing for TS is potentially useful in several settings:

- First, it can be helpful in confirming a clinical diagnosis of TS, especially in young patients in whom many clinical signs and symptoms have yet to develop.
- Second, in many families with a history of TS in which there is a sporadic case of TS in a new child, genetic testing can provide reassurance to parents, children, and other family members that they do not carry the TS gene mutation.
- Third, DNA testing is useful for prenatal diagnosis.

TREATMENT

Rx

The management of TSC is presently symptomatic.

NONPHARMACOLOGIC THERAPY

Genetic counseling should be offered to families with affected members, even though accurate counseling remains difficult because of the variability of gene expression.

ACUTE GENERAL Rx/CHRONIC Rx

- Treatment methods currently available for patients with disfiguring facial angiofibromas include cryosurgery, curettage, dermabrasion, chemical peeling, excision, and laser therapy.
- Some patients have been treated successfully with antiepileptic medications; unfortunately, there are multiple cases of intractable seizure where medical treatment is ineffective. In some cases of intractable epilepsy, neurosurgical intervention becomes a life-saving option.
- In such drug-resistant cases of TS, the early administration of vigabatrin (α-vinyl-gamma aminobutyric acid), a selective irreversible inhibitor of GABA-transaminase, has been proven to result in 80% to 100% cessation rates

Section I DISEASES AND DISORDERS

TABLE 1-51 Cutaneous Manifestations Associated with Tuberous Sclerosis Complex (TSC)

Cutaneous Lesions	Descriptions	Age of Onset	Prevalence	Diagnostic Classification
Hypomelanotic macules ("ash leaf" spots) or Fitzpatrick patches	Leaf-shaped or polygonal white spots enhanced by Wood's lamp examination; more common on the trunk and buttocks	Earliest cutaneous lesion; usually present at birth or infancy	97.2%	Major
Facial angiofibromas	Red to pink papules with a smooth surface, symmetrically distributed over the centrofacial areas, sparing the upper lips	Second to fifth year of life; become more prominent with age	74.5%	Major
Shagreen patches	Slightly elevated patch or plaque, usually found on the dorsal body surfaces, especially the lumbosacral area; its rough surface resembles an orange peel; represents a connective tissue nevus, sometimes called collagenoma	Rare during infancy; tend to increase in size and number with age	48.1%	Major
Molluscum pendulum	Multiple soft pedunculated skin growths on neck; rarely in axilla or groin	More common during first decade of life; rare during infancy	22.6%	Minor
Forehead fibrous plaque	Yellowish-brown or skin-colored plaques of variable size and shape, usually located on the forehead or scalp	Common at any age and can be seen at birth or early infancy	18.9%	Major
Periungual fibromas	Skin-colored or reddish nodules seen on the lateral nail groove, nail plate, or along the proximal nail folds; more commonly found on the toes than on the fingers	Present at puberty or soon after; become more common with age	15.1%	Major
"Confetti-like" macules	Multiple 1-2 mm white spots symmetrically distributed over extremities	Second decade or adulthood	2.8%	Minor

of infantile spasms. Vigabatrin is marketed in many European countries, but remains unavailable in the U.S. and has not been approved by the FDA.

- Embolization and/or renal sparing surgery are treatment options for renal angiomyolipomas.
- Oopherectomy, medroxyprogesterone, and tamoxifen use have been advocated in patients with LAM, but therapeutic benefit is unclear. Lung transplantation is reserved for patients with end-stage LAM.
- Most rhabdomyomas tend to regress with increasing age, although tumour growth has been documented in some at puberty. Surgery is recommended only for life-threatening situations, such as hemodynamic compromise.
- Oral rapamycin or sirolimus therapy can induce regression of brain astrocytomas associated with TS. Ongoing therapeutic trials with rapamycin in lymphangioleiomyomatosis appear promising.

REFERRAL

A multidisciplinary team including genetics, neurology, ophthalmology, nephrology, dermatology, neurosurgery, and plastic surgery should evaluate children suspected of having TS.

PEARLS & CONSIDERATIONS

PREVENTION

It is speculated that if one could establish the prenatal diagnosis of TS and begin using rapamycin early, one might prevent the development of TS manifestations.

SUGGESTED READINGS

Hurst JS, Wilcoski S: Recognizing an index case of tuberous sclerosis, *Am Fam Physician* 61(3):703-708, 2001.

Schwartz RA: Tuberous sclerosis complex: advances in diagnosis, genetics, and management, *J Am Acad Dermatology,* 57(2):189-202, 2007.

AUTHOR: **RUBY SATPATHY, M.D.**

BASIC INFORMATION

DEFINITION

Acute tubular necrosis refers to intrinsic tubular damage induced by hypoperfusion to renal parenchymal cells, particularly tubular epithelium, that results in sodium loss and FE_{Na} >1% (fractional excretion of sodium).

SYNONYMS

Ischemic or nephrotoxic ARF

ICD-9CM CODES

584.5 With lesion of tubular necrosis
Renal failure with (acute) tubular necrosis
Tubular necrosis: NOS, acute
997.5 Urinary complications
Tubular necrosis (acute) specified as due to procedure

EPIDEMIOLOGY & DEMOGRAPHICS

- Accounts for 90% of intrinsic renal failure.
- Most common cause of intrinsic renal failure among hospitalized patients, including pediatric and adult, especially on surgical services in patients undergoing major cardiovascular surgery or in intensive care units in patients suffering severe trauma, hemorrhage, sepsis, or volume depletion.

PHYSICAL FINDINGS & CLINICAL PRESENTATION

No apparent physical findings. Clinical features include recent hemorrhage, hypotension, or surgery thereby suggesting ischemic ARF. Recent radiocontrast study, nephrotoxic drugs, history suggestive of rhabdomyolysis, hemolysis, or myeloma may suggest toxin-mediated ARF.

- Three phases of ischemic ARF:
  1. Initiation phase (hours to days)—renal hypoperfusion, evolving ischemia.
  2. Maintenance phase (1 to 2 wk)—renal cell injury established, GFR stabilizes at its nadir (5 to 10 ml/min), urine output at its lowest, uremic complications arise.
  3. Recovery phase (>2 wk)—renal parenchymal cell repair and regeneration, gradual return of GFR to premorbid levels; may be complicated by a marked diuretic phase due to excretion of retained salt and water and other solutes, continued use of diuretics, or delayed recovery of epithelial cell function (solute and water reabsorption) relative to glomerular filtration.

PATHOLOGIC FINDINGS

- Ischemic ARF—patchy and focal necrosis of tubule epithelium with detachment from its basement membrane and occlusion of tubule lumens with casts composed of epithelial cells, cellular debris, Tamm-Horsfall mucoprotein (represents the matrix of all urinary casts), and pigments. Also present is leukocyte accumulation in vasa recta (capillaries that return the NaCl and water reabsorbed in the loop of Henle and medullary collecting tubule to the systemic circulation). Morphology of glomeruli and renal vasculature remain normal. Necrosis most severe in pars recta (straight portion of proximal tubule and thick ascending limb of loop of Henle).
- Nephrotoxic ARF—morphologic changes in convoluted and straight portion of proximal tubule. Tubule cell necrosis less pronounced than in ischemic ARF.

ETIOLOGY

Hypotension or shock, prolonged prerenal azotemia, postoperative sepsis syndrome, rhabdomyolysis, hemolysis (hypercalcemia, hemoglobin, urate, oxalate, myeloma light chains), antimicrobial drugs (acyclovir, foscarnet, aminoglycosides, amphotericin B, pentamidine), radiocontrast (contrast nephropathy), chemotherapy (cisplatin, ifosfamide).

DIAGNOSIS

DIFFERENTIAL DIAGNOSIS

Allergic interstitial nephritis, acute bilateral pyelonephritis

WORKUP

LABORATORY TESTS

- Urinalysis for specific gravity (SG), U_{Na}, P_{Cr}, P_{Na}, U_{Cr}
- Calculate fractional excretion of sodium (FE_{Na}) = $[(U_{Na} \times P_{Cr}) / (P_{Na} \times U_{Cr})] \times 100$

LABORATORY FINDINGS

FE_{Na} >1%
U_{Na} >20 mmol/L
SG <1.015

IMAGING STUDIES

Not necessary

TREATMENT

ACUTE GENERAL Rx

Should focus on providing etiology-specific supportive care or correction of primary hemodynamic abnormality. No specific therapies for established ATN. Peritoneal or hemodialysis for replacement of renal function until regeneration and repair restore renal function.

DISPOSITION

Recovery typically takes 1 to 2 wk after normalization of renal perfusion as it requires repair and regeneration of renal cells.

REFERRAL

Renal consultation for severe cases of ATN requiring dialysis.

PEARLS & CONSIDERATIONS

COMMENTS

Prevention is paramount.

PREVENTION

Aggressive restoration of intravascular volume in surgical/trauma patients to prevent ischemic ARF. Tailoring dosage of potential nephrotoxins to body size and GFR to limit renal injury.

SUGGESTED READINGS

Barletta et al: Acute renal failure in children and infants, *Curr Opin Crit Care* 10(6):499-504, 2004.
Lameire N et al: Acute renal failure, *Lancet* 365:417-430, 2005.
Lameire N: The pathophysiology of acute renal failure, *Crit Care Clin* 21(2):197-210, 2005.

AUTHOR: **CHAITANYA V. REDDY, D.O.**

BASIC INFORMATION

DEFINITION

Tularemia is a zoonosis caused by small, facultative gram-negative intracellular coccobacillus *Francisella tularensis.* Clinical manifestations range from asymptomatic illness to septic shock and death.

SYNONYMS

Rabbit fever
Deerfly fever
O'Hara's disease

ICD-9CM CODES
021.9 Tularemia

EPIDEMIOLOGY & DEMOGRAPHICS

INCIDENCE (IN U.S.): Highest overall incidence in Arkansas, Missouri, and Okalahoma. It also found in Canada, Mexico, and European countries, Turkey, Israel, China and Japan.
PEAK INCIDENCE: June through August and in December
PREDOMINANT SEX: Male
PREDOMINANT AGE: Occurs at any age

PHYSICAL FINDINGS & CLINICAL PRESENTATION

Physical Findings

- Incubation period is 3 to 5 days but may range from 1 to 21 days.
- Most common initial signs and symptoms:
  1. Fever
  2. Chills
  3. Headache
  4. Malaise
  5. Anorexia
  6. Fatigue
  7. Cough
  8. Myalgias
  9. Chest discomfort
  10. Vomiting
  11. Abdominal pain
  12. Diarrhea
  13. Conjunctivitis
  14. Lymphadenitis

Clinical Presentation

- Ulceroglandular and glandular: account for 75% to 80% of cases. Fever and a single erythematous papuloulcerative lesion with a central Eschar accompanied by tender lymphadenopathy.
- Oculoglandular: accounts for 1% to 2% of cases. Painful inflamed conjunctiva with numerous yellowish nodules and pinpoint ulcers. Purulent conjunctivitis with regional lymphadenopathy. Corneal perforation may occur.
- Oropharyngeal and gastrointestinal: account for 1% to 4% of cases. Acute exudative membranes pharyngitis associated with cervical lymphadenopathy. Ulcerative intestinal lesion associated with mesenteric lymphadenopathy, diarrhea, abdominal pain, nausea, vomiting, and GI bleeding.
- Pulmonary: occurs often in the elderly and has a higher mortality. Symptoms include nonproductive cough, dyspnea, or pleuritic chest pain.
- Typhoidal: 10% of all cases of tularemia. Rare in U.S. Symptoms include high continuous fever, signs of endotoxemia, and severe headache. Mortality can approach 30%.

COMPLICATIONS

1. Intravascular coagulation
2. Renal failure
3. Rhabdomyolysis
4. Jaundice
5. Hepatitis
6. Meningitis
7. Encephalitis
8. Pericarditis
9. Peritonitis
10. Osteomyelitis
11. Splenic rupture
12. Thrombophlebitis
13. Myositis and septicemia

ETIOLOGY

- Caused by infection with *F. tularensis.*
- Two main biovars of *F. tularensis:* Type A and Type B. Type A produces severe disease in humans. Type B produces milder subclinical infection.
- Transmitted by ticks, tabanid flies, and mosquitoes. Also acquired by inhalation and ingestion.
- Cases also occur after exposure to animals (wild rabbit, squirrels, birds, sheep, beavers, muskrats, and domestic dogs and cats) or animal products.
- Laboratory acquisition is possible.
- Pathogenesis: after inoculation into the skin the organism multiplies locally within 2 to 5 days, then it produces erythematous tender or pruritic papule. The papule rapidly enlarges and forms an ulcer with a black base. The bacteria spread to the regional lymph nodes producing lymphadenopathy, and with bacteremia may spread to distant organs.

DIAGNOSIS

DIFFERENTIAL DIAGNOSIS

- Rickettsial infections
- Meningococcal infections
- Cat-scratch disease
- Infectious mononucleosis
- Atypical pneumonia
- Group A strep pharyngitis
- Typhoid fever
- Fungal infection—sporotrichosis
- Anthrax
- Plague
- Bacterial skin infections

WORKUP

- CBC
- Chest x-ray examination
- Cultures of blood, lymph node, pleural fluid, wounds, sputum, and gastric aspirate
- Antigen detection in urine
- PCR
- Serology

LABORATORY TESTS

- WBC count and ESR normal or elevated.
- Rarely seen on Gram-stained smears or tissue biopsies.
- Antibodies to *F. tularensis* demonstrated by tube agglutination, micro agglutination, hem agglutination, and ELISA; definitive serologic diagnosis requires a fourfold or greater rise in titer between acute and convalescent specimens.
- Polymerase chain reaction (PCR) to facilitate early diagnosis.

IMAGING STUDIES

Chest x-ray examination to show bilateral patchy infiltrate, lobar parenchymal infiltrate, cavitary lesion, pleural effusion, or emphysema

TREATMENT

ACUTE GENERAL Rx

Immediate therapy to limit extent of acute illness and complication

- Streptomycin 10 mg/kg IM q12h (daily dose should not exceed 2 g) or gentamicin 3 to 5 mg/kg q8h.
- Tetracycline 500 mg po qid or doxycycline 100 mg po bid or chloramphenicol 25 to 50 mg/kg q6h (do not exceed 6 g).
- Quinolones offer new options for the treatment of tularemia.
- Combination antibiotics required for tularemic meningitis—chloramphenicol plus streptomycin.

Surgical therapies are limited to drainage of abscessed lymph nodes and chest tube drainage of empyemas.

PROGNOSIS

The mortality rate of severe untreated infection (tularemic pneumonia and typhoidal tularemia) can be as high as 30%. Overall mortality associated with tularemia is 2% to 4% with appropriate treatment. Lifelong immunity usually follows tularemia.

DISPOSITION

Follow-up as outpatient

PREVENTION

- Educate the public to prevent sick or dead animals.
- Use insect repellants.

- Remove ticks promptly.
- Drink only potable water.
- Adequately cook wild meats.
- Tularemia vaccine has been developed but is not commercially available in U.S.; however, it is available from the Centers for Disease Control and Prevention (CDC). Vaccination of high-risk individuals working with large quantities of cultured organism is recommended.
- Avoid skinning wild animals, especially rabbits; wear gloves while handling animal carcasses.
- Do not use wells or other water that is contaminated by dead animals.
- Hospitalized patients with tularemia do not need special isolation. Standard universal precautions for contaminated secretion are adequate when handling drainage from wounds.
- Laboratory personnel should be notified of potential danger.

REFERRAL

For consultation with infectious diseases specialist in suspected cases.

A cluster of tularemia cases, particularly in an urban area or nonendemic regions, should prompt concern over the possibility of bioterrorism; the local public health authorities should be contacted immediately to investigate the possibility of deliberate release of tularemia as a weapon of terror.

PEARLS & CONSIDERATIONS

- Alert the microbiology laboratory to the possibility of tularemia.
- Do not use doxycycline or tetracycline in children or pregnant women.
- Because of its highly contagious nature with low inoculums, tularemia is considered an agent that could be used by terrorists. It is classified as a category A critical biologic agent by the CDC.

SUGGESTED READINGS

Centers for Disease Control and Prevention: Tularemia transmitted by insect bites—Wyoming, 2001-2003, *MMWR Morb Mortal Wkly Rep* 54(7):170, 2005.

Daya M, Nakamura Y: Pulmonary disease from biological agents: anthrax, plague, Q fever, and tularemia, *Crit Care Clin* 21(4):747-763, 2005.

Duckett NS et al: Intranasal interleukin-12 treatment for protection against respiratory infection with the *Francisella tularensis* live vaccine strain, *Infect Immun* 73(4):2306-2311, 2005.

Schmitt P et al: A novel screening ELISA and a confirmatory Western blot useful for diagnosis and epidemiological studies of tularemia, *Epidemiol Infect* 133(4):759-766, 2005.

Staples JE et al: Epidemiologic and molecular analysis of human tularemia, United States, 1964-2004, *Emerg Infect Dis* 12(7):1113, 2006.

AUTHORS: **GLENN G. FORT, M.D., M.P.H., DENNIS J. MIKOLICH, M.D.,** and **VASANTHI ARUMUGAM, M.D.**

BASIC INFORMATION

DEFINITION

Turner's syndrome refers to a pattern of malformation characterized by short stature, ovarian hypofunction, loose nuchal skin, and cubitus valgus as described by Turner in 1938. An associated 45,X chromosome constitution was recognized by Ford et al in 1959.

ICD-9CM CODES
758.6 Syndrome, Turner's

EPIDEMIOLOGY & DEMOGRAPHICS

INCIDENCE: 1 case out of every 2500 to 5000 live births

PHYSICAL FINDINGS & CLINICAL PRESENTATION

- Turner's phenotype is recognizable at any point on the developmental spectrum.
- In spontaneous abortuses the most common sex chromosome abnormality detected (45,X chromosome constitution) is found in 75% of affected individuals and accounts for 20% of such cases.
- In fetuses, it is suspected because of such ultrasonographic manifestations as thickening of the nuchal folds, frank nuchal cystic hygromas, or mild shortness of the femora at midtrimester.
- In infants:
  1. At birth may display loose nuchal skin (pterygium colli) and edema on the dorsa of hands and feet
  2. Canthal folds reflecting midface hypoplasia and redundant skin in the periorbital region
  3. Nipples appearing widely spaced
  4. Heart and cardiovascular system: murmur of aortic stenosis or bicuspid aortic valve or diminished femoral pulses suggestive of aortic coarctation
  5. Renal ultrasonography: renal ectopia such as pelvic kidney or horseshoe kidneys
- In older children:
  1. Slow linear growth
  2. Short stature—may be improved with growth hormone therapy (Fig. 1-283)
  3. Delayed or absent menses—secondary sex characteristics possibly normalized with estrogen replacement therapy
  4. Intelligence is often normal, but delays in spatial perception or visual motor integration are commonly observed; frank mental retardation is rare

ETIOLOGY

- Phenotype caused by absence of the second sex chromosome, whether X or Y
- 45,X chromosome constitution in about 50% of affected individuals
- Other chromosome aberrations (40% of cases): isochromosome Xq (46,X,i[Xq]) or mosaicism (XX/X)
- With deletions involving the short (or "p") arm of the X chromosome: short stature but little ovarian hypofunction
- Deletions involving Xq13-q27: ovarian failure
- Usually a deficiency of paternal contribution of sex chromosome, reflecting paternal nondisjunction

DIAGNOSIS

DIFFERENTIAL DIAGNOSIS

- Noonan syndrome, an autosomally dominant inherited disorder also characterized by loose nuchal skin, midface hypoplasia, canthal folds, and stenotic cardiac valvular defects and affecting males and females equally; also have normal chromosome constitutions
- Other conditions in the differential diagnosis of loose skin, whether or not associated with edema:
  1. Fetal hydantoin syndrome (loose nuchal skin, midface hypoplasia, distal digital hypoplasia)
  2. Disorders of chromosome constitution (trisomy 21, tetrasomy 12p mosaicism)
  3. Congenital lymphedema (Milroy edema)

WORKUP

- Giemsa banded karyotype to confirm clinical diagnosis
- Once diagnosis is established: cardiologic consultation for evaluation for cardiac valvular abnormalities or aortic coarctation
- Renal ultrasonography
- Endocrine evaluations in older patients with short stature or amenorrhea
- Psychometrics to document known or suspected learning disabilities

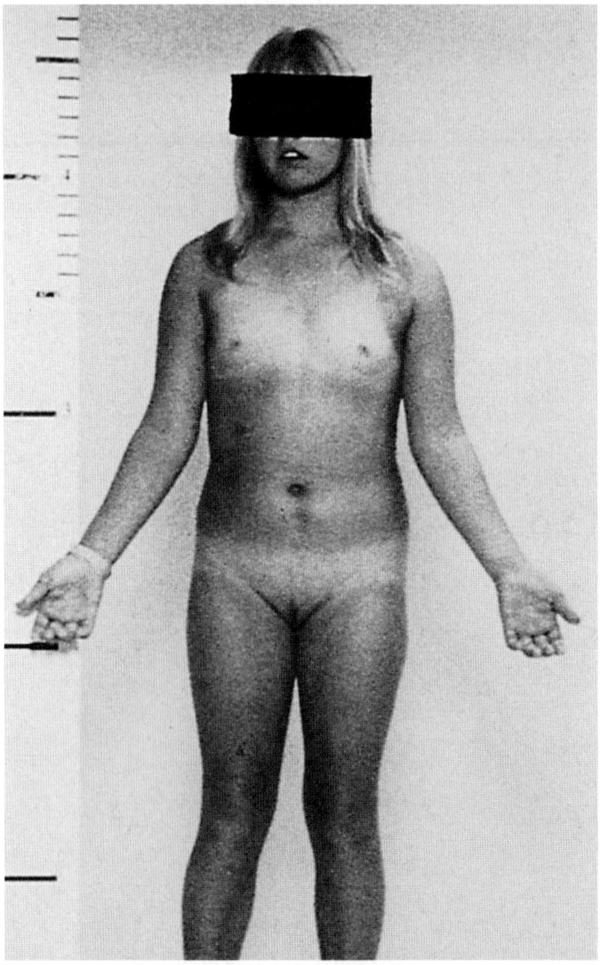

FIGURE 1-283 A 17-year-old patient with Turner's syndrome demonstrating short stature, poor sexual development, and increased carrying angles at elbows. Patient also has webbing of the neck. (From Mishell D [ed]: *Comprehensive gynecology,* ed 3, St Louis, 1997, Mosby.)

LABORATORY TESTS

- As noted, routine Giemsa banded karyotype on peripheral lymphocytes to confirm the clinical impression in all suspected cases of Turner's syndrome
- Recognition of associated medical problems, such as hypergonadotropic hypogonadism or autoimmune thyroiditis prompting periodic evaluation of these potential areas

IMAGING STUDIES

- Echocardiogram
- Renal ultrasonography
- Abdominal ultrasonography for evaluation of ovarian and uterine size and morphology
- MRI of brain (especially in cases with known or suspected neurologic impairment)
- Radiographs (for evaluation of carpal/metacarpal abnormalities, radioulnar synostosis)
- Bone age (for evaluation of short stature)

TREATMENT

Rx

Recognition of the multisystem involvement of Turner's syndrome necessitates multiple medical specialists working in concert with the primary care provider to maximize and improve outcome while minimizing unnecessary or redundant testing.

NONPHARMACOLOGIC THERAPY

General medical care guided by normal medical standards with special attention paid to identifying such age-related problems as developmental delays, learning disabilities, slow growth, or amenorrhea.

ACUTE GENERAL Rx

Specific treatment geared to the specific medical problem (e.g., cardiac or renal dysfunction)

CHRONIC Rx

- Estrogen replacement therapy in early adolescence
- Some benefit from recombinant human growth hormone therapy

REFERRAL

- To geneticist: clinical diagnosis, differential diagnosis, recurrence risk counseling, cytogenetic tests
- To endocrinologist (pediatric): evaluation of short stature, estrogen or growth hormone replacement therapy
- To cardiologist: for cardiac valvular abnormalities or aortic coarctation

PEARLS & CONSIDERATIONS

!

COMMENTS

- Although newer studies are optimistic regarding outcomes, previous reports suffered from retrospective observations, case reports, and ascertainment bias, contributing to a generally poor interaction between physician and patient.
- Affected individuals and families often benefit from the contemporary experiences and expertise of members of genetic support groups. The Turner Syndrome Association (phone: 612-379-3607 or 800-365-9944; Internet: http://www.turner-syndrome-us.org) and the Alliance of Genetic Support Groups (phone: 800-336-4363; Internet: http://medhelp.org/www/agsg.htm) are valuable resources.

EVIDENCE

EBM

Evidence shows that recombinant human growth hormone (hGH) increases short-term growth in girls with Turner's syndrome by approximately 3 cm in the first year of treatment and approximately 2 cm/year after 2 years. There is little evidence of serious short-term adverse effects in these trials or of the effects of hGH on final height.[1] Ⓐ

Evidence-Based Reference

1. Cave CB, Bryant J, Milne R: Recombinant growth hormone in children and adolescents with Turner syndrome, *Cochrane Database Syst Rev* 1, 2003. Ⓐ

SUGGESTED READINGS

Conniff C: Turner's syndrome, *Adolesc Med* 13(2):359, 2002.

Elsheikh M et al: Turner's syndrome in adulthood, *Endocr Rev* 23(1):120, 2002.

AUTHORS: **LUTHER K. ROBINSON, M.D.,** and **RUBEN ALVERO, M.D.**

BASIC INFORMATION

DEFINITION

Typhoid fever is a systemic infection caused by *Salmonella typhi.*

SYNONYMS

Typhoid
Enteric fever

ICD-9CM CODES
002.0 Typhoid fever

EPIDEMIOLOGY & DEMOGRAPHICS

INCIDENCE (IN U.S.): Approximately 500 cases of *S. typhi* infections are reported annually.

PHYSICAL FINDINGS & CLINICAL PRESENTATION

- Incubation period of a few days to several weeks.
- Usual manifestations:
  1. Prolonged fever
  2. Myalgias
  3. Headache
  4. Cough
  5. Sore throat
  6. Malaise
  7. Anorexia, at times with abdominal pain and hepatosplenomegaly
  8. Diarrhea or constipation may occur early in the course of illness
  9. Rose spots, which are faint, maculopapular, blanching lesions, may sometimes be seen on the chest or abdomen
- In the untreated patient, fever may last 1 to 2 mo. The main complication of untreated disease is GI bleeding as a result of perforation from ulceration of Peyer's patches in the ileum. Mental status changes and shock are rare complications. The relapse rate is approximately 10%.

ETIOLOGY

- *Salmonella typhi.*
- *S. paratyphi.*
- *S. typhi* or *S. paratyphi* found only in humans.
- Acquisition of disease by ingestion of food or water contaminated by other humans.
- In the U.S. most cases are acquired either during foreign travel or by ingestion of food prepared by chronic carriers, many of whom acquired the organism outside of the U.S.

DIAGNOSIS

DIFFERENTIAL DIAGNOSIS

- Malaria
- Tuberculosis
- Brucellosis
- Amebic liver abscess

WORKUP

- Blood, stool, and urine cultures are helpful.
- Cultures should be repeated if initially negative.
- Blood cultures are more likely to be positive early in the course of illness.
- Stool and urine cultures are more commonly positive in the second and third weeks of illness.
- Bone marrow biopsy cultures are 90% positive, although this procedure is usually not necessary.
- Serology using Widal test is helpful in retrospect, showing a fourfold increase in convalescent titers.

LABORATORY TESTS

- Neutropenia is common.
- Transaminitis is possible.
- Culture:
  1. Blood
  2. Body fluids
  3. Biopsy specimens

TREATMENT

ACUTE GENERAL Rx

- Ciprofloxacin 500 mg PO bid or 400 mg IV bid for 14 days
- Ceftriaxone 2 g IV qd for 14 days
- If organism sensitive
  1. SMX/TMP, 1 to 2 DS tabs PO bid *or*
  2. Amoxicillin, 2 g PO q8h to complete 14 days
- Dexamethasone, 3 mg/kg IV initially, followed by 1 mg/kg IV q6h for 8 doses for patients with septic shock or mental status changes

CHRONIC Rx

- Carrier states possible
- More common in age >60 yr and in persons with gallstones
- Usual site of colonization: gallbladder
- Treatment in those with persistently positive stool cultures and in food-handlers
- Suggested regimens for eradication of carrier state
  1. Ciprofloxacin 500 mg PO bid for 4 wk
  2. SMX/TMP 1 to 2 tabs PO bid for 6 wk (if susceptible)
  3. Amoxicillin, 2 g PO q8h for 6 wk (if susceptible)
- Cholecystectomy possibly required in carriers with gallstones who fail medical therapy

DISPOSITION

- Treated patients usually respond to therapy, with a small percentage becoming chronic carriers.
- The relapse rate is approximately 10%.
- Untreated patients may have serious complications.

REFERRAL

- Failure of therapy
- Chronic carrier

PEARLS & CONSIDERATIONS

COMMENTS

- Oral and parenteral vaccines are available for travelers to areas of high risk.
- Vaccines are about 70% effective.
- Immunity wanes after several years.
- Parenteral preparations are accompanied by frequent side effects:
  1. Pain at injection site
  2. Fever
  3. Malaise
  4. Headaches

EVIDENCE

Antimicrobial resistance has increased and a quinolone or a third-generation cephalosporin may be the best choice for empiric therapy of typhoid.

In a randomized controlled trial (RCT), 20 patients with blood culture-positive typhoid fever were openly randomized to receive ciprofloxacin and 22 to receive ceftriaxone. Six patients in the ceftriaxone group but none in the ciprofloxacin group had an outcome classed as treatment failure. All six in the ceftriaxone group who experienced treatment failure were switched to ciprofloxacin and became afebrile and asymptomatic within 48 hours.[1] Ⓑ

In an RCT of a 10-day compared with a 14-day regimen of ciprofloxacin in 69 patients with enteric fever, 52.2% of whom had infection with multidrug-resistant strains of *Salmonella typhi* or *S. paratyphi,* a 100% cure rate was observed for both regimens. Relapse occurred in two patients (on the 14-day regimen).[2] Ⓑ

In an RCT, 64 patients with positive blood or stool cultures for *Salmonella typhi* or *S. paratyphi* were randomized to receive azithromycin (36) or ciprofloxacin (28). Twenty-one patients had multidrug-resistant infection (to ampicillin, chloramphenicol, and trimethoprim-sulfamethoxazole). All patients in both groups improved and were cured.[3] Ⓑ

Of 64 children with uncomplicated typhoid fever and blood cultures positive for *Salmonella typhi,* all susceptible to azithromycin and ceftriaxone, 31 of 34 treated with azithromycin and 29 of 30 treated with ceftriaxone were cured.[4] Ⓑ

Vaccination is recommended when traveling in high-risk endemic areas. The World Health Organization and the Centers for Disease Control and Prevention recommend vaccination when traveling to areas where typhoid fever is endemic.[5] C A systematic review of 17 studies involving nearly 2 million people found that the older whole-cell vaccines produced more prolonged protection than either the Ty21a or Vi vaccine but were associated with higher toxicity.[6] A

Evidence-Based References

1. Wallace MR et al: Ciprofloxacin versus ceftriaxone in the treatment of multiresistant typhoid fever, *Eur J Clin Microbiol Infect Dis* 12:907, 1993. B
2. Alam MN et al: Efficacy of ciprofloxacin in enteric fever: comparison of treatment duration in sensitive and multidrug-resistant *Salmonella*, *Am J Trop Med Hyg* 53:306, 1995. B
3. Girgis NI et al: Azithromycin versus ciprofloxacin for treatment of uncomplicated typhoid fever in a randomized trial in Egypt that included patients with multidrug resistance, *Antimicrob Agents Chemother* 43:1441, 1999. B
4. Frenck RW Jr et al: Azithromycin versus ceftriaxone for the treatment of uncomplicated typhoid fever in children, *Clin Infect Dis* 31:1134, 2000. B
5. Centers for Disease Control and Prevention: Typhoid immunization: recommendations of the Advisory Committee on Immunization Practices, *MMWR Recomm Rep* 43(RR-14):1, 1994. C
6. Engels EA, Lau J: Vaccines for preventing typhoid fever, *Cochrane Database Syst Rev* 4, 1998. A

SUGGESTED READINGS

Bhan MK, Bahl R, Bhatnagar S: Typhoid and paratyphoid fever, *Lancet* 366:749, 2005.

Connor BA, Schwartz E: Typhoid and paratyphoid fever in travelers, *Lancet Infect Dis* 5(10):623, 2005.

House D et al: Use of paired serum samples for serodiagnosis of typhoid fever, *J Clin Microbiol* 43(9):4889, 2005.

Huang DB, DuPont HL: Problem pathogens: extra-intestinal complications of *Salmonella enterica* serotype Typhi infection, *Lancet Infect Dis* 5(6):341, 2005.

Kadhiravan T et al: Clinical outcomes in typhoid fever: adverse impact of infection with nalidixic acid-resistant *Salmonella typhi*, *BMC Infect Dis* 5(1):37, 2005.

Phongmany S et al: A randomized comparison of oral chloramphenicol versus ofloxacin in the treatment of uncomplicated typhoid fever in Laos, *Trans R Soc Trop Med Hyg* 99(6):451, 2005.

Steinberg EB et al: Typhoid fever in travelers: who should be targeted for prevention? *Clin Infect Dis* 39(2):186, 2004.

Vollaard AM et al: Helicobacter pylori infection and typhoid fever in Jakarta, Indonesia, *Epidemiol Infect* 134(1):163, 2006.

AUTHORS: **GLENN G. FORT, M.D., M.P.H., DENNIS J. MIKOLICH, M.D.,** and **MAURICE POLICAR, M.D.**

BASIC INFORMATION

DEFINITION

Ulcerative colitis is a chronic inflammatory bowel disease of undetermined etiology.

SYNONYMS

Inflammatory bowel disease (IBD)
Idiopathic proctocolitis

ICD-9CM CODES
556.9 Ulcerative colitis

EPIDEMIOLOGY & DEMOGRAPHICS

INCIDENCE:

- 50 to 150 cases/100,000 persons; most common between age 14 and 38 yr.
- Appendectomy for an inflammatory condition (appendicitis or lymphadenitis) but not for nonspecific abdominal pain is associated with a low risk of subsequent ulcerative colitis. This inverse relation is limited to patients who undergo surgery before the age of 20 yr.

PHYSICAL FINDINGS & CLINICAL PRESENTATION

- Patients with ulcerative colitis often present with bloody diarrhea accompanied by tenesmus, fever, dehydration, weight loss, anorexia, nausea, and abdominal pain.
- Abdominal distention and tenderness.
- Bloody diarrhea.
- Fever, evidence of dehydration.
- Evidence of extraintestinal manifestations may be present: liver disease, sclerosing cholangitis, iritis, uveitis, episcleritis, arthritis, erythema nodosum, pyoderma gangrenosum, aphthous stomatitis.

DIAGNOSIS

DIFFERENTIAL DIAGNOSIS

- Crohn's disease
- Bacterial infections
  1. Acute: *Campylobacter, Yersinia, Salmonella, Shigella, Chlamydia, Escherichia coli, Clostridium difficile,* gonococcal proctitis
  2. Chronic: Whipple's disease, TB, enterocolitis
- Irritable bowel syndrome
- Protozoal and parasitic infections (amebiasis, giardiasis, cryptosporidiosis)
- Neoplasm (intestinal lymphoma, carcinoma of colon)
- Ischemic bowel disease
- Diverticulitis
- Celiac sprue, collagenous colitis, radiation enteritis, endometriosis, gay bowel syndrome

WORKUP

Diagnostic workup includes:

- Comprehensive history, physical examination
- Laboratory tests (see following section)
- Colonoscopy to establish the presence of mucosal inflammation: typical endoscopic findings in ulcerative colitis are friable mucosa, diffuse, uniform erythema replacing the usual mucosal vascular pattern, and pseudopolyps; rectal involvement is invariably present if the disease is active

LABORATORY TESTS

- Anemia, high sedimentation rate (in severe colitis) are common.
- Potassium, magnesium, calcium, albumin may be decreased.
- Antineutrophil cytoplasmic antibodies (ANCA) with a perinuclear staining pattern (pANCA) can be found in >45% of patients; there is an increased frequency in treatment-resistant left-sided colitis, suggesting a possible association between these antibodies and a relative resistance to medical therapy in patients with ulcerative colitis.

IMAGING STUDIES

Image studies are generally not indicated. Air-contrast barium enema, when used, may reveal continuous involvement (including the rectum), pseudopolyps, decreased mucosal pattern, and fine superficial ulcerations.

TREATMENT

NONPHARMACOLOGIC THERAPY

- Correct nutritional deficiencies; TPN with bowel rest may be necessary in severe cases; folate supplementation may reduce the incidence of dysplasia and cancer in chronic ulcerative colitis.
- Avoid oral feedings during acute exacerbation to decrease colonic activity; a low-roughage diet may be helpful in *early* relapse.
- Psychotherapy is useful in most patients. Referral to self-help groups is also important because of the chronicity of the disease and the young age of the patients.

ACUTE GENERAL Rx

The therapeutic options vary with the degree of disease (mild, severe, fulminant) and areas of involvement (distal, extensive):

- Mild or moderate disease can be treated with mesalamine (Rowasa). It can be administered as an enema (40 mg once daily at bedtime for 3 to 6 wk) or suppository (500 mg bid) for patients with distal colonic disease. Oral forms in which the 5-ASA is in a slow-release or pH-dependent matrix (Pentasa 1 g qid, Asacol 800 mg PO tid) can deliver therapeutic concentrations to the more proximal small bowel or distal ileum.
- Olsalazine (Dipentum) is often useful for maintenance of remission of ulcerative colitis in patients intolerant to sulfasalazine. Usual dose is 500 mg bid taken with food.
- Balsalazide (Colazal) is indicated for mild to moderately active ulcerative colitis. Usual dose is three 750 mg capsules tid.
- Severe disease usually responds to oral corticosteroids (e.g., prednisone 40 to 60 mg/day); corticosteroid suppositories or enemas are also useful for distal colitis.
- Fulminant disease generally requires hospital admission and parenteral corticosteroids (e.g., IV hydrocortisone 100 mg q6h); when bowel movements have returned to normal and the patient is able to eat normally, oral prednisone is resumed. IV cyclosporine can also be used in severe refractory cases; renal toxicity is a potential complication.
- Surgery is indicated in patients who fail to respond to intensive medical therapy. Colectomy is usually curative in these patients and also eliminates the high risk of developing adenocarcinoma of the colon (10% to 20% of patients develop it after 10 yr with the disease); newer surgical techniques allow for the preservation of the sphincter.

CHRONIC Rx

- Colonoscopic surveillance and multiple biopsies should be instituted approximately 10 yr after diagnosis because of the increased risk of colon carcinoma.
- Erythropoietin is useful in patients with anemia refractory to treatment with iron and vitamins.

DISPOSITION

The clinical course is variable; 15% to 20% of patients will eventually require colectomy; >75% of patients treated medically will experience relapse.

REFERRAL

- GI consultation for initial diagnostic sigmoidoscopy/colonoscopy in suspected cases
- Surgical referral for patients with severe disease unresponsive to medical therapy

EVIDENCE

There is evidence that sulfasalazine and other 5-ASA preparations are effective in the management of acute ulcerative colitis and in the maintenance of remission.

A systematic review compared the newer 5-ASA preparations with sulfasalazine in the management of active ulcerative colitis. The review found that the newer 5-ASA agents were superior to placebo and had a tendency toward a therapeutic benefit over sulfasalazine. Although both 5-ASA agents and sulfasalazine are equally effective, sulfasalazine is associated with more side effects.[1] Ⓐ

In another systematic review the relative merits of 5-ASA preparations and sulfasalazine were compared in the maintenance of remission in ulcerative colitis. Although both sulfasalazine and 5-ASA preparations were superior to placebo in maintenance therapy, sulfasalazine had a significantly therapeutic superiority over 5-ASA preparations. This review found that sulfasalazine and 5-ASA had similar rates of adverse effects.[2] Ⓐ

There is evidence that topical mesalamine is effective in maintaining remission in ulcerative colitis.

A meta-analysis of controlled trials for treatment options in ulcerative colitis found that topical mesalamine was more effective than either oral 5-ASA preparations or steroids in inducing remission of active left-sided ulcerative colitis and proctitis.[3] Ⓐ

A randomized controlled trial (RCT) compared oral mesalamine (daily) and mesalamine enemas (twice weekly) vs. oral mesalamine and placebo enema, in the maintenance of remission in ulcerative colitis, over 12 months. The trial found that the use of both oral and topical mesalamine was more effective in maintaining remission than oral mesalamine alone.[4] Ⓑ

Another RCT compared the use of a single 500-mg mesalamine suppository vs. placebo as the sole therapy for the maintenance of remission in ulcerative proctitis. The study found that the time to relapse was significantly longer in the treatment group and, after both 12 and 24 months, the number of patients who remained in remission was significantly greater for those patients treated with mesalamine.[5] Ⓑ

There is clinical consensus that steroid therapy has an important role in the management of ulcerative colitis.

The American College of Gastroenterology guidelines recommend that patients with active disease, who are refractory to oral aminosalicylates, topical mesalamine, or topical steroid therapy, may require treatment with oral prednisone (in doses up to 40 to 60 mg/day).[6] Ⓒ

Patients with severe colitis refractory to maximal oral treatment with prednisone, oral aminosalicylates, and topical medications, or the patient who presents with toxicity, should be hospitalized for a course of intravenous steroids.[6] Ⓒ

Clinical consensus supports the use of 6-mercaptopurine and azathioprine in the management of ulcerative colitis.

6-mercaptopurine and azathioprine are effective for patients with ulcerative colitis who do not respond to oral prednisone but who are not so acutely ill as to intravenous therapy.[6] Ⓒ

In patients who require treatment with intravenous steroids or cyclosporine-A, long-term remission is significantly enhanced with the addition of long-term maintenance with 6-mercaptopurine.[6] Ⓒ

There is evidence that cyclosporine-A is effective in the management of severe ulcerative colitis.

A systematic review identified two randomized controlled trials (RCTs) that investigated the efficacy of cyclosporine-A in the treatment of severe ulcerative colitis.[7] Ⓐ

One RCT compared cyclosporine-A vs. placebo in 20 patients with severe ulcerative colitis defined as steroid refractory. This study found that cyclosporine-A treatment resulted in a significant increase in clinical response compared with placebo.[7] Ⓐ

The second RCT compared cyclosporine-A vs. methylprednisalone in patients with severe ulcerative colitis and found that both therapies were equally effective in inducing a clinical response.[7] Ⓐ

Clinical consensus supports the use of surgery in severe ulcerative colitis.

The American College of Gastroenterology guidelines recommend that absolute indications for surgery are exsanguinating hemorrhage, perforation, and documented or strongly suspected carcinoma. Other indications for surgery are severe colitis unresponsive to conventional maximal medical therapy and the patient with less severe, but medically intractable symptoms or intolerable side effects of medication.[6] Ⓒ

There is limited evidence that transdermal nicotine patches are effective in achieving clinical improvement and remission in patients with mild to moderate ulcerative colitis.

An RCT compared the use of nicotine transdermal patches vs. placebo over 4 weeks in 64 patients with mild to moderate ulcerative colitis. The study found that treatment with transdermal nicotine patches produced a significant clinical response compared with placebo.[8] Ⓑ

Evidence-Based References

1. Sutherland L, MacDonald JK: Oral 5-aminosalicylic acid for induction of remission in ulcerative colitis, *Cochrane Database Syst Rev* 3, 2003. Ⓐ
2. Sutherland L et al: Oral 5-aminosalicylic acid for maintenance of remission in ulcerative colitis, *Cochrane Database Syst Rev* 4, 2002. Ⓐ
3. Cohen RD et al: A meta-analysis and overview of the literature on treatment options for left-sided ulcerative colitis and ulcerative proctitis, *Am J Gastroenterol* 95:1263, 2000. Ⓐ
4. d'Albasio G et al: Combined therapy with 5-aminosalicylic acid tablets and enemas for maintaining remission in ulcerative colitis: a randomized double-blind study, *Am J Gastroenterol* 92:1143, 1997. Ⓑ
5. Hanauer S et al: Long-term use of mesalamine (Rowasa) suppositories in remission maintenance of ulcerative proctitis, *Am J Gastroenterol* 95:1749, 2000. Ⓑ
6. Kornbluth A, Sachar DB, Practice Parameters Committee of the American College of Gastroenterology: Ulcerative colitis practice guidelines in adults (update): American College of Gastroenterology, Practice Parameters Committee, *Am J Gastroenterol* 99:1371, 2004. Ⓒ
7. Shibolet O et al: Cyclosporine A for induction of remission in severe ulcerative colitis, *Cochrane Database Syst Rev* 1, 2005. Ⓐ
8. Sandborn WJ et al: Transdermal nicotine for mildly to moderately active ulcerative colitis. A randomized, double-blind, placebo-controlled trial, *Ann Intern Med* 126:364, 1997. Ⓑ

AUTHOR: **FRED F. FERRI, M.D.**

BASIC INFORMATION

DEFINITION

Urethritis is a well-defined clinical syndrome manifested by dysuria, a urethral discharge, or both.

ICD-9CM CODES
597.80 Urethritis, unspecified
098.20 Gonococcal

EPIDEMIOLOGY & DEMOGRAPHICS

- The major single specific etiology of acute urethritis is *Neisseria gonorrhoeae,* producing GCU. Urethritis of all other etiologies is called *nongonococcal urethritis* (NGU).
- NGU is twice as common as GCU in the U.S. NGU is the most common STD syndrome occurring in men, accounting for 6 million office visits annually. NGU is more frequently encountered in higher socioeconomic groups. GCU is more common in homosexual males than heterosexual males with acute urethritis.
- The gonococcus is a gram-negative, kidney-shaped diplococcus with flattened opposed margins. The urethra is the most common site of infection in all men. In heterosexual men, the pharynx is infected in 7%, and in homosexual men, the pharynx is infected in 40% and the rectum in 25%. A single episode of intercourse with an infected partner carries a transmission risk of 20% for males; female partners of an infected male will contract the disease 80% of the time.

PHYSICAL FINDINGS & CLINICAL PRESENTATION

SYMPTOMS OF GONOCOCCAL URETHRITIS: Urethral discharge and dysuria are the most common symptoms. There is complaint of urethral itching. Prostatic involvement can cause frequency, urgency, and nocturia. It can involve the epididymis through spreading down the vas deferens, causing acute epididymitis.
INCUBATION PERIOD: 3 to 10 days. Without treatment urethritis persists for 3 to 7 wk, with 95% of men becoming asymptomatic after 3 mo. GCU is asymptomatic in up to 60% of contacts.
SIGNS OF GONOCOCCAL URETHRITIS: Yellow-brown discharge, meatal edema, urethral tenderness to palpation. Rectal bleeding with pus is seen with gonococcal proctitis. Periurethritis leading to urethral stenosis can occur. Disseminated infection can occur. Tenosynovitis and arthritis can occur. Rarely, hepatitis, myocarditis, endocarditis, and meningitis can occur.

DIAGNOSIS

DIFFERENTIAL DIAGNOSIS

- NGU
- Herpes simplex virus

LABORATORY TESTS

- Calcium alginate or rayon swab on a metal shaft (*not* cotton-tipped swabs, which are bactericidal) of the urethra should be done anywhere from 2 to 4 hr after voiding to prevent bacterial washout with voiding.
- Cultures of the pharynx and rectum when indicated.
- Gram staining should be done. Modified Thayer-Martin media is used.
- On examination of the urethral smear, the presence of small numbers of PMNs provides objective evidence of urethritis. The complete absence of PMNs on a urethral smear argues against urethritis. If in addition to the PMNs there are gram-negative, intracellular diplococci, the diagnosis of gonorrhea is established.

TREATMENT

NONPHARMACOLOGIC THERAPY

BEHAVIORAL MANAGEMENT: Avoid intercourse until cure has been attained and sexual partners have been evaluated and treated.

ACUTE GENERAL Rx

FOR UNCOMPLICATED URETHRAL, CERVICAL, AND RECTAL GCU: Ceftriaxone 125 mg IM + doxycycline 100 mg bid × 7 days. Alternative therapy: ciprofloxacin 500 mg PO × 1 day; ofloxacin 400 mg PO × 1 day (all of these to be followed by 7 days of doxycycline 100 mg PO bid).

- In uncomplicated gonococcal infections, single-drug regimens using selected fluoroquinolones, selected cephalosporins, or spectinomycin are highly effective and safe.
- Resistance to penicillins, sulphonamides, and tetracyclines is now widespread.
- Dual treatment for gonococcal and chlamydial infections is based on theory and expert opinion rather than on evidence from clinical trials.

FOR EPIDIDYMITIS: Ceftriaxone 250 mg IM followed by doxycycline 100 mg PO bid × 10 days. Alternative therapy: ofloxacin 300 mg PO bid × 10 days.

CHRONIC Rx

POSTGONOCOCCAL URETHRITIS (PGU): Reinfection is the most common cause of recurrence. Repeat swab and culture of the urethra, pharynx, and rectum (where applicable) are mandatory. Persistence of PMNs with the absence of gram-negative intracellular diplococci suggests a diagnosis of postgonococcal urethritis. This occurs when GCU is treated with a regimen that is ineffective against coincident chlamydial infection; it represents NGU following GCU. The syndrome should be treated as NGU. Persistence of *N. gonorrhoeae* by smear or culture requires treatment for *N. gonorrhoeae.*

PEARLS & CONSIDERATIONS

COMMENTS

- CAUTION: Tetracyclines and fluoroquinolones are *contraindicated* in pregnancy. *Chlamydia* infection in pregnancy can be treated with amoxicillin 500 mg PO tid for 7 days or with clindamycin 450 mg PO tid for 10 days.
- *Posttreatment cultures are required.*

EVIDENCE

A single dose of oral cefixime is as effective as a single intramuscular dose of ceftriaxone in the treatment of genital gonococcal infection.[1] (A)

Single-dose regimens of oral cefuroxime and oral ciprofloxacin are both equally effective in eradicating penicillinase-producing Neisseria gonorrhea from males and females with uncomplicated gonorrheal infections.[2] (B)

In the treatment of genital gonococcal infection in pregnancy, amoxicillin plus probenecid, spectinomycin, and ceftriaxone produce similar overall cure rates.[3] (B)

Evidence-Based References

1. Brocklehurst P: Antibiotics for gonorrhoea in pregnancy. In: Cochrane Library 2, Chichester, UK, 2004, John Wiley. Reviewed in: *Clin Evid* 11:2104, 2004. (A)
2. Thorpe EM: Comparison of single dose cefuroxime axetil with ciprofloxacin in treatment of uncomplicated gonorrhoea caused by penicillinase producing and non-penicillinase producing N. gonorrhoeae strains, *Antimicrob Agents Chemother* 40:2775, 1996. (B)
3. Cavenee M, Farris J, Spalding T: Treatment of gonorrhea in pregnancy, *Am J Obstet Gynecol* 185:629, 2001. Reviewed in: *Clin Evid* 11:2104, 2004. (B)

AUTHORS: **PHILIP J. ALIOTTA, M.D., M.S.H.A.,** and **RUBEN ALVERO, M.D.**

BASIC INFORMATION

DEFINITION

Nongonococcal urethritis is urethral inflammation caused by any of several organisms.

SYNONYMS

NGU

ICD-9CM CODES
099.40 Nongonococcal
099.41 Chlamydial

EPIDEMIOLOGY & DEMOGRAPHICS

- Occurrence is 50% in STD clinics.
- NGU most commonly affects men in higher socioeconomic class, affecting heterosexual men more frequently than homosexual men.
- NGU carries a greater morbidity than GCU.
- Asymptomatic infection occurs in 28% of the contacts of women with chlamydial cervical infection.

PHYSICAL FINDINGS & CLINICAL PRESENTATION

INCUBATION PERIOD: 2 to 35 days
SYMPTOMS: Dysuria, whitish-to-clear urethral discharge, and urethral itching. The onset of symptoms in NGU is less acute than GCU.
SIGNS: Whitish-to-clear urethral discharge, meatal edema, and erythema. Infected women manifest pyuria, and the disease can present as acute urethral syndrome.

COMPLICATIONS

Epididymitis in heterosexual men may be linked to nonbacterial prostatitis, proctitis in homosexual men, and Reiter's syndrome.

ETIOLOGY

- Most common agent is *Chlamydia* spp., an obligate intracellular parasite possessing both DNA and RNA, replicating by binary fission. It causes 20%-50% of NGU cases. Two species exist:
  1. *Chlamydia psittaci*
  2. *Chlamydia trachomatis* with its 15 serotypes
     a. Serotypes A-C cause hyperendemic blinding trachoma.
     b. Serotypes D-K cause genital tract infection.
     c. Serotypes L1-L3 cause lymphogranuloma venereum.
- Other causes of NGU: *Ureaplasma urealyticum* causing 15% to 30% of the cases of NGU, *Trichomonas vaginalis,* and herpes simplex virus. The cause of 20% of the cases of NGU has not been identified.

DIAGNOSIS

DIFFERENTIAL DIAGNOSIS

- GCU
- Herpes simplex virus
- Trichomoniasis

LABORATORY TESTS

- Requires demonstration of urethritis and exclusion of infection with *N. gonorrhoeae.*
- The appearance of PMNs on urethral smear confirms the diagnosis of urethritis. Because *Chlamydia* is an intracellular parasite of the columnar epithelium, the best specimen for culture is an endourethral swab taken from an area 2 to 4 cm inside the urethra. The organism can only be grown in tissue culture, which is expensive.
- New techniques have been developed and are useful in making the diagnosis: nucleic acid hybridization, enzyme-linked immunosorbent assay (ELISA), and direct immunofluorescence.
- For culture, a Dacron-tipped swab is used; avoid calcium alginate or cotton swabs.

TREATMENT

Because it is impossible to differentiate among the common etiologies of NGU, the condition is treated syndromically, including in the initial treatment regimen those drugs effective against the common causative agents.

- Recommended: azithromycin 1000 mg as a single dose or doxycycline 100 mg PO bid for 7 days
- Other drugs: tetracycline 500 mg PO qid for 7 days
- Alternative regimens: erythromycin base 500 mg PO qid for 7 days, ofloxacin 300 mg PO bid for 7 days, levofloxacin 500 mg PO daily for 7 days

In pregnant women:

- Both amoxicillin and erythromycin are likely effective in achieving microbiologic cure.
- Clindamycin and erythromycin have a similar effect on cure rates.
- A single dose of azithromycin is more effective in achieving microbiologic cure of *C. trachomatis* than a 7-day course of erythromycin.

In men and nonpregnant women:

- Multiple-dose regimens of tetracyclines and macrolides achieve microbiologic cure in at least 95% of patients.
- Erythromycin daily dose of 2 g is likely beneficial.
- Ciprofloxacin is less effective in the treatment of *C. trachomatis* infection when compared with doxycycline.
- A single dose of azithromycin is as successful at curing *C. trachomatis* as a 7-day course of doxycycline.

PEARLS & CONSIDERATIONS

COMMENTS

- CAUTION: Tetracyclines and fluoroquinolones are *contraindicated* in pregnancy. *Chlamydia* infection in pregnancy can be treated with amoxicillin 500 mg PO tid for 7 days or with clindamycin 450 mg PO tid for 10 days.
- *Posttreatment cultures are required.*

EVIDENCE

Treatment of *Chlamydia trachomatis.*

Both 1 g azithromycin and a 7-day course of doxycycline (100 mg twice daily) produce high clinical cure rates within 2 weeks in the treatment of genital chlamydial infection in men and nonpregnant women.[1] Ⓐ

In the treatment of genital chlamydial infection in pregnant women, a single dose of azithromycin 1g is highly effective and well tolerated, being equally as effective as a 7-day course of amoxicillin and significantly more effective than a 7-day course of erythromycin.[2-4] Ⓐ Ⓑ

Evidence-Based References

1. Lau C-Y, Qureshi AK: Azithromycin versus doxycycline for genital chlamydial infections: a meta-analysis of randomised clinical trials, *Sex Transm Dis* 29:497, 2002. Reviewed in: *Clin Evid* 12:2200, 2004. Ⓐ
2. Brocklehurst P, Rooney G: Interventions for treating genital chlamydia trachomatis infection in pregnancy. In: Cochrane Library 2, Chichester, UK, 2004, John Wiley. Reviewed in: *Clin Evid* 11:2064, 2004. Ⓑ
3. Jacobson JF et al: A randomized controlled trial comparing amoxicillin and azithromycin for the treatment of chlamydia trachomatis in pregnancy, *Am J Obstet Gynecol* 184: 1352, 2001. Reviewed in: *Clin Evid* 11:2064, 2004. Ⓐ
4. Kacmar J et al: A randomized trial of azithromycin versus amoxicillin for the treatment of Chlamydia trachomatis in pregnancy, *Infect Dis Obstet Gynecol* 9:197, 2001. Reviewed in: *Clin Evid* 11:2064, 2004. Ⓐ

AUTHORS: **PHILIP J. ALIOTTA, M.D., M.S.H.A.,**
and **RUBEN ALVERO, M.D.**

BASIC INFORMATION

DEFINITION

Urinary tract infection (UTI) is a term that encompasses a broad range of clinical entities that have in common a positive urine culture. A conventional threshold is growth of >100,000 colony-forming units per ml from a midstream-catch urine sample. In symptomatic patients, a smaller number of bacteria (between 100 and 10,000 colony-forming units per ml of midstream urine) is recognized as an infection.

SYNONYMS

UTI

ICD-9CM CODES
595.0 Acute cystitis
595.3 Trigonitis
595.2 Chronic cystitis
590.1 Acute pyelonephritis
590.0 Chronic pyelonephritis
590.8 Nonspecific pyelonephritis

CLASSIFICATION

FIRST INFECTION: The first documented UTI; tends to be uncomplicated and is easily treated.

UNRESOLVED BACTERIURIA: UTI in which the urinary tract is not sterilized during therapy. Main causes are bacterial resistance, patient noncompliance with medication, resistance, mixed bacterial infection, rapid reinfection, azotemia, infected stones, Munchausen's, and papillary necrosis.

BACTERIAL PERSISTENCE: UTI in which the urine cultures become sterile during therapy, but a persistent source of infection from a site within the urinary tract that was excluded from the high urinary concentrations gives rise to reinfection by the same organism. Causes: infected stone, chronic bacterial prostatitis, atrophic infected kidney, vesicovaginal or enterovesical fistulas, obstructive uropathy, infected pyelocalyceal diverticula, infected ureteral stump following nephrectomy, infected necrotic papillae from papillary necrosis, infected urachal cysts, infected medullary sponge kidney, urethral diverticula, and foreign bodies.

REINFECTION: UTI in which a new infection occurs with new pathogens at variable intervals after a previous infection has been eradicated.

Relapse: The less common form of recurrent infection; occurs within 2 wk of treatment when the same organism reappears in the same site as the previous infection. Relapsing infections of the urinary tract most commonly occur in pyelonephritis, kidney obstruction from a stone, and prostatitis.

EPIDEMIOLOGY & DEMOGRAPHICS

INCIDENCE:

In Neonates: More common in boys as a result of anatomic abnormalities.

In Preschool Children: More common in girls (4.5% vs. 0.5% for boys).

In Adulthood: More common in women, with a 1% to 3% prevalence in nonpregnant women. In pregnancy at 12 wk, the incidence of asymptomatic bacteriuria is similar to nonpregnant women, at 2% to 10%. However, 70% to 80% of women with asymptomatic bacteriuria develop acute pyelonephritis, especially in the second and third trimesters, and suffer a pyelonephritic recurrence rate of 10%. In adults, 65 yr and older, at least 10% of men and 20% of women have bacteriuria.

PHYSICAL FINDINGS & CLINICAL PRESENTATION

- UTI presentation is inconsistent and cannot be relied upon to diagnose UTI accurately or to localize the site of infection. Patients complain of:
  1. Urinary frequency, urgency
  2. Dysuria
  3. Urge incontinence
  4. Suprapubic pain
  5. Gross or microscopic hematuria
- When negative cultures are associated with significant pyuria, vaginal discharge, or hematuria, infections with *Chlamydia trachomatis, Neisseria gonorrhoeae,* and *Trichomonas vaginalis* should be considered.
- Acute pyelonephritis (PN) presents with fever, flank or abdominal pain, chills, malaise, vomiting, and diarrhea. It is these systemic symptoms that distinguish pyelonephritis from cystitis. Complications of acute pyelonephritis are renal abscess, perinephric abscess, emphysematous pyelonephritis, and pyonephrosis.

ETIOLOGY & PATHOGENESIS

- Four major pathways:
  1. Ascending from the urethra
  2. Lymphatic
  3. Hematogenous
  4. Direct extension from another organ system
- Other risk factors: neurologic diseases, renal failure, diabetes; anatomic abnormalities: bladder outlet obstruction, urethral stricture, vesicoureteral reflux, fistula, urinary diversion, megacystis, and infected stones; age; pregnancy; instrumentation, poor patient compliance, poor hygiene, infrequent voider, diaphragm contraceptives, tampon use, douches, and catheters

Catheters: All patients who require a long-term Foley catheter eventually develop significant levels of bacteriuria. Treatment is reserved for those individuals who become symptomatic (i.e., leukocytosis, fever, chills, malaise, loss of appetite, etc.) Using prophylactic antibiotics to treat patients who have chronic catheters is to be discouraged because of the risk of acquiring bacteria that are resistant to antibiotic therapy.

- Once bacteria reach the urinary tract, three factors determine whether the infection occurs (Box 1-14):
  1. Virulence of the microorganism
  2. Inoculum size
  3. Adequacy of the host defense mechanisms
- These factors also determine the anatomic level of the UTI.

Urinary Pathogens: In >95% of UTIs the infecting organism is a member of the Enterobacteriaceae, *Pseudomonas aeruginosa,* enterococci, or, in young women, *Staphylococcus saprophyticus*. In contrast, the organisms that commonly colonize the distal urethra and skin of both men and women and the vagina of women are *Staphylococcus epidermidis,* diphtheroids,

BOX 1-14 Bacterial Factors

1. The size of the inoculum
2. The virulence of the infecting organism:
   a. Virulence factors:
      i. P-fimbriae facilitate the adherence of bacteria to biologic surfaces.
      ii. K-antigens facilitate adherence and protect the organisms from the host-immune response.
      iii. O-antigens are an important source of the systemic reactions, such as fever and shock, that occur with bacterial infections.
      iv. H antigens are associated with flagella and are related to bacterial locomotion.
      v. Hemolysin may potentiate tissue damage and facilitate local bacterial growth.
      vi. Urease alkalinizes the urine and facilitates stone formation, thus potentiating infection.
   b. Biofilms harbor bacteria on prosthetic devices and may be a source of recurrent infections.
   c. The presence of sialosyl galactosyl globoside (SGG) on the surface of kidney cells. This compound is a highly powerful receptor for *E. coli* bacteria.
   d. Women with a deficiency in human beta-defensin-1 (HBD-1) are at greater risk for urinary tract infection.
3. Adequacy of host defense mechanisms

lactobacilli, *Gardnerella vaginalis,* and a variety of anaerobes that rarely cause UTI. Generally, the isolation of two or more bacterial species from a urine culture signifies a contaminated specimen, unless the patient is being managed with an indwelling catheter or urinary diversion or has a chronic complicated infection.

Defense Mechanisms against Cystitis: Low pH and high osmolarity, mucopolysaccharide glycosaminoglycan protective layer, normal bladder that empties completely and has no incontinence, and the presence of estrogen

DIAGNOSIS (Dx)

DIFFERENTIAL DIAGNOSIS

- Interstitial cystitis
- Vaginitis
- Urethritis (gonococcal, nongonococcal, *Trichomonas*)
- Frequency-urgency syndrome, prostatitis (acute and chronic)
- Obstructive uropathy
- Infected stones
- Fistulas
- Papillary necrosis
- Vesicoureteral reflux

LABORATORY TESTS

- Urinalysis with microscopic evaluation of clean-catch urine for bacteria and pyuria
- Urine C&S
- CBC with differential (shows leukocytosis)
- Antibody-coated bacteria are seen with pyelonephritis

IMAGING STUDIES

- Warranted only if renal infection or genitourinary abnormality is suspected
- KUB, VCUG, renal sonogram, IVP, CT scan, and nuclear scan
- Specialty examination: cystoscopy with occasional retrograde pyelography to rule out obstructive uropathy; stenting the obstruction possibly required

TREATMENT (Rx)

NONPHARMACOLOGIC THERAPY

- Hot sitz baths, anticholinergics, urinary analgesics
- For pyelonephritis: bed rest, analgesics, antipyretics, and IV hydration

ACUTE GENERAL Rx

- Conventional therapy of 7 days; short-term therapy of 1, 3, or 5 days.
- Agents of choice: amoxicillin/clavulanate, cephalosporins, fluoroquinolones, nitrofurantoin, and trimethoprim with sulfonamide.
- For pyelonephritis: hospitalization until afebrile and stable, then at home via home care agency with IV antibiotic composed of aminoglycoside plus cephalosporin × 1 wk followed by oral agents (based on sensitivity) for 2 wk. Moderate forms of pyelonephritis have been successfully treated with fluoroquinolone therapy for 21 days, without requiring hospitalization. Most important, complicating factors such as obstructive uropathy or infected stones must be identified and treated.
- Section III, "Urinary Tract Infection," describes an approach to the management of UTI.

PEARLS & CONSIDERATIONS (!)

COMMENTS

- *Asymptomatic bacteriuria:* occurs in both anatomically normal and abnormal urinary tracts. This can clear spontaneously, persist, or lead to symptomatic kidney infection. Treatment is recommended in patients with vesicoureteral reflux, stones, obstructive uropathy, parenchymal renal disease, diabetes mellitus, and pregnant or immunocompromised patients.
- *Pregnancy:* 20% to 40% of pregnant women with untreated bacteriuria develop pyelonephritis. This is associated with prematurity and low-birth-weight infants. Confirmed significant bacteriuria should be treated with an aminopenicillin and cephalosporin.
- *Recurrent UTI:* caused by an unresolved infection, vaginal colonization of the originally infecting organism, or reinfection with a new strain. Management of recurrent UTI includes continuous antibiotic prophylaxis, intermittent self-treatment, and postcoital prophylaxis. Prophylaxis is recommended for women who experience two or more symptomatic UTIs over a 6-mo period or three or more episodes over a 12-mo period.
  1. Changes after menopause: lower levels of lactobacilli, decreased estrogen, senile atrophy of the genitalia, and loss of bladder elasticity (compliance).
  2. Biologic factors altering defense systems: the presence of sialosyl galactosyl globoside (SGG) on the surface of the kidney acts as a powerful receptor for *E. coli* and increases the risk for UTI; the presence of the blood group P1 causes increased binding of *E. coli* that is resistant to normal infection-fighting mechanisms in the body and it is believed that some individuals are deficient in a compound called *human beta-defensin-1* (HBD-1), a naturally occurring antibiotic that fights *E. coli* within the urinary tract.

Resistance:

- Because of the overuse of antibiotics, organisms once sensitive to a number of agents are now increasingly more resistant, making effective management of UTI and pyelonephritis more difficult and potentially more dangerous. Most important has been the increasing resistance to TMP-SMX, the current primary care provider drug of choice for acute uncomplicated UTI in women.
- When choosing a treatment regimen physicians should consider such factors as:
  1. In-vitro susceptibility
  2. Adverse effects
  3. Cost effectiveness
  4. Resistance rates in the respective communities

EVIDENCE (EBM)

A systematic review examined the optimal duration of antibiotic treatment for uncomplicated UTIs in elderly women. The comparison of short (3 to 6 days) and longer (7 to 14 days) treatments did not show any significant difference, but the methodologic quality and sample size of all the trials were low.[1] Ⓑ

A systematic review of RCTs examining which treatment is most effective for symptomatic UTIs during pregnancy found no significant differences between treatments with regard to cure rates, recurrent infection, and incidence of preterm delivery.[2] Ⓑ

A systematic review and a subsequent RCT in women with uncomplicated acute pyelonephritis have found no consistent differences in cure rates between oral trimethoprim/sulfamethoxazole (TMP/SMX), amoxicillin/clavulanic acid, or ciprofloxacin.[3,4] Ⓐ

Evidence-Based References

1. Lutters M, Vogt N: Antibiotic duration for treating uncomplicated, symptomatic lower urinary tract infections in elderly women (Cochrane Review). In: Cochrane Library 1, Chichester, UK, 2004, John Wiley. Ⓑ
2. Vazquez JC, Villar J: Treatments for symptomatic urinary tract infections during pregnancy (Cochrane Review). In: Cochrane Library 1, Chichester, UK, 2004, John Wiley. Ⓑ
3. Pinson AG et al: Oral antibiotic therapy for acute pyelonephritis: a methodologic review of the literature, *J Gen Intern Med* 7:544, 1992. Reviewed in: *Clin Evid* 10:2204, 2003. Ⓐ
4. Richard GA et al: Levofloxacin versus ciprofloxacin versus lomefloxacin in acute pyelonephritis, *Urology* 52:5155, 1998. Reviewed in: *Clin Evid* 10:2204, 2003. Ⓐ

AUTHORS: **PHILIP J. ALIOTTA, M.D., M.S.H.A.,** and **RUBEN ALVERO, M.D.**

BASIC INFORMATION

DEFINITION

Urolithiasis is the presence of calculi within the urinary tract. The five major types of urinary stones are calcium oxalate (>50%), calcium phosphate (10% to 20%), uric acid (8%), struvite (15%), and cystine (3%).

SYNONYMS

Nephrolithiasis
Renal colic

ICD-9CM CODES
592.9 Urinary calculus

EPIDEMIOLOGY & DEMOGRAPHICS

- Urinary stone disease afflicts 250,000 to 750,000 Americans/yr.
- Male:female ratio is 4:1. After the sixth decade, the ratio is 1.5:1.
- Incidence of symptomatic nephrolithiasis is greatest during the summer (resulting from increased humidity and temperatures with increased risk of dehydration and concentrated urine).
- Calcium oxalate or mixed calcium oxalate/calcium phosphate stones account for 70% of urolithiasis.

PHYSICAL FINDINGS & CLINICAL PRESENTATION

Stones may be asymptomatic or may cause the following signs and symptoms from obstruction:

- Sudden onset of flank tenderness
- Nausea and vomiting
- Patient in constant movement, attempting to lessen the pain (patients with an acute abdomen are usually still because movement exacerbates the pain)
- Pain may be referred to the testes or labium (progression of stone down the urinary ureter)
- Fever and chills accompanying the acute colic if there is superimposed infection
- Pain may radiate anteriorly over to the abdomen and result in intestinal ileus

ETIOLOGY

- Increased absorption of calcium in the small bowel: type I absorptive hypercalciuria (independent of calcium intake)
- Idiopathic hypercalciuria nephrolithiasis is the most common diagnosis for patients with calcium stones; the diagnosis is made only if there is no hypercalcemia and no known cause for hypercalciuria
- Increased vitamin D synthesis (e.g., secondary to renal phosphate loss: type III absorptive hypercalciuria)
- Renal tubular malfunction with inadequate reabsorption of calcium and resulting hypercalciuria
- Heterozygous mutations in the NPT2a gene result in hypophosphatemia and urinary phosphate loss
- Hyperparathyroidism with resulting hypercalcemia
- Elevated uric acid level (metabolic defects, dietary excess)
- Chronic diarrhea (e.g., inflammatory bowel disease) with increased oxalate absorption
- Type I (distal tubule) renal tubular acidosis (<1% of calcium stones)
- Chronic hydrochlorothiazide treatment
- Chronic infections with urease-producing organisms (e.g., *Proteus, Providencia, Pseudomonas, Klebsiella*). Struvite, or magnesium ammonium phosphate crystals, are produced when the urinary tract is colonized by bacteria, producing elevated concentrations of ammonia
- Abnormal excretion of cystine
- Chemotherapy for malignancies

DIAGNOSIS

DIFFERENTIAL DIAGNOSIS

- Urinary tract infection
- Pyelonephritis
- Diverticulitis
- PID
- Ovarian pathology
- Factitious (drug addicts)
- Appendicitis
- Small bowel obstruction
- Ectopic pregnancy
- The differential diagnosis of obstructive uropathy is described in Section II

WORKUP

- Laboratory and imaging studies. Stone analysis should be performed on recovered stones.
- A clinical algorithm for evaluation of nephrolithiasis is described in Section III.
- Box 1-15 describes past medical history significant for urolithiasis.

LABORATORY TESTS

- Urinalysis: hematuria may be present; however, its absence does not exclude urinary stones. Evaluation of urinary pH is of value in identification of type of stone (pH >7.5 is associated with struvite stones, whereas pH <5 generally is seen with uric acid or with cystine stones).
- Urine C&S should be obtained for all patients.
- Serum chemistries should include calcium, electrolytes, phosphate, and uric acid.
- Additional tests: 24-hr urine collection for calcium, uric acid, phosphate, oxalate, and citrate excretion is generally reserved for patients with recurrent stones.

IMAGING STUDIES

- Plain films of the abdomen can identify radioopaque stones (calcium, uric acid stones).
- Renal sonogram may be helpful.
- IVP demonstrates the size and location of the stone, as well as degree of obstruction.
- Unenhanced (noncontrast) helical CT scan does not require contrast media and can visualize the calculus (identified by the "rim sign" or "halo" repre-

BOX 1-15 Past Medical History Significant for Urolithiasis

Diseases associated with disturbances of calcium metabolism: primary hyperparathyroidism, Wilson's disease, medullary sponge kidney, osteoporosis, immobilization, sarcoidosis, osteolytic metastases, plasmacytoma, neuroendocrine tumors, Paget's disease
Dietary history: purine gluttony, calcium excess, milk alkali, oxalate excess, sodium excess, low citrus fruit intake
Medications: uricosurics, diuretics, analgesics, vitamins C and D, antacids (especially phosphorus-binding agents), acetazolamide, calcium channel blockers, triamterene, theophylline, protease inhibitors (indinavir), sulfonamides
Diseases associated with disturbances of oxalate metabolism: primary hyperoxaluria types I and II, Crohn's disease, ulcerative colitis, intestinal bypass surgery (especially jejunoileal bypass), ileal resection
Diseases associated with disturbances of purine metabolism
Intrinsic metabolic disorders—anemia, neoplastic disorders (especially leukemias), intoxication, myocardial infarction, irradiation, cytotoxic chemotherapy
Enzyme deficiency—primary gout, Lesch-Nyhan syndrome
Altered excretion—renal insufficiency, metabolic acidosis
Infectious history: organisms (particularly Proteus and Klebsiella), febrile upper tract involvement and dates if hospitalized.

From Nseyo UO (ed): *Urology for primary care physicians,* Philadelphia, 1999, WB Saunders.

senting the edematous ureteral wall around the stone). It is fast, accurate (sensitivity 15% to 100%, specificity 94% to 96%), and readily identifies all stone types in all locations. This modality is being used increasingly in the initial assessment of renal colic.

TREATMENT

NONPHARMACOLOGIC THERAPY

- Increase in water or other fluid intake (doubling of previous fluid intake unless patient has a history of CHF or fluid overload)
- Normal dietary calcium intake is recommended. If one does not consume enough calcium, less is available to bind to dietary oxalate; as a result, more oxalate reaches the colon, is absorbed into the bloodstream, and is excreted as calcium oxalate, setting the stage for calcium urolithiasis
- Sodium restriction (to decrease calcium excretion), decreased protein intake to 1 g/kg/day (to decrease uric acid, calcium, and oxalate excretion)
- Increase in bran (may decrease bowel transit time with increased binding of calcium and subsequent decrease in urinary calcium)

ACUTE GENERAL Rx

- Pain control (use of narcotics is generally indicated because of the severity of pain)
- Specific therapy tailored to the stone type:
  1. Uric acid calculi: control of hyperuricosuria with allopurinol 100 to 300 mg/day; increase urinary pH with potassium citrate, 10-mEq tablets tid
  2. Calcium stones:
     a. HCTZ 25 to 50 mg qd in patients with type I absorptive hypercalciuria
     b. Decrease bowel absorption of calcium with cellulose phosphate 10 g/day in patients with type I absorptive hypercalciuria
     c. Orthophosphates to inhibit vitamin B synthesis in patients with type III absorptive hypercalciuria
     d. Potassium citrate supplementation in patients with hypocitraturic calcium nephrolithiasis
     e. Purine dietary restrictions or allopurinol in patients with hyperuricosuric calcium nephrolithiasis
  3. Struvite stones:
     a. Most of the stones are large and cause obstruction and bleeding.
     b. ESWL and percutaneous nephrolithotomy are generally necessary.
     c. Prolonged use of antibiotics directed against the predominant urinary tract organism may be beneficial to prevent recurrence.
  4. Cystine stones: Hydration and alkalization of the urine to pH >6.5, penicillamine, and tiopronin can also be used to reduce the formation of cystine; captopril is also beneficial and causes fewer side effects
- Surgical treatment in patients with severe pain unresponsive to medication and patients with persistent fever or nausea or significant impediment of urine flow:
  a. Ureteroscopic stone extraction
  b. Extracorporeal shock wave lithotripsy (ESWL) for most renal stones
- In 1997 the American Urological Association issued the following guidelines for the treatment of ureteral stones:
  1. Proximal ureteral stones <1 cm in diameter: options are ESWL, percutaneous nephroureterolithotomy, and ureteroscopy
  2. Proximal ureteral stones >1 cm in diameter: options are ESWL, percutaneous nephroureterolithotomy, and ureteroscopy. Placement of a ureteral stent should be considered if the stone is causing high-grade obstruction
  3. Distal ureteral stones <1 cm in diameter: most of these pass spontaneously. ESWL and ureteroscopy are two accepted modes of therapy
  4. Distal ureteral stones >1 cm in diameter: watchful waiting, ESWL, ureteroscopy (following stone fragmentation)
- Section III describes an approach to the management of ureteral calculi.

CHRONIC Rx

Maintenance of proper hydration and dietary restrictions (see "Acute General Rx")

DISPOSITION

- >50% of patients will pass the stone within 48 hr.
- Stones will recur in approximately 50% of patients within 5 yr if no medical treatment is provided.

REFERRAL

Urology referral in complicated or recurrent urolithiasis; most patients with small uncomplicated ureteral or renal calculi can be followed as outpatient, whereas patients with persistent vomiting, suspected UTI, pain unresponsive to oral analgesics, or obstructing calculus associated with solitary kidney should be admitted

PEARLS & CONSIDERATIONS

COMMENTS

- Early identification and aggressive treatment of urinary tract infections is indicated in all patients with struvite stones.
- Alkalinization of urine (pH >7.5 with penicillamine) is useful in patients with recurrent cystine stones.
- An algorithmic approach to the management of ureteral calculi is described in Section III.

SUGGESTED READINGS

Borghi L et al: Comparison of two diets for the prevention of recurrent stones in idiopathic hypercalciuria, *N Engl J Med* 346:77, 2002.

Pietrow PK, Karellas ME: Medical management of common urinary calculi, *Am Fam Physician* 74:86, 2006.

Prie D et al: Nephrolithiasis and osteoporosis associated with hypophosphatemia caused by mutations in the type 2a sodium-phosphate cotransporter, *N Engl J Med* 347:983, 2002.

Worster A et al: The accuracy of noncontrast helical computed tomography versus intravenous pyelography in the diagnosis of suspected acute urolithiasis: a meta-analysis, *Ann Intern Med* 40:280, 2002.

AUTHOR: **FRED F. FERRI, M.D.**

BASIC INFORMATION

DEFINITION

Urticaria is a pruritic rash involving the epidermis and the upper portions of the dermis, resulting from localized capillary vasodilation and followed by transudation of protein-rich fluid in the surrounding tissue and manifesting clinically with the presence of hives.

SYNONYMS

Hives
Wheals

ICD-9CM CODES
708.8 Other unspecified urticaria

EPIDEMIOLOGY & DEMOGRAPHICS

- At least 20% of the population will have one episode of hives during their lifetime.
- Incidence is increased in atopic patients.
- The etiology of chronic urticaria (hives lasting longer than 6 wk) is determined in only 5% to 20% of cases.

PHYSICAL FINDINGS & CLINICAL PRESENTATION

- Presence of elevated, erythematous, or white nonpitting plaques that change in size and shape over time; they generally last a few hours and disappear without a trace.
- Annular configuration with central pallor (Fig. 1-284).

ETIOLOGY

- Foods (e.g., shellfish, eggs, strawberries, nuts)
- Drugs (e.g., penicillin, aspirin, sulfonamides)
- Systemic diseases (e.g., SLE, serum sickness, autoimmune thyroid disease, polycythemia vera)
- Food additives (e.g., salicylates, benzoates, sulfites)
- Infections (viral infections, fungal infections, chronic bacterial infections)
- Physical stimuli (e.g., pressure urticaria, exercise-induced, solar urticaria, cold urticaria)
- Inhalants (e.g., mold spores, animal danders, pollens)
- Contact (nonimmunologic) urticaria (e.g., caterpillars, plants)
- Other: hereditary angioedema, urticaria pigmentosa, pregnancy, cold urticaria, hair bleaches, chemicals, saliva, cosmetics, perfumes, pemphigoid, emotional stress

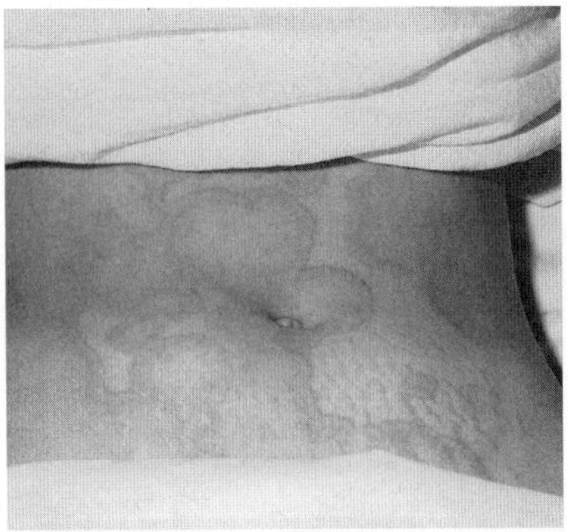

FIGURE 1-284 Wheal (urticaria). Note central cleaning, giving annular configuration. (From Noble J et al: *Textbook of primary care medicine,* ed 3, St Louis, 2001, Mosby.)

DIAGNOSIS

DIFFERENTIAL DIAGNOSIS

- Erythema multiforme
- Erythema marginatum
- Erythema infectiosum
- Urticarial vasculitis
- Herpes gestationis
- Drug eruption
- Multiple insect bites
- Bullous pemphigoid

WORKUP

- It is useful to determine whether hives are acute or chronic; a medical history focused on various etiologic factors is necessary before embarking on extensive laboratory testing.
- A diagnostic approach to chronic urticaria is described in Section III.

LABORATORY TESTS

- CBC with differential
- Stool for ova and parasites in patients with suspected parasitic infestations
- ANA, ESR, TSH, LFTs, eosinophil count are indicated only in selected patients
- Measurement of C_4 in patients who present with angioedema alone
- Skin biopsy is helpful in patients with fever, arthralgias, and elevated ESR

TREATMENT

NONPHARMACOLOGIC THERAPY

- Remove suspected etiologic agents (e.g., stop aspirin and all nonessential drugs), restrict diet (e.g., elimination of tomatoes, nuts, eggs, shellfish).
- Elimination of yeast should be attempted in patients with chronic urticaria (*Candida albicans* sensitivity may be a factor in patients with chronic urticaria).

ACUTE GENERAL Rx

- Oral antihistamines: use of nonsedating antihistamines (e.g., loratadine [Claritin] 10 mg qd or cetirizine [Zyrtec] 10 mg qd) is preferred over first-generation antihistamines (e.g., hydroxyzine, diphenhydramine).
- Doxepin (a tricyclic antidepressant) that blocks both H_1 and H_2 receptors 25 to 75 mg qhs may be effective in patients with chronic urticaria.
- Oral corticosteroids should be reserved for refractory cases (e.g., prednisone 20 mg qd or 20 mg bid).
- H_2 receptor antagonists (cimetidine, ranitidine, famotidine) can be added to H_1 antagonists in refractory cases.

CHRONIC Rx

- Use of nonsedating antihistamines, doxepin, and/or oral corticosteroids (see "Acute General Rx")
- Low dose of the immunosuppressant cyclosporine (2.5 to 3 mg/kg body weight/day) has been shown to be effective and corticosteroid sparing in chronic urticaria
- There is insufficient data to support use of leukotriene antagonists (zafirlukast, montelukast) in patients with chronic urticaria

DISPOSITION

- Most cases of urticaria resolve within 6 wk.
- Only 25% of patients with a history of chronic urticaria are completely cured after 5 yr.

PEARLS & CONSIDERATIONS

COMMENTS

Local treatment (e.g., starch baths or Aveeno baths) may be helpful in selected patients; however, local treatment is generally not rewarding.

SUGGESTED READINGS

Kaplan AP: Chronic urticaria and angioedema, *N Engl J Med* 346:157, 2002.
Muller BA: Urticaria and angioedema: A practical approach, *Am Fam Physician* 69:1123, 2004.

AUTHOR: **FRED F. FERRI, M.D.**

BASIC INFORMATION

DEFINITION

Uterine malignancy includes tumors from the endometrium (discussed elsewhere in this text) and sarcomas. Uterine sarcoma is an abnormal proliferation of cells originating from the mesenchymal, or connective tissue, elements of the uterine wall.

SYNONYMS

Leiomyosarcomas
Endometrial stromal sarcoma
Malignant mixed müllerian tumors
Adenosarcomas

ICD-9CM CODES
182.0 Malignant neoplasm of body of uterus (corpus uteri), except isthmus
182.1 Malignant neoplasm of body of uterus, isthmus
182.8 Malignant neoplasm of body of uterus, other specified sites of body of uterus

EPIDEMIOLOGY & DEMOGRAPHICS

INCIDENCE: 17.1 cases/1 million females. Endometrial cancer remains the most common gynecological malignancy in the U.S.

PREVALENCE: Uterine sarcoma accounts for 4.3% of all cancers of the uterine corpus and is the most lethal gynecologic malignancy.

MEAN AGE AT DIAGNOSIS: The age at diagnosis is variable. Mean age at diagnosis is 52 yr.

RISK FACTORS: Similar to endometrial carcinoma

PHYSICAL FINDINGS & CLINICAL PRESENTATION

- Abnormal vaginal bleeding is the most common symptom
- May also present as pelvic pain or pressure and pelvic mass on examination
- May appear as tumor protruding through the cervix
- Vaginal discharge may also be a presenting symptom
- Rapidly enlarging uterus

ETIOLOGY

- The exact etiology is unknown.
- Prior pelvic radiation is a risk factor for sarcoma.
- Black women may be at higher risk.

DIAGNOSIS

DIFFERENTIAL DIAGNOSIS

Leiomyoma

WORKUP

Diagnosis is made histologically by biopsy for abnormal bleeding.

LABORATORY TESTS

Chest radiography, CT scans, and MRI are used to evaluate spread.

IMAGING STUDIES

- Chest radiography is usually done as routine preoperative testing.
- CT scans and MRI are good for assessing tumor spread once diagnosis is made.

TREATMENT

NONPHARMACOLOGIC THERAPY

- Surgical excision is the mainstay of treatment.
- Grade and stage of tumor affect prognosis (Fig. 1-285).
- The benefit of adjuvant radiotherapy in stage I endometrial adenocarcinoma to improve pelvic disease control and improve survival remains controversial despite several phase 3 trials.
- Chemotherapeutic agents have produced only partial and short-term responses.

DISPOSITION

- Survival varies with each type of sarcoma but is generally very poor.
- Five-year survival for leiomyosarcoma ranges from 48% for stage I to 0% for stage IV.
- Five-year survival for malignant mixed mesodermal tumor ranges from 36% for stage I to 6% for stage IV.

REFERRAL

Uterine sarcoma should be managed by a gynecologic oncologist and radiation oncologist.

SUGGESTED READINGS

Elima Y et al: Para-aortic lymph node metastasis in relation to serum CA 125 levels and nuclear grade in endometrial carcinoma, *Acta Obstet Gynecol Scond* 81(5):458, 2002.
Lee CM et al: Frequency and effect of adjuvant radiation therapy among women with Stage I endometrial adenocarcinoma, *JAMA* 295:389, 2006.
Pitsm G et al: Stage II endometrial carcinoma: prognostic factors and risk classification in 170 patients, *Intern J Radiat Oncol Biol Physics* 53(4):862, 2002.

AUTHORS: **GIL FARKASH, M.D.,** and **RUBEN ALVERO, M.D.**

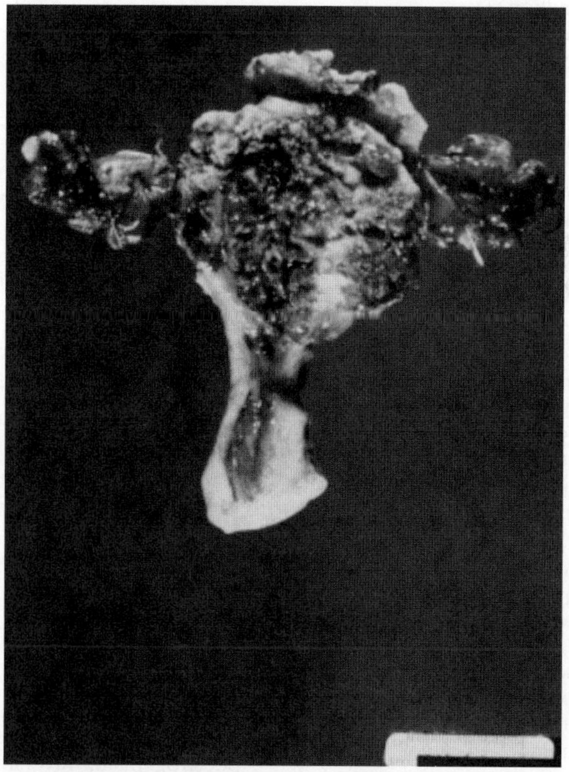

FIGURE 1-285 This grade 3 adenocarcinoma demonstrates extensive myometrial invasion. The tumor has penetrated the uterine serosa and extends onto the fundus and into the upper left broad ligament. (From Copeland LJ: *Textbook of gynecology,* ed 2, Philadelphia, 2000, WB Saunders.)

BASIC INFORMATION

DEFINITION

Uterine myomas are benign tumors of muscle cell origin. They are discrete nodular tumors that vary in size and number and that may be found as subserosal, intramucosal, or submucosal masses within the uterus or may be found in the cervix or broad ligament or on a pedicle.

SYNONYMS

Leiomyomas, fibroids

ICD-9CM CODES
218.9 Leiomyomas, fibroids

EPIDEMIOLOGY & DEMOGRAPHICS

- Estimated presence in at least 20% of all reproductive age women
- The most common benign uterine tumor
- More common in black than in white women
- Asymptomatic fibroids may be present in 40% to 50% of women >40 yr of age
- May occur singly but are often multiple
- Fewer than half of all fibroids are estimated to produce symptoms
- Frequently diagnosed incidentally on pelvic examination
- There is increased familial incidence
- Potential to enlarge during pregnancy, as well as to regress after menopause
- Infrequent primary cause of infertility in <3% of infertile patients
- Symptomatic myomas are the primary indication for approximately 30% of all hysterectomies.

PHYSICAL FINDINGS & CLINICAL PRESENTATION

- Enlarged, irregular uterus on pelvic examination.
- Presenting symptoms:
  1. Menorrhagia (most common)
  2. Chronic pelvic pain (dysmenorrhea, dyspareunia, pelvic pressure)
  3. Acute pain (torsion of pedunculated myoma, infarction, and degeneration)
  4. Urinary symptoms (frequency from bladder pressure, partial ureteral obstruction, complete ureteral obstruction)
  5. Rectosigmoid compression with constipation or intestinal obstruction
  6. Prolapse through cervix of pedunculated submucosal tumor
  7. Venous stasis of lower extremities
  8. Polycythemia
  9. Ascites

ETIOLOGY

Incompletely understood. It is suggested that myomas arise from an original single smooth muscle cell in the myometrium. Each individual myoma is monoclonal. All the cells are derived from one progenitor myocyte. Malignant degeneration of preexisting leiomyoma is extremely uncommon (<0.5%).

DIAGNOSIS

DIFFERENTIAL DIAGNOSIS

Leiomyosarcoma, ovarian mass (neoplastic, nonneoplastic, endometrioma), inflammatory mass, pregnancy

WORKUP

- Complete pelvic examination, rectovaginal examination, Pap test
- Estimation of size of mass in centimeters
- Endometrial sampling may be indicated (biopsy or D&C) when abnormal bleeding and pelvic mass are present
- If urinary symptoms are prominent, cystometry, cystoscopy to rule out bladder lesions, IVP to rule out impingement on urinary system

LABORATORY TESTS

- Pregnancy test
- Pap smear
- CBC, ESR
- Fecal occult blood

IMAGING STUDIES

- Pelvic ultrasound (transvaginal may have higher diagnostic accuracy) is useful.
- CT scan is helpful in planning treatment if malignancy is strongly suspected.
- Hysteroscopy may provide direct evidence of intrauterine pathology or submucosal leiomyoma that distorts uterine cavity.

TREATMENT

Management should be based on primary symptoms and may include observation with close follow-up, temporizing surgical therapies, medical management, or definitive surgical procedures.

NONSURGICAL Rx

- Patient observation and follow-up with periodic repeat pelvic examinations to ensure that tumors are not growing rapidly.
- GnRH agonist use results in 40% to 60% reduction in uterine volume. Hypoestrogenism, reversible bone loss, hot flushes associated with use. Limit to short-term use and consider low-dose hormonal replacement to minimize hypoestrogenic effects.
- Regrowth occurs in about 50% of women treated a few months after cessation.
- Indications for GnRH:
  1. Fertility preservation in women with large myomas before attempting conception or preoperative myectomy treatment
  2. Anemia treatment to normalize hemoglobin before surgery
  3. Women approaching menopause to avoid surgery
  4. Preoperative for large myomas to make vaginal hysterectomy, hysteroscopic resection/ablation, or laparoscopic destruction more feasible
  5. Women with medical contraindications for surgery
  6. Personal or medical indications for delaying surgery
- Progestational agents may also result in decrease in uterine size and amenorrhea, allowing iron therapy to treat anemia with limited success.
- Other drugs used and under investigation:
  1. Danazol: androgen and multienzyme inhibitor of steroidogenesis.
  2. Mifepristone: antiprogestogen, shown to reduce the fibroid volume of 40% to 50% with amenorrhea.
  3. Raloxifene: SERM, either alone or with a GnRHa, shown to reduce the fibroid volume 70% up to 1 yr but only in postmenopausal women.
  4. Fadrozole: aromatase inhibitor, reported to have produced a 71% reduction in volume.

SURGICAL Rx

- Indications
  1. Abnormal uterine bleeding with anemia, refractory to hormonal therapy
  2. Chronic pain with severe dysmenorrhea, dyspareunia, or lower abdominal pressure/pain
  3. Acute pain, torsion, or prolapsing submucosal fibroid
  4. Urinary symptoms or signs such as hydronephrosis
  5. Rapid uterine enlargement premenopausal or any growth after menopause
  6. Infertility or recurrent pregnancy loss with leiomyoma as only finding
  7. Enlarged uterus with compression symptoms or discomfort
- Procedures
  1. Hysterectomy (definitive procedure)
  2. Abdominal myomectomy (to preserve fertility)
  3. Vaginal myomectomy for prolapsed pedunculated submucous fibroid
  4. Hysteroscopic resection
  5. Laparoscopic myomectomy
  6. Uterine artery embolization

COMPLICATIONS
- Red degeneration
- Leiomyosarcoma (<0.1%)

REFERRAL

Consultation with gynecologic oncologist if suspicion of malignancy

EVIDENCE

EBM

Two small randomized controlled trials (RCTs), one comparing ibuprofen with placebo and the other comparing naproxen with placebo in women with menorrhagia and fibroids, found no significant difference in blood loss between the nonsteroidal antiinflammatory studied and placebo.[1,2] Ⓐ

One systematic review, studying women with menorrhagia, found that nonsteroidal anti-inflammatories including mefenamic acid, naproxen, ibuprofen, and diclofenac and meclofenamic acid all significantly reduced mean menstrual blood loss compared with placebo. This review studied women with menorrhagia rather than fibroids.[3] Ⓐ

We are unable to cite any evidence that meets our criteria concerning the use of danazol in women with fibroids. Two systematic reviews found that danazol significantly improved menstrual loss vs. placebo in women suffering from menorrhagia (but not specifically with associated fibroids). Authors of one review add that the use of danazol may be limited by its side effect profile.[3,4] Ⓐ

We are also unable to cite any evidence that meets our criteria concerning the treatment of women with fibroids with progestogens. One systematic review found that luteal-phase progestogens were significantly worse at reducing menstrual loss compared with danazol, tranexamic acid, and progesterone-releasing intrauterine devices in women with menorrhagia (not specifically with associated fibroids).[5] Ⓐ

Also an RCT included in a systematic review found no significant difference in reduction in menstrual blood loss between oral norethisterone (21 days/cycle) vs. levonorgestrel-releasing intrauterine device in women with menorrhagia, again not specifically with associated fibroids.[5] Ⓐ

A systematic review of pretreatment with gonadotropin-releasing hormone analogs, 3 to 4 months before uterine fibroid surgery, showed a reduction in tumor size and greater ease of surgery, as well as significant improvement in preoperative and postoperative hemoglobin and hematocrit.[6] Ⓐ

There is limited evidence from one RCT to suggest that laparoscopically assisted vaginal hysterectomy is associated with shorter recovery times and less postoperative pain than total abdominal hysterectomy for fibroids.[7] Ⓐ

One RCT comparing thermal balloon ablation with rollerball endometrial ablation in women pretreated with 2 months of gondarelin analogues found no significant difference in hysterectomy or amenorrhea rates, bleeding, or hemoglobin at 1 year, although operating time was reduced in the thermal balloon group.[8] Ⓐ

Limited evidence from two RCTs suggest there is less postoperative pain and fever, a smaller drop in hemoglobin, and shorter recovery times associated with laparoscopic myomectomy than with abdominal myomectomy for fibroids.[9,10] Ⓐ

We were unable to find any RCTs concerning the use of uterine artery embolization. However, guidelines advise that it is generally safe in appropriately selected patients.[11] Ⓒ

Evidence-Based References

1. Ylikorkala O, Pekonen F: Naproxen reduces idiopathic but not fibromyoma-induced menorrhagia, *Obstet Gynecol* 68:10, 1986. Reviewed in: *Clin Evid* 10:2092, 2003. Ⓐ
2. Makarainen L, Ylikorkala O: Primary and myoma-associated menorrhagia: role of prostaglandins and effects of ibuprofen, *Br J Obstet Gynecol* 93:974, 1986. Reviewed in: *Clin Evid* 10:2092, 2003. Ⓐ
3. Working Party of the National Health Committee New Zealand: Guidelines for the management of heavy menstrual bleeding, Wellington, 1998, Ministry of Health. Reviewed in: *Clin Evid* 10:2151, 2003. Ⓐ
4. Beaumont H et al: Danazol for heavy menstrual bleeding, *Cochrane Database Syst Rev* 2, 2002 (Cochrane Review). Ⓐ
5. Letharby A, Irvine G, Cameron I: Cyclical progestogens for heavy menstrual bleeding (Cochrane review). Reviewed in: Cochrane Library 1, Chichester, UK, 2004, John Wiley. Ⓐ
6. Lethaby A, Vollenhoven B, Sowter M: Preoperative GnRH analogue therapy before hysterectomy or myomectomy for uterine fibroids (Cochrane Review). Reviewed in: Cochrane Library 1, Chichester, UK, 2004, John Wiley. Ⓐ
7. Ferrari MM et al: Identifying the indications for laparoscopically assisted vaginal hysterectomy: a prospective, randomised comparison with abdominal hysterectomy in patients with symptomatic uterine fibroids, *Br J Obstet Gynaecol* 107:620, 2000. Reviewed in: *Clin Evid* 10:2092, 2003. Ⓐ
8. Soysal ME, Soysal SK, Vicdan K: Thermal balloon ablation in myoma-induced menorrhagia under local anesthesia, *Gynecol Obstet Invest* 51:128, 2001. Reviewed in: *Clin Evid* 10:2092, 2003. Ⓐ
9. Mais V et al: Laparoscopic versus abdominal myomectomy: a prospective, randomized trial to evaluate benefits in early outcome, *Am J Obstet Gynecol* 174:654, 1996. Reviewed in: *Clin Evid* 10:2092, 2003. Ⓐ
10. Seracchioli R et al: Fertility and obstetric outcome after laparoscopic myomectomy of large myomata: a randomised comparison with abdominal myomectomy, *Hum Reprod* 15:2663, 2000. Reviewed in: *Clin Evid* 10:2092, 2003. Ⓐ
11. Institute for Clinical Systems Improvement (ICSI): *Technology Assessment Report. Uterine Artery Embolization for Uterine Fibroids,* Bloomington, MN, 2003, ICSI. Ⓒ

SUGGESTED READINGS

DeWaay DJ et al: Natural history of uterine polyps and leiomyomata, *Obstet Gynecol* 100:3, 2002.

Olive DL, Lindheim SR, Pritts EA: Non-surgical management of leiomyoma, *Curr Opin Obstet Gynecol* 16(3):239, 2004.

AUTHORS: **ARUNDATHI G. PRASAD, M.D.,** and **RUBEN ALVERO, M.D.**

BASIC INFORMATION

DEFINITION

Uterine prolapse refers to the protrusion of the uterus into or out of the vaginal canal. In a *first-degree uterine prolapse,* the cervix is visible when the perineum is depressed. In a *second-degree uterine prolapse,* the uterine cervix has prolapsed through the vaginal introitus, with the fundus remaining within the pelvis proper. In a *third-degree uterine prolapse* (i.e., *complete uterine prolapse, uterine procidentia*), the entire uterus is outside the introitus.

SYNONYMS

Genital prolapse
Uterine descensus
Pelvic organ prolapse

ICD-9CM CODES
618.8 Genital prolapse
618.1 Uterine descensus
618.8 Pelvic organ prolapse

EPIDEMIOLOGY & DEMOGRAPHICS

PREVALENCE: Most prevalent in postmenopausal multiparous women.
RISK FACTORS:
- Pregnancy
- Labor
- Vaginal childbirth
- Obesity
- Chronic coughing
- Constipation
- Pelvic tumors
- Ascites
- Strenuous physical exertion
- Caucasian race

GENETICS: Increased incidence in women with spina bifida occulta.

PHYSICAL FINDINGS & CLINICAL PRESENTATION

- Pelvic pressure
- Bearing-down sensation
- Bilateral groin pain
- Sacral backache
- Coital difficulty
- Protrusion from vagina
- Spotting
- Ulceration
- Bleeding
- Examination of patient in lithotomy, sitting, and standing positions and before, during, and after a maximum Valsalva effort
- Erosion or ulceration of the cervix possible in the most dependent area of the protrusion

ETIOLOGY

- Vaginal childbirth and chronic increases in intraabdominal pressure leading to detachments, lacerations, and denervations of the vaginal support system
- Further weakening of pelvic support system by hypoestrogenic atrophy
- Some cases from congenital or inherited weaknesses within the pelvic support system
- Neonatal uterine prolapse mostly coexistent with congenital spinal defects

DIAGNOSIS

DIFFERENTIAL DIAGNOSIS

- Occasionally, elongated cervix; body of the uterus remains undescended.
- Diagnosis is based on history and physical examination. Currently there is only one genital tract prolapse classification system that has attained international acceptance & recognition, the patient pelvic organ prolapse quantification (POP-Q). See Boxes 1-16 and 1-17.

WORKUP

- If erosion or ulceration of the cervix is present, a Pap smear followed by a cervical biopsy should be performed if indicated.
- If urinary symptoms are significant, further urodynamic workup is indicated, looking for concurrent cystourethrocele, cystocele, enterocele, or rectocele.

LABORATORY TESTS

Urine culture

IMAGING STUDIES

Ultrasound if concurrent fibroids need further evaluation

TREATMENT

NONPHARMACOLOGIC THERAPY

- Prophylactic measures
  1. Diagnosis and treatment of chronic respiratory and metabolic disorders
  2. Correction of constipation
  3. Weight control, nutrition, and smoking cessation counseling
  4. Teaching of pelvic muscle exercises
- Supportive pessary therapy
  1. Ring-type pessary useful for first- or second-degree prolapse
  2. Gellhorn pessary preferred for more advanced prolapse
  3. Use of pessaries in conjunction with continuous hormone replacement therapy, unless contraindicated
  4. Perineorrhaphy under local anesthesia possibly needed to support the pessary if the vaginal outlet is very relaxed

ACUTE GENERAL Rx

- Patients who are only infrequently symptomatic: insertion of a tampon or diaphragm for temporary relief when prolonged standing is anticipated
- Neonatal uterine prolapse: simple digital reduction or the use of a small pessary

CHRONIC Rx

- Hormone replacement therapy at the time of menopause helps preserve tissue strength, maintain elasticity of the

BOX 1-16 Staging of Pelvic Organ Prolapse Based on POP-Q Examination

Stage 0	No prolapse.
Stage I	Most distal prolapse more than 1 cm above hymenal ring.
Stage II	Most distal point is 1 cm or less above hymenal ring.
Stage III	Most distal point is more than 1 cm below the hymenal ring but not further than 2 cm less the total vaginal length i.e. $> +1$ cm but $< +$ (TVL-2) cm.
Stage IV	Complete vaginal eversion.

From Pemberton J (ed): *The pelvic floor,* Philadelphia, 2002, WB Saunders.

BOX 1-17 Points of Reference for POP-Q

Point A Three cm above the hymen on anterior vaginal wall (Aa) or posterior vaginal wall (Ap). Point Aa roughly corresponds with the urethrovesical junction. These points can range from −3 cm (no prolapse) to +3 cm (maximal prolapse).
Point B The lowest extent of the segment of vagina between point A and the apex of the vagina. Unlike points A they are not fixed but will be the same as A if point A is the most protruding point. In maximal prolapse it will be the same as point C.
Point C The most distal part of the cervix or vaginal vault.
Point D The posterior fornix, which is thus omitted in women with prior hysterectomy.
Genital hiatus From midline external urethral meatus to inferior hymenal ring.
Perineal body From inferior hymenal ring to middle of anal orifice.
Vaginal length This should be measured without undue stretching of the vagina.

From Pemberton J (ed): *The pelvic floor,* Philadelphia, 2002, WB Saunders.

vagina, and promote the durability of surgical repairs.

- Gold standard for therapy is vaginal hysterectomy.
- Vaginal apex should be well suspended, but a prophylactic sacrospinous ligament fixation is not routinely required.
- If occult enterocele present, McCall culdoplasty is performed.
- If vaginal approach to hysterectomy is contraindicated, abdominal hysterectomy is performed; vaginal apex likewise well supported.
- Colpocleisis is considered for the elderly patient who is sexually inactive and is a high-risk patient from a surgical point of view; can be done rapidly under local anesthesia with mild sedation if necessary.
- For symptomatic women who desire childbearing: management with pessaries or pelvic muscle exercises is recommended; if surgical correction is required, transvaginal sacrospinous fixation is the preferred method.
- Other surgical options are sling operations and sacral cervicopexy.

DISPOSITION

If untreated, uterine prolapse progressively worsens.

REFERRAL

To a gynecologist/urologist if pessary fitting or surgical intervention is needed

PEARLS & CONSIDERATIONS

COMMENTS

Surgery contraindicated in mild or asymptomatic uterine prolapse because the patient will seldom benefit from the operation although exposed to its risks.

EVIDENCE

We are unable to cite any evidence for the effect of topical estrogens, oral estrogens, or oral estrogens plus progestogens on uterine prolapse specifically. However, there is evidence for the benefit of some of these treatments when used for other genitourinary symptoms that may be associated with prolapse.

A systematic review found that both topical and oral estrogens improved urogenital menopausal symptoms vs. placebo or no treatment.[1] Ⓐ

An RCT of 84 women treated for 24 weeks found that an estrogen ring significantly decreased menopausal dyspareunia compared with placebo.[2] Ⓐ

A systematic review concluded that estrogen creams, pessaries, tablets, and the estradiol vaginal ring appeared to be equally effective for the symptoms of vaginal atrophy.[3] Ⓐ

The benefits of hormone replacement therapy (HRT) need to be balanced against the harms associated with its use.

Unopposed estrogen significantly increases the risk of endometrial hyperplasia compared with placebo.[4] Ⓐ

The Women's Health Initiative trial, including the subgroup treated with combined estrogen and progestogen replacement therapy, was discontinued after 5.2 years' follow-up due to increased risk of invasive breast cancer, coronary events, stroke, and pulmonary embolism vs. placebo.[5] Ⓐ

A meta-analysis of four large RCTs on the effects of long-term HRT reported a relative risk of developing breast cancer of 1.27, pulmonary embolism of 2.16, and coronary heart disease of 1.11 in those receiving HRT.[6] Ⓐ

We are unable to cite any evidence for the effect of surgery on uterine prolapse. There is evidence for the benefit of surgery in symptoms of stress incontinence that could be associated with prolapse.

We are unable to cite any evidence concerning hysterectomy or the use of pessaries in the treatment of uterine prolapse.

Although there is evidence for the benefit of pelvic floor exercises in the treatment of urinary incontinence, we are unable to cite any evidence on their use for treatment of uterine prolapse specifically.

Evidence-Based References

1. Cardozo L et al: A systematic review of estrogens for recurrent urinary tract infections: third report of the hormones and urogenital therapy committee, *Int Urogynecol J Pelvic Floor Dysfunct* 12:15, 2001. Reviewed in: *Clin Evid* 12:2624, 2004. Ⓐ
2. Casper F, Petri E: Local treatment of urogenital atrophy with an estradiol-releasing vaginal ring: a comparative and a placebo-controlled multicenter study. Vaginal Ring Study Group, *Int Urogynecol J Pelvic Floor Dysfunct* 10:171, 1999. Reviewed in: *Clin Evid* 11:2459, 2004. Ⓐ
3. Suckling J, Lethaby A, Kennedy R: Local oestrogen for vaginal atrophy in postmenopausal women, *Cochrane Database Syst Rev* 4, 2003 (Cochrane Review). Ⓐ
4. Lethaby A et al: Hormone replacement therapy in postmenopausal women: endometrial hyperplasia and irregular bleeding. In: Cochrane Library 2:2004, Chichester, UK, John Wiley. Reviewed in: *Clin Evid* 11:2459, 2004. Ⓐ
5. Writing group for the Women's Health Initiative Investigators: Risk and benefits of estrogen plus progestin in healthy postmenopausal women. Principal results from the Women's Health Initiative randomized controlled trial, *JAMA* 288:321, 2002. Reviewed in: *Clin Evid* 11:1450, 2004. Ⓐ
6. Beral V, Banks E, Reeves G: Evidence from randomized controlled trials on the long-term effects of hormone replacement therapy, *Lancet* 360:942, 2002. Reviewed in: *Clin Evid* 11:2459, 2004. Ⓐ

SUGGESTED READING

Thaker R: Management of uterine prolapse, *BMJ* 324:1258, 2002.

AUTHORS: **ARUNDATHI G. PRASAD, M.D.**, and **RUBEN ALVERO, M.D.**

BASIC INFORMATION

DEFINITION

Uveitis is inflammation of the uveal tract, including the iris, ciliary body, and choroid. It may also involve other closed structures such as the sclera, retina, and vitreous humor.

SYNONYMS

Anterior uveitis
Posterior uveitis
Acute or chronic uveitis
Granulomatous or nongranulomatous uveitis
Iritis
Chroiditis
Pars planitis
Iridocyclitis

ICD-9CM CODES
364.3 Unspecified iridocyclitis, uveitis

EPIDEMIOLOGY & DEMOGRAPHICS

INCIDENCE (IN U.S.): Common; busy ophthalmologist will see two or more cases per week.
PEAK INCIDENCE: Middle age or older; uveitis in childhood rare; equal in boys and girls; 25% idiopathic and 75% related to toxoplasmosis, juvenile rheumatoid arthritis, pars planitis, toxicaris canis, or Behçet's disease
PREVALENCE (IN U.S.): 17 cases/100,000 persons
PREDOMINANT SEX: None
PREDOMINANT AGE: 38 yr

PHYSICAL FINDINGS & CLINICAL PRESENTATION

- Symptoms of uveitis depend on the site of involvement and whether process is acute or insidious:
  - Acute anterior uveitis: pain and photophobia. Vision may not be affected initially.
  - Posterior uveitis: floaters, hazy vision. Involvement of the retina may produce blind spots or flashing lights.
  - Insidious anterior uveitis: symptoms may not be present until scarring cataracts and loss of vision occur.
- Photophobia
- Blurred visual acuity
- Irregular pupil
- Hazy cornea
- Abnormal cells and flare in anterior chamber or vitreous humor
- Retinal hemorrhage, vascular sheathing
- Conjunctival injection
- Ciliary flush
- Keratitic precipitates (precipitates on the cornea)
- Hazy vitreous
- Retinal inflammation
- Iris nodules
- Glaucoma
- Rheumatoid arthritis
- Scleritis
- Systemic symptoms related to etiology

ETIOLOGY

- Infections: herpes simplex virus, cytomegalovirus, toxoplasmosis, tuberculosis, syphilis, HIV
- Systemic disorders: sarcoidosis, Behçet's syndrome, HLA-B27 associated diseases (e.g., ankylosing spondylitis, reactive arthritis), inflammatory bowel disease, juvenile idiopathic arthritis
- Idiopathic

DIAGNOSIS

DIFFERENTIAL DIAGNOSIS

- Glaucoma
- Conjunctivitis
- Retinal detachment
- Retinopathy
- Keratitis
- Scleritis
- Episcleritis
- Masquerating syndromes: lymphoma, uveal melanoma, metastases (breast, lung, renal), leukemia, retinitis pigmentosa, retinoblastoma

WORKUP

- Associated with arthritis, syphilis, tuberculosis, granulomatous disease, collagen-vascular disease, allergies, AIDS, sarcoid, Behçet's disease, histoplasmosis, toxoplasmosis, and toxicaris canis
- Slit lamp examination, indirect ophthalmoscopy

LABORATORY TESTS

- CBC
- Laboratory tests for specific inflammatory causes cited previously in "Workup" (e.g., ANA, ESR, VDRL, HLA-B27, PPD, Lyme titer)
- Visual field testing

IMAGING STUDIES

- Chest x-ray in suspected sarcoidosis, TB, histoplasmosis
- Sacroiliac x-ray in suspected ankylosing spondylitis

TREATMENT

NONPHARMACOLOGIC THERAPY

- Treat the underlying disease. Treatment is often multidisciplinary (ophthalmologist, internist, rheumatologist, ID specialist).
- Treat photophobia and local pain.

ACUTE GENERAL Rx

- Corticosteroids are the mainstay of therapy for noninfectious causes. The route of administration depends on the location of inflammation, the severity, and the presence of systemic disease. Cycloplegic drops (cyclopentolate [Cyclogyl]) or cycloplegic agents (homatropine hydrobromide [Optic] 1gtt q3 to 4h while awake) and topical steroids (prednisone acetate 1% 1 gtt qh during day, prn at night until favorable response, then q4 to 6h); avoid topical corticosteroids in infectious uveitis. Periocular corticosteroid injections can be used for posterior disease. They have the advantage of achieving high intraocular levels of steroids without the systemic side effects of oral corticosteroids.
- Antibiotics for bacterial infections and antiviral agents, when infection is suspected, should be started to prevent retinal damage.
- Systemic steroids if appropriate for the underlying disease. Systemic corticosteroid therapy is generally reserved for patients with systemic disorders and those with bilateral disease that is refractory to local medication or those with major ocular disability or retinitis.
- Antimetabolites when indicated. Immunosuppressive medications used in steroid-dependent or refractory uveitis include methotrexate, sulfasalazine, azathioprine, cyclosporine, and tacrolimus. These medications can have significant toxicity and should be prescribed only by physicians experienced with their use.

CHRONIC Rx

- Topical steroids and cycloplegics.
- Treat underlying cause.

DISPOSITION

Urgent referral to ophthalmologist for diagnosis and treatment.

REFERRAL

- Eye problem should be followed early on by an ophthalmologist.
- Underlying medical disease should be treated by the primary care physician.

PEARLS & CONSIDERATIONS

COMMENTS

- In 90% of cases, the condition is idiopathic.
- Associated causes are found approximately 10% of the time, usually chronic and recurrent.
- Chronic glaucoma, cataracts, retinal degeneration, and other severe eye problems occur with the disease and the treatment.

SUGGESTED READINGS

Hajj-Ali RA, Lowder C, Mandell BF: Uveitis in the internist's office: are a patient's eye symptoms serious? *Cleve Clin J Med* 72:329-339, 2005.

Kadayifcilar S, Eldem B, Tumer B: Uveitis in childhood, *J Pediatr Ophthalmol Strabismus* 40(6):335, 2003.

AUTHOR: **MELVYN KOBY, M.D.**

BASIC INFORMATION

DEFINITION

Bleeding per vagina at any time during pregnancy must be regarded as abnormal and is associated with an increased likelihood of pregnancy complications.

SYNONYMS

Hemorrhage

ICD-9CM CODES
634.9 Spontaneous abortion
633.9 Ectopic pregnancy
630/631 Molar pregnancy
622.7 Cervical polyps
180.9/180.0/180.8 Cervical dysplasia/cancer
616.0 Cervicitis
616.10 Vulvovaginitis
184.0 Vaginal cancer
644.2 Premature labor term labor
641.1 Placenta previa
641.2 Placental abruption

EPIDEMIOLOGY & DEMOGRAPHICS

- Common in U.S.; 20% to 25% of patients have vaginal spotting/bleeding in first trimester; of those, miscarriage occurs in 50%.
- Occurs in women of childbearing age.
- Between 1% and 2% of all pregnancies in the U.S. are ectopic.
- After one ectopic pregnancy, the chance of another is 7% to 15%.
- Ectopic pregnancy is the leading cause of maternal mortality in the first trimester.
- Average reported frequency for placental abruption is about 1 in 150 deliveries (0.3%).
- Incidence of placenta previa is <1 in 200 deliveries (0.5%).

PHYSICAL FINDINGS & CLINICAL PRESENTATION

- Bleeding: ranges from scant to life-threatening with hemodynamic instability
- Color: brown to bright red
- Can be painless or painful (cramps, back pain, severe abdominal pain)
- Fetal compromise: ranges from none to fetal demise

ETIOLOGY

- Influenced by gestational age
- Vaginal
- Cervical
- Uterine

DIAGNOSIS

DIFFERENTIAL DIAGNOSIS

- Any gestational age:
  1. Cervical lesions: polyps, decidual reaction, neoplasia
  2. Vaginal trauma
  3. Cervicitis/vulvovaginitis
  4. Postcoital trauma
  5. Bleeding dyscrasias
- Gestation <20 wk:
  1. Spontaneous abortion
  2. Presence of intrauterine device
  3. Ectopic pregnancy
  4. Molar pregnancy
  5. Implantation bleeding
  6. Low-lying placenta
- Gestation >20 wk:
  1. Molar pregnancy
  2. Placenta previa
  3. Placental abruption
  4. Vasa previa
  5. Marginal separation of the placenta
  6. Bloody show at term
  7. Preterm labor
- Section II describes the differential diagnosis of vaginal bleeding in pregnancy.

WORKUP

- Gestation <20 wk (Section III, "Bleeding, Early Pregnancy")
  1. Pelvic examination
  2. Culdocentesis
  3. Laparoscopy
  4. Laparotomy
  5. Ultrasound to verify viable intrauterine pregnancy
- Gestation >20 wk:
  1. Ultrasound to locate placenta before pelvic examination
  2. If placenta previa, no speculum or bimanual examination
  3. If preterm labor, appropriate evaluation done

LABORATORY TESTS

- Urine pregnancy test: if positive, get quantitative β human chorionic gonadotropin (hCG)
  1. Early pregnancy: follow serially every 48 hr
  2. Normal pregnancy: hCG doubles approximately every 48 hr
  3. Spontaneous abortion: hCG levels will fall
  4. Ectopic pregnancy: hCG level will rise inappropriately
  5. Molar pregnancy: hCG level is extremely high
- CBC
- Blood type and screen (Rh-negative patients need RhoGAM)
- Coagulation profile (useful in missed abortion and abruption)
- Cervical cultures/wet mount
- Pap smear for cervical malignancy; caution with biopsy, because cervix can bleed extensively

IMAGING STUDIES

Ultrasound:

- 5 to 6 wk: gestational sac (transvaginally); hCG >2500 mIU/ml (third IS) or >1000 mIU/ml (second IS)
- 8 to 9 wk: fetal cardiac activity
- Molar pregnancy: characteristic cluster of cysts
- Location of placenta
- Degree of placental separation: difficult to assess

TREATMENT

NONPHARMACOLOGIC THERAPY

- Pelvic rest: no coitus, douching, or tampons
- Bed rest, if >20 wk
- Counseling: genetic, bereavement

ACUTE GENERAL Rx

- Hemodynamic stabilization
- Emergency D&C, laparotomy, or cesarean section as necessary

CHRONIC Rx

Depends on diagnosis

DISPOSITION

Depends on diagnosis

REFERRAL

- If patient is unstable and needs emergency ob/gyn management and/or surgery
- If patient has diagnosis of ectopic or molar pregnancy, because immediate surgical treatment is indicated
- Perinatal consultation for high-risk pregnancy

EVIDENCE

Administration of anti-D immunoglobulin to Rhesus-negative women at 24 weeks and 34 weeks gestation during the first pregnancy reduces the risk of Rhesus-D alloimmunization from 1.5% to 0.2%.[1] Ⓐ

Evidence-Based Reference

1. Crowther CA: Anti-D administration in pregnancy for preventing Rhesus alloimmunization. In: Cochrane Library, 2, 2004. Chichester, UK: John Wiley. Ⓐ

SUGGESTED READING

Coppola PT, Coppola M: Vaginal bleeding in the first 20 weeks of pregnancy, *Emerg Med Clin North Am* 21(3):667, 2003.

AUTHORS: **GEORGE T. DANAKAS, M.D.,** and **RUBEN ALVERO, M.D.**

BASIC INFORMATION

DEFINITION

Vaginal malignancy is an abnormal proliferation of vaginal epithelium demonstrating malignant cells below the basement membrane.

SYNONYMS

Squamous cell carcinoma of the vagina
Adenocarcinoma of the vagina
Melanoma of the vagina
Sarcoma of the vagina
Endodermal sinus tumor

ICD-9CM CODES
184.0 Vagina, vaginal neoplasm

EPIDEMIOLOGY & DEMOGRAPHICS

INCIDENCE: 0.42 cases/100,000 persons
PREVALENCE: Vaginal cancer is the second rarest gynecologic cancer. It comprises 2% of malignancies of the female genital tract.
MEAN AGE AT DIAGNOSIS: Predominantly a disease of menopause. Mean age at diagnosis is 60 yr old.

PHYSICAL FINDINGS & CLINICAL PRESENTATION

- Majority of cases are asymptomatic
- Postmenopausal vaginal bleeding and/or vaginal discharge are the most common symptoms
- May also present as pelvic pain or pressure, dyspareunia, dysuria, malodor, or postcoital bleeding
- May present as a vaginal lesion or abnormal Pap smear

ETIOLOGY

- The exact etiology is unknown.
- Vaginal intraepithelial neoplasia is thought to be a precursor for squamous cell carcinoma of the vagina.
- Chronic pessary use has been associated with vaginal malignancy.
- Prior pelvic radiation may be a risk factor.
- Clear-cell adenocarcinoma is related to in utero diethylstilbestrol exposure.

DIAGNOSIS

DIFFERENTIAL DIAGNOSIS

- Extension from other primary carcinoma more common than primary vaginal cancer
- Vaginitis

WORKUP

- Diagnosis is made histologically by biopsy.
- Colposcopy and biopsy should follow suspicious Pap smear.
- Cystoscopy, proctosigmoidoscopy, chest radiography, IV urography, and barium enema may be used for clinical staging.
- CT scan and MRI are being used to evaluate spread.
- Staging I to IV (Fig. 1-286).

IMAGING STUDIES

- Chest radiography, IV urography, and barium enema are used for staging.
- CT scan and MRI are good for assessing tumor spread.

TREATMENT

NONPHARMACOLOGIC THERAPY

- Radiation therapy is the mainstay of treatment.
- Stage I tumors that are small and confined to the posterior, upper third of the vagina may be treated with radical surgery.
- Other stages require a whole-pelvis, interstitial, and/or intracavitary radiation therapy.
- Chemotherapy is used in conjunction with radiotherapy in rare select cases.

DISPOSITION

Five-year survival ranges from 80% for stage I to 17% for stage IV.

REFERRAL

Vaginal cancer should be managed by a gynecologic oncologist and radiation oncologist.

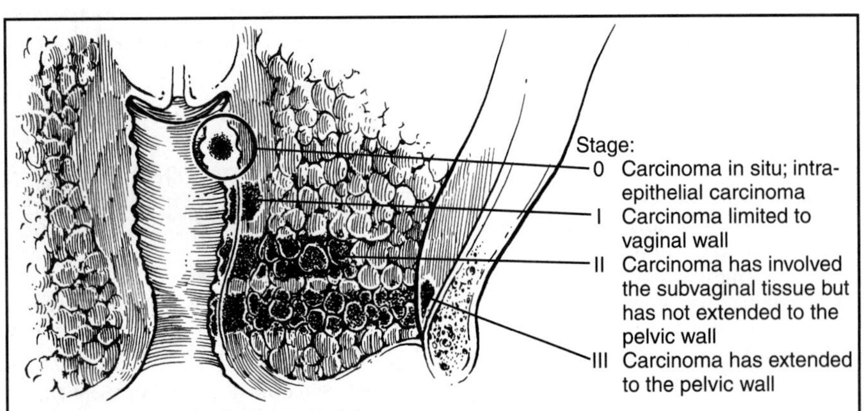

FIGURE 1-286 Staging system for vaginal cancer. Metastatic disease that involves the bladder or rectum is stage IV-a. Metastatic disease beyond the pelvis is stage IV-b. (From Copeland LJ: *Textbook of gynecology,* ed 2, Philadelphia, 2000, WB Saunders.)

EVIDENCE

A retrospective review of 121 women with vaginal intraepithelial neoplasia (VAIN) found recurrence rates following partial vaginectomy, laser, and 5-fluorouracil of 0, 38, and 59%, respectively, after at least 7 months' follow-up.[1] Ⓑ

A retrospective review of 71 patients with primary vaginal carcinoma treated with interstitial iridium-192 with or without external beam radiotherapy found that interstitial irradiation resulted in local control in the majority of patients with primary vaginal carcinoma with acceptable morbidity.[2] Ⓑ

A retrospective review of 84 patients with primary invasive vaginal cancer managed at one institution over a 25-year period found that patients with stage I and II squamous cell vaginal carcinoma managed by initial surgery followed by selective radiotherapy had good outcomes in terms of survival and local tumor control.[3] Ⓑ

Evidence-Based References

1. Dodge JA et al: Clinical features and risk of recurrence among patients with vaginal intraepithelial neoplasia, *Gynecol Oncol* 83:363, 2001. Ⓑ
2. Tewari KS et al: Primary invasive carcinoma of the vagina: treatment with interstitial brachytherapy, *Cancer* 91:758, 2001. Ⓑ
3. Tjalma WA et al: The role of surgery in invasive squamous carcinoma of the vagina, *Gynecol Oncol* 81:360, 2001. Ⓑ

SUGGESTED READING

Kim H et al: Case report: magnetic resonance imaging of vaginal malignant melanoma, *J Comput Assist Tomogr* 27(3):357, 2003.

AUTHORS: **GIL FARKASH, M.D.,** and **RUBEN ALVERO, M.D.**

BASIC INFORMATION

DEFINITION

Vaginismus refers to the involuntary spasm of the vaginal, introital, and/or levator ani muscles, preventing penetration or causing painful intercourse.

ICD-9CM CODES
300.11 Hysterical vaginismus
306.51 Psychogenic or functional vaginismus
625.1 Reflex vaginismus

EPIDEMIOLOGY & DEMOGRAPHICS

INCIDENCE: Estimated at about 11.7% to 42% of women presenting to sexual dysfunction clinics

PREVALENCE: Affects approximately 1:200 women

PREDOMINANT SEX: Affects only females

RISK FACTORS: Any previous sexual trauma, including incest or rape

PHYSICAL FINDINGS & CLINICAL PRESENTATION

- Fear of pain with coitus
- Dyspareunia
- Orgasmic dysfunction

ETIOLOGY

- Learned conditioned response to real or imagined painful vaginal experience (e.g., traumatic speculum examination, incest, rape)
- Vaginitis
- PID
- Endometriosis
- Anatomic anomalies
- Atrophic vaginitis
- Mucosal tears
- Inadequate lubrication
- Focal vulvitis
- Painful hymenal tags
- Scarring secondary to episiotomy
- Skin disorders
- Topical allergies
- Postherpetic neuralgia

DIAGNOSIS

WORKUP

- Thorough history (including sexual history)
- Careful pelvic examination
- Behavioral therapy

TREATMENT

NONPHARMACOLOGIC THERAPY

- Deconditioning the response by systematic self-administered progressive dilation techniques using fingers or dilators
- Behavioral and/or psychosexual therapy

ACUTE GENERAL Rx

- Botulinum toxin therapy given locally has been shown to relieve the perineal muscle spasms associated with vaginismus, allowing resumption of intercourse.
  1. Acts by preventing neuromuscular transmission, causing muscle weakness
  2. Considered experimental treatment for vaginismus at this time
- Cause should be determined by history and explained to the patient so that she understands the mechanics of the muscle spasms.
- Patient must be motivated to desire painless vaginal insertion for such reasons as pleasurable coitus, tampon insertion, or gynecologic examination.
- Patient (and her partner) must be willing to patiently undergo the process of systematic desensitization and counseling.

DISPOSITION

A high percentage of successfully treated patients

REFERRAL

To a gynecologist or sex therapist

PEARLS & CONSIDERATIONS

COMMENTS

- May uncover early sexual abuse or an aversion to sexuality in general.
- To American Association of Sex Educators, Counselors and Therapists, 11 Dupont Circle, NW, Washington, DC, 20036.
- To Sex Information and Education Council of the U.S. (SIECUS), 85th Avenue, New York, NY 10022.

SUGGESTED READINGS

Heim LJ: Evaluation and differential diagnosis of dyspareunia, *Am Fam Physician* 63(8): 1535, 2001.
McGuire H, Hawton K: Interventions for vaginismus, [update of Cochrane Database Syst Rev 2:CD001760, 2001], 1:CD001760, 2003.

AUTHORS: **BETH J. WUTZ, M.D.,** and **RUBEN ALVERO, M.D.**

BASIC INFORMATION

DEFINITION

Bacterial vaginosis (BV) is a thin, gray, homogenous, malodorous vaginal discharge that results from a shift in the vaginal flora from a predominance of lactobacilli to high concentrations of anaerobic bacteria.

SYNONYMS

Before 1955: nonspecific vaginitis
1955: *Haemophilus vaginalis* vaginitis
1963: *Corynebacterium vaginalis* vaginitis
1980: *Gardnerella vaginalis* vaginitis
1990: Bacterial vaginosis

ICD-9CM CODES
616.10 Vaginitis, bacterial

EPIDEMIOLOGY & DEMOGRAPHICS

- Most common vaginal infection
- *Gardnerella, Mycoplasma,* and *Mobiluncus* are harbored in the urethra of male partners; however,
  1. Male partners are asymptomatic.
  2. There is no improved cure rate or lower reinfection rate if the infected patient's male partner is treated.
  3. Abstinence from intercourse or condom use while the patient completes her treatment regimen may improve cure rates and lessen recurrences.

PHYSICAL FINDINGS & CLINICAL PRESENTATION

- 50% of patients are asymptomatic
- A thin, dark, or dull gray homogenous discharge that adheres to the vaginal walls
- An offensive, "fishy" odor that is accentuated after intercourse or menses
- Pruritus (only in 13%)

ETIOLOGY

- *Gardnerella vaginalis* is detected in 40% to 50% of vaginal secretions.
  1. Increase in vaginal pH caused by decrease in hydrogen peroxide–producing lactobacilli
  2. Anaerobes predominate and produce amines
- Amines, when alkalinized by semen, menstrual blood, the use of alkaline douches, or the addition of 10% KOH, volatilize and cause the unpleasant "fishy" odor.
- In BV:
  1. *Bacteroides* (anaerobes) species are increased 1000× the usual concentration.
  2. *G. vaginalis* are 100× normal.
  3. *Peptostreptococcus* are 10× normal.
  4. *Mycoplasma hominis* and Enterobacteriacea members are present in increased concentrations.

DIAGNOSIS

WORKUP

Seattle Group Criteria:
- Detecting three of the four following signs will diagnose 90% correctly, with <10% false positives:
  1. Thin, gray, homogenous, malodorous discharge that adheres to the vaginal walls
  2. Elevated pH >4.5
  3. Positive KOH whiff test
  4. Clue cells present on wet mount
- Cultures are unnecessary.
- Pap smear will not identify *G. vaginalis.*
- Gram stain of vaginal secretions will reveal clue cells and abnormal mixed bacteria (Fig. 1-287).

TREATMENT

ACUTE GENERAL Rx

RECOMMENDED REGIMENS (EQUAL EFFICACY):
1. Metronidazole 500 mg PO bid for 7 days
2. 0.75% metronidazole gel in vagina bid for 5 days
3. 2% clindamycin cream qd for 7 days

ALTERNATE REGIMENS (LOWER EFFICACY FOR BV):
1. Clindamycin ovules 100 g intravaginally qhs for 3 days
2. Clindamycin 300 mg PO bid for 7 days (increased incidence of diarrhea)
3. Metronidazole ER 750 mg PO qd for 7 days
4. Metronidazole 2 g PO single dose (higher relapse rate)

Patients should be advised to avoid alcohol while taking metronidazole and for 24 hr thereafter.

TREATMENT IN PREGNANCY:
All pregnant patients proven to have BV should be treated because of its association with preterm labor, chorioamnionitis, and PROM.

RECOMMENDED REGIMENS:
1. Metronidazole 250 mg PO tid for 7 days
2. Clindamycin 300 mg PO bid for 7 days
- Existing data do not support the use of topical agents during pregnancy.
- Multiple studies and meta-analysis have not demonstrated associations between metronidazole use during pregnancy and teratogenic effects in newborns.

RECURRENT BV:
- Condom use may help reduce the risk of recurrence.
- Concurrent treatment of male partner is controversial. Consider treating the male partner if there is recurrent vaginitis or any suspicion of associated upper genital tract infection.

PEARLS & CONSIDERATIONS

- Bacterial vaginosis has been associated with PID, cystitis, posthysterectomy vaginal cuff cellulitis, postabortal infection, preterm delivery, premature rupture of membranes (PROM), amnionitis, chorioamnionitis, and postpartum endometritis. New evidence also shows BV increases women's risk of acquiring HIV.
- Higher cumulative cure rates have been found at 3 to 4 weeks for a 7-day regimen of metronidazole (500 mg twice daily) than with a single dose (2 g).

EVIDENCE

See Section I, "Vulvovaginitis, Bacterial."

SUGGESTED READING

Mitchell H: Vaginal discharge-causes, diagnosis, and treatment, *BMJ* 328(7451):1306, 2004.

AUTHORS: **ARUNDATHI G. PRASAD, M.D.,** and **RUBEN ALVERO, M.D.**

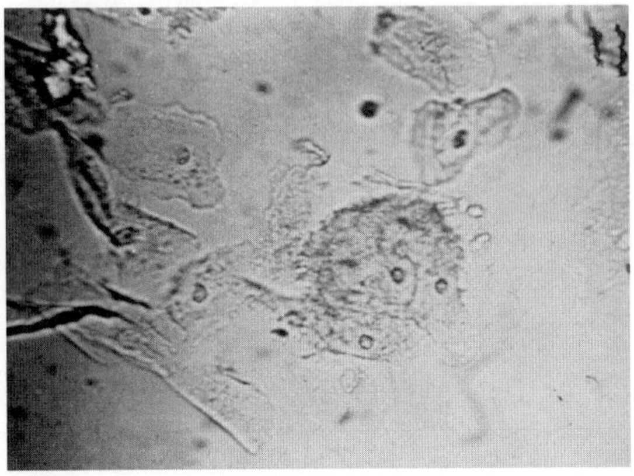

FIGURE 1-287 Clue cells characteristic of bacterial vaginosis, squamous epithelial cells whose borders are obscured by bacteria. (From Carlson K [ed]: *Primary care of women,* St Louis, 1995, Mosby.)

BASIC INFORMATION

DEFINITION

Varicella is a common viral illness characterized by acute onset of generalized vesicular rash and fever.

SYNONYMS

Chickenpox

ICD-9CM CODES
052.9 Varicella

EPIDEMIOLOGY & DEMOGRAPHICS

- Varicella is extremely contagious. More than 90% of unvaccinated contacts become infected.
- The incubation period of chickenpox ranges from 9 to 21 days.
- Peak incidence is in the springtime.
- The predominant age is 5 to 10 yr.
- Infectious period begins 2 days before onset of clinical symptoms and lasts until all lesions have crusted.
- Most patients will have lifelong immunity following an attack of chickenpox; protection from chickenpox following varicella vaccine is approximately 6 yr.

PHYSICAL FINDINGS & CLINICAL PRESENTATION

- Findings vary with the clinical course. Initial symptoms consist of fever, chills, backache, generalized malaise, and headache.
- Symptoms are generally more severe in adults.
- Initial lesions generally occur on the trunk (centripetal distribution) and occasionally on the face; these lesions consist primarily of 3- to 4-mm red papules with an irregular outline and a clear vesicle on the surface (dew drops on a rose petal appearance).
- Intense pruritus generally accompanies this stage.
- New lesion development generally ceases by the fourth day with subsequent crusting by the sixth day.
- Lesions generally spread to the face and the extremities (centrifugal spread).
- Patients generally present with lesions at different stages at the same time.
- Crusts generally fall off within 5 to 14 days.
- Fever is usually highest during the eruption of the vesicles; temperature generally returns to normal following disappearance of vesicles.
- Signs of potential complications (e.g., bacterial skin infections, neurologic complications, pneumonia, hepatitis) may be present on physical examination.
- Mild constitutional symptoms (e.g., anorexia, myalgias, headaches, restlessness) may be present (most common in adults).
- Excoriations may be present if scratching is prominent.

ETIOLOGY

Varicella-zoster virus (VZV) is a human herpes virus III that can manifest with either varicella or herpes zoster (i.e., shingles, which is a reactivation of varicella).

DIAGNOSIS

DIFFERENTIAL DIAGNOSIS

- Other viral infection
- Impetigo
- Scabies
- Drug rash
- Urticaria
- Dermatitis herpetiformis
- Smallpox

WORKUP

Diagnosis is usually made based on patient's history and clinical presentation.

LABORATORY TESTS

- Laboratory evaluation is generally not necessary.
- CBC may reveal leukopenia and thrombocytopenia.
- Serum varicella titers (significant rise in serum varicella IgG antibody level), skin biopsy, or Tzanck smear are used only when diagnosis is in question.

TREATMENT

NONPHARMACOLOGIC THERAPY

- Use antipruritic lotions for symptomatic relief.
- Avoid scratching to prevent excoriations and superficial skin infections.
- Use a mild soap for bathing; hands should be washed often.

ACUTE GENERAL Rx

- Use acetaminophen for fever and myalgias; aspirin should be avoided because of the increased risk of Reye's syndrome.
- Oral acyclovir (20 mg/kg qid for 5 days) initiated at the earliest sign (within 24 hr of illness) is useful in healthy, nonpregnant individuals 13 yr of age or older to decrease the duration and severity of signs and symptoms. Immunocompromised hosts should be treated with IV acyclovir 500 mg/m^2 or 10 mg/kg q8h IV for 7 to 10 days.
- Varicella is most contagious from 2 days before to a few days after the onset of the rash. Varicella vaccine is available for children and adults; protection lasts at least 6 yr. Healthy, nonimmune adults and children exposed to varicella-zoster virus should receive prophylaxis with live attenuated varicella vaccine (Varivax). Patients with HIV or other immunocompromised patients should not receive the live attenuated vaccine.
- Exposed patients with contraindications to varicella vaccine can be treated with varicella-zoster immunoglobulin (VariZIG). It is effective in preventing varicella in susceptible individuals. Dose is 12.5 U/kg IM (up to a maximum of 625 U). VZIG must be administered as early as possible after presumed exposure (within 4 days). If VariZIG cannot be obtained and administered within 4 days, providers should consider the use of intravenous immune globulin (IVIG) within 4 days of exposure.
- Pruritus from chickenpox can be controlled with antihistamines (e.g., hydroxyzine 25 mg q6h) and oral antipruritic lotions (e.g., calamine).
- Oral antibiotics are not routinely indicated and should be used only in patients with secondary infection and infected lesions (most common infective organisms are *Streptococcus* sp. and *Staphylococcus* sp.).

DISPOSITION

- The course is generally benign in immunocompetent adults and children.
- Infants who develop chickenpox are incapable of controlling the infection and should be given varicella-zoster immunoglobulin or γ-globulin if VZIG is not available.

PEARLS & CONSIDERATIONS

COMMENTS

- VZIG can be obtained from the nearest regional Red Cross Blood Center or the Centers for Disease Control and Prevention in Atlanta, Georgia.
- Varicella immunization is recommended for all who have not had chickenpox; dosage for adults and adolescents (>13 yr old) is two 0.5-ml doses 4 to 8 wk apart.

EVIDENCE

There is evidence that oral acyclovir reduces the symptoms of chickenpox in otherwise healthy people if started early, but its clinical importance in this area remains controversial.

The reviewers note that the clinical importance of acyclovir in otherwise healthy children remains controversial.[1] Ⓐ

Evidence-Based Reference

1. Klassen TP et al: Acyclovir for treating varicella in otherwise healthy children and adolescents, *Cochrane Database Syst Rev* 2:CD002980, 2004. Ⓐ

AUTHOR: **FRED F. FERRI, M.D.**

BASIC INFORMATION

DEFINITION

Varicose veins are dilated networks of the subcutaneous venous system that result from valvular incompetence.

SYNONYMS

Chronic venous insufficiency
Stasis skin changes

ICD-9CM CODES
454.9 Varicose veins

EPIDEMIOLOGY & DEMOGRAPHICS

PREVALENCE:
- Approximately 30% of adults, with increasing incidence with age
- Increased incidence during pregnancy, especially with advanced maternal age

PREDOMINANT SEX: Female > male

GENETICS:
- Familial tendency
- Evidence for dominant, recessive, and multifactorial types of inheritance

RISK FACTORS:
- Advancing age
- Prolonged standing
- Pregnancy
- Obesity
- Use of oral contraceptives

PHYSICAL FINDINGS & CLINICAL PRESENTATION

- Visible tortuous veins in the territory of either the long saphenous vein (most common), short saphenous vein, or both
- Dull ache, burning, or cramping in leg muscles
- Worsening discomfort with standing, warm temperatures, or menses
- Blowouts-localized dilatations
- Tortuous dilation of superficial veins
- Dermatitis, hyper/hypopigmentation, edema, eczema
- Varicose ulcer, sometimes with superficial infection

ETIOLOGY

- Normally, blood flow directed from the superficial venous system to the deep venous system via communication of perforating vessels
- Best thought of as "venous hypertension"
- Valvular incompetence in perforator veins of lower extremity leading to reverse flow of fluid from high-pressure deep venous system to low-pressure superficial venous system, resulting in dilation of superficial veins, leg edema, and pain
- Rarely associated with deep vein thrombophlebitis
- Exacerbated by restrictive clothing

DIAGNOSIS

DIFFERENTIAL DIAGNOSIS

Conditions that can lead to superficial venous stasis other than primary valvular insufficiency include:
- Arterial occlusive disease
- Diabetes
- Deep vein thrombophlebitis
- Peripheral neuropathies
- Unusual infections
- Carcinoma

WORKUP

- Mainly a clinical diagnosis—Trendelenburg test
- Arterial studies to rule out arterial insufficiency before initiating therapy for venous insufficiency

LABORATORY TESTS

Not useful

IMAGING STUDIES

Duplex ultrasound
- Gold standard for evaluation of varicose veins
- Quantitation of flow through venous valves under direct visualization
- Allows precise anatomic identification of source of venous reflux
- Rarely ascending venography and varicography for unusually located varices and recurrence after surgical treatment.

TREATMENT

NONPHARMACOLOGIC THERAPY

- Leg elevation and rest
- Graded compression stockings: used early in morning before edema accumulates and removed before going to bed
- Weight loss
- Avoidance of occlusive clothing

ACUTE GENERAL Rx

- For associated stasis dermatitis: topical corticosteroids
- Treatment of secondary infection with appropriate antibiotics

CHRONIC Rx

- Compression sclerotherapy: injection of 1% to 3% solution of sodium tetradecyl sulfate or 5% ethanolamine oleate
- Surgery: indications include the following:
  1. Persistent varicosities with conservative treatment
  2. Failed sclerotherapy
  3. Previous or impending bleeding from ulcerated varicosities
  4. Disabling pain
  5. Cosmetic concerns
- Surgical methods include (must be combined with compressive therapy):
  1. Saphenous vein ligation
  2. Ligation of incompetent perforating veins
  3. Saphenous vein stripping with or without avulsion of varicosities
  4. Ambulatory "miniphlebectomies": avulsion of superficial varicosities with saphenous vein stripping
  5. New treatments: endovenous obliteration using radiofrequency (diathermy) or laser as an alternative to traditional stripping of the long saphenous vein and powered phlebectomy for avulsing calf varicosities.

COMPLICATIONS:
- Hemorrhage
- Thrombophlebitis
- Atrophie blanche
- Varicose eczema
- Lipodermatosclerosis
- Venous ulceration

DISPOSITION

A chronic condition in which a combination of compressive and surgical therapy can adequately control varicosities

REFERRAL

- To dermatologist for dermatitis complications
- To surgeon for failed conservative management or varicose veins with complications

EVIDENCE

An RCT of endovenous radiofrequency obliteration vs. ligation and stripping demonstrated equivalent success rates, but significant advantages were demonstrated (e.g., shorter return to work and less pain experienced) in the radiofrequency obliteration group.[1] (B)

A systematic review found that compression was more effective than no compression for the healing of venous leg ulcers.[2] (A)

Evidence-Based References

1. Lurie F et al: Prospective randomized study of endovenous radiofrequency obliteration (closure procedure) versus ligation and stripping in a selected patient population (EVOLVeS Study), *J Vasc Surg* 38:207, 2003. (B)
2. Cullum N et al: Compression for venous leg ulcers (Cochrane Review). In: Cochrane Library 1, Chichester, UK, 2004, John Wiley. (A)

SUGGESTED READINGS

Crane J, Cheshire N: Recent developments in vascular surgery, *BMJ* 327(7420):911, 2003.
Hagen MD, Johnson ED: What treatments are effective for varicose veins? *J Fam Pract* 52(4):329, 2003.

AUTHORS: **ARUNDATHI G. PRASAD, M.D.,** and **RUBEN ALVERO, M.D.**

BASIC INFORMATION

DEFINITION

A varicocele is a collection of dilated and tortuous veins in the pampiniform plexus surrounding the spermatic cord in the scrotum.

SYNONYM

Sometimes referred to as a "bag of worms"

ICD-9CM CODES
456.4

EPIDEMIOLOGY AND DEMOGRAPHICS

PREVALENCE: A varicocele is present in up to 20% of all males. It occurs in approximately 30% of infertile men. However, only 10% to 15% of males with varicoceles have fertility problems.

RISK FACTORS: There is no reliable data on epidemiological risk factors for varicocele, such as a family history or environmental exposures.

PHYSICAL FINDINGS & CLINICAL PRESENTATION

Patients may report a mass lying posterior to and above the testis. When the patient is supine, dilation of the veins is generally decreased. Dilation and tortuosity of the veins increases when the patient is upright and when the patient performs a Valsalva maneuver.

The majority of cases occur more commonly on the left side because the left spermatic vein enters the left renal vein at a 90-degree angle, whereas the right testicular vein drains directly into the vena cava.

ETIOLOGY

Varicoceles are caused by dysfunction of the valves in the spermatic vein, which allows pooling of blood in the pampiniform plexus.

DIAGNOSIS

DIFFERENTIAL DIAGNOSIS

- Hydrocele
- Spermatocele
- Epidydimal orchitis
- Testicular tumor

WORKUP

Patient should be examined in an upright position and a supine position.

LABORATORY TESTS

Semen analysis if a varicocele is detected and the patient is infertile.

IMAGING STUDIES

Doppler ultrasound, with or without high-resolution color flow, is the most common and least invasive technique to confirm a varicocele and differentiate it from other scrotal abnormalities.

TREATMENT

Once a varicocele is identified, providers must document bilateral testicular size at regular intervals. If the testicle on the affected side is small, spermatogenesis may have been adversely affected.

SURGERY

- Varicocelectomy is performed by ligation of the veins of the pampiniform plexus through an inguinal incision or by ligating the internal spermatic vein in the retroperitoneum. This is generally performed as an ambulatory surgery.
- The goal of varicocelectomy is to maximize chances for fertility.
- Surgical treatment is indicated when there is significant disparity in testicular size or pain. Also, surgery should be performed if the contralateral testis is diseased or absent. Surgery may be considered if the varicocele is large, even without a disparity in testicular size.
- Postoperatively the involved testis typically enlarges and catches up to the uninvolved side in 1 to 2 yr. Semen parameters also improve significantly in 65% of patients.
- The success rate of surgical repair is close to 98% and that of percutaneous repair is significantly lower.

PEARLS & CONSIDERATIONS

COMMENTS

- A varicocele in a boy less than 10 yr of age or on the right side may be indicative of an abdominal or retroperitoneal mass. Ultrasound should be performed.
- The sudden occurrence of a left-sided varicocele in an older man indicates occlusion of the spermatic vein and should prompt evaluation for a renal tumor.

SUGGESTED READINGS

Behrman R et al: *Nelson textbook of pediatrics,* ed 16, Philadelphia, 2000, WB Saunders, pp 1652-1654.

Diamond DA: Adolescent varicocele, *Curr Opin Urol* 17(4):263-267, 2007.

Nseyo U et al: *Urology for primary care physicians,* Philadelphia, 1999, WB Saunders, pp 339-346.

AUTHORS: **ELIZABETH NOWAK, D.O.,** and **JANICE PATACSIL-TRULL, M.D.**

BASIC INFORMATION

DEFINITION

Venous ulcers are shallow wounds with irregular borders that usually occur on the lower extremities above or over the malleoli. These ulcerations develop due to high venous pressures caused by incompetent valves or obstructed veins.

SYNONYMS

Stasis ulcers, peripheral venous insufficiency, venous leg ulcers

ICD-9CM CODES
459.3 Chronic venous hypertension, including stasis edema
459.81 Peripheral venous insufficiency
707.1 Ulcer of the lower limb

EPIDEMIOLOGY & DEMOGRAPHICS

PEAK PREVALENCE: Occurs between 60 and 80 years of age, women > men.
RISK FACTORS: Smoking, obesity, diabetes mellitus, phlebitis, increasing age, family history of varicose veins, history of DVT.

PHYSICAL FINDINGS & CLINICAL PRESENTATION

- Patients with venous stasis often have chronic skin changes on their lower limbs, including hyperpigmentation, hyperkeratosis, and dependent edema. Skin color changes are due to the extravasation of red blood cells and the resultant deposition of hemosiderin.
- Venous dermatitis or stasis dermatitis is common in these patients and is characterized by pruritic, red, and scaly eczematous changes.
- Smooth white plaques of atrophic sclerosis are known as atrophie blanche and can be a clue that the patient has venous disease.
- Venous ulcers are shallow, full-thickness ulcers, with irregular borders and areas of granulation tissue. Necrosis is extremely rare.
- Patients often report a long history of dependent lower-extremity edema, and aching pain in the legs that is often worse after standing for long periods.

ETIOLOGY

Venous stasis develops from valvular incompetence or obstruction, resulting in venous hypertension. Some authors propose that venous hypertension leads to malformation of capillaries causing leakage of fluid and reduced blood flow to the skin. The resultant hypoxic tissue is prone to ulceration after minor trauma. The underlying vascular deficiency also impedes wound healing.

DIAGNOSIS

DIFFERENTIAL DIAGNOSIS

- Peripheral arterial disease (with ischemia and necrosis)
- Diabetic ulceration (often secondary to neuropathy)
- Decubitus ulceration (due to pressure over a bony prominence)
- Vasculitis (with erythema and bullae)
- Necrotic ulceration from infection
- Basal cell carcinoma or squamous cell carcinoma

WORKUP

- The majority of patients can be diagnosed clinically from the physical exam; however up to 25% of patients have concomitant arterial disease. In these patients an ankle-brachial index should be performed. Arterial insufficiency is suggested by an ABI of <1.0.
- Patients with lower-extremity ulcers should also be evaluated for diabetes.
- If vasculitis is suspected, a biopsy of the edge of the ulcer can confirm the diagnosis.
- Any wound that is present for more than 3 months should be biopsied to rule out malignancy.

IMAGING STUDIES

If the ulcer appears infected consider plain x-ray films to evaluate for osteomyelitis.

TREATMENT

NONPHARMACOLOGIC THERAPY

- The goal of therapy is to improve venous return to the heart, thus decreasing edema, inflammation, and tissue ischemia.
- First line treatment includes compression bandages and elevation of the leg above the heart for at least 30 minutes three to four times a day. Bandages are used under compression stockings to provide a clean, moist environment to promote healing. Highly exudative wounds require absorbent dressings, whereas dry wounds may need a more occlusive dressing. There is no conclusive evidence that supports one type of dressing over another.
- Smaller ulcers can be treated using compression stockings. Knee-high stockings with graded pressure providing at least 35 to 40 mm Hg of pressure at the ankle and 20 to 25 mm Hg at the knee are most effective.
- Compression with either bandages or stockings is to be used only after arterial disease has been excluded as it can cause limb ischemia.
- Surgical intervention is not routine; however, options include sclerotherapy, replacement of venous valves, ligation, and stripping of veins. Skin grafts are also an option for nonhealing wounds.

ACUTE GENERAL Rx

- Moist occlusive dressings and certain topical agents can aid in the healing of venous ulcers.
- Dressings can be nonadherent (Telfa), occlusive (Tegaderm, DuoDerm), or medicated like the Unna boot. Occlusive bandages have the advantage of reducing pain and can be changed by the patient every 5 to 7 days. These bandages do not increase the rate of wound infection if used appropriately.
- Daily aspirin (300 mg) is recommended to accelerate healing.
- Underlying systemic hypertension and diabetes should be aggressively treated.
- Pentoxifylline (Trental) may improve healing through its antithrombotic effects as well as fibrinolytic properties. Pentoxifylline 800 mg tid has been shown to be an effective adjuvant to compression therapy.
- Antiseptics such as iodine cause cellular toxicity and should not be used on ulcers. In addition, silver sulfadiazine (Silvadene), neomycin, and bacitracin are common causes of contact dermatitis and skin irritation and are not recommended.
- Systemic antibiotics are not indicated unless there are obvious signs of infection including erythema, heat, purulent drainage, and pain.
- Prevention includes continued use of compression stockings, leg elevation, smoking cessation, and weight loss.

COMPLEMENTARY & ALTERNATIVE MEDICINE

Horse chestnut seed extract (50 mg bid) has been shown to reduce the edema associated with venous stasis. It can be used in patients who cannot tolerate compression therapy (see "Suggested Reading").

DISPOSITION

Overall prognosis is poor. Although 50% of ulcers will heal after 4 months, 20% are nonhealing after 2 years of treatment and 8% after 8 years. Recurrence is common.

REFERRAL

- Referral to a wound clinic should be considered in patients with large (>5×5 cm) or long-standing wounds.
- All patients should be evaluated after 1 month of therapy. If the wound shows little to no progress in healing, referral is also suggested.

SUGGESTED READING

Palfreyman SJ et al: Dressings for healing venous leg ulcers (Cochrane Review), *Cochrane Database of Syst Rev* 3:CD001103, 2006.

AUTHOR: **KELLY BOSSENBROEK, M.D.**

BASIC INFORMATION

DEFINITION

- Ventricular septal defect (VSD) refers to an abnormal communication through the septum separating the right and left ventricles.
- VSDs may be large or small, single or multiple.
- VSDs are located at various anatomic regions of the septum and classified as:
  1. Membranous (75% to 80%): most common type, defect extends into the membranous portion of the interventricular septum.
  2. Muscular or trabecular (5% to 20%): defect entirely surrounded by muscular tissue.
  3. Canal or inlet (8%): defect commonly lies beneath the septal leaflet of the tricuspid valve; often seen in patients with Down's syndrome.
  4. Subarterial, outlet, infundibular, or supracristal (5% to 7%): least common type, defect usually found beneath the aortic valve and may lead to aortic regurgitation.

SYNONYMS

VSD

ICD-9CM CODES
745.4 Ventricular septal defect

EPIDEMIOLOGY & DEMOGRAPHICS

- VSD was first described by Dalrymple in 1847.
- VSDs are some of the most common congenital heart abnormalities (along with bicuspid aortic valve and mitral valve prolapse), accounting for 30% of all congenital cardiac defects.
- VSD accounts for about 25% of all congenital heart defects in children and 10% in adults (decrease due to spontaneous closure of many VSDs by adulthood).
- Prevalence is 1.17 per 1000 live births and 0.5 per 1000 adults.
- Found with equal frequency in males and females.
- VSD may be associated with:
  1. Atrial septal defect (35%)
  2. Patent ductus arteriosus (22%)
  3. Coarctation of the aorta (17%)
  4. Subvalvular aortic stenosis (4%)
  5. Subpulmonic stenosis
- Multiple VSDs are more prevalent in patients with tetralogy of Fallot and double outlet right ventricular defects.

PHYSICAL FINDINGS & CLINICAL PRESENTATION

- Clinical presentation depends on the direction and volume of the VSD shunt, which is dictated by the size of the defect and the ratio of the pulmonary to systemic vascular resistance.
- Infants may be asymptomatic at birth because of elevated pulmonary artery resistance. Over the first few weeks of life, pulmonary arterial resistance decreases, allowing more left-to-right shunting through the VSD, with subsequent increased flow into the lungs, left atrium, and left ventricle, causing left ventricular volume overload. Tachypnea, failure to thrive, and congestive heart failure will then ensue.
- In adults with VSD, the shunt is left to right in the absence of pulmonary stenosis and pulmonary hypertension, and patients typically manifest with symptoms of heart failure (e.g., shortness of breath, orthopnea, and dyspnea on exertion).
- A spectrum of physical findings may be seen including:
  1. Holosystolic murmur heard best along the left sternal border
  2. Systolic thrill
  3. Mid-diastolic rumble heard at the apex
  4. S_3
  5. Rales
- With the development of pulmonary hypertension:
  1. Augmented pulmonic component of S_2
  2. Cyanosis, clubbing, right ventricular heave, and signs of right heart failure (seen in Eisenmenger's complex with reversal of the shunt in a right-to-left direction)

ETIOLOGY

- Usually congenital (the focus of our review), but may occur post-myocardial infarction.
- After acute myocardial infarction: rupture of the intraventricular septum typically occurs 3 to 5 days after the event, and occurs in up to 2% of the cases.

DIAGNOSIS

The diagnosis of VSD is suspected by physical examination. Imaging studies, particularly transthoracic echocardiography with color Doppler, establish the diagnosis.

DIFFERENTIAL DIAGNOSIS

Based on physical examination, the diagnosis of VSD may be confused with other causes of systolic murmurs such as mitral regurgitation, tricuspid regurgitation, aortic stenosis, pulmonary stenosis, and hypertrophic cardiomyopathy.

WORKUP

Any person that is suspected of having a VSD should have an ECG, a chest x-ray, and an echocardiogram.

LABORATORY TESTS

- Laboratory tests are not specific, but may offer insight into the severity of the disease.
- CBC may show polycythemia, especially in patients with Eisenmenger's complex.
- Arterial blood gases may show hypoxemia.

IMAGING STUDIES

- ECG findings vary according to the size of the VSD and whether pulmonary hypertension is present. In large VSDs with pulmonary hypertension, right axis deviation is seen along with evidence of right ventricular hypertrophy.
- Chest x-ray findings in patients with VSD include:
  1. Cardiomegaly results from volume overload and directly relates to the magnitude of the shunt
  2. Enlargement of the proximal pulmonary arteries along with redistribution and pruning of the distal pulmonary vessels resulting from sustained pulmonary hypertension (Fig. 1-288, *A*)
- Echocardiography is the imaging modality of choice in the diagnosis of VSD.
  1. Two-dimensional echo and color Doppler displays the size and location of the VSD (Fig. 1-288, *B*).
  2. Continuous wave Doppler not only approximates the gradient between the left and right ventricle, but also estimates the pulmonary artery pressure.
  3. Magnitude of shunt can be determined by calculation of pulmonary to systemic flow ratio on echo.
- Cardiac catheterization may confirm echocardiography findings in the measurement of right heart pressures and the calculation of the pulmonary to systemic flow ratio.
- Ventriculography may help to locate the VSD.

TREATMENT

The decision to close a VSD depends on its type, size, and shunt severity, as well as the patient's pulmonary vascular resistance, functional capacity, and associated valvular abnormalities.

NONPHARMACOLOGIC THERAPY

- In young children, small asymptomatic VSDs with a pulmonary to systemic blood flow ratio of ≤1.5:1 and no evi-

dence of pulmonary hypertension can be observed.
- Oxygen and low-salt diet is recommended in patients with congestive heart failure.

ACUTE GENERAL Rx

Surgery is indicated in:
- Infants with congestive heart failure
- Children between the ages of 1 and 6 with persistent VSD and a pulmonary to systemic blood flow ratio >2:1
- Adults with VSD and flow ratios >1.5:1, pulmonary artery systolic pressure >50 mm Hg, increased LV and LA size, or deteriorating left ventricular function in the absence of irreversible pulmonary hypertension
- Percutaneous transcatheter closure by Amplatzer occluder devices have been used with success for muscular VSD closure in small studies of congenital VSDs and anecdotally in postinfarct VSDs.

CHRONIC Rx

See "Acute General Rx."

DISPOSITION

- The natural history of isolated VSD depends on the type of defect, its size, and associated abnormalities.
- Approximately 75% to 80% of small VSDs close spontaneously by age 10 yr.
- In patients with large VSDs, only 10% to 15% will close spontaneously.
- Large VSDs left untreated may lead to arrhythmias, congestive heart failure, pulmonary hypertension, and Eisenmenger's complex.
- Eisenmenger's complex carries a poor prognosis, with most patients dying before the age of 40 yr.

REFERRAL

All infants and children diagnosed with VSD should be referred to a pediatric cardiologist. Adults with VSD should be referred to an adult cardiologist. Cardiothoracic surgeons experienced in congenital heart disease surgery should be consulted if surgery is indicated.

PEARLS & CONSIDERATIONS

COMMENTS

- A loud murmur does not imply a large VSD. Small, hemodynamically insignificant VSDs can cause loud murmurs.
- In Eisenmenger's complex, the right-to-left shunting across the VSD is usually not associated with an audible murmur.
- Risk of patients with unrepaired VSD developing infective endocarditis is 4%. The risk is higher if aortic insufficiency is present.
- Endocarditis prophylaxis is no longer indicated 6 months after a VSD repair without residual shunt, as per the updated 2007 AHA guidelines.

SUGGESTED READINGS

Butera G et al: Percutaneous closure of ventricular septal defects: state of the art, *J Cardiovasc Med (Hagerstown)* 8(1):39, 2007.

Minette MS, Sahn DJ: Ventricular septal defects, *Circulation* 114(20):2190, 2006.

Turner SW et al: The natural history of ventricular septal defects, *Arch Dis Child* 81(5):413, 1999.

Wilson W et al: Prevention of infective endocarditis: guidelines from the American Heart Association, *Circulation* 115:739, 2007.

AUTHORS: **CRAIG J. McMACKIN, M.D.**, and **WEN-CHIH WU, M.D.**

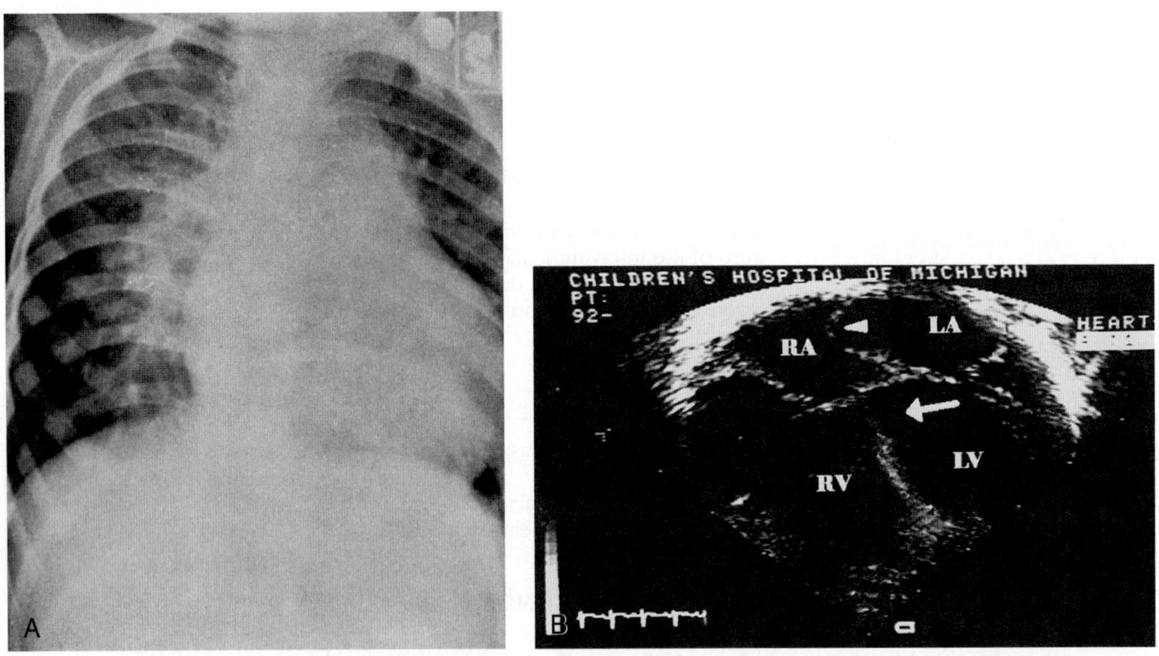

FIGURE 1-288 **A,** Chest roentgenogram of a child with a large VSD, large pulmonary blood flow, and pulmonary hypertension, but only mild elevation of PVR. This is reflected in the evidence of left and right ventricular enlargement, enlargement of the main pulmonary artery, and marked increase in pulmonary blood flow. **B,** Apical four-chamber echocardiographic view of ventricular septal defect *(large arrow)*. Small arrow points to interatrial septum. *LA,* Left atrium; *LV,* left ventricle; *RA,* right atrium; *RV,* right ventricle. (**A** From Pacifico AD et al: Surgical treatment of ventricular septal defect. In Sabiston DC Jr, Spencer FC [eds]: *Surgery of the chest,* ed 5, Philadelphia, 1990, WB Saunders. **B** Courtesy Richard Humes, M.D., Associate Professor of Pediatrics, Director of Echocardiography Laboratory, Children's Hospital of Michigan, Detroit.)

BASIC INFORMATION

DEFINITION

Vertebral compression fractures are defined as fractures of spinal vertebrae in which a bony surface is driven toward another bony surface. These fractures are classified as a radiographic reduction in vertebral body height of more than 15% to 20%.

SYNONYMS

Thoracolumbar vertebral compression fractures
Osteoporotic fractures

ICD9-CM CODES
805.8 Compression fracture, spine
805.4 Compression fracture, lumbar vertebra
805.2 Compression fracture, thoracic vertebra
733.13 Compression fracture, L2 vertebra

EPIDEMIOLOGY & DEMOGRAPHICS

Approximately 700,000 vertebral compression fractures (VCFs) occur in the U.S. each year, affecting approximately 25% of postmenopausal women. The prevalence increases with age, reaching a peak of 40% in women greater than 80 years of age. Compression fractures are also a major concern among men, though VCF rates are lower.

RISK FACTORS:

- Modifiable: tobacco or alcohol use, osteoporosis, estrogen deficiency (early menopause, bilateral ovariectomy, premenopausal amenorrhea for more than 1 year), frailty, impaired vision, abusive situations, inadequate physical activity, low BMI, and dietary deficiency of vitamin D or calcium
- Nonmodifiable: advanced age, female, dementia, Caucasian, history of fractures in adulthood and among first-degree relatives, falls

PHYSICAL FINDINGS & CLINICAL PRESENTATION

- Asymptomatic: most VCFs are asymptomatic, except for height loss or kyphosis (dowager hump). Kyphosis is often a sign of multiple VCF.
- Symptomatic: often present as acute back pain after activity (e.g., bending, lifting) or coughing; neck strain and rib pain may also be present.

ETIOLOGY

- Vertebral compression fractures take place when the combination of bending and axial loads on the spine exceed the strength of the vertebral body.
- Primary etiology is osteoporosis.

DIAGNOSIS

DIFFERENTIAL DIAGNOSIS

- Hyperparathyroidism
- Osteomalacia
- Granulomatous diseases (e.g., tuberculosis)
- Hematologic/oncologic diseases (e.g., multiple myeloma, malignancy)

WORKUP

- Only one third of VCFs are diagnosed.
- VCF can be clinical suspected from history and physical alone.
- There may or may not be a specific injury or remembered event.

LABORATORY TESTS

Tests to rule out infection or cancer may be helpful, such as ESR, CBC, alkaline phosphatase, and C-reactive protein, but can be reserved for individuals for whom there is a clinical suspicion.

IMAGING STUDIES

- Plain frontal and lateral radiographs (x-rays) are the initial imaging method (Fig. 1-289) and may be sufficient, particularly when no neurologic abnormalities are present. MRI and CT scans may be uncomfortable or painful for the patient, especially in the acute phase.
- Computed tomography (CT scans), though not routinely necessary, can be helpful for visualizing fractures not seen on plain films, evaluating the integrity of the posterior vertebral wall, ruling out other causes of back pain, detecting spinal canal narrowing, and assessing instability.
- Magnetic resonance imaging (MRI) may be useful when spinal cord compression is suspected, if neurologic symptoms are present, or to distinguish malignancy from osteoporosis (such as in patients younger than 55 years of age with a VCR after minimum or no trauma).
- Bone density studies may be helpful in determining the severity of osteoporosis, a key risk fracture for predicting future fractures.

TREATMENT

NONPHARMACOLOGIC THERAPY

- Physical therapy.
- External back braces.
- Exercise programs—getting the person active as soon as possible is extremely important both short and long term.

ACUTE GENERAL Rx

- Analgesics for pain control, including acetaminophen and opioids (oral or parenteral). Prevention of constipation is important with opioids.
- Nonsteroidal anti-inflammatory drugs are helpful but must be used with caution in the elderly or when contraindicated.
- Muscle relaxants used judiciously.
- Carefully selected patients who do not respond to conservative therapy or who have severe pain may be considered for percutaneous vertebroplasty (acrylic bone cement is injected into the affected vertebral body in an effort to stabilize the fracture and reduce pain) and kyphoplasty (a high-pressure inflatable bone tamp or balloon is expanded before injection of bone cement into the cavity in the fractured vertebral body). Although potentially useful procedures, prospective studies will need to be performed comparing long-term outcomes and risks to conventional treatment.

CHRONIC Rx

Osteoporosis should be treated: reduction of risk factors (e.g., smoking and alcohol), diet exercise, calcium and vitamin D supplements, and consideration of medications that treat osteoporosis (e.g., bisphosphonates).

REFERRAL

Referral is indicated for neurologic abnormalities, unremitting pain, instability, continued disability, or when the investigation of the cause of the fracture reveals serious underlying pathology.

PEARLS & CONSIDERATIONS

COMMENTS

- Vertebral compression fractures should be suspected in anyone older than 50 years of age with the acute onset of low back pain.
- Solitary vertebral fractures higher than T7 are unusual and may be suspicious for other pathologic etiologies.
- Diagnosing and treating osteoporosis reduces the incidence of VCRs.
- Getting people with VCF physically active as soon as possible will be efficacious both acutely and in the long term.
- In general, VCF can perhaps be best managed through a partnership of the patient, the primary care physician, orthopedist, physical therapist, dietician, and social worker.

PREVENTION

Reducing the effects of modifiable risk factors is key.

SUGGESTED READINGS

Banerjee S et al: Back stab: percutaneous vertebroplasty in severe back pain, *Can Fam Physician* 53(7):1169, 2007.

Brunton S et al: Vertebral compression fractures in primary care: recommendations from a consensus panel, *J Fam Pract* 54(9):781-788, 2005.

Garfin SR, Reilley MA: Minimally invasive treatment of osteoporotic vertebral body compression fractures, *Spine J* 1:76-80, 2002.

Mazanec DJ et al: Vertebral compression fractures: manage aggressively to prevent sequelae, *Cleve Clin J Med* 70(2):147-156, 2003.

Old JL, Calvert M: Vertebral compression fractures in the elderly, *Am Fam Physician* 69:111-116, 2004.

AUTHOR: **JEFFREY BORKAN, M.D., PH.D**

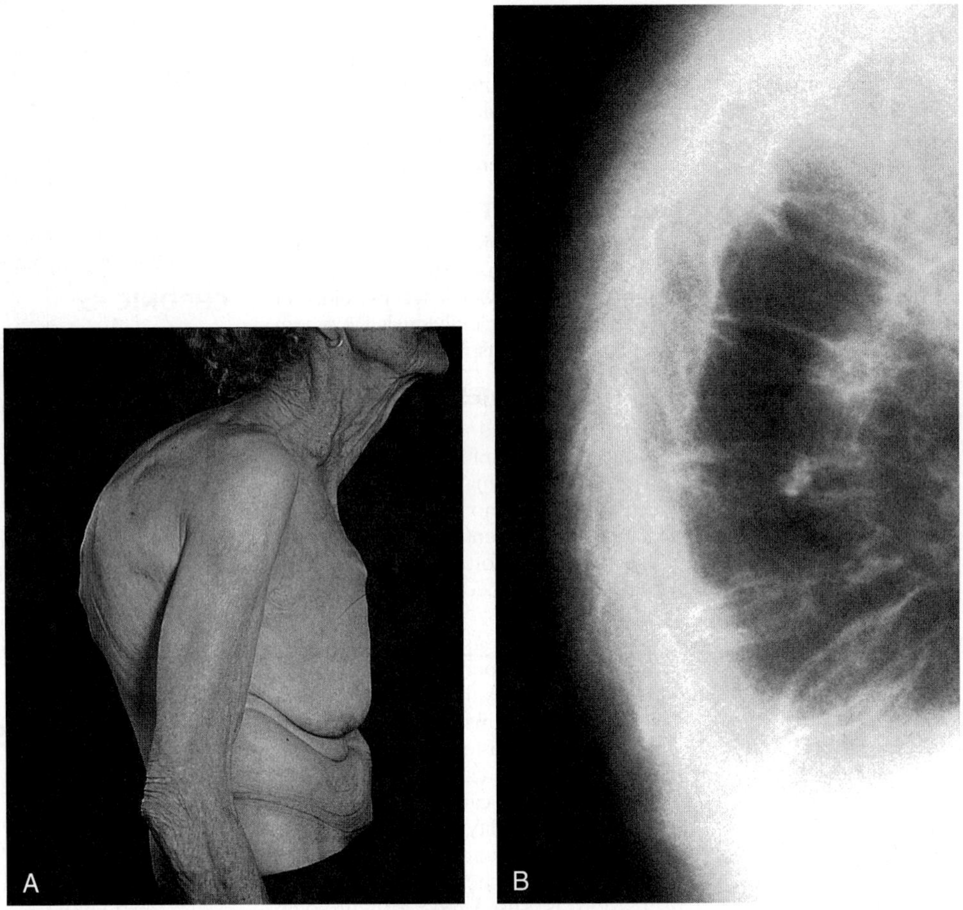

FIGURE 1-289 Dowager's hump. A, Marked thoracic kyphosis due to multiple osteoporotic fractures in an elderly woman with **(B)** corresponding radiograph. (From Hochberg MC, Silman AJ, Smolen JS, Weinblatt ME, Weisman MH [eds]: *Rheumatology,* ed 3, St. Louis, 2003, Mosby.)

BASIC INFORMATION

DEFINITION

Vestibular neuronitis is a syndrome of sudden-onset, often severe, prolonged vertigo of peripheral origin.

SYNONYMS

Labyrinthitis, vestibular neuronitis, acute neuritis

ICD-9CM CODES
078.81 Vestibular neuronitis
386.12 Neuronitis, vestibular

EPIDEMIOLOGY & DEMOGRAPHICS

Viral origin supported by the fact that it occurs in epidemics, may affect several family members, and occurs more commonly in spring and early summer. Male-to-female ratio is similar. Thought to result from selective inflammation of the vestibular nerve; etiology presumed to be viral. There is selective damage to the superior part of the vestibular labyrinth, supplied by the superior division of the vestibular nerve.

PHYSICAL FINDINGS & CLINICAL PRESENTATION

- Course: develops over period of hours, resolves over periods of days, though with frequent long-term sequela; may have viral prodrome.
- Symptoms of vertigo, spontaneous peripheral nystagmus, positive head-thrust test, imbalance. Patient reports intense sensation of rotation, difficulty standing and walking, tends to veer toward affected side, autonomic symptoms with pallor, sweating, nausea and vomiting.

ETIOLOGY

Thought to be viral in origin, possibly thought to be due to herpes zoster, but trial of valacyclovir with and without methylprednisolone showed no efficacy for valacyclovir, but efficacy for the steroid.

DIAGNOSIS

DIFFERENTIAL DIAGNOSIS

Labyrinthitis: similar etiology, but includes hearing loss
- Labyrinthine infarction
- Perilymph fistula
- Brainstem and cerebellar infarction
- Migraine-associated vertigo
- Multiple sclerosis

WORKUP

Head-thrust test: grasp patient's head, apply brief small-amplitude rapid head turn, first to one side and then the other; patient fixates on examiner's nose: positive test is lack of corrective eye movements "saccades" on affected side.

LABORATORY TESTS

- ENG: testing of the vestibular apparatus with physical challenges, unilateral lack of caloric response
- Audiogram: normal

IMAGING STUDIES

Brain imaging: CT or MRI—normal

TREATMENT

NONPHARMACOLOGIC THERAPY

Vestibular exercises, when tolerated, will accelerate recovery.

ACUTE GENERAL Rx

- Methylprednisolone: 100 mg days 1 to 3, 80 mg days 4 to 6, 60 mg days 7 to 9, 40 mg days 10 to 12, 20 mg days 13 to 15, 10 mg days 14 to 16, 5 mg days 18 to 20
- Antihistamines: meclizine, dimenhydrinate, promethazine
- Anticholinergics: scopolamine
- Antidopaminergics: droperidol, prochlorperazine
- AntiGABA agents: diazepam, valium

CHRONIC Rx

- Vestibular rehabilitation exercises
- AntiGABA agents
- Antihistamines

DISPOSITION

Most patients able to be treated as outpatients, but if dehydrated due to severe vomiting may require brief parenteral therapy.

REFERRAL

- ENT: if diagnosis uncertain, additionally these patients are at risk for BPPV subsequently, also symptoms may linger.
- Neurology: if question of central origin or migraine.

PEARLS & CONSIDERATIONS

COMMENTS

Utility of steroids questioned until study reported in *NEJM* 7/04 demonstrated steroids improve recovery of vestibular function. Often damage to labyrinth is permanent, but compensated. These patients are at risk to develop BPPV due to damaged vestibular apparatus. Patients recover from dramatic acute symptoms, but subtle vestibular deficits may linger for prolonged period, if not indefinitely.

PREVENTION

None

PATIENT/FAMILY EDUCATION

Vestibular Disorders Association: http://www.vestibular.org

SUGGESTED READINGS

Baloh RW: Vestibular neuritis, *N Eng J Med* 348:1027-1032, 2003.

Strupp M et al: Methylprednisolone, valacyclovir or the combination for vestibular neuritis, *N Eng J Med* 351(4):354-361, 2004.

Timothy Hain, M.D., director of Balance Center at Northwestern University, maintains http://www.tchain.com.

AUTHOR: **JUDITH NUDELMAN, M.D.**

BASIC INFORMATION

DEFINITION

Vitiligo is the acquired loss of epidermal pigmentation characterized histologically by the absence of epidermal melanocytes.

ICD-9CM CODES
709.1 Vitiligo

EPIDEMIOLOGY & DEMOGRAPHICS

PREVALENCE: 1% of the population

PREDOMINANT AGE: Can begin at any age, but age at onset is under 20 yr for half the patients

GENETICS: Positive family history in 25%-30%

PHYSICAL FINDINGS & CLINICAL PRESENTATION

- Hypopigmented and depigmented lesions (Fig. 1-290) favor sun-exposed regions, intertriginous areas, genitalia, and sites over bony prominences (type A vitiligo).
- Areas around body orifices are also frequently involved.
- The lesions tend to be symmetric.
- Occasionally the lesions are linear or pseudodermatomal (type B vitiligo).
- Vitiligo lesions may occur at trauma sites (Koebner's phenomenon).
- The hair in affected areas may be white.
- The margins of the lesions are usually well demarcated, and when a ring of hyperpigmentation is seen, the term *trichrome vitiligo* is used.
- The term *marginal inflammatory vitiligo* is used to describe lesions with raised borders.
- Initially the disease is limited, but the lesions tend to become more extensive over the years.
- Type B vitiligo is more common in children.
- Vitiligo may begin around pigmented nevi, producing a halo (Sutton's nevus); in such cases the central nevus often regresses and disappears over time.

ETIOLOGY & PATHOGENESIS

Three pathophysiologic theories:
- Autoimmune theory (autoantibodies against melanocytes)
- Neural theory (neurochemical mediator selectively destroys melanocytes)
- Self-destructive process whereby melanocytes fail to protect themselves against cytotoxic melanin precursors

Although vitiligo is considered to be an acquired disease, 25% to 30% is familial; the mode of transmission is unknown (polygenic or autosomal dominant with incomplete penetrance and variable expression).

Associated disorders:
- Alopecia areata
- Type 1 diabetes mellitus
- Adrenal insufficiency
- Hyper- and hypothyroidism
- Mucocutaneous candidiasis
- Pernicious anemia
- Polyglandular autoimmune syndromes
- Melanoma

DIAGNOSIS

DIFFERENTIAL DIAGNOSIS (OTHER HYPOPIGMENTATION DISORDERS)

Acquired:
- Chemical-induced
- Halo nevus
- Idiopathic guttate hypomelanosis
- Leprosy
- Leukoderma associated with melanoma
- Pityriasis alba
- Postinflammatory hypopigmentation
- Tinea versicolor
- Vogt-Koyanagi syndrome (vitiligo, uveitis, and deafness)

Congenital:
- Albinism, partial (piebaldism)
- Albinism, total
- Nevus anemicus
- Nevus depigmentosus
- Tuberous sclerosis

WORKUP

- Physical examination
- Wood's light examination may enhance lesions in light-skinned individuals

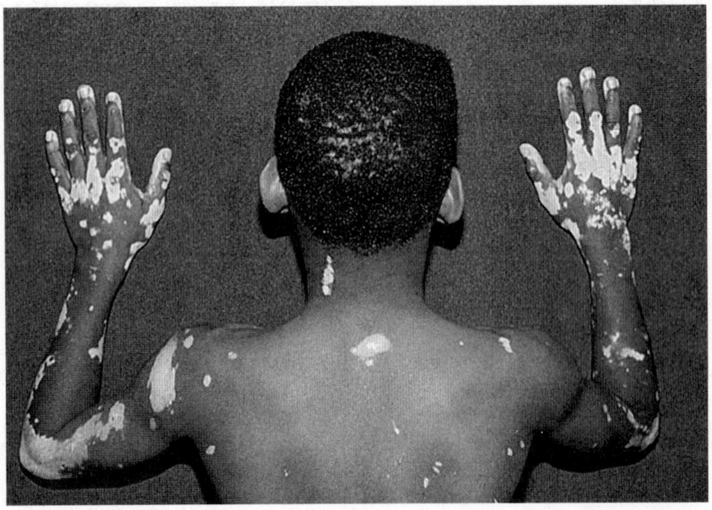

FIGURE 1-290 Multiple, sharply demarcated, symmetric, depigmented areas of vitiligo. (From Behrman RE: *Nelson textbook of pediatrics,* Philadelphia, 2006, WB Saunders.)

TREATMENT

- Treatment indicated primarily for cosmetic purposes when depigmentation causes emotional or social distress. Depigmentation is more noticeable in darker complexions.
- Cosmetic masking agents (Dermablend, Covermark) or stains (Dy-O-Derm, Vita-Dye).
- Sunless tanning lotions (dihydroxyacetone).
- Repigmentation (achieved by activation and migration of melanocytes from hair follicles; therefore skin with little or no hair responds poorly to treatment).
- PUVA (psoralen phototherapy): oral or topical psoralen administration followed by phototherapy with UVA (150 to 200 treatments required over 1 to 2 yr).
- Psoralens and sunlight (Puvasol).
- Topical midpotency steroids (e.g., triamcinolone 0.1% or desonide 0.05% cream qd for 3 to 4 mo).
- Intralesional steroid injection.
- Systemic steroids (betamethasone 5 mg qd on two consecutive days per wk for 2 to 4 mo).
- Total depigmentation (in cases of extensive vitiligo) with 20% monobenzyl ether or hydroquinone. This is a permanent procedure, and patients will require lifelong protection from sun exposure.
- Topical immunomodulators (tacrolimus, pimecromilus) can also induce repigmentation of vitiliginous skin lesions. Their potential for systemic immunosuppression or increased risk of skin or other malignancies remains to be defined.
- Calcipotriol, a synthetic analog of vitamin D_3, has also been used in combination with UV light or clobetasol, with limited results.

SUGGESTED READING

Grimes PE: New insights and new therapies in vitiligo, *JAMA* 293:730, 2005.

AUTHORS: **FRED F. FERRI, M.D.,** and **TOM J. WACHTEL, M.D.**

BASIC INFORMATION

DEFINITION

Von Hippel-Lindau disease (VHL) is a rare autosomal dominant inherited disease characterized by the formation of hemangioblastomas, cysts, and malignancies involving multiple organs and systems.

SYNONYMS Hippel-Lindau syndrome, cerebelloretinal hemangioblastomatosis, retinocerebellar angiomatosis

ICD-9CM CODES
759.6 von Hippel-Lindau disease

EPIDEMIOLOGY & DEMOGRAPHICS

- The incidence of VHL is 1 case/36,000 people.
- Mean age at diagnosis is 26 years because of clinical manifestations, but it can occur from infancy to the seventh decade of life.
- In the U.S. approximately 7000 people are affected.
- Affected individuals are at risk of developing renal cell carcinoma, pheochromocytoma, pancreatic islet cell tumor, endolymphatic sac tumor, and hemangioblastomas of the cerebellum and retina.

PHYSICAL FINDINGS & CLINICAL PRESENTATION

- Retinal angiomas (60%)
  1. Usually occurs by age 25
  2. Often multifocal and bilateral
  3. Detached retina
  4. Glaucoma
  5. Blindness
- CNS hemangioblastomas (59%)
  1. Cerebellum is the most common site followed by the spine and medulla
  2. Usually multiple, and mean age at diagnosis is 25 years
  3. Headache, ataxia, slurred speech, nystagmus, vertigo, nausea, and vomiting
- Renal cysts (~60%) and clear cell renal cell carcinoma (25% to 45%)
  1. Usually occurs by the age of 40
  2. May be asymptomatic or cause abdominal and flank pain
  3. Renal cell carcinoma is bilateral in 75% of patients
- Pancreatic cysts
  1. Usually asymptomatic
  2. Large cysts can cause biliary obstructive symptoms
  3. Diarrhea and diabetes may develop if enough of the pancreas is replaced by cysts
- Pheochromocytoma (7% to 18%)
  1. Bilateral in 50% to 80% of cases
  2. Hypertension, palpitations, sweating, and headache
  3. Commonly occurs with pancreatic islet cell tumors
- Papillary cystadenoma of the epididymis (10% to 25% of men with VHL)
  1. Palpable scrotal mass
  2. May be unilateral or bilateral
- Papillary cystadenoma of the broad ligaments (unknown incidence)
  1. Usually asymptomatic
  2. Reported symptoms include pain, dyspareunia, menorrhagia
- Endolymphatic sac tumors of the middle ear
  1. Ataxia
  2. Loss of hearing
  3. Facial paralysis

ETIOLOGY

VHL disease is primarily caused by a mutation of the von Hippel-Lindau gene located on the short arm of chromosome 3. The VHL disease gene codes for a cytoplasmic protein that functions in tumor suppression.

DIAGNOSIS

- Established in presence of a positive family history, a single retinal or cerebellar hemangioblastoma, or a visceral lesion (e.g., renal cell carcinoma, pheochromocytoma, pancreatic cysts or tumor).
- If no clear family history is present, two or more hemangioblastomas or one hemangioblastoma with a visceral lesion are required to make the diagnosis.
- Screening family members is essential in the early detection of VHL disease.

WORKUP

Screening laboratory, ophthalmoscopic, and imaging studies to look for sites of involvement.

LABORATORY TESTS

- CBC may reveal erythrocytosis requiring periodic phlebotomies
- Electrolytes, BUN, and creatinine
- Urine for norepinephrine, epinephrine, and vanillylmandelic acid looking for pheochromocytoma

IMAGING STUDIES

- Indirect and direct ophthalmoscopy, fluorescein angiography, and tonometry are studies used in screening for retinal angiomas and glaucoma.
- CT scan of the abdomen is used in the screening, detection, and monitoring of patients with renal cysts or tumors, pheochromocytomas, pancreatic cysts, and tumors.
  1. Renal cysts grow on average 0.5 cm/yr.
  2. Renal tumors grow on average 1.5 cm/yr.
  3. CT scans are done every 6 mo for the first 2 yr and every yr for life in patients who have had surgery for renal cell carcinoma.
- MRI with gadolinium is used for screening and evaluation of CNS and spinal hemangioblastomas, endolymphatic sac tumors, and pheochromocytomas.
- Angiography may be done before CNS surgery.

TREATMENT

NONPHARMACOLOGIC THERAPY

Genetic counseling

ACUTE GENERAL Rx

- Laser photocoagulation and cryotherapy is used in patients with retinal angiomas to prevent blindness.
- For cerebellar hemangioblastomas the treatment is surgery. External-beam radiation and stereotactic radiosurgery can also be done.
- For renal tumors, surgery is delayed until one of the renal tumors reaches 3 cm in diameter. Nephron-sparing surgery is the preferred approach.
- Nephrectomy is indicated in patients with end-stage renal disease requiring dialysis because of the malignant potential of the disease.
- Pancreatic islet cell tumors usually require surgical removal.
- Adrenalectomy for pheochromocytoma.

CHRONIC Rx

- Dialysis has been delayed in many patients because of nephron-sparing surgery.
- Renal transplantation is usually delayed for 1 yr after bilateral nephrectomy for renal tumors to ensure that no metastases have occurred.

DISPOSITION Median life expectancy is 49 yr of age.

REFERRAL

Geneticist, neurosurgeon, urologist, nephrologist, ophthalmologist, otolaryngologist, neurologist, endocrinologist, and radiation oncologist.

PEARLS & CONSIDERATIONS

The most common cause of death is renal cell carcinoma.

COMMENTS

More information for patients can be obtained at von Hippel-Lindau Family Alliance.

SUGGESTED READINGS

Couch V et al: von Hippel-Lindau Disease, *Mayo Clin Proc* 75:265, 2000.

Evans JP et al: von Hippel-Lindau disease, *eMedcine,* 2006.

Lonser RR et al: Von Hippel-Lindau disease, *Lancet* 361:2059, 2003.

AUTHOR: **WEN-Y. WU-CHEN, M.D.**

BASIC INFORMATION

DEFINITION

Von Willebrand's disease is a congenital disorder of hemostasis characterized by defective or deficient von Willebrand factor (vWF). There are several subtypes of von Willebrand's disease. The most common type (80% of cases) is type I, which is caused by a quantitative decrease in von Willebrand factor; type IIA and type IIB are results of qualitative protein abnormalities; type III is a rare autosomal recessive disorder characterized by a near complete quantitative deficiency of vWF. *Acquired von Willebrand's disease (AvWD)* is a rare disorder that usually occurs in elderly patients and usually presents with mucocutaneous bleeding abnormalities and no clinically meaningful family history. It is often accompanied by a hematoproliferative or autoimmune disorder. Successful treatment of the associated illness can reverse the clinical and laboratory manifestations.

SYNONYMS

Pseudohemophilia

ICD-9CM CODES
286.4 von Willebrand's disease

EPIDEMIOLOGY & DEMOGRAPHICS

- Autosomal dominant disorder
- Most common inherited bleeding disorder
- Prevalence is 1% to 2 % in general population, according to screening studies; estimates based on referral for symptoms of bleeding suggest a prevalence of 30 to 100 cases per million

PHYSICAL FINDINGS & CLINICAL PRESENTATION

- Generally normal physical examination
- Mucosal bleeding (gingival bleeding, epistaxis) and GI bleeding may occur
- Easy bruising
- Postpartum bleeding, bleeding after surgery or dental extraction, menorrhagia

ETIOLOGY

Quantitative or qualitative deficiency of vWF (see "Definition")

DIAGNOSIS

DIFFERENTIAL DIAGNOSIS

Platelet function disorders, clotting factor deficiencies

WORKUP

- Laboratory evaluation (see "Laboratory Tests")
- Initial testing includes PTT (increased), platelet count (normal), and bleeding time (prolonged)
- Subsequent tests include vWF level (decreased), factor VIII:C (decreased), and ristocetin agglutination (increased in type II B) (Table 1-52)

LABORATORY TESTS

- Normal platelet number and morphology
- Prolonged bleeding time
- Decreased factor VIII coagulant activity
- Decreased von Willebrand factor antigen or ristocetin cofactor
- Normal platelet aggregation studies
- Type II A von Willebrand can be distinguished from type I by absence of ristocetin cofactor activity and abnormal multimer
- Type IIB von Willebrand is distinguished from type I by abnormal multimer

TREATMENT

NONPHARMACOLOGIC THERAPY

- Avoidance of aspirin and other NSAIDs.
- Evaluation for likelihood of bleeding (with measurement of bleeding time) before surgical procedures. When a patient undergoes surgery or receives repeated therapeutic doses of concentrates, factor VIII activity should be assayed every 12 hr on the day a dose is administered and every 24 hr thereafter.

GENERAL Rx

- The mainstay of treatment in von Willebrand's disease is the replacement of the deficient protein at the time of spontaneous bleeding, or before invasive procedures are performed.
- Desmopressin acetate (DDAVP) is useful to release stored vWF from endothelial cells. It is used to cover minor procedures and traumatic bleeding in mild type I von Willebrand's disease. Dose is 0.3 μg/kg in 100 ml of normal saline solution IV infused >20 min. DDAVP is also available as a nasal spray (dose of 150 μg spray administered to each nostril) as a preparation for minor surgery and management of minor bleeding episodes. DDAVP is not effective in type IIA von Willebrand's disease and is potentially dangerous in type IIB (increased risk of bleeding and thrombocytopenia).
- In patients with severe disease, replacement therapy in the form of cryoprecipitate is the method of choice. The standard dose is 1 bag of cryoprecipitate per 10 kg of body weight.
- Factor VIII concentrate rich in vWF (Humate-P, Armour) is useful to correct bleeding abnormalities in type IIA, IIB and type III von Willebrand's disease without alloantibodies. Alloantibodies that inactivate von Willebrand factor and form circulating immune complexes develop in 15% of patients with type III von Willebrand's disease who have received multiple transfusions. In these patients, recombinant factor VIII is preferred because autoantibodies can elicit life-threatening anaphylactic reactions because of complement activation by immune complexes.
- Life-threatening hemorrhage unresponsive to therapy with cryoprecipitate or factor VIII concentrate may require transfusion of normal platelets.

SUGGESTED READING

Mannucci PM: Treatment of von Willebrand's disease, *N Engl J Med* 351:683, 2004.

AUTHOR: **FRED F. FERRI, M.D.**

TABLE 1-52 Genetic and Laboratory Findings in von Willebrand's Disease

PARAMETER							
Type	BT	VIII-c	vw-Ag	R-cof	Ripa	Multimer Structure	Mode of Inheritance
I (classic)	P	R	R	R	R	N	AD
II							
A	P	N/R	N/R	R	R	Abn	AD
B	P	N/R	N/R	N/R	I	Abn	AD
III	P	R	R	R	R	Variable	AR

From Behrman RE: *Nelson textbook of pediatrics,* ed 17, Philadelphia, 2004, WB Saunders.
Abn, Abnormal; *AD,* autosomal dominant; *AR,* autosomal recessive; *BT,* bleeding time; *I,* increased; *N,* normal; *N/R,* normal or reduced; *P,* prolonged; *R,* reduced; *R-Cof,* ristocetin cofactor; *RIPA,* ristocetin-induced platelet aggregation (agglutination); *vW-Aq,* von Willebrand antigen (protein); *VIII-C,* factor VIII coagulant activity.

BASIC INFORMATION

DEFINITION

Vulvar cancer is an abnormal cell proliferation arising on the vulva and exhibiting malignant potential. The majority are of squamous cell origin; however, other types include adenocarcinoma, basal cell carcinoma, sarcoma, and melanoma.

SYNONYMS

Squamous cell carcinoma of the vulva (90%)
Basal cell carcinoma of the vulva
Adenocarcinoma of the vulva
Melanoma of the vulva
Bartholin gland carcinoma
Verrucous carcinoma of the vulva
Vulvar sarcoma

ICD-9CM CODES
184.4 Vulvar neoplasm

EPIDEMIOLOGY & DEMOGRAPHICS

INCIDENCE: 1.8 cases/100,000 persons
PREVALENCE: Vulvar cancer is uncommon. It comprises 4% of malignancies of the female genital tract. It is the fourth most common gynecologic malignancy.
MEAN AGE AT DIAGNOSIS: Predominantly a disease of menopause. Mean age at diagnosis is 65 yr.

PHYSICAL FINDINGS & CLINICAL PRESENTATION

- Vulvar pruritus or pain is present.
- May produce a malodor or discharge or present as bleeding.
- Raised lesion, may have fleshy, ulcerated, leukoplakic, or warty appearance; may have multifocal lesions.
- Lesions are usually located on labia majora, but may be seen on labia minora, clitoris, and perineum.
- The lymph nodes of groin may be palpable.

ETIOLOGY

- The exact etiology is unknown.
- Vulvar intraepithelial neoplasia has been reported in 20% to 30% of invasive squamous cell carcinoma of the vulva, but the malignant potential is unknown.
- Human papillomavirus is found in 30% to 50% of vulvar carcinoma, but its exact role is unclear.
- Chronic pruritus, wetness, industrial wastes, arsenicals, hygienic agents, and vulvar dystrophies have been implicated as causative agents.

DIAGNOSIS

DIFFERENTIAL DIAGNOSIS

- Lymphogranuloma inguinale
- Tuberculosis
- Vulvar dystrophies
- Vulvar atrophy
- Paget's disease

WORKUP

- Diagnosis is made histologically by biopsy
- Thorough examination of the lesion and assessment of spread
- Possible colposcopy of adjacent areas
- Cytologic smear of vagina and cervix
- Cystoscopy and proctosigmoidoscopy may be necessary

IMAGING STUDIES

- Chest radiography
- CT scan and MRI for assessing local tumor spread

TREATMENT

NONPHARMACOLOGIC THERAPY

- Treatment is individualized depending on the stage of the tumor.
- Stage I tumors with <1 mm stromal invasion are treated with complete local excision without groin node dissection.
- Stage I tumors with >1 mm stromal invasion are treated with complete local excision with groin node dissection.
- Stage II tumors require radical vulvectomy with bilateral groin node dissection.
- Advanced-stage disease may require the addition of radiation and chemotherapy to the surgical regimen.
- Section III describes a treatment algorithm for management of vulvar cancer.

DISPOSITION

Five-year survival ranges from 90% for stage I to 15% for stage IV.

REFERRAL

Vulvar cancer should be managed by a gynecologic oncologist and radiation oncologist.

EVIDENCE

The relative rarity of vulvar malignancy means that randomized controlled trials of therapeutic modalities are uncommon; most studies are retrospective reviews and observational studies.

Surgery remains the standard treatment for early vulval cancer.

A systematic review that compared individualized treatment with standard extensive surgery in terms of effectiveness and safety identified two observational studies suitable for inclusion. Even so, on the basis of the available evidence, the reviewers felt able to draw a number of conclusions, as below.[1]

Patients with T1-2 tumor can be safely treated with a radical local vulvar excision.[1] Ⓑ

Patients with cT1-2N0M0 cancer can probably be safely treated by the triple incision technique rather than by en-bloc dissection, because the incidence of skin bridge recurrence is low after triple incision surgery.[1] Ⓑ

Patients with a lateral cT1N0M0 tumor can probably be treated safely with an ipsilateral groin lymph node dissection.[1] Ⓑ

Femoral lymph node dissection should not be omitted, even in patients with a very favorable prognosis.[1] Ⓑ

In patients with early vulvar cancer, primary radiotherapy to the groin is associated with a greater risk of recurrence but lower morbidity than primary surgery to the groin.

Recurrence of tumor after primary radiotherapy to the inguinofemoral lymph nodes appears to be more common after primary radiotherapy than after surgery.[1] Ⓐ

However, morbidity after radiotherapy is lower than after surgery, both in the short term and the long term.[1] Ⓐ

Uncontrolled clinical trials suggest that primary radiotherapy in early vulvar cancer results in fewer recurrences in the groin than a wait-and-see policy.[1] Ⓑ

Evidence-Based Reference

1. Ansink A, van der Velden J, Collingwood M: Surgical interventions for early squamous cell carcinoma of the vulva, *Cochrane Database Syst Rev* 4, 1999. ⒶⒷ

SUGGESTED READINGS

Canavan TP, Cohen D: Vulvar cancer, *Am Fam Physician* 66(7):1269, 2002.
Coleman RL, Santoso JT: Vulvar carcinoma, *Curr Treat Opt Oncol* 1(2):177, 2000.
Grandys EC Jr, Aroris JV: Innovations in the management of vulvar carcinoma, *Curr Opin Obstet Gynecol* 12(1):15, 2000.

AUTHORS: **GIL FARKASH, M.D.,** and **RUBEN ALVERO, M.D.**

BASIC INFORMATION

DEFINITION

Bacterial vulvovaginitis is inflammation affecting the vagina, only rarely affecting the vulva, caused by anaerobic and aerobic bacteria.

SYNONYMS

Bacterial vaginosis
Gardnerella vaginalis
Haemophilus vaginalis
Corynebacterium vaginalis

ICD-9CM CODES
616.10 Vulvovaginitis

EPIDEMIOLOGY & DEMOGRAPHICS

- Most prevalent form of vaginal infection of reproductive age women in the U.S.
- 32% to 64% in patients visiting STD clinics
- 12% to 25% in other clinic populations
- 10% to 26% in patients visiting obstetric clinics
- May be associated with adverse pregnancy outcomes: premature rupture of membranes, preterm labor, preterm birth
- Organisms frequently found in postpartum or postcesarean endometritis

PHYSICAL FINDINGS & CLINICAL PRESENTATION

- >50% of all women may be without symptoms.
- Unpleasant, fishy, or musty vaginal odor in about 50% to 70% of all patients. Odor exacerbated immediately after intercourse or during menstruation.
- Vaginal discharge is increased.
- Vaginal itching and irritation occur.

ETIOLOGY

- Synergistic polymicrobial infection characterized by an overgrowth of bacteria normally found in the vagina
- Anaerobics: *Bacteroides* spp., *Peptostreptococcus* spp., *Mobiluncus* spp.
- Facultative anaerobes: *G. vaginalis, Mycoplasma hominis*
- Concentration of anaerobic bacteria increased to 100 to 1000 times normal
- Lactobacilli are absent or greatly reduced

DIAGNOSIS

DIFFERENTIAL DIAGNOSIS

- Fungal vaginitis
- *Trichomonas* vaginitis
- Atrophic vaginitis
- Cervicitis

WORKUP

- Pelvic examination
- Speculum examination
- Normal saline and 10% KOH slide of discharge
- Amsel criteria for diagnosis (three of four should be present):
  1. pH >4.5
  2. Clue cells (epithelial cells covered with bacteria) on saline solution slide
  3. Positive whiff test on 10% KOH
  4. Homogeneous, white, adherent discharge
- Section III, "Vaginal Discharge," describes the evaluation of discharge

TREATMENT

ACUTE GENERAL Rx

- Metronidazole 500 mg PO bid × 7 days, >90% cure rate
- Metronidazole 2 g PO × 1 day, 67% to 92% cure rate
- Metronidazole gel 5 g, intravaginal bid × 5 days
- Clindamycin 2% cream 5 g, intravaginal qd × 7 days
- Clindamycin 300 mg PO bid × 7 days in pregnancy

CHRONIC Rx

Clindamycin 300 mg PO bid × 7 days; cure rate similar to those achieved with metronidazole

Related to adverse pregnancy outcomes

- Metronidazole 250 mg PO bid × 7 days
- Metronidazole zympoxidase
- Clindamycin 300 mg PO bid × 7 days
- Good hygiene: avoidance of douching, harsh shower gels, bubble baths; cotton underwear

DISPOSITION

- Reevaluate if not cured with treatment
- Recurrence fairly common

REFERRAL

Refer to obstetrician/gynecologist for recurrence or pregnant patient with bacterial vaginosis

PEARLS & CONSIDERATIONS

COMMENTS

Treating sexual partners has failed to demonstrate a benefit.

EVIDENCE

Higher cumulative cure rates have been found at 3 to 4 weeks for a 7-day regimen of metronidazole (500 mg twice daily) than with a single dose (2 g).[1] Ⓐ

The limited evidence comparing oral vs. intravaginal treatment and metronidazole vs. clindamycin concludes that there is little difference in outcome between the two agents.[2] Ⓐ

Good-quality trials have shown that antibiotic therapy is effective at eradicating bacterial vaginosis during pregnancy. However, evidence does not support treating asymptomatic women to prevent preterm birth, but for women with previous preterm delivery, it may reduce the risk of preterm rupture of membranes and low birth weight.[3] Ⓐ

Evidence-Based References

1. Joesoef MR, Schmid GP: Bacterial vaginosis: review of treatment options and potential clinical indications for therapy, *Clin Infect Dis* 28(suppl 1):S57, 1999. Reviewed in: *Clin Evid* 13:1968, 2005. Ⓐ
2. Joesoef MR, Schmid G: Bacterial vaginosis. In: *Clin Evid* 13:1968, London, 2005, BMJ Publishing Group. Ⓐ
3. McDonald H et al: Antibiotics for treating bacterial vaginosis in pregnancy (Cochrane Review), *Cochrane Database Syst Rev* 1, 2005. Ⓐ

SUGGESTED READING

Centers for Disease Control and Prevention: 2002 Guidelines for treatment of sexually transmitted diseases, *MMWR, Morb Mortal Wkly Rep,* 51 (RR-6), 2002.

AUTHORS: **JULIE ANNE SZUMIGALA, M.D.,** and **RUBEN ALVERO, M.D.**

BASIC INFORMATION

DEFINITION

Estrogen-deficient vulvovaginitis is the irritation and/or inflammation of the vulva and vagina because of progressive thinning and atrophic changes secondary to estrogen deficiency (Fig. 1-291).

SYNONYMS

Atrophic vaginitis

ICD-9CM CODES
616.10 Vulvovaginitis

EPIDEMIOLOGY & DEMOGRAPHICS

- Seen most often in postmenopausal women
- Average age of menopause is 52 yr
- In 1990, there were 36 million women 50 yr of age or older

PHYSICAL FINDINGS & CLINICAL PRESENTATION

- Thinning of pubic hair, labia minora and majora
- Decreased secretions from the vestibular glands, with vaginal dryness
- Regression of subcutaneous fat
- Vulvar and vaginal itching
- Dyspaereunia
- Dysuria and urinary frequency
- Vaginal spotting

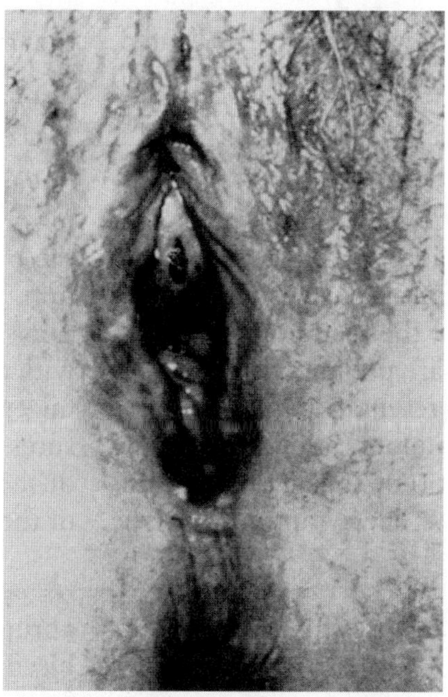

FIGURE 1-291 Advanced postmenopausal atrophy of the vulva in a 72-year-old woman. (From Symonds EM, Macpherson MBA: *Color atlas of obstetrics and gynecology,* St Louis, 1994, Mosby.)

ETIOLOGY

Estrogen deficiency

DIAGNOSIS

DIFFERENTIAL DIAGNOSIS

- Infectious vulvovaginitis
- Squamous cell hyperplasia
- Lichen sclerosus
- Vulvar malignancy
- Vaginal malignancy
- Cervical and endometrial malignancy

WORKUP

- Pelvic examination
- Speculum examination
- Pap smear
- Possible endometrial biopsy if bleeding

LABORATORY TESTS

FSH and estradiol: generally after menopause, estradiol <15 pg and FSH >40 mIU/ml

TREATMENT

ACUTE GENERAL Rx

- Premarin 0.625 mg PO qd.
- Estraderm patch 0.05 mg × 2 per week.
- If uterus present:
  1. Estrogen + 2.5 mg PO Provera qd *or*
  2. Estrogen + 10 mg PO Provera × 10 days each mo
- Conjugated estrogen vaginal cream intravaginally. Estradiol vaginal cream 0.01%.
  2 to 4 g/day × 2 wk then
  1 to 2 g/day × 2 wk then
  1 to 2 g × 3 days/wk
- Vagifen (estradiol vaginal tablets) 25 mg inserted intravaginally daily for 2 wk then twice weekly. May take up to 12 wk to feel the full benefits of the medication.
- Conjugated estrogen vaginal cream: 2-4 g qd (3 wk on, 1 wk off) for 3 to 5 mo.

CHRONIC Rx

See "Acute General Rx." May discontinue vaginal estrogen cream once symptoms alleviate.

DISPOSITION

The symptoms should be improved with the therapy. Caution for vaginal bleeding if uterus present

REFERRAL

To obstetrician/gynecologist if vaginal bleeding

EVIDENCE

A systematic review comparing intravaginal creams, pessaries/tablets, and the estradiol-releasing vaginal ring in postmenopausal women found significant differences favoring the cream, ring, and tablets compared with placebo or moisturizing gel. Creams, tablets, and the estradiol ring were equally effective. Some trials noted significant side effects with the cream (uterine bleeding, breast pain, perineal pain, endometrial overstimulation).[1] Ⓐ

Estrogen therapy effectively decreases the frequency and severity of menopausal hot flashes as well as those symptoms related to vaginal and urethral atrophy. There is little to choose between the available estrogens now licensed, although some patients have ethical objections to conjugated equine estrogens, which are derived from the urine of pregnant mares. There is no evidence that estriol would be any safer in terms of risk of heart disease, heart attacks, strokes, or breast cancer.[2,3] Ⓑ

Evidence-Based References

1. Suckling J, Lethaby A, Kennedy R: Local oestrogen for vaginal atrophy in postmenopausal women (Cochrane Review), *Cochrane Database Syst Rev* 4, 2003. Ⓐ
2. Grady D et al; HERS Research Group: Cardiovascular disease outcomes during 6.8 years of hormone therapy: Heart and Estrogen/progestin Replacement Study follow-up (HERS II), *JAMA* 288:49, 2002. Ⓑ
3. Hulley S et al; HERS Research Group: Noncardiovascular disease outcomes during 6.8 years of hormone therapy: Heart and Estrogen/progestin Replacement Study follow-up (HERS II), *JAMA* 288:58, 2002. Ⓑ

AUTHORS: **JULIE ANNE SZUMIGALA, M.D.,** and **RUBEN ALVERO, M.D.**

BASIC INFORMATION

DEFINITION

Fungal vulvovaginitis is the inflammation of vulva and vagina caused by *Candida* spp.

SYNONYMS

Monilial vulvovaginitis

ICD-9CM CODES
112.1 Vulvovaginitis, monilial

EPIDEMIOLOGY & DEMOGRAPHICS

- Second most common cause of vaginal infection.
- Approximately 13 million people were affected in 1990.
- 75% of women will have at least one episode during their childbearing years, and approximately 40% to 50% of these will experience a second attack.
- No symptoms in 20% to 40% of women who have positive cultures.

PHYSICAL FINDINGS & CLINICAL PRESENTATION

- Intense vulvar and vaginal pruritus
- Edema and erythema of vulva
- Thick, curdlike vaginal discharge
- Adherent, dry, white, curdy patches attached to vaginal mucosa

ETIOLOGY

- *Candida albicans* is responsible for 80%-95% of vaginal fungal infections.
- *Candida tropicalis* and *Torulopsis glabrata (Candida glabrata)* are the most common nonalbicans *Candida* species that can induce vaginitis.

PREDISPOSING HOST FACTORS

- Pregnancy
- Oral contraceptives (high-estrogen)
- Diabetes mellitus
- Antibiotics
- Immunosuppression (e.g., HIV)
- Tight, poorly ventilated, nylon underclothing, with increased local perineal moisture and temperature

DIAGNOSIS

DIFFERENTIAL DIAGNOSIS

- Bacterial vaginosis
- *Trichomonas* vaginitis
- Atrophic vaginitis
- Section II describes the differential diagnosis of vaginal discharges and infections

WORKUP

- Pelvic examination
- Speculum examination
- Hyphae or budding spores on 10% KOH preparation (positive in 50% to 70% of individuals with yeast infection)
- Section III, "Vaginal Discharge," describes the evaluation of discharge

LABORATORY TESTS

Culture, especially recurrence for identification

TREATMENT

ACUTE GENERAL Rx

- Cure rate of the various azole derivatives 85% to 90%; little evidence of superiority of one azole agent over another
- No significant differences in persistent symptoms with oral or vaginal treatment
- Fluconazole (oral) associated with increased frequency of mild nausea, headache, abdominal pain
- Cure rate of polyene (Nystatin) cream and suppositories, 75% to 80%
- Miconazole 200-mg suppository (Monistat 3), one suppository × 3 or 2% vaginal cream (Monistat 7), one applicator full intravaginally qhs × 7
- Clotrimazole 200-mg vaginal tablet, one tablet intravaginally qhs × 3 or 100-mg vaginal tablet (Gyne-Lotrimin, Mycelex-G) one tablet intravaginally qhs × 7, or 1% vaginal cream intravaginally qhs × 7
- Butoconazole 2% cream (Femstat) one applicator intravaginally qhs × 3
- Terconazole 80-mg suppository or 0.8% vaginal cream (Terazol 3), one suppository or one applicator intravaginally qhs × 3 or 0.4% vaginal cream (Terazol 7), one applicator intravaginally qhs × 7
- Gynecazole-1 vaginal cream one applicator intravaginally × 1
- Tioconazole 6.5% ointment (Vagi-stat), one applicator intravaginally × 1
- Fluconazole (Diflucan) 150 mg PO × 1

CHRONIC Rx (FOUR OR MORE SYMPTOMATIC EPISODES/YR)

- Resistance or recurrence
  1. 14- to 21-day course of 7-day regimens mentioned in "Acute General Rx"
  2. Fluconazole (Diflucan) 150 mg PO × 1
  3. Ketoconazole (Nizoral) 200 mg PO bid × 5 to 14 days
  4. Itraconazole (Sporanox) 200 mg PO qd × 3 days
  5. Boric acid 600-mg capsule intravaginally bid × 14 days
- Prophylactic regimens
  1. Clotrimazole one 500-mg vaginal tablet each month
  2. Ketoconazole 200 mg PO bid × 5 days each month
  3. Fluconazole 150 mg PO × 1 each month
  4. Miconazole 100-mg vaginal tablet × 2 weekly

DISPOSITION

- If symptoms do not resolve completely with treatment, or if they recur within a 2- to 3-mo period, further evaluation is indicated.
- Reexamination and possibly culture are necessary.
- Positive culture in absence of symptoms should not lead to treatment. Approximately 30% of women harbor *Candida* spp. and other species in the vagina.

REFERRAL

To obstetrician/gynecologist for recurrence

PEARLS & CONSIDERATIONS

COMMENTS

- No evidence that treating a woman's male sexual partner significantly improves woman's infection or reduces their rate of relapse.

EVIDENCE

Vulvovaginal candidiasis

Several randomized controlled trials (RCTs) found that topical imidazoles were more effective than placebo for the treatment of vulvovaginal candidiasis in nonpregnant women.[1] Ⓐ

An RCT compared intravaginal nystatin vs. placebo in nonpregnant women with symptomatic vulvovaginal candidiasis. Nystatin significantly reduced the number of patients reporting a poor symptomatic response after 2 weeks.[2] Ⓐ

A systematic review found that topical imidazole therapy was more effective than nystatin in the management of vaginal candidiasis in pregnancy. Treatment for 7 days may be necessary during pregnancy.[3] Ⓐ

A systematic review compared oral vs. topical azoles in nonpregnant women with vulvovaginal candidiasis. Both routes of administration were found to be equally effective in terms of clinical and mycologic cure.[4] Ⓐ

Evidence-Based References

1. Spence D: Candidiasis (vulvovaginal). In: *Clin Evid* 10:2044, London, 2003, BMJ Publishing Group. Ⓐ
2. Isaacs JH: Nystatin vaginal cream in monilial vaginitis, *Illinois Med J* 3:240, 1973. 10:2044, 2003. Ⓐ
3. Young GL, Jewell D: Topical treatment for vaginal candidiasis (thrush) in pregnancy. In: Cochrane Library 1, Chichester, UK, 2004, John Wiley. Ⓐ
4. Watson MC et al: Oral versus intra-vaginal imidazole and triazole anti-fungal treatment of uncomplicated vulvovaginal candidiasis (thrush). In: Cochrane Library 1, Chichester, UK, 2004, John Wiley. Ⓐ

AUTHORS: **JULIE ANNE SZUMIGALA, M.D.,** and **RUBEN ALVERO, M.D.**

BASIC INFORMATION

DEFINITION

Prepubescent vulvovaginitis is an inflammatory condition of vulva and vagina.

ICD-9CM CODES
616.10 Vulvovaginitis

EPIDEMIOLOGY & DEMOGRAPHICS

- Most common gynecologic problem of the premenarcheal female.
- Prepubertal girl is susceptible to irritation and trauma because of the absence of protective hair and labial fat pads and the lack of estrogenization with atrophic vaginal mucosa.
- Symptoms of vulvovaginitis and introital irritation and discharge account for 80% to 90% of gynecologic visits.
- Nonspecific etiology in approximately 75% of children with vulvovaginitis.
- Majority of vulvovaginitis in children involves a primary irritation of the vulva with secondary involvement of the lower one third of the vagina.

PHYSICAL FINDINGS & CLINICAL PRESENTATION

- Vulvar pain, dysuria, pruritus
  1. Discharge is not a primary symptom.
  2. If present, vaginal discharge may be foul smelling or bloody.

ETIOLOGY

- Infections
  1. Bacterial
  2. Protozoal
  3. Mycotic
  4. Viral
- Endocrine disorders
- Labial adhesions
- Poor hygiene
- Sexual abuse
- Allergic substance
- Trauma
- Foreign body
- Masturbation
- Constipation
- Section II describes the differential diagnosis of vaginal discharge in prepubertal girls

DIAGNOSIS

DIFFERENTIAL DIAGNOSIS

- Physiologic leukorrhea
- Foreign body
- Bacterial vaginosis
- Gonorrhea
- Fungal vulvovaginitis
- *Trichomonas* vulvovaginitis
- Sexual abuse
- Pinworms

WORKUP

- Pelvic, genital examination
- Speculum examination
- Rectal examination
- KOH and normal saline preparation of discharge
- Section III, "Vaginal Discharge," describes the evaluation of discharge

LABORATORY TESTS

- Urinalysis to rule out UTI and diabetes
- Cultures including STDs

TREATMENT

NONPHARMACOLOGIC THERAPY

- Avoid tight clothing
- Perineal hygiene
- Avoid irritant chemicals
- Reassurance

ACUTE GENERAL Rx

- Group A β *Streptococcus* and *Streptococcus pneumoniae:* penicillin V potassium 125 to 250 mg PO qid × 10 days
- *Chlamydia trachomatis:* erythromycin 50 mg/kg/day PO × 10 days
  1. Children >8 yr of age, doxycycline 100 mg bid PO × 7 days
- *Neisseria gonorrhoeae:* ceftriaxone 125 mg IM × 1 day
  1. Children >8 yr of age should also be given doxycycline 100 mg bid PO × 7 days
- *Staphylococcus aureus:* amoxicillin-clavulanate 20 to 40 mg/kg/day PO × 7 to 10 days
- *Haemophilus influenzae:* amoxicillin 20 to 40 mg/kg/day PO × 7 days
- *Trichomonas:* metronidazole 125 mg (15 mg/kg/day) tid PO × 7 to 10 days
- Pinworms: mebendazole 100-mg tablet chewable, repeat in 2 wk
- Labial agglutination: spontaneous resolution or topical estrogen cream for 7 to 10 days

CHRONIC Rx

See "Referral."

DISPOSITION

Further education:
- Young child: hygiene
- Adolescent: pregnancy prevention and "safe sex"

REFERRAL

- To obstetrician/gynecologist
- To pediatrician

SUGGESTED READING

Van Neer PA, Korver CR: Constipation presenting as recurrent vulvovaginitis in prepubertal children, *J Am Acad Dermatol* 43(4):718, 2000.

AUTHORS: **JULIE ANNE SZUMIGALA, M.D.,** and **RUBEN ALVERO, M.D.**

BASIC INFORMATION

DEFINITION

Trichomonas vulvovaginitis is the inflammation of vulva and vagina caused by *Trichomonas* spp.

SYNONYMS

Trichomonas *vaginalis*

ICD-9CM CODES
131.01 Vulvovaginitis, trichomonal

EPIDEMIOLOGY & DEMOGRAPHICS

- Acquired through sexual contact
- Diagnosed in:
  1. 50% to 75% of prostitutes
  2. 5% to 15% of women visiting gynecology clinics
  3. 7% to 32% of women in STD clinics
  4. 5% of women in family planning clinics

PHYSICAL FINDINGS & CLINICAL PRESENTATION

- Profuse, yellow, malodorous vaginal discharge and severe vaginal itching
- Vulvar itching
- Dysuria
- Dyspareunia
- Intense erythema of the vaginal mucosa
- Cervical petechiae ("strawberry cervix")
- Asymptomatic in approximately 50% of women and 90% of men

ETIOLOGY

Single-cell parasite known as *trichomonad*

RISK FACTORS

- Multiple sexual partners
- History of previous STDs

DIAGNOSIS

DIFFERENTIAL DIAGNOSIS (Table 1-53)

- Bacterial vaginosis
- Fungal vulvovaginitis
- Cervicitis
- Atrophic vulvovaginitis

WORKUP

- Pelvic examination
- Speculum examination
- Mobile trichomonads seen on normal saline preparation: 70% sensitivity
- Elevated pH (>5) of vaginal discharge
- Culture is most sensitive commercially available method
- A large number of inflammatory cells on normal saline preparation
- Section III describes the evaluation of vaginal discharge

LABORATORY TESTS

- Culture (modified Diamond media): 90% sensitivity
- Direct enzyme immunoassay
- Fluorescein-conjugated monoclonal antibody test
- Pap test 40% detected

TREATMENT

NONPHARMACOLOGIC THERAPY

Condom use

ACUTE GENERAL Rx

Metronidazole (Flagyl) 2 g PO × 1 or 500 mg PO bid × 7 days *or* Tindamax (tinidazole) single 2 g oral dose in both sexes

CHRONIC Rx

- Metronidazole gel: less likely to achieve therapeutic levels; therefore not recommended
- Metronidazole (retreat): 500 mg PO bid × 7 days
- Treatment of future recurrences: Metronidazole 2 g PO qd × 3 to 5 days
- Allergy, intolerance, or adverse reactions: Alternatives to metronidazole are not available. Patients who are allergic to metronidazole can be managed by desensitization
- Pregnancy
  1. Associated with adverse outcomes (i.e., PROM)
  2. Metronidazole 2 g PO × 1 day

DISPOSITION

Trichomonas infection is considered an STD; therefore treatment of the sexual partner is necessary.

REFERRAL

To obstetrician/gynecologist for recurrence and pregnancy

EVIDENCE

A single oral dose of any nitroimidazole is effective in achieving parasitologic cure at short-term follow-up.[1] Ⓐ

Treatment of sexual partners may significantly reduce reinfection rates of Trichomonas vaginalis.[2] Ⓐ

The effects of metronidazole treatment on pregnancy outcomes remains uncertain and therefore treatment in pregnancy should be reserved for symptomatic infections only.[3] Ⓐ

Evidence-Based References

1. Forna F, Gülmezoglu AM: Interventions for treating trichomoniasis in women. In: Cochrane Library 3, Chichester, UK, 2004, John Wiley. Ⓐ
2. Lyng J, Christensen J: A double-blind study of the value of treatment with a single dose tinidazole of partners to females with trichomoniasis, *Acta Obstet Gynecol Scand* 60:199, 1981. Ⓐ
3. Gülmezoglu AM: Interventions for trichomoniasis in pregnancy. In: Cochrane Library 3, Chichester, UK, 2004, John Wiley. Ⓐ

TABLE 1-53 **Differential Diagnosis of Vaginitis**

Characteristics of Vaginal Discharge	*C. Albicans* Vaginitis	*T. Vaginalis* Vaginitis	Bacterial Vaginosis
pH	4.5	>5.0	>5.0
White curd	Usually	No	No
Odor with KOH	No	Yes	Yes
Clue cells	No	No	Usually
Motile trichomonads	No	Usually	No
Yeast cells3	Yes	No	No

From Goldman L, Ausiello D (eds): *Cecil textbook of medicine,* ed 22, Philadelphia, 2004, WB Saunders.

SUGGESTED READING

Workowski KA, Levine WC: Sexually transmitted diseases treatment guidelines, *MMWR Recomm Rep* 55:11, 2006.

AUTHORS: **JULIE ANNE SZUMIGALA, M.D.,** and **RUBEN ALVERO, M.D.**

BASIC INFORMATION

DEFINITION

Waldenström's macroglobulinemia (WM) is a plasma cell dyscrasia characterized by the presence of immunoglobulin (IgM) monoclonal macroglobulins.

SYNONYMS

WM
Monoclonal macroglobulinemia

ICD-9CM CODES
273.3 Waldenström's macroglobulinemia

EPIDEMIOLOGY & DEMOGRAPHICS

- Accounts for 2% of all hematologic cancers
- 1500 people diagnosed each year in the U.S.
- Overall incidence: 3 per million per year; 0.61/100,000 in men, 0.36/ 100,000 in women
- Median age varies between 63 and 68 yr
- More common among men than women and among whites than blacks

PHYSICAL FINDINGS & CLINICAL PRESENTATION

- Weakness
- Fatigue
- Weight loss
- Headache, dizziness, vertigo, deafness, and seizures (hyperviscosity syndrome)
- Easy bleeding (e.g., epistaxis)
- Retinal vein link-sausage shaped
- Lymphadenopathy (15%)
- Hepatomegaly (20%)
- Most commonly encountered neurological presentation is symmetric polyneuropathy
- Splenomegaly (15%)
- Purpura
- Peripheral neuropathy (5%)

ETIOLOGY

- The exact cause of WM is not known.
- Multiple reports suggest familial clustering, which indicates a genetic defect. In one study, chromosomal deletions in 6q21-22.1 were confirmed in 42% of WM patients, regardless of family history. In another study, the strongest evidence of linkage was found on chromosomes 1q and 4q.
- The main risk factor for development of WM is having IgM monoclonal gammopathy of unknown significance (MGUS).
- Radiation exposure, occupational chemicals, and chronic inflammatory stimulation have been suggested but there is insufficient evidence to substantiate these hypotheses.

DIAGNOSIS

The diagnosis of WM is usually established by laboratory blood tests and by bone marrow biopsy.

DIFFERENTIAL DIAGNOSIS

- MGUS
- Multiple myeloma
- Chronic lymphocytic leukemia
- Hairy-cell leukemia
- Lymphoma

WORKUP

In any patient suspected of having WM, specific blood tests (CBC, erythrocyte sedimentation rate [ESR], serum or urine protein electrophoresis [SPEP or UPEP, respectively], IgM level, beta 2-microglobulin, serum viscosity) should be ordered. Bone marrow biopsy will confirm the diagnosis.

LABORATORY TESTS

- CBC with differential:
  1. Anemia is a common finding, with a median hemoglobin value of approximately 10 g/dl. WBC count is usually normal; thrombocytopenia can occur.
  2. Peripheral smear may reveal malignant lymphoid cells in terminal patients.
- Elevated ESR.
- SPEP: homogeneous M spike
- Immunoelectrophoresis: confirms IgM
- Urine immunoelectrophoresis: monoclonal light chains are usually kappa chains. Bence Jones protein can be seen, but is not the typical finding in WM
- IgM levels are high, generally >3 g/dl
- Beta 2-microglobulin: elevated in 55%, high levels are associated with poor prognosis.
- Serum viscosity: symptoms usually occur when the serum viscosity is four times the viscosity of normal serum; classical feature although present in only 15% of cases.
- Cryoglobulins, rheumatoid factor, or cold agglutinins may be present
- Bone marrow biopsy: lymphoplasmacytoid cells are characteristic.

IMAGING STUDIES

Chest x-ray can be obtained to rule out pulmonary involvement.

TREATMENT

- Because of the incurable nature of WM, the aim of treatment is to relieve symptoms and reduce the risk of organ damage. Considerations for the initiation of treatment include the following: hemoglobin concentration less than 100 × 10^9/L, significant adenopathy or organomegaly, symptomatic hyperviscosity, severe neuropathy, amyloidosis, cryoglobulinemia, cold-agglutinin disease, or evidence of disease transformation.
- Treatment is directed at both hyperviscocity and the lymphoproliferative disorder itself.

NONPHARMACOLOGIC THERAPY

Asymptomatic patients do not require treatment, and these patients should be monitored periodically for the onset of symptoms or changes in blood tests (e.g., worsening anemia, thrombocytopenia, rising IgM, and serum viscosity).

ACUTE GENERAL Rx

1. Plasmapharesis is the treatment used to alleviate symptoms of hyperviscocity.
2. Treatment of the lymphoproliferative disorder includes the age of combination therapy:
   a. Rituximab, a monoclonal anti-CD 20 antibody, in combination with nucleoside analogs.
   b. Nucleoside analogs and alkylator agents (chlorambucil).
   c. Combination chemotherapy such as CHOP (cyclophosphamide, vincristine, prednisone, doxorubicin): studies suggest combination therapy is on par if not better than single-agent therapy.

CHRONIC Rx

- Refractory patients can be retried on original therapy if length of response from initial therapy is greater than 2 yr. If the response from the initial therapy was <2 yr, alternative first-line agents such as fludarabine or cladribine can be used.
- Other treatment options: interferon alpha, thalidomide, and autologous stem cell transplantation.

DISPOSITION

- The onset of WM is slow and insidious. Most patients die from progression of the disease with hyperviscosity, hemorrhage, and infection, or from congestive heart failure.
- Some patients develop acute myelogenous leukemia, immunoblastic sarcoma, or chronic myelogenous leukemia as a preterminal event.
- Median survival in patients with WM is about 4 yr.
- Approximately 10% of patients will achieve complete remission, with prognosis being more favorable (median survival 11 yr).
- A staging system using serum beta 2-microglobulin concentration, hemoglobin concentration, and serum IgM concentration before treatment pro-

vides insight into prognosis and survival.
- Other factors can negatively affect the survival: age >65, male gender, the presence of organomegaly and the presence of cytopenias.

REFERRAL

If WM is suspected, a hematology consultation is helpful in guiding future workup, treatment, and monitoring.

PEARLS & CONSIDERATIONS

COMMENTS

- WM was first described in 1944 by the Swedish physician Jan Gosta Waldenström.
- Amyloidosis is rare, occurring in 5% of patients with WM.

SUGGESTED READINGS

Dimopoulos MA, Anagnostopoulos A: Waldenström's macroglobulinemia, *Best Pract Res Clin Haematol* 18(4):747, 2005.

Gertz MA: Waldenström macroglobulinemia: a review of therapy, *Am J Hematol* 79(2):147, 2005.

Fonseca R, Hayman S: Waldenström macroglobulinaemia, *Br J Haematol* 138:700, 2007.

Vijay A, Gertz MA: Waldenström macroglobulinemia, *Blood* 109(12):5096, 2007.

AUTHOR: **RAMI ELTIBI, M.D.**

BASIC INFORMATION

DEFINITION

Warts are benign epidermal neoplasms caused by human papillomavirus (HPV).

SYNONYMS

Verruca vulgaris (common warts)
Verruca plana (flat warts)
Condyloma acuminatum (venereal warts)
Verruca plantaris (plantar warts)
Mosaic warts (cluster of many warts)

ICD-9CM CODES
078.10 Viral warts
0.78.19 Venereal wart (external genital organs)

EPIDEMIOLOGY & DEMOGRAPHICS

- Common warts occur most frequently in children and young adults.
- Anogenital warts are most common in young, sexually active patients. Genital warts are the most common viral STD in the U.S., with up to 24 million Americans carrying the virus that causes them.
- Common warts are longer lasting and more frequent in immunocompromised patients (e.g., lymphoma, AIDS, immunosuppressive drugs).
- Plantar warts occur most frequently at points of maximal pressure (over the heads of the metatarsal bones or on the heels).

PHYSICAL FINDINGS & CLINICAL PRESENTATION

- Common warts (Fig. 1-292) have an initial appearance of a flesh-colored papule with a rough surface; they subsequently develop a hyperkeratotic appearance with black dots on the surface (thrombosed capillaries); they may be single or multiple and are most common on the hands.
- Warts obscure normal skin lines (important diagnostic feature). Cylindrical projections from the wart may become fused, forming a mosaic pattern.
- Flat warts generally are pink or light yellow, slightly elevated, and often found on the forehead, back of hands, mouth, and beard area; they often occur in lines corresponding to trauma (e.g., a scratch); are often misdiagnosed (particularly when present on the face) and inappropriately treated with topical corticosteroids.
- Filiform warts have a fingerlike appearance with various projections; they are generally found near the mouth, beard, or periorbital and paranasal regions.
- Plantar warts are slightly raised and have a roughened surface; they may cause pain when walking; as they involute, small hemorrhages (caused by thrombosed capillaries) may be noted.
- Genital warts are generally pale pink with several projections and a broad base. They may coalesce in the perineal area to form masses with a cauliflower-like appearance.
- Genital warts on the cervical epithelium can produce subclinical changes that may be noted on Pap smear or colposcopy.

ETIOLOGY

- Human papillomavirus (HPV) infection; >60 types of viral DNA have been identified. Transmission of warts is by direct contact.
- Genital warts are usually caused by HPV types 6 or 11.

DIAGNOSIS

DIFFERENTIAL DIAGNOSIS

- Molluscum contagiosum
- Condyloma latum
- Acrochordon (skin tags) or seborrheic keratosis
- Epidermal nevi
- Hypertrophic actinic keratosis
- Squamous cell carcinomas
- Acquired digital fibrokeratoma
- Varicella zoster virus in patients with AIDS
- Recurrent infantile digital fibroma
- Plantar corns (may be mistaken for plantar warts)

WORKUP

- Diagnosis is generally based on clinical findings.
- Suspect lesions should be biopsied.

LABORATORY TESTS

Colposcopy with biopsy of patients with cervical squamous cell changes

TREATMENT

NONPHARMACOLOGIC THERAPY

- Importance of use of condoms to reduce transmission of genital warts should be emphasized.
- Watchful waiting is an acceptable option in the treatment of warts, because many warts will disappear without intervention over time.
- Plantar warts that are not painful do not need treatment.

GENERAL Rx

- Common warts:
  1. Application of topical salicylic acid 17% (e.g., Duofilm). Soak area for 5 min in warm water and dry. Apply thin layer once or twice daily for up to 12 wk, avoiding normal skin. Bandage.
  2. Liquid nitrogen, electrocautery are also common methods of removal.
  3. Blunt dissection can be used in large lesions or resistant lesions.

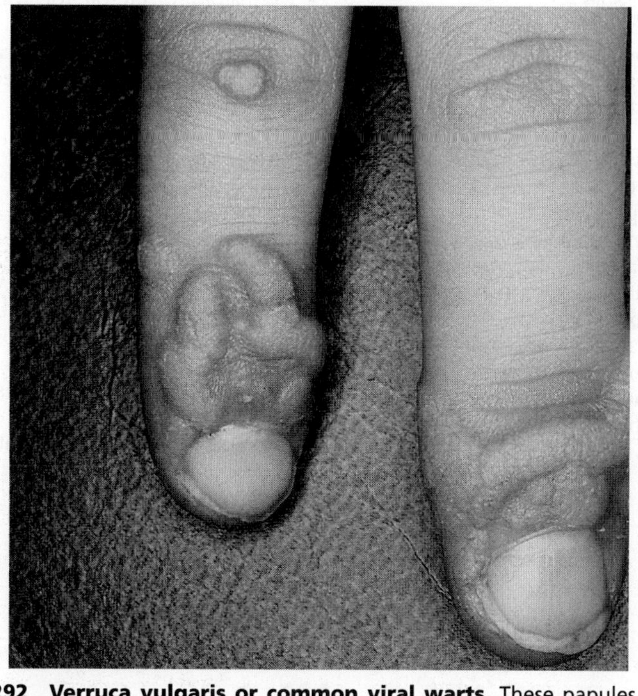

FIGURE 1-292 Verruca vulgaris or common viral warts. These papules often have verrucous surface changes. (From Callen JP: *Color atlas of dermatology,* ed 2, Philadelphia, 2000, WB Saunders.)

4. Duct tape occlusion is also effective for treating common warts. It is cut to cover warts and left in place for 6 days. It is removed after 6 days and the warts are soaked in water and then filed with pumice stones. New tape is applied 12 hr later. This treatment can be repeated until warts resolve.
- Filiform warts: surgical removal is necessary.
- Flat warts: generally more difficult to treat.
  1. Tretinoin cream applied at hs over the involved area for several weeks may be effective
  2. Application of liquid nitrogen
  3. Electrocautery
  4. 5-Fluorouracil cream (Efudex 5%) applied once or twice a day for 3 to 5 wk is also effective. Persistent hyperpigmentation may occur following Efudex use
- Plantar warts:
  1. Salicylic acid therapy (e.g., Occlusal-HP). Soak wart in warm water for 5 min, remove loose tissue, dry. Apply to area, allow to dry, reapply. Use once or twice daily; maximum 12 wk. Use of 40% salicylic acid plasters (Mediplast) is also a safe, nonscarring treatment; it is particularly useful in treating mosaic warts covering a large area.
  2. Blunt dissection is also a fast and effective treatment modality.
  3. Laser therapy can be used for plantar warts and recurrent warts; however, it leaves open wounds that require 4 to 6 wk to fill with granulation tissue.
  4. Interlesional bleomycin is also effective but generally used when all other treatments fail.
- Genital warts:
  1. Can be effectively treated with 20% podophyllin resin in compound tincture of benzoin applied with a cotton tip applicator by the treating physician and allowed to air dry. The treatment can be repeated weekly if necessary.
  2. Podofilox (Condylox 0.5% gel) is now available for application by the patient. Local adverse effects include pain, burning, and inflammation at the site.
  3. Cryosurgery with liquid nitrogen delivered with a probe or as a spray is effective for treating smaller genital warts.
  4. Carbon dioxide laser can also be used for treating primary or recurrent genital warts (cure rate >90%).
  5. Imiquimod (Aldara) cream, 5% is a patient-applied immune response modifier effective in the treatment of external genital and perianal warts (complete clearing of genital warts in >70% of females and >30% of males in 4 to 16 wk). Sexual contact should be avoided while the cream is on the skin. It is applied three times/wk before normal sleeping hours and is left on the skin for 6 to 10 hr.
- Application of trichloroacetic acid (TCA) or bichloracetic acid (BCA) 80% to 90% is also effective for external genital warts. A small amount should be applied only to warts and allowed to dry, at which time a white "frosting" develops. This treatment can be repeated weekly if necessary.

DISPOSITION

- Warts can be effectively treated with the previous modalities, with complete resolution in the majority of patients; however, recurrence rate is high.
- Cervical carcinomas and precancerous lesions in women are associated with genital papillomavirus infection.
- Squamous cell anal cancer is also associated with a history of genital warts.

REFERRAL

- Dermatology referral for warts resistant to conservative therapy
- Surgical referral in selected cases
- STD counseling for patients with anogenital warts

PEARLS & CONSIDERATIONS

COMMENTS

- Subungual and periungual warts are generally more resistant to treatment. Dermatology referral for cryosurgery is recommended in resistant cases.
- Examination of sex partners is not necessary for the management of genital warts because no data indicate that reinfection plays a role.

EVIDENCE (EBM)

Genital

Podofilox has been shown to be more effective than placebo after 16 weeks of treatment.[1] Ⓐ

No significant difference has been found between podofilox and podophyllin resin in terms of genital wart clearance.[1] Ⓐ

Imiquimod is more effective than placebo in clearing genital warts and reducing recurrences in non-HIV-infected patients.[2] Ⓐ

Palmar-Plantar

Salicylic acid is an effective treatment for cutaneous warts.

Topical treatments containing salicylic acid are clearly better than placebo for the treatment of cutaneous warts.[3] Ⓐ

The reviewers note that there is some evidence that cryotherapy is of only equivalent efficacy to simpler, safer treatments, including topical salicylic acid.[3] Ⓑ

Cryotherapy is significantly less effective than treatment with duct tape at producing complete resolution.[4] Ⓑ

There is no significant difference between cryotherapy at intervals of 2 weeks, 3 weeks, or 4 weeks in terms of wart clearance.[3] Ⓐ

There is no significant difference between no further treatment vs. prolonging cryotherapy for a further 3 months (after 6 months of therapy) in terms of the proportion of patients with clearance of warts.[3] Ⓐ

Evidence-Based References

1. Wiley DJ: Genital warts. In: *Clin Evid* 9, web version only, London, 2003, BMJ Publishing Group. Ⓐ
2. Moore RA et al: Imiquimod for the treatment of genital warts: a quantitative systematic review, *BMC Infect Dis* 1:3, 2001. Reviewed in: *Clin Evid* 10, 2003, web version only. Ⓐ
3. Gibbs S et al: Local treatments for cutaneous warts (Cochrane Review). In: The Cochrane Library 2, Oxford, 2003, Update Software. Reviewed In: *Clin Evid* 9:1868, 2003. ⒶⒷ
4. Focht DR, Spicer C, Fairchok MP: The efficacy of duct tape vs cryotherapy in the treatment of verruca vulgaris (the common wart), *Arch Pediatr Adolesc Med* 156:971, 2002. Ⓑ

SUGGESTED READING

Bacelieri R, Johnson SM: Cutaneous warts: an evidence-based approach to therapy, *Am Fam Physician* 72:647, 2005.

AUTHOR: **FRED F. FERRI, M.D.**

BASIC INFORMATION

DEFINITION

Wegener granulomatosis is a multisystem disease generally consisting of the classic triad of:

1. Necrotizing granulomatous lesions in the upper or lower respiratory tract
2. Generalized focal necrotizing vasculitis involving both arteries and veins
3. Focal glomerulonephritis of the kidneys

"Limited forms" of the disease can also occur and may evolve into the classic triad; Wegener granulomatosis can be classified using the "ELK" classification, which identifies the three major sites of involvement: *E,* ears, nose, and throat or respiratory tract; *L,* lungs; *K,* kidneys.

ICD-9CM CODES
446.4 Wegener's granulomatosis

EPIDEMIOLOGY & DEMOGRAPHICS

INCIDENCE: 3/100,000 persons, equal in men and women
MEAN AGE AT ONSET: 41 yr

PHYSICAL FINDINGS & CLINICAL PRESENTATION

- Clinical manifestations often vary with the stage of the disease and degree of organ involvement. 90% of patients present with symptoms involving the upper or lower airways or both.
- Frequent manifestations are:
  1. Upper respiratory tract: chronic sinusitis, chronic otitis media, mastoiditis, nasal crusting, obstruction and epistaxis, nasal septal perforation, nasal lacrimal duct stenosis, saddle nose deformities (resulting from cartilage destruction)
  2. Lung: hemoptysis, multiple nodules, diffuse alveolar pattern
  3. Kidney: renal insufficiency, glomerulonephritis
  4. Skin: necrotizing skin lesions
  5. Nervous system: mononeuritis multiplex, cranial nerve involvement
  6. Joints: monarthritis or polyarthritis (nondeforming), usually affecting large joints
  7. Mouth: chronic ulcerative lesions of the oral mucosa, "mulberry" gingivitis
  8. Eye: proptosis, uveitis, episcleritis, retinal and optic nerve vasculitis

ETIOLOGY

Unknown

DIAGNOSIS

DIFFERENTIAL DIAGNOSIS

- Other granulomatous lung diseases (e.g., sarcoidosis, lymphomatoid granulomatosis, Churg-Strauss syndrome, necrotizing sarcoid granulomatosis, bronchocentric granulomatosis, sarcoidosis); the differential diagnosis of granulomatous lung disease is described in Section II
- Neoplasms (especially lymphoproliferative disease)
- Goodpasture's syndrome
- Bacterial or fungal sinusitis
- Midline granuloma
- Viral infections
- Other causes of glomerulonephritis (e.g., poststreptococcal nephritis)

WORKUP

- Wegener granulomatosis should be suspected in anyone presenting with sinus disease that does not respond to conventional treatment, pulmonary hemorrhage, glomerulonephritis, mononeuritis multiplex resulting in wrist or foot drop, progressive migratory arthralgias or arthritis, and unexplained multisystem disease.
- Chest x-ray, laboratory evaluation, PFTs, and tissue biopsy.

LABORATORY TESTS

- Positive test for cytoplasmic pattern of ANCA (c-ANCA).
- Anemia, leukocytosis.
- Urinalysis: may reveal hematuria, RBC casts, and proteinuria.
- Elevated serum creatinine, decreased creatinine clearance.
- Increased ESR, positive rheumatoid factor, and elevated C-reactive protein may be found.

IMAGING STUDIES

- Chest x-ray: may reveal bilateral multiple nodules, cavitated mass lesions, pleural effusion (20%). Up to one third of patients without pulmonary signs or symptoms have an abnormal chest x-ray.
- PFTs: useful in detecting stenosis of the airways.
- Biopsy of one or more affected organs should be attempted; the most reliable source for tissue diagnosis is the lung. Lesions in the nasopharynx (if present) can be easily biopsied but biopsy is positive in only 20%. Biopsy of radiographically abnormal pulmonary parenchyma provides the highest yield (>90%).

TREATMENT

NONPHARMACOLOGIC THERAPY

- Ensure proper airway drainage.
- Give nutritional counseling.

ACUTE GENERAL Rx

- Prednisone 60 to 80 mg/day and cyclophosphamide 2 mg/kg are generally effective and are used to control clinical manifestations; once the disease comes under control, prednisone is tapered and cyclophosphamide is continued. Other potentially useful agents in patients intolerant to cyclophosphamide are methotrexate, azathioprine, and mycophenolate mofetil.
- TMP-SMX therapy may represent a useful alternative in patients with lesions limited to the upper or lower respiratory tracts in absence of vasculitis or nephritis. Treatment with TMP-SMX (160 mg/800 mg bid) also reduces the incidence of relapses in patients with Wegener granulomatosis in remission. It is also useful in preventing *Pneumocystis carinii* pneumonia, which occurs in 10% of patients receiving induction therapy. When used for prophylaxis, dose of TMP-SMX (160 mg/800 mg) is 1 tablet three times/wk.

DISPOSITION

Five-year survival with aggressive treatment is approximately 80%; without treatment 2-yr survival is <20%.

REFERRAL

Surgical referral for biopsy

PEARLS & CONSIDERATIONS

COMMENTS

- Methotrexate (20 mg/wk) represents an alternative to cyclophosphamide in patients who do not have immediately life-threatening disease.
- C-ANCA levels should not dictate changes in therapy, because they correlate erratically with disease activity.
- The incidence of venous thrombotic events in Wegener granulomatosis is significantly higher than the general population. Clinicians should maintain a heightened awareness of the risks of venous thrombosis and a lower threshold for evaluating patients for possible DVT or pulmonary embolism.

SUGGESTED READINGS

Finkielman JD et al: Antiproteinase 3 antineutrophil cytoplasmic antibodies and disease activity in Wegener granulomatosis, *Ann Intern Med* 147(9):611-619.
Langford CA: Update on Wegener granulomatosis, *Cleve Clin J Med* 72:689-697, 2005.
Merkel PA et al: Brief communication: high incidence of venous thrombotic events among patients with Wegener granulomatosis: the Wegener's Clinical Occurrence of Thrombosis (WeCLOT) study, *Ann Intern Med* 142:620-626, 2005.

AUTHOR: **FRED F. FERRI, M.D.**

BASIC INFORMATION

DEFINITION

Wernicke's encephalopathy is the syndrome of acute extraocular muscle dysfunction, confusion, and ataxia, resulting from thiamine deficiency.

SYNONYMS

Korsakoff's syndrome
Wernicke-Korsakoff syndrome
Alcoholic polyneuritic psychosis

ICD-9CM CODES
265.1 Wernicke's encephalopathy, disease, or syndrome

EPIDEMIOLOGY & DEMOGRAPHICS

- Most commonly associated with alcohol abuse; consider in other conditions where malabsorption or altered metabolism may occur (e.g., hyperemesis gravidarum, gastric bypass)
- Slightly more common in males
- Age of onset evenly distributed between ages 30 and 70

PHYSICAL FINDINGS & CLINICAL PRESENTATION

- Disturbance of extraocular motility, including nystagmus, abducens nerve palsy, and disorders of conjugate gaze.
- Encephalopathy.
- Ataxia of gait.
- Peripheral neuropathy may be seen in addition to the typical findings described previously.

ETIOLOGY

Thiamine deficiency from alcohol abuse or other malnourished state. It may be iatrogenic from prolonged dextrose infusion without thiamine supplementation.

DIAGNOSIS

DIFFERENTIAL DIAGNOSIS

- Thiamine deficiency, including alcohol abuse, malnutrition, or iatrogenic cause
- Stroke, mass lesion, or trauma affecting upper brainstem, thalamus, and associated structures

WORKUP

Patients must be evaluated with a high index of suspicion, and treated rapidly, even in advance of laboratory results.

LABORATORY TESTS

- CBC.
- Serum chemistries.
- Serum pyruvate is elevated.
- Whole-blood or erythrocyte transketolase are decreased; rapid resolution to normal in 24 hr with thiamine repletion.

IMAGING STUDIES

- MRI may show T2 hyperintense diencephalic and mesencephalic lesions acutely, but there is no definitive radiologic study for diagnosis.
- CT scan may show cerebral atrophy from chronic alcoholism.

TREATMENT

NONPHARMACOLOGIC THERAPY

Alcoholics Anonymous

ACUTE GENERAL Rx

- 100 mg thiamine IV or IM immediately; typically thiamine IV for 3 to 5 days, then oral.
- Avoid dextrose-containing fluids until thiamine repleted.
- Prophylactic treatment for delirium tremens if alcoholic.

CHRONIC Rx

- Attempt to treat alcoholism or underlying malnourished state.
- Chronic oral thiamine repletion; typical dose 5 mg/day.
- Case reports suggest donepezil may help chronic memory problems.
- Inadequately treated disease may progress to Korsakoff's psychosis (see relevant entry).

DISPOSITION

Enter substance abuse program after acute phase. Long-term care is determined by level of recovery.

REFERRAL

Neurology should be consulted if symptoms do not resolve after thiamine therapy.

PEARLS & CONSIDERATIONS

COMMENTS

- Give thiamine if the disease is even suspected.
- Prognosis is generally poor, with 10%-20% mortality even with treatment. Most patients will be left with impaired learning and memory, which may be subtle.
- A preventable cause is prolonged dextrose-containing IV fluids without supplemental thiamine.

EVIDENCE

Thiamine has been established as the treatment of choice for over 50 years. The evidence for its benefit is based on case reports and clinical experience. No randomized controlled trials (RCTs) are available to guide clinicians in the dosage, route, or duration of therapy in the acute presentation of the syndrome.

A recent RCT that looked at alcoholics without frank clinical evidence of Korsakoff's psychosis showed that those treated with the highest dose of thiamine showed neuropsychologic evidence of improvement in working memory, suggesting that even "asymptomatic" alcoholics may benefit from thiamine supplementation.[1,2]

Evidence-Based References

1. Ambrose ML et al: Thiamine treatment and working memory function of alcohol-dependent people: preliminary findings, *Alcohol Clin Exp Res* 25(1):112-116, 2001.
2. Day E et al: Thiamine for Wernicke-Korsakoff syndrome in people at risk from alcohol abuse, *Cochrane Database Syst Rev* 1:CD004033, 2004.

SUGGESTED READINGS

Cochrane et al: Acetylcholinesterase inhibitors for the treatment of Wernicke-Korsakoff syndrome—three further cases show response to donepezil, *Alcohol Alcohol* 40(2):151-154, 2005.

Cook CC: Prevention and treatment of Wernicke-Korsakoff syndrome, *Alcohol Alcohol Suppl* 35(suppl 1):19, 2000.

Harper C: Thiamine (vitamin B1) deficiency and associated brain damage is still common throughout the world and prevention is simple and safe! *Eur J Neurol* 13(10):1078, 2006.

Martin PR et al: The role of thiamine deficiency in alcoholic brain disease, *Alcohol Res Health* 27(2):134-142, 2003.

Sechi G, Serra A: Wernicke's encephalopathy: new clinical settings and recent advances in diagnosis and management, *Lancet Neurol* 6(5):442, 2007.

Zubaran C, Fernandes JG, Rodnight R: Wernicke-Korsakoff syndrome, *Postgrad Med J* 73(855):27, 1997.

AUTHOR: **DANIEL MATTSON, M.D., M.SC.(MED.)**

BASIC INFORMATION

DEFINITION

West Nile virus infection is an illness affecting the central nervous system (CNS) caused by the mosquito-borne West Nile virus.

SYNONYMS

West Nile virus fever
West Nile virus encephalitis
Neuroinvasive West Nile virus infection
Nonneuroinvasive West Nile virus infection

ICD-9CM CODES
066.4 West Nile virus infection

EPIDEMIOLOGY & DEMOGRAPHICS

- Before 1999, West Nile virus (WNV) infection was confined to areas in the Middle East, with occasional outbreaks in Europe. The infection began being diagnosed in the Western hemisphere in 1999. First seen in the northeast and mid-Atlantic states, West Nile virus infection has spread steadily, each year, to new regions of the U.S., with a general westward migration pattern. In the year 2003, a record number of cases were reported from the U.S., with over 7000 cases reported resulting in several hundred deaths. Most deaths occur in elderly patients with WNV encephalitis. In 2003, the midwestern states of Illinois, Ohio, Michigan, and Louisiana were hardest hit. In 2004 and 2005, the incidence of WNV infection diminished gradually as it spread to the western states. Human cases of WNV infection have now been reported across all the contiguous continental U.S. (sparing only Hawaii and Alaska). More than 4200 neuroinvasive and nonneuroinvasive cases were reported in the U.S. in 2006.
- The virus is carried by a number of species of birds, as well as horses and several other animals. It is transmitted to humans through the bite of an infected mosquito. For this reason, West Nile virus infection is seen primarily from mid-summer to mid-autumn, the period of maximum mosquito intensity.
- The majority of severe cases have been reported among individuals >50 yr of age. There is no gender predilection.
- Person-to-person transmission is fortunately rare but has been reported to occur by blood transfusion, organ transplantation, breastfeeding, and perhaps by perinatal transmission; the blood supply is now routinely tested by nucleic acid testing methods to reduce the risk of transmission-acquired WNV in the U.S.

PHYSICAL FINDINGS & CLINICAL PRESENTATION

- Less than 20% of infected individuals develop symptomatic disease. The initial phase of illness is nonspecific, with abrupt onset of fever accompanied by malaise, eye pain, anorexia, headache, and, occasionally, rash and lymphadenopathy. Less commonly, myocarditis, hepatitis, or pancreatitis may occur.
- In approximately 1 in 150 cases, especially among elderly patients, severe neurologic sequelae will occur. Most common among these are ataxia, cranial nerve palsies, optic neuritis, seizures, myelitis, and polyradiculitis.

ETIOLOGY

The West Nile virus is a member of the flavivirus group, along with the yellow fever, dengue, St. Louis, and Japanese encephalitis viruses. It has a large reservoir in nature, infecting many species of birds, as well as certain mammals, and is thought to be spread to humans exclusively by various species of mosquito. Neurologic disease is caused by direct invasion of the CNS.

DIAGNOSIS

Dx

DIFFERENTIAL DIAGNOSIS

- Meningitis or encephalitis caused by more common viruses (e.g., enteroviruses, herpes simplex)
- Bacterial meningitis
- Vasculitis
- Fungal meningitis (e.g., cryptococcal infection)
- Tuberculous meningitis

LABORATORY TESTS

- CBC, electrolytes (hyponatremia common)
- Spinal tap and CSF examination: typically demonstrates lymphocytic pleocytosis with normal level of glucose and elevated level of protein
- CSF West Nile virus IgM antibody level: rare false-positive results in persons recently vaccinated to Japanese encephalitis or yellow fever viruses

IMAGING STUDIES

CT or MRI studies of the brain to exclude mass lesions; cerebral edema

TREATMENT

Rx

NONPHARMACOLOGIC THERAPY

Hospitalization, intravenous hydration, ventilator support may be necessary.

ACUTE GENERAL Rx

No specific therapy has been established in clinical trials. Ribavirin and interferon alpha-2b have been shown to have in vitro activity against the virus. Intravenous immune globulin from convalescent patient plasma is under study but no controlled trials have been reported as yet.

CHRONIC Rx

Chronic rehabilitation therapy usually necessary for patients with severe neurologic impairment. Mental status defects following WNV neuroinvasive disease appear to be more common and severe than initially recognized.

DISPOSITION

Chronic rehabilitation as needed following recovery from acute infection

REFERRAL

- Infectious disease consultant
- Public health authorities

PEARLS & CONSIDERATIONS

COMMENTS

- Diagnosis requires a high index of suspicion, because disease course may be nonspecific and may mimic other, more common disorders.
- Specific laboratory diagnostic studies are available only through public health laboratories.
- Best means of prevention is reduction in mosquito population by draining of stagnant water deposits and, if necessary, insecticide spraying.
- Individuals may reduce risk by covering arms and legs in areas where mosquitoes are likely to be found and using insect repellent containing DEET.

EVIDENCE

EBM

We are unable to cite evidence that meets our criteria.

SUGGESTED READINGS

Carson PJ et al: Long-term clinical and neuropsychological outcomes of West Nile virus infection, *Clin Infect Dis* 43(6):723, 2006.

CDC: Update: West Nile virus activity—United States, 2005, *MMWR* 54(34):851-852, 2005.

Gottfried K, Quinn R, Jones T: Clinical description and follow-up investigation of human West Nile Virus cases, *South Med J* 98(6):603-606, 2005.

Haaland KY et al: Mental status after West Nile virus infection, *Emerg Infect Dis* 12(8):1260, 2006.

Higgs S et al: Nonviremic transmission of West Nile virus, *Proc Natl Acad Sci U S A* 102(25):8871-8874, 2005.

Stramer SL et al: West Nile virus among blood donors in the United States, 2003 and 2004, *N Engl J Med* 353(5):451-459, 2005.

AUTHORS: **GLENN G. FORT, M.D., M.P.H., DENNIS J. MIKOLICH, M.D.,** and **JOSEPH R. MASCI, M.D.**

BASIC INFORMATION

DEFINITION

Whiplash refers to a hyperextension injury to the neck, often the result of being struck from behind by a fast-moving vehicle.

SYNONYMS

Acceleration flexion-extension neck injury

ICD-9CM CODES
847.0 Whiplash injury or syndrome

EPIDEMIOLOGY & DEMOGRAPHICS

- Whiplash occurs in more than 1 million people each year.
- Most injuries (40%) are the result of rear-end motor vehicle accidents.
- Whiplash occurs at all ages, in both sexes, and at all socioeconomic levels.
- Incidence is 4 per 1000 persons and is higher in women than men.
- Nearly 50% of patients with whiplash seek legal advice.
- Whiplash is also seen in shaken baby syndrome.

PHYSICAL FINDINGS & CLINICAL PRESENTATION

- Most present with a history of being involved in a motor vehicle accident and rear-ended by another vehicle
- Pain not present initially but usually develops hours to a few days later
- Neck tightness and stiffness
- Occipital headache
- Shoulder, arm, and back pain
- Numbness in the arms
- Tinnitus
- TMJ pain
- Dysphagia (retropharyngeal hematoma)
- Decreased range of motion of the neck
- Depressive symptoms

ETIOLOGY

- The mechanism of injury is due to the sudden acceleration of the body forward, forcing the neck to hyperextend backward, causing injury to ligaments, muscles, bone, and/or intervertebral disk. At the end of the accident the head is thrust forward in a flexion position, sometimes causing injury to C5-C6-C7.
- Motor vehicle accidents, trauma from falls, contact sports, physical abuse, and altercations are all possible causes of whiplash.
- The incidence of whiplash injury following polytrauma is low.
- Low-velocity crashes constitute a major cause of whiplash injury.

DIAGNOSIS

DIFFERENTIAL DIAGNOSIS

- Osteoarthritis
- Cervical disk disease
- Fibrositis
- Neuritis
- Torticollis
- Spinal cord tumor
- TMJ syndrome
- Tension headache
- Migraine headache

WORKUP

Any patient who presents with symptoms of whiplash and musculoskeletal or neurologic signs merits a workup to exclude cervical spine fractures or herniated disk disease.

LABORATORY TESTS

Laboratory studies are not helpful.

IMAGING STUDIES

- Plain C-spine films (AP, lateral, and odontoid views)
- Flexion/extension x-rays
- CT scan to exclude fracture
- MRI

TREATMENT

NONPHARMACOLOGIC THERAPY

- Soft cervical collar for no longer than 72 hr
- Moist heat 15 to 20 min 4 to 6 times per day
- Continue with usual activities

ACUTE GENERAL Rx

- Analgesics
  1. Ibuprofen 800 mg PO tid
  2. Naproxen 500 mg PO bid
  3. Acetaminophen 1 g PO qid
- Muscle relaxants (short-term use)
  1. Cyclobenzaprine 10 mg PO tid
  2. Methocarbamol 1 g PO qid
  3. Carisoprodol 350 mg PO qid

CHRONIC Rx

NSAIDs can be used long term.

DISPOSITION

- Most patients recover from the acute whiplash injury within weeks.
- 20% to 40% may develop chronic whiplash syndrome (symptoms of headache, neck pain, and psychiatric complaints that persist for 6 mo).
- Older age, female gender, lawyer involvement, and being at work before entry to the clinic were found to be prognostic factors associated with a negative outcome.

REFERRAL

Orthopedic

PEARLS & CONSIDERATIONS

COMMENTS

- Nearly one third of all personal injury cases involve cervical injuries.
- There is no dose-response relationship between trauma severity and incidence of whiplash injury.
- The entity of chronic whiplash syndrome remains elusive. Some authorities argue that financial motivation is a factor leading to persistent neck symptoms. Other studies do not substantiate this, countering a true chronic injury to the soft tissues of the neck.

EVIDENCE

High-dose methylprednisolone has been shown to be effective in improving outcomes after acute spinal cord injury, provided that it can be administered within 8 hours of injury and continued for 23 hours.[1] Ⓐ

Two systematic reviews found a general lack of evidence supporting treatments used in acute whiplash injury.[2,3]

One of the reviews found that early mobilization resulted in better pain relief and improved range of motion at 4 and 8 weeks compared with immobilization, analgesics, rest, and education.[2] Ⓐ

The other review found a trend toward active interventions being more effective than passive.[3] Ⓐ

Active mobilization was shown to be significantly more effective than rest plus a collar in one randomized controlled trial, but only when commenced immediately after the injury.[4] Ⓐ

A meta-analysis in people with chronic neck or back pain with acute spasm found cyclobenzaprine significantly improved symptoms compared with placebo after 2 weeks.[5] Ⓑ

A randomized, parallel-group trial showed that immobilization, "act-as-usual," and mobilization had similar effects regarding prevention of pain, disability, and work capability 1 year after a whiplash injury.[6]

Evidence-Based References

1. Bracken MB: Steroids for acute spinal cord injury, *Cochrane Database Syst Rev* 2:2002. Ⓐ
2. Spitzer WO et al: Scientific monograph of the Quebec Task Force on whiplash-associated disorders: redefining 'whiplash' and its management, *Spine* 20(suppl 8):1, 1995. Reviewed in: *Clin Evid* 13:2005. Ⓐ

3. Verhagen AP et al: Conservative treatments for whiplash, *Cochrane Database Syst Rev* 1:2004. Ⓐ
4. Rosenfeld M, Gunnarsson R, Borenstein P: Early intervention in whiplash-associated disorders: a comparison of two treatment protocols, *Spine* 25:1782, 2000. Reviewed in: *Clin Evid* 10:1377, 2003. Ⓐ
5. Aker PD et al: Conservative management of mechanical neck pain: systematic overview and meta-analysis, *BMJ* 313:1291, 1996. Reviewed in: *Clin Evid* 10:1377, 2003. Ⓑ
6. Kongsted A et al: Neck collar, "act-as-usual" or active mobilization for whiplash injury? A randomized parallel-group trial, *Spine* 32(6):618, 2007.

SUGGESTED READINGS

Carroll LJ et al: Frequency, timing, and course of depressive symptomatology after whiplash, *Spine* 31(16):E551, 2006.

Dufton JA et al: Prognostic factors associated with minimal improvement following acute whiplash-associated disorders, *Spine* 31(20): E759, 2006.

Giannoudis PV et al: Incidence and outcome of whiplash injury after multiple trauma, *Spine* 32(7):776, 2007

Rodriquez AA, Barr KP, Burns SP: Whiplash: pathophysiology, diagnosis, treatment, and prognosis, *Muscle Nerve* 29(6):768, 2004.

Sterner Y, Gerdle B: Acute and chronic whiplash disorders—a review, *J Rehabil Med* 36(5):193, 2004.

AUTHOR: **JORGE VILLAFUERTE, M.D.**

BASIC INFORMATION

DEFINITION

Whipple's disease is a multisystem illness characterized by malabsorption and its consequences, lymphadenopathy, arthritis, cardiac involvement, ocular symptoms and neurologic problems, caused by the gram-positive bacillus *Tropheryma whippeli*.

SYNONYMS

Intestinal lipodystrophy (name used by Dr. Whipple in 1907)

ICD-9CM CODES
040.2 Whipple's disease

EPIDEMIOLOGY & DEMOGRAPHICS

- Uncommon illness (only about 1000 cases have been reported to date)
- Peak age: 30 to 60 yr of age; mean age at diagnosis is 50
- More frequent in men than women and in Caucasians
- Specific environmental factors have not been associated with Whipple's disease.

PHYSICAL FINDINGS & CLINICAL PRESENTATION

PHYSICAL FINDINGS:

- Abdominal distention, sometimes with tenderness and less commonly fullness or mass, which represents enlarged mesenteric lymph nodes
- Signs of weight loss, cachexia
- Clubbing
- Lymphadenopathy
- Inflamed joints
- Heart murmur or rub
- Sensory loss or motor weakness related to peripheral neuropathy
- Abnormal mental status examination
- Pallor

CLINICAL PRESENTATION: Whipple's disease is characterized by 2 stages: a prodromal stage and a much later steady-state stage. The prodromal stage is marked by protean symptoms and chronic arthralgias and arthritis. The steady-state stage, which follows the prodromal stage by an average time of 6 years, is manifested with weight loss, diarrhea, or both. When the disease presents with extraintestinal symptoms (e.g., arthralgia), few clinicians will suspect the diagnosis unless or until GI symptoms are present. Weight loss, diarrhea, and arthropathies are found together in 75% of patients at time of diagnosis. The GI manifestations are those seen in malabsorption of any cause:

- Diarrhea: 5 to 10 semiformed, malodorous steatorrheic stools per day
- Abdominal bloating and cramps
- Anorexia

Extraintestinal manifestations of malabsorption:

- Weight loss, fatigue
- Anemia
- Bleeding diathesis
- Edema and ascites
- Osteomalacia

Extraintestinal involvement:

- Arthritis (intermittent, migratory, affecting small, large, and axial joints)
- Pleuritic chest pain and cough
- Pericarditis, endocarditis
- Dementia, ophthalmoplegia, myoclonus, and many other symptoms, because any portion of the central nervous system may be a disease site
- Fever

ETIOLOGY & PATHOGENESIS

- Infectious disease caused by *Tropheryma whippeli,* an actinobacter.
- The bacillus has never been cultured, nor has direct transmission from patient to patient ever been documented; however, the agent can be seen in tissue samples by electron microscopy and identified by polymerase chain reaction (PCR).
- Predictable response to appropriate antibiotic therapy confirms the pathogenic role of the infection.
- Tissue infiltration by macrophages is believed to be the mechanism of specific organ dysfunction and symptoms.
- Subtle defects of the cell-mediated immunity exist in active and inactive Whipple's disease that may predispose certain individuals to clinical manifestations. HLA-B27 positivity is found in 26% of patients (four times higher than expected).

DIAGNOSIS (Dx)

DIFFERENTIAL DIAGNOSIS

Malabsorption/maldigestion:

- Celiac disease
- *Mycobacterium avium-intracellulare* intestinal infection in patients with AIDS
- Intestinal lymphoma
- Abetalipoproteinemia
- Amyloidosis
- Systemic mastocytosis
- Radiation enteritis
- Crohn's disease
- Short bowel syndrome
- Pancreatic insufficiency
- Intestinal bacterial overgrowth
- Lactose deficiency
- Postgastrectomy syndrome
- Other cause of diarrhea (see Section III, "Diarrhea, Acute" and "Diarrhea, Chronic")
- Seronegative inflammatory arthritis (see Section II for differential diagnosis)
- Pericarditis and pleuritis
- Lymphadenitis
- Neurologic disorders

WORKUP

Laboratory tests and imaging studies are useful; however, the diagnosis of Whipple's disease is usually made by upper endoscopy and biopsy. Endoscopic findings reveal a pale yellow shaggy mucosa alternating with an erythematous, erosive, or friable mucosa in the duodenum or jejunum.

LABORATORY TESTS

- Anemia (iron, folate, or vitamin B_{12} deficiency)
- Hypokalemia
- Hypocalcemia
- Hypomagnesemia
- Hypoalbuminemia
- Prolonged prothrombin time
- Low serum carotene
- Low cholesterol
- Leukocytosis
- Steatorrhea demonstrated by a Sudan fecal fat stain
- 72-Hr stool collection demonstrating more than 7 g/24 hr of fat in the stool is impractical to perform, especially in ambulatory patients
- Defective d-xylose absorption

IMAGING STUDIES

Small bowel x-rays after barium ingestion often show thickening of mucosal folds.

BIOPSY

Infiltration of the intestinal lamina propria by PAS-positive macrophages containing gram-positive, acid-fast negative bacilli, associated with lymphatic dilation (diagnostic); PCR of the involved tissue in uncertain cases. If PAS staining of the small bowel biopsy specimen is positive and the PCR assay is negative, the diagnosis of Whipple's disease must be confirmed; this can be done by immunohistochemical testing with an antibody to *T. whippeli*. If this test is positive, Whipple's disease is confirmed.

TREATMENT (Rx)

- Antibiotics: TMP/SMX DS bid for 12 to 24 months, usually preceded by parenteral administration of streptomycin (1 g/day) together with penicillin G (1.2 million U/day) or ceftriaxone (2 g/day) for 2 weeks.
- Alternative regimen consists of doxycycline (200 mg/day) plus hydroxychloroquine (200 mg tid).
- Treat specific vitamin, mineral, and nutrient deficiencies.
- Patients with a neurologic recurrence of Whipple's disease have a poor prognosis. Interferon gamma has been proposed for treatment of recurrent CNS disease.

SUGGESTED READING

Fenollar F et al: Whipple's disease, *N Engl J Med* 356:55, 2007.

AUTHORS: **FRED F. FERRI, M.D.,** and **TOM J. WACHTEL, M.D.**

BASIC INFORMATION

DEFINITION

Wilson's disease is a disorder of copper transport with inadequate biliary copper excretion, leading to an accumulation of the metal in liver, brain, kidneys, and corneas.

SYNONYMS

Progressive hepatolenticular degeneration

ICD-9CM CODES
275.1 Wilson's disease

EPIDEMIOLOGY & DEMOGRAPHICS

PREVALENCE: 1 in 30,000
PREDOMINANT SEX: Affects men and women equally (autosomal recessive gene)
ONSET OF SYMPTOMS: 3 to 40 yr of age

PHYSICAL FINDINGS & CLINICAL PRESENTATION

Hepatic presentation:
- Acute hepatitis with malaise, anorexia, nausea, jaundice, elevated transaminase, prolonged prothrombin time; rarely fulminant hepatic failure
- Chronic active (or autoimmune) hepatitis with fatigue, malaise, rashes, arthralgia, elevated transaminase, elevated serum IgG, positive ANA and anti–smooth muscle antibody
- Chronic liver disease/cirrhosis with hepatosplenomegaly, ascites, low serum albumin, prolonged prothrombin time, portal hypertension

Neurologic presentation:
- Movement disorder: tremors, ataxia
- Spastic dystonia: masklike facies, rigidity, gait disturbance, dysarthria, drooling, dysphagia

Ophthalmic:
- Kaiser-Fleisher ring
- Sunflower cataracts

Psychiatric presentation:
- Depression, obsessive-compulsive disorder, psychopathic behaviors, neuroses

Other organs:
- Hemolytic anemia
- Renal disease (i.e., Fanconi's syndrome with hematuria, phosphaturia, renal tubular acidosis, vitamin D–resistant rickets)
- Cardiomyopathy
- Arthritis
- Hypoparathyroidism
- Hypogonadism

PHYSICAL FINDINGS:
- Ocular: the Kayser-Fleischer ring is a gold-yellow ring seen at the periphery of the iris (Fig. 1-293); these should be sought using slit-lamp examination by a skilled examiner
- Stigmata of acute or chronic liver disease
- Neurologic abnormalities: see previous

ETIOLOGY & PATHOGENESIS

- Dietary copper is transported from the intestine to the liver where normally it is metabolized into ceruloplasmin. In Wilson's disease, defective incorporation of copper into ceruloplasmin and a decrease of biliary copper excretion lead to accumulation of this mineral.
- The gene for Wilson's disease is located in chromosome 13.

DIAGNOSIS

DIFFERENTIAL DIAGNOSIS

- Hereditary hypoceruloplasminemia
- Menkes' disease
- Consider the diagnosis of Wilson's disease in all cases of acute or chronic liver disease where another cause has not been established
- Consider Wilson's disease in patients with movement disorders or dystonia even without symptomatic liver disease

LABORATORY TESTS

- Abnormal LFTs (note that AST may be higher than ALT)
- Low serum ceruloplasmin level (<200 mg/L)
- Low serum copper (<65 μg/L)
- 24-hr urinary copper excretion greater than 100 μg (normal <30 μg); increases to greater than 1200 μg/24 hr after 500 mg of d-penicillamine (normal <500 μg/24 hr)
- Low serum uric acid and phosphorus
- Abnormal urinalysis (hematuria)

BIOPSY

- Early:
  Steatosis, focal necrosis, glycogenated hepatocyte nuclei
  May reveal inflammation and piecemeal necrosis
- Late: cirrhosis
- Hepatic copper content (>250 μg/g of dry weight) (normal is 20 to 50 μg)
- Histochemical confirmation of excess copper can be helpful in diagnosis, but if absent, does not exclude Wilson's disease. The lack of immunoreactivity to copper-binding protein can occur because of the diffuse presence of copper in the cytoplasm and because of the assay's low sensitivity. Rhodamine and rubeanic acid stains can show dense granular lysosomal copper deposition in hepatocytes at the stage of cirrhotic nodular regeneration.

TREATMENT

- Penicillamine: (chelator therapy)
  0.75 to 1.5 g/day divided bid (with pyridoxine 25 mg/day)
  Monitor CBC and urinalysis weekly
- Trientine: (triethylene tetramine) (chelator therapy)
  1 to 2 g/day divided tid
  Monitor CBC
- Zinc: (inhibits intestinal copper absorption)
  50 mg tid
  Monitor zinc level
- Ammonium tetrathiomolybdate for neurologic symptoms
- Antioxidants
- Liver transplant (for severe hepatic failure unresponsive to chelation); liver transplantation corrects the underlying pathophysiology and can be lifesaving

PROGNOSIS

Good with early chelation treatment

REFERRAL

To gastroenterologist, neurologist

COMMENTS

Family screening of first-degree relatives must be undertaken. Genetic diagnosis is also useful in patients with indeterminate clinical and biochemical features.

SUGGESTED READING

Ala A et al: Wilson's disease, *Lancet* 369:397, 2007.

AUTHORS: **FRED F. FERRI, M.D.**, and **TOM J. WACHTEL, M.D.**

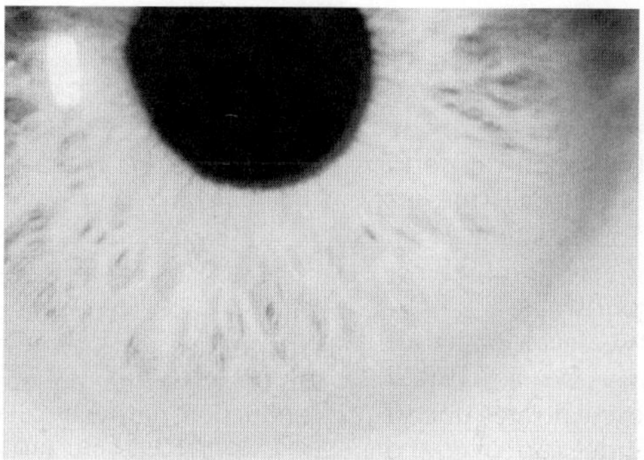

FIGURE 1-293 Wilson's disease. A Kayser-Fleisher ring, which is a gold-yellow ring, extends to the limbus without a clear interval. (From Palay D [ed]: *Ophthalmology for the primary care physician*, St Louis, 1997, Mosby.)

BASIC INFORMATION

DEFINITION

Wolff-Parkinson-White syndrome is an electrocardiographic abnormality associated with earlier than normal ventricular depolarization following the atrial impulse and predisposing the affected person to tachyarrhythmias.

SYNONYMS

Preexcitation syndrome

ICD-9CM CODES
426.7 Wolff-Parkinson-White syndrome
426.81 Lown-Ganong-Levine syndrome

EPIDEMIOLOGY & DEMOGRAPHICS

- Prevalence: 1.5 cases/1000 persons
- Prevalence higher in males and decreases with age
- Most patients with WPW syndrome have normal hearts, but associations with mitral valve prolapse, cardiomyopathies, and Ebstein's anomaly have been reported

PHYSICAL FINDINGS & CLINICAL PRESENTATION

Paroxysmal tachycardias
- 10% of WPW patients aged 20 to 40 yr
- 35% of WPW patients aged >60 yr

The type of tachycardia is:
- Reciprocating tachycardia at 150 to 250 beats per minute (80%)
- Atrial fibrillation (15%)
- Atrial flutter (5%)
- Ventricular tachycardia: rare
- Sudden death is rare (<1/1000 cases)

ETIOLOGY & PATHOGENESIS

- Existence of accessory pathways (Kent bundles).
- If the accessory pathway is capable of anterograde conduction, two parallel routes of AV conduction are possible, one subject to delay through the AV mode, the other without delay through the accessory pathway. The resulting QRS complex is a fusion beat with the "delta" wave representing ventricular activation through the accessory pathway (Fig. 1-294).
- Tachycardias occur when, because of different refractory periods, conduction is anterograde in one pathway (usually the normal AV pathway) and retrograde in the other (usually the accessory pathway). Some patients (5% to 10%) with WPW syndrome have multiple accessory pathways.
- In patients with WPW, development of atrial fibrillation may be associated with very rapid ventricular rates due to atrial ventricular conduction over the anomalous AV pathway.

DIAGNOSIS

Three basic features characterize the ECG abnormalities in WPW syndrome (Fig. 1-295):
- PR interval <120 msec
- QRS complex >120 msec with a slurred, slowly rising onset of QRS in some lead (delta wave)
- ST-T wave changes

Variants
- Lown-Ganong-Levine syndrome: atriohisian pathway with short PR interval and normal QRS complex on ECG (no delta wave)
- Atriofascicular accessory pathways: duplication of the AV node, with normal baseline ECG

TREATMENT

- No treatment in the absence of tachyarrhythmias.
- Symptomatic tachyarrhythmias.
- Acute episode: adenosine, verapamil, or diltiazem can be used to terminate an episode of reciprocal tachycardia.
- Digitalis should not be used because it can reduce refractoriness in the accessory pathway and accelerate the tachycardia. Cardioversion should be used in the presence of hemodynamic impairment.
- Treatment of atrial fibrillation: in patients with WPW, administration of AV nodal-blocking agents will not slow the ventricular rate because AV bypass tracts capable of rapid conduction do not respond to AV blocking agents. Procainamide is the drug of choice to control ventricular rate and restore sinus rhythm in patients with WPW who have atrial fibrillation.

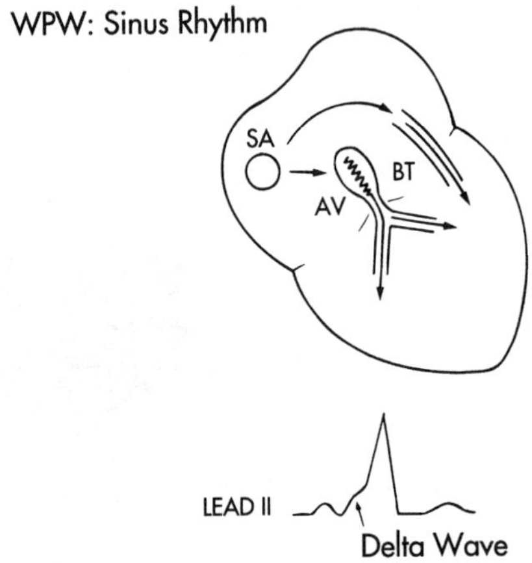

FIGURE 1-294 With Wolff-Parkinson-White syndrome an abnormal accessory conduction pathway called a bypass tract (BT) connects the atria and ventricles. (From Goldberger AL [ed]: *Clinical electrocardiography: a simplified approach,* ed 6, St Louis, 1999, Mosby.)

- Prevention:
  Empiric trials or serial electrophysiologic drug testing of:
  1. Quinidine and propranolol
  2. Procainamide and verapamil
  3. Amiodarone
  4. Sotalol
- Electrical or surgical ablation of the accessory pathway (see below)

EVIDENCE

In a literature review of studies of children receiving hospital treatment in the U.S. for Wolff-Parkinson-White (WPW) syndrome, catheter ablation was found to have lower cost, mortality, and morbidity than either medical management or surgery. The authors concluded that it is the treatment of choice for the child aged 5 years or older with WPW and supraventricular tachycardia.[1,2] Ⓑ

Evidence-Based References

1. Garson A, Kanter RJ: Management of the child with Wolff-Parkinson-White syndrome and supraventricular tachycardia: model for cost effectiveness, *J Cardiovasc Electrophysiol* 8(11):1320, 1997. Reviewed in: The NHS Economic Evaluation Database, 1997. Ⓑ
2. Pappone C et al: Radiofrequency ablation in children with asymptomatic WPW, *N Engl J Med* 351:1197, 2004.

SUGGESTED READING

Pappone C et al: A randomized study of prophylactic catheter ablation in asymptomatic patients with the WPW syndrome, *N Engl J Med* 349:1803, 2003.

AUTHORS: **FRED F. FERRI, M.D.**, and **TOM J. WACHTEL, M.D.**

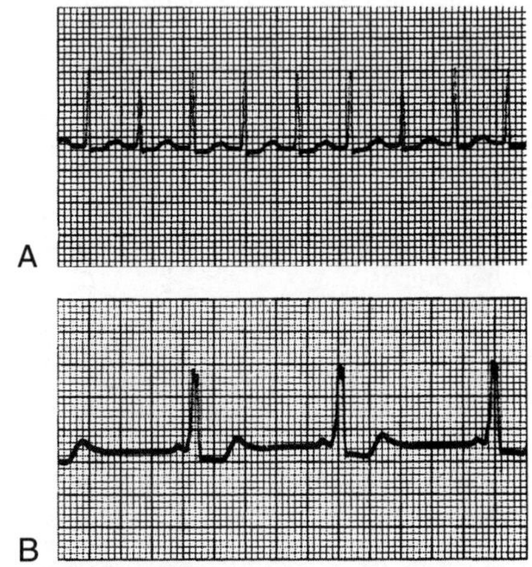

FIGURE 1-295 **A,** SVT in a child with Wolff-Parkinson-White (WPW) syndrome. Note the normal QRS complexes during the tachycardia. **B,** Later the typical features of WPW syndrome are apparent (short P-R interval, delta wave, and wide QRS). (From Behrman RE: *Nelson textbook of pediatrics,* ed 17, Philadelphia, 2004, WB Saunders.)

BASIC INFORMATION

DEFINITION

Yellow fever is an infection, primarily of the liver, with systemic manifestations caused by the yellow fever virus (YFV). The clinical spectrum ranges from asymptomatic infection to life-threatening disease.

SYNONYMS

Tropical hemorrhagic fever from Yellow Fever Virus

ICD-9CM CODES
060.9 Yellow fever

EPIDEMIOLOGY & DEMOGRAPHICS

GEOGRAPHIC DISTRIBUTION

- South America and Africa, in countries between +15 and –15 degrees latitude.
- From 1985 to 1999, more than 20,000 cases and 7000 deaths were reported to the World Health Organization, with more than 90% of cases in Africa.

INCIDENCE: Approximate attack rates of 3% in Africa and Amazon.

PREVALENCE: Endemic areas: 20% of population.

PREDOMINANT SEX: In Africa and Amazon, male agricultural workers.

PHYSICAL FINDINGS & CLINICAL PRESENTATION

- Most subclinical.
- Onset sudden after incubation period of 3 to 6 days.
- Viremic (early) phase:
  1. Fever, chills
  2. Severe headache
  3. Lumbosacral pain
  4. Myalgias, nausea, malaise
  5. Conjunctivitis
  6. Relative bradycardia (Faget's sign)
- After brief recovery, toxic phase:
  1. Jaundice
  2. Oliguria
  3. Albuminuria
  4. Hemorrhage
  5. Encephalopathy
  6. Shock
  7. Acidosis
- Case fatality rate 25% to 50%.

ETIOLOGY

- Yellow fever virus *(L. flavus)*
  1. Flavivirus infects hepatic cells.
  2. Late in infection, cytopathic effects (antibody- and cell-mediated) produce pathology.
- Vector
  1. *Aedes aegypti* (urban).
  2. *Aedes* spp., Haemagogus (especially in Amazon) mosquitos (sylvan).
  3. Primary hosts humans and simian species.
  4. Exists in two transmission cycles:
     a. Sylvatic or jungle cycle involving mosquitos and nonhuman primates.
     b. Urban cycle involving mosquitos and humans.

PATHOGENESIS & PATHOLOGY

- Virus replication begins at site of mosquito bite, spreading to lymphatic channels and regional lymph nodes. Viremic spread to other organs, especially liver, spleen, and bone marrow.
- Shock and fatal illness result from direct damage to organs and vasoactive cytokines.
- Viral antigen found in hepatocytes, kidneys, and myocardium.
- Midzone of liver lobules primarily affected.
- Hemorrhages of mucosal surfaces of gastrointestinal tract.

DIAGNOSIS

DIFFERENTIAL DIAGNOSIS

- Viral hepatitis
- Leptospirosis
- Malaria
- Typhoid fever
  1. Typhus
  2. Relapsing fever
- Other hemorrhagic fevers

LABORATORY TESTS

- CBC
  1. Mild leukopenia
  2. Thrombocytopenia
  3. Anemia
- LFTs
  1. AST levels exceed ALT levels.
  2. Alkaline phosphatase normal or slightly elevated.
  3. Elevated bilirubin levels.
- Elevated BUN and creatinine
- Proteinuria
- Coagulation studies
  1. Demonstrate abnormal prothrombin time *or*
  2. Reveal DIC
- Terminal hypoglycemia
- CSF
  1. Pleocytosis
  2. Elevated protein count
- Specific diagnosis confirmed by:
  1. Viral isolation from blood
  2. Viral antigen in serum (ELISA)
  3. Viral RNA by PCR
  4. IgM-capture ELISA
     a. Preferred serologic test.
     b. Appears within 5 to 7 days.
     c. Rising Ab confirmed by paired sera.
     d. Cross-reactivity with other flavivirus infections.
  5. Immunohistochemical staining of postmortem liver biopsy specimens

TREATMENT

ACUTE GENERAL Rx

- Acetaminophen (for headache and fever) and H2 blockers (GI bleeding)
- Blood transfusion, volume replacement for hemorrhage and shock
- Dialysis for renal failure
- Avoidance of sedatives and drugs dependent on hepatic metabolism

DISPOSITION

Follow up until hepatic, renal, CNS disease resolved

REFERRAL

To infectious diseases expert for accurate diagnosis and management

PEARLS & CONSIDERATIONS

PREVENTION

- Yellow fever is preventable.
- Recovery from yellow fever confers lasting immunity.
- Live, attenuated yellow fever vaccine provides protective immunity in 95% of vaccinees within 10 days of vaccination. Reimmunization at 10-yr intervals for travelers.
- Vaccine contraindicated in:
  1. Infants <6 months (postvaccinal encephalitis)
  2. Immunosuppressed patients
  3. Pregnant women and nursing mothers
  4. Patients with egg hypersensitivity
- Adverse effects of vaccine:
  1. General
     a. Mild headaches, myalgias, low-grade fevers (25% vaccinees in clinical trials).
     b. Immediate hypersensitivity reaction (history of egg allergy).
  2. Vaccine-associated neurotropic disease (postvaccine encephalitis)
     a. Primarily among infants.
     b. Adult cases only in first-time vaccine recipients.
  3. Vaccine-associated viscerotropic disease
     a. Disease syndrome resembling wild-type yellow fever, often fatal.
     b. All cases in first-time vaccinees.

SUGGESTED READINGS

Doblas A et al: Yellow fever vaccine–associated viscerotropic disease and death in Spain, *J Clin Virol* 36(2):156, 2006.

Gerasimon G, Lowry K: Rare case of fatal yellow fever vaccine-associated viscerotropic disease, *South Med J* 98(6):653, 2005.

Lourenco-de-Oliveira R et al: *Ades aegypti* in Brazil: genetically differentiated populations with high susceptibility to dengue and yellow fever viruses, *Trans R Soc Trop Med Hyg* 98(1):43, 2004.

Massad E et al: Yellow fever vaccination: how much is enough? *Vaccine* 23(30):3908, 2005.

Monath TP: Yellow fever vaccine, *Expert Rev Vaccines* 4(4):553, 2005.

Pugachev KV, Guirakhoo F, Monath TP: New developments in flavivirus vaccines with special attention to yellow fever, *Curr Opin Infect Dis* 18(5):387, 2005.

AUTHORS: **STEVEN M. OPAL, M.D.,** and **MARILYN FABBRI, M.D.**

BASIC INFORMATION

DEFINITION

Zenker's diverticulum refers to the acquired physiologic obstruction of the esophageal introitus that results from mucosal herniation posteriorly between the cricopharyngeus muscle and the inferior pharyngeal constrictor muscle (Fig. 1-296).

SYNONYMS

Pharyngoesophageal diverticulum
Pulsion diverticulum

ICD-9CM CODES
530.6 Zenker's diverticulum (esophagus)

EPIDEMIOLOGY & DEMOGRAPHICS

- Rare disease: <1% of all barium swallows
- Commonly seen in people over 50 yr of age (most common in women and elderly)
- Peak incidence is seventh to ninth decades
- Associated with gastroesophageal reflux disease (GERD) and hiatal hernia

PHYSICAL FINDINGS & CLINICAL PRESENTATION

Small Zenker's diverticulum may be asymptomatic. As they become larger, symptoms include:
- Dysphagia to solids and liquids
- Regurgitation of undigested food
- Sensation of globus or fullness in the neck
- Cough
- Halitosis
- Aspiration pneumonia
- Weight loss
- Voice changes
- Sialorrhea (excessive drooling)

ETIOLOGY

- The specific cause is not known. The leading hypothesis suggests a discoordination of the swallowing muscles (specifically, incomplete relaxation of the cricopharyngeus muscle) that leads to an increased pressure on the mucosa of the hypopharynx, resulting in a progressive distention of that mucosa in its weakest area (posterior wall in "Killian's triangle," the point between the oblique fibers of the inferior pharyngeal muscle and the horizontal fibers of the cricopharyngeus muscle). The end result is the formation of a false diverticulum where food elements and secretions may be lodged, causing the symptoms listed previously.
- Zenker's diverticulum may also occur after anterior spinal surgery or cervical spine injury.

DIAGNOSIS

- Clinical presentation and barium swallow typically make the diagnosis of Zenker's diverticulum.
- Neck ultrasound can also be used.

DIFFERENTIAL DIAGNOSIS

The differential diagnosis is similar to anyone presenting with dysphagia:
- Achalasia
- Esophageal spasm
- Esophageal carcinoma
- Esophageal webs
- Peptic stricture
- Lower esophageal (Schatzki) ring
- Foreign bodies
- Central nervous system disorders (stroke, Parkinson's disease, amyotrophic lateral sclerosis, multiple sclerosis, myasthenia gravis, muscular dystrophies)
- Dermatomyositis
- Infection

WORKUP

Barium swallow is the test of choice. Upper endoscopy runs the risk of perforation. Manometry motility studies are usually not indicated.

LABORATORY TESTS

Not specific.

IMAGING STUDIES

- Barium swallow: demonstrates a herniated sac with a narrow diverticular neck that typically originates proximal to the cricopharyngeus at the level of C5-C6 (Fig. 1-297).
- Endoscopy is only indicated if barium studies show mucosal irregularities to rule out neoplasia.
- Oropharyngeal-esophageal scintigraphy has recently been shown to be an effective, sensitive, and simple diagnostic study for both qualitative and quantitative analyses.
- A chest x-ray is performed in cases of suspected aspiration pneumonia.

TREATMENT

NONPHARMACOLOGIC THERAPY

- Soft mechanical diet can be tried in patients with symptoms of dysphagia.
- Avoid seeds, skins, and nuts.

ACUTE GENERAL Rx

- Surgical repair is the conventional treatment for symptomatic patients (dysphagia, cough, aspiration) with excellent relief of symptoms in nearly all patients and low procedural mortality (<1.5%). Procedures include:
  1. Cervical diverticulectomy with cricopharyngeal myotomy (most common approach)
  2. Diverticulopexy or diverticular inversion with cricopharyngeal myotomy
  3. Diverticulectomy alone
  4. Cricopharyngeal myotomy alone
- Endoscopic techniques (esophagodiverticulotomy) have largely replaced conventional surgery and include:
  1. Endoscopic stapler diverticulotomy (may be the initial treatment of choice)

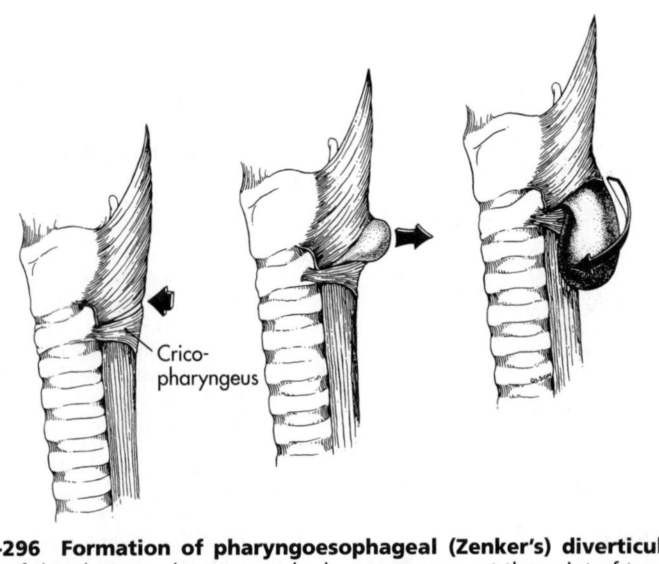

FIGURE 1-296 Formation of pharyngoesophageal (Zenker's) diverticulum. *Left,* Herniation of the pharyngeal mucosa and submucosa occurs at the point of transition *(arrow)* between the oblique fibers of the thyropharyngeus muscle and the more horizontal fibers of the cricopharyngeus muscle. *Center and right,* As the diverticulum enlarges, it dissects toward the left side and downward into the superior mediastinum in the prevertebral space. (From Sabiston D: *Textbook of surgery,* ed 15, Philadelphia, 1997, WB Saunders.)

2. Microendoscopic carbon dioxide laser surgical diverticulotomy
3. Diverticula <3 cm is a contraindication to endosurgical approach
4. Head-to-head comparison with surgical repairs showed endocscopic techniques to be similar in results, relief of symptoms, and patient satisfaction

CHRONIC Rx

In patients not having surgery, treatment is directed toward any complications that may occur:

- Antibiotics for aspiration pneumonia
- H_2 antagonists for ulcerations that can develop within the diverticulum
- Botulinum toxin for temporary relief of dysphagia

DISPOSITION

- If left untreated, progressive enlargement of the diverticulum occurs.
- The risk of complications (e.g., aspiration pneumonia) increases with the size of the diverticulum.
- Postsurgical recurrence can occur (4%); however, these are usually asymptomatic.

REFERRAL

Any patient with dysphagia requires a gastroenterology consultation. A thoracic surgical, ENT, or head and neck surgeon may be consulted if surgery is considered.

PEARLS & CONSIDERATIONS

COMMENTS

The association with cancer is rare (0.4%).

SUGGESTED READINGS

Bonavina L et al: Long-term results of endosurgical and open surgical approach for Zenker diverticulum, *World J Gastroenterol* 14;13(18):2586, 2007.

Gustantini M et al: Esophageal diverticula, *Best Pract Res Clin Gastroenterology* 18(1):3, 2004.

Manni J et al: The endoscopic stapler diverticulotomy for Zenker's diverticulum, *Eur Arch Otorhinolaryngol* 261(2):68, 2004.

Ruiz-Tovar J et al:. 20 years experience in the management of Zenker's diverticulum in a third-level hospital, *Rev Esp Enferm Dig* 98(6):429, 2006.

Wirth D et al: Outcome and quality of life after open surgery versus endoscopic stapler-assisted esophagodiverticulostomy for Zenker's diverticulum, *Dis Esophagus* 19(4): 294, 2006.

AUTHOR: **ABDULBAKI ABDULRAHMAN, M.D.**

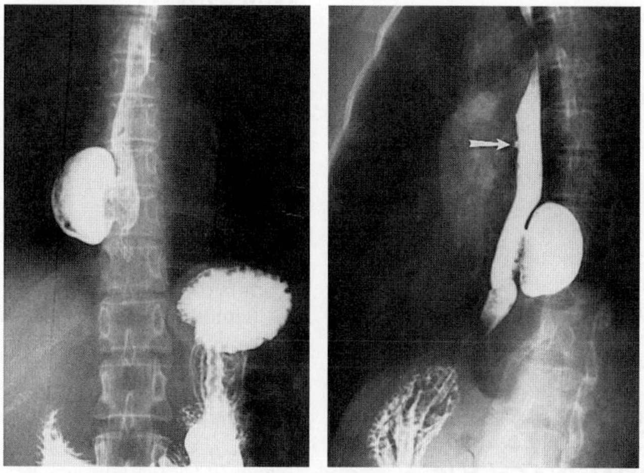

FIGURE 1-297 Posteroanterior *(left)* and oblique *(right)* views from barium esophagogram showing both a typical diverticulum of the junction of the mid-esophagus and distal esophagus and a small traction diverticulum *(arrow)* of the mid-esophagus. (From Sabiston D: *Textbook of surgery,* ed 15, Philadelphia, 1997, Saunders.)

BASIC INFORMATION

DEFINITION

Zollinger-Ellison (ZE) syndrome is a hypergastrinemic state caused by a pancreatic or extrapancreatic non–beta islet cell tumor (gastrinoma) and resulting in peptic acid disease.

SYNONYMS

Gastrinoma

ICD-9CM CODES
251.5 Zollinger-Ellison syndrome

EPIDEMIOLOGY & DEMOGRAPHICS

- Incidence is unknown, but 0.1% of all duodenal ulcers are believed to be caused by ZE.
- Occurs in both genders and at any age (most common in 30 to 50 yr of age).
- Two thirds of gastrinomas are sporadic, and one third are associated with multiple endocrine neoplasia type 1 (MEN-1), an autosomal dominant genetic disorder that also includes hyperparathyroidism and pituitary tumors.
- About 60% of gastrinomas are malignant.

PHYSICAL FINDINGS & CLINICAL PRESENTATION

- The vast majority of patients (95%) present with symptoms of peptic ulcer (see Section I, "Peptic Ulcer Disease").
- 60% of patients have symptoms related to gastroesophageal reflux disease (see Section I, "Gastroesophageal Reflux Disease").
- One third of patients with ZE have diarrhea and, less commonly, steatorrhea.

The following circumstances warrant suspicion of ZE syndrome:

- Ulcers distal to the first portion of the duodenum
- Multiple peptic ulcers
- Ineffective treatment for peptic ulcer disease with the usual drug doses and schedules
- Peptic ulcer and diarrhea
- Familial history of peptic ulcer
- Patients with a personal or family history suggesting parathyroid or pituitary tumors of dysfunction
- Peptic ulcer and urinary tract calculi
- Patients with peptic ulcer who are negative for *H. pylori* and do not have a history of NSAID use

ETIOLOGY

- The pathophysiologic manifestations of ZE syndrome are related to the effects of hypergastrinemia. Gastrin stimulates gastric acid secretion, which in turn is responsible for the development of duodenal ulcers and diarrhea. Gastrin also promotes gastric mucosal epithelial cell growth and resulting parietal cell hyperplasia.
- Gastrinomas are usually small (0.1 to 2 cm) but sometimes large (>20 cm) tumors.
- 60% of gastrinomas are malignant, with liver and regional lymph nodes the most common site of metastases. Histology is not a good predictor of the biology of gastrinomas.
- 60% of patients with MEN-1 have gastrinomas.
- 10% of patients with ZE syndrome have islet cell hyperplasia rather than gastrinomas; in 10% to 20% of patients with gastrinoma the tumors cannot be located because of small size.

DIAGNOSIS

DIFFERENTIAL DIAGNOSIS

- Peptic ulcer disease (see Section I, "Peptic Ulcer Disease")
- Gastroesophageal reflux disease (see Section I, "Gastroesophageal Reflux Disease")
- Diarrhea (see Section III, "Diarrhea, Acute" and "Diarrhea, Chronic")

WORKUP

- Diagnosis of peptic ulcer
  - UGI series (may also show prominent gastric rugal folds)
  - Endoscopy
- Gastric acid secretion
- Serum gastrin level (fasting) >150 pg/ml (causes of false-positive: pernicious anemia, renal failure, retained gastric antrum syndrome, diabetes mellitus, rheumatoid arthritis)
- Provocative gastrin level tests
  - Secretin stimulation
  - Calcium stimulation
  - Standard test meal stimulation
- Gastrinoma localization
  - Arteriography
  - Abdominal sonography
  - Abdominal CT scan
  - Abdominal MRI
  - Selective portal vein branch gastrin level
  - Octreotide scan

TREATMENT

- Surgical resection of the gastrinoma (NOTE: 90% of gastrinomas can be located, resulting in a 40% overall cure rate)
- Total gastrectomy or vagotomy (palliative in some patients)
- Medical treatment
  - Proton pump inhibitors (e.g., omeprazole or lansoprazole)
  - Somatostatin or octreotide
  - Chemotherapy for metastatic gastrinoma with streptozotocin, 5-FU, and doxorubicin

PROGNOSIS

Five-year survival:

- Two thirds of all patients
- 20% with liver metastases
- 90% without liver metastases

REFERRAL

To gastroenterologist

SUGGESTED READING

Norten JA et al: Surgery to cure Zollinger-Ellison syndrome, *N Engl J Med* 341:635, 1999.

AUTHORS: **FRED F. FERRI, M.D.,** and **TOM J. WACHTEL, M.D.**

Section II

Differential Diagnosis

ABDOMINAL DISTENTION

ICD-9CM # 787.3

NONMECHANICAL OBSTRUCTION

Excessive intraluminal gas.
Intraabdominal infection.
Trauma.
Retroperitoneal irritation (renal colic, neoplasms, infections, hemorrhage).
Vascular insufficiency (thrombosis, embolism).
Mechanical ventilation.
Extraabdominal infection (sepsis, pneumonia, empyema, osteomyelitis of spine).
Metabolic/toxic abnormalities (hypokalemia, uremia, lead poisoning).
Chemical irritation (perforated ulcer, bile, pancreatitis).
Peritoneal inflammation.
Severe pain, pain medications.

MECHANICAL OBSTRUCTION

Neoplasm (intraluminal, extraluminal).
Adhesions, endometriosis.
Infection (intraabdominal abscess, diverticulitis).
Gallstones.
Foreign body, bezoars.
Pregnancy.
Hernias.
Volvulus.
Stenosis at surgical anastomosis, radiation stenosis.
Fecaliths.
Inflammatory bowel disease.
Gastric outlet obstruction.
Hematoma.
Other: parasites, superior mesenteric artery (SMA) syndrome, pneumatosis intestinalis, annular pancreas, Hirschsprung's disease, intussusception, meconium.

ABDOMINAL PAIN, ADOLESCENCE[23]

ICD-9CM # 789.67

Acute gastroenteritis.
Appendicitis.
Inflammatory bowel disease.
Peptic ulcer disease.
Cholecystitis.
Neoplasm.
Diabetic ketoacidosis.
Functional abdominal pain.
Pelvic inflammatory disease.
Pregnancy.
Pyelonephritis.
Renal stone.
Trauma.

ABDOMINAL PAIN, CHILDHOOD[23]

ICD-9CM # 789.67

Acute gastroenteritis.
Appendicitis.
Constipation.
Cholecystitis, acute.
Intestinal obstruction.
Pancreatitis.
Neoplasm.
Inflammatory bowel disease.
Other:
  Functional abdominal pain.
  Pyelonephritis.
  Pneumonia.
  Diabetic ketoacidosis.
  Heavy metal poisoning.
  Sickle cell crisis.
  Trauma.

ABDOMINAL PAIN, DIFFUSE

ICD-9CM # 789.67

Early appendicitis.
Aortic aneurysm.
Gastroenteritis.
Intestinal obstruction.
Diverticulitis.
Peritonitis.
Mesenteric insufficiency or infarction.
Pancreatitis.
Inflammatory bowel disease.
Irritable bowel.
Mesenteric adenitis.
Metabolic: toxins, lead poisoning, uremia, drug overdose, diabetic ketoacidosis (DKA), heavy metal poisoning.
Sickle cell crisis.
Pneumonia (rare).
Trauma.
Urinary tract infection, pelvic inflammatory disease (PID).
Other: acute intermittent porphyria, tabes dorsalis, periarteritis nodosa, Henoch-Schönlein purpura, adrenal insufficiency.

ABDOMINAL PAIN, EPIGASTRIC

ICD-9CM # 789.66

Gastric: peptic ulcer disease (PUD), gastric outlet obstruction, gastric ulcer.
Duodenal: PUD, duodenitis.
Biliary: cholecystitis, cholangitis.
Hepatic: hepatitis.
Pancreatic: pancreatitis.
Intestinal: high small bowel obstruction, early appendicitis.
Cardiac: angina, MI, pericarditis.
Pulmonary: pneumonia, pleurisy, pneumothorax.
Subphrenic abscess.
Vascular: dissecting aneurysm, mesenteric ischemia.

ABDOMINAL PAIN, INFANCY[23]

ICD-9CM # 789.67

Acute gastroenteritis.
Appendicitis.
Intussusception.
Volvulus.
Meckel diverticulum.
Other:
  Colic.
  Trauma.

ABDOMINAL PAIN, LEFT LOWER QUADRANT

ICD-9CM # 789.64

Intestinal: diverticulitis, intestinal obstruction, perforated ulcer, inflammatory bowel disease, perforated descending colon, inguinal hernia, neoplasm, appendicitis.
Reproductive: ectopic pregnancy, ovarian cyst, torsion of ovarian cyst, tuboovarian abscess, mittelschmerz, endometriosis, seminal vesiculitis.
Renal: renal or ureteral calculi, pyelonephritis, neoplasm.
Vascular: leaking aortic aneurysm.
Psoas abscess.
Trauma.

ABDOMINAL PAIN, LEFT UPPER QUADRANT

ICD-9CM # 789.32

Gastric: PUD, gastritis, pyloric stenosis, hiatal hernia.
Pancreatic: pancreatitis, neoplasm, stone in pancreatic duct or ampulla.
Cardiac: MI, angina pectoris.
Splenic: splenomegaly, ruptured spleen, splenic abscess, splenic infarction.
Renal: calculi, pyelonephritis, neoplasm.
Pulmonary: pneumonia, empyema, pulmonary infarction.
Vascular: ruptured aortic aneurysm.
Cutaneous: herpes zoster.
Trauma.
Intestinal: high fecal impaction, perforated colon, diverticulitis.

ABDOMINAL PAIN, NONSURGICAL CAUSES

ICD-9CM # 789.9

Irritable bowel syndrome.
Urinary tract infection, pyelonephritis, salpingitis, pelvic inflammatory disease (PID).
Gastroenteritis, gastritis, peptic ulcer.
Diverticular spasm.
Hepatitis, mononucleosis.
Pancreatitis.
Inferior wall myocardial infarction.
Basilar pneumonia, pulmonary embolism.
Diabetic ketoacidosis.
Strain or hematoma of rectus muscle.
Ruptured Graafian follicle.
Herpes zoster.
Nerve root compression.
Sickle cell crisis.
Acute adrenal insufficiency.
Others: acute porphyria, familial Mediterranean fever, tabes dorsalis.

ABDOMINAL PAIN, PERIUMBILICAL

ICD-9CM # 789.65

Intestinal: small bowel obstruction or gangrene, early appendicitis.
Vascular: mesenteric thrombosis, dissecting aortic aneurysm.
Pancreatic: pancreatitis.
Metabolic: uremia, DKA.
Trauma.

ABDOMINAL PAIN, POORLY LOCALIZED[23]

ICD-9CM # 789.60

EXTRAABDOMINAL

Metabolic

DKA, acute intermittent porphyria, hyperthyroidism, hypothyroidism, hypercalcemia, hypokalemia, uremia, hyperlipidemia, hyperparathyroidism.

Hematologic

Sickle cell crisis, leukemia or lymphoma, Henoch-Schönlein purpura.

Infectious

Infectious mononucleosis, Rocky Mountain spotted fever, acquired immunodeficiency syndrome (AIDS), streptococcal pharyngitis (in children), herpes zoster.

Drugs and toxins

Heavy metal poisoning, black widow spider bites, withdrawal syndromes, mushroom ingestion.

Referred pain

Pulmonary: pneumonia, pulmonary embolism, pneumothorax.
Cardiac: angina, myocardial infarction, pericarditis, myocarditis.
Genitourinary: prostatitis, epididymitis, orchitis, testicular torsion.
Musculoskeletal: rectus sheath hematoma.

Functional

Somatization disorder, malingering, hypochondriasis, Munchausen syndrome.

INTRAABDOMINAL

Early appendicitis, gastroenteritis, peritonitis, pancreatitis, abdominal aortic aneurysm, mesenteric insufficiency or infarction, intestinal obstruction, volvulus, ulcerative colitis.

ABDOMINAL PAIN, PREGNANCY[23]

ICD-9CM # 789.67

GYNECOLOGIC (GESTATIONAL AGE IN PARENTHESES)

Miscarriage	(<20 wk; 80% <12 wk)
Septic abortion	(<20 wk)
Ectopic pregnancy	(<14 wk)
Corpus luteum cyst rupture	(<12 wk)
Ovarian torsion	(Especially <24 wk)
Pelvic inflammatory disease	(<12 wk)
Chorioamnionitis	(>16 wk)
Abruptio placentae	(>16 wk)

NONGYNECOLOGIC

Appendicitis	(Throughout)
Cholecystitis	(Throughout)
Hepatitis	(Throughout)
Pyelonephritis	(Throughout)
Preeclampsia	(>20 wk)

ABDOMINAL PAIN, RIGHT LOWER QUADRANT

ICD-9CM # 789.63

Intestinal: acute appendicitis, regional enteritis, incarcerated hernia, cecal diverticulitis, intestinal obstruction, perforated ulcer, perforated cecum, Meckel diverticulitis.
Reproductive: ectopic pregnancy, ovarian cyst, torsion of ovarian cyst, salpingitis, tuboovarian abscess, mittelschmerz, endometriosis, seminal vesiculitis.
Renal: renal and ureteral calculi, neoplasms, pyelonephritis.
Vascular: leaking aortic aneurysm.
Psoas abscess.
Trauma.
Cholecystitis.

ABDOMINAL PAIN, RIGHT UPPER QUADRANT

ICD-9CM # 789.61

Biliary: calculi, infection, inflammation, neoplasm.
Hepatic: hepatitis, abscess, hepatic congestion, neoplasm, trauma.
Gastric: PUD, pyloric stenosis, neoplasm, alcoholic gastritis, hiatal hernia.
Pancreatic: pancreatitis, neoplasm, stone in pancreatic duct or ampulla.
Renal: calculi, infection, inflammation, neoplasm, rupture of kidney.
Pulmonary: pneumonia, pulmonary infarction, right-sided pleurisy.
Intestinal: retrocecal appendicitis, intestinal obstruction, high fecal impaction, diverticulitis.
Cardiac: myocardial ischemia (particularly involving the inferior wall), pericarditis.
Cutaneous: herpes zoster.
Trauma.
Fitz-Hugh-Curtis syndrome (perihepatitis).

ABDOMINAL PAIN, SUPRAPUBIC

ICD-9CM # 789.85

Intestinal: colon obstruction or gangrene, diverticulitis, appendicitis.
Reproductive system: ectopic pregnancy, mittelschmerz, torsion of ovarian cyst, PID, salpingitis, endometriosis, rupture of endometrioma.
Cystitis, rupture of urinary bladder.

ABORTION, RECURRENT

ICD-9CM # 761.8

Congenital anatomic abnormalities.
Adhesions (uterine synechiae).
Uterine fibroids.
Endometriosis.
Endocrine abnormalities (luteal phase insufficiency, hypothyroidism, uncontrolled diabetes mellitus).
Parenteral chromosome abnormalities.
Maternal infections (cervical mycoplasma, ureaplasma, chlamydia).
DES exposure, heavy metal exposure.
Thrombocytosis.
Allogenic immunity, autoimmunity, lupus anticoagulant.

ACHES AND PAINS, DIFFUSE[21]

ICD-9CM # 719.49

Postviral arthralgias/myalgias.
Bilateral soft tissue rheumatism.
Overuse syndromes.
Fibrositis.
Hypothyroidism.
Metabolic bone disease.
Paraneoplastic syndrome.
Myopathy (polymyositis, dermatomyositis).
RA.
Sjögren's syndrome.
Polymyalgia rheumatica.
Hypermobility.
Benign arthralgias/myalgias.
Chronic fatigue syndrome.
Hypophosphatemia.

ACIDOSIS, LACTIC

ICD-9CM # 276.2

TISSUE HYPOXIA

Shock (hypovolemic, cardiogenic, endotoxic).
Respiratory failure (asphyxia).
Severe CHF.
Severe anemia.
Carbon monoxide or cyanide poisoning.

ASSOCIATED WITH SYSTEMIC DISORDERS

Neoplastic diseases (e.g., leukemia, lymphoma).
Liver or renal failure.
Sepsis.
Diabetes mellitus.
Seizure activity.
Abnormal intestinal flora.
Alkalosis.
HIV.

SECONDARY TO DRUGS OR TOXINS

Salicylates.
Ethanol, methanol, ethylene glycol.
Fructose or sorbitol.
Biguanides (phenformin, metformin [usually occurring in patients with renal insufficiency]).
Isoniazid.

Streptozocin.
Nucleoside reverse transcriptase inhibitors (zidovudine, didanosine, stavudine).

HEREDITARY DISORDERS

G6PD deficiency and others.

ACIDOSIS, METABOLIC

ICD-9CM # 276.2

METABOLIC ACIDOSIS WITH INCREASED AG (AG ACIDOSIS)

Lactic acidosis.
Ketoacidosis (diabetes mellitus, alcoholic ketoacidosis).
Uremia (chronic renal failure).
Ingestion of toxins (paraldehyde, methanol, salicylate, ethylene glycol).
High-fat diet (mild acidosis).

METABOLIC ACIDOSIS WITH NORMAL AG (HYPERCHLOREMIC ACIDOSIS)

Renal tubular acidosis (including acidosis of aldosterone deficiency).
Intestinal loss of HCO_3^- (diarrhea, pancreatic fistula).
Carbonic anhydrase inhibitors (e.g., acetazolamide).
Dilutional acidosis (as a result of rapid infusion of bicarbonate-free isotonic saline).
Ingestion of exogenous acids (ammonium chloride, methionine, cystine, calcium chloride).
Ileostomy.
Ureterosigmoidostomy.
Drugs: amiloride, triamterene, spironolactone, β-blockers.

ACIDOSIS, RESPIRATORY

ICD-9CM # 276.2

Pulmonary disease (COPD, severe pneumonia, pulmonary edema, interstitial fibrosis).
Airway obstruction (foreign body, severe bronchospasm, laryngospasm).
Thoracic cage disorders (pneumothorax, flail chest, kyphoscoliosis).
Defects in muscles of respiration (myasthenia gravis, hypokalemia, muscular dystrophy).
Defects in peripheral nervous system (amyotrophic lateral sclerosis, poliomyelitis, Guillain-Barré syndrome, botulism, tetanus, organophosphate poisoning, spinal cord injury).
Depression of respiratory center (anesthesia, narcotics, sedatives, vertebral artery embolism or thrombosis, increased intracranial pressure).
Failure of mechanical ventilator.

ACUTE SCROTUM

ICD-9CM # 608.9

Testicular torsion.
Epididymitis.
Testicular neoplasm.
Orchitis.

ADNEXAL MASS[23]

ICD-9CM # CODE VARIES WITH SPECIFIC DISORDER

Ovary (neoplasm, endometriosis, functional cyst).
Fallopian tube (ectopic pregnancy, neoplasm, tuboovarian abscess, hydrosalpinx, paratubal cyst).
Uterus (fibroid, neoplasm).
Retroperitoneum (neoplasm, abdominal wall hematoma or abscess).
Urinary tract (pelvic kidney, distended bladder, urachal cyst).
Inflammatory bowel disease.
GI tract neoplasm.
Diverticular disease.
Appendicitis.
Bowel loop with feces.

ADRENAL MASSES[33]

ICD-9CM # 194.0 ADRENOCORTICAL CARCINOMA
255.8 ADRENAL HYPERPLASIA

UNILATERAL ADRENAL MASSES

Functional lesions
Adrenal adenoma.
Adrenal carcinoma.
Pheochromocytoma.
Primary aldosteronism, adenomatous type.
Nonfunctional lesions
Incidentaloma of adrenal.
Ganglioneuroma.
Myelolipoma.
Hematoma.
Adenolipoma.
Metastasis.

BILATERAL ADRENAL MASSES

Functional lesions
ACTH-dependent Cushing's syndrome.
Congenital adrenal hyperplasia.
Pheochromocytoma.
Conn's syndrome, hyperplastic variety.
Micronodular adrenal disease.
Idiopathic bilateral adrenal hypertrophy.
Nonfunctional lesions
Infection (tuberculosis, fungi).
Infiltration (leukemia, lymphoma).
Replacement (amyloidosis).
Hemorrhage.
Bilateral metastases.

ADYNAMIC ILEUS[23]

ICD-9CM # 560.1

Abdominal trauma.
Infection (retroperitoneal, pelvic, intrathoracic).
Laparotomy.
Metabolic disease (hypokalemia).
Renal colic.
Skeletal injury (rib fracture, vertebral fracture).
Medications (e.g., narcotics).

AEROPHAGIA (BELCHING, ERUCTATION)

ICD-9CM # 787.3

Anxiety disorders.
Rapid food ingestion.
Carbonated beverages.
Nursing infants (especially when nursing in horizontal position).
Eating or drinking in supine position.
Gum chewing.
Poorly fitting dentures, orthodontic appliances.
Hiatal hernia, gastritis, nonulcer dyspepsia.
Cholelithiasis, cholecystitis.
Ingestion of legumes, onions, peppers.

AIRWAY OBSTRUCTION, PEDIATRIC AGE[17]

ICD-9CM # 496 OBSTRUCTION DUE TO BRONCHOSPASM
934.9 OBSTRUCTION DUE TO FOREIGN BODY
478.75 OBSTRUCTION DUE TO LARYNGOSPASM
506.9 OBSTRUCTION DUE TO INHALATION OF FUMES OR VAPORS

CONGENITAL CAUSES

Craniofacial dysmorphism.
Hemangioma.
Laryngeal cleft/web.
Laryngoceles, cysts.
Laryngomalacia.
Macroglossia.
Tracheal stenosis.
Vascular ring.
Vocal cord paralysis.

ACQUIRED INFECTIOUS CAUSES

Acute laryngotracheobronchitis.
Epiglottitis.
Laryngeal papillomatosis.
Membranous croup (bacterial tracheitis).
Mononucleosis.
Retropharyngeal abscess.
Spasmodic croup.
Diphtheria.

ACQUIRED NONINFECTIOUS CAUSES

Anaphylaxis.
Foreign body aspiration.
Supraglottic hypotonia.
Thermal/chemical burn.
Trauma.
Vocal cord paralysis.
Angioneurotic edema.

AKINETIC/RIGID SYNDROME[1]

ICD-9CM # CODE NOT AVAILABLE

Parkinsonism (idiopathic, drug-induced).
Catatonia (psychosis).
Progressive supranuclear palsy.
Multisystem atrophy (Shy-Drager syndrome, olivopontocerebellar atrophy).
Diffuse Lewy-body disease.
Toxins (MPTP, manganese, carbon monoxide).
Huntington's disease and other hereditary neurodegenerative disorders.

ALKALOSIS, METABOLIC

ICD-9CM # 276.3

CHLORIDE-RESPONSIVE

Vomiting.
Nasogastric (NG) suction.
Diuretics.
Posthypercapnic alkalosis.
Stool losses (laxative abuse, cystic fibrosis, villous adenoma).
Massive blood transfusion.
Exogenous alkali administration.

CHLORIDE-RESISTANT

Hyperadrenocorticoid states (Cushing's syndrome, primary hyperaldosteronism, secondary mineralocorticoidism [licorice, chewing tobacco]).
Hypomagnesemia.
Hypokalemia.
Bartter's syndrome.

ALKALOSIS, RESPIRATORY

ICD-9CM # 276.3

Hypoxemia (pneumonia, pulmonary embolism, atelectasis, high-altitude living).
Drugs (salicylates, xanthenes, progesterone, epinephrine, thyroxine, nicotine).
Central nervous system (CNS) disorders (tumor, cerebrovascular accident [CVA], trauma, infections).
Psychogenic hyperventilation (anxiety, hysteria).
Hepatic encephalopathy.
Gram-negative sepsis.
Hyponatremia.
Sudden recovery from metabolic acidosis.
Assisted ventilation.

ALOPECIA[12,25]

ICD-9CM # 704.00 ALOPECIA NOS
704.01 ALOPECIA, ANDROGENIC
704.01 ALOPECIA AREATA
757.4 ALOPECIA, CONGENITAL
316 ALOPECIA, PSYCHOGENIC

SCARRING ALOPECIA

Congenital (aplasia cutis).
Tinea capitis with inflammation (kerion).
Bacterial folliculitis.
Discoid lupus erythematosus.
Lichen planopilaris.
Folliculitis decalvans.
Neoplasm.
Trauma.

NONSCARRING ALOPECIA

Cosmetic treatment.
Tinea capitis.
Structural hair shaft disease.
Trichotillomania (hair pulling).
Anagen arrest.
Telogen arrest.
Alopecia areata.
Androgenetic alopecia.

ALVEOLAR CONSOLIDATION

ICD-9CM # 514

Infection.
Neoplasm (bronchoalveolar carcinoma, lymphoma).
Aspiration.
Trauma.
Hemorrhage (Wegener's Goodpasture, bleeding diathesis).
ARDS.
CHF.
Renal failure.
Eosinophilic pneumonia.
Bronchiolitis obliterans.
Pulmonary alveolar proteinosis.

ALVEOLAR HEMORRHAGE[25]

ICD-9CM # 770.3

Hematologic disorders (coagulopathies, thrombocytopenia).
Goodpasture syndrome (antibasement-membrane antibody disease).
Wegener's vasculitis.
Immune complex-mediated vasculitis.
Idiopathic pulmonary hemosiderosis.
Drugs (penicillamine).
Lymphangiogram contrast.
Mitral stenosis.

AMENORRHEA

ICD-9CM # 626.0

PREGNANCY

EARLY MENOPAUSE

Hypothalamic dysfunction: defective synthesis or release of LHRH, anorexia nervosa, stress, exercise.
***Pituitary dysfunction*:** neoplasm, postpartum hemorrhage, surgery, radiotherapy.
***Ovarian dysfunction*:** gonadal dysgenesis, 17-a-hydroxylase deficiency, premature ovarian failure, polycystic ovarian disease, gonadal stromal tumors.

UTEROVAGINAL ABNORMALITIES

Congenital: imperforate hymen, imperforate cervix, imperforate or absent vagina, müllerian agenesis.
Acquired: destruction of endometrium with curettage (Asherman's syndrome), closure of cervix or vagina caused by traumatic injury, hysterectomy.

OTHER

Metabolic diseases (liver, kidney), malnutrition, rapid weight loss, exogenous obesity, endocrine abnormalities (Cushing's syndrome, Graves' disease, hypothyroidism).

AMNESIA

ICD-9CM # 292.83 DRUG INDUCED
300.12 HYSTERICAL
780.9 RETROGRADE
437.7 TRANSIENT GLOBAL

Degenerative diseases (e.g., Alzheimer's, Huntington's disease).
CVA (especially when involving thalamus, basal forebrain, and hippocampus).
Head trauma.
Postsurgical (e.g., mammillary body surgery, bilateral temporal lobectomy).
Infections (herpes simplex encephalitis, meningitis).
Wernicke-Korsakoff syndrome.
Cerebral hypoxia.
Hypoglycemia.
CNS neoplasms.
Creutzfeldt-Jakob disease.
Medications (e.g., midazolam and other benzodiazepines).
Psychosis.
Malingering.

ANAL INCONTINENCE[23]

ICD-9CM # 787.6

TRAUMATIC

Nerve injured in surgery.
Spinal cord injury.
Obstetric trauma.
Sphincter injury.

NEUROLOGIC

Spinal cord lesions.
Dementia.
Autonomic neuropathy (e.g., diabetes mellitus).
Obstetrics: pudendal nerve stretched during surgery.
Hirschsprung's disease.

MASS EFFECT

Carcinoma of anal canal.
Carcinoma of rectum.
Foreign body.
Fecal impaction.
Hemorrhoids.

MEDICAL

Procidentia.
Inflammatory disease.
Diarrhea.
Laxative abuse.

PEDIATRIC

Congenital.
Meningocele.
Myelomeningocele.
Spina bifida.
After corrective surgery for imperforate anus.
Sexual abuse.
Encopresis.

ANAPHYLAXIS[18]

ICD-9CM # 995.0

PULMONARY

Laryngeal edema.
Epiglottitis.
Foreign body aspiration.
Pulmonary embolus.
Asphyxiation.
Hyperventilation.

CARDIOVASCULAR

Myocardial infarction.
Arrhythmia.
Hypovolemic shock.
Cardiac arrest.

CNS

Vasovagal reaction.
CVA.
Seizure disorder.
Drug overdose.

ENDOCRINE

Hypoglycemia.
Pheochromocytoma.
Carcinoid syndrome.
Catamenial (progesterone-induced anaphylaxis).

PSYCHIATRIC

Vocal cord dysfunction syndrome.
Munchausen's disease.
Panic attack/globus hystericus.

OTHER

Hereditary angioedema.
Cord urticaria.
Idiopathic urticaria.
Mastocytosis.
Serum sickness.
Idiopathic capillary leak syndrome.
Sulfite exposure.
Scombroid poisoning (tuna, blue fish, mackerel).

ANDROGEN EXCESS, REPRODUCTIVE-AGE WOMAN

ICD-9CM # CODE VARIES WITH SPECIFIC DISORDER

Polycystic ovary syndrome.
Idiopathic.
Medications (e.g., anabolizing agents, testosterone, danazol).
Pregnancy (luteoma, hyperreactio luteinalis).
Sertoli-Leydig ovarian neoplasm.
Adrenal adenoma or hyperplasia.
Cushing's syndrome.
Glucocorticoid resistance.
Hypothyroidism.
Hyperprolactinemia.

ANEMIA, DRUG-INDUCED[15]

ICD-9CM # 283.0

DRUGS THAT MAY INTERFERE WITH RED CELL PRODUCTION BY INDUCING MARROW SUPPRESSION OR APLASIA

Alcohol.
Antineoplastic drugs.
Antithyroid drugs.
Antibiotics.
Oral hypoglycemic agents.
Phenylbutazone.
Azidothymidine (AZT).

DRUGS THAT INTERFERE WITH VITAMIN B_{12}, FOLATE, OR IRON ABSORPTION OR UTILIZATION

Nitrous oxide.
Anticonvulsant drugs.
Antineoplastic drugs.
Isoniazid, cycloserine A.

DRUGS CAPABLE OF PROMOTING HEMOLYSIS

Immune mediated
Penicillins.
Quinine.
Alpha-methyldopa.
Procainamide.
Mitomycin C.
Oxidative stress
Antimalarials.
Sulfonamide drugs.
Nalidixic acid.

DRUGS THAT MAY PRODUCE OR PROMOTE BLOOD LOSS

Aspirin.
Alcohol.
Nonsteroidal anti-inflammatory agents.
Corticosteroids.
Anticoagulants.

ANEMIA, LOW RETICULOCYTE COUNT[1]

ICD-9CM # 285.9

MICROCYTIC ANEMIA (MCV <80)

Iron deficiency.
Thalassemia minor.
Sideroblastic anemia.
Lead poisoning.

MACROCYTIC ANEMIA (MCV >100)

Megaloblastic anemias.
Folate deficiency.
Vitamin B_{12} deficiency.
Drug-induced megaloblastic anemia.
Nonmegaloblastic macrocytosis.
Liver disease.
Hypothyroidism.

NORMOCYTIC ANEMIA (MCV 80-100)

Early iron deficiency.
Aplastic anemia.
Myelophthisic disorders.
Endocrinopathies.
Anemia of chronic disease.
Uremia.
Mixed nutritional deficiency.

ANEMIA, MEGALOBLASTIC[33]

ICD-9CM # 281.0 PERNICIOUS ANEMIA
281.1 B_{12} DEFICIENCY
281.2 FOLATE DEFICIENCY
281.3 B_{12} WITH FOLATE DEFICIENCY
281.4 PROTEIN OR AMINO ACID DEFICIENCY
281.8 NUTRITIONAL
281.9 NOS

COBALAMIN (CBL) DEFICIENCY

Nutritional Cbl deficiency (insufficient Cbl intake): vegetarians, vegans, breast-fed infants of mothers with pernicious anemia.
Abnormal intragastric events (inadequate proteolysis of food Cbl): atrophic gastritis, partial gastrectomy with hypochlorhydria.
Loss/atrophy of gastric oxyntic mucosa (deficient IF molecules): total or partial gastrectomy, pernicious anemia (PA), caustic destruction (lye).
Abnormal events in small bowel lumen:
Inadequate pancreatic protease (R-Cbl not degraded, Cbl not transferred to IF).
- Insufficiency of pancreatic protease—pancreatic insufficiency.
- Inactivation of pancreatic protease—Zollinger-Ellison syndrome.

Usurping of luminal Cbl (inadequate Cbl binding to IF).
- By bacteria—stasis syndromes (blind loops, pouches of diverticulosis, strictures, fistulas, anastomoses); impaired bowel motility (scleroderma, pseudoobstruction), hypogammaglobulinemia.
- By *Diphyllobothrium latum*.

Disorders of ileal mucosa/IF receptors (IF-Cbl not bound to IF receptors):
Diminished or absent IF receptors—ileal bypass/resection/fistula.
Abnormal mucosal architecture/function—tropical/nontropical sprue, Crohn's disease, TB ileitis, infiltration by lymphomas, amyloidosis.
IF-/post IF-receptor defects—Imerslund-Graesbeck syndrome, TC II deficiency.

Drug-induced effects (slow K, biguanides, cholestyramine, colchicine, neomycin, PAS).

DISORDERS OF PLASMA CBL TRANSPORT (TC II-CBL NOT DELIVERED TO TC II RECEPTORS)

Congenital TC II deficiency, defective binding of TC II-Cbl to TC II receptors (rare).

METABOLIC DISORDERS (CBL NOT UTILIZED BY CELL)

Inborn enzyme errors (rare).

Acquired disorders: (Cbl oxidized to cob[III]alamin)—N_2O inhalation.

FOLATE DEFICIENCY

Nutritional causes

Decreased dietary intake—poverty and famine (associated with kwashiorkor, marasmus), institutionalized individuals (psychiatric/nursing homes), chronic debilitating disease/goats' milk (low in folate), special diets (slimming), cultural/ethnic cooking techniques (food folate destroyed) or habits (folate-rich foods not consumed).

Decreased diet and increased requirements:

- Physiologic: pregnancy and lactation, prematurity, infancy.
- Pathologic: intrinsic hematologic disease (autoimmune hemolytic disease), drugs, malaria; hemoglobinopathies (SS, thalassemia), RBC membrane defects (hereditary spherocytosis, paroxysmal nocturnal hemoglobinopathy); abnormal hematopoiesis (leukemia/lymphoma, myelodysplastic syndrome, agnogenic myeloid metaplasia with myelofibrosis); infiltration with malignant disease; dermatologic (psoriasis).

Folate malabsorption

With normal intestinal mucosa:

- Some drugs (controversial).
- Congenital folate malabsorption (rare).

With mucosal abnormalities—tropical and nontropical sprue, regional enteritis.

Defective cellular folate uptake—familial aplastic anemia (rare)

Inadequate cellular utilization

Folate antagonists (methotrexate).

Hereditary enzyme deficiencies involving folate.

Drugs (multiple effects on folate metabolism)

Alcohol, sulfasalazine, triamterine, pyrimethamine, trimethoprim-sulfamethoxazole, diphenylhydantoin, barbiturates.

MISCELLANEOUS MEGALOBLASTIC ANEMIAS (NOT CAUSED BY CBL OR FOLATE DEFICIENCY)

Congenital disorders of DNA synthesis (rare)

Orotic aciduria, Lesch-Nyhan syndrome, congenital dyserythropoietic anemia.

Acquired disorders of DNA synthesis

Thiamine-responsive megaloblastosis (rare).

Malignancy—erythroleukemia—refractory sideroblastic anemias—all antineoplastic drugs that inhibit DNA synthesis.

Toxic—alcohol.

ANERGY, CUTANEOUS[33]

ICD-9CM # 279.9

IMMUNOLOGIC

Acquired (AIDS, acute leukemia, carcinoma, CLL, Hodgkin's lymphoma, NHL).

Congenital (ataxia-telangiectasia, Di George's syndrome, severe combined immunodeficiency, Wiskott-Aldrich syndrome).

INFECTIONS

Bacterial (bacterial pneumonia, brucellosis).

Disseminated mycotic infections.

Mycobacterial (lepromatous leprosy, TB).

Viral (varicella, hepatitis, influenza, mononucleosis, measles, mumps).

IMMUNOSUPPRESSIVE MEDICATIONS

Systemic corticosteroids.

Methotrexate, cyclophosphamide.

Rifampin.

OTHER

Alcoholic cirrhosis, biliary cirrhosis, sarcoidosis, rheumatic disease.

Diabetes, Crohn's disease, uremia.

Anemia, pyridoxine deficiency, sickle cell anemia.

Burns, malnutrition, pregnancy, old age, surgery.

ANEURYSMS, THORACIC AORTA

ICD-9CM # 441.2

Trauma.

Infection.

Inflammatory (syphilis, Takayasu's disease).

Collagen vascular disease (rheumatoid arthritis, ankylosing spondylitis).

Annuloaortic ectasia (Marfan's syndrome, Ehlers-Danlos syndrome).

Congenital.

Coarctation.

Cystic medial necrosis.

ANHYDROSIS

ICD-9CM # 705.1

Drugs (anticholinergics).

Dehydration.

Hysteria.

Obstruction of sweat ducts (e.g., inflammation, miliaria).

Local radiant heat or pressure.

CNS lesions (medulla, hypothalamus, pons).

Spinal cord lesions.

Lesions of sympathetic nerves.

Congenital sweat gland disturbances.

ANION GAP INCREASE

ICD-9CM # 276.9

Uremia.

Ketoacidosis (diabetic, starvation, alcoholic).

Lactic acidosis.

Ethylene glycol poisoning.

Salicylate overdose.

Methanol poisoning.

ANISOCORIA

ICD-9CM # 379.41

Mydriatic or miotic drugs.

Prosthetic eye.

Inflammation (keratitis, iridocyclitis).

Infections (herpes zoster, syphilis, meningitis, encephalitis, TB, diphtheria, botulism).

Subdural hemorrhage.

Cavernous sinus thrombosis.

Intracranial neoplasm.

Cerebral aneurysm.

Glaucoma.

CNS degenerative diseases.

Internal carotid ischemia.

Toxic polyneuritis (alcohol, lead).

Adie's syndrome.

Horner's syndrome.

Diabetes mellitus (DM).

Trauma.

Congenital.

ANOVULATION

ICD-9CM # 628.0

Anorexia and bulimia.

Strenuous exercise.

Weight loss/malnutrition.

Empty sella syndrome.

Pituitary disorders (infarction, infection, trauma, irradiation, surgery, microadenomas, macroadenomas).

Idiopathic hypopituitarism.

Drug induced.

Thyroid dysfunction (hypothyroidism, hyperthyroidism).

Systemic diseases (e.g., liver disease).

Adrenal hyperfunction (Cushing's syndrome, congenital adrenal hyperplasia).

Polycystic ovarian syndrome.

Isolated gonadotropin deficiency.

APPETITE LOSS IN INFANTS AND CHILDREN[17]

ICD-9CM # 783.0 APPETITE LOSS
307.59 APPETITE LOSS, PSYCHOGENIC ORIGIN

ORGANIC DISEASE

Infection (acute or chronic)

Neurologic

Congenital degenerative disease.

Hypothalamic lesion.

Increased intracranial pressure (including a brain tumor).
Swallowing disorders (neuromuscular).

Gastrointestinal

Oral lesions (e.g., thrush or herpes simplex).
Gastroesophageal reflux.
Obstruction (especially with gastric or intestinal distention).
Inflammatory bowel disease.
Celiac disease.
Constipation.

Cardiac

Congestive heart failure (especially associated with cyanotic lesions).

Metabolic

Renal failure and/or renal tubule acidosis.
Liver failure.
Congenital metabolic disease.
Lead poisoning.

Nutritional

Marasmus.
Iron deficiency.
Zinc deficiency.

Fever

Rheumatoid arthritis.
Rheumatic fever.

Drugs

Morphine.
Digitalis.
Antimetabolites.
Methylphenidate.
Amphetamines.

Miscellaneous

Prolonged restriction of oral feedings, beginning in the neonatal period.
Systemic lupus erythematosus.
Tumor.

PSYCHOLOGIC FACTORS

Anxiety, fear, depression, mania (limbic influence on the hypothalamus).
Avoidance of symptoms associated with meals (abdominal pain, diarrhea, bloating, urgency, dumping syndrome).
Anorexia nervosa.
Excessive weight loss and food aversion in athletes, simulating anorexia nervosa.

ARTERIAL OCCLUSION[13]

ICD-9CM # 444.22 ARTERIAL OCCLUSION, LOWER EXTREMITIES
444.21 ARTERIAL OCCLUSION, UPPER EXTREMITIES

Thromboembolism (post-MI, mitral stenosis, rheumatic valve disease, atrial fibrillation, atrial myxoma, marantic endocarditis, bacterial endocarditis, Libman-Sacks endocarditis).
Atheroembolism (microemboli composed of cholesterol, calcium, and platelets from proximal atherosclerotic plaques).
Arterial thrombosis (endothelial injury, altered arterial blood flow, trauma, severe atherosclerosis, acute vasculitis).
Vasospasm.
Trauma.
Hypercoagulable states.
Miscellaneous (irradiation, drugs, infections, necrotizing).

ARTHRITIS AND ABDOMINAL PAIN

ICD-9CM # CODE VARIES WITH SPECIFIC DISORDER

Viral syndrome.
Inflammatory bowel disease.
Celiac disease.
Vasculitis.
SLE.
Rheumatoid arthritis.
Scleroderma.
Amyloidosis.
Chronic hepatitis C.
Whipple's disease.
Polyarteritis nodosa.
Behçet's disease.
Familial Mediterranean fever.
Blind loop syndrome.

ARTHRITIS AND DIARRHEA

ICD-9CM # CODE VARIES WITH SPECIFIC DISORDER

Viral syndrome.
Inflammatory bowel disease.
Celiac disease.
Whipple's disease.
Enterogenic (bacterial) reactive arthritis.
Collagenous colitis.
Behçet's disease.
Hyperthyroidism.
Spondyloarthropathy.
Blind loop syndrome.

ARTHRITIS AND EYE LESIONS[6]

ICD-9CM # CODE VARIES WITH SPECIFIC DIAGNOSIS

SLE.
Sjögren's syndrome.
Behçet's syndrome.
Sarcoidosis.
SBE.
Lyme disease.
Wegener's granulomatosis.
Giant cell arteritis.
Takayasu's arteritis.
Rheumatoid arthritis, JRA.
Scleroderma.
Inflammatory bowel disease.
Whipple's disease.
Ankylosing spondylitis.
Reactive arthritis.
Psoriatic arthritis.

ARTHRITIS AND HEART MURMUR[6]

ICD-9CM # CODE VARIES WITH SPECIFIC DIAGNOSIS

Subacute bacterial endocarditis (SBE).
Cardiac myxoma.
Ankylosing spondylitis.
Reactive arthritis.
Acute rheumatic fever.
Rheumatoid arthritis (RA).
SLE with Libman-Sacks endocarditis.
Relapsing polychondritis.

ARTHRITIS AND MUSCLE WEAKNESS[8]

ICD-9CM # CODE VARIES WITH SPECIFIC DIAGNOSIS

RA.
Ankylosing spondylitis.
Polymyositis.
Dermatomyositis.
SLE, scleroderma, mixed connective tissue disease.
Sarcoidosis.
HIV-associated arthritis.
Whipple's disease.

ARTHRITIS AND RASH[6]

ICD-9CM # CODE VARIES WITH SPECIFIC DIAGNOSIS

Chronic urticaria.
Vasculitic urticaria.
SLE.
Dermatomyositis.
Polymyositis.
Psoriatic arthritis.
Reactive arthritis.
Chronic sarcoidosis.
Serum sickness.
Sweet's syndrome.
Leprosy.

ARTHRITIS AND SUBCUTANEOUS NODULES[6]

ICD-9CM # CODE VARIES WITH SPECIFIC DIAGNOSIS

RA.
Gout.
Pseudogout (rare).
Sarcoidosis.
Light chain (LA) amyloidosis (primary, multiple myeloma).
Acute rheumatic fever (ARF).
Hemochromatosis.
Whipple's disease.
Multicentric reticulohistiocytosis.

ARTHRITIS AND WEIGHT LOSS[6]

ICD-9CM # CODE VARIES WITH SPECIFIC DIAGNOSIS

Severe RA.
RA with vasculitis.

Reactive arthritis.
RA or psoriatic arthritis or ankylosing spondylitis with amyloidosis.
Cancer.
Enteropathic arthritis (Crohn's, ulcerative colitis).
HIV infection.
Whipple's disease.
Blind loop syndrome.
Scleroderma with intestinal bacterial overgrowth.

ARTHRITIS, AXIAL SKELETON

ICD-9CM # 720.0 ARTHRITIS, RHEUMATOID, SPINE
696.0 ARTHRITIS, PSORIATIC
715.9 ARTHRITIS, DEGENERATIVE, NOS
720.0 ANKYLOSING SPONDYLITIS

RA.
Psoriatic arthritis.
Reiter's syndrome.
Ankylosing spondylitis.
Juvenile RA.
Degenerative disease of the nucleus pulposus.
Spondylosis deformans.
Diffuse idiopathic skeletal hyperostosis (DISH).
Alkaptonuria.
Infection.

ARTHRITIS, FEVER, AND RASH[6]

ICD-9CM # CODE VARIES WITH SPECIFIC DIAGNOSIS

Rubella, parvovirus B-19.
Gonococcemia, meningococcemia.
Secondary syphilis, Lyme borreliosis.
Adult acute rheumatic fever, adult Still's disease, adult Kawasaki disease.
Vasculitic urticaria.
Acute sarcoidosis.
Familial Mediterranean fever.
Hyperimmunoglobulinemia D and periodic fever syndrome.

ARTHRITIS, MONOARTICULAR AND OLIGOARTICULAR[2]

ICD-9CM # 715.3 OSTEOARTHRITIS, LOCALIZED
711.9 INFECTIOUS ARTHRITIS
716.6 MONOARTICULAR ARTHRITIS
5TH DIGIT TO BE ADDED TO THE ABOVE DEPENDING ON SITE OF ARTHRITIS
0. SITE UNSPECIFIED
1. SHOULDER REGION
2. UPPER ARM
3. FOREARM
4. HAND
5. PELVIC REGION AND THIGH
6. LOWER LEG
7. ANKLE AND/OR FOOT
8. OTHER SPECIFIED EXCEPT SPINE

Septic arthritis (*S. aureus, Neisseria gonorrhea, Meningococci, Streptococci, S. pneumoniae,* enteric gram-neg bacilli).
Crystalline-induced arthritis (gout, pseudogout, calcium oxalate, hydroxyapatite and other basic calcium/phosphate crystals).
Traumatic joint injury.
Hemarthrosis.
Monoarticular or oligoarticular flare of an inflammatory polyarticular rheumatic disease (RA, psoriatic arthritis, Reiter's syndrome, SLE).

ARTHRITIS, PEDIATRIC AGE[17]

ICD-9CM # 711.9 INFECTIOUS ARTHRITIS
714.30 JUVENILE CHRONIC OR UNSPECIFIED
714.31 JUVENILE RHEUMATOID POLYARTICULAR ACUTE
714.32 JUVENILE RHEUMATOID PAUCIARTICULAR
714.33 JUVENILE RHEUMATOID MONO-ARTICULAR

RHEUMATIC DISEASES OF CHILDHOOD

Acute rheumatic fever.
Systemic lupus erythematosus.
Juvenile ankylosing spondylitis.
Polymyositis and dermatomyositis.
Vasculitis.
Scleroderma.
Psoriatic arthritis.
Mixed connective tissue disease and overlap syndromes.
Kawasaki disease.
Behçet's syndrome.
Familial Mediterranean fever.
Reiter's syndrome.
Reflex sympathetic dystrophy.
Fibromyalgia (fibrositis).

INFECTIOUS DISEASES

Bacterial arthritis.
Viral or postviral arthritis.
Fungal arthritis.
Osteomyelitis.
Reactive arthritis.

NEOPLASTIC DISEASES

Leukemia.
Lymphoma.
Neuroblastoma.
Primary bone tumors.

NONINFLAMMATORY DISORDERS

Trauma.
Avascular necrosis syndromes.
Osteochondroses.
Slipped capital femoral epiphysis.
Diskitis.
Patellofemoral dysfunction (chondromalacia patellae).
Toxic synovitis of the hip.
Overuse syndromes.

GENETIC OR CONGENITAL SYNDROMES

HEMATOLOGIC DISORDERS

Sickle cell disease.
Hemophilia.

INFLAMMATORY BOWEL DISEASE

MISCELLANEOUS

Growing pains.
Psychogenic arthralgias (conversion reactions).
Hypermobility syndrome.
Villonodular synovitis.
Foreign body arthritis.

ARTHRITIS, POLYARTICULAR

ICD-9CM # 715.09 GENERALIZED OSTEO-ARTHRITIS, MULTIPLE SITES
716.89 ARTHRITIS, MULTIPLE SITES
714.31 JUVENILE RHEUMATOID, POLYARTICULAR, ACUTE

RA, juvenile (rheumatoid) polyarthritis.
SLE, other connective tissue diseases, erythema nodosum, palindromic rheumatism, relapsing polychondritis.
Psoriatic arthritis, ankylosing spondylitis.
Sarcoidosis.
Lyme arthritis, bacterial endocarditis, *Neisseria gonorrhoeae* infection, rheumatic fever, Reiter's disease.
Crystal deposition disease.
Hypersensitivity to serum or drugs.
Hepatitis B, HIV, rubella, mumps.
Other: serum sickness, leukemias, lymphomas, enteropathic arthropathy, Whipple's disease, Behçet's syndrome, Henoch-Schönlein purpura, familial Mediterranean fever, hypertrophic pulmonary osteoarthropathy.

ASCITES

ICD-9CM # 789.5 ASCITES NOS
197.6 ASCITES, CANCEROUS (MALIGNANT)
457.8 ASCITES, CHYLOUS

Hypoalbuminemia: nephrotic syndrome, protein-losing gastroenteropathy, starvation.
Cirrhosis.
Hepatic congestion: CHF, constrictive pericarditis, tricuspid insufficiency, hepatic vein obstruction (Budd-Chiari syndrome), inferior vena cava or portal vein obstruction.
Peritoneal infections: TB and other bacterial infections, fungal diseases, parasites.
Neoplasms: primary hepatic neoplasms, metastases to liver or peritoneum, lymphomas, leukemias, myeloid metaplasia.
Lymphatic obstruction: mediastinal tumors, trauma to the thoracic duct, filariasis.
Ovarian disease: Meigs' syndrome, struma ovarii.
Chronic pancreatitis or pseudocyst: pancreatic ascites.
Leakage of bile: bile ascites.
Urinary obstruction or trauma: urine ascites.
Myxedema.
Chylous ascites.

ASTHMA, CHILDHOOD[4]

ICD-9CM # 493.0 USE 5TH DIGIT
0. WITHOUT MENTION OF STATUS ASTHMATICUS
1. WITH STATUS ASTHMATICUS

INFECTIONS

Bronchiolitis (RSV).
Pneumonia.
Croup.
Tuberculosis, histoplasmosis.
Bronchiectasis.
Bronchiolitis obliterans.
Bronchitis.
Sinusitis.

ANATOMIC, CONGENITAL

Cystic fibrosis.
Vascular rings.
Ciliary dyskinesia.
B lymphocyte immune defect.
Congestive heart failure.
Laryngotracheomalacia.
Tumor, lymphoma.
H-type tracheoesophageal fistula.
Repaired tracheoesophageal fistula.
Gastroesophageal reflux.

VASCULITIS, HYPERSENSITIVITY

Allergic bronchopulmonary aspergillosis.
Allergic alveolitis, hypersensitivity pneumonitis.
Churg-Strauss syndrome.
Periarteritis nodosa.

OTHER

Foreign body aspiration.
Pulmonary thromboembolism.
Psychogenic cough.
Sarcoidosis.
Bronchopulmonary dysplasia.
Vocal cord dysfunction.

ATAXIA

ICD-9CM # 781.3 ATAXIA NOS
303.0 ALCOHOLIC, ACUTE
303.9 ALCOHOLIC, CHRONIC
334.3 CEREBELLAR
331.89 CEREBRAL
334.0 FRIEDREICH'S
300.11 HYSTERICAL

Vertebral-basilar artery ischemia.
Diabetic neuropathy.
Tabes dorsalis.
Vitamin B_{12} deficiency.
Multiple sclerosis and other demyelinating diseases.
Meningomyelopathy.
Cerebellar neoplasms, hemorrhage, abscess, infarct.
Nutritional (Wernicke's encephalopathy).
Paraneoplastic syndromes.
Parainfectious: Guillain-Barré syndrome, acute ataxia of childhood and young adults.
Toxins: phenytoin, alcohol, sedatives, organophosphates.
Wilson's disease (hepatolenticular degeneration).
Hypothyroidism.
Myopathy.
Cerebellar and spinocerebellar degeneration: ataxia/telangiectasia, Friedreich's ataxia.
Frontal lobe lesions: tumors, thrombosis of anterior cerebral artery, hydrocephalus.
Labyrinthine destruction: neoplasm, injury, inflammation, compression.
Hysteria.
AIDS.

ATELECTASIS

ICD-9CM # 518.0

Lung neoplasm (primary or metastatic).
Infection (pneumonia, TB, fungal, histoplasmosis).
Postoperative (lower lobes).
Sarcoidosis.
Mucoid impaction.
Foreign body.
Postinflammatory (middle lobe syndrome).
Pneumothorax.
Pleural effusion.
Pneumoconiosis.
Interstitial fibrosis.
Bulla.
Mediastinal or adjacent mass.

ATRIUM ENLARGEMENT, RIGHT ATRIUM

ICD-9CM # CODE VARIES WITH SPECIFIC DISORDER

Right ventricular failure.
Atrial septal defect.
Tricuspid regurgitation.
Tricuspid stenosis.
Pulmonary hypertension.
Restrictive cardiomyopathy.
Right atrial myxoma.
Ebstein's anomaly.
Anomalous pulmonary venous drainage to the right atrium.
Endomyocardial fibrosis.
Sinus of Valsalva fistula.
Arrhythmogenic right ventricular dysplasia.

AV NODAL BLOCK[13]

ICD-9CM # 426.10 AV BLOCK (INCOMPLETE, PARTIAL)
426.0 AV BLOCK, COMPLETE

Idiopathic fibrosis (Lenegre's disease).
Sclerodegenerative processes (e.g., Lev's disease with calcification of the mitral and aortic annuli).
AV node radiofrequency ablation procedure.
Medications (e.g., digoxin, beta blockers, calcium channel blockers, class III antiarrhythmics).
Acute inferior wall MI.
Myocarditis.
Infections (endocarditis, Lyme disease).
Infiltrative diseases (e.g., hemochromatosis, sarcoidosis, amyloidosis).
Trauma (including cardiac surgical procedures).
Collagen vascular diseases.
Aortic root diseases (e.g., spondylitis).
Electrolyte abnormalities (e.g., hyperkalemia).

BACK PAIN

ICD-9CM # 724.5 BACK PAIN (POSTURAL)
724.2 LOW BACK PAIN
307.89 BACK PAIN PSYCHOGENIC
724.8 STIFF BACK
847.9 BACK STRAIN
724.6 BACKACHE, SACROILIAC

Trauma: injury to bone, joint, or ligament.
Mechanical: pregnancy, obesity, fatigue, scoliosis.
Degenerative: osteoarthritis.

Infections: osteomyelitis, subarachnoid or spinal abscess, TB, meningitis, basilar pneumonia.
Metabolic: osteoporosis, osteomalacia.
Vascular: leaking aortic aneurysm, subarachnoid or spinal hemorrhage/infarction.
Neoplastic: myeloma, Hodgkin's disease, carcinoma of pancreas, metastatic neoplasm from breast, prostate, lung.
GI: penetrating ulcer, pancreatitis, cholelithiasis, inflammatory bowel disease.
Renal: hydronephrosis, calculus, neoplasm, renal infarction, pyelonephritis.
Hematologic: sickle cell crisis, acute hemolysis.
Gynecologic: neoplasm of uterus or ovary, dysmenorrhea, salpingitis, uterine prolapse.
Inflammatory: ankylosing spondylitis, psoriatic arthritis, Reiter's syndrome.
Lumbosacral strain.
Psychogenic: malingering, hysteria, anxiety.
Endocrine: adrenal hemorrhage or infarction.

BACK PAIN, VISCEROGENIC ORIGIN

ICD-9CM # CODE VARIES WITH SPECIFIC DISORDER

Urolithiasis.
Aortic aneurysm.
Colorectal carcinoma.
Endometriosis.
Tubal pregnancy.
Prostatitis.
Peptic ulcer.
Pancreatitis.
Diverticular spasm.
Metastatic neoplasm (e.g., bladder, uterus, ovary, kidney).

BALLISM*

ICD-9CM # 333.5

Cerebral infarction or hemorrhage.
Medications (e.g., dopamine agonists, phenytoin).
CNS neoplasm (primary or metastatic).
Nonketotic hyperosmolar state.

*Violent, flinging, nonpatterned rapid movements

BLEEDING, LOWER GI

ICD-9CM # 578.9

(ORIGINATING BELOW THE LIGAMENT OF TREITZ)

Small Intestine

Ischemic bowel disease (mesenteric thrombosis, embolism, vasculitis, trauma).
Small bowel neoplasm: leiomyomas, carcinoids.
Hereditary hemorrhagic telangiectasia (Rendu-Osler-Weber syndrome).
Meckel diverticulum and other small intestine diverticula.
Aortoenteric fistula.
Intestinal hemangiomas: blue rubber-bleb nevi, intestinal hemangiomas, cutaneous vascular nevi.
Hamartomatous polyps: Peutz-Jeghers syndrome (intestinal polyps, mucocutaneous pigmentation).
Infections of small bowel: tuberculous enteritis, enteritis necroticans.
Volvulus.
Intussusception.
Lymphoma of small bowel, sarcoma, Kaposi's sarcoma.
Irradiation ileitis.
AV malformation of small intestine.
Inflammatory bowel disease.
Polyarteritis nodosa.
Other: pancreatoenteric fistulas, Henoch-Schönlein purpura, Ehlers-Danlos syndrome, systemic lupus erythematosus, amyloidosis, metastatic melanoma.

Colon

Carcinoma (particularly left colon).
Diverticular disease.
Inflammatory bowel disease.
Ischemic colitis.
Colonic polyps.
Vascular abnormalities: angiodysplasia, vascular ectasia.
Radiation colitis.
Infectious colitis.
Uremic colitis.
Aortoenteric fistula.
Lymphoma of large bowel.
Hemorrhoids.
Anal fissure.
Trauma, foreign body.
Solitary rectal/cecal ulcers.
Long-distance running.

BLEEDING, LOWER GI, PEDIATRIC[2]

ICD-9CM # 578.9

<3 MONTHS

Swallowed maternal blood.
Infectious colitis.
Milk allergy.
Bleeding diathesis.
Intussusception.
Midgut volvulus.
Meckel diverticulum.
Necrotizing enterocolitis.

<2 YEARS OLD

Anal fissure.
Infectious colitis.
Milk allergy.
Colitis.
Intussusception.
Meckel diverticulum.
Polyp.
Duplication.
Hemolytic uremic syndrome.
Inflammatory bowel disease.
Pseudomembranous enterocolitis.

<5 YEARS OLD

Infectious colitis.
Anal fissure.
Polyp.
Intussusception.
Meckel diverticulum.
Henoch-Schönlein purpura.
Hemolytic uremic syndrome.
Inflammatory bowel disease.
Pseudomembranous enterocolitis.

5-18 YEARS

Infectious colitis.
Inflammatory bowel disease.
Pseudomembranous enterocolitis.
Polyp.
Hemolytic-uremic syndrome.
Hemorrhoid.

BLEEDING, UPPER GI

ICD-9CM # 578.9

(ORIGINATING ABOVE THE LIGAMENT OF TREITZ)

Oral or pharyngeal lesions: swallowed blood from nose or oropharynx.
Swallowed hemoptysis
Esophageal: varices, ulceration, esophagitis, Mallory-Weiss tear, carcinoma, trauma.
Gastric: peptic ulcer (including Cushing and Curling's ulcers), gastritis, angiodysplasia, gastric neoplasms, hiatal hernia, gastric diverticulum, pseudoxanthoma elasticum, Rendu-Osler-Weber syndrome.
Duodenal: peptic ulcer, duodenitis, angiodysplasia, aortoduodenal fistula, duodenal diverticulum, duodenal tumors, carcinoma of ampulla of Vater, parasites (e.g., hookworm), Crohn's disease.
Biliary: hematobilia (e.g., penetrating injury to liver, hepatobiliary malignancy, endoscopic papillotomy).

BLEEDING, UPPER GI, PEDIATRIC[2]

ICD-9CM # 578.9

<3 MONTHS OLD

Swallowed maternal blood.
Gastritis.
Ulcer, stress.
Bleeding diathesis.
Foreign body (NG tube).
Vascular malformation.
Duplication.

<2 YEARS OLD

Esophagitis.
Gastritis.
Ulcer.
Pyloric stenosis.

Mallory-Weiss syndrome.
Vascular malformation.
Duplication.

<5 YEARS OLD

Esophagitis.
Gastritis.
Ulcer.
Esophageal varices.
Foreign body.
Mallory-Weiss syndrome.
Hemophilia.
Vascular malformations.

5-18 YEARS OLD

Esophagitis.
Gastritis.
Ulcer.
Esophageal varices.
Mallory-Weiss syndrome.
Inflammatory bowel disease.
Hemophilia.
Vascular malformation.

BLINDNESS, GERIATRIC AGE

ICD-9CM # 369.4

Cataracts.
Glaucoma.
Diabetic retinopathy.
Macular degeneration.
Trauma.
CVA.
Corneal scarring.

BLINDNESS, MONOCULAR, TRANSIENT

ICD-9CM # 369.67

Migraine (vasospasm).
Embolic cerebrovascular disease.
Intermittent angle-closure glaucoma.
Partial retinal vein occlusion.
Hyphema.
Optic disc edema.
Giant cell arteritis.
Psychogenic.
Hypotension.
Hypercoagulopathy disorders.
Multiple sclerosis.

BLINDNESS, PEDIATRIC AGE[20]

ICD-9CM # CODE VARIES WITH SPECIFIC DISORDER

CONGENITAL

Optic nerve hypoplasia or aplasia.
Optic coloboma.
Congenital hydrocephalus.
Hydranencephaly.
Porencephaly.
Micrencephaly.
Encephalocele, particularly occipital type.
Morning glory disc.
Aniridia.
Anterior microphthalmia.
Peter's anomaly.
Persistent pupillary membrane.
Glaucoma.
Cataracts.
Persistent hyperplastic primary vitreous.

PHAKOMATOSES

Tuberous sclerosis.
Neurofibromatosis (special association with optic glioma).
Sturge-Weber syndrome.
von Hippel–Lindau disease.

TUMORS

Retinoblastoma.
Optic glioma.
Perioptic meningioma.
Craniopharyngioma.
Cerebral glioma.
Posterior and intraventricular tumors when complicated by hydrocephalus.
Pseudotumor cerebri.

NEURODEGENERATIVE DISEASES

Cerebral storage disease.
Gangliosidoses, particularly Tay-Sachs disease (infantile amaurotic familial idiocy), Sandhoff's variant, generalized gangliosidosis.
Other lipidoses and ceroid lipofuscinoses, particularly the late-onset amaurotic familial idiocies such as those of Jansky-Bielschowsky and of Batten-Mayou-Spielmeyer-Vogt.
Mucopolysaccharidoses, particularly Hurler's syndrome and Hunter's syndrome.
Leukodystrophies (dysmyelination disorders), particularly metachromatic leukodystrophy and Canavan's disease.
Demyelinating sclerosis (myelinoclastic diseases), especially Schilder's disease and Devic's neuromyelitis optica.
Special types: Dawson's disease, Leigh's disease, Bassen-Kornzweig syndrome, Refsum's disease.
Retinal degenerations: retinitis pigmentosa and its variants, Leber's congenital type.
Optic atrophies: congenital autosomal recessive type, infantile and congenital autosomal dominant types, Leber's disease, and atrophies associated with hereditary ataxias—the types of Behr, of Marie, and of Sanger-Brown.

INFECTIOUS PROCESSES

Encephalitis, especially in the prenatal infection syndromes caused by *Toxoplasma gondii,* cytomegalovirus, rubella virus, *Treponema pallidum,* herpes simplex.
Meningitis; arachnoiditis.
Chorioretinitis.
Endophthalmitis.
Keratitis.

HEMATOLOGIC DISORDERS

Leukemia with central nervous system involvement.

VASCULAR AND CIRCULATORY DISORDERS

Collagen vascular diseases.
Arteriovenous malformations—intracerebral hemorrhage, subarachnoid hemorrhage.
Central retinal occlusion.

TRAUMA

Contusion or avulsion of optic nerves, chiasm, globe, cornea.
Cerebral contusion or laceration.
Intracerebral, subarachnoid, or subdural hemorrhage.

DRUGS AND TOXINS

Other

Retinopathy of prematurity.
Sclerocornea.
Conversion reaction.
Optic neuritis.
Osteopetrosis.

BLISTERS, SUBEPIDERMAL

ICD-9CM # 919.2

Burns.
Porphyria cutanea tarda.
Bullous pemphigoid.
Bullous drug reaction.
Arthropod bite reaction.
Toxic epidermal necrosis.
Dermatitis herpetiformis.
Polymorphous light eruption.
Variegate porphyria.
Lupus erythematosus.
Epidermolysis bullosa.
Pseudoporphyria.
Acute graft-versus-host reaction.
Linear IgA disease.
Leukocytoclastic vasculitis.
Pressure necrosis.
Urticaria pigmentosa.
Amyloidosis.

BONE LESIONS, PREFERENTIAL SITE OF ORIGIN[32]

ICD-9CM # 170.0 SKULL AND FACE
170.1 MANDIBLE
170.2 VERTEBRAL COLUMN
170.3 RIBS, STERNUM, CLAVICLE
170.4 SCAPULA, LONG BONES UPPER LIMB
170.5 SHORT BONES AND UPPER LIMB
170.6 PELVIC BONES, SACRUM COCCYX
170.7 LONG BONES LOWER LIMB
170.8 SHORT BONES LOWER LIMB
170.9 BONE CANCER NOS
198.5 BONE CANCER, METASTATIC

EPIPHYSIS

Chondroblastoma.
Giant-cell tumor—after fusion of growth plate.
Langerhans' cell histiocytosis.
Clear cell chondrosarcoma.
Osteosarcoma.

METAPHYSIS

Parosteal sarcoma.
Chondrosarcoma.
Fibrosarcoma.
Nonossifying fibroma.
Giant-cell tumor—before fusion of growth plate.
Unicameral bone cyst.
Aneurysmal bone cyst.

DIAPHYSIS

Myeloma.
Ewing's tumor.
Reticulum cell sarcoma.

METADIAPHYSEAL

Fibrosarcoma.
Fibrous dysplasia.
Enchondroma.
Osteoid osteoma.
Chondromyofibroma.

BONE MARROW FIBROSIS[12]

ICD-9CM # 289.9

MYELOID DISORDERS

Myelofibrosis with myeloid metaplasia.
Metastatic cancer.
Chronic myeloid leukemia.
Myelodysplastic syndrome.
Atypical myeloid disorder.
Acute megakaryocytic leukemia.
Other acute myeloid leukemias.
Gray platelet syndrome.

LYMPHOID DISORDERS

Hairy cell leukemia.
Multiple myeloma.
Lymphoma.

NONHEMATOLOGIC DISORDERS

Connective tissue disorder.
Infections (tuberculosis, kala-azar).
Vitamin D–deficiency rickets.
Renal osteodystrophy.

BONE MINERAL DENSITY, INCREASED

ICD-9CM # 733.99

Paget's disease of bone.
Skeletal metastases.
Diffuse idiopathic skeletal hyperostosis (DISH).
Osteonecrosis.
Sarcoidosis.
Hypoparathyroidism, pseudohypoparathyroidism.
Milk-alkali syndrome.
Osteopetrosis.
Hypervitaminosis, A or D.
Dysplasias (craniodiaphyseal, craniometaphyseal, frontometaphyseal).
Endosteal hyperostosis.
Fluorosis.
Heavy metal poisoning.
Ionizing radiation.
Other: lymphoma, leukemia, mastocytosis, multiple myeloma, polycythemia vera.

BONE PAIN

ICD-9CM # CODE NOT AVAILABLE

Trauma.
Neoplasm (primary or metastatic).
Osteoporosis with compression fracture.
Paget's disease of bone.
Infection (osteomyelitis, septic arthritis).
Osteomalacia.
Viral syndrome.
Sickle cell disease.
Anxiety.

BONE RESORPTION[32]

ICD-9CM # 733.90 BONE DISORDER

DISTAL CLAVICLE

Hyperparathyroidism.
Rheumatoid arthritis.
Scleroderma.
Posttraumatic osteolysis.
Progeria.
Pycnodysostosis.
Cleidocranial dysplasia.

INFERIOR ASPECT OF RIBS

Vascular impression, associated with but not limited to coarctation of the aorta.
Hyperparathyroidism.
Neurofibromatosis.

TERMINAL PHALANGEAL TUFTS

Scleroderma.
Raynaud's phenomenon.
Vascular disease.
Frostbite, electrical burns.
Psoriasis.
Tabes dorsalis.
Hyperparathyroidism.

GENERALIZED RESORPTION

Paraplegia.
Myositis ossificans.
Osteoporosis.

BRADYCARDIA, SINUS[13]

ICD-9CM # 427.89

Idiopathic.
Degenerative processes (e.g., Lev's disease, Lenegre's disease).
Medications
Beta blockers.
Some calcium channel blockers (diltiazem, verapamil).
Digoxin (when vagal tone is high).
Class I antiarrhythmic agents (e.g., procainamide).
Class III antiarrhythmic agents (amiodarone, sotalol).
Clonidine.
Lithium carbonate.
Acute myocardial ischemia and infarction
Right or left circumflex coronary artery occlusion or spasm.
High vagal tone (e.g., athletes).

BREAST INFLAMMATORY LESION[10]

ICD-9CM # 611.0 ACUTE MASTITIS
610.1 CHRONIC CYSTIC MASTITIS
771.5 NEONATAL INFECTIVE MASTITIS
778.7 NEONATAL NONINFECTIVE MASTITIS

Mastitis (*S. aureus, Beta-hemolytic Strep*).
Trauma.
Foreign body (sutures, breast implants).
Granuloma (TB, fungal).
Fat necrosis post biopsy.
Necrosis or infarction (anticoagulant therapy, pregnancy).
Breast malignancy.

BREAST MASS

ICD-9CM # 611.72

Fibrocystic breasts.
Benign tumors (fibroadenoma, papilloma).
Mastitis (acute bacterial mastitis, chronic mastitis).
Malignant neoplasm.
Fat necrosis.
Hematoma.
Duct ectasia.
Mammary adenosis.

BREATH ODOR[31]

ICD-9CM # 784.9 HALITOSIS

Sweet, fruity: DKA, starvation ketosis.
Fishy, stale: uremia (trimethylamines).
Ammonia-like: uremia (ammonia).
Musty fish, clover: fetor hepaticus (hepatic failure).
Foul, feculent: intestinal obstruction/diverticulum.
Foul, putrid: nasal/sinus pathology (infection, foreign body, cancer), respiratory infections (empyema, lung abscess, bronchiectasis).
Halitosis: tonsillitis, gingivitis, respiratory infections, Vincent's angina, gastroesophageal reflux, achalasia.
Cinnamon: pulmonary TB.

BREATHING, NOISY[31]

ICD-9CM # 786.09 BREATHING, LABORED
789.09 SNORING, WHEEZING
786.1 STRIDOR

Infection: upper respiratory infection, peritonsillar abscess, retropharyngeal abscess, epiglottitis, laryngitis, tracheitis, bronchitis, bronchiolitis.
Irritants and allergens: hyperactive airway, asthma (reactive airway disease), rhinitis, angioneurotic edema.
Compression from outside of the airway: esophageal cysts or foreign body, neoplasms, lymphadenopathy.
Congenital malformation and abnormality: vascular rings, laryngeal webs, laryngomalacia, tracheomalacia, hemangiomas within the upper airway, stenoses within the upper airway, cystic fibrosis.
Acquired abnormality (at every level of the airway): nasal polyps, hypertrophied adenoids and/or tonsils, foreign body, intraluminal tumors, bronchiectasis.
Neurogenic disorder: vocal cord paralysis.

BULLOUS DISEASES

ICD-9CM # 694.9 BULLOUS DERMATOSES
694.5 BULLOUS PEMPHIGOID
694.4 PEMPHIGUS VULGARIS
694.4 PEMPHIGUS FOLIACEUS

Bullous pemphigoid.
Pemphigus vulgaris.
Pemphigus foliaceus.
Paraneoplastic pemphigus.
Cicatricial pemphigoid.
Erythema multiforme.
Dermatitis herpetiformis.
Herpes gestationis.
Impetigo.
Erosive lichen planus.
Linear IgA bullous dermatosis.
Epidermolysis bullosa acquisita.

CALCIFICATION ON CHEST X-RAY

ICD-9CM # 722.92

Lung neoplasm (primary or metastatic).
Silicosis.
Idiopathic pulmonary fibrosis.
Tuberculosis.
Histoplasmosis.
Disseminated varicella infection.
Mitral stenosis (end-stage).
Secondary hyperparathyroidism.

CALCIFICATIONS, CUTANEOUS

ICD-9CM # 709.3

Calcification, Raynaud's phenomenon, esophageal dysmotility, sclerodactyly, and telangiectasia (CREST) syndrome.
Trauma.
Pancreatitis or pancreatic cancer.
Chronic renal failure.
Sarcoidosis.
Hyperparathyroidism.
Milk-alkali syndrome.
Hypervitaminosis D.
Panniculitis.
Idiopathic.
Iatrogenic (e.g., application of calcium alginate dressing to skin).
Multiple myeloma.
Dermatomyositis.
Parasitic infections.
Leukemia.
Lymphoma.

CALCIUM STONES

ICD-9CM # 592.9

Medications (e.g., antacids, loop diuretics, vitamin D, acetazolamide, glucocorticoids).
Primary hyperparathyroidism.
Hypercalcemia from malignancy.
Sarcoidosis.
Prolonged immobilization.
Hyperoxaluria (e.g., Crohn's disease, celiac disease, chronic pancreatitis).
Hyperuricosuria (e.g., hyperuricemia, excessive dietary purine, allopurinol, probenecid).
Renal tubular acidosis.
Milk-alkali syndrome.
Thyrotoxicosis.
Hypocitraturia (e.g., metabolic acidosis, hypomagnesemia, hypokalemia).

CARDIAC ARREST, NONTRAUMATIC[23]

ICD-9CM # 427.5 CARDIAC ARREST NOS

Cardiac (coronary artery disease, cardiomyopathies, structural abnormalities, valve dysfunction, arrhythmias).
Respiratory (upper airway obstruction, hypoventilation, pulmonary embolism, asthma, COPD exacerbation, pulmonary edema).
Circulatory (tension pneumothorax, pericardial tamponade, PE, hemorrhage, sepsis).
Electrolyte abnormalities (hypokalemia or hyperkalemia, hypomagnesemia or hypermagnesemia, hypocalcemia).
Medications (tricyclic antidepressants, digoxin, theophylline, calcium channel blockers).
Drug abuse (cocaine, heroin, amphetamines).
Toxins (carbon monoxide, cyanide).
Environmental (drowning/near-drowning, electrocution, lightning, hypothermia or hyperthermia, venomous snakes).

CARDIAC DEATH, SUDDEN[1]

ICD-9CM # CODE VARIES WITH SPECIFIC DISORDER

Noncardiac.
- CNS hemorrhage.
- Massive pulmonary embolus.
- Drug overdose.
- Hypoxia secondary to lung disease.
- Aortic dissection or rupture.

Cardiac.
- Ventricular tachycardia.
- Bradyarrhythmia, sick sinus syndrome.
- Aortic stenosis.
- Tetralogy of Fallot.
- Pericardial tamponade.
- Cardiac tumors.
- Complications of infective endocarditis.
- Hypertrophic cardiomyopathy (arrhythmia or obstruction).
- Myocardial ischemia.
  - Atherosclerosis.
  - Prinzmetal's angina.
  - Kawasaki's arteritis.

CARDIAC ENLARGEMENT[13]

ICD-9CM # 429.3 CARDIOMEGALY, IDIOPATHIC
746.89 CARDIOMEGALY, CONGENITAL
402.0 CARDIOMEGALY, MALIGNANT
402.1 CARDIOMEGALY, BENIGN

CARDIAC CHAMBER ENLARGEMENT

Chronic volume overload
Mitral or aortic regurgitation.
Left-to-right shunt (PDA, VSD, AV fistula).
Cardiomyopathy
Ischemic.
Nonischemic.
Decompensated pressure overload
Aortic stenosis.
Hypertension.
High-output states
Severe anemia.
Thyrotoxicosis.
Bradycardia
Severe sinus bradycardia.
Complete heart block.

LEFT ATRIUM

LV failure of any cause.
Mitral valve disease.
Myxoma.

RIGHT VENTRICLE

Chronic volume overload.
Tricuspid or pulmonic regurgitation.
Left-to-right shunt (ASD).

Decompensated pressure overload:
- Pulmonic stenosis.
- Pulmonary artery hypertension:
  - Primary.
  - Secondary (PE, COPD).
- Pulmonary venoocclusive disease.

RIGHT ATRIUM

RV failure of any cause.
Tricuspid valve disease.
Myxoma.
Ebstein's anomaly.

MULTICHAMBER ENLARGEMENT

Hypertrophic cardiomyopathy.
Acromegaly.
Severe obesity.

PERICARDIAL DISEASE

Pericardial effusion with or without tamponade.
Effusive constrictive disease.
Pericardial cyst, loculated effusion.

PSEUDOCARDIOMEGALY

Epicardial fat.
Chest wall deformity (pectus excavatum, straight back syndrome).
Low lung volumes.
AP chest x-ray.
Mediastinal tumor, cyst.

CARDIAC MURMURS

ICD-9CM # CODE VARIES WITH SPECIFIC DISORDER

SYSTOLIC

Mitral regurgitation (MR).
Tricuspid regurgitation (TR).
Ventricular septal defect (VSD).
Aortic stenosis (AS).
Idiopathic hypertrophic subaortic stenosis (IHSS).
Pulmonic stenosis (PS).
Innocent murmur of childhood.
Coarctation of aorta.
Mitral valve prolapse (MVP).

DIASTOLIC

Aortic regurgitation (AR).
Atrial myxoma.
Mitral stenosis (MS).
Pulmonary artery branch stenosis.
Tricuspid stenosis (TS).
Graham Steell murmur (diastolic decrescendo murmur heard in severe pulmonary hypertension).
Pulmonic regurgitation (PR).
Severe mitral regurgitation (MR).
Austin Flint murmur (diastolic rumble heard in severe AR).
Severe VSD and patent ductus arteriosus.

CONTINUOUS

Patent ductus arteriosus.
Pulmonary AV fistula.

CARDIOEMBOLISM

ICD-9CM # 410.9

Acute MI.
Atrial fibrillation.
Left ventricular aneurysm.
Valvular heart disease (e.g., rheumatic mitral valve disease, mitral valve prolapse).
Dilated cardiomyopathy.
Atrial septal defect.
Patent foramen ovale.
Cardioversion for atrial fibrillation.
Infective endocarditis.
Atrial septal aneurysm.
Sick sinus syndrome and cardiac arrhythmias.
Nonbacterial thrombotic endocarditis.
Prosthetic heart valves.
Atrial myxoma and other intracardiac tumors.
Cyanatic heart disease.
Balloon angioplasty.
Coronary artery bypass grafting.
Aneurysms of sinus of Valsalva.
Others: VVI pacing, ventricular support devices, heart transplantation, intracardiac defects with paradoxical embolism.

CARDIOGENIC SHOCK

ICD-9CM # 785.51

Myocardial infarction.
Arrhythmias.
Pericardial effusion/tamponade.
Chest trauma.
Valvular heart disease.
Myocarditis.
Cardiomyopathy.
CHF, end-stage.

CAVITARY LESION ON CHEST X-RAY[14]

ICD-9CM # 793.1 CHEST X-RAY LUNG SHADOW

NECROTIZING INFECTIONS

Bacteria: anaerobes, *Staphylococcus aureus,* enteric gram-negative bacteria, *Pseudomonas aeruginosa, Legionella* species, *Haemophilus influenzae, Streptococcus pyogenes, Streptococcus pneumoniae* (?), *Rhodococcus, Actinomyces.*
Mycobacteria: *Mycobacterium tuberculosis, Mycobacterium kansasii,* MAI.
Bacteria-like: *Nocardia* species.
Fungi: *Coccidioides immitis, Histoplasma capsulatum, Blastomyces hominis, Aspergillus* species, *Mucor* species.
Parasitic: *Entamoeba histolytica, Echinococcus, Paragonimus westermani.*

CAVITARY INFARCTION

Bland infarction (with or without superimposed infection).
Lung contusion.

SEPTIC EMBOLISM

S. aureus, anaerobes, others.

VASCULITIS

Wegener's granulomatosis, periarteritis.

NEOPLASMS

Bronchogenic carcinoma, metastatic carcinoma, lymphoma.

MISCELLANEOUS LESIONS

Cysts, blebs, bullae, or pneumatocele with or without fluid collections.
Sequestration.
Empyema with air-fluid level.
Bronchiectasis.

CEREBRAL INFARCTION SECONDARY TO INHERITED DISORDERS

ICD-9CM # 434.91

Homocystinuria.
Marfan's syndrome.
Ehlers-Danlos syndrome.
Rendu-Osler-Weber syndrome.
Pseudoxanthoma elasticum.
Fabry's disease.

CEREBROVASCULAR DISEASE, ISCHEMIC[35]

ICD-9CM # 437.9

VASCULAR DISORDERS

Large-vessel atherothrombotic disease.
Lacunar disease.
Arterial-to-arterial embolization.
Carotid or vertebral artery dissection.
Fibromuscular dysplasia.
Migraine.
Venous thrombosis.
Radiation.
Complications of arteriography.
Multiple, progressive intracranial arterial occlusions.

INFLAMMATORY DISORDERS

Giant cell arteritis.
Polyarteritis nodosa.
Systemic lupus erythematosus.
Granulomatous angiitis.
Takayasu's disease.
Arteritis associated with amphetamine, cocaine, or phenylpropanolamine.
Syphilis, mucormycosis.
Sjögren's syndrome.
Behçet's syndrome.

CARDIAC DISORDERS

Rheumatic heart disease.
Mural thrombus.
Arrhythmias.
Mitral valve prolapse.
Prosthetic heart valve.
Endocarditis.
Myxoma.
Paradoxical embolus.

HEMATOLOGIC DISORDERS

Thrombotic thrombocytopenic purpura.
Sickle cell disease.
Hypercoagulable states.
Polycythemia.
Thrombocytosis.
Leukocytosis.
Lupus anticoagulant.

CHEST PAIN, CHILDREN[4]

ICD-9CM # 786.50 CHEST PAIN NOS
786.59 CHEST PRESSURE
786.52 CHEST PAIN, PLEURITIC

MUSCULOSKELETAL (COMMON)

Trauma (accidental, abuse).
Exercise, overuse injury (strain, bursitis).
Costochondritis (Tietze's syndrome).
Herpes zoster (cutaneous).
Pleurodynia.
Fibrositis.
Slipping rib.
Sickle cell anemia vaso-occlusive crisis.
Osteomyelitis (rare).
Primary or metastatic tumor (rare).

PULMONARY (COMMON)

Pneumonia.
Pleurisy.
Asthma.
Chronic cough.
Pneumothorax.
Infarction (sickle cell anemia).
Foreign body.
Embolism (rare).
Pulmonary hypertension (rare).
Tumor (rare).

GASTROINTESTINAL (LESS COMMON)

Esophagitis (gastroesophageal reflux).
Esophageal foreign body.
Esophageal spasm.
Cholecystitis.
Subdiaphragmatic abscess.
Perihepatitis (Fitz-Hugh-Curtis syndrome).
Peptic ulcer disease.

CARDIAC (LESS COMMON)

Pericarditis.
Postpericardiotomy syndrome.
Endocarditis.
Mitral valve prolapse.
Aortic or subaortic stenosis.
Arrhythmias.
Marfan's syndrome (dissecting aortic aneurysm).
Anomalous coronary artery.
Kawasaki disease.
Cocaine, sympathomimetic ingestion.
Angina (familial hypercholesterolemia).

IDIOPATHIC (COMMON)

Anxiety, hyperventilation.
Panic disorder.

OTHER (LESS COMMON)

Spinal cord or nerve root compression.
Breast-related pathologic condition.
Castleman's disease (lymph node neoplasm).

CHEST PAIN (NONPLEURITIC)[8]

ICD-9CM # 786.50 CHEST PAIN NOS
786.59 CHEST DISCOMFORT

Cardiac: myocardial ischemia/infarction, myocarditis.
Esophageal: spasm, esophagitis, ulceration, neoplasm, achalasia, diverticula, foreign body.
Referred pain from subdiaphragmatic GI structures.
Gastric and duodenal: hiatal hernia, neoplasm, PUD.
Gallbladder and biliary: cholecystitis, cholelithiasis, impacted stone, neoplasm.
Pancreatic: pancreatitis, neoplasm.
Dissecting aortic aneurysm.
Pain originating from skin, breasts, and musculoskeletal structures: herpes zoster, mastitis, cervical spondylosis.
Mediastinal tumors: lymphoma, thymoma.
Pulmonary: neoplasm, pneumonia, pulmonary embolism/infarction.
Psychoneurosis.
Chest pain associated with mitral valve prolapse.

CHEST PAIN (PLEURITIC)

ICD-9CM # 786.52 CHEST PAIN, PLEURITIC

Cardiac: pericarditis, postpericardiotomy/Dressler's syndrome.
Pulmonary: pneumothorax, hemothorax, embolism/infarction, pneumonia, empyema, neoplasm, bronchiectasis, pneumomediastinum, TB, carcinomatous effusion.
GI: liver abscess, pancreatitis, esophageal rupture, Whipple's disease with associated pericarditis or pleuritis.
Subdiaphragmatic abscess.
Pain originating from skin and musculoskeletal tissues: costochondritis, chest wall trauma, fractured rib, interstitial fibrositis, myositis, strain of pectoralis muscle, herpes zoster, soft tissue and bone tumors.
Collagen vascular diseases with pleuritis.
Psychoneurosis.
Familial Mediterranean fever.

CHOLESTASIS[12]

ICD-9CM # 574.71

EXTRAHEPATIC

Choledocholithiasis.
Bile duct stricture.
Cholangiocarcinoma.
Pancreatic carcinoma.
Chronic pancreatitis.
Papillary stenosis.
Ampullary cancer.
Primary sclerosing cholangitis.
Choledochal cysts.
Parasites (e.g., ascaris, clonorchis).
AIDS.
Cholangiography.
Biliary atresia.
Portal lymphadenopathy.
Mirizzi's syndrome.

INTRAHEPATIC

Viral hepatitis.
Alcoholic hepatitis.
Drug induced.
Ductopenia syndromes.
Primary biliary cirrhosis.
Benign recurrent intrahepatic cholestasis.
Byler's disease.
Primary sclerosing cholangitis.
Alagille's syndrome.
Sarcoid.
Lymphoma.
Postoperative.
Total parenteral nutrition.
Alpha-1-antitrypsin deficiency.

CHOREA

ICD-9CM # 333.5

Medications (e.g., neuroleptics, tricyclics, antiparkinsonian drugs).
Cerebral palsy.
Huntington's disease.
Benign hereditary chorea.
Thyroid disorder (hyperthyroidism, hypothyroidism).
Friedrich's ataxia.
Ataxia-telangiectasia.
Hypoglycemia, hyperglycemia.
Electrolyte abnormalities (hyponatremia, hypocalcemia, hypomagnesemia, hypernatremia).
Vitamin B_{12} deficiency.
Systemic lupus erythematosus.
Wilson's disease.
Alcohol.
Cocaine.
Carbon monoxide poisoning.
Mercury poisoning.

CHOREOATHETOSIS[25]

ICD-9CM # 275.1 CHOREO-ATHETOSIS-AGITANS SYNDROME
33.5 CHOREO-ATHETOSIS PAROXYSMAL

SYSTEMIC DISEASES

Systemic lupus erythematosus.
Polycythemia.
Thyrotoxicosis.
Rheumatic fever.
Cirrhosis of the liver (acquired hepatocerebral degeneration).
Diabetes mellitus.
Wilson's disease.

PRIMARY DEGENERATIVE BRAIN DISEASES

Huntington's chorea.
Olivopontocerebellar atrophies.
Neuroacanthocytosis.

FOCAL BRAIN DISEASES

Hemichorea.
Stroke.
Tumor.
Arteriovenous malformation.

DRUG-INDUCED CHOREOATHETOSIS

Parkinson's disease drugs
Levodopa.
Epilepsy drugs
Phenytoin.
Carbamazepine.
Phenobarbital.
Gabapentin.
Valproate.
Psychostimulant drugs
Cocaine.
Amphetamine.
Methamphetamine.
Dextroamphetamine.
Methylphenidate.
Pemoline.
Psychotropic drugs
Lithium.
Tricyclic antidepressant drugs.
Oral contraceptive drugs
Cimetidine.

CHYLOTHORAX

ICD-9CM # 457.8

Post lymph node dissection of neck or chest.
Subclavian venous catheterization.
Thoracic aneurysm repair.
Trauma to chest and neck.
Mediastinal tumor resection.
Esophagectomy, pneumonectomy.
Lymphangitis, mediastinitis.
Neoplasms (lymphoma, carcinoma of esophagus, lung, mediastinal malignancies).
Sympathectomy.
Venous thrombosis.
Congenital.

CLUBBING

ICD-9CM # 781.5 CLUBBING FINGER

Pulmonary neoplasm (lung, pleura).
Other neoplasm (GI, liver, Hodgkin's, thymus, osteogenic sarcoma).
Pulmonary infectious process (empyema, abscess, bronchiectasis, TB, chronic pneumonitis).
Extrapulmonary infectious process (subacute bacterial endocarditis, intestinal TB, bacterial or amebic dysentery, arterial graft sepsis).
Pneumoconiosis.
Cystic fibrosis.
Sarcoidosis.
Cyanotic congenital heart disease.
Endocrine (Graves' disease, hyperparathyroidism).
Inflammatory bowel disease.
Celiac disease.
Chronic liver disease, cirrhosis (particularly biliary and juvenile).
Pulmonary AV malformations.
Idiopathic.
Thyroid acropachy.
Hereditary (pachydermoperiostosis).
Chronic trauma (jackhammer operators, machine workers).

COLOR CHANGES, CUTANEOUS[31]

ICD-9CM # 709.00 PIGMENTATION ANOMALY

BROWN

Generalized: pituitary, adrenal, liver disease, ACTH-producing tumor (e.g., oat cell lung carcinoma).
Localized: nevi, neurofibromatosis.

WHITE

Generalized: albinism.
Localized: vitiligo, Raynaud's syndrome.

RED (ERYTHEMA)

Generalized: fever, polycythemia, urticaria, viral exanthems.
Localized: inflammation, infection, Raynaud's syndrome.

YELLOW

Generalized: liver disease, chronic renal disease, anemia.
Generalized (except sclera): hypothyroidism, increased intake of vegetables containing carotene.
Localized: resolving hematoma, infection, peripheral vascular insufficiency.

BLUE

Lips, mouth, nail beds: cardiovascular and pulmonary diseases, Raynaud's.

COMA

ICD-9CM # 780.01

Vascular: hemorrhage, thrombosis, embolism.
CNS infections: meningitis, encephalitis, cerebral abscess.
Cerebral neoplasms with herniation.
Head injury: subdural hematoma, cerebral concussion, cerebral contusion.
Drugs: narcotics, sedatives, hypnotics.
Ingestion or inhalation of toxins: CO, alcohol, lead.
Metabolic disturbances.
Hypoxia.
Acid-base disorders.
Hypoglycemia, hyperglycemia.
Hepatic failure.
Electrolyte disorders.
Uremia.
Hypothyroidism.
Hypothermia, hyperthermia.
Hypotension, malignant hypertension.
Postictal.

COMA, NORMAL COMPUTED TOMOGRAPHY[1]

ICD-9CM # 780.01

MENINGEAL DISORDERS

Subarachnoid hemorrhage (uncommon).
Bacterial meningitis.
Encephalitis.
Subdural empyema.

EXOGENOUS TOXINS

Sedative drugs and barbiturates.
Anesthetics and γ-hydroxybutyrate.*
Alcohols.
Stimulants:
 Phencyclidine.†
 Cocaine and amphetamine.‡
Psychotropic drugs:
 Cyclic antidepressants.
 Phenothiazines.
 Lithium.
Anticonvulsants.
Opioids.
Clonidine.§
Penicillins.
Salicylates.
Anticholinergics.
Carbon monoxide, cyanide, and methemoglobinemia.

ENDOGENOUS TOXINS/ DEFICIENCIES/DERANGEMENTS

Hypoxia and ischemia.
Hypoglycemia.
Hypercalcemia.
Osmolar:
 Hyperglycemia.
 Hyponatremia.
 Hypernatremia.
Organ system failure.
 Hepatic encephalopathy.
 Uremic encephalopathy.
 Pulmonary insufficiency (carbon dioxide narcosis).

SEIZURES

Prolonged postictal state.
Spike-wave stupor.

HYPOTHERMIA OR HYPERTHERMIA

Brainstem ischemia.
Basilar artery stroke.
Brainstem or cerebellar hemorrhage.
Conversion or malingering.

---

*General anesthetic, similar to γ-aminobutyric acid; recreational drug and body building aid. Rapid onset, rapid recovery often with myoclonic jerking and confusion. Deep coma (2-3 hr; Glasgow Coma Scale = 3) with maintenance of vital signs.

†Coma associated with cholinergic signs: lacrimation, salivation, bronchorrhea, and hyperthermia.

‡Coma after seizures or status (i.e., a prolonged postictal state).

§An antihypertensive agent active through the opiate receptor system; frequent overdose when used to treat narcotic withdrawal.

COMA, PEDIATRIC POPULATION[28]

ICD-9CM # 780.01

ANOXIA

Birth asphyxia.
Carbon monoxide poisoning.
Croup/epiglottitis.
Meconium aspiration.

INFECTION

Hemolysis.
Blood loss.
Hydrops fetalis.
Infection.
Meningoencephalitis.
Sepsis.
Postimmunization encephalitis.

INCREASED INTRACRANIAL PRESSURE

Anoxia.
Inborn metabolic errors.
Toxic encephalopathy.
Reye's syndrome.
Head trauma/intracranial bleed.
Hydrocephalus.
Posterior fossa tumors.

HYPERTENSIVE ENCEPHALOPATHY

Coarctation of aorta.
Nephritis.
Vasculitis.
Pheochromocytoma.

ISCHEMIA

Hypoplastic left heart.
Shunting lesions.
Aortic stenosis.
Cardiovascular collapse (any cause).

PURPURIC CAUSES

Disseminated intravascular coagulation.
Hemolytic-uremic syndrome.
Leukemia
Thrombotic purpura.

HYPERCAPNIA

Cystic fibrosis.
Bronchopulmonary dysplasia.
Congenital lung anomalies.

NEOPLASM

Medulloblastoma.
Glioma of brainstem.
Posterior fossa tumors.

DRUGS/TOXINS

Maternal sedation.
Alcohol.
Any drug.
Lead.
Salicylism.
Arsenic.
Pesticides.

ELECTROLYTE ABNORMALITIES

Hypernatremia (diarrhea, dehydration, salt poisoning).
Hyponatremia (SIADH, androgenital syndrome, gastroenteritis).
Hyperkalemia (renal failure, salicylism, androgenitalism).
Hypokalemia (diarrhea, hyperaldosteronism, salicylism, DKA).
Hypocalcemia (vitamin D deficiency, hyperparathyroidism).
Severe acidosis (sepsis, cold injury, salicylism, DKA).

HYPOGLYCEMIA

Birth injury or stress.
Diabetes.
Alcohol.
Salicylism.
Hyperinsulinemia.
Iatrogenic.

POSTSEIZURE

Renal causes
Nephritis.
Hypoplastic kidneys.
Hepatic causes
Acute hepatitis.
Fulminant hepatic failure.
Inborn metabolic errors.
Bile duct atresia.

CONJUNCTIVAL NEOPLASM

ICD-9CM # CODE VARIES WITH SPECIFIC DISORDER

MALIGNANT

Squamous cell carcinoma.
Melanoma.
Sebaceous carcinoma.
Kaposi's sarcoma.
Metastatic neoplasms.

BENIGN

Melanocytic nevus.
Squamous papilloma.
Hemangioma.
Lymphangioma.
Myxoma.

CONSTIPATION

ICD-9CM # 564.0

Intestinal obstruction.
Fecal impaction.
Diverticular disease.
GI neoplasm.
Strangulated femoral hernia.
Gallstone ileus.
Tuberculous stricture.
Adhesions.
Ameboma.
Volvulus.
Intussusception.
Inflammatory bowel disease.
Hematoma of bowel wall, secondary to trauma or anticoagulants.
Poor dietary habits: insufficient bulk in diet, inadequate fluid intake.
Change from daily routine: travel, hospital admission, physical inactivity.
Acute abdominal conditions: renal colic, salpingitis, biliary colic, appendicitis, ischemia.
Hypercalcemia or hypokalemia, uremia.
Irritable bowel syndrome, pregnancy, anorexia nervosa, depression.
Painful anal conditions: hemorrhoids, fissure, stricture.
Decreased intestinal peristalsis: old age, spinal cord injuries, myxedema, diabetes, multiple sclerosis, parkinsonism and other neurologic diseases.
Drugs: codeine, morphine, antacids with aluminum, verapamil, anticonvulsants, anticholinergics, disopyramide, cholestyramine, alosetron, iron supplements.
Hirschsprung's disease, meconium ileus, congenital atresia in infants.

CORNEAL SENSATION, DECREASED

ICD-9CM # 371.89

Herpes (simplex, zoster).
Contact lens wear.
Topical agents (NSAIDs, anesthetics, beta blockers).
Diabetes.
Eye trauma.
Postsurgery.

COUGH

ICD-9CM # 786.2

Infectious process (viral, bacterial).
Postinfectious.
"Smoker's cough."
Rhinitis (allergic, vasomotor, postinfectious).
Asthma.
Exposure to irritants (noxious fumes, smoke, cold air).
Drug-induced (especially ACE inhibitors, β-blockers).
GERD.
Interstitial lung disease.
Lung neoplasms.
Lymphomas, mediastinal neoplasms.
Bronchiectasis.
Cardiac (CHF, pulmonary edema, mitral stenosis, pericardial inflammation).
Recurrent aspiration.
Inflammation of larynx, pleura, diaphragm, mediastinum.
Cystic fibrosis.
Anxiety.
Other: pulmonary embolism, foreign body inhalation, aortic aneurysm, Zenker's diverticulum, osteophytes, substernal thyroid, thyroiditis, PMR.

CUTANEOUS INFECTIONS, ATHLETES

ICD-9CM # 686.9

Tinea pedis.
Tinea cruris.
Molluscum contagiosum.

Herpes simplex.
Verruca vulgaris.
Folliculitis.
Impetigo.
Furuncles.
Otitis externa.
Erythrasma.

CYANOSIS

ICD-9CM # 782.5 CYANOSIS NOS
770.8 CYANOSIS, NEWBORN

Congenital heart disease with right-to-left shunt.
Pulmonary embolism.
Hypoxia.
Pulmonary edema.
Pulmonary disease (oxygen diffusion and alveolar ventilation abnormalities).
Hemoglobinopathies.
Decreased cardiac output.
Vasospasm.
Arterial obstruction.
Pulmonary AV fistulas.
Elevated hemidiaphragm.
Neoplasm (bronchogenic carcinoma, mediastinal neoplasm, intrahepatic lesion).
Substernal thyroid.
Infectious process (pneumonia, empyema, TB, subphrenic abscess, hepatic abscess).
Atelectasis.
Idiopathic.
Eventration.
Phrenic nerve dysfunction (myelitis, myotonia, herpes zoster).
Trauma to phrenic nerve or diaphragm (e.g., surgery).
Aortic aneurysm.
Intraabdominal mass.
Pulmonary infarction.
Pleurisy.
Radiation therapy.
Rib fracture.
Superior vena cava syndrome.

DAYTIME SLEEPINESS

ICD-9CM # CODE VARIES WITH SPECIFIC DISORDER

Sleep deprivation.
Medication induced (e.g., benzodiazepines, beta blockers, narcotics, sedative antidepressants, gabapentin).
Depression.
Obstructive sleep apnea.
Medical illness (e.g., severe anemia, hypothyroidism, COPD, hepatic failure, renal insufficiency, CHF, electrolyte disturbances).
Circadian rhythm abnormalities (e.g., jet lag, shift work sleep disorder).
Restless legs syndrome.
Posttrauma.
Narcolepsy.
Neurologic disorders (e.g., neurodegenerative disorders, parkinsonism, multiple sclerosis, lesions affecting thalamus, hypothalamus, or brainstem).

DELIRIUM[23]

ICD-9CM # 780.09 DELIRIUM NOS
293.0 ACUTE DELIRIUM

PHARMACOLOGIC AGENTS

Anxiolytics (benzodiazepines).
Antidepressants (e.g., amitriptyline, doxepin, imipramine).
Cardiovascular agents (e.g., methyldopa, digitalis, reserpine, propranolol, procainamide, captopril, disopyramide).
Antihistamine.
Cimetidine.
Corticosteroids.
Antineoplastics.
Drugs of abuse (alcohol, cannabis, amphetamines, cocaine, hallucinogens, opioids, sedative-hypnotics, phencyclidine).

METABOLIC DISORDERS

Hypercalcemia.
Hypercarbia.
Hypoglycemia.
Hyponatremia.
Hypoxia.

INFLAMMATORY DISORDERS

Sarcoidosis.
SLE.
Giant cell arteritis.

ORGAN FAILURE

Hepatic encephalopathy.
Uremia.

NEUROLOGIC DISORDERS

Alzheimer's disease.
CVA.
Encephalitis (including HIV).
Encephalopathies.
Epilepsy.
Huntington's disease.
Multiple sclerosis.
Neoplasms.
Normal pressure hydrocephalus.
Parkinson's disease.
Pick's disease.
Wilson's disease.

ENDOCRINE DISORDERS

Addison's disease.
Cushing's disease.
Panhypopituitarism.
Parathyroid disease.
Postpartum psychosis.
Recurrent menstrual psychosis.
Sydenham's chorea.
Thyroid disease.

DEFICIENCY STATES

Niacin.
Thiamine, Vitamin B_{12}, and folate.

DELIRIUM, DIALYSIS PATIENT[23]

ICD-9CM # 293.0 ACUTE DELIRIUM
293.9 ENCEPHALOPATHY FROM DIALYSIS

STRUCTURAL

Cerebrovascular accident (particularly hemorrhage).
Subdural hematoma.
Intracerebral abscess.
Brain tumor.

METABOLIC

Disequilibrium syndrome.
Uremia.
Drug effects.
Meningitis.
Hypertensive encephalopathy.
Hypotension.
Postictal state.
Hypernatremia or hyponatremia.
Hypercalcemia.
Hypermagnesemia.
Hypoglycemia.
Severe hyperglycemia.
Hypoxemia.
Dialysis dementia.

DEMYELINATING DISEASES[35]

ICD-9CM # 341.9

MULTIPLE SCLEROSIS

Relapsing and chronic progressive forms.
Acute multiple sclerosis.
Neuromyelitis optica (Devic's disease).

DIFFUSE CEREBRAL SCLEROSIS

Schilder's encephalitis periaxialis diffusa.
Baló's concentric sclerosis.

ACUTE DISSEMINATED ENCEPHALOMYELITIS

After measles, chickenpox, rubella, influenza, mumps.
After rabies or smallpox vaccination.

NECROTIZING HEMORRHAGIC ENCEPHALITIS

Hemorrhagic leukoencephalitis.

LEUKODYSTROPHIES

Krabbe's globoid leukodystrophy.
Metachromatic leukodystrophy.
Adrenoleukodystrophy.
Adrenomyeloneuropathy.
Pelizaeus-Merzbacher leukodystrophy.
Canavan's disease.
Alexander's disease.

DIARRHEA, TUBE-FED PATIENT[12]

ICD-9CM # 564.4

COMMON CAUSES UNRELATED TO TUBE FEEDING

Elixir medications containing sorbitol.
Magnesium-containing antacids.
Antibiotic-induced sterile gut.
Pseudomembranous colitis.

POSSIBLE CAUSES RELATED TO TUBE FEEDING

Inadequate fiber to form stool bulk.
High fat content of formula (in the presence of fat malabsorption syndrome).
Bacterial contamination of enteral products and delivery systems (causal association with diarrhea not documented).
Rapid advancement in rate (after the GI tract is unused for prolonged periods).

UNLIKELY CAUSES RELATED TO TUBE FEEDING

Formula hyperosmolality (proven not to be the cause of diarrhea).
Lactose (absent from nearly all enteral feeding formulas).

DIPLOPIA, BINOCULAR

ICD-9CM # 368.2

Cranial nerve palsy (3rd, 4th, 6th).
Thyroid eye disease.
Myasthenia gravis.
Decompensated strabismus.
Orbital trauma with blow-out fracture.
Orbital pseudotumor.
Cavernous sinus thrombosis.

DIPLOPIA, MONOCULAR

ICD-9CM # 368.2

Postoperative corrected long-standing tropia.
Defective contact lenses.
Poorly fitting bifocals.
Trauma to iris.
Corneal disorder (e.g., dry eye, astigmatism).
Cataracts.
Lens subluxation.
Nystagmus.
Eyelid twitching.
Foreign body in aqueous or vitreous media.
Migraine.
Lesions of occipital cortex.
Psychogenic.

DIPLOPIA, VERTICAL

ICD-9CM # 368.2

Myasthenia.
Superior oblique palsy.
Myositis or pseudotumor with orbital involvement.
Lymphoma or metastases affecting the orbits.
Brainstem or cerebellar lesions.
Hydrocephalus.
Third nerve palsy.
Botulism.
Wernicke's encephalopathy.
Dysthyroid orbitopathy (muscle infiltration).

DIZZINESS

ICD-9CM # 780.4

Viral syndrome.
Anxiety, hyperventilation.
Benign positional paroxysmal vertigo.
Medications (e.g., sedatives, antihypertensives, analgesics).
Withdrawal from medications (e.g., benzodiazepines, SSRIs).
Alcohol or drug abuse.
Postural hypotension.
Hypoglycemia, hyperglycemia.
Hematologic disorders (e.g., anemia, polycythemia, leukemia).
Head trauma.
Meniere's disease.
Vertebrobasilar ischemia.
Cervical osteoarthritis.
Cardiac abnormalities (arrhythmias, cardiomyopathy, CHF, pericarditis).
Multiple sclerosis.
Peripheral vestibulopathy.
Air or sea travel.
Electrolyte abnormalities.
Eye problems (cornea, lens, retina).
Migraine.
Brainstem infarct.
Autonomic neuropathy.
Chronic otomastoiditis.
Complex partial seizures.
Ramsey Hunt syndrome.
Arteritis.
Syncope and presyncope.
Perilymph fistula.
Cerebellopontine tumor.
Hepatic or renal disease.

DRY EYE

ICD-9CM # 375.15

Contacts.
Medications (antihistamines, clonidine, beta blockers, ibuprofen, scopolamine).
Keratoconjunctivitis sicca.
Trauma.
Environmental causes (air conditioning in patient with contacts).

DYSPAREUNIA[10]

ICD-9CM # 625.0 DYSPAREUNIA
608.89 DYSPAREUNIA, MALE
302.76 DYSPAREUNIA, PSYCHOGENIC

INTROITAL

Vaginismus.
Intact or rigid hymen.
Clitoral problems.
Vulvovaginitis.
Vaginal atrophy: hypoestrogen.
Vulvar dystrophy.
Bartholin or Skene gland infection.
Inadequate lubrication.
Operative scarring.

MIDVAGINAL

Urethritis.
Trigonitis.
Cystitis.
Short vagina.
Operative scarring.
Inadequate lubrication.

DEEP

Endometriosis.
Pelvic infection.
Uterine retroversion.
Ovarian pathology.
Gastrointestinal.
Orthopedic.
Abnormal penile size or shape.

DYSPHAGIA

ICD-9CM # 787.2

Esophageal obstruction: neoplasm, foreign body, achalasia, stricture, spasm, esophageal web, diverticulum, Schatzki's ring.
Peptic esophagitis with stricture, Barrett's stricture.
External esophageal compression: neoplasms (thyroid neoplasm, lymphoma, mediastinal tumors), thyroid enlargement, aortic aneurysm, vertebral spurs, aberrant right subclavian artery (dysphagia lusoria).
Hiatal hernia, GERD.
Oropharyngeal lesions: pharyngitis, glossitis, stomatitis, neoplasms.
Hysteria: globus hystericus.
Neurologic and/or neuromuscular disturbances: bulbar paralysis, myasthenia gravis, ALS, multiple sclerosis, parkinsonism, CVA, diabetic neuropathy.
Toxins: poisoning, botulism, tetanus, postdiphtheritic dysphagia.
Systemic diseases: scleroderma, amyloidosis, dermatomyositis.
Candida and herpes esophagitis.
Presbyesophagus.

DYSPNEA

ICD-9CM # 786.00

Upper airway obstruction: trauma, neoplasm, epiglottitis, laryngeal edema, tongue retraction, laryngospasm, abductor paralysis of vocal cords, aspiration of foreign body.
Lower airway obstruction: neoplasm, COPD, asthma, aspiration of foreign body.
Pulmonary infection: pneumonia, abscess, empyema, TB, bronchiectasis.
Pulmonary hypertension.
Pulmonary embolism/infarction.
Parenchymal lung disease.
Pulmonary vascular congestion.
Cardiac disease: ASHD, valvular lesions, cardiac dysrhythmias, cardiomyopathy, pericardial effusion, cardiac shunts.

Space-occupying lesions: neoplasm, large hiatal hernia, pleural effusions.
Disease of chest wall: severe kyphoscoliosis, fractured ribs, sternal compression, morbid obesity.
Neurologic dysfunction: Guillain-Barré syndrome, botulism, polio, spinal cord injury.
Interstitial pulmonary disease: sarcoidosis, collagen vascular diseases, DIP, Hamman-Rich pneumonitis, etc.
Pneumoconioses: silicosis, berylliosis, etc.
Mesothelioma.
Pneumothorax, hemothorax, pleural effusion.
Inhalation of toxins.
Cholinergic drug intoxication.
Carcinoid syndrome.
Hematologic: anemia, polycythemia, hemoglobinopathies.
Thyrotoxicosis, myxedema.
Diaphragmatic compression caused by abdominal distention, subphrenic abscess, ascites.
Lung resection.
Metabolic abnormalities: uremia, hepatic coma, DKA.
Sepsis.
Atelectasis.
Psychoneurosis.
Diaphragmatic paralysis.
Pregnancy.

DYSURIA

ICD-9CM # 788.1 DYSURIA
306.53 DYSURIA, PSYCHOGENIC

Urinary tract infection.
Estrogen deficiency (in postmenopausal female).
Vaginitis.
Genital infection (e.g., herpes, condyloma).
Interstitial cystitis.
Chemical irritation (e.g., deodorant aerosols, douches).
Meatal stenosis or stricture.
Reiter's syndrome.
Bladder neoplasm.
GI etiology (diverticulitis, Crohn's disease).
Impaired bladder or sphincter action.
Urethral carbuncle.
Chronic fibrosis posttrauma.
Radiation therapy.
Prostatitis.
Urethritis (gonococcal, *Chlamydiae*).
Behçet's syndrome.
Stevens-Johnson syndrome.

EARACHE[30]

ICD-9CM # 388.70 EARACHE
388.72 EAR PAIN, REFERRED

Otitis media.
Serous otitis media.
Eustachitis.
Otitis externa.
Otitic barotrauma.
Mastoiditis.
Foreign body.
Impacted cerumen.
Referred otalgia, as with TMJ dysfunction, dental problems, and tumors.

ECTOPIC ACTH SECRETION[12]

ICD-9CM # 255.0

Small cell carcinoma of lung.
Endocrine tumors of foregut origin.
- Thymic carcinoid.
- Islet cell tumor.
- Medullary carcinoid, thyroid.
- Bronchial carcinoid.

Pheochromocytoma.
Ovarian tumors.

EDEMA, CHILDREN[17]

ICD-9CM # 782.3 EDEMA NOS

CARDIOVASCULAR

Congestive heart failure.
Acute thrombi or emboli.
Vasculitis of many types.

RENAL

Nephrotic syndrome.
Glomerulonephritis of many types.
End-stage renal failure.

ENDOCRINE OR METABOLIC

Thyroid disease.
Starvation.
Hereditary angioedema.

IATROGENIC

Drugs (diuretics and steroids).
Water or salt overload.

HEMATOLOGIC

Hemolytic disease of the newborn.

GASTROINTESTINAL

Hepatic cirrhosis.
Protein-losing enteritis.
Lymphangiectasis.
Cystic fibrosis.
Celiac disease.
Enteritis of many types.

LYMPHATIC ABNORMALITIES

Congenital (gonadal dysgenesis).
Acquired.

EDEMA, GENERALIZED

ICD-9CM # 782.3 EDEMA NOS

Congestive heart failure (CHF).
Cirrhosis.
Nephrotic syndrome.
Pregnancy.
Idiopathic.
Acute nephritic syndrome.
Myxedema.
Medications (NSAIDs, estrogens, vasodilators).

EDEMA, LEG, UNILATERAL[23]

ICD-9CM # 782.3

WITH PAIN

DVT.
Postphlebitic syndrome.
Popliteal cyst rupture.
Gastrocnemius rupture.
Cellulitis.
Psoas or other abscess.

WITHOUT PAIN

DVT.
Postphlebitic syndrome.
Other venous insufficiency (after saphenous vein harvest, varicosities).
Lymphatic obstruction/lymphedema (carcinoma, lymphoma, sarcoidosis, filariasis, retroperitoneal fibrosis).

EDEMA OF LOWER EXTREMITIES

ICD-9CM # 782.3

CHF (right-sided).
Hepatic cirrhosis.
Nephrosis.
Myxedema.
Lymphedema.
Pregnancy.
Abdominal mass: neoplasm, cyst.
Venous compression from abdominal aneurysm.
Varicose veins.
Bilateral cellulitis.
Bilateral thrombophlebitis.
Vena cava thrombosis, venous thrombosis.
Retroperitoneal fibrosis.

EJECTION SOUND OR CLICK

ICD-9CM # 785.3

Aortic regurgitation.
Aortic root dilatation.
Systemic hypertension.
Chronic pulmonary hypertension.
Tetralogy of Fallot.
Atrial septal defect.
Pulmonary valve stenosis.
Aortic aneurysm.

ELBOW PAIN

ICD-9CM # 719.42

Trauma.
Infection.
Inflammatory arthritis.
Lateral or medial epicondylitis.
Entrapment neuropathy.
Olecranon bursitis.
Osteoarthritis.
Gout.
Cervical disease (referred pain).
Shoulder disease (referred pain).
Partial subluxation.
Synovial osteochondromatosis.
Loose body.

ELEVATED HEMIDIAPHRAGM

ICD-9CM # 519.4 DIAPHRAGM DISORDER
519.4 DIAPHRAGM PARALYSIS
756.6 DIAPHRAGM EVENTRATION, CONGENITAL

Neoplasm (bronchogenic carcinoma, mediastinal neoplasm, intrahepatic lesion).
Substernal thyroid.
Infectious process (pneumonia, empyema, TB, subphrenic abscess, hepatic abscess).
Atelectasis.
Idiopathic.
Eventration.
Phrenic nerve dysfunction (myelitis, myotonia, herpes zoster).
Trauma to phrenic nerve or diaphragm (e.g., surgery).
Aortic aneurysm.
Intraabdominal mass.
Pulmonary infarction.
Pleurisy.
Radiation therapy.
Rib fracture.

EMBOLI, ARTERIAL[23]

ICD-9CM # 444.22 EMBOLISM, ARTERY, LOWER EXTREMITY
444.21 EMBOLISM, ARTERY, UPPER EXTREMITY

Myocardial infarction with mural thrombi.
Atrial fibrillation.
Cardiomyopathies.
Prosthetic heart valves.
CHF.
Endocarditis.
Left ventricular aneurysm.
Left atrial myxoma.
Sick sinus syndrome.
Paradoxical embolus from venous thrombosis.
Aneurysms of large blood vessels.
Atheromatous ulcers of large blood vessels.

EMESIS, PEDIATRIC AGE[17]

ICD-9CM # 787.03

INFANCY

Gastrointestinal tract

Congenital:

Regurgitation—chalasia, gastroesophageal reflux.
Atresia—stenosis (tracheoesophageal fistula, prepyloric diaphragm, intestinal atresia).
Duplication.
Volvulus (errors in rotation and fixation, Meckel diverticulum).
Congenital bands.
Hirschsprung's disease.
Meconium ileus (cystic fibrosis), meconium plug.

Acquired:

Acute infectious gastroenteritis, food poisoning (staphylococcal, clostridial).
Pyloric stenosis.
Gastritis, duodenitis.
Intussusception.
Incarcerated hernia—inguinal, internal secondary to old adhesions.
Cow's milk protein intolerance, food allergy, eosinophilic gastroenteritis.
Disaccharidase deficiency.
Celiac disease—presents after introduction of gluten in diet; inherited risk.
Adynamic ileus—the mediator for many nongastrointestinal causes.
Neonatal necrotizing enterocolitis.
Chronic granulomatous disease with gastric outlet obstruction.

Nongastrointestinal tract

Infectious—otitis, urinary tract infection, pneumonia, upper respiratory tract infection, sepsis, meningitis.
Metabolic—aminoaciduria and organic aciduria, galactosemia, fructosemia, adrenogenital syndrome, renal tubular acidosis, diabetic ketoacidosis, Reye's syndrome.
Central nervous system—trauma, tumor, infection, diencephalic syndrome, rumination, autonomic responses (pain, shock).
Medications—anticholinergics, aspirin, alcohol, idiosyncratic reaction (e.g., codeine).

CHILDHOOD

Gastrointestinal tract

Peptic ulcer—vomiting is a common presentation in children younger than 6 yr old.
Trauma—duodenal hematoma, traumatic pancreatitis, perforated bowel.
Pancreatitis—mumps, trauma, cystic fibrosis, hyperparathyroidism, hyperlipidemia, organic acidemias.
Crohn's disease.
Idiopathic intestinal pseudoobstruction.
Superior mesenteric artery syndrome.

Nongastrointestinal tract

Central nervous system—cyclic vomiting, migraine, anorexia nervosa, bulimia.

ENCEPHALOMYELITIS, NONVIRAL CAUSES[22]

ICD-9CM # CODE VARIES WITH SPECIFIC DISORDER

Subacute bacterial endocarditis.
Rocky Mountain spotted fever.
Typhus.
Ehrlichia.
Q fever.
Chlamydia.
Mycoplasma.
Legionella.
Brucellosis.
Listeria.
Whipple's disease.
Cat-scratch disease.
Syphilis (meningovascular).
Relapsing fever.
Lyme disease.
Leptospirosis.
Nocardia.
Actinomycosis.
Tuberculosis.
Cryptococcus.
Histoplasma.
Toxoplasma.
Plasmodium falciparum.
Trypanosomiasis.
Behçet's disease.
Vasculitis.
Carcinoma.
Drug reactions.

ENCEPHALOPATHY, METABOLIC[33]

ICD-9CM # 291.2 ALCOHOLIC ENCEPHALOPATHY
572.2 HEPATIC ENCEPHALOPATHY
251.2 HYPOGLYCEMIC ENCEPHALOPATHY
349.82 TOXIC ENCEPHALOPATHY
984.9 LEAD ENCEPHALOPATHY
293.9 ENCEPHALOPATHY

Substrate deficiency: hypoxia/ischemia, carbon monoxide poisoning, hypoglycemia.
Cofactor deficiency: thiamine, vitamin B_{12}, pyridoxine (INH administration).
Electrolyte disorders: hyponatremia, hypercalcemia, carbon dioxide narcosis, dialysis, hypermagnesemia, disequilibrium syndrome.
Endocrinopathies: DKA, hyperosmolar coma, hypothyroidism, hyperadrenocorticism, hyperparathyroidism.
Endogenous toxins: liver disease, uremia, porphyria.
Exogenous toxins: drug overdose (sedative/hypnotics, ethanol, narcotics, salicylates, tricyclic antidepressants), drug withdrawal, toxicity of therapeutic medications, industrial toxins (e.g., organophosphates, heavy metals), sepsis.
Heat stroke.
Epilepsy (postictal).

ENTHESOPATHY

ICD-9CM # CODE NOT AVAILABLE

Viremia or bacteremia.
Ankylosing spondylitis.
Psoriatic arthritis.
Drug-induced (quinolones, etretinate).
Reactive arthritis.
Disseminated idiopathic skeletal hyperostosis (DISH).
Reiter's syndrome.

EPILEPSY

ICD-9CM # 345.9 EPILEPSY NOS

Psychogenic spells.
Transient ischemic attack.
Hypoglycemia.
Syncope.
Narcolepsy.
Migraine.
Paroxysmal vertigo.
Arrhythmias.
Drug reaction.

EPISTAXIS

ICD-9CM # 784.7

Trauma.
Medications (nasal sprays, NSAIDs, anticoagulants, antiplatelets).
Nasal polyps.
Cocaine use.
Coagulopathy (hemophilia, liver disease, DIC, thrombocytopenia).
Systemic disorders (hypertension, uremia).
Infections.
Anatomic malformations.
Rhinitis.
Nasal polyps.
Local neoplasms (benign and malignant).
Desiccation.
Foreign body.

ERECTILE DYSFUNCTION, ORGANIC[28]

ICD-9CM # 607.84

Neurogenic abnormalities: Somatic nerve neuropathy, central nervous system abnormalities.
Psychogenic causes: Depression, performance anxiety, marital conflict.
Endocrine causes: Hyperprolactinemia, hypogonadotropic hypogonadism, testicular failure, estrogen excess.
Trauma: Pelvic fracture, prostate surgery, penile fracture.
Systemic disease: Diabetes mellitus, renal failure, hepatic cirrhosis.
Medications: Diuretics, antidepressants, H2 blockers, exogenous hormones, alcohol, antihypertensives, nicotine abuse, finasteride, etc.
Structural abnormalities: Peyronie's disease.

EROSIONS, GENITALIA

ICD-9CM # 599.84

Candidiasis.
Intraepithelial neoplasia.
Squamous cell carcinoma.
Lichen planus.
Pemphigus vulgaris.
Erythema multiforme.
Lichen sclerosus.
Bullous pemphigoid.
Extramammary Paget's disease.
Impetigo.

ERYTHRODERMA

ICD-9CM # SECONDARY 695.9
 # MACULOPAPULAR 696.2
 # PSORIATICUM 696.1
 # EXFOLIATIVE 695.89
 # NEONATORUM 778.8

Drug reaction (e.g., allopurinol, ampicillin, phenytoin, vancomycin, dapsone, omeprazole, carbamazepine).
Atopic dermatitis.
Psoriasis.
Contact dermatitis.
Idiopathic.
Pityriasis rubra.
Chronic actinic dermatitis.
Bullous pemphigoid.
Paraneoplastic.
Cutaneous T-cell lymphoma.
Connective tissue disease.
Hypereosinophilia syndrome.

ESOPHAGEAL PERFORATION[23]

ICD-9CM # 530.4 PERFORATION, NONTRAUMATIC
862.22 INJURY, TRAUMATIC

Trauma.
Caustic burns.
Iatrogenic.
Foreign bodies.
Spontaneous rupture (Boerhaave's syndrome).
Postoperative breakdown of anastomosis.

ESOPHAGITIS[22]

ICD-9CM # 530.12

Infectious:
- Candidiasis.
- Cytomegalovirus.
- Herpes simplex virus.
- HIV infection, acute.

Noninfectious:
- Gastroesophageal reflux.
- Mucositis from cancer chemotherapy.
- Mucositis from radiation therapy.
- Aphthous ulcers.

ESOTROPIA

ICD-9CM # NONACCOMODATIVE 378.00
 # ACCOMMODATIVE 378.35
 # ALTERNATING 378.05

Congenital.
Accomodative esotropia.
Myasthenia gravis.
Abducens palsy.
Pseudo-sixth nerve palsy.
Medial rectus entrapment (e.g., blowout fracture).
Posterior internuclear ophthalmoplegia.
Wernicke's encephalopathy.
Thyroid myopathy.
Chiari malformation.

EXANTHEMS[25]

ICD-9CM # 782.1

Measles.
Rubella.
Erythema infectiosum (fifth disease).
Roseola exanthema.
Varicella.
Enterovirus.
Adenovirus.
Epstein-Barr virus.
Kawasaki disease.
Staphylococcal scalded skin.
Scarlet fever.
Meningococcemia.
Rocky Mountain spotted fever.

EYELID NEOPLASM

ICD-9CM # CODE VARIES WITH SPECIFIC DISORDER

MALIGNANT

Melanoma.
Basal cell carcinoma.
Squamous cell carcinoma.
Bowen's disease.
Sebaceous cell carcinoma.
Metastatic lymphoma/leukemia.

BENIGN

Melanocytic nevus.
Pilar, eccrine, or apocrine tumor.
Neurofibroma.
Keratosis.
Squamous papilloma.
Keratoacanthoma.

EYELID RETRACTION

ICD-9CM # 374.89

Congenital.
Graves' ophthalmopathy.
Myasthenia gravis.
Postsurgical.
Guillain-Barré.
Cerebellar disease.
Horizontal gaze palsy.
Partial palsy of superior rectus muscle.
Encephalitis.
Closed head injury.
Disseminated sclerosis.
Eye trauma.
Contact lens wear.
Proptosis.
Eyelid neoplasm.
Atopic dermatitis.
Herpes zoster ophthalmicus.
Botulinum toxin injection.
Cyclic oculomotor paralysis.
Spheroid wing meningioma.
Hepatic cirrhosis.
Down syndrome.
Essential hypertension.
Meningitis.
Paget's disease of bone.

EYE PAIN

ICD-9CM # 379.91

Foreign body.
Herpes zoster.
Trauma.
Conjunctivitis.
Iritis.
Iridocyclitis.
Uveitis.
Blepharitis.
Ingrown lashes.
Orbital or periorbital cellulitis/abscess.
Sinusitis.
Headache.
Glaucoma.
Inflammation of lacrimal gland.
Tic douloureux.
Cerebral aneurysm.
Cerebral neoplasm.
Entropion.
Retrobulbar neuritis.
UV light.
Dry eyes.
Irritation or inflammation from eye drops, dust, cosmetics, etc.

FACIAL PAIN

ICD-9CM # 784.0

Infection, abscess.
Postherpetic neuralgia.
Trauma, posttraumatic neuralgia.
Tic douloureux.
Cluster headache, "lower-half headache."
Geniculate neuralgia.
Anxiety, somatization syndrome.
Glossopharyngeal neuralgia.
Carotidynia.

FACIAL PARALYSIS[25]

ICD-9CM # 351.0 FACIAL (7TH NERVE) PALSY

INFECTION

Bacterial: otitis media, mastoiditis, meningitis, Lyme disease.
Viral: herpes zoster, mononucleosis, varicella, rubella, mumps, Bell's palsy.
Mycobacterial: TB, meningitis, leprosy.
Miscellaneous: syphilis, malaria.

TRAUMA

Temporal bone fracture, facial laceration.
Surgery.

NEOPLASM

Malignant: squamous cell carcinoma, basal cell and adenocystic tumors, leukemia, parotid neoplasms, metastic tumors.
Benign: facial nerve neuroma, vestibular schwannoma, congenital cholesteatoma.

IMMUNOLOGIC

Guillain-Barré syndrome, periarteritis nodosa.
Reaction to tetanus antiserum.

METABOLIC

Pregnancy.
Hypothyroidism.
DM.

FAILURE TO THRIVE

ICD-9CM # 783.4

MALABSORPTION

Cow's milk protein allergy.
Cystic fibrosis.
Celiac disease.
Biliary atresia.

INSUFFICIENT CALORIC INTAKE

Parental neglect.
Feeding difficulties (CNS lesion, severe reflux, oromotor abnormalities).
Use of diluted formula preparation.
Food shortage (poverty).

INCREASED NEEDS

Hyperthyroidism.
Congenital heart defects.
Malignancy.
Renal or hepatic disease.
HIV.

IMPROPER UTILIZATION

Storage disorders.
Amino acid disorders.
Trisomy 13, 21, 18.

FATIGUE

ICD-9CM # 780.7 FATIGUE NOS
300.5 FATIGUE PSYCHOGENIC
780.7 CHRONIC FATIGUE SYNDROME

Depression.
Anxiety, emotional stress.
Inadequate sleep.
Prolonged physical activity.
Pregnancy and postpartum period.
Anemia.
Hypothyroidism.
Medications (β-blockers, anxiolytics, antidepressants, sedating antihistamines, clonidine, methyldopa).
Viral or bacterial infections.
Sleep apnea syndrome.
Dieting.
Renal failure, CHF, COPD, liver disease.

FATTY LIVER

ICD-9CM # 571.8

Obesity.
Alcohol abuse.
Diabetes mellitus.
Acute fatty liver of pregnancy.
Medications (tetracycline, valproic acidglucocorticoids, amiodarone, estrogen, methotrexate).
Reye's syndrome.
Wilson's disease.
Nonalcoholic steatosis.

FEVER AND JAUNDICE

ICD-9CM # 789.6 FEVER
782.4 JAUNDICE

Cholecystitis.
Hepatic abscess (pyogenic, amebic).
Ascending cholangitis.
Pancreatitis.
Malaria.
Neoplasm (hepatic pancreatic, biliary tract, metastatic).
Mononucleosis.
Viral hepatitis.
Sepsis.
Babesiosis.
HIV (cryptosporidium).
Biliary ascariasis.
Toxic shock syndrome.
Yersinia infection, leptospirosis, Yellow fever, Dengue fever, relapsing fever.

FEVER AND RASH

ICD-9CM # 782.1 EXANTHEM
57.9 EXANTHEM VIRAL
789.6 FEVER

Drug hypersensitivity: penicillin, sulfonamides, thiazides, anticonvulsants, allopurinol.
Viral infection: measles, rubella, varicella, erythema infectiosum, roseola, enterovirus infection, viral hepatitis, infectious mononucleosis, acute HIV.
Other infections: meningococcemia, staphylococcemia, scarlet fever, typhoid fever, Pseudomonas bacteremia, Rocky Mountain spotted fever, Lyme disease, secondary syphilis, bacterial endocarditis, babesiosis, brucellosis, listeriosis.
Serum sickness.
Erythema multiforme.
Erythema marginatum.
Erythema nodosum.
SLE.
Dermatomyositis.
Allergic vasculitis.
Pityriasis rosea.
Herpes zoster.

FEVER IN RETURNING TRAVELERS AND IMMIGRANTS[25]

ICD-9CM # CODE VARIES WITH SPECIFIC DISORDER

Differential Diagnosis of Some Selected Systemic Febrile Illnesses to Consider in Returned Travelers and Immigrants.*

COMMON

Acute respiratory tract infection (worldwide).
Gastroenteritis (worldwide) [foodborne, waterborne, fecal-oral].

Enteric fever, including typhoid (worldwide) [food, water].
Urinary tract infection (worldwide) [sexual contact].
Drug reactions [antibiotics, prophylactic agents, other] {rash frequent}.
Malaria (tropics, limited areas of temperate zones) [mosquitoes].
Arboviruses (Africa; tropics) [mosquitoes, ticks, mites].
Dengue (Asia, Caribbean, Africa) [mosquitoes].
Viral hepatitis (worldwide).
Hepatitis A (worldwide) [food, fecal-oral].
Hepatitis B (worldwide, especially Asia, sub-Saharan Africa) [sexual contact] {long incubation period}.
Hepatitis C (worldwide) [blood or sexual contact].
Hepatitis E (Asia, North Africa, Mexico, ?others) [food, water].
Tuberculosis (worldwide) [airborne, milk] {long period to symptomatic infection}.
Sexually transmitted diseases (worldwide) [sexual contact].

LESS COMMON

Filariasis (Asia, Africa, South America) [biting insects] {long incubation period, eosinophilia}.
Measles (developing world) [airborne] {in susceptible individual}.
Amebic abscess (worldwide) [food].
Brucellosis (worldwide) [milk, cheese, food, animal contact].
Listeriosis (worldwide) [foodborne] {meningitis}.
Leptospirosis (worldwide) [animal contact, open fresh water] {jaundice, meningitis}.
Strongyloidiasis (warm and tropical areas) [soil contact] {eosinophilia}.
Toxoplasmosis (worldwide) [undercooked meat].

RARE

Relapsing fever (western Americas, Asia, northern Africa) [ticks, lice].
Hemorrhagic fevers (worldwide) [arthropod and nonarthropod transmitted].
Yellow fever (tropics) [mosquitoes] {hepatitis}.
Hemorrhagic fever with renal syndrome (Europe, Asia, North America) [rodent urine] {renal impairment}.
Hantavirus pulmonary syndrome (western North America, ?other) [rodent urine] {respiratory distress syndrome}.
Lassa fever (Africa) [rodent excreta, person to person] {high mortality rate}
Other—chikungunya, Rift Valley, Ebola-Marburg, etc. (various) [insect bites, rodent excreta, aerosols, person to person] {often severe}.
Rickettsial infections {Rashes and eschars}.
Leishmaniasis, visceral (Middle East, Mediterranean, Africa, Asia, South America) [biting flies] {long incubation period}.
Acute schistosomiasis (Africa, Asia, South America, Caribbean) [fresh water].
Chagas' disease (South and Central America) [reduviid bug bites] {often asymptomatic}.
African trypanosomiasis (Africa) [tsetse fly bite] {neurologic syndromes, sleeping sickness}.
Bartonellosis (South America) [sandfly bite; cb] {skin nodules}.
HIV infection/AIDS (worldwide) [sexual and blood contact].
Trichinosis (worldwide) [undercooked meat] {eosinophilia}.
Plague (temperate and tropical plains) [animal exposures and fleas].
Tularemia (worldwide) [animal contact, fleas, aerosols] {ulcers, lymph nodes}.
Anthrax (worldwide) [animal, animal product contact] {ulcers}.
Lyme disease (North America, Europe) [tick bites] {arthritis, meningitis, cardiac abnormalities}.

*Diagnoses for which particular symptoms are indicative are in italics. Exposure to regions of the world that are most likely to be significant to the diagnosis are presented in (parentheses). Vectors, risk behaviors, and sources associated with acquisition are presented in [brackets]. Special clinical characteristics are listed within {braces}.

FINGER LESIONS, INFLAMMATORY

ICD-9CM # CODE VARIES WITH SPECIFIC DISORDER

Paronychia.
Herpes simplex type 1 (herpetic whitlow).
Dyshidrotic eczema (pompholyx).
Herpes zoster.
Bacterial endocarditis (Osler's nodes).
Psoriatic arthritis.

FLATULENCE AND BLOATING[30]

ICD-9CM # 787.3

Ingestion of nonabsorbable carbohydrates.
Ingestion of carbonated beverages.
Malabsorption: pancreatic insufficiency, biliary disease, celiac disease, bacterial overgrowth in small intestine.
Lactase deficiency.
Irritable bowel syndrome.
Anxiety disorders.
Food poisoning, giardiasis.

FLUSHING[24]

ICD-9CM # 782.62

Physiologic flushing: menopause, ingestion of monosodium glutamate (Chinese restaurant syndrome), ingestion of hot drinks.
Drugs: alcohol (with or without disulfiram, metronidazole, or chlorpropamide), nicotinic acid, diltiazem, nifedipine, levodopa, bromocriptine, vancomycin, amyl nitrate.
Neoplastic disorders: carcinoid syndrome, Vipoma syndrome, medullary carcinoma of thyroid, systemic mastocytosis, basophilic chronic myelocytic leukemia, renal cell carcinoma.
Anxiety.
Agnogenic flushing.

FOOT DERMATITIS

ICD-9CM # CODE VARIES WITH SPECIFIC DISORDER

Tinea pedis.
Dyshidrotic eczema.
Tylosis (mechanically induced hyperkeratosis, fissuring, and dryness).
Allergic contact dermatitis.
Psoriasis.
Peripheral vascular insufficiency.
Neuropathic foot ulcers (diabetes mellitus, poorly fitting shoes).
Acquired plantar keratoderma.
Sezary's syndrome.

FOOTDROP

ICD-9CM # CODE VARIES WITH SPECIFIC DISORDER

Peripheral neuropathy.
L5 radiculopathy.
Peroneal nerve compression.
Sciatic nerve palsy.
Scapuloperoneal syndromes.
Spasticity.
Peroneal nerve compression.
Myopathy.
Dystonia.

FOOT LESION, ULCERATING

ICD-9CM # 917.9

Cellulitis.
Plantar wart.
Squamous cell carcinoma.
Actinomycosis (Madura foot).
Plantar fibromatosis.
Pseudoepitheliomatous hyperplasia.

FOOT PAIN

ICD-9CM # CODE VARIES WITH SPECIFIC DIAGNOSIS

Trauma (fractures, musculoskeletal and ligamentous strain).
Inflammation (Plantar fasciitis, Achilles tendonitis or bursitis, calcaneal apophysitis).
Arterial insufficiency, Raynaud's phenomenon, thromboangiitis obliterans.
Gout, pseudogout.
Calcaneal spur.
Infection (cellulitis, abscess, lymphangitis, gangrene).
Decubitus ulcer.
Paronychia, ingrown toenail.
Thrombophlebitis, postphlebitic syndrome.

FOREARM AND HAND PAIN

ICD-9CM # 959.3 FOREARM INJURY
959.4 HAND INJURY

Epicondylitis.
Tenosynovitis.
Osteoarthritis.
Cubital tunnel syndrome.
Carpal tunnel syndrome.
Trauma.
Herpes zoster.
Peripheral vascular insufficiency.
Infection (cellulitis, abscess).

GAIT ABNORMALITY

ICD-9CM # 781.2 GAIT ABNORMALITY

Parkinsonism.
Degenerative joint disease (hips, back, knees).
Multiple sclerosis.
Trauma, foot pain.
CVA.
Cerebellar lesions.
Infections (tabes, encephalitis, meningitis).
Sensory ataxia.
Dystonia, cerebral palsy, neuromuscular disorders.
Metabolic abnormalities.

GALACTORRHEA[25]

ICD-9CM # 611.6

Prolonged suckling.
Drugs (INH, phenothiazines, reserpine derivatives, amphetamines, spironolactone and tricyclic antidepressants).
Major stressors (surgery, trauma).
Hypothyroidism.
Pituitary tumors.

GASTRIC EMPTYING, DELAYED[1]

ICD-9CM # 536.8 GASTRIC MOTILITY DISORDER

MECHANICAL OBSTRUCTION

Duodenal or pyloric channel ulcer.
Pyloric stricture.
Tumor of the distal stomach.

FUNCTIONAL OBSTRUCTION (GASTROPARESIS)

Drugs: anticholinergics, beta-adrenergics, opiates.
Electrolyte imbalance: hypokalemia, hypocalcemia, hypomagnesemia.
Metabolic disorders: DM, hypoparathyroidism, hypothyroidism, pregnancy.
Vagotomy.
Viral infections.
Neuromuscular disorders (myotonic dystrophy, autonomic neuropathy, scleroderma, polymyositis).
Gastric pacemaker (i.e., tachygastria).
Brainstem tumors.
GERD.
Psychiatric disorders: anorexia nervosa, psychogenic vomiting.
Idiopathic.

GASTRIC EMPTYING, RAPID

ICD-9CM # 536.8 GASTRIC MOTILITY DISORDER

Pancreatic insufficiency.
Dumping syndrome.
Peptic ulcer.
Celiac disease.
Promotility agents.
Zollinger-Ellison disease.

GENITAL DISCHARGE, FEMALE[10]

ICD-9CM # 629.9

Physiologic discharge: cervical mucus, vaginal transudation, bacteria, squamous epithelial cells.
Individual variation.
Pregnancy.
Sexual response.
Menstrual cycle variation.
Infection.
Foreign body: tampon, cervical cap, other.
Neoplasm.
Fistula.
IUD.
Cervical ectropion.
Spermicide.
Nongenital causes: urinary incontinence, urinary tract fistula, Crohn's disease, rectovaginal fistula.

GENITAL SORES[1]

ICD-9CM # 054.10 GENITAL HERPES
91.0 GENITAL SYPHILIS
078.11 CONDYLOMA ACUMINATUM
099.0 CHANCROID
099.2 GRANULOMA INGUINALE
099.1 LYMPHOGRANULOMA VENEREUM
629.8 ULCER, GENITAL SITE, FEMALE
608.89 ULCER, GENITAL SITE, MALE

Herpes genitalis.
Syphilis.
Chancroid.
Lymphogranuloma venereum.
Granuloma inguinale.
Condyloma acuminatum.
Neoplastic lesion.
Trauma.

GLUCOCORTICOID DEFICIENCY[12]

ICD-9CM # 255.4

ACTH-independent causes.
TB.
Autoimmune (idiopathic).
Other rare causes:
- Fungal infection.
- Adrenal hemorrhage.
- Metastases.
- Sarcoidosis.
- Amyloidosis.
- Adrenoleukodystrophy.
- Adrenomyeloneuropathy.
- HIV infection.
- Congenital adrenal hyperplasia.
- Medications (e.g., ketoconazole).

ACTH-dependent causes:
Hypothalamic-pituitary-adrenal suppression.
- Exogenous.
  - Glucocorticoid.
  - ACTH.
- Endogenous—cure of Cushing's syndrome.

Hypothalamic-pituitary lesions.
- Neoplasm.
  - Primary pituitary tumor.
  - Metastatic tumor.
- Craniopharyngioma.
- Infection.
  - Tuberculosis.
  - Actinomycosis.
  - Nocardiosis.
- Sarcoid.
- Head trauma.
- Isolated ACTH deficiency.

GOITER

ICD-9CM # 240.9 GOITER, UNSPECIFIED
241.9 GOITER, ADENOMATOUS
246.1 GOITER, CONGENITAL
240.9 GOITER, NONTOXIC DIFFUSE
241.1 GOITER, NONTOXIC MULTINODULAR
240.0 SIMPLE GOITER
242.1 THYROTOXIC GOITER

Thyroiditis.
Toxic multinodular goiter.
Graves' disease.
Medications (PTU, methimazole, sulfonamides, sulfonylureas, ethionamide, amiodarone, lithium, etc.).
Iodine deficiency.
Sarcoidosis, amyloidosis.
Defective thyroid hormone synthesis.
Resistance to thyroid hormone.

GRANULOMATOUS DERMATITIDES

ICD-9CM # CODE VARIES WITH SPECIFIC DISORDER

Granuloma annulare.
Sarcoidosis.
Necrobiosis lipoidica diabeticorum.
Cutaneous Crohn's disease.
Rheumatoid nodules.
Annular elastolytic giant cell granuloma (actinic granuloma).
Foreign body granuloma.

GRANULOMATOUS DISORDERS[29]

**ICD-9CM # 446.4 GRANULOMATOSIS
288.1 GRANULOMATOUS DISEASE**

INFECTIONS

Fungi
Histoplasma.
Coccidioides.
Blastomyces.
Sporothrix.
Aspergillus.
Cryptococcus.
Protozoa
Toxoplasma.
Leishmania.
Metazoa
Toxocara.
Schistosoma.
Spirochetes
Treponema pallidum.
T. pertenue.
T. carateum.
Mycobacteria
M. tuberculosis.
M. leprae.
M. kansasii.
M. marinum.
M. avian.
Bacille Calmette-Guérin (BCG) vaccine.
Bacteria
Brucella.
Yersinia.
Other infections
Cat scratch.
Lymphogranuloma.

NEOPLASIA

Carcinoma.
Reticulosis.
Pinealoma.
Dysgerminoma.
Seminoma.
Reticulum cell sarcoma.
Malignant nasal granuloma.

CHEMICALS

Beryllium.
Zirconium.
Silica.
Starch.

IMMUNOLOGIC ABERRATIONS

Sarcoidosis.
Crohn's disease.
Primary biliary cirrhosis.
Wegener's granulomatosis.
Giant-cell arteritis.
Peyronie's disease.
Hypogammaglobulinemia.
Systemic lupus erythematosus.
Lymphomatoid granulomatosis.
Histiocytosis X.
Hepatic granulomatous disease.
Immune complex disease.
Rosenthal-Melkersson syndrome.
Churg-Strauss allergic granulomatosis.

LEUKOCYTE OXIDASE DEFECT

Chronic granulomatous disease of childhood.

EXTRINSIC ALLERGIC ALVEOLITIS

Farmer's lung.
Bird fancier's.
Mushroom worker's.
Suberosis (cork dust).
Bagassosis.
Maple bark stripper's.
Paprika splitter's.
Coffee bean.
Spatlese lung.

OTHER DISORDERS

Whipple's disease.
Pyrexia of unknown origin.
Radiotherapy.
Cancer chemotherapy.
Panniculitis.
Chalazion.
Sebaceous cyst.
Dermoid.
Sea urchin spine injury.

GRANULOMATOUS LIVER DISEASE

ICD-9CM # 572.8

Sarcoidosis.
Wegener's granulomatosis.
Vasculitis.
Inflammatory bowel disease.
Allergic granulomatosis.
Erythema nodosum.
Infections (fungal, viral, parasitic).
Primary biliary cirrhosis.
Lymphoma.
Hodgkin's disease.
Drugs (e.g., allopurinol, hydralazine, sulfonamides, penicillins).
Toxins (copper sulfate, beryllium).

GROIN MASSES

ICD-9CM # 959.1

Hernia (inguinal, femoral).
Hydrocele.
Varicocele.
Sebaceous cyst.
Hydradenitis of inguinal apocrine glands.
Neoplasm: lymphoma, metastases.
Lipoma.
Hematoma.
Reactive inguinal adenopathy, femoral adenitis.
Folliculitis, psoas abscess.
Epididymitis, testicular torsion, ectopic testes.
Aneurysm or pseudoaneurysm of femoral artery.

GROIN PAIN, ACTIVE PATIENT[34]

**ICD-9CM # 959.1 GROIN INJURY
848.8 GROIN PAIN**

MUSCULOSKELETAL

Avascular necrosis of the femoral head.
Avulsion fracture (lesser trochanter, anterior superior iliac spine, anterior inferior iliac spine).
Bursitis (iliopectineal, trochanteric).
Entrapment of the ilioinguinal or iliofemoral nerve.
Gracilis syndrome.
Muscle tear (adductors, iliopsoas, rectus abdominis, gracilis, sartorius, rectus femoris).
Myositis ossificans of the hip muscles.
Osteitis pubis.
Osteoarthritis of the femoral head.
Slipped capital femoral epiphysis.
Stress fracture of the femoral head or neck and pubis.
Synovitis.

HERNIA-RELATED

Avulsion of the internal oblique muscle in the conjoined tendon.
Defect at the insertion of the rectus abdominis muscle.
Direct inguinal hernia.
Femoral ring hernia.
Indirect inguinal hernia.
Inguinal canal weakness.

UROLOGIC

Epididymitis.
Fracture of the testis.
Hydrocele.
Kidney stone.
Posterior urethritis.
Prostatis.
Testicular cancer.
Torsion of the testis.
Urinary tract infection.
Varicocele.

GYNECOLOGIC

Ectopic pregnancy.
Ovarian cyst.
Pelvic inflammatory disease.
Torsion of the ovary.
Vaginitis.

LYMPHATIC ENLARGEMENT IN GROIN

GYNECOMASTIA

ICD-9CM # 611.1 GYNECOMASTIA, NONPUERPERAL

Physiologic (puberty, newborns, aging).
Drugs (estrogen and estrogen precursors, digitalis, testosterone and exogenous androgens, clomiphene, cimetidine, spironolactone, ketoconazole, amiodarone, ACE inhibitors, isoniazid, phenytoin, methyldopa, metoclopramide, phenothiazine).
Increased prolactin level (prolactinoma).
Liver disease.
Adrenal disease.
Thyrotoxicosis.
Increased estrogen production (hCG-producing tumor, testicular tumor, bronchogenic carcinoma).
Secondary hypogonadism.
Primary gonadal failure (trauma, castration, viral orchitis, granulomatous disease).

Defects in androgen synthesis.
Testosterone deficiency.
Klinefelter's syndrome.

HALITOSIS

ICD-9CM # 784.9

Tobacco use.
Alcohol use.
Dry mouth (mouth breathing, inadequate fluid intake).
Foods (onion, garlic, meats, nuts).
Disease of mouth or nose (infections, cancer, inflammation).
Medications (antihistamines, antidepressants).
Systemic disorders (diabetes, uremia).
GI disorders (esophageal diverticula, hiatal hernia, GERD, achalasia).
Sinusitis.
Pulmonary disorders (bronchiectasis, pneumonia, neoplasms, TB).

HAND PAIN AND SWELLING[6]

ICD-9CM # CODE VARIES WITH SPECIFIC DIAGNOSIS

Trauma.
Gout.
Pseudogout.
Cellulitis.
Lymphangitis.
DVT of upper extremity.
Thrombophlebitis.
Rheumatoid arthritis.
Remitting seronegative symmetrical synovitis with pitting edema (RS3PE).
Polymyalgia rheumatica.
Mixed connective tissue disease.
Scleroderma.
Rupture of the olecranon bursa.
Metzger's syndrome (neoplasia).
The puffy hand of drug addiction.
Reflex sympathetic dystrophy.
Eosinophilic fasciitis.
Sickle cell (hand-foot syndrome).
Leprosy.
Factitial (the rubber band syndrome).

HEADACHE[11]

ICD-9CM # 784.0 HEADACHE NOS
307.81 HEADACHE, TENSION
346.2 HEADACHE, CLUSTER
346.9 HEADACHE, MIGRAINE
784.0 HEADACHE, VASCULAR

Vascular: migraine, cluster headaches, temporal arteritis, hypertension, cavernous sinus thrombosis.
Musculoskeletal: neck and shoulder muscle contraction, strain of extraocular and/or intraocular muscles, cervical spondylosis, temporomandibular arthritis.
Infections: meningitis, encephalitis, brain abscess, sepsis, sinusitis, osteomyelitis, parotitis, mastoiditis.
Cerebral neoplasm.
Subdural hematoma.
Cerebral hemorrhage/infarct.
Pseudotumor cerebri.
Normal pressure hydrocephalus (NPH).
Postlumbar puncture.
Cerebral aneurysm, arteriovenous malformations.
Posttrauma.
Dental problems: abscess, periodontitis, poorly fitting dentures.
Trigeminal neuralgia, glossopharyngeal neuralgia.
Otitis and other ear diseases.
Glaucoma and other eye diseases.
Metabolic: uremia, carbon monoxide inhalation, hypoxia.
Pheochromocytoma, hypoglycemia, hypothyroidism.
Effort induced: benign exertional headache, cough, headache, coital cephalalgia.
Drugs: alcohol, nitrates, histamine antagonists.
Paget's disease of the skull.
Emotional, psychiatric.

HEADACHE AND FACIAL PAIN[33]

ICD-9CM # 784.0 HEADACHE NOS
784.0 FACIAL PAIN

VASCULAR HEADACHES

Migraine

Migraine with headaches and inconspicuous neurologic features:
- Migraine without aura ("common migraine").

Migraine with headaches and conspicuous neurologic features:
- With transient neurologic symptoms: Migraine with typical aura ("classic migraine").
  Sensory, basilar, and *hemiplegic migraine.*
- With prolonged or permanent neurologic features ("complicated migraine"):
  Ophthalmoplegic migraine.
  Migrainous infarction.

Migraine without headaches but with conspicuous neurologic features ("migraine equivalents"):
- Abdominal migraine.
- Benign paroxysmal vertigo of childhood.
- Migraine aura without headache ("isolated auras," transient migrainous accompaniments).

Cluster headaches

Episodic cluster headache ("cyclic cluster headaches").
Chronic cluster headaches.
Chronic paroxysmal hemicrania.

Other vascular headaches

Headaches of reactive vasodilation (fever, drug-induced, postictal, hypoglycemia, hypoxia, hypercarbia, hyperthyroidism).
Headaches associated with arterial hypertension:
- Chronic severe hypertension (diastolic 120 mm Hg).
- Paroxysmal severe hypertension (pheochromocytoma, some coital headaches).

Headaches caused by cranial arteritis:
- Giant cell arteritis ("temporal arteritis").
- Other vasculitides.

HEADACHES ASSOCIATED WITH DEMONSTRABLE MUSCLE SPASM

Headache caused by posturally induced or perilesional muscle spasm:
- Headaches of sustained or impaired posture (e.g., prolonged close work, driving).
- Headaches associated with cervical spondylosis and other diseases of cervical spine.
- Myofascial pain dysfunction syndrome (headache or facial pain associated with disorders of teeth, jaws, and related structures, or "TMJ syndrome").

Headaches caused by psychophysiologic muscular contraction ("muscle contraction headaches," or tension-type headache associated with disorder of pericranial muscles).

HEADACHES AND FACIAL PAIN WITHOUT DEMONSTRABLE PHYSICAL SUBSTRATE

Headaches of uncertain etiology:
- "Tension headaches" (tension-type headache unassociated with disorder of pericranial muscles).
- Some forms of posttraumatic headache.

Psychogenic headaches (e.g., hypochondriacal, conversional, delusional, malingered).
Facial pain of uncertain etiology ("atypical facial pain").

COMBINED TENSION-MIGRAINE HEADACHES

Episodic migraine superimposed on chronic tension headaches.
Chronic daily headaches:
- Associated with analgesic and/or ergotamine overuse ("rebound headaches").
- Not associated with drug overuse.

HEADACHES AND HEAD PAINS CAUSED BY DISEASES OF EYES, EARS, NOSE, SINUSES, TEETH, OR SKULL

HEADACHES CAUSED BY MENINGEAL INFLAMMATION

Subarachnoid hemorrhage.
Meningitis and meningoencephalitis.
Others (e.g., meningeal carcinomatosis).

HEADACHES ASSOCIATED WITH ALTERED INTRACRANIAL PRESSURE ("TRACTION HEADACHES")

Increased intracranial pressure

Intracranial mass lesions (neoplasm, hematoma, abscess, etc.).
Hydrocephalus.
Benign intracranial hypertension.
Venous sinus thrombosis.

Decreased intracranial pressure

Post–lumbar puncture headaches.
Spontaneous hypoliquorrheic headaches.

HEADACHES AND HEAD PAINS CAUSED BY CRANIAL NEURALGIAS

Presumed irritation of superficial nerves

Occipital neuralgia.
Supraorbital neuralgia.

Presumed irritation of intracranial nerves

Trigeminal neuralgia ("tic douloureux").
Glossopharyngeal neuralgia.

HEAD AND NECK, SOFT TISSUE MASSES

ICD-9CM # CODE VARIES WITH SPECIFIC DIAGNOSIS

Lipoma.
Pilar cyst.
Epidermal inclusion cyst.
Dermoid cyst.
Bone cyst.
Hemangioma.
Eosinophilic granuloma.
Other: facial nerve neuroma, teratoma, rhabdomyoma, rhabdomyosarcoma, branchial cleft cyst.

HEARING LOSS, ACUTE[23]

ICD-9CM # 388.2

Infectious: mumps, measles, influenza, herpes simplex, herpes zoster, CMV, mononucleosis, syphilis.
Vascular: macroglobulinemia, sickle cell disease, Berger's disease, leukemia, polycythemia, fat emboli, hypercoagulable states.
Metabolic: diabetes, pregnancy, hyperlipoproteinemia.
Conductive: cerumen impaction, foreign bodies, otitis media, otitis externa, barotrauma, trauma.
Medications: aminoglycosides, loop diuretics, antineoplastics, salicylates, vancomycin.
Neoplasm: acoustic neuroma, metastatic neoplasm.

HEARTBURN AND INDIGESTION[30]

ICD-9CM # 787.1 HEARTBURN
536.8 INDIGESTION

Reflux esophagitis.
Gastritis.
Nonulcer dyspepsia.
Functional GI disorder (anxiety disorder, social/environmental stresses).
Excessive intestinal gas (ingestion of flatulogenic foods, GI stasis, constipation).
Gas entrapment (hepatitis or splenic flexure syndrome).
Neoplasm (adenocarcinoma of stomach or esophagus, lymphoma).
Gallbladder disease.

HEART FAILURE, PREGNANCY

ICD-9CM # 428.90

Congenital valvular heart disease exacerbated by pregnancy.
Peripartum cardiomyopathy.
Untreated thyrotoxicosis.
Hypothyroidism.
Pulmonary hypertension.
Myocardial infarction.

HEEL PAIN

ICD-9CM # CODE VARIES WITH SPECIFIC DIAGNOSIS

Achilles tendonitis/tendinopathy (insertional, noninsertional).
Retrocalcaneal bursitis (superficial, deep).
Plantar fasciopathy.
Neuropathy (tarsal tunnel, posterior tibial nerve [medial calcaneal branch], abductor digiti quinti).
Calcaneal stress fracture.
Puncture wound, foreign body.
Cellulitis.
Spondyloarthropathy.
Fat pad atrophy.
Soft tissue tumor.
S1 radiculopathy.
Paget's disease of bone.
Haglund deformity.
Primary or metastatic bone tumor.

HEEL PAIN, PLANTAR[21]

ICD-9CM # 729.5

SKIN

Keratoses.
Verruca.
Ulcer.
Fissure.

CONNECTIVE TISSUE

Fat

Atrophy.
Panniculitis.

Dense connective tissue

Inflammatory fasciitis.
Fibromatosis.
Enthesopathy.
Bursitis.

Bone (calcaneus)

Stress fracture.
Paget's disease.
Benign bone cyst/tumor.
Malignant bone tumor.
Metabolic bone disease (osteopenia).

Nerve

Tarsal tunnel.
Plantar nerve entrapment.
S1 nerve root radiculopathy.
Painful peripheral neuropathy.

INFECTION

Dermatomycoses.
Acute osteomyelitis.
Plantar abscess.

MISCELLANEOUS

Foreign body.
Nonunion calcaneus fracture.
Psychogenic.
Idiopathic.

HEMARTHROSIS

ICD-9CM # 848.9 HEMARTHROSIS (SPRAIN) NOS

Trauma.
Anticoagulant therapy.
Thrombocytopenia, thrombocytosis.
Bleeding disorders (e.g., von Willebrand's disease).
Charcot's joint.
Idiopathic.
Other: pigmented villonodular synovitis, hemangioma, synovioma, AV fistula, ruptured aneurysm.

HEMATURIA

ICD-9CM # 599.7 HEMATURIA, BENIGN (ESSENTIAL)

Use the mnemonic TICS:
T (trauma): blow to kidney, insertion of Foley catheter or foreign body in urethra, prolonged and severe exercise, very rapid emptying of overdistended bladder.
(tumor): hypernephroma, Wilms' tumor, papillary carcinoma of the bladder, prostatic and urethral neoplasms.
(toxins): turpentine, phenols, sulfonamides and other antibiotics, cyclophosphamide, NSAIDs.
I (infections): glomerulonephritis, TB, cystitis, prostatitis, urethritis, *Schistosoma haematobium,* yellow fever, blackwater fever.
(inflammatory processes): Goodpasture's syndrome, periarteritis, postirradiation.
C (calculi): renal, ureteral, bladder, urethra.
(cysts): simple cysts, polycystic disease.
(congenital anomalies): hemangiomas, aneurysms, AVM.

S (surgery): invasive procedures, prostatic resection, cystoscopy.
(sickle cell disease and other hematologic disturbances): hemophilia, thrombocytopenia, anticoagulants.
(somewhere else): bleeding genitals, factitious (drug addicts).

HEMATURIA, DIFFERENTIAL BASED ON AGE AND SEX

ICD-9CM # 599.7 HEMATURIA BENIGN (ESSENTIAL)
OTHER CODES FOR HEMATURIA VARY WITH CAUSE OF HEMATURIA

0-20 YR

Acute urinary tract infections.
Acute glomerulonephritis.
Congenital urinary tract anomalies with obstruction.
Trauma to genitals.

20-40 YR

Acute urinary tract infection.
Trauma to genitals.
Urolithiasis.
Bladder cancer.

40-60 YR (WOMEN)

Acute urinary tract infection.
Bladder cancer.
Urolithiasis.

40-60 YR (MEN)

Acute urinary tract infection.
Bladder cancer.
Urolithiasis.

60 YR AND OLDER (WOMEN)

Acute urinary tract infection.
Bladder cancer.
Vaginal trauma or irritation.
Urolithiasis.

60 YR AND OLDER (MEN)

Acute urinary tract infection.
Benign prostatic hyperplasia.
Bladder cancer.
Urolithiasis.
Trauma.

HEMIPARESIS/HEMIPLEGIA

ICD-9CM # 436.0 ACQUIRED DUE TO ACUTE CVA, FLACCID
436.1 ACQUIRED DUE TO CVA, ACUTE, SPASTIC

CVA.
Transient ischemic attack.
Cerebral neoplasm.
Multiple sclerosis or other demyelinating disorder.
CNS infection.
Migraine.
Hypoglycemia
Subdural hematoma.
Vasculitis.
Todd's paralysis.
Epidural hematoma.
Metabolic (hyperosmolar state, electrolyte imbalance).
Psychiatric disorders.
Congenital disorders.
Leukodystrophies.

HEMOLYSIS AND HEMOGLOBINURIA

ICD-9CM # 773.2 HEMOLYSIS
791.2 HEMOGLOBINURIA

Erythrocyte trauma (prosthetic cardiac valves, marching and severe trauma, extensive burns).
Infections (malaria, *Bartonella, Clostridium Welchii*).
Brown recluse spider bite.
Incompatible blood transfusions.
Hemolytic uremic syndrome.
Thrombotic thrombocytopenic purpura (TTP).
Paroxysmal nocturnal hemoglobinuria (PNH).
Drugs (penicillins, quinidine, methyldopa, sulfonamides, nitrofurantoin).
Erythrocyte enzyme deficiencies (e.g., exposure to fava beans in patients with glucose-6-phosphate dehydrogenase deficiency).

HEMOLYSIS, INTRAVASCULAR

ICD-9CM # 283.2

Infections.
Exertional hemolysis (e.g., prolonged march).
Valve hemolysis.
Microangiopathic hemolytic anemia.
Osmotic and chemical agents.
Thermal injury.
Cold agglutinins.
Venoms (snakes, spiders).
Paroxysmal nocturnal hemoglobinuria (PNH).

HEMOLYSIS, MECHANICAL

ICD-9CM # 283.19

Prosthetic heart valves.
Aortic stenosis.
Malignant hypertension.
Metastatic adenocarcinoma.
Traumatic exercise.
Renal transplants.
Renal cortical necrosis.
Glomerulonephritis.
Thrombotic thrombocytopenic purpura (TTP), hemolytic-uremic syndrome (HUS).
Renal vasculitis.
Scleroderma.
Diabetes.

HEMOPERITONEUM

ICD-9CM # 568.81

Ruptured Graafian follicle.
Ruptured spleen.
Ectopic pregnancy.
Traumatic laceration of liver.
Ruptured aneurysm.
Ruptured bladder.
Traumatic laceration of bowel, pancreas, uterus.

HEMOPTYSIS

ICD-9CM # 786.3

CARDIOVASCULAR

Pulmonary embolism/infarction.
Left ventricular failure.
Mitral stenosis.
AV fistula.
Severe hypertension.
Erosion of aortic aneurysm.

PULMONARY

Neoplasm (primary or metastatic).
Infection.
Pneumonia: *Streptococcus pneumoniae, Klebsiella pneumoniae, Staphylococcus aureus, Legionella pneumophila.*
Bronchiectasis.
Abscess.
TB.
Bronchitis.
Fungal infections (aspergillosis, coccidioidomycosis).
Parasitic infections (amebiasis, ascariasis, paragonimiasis).
Vasculitis: Wegener's granulomatosis, Churg-Strauss syndrome, Henoch-Schönlein purpura.
Goodpasture's syndrome.
Trauma (needle biopsy, foreign body, right-sided heart catheterization, prolonged and severe cough).
Cystic fibrosis, bullous emphysema.
Pulmonary sequestration.
Pulmonary AV fistula.
SLE.
Idiopathic pulmonary hemosiderosis.
Drugs: aspirin, anticoagulants, penicillamine.
Pulmonary hypertension.
Mediastinal fibrosis.

OTHER

Epistaxis, trauma.
Laryngeal bleeding (laryngitis, laryngeal neoplasm).
Hematologic disorders (clotting abnormalities, DIC, thrombocytopenia).

HEPATIC CYSTS[33]

ICD-9CM # 751.62 HEPATIC CYST, CONGENITAL
122.8 ECHINOCOCCUS INFECTION, LIVER

CONGENITAL HEPATIC CYSTS

Parenchymal: solitary cyst, polycystic disease.
Ductal: localized dilatation, multiple cystic dilatations of intrahepatic ducts (Caroli's disease).

ACQUIRED HEPATIC CYSTS

Inflammatory cysts: retention cysts, echinococcal cyst, amebic cyst.
Neoplastic cyst.
Peliosis hepatis.

HEPATIC GRANULOMAS[1]

ICD-9CM # 572.8

INFECTIONS

Bacterial, spirochetal: TB and atypical mycobacterial infections, tularemia, brucellosis, leprosy, syphilis, Whipple's disease, listeriosis.
Viral: mononucleosis, CMV.
Rickettsial: Q fever.
Fungal: coccidioidomycosis, histoplasmosis, cryptococcal infections, actinomycosis, aspergillosis, nocardiosis.
Parasitic: schistosomiasis, clonorchiasis, toxocariasis, ascariasis, toxoplasmosis, amebiasis.

HEPATOBILIARY DISORDERS

Primary biliary cirrhosis, granulomatous hepatitis, jejunoileal bypass.

SYSTEMIC DISORDERS

Sarcoidosis, Wegener's granulomatosis, inflammatory bowel disease, Hodgkin's disease, lymphoma.

DRUGS/TOXINS

Beryllium, parenteral foreign material (starch, talc, silicone, etc.), phenylbutazone, a-methyldopa, procainamide, allopurinol, phenytoin, nitrofurantoin, hydralazine.

HEPATITIS, ACUTE[22]

ICD-9CM # CODE VARIES WITH SPECIFIC DISORDER

Infectious:
- Hepatitis A, B, C, D, G.
- Epstein-Barr virus.
- Cytomegalovirus.
- Herpes simplex virus.
- Yellow fever.
- Leptospirosis.
- Q fever.
- HIV.
- Brucellosis.
- Lyme disease.
- Syphilis.

Noninfectious:
- Drug induced.
- Autoimmune.
- Ischemic.
- Acute fatty liver of pregnancy.
- Acute Budd-Chiari syndrome.
- Wilson's disease.

HEPATITIS, CHRONIC[22]

ICD-9CM # 571.40 HEPATITIS, NONINFECTIOUS, CHRONIC
072.22 HEPATITIS B, CHRONIC
070.44 HEPATITIS C, CHRONIC

Chronic viral hepatitis:
- Hepatitis B.
- Hepatitis C.
- Hepatitis D.

Autoimmune hepatitis and variant syndromes.
Hereditary hemochromatosis.
Wilson's disease.
α-Antitrypsin deficiency.
Fatty liver and nonalcoholic steatohepatitis.
Alcoholic liver disease.
Drug-induced liver disease.
Hepatic granulomas:
- Infectious.
- Drug induced.
- Neoplastic.
- Idiopathic.

HEPATOMEGALY

ICD-9CM # 789.1

FREQUENT JAUNDICE

Infectious hepatitis.
Toxic hepatitis.
Carcinoma: liver, pancreas, bile ducts, metastatic neoplasm to liver.
Cirrhosis.
Obstruction of common bile duct.
Alcoholic hepatitis.
Biliary cirrhosis.
Cholangitis.
Hemochromatosis with cirrhosis.

INFREQUENT JAUNDICE

CHF.
Amyloidosis.
Liver abscess.
Sarcoidosis.
Infectious mononucleosis.
Alcoholic fatty infiltration.
Nonalcoholic steatohepatitis
Lymphoma.
Leukemia.
Budd-Chiari syndrome.
Myelofibrosis with myeloid metaplasia.
Familial hyperlipoproteinemia type 1.
Other: amebiasis, hydatid disease of liver, schistosomiasis, kala-azar *(Leishmania donovani)*, Hurler's syndrome, Gaucher's disease, kwashiorkor.

HERMAPHRODITISM[4]

ICD-9CM # 752.7 HERMAPHRODITISM, CONGENITAL

FEMALE PSEUDOHERMAPHRODITISM

Androgen exposure:
- Fetal source:
  - 21-Hydroxylase (P450 c21) deficiency.
  - 11β-Hydroxylase (P450 c11) deficiency.
  - 3β-Hydroxysteroid dehydrogenase II (3β-HSD II) deficiency.
  - Aromatase (P450arom) deficiency.
- Maternal source.
- Virilizing ovarian tumor.
- Virilizing adrenal tumor.
- Androgenic drugs.

Undetermined origin:
- Associated with genitourinary and gastrointestinal tract defects.

MALE PSEUDOHERMAPHRODITISM

Defects in testicular differentiation:
- Denys-Drash syndrome (mutation in WT1 gene).
- WAGR syndrome (*W*ilms tumor, *a*niridia, *g*enitourinary malformation, *r*etardation).
- Deletion of 11p13.
- Camptomelic syndrome (autosomal gene at 17q24.3- q25.1) and SOX 9 mutation.
- XY pure gonadal dysgenesis (Swyer syndrome).
  - Mutation in SRY gene.
  - Unknown cause.
- XY gonadal agenesis.

Deficiency of testicular hormones:
- Leydig cell aplasia.
- Mutation in LH receptor.
- Lipoid adrenal hyperplasia (P450 scc) deficiency; mutation in StAR (steroidogenic acute regulatory protein).
- 3b-HSDII deficiency.
- 17-Hydroxylase/17, 20-lyase (P450 c17) deficiency.
- Persistent müllerian duct syndrome.
  - Gene mutations, müllerian-inhibiting substance (MIS).
  - Receptor defects for mis.

Defect in androgen action:
- 5α-Reductase II mutations.
- Androgen receptor defects:
  - Complete androgen insensitivity syndrome.
  - Partial androgen insensitivity syndrome.
  - (Reifenstein and other syndromes).
  - Smith-Lemli-Opitz syndrome.
    - Defect in conversion of 7-dehydrocholesterol to cholesterol.

TRUE HERMAPHRODITISM

XX.
XY.
XX/XY chimeras.

HICCUPS[18]

ICD-9CM # 786.8

TRANSIENT HICCUPS

Sudden excitement, emotion.
Gastric distention.
Esophageal obstruction.
Alcohol ingestion.
Sudden change in temperature.

PERSISTENT OR CHRONIC HICCUPS

Toxic/metabolic: uremia, DM, hyperventilation, hypocalcemia, hypokalemia, hyponatremia, gout, fever.
Drugs: benzodiazepines, steroids, a-methyldopa, barbiturates.
Surgery/general anesthesia.
Thoracic/diaphragmatic disorders: pneumonia, lung cancer, asthma, pleuritis, pericarditis, myocardial infarction, aortic aneurysm, esophagitis, esophageal obstruction, diaphragmatic hernia or irritation.
Abdominal disorders: gastric ulcer or cancer, hepatobiliary or pancreatic disease, IBD, bowel obstruction, intraabdominal or subphrenic abscess, prostatic infection or cancer.
Central nervous system disorders: traumatic, infectious, vascular, structural.
Ear, nose, and throat disorders: pharyngitis, laryngitis, tumor, irritation of auditory canal.
Psychogenic disorders.
Idiopathic disorders.

HIP PAIN, CHILDREN[23]

ICD-9CM # 959.6 HIP INJURY
719.95 HIP JOINT DISORDER
843.9 HIP STRAIN

TRAUMA

Hip or pelvis fractures.
Overuse injuries.

INFECTION

Septic arthritis.
Osteomyelitis.

INFLAMMATION

Transient synovitis.
Juvenile rheumatoid arthritis.
Rheumatic fever.

NEOPLASM

Leukemia.
Osteogenic or Ewing's sarcoma.
Metastatic disease.

HEMATOLOGIC DISORDERS

Hemophilia.
Sickle cell anemia.

MISCELLANEOUS

Legg-Calvé-Perthes disease.
Slipped capital femoral epiphysis.

HIRSUTISM

ICD-9CM # 704.1

Idiopathic: familial, possibly increased sensitivity to androgens.
Menopause.
Polycystic ovarian syndrome.
Drugs: androgens, anabolic steroids, methyltestosterone, minoxidil, diazoxide, phenytoin, glucocorticoids, cyclosporine.
Congenital adrenal hyperplasia.
Adrenal virilizing tumor.
Ovarian virilizing tumor: arrhenoblastoma, hilus cell tumor.
Pituitary adenoma.
Cushing's syndrome.
Hypothyroidism (congenital and juvenile).
Acromegaly.
Testicular feminization.

HIV INFECTION, ANORECTAL LESIONS[23]

ICD-9CM # 042 HIV INFECTION, SYMPTOMATIC
V08 HIV INFECTION, ASYMPTOMATIC

COMMON CONDITIONS

Anal fissure.
Abscess and fistula.
Hemorrhoids.
Pruritus ani.
Pilonidal disease.

COMMON STDS

Gonorrhea.
Chlamydia.
Herpes.
Chancroid.
Syphilis.
Condylomata acuminata.

ATYPICAL CONDITIONS

Infectious: TB, CMV, actinomycosis, cryptococcus.
Neoplastic: lymphoma, Kaposi's sarcoma, squamous cell carcinoma.
Other: idiopathic and ulcer.

HIV INFECTION, CHEST RADIOGRAPHIC ABNORMALITIES[23]

ICD-9CM # 042 HIV INFECTION, SYMPTOMATIC
V08 HIV INFECTION, ASYMPTOMATIC

DIFFUSE INTERSTITIAL INFILTRATION

Pneumocystis carinii.
Cytomegalovirus.
Mycobacterium tuberculosis.
Mycobacterium avium complex.
Histoplasmosis.
Coccidioidomycosis.
Lymphoid interstitial pneumonitis.

FOCAL CONSOLIDATION

Bacterial pneumonia.
Mycoplasma pneumoniae.
Pneumocystis carinii.
Mycobacterium tuberculosis.
Mycobacterium avium complex.

NODULAR LESIONS

Kaposi's sarcoma.
Mycobacterium tuberculosis.
Mycobacterium avium complex.
Fungal lesions.
Toxoplasmosis.

CAVITARY LESIONS

Pneumocystis carinii.
Mycobacterium tuberculosis.
Bacterial infection.

PLEURAL EFFUSION

Kaposi's sarcoma.
(Small effusion may be associated with any infection).

ADENOPATHY

Kaposi's sarcoma.
Lymphoma.
Mycobacterium tuberculosis.
Cryptococcus.

PNEUMOTHORAX

Kaposi's sarcoma.

HIV INFECTION, COGNITIVE IMPAIRMENT[22]

ICD-9CM # 042 HIV INFECTION, SYMPTOMATIC

EARLY TO MID-STAGE HIV DISEASE

Depression.
Alcohol and substance abuse.
Medication-induced cognitive impairment.
Metabolic encephalopathies.
HIV-related cognitive impairment.

ADVANCED HIV DISEASE ($CD4^+$ <100/MM^3)

Opportunistic infection of CNS.
Neurosyphilis.
CNS lymphoma.
Progressive multifocal leukoencephalopathy.
Depression.
Metabolic encephalopathies.
Medication-induced cognitive impairment.
Stroke.
HIV dementia.

HIV INFECTION, CUTANEOUS MANIFESTATIONS[18]

ICD-9CM # 042 HIV INFECTION, SYMPTOMATIC
V08 HIV INFECTION, ASYMPTOMATIC

BACTERIAL INFECTION

Bacillary angiomatosis: Numerous angiomatous nodules associated with fever, chills, weight loss.

Staphylococcus aureus: Folliculitis, ecthyma, impetigo, bullous impetigo, furuncles, carbuncles.
Syphilis: May occur in different forms (primary, secondary, tertiary); chancre may become painful because of secondary infection.

FUNGAL INFECTION

Candidiasis: Mucous membranes (oral, vulvovaginal), less commonly candida intertrigo or paronychia.
Cryptococcoses: Papules or nodules that strongly resemble molluscum contagiosum; other forms include pustules, purpuric papules, and vegetating plaques.
Seborrheic dermatitis: Scaling and erythema in the hair-bearing areas (eyebrows, scalp, chest, and pubic area).

ARTHROPOD INFESTATIONS

Scabies: Pruritus with or without rash, usually generalized but can be limited to a single digit.

VIRAL INFECTION

Herpes simplex: Vesicular lesion in clusters; perianal, genital, orofacial, or digital; can be disseminated.
Herpes zoster: Painful dermatomal vesicles that may ulcerate or disseminate.
HIV: Discrete erythematous macules and papules on the upper trunk, palms, and soles are the most characteristic cutaneous finding of acute HIV infection.
Human papillomavirus: Genital warts (may become unusually extensive).
Kaposi's sarcoma (herpesvirus): Erythematous macules or papules; enlarge at varying rates; violaceous nodules or plaques; occasionally painful.
Molluscum contagiosum: Discrete umbilicated papules commonly on the face, neck, and intertriginous sites (axilla, groin, or buttocks).

NONINFECTIOUS

Drug reactions: More frequent and severe in HIV patients.
Nutritional deficiencies: Mainly seen in children and patients with chronic diarrhea; diffuse skin manifestations, depending upon the deficiency.
Psoriasis: Scaly lesions; diffuse or localized; can be associated with arthritis.
Vasculitis: Palpable purpuric eruption (can resemble septic emboli).

HIV INFECTION, ESOPHAGEAL DISEASE

ICD-9CM # CODE VARIES WITH SPECIFIC DIAGNOSIS

Candida infection.
Cytomegalovirus infection.
Aphthous ulcer.
Herpes simplex.

HIV INFECTION, HEPATIC DISEASE[22]

ICD-9CM # 042 HIV INFECTION, SYMPTOMATIC

VIRUSES

Hepatitis A.
Hepatitis B.
Hepatitis C.
Hepatitis D (with HBV).
Epstein-Barr virus.
Cytomegalovirus.
Herpes simplex virus.
Adenovirus.
Varicella-zoster virus.

MYCOBACTERIA

Mycobacterium avium complex.
Mycobacterium tuberculosis.

FUNGI

Histoplasma capsulatum.
Cryptococcus neoformans.
Coccidioides immitis.
Candida albicans.
Pneumocystis carinii.
Penicillium marneffei.

PROTOZOA

Toxoplasma gondii.
Cryptosporidium parvum.
Microsporida spp.
Schistosoma.

BACTERIA

Bartonella henselae (peliosis hepatis).

MALIGNANCY

Kaposi's sarcoma (HHV-8).
Non-Hodgkin's lymphoma.
Hepatocellular carcinoma.

MEDICATIONS

Zidovudine.
Didanosine.
Ritonavir.
Other HIV-1 protease inhibitors.
Fluconazole.
Macrolide antibiotics.
Isoniazid.
Rifampin.
Trimethoprim-sulfamethoxazole.

HIV INFECTION, LOWER GI TRACT DISEASE[22]

ICD-9CM # 042 HIV INFECTION, SYMPTOMATIC

CAUSES OF ENTEROCOLITIS

Bacteria
Campylobacter jejuni and other spp.
Salmonella spp.
Shigella flexneri.
Aeromonas hydrophila.
Plesiomonas shigelloides.
Yersinia enterocolitica.
Vibrio spp.
Mycobacterium avium complex.
Mycobacterium tuberculosis.
Escherichia coli (enterotoxigenic, enteroadherent).
Bacterial overgrowth.
Clostridium difficile (toxin).
Parasites
Cryptosporidium parvum.
Microsporida *(Enterocytozoon bieneusi, Septata intestinalis).*
Isospora belli.
Entamoeba histolytica.
Giardia lamblia.
Cyclospora cayetanensis.
Viruses
Cytomegalovirus.
Adenovirus.
Calicivirus.
Astrovirus.
Picobirnavirus.
Human immunodeficiency virus.
Fungi
Histoplasma capsulatum.

CAUSES OF PROCTITIS

Bacteria
Chlamydia trachomatis.
Neisseria gonorrhoeae.
Treponema pallidum.
Viruses
Herpes simplex.
Cytomegalovirus.

HIV INFECTION, OCULAR MANIFESTATIONS[33]

ICD-9CM # 042 HIV INFECTION, SYMPTOMATIC
V08 HIV INFECTION, ASYMPTOMATIC

EYELIDS

Molluscum contagiosum.
Kaposi's sarcoma.

CORNEA/CONJUNCTIVA

Keratoconjunctivitis sicca.
Bacterial/fungal ulcerative keratitis.
Herpes simplex.
Herpes zoster ophthalmicus.
Conjunctival microvasculopathy.
Kaposi's sarcoma.

RETINA, CHOROID, AND VITREOUS

Microvasculopathy.
Endophthalmitis.
Cytomegalovirus retinitis.
Acute retinal necrosis.
Syphilis.
Toxoplasmosis.
Pneumocystis choroidopathy.
Cryptococcosis.
Mycobacterial infection.
Intraocular lymphoma.
Candidiasis.
Histoplasmosis.

DRUGS ASSOCIATED WITH OCULAR TOXICITY

Rifabutin.
Didanosine.

NEUROOPHTHALMIC

Disc edema.
Primary or secondary optic neuropathy.
Cranial nerve palsies.

ORBITAL

Lymphoma.
Infection.
Pseudotumor.

HIV INFECTION, PULMONARY DISEASE[22]

ICD-9CM # 042 HIV INFECTION, SYMPTOMATIC

MYCOBACTERIAL

M. tuberculosis.
M. kansasii.
M. avium complex.
Other nontuberculous mycobacteria.

OTHER BACTERIAL

Streptococcus pneumoniae.
Staphylococcus aureus.
Haemophilus influenzae.
Enterobacteriaceae.
Pseudomonas aeruginosa.
Moraxella catarrhalis.
Group A *Streptococcus.*
Nocardia species.
Rhodococcus equi.
Chlamydia pneumoniae.

FUNGAL

Pneumocystis carinii.
Cryptococcus neoformans.
Histoplasma capsulatum.
Coccidioides immitis.
Aspergillus species.
Blastomyces dermatitidis.
Penicillium marneffei.

VIRAL

Cytomegalovirus.
Herpes simplex virus.
Adenovirus.
Respiratory syncytial virus.
Influenza viruses.
Parainfluenza virus.

OTHER

Toxoplasma gondii.
Strongyloides stercoralis.
Kaposi's sarcoma.
Lymphoma.
Lung cancer.
Lymphocytic interstitial pneumonitis.
Nonspecific interstitial pneumonitis.
Bronchiolitis obliterans with organizing pneumonia.
Pulmonary hypertension.
Emphysema-like or bullous disease.
Pneumothorax.
Congestive heart failure.
Diffuse alveolar damage.
Pulmonary embolus.

HOARSENESS

ICD-9CM # 784.49

Allergic rhinitis.
Infections (laryngitis, epiglottitis, tracheitis, croup).
Vocal cord polyps.
Voice strain.
Irritants (tobacco smoke).
Vocal cord trauma (intubation, surgery).
Neoplastic involvement of vocal cord (primary or metastatic).
Neurologic abnormalities (multiple sclerosis, ALS, parkinsonism).
Endocrine abnormalities (puberty, menopause, hypothyroidism).
Other (laryngeal webs or cysts, psychogenic, muscle tension abnormalities).

HYDROCEPHALUS

ICD-9CM # 331.4

Head trauma.
Brain neoplasm (primary or metastatic).
Spinal cord tumor.
Cerebellar infarction.
Exudative or granulomatous meningitis.
Cerebellar hemorrhage.
Subarachnoid hemorrhage.
Aqueductal stenosis.
Third ventricle colloid cyst.
Hindbrain malformation.
Viral encephalitis.
Metastases to leptomeninges.

HYPERCALCEMIA

ICD-9CM # 275.42 HYPERCALCEMIA DISORDER

Malignancy: increased bone resorption via osteoclast-activating factors, secretion of PTH-like substances, prostaglandin E2, direct erosion by tumor cells, transforming growth factors, colony-stimulating activity. Hypercalcemia is common in the following neoplasms:
 Solid tumors: breast, lung, pancreas, kidneys, ovary.
 Hematologic cancers: myeloma, lymphosarcoma, adult T-cell lymphoma, Burkitt's lymphoma.
Hyperparathyroidism: increased bone resorption, GI absorption, and renal absorption; etiology:
 Parathyroid hyperplasia, adenoma.
 Hyperparathyroidism or renal failure with secondary hyperparathyroidism.
 Granulomatous disorders: increased GI absorption (e.g., sarcoidosis).
 Paget's disease: increased bone resorption, seen only during periods of immobilization.
 Vitamin D intoxication, milk-alkali syndrome; increased GI absorption.
 Thiazides: increased renal absorption.
Other causes: familial hypocalciuric hypercalcemia, thyrotoxicosis, adrenal insufficiency, prolonged immobilization, vitamin A intoxication, recovery from acute renal failure, lithium administration, pheochromocytoma, disseminated SLE.

HYPERCALCEMIA, MALIGNANCY-INDUCED

ICD-9CM # 275.42

Lung carcinoma	(6% frequency, 35% of hypercalcemic cases)
Breast carcinoma	(10% frequency, 25% of hypercalcemic cases)
Multiple myeloma	(33% frequency, 10% of hypercalcemic cases)
Lymphoma	(4% of hypercalcemic cases)
Genitourinary cancer	(6% of hypercalcemic cases)

HYPERCAPNIA, PERSISTENT[33]

ICD-9CM # 786.09

Hypercapnia with normal lungs: CNS disturbances (CVA, parkinsonism, encephalitis), metabolic alkalosis, myxedema, primary alveolar hypoventilation, spinal cord lesions.
Diseases of the chest wall (e.g., kyphoscoliosis, ankylosing spondylitis).
Neuromuscular disorders (e.g., myasthenia gravis, Guillain-Barré syndrome, amyotrophic lateral sclerosis, muscular dystrophy, poliomyelitis).
COPD.

HYPERGASTRINEMIA

ICD-9CM # CODE VARIES WITH SPECIFIC DISORDER

Decreased gastrin release inhibition from medications (proton pump inhibitors [PPIs], H_2 receptor antagonists), vagotomy.
Chronic renal failure.
Hypochlorhydria due to atrophic gastritis, gastric carcinoma, pernicious anemia.
Gastrinoma (Zollinger-Ellison syndrome).
Pyloric obstruction.
Hyperplasia of antral G cells.
Rheumatoid arthritis.

HYPERHIDROSIS[4]

ICD-9CM # 780.8 HYPERHIDROSIS

CORTICAL

Emotional.
Familial dysautonomia.
Congenital ichthyosiform erythroderma.
Epidermolysis bullosa.
Nail-patella syndrome.
Jadassohn-Lewandowsky syndrome.
Pachyonychia congenita.
Palmoplantar keratoderma.

HYPOTHALAMIC

Drugs
Antipyretics.
Emetics.
Insulin.
Meperidine.
Exercise
Infection
Defervescence.
Chronic illness.
Metabolic
Debility.
Diabetes mellitus.
Hyperpituitarism.
Hyperthyroidism.
Hypoglycemia.
Obesity.
Porphyria.
Pregnancy.
Rickets.
Infantile scurvy.
Cardiovascular
Heart failure.
Shock.
Vasomotor
Cold injury.
Raynaud phenomenon.
Rheumatoid arthritis.
Neurologic
Abscess.
Familial dysautonomia.
Postencephalitic.
Tumor.
Miscellaneous
Chédiak-Higashi syndrome.
Compensatory.
Phenylketonuria.
Pheochromocytoma.
Vitiligo.
Medullary
Physiologic gustatory sweating.
Encephalitis.
Granulosis rubra nasi.
Syringomyelia.
Thoracic sympathetic trunk injury.
Spinal
Cord transection.
Syringomyelia.
Changes in blood flow
Mallucci syndrome.
Arteriovenous fistula.
Klippel-Trenaunay syndrome.
Glomus tumor.
Blue rubber bleb nevus syndrome.

HYPERKALEMIA

ICD-9CM # 276.7

Pseudohyperkalemia.
- Hemolyzed specimen.
- Severe thrombocytosis (platelet count 0.106 ml).
- Severe leukocytosis (white blood cell count 0.105 ml).
- Fist clenching during phlebotomy.

Excessive potassium intake (often in setting of impaired excretion).
- Potassium replacement therapy.
- High-potassium diet.
- Salt substitutes with potassium.
- Potassium salts of antibiotics.

Decreased renal excretion.
- Potassium-sparing diuretics (e.g., spironolactone, triamterene, amiloride).
- Renal insufficiency.
- Mineralocorticoid deficiency.
- Hyporeninemic hypoaldosteronism (DM).
- Tubular unresponsiveness to aldosterone (e.g., SLE, multiple myeloma, sickle cell disease).
- Type 4 RTA.
- ACE inhibitors.
- Heparin administration.
- NSAIDs.
- Trimethoprim-sulfamethoxazole.
- β-Blockers.
- Pentamidine.

Redistribution (excessive cellular release).
- Acidemia (each 0.1 decrease in pH increases the serum potassium by 0.4 to 0.6 mEq/L). Lactic acidosis and ketoacidosis cause minimal redistribution.
- Insulin deficiency.
- Drugs (e.g., succinylcholine, markedly increased digitalis level, arginine, β-adrenergic blockers).
- Hypertonicity.
- Hemolysis.
- Tissue necrosis, rhabdomyolysis, burns.
- Hyperkalemic periodic paralysis.

HYPERKINETIC MOVEMENT DISORDERS[27]

ICD-9CM # 314.8 HYPERKINETIC SYNDROME
275.1 CHOREOATHETOSIS
335.5 HEMIBALLISM
333.7 DYSTONIA DUE TO DRUGS
333.6 DYSTONIA, IDIOPATHIC

Chorea, choreoathetosis: drug-induced, Huntington's chorea, Sydenham's chorea.
Tardive dyskinesia (e.g., phenothiazines).
Hemiballismus (lacunar CVA near subthalamic nuclei in basal ganglia, metastatic lesions, toxoplasmosis [in AIDS]).
Dystonia (idiopathic, familial, drug-induced [prochlorperazine, metoclopramide]), Wilson's disease.
Liver failure.
Thyrotoxicosis.
SLE, polycythemia.

HYPERMAGNESEMIA

ICD-9CM # 275.2

Renal failure (decreased GFR).
Decreased renal excretion secondary to salt depletion.
Abuse of antacids and laxatives containing magnesium in patients with renal insufficiency.
Endocrinopathies (deficiency of mineralocorticoid or thyroid hormone).
Increased tissue breakdown (rhabdomyolysis).
Redistribution: acute DKA, pheochromocytoma.
Other: lithium, volume depletion, familial hypocalciuric hypercalcemia.

HYPERPHOSPHATEMIA

ICD-9CM # 275.3

Excessive phosphate administration.
Excessive oral intake or IV administration.
Laxatives containing phosphate (phosphate tablets, phosphate enemas).
Decreased renal phosphate excretion.
Acute or chronic renal failure.
Hypoparathyroidism or pseudohypoparathyroidism.
Acromegaly, thyrotoxicosis.
Biphosphonate therapy.
Tumor calcinosis.
Sickle cell anemia.
Transcellular shift out of cells.
Chemotherapy of lymphoma or leukemia, tumor lysis syndrome, hemolysis.
Acidosis.
Rhabdomyolysis, malignant hyperthermia.
Artifact: in vitro hemolysis.
Pseudohyperphosphatemia: hyperlipidemia, paraproteinemia, hyperbilirubinemia.

HYPERPIGMENTATION[5]

ICD-9CM # 709.00

Addison's disease.*
Arsenic ingestion.
ACTH or MSH producing tumors (e.g., oat cell carcinoma of the lung).*
Drug induced (i.e., antimalarials, some cytotoxic agents).
Hemochromatosis ("bronze" diabetes).
Malabsorption syndrome (Whipple's disease and celiac sprue).
Melanoma.
Melanotropic hormone injection.*
Pheochromocytoma.
Porphyrias (porphyria cutanea tarda and variegate porphyria).
Pregnancy.

Progressive systemic sclerosis and related conditions.
PUVA therapy (psoralen administration) for psoriasis and vitiligo.*

ACTH, Adrenocorticotropic hormone; *MSH,* melanocyte-stimulating hormone; *PUVA,* psoralen plus ultraviolet A.
*Accentuation on sun-exposed surfaces.

HYPERSPLENISM, ASSOCIATED CONDITIONS

ICD-9CM # 289.4

Cirrhosis.
Portal vein thrombosis.
Myeloproliferative diseases.
Lymphomas.
Leukemias.
Splenic vein thrombosis.
Autoimmune disease.
Sickle cell disease.
Thalassemias.
Gaucher's disease.
Niemann-Pick disease.

HYPERTRICHOSIS[7]

ICD-9CM # 704.1 HYPERTRICHOSIS NOS
757.4 HYPERTRICHOSIS, CONGENITAL

DRUGS

Dilantin.
Streptomycin.
Hexachlorobenzene.
Penicillamine.
Diazoxide.
Minoxidil.
Cyclosporine.

SYSTEMIC ILLNESS

Hypothyroidism.
Anorexia nervosa.
Malnutrition.
Porphyria.
Dermatomyositis.

IDIOPATHIC

HYPERTROPHIC OSTEOARTHROPATHY

ICD-9CM # 731.2

Idiopathic.
Pulmonary disease (e.g., pulmonary fibrosis, cystic fibrosis, sarcoidosis).
Bronchogenic carcinoma.
AIDS.
GI neoplasm (e.g., esophagus, colon).
Hepatic neoplasm, cirrhosis.
Cardiovascular diseases, aortic aneurysm, aortic prosthesis.
Congenital cyanotic heart disease, patent ductus arteriosus.
Pulmonary infections, bacterial endocarditis, amebic dysentery.
Inflammatory bowel disease.
Connective tissue diseases.
Lymphomas.
Thyroid acropachy.

HYPERVENTILATION, PERSISTENT[33]

ICD-9CM # 786.01

Fibrotic lung disease.
Metabolic acidosis (e.g., diabetes, uremia).
CNS disorders (midbrain and pontine lesions).
Hepatic coma.
Salicylate intoxication.
Fever.
Sepsis.
Psychogenic (e.g., anxiety).

HYPOCALCEMIA

ICD-9CM # 275.41

Renal insufficiency: hypocalcemia caused by:
- Increased calcium deposits in bone and soft tissue secondary to increased serum PO423 level.
- Decreased production of 1,25-dihydroxyvitamin D.
- Excessive loss of 25-OHD (nephrotic syndrome).

Hypoalbuminemia: each decrease in serum albumin (g/L) will decrease serum calcium by 0.8 mg/dl but will not change free (ionized) calcium.
Vitamin D deficiency:
- Malabsorption (most common cause).
- Inadequate intake.
- Decreased production of 1,25-dihydroxyvitamin D (vitamin D-dependent rickets, renal failure).
- Decreased production of 25-OHD (parenchymal liver disease).
- Accelerated 25-OHD catabolism (phenytoin, phenobarbital).
- End-organ resistance to 1,25-dihydroxyvitamin D.

Hypomagnesemia: hypocalcemia caused by:
- Decreased PTH secretion.
- Inhibition of PTH effect on bone.

Pancreatitis, hyperphosphatemia, osteoblastic metastases: hypocalcemia is secondary to increased calcium deposits (bone, abdomen).
Pseudohypoparathyroidism (PHP): autosomal recessive disorder characterized by short stature, shortening of metacarpal bones, obesity, and mental retardation; the hypocalcemia is secondary to congenital end-organ resistance to PTH.
Idiopathic hypoparathyroidism, surgical removal of parathyroids (e.g., neck surgery).
"Hungry bones syndrome": rapid transfer of calcium from plasma into bones after removal of a parathyroid tumor.
Sepsis.
Massive blood transfusion (as a result of EDTA in blood).

HYPOCAPNIA

ICD-9CM # 786.01

Hyperventilation.
Pneumonia, pneumonitis.
Fever, sepsis.
Medications (salicylates, β-adrenergic agonists, progesterone, methylxanthines).
Pulmonary disease (asthma, interstitial fibrosis).
Pulmonary embolism.
Hepatic failure.
Metabolic acidosis.
High altitude.
CHF.
Pregnancy.
Pain.
CNS lesions.

HYPOGLYCEMIA

ICD-9CM # SPONTANEOUS 251.2
 # DIABETIC 250.3
 # DUE TO INSULIN 251.0
 # POSTOPERATIVE 579.3
 # REACTIVE 251.2

Oral hypoglycemics (therapeutic, factitious).
Exogenous insulin (therapeutic, factitious).
Postoperative gastric emptying (alimentary hyperinsulinism).
Severe malnutrition.
Liver disease.
Hypermetabolic state (sepsis).
Ketotic hypoglycemia.
Insulinoma.
Antibodies to endogenous insulin.
Hormone deficiencies (glucagon, growth hormone, hypoadrenalism).
Enzyme disorders in metabolism of glycogen, hexose, glycolysis, and Krebs cycle.
Idiopathic.

HYPOGONADISM

ICD-9CM # 256.3 FEMALE
257.2 MALE
256.3 OVARIAN
253.4 PITUITARY
257.2 TESTICULAR

HYPERGONADOTROPIC HYPOGONADISM

Hormone resistance (androgen, LH insensitivity).
Gonadal defects (e.g., Klinefelter's syndrome, myotonic dystrophy).
Drug induced (e.g., spironolactone, cytotoxins).
Alcoholism, radiation-induced.
Mumps orchitis.
Anatomic defects, castration.

HYPOGONADOTROPIC HYPOGONADISM

Pituitary lesions (neoplasms, granulomas, infarction, hemochromatosis, vasculitis).

Section II DIFFERENTIAL DIAGNOSIS

Drug-induced (e.g., glucocorticoids).
Hyperprolactinemia.
Genetic disorders (Laurence-Moon-Biedl syndrome, Prader-Willi).
Delayed puberty.
Other: chronic disease, nutritional deficiency, Kallmann's syndrome, idiopathic isolated LH or FSH deficiency.

HYPOKALEMIA

ICD-9CM # 276.8

Cellular shift (redistribution) and undetermined mechanisms.
Alkalosis (each 0.1 increase in pH decreases serum potassium by 0.4 to 0.6 mEq/L).
Insulin administration.
Vitamin B_{12} therapy for megaloblastic anemias, acute leukemias.
Hypokalemic periodic paralysis: rare familial disorder manifested by recurrent attacks of flaccid paralysis and hypokalemia.
β-Adrenergic agonists (e.g., terbutaline), decongestants, bronchodilators, theophylline, caffeine.
Barium poisoning, toluene intoxication, verapamil intoxication, chloroquine intoxication.
Correction of digoxin intoxication with digoxin antibody fragments (Digibind).
Increased renal excretion.
  Drugs:
    Diuretics, including carbonic anhydrase inhibitors (e.g., acetazolamide).
    Amphotericin B.
    High-dose sodium penicillin, nafcillin, ampicillin, or carbenicillin.
    Cisplatin.
    Aminoglycosides.
    Corticosteroids, mineralocorticoids.
    Foscarnet sodium.
  RTA: distal (type 1) or proximal (type 2).
    Diabetic ketoacidosis (DKA), ureteroenterostomy.
    Magnesium deficiency.
    Postobstruction diuresis, diuretic phase of ATN.
    Osmotic diuresis (e.g., mannitol).
    Bartter's syndrome: hyperplasia of juxtaglomerular cells leading to increased renin and aldosterone, metabolic alkalosis, hypokalemia, muscle weakness, and tetany (seen in young adults).
    Increased mineralocorticoid activity (primary or secondary aldosteronism), Cushing's syndrome.
    Chronic metabolic alkalosis from loss of gastric fluid (increased renal potassium secretion).
GI loss.
  Vomiting, nasogastric suction.
    Diarrhea.
    Laxative abuse.
    Villous adenoma.
    Fistulas.
    Inadequate dietary intake (e.g., anorexia nervosa).
    Cutaneous loss (excessive sweating).
    High dietary sodium intake, excessive use of licorice.

HYPOMAGNESEMIA

ICD-9CM # 275.2

GI and nutritional
Defective GI absorption (malabsorption).
Inadequate dietary intake (e.g., alcoholics).
Parenteral therapy without magnesium.
Chronic diarrhea, villous adenoma, prolonged nasogastric suction, fistulas (small bowel, biliary).
Excessive renal losses
Diuretics.
RTA.
Diuretic phase of ATN.
Endocrine disturbances (DKA, hyperaldosteronism, hyperthyroidism, hyperparathyroidism), SIADH, Bartter's syndrome, hypercalciuria, hypokalemia.
Cisplatin, alcohol, cyclosporine, digoxin, pentamidine, mannitol, amphotericin B, foscarnet, methotrexate.
Antibiotics (gentamicin, ticarcillin, carbenicillin).
Redistribution: hypoalbuminemia, cirrhosis, administration of insulin and glucose, theophylline, epinephrine, acute pancreatitis, cardiopulmonary bypass.
Miscellaneous: sweating, burns, prolonged exercise, lactation, "hungry-bones" syndrome.

HYPONATREMIA

ICD-9CM # 276.1

Renal loss from renal disease, diuretics.
GI loss (diarrhea, vomiting, suction).
Hypertonic hyponatremia (e.g., increased serum osmolality from hyperglycemia).
Transcutaneous loss (extensive burns, excessive sweating).
Fluid sequestration (e.g., ascites).
Osmotic diuresis (e.g., mannitol, glucose).
Dilutional (psychogenic polydipsia, iatrogenic).
Syndrome of inappropriate antidiuretic hormone secretion.
Edema with water and sodium retention.
Artifact (e.g., severe hyperlipidemia).
Laboratory error.
Adrenal insufficiency.

HYPOPHOSPHATEMIA

ICD-9CM # 275.3

Decreased intake (prolonged starvation [alcoholics], hyperalimentation, or IV infusion without phosphate).
Malabsorption.
Phosphate-binding antacids.
Renal loss:
  RTA.
  Fanconi syndrome, vitamin D-resistant rickets.
  ATN (diuretic phase).
  Hyperparathyroidism (primary or secondary).
  Familial hypophosphatemia.
  Hypokalemia, hypomagnesemia.
  Acute volume expansion.
  Glycosuria, idiopathic hypercalciuria.
  Acetazolamide.
Transcellular shift into cells:
  Alcohol withdrawal.
  DKA (recovery phase).
  Glucose-insulin or catecholamine infusion.
  Anabolic steroids.
  Total parenteral nutrition.
  Theophylline overdose.
  Severe hyperthermia; recovery from hypothermia.
  "Hungry bones" syndrome.

HYPOPIGMENTATION

ICD-9CM # 709.00

Vitiligo.
Tinea versicolor.
Atopic dermatitis.
Chemical leukoderma.
Idiopathic hypomelanosis.
Sarcoidosis.
SLE.
Scleroderma.
Oculocutaneous albinism.
Phenylketonuria.
Nevoid hypopigmentation.

HYPOTENSION, POSTURAL

ICD-9CM # 458.0

Antihypertensive medications (especially α-blockers, diuretics, ACE inhibitors).
Volume depletion (hemorrhage, dehydration).
Impaired cardiac output (constrictive pericarditis, aortic stenosis).
Peripheral autonomic dysfunction (DM, Guillain Barré).
Idiopathic orthostatic hypotension.
Central autonomic dysfunction (Shy-Grager syndrome).
Peripheral venous disease.
Adrenal insufficiency.

IMPOTENCE[24]

ICD-9CM # 302.72 PSYCHOSEXUAL
607.84 ORGANIC
997.99 ORGANIC POST-PROSTATECTOMY

Psychogenic.
Endocrine: hyperprolactinemia, DM, Cushing's syndrome, hypothyroidism or hyperthyroidism, abnormality of hypothalamic-pituitary-testicular axis.

Vascular: arterial insufficiency, venous leakage, AV malformation, local trauma.
Medications.
Neurogenic: autonomic or sensory neuropathy, spinal cord trauma or tumor, CVA, multiple sclerosis, temporal lobe epilepsy.
Systemic illness: renal failure, COPD, cirrhosis of liver, myotonic dystrophy.
Peyronie's disease.
Prostatectomy.

INFERTILITY, FEMALE[12]

ICD-9CM # 628.9

FALLOPIAN TUBE PATHOLOGY

PID or puerperal infection.
Congenital anomalies.
Endometriosis.
Secondary to past peritonitis of nongenital origin.
Amenorrhea and anovulation.
Minor anovulatory disturbances.

CERVICAL AND UTERINE FACTORS

Leiomyomas and polyps.
Uterine anomalies.
Intrauterine synechiae (Asherman's syndrome).
Destroyed endocervical glands (postsurgery or postinfection).

VAGINAL FACTORS

Congenital absence of vagina.
Imperforate hymen.
Vaginismus.
Vaginitis.

IMMUNOLOGIC FACTORS

Sperm-immobilizing antibodies.
Sperm-agglutinating antibodies.

NUTRITIONAL AND METABOLIC FACTORS

Thyroid disorders.
Diabetes mellitus.
Severe nutritional disturbances.

INFERTILITY, MALE[12]

ICD-9CM # 606.9

DECREASED PRODUCTION OF SPERMATOZOA

Varicocele.
Testicular failure.
Endocrine disorders.
Cryptorchidism.
Stress, smoking, caffeine, nicotine, recreational drugs.

DUCTAL OBSTRUCTION

Epididymal (postinfection).
Congenital absence of vas deferens.
Ejaculatory duct (postinfection).
Postvasectomy.

INABILITY TO DELIVER SPERM INTO VAGINA

Ejaculatory disturbances.
Hypospadias.
Sexual problems (i.e., impotence), medical or psychological.

ABNORMAL SEMEN

Infection.
Abnormal volume.
Abnormal viscosity.
Abnormal sperm motion.

IMMUNOLOGIC FACTORS

Sperm-immobilizing antibodies.
Sperm-agglutinating antibodies.

INSOMNIA[30]

ICD-9CM # 780.52 INSOMNIA NOS
307.42 INSOMNIA, CHRONIC ASSOCIATED WITH ANXIETY OR DEPRESSION
780.51 INSOMNIA WITH SLEEP APNEA

Anxiety disorder, psychophysiologic insomnia.
Depression.
Drugs (e.g., caffeine, amphetamines, cocaine), hypnotic-dependent sleep disorder.
Pain, fibromyalgia.
Inadequate sleep hygiene.
Restless leg syndrome.
Obstructive sleep apnea.
Sleep bruxism.
Medical illness (e.g., GERD, sleep-related asthma, parkinsonism and movement disorders).
Narcolepsy.
Other: periodic leg movement of sleep, central sleep apnea, REM behavioral disorder.

INTESTINAL PSEUDOOBSTRUCTION[33]

ICD-9CM # 560.1 ADYNAMIC INTESTINAL OBSTRUCTION
564.9 INTESTINAL DISORDER, FUNCTIONAL

"PRIMARY" (IDIOPATHIC INTESTINAL PSEUDOOBSTRUCTION)

Hollow visceral myopathy:
- Familial.
- Sporadic.

Neuropathic:
- Abnormal myenteric plexus.
- Normal myenteric plexus.

SECONDARY

Scleroderma.
Myxedema.
Amyloidosis.
Muscular dystrophy.
Hypokalemia.
Chronic renal failure.
Diabetes mellitus.
Drug toxicity caused by:
- Anticholinergics.
- Opiate narcotics.

Ogilvie's syndrome.

INTRACEREBRAL HEMORRHAGE, NONHYPERTENSIVE CAUSES

ICD-9CM # 431

Trauma.
Anticoagulation.
Intracranial tumors.
Vascular malformations.
Bleeding disorders.
Vasculitides (e.g., polyarteritis nodosa, granulomatous angiitis).
Cocaine and other sympathomimetic agents.
Cerebral amyloid angiopathy.

INTRACRANIAL LESION

ICD-9CM # 348.8

Tumor (primary or metastatic).
Abscess.
Stroke.
Intracranial hemorrhage.
Angioma.
Multiple sclerosis (initial single lesion).
Granuloma.
Herpes encephalitis.
Artifact.

INTRAOCULAR NEOPLASM

ICD-9CM # CODE VARIES WITH SPECIFIC DISORDER

MALIGNANT

Retinoblastoma.
Melanoma.
Reticulum cell sarcoma.
Metastatic tumor.

BENIGN

Melanocytic nevus.
Hemangioma.
Reactive lymphoid hyperplasia.

IRON OVERLOAD

ICD-9CM # 790.6 IRON, ABNORMAL BLOOD LEVEL
275, IRON, METABOLISM DISORDER

Hereditary hemochromatosis.
Chronic iron supplementation (PO, IM, transfusions).
Nonalcoholic steatohepatitis.

Chronic viral hepatitis.
Alcoholic liver disease.
Chronic anemias (e.g., sideroblastic anemia, thalassemia major).
Porphyria cutanea tarda.

ISCHEMIC COLITIS, NONOCCLUSIVE[18]

ICD-9CM # 557.1

ACUTE DIMINUTION OF COLONIC INTRAMURAL BLOOD FLOW

Small vessel obstruction
Collagen-vascular disease.
Vasculitis, diabetes.
Oral contraceptives.
Nonocclusive hypoperfusion
Hemorrhage.
CHF, MI, Arrhythmias.
Sepsis.
Vasoconstricting agents: vasopressin, ergot.
Increased viscosity: polycythemia, sickle cell disease, thrombocytosis.

INCREASED DEMAND ON MARGINAL BLOOD FLOW

Increased motility
Mass lesion, stricture.
Constipation.
Increased intraluminal pressure
Bowel obstruction.
Colonoscopy.
Barium enema.

ISCHEMIC NECROSIS OF CARTILAGE AND BONE[12]

ICD-9CM # 733.90

ENDOCRINE/METABOLIC

Ethanol abuse.
Glucocorticoid therapy.
Cushing's disease.
Diabetes mellitus.
Hyperuricemia.
Osteomalacia.
Hyperlipidemia.

STORAGE DISEASES (E.G., GAUCHER'S DISEASE)

Hemoglobinopathies (e.g., sickle cell disease).
Trauma (e.g., dislocation, fracture).
HIV infection.
Dysbaric conditions (e.g., caisson disease).
Collagen-vascular disorders.
Irradiation.
Pancreatitis.
Organ transplantation.
Hemodialysis.
Burns.
Intravascular coagulation.
Idiopathic, familial.

JAUNDICE

ICD-9CM # 782.4 JAUNDICE NOS
576.8 JAUNDICE, OBSTRUCTIVE
277.4 BILIRUBIN EXCRETION DISORDERS

PREDOMINANCE OF DIRECT (CONJUGATED) BILIRUBIN

Extrahepatic obstruction.
Common duct abnormalities: calculi, neoplasm, stricture, cyst, sclerosing cholangitis.
Metastatic carcinoma.
Pancreatic carcinoma, pseudocyst.
Ampullary carcinoma.
Hepatocellular disease: hepatitis, cirrhosis.
Drugs: estrogens, phenothiazines, captopril, methyltestosterone, labetalol.
Cholestatic jaundice of pregnancy.
Hereditary disorders: Dubin-Johnson syndrome, Rotor's syndrome.
Recurrent benign intrahepatic cholestasis.

PREDOMINANCE OF INDIRECT (UNCONJUGATED) BILIRUBIN

Hemolysis: hereditary and acquired hemolytic anemias.
Inefficient marrow production.
Impaired hepatic conjugation: chloramphenicol.
Neonatal jaundice.
Hereditary disorders: Gilbert's syndrome, Crigler-Najjar syndrome.

JOINT PAIN, ANTERIOR HIP, MEDIAL THIGH, KNEE[25]

ICD-9CM # 719.4 ADD 5TH DIGIT
0 SITE NOS
1 SHOULDER REGION
2 UPPER ARM (ELBOW, HUMERUS)
3 FOREARM (RADIUS, WRIST, ULNA)
4 HAND
5 PELVIC REGION AND THIGH
6 LOWER LEG (FIBULA, PATELLA, TIBIA)
7 ANKLE AND/OR FOOT

ACUTE

Acute rheumatic fever.
Adductor muscle strain.
Avascular necrosis.
Crystal arthritis.
Femoral artery (pseudo) aneurysm.
Fracture (femoral neck or intertrochanteric).
Hemarthrosis.
Hernia.
Herpes zoster.
Iliopectineal bursitis.
Iliopsoas tendinitis.
Inguinal lymphadenitis.
Osteomalacia.
Painful transient osteoporosis of hip.
Septic arthritis.

SUBACUTE AND CHRONIC

Adductory muscle strain.
Amyloidosis.
Acute rheumatic fever.
Femoral artery aneurysm.
Hernia (inguinal or femoral).
Iliopectineal bursitis.
Iliopsoas tendinitis.
Inguinal lymphadenopathy.
Osteochondromatosis.
Osteomyelitis.
Osteitis deformans (Paget's disease).
Osteomalacia (pseudofracture).
Postherpetic neuralgia.
Sterile synovitis (e.g., rheumatoid arthritis, psoriatic, systemic lupus erythematosus).

JOINT PAIN, HIP, LATERAL THIGH[25]

ICD-9CM # 959.6 HIP INJURY
719.95 HIP JOINT DISORDER
843.9 HIP STRAIN

ACUTE

Herpes zoster.
Iliotibial tendinitis.
Impacted fracture of femoral neck.
Lateral femoral cutaneous neuropathy (meralgia paresthetica).
Radiculopathy: L4-5.
Trochanteric avulsion fracture (greater trochanter).
Trochanteric bursitis.
Trochanteric fracture.

SUBACUTE AND CHRONIC

Lateral femoral cutaneous neuropathy (meralgia paresthetica).
Osteomyelitis.
Postherpetic neuralgia.
Radiculopathy: L4-5.
Tumors.

JOINT PAIN, POLYARTICULAR

ICD-9CM # 719.40

Osteoarthritis.
Rheumatoid arthritis.
Fibromyalgia.
Viral syndrome (e.g., human parvovirus B19 infection).
Systemic lupus erythematosus.
Psoriatic arthritis.
Ankylosing spondylitis.

JOINT PAIN, POSTERIOR HIPS, THIGH, BUTTOCKS[25]

ICD-9CM # 719.4 ADD 5TH DIGIT
0 SITE NOS
1 SHOULDER REGION
2 UPPER ARM (ELBOW, HUMERUS)
3 FOREARM (RADIUS, WRIST, ULNA)

4 HAND
5 PELVIC REGION AND THIGH
6 LOWER LEG (FIBULA, PATELLA, TIBIA)
7 ANKLE AND/OR FOOT

ACUTE

Gluteal muscle strain.
Herpes zoster.
Ischial bursitis.
Ischial or sacral fracture.
Osteomalacia (pseudofracture).
Sciatic neuropathy.
Radiculopathy: L5-S1.

SUBACUTE AND CHRONIC

Gluteal muscle strain.
Ischial bursitis.
Lumbar spinal stenosis.
Osteoarthritis of hip.
Osteitis deformans (Paget's disease).
Osteomyelitis.
Osteochondromatosis.
Osteomalacia (pseudofracture).
Postherpetic neuralgia.
Radiculopathy: L5-S1.
Tumors.

JOINT SWELLING

ICD-9CM # 719.0 ADD 5TH DIGIT
0 SITE NOS
1 SHOULDER REGION
2 UPPER ARM (ELBOW, HUMERUS)
3 FOREARM (RADIUS, WRIST, ULNA)
4 HAND
5 PELVIC REGION AND THIGH
6 LOWER LEG (FIBULA, PATELLA, TIBIA)
7 ANKLE AND/OR FOOT

Trauma.
Osteoarthritis.
Gout.
Pyogenic arthritis.
Pseudogout.
Rheumatoid arthritis.
Viral syndrome.

JUGULAR VENOUS DISTENTION

ICD-9CM # 459.89 INCREASED VENOUS PRESSURE

Right-sided heart failure.
Cardiac tamponade.
Constrictive pericarditis.
Goiter.
Tension pneumothorax.
Pulmonary hypertension.
Cardiomyopathy (restrictive).
Superior vena cava syndrome.
Valsalva maneuver.
Right atrial myxoma.
COPD.

KERATITIS, NONINFECTIOUS

ICD-9CM # 370.9

Collagen vascular disease.
Atopic keratoconjunctivitis.
Chemical injury.
Thermal injury.
Ectropion/entropion.
Lid defects.
Exophthalmos.
Keratoconjuctivitis sicca.
Erythema multiforme.
Mucous membrane pemphigoid.
Diabetes mellitus (delayed epithelial healing).
Neuroparalytic (cranial nerve VII).
Neurotrophic (diabetes, cranial nerve V).

KNEE PAIN[25]

ICD-9CM # 844.1 COLLATERAL LIGAMENT SPRAIN, MEDIAL
844.2 CRUCIATE LIGAMENT SPRAIN
716.96 KNEE INFLAMMATION
959.7 KNEE INJURY
718.86 KNEE INSTABILITY
836.1 LATERAL MENISCUS TEAR
836.0 MEDIAL MENISCUS TEAR
844.8 PATELLAR SPRAIN
719.56 KNEE STIFFNESS
719.06 KNEE SWELLING

DIFFUSE

Articular.
Anterior.
Prepatellar bursitis.
Patellar tendon enthesopathy.
Chondromalacia patellae.
Patellofemoral osteoarthritis.
Cruciate ligament injury.
Medial plica syndrome.

MEDIAL

Anserine bursitis.
Spontaneous osteonecrosis.
Osteoarthritis.
Medial meniscal tear.
Medial collateral ligament bursitis.
Referred pain from hip and L3.
Fibromyalgia.

LATERAL

Iliotibial band syndrome.
Meniscal cyst.
Lateral meniscal tear.
Collateral ligament.
Peroneal tenosynovitis.

POSTERIOR

Popliteal cyst (Baker's cyst).
Tendinitis.
Aneurysms, ganglions, sarcoma.

LEFT AXIS DEVIATION[19]

ICD-9CM # 426.3 LEFT BUNDLE BRANCH BLOCK
426.2 LEFT BUNDLE BRANCH HEMIBLOCK
429.3 LEFT VENTRICULAR HYPERTROPHY

Normal variation.
Left anterior fascicular block (hemiblock).
Left bundle branch block.
Left ventricular hypertrophy.
Mechanical shifts causing a horizontal heart, high diaphragm, pregnancy, ascites.
Some forms of ventricular tachycardia.
Endocardial cushion defects and other congenital heart disease.

LEFT BUNDLE BRANCH BLOCK

ICD-9CM # 426.3

Ischemic heart disease.
Electrolyte abnormalities (e.g., hyperkalemia).
Cardiomyopathy.
Idiopathic.
LVH.
Pulmonary embolism.
Cardiac trauma.
Bacterial endocarditis.

LEG CRAMPS, NOCTURNAL

ICD-9CM # 729.82 MUSCLE CRAMPS

Diabetic neuropathy.
Medications.
Electrolyte abnormalities (hypokalemia, hyponatremia, hypocalcemia, hyperkalemia, hypophosphatemia).
Respiratory alkalosis.
Uremia.
Hemodialysis.
Peripheral nerve injury.
ALS.
Alcohol use.
Heat cramps.
Vitamin B_{12} deficiency.
Hyperthyroidism.
Contractures.
DVT.
Hypoglycemia.
Peripheral vascular insufficiency.
Baker's cyst.

LEG LENGTH DISCREPANCIES[20]

ICD-9CM # 736.81 LEG LENGTH DISCREPANCY, ACQUIRED
755.30 LEG LENGTH DISCREPANCY, CONGENITAL

CONGENITAL

Proximal femoral local deficiency.
Coxa vara.

Hemiatrophy-hemihypertrophy (anisomelia).
Development dysplasia of the hip.

DEVELOPMENTAL

Legg-Calvé-Perthes disease.

NEUROMUSCULAR

Polio.
Cerebral palsy (hemiplegia).

INFECTIOUS

Pyogenic osteomyelitis with physeal damage.

TRAUMA

Physeal injury with premature closure.
Overgrowth.
Malunion (shortening).

TUMOR

Physeal destruction.
Radiation-induced physeal injury.
Overgrowth.

LEG MOVEMENT WHEN STANDING, INVOLUNTARY

ICD-9CM # CODE VARIES WITH SPECIFIC DISORDER

Benign essential tremor.
Orthostatic tremor.
Spastic ataxia.
Cerebellar truncal tremor.
Postanoxic myoclonus.

LEG PAIN WITH EXERCISE

ICD-9CM # 729.82 MUSCLE CRAMPS

Shin splints.
Arteriosclerosis obliterans.
Neurogenic (spinal cord compression or ischemia).
Venous claudication.
Popliteal cyst.
DVT.
Thromboangiitis obliterans.
Adventitial cysts.
Popliteal artery entrapment syndrome.
McArdle syndrome.

LEG ULCERS[25]

ICD-9CM # 440.23 LOWER LIMB, ARTERIOSCLEROTIC
707.1 LOWER LIMB, CHRONIC
707.1 LOWER LIMB, NEUROGENIC
250.70 LOWER LIMB, CHRONIC DIABETES MELLITUS TYPE II
250.71 LOWER LIMB, CHRONIC, DIABETES MELLITUS TYPE I

VASCULAR

Arterial: arteriosclerosis, thromboangiitis obliterans, AV malformation, cholesterol emboli.
Venous: superficial varicosities, incompetent perforators, DVT, lymphatic abnormalities.

VASCULITIS HEMATOLOGIC

Sickle cell anemia, thalassemia, polycythemia vera, leukemia, cold agglutinin disease.
Macroglobulinemia, protein C and protein S deficiency, cryoglobulinemia, lupus anticoagulant, antiphospholipid syndrome.

INFECTIOUS

Fungus: Blastomycosis, coccidioidomycosis, histoplasmosis, sporotrichosis.
Bacterial: Furuncle, ecthyma, septic emboli.
Protozoal: leishmaniasis.

METABOLIC

Necrobiosis lipoidica diabeticorum.
Localized bullous pemphigoid.
Gout, calcinosis cutis, Gaucher's disease.

TUMORS

Basal cell carcinoma, squamous cell carcinoma, melanoma.
Mycosis fungoides, Kaposi's sarcoma, metastatic neoplasms.

TRAUMA

Burns, cold injury, radiation dermatitis.
Insect bites.
Factitial, excessive pressure.

NEUROPATHIC

Diabetic trophic ulcers.
Tabes dorsalis, syringomyelia.

DRUGS

Warfarin, IV colchicine extravasation, methotrexate, halogens, ergotism, hydroxyurea.

PANNICULITIS

Weber-Christian disease.
Pancreatic fat necrosis, alpha-antitrypsinase deficiency.

LEPTOMENINGEAL LESIONS

ICD-9CM # CODE VARIES WITH SPECIFIC DISORDER

Metastases.
Multiple sclerosis.
Bacterial or viral meningitis.
Vasculitis.
Lyme disease.
Tuberculosis.
Fungal infections (e.g., Cryptococcus).
Sarcoidosis.
Wegener's granulomatosis.
Neurocysticercosis.
Rheumatoid nodules.
Histiocytosis.

LEUKOCORIA

ICD-9CM # 379.90

Cataract.
Retinal detachment.
Retinoblastoma.
Retinal telangiectasia.
Retrolenticular vascularized membrane.
Familial exudative vitreoretinopathy.

LIMP

ICD-9CM # 781.2 GAIT ABNORMALITY
719.75 GAIT DISORDER DUE TO JOINT ABNORMALITY IN HIP, BUTTOCK, OR FEMUR
719.76 GAIT DISORDER DUE TO JOINT ABNORMALITY IN LOWER LEG
719.77 GAIT DISORDER DUE TO JOINT ABNORMALITY IN ANKLE AND/ OR FOOT
300.11 HYSTERICAL GAIT DISORDER

Degenerative joint disease, osteochondritis dissecans, chondromalacia patellae.
Trauma to extremities, vertebral disc, hips.
Poorly fitting shoes, foreign body in shoe, unequal leg length.
Splinter in foot.
Joint infection (septic arthritis, osteomyelitis), viral arthritis.
Abdominal pain (e.g., appendicitis, incarcerated hernia), testicular torsion.
Polio, neuromuscular disorders, Guillain-Barré syndrome, multiple sclerosis.
Osgood-Schlatter disease.
Legg-Calvé-Perthes disease.
Factitious, somatization syndrome.
Neoplasm (local or metastatic).
Other: diskitis, periostitis, sickle cell disease, hemophilia.

LIMPING, PEDIATRIC AGE[20]

ICD-9CM # 781.2 GAIT ABNORMALITY

TODDLER (1-3 YR)

Infection:
- Septic arthritis:
  - Hip.
  - Knee.
- Osteomyelitis.
- Diskitis.

Occult trauma:
- Toddler's fracture.

Neoplasia.

CHILDHOOD (4-10 YR)

Infection:
- Septic arthritis:
  - Hip.
  - Knee.
- Osteomyelitis.
- Diskitis.
- Transient synovitis, hip.

LCPD.
Tarsal coalition.
Rheumatologic disorder:
- JRA.

Trauma.
Neoplasia.

ADOLESCENCE (11+ YR)

SCFE.
Rheumatologic disorder:
- JRA.

Trauma.
Tarsal coalition.
Hip dislocation (DDH).
Neoplasia.

DDH, Developmental dysplasia of the hip; *JRA,* juvenile rheumatoid arthritis; *LCPD,* Legg-Calvé-Perthes disease; *SCFE,* slipped capital femoral epiphysis.

LIVEDO RETICULITIS

ICD-9CM # CODE NOT AVAILABLE

Emboli (SBE, left atrial myxoma, cholesterol emboli).
Thrombocythemia or polycythemia.
Antiphospholipid antibody syndrome.
Cryoglobulinemia, cryofibrinogenemia.
Leukocytoclastic vasculitis.
SLE, rheumatoid arthritis, dermatomyositis.
Pancreatitis.
Drugs (quinine, quinidine, amantadine, catecholamines).
Physiologic (cutis marmorata).
Congenital.

LIVER LESIONS, BENIGN, OFTEN CONFUSED WITH MALIGNANCY

ICD-9CM # 573.8

Fatty infiltration.
Adenoma.
Hemangioma.
Cysts.
Flow artifacts.
Focal nodular hyperplasia.
Nonenhanced vessels.

LOW-VOLTAGE ECG

ICD-9CM # 794.31

Hypothyroidism.
Obesity.
Pericardial effusion.
Anasarca.
Pleural effusion.
Pneumothorax.
Amyloidosis.
Aortic stenosis.

LYMPHADENOPATHY[12]

ICD-9CM # 785.6

GENERALIZED

AIDS.
Lymphoma: Hodgkin's disease, non-Hodgkin's lymphoma.
Leukemias, reticuloendotheliosis.
Infectious mononucleosis, CMV, and other viral infections.
Diffuse skin infection: generalized furunculosis, multiple tick bites.
Parasitic infections: toxoplasmosis, filariasis, leishmaniasis, Chagas' disease.
Serum sickness.
Collagen vascular diseases (RA, SLE).
Dengue (arbovirus infection).
Sarcoidosis and other granulomatous diseases.
Drugs: INH, hydantoin derivatives, antithyroid and antileprosy drugs.
Secondary syphilis.
Hyperthyroidism, lipid-storage diseases.

LOCALIZED

Cervical nodes
Infections of the head, neck, ears, sinuses, scalp, pharynx.
Mononucleosis.
Lymphoma.
TB.
Malignancy of head and neck.
Rubella.
Scalene/supraclavicular nodes
Lymphoma.
Lung neoplasm.
Bacterial or fungal infection of thorax or retroperitoneum.
GI malignancy.
Axillary nodes
Infections of hands and arms.
Cat-scratch disease.
Neoplasm (lymphoma, melanoma, breast carcinoma).
Brucellosis.
Epitrochlear nodes
Infections of the hand.
Lymphoma.
Tularemia.
Sarcoidosis, secondary syphilis (usually bilateral).
Inguinal nodes
Infections of leg or foot, folliculitis (pubic hair).
LGV, syphilis.
Lymphoma.
Pelvic malignancy.
Pasteurella pestis.
Hilar nodes
Sarcoidosis.
TB.
Lung carcinoma.
Fungal infections, systemic.
Mediastinal nodes
Sarcoidosis.
Lymphoma.
Lung neoplasm.
TB.
Mononucleosis.
Histoplasmosis.
Abdominal/retroperitoneal nodes
Lymphoma.
TB.
Neoplasm (ovary, testes, prostate and other malignancies).

LYMPHANGITIS[22]

ICD-9CM # 457.2

Acute:
- Group A streptococci.
- *Staphylococcus aureus.*
- *Pasteurella multicida.*

Chronic:
- *Sporothrix schenckii* (sporotrichosis).
- *Mycobacterium marinum* (swimming pool granuloma).
- *Mycobacterium kansasii.*
- *Nocardia brasiliensis.*
- *W. bancrofti.*

LYMPHOCYTOSIS, ATYPICAL[22]

ICD-9CM # 288.8

Epstein-Barr virus primary infection (infectious mononucleosis).
Cytomegalovirus primary infection (heterophile-negative mono).
Human herpesvirus 6 primary infection (roseola).
Primary HIV infection.
Toxoplasmosis.
Acute viral hepatitis.
Rubella, mumps.
Drug reactions (e.g., phenytoin, sulfa).

MEDIASTINAL MASSES OR WIDENING ON CHEST X-RAY

ICD-9CM # 785.6 ADENOPATHY
519.3 DISEASE NEC
793.2 SHIFT (CXR)

Lymphoma: Hodgkin's disease and non-Hodgkin's lymphoma.
Sarcoidosis.
Vascular: aortic aneurysm, ectasia or tortuosity of aorta or bronchocephalic vessels.
Carcinoma: lungs, esophagus.
Esophageal diverticula.
Hiatal hernia.
Achalasia.
Prominent pulmonary outflow tract: pulmonary hypertension, pulmonary embolism, right-to-left shunts.
Trauma: mediastinal hemorrhage.
Pneumomediastinum.
Lymphadenopathy caused by silicosis and other pneumoconioses.
Leukemias.
Infections: TB, viral (rare), *Mycoplasma* (rare), fungal, tularemia.
Substernal thyroid.
Thymoma.
Teratoma.
Bronchogenic cyst.

Pericardial cyst.
Neurofibroma, neurosarcoma, ganglioneuroma.

MEDIASTINITIS, ACUTE[22]

ICD-9CM # 519.2

Esophageal perforation.
Iatrogenic.
EGD, esophageal dilation, esophageal variceal sclerotherapy, nasogastric tube, Sengstaken-Blackmore tube, endotracheal intubation, esophageal surgery, paraesophageal surgery, transesophageal echocardiography, anterior stabilization of cervical vertebral bodies.
Swallowed foreign bodies.
Trauma.
Spontaneous perforation (e.g., emesis, carcinoma).
Head and neck infections (e.g., tonsillitis, pharyngitis, parotitis, epiglottitis, odontogenic).
Infections originating at another site (e.g., TB, pneumonia, pancreatitis, osteomyelitis of sternum, clavicle, ribs).
Cardiothoracic surgery (median sternotomy) (e.g., CABG, valve replacement, other types of cardiothoracic surgery).

MELANONYCHIA

ICD-9CM # CODE VARIES WITH SPECIFIC DISORDER

Pregnancy.
Trauma.
Medications (e.g., AZT, 5-fluorouracil, doxorubicin, psoralens).
Nail matrix nevus.
HIV infection.
Onychomycosis.
Melanocyte hyperplasia.
Verrucae.
Pustular psoriasis.
Lichen planus.
Basal cell carcinoma.
Nail matrix melanoma.
Subungual keratosis.
Addison's disease.
Bowen's disease.

MEMORY LOSS SYMPTOMS, ELDERLY PATIENTS

ICD-9CM # CODE VARIES WITH SPECIFIC DISORDER

Age-related mild cognitive impairment.
Depression (pseudodementia).
Medications (e.g., anticholinergics, sedatives).
Hypothyroidism.
Chronic hypoxia.
Cerebrovascular infarcts.
Alzheimer's disease.
Hepatic disease.
Chronic renal failure.
Hyperthyroidism.
Frontotemporal dementia.
Lewy body dementia.

MENINGITIS, CHRONIC[23]

ICD-9CM # 322.2

TB.
Fungal CNS infection.
Tertiary syphilis.
CNS neoplasm.
Metabolic encephalopathies.
Multiple sclerosis.
Chronic subdural hematoma.
SLE cerebritis.
Encephalitides.
Sarcoidosis.
NSAIDs.
Behçet's syndrome.
Anatomic defects (traumatic, congenital, postoperative).
Granulomatous angiitis.

MENINGITIS, RECURRENT[22]

ICD-9CM # CODE VARIES WITH SPECIFIC DISORDER

Drug induced (with rechallenge).
Parameningeal focus.
Infection (sinusitis, mastoiditis, osteomyelitis, brain abscess).
Tumor (epidermoid cyst, craniopharyngioma).
Posttraumatic (bacterial).
Mollaret's meningitis.
Systemic lupus erythematosus.
Herpes simplex virus.

MESENTERIC ISCHEMIA, NONOCCLUSIVE[23]

ICD-9CM # 557.0 MESENTERIC ARTERY EMBOLISM OR INFARCTION
557.1 MESENTERIC ARTERY INSUFFICIENCY, CHRONIC
902.39 MESENTERIC VEIN INJURY

Cardiovascular disease resulting in low-flow states (CHF, cardiogenic shock, post cardiopulmonary bypass, dysrhythmias).
Septic shock.
Drug induced (cocaine, vasopressors, ergot alkaloid poisoning).

MESENTERIC VENOUS THROMBOSIS[23]

ICD-9CM # 557.0

Hypercoagulable states (protein C or S deficiency, antithrombin III deficiency, Factor V Leyden, malignancy, polycythemia vera, sickle cell disease, homocystinemia, lupus anticoagulant, cardiolipin antibody).
Trauma (operative venous injury, abdominal trauma, postsplenectomy).
Inflammatory conditions (pancreatitis, diverticulitis, appendicitis, cholangitis).
Other: CHF, renal failure, portal hypertension, decompression sickness.

METASTATIC NEOPLASMS

ICD-9CM # 198.5 BONE AND BONE MARROW
198.3 BRAIN AND SPINAL CORD
197.7 LIVER
197.0 LUNG

To: Bone	To: Brain
Breast	Lung
Lung	Breast
Prostate	Melanoma
Thyroid	GU tract
Kidney	Colon
Bladder	Sinuses
Endometrium	Sarcoma
Cervix	Skin
Melanoma	Thyroid

To: Liver	To: Lung
Colon	Breast
Stomach	Colon
Pancreas	Kidney
Breast	Testis
Lymphomas	Stomach
Bronchus	Thyroid
Lung	Melanoma
Sarcoma	
Choriocarcinoma	
Kidney	

MICROCEPHALY[4]

ICD-9CM # 742.1 MICROCEPHALUS

PRIMARY (GENETIC)

Familial (autosomal recessive).
Autosomal dominant.
Syndromes:
Down (21-trisomy).
Edward (18-trisomy).
Cri-du-chat (5 p-).
Cornelia de Lange.
Rubinstein-Taybi.
Smith-Lemli-Opitz.

SECONDARY (NONGENETIC)

Radiation.
Congenital infections:
Cytomegalovirus.
Rubella.
Toxoplasmosis.
Drugs:
Fetal alcohol.
Fetal hydantoin.
Meningitis/encephalitis.
Malnutrition.
Metabolic.
Hyperthermia.
Hypoxic-ischemic encephalopathy.

MICROPENIS[24]

ICD-9CM # 752.69 PENILE AGENESIS OR ATRESIA
607.89 PENILE ATROPHY
752.64 MICROPENIS (CONGENITAL)

HYPOGONADOTROPIC HYPOGONADISM (HYPOTHALAMIC OR PITUITARY DEFICIENCIES)

Kallmann's syndrome: autosomal dominant; associated with hyposmia.
Prader-Willi syndrome: hypotonia, mental retardation, obesity, small hands and feet.
Rud syndrome: hyposomia, ichthyosis, mental retardation.
De Morsier's syndrome (septooptic dysplasia): hypopituitarism, hypoplastic optic discs, absent septum pellucidum.

HYPERGONADOTROPIC HYPOGONADISM

Primary testicular defect: disorders of testicular differentiation or inborn errors of testosterone synthesis.
Klinefelter syndrome.
Other X polysomies (i.e., XXXXY, XXXY).
Robinow's syndrome: brachymesomelic dwarfism, dysmorphic facies.

PARTIAL ANDROGEN INSENSITIVITY

IDIOPATHIC

Defective morphogenesis of the penis.

MIOSIS

ICD-9CM # 379.42 MIOSIS PERSISTENT NOT DUE TO MIOTICS

Medications (e.g., morphine, pilocarpine).
Neurosyphilis.
Congenital.
Iritis.
CNS pontine lesion.
CNS infections.
Cavernous sinus thrombosis.
Inflammation/irritation of cornea or conjunctiva.

MONOARTHRITIS, ACUTE

ICD-9CM # 716.60

Overuse.
Trauma.
Gout.
Pseudogout.
Osteoarthritis.
Infectious arthritis (e.g., gonococcal, Lyme disease, viral, mycobacteria, fungi).
Osteomyelitis.
Avascular necrosis of bone.
Hemarthrosis.
Bowel disease associated arthritis.
Bone malignancy.
Psoriatic arthritis.
Juvenile rheumatoid arthritis.
Sarcoidosis.
Hemoglobinopathies.
Vasculitic syndromes.
Behçet's syndrome.
Foreign body synovitis.
Hypertrophic pulmonary osteoarthropathy.
Amyloidosis, familial Mediterranean fever.

MONONEUROPATHY

ICD-9CM # 355.9

Herpes zoster.
Herpes simplex.
Vasculitis.
Trauma, compression.
Diabetes.
Postinfectious or inflammatory.

MUSCLE WEAKNESS

ICD-9CM # 728.9

Physical deconditioning.
Impaired cardiac output (e.g., mitral stenosis, mitral regurgitation).
Uremia, liver failure.
Electrolyte abnormalities (hypokalemia, hyperkalemia, hypophosphatemia, hypercalcemia), hypoglycemia.
Drug-induced (e.g., statin myopathy).
Muscular dystrophies.
Steroid myopathy.
Alcoholic myopathy.
Myasthenia gravis, Lambert-Eaton syndrome.
Infections (polio, botulism, HIV, hepatitis, diphtheria, tick paralysis, neurosyphilis, brucellosis, TB, trichinosis).
Pernicious anemia, other anemias, beriberi.
Psychiatric illness (depression, somatization syndrome).
Organophosphate or arsenic poisoning.
Inflammatory myopathies (e.g., collagen vascular disease, RA, sarcoidosis).
Endocrinopathies (e.g., adrenal insufficiency, hypothyroidism), diabetic neuropathy.
Other: motor neuron disease, mitochondrial myopathy, L-tryptophan (eosinophilia-myalgia), rhabdomyolysis, glycogen storage disease, lipid storage disease.

MUSCLE WEAKNESS, LOWER MOTOR NEURON VERSUS UPPER MOTOR NEURON[35]

ICD-9CM # 728.9

LOWER MOTOR NEURON

Weakness, usually severe.
Marked muscle atrophy.
Fasciculations.
Decreased muscle stretch reflexes.
Clonus not present.
Flaccidity.
No Babinski sign.
Asymmetric and may involve one limb only in the beginning to become generalized as the disease progresses.

UPPER MOTOR NEURON

Weakness, usually less severe.
Minimal disuse muscle atrophy.
No fasciculations.
Increased muscle stretch reflexes.
Clonus may be present.
Spasticity.
Babinski sign.
Often initial impairment of only skilled movements.
In the limbs the following muscles may be the only ones weak or weaker than the others: triceps; wrist and finger extensors; interossei; iliopsoas; hamstrings; and foot dorsiflexors, inverters and extroverters.

MYDRIASIS

ICD-9CM # 379.43 MYDRIASIS PERSISTENT NOT DUE TO MYDRIATICS

Coma.
Medications (cocaine, atropine, epinephrine, etc.).
Glaucoma.
Cerebral aneurysm.
Ocular trauma.
Head trauma.
Optic atrophy.
Cerebral neoplasm.
Iridocyclitis.

MYELIN DISORDERS

ICD-9CM # CODE VARIES WITH SPECIFIC DISORDER

Multiple sclerosis.
Vitamin B_{12} deficiency.
Radiation.
Hypoxia.
Toxicity from carbon monoxide, alcohol, mercury.
Progressive multifocal encephalopathy.
Acute disseminated encephalomyelitis.
Acute hemorrhagic leukoencephalopathy.
Phenylketonuria.
Adrenoleukodystrophy.
Krabbe's disease.

MYELOPATHY AND MYELITIS[33]

ICD-9CM # 722.70 MYELOPATHY, DISCOGENIC INTERVERTEBRAL NOS
336.9 MYELOPATHY, NONDISCOGENIC UNSPECIFIED

INFLAMMATORY

Infectious: spirochetal TB, zoster, rabies, HIV, polio, rickettsial, fungal, parasitic.

Noninfectious: idiopathic transverse myelitis, multiple sclerosis.

TOXIC/METABOLIC

DM, pernicious anemia, chronic liver disease, pellagra, arsenic.

TRAUMA COMPRESSION

Spinal neoplasm, cervical spondylosis, epidural abscess, epidural hematoma.

VASCULAR

AV malformation, SLE, periarteritis nodosa, dissecting aortic aneurysm.

PHYSICAL AGENTS

Electrical injury, irradiation.

NEOPLASTIC

Spinal cord tumors, paraneoplastic myelopathy.

MYOCARDIAL ISCHEMIA[33]

ICD-9CM # 414.8 ISCHEMIA (CHRONIC)
411.89 ISCHEMIA, ACUTE WITHOUT MI

Atherosclerotic obstructive coronary artery disease.
Nonatherosclerotic coronary artery disease:
- Coronary artery spasm.
- Congenital coronary artery anomalies:
  - Anomalous origin of coronary artery from pulmonary artery.
  - Aberrant origin of coronary artery from aorta or another coronary artery.
  - Coronary arteriovenous fistula.
  - Coronary artery aneurysm.

Acquired disorders of coronary arteries:
- Coronary artery embolism.
- Dissection:
  - Surgical.
  - During percutaneous coronary angioplasty.
  - Aortic dissection.
  - Spontaneous (e.g., during pregnancy).
- Extrinsic compression:
  - Tumors.
  - Granulomas.
  - Amyloidosis.
- Collagen-vascular disease:
  - Polyarteritis nodosa.
  - Temporal arteritis.
  - Rheumatoid arthritis.
  - Systemic lupus erythematosus.
  - Scleroderma.
- Miscellaneous disorders:
  - Irradiation.
  - Trauma.
  - Kawasaki disease.
- Syphilis.

Hereditary disorders:
- Pseudoxanthoma elasticum.
- Gargoylism.
- Progeria.
- Homocystinuria.
- Primary oxaluria.

"Functional" causes of myocardial ischemia in absence of anatomic coronary artery disease:
- Syndrome X.
- Hypertrophic cardiomyopathy.
- Dilated cardiomyopathy.
- Muscle bridge.
- Hypertensive heart disease.
- Pulmonary hypertension.
- Valvular heart disease; aortic stenosis, aortic regurgitation.

MYOCLONUS

ICD-9CM # 333.2

Physiologic (e.g., exercise or anxiety induced).
Renal failure.
Hepatic failure.
Hyponatremia.
Hypoglycemia or severe hyperglycemia.
Postdialysis.
Epileptic myoclonus.
Postencephalitis.
CNS lesion (stroke, neoplasm).
CNS trauma.
Parkinson's disease.
Medications (e.g., tricyclics, L-dopa).
Friedrich's ataxia.
Ataxia telangiectasia.
Wilson's disease.
Huntington's disease.
Progressive supranuclear palsy.
Heavy metal poisoning.
Benign familial.

MYOPATHIES, INFECTIOUS

ICD-9CM # 359.8

HIV.
Viral myositis.
Trichinosis.
Toxoplasmosis.
Cysticercosis.

MYOPATHIES, INFLAMMATORY

ICD-9CM # 359.9

SLE, rheumatoid arthritis.
Sarcoidosis.
Paraneoplastic syndrome.
Polymyositis, dermatomyositis.
Polyarteritis nodosa.
Mixed connective tissue disease.
Scleroderma.
Inclusion body myositis.
Sjögren's syndrome.
Cimetidine, D-penicillamine.

MYOPATHIES, TOXIC[1]

ICD-9CM # 359.4

Inflammatory: cimetidine, D-penicillamine.
Noninflammatory necrotizing or vacuolar: cholesterol-lowering agents, chloroquine, colchicine.
Acute muscle necrosis and myoglobinuria: cholesterol-lowering drugs, alcohol, cocaine.
Malignant hyperthermia: halothane, ethylene, others; succinylcholine.
Mitochondrial: zidovudine.
Myosin loss: nondepolarizing neuromuscular blocking agents; glucocorticoids.

MYOSITIS, INFLAMMATORY[1]

ICD-9CM # 729.1

INFECTIOUS

Viral myositis:
- Retroviruses (HIV, HTLV-I).
- Enteroviruses (echovirus, Coxsackievirus).
- Other viruses (influenza, hepatitis A and B, Epstein-Barr virus).

Bacterial: pyomyositis.
Parasites: trichinosis, cysticercosis.
Fungi: candidiasis.

IDIOPATHIC

Granulomatous myositis (sarcoid, giant cell).
Eosinophilic myositis.
Eosinophilia-myalgia syndrome.

ENDOCRINE/METABOLIC DISORDERS

Hypothyroidism.
Hyperthyroidism.
Hypercortisolism.
Hyperparathyroidism.
Hypoparathyroidism.
Hypocalcemia.
Hypokalemia.

METABOLIC MYOPATHIES

Myophosphorylase deficiency (McArdle's disease).
Phosphofructokinase deficiency.
Myoadenylate deaminase deficiency.
Acid maltase deficiency.
Lipid storage diseases.
Acute rhabdomyolysis.

DRUG-INDUCED MYOPATHIES

Alcohol.
D-Penicillamine.
Zidovudine.
Colchicine.
Chloroquine, hydroxychloroquine.
Lipid-lowering agents.
Cyclosporine.
Cocaine, heroin, barbiturates.
Corticosteroids.

NEUROLOGIC DISORDERS

Muscular dystrophies.
Congenital myopathies.
Motor neuron disease.
Guillain-Barré syndrome.
Myasthenia gravis.

NAIL CLUBBING

ICD-9CM # 703.9

COPD.
Pulmonary malignancy.
Cirrhosis.
Inflammatory bowel disease.
Chronic bronchitis.
Congenital heart disease.
Endocarditis.
AV malformations.
Asbestosis.
Trauma.
Idiopathic.

NAIL, HORIZONTAL WHITE LINES (BEAU'S LINES)

ICD-9CM # 703.8

Malnutrition.
Idiopathic.
Trauma.
Prolonged systemic illnesses.
Pemphigus.
Raynaud's disease.

NAIL KOILONYCHIA

ICD-9CM # 703.8

Trauma.
Iron deficiency.
SLE.
Hemochromatosis.
Raynaud's disease.
Nail-patella syndrome.
Idiopathic.

NAIL ONYCHOLYSIS

ICD-9CM # 703.8

Infection.
Trauma.
Psoriasis.
Connective tissue disorders.
Sarcoidosis.
Hyperthyroidism.
Amyloidosis.
Nutritional deficiencies.

NAIL PITTING

ICD-9CM # 703.8

Psoriasis.
Alopecia areata.
Reiter's syndrome.
Trauma.
Idiopathic.

NAIL SPLINTER HEMORRHAGE

ICD-9CM # 703.8

SBE.
Trauma.
Malignancies.
Oral contraceptives.
Pregnancy.
SLE.
Antiphospholipid syndrome.
Psoriasis.
Rheumatoid arthritis.
Peptic ulcer disease.

NAIL STRIATIONS

ICD-9CM # 703.8

Psoriasis.
Alopecia areata.
Trauma.
Atopic dermatitis.
Vitiligo.

NAIL TELANGIECTASIA

ICD-9CM # 703.8

Rheumatoid arthritis.
Scleroderma.
Trauma.
SLE.
Dermatomyositis.

NAIL WHITENING (TERRY'S NAILS)

ICD-9CM # 703.8

Malnutrition.
Trauma.
Liver disease (cirrhosis, hepatic failure).
Diabetes mellitus.
Hyperthyroidism.
Idiopathic.

NAIL YELLOWING

ICD-9CM # 703.8

Tobacco abuse.
Nephrotic syndrome.
Chronic infections (TB, sinusitis).
Bronchiectasis.
Lymphedema.
Raynaud's disease.
Rheumatoid arthritis.
Pleural effusions.
Thyroiditis.
Immunodeficiency.

NAUSEA AND VOMITING

ICD-9CM # 787.01

Infections (viral, bacterial).
Intestinal obstruction.
Metabolic (uremia, electrolyte abnormalities, DKA, acidosis, etc.).
Severe pain.
Anxiety, fear.
Psychiatric disorders (bulimia, anorexia nervosa).
Pregnancy.
Medications (NSAIDs, erythromycin, morphine, codeine, aminophylline, chemotherapeutic agents, etc.).
Withdrawal from substance abuse (drugs, alcohol).
Head trauma.
Vestibular or middle ear disease.
Migraine headache.
CNS neoplasms.
Radiation sickness.
PUD.
Carcinoma of GI tract.
Reye's syndrome.
Eye disorders.
Abdominal trauma.

NECK AND ARM PAIN

ICD-9CM # 723.1 NECK PAIN
847.0 NECK STRAIN
959.09 NECK INJURY
959.2 ARM INJURY
840.9 ARM STRAIN

Cervical disc syndrome.
Trauma, musculoskeletal strain.
Rotator cuff syndrome.
Bicipital tendonitis.
Glenohumeral arthritis.
Acromioclavicular arthritis.
Thoracic outlet syndrome.
Pancoast tumor.
Infection (cellulitis, abscess).
Angina pectoris.

NECK MASS[25]

ICD-9CM # 784.2

CONGENITAL ANOMALIES

Thyroglossal duct cyst.
Bronchial apparatus anomalies.
Teratomas.
Ranula.
Dermoid cysts.
Hemangioma.
Laryngoceles.
Cystic hygroma.

NONNEOPLASTIC INFLAMMATORY ETIOLOGIES

Folliculitis.
Adenopathy secondary to peritonsillar abscess.
Retropharyngeal or parapharyngeal abscess.
Salivary gland infections.
Viral infections (mononucleosis, HIV, CMV).
TB.
Cat-scratch disease.
Toxoplasmosis.
Actinomyces.
Atypical mycobacterium.
Jugular vein thrombus.

NEOPLASM (PRIMARY OR METASTATIC)

Lipoma.

NECK PAIN[25]

ICD-9CM # 723.1 NECK PAIN (NONDISCOGENIC)
959.09 NECK INJURY

INFLAMMATORY DISEASES

Rheumatoid arthritis (RA).
Spondyloarthropathies.
Juvenile RA.

NONINFLAMMATORY DISEASE

Cervical osteoarthritis.
Diskogenic neck pain.
Diffuse idiopathic skeletal hyperostosis.
Fibromyalgia or myofascial pain.

INFECTIOUS CAUSES

Meningitis.
Osteomyelitis.
Infectious diskitis.

NEOPLASMS

Primary.
Metastatic.

REFERRED PAIN

Temporomandibular joint pain.
Cardiac pain.
Diaphragmatic irritation.
Gastrointestinal sources (gastric ulcer, gallbladder, pancreas).

NEPHRITIC SYNDROME, ACUTE[1]

ICD-9CM # 580.89

LOW SERUM COMPLEMENT LEVEL

Acute postinfectious glomerulonephritis.
Membranoproliferative glomerulonephritis.
SLE.
Subacute bacterial endocarditis.
Visceral abscess "shunt" nephritis.
Cryoglobulinemia.

NORMAL SERUM COMPLEMENT LEVEL

IgA nephropathy.
Idiopathic rapidly progressive glomerulonephritis.
Antiglomerular basement membrane disease.
Polyarteritis nodosa.
Wegener's glomerulonephritis.
Henoch-Schönlein purpura.
Goodpasture's syndrome.

NEPHROCALCINOSIS

ICD-9CM # 275.49

Sarcoidosis.
Hyperparathyroidism.
Chronic glomerulonephritis.
Milk-alkali syndrome.
Distal renal tubular acidosis.
Medullary sponge kidney.
Bartter's syndrome.
Hypervitaminosis D.
Idiopathic hypercalciuria.
Hyperoxaluria.
Cortical necrosis.
Tuberculosis.
Idiopathic hypercalciuria.
Rapidly progressive osteoporosis.

NEUROGENIC BLADDER[26]

ICD-9CM # 396.54

SUPRATENTORIAL

CVA.
Parkinson's disease.
Alzheimer's disease.
Cerebral palsy.

SPINAL CORD

Spinal cord injury.
Spinal stenosis.
Central cord syndrome.
ALS.
Multiple sclerosis.
Myelodysplasia.

PERIPHERAL NEUROPATHY

Diabetes.
Alcohol.
Shingles.
Syphilis.

NEUROLOGIC DEFICIT, FOCAL[23]

**ICD-9CM # 436 CVA
435.9 TIA**

TRAUMATIC: INTRACRANIAL, INTRASPINAL

Subdural hematoma.
Intraparenchymal hemorrhage.
Epidural hematoma.
Traumatic hemorrhagic necrosis.

INFECTIOUS

Brain abscess.
Epidural and subdural abscesses.
Meningitis.

NEOPLASTIC

Primary central nervous system tumors.
Metastatic tumors.
Syringomyelia.
Vascular.
Thrombosis.
Embolism.
Spontaneous hemorrhage: arteriovenous malformation, aneurysm, hypertensive.

METABOLIC

Hypoglycemia.
B_{12} deficiency.
Postseizure.
Hyperosmolar nonketotic.

OTHER

Migraine.
Bell's palsy.
Psychogenic.

NEUROLOGIC DEFICIT, MULTIFOCAL[23]

**ICD-9CM # 436 CVA
435.9 TIA**

Acute disseminated encephalomyelitis: Postviral or postimmunization.
Infectious encephalomyelitis: Poliovirus, enteroviruses, arbovirus, herpes zoster, Epstein-Barr virus.
Granulomatous encephalomyelitis: Sarcoid.
Autoimmune: Systemic lupus erythematosus.
Other: Familial spinocerebellar degenerations.

NEUROPATHIC BLADDER

ICD-9CM # 596.59

Diabetes.
Stroke.
Multiple sclerosis.
Parkinson's disease.
Dementia.
Encephalopathy.
Brain trauma.
Spinal cord trauma.
Pelvic surgery.
Spina bifida.

NEUROPATHIES WITH FACIAL NERVE INVOLVEMENT

ICD-9CM # CODE VARIES WITH SPECIFIC DISORDER

Sarcoidosis.
HIV.
Lyme disease.
Guillain-Barré.
Others: Chronic inflammatory polyneuropathy, Tangier disease, amyloidosis.

NEUROPATHIES, PAINFUL[35]

**ICD-9CM # 355.9 NEUROPATHY NOS
357.5 ALCOHOLIC
357.8 CHRONIC PROGRESSIVE OR RELAPSING
356.2 CONGENITAL SENSORY
356.0 DEJERINE-SOTTAS
356.60 DIABETIC POLYNEUROPATHY, TYPE II
356.61 DIABETIC POLYNEUROPATHY TYPE I**

MONONEUROPATHIES

Compressive neuropathy (carpal tunnel, meralgia paresthetica).
Trigeminal neuralgia.
Ischemic neuropathy.
Polyarteritis nodosa.
Diabetic mononeuropathy.
Herpes zoster.
Idiopathic and familial brachial plexopathy.

POLYNEUROPATHIES

Diabetes mellitus.
Paraneoplastic sensory neuropathy.
Nutritional neuropathy.
Multiple myeloma.
Amyloid.
Dominantly inherited sensory neuropathy.
Toxic (arsenic, thallium, metronidazole).
AIDS-associated neuropathy.
Tangier disease.
Fabry's disease.

NIPPLE LESIONS

ICD-9CM # CODE VARIES WITH SPECIFIC DISORDER

Contact dermatitis.
Trauma.
Paget's disease.
Sebaceous hyperplasia.
Neurofibroma.
Accessory nipple.
Papillary adenoma.
Nevoid hyperkeratosis.
Cellulitis.

NODULAR LESIONS, SKIN

ICD-9CM # 782.2

Lipoma.
Cherry angioma.
Angiokeratoma.
Hemangioma.
Classic Kaposi's sarcoma.
Nodular melanoma.
Pyogenic granuloma.
Angiosarcoma.
Eccrine poroma.

NODULES, PAINFUL

ICD-9CM # CODE VARIES WITH SPECIFIC DISORDER

Arthropod bite or sting.
Erythema nodosum.
Glomus tumor.
Neuroma.
Leiomyoma.
Angiolipoma.
Dermatofibroma.
Osler's node.
Blue rubber bleb nevus.
Vasculitis.
Sweet's syndrome.

NYSTAGMUS

**ICD-9CM # 379.50 NYSTAGMUS NOS
386.11 BENIGN POSITIONAL
386.2 CENTRAL POSITIONAL
379.59 CONGENITAL**

Medications (meperidine, barbiturates, phenytoin, phenothiazines, etc.).
Multiple sclerosis.
Congenital.
Neoplasm (cerebellar, brainstem, cerebral).
Labyrinthine or vestibular lesions.
CNS infections.
Optic atrophy.
Other: Arnold-Chiari malformation, syringobulbia, chorioretinitis, meningeal cysts.

NYSTAGMUS, MONOCULAR

ICD-9CM # 379.50

Amblyopia.
Strabismus.
Multiple sclerosis.
Monocular blindness.
Internuclear ophthalmoplegia.
Lid fasciculations.
Brainstem infarct.

OPHTHALMOPLEGIA[1]

**ICD-9CM # 378.9 OPHTHALMOPLEGIA NOS
378.52 CEREBELLAR ATAXIA SYNDROME
376.22 EXOPHTHALMIC**

BILATERAL

Botulism.
Myasthenia gravis.
Wernicke's encephalopathy.
Acute cranial polyneuropathy.
Brainstem stroke.

UNILATERAL

Carotid-posterior (3rd cranial nerve, pupil involved communicating aneurysm).
Diabetic-idiopathic (3rd or 6th cranial nerve, pupil spared).
Myasthenia gravis.
Brainstem stroke.

OPSOCLONUS*

ICD-9CM # 379.59

Multiple sclerosis.
Encephalitis.
CNS lymphoma.
Hydrocephalus.
Pontine hemorrhage.
Thalamic disorder (glioma, hemorrhage).
Hyperosmolar coma.
Carcinoma, paraneoplastic.
Cocaine.
Medications (e.g., phenytoin, haloperidol, amitriptyline, diazepam, vidarabine).

*Spontaneous, multivector, chaotic eye movement

ORAL MUCOSA, ERYTHEMATOUS LESIONS[8]

**ICD-9CM # 528.3 ORAL ABSCESS
528.9 ORAL DISEASE (SOFT TISSUE)
528.8 HYPERPLASIA (TONGUE)**

Allergy.
Erythroplakia.
Candidiasis.
Geographic tongue.
Stomatitis areata migrans.
Plasma cell gingivitis.
Pemphigus vulgaris.

ORAL MUCOSA, PIGMENTED LESIONS[8]

**ICD-9CM # 528.3 ORAL ABSCESS
528.9 ORAL DISEASE (SOFT TISSUE)
528.8 HYPERPLASIA (TONGUE)**

Racial pigmentation.
Oral melanotic macule.
Peutz-Jeghers syndrome.
Neurofibromatosis.
Albright's syndrome.
Addison's disease.
Chloasma.
Drug reaction: quinacrine, Minocin, chlorpromazine, Myleran.
Amalgam tattoo.
Lead line.
Smoker's melanosis.
Nevi.
Melanoma.

ORAL MUCOSA, PUNCTATE EROSIVE LESIONS[8]

**ICD-9CM # 528.3 ORAL ABSCESS
528.9 ORAL DISEASE (SOFT TISSUE)
528.8 HYPERPLASIA (TONGUE)**

Viral lesion: Herpes simplex, coxsackievirus (A, B, A16), herpes zoster.
Aphthous stomatitis.
Sutton's disease (giant aphthae).
Behçet's syndrome.
Reiter's syndrome.
Neutropenia.
Acute necrotizing ulcerative gingivostomatitis (ANUG).
Drug reaction.
Inflammatory bowel disease.
Contact allergy.

ORAL MUCOSA, WHITE LESIONS[8]

**ICD-9CM # 528.3 ORAL ABSCESS
528.9 ORAL DISEASE (SOFT TISSUE)
528.8 HYPERPLASIA (TONGUE)**

Leukoplakia.
White, hairy leukoplakia.
Squamous cell carcinoma.
Lichen planus.
Stomatitis nicotinica.
Benign intraepithelial dyskeratosis.
White spongy nevus.
Leukoedema.
Darier-White disease.
Pachyonychia congenital.
Candidiasis.
Allergy.
SLE.

ORAL VESICLES AND ULCERS[1]

ICD-9CM # 528.9

Aphthous stomatitis.
Primary herpes simplex infection.
Vincent's stomatitis.
Syphilis.
Coxsackievirus A (herpangina).
Fungi (histoplasmosis).
Behçet's syndrome.
Systemic lupus erythematosus.
Reiter's syndrome.
Crohn's disease.
Erythema multiforme.
Pemphigus.
Pemphigoid.

ORBITAL LESIONS, CALCIFIED

ICD-9CM # 376.89

Chronic inflammation.
Phlebolith.
Dermoid cyst.
Mucocele walls.
Tumors (lacrimal gland, fibro-osseous).
Meningioma (optic sheath).
Lymphangioma.
Orbital varix.

ORBITAL LESIONS, CYSTIC

ICD-9CM # 376.9

Sweat gland cyst.
Dermoid cyst.
Lacrimal gland cyst.
Abscess.
Conjunctival cyst.
Lymphangioma.
Schwannoma.

ORGASM DYSFUNCTION[10]

ICD-9CM # 302.73 ORGASM INHIBITED FEMALE PSYCHOSEXUAL
302.74 ORGASM INHIBITED MALE PSYCHOSEXUAL

Anorgasmia: inadequate stimulation or learning.
Spinal cord lesion or injury.
Multiple sclerosis.
Alcoholic neuropathy.
Amyotrophic lateral sclerosis.
Spinal cord accident.
Spinal cord trauma.
Peripheral nerve damage.
Radical pelvic surgery.
Herniated lumbar disk.
Hypothyroidism.
Addison's disease.
Cushing's disease.
Acromegaly.
Hypopituitarism.
Pharmacologic agents (e.g., SSRIs, β-blockers).
Psychogenic.

OSTEOPOROSIS, SECONDARY CAUSES

ICD-9CM # 733.00

Medication induced (e.g., glucocorticoids, anticonvulsants, heparin, LHRH agonists or antagonists).
Hyperparathyroidism.
Hyperthyroidism.
Prolonged immobilization.
Chronic renal failure.
Sickle cell disease.
Multiple myeloma.
Myeloproliferative diseases.
Leukemias and lymphomas.
Acromegaly.
Prolactinoma.
Diabetes mellitus.
Total parenteral nutrition.
Malabsorption.
Chronic hypophosphatemia.
Connective tissue disorders (e.g., osteogenesis imperfecta, Marfan's syndrome, Ehlers-Danlos).
Hepatobiliary disease.
Postgastrectomy.
Aluminum containing antacids.
Systemic mastocytosis.
Homocystinuria.

OVULATORY DYSFUNCTION[18]

ICD-9CM # 628.0 ANOVULATORY CYCLE
626.5 OVULATION PAIN

HYPERANDROGENIC ANOVULATION

Polycystic ovarian syndrome.
Late-onset congenital adrenal hyperplasias.
Ovarian hyperthecosis.
Androgen-producing ovarian tumors.
Androgen-producing adrenal tumors.
Cushing's syndrome.

HYPOESTROGENIC ANOVULATION (HYPOTHALAMIC OR PITUITARY ETIOLOGY)

Hypogonadotropic hypoestrogenic states

Reversible:
Functional hypothalamic amenorrheas:
- Eating disorders (anorexia nervosa, excessive weight loss).
- Excessive athletic training.

Neoplastic:
- Craniopharyngioma.
- Pituitary stalk compression.

Infiltrative diseases:
- Histiocytosis-X.
- Sarcoidosis.

Hypophysitis.
Pituitary adenomas:
- Hyperprolactinemia.
- Euprolactinemic galactorrhea.

Endocrinopathies:
- Hypothyroidism/hyperthyroidism.
- Cushing's disease.

Irreversible:
- Kallmann's syndrome.
- Isolated gonadotropin deficiency (hypothalamic or pituitary origin).
- Panhypopituitarism/pituitary insufficiency:
  - Sheehan's syndrome, pituitary apoplexy.
  - Pituitary irradiation or ablation.

Hypergonadotropic hypoestrogenic states

Physiologic states:
- Menopause.
- Perimenopause.

Premature ovarian failure.
Immune-related:
- Radiation/chemotherapy-induced.

Ovarian dysgenesis.
Turner's syndrome.
46XX with mutations of X.
Androgen insensitivity syndrome.

MISCELLANEOUS

Endometriosis.
Luteal phase defect.

PAIN, MIDFOOT

ICD-9CM # 719.47

MEDIAL ASPECT

Tendonitis of posterior tibialis.
Tendonitis of flexor digitorum longus.
Tendonitis of flexor hallucis longus.
Infection (osteomyelitis, septic arthritis, cellulitis) of foot.
Peripheral vascular insufficiency.
Fracture.
Osteoarthritis.
Gout, pseudogout.
Neuropathy.
Tumor.

LATERAL ASPECT

Peroneus longus tendonitis.
Peroneus brevis tendonitis.
Infection (osteomyelitis, septic arthritis, cellulitis) of foot.
Peripheral vascular insufficiency.
Fracture.
Osteoarthritis.
Gout, pseudogout.
Neuropathy.
Tumor.

PAIN, PLANTAR ASPECT, HEEL

ICD-9CM # 719.47

Plantar fasciitis.
Tarsal tunnel syndrome.
Neuroma.
Infection (osteomyelitis, septic arthritis, cellulitis) of foot.
Peripheral vascular insufficiency.
Fracture.
Bone cyst.
Osteoarthritis.
Gout, pseudogout.

Neuropathy.
Tumor.
Heel pad atrophy.
Plantar fascia rupture.

PAIN, POSTERIOR HEEL

ICD-9CM # 729.5

Achilles tendonitis.
Retrocalcaneal bursitis.
Retroachilles bursitis.
Infection (osteomyelitis, septic arthritis, cellulitis) of foot.
Peripheral vascular insufficiency.
Fracture.
Osteoarthritis.
Gout, pseudogout.
Neuropathy.
Tumor.

PALINDROMIC RHEUMATISM[6]

ICD-9CM # 719.3 USE 5TH DIGIT
0. SITE UNSPECIFIED
1. SHOULDER REGION
2. UPPER ARM (ELBOW, HUMERUS)
3. FOREARM (RADIUS, WRIST, ULNA)
4. HAND (CARPAL, METACARPAL, FINGERS)
5. PELVIC REGION AND THIGH
6. LOWER LEG
7. ANKLE AND FOOT
8. OTHER
9. MULTIPLE

Palindromic rheumatoid arthritis.
Essential palindromic rheumatism.
Crystal synovitis (gout, CPPD, pseudogout, calcific periarthritis).
Lyme borreliosis, stages 2 and 3.
Sarcoidosis.
Whipple's disease.
Acute rheumatic fever.
Reactive arthritis (rare).

PALPITATIONS[30]

ICD-9CM # 785.1 PALPITATIONS

Anxiety.
Electrolyte abnormalities (hypokalemia, hypomagnesemia).
Exercise.
Hyperthyroidism.
Ischemic heart disease.
Ingestion of stimulant drugs (cocaine, amphetamines, caffeine).
Medications (digoxin, β-blockers, calcium channel antagonists, hydralazines, diuretics, minoxidil).
Hypoglycemia in type 1 DM.
Mitral valve prolapse.
Wolff-Parkinson-White (WPW) syndrome.
Sick sinus syndrome.

PANCREATIC CALCIFICATIONS

ICD-9CM # 577.8

Chronic pancreatitis.
Hyperparathyroidism.
Metastatic neoplasm.
Pseudocyst.
Hereditary pancreatitis.
Cystoadenoma.
Cystoadenocarcinoma.
Cavernous lymphangioma.
Hemorrhage.
Acute pancreatitis (saponification).

PANCYTOPENIA[33]

ICD-9CM # 284.8

PANCYTOPENIA WITH HYPOCELLULAR BONE MARROW

Acquired aplastic anemia.
Constitutional aplastic anemia.
Exposure to chemical or physical agents, including ionizing irradiation and chemotherapeutic agents.
Some hematologic malignancies, including myelodysplasia and aleukemic leukemia.

PANCYTOPENIA WITH NORMAL OR INCREASED CELLULARITY OF HEMATOPOIETIC ORIGIN

Some hematologic malignancies, including myelodysplasia, and some leukemias, lymphomas, and myelomas.
Paroxysmal nocturnal hemoglobinuria.
Hypersplenism.
Vitamin B_{12}, folate deficiencies.
Overwhelming infection.

PANCYTOPENIA WITH BONE MARROW REPLACEMENT

Tumor metastatic to marrow.
Metabolic storage diseases.
Osteopetrosis.
Myelofibrosis.

PAPILLEDEMA

ICD-9CM # 377.00 PAPILLEDEMA NOS
377.02 WITH DECREASED OCULAR PRESSURE
377.01 WITH INCREASED INTRACRANIAL PRESSURE
377.03 WITH RETINAL DISORDER

CNS infections (viral, bacterial, fungal).
Medications (lithium, cisplatin, corticosteroids, tetracycline, etc.).
Head trauma.
CNS neoplasm (primary or metastatic).
Pseudotumor cerebri.
Cavernous sinus thrombosis.
SLE.
Sarcoidosis.
Subarachnoid hemorrhage.
Carbon dioxide retention.
Arnold-Chiari malformation and other developmental or congenital malformations.
Orbital lesions.
Central retinal vein occlusion.
Hypertensive encephalopathy.
Metabolic abnormalities.

PAPULOSQUAMOUS DISEASES[12]

ICD-9CM # 709.8

Psoriasis.
Pityriasis rubra pilaris.
Pityriasis rosea.
Lichen planus.
Lichen nitidus.
Secondary syphilis.
Pityriasis lichenoides.
Parapsoriasis.
Mycosis fungoides.
Dermatophytosis.
Tinea versicolor.

PARANEOPLASTIC NEUROLOGIC SYNDROMES

ICD-9CM # CODE VARIES WITH SPECIFIC DISORDER

Lambert-Eaton myasthenic syndrome.
Myasthenia gravis.
Guillain-Barré syndrome.
Amyotrophic lateral sclerosis.
Dermatomyositis.
Carcinoid myopathy.
Cerebellar degeneration.
Encephalomyelitis.
Optic neuritis, uveitis, retinopathy.
Stiff-man syndrome.
Autonomic neuropathy.
Brachial neuritis.
Sensory neuropathy.
Progressive multifocal leukoencephalopathy.

PARANEOPLASTIC SYNDROMES, ENDOCRINE[33]

ICD-9CM # CODE VARIES WITH SPECIFIC DISORDER

Hypercalcemia.
Syndrome of inappropriate secretion of antidiuretic hormone.
Hypoglycemia.
Zollinger-Ellison syndrome.
Ectopic secretion of human chorionic gonadotropin.
Cushing's syndrome.

PARANEOPLASTIC SYNDROMES, NONENDOCRINE[33]

ICD-9CM # CODE VARIES WITH SPECIFIC DISORDER

CUTANEOUS

Dermatomyositis.
Acanthosis nigricans.
Sweet's syndrome.
Erythema gyratum repens.
Systemic nodular panniculitis (Weber-Christian disease).

RENAL

Nephrotic syndrome.
Nephrogenic diabetes insipidus.

NEUROLOGIC

Subacute cerebellar degeneration.
Progressive multifocal leukoencephalopathy.
Subacute motor neuropathy.
Sensory neuropathy.
Ascending acute polyneuropathy (Guillain-Barré syndrome).
Myasthenic syndrome (Eaton-Lambert syndrome).

HEMATOLOGIC

Microangiopathic hemolytic anemia.
Migratory thrombophlebitis (Trousseau's syndrome).
Anemia of chronic disease.

RHEUMATOLOGIC

Polymyalgia rheumatica.
Hypertrophic pulmonary osteoarthropathy.

PARAPLEGIA

ICD-9CM # 344.1 PARAPLEGIA, ACQUIRED
343.0 PARAPLEGIA, CONGENITAL
438.50 PARAPLEGIA, LATE EFFECT OF CVA

Trauma: penetrating wounds to motor cortex, fracture-dislocation of vertebral column with compression of spinal cord or cauda equina, prolapsed disk, electrical injuries.
Neoplasm: parasagittal region, vertebrae, meninges, spinal cord, cauda equina, Hodgkin's disease, NHL, leukemic deposits, pelvic neoplasms.
Multiple sclerosis and other demyelinating disorders.
Mechanical compression of spinal cord, cauda equina, or lumbosacral plexus: Paget's disease, kyphoscoliosis, herniation of intervertebral disk, spondylosis, ankylosing spondylitis, RA, aortic aneurysm.
Infections: spinal abscess, syphilis, TB, poliomyelitis, leprosy.
Thrombosis of superior sagittal sinus.
Polyneuritis: Guillain-Barré syndrome, diabetes, alcohol, beriberi, heavy metals.
Heredofamilial muscular dystrophies.
ALS.
Congenital and familial conditions: syringomyelia, myelomeningocele, myelodysplasia.
Hysteria.

PARESTHESIAS

ICD-9CM # 782.0

Multiple sclerosis.
Nutritional deficiencies (thiamin, vitamin B_{12}, folic acid).
Compression of spinal cord or peripheral nerves.
Medications (e.g., INH, lithium, nitrofurantoin, gold, cisplatin, hydralazine, amitriptyline, sulfonamides, amiodarone, metronidazole, dapsone, disulfiram, chloramphenicol).
Toxic chemicals (e.g., lead, arsenic, cyanide, mercury, organophosphates).
DM.
Myxedema.
Alcohol.
Sarcoidosis.
Neoplasms.
Infections (HIV, Lyme disease, herpes zoster, leprosy, diphtheria).
Charcot-Marie-Tooth syndrome and other hereditary neuropathies.
Guillain-Barré neuropathy.

PARKINSONISM-PLUS SYNDROMES

ICD-9CM # CODE VARIES WITH SPECIFIC DISORDER

Parkinson's disease.
Shy-Drager syndrome.
Corticobasal degeneration.
Olivo-ponto-cerebellar atrophy.
Dementia with Lewy bodies.
Progressive supranuclear palsy.
Striatonigral degeneration.

PAROTID SWELLING[3]

ICD-9CM # 527.2 ALLERGIC PAROTITIS
72.9 INFECTIOUS PAROTITIS
527.8 SALIVARY GLAND OBSTRUCTION
527.5 SALIVARY GLAND OBSTRUCTION WITH CALCULUS
527.8 SALIVARY GLAND STRICTURE
527.3 SALIVARY GLAND ABSCESS
235.1 SALIVARY GLAND NEOPLASM

INFECTIOUS

Mumps.
Parainfluenza.
Influenza.
Cytomegalovirus infection.
Coxsackievirus infection.
Lymphocytic choriomeningitis.
Echovirus infection.
Suppuration (bacterial).
Actinomyces infection.
Mycobacterial infection.
Cat-scratch disease.

NONINFECTIOUS

Drug hypersensitivity (thiouracil, phenothiazines, thiocyanate, iodides, copper, isoprenaline, lead, mercury, phenylbutazone).
Sarcoidosis.
Tumors, mixed.
Hemangioma, lymphangioma.
Sialectasis.
Sjögren's syndrome.
Mikulicz's syndrome (scleroderma, mixed connective tissue disease, systemic lupus erythematosus).
Recurrent idiopathic parotitis.
Pneumoparotitis.
Trauma.
Sialolithiasis.
Foreign body.
Cystic fibrosis.
Malnutrition (marasmus, alcohol cirrhosis).
Dehydration.
Diabetes mellitus.
Waldenström's macroglobulinemia.
Reiter's syndrome.
Amyloidosis.

NONPAROTID SWELLING

Hypertrophy of masseter muscle.
Lymphadenopathy.
Rheumatoid mandibular joint swelling.
Tumors of jaw.
Infantile cortical hyperostosis.

PELVIC MASS

ICD-9CM # 789.39

Hemorrhagic ovarian cyst.
Simple ovarian cyst (follicle or corpus luteum).
Ovarian carcinoma, carcinoma of fallopian tube, colorectal carcinoma, metastatic carcinoma, prostate carcinoma, bladder carcinoma, lymphoma, Hodgkin's disease.
Cystadenoma, teratoma, endometrioma.
Leiomyoma.
Leiomyosarcoma.
Diverticulitis, diverticular abscess.
Appendiceal abscess, tuboovarian abscess.
Ectopic pregnancy, intrauterine pregnancy.
Paraovarian cyst.
Hydrosalpinx.

PELVIC PAIN, CHRONIC[7]

ICD-9CM # 625.9 PELVIC PAIN, FEMALE
789.09 PELVIC PAIN, MALE

GYNECOLOGIC DISORDERS

Primary dysmenorrhea.
Endometriosis.
Adenomyosis.
Adhesions.
Fibroids.
Retained ovary syndrome after hysterectomy.
Previous tubal ligation.
Chronic pelvic infection.

MUSCULOSKELETAL DISORDERS

Myofascial pain syndrome.

GASTROINTESTINAL DISORDERS

Irritable bowel syndrome.
Inflammatory bowel disease.

URINARY TRACT DISORDERS

Interstitial cystitis.
Nonbacterial urethritis.

PELVIC PAIN, GENITAL ORIGIN[23]

ICD-9CM # 625.9 PELVIC PAIN, FEMALE
789.09 PELVIC PAIN, MALE

PERITONEAL IRRITATION

Ruptured ectopic pregnancy.
Ovarian cyst rupture.
Ruptured tuboovarian abscess.
Uterine perforation.

TORSION

Ovarian cyst or tumor.
Pedunculated fibroid.

INTRATUMOR HEMORRHAGE OR INFARCTION

Ovarian cyst.
Solid ovarian tumor.
Uterine leiomyoma.

INFECTION

Endometritis.
Pelvic inflammatory disease.
Trichomonas cervicitis or vaginitis.
Tuboovarian abscess.

PREGNANCY-RELATED

First Trimester
Ectopic pregnancy.
Abortion.
Corpus luteum hematoma.
Late Pregnancy
Placental problems.
Preeclampsia.
Premature labor.

MISCELLANEOUS

Endometriosis.
Foreign objects.
Pelvic adhesions.
Pelvic neoplasm.
Primary dysmenorrhea.

PENILE RASH

ICD-9CM # 782.1

Herpes simplex 2.
Balanitis (candida).
Condyloma acuminata.
Molluscum contagiosum.
Scabies.
Pediculosis pubis.
Pearly penile papules.
Lichen nitidus.
Fox-Forcyte disease (follicular papules).

PERICARDIAL EFFUSION

ICD-9CM # 420.90

Pericarditis.
Uremia.
Myxedema.
Neoplasm (leukemia, lymphoma, metastatic).
Hemorrhage (trauma, leakage of thoracic aneurysm).
SLE, Rheumatoid disease.
Myocardial infarction.

PERIODIC PARALYSIS, HYPERKALEMIC

ICD-9CM # 344.9

Chronic renal failure.
Renal insufficiency with excessive potassium supplementation.
Potassium-sparing diuretics.
Endocrinopathies (hypoaldosteronism, adrenal insufficiency).

PERIODIC PARALYSIS, HYPOKALEMIC

ICD-9CM # 344.9

Chronic diarrhea (laxative abuse, sprue, villous adenoma).
Potassium depleting diuretics.
Medications (amphotericin B, corticosteroids).
Chronic licorice ingestion.
Thyrotoxicosis.
Renal tubular acidosis.
Conn's syndrome.
Barter's syndrome.
Barium intoxication.

PERITONEAL CARCINONOMATOSIS[12]

ICD-9CM # 197.6

PRIMARY DISORDERS OF THE PERITONEUM: MESOTHELIOMA

Metastatic spread from
Stomach.
Colon.
Pancreas.
Carcinoid.
Other intraabdominal organs
Ovary.
Pseudomyxoma peritonei.
Extraabdominal primary tumors
Breast.
Lung.
Hematologic malignancy
Lymphoma.

PERITONEAL EFFUSION[16]

ICD-9CM # 792.9

TRANSUDATES

Increased hydrostatic pressure or decreased plasma oncotic pressure.
Congestive heart failure.
Hepatic cirrhosis.
Hypoproteinemia.

EXUDATES

Increased capillary permeability or decreased lymphatic resorption.
Infections (TB, spontaneous bacterial peritonitis, secondary bacterial peritonitis).
Neoplasms (hepatoma, metastatic carcinoma, lymphoma, mesothelioma).
Trauma.
Pancreatitis.
Bile peritonitis (e.g., ruptured gallbladder).

CHYLOUS EFFUSION

Damage or obstruction to thoracic duct.
Trauma.
Lymphoma.
Carcinoma.
Tuberculosis.
Parasitic infection.

PHOTODERMATOSES[12]

ICD-9CM # 692.72

Polymorphous light eruption.
Chronic actinic dermatitis.
Solar urticaria.
Phototoxicity and photoallergy.
Porphyrias.

PHOTOSENSITIVITY

ICD-9CM # 692.72

Solar urticaria.
Photoallergic reaction.
Phototoxic reaction.
Polymorphous light eruption.
Porphyria cutanea tarda.
SLE.
Drug induced (e.g., tetracyclines).

PLEURAL EFFUSIONS

ICD-9CM # 511.9 PLEURAL EFFUSION, UNSPECIFIED

EXUDATIVE

Neoplasm: bronchogenic carcinoma, breast carcinoma, mesothelioma, lymphoma, ovarian carcinoma, multiple myeloma, leukemia, Meigs' syndrome.

Infections: viral pneumonia, bacterial pneumonia, *Mycoplasma,* TB, fungal and parasitic diseases, extension from subphrenic abscess.
Trauma.
Collagen vascular diseases: SLE, RA, scleroderma, polyarteritis, Wegener's granulomatosis.
Pulmonary infarction.
Pancreatitis.
Postcardiotomy/Dressler's syndrome.
Drug-induced lupus erythematosus (hydralazine, procainamide).
Postabdominal surgery.
Ruptured esophagus.
Chronic effusion secondary to congestive failure.

TRANSUDATIVE

CHF.
Hepatic cirrhosis.
Nephrotic syndrome.
Hypoproteinemia from any cause.
Meigs' syndrome.

PLEURAL EFFUSIONS, MALIGNANCY-ASSOCIATED

ICD-9CM # 197.2

Lung cancer	(30% to 40%)
Breast cancer	(20% to 25%)
Lymphoma	(10% to 15%)
Leukemia	(5 % to 10%)
GI tract	(5%)
GU tract	(5%)
Reproductive	(3%)

PNEUMONIA, RECURRENT

ICD-9CM # 482.9 BACTERIAL PNEUMONIA
480.9 VIRAL PNEUMONIA
484.1 FUNGAL PNEUMONIA
485 SEGMENTAL PNEUMONIA

Mechanical obstruction from neoplasm.
Chronic aspiration (tube feeding, alcoholism, CVA, neuromuscular disorders, seizure disorder, inability to cough).
Bronchiectasis.
Kyphoscoliosis.
COPD, CHF, asthma, silicosis, pulmonary fibrosis, cystic fibrosis.
Pulmonary TB, chronic sinusitis.
Immunosuppression (HIV, corticosteroids, leukemia, chemotherapy, splenectomy).

POLYCYTHEMIA

ICD-9CM # 790.0

Tobacco abuse.
Chronic lung disease.
High altitude.
Sleep apnea.
Right-to-left cardiac shunts.
Erythropoietin administration.
Androgens/anabolic steroids.
Polycystic kidney disease.
Renal cell carcinoma.
Hepatocellular carcinoma.
Polycythemia vera.
Carbon monoxide exposure.
Primary familial and congenital polycythemia.
High-oxygen–affinity hemoglobins.
Uterine leiomyoma, meningioma, pheochromocytoma, parathyroid carcinoma.
Cobalt exposure.

POLYNEUROPATHY[35]

ICD-9CM # 357.9

PREDOMINANTLY MOTOR

Guillain-Barré syndrome.
Porphyria.
Diphtheria.
Lead.
Hereditary sensorimotor neuropathy, types I and II.
Paraneoplastic neuropathy.

PREDOMINANTLY SENSORY

Diabetes.
Amyloidosis.
Leprosy.
Lyme disease.
Paraneoplastic neuropathy.
Vitamin B_{12} deficiency.
Hereditary sensory neuropathy, types I-IV.

PREDOMINANTLY AUTONOMIC

Diabetes.
Amyloidosis.
Alcoholic neuropathy.
Familial dysautonomias.

MIXED SENSORIMOTOR

Systemic diseases: Renal failure, hypothyroidism, acromegaly, rheumatoid arthritis, periarteritis nodosa, systemic lupus erythematosus, multiple myeloma, macroglobulinemia, remote effect of malignancy.
Medications: Isoniazid, nitrofurantoin, ethambutol, chloramphenicol, chloroquine, vincristine, vinblastine, dapsone, disulfiram, diphenylhydantoin, cisplatin, 1-tryptophan.
Environmental toxins: *N*-hexane, methyl *N*-butyl ketone, acrylamide, carbon disulfide, carbon monoxide, hexachlorophene, organophosphates.
Deficiency disorders: Malabsorption, alcoholism, vitamin B_1 deficiency, Refsum's disease, metachromatic leukodystrophy.

POLYNEUROPATHY, DRUG-INDUCED[35]

ICD-9CM # 357.6

DRUGS IN ONCOLOGY

Vincristine.
Procarbazine.
Cisplatin.
Misonidazole.
Metronidazole (Flagyl).
Taxol.

DRUGS IN INFECTIOUS DISEASES

Isoniazid.
Nitrofurantoin.
Dapsone.
ddC (dideoxycytidine).
ddI (dideoxyinosine).

DRUGS IN CARDIOLOGY

Hydralazine.
Perhexiline maleate.
Procainamide.
Disopyramide.

DRUGS IN RHEUMATOLOGY

Gold salts.
Chloroquine.

DRUGS IN NEUROLOGY AND PSYCHIATRY

Diphenylhydantoin.
Glutethimide.
Methaqualone.

MISCELLANEOUS

Disulfiram (Antabuse).
Vitamin: pyridoxine (megadoses).

POLYNEUROPATHY, SYMMETRIC[35]

ICD-9CM # 357.9

ACQUIRED NEUROPATHIES

Toxic:
- Drugs.
- Industrial toxins.
- Heavy metals.
- Abused substances.

Metabolic/endocrine:
- Diabetes.
- Chronic renal failure.
- Hypothyroidism.
- Polyneuropathy of critical illness.

Nutritional deficiency:
- Vitamin B_{12} deficiency.
- Alcoholism.
- Vitamin E deficiency.

Paraneoplastic:
- Carcinoma.
- Lymphoma.

Plasma cell dyscrasia:
- Myeloma, typical, atypical, and solitary forms.
- Primary systemic amyloidosis.

Idiopathic chronic inflammatory demyelinating polyneuropathies.
Polyneuropathies associated with peripheral nerve autoantibodies.
Acquired immunodeficiency syndrome.

INHERITED NEUROPATHIES

Neuropathies with biochemical markers

Refsum's disease.
Bassen-Kornzweig disease.

Tangier disease.
Metachromatic leukodystrophy.
Krabbe's disease.
Adrenomyeloneuropathy.
Fabry's disease.
Neuropathies without biochemical markers or systemic involvement
Hereditary motor neuropathy.
Hereditary sensory neuropathy.
Hereditary sensorimotor neuropathy.

POLYURIA

ICD-9CM # 788.42

DM.
Diabetes insipidus.
Primary polydipsia (compulsive water drinking).
Hypercalcemia.
Hypokalemia.
Postobstructive uropathy.
Diuretic phase of renal failure.
Drugs: diuretics, caffeine, alcohol, lithium.
Sickle cell trait or disease, chronic pyelonephritis (failure to concentrate urine).
Anxiety, cold weather.

POPLITEAL SWELLING

ICD-9CM # 459.2 VENOUS OBSTRUCTION
747.4 VEIN ANOMALY, LOWER LIMB VESSEL
442.3 ARTERY ANEURYSM
904.41 ARTERY INJURY
447.8 ENTRAPMENT SYNDROME
727.51 BAKER'S CYST
451.2 PHLEBITIS, LOWER EXTREMITY
727.67 RUPTURE OF ACHILLES TENDON

Phlebitis (superficial).
Lymphadenitis.
Trauma: fractured tibia or fibula, contusion, traumatic neuroma.
DVT.
Ruptured varicose vein.
Baker's cyst.
Popliteal abscess.
Osteomyelitis.
Ruptured tendon.
Aneurysm of popliteal artery.
Neoplasm: lipoma, osteogenic sarcoma, neurofibroma, fibrosarcoma.

PORTAL HYPERTENSION[1]

ICD-9CM # 572.3

INCREASED RESISTANCE TO FLOW

Presinusoidal
Portal or splenic vein occlusion (thrombosis, tumor).
Schistosomiasis.
Congenital hepatic fibrosis.
Sarcoidosis.
Sinusoidal
Cirrhosis (all causes).
Alcoholic hepatitis.
Postsinusoidal
Venoocclusive disease.
Budd-Chiari syndrome.
Constrictive pericarditis.

INCREASED PORTAL BLOOD FLOW

Splenomegaly not caused by liver disease.
Arterioportal fistula.

POSTMENOPAUSAL BLEEDING

ICD-9CM # 627.1

Hormone replacement therapy.
Neoplasm (uterine, ovarian, cervical, vaginal, vulvar).
Atrophic vaginitis.
Vaginal infection.
Polyp.
Extragenital (GI, urinary).
Tamoxifen.
Trauma.

POSTURAL HYPOTENSION, NONNEUROLOGIC CAUSES

ICD-9CM # 458.0

Diuretics and hypertensive agents.
GI hemorrhage.
Alcohol.
Excessive heat.
Rapid volume loss from diarrhea, vomiting.
Hemodialysis.
Extensive burns.
Pyrexia.
Aortic stenosis (impaired output).
Constrictive pericarditis, atrial myxoma (impaired cardiac filling).
Adrenal insufficiency.
Diabetes insipidus.
Vasodilatory agents (e.g., nitrates).

PREMATURE GRAYING, SCALP HAIR

ICD-9CM # CODE VARIES WITH SPECIFIC DISORDER

Chemical exposure (e.g., phenol/catechol derivatives, sulfhydryls, arsenic).
Physical agents (e.g., ionizing radiation, lasers).
Hyperthyroidism.
Vitamin B_{12} deficiency.
Down's syndrome.
Chronic and severe protein deficiency.
Vitiligo.
Idiopathic.
Myotonic dystrophy.
Ataxia telangiectasia.
Progeria.
Wermer's syndrome.

PROPTOSIS[27]

ICD-9CM # 376.30

Thyrotoxicosis.
Orbital pseudotumor.
Optic nerve tumor.
Cavernous sinus AV fistula, cavernous sinus thrombosis.
Cellulitis.
Metastatic tumor to orbit.

PROTEINURIA

ICD-9CM # 791.0

Nephrotic syndrome as a result of primary renal diseases.
Malignant hypertension.
Malignancies: multiple myeloma, leukemias, Hodgkin's disease.
CHF.
DM.
SLE, RA.
Sickle cell disease.
Goodpasture's syndrome.
Malaria.
Amyloidosis, sarcoidosis.
Tubular lesions: cystinosis.
Functional (after heavy exercise).
Pyelonephritis.
Pregnancy.
Constrictive pericarditis.
Renal vein thrombosis.
Toxic nephropathies: heavy metals, drugs.
Radiation nephritis.
Orthostatic (postural) proteinuria.
Benign proteinuria: fever, heat, or cold exposure.

PRURITUS

ICD-9CM # 698.9 PRURITUS NOS
697.0 PRURITUS ANI
698.1 PRURITUS, GENITAL ORGANS

Dry skin.
Drug-induced eruption, fiberglass exposure.
Scabies.
Skin diseases.
Myeloproliferative disorders: mycosis fungoides, Hodgkin's lymphoma, multiple myeloma, polycythemia vera.
Cholestatic liver disease.
Endocrine disorders: DM, thyroid disease, carcinoid, pregnancy.
Carcinoma: breast, lung, gastric.
Chronic renal failure.
Iron deficiency.
AIDS.
Neurosis.
Sjögren's syndrome.

PRURITUS ANI[23]

ICD-9CM # 697.0

FECAL IRRITATION

Poor hygiene.

Anorectal conditions (fissure, fistula, hemorrhoids, skin tags, perianal clefts).
Spicy foods, citrus foods, caffeine, colchicine, quinidine.

CONTACT DERMATITIS

Anesthetic agents, topical corticosteroids, perfumed soap.

DERMATOLOGIC DISORDERS

Psoriasis, seborrhea, lichen simplex or sclerosus.

SYSTEMIC DISORDERS

Chronic renal failure, myxedema, DM, thyrotoxicosis, polycythemia vera, Hodgkin's disease.

SEXUALLY TRANSMITTED DISEASES

Syphilis, herpes simplex virus, human papillomavirus.

OTHER INFECTIOUS AGENTS

Pinworms.
Scabies.
Bacterial infection, viral infection.

PSEUDOHERMAPHRODITISM, FEMALE

ICD-9CM # ADRENAL 255.2
 # WITHOUT ADRENOCORTICAL DISORDER 752.7

Congenital adrenal hyperplasia.
Maternal use of testosterone or related steroids.
Virilizing ovarian or adrenal tumor.
Virilizing luteoma of pregnancy.
Disturbances in differentiation of urogenital structures, non-androgen related.
Maternal virilizing adrenal hyperplasia.
Fetal P450 aromatase deficiency.

PSEUDOHERMAPHRODITISM, MALE

ICD-9CM # ADRENAL 255.2
 # WITHOUT ADRENOCORTICAL DISORDER 752.7

Maternal ingestion of progestagens.
End-organ resistance to androgenic hormones.
5-Alpha-reductase-2 deficiency.
XY gonadal dysgenesis.
Testicular regression syndrome.
Defects in testosterone metabolism by peripheral tissues.
Testosterone biosynthesis defects.

PSEUDOINFARCTION[19]

ICD-9CM # CODE NOT AVAILABLE

Cardiac tumors, primary and secondary.
Cardiomyopathy (particularly hypertrophic and dilated).
Chagas' disease.
Chest deformity.
COPD (particularly emphysema).
HIV infection.
Hyperkalemia.
Left anterior fascicular block.
Left bundle branch block.
Left ventricular hypertrophy.
Myocarditis and pericarditis.
Normal variant.
Pneumothorax.
Poor R wave progression, rotational changes, and lead placement.
Pulmonary embolism.
Trauma to chest (nonpenetrating).
Wolff-Parkinson-White syndrome.
Rare causes: pancreatitis, amyloidosis, sarcoidosis, scleroderma.

PSYCHOSIS[25]

ICD-9CM # 298.9 PSYCHOSIS NOS
298.90 PSYCHOSIS, AFFECTIVE
291.0 PSYCHOSIS, ALCOHOLIC
290.41 PSYCHOSIS, ACUTE ARTERIOSCLEROTIC

PRIMARY

Schizophrenia related.*
Major depression.
Dementia.
Bipolar disorder.

SECONDARY

Drug use.†
Drug withdrawal.‡
Drug toxicity.§
Charles Bonnet syndrome.
Infections (pneumonia).
Electrolyte imbalance.
Syphilis.
Congestive heart failure.
Parkinson's disease.
Trauma to temporal lobe.
Postpartum psychosis.
Hypothyroidism/hyperthyroidism.
Hypomagnesemia.
Epilepsy.
Meningitis.
Encephalitis.
Brain abscess.
Herpes encephalopathy.
Hypoxia.
Hypercarbia.
Hypoglycemia.
Thiamine deficiency.
Postoperative states.

*Includes schizophrenia, schizophreniaform disorder, brief reactive psychosis.
†Includes hypnotics, glucocorticoids, marijuana, phencyclidine, atropine, dopaminergic agents (e.g., amantadine, bromocriptine, l-dopa), immunosuppressants.
‡Includes alcohol, barbiturates, benzodiazepines.
§Includes digitalis, theophylline, cimetidine, anticholinergics, glucocorticoids, catecholaminergic agents.

PTOSIS

ICD-9CM # 374.30 PTOSIS NOS
743.61 CONGENITAL
374.33 MECHANICAL
374.32 MYOGENIC
374.31 PARALYTIC

Third nerve palsy.
Myasthenia gravis.
Horner's syndrome.
Senile ptosis.

PUBERTY, DELAYED[24]

ICD-9CM # 259.0

NORMAL OR LOW SERUM GONADOTROPIN LEVELS

Constitutional delay in growth and development.
Hypothalamic and/or pituitary disorders:
- Isolated deficiency of growth hormone.
- Isolated deficiency on Gn-RH.
- Isolated deficiency of LH and/or FSH.
- Multiple anterior pituitary hormone deficiencies.
- Associated with congenital anomalies: Kallmann's syndrome; Prader-Willi syndrome; Laurence-Moon-Biedl syndrome; Friedreich's ataxia.
- Trauma.
- Postinfection.
- Hyperprolactinemia.
- Postirradiation.
- Infiltrative disease (histiocytosis).
- Tumor.
- Autoimmune hypophysitis.
- Idiopathic.

Functional:
- Chronic endocrinologic or systemic disorders.
- Emotional disorders.
- Drugs: cannabis.

INCREASED SERUM GONADOTROPIN LEVELS

Gonadal abnormalities:
- Congenital:
  - Gonadal dysgenesis.
  - Klinefelter's syndrome.
  - Bilateral anorchism.
  - Resistant ovary syndrome.
  - Myotonic dystrophy in males.
  - 17-Hydroxylase deficiency in females.
  - Galactosemia.
- Acquired:
  - Bilateral gonadal failure resulting from trauma or infection or after surgery, irradiation, or chemotherapy.
  - Oophoritis: isolated or with other autoimmune disorders.

Uterine or vaginal disorders:
- Absence of uterus and/or vagina.
- Testicular feminization: complete or incomplete androgen insensitivity.

PUBERTY, PRECOCIOUS

ICD-9CM # 255.2

Idiopathic.
Congenital virilizing adrenal hyperplasia.
Hypothalamic tumors.
Head trauma.
Hydrocephalus.
Degenerative CNS disease.
Arachnoid cyst.
Sex chromosome abnormalities (e.g., 47, XXY, 48, XXXY).
Perinatal asphyxia.
CNS infection (e.g., meningitis, encephalitis).

PULMONARY CRACKLES

ICD-9CM # CODE NOT AVAILABLE

Pneumonia.
Left ventricular failure.
Asbestosis, silicosis, interstitial lung disease.
Chronic bronchitis.
Alveolitis (allergic, fibrosing).
Neoplasm.

PULMONARY LESIONS

ICD-9CM # 518.3 PULMONARY INFILTRATE
518.89 PULMONARY NODULE
508.9 PULMONARY DISORDER DUE TO UNSPECIFIED EXTERNAL AGENT
861.20 PULMONARY INJURY NOS

TB.
Legionella pneumonia.
Mycoplasma pneumonia.
Viral pneumonia.
Pneumocystis carinii.
Hypersensitivity pneumonitis
Aspiration pneumonia.
Fungal disease (aspergillosis, histoplasmosis).
ARDS associated with pneumonia.
Psittacosis.
Sarcoidosis.
Septic emboli.
Metastatic cancer.
Multiple pulmonary emboli.
Rheumatoid nodules.

PULMONARY NODULE, SOLITARY

ICD-9CM # 518.89

Bronchogenic carcinoma.
Granuloma from histoplasmosis.
TB granuloma.
Granuloma from coccidioidomycosis.
Metastatic carcinoma.
Bronchial adenoma.
Bronchogenic cyst.
Hamartoma.
AV malformation.
Other: fibroma, intrapulmonary lymph node, sclerosing hemangioma, bronchopulmonary sequestration.

PULSELESS ELECTRICAL ACTIVITY

ICD-9CM # CODE NOT AVAILABLE

Hypovolemia.
Hypoxia.
Hyperkalemia.
Acidosis.
Cardiac tamponade.
Tension pneumothorax.
Pulmonary embolus.
Drug overdose.
Hypothermia.

PUPILLARY DILATATION, POOR RESPONSE TO DARKNESS

ICD-9CM # CODE VARIES WITH SPECIFIC DISORDER

Drugs (narcotics, general anesthetics, cholinergics).
Acute trauma (spasm from prostaglandin release).
Inflammation, infection (interruption of inhibitory fibers to the Edinger-Westphal nucleus).
Old age (loss of inhibition at midbrain from reticular activating formation).
Horner's syndrome (sympathetic neuron interruption).
Adie's syndrome tonic pupil.
Lymphoma.
Congenital miosis.

PURPURA

ICD-9CM # 287.2 PURPURA NOS
287.0 AUTOIMMUNE
287.0 HENOCH-SCHÖNLEIN
287.3 IDIOPATHIC THROMBOCYTOPENIC
446.6 THROMBOCYTOPENIC

THROMBOTIC

Trauma.
Septic emboli, atheromatous emboli.
DIC.
Thrombocytopenia.
Meningococcemia.
Rocky Mountain spotted fever.
Hemolytic-uremic syndrome.
Viral infection: echo, coxsackie.
Scurvy.
Other: left atrial myxoma, cryoglobulinemia, vasculitis, hyperglobulinemic purpura.

QT INTERVAL PROLONGATION[19]

ICD-9CM # 794.31

Drugs:
- Class I antiarrhythmics (e.g., disopyramide, procainamide, quinidine).
- Class III antiarrhythmics.
- Tricyclic antidepressants.
- Phenothiazines.
- Astemizole.
- Terfenadine.
- Adenosine.
- Antibiotics (e.g., erythromycin and other macrolides).
- Antifungal agents.
- Pentamidine, chloroquine.

Ischemic heart disease.
Cerebrovascular disease.
Rheumatic fever.
Myocarditis.
Mitral valve prolapse.
Electrolyte abnormalities.
Hypocalcemia.
Hypothyroidism.
Liquid protein diets.
Organophosphate insecticides.
Congenital prolonged QT syndrome.

RECTAL PAIN

ICD-9CM # 569.42

Anal fissure.
Thrombosed hemorrhoid.
Anorectal abscess.
Foreign bodies.
Fecal impaction.
Endometriosis.
Neoplasms (primary or metastatic).
Pelvic inflammatory disease.
Inflammation of sacral nerves.
Compression of sacral nerves.
Prostatitis.
Other: proctalgia fugax, uterine abnormalities, myopathies, coccygodynia.

RED EYE

ICD-9CM # 379.93

Infectious conjunctivitis (bacterial, viral).
Allergic conjunctivitis.
Acute glaucoma.
Keratitis (bacterial, viral).
Iritis.
Trauma.

RED HOT JOINT

ICD-9CM # CODE VARIES WITH SPECIFIC DISORDER

Trauma.
Gout.
Infection (septic joint).
Pseudogout (calcium pyrophosphate dehydrate crystal deposition).
Psoriatic arthropathy.
Reactive arthritis.
Palindromic rheumatism.

RENAL ARTERY OCCLUSION, CAUSES

ICD-9CM # 593.81

Atrial fibrillation.
Angiography or stent placement.
Abdominal aortic surgery.
Trauma.
Renal artery aneurysm/dissection.
Vasculitis.
Thrombosis in patient with fibromuscular dysplasia.
Atherosclerosis.
Septic embolism.
Mural thrombus thromboembolism.
Atrial myxoma thromboembolism.
Mitral stenosis thromboembolism.
Prosthetic valve thromboembolism.
Renal cell carcinoma.

RENAL CYSTIC DISORDERS

ICD-9CM # CODE VARIES WITH SPECIFIC DISORDER

Simple cysts.
Acquired cystic kidney disease.
Autosomal dominant polycystic kidney disease.
Autosomal recessive polycystic kidney disease.
Medullary cystic disease.
Medullary sponge kidney.

RENAL FAILURE, INTRINSIC OR PARENCHYMAL CAUSES[33]

ICD-9CM # 584. ACUTE, USE 4TH DIGIT
5. WITH ACUTE TUBULAR NECROSIS
6. WITH CORTICAL NECROSIS
7. WITH MEDULLARY NECROSIS
8. WITH OTHER UNSPECIFIED PATHOLOGIC CONDITION IN KIDNEY
9. RENAL FAILURE UNSPECIFIED
585 RENAL FAILURE, CHRONIC

ABNORMALITIES OF THE VASCULATURE

Renal arteries: atherosclerosis, thromboembolism, arteritis.
Renal veins: thrombosis.
Microvasculature: vasculitis, thrombotic microangiopathy.

ABNORMALITIES OF GLOMERULI (ACUTE GLOMERULONEPHRITIS)

Antiglomerular membrane disease (Goodpasture's syndrome).
Immune complex glomerulonephritis: SLE, postinfectious, idiopathic, membranoproliferative.

ABNORMALITIES OF INTERSTITIUM (ACUTE INTERSTITIAL NEPHRITIS)

Drugs (e.g., antibiotics, NSAIDs, diuretics, anticonvulsants, allopurinol).
Infectious pyelonephritis.
Infiltrative: lymphoma, leukemia, sarcoidosis.

ABNORMALITIES OF TUBULES

Physical obstruction (uric acid, oxalate, light chains).
Acute tubular necrosis:
- Ischemic.
- Toxic (antibiotics, chemotherapy, immunosuppressives, radiocontrast dyes, heavy metals, myoglobin, hemolysed RBCs).

RENAL FAILURE, POSTRENAL CAUSES[33]

ICD-9CM # 584. ACUTE, USE 4TH DIGIT
5. WITH ACUTE TUBULAR NECROSIS
6. WITH CORTICAL NECROSIS
7. WITH MEDULLARY NECROSIS
8. WITH OTHER UNSPECIFIED PATHOLOGIC CONDITION IN KIDNEY
9. RENAL FAILURE UNSPECIFIED
585 RENAL FAILURE, CHRONIC

URETER AND RENAL PELVIS

Intrinsic obstruction:
- Blood clots.
- Stones.
- Sloughed papillae: diabetes, sickle cell disease, analgesic nephropathy.
- Inflammatory: fungus ball.

Extrinsic obstruction:
- Malignancy.
- Retroperitoneal fibrosis.
- Iatrogenic: inadvertent ligation of ureters.

BLADDER

Prostatic hypertrophy or malignancy.
Neuropathic bladder.
Blood clots.
Bladder cancer.
Stones.

URETHRAL

Strictures.
Congenital valves.

RENAL FAILURE, PRERENAL CAUSES[33]

ICD-9CM # 584. ACUTE, USE 4TH DIGIT
5. WITH ACUTE TUBULAR NECROSIS
6. WITH CORTICAL NECROSIS
7. WITH MEDULLARY NECROSIS
8. WITH OTHER UNSPECIFIED PATHOLOGIC CONDITION IN KIDNEY
9. RENAL FAILURE UNSPECIFIED
585 RENAL FAILURE, CHRONIC

DECREASED CARDIAC OUTPUT

CHF.
Arrhythmias.
Pericardial constriction or tamponade.
Pulmonary embolism.

HYPOVOLEMIA

GI tract loss (vomiting, diarrhea, nasogastric suction).
Blood losses (trauma, GI tract surgery).
Renal losses (diuretics, mineralocorticoid deficiency, postobstructive diuresis).
Skin losses (burns).

VOLUME REDISTRIBUTION (DECREASE IN EFFECTIVE BLOOD VOLUME)

Hypoalbuminemic states (cirrhosis, nephrosis).
Sequestration of fluid in "third" space (ischemic bowel, peritonitis, pancreatitis).
Peripheral vasodilation (sepsis, vasodilators, anaphylaxis).

ALTERED RENAL VASCULAR RESISTANCE

Increase in afferent vascular resistance (NSAIDs, liver disease, sepsis, hypercalcemia, cyclosporine).
Decrease in efferent arteriolar tone (ACE inhibitors).

RENAL VEIN THROMBOSIS, CAUSES

ICD-9CM # 453.3

Nephrotic syndrome.
Renal cell carcinoma.
Aortic aneurysm causing compression.
Lymphadenopathy.
Retroperitoneal fibrosis.
Estrogen therapy.
Pregnancy.
Renal cell carcinoma with vein invasion.
Severe dehydration.

RESPIRATORY FAILURE, HYPOVENTILATORY[25]

ICD-9CM # 518.81 RESPIRATORY FAILURE

ABNORMAL RESPIRATORY CAPACITY (NORMAL RESPIRATORY WORKLOADS)

Acute depression of central nervous system:
  Various causes.
Chronic central hypoventilation syndromes:
  Obesity-hypoventilation syndrome.
  Sleep apnea syndrome.
  Hypothyroidism.
  Shy-Drager syndrome (multisystem atrophy syndrome).
Acute toxic paralysis syndromes:
  Botulism.
  Tetanus.
  Toxic ingestion or bites.
  Organophosphate poisoning.
Neuromuscular disorders (acute and chronic):
  Myasthenia gravis.
  Guillain-Barré syndrome.
  Drugs.
  Amyotrophic lateral sclerosis.
  Muscular dystrophies.
  Polymyositis.
  Spinal cord injury.
  Traumatic phrenic nerve paralysis.

ABNORMAL PULMONARY WORKLOADS

Chronic obstructive pulmonary disease:
  Chronic bronchitis.
  Asthmatic bronchitis.
  Emphysema.
Asthma and acute bronchial hyperreactivity syndromes.
Upper airway obstruction.
Interstitial lung diseases.

ABNORMAL EXTRAPULMONARY WORKLOADS

Chronic thoracic cage disorders:
  Severe kyphoscoliosis.
  After thoracoplasty.
  After thoracic cage injury.
Acute thoracic cage trauma and burns.
Pneumothorax.
Pleural fibrosis and effusions.
Abdominal processes.

RETINOPATHY, HYPERTENSIVE

ICD-9CM # 362.11

Retinal venous obstruction.
Diabetic retinopathy.
Ocular ischemic syndrome.
Hyperviscosity.
Tortuosity of retinal artery.

RIGHT AXIS DEVIATION[19]

ICD-9CM # CODE VARIES WITH SPECIFIC DIAGNOSIS

Normal variation.
Right ventricular hypertrophy.
Left posterior fascicular block.
Lateral myocardial infarction.
Pulmonary embolism.
Dextrocardia.
Mechanical shifts or emphysema causing a vertical heart.

SALIVARY GLAND ENLARGEMENT

ICD-9CM # 527.1

Neoplasm.
Sialolithiasis.
Infection (mumps, bacterial infection, HIV, TB).
Sarcoidosis.
Idiopathic.
Acromegaly.
Anorexia/bulimia.
Chronic pancreatitis.
Medications (e.g., phenylbutazone).
Cirrhosis.
Diabetes mellitus.

SALIVARY GLAND SECRETION, DECREASED

ICD-9CM # 527.7

Medications (antihistamines, antidepressants, neuroleptics, antihypertensives).
Dehydration.
Anxiety.
Sjögren's syndrome.
Sarcoidosis.
Mumps.
Amyloidosis.
CNS disorders.
Head and neck radiation.

SCROTAL PAIN[25]

ICD-9CM # 878.2 SCROTAL INJURY, TRAUMATIC
608.9 SCROTAL DISORDER NOS
608.4 SCROTAL CELLULITIS
608.83 SCROTAL HEMORRHAGE, NONTRAUMATIC
608.4 SCROTAL NODULE, INFLAMMATORY

Torsion:
  Appendages.
  Spermatic cord.
Infection:
  Orchitis.
  Abscess.
  Epididymitis.
Neoplasia:
  Benign.
  Malignant.
Incarcerated hernia.
Trauma.
Hydrocele.
Spermatocele.
Varicocele.

SCROTAL SWELLING

ICD-9CM # 608.86

Hydrocele.
Varicocele.
Neoplasm.
Acute epididymitis.
Orchitis.
Trauma.
Hernia.
Torsion of spermatic cord.
Torsion of epididymis.
Torsion of testis.
Insect bite.
Folliculitis.
Sebaceous cyst.
Thrombosis of spermatic vein.
Other: lymphedema, dermatitis, fat necrosis, Henoch-Schönlein purpura, idiopathic scrotal edema.

SEIZURE

ICD-9CM # 780.39

Syncope.
Alcohol abuse/withdrawal.
TIA.
Hemiparetic migraine.
Psychiatric disorders.
Carotid sinus hypersensitivity.
Hyperventilation, prolonged breath holding.
Hypoglycemia.
Narcolepsy.
Movement disorders (tics, hemiballismus).
Hyponatremia.
Brain tumor (primary or metastatic).
Tetanus.
Strychnine, phencyclidine poisoning.

SEIZURE, PEDIATRIC[2]

ICD-9CM # 780.39 INFANTILE SEIZURES
779.0 SEIZURES, NEWBORN

FIRST MONTH OF LIFE

First day

Hypoxia.
Drugs.
Trauma.
Infection.
Hyperglycemia.
Hypoglycemia.
Pyridoxine deficiency.

Day 2-3
Infection.
Drug withdrawal.
Hypoglycemia.
Hypocalcemia.
Developmental malformation.
Intracranial hemorrhage.
Inborn error of metabolism.
Hyponatremia or hypernatremia.
Day >4
Infection.
Hypocalcemia.
Hyperphosphatemia.
Hyponatremia.
Developmental malformation.
Drug withdrawal.
Inborn error of metabolism.

1 TO 6 MONTHS

As above.

6 MONTHS TO 3 YEARS

Febrile seizures.
Birth injury.
Infection.
Toxin.
Trauma.
Metabolic disorder.
Cerebral degenerative disease.

>3 YEARS

Idiopathic.
Infection.
Trauma.
Cerebral degenerative disease.

SEXUALLY TRANSMITTED DISEASES, ANORECTAL REGION[23]

ICD-9CM # 569.49 INFECTION AND REGION

ULCERATIVE

Lymphogranuloma venereum.
Herpes simplex virus.
Early (primary) syphilis.
Chancroid *(Haemophilus ducreyi)*.
Cytomegalovirus.
Idiopathic (usually HIV positive).

NONULCERATIVE

Condyloma acuminatum.
Gonorrhea.
Chlamydia *(Chlamydia trachomitis)*.
Syphilis.

SEXUAL PRECOCITY[36]

ICD-9CM # 259.1

TRUE PRECOCIOUS PUBERTY

Premature reactivation of LHRH pulse generator.

INCOMPLETE SEXUAL PRECOCITY

(Pituitary Gonadotropin Independent).
Males
Chorionic gonadotropin-secreting tumor.
Leydig cell tumor.
Familial testotoxicosis.
Virilizing congenital adrenal hyperplasia.
Virilizing adrenal tumor.
Premature adrenarche.
Females
Granulosa cell tumor (follicular cysts may be manifested similarly).
Follicular cyst.
Feminizing adrenal tumor.
Premature thelarche.
Premature adrenarche.
Late-onset virilizing congenital adrenal hyperplasia.
In both sexes
McCune-Albright syndrome.
Primary hypothyroidism.

SHOULDER PAIN

ICD-9CM # 952.2 SHOULDER INJURY
718.81 SHOULDER INSTABILITY
726.19 SHOULDER LIGAMENT OR MUSCLE INSTABILITY
840.9 SHOULDER STRAIN, SITE UNSPECIFIED

WITH LOCAL FINDINGS IN SHOULDER

Trauma: contusion, fracture, muscle strain, trauma to spinal cord.
Arthrosis, arthritis, RA, ankylosing spondylitis.
Bursitis, synovitis, tendinitis, tenosynovitis.
Aseptic (avascular) necrosis.
Local infection: septic arthritis, osteomyelitis, abscess, herpes zoster, TB.

WITHOUT LOCAL FINDINGS IN SHOULDER

Cardiovascular disorders: ischemic heart disease, pericarditis, aortic aneurysm.
Subdiaphragmatic abscess, liver abscess.
Cholelithiasis, cholecystitis.
Pulmonary lesions: apical bronchial carcinoma, pleurisy, pneumothorax, pneumonia.
GI lesions: PUD, gastric neoplasm, peptic esophagitis.
Pancreatic lesions: carcinoma, calculi, pancreatitis.
CNS abnormalities: neoplasm, vascular abnormalities.
Multiple sclerosis.
Syringomyelia.
Polymyositis/dermatomyositis.
Psychogenic.
Polymyalgia rheumatica.
Ectopic pregnancy.

SHOULDER PAIN BY LOCATION

ICD-9CM # 952.2 SHOULDER INJURY
726.19 SHOULDER LIGAMENT OR MUSCLE INSTABILITY
840.8 SHOULDER SEPARATION

TOP OF SHOULDER (C4)

Cervical source.
Acromioclavicular.
Sternoclavicular.
Diaphragmatic.

SUPEROLATERAL (C5)

Rotator cuff tendinitis.
Impingement.
Adhesive capsulitis.
Glenohumeral arthritis.

ANTERIOR

Bicipital tendinitis and rupture.
Glenoid labral tear.
Adhesive capsulitis.
Glenohumeral arthritis.
Osteonecrosis.

AXILLARY

Neoplasm (Pancoast's, mediastinal).
Herpes zoster.

SMALL BOWEL OBSTRUCTION[23]

ICD-9CM # 751.1 SMALL INTESTINE OBSTRUCTION, CONGENITAL
560.81 SMALL INTESTINE OBSTRUCTION DUE TO ADHESION

INTRINSIC

Congenital (atresia, stenosis).
Inflammatory (Crohn's, radiation enteritis).
Neoplasms (metastatic or primary).
Intussusception.
Traumatic (hematoma).

EXTRINSIC

Hernias (internal and external).
Adhesions.
Volvulus.
Compressing masses (tumors, abscesses, hematomas).

INTRALUMINAL

Foreign body.
Gallstones.
Bezoars.
Barium.
Ascaris infestation.

SMALL INTESTINE ULCERATION

ICD-9CM # 569.82

Inflammatory bowel disease.
Celiac disease.
Vasculitis, systemic lupus erythematosus (SLE), Behçet's syndrome.
Uremia.
Infections *(Campylobacter,* tuberculosis [TB], *Yersinia,* parasites, typhoid, cytomegalovirus [CMV], *Clostridium).*
Mesenteric insufficiency.
Neoplasms.
Radiation.
Drugs (salicylates, potassium, indomethacin, antimetabolites).
Meckel diverticulum.
Zollinger-Ellison syndrome.
Lymphocytic enterocolitis.
Stomal ulceration.

SMELL DISTURBANCE

ICD-9CM # CODE VARIES WITH SPECIFIC DISORDER

Upper respiratory tract infection.
Nasal or paranasal sinus disease.
Exposure to noxious vapors.
Head trauma.
Idiopathic.
Dental caries, periodontal disease.
Medications.

SORE THROAT[30]

ICD-9CM # 426 PHARYNGITIS
075 MONONUCLEOSIS
472.1 CHRONIC PHARYNGITIS
487.1 PHARYNGITIS, INFLUENZAL
074.0 COXSACKIE VIRUS PHARYNGITIS

WITHOUT PHARYNGEAL ULCERS

Viral pharyngitis.
Allergic pharyngitis.
Infectious mononucleosis.
Streptococcal pharyngitis.
Gonococcal pharyngitis.
Sinusitis with postnasal drip.

WITH PHARYNGEAL ULCERS

Herpangina.
Herpes simplex.
Candidiasis.
Fusospirochetal infection (Vincent's angina).

SPASTIC PARAPLEGIAS

ICD-9CM # 344.1

Cervical spondylosis.
Friedreich's ataxia.
Multiple sclerosis.
Spinal cord tumor.
HIV.
Tertiary syphilis.
Vitamin B_{12} deficiency.
Spinocerebellar ataxias.
Syringomyelia.
Spinal cord AV malformations.
Adrenoleukodystrophy.

SPINAL CORD COMPRESSION, EPIDURAL

ICD-9CM # CODE VARIES WITH SPECIFIC DISORDER

Osteoarthritis.
Meningioma.
Spinal epidural abscess.
Spinal epidural hematoma.
Spinal epidural vascular malformations.
Rheumatoid arthritis.
Metastatic cancer (vertebral, intramedullary, leptomeninges).
Radiation myelopathy.
Neurofibroma.
Sarcoidosis.
Paraneoplastic myelopathy.
Histiocytosis.

SPINAL CORD DYSFUNCTION

ICD-9CM # 336.9 SPINAL CORD COMPRESSION
336.9 SPINAL CORD DISEASE NOS
742.9 SPINAL CORD DISEASE, CONGENITAL
281.1 SPINAL CORD DEGENERATION, B_{12} DEFICIENCY ANEMIA
336.8 SPINAL CORD ATROPHY, ACUTE
336.10 SPINAL CORD ATROPHY, ADULT

Trauma.
Multiple sclerosis.
Transverse myelitis.
Neoplasm (primary, metastatic).
Syringomyelia.
Spinal epidural abscess.
HIV myelopathy.
Diskitis.
Spinal epidural hematoma.
Spinal cord infarction.
Spinal AV malformation.
Subarachnoid hemorrhage.

SPINAL CORD ISCHEMIC SYNDROMES

ICD-9CM # CODE VARIES WITH SPECIFIC DISORDER

Systemic hypotension.
Venous or arterial occlusion.
Arterial dissection.
Thromboembolism.
Endovascular procedures.
Vasculitis.
Fibrocartilaginous embolism.
Regional hemodynamic compromise.

SPINAL TUMORS[12]

ICD-9CM # 299.7

EXTRADURAL

Metastases.
Primary bone tumors arising in spine.

INTRADURAL EXTRAMEDULLARY

Meningiomas.
Neurofibromas.
Schwannomas.
Lipomas.
Arachnoid cysts.
Epidermoid cysts.
Metastasis.

INTRAMEDULLARY

Ependymoma.
Glioma.
Hemangioblastoma.
Lipoma.
Metastases.

SPLENOMEGALY

ICD-9CM # 789.2 SPLENOMEGALY UNSPECIFIED
289.51 CHRONIC CONGESTIVE
759.0 CONGENITAL
789.2 UNKNOWN ORIGIN

Hepatic cirrhosis.
Neoplastic involvement: CML, CLL, lymphoma, multiple myeloma.
Bacterial infections: TB, infectious endocarditis, typhoid fever, splenic abscess.
Viral infections: infectious mononucleosis, viral hepatitis, HIV.
Gaucher's disease and other lipid storage diseases.
Sarcoidosis.
Parasitic infections (malaria, kala-azar, histoplasmosis).
Hereditary and acquired hemolytic anemias.
Idiopathic thrombocytopenic purpura (ITP).
Collagen vascular disorders: SLE, RA (Felty's syndrome), polyarteritis nodosa.
Serum sickness, drug hypersensitivity reaction.
Splenic cysts and benign tumors: hemangioma, lymphangioma.
Thrombosis of splenic or portal vein.
Polycythemia vera, myeloid metaplasia.

STEATOHEPATITIS

ICD-9CM # 571.8

Alcohol abuse.
Obesity.
Diabetes mellitus.
Parenteral nutrition.
Medications (high-dose estrogen, amiodarone, corticosteroids, methotrexate, nifedipine).
Jejunoileal bypass.

Abetalipoproteinemia.
Wilson's disease, Weber-Christian disease.

STOMATITIS, BULLOUS

ICD-9CM # 528.0

Erythema multiforme.
Erosive lichen planus.
Bullous pemphigoid.
SLE.
Pemphigus vulgaris.
Mucous membrane pemphigoid.

STRIDOR, PEDIATRIC AGE[4]

ICD-9CM # 786.1 STRIDOR
748.3 STRIDOR LARYNGEAL CONGENITAL

RECURRENT

Allergic (spasmodic) croup.
Respiratory infections in a child with otherwise asymptomatic anatomic narrowing of the large airways.
Laryngomalacia.

PERSISTENT

Laryngeal obstruction:
- Laryngomalacia.
- Papillomas, other tumors.
- Cysts and laryngoceles.
- Laryngeal webs.
- Bilateral abductor paralysis of the cords.
- Foreign body.

Tracheobronchial disease:
- Tracheomalacia.
- Subglottic tracheal webs.

Endotracheal, endobronchial tumors.
Subglottic tracheal stenosis.
Congenital.
Acquired.
Extrinsic masses.
Mediastinal masses.
Vascular ring.
Lobar emphysema.
Bronchogenic cysts.
Thyroid enlargement.
Esophageal foreign body.
Tracheoesophageal fistulas.
Other.
Gastroesophageal reflux.
Macroglossia, Pierre Robin syndrome.
Cri du chat syndrome.
Hysterical stridor.
Hypocalcemia.

STROKE[33]

ICD-9CM # 436 ACUTE STROKE

Hypoglycemia.
Drug overdose or intoxication.
Hysterical conversion reaction.
Hyperventilation.
Metabolic encephalopathy.
Migraine.
Syncope.
Transient global amnesia.
Seizures.
Vestibular vertigo.

STROKE, PEDIATRIC AGE[20]

ICD-9CM # 436 STROKE, ACUTE

CARDIAC DISEASE

Congenital:
- Aortic stenosis.
- Mitral stenosis; mitral prolapse.
- Ventricular septal defects.
- Patent ductus arteriosus.
- Cyanotic congenital heart disease involving right-to-left shunt.

Acquired:
- Endocarditis (bacterial, SLE).
- Kawasaki disease.
- Cardiomyopathy.
- Atrial myxoma.
- Arrhythmia.
- Paradoxical emboli through patent foramen ovale.
- Rheumatic fever.
- Prosthetic heart valve.

HEMATOLOGIC ABNORMALITIES

Hemoglobinopathies:
- Sickle cell (SS) disease.
- Sickle (SC) disease.

Polycythemia.
Leukemia/lymphoma.
Thrombocytopenia.
Thrombocytosis.
Disorders of coagulation:
- Protein C deficiency.
- Protein S deficiency.
- Factor V Leiden.
- Antithrombin III deficiency.
- Lupus anticoagulant.
  - Oral contraceptive pill use.
  - Pregnancy and the postpartum state.
  - Disseminated intravascular coagulation.
  - Paroxysmal nocturnal hemoglobinuria.
  - Inflammatory bowel disease (thrombosis).

INFLAMMATORY DISORDERS

Meningitis:
- Viral.
- Bacterial.
- Tuberculosis.

Systemic infection:
- Viremia.
- Bacteremia.
- Local head and neck infections.

Drug-induced inflammation:
- Amphetamine.
- Cocaine.

Autoimmune disease:
- Systemic lupus erythematosus.
- Juvenile rheumatoid arthritis.
- Takayasu's arteritis.
- Mixed connective tissue disease.
- Polyarteritis nodosum.
- Primary CNS vasculitis.
- Sarcoidosis.
- Behçet's syndrome.
- Wegener's granulomatosis.

METABOLIC DISEASE ASSOCIATED WITH STROKE

Homocystinuria.
Pseudoxanthoma elasticum.
Fabry's disease.
Sulfite oxidase deficiency.
Mitochondrial disorders:
- MELAS.
- Leigh syndrome.

Ornithine transcarbamylase deficiency.

INTRACEREBRAL VASCULAR PROCESSES

Ruptured aneurysm.
Arteriovenous malformation.
Fibromuscular dysplasia.
Moyamoya disease.
Migraine headache.
Postsubarachnoid hemorrhage vasospasm.
Hereditary hemorrhagic telangiectasia.
Sturge-Weber syndrome.
Carotid artery dissection.
Postvaricella.

TRAUMA AND OTHER EXTERNAL CAUSES

Child abuse.
Head trauma/neck trauma.
Oral trauma.
Placental embolism.
ECMO therapy.

CNS, Central nervous system; *ECMO,* extracorporeal membrane oxygenation; *MELAS,* mitochondrial encephalomyopathy, lactic acidosis, and stroke.

STROKE, YOUNG ADULT, CAUSES[1]

ICD-9CM # 436

Cardiac factors (ASD, MVP, patent foramen ovale).
Inflammatory factors (SLE, polyarteritis nodosa).
Infections (endocarditis, neurosyphilis).
Drugs (cocaine, heroin, oral contraceptives, decongestants).
Arterial dissection.
Hematolic factors (DIC, TTP, deficiency of protein S, protein C, antithrombin III).
Migraine.
Postpartum angiopathy.
Others: premature atherosclerosis, fibromuscular dysplasia.

ST SEGMENT ELEVATIONS, NONISCHEMIC

ICD-9CM #794.31

Early repolarization.
Acute pericarditis.
LVH.
Normal pattern variant.
LBBB.
Pulmonary embolism.
Hyperkalemia.
Postcardioversion.

SUDDEN DEATH, PEDIATRIC AGE[4]

ICD-9CM # CODE VARIES WITH SPECIFIC DISORDER

SIDS AND SIDS "MIMICS"

SIDS.
Long Q-T syndromes.
Inborn errors of metabolism.
Child abuse.
Myocarditis.
Duct-dependent congenital heart disease.

CORRECTED OR UNOPERATED CONGENITAL HEART DISEASE

Aortic stenosis.
Tetralogy of Fallot.
Transposition of great vessels (postoperative atrial switch).
Mitral valve prolapse.
Hypoplastic left heart syndrome.
Eisenmenger's syndrome.

CORONARY ARTERIAL DISEASE

Anomalous origin.
Anomalous tract.
Kawasaki disease.
Periarteritis.
Arterial dissection.
Marfan's syndrome.
Myocardial infarction.

MYOCARDIAL DISEASE

Myocarditis.
Hypertrophic cardiomyopathy.
Dilated cardiomyopathy.
Arrhythmogenic right ventricular dysplasia.

CONDUCTION SYSTEM ABNORMALITY/ARRHYTHMIA

Long Q-T syndromes.
Proarrhythmic drugs.
Preexcitation syndromes.
Heart block.
Commotio cordis.
Idiopathic ventricular fibrillation.
Heart tumor.

MISCELLANEOUS

Pulmonary hypertension.
Pulmonary embolism.
Heat stroke.
Cocaine.
Anorexia nervosa.
Electrolyte disturbances.

SIDS, Sudden infant death syndrome.

SUDDEN DEATH, YOUNG ATHLETE

ICD-9CM # CODE VARIES WITH SPECIFIC DIAGNOSIS

Hyperthrophic cardiomyopathy.
Coronary artery anomalies.
Myocarditis.
Ruptured aortic aneurysm (Marfan's syndrome).
Arrhythmias.
Aortic valve stenosis.
Asthma.
Trauma (cerebral, cardiac).
Drug and alcohol abuse.
Heat stroke.
Cardiac sarcoidosis.
Atherosclerotic coronary artery disease.
Dilated cardiomyopathy.

SWOLLEN LIMB

ICD-9CM # 729.81 SWOLLEN ARM OR HAND
729.81 SWOLLEN LEG OR FOOT

Trauma.
Insect bite.
Abscess.
Lymphedema.
Thrombophlebitis.
Lipoma.
Neurofibroma.
Postphlebitic syndrome.
Myositis ossificans.
Nephrosis, cirrhosis, CHF.
Hypoalbuminemia.
Varicose veins.

TALL STATURE[24]

ICD-9CM # 253.0 GROWTH HORMONE OVERPRODUCTION, GIGANTISM

CONSTITUTIONAL (FAMILIAL OR GENETIC)—MOST COMMON CAUSE

ENDOCRINE CAUSES

Growth hormone excess—gigantism.
Sexual precocity (tall as children, short as adults):
- True sexual precocity.
- Pseudosexual precocity.

Androgen deficiency:
- Klinefelter's syndrome.
- Bilateral anorchism.

GENETIC CAUSES

Klinefelter's syndrome.
Syndromes of XYY, XXYY.

MISCELLANEOUS SYNDROMES AND DISORDERS

Cerebral gigantism or Sotos' syndrome: prominent forehead, hypertelorism, high arched palate, dolichocephaly, mental retardation, large hands and feet, and premature eruption of teeth. Large at birth, with most rapid growth in first 4 years of life.
Marfan's syndrome: disorder of mesodermal tissues, subluxation of the lenses, arachnodactyly, and aortic aneurysm.
Homocystinuria: same phenotype as Marfan's syndrome.
Obesity: tall as infants, children, and adolescents.
Total lipodystrophy: large hands and feet, generalized loss of subcutaneous fat, insulin-resistant diabetes mellitus, and hepatomegaly.
Beckwith-Wiedemann syndrome: neonatal tallness, omphalocele, macroglossia, and neonatal hypoglycemia.
Weaver-Smith syndrome: excessive intrauterine growth, mental retardation, megalocephaly, widened bifrontal diameter, hypertelorism, large ears, micrognathia, camptodactyly, broad thumbs, and limited extension of elbows and knees.
Marshall-Smith syndrome: excessive intrauterine growth, mental retardation, blue sclerae, failure to thrive, and early death.

TARDIVE DYSKINESIA[11]

ICD-9CM # 781.3 DYSKINESIA
300.11 HYSTERICAL DYSKINESIA
333.82 OROFACIAL DYSKINESIA
307.9 PSYCHOGENIC DYSKINESIA

DIFFERENTIAL DIAGNOSIS:

Medications (antidepressants, anticholinergics, amphetamines, lithium, l-dopa, phenytoin).
Brain neoplasms.
Ill-fitting dentures.
Huntington's disease.
Idiopathic dystonias (tics, blepharospasm, aging).
Wilson's disease.
Extrapyramidal syndrome (postanoxic or postencephalitic).
Torsion dystonia.

TASTE AND SMELL LOSS[1]

ICD-9CM # 781.1 SMELL AND TASTE DISTURBANCE OF SENSATION

TASTE

Local: radiation therapy.
Systemic: cancer, renal failure, hepatic failure, nutritional deficiency (vitamin B_{12}, zinc), Cushing's syndrome, hypothyroidism, DM, infection (influenza), drugs (antirheumatic and antiproliferative).
Neurologic: Bell's palsy, familial dysautonomia, multiple sclerosis.

SMELL

Local: allergic rhinitis, sinusitis, nasal polyposis, bronchial asthma.
Systemic: renal failure, hepatic failure, nutritional deficiency (vitamin B_{12}), Cushing's syndrome, hypothyroidism, DM, infection (viral hepatitis, influenza), drugs (nasal sprays, antibiotics).
Neurologic: head trauma, multiple sclerosis, Parkinson's disease, frontal brain tumor.

TELANGIECTASIA

ICD-9CM # 448.9

Oral contraceptive agents.
Pregnancy.
Rosacea.
Varicose veins.
Trauma.
Drug induced (corticosteroids, systemic or topical).
Spider telangiectases.
Hepatic cirrhosis.
Mastocytosis.
SLE, dermatomyositis, systemic sclerosis.

TENDINOPATHY[23]

ICD-9CM # 727.9

INTRINSIC FACTORS

Anatomic factors
Malalignment.
Muscle weakness or imbalance.
Muscle inflexibility.
Decreased vascularity.
Systemic factors
Inflammatory conditions (e.g., SLE).
Pregnancy.
Quinolone-induced tendinopathy.
Age-related factors
Tendon degeneration.
Increased tendon stiffness.
Tendon calcification.
Decreased vascularity.

EXTRINSIC FACTORS

Repetitive mechanical load
Excessive duration.
Excessive frequency.
Excessive intensity.
Poor technique.
Workplace factors.
Equipment problems
Footwear.
Athletic field surface.
Equipment factors (e.g., racquet size).
Protective gear.

TESTICULAR FAILURE[9]

ICD-9CM # 257.1 TESTICULAR FAILURE

PRIMARY

Klinefelter's syndrome (XXY).
XYY.
Vanishing testes syndrome (in utero or early postnatal torsion).
Noonan's syndrome.
Varicocele.
Myotonic dystrophy.
Orchitis (mumps, gonorrhea).
Cryptorchidism.
Chemical exposure.
Irradiation to testes.
Spinal cord injury.
Polyglandular failure.
Idiopathic oligospermia or azoospermia.
Germinal cell aplasia (Sertoli cell–only syndrome).
Idiopathic testicular failure.
Testicular torsion.
Testicular trauma.
Diethylstilbestrol (maternal use during pregnancy resulting in in utero estrogen exposure).
Testicular tumor with subsequent irradiation therapy, chemotherapy, or surgery (retroperitoneal lymph node dissection or orchiectomy).

SECONDARY

Delayed puberty.
Kallmann's syndrome.
Isolated gonadotropin deficiency.
Prader-Labhart-Willi syndrome.
Lawrence-Moon-Biedl syndrome.
Central nervous system irradiation.
Prepubertal panhypopituitarism.
Postpubertal panhypopituitarism.
Hypogonadism secondary to hyperprolactinemia.
Adrenogenital syndrome.
Chronic liver disease.
Chronic renal failure/uremia.
Hemochromatosis.
Cushing's syndrome.
Malnutrition.
Massive obesity.
Sickle cell anemia.
Hyper/hypothyroidism.
Anabolic steroid use.

TESTICULAR PAIN

ICD-9CM # 608.9

Testicular torsion.
Trauma.
Epididymitis.
Orchitis.
Neoplasm.
Urolithiasis.
Inguinal hernia.
Infection (cellulitis, abscess, folliculitis).
Anxiety.

TESTICULAR SIZE VARIATIONS[9]

ICD-9CM # 608.3 TESTICULAR ATROPHY
608.89 TESTICULAR MASS
257.2 HYPOGONADISM

SMALL TESTES

Hypothalamic-pituitary dysfunction.
Gonadotropin deficiency.
Growth hormone deficiency.
Normal variant.
Primary hypogonadism.
Autoimmune destruction, chemotherapy, cryptorchidism, irradiation, Klinefelter's syndrome, orchiditis, testicular regression syndrome, torsion, trauma.

LARGE TESTES

Adrenal rest tissue.
Compensatory.
Fragile X syndrome.
Idiopathic.
Tumor.

TETANUS[23]

ICD-9CM # 037

Acute abdomen.
Black widow spider bite.
Dental abscess.
Dislocated mandible.
Dystonic reaction.
Encephalitis.
Head trauma.
Hyperventilation syndrome.
Hypocalcemia.
Meningitis.
Peritonsillar abscess.
Progressive fluctuating muscular rigidity (stiff-man syndrome).
Psychogenic.
Rabics.
Sepsis.
Subarachnoid hemorrhage.
Status epilepticus.
Strychnine poisoning.
Temporomandibular joint syndrome.

THROMBOCYTOPENIA

ICD-9CM # 287.3 CONGENITAL OR PRIMARY
287.4 SECONDARY
287.5 THROMBOCYTOPENIA NOS

INCREASED DESTRUCTION

Immunologic
Drugs: quinine, quinidine, digitalis, procainamide, thiazide diuretics, sulfonamides, phenytoin, aspirin, penicillin, heparin, gold, meprobamate, sulfa drugs, phenylbutazone, nonsteroidal anti-inflammatory drugs (NSAIDs), methyldopa, cimetidine, furosemide, INH, cephalosporins, chlorpropamide, organic arsenicals, chloroquine, platelet glycoprotein IIb/IIIa receptor inhibitors, ranitidine, indomethacin, carboplatin, ticlopidine, clopidogrel.
Idiopathic thrombocytopenic purpura (ITP).
Transfusion reaction: transfusion of platelets with plasminogen activator (PLA) in recipients without PLA-1.
Fetal/maternal incompatibility.
Collagen vascular diseases (e.g., systemic lupus erythematosus [SLE]).
Autoimmune hemolytic anemia.
Lymphoreticular disorders (e.g., CLL).
Nonimmunologic
Prosthetic heart valves.
Thrombotic thrombocytopenic purpura (TTP).
Sepsis.
DIC.
Hemolytic-uremic syndrome (HUS).
Giant cavernous hemangioma.

DECREASED PRODUCTION

Abnormal marrow.
Marrow infiltration (e.g., leukemia, lymphoma, fibrosis).
Marrow suppression (e.g., chemotherapy, alcohol, radiation).
Hereditary disorders.
Wiskott-Aldrich syndrome: X-linked disorder characterized by thrombocytopenia, eczema, and repeated infections.
May-Hegglin anomaly: increased megakaryocytes but ineffective thrombopoiesis.
Vitamin deficiencies (e.g., vitamin B_{12}, folic acid).

SPLENIC SEQUESTRATION, HYPERSPLENISM

DILUTIONAL, AS A RESULT OF MASSIVE TRANSFUSION

THROMBOCYTOSIS

ICD-9CM # 289.9 THROMBOCYTOSIS, ESSENTIAL

Iron deficiency.
Posthemorrhage.
Neoplasms (GI tract).
CML.
Polycythemia vera.
Myelofibrosis with myeloid metaplasia.
Infections.
After splenectomy.
Postpartum.
Hemophilia.
Pancreatitis.
Cirrhosis.
Idiopathic.

THYROMEGALY

ICD-9CM # CODE VARIES WITH SPECIFIC DIAGNOSIS

Goiter.
Graves' disease.
Thyroiditis (lymphocytic, granulomatous, suppurative).
Toxic adenoma.
Neoplasm (primary, metastatic).

TICK-RELATED INFECTIONS

ICD-9CM # 082.0 ROCKY MOUNTAIN SPOTTED FEVER
066.1 COLORADO TICK FEVER
088.82 BABESIOSIS
082.8 EHRLICHIOSIS
088.81 LYME DISEASE

Lyme disease.
Rocky Mountain spotted fever.
Babesiosis.
Tularemia.
Q fever.
Colorado tick fever.
Ehrlichiosis.
Relapsing fever.

TICS

ICD-9CM # 307.20

Tourette's syndrome.
Physiologic tic.
Anxiety disorder.
Huntington's disease.
Medications (e.g., antipsychotics, carbamazepine, phenytoin, phenobarbital).
Encephalitis.
Head trauma.
Schizophrenia.
Carbon monoxide poisoning.
Stroke.
Sydenham's chorea.
Creutzfeldt-Jakob disease.

TORSADES DE POINTES[19]

ICD-9CM # CODE NOT AVAILABLE

Antiarrhythmics known to increase the QT interval (e.g., quinidine, procainamide, amiodarone, disopyramide, sotalol).
Tricyclic antidepressants and phenothiazines.
Histamine (H1) antagonists (e.g., astemizole, terfenadine).
Antiviral and antifungal agents and antibiotics.
Hypokinemia.
Hypomagnesemia.
Insecticide poisoning.
Bradyarrhythmias.
Congenital long QT syndrome.
Subarachnoid hemorrhage.
Chloroquinine, pentamidine.
Cocaine abuse.

TREMOR

ICD-9CM # 781.0 TREMOR NOS
333.1 BENIGN ESSENTIAL TREMOR
333.1 FAMILIAL TREMOR

TREMOR PRESENT AT REST

Parkinsonism.
CNS neoplasms.
Tardive dyskinesia.

POSTURAL TREMOR (PRESENT DURING MAINTENANCE OF A POSTURE)

Essential senile tremor.

ACTION TREMOR (PRESENT WITH MOVEMENT)

Anxiety.
Medications (bronchodilators, caffeine, corticosteroids, lithium, etc.).
Endocrine disorders (hyperthyroidism, pheochromocytoma, carcinoid).
Withdrawal from substance abuse.

TUBULOINTERSTITIAL DISEASE, ACUTE[12]

ICD-9CM # 584.5

DRUGS

Antibiotics, penicillins, cephalosporins, rifampin.
Sulfonamides: cotrimoxazole, sulfamethoxazole.
NSAIDs: propionic acid derivatives.
Miscellaneous: phenytoin, thiazides, allopurinol, cimetidine, ifosfamide.

INFECTIONS

Invasion of renal parenchyma.
Reaction to systemic infections: streptococcal, diphtheria, hantavirus.

SYSTEMIC DISEASES

Immune mediated: lupus, transplanted kidney, cryoglobulinemias.
Metabolic: urate, oxalate.
Neoplastic: lymphoproliferative diseases.

IDIOPATHIC

TUBULOINTERSTITIAL KIDNEY DISEASE[12]

ICD-9CM # 584.5

Ischemic and toxic acute tubular necrosis.
Allergic interstitial nephritis.
Interstitial nephritis secondary to immune complex-related collagen vascular disease (e.g., SLE, Sjögren's).
Granulomatous diseases (sarcoidosis, uveitis).
Pigment-related tubular injury (myoglobinuria, hemoglobinuria).
Hypercalcemia with nephrocalcinosis.
Tubular obstruction (drugs such as indinavir, uric acid in tumor lysis syndrome).
Myeloma kidney or cast nephropathy.
Infection-related interstitial nephritis: *legionella, leptospira*.
Infiltrative diseases (e.g., lymphoma).

URETHRAL DISCHARGE AND DYSURIA

ICD-9CM # 788.7 URETHRAL DISCHARGE
599.9 URETHRAL DISCHARGE BLOODY
788.1 DYSURIA

Urethritis (gonococcal, chlamydial, trichomonal).
Cystitis.
Prostatitis.
Vaginitis (candidiasis, chemical).
Meatal stenosis.
Interstitial cystitis.
Trauma (foreign body, masturbation, horseback or bike riding).

URIC ACID STONES

ICD-9CM # 792.9

Hyperuricemia.
Excessive dietary purine.
Medications (salicylates, allopurinol, probenecid).
Urine pH <5.5 (e.g., diarrhea, high animal protein diet).
Decreased urine output (dehydration, malabsorption, diarrhea, inadequate fluid intake).
Tumor lysis.
Hemolytic anemia.
Myeloproliferative disorders.

URINARY RETENTION, ACUTE

ICD-9CM # 788.20

Mechanical obstruction: urethral stone, foreign body, urethral stricture, BPH, prostate carcinoma, prostatitis, trauma with hematoma formation.
Neurogenic bladder.
Neurologic disease (MS, parkinsonism, tabes dorsalis, CVA).
Spinal cord injury.
CNS neoplasm (primary or metastatic).
Spinal anesthesia.
Lower urinary tract instrumentation.
Medications (antihistamines, antidepressants, narcotics, anticholinergics).
Abdominal or pelvic surgery.
Alcohol toxicity.
Pregnancy.
Anxiety.
Encephalitis.
Postoperative pain.
Encephalitis.
Spina bifida occulta.

URINE, RED[26]

ICD-9CM # CODE VARIES WITH SPECIFIC DIAGNOSIS

WITH A POSITIVE DIPSTICK

Hematuria.
Hemoglobinuria: negative urinalysis.
Myoglobinuria: negative urinalysis.

WITH A NEGATIVE DIPSTICK

Drugs
Aminosalicylic acid.
Deferoxamine mesylate.
Ibuprofen.
Phenacetin.
Phenolphthalein.
Phensuximide.
Rifampin.
Anthraquinone laxatives.
Doxorubicin.
Methyldopa.
Phenazopyridine.
Phenothiazine.
Phenytoin.
Dyes
Azo dyes.
Eosin.
Foods
Beets, berries, maize.
Rhodamine B.
Metabolic
Porphyrins.
Serratia marcescens (red diaper syndrome).
Urate crystalluria.

UROPATHY, OBSTRUCTIVE[33]

ICD-9CM # 599.6

INTRINSIC CAUSES

Intraluminal
Intratubular deposition of crystals (uric acid, sulfas).
Stones.
Papillary tissue.
Blood clots.
Intramural
Functional.
Ureter (ureteropelvic or ureterovesical dysfunction).
Bladder (neurogenic): spinal cord defect or trauma, diabetes, multiple sclerosis, Parkinson's disease, cerebrovascular accidents.
Bladder neck dysfunction.
Anatomic
Tumors.
Infection, granuloma.
Strictures.

EXTRINSIC CAUSES

Originating in the reproductive system
Prostate: benign hypertrophy or cancer.
Uterus: pregnancy, tumors, prolapse, endometriosis.
Ovary: abscess, tumor, cysts.
Originating in the vascular system
Aneurysms (aorta, iliac vessels).
Aberrant arteries (ureteropelvic junction).
Venous (ovarian veins, retrocaval ureter).
Originating in the gastrointestinal tract
Crohn's disease.
Pancreatitis.
Appendicitis.
Tumors.
Originating in the retroperitoneal space
Inflammations.
Fibrosis.
Tumor, hematomas.

UTERINE BLEEDING, ABNORMAL[10]

ICD-9CM # 626.9

PREGNANCY

Threatened abortion.
Incomplete abortion.
Complete abortion.
Molar pregnancy.
Ectopic pregnancy.
Retained products of conception.

OVULATORY

Vulva: infection, laceration, tumor.
Vagina: infection, laceration, tumor, foreign body.
Cervix: polyps, cervical erosion, cervicitis, carcinoma.
Uterus: fibroids (submucous fibroids most likely to cause abnormal bleeding), polyps, adenomyosis, endometritis, intrauterine device, atrophic endometrium.
Pregnancy complications: ectopic pregnancy; threatened, incomplete, complete abortion; retained products of conception.
Abnormality of clotting system.
Midcycle bleeding.
Halban's disease (persistent corpus luteum).
Menorrhagia.
Pelvic inflammatory disease.

ANOVULATORY

Physiologic causes:
- Puberty.
- Perimenopausal.

Pathologic causes:
- Ovarian failure (FSH over 40 IU/ml).
- Hyperandrogenism.
- Hyperprolactinemia.
- Obesity.
- Hypothalamic dysfunction (polycystic ovaries); LH/FSH ratio greater than 2 to 1.
- Hyperplasia.
- Endometrial carcinoma.
- Estrogen-producing tumors.
- Hypothyroidism.

VAGINAL BLEEDING, PREGNANCY[7]

ICD-9CM # 626.6 IRREGULAR VAGINAL BLEEDING

FIRST TRIMESTER

Implantation bleeding.
Abortion.
Threatened.
Complete.
Incomplete.
Missed.
Ectopic pregnancy.
Neoplasia.
Hydatidiform mole.
Cervix.

THIRD TRIMESTER

Placenta previa.
Placental abruption.
Premature labor.
Choriocarcinoma.

VAGINAL DISCHARGE, PREPUBERTAL GIRLS[17]

ICD-9CM # 623.5 VAGINAL DISCHARGE

Irritative (bubble baths, sand).
Poor perineal hygiene.
Foreign body.
Associated systemic illness (group A streptococci, chickenpox).
Infections.
Escherichia coli with foreign body.
Shigella organisms.
Yersinia organisms.
Infections (consider sexual abuse).
Chlamydia trachomatis.
Neisseria gonorrhoeae.
Trichomonas vaginalis.
Tumor (rare).

VASCULITIS, CLASSIFICATION[23]

ICD-9CM # 447.6

LARGE VESSEL DISEASE

Arteritis
Giant cell arteritis.
Takayasu's arteritis.
Arteritis associated with Reiter's syndrome, ankylosing spondylitis.

MEDIUM AND SMALL VESSEL DISEASE

Polyarteritis nodosa
Primary (idiopathic).
Associated with viruses (Hepatitis B or C, CMV, HIV, herpes zoster).
Associated with malignancy (hairy cell leukemia).
Familial Mediterranean fever.
Granulomatous vasculitis
Wegener's granulomatosis.
Lymphomatoid granulomatosis.
Behçet's disease
Kawasaki disease (mucocutaneous lymph node syndrome)

PREDOMINANTLY SMALL VESSEL DISEASE

Hypersensitivity vasculitis (leukocytoclastic vasculitis)
Henoch-Schönlein purpura.
Mixed cryoglobulinemia.
Serum sickness.
Vasculitis associated with connective tissue diseases (SLE, Sjögren's syndrome).
Vasculitis associated with specific syndromes:
Primary biliary cirrhosis.
Lyme disease.
Chronic active hepatitis.
Drug-induced vasculitis.
Churg-Strauss syndrome
Goodpasture's syndrome
Erythema nodosum
Panniculitis
Buerger's disease (thrombophlebitis obliterans)

VASCULITIS (DISEASES THAT MIMIC VASCULITIS)[25]

ICD-9CM # CODE VARIES WITH SPECIFIC DISEASE

EMBOLIC DISEASE

Infectious or marantic endocarditis.
Cardiac mural thrombus.
Atrial myxoma.
Cholesterol embolization syndrome.

NONINFLAMMATORY VESSEL WALL DISRUPTION

Atherosclerosis.
Arterial fibromuscular dysplasia.
Drug effects (vasoconstrictors, anticoagulants).
Radiation.
Genetic disease (neurofibromatosis, Ehlers-Danlos syndrome).
Amyloidosis.
Intravascular malignant lymphoma.

DIFFUSE COAGULATION

Disseminated intravascular coagulation.
Thrombotic thrombocytopenic purpura.
Hemolytic-uremic syndrome.
Protein C and S deficiencies, factor V/Leiden mutation.
Antiphospholipid syndrome.

VENTILATION–PERFUSION MISMATCH ON LUNG SCAN

ICD-9CM # CODE VARIES WITH SPECIFIC DISORDER

Pulmonary embolism.
Emphysema.
Irradiation.
Pulmonary hypertension.
AV malformations.
Pulmonary thrombosis.
External compression of pulmonary artery (neoplasm, cysts, fibrosing mediastinitis).
Vasculitis.
Tuberculosis.
Pulmonary thrombosis.
Congenital (pulmonary artery hypoplasia, congenital heart disease with upper lobe diversion).
Sequestered segment.
Parasitic lung disease.
Intraluminal obstruction from catheter fragments.

VENTRICULAR FAILURE

ICD-9CM # 429.9 VENTRICULAR DYSFUNCTION

LEFT VENTRICULAR FAILURE

Systemic hypertension.
Valvular heart disease (AS, AR, MR).
Cardiomyopathy, myocarditis.
Bacterial endocarditis.
Myocardial infarction.
Idiopathic hypertrophic subaortic stenosis.

RIGHT VENTRICULAR FAILURE

Valvular heart disease (mitral stenosis).
Pulmonary hypertension.
Bacterial endocarditis (right-sided).
Right ventricular infarction.

BIVENTRICULAR FAILURE

Left ventricular failure.
Cardiomyopathy.
Myocarditis
Arrhythmias.
Anemia.
Thyrotoxicosis.
Arteriovenous fistula.
Paget's disease.
Beri-beri.

VERRUCOUS LESIONS

ICD-9CM # CODE VARIES WITH SPECIFIC DISORDER

Warts.
Seborrheic keratosis.
Lichen simplex.
Acanthosis nigricans.
Scabies (Norwegian, crusted).
Verrucous carcinoma.
Nevus sebaceous.
Deep fungal infection.

VERTIGO

ICD-9CM # 780.4 VERTIGO NOS
386.11 BENIGN PAROXYSMAL POSITIONAL
386.2 CENTRAL ORIGIN
386.10 PERIPHERAL
386.12 VESTIBULAR (NEURONITIS)

PERIPHERAL

Otitis media.
Acute labyrinthitis.
Vestibular neuronitis.
Benign positional vertigo.
Meniere's disease.
Ototoxic drugs: streptomycin, gentamicin.
Lesions of the eighth nerve: acoustic neuroma, meningioma, mononeuropathy, metastatic carcinoma.
Mastoiditis.

CNS OR SYSTEMIC

Vertebrobasilar artery insufficiency.
Posterior fossa tumor or other brain tumors.
Infarction/hemorrhage of cerebral cortex, cerebellum, or brainstem.
Basilar migraine.
Metabolic: drugs, hypoxia, anemia, fever.
Hypotension/severe hypertension.
Multiple sclerosis.
CNS infections: viral, bacterial.
Temporal lobe epilepsy.
Arnold-Chiari malformation, syringobulbia.
Psychogenic: ventilation, hysteria.

VESICULOBULLOUS DISEASES[12]

ICD-9CM # 709.8

IMMUNOLOGICALLY MEDIATED DISEASES

Bullous pemphigoid.
Herpes gestationis.
Mucous membrane pemphigoid.
Epidermolysis bullosa acquisita.
Dermatitis herpetiformis.
Pemphigus (vulgaris, foliaceus, paraneoplastic).

HYPERSENSITIVITY DISEASES

Erythema multiforme minor.
Erythema multiforme major (Stevens-Johnson syndrome).
Toxic epidermal necrolysis.

METABOLIC DISEASES

Porphyria cutanea tarda.
Pseudoporphyria.
Diabetic blisters.

INHERITED GENETIC DISORDERS

Epidermolysis bullosa.
- Simplex.
- Junctional.
- Dystrophic.

INFECTIOUS DISEASES

Impetigo.
Staphylococcal scalded skin syndrome.
Herpes simplex.
Varicella.
Herpes zoster.

VISION LOSS, ACUTE, PAINFUL

ICD-9CM # 368.11 VISION LOSS, SUDDEN

Acute angle-closure glaucoma.
Corneal ulcer.
Uveitis.
Endophthalmitis.
Factitious.
Somatization syndrome.
Trauma.

VISION LOSS, ACUTE, PAINLESS

ICD-9CM # 368.11 VISION LOSS, SUDDEN

Retinal artery occlusion.
Optic neuritis.
Retinal vein occlusion.
Vitreous hemorrhage.
Retinal detachment.
Exudative macular degeneration.
CVA.
Ischemic optic neuropathy.
Factitious.
Somatization syndrome, anxiety reaction.

VISION LOSS, CHILDREN

ICD-9CM # 368.9

Craniopharyngioma.
Hereditary optic atrophy.
Optic nerve glioma.
Glioma of chiasm.
Albinism.
Optic nerve hypoplasia.

VISION LOSS, CHRONIC, PROGRESSIVE

ICD-9CM # 369.9 VISION LOSS NOS

Cataract.
Macular degeneration.
Cerebral neoplasm.
Refractive error.
Open-angle glaucoma.

VISION LOSS, MONOCULAR, TRANSIENT

ICD-9CM # 369.9

Thromboembolism.
Vasculitis.
Migraine (vasospasm).
Anxiety reaction.
CNS tumor.
Temporal arteritis.
Multiple sclerosis.

VOCAL CORD PARALYSIS

ICD-9CM # 478.30 UNSPECIFIED
478.31 UNILATERAL PARTIAL
478.32 UNILATERAL COMPLETE
478.33 BILATERAL PARTIAL
478.34 BILATERAL COMPLETE

Neoplasm: primary or metastatic (e.g., lung, thyroid, parathyroid, mediastinum).
Neck surgery (parathyroid, thyroid, carotid endarterectomy, cervical spine).
Idiopathic.
Viral, bacterial, or fungal infection.
Trauma (intubation, penetrating neck injury).
Cardiac surgery.
Rheumatoid arthritis.
Multiple sclerosis.
Parkinsonism.
Toxic neuropathy.
CVA.
CNS abnormalities: hydrocephalus, Arnold-Chiari malformation, meningomyelocele.

VOLUME DEPLETION[1]

ICD-9CM # 276.5

Gastrointestinal losses:
- Upper: bleeding, nasogastric suction, vomiting.
- Lower: bleeding, diarrhea, enteric or pancreatic fistula, tube drainage.

Renal losses:
- Salt and water: diuretics, osmotic diuresis, postobstructive diuresis, acute tubular necrosis (recovery phase), salt-losing nephropathy, adrenal insufficiency, renal tubular acidosis.

Water loss: diabetes insipidus.
Skin and respiratory losses:
- Sweat, burns, insensible losses.

Sequestration without external fluid loss:
- Intestinal obstruction, peritonitis, pancreatitis, rhabdomyolysis, internal bleeding.

VOLUME EXCESS[1]

ICD-9CM # CODE VARIES WITH SPECIFIC DIAGNOSIS

PRIMARY RENAL SODIUM RETENTION (INCREASED EFFECTIVE CIRCULATING VOLUME)

Renal failure, nephritic syndrome, acute glomerulonephritis.
Primary hyperaldosteronism.
Cushing's syndrome.
Liver disease.

SECONDARY RENAL SODIUM RETENTION (DECREASED EFFECTIVE CIRCULATING VOLUME)

Heart failure.
Liver disease.
Nephrotic syndrome (minimal change disease).
Pregnancy.

VOMITING

ICD-9CM # 787.03

GI disturbances:
Obstruction: esophageal, pyloric, intestinal.
Infections: viral or bacterial enteritis, viral hepatitis, food poisoning, gastroenteritis.
Pancreatitis.
Appendicitis.
Biliary colic.
Peritonitis.
Perforated bowel.
Diabetic gastroparesis.
Other: gastritis, PUD, IBD, GI tract neoplasms.
Drugs: morphine, digitalis, cytotoxic agents, bromocriptine.
Severe pain: MI, renal colic.
Metabolic disorders: uremia, acidosis/alkalosis, hyperglycemia, DKA, thyrotoxicosis.
Trauma: blows to the testicles, epigastrium.
Vertigo.
Reye's syndrome.
Increased intracranial pressure.
CNS disturbances: trauma, hemorrhage, infarction, neoplasm, infection, hypertensive encephalopathy, migraine.
Radiation sickness.
Nausea and vomiting of pregnancy, hyperemesis gravidarum.
Motion sickness.

Bulimia, anorexia nervosa.
Psychogenic: emotional disturbances, offensive sights or smells.
Severe coughing.
Pyelonephritis.
Boerhaave's syndrome.
Carbon monoxide poisoning.

VULVAR LESIONS[10]

ICD-9CM # 625.8 VULVAR MASS
098.0 VULVAR ULCER, GONOCOCCAL
091.0 VULVAR ULCER, SYPHILITIC
616.51 BEHÇET'S
624.0 LEUKOPLAKIA
624.8 DYSPLASIA
233.3 CARCINOMA
616.9 INFLAMMATORY LESION
624.4 VULVAR SCAR (OLD)
624.1 VULVAR ATROPHY

RED LESION

Infection/infestation

Fungal infection:
- Candida.
- Tinea cruris.
- Intertrigo.
- Pityriasis versicolor.

Sarcoptes scabiei.
Erythrasma: *Corynebacterium minutissimum.*
Granuloma inguinale: *Calymmatobacterium granulomatis.*
Folliculitis: *Staphylococcus aureus.*
Hidradenitis suppurativa.
Behçet's syndrome.

Inflammation

Reactive vulvitis.
Chemical irritation:
- Detergent.
- Dyes.
- Perfume.
- Spermicide.
- Lubricants.
- Hygiene sprays.
- Podophyllum.
- Topical 5-FU.
- Saliva.
- Gentian violet.
- Semen.

Mechanical trauma: scratching.
Vestibular adenitis.
Essential vulvodynia.
Psoriasis.
Seborrheic dermatitis.

Neoplasm

Vulvar intraepithelial neoplasia (VIN):
- Mild dysplasia.
- Moderate dysplasia.
- Severe dysplasia.
- Carcinoma-in-situ.

Vulvar dystrophy.
Bowen's disease.
Invasive cancer:
- Squamous cell carcinoma.
- Malignant melanoma.
- Sarcoma.
- Basal cell carcinoma.
- Adenocarcinoma.
- Paget's disease.
- Undifferentiated.

WHITE LESION

Vulvar dystrophy:
- Lichen sclerosus.
- Vulvar dystrophy.
- Vulvar hyperplasia.
- Mixed dystrophy.

VIN.
Vitiligo.
Partial albinism.
Intertrigo.
Radiation treatment.

DARK LESION

Lentigo.
Nevi (mole).
Neoplasm (see Neoplasm, Vulvar, below).
Reactive hyperpigmentation.
Seborrheic keratosis.
Pubic lice.

ULCERATIVE LESION

Infection

Herpes simplex.
Vaccinia.
Treponema pallidum.
Granuloma inguinale.
Pyoderma.
Tuberculosis.

Noninfection

Behçet's disease.
Crohn's disease.
Pemphigus.
Pemphigoid.
Hidradenitis suppurativa (see Neoplasm, Vulvar, below).

Neoplasm

Basal cell carcinoma.
Squamous cell carcinoma.
Vulvar tumor <1 cm:
- Condyloma acuminatum.
- Molluscum contagiosum.
- Epidermal inclusion.
- Vestibular cyst.
- Mesenephric duct.
- VIN.
- Hemangioma.
- Hidradenoma.
- Neurofibroma.
- Syringoma.
- Accessory breast tissue.
- Acrochordon.
- Endometriosis.
- Fox-Fordyce disease.
- Pilonidal sinus.

Vulvar tumor >1 cm:
- Bartholin cyst or abscess.
- Lymphogranuloma venereum.
- Fibroma.
- Lipoma.
- Verrucous carcinoma.
- Squamous cell carcinoma.
- Hernia.
- Edema.
- Hematoma.
- Acrochordon.
- Epidermal cysts.
- Neurofibromatosis.
- Accessory breast tissue.

WEAKNESS, ACUTE, EMERGENT[23]

ICD-9CM # 780.7

Demyelinating disorders (Guillain-Barré, chronic inflammatory demyelinating polyneuropathy [CIDP]).
Myasthenia gravis.
Infectious (poliomyelitis, diphtheria).
Toxic (botulism, tick paralysis, paralytic shellfish toxin, puffer fish, newts).
Metabolic (acquired or familial hypokalemia, hypophosphatemia, hypermagnesemia).
Metals poisoning (arsenic, thallium).
Porphyria.

WEAKNESS, GRADUAL ONSET

ICD-9CM # 780.7

Depression.
Malingering.
Anemia.
Hypothyroidism.
Medications (e.g., sedatives, antidepressants, narcotics).
CHF.
Renal failure.
Liver failure.
Respiratory insufficiency.
Alcoholism.
Nutritional deficiencies.
Disorders of motor unit.
Basal ganglia disorders.
Upper motor neuron lesions.

WEAKNESS, NONNEUROMUSCULAR CAUSES

ICD-9CM # 780.79

Anxiety disorder.
Infectious process.
Anemia.
Renal insufficiency.
Hyperventilation.
Malignancy.
Hypothyroidism.
Hypotension.
Hypercapnia.
Hypoglycemia.
Cardiac arrhythmias.
Hepatic insufficiency.
Electrolyte imbalance.
Malnutrition.
Cerebrovascular insufficiency.

WEIGHT GAIN

ICD-9CM # 783.1 ABNORMAL WEIGHT GAIN
278.00 OBESITY

Sedentary lifestyle.
Fluid overload.
Discontinuation of tobacco abuse.

Endocrine disorders (hypothyroidism, hyperinsulinism associated with maturity-onset DM, Cushing's syndrome, hypogonadism, insulinoma, hyperprolactinemia, acromegaly).
Medications (nutritional supplements, oral contraceptives, glucocorticoids, etc.).
Anxiety disorders with compulsive eating.
Laurence-Moon-Biedl syndrome, Prader-Willi syndrome, other congenital diseases.
Hypothalamic injury (rare; <100 cases reported in medical literature).

WEIGHT LOSS

ICD-9CM # 783.2 ABNORMAL WEIGHT LOSS

Malignancy.
Psychiatric disorders (depression, anorexia nervosa).
New-onset DM.
Malabsorption.
COPD.
AIDS.
Uremia, liver disease.
Thyrotoxicosis, pheochromocytoma, carcinoid syndrome.
Addison's disease.
Intestinal parasites.
Peptic ulcer disease.
Inflammatory bowel disease.
Food faddism.
Postgastrectomy syndrome.

WHEEZING

ICD-9CM # 786.09

Asthma.
COPD.
Interstitial lung disease.
Infections (pneumonia, bronchitis, bronchiolitis, epiglottitis).
Cardiac asthma.
GERD with aspiration.
Foreign body aspiration.
Pulmonary embolism.
Anaphylaxis.
Obstruction airway (neoplasm, goiter, edema or hemorrhage from trauma, aneurysm, congenital abnormalities, strictures, spasm).
Carcinoid syndrome.

WHEEZING, PEDIATRIC AGE[4]

ICD-9CM # 786.09 WHEEZING

Reactive airways disease.
Atopic asthma.
Infection-associated airway reactivity.
Exercise-induced asthma.
Salicylate-induced asthma and nasal polyposis.
Asthmatic bronchitis.
Other hypersensitivity reactions:
  Hypersensitivity pneumonitis.
  Tropical eosinophilia.
  Visceral larva migrans.
  Allergic bronchopulmonary aspergillosis.
Aspiration:
  Foreign body.
  Food, saliva, gastric contents.
  Laryngotracheoesophageal cleft.
  Tracheoesophageal fistula, H-type.
  Pharyngeal incoordination or neuromuscular weakness.
Cystic fibrosis.
Primary ciliary dyskinesia.
Cardiac failure.
Bronchiolitis obliterans.
Extrinsic compression of airways:
  Vascular ring.
  Enlarged lymph node.
  Mediastinal tumor.
  Lung cysts.
Tracheobronchomalacia.
Endobronchial masses.
Gastroesophageal reflux.
Pulmonary hemosiderosis.
Sequelae of bronchopulmonary dysplasia.
"Hysterical" glottic closure.
Cigarette smoke, other environmental insults.

WRIST PAIN

ICD-9CM # 959.3

MECHANICAL

Osteoarthritis.
Ligament tear.
Fracture.
Ganglion.
De Quervain's tenosynovitis.
Avascular necrosis (scaphoid, lunate).
Nonunion of scaphoid or lunate.
Neoplasm.

METABOLIC

Pregnancy.
Diabetes.
Gout.
Pseudogout.
Paget's disease.
Acromegaly.
Hypothyroidism.
Hyperparathyroidism.

INFECTIOUS

Osteomyelitis.
Septic arthritis.
Cat-scratch disease.
Tick bite (Lyme disease, babesiosis).
Tuberculosis.

NEUROLOGIC

Peripheral neuropathy.
Nerve injury (median, ulnar, radial nerve).
Thoracic outlet compression syndrome.
Distal posterior interosseous nerve syndrome.

RHEUMATOLOGIC

Psoriasis.
Rheumatoid arthritis.
Systemic lupus erythematosus (SLE), mixed connective tissue disorder (MCTD).
Scleroderma.

MISCELLANEOUS

Granulomatous (sarcoidosis).
Amyloidosis.
Multiple myeloma.
Leukemia.

XEROPHTHALMIA[25]

ICD-9CM # 372.53 XEROPHTHALMIA

MEDICATIONS

Tricyclic antidepressants: amitriptyline (Elavil), doxepin (Sinequan).
Antihistamines: diphenhydramine (Benadryl), chlorpheniramine (Chlor-Trimeton), promethazine (Phenergan), and many cold and decongestant preparations.
Anticholinergic agents: antiemetics such as scopolamine, antispasmodic agents such as oxybutynin chloride (Ditropan).

ABNORMALITIES OF EYELID FUNCTION

Neuromuscular disorders.
Aging.
Thyrotoxicosis.

ABNORMALITIES OF TEAR PRODUCTION

Hypovitaminosis A.
Stevens-Johnson syndrome.
Familial diseases affecting sebaceous secretions.

ABNORMALITIES OF CORNEAL SURFACES

Scarring from past injuries and herpes simplex infection.

XEROSTOMIA[25]

ICD-9CM # 527.7

MEDICATIONS

Tricyclic antidepressants: amitriptyline (Elavil), doxepin (Sinequan).
Antihistamines: diphenhydramine (Benadryl), chlorpheniramine (Chlor-Trimeton), promethazine (Phenergan), and many cold and decongestant preparations.
Anticholinergic agents: antiemetics such as scopolamine, antispasmodic agents such as oxybutynin chloride (Ditropan).

DEHYDRATION

Debility.
Fever.

POLYURIA

Alcohol intake.
Arrhythmia.
Diabetes.

PREVIOUS HEAD AND NECK IRRADIATION

SYSTEMIC DISEASES

Sjögren's syndrome.
Sarcoidosis.
Amyloidosis.
Human immunodeficiency virus (HIV) infection.
Graft-vs.-host disease.

REFERENCES

1. Andreoli TE (ed): *Cecil essentials of medicine,* ed 5, Philadelphia, 2001, WB Saunders.
2. Barkin RM, Rosen P: *Emergency pediatrics: a guide to ambulatory care,* ed 5, St Louis, 1998, Mosby.
3. Baude AI: *Infectious diseases and medical microbiology,* ed 2, Philadelphia, 1986, WB Saunders.
4. Behrman RE: *Nelson textbook of pediatrics,* ed 16, Philadelphia, 2000, WB Saunders.
5. Callen JP: *Color atlas of dermatology,* ed 2, Philadelphia, 2000, WB Saunders.
6. Canoso J: *Rheumatology in primary care,* Philadelphia, 1997, WB Saunders.
7. Carlson KJ: *Primary care of women,* ed 2, St Louis, 2000, Mosby.
8. Conn R: *Current diagnosis,* ed 9, Philadelphia, 1997, WB Saunders.
9. Copeland LJ: *Textbook of gynecology,* ed 2, Philadelphia, 2000, WB Saunders.
10. Danakas G (ed): *Practical guide to the care of the gynecologic/obstetric patient,* St Louis, 1997, Mosby.
11. Goldberg RJ: *The care of the psychiatric patient,* ed 3, St Louis, 2006, Mosby.
12. Goldman L, Ausiello D: *Cecil textbook of medicine,* ed 21, Philadelphia, 2004, WB Saunders.
13. Goldman L, Braunwauld E (eds): *Primary cardiology,* Philadelphia, 1998, WB Saunders.
14. Gorbach SL: *Infectious diseases,* ed 2, Philadelphia, 1998, WB Saunders.
15. Harrington J: *Consultation in internal medicine,* ed 2, St Louis, 1997, Mosby.
16. Henry JB: *Clinical diagnosis and management by laboratory methods,* ed 20, Philadelphia, 2001, WB Saunders.
17. Hoekelman R: *Primary pediatric care,* ed 3, St Louis, 1997, Mosby.
18. Kassirer J (ed): *Current therapy in adult medicine,* ed 4, St Louis, 1998, Mosby.
19. Khan MG: *Rapid ECG interpretation,* Philadelphia, 2003, WB Saunders.
20. Kliegman R: *Practical strategies in pediatric diagnosis and therapy,* Philadelphia, 1996, WB Saunders.
21. Klippel J (ed): *Practical rheumatology,* London, 1995, Mosby.
22. Mandell GL: *Mandell, Douglas, and Bennett's principles and practice of infectious diseases,* ed 6, New York, 2005, Churchill Livingstone.
23. Marx J (ed): *Rosen's emergency medicine: concepts and clinical practice,* ed. 5, St Louis, 2002, Mosby.
24. Moore WT, Eastman RC: *Diagnostic endocrinology,* ed 2, St Louis, 1996, Mosby.
25. Noble J (ed): *Primary care medicine,* ed 3, St Louis, 2001, Mosby.
26. Nseyo UO: *Urology for primary care physicians,* Philadelphia, 1999, WB Saunders.
27. Palay D (ed): *Ophthalmology for the primary care physician,* St Louis, 1997, Mosby.
28. Rakel RE: *Principles of family practice,* ed 6, Philadelphia, 2002, WB Saunders.
29. Schwarz MI: *Interstitial lung disease,* ed 2, St Louis, 1993, Mosby.
30. Seller RH: *Differential diagnosis of common complaints,* ed 4, Philadelphia, 2000,WB Saunders.
31. Siedel HM (ed): *Mosby's guide to physical examination,* ed 4, St Louis, 1999, Mosby.
32. Specht N: *Practical guide to diagnostic imaging,* St Louis, 1998, Mosby.
33. Stein JH (ed): *Internal medicine,* ed 5, St Louis, 1998, Mosby.
34. Swain R, Snodgrass: *Phys Sportmed* 23:56, 1995.
35. Wiederholt WC: *Neurology for non-neurologists,* ed 4, Philadelphia, 2000, WB Saunders.
36. Wilson JD: *Williams textbook of endocrinology,* ed 9, Philadelphia, 1998, WB Saunders.

Section III

Clinical Algorithms

PLEASE NOTE: These algorithms are designed to assist clinicians in the evaluation and treatment of patients. They may not apply to all patients with a particular disorder and are not intended to replace the clinician's individual judgment.

ICD-9CM # 995.5 Child maltreatment syndrome

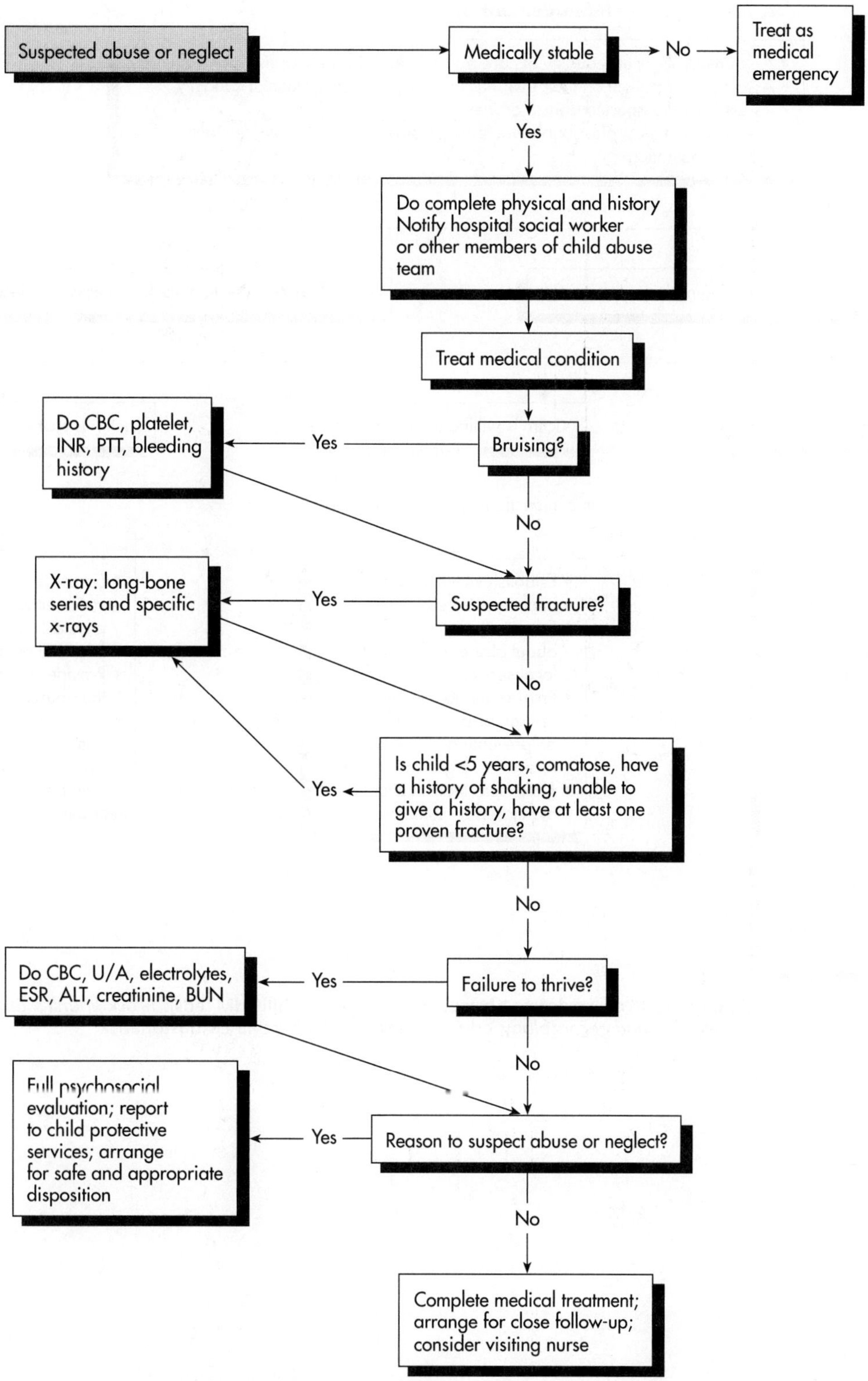

Note: Refer to Section I for additional information on this topic.

FIGURE 3-1 Management of suspected child abuse. *CBC,* Complete blood count; *ESR,* erythrocyte sedimentation rate; *INR,* international normalized ratio; *PTT,* partial thromboplastin time; *U/A,* urinalysis. (Modified from Marx J [ed]: *Rosen's emergency medicine,* ed 6, St Louis, 2006, Mosby.)

Management of Geriatric Abuse

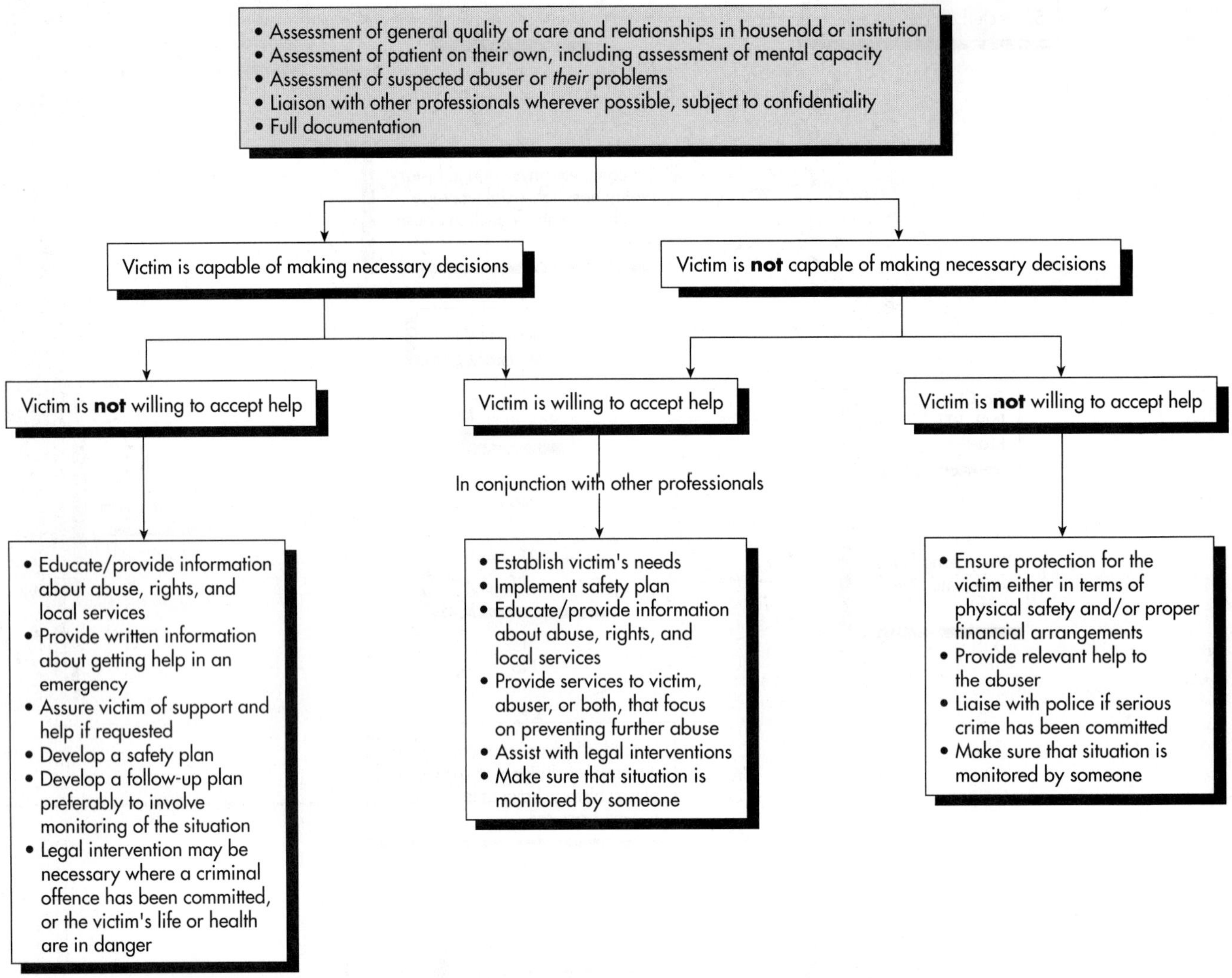

FIGURE 3-2 Management of geriatric abuse. (From Tallis RC, Fillit HM [eds]: *Brocklehurst's textbook of geriatric medicine and gerontology,* ed 6, London, 2003, Churchill Livingstone.)

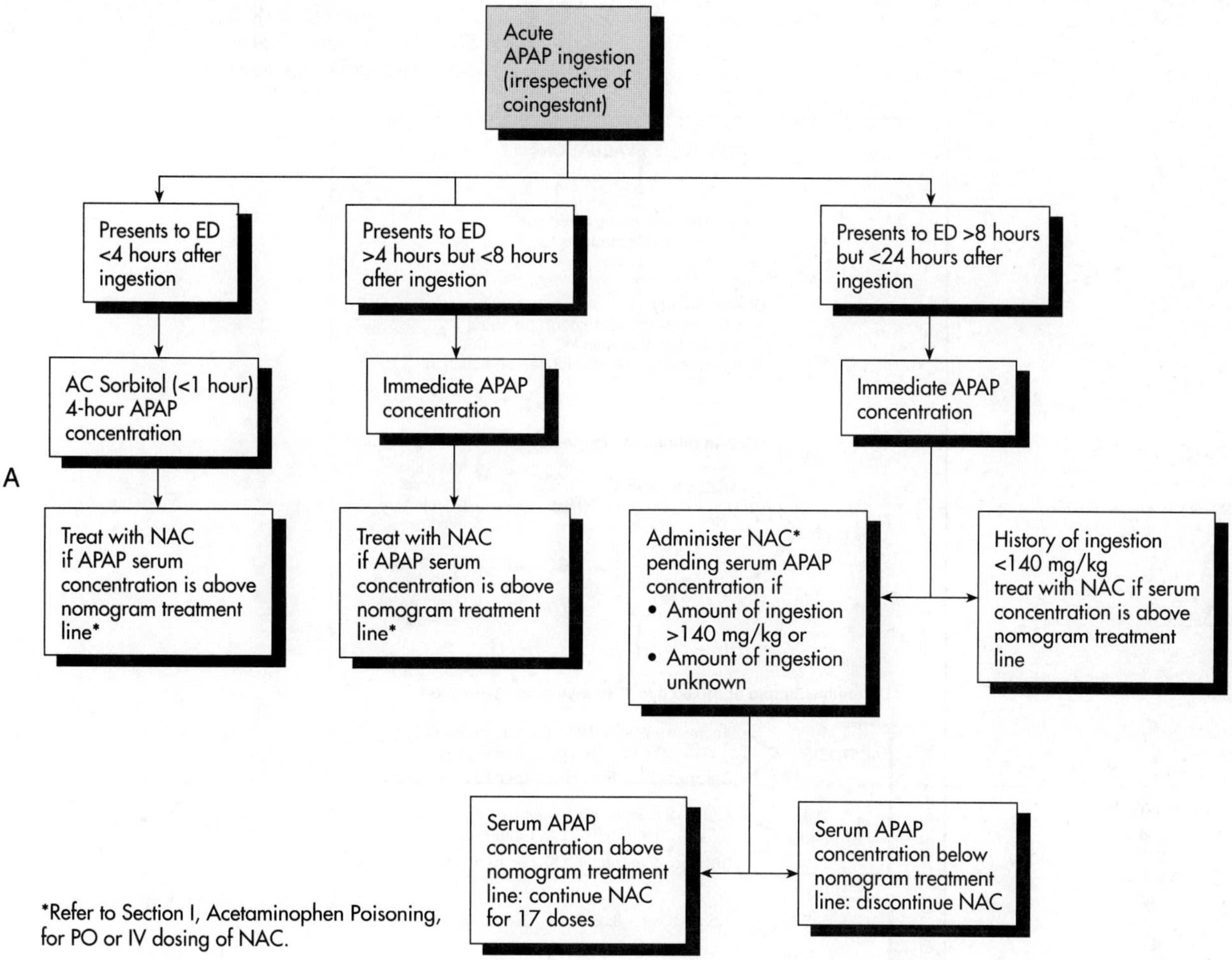

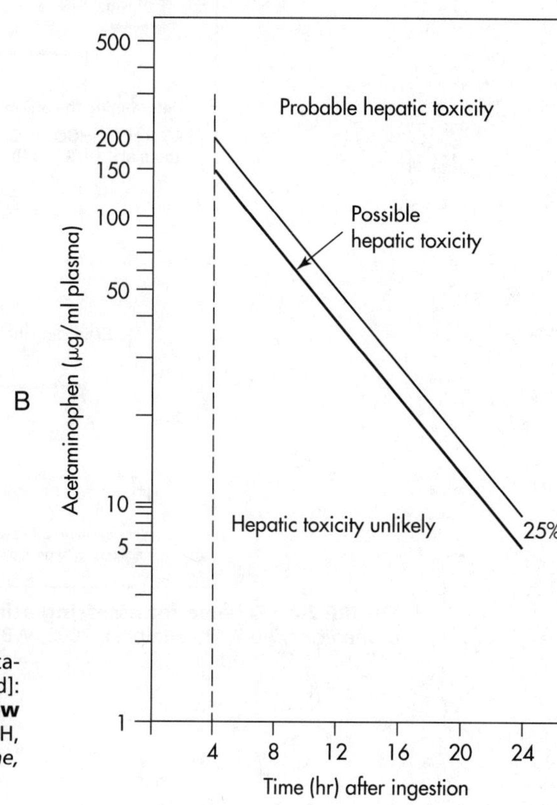

FIGURE 3-3 A, Treatment of acetaminophen ingestion. *APAP,* Acetaminophen; *ED,* emergency department; *NAC, N*-acetylcysteine. (From Marx J [ed]: *Rosen's emergency medicine,* ed 5, St Louis, 2002, Mosby.) **B, Rumack-Matthew nomogram for acetaminophen poisoning.** (Modified from Rumack BH, Matthew H: *Pediatrics* 55:871, 1975. In Marx J [ed]: *Rosen's emergency medicine,* ed 6, St Louis, 2006, Mosby.)

ICD-9CM # 276.2 Lactic acidosis
276.2 Metabolic acidosis
276.2 Respiratory acidosis
276.3 Respiratory alkalosis
276.3 Metabolic alkalosis

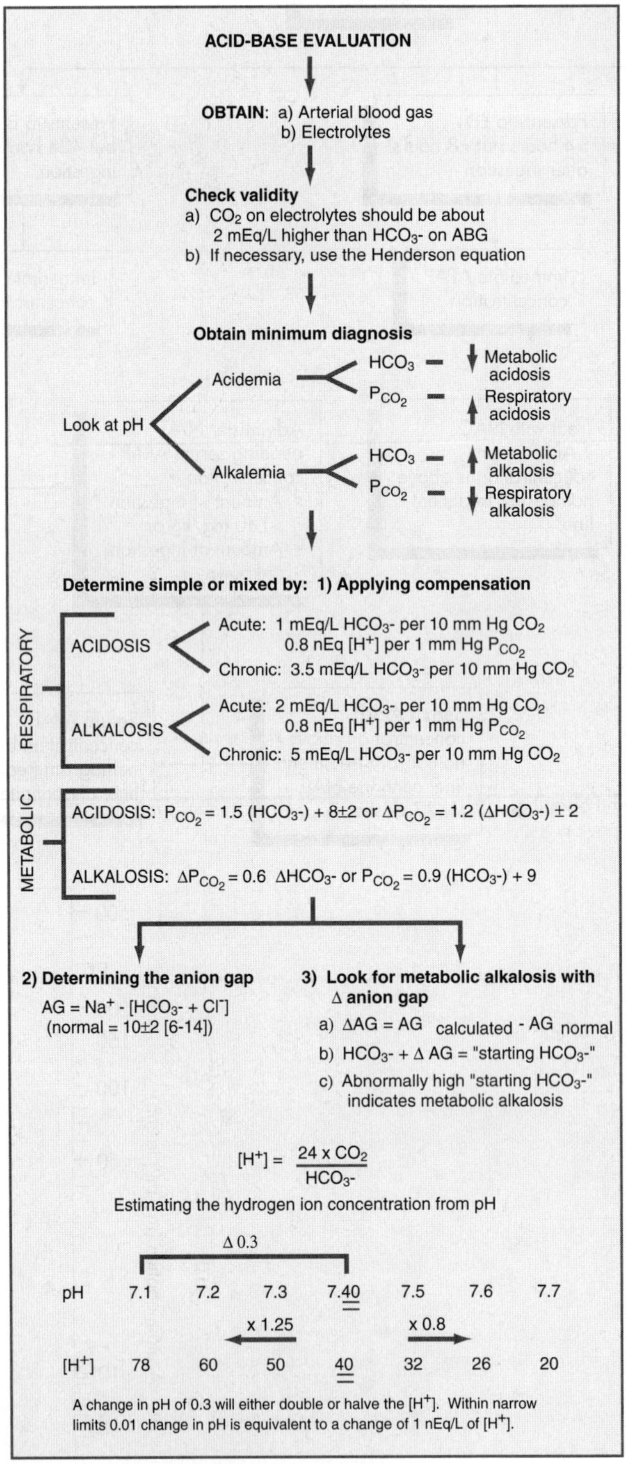

FIGURE 3-4 Scheme for assessing acid-base homeostasis. (From Andreoli TE [ed]: *Cecil essentials of medicine,* ed 7, Philadelphia, 2008, WB Saunders.)

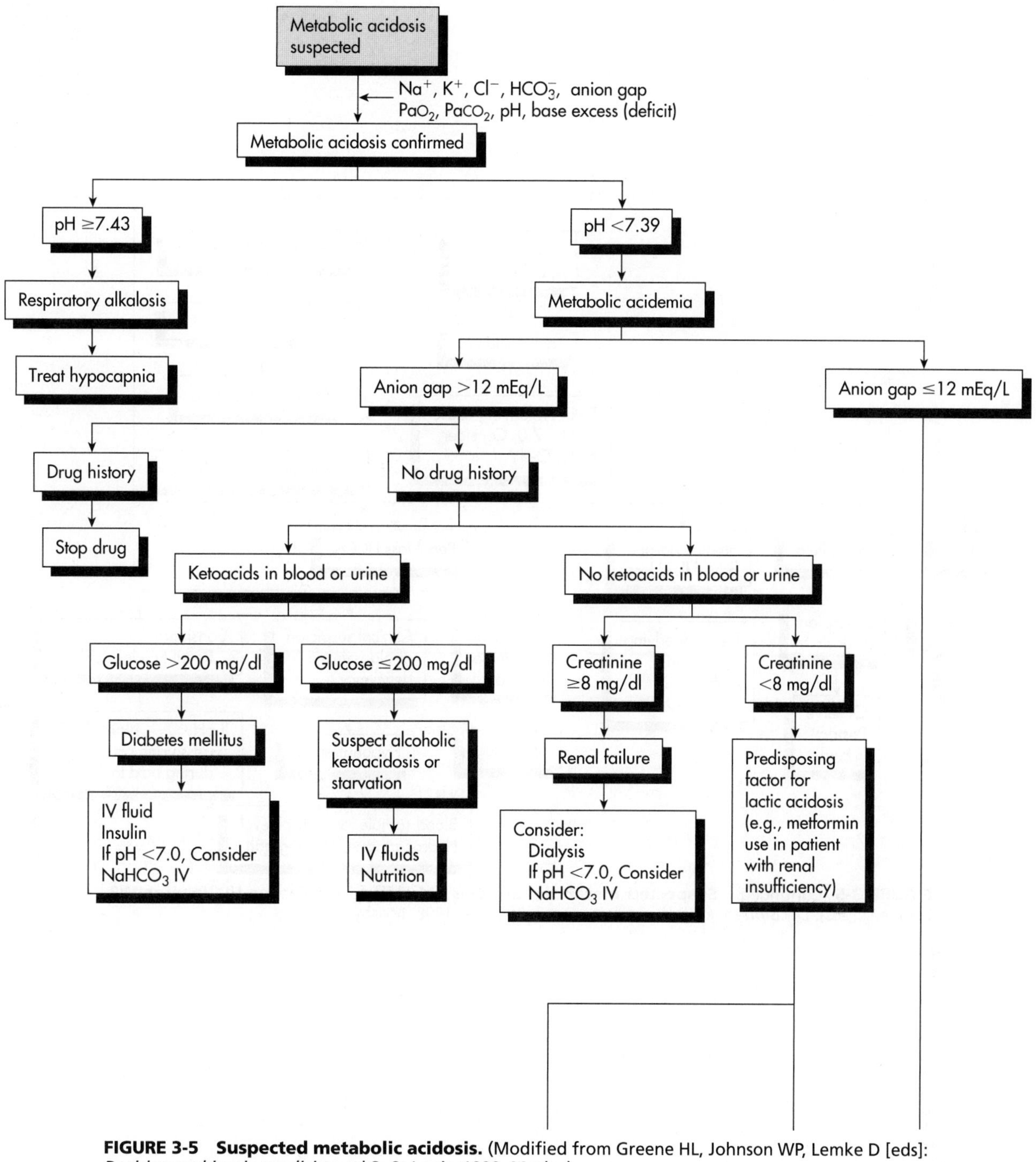

FIGURE 3-5 Suspected metabolic acidosis. (Modified from Greene HL, Johnson WP, Lemke D [eds]: *Decision making in medicine,* ed 2, St Louis, 1998, Mosby.)

Continued on following page

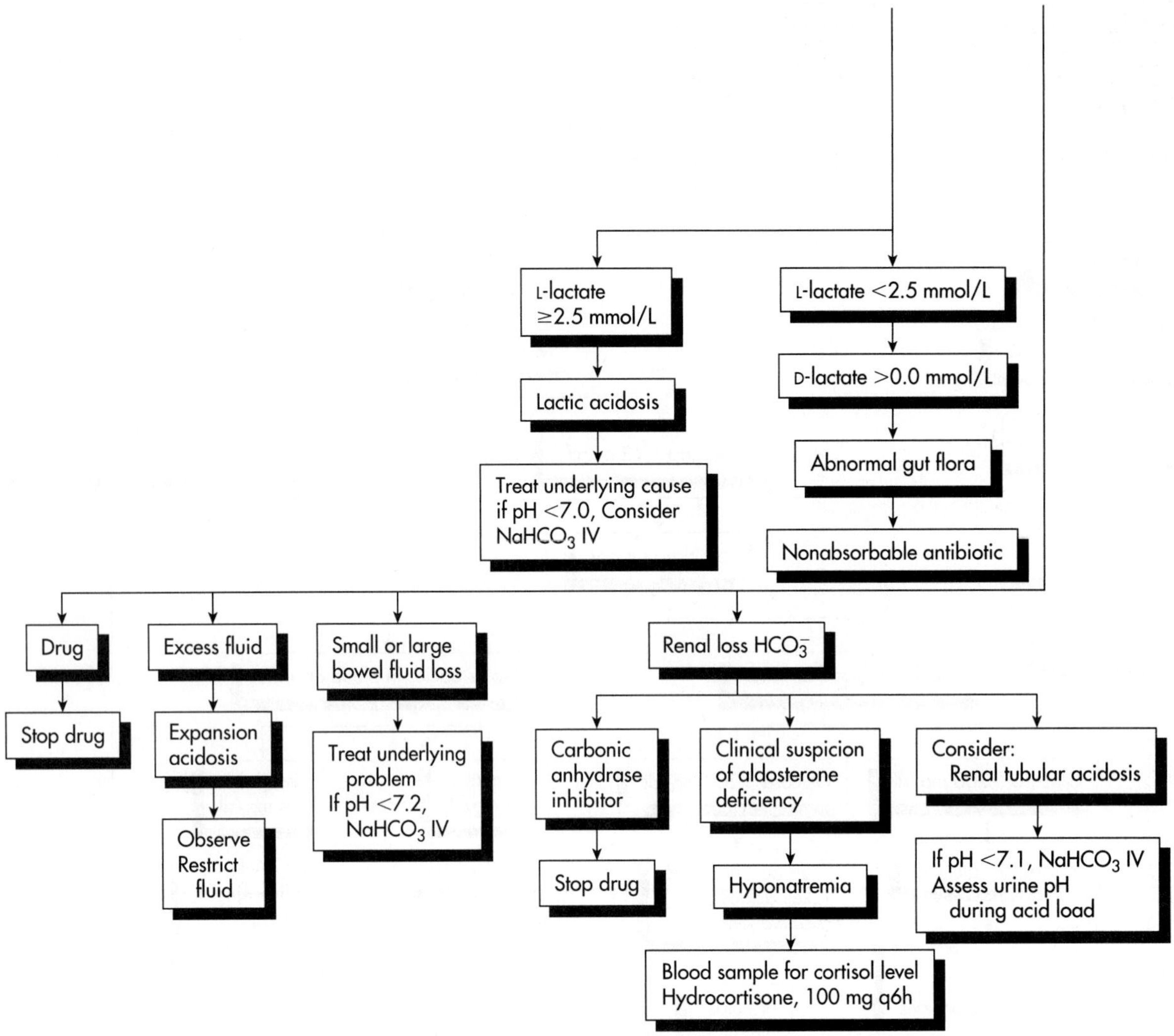

FIGURE 3-5 (Continued) **Suspected metabolic acidosis**. (Modified from Greene HL, Johnson WP, Lemke D [eds]: *Decision making in medicine*, ed 2, St Louis, 1998, Mosby.)

ACIDOSIS, RESPIRATORY, ACUTE

ICD-9CM # 276.2

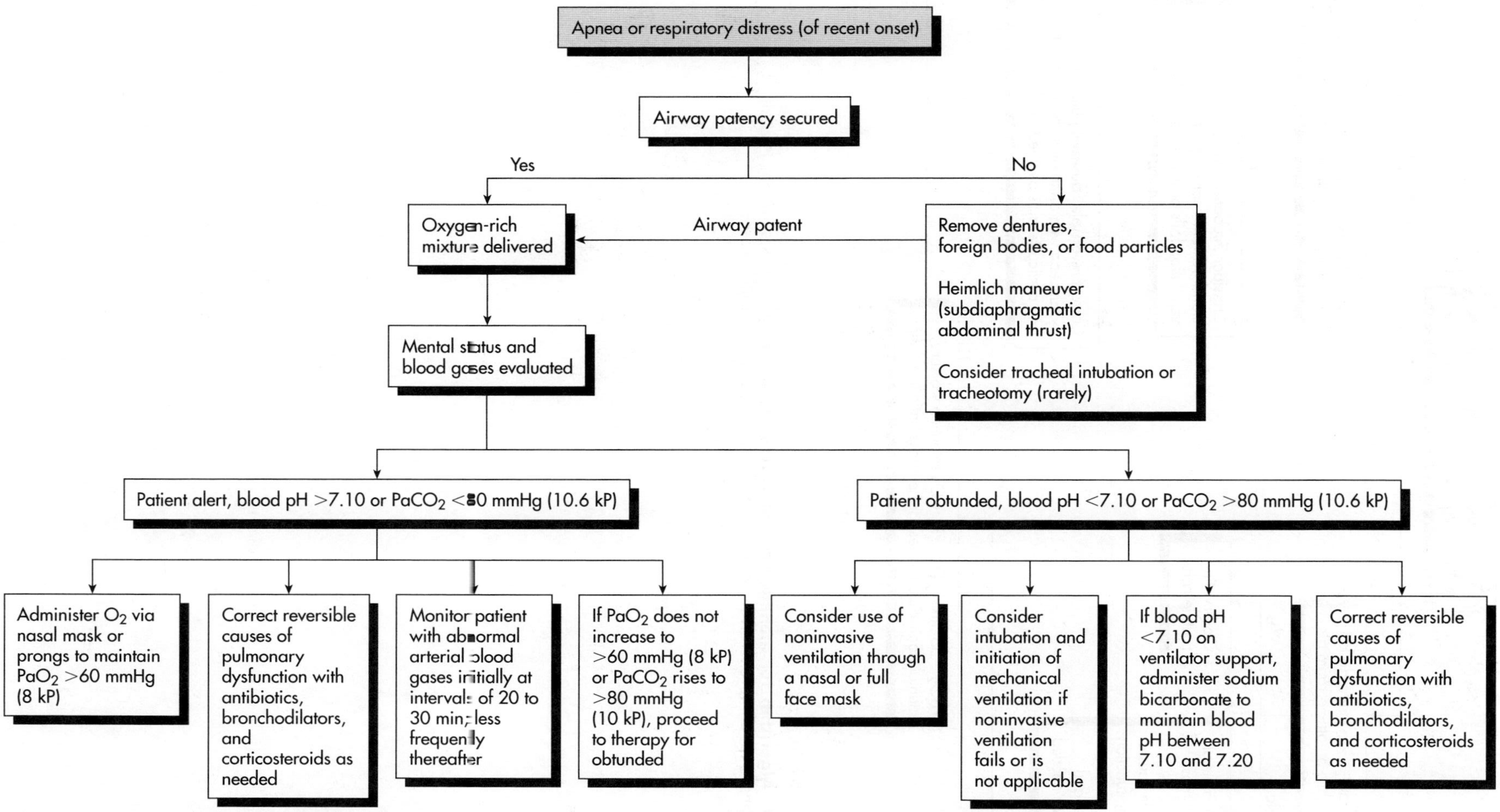

FIGURE 3-6 Algorithm for management of acute respiratory acidosis. (From Feehally J, Floege J, Johnson RJ: *Comprehensive clinical nephrology,* ed 3, St Louis, 2007, Mosby.)

ICD-9CM # 276.2

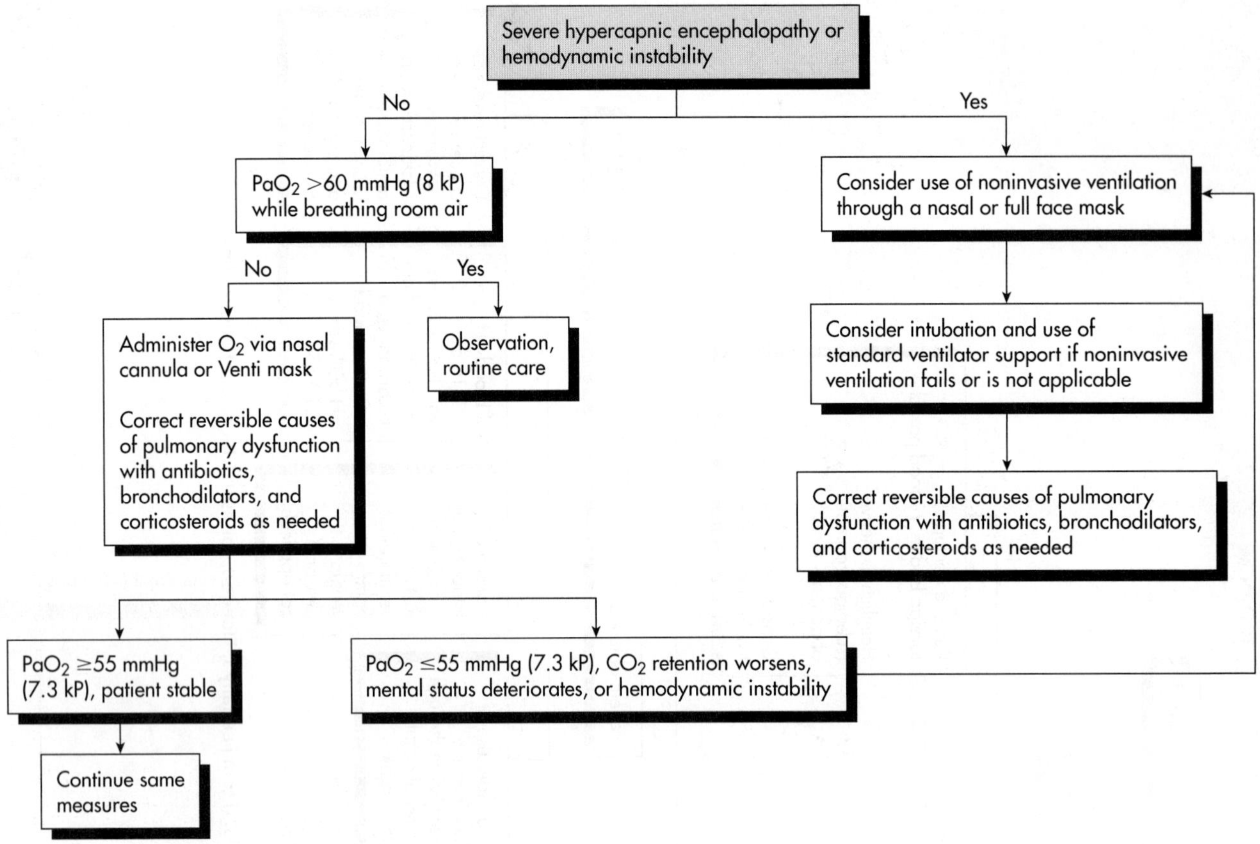

FIGURE 3-7 Algorithm for management of chronic respiratory acidosis. (From Feehally J, Floege J, Johnson RJ: *Comprehensive clinical nephrology,* ed 3, St Louis, 2007, Mosby.)

ICD-9CM # 518.82

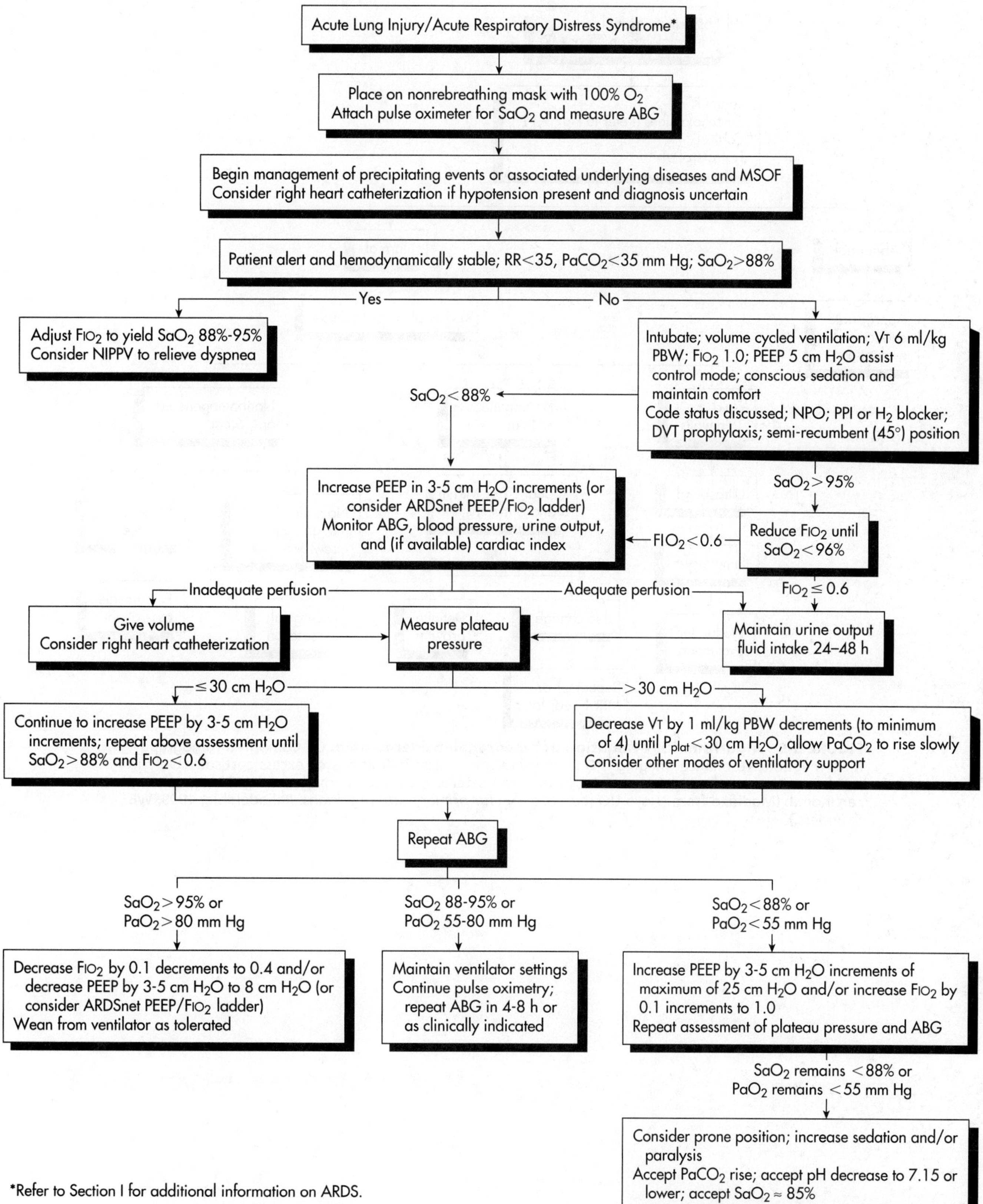

*Refer to Section I for additional information on ARDS.

FIGURE 3-8 An algorithm for the initial management of acute respiratory distress syndrome. *ABG,* Arterial blood gas analysis; *ARDS,* acute respiratory distress syndrome; *CO,* carbon dioxide; *DVT,* deep venous thrombosis; *FIO_2,* inspired oxygen concentration; *MSOF,* multisystem organ failure; *NIPPV,* noninvasive intermittent positive pressure ventilation; *O_2,* oxygen; *$PaCO_2$,* arterial partial pressure of carbon dioxide; *PaO_2,* arterial partial pressure of oxygen; *PBW,* predicted body weight; *PEEP,* positive end-expiratory pressure; *P_{plat},* plateau pressure; *RR,* respiratory rate; *SaO_2,* arterial oxygen saturation; *VT,* tidal volume. (Modified from Goldman L, Ausiello D [eds]: *Cecil textbook of medicine,* ed 23, Philadelphia, 2008, WB Saunders.)

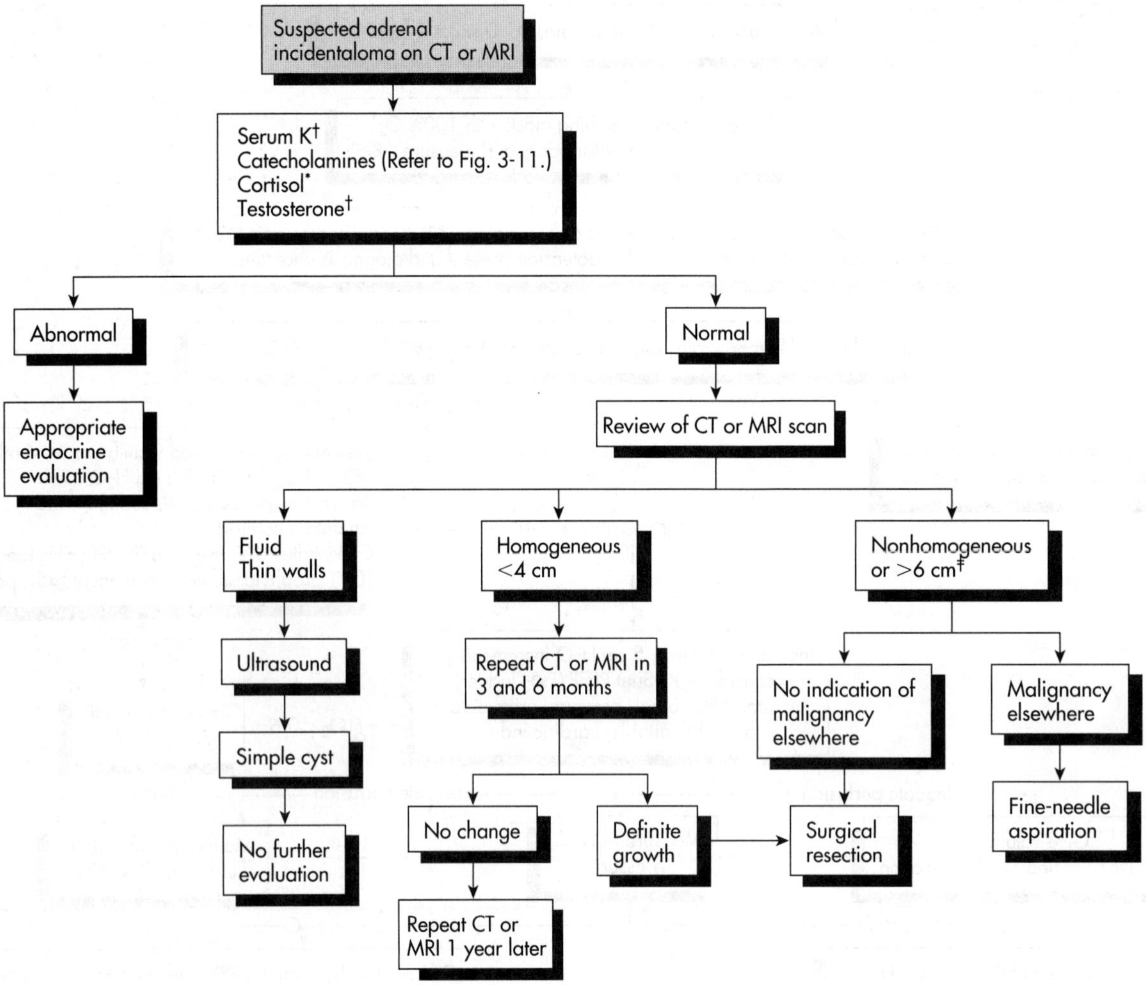

FIGURE 3-9 Algorithm for evaluation of an adrenal incidentaloma. *CT,* Computed tomography; *MRI,* magnetic resonance imaging. *Only if there are clinical indications of excess cortisol. †Only in women with hirsutism. ‡Measure dehydroepiandrosterone sulfate, a marker of primary adrenal carcinoma. (Modified from Nseyo UO [ed]: *Urology for primary care physicians,* Philadelphia, 1999, WB Saunders.)

ICD-9CM # 255.4 Addison's disease

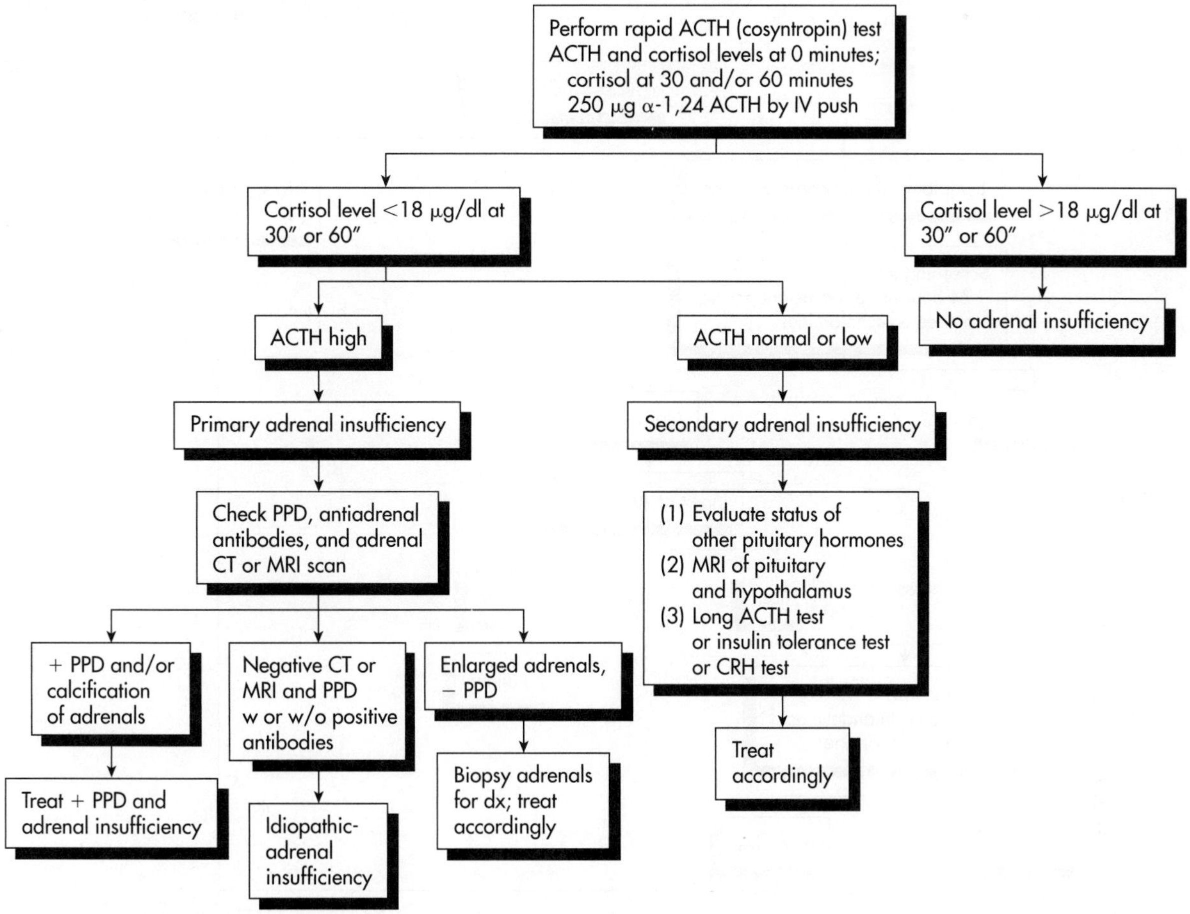

FIGURE 3-10 Evaluation of adrenal insufficiency. *ACTH,* Adrenocorticotropic hormone; *CRH,* corticotropin-releasing hormone; *CT,* computed tomography; *MRI,* magnetic resonance imaging; *PPD,* purified protein derivative. (Modified from Noble J: *Primary care medicine,* ed 3, St Louis, 2001, Mosby.)

ICD-9CM # 194.0 Adrenal cortical carcinoma site NOS M8370/3
255.8 Adrenal hyperplasia

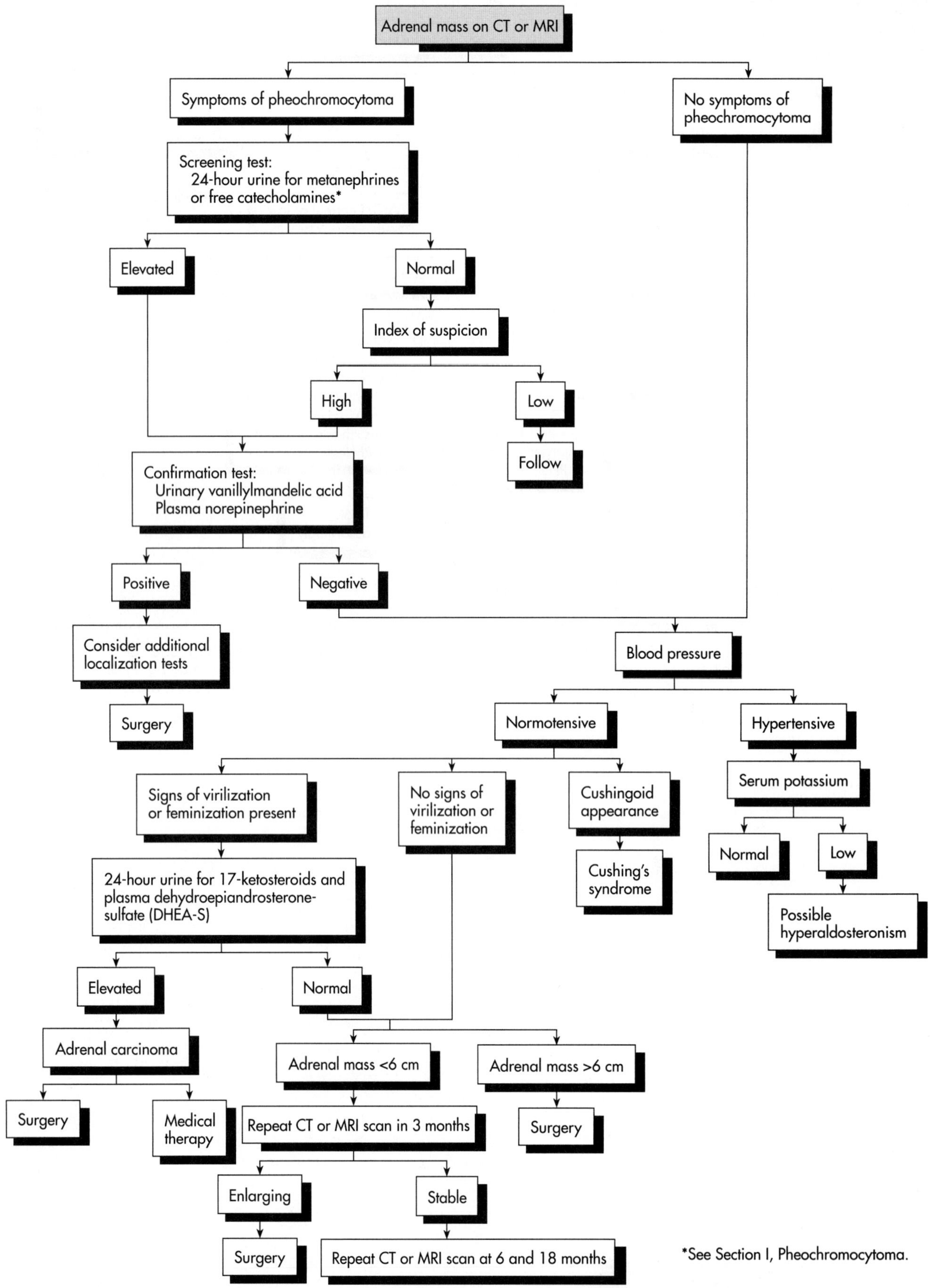

FIGURE 3-11 Evaluation of adrenal mass. *CT,* Computed tomography; *MRI,* magnetic resonance imaging. (From Greene HL, Johnson WP, Lemcke D [eds]: *Decision making in medicine,* ed 2, St Louis, 1998, Mosby.)

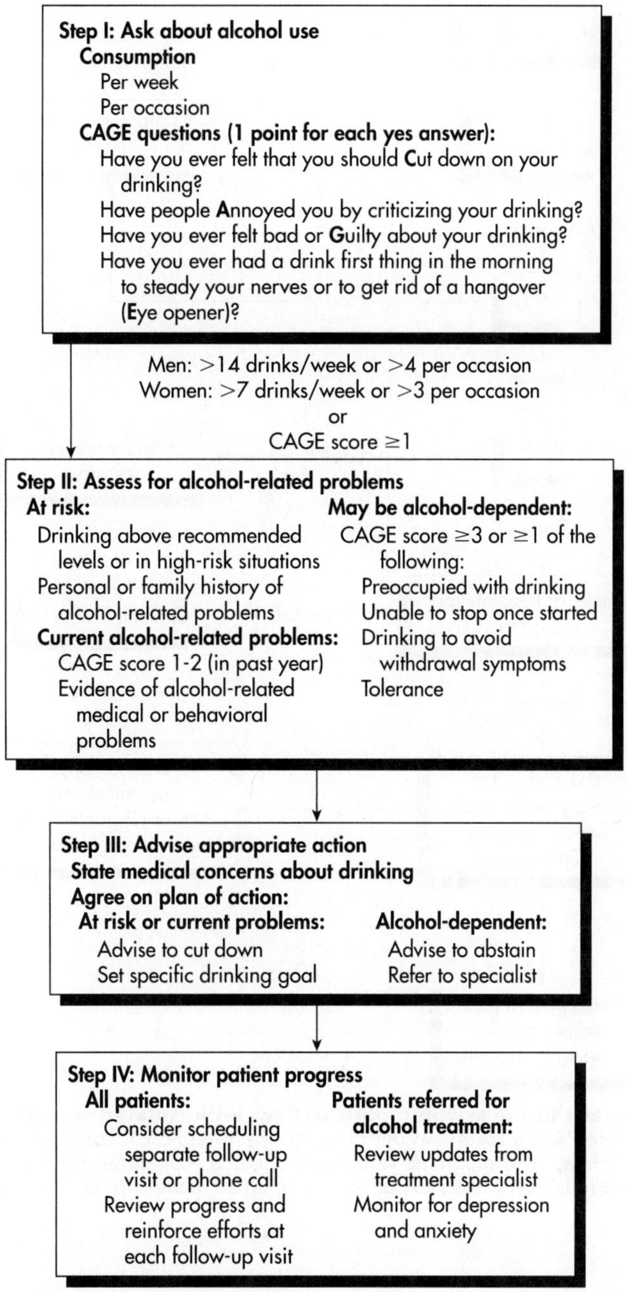

FIGURE 3-12 Screening and brief intervention for alcohol problems in clinical practice. (From Goldman L, Ausiello D [eds]: *Cecil textbook of medicine,* ed 23, Philadelphia, 2008, WB Saunders.)

ICD-9CM # 790.4

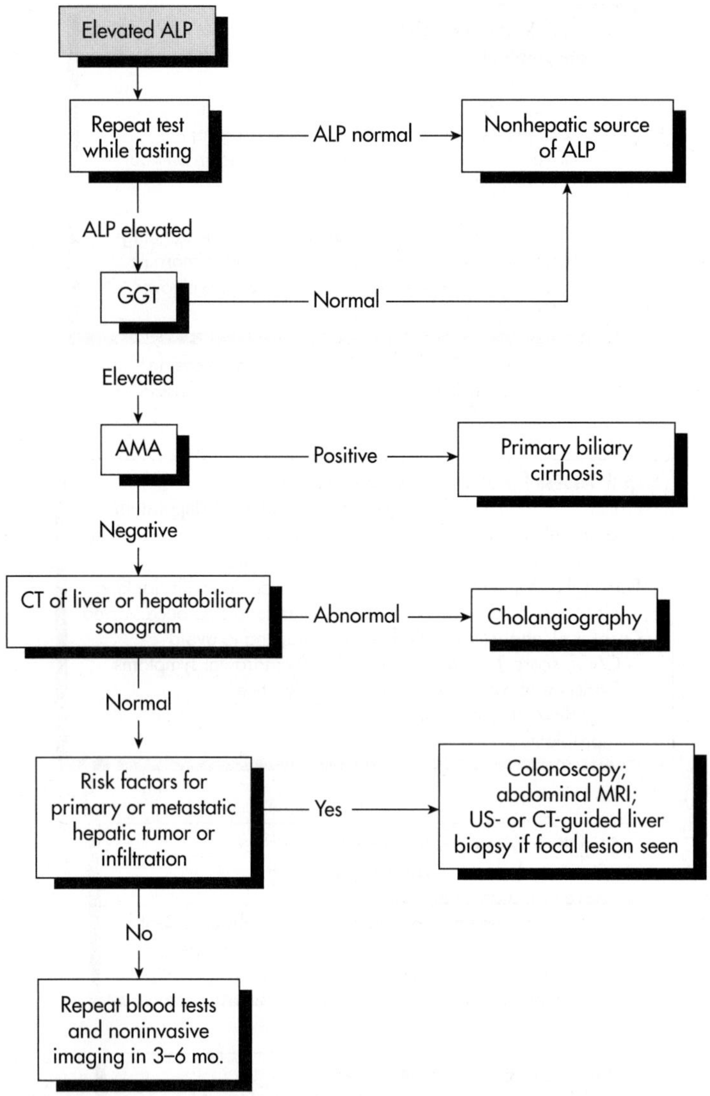

FIGURE 3-13 Approach to the asymptomatic patient with isolated elevated levels of serum alkaline phosphatase (ALP). *AMA,* Antimitochondrial antibody; *CT,* computed tomography; *GGT,* γ-glutayml transpeptidase; *MRI,* magnetic resonance imaging; *US,* ultrasonography. (Modified from Goldman L, Ausiello D [eds]: *Cecil textbook of medicine,* ed 23, Philadelphia, 2008, WB Saunders.)

ICD-9CM # 273.6

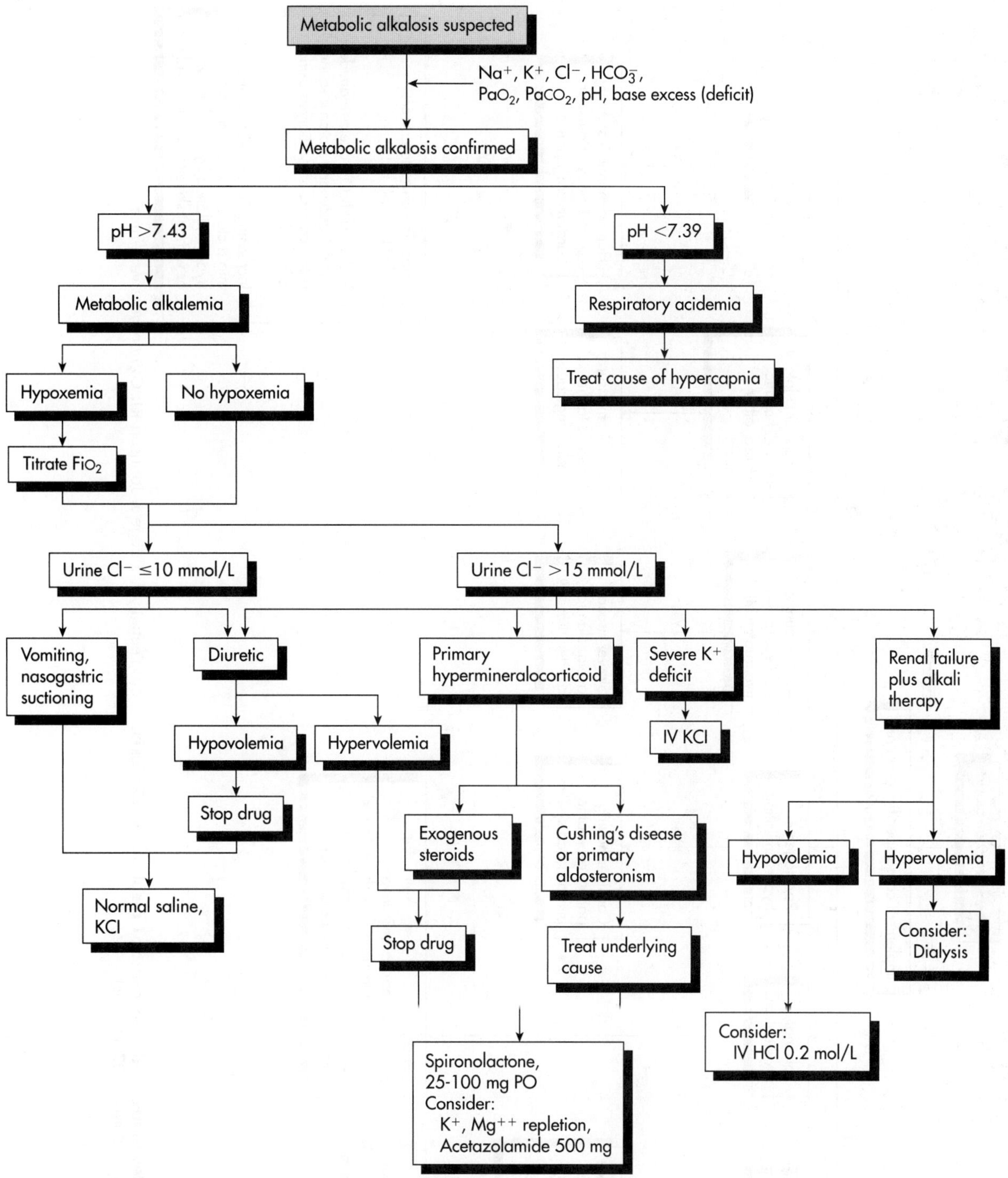

FIGURE 3-14 Suspected metabolic alkalosis. (From Greene HL, Johnson WP, Lemke D [eds]: *Decision making in medicine,* ed 2, St Louis, 1998, Mosby.)

ALKALOSIS, RESPIRATORY

ICD-9CM # 276.3

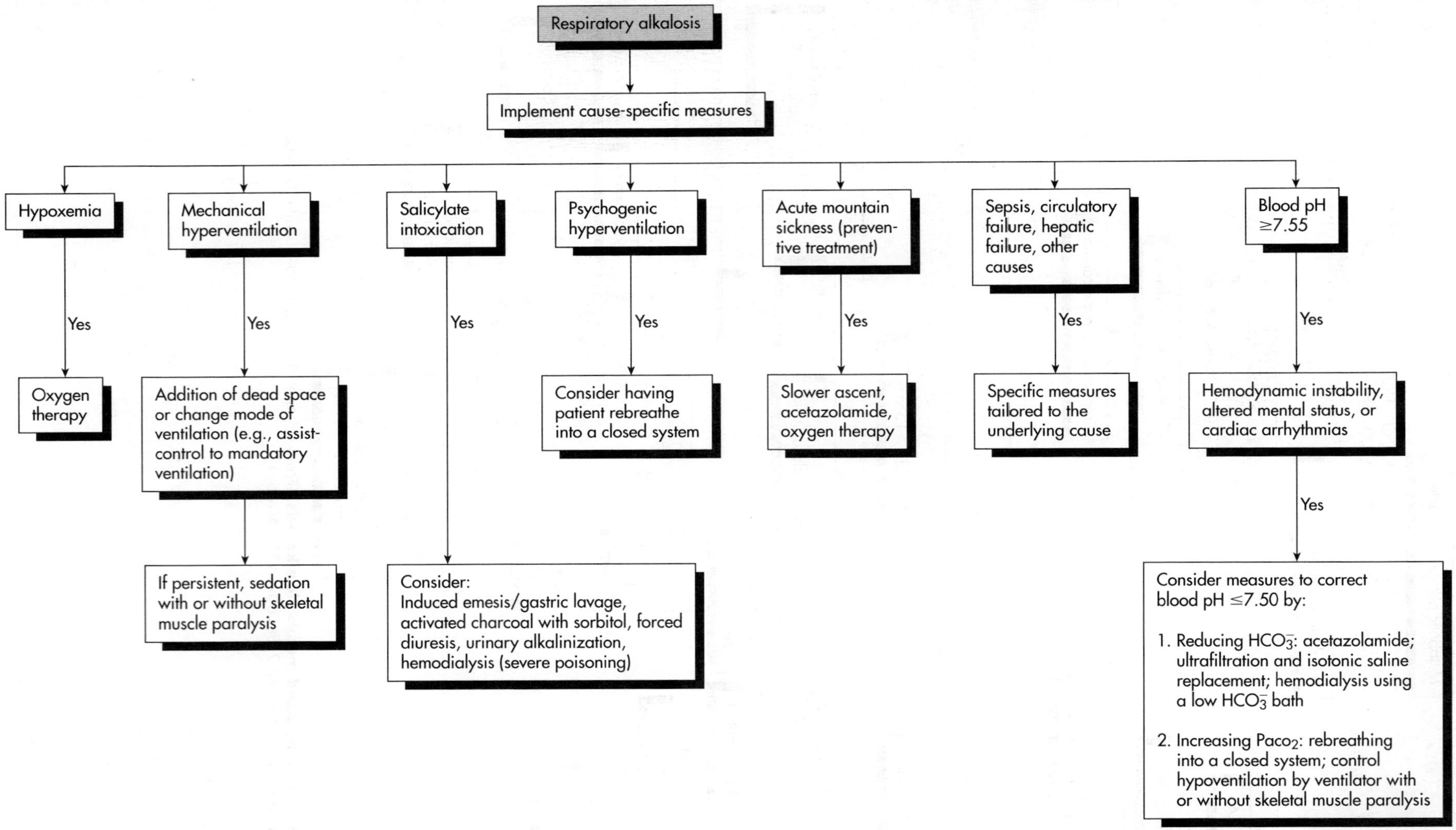

FIGURE 3-15 Recommended treatment of respiratory alkalosis. (From Feehally J, Floege J, Johnson RJ: *Comprehensive clinical nephrology,* ed 3, St Louis, 2007, Mosby.)

ICD-9CM # 704.00

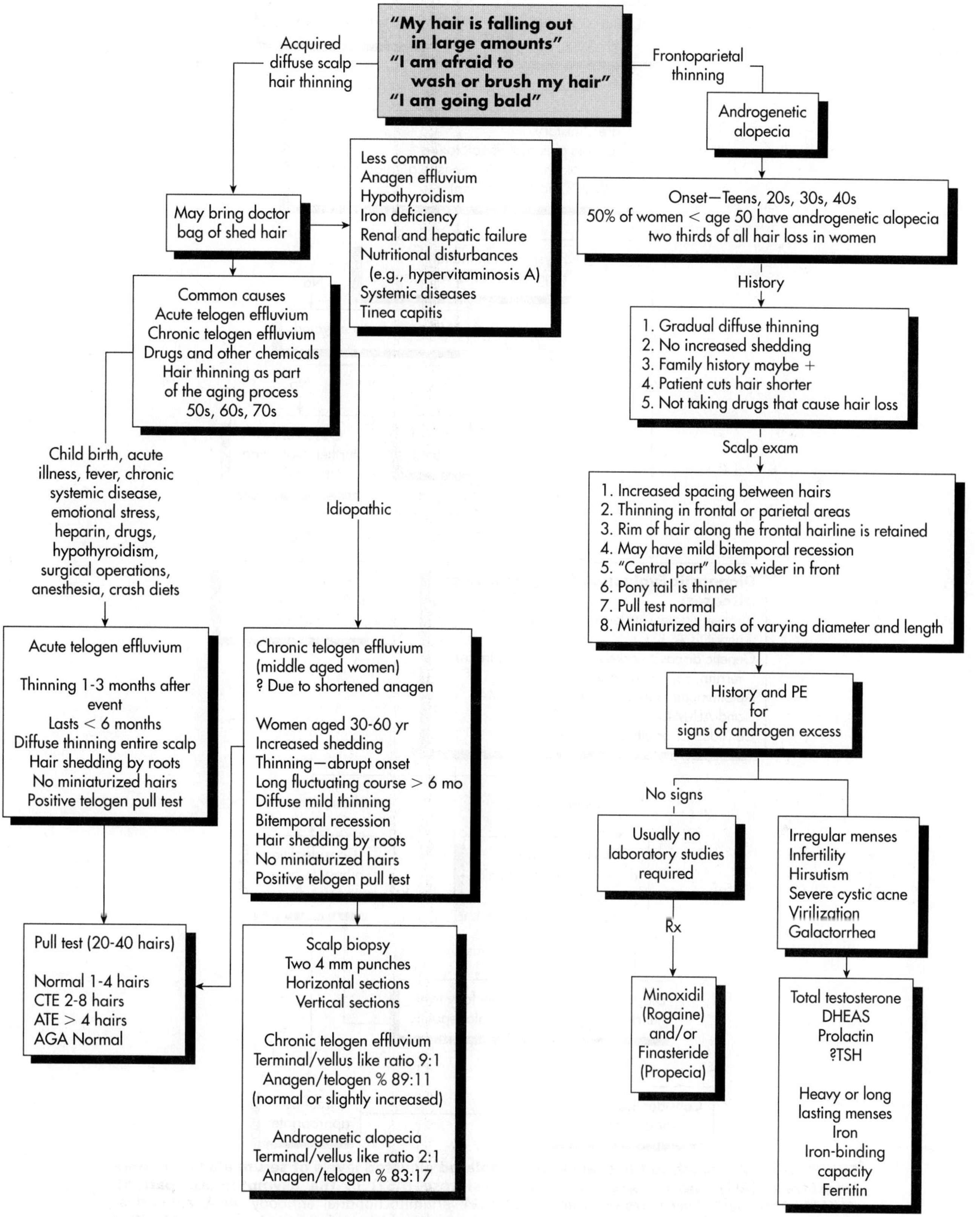

FIGURE 3-16 Evaluation and treatment of alopecia in females. *CTE,* Chronic telogen effluvium; *AGA,* androgenetic alopecia; *ATE,* acute telogen effluvium. (Modified from Habif TA: *Clinical dermatology,* ed 4, St Louis, 2004, Mosby.)

ICD-9CM # 573.9

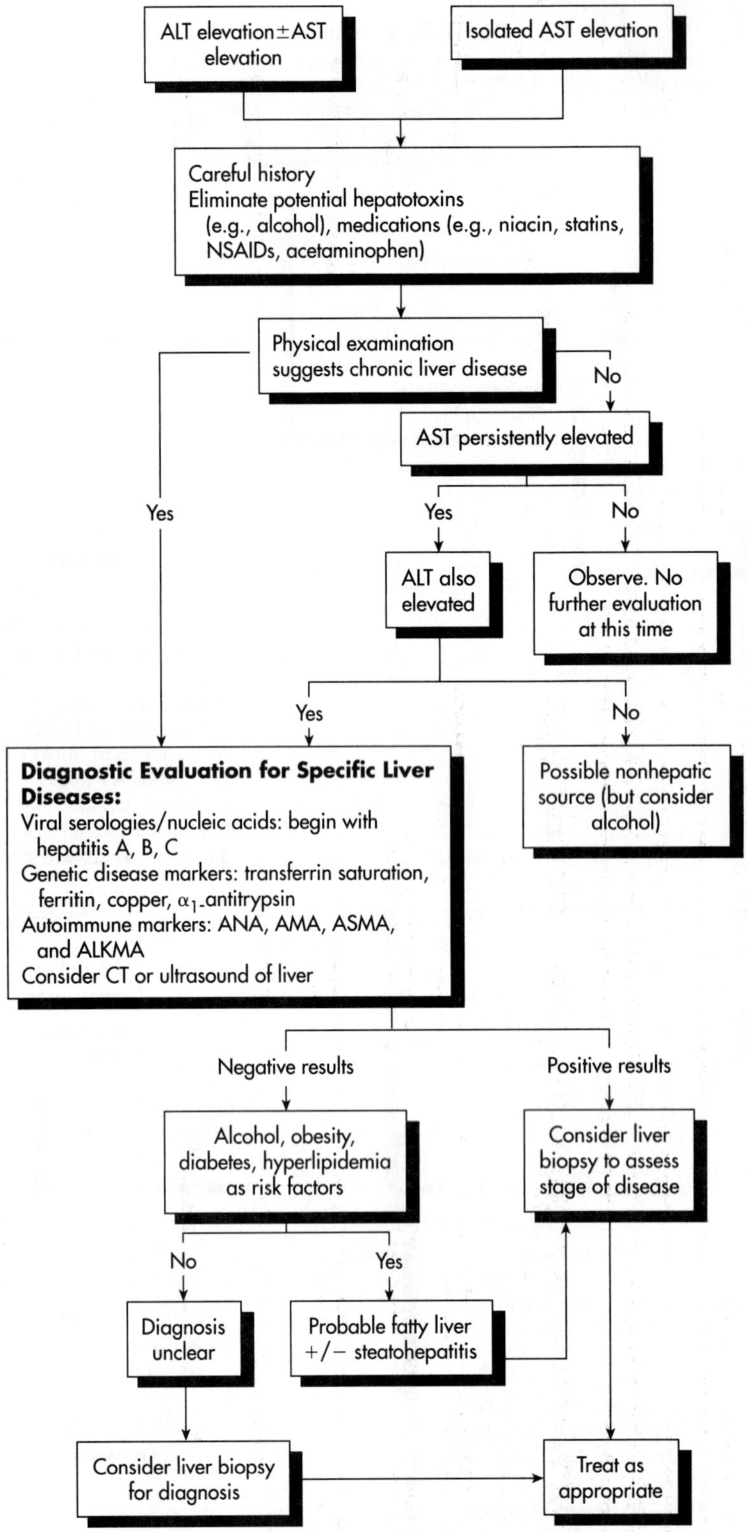

FIGURE 3-17 Approach to the evaluation of isolated elevated levels of serum alanine aminotransferase (ALT) and/or aspartate aminotransferase (AST) in the asymptomatic patient. *ALKMA,* Anti–liver/kidney microsomal antibody; *AMA,* antimitochondrial antibody; *ANA,* antinuclear antibody; *ASMA,* anti–smooth muscle antibody; *NSAIDs,* nonsteroidal anti-inflammatory drugs. (Modified from Goldman L, Ausiello D [eds]: *Cecil textbook of medicine,* ed 23, Philadelphia, 2008, WB Saunders.)

ICD-9CM # 626.0

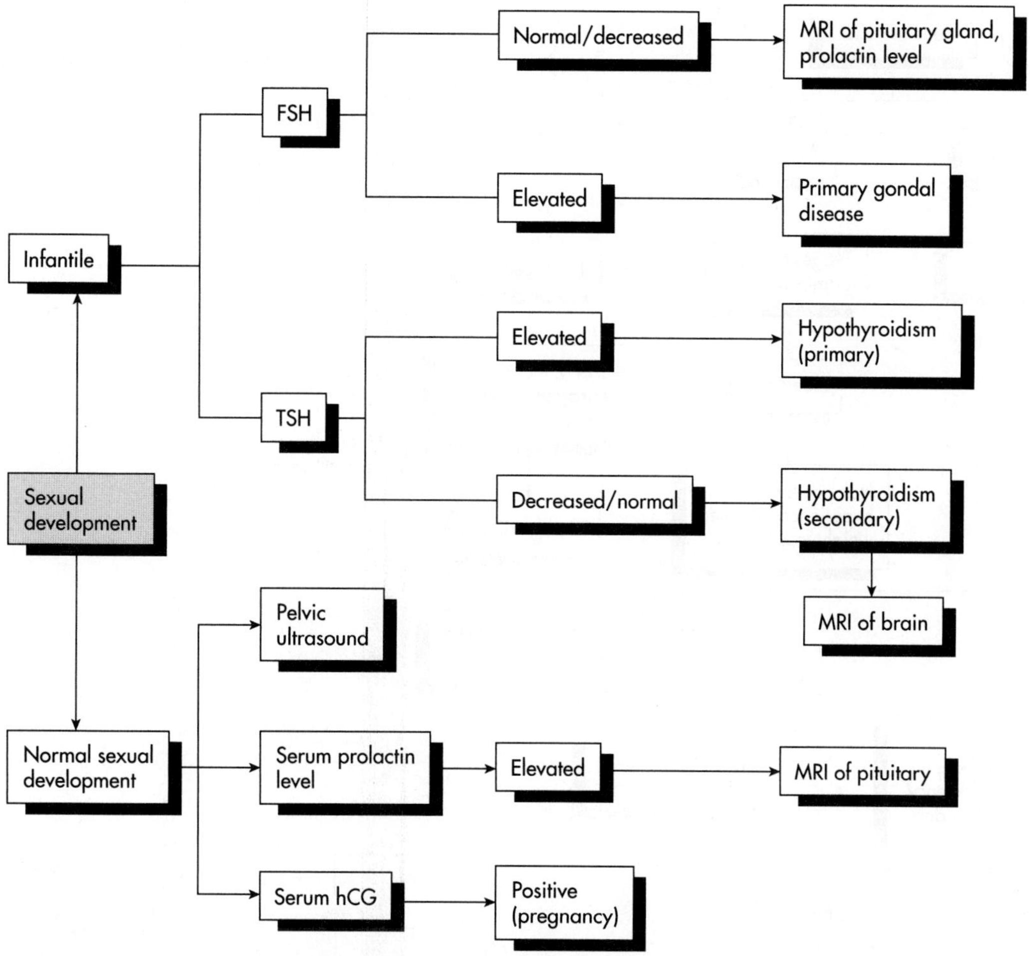

FIGURE 3-18 Evaluation of primary amenorrhea. *FSH,* Follicle-stimulation hormone; *MRI,* magnetic resonance imaging; *TSH,* thyroid stimulating hormone. (From Ferri FF: *Ferri's best test: a practical guide to clinical laboratory medicine and diagnostic imaging,* ed 2, Philadelphia, 2009, Elsevier Mosby.)

BOX 3-1 **Amenorrhea, Primary**

Diagnostic imaging	Lab evaluation
Best test	***Best tests***
MRI of pituitary/hypothalamus with gadolinium when hypothalamic/pituitary lesion is suspected	FSH Prolactin TSH
Ancillary tests	***Ancillary tests***
Pelvic ultrasound	Serum hCG

From Ferri FF: *Ferri's best test: a practical guide to clinical laboratory medicine and diagnostic imaging,* ed 2, Philadelphia, 2009, Elsevier Mosby.

FSH, Follicle-stimulating hormone; *MRI,* magnetic resonance imaging; *TSH,* thyroid-stimulating hormone.

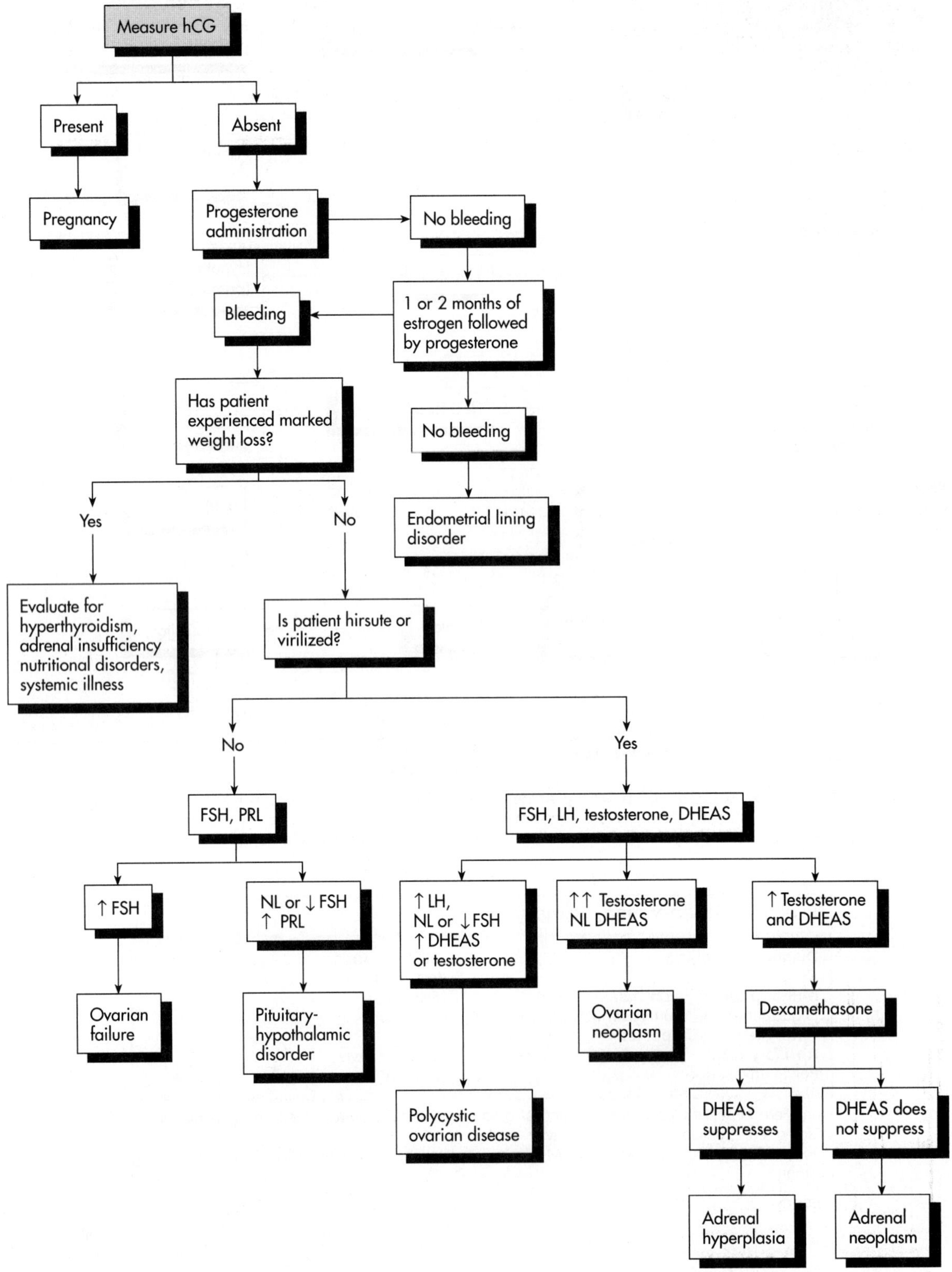

FIGURE 3-19 Evaluation of secondary amenorrhea. *DHEAS,* Dehydroepiandrosterone-sulfate; *FSH,* follicle-stimulating hormone; *hCG,* human chorionic gonadotropin; *LH,* luteinizing hormone; *NL,* normal; *PRL,* prolactin; ↑, increased; ↑↑, markedly increased; ↓, decreased. (From Andreoli TE [ed]: *Cecil essentials of medicine,* ed 7, Philadelphia, 2008, WB Saunders.)

ICD-9CM # 277.3

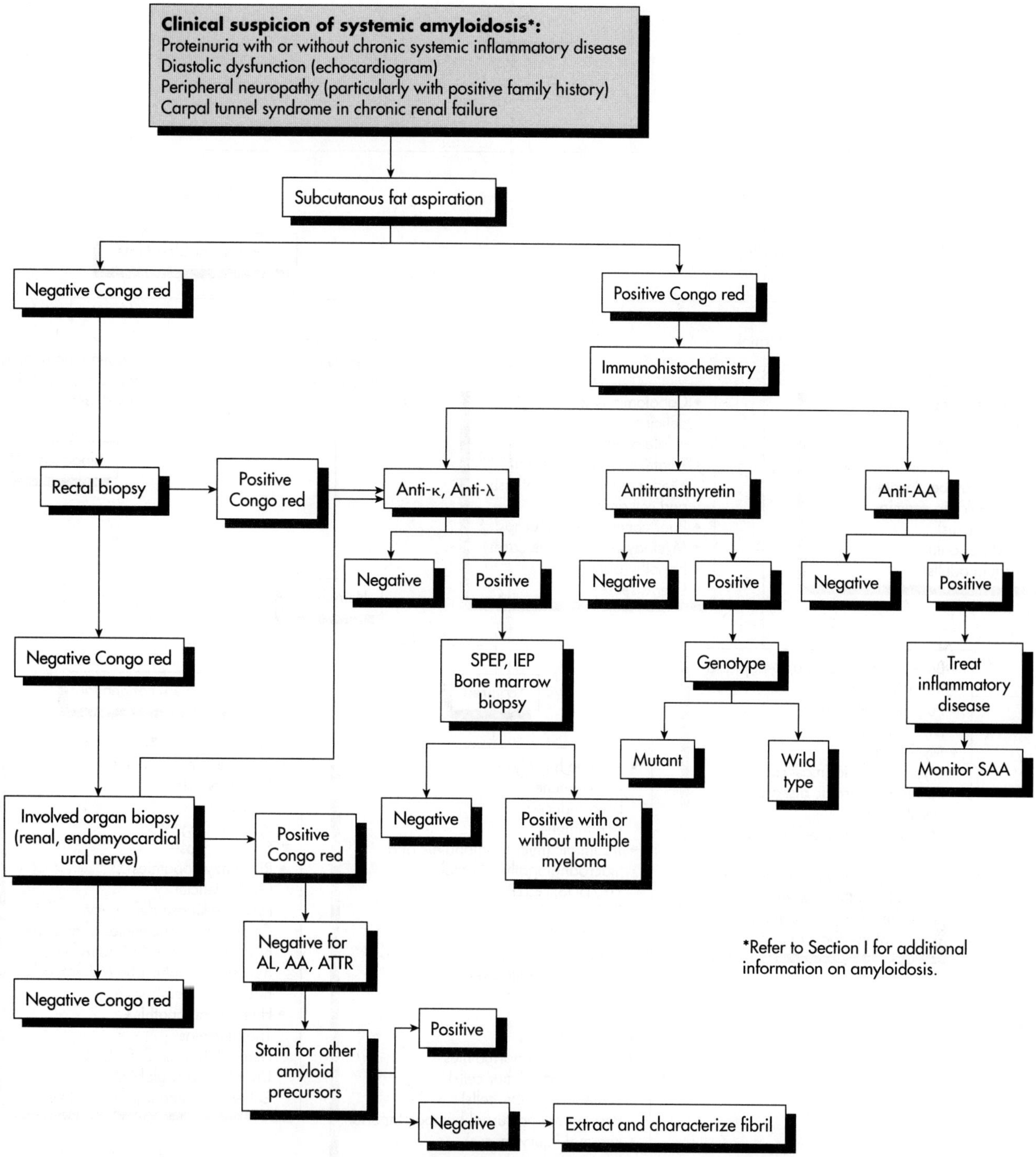

FIGURE 3-20 Approach to the patient with possible systemic amyloidosis. *IEP,* Immunoelectrophoresis; *SPEP,* serum protein electrophoresis. (Modified from Goldman L, Ausiello D [eds]: *Cecil textbook of medicine,* ed 23, Philadelphia, 2008, WB Saunders.)

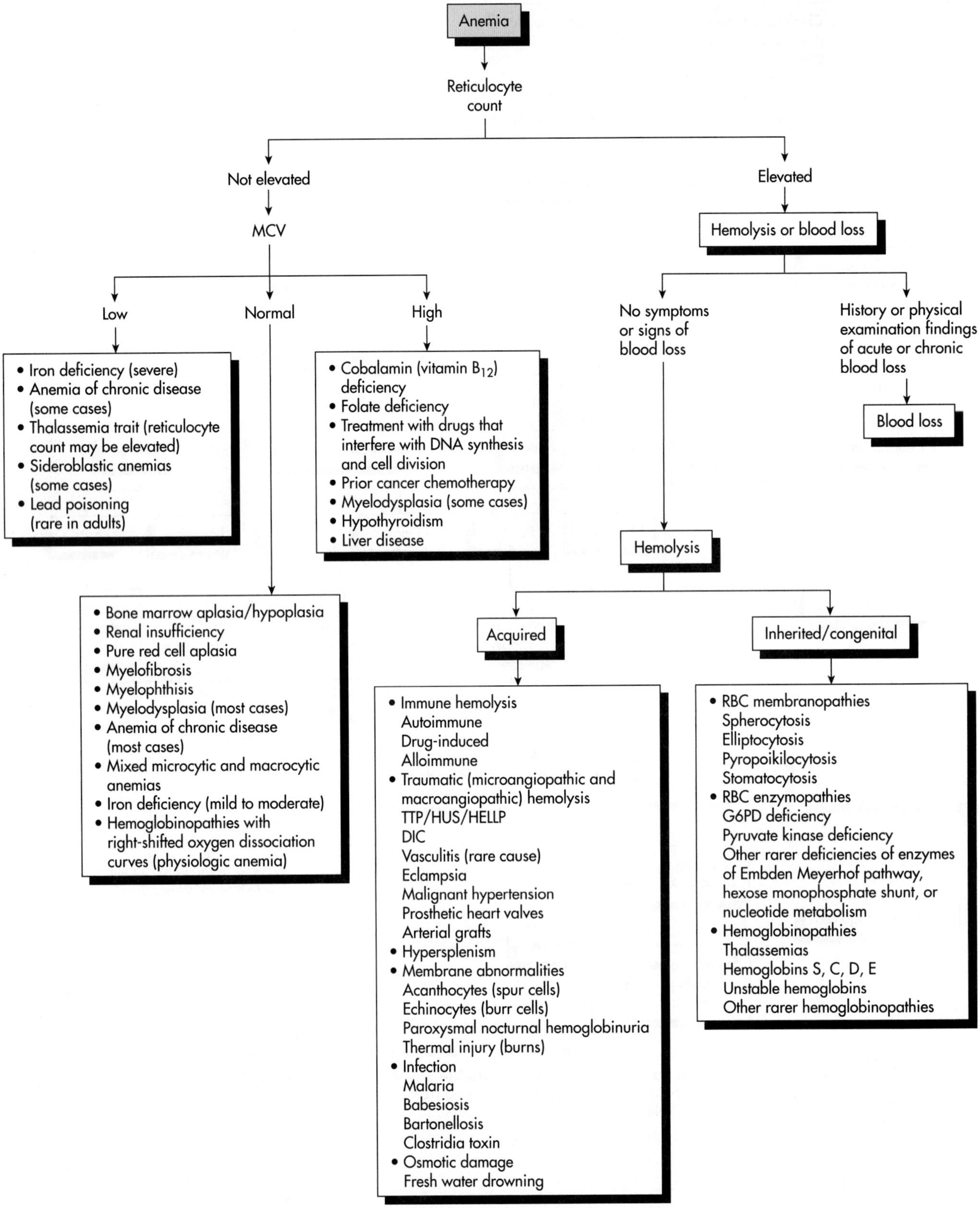

FIGURE 3-21 Algorithm for diagnosis of anemias. *DIC,* Disseminated intravascular coagulation; *HELLP, h*epatomegaly-elevated *l*iver (function tests)-*l*ow *p*latelets; *HUS,* hemolytic-uremic syndrome; *MCV,* mean corpuscular volume; *RBC,* red blood cell; *TTP,* thrombotic thrombocytopenic purpura. (From Goldman L, Ausiello D [eds]: *Cecil textbook of medicine,* ed 23, Philadelphia, 2008, WB Saunders.)

ICD-9CM # 285.9

Treatment Algorithm for ACD

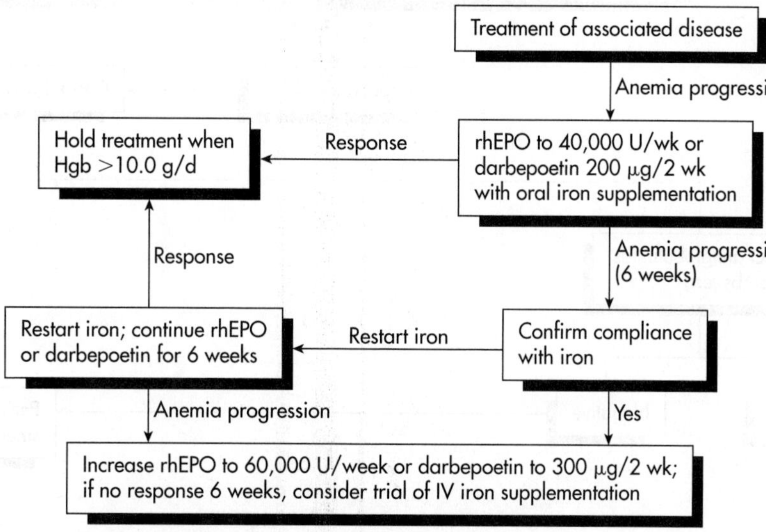

FIGURE 3-22 Treatment algorithm for anemia of chronic disease (ACD). (Modified from Young NS, Gerson SL, High KA [eds]: *Clinical hematology,* St Louis, 2006, Mosby.)

Differential Diagnosis of Anemia with Low Serum Iron

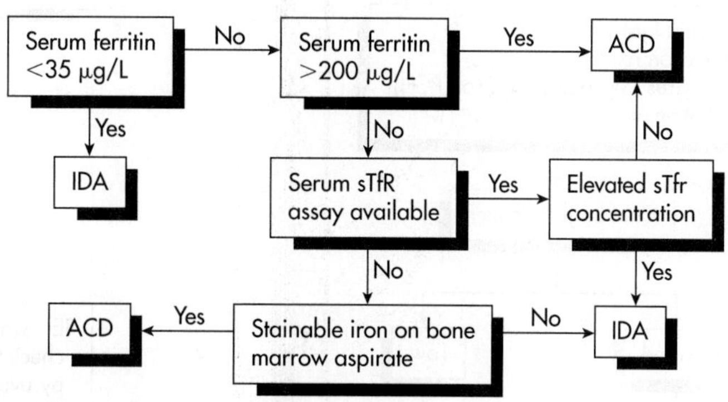

FIGURE 3-23 Differential diagnosis of anemia with low serum iron. *IDA,* Iron deficiency anemia; *sTfR,* soluble transferrin receptor. (From Young NS, Gerson SL, High KA [eds]: *Clinical hematology,* St Louis, 2006, Mosby.)

TABLE 3-1 Laboratory Characteristics of ACD, IDA, and IDA with Inflammation

	ACD	Iron Deficiency Anemia	Iron Deficiency Anemia with Inflammation
Mean corpuscular volume	72-100 fL	<85 fL	<100 fL
Mean corpuscular hemoglobin concentration	<36 gm/dl	<32 gm/dl	<32 gm/dl
Serum iron	Decreased	Decreased	Decreased
Serum total iron-binding capacity (TIBC)	Typical below mid-normal range	Elevated	Less than upper limit of normal range
TIBC saturation	2-20%	<15% (usually <10%)	<15%
Serum ferritin	>35 μg/ml	<35 ng/ml	<200 ng/ml
Serum soluble transferring receptor concentration	Normal (may be increased if serum ferritin > 200 μg/L)	Increased	Increased
Stainable iron in bone marrow	Present	Absent	Absent

From Young NS, Gerson SL, High KA (eds): *Clinical hematology,* St Louis, 2006, Mosby.

ICD-9CM # 283.9

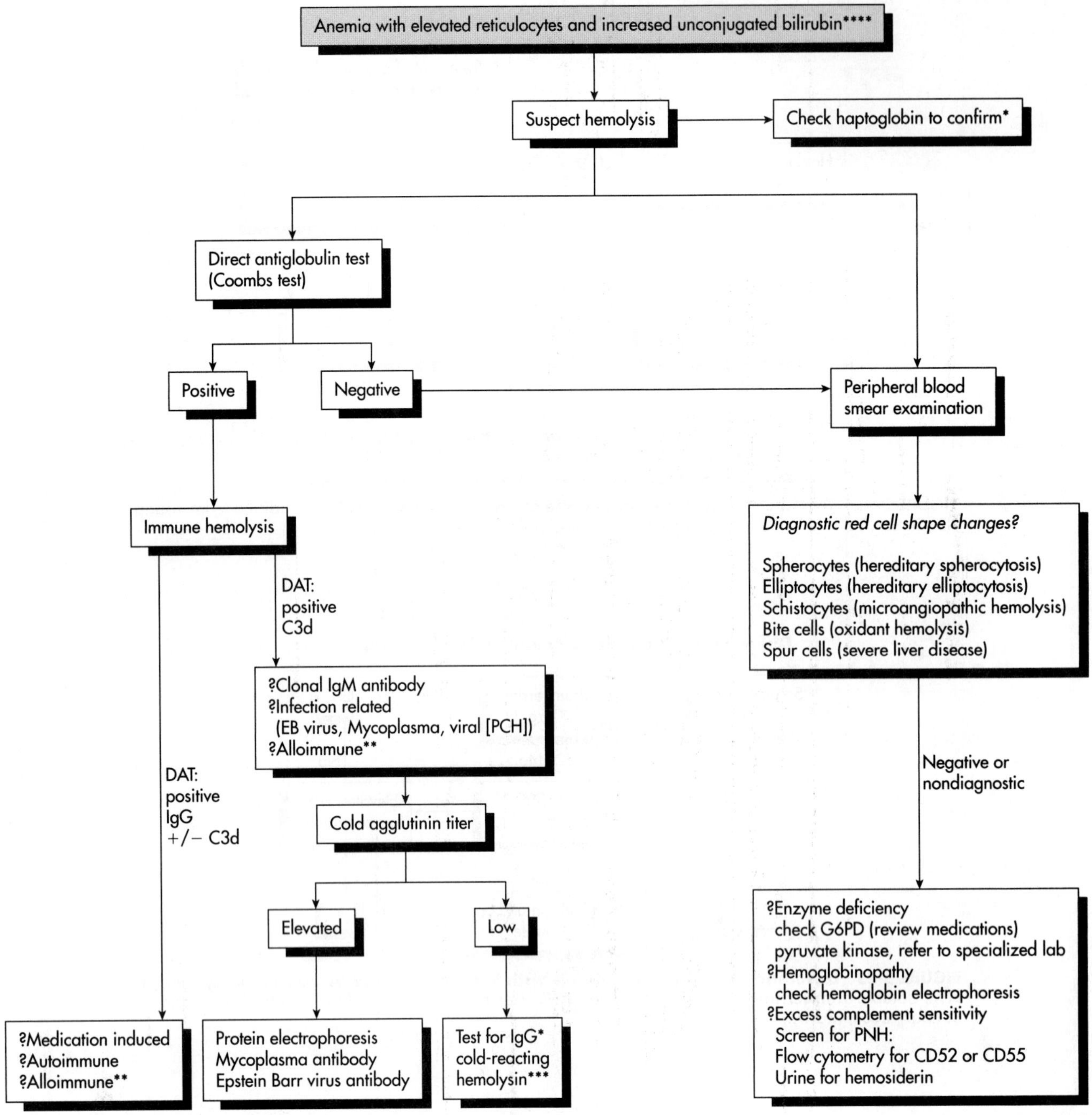

*Other parameters that may be useful: serum lactic dehydrogenase which is markedly increased in intravascular hemolysis and plasma hemoglobin which is elevated in severe hemolysis.
**Hemolytic transfusion reactions, mismatched red blood cell transplants
***Donath-Landsteiner test
****Refer to Section I, Anemia, Autoimmune Hemolytic, for additional information on this topic.

FIGURE 3-24 Anemia with elevated reticulocytes and increased unconjugated bilirubin. *DAT,* Direct antiglobulin test; *EB,* Epstein-Barr; *G6PD,* glucose-6-phosphate dehydrogenase; *PCH,* paroxysmal cold hemoglobinuria; *PNH,* paroxysmal nocturnal hemoglobinuria; *rbc,* red blood cell. (From Young NS, Gerson SL, High KA [eds]: *Clinical hematology,* St Louis, 2006, Mosby.)

ANEMIA, MACROCYTIC

ICD-9CM # 281.9

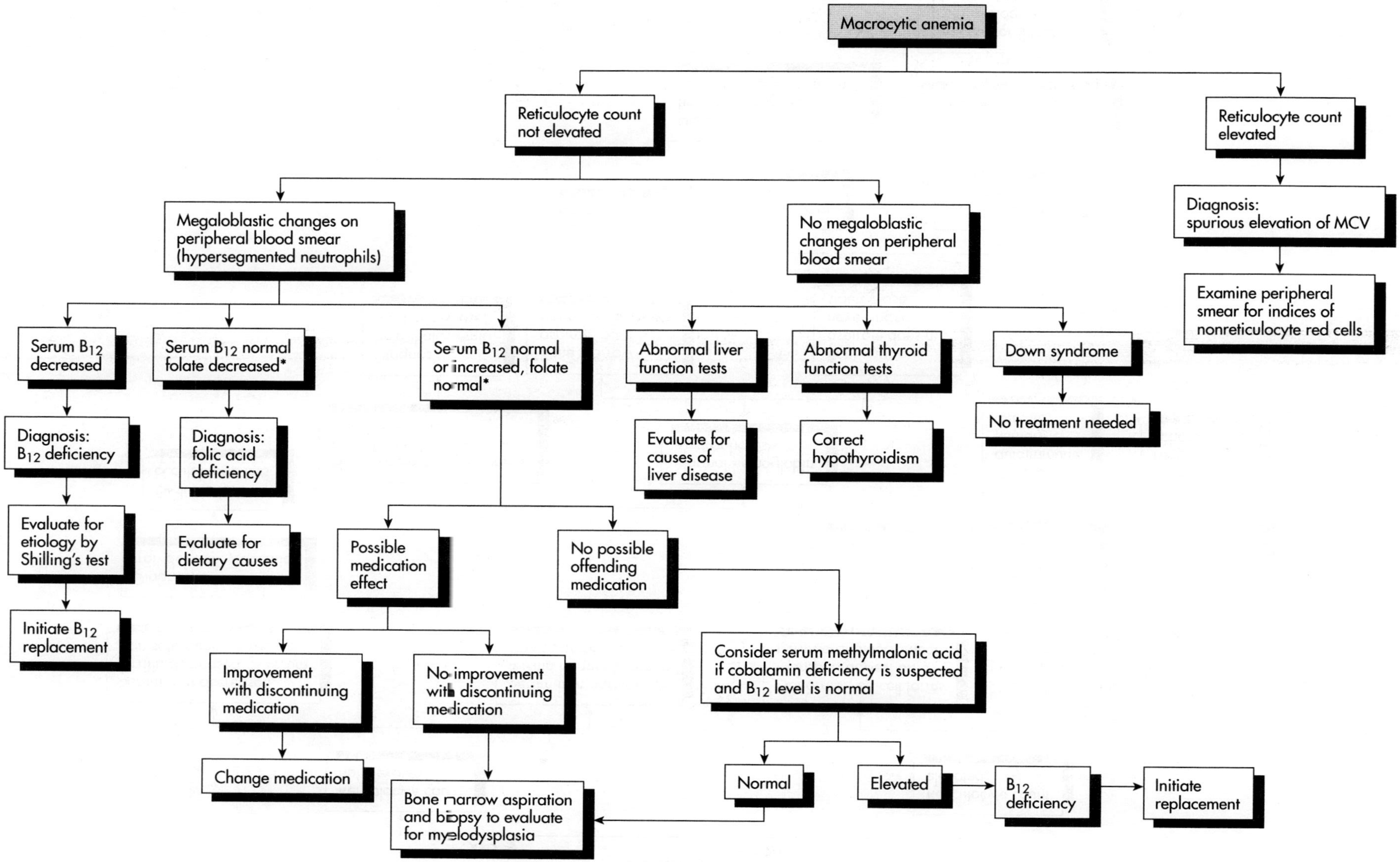

*Measure both serum and RBC folate levels.

FIGURE 3-25 Differential diagnosis of macrocytic anemia. (Modified from Rakel RE [ed]: *Principles of family practice,* ed 7, Philadelphia, 2007, WB Saunders.)

ANEMIA, MICROCYTIC

ICD-9CM # 282.4

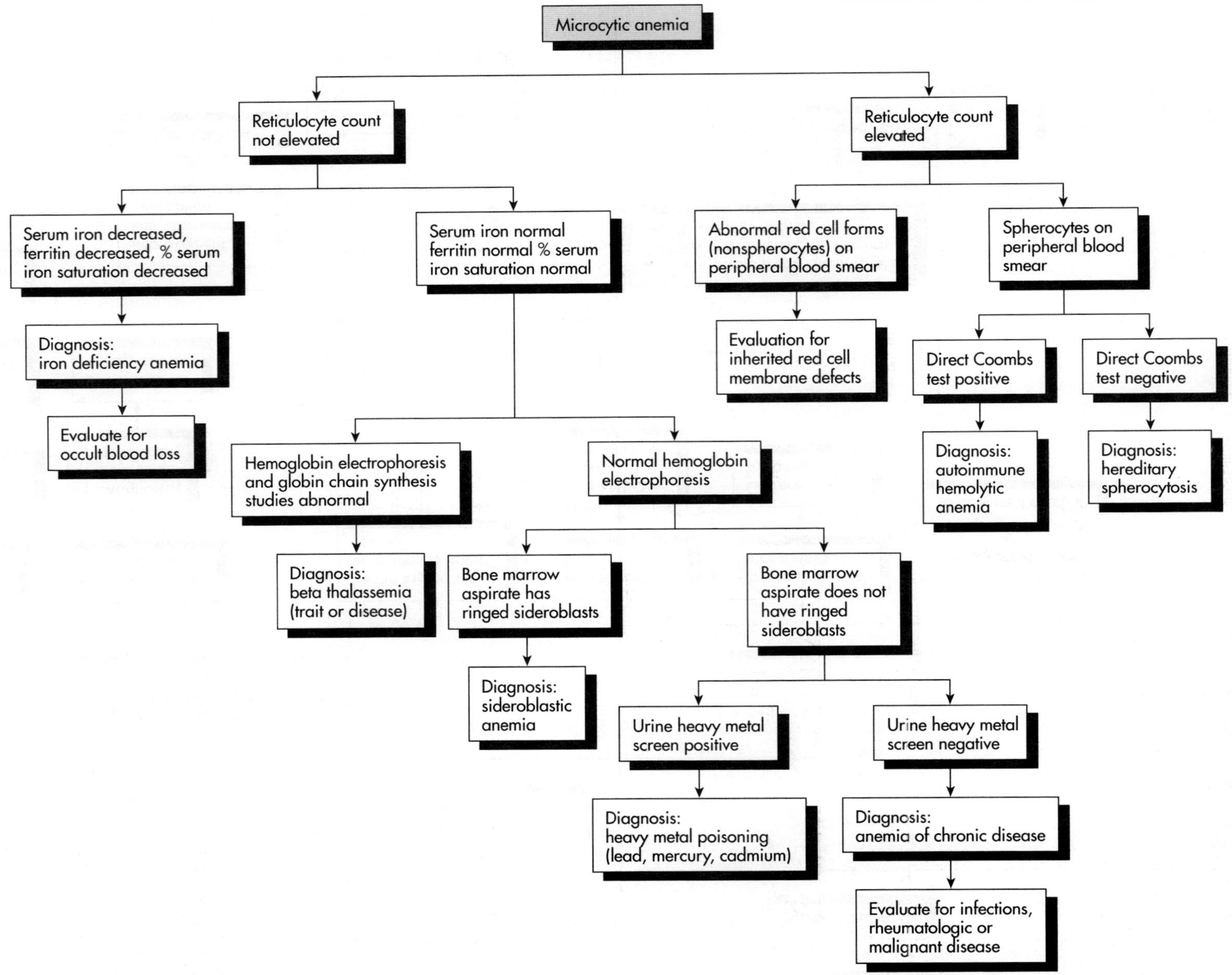

FIGURE 3-26 Differential diagnosis of microcytic anemia. (Modified from Rakel RE [ed]: *Principles of family practice,* ed 7, Philadelphia, 2007, WB Saunders.)

ANEMIA WITH RETICULOCYTOSIS

ICD-9CM # 790.99

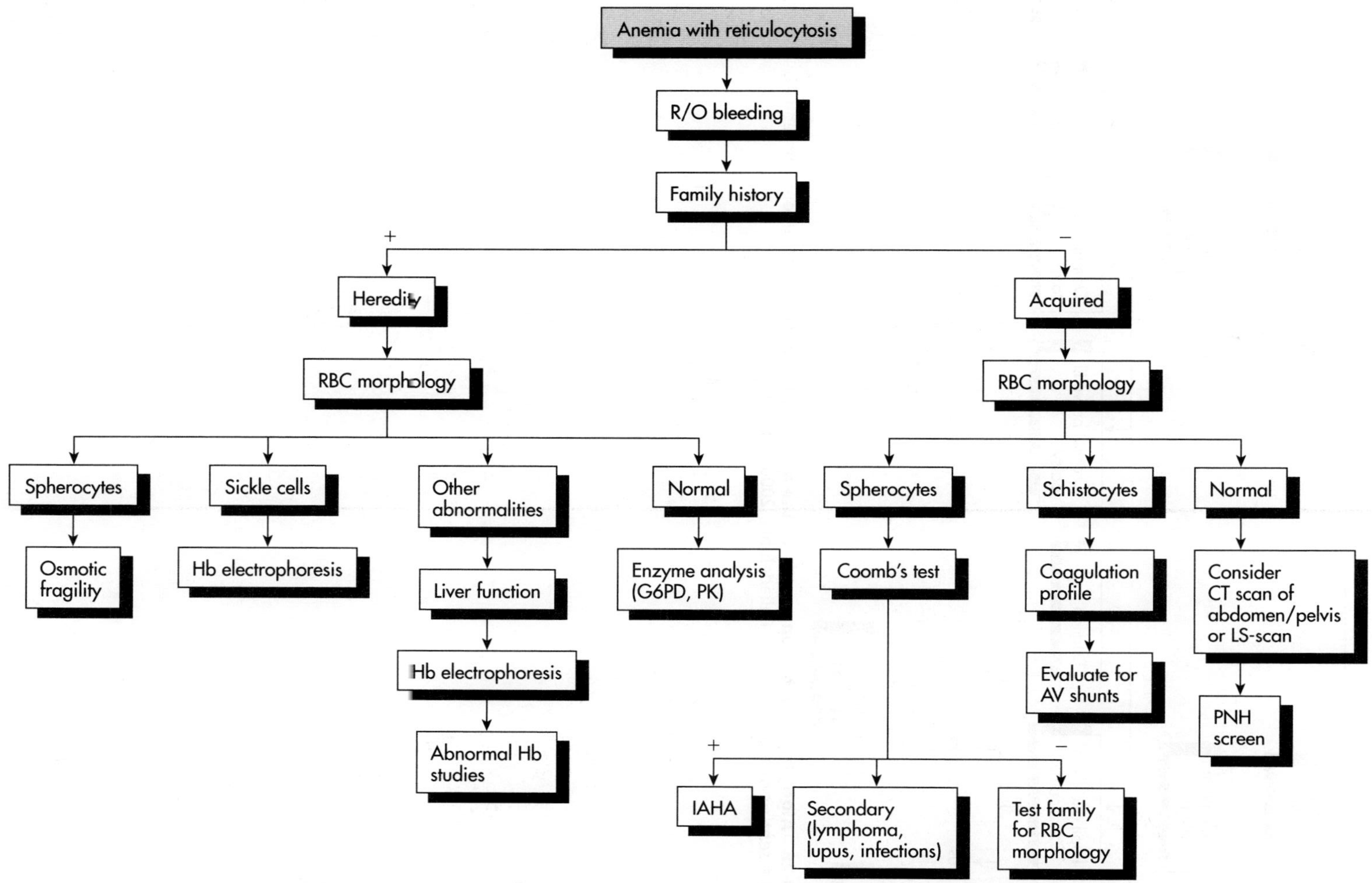

FIGURE 3-27 Evaluations of patients with hemolytic anemia. *AV,* Arteriovenous; *Hb,* hemoglobin; *IAHA,* idiopathic autoimmune hemolytic anemia; *LS,* liver spleen; *PK,* pyruvate kinase; *PNH,* paroxysmal nocturnal hemoglobinuria; *RBC,* red blood cell.

ICD-9CM # 379.41

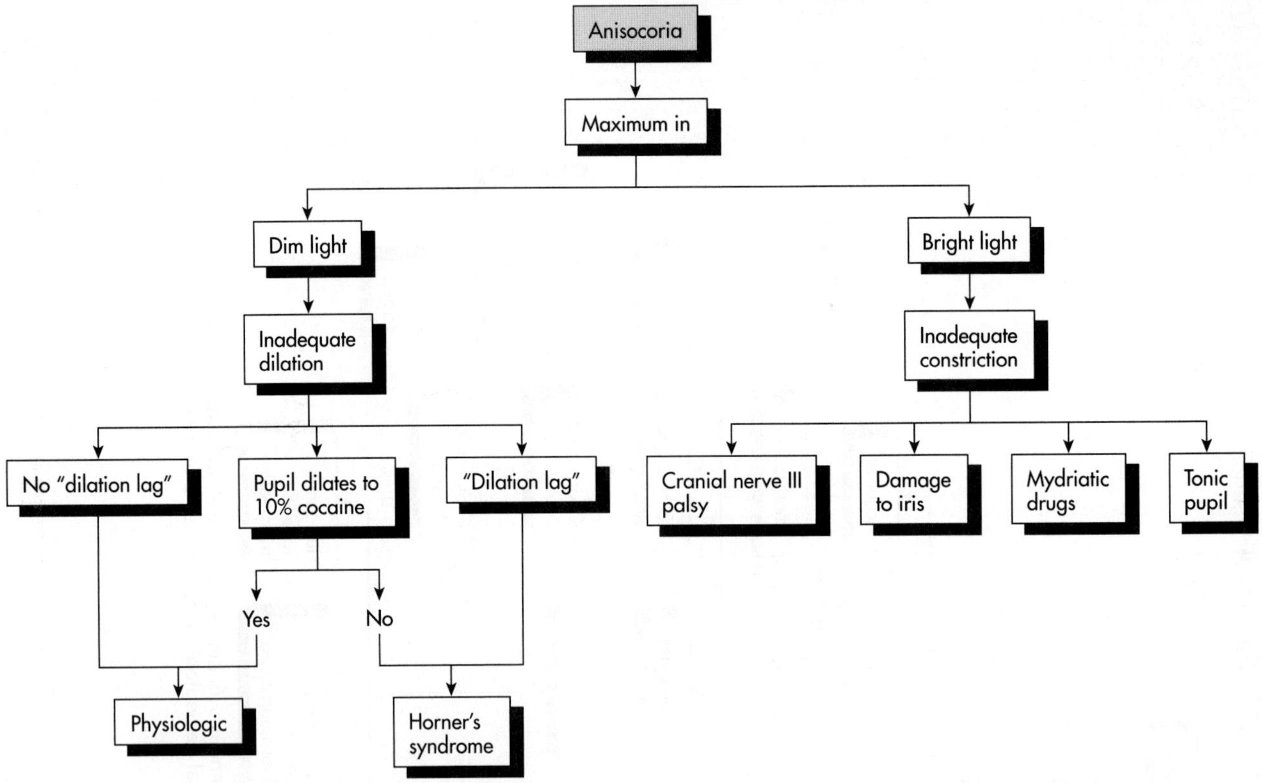

FIGURE 3-28 Algorithm for the approach to unequal pupils (anisocoria). (From Andreoli TE [ed]: *Cecil essentials of medicine,* ed 7, Philadelphia, 2008, WB Saunders.)

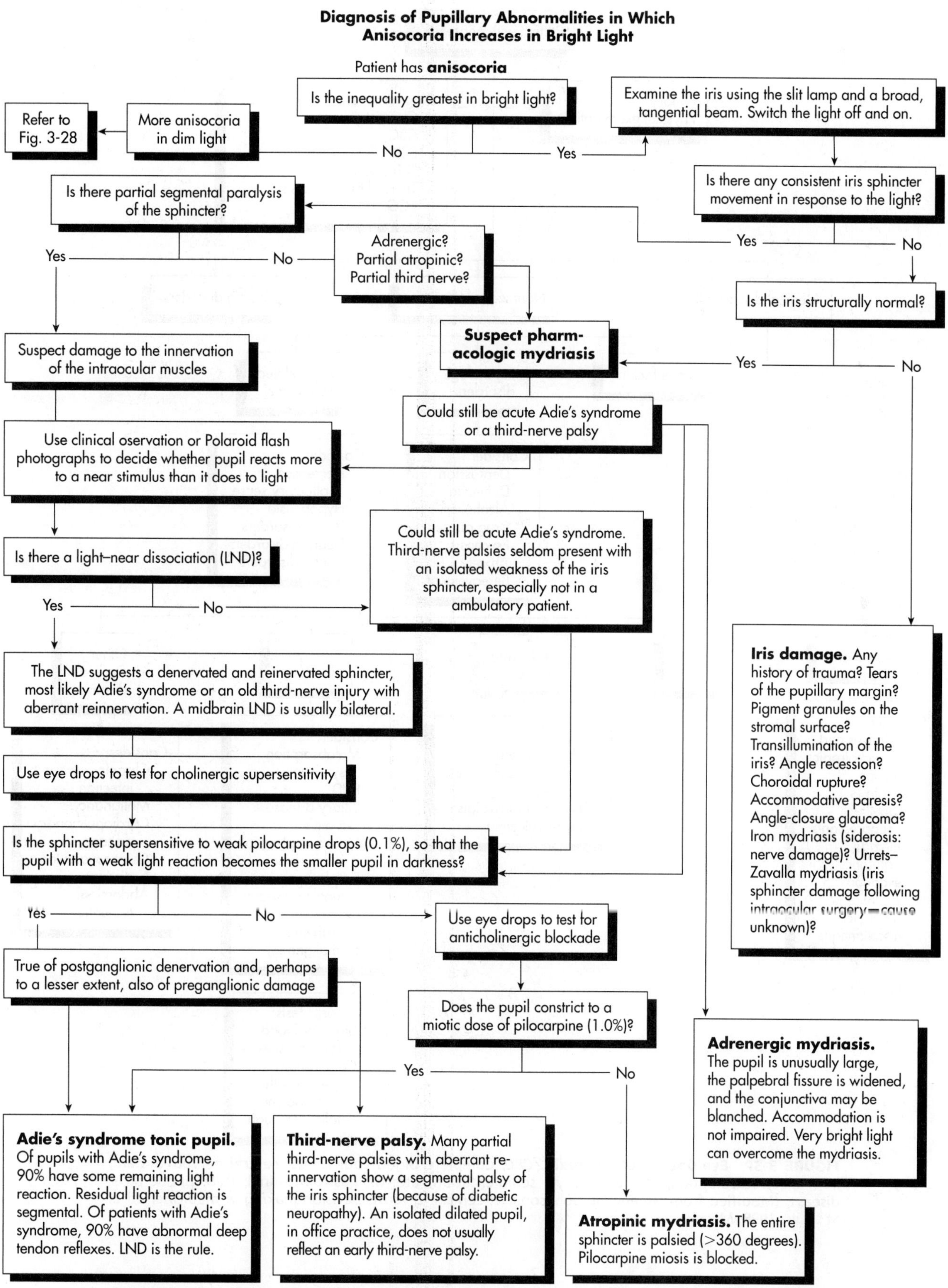

FIGURE 3-29 Diganosis of pupillary abnormalities in which anisocoria increases in bright light. Initial pupillary inequality is greater in bright light than in darkness, which indicates that the sphincter of the large pupil is weak or that a parasympathetic lesion is present on that side. (From Yanoff M, Duker JS: *Ophthalmology,* ed 2, St Louis, 2004, Mosby.)

ICD-9CM # 783.0

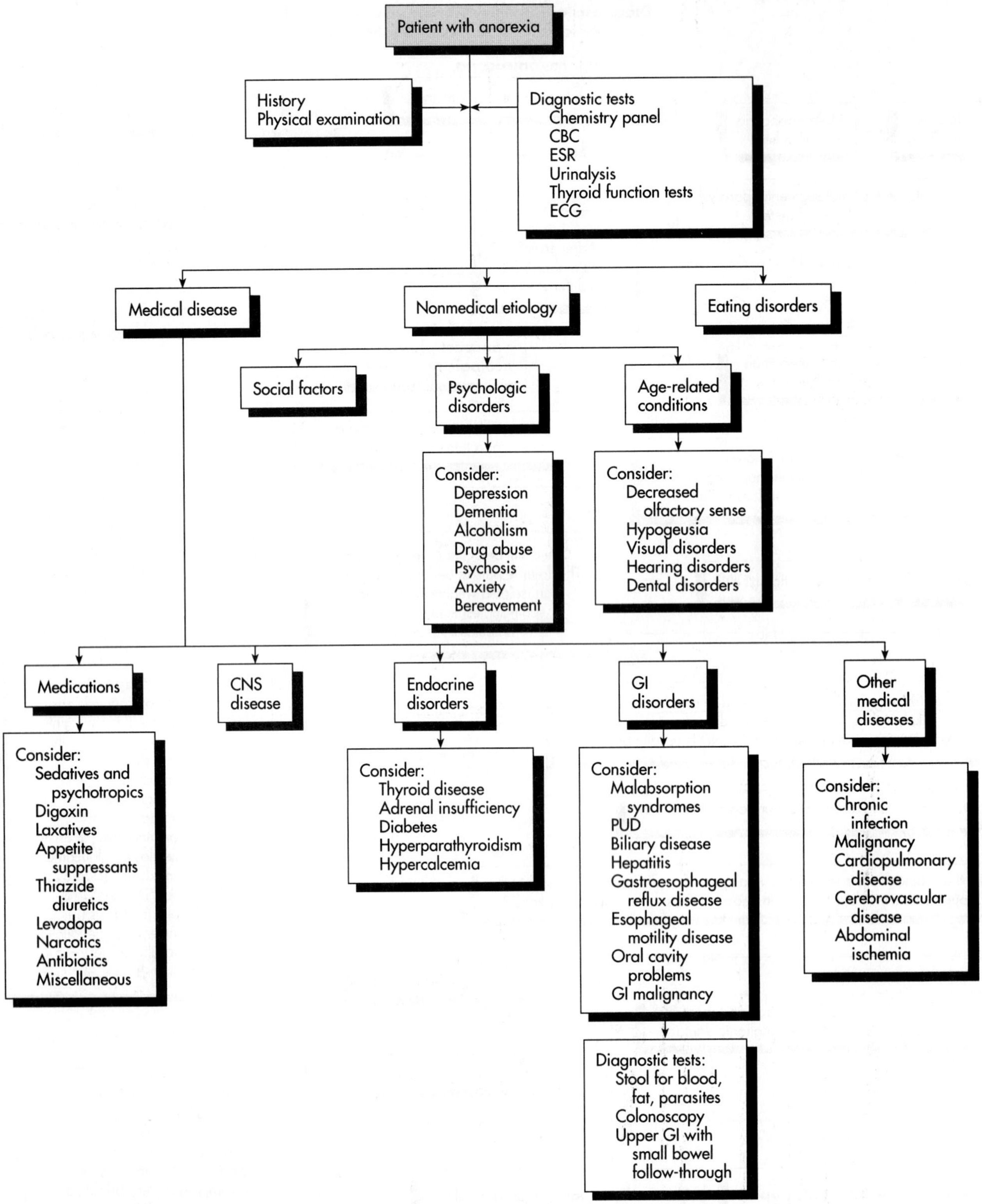

FIGURE 3-30 Evaluation of anorexia. *CBC,* Complete blood count; *CNS,* central nervous system; *ECG,* electrocardiogram; *ESR,* erythrocyte sedimentation rate; *GI,* gastrointestinal; *PUD,* peptic ulcer disease. (Modified from Greene HL, Johnson WP, Lemcke D [eds]: *Decision making in medicine,* ed 2, St Louis, 1998, Mosby.)

ICD-9CM # 795.79

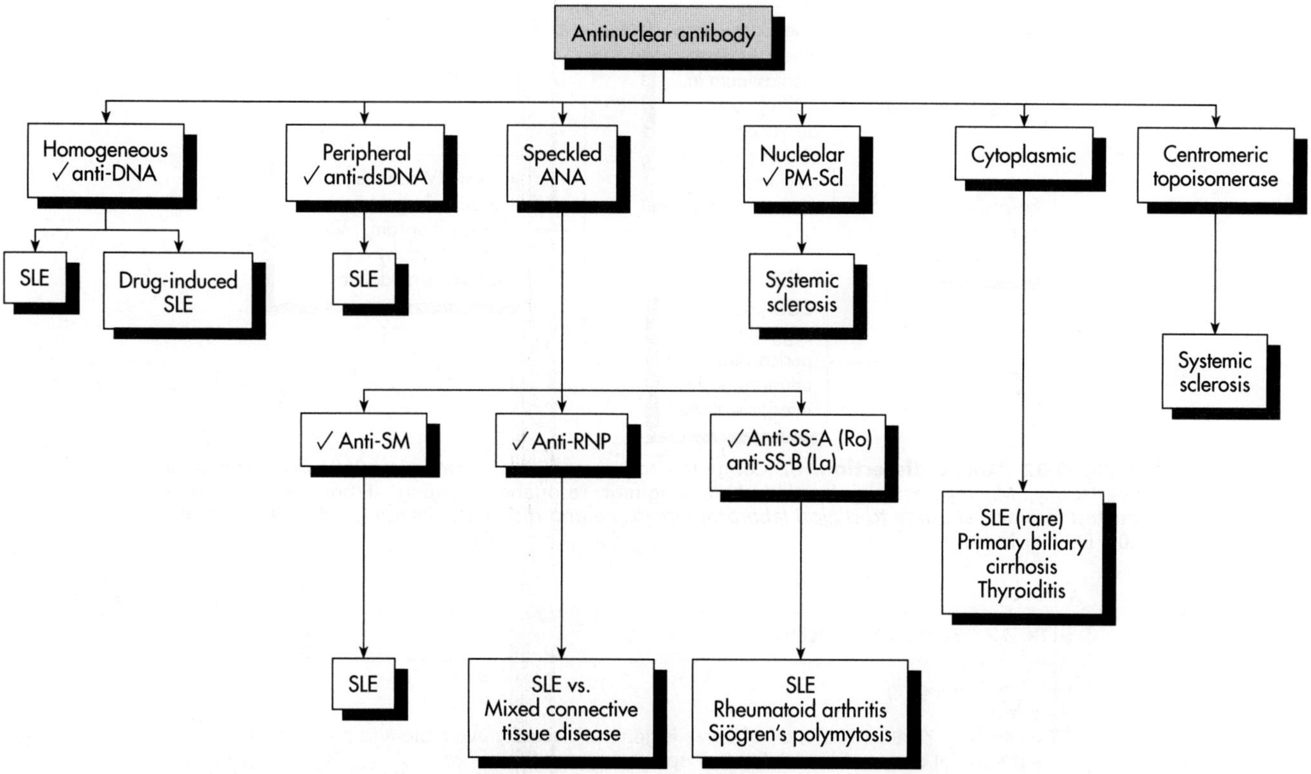

FIGURE 3-31 Diagnostic tests and diagnoses to consider from antinuclear antibody pattern. *ANA,* Antinuclear antibody; *SLE,* systemic lupus erythematosus. (From Carlson KJ et al: *Primary care of women,* ed 2, St Louis, 2002, Mosby.)

ICD-9CM # 441.00

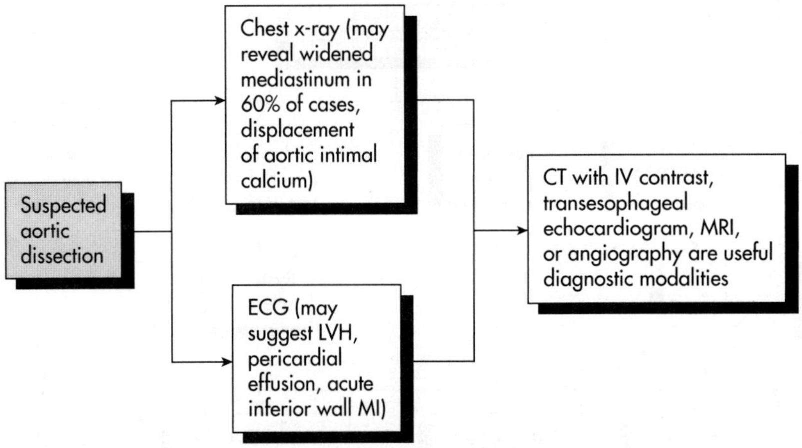

FIGURE 3-32 Aortic dissection. *CT,* Computed tomography; *IV,* intravenous; *LVH,* left ventricular hypertrophy; *MI,* myocardial infarction; *MRI,* magnetic resonance imaging. (From Ferri FF: *Ferri's best test: a practical guide to clinical laboratory medicine and diagnostic imaging,* ed 2, Philadelphia, 2009, Elsevier Mosby.)

BOX 3-2 Aortic Dissection

Diagnostic imaging
Best test
CT (sensitivity 83% to 100%; CT of aorta is generally readily available and performed as the initial diagnostic modality in suspected aortic dissection)
Ancillary tests
MRI (sensitivity 90% to 100%; difficult test for unstable, intubated patient)
Transesophageal echocardiogram (sensitivity 97% to 100%; can also detect aortic insufficiency and pericardial effusion)
Aortography (sensitivity 80% to 90%; involves IV contrast; allows visualization of coronary arteries)

Lab evaluation
Best test
None
Ancillary tests
CBC
BUN, creatinine

From Ferri FF: *Ferri's best test: a practical guide to clinical laboratory medicine and diagnostic imaging,* ed 2, Philadelphia, 2009, Elsevier Mosby.
BUN, Blood urea nitrogen; *CBC,* complete blood count; *CT,* computed tomography; *MRI,* magnetic resonance imaging.

ICD-9CM # 424.1

Initial Diagnostic Evaluation of Patients with Suspected Aortic Stenosis[††]

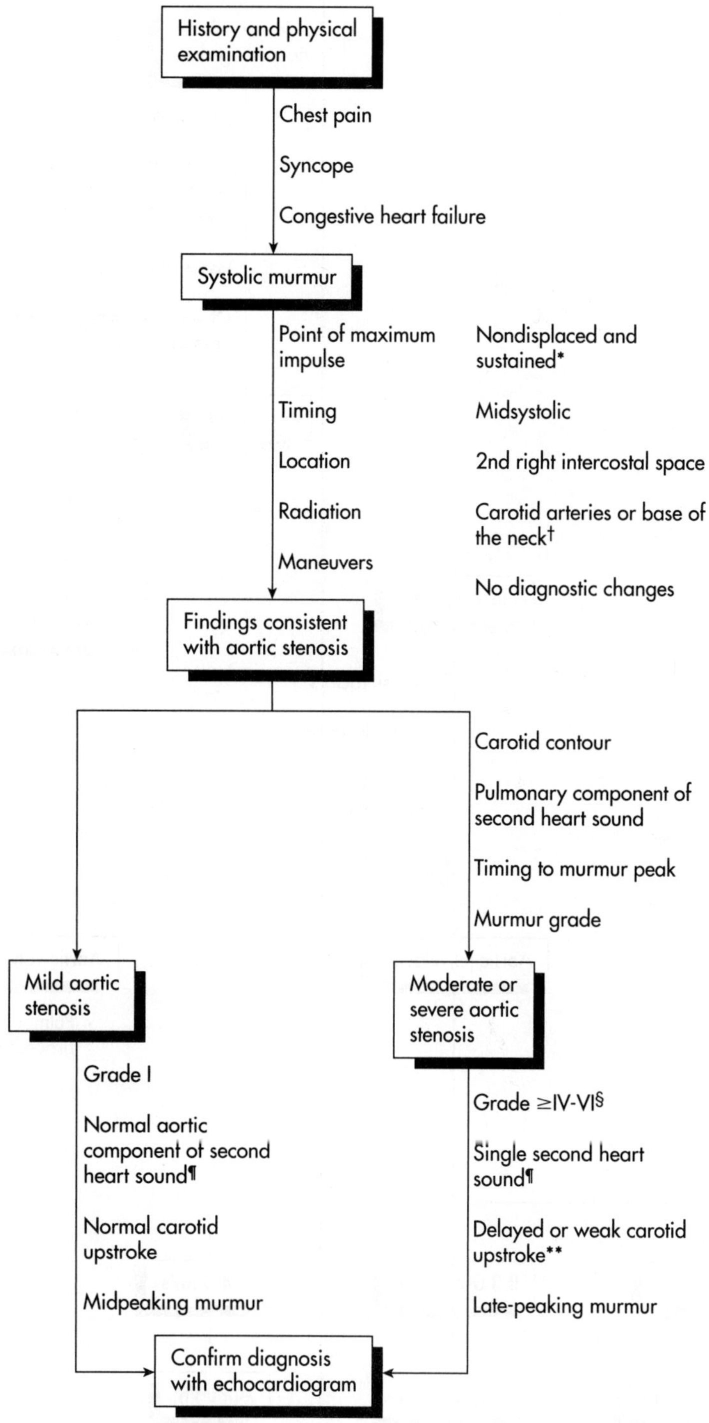

*May be displaced in the setting of left ventricular systolic dysfunction.
†Radiation to apex with Gallavardin phenomenon.
§Grade I: severe stenosis unlikely; grade IV: highly specific for severe stenosis.
¶Normal aortic component of second heart sound implies normal valve closure and absence of severe stenosis.
**Carotid upstroke may be normal in severe aortic stenosis in those patients with long-standing hypertension secondary to decreased arterial wall compliance.
††See Section I for additional information on this topic.

FIGURE 3-33 Aortic stenosis, diagnostic approach and management. Initial diagnostic evaluation of patients with suspected aortic stenosis. (From Crawford MH, DiMarco JP, Paulus WJ [eds]: *Cardiology,* ed 2, St Louis, 2004, Mosby.)

Continued on following page

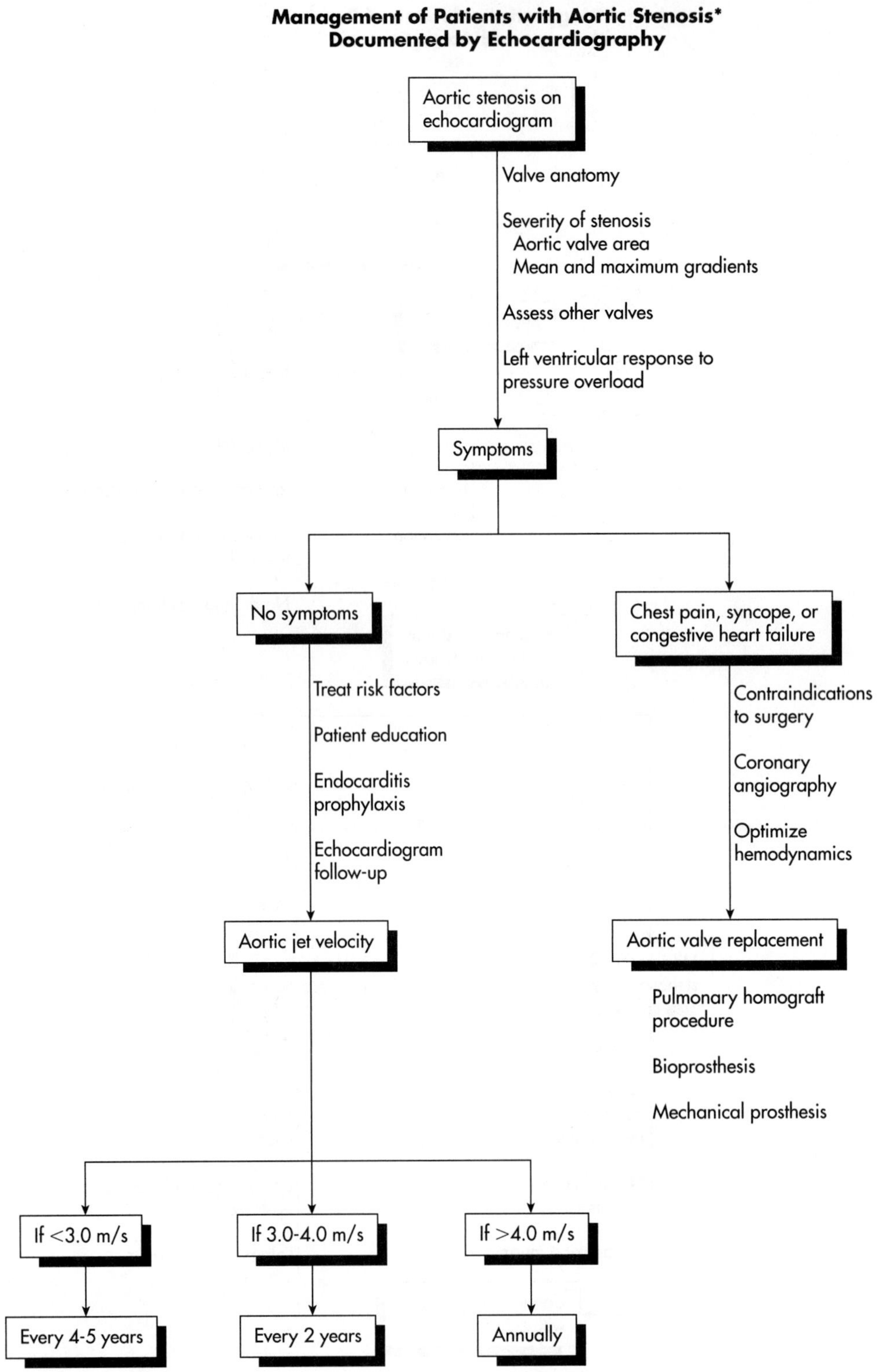

*See Section I for additional information on this topic.

FIGURE 3-34 Aortic stenosis, diagnostic approach and management. Management of patients with aortic stenosis documented by echocardiography. (From Crawford MH, DiMarco JP, Paulus WJ [eds]: *Cardiology,* ed 2, St Louis, 2004, Mosby.)

ICD-9CM # 719.40 Arthralgia site NOS
719.41 Arthralgia, shoulder region
719.42 Arthralgia, upper arm
719.43 Arthralgia, forearm
719.44 Arthralgia, hand
719.45 Arthralgia, pelvic region and thigh
719.46 Arthralgia, lower leg
719.47 Arthralgia, ankle and/or foot

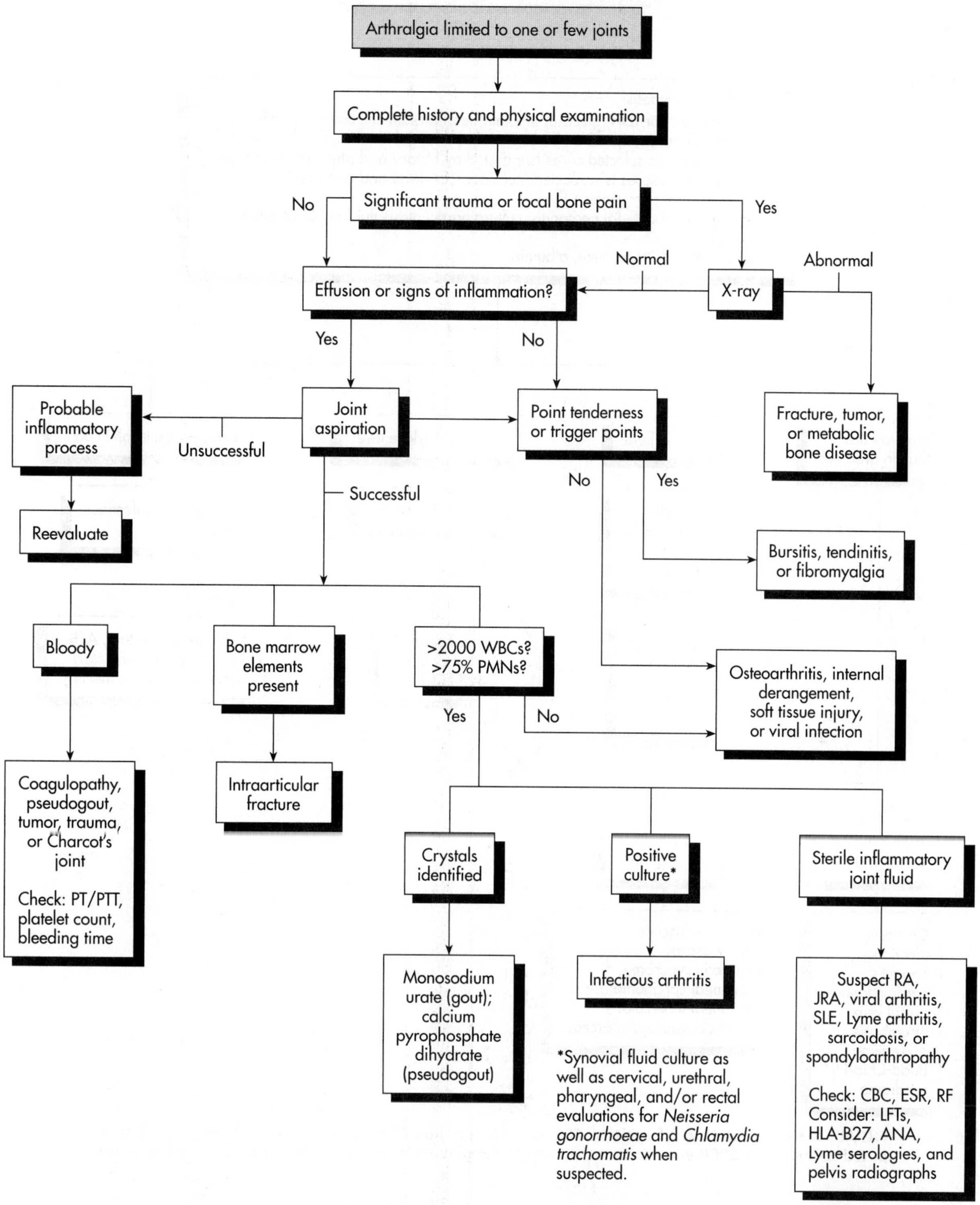

FIGURE 3-35 A diagnostic approach to arthralgia in a few joints. *ANA,* Antinuclear antibodies; *CBC,* complete blood count; *ESR,* erythrocyte sedimentation rate; *JRA,* juvenile rheumatoid arthritis; *LFTs,* liver function tests; *PMNs,* polymorphonuclear neutrophils; *PT,* prothrombin time; *PTT,* partial thromboplastin time; *RA,* rheumatoid arthritis; *RF,* rheumatoid factor; *SLE,* systemic lupus erythematosus; *WBCs,* white blood cells. (Modified from American College of Rheumatology Ad Hoc Committee on Clinical Guidelines: *Arthritis Rheum* 39:1, 1996.)

ICD-9CM # 789.5 Ascites NOS
197.6 Ascites, cancerous (malignant) M8000/6
457.8 Chylous
014.0 Tuberculous

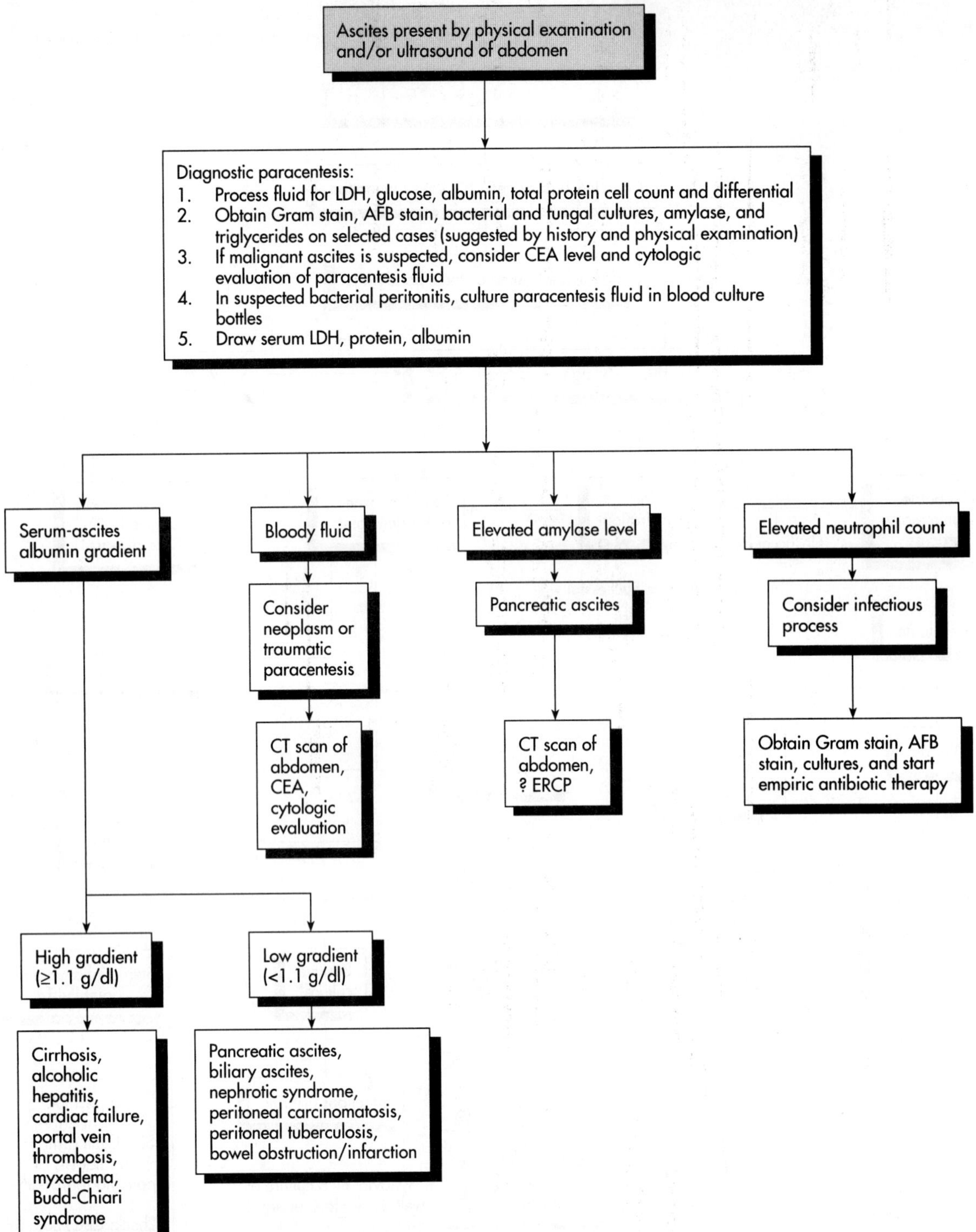

FIGURE 3-36 Evaluation of ascites. *AFB,* Acid-fast bacillus; *CEA,* carcinoembryonic antigen; *CT,* computed tomography; *ERCP,* endoscopic retrograde cholangiopancreatography; *LDH,* lactate dehydrogenase.

ICD-9CM # 197.6

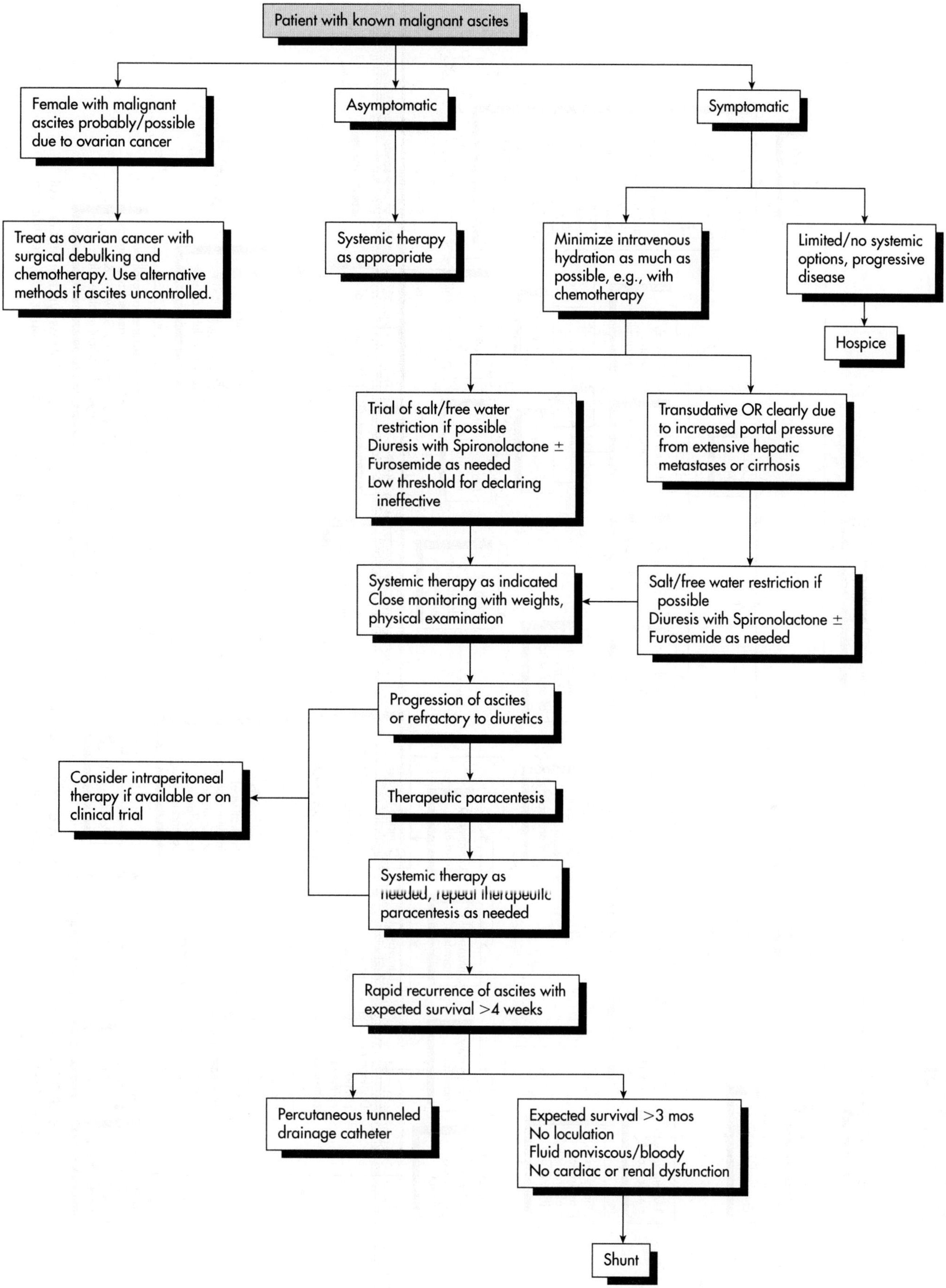

FIGURE 3-37 Ascites, malignant, treatment approach. (From Abeloff MD: *Clinical oncology,* ed 3, Philadelphia, 2004, Elsevier.)

ASPIRATION, GASTRIC CONTENTS

ICD-9CM # 507.0

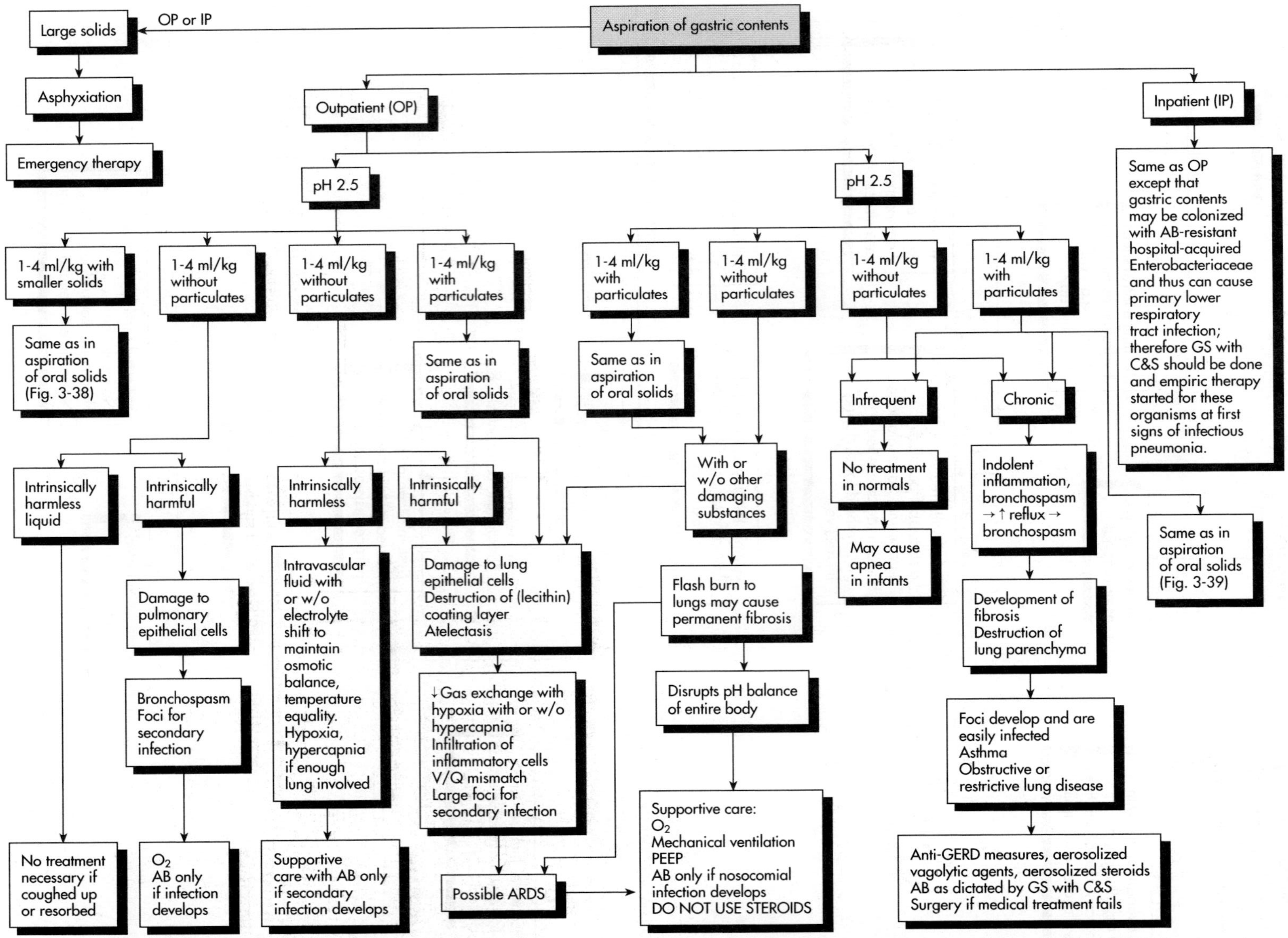

FIGURE 3-38 Management of aspiration of gastric contents. *AB,* Antibiotics; *ARDS,* acute respiratory distress syndrome; *C&S,* culture and sensitivity; *GERD,* gastroesophageal reflux disease; *GS,* Gram's stain; *PEEP,* positive end-expiratory pressure; *V/Q,* ventilation-perfusion. (From Kassirer J [ed]: *Current therapy in adult medicine,* ed 4, St Louis, 1998, Mosby.)

ASPIRATION, ORAL CONTENTS

ICD-9CM # 507.0

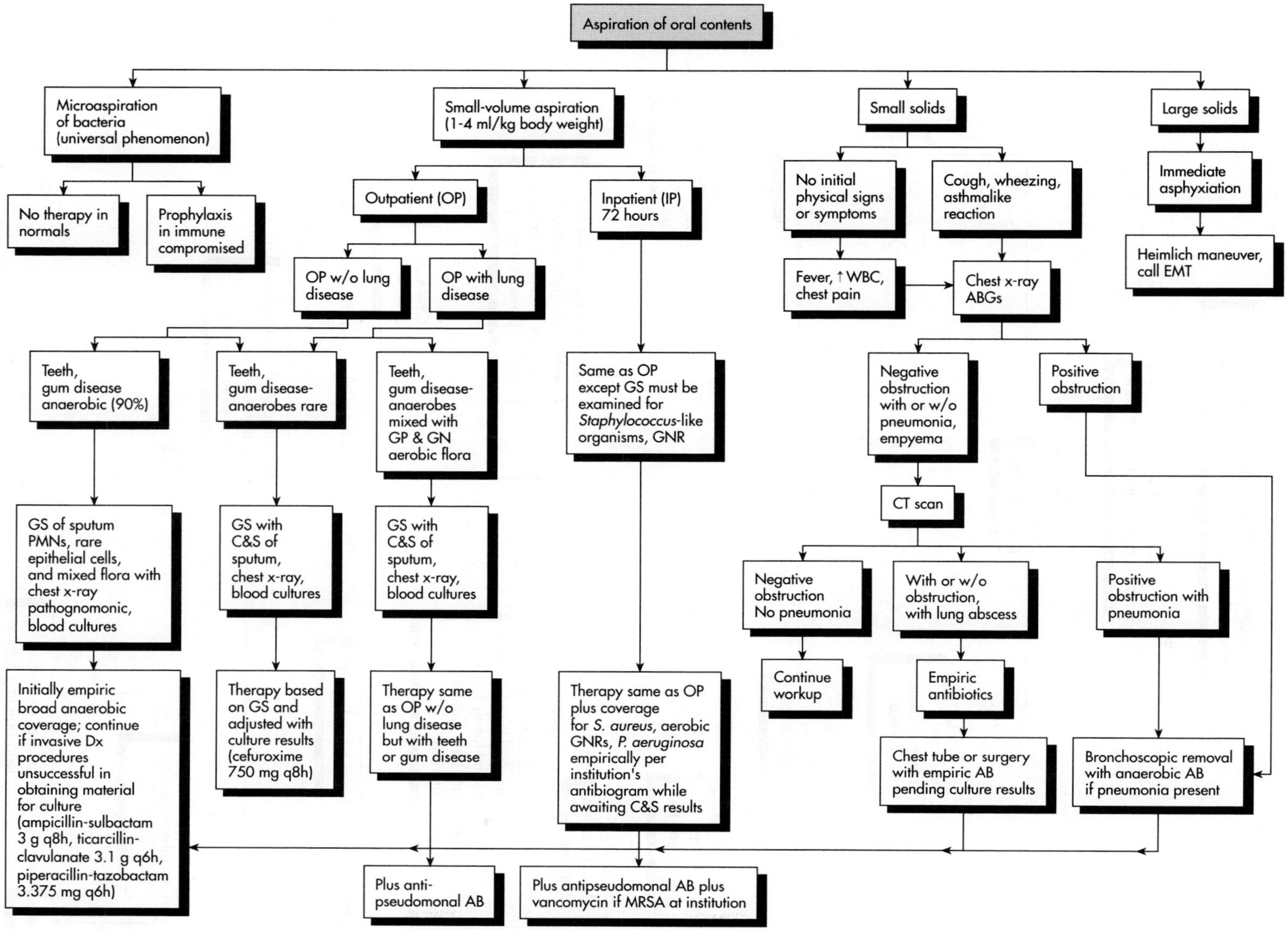

FIGURE 3-39 Management of aspiration of oral contents. *AB,* Antibiotics; *ABG,* arterial blood gases; *C&S,* culture and sensitivity; *CT,* computed tomography; *Dx,* diagnostic; *EMT,* emergency medical technician; *GN,* gram-negative; *GNRs,* gram-negative rods; *GP,* gram-positive; *GS,* Gram stain; *MRSA,* methicillin-resistant *Staphylococcus aureus; PMNs,* polymorphonuclear leukocytes; *WBC,* white blood cells. (From Kassirer J [ed]: *Current therapy in adult medicine,* ed 4, St Louis, 1998, Mosby.)

ICD-9CM # 493.9 Asthma, unspecified
493.1 Intrinsic asthma
493.0 Extrinsic asthma

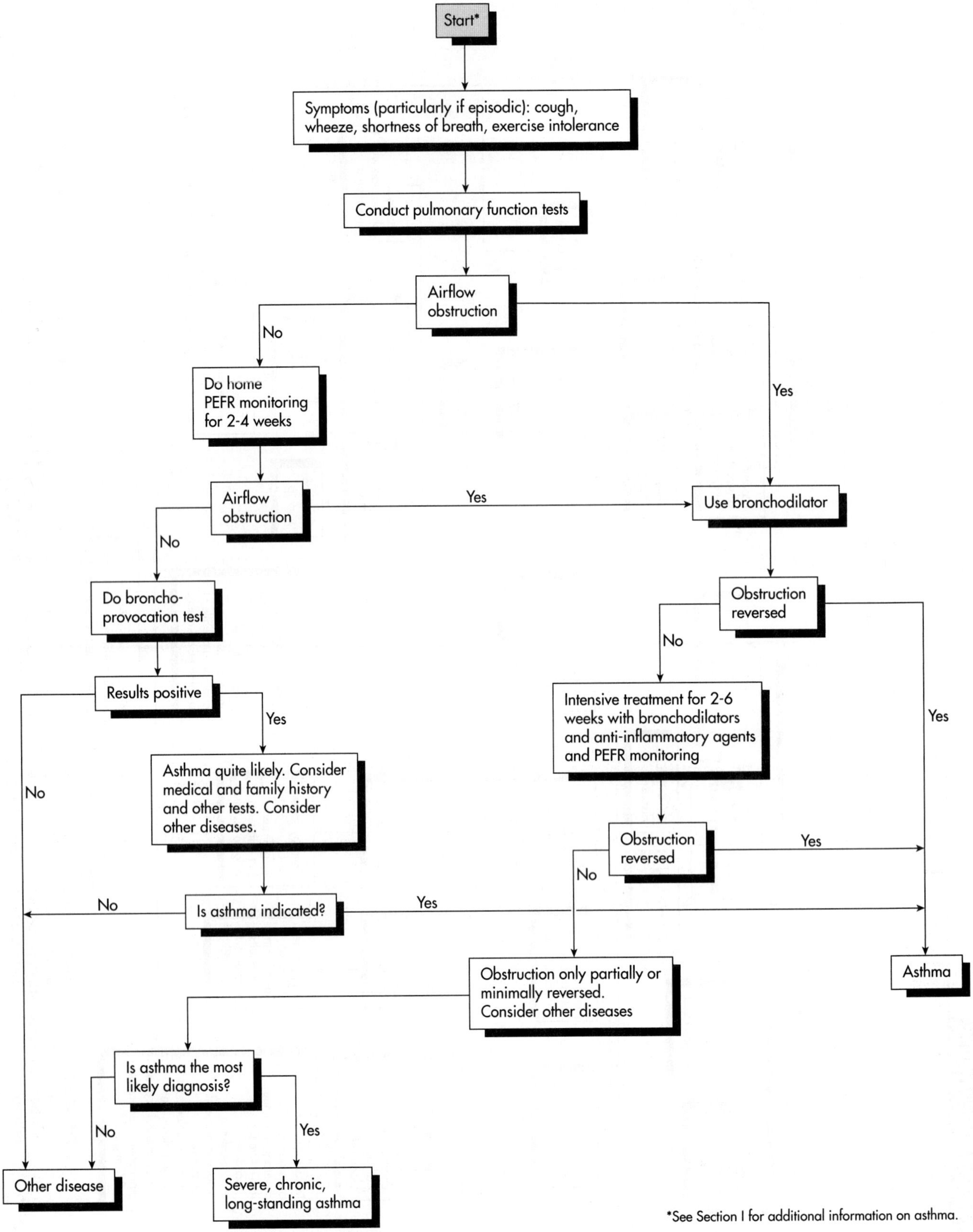

*See Section I for additional information on asthma.

FIGURE 3-40 Algorithm for diagnosing asthma. *PEFR,* Peak expiratory flow rates. (From Fireman P: *Atlas of allergies and immunology,* ed 3, St Louis, 2006, Mosby.)

ASTHMA, EMERGENCY DEPARTMENT AND HOSPITAL-BASED CARE

ICD-9CM # 493.9 Asthma, unspecified
493.1 Intrinsic asthma
493.0 Extrinsic asthma

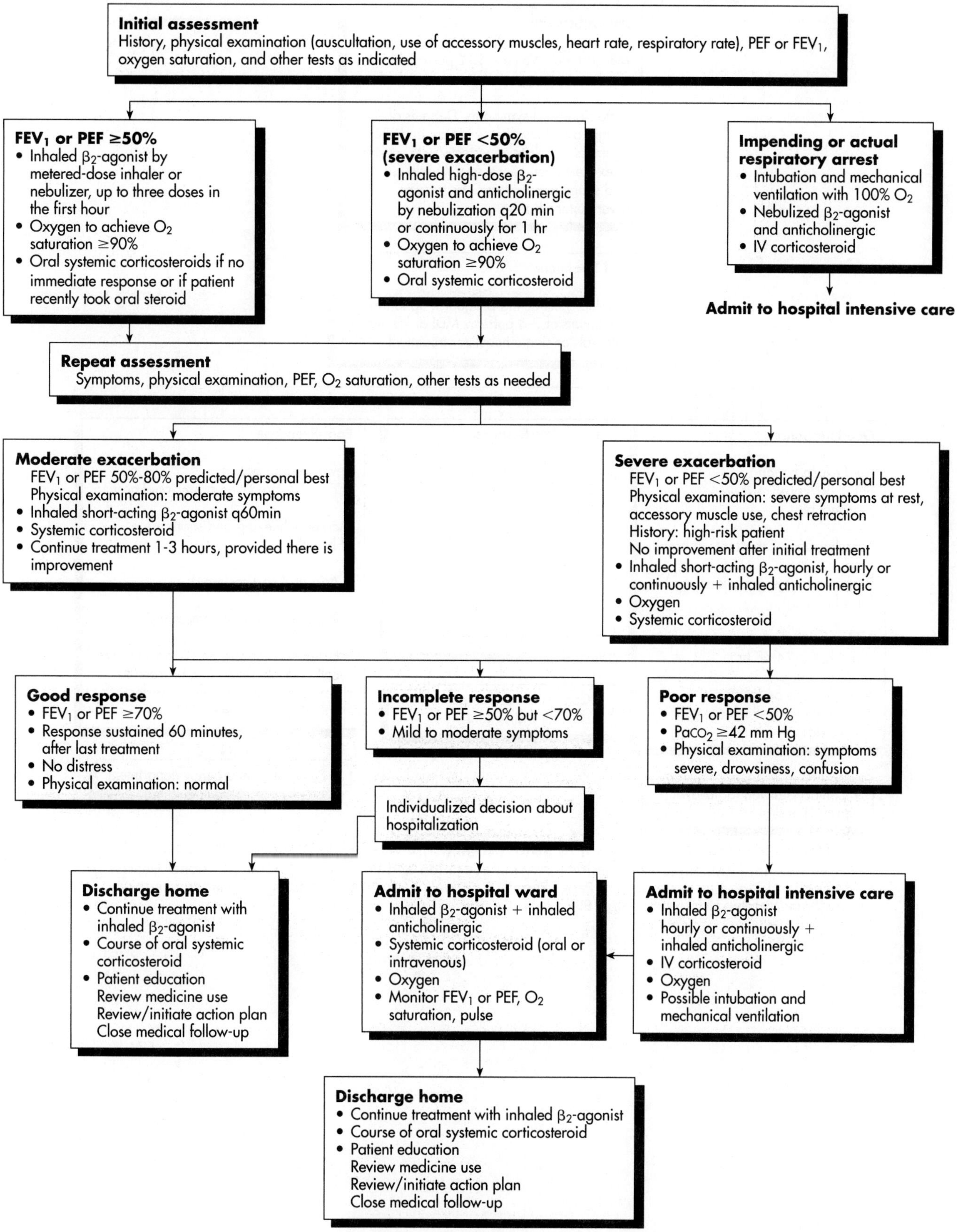

FIGURE 3-41 Management of asthma exacerbations: emergency department and hospital-based care. *FEV_1*, Forced expiratory volume in 1 second; *PEF*, peak expiratory flow. (From National Asthma Education and Prevention Program: *Guidelines for the diagnosis and management of asthma,* NIH Pub No 97-4051A, Bethesda, MD, 1997, National Institutes of Health, National Heart, Lung, and Blood Institute.)

ICD-9CM # 493.9 Asthma, unspecified
493.1 Intrinsic asthma
493.0 Extrinsic asthma

Assess Severity

Measure PEF: Value <50% personal best or predicted suggests severe exacerbation

Note signs and symptoms: Degrees of cough, breathlessness, wheeze, and chest tightness correlate imperfectly with severity of exacerbation. Accessory muscle use and suprasternal retractions suggest severe exacerbation

Initial Treatment

- Inhaled short-acting β-agonist: up to three treatments of 2-4 puffs by MDI at 20-minute intervals or single nebulizer treatment

Good Response

Mild exacerbation
PEF >80% predicted or personal best

No wheezing or shortness of breath

Response to β_2-agonist sustained for 4 hr

- May continue β_2-agonist every 3-4 hr for 24-48 hr
- For patients on inhaled corticosteroids, double dose for 7-10 days

→ • Contact clinician for follow-up instructions

Incomplete Response

Moderate exacerbation
PEF 50%-80% predicted or personal best

Persistent wheezing or shortness of breath

- Add oral corticosteroid
- Continue β_2-agonist

→ • Contact clinician urgently (this day) for instructions

Poor Response

Severe exacerbation
PEF <50% predicted or personal best

Marked wheezing and shortness of breath

- Add oral corticosteroid
- Repeat β_2-agonist immediately
- If distress is severe and nonresponsive, call your physician and proceed to emergency department; consider calling ambulance or 911

→ • Proceed to emergency department

FIGURE 3-42 Home management of acute asthma. *MDI,* Metered-dose inhaler; *PEF,* peak expiratory flow rate. (Modified from National Asthma Education and Prevention Program, National Heart, Lung, and Blood Institute, Expert Panel Report 2: *Guidelines for the diagnosis and management of asthma,* NIH Pub No 97-4051, July 1997.)

ICD-9CM # 781.3 Ataxia NOS
303.9 Alcoholic, chronic
334.3 Cerebellar
331.89 Cerebral
334.0 Friedreich's

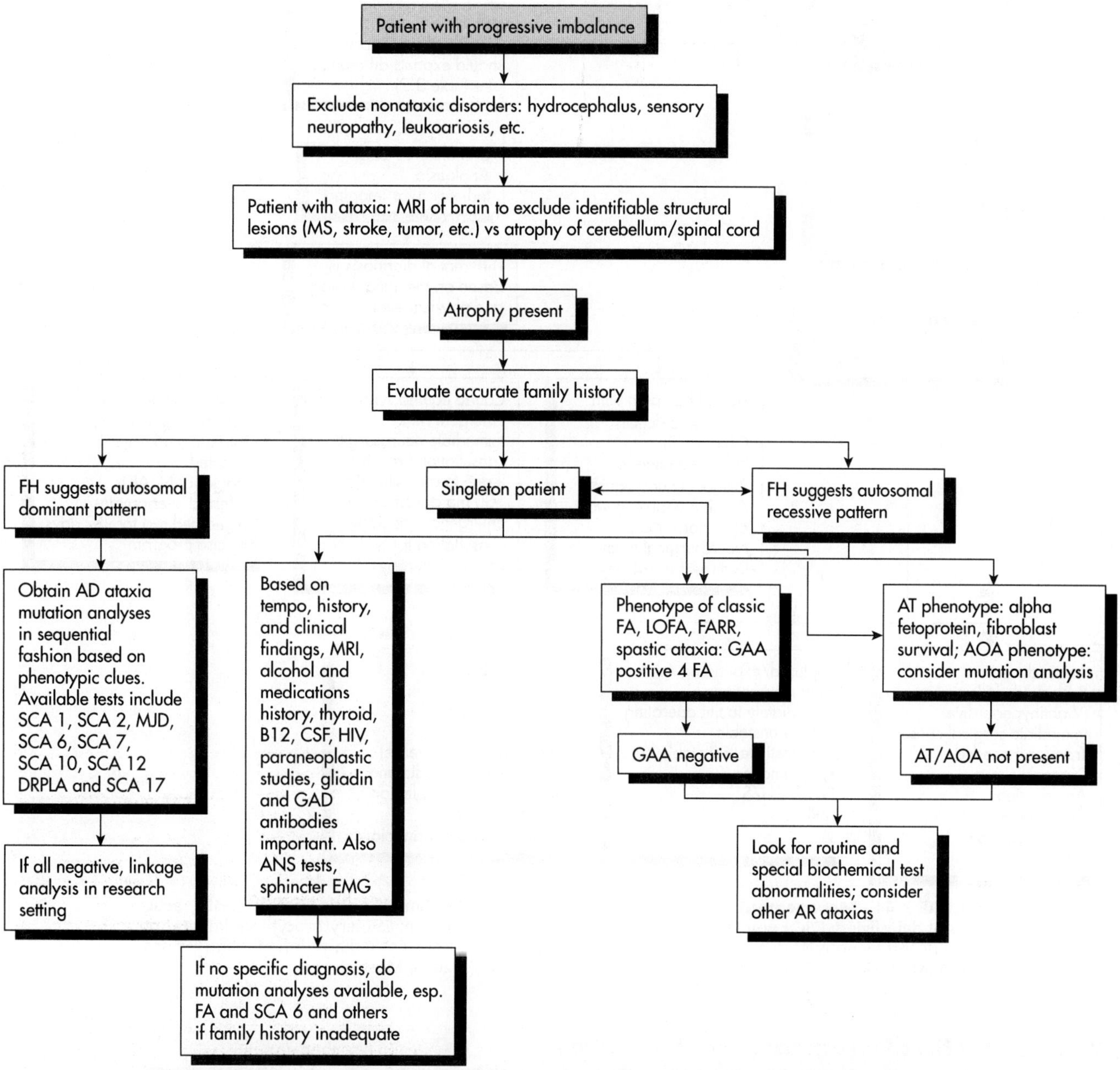

FIGURE 3-43 An algorithm for a diagnostic approach to patients with progressive ataxia. *AOA,* Ataxia with oculomotor apraxia; *AT,* ataxia-telengiectasia; *CSF,* cerebrospinal fluid; *DRPLA,* dentatorubral-pallidoluysian atrophy; *EMG,* electromyelography; *FA,* Friedreich's ataxia; *FH,* family history; *GAD,* glutamate decarboxylase; *HIV,* human immunodeficiency virus; *MRI,* magnetic resonance imaging; *MS,* multiple sclerosis; *SCA,* spinocerebellar ataxia. (From Bradley WG, Daroff RB, Fenichel GM, Jankovic J [eds]: *Neurology in clinical practice,* ed 4, Philadelphia, 2004, Butterworth Heinemann.)

ICD-9CM # 847.9

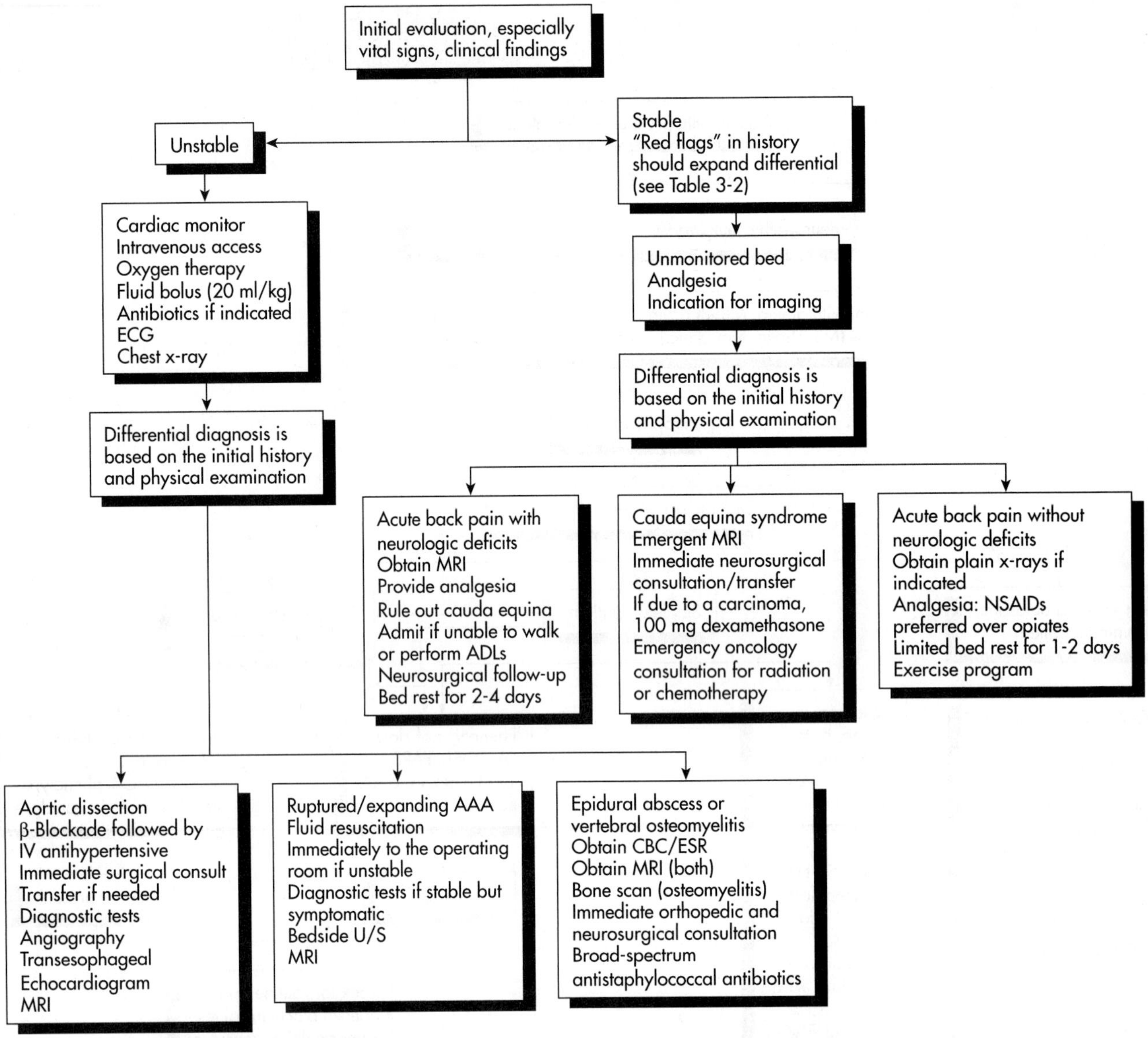

FIGURE 3-44 Management of acute low back pain. *AAA,* Abdominal aortic aneurysm; *ADL,* activities of daily living; *CBC,* complete blood count; *ECG,* electrocardiogram; *ESR,* erythrocyte sedimentation rate; *IV,* intravenous; *MRI,* magnetic resonance imaging; *NSAIDs,* nonsteroidal anti-inflammatory drugs. (From Marx JA [ed]: *Rosen's emergency medicine,* ed 6, St Louis, 2006, Mosby.)

TABLE 3-2 Red Flags for Potentially Serious Conditions

Possible Fracture	Possible Tumor or Infection	Possible Cauda Equina Syndrome
From Medical History		
Major trauma, such as vehicle accident or fall from height	Age over 50 or under 20 yr	Saddle anesthesia
Minor trauma or even strenuous lifting (in older or potentially osteoporotic patient)	History of cancer	Recent onset of bladder dysfunction, such as urinary retention, increased frequency, or overflow incontinence
	Constitutional symptoms, such as recent fever or chills or unexplained weight loss	Severe or progressive neurologic deficit in the lower extremity
	Risk factors for spinal infection: recent bacterial infection (e.g., urinary tract infection); intravenous drug abuse; or immune suppression (from steroids, transplant, or human immunodeficiency virus)	
	Pain that worsens when supine; severe nighttime pain	

ICD-9CM # 782.4

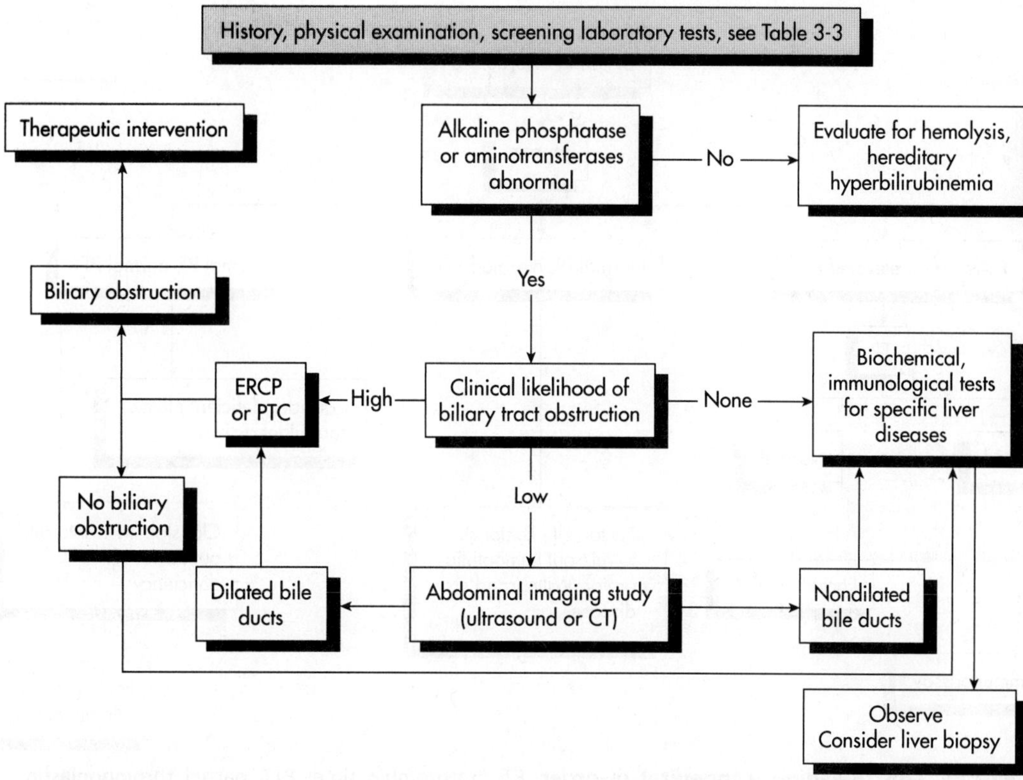

FIGURE 3-45 Diagnosis algorithm for the evaluation of hyperbilirubinemia and other liver test abnormalities and/or signs and symptoms suggestive of liver disease. *CT,* Computed tomography; *ERCP,* endoscopic retrograde cholangiopancreatography; *PTC,* percutaneous cholangiogram. (From Goldman L, Ausiello D [eds]: *Cecil textbook of medicine,* ed 23, Philadelphia, 2008, WB Saunders. Modified from Lidofsky SD, Scharschmidt BF: Jaundice, *in* Feldman M, Scharschmidt BF, Sleisenger MH [eds] *Gastrointestinal and liver disease,* ed 6, Philadelphia, 1998, WB Saunders.)

TABLE 3-3 **Obstructive Jaundice Versus Cholestatic Liver Disease**

Feature	Suggests Obstructive Jaundice	Suggests Parenchymal Liver Disease
History	Abdominal pain Fever, rigors Prior biliary surgery Older age Acholic stools	Anorexia, malaise, myalgias, suggestive of viral prodrome Known infectious exposure Receipt of blood products, use of intravenous drugs Exposure to known hepatotoxin Family history of jaundice
Physical examination	High fever Abdominal tenderness Palpable abdominal mass Abdominal scar	Ascites Other stigmata of liver disease (e.g., prominent abdominal veins, gynecomastia, spider angiomata, asterixis, encephalopathy, Kayser-Fleischer rings)
Laboratory studies	Predominant elevation of serum bilirubin and alkaline phosphatase Prothrombin time that is normal or normalizes with vitamin K administration Elevated serum amylase	Predominant elevation of serum aminotransferases Prolonged prothrombin time that does not correct with vitamin K administration Blood tests indicative of specific liver disease

From Goldman L, Ausiello D (eds): *Cecil textbook of medicine,* ed 23, Philadelphia, 2008, WB Saunders.

Section III CLINICAL ALGORITHMS

ICD-9CM # 286.9

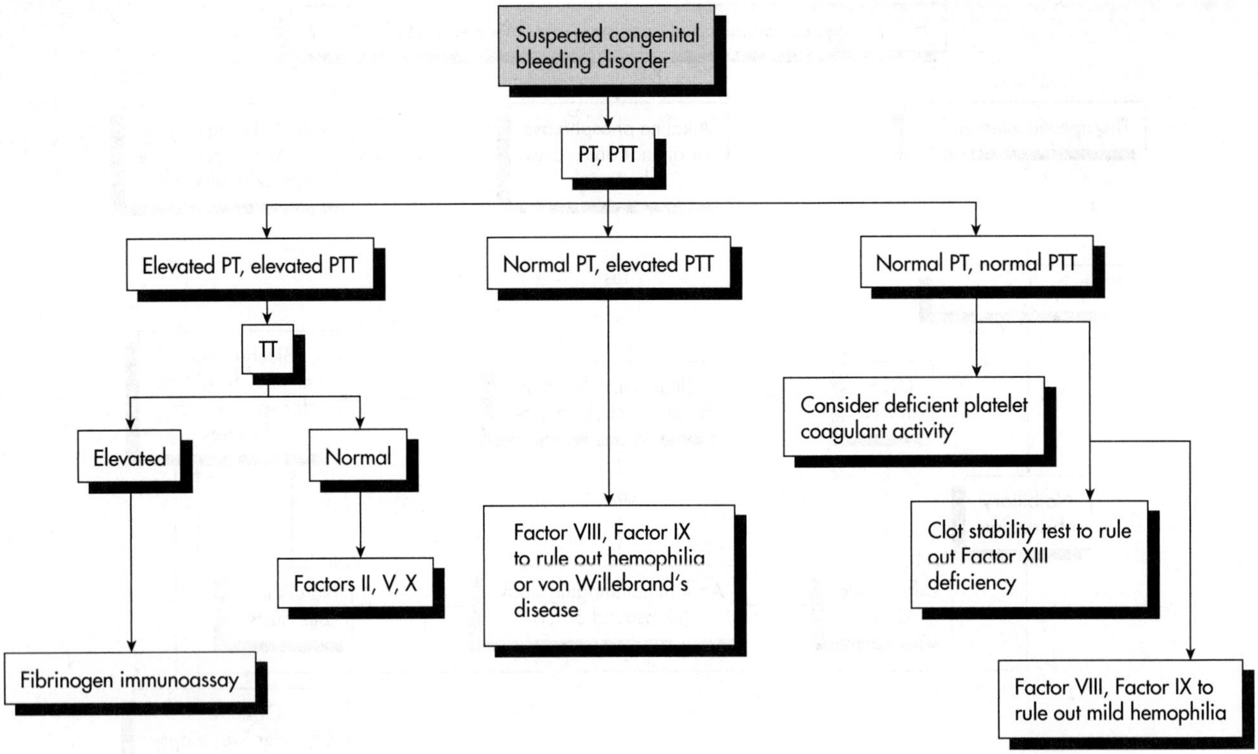

FIGURE 3-46 Bleeding, congenital disorder. *PT,* Prothrombin time; *PTT,* partial thromboplastin time; *TT,* thrombin time.

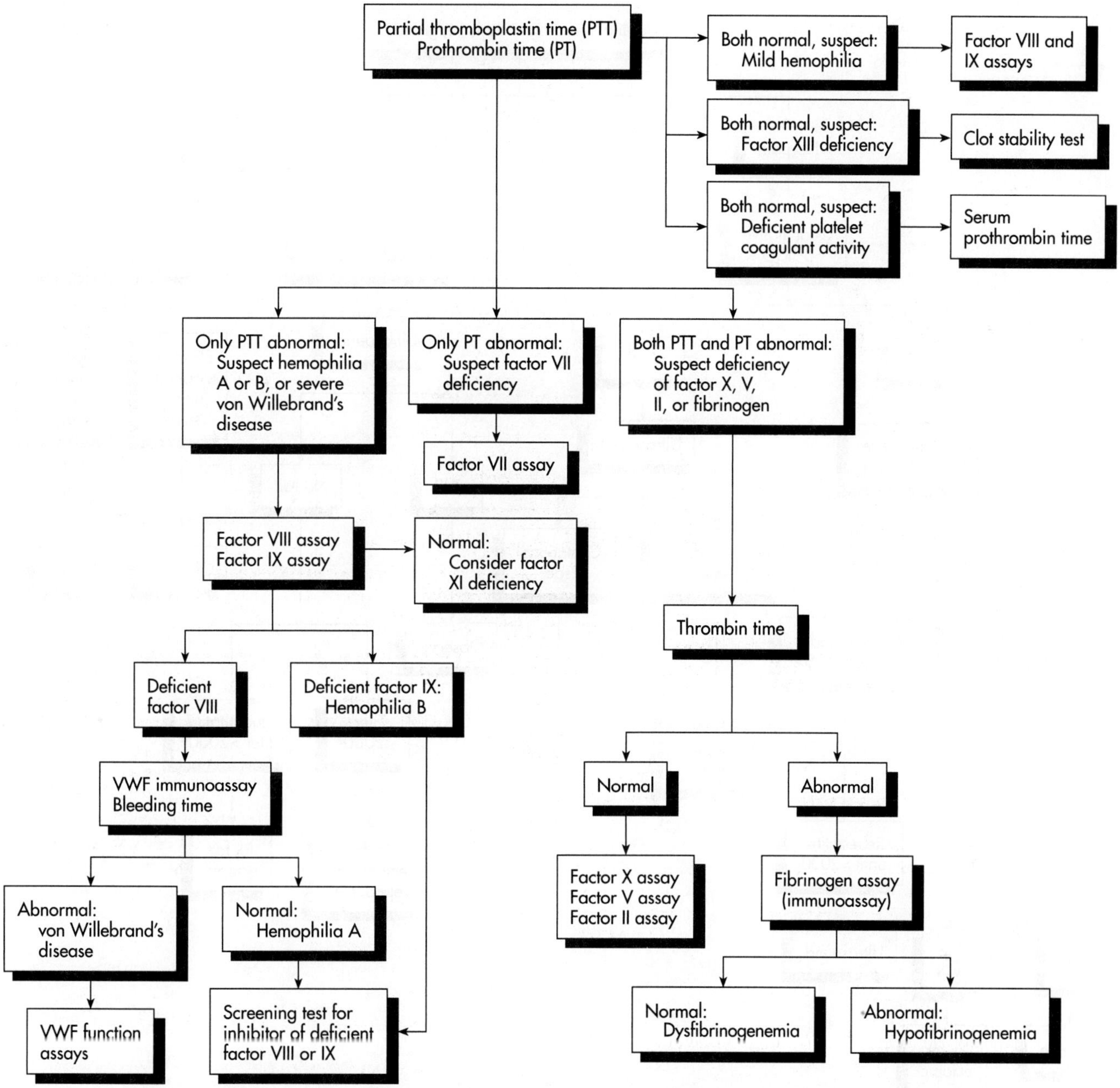

FIGURE 3-47 Laboratory evaluation of a patient with a bleeding disorder in whom the history and physical examination suggest a congenital coagulation disorder. *VWF,* von Willebrand factor. (From Stein JH [ed]: *Internal medicine,* ed 5, St Louis, 1998, Mosby.)

ICD-9CM # 641.9 Vaginal bleeding NOS in pregnancy

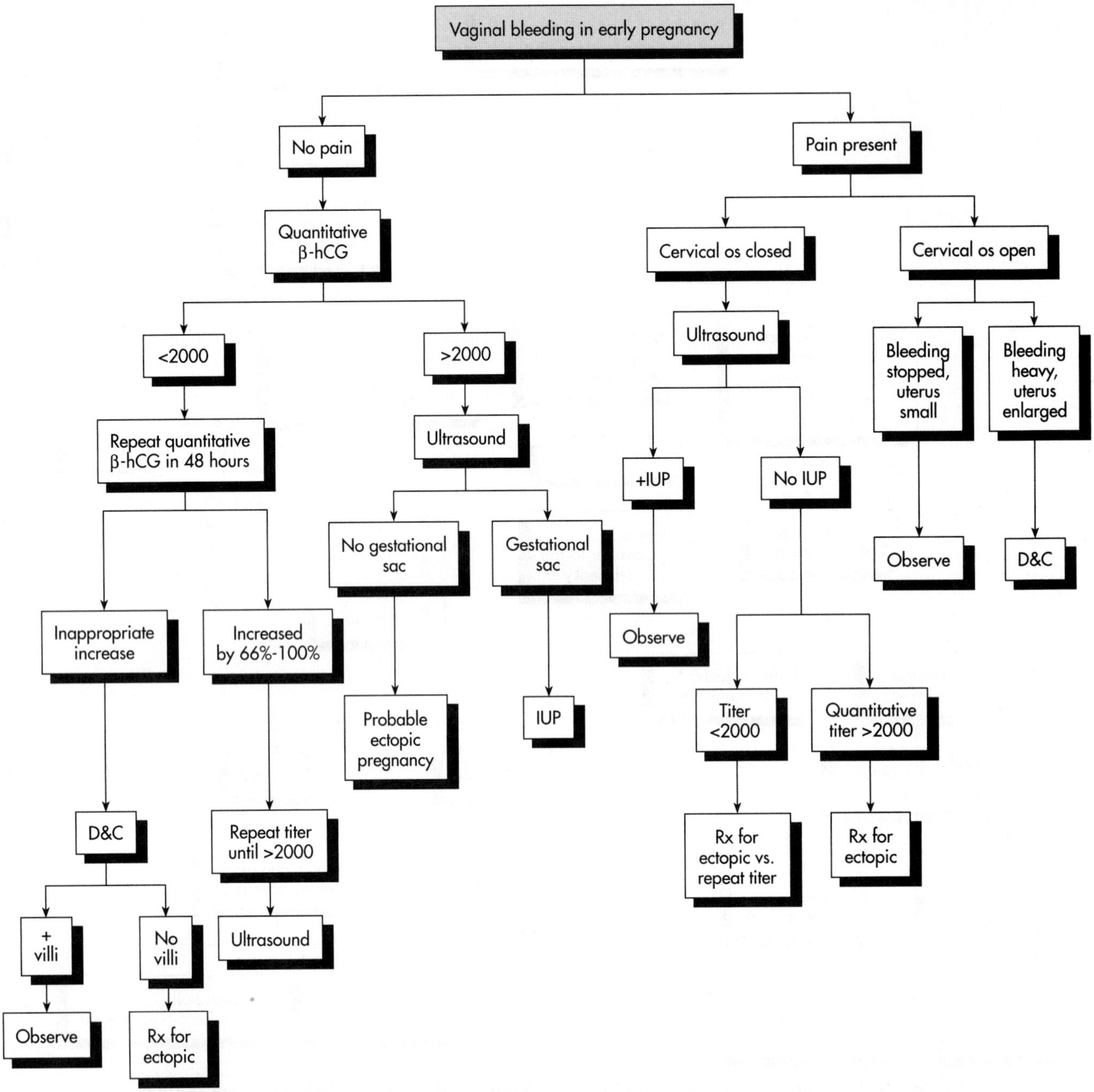

FIGURE 3-48 Diagnosis of vaginal bleeding in early pregnancy. *D&C,* Dilation and curettage; *β-hCG,* β-human chorionic gonadotropin; *IUP,* intrauterine pregnancy. (From Carlson KJ et al: *Primary care of women,* ed 2, St Louis, 2002, Mosby.)

ICD-9CM # 578.9

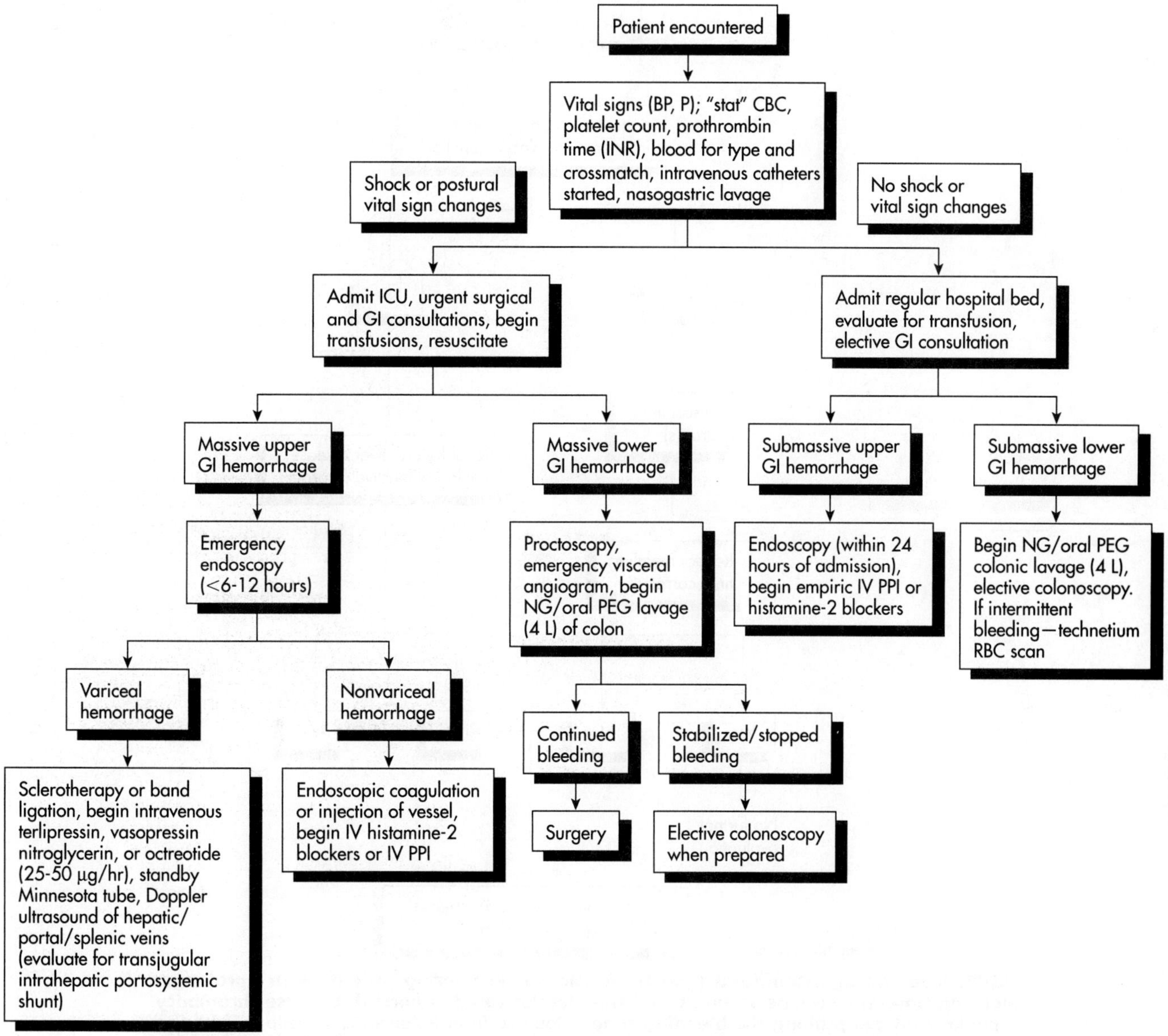

FIGURE 3-49 Approach to the patient with gastrointestinal hemorrhage. *BP,* Blood pressure; *CBC,* complete blood count; *GI,* gastrointestinal; *ICU,* intensive care unit; *IV,* intravenous; *NG,* nasogastric; *P,* weight; *PEG,* percutaneous endoscopic gastrostomy; *PPI,* proton pump inhibitor; *RBC,* red blood cell. (Modified from Goldman L, Ausiello D [eds]: *Cecil textbook of medicine,* ed 23, Philadelphia, 2008, WB Saunders.)

ICD-9CM # 790.92

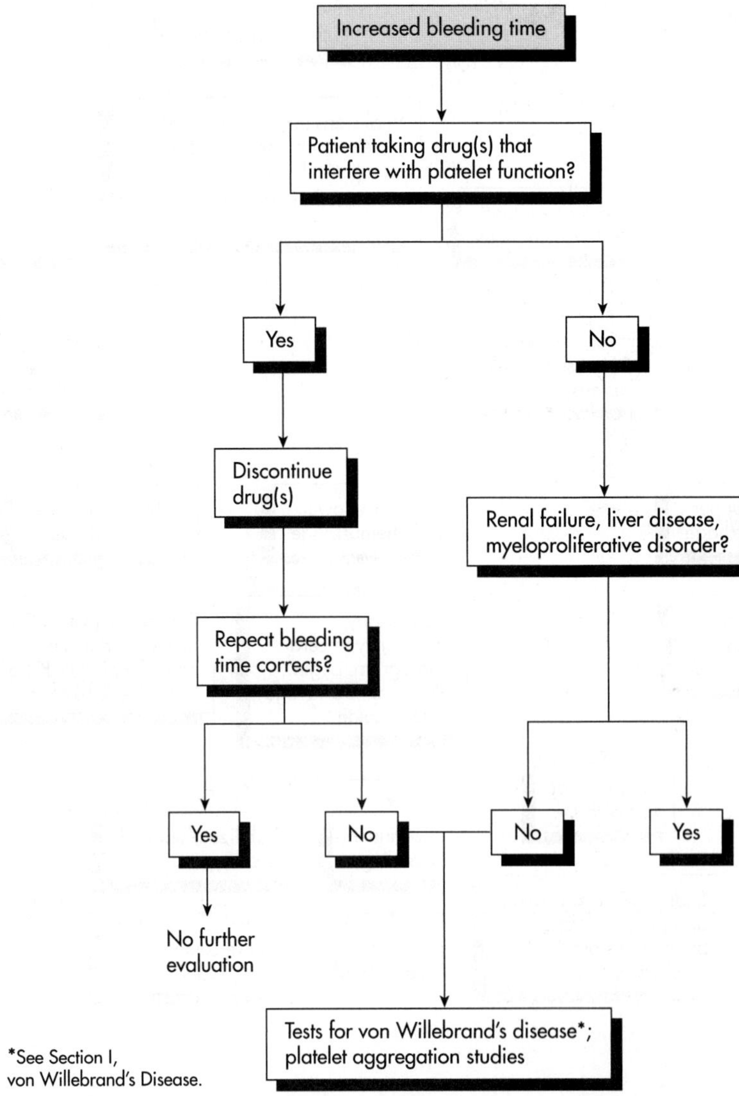

FIGURE 3-50 An algorithm for diagnostic decisions in evaluating patients with a prolonged bleeding time. The scheme assumes that the platelet count is normal, because thrombocytopenia itself can prolong the bleeding time. (Modified from Goldman L, Ausiello D [eds]: *Cecil textbook of medicine,* ed 23, Philadelphia, 2008, WB Saunders.)

ICD-9CM # 623.8 Vaginal bleeding NOS

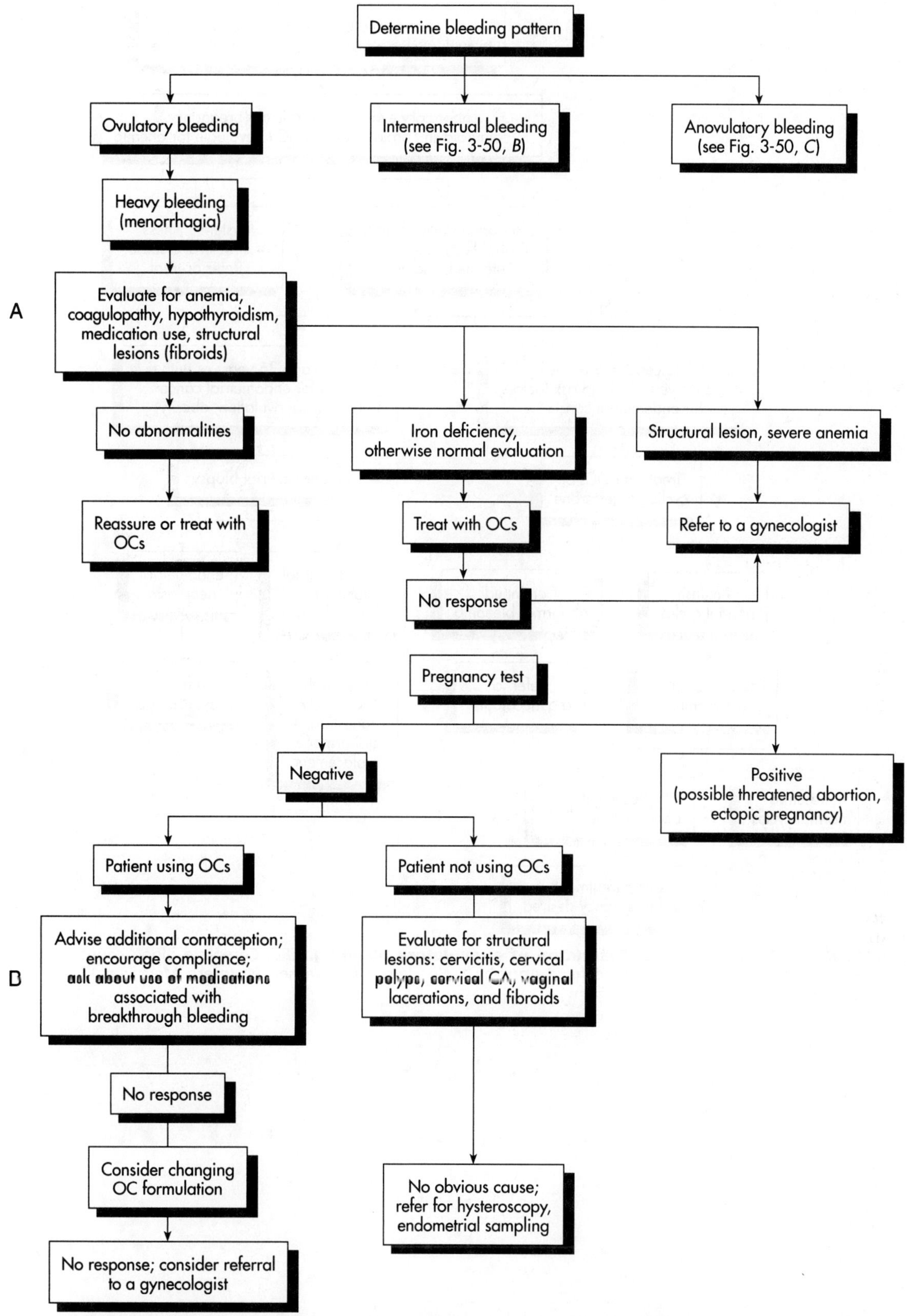

FIGURE 3-51 A, Evaluation of ovulatory bleeding. B, Evaluation of intermenstrual bleeding. *OCs,* Oral contraceptives. (Modified from Appleby J, Henderson M, Wathen PI: *Intern Med* Sept:17, 1996.)

Continued on following page

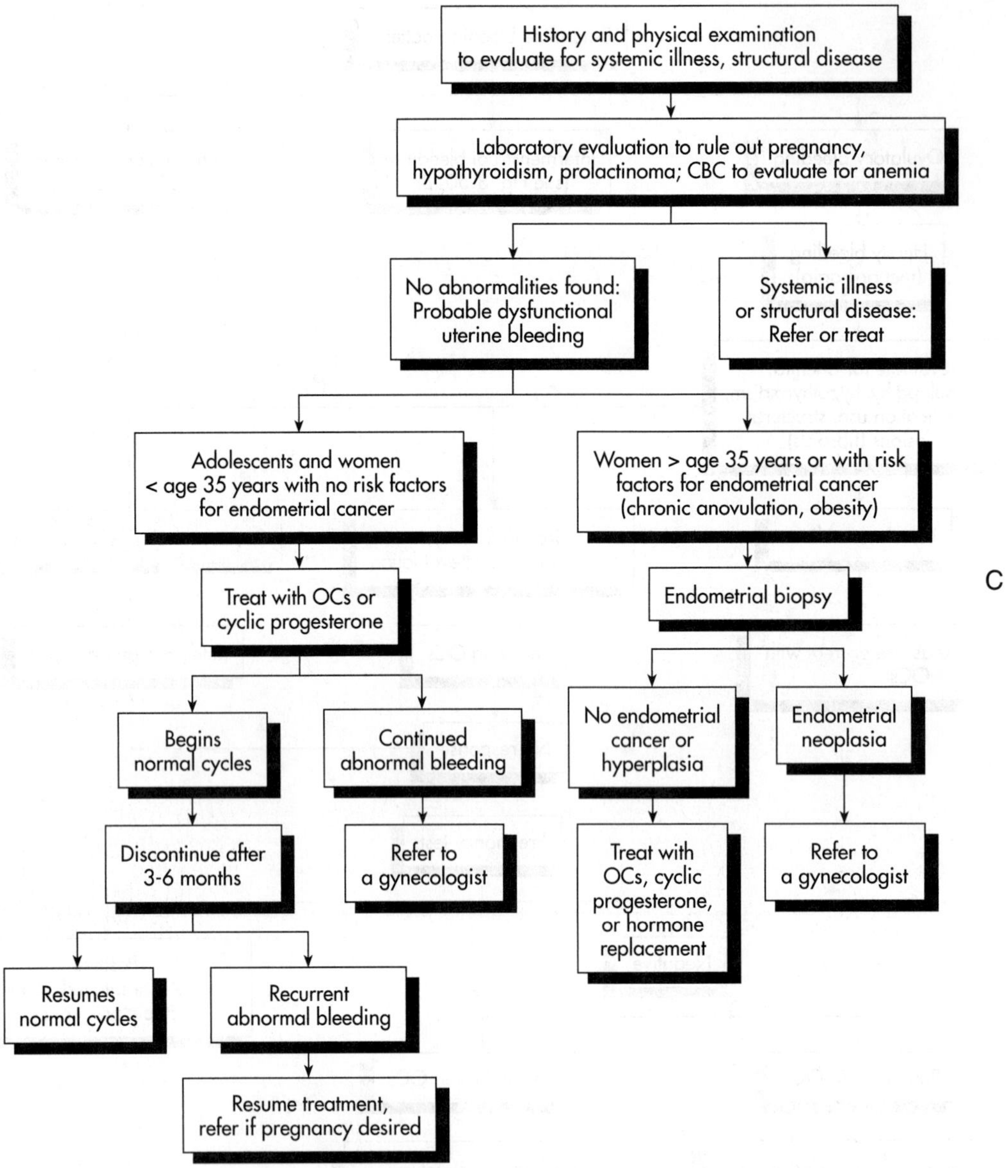

FIGURE 3-51 (Continued) **C, Evaluation of anovulatory bleeding.** *CBC,* Complete blood count; *OCs,* oral contraceptives. (Modified from Appleby J, Henderson M, Wathen PI: *Intern Med* Sept:17, 1996.)

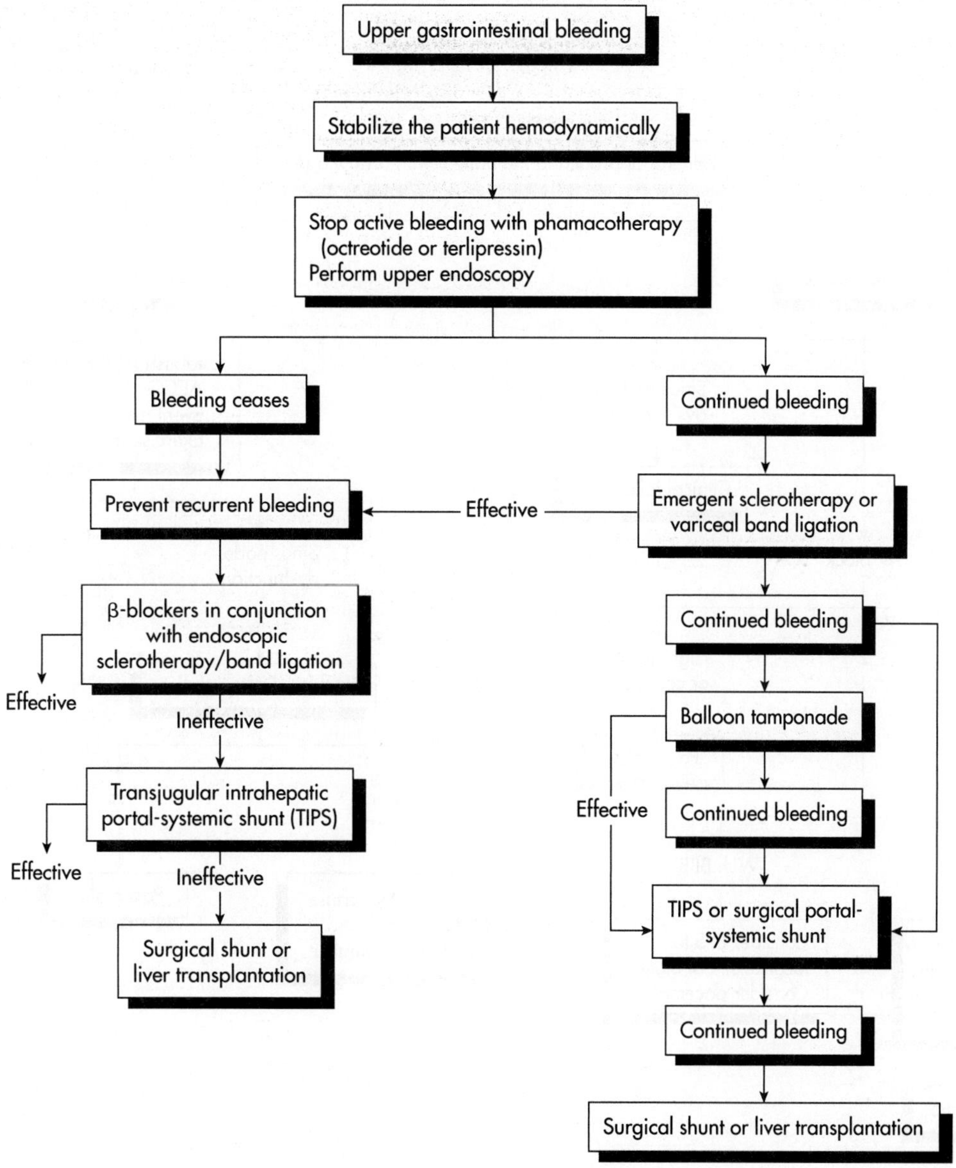

FIGURE 3-52 Management algorithm for variceal bleeding. (From Goldman L, Ausiello D [eds]: *Cecil textbook of medicine*, ed 23, Philadelphia, 2008, WB Saunders.)

ICD-9CM # 427.89 Unspecified bradycardia
427.81 Chronic bradycardia
770.8 Newborn bradycardia
427.89 Postoperative bradycardia
337 Reflex bradycardia
427.89 Sinus bradycardia

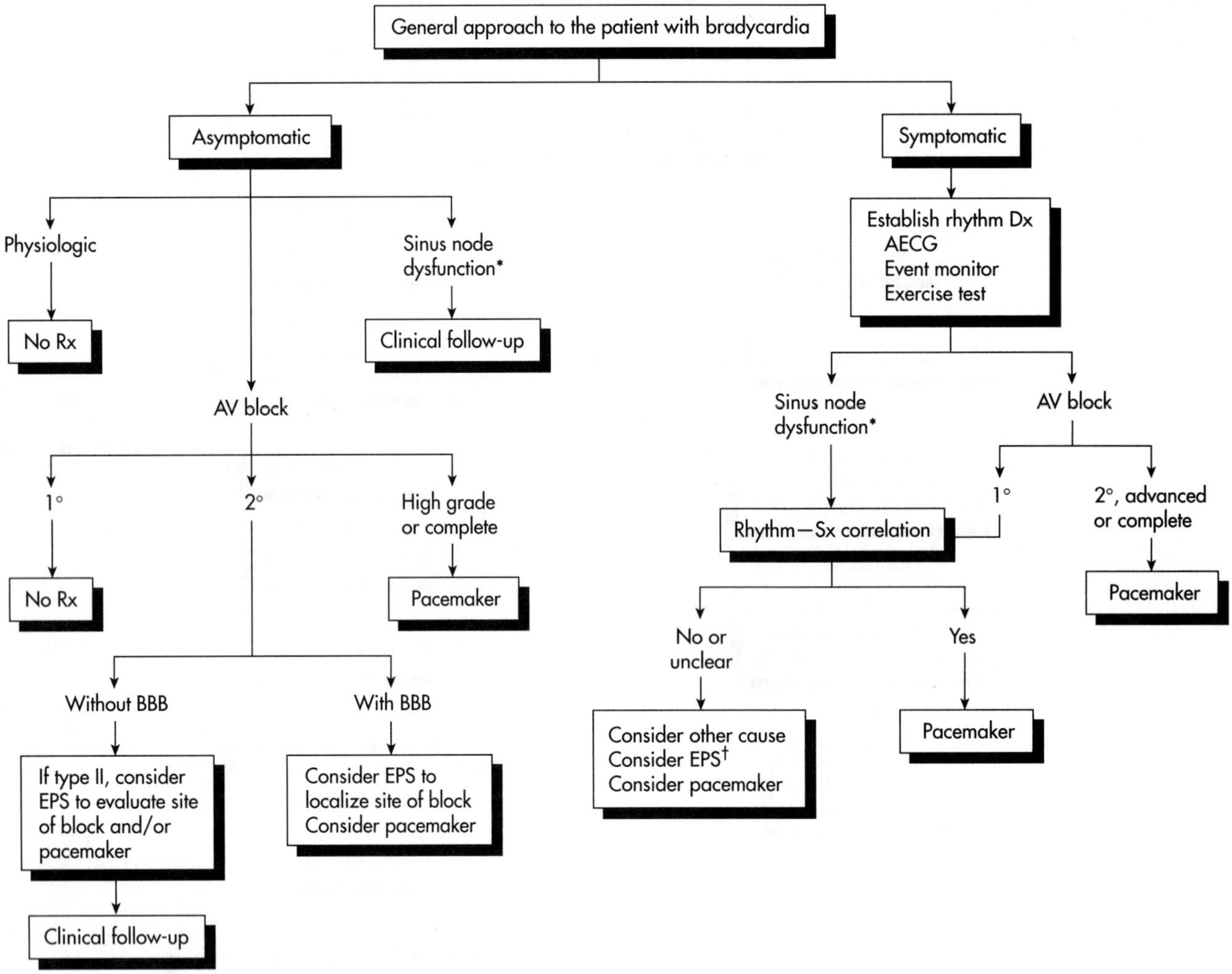

*Includes bradycardia-tachycardia syndrome.
†EPS includes sinus node function and ventricular arrhythmia induction studies.

FIGURE 3-53 General approach to the patient with bradycardia. *AECG,* Ambulatory electrocardiography; *AV,* atrioventricular; *BBB,* bundle branch block; *Dx,* diagnostic; *EPS,* electrophysiologic study; *Rx,* treatment; *Sx,* symptoms; 1°, first-degree; 2°, second-degree. (From Goldman L, Braunwald E [eds]: *Primary cardiology,* ed 2, Philadelphia, 2003, WB Saunders.)

ICD-9CM # 676.8

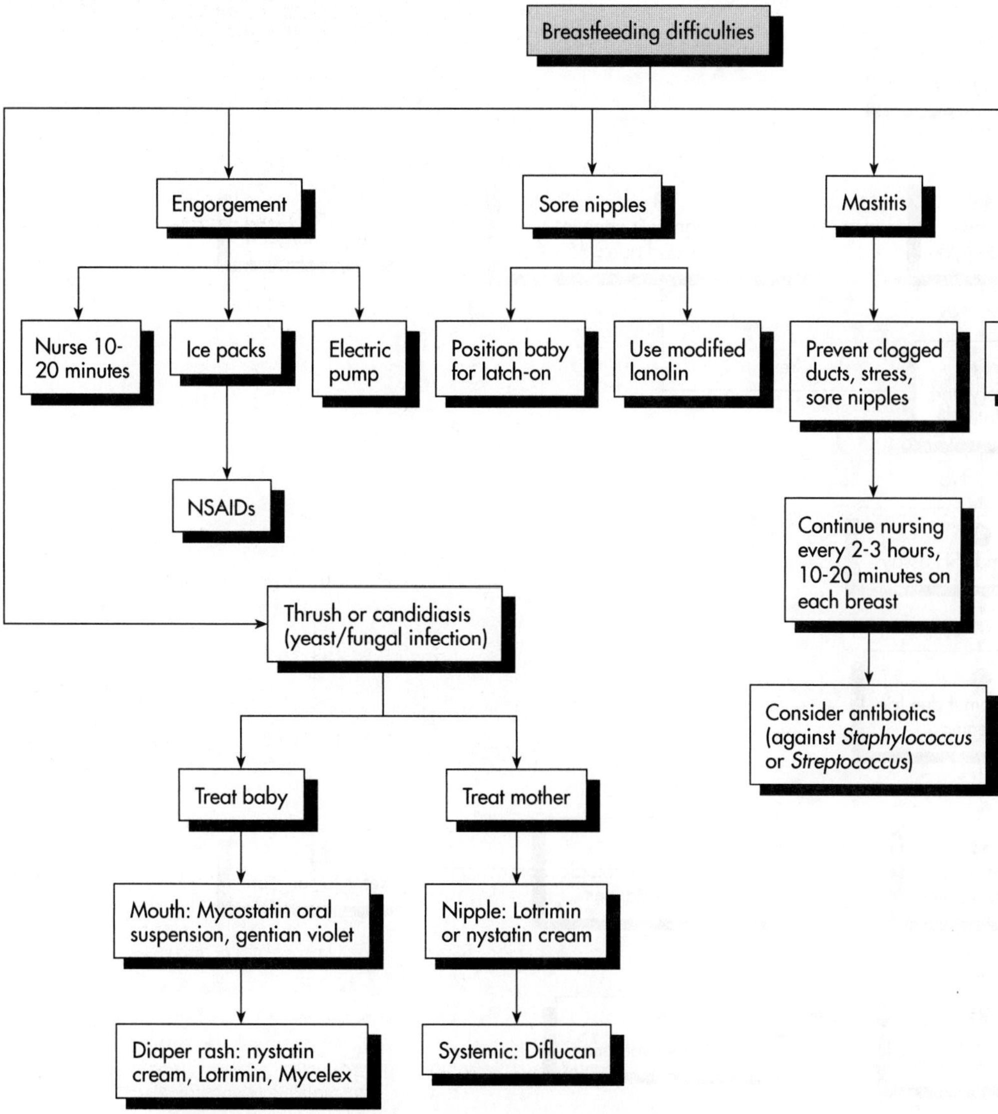

FIGURE 3-54 Management of breastfeeding difficulties. *NSAIDs,* nonsteroidal anti-inflammatory drugs. (Modified from Zuspan FP [ed]: *Handbook of obstetrics, gynecology, and primary care,* St Louis, 1998, Mosby.)

ICD-9CM # 611.79

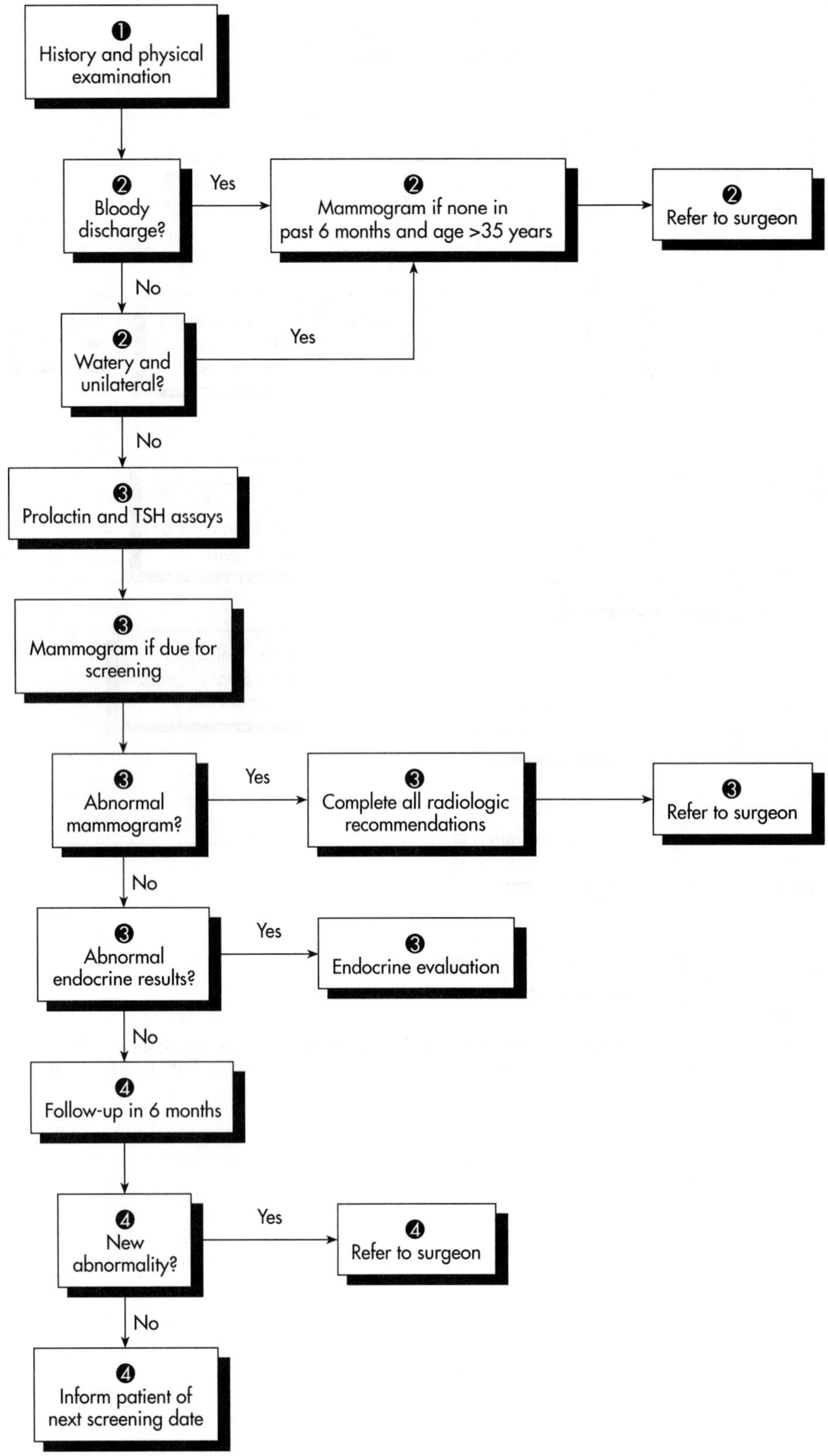

*Without palpable mass.

FIGURE 3-55 Breast cancer screening and evaluation. (From Institute for Clinical Systems Integration, Minneapolis: *Postgrad Med* 100:182, 1996.)

FIGURE 3-55 (Continued)

1. **History and physical examination.*** Patients who present with a complaint of nipple discharge should be evaluated with breast-related history taking and a physical examination. History taking is aimed at uncovering and characterizing any other breast-related symptom. A risk assessment should also be undertaken for identified risk factors, including patient age over 50 years, any past personal history of breast cancer, history of hyperplasia on previous breast biopsies, and family history of breast cancer in first-degree relatives (mother, sister, daughter). Physical examination should include inspection of the breast for any evidence of ulceration or contour changes and inspection of the nipple for Paget's disease. Palpation should be performed with the patient in both the upright and the supine positions to determine the presence of any palpable mass.
2. **Bloody discharge?** If the discharge appears frankly bloody, the patient should be referred to a surgeon for evaluation. At the time of referral, a mammogram of the involved breast should be obtained if the patient is over 35 years of age and has not had a mammogram within the preceding 6 months. Similarly, patients with a watery, unilateral discharge should be referred to a surgeon for evaluation and possible biopsy.
3. **Endocrine tests. Mammogram.** If the discharge appears frankly milky or is bilateral, serum prolactin and serum thyroid-stimulating hormone (TSH) assays should be performed to rule out the presence of an endocrinologic basis for the symptoms. At the time of that visit, a mammogram should also be performed if the patient is due for routine mammographic screening according to the recommended intervals. A patient with an abnormal mammogram should be further evaluated radiologically to better characterize the lesion and then be referred to a surgeon if appropriate. Make certain that all recommended additional views, ultrasound examinations, and follow-up studies have been obtained before referral to a surgeon. Should the mammogram appear normal, results of the assays for TSH and prolactin should be reviewed. If the results are abnormal the patient should undergo appropriate evaluation for etiology, either by a primary care physician or by an endocrinologist.
4. **Six-month follow-up results.** If results of the mammogram and the endocrinologic screening studies are normal, the patient should return for a follow-up visit in 6 months to ensure that there has been no specific change in the character of the discharge, such as development of frank bleeding or Paget's disease, that would warrant surgical evaluation. If the evaluation at that follow-up visit fails to reveal any palpable or visible abnormalities, the patient should be returned to the routine screening process with studies performed at the recommended intervals.

---

*ICSI health care guidelines are designed to assist clinicians by providing an analytic framework for the evaluation and treatment of patients. They are not intended either to replace a clinician's judgment or to establish a protocol for all patients with a particular condition. A guideline will rarely establish the only approach to a problem. In addition, guidelines are "living documents" that are expected to be imperfect and are subject to annual review and revision.

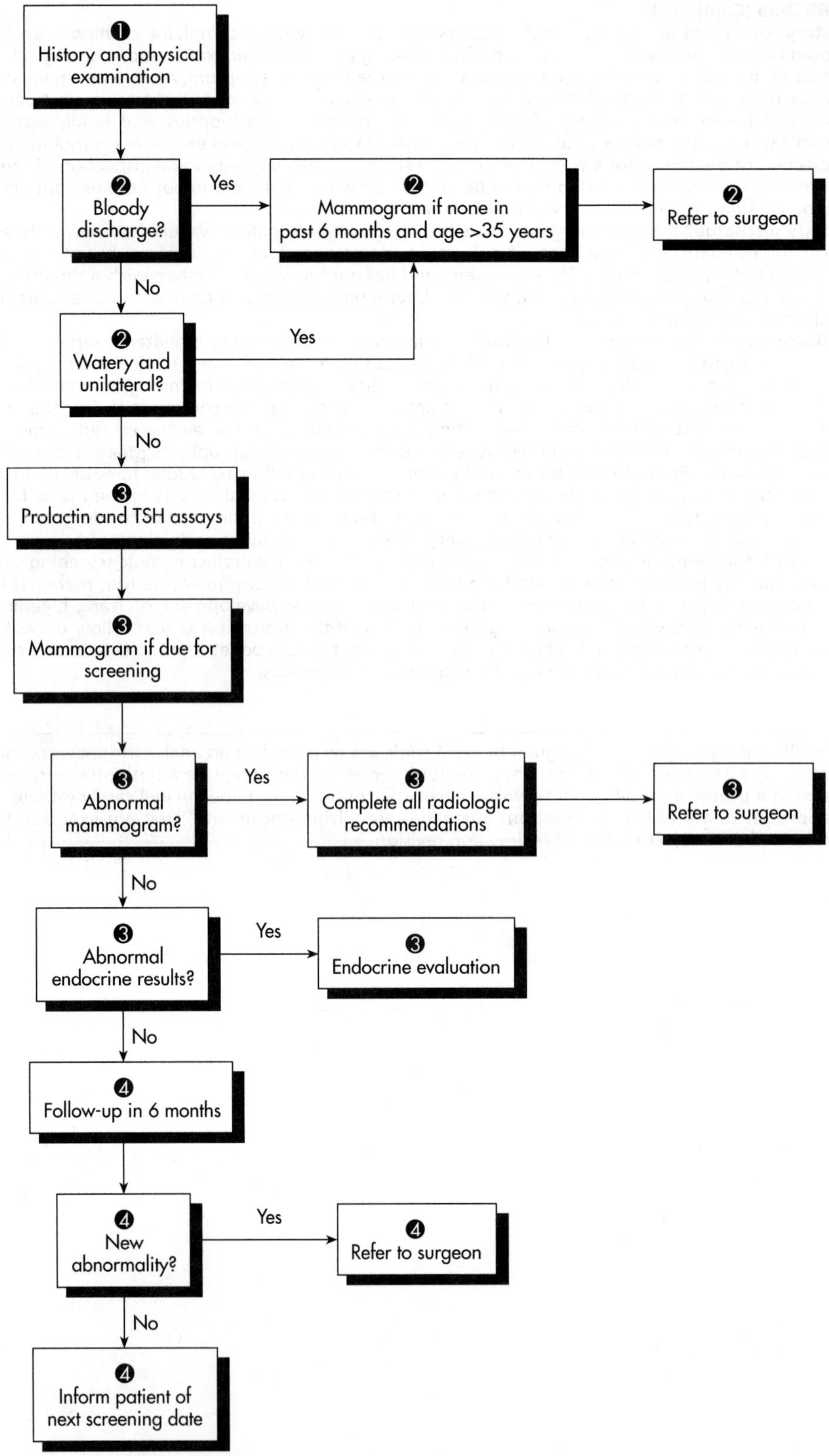

FIGURE 3-56 Breast cancer screening and evaluation. (From Institute for Clinical Systems Integration, Minneapolis: *Postgrad Med* 100:182-187, 1996.)

FIGURE 3-56 (Continued)

1. **Screening mammogram.*** Patients are most commonly referred to a radiologist for screening mammography. Occasionally, however, patients are referred for diagnostic mammography based on symptoms or findings on breast exam. In the event of an abnormal finding on the mammogram, complete evaluation under the direction of a radiologist is recommended. It is the responsibility of the radiologist to complete the radiologic assessment so that the best possible characterization of the abnormality can be provided in an expeditious fashion to the primary care physician who ordered the original study. Any recommendations for referral to a surgeon for possible biopsy should be made directly to the primary care physician. The ultimate responsibility to make the referral will rest with the primary care physician.
2. **Abnormal mammogram. Sorting abnormalities. Suspicious for cancer?** On obtaining an abnormal finding on a mammogram, the radiologist determines whether further mammographic images are required for completion of the evaluation process. This may include a repeated image of the involved breast at 6 months to document stability of a low-risk, probably benign lesion. Alternatively, spot compression, magnification, or both may be necessary to obtain further characterization of indeterminate breast lesions. These additional studies should be done with the radiologist present to reduce the risk of patient recall for further studies necessary to evaluate the same lesion.
   On completion of these views, each and every abnormality uncovered for each independent lesion of the breast studied should be sorted according to the nature of the abnormality. The radiologist should classify the lesion as representing either suspicious microcalcifications, architectural distortion, or a soft-tissue mass. For any lesions identified as demonstrating microcalcifications that suggest cancer, biopsy will be recommended. It is up to the primary care physician to make the referral to a surgeon for biopsy. If a soft-tissue mass is identified on the mammogram, it should be studied further to determine its relative risk for malignancy. Any suspect lesions identified as having associated microcalcifications, architectural distortion, or interval growth when compared with the previous mammogram should likewise be referred to a surgeon for possible biopsy.
3. **Ultrasound results.** When the mass is not immediately suggestive of cancer, an ultrasound should be performed to determine whether the lesion is solid. A solid mass should be further characterized for its level of benignity according to three criteria:
   - Size less than 15 mm
   - Three or fewer lobulations
   - More than 50% of the margin of the lesion appearing well circumscribed in any view

   Patients who have lesions that fit all three criteria may be observed and then evaluated with a 6-month follow-up study. Any lesion that does not fit all three criteria for benignity should be characterized as indeterminate, and biopsy should be considered. Likewise, any solid mass that is palpable should be referred to a surgeon for possible open biopsy. Finally, any lesion that appears to be new since the last screening mammogram should be considered for biopsy.
4. **Aspiration and results.** If the ultrasound of the soft-tissue mass demonstrates that it is a cystic lesion, the cyst should be further categorized by the criteria listed in the algorithm: irregular wall, as seen on ultrasonography; internal echoes; complex, septated appearance; and palpability within the region of the ultrasound-proven cyst. A positive finding for any of these criteria would be an indication for ultrasound-directed aspiration of the cyst. Aspiration should also be offered if the patient requests it.
   After cyst aspiration, a single-view mammogram should be obtained to demonstrate complete resolution of the lesion. If the lesion is sufficiently complex, a cyst pneumogram may be performed. Should any residual mass be present or if the cyst pneumogram findings are abnormal, biopsy should be recommended. If, on the other hand, the mass is a simple cyst that does not fit any of the previously listed criteria, the patient should be returned to the screening process, and completion of this evaluation should be reported to the ordering health care provider.

---

*ICSI health care guidelines are designed to assist clinicians by providing an analytic framework for the evaluation and treatment of patients. They are not intended either to replace a clinician's judgment or to establish a protocol for all patients with a particular condition. A guideline will rarely establish the only approach to a problem. In addition, guidelines are "living documents" that are expected to be imperfect and are subject to annual review and revision.

ICD-9CM # 611.72 Breast mass or lump, nonpuerperal

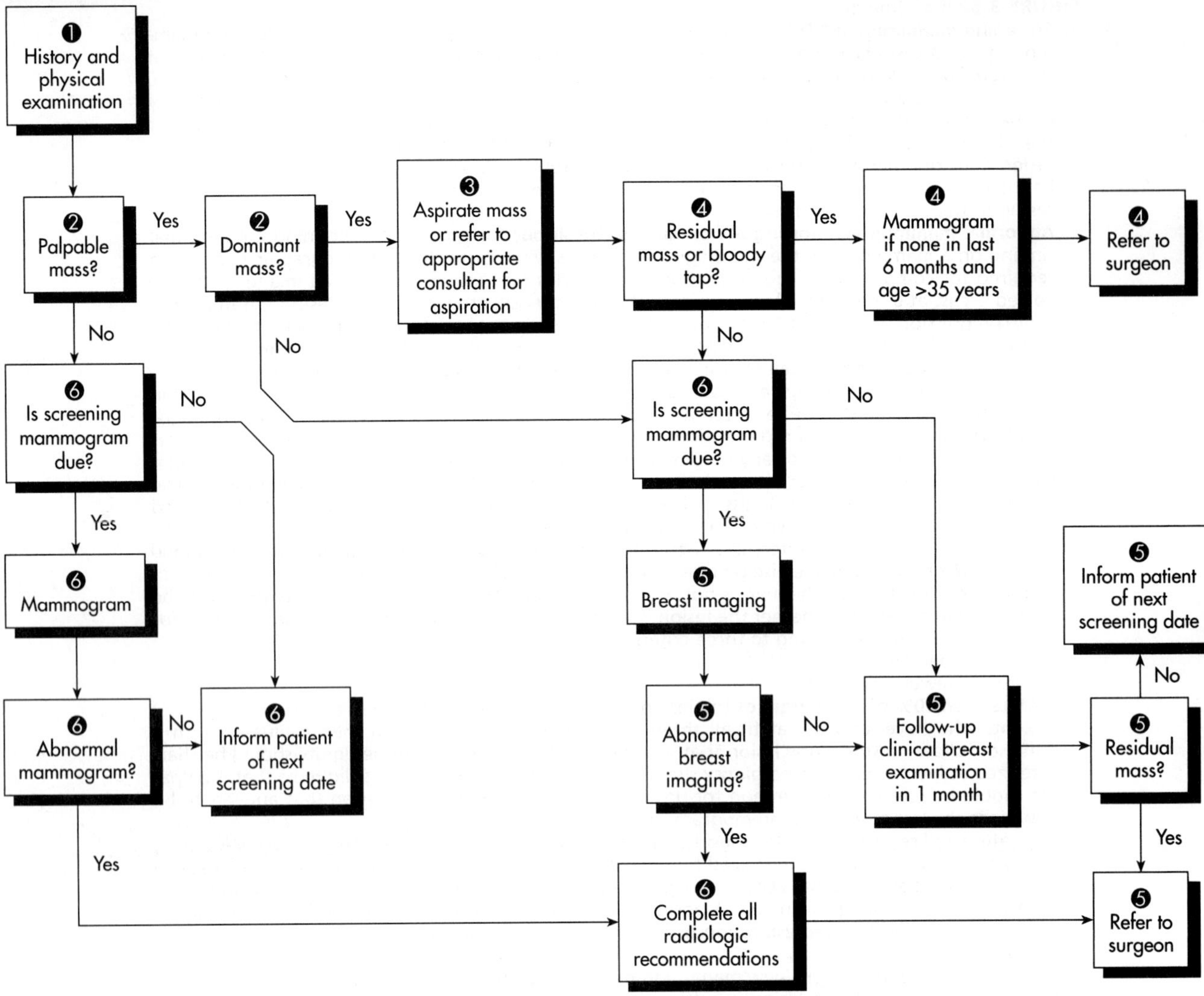

FIGURE 3-57 Breast cancer screening and evaluation. (From Institute for Clinical Systems Integration, Minneapolis: *Postgrad Med* 100:182, 1996.)

1. **History and physical examination.*** Primary care evaluation is initiated with history taking aimed at uncovering and characterizing any breast-related symptom. A risk assessment should also be undertaken for identified risk factors, including patient age over 50 years, any past personal history of breast cancer, history of hyperplasia on previous breast biopsies, and family history of breast cancer in first-degree relatives (mother, sister, daughter). Physical examination should include inspection of the breast for any evidence of ulceration or contour changes and inspection of the nipple for Paget's disease. Palpation should be performed with the patient in both the upright and supine positions to determine the presence of any palpable mass.
2. **Palpable mass? Dominant mass?** A dominant mass is a palpable finding that is discrete and clearly different from the surrounding parenchyma. If a palpable mass is identified, it should be determined whether it represents a dominant (i.e., discrete) mass, which requires immediate evaluation. The primary care physician or appropriate consultant should attempt to aspirate any dominant mass because a simple cyst may be uncovered, in which case aspiration completes the evaluation process.
3. **Aspirate mass or refer for aspiration.** Aspiration of a dominant palpable mass should be performed by the primary care physician or by the appropriate consultant. The breast skin is prepped with alcohol. Then, with the lesion immobilized by the nonoperating hand, an 18- to 25-gauge needle mounted on a 10-ml syringe is directed to the central portion of the mass for a single attempt at aspiration. Successful aspiration of a simple cyst would yield a nonbloody fluid with complete resolution of the dominant mass. Typical watery fluid may be discarded. However, cyst fluid that is bloody or unusually tenacious should be examined cytologically.

FIGURE 3-57 (Continued)

4. **Residual mass or bloody tap? Mammogram if none in past 6 months. Refer to surgeon.** Should the mass remain after the attempt at aspiration or should frank blood be aspirated during the process, the presence of a malignant process cannot be ruled out. Patients with a residual mass or bloody tap should be referred to a surgeon for possible biopsy. Before the referral, a mammogram should be obtained for any patient over age 35 years who has not had a mammogram within the preceding 6 months. In patients 35 years and under, obtaining any other breast-imaging studies should be left to the discretion of the surgeon or radiologist.
5. **Is screening mammogram due? Breast imaging. Follow-up clinical breast examination. Refer to surgeon.** Should physical examination demonstrate a palpable mass that is not clearly a discrete and dominant mass, its size, location, and character should be documented in anticipation of a follow-up examination. A screening mammogram should be obtained if one has not been done within the recommended interval. If no mammogram is required or if a required mammogram demonstrates no abnormality, a follow-up examination in 1 month is indicated. Should any residual mass be identified, the patient should be referred to a surgeon for possible biopsy. Patients with a persisting nondominant palpable mass that does not resolve within 1 month and those with any recurring cystic mass should be referred for surgical evaluation. If no mass is apparent at the time of the follow-up examination, the patient should then be informed of the appropriate date for her next screening examination, according to the recommended intervals.
6. **Screening mammogram and results.** After completion of the physical examination, the appropriateness of a routine screening mammogram should be determined. If a mammogram is done, the radiologist should provide the results to the primary care physician for reporting to the patient. Should any abnormalities be uncovered, it will be the responsibility of the radiologist to complete any additional imaging studies required for the complete radiographic characterization of the lesion. The radiologist should make certain that all recommended additional views, follow-up studies, and ultrasound examinations have been completed before referral to a surgeon. However, it is important that the primary care physician who ordered the mammogram review the results of these studies to understand fully the opinion of the radiologist and to ensure that all recommendations of the radiologist have been completed. Should the radiologist recommend that surgical consultation is warranted, it will be the responsibility of the primary care physician to establish this referral.

NOTE: *The importance of communication between the surgical consultant and the primary care physician cannot be overstated. Biopsy results should be reported both to the surgeon and to the primary care physician. More important, patients who do not require biopsy after surgical consultation should be returned to the routine screening process. This process is under the supervision of the primary care physician. Therefore it is absolutely necessary for the primary care physician to know when the patient reenters the routine screening population. In the event that new symptoms arise during the screening interval, the patient should be evaluated by the primary care physician using the primary care evaluation process of this guideline.*

---

*ICSI health care guidelines are designed to assist clinicians by providing an analytic framework for the evaluation and treatment of patients. They are not intended either to replace a clinician's judgment or to establish a protocol for all patients with a particular condition. A guideline will rarely establish the only approach to a problem. In addition, guidelines are "living documents" that are expected to be imperfect and are subject to annual review and revision.

ICD-9CM # 259.2 Carcinoid syndrome

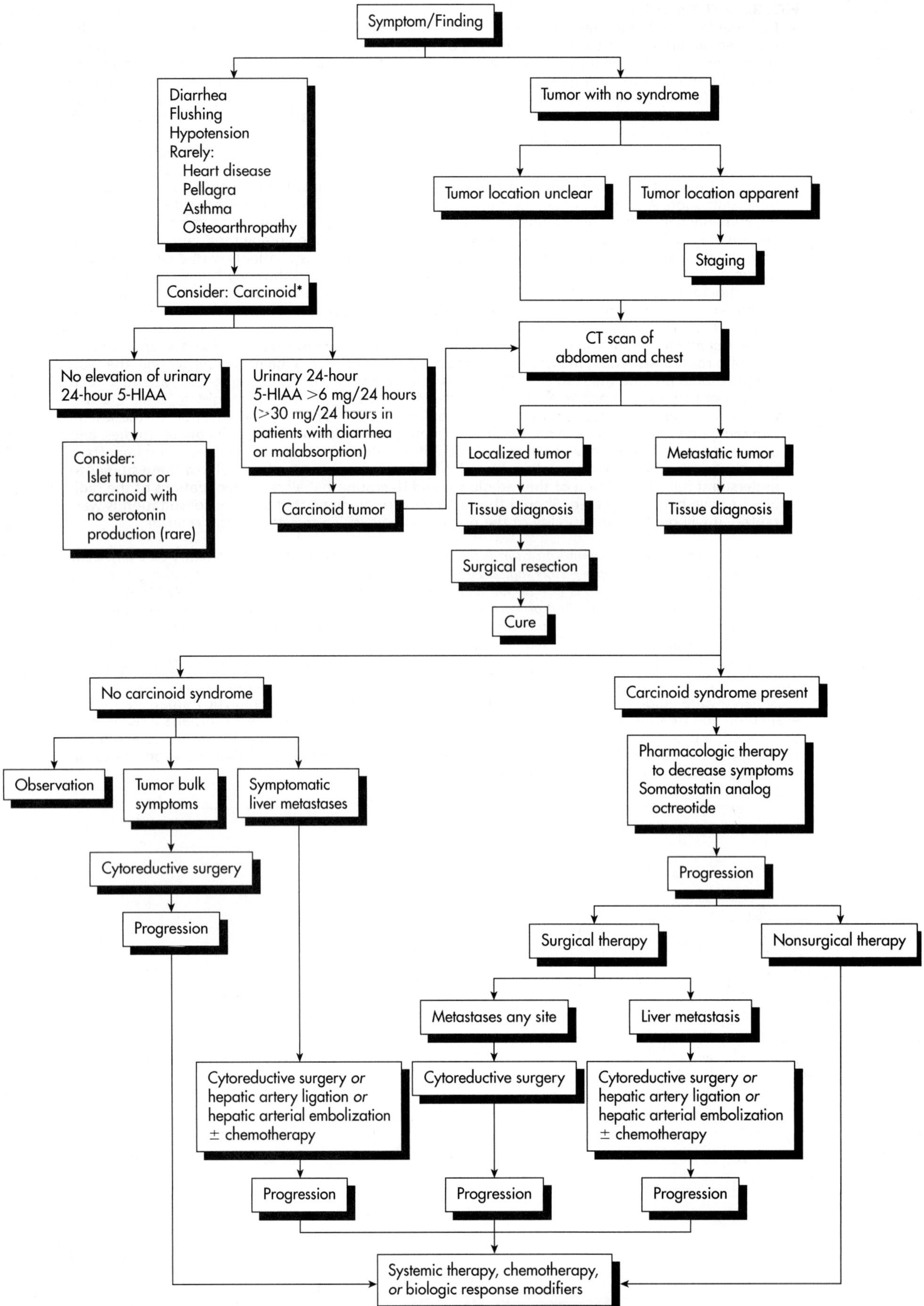

*See Section I for additional information on this topic.

FIGURE 3-58 Diagnosis and treatment of carcinoid tumors. *5-HIAA,* 5-Hydroxyindoleacetic acid. (Modified from Abeloff MD: *Clinical oncology,* ed 3, New York, 2004, Churchill Livingstone.)

ICD-9CM # 429.3 Idiopathic cardiomegaly
746.89 Congenital cardiomegaly
402.0 Hypertensive cardiomegaly, malignant
402.1 Hypertensive cardiomegaly, benign
402.11 Hypertensive cardiomegaly with congestive heart failure

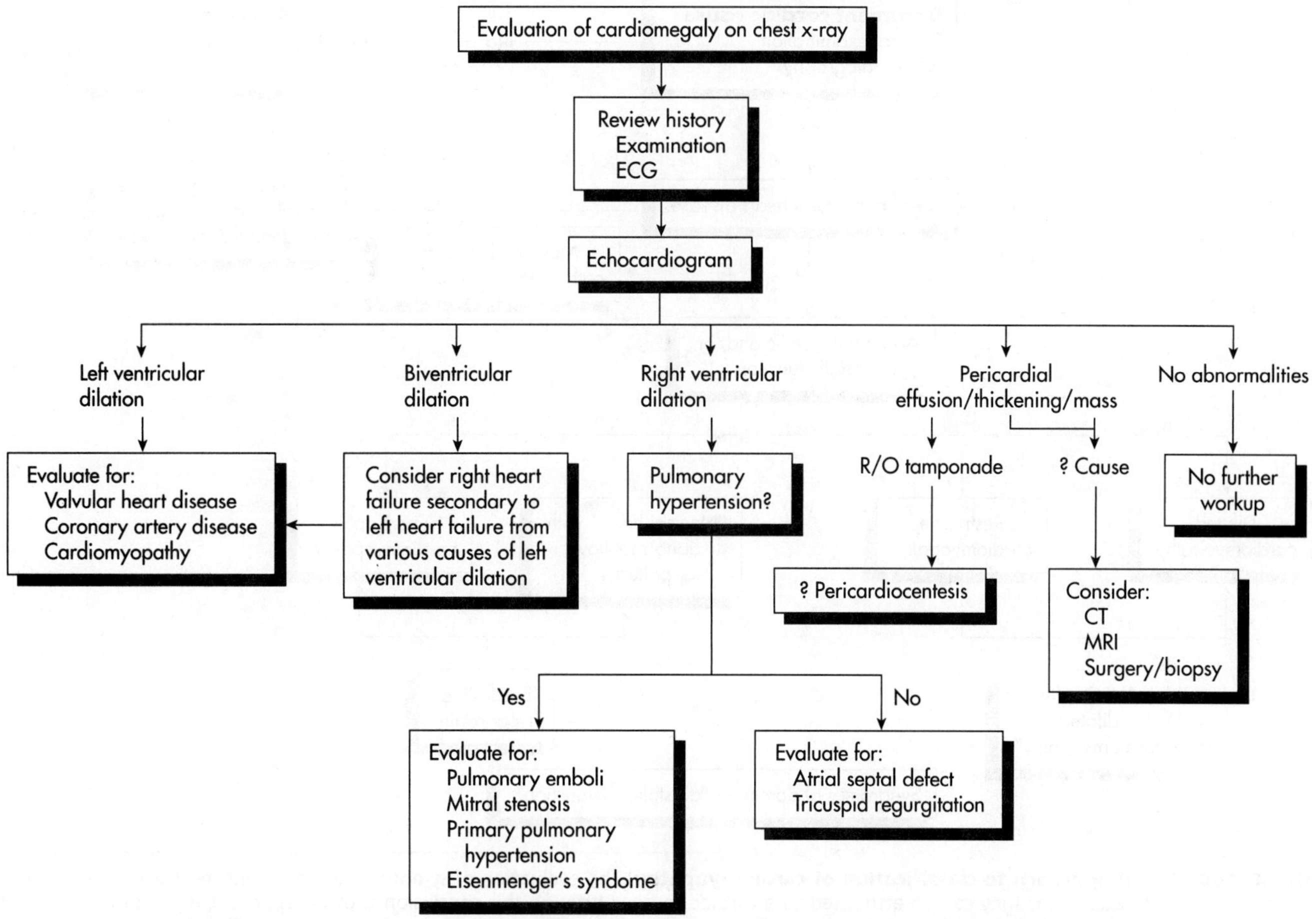

FIGURE 3-59 Approach to the patient with cardiomegaly. When cardiomegaly is found on the chest radiograph, the history and physical examination should be reviewed and an electrocardiogram (ECG) performed before obtaining a two-dimensional Doppler echocardiographic study. Cardiomegaly may be explained by left ventricular dilation, biventricular dilation, right ventricular dilation, or pericardial abnormalities, or it may be found to be spurious on the echocardiogram. Rarely, isolated abnormalities of the atrium, particularly the left atrium, may cause abnormalities on the chest radiograph but will not cause true cardiomegaly. Depending on the echocardiographic findings, further tests can help elucidate the cause of echocardiographically confirmed cardiomegaly. *CT,* Computer tomography; *MRI,* magnetic resonance imaging; *R/O,* rule out. (From Goldman L, Braunwald E [eds]: *Primary cardiology,* ed 2, Philadelphia, 2003, WB Saunders.)

ICD-9CM # 425.4

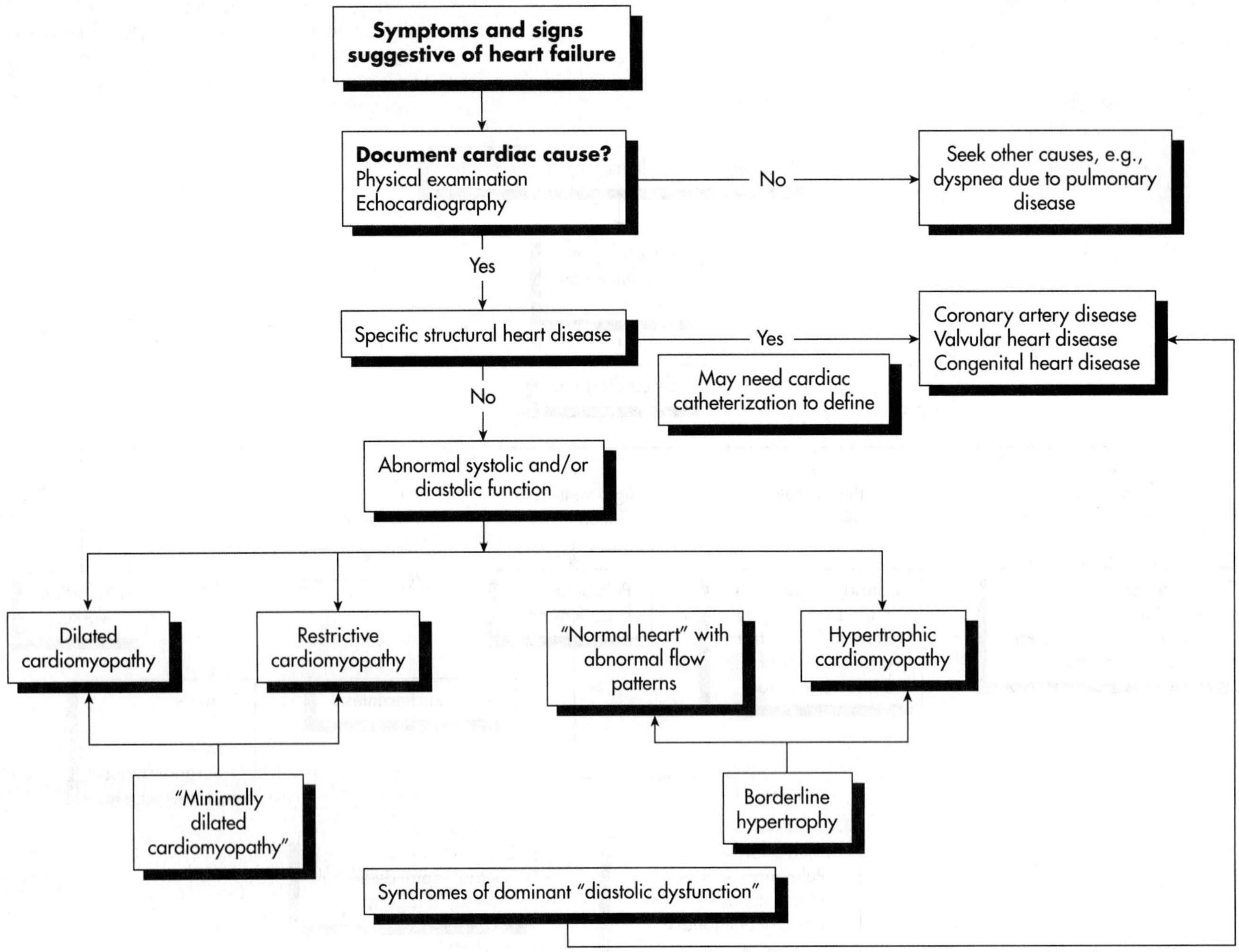

FIGURE 3-60 Initial approach to classification of cardiomyopathy. The evaluation of symptoms or signs consistent with heart failure first includes confirmation that they can be attributed to a cardiac cause. Although this conclusion is often apparent from routine physical examination, echocardiography serves to confirm cardiac disease and provides clues to the presence of other cardiac disease, such as focal abnormalities, suggesting primary valve disease or congenital heart disease. Having excluded these conditions, cardiomyopathy is generally considered to be dilated, restrictive, or hypertrophic. Patients with apparently normal cardiac structure and contraction are occasionally found to demonstrate abnormal intracardiac flow patterns consistent with diastolic dysfunction but should also be evaluated carefully for other causes of their symptoms. Most patients with so-called diastolic dysfunction also demonstrate at least borderline criteria for left ventricular hypertrophy, frequently in the setting of chronic hypertension and diabetes. A moderately decreased ejection fraction without marked dilation or a pattern of restrictive cardiomyopathy is sometimes referred to as "minimally dilated cardiomyopathy" which may represent either a distinct entity or a transition between acute and chronic disease. (From Goldman L, Ausiello D [eds]: *Cecil textbook of medicine,* ed 23, Philadelphia, 2008, WB Saunders.)

TABLE 3-4 **Profiles of Symptomatic Cardiomyopathy**

	Dilated	Restrictive	Hypertrophic
Ejection fraction (normal >55%)	<30%	25-50%	>60%
Left ventricular diastolic dimension (normal <55 mm)	≥60 mm	<60 mm	Often decreased
Left ventricular wall thickness	Decreased	Normal or increased	Markedly increased
Atrial size	Increased	Increased; may be massive	Increased
Valvular regurgitation	Mitral first during decompensation; tricuspid regurgitation in late stages	Frequent mitral and tricuspid regurgitation, rarely severe	Mitral regurgitation
Common first symptoms*	Exertional intolerance	Exertional intolerance, fluid retention	Exertional intolerance; may have chest pain
Congestive symptoms*	Left before right, except right prominent in young adults	Right often exceeds left	Primary exertional dyspnea
Risk for arrhythmia	Ventricular tachyarrhythmias; conduction block in Chagas' disease, giant cell myocarditis, and some families; atrial fibrillation	Ventricular tachyarrhythmias uncommon except in sarcoidosis; conduction block in sarcoidosis and amyloidosis, atrial fibrillation	Ventricular tachyarrhythmias, atrial fibrillation

From Goldman L, Ausiello D [eds]: *Cecil textbook of medicine,* ed 23, Philadelphia, 2008, WB Saunders.

*Left-sided symptoms of pulmonary congestion: dyspnea on exertion, orthopnea, paroxysmal nocturnal dyspnea. Right-sided symptoms of systemic venous congestion: discomfort on bending, hepatic and abdominal distention, peripheral edema.

ICD-9CM # 425.1

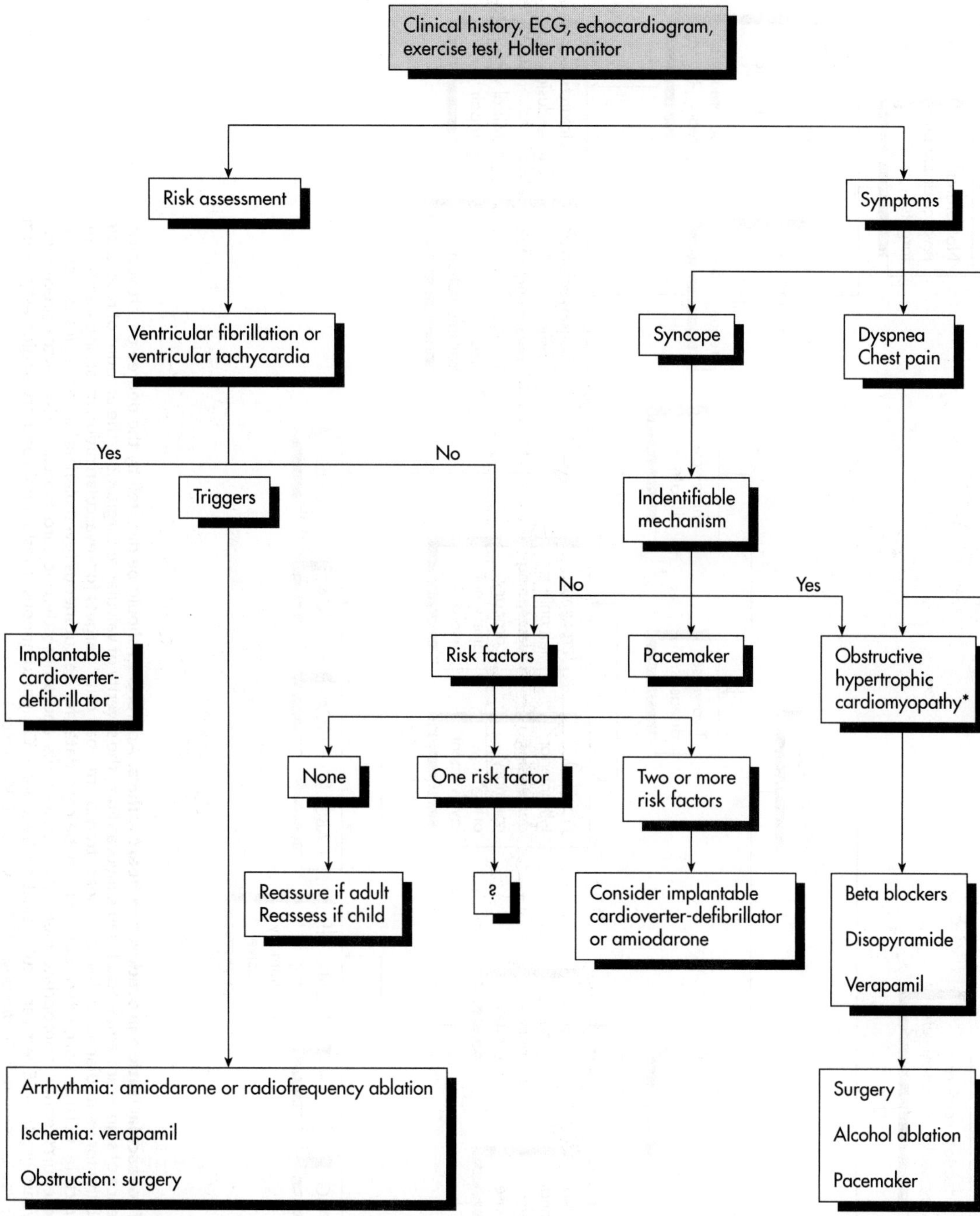

*Refer to Section I for additional information on this topic.

FIGURE 3-61 Suggested management of symptoms and risk in patients who have hypertrophic cardiomyopathy. *ECG,* Electrocardiogram. (From Crawford MH, DiMarco JP, Paulus WJ [eds]: *Cardiology,* ed 2, St Louis, 2004, Mosby.)

ICD-9CM # 414.8

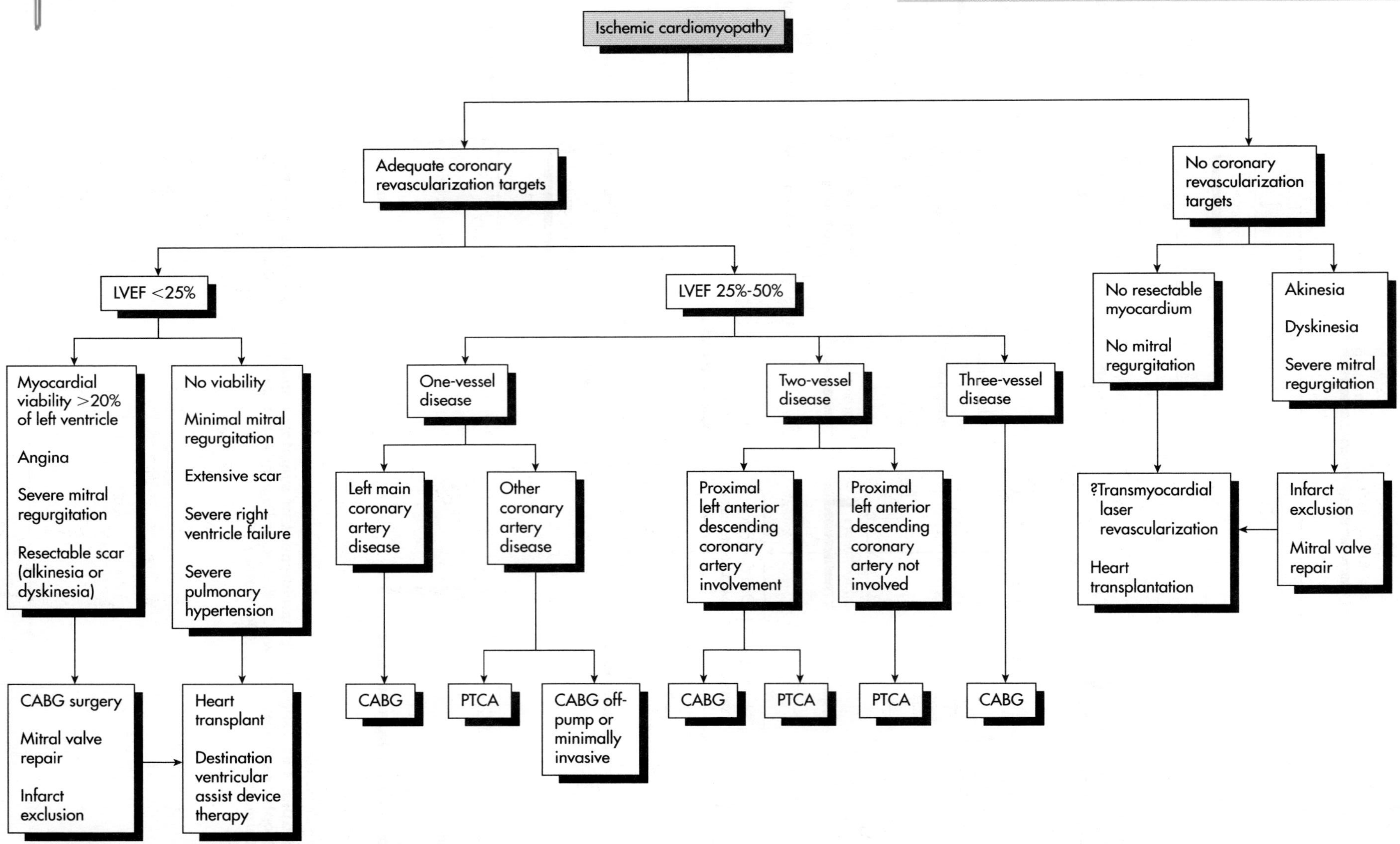

FIGURE 3-62 Choice of revascularization procedures in heart failure. Approaches should be dictated by the degree of left ventricular dysfunction, the presence of significant amounts of viable myocardium, the severity of valvular regurgitation, the amount of resectable myocardial scar, and suitability for ventriular assist device of heart transplant "bail out." Targets for revascularization must also be present. These considerations will dictate, in large part, which patients may be candidates for percutaneous revascularization strategies as well. All patients regardless of procedure require appropriate medication treatments and atherosclerotic cardiovascular risk factor prevention. *CABG,* Coronary artery bypass graft; *LVEF,* left ventricular ejection fraction; *PTCA,* percutaneous transluminal coronary angioplasty. (From Crawford MH, DiMarco JP, Paulus WJ [eds]: *Cardiology,* ed 2, St Louis, 2004, Mosby.)

ICD-9CM # 437.1 Cerebral ischemia (chronic)
435.9 Cerebral ischemia intermittent (transient)

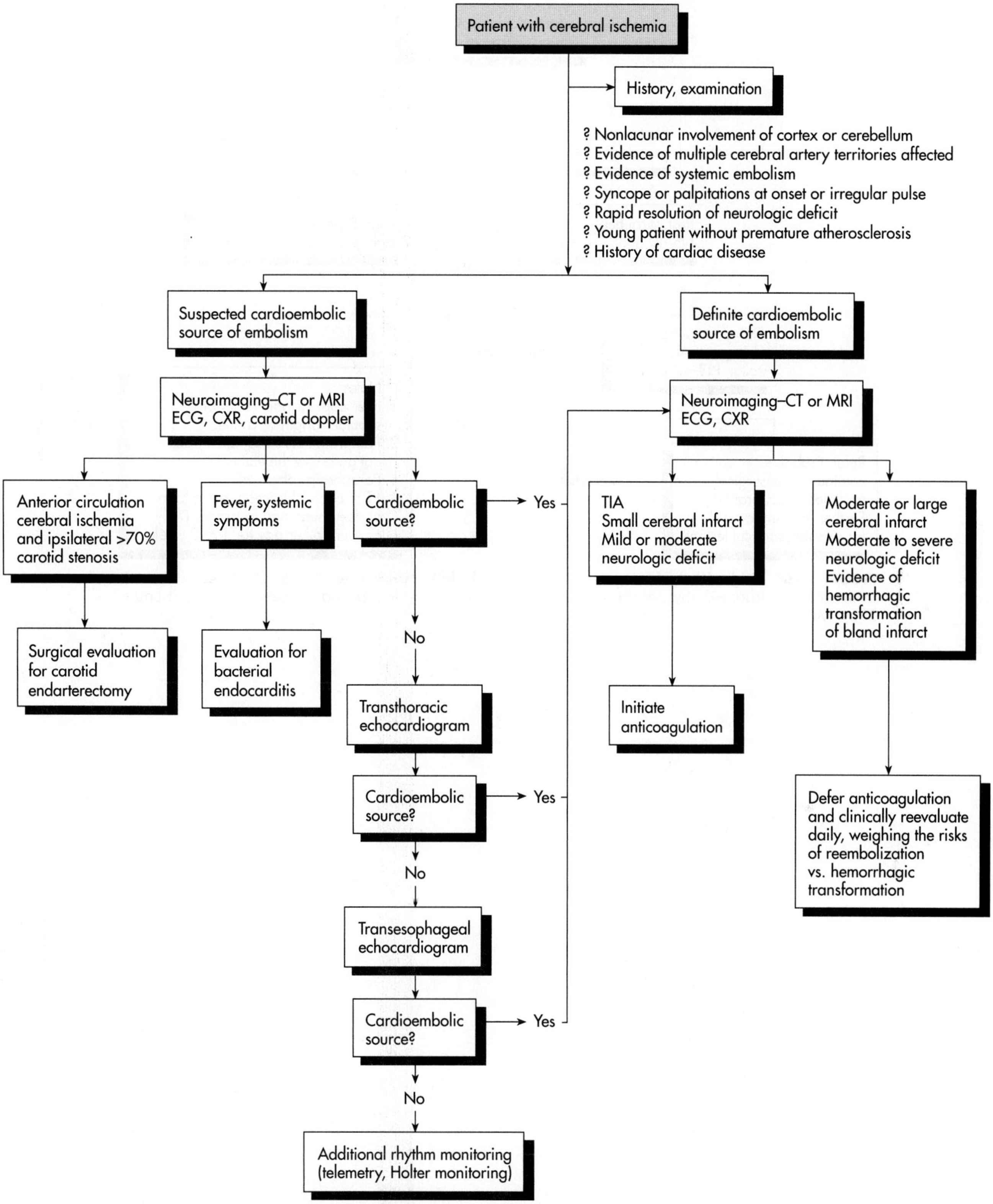

FIGURE 3-63 Evaluation of patients with cerebral ischemia for a cardioembolic source. *CT,* Computed tomography; *CXR,* chest radiograph; *ECG,* electrocardiogram; *MRI,* magnetic resonance imaging; *TIA,* transient ischemic attack. (Modified from Johnson R [ed]: *Current therapy in neurologic disease,* ed 5, St Louis, 1997, Mosby.)

ICD-9CM # 722.4 Degenerative intervertebral cervical disk
722.71 Degenerative cervical disk with myelopathy

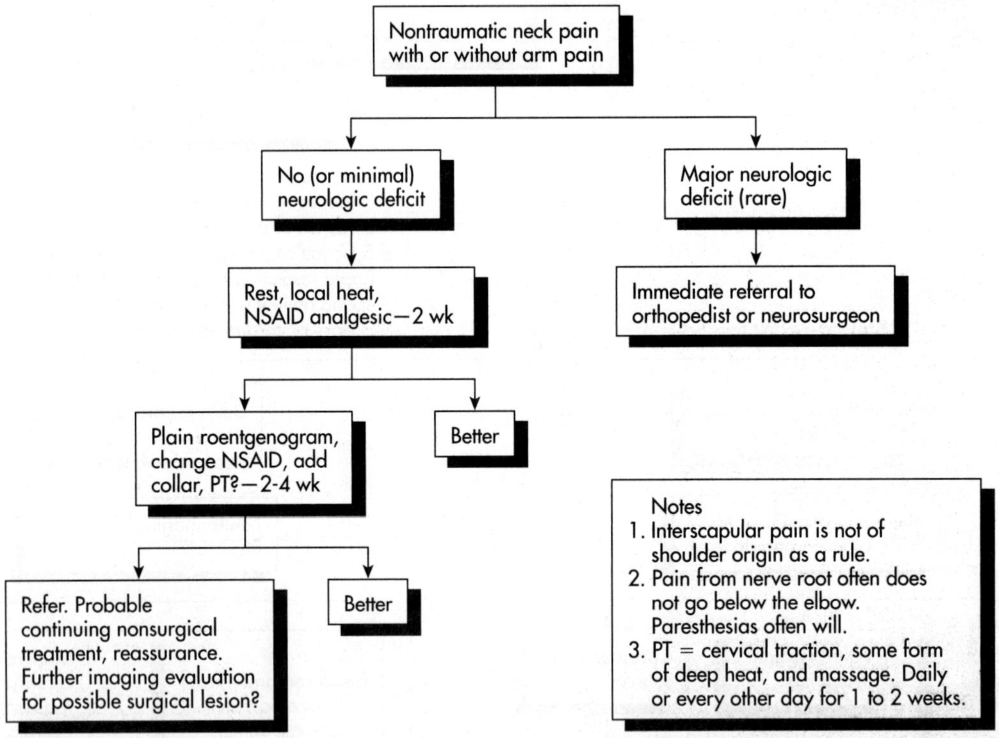

FIGURE 3-64 Algorithm for suspected cervical disk syndrome. *NSAID,* Nonsteroidal anti-inflammatory drug; *PT,* physical therapy. (From Mercier LR [ed]: *Practical orthopaedics,* ed 6, St Louis, 2004, Mosby.)

ICD-9CM # 496 COPD
492.8 Emphysema

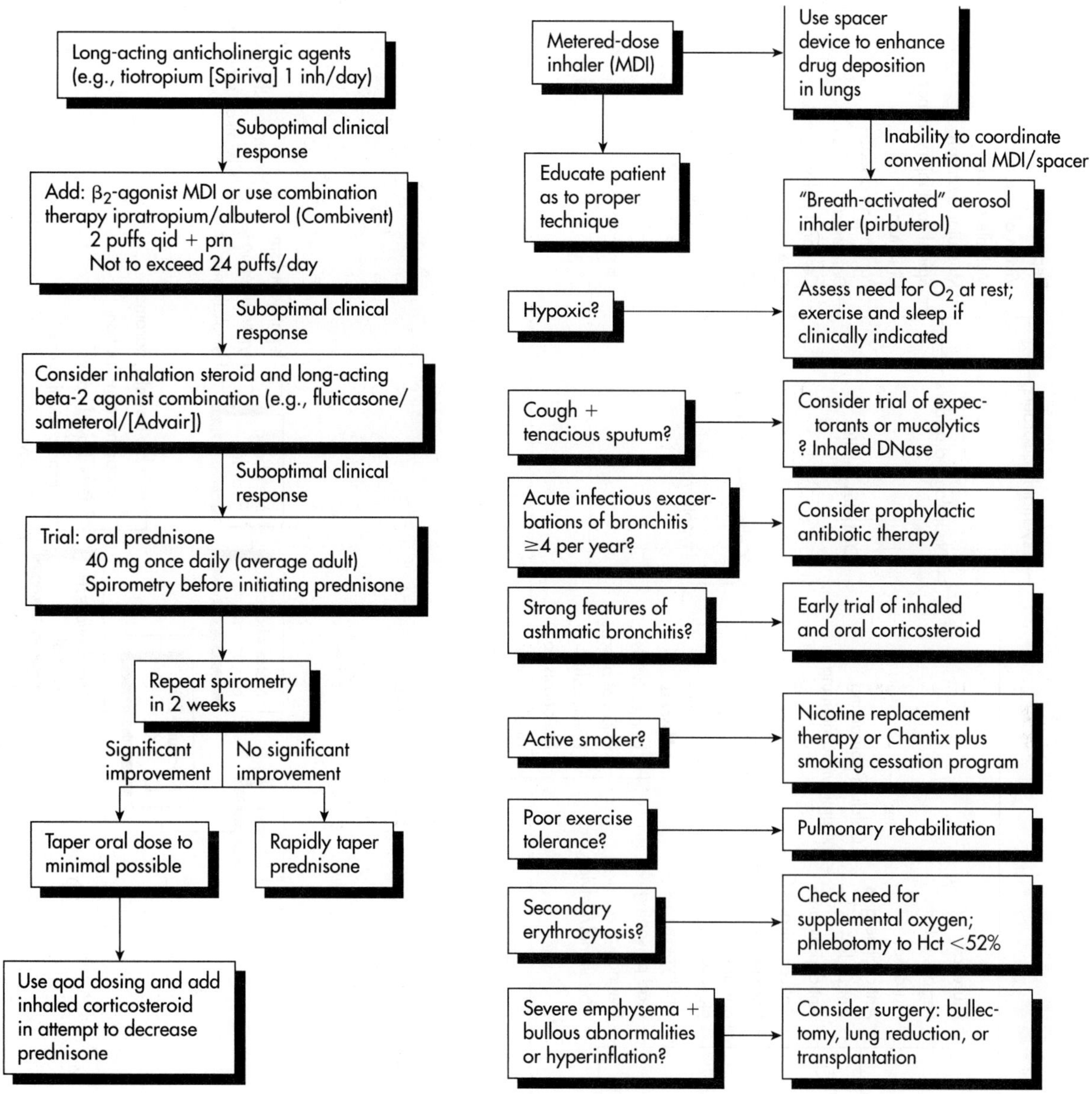

Note: Refer to Section I for additional information on this topic.

FIGURE 3-65 Managed care guide: pharmacotherapy and general management approaches for chronic obstructive pulmonary disease (COPD). *DNase,* Deoxyribonuclease; *Hct,* hematocrit; *prn,* as needed; *qid,* four times a day; *qod,* every other day. (Modified from Noble J: *Primary care medicine,* ed 3, St Louis, 2001, Mosby.)

CONSTIPATION

ICD-9CM # 564.0

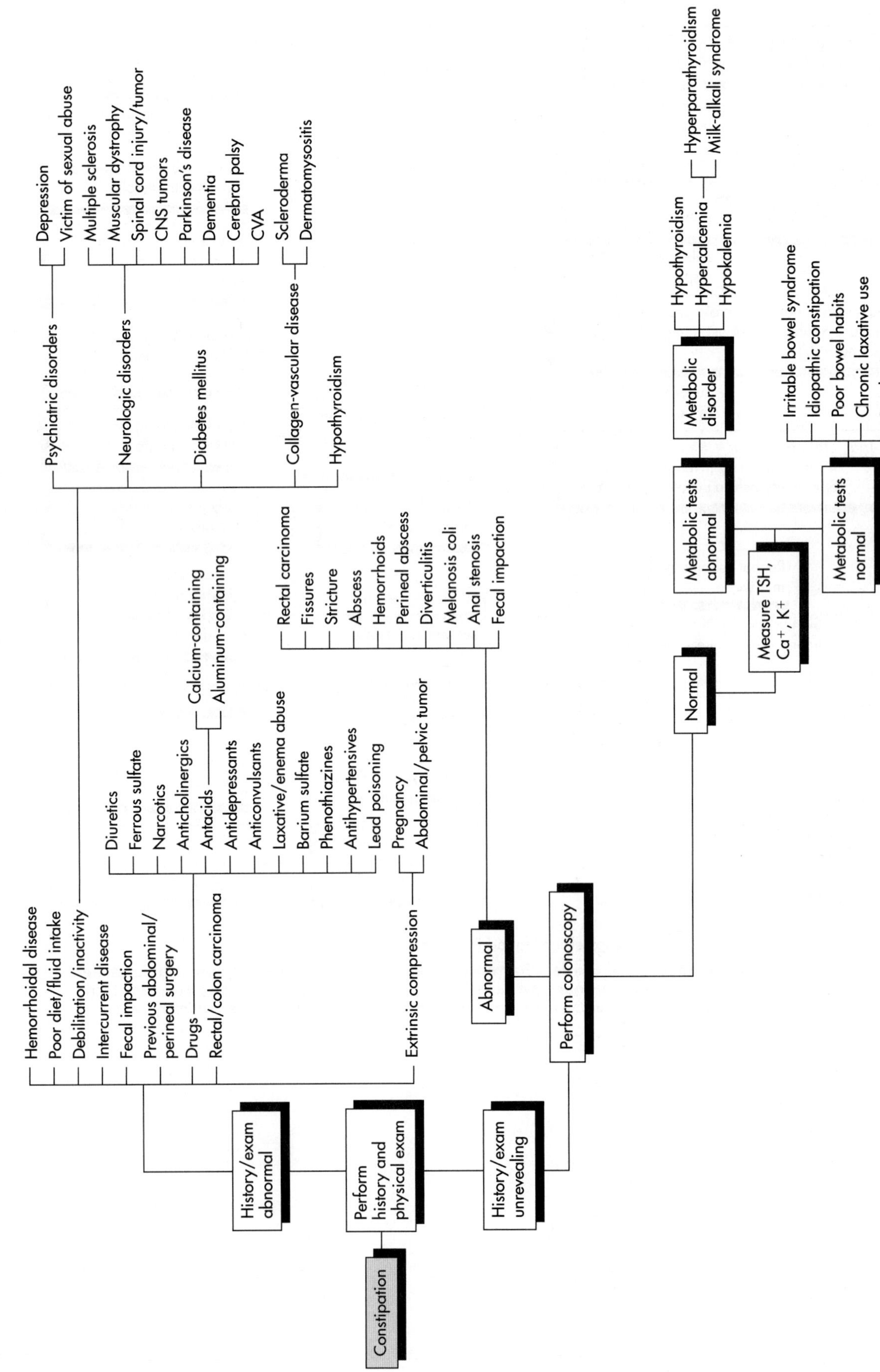

FIGURE 3-66 Constipation. *BE,* Barium enema; *CNS,* central nervous system; *CVA,* cerebral vascular accident; *TSH,* thyroid-stimulating hormone. (From Healey PM: *Common medical diagnosis,* ed 3, Philadelphia, 2000, WB Saunders.)

ICD-9CM # V25.09

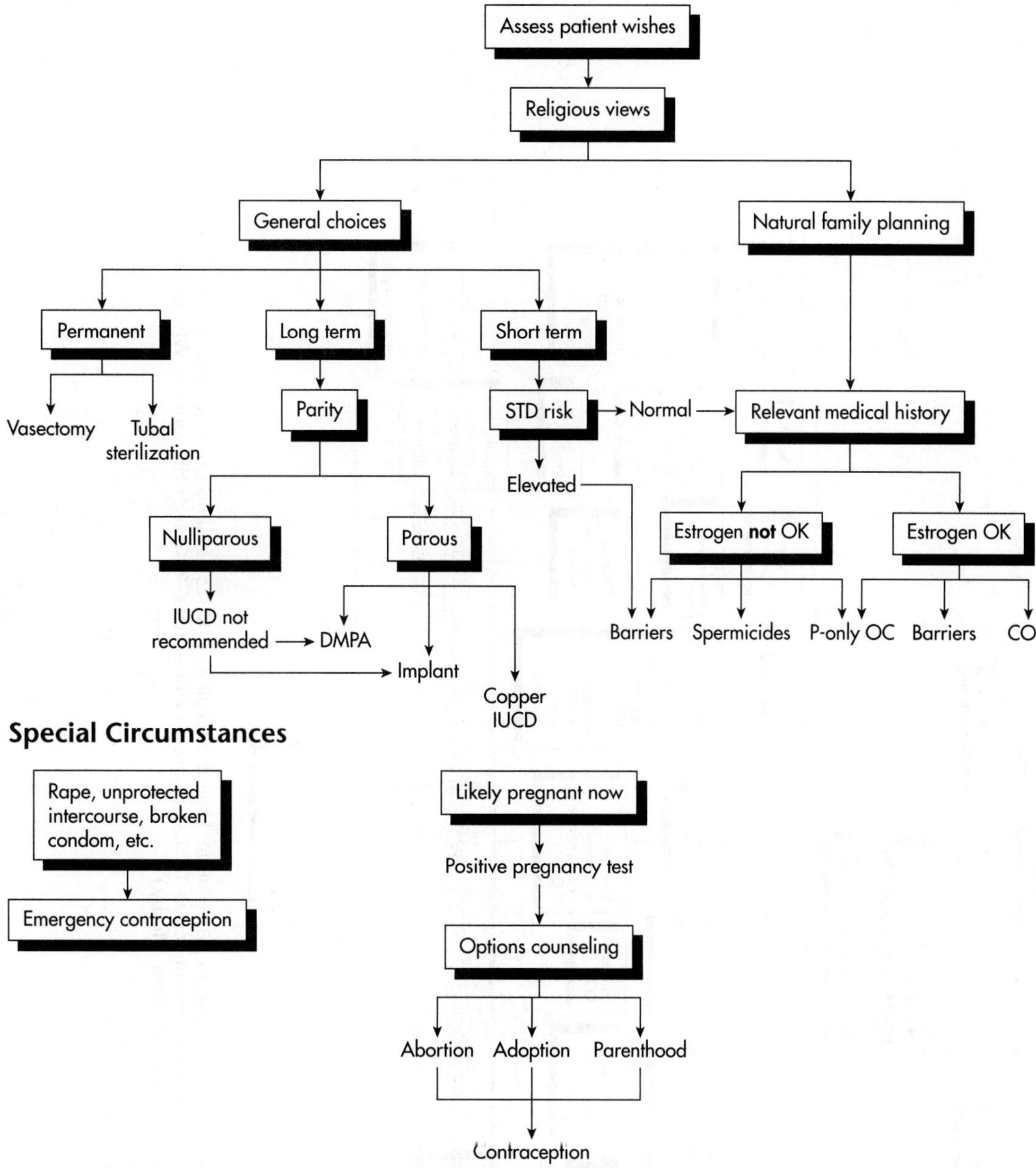

FIGURE 3-67 Helping couples select a contraceptive method. *COC,* Combination estrogen-progestin oral contraceptive; *DMPA,* depot medroxyprogesterone acetate; *IUCD,* intrauterine contraceptive device; *P-only OC,* progestin-only oral contraceptive; *STD,* sexually transmitted disease. (From Copeland LJ: *Textbook of gynecology,* ed 2, Philadelphia, 2000, WB Saunders.)

ICD-9CM # V25.01 Prescription or use, oral contraceptive

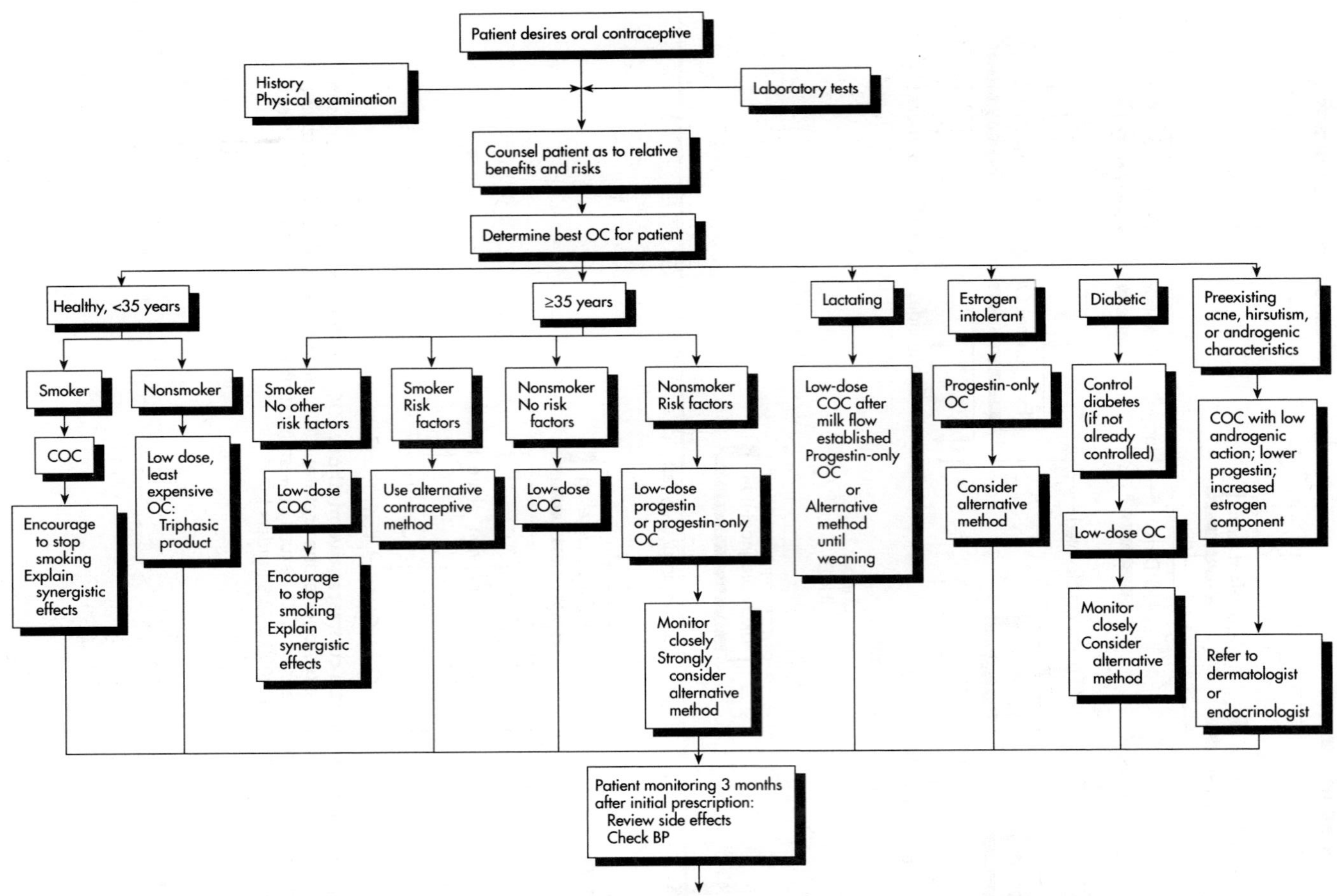

FIGURE 3-68 Contraceptive use. *BP,* Blood pressure; *BTB,* breakthrough bleeding; *COC,* combination oral contraceptives; *CVA,* cerebrovascular accident; *OC,* oral contraceptive. (From Robles TA: Use of oral contraceptives. In Greene HL, Johnson WP, Lemcke D [eds]: *Decision making in medicine,* ed 2, St Louis, 1998, Mosby.)

CONTRACEPTIVE USE, ORAL—cont'd

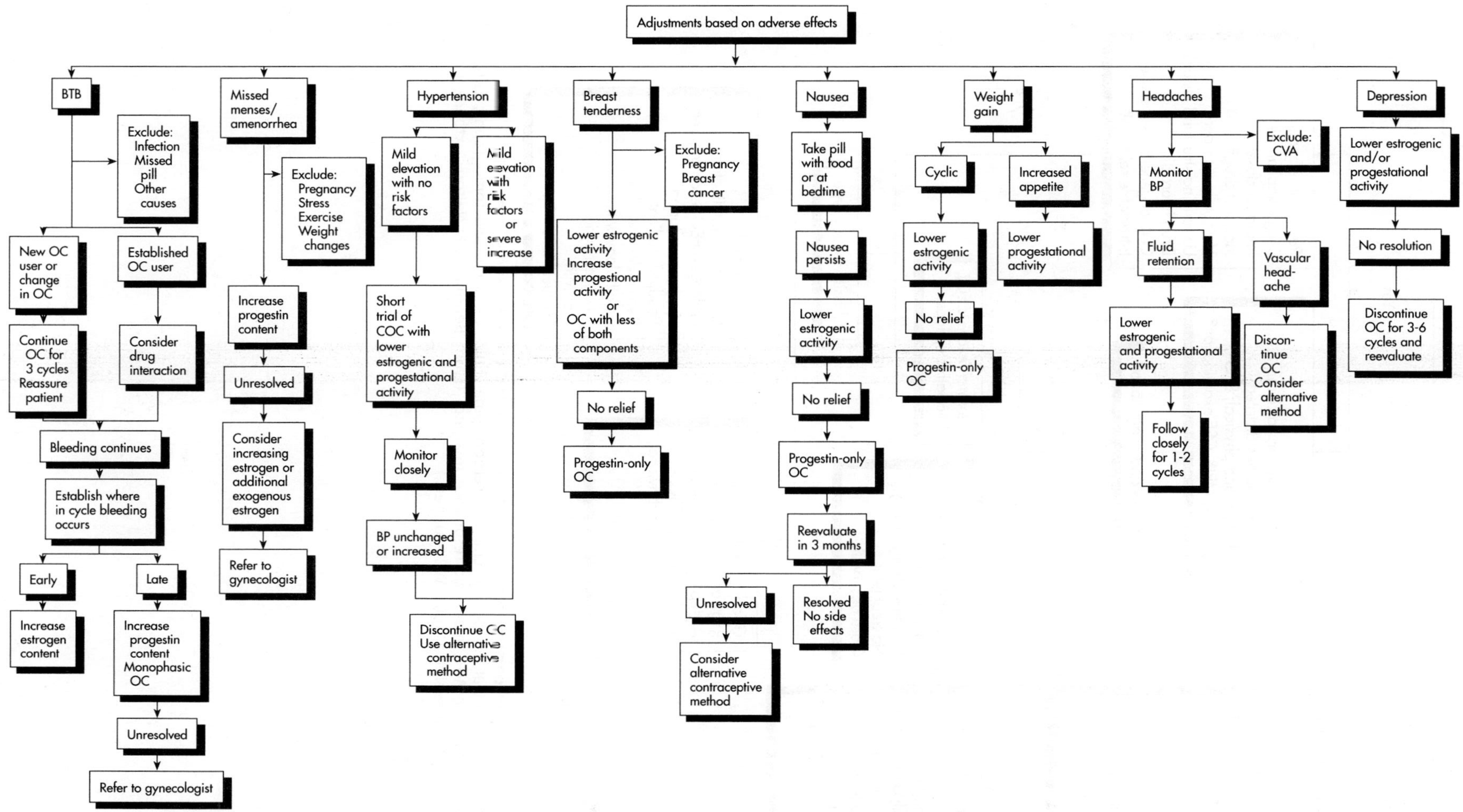

FIGURE 3-68 (Continued) **Contraceptive use.** *BP,* Blood pressure; *BTB,* breakthrough bleeding; *COC,* combination oral contraceptives; *CVA,* cerebrovascular accident; *OC,* oral contraceptive. (From Robles TA: Use of oral contraceptives. In Greene HL, Johnson WP, Lemcke D [eds]: *Decision making in medicine,* ed 2, St Louis, 1998, Mosby.)

ICD-9CM # 780.39

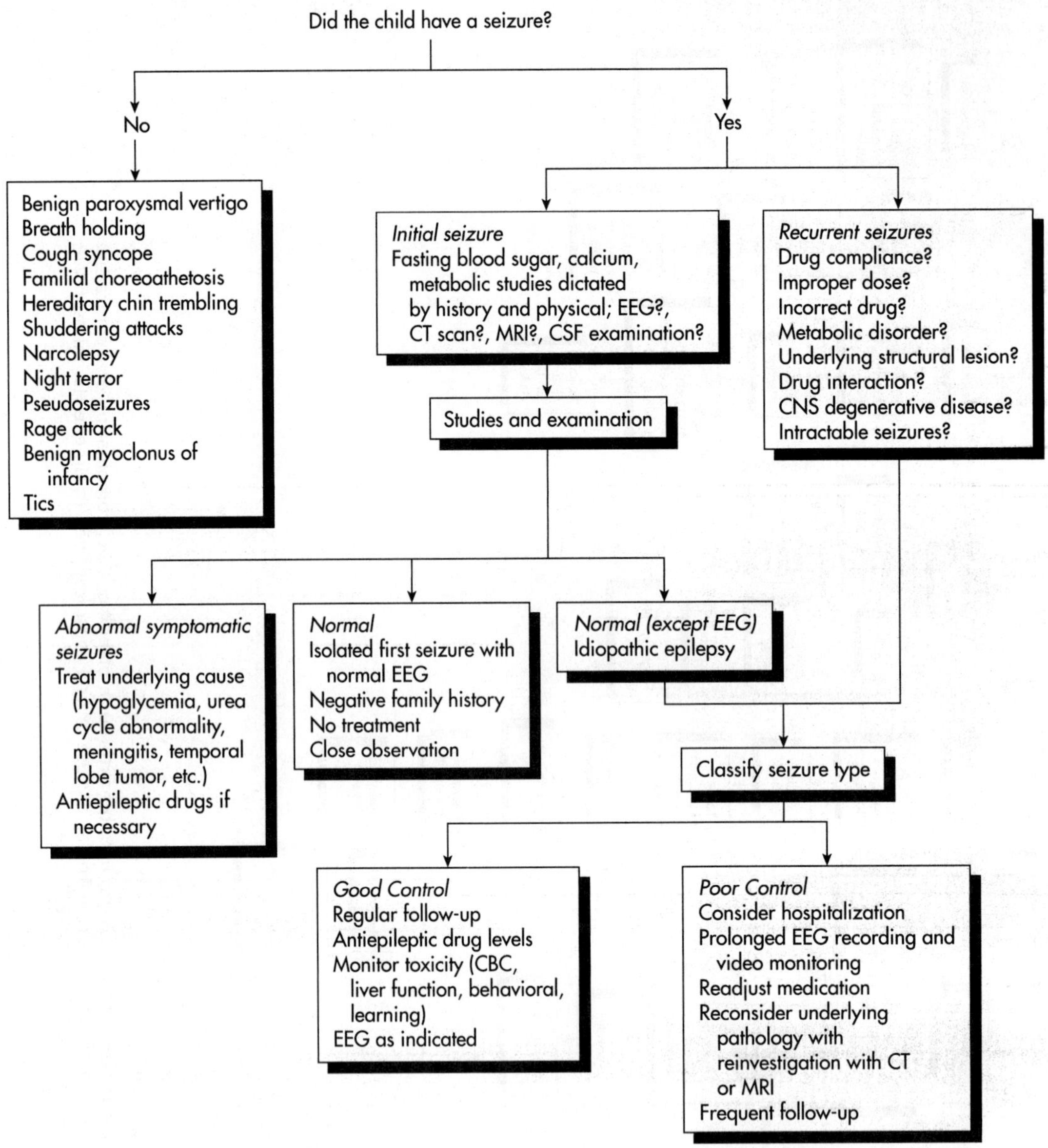

FIGURE 3-69 An approach to the child with a suspected convulsive disorder. *CBC,* Complete blood count; *CNS,* central nervous system; *CSF,* cerebrospinal fluid; *CT,* computed tomography; *EEG,* electroencephalogram; *MRI,* magnetic resonance imaging. (From Behrman RE: *Nelson textbook of pediatrics,* ed 18, Philadelphia, 2007, WB Saunders.)

ICD-9CM # 918.1 Corneal abrasion
743.9 Corneal anomalies NOS

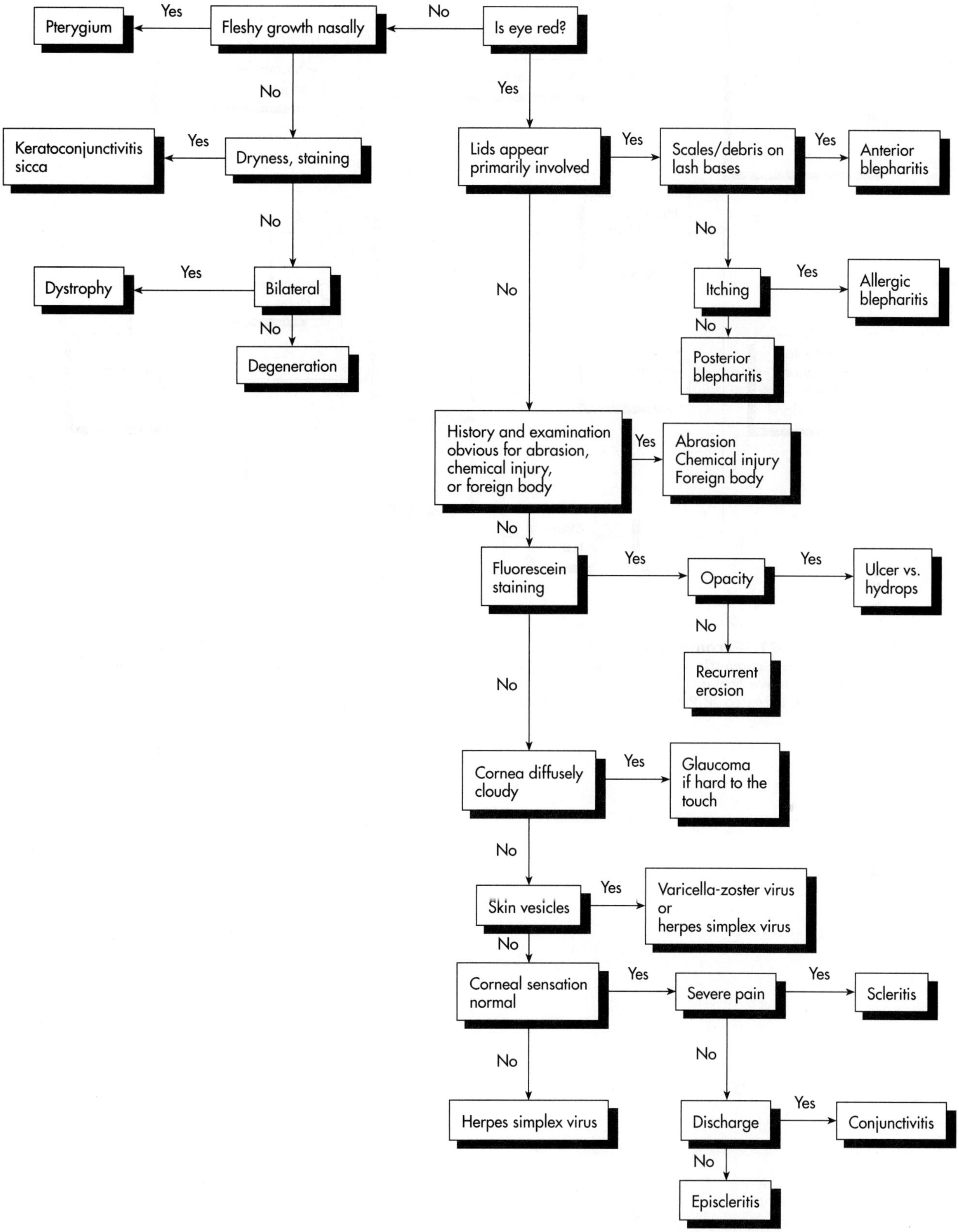

FIGURE 3-70 Approach to the patient with corneal disorders. (From Noble J [ed]: *Primary care medicine,* ed 3, St Louis, 2001, Mosby.)

ICD-9CM # 414.00

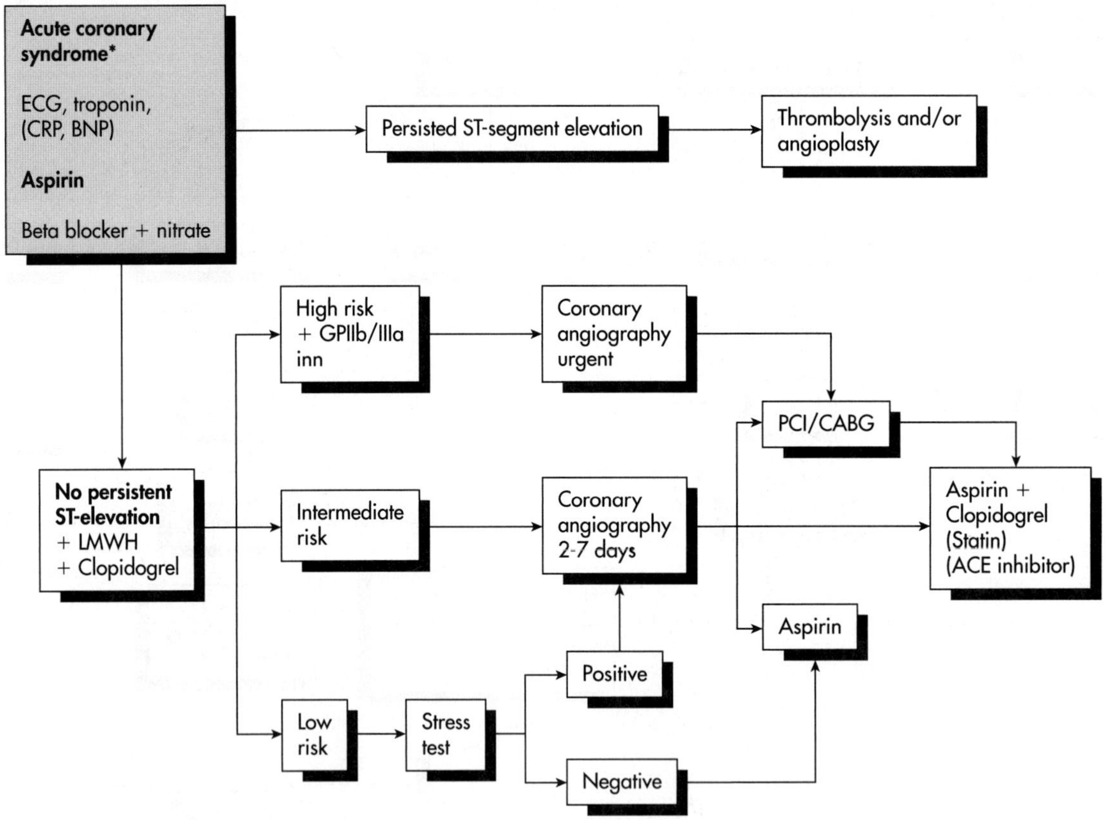

*Refer to Section I for additional information on this topic.

FIGURE 3-71 Recommended treatment strategy for unstable coronary artery disease. *ACE,* Angiotensin-converting enzyme; *BNP,* brain natriuretic peptide; *CABG,* coronary artery bypass grafting; *CRP,* C-reactive protein; *ECG,* electrocardiogram; *PCI,* percutaneous coronary intervention. (From Crawford MH, DiMarco JP, Paulus WJ [eds]: *Cardiology,* ed 2, St Louis, 2004, Mosby.)

ICD-9CM # 786.2

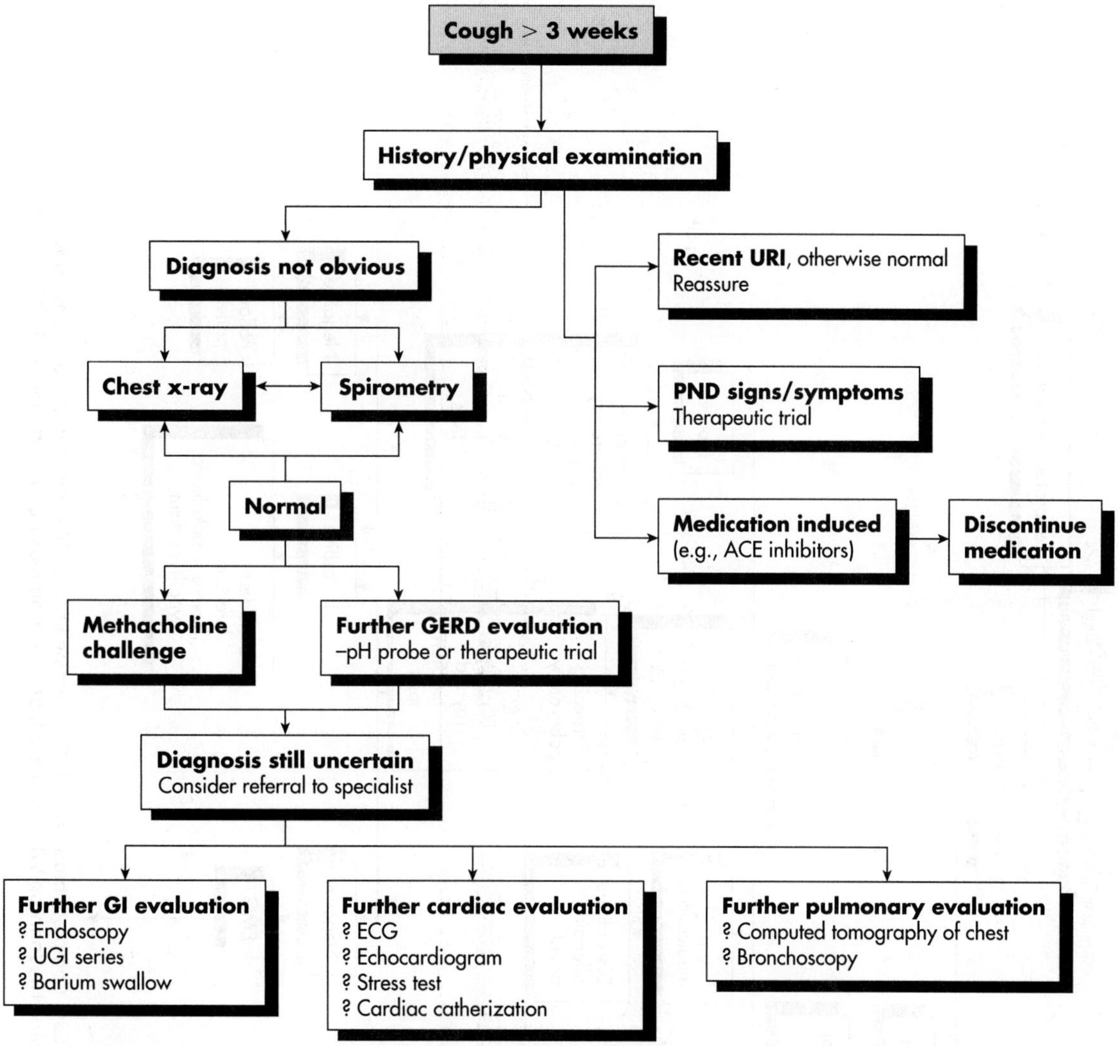

FIGURE 3-72 Diagnostic approach to chronic cough. *ECG,* Electrocardiogram; *GERD,* gastroesophageal reflux disease; *PND,* paroxysmal nocturnal dyspnea; *UGI,* upper gastrointestinal tract; *URI,* upper respiratory infection. (From Carlson KJ et al: *Primary care of women,* ed 2, St Louis, 2002, Mosby.)

CREATINE KINASE ELEVATION

ICD-9CM # V72.6

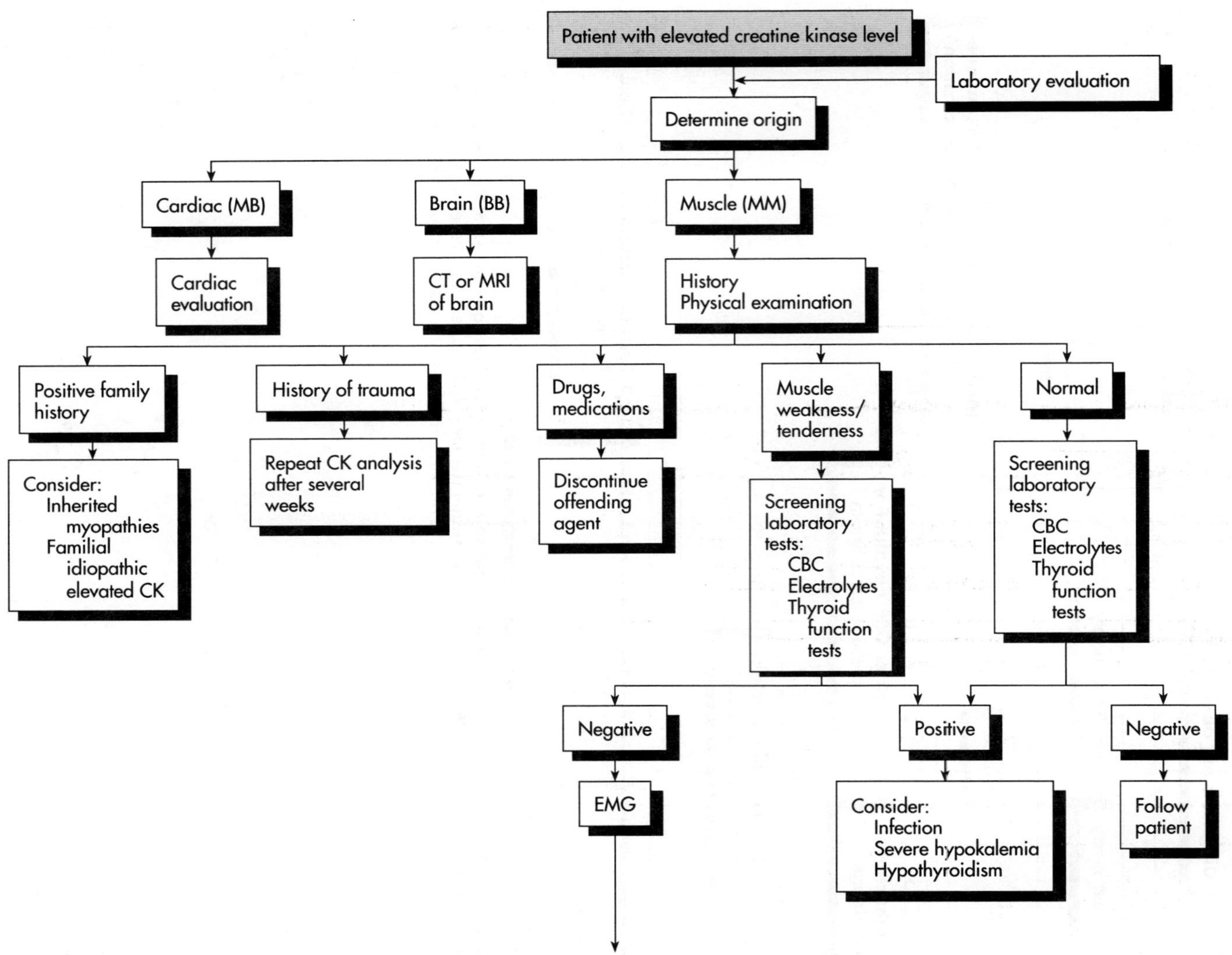

FIGURE 3-73 Evaluation of creatine kinase elevation. *CBC,* Complete blood count; *CK,* creatine kinase; *CT,* computed tomography; *EMG,* electromyography; *MRI,* magnetic resonance imaging. (From Greene HL, Johnson WP, Lemcke D [eds]: *Decision making in medicine,* ed 2, St Louis, 1998, Mosby.)

CREATINE KINASE ELEVATION—cont'd

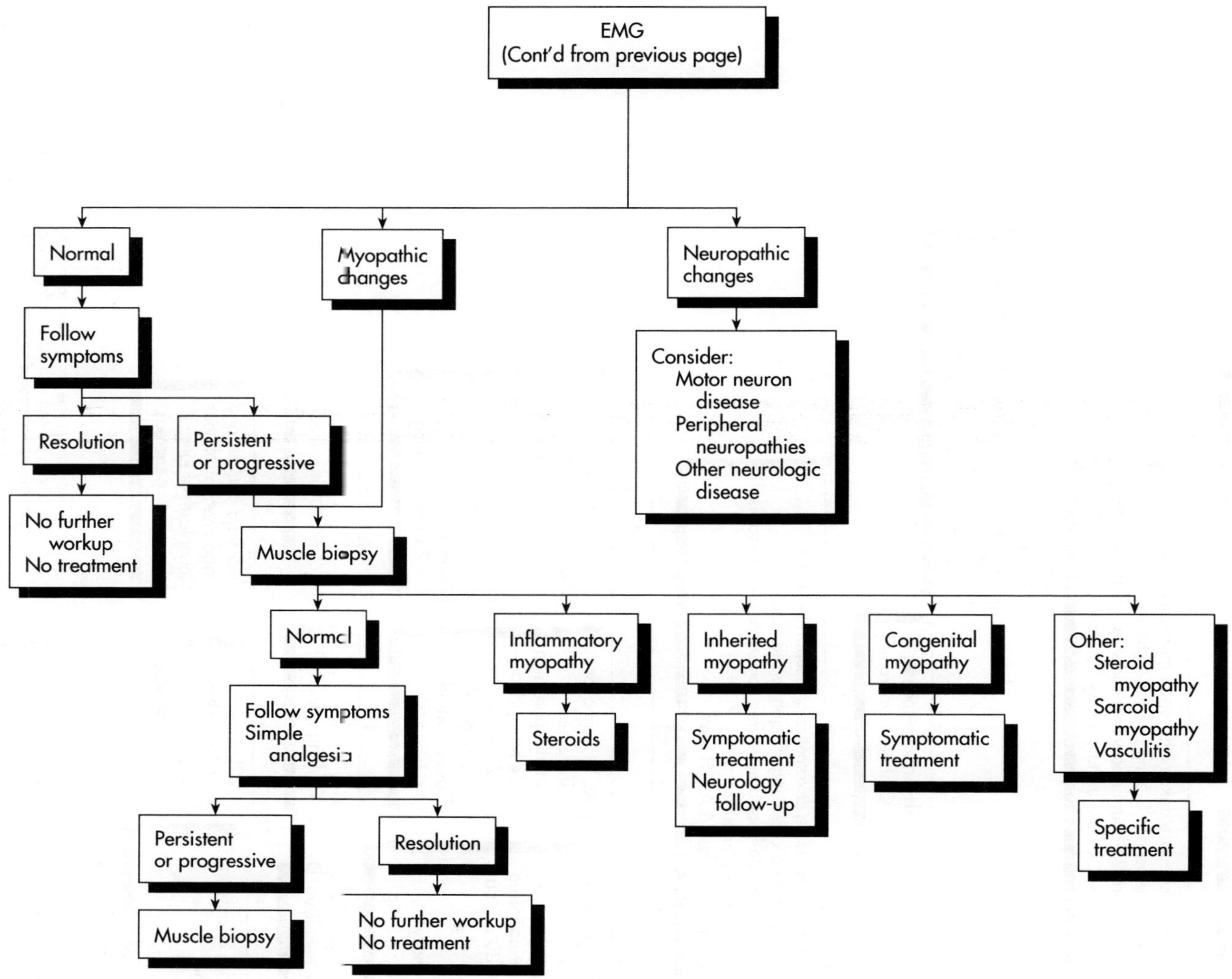

FIGURE 3-73 (Continued) **Evaluation of creatine kinase elevation.** *CBC,* Complete blood count; *CK,* creatine kinase; *CT,* computed tomography; *EMG,* electromyography; *MRI,* magnetic resonance imaging. (From Greene HL, Johnson WP, Lemcke D [eds]: *Decision making in medicine,* ed 2, St Louis, 1998, Mosby.)

ICD-9CM # 255.0

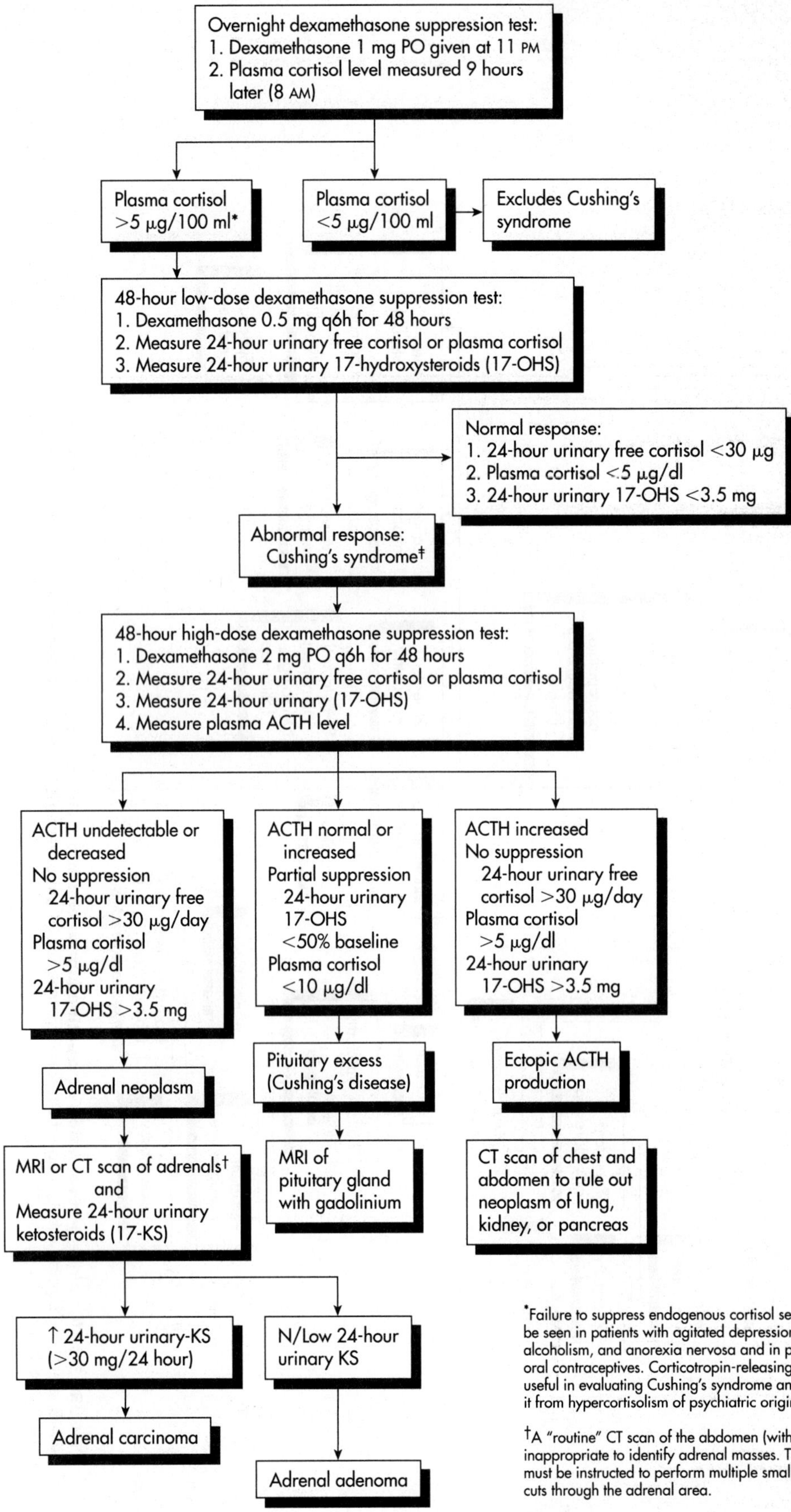

*Failure to suppress endogenous cortisol secretion can also be seen in patients with agitated depression, severe stress, alcoholism, and anorexia nervosa and in patients taking oral contraceptives. Corticotropin-releasing factor (CRF) is useful in evaluating Cushing's syndrome and in differentiating it from hypercortisolism of psychiatric origin.

†A "routine" CT scan of the abdomen (with cuts >1 cm) is inappropriate to identify adrenal masses. The radiographer must be instructed to perform multiple small tomographic cuts through the adrenal area.

‡Refer to Section I for additional information on this topic.

FIGURE 3-74 Cushing's syndrome. *ACTH,* Adrenocorticotropic hormone; *CT,* computed tomography; *MRI,* magnetic resonance imaging; *PO,* by mouth. (From Ferri F: *Practical guide to the care of the medical patient,* ed 7, St Louis, 2007, Mosby.)

ICD-9CM # variable with specific disorder

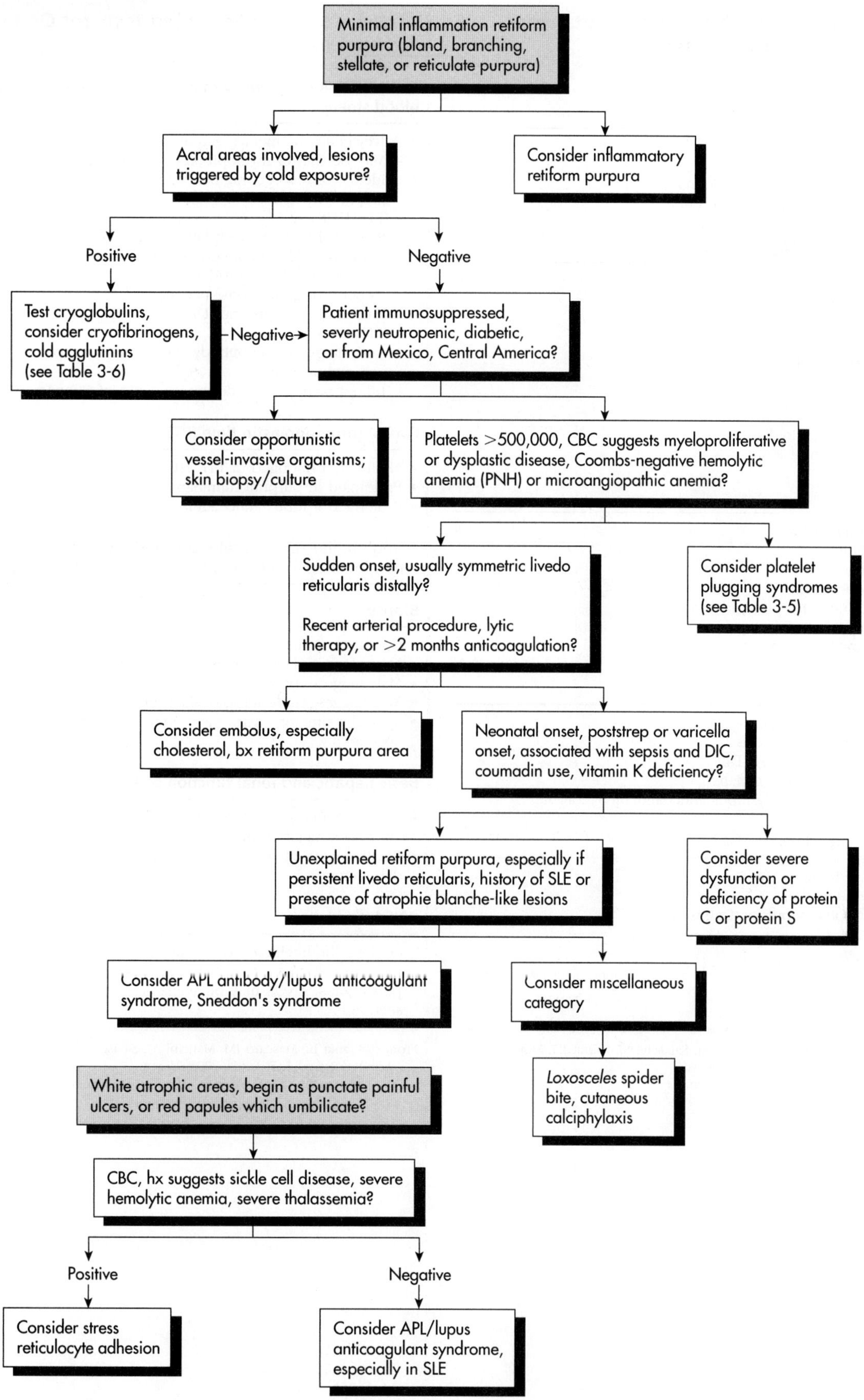

FIGURE 3-75 Cutaneous microvascular occlusion syndromes. *APL,* Antiphospholipid; *CBC,* complete blood count; *DIC,* disseminated intravascular coagulation; *PNH,* paroxysmal nocturnal hemoglobinuria; *SLE,* systemic lupus erythematosus. (From Bolognia JL, Mascaro JM, Mancini AJ, Salasche SJ, Saurat JH, Stingl G [eds]: *Dermatology,* ed 2, St Louis, 2008, Mosby.)

Continued on following page

TABLE 3-5 Differential Diagnosis of Cutaneous Microvascular Occlusion Based on Pathophysiology

Platelet plugging

- Heparin necrosis
- Myeloproliferative thrombocytosis
- Paroxysmal nocturnal hemoglobinuria
- Thrombotic thrombocytopenic purpura

Cold-related gelling or agglutination

- Cryoglobulinemia
- Cryofibrinogenemia
- Cold agglutinins

Vessel-invasive organisms

- Ecthyma gangrenosum
- Opportunitstic fungi
- Disseminated strongyloidiasis
- Lucio phenomenon of leprosy

Embolization

- Cholesterol embolus
- Oxalate embolus
- Atrial myxoma
- Marantic endocarditis
- Libman–Sacks/antiphospholipid antibody
- Crystal globulin vasculopathy
- Hypereosinophilic syndrome

Systemic coagulopathies

- Neonatal purpura fulminans
- Coumadin (warfarin) necrosis
- Purpura fulminans of sepsis/DIC
- Postinfectious purpura fulminans
- Antiphospholipid antibody/lupus anticoagulant syndrome

Vascular coagulopathies

- Sneddon's syndrome
- Livedoid vasculopathy
- Malignant atrophic papulosis/Degos' disease

Miscellaneous

- Stress reticulocyte adhesion
- Cutaneous calciphylaxis

From Bolognia JL, Mascaro JM, Mancini AJ, Salasche SJ, Saurat JH, Stingl G [eds]: *Dermatology,* ed 2, St Louis, 2008, Mosby.

DIC, Disseminated intravascular coagulation.

TABLE 3-6 Basic Screening Tests for Occlusive Syndrome

Complete blood count with differential, platelet count, and blood smear

- Polycythemia or anemia, granulocytosis, thrombocytosis, poikilocytosis
  - May be sign of myeloproliferative or myelodysplastic diseases
- Evidence of red cell fragmentation (schistocytes) and microangiopathy, consider:
  - TTP/HUS
  - Purpura fulminans with DIC, occasionally
  - Antiphospholipid antibody syndrome, occasionally
- Thrombocytopenia, consider:
  - Heparin necrosis, some patients
  - Purpura fulminans with DIC
  - TTP/HUS
  - Antiphospholipid antibody syndrome, some patients
- Severe neutropenia
  - Immunocompromised; opportunistic infections very likely

Partial thromboplastin time (PTT)

- Minimally prolonged in TTP/HUS
- Prolonged in purpura fulminans and DIC
- Prolonged if lupus anticoagulant activity present, and assay sensitive

Cryoglobulins (occasionally cryofibrinogen and cold agglutinins) when location and history suggest cold occlusion syndrome

Biopsy

- Confirms occlusion versus other mechanisms of vessel injury
- May suggest platelet plugs instead of fibrin thrombi
- May suggest cryoglobulin gelling
- May suggest cholesterol, oxalate, or crystal globulin occlusion
- Special stains for organisms in immunocompromised hosts, when appropriate

Basic hepatic and renal function screens

- Hepatic function can affect vitamin K-dependent factors and coumadin metabolism
- Renal disease moves cutaneous calciphylaxis higher in the differential diagnosis

ANCA

To reduce the likelihood of the uncommon noninflammatory retiform purpura presentation of Wegener's granulomatosis or microscopic polyangiitis. ANCA may be available before permanent histology sections.

From Bolognia JL, Mascaro JM, Mancini AJ, Salasche SJ, Saurat JH, Stingl G [eds]: *Dermatology,* ed 2, St Louis, 2008, Mosby.

ANCA, Antineutrophil cytoplasmic antibody; *HUS,* hemolytioc uremic syndrome; *TTP,* thrombotic thrombocytopenic purpura.

CYANOSIS

ICD-9CM # 782.5 Cyanosis NOS

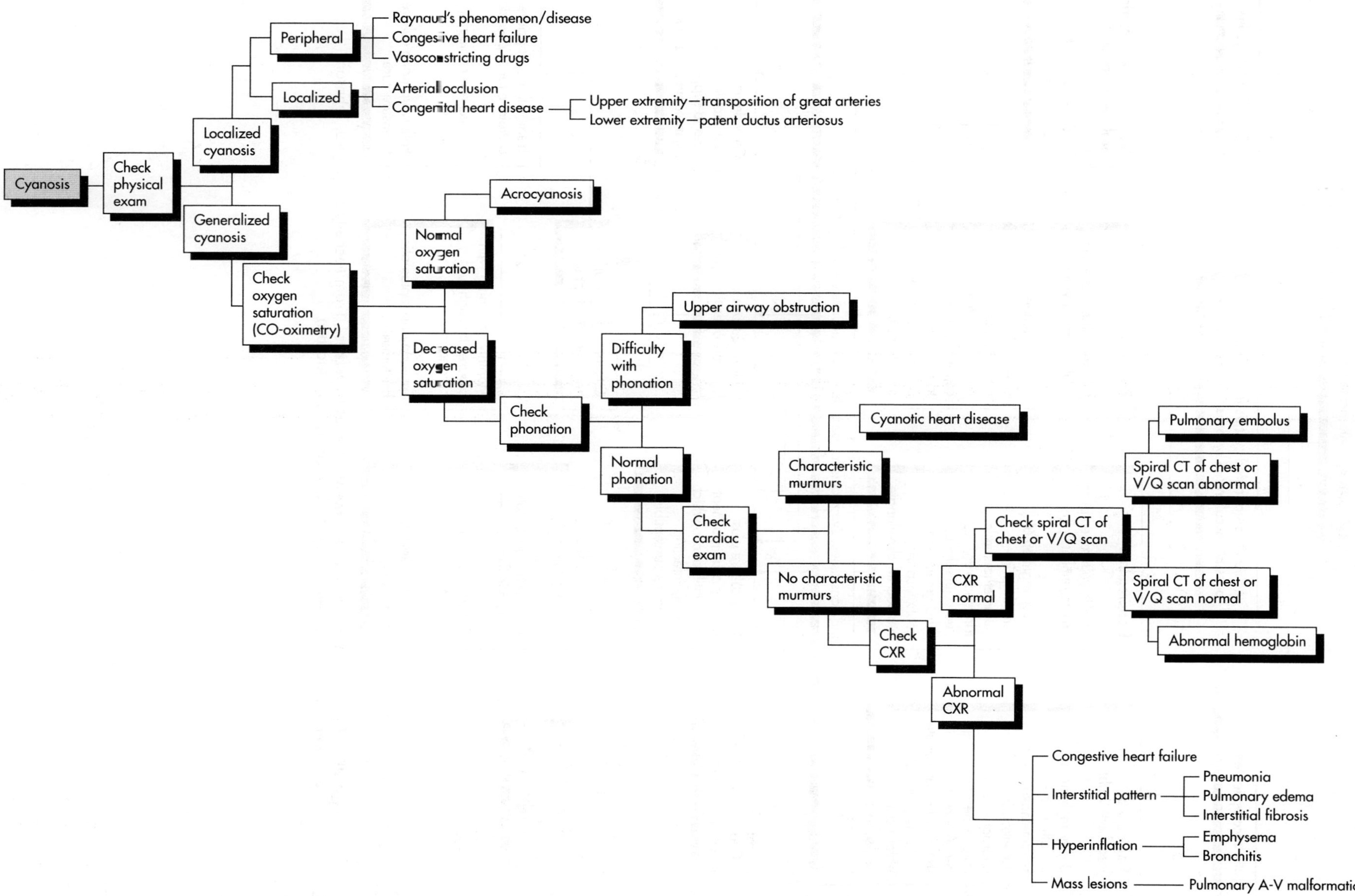

FIGURE 3-76 Cyanosis. *A-V,* Arteriovenous; *CXR,* chest x-ray; *V/Q,* ventilation-perfusion. (From Healey PM: *Common medical diagnosis: an algorithmic approach,* ed 3, Philadelphia, 2000, WB Saunders.)

ICD-9CM # 595.0

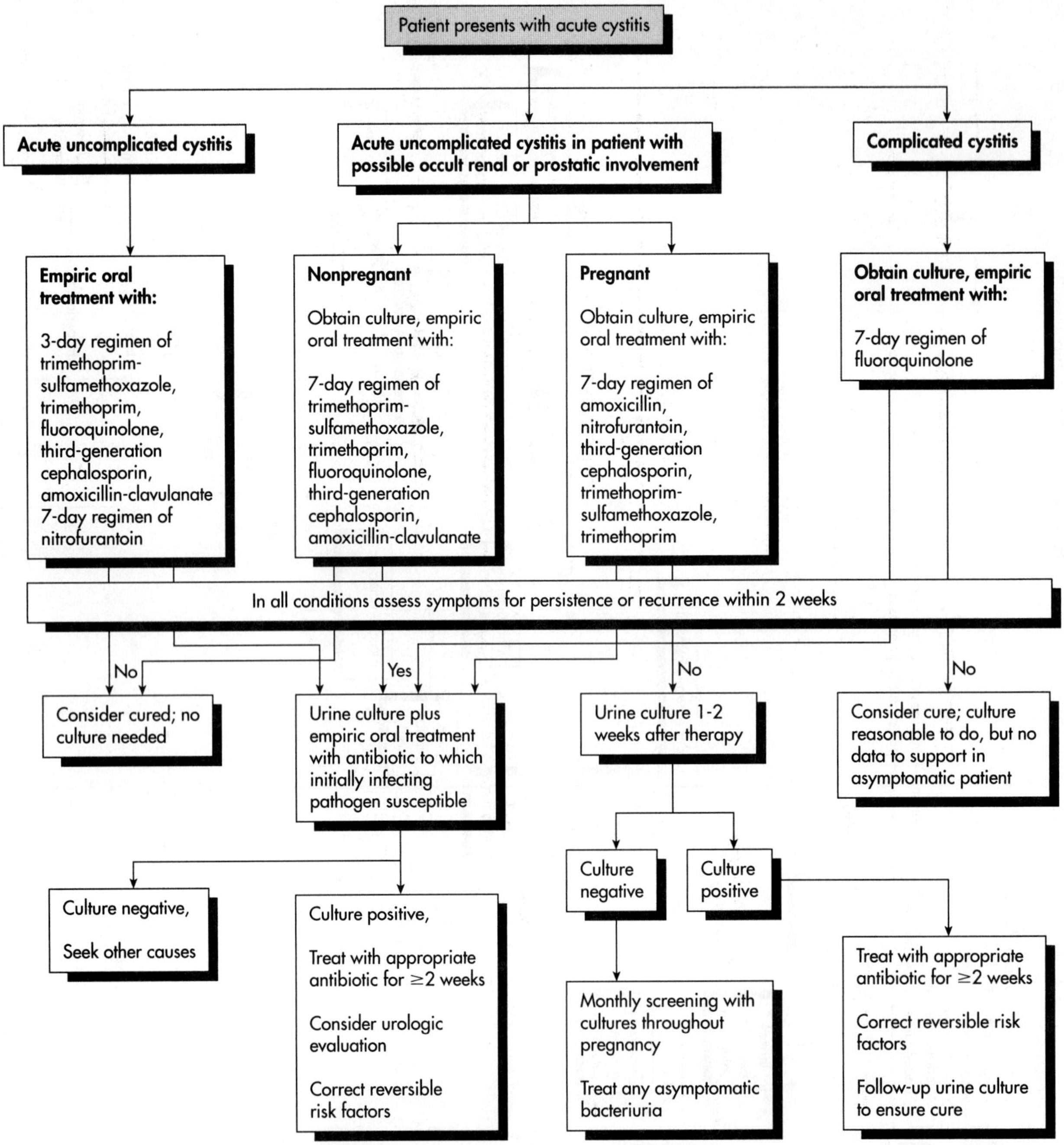

FIGURE 3-77 Algorithm for management of acute cystitis. (From Feehally J, Floege J, Johnson RJ: *Comprehensive clinical nephrology,* ed 3, St Louis, 2007, Mosby.)

ICD-9CM # 451.1 Thrombosis of deep veins of lower extremities
451.83 Thrombosis of deep veins of upper extremities

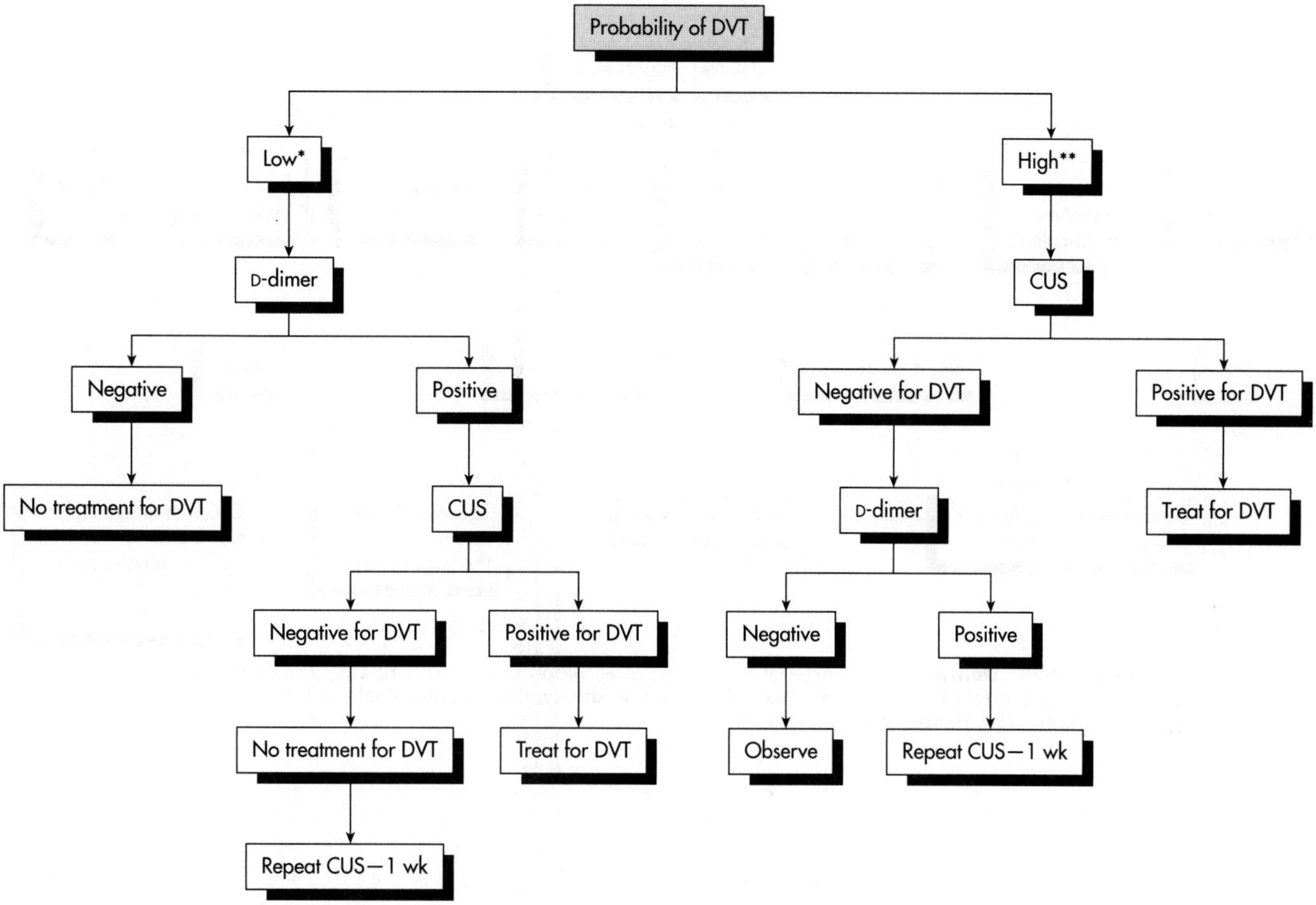

*Low probability
None of features of high probability and an alternative diagnosis likely

**High probability
1. History of active cancer
2. History of prolonged immobilization
3. History recent surgery
4. History recent leg trauma
5. Previous history of thromboembolic disease
6. Family history of thromboembolic disease
7. BCP use
8. History recent long travel
9. Exam positive for swelling and tenderness compared to other extremity

FIGURE 3-78 Diagnostic approach to deep vein thrombosis. *CUS,* Compressive ultrasound; *DVT,* deep vein thrombosis.

ICD-9CM # 293.0

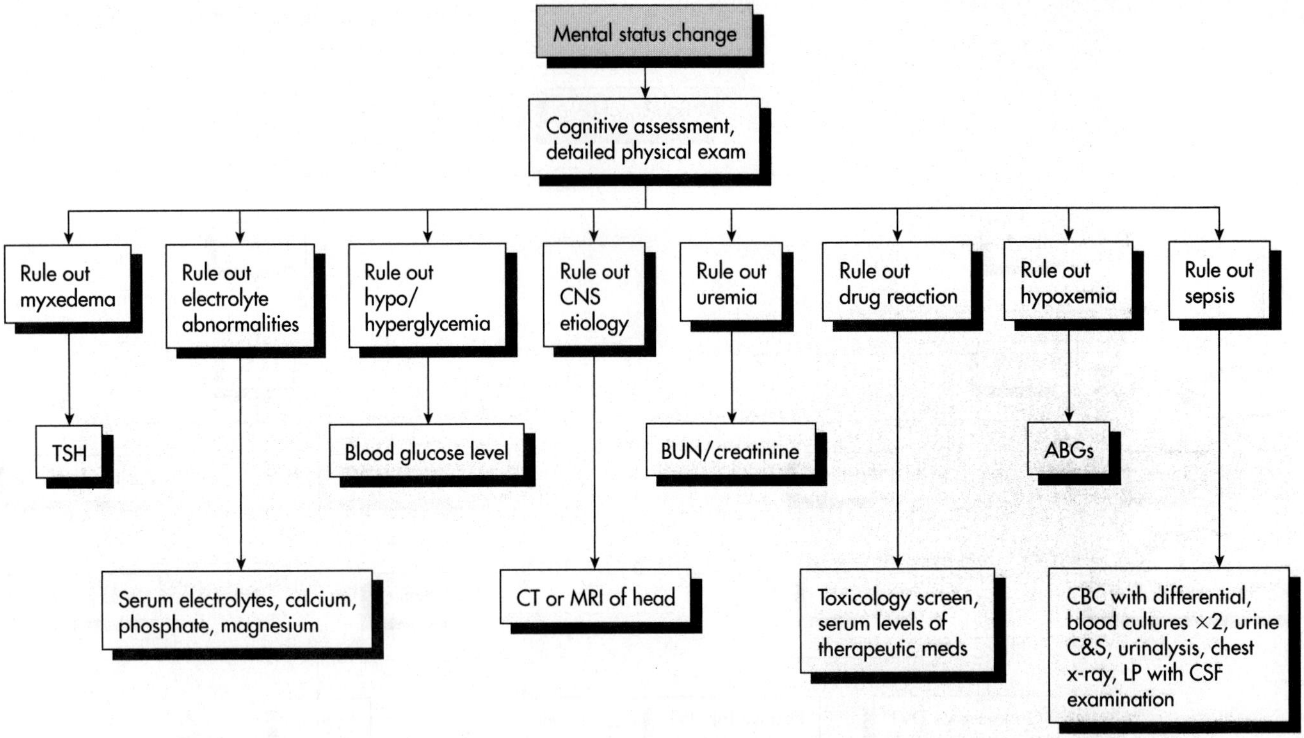

FIGURE 3-79 Delirium. *ABG,* Arterial blood gas; *BUN,* blood urea nitrogen; *CBC,* complete blood count; *CNS,* central nervous system; *C&S,* culture and sensitivity; *CSF,* cerebrospinal fluid; *CT,* computed tomography; *TSH,* thyroid-stimulating hormone.

ICD-9CM # 293.0 Delirium, acute
292.81 Delirium, drug induced
293.1 Delirium, subacute
293.81 Delirium, transient organic with delusions
293.82 Delirium, transient organic with hallucinations

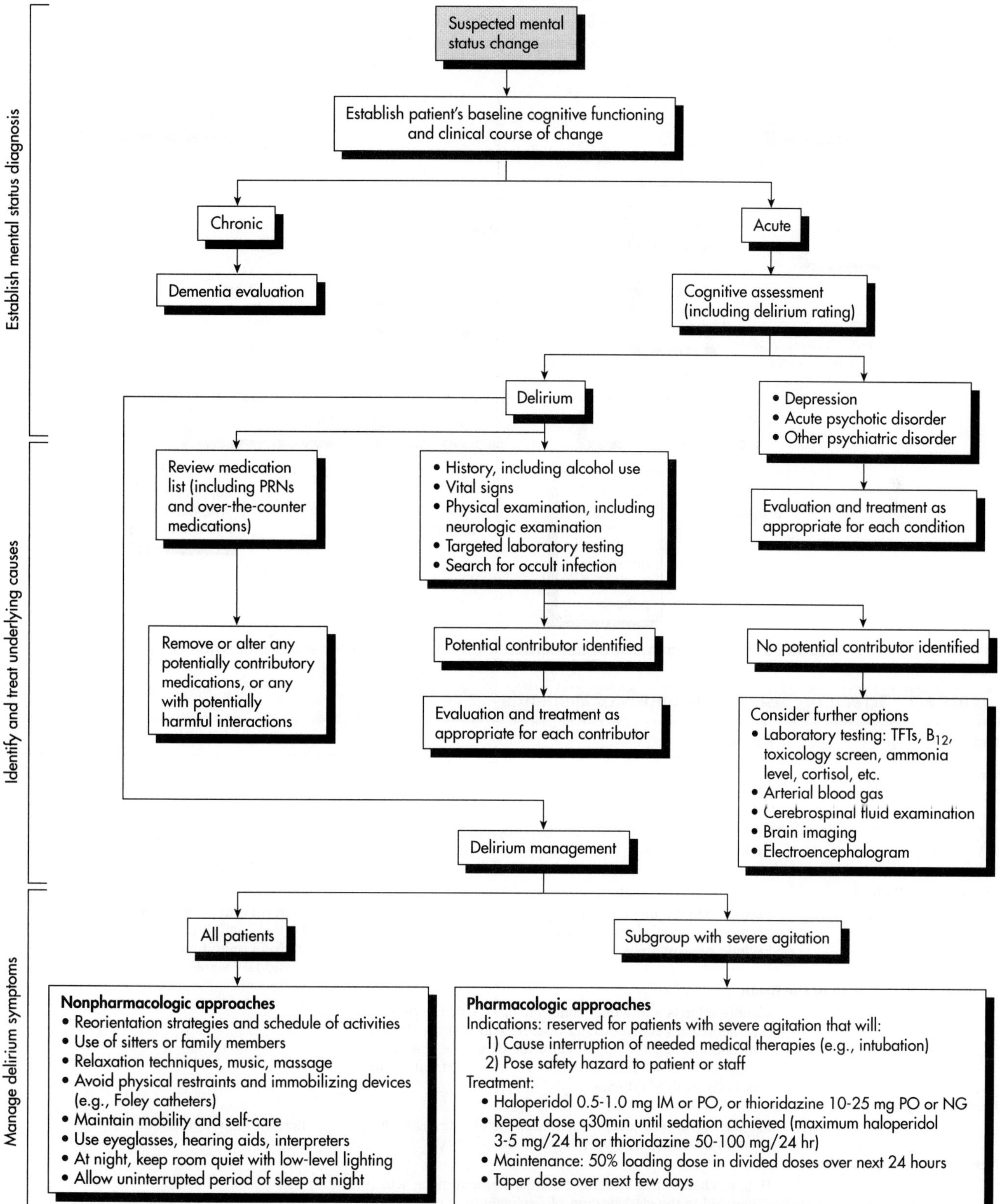

FIGURE 3-80 Algorithm for evaluation of suspected mental status change in an older patient. *IM,* Intramuscular; *NG,* nasogastric; *PO,* by mouth; *PRNs,* as needed; *TFTs,* thyroid function tests. (From Goldman L, Ausiello D [eds]: *Cecil textbook of medicine,* ed 23, Philadelphia, 2008, WB Saunders.)

ICD-9CM # 290.10 Dementia, presenile
290.0 Dementia, senile
437.0 Dementia, arteriosclerotic

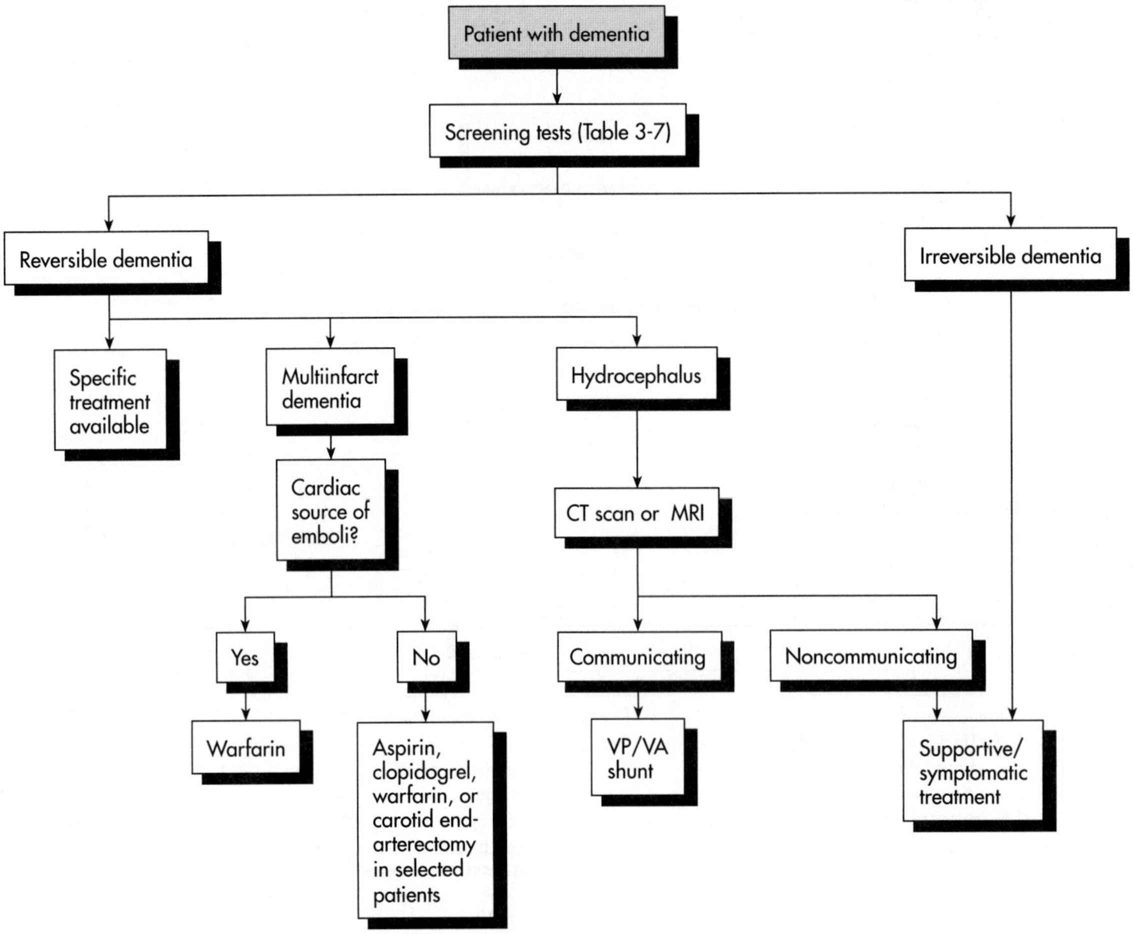

FIGURE 3-81 Management of dementia. *VA,* Ventriculoatrial; *VP,* ventriculoperitoneal.

TABLE 3-7 Screening Tests for Diagnosis of Dementia

Test	Rationale	Remarks
Blood Test		
Complete blood count	Assess general nutritional status	
Serum B_{12} level	Exclude vitamin B_{12} deficiency	Consider Schilling's test if B_{12} level is low
TSH + free T_4 *or* TSH + FTI	Exclude primary and secondary hypothyroidism	
HIV serology	Exclude HIV infection	Perform only if indicated; consent from patient required
Cerebrospinal Fluid		
Cell count/protein level	Exclude chronic meningitis	Perform only if indicated
Cytology	Exclude carcinomatous meningitis	Perform only if indicated
VDRL	Exclude neurosyphilis	Perform only if indicated; check serum TPHA and HIV serology if CSF VDRL is positive
CT Scan/MRI/PET Scan of the Brain	Identify infarcts and white matter changes; exclude presence of neoplasm, demyelinating disease, and hydrocephalus; location of atrophy may suggest the diagnosis (e.g., parahippocampal atrophy in Alzheimer's disease, frontotemporal atrophy in Pick's disease)	
Electroencephalogram	Exclude metabolic encephalopathies; useful if Creutzfeldt-Jakob disease or status epilepticus is suspected	Perform only if indicated
Neuropsychologic Evaluation	Help to characterize pattern of cognitive impairment, which may aid in the classification of dementia; rule out pseudodementia from depression	

Modified from Johnson RT, Griffin JW: *Current therapy in neurologic disease,* ed 5, St Louis, 1997, Mosby.
CSF, Cerebrospinal fluid; *CT,* computed tomography; *FTI,* free thyroxine index; *HIV,* human immunodeficiency virus; *MRI,* magnetic resonance imaging; *PET,* positron emission tomography; T_4, thyroxine; *TPHA,* Treponema pallidum hemagglutination assay; *TSH,* thyroid-stimulating hormone; *VDRL,* Venereal Disease Research Laboratory test.

ICD-9CM # 296.2 Major depressive disorder, single episode

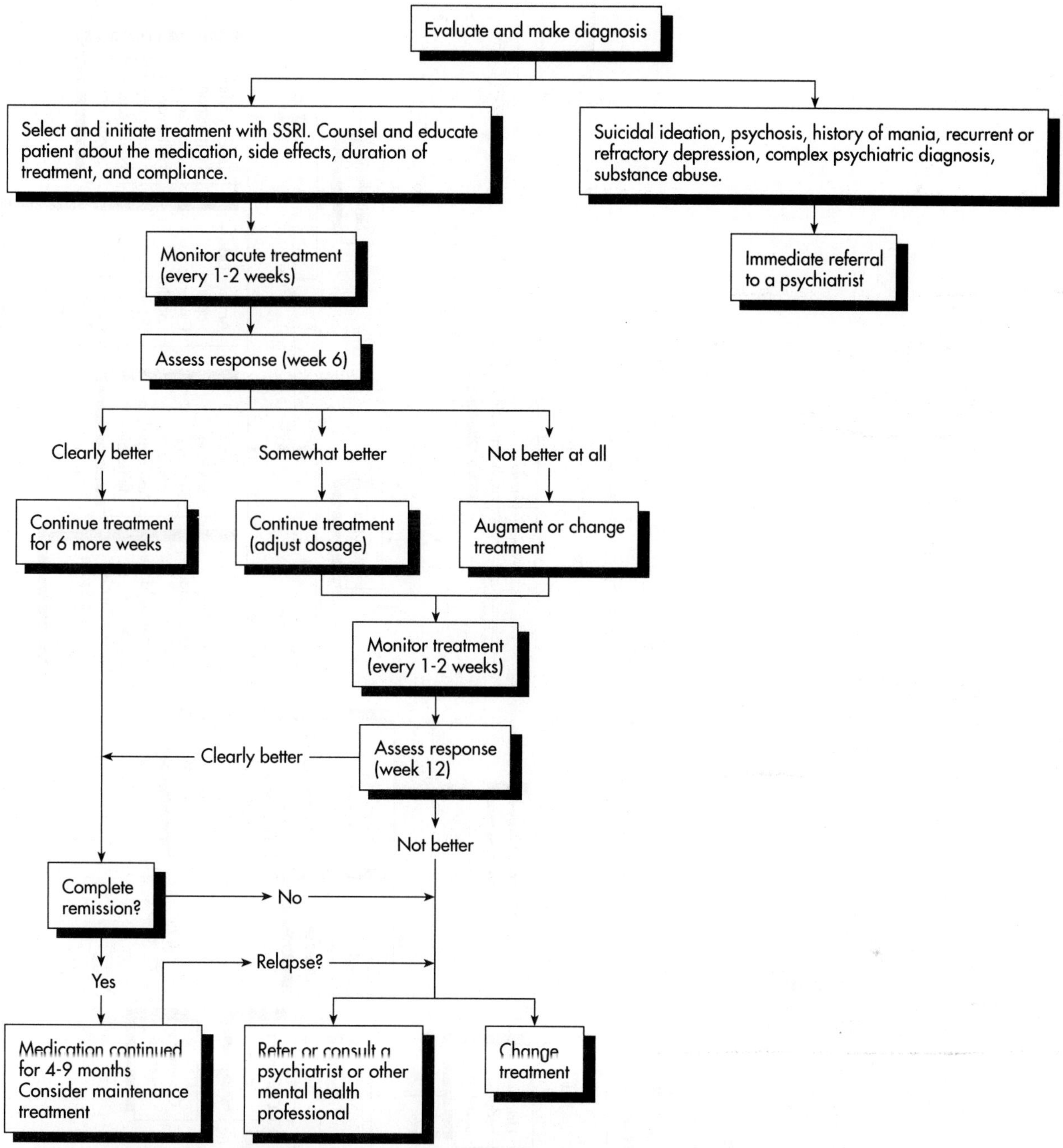

FIGURE 3-82 Guidelines for the treatment of depression in the primary care setting. *SSRI,* Selective serotonin reuptake inhibitor. NOTE: Time of assessment (weeks 6 and 12) rests on very modest data. It may be necessary to revise the treatment plan earlier for patients who fail to respond. (From AHCPR Quick Reference Guide of Clinicians, No. 5: Depression in primary care: *Detection, diagnosis and treatment,* 1993; and American Psychiatric Association: *Diagnostic and statistical manual of mental disorders,* ed 4, Washington, DC, 1994, American Psychiatric Association.)

DEVELOPMENTAL DELAY

ICD-9CM # 783.4 Developmental delay, physiological

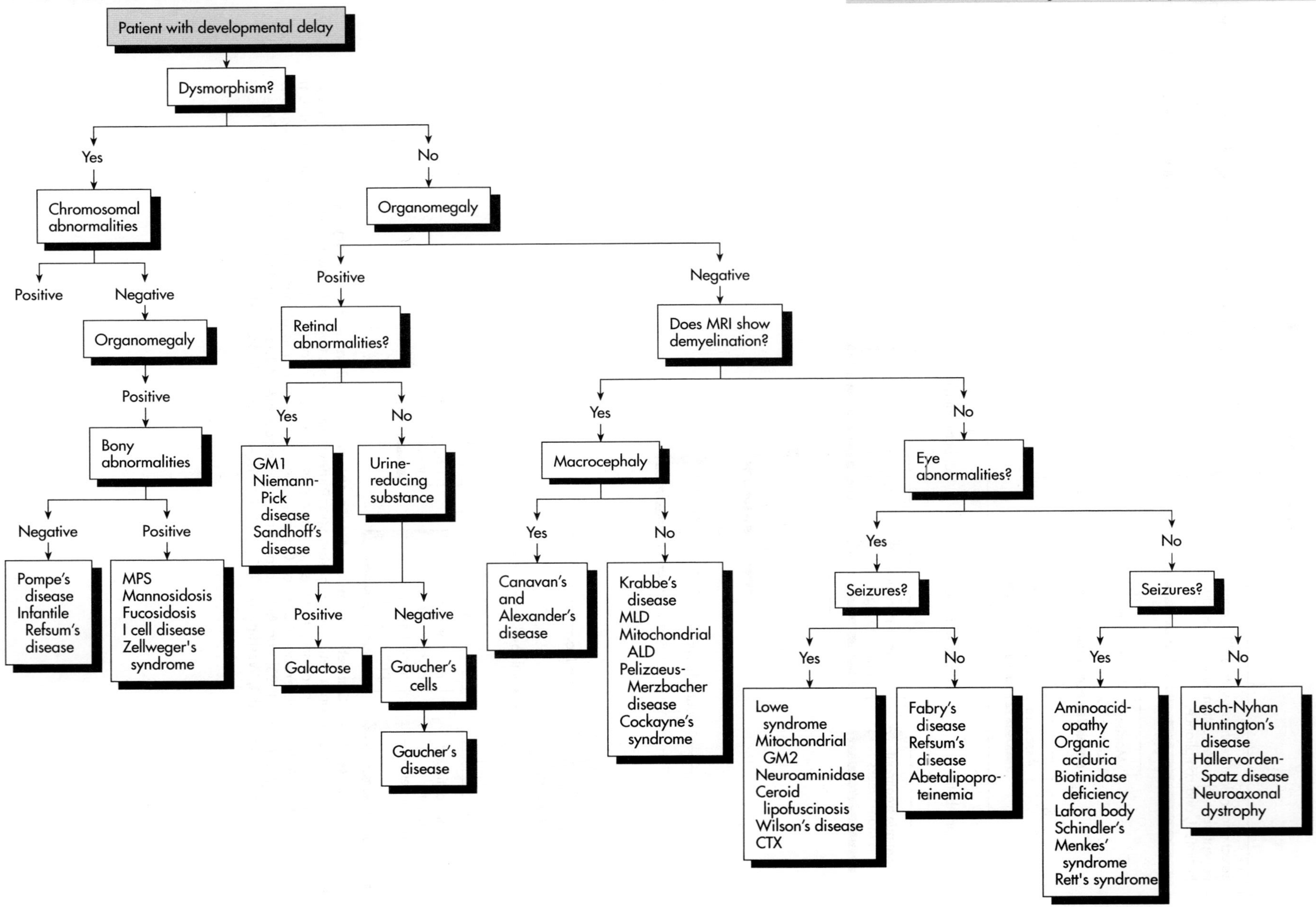

FIGURE 3-83 Workup for developmental delay. *ALD,* Adrenoleukodystrophy; *CTX,* cerebrotendinous xanthomatosis; *MLD,* metachromatic leukodystrophy; *MPS,* mucopolysaccharidosis; *MRI,* magnetic resonance imaging. (From Johnson RT, Griffin JW: *Current therapy in neurologic disease,* ed 5, St Louis, 1997, Mosby.)

ICD-9CM # 253.5

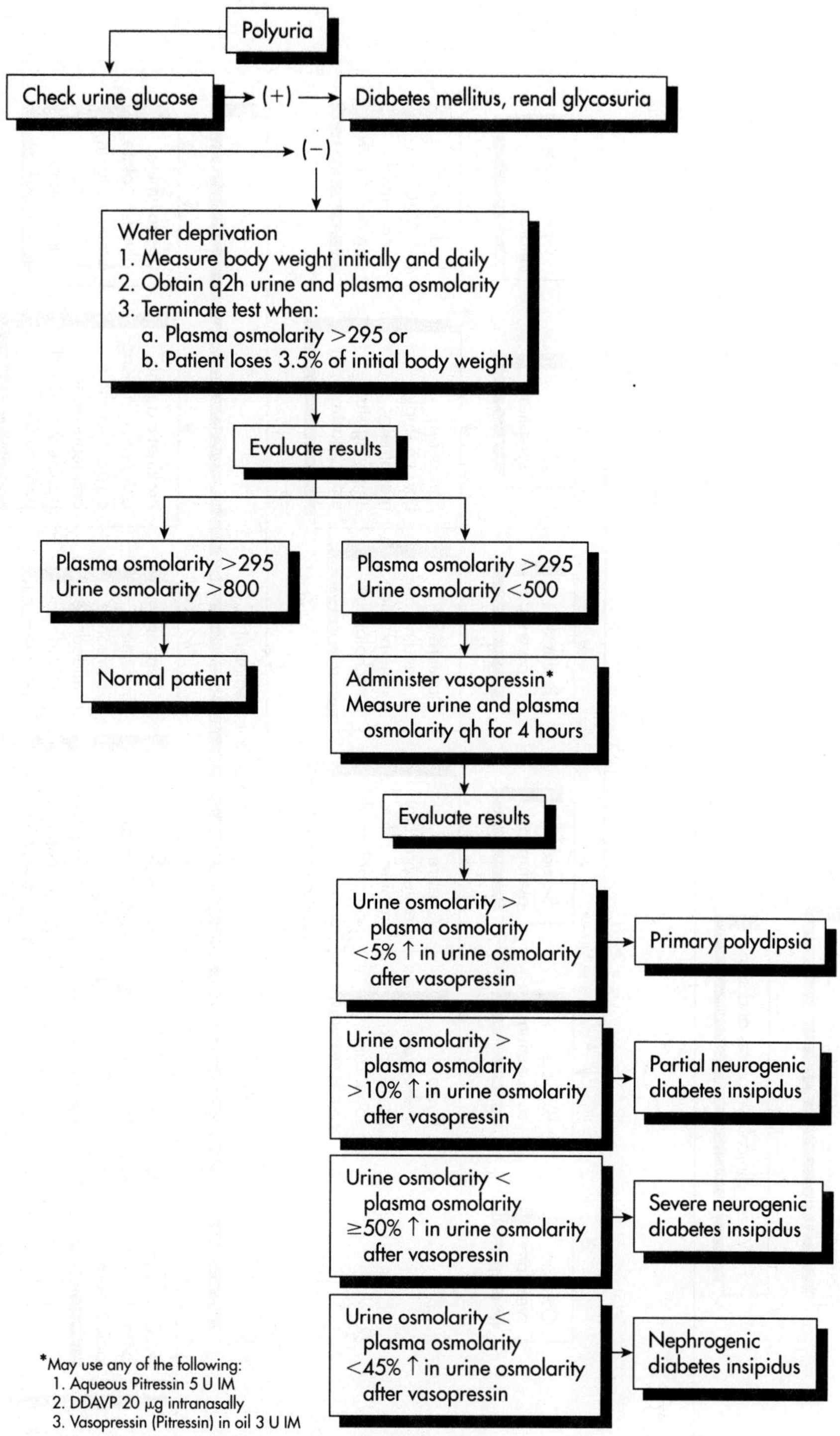

Note: Refer to Section I for additional information on this topic.

FIGURE 3-84 Diagnostic flowchart for diabetes insipidus. (From Ferri F: *Practical guide to the care of the medical patient,* ed 7, St Louis, 2007, Mosby.)

DIABETIC AUTONOMIC NEUROPATHY

ICD-9CM # 250.6

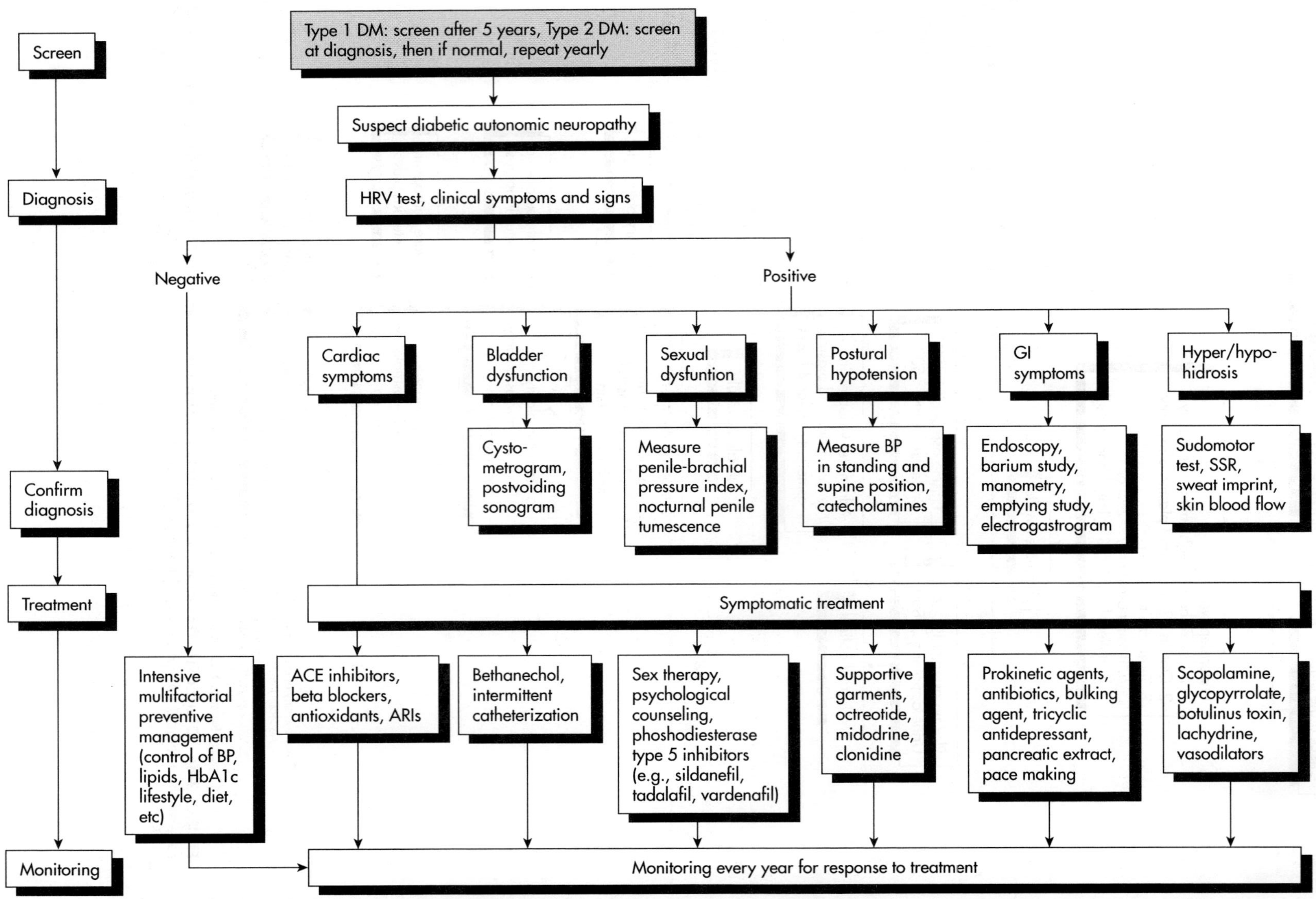

FIGURE 3-85 Diagnosis and treatment algorithm of diabetic autonomic neuropathy. *ACE,* Angiotensin-converting enzyme; *ARI,* aldose reductase inhibitor; *BP,* blood pressure; *DM,* diabetes mellitus; *GI,* gastrointestinal; *HRV,* heart rate variability; *PGE₁,* prostaglandin E₁; *SSR,* sympathetic skin response. (Modified from Larsen PR, Kronenberg HM, Memlmed S, Polansky, KS [eds]: *Williams textbook of endocrinology,* ed 11, Philadelphia, 2008, Saunders.)

DIABETIC KETOACIDOSIS/HYPEROSMOLAR HYPERGLYCEMIC STATE

ICD-9CM # 250.1 Diabetic ketoacidosis
250.2 Hyperosmolar hyperglycemic state

Adult patient with DKA or HHS

Complete initial evaluation, including (but not limited to):
- Medical history and physical examination
- Complete blood count with differential
- Fingerstick blood glucose
- Serum chemistries ("Chem-10" plus serum ketones)
- Urine for urinalysis and ketones
- Cultures as indicated (wound, blood, urine, etc.)
- Chest ± Abdominal x-ray
- 12-lead electrocardiogram

Concurrently, begin empiric fluid resuscitation with 0.9% NaCl at 1000 ml/hr
Consider volume expanders if hypovolemic shock is present
Continue fluid resuscitation until volume status and cardiovascular parameters (pulse, blood pressure) have been restored

IV fluids
Based on corrected serum sodium*
If high/normal, use 0.45% NaCl
If low/normal, use 0.9% NaCl
Continue IV fluids at 250-1000 ml/hr, depending on volume status, cardiovascular history, and cardiovascular status (pulse, BP)

Insulin therapy
Regular insulin bolus, 0.15 U/kg
IV infusion, 0.10 U/kg hr
Check serum glucose hourly—should fall by 50-80 mg/dl/hr.
If serum glucose falling too rapidly, back off on insulin infusion
If serum glucose rising or falling too slowly, increase insulin infusion rate by 50%-100%

When serum glucose reaches 250-300 mg/dl:
Add dextrose to IV fluids. Continue IV fluids at 150-250 ml/hr, and adjust insulin infusion to maintain serum glucose of 200-250 mg/dl until metabolic control is achieved:
For DKA, continue until anion gap has closed and acidosis has resolved
For HHS, continue until plasma osmolality drops below 310 mOsm/kg
Begin more exhaustive search for precipitant of metabolic decompensation

Continuing management:
Follow and replete serum electrolytes (including divalent cations) q2-4h until stable
After resolution of hyperglycemic state, follow blood glucose q4h and initiate sliding scale regular insulin coverage
Convert IV insulin to subcutaneous injections (or resumption of prior therapy), ensuring adequate overlap if treating patients without endogenous insulin secretion
Begin clear liquid diet and advance as tolerated. Encourage resumption of ambulation and activity
Review and update diabetes education, with special attention to prevention of further hyperglycemic crises

Potassium (K^+) repletion
Obtain baseline serum potassium
Obtain 12-lead ECG

$[K^+] \geq 5.5$ mEq/L → Hold K^+ therapy → Treat hyperkalemia if ECG changes present → Recheck $[K^+]$ in 2 hr

$[K^+] < 5.5$ mEq/L and adequate urine output → Add K^+ to IV fluids (Use KCl and/or KPhos)
$[K^+]$ = 4.5-5.4: add 20 mEq/L IVF
$[K^+]$ = 3.5-4.4: add 30 mEq/L IVF
$[K^+] < 3.5$: add 40 mEq/L IVF

Follow serum $[K^+]$ every 2-4 hours until stable: anticipate rapid drop of serum $[K^+]$ during therapy, due to dilution and intracelular shifting
Ensure adequate urine output to avoid over-repletion and hyperkalemia
Continue K^+ repletion until serum $[K^+]$ is stable at between 4-5 mEq/L
If refractory hypokalemia, ensure concurrent magnesium repletion
Repletion may need to be continued for several days, as total body losses may reach up to 500 mEq

Bicarbonate therapy
Obtain ABG
Obtain baseline serum bicarbonate

$pH < 6.9$ → 88 mEq/L (2 amps) $NaHCO_3$ over 2 hr
$6.9 \leq pH < 7.0$ → 44 mEq/L (1 amp) $NaHCO_3$ over 1 hr
$pH \geq 7.0$ → Assess need for bicarbonate

Repeat ABG after bicarbonate administration
Repeat $NaHCO_3$ therapy until $pH \geq 7.0$, then discontinue therapy
Follow serum bicarbonate q4h until stable

*Sodium correction: Serum sodium should be corrected for hyperglycemia. For every 100 mg/dl of glucose elevation above 100 mg/dl, add 1.6 mEq/L to the measured sodium value; this will yield the correction serum sodium concentration.

Note: Refer to Section I for additional information on these topics.

FIGURE 3-86 Management of diabetic ketoacidosis (DKA) and hyperosmolar hyperglycemic state (HHS). *ABG*, Arterial blood gas; *DKA*, diabetic ketoacidosis; *ECG*, electrocardiograph; *HHS*, hyperosmolar hyperglycemic state. (From Goldman L, Ausiello D [eds]: *Cecil textbook of medicine*, ed 23, Philadelphia, 2008, WB Saunders.)

ICD-9CM # 787.91

1. Physical examination

Hydrate as necessary

2. Stool examination

Inflammatory cells

Present: suggests mucosal disease
a. IBD
b. Invasive bacterial infections (such as *Shigella* spp., *Salmonella* spp., amebiasis, *Campylobacter*)

Absent: suggests viral gastroenteritis, toxin (*Staphylococcus, Escherichia coli, Aeromonas*, or *Plesiomonas* spp.), or drug-related diarrhea or IBS

Ova and parasites

Blood: if present, consider:

a. IBD
b. Bacterial infections:
Salmonella spp.
Shigella spp.
Amebiasis
Campylobacter
Clostridium difficile toxin
E. coli O157:H7

3. Culture stool

Positive culture result

Treat appropriately, except for *Salmonella* infections in which treatment may prolong the carrier state

Negative culture result

See step 5 in Fig. 3-87

4. Flexible sigmoidoscopy

Abnormal mucosa

a. Pseudomembranes: check for *C. difficile* toxin: treat with metronidazole or vancomycin
b. Ulcerations/granularity
(1) Proctitis only: culture for *Chlamydia trachomatis, Neisseria gonorrhoeae;* Gram stain and culture urethra and pharynx; biopsy as in (2)
(2) More extensive: culture; biopsy to look for amebae, granulomas, or nonspecific finding of IBD

Normal mucosa

Wait for culture results

5. Negative stool culture result

Inflammatory cells in stool

IBD likely

a. Severely ill: rule out toxic megacolon; analyze blood cultures; abdominal x-ray; treat as IBD
b. Not severely ill: barium studies or colonoscopy after careful and gentle preparation

No inflammatory cells in stool

a. If history is appropriate, with travel to endemic areas, or if patient has hypogammaglobulinemia, evaluate duodenal aspirate for *Giardia*
b. Stop all drugs, stop milk products, rule out malabsorption, observe, and treat symptomatically; if symptoms persist or recur, perform barium studies or colonoscopy

FIGURE 3-87 Diagnostic steps in the assessment of acute diarrhea. *IBD,* Inflammatory bowel disease; *IBS,* irritable bowel syndrome. (Modified from Stein JH [ed]: *Internal medicine,* ed 5, St Louis, 1998, Mosby.)

ICD-9CM # 787.91

1. Diagnostic steps 1 to 4 as in Fig. 3-87

a. Results diagnostic for infectious diarrhea (uncommon in chronic diarrhea except for *Clostridium difficile* after antibiotics), inflammatory bowel disease, or overt drug-induced diarrhea
b. Results nondiagnostic; usually without inflammatory cells in stool

2. Stool volume

a. Small volume: usually seen in infectious diarrhea or inflammatory bowel disease (consider colonoscopy), but can also be seen in malabsorption syndromes and irritable bowel syndrome
b. Large volume: suggests malabsorption syndromes, secretory diarrhea, or laxative abuse

3. Stool Sudan stain

Positive

Suggests malabsorption syndrome, pancreatic insufficiency, bile salt insufficiency, or mucosal disease

Negative

See step 4

4. Oral intake stopped

Diarrhea continues

a. Secretory diarrhea: stool osmolality = stool $(Na^+ + K^+) \times 2$
b. Nasogastric suction
   (1) Diarrhea stops
      (a) Zollinger-Ellison syndrome: gastric analysis, gastrin, secretin stimulation
      (b) Laxative abuse: see step 5
   (2) Diarrhea continues
      (a) Secretory diarrhea: plasma VIP, calcitonin, urinary 5-HIAA abdominal ultrasound, computed tomography and/or selective mesenteric angiogram to identify tumor
      (b) Laxative abuse: see step 5

Diarrhea stops

a. Malabsorption syndromes: stool osmolality > plasma osmolality
b. Laxative ingestion: see step 5
c. Congenital chloridorrhea
   (1) Stool electrolytes: chloride concentration greater than the sum of sodium and potassium concentrations in stool water
   (2) No fecal osmotic gap

5. Laxative abuse detection

a. Screening tests
   (1) Detailed history
   (2) Colonoscopy and biopsy for melanosis coli
   (3) Barium enema: dilated, hypomotile "cathartic colon"
b. Specific tests (if available)
   (1) Urine screening test for senna
   (2) Chromatographic test for bisacodyl
   (3) Stool test for fecal sulfate and phosphate
   (4) Magnesium concentration in fecal water (atomic absorption spectrophotometry)

6. Radiologic studies

Perform barium studies only after stool examination, culture, and studies requiring quantitative measurements of the stool have been completed.

FIGURE 3-88 Diagnostic approach to the patient with chronic diarrhea (patients who are HIV negative). *5-HIAA,* 5-Hydroxyindoleacetic acid; *VIP,* vasoactive intestinal polypeptide. (Modified from Stein JH [ed]: *Internal medicine,* ed 5, St Louis, 1998, Mosby.)

DIARRHEA, CHRONIC, IN PATIENTS WITH HIV INFECTION

ICD-9CM # 787.1 Diarrhea, chronic

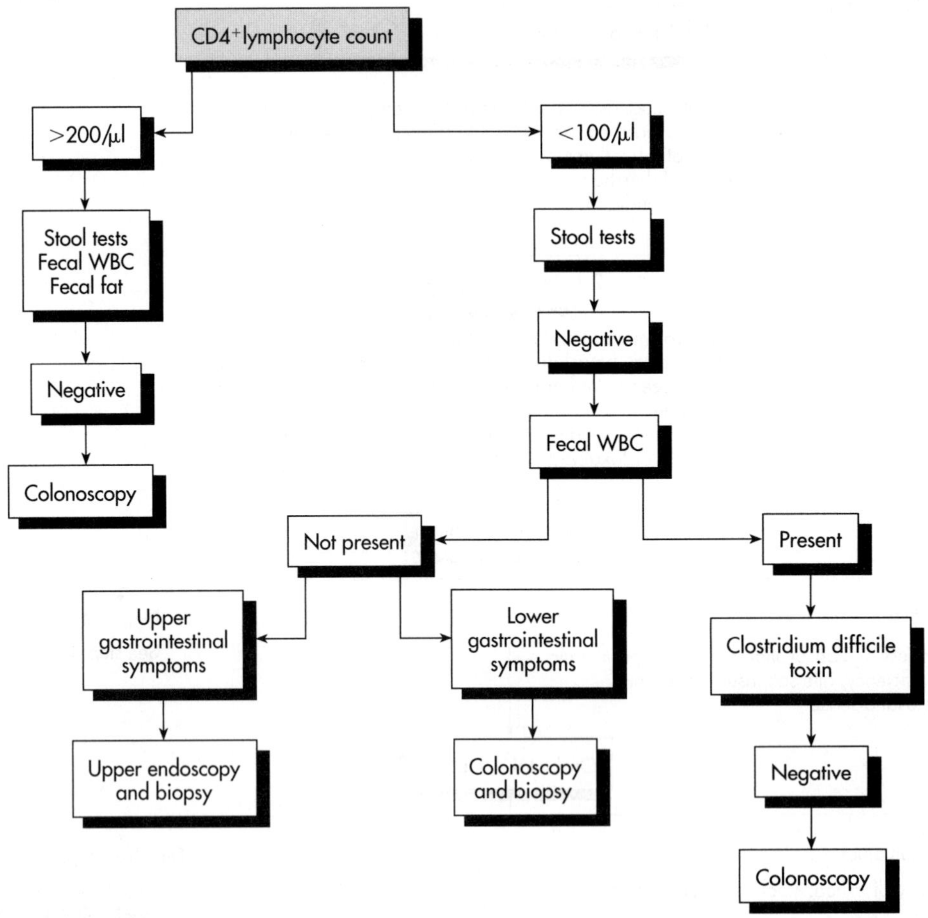

FIGURE 3-89 Approach to evaluating chronic diarrhea in patients with HIV infection. *WBC,* White blood cell count. (Modified from Wilcox CM: *Gastrointest Dis Today* 5:9, 1996.)

TABLE 3-8 Common Gastrointestinal Pathogens Associated with HIV Infection

Pathogen	CD4+ Cells/μl	Stool Volume and Frequency	Abdominal Pain	Weight Loss	Fever	Fecal Leukocytes
Cytomegalovirus*	<100	Mild to moderate	++	++	++	+
Cryptosporidiosis	<100	Moderate to severe	−	++	−	−
Microsporidiosis	<100	Mild to moderate	−	+	−	−
Mycobacterium avium complex†	<100	Mild to moderate	+	+++	+++	−

From Wilcox CM: *Gastrointest Dis Today* 5:9, 1996.
*Can have proctitis symptoms when involving the distal colon.
†Typical presentation is fever and wasting; diarrhea is usually secondary.
+++, Very common; ++, frequent; +, can occur; −, absent.

DILATED PUPIL

ICD-9CM # 379.43 Pupil dilation

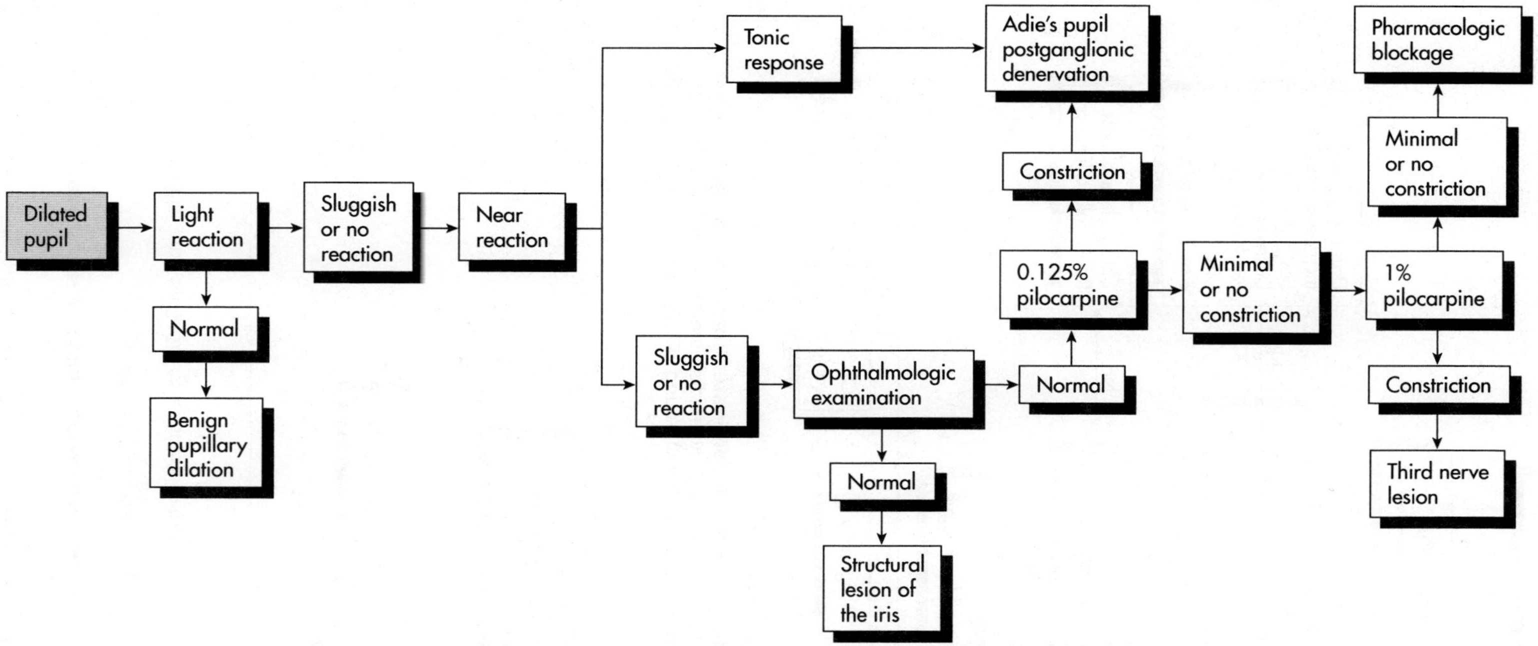

FIGURE 3-90 Use of pilocarpine to help differentiate between different causes of a dilated pupil. (From Goldman L, Ausiello D [eds]: *Cecil textbook of medicine,* ed 23, Philadephia, 2008, WB Saunders.)

ICD-9CM # 286.6

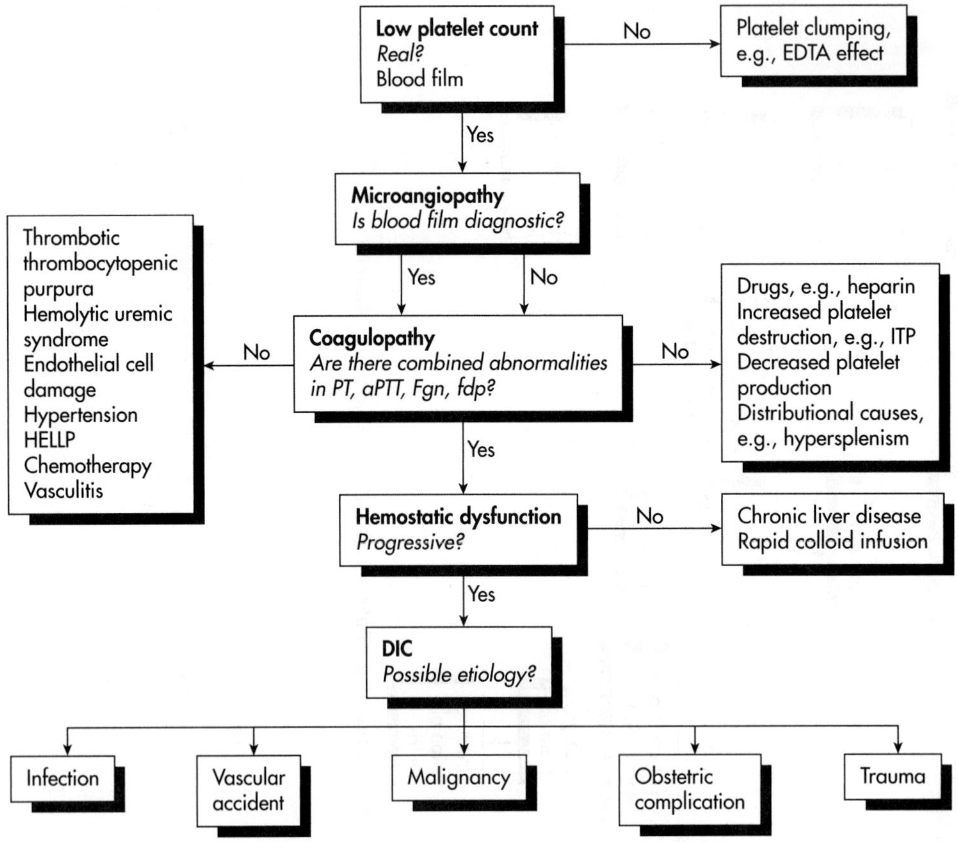

Note: Refer to Section I for additional information on this topic.

FIGURE 3-91 Differential diagnostic algorithm for disseminated intravascular coagulation (DIC). *aPTT,* Activated partial thromboplastin time; *EDTA,* ethylenediaminetetraacetic acid; *ITP,* idiopathic thrombocytopenic purpura; *PT,* prothrombin time. (From Young NS, Gerson SL, High KA [eds]: *Clinical hematology,* St Louis, 2006, Mosby.)

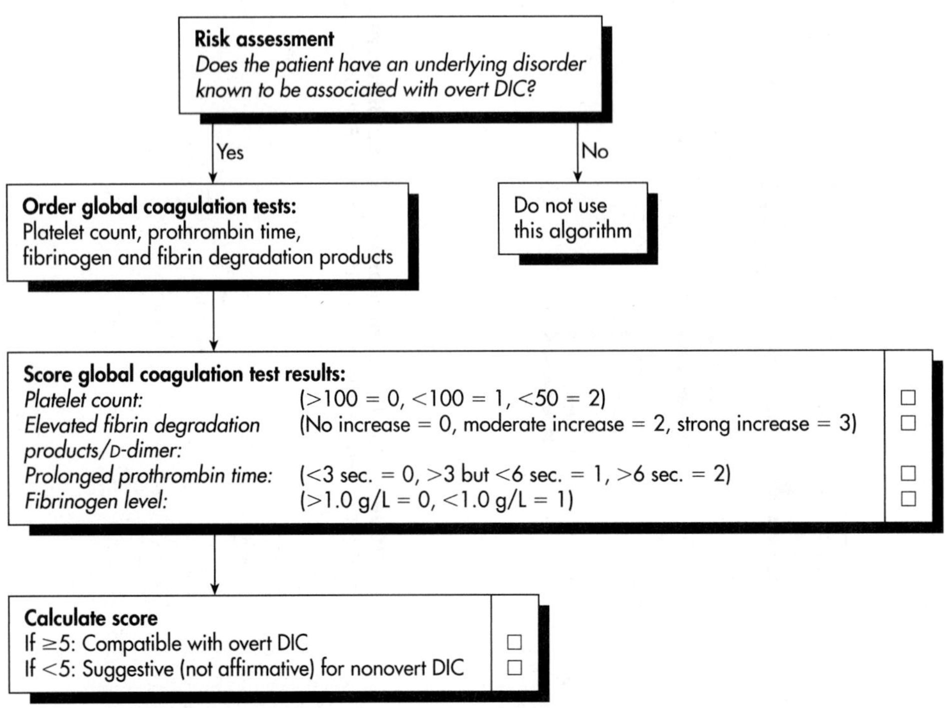

Note: Refer to Section I for additional information on this topic.

FIGURE 3-92 Laboratory testing and diagnosis of overt disseminated intravascular coagulation (DIC). (From Young NS, Gerson SL, High KA [eds]: *Clinical hematology,* St Louis, 2006, Mosby.)

ICD-9CM # 563.3 Dyspepsia atonic
536.8 Dyspepsia disorders other unspecified function of stomach
306.4 Dyspepsia, psychogenic

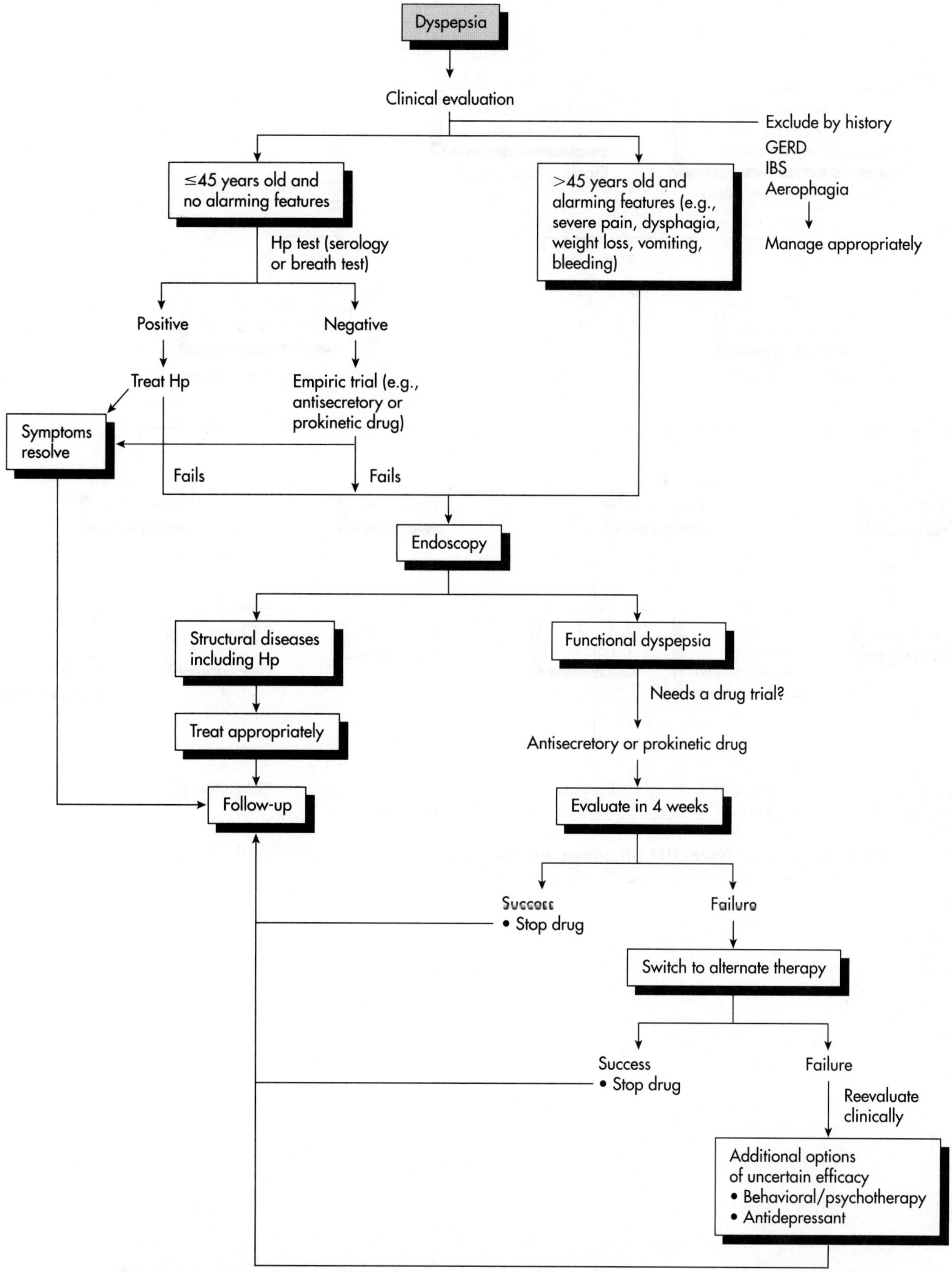

FIGURE 3-93 Algorithm for the evaluation of dyspepsia. *GERD,* Symptomatic gastroesophageal reflux disease; *Hp, Helicobacter pylori; IBS,* irritable bowel syndrome. (From Goldman L, Ausiello D [eds]: *Cecil textbook of medicine,* ed 23, Philadelphia, 2008, WB Saunders.)

ICD-9CM # 787.2

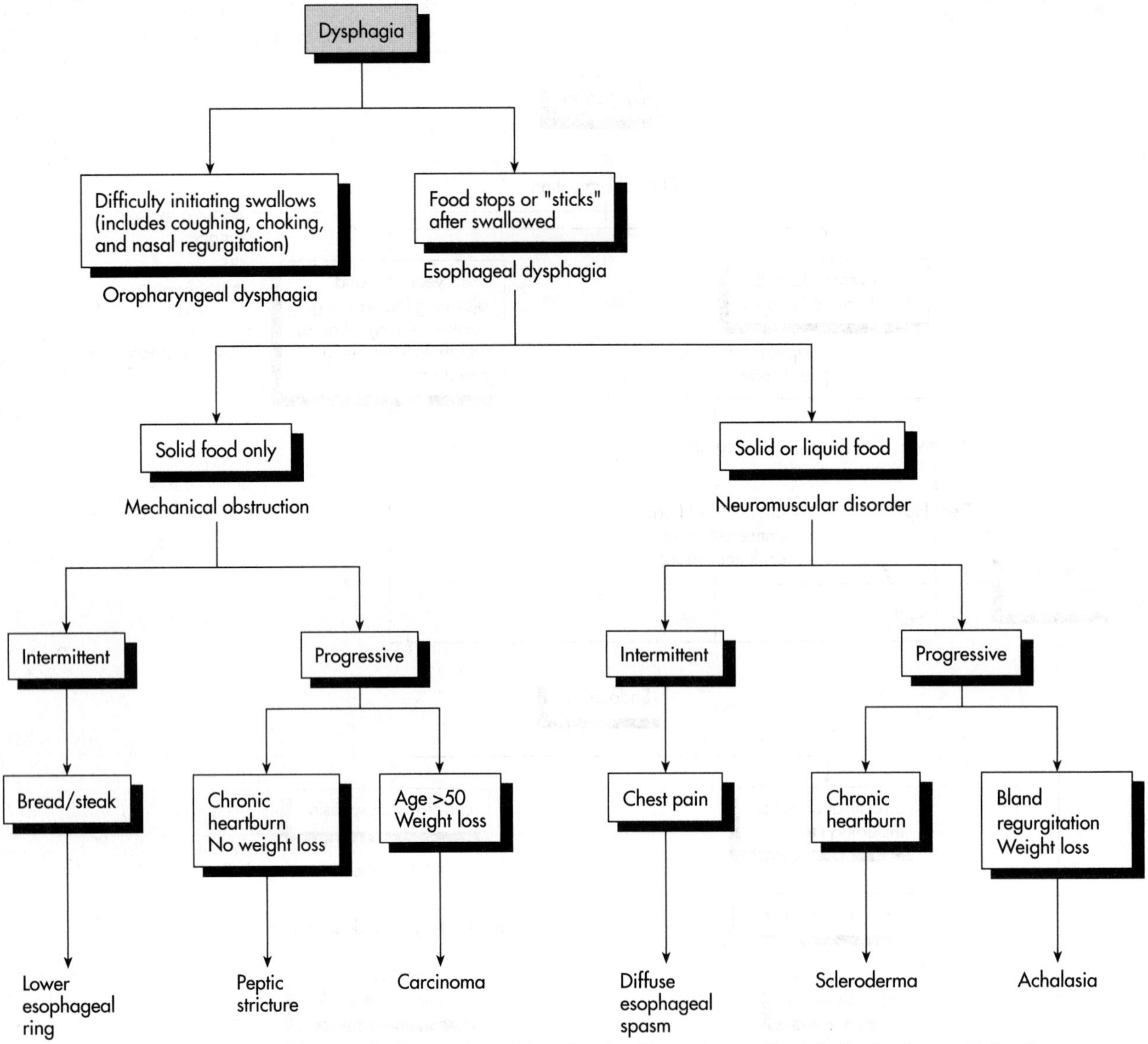

FIGURE 3-94 Differential diagnosis of dysphagia. (From Andreoli TE [ed]: *Cecil essentials of medicine,* ed 7, Philadelphia, 2008, WB Saunders.)

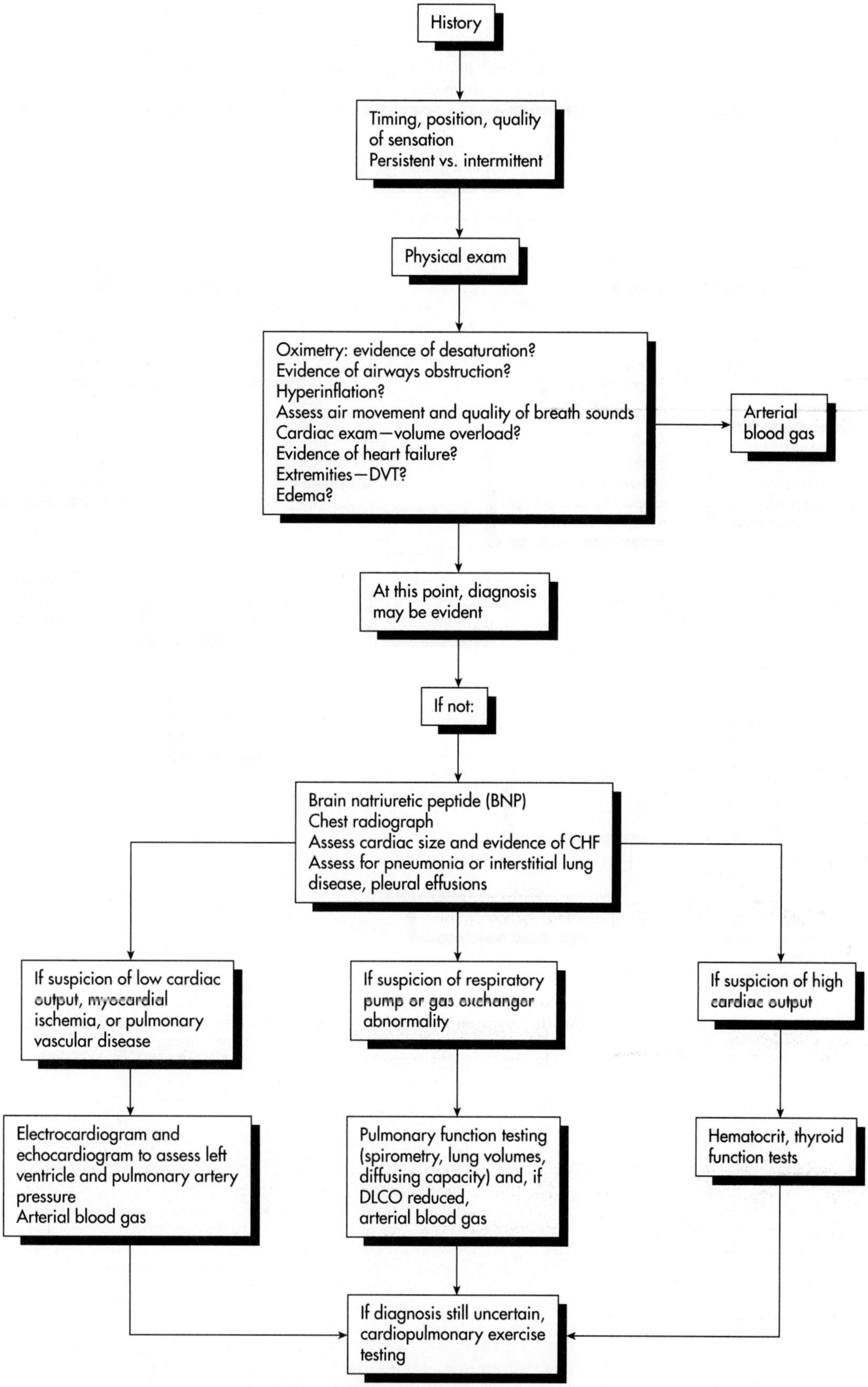

FIGURE 3-95 Algorithm for the evaluation of the patient with dyspnea. The pace and completeness with which one approaches this framework depends on the intensity and acuity of the patient's symptoms. In a patient with severe, acute dyspnea, for example, an arterial blood gas measurement may be one of the first laboratory evaluations, whereas this measurement might not be obtained until much later in the workup in a patient with chronic breathlessness of unclear cause. A therapeutic trial of a medication, for example, a bronchodilator, may be instituted at any point if one is fairly confident of the diagnosis based on the data available at that time. *CHF,* Congestive heart failure; *DLCO,* diffusing capacity of the lung for carbon monoxide; *DVT,* deep venous thrombosis. (From Schwartzstein RM, Feller-Kopman D: Approach to the patient with dyspnea. In Braunwald E, Goldman L [eds]: *Primary cardiology,* ed 2, Philadelphia, 2003, WB Saunders.)

ICD-9CM # 788.1 Dysuria
788.7 Urethral discharge
623.5 Vaginal discharge

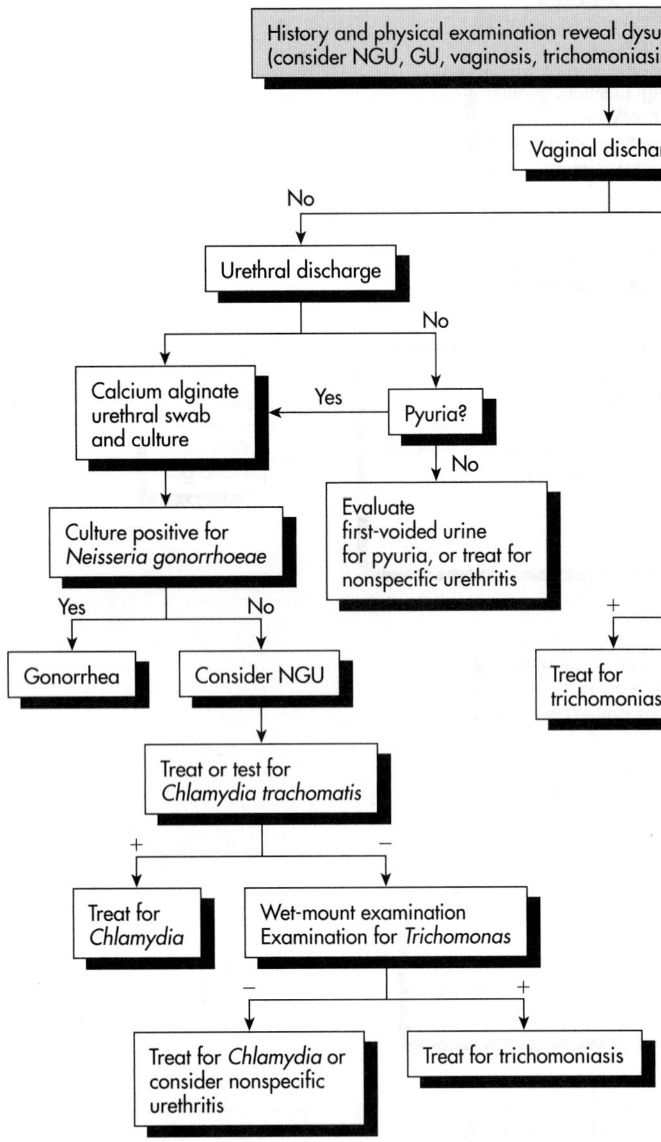

FIGURE 3-96 Evaluation of patients with dysuria and/or urethral/vaginal discharge. *GU,* Gonococcal urethritis; *KOH,* potassium hydroxide; *NGU,* nongonococcal urethritis. (Modified from Nseyo UO [ed]: *Urology for primary care physicians,* Philadelphia, 1999, WB Saunders.)

ICD-9CM # 633.01

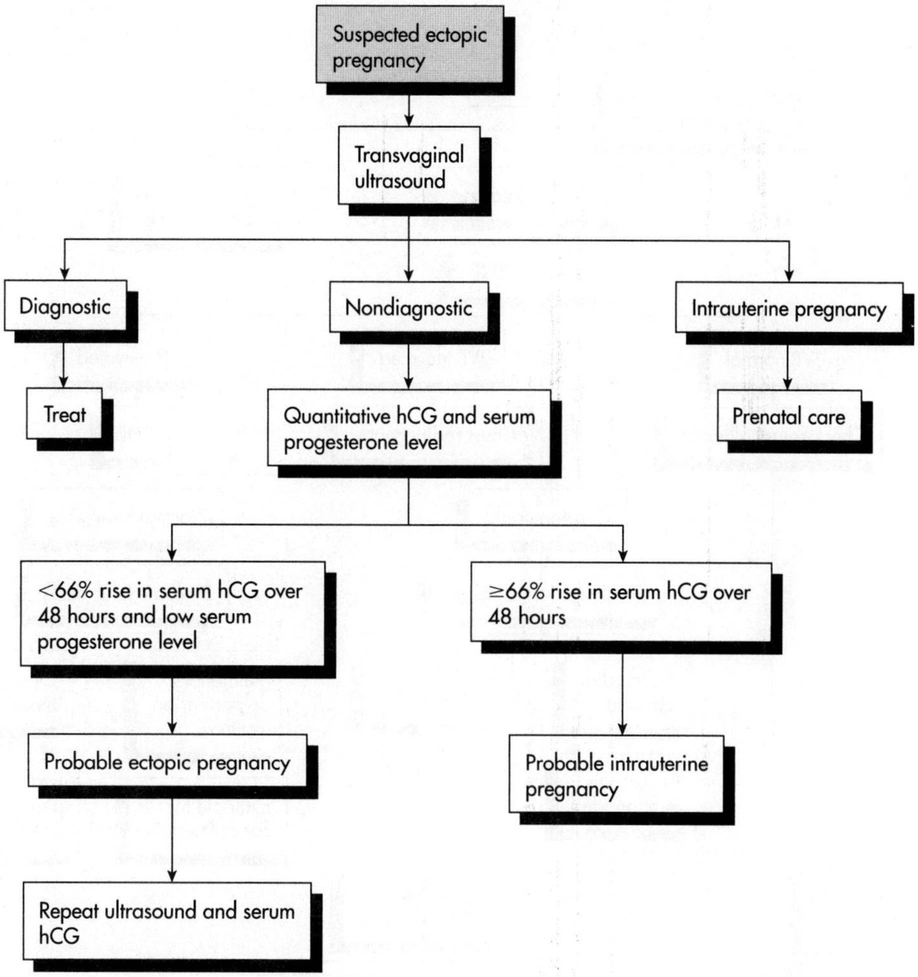

FIGURE 3-97 Ectopic pregnancy. *hCG,* Human chorionic gonadotropin.

ICD-9CM # 782.3 Edema NOS
782.3 Edema, lower extremities

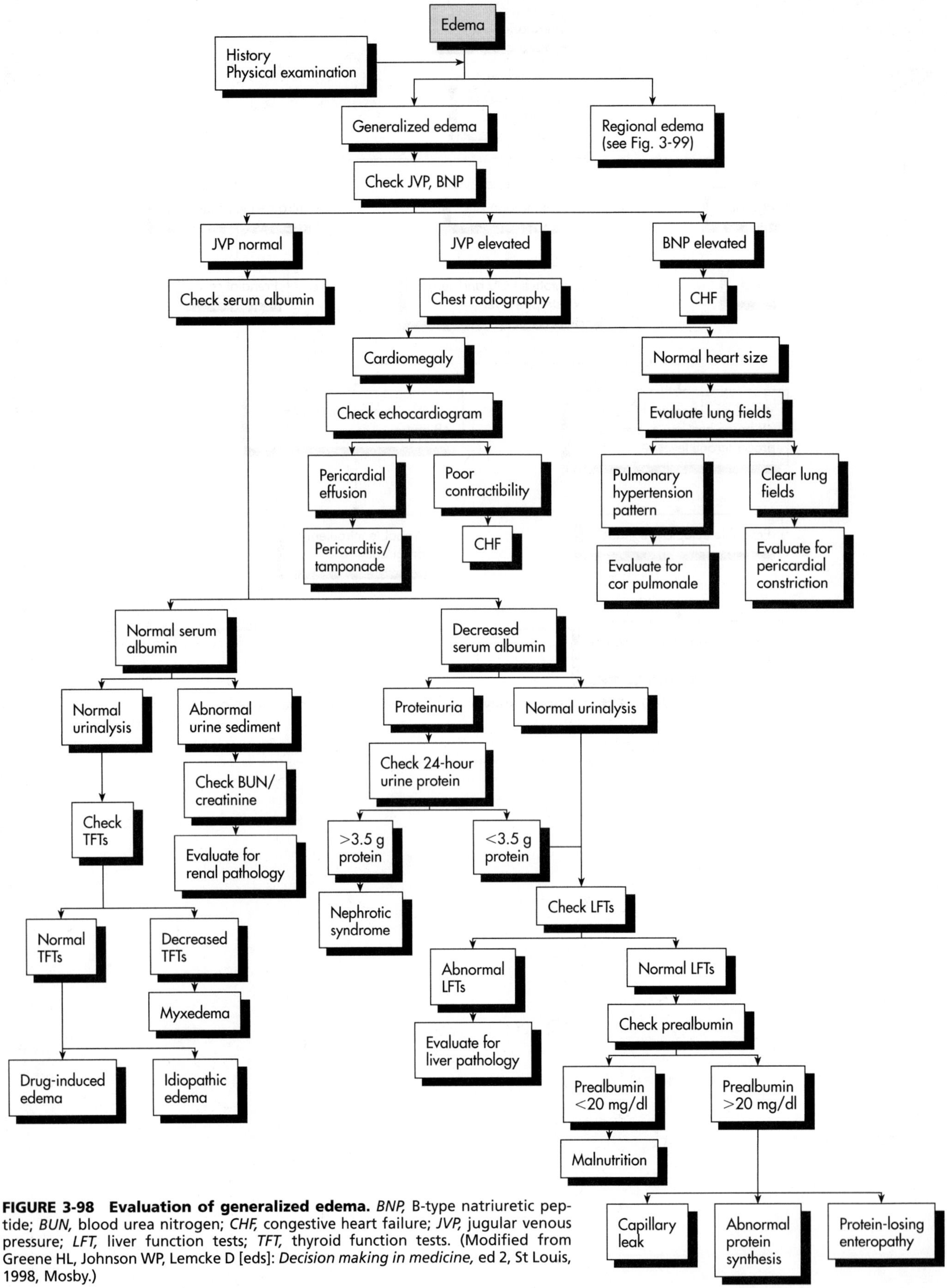

FIGURE 3-98 Evaluation of generalized edema. *BNP,* B-type natriuretic peptide; *BUN,* blood urea nitrogen; *CHF,* congestive heart failure; *JVP,* jugular venous pressure; *LFT,* liver function tests; *TFT,* thyroid function tests. (Modified from Greene HL, Johnson WP, Lemcke D [eds]: *Decision making in medicine,* ed 2, St Louis, 1998, Mosby.)

EDEMA, REGIONAL

ICD-9CM # 250.6

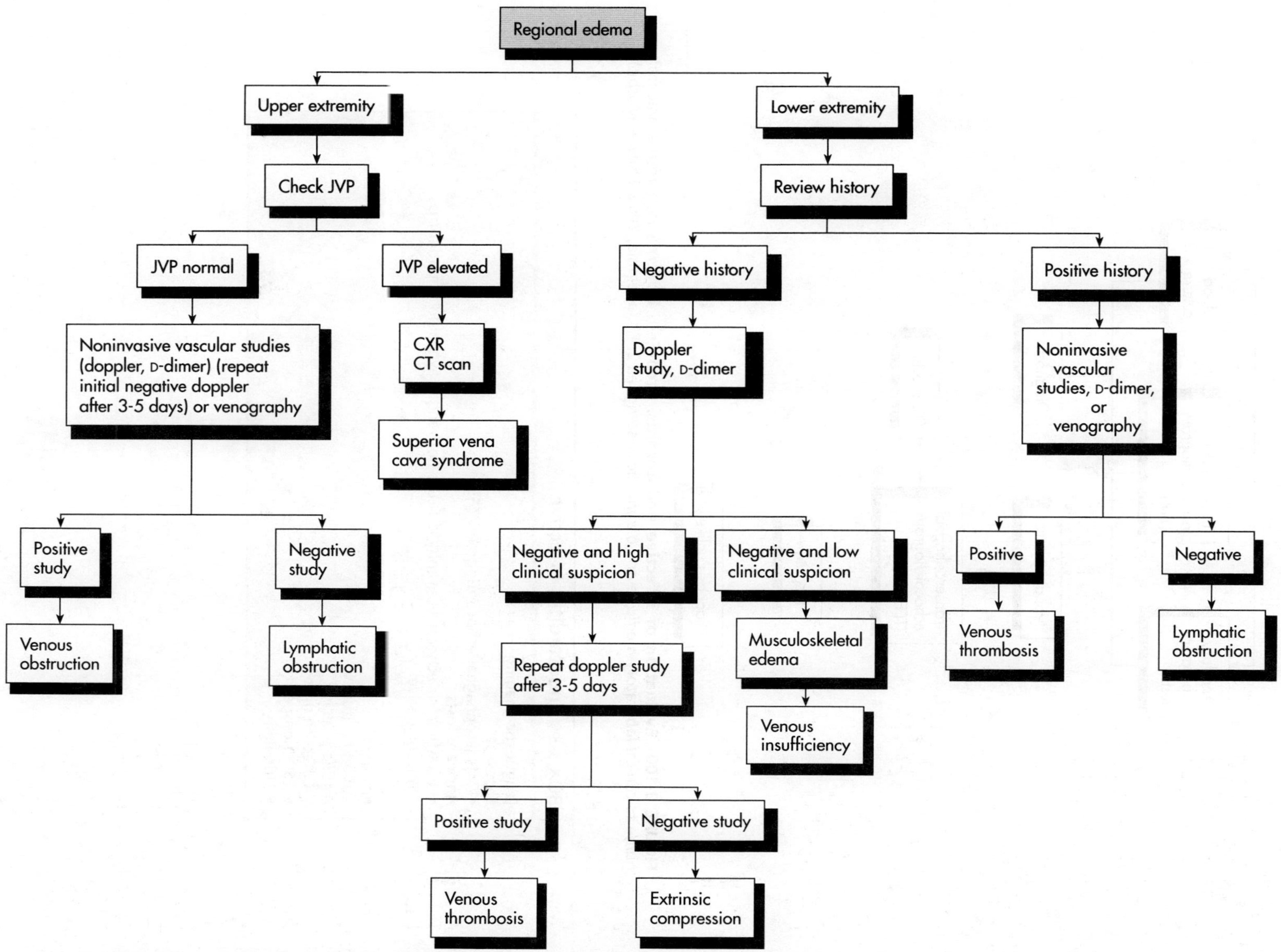

FIGURE 3-99 Evaluation of regional edema. *CT,* Computed tomography; *CXR,* chest x-ray examination; *JVP,* jugular venous pressure. (Modified from Greene HL, Johnson WP, Lemcke D [eds]: *Decision making in medicine,* ed 2, St Louis, 1998, Mosby.)

ICD-9CM # 421.0 Infective endocarditis
996.61 Prosthetic valve endocarditis

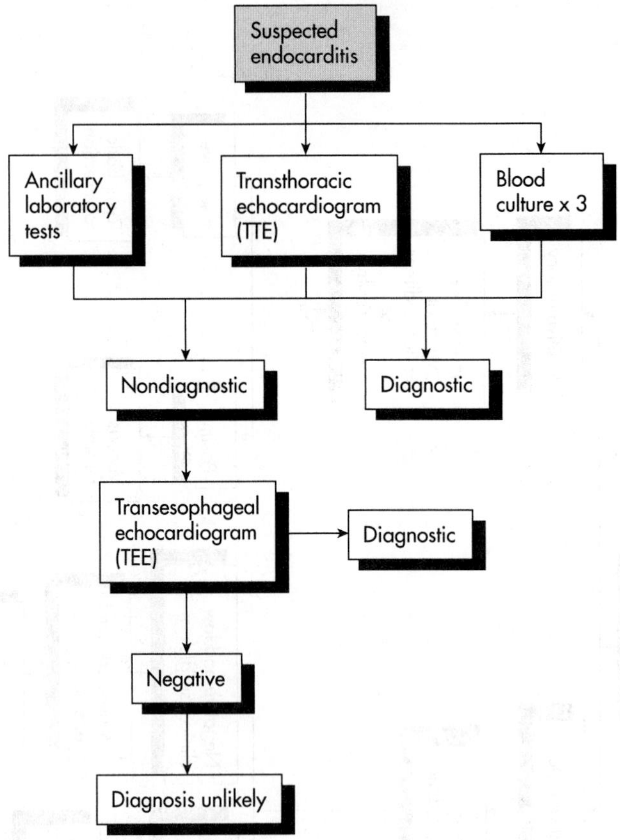

FIGURE 3-100 Evaluation of infective endocarditis. (From Ferri FF: *Ferri's best test: a practical guide to clinical laboratory medicine and diagnostic imaging,* ed 2, Philadelphia, 2009, Elsevier Mosby.)

BOX 3-3 **Endocarditis, Infective**

Diagnostic imaging
Best test
- Transesophageal echocardiogram (TEE)

Ancillary tests
- Transthoracic echocardiography if TEE is not readily available or patient is uncooperative

Lab evaluation
Best test
- Blood culture × 3

Ancillary tests
- CBC with differential
- ESR (nonspecific)
- Urinalysis

ICD-9CM # 788.30

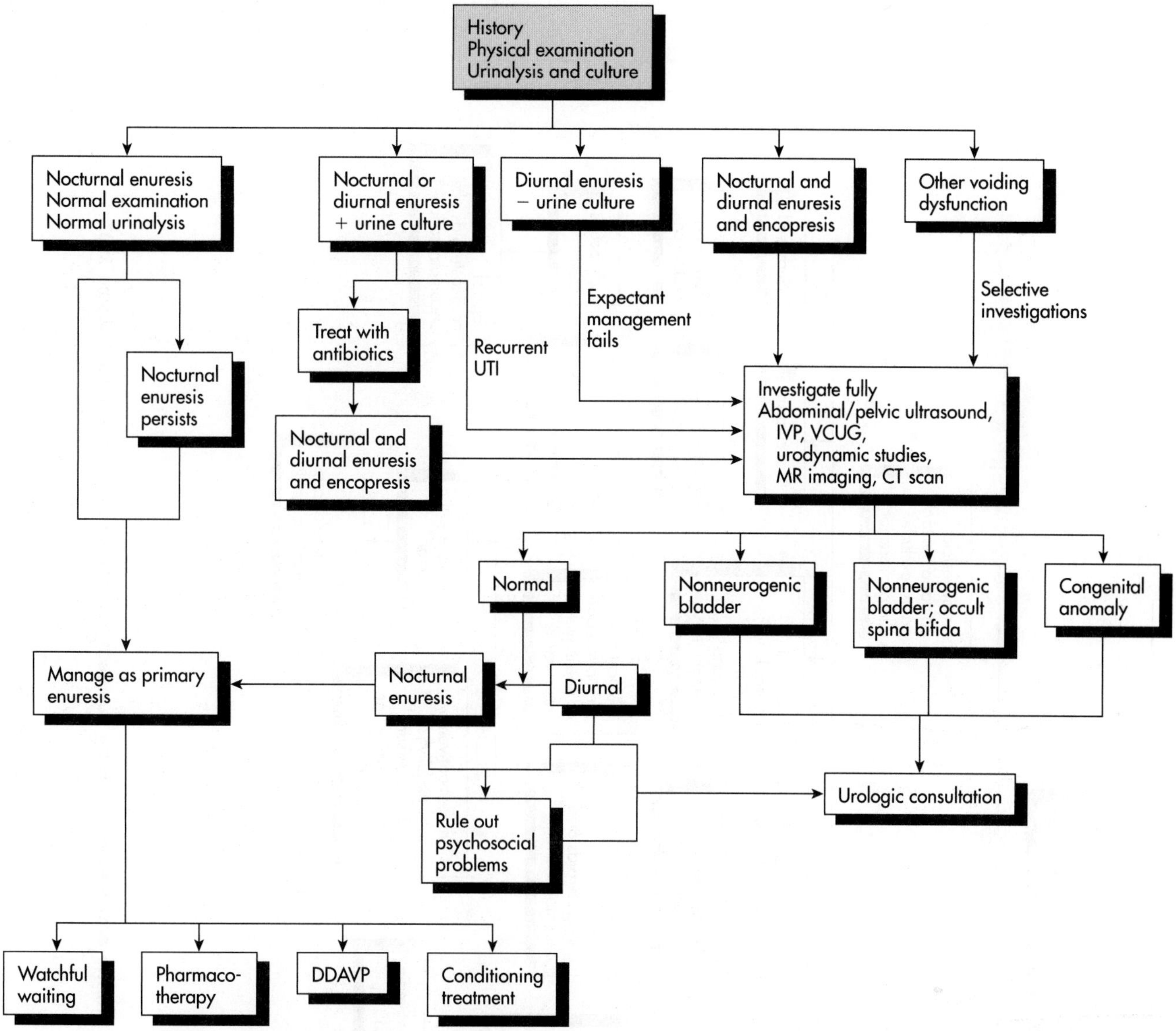

FIGURE 3-101 Algorithm of management of pediatric enuresis and voiding dysfunction. *CT,* Computed tomography; *DDAVP,* desmopressin acetate; *IVP,* intravenous pyelogram; *MR,* magnetic resonance; *UTI,* urinary tract infection; *VCUG,* voiding cystourethrogram. (From Nseyo UO [ed]: *Urology for primary care physicians,* Philadelphia, 1999, WB Saunders.)

ENVENOMATION, MARINE

ICD-9CM # 989.5

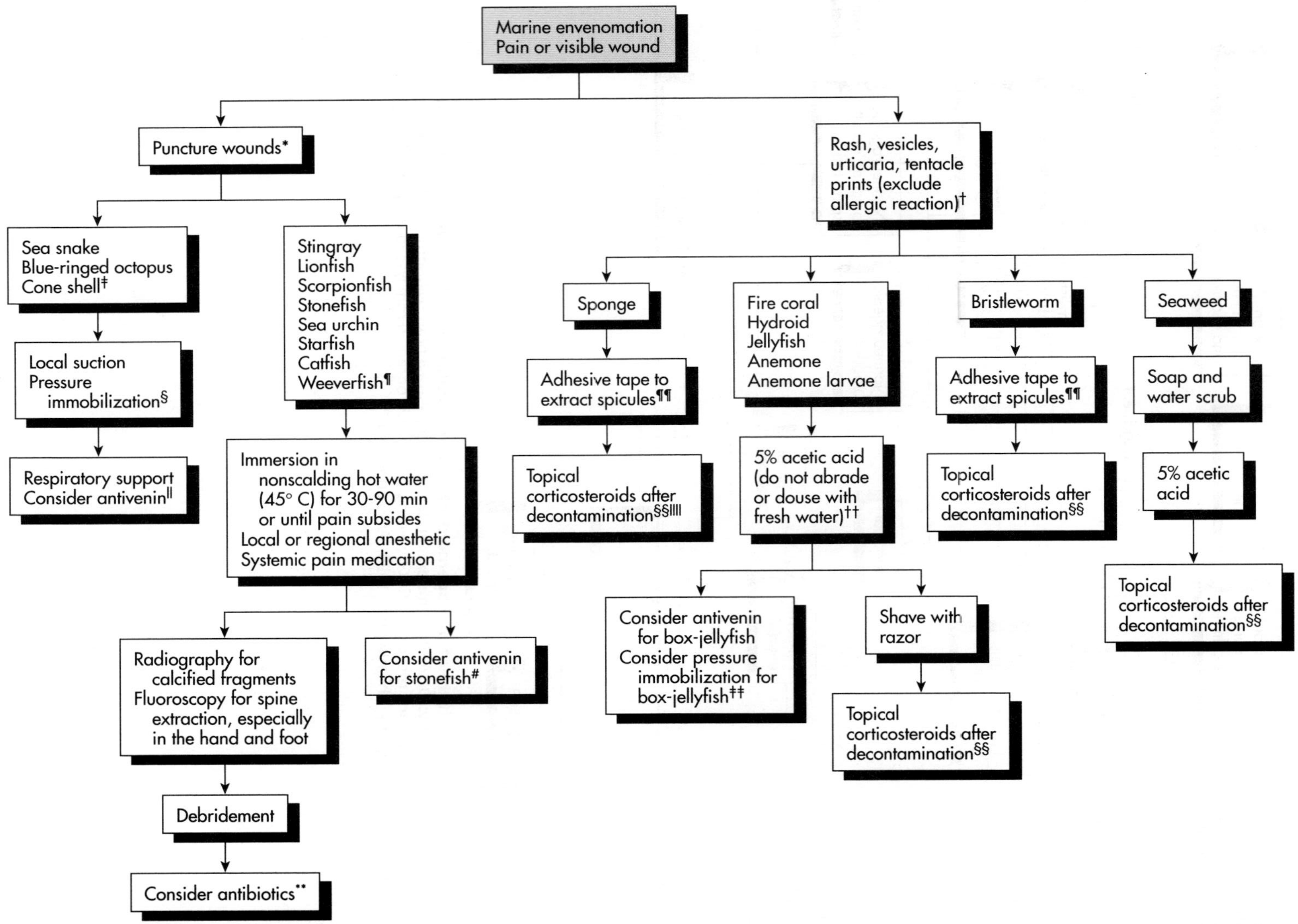

FIGURE 3-102 Algorithmic approach to marine envenomation. (From Auerbach PS: *Wilderness medicine*, ed 5, St Louis, 2007, Mosby.)

FIGURE 3-102 (Continued)

*A gaping laceration, particularly of the lower extremity, with cyanotic edges suggests a stingray wound. Multiple punctures in an erratic pattern with or without purple discoloration or retained fragments are typical of a sea urchin sting. One to eight (usually two) fang marks are usually present after a sea snake bite. A single ischemic puncture wound with an erythematous halo and rapid swelling suggests scorpionfish envenomation. Blisters often accompany a lionfish sting. Painless punctures with paralysis suggest the bite of a blue-ringed octopus; the site of a cone shell sting is punctate, painful, and ischemic in appearance.

†Wheal and flare reactions are nonspecific. Rapid (within 24 hours) onset of skin necrosis suggests an anemone sting. "Tentacle prints" with cross-hatching or a frosted appearance are pathognomonic for box-jellyfish (*Chironex fleckeri*) envenomation. Ocular or intraoral lesions may be caused by fragmented hydroids or coelenterate tentacles. An allergic reaction must be treated promptly.

‡Sea snake venom causes weakness, respiratory paralysis, myoglobinuria, myalgias, blurred vision, vomiting, and dysphagia. The blue-ringed octopus injects tetrodotoxin, which causes rapid neuromuscular paralysis.

§If *immediately* available (which is rarely the case), local suction can be applied without incision using a plunger device, such as The Extractor (Sawyer Products, Safety Harbor, Fla.). As soon as possible, venom should be sequestered locally with a proximal venous-lymphatic occlusive band of constriction or (preferably) the pressure immobilization technique, in which a cloth pad is compressed directly over the wound by an elastic wrap that should encompass the entire extremity at a pressure of 9.33 kPa (70 mm Hg) or less. Incision and suction are not recommended.

||Early ventilatory support has the greatest influence on outcome. The minimal initial dose of sea snake antivenin is 1 to 3 vials; up to 10 vials may be required.

¶The wounds range from large lacerations (stingrays) to minute punctures (stonefish). Persistent pain after immersion in hot water suggests a stonefish sting or a retained fragment of spine. The puncture site can be identified by forcefully injecting 1% to 2% lidocaine or another local anesthetic agent without epinephrine near the wound and observing the egress of fluid. Do not attempt to crush the spines of sea urchins if they are present in the wound. Spine dye from already-extracted sea urchin spines will disappear (be absorbed) in 24 to 36 hours.

#The initial dose of stonefish antivenin is one vial per two puncture wounds.

**The antibiotics chosen should cover *Staphylococcus*, *Streptococcus*, and microbes of marine origin, such as *Vibrio.*

††Acetic acid 5% (vinegar) is a good all-purpose decontaminant and is mandated for the sting from a box-jellyfish. Alternatives, depending on the geographic region and indigenous jellyfish species, include isopropyl alcohol, bicarbonate (baking soda), ammonia, papain, and preparations containing these agents.

‡‡The initial dose of box-jellyfish antivenin is one ampule intravenously or three ampules intramuscularly.

§§If inflammation is severe, steroids should be given systematically (beginning with at least 60 to 100 mg of prednisone or its equivalent) and the dose tapered over a period of 10 to 14 days.

||||An alternative is to apply and remove commercial facial peel materials.

¶¶An alternative is to apply and remove commercial facial peel materials followed by topical soaks of 30 ml of 5% acetic acid (vinegar) diluted in 1 L of water for 15 to 30 minutes several times a day until the lesions begin to resolve. Anticipate surface desquamation in 3 to 6 weeks.

EOSINOPHILIC DERMATOSES

ICD-9CM # 691.8

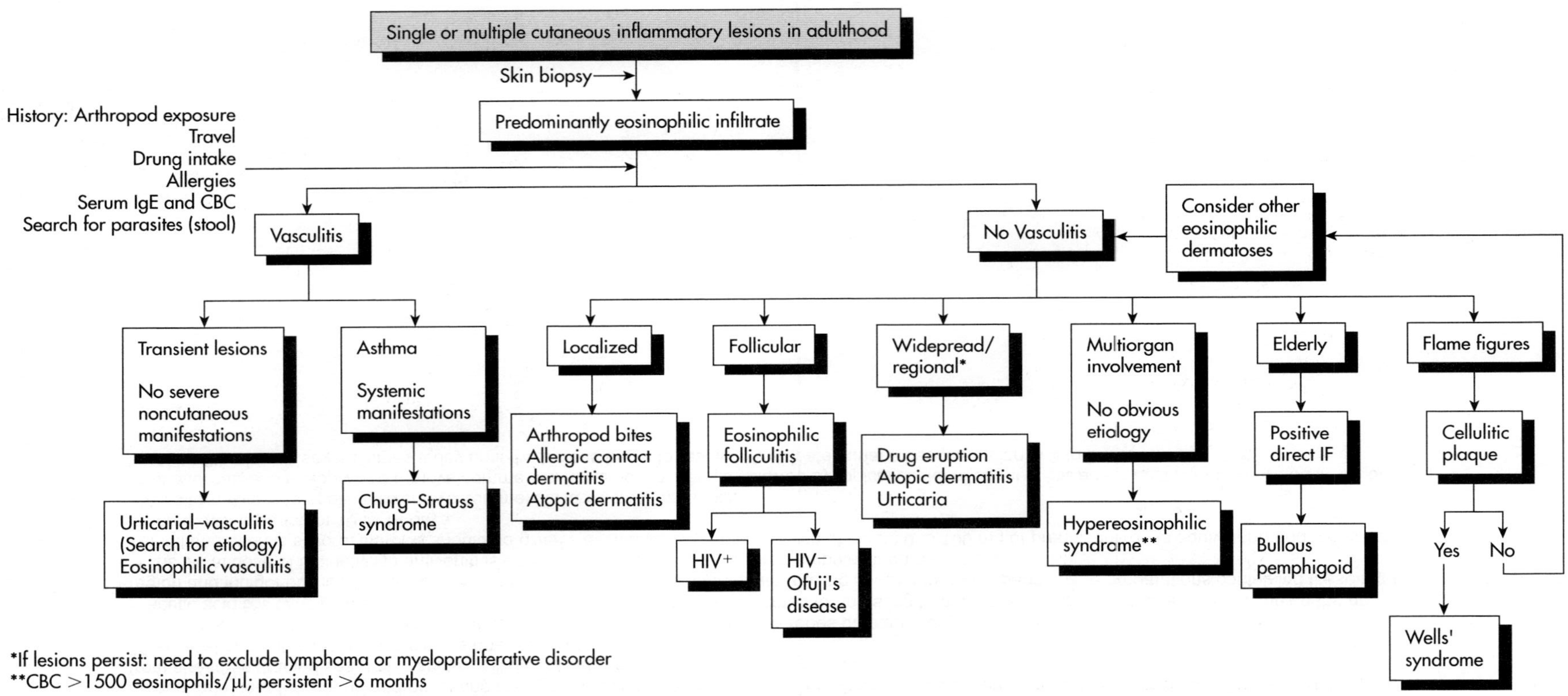

*If lesions persist: need to exclude lymphoma or myeloproliferative disorder
**CBC >1500 eosinophils/μl; persistent >6 months

FIGURE 3-103 Evaluation of adult patients with eosinophilic dermatoses. Histologically, these dermatoses are characterized by a prominent eosinophilic infiltrate. *CBC,* Complete blood count; *HIV,* human immunodeficiency virus; *IF,* intrinsic factor; *IgE,* immunoglobulin E. (From Bolognia JL, Mascaro JM, Mancini AJ, Salasche SJ, Saurat JH, Stingl G [eds]: *Dermatology,* ed 2, St Louis, 2008, Mosby.)

ICD-9CM # 464.30

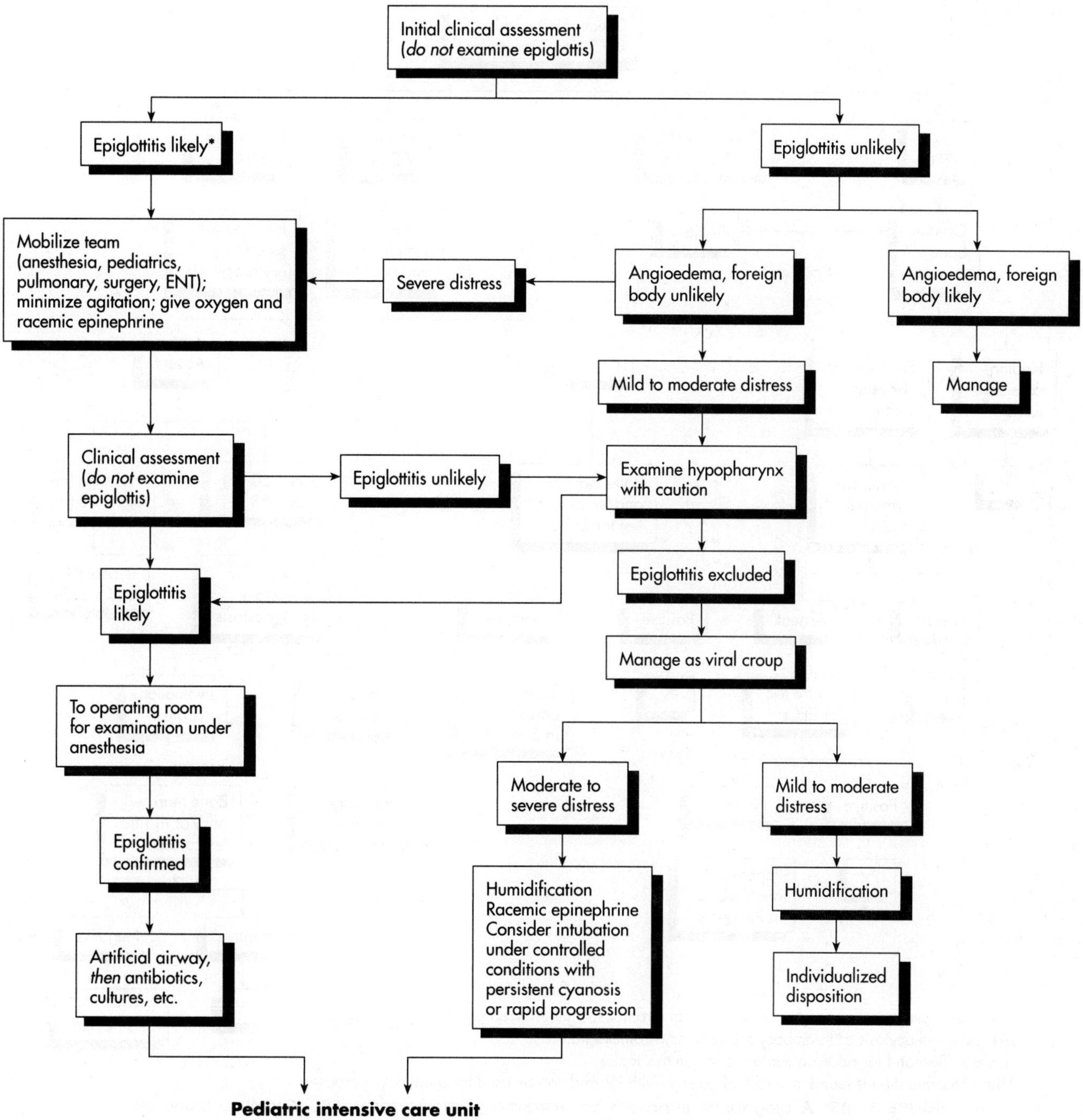

*Refer to Section I for additional information on this topic.

FIGURE 3-104 Optimal assessment and management of upper airway obstruction caused by epiglottitis or severe croup. Care must be individualized to reflect resources and logistic issues within a given institution. *ENT,* Ear, nose, throat. (From Barkin RM, Rosen P: *Emergency pediatrics,* St Louis, 1999, Mosby.)

ICD-9CM # 289.0 Polycythemia, acquired

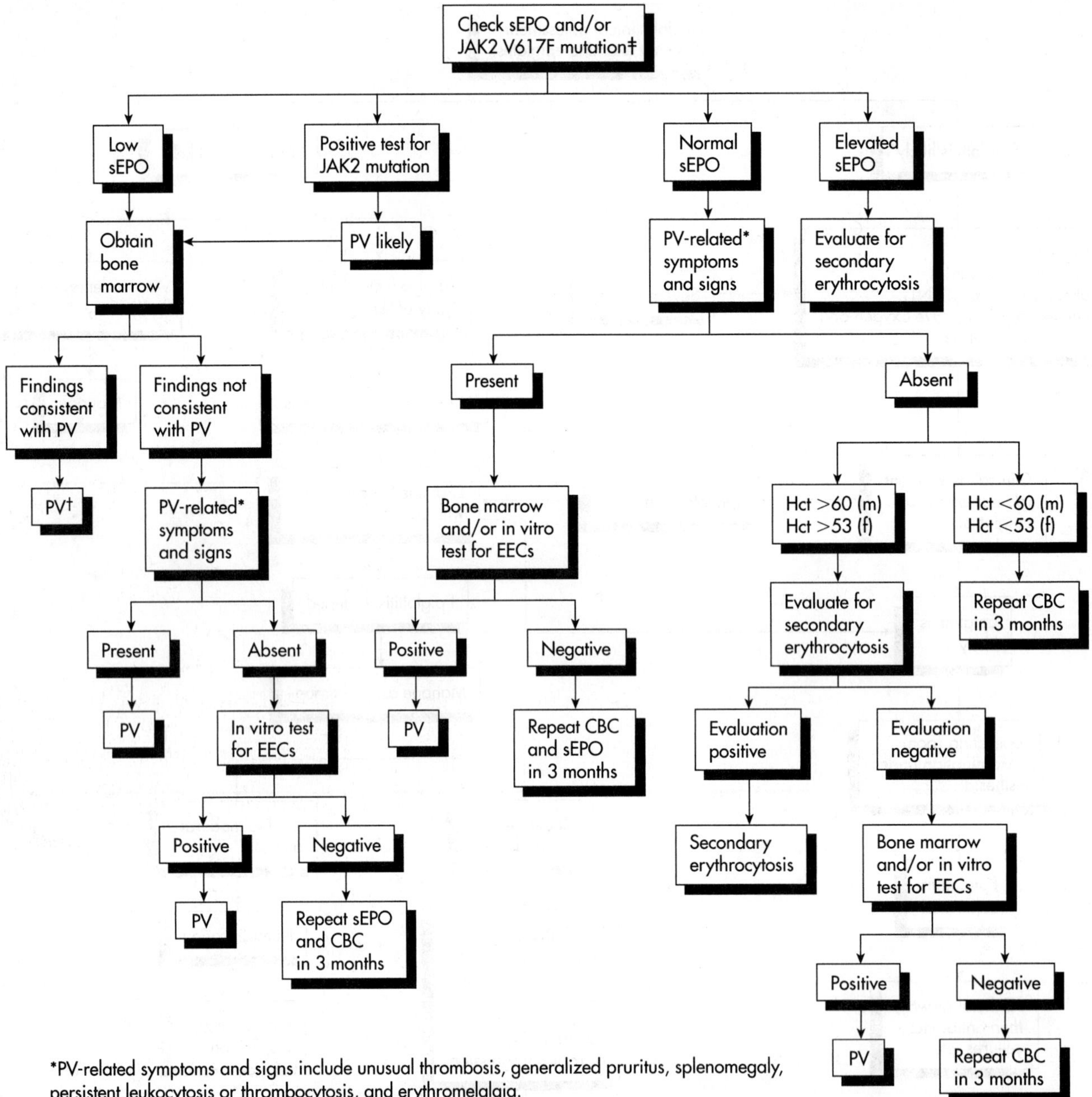

*PV-related symptoms and signs include unusual thrombosis, generalized pruritus, splenomegaly, persistent leukocytosis or thrombocytosis, and erythromelalgia.

†Refer to Section I for additional information on this topic.

‡The JAK2 mutation is found in >95% of patients with PV and can be used for diagnostic purposes.

FIGURE 3-105 A diagnostic approach to acquired erythrocytosis. *CBC,* Complete blood cell count; *EEC,* endogenous (spontaneous) erythroid colonies; *f,* female; *Hct,* hematocrit; *m,* male; *PV,* polycythemia vera; *sEPO,* serum erythropoietin level. (From Goldman L, Ausiello D [eds]: *Cecil textbook of medicine,* ed 23, Philadelphia, 2008, WB Saunders.)

ERYTHRODERMA

ICD-9CM # 695.9 Secondary
695.89 Exfoliative
696.2 Maculopapular
696.1 Psoriaticum
695.89 Infantum

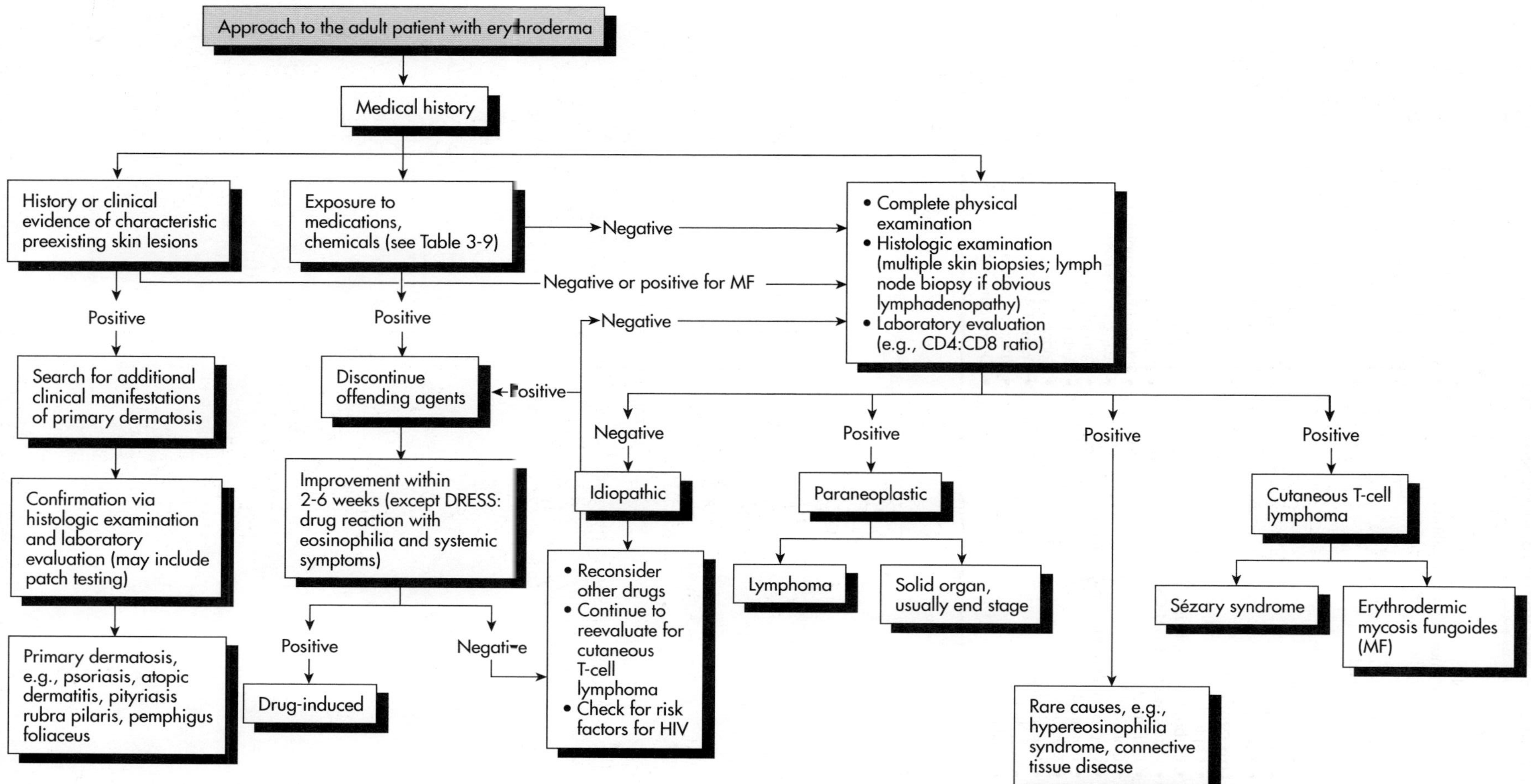

FIGURE 3-106 Approach to the differential diagnosis of adult erythroderma. (From Bolognia JL, Mascaro JM, Mancini AJ, Salasche SJ, Saurat JH, Stingl G [eds]: *Dermatology,* ed 2, St Louis, 2008, Mosby.)

Continued on following page

TABLE 3-9 **Drugs Associated with Erythroderma**

Common

- Allopurinol
- Ampicillin/amoxicillin/penicillin G
- Carbamazepine/oxcarbazepine
- Dapsone
- Omeprazole/lansoprazole
- Phenobarbital
- Phenothiazines
- Phenytoin
- Sulfasalazine
- Sulfonamides
- Vancomycin

Less common

- Captopril
- Carboplatin/cisplatin
- Cytokines (IL-2/GM-CSF)
- Diflunisal
- Gold
- Hydroxychloroquine/mefloquine
- Isoniazid
- Mercury
- Minocycline
- Nifedipine
- Thalidomide

Rare

- Amiodarone
- Aztreonam
- Cimetidine
- Chlorpromazine
- Clofazimine
- Codeine
- Diltiazem
- Erythropoietin
- Fluorouracil
- Indinavir sulfate
- Lithium
- Mitomycin C
- Pentostatin
- Piroxicam
- Practolol
- Ranitidine
- Rifampin (rifampicin)
- Tear gas (CS gas)
- Teicoplanin
- Terbinafine
- Tobramycin
- Tramadol
- Vinca alkaloids
- Zidovudine

FATIGUE

ICD-9CM # 780.7 Fatigue, general

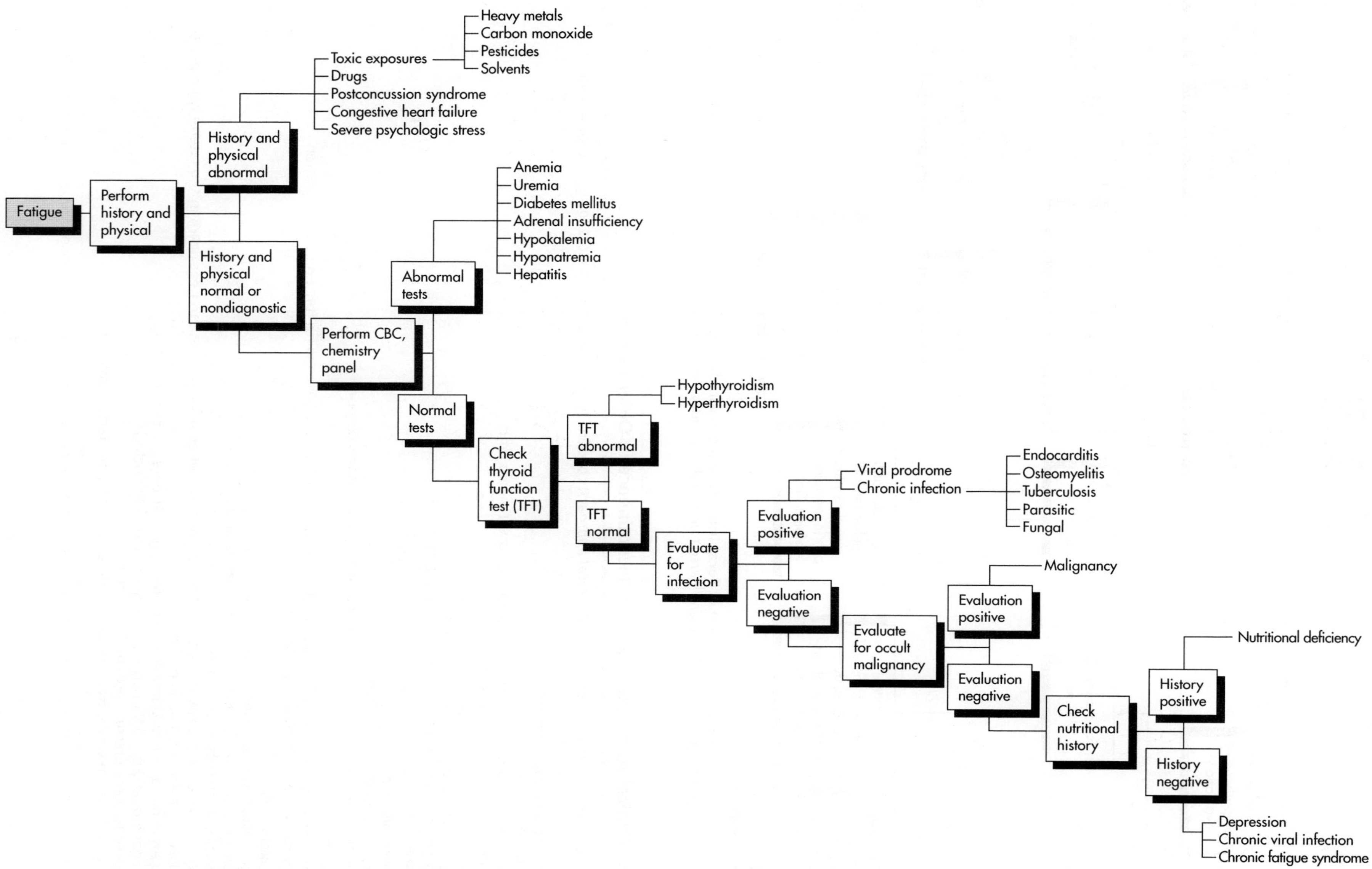

FIGURE 3-107 Evaluation of fatigue. *CBC,* Complete blood count. (From Healey PM: *Common medical diagnosis: an algorithmic approach,* ed 3, Philadelphia, 2000, WB Saunders.)

ICD-9CM # 787.6

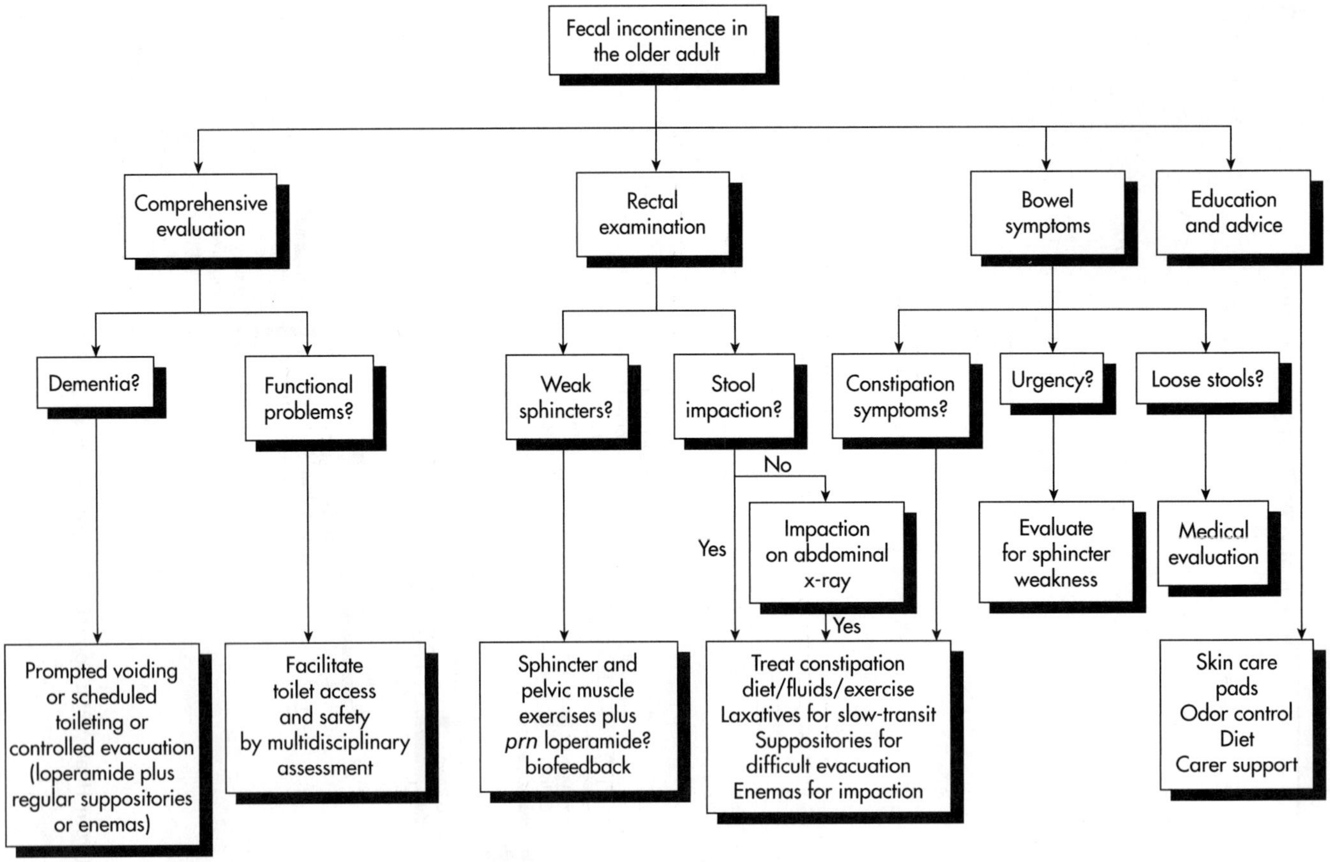

FIGURE 3-108 Evaluation of fecal incontinence. (From Tallis RC, Fillit HM [eds]: *Brocklehurst's textbook of geriatric medicine and gerontology,* ed 6, London, 2003, Churchill Livingstone.)

BOX 3-4 Clinical Assessment of Fecal Incontinence in Older People

Emphasis in older people is on a *structured clinical approach* to identify all contributing factors for fecal incontinence

History
- Duration of fecal incontinence
- Frequency of episodes
- Type (constant soiling, small amounts, complete bowel movement)
- Stool consistency (diarrhea, hard stool)
- Unconscious leakage or symptoms of urgency
- Constipation symptoms/current laxative use
- Systemic illness (confusion, depression, weight loss, anemia)
- Antibiotic use

General examination
- Cognitive and mood assessment
- Neurological profile (stroke, autonomic neuropathy, Parkinson's disease)

Toilet access
- Evaluate ability to use toilet based on muscle strength coordination, vision, limb function, and cognition
- Place in context of current living environment

Specific examination

Abdominal inspection for distension and tenderness
- Perineal inspection for skin breakdown, dermatitis, surgical scars
- Perianal sensation/cutaneous anal reflex
- Observe for excessive downward motion of the pelvic floor when asking patient to bear down in the lateral lying position
- Digital examination for stool impaction
- Digital examination for evaluation of impaired sphincter tone
  - Anal gaping, and/or easy insertion of finger (internal sphincter)
  - Reduced squeeze pressure (external sphincter)
- Ask patient to strain while sitting on commode and observe for rectal prolapse

From Tallis RC, Fillit HM (eds): *Brocklehurst's textbook of geriatric medicine and gerontology,* ed 6, London, 2003, Churchill Livingstone.

FEVER OF UNDETERMINED ORIGIN

ICD-9CM # 780.6 Pyrexia of undetermined origin

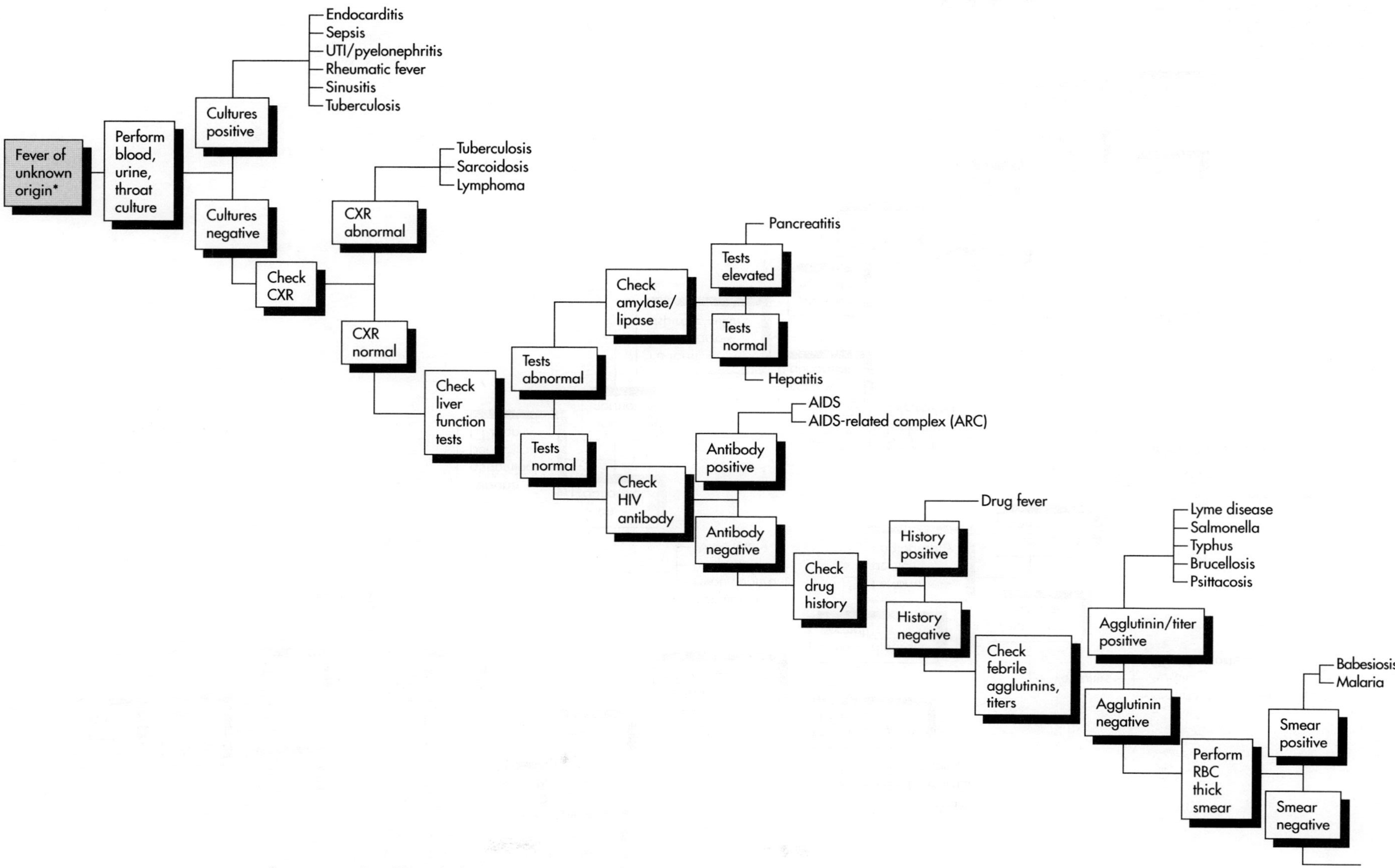

*Refer to Section I for additional information on this topic.

FIGURE 3-109 Approach to the patient with fever of undetermined origin. *AIDS,* Acquired immunodeficiency syndrome; *ANA,* antinuclear antibody; *CT,* computed tomography; *CSR,* chest x-ray; *ESR,* erythrocyte sedimentation rate; *GI,* gastrointestinal; *HIV,* human immunodeficiency virus; *RBC,* red blood cell; *UTI,* urinary tract infection. (From Healey PM: *Common medical diagnosis: an algorithmic approach,* ed 3, Philadelphia, 2000, WB Saunders.)

Continued on following page

FEVER OF UNDETERMINED ORIGIN—cont'd

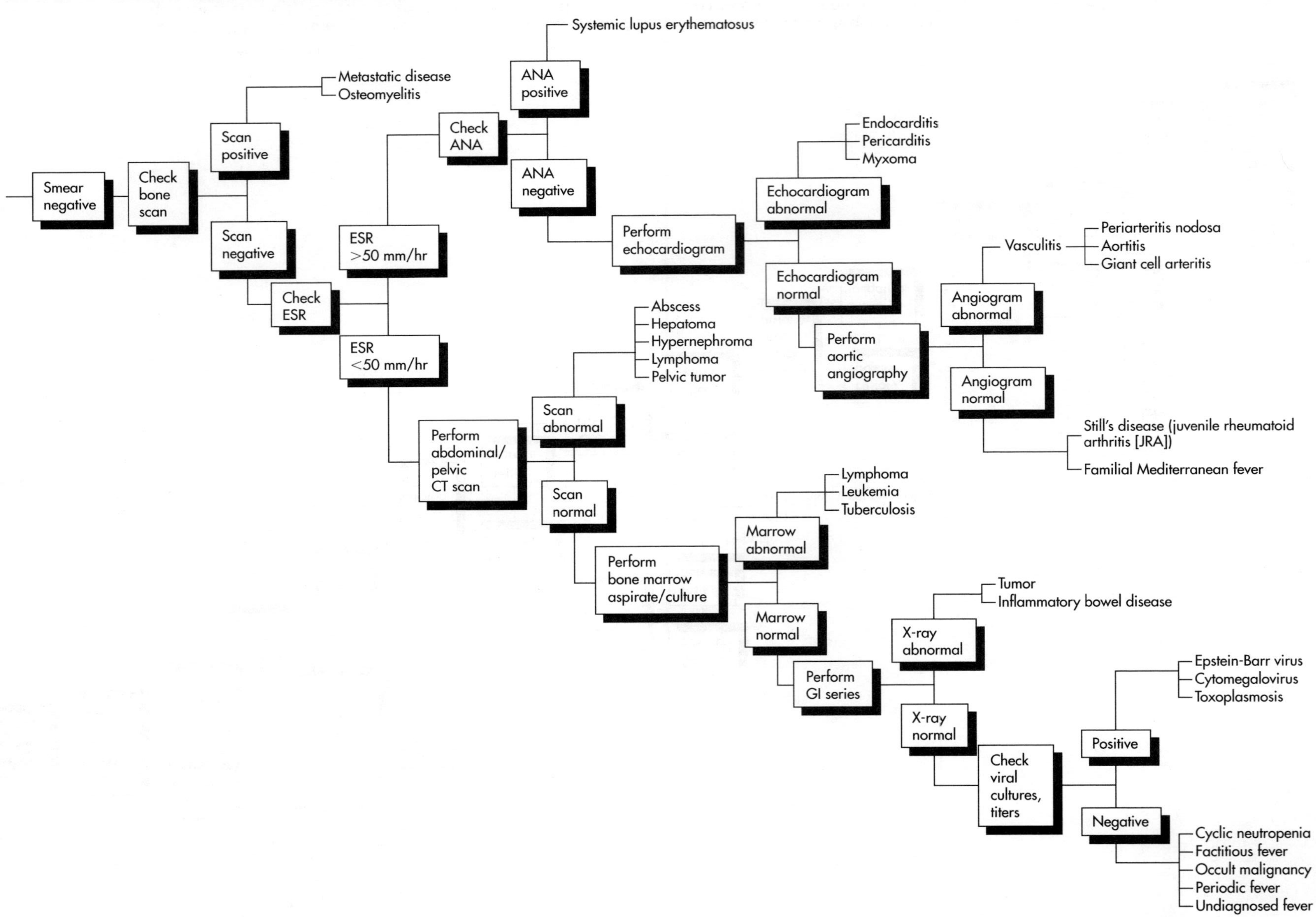

FIGURE 3-109 (Continued) *AIDS,* Acquired immunodeficiency syndrome; *ANA,* antinuclear antibody; *CT,* computed tomography; *CSR,* chest x-ray; *ESR,* erythrocyte sedimentation rate; *GI,* gastrointestinal; *HIV,* human immunodeficiency virus; *RBC,* red blood cell; *UTI,* urinary tract infection. (From Healey PM: *Common medical diagnosis: an algorithmic approach,* ed 3, Philadelphia, 2000, WB Saunders.)

ICD-9CM # 729.1

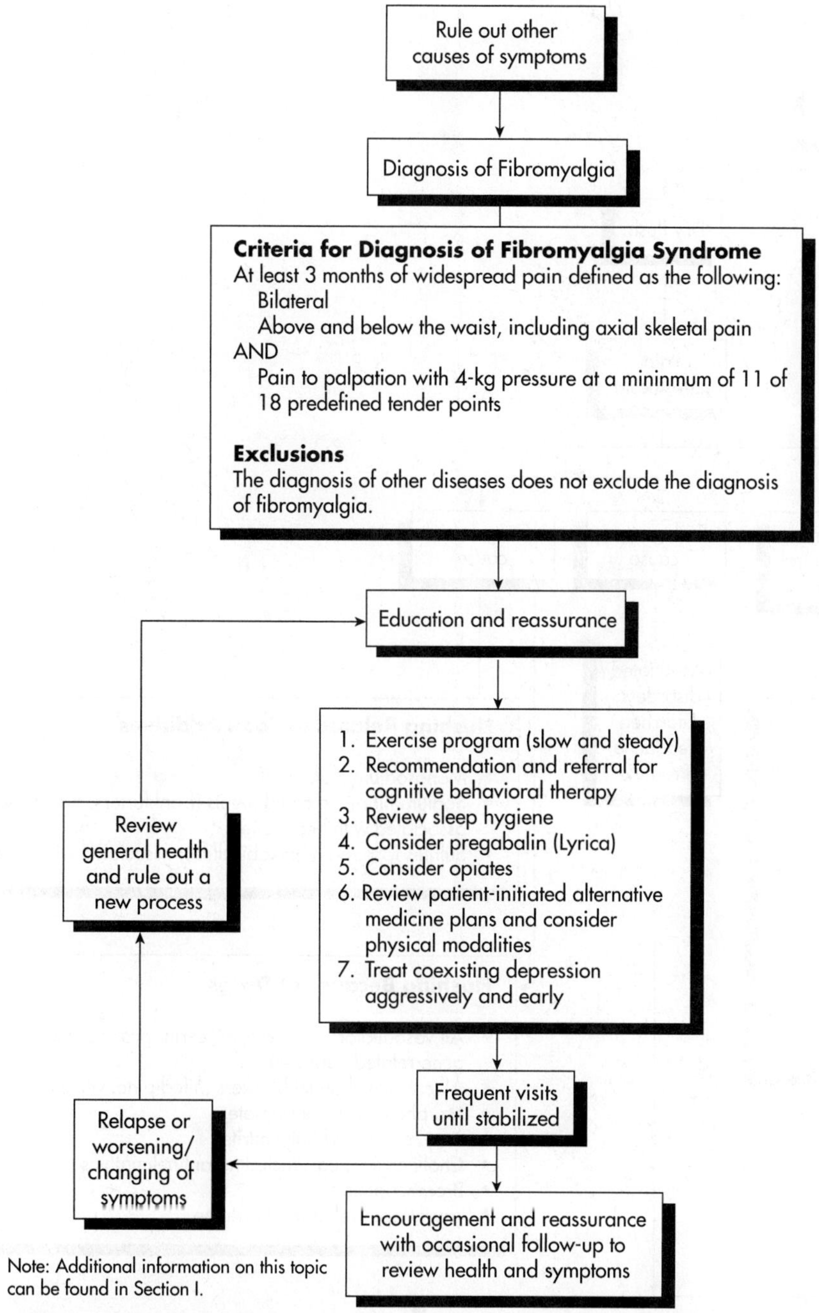

FIGURE 3-110 Treatment algorithim for fibromyalgia. (Modified from Harris ED, Budd RC, Firestein GS, Genovese MC, Sergent JS, Ruddy S, et al: *Kelley's textbook of rheumatology,* ed 7, Philadelphia, 2005, Saunders.)

ICD-9CM # 782.62

Flushing

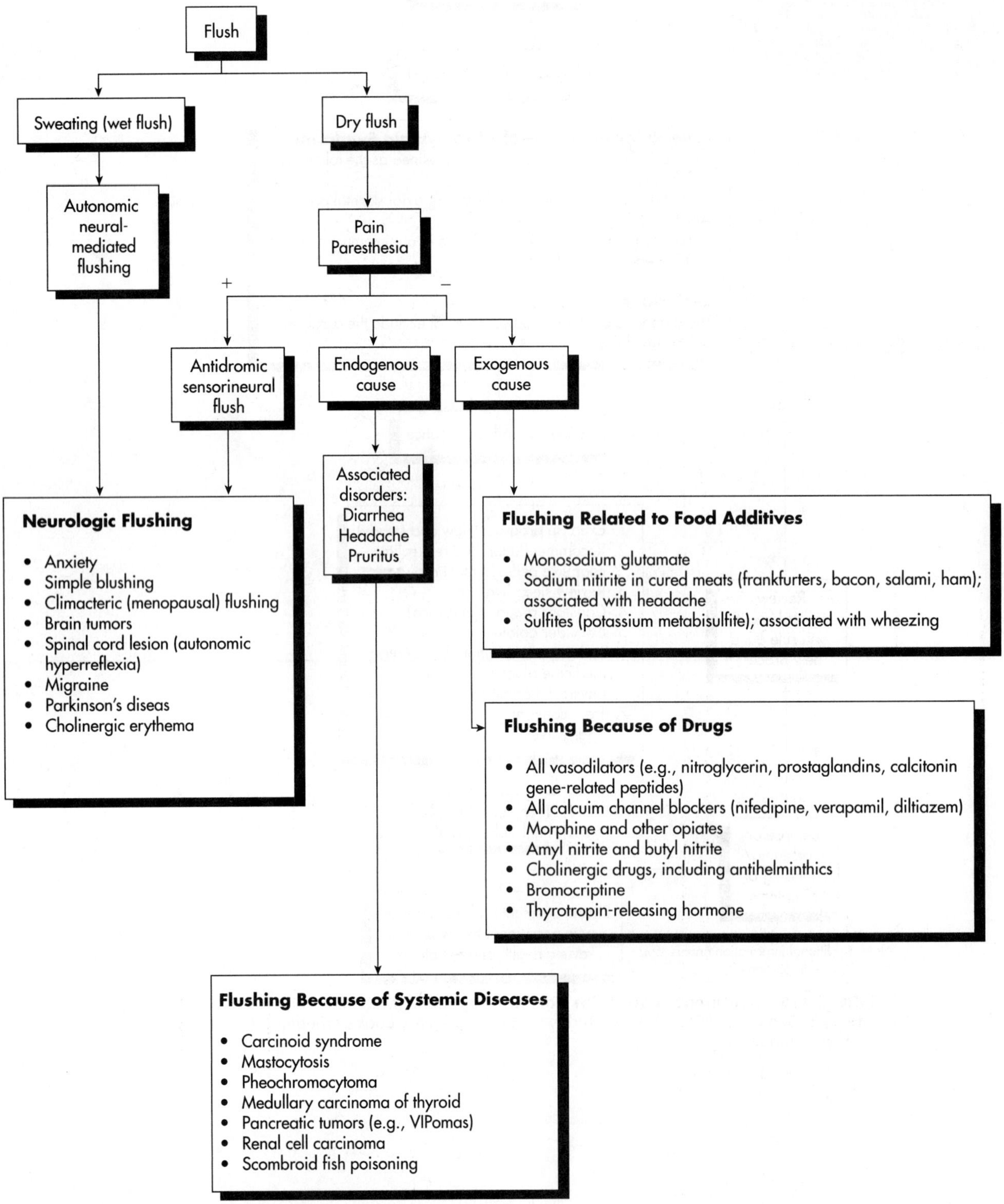

FIGURE 3-111 Evaluation of patients with flushing. (From Bolognia JL, Mascaro JM, Mancini AJ, Salasche SJ, Saurat JH, Stingl G [eds]: *Dermatology,* ed 2, St Louis, 2008, Mosby.)

ICD-9CM # 829.0 Fracture bone(s) NOS closed
829.1 Fracture bone(s) NOS open

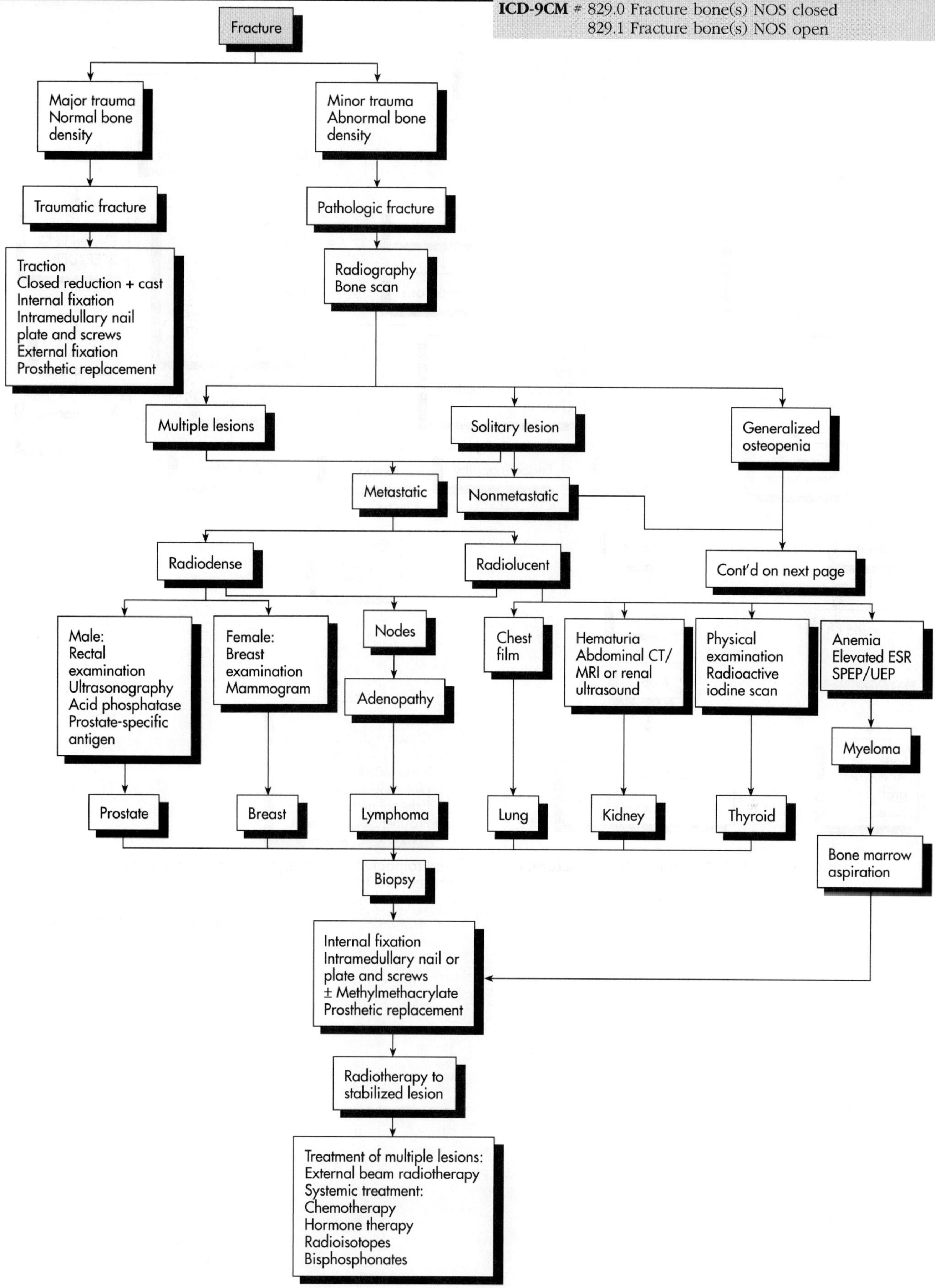
Fracture
Major trauma
Normal bone
density
Minor trauma
Abnormal bone
density
Traumatic fracture
Pathologic fracture
Traction
Closed reduction + cast
Internal fixation
Intramedullary nail
plate and screws
External fixation
Prosthetic replacement
Radiography
Bone scan
Multiple lesions
Solitary lesion
Generalized
osteopenia
Metastatic
Nonmetastatic
Radiodense
Radiolucent
Cont'd on next page
Male:
Rectal
examination
Ultrasonography
Acid phosphatase
Prostate-specific
antigen
Female:
Breast
examination
Mammogram
Nodes
Adenopathy
Chest
film
Hematuria
Abdominal CT/
MRI or renal
ultrasound
Physical
examination
Radioactive
iodine scan
Anemia
Elevated ESR
SPEP/UEP
Myeloma
Prostate
Breast
Lymphoma
Lung
Kidney
Thyroid
Bone marrow
aspiration
Biopsy
Internal fixation
Intramedullary nail or
plate and screws
± Methylmethacrylate
Prosthetic replacement
Radiotherapy to
stabilized lesion
Treatment of multiple lesions:
External beam radiotherapy
Systemic treatment:
Chemotherapy
Hormone therapy
Radioisotopes
Bisphosphonates

FIGURE 3-112 Bone fracture. *CT,* Computed tomography; *ESR,* erythrocyte sedimentation rate; *MRI,* magnetic resonance imaging; *SPEP,* serum protein electrophoresis; *UEP,* urine electrophoresis. (From Greene HL, Johnson WP, Lemcke D [eds]: *Decision making in medicine,* ed 2, St Louis, 1998, Mosby.)

Continued on following page

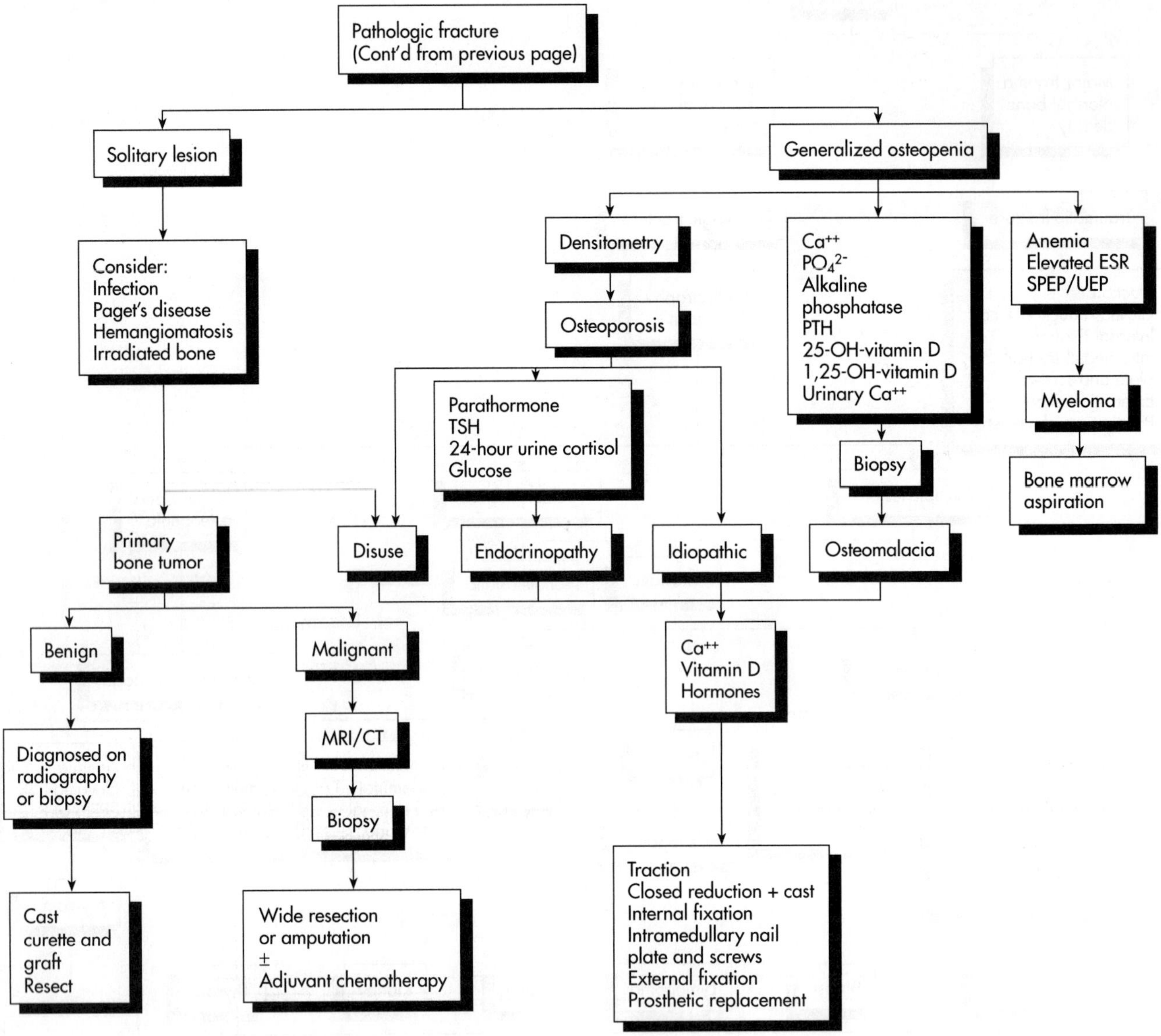

FIGURE 3-112 (Continued) **Bone fracture.** *CT,* Computed tomography; *ESR,* erythrocyte sedimentation rate; *MRI,* magnetic resonance imaging; *SPEP,* serum protein electrophoresis; *UEP,* urine electrophoresis. (From Greene HL, Johnson WP, Lemcke D [eds]: *Decision making in medicine,* ed 2, St Louis, 1998, Mosby.)

GENITALIA, AMBIGUOUS

ICD-9CM # 752.7

1. History: family history, pregnancy (hormones, virilization inspection)
   Palpation of inguinal region and labioscrotal folds; rectal examination
   Karyotype analysis
   Initial studies: plasma 17-hydroxyprogesterone, androstenedione, dehydroepiandrosterone, testosterone, and dihydrotestosterone
   Serum electrolytes
   Sonogram or MRI of kidneys, ureters, and pelvic contents
   Provisional Dx

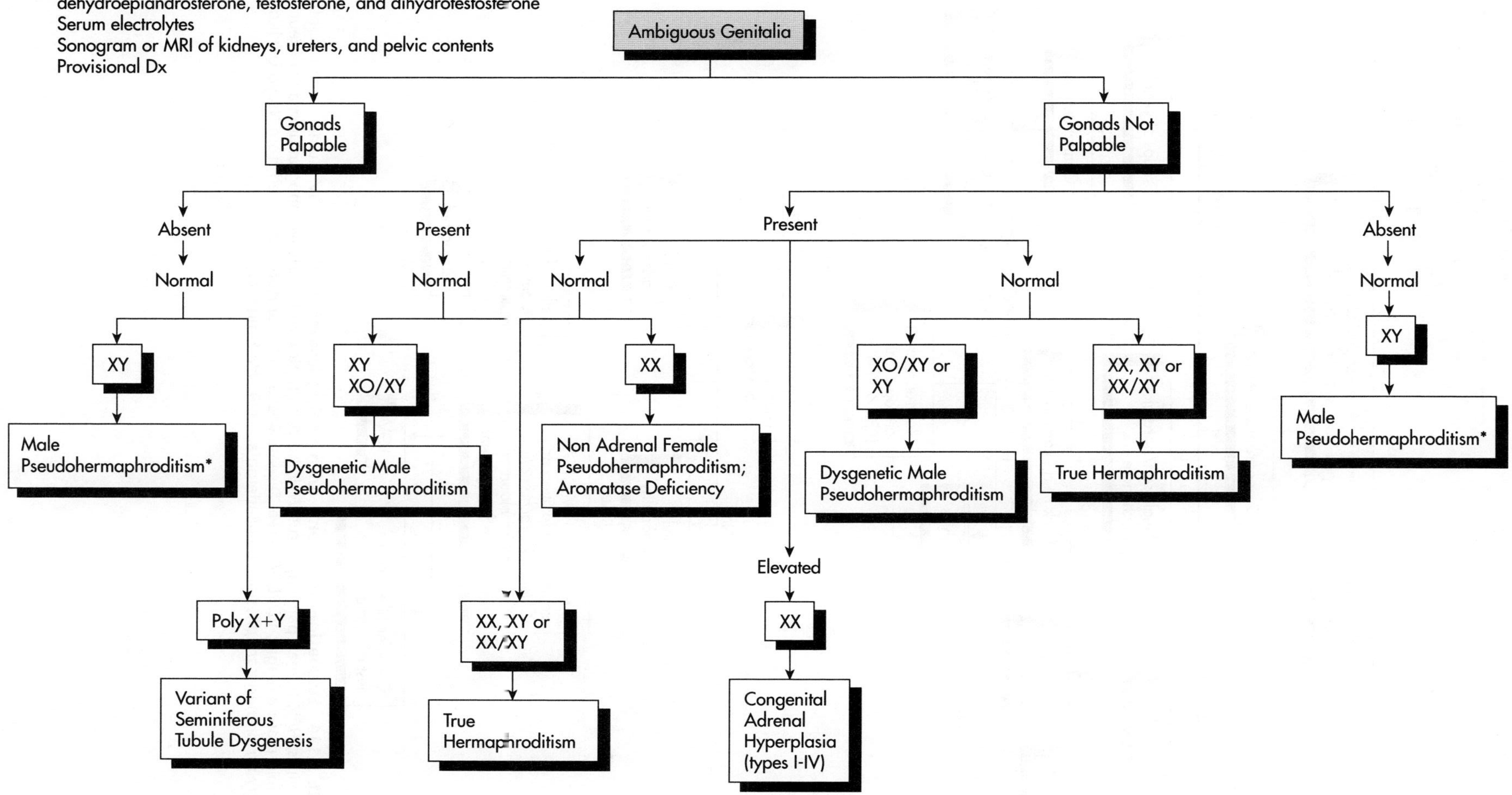

2. "Vaginogram" (urogenital sinogram): selected cases
   Endoscopy, laparotomy, gonadal biopsy: restricted to male pseudohermaphrodites, true hermaphrodites, and selected instances of nonadrenal femal pseudohermaphroditism

*Plasma 17-hydroxyprogesterone levels may be modestly elevated in patients with CYP11 (Type III), 3β-hydroxysteroid dehydrogenase deficiency (Type IV) and are "low" in patients with CYP17 (Type V) and CYP11A1 deficiency (Type VI)

FIGURE 3-113 Steps in the diagnosis of intersexuality in infancy and childhood. Step 1 involves initial work-up and provisional diagnosis. Step 2 is used in selected cases. *MRI,* Magnetic resonance imaging. (From Larsen PR, Kronenberg HM, Memlmed S, Polansky, KS [eds]: *Williams textbook of endocrinology,* ed 11, Philadelphia, 2008, Saunders.)

ICD-9CM # 054.10 Genital herpes
91.0 Genital syphilis
078.11 Condyloma acuminatum
099.0 Chancroid
099.2 Granuloma inguinale
099.1 Lymphogranuloma venereum
629.8 Ulcer, genital site, female
608.89 Ulcer, genital site, male

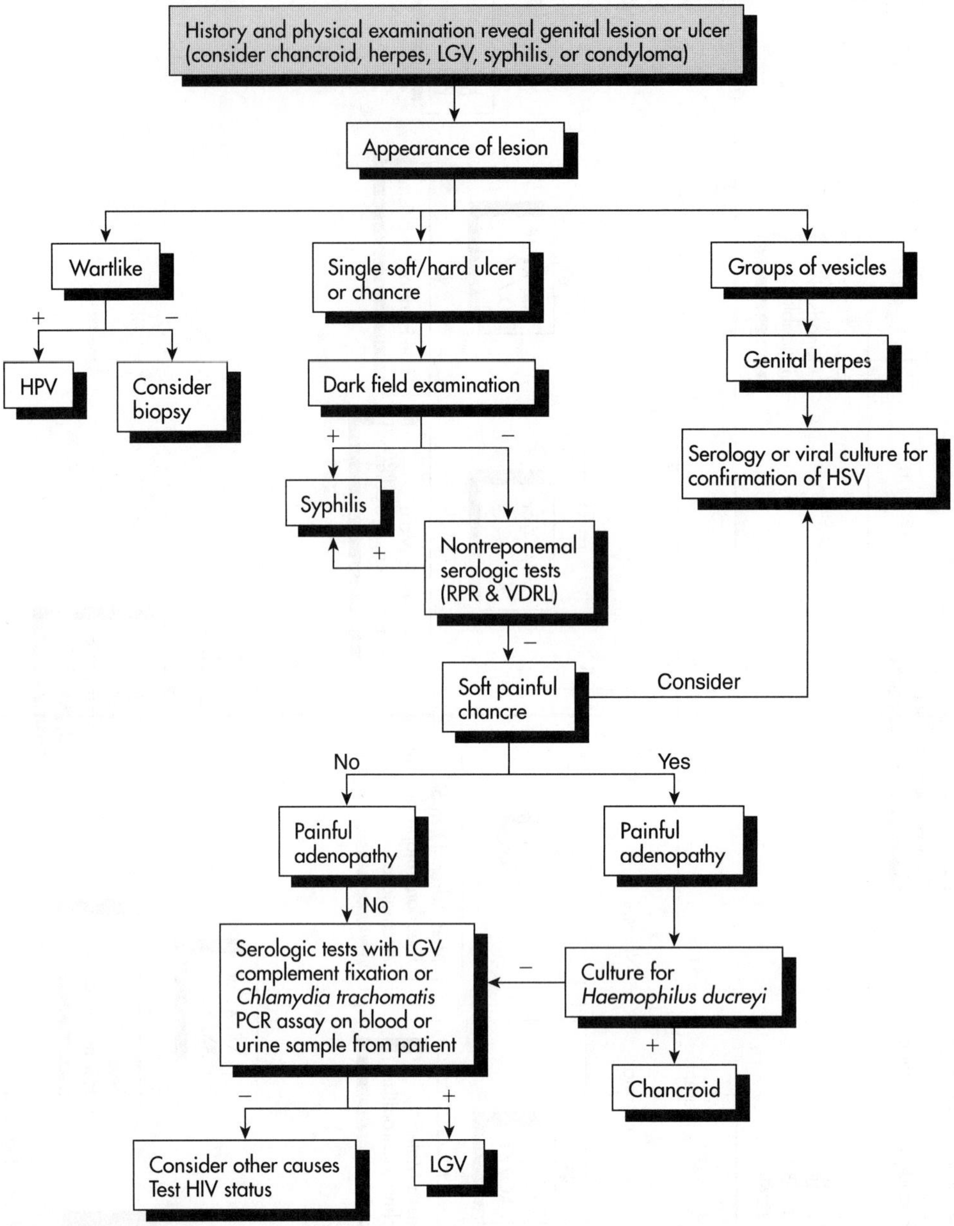

FIGURE 3-114 Evaluation of patients with genital lesions or ulcers. *HIV,* Human immunodeficiency virus; *HPV,* human papillomavirus; *HSV,* herpes simplex virus; *LGV,* lymphogranuloma venereum; *RPR,* rapid plasma reagin; *VDRL,* Venereal Disease Research Laboratory. (Modified from Nseyo UO [ed]: *Urology for primary care physicians,* Philadelphia, 1999, WB Saunders.)

ICD-9CM # 240.9 Goiter, unspecified
240.0 Goiter, simple
241.9 Goiter, adenomatous
246.1 Goiter, congenital
242.1 Goiter, uninodular with thyrotoxicosos
242.2 Goiter, multinodular with thyrotoxicosos

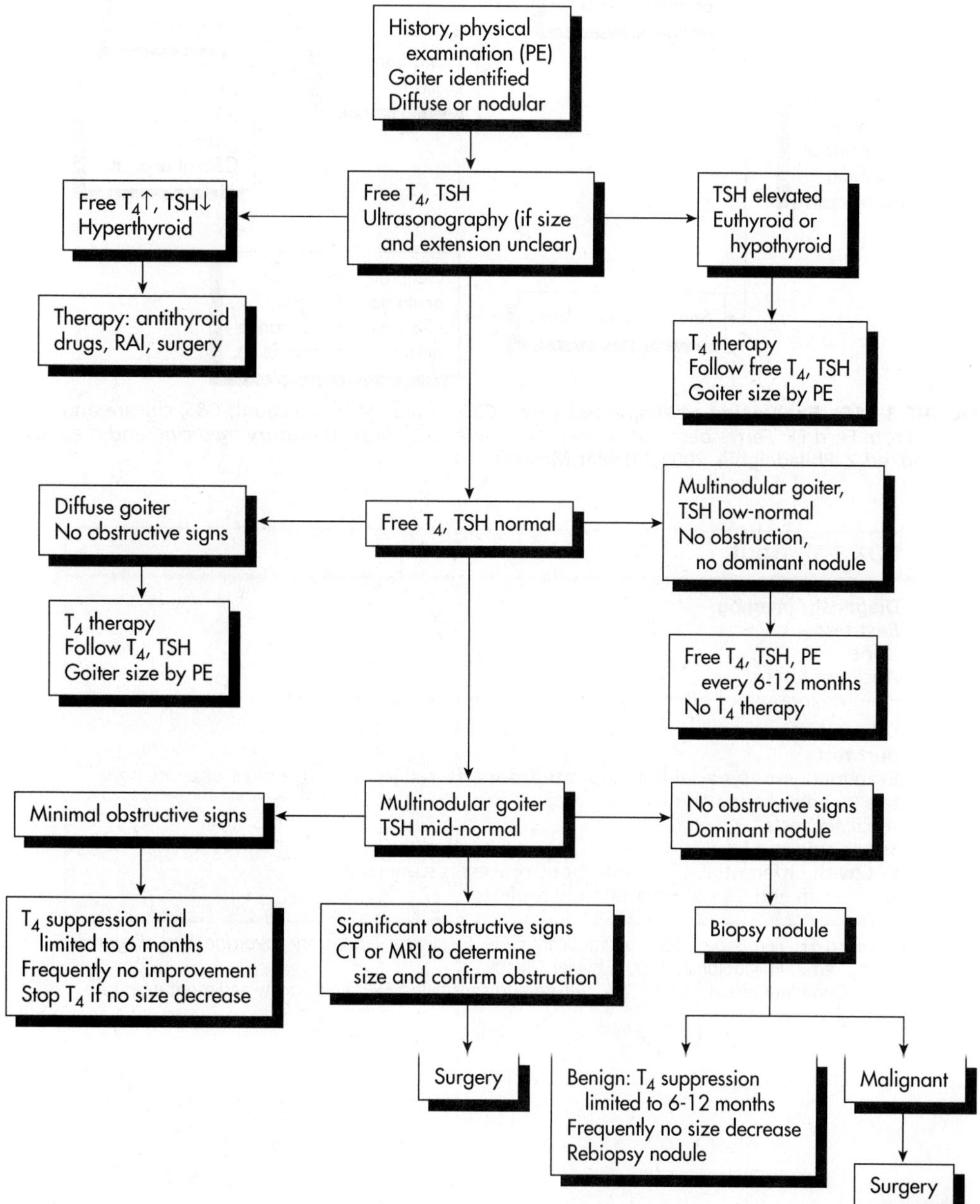

FIGURE 3-115 Evaluation and management of patients with nontoxic diffuse and nodular goiter and undetermined thyroid status. *CT,* Computed tomography; *MRI,* magnetic resonance imaging; *RAI,* radioactive iodine; *TSH,* thyroid-stimulating hormone. (From Goldman L, Ausiello D [eds]: *Cecil textbook of medicine,* ed 23, Philadelphia, 2008, WB Saunders.)

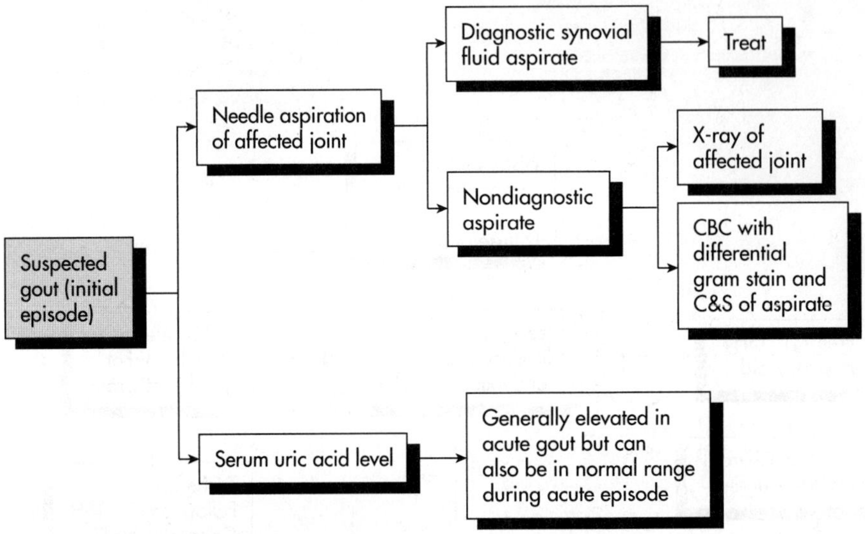

FIGURE 3-116 Evaluation of suspected gout. *CBC,* Complete blood count; *C&S,* culture and sensitivity. (From Ferri FF: *Ferri's best test: a practical guide to clinical laboratory medicine and diagnostic imaging,* ed 2, Philadelphia, 2009, Elsevier Mosby.)

BOX 3-5 **Gout**

Diagnostic imaging
Best test
None
Ancillary tests
Plain radiograph of affected joint when diagnosis is unclear

Lab evaluation
Best test
Examination of synovial fluid aspirate from affected joint for presence of urate crystals (needle-shaped and birefringent)
Ancillary tests
Serum uric acid level
CBC with differential, ESR if infectious process is suspected
Gram stain and C&S of synovial fluid aspirate

From Ferri FF: *Ferri's best test: a practical guide to clinical laboratory medicine and diagnostic imaging,* ed 2, Philadelphia, 2009, Elsevier Mosby.
CBC, Complete blood count; *C&S,* culture and sensitivity; *ESR,* erythrocyte sedimentation rate.

ICD-9CM # Variable with specific diagnosis

Noninfectious Granulomas: Paradigm for Histologic Diagnosis

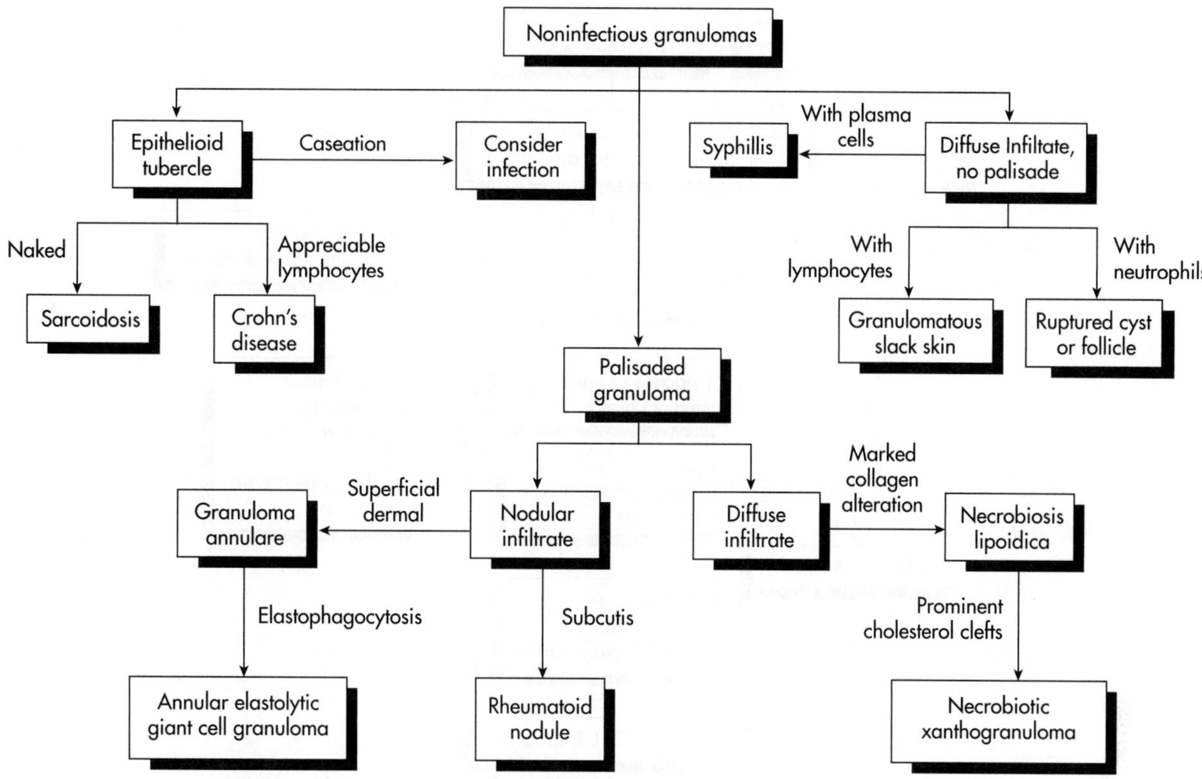

FIGURE 3-117 Noninfectious granulomas. Paradigm for histologic diagnosis.

TABLE 3-10 Clinical Features of the Major Granulomatous Dermatitides

	Sarcoidosis	Classic GA*	NLD	AEGCG	Crohn's Disease	Rheumatoid Nodule
Average age (years)	25-35, 45-65	<30		40	35	30-40
Sex	Female	Female	Female	Female	Female	Female
Racial predilection in United States	African American	None	None	Caucasian	None	None
Site	Symmetric on face, neck, upper trunk, extremities	Hands, feet, extremities	Anterior and lateral distal lower extremities	Face, neck, forearms	Genital areas, lower > upper extremities	Juxtaarticular areas, elbows, hands, ankles, feet
Appearance	Red to red-brown papules and plaques	Papules coalescing into annular plaques	Plaques with elevated borders, telangiectasias centrally	Annular plaques	Dusky erythema and swelling, ulceration	Skin-colored, firm, mobile subcutaneous nodules
Size of lesions	1-5 cm	1-2 mm papules, <5 cm annular plaques	>10 cm	1-6 cm	Variable	1-3 cm
Number of lesions	Variable	1-10	1-10	1-10	1-5	1-10
Associations	Systemic manifestations of sarcoidosis	Rare diabetes mellitus, malignancy	Diabetes mellitus	Actinic damage	Intestinal Crohn's disease	Rheumatoid arthritis
Special clinical characteristics	Occasional central atrophy and hypopigmentation	Central hyperpigmentation	Yellow-brown atrophic centers, ulceration	Central atrophy and hypopigmentation	Draining sinuses and fistulae	Occasional ulceration, especially at site of trauma

From Bolognia JL, Mascaro JM, Mancini AJ, Salasche SJ, Saurat JH, Stingl G [eds]: *Dermatology,* ed 2, St Louis, 2008, Mosby.
AEGCG, Annular elastolytic giant cell granuloma; *GA,* granuloma annulare; *NLD,* necrobiosis lipoidica diabeticorum.
*Clinical variants include generalized, micropapular, nodular, perforating, subcutaneous, and patch GA.

ICD-9CM # 611.1 Gynecomastia nonpuerperal

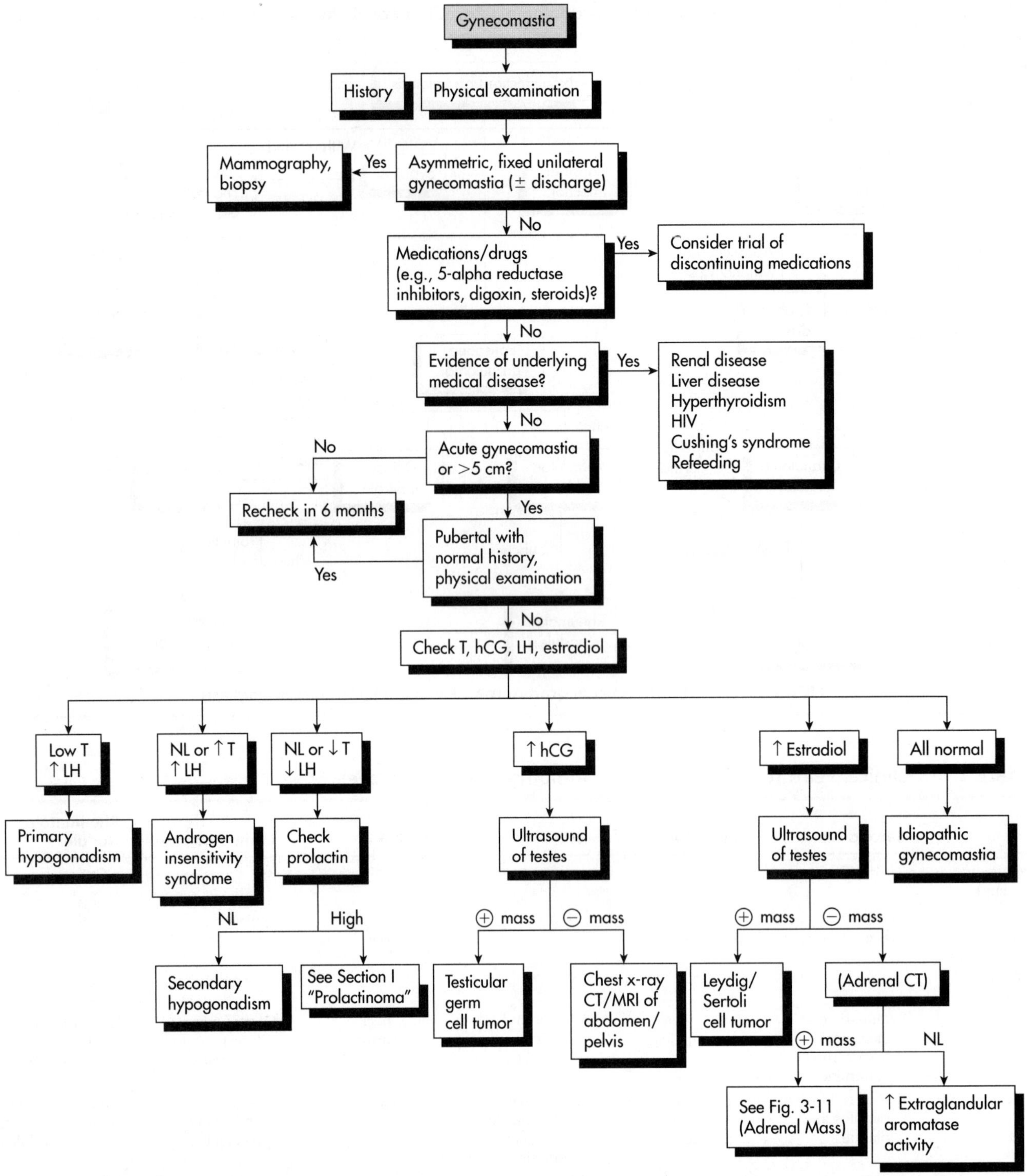

FIGURE 3-118 Evaluation of gynecomastia. *CT,* Computed tomography; *hCG,* human chorionic gonadotropin; *HIV,* human immunodeficiency syndrome; *LH,* luteinizing hormone; *MRI,* magnetic resonance imaging; *NL,* normal limits; *T,* testosterone. (Modified from Noble J: *Primary care medicine,* ed 3, St Louis, 2001, Mosby.)

ICD-9CM # 389.00 Hearing loss, conductive
389.10 Hearing loss, sensorineural

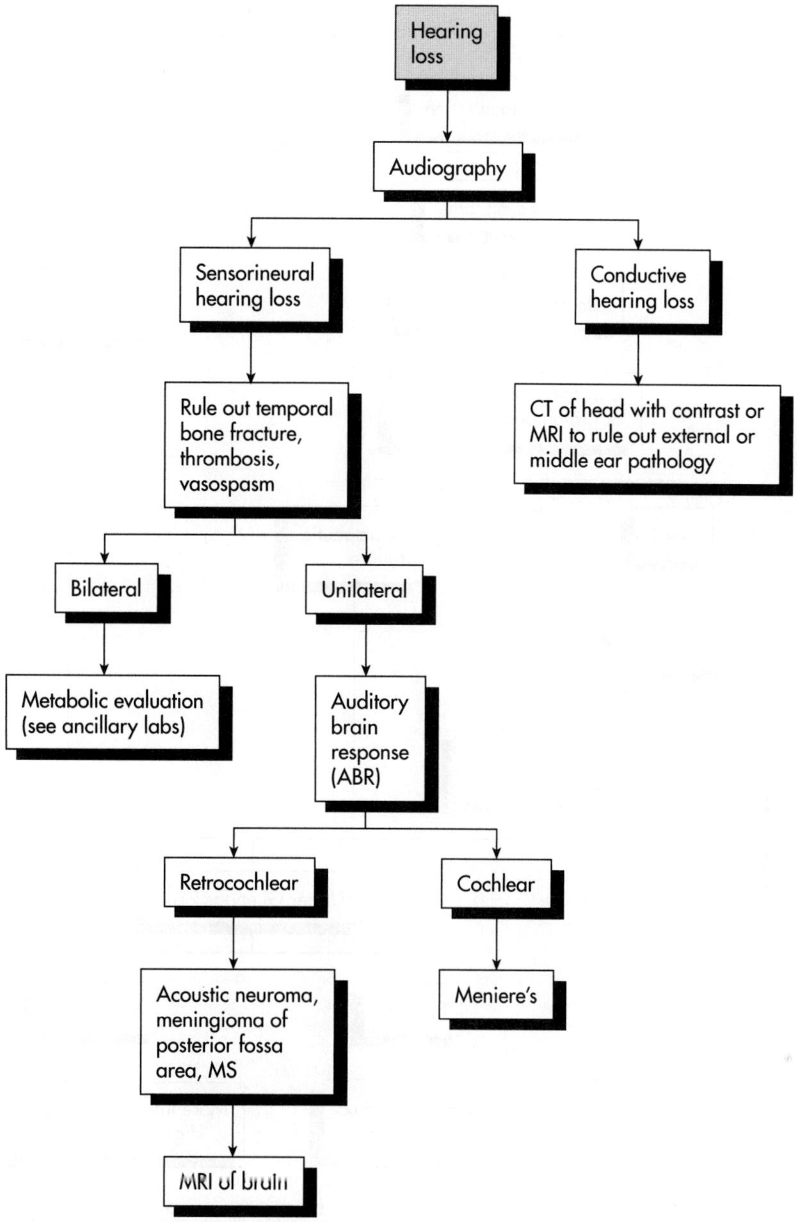

FIGURE 3-119 Evaluation of hearing loss. *CT,* Computed tomography; *MRI,* magnetic resonance imaging. (From Ferri FF: *Ferri's best test: a practical guide to clinical laboratory medicine and diagnostic imaging,* ed 2, Philadelphia, 2009, Elsevier Mosby.)

BOX 3-6 **Hearing Loss**

Diagnostic imaging	Lab evaluation
Best test	***Best test***
None	None
Ancillary tests	***Ancillary tests***
CT of head with contrast or MRI with contrast	CBC
CT of temporal bone without contrast	ALT, AST
	ANA, VDRL
	TSH

From Ferri FF: *Ferri's best test: a practical guide to clinical laboratory medicine and diagnostic imaging,* ed 2, Philadelphia, 2009, Elsevier Mosby.

ALT, Alanine aminotransferase; *ANA,* antibody to nuclear antigens; *AST,* angiotension sensitivity test; *CBC,* complete blood count; *CT,* computed tomography; *TSH,* thyroid-stimulating hormone; *VDRL,* Venereal Disease Research Laboratory test.

ICD-9CM # 787.1

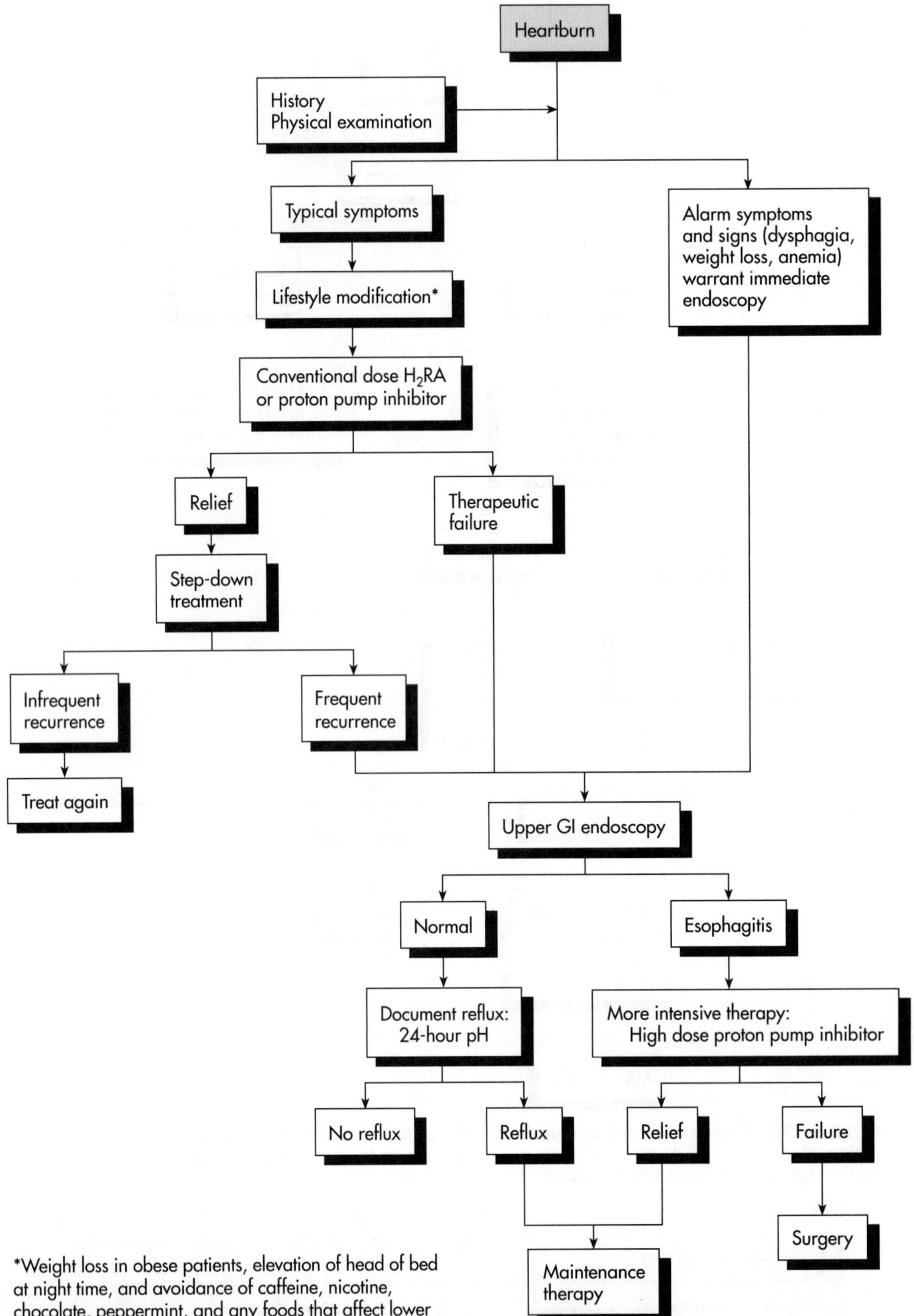

*Weight loss in obese patients, elevation of head of bed at night time, and avoidance of caffeine, nicotine, chocolate, peppermint, and any foods that affect lower esophageal sphincter.

FIGURE 3-120 Treatment of a patient with heartburn. *GI,* Gastrointestinal; *H_2RA,* H_2 receptor antagonist. (Modified from Sampliner RE: Heartburn. In Greene HL, Johnson WP, Lemcke D [eds]: *Decision making in medicine,* ed 2, St Louis, 1998, Mosby.)

ICD-9CM # 599.7

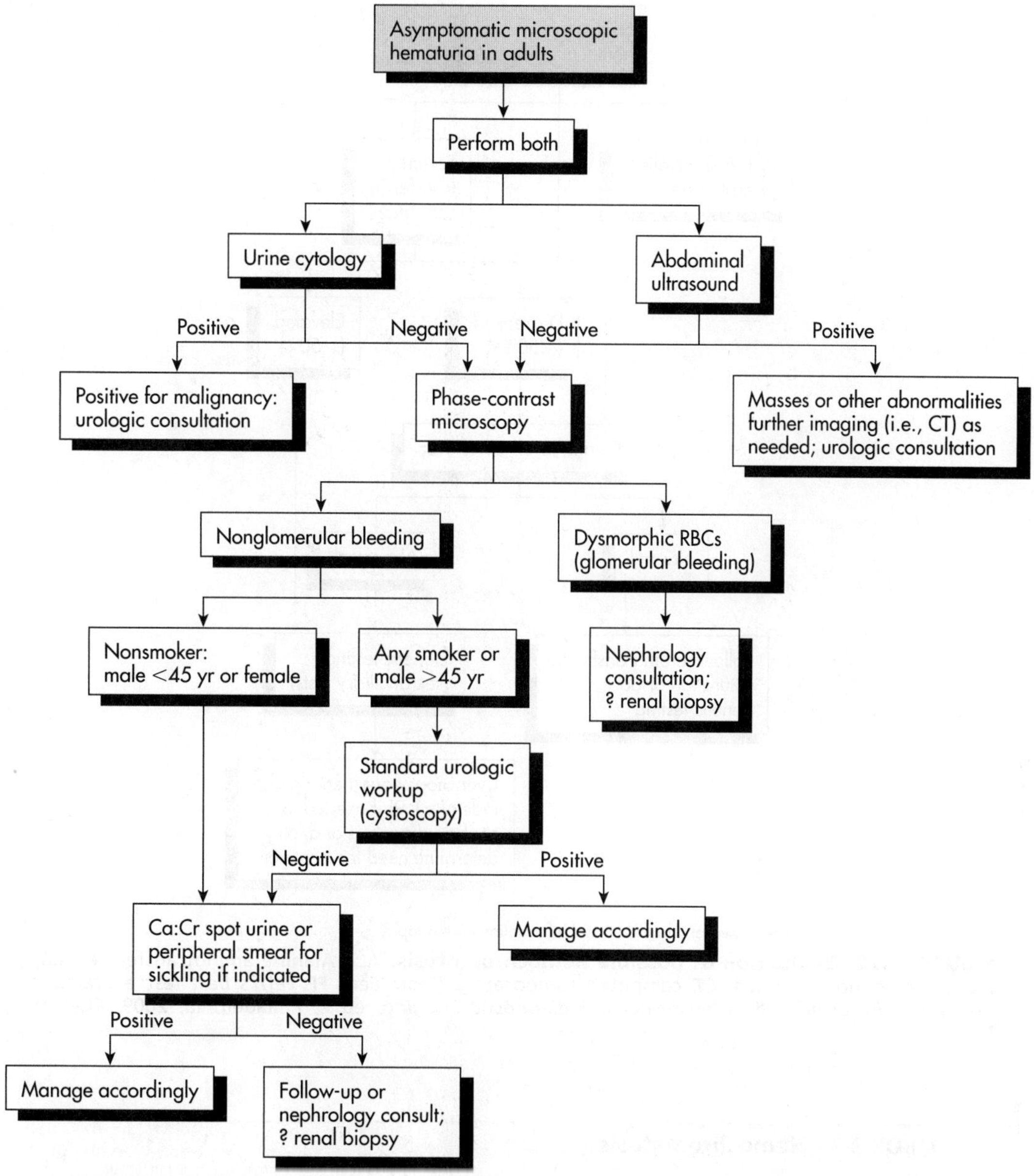

FIGURE 3-121 Suggested algorithm for the evaluation of adult asymptomatic microscopic hematuria. These patients must have no symptoms referable to the hematuria and a negative urinalysis except for red blood cells (RBCs). Adults with gross hematuria require a full urologic evaluation. *Ca:Cr,* Calcium:creatinine ratio. (Modified from Nseyo UO [ed]: *Urology for primary care physicians,* Philadelphia, 1999, WB Saunders.)

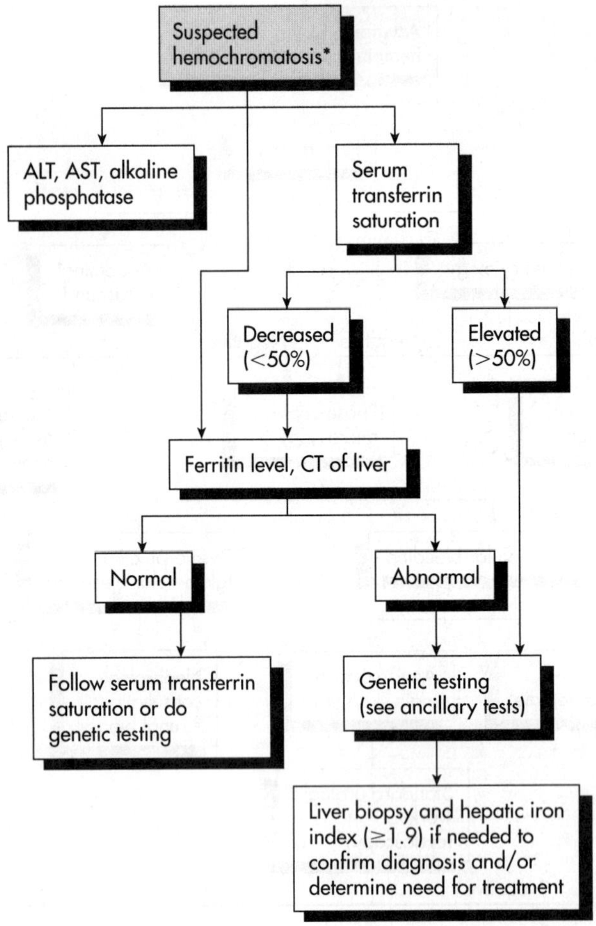

*Refer to Section I for additional information on this topic.

FIGURE 3-122 Evaluation of possible hemochromotosis. *ALT,* Alanine aminotransferase; *AST,* aspartate aminotransferase; *CT,* computed tomography. (From Ferri FF: *Ferri's best test: a practical guide to clinical laboratory medicine and diagnostic imaging,* ed 2, Philadelphia, 2009, Elsevier Mosby.)

BOX 3-7 **Hemochromatosis**

Diagnostic imaging

Best test

None

Ancillary tests

Noncontrast CT or MRI of liver is useful for excluding other causes of elevated liver enzymes. Imaging of liver may reveal increased density of liver tissue and is also useful in screening for hepatoma (increased risk in patients with cirrhosis)

Lab evaluation

Best tests

Plasma transferring saturation is best screening test

Plasma ferritin is also a good indicator of total body iron stores but may be elevated in many other conditions (e.g., inflammation, malignancy)

Measurement of hepatic iron index (hepatic iron concentration/age) in liver biopsy specimen can confirm diagnosis

Ancillary tests

ALT, AST, alkaline phosphatase

Genetic testing (HFE phenotyping for C282Y and H63D mutations)

From Ferri FF: *Ferri's best test: a practical guide to clinical laboratory medicine and diagnostic imaging,* ed 2, Philadelphia, 2009, Elsevier Mosby.

ALT, Alanine aminotransferase; *AST,* aspartate aminotransferase; *CT,* computed tomography; *MRI,* magnetic resonance imaging.

HEMOPTYSIS

ICD-9CM # 786.3

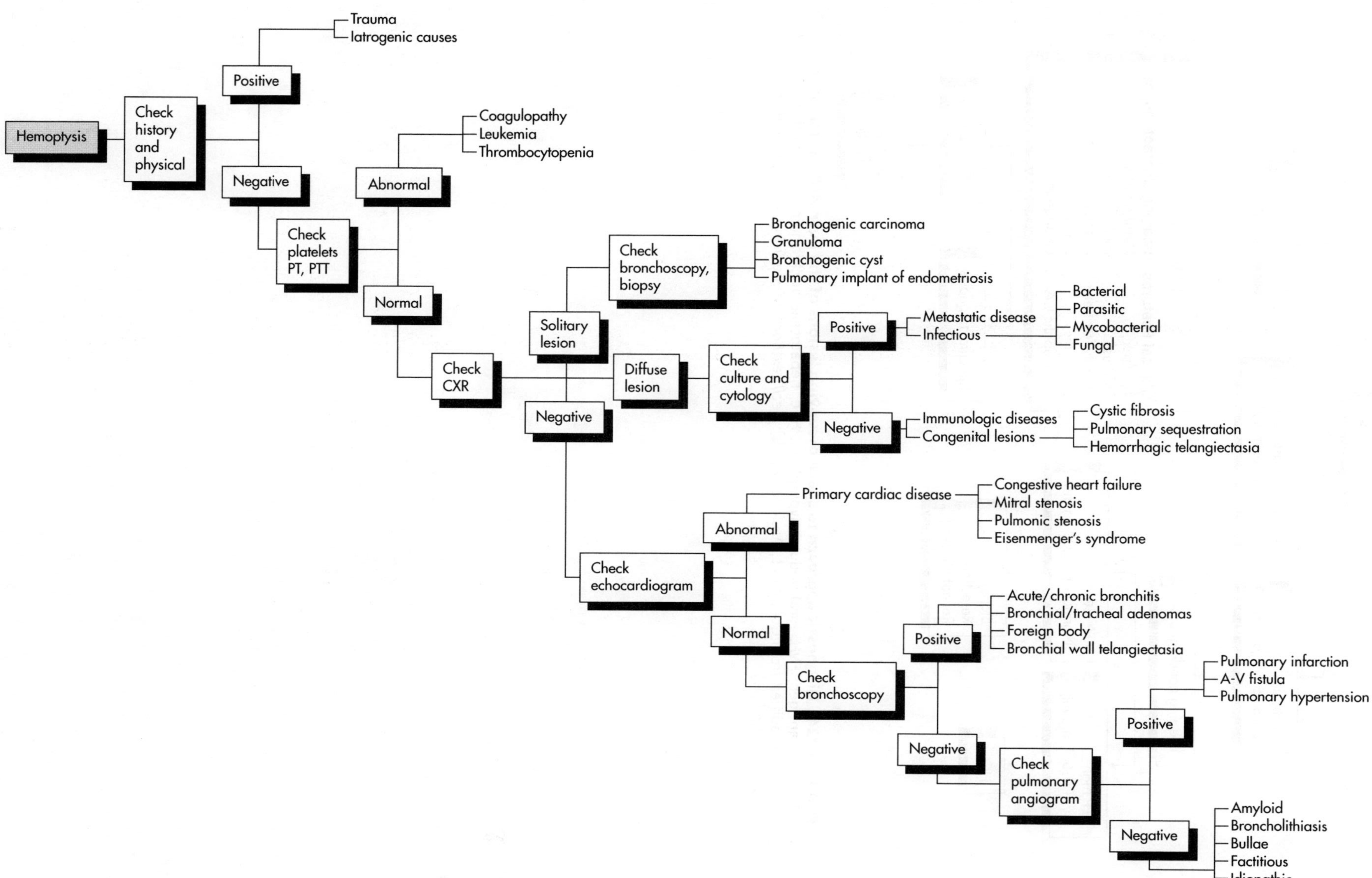

FIGURE 3-123 Evaluation of hemoptysis. *A-V,* Arteriovenous; *CXR,* chest x-ray; *PT,* prothrombin time; *PTT,* partial thromboplastin time. (From Healey PM: *Common medical diagnosis: an algorithmic approach,* ed 3, Philadelphia, 2000, WB Saunders.)

ICD-9CM # 751.60

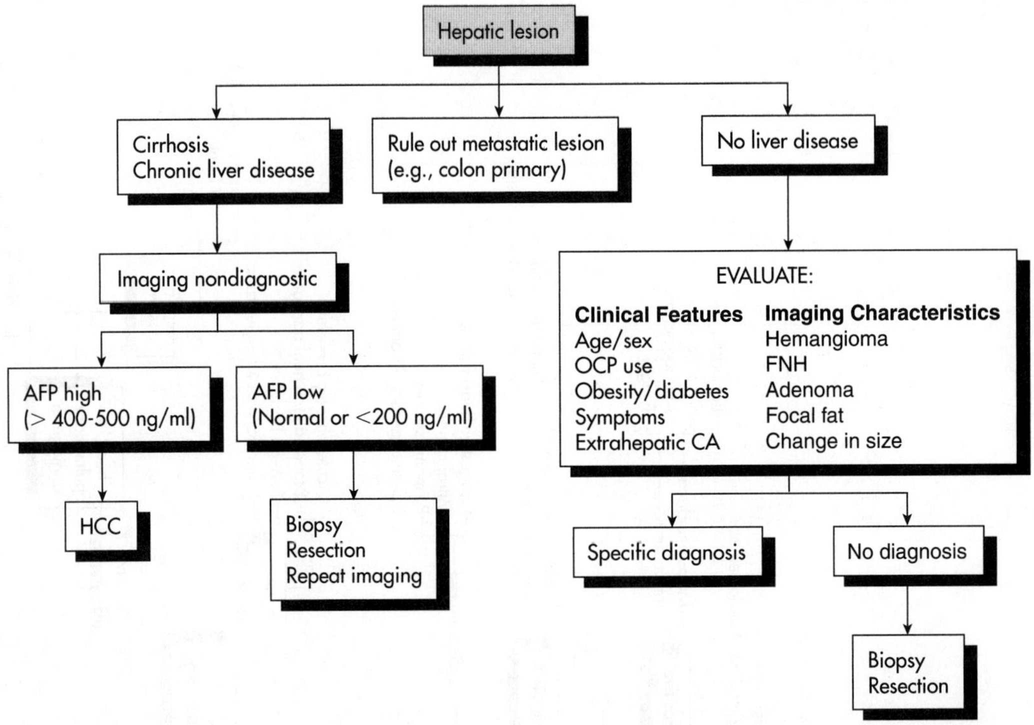

FIGURE 3-124 Diagnostic approach to space occupying lesions of the liver. *AFP,* α-Fetoprotein; *CA,* cancer antigen; *FNH,* focal nodular hyperplasia; *HCC,* hepatocellular carcinoma; *OCP,* oral contraceptives. (Modified from Goldman L, Ausiello D [eds]: *Cecil textbook of medicine,* ed 23, Philadelphia, 2008, WB Saunders.)

ICD-9CM # 070.9

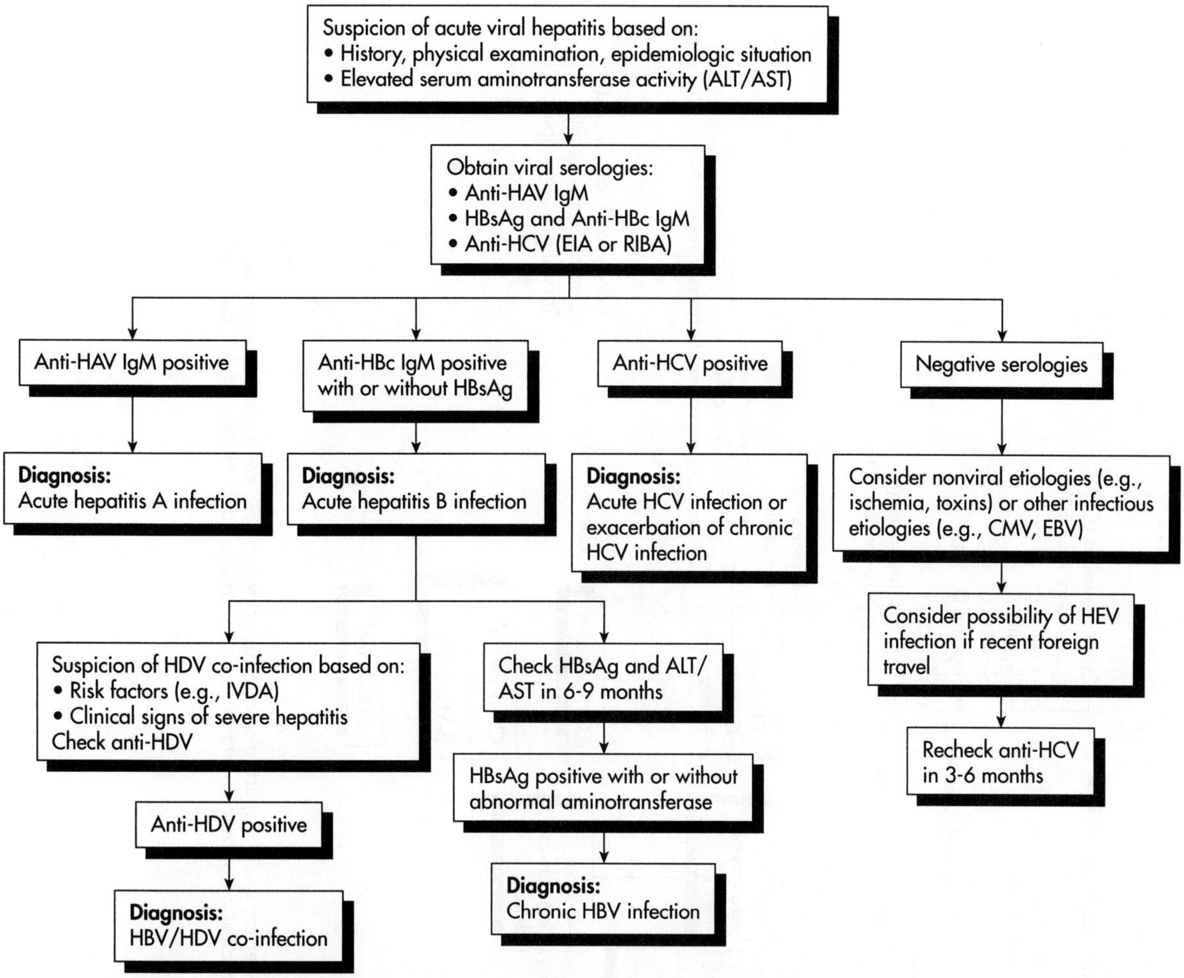

FIGURE 3-125 A flow diagram showing the use of specific serologic tests for the diagnosis of acute viral hepatitis in relation to the clinical and epidemiologic setting. Co-infections and superinfections of chronic hepatitis B or C patients should always be considered in cases that do not fit well with the clinical or serologic picture. *CMV,* Cytomegalovirus; *EBV,* Epstein-Barr virus; *EIA,* enzyme immunoassay; *HBV,* hepatitis B virus; *HCV,* hepatitis C virus; *HDV,* hepatitis D virus; *HEV,* hepatoencephalomyelitis virus; *IVDA,* intravenous drug abuse; *RIBA,* recombinant immunoblot assay. (From Mandell GL: *Mandell, Douglas, and Bennett's principles and practice of infectious diseases,* ed 6, New York, 2005, Churchill Livingstone.)

HEPATOMEGALY

ICD-9CM # 789.1

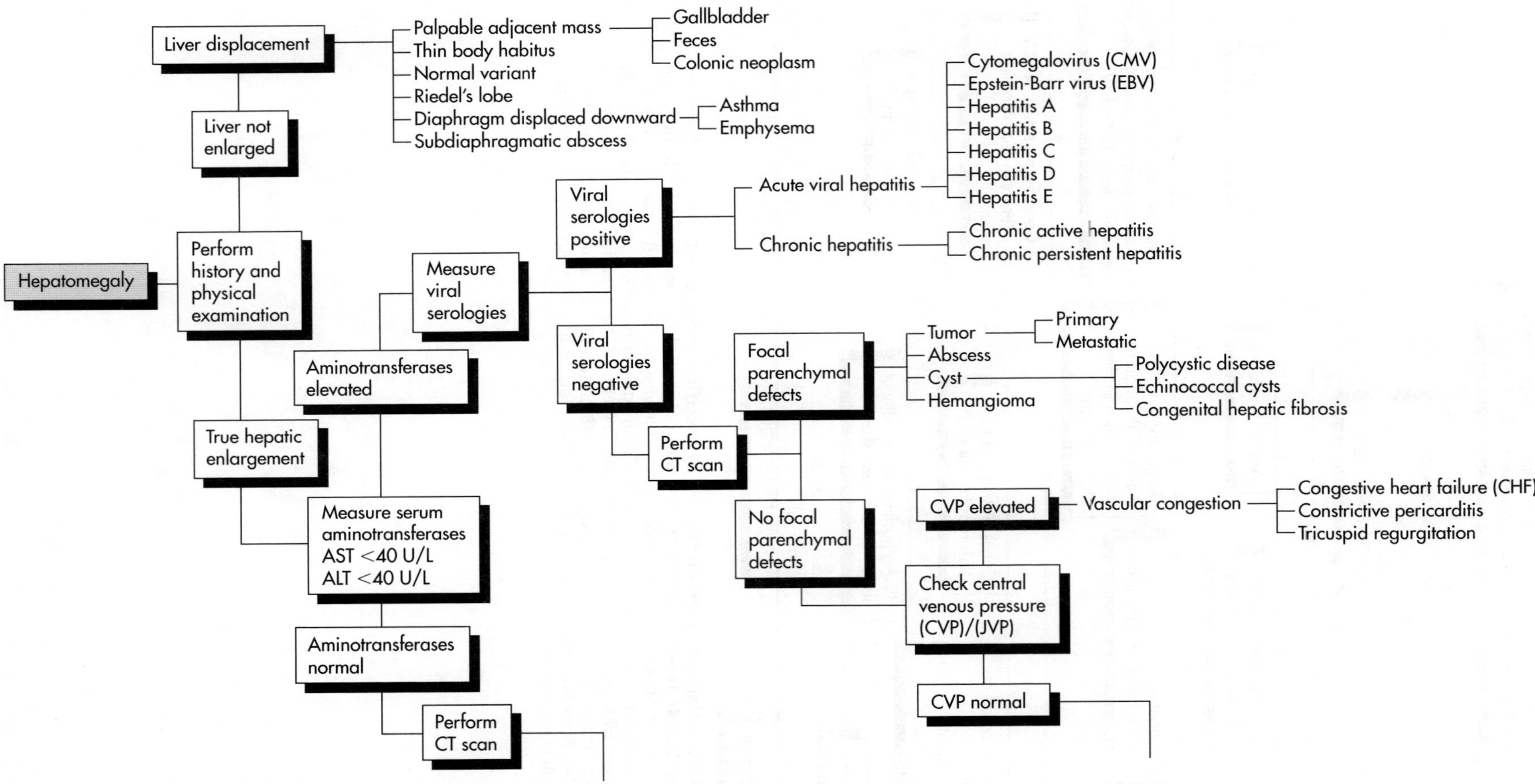

Figure 3-126 Hepatomegaly. *ALT,* Alanine aminotransferase; *AST,* aspartate aminotransferase; *CT,* computed tomography; *JVP,* jugular venous pressure. (From Healey PM: *Common medical diagnosis: an algorithmic approach,* ed 3, Philadelphia, 2000, WB Saunders.)

HEPATOMEGALY—cont'd

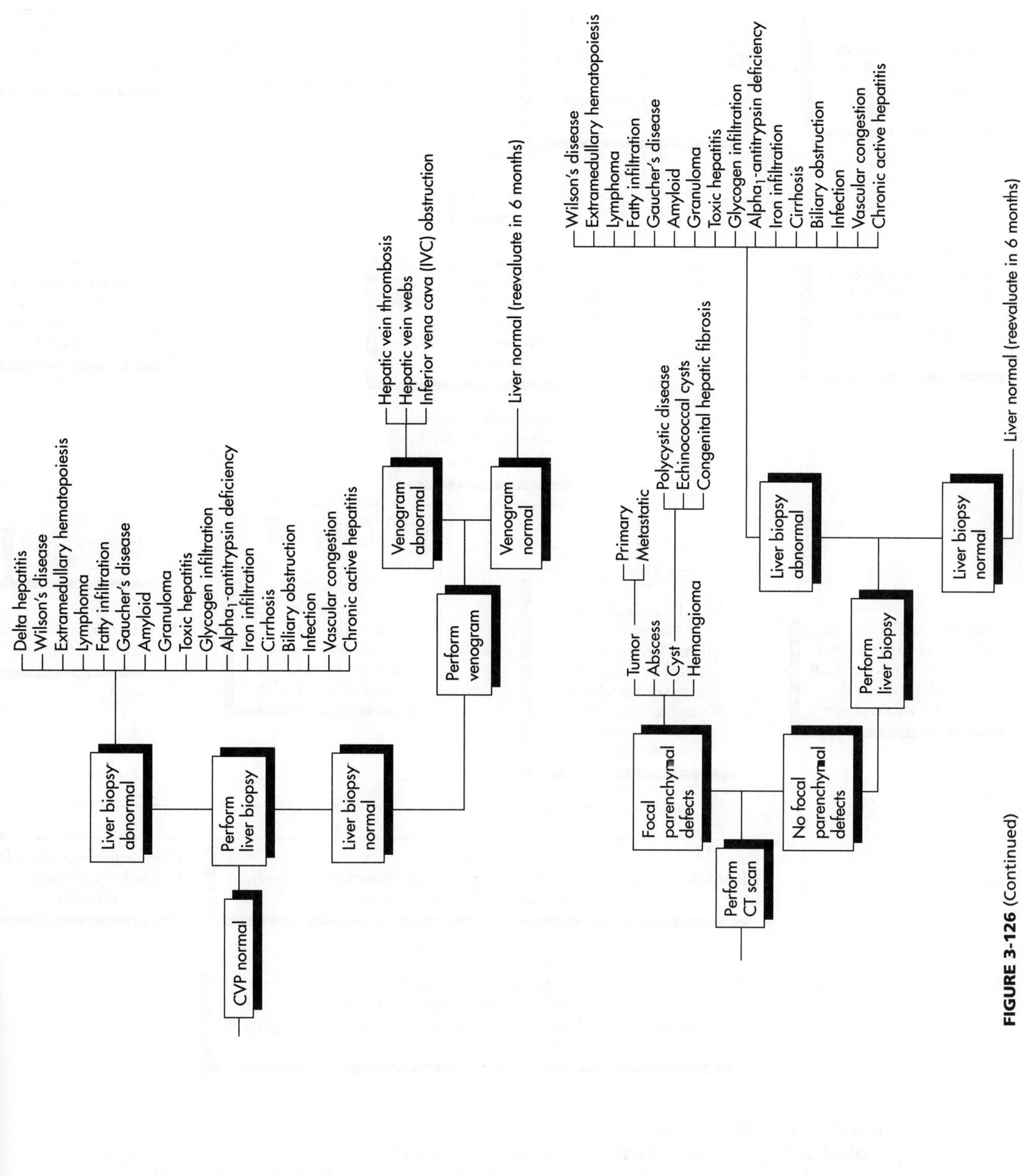

FIGURE 3-126 (Continued)

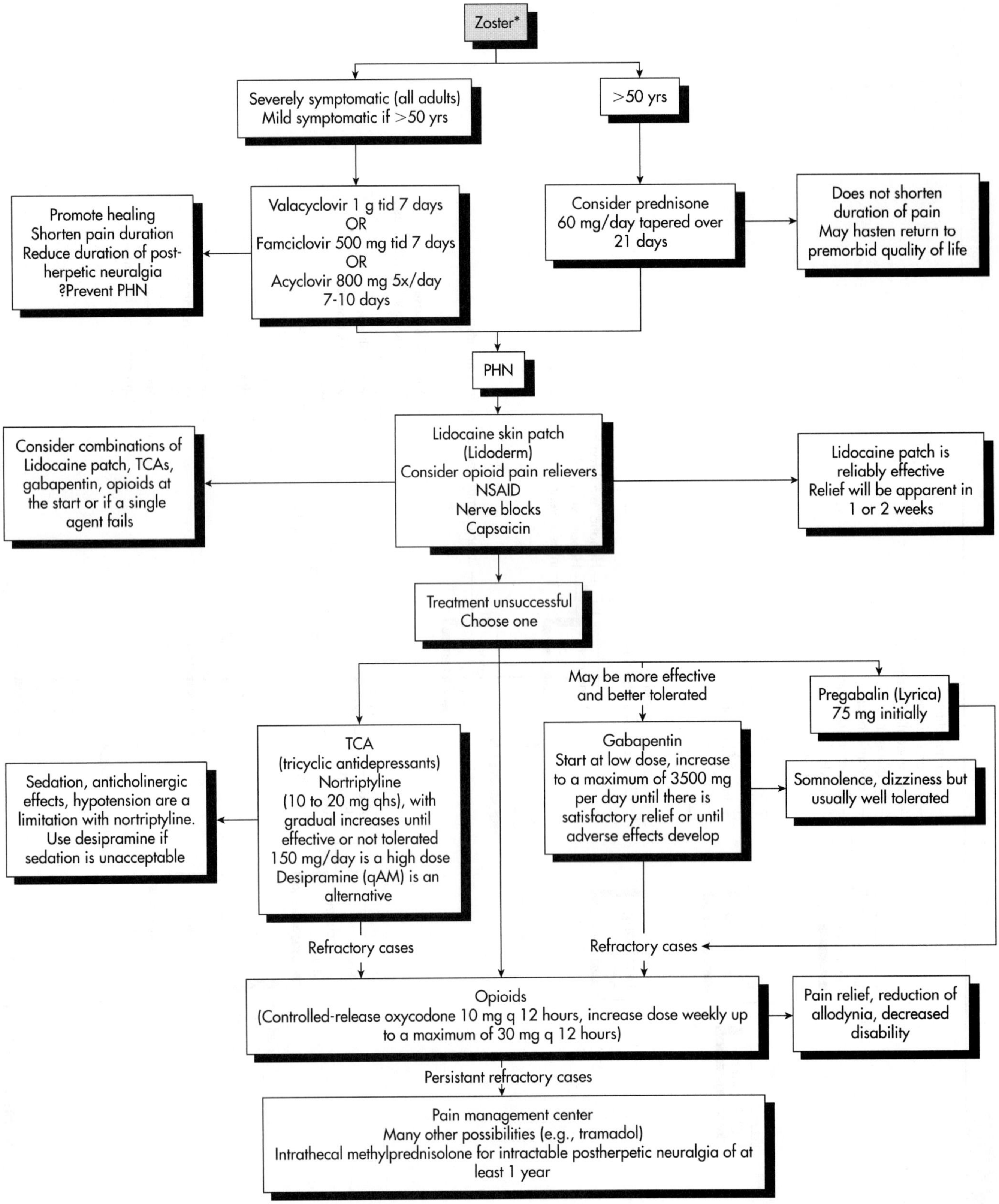

*Refer to Section I for additional information on this topic.

FIGURE 3-127 Treatment of herpes zoster and postherpetic neuralgia. *PHN,* Postherpetic neuralgia; *TCA,* tricyclic antidepressant; *NSAID,* nonsteroidal anti-inflammatory drug. (Modified from Habif TA: *Clinical dermatology,* ed 4, St Louis, 2004, Mosby.)

HIGH-ALTITUDE PULMONARY EDEMA

ICD-9CM # 289 Mountain sickness, acute
993.2 High altitude, effects

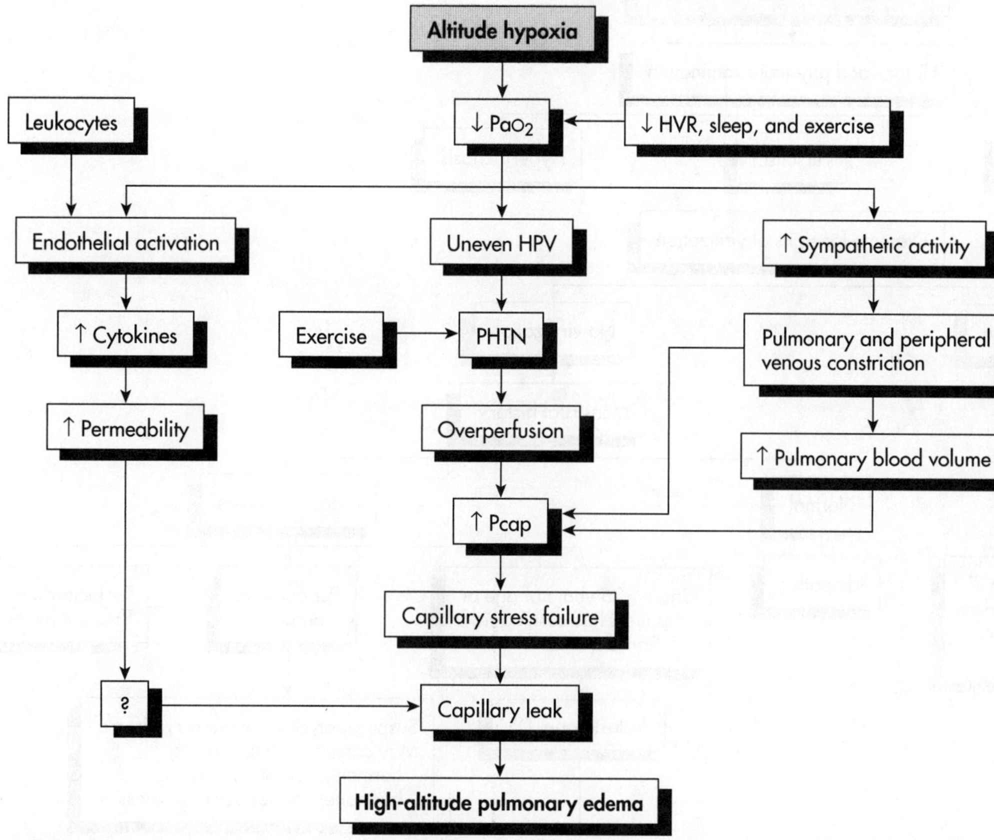

FIGURE 3-128 Proposed pathophysiology of high-altitude pulmonary edema. *HPV,* Hypoxic pulmonary vasoconstriction; *HVR,* hypoxic ventilatory response; *Pcap,* capillary pressure; *PHTN,* pulmonary hypertension. (From Auerbach PS: *Wilderness medicine,* ed 5, St Louis, 2007, Mosby.)

ICD-9CM # 704.1

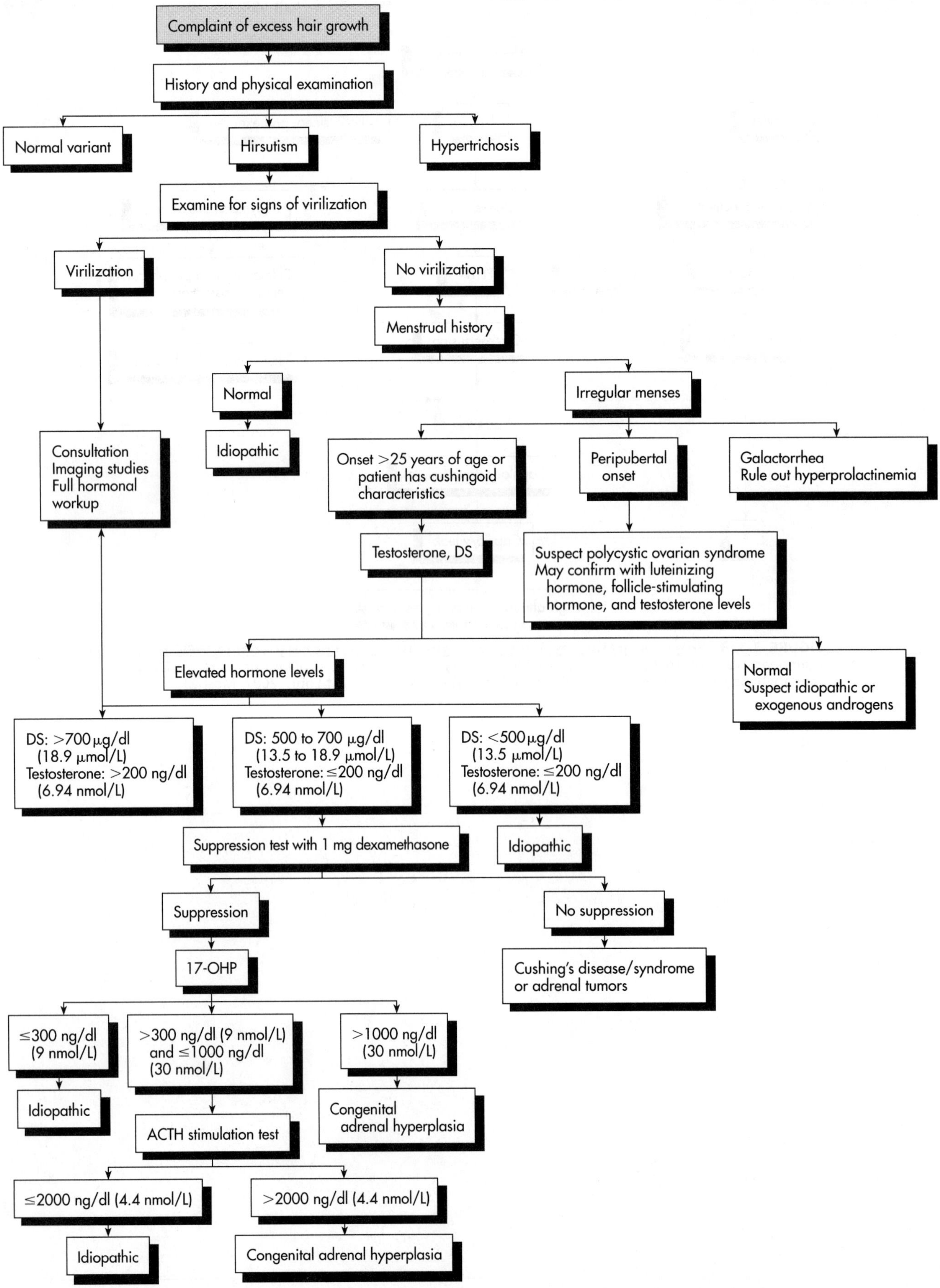

FIGURE 3-129 Algorithm showing the evaluation and treatment of hirsutism. *ACTH,* Adrenocorticotropic hormone; *DS,* dehydroepiandrosterone; *17-OHP,* 17-hydroxyprogesterone. (From Gilchrist VJ, Hecht BR: *Am Fam Physician* 52:1837, 1995.)

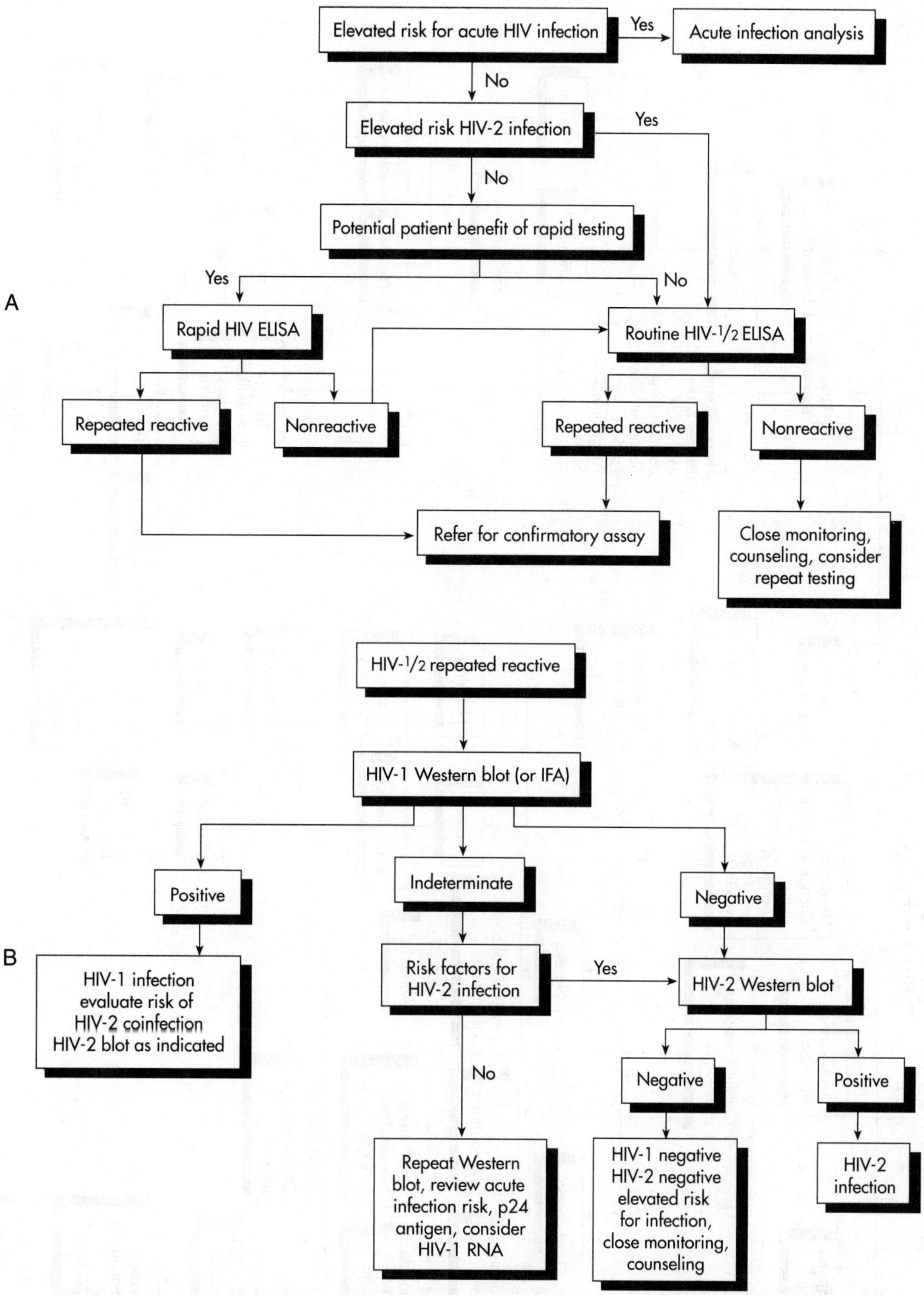

FIGURE 3-130 Algorithm for HIV detection in patients at risk for HIV infection. Note that in the absence of documented infection, all individuals with HIV risk factors should be monitored and followed as indicated with routine testing. **A,** Screening algorithm. HIV screening should be considered for all patients at elevated risk for infection. The choice of screening test may be guided by clinical circumstances. **B,** Confirmation algorithm. Negative and indeterminate results require discussion and consideration for alternative possibilities, especially the presence of acute HIV infection. (From Mandell GL, Bennett JE, Dolin R: *Principles and practice of infectious diseases,* ed 6, Philadelphia, 2005, Churchill Livingstone.)

HIV-INFECTED PATIENT, ACUTELY ILL

ICD-9CM # 789.1

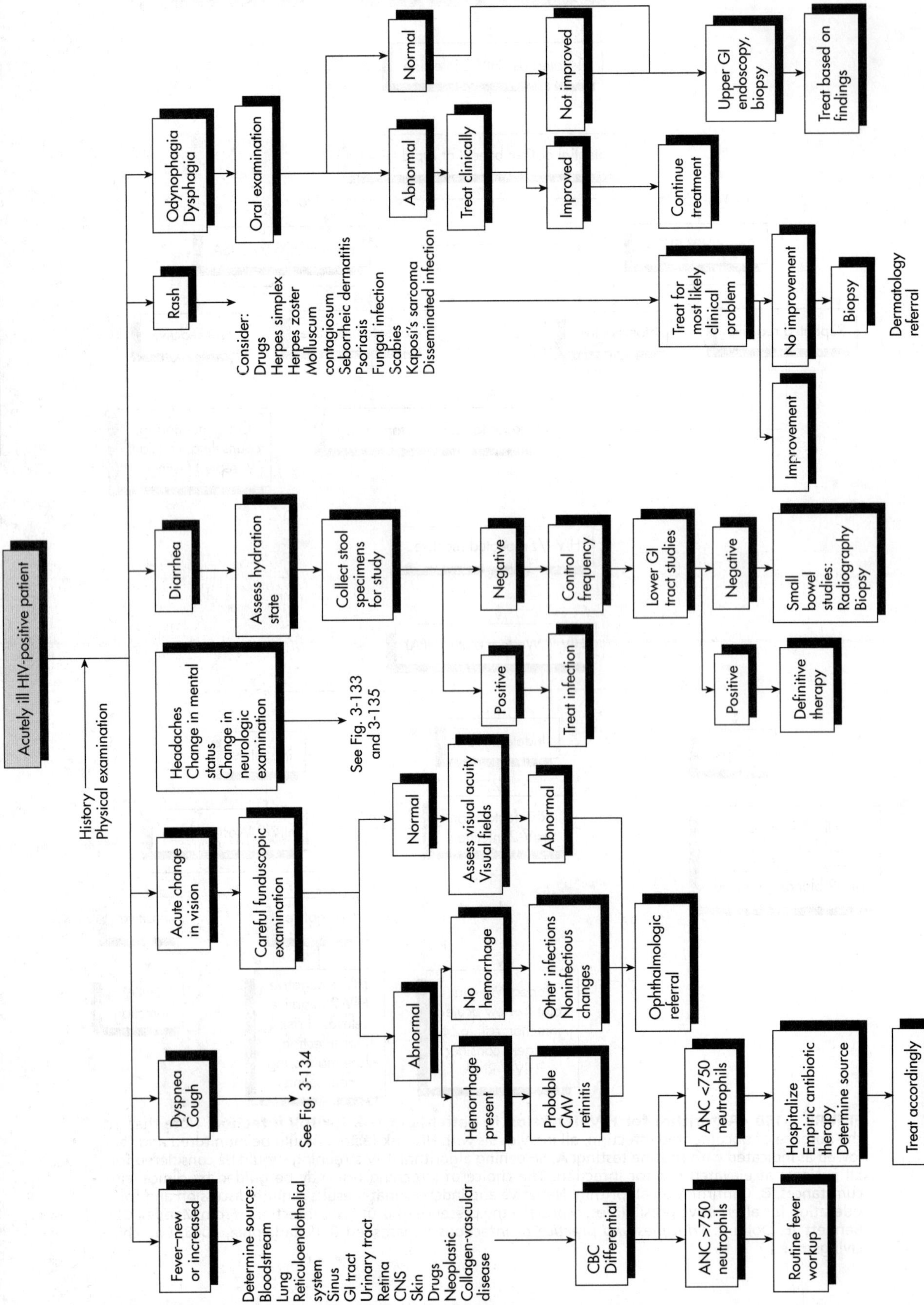

FIGURE 3-131 Acutely ill HIV-positive patient. *ANC,* Absolute neutrophil count; *CBC,* complete blood count; *CMV,* cytomegalovirus; *CNS,* central nervous system; *GI,* gastrointestinal. (Modified from Greene HL, Johnson WP, Lemcke D [eds]: *Decision making in medicine,* ed 2, St Louis, 1998, Mosby.)

HIV-INFECTED PATIENT, CARDIAC DYSFUNCTION

ICD-9CM # 861.00

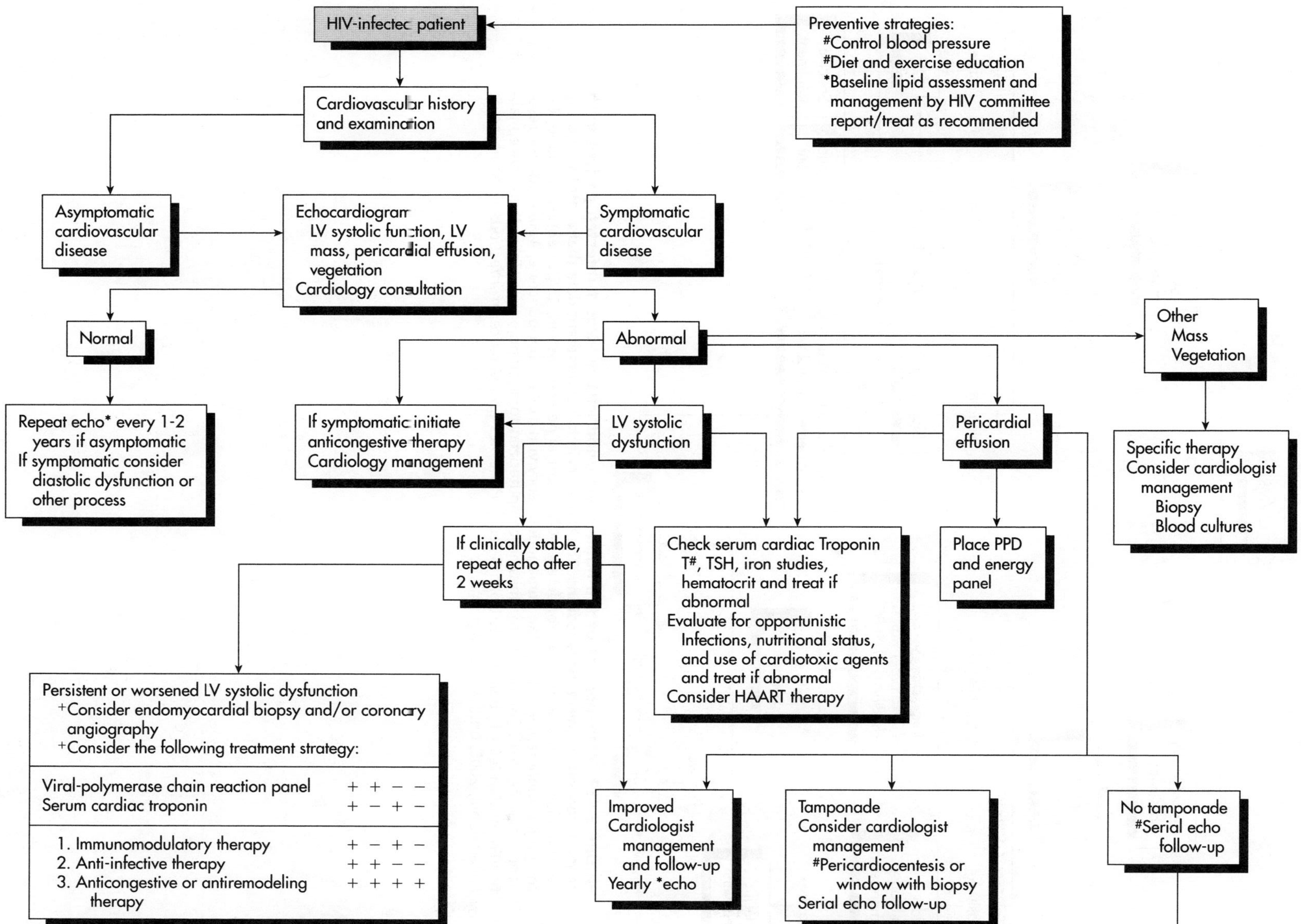

Legend:
*Evidence based
#Non-HIV standard of care data
+Thought for future research

FIGURE 3-132 :ardiac dysfunction in HIV-infected patients. *HAART,* Highly active antiretroviral therapy; *LV,* left ventricular; *PPD,* purified protein derivative; *TSH,* thyroid stimulating hormone. (From Dolin R, Masur H, Saag MS [eds]: *A DS therapy,* ed 2, New York, 2003, Churchill Livingstone.)

ICD-9CM # 042

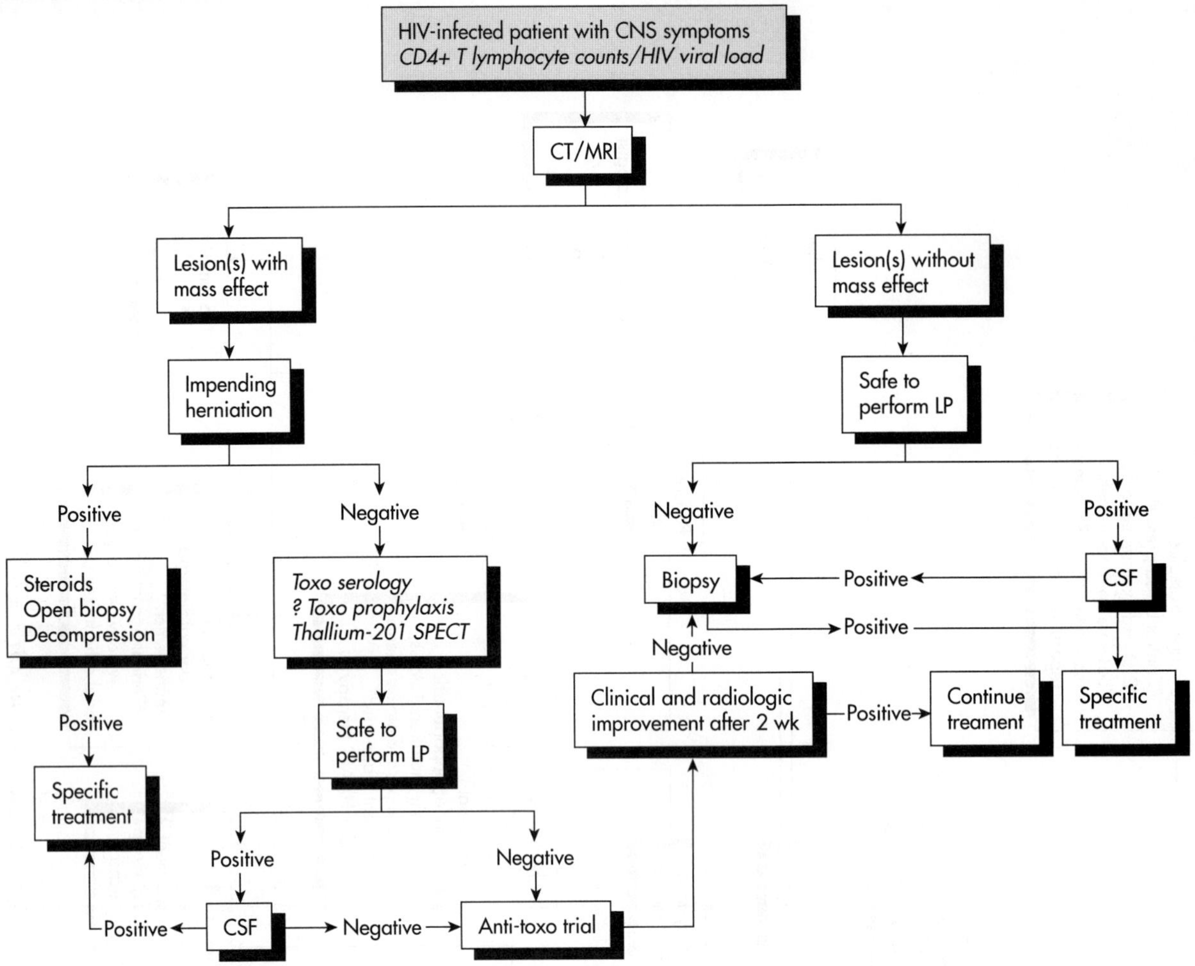

FIGURE 3-133 Management of the human immunodficiency virus 1–infected patient with central nervous system mass lesions. The elements in italics represent data that contribute to the decision-making process (see text for details). *CNS,* Central nervous system; *CSF,* cerebrospinal fluid; *CT,* computed tomography; *HIV,* human immunodeficiency virus; *LP,* lumbar puncture; *MRI,* magnetic resonance imaging; *SPECT,* single photo emission computerized tomography; *toxo, Toxoplasma* encephalitis. (From Mandell GL, Bennett JE, Dolin R [eds]: *Principles and practice of infectious diseases,* ed 6, Philadelphia, 2005, Churchill Livingstone.)

HIV-INFECTED PATIENT WITH RESPIRATORY COMPLAINTS

ICD-9CM # 042 HIV infection, symptomatic

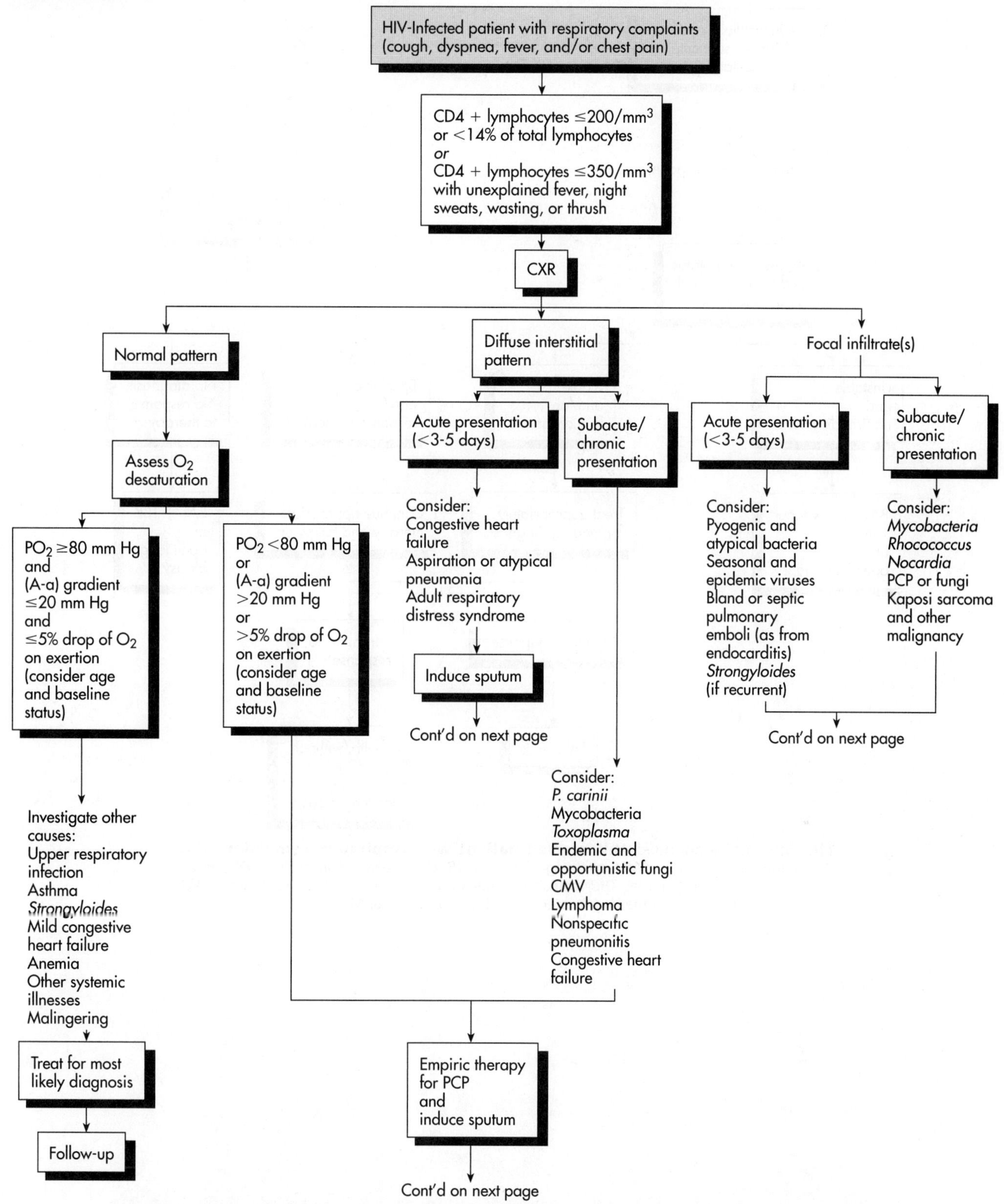

FIGURE 3-134 HIV-infected patient with respiratory complaints. *BAL,* Bronchoalveolar lavage; *CMV,* cytomegalovirus; *CXR,* chest x-ray examination; *PCP, Pneumocystis carinii* pneumonia; *TBB,* transbronchial biopsy. (From Greene HL, Johnson WP, Lemcke D [eds]: *Decision making in medicine,* 2, St Louis, 1998, Mosby.)

Continued on following page

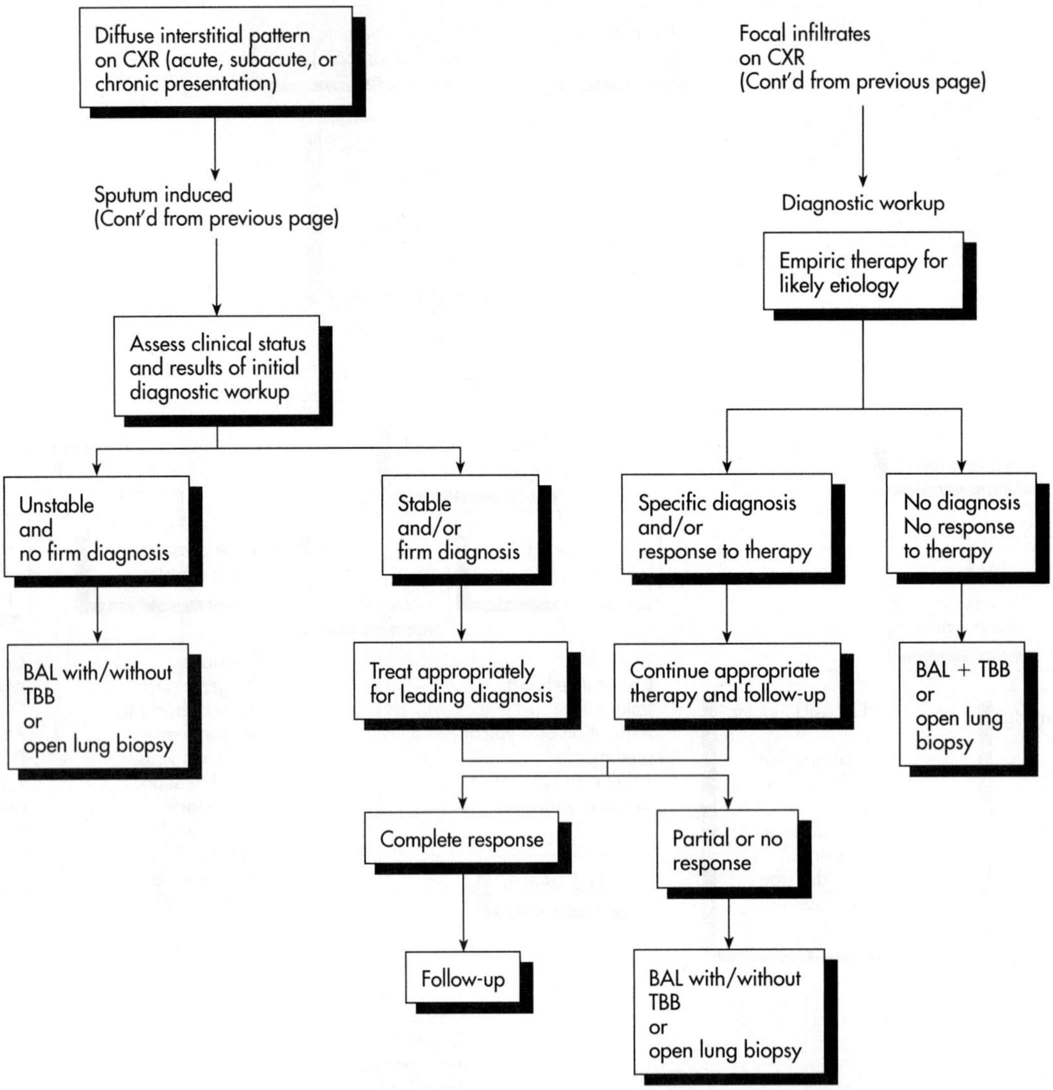

FIGURE 3-134 (Continued) **HIV-infected patient with respiratory complaints.** *BAL,* Bronchoalveolar lavage; *CMV,* cytomegalovirus; *CXR,* chest x-ray examination; *PCP, Pneumocystis carinii* pneumonia; *TBB,* transbronchial biopsy. (From Greene HL, Johnson WP, Lemcke D [eds]: *Decision making in medicine,* 2, St Louis, 1998, Mosby.)

HIV-INFECTED PATIENT WITH SUSPECTED CENTRAL NERVOUS SYSTEM INFECTION

ICD-9CM # 042 HIV infection, symptomatic

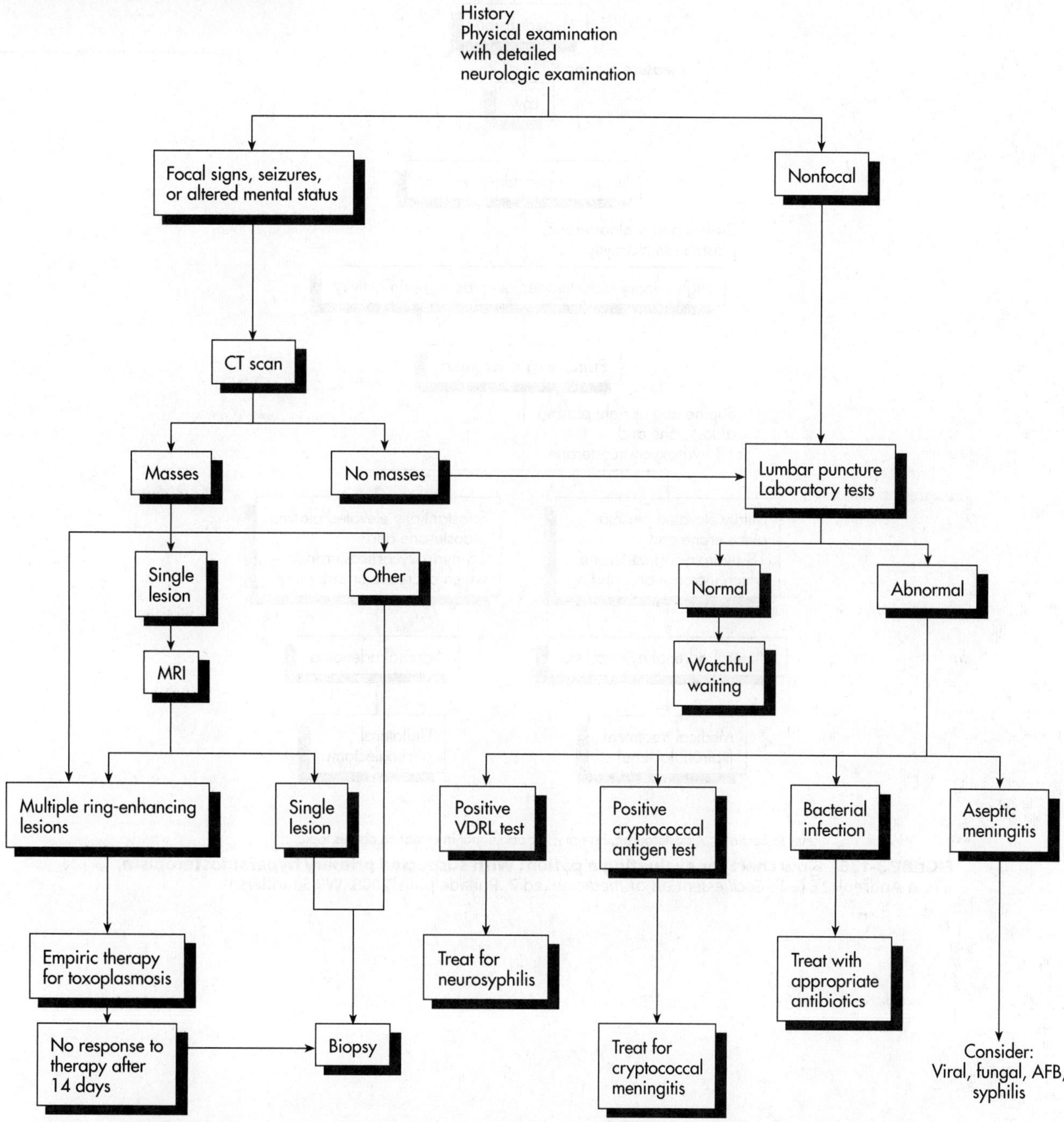

FIGURE 3-135 HIV-positive patient with suspected central nervous system infection. *AFB,* Acid-fast bacilli; *CNS,* central nervous system; *CT,* computed tomography; *MRI,* magnetic resonance imaging; *VDRL,* Venereal Disease Research Laboratory. (From Greene HL, Johnson WP, Lemcke D [eds]: *Decision making in medicine,* ed 2, St Louis, 1998, Mosby.)

ICD-9CM # 255.1 Primary aldosteronism

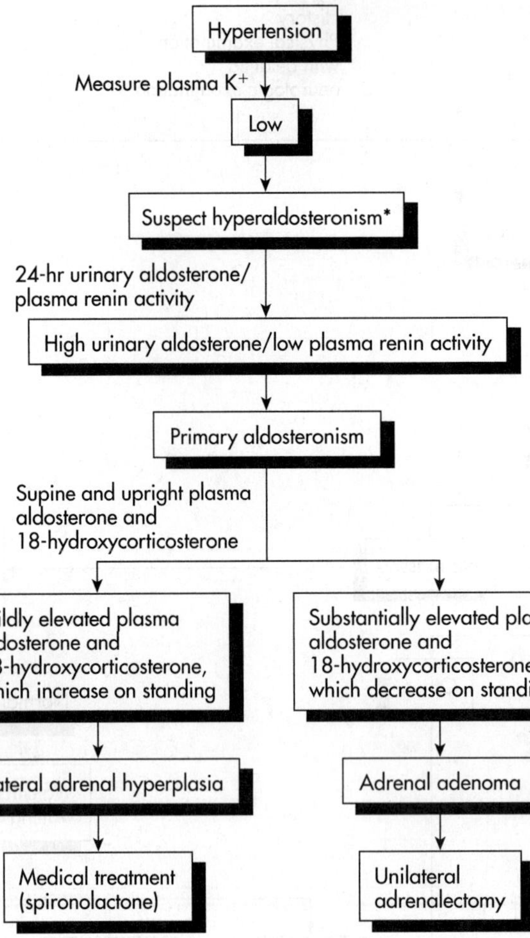

*Refer to Section I, Aldosteronism, Primary, for additional information on this topic.

FIGURE 3-136 Flow chart for evaluating a patient with suspected primary hyperaldosteronism. (From Andreoli TE [ed]: *Cecil essentials of medicine,* ed 7, Philadelphia, 2008, WB Saunders.)

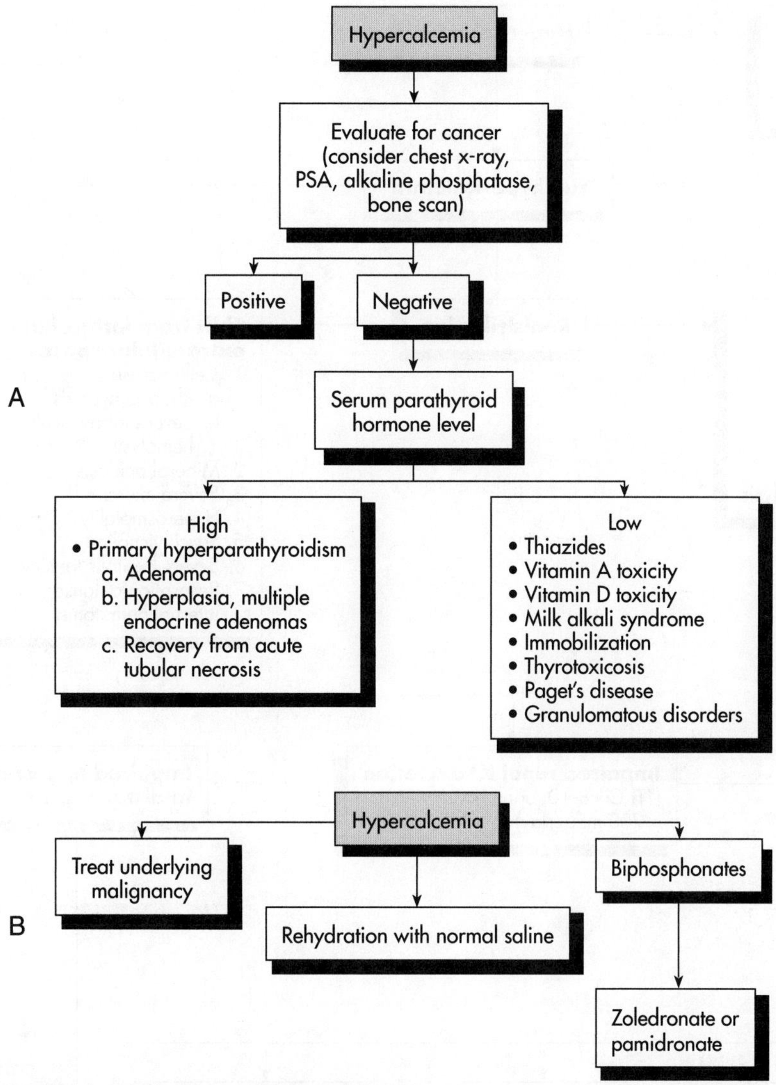

FIGURE 3-137 A, Evaluation of hypercalcemia. *PSA,* Prostate-specific antigen. **B, Therapy for hypercalcemia.** *IM,* Intramuscularly; *IV,* intravenously.

ICD-9CM # 276.7

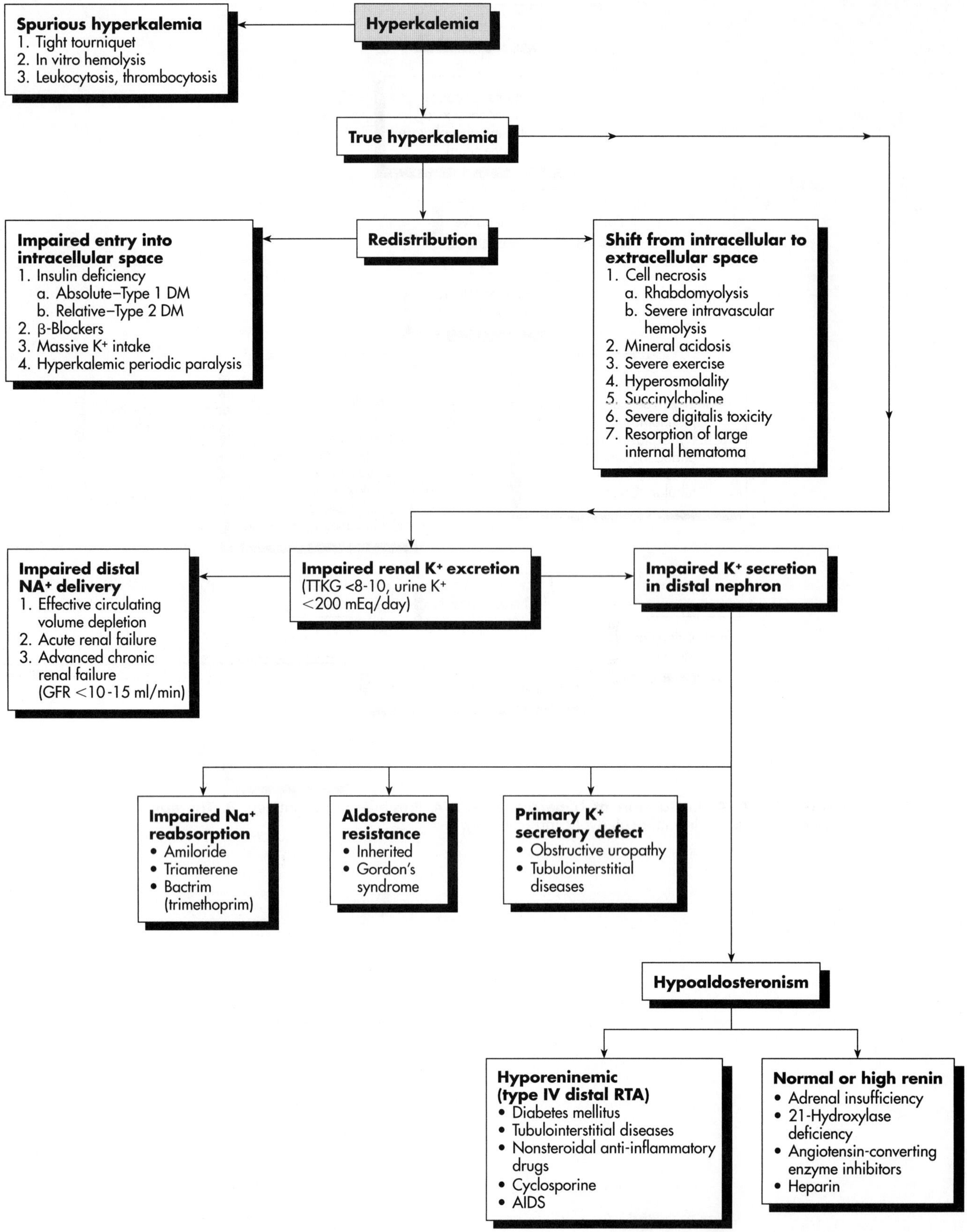

Hyperkalemia
Spurious hyperkalemia
1. Tight tourniquet
2. In vitro hemolysis
3. Leukocytosis, thrombocytosis
True hyperkalemia
Redistribution
Impaired entry into intracellular space
1. Insulin deficiency
a. Absolute–Type 1 DM
b. Relative–Type 2 DM
2. β-Blockers
3. Massive K+ intake
4. Hyperkalemic periodic paralysis
Shift from intracellular to extracellular space
1. Cell necrosis
a. Rhabdomyolysis
b. Severe intravascular hemolysis
2. Mineral acidosis
3. Severe exercise
4. Hyperosmolality
5. Succinylcholine
6. Severe digitalis toxicity
7. Resorption of large internal hematoma
Impaired distal NA+ delivery
1. Effective circulating volume depletion
2. Acute renal failure
3. Advanced chronic renal failure (GFR <10-15 ml/min)
Impaired renal K+ excretion (TTKG <8-10, urine K+ <200 mEq/day)
Impaired K+ secretion in distal nephron
Impaired Na+ reabsorption
• Amiloride
• Triamterene
• Bactrim (trimethoprim)
Aldosterone resistance
• Inherited
• Gordon's syndrome
Primary K+ secretory defect
• Obstructive uropathy
• Tubulointerstitial diseases
Hypoaldosteronism
Hyporeninemic (type IV distal RTA)
• Diabetes mellitus
• Tubulointerstitial diseases
• Nonsteroidal anti-inflammatory drugs
• Cyclosporine
• AIDS
Normal or high renin
• Adrenal insufficiency
• 21-Hydroxylase deficiency
• Angiotensin-converting enzyme inhibitors
• Heparin

FIGURE 3-138 Diagnostic approach to hyperkalemia. *AIDS,* Acquired immunodeficiency syndrome; *DM,* diabetes mellitus; *GFR,* glomerular filtration rate; *RTA,* renal tubular acidosis; *TTKG,* transtubular potassium gradient. (From Andreoli TE [ed]: *Cecil essentials of medicine,* ed 7, Philadelphia, 2008, WB Saunders.)

HYPERKALEMIA, EVALUATION AND TREATMENT

ICD-9CM # 276.7

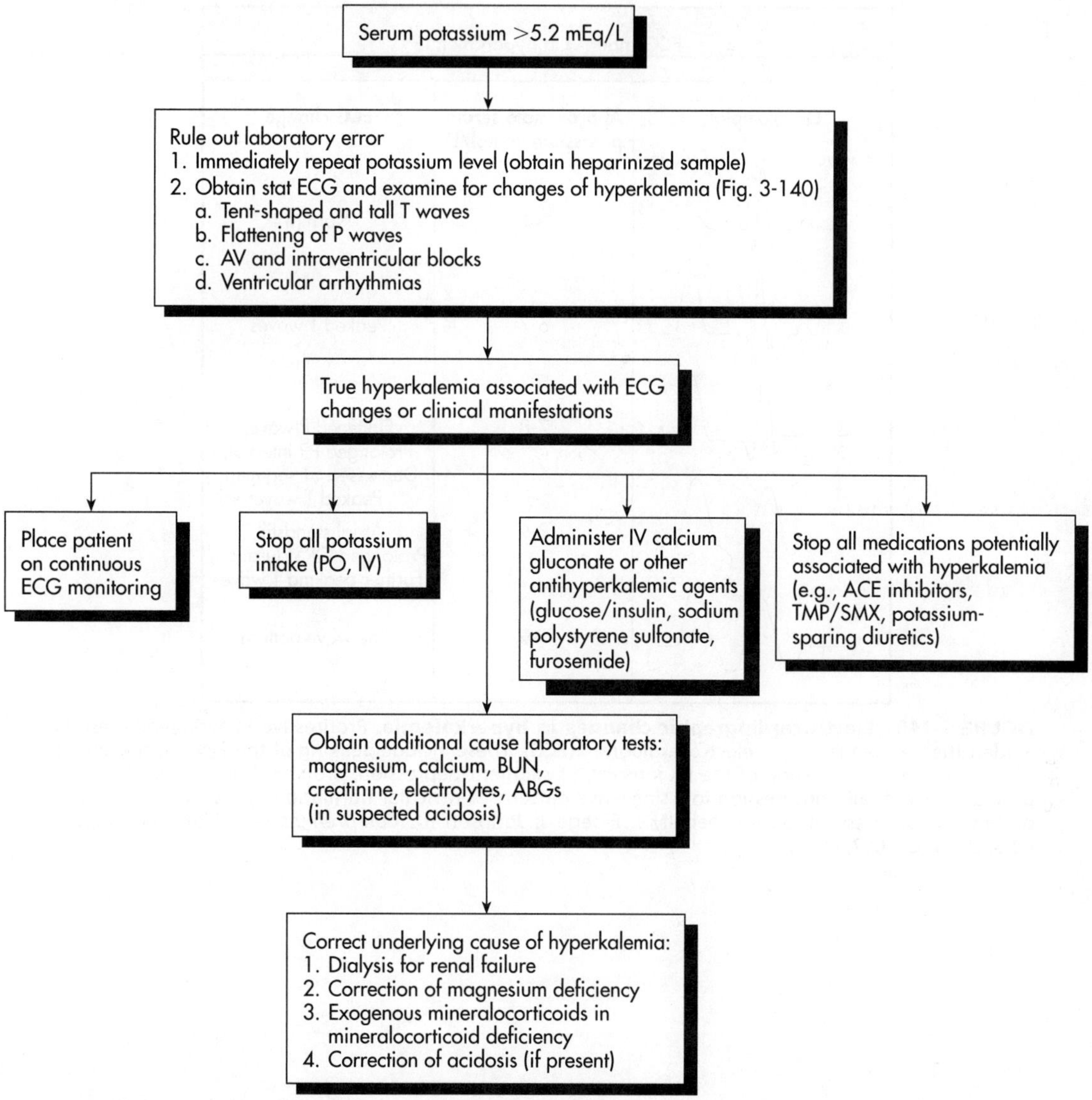

FIGURE 3-139 Evaluation and treatment of hyperkalemia. *ABGs,* Arterial blood gases; *ACE,* angiotensin-converting enzyme; *AV,* atrioventricular; *BUN,* blood urea nitrogen; *ECG,* electrocardiogram; *IV,* intravenous; *PO,* oral; *TMP/SMX,* trimethoprim-sulfamethoxazole. (From Ferri F: *Practical guide to the care of the medical patient,* ed 7, St Louis, 2007, Mosby.)

Continued on following page

ECG changes in hyperkalemia

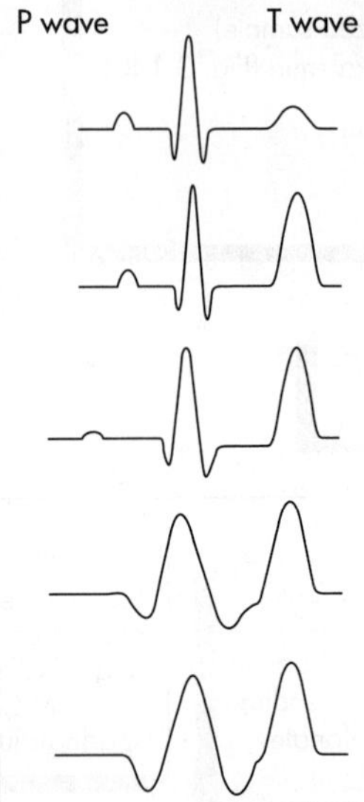

QRS complex	Approximate serum potassium (mmol/L)	ECG change
	~4	Normal
	6-7	Peaked T waves
	7-8	Flattened P wave, Prolonged PR interval, Depressed ST segment, Peaked T wave
	8-9	Atrial standstill, Prolonged QRS duration, Further peaking T waves
	>9	Sine wave pattern

FIGURE 3-140 Electrocardiographic changes in hyperkalemia. Progressive hyperkalemia results in identifiable changes in the electrocardiogram (ECG). These include peaking of the T wave, flattening of the P wave, prolongation of the PR interval, ST segment depression, prolongation of the QRS complex, and, eventually, progression to a sine wave pattern. Ventricular fibrillation may occur at any time during this progression. (From Feehally J, Floege J, Johnson RJ: *Comprehensive clinical nephrology,* ed 3, St Louis, 2007, Mosby.)

HYPERMAGNESEMIA

ICD-9CM # 275.2

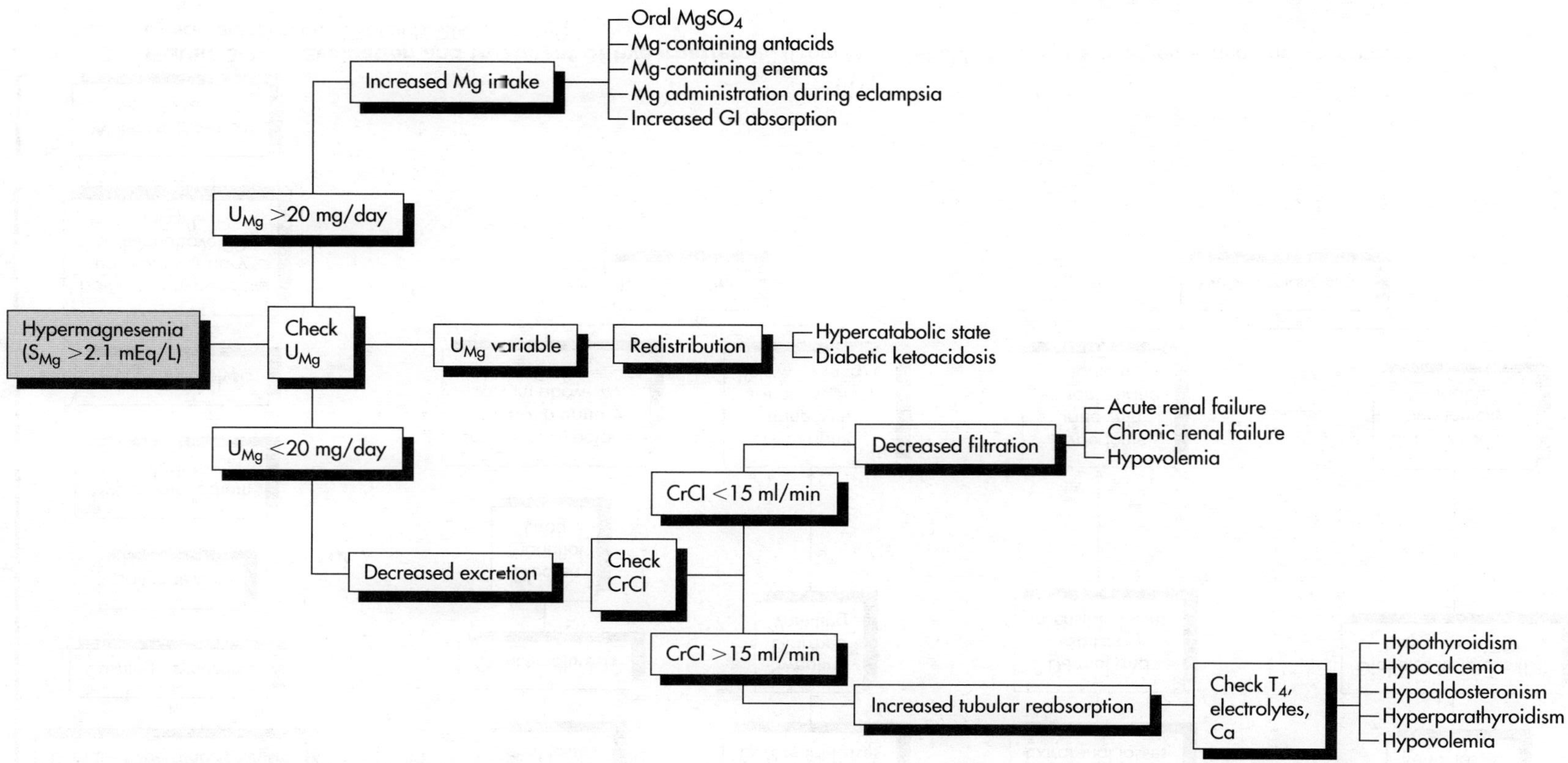

FIGURE 3-141 **Hypermagnesemia** *CrCl,* Creatinine clearance; *GI,* gastrointestinal; *MgSO,* magnesium sulfate. (From Healey PM: *Common medical diagnosis: an algorithmic approach,* ed 3, Philadelphia, 2000, WB Saunders.)

HYPERNATREMIA

ICD-9CM # 276.0

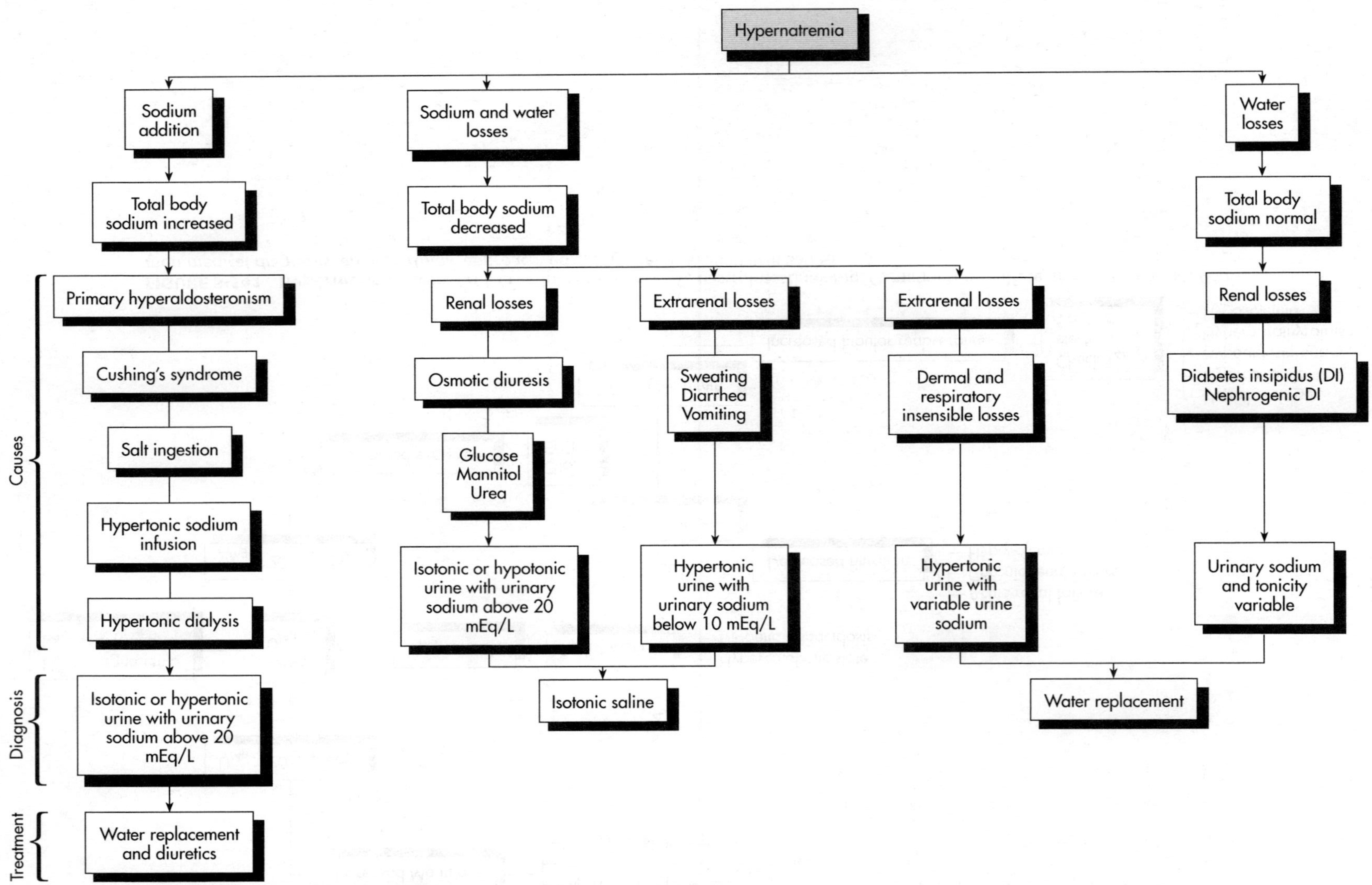

FIGURE 3-142 Evaluation and treatment of hypernatremia. (From Marx J et al [eds]: *Rosen's emergency medicine: concepts and clinical practice,* ed 6, St Louis, 2006, Mosby.)

HYPERPHOSPHATEMIA

ICD-9CM # 995.5 Child Maltreatment Syndrome

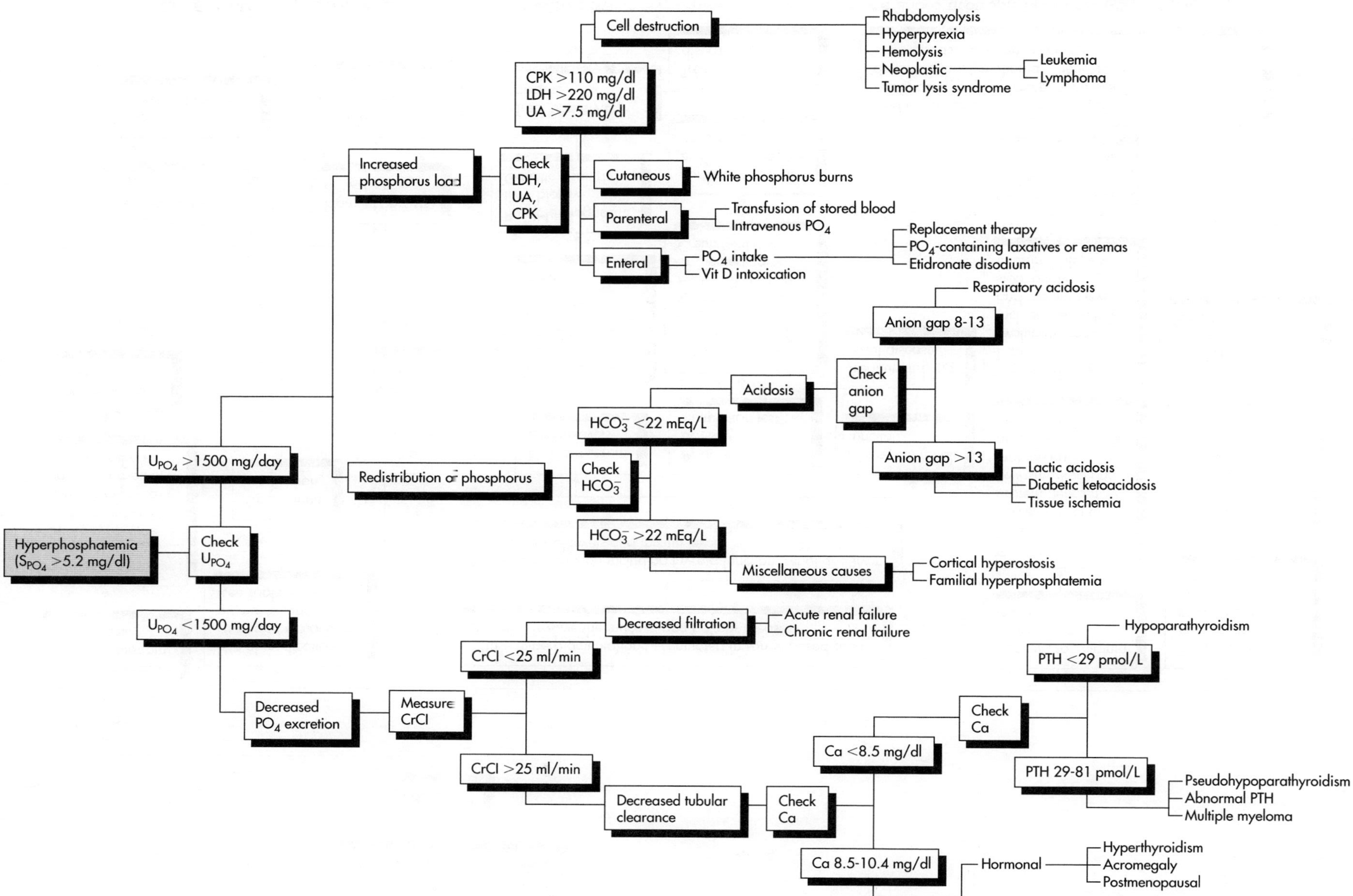

FIGURE 3-143 Approach to hyperphosphatemia. *CT,* Computerized tomography; *MRI,* magnetic resonance imaging; *T,* thyroxine; *TSH,* thyroid-stimulating hormone. (From Healey PM: *Common medical diagnosis: An algorithmic approach,* ed 3, Philadelphia, 2000, WB Saunders.)

HYPERPIGMENTATION

ICD-9CM # 709.00

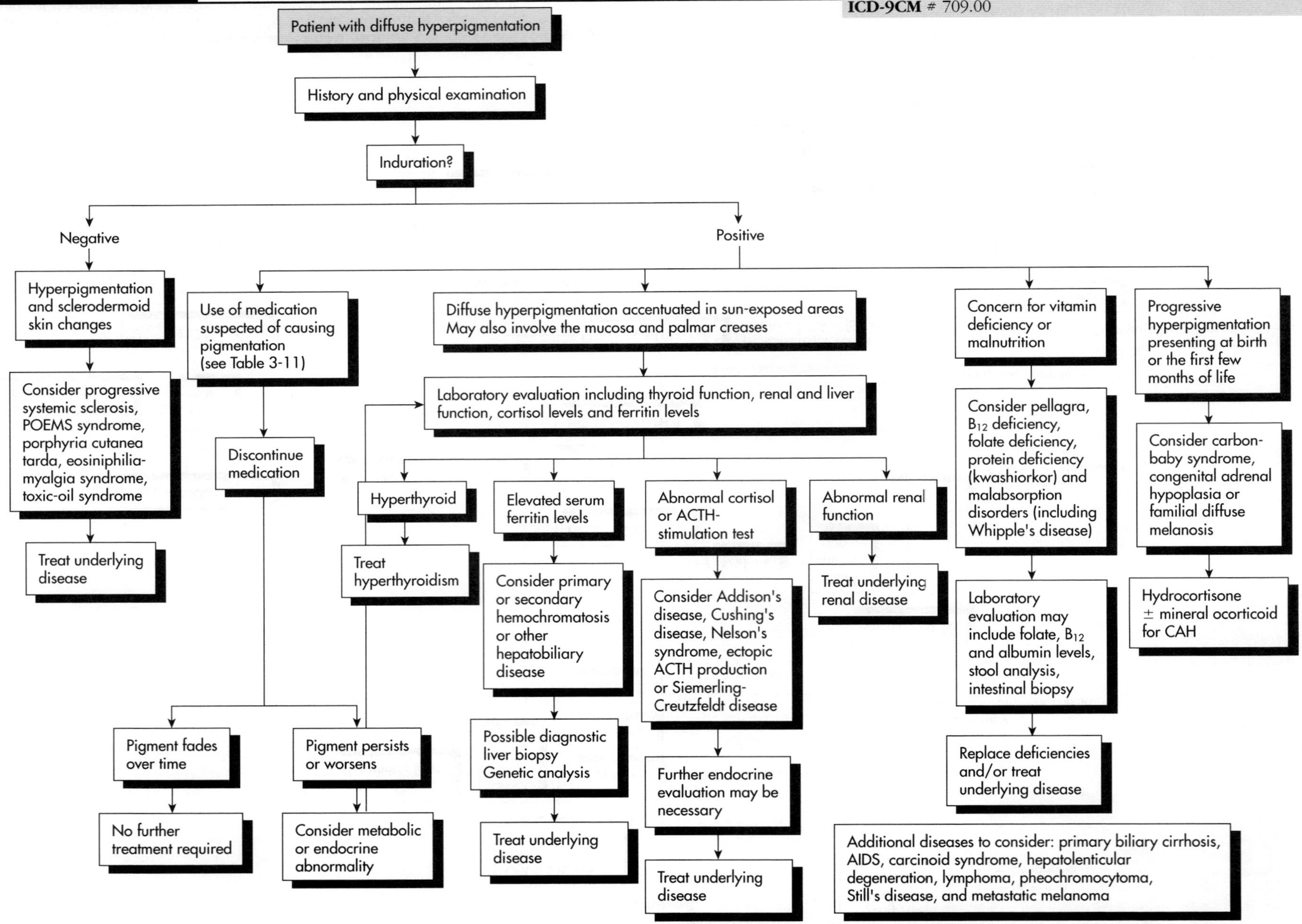

FIGURE 3-144 Approach to the adult patient with diffuse hyperpigmentation. *ACTH,* Adrenocorticotropic hormone; *AIDS,* acquired immunodeficiency syndrome; *CAH,* congenital adrenal hyperplasia; POEMS, polyneuropathy, organomegaly, endocrinopathies, monoclonal gammopathy, skin changes. (From Bolognia JL, Mascaro JM, Mancini AJ, Salasche SJ, Saurat JH, Stingl G [eds]: *Dermatology,* ed 2, St Louis, 2008, Mosby.)

TABLE 3-11 **Drugs and Chemicals Associated with Hyperpigmentation**

DRUG OR CHEMICAL	CLINICAL FEATURES	HISTOPATHOLOGY/COMMENT
Cancer chemotherapeutic agents		
BCNU (Topical)	• Hyperpigmentation at site of application (no reaction seen with parenteral administration)	• Hyperplasia of basal melanocytes consistent with postinflammatory hyperpigmentation
Bleomycin	• Linear, flagellate bands, associated with minor trauma • Nails may be involved • Hyperpigmentation overlying joints	• Increased epidermal melanin • Little dermal pigment incontinence • No increase in epidermal melanocytes
Busulfan	• Generalized hyperpigmentation resembling Addison's disease; sometimes seen in association with drug-induced pulmonary fibrosis	• Increased melanin in basal keratinocytes and in dermal macrophages
Cyclophosphamide	• Diffuse hyperpigmentation of the skin and mucous membranes • Localized pigment of the nails (transverse or longitudinal bands), palms and soles, or teeth	• Pigmentation usually regresses within 6 to 12 months after therapy is discontinued
Dactinomycin	• Generalized hyperpigmentation, most prominent on the face	• Pigmentation fades after treatment discontinued
Daunorubicin	• Hyperpigmentation of light-exposed areas • Transverse brown-black nail bands	• Structurally similar to doxorubicin
Doxorubicin	• Pigmentation of the nails; hyperpigmentation of the palmar creases, palms, soles, buccal mucosa, dorsae of the knuckles and tongue	• Increased epidermal melanin • Increased number of melanocytes
5-Fluorouracil	• Hyperpigmentation in sun-exposed areas • Increased pigmentation of skin overlying veins used for infusion, dorsae of the hands and trunk	• Synergistic hyperpigmentation of irradiation portal sites
Hydroxyurea	• Reversible hyperpigmentation over pressure points and the back • Nails may be involved	• Lichenoid eruption with secondary hyperpigmentation
Mechlorethamine (nitrogen mustard)	• Topical use for cutaneous lymphoma may result in generalized hyperpigmentation • More intense in lesional skin	• Disaggregation of melanosomes within keratinocytes • Increased number of melanocytes
Methotrexate	• Uniform hyperpigmentation in sun-exposed areas	• Uncommon • May be postinflammatory hyperpigmentation secondary to photosensitivity reaction
Antimalarials		
Amino quinolones (chloroquine, hydroxychloroquine, amodiaquine)	• Yellow-brown or gray to blue-black pigment, usually in pretibial areas; face, hard palate, and subungual areas may be involved	• Dyspigmentation in up to 25% of patients • Dermal deposition of melanin-drug complexes; hemosiderin around capillaries • May fade, but rarely resolves, upon discontinuation of drug
Heavy metals		
Arsenic	• Areas of bronze hyperpigmentation ± superimposed raindrops • Keratoses on the palms and soles associated with pigmentation	• May appear 1–20 years after exposure • Dermal and epidermal deposition of arsenic • Increased epidermal melanin synthesis
Bismuth	• Generalized blue-gray discoloration of face, neck, dorsal hands • Oral mucosa and gingivae may be involved	• Bismuth granules in the papillary and reticular dermis
Gold	• Permanent blue-gray discoloration in sun-exposed areas, mostly around the eyes (chrysiasis)	• Gold particles within macrophage lysosomes in the dermis
Iron	• Permanent brown pigment at injection or application sites	• Pigment coats collagen fibers and is deposited in dermal macrophages
Lead	• 'Lead line' in gingival margin • Nail pigmentation	• Lead line is due to subepithelial deposition of lead granules
Mercury	• Slate-gray pigmentation, particularly in skin folds	• Brown-black granules free in dermis, in association with elastic fibers, and within macrophages
Silver	• Generalized slate-gray pigmentation, increased in sun-exposed areas • Nails and sclerae may also be involved • Localized at sites of application	• Silver granules in the basement membrane and on the membrana propria of eccrine glands

Continued on following page

TABLE 3-11 Drugs and Chemicals Associated with Hyperpigmentation—cont'd

DRUG OR CHEMICAL	CLINICAL FEATURES	HISTOPATHOLOGY/COMMENT
Hormones		
Oral contraceptives	• Melasma; increased pigment of nipples and nevi	• Increased melanocytes and increased melanin synthesis
ACTH/MSH	• Diffuse brown or bronze pigmentation; seen in Addison's disease and Cushing's syndrome	• Increased melanin synthesis
Miscellaneous compounds		
Amiodarone	• Slate-gray to violaceous discoloration of sun-exposed skin	• Yellow-brown granules in dermis, mostly perivascular • Lysosomal inclusions with a lipid-like substance
Azidothymidine (zidovudine, AZT)	• Nail and mucocutaneous hyperpigmentation	• Skin biopsy shows increased epidermal and dermal melanin
Clofazimine	• Diffuse red to red-brown discoloration of skin • Violet-brown to bluish discoloration, especially lesional skin	• Redness secondary to drug in fat • Phagolysosomes with lipofuscin material
Dioxins	• Chloracne most common skin finding • Hyperpigmentation may occur in sun-exposed areas	• Rare, except in accidental exposure
Hydroquinone	• Hyperpigmentation in areas of application due to exogenous ochronosis	• Yellow-brown banana-shaped fibers in papillary dermis
Minocycline	• Blue-black discoloration in old acne scars or sites of inflammation as well as lower extremities • May also involve nails, sclerae, oral mucosa, bones and teeth • Generalized 'muddy brown' pigmentation pattern in some patients	• Iron-containing granules and/or increased melanin, depending on clinical type
Psoralens	• Increased pigmentation after exposure to UVA light (PUVA)	• Proliferation of follicular melanocytes • Increased synthesis and transfer of melanin
Psychotropic drugs (phenothiazine, chlorpromazine, imipramine, despiramine)	• Slate-gray discoloration in sun-exposed areas	• Golden-brown granules in the upper dermis • Electron-dense inclusion bodies

From Bolognia JL, Mascaro JM, Mancini AJ, Salasche SJ, Saurat JH, Stingl G [eds]: *Dermatology,* ed 2, St Louis, 2008, Mosby.

ICD-9CM # 253.1

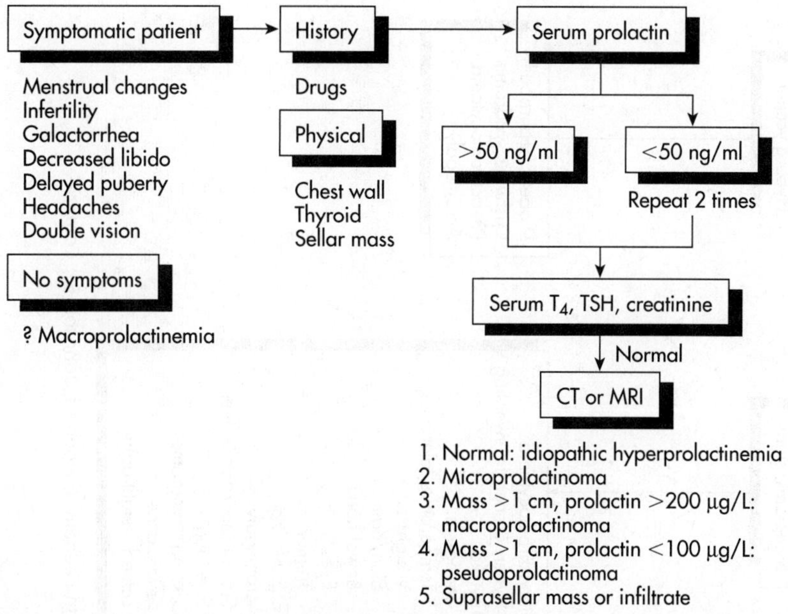

FIGURE 3-145 Approach to hyperprolactinemia. *CT,* Computed tomography; *MRI,* magnetic resonance imaging; *T,* thyroxine; *TSH,* thyroid-stimulating hormone. (From Copeland LJ: *Textbook of gynecology,* ed 2, Philadelphia, 2000, WB Saunders.)

HYPERTENSION, ENDOCRINE INVESTIGATION

ICD-9CM # 401.1

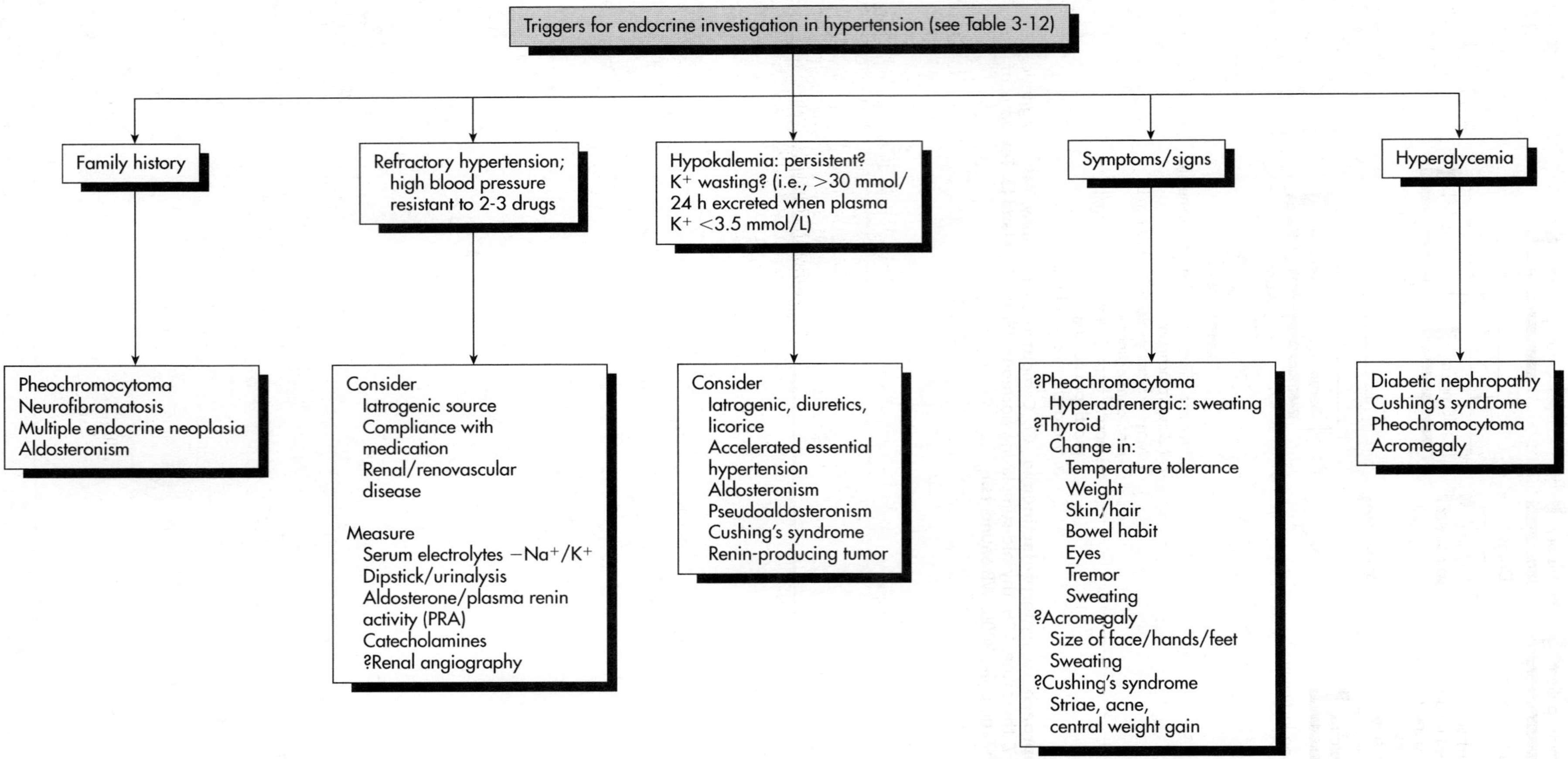

FIGURE 3-146 Clinical observations suggesting endocrine investigation in hypertension. (From Feehally J, Floege J, Johnson RJ: *Comprehensive clinical nephrology,* ed 3, St Louis, 2007, Mosby.)

TABLE 3-12 Causes of Endocrine Hypertension

Pituitary	Thyroid
Cushing's disease	Hypothyroidism
Acromegaly	Hyperthyroidism
Adrenal cortex	Renin-secreting tumors
Primary aldosteronism	Others
Pseudoaldosteronism	Hyperparathyroidism?
Cushing's syndrome	Endothelioma
Adrenal medulla	
Pheochromocytoma	

From Feehally J, Floege J, Johnson RJ: *Comprehensive clinical nephrology,* ed 3, St Louis, 2007, Mosby.

ICD-9CM # 401.0

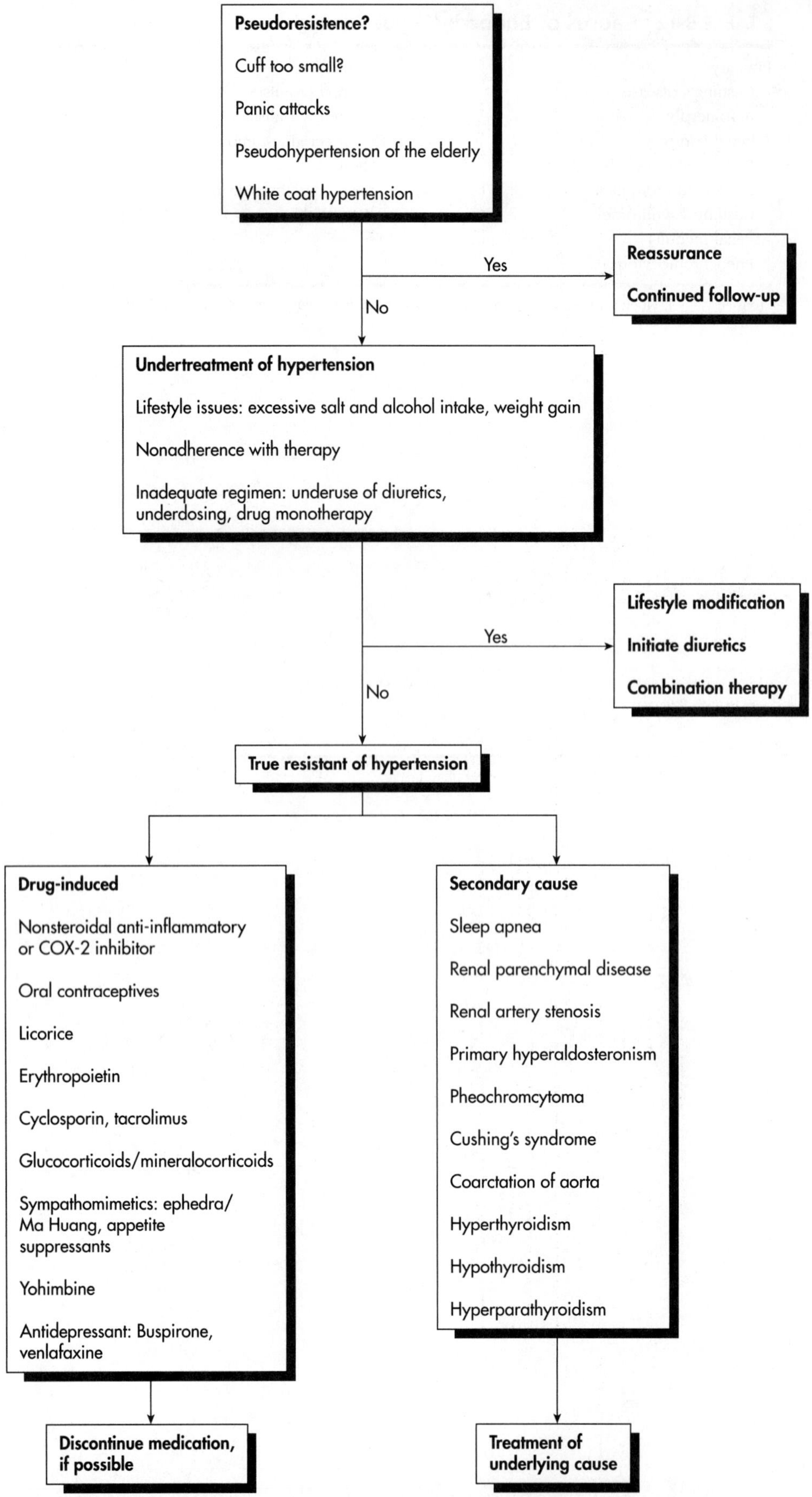

FIGURE 3-147 Approach to the patient with "resistant" hypertension. (From Crawford MH, DiMarco JP, Paulus WJ [eds]: *Cardiology,* ed 2, St. Louis, 2004, Mosby.)

ICD-9CM # 401.1 Essential hypertension
401.0 Malignant hypertension due to renal artery stenosis
642 Hypertension complicating pregnancy
405.01 Malignant hypertension secondary to renal artery stenosis
437.2 Hypertensive encephalopathy

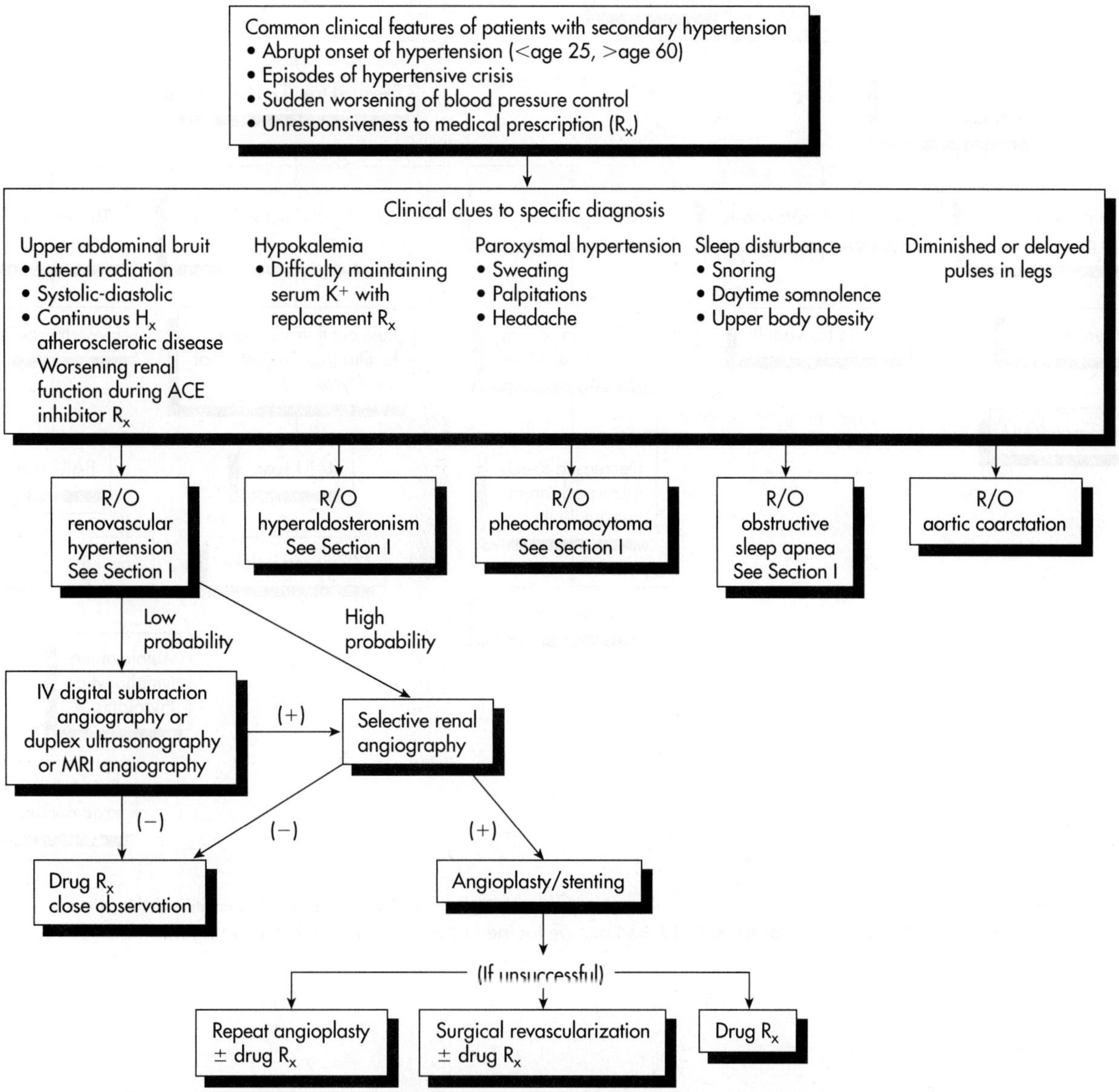

FIGURE 3-148 Algorithm for identifying patients for evaluation of secondary causes of hypertension. *ACE,* Angiotension-converting enzyme; *Hx,* history; *K+,* potassium; *R/O,* rule out. (Modified from Goldman L, Ausiello D [eds]: *Cecil textbook of medicine,* ed 23, Philadelphia, 2008, WB Saunders.)

ICD-9CM # 242.9

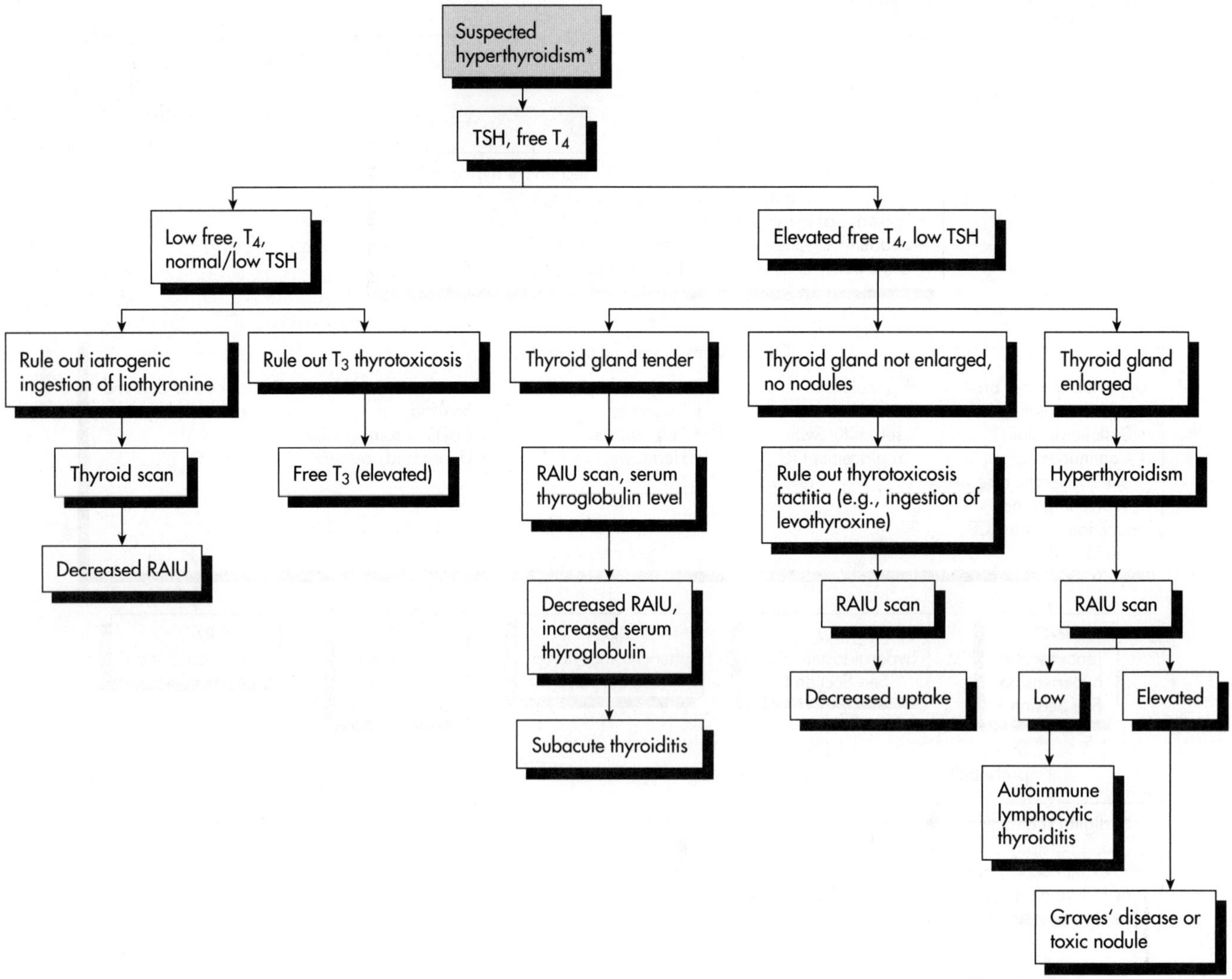

*Refer to Section I for additional information on this topic.

FIGURE 3-149 Hyperthyroidism. *RAIU,* Radioactive iodine uptake; *TSH,* thyroid-stimulating hormone.

ICD-9CM # 790.6

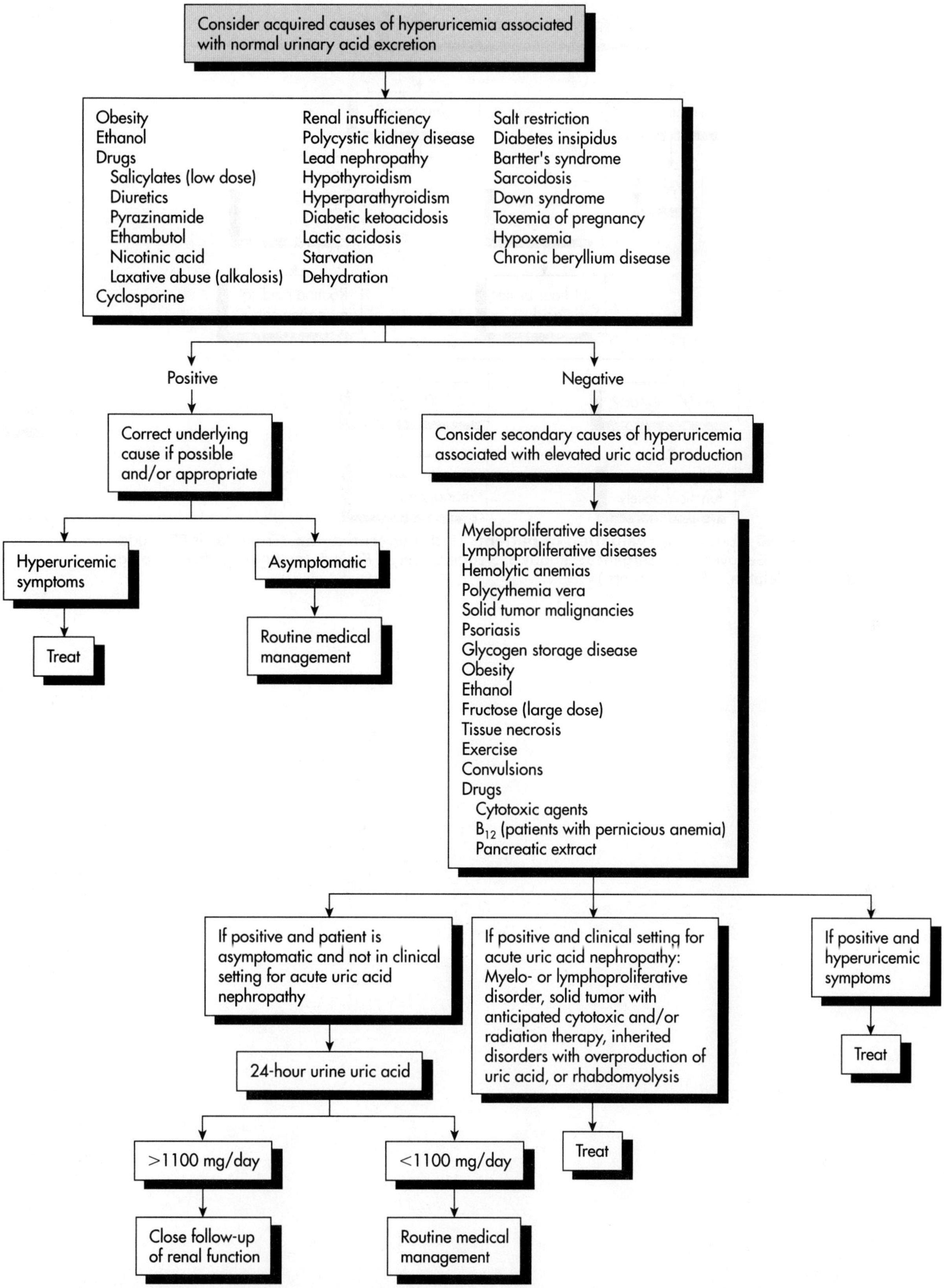

FIGURE 3-150 Evaluation of patients with hyperuricemia. (From Harris ED, Budd RC, Firestein GS, Genovese MC, Sergent JS, Ruddy S, Sledge CB [eds]: *Kelley's textbook of rheumatology,* ed 7, Philadelphia, 2005, Saunders.)

Continued on following page

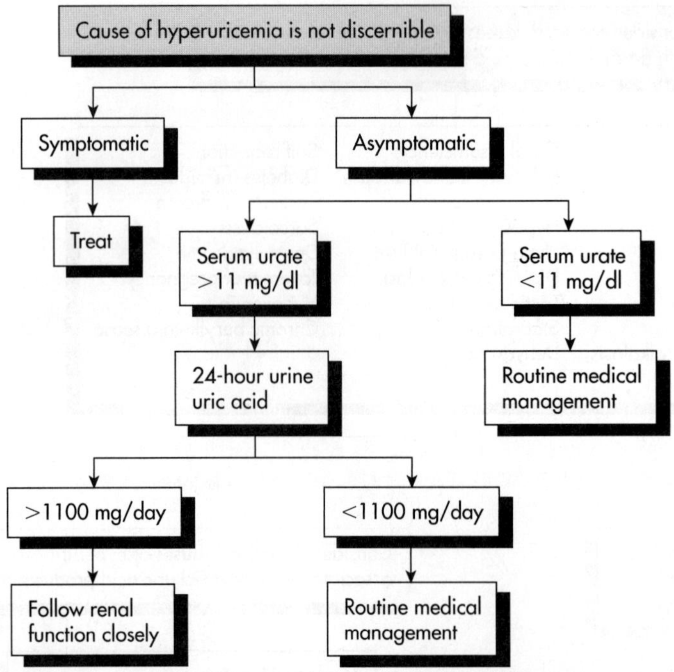

FIGURE 3-150 (Continued) **Evaluation of patients with hyperuricemia.** (From Harris ED, Budd RC, Firestein GS, Genovese MC, Sergent JS, Ruddy S, Sledge CB [eds]: *Kelley's textbook of rheumatology,* ed 7, Philadelphia, 2005, Saunders.)

ICD-9CM # 275.41

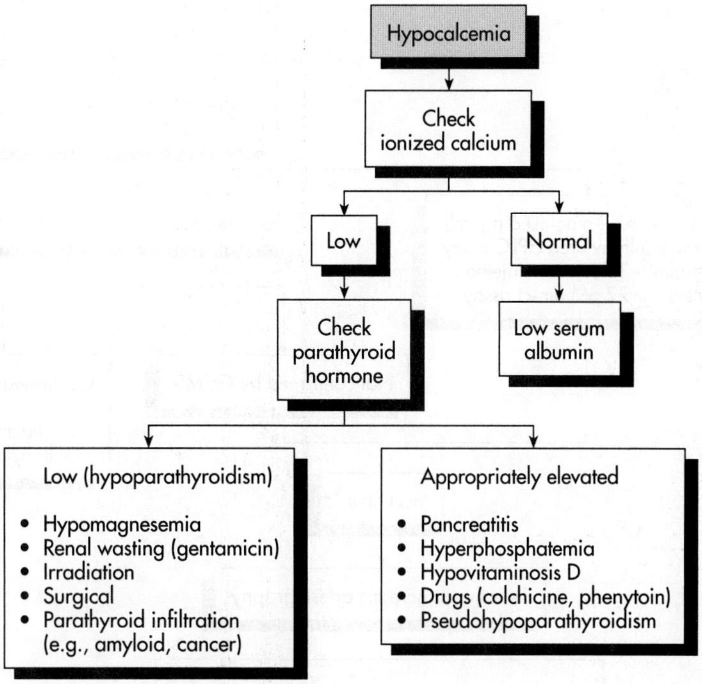

FIGURE 3-151 Evaluation of hypocalcemia. (From Wachtel TJ, Stein MD: *Practical guide to the care of the ambulatory patient,* ed 2, St Louis, 2000, Mosby.)

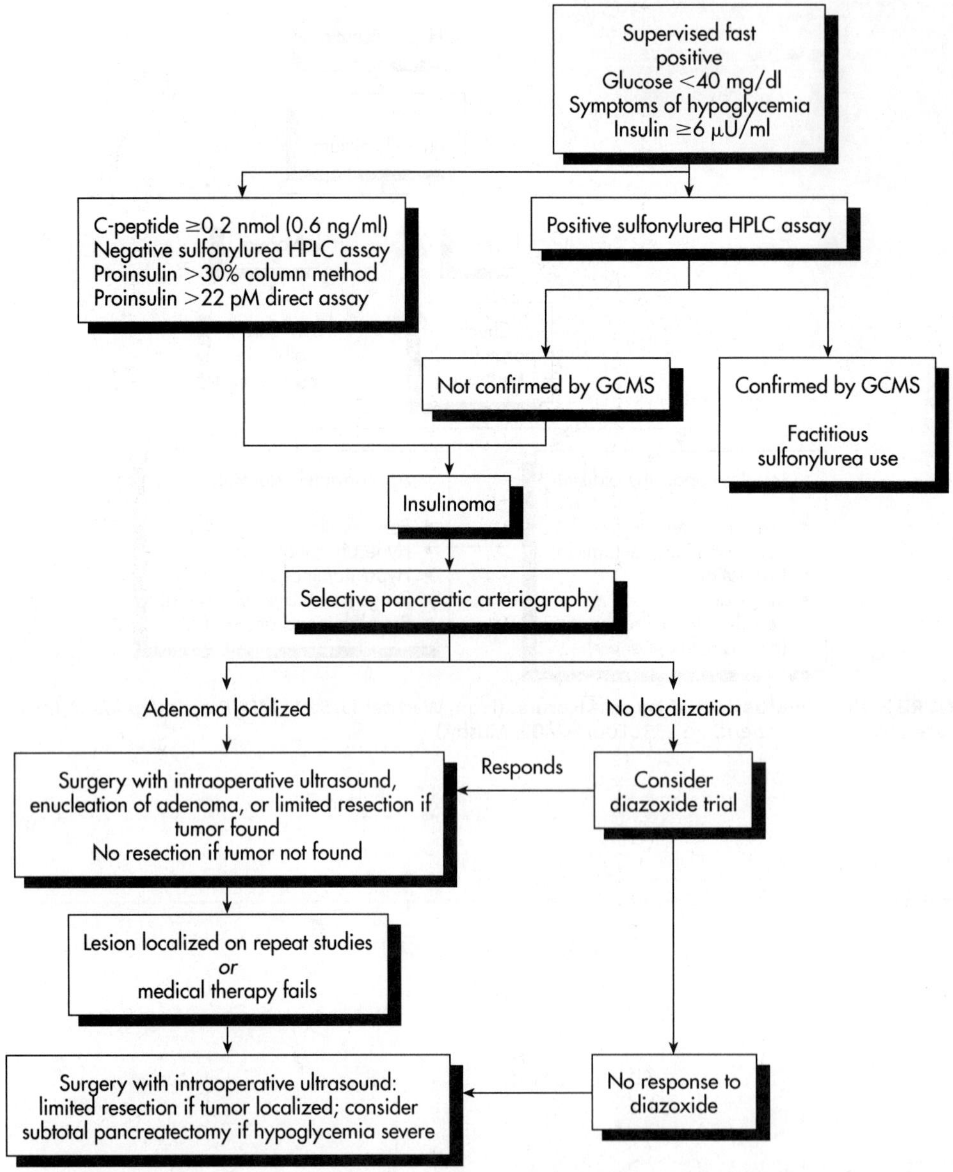

FIGURE 3-152 Diagnostic evaluation of patients with documented hypoglycemia and elevated insulin. *GCMS,* Gas chromatography mass spectrometry; *HPLC,* high-pressure liquid chromatography. (Modified from Moore WT, Eastman RC: *Diagnostic endocrinology,* ed 2, St Louis, 1996, Mosby.)

ICD-9CM # 256.3 Hypogonadism, female
257.2 Hypogonadism, male

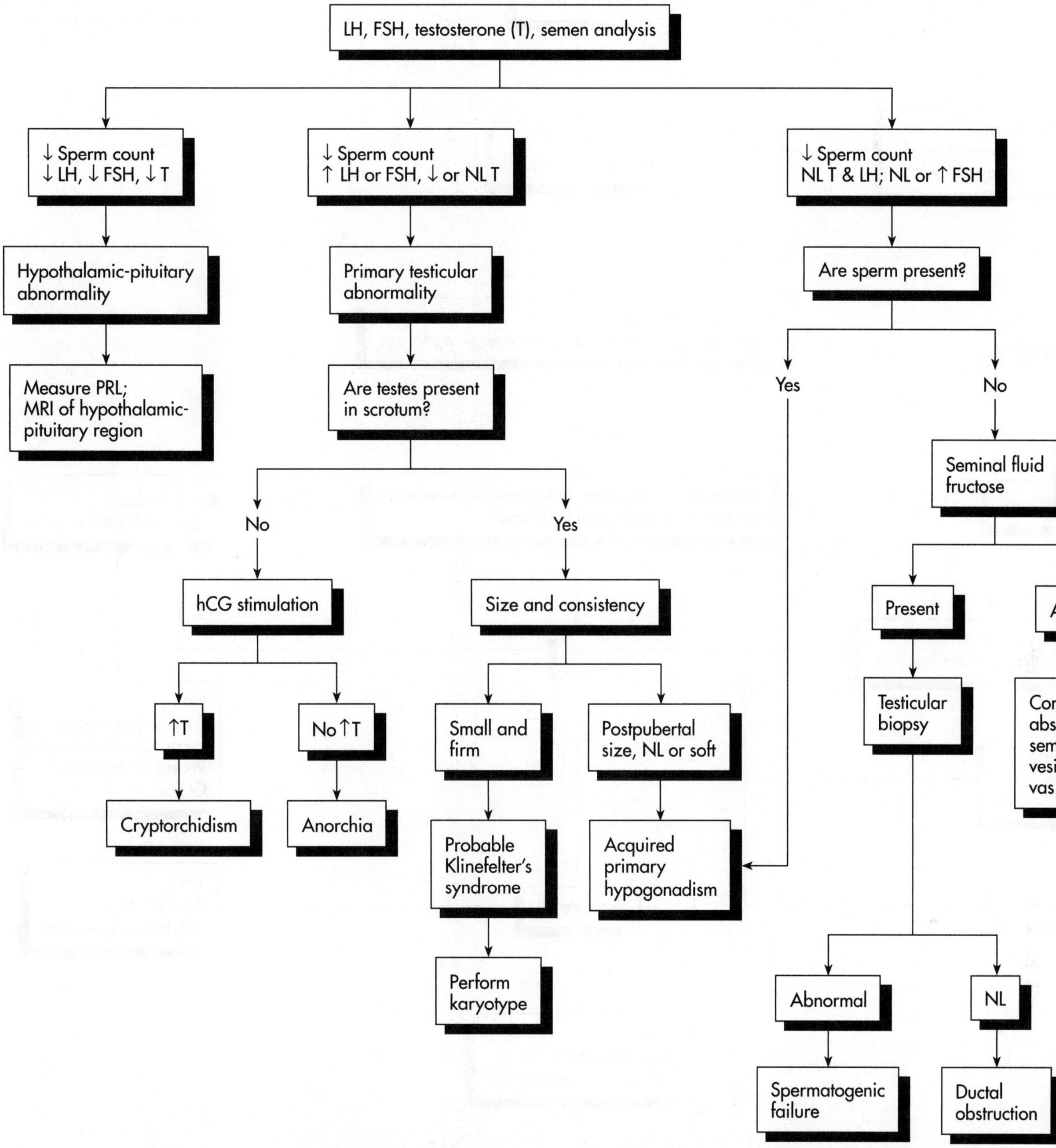

FIGURE 3-153 Laboratory evaluation of hypogonadism. *FSH,* Follicle-stimulating hormone; *hCG,* human chorionic gonadotropin; *LH,* luteinizing hormone; *MRI,* magnetic resonance imaging; *NL,* normal; *PRL,* prolactin; ↑, elevated; ↓, decreased or low. (From Andreoli TE [ed]: *Cecil essentials of medicine*, ed 7, Philadelphia, 2008, WB Saunders.)

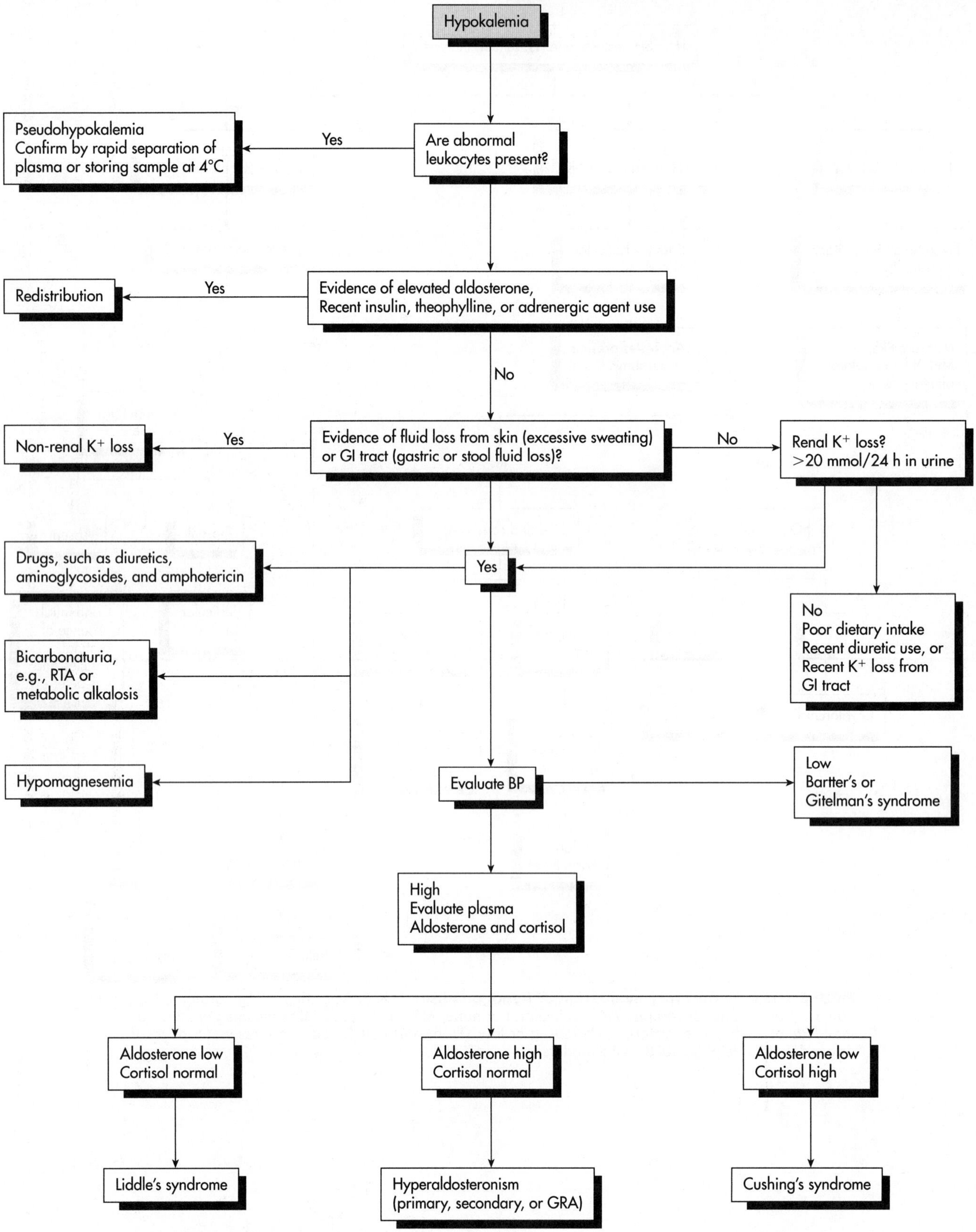

FIGURE 3-154 Diagnostic evaluation of hypokalemia. *GRA,* Glucose remediable aldosteronism; *RTA,* renal tubular acidosis. (From Feehally J, Floege J, Johnson RJ: *Comprehensive clinical nephrology,* ed 3, St Louis, 2007, Mosby.)

ICD-9CM # 275.2

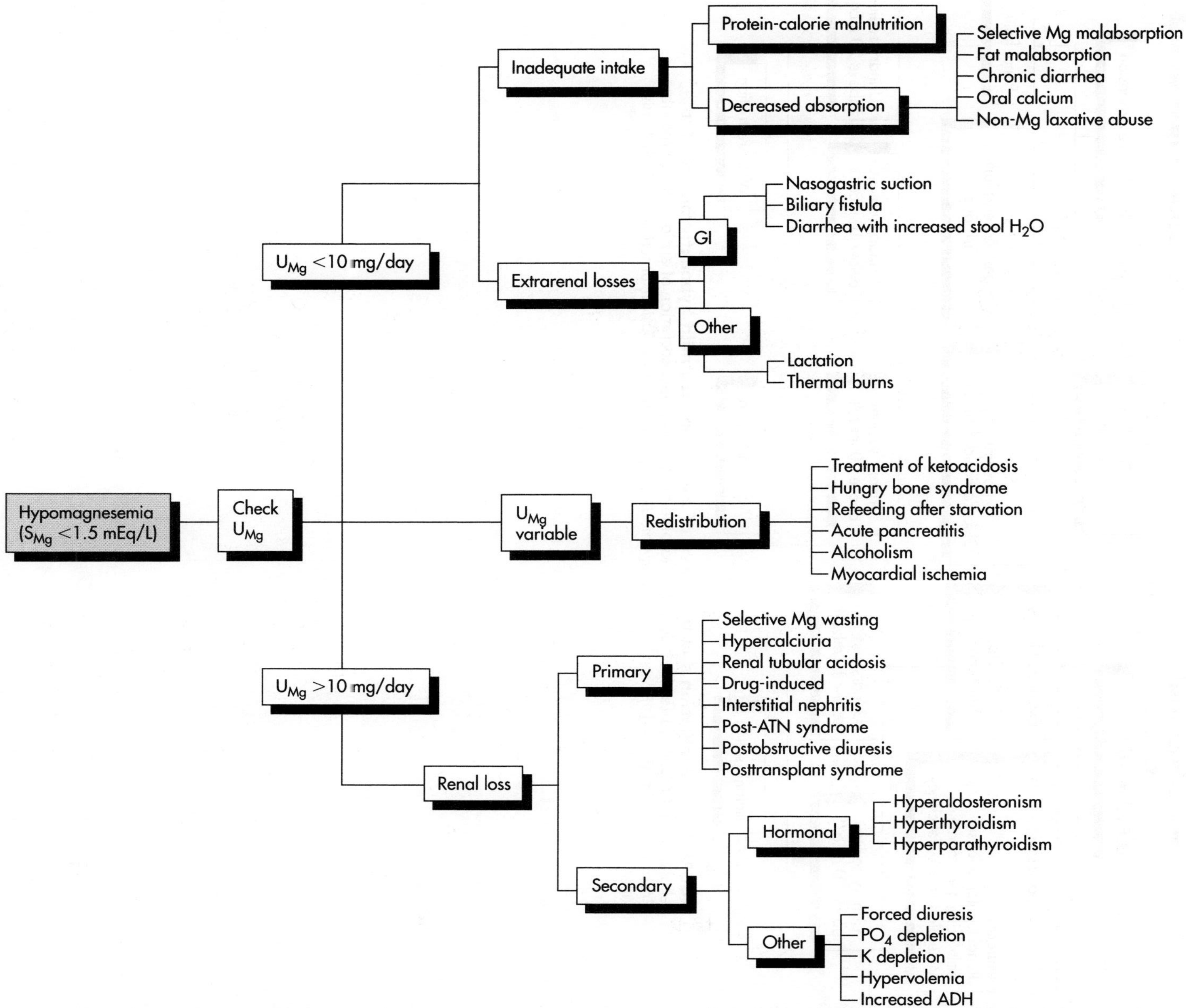

FIGURE 3-155 Hypomagnesemia. *ADH,* Antidiuretic hormone; *GI,* gastrointestinal; *post-ATN,* post acute tubular necrosis. (From Healy PM: *Common medical diagnosis an algorithmic approach,* ed 3, Philadelphia, 2000, WB Saunders.)

ICD-9CM # 276.1

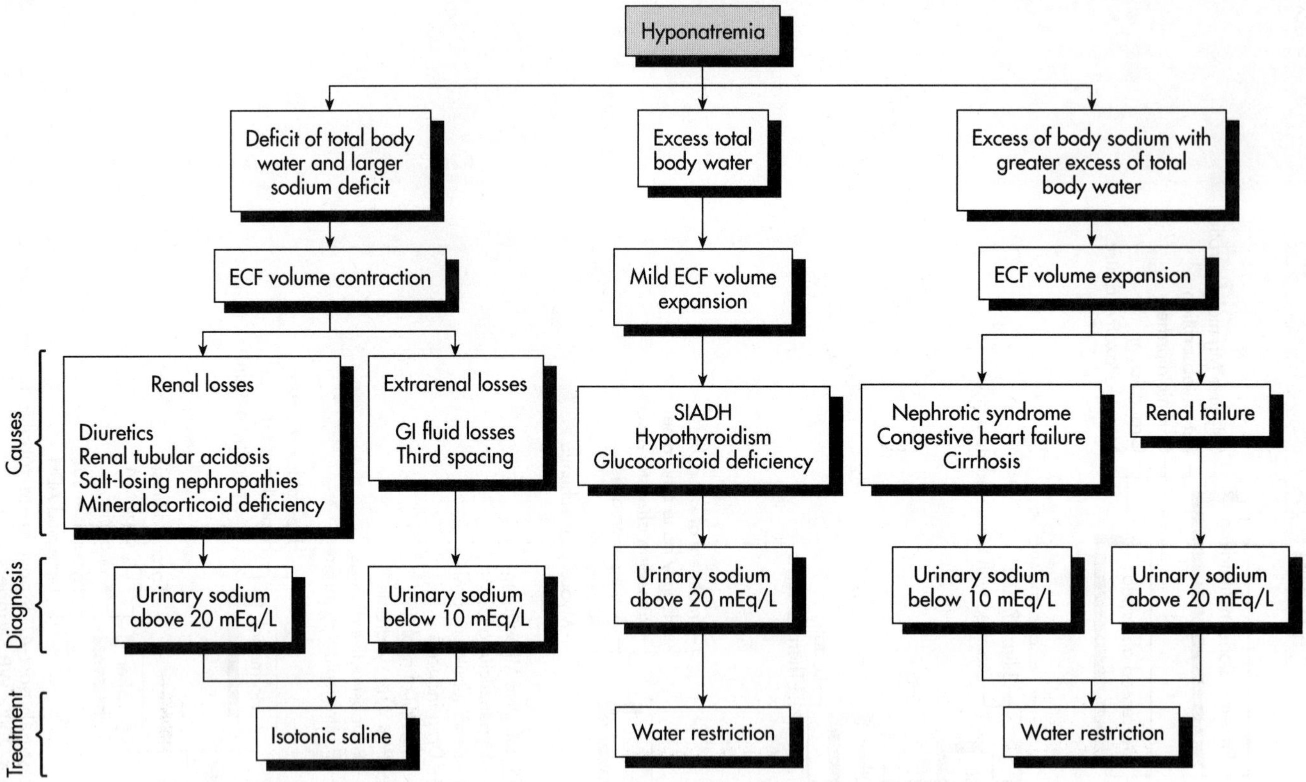

FIGURE 3-156 Evaluation and treatment of asymptomatic, mild hyponatremia. *ECF,* Extracellular fluid; *GI,* gastrointestinal; *SIADH,* syndrome of inappropriate secretion of antidiuretic hormone. (From Marx J et al [eds]: *Rosen's emergency medicine: concepts and clinical practice,* ed 6, St Louis, 2006, Mosby.)

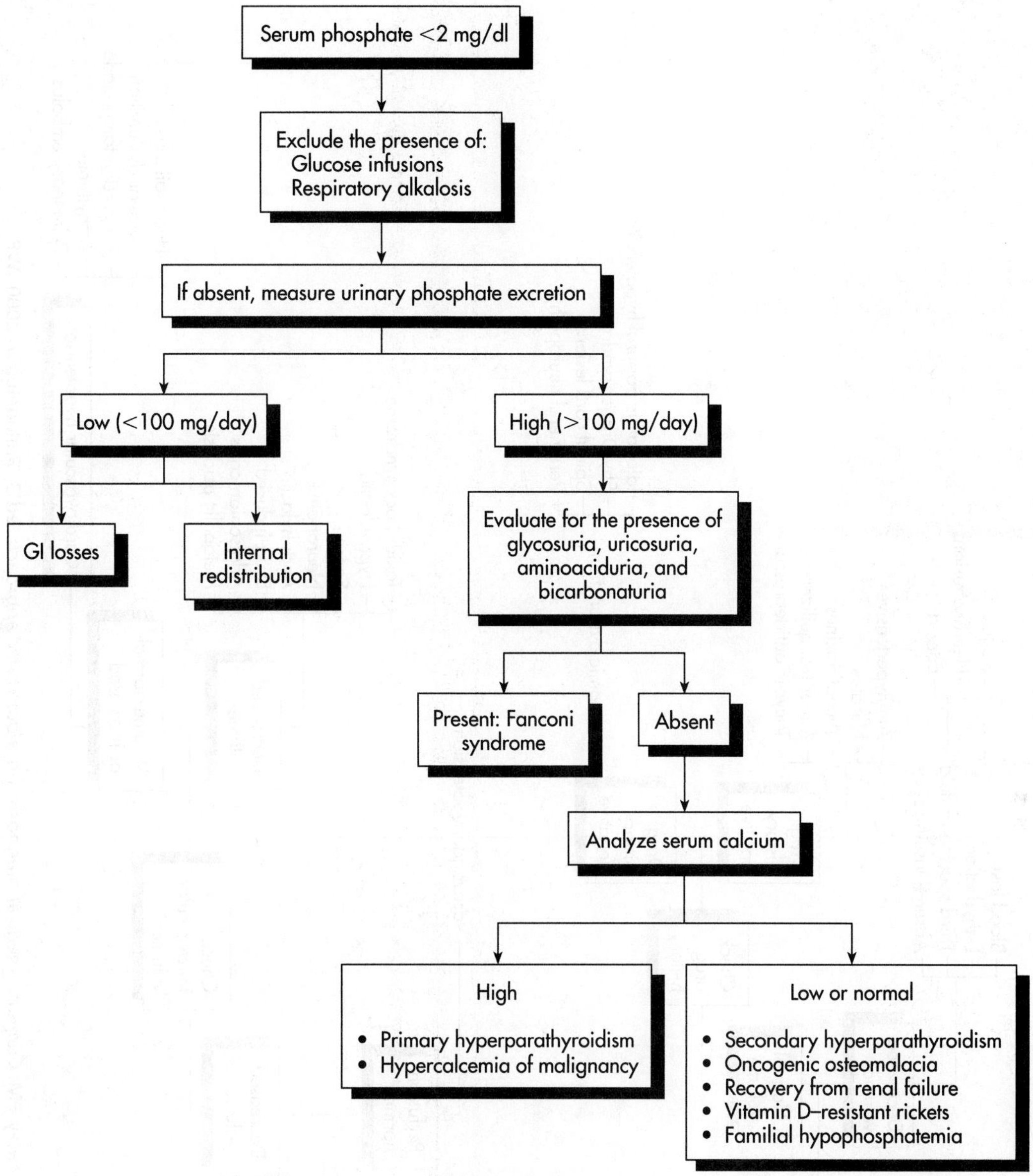

FIGURE 3-157 Diagnostic workup of hypophosphatemia. *GI,* Gastrointestinal. (From Stein JH [ed]: *Internal medicine,* ed 5, St Louis, 1998, Mosby.)

HYPOTENSION

ICD-9CM # 458.9 Hypotension, NOS
458.1 Hypotension, chronic
458.2 Hypotension, iatrogenic
458.0 Hypotension, orthostatic or postural

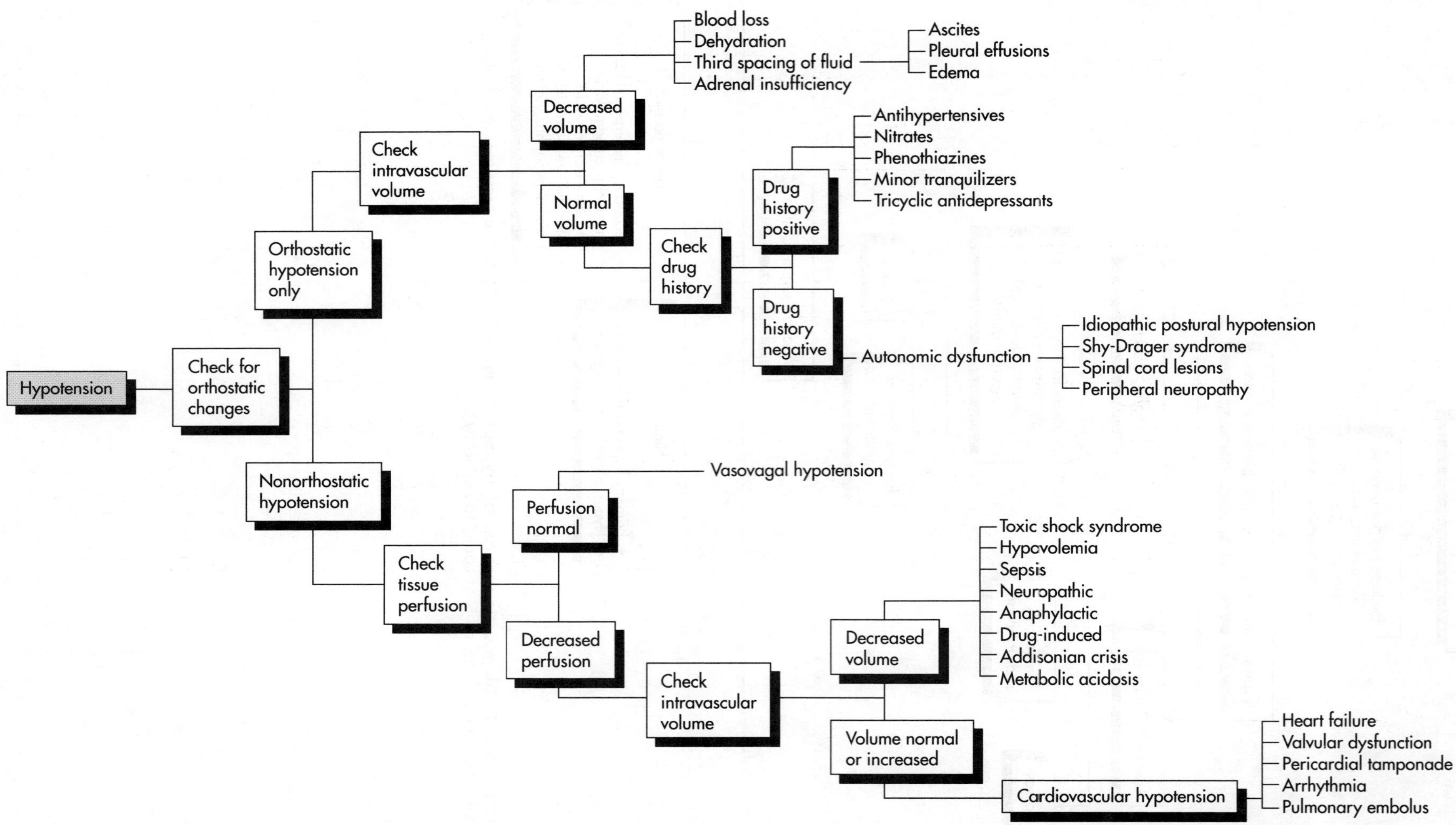

FIGURE 3-158 Hypotension. (From Healey PM: *Common medical diagnosis: an algorithmic approach,* ed 3, Philadelphia, 2000, WB Saunders.)

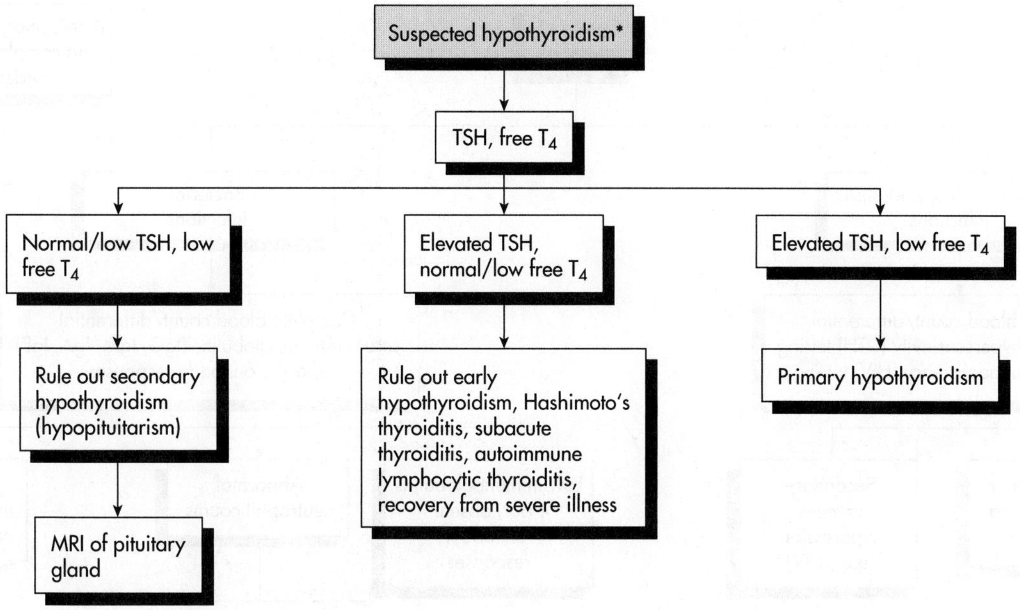

*Refer to Section I for additional information on this topic.

FIGURE 3-159 Hypothyroidism. *MRI,* Magnetic resonance imaging; *TSH,* thyroid-stimulating hormone.

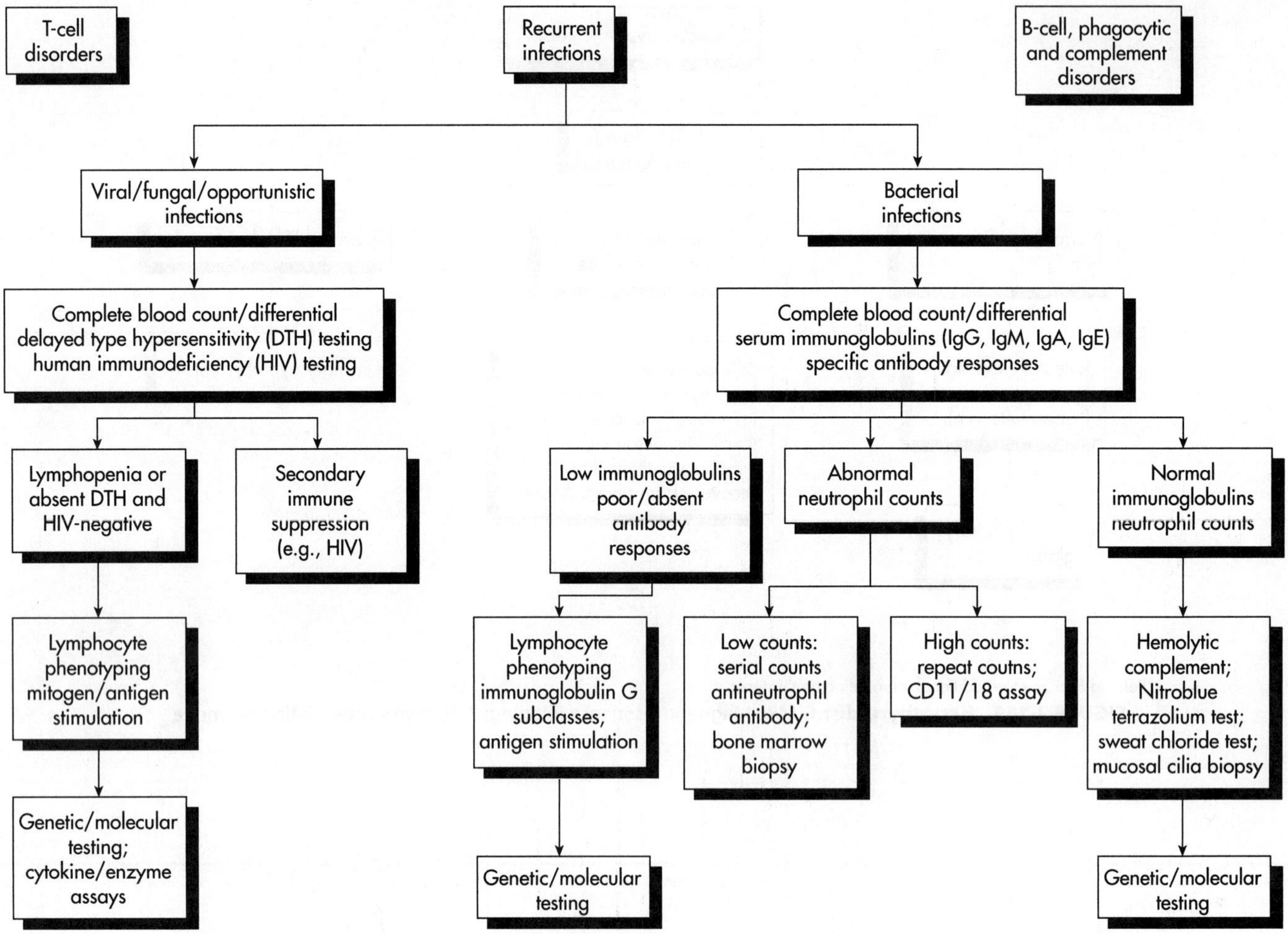

FIGURE 3-160 A diagnostic testing algorithm for primary immunodeficiency diseases. (From *MMWR* 53[RR-1], 2004.)

ICD-9CM # 628.9 Infertility, female, unspecified
606.9 Infertility, male, unspecified

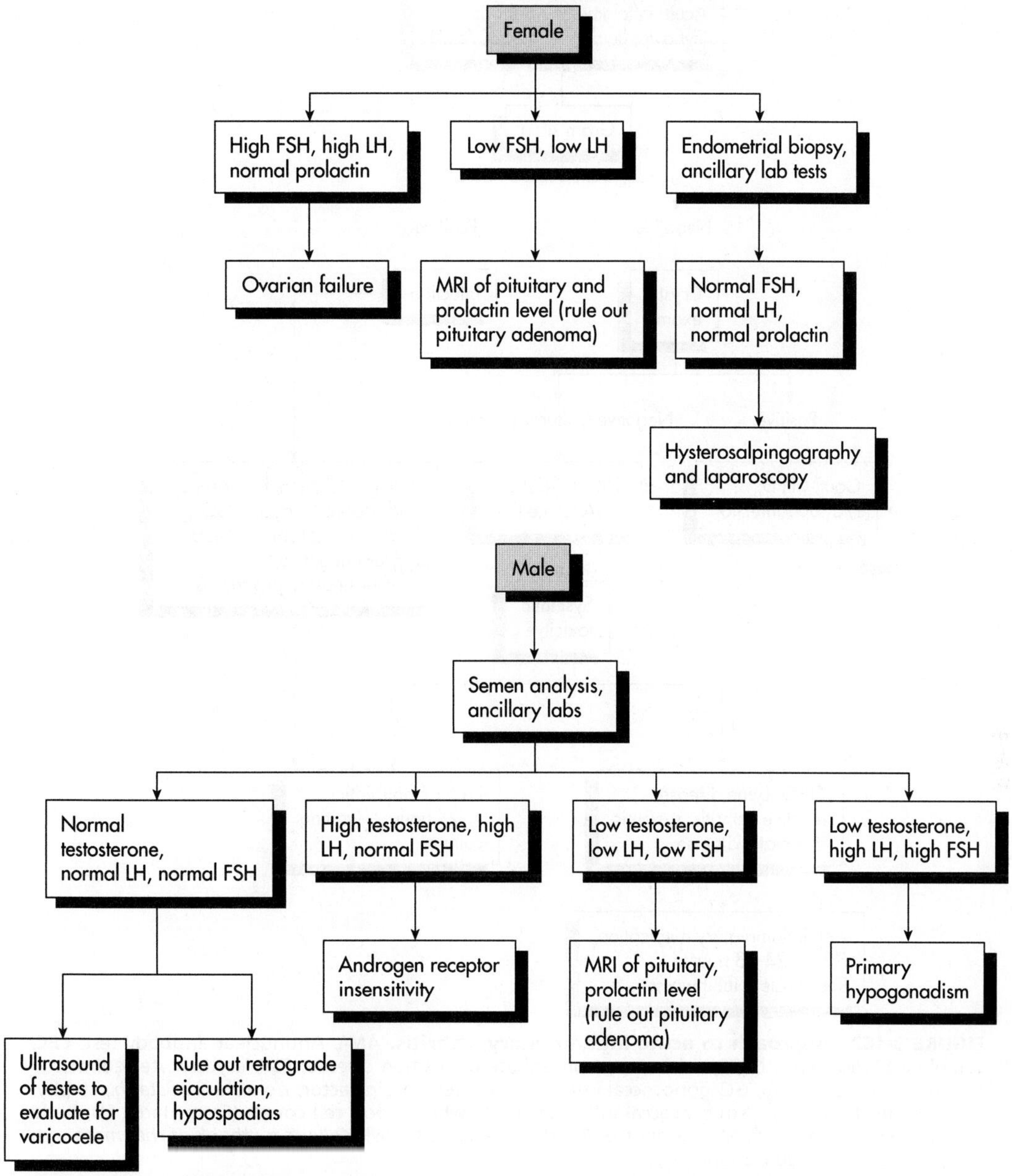

FIGURE 3-161 Approach to infertility diagnosis and management. *FSH,* Follicle-stimulating hormone; *LH,* luteinizing hormone; *MRI,* magnetic resonance imaging. (From Ferri FF: *Ferri's best test: a practical guide to clinical laboratory medicine and diagnostic imaging,* ed 2, Philadelphia, 2009, Elsevier Mosby.)

BOX 3-8 **Infertility**

Diagnostic imaging
Best test
None
Ancillary tests
MRI of pituitary with contrast
Hysterosalpingography
Testicular ultrasound

Lab evaluation
Best tests
Male: semen analysis
Female: endometrial biopsy
Ancillary tests
FSH, LH
Prolactin
Serum testosterone (male)
TSH
CBC, ESR, FBS
Urinalysis, VDRL, *Mycoplasma* culture, chlamidiae serology

Ferri FF: *Ferri's best test: a practical guide to clinical laboratory medicine and diagnostic imaging,* ed 2, Philadelphia, 2009, Elsevier Mosby.

CBC, Complete blood count; *ESR,* erythrocyte sedimentation rate; *FBS,* fasting blood sugar; *FSH,* follicle-stimulating hormone; *LH,* luteinizing hormone; *MRI,* magnetic resonance imaging; *VDRL,* Venereal Disease Research Laboratory (test).

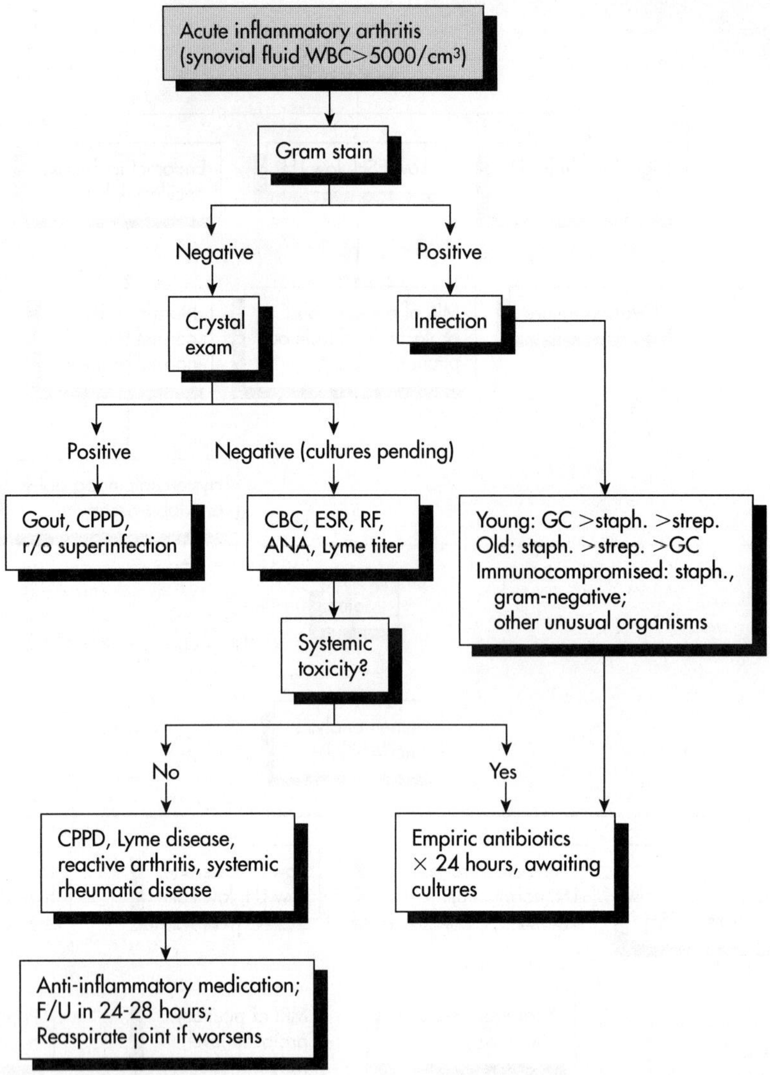

FIGURE 3-162 Approach to acute inflammatory arthritis. *ANA,* Antinuclear antibody test; *CBC,* complete blood count; *CPPD;* calcium pyrophosphate deposition disease; *ESR,* erythrocyte sedimentation rate; *F/U,* follow-up; *GC,* gonococcal infection; *RF,* rheumatoid factor; *r/o,* rule out; *staph.,* staphylococcal infection; *strep.,* streptococcal infection; *WBC,* white blood cell count. (From Harris ED, Budd RC, Firestein GS, Genovese MC, Sergent JS, Ruddy S, Sledge CB [eds]: *Kelley's textbook of rheumatology,* ed 7, Philadelphia, 2005, Saunders.)

ICD-9CM # 564.1

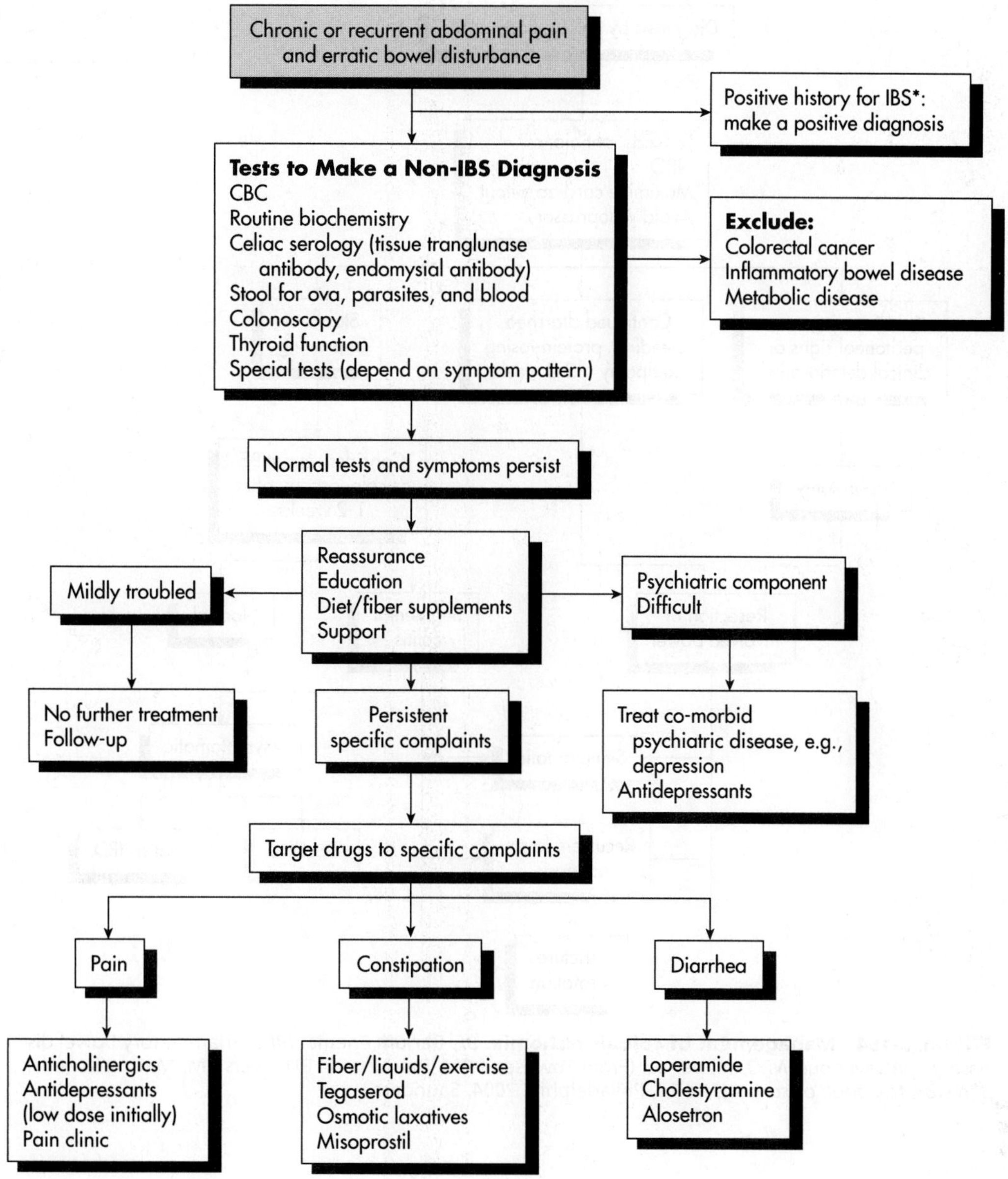

*Refer to Section I for additional information on this topic.

FIGURE 3-163 Evaluation of suspected irritable bowel syndrome (IBS). *CBC,* Complete blood count. (Modified from Goldman L, Ausiello D [eds]: *Cecil textbook of medicine,* ed 23, Philadelphia, 2008, WB Saunders.)

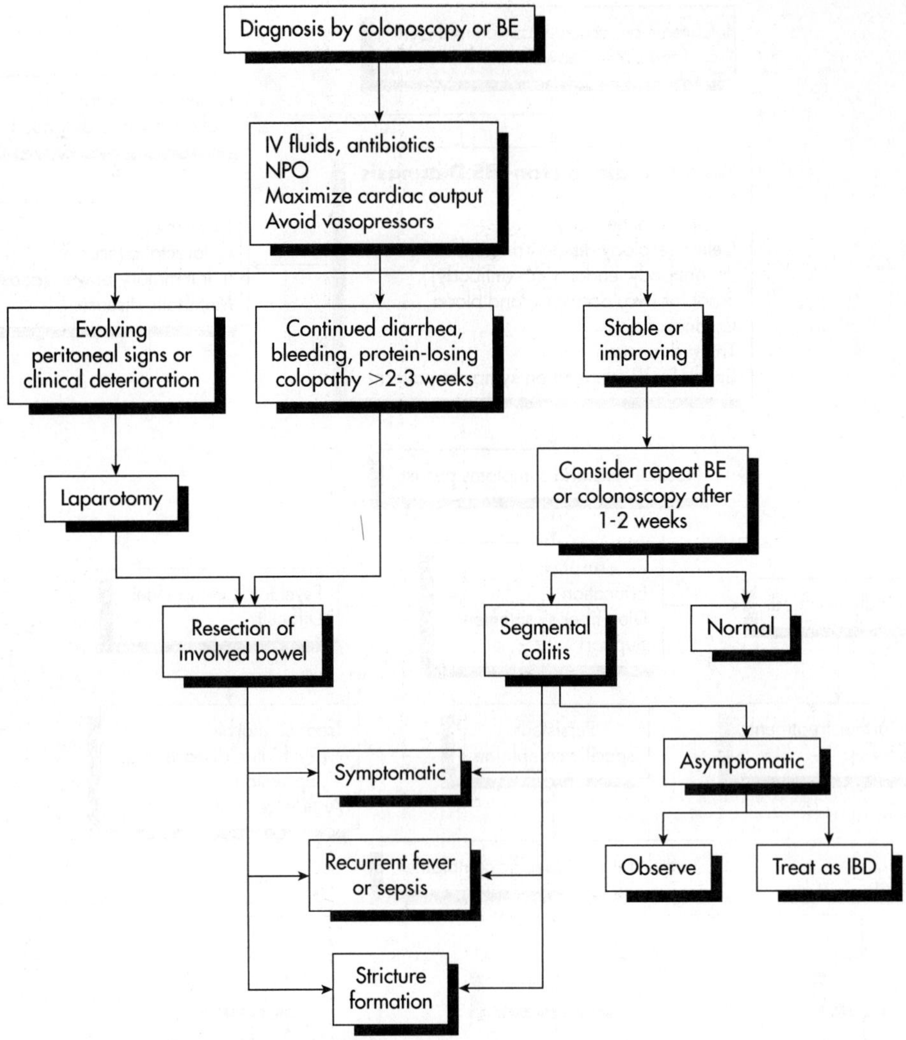

FIGURE 3-164 Management of colonic ischemia. *BE,* Barium enema; *IBD,* inflammatory bowel disease; *IV,* intravenous; *NPO,* nil per os. (From Townsend CM, Beauchamp RD, Evers BM, Mattox KL [eds]: *Sabiston textbook of surgery,* ed 17, Philadelphia, 2004, Saunders.)

JAUNDICE AND HEPATOBILIARY DISEASE

ICD-9CM # 782.4 Jaundice NOS
277.4 Bilirubin excretion disorders
576.8 Jaundice, obstructive

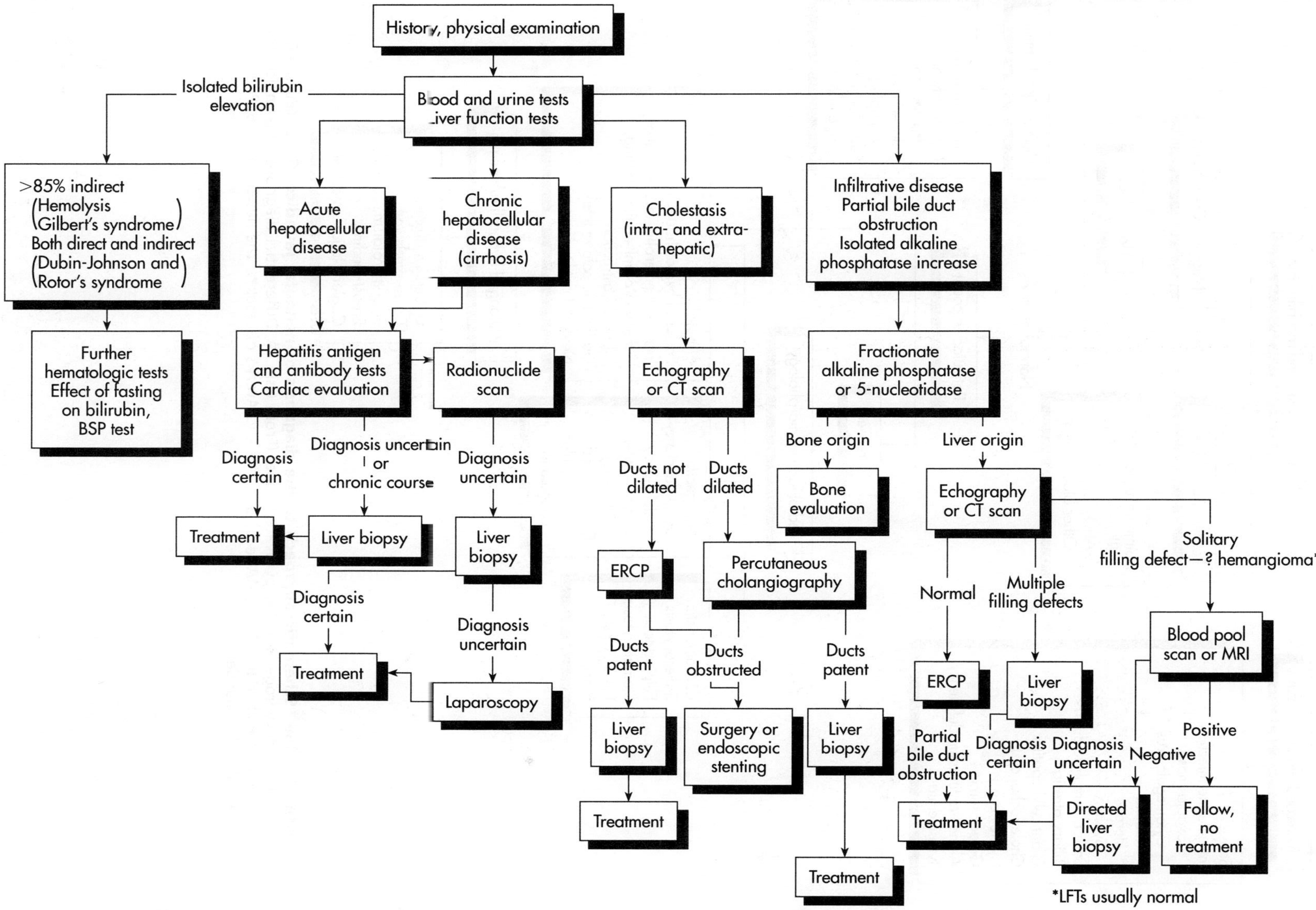

FIGURE 3-165 Evaluation of jaundice and hepatobiliary disease. *BSP,* Bromsulphalein; *CT,* computed tomography; *ERCP,* endoscopic retrograde cholangiopancreatography; *LFTs,* liver function tests; *MRI,* magnetic resonance imaging. (From Stein JH [ed]: *Internal medicine,* ed 5, St Louis, 1998, Mosby.)

ICD-9CM # 774.6 Jaundice neonatal, NOS
773.1 ABO reaction perinatal
774.1 Hemolytic perinatal
773.0 RH reaction perinatal
751.61 Bile duct obstruction, congenital

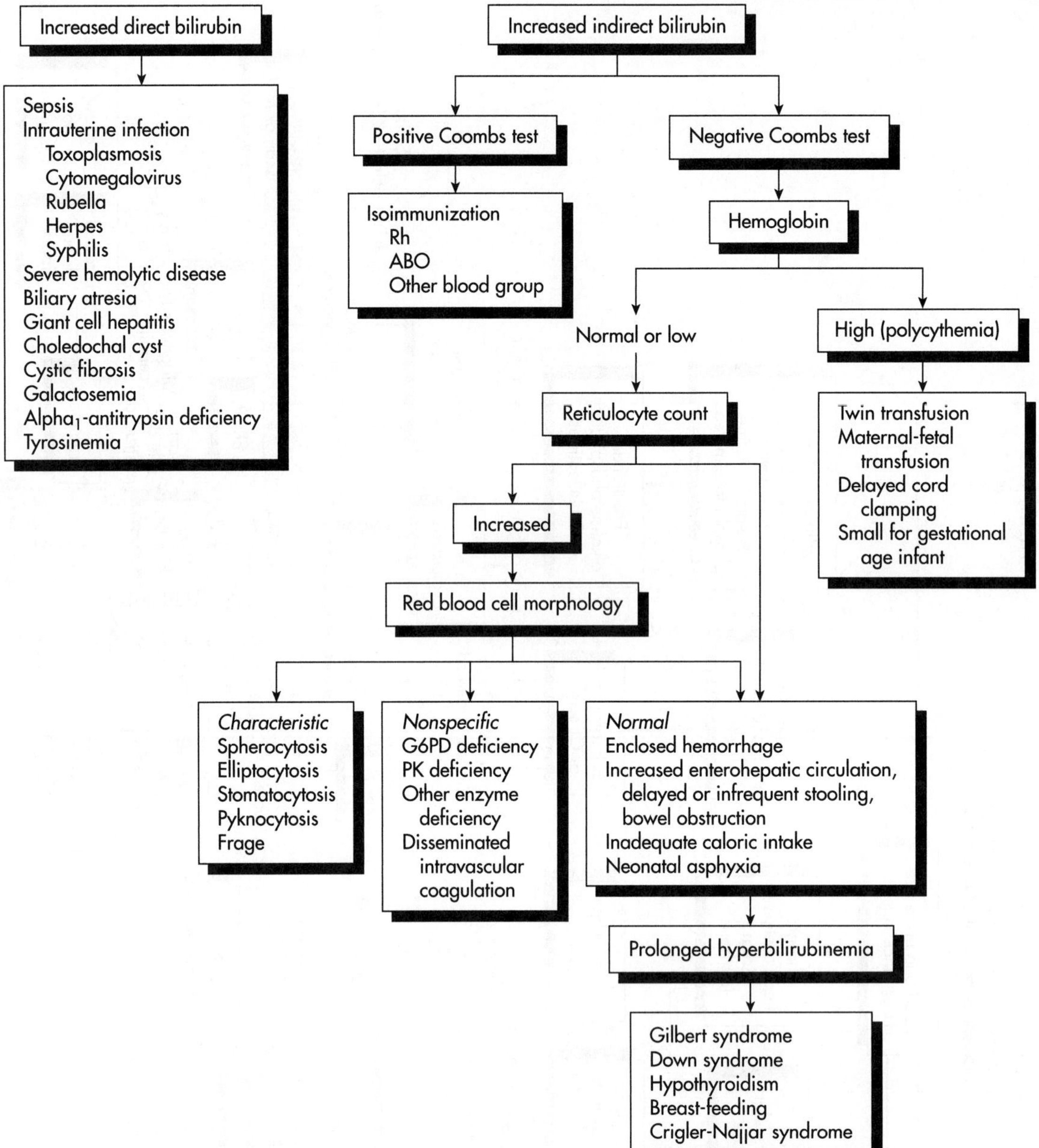

FIGURE 3-166 Schematic approach to the diagnosis of neonatal jaundice. *G6PD,* Glucose-6-phosphate dehydrogenase; *PK,* pyruvate kinase. (From Oski FA: Differential diagnosis of jaundice. In Taeusch HW, Ballard RA, Avery MA [eds]: *Schaffer and Avery's diseases of the newborn,* ed 6, Philadelphia, 1991, WB Saunders.)

ICD-9CM # 719.0

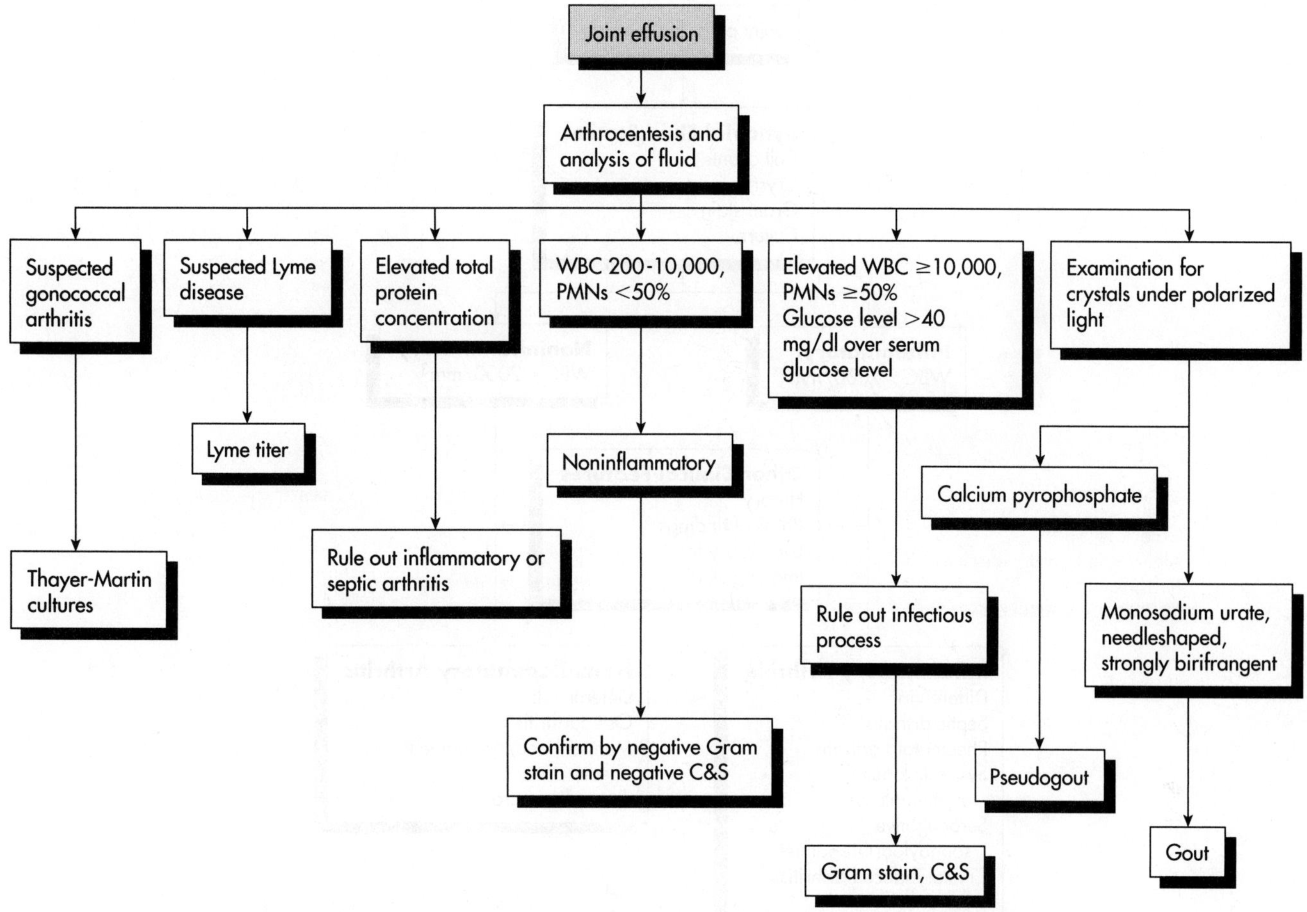

FIGURE 3-167 Joint effusion. *C&S,* Culture and sensitivity; *WBC,* white blood cell count.

ICD-9CM # 719.00

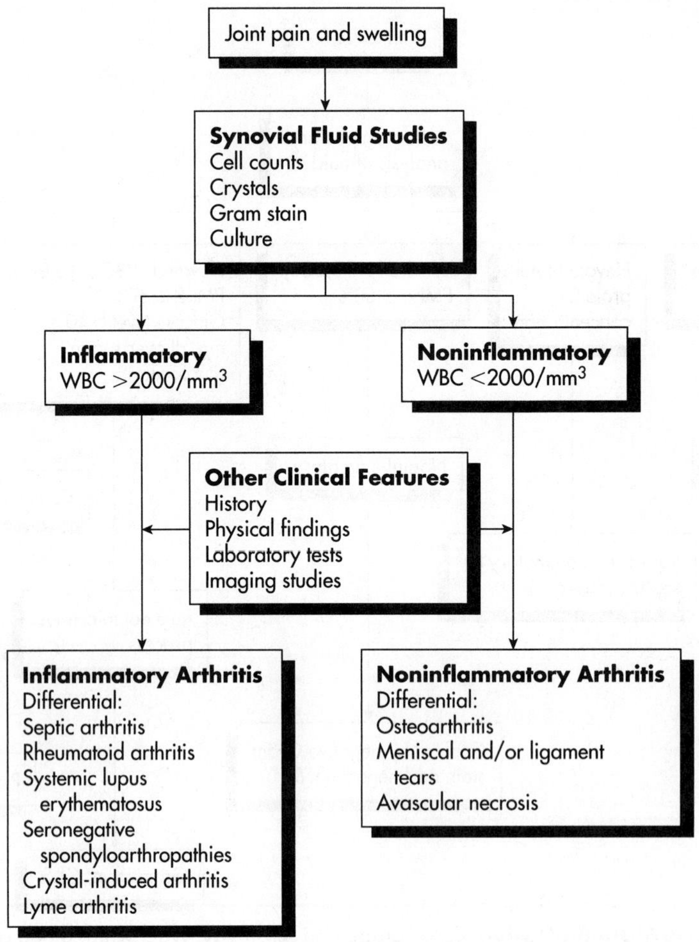

FIGURE 3-168 Diagnostic approach for swollen joints. *WBC,* White blood cell count. (From Goldman L, Ausiello D [eds]: *Cecil textbook of medicine,* ed 23, Philadelphia, 2008, WB Saunders.)

ICD-9CM # 716.96 Knee inflammation
959.7 Knee injury
719.56 Knee stiffness
719.06 Knee swelling

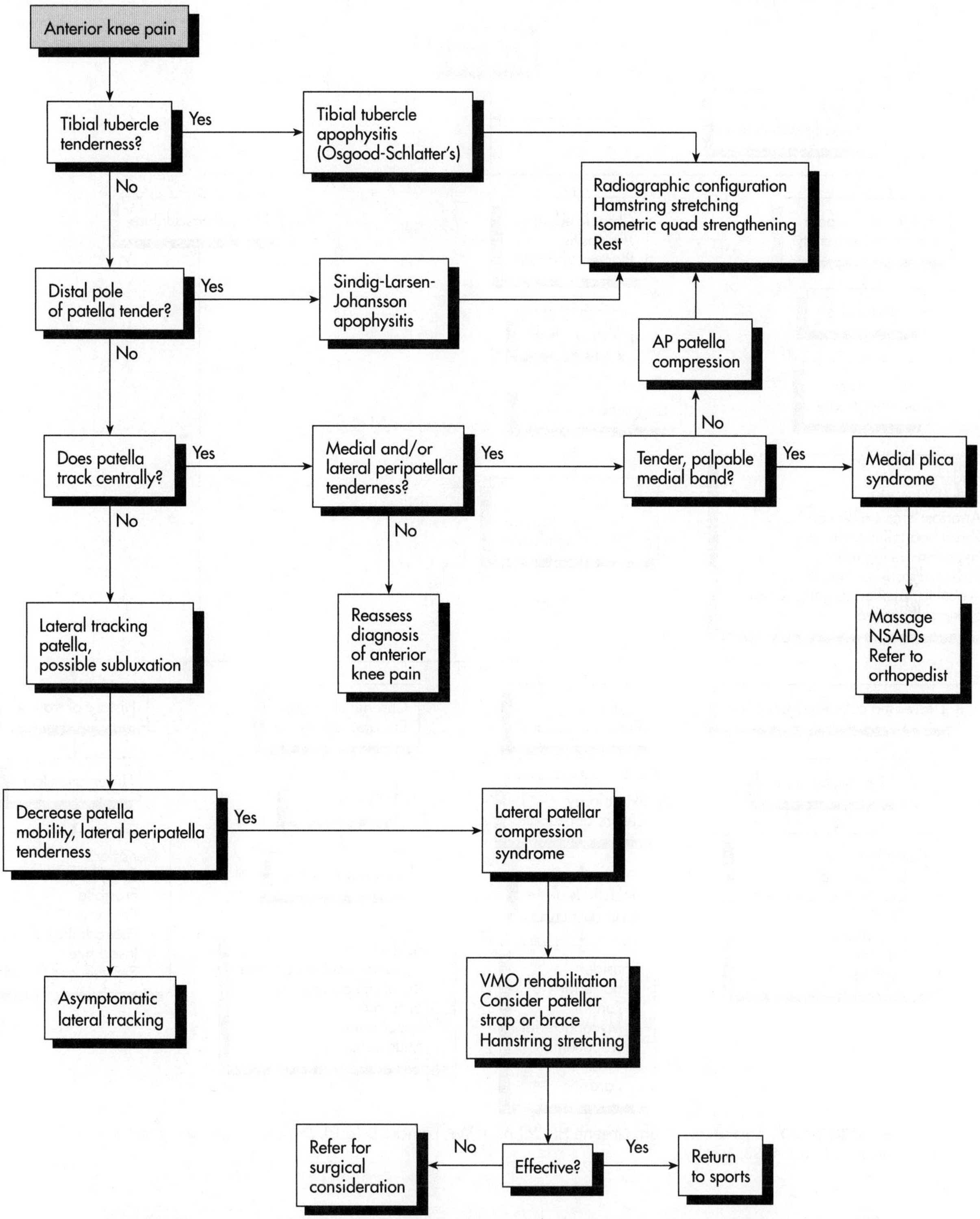
Anterior knee pain
Tibial tubercle tenderness?
Yes
Tibial tubercle apophysitis (Osgood-Schlatter's)
Radiographic configuration
Hamstring stretching
Isometric quad strengthening
Rest
No
Distal pole of patella tender?
Yes
Sindig-Larsen-Johansson apophysitis
AP patella compression
No
Does patella track centrally?
Yes
Medial and/or lateral peripatellar tenderness?
Yes
Tender, palpable medial band?
Yes
Medial plica syndrome
No
No
No
Lateral tracking patella, possible subluxation
Reassess diagnosis of anterior knee pain
Massage
NSAIDs
Refer to orthopedist
Decrease patella mobility, lateral peripatella tenderness
Yes
Lateral patellar compression syndrome
VMO rehabilitation
Consider patellar strap or brace
Hamstring stretching
Asymptomatic lateral tracking
Refer for surgical consideration
No
Effective?
Yes
Return to sports

FIGURE 3-169 Evaluation and management of knee extensor mechanism pain. Focused treatment based on specific etiology will prevent recurrence. *AP,* Anteroposterior; *NSAIDs,* nonsteroidal anti-inflammatory drugs; *VMO,* vastus medialis obliquus muscle. (From Scudieri G [ed]: *Sports medicine, principles of primary care,* St Louis, 1997, Mosby.)

ICD-9CM # 440.23 Ulcer, lower limb, arteriosclerotic
707.1 Ulcer, lower limb, chronic
707.1 Ulcer, lower limb, neurogenic
707.9 Ulcer, non-healing
707.0 Pressure ulcer

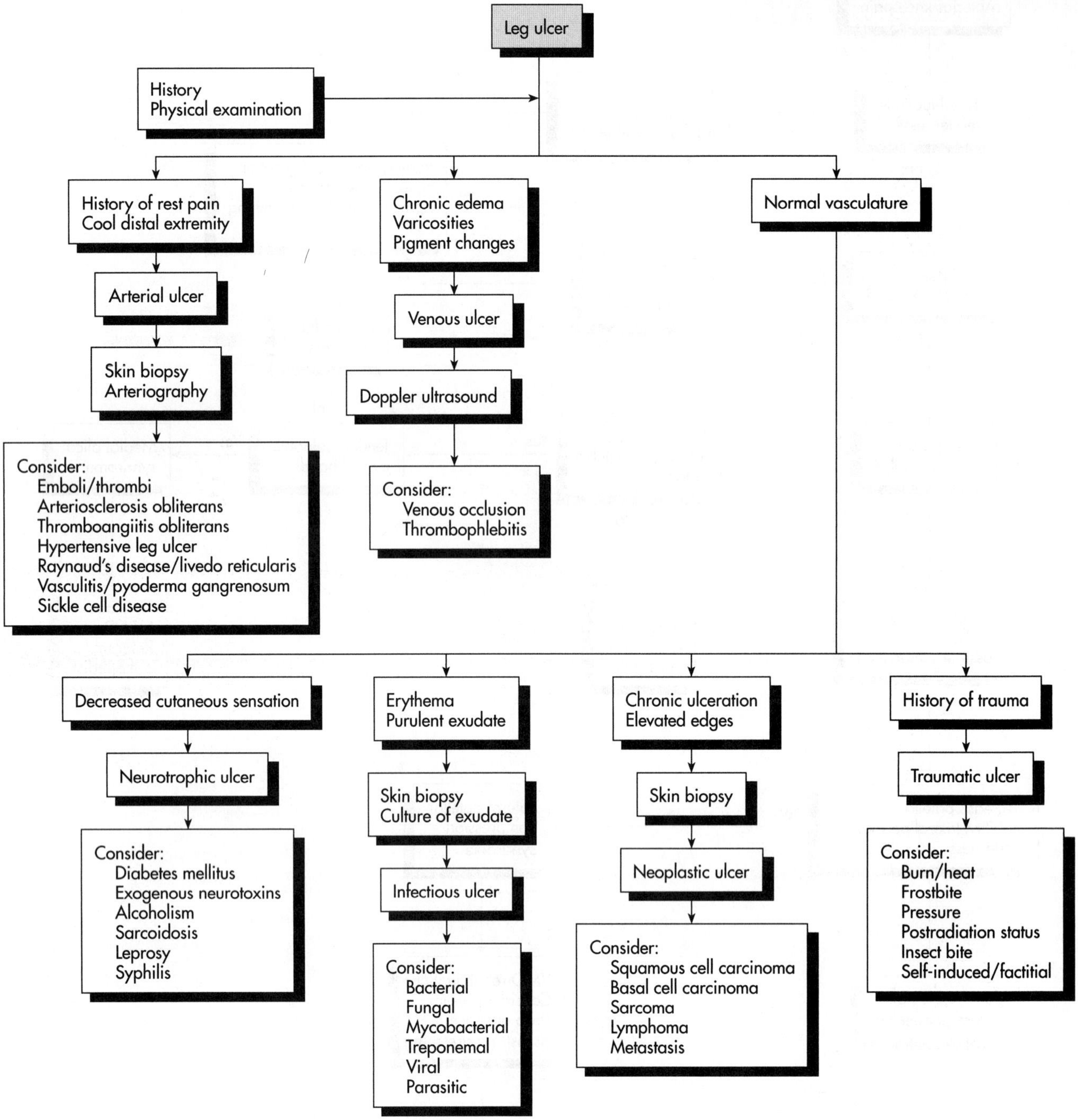

FIGURE 3-170 Leg ulcer. (From Greene HL, Johnson WP, Lemcke D [eds]: *Decision making in medicine*, ed 2, St Louis, 1998, Mosby.)

ICD-9CM # 573.9

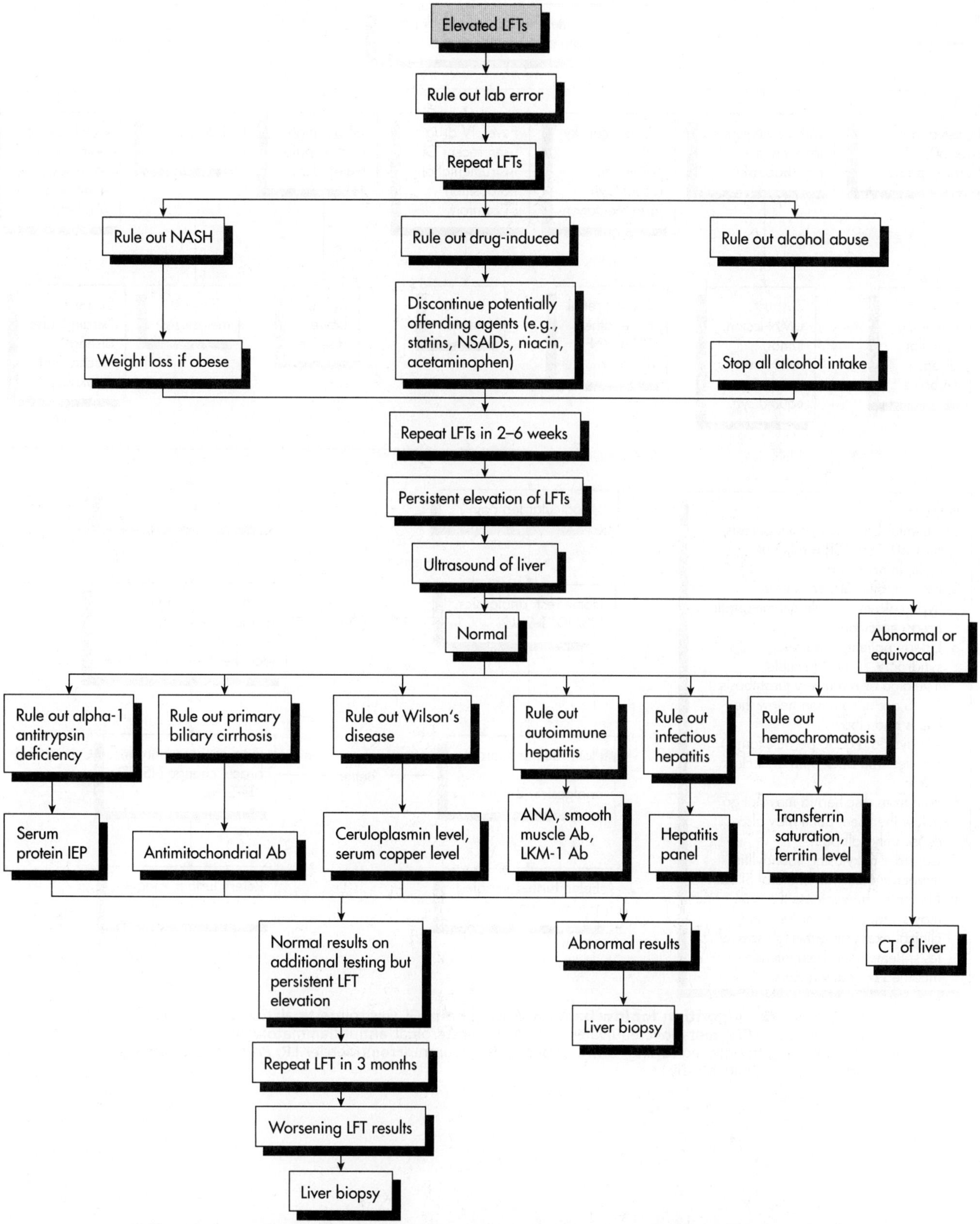

FIGURE 3-171 Liver function test elevations. *Ab,* Antibody; *ANA,* antibody to nuclear antigens; *CT,* computed tomography; *IEP,* immuno-electrophoresis; *LFT,* liver function test; *LKM,* liver-kidney microsome; *NASH,* nonalcoholic steatohepatitis; *NSAIDs,* nonsteroidal anti-inflammatory drugs.

LOW BACK AND/OR LEG PAIN

ICD-9CM # 724.2

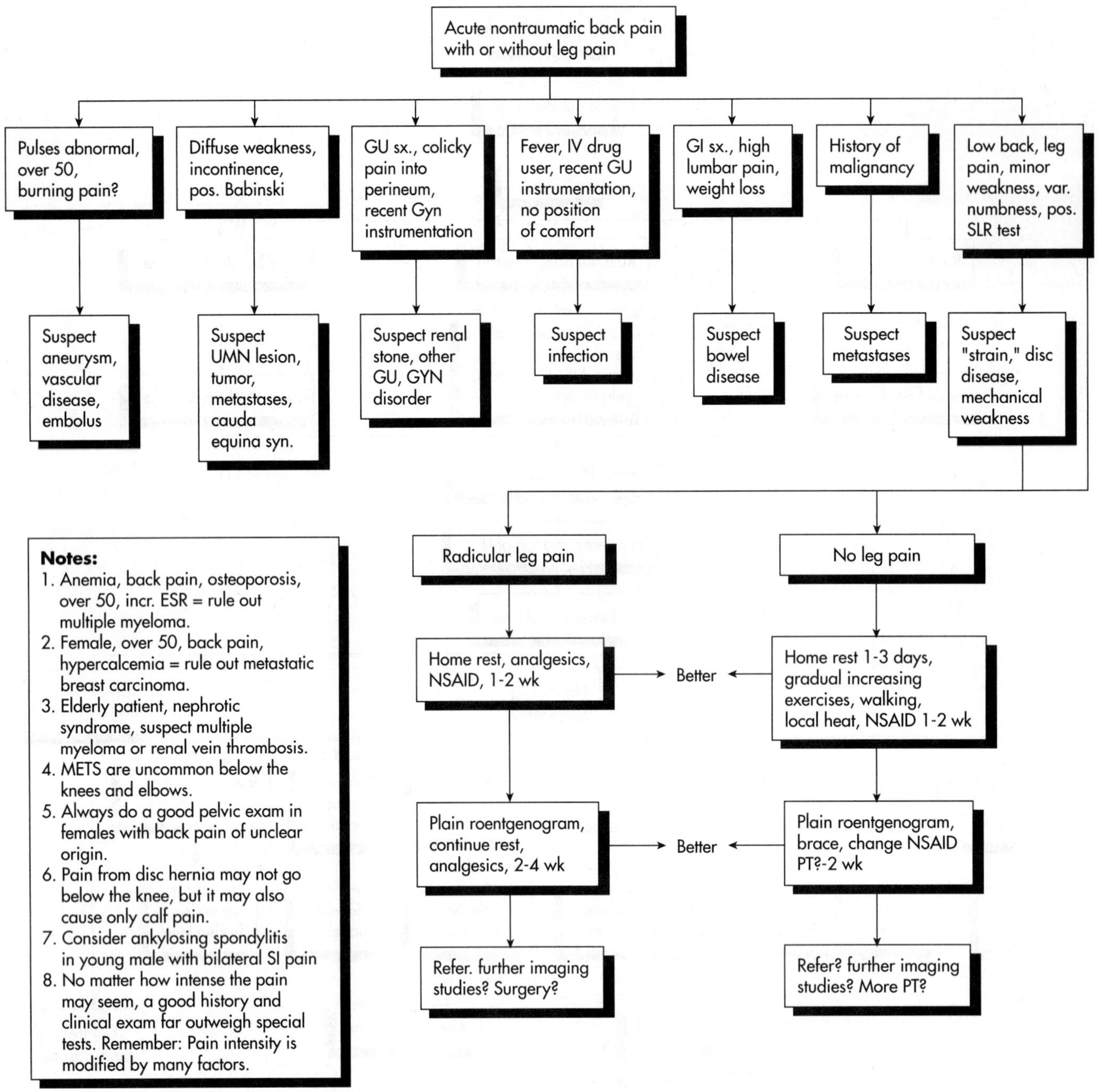

FIGURE 3-172 Algorithm for low back and/or leg pain. *GI,* Gastrointestinal; *GU,* genitourinary; *IV,* intravenous; *METS,* metabolic equivalents; *NSAID,* nonsteroidal anti-inflammatory drug; *PT,* physical therapy; *SLR,* straight-leg raising; *UMN,* upper motor neuron. (From Mercier LR: *Practical orthopedics,* ed 2, St Louis, 2000, Mosby.)

ICD-9CM # 785.6

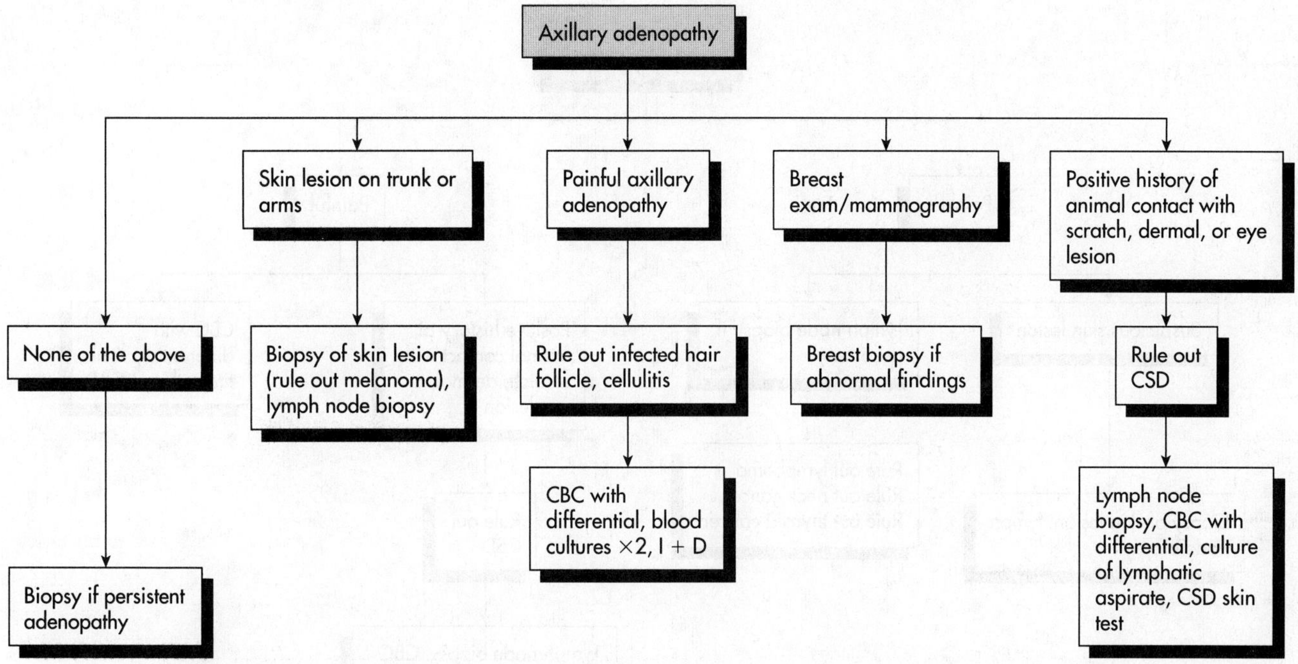

FIGURE 3-173 Lymphadenopathy, axillary. *CBC,* Complete blood count; *CSD,* cat-scratch disease.

ICD-9CM # 785.6

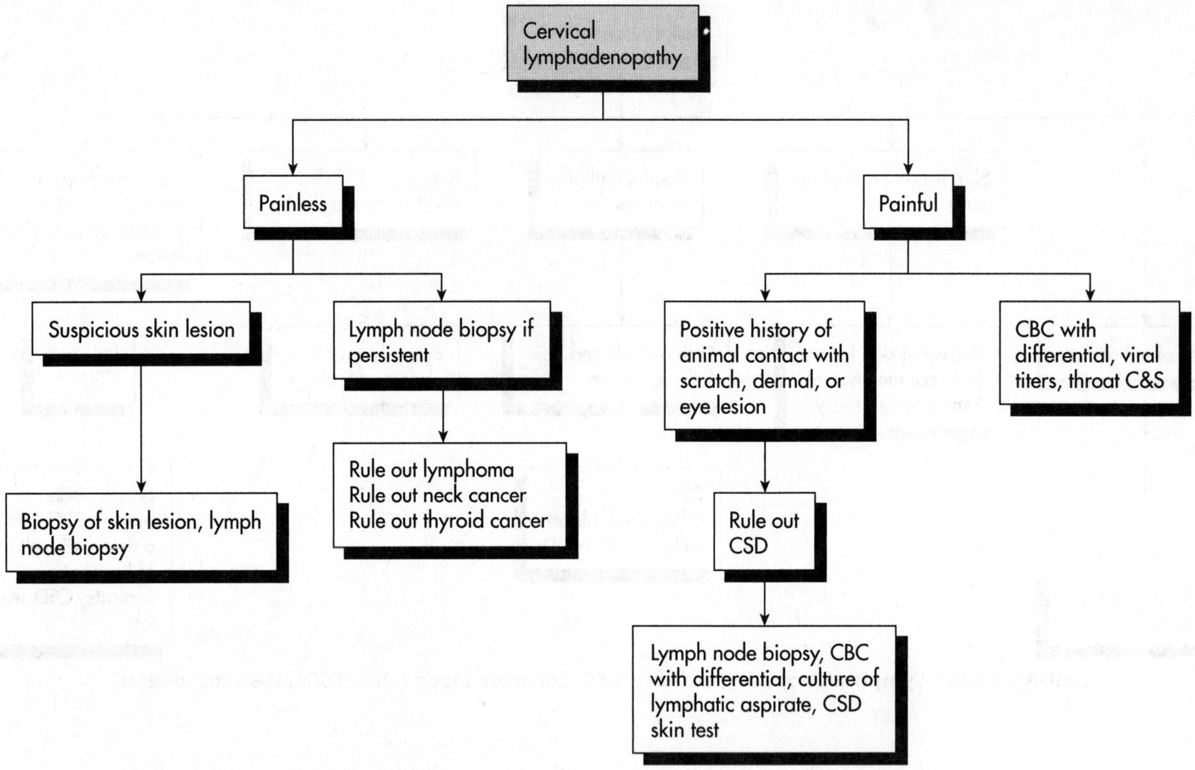

FIGURE 3-174 Lymphadenopathy, cervical. *CBC,* Complete blood count; *C&S,* culture and sensitivity; *CSD,* cat-scratch disease.

ICD-9CM # 785.6

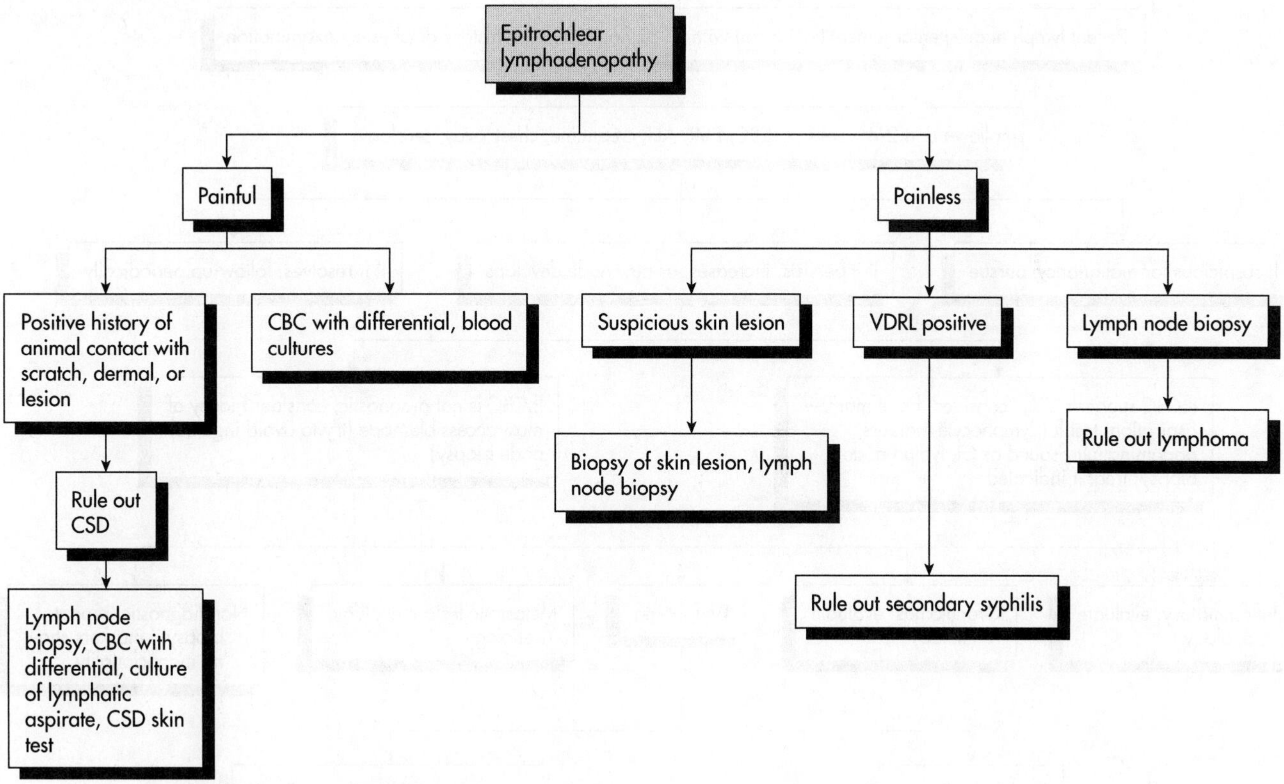

FIGURE 3-175 Lymphadenopathy, epitrochlear. *CBC,* Complete blood count; *CSD,* cat-scratch disease; *VDRL,* Venereal Disease Research Laboratory.

ICD-9CM # 785.6 Lymphadenopathy, unknown etiology

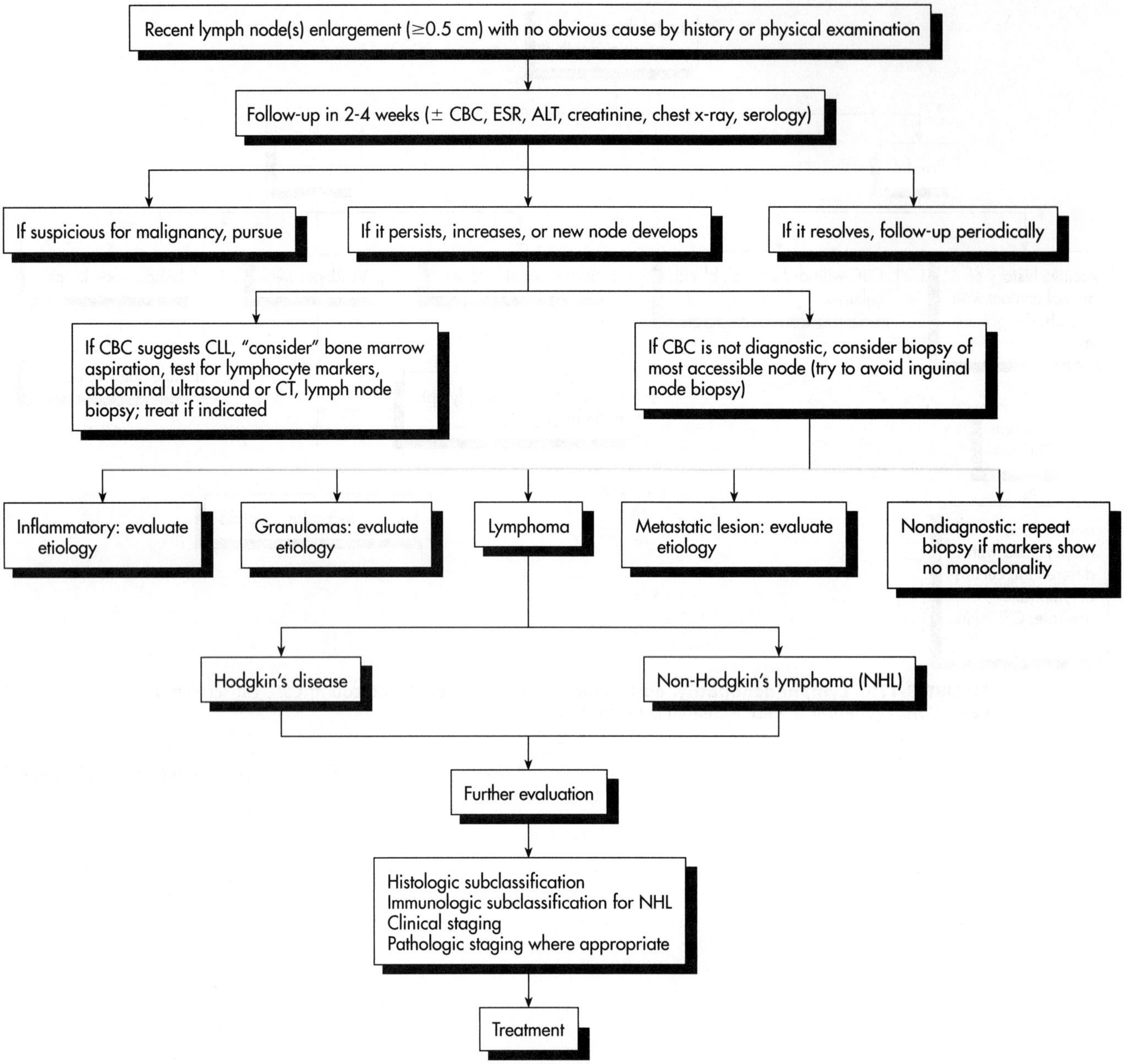

FIGURE 3-176 Workup of lymphadenopathy. *ALT,* Alanine aminotransferase; *CBC,* complete blood count; *CLL,* chronic lymphocytic leukemia; *CT,* computed tomography; *ESR,* erythrocyte sedimentation rate. (Modified from Noble J [ed]: *Primary care medicine*, ed 3, St Louis, 2001, Mosby.)

ICD-9CM # 785.6

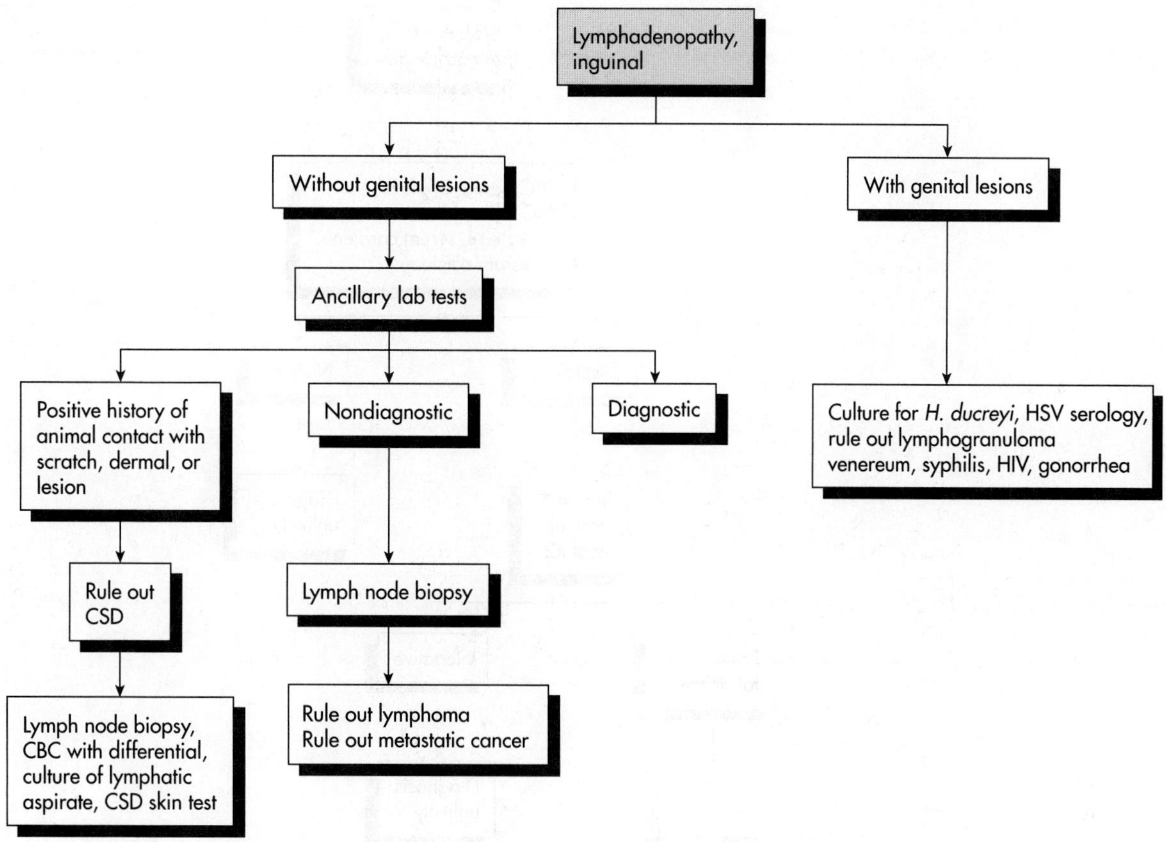

FIGURE 3-177 Lymphadenopathy, inguinal. *CBC,* Complete blood count; *CSD,* cat-scratch disease; *HSV,* herpes simplex virus.

ICD-9CM # 579.9

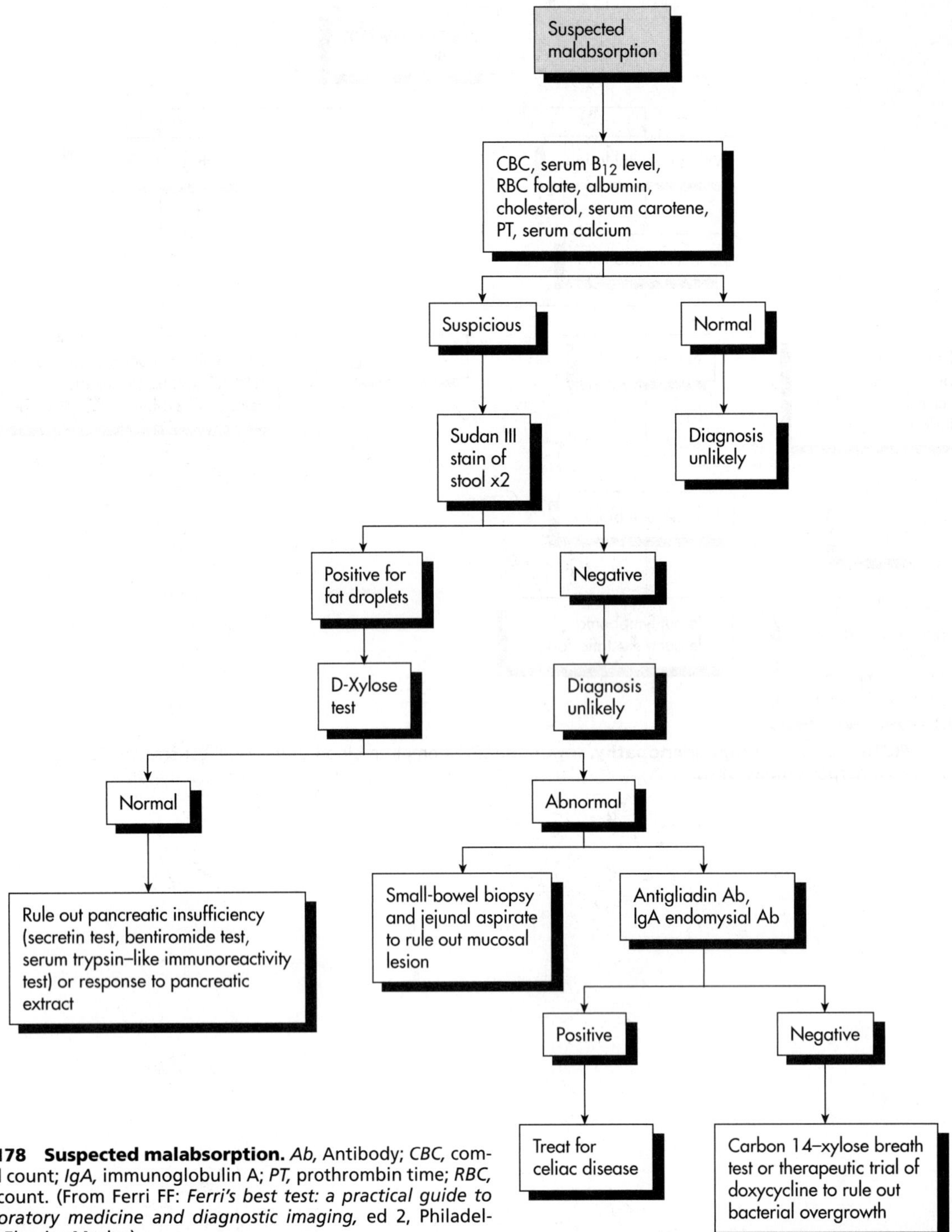

FIGURE 3-178 Suspected malabsorption. *Ab,* Antibody; *CBC,* complete blood count; *IgA,* immunoglobulin A; *PT,* prothrombin time; *RBC,* red blood count. (From Ferri FF: *Ferri's best test: a practical guide to clinical laboratory medicine and diagnostic imaging,* ed 2, Philadelphia, 2009, Elsevier Mosby.)

BOX 3-9 Malabsorption, Suspected

Diagnostic imaging
Best test
Small-bowel series
Ancillary test
CT of pancreas with IV contrast

Lab evaluation
Best test
Biopsy of small bowel

Ancillary tests
Albumin, total protein
ALT, AST, PT
Serum lytes, BUN, creatinine
Sudan III stain of stool for fecal leukocytes
CBC, RBC folate, serum iron, serum carotene, cholesterol, serum calcium
Hydrogen 14-C xylose breath test
D-Xylose test, secretin test
Quantitative fecal test
Antigliadin antibody, IgA endomysial antibody

From Ferri FF: *Ferri's best test: a practical guide to clinical laboratory medicine and diagnostic imaging,* ed 2, Philadelphia, 2009, Elsevier Mosby.

ALT, Alanine aminotransferase; *AST,* aspartate aminotransferase; *BUN,* blood urea nitrogen; *CBC,* complete blood count; *CT,* computed tomography; *IgA,* immunoglobulin A; *IV,* intravenous; PT, prothrombin time; *RBC,* red blood count.

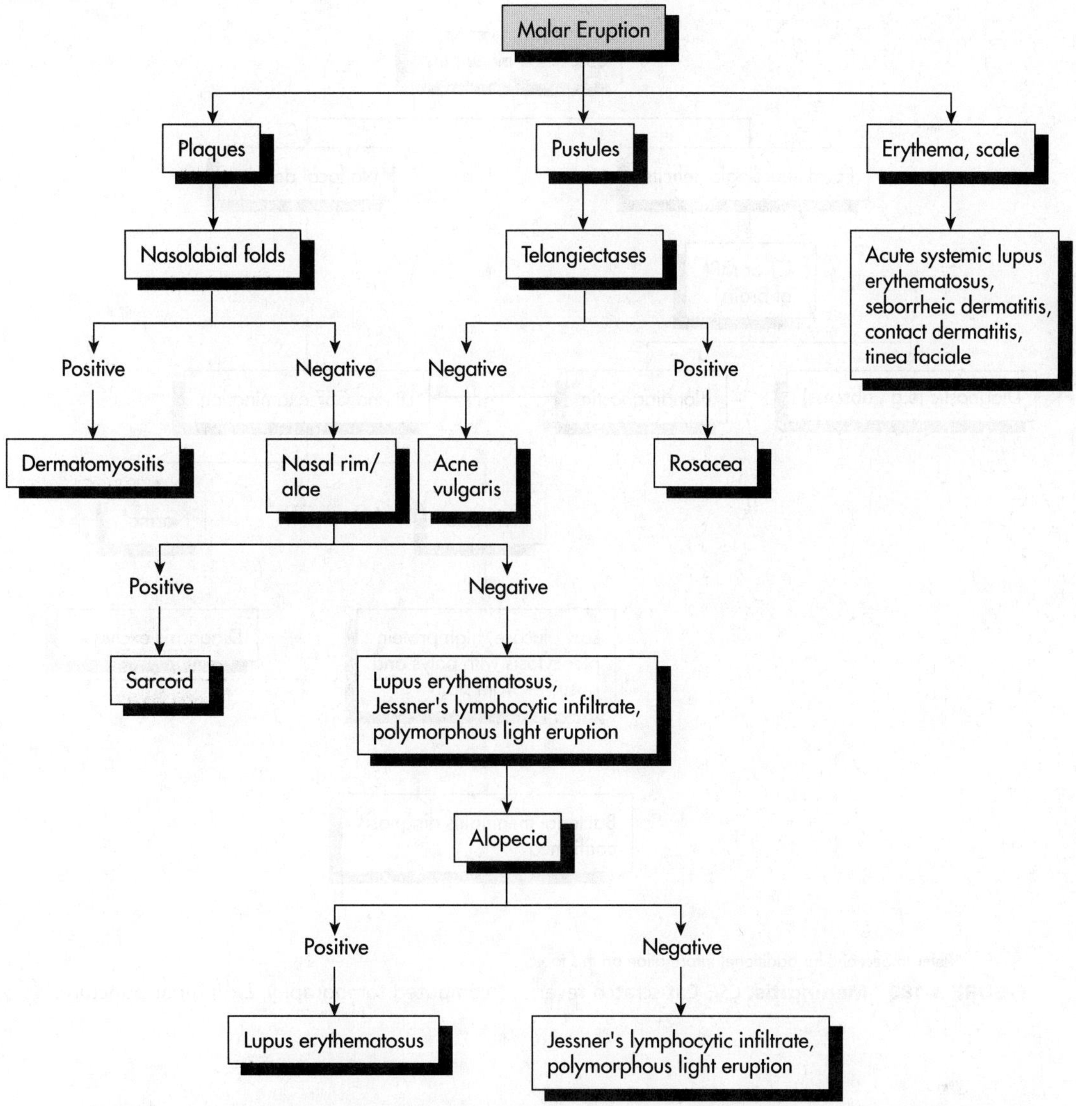

FIGURE 3-179 Clinical algorithm for diagnosis of a malar eruption, which must be confirmed by appropriate cultures, serology, and biopsy. (From Harris ED, Budd RC, Firestein GS, Genovese MC, Sergent JS, Ruddy S, Sledge CB [eds]: *Kelley's textbook of rheumatology,* ed 7, Philadelphia, 2005, Saunders.)

ICD-9CM # 320 Bacterial meningitis
047.8 Meningitis, aseptic

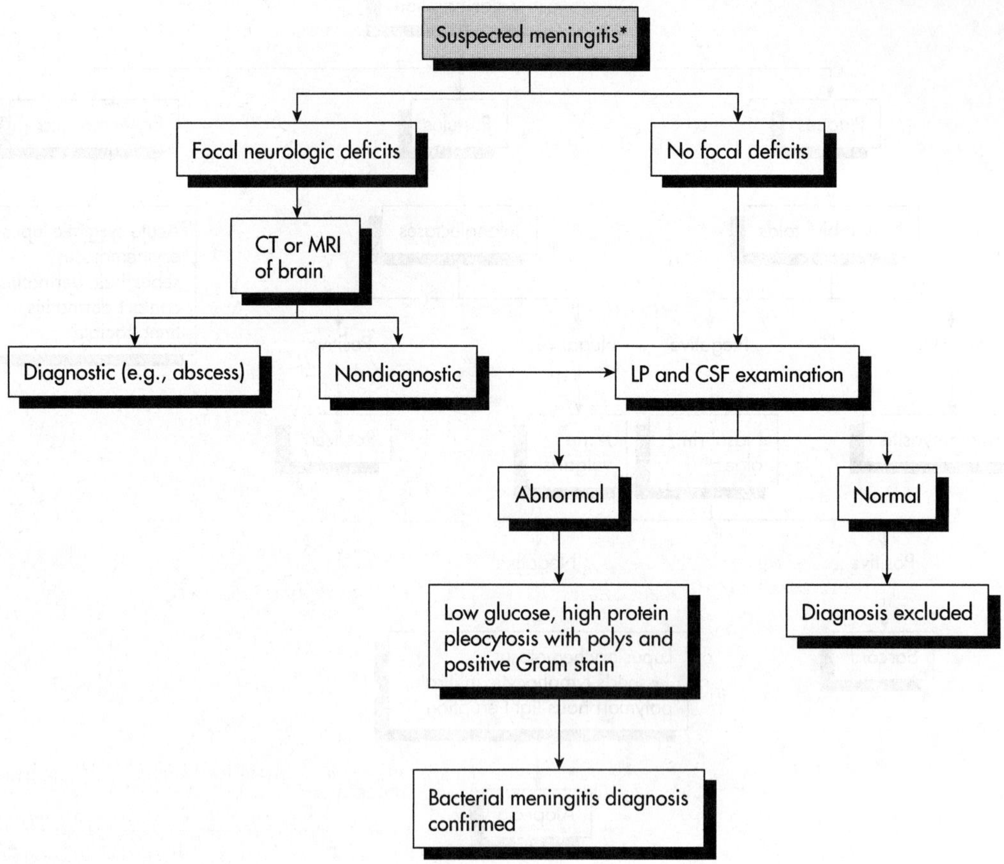

*Refer to Section I for additional information on this topic.

FIGURE 3-180 Meningitis. *CSF,* Cat-scratch fever; *CT,* computed tomography; *LP,* lumbar puncture.

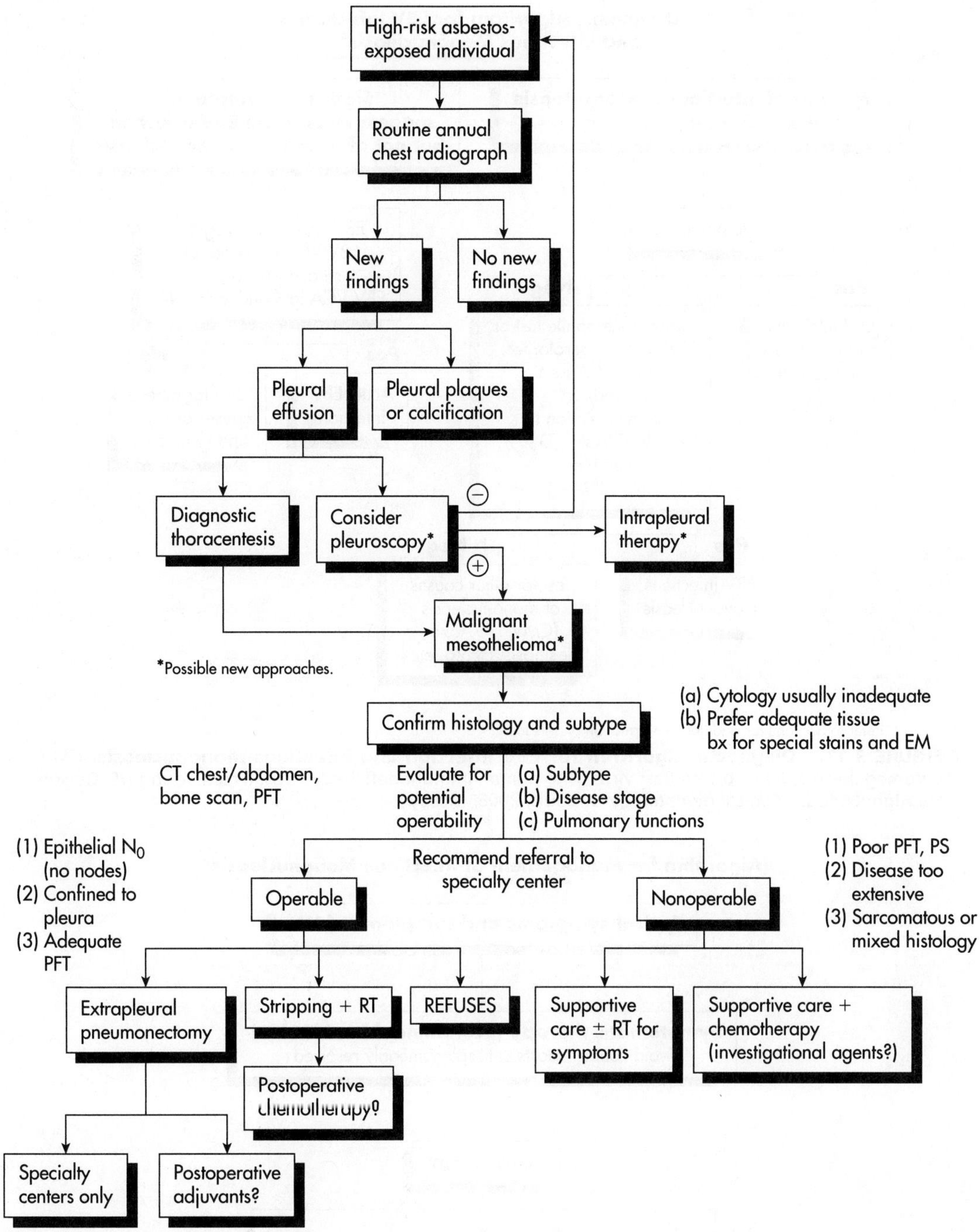

*Refer to Section I for additional information on this topic.

FIGURE 3-181 Evaluation and treatment of mesothelioma. *bx,* Biopsy; *CT,* computed tomography; *EM,* electron microscopy; *PFT,* pulmonary function test; *PS,* pleural sclerosis; *RT,* respiratory therapy. (From Abeloff MD: *Clinical oncology,* ed 3, New York, 2004, Churchill Livingstone.)

ICD-9CM # 075

Diagnostic Algorithm for EBV Infection and Infectious Mononucleosis*

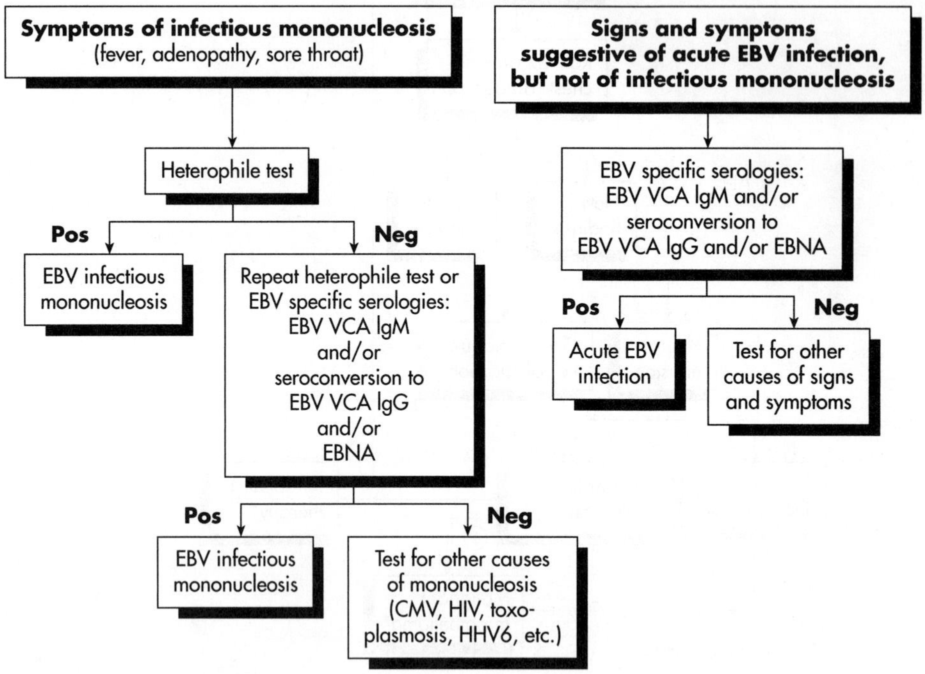

*Refer to Section I for additional information on this topic.

FIGURE 3-182 Diagnostic algorithm for EBV infection and infectious mononucleosis. *CMV,* Cytomegalovirus; *EBV,* Epstein-Barr virus; *HIV,* human immunodeficiency virus. (From Young NS, Gerson SL, High KA [eds]: *Clinical hematology,* St Louis, 2006, Mosby.)

Algorithm for Management of Infectious Mononucleosis*

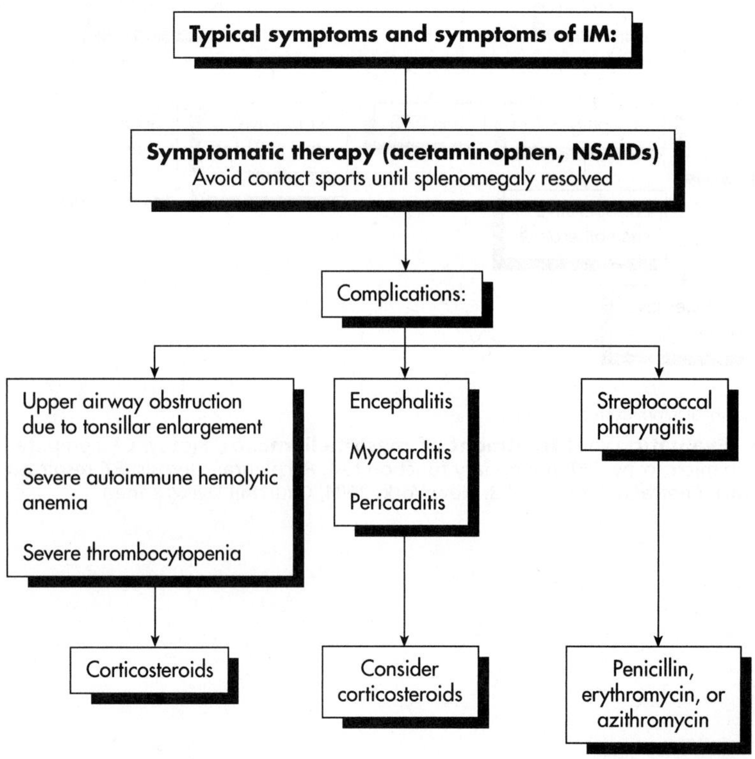

*Refer to Section I for additional information on this topic.

FIGURE 3-183 Algorithm for management of infectious mononucleosis. *IM,* Infectious mononucleosis; *NSAIDs,* nonsteroidal anti-inflammatory drugs. (From Young NS, Gerson SL, High KA [eds]: *Clinical hematology,* St Louis, 2006, Mosby.)

MULTIPLE MYELOMA

ICD-9CM # 203.0

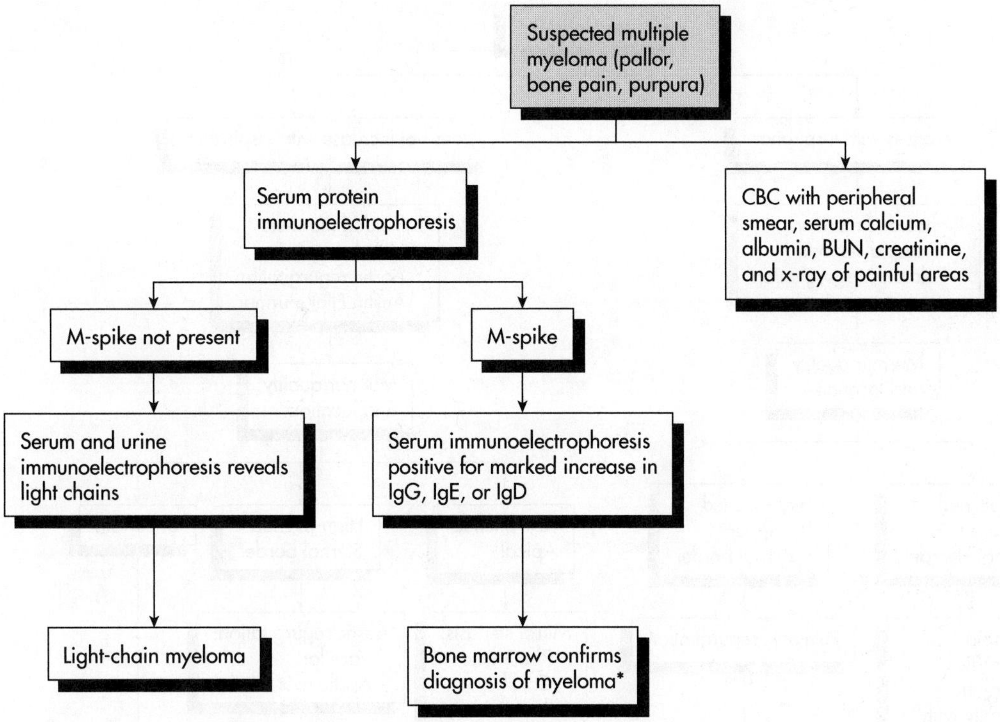

*Refer to Section I for additional information on this topic.

FIGURE 3-184 Multiple myeloma. *CBC,* Complete blood count; *Ig,* immunoglobulin.

ICD-9CM # 785.2 Murmur heart

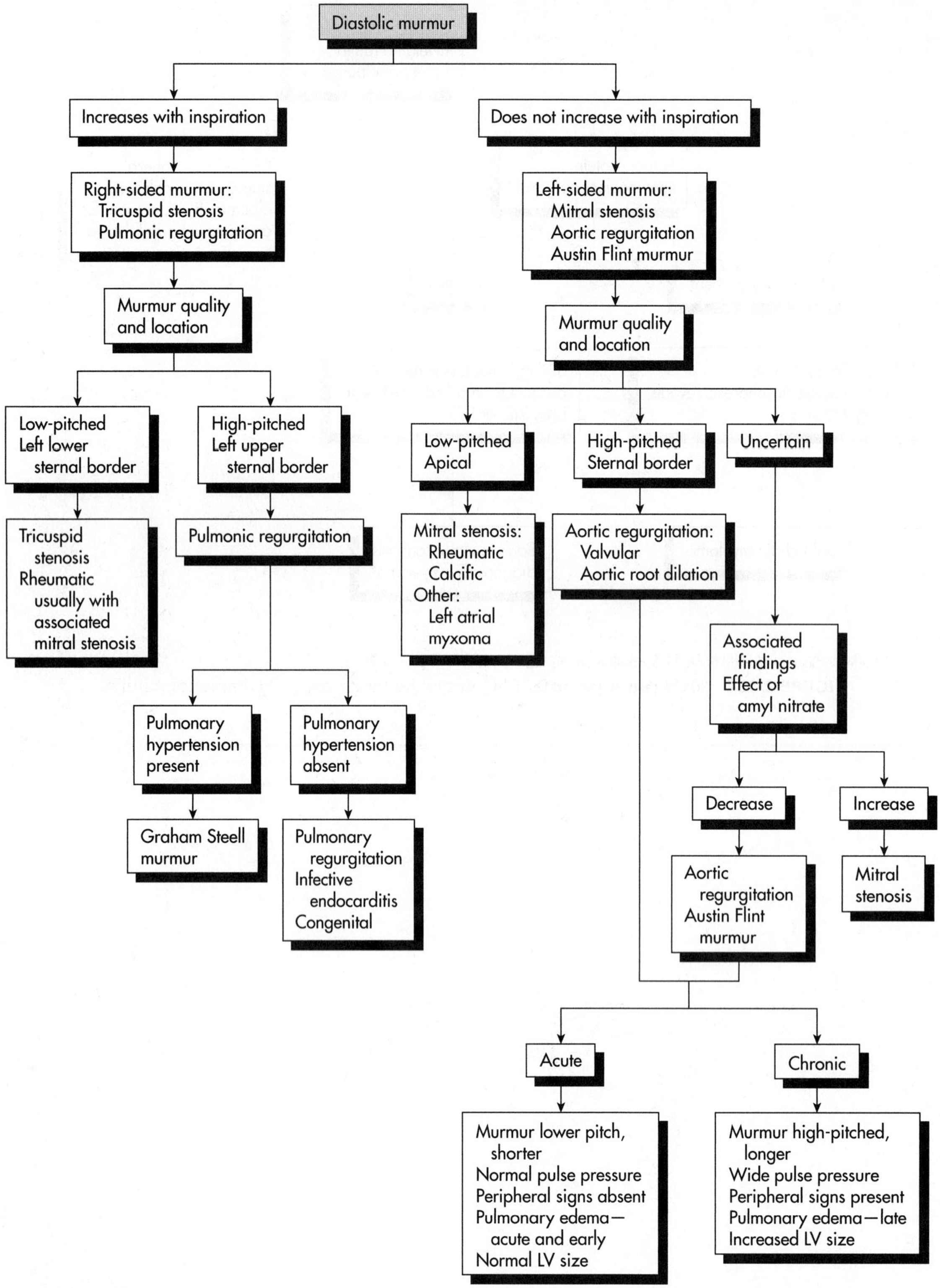

FIGURE 3-185 Diastolic murmur. *LV,* Left ventricle. (From Greene HL, Johnson WP, Lemke D [eds]: *Decision making in medicine,* ed 2, St Louis, 1998, Mosby.)

ICD-9CM # 785.2 Murmur heart

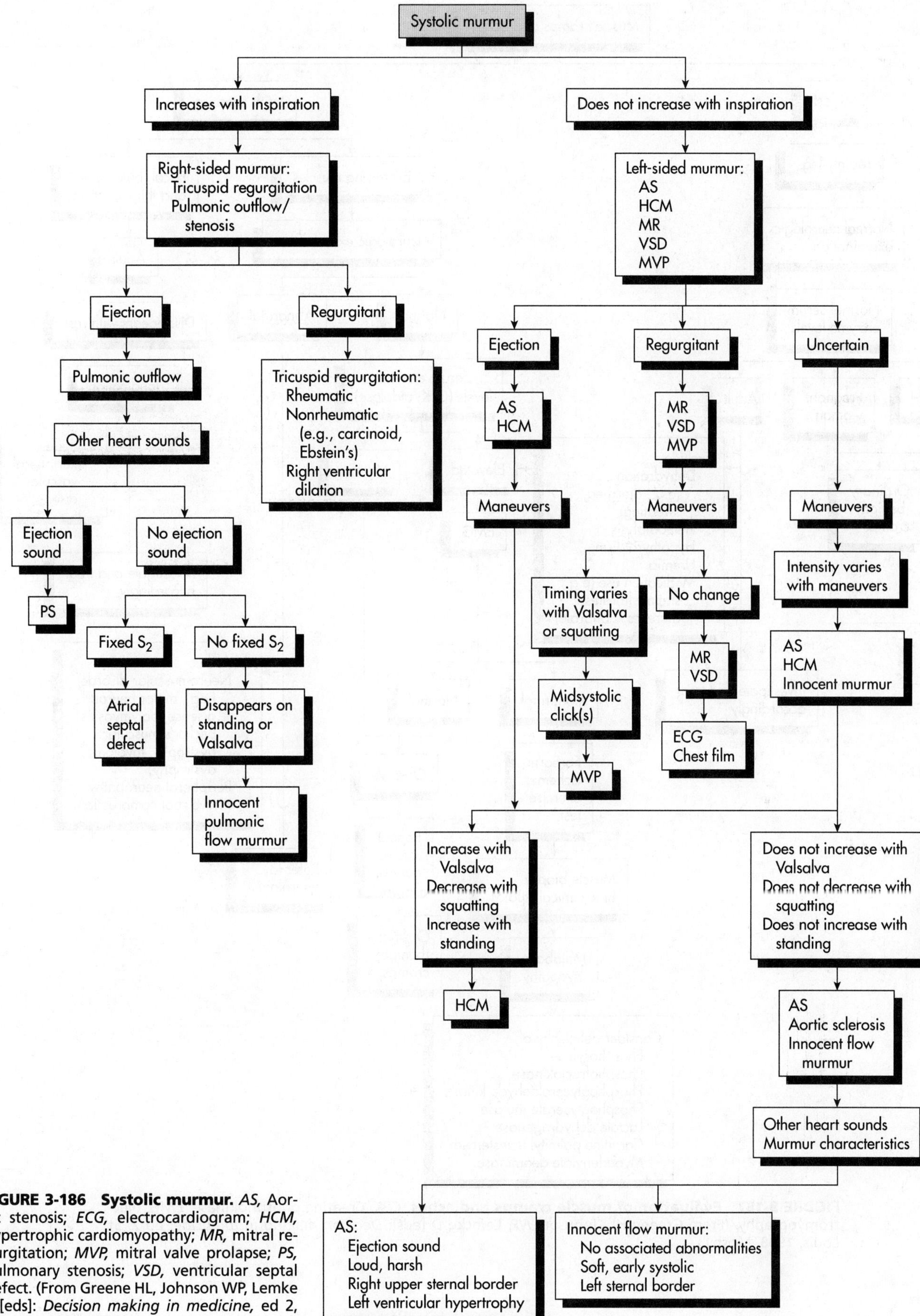

FIGURE 3-186 Systolic murmur. *AS,* Aortic stenosis; *ECG,* electrocardiogram; *HCM,* hypertrophic cardiomyopathy; *MR,* mitral regurgitation; *MVP,* mitral valve prolapse; *PS,* pulmonary stenosis; *VSD,* ventricular septal defect. (From Greene HL, Johnson WP, Lemke D [eds]: *Decision making in medicine,* ed 2, St Louis, 1998, Mosby.)

ICD-9CM # 729.82

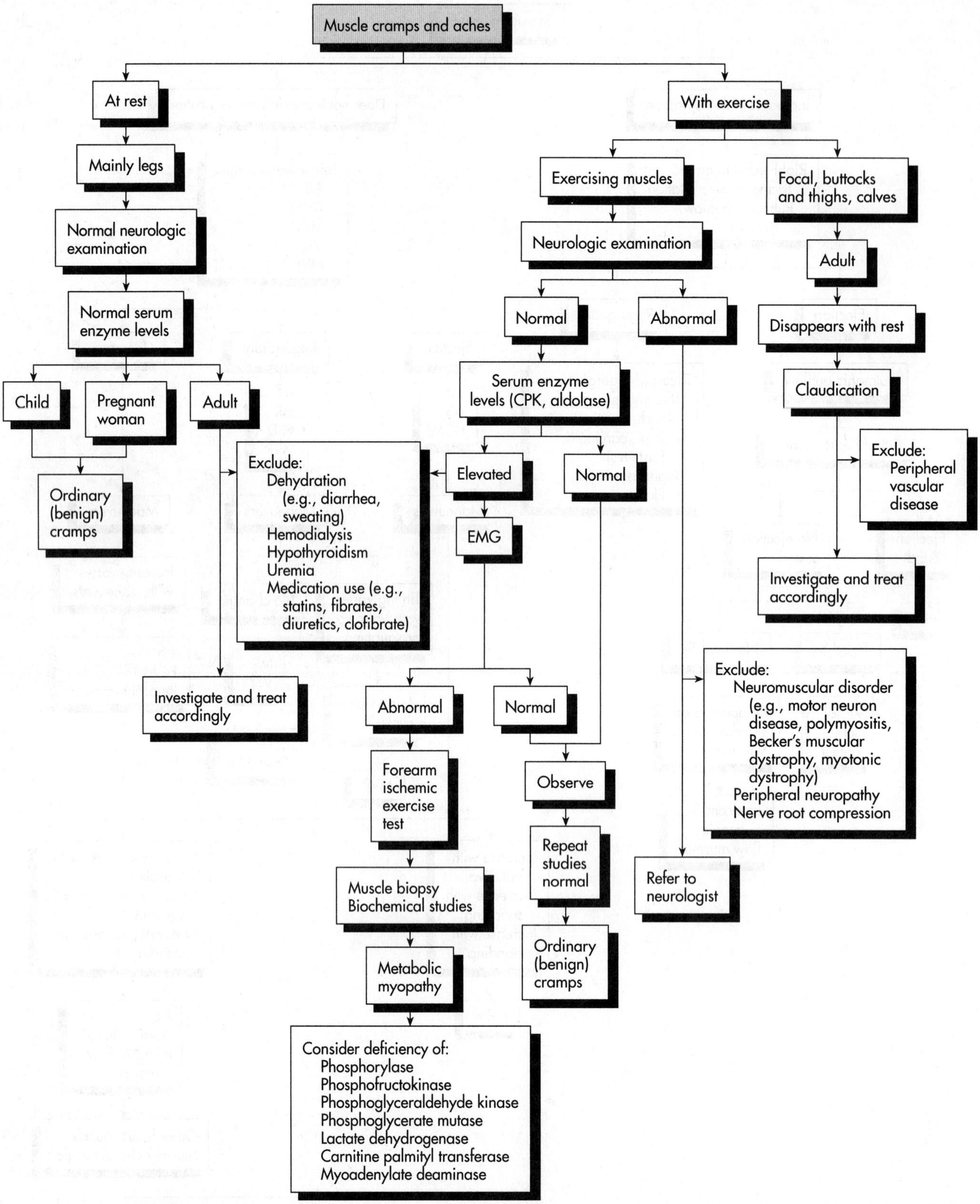

FIGURE 3-187 Evaluation of muscle cramps and aches. *CPK,* Creatine phosphokinase; *EMG,* electromyography. (From Greene HL, Johnson WP, Lemcke D [eds]: *Decision making in medicine,* ed 2, St Louis, 1998, Mosby.)

MUSCLE WEAKNESS

ICD-9CM # 782.9

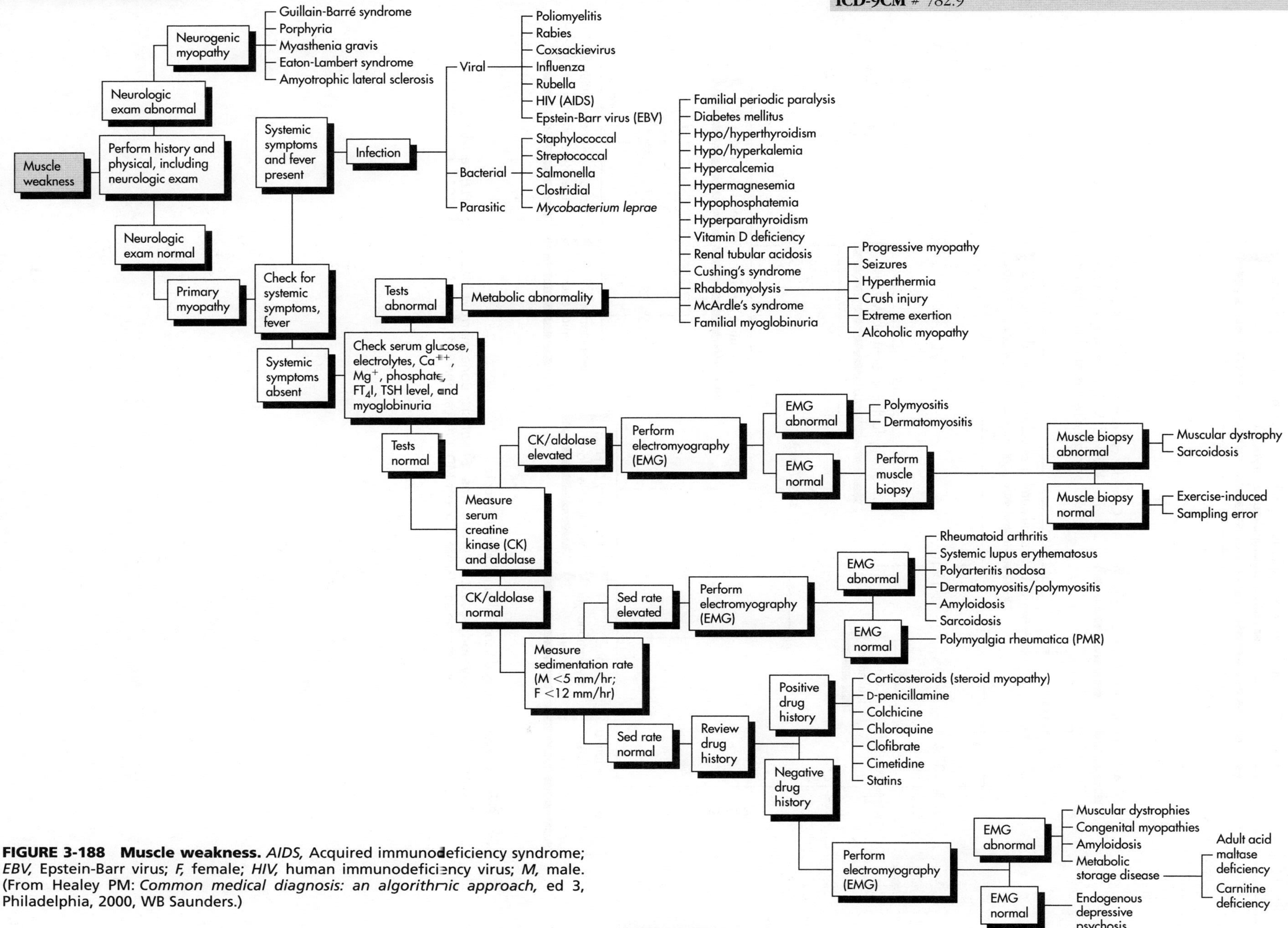

FIGURE 3-188 Muscle weakness. *AIDS,* Acquired immunodeficiency syndrome; *EBV,* Epstein-Barr virus; *F,* female; *HIV,* human immunodeficiency virus; *M,* male. (From Healey PM: *Common medical diagnosis: an algorithmic approach,* ed 3, Philadelphia, 2000, WB Saunders.)

ICD-9CM # 238.7

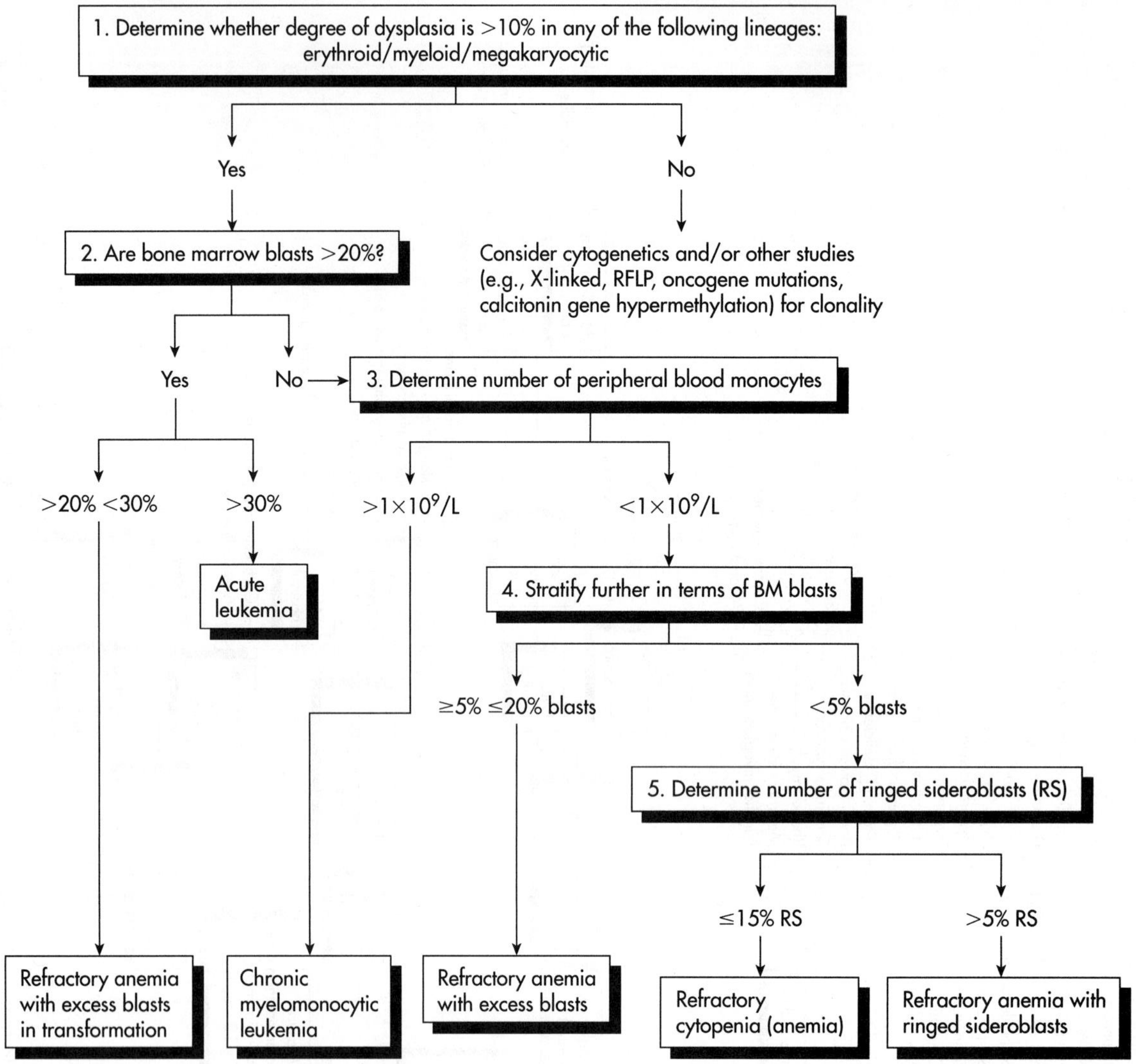

Note: Refer to Section I for additional information on this topic.

FIGURE 3-189 Myelodysplastic syndromes. *BM blasts,* Bone marrow blastocyst; *RFLP,* restriction fragment length polymorphism. (From Abeloff MD: *Clinical oncology,* ed 3, New York, 2004, Churchill Livingstone.)

MYOCARDIAL ISCHEMIA, SUSPECTED

ICD-9CM # 290.10 Dementia, presenile
290.0 Dementia, senile
437.0 Dementia, arteriosclerotic

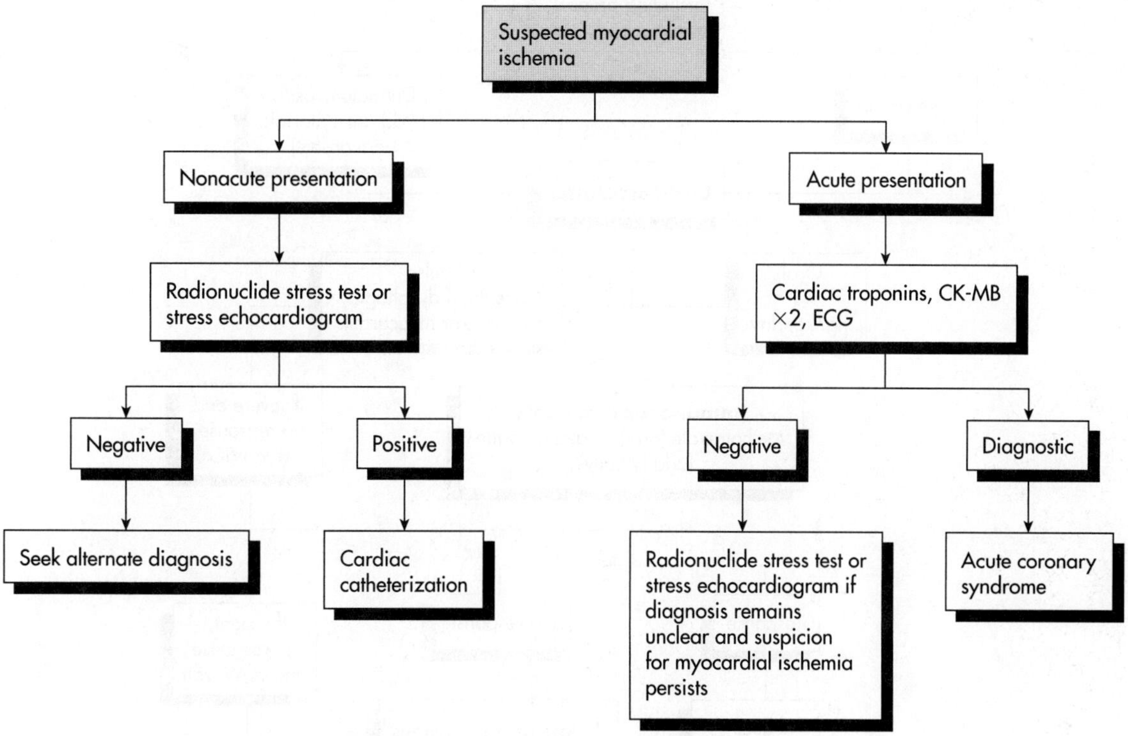

FIGURE 3-190 Myocardial ischemia, suspected. *CK-MB,* Myocardial muscle creatine kinase isoenzyme; *ECG,* electrocardiogram.

ICD-9CM # 729.1

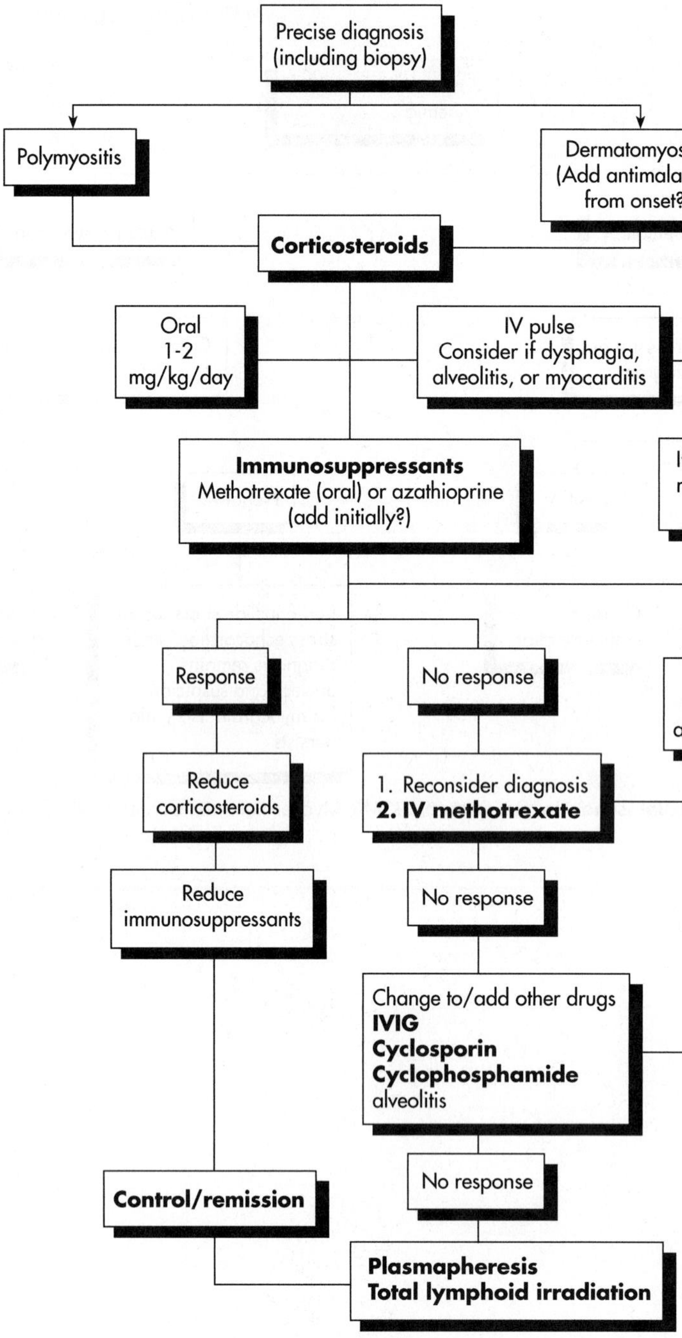

FIGURE 3-191 Drug management of myositis. Tentative algorithm for drug management of polymyositis and dermatomyositis. *IV,* Intravenous; *IVIG,* IV immunoglobulins. (From Hochberg MC, Silman AJ, Smolen JS, Weinblatt ME, Weisman MH: *Rheumatology,* ed 3, St Louis, 2003, Mosby.)

ICD-9CM # 703.8

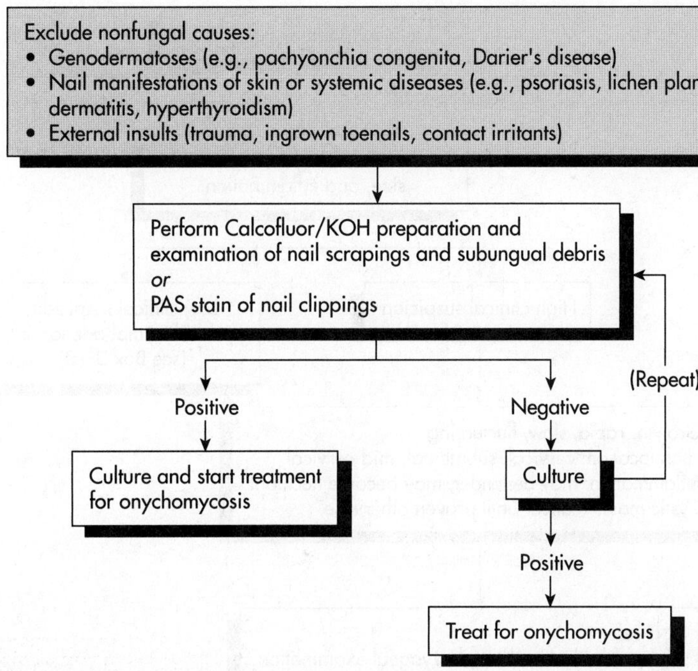

FIGURE 3-192 Diagnostic algorithm for dystrophy of one or more nails. An organized approach is essential in correctly and efficiently diagnosing onychomycosis. (From Bolognia JL, Mascaro JM, Mancini AJ, Salasche SJ, Saurat JH, Stingl G]eds]: *Dermatology,* ed 2, St Louis, 2008, Mosby.)

ICD-9CM # 784.2

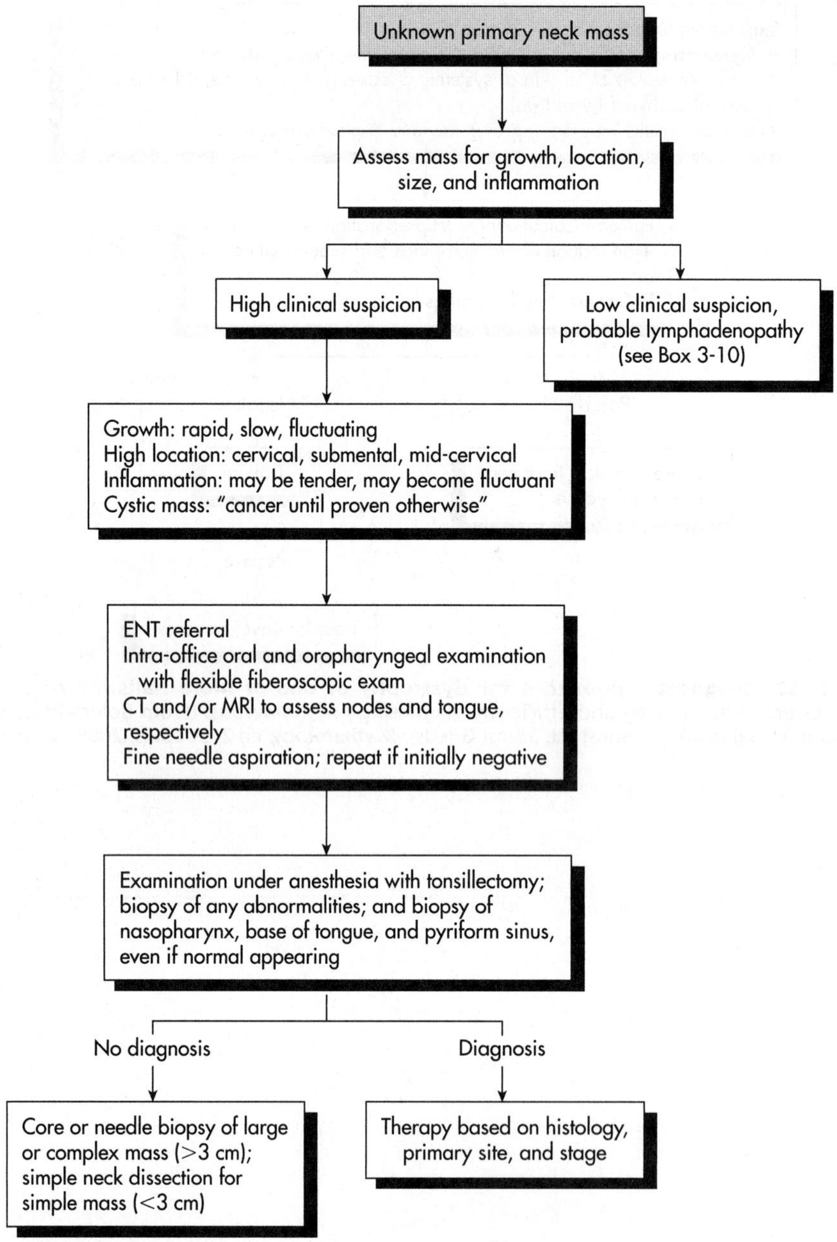

FIGURE 3-193 Evaluation of an unknown primary neck mass. *CT,* Computed tomography; *ENT,* ear, nose, and throat; *MRI,* magnetic resonance imaging. (From Goldman L, Ausiello D [eds]: *Cecil textbook of medicine,* ed 23, Philadelphia, 2008. WB Saunders.)

BOX 3-10 An Approach to the Patient with Lymphadenopathy

1. Does the patient have a known illness that causes lymphadenopathy? Treat and monitor for resolution.
2. Is there an obvious infection to explain the lymphadenopathy (e.g., infectious mononucleosis)? Treat and monitor for resolution.
3. Are the nodes very large and/or very firm and thus suggestive of malignancy? Perform a biopsy.
4. Is the patient very concerned about malignancy and unable to be reassured that malignancy is unlikely? Perform a biopsy.
5. If none of the preceding are true, perform a complete blood cell count and if it is unrevealing, monitor for a predetermined period (usually 2 to 6 weeks). If the nodes do not regress or if they increase in size, perform a biopsy.

From Goldman L, Ausiello D (eds): *Cecil textbook of medicine,* ed 23, Philadelphia, 2008, WB Saunders.

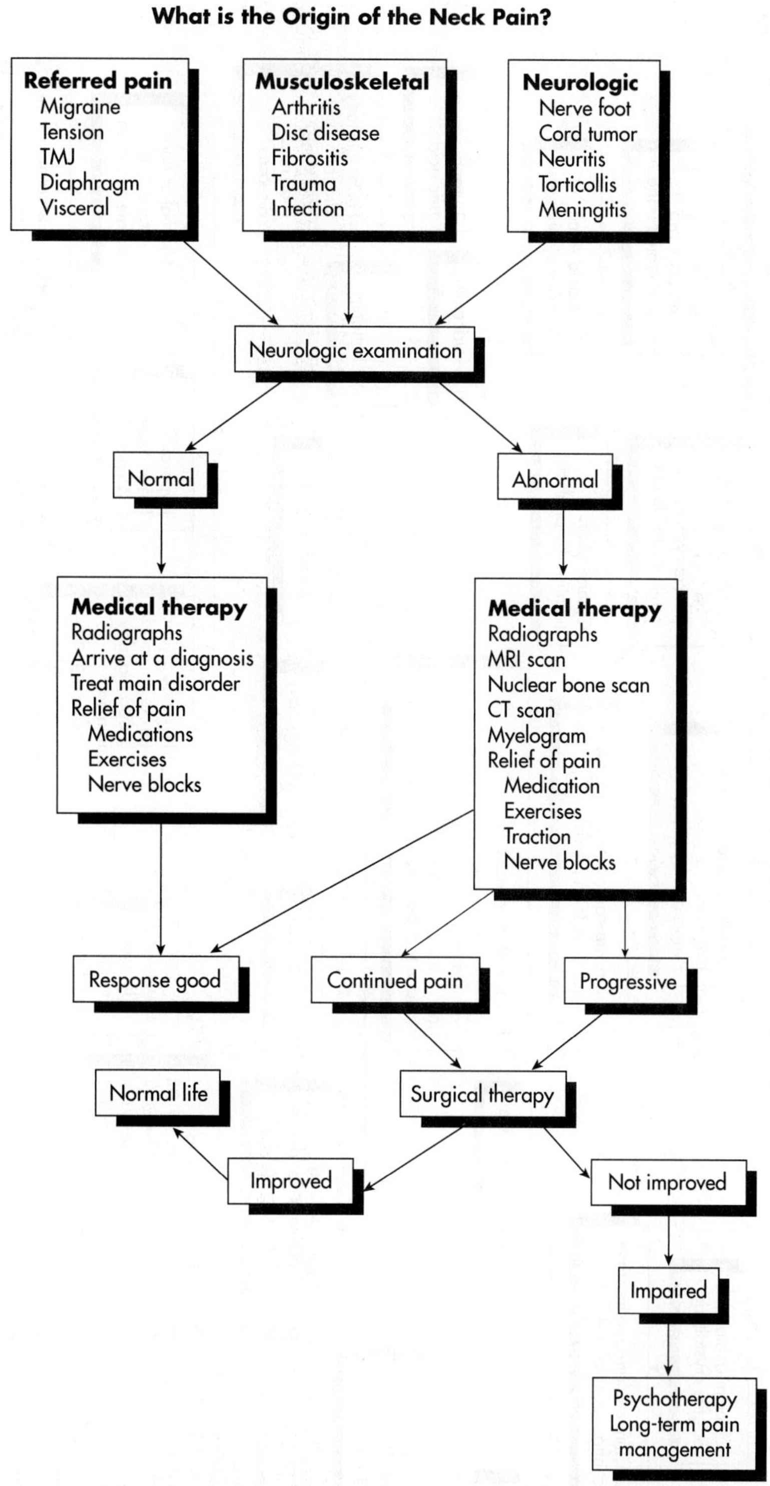

FIGURE 3-194 Neck pain algorithm for diagnosis and treatment. *CT,* Computed tomography; *MRI,* magnetic resonance imaging; *TMJ,* temporomandibular joint. (From Nakano KK: Neck and back pain. In Stein JH [ed]: *Internal medicine,* ed 5, St Louis, 1998, Mosby, pp 963-971.)

NEPHROLITHIASIS

ICD-9CM # 592.9 Urinary calculus

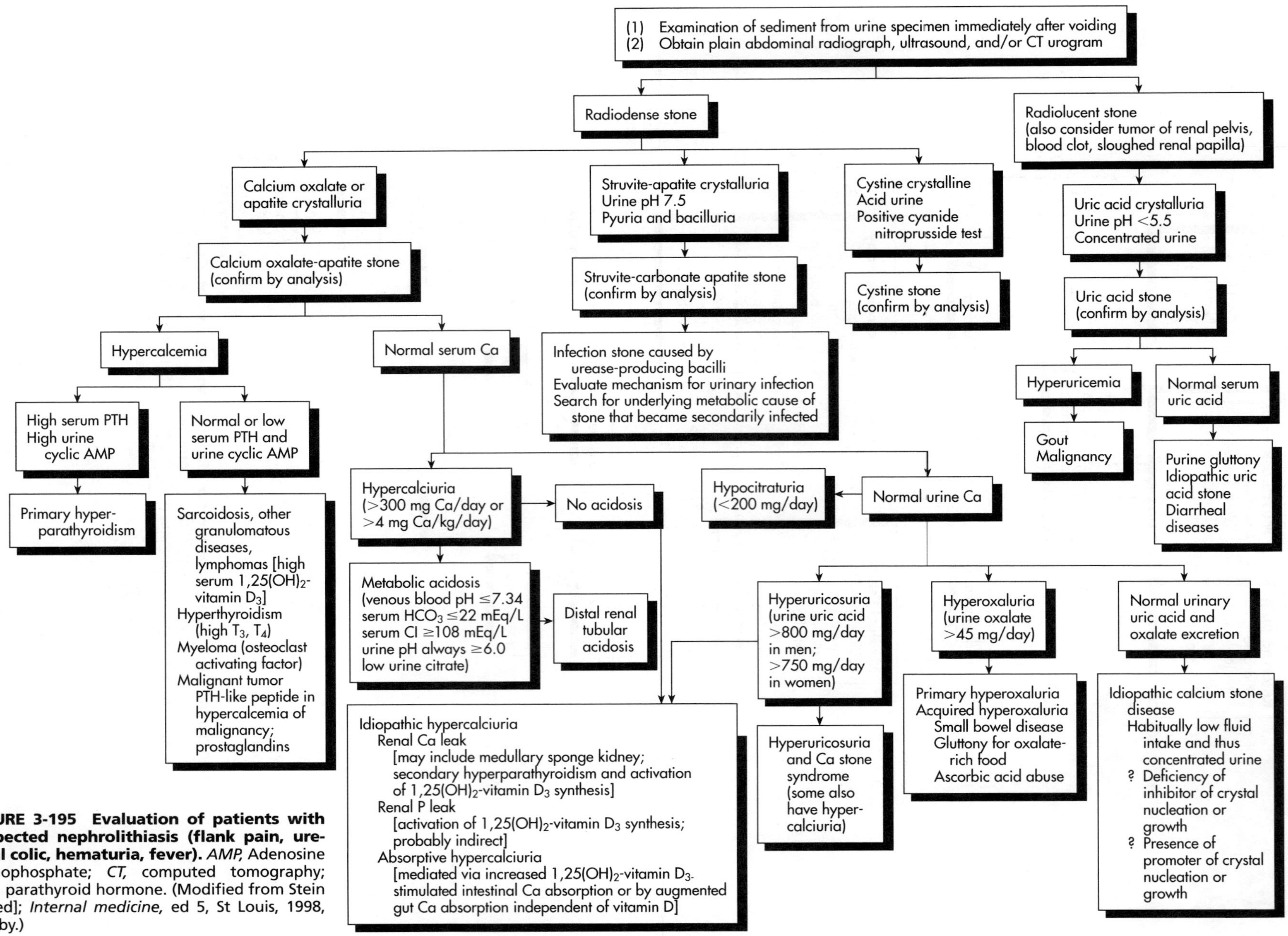

FIGURE 3-195 Evaluation of patients with suspected nephrolithiasis (flank pain, ureteral colic, hematuria, fever). *AMP,* Adenosine monophosphate; *CT,* computed tomography; *PTH,* parathyroid hormone. (Modified from Stein JH [ed]; *Internal medicine,* ed 5, St Louis, 1998, Mosby.)

ICD-9CM # 729.2

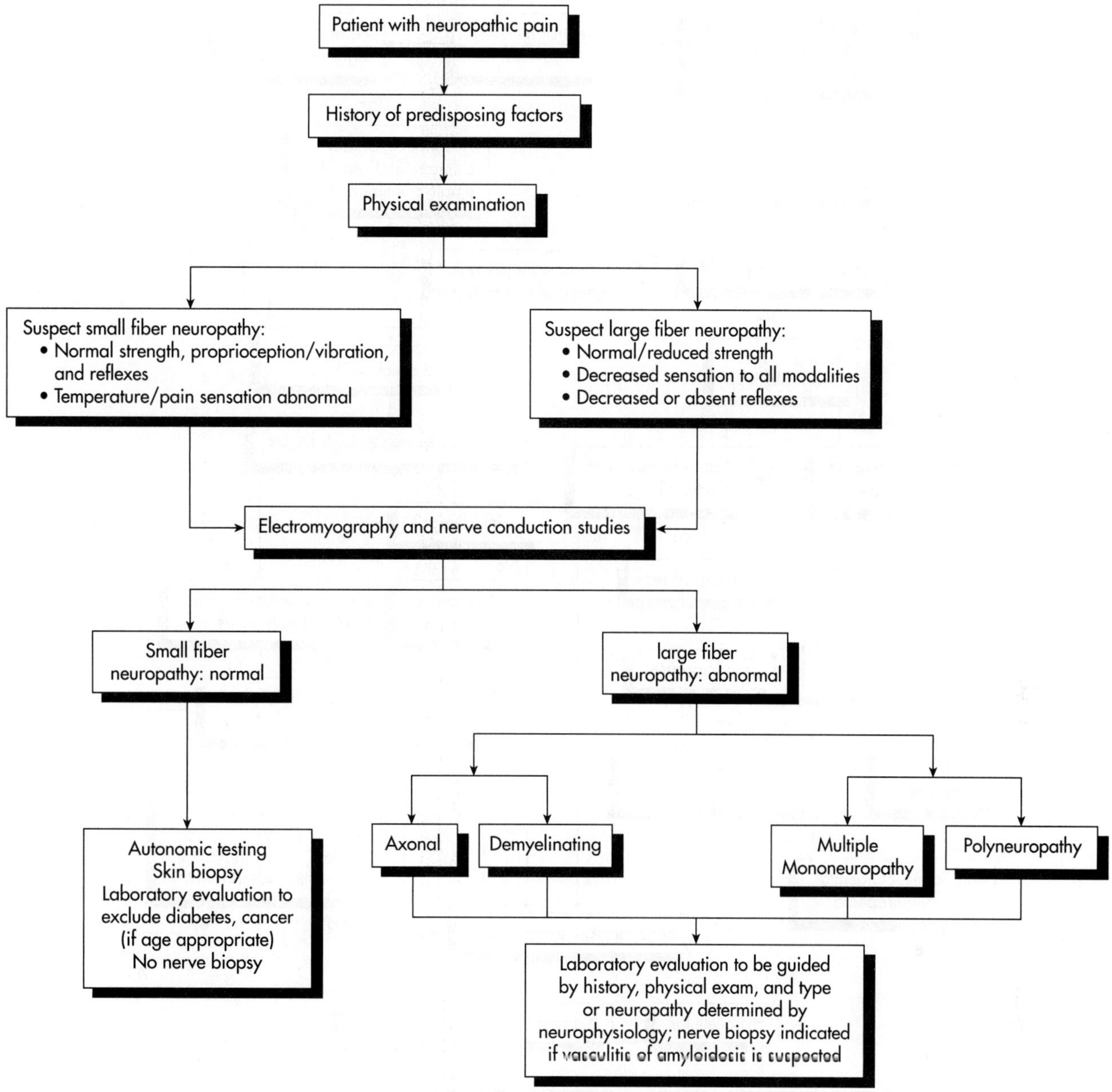

FIGURE 3-196 Neuropathic pain, diagnostic approach.

ICD-9CM # 288.0

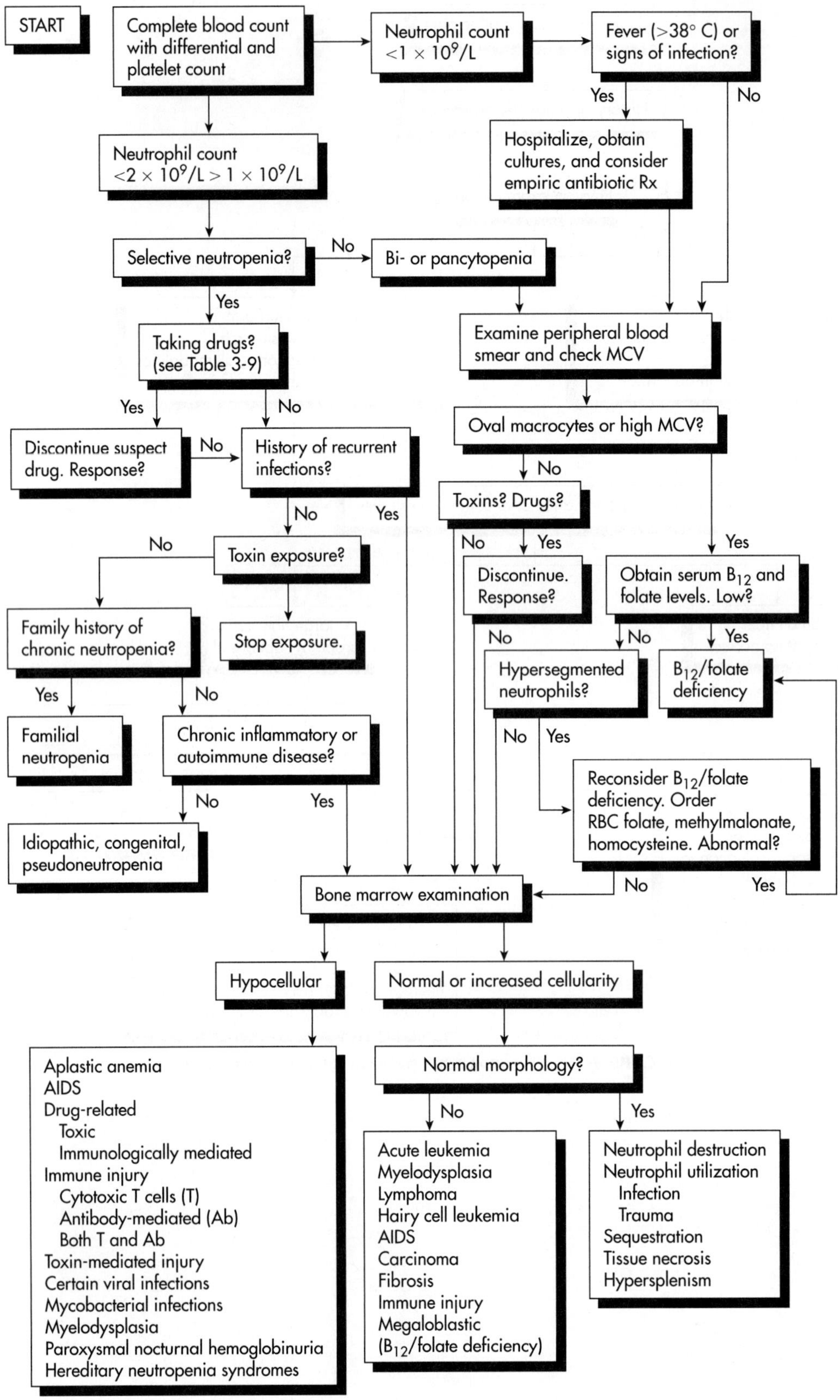

FIGURE 3-197 A practical algorithm for the evaluation of patients with neutropenia. The fundamental diagnostic principle is that for patients with severe neutropenia or for those with bicytopenia or pancytopenia, bone marrow examination will likely be necessary unless the following diagnoses are made: (1) a nutritional (folate or vitamin B_{12}) deficiency or (2) drug- or toxin-induced neutropenia in a patient whose neutropenia resolves after discontinuation of the offending agent. *AIDS,* Acquired immunodeficiency syndrome; *MCV,* mean corpuscular volume; *RBC,* red blood cell. (From Goldman L, Ausiello D [eds]: *Cecil textbook of medicine,* ed 23, Philadelphia, 2008, WB Saunders.)

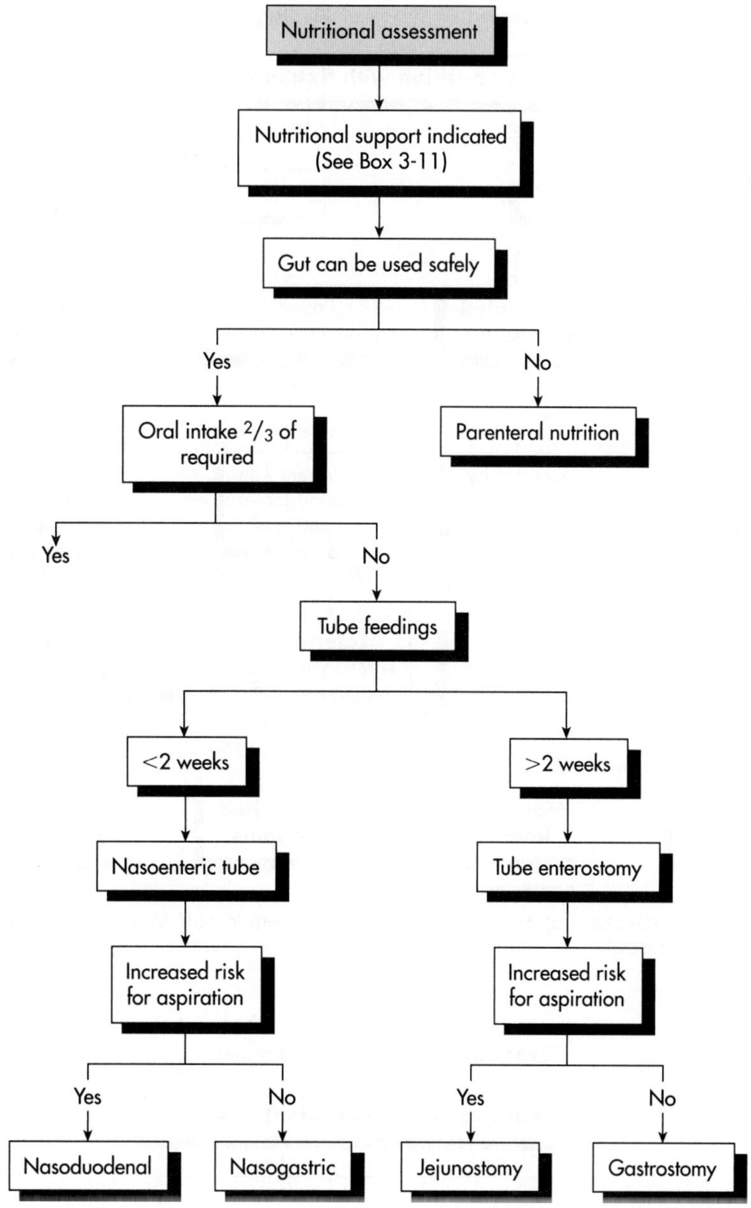

FIGURE 3-198 Decision approach for the type and route of nutritional support. (From Goldman L, Ausiello D [eds]: *Cecil textbook of medicine,* ed 23, Philadelphia, 2008, WB Saunders.)

BOX 3-11 **Indications for the Use of Enteral Nutrition in Adult Medical Patients**
Protein-energy malnutrition with anticipated significantly decreased oral intake for at least 7 days
Anticipated significantly decreased oral intake for 10 days
Severe dysphagia
Massive small bowel resection (used in combination with total parenteral nutrition)
Low-output (<500 ml/day) enterocutaneous fistula

From Goldman L, Ausiello D (eds): *Cecil textbook of medicine,* ed 23, Philadelphia, 2008, WB Saunders.

ICD-9CM # 379.50

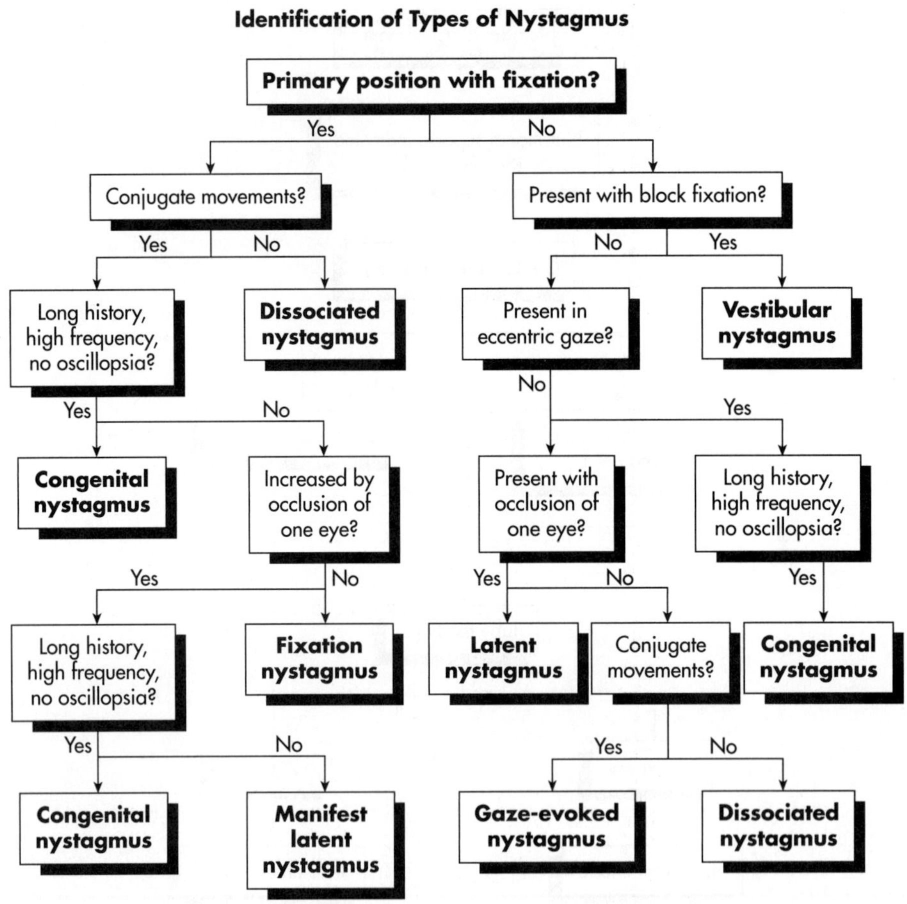

FIGURE 3-199 Identification of types of nystagmus. (From Yanoff M, Duker JS: *Ophthalmology,* ed 2, St Louis, 2004, Mosby.)

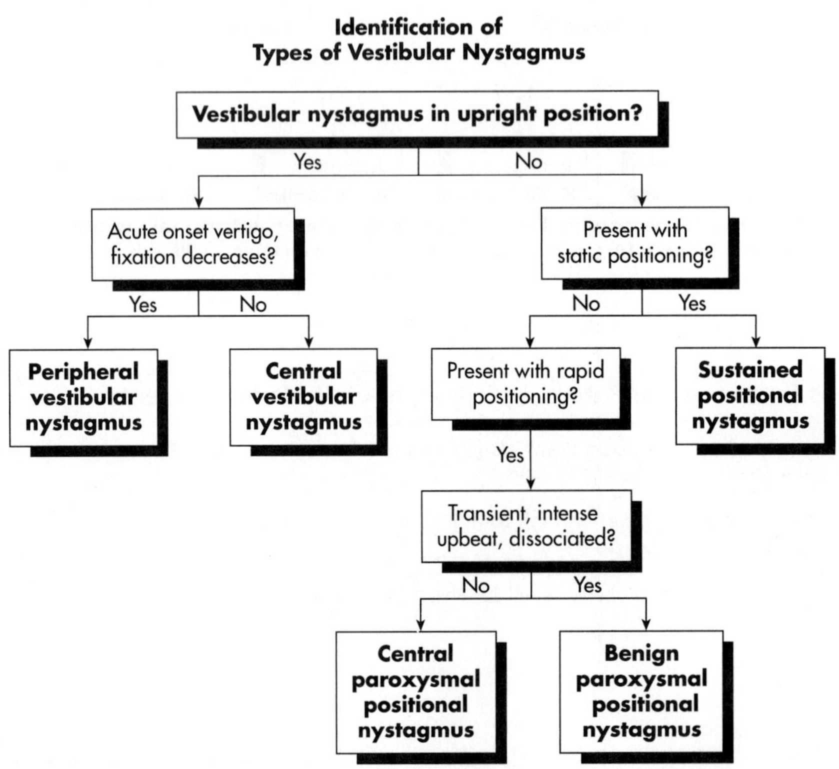

FIGURE 3-200 Identification of types of vestibular nystagmus. (From Yanoff M, Duker JS: *Ophthalmology,* ed 2, St Louis, 2004, Mosby.)

TABLE 3-13 Characteristics and Localizations of Vestibular Nystagmus

Nystagmus	Characteristics	Localization
Spontaneous peripheral vestibular	Jerk, horizontal, small torsional, inhibited by fixation	Labyrinth, eighth nerve (acute)
Central vestibular (fixation) nystagmus	Jerk, pendular, horizontal, vertical, torsional, not inhibited by fixation	Brainstem, cerebellum
Sustained positional vestibular	Jerk, horizontal, small torsional, direction fixed, direction changing (static positioning)	Labyrinth, eighth nerve or brainstem, cerebellum
Benign paroxysmal positional	Jerk, dissociated upbeat, latency, not inhibited by fixation, fatigue (Nylen–Barany maneuver)	Posterior vertical canal
Central paroxysmal positional	Jerk, symmetric, upbeat, downbeat	Brainstem, cerebellum

From Yanoff M, Duker JS: *Ophthalmology,* ed 2, St Louis, 2004, Mosby.

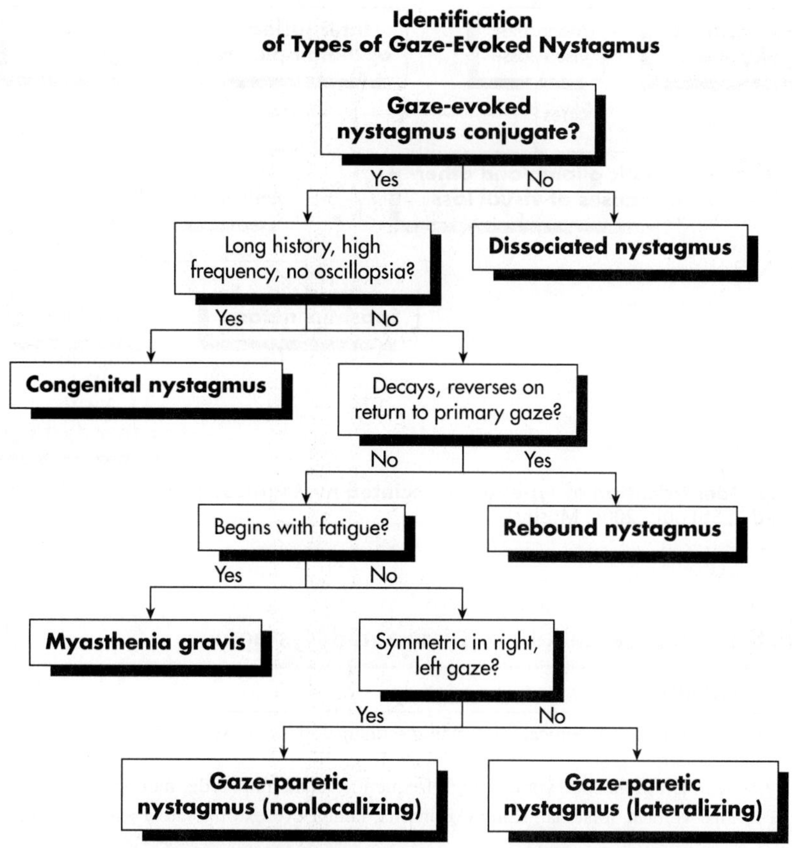

FIGURE 3-201 Identification of types of gaze-evoked nystagmus. (From Yanoff M, Duker JS: *Ophthalmology,* ed 2, St Louis, 2004, Mosby.)

TABLE 3-14 Characteristics and Localizations of Gaze-Evoked Nystagmus

Nystagmus	Characteristics	Localization
Physiologic, endpoint	Jerk, small amplitude, intermittent, extremes of horizontal and up gaze	Physiologic
Gaze-paretic (symmetric)	Jerk (decreasing velocity slow components) at 30° eccentric gaze	Nonlocalizing (drugs, mental fatigue)
Gaze-paretic (asymmetric)	Jerk (decreasing velocity slow components), horizontal, at 30° eccentric gaze, larger amplitude toward side of lesion	Lesions of brainstem, cerebellum, cerebral hemisphere
Rebound	Jerk, horizontal, decreases and direction can reverse in eccentric gaze, transient jerk nystagmus on return to primary gaze, fast components beating toward eccentric gaze	Cerebellum
Myasthenia gravis	Jerk, horizontal or vertical, gradual onset in prolonged eccentric gaze	Myoneural junction (fatigue—increasing transmission block)

From Yanoff M, Duker JS: *Ophthalmology,* ed 2, St Louis, 2004, Mosby.

Continued on following page

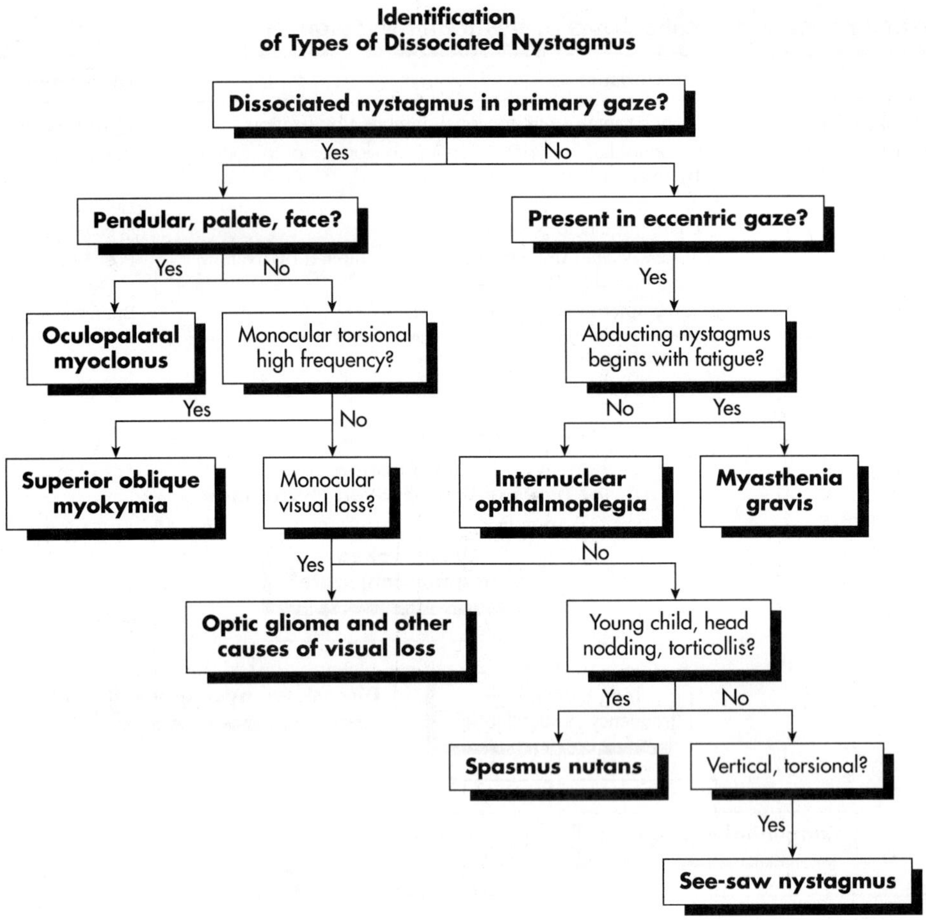

FIGURE 3-202 Identification of types of dissociated nystagmus. (From Yanoff M, Duker JS: *Ophthalmology,* ed 2, St Louis, 2004, Mosby.)

TABLE 3-15 Characteristics and Localizations of Dissociated Nystagmus

Nystagmus	Characteristics	Localization
Acquired pendular in adults	Pendular, horizontal, vertical, torsional, disconjugate (coexisting palatal myoclonus)	Brainstem, cerebellum
Superior oblique myokymia	Pendular, jerk, torsional, vertical, high frequency, small amplitude, monocular	Trochlear nucleus
See-saw	Pendular vertical, torsional, rising eye intorts, falling eye extorts; rarely jerk	Midbrain (interstitial nucleus of Cajal)
Abducting 'nystagmus' of internuclear ophthalmoplegia	Jerk, horizontal, decreasing velocity slow components, larger in abducting eye	Medial longitudinal fasciculus in pons, midbrain horizontal gaze
Abducting nystagmus of myasthenia gravis	Gaze-paretic nystagmus in horizontal gaze, greater paresis of medial rectus muscle	Myoneural junction—myasthenia gravis

From Yanoff M, Duker JS: *Ophthalmology,* ed 2, St Louis, 2004, Mosby.

OBESITY, ENDOCRINE EVALUATION

ICD-9CM # 278.01

Endocrine Evaluation of Obesity

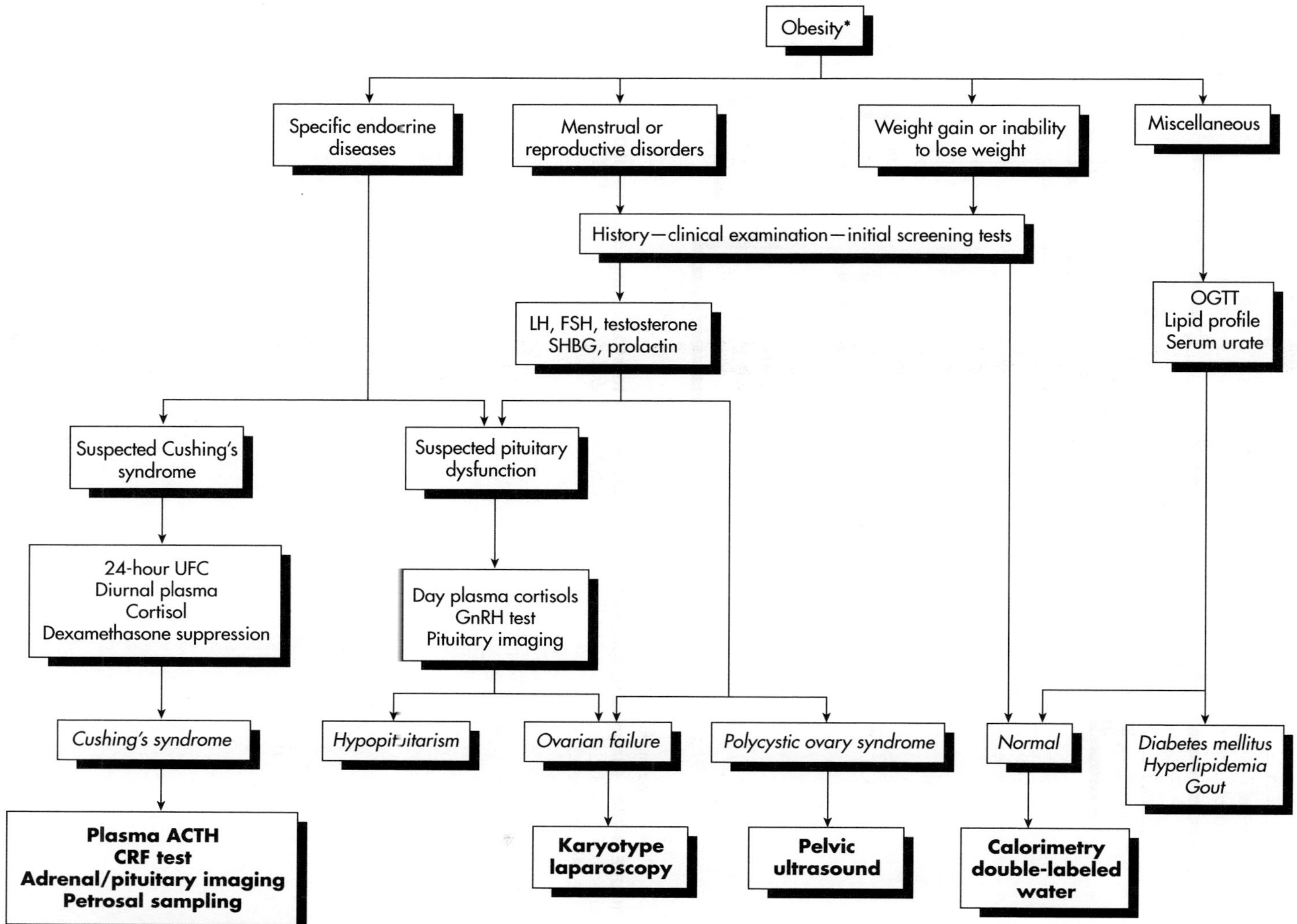

*Refer to Section I for additional information on this topic.

FIGURE 3-203 Endocrine evaluation of obesity. *ACTH,* Adrenocortiotropic hormone; *CRF,* corticotropin-releasing factor; *FSH,* follicle-stimulating hormone; *LH,* luteinizing hormone; *OGTT,* oral glucose tolerance test; *SHBG,* sex hormone-binding globulin; *UFC,* urinary free cortisol. (From Besser CM, Thorner MO: *Comprehensive clinical endocrinology,* ed 3, St Louis, Mosby, 2002.)

ICD-9CM # 515

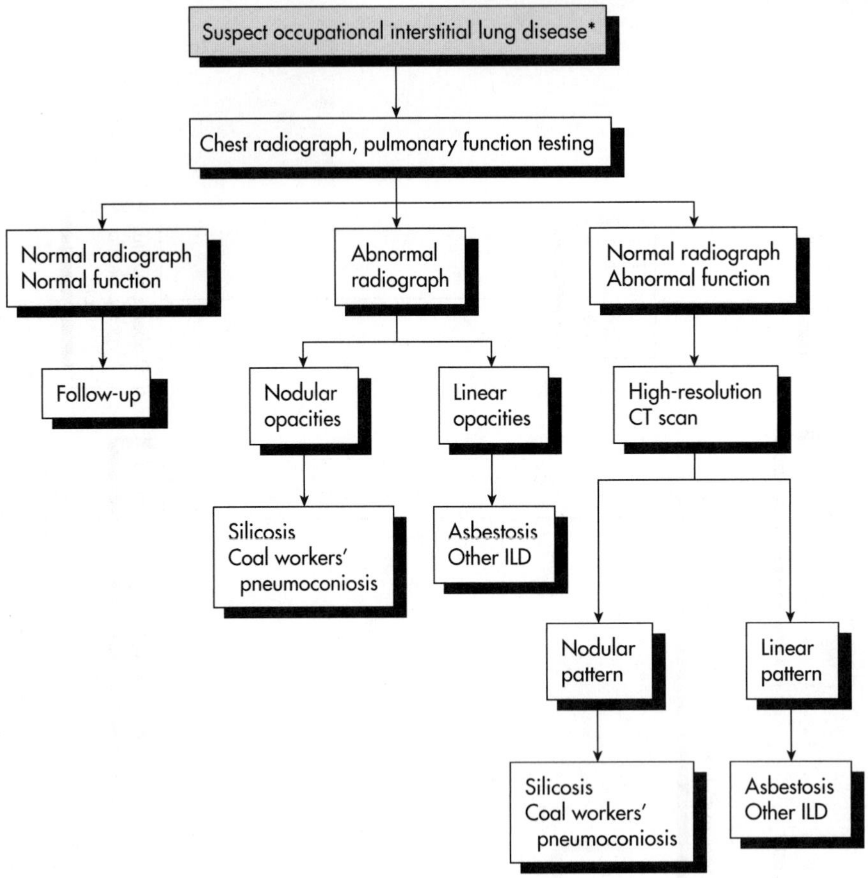

*Refer to Section I for additional information on this topic.

FIGURE 3-204 Diagnostic approach to occupational interstitial lung disease (ILD). *CT,* Computed tomography. (From Goldman L, Ausiello D [eds]): *Cecil textbook of medicine,* ed 23, Philadelphia, 2008, WB Saunders.)

OLIGURIA

ICD-9CM # 788.5

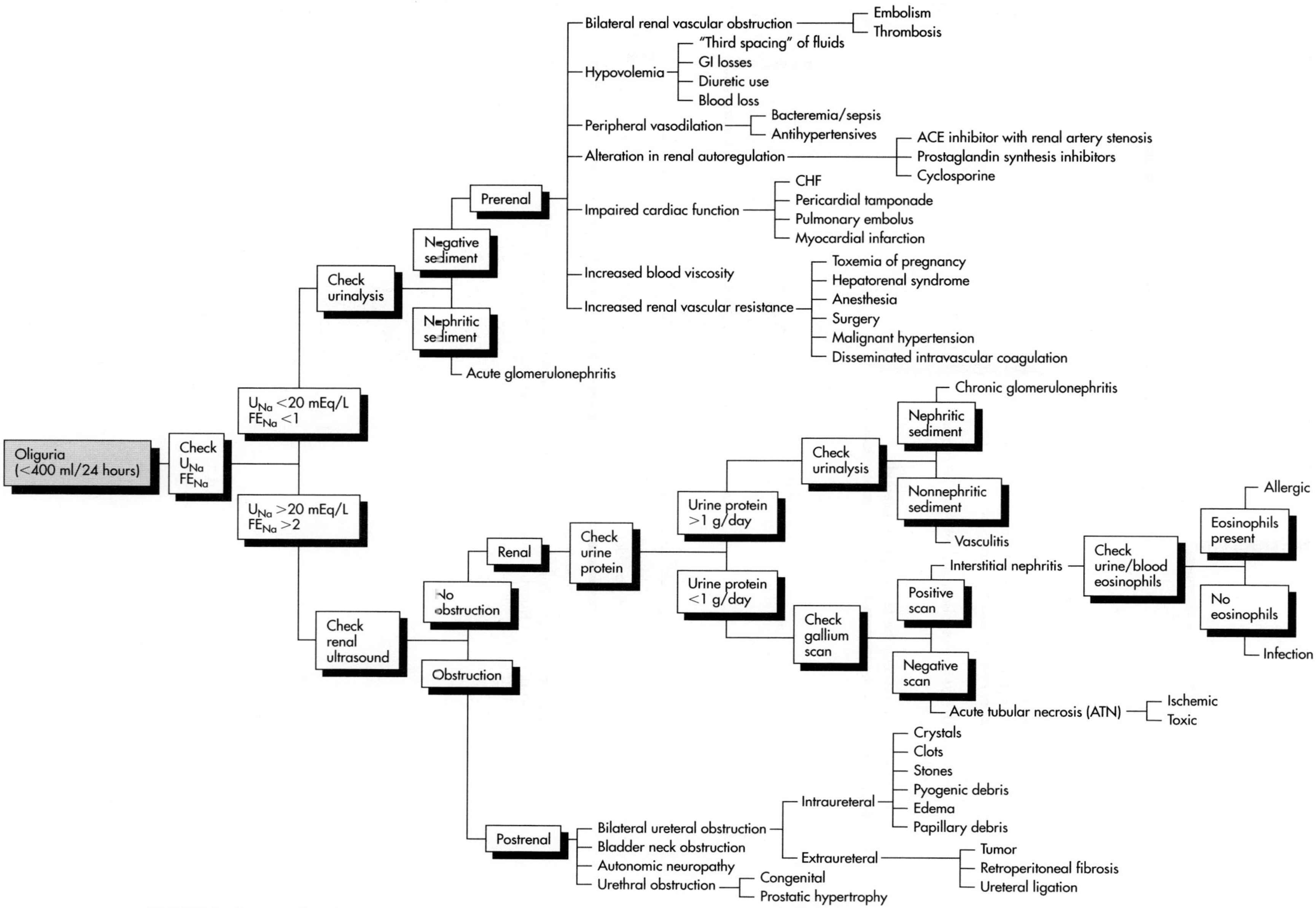

FIGURE 3-205 Evaluation of oliguria. *ACE,* Angiotensin-converting enzyme; *CHF,* congestive heart failure; *GI,* gastrointestinal. (From Healey PM: *Common medical diagnosis: an algorithmic approach,* ed 3, Philadelphia, 2000, WB Saunders.)

ICD-9CM # 715.9

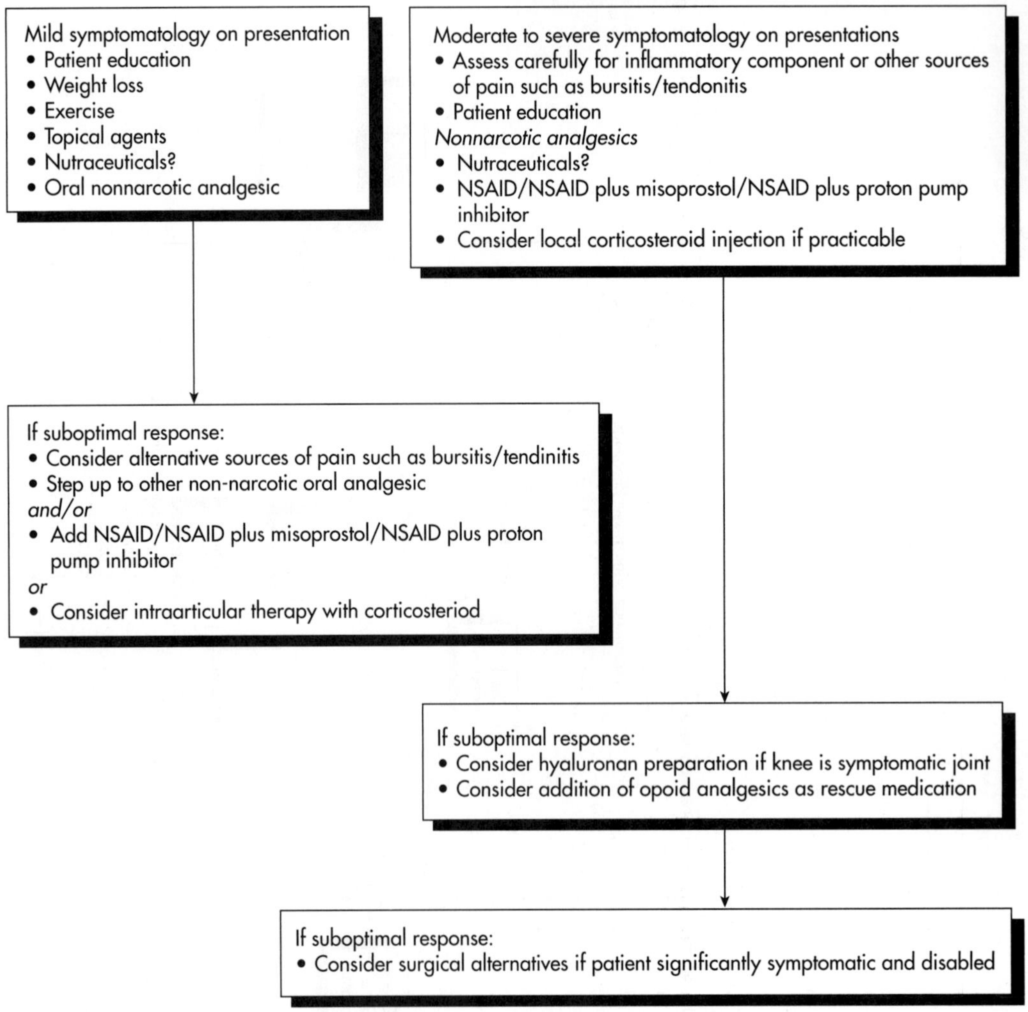

Note: Refer to Section I for additional information on this topic.

FIGURE 3-206 Flow chart for the management of osteoarthritis. *NSAID,* Nonsteroidal anti-inflammatory drug. (From Hochberg MC, Silman AJ, Smolen JS, Weinblatt ME, Weisman MH: *Rheumatology,* ed 3, St Louis, 2003, Mosby.)

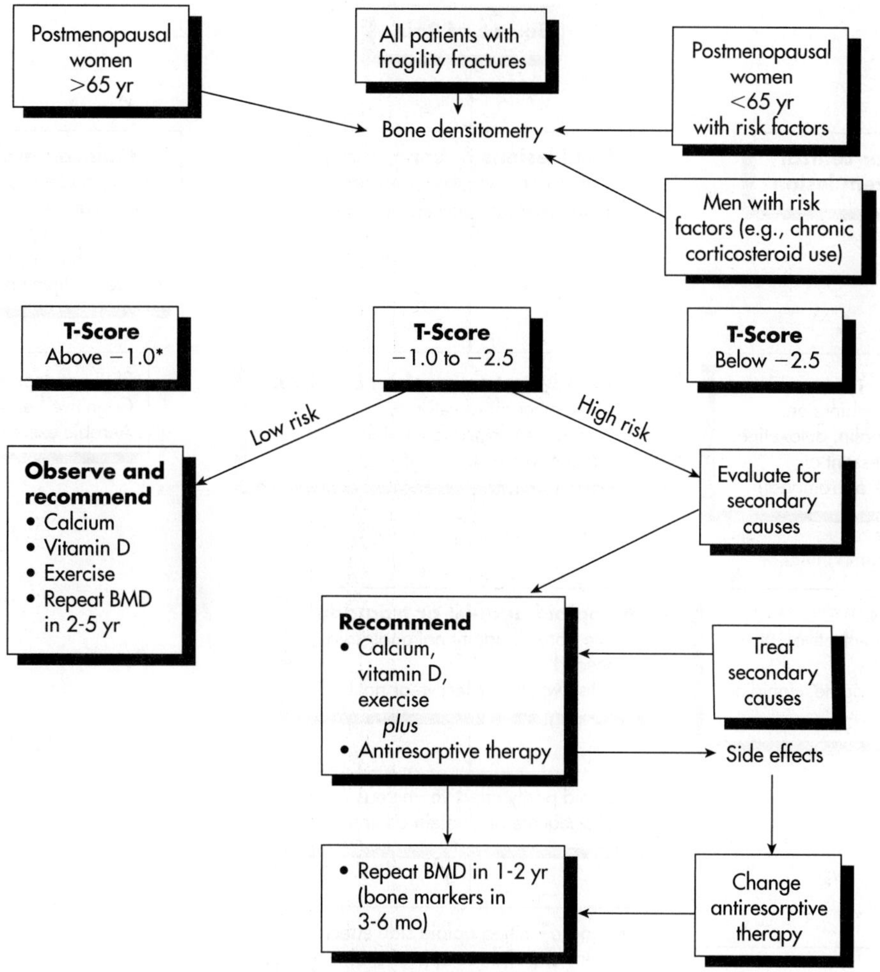

*Patients with fragility fractures and a T-score above −1.0 should be evaluated for other causes of pathologic fracture.

Note: Section I contains additional information on this topic.

FIGURE 3-207 Diagnosis and management of osteoporosis. The diagram outlines an approach based largely on evidence from studies of postmenopausal white women, with dual-energy x-ray absorptiometry used to measure bone mineral density (BMD). Its application to other populations, including patients with secondary osteoporosis and other methods of assessing BMD, is not established. (Modified from Larsen PR, Kronenberg HM, Memlmed S, Polansky KS: *Williams textbook of endocrinology,* ed 11, Philadelphia, 2008, Saunders.)

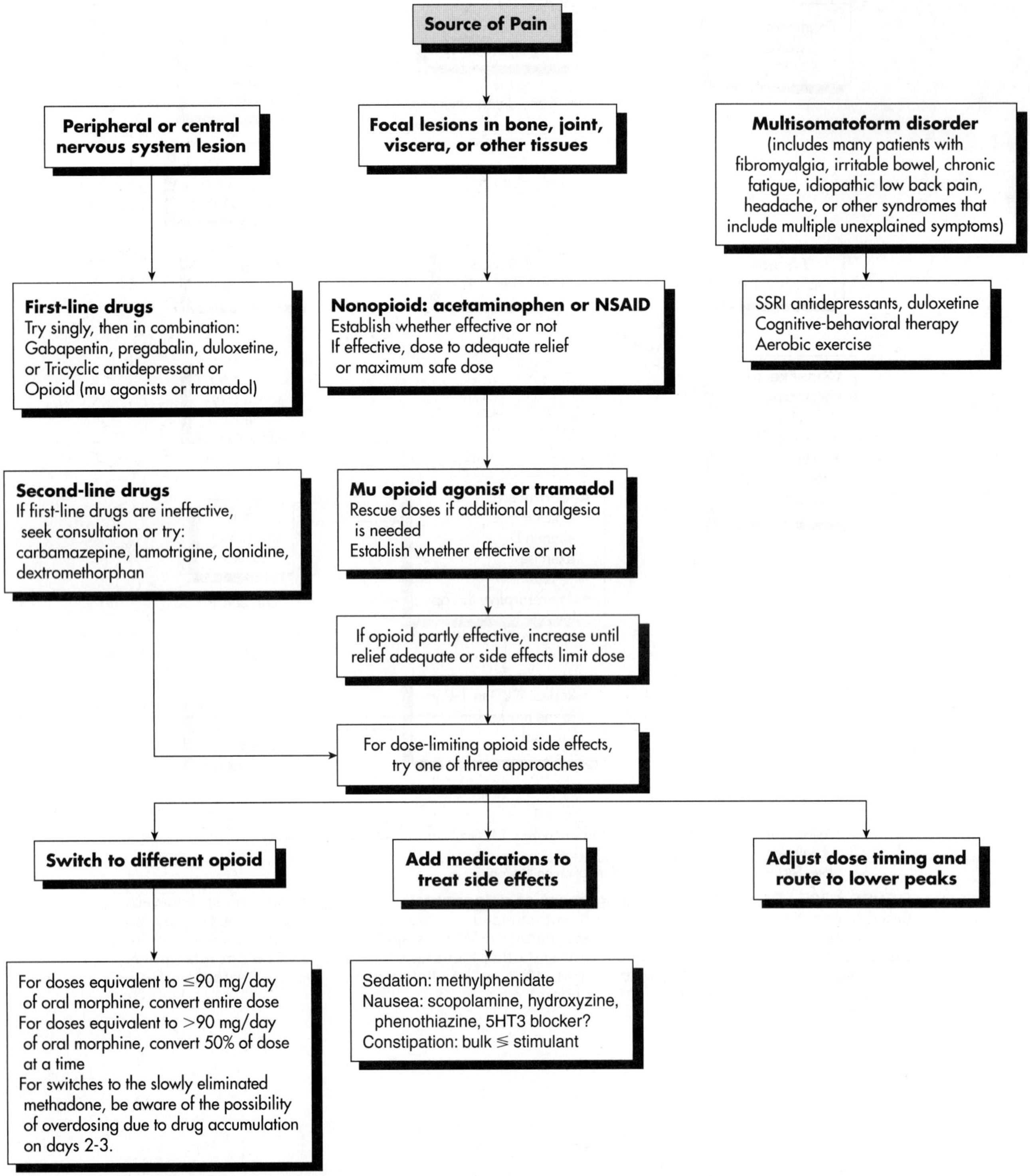

FIGURE 3-208 Algorithm for the treatment of pain. *COX,* Cyclooxygenese; *NSAID,* nonsteroidal anti-inflammatory drug; *SSRI,* selective serotonin reuptake inhibitor. (Modified from Goldman L, Ausiello D [eds]: *Cecil textbook of medicine,* ed 23, Philadelphia, 2008, WB Saunders.)

ICD-9CM # 785.1

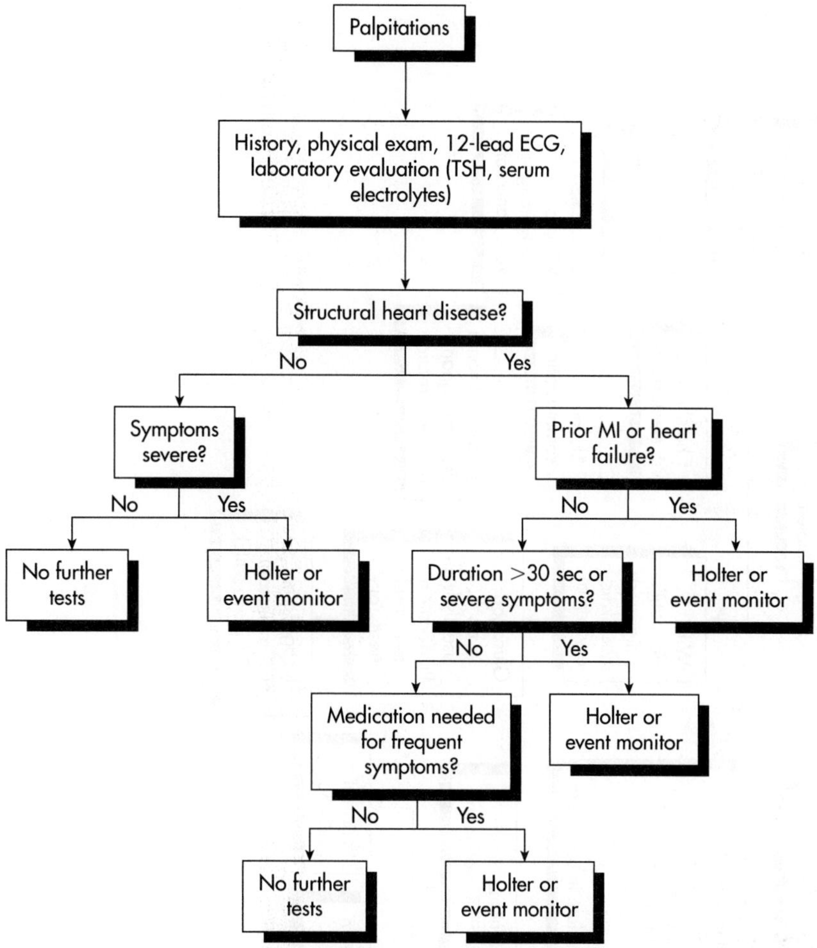

FIGURE 3-209 Diagnostic approach to the patient with palpitations. *ECG,* Electrocardiogram; *MI,* myocardial infarction; *TSH,* thyroid-stimulating hormone. (From Hiatky MA: Approach to the patient with palpitations. In Braunwald E, Goldman L [eds]: *Primary cardiology,* ed 2, Philadelphia, 2003, WB Saunders.)

PANCREATIC ISLET CELL TUMORS

ICD-9CM # 211.7

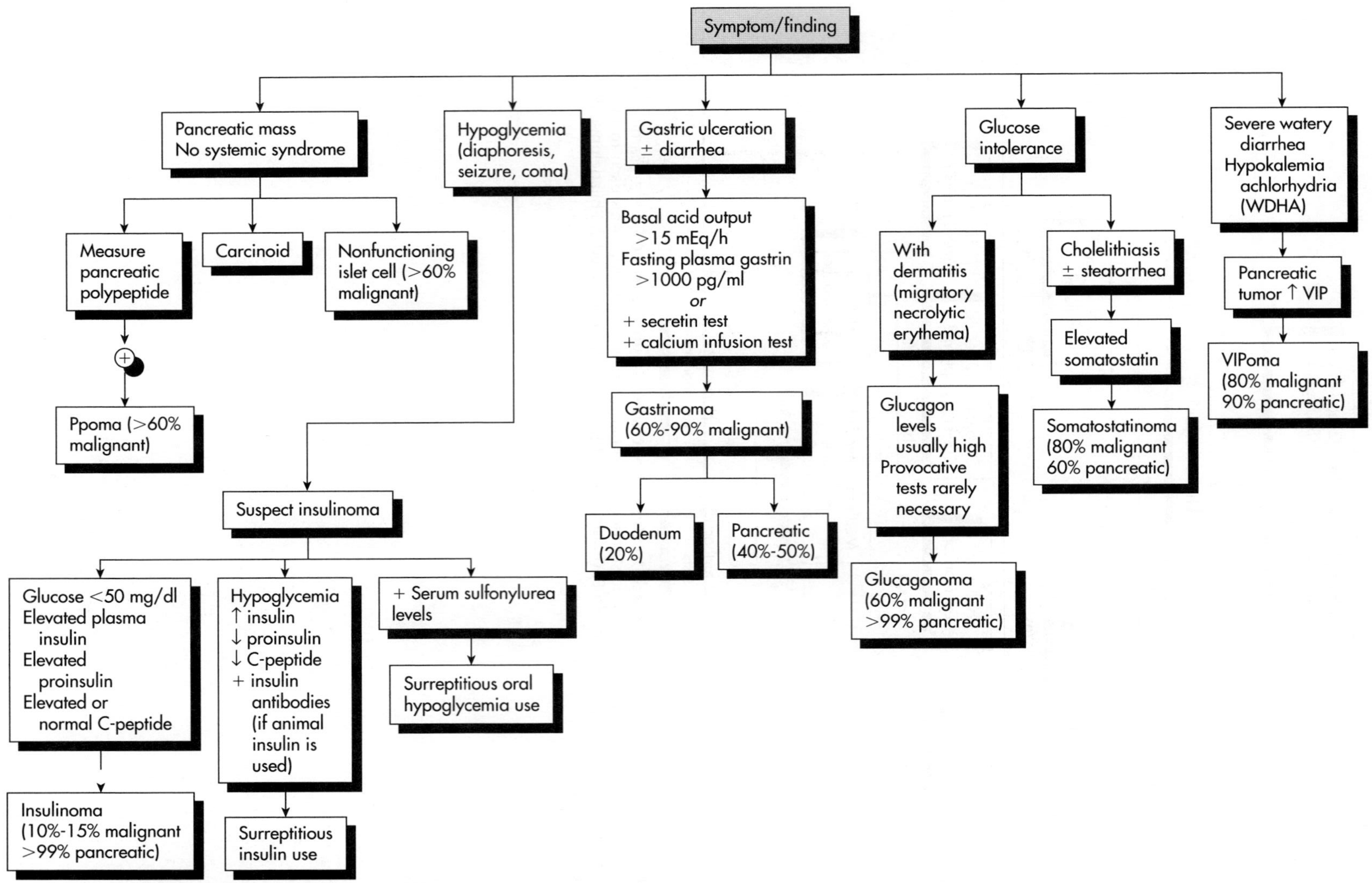

FIGURE 3-210 Diagnosis of pancreatic islet cell tumors. *Ppoma,* Islet cell tumor secreting pancreatic polypeptide; *VIP,* vasoactive intestinal peptide; *VIPoma,* islet cell tumor secreting vasoactive intestinal peptide. (Modified from Abeloff MD: *Clinical oncology,* ed 3, New York, 2004, Churchill Livingstone.)

ICD-9CM # 789.36

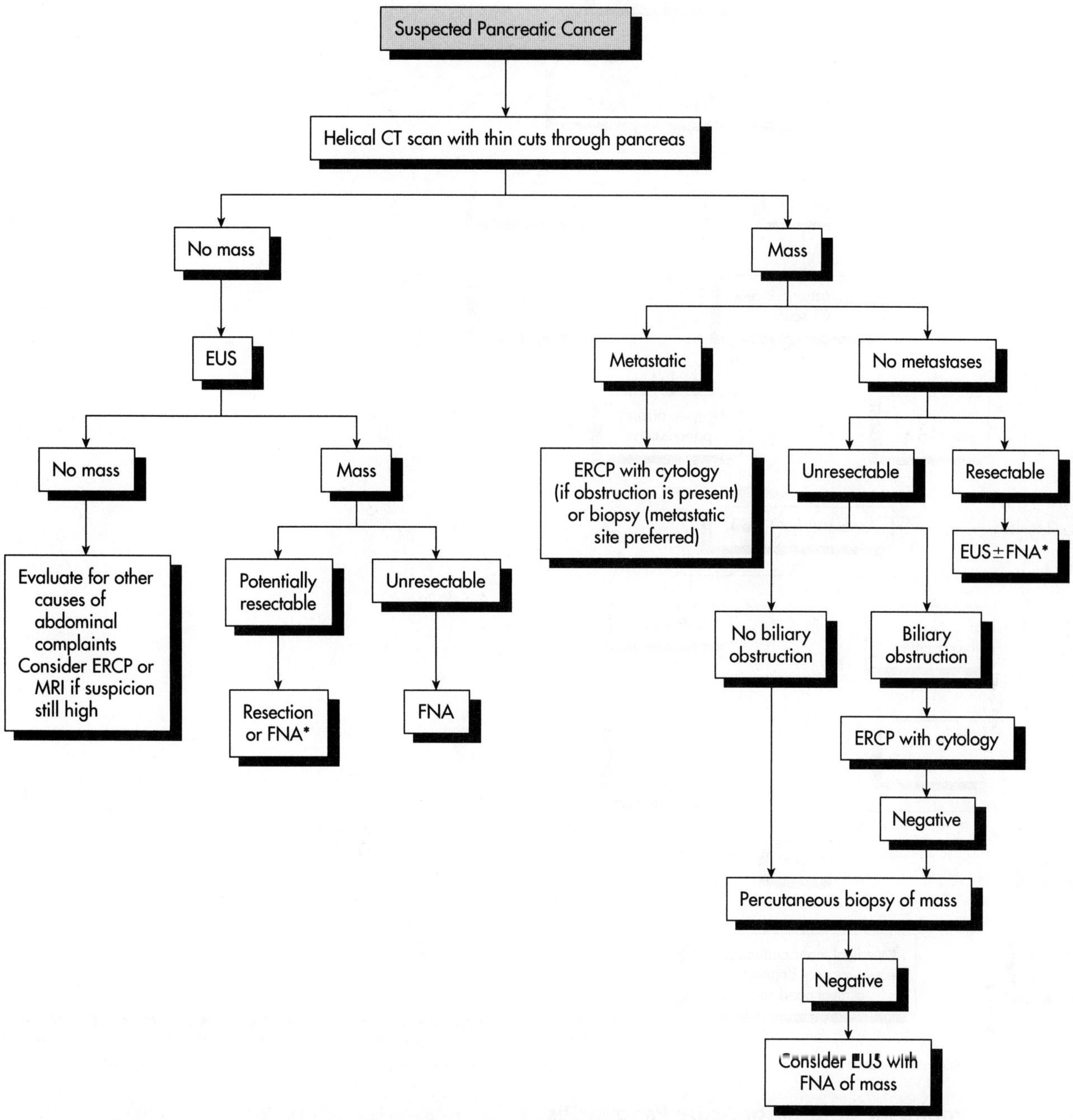

FIGURE 3-211 Diagnostic algorithm for pancreatic cancer. Intraoperative fine-needle aspiration (FNA) if found inoperable during surgery. *CT,* Computed tomographic scan; *ERCP,* endoscopic retrograde cholangiopancreatography; *EUS,* endoscopic ultrasonography; *MRI,* magnetic resonance imaging. (From Goldman L, Ausiello D [eds]: *Cecil textbook of medicine,* ed 23, Philadelphia, 2008, WB Saunders.)

ICD-9CM # 577.0

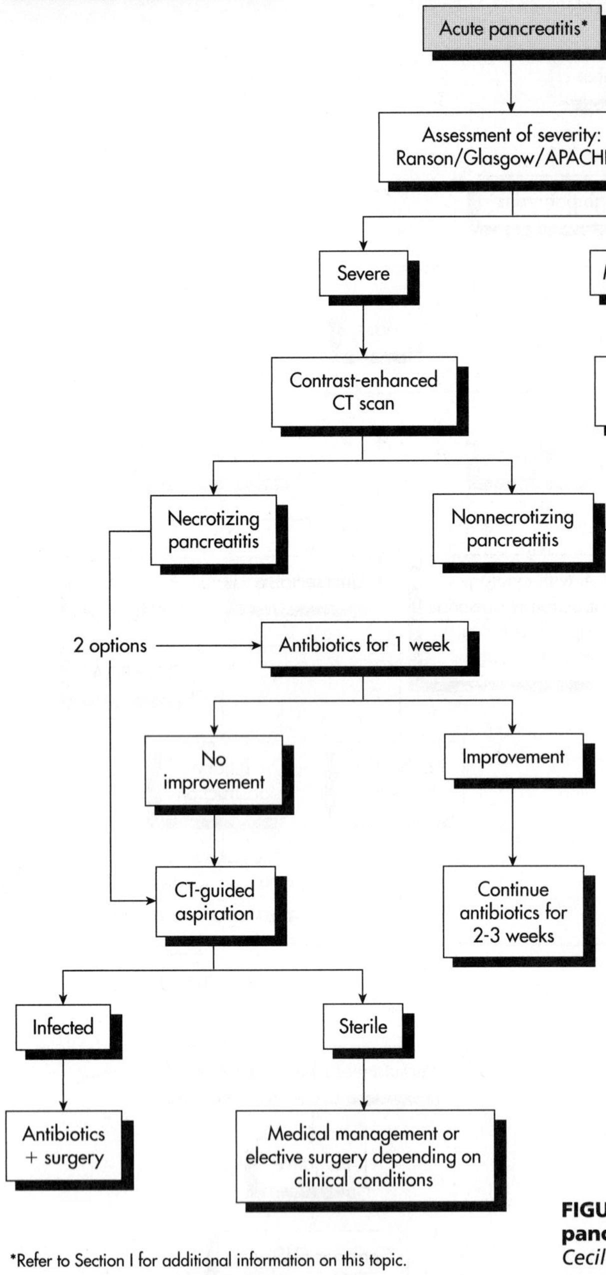

FIGURE 3-212 Approach to the patient with suspected or proven acute pancreatitis. *CT,* Computed tomography. (From Goldman L, Ausiello D [eds]: *Cecil textbook of medicine,* ed 23, Philadelphia, 2008, WB Saunders.)

TABLE 3-16 Prognostic Criteria for Acute Pancreatitis

Ranson Criteria*	Simplified Glasgow Criteria†	Computed Tomography Criteria‡
On admission	Within 48 hr of admission	Normal
Age >55 yr	Age >55 yr	Enlargement
WBC >16,000/μL	WBC >15,000/μL	Pancreatic inflammation
AST >250 U/L	LDH >600 U/L	Single fluid collection
LDH >350 U/L	Glucose >180 mg/dl	Multiple fluid collection
Glucose >200 mg/dl	Albumin <3.2 g/dl	
48 hr after admission	Ca^{2+} <8 mg/dl	
hematocrit	Arterial Po_2 <60 mm Hg	
decrease by >10%	BUN >45 mg/dl	
BUN increase by >5 mg/dl		
Ca^{2+} <8 mg/dl		
Arterial Po_2 <60 mm Hg		
Base deficit >4 mEq/L		
Fluid sequestration >6 L		

From Goldman L, Ausiello D (eds): *Cecil textbook of medicine,* ed 23, Philadelphia, 2008, WB Saunders.

AST, Aspartate aminotransferase; *BUN,* blood urea nitrogen; *LDH,* lactate dehydrogenase; *WBC,* white blood cells.

*Three or more Ranson's criteria predict a complicated clinical course. Data from Ranson JH, Rifkind KM, Turner JW: Prognostic signs and nonoperative peritoneal lavage in acute pancreatitis. Surg Gynecol Obstet 1976:143:209-219.

†Data from Blamey SL et al: Prognostic factors in acute pancreatitis, *Gut* 25:1340, 1984.

‡Grades A and B represent mild disease with no risk of infection or death. Grade C represents moderately severe disease with a minimal likelihood of infection and essentially no risk of mortality. Grades D and E represent severe pancreatitis with an infection rate of 30% to 50% and mortality rate of 15%. Data from Balthazar EJ et al: Acute pancreatitis value of CT in establishing prognosis, *Radiology* 174:331, 1990.

ICD-9CM # 577.1

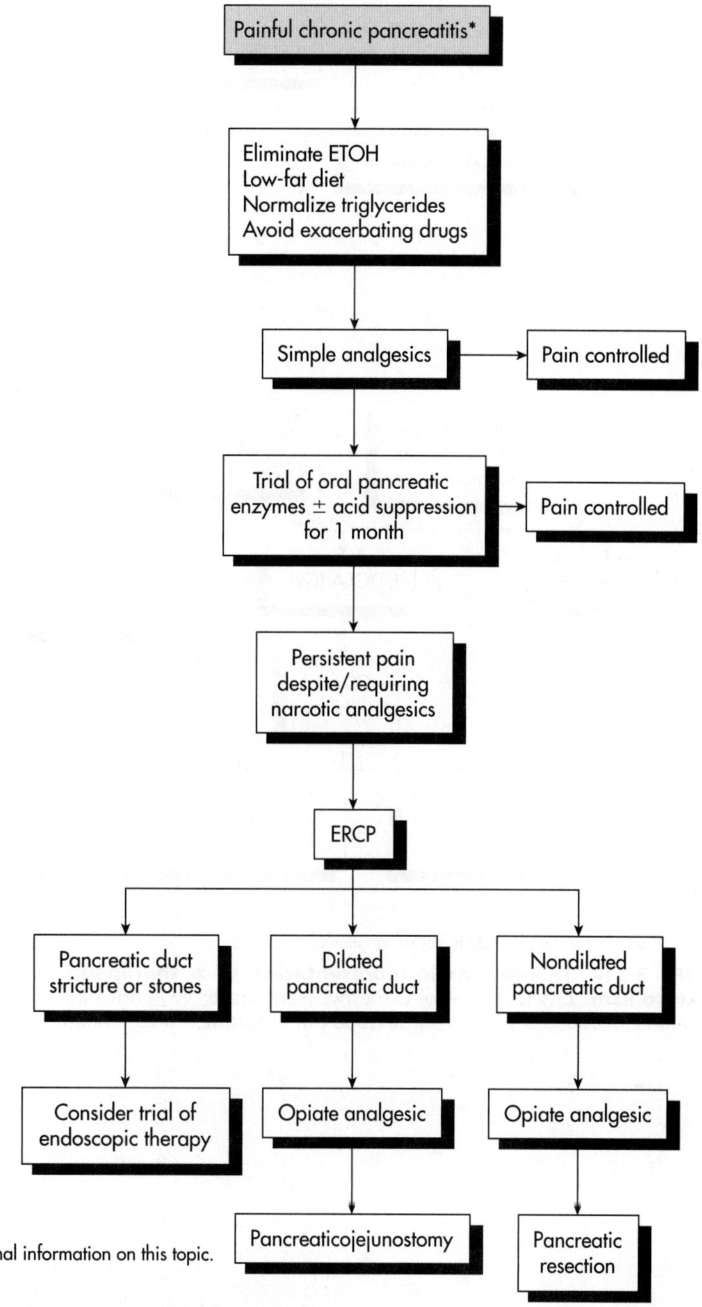

*Refer to Section I for additional information on this topic.

FIGURE 3-213 Approach to the patient with painful chronic pancreatitis. *ERCP,* Endoscopic retrograde cholangiopancreatography; *ETOH,* alcohol. (From Goldman L, Ausiello D [eds]: *Cecil textbook of medicine,* ed 23, Philadelphia, 2008, WB Saunders.)

ICD-9CM # 332.0 Idiopathic Parkinson's disease
332.1 Parkinson's disease, secondary

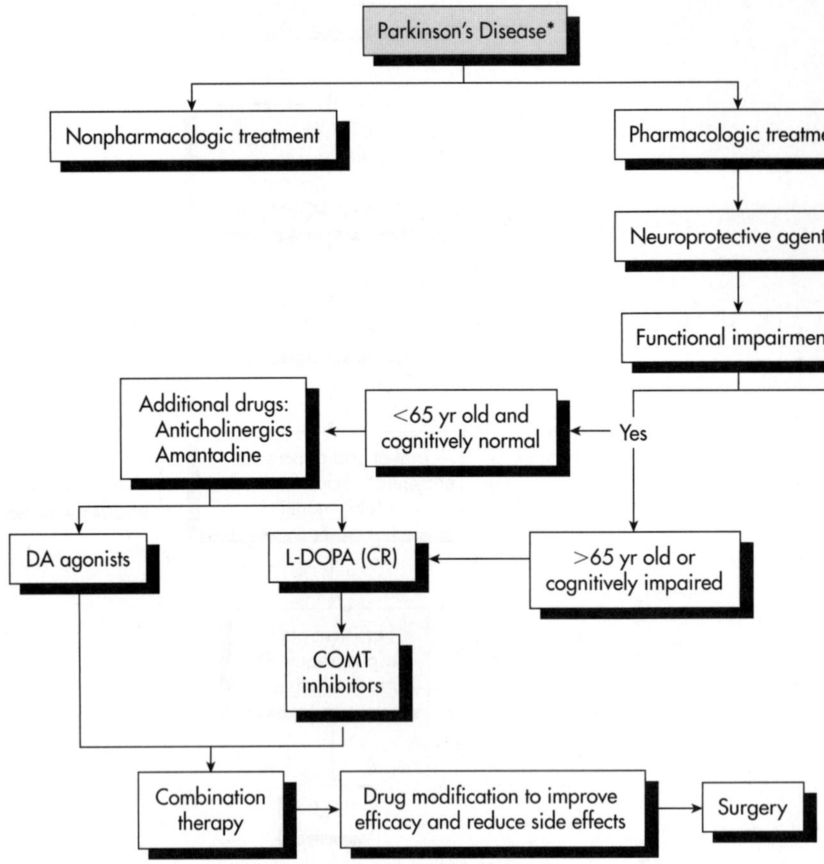

*Refer to Section I for additional information on this topic.

FIGURE 3-214 Diagrammatic representation of a therapeutic approach to patients with parkinsonism. *COMT,* Catechol-O-methyl transferase; *CR,* controlled release; *DA,* dopamine. (From Goldman L, Ausiello D [eds]: *Cecil textbook of medicine,* ed 23, Philadelphia, 2008, WB Saunders.)

ICD-9CM # 301.9 Personality disorder NOS
301.51 Munchausen syndrome

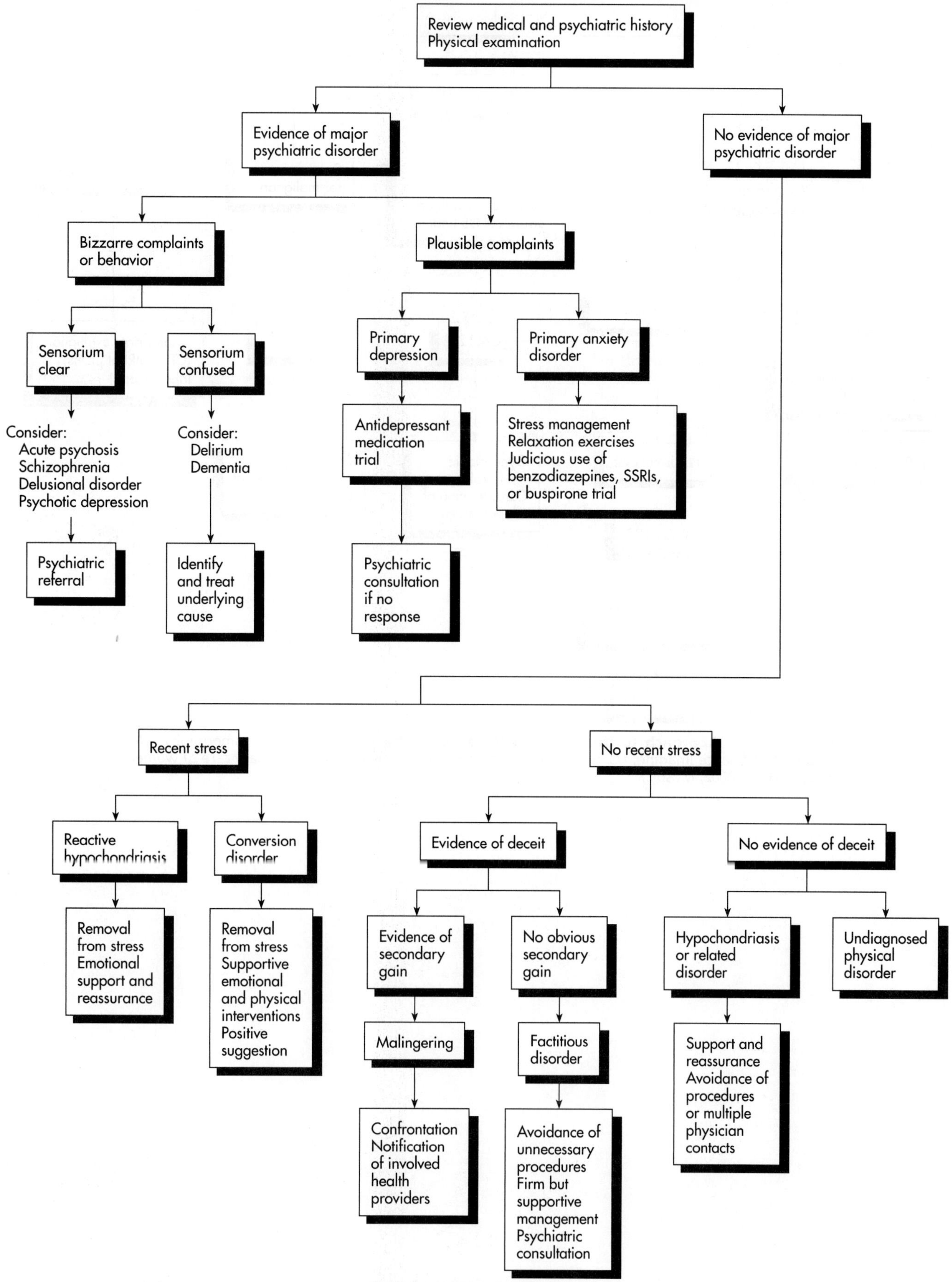

FIGURE 3-215 Patient with ill-defined physical complaints. Previous or recent evaluations are noncontributory. *SSRIs,* Selective serotonin reuptake inhibitors. (From Greene H, Johnson WP, Lemcke D [eds]: *Decision making in medicine,* ed 2, St Louis, 1998, Mosby.)

ICD-9CM # 789.39

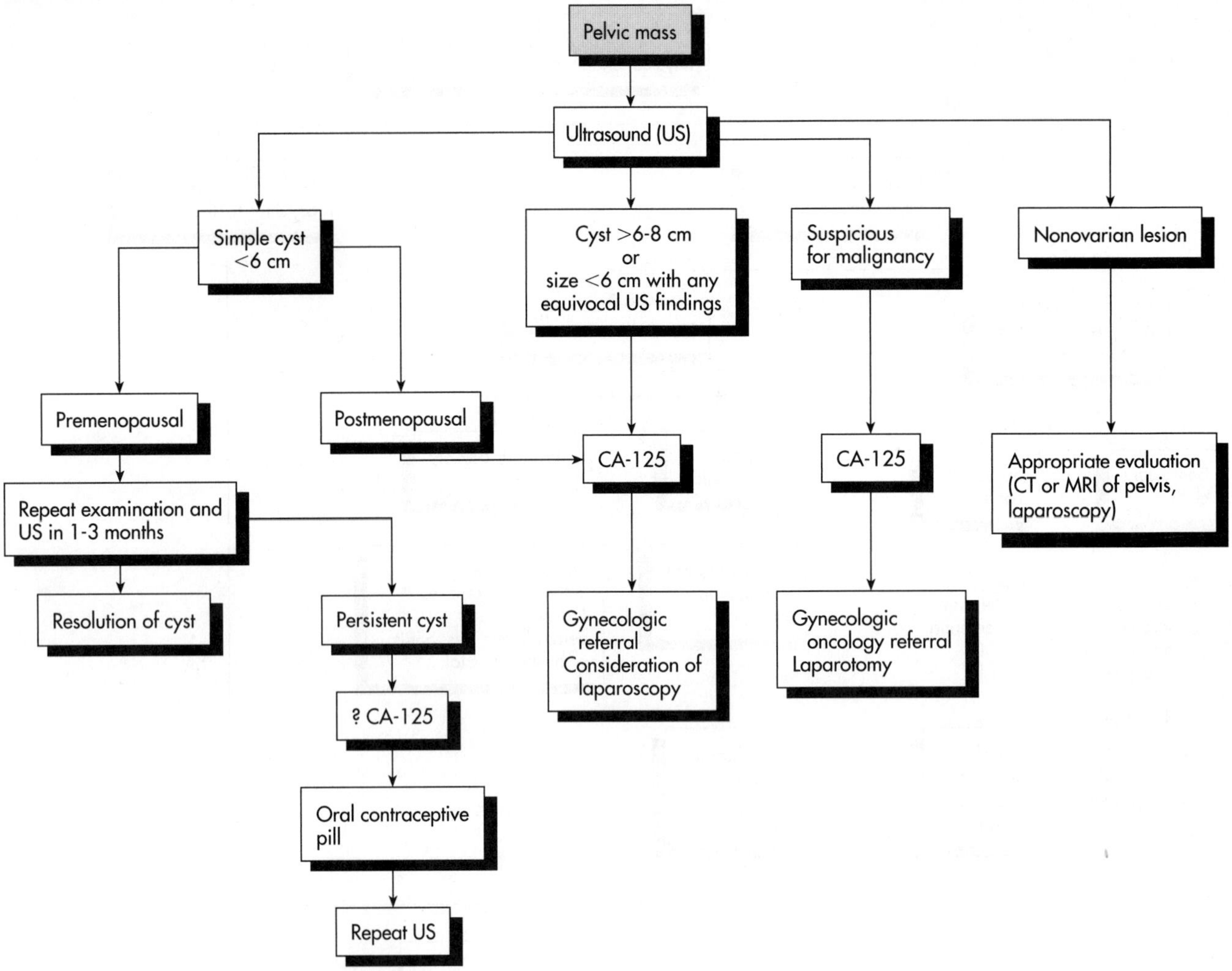

FIGURE 3-216 Approach to the patient with a pelvic mass. *CT,* Computed tomography; *MRI,* magnetic resonance imaging; *US,* ultrasound. (Modified from Carlson KJ et al: *Primary care of women,* ed 2, St Louis, 2002, Mosby.)

PELVIC PAIN, REPRODUCTIVE-AGE WOMAN

ICD-9CM # 625.9

1. Rapid history and external abdominal examination

- **If surgical abdomen**: Consider early ob/gyn/surgery consultation
  - Rupture (ectopic, cyst, abscess)
  - Torsion (adnexal, fibroid)
  - Perforation (uterine)
  - Appendicitis

2. Vital signs

- **If unstable**: Establish venous access and administer fluid bolus
  Spin Hct, type and crossmatch blood as needed
  Consider early ob/gyn/surgery consult without ultrasound
  - Rupture (ectopic, cyst)
  - Septic (abortion, abscess)
  - Placental (previa, abruptio)

3. Complete history and physical examination, and perform pelvic examination

- **If obvious abortion**: Consult obstetrician and consider ultrasound
  - Abortion (incomplete, septic)
- **If late pregnancy**: Forego pelvic exam
  Check for fetal heart tones
  Consider ultrasound followed by ob/gyn consultation
  - Placenta previa or abruptio
  - Premature labor contractions

4. Laboratory diagnostic workup (pregnancy test, CBC, UA/micro)

- **If pregnant**: Consider ultrasound followed by ob/gyn consultation
  - R/I viable intrauterine gestation
  - R/O ectopic pregnancy, abortion, placental problems
  - R/O free intraperitoneal fluid, abscess formation
- **If not pregnant**: Consider ultrasound and ob/gyn/surgery consultation
  - R/O gynecologic surgical problems
  - Ovarian cyst rupture, hemorrhage
  - Tubo-ovarian abscess rupture
  - Adnexal or fibroid torsion
  - Uterine perforation

  - Consider nonsurgical gynecologic problems
  - PID, pelvic adhesions, endometriosis, neoplasm, menstrual

  - R/O general surgery problems
  - Appendicitis and complications
  - Other, GI, GU, vascular, orthopedic surgery problems

  - Consider nonsurgical nongynecologic problems
  - Systemic illnesses

FIGURE 3-217 Evaluation and management of reproductive-age women with acute pelvic pain. *CBC,* Complete blood count; *GI,* gastrointestinal; *GU,* genitourinary; *Hct,* hematocrit; *PID,* pelvic inflammatory disease; *UA/micro,* urinalysis with microscopy. (From Marx JA (ed): *Rosen's emergency medicine,* ed 6, St Louis, 2006, Mosby.)

ICD-9CM # 420.90

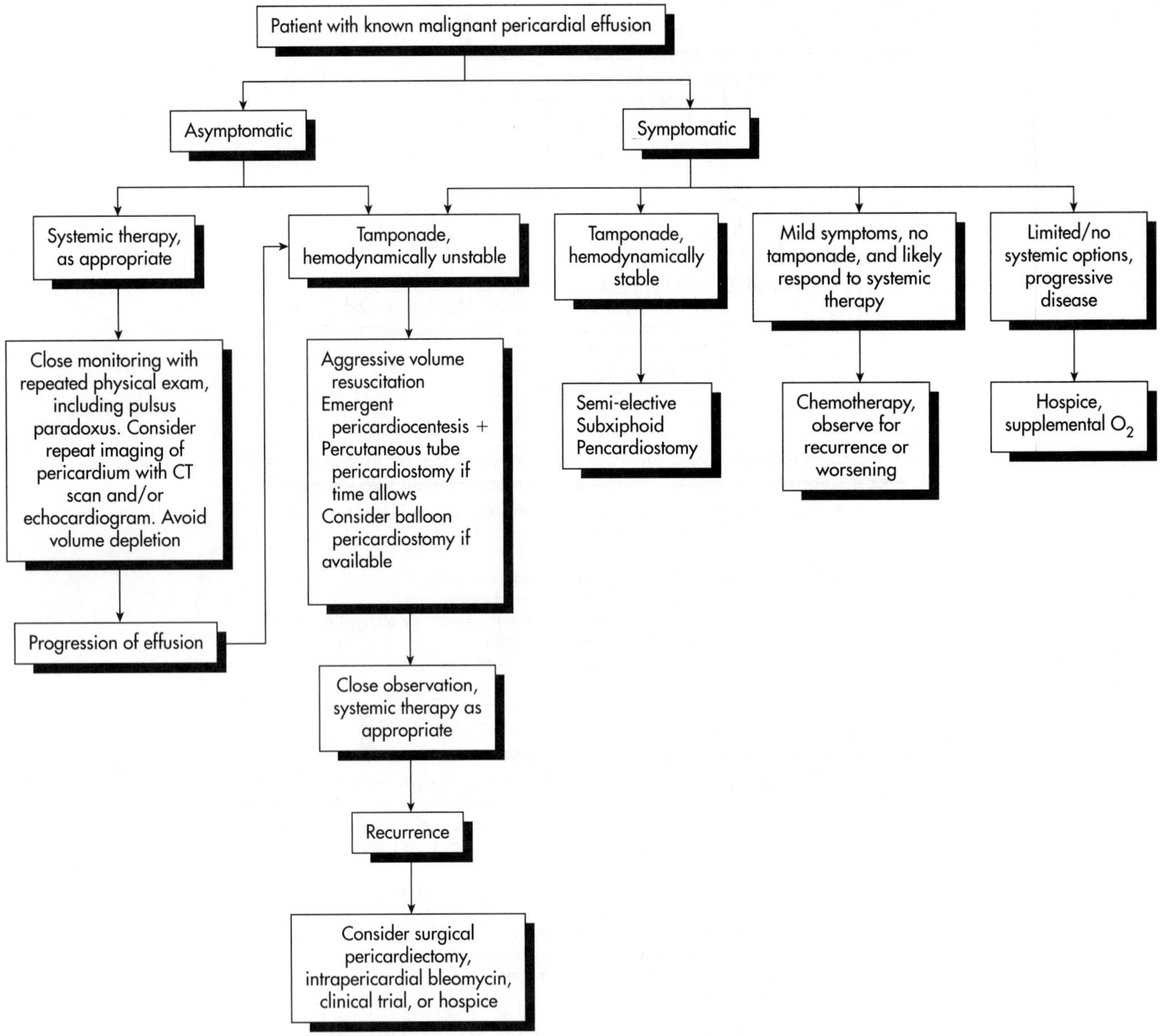

FIGURE 3-218 Treatment approach to patient with known malignant pericardial effusion. *CT,* Computed tomography. (From Abeloff MD: *Clinical oncology,* ed 3, Philadelphia, 2004, Elsevier.)

ICD-9CM # 356.9 Peripheral nerve neuropathy
355.10 Lower extremity neuropathy
354.11 Upper extremity neuropathy

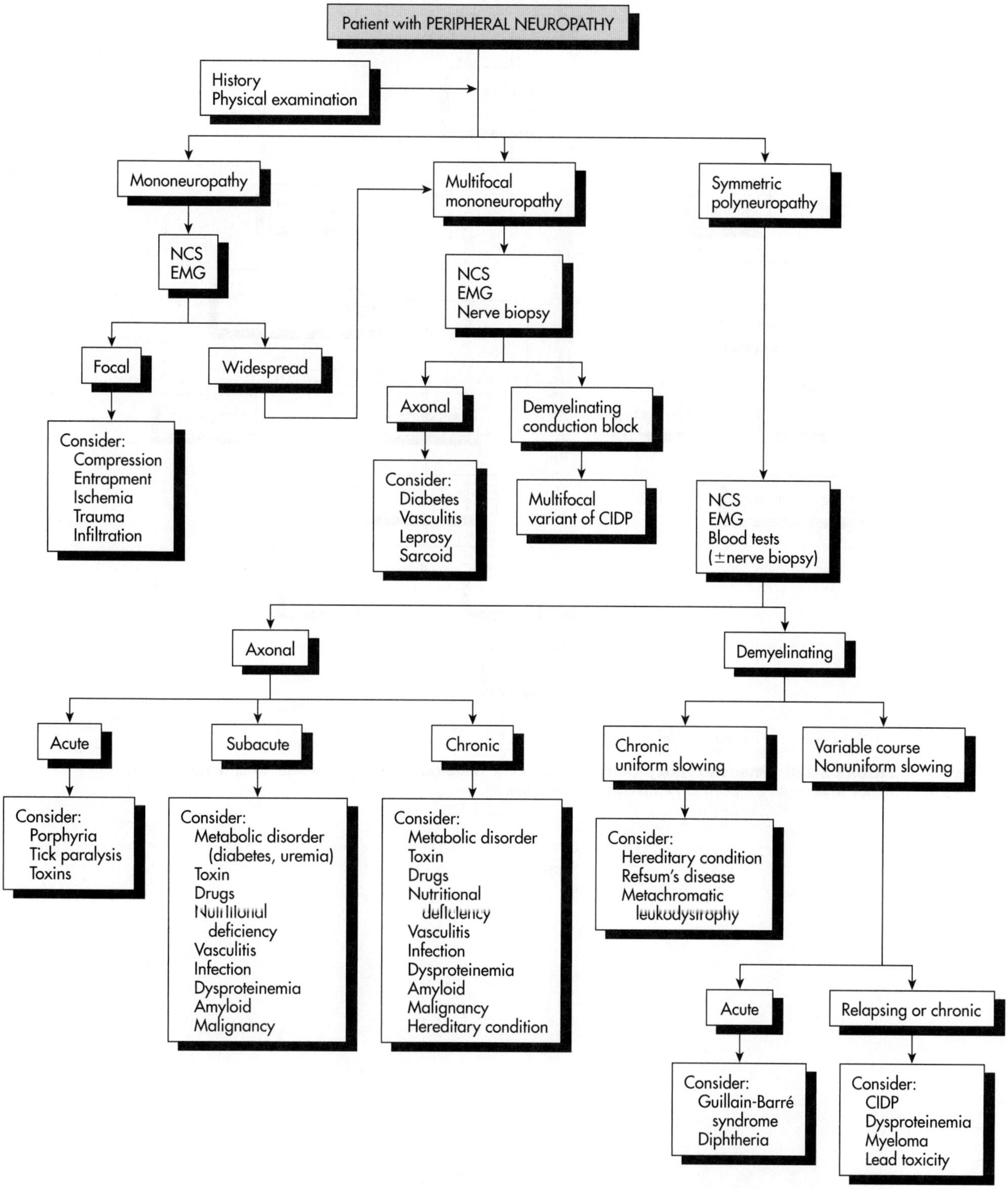

FIGURE 3-219 Approach to the patient with peripheral neuropathy. *CIDP,* Chronic inflammatory demyelinating polyradioneuropathy; *EMG,* electromyogram; *NCS,* nerve conduction studies. (From Greene HL, Johnson WP, Lemcke DL: *Decision making in medicine,* ed 2, St Louis, 1988, Mosby.)

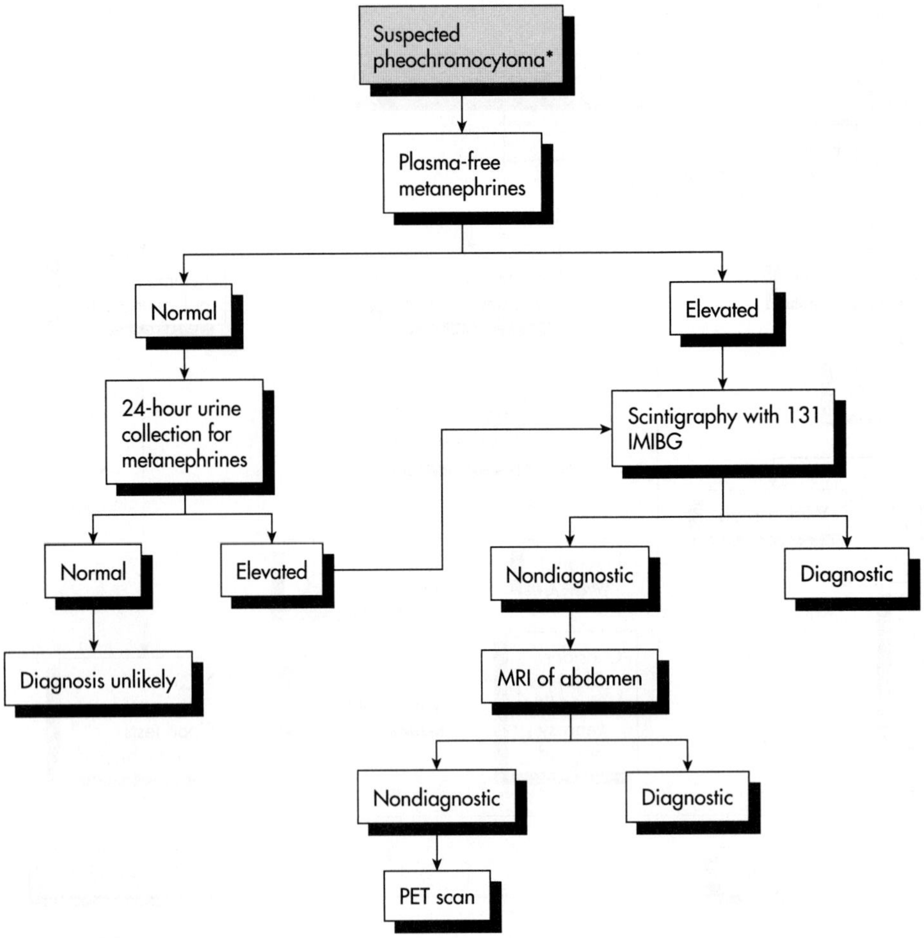

*Refer to Section I for additional information on this topic.

FIGURE 3-220 Pheochromocytoma. *IMIBG,* Iodine metaiodobenzyl guanidine; *MRI,* magnetic resonance imaging; *PET,* positron emission tomography.

PHOTOSENSITIVITY

ICD-9CM # 692.72

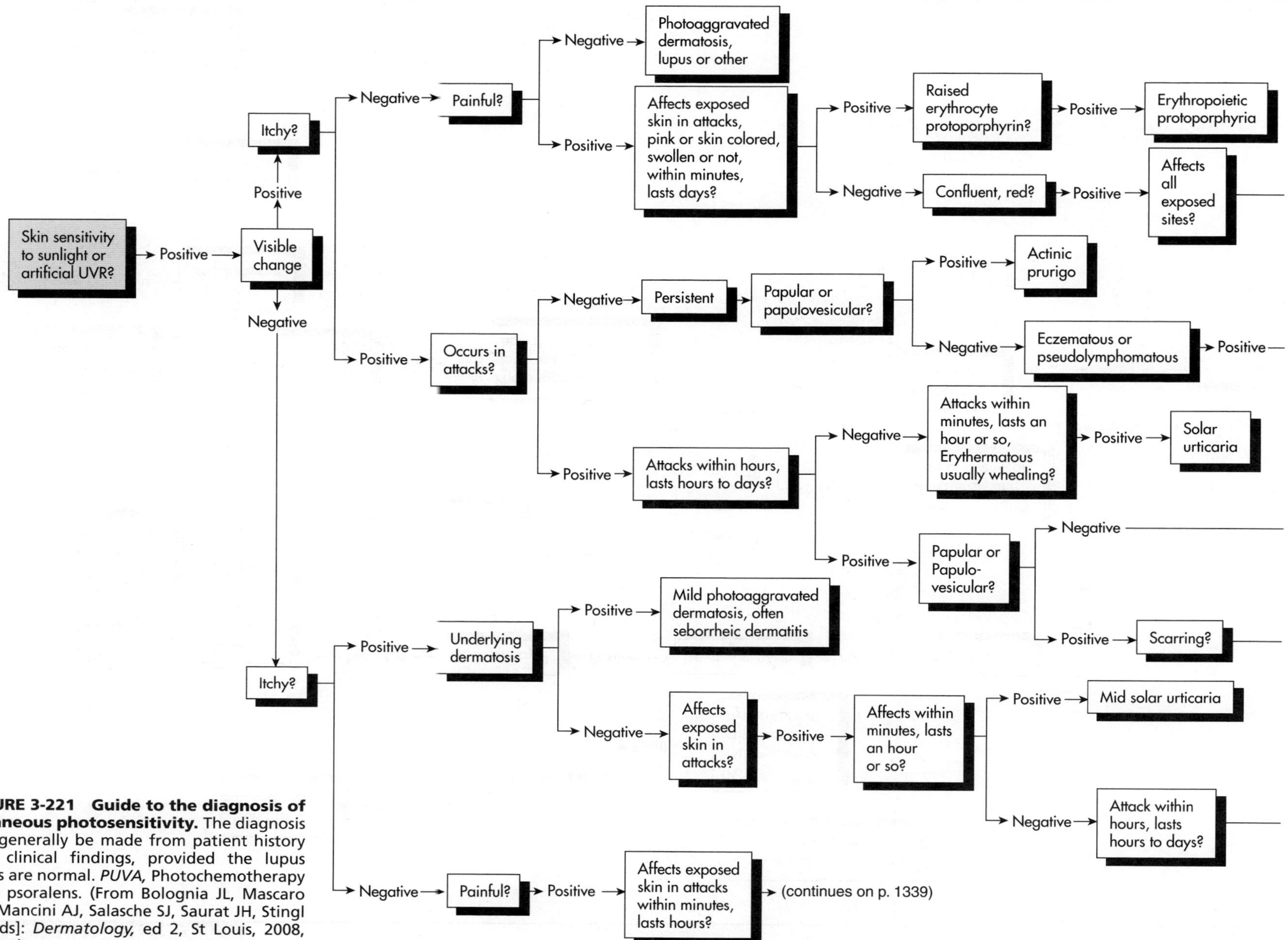

FIGURE 3-221 Guide to the diagnosis of cutaneous photosensitivity. The diagnosis can generally be made from patient history and clinical findings, provided the lupus titers are normal. *PUVA,* Photochemotherapy with psoralens. (From Bolognia JL, Mascaro JM, Mancini AJ, Salasche SJ, Saurat JH, Stingl G [eds]: *Dermatology,* ed 2, St Louis, 2008, Mosby.)

Continued on following page

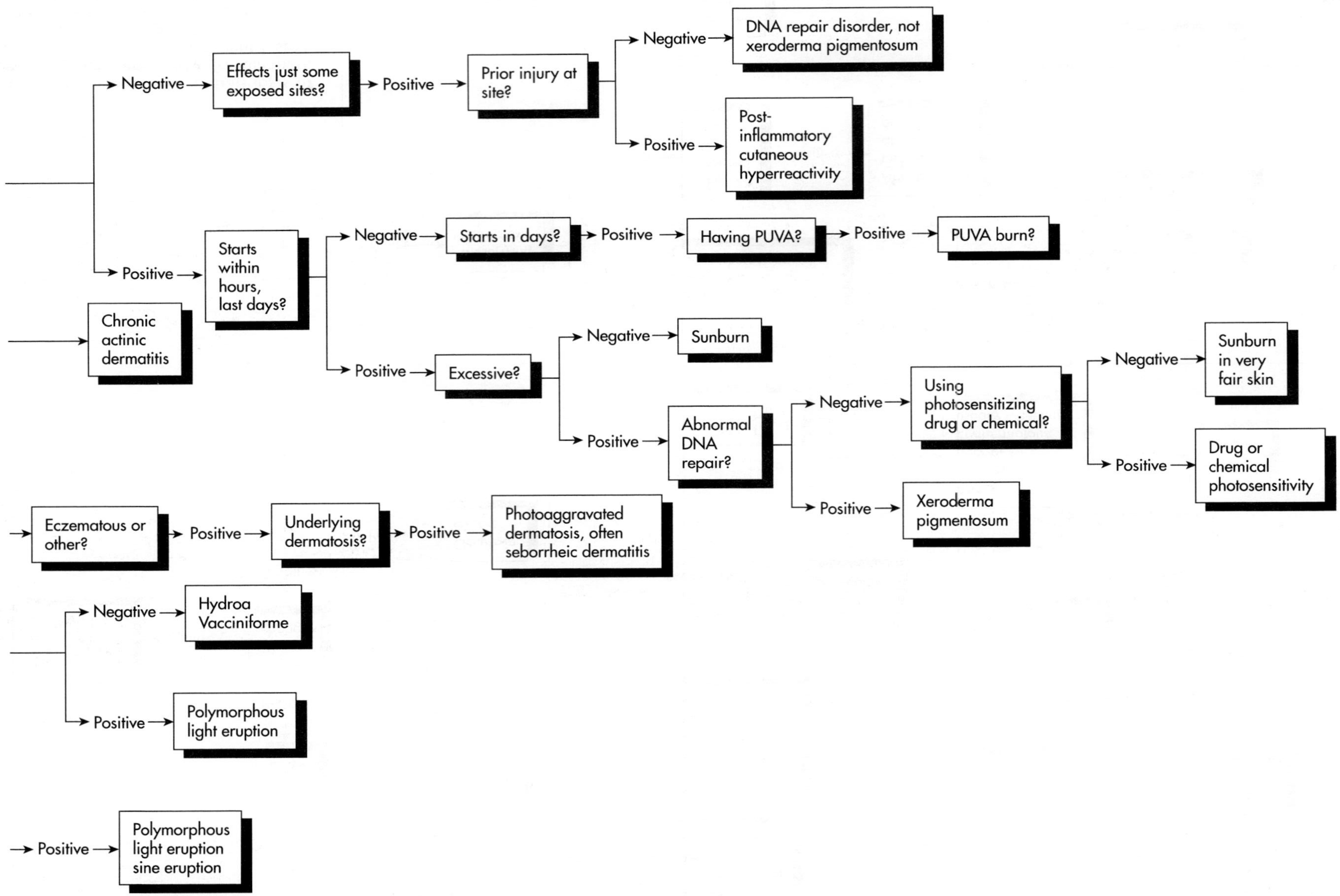

FIGURE 3-221 (Continued) **Guide to the diagnosis of cutaneous photosensitivity.** The diagnosis can generally be made from patient history and clinical findings, provided the lupus titers are normal. *PUVA,* Photochemotherapy with psoralens. (From Bolognia JL, Mascaro JM, Mancini AJ, Salasche SJ, Saurat JH, Stingl G [eds]: *Dermatology,* ed 2, St Louis, 2008, Mosby.)

PHOTOSENSITIVITY—cont'd

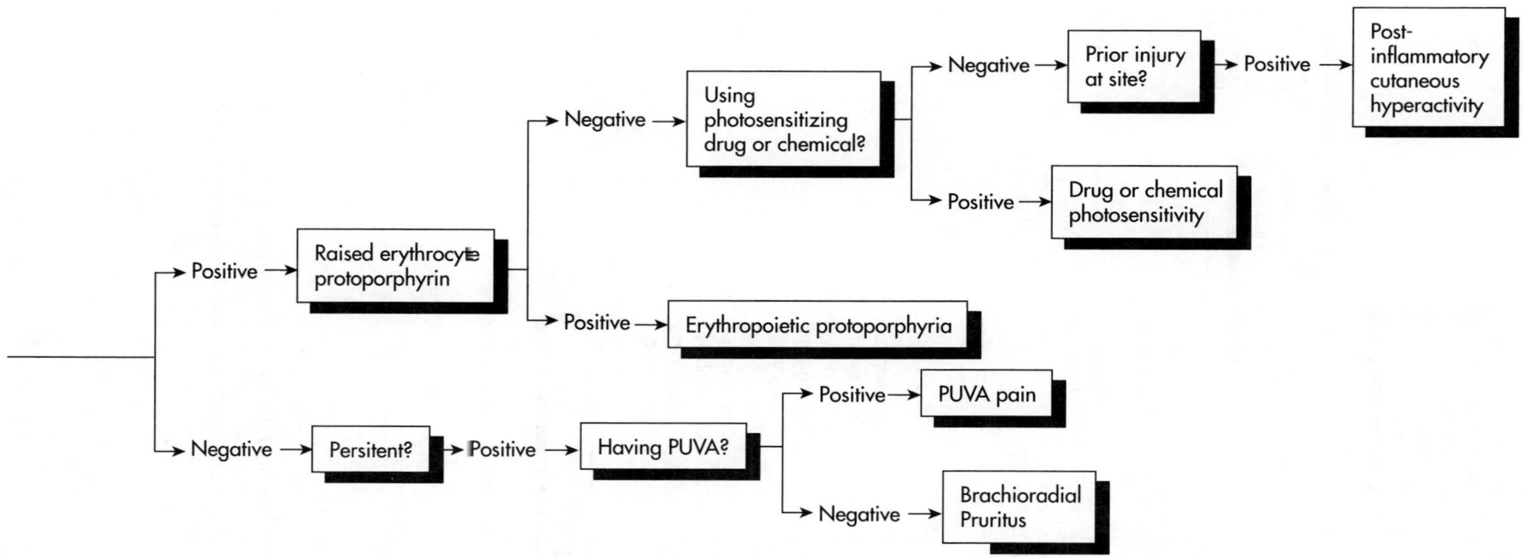

FIGURE 3-221 (Continued)

ICD-9CM # 253 Pituitary adenoma
253.0 Acromegaly
253.1 Prolactinoma

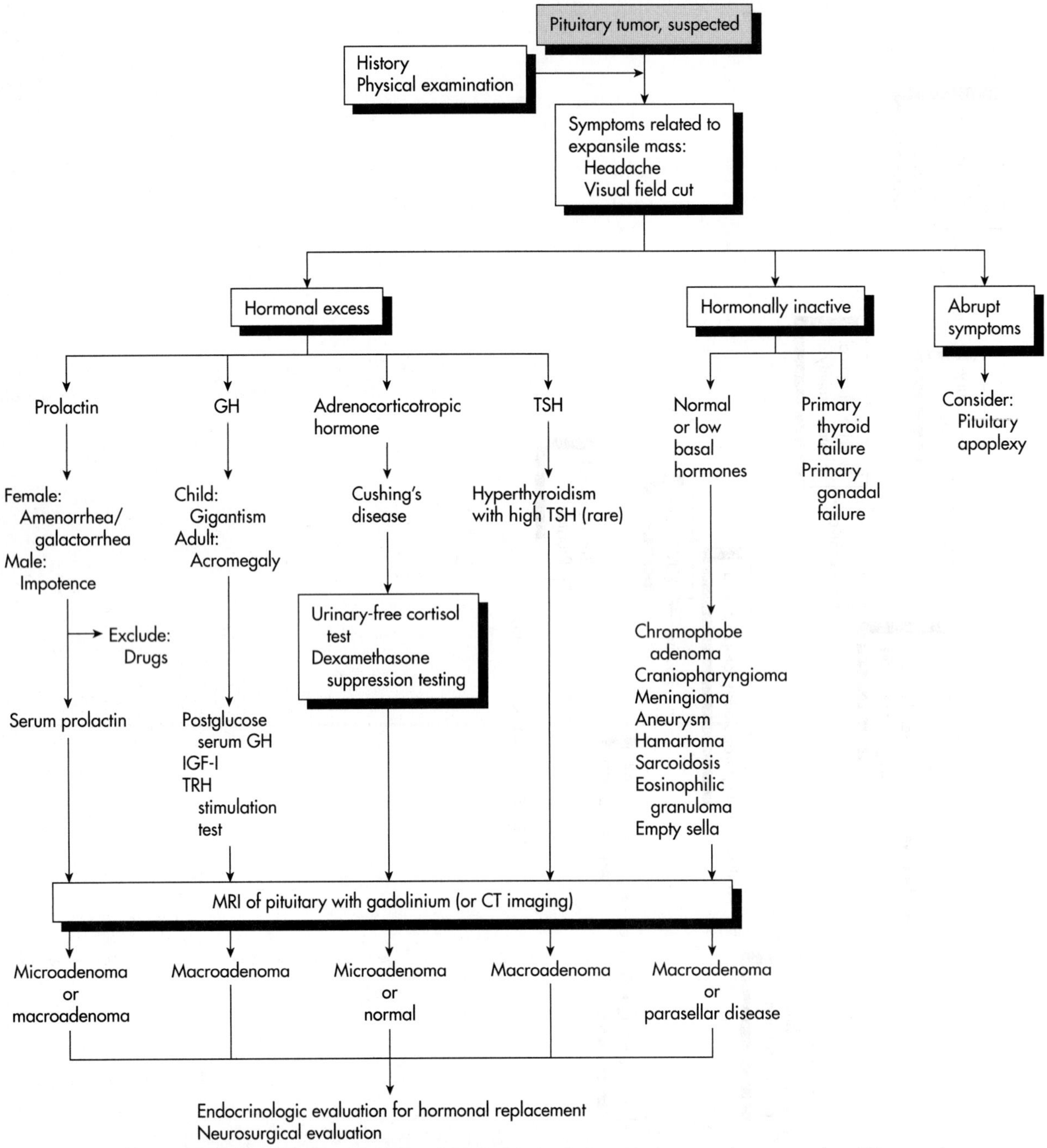

FIGURE 3-222 Evaluation of suspected pituitary tumor. *CT,* Computed tomography; *GH,* growth hormone; *IGF-I,* one of the insulin-like growth factors; *MRI,* magnetic resonance imaging; *TRH,* thyrotropin-releasing hormone; *TSH,* thyroid-stimulating hormone. (From Greene HL, Johnson WP, Lemcke D: *Decision making in medicine,* ed 2, St Louis, 1998, Mosby.)

ICD-9CM # 197.2

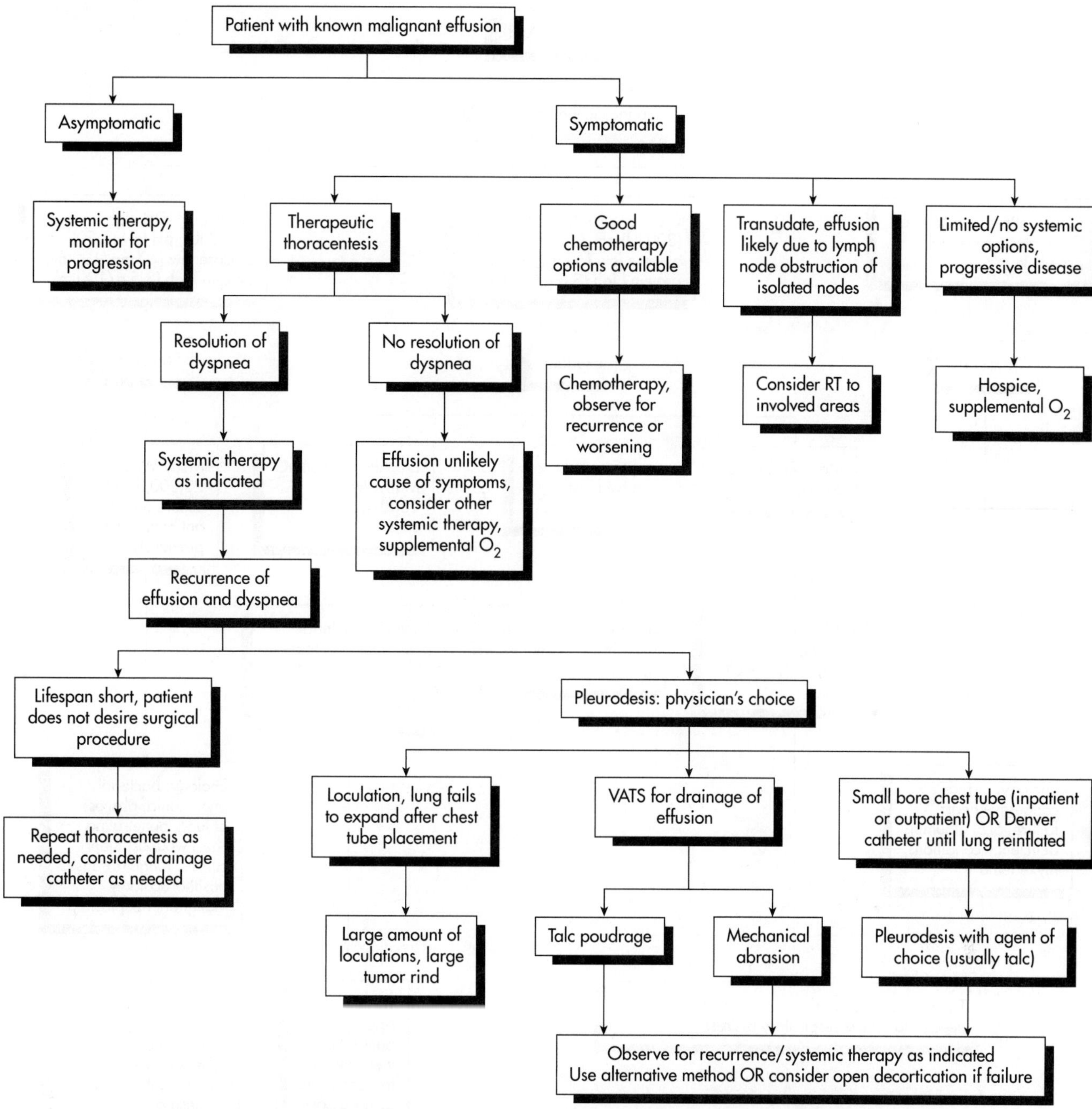

FIGURE 3-223 Treatment approach to patient with known malignant effusion. *RT,* Radiation therapy; *VATS,* video-assisted thoracic surgery. (From Abeloff MD: *Clinical oncology,* ed 3, Philadelphia, 2004, Elsevier.)

ICD-9CM # 511.9 Pleural effusion, unspecified

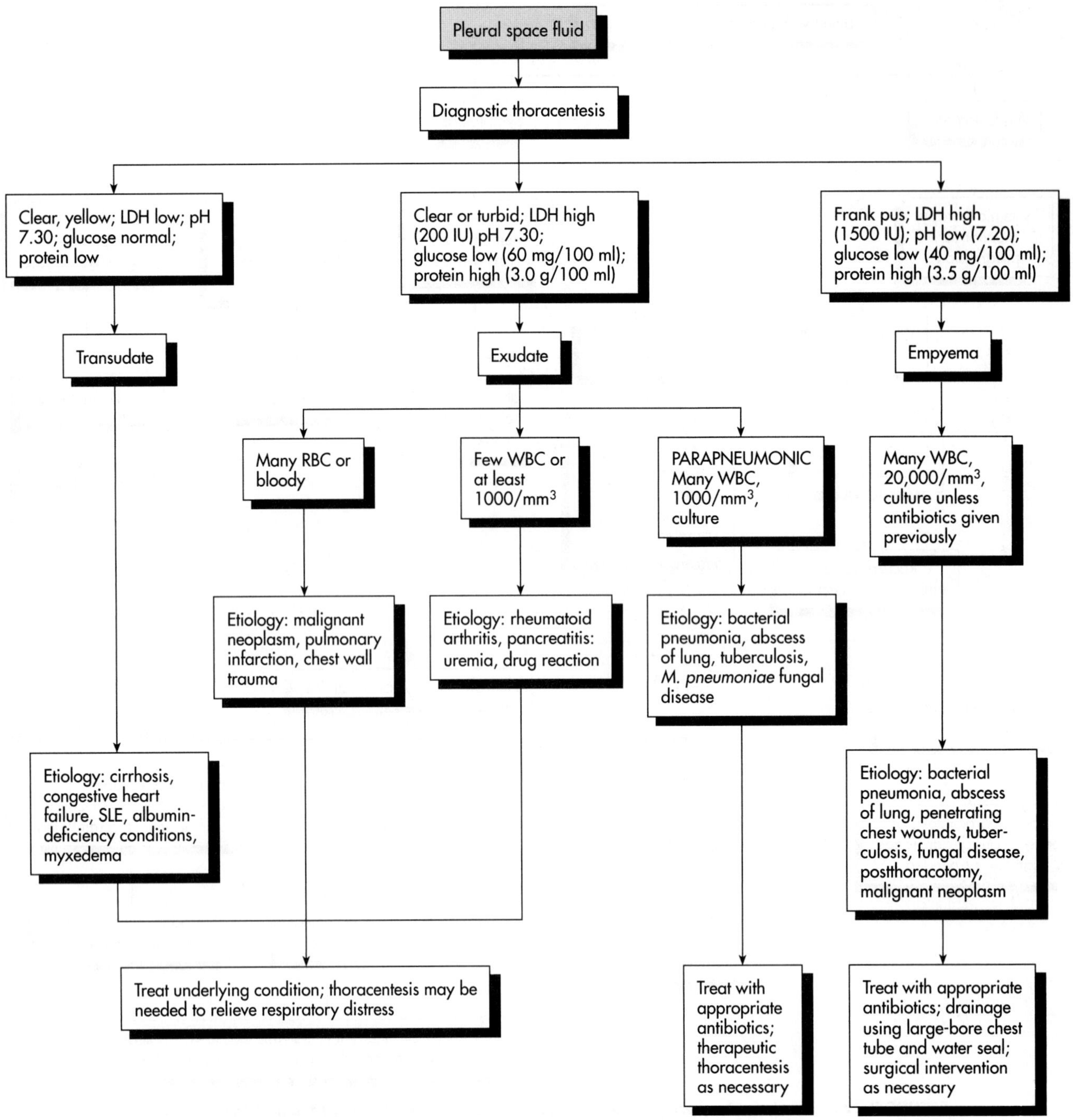

FIGURE 3-224 Evaluation, common etiologies, and management of pleural effusion and empyema. *LDH,* Lactate dehydrogenase; *RBC,* red blood cells; *SLE,* systemic lupus erythematosus; *WBC,* white blood cells. (From Kassirer J [ed]: *Current therapy in adult medicine,* ed 4, St Louis, 1998, Mosby.)

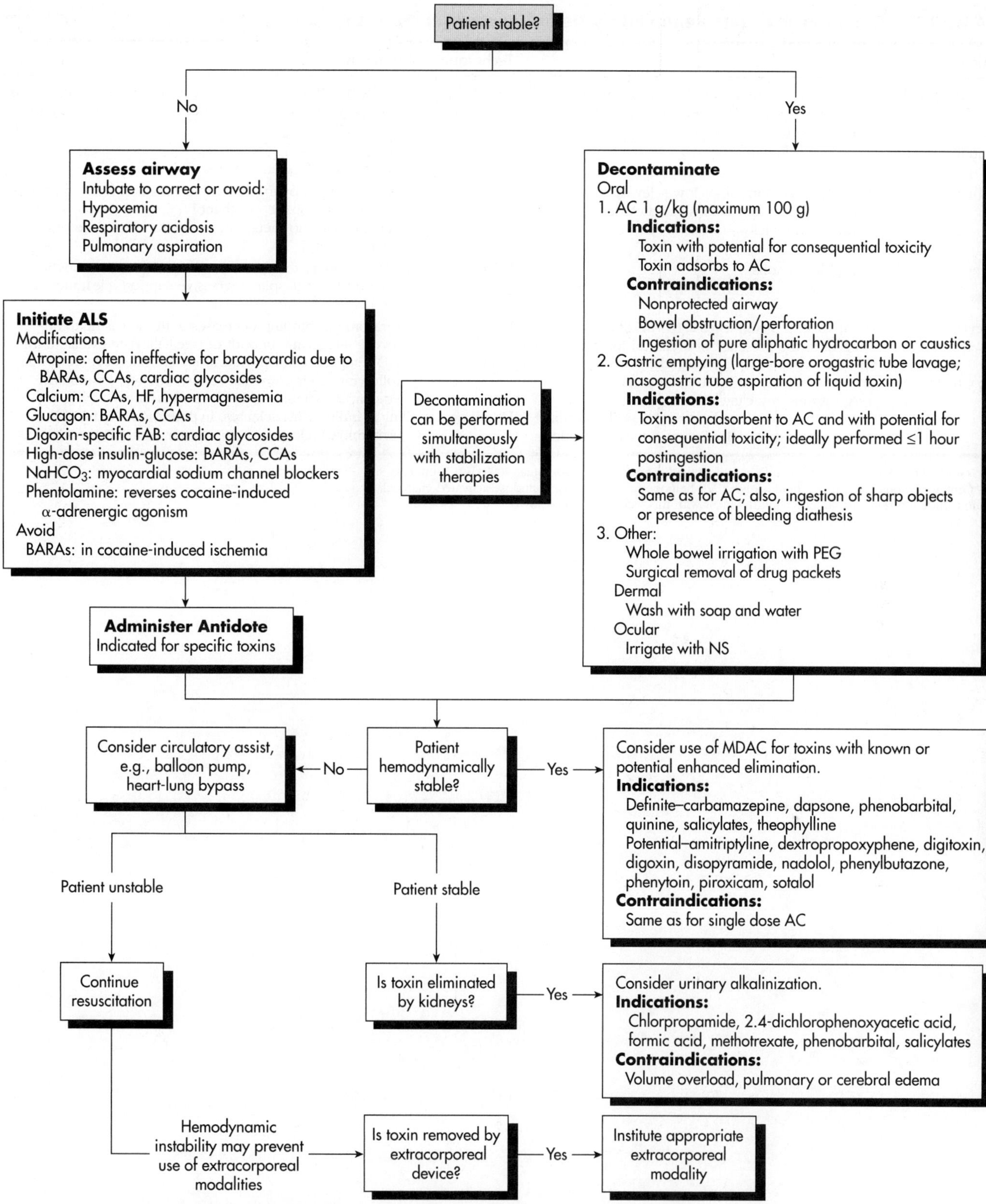

FIGURE 3-225 Algorithm for the management of acute poisoning. See also Table 3-16. *AC,* activated charcoal; *BARAs,* beta-adrenergic receptor antagonists; *CCAs,* L-type calcium channel antagonists; *HF,* hydrolluoric acid; *MDAC,* multidose activated charcoal; *NS,* 0.9% saline solution; *PEG,* nonabsorbable polyethylene glycol solution. (From Goldman L, Ausiello D [eds]: *Cecil textbook of medicine,* ed 23, Philadelphia, 2008, WB Saunders.)

Continued on following page

TABLE 3-17 Common Toxicants Removed by Hemodialysis/Hemoperfusion

Toxicant	Indications	Technique	Comments
Ethylene glycol	Serum level ≥50 ml/dl, or lower levels with concomitant metabolic acidosis and evidence of end-organ toxicity	HD	May not be required in patient with normal creatinine clearance and acid-base status who is receiving fomepizole
Lithium*	Clinical indications	HD	Clinical indication is CNS toxicity (e.g., decreased mental status, ataxia, coma, seizures)
Methanol	Serum level ≥50 ml/dl, or lower levels with concomitant metabolic acidosis and evidence of end-organ toxicity	HD	Usually required owing to slow elimination half-life in presence of fomepizole or ethanol (30.3 to 54.4 hr), even in patients with no metabolic acidosis or evidence of end-organ toxicity
Phenobarbital	Clinical indications	HP/HD	Rarely necessary except when the patient is hemodynamically unstable despite aggressive support; clearance rates are better with HD than HP
Salicylates	*Acute toxicity:* serum level ≥100 ml/dl or <100 mg/dl in the presence of a clinical indication *Chronic toxicity:* any clinical indication	HD	Serum protein binding decreases with increasing toxic levels, increasing amount of free salicylate available for HD removal; clinical indications are one or more of the following: altered mental status, seizures, pulmonary edema, intractable acidosis, renal failure
Theophylline	*Acute toxicity:* serum level ≥90 µg/ml or <90 µg/ml plus any clinical indication *Chronic toxicity:* serum level ≥40 µg/dl and not declining despite MDAC; any clinical indication	HP/HD	Clinical indications: seizures, hypotension, ventricular arrhythmias; clearance rates better with HD than HP

From Goldman L, Ausiello D [eds]: *Cecil textbook of medicine,* ed 23, Philadelphia, 2008, WB Saunders.
CNS, Central nervous system; *HD,* hemodialysis; *HP,* hemoperfusion; *MDAC,* multidose activated charcoal.
*Hemodiafiltration removes lithium; clinical benefit with this technique is unknown.

ICD-9CM # 776.4

Diagnostic Algorithm for Polycythemia

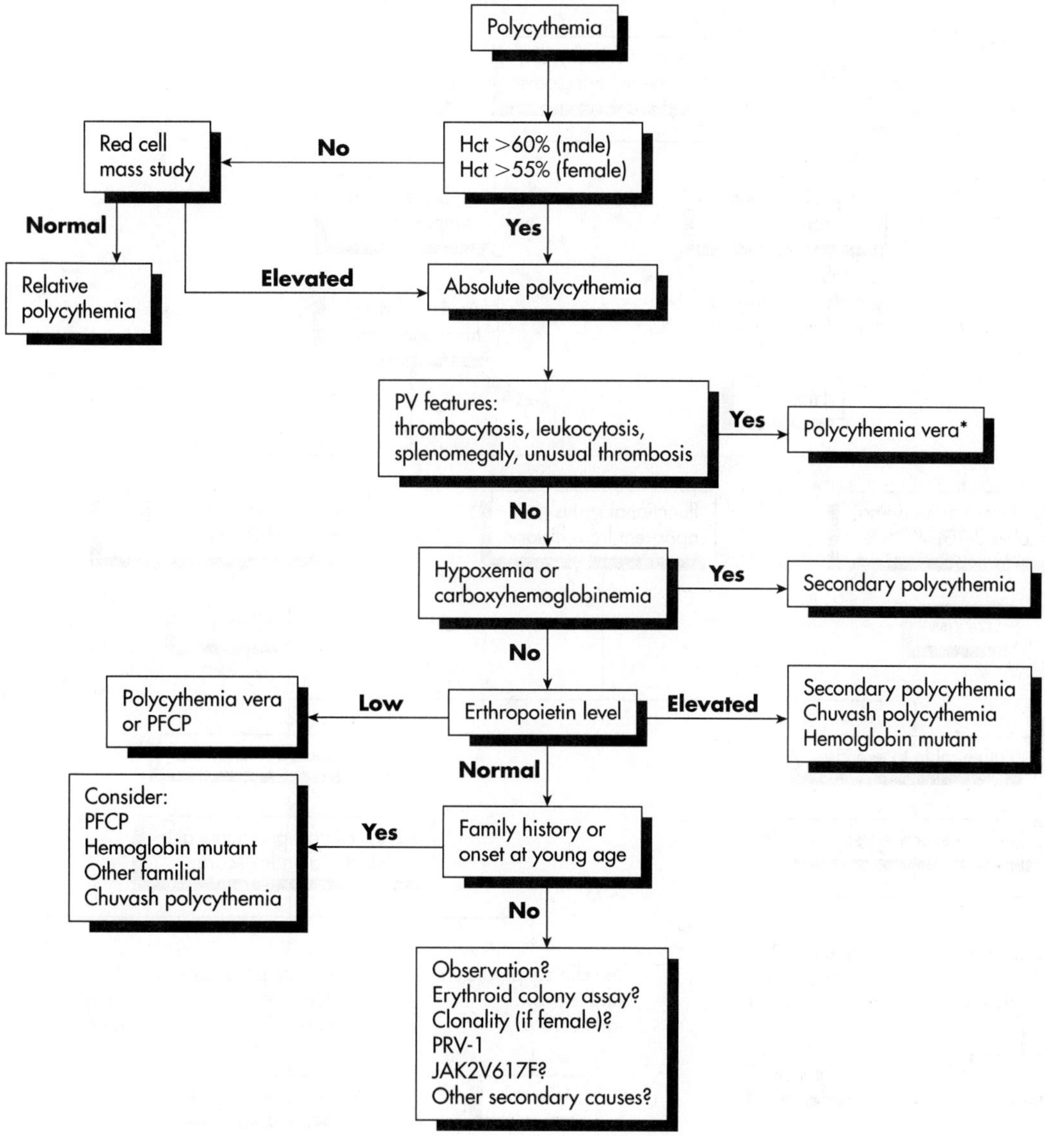

*Refer to Section I for additional information on this topic.

FIGURE 3-226 Diagnostic algorithm for polycythemia. *JAK2V617F,* JAK-2 mutation; *PFCP,* primary familial and congenital polycythemia; *PRV-1,* polycythemia rubra vera 1. (From Young NS, Gerson SL, High KA [eds]: *Clinical hematology,* St Louis, 2006, Mosby.)

PREOPERATIVE EVALUATION, PATIENT WITH CORONARY HEART DISEASE

ICD-9CM # 411.89 Coronary insufficiency, acute
411.8 Coronary insufficiency, chronic
411.1 Coronary insufficiency or intermediate syndrome

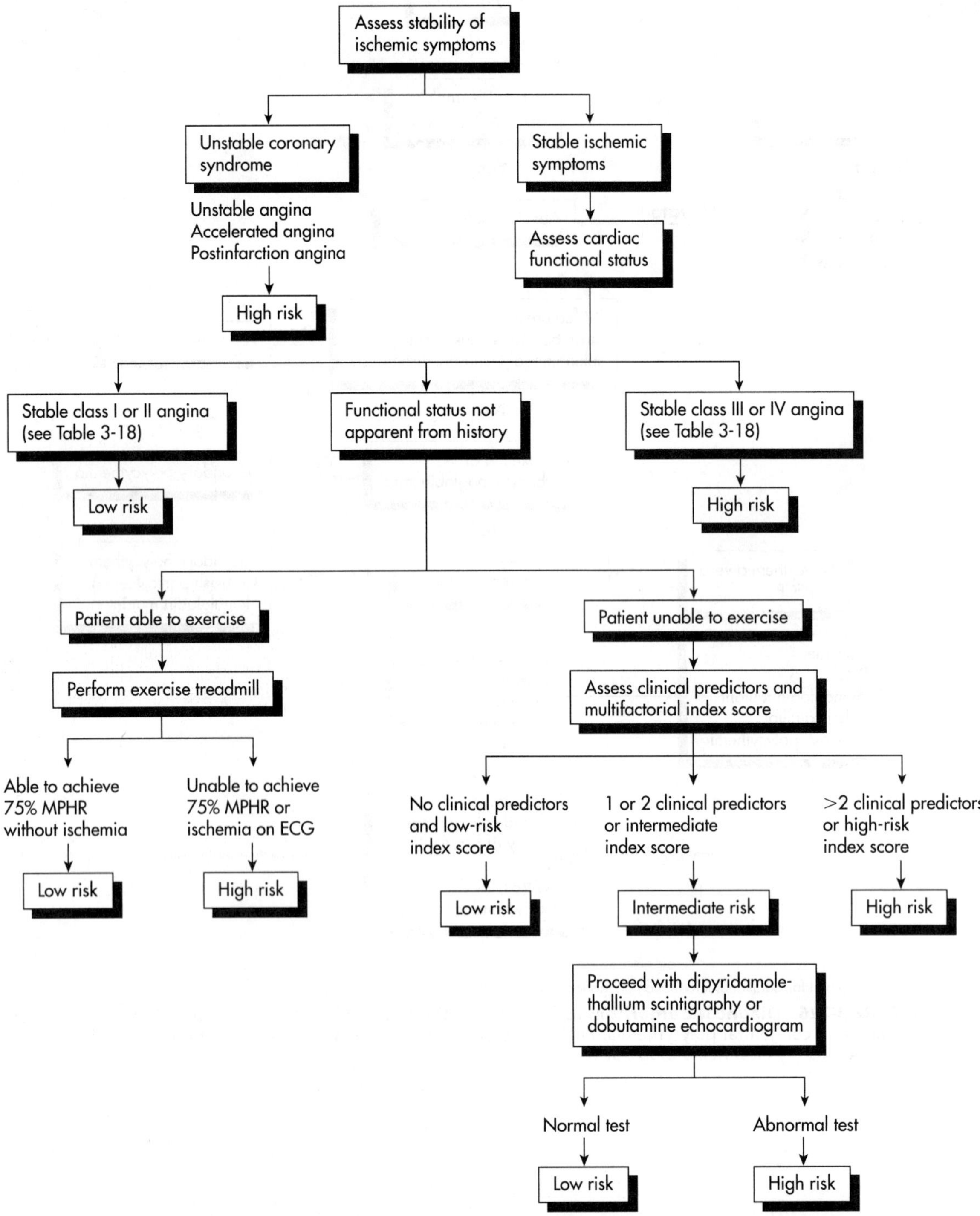

FIGURE 3-227 Preoperative evaluation of patients with known or suspected coronary artery disease. (From Goldman L, Braunwald E [eds]: *Primary cardiology*, ed 2, Philadelphia, 2003, WB Saunders.)

TABLE 3-18 New York Heart Association Functional Classification

Class I	No limitation	Ordinary physical activity does not cause symptoms
Class II	Slight limitation	Comfortable at rest Ordinary physical activity causes symptoms
Class III	Marked limitation	Comfortable at rest Less than ordinary activity causes symptoms
Class IV	Inability to carry on any physical activity	Symptoms present at rest

ICD-9CM # 253.1

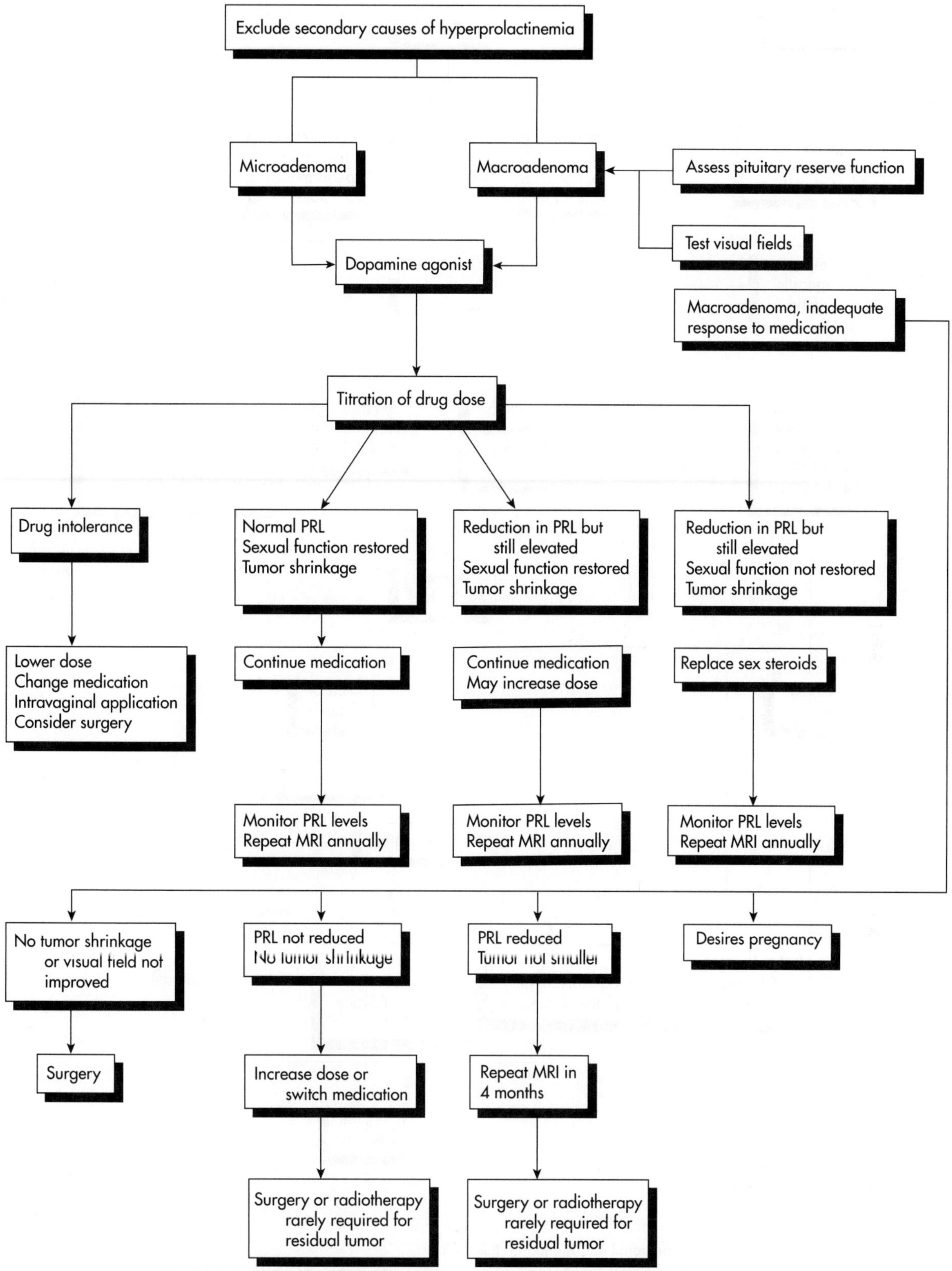

Note: Refer to Section I for additional information on this topic.

FIGURE 3-228 Prolactinoma management. After secondary causes of hyperprolactinemia have been excluded, subsequent management decisions are based on clinical imaging and biochemical criteria. *MRI,* Magnetic resonance imaging; *PRL,* prolactin. (From Larsen PR, Kronenberg HM, Memlmed S, Polansky KS: *Williams textbook of endocrinology,* ed 11, Philadelphia, 2008, Saunders.)

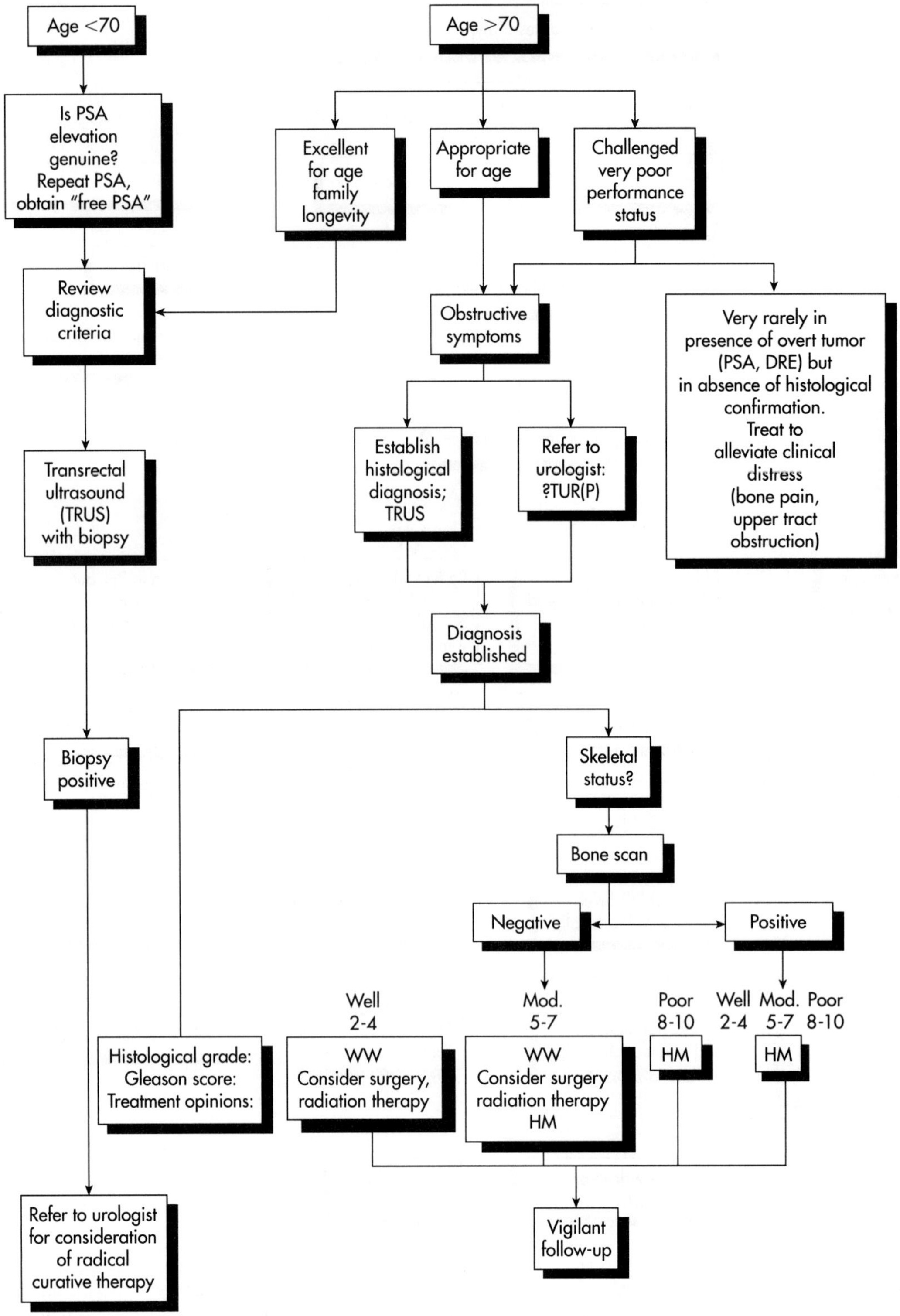

Note: Refer to Section I for additional information on this topic.

FIGURE 3-229 Assessment and treatment of a patient with prostate cancer suspected on the grounds of a digital rectal exam and PSA. *DRE,* Digital rectal examination; *HM,* hormonal manipulation; *PSA,* prostate specific antigen; *TUR(P),* transurethral resection (prostate); *WW,* watchful waiting. (Modified from Tallis RC, Fillit HM [eds]: *Brocklehurst's textbook of geriatric medicine and gerontology,* ed 6, London, 2003, Churchill Livingstone.)

ICD-9CM # 600 Benign prostatic hyperplasia

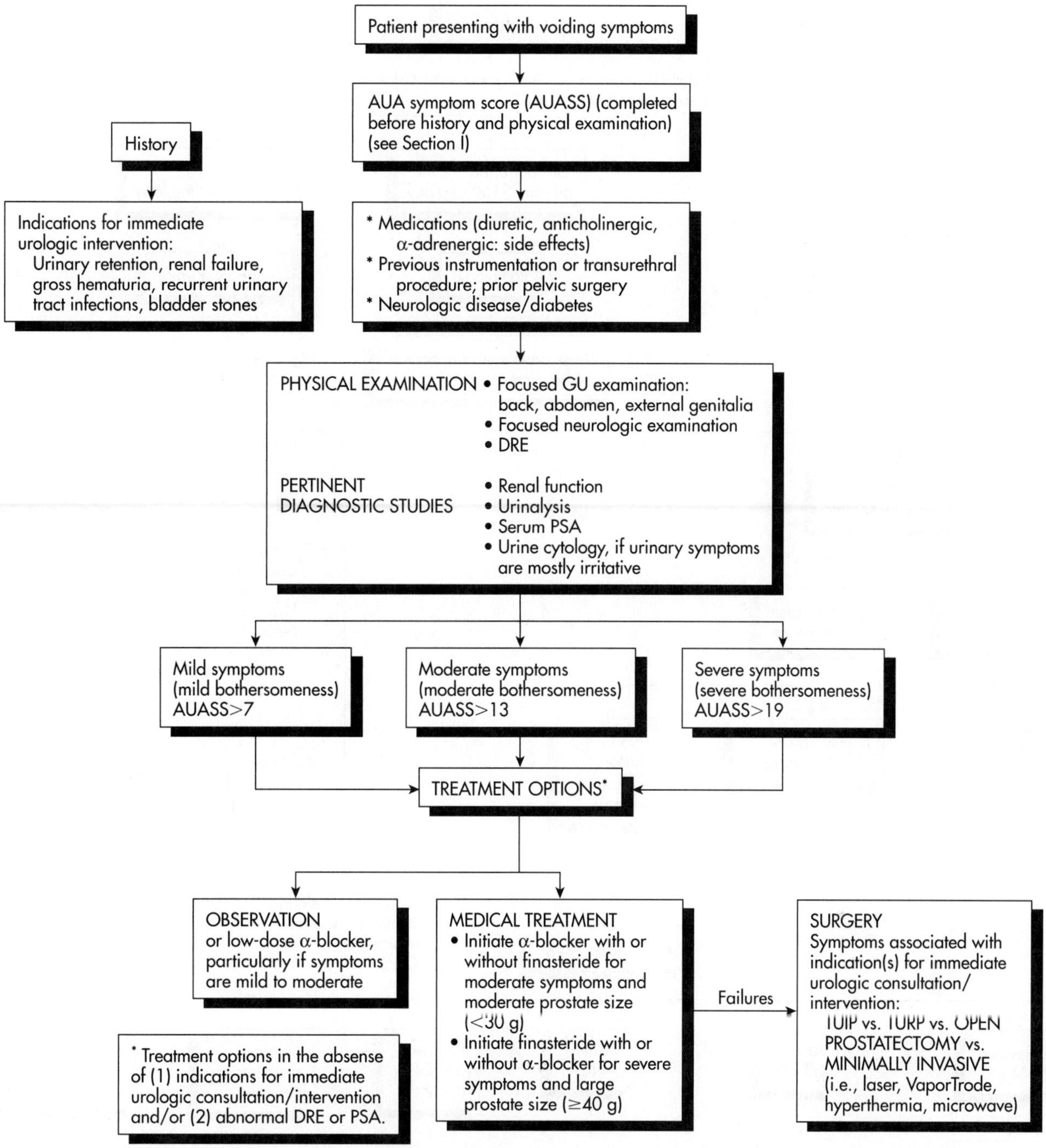

Note: Refer to Section I for additional information on this topic.

FIGURE 3-230 Critical pathway for patients with benign prostatic hypertrophy. *AUA,* American Urological Association; *DRE,* digital rectal examination; *GU,* genitourinary; *PSA,* prostate-specific antigen; *TUIP,* transurethral incision of the prostate; *TURP,* transurethral resection of the prostate. (From Nseyo UO [ed]: *Urology for primary care physicians,* Philadelphia, 1999, WB Saunders.)

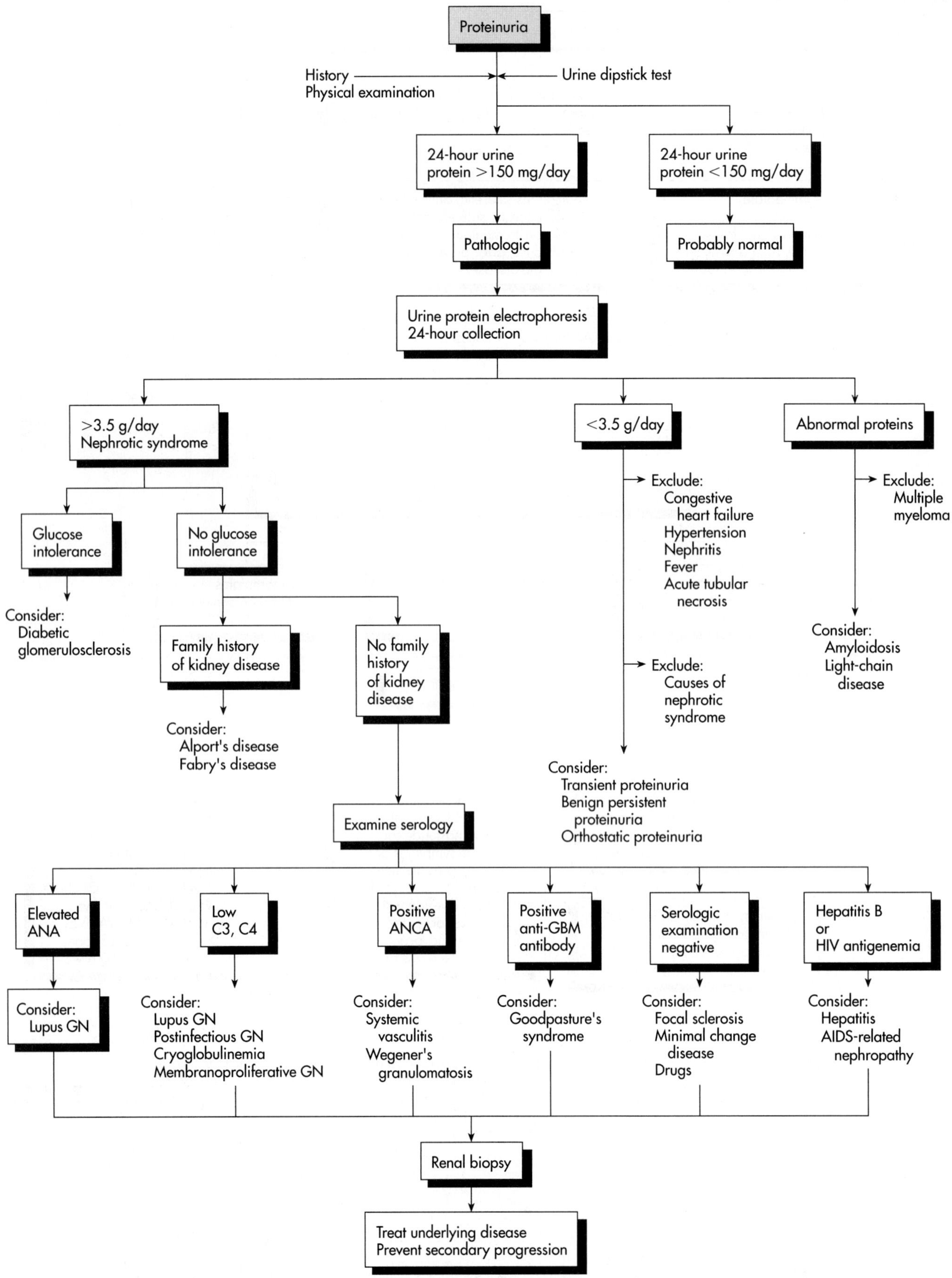

FIGURE 3-231 Proteinuria. *AIDS,* Acquired immunodeficiency syndrome; *ANA,* antinuclear antibody; *ANCA,* antineutrophil cytoplasmic autoantibody; *anti-GBM,* anti–glomerular basement membrane; *GN,* glomerulonephritis. (From Greene HL, Johnson WP, Lemcke D [eds]: *Decision making in medicine,* ed 2, St Louis, 1998, Mosby.)

PRURITUS, GENERALIZED

ICD-9CM # 698.9 Pruritus NOS

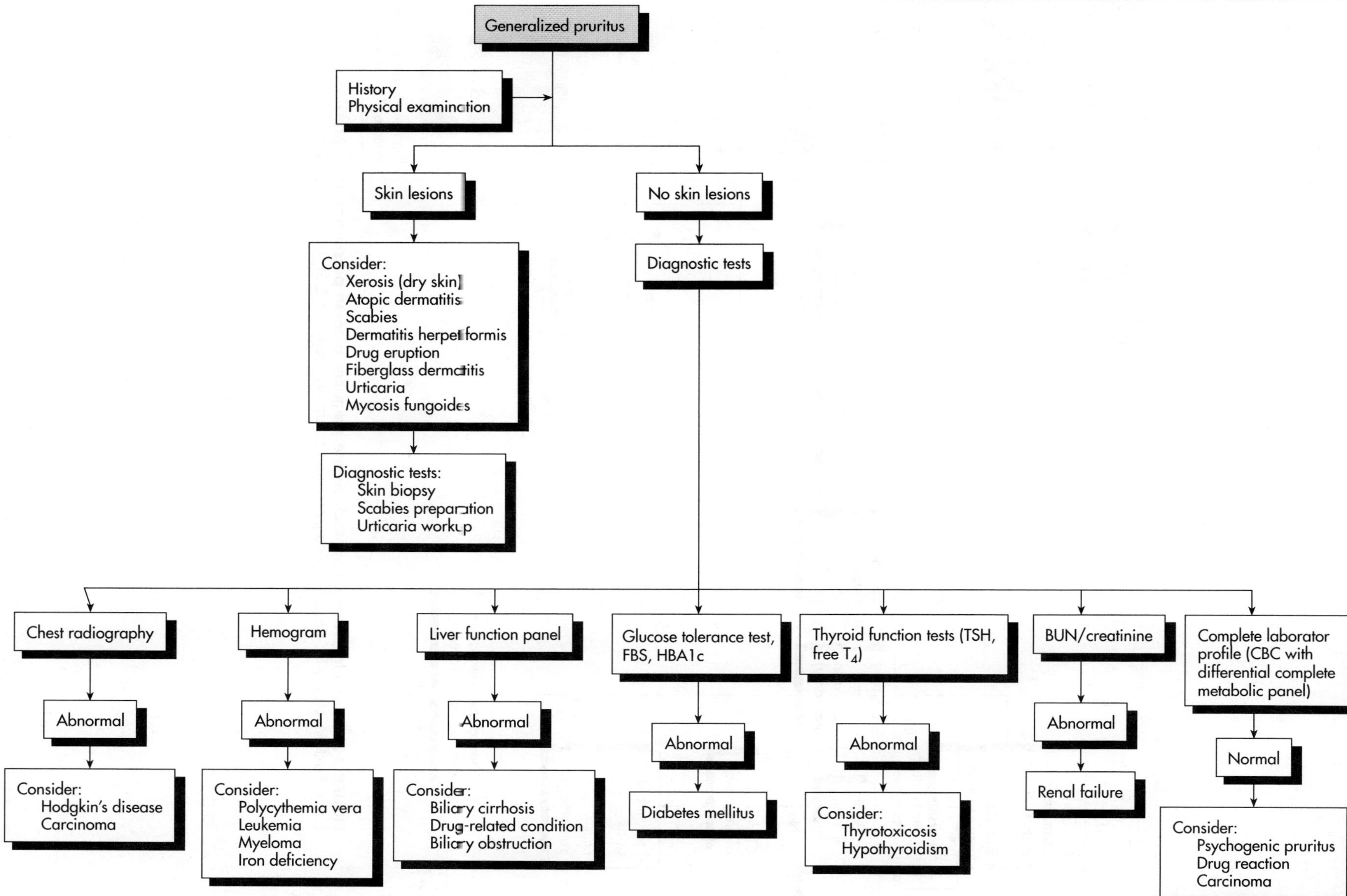

FIGURE 3-232 Evaluation of generalized pruritus. *BUN,* Blood urea nitrogen; *CBC,* complete blood count; *FBS,* fasting blood sugar; *HBA1c,* hemoglobin A1c; T_4, thyroxine; *TSH,* thyroid-stimulating hormone. (From Greene HL, Johnson WP, Lemcke D [eds]: *Decision making in medicine*, ed 2, St Louis, 1998, Mosby.)

ICD-9CM # 698.9

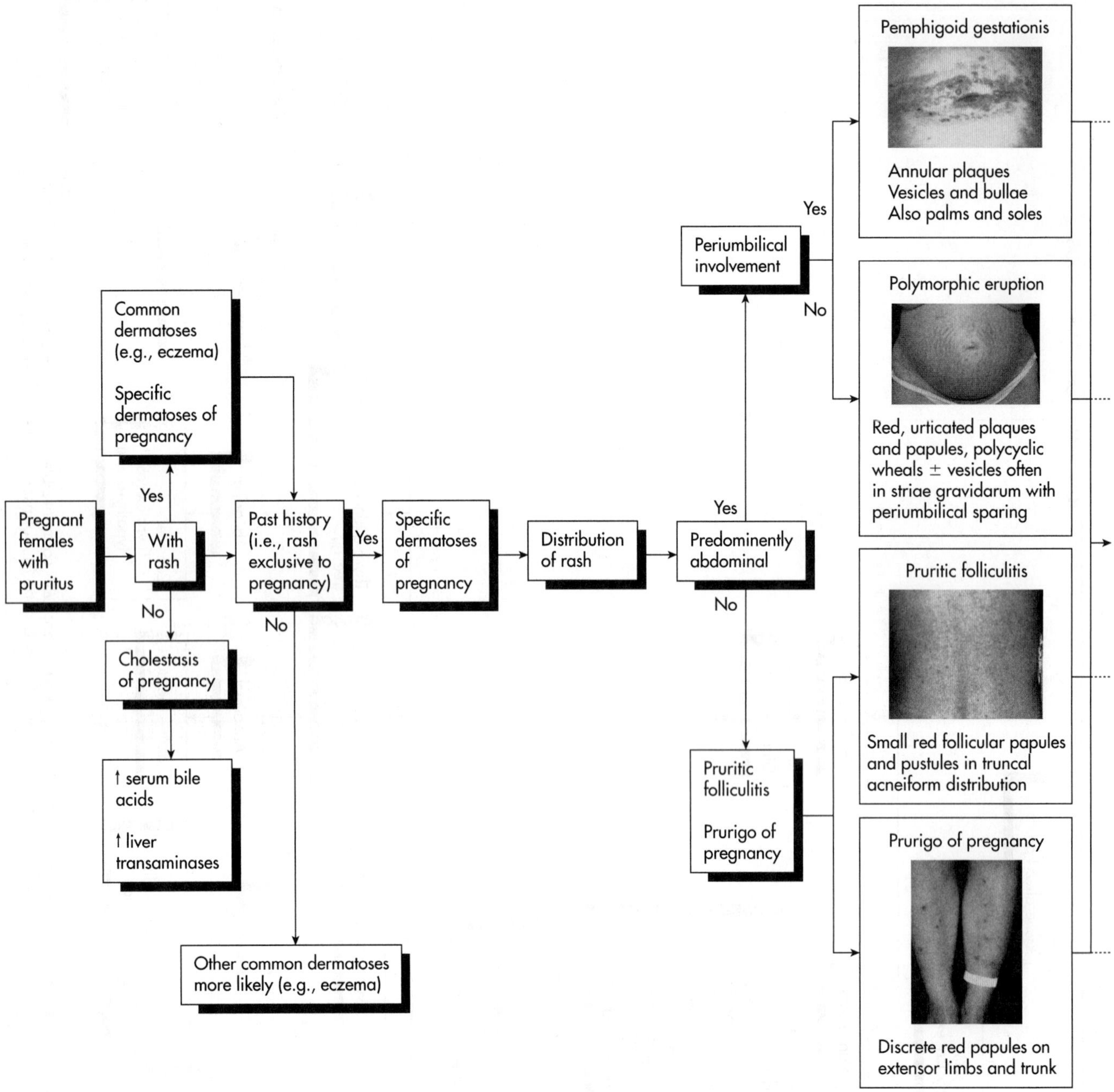

FIGURE 3-233 An algorithmic approach to the pregnant woman presenting with pruritus. (From Black M, McKay M: *Obstetrics and gynecological dermatology,* ed 2, St. Louis, 2002, Mosby.)

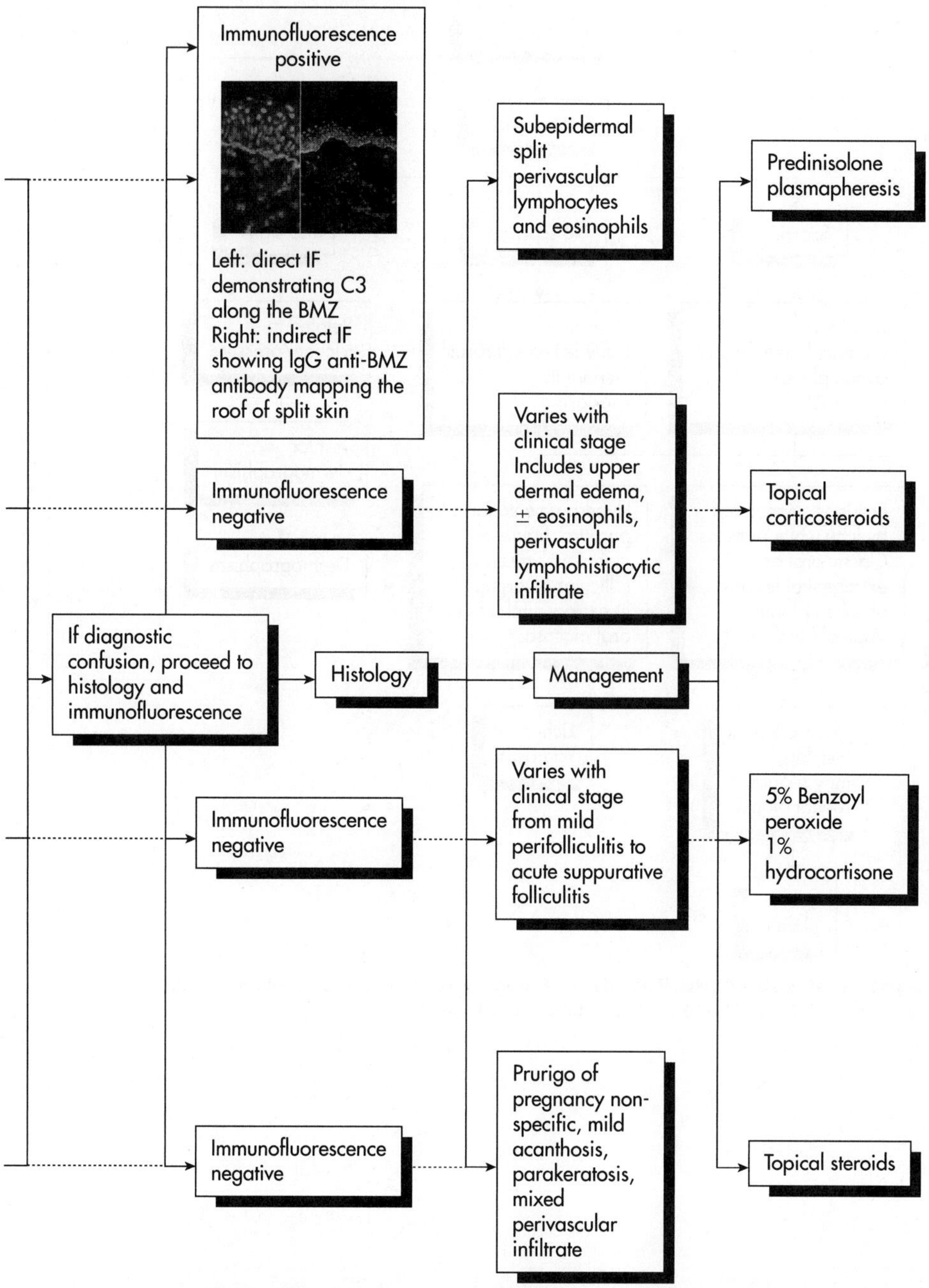

FIGURE 3-233 (Continued) **An algorithmic approach to the pregnant woman presenting with pruritus.** (From Black M, McKay M: *Obstetrics and gynecological dermatology,* ed 2, St. Louis, 2002, Mosby.)

ICD-9CM # 698.1

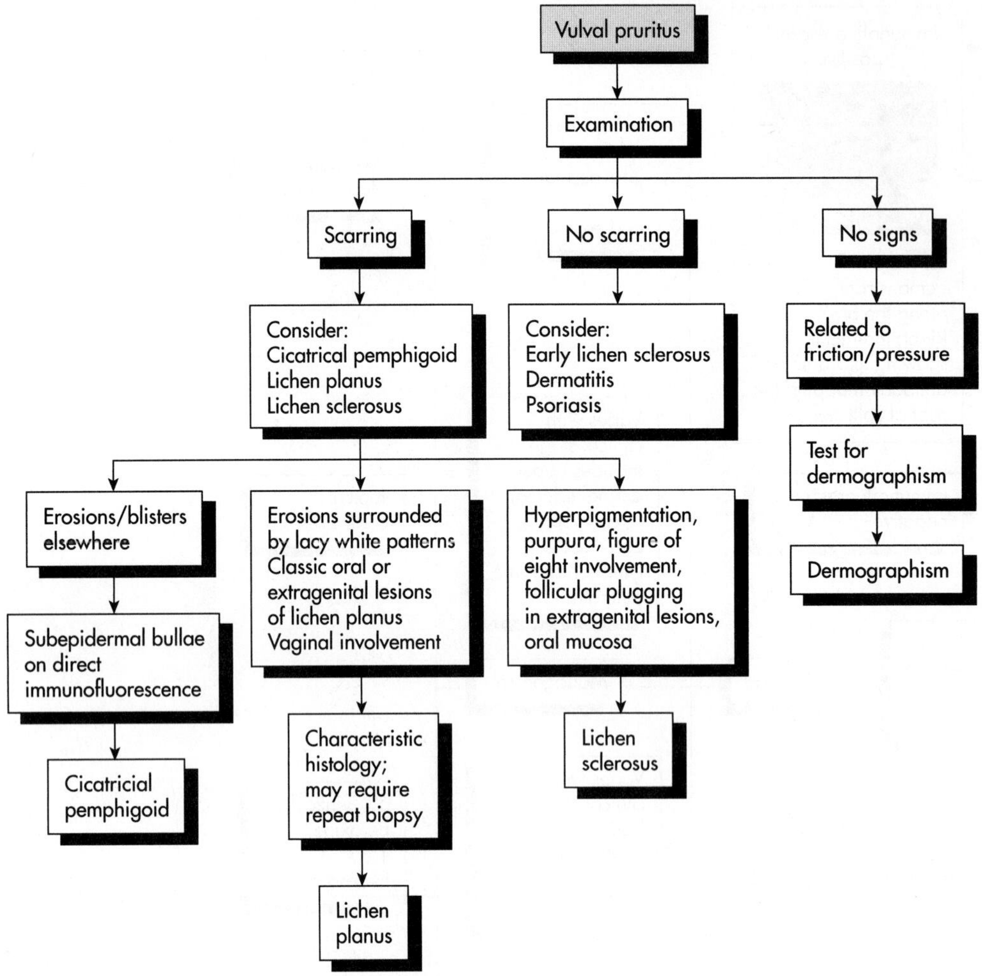

FIGURE 3-234 The diagnosis of vulvar pruritus. (From Bolognia JL, Mascaro JM, Mancini AJ, Salasche SJ, Saurat JH, Stingl G [eds]: *Dermatology,* ed 2, St Louis, 2008, Mosby.)

ICD-9CM # 275.49

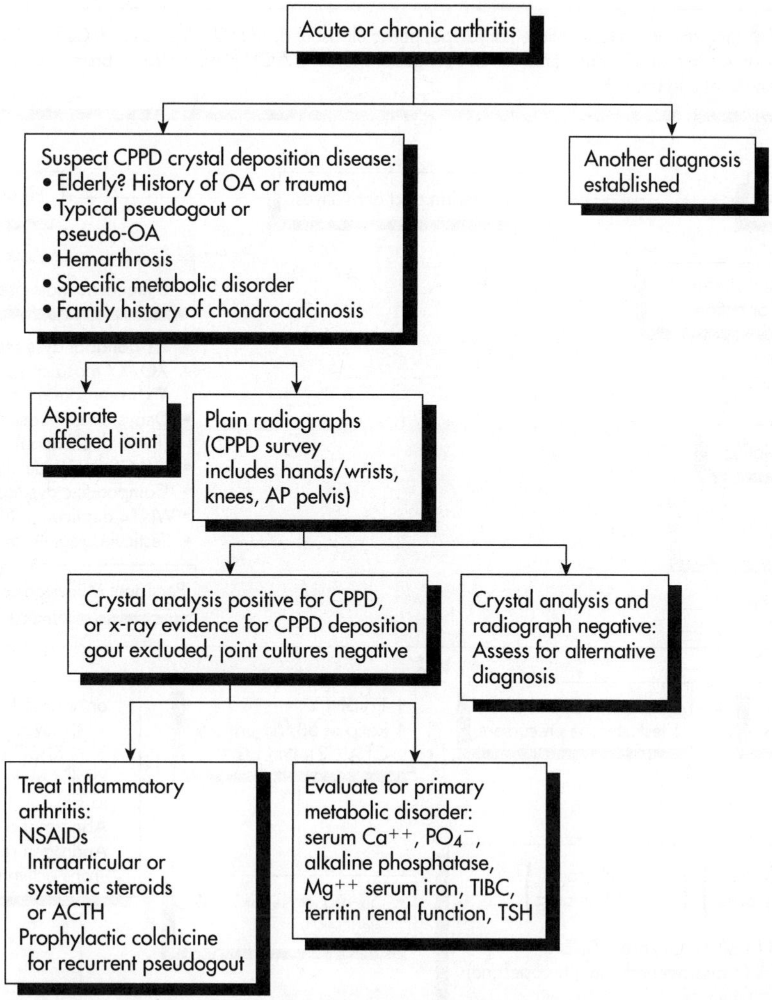

FIGURE 3-235 Algorithm for evaluation and treatment of calcium pyrophosphate dihydrate deposition disease. *ACTH,* Adrenocorticotropic hormone; *AP,* anteroposterior; *CPPD,* calcium pyrophosphate deposition; *OA,* osteoarthritis; *TIBC,* total iron-binding capacity; *TSH,* thyroid-stimulating hormone. (From Harris ED, Budd RC, Firestein GS, Genovese MC, Sergent JS, Ruddy S, et al: *Kelley's textbook of rheumatology,* ed 7, Philadelphia, 2005, Saunders.)

ICD-9CM # 752.7

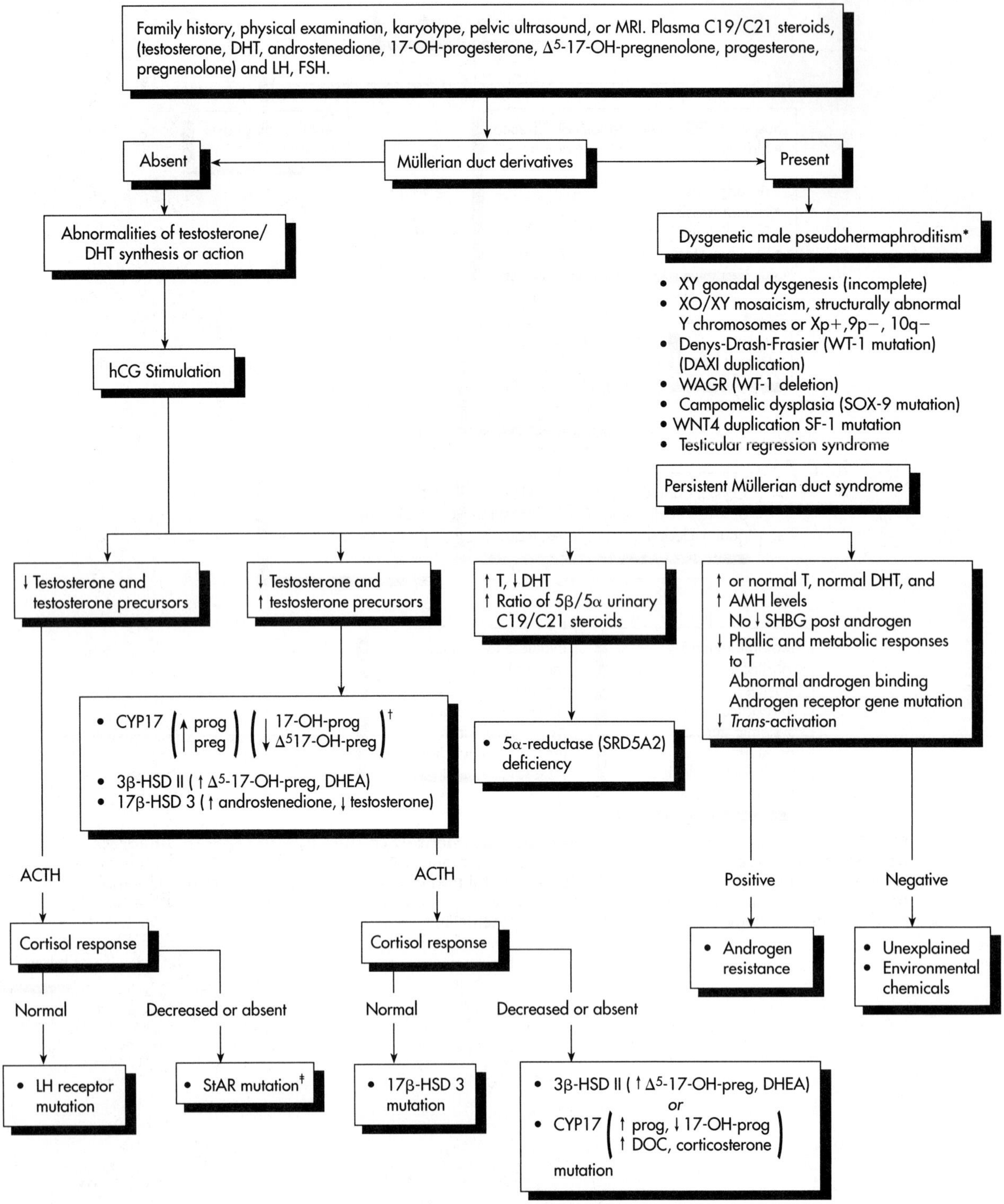

*Patients with dysgenetic male pseudohermaphroditism may manifest varying degress of testicular dysgenesis with either complete or partial testosterone/DHT and/or AMH deficiency. Therefore, not all patients may manifest either ambiguous genitalia or the presence of müllerian ducts.

†CYP17 (P450??) catalyzes the 17-hydroxylation of progesterone and pregnenolone to 17-hydroxyprogesterone and Δ^5-17-hydroxypregnenolone as well as the scission (lyase) of 17-hydroxypregnenolone to DHEA. Patients with 17, 20-lyase deficiency have elevated levels of 17-hydroxyprogesterone and Δ^5-17-hydroxypregnenolone in relation to androstenedione and DHEA wither before or after hCG stimulation.

‡The StAR (steroidogenic acute regulatory) protein is involved in the transport of cholesterol from the outer to the inner mitochondrial membrane where the enzyme CYP11A1(P450??) resides. Patients with a mutation in the CYP11A1 enzymatic activity in intact. They manifest congenital lipoid adrenal hyperplasia.

FIGURE 3-236 Steps in the differential diagnosis of male pseudohermaphroditism. *3β-HSD 11,* 3β-hydroxysteroid dehydrogenase/Δ^5-isomerase; 17β-HSD 3, 17β-hydroxysteroid dehydrogenase (oxido-reductase) type 3; *ACTH,* adrenocorticotropic hormone; *AMH,* antimüllerian hormone; *CYP17,* 17α-hydroxylase/17,20-lyase; *DHEA,* dehydroepiandrosterone; *DHT,* dihydrotestosterone; *FSH,* follicle-stimulating hormone; *LH,* luteinizing hormone; *MRI,* magnetic resonance imaging; *SHBG,* sex hormone-binding globulin; *SF1,* steroidogenic factor-1; *T,* testosterone; *WAGR,* Wilms tumor, aniridia, genital anomalies, and mental retardation. (From Larsen PR, Kronenberg HM, Memlmed S, Polansky KS: *Williams textbook of endocrinology,* ed 11, Philadelphia, 2008, Saunders.)

ICD-9CM # 301.9 Psychosomatic personality disorder

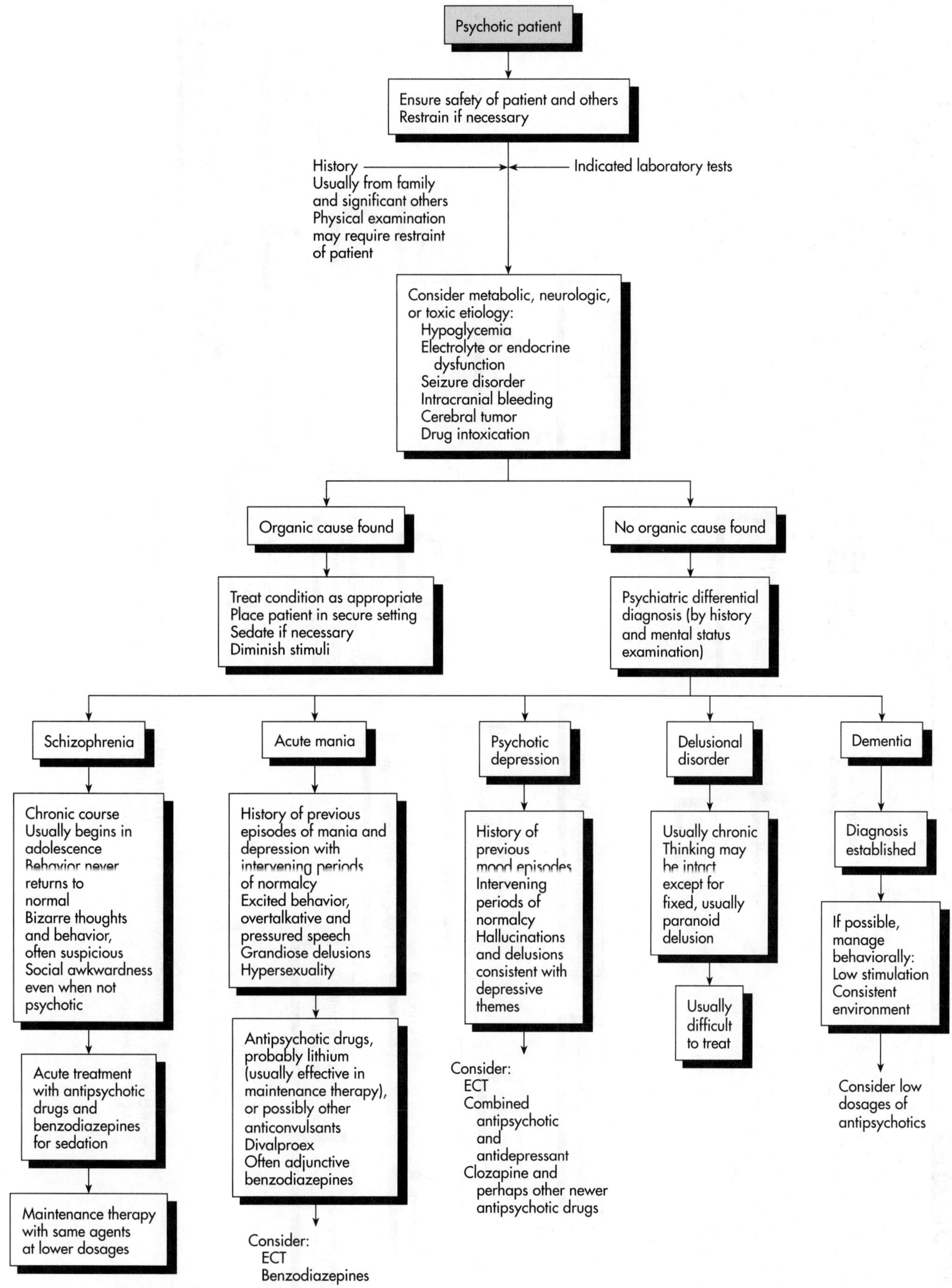

FIGURE 3-237 Evaluation of psychotic patient. *ECT,* Electroconvulsive therapy. (From Greene HL, Johnson WP, Lemcke D [eds]: *Decision making in medicine,* ed 2, St Louis, 1998, Mosby.)

PUBERTY, DELAYED

ICD-9CM # 259.0

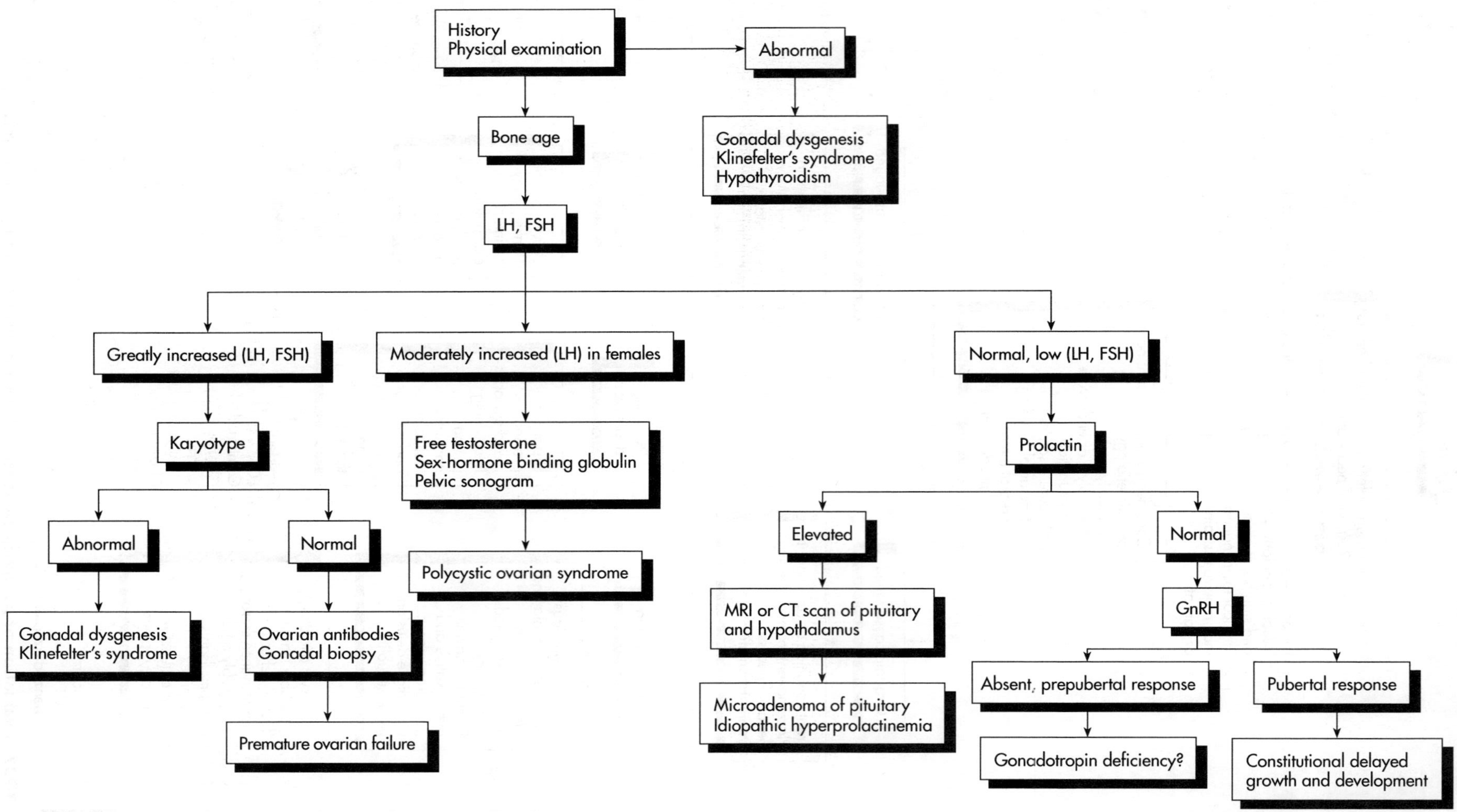

FIGURE 3-238 Evaluation of patient with delayed puberty. *CT,* Computed tomography; *FSH,* follicle-stimulating hormone; *GnRH,* gonadotropin-releasing hormone; *LH,* luteinizing hormone; *MRI,* magnetic resonance imaging. (From Moore WT, Eastman RC: *Diagnostic endocrinology,* ed 2, St Louis, 1996, Mosby.)

ICD-9CM # 259.1 Puberty precocious NOS

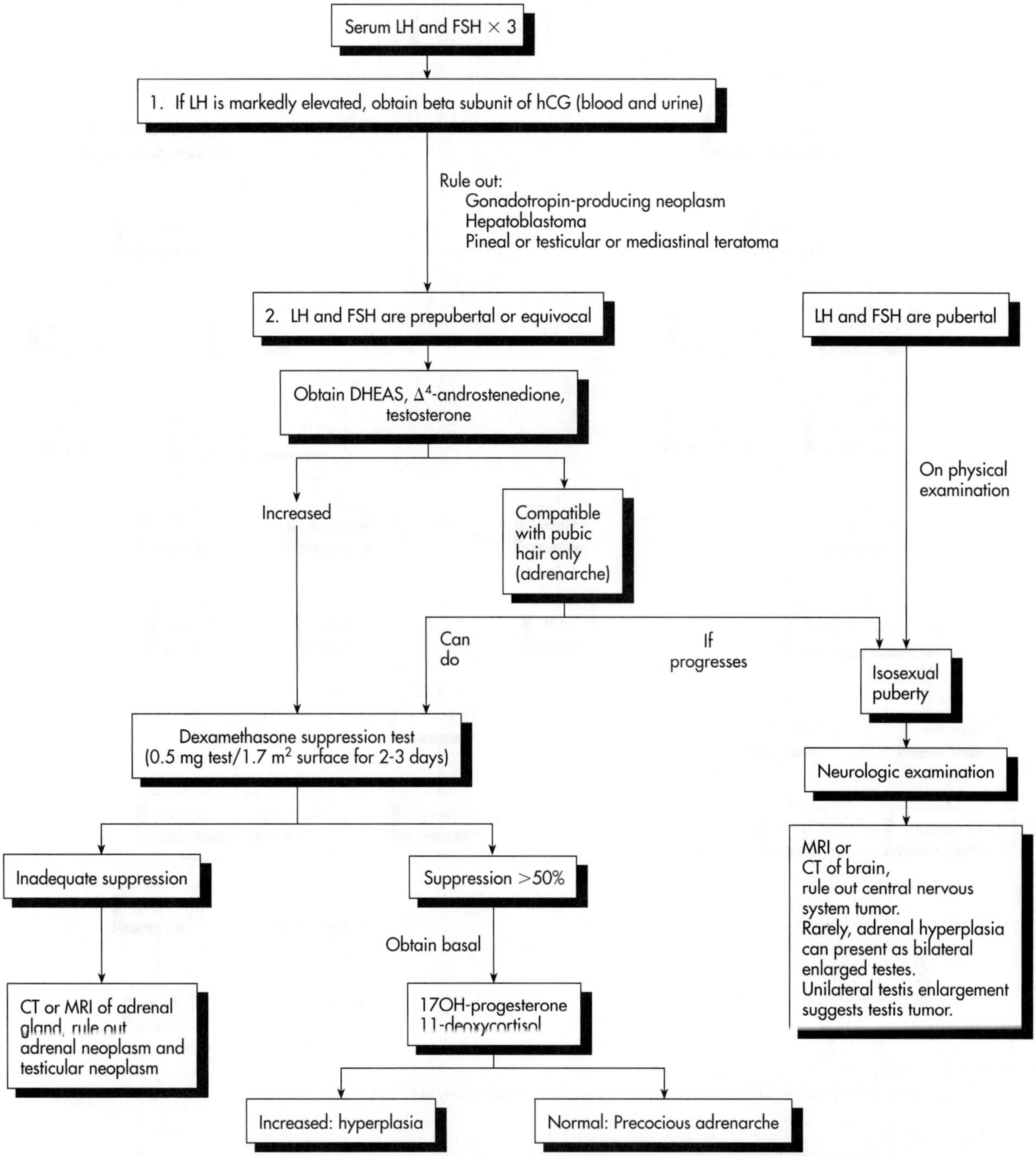

FIGURE 3-239 Evaluation of precocious puberty, excluding factitious and iatrogenic causes. *CT,* Computed tomography; *DHEAS,* dehydroepiandrosterone sulfate; *FSH,* follicle-stimulating hormone; *hCG,* human chorionic gonadotropin; *LH,* luteinizing hormone; *MRI,* magnetic resonance imaging. (Modified from Odell WD: The physiology of puberty: disorders of the pubertal process. In DeGroot LJ et al [eds]: *Endocrinology,* vol 3, New York, 1979, Grune & Stratton.)

ICD-9CM # 415.1

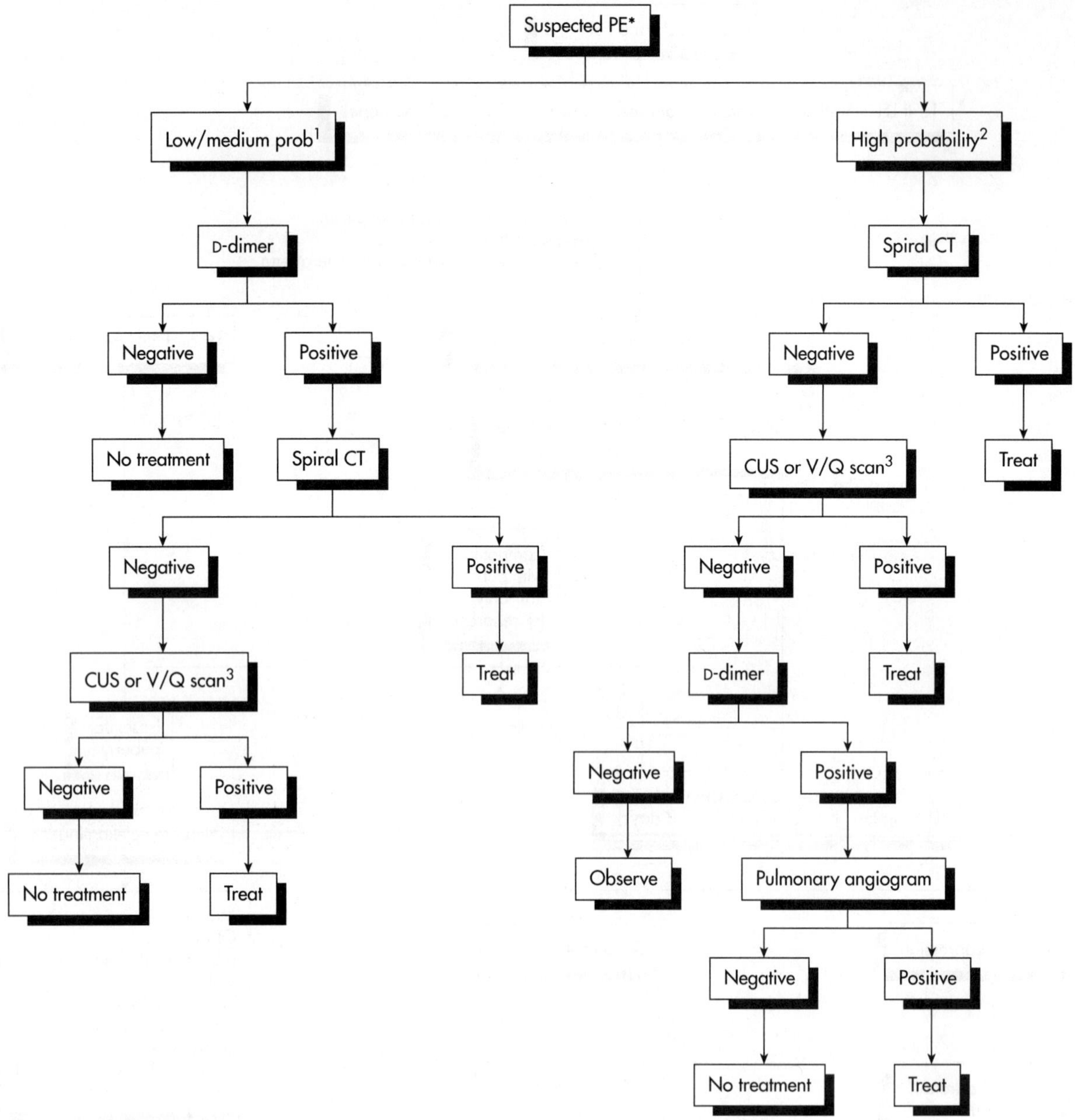

- [1]*Low probability*
  Likely alternative diagnosis established for symptoms and signs listed below, but PE still suspected

- [2]*High probability*
  No alternative diagnosis for the following:
  1. New onset dyspnea with/without hypoxia
  2. Pleuritic chest pain
  3. Hypoxia: increased A-a gradient
  4. Shock
  5. Syncope
  6. Hemoptysis

- [3]If chest x-ray is normal

*Refer to Section I for additional information on this topic.

FIGURE 3-240 Diagnostic approach to pulmonary embolism. *CT,* Computed tomography; *CUS,* compressive ultrasound of lower extremities; *PE,* pulmonary embolism; *V/Q,* ventilation/perfusion.

ICD-9CM # 518.89

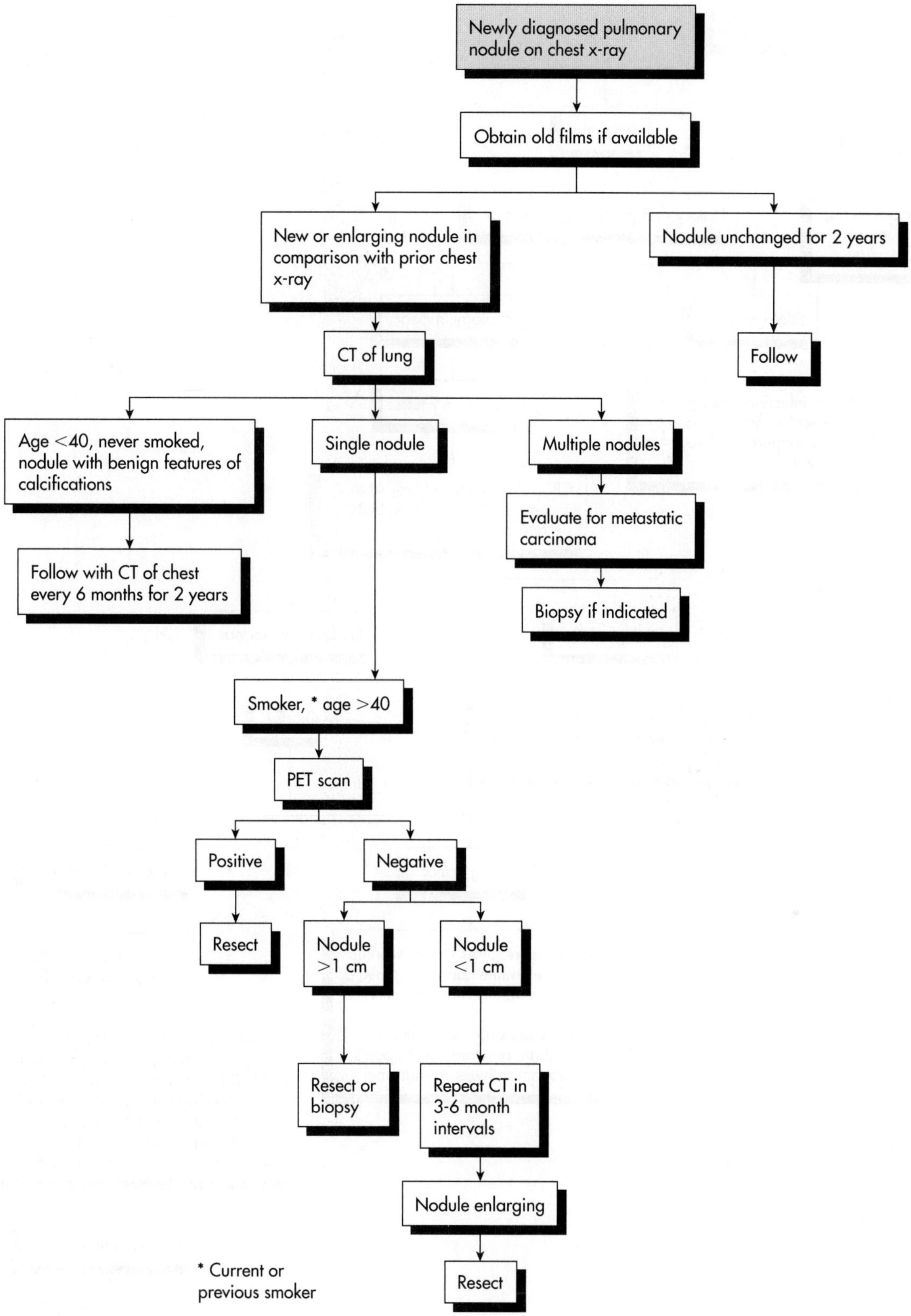

FIGURE 3-241 Pulmonary nodule. *CT,* Computed tomography; *PET,* positron emission tomography.

ICD-9CM # 287.2 Purpura, NOS

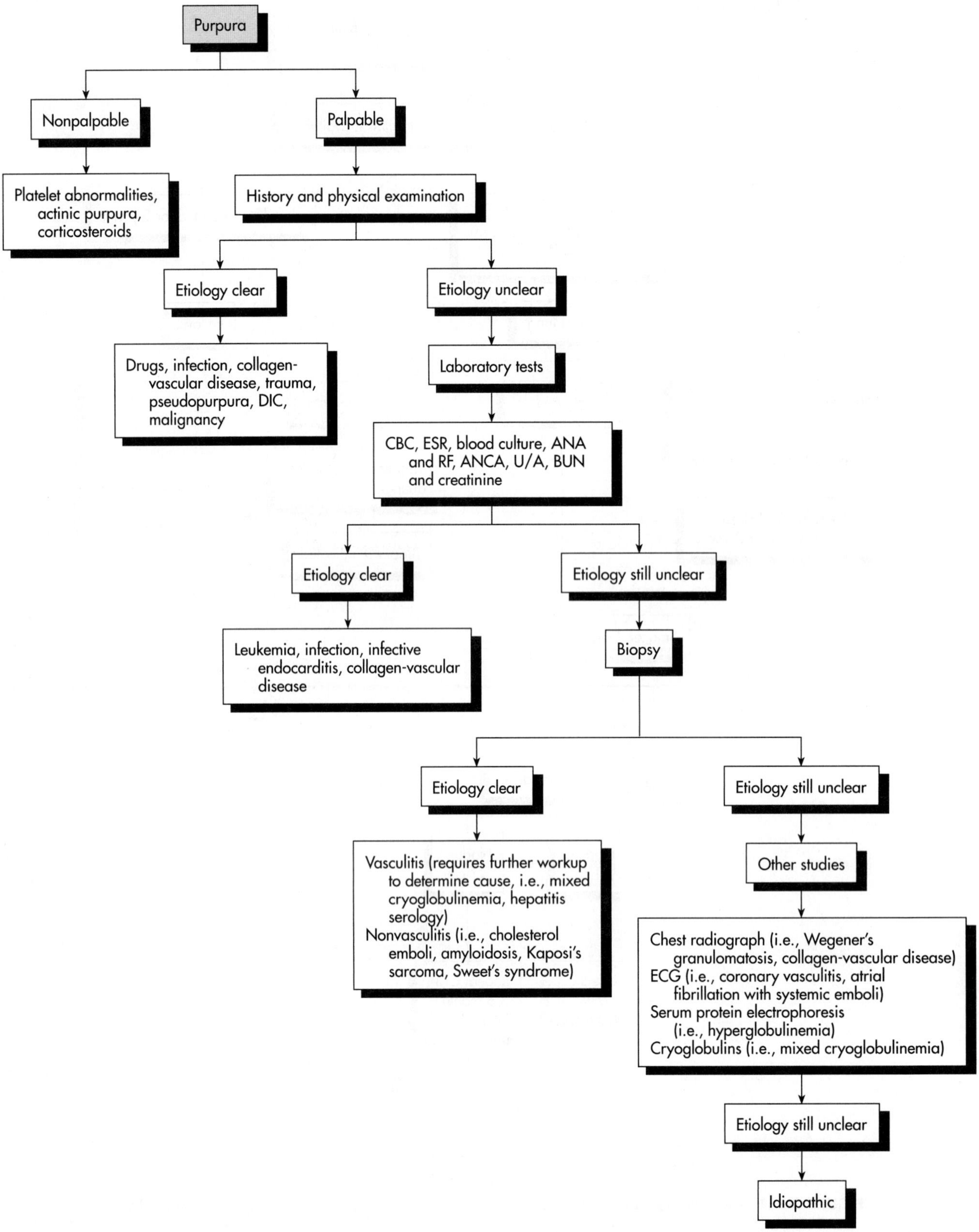

FIGURE 3-242 Diagnostic algorithm for palpable purpura. *AIDS, Acquired immunodeficiency syndrome; ANA,* antinuclear antibody; *ANCA,* antineutrophil cytoplasmic antibody test; *BUN,* blood urea nitrogen; *CBC,* complete blood cell count; *DIC,* disseminated intravascular coagulation; *ECG,* electrocardiogram; *ESR,* erythrocyte sedimentation rate; *MCV,* mean corpuscular volume; *RF,* rheumatoid factor; *U/A,* urinalysis. (From Stevens GL, Adelman HM, Wallach PM: *Am Fam Physician* 52:1355, 1995.)

ICD-9CM # 379.93

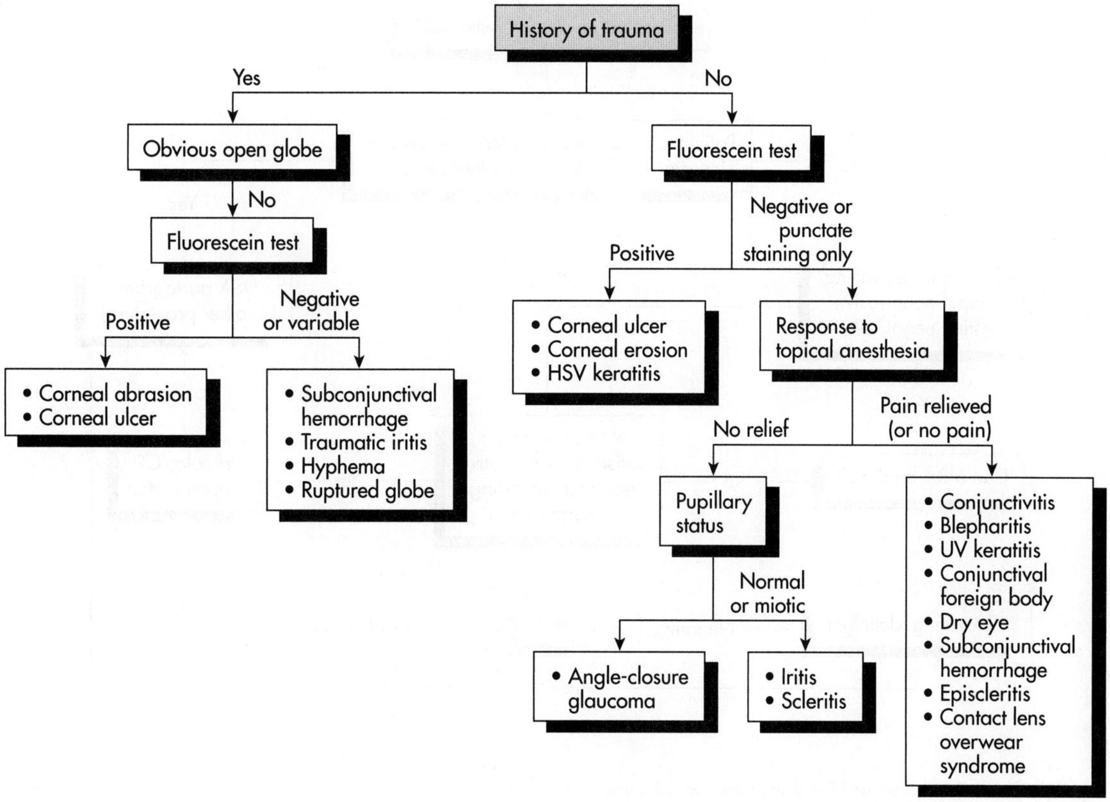

FIGURE 3-243 Algorithm showing diagnostic procedure for the acute red eye. *HSV,* Herpes simplex virus; *UV,* ultraviolet. (From Auerbach PS: *Wilderness medicine,* ed 5, St Louis, 2007, Mosby.)

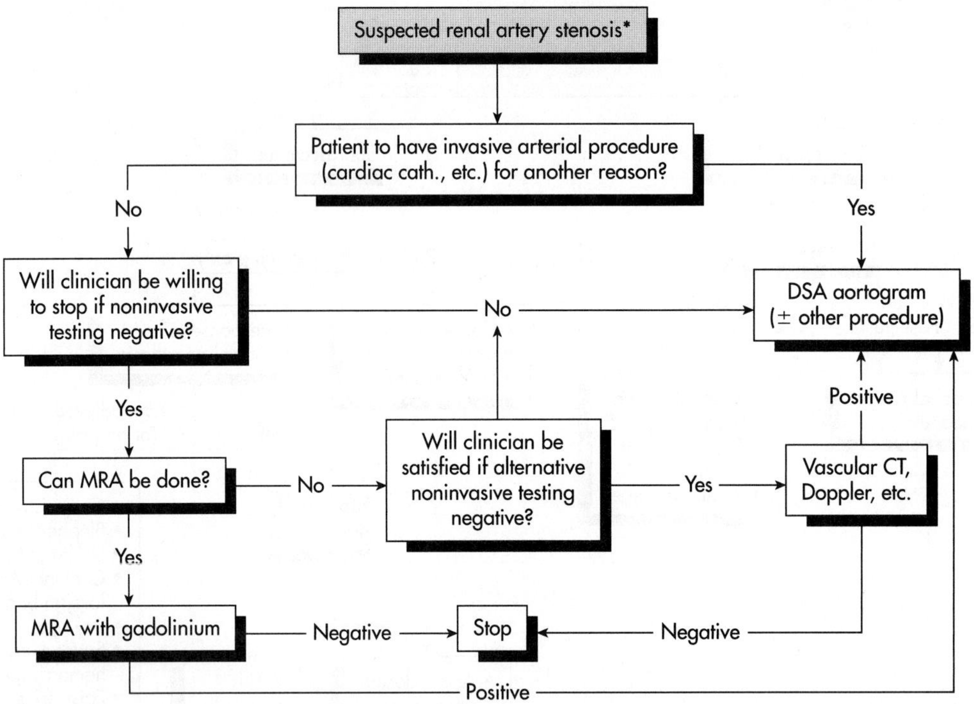

*Refer to Section I for additional information on this topic.

FIGURE 3-244 Approach to the anatomical evaluation of renal artery stenosis. Once stenosis is suspected, if the patient is to have another invasive arterial procedure, noninvasive imaging is deferred and a low-volume digital substraction aortogram (DSA) is done at the time of that procedure. In other cases, the clinician should assess whether a negative noninvasive test would be sufficient evidence to acquit the renal arteries. If so, noninvasive testing should be performed. If not, consideration should be given to DSA and selective angiography. *Cath,* Catherization; *CT,* computed tomography; *MRA,* magnetic resonance angiography. (From Zipes DP, Libby P, Bonow RO, Braunwauld E [eds]: *Braunwald's heart disease,* ed 7, Philadelphia, 2005, Elsevier.)

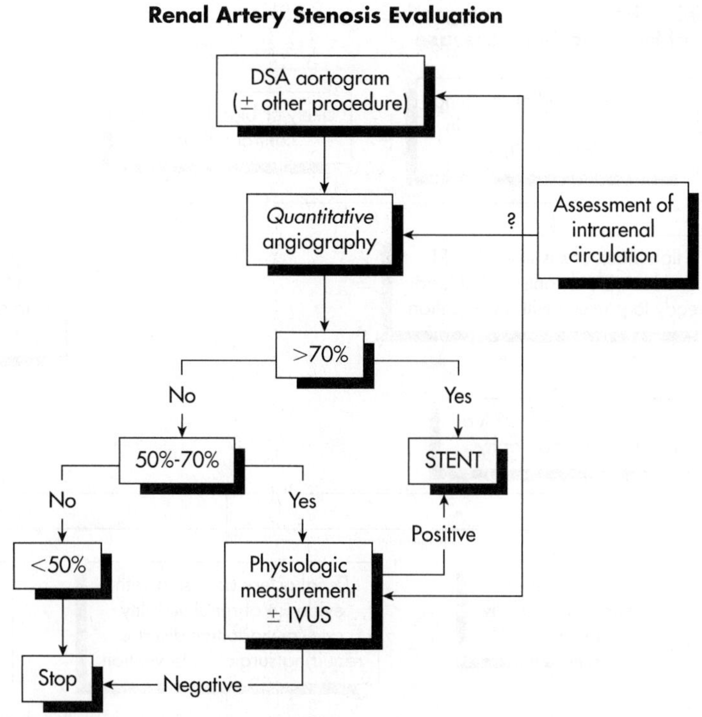

FIGURE 3-245 Approach to the angiographic evaluation and treatment of renal artery stenosis. Once a digital substraction aortogram (DSA) is performed, confirming the presence of renovascular disease, quantitative angiography and objective evaluation of the severity of stenosis should be performed. Very severe (>70% diameter stenosis) lesions are subjected to revascularization, and mild lesions (<50% diameter stenosis) are not. It is believed that the intermediate lesion should be assessed with physiological evaluation and/or an additional anatomical documentation of severity, such as intravascular ultrasound (IVUS). The absence of tranlesional flow acceleration or a pressure gradient should mitigate the desire to intervene. (From Zipes DP, Libby P, Bonow RO, Braunwauld E [eds]: *Braunwald's heart disease,* ed 7, Philadelphia, 2005, Elsevier.)

ICD-9CM # 593.81

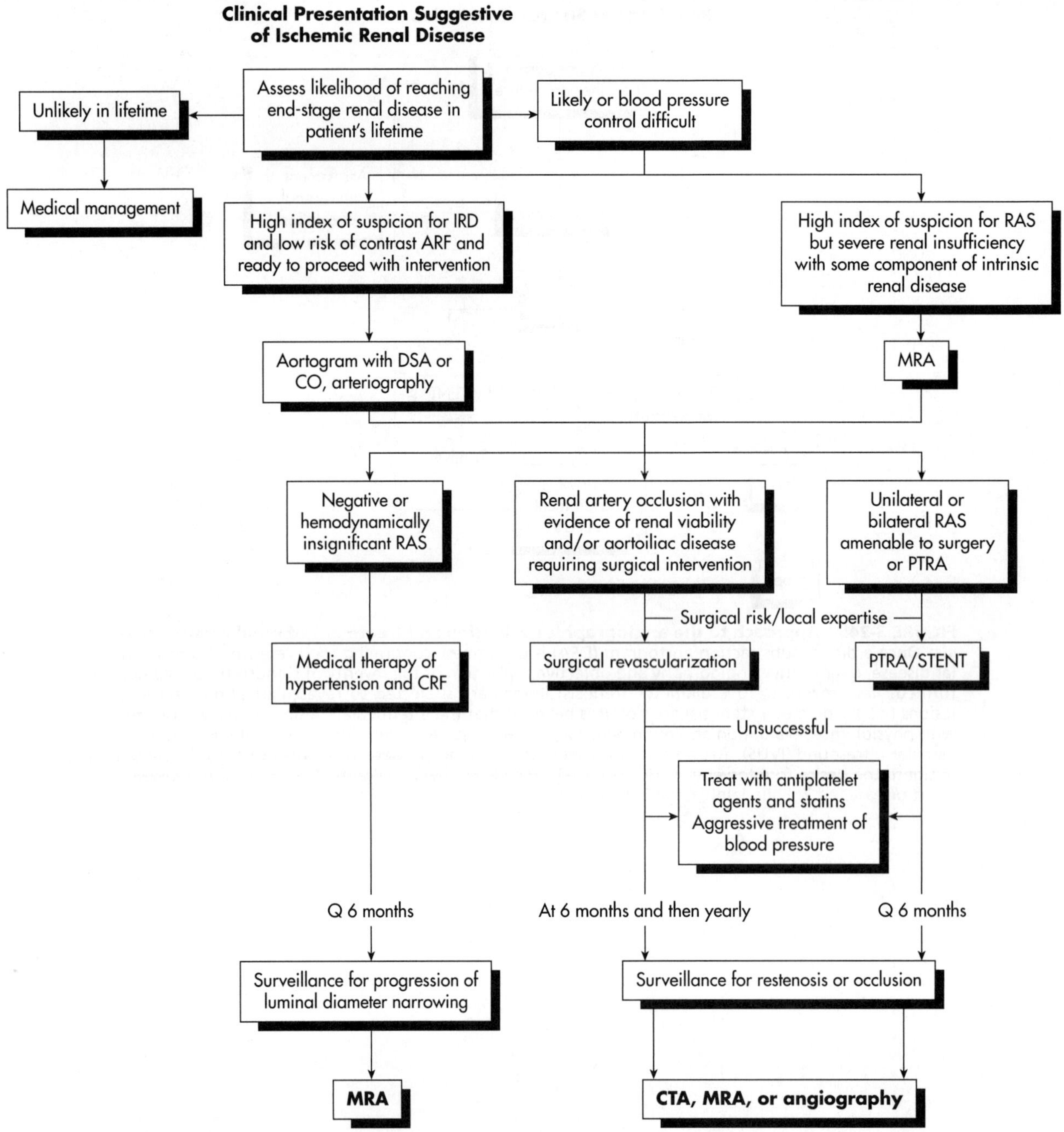

FIGURE 3-246 Clinical presentation suggestive of ischemic renal disease. *ARF,* acute renal failure; *CTA,* computed tomography angiography; *CRF,* chronic renal failure; *DSA,* digital substraction angiogram; *IRD,* ischemic renal disease; *MRA,* magnetic resonance angiography; *PTRA,* percutaneuos transluminal renal angioplasty; *RAS,* renal artery stenosis; *RDS,* respiratory distress syndrome. (Modified from Feehally J, Floege J, Johnson RJ: *Comprehensive clinical nephrology,* ed 3, St Louis, 2007, Mosby.)

ICD-9CM # 584.9 Acute renal failure, unspecified

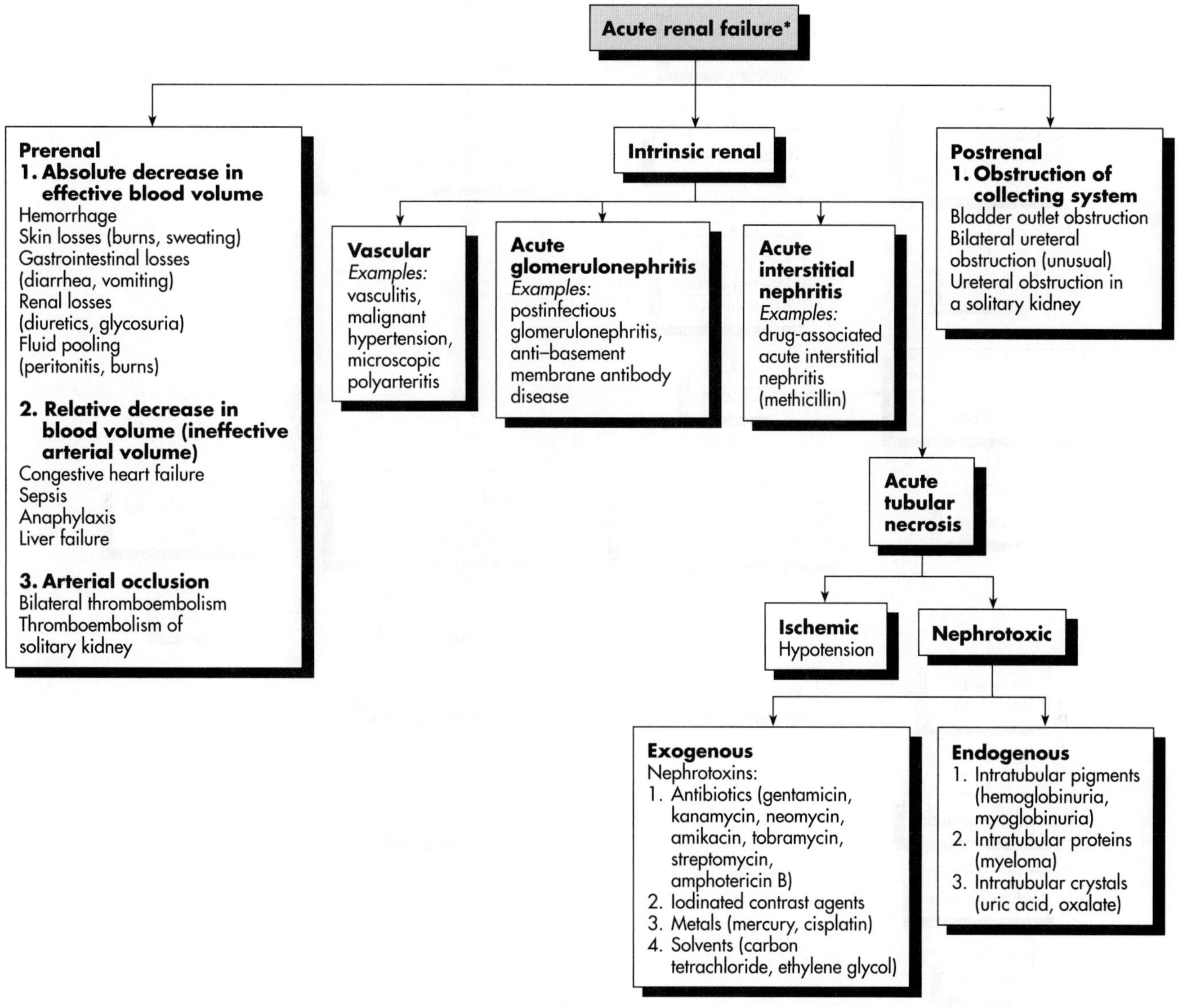

*Refer to Section I for additional information on this topic.

FIGURE 3-247 Causes of acute renal failure. (From Andreoli TE [ed]: *Cecil essentials of medicine*, ed 7, Philadelphia, 2008, WB Saunders.)

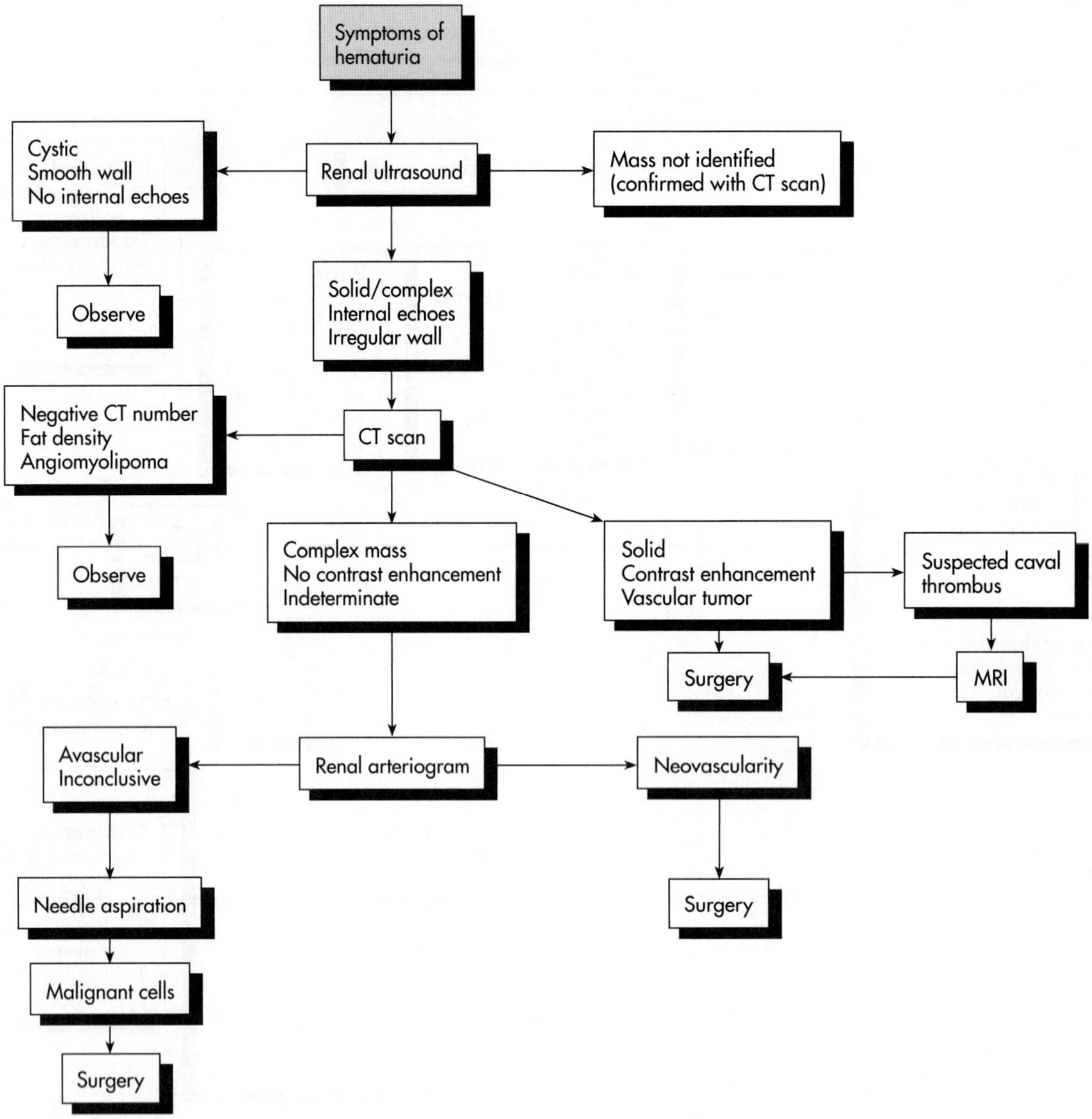

FIGURE 3-248 Evaluation of a patient with a renal mass. *CT,* Computed tomography; *MRI,* magnetic resonance imaging. (Modified from Williams RD: Tumors of the kidney, ureter, and bladder. In Goldman L, Ausiello D [eds]: *Cecil textbook of medicine,* ed 23, Philadelphia, 2008, WB Saunders.)

RESPIRATORY DISTRESS

ICD-9CM # 786.09 Respiratory distress NOS
518.82 Respiratory distress, acute

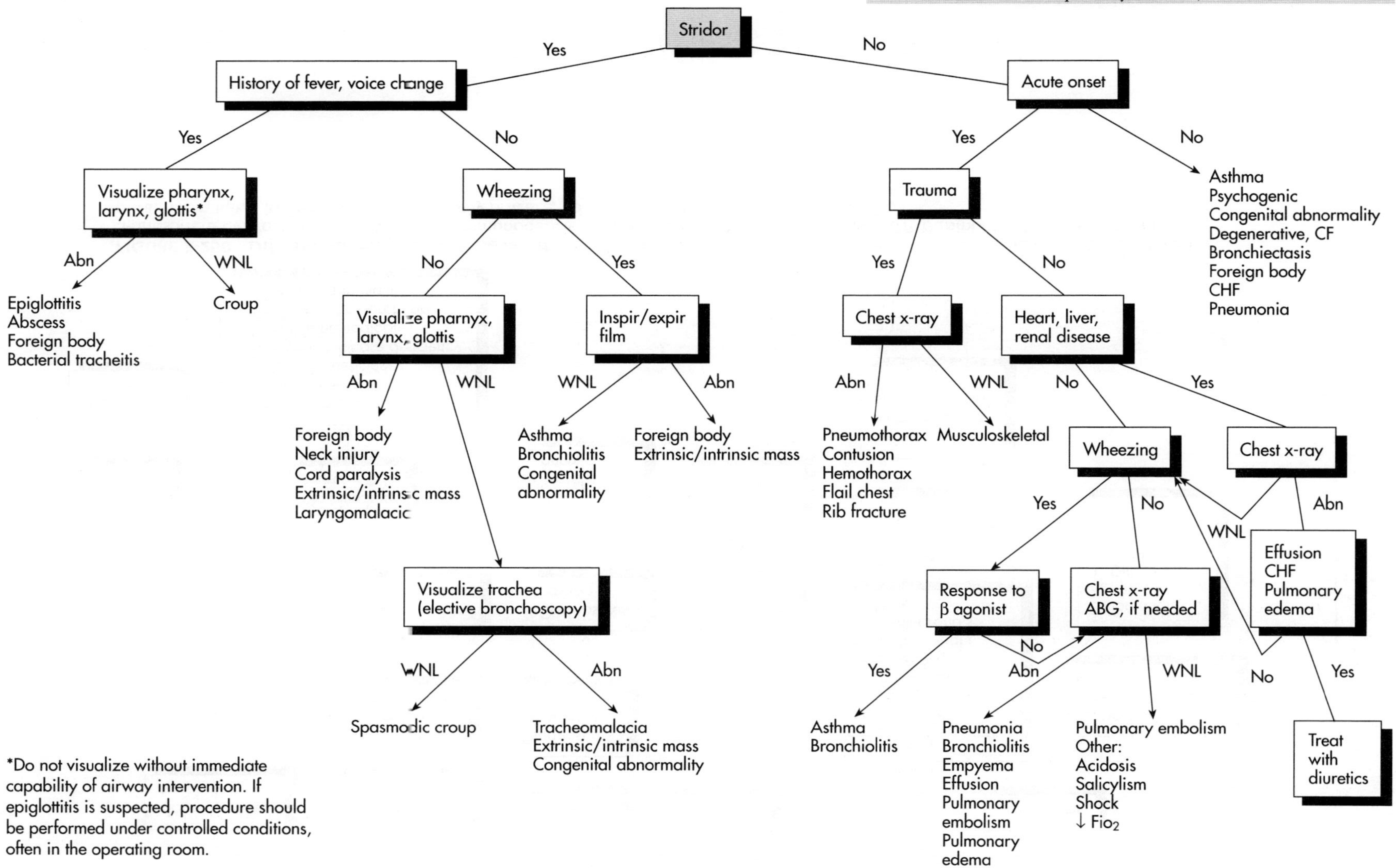

*Do not visualize without immediate capability of airway intervention. If epiglottitis is suspected, procedure should be performed under controlled conditions, often in the operating room.

FIGURE 3-249 Respiratory distress pediatric patient. *ABG,* Arterial blood gas; *Abn,* abnormal; *CF,* cystic fibrosis; *CHF,* congestive heart failure; *WNL,* within normal limits. (From Barkin RM, Rosen P: *Emergency pediatrics,* St Louis, 1999, Mosby.)

RETICULOCYTE COUNT, ELEVATED

ICD-9CM # 790.99

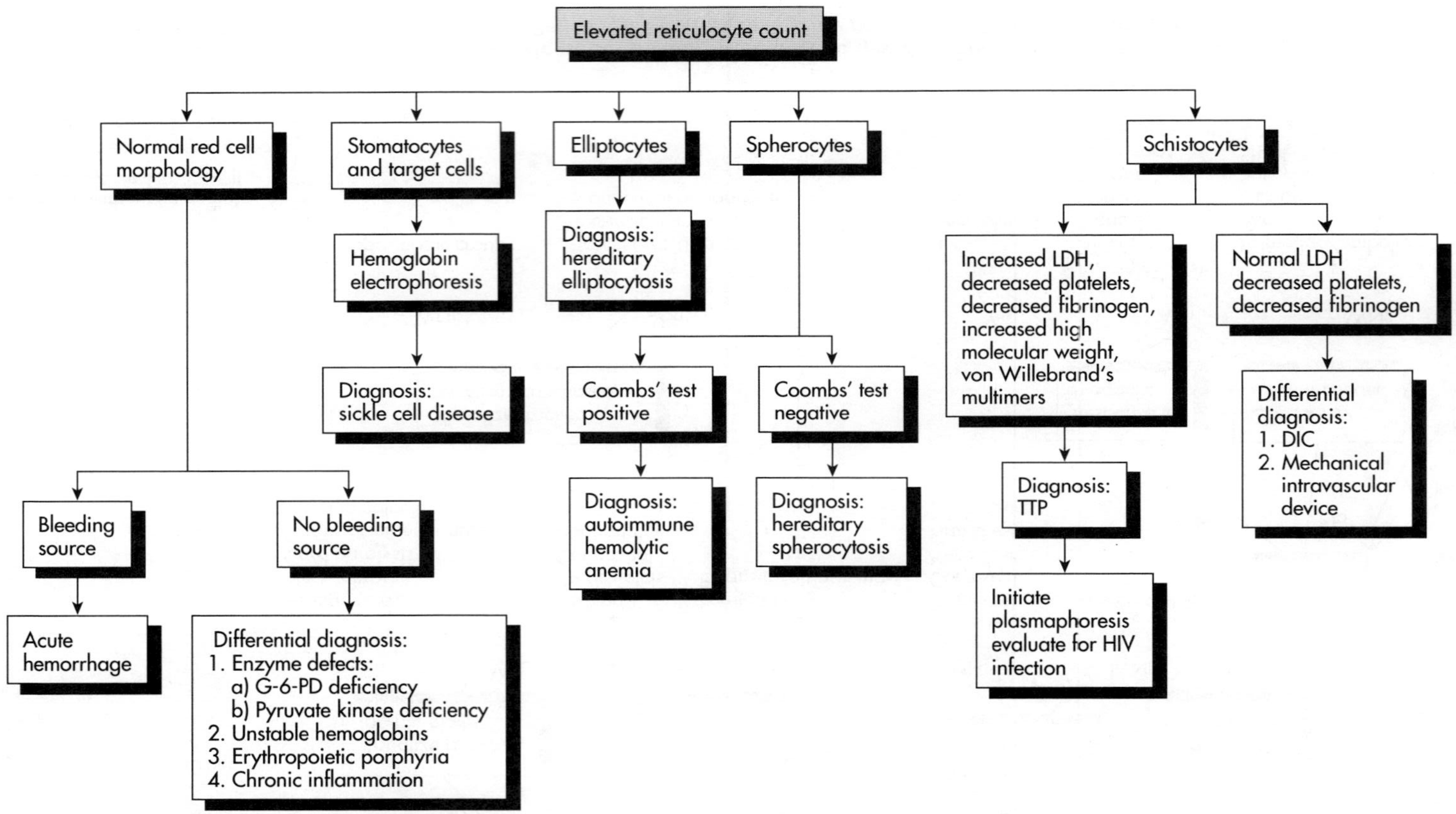

FIGURE 3-250 Differential diagnosis of elevated reticulocyte count. *DIC,* Disseminated intravascular coagulation; *G6PD,* glucose-6-phosphate dehydrogenase; *HIV,* human immunodeficiency virus; *LDH,* lactic dehydrogenase; *TTP,* thrombotic thrombocytopenic purpura. (From Rakel RE [ed]: *Principles of family practice,* ed 7, Philadelphia, 2007, WB Saunders.)

ICD-9CM # 478.1

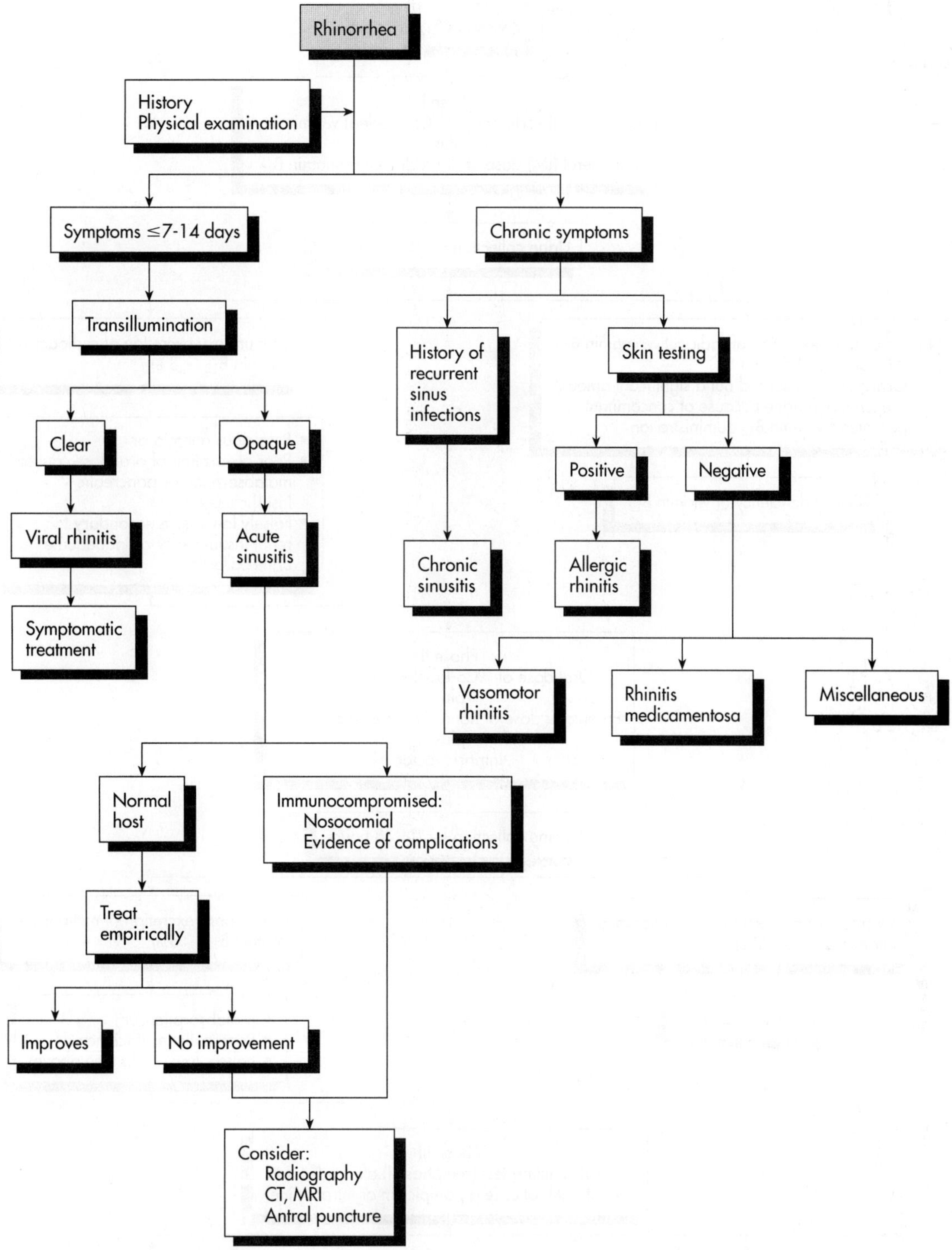

FIGURE 3-251 Approach to a patient with rhinorrhea. *CT,* Computed tomography; *MRI,* magnetic resonance imaging. (From Noble J [ed]: *Primary care medicine,* ed 3, St Louis, 2001, Mosby.)

ICD-9CM # 281.0

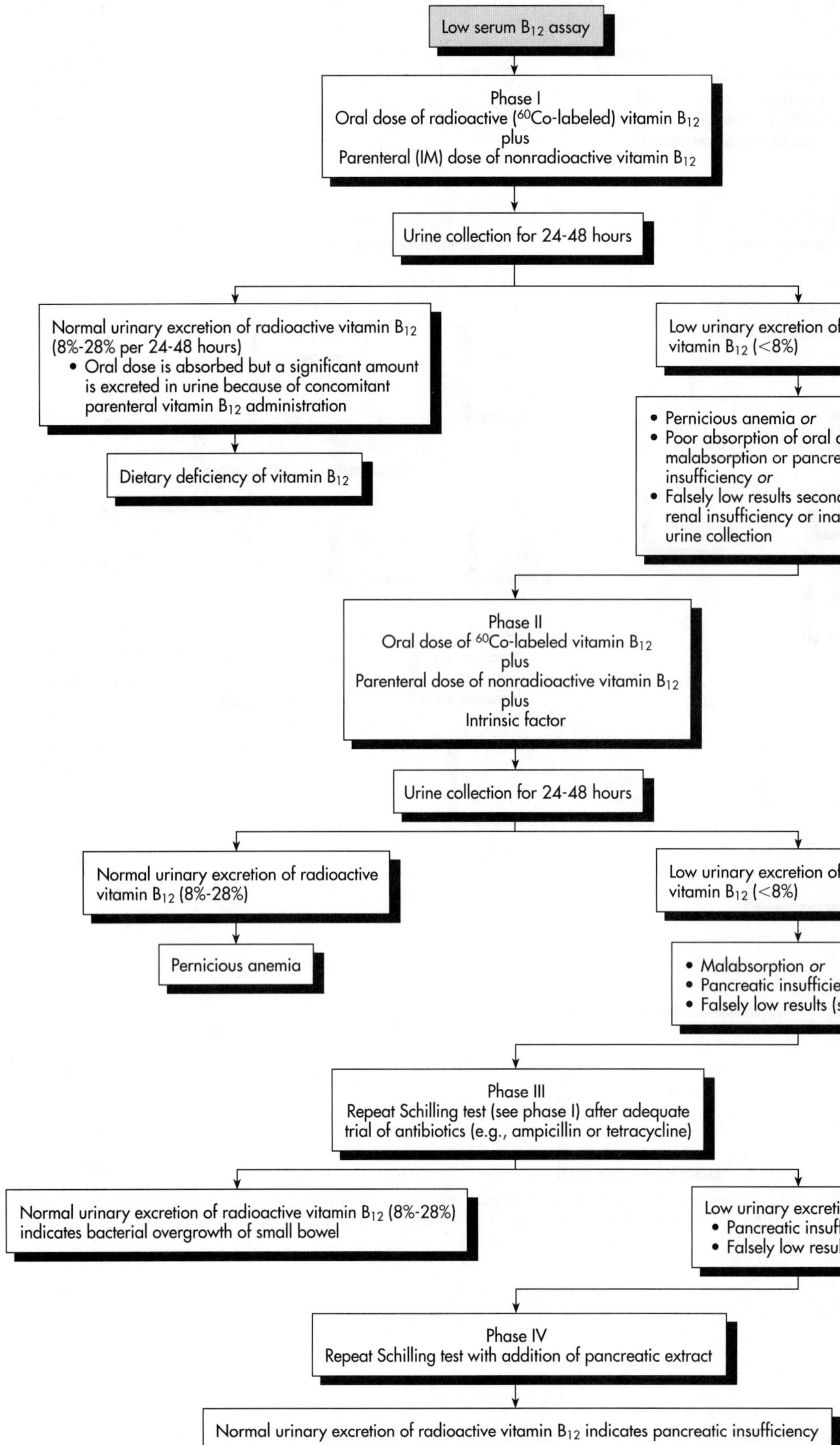

FIGURE 3-252 Schilling test. *IM,* Intramuscular. (From Ferri FF: *Practical guide to the care of the medical patient,* ed 7, St Louis, 2007, Mosby.)

ICD-9CM # 737.30 Idiopathic scoliosis
737.39 Paralytic scoliosis
754.2 Congenital scoliosis
724.3 Sciatic scoliosis
737.43 Associated with neurofibromatosis

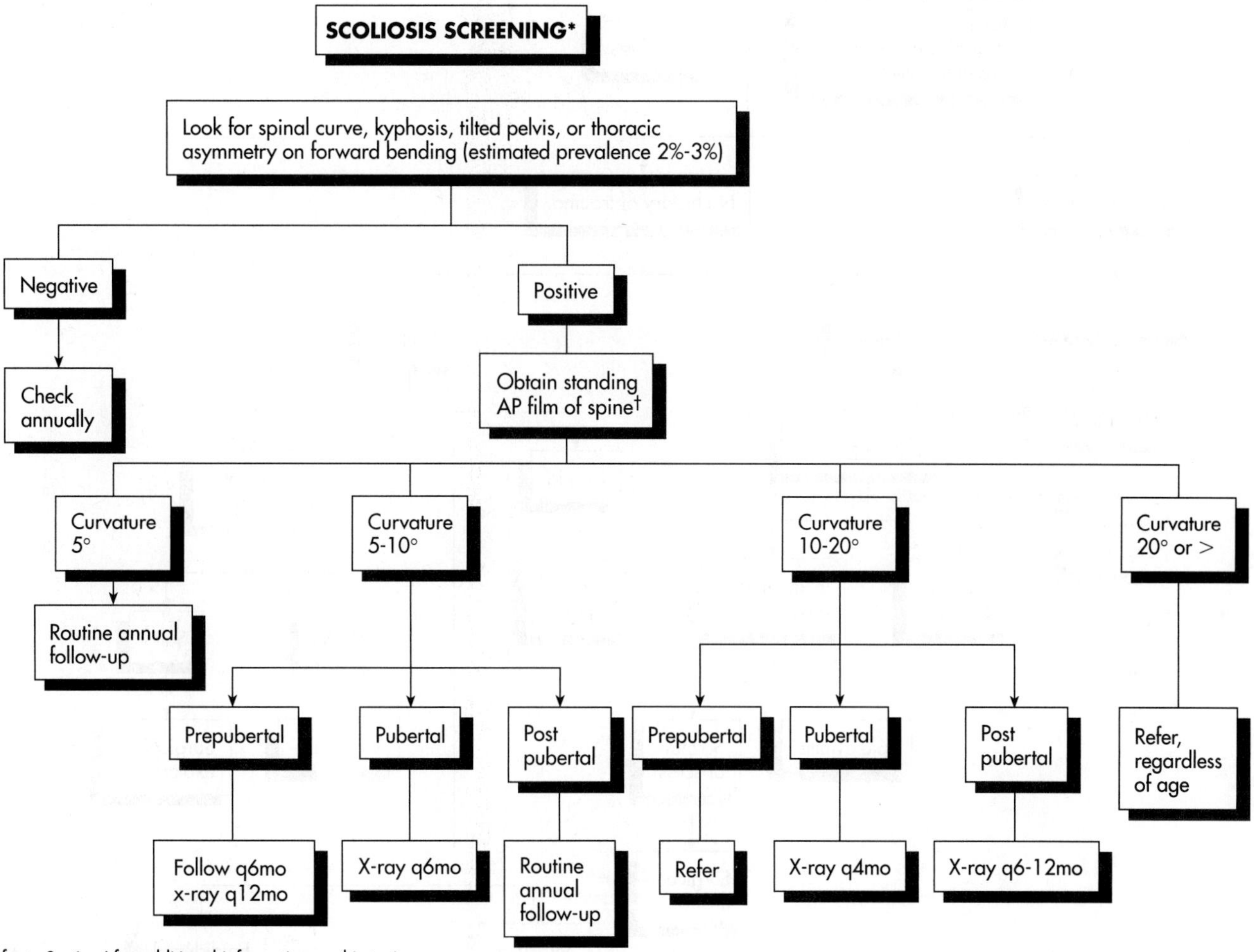

*Refer to Section I for additional information on this topic.
†Cobb method of angle measurement

1. Find the lowest vertebra whose bottom tilts toward concavity of curve.
2. Erect a perpendicular line from extension of bottom surface.
3. Find highest vertebra as in #1 and erect perpendicular from extension of top surface.
4. Measure intersecting angle = angle of scoliosis.

FIGURE 3-253 Scoliosis screening and follow-up. *AP,* Anteroposterior. (From Driscoll C [ed]: *The family practice desk reference,* ed 3, St Louis, 1996, Mosby.)

ICD-9CM # 608.89

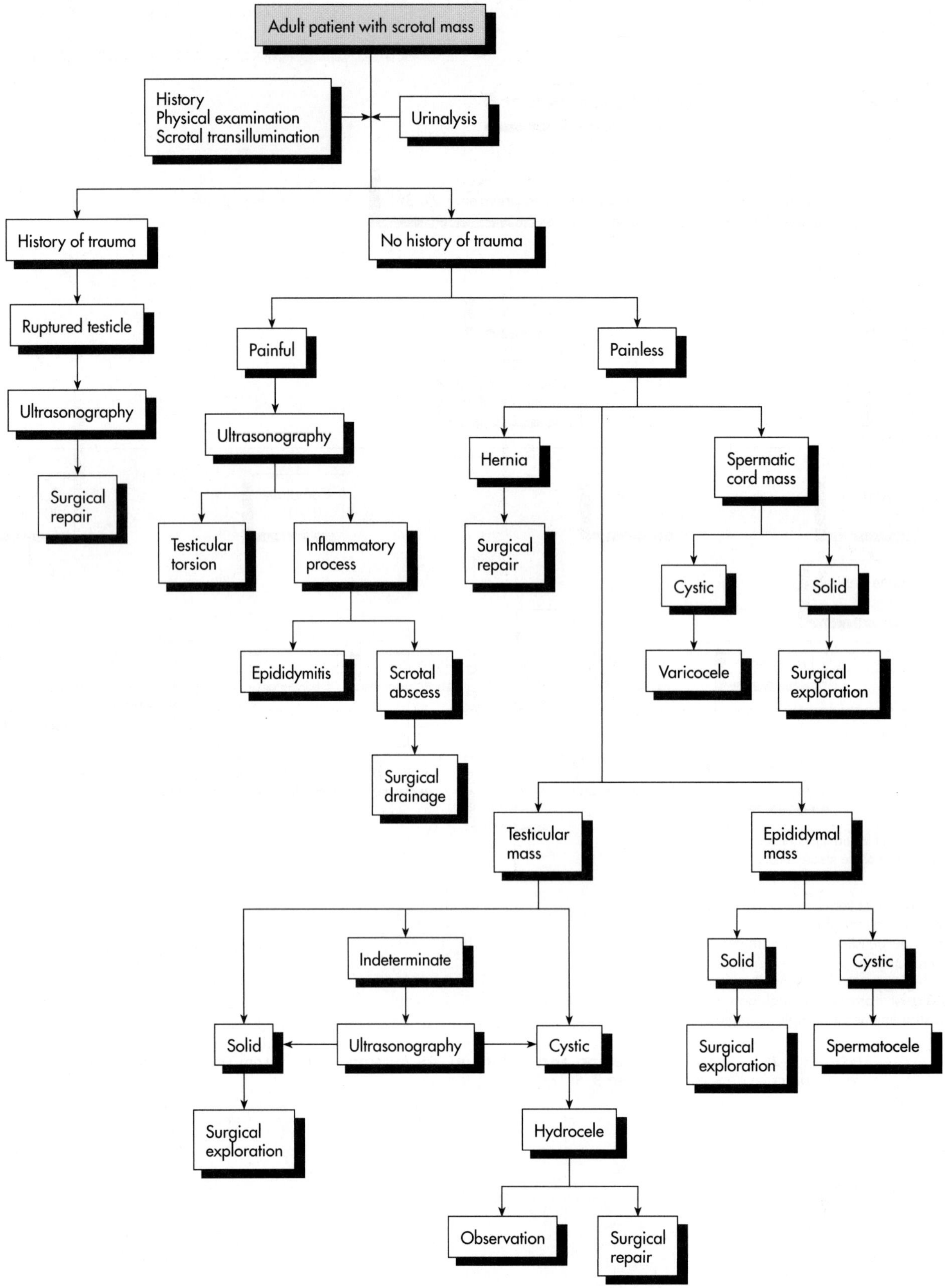

FIGURE 3-254 Evaluation of scrotal mass. (From Greene HL, Johnson WP, Lemcke D [eds]: *Decision making in medicine*, ed 2, St Louis, 1998, Mosby.)

ICD-9CM # 038.9

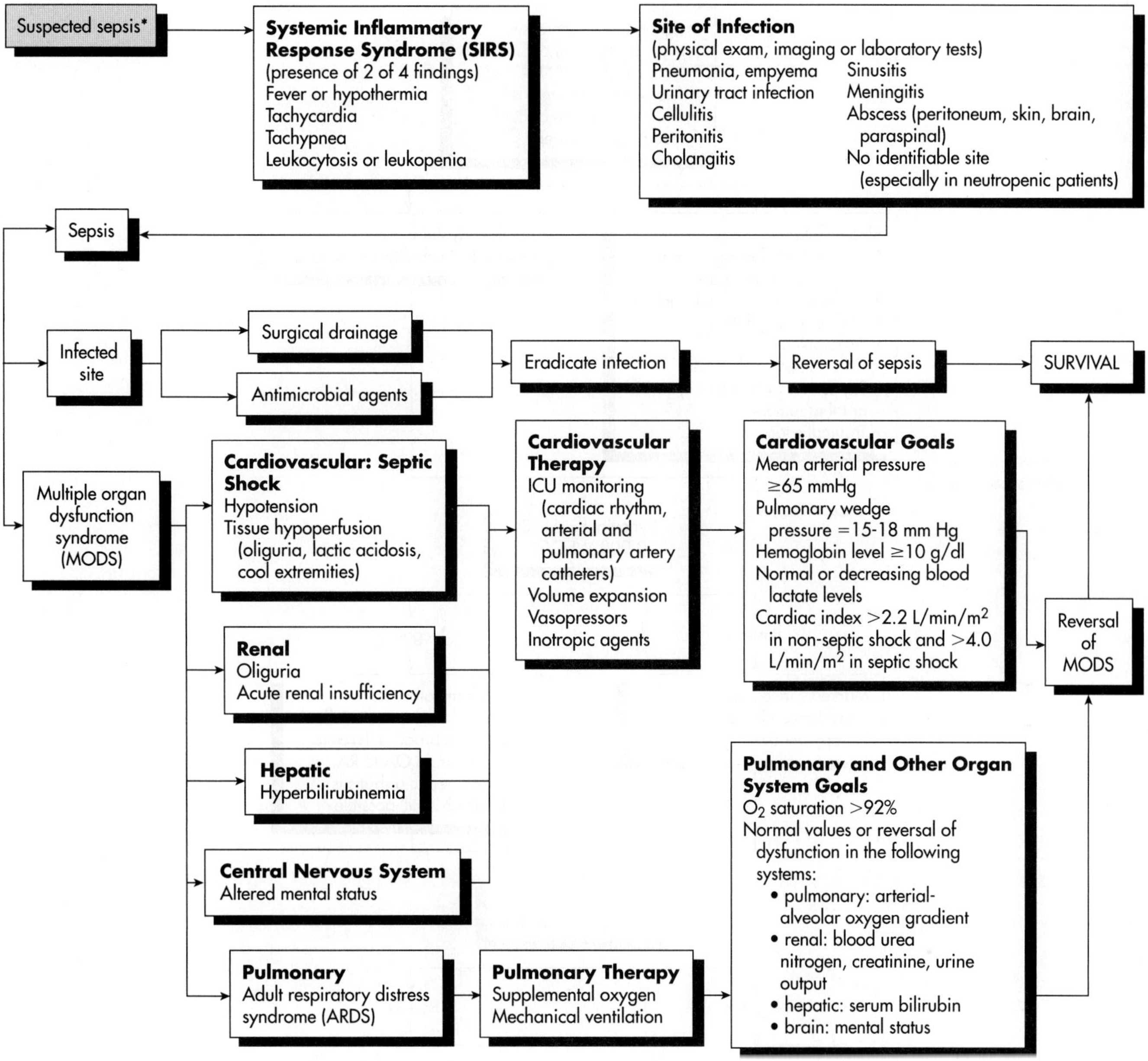

*Refer to Section I for additional information on this topic.

FIGURE 3-255 Diagnostic evaluation and management of sepsis and septic shock. (From Goldman L, Ausiello D [eds]: *Cecil textbook of medicine*, ed 23, Philadelphia, 2008, WB Saunders.)

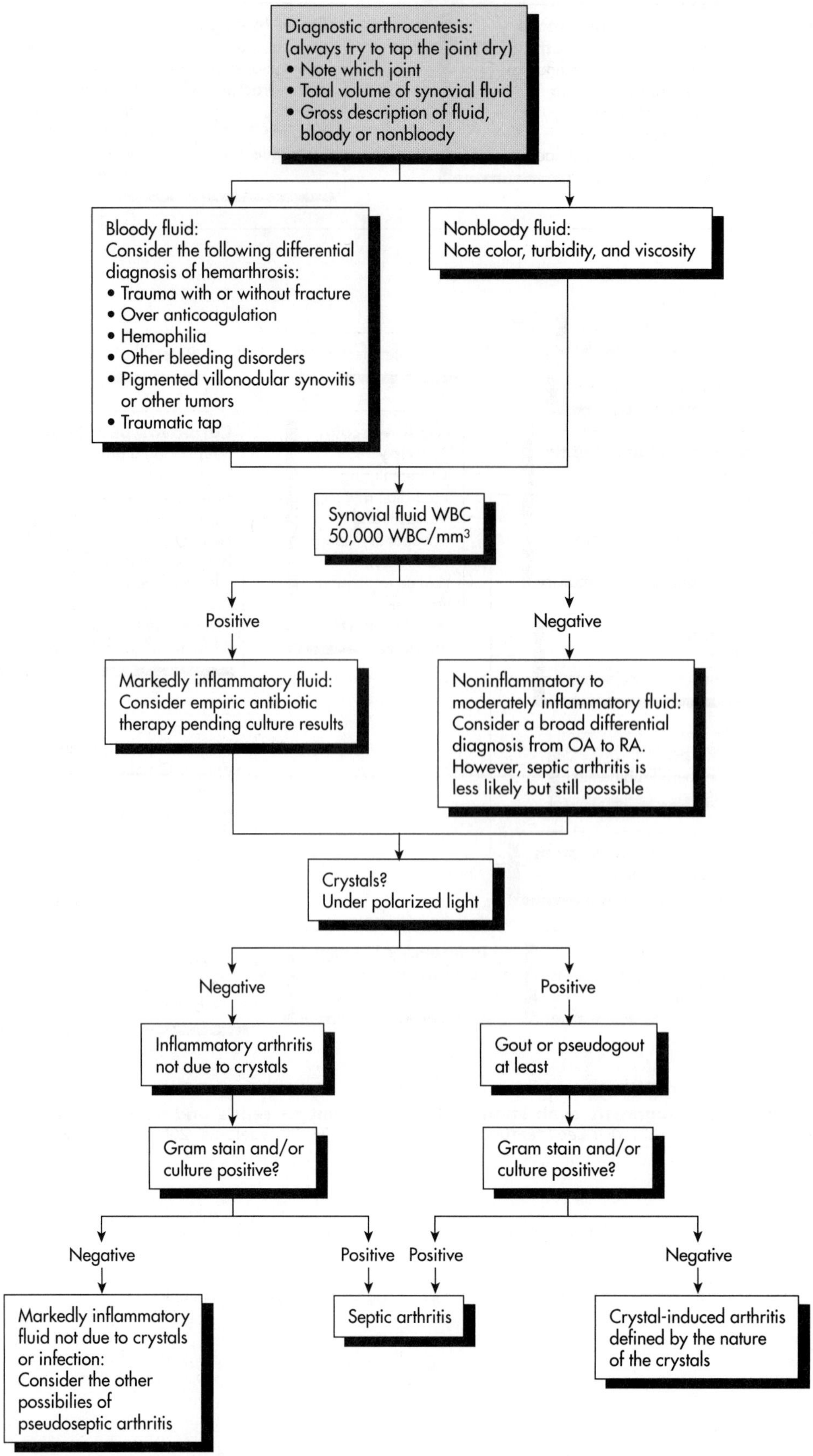

FIGURE 3-256 Algorithm for synovial fluid analysis in septic arthritis. *OA,* Osteoarthritis; *RA,* rheumatoid arthritis. (From Harris ED, Budd RC, Firestein GS, Genovese MC, Sergent JS, Ruddy S, Sledge CB [eds]: *Kelley's textbook of rheumatology,* ed 7, Philadelphia, 2005, Saunders.)

SEXUAL DYSFUNCTION

ICD-9CM # 309.2 Sexual disorder (psychosexual)
V41.7 Sexual function problem

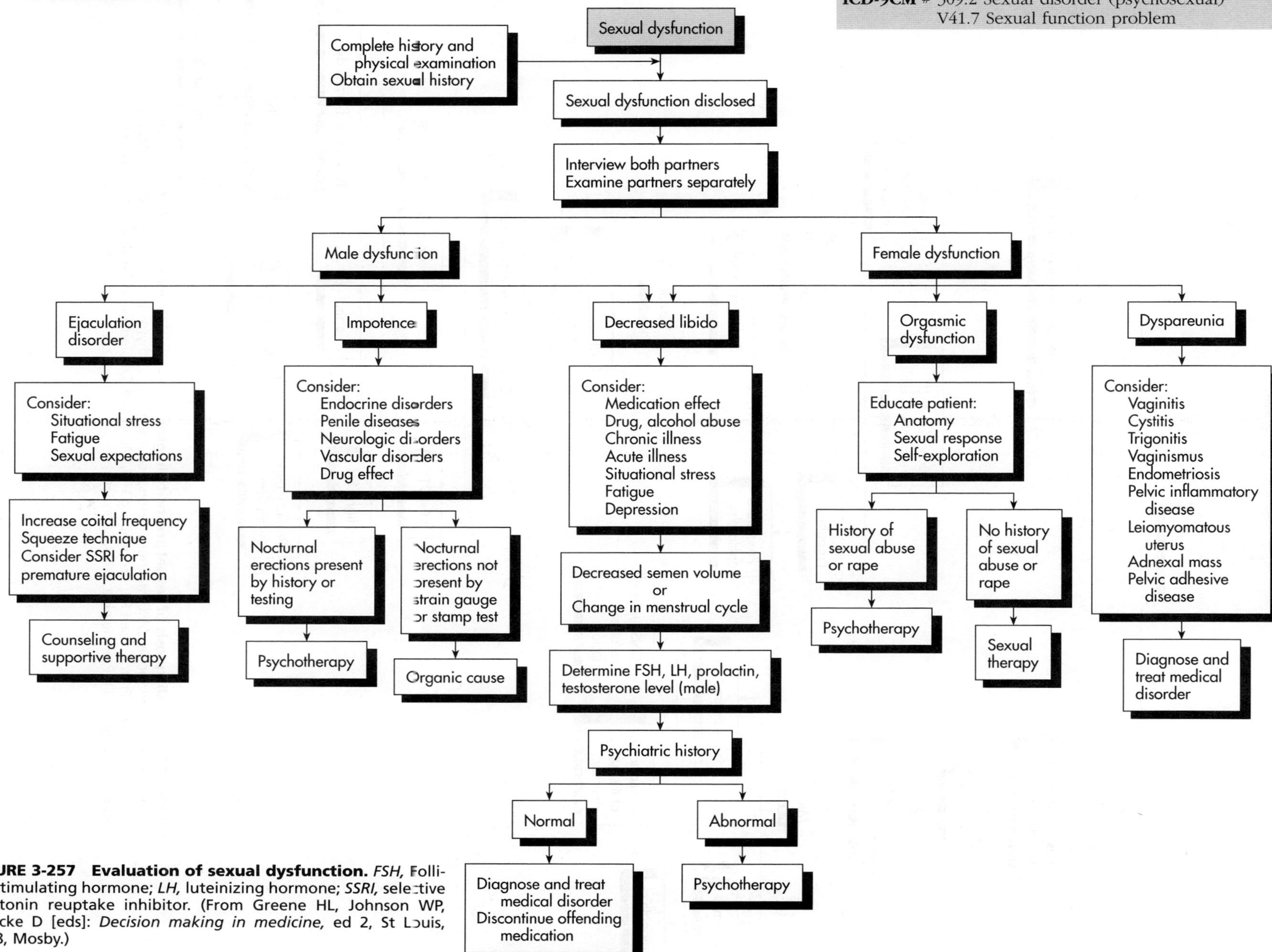

FIGURE 3-257 Evaluation of sexual dysfunction. *FSH,* Follicle-stimulating hormone; *LH,* luteinizing hormone; *SSRI,* selective serotonin reuptake inhibitor. (From Greene HL, Johnson WP, Lemcke D [eds]: *Decision making in medicine,* ed 2, St Louis, 1998, Mosby.)

ICD-9CM # 259.1

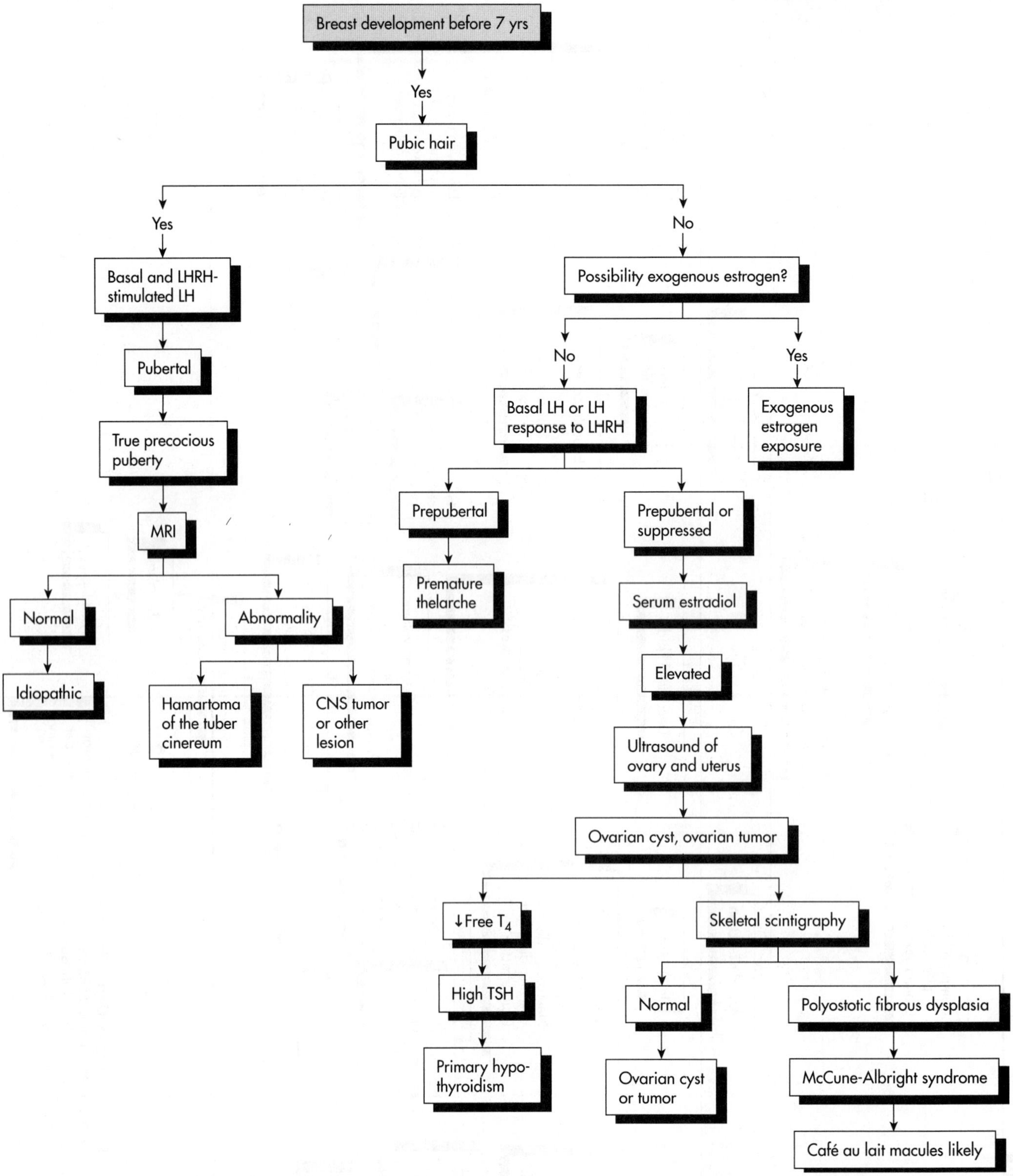
Breast development before 7 yrs
Yes
Pubic hair
Yes
No
Basal and LHRH-stimulated LH
Pubertal
True precocious puberty
MRI
Normal
Idiopathic
Abnormality
Hamartoma of the tuber cinereum
CNS tumor or other lesion
Possibility exogenous estrogen?
No
Yes
Exogenous estrogen exposure
Basal LH or LH response to LHRH
Prepubertal
Premature thelarche
Prepubertal or suppressed
Serum estradiol
Elevated
Ultrasound of ovary and uterus
Ovarian cyst, ovarian tumor
↓Free T_4
High TSH
Primary hypothyroidism
Skeletal scintigraphy
Normal
Ovarian cyst or tumor
Polyostotic fibrous dysplasia
McCune-Albright syndrome
Café au lait macules likely

FIGURE 3-258 The diagnosis of sexual precocity in girls. *LH,* Luteinizing hormone; *LHRH,* luteinizing hormone-releasing hormone; *MRI,* magnetic resonance imaging; *T_4,* thyroxine; *TSH,* thyroid-stimulating hormone; *yrs,* years. (From Larsen PR, Kronenberg HM, Memlmed S, Polansky, KS [eds]: *Williams textbook of endocrinology,* ed 11, Philadelphia, 2008, Saunders.)

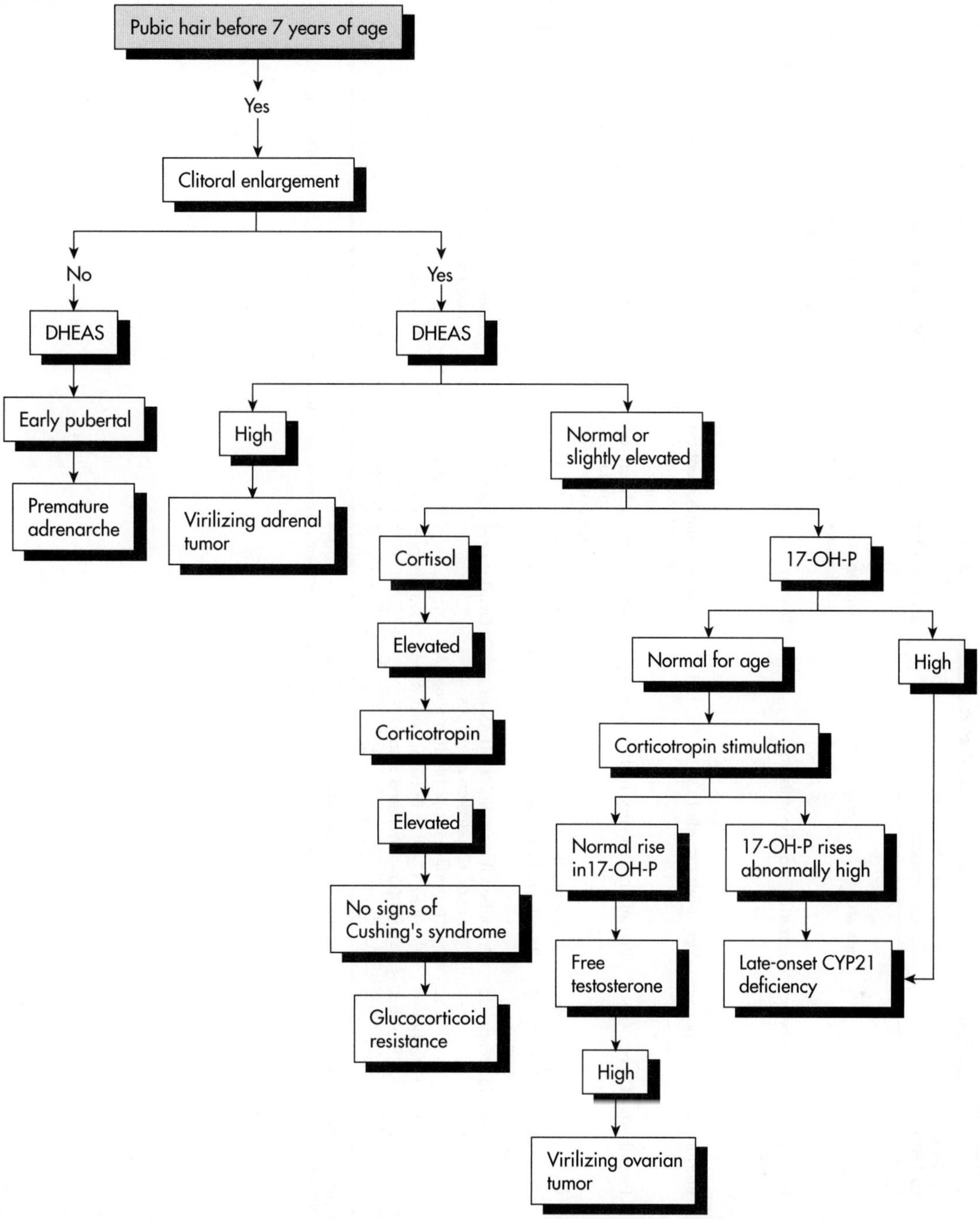
Pubic hair before 7 years of age
Yes
Clitoral enlargement
No
Yes
DHEAS
DHEAS
Early pubertal
Premature adrenarche
High
Virilizing adrenal tumor
Normal or slightly elevated
Cortisol
Elevated
Corticotropin
Elevated
No signs of Cushing's syndrome
Glucocorticoid resistance
17-OH-P
Normal for age
High
Corticotropin stimulation
Normal rise in17-OH-P
17-OH-P rises abnormally high
Free testosterone
High
Virilizing ovarian tumor
Late-onset CYP21 deficiency

FIGURE 3-259 The evaluation of pubic hair in normal phenotypic girls before 7 years. *DHEA,* Dehydroepiandrosterone; *17-OH-P,* 17-hydroxy progesterone. (From Larsen PR, Kronenberg HM, Memlmed S, Polansky, KS [eds]: *Williams textbook of endocrinology,* ed 11, Philadelphia, 2008, Saunders.)

Continued on following page

SEXUAL PRECOCITY, FEMALE PUBIC HAIR DEVELOPMENT—cont'd

TABLE 3-19 **Differential Diagnosis of Sexual Precocity**

	Plasma Gonadotropins	LH Response to LHRH	Serum Sex Steroid Concentration	Gonadal Size	Miscellaneous
In Both Sexes					
McCune-Albright syndrome	Suppressed	Suppressed	Sex steroids pubertal or higher	Ovarian (on ultrasound); slight testicular enlargement	Skeletal survey for polyostotic fibrous dysplasia and skin examination for café au lait spots
Primary hypothyroidism	LH prepubertal; FSH may be slightly elevated	Prepubertal FSH may be increased	Estradiol may be pubertal	Testicular enlargement; ovaries cystic	TSH and prolactin elevated; T_4 low
Females					
Granulosa cell tumor (follicular cysts may present similarly)	Suppressed	Prepubertal LH response	Very high estradiol	Ovarian enlargement on physical examination, CT, or ultrasonography	Tumor often palpable on abdominal examination
Follicular cyst	Suppressed	Prepubertal LH response	Prepubertal to very high estradiol	Ovarian enlargement on physical examination, CT, or ultrasonography	Single or recurrent episodes of menses and/or breast development; exclude McCune-Albright syndrome
Feminizing adrenal tumor	Suppressed	Prepubertal LH response	High estradiol and DHEAS values	Ovaries prepubertal	Unilateral adrenal mass
Premature thelarche	Prepubertal	Prepubertal LH, pubertal estradiol response	Prepubertal or early	Ovaries prepubertal	Onset usually before 3 years of age
Premature adrenarche	Prepubertal	Prepubertal LH response	Prepubertal estradiol; DHEAS or urinary 17-ketosteroid values appropriate for pubic hair stage 2	Ovaries prepubertal	Onset usually after 6 years of age; more frequent in brain-injured children
Late-onset virilizing congenital adrenal hyperplasia	Prepubertal	Prepubertal LH response	Elevated 17-OHP in basal or corticotropin-stimulated state	Ovaries prepubertal	Autosomal recessive

From Larson PR, Kronenberg HM, Memlmed S, Polansky, KS [eds]: *Williams textbook of endocrinology,* ed 11, Philadelphia, 2008, Saunders.
CNS, Central nervous system; *CT,* computed tomography; *DHEAS,* dehydroepiandrosterone sulfate; *hCG,* human chorionic gonadotropin; *LH,* luteinizing hormone; *MRI,* magnetic resonance imaging; *17-OHP,* 17-hydroxyprogesterone; T_4, thyroxine; *TSH,* thyrotropin.

SEXUAL PRECOCITY, MALE

ICD-9CM # 259.1

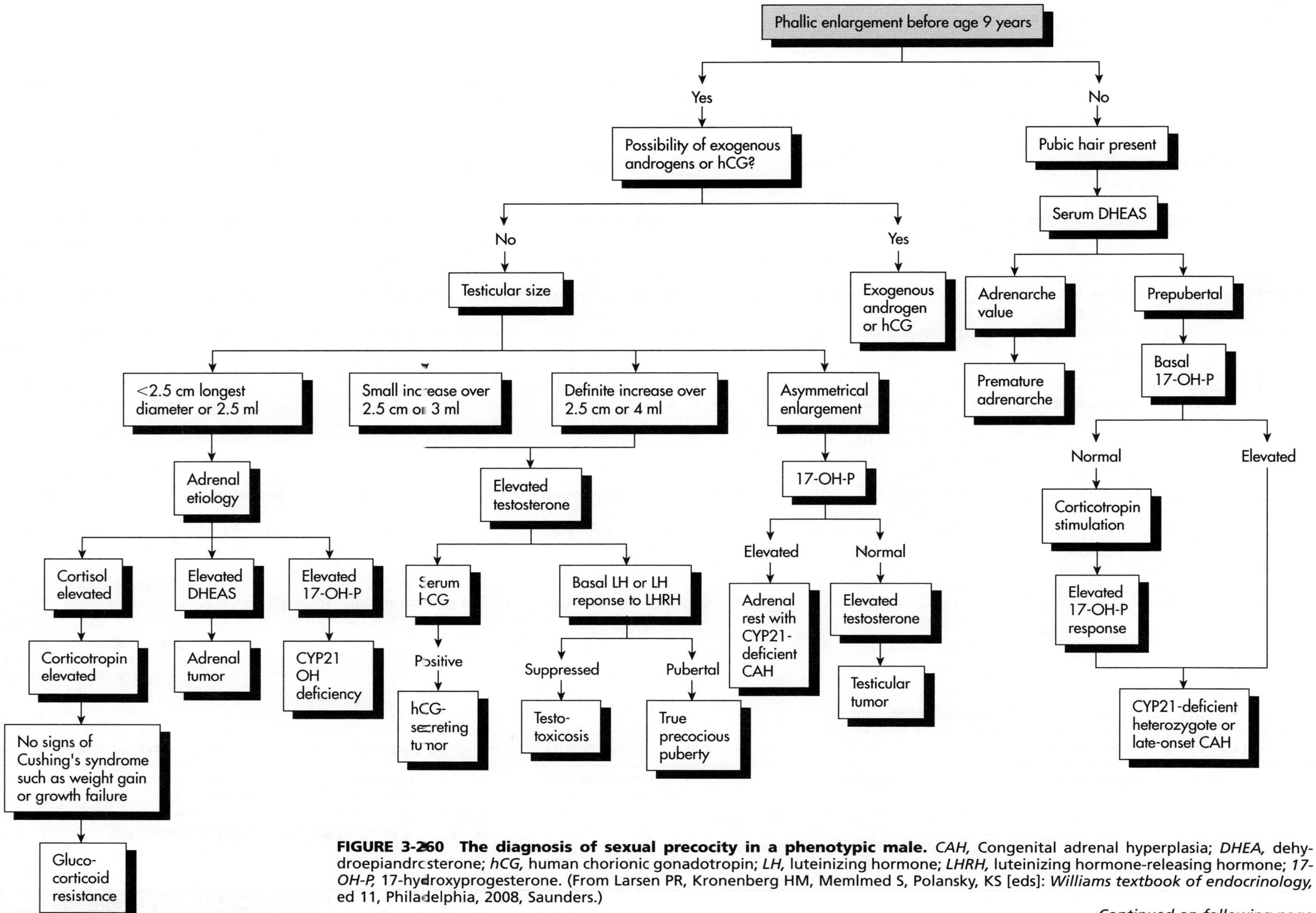

FIGURE 3-260 The diagnosis of sexual precocity in a phenotypic male. *CAH,* Congenital adrenal hyperplasia; *DHEA,* dehydroepiandrosterone; *hCG,* human chorionic gonadotropin; *LH,* luteinizing hormone; *LHRH,* luteinizing hormone-releasing hormone; *17-OH-P,* 17-hydroxyprogesterone. (From Larsen PR, Kronenberg HM, Memlmed S, Polansky, KS [eds]: *Williams textbook of endocrinology,* ed 11, Philadelphia, 2008, Saunders.)

Continued on following page

SEXUAL PRECOCITY MALE—cont'd

TABLE 3-20 Differential Diagnosis of Sexual Precocity

	Plasma Gonadotropins	LH Response to LHRH	Serum Sex Steroid Concentration	Gonadal Size	Miscellaneous
True Precocious Puberty (premature reactivation of LHRH pulse generator)	Prominent LH pulses, initially during sleep	Pubertal LH response	Pubertal values of testosterone or estradiol	Normal pubertal testicular enlargement or ovarian and uterine enlargement (by ultrasonography)	MRI of brain to rule out CNS tumor or other abnormality; skeletal survey for McCune-Albright syndrome
Incomplete Sexual Precocity (pituitary gonadotropin-independent)					
Males					
Chorionic gonadotropin-secreting tumor in males	High hCG, low LH	Prepubertal LH response	Pubertal value of testosterone	Slight to moderate uniform enlargement of testes	Hepatomegaly suggests hepatoblastoma; CT scan of brain if chorionic gonadotropin-secreting CNS tumor suspected
Leydig cell tumor in males	Suppressed	No LH response	Very high testosterone	Irregular assymmetrical enlargement of testes	
Familial testotoxicosis	Suppressed	No LH response	Pubertal values of testosterone	Testes symmetrical and larger than 2.5 cm but smaller than expected for pubertal development; spermatogenesis occurs	Familial; probably sex-limited, autosomal dominant trait
Virilizing congenital adrenal hyperplasia	Prepubertal	Prepubertal LH response	Elevated 17-OHP in CYP21 deficiency or elevated 11-deoxycortisol in CYP11B1 deficiency	Testes prepubertal	Autosomal recessive, may be congenital or late-onset form, may have salt loss in CYP21 deficiency or hypertension in CYP11B1 deficiency
Virilizing adrenal tumor	Prepubertal	Prepubertal LH response	High DHEAS and androstenedione values	Testes prepubertal	CT, MRI, or ultrasonography of abdomen
Premature adrenarche	Prepubertal	Prepubertal LH response	Prepubertal testosterone, DHEAS, or urinary 17-ketosteroid values appropriate for pubic hair stage 2	Testes prepubertal	Onset usually after 6 years of age; more frequent in CNS-injured children
In Both Sexes					
McCune-Albright syndrome	Suppressed	Suppressed	Sex steroids pubertal or higher	Ovarian (on ultrasound); slight testicular enlargement	Skeletal survey for polyostotic fibrous dysplasia and skin examination for café au lait spots
Primary hypothyroidism	LH prepubertal; FSH may be slightly elevated	Prepubertal FSH may be increased	Estradiol may be pubertal	Testicular enlargement; ovaries cystic	TSH and prolactin elevated; T_4 low

From Larson PR, Kronenberg HM, Memlmed S, Polansky, KS [eds]: *Williams textbook of endocrinology,* ed 11, Philadelphia, 2008, Saunders.

CNS, Central nervous system; *CT,* computed tomography; *DHEAS,* dehydroepiandrosterone sulfate; *hCG,* human chorionic gonadotropin; *LH,* luteinizing hormone; *MRI,* magnetic resonance imaging; *17-OHP,* 17-hydroxyprogesterone; T_4, thyroxine; *TSH,* thyrotropin.

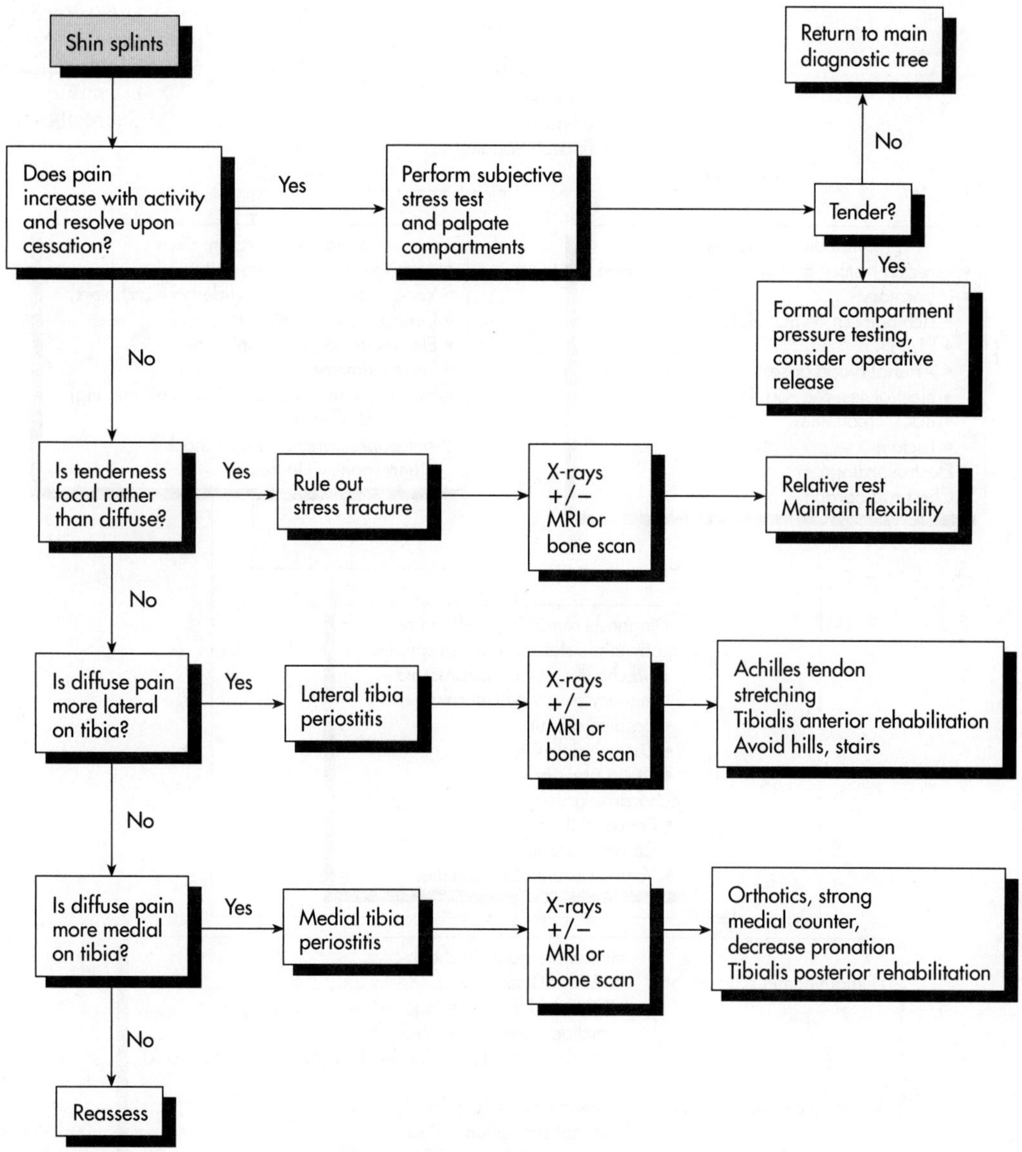

FIGURE 3-261 Evaluation and management of shin splints. *MRI,* Magnetic resonance imaging. (Modified from Scudieri G [ed]: *Sports medicine, principles of primary care,* St Louis, 1997, Mosby.)

ICD-9CM # 785.50 Shock NOS
995.0 Shock anaphylactic
785.51 Shock cardiogenic
785.59 Shock septic
958.4 Shock traumatic
977.9 Shock due to drug, medicine incorrectly administered

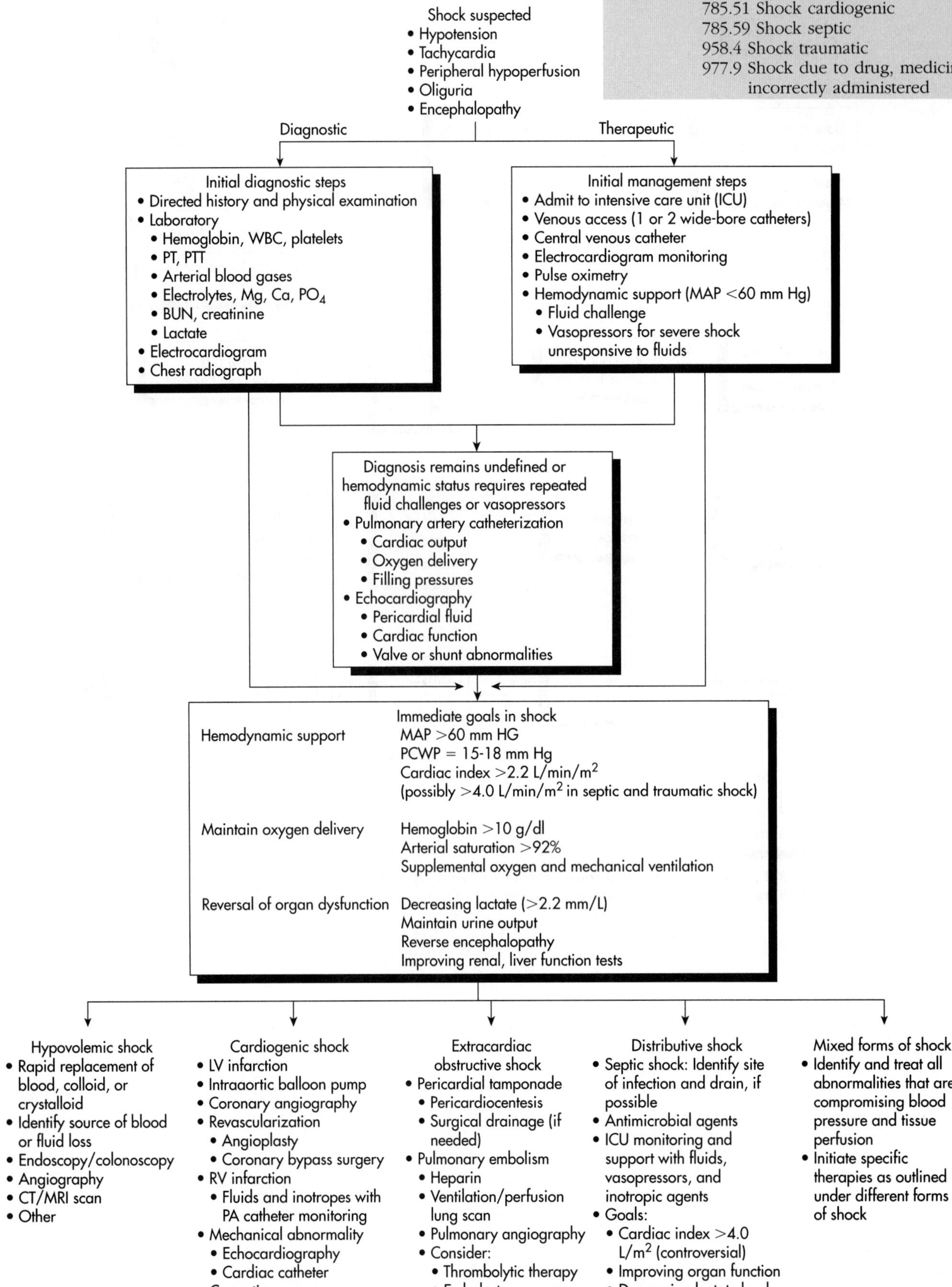

FIGURE 3-262 An approach to the diagnosis and treatment of shock. *BUN,* Blood urea nitrogen; *CT,* computed tomography; *LV,* left ventricular; *MAP,* mean arterial pressure; *MRI,* magnetic resonance imaging; *PA,* pulmonary arterial; *PCWP,* pulmonary capillary wedge pressure, *PT,* prothrombin time; *PTT,* partial thromboplastin time; *RV,* right ventricular; *WBC,* white blood cell count. (From Goldman L, Ausiello D [eds]: *Cecil textbook of medicine,* ed 23, Philadelphia, 2008, WB Saunders.)

SHOULDER PAIN

ICD-9CM # variable with specific disorder

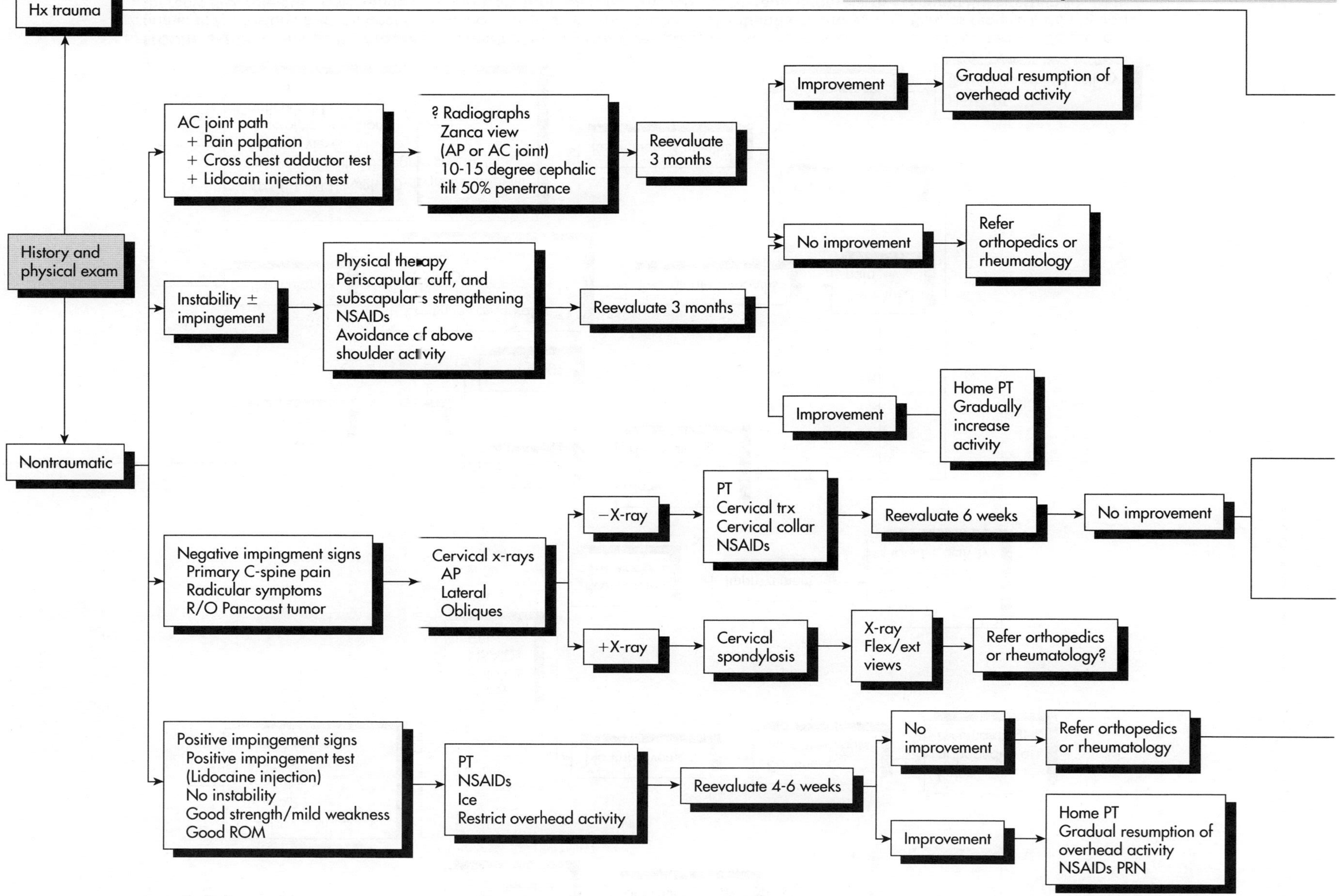

FIGURE 3-263 Algorithmic evaluation of shoulder pain. *AC,* Acromioclavicular; *AP,* anteroposterior; *GH,* glenohumeral; *Hx,* history; *MRI,* magnetic resonance imaging; *NSAID,* nonsteroidal anti-inflammatory drug; *PRN,* as required; *PT,* physical therapy; *R/O,* rule out; *ROM,* range of motion; *Sx,* symptoms; *trx,* traction; *Tx,* therapy. (From Harris ED, Budd RC, Firestein GS, Genovese MC, Sergent JS, Ruddy S, Sledge CB [eds]: *Kelley's textbook of rheumatology,* ed 7, Philadelphia, Saunders.)

Continued on following page

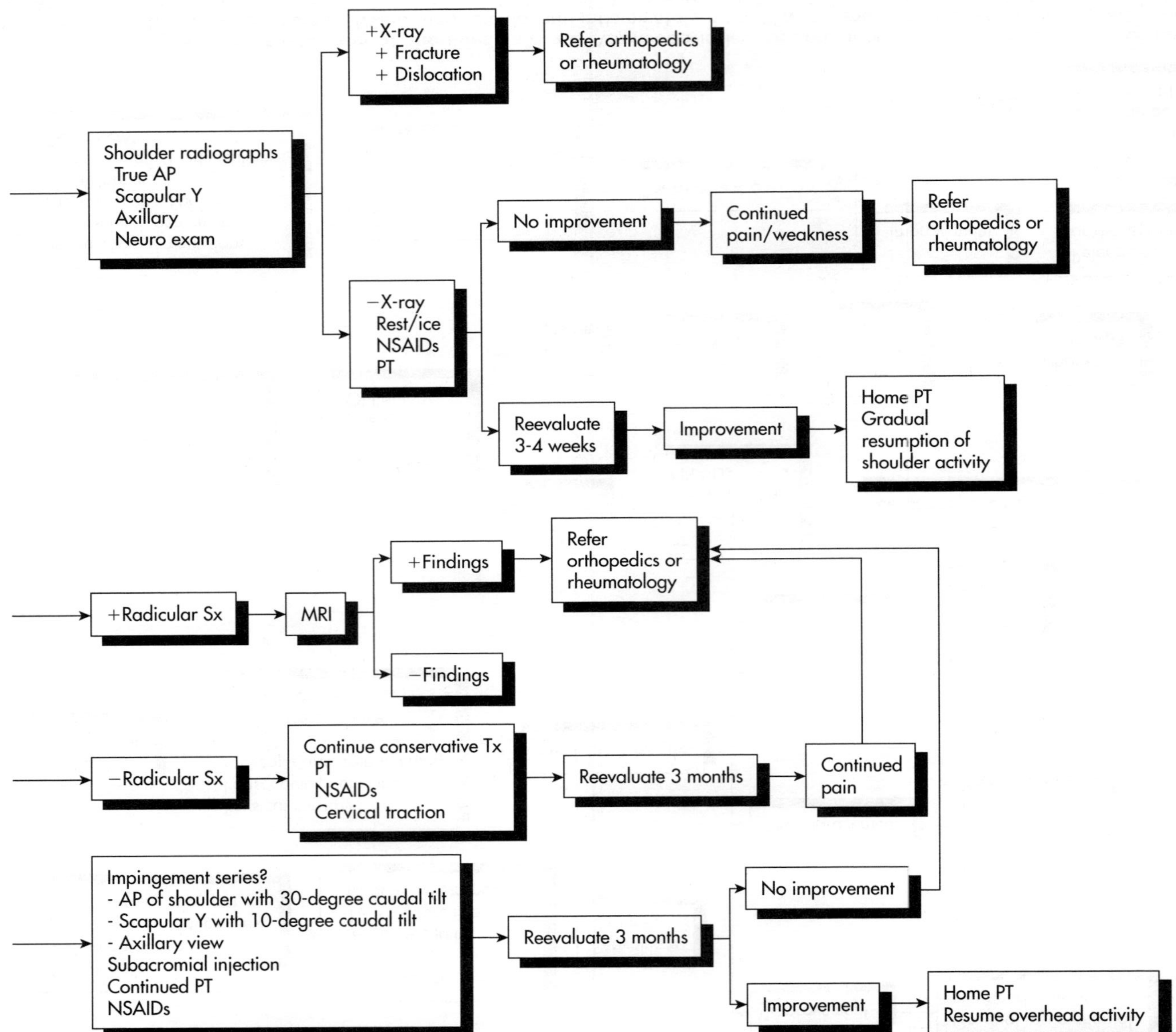

FIGURE 3-263 (Continued) **Algorithmic evaluation of shoulder pain.** *AC,* Acromioclavicular; *AP,* anteroposterior; *GH,* glenohumeral; *Hx,* history; *MRI,* magnetic resonance imaging; *NSAID,* nonsteroidal anti-inflammatory drug; *PRN,* as required; *PT,* physical therapy; *R/O,* rule out; *ROM,* range of motion; *Sx,* symptoms; *trx,* traction; *Tx,* therapy. (From Harris ED, Budd RC, Firestein GS, Genovese MC, Sergent JS, Ruddy S, Sledge CB [eds]: *Kelley's textbook of rheumatology,* ed 7, Philadelphia, Saunders.)

SHOULDER PAIN—cont'd

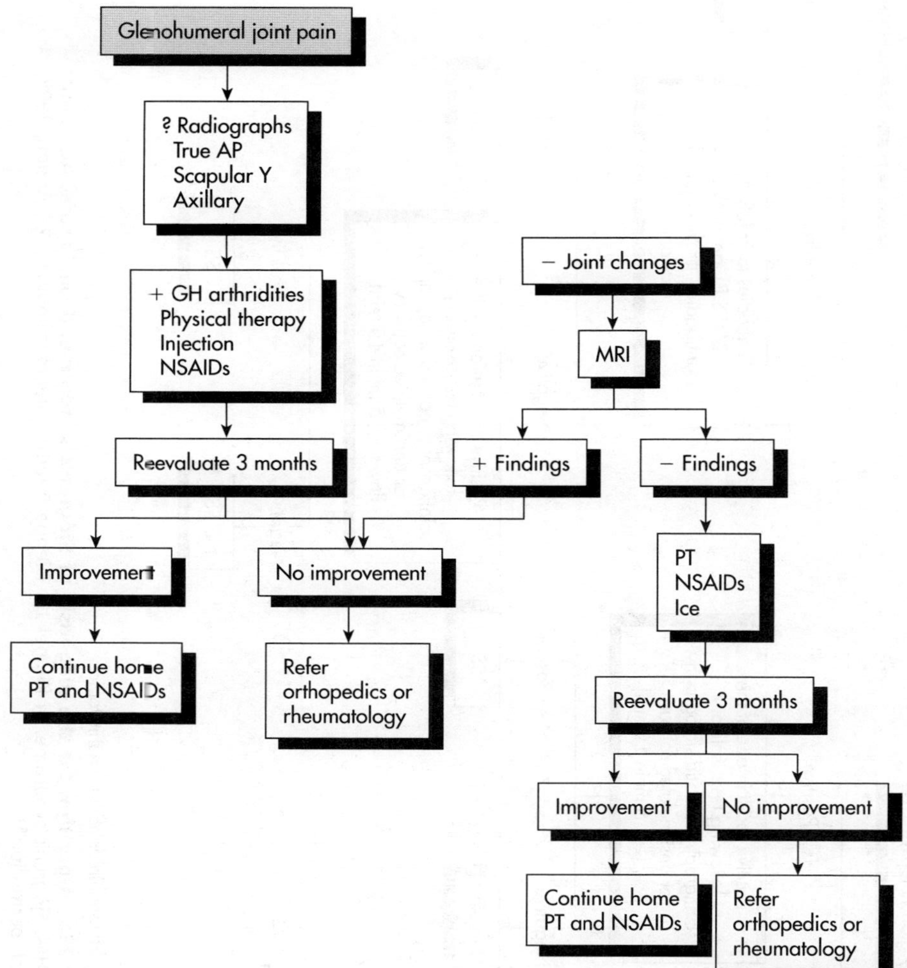

FIGURE 3-263 (Continued)

ICD-9CM # 710.2

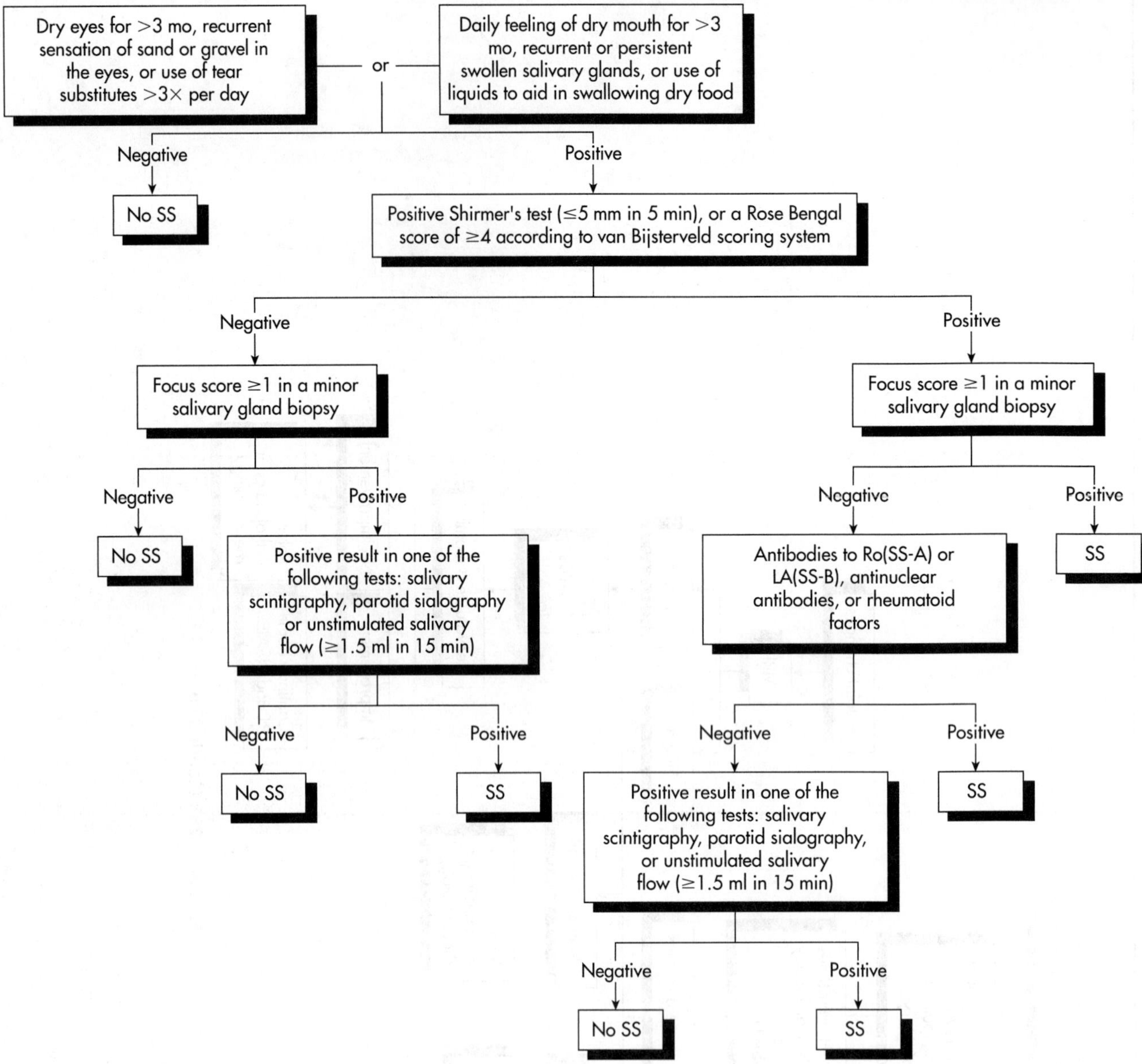

Note: Refer to Section I for additional information on this topic.

FIGURE 3-264 Algorithm for the diagnosis of Sjögren's syndrome. (From Tzoufas AG, Moutsopoulos HM: Sjögren's syndrome. In Klippel JH, Dieppe P [eds]: *Rheumatology,* ed 2, London, 1998, Mosby, with permission.)

ICD-9CM # 709.8

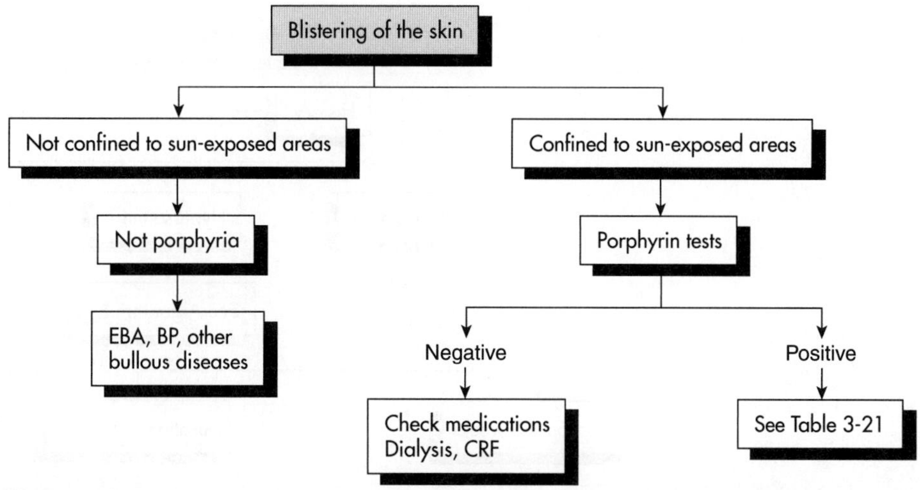

FIGURE 3-265 An approach to the patient with blistering of the skin. *BP,* Bullous pemphigoid; *CRF,* chronic renal failure; *EBA,* epidermolysis bullosa acquisita. (From Bolognia JL, Mascaro JM, Mancini AJ, Salasche SJ, Saurat JH, Stingl G [eds]: *Dermatology,* ed 2, St Louis, 2008, Mosby.)

TABLE 3-21 Investigative Tests Used in the Diagnosis of Porphyria

Porphyria	Enzyme	Urine	Stool	Plasma	RBC
Porphyria cutanea tarda	Uroporphyrinogen decarboxylase	URO+++ COPRO+ 7COOH III>I	ISO-COPRO++ 7COOH	+	−
Erythropoietic protoporphyria	Ferrochelatase	Normal	PROTO+	+	free PROTO++
Congenital erythropoietic porphyria	Uroporphyrinogen III synthase	URO I+ COPRO I+	COPRO I+	+	URO I+ COPRO I+ PROTO+
Acute intermittent porphyria	Porphobilinogen deaminase	*ALA+++ *PBG+++	*ALA+ *PBG+	−	−
Variegate porphyria	Protoporphyrinogen oxidase	*ALA++ *PBG++ URO+ COPRO++	COPRO+ PROTO++ PORPH X+++	625–7 nm peak	−
Heriditary coproporphyria	Coproporphyrinogen oxidase	*ALA++ *PBG++ COPRO++ URO+	COPRO+	+	−
Aminolevulinic acid (ALA) dehydratase-deficient porphyria	ALA dehydratase	ALA+++ COPROIII	−	−	Zn PROTO+
Hepatoerythropoietic porphyria	Uroporphyrinogen decarboxylase	URO+++ COPRO+ 7COOH III>I	ISO-COPRO++ 7COOH	+	Zn and free PROTO++
Tyrosinemia	ALA dehydratase	ALA	−	−	−
Iron deficiency	Ferrochelatase	−	−	−	Zn PROTO++
Lead poisoning	ALA dehydratase Coproporphyrinogen oxidase Ferrochelatase	ALA+++ COPRO±	−	−	Zn PROTO+

From Bolognia JL, Mascaro JM, Mancini AJ, Salasche SJ, Saurat JH, Stingl G (eds): *Dermatology,* ed 2, St Louis, 2008, Mosby.
COPRO, Coproporphyrin; *ISO-COPRO,* isocoproporphyrin; *PROTO,* protoporphyrin; *RBC,* red blood cells; *URO,* uroporphyrin; +, positive; −, negative; *, during acute attack.

ICD-9CM # 780.50 Sleep disorder, unspecified cause

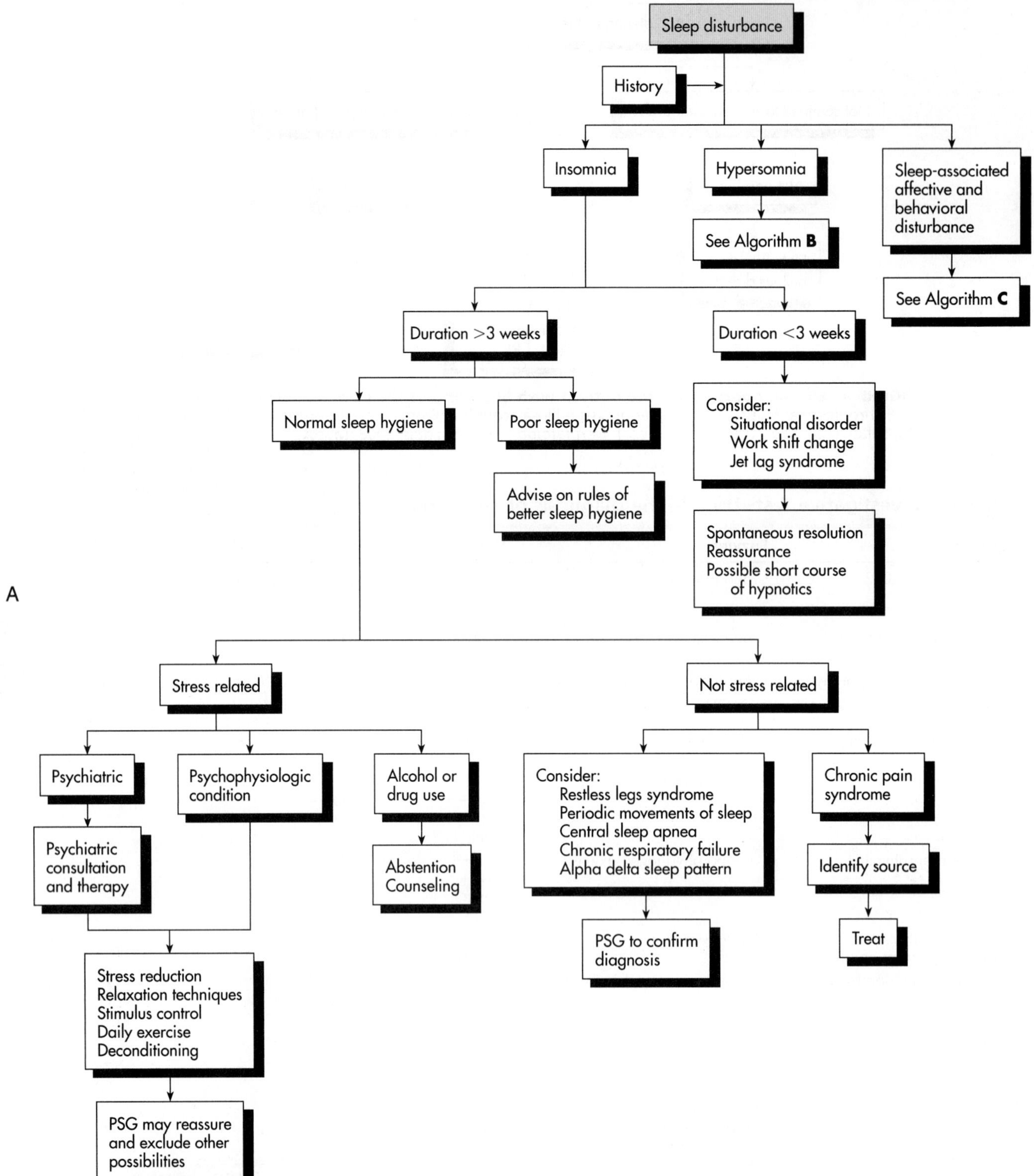

FIGURE 3-266 A, Patient with sleep disturbance. *MSLT,* Multiple sleep latency tests; *PSG,* polysomnography. (From Greene HL, Johnson WP, Lemcke D [eds]: *Decision making in medicine,* ed 2, St Louis, 1998, Mosby.)

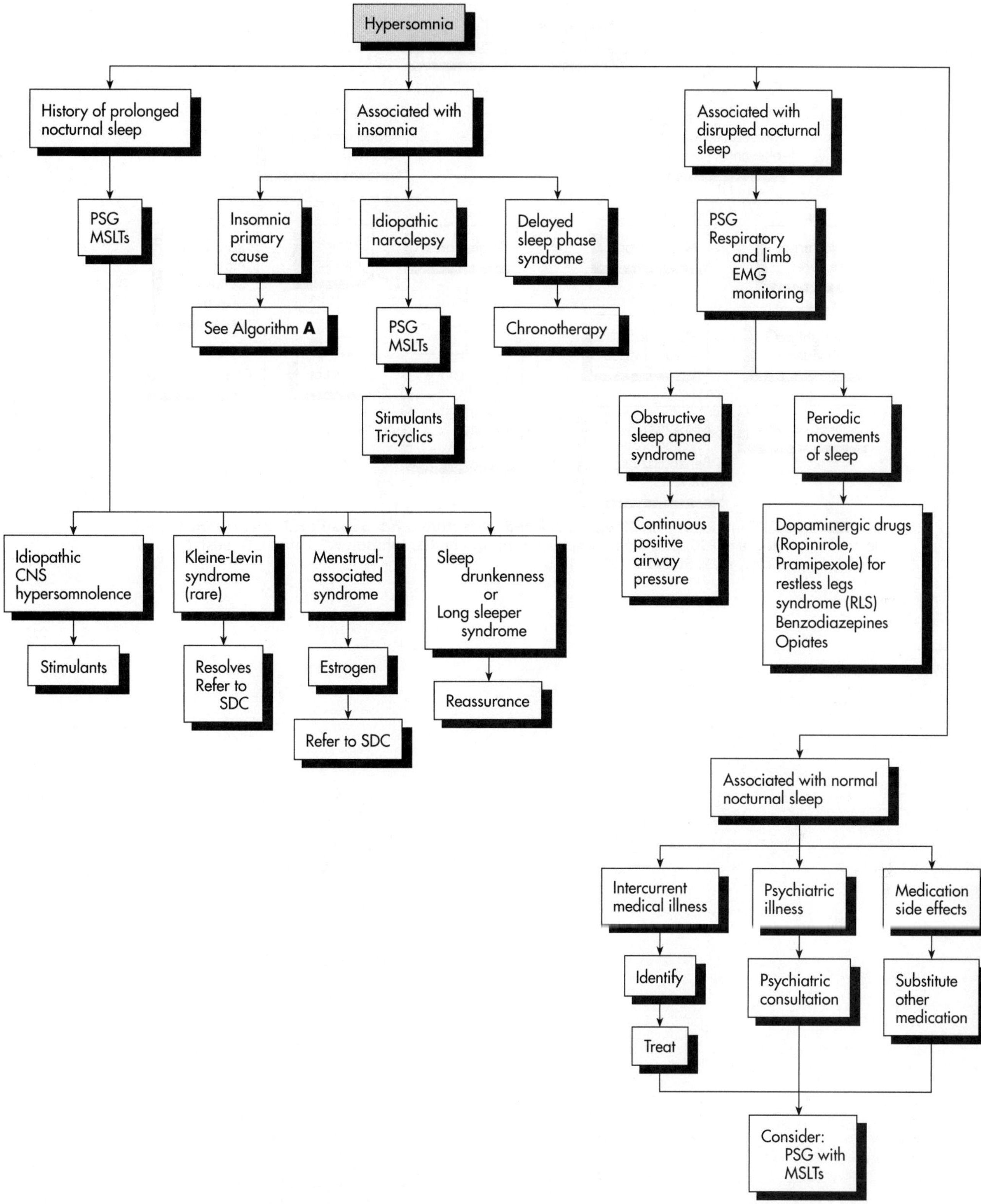

FIGURE 3-266 (Continued) **B, Hypersomnia.** *CNS,* Central nervous system; *EMG,* electromyelogram; *MSLTs,* multiple sleep latency tests; *PSG,* polysomnography; *SDC,* sleep disorders clinic. (From Greene HL, Johnson WP, Lemcke D [eds]: *Decision making in medicine,* ed 2, St Louis, 1998, Mosby.)

Continued on following page

C

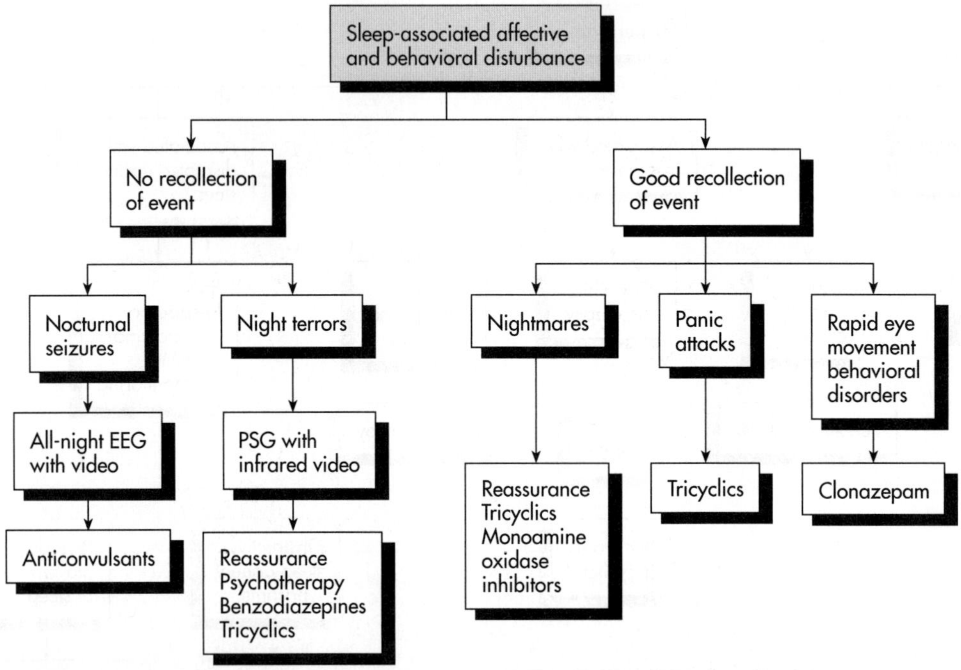

FIGURE 3-266 (Continued) **C, Sleep-associated affective and behavioral disturbance.** *EEG,* Electroencephalogram; *PSG,* polysomnography. (From Greene HL, Johnson WP, Lemcke D [eds]: *Decision making in medicine,* ed 2, St Louis, 1998, Mosby.)

ICD-9CM # 192.2

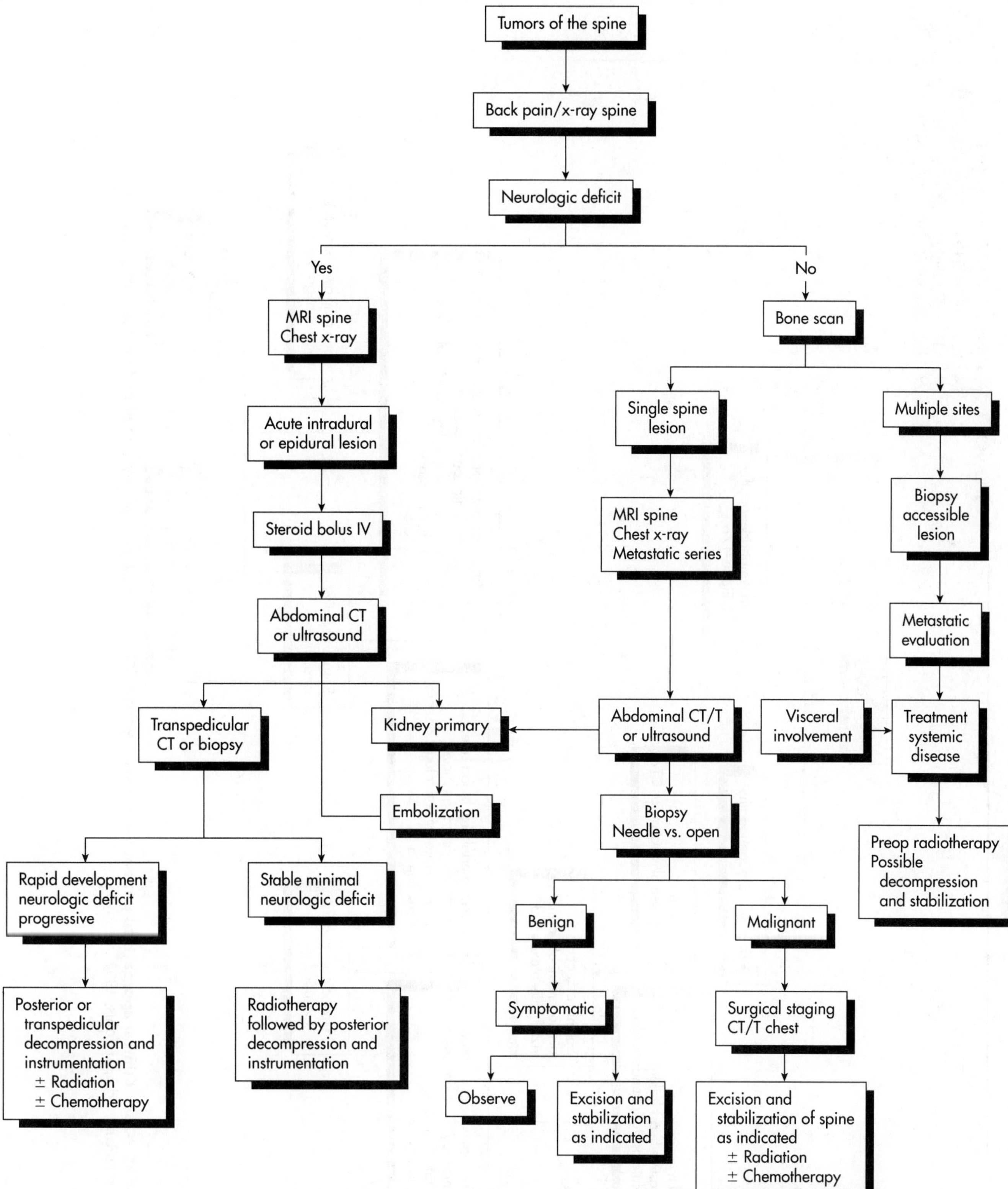

FIGURE 3-267 Diagnostic and therapeutic approach to tumors of the spine. *CT,* Computed tomography; *IV,* intravenous; *MRI,* magnetic resonance imaging. (From Abeloff MD: *Clinical oncology,* ed 3, Philadelphia, 2004, Elsevier.)

SPLENOMEGALY

ICD-9CM # 789.2 Splenomegaly, unspecified
289.51 Splenomegaly, chronic congestive
759.0 Splenomegaly, congenital
789.2 Splenomegaly, unknown etiology

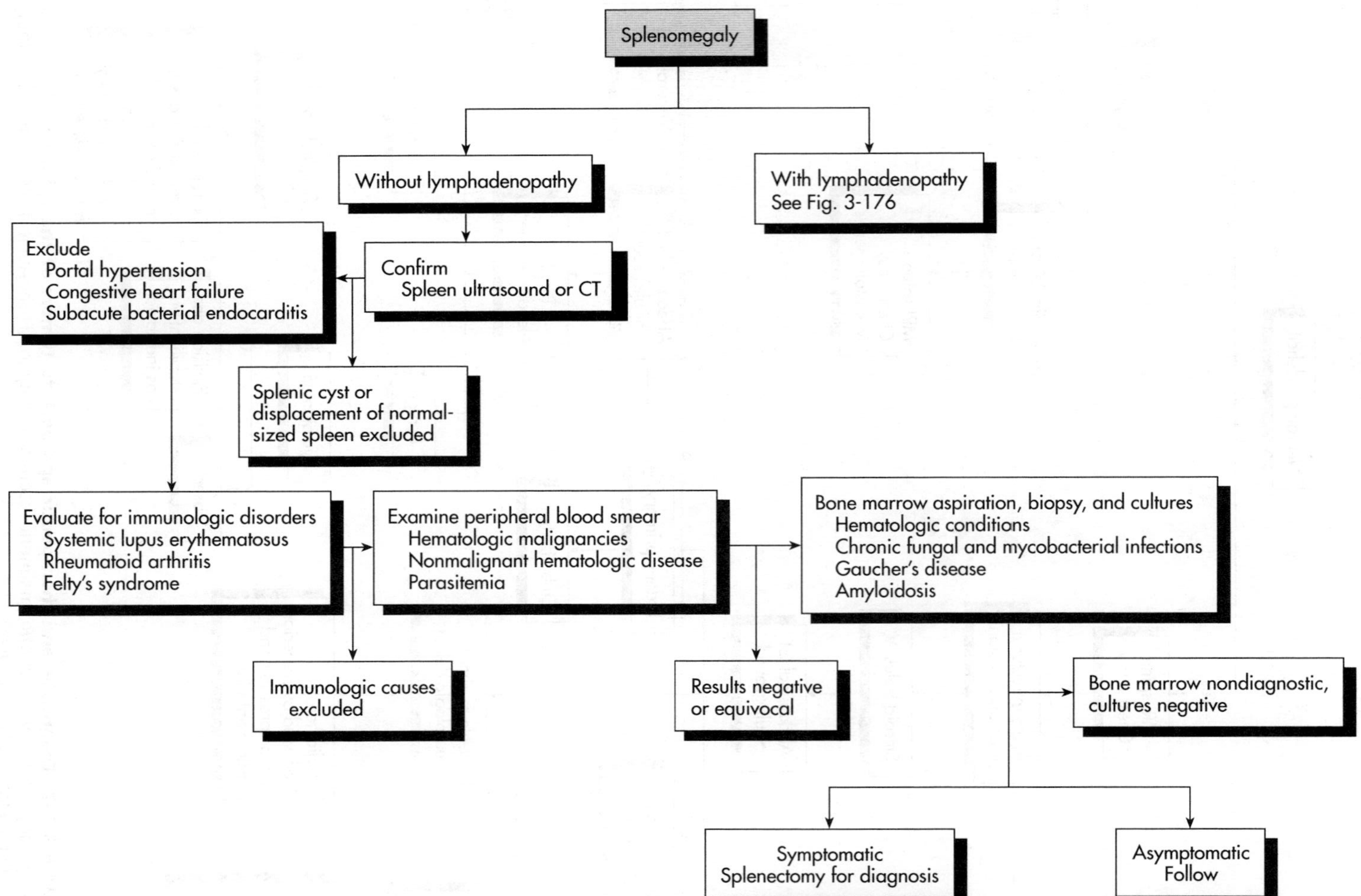

FIGURE 3-268 Clinical approach to patient with splenomegaly. *CT,* Computed tomography. (Modified from Stein JH [ed]: *Internal medicine,* ed 5, St Louis, 1998, Mosby.)

ICD-9CM # 720.7

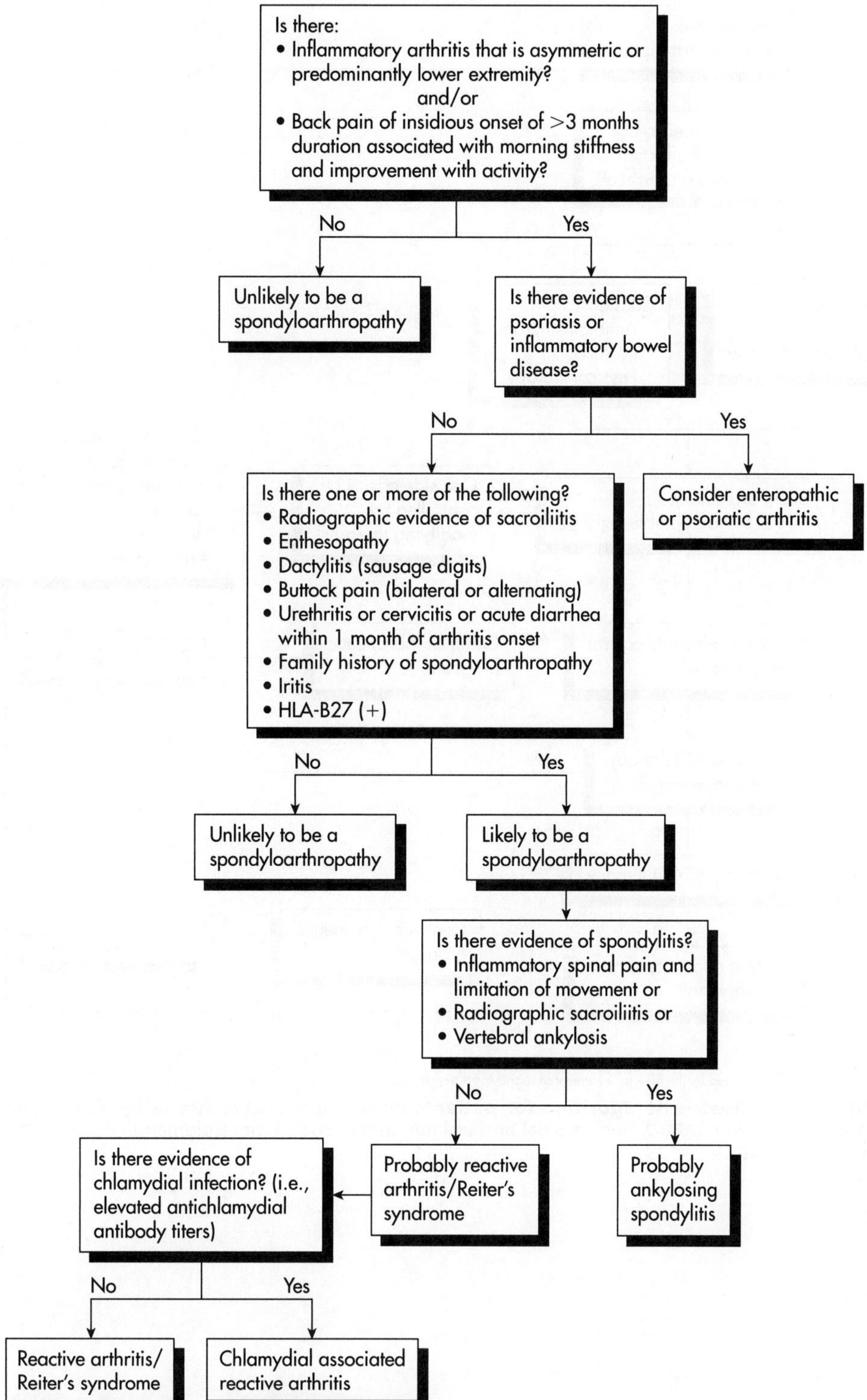

FIGURE 3-269 Algorithm for diagnosis of the spondyloarthropathies. (From Goldman L, Ausiello D: *Cecil textbook of medicine,* ed 23, Philadelphia, 2008, WB Saunders.)

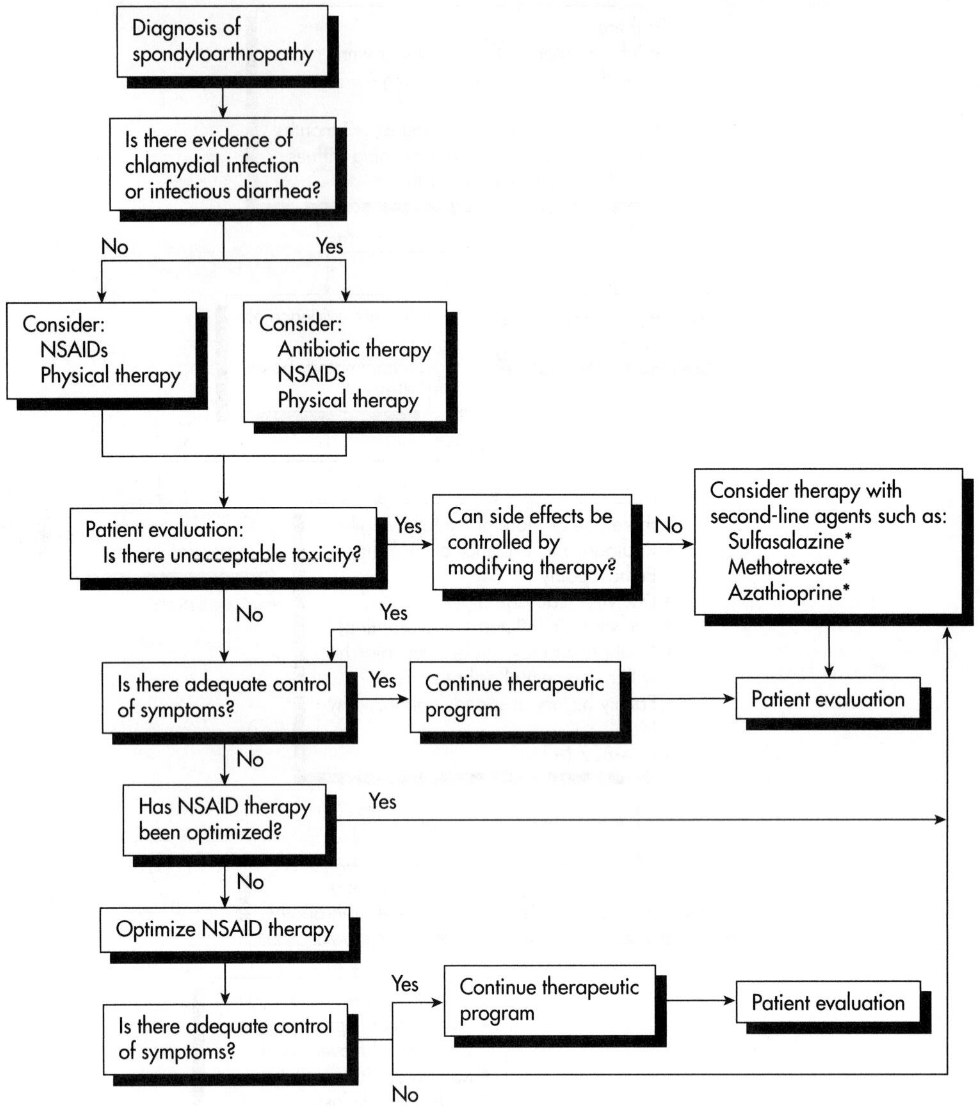

*Not approved by the FDA for treatment of spondyloarthropathies.

FIGURE 3-270 Treatment algorithm for patients with a spondyloarthropathy. *FDA,* Food and Drug Administration; *NSAID,* nonsteroidal anti-inflammatory drug. (From Goldman L, Ausiello D: *Cecil textbook of medicine,* ed 23, Philadelphia, 2008, WB Saunders.)

ICD-9CM # 721.0

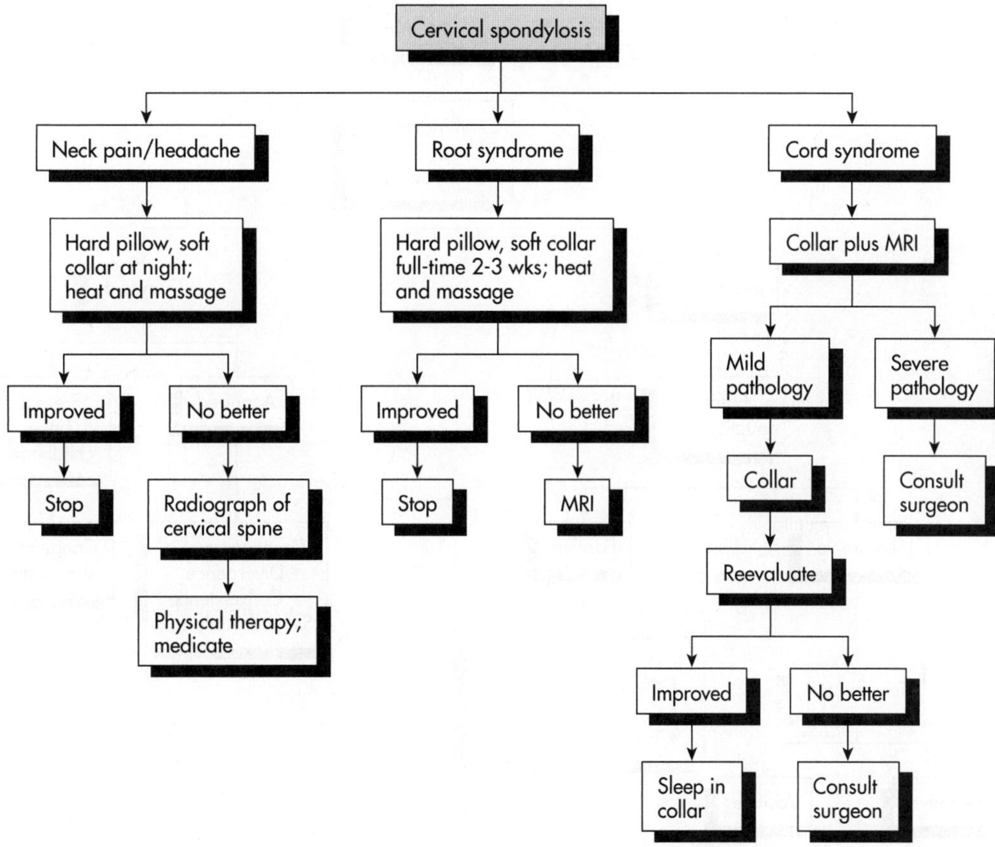

FIGURE 3-271 Algorithm for the treatment of cervical spondylosis. *MRI,* Magnetic resonance imaging. (From Ronthal M, Rachlin JR: Cervical spondylosis. In Johnson RT, Griffin JW [eds]: *Current therapy in neurologic disease,* ed 5, St Louis, 1997, Mosby.)

ICD-9CM # 378.9

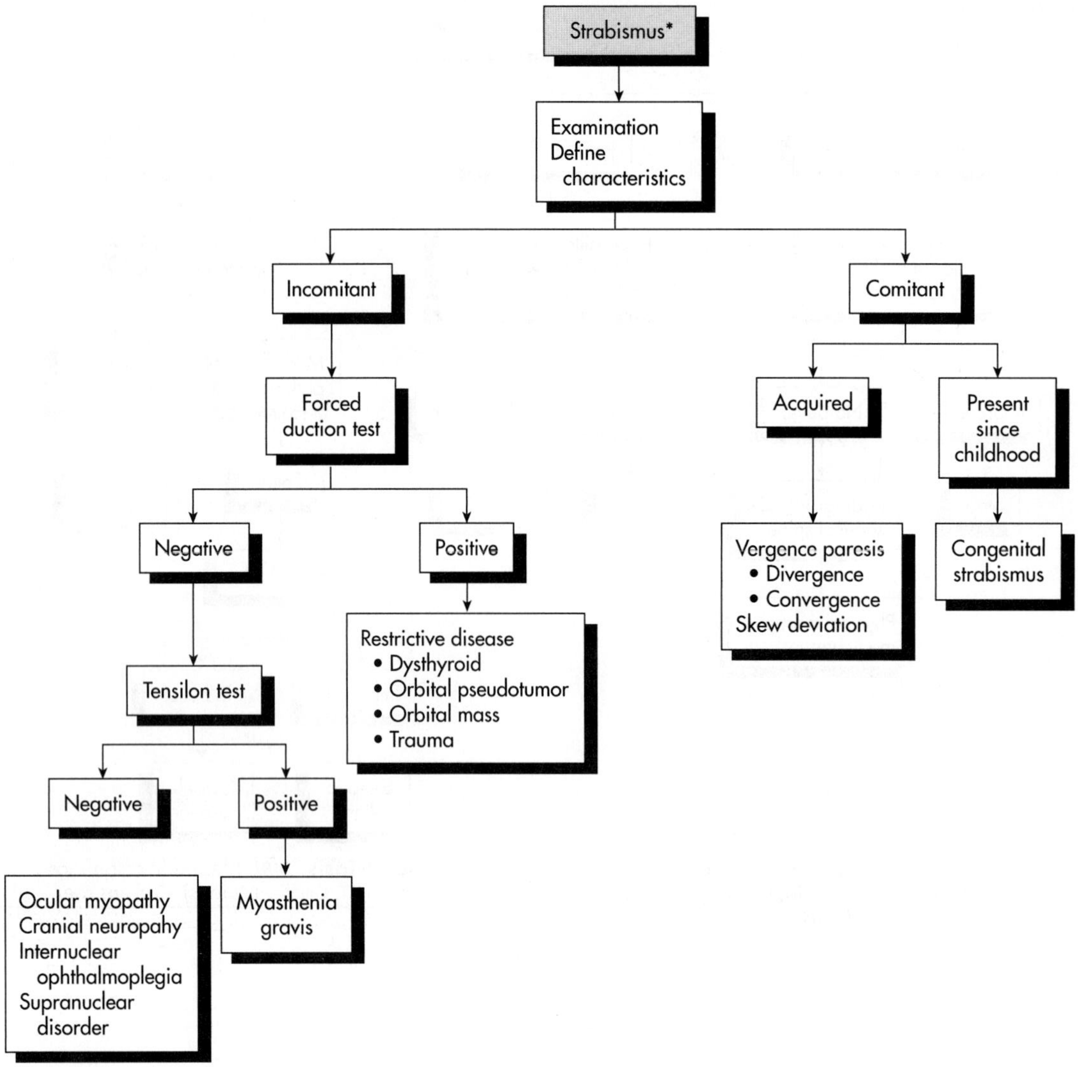
Strabismus*
Examination
Define characteristics
Incomitant
Comitant
Forced duction test
Acquired
Present since childhood
Negative
Positive
Vergence paresis
• Divergence
• Convergence
Skew deviation
Congenital strabismus
Restrictive disease
• Dysthyroid
• Orbital pseudotumor
• Orbital mass
• Trauma
Tensilon test
Negative
Positive
Ocular myopathy
Cranial neuropahy
Internuclear ophthalmoplegia
Supranuclear disorder
Myasthenia gravis

*Refer to Section I for additional information on this topic.

FIGURE 3-272 Diagnostic tests that help differentiate between common causes of strabismus. (From Goldman L, Ausiello D [eds]: *Cecil textbook of medicine,* ed 23, Philadelphia, 2008, WB Saunders.)

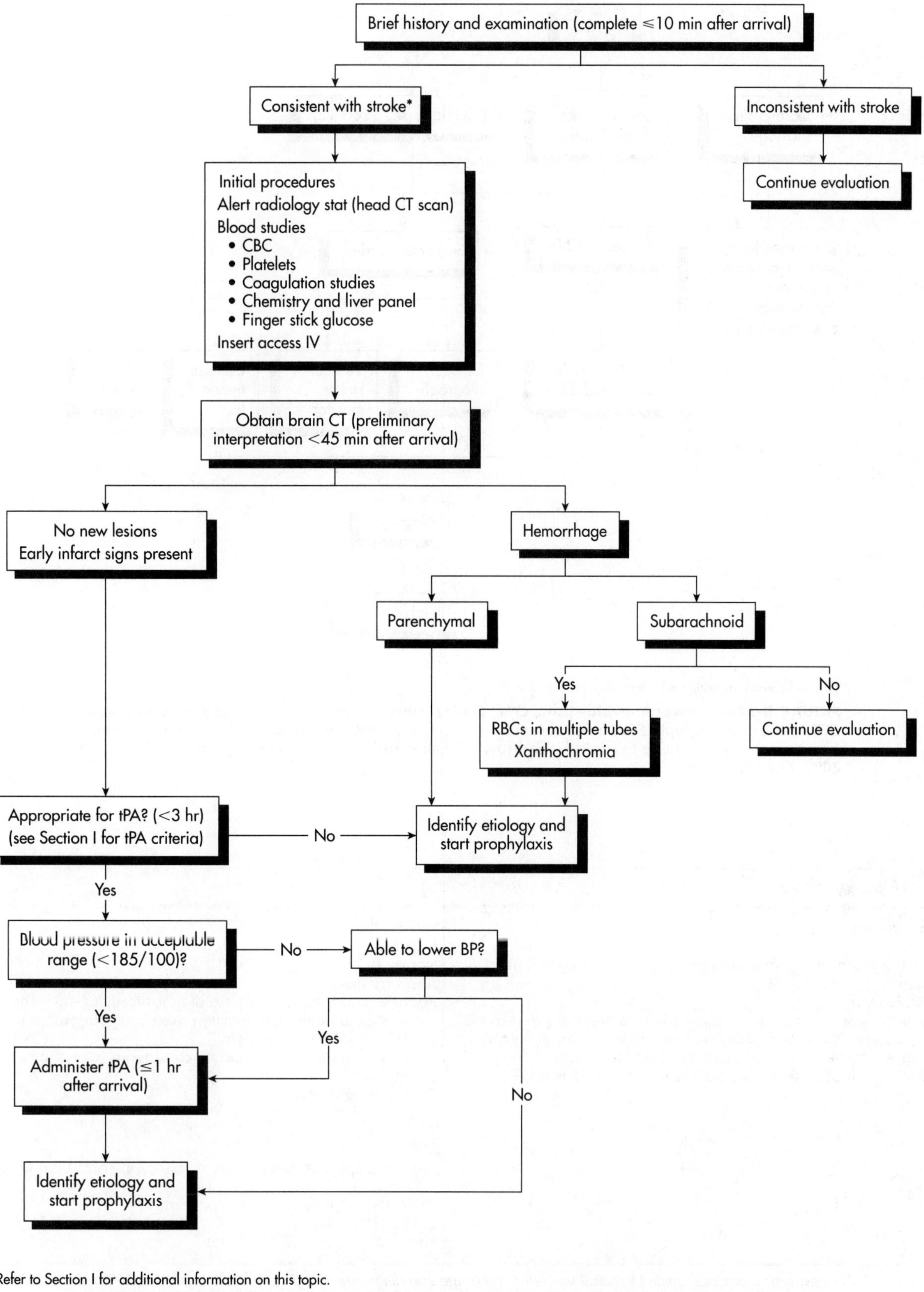

*Refer to Section I for additional information on this topic.

FIGURE 3-273 Algorithm for the emergency evaluation of a patient with suspected stroke. *BP,* Blood pressure; *CBC,* complete blood count; *CT,* computed tomography; *RBCs,* red blood cells; *tPA,* tissue plasminogen activator. (From Goldman L, Ausiello D [eds]: *Cecil textbook of medicine,* ed 23, Philadelphia, 2008, WB Saunders.)

ICD-9CM # 720.2

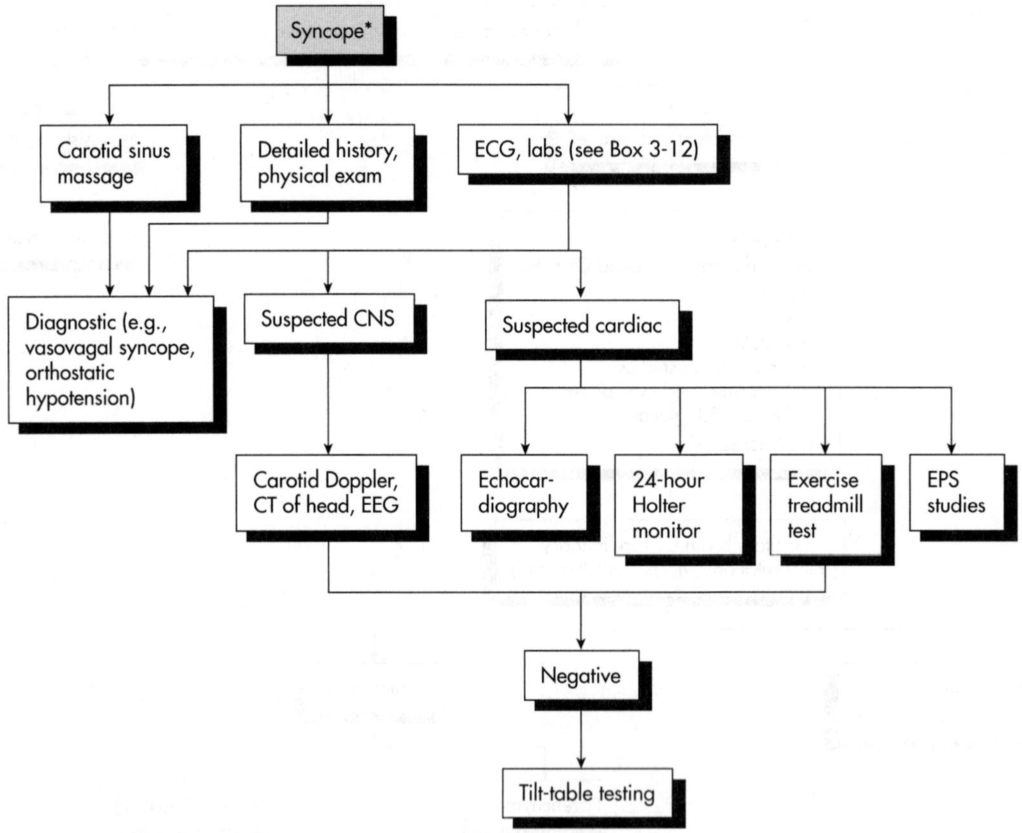

*Refer to Section I for additional information on this topic.

FIGURE 3-274 Syncope evaluation. *CNS,* Central nervous system; *CT,* computed tomography; *ECG,* electrocardiograph; *EEG,* electroencephalograph; *EPS,* electrophysiologic. (From Ferri FF: *Ferri's best test: a practical guide to clinical laboratory medicine and diagnostic imaging,* ed 2, Philadelphia, 2009, Elsevier Mosby.)

BOX 3-12 Syncope

Diagnostic imaging

Best test

None. Diagnostic imaging should be guided by history and physical exam

Ancillary tests

Echocardiography is useful in patients with a heart murmur to r/o aortic stenosis, hypertrophic cardiomyopathy, or atrial myxoma

If seizure is suspected, CT of head and EEG are indicated

Spiral CT of chest or ventilation/perfusion scan if PE is suspected

Lab evaluation

Best test

None

Ancillary tests

Routine blood tests rarely yield diagnostically useful information and should be done only when specifically suggested by history and physical exam

Serum pregnancy test should be considered in women of child-bearing age

CBC, lytes, BUN, creatinine

Serum calcium, magnesium

ABGs

ECG

Cardiac troponins, isoenzymes if history of chest pain before syncope

Toxicology screen in selected patients

Cardiac stress test

Electrophysiologic (EPS) studies

From Ferri FF: *Ferri's best test: a practical guide to clinical laboratory medicine and diagnostic imaging,* ed 2, Philadelphia, 2009, Elsevier Mosby.

ABG, Arterial blood gas; *BUN,* blood urea nitrogen; *CBC,* complete blood count; *CT,* computed tomography; *ECG,* electrocardiograph; *EEG,* electroencephalograph.

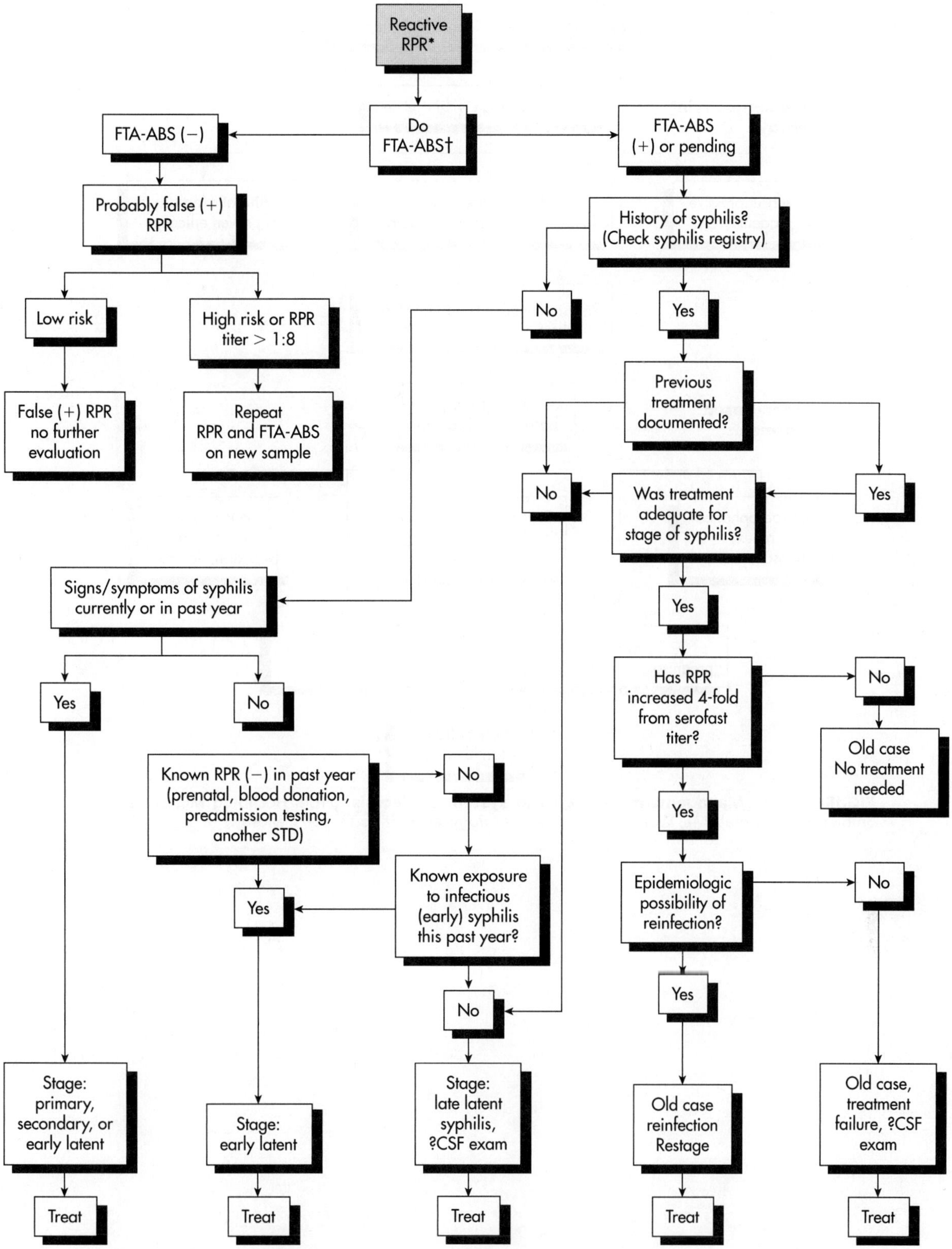

FIGURE 3-275 Interpretation of reactive serologic tests for syphilis. *CSF,* cerebrospinal fluid; *FTA-ABS,* fluorescent treponemal antibody absorption; *RPR,* rapid plasma reagent; *STD,* sexually transmitted disease. (From Habif TA: *Clinical dermatology,* ed 4, St Louis, 2004, Mosby.)

ICD-9CM # 710.1

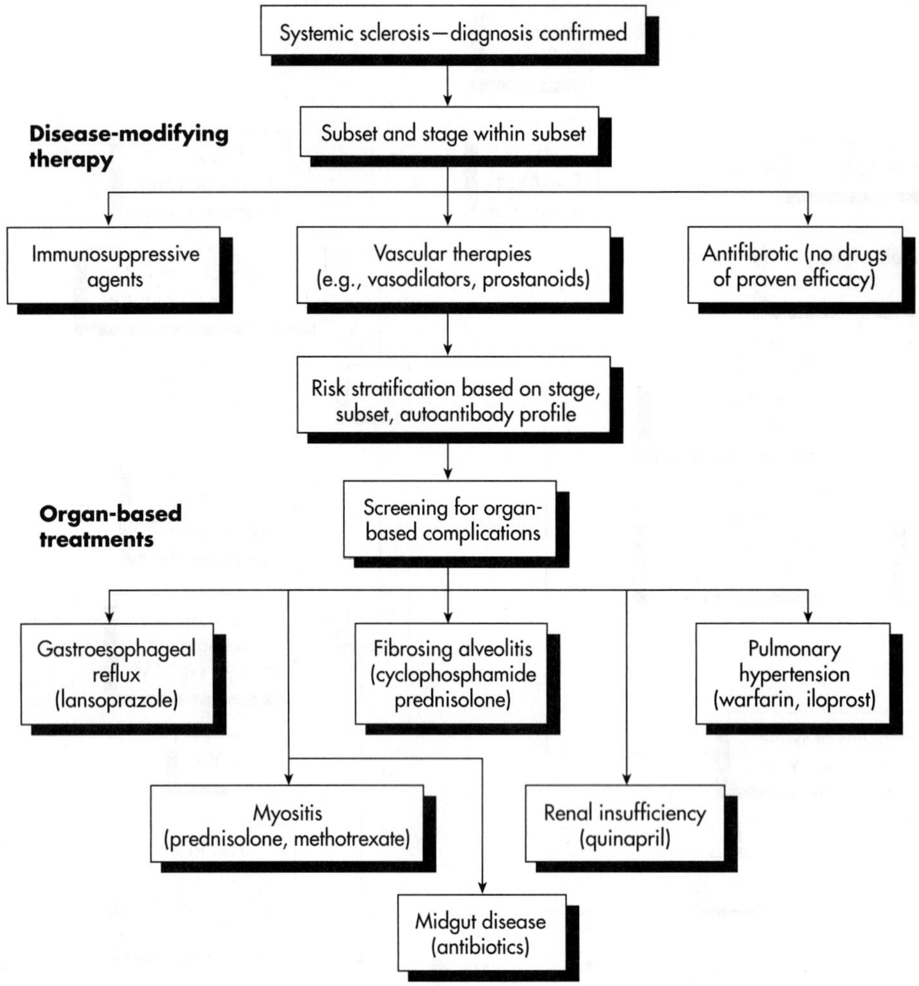

FIGURE 3-276 Management strategies in systemic sclerosis. (From Hochberg MC, Silman AJ, Smolen JS, Weinblatt ME, Weisman MH: *Rheumatology,* ed 3, St Louis, 2003, Mosby.)

ICD-9CM # 785.0

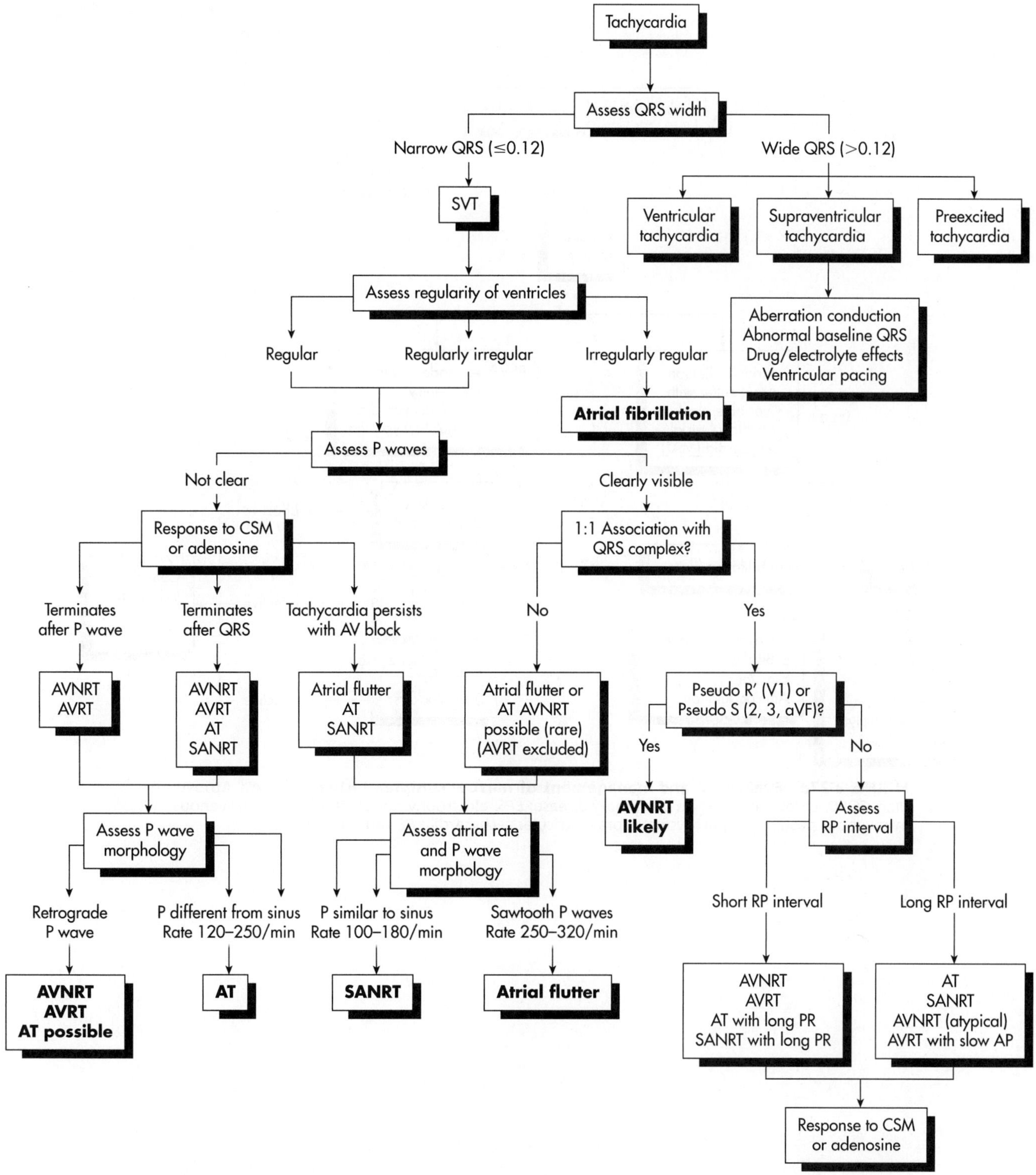

FIGURE 3-277 Stepwise approach to the diagnosis of type of tachycardia based on 12-lead electrocardiogram during the episode. The initial step is to determine whether the tachycardia has a wide or narrow QRS complex. For wide-complex tachycardia, see Figure 3-265; the remainder of the algorithm is helpful in diagnosiing the type of narrow-complex tachycardia. *AP,* Accessory pathway; *AT,* atrial tachycardia; *AV,* atrioventricular; *AVNRT,* AV nodal reentrant tachycardia; *AVRT,* AV reciprocating tachycardia; *CSM,* carotid sinus massage; *SANRT,* sinoatrial nodal reentry tachycardia; *SVT,* supraventricular tachycardia. (From Zipes DP, Libby P, Bonow RO, Braunwald E [eds]: *Braunwald's heart disease,* ed 7, Philadelphia, 2005, Elsevier.)

ICD-9CM # 427.2 Paroxysmal tachycardia
427.0 Supraventricular paroxysmal tachycardia
427.42 Ventricular flutter
427.1 Ventricular paroxysmal tachycardia
427.89 Atrial tachycardia

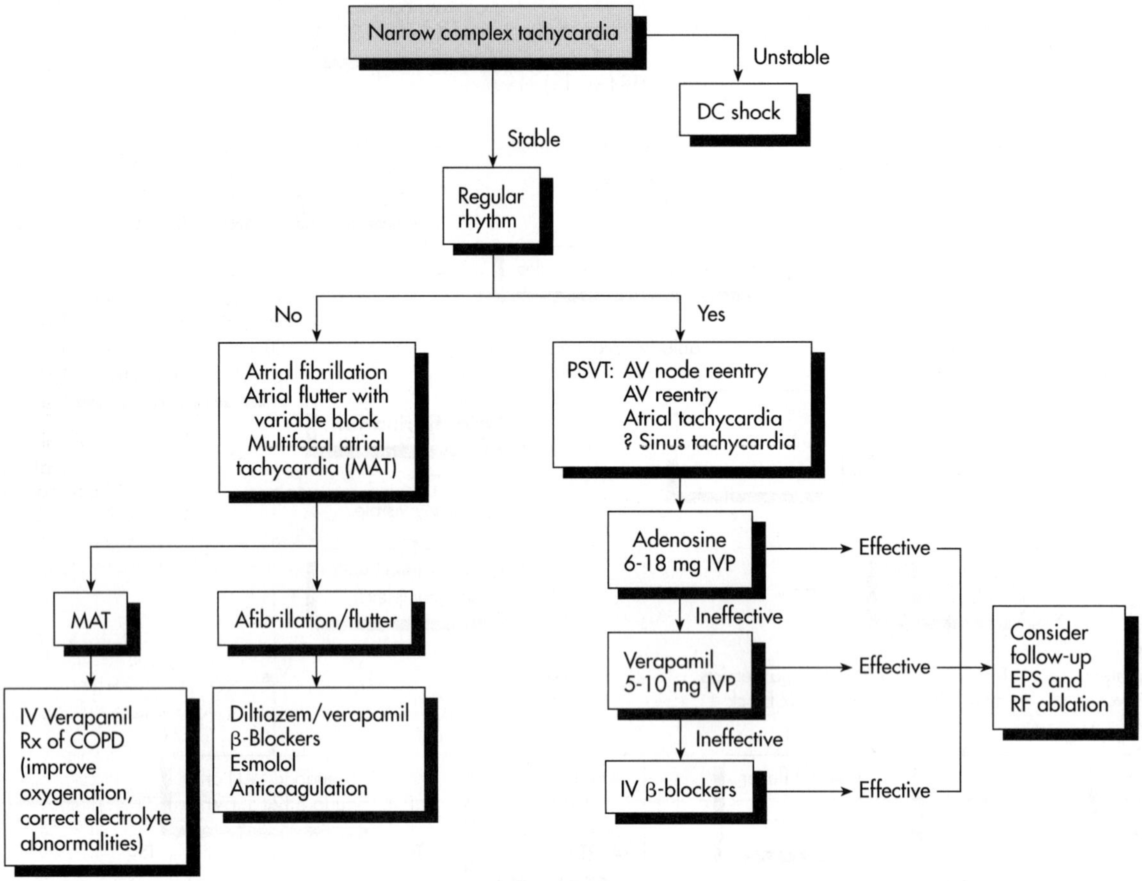

FIGURE 3-278 Evaluation and management of narrow complex tachycardia. *AV,* Atrioventricular; *COPD,* chronic obstructive pulmonary disease; *EPS,* electrophysiologic studies; *IV,* intravenous; *IVP,* intravenous push; *PSVT,* paroxysmal supraventricular tachycardia; *RF,* radiofrequency.

ICD-9CM # 427.2 Paroxysmal tachycardia
427.0 Supraventricular paroxysmal tachycardia
427.42 Ventricular flutter
427.1 Ventricular paroxysmal tachycardia
427.89 Atrial tachycardia

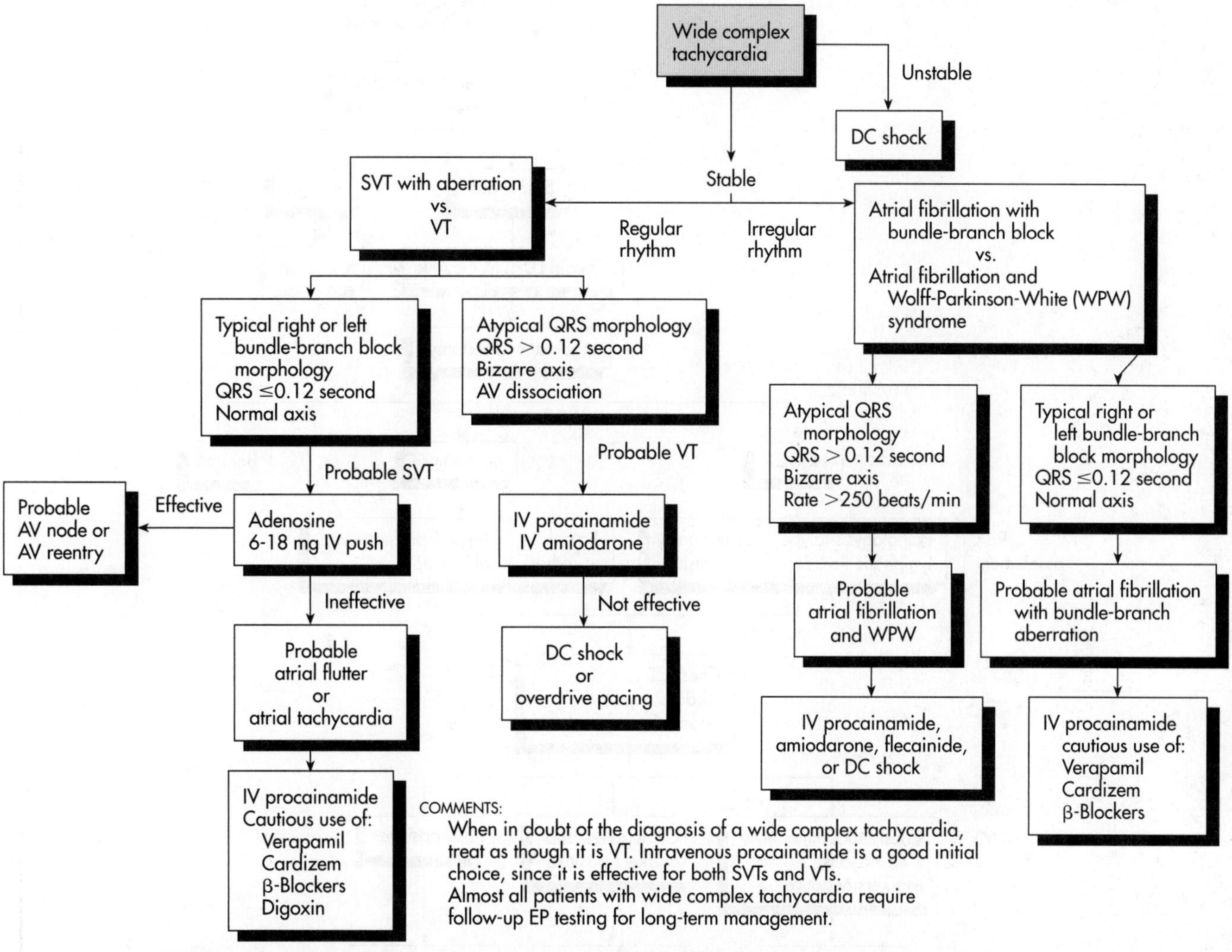

COMMENTS:
When in doubt of the diagnosis of a wide complex tachycardia, treat as though it is VT. Intravenous procainamide is a good initial choice, since it is effective for both SVTs and VTs.
Almost all patients with wide complex tachycardia require follow-up EP testing for long-term management.

FIGURE 3-279 Evaluation and management of wide complex tachycardia. *AV,* Atrioventricular; *EP,* electrophysiologic; *IV,* intravenous; *SVT,* supraventricular tachycardia; *VT,* ventricular tachycardia. (From Driscoll CE et al: *The family practice desk reference,* ed 3, St Louis, 1996, Mosby.)

ICD-9CM # 186.9 Testicular neoplasm
M906/3 (seminoma)
M9101/3 (embryonal carcinoma or teratoma)
M9100/3 (choriocarcinoma)

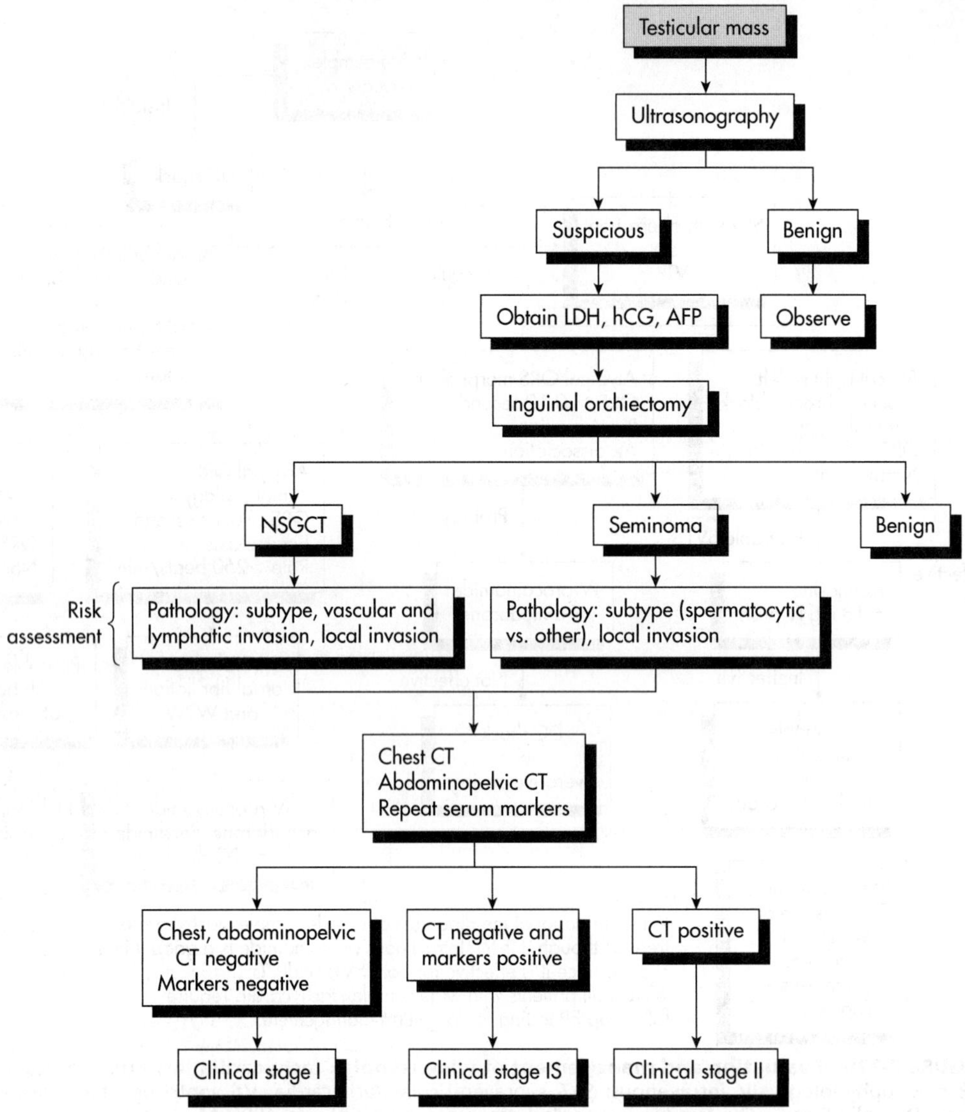

FIGURE 3-280 Diagnosis, staging, and risk assessment of patients with testicular germ cell tumor. *AFP,* Alpha-fetoprotein; *CT,* computed tomography; *hCG,* human chorionic gonadotropin; *LDH,* lactic dehydrogenase; *NSGCT,* nonseminoma germ cell tumor. (From Abeloff MD: *Clinical oncology,* ed 3, New York, 2004, Churchill Livingstone.)

ICD-9CM # 353.0

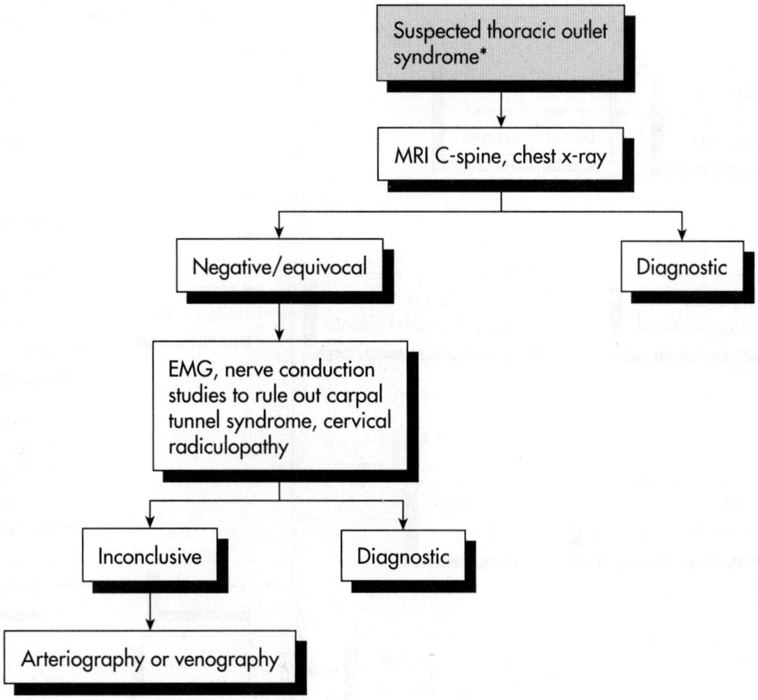

*Refer to Section I for additional information on this topic.

FIGURE 3-281 Thoracic outlet syndrome. *EMG,* Electromyogram; *MRI,* magnetic resonance imaging.

ICD-9CM # 287.3 Congenital or primary
287.4 Secondary
287.5 Thrombocytopenia NOS

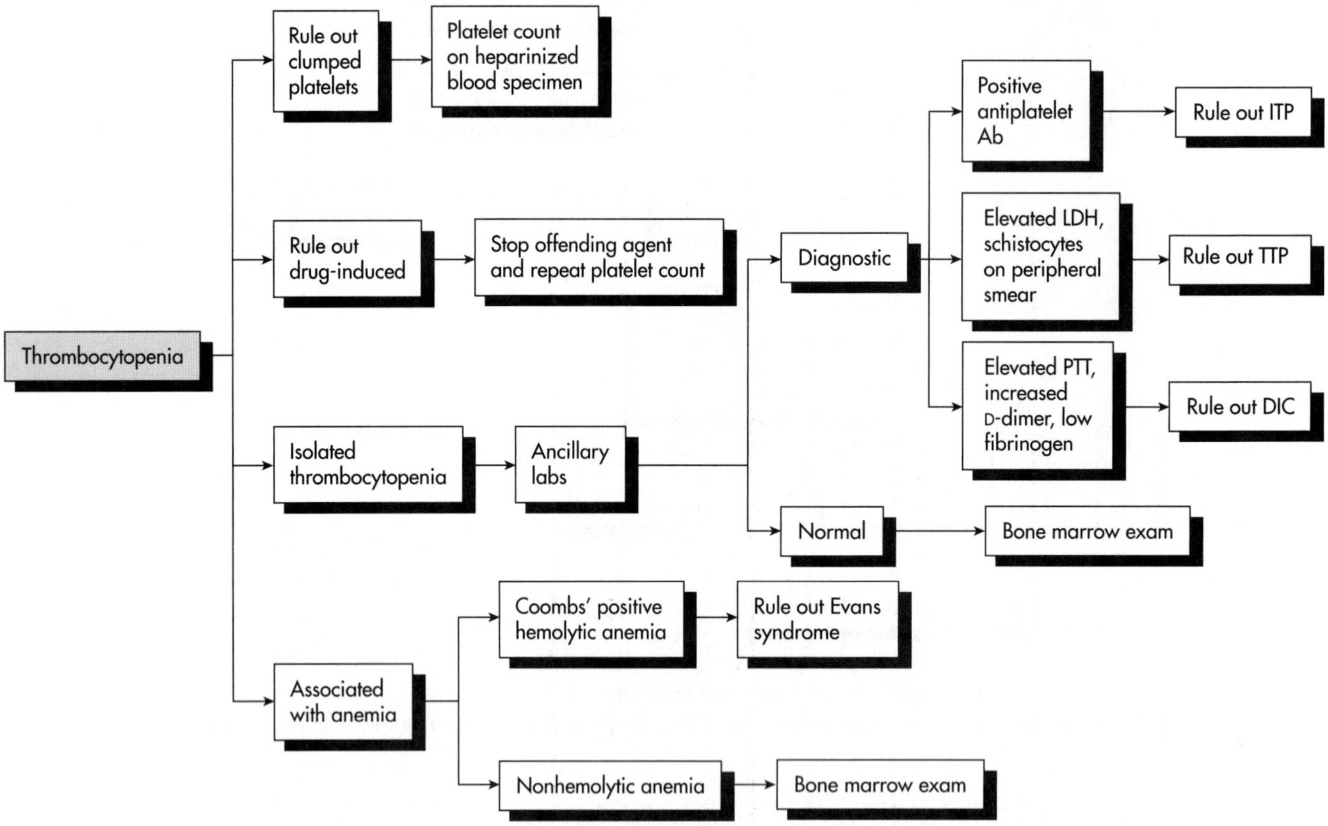

FIGURE 3-282 Evaluation of thrombocytopenia. *DIC,* Disseminated intravascular coagulation; *ITP,* idiopathic thrombocytopenic purpura; *LDH,* lactic dehydrogenase; *PPT,* partial thromboplastin time; *TTP,* thrombotic thrombocytopenic purpura. (From Ferri FF: *Ferri's best test: a practical guide to clinical laboratory medicine and diagnostic imaging,* ed 2, Philadelphia, 2009, Elsevier Mosby.)

BOX 3-13 **Thrombocytopenia**

Diagnostic imaging	Lab evaluation
Best Test	***Best Test***
None	Bone marrow exam
Ancillary test	***Ancillary tests***
CT of abdomen if splenomegaly is present	CBC, PT, PTT
	LDH
	HIV, ANA
	Antiplatelet Ab
	D-dimer
	Coombs' tests

From Ferri FF: *Ferri's best test: a practical guide to clinical laboratory medicine and diagnostic imaging,* ed 2, Philadelphia, 2009, Elsevier Mosby.

ANA, Antibody to nuclear antigens; *CBC,* complete blood count; *CT,* computed tomography; *HIV,* human immunodeficiency virus; *LDH,* lactic dehydrogenase; *PT,* prothrombin time; *PTT,* partial thromboplastin time.

ICD-9CM # 289.9

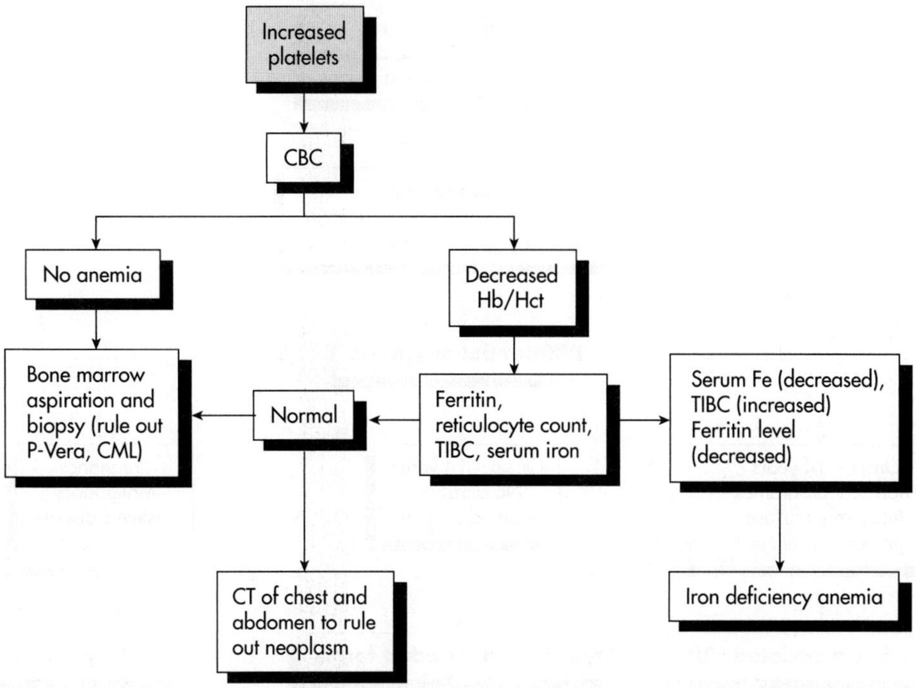

FIGURE 3-283 Thrombocytosis diagnosis. *CBC,* Complete blood count; *CML,* chronic myelogenous leukemia; *CT,* computed tomography; *Fe,* iron; *Hb/Hct,* hemoglobin/hematocrit; *TIBC,* total iron-binding capacity. (From Ferri FF: *Ferri's best test: a practical guide to clinical laboratory medicine and diagnostic imaging,* ed 2, Philadelphia, 2009, Elsevier Mosby.)

BOX 3-14 **Thrombocytosis**

Diagnostic imaging	Lab evaluation
Best Test	***Best Test***
None	Bone marrow exam
Ancillary test	***Ancillary tests***
CT of chest and abdomen	CBC
	Reticulocyte count
	Stool for OB ×3
	Serum ferritin, TIBC, iron

From Ferri FF: *Ferri's best test: a practical guide to clinical laboratory medicine and diagnostic imaging,* ed 2, Philadelphia, 2009, Elsevier Mosby.

CBC, Complete blood count; *CT,* computed tomography; *OB,* occult blood; *TIBC,* total iron-binding capacity.

ICD-9CM # 453.9

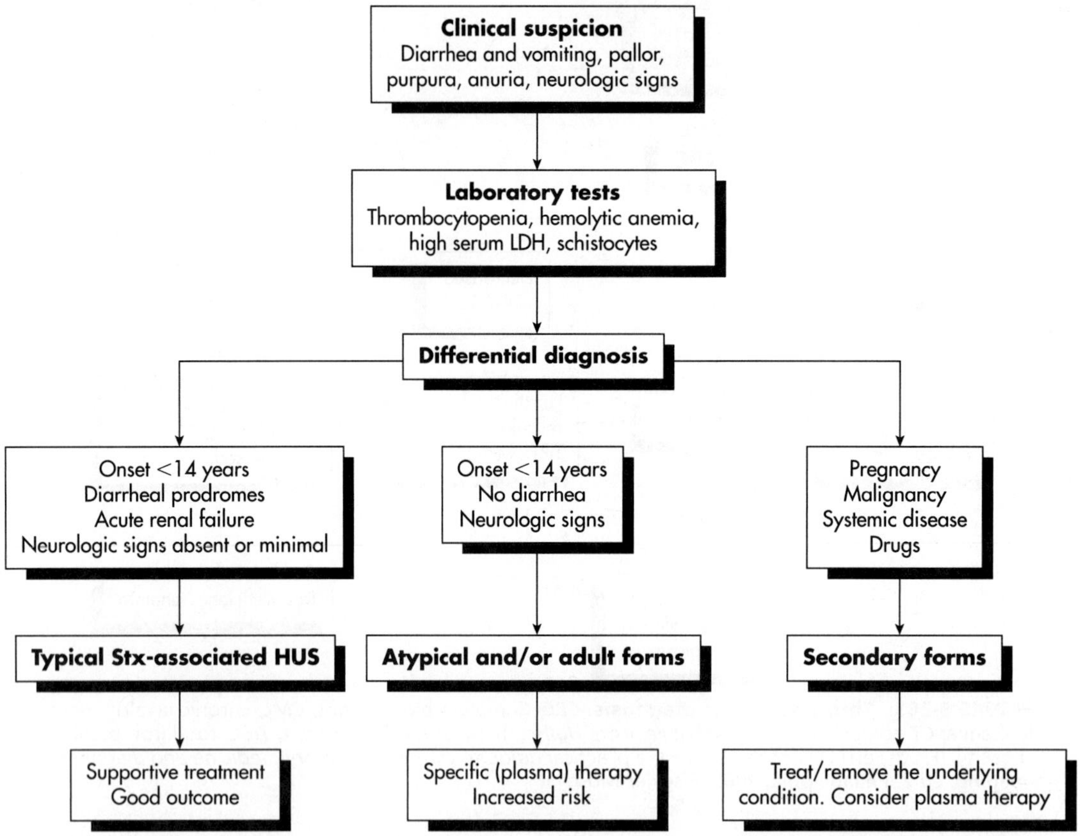

FIGURE 3-284 Algorithm for the differential diagnosis of thrombotic microangiopathies. Patients with suggestive symptoms should be investigated for specific signs of microangiopathic hemolysis. In adults, secondary forms of the disease must be ruled out. Early diagnosis may help establish the most appropriate therapy. In children with Shiga toxin–associated hemolytic-uremic syndrome (HUS), supportive treatment is mandatory. Specific therapies should be considered only in adults and in atypical forms. In secondary forms, treating and/or removing the underlying disease is fundamental. *LDH,* Lactate dehydrogenase. (From Feehally J, Floege J, Johnson RJ: *Comprehensive clinical nephrology,* ed 3, St. Louis, 2007, Mosby.)

THROMBOTIC THROMBOCYTOPENIC PURPURA AND HEMOLYTIC-UREMIC SYNDROME

ICD-9CM # 446.6 Thrombotic thrombocytic purpura
ICD-9CM # 283.11 Hemolytic-uremic syndrome

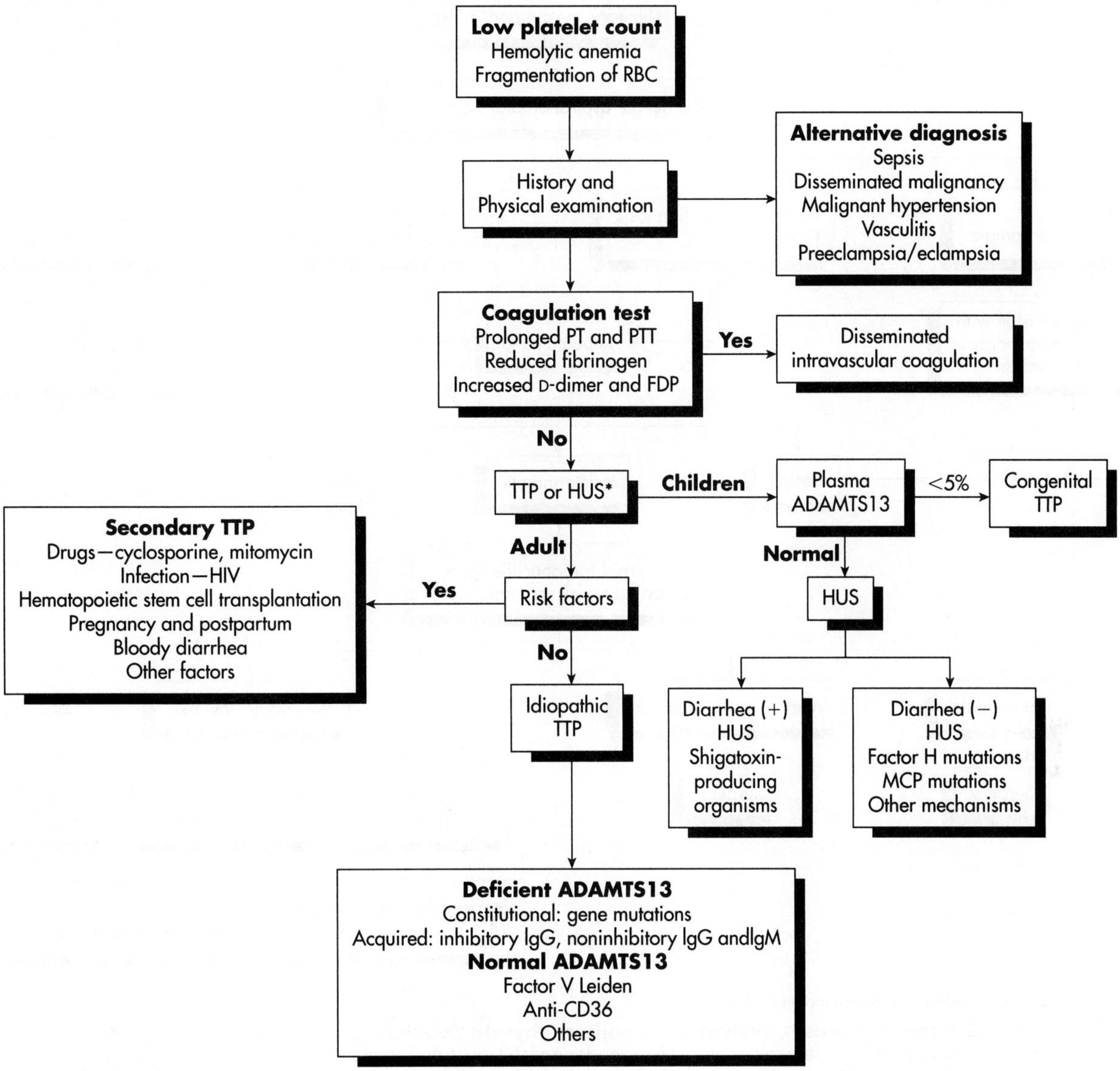

*Refer to Section I for additional information on this topic.

FIGURE 3-285 Algorithm for diagnosis of thrombotic thrombocytopenic purpura (TTP) and hemolytic-uremic syndrome (HUS). *MCP,* Membrane cofactor protein; *PT,* prothrombin time; *PTT,* partial thromboplastin time; *RBC,* red blood cell count. (From Young NS, Gerson SL, High KA [eds]: *Clinical hematology,* St Louis, 2006, Mosby.)

ICD-9CM # 241.0 Nodule, thyroid

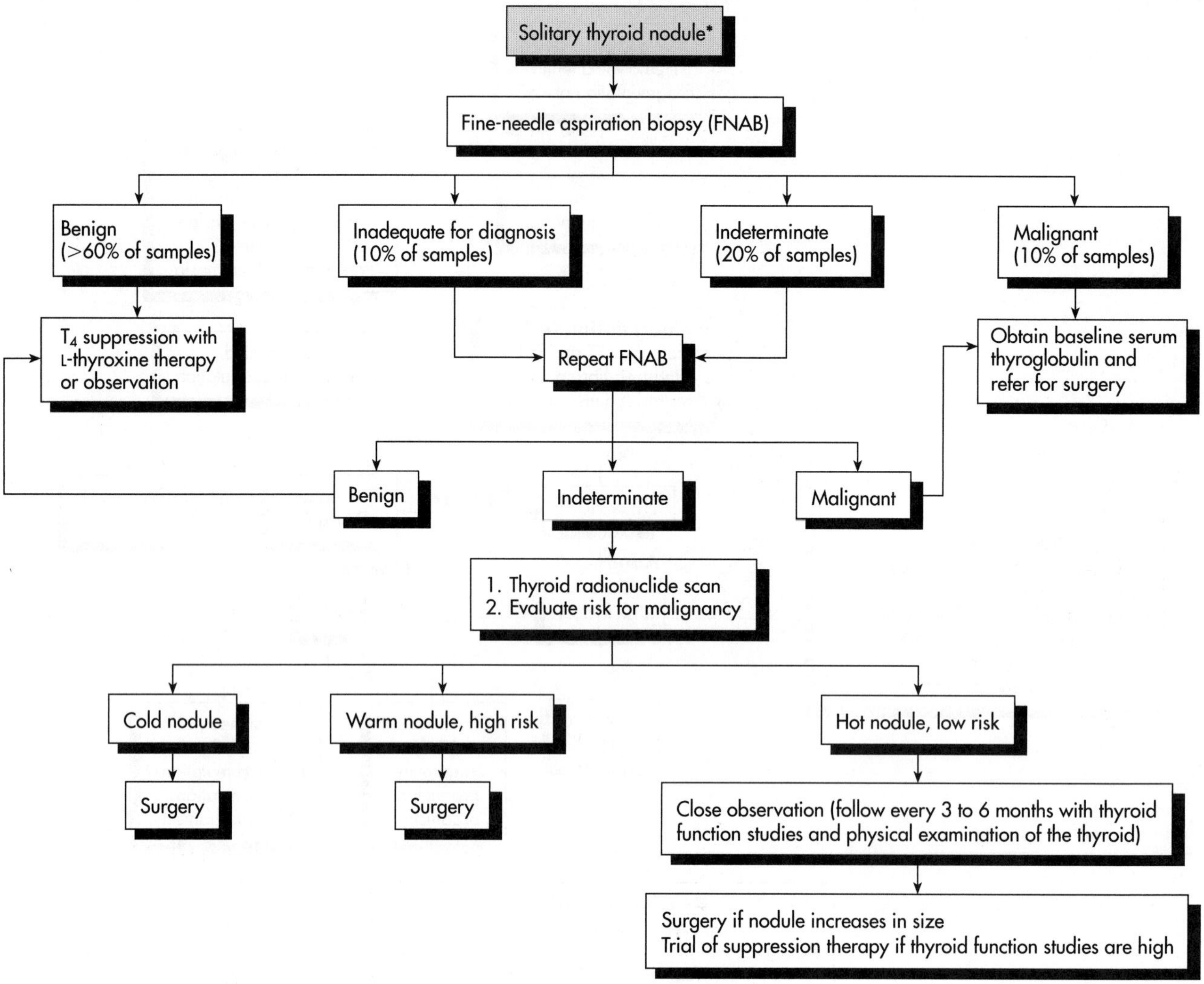

*Refer to Section I for additional information on this topic.

FIGURE 3-286 Diagnostic evaluation of solitary thyroid nodule. High risk for malignancy: nodule >2 cm, age <40 yr, male sex, regional lymphadenopathy, fixation to adjacent tissues, history of prior head and neck irradiation. (From Ferri F: *Practical guide to the care of the medical patient,* ed 7, St Louis, 2007, Mosby.)

ICD-9CM # 245.0 Acute thyroiditis

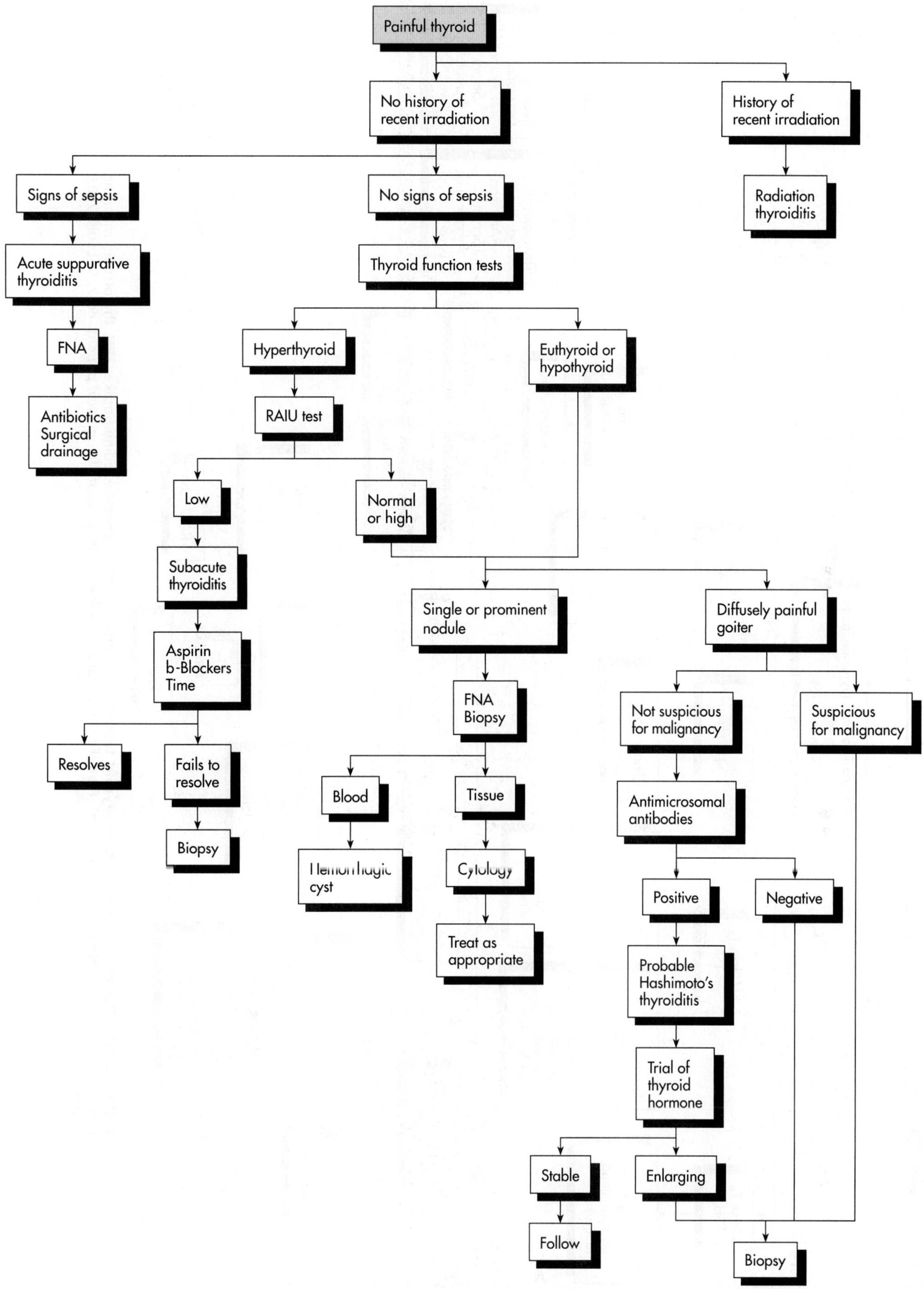

FIGURE 3-287 Painful thyroid. *FNA,* Fine-needle aspiration; *RAIU,* radioactive iodine uptake. (From Greene HL, Johnson WP, Lemcke D [eds]: *Decision making in medicine,* ed 2, St Louis, 1998, Mosby.)

THYROID TESTING

ICD-9CM # V77.0

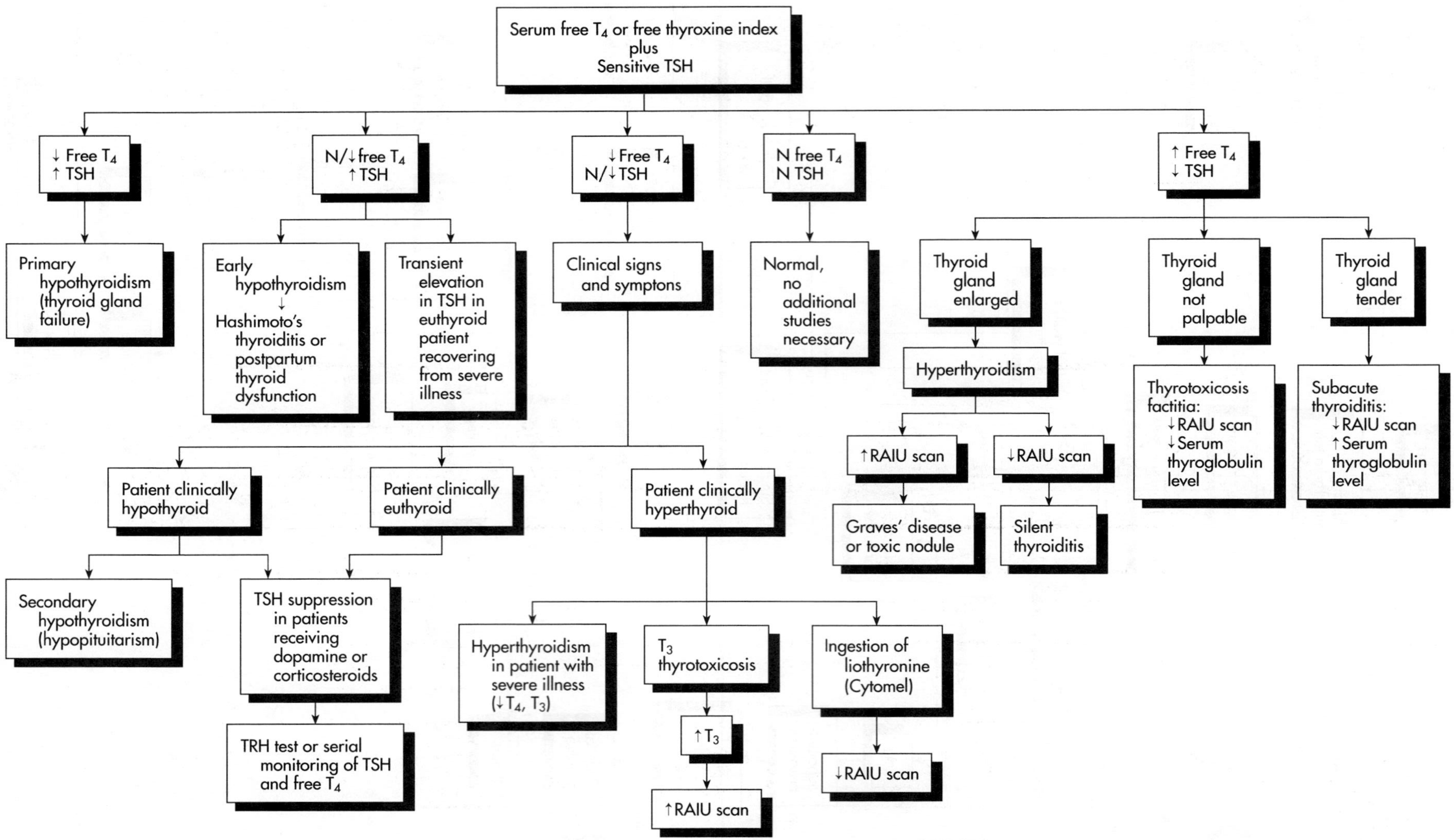

FIGURE 3-288 Diagnostic approach to thyroid testing. *N,* Normal; *RAIU,* radioactive iodine uptake; *TRH,* thyrotropin-releasing hormone; *TSH,* thyroid-stimulating hormone. (From Ferri FF: *Practical guide to the care of the medical patient,* ed 7, St Louis, 2007, Mosby.)

ICD-9CM # 388.30

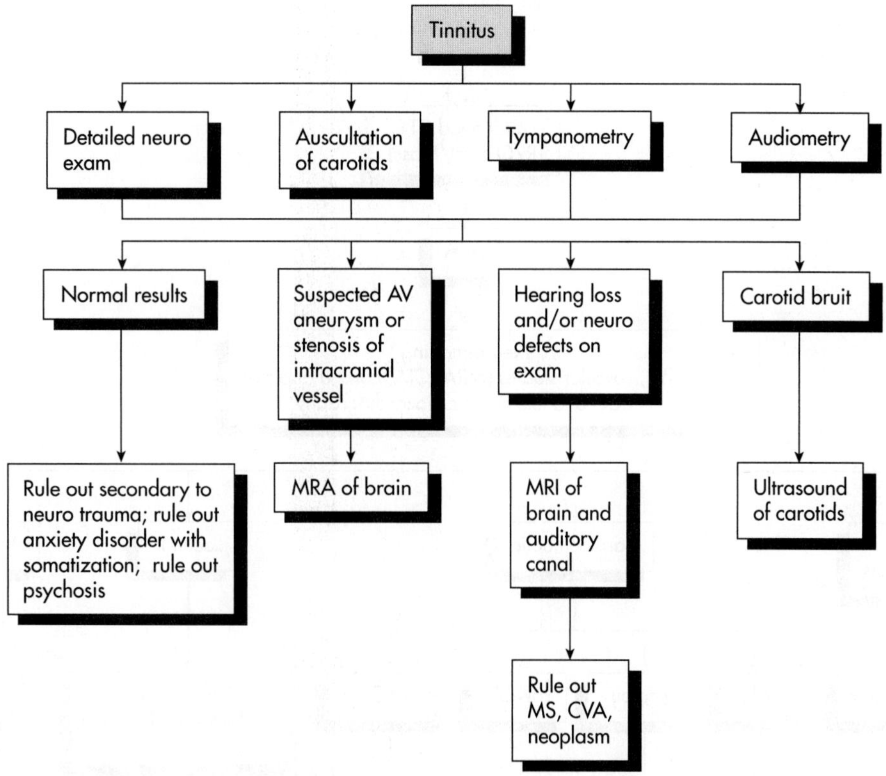

FIGURE 3-289 Tinnitus evaluation. *AV,* Atrioventricular; *CVA,* cerebrovascular accident; *MRA,* magnetic resonance angiography; *MRI,* magnetic resonance imaging; *MS,* multiple sclerosis. (From Ferri FF: *Ferri's best test: a practical guide to clinical laboratory medicine and diagnostic imaging,* ed 2, Philadelphia, 2009, Elsevier Mosby.)

BOX 3-15 Tinnitus

Diagnostic imaging	Lab evaluation
Best Test	***Best Test***
None	None
Ancillary tests	***Ancillary tests***
Carotid Doppler ultrasound	CBC
MRI of brain and auditory canals	Lipid panel
Brain MRA	

From Ferri FF: *Ferri's best test: a practical guide to clinical laboratory medicine and diagnostic imaging,* ed 2, Philadelphia, 2009, Elsevier Mosby.

CBC, Complete blood count; *MRA,* magnetic resonance angiography; *MRI,* magnetic resonance imaging.

ICD-9CM # 435.9 Unspecified transient cerebral ischemia

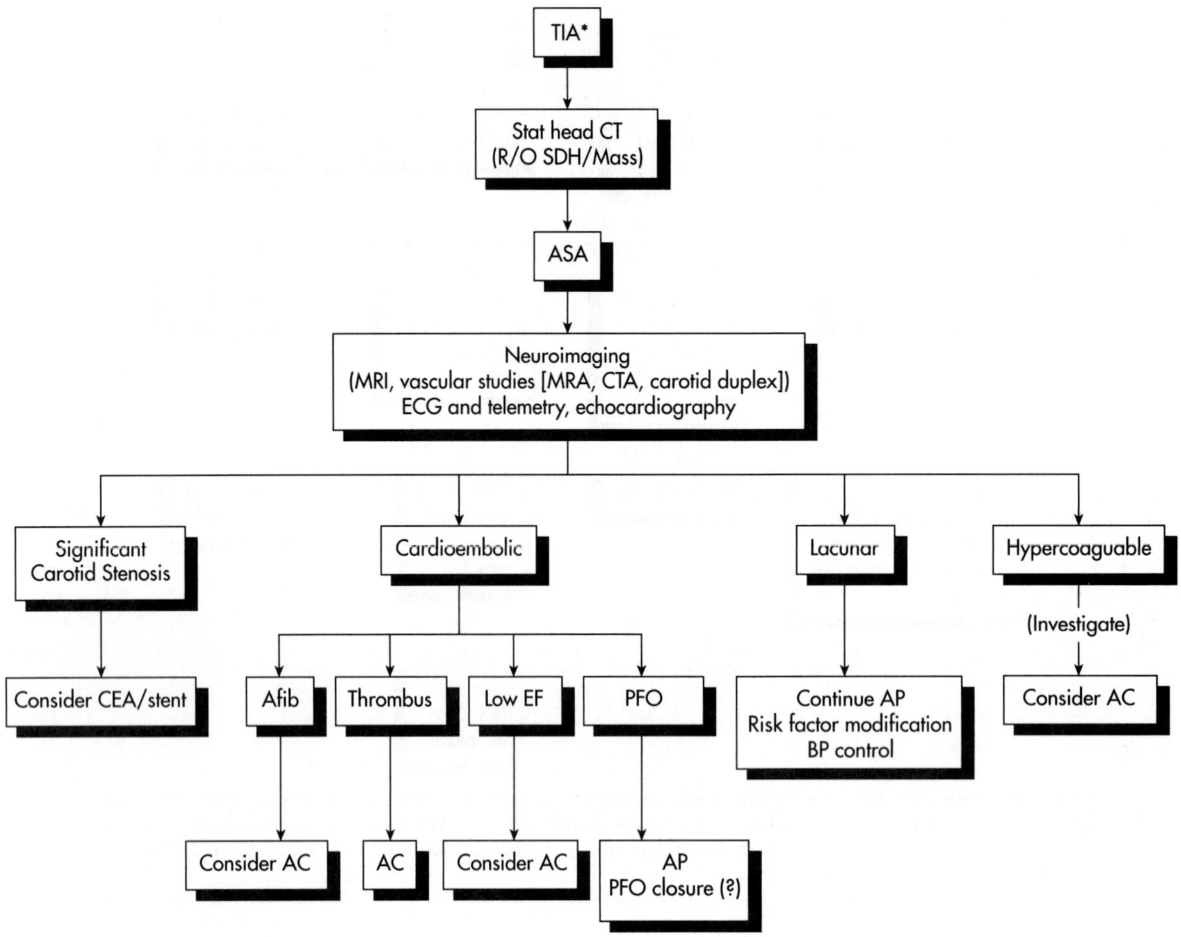

*Refer to Section I for additional information on this topic.

FIGURE 3-290 Transient ischemic attack. *AC,* Anticoagulation; *AP,* antiplatelet; *ASA,* aspirin; *BP,* blood pressure; *CEA,* carotid endarterectomy; *EF,* ejection fraction; *PFO,* patent foramen ovale; *TIA,* transient ischemic attack.

ICD-9CM # 780.09

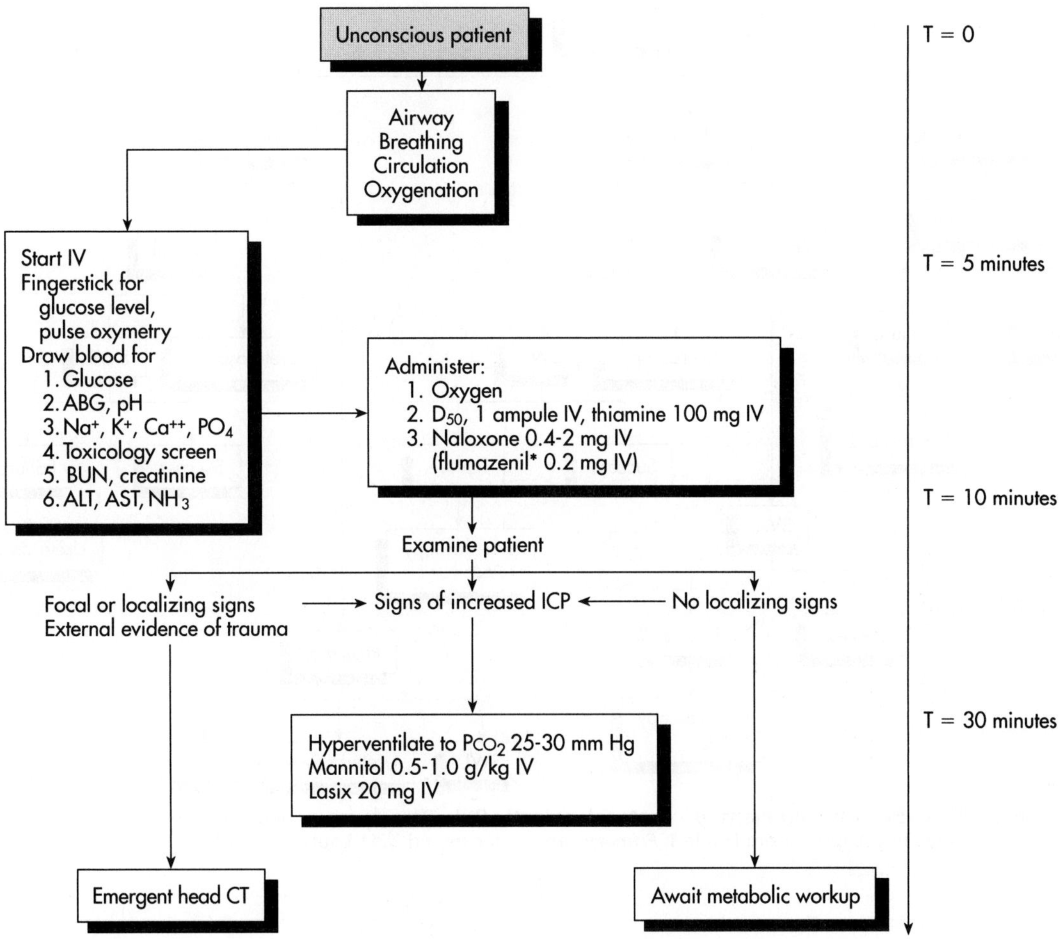

* Use of flumazenil should not be considered routine because it can precipitate seizures in certain subsets of patients.

FIGURE 3-291 Approach to the unconscious patient. *ABG,* Arterial blood gas; *ALT,* alanine aminotransferase; *AST,* aspartate aminotransferase; *BUN,* blood urea nitrogen; *CT,* computed tomography; *ICP,* intracranial pressure. (Modified from Johnson RT, Griffin JW: *Current therapy in neurologic disease,* ed 5, St Louis, 1997, Mosby.)

ICD-9CM # 592.9 Urinary calculus

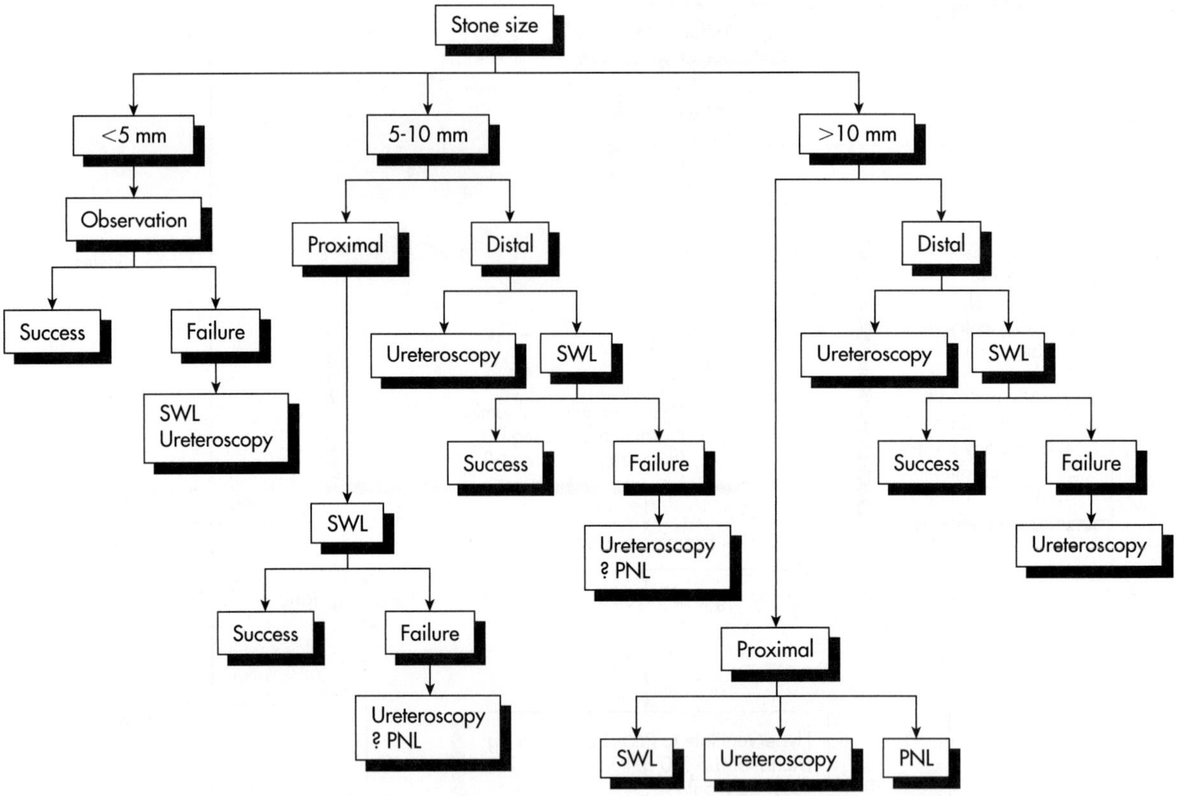

FIGURE 3-292 Management of ureteral calculi. *PNL,* Percutaneous nephrostolithotomy; *SWL,* shock wave lithotripsy. (From Noble J: *Primary care medicine,* ed 3, St Louis, 2001, Mosby.)

ICD-9CM # 788.7

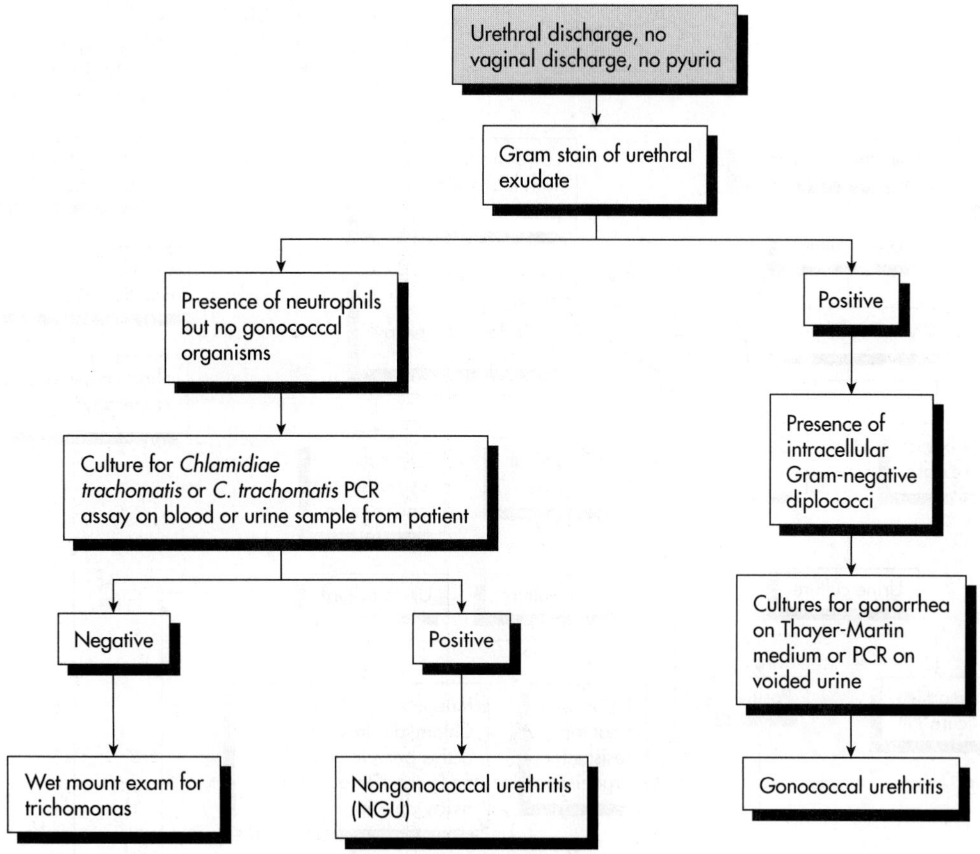

FIGURE 3-293 Urethral discharge.

ICD-9CM # 595.0 Acute cystitis
595.3 Trigonitis
595.2 Chronic cystitis
590.1 Acute pyelonephritis
590.0 Chronic pyelonephritis
590.8 Nonspecific pyelonephritis

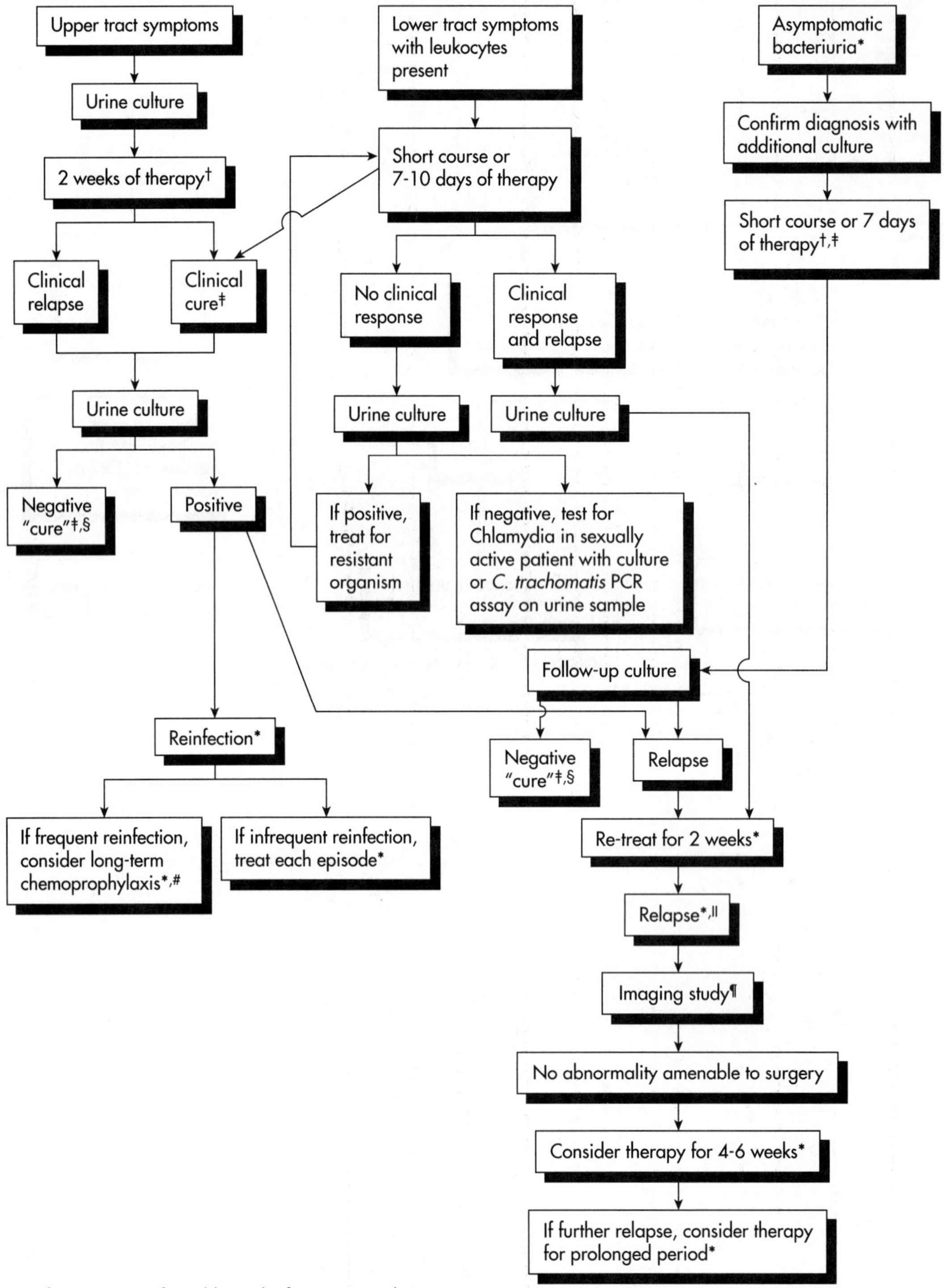

Note: Refer to Section I for additional information on this topic.

* Consider no therapy in nonpregnant adults without obstructive uropathy or symptoms of urinary tract infection.
† Consider imaging studies in all children and men with correction of significant lesions.
‡ Follow-up culture is required only in pregnancy, in children, and in adults with obstructive uropathy.
§ Obtain follow-up cultures monthly in pregnant women and at 6 weeks and 6 months in children.
|| Evaluate men for chronic bacterial prostatitis.
¶ Delay 2 months postpartum in pregnant women.
# Consider imaging studies after three to four reinfections in women.

FIGURE 3-294 Approach to the management of urinary tract infection. (Modified from Mandell GL: *Mandell, Douglas, and Bennett's principles and practice of infectious diseases,* ed 6, New York, 2005, Churchill Livingstone.)

ICD-9CM # 599.6

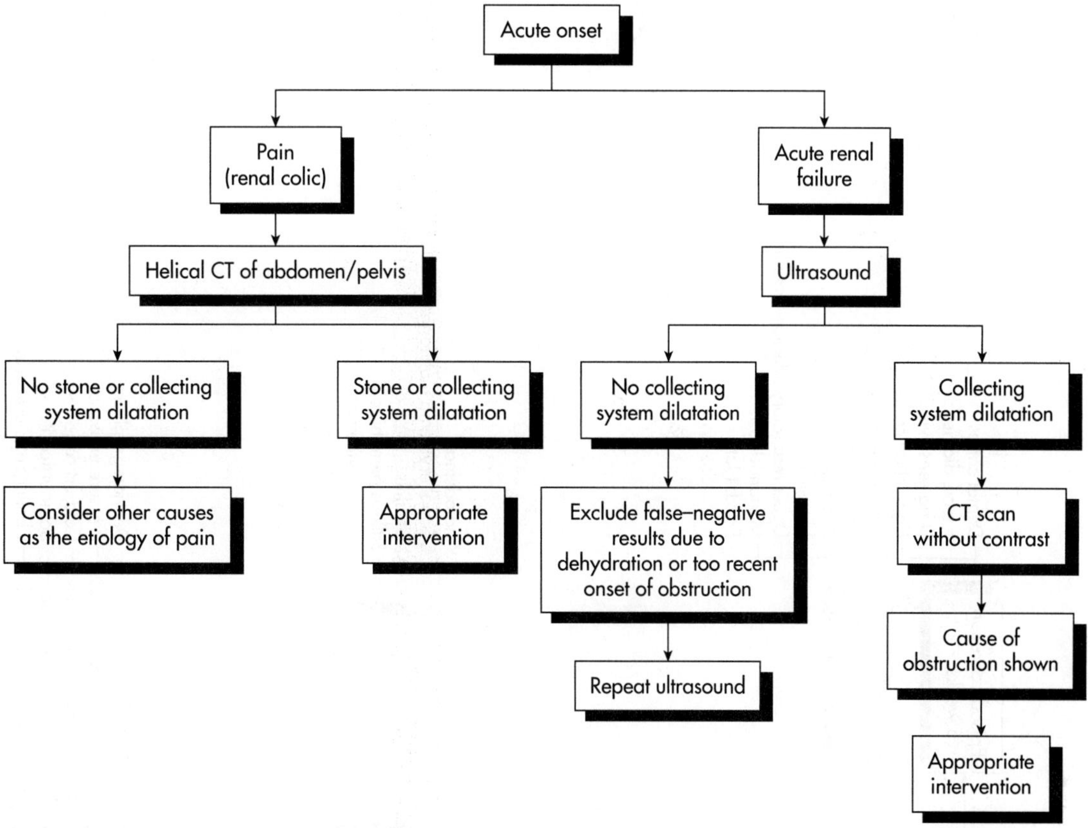

FIGURE 3-295 Scheme of a diagnostic approach to urinary tract obstruction. *CT,* Computed tomography; *IVP,* intravenous pyelography; *KUB,* kidney, ureter, bladder (a flat film of the abdomen without contrast medium). (Modified from Goldman L, Ausiello D [eds]: *Cecil textbook of medicine,* ed 23, Philadelphia, 2008, WB Saunders.)

BOX 3-16 **Diagnostic Tests Used in Obstructive Uropathy**

Upper Urinary Tract Obstruction
Sonography (ultrasound)
Plain films of the abdomen (KUB)
Excretory or intravenous pyelography (very rarely needed)
Retrograde pyelography
Isotopic renography
Computed tomography (helical CT)
Magnetic resonance imaging
Pressure flow studies (the Whitaker test)

Lower Urinary Tract Obstruction
Some of the tests listed above
Cystoscopy
Voiding cystourethrogram
Retrograde urethrography
Urodynamic tests
- Debimetry
- Cystometrography
- Electromyography
- Urethral pressure profile

KUP, Kidneys, ureter, bladder.

URTICARIA, EVALUATION

ICD-9CM # 708.8 Other unspecified urticaria

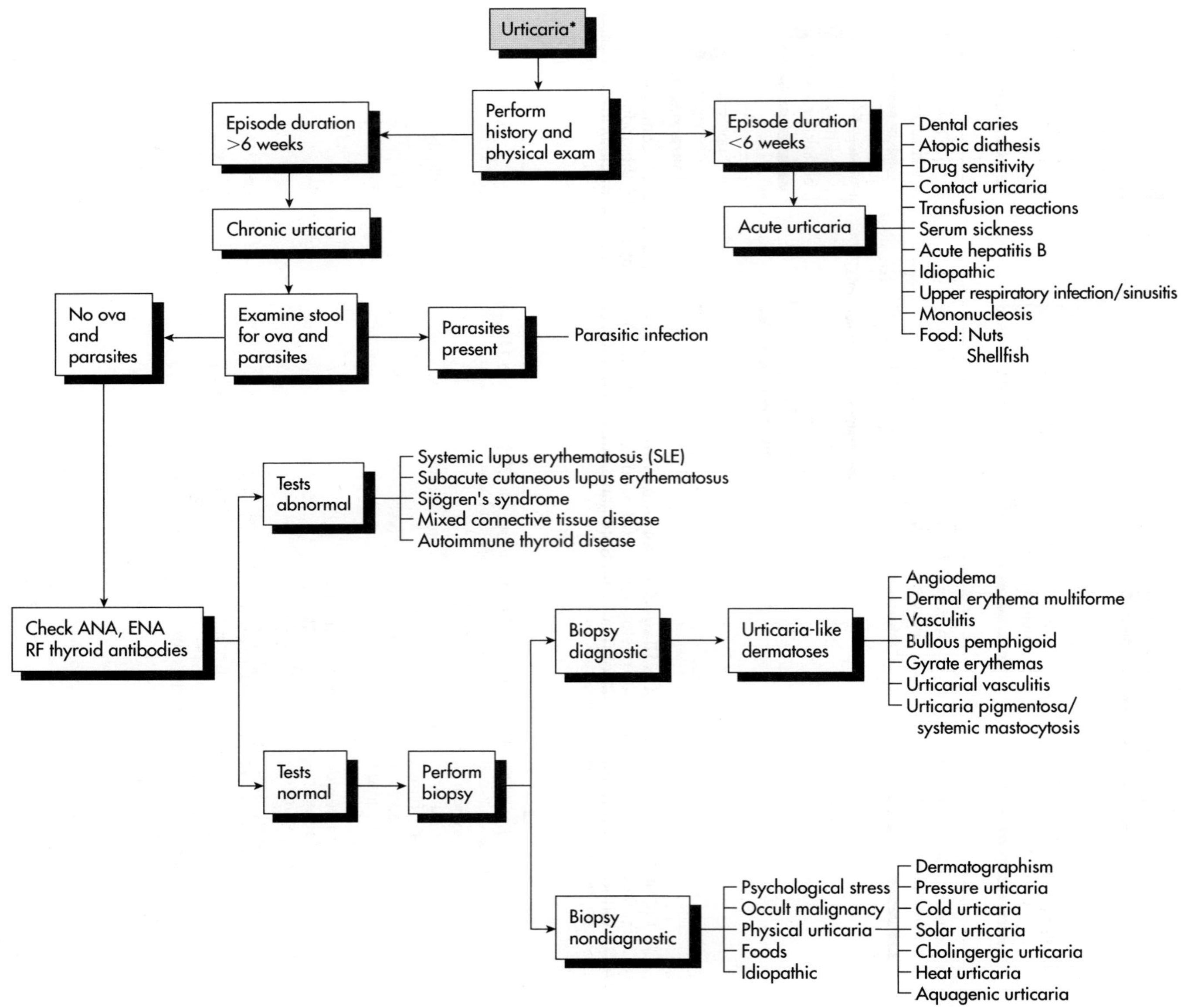

*Refer to Section I for additional information on this topic.

FIGURE 3-296 Evaluation of urticaria. *ANA,* Antibody to nuclear antigens; *ENA,* extractable nuclear antigens; *RF,* rheumatoid factor. (From Healy PM, Jacobson EJ: *Common medical diagnoses,* ed 3, Philadelphia, 2000, WB Saunders.)

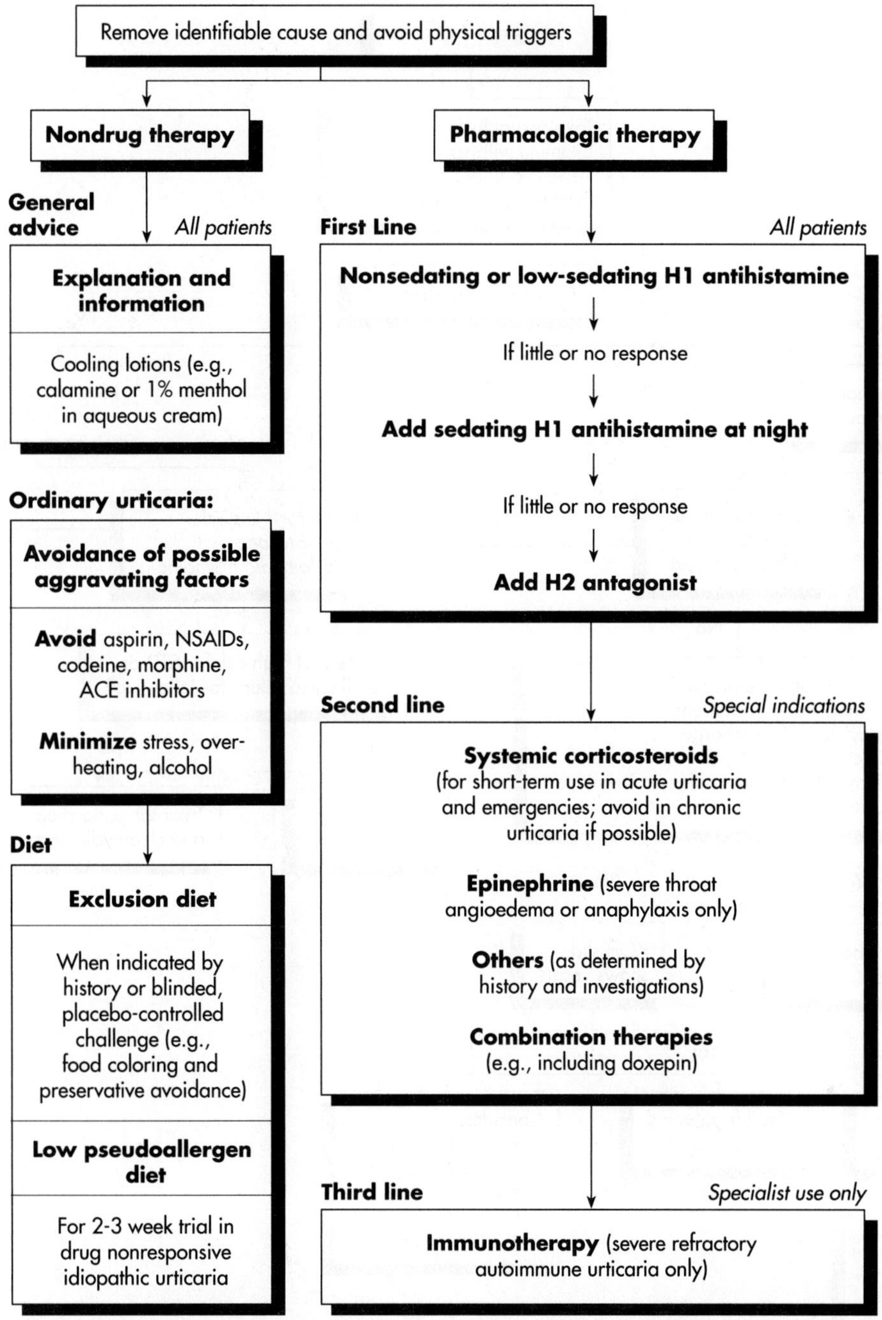

FIGURE 3-297 Management of ordinary and physical chronic uticaria. *ACE,* Angiotensin-converting enzyme; *NSAID,* nonsteroidal anti-inflammatory drug. (From Bolognia JL, Mascaro JM, Mancini AJ, Salasche SJ, Saurat JH, Stingl G: *Dermatology,* ed 2, St Louis, 2008, Mosby.)

ICD-9CM # 623.5

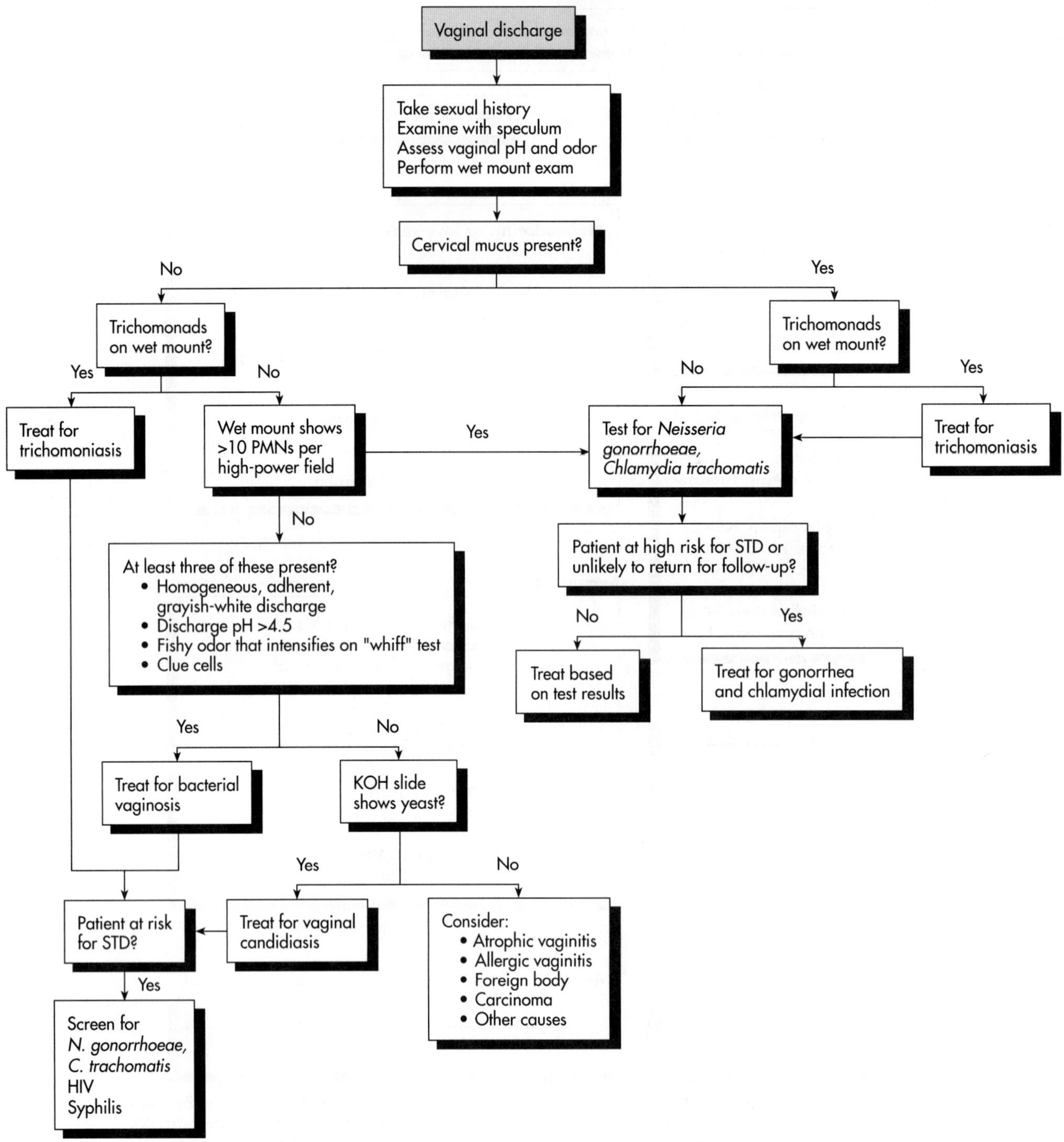

FIGURE 3-298 Evaluation of vaginal discharge. *HIV,* Human immunodeficiency virus; *KOH,* potassium hydroxide; *PMN,* polymorphonuclear leukocyte; *STD,* sexually transmitted disease. (From Fox KK, Behets FMT: *Postgrad Med* 98:87, 1995.)

ICD-9CM # 618.0

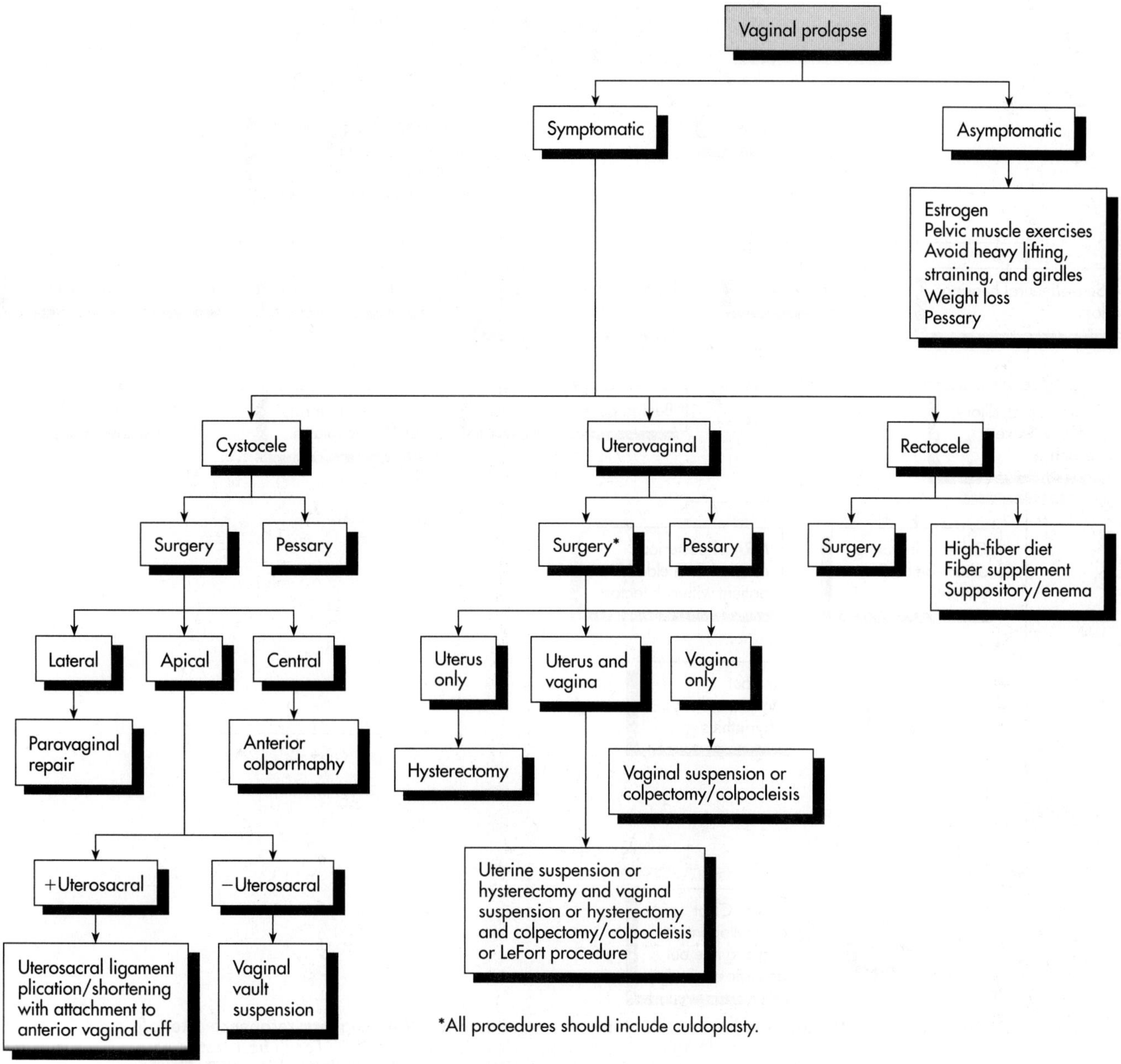

FIGURE 3-299 Management of vaginal prolapse. (From Zuspan FP [ed]: *Handbook of obstetrics, gynecology, and primary care,* St Louis, 1998, Mosby.)

ICD-9CM # 780.4

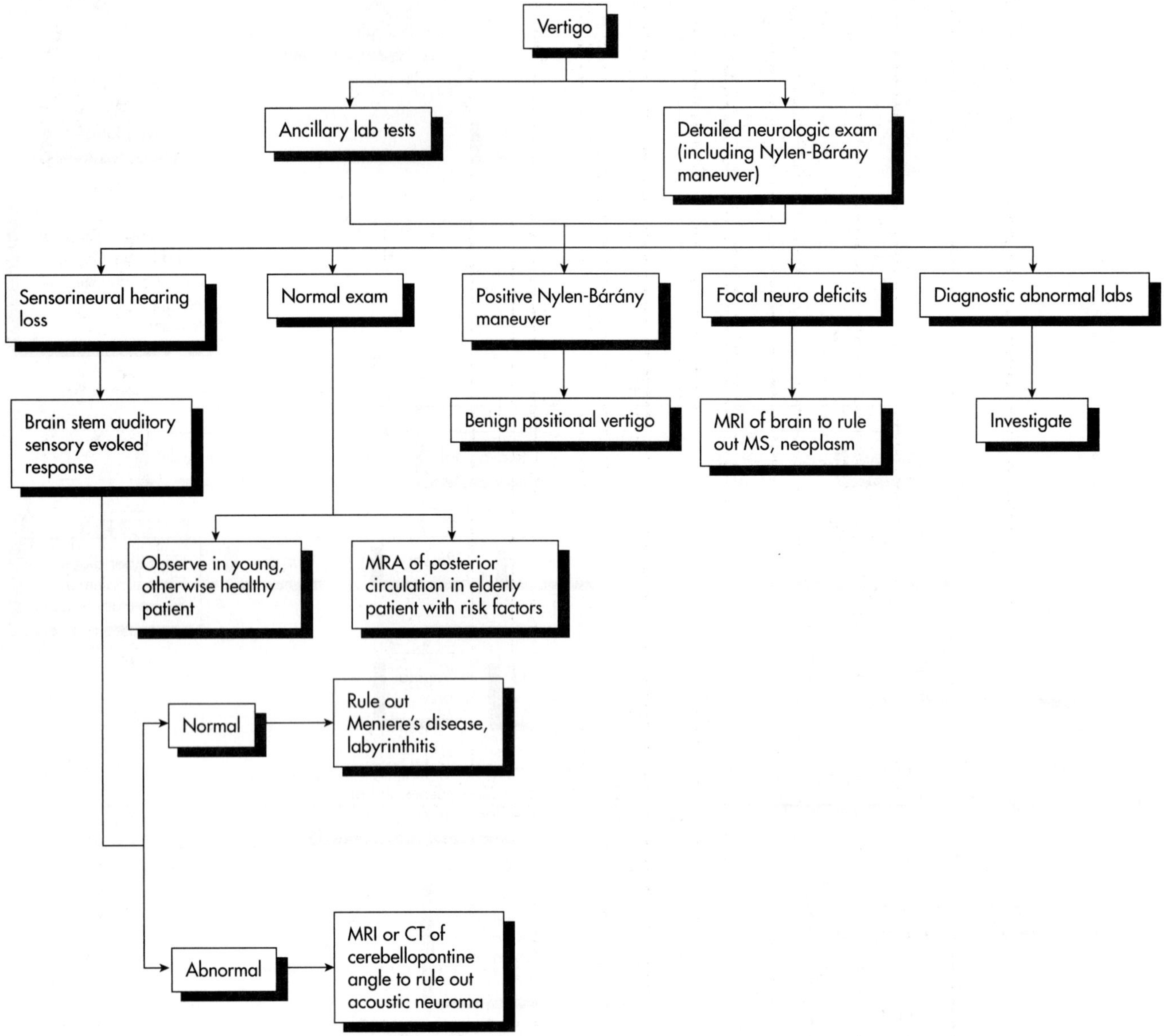

FIGURE 3-300 Vertigo evaluation. *CT,* Computed tomography; *MRA,* magnetic resonance arteriography; *MRI,* magnetic resonance imaging; *MS,* multiple sclerosis. (From Ferri FF: *Ferri's best test: a practical guide to clinical laboratory medicine and diagnostic imaging,* ed 2, Philadelphia, 2009, Elsevier Mosby.)

BOX 3-17 **Vertigo**

Diagnostic imaging
Best test
MRI of brain
Ancillary tests
MRA of posterior circulation
CT of cerebellopontine region if MRI is contraindicated

Lab evaluation
Best test
None
Ancillary tests
CBC with differential
Serum glucose, creatinine, ALT, electrolytes

From Ferri FF: *Ferri's best test: a practical guide to clinical laboratory medicine and diagnostic imaging,* ed 2, Philadelphia, 2009, Elsevier Mosby.

Alt, Alanine aminotransferase; *CBC,* complete blood count; *CT,* computed tomography; *MRA,* magnetic resonance arteriography; *MRI,* magnetic resonance imaging.

ICD-9CM # 184.4 Vulvar neoplasm

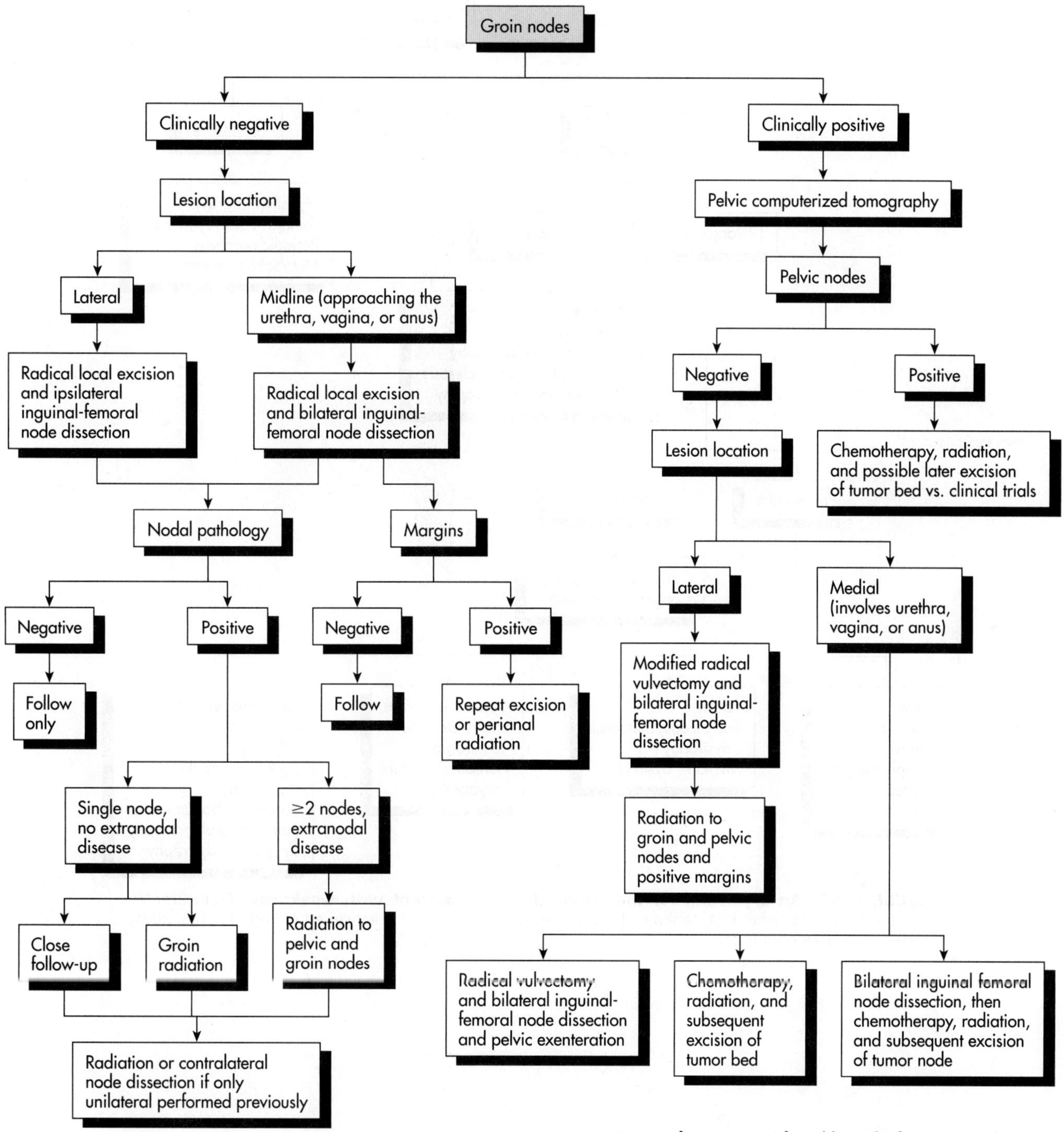

Note: Refer to Section I for additional information on this topic.

FIGURE 3-301 Treatment algorithm for management of patients with vulvar cancer. (From Copeland LJ: *Textbook of gynecology,* ed 2, Philadelphia, 2000, WB Saunders.)

ICD-9CM # 780.79

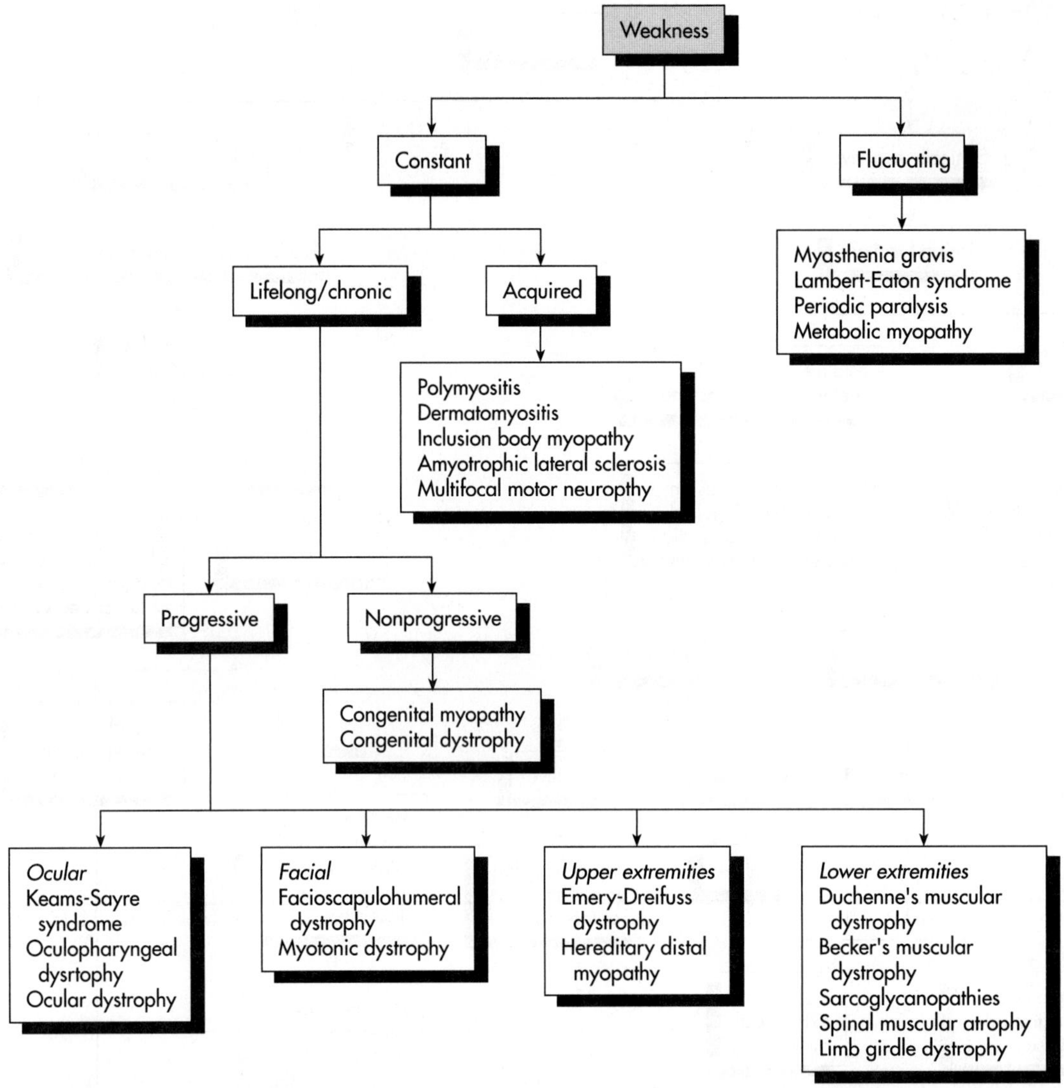

FIGURE 3-302 An algorithm for the approach to the patient with weakness. (From Bradley WG, Daroff RB, Fenichel GM, Jankovic J [eds]: *Neurology in clinical practice,* ed 4, Philadelphia, 2004, Butterworth Heinemann.)

WEIGHT GAIN

ICD-9CM # 783.1 Abnormal weight gain
278.00 Obesity

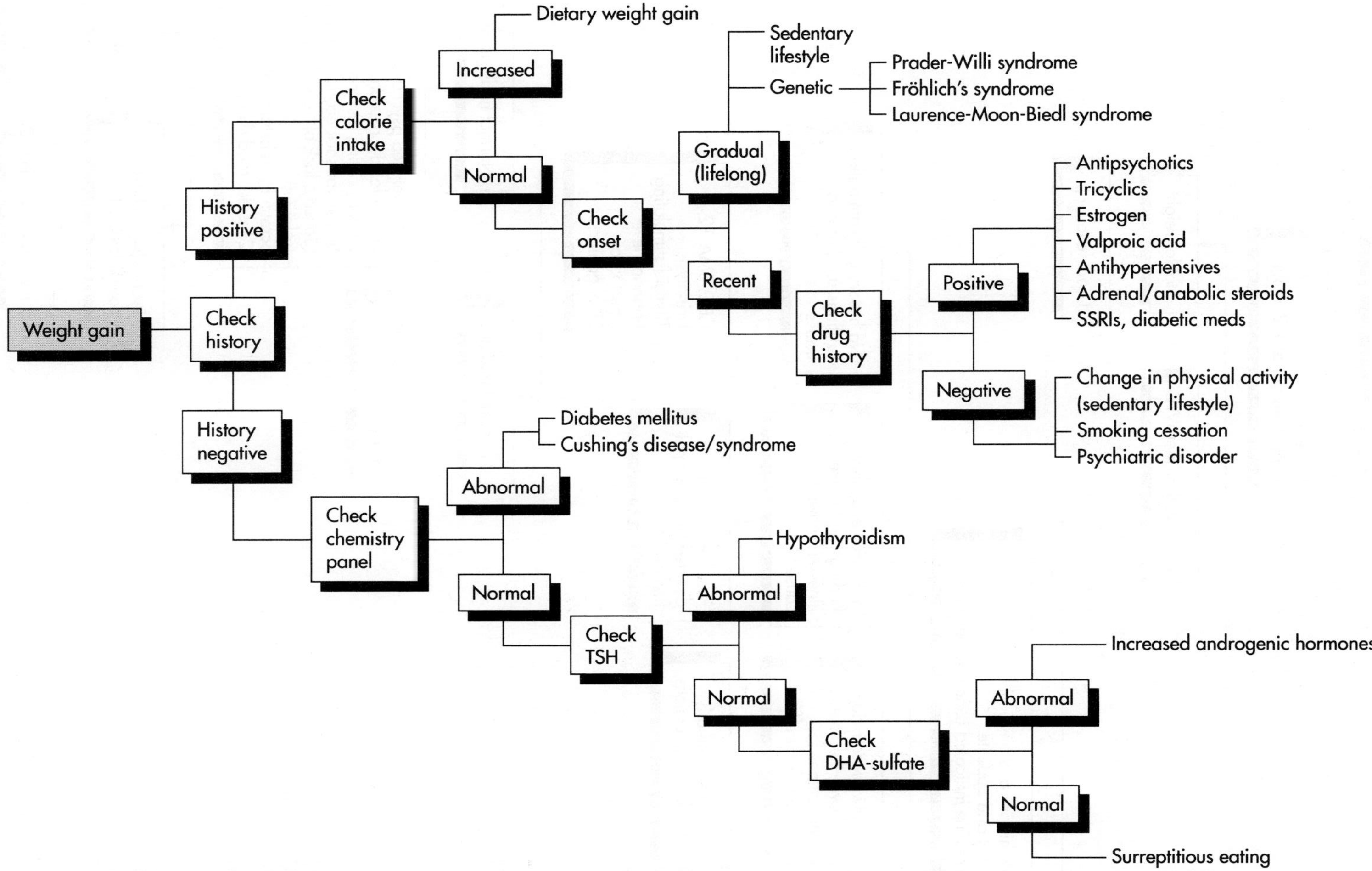

FIGURE 3-303 Weight gain. *DHA,* Dehydroepiandrosterone; *SSRIs,* serotonin reuptake inhibitors; *TSH,* thyroid-stimulating hormone. (Modified from Healey PM: *Common medical diagnosis: an algorithmic approach,* ed 3, Philadelphia, 2000, WB Saunders.)

ICD-9CM # 783.21

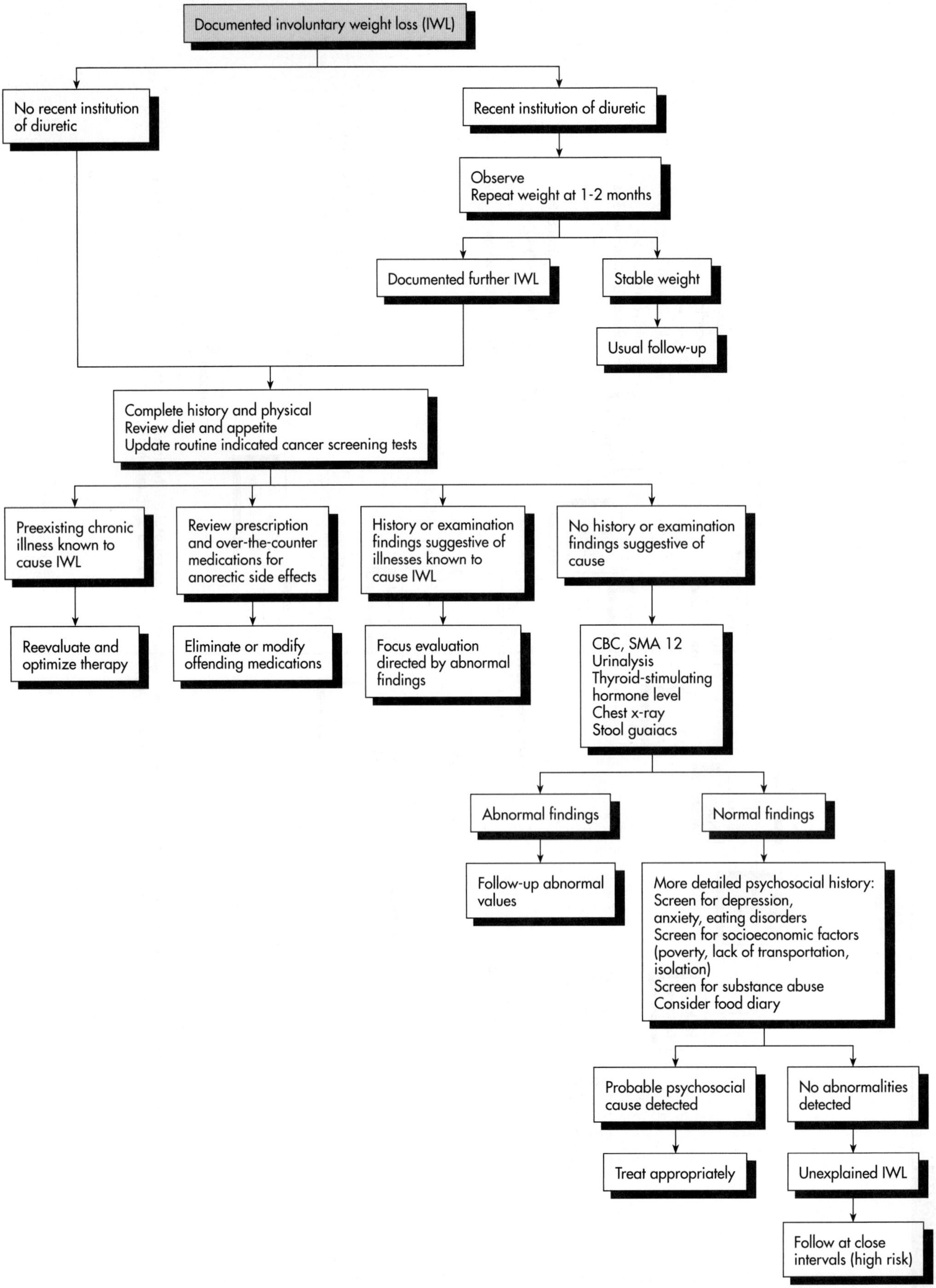

FIGURE 3-304 Involuntary weight loss. *CBC,* Complete blood count. (From Greene HL, Johnson WP, Lemcke D [eds]: *Decision making in medicine,* ed 2, St Louis, 1998, Mosby.)

Section IV

Laboratory Tests and Interpretation of Results

This section contains more than 200 commonly performed laboratory tests. In general, the tests are approached with the following format:

1. Laboratory test.
2. Normal range in adult patients. Normal values are given using the present (traditional) reference interval, followed by the Système Internationale (SI) reference interval, the conversion factor (CF), and the suggested minimum increment (SMI).
3. Common abnormalities, such as positive test, increased or decreased value.
4. Causes of abnormal result.

The normal ranges may differ slightly, depending on the laboratory. The reader should be aware of the "normal range" of the particular laboratory performing the test. Every attempt has been made to present current laboratory test data, with emphasis on practical considerations.

ACE LEVEL; *see* ANGIOTENSIN-CONVERTING ENZYME

ACETONE (serum or plasma)

Normal: Negative
Elevated in: DKA, starvation, isopropanol ingestion

ACETYLCHOLINE RECEPTOR (AChR) ANTIBODY

Normal: <0.03 nmol/L
Elevated in: Myasthenia gravis. Changes in AChR concentration correlate with the clinical severity of myasthenia gravis following therapy and during therapy with prednisone and immunosuppressants. False-positive AChR antibody results may be found in patients with Eaton-Lambert syndrome.

ACID-BASE REFERENCE VALUES; *see* Tables 4-1 and 4-2

ACID PHOSPHATASE (serum)

Normal range: 0-5.5 U/L (0-90 nkat/L [CF: 16.67; SMI: 2 nkat/L])
Elevated in: Carcinoma of prostate, other neoplasms (breast, bone), Paget's disease, osteogenesis imperfecta, malignant invasion of bone, Gaucher's disease, multiple myeloma, myeloproliferative disorders, benign prostatic hypertrophy, prostatic palpation or surgery, hyperparathyroidism, liver disease, chronic renal failure, idiopathic thrombocytopenic purpura, bronchitis

ACID SERUM TEST; *see* HAM TEST

TABLE 4-1 **Commonly Used Acid-Base Reference Values for Arterial and Venous Plasma or Serum (Averaged from Various Sources)**

	ARTERIAL		VENOUS	
	Conventional Units	**SI Units***	**Conventional Units**	**SI Units***
pH	7.40 (7.35-7.45)	7.40 (7.35-7.45)	7.37 (7.32-7.42)	7.37 (7.32-7.42)
P_{CO_2}	40 mm Hg (35-45)	5.33 kPa (4.67-6.10)	45 mm Hg (45-50)	6.10 kPa (5.33-6.67)
P_{O_2}	80-100 mm Hg	10.66-13.33 kPa	40 mm Hg (37-43)	5.33 kPa (4.93-5.73)
HCO_3 (CO_2 combining power)	24 mEq/L (20-28)	24 mmol/L (20-28)	26 mEq/L (22-30)	26 mmol/L (22-30)
CO_2 content	25 mEq/L (22-28)	25 mmol/L (22-28)	27 mEq/L (24-30)	27 mmol/L (24-30)

From Ravel R: *Clinical laboratory medicine,* ed 6, St Louis, 1995, Mosby.
*International system.

TABLE 4-2 **Summary of Laboratory Findings in Primary Uncomplicated Respiratory and Metabolic Acid-Base Disorders***

Disorder	P_{CO_2}	pH	Base Excess
Acute primary respiratory hypoactivity (respiratory acidosis)	Increase	Decrease	Normal/positive
Acute primary respiratory hyperactivity (respiratory alkalosis)	Decrease	Increase	Normal/negative
Uncompensated metabolic acidosis	Normal	Decrease	Negative
Uncompensated metabolic alkalosis	Normal	Increase	Positive
Partially compensated metabolic acidosis	Decrease	Decrease	Negative
Partially compensated metabolic alkalosis	Increase	Increase	Positive
Chronic primary respiratory hypoactivity (compensated respiratory acidosis)	Increase	Normal	Positive
Fully compensated metabolic alkalosis	Increase	Normal	Positive
Chronic primary respiratory hyperactivity (compensated respiratory alkalosis)	Decrease	Normal	Negative
Fully compensated metabolic acidosis	Decrease	Normal	Negative

From Ravel R: *Clinical laboratory medicine,* ed 6, St Louis, 1995, Mosby.
*Base excess results refer to negative (−) values more than 22 and positive (+) values more than +2.

ACTIVATED PARTIAL THROMBOPLASTIN TIME (APTT, aPTT); *see* PARTIAL THROMBOPLASTIN TIME

ALANINE AMINOTRANSFERASE (ALT, SGPT)

Normal range: 0-35 U/L (0.058 μkat/L [CF: 0.02 μkat/L])
Elevated in: Liver disease (hepatitis, cirrhosis, Reye's syndrome), hepatic congestion, infectious mononucleosis, myocardial infarction, myocarditis, severe muscle trauma, dermatomyositis/polymyositis, muscular dystrophy, drugs (antibiotics, narcotics, antihypertensive agents, heparin, labetalol, statins, NSAIDs, amiodarone, chlorpromazine, phenytoin), malignancy, renal and pulmonary infarction, convulsions, eclampsia, shock liver

ALBUMIN (serum)

Normal range: 4-6 g/dl (40-60 g/L [CF: 10; SMI: 1 g/L])
Elevated in: Dehydration (relative increase)
Decreased in: Liver disease, nephrotic syndrome, poor nutritional status, rapid IV hydration, protein-losing enteropathies (inflammatory bowel disease), severe burns, neoplasia, chronic inflammatory diseases, pregnancy, oral contraceptives, prolonged immobilization, lymphomas, hypervitaminosis A, chronic glomerulonephritis

ALDOLASE (serum)

Normal range: 0-6 U/L (0-100 nkat/L [CF: 16.67; SMI: 20 nkat/L])
Elevated in: Muscular dystrophy, rhabdomyolysis, dermatomyositis/polymyositis, trichinosis, acute hepatitis and other liver diseases, myocardial infarction, prostatic carcinoma, hemorrhagic pancreatitis, gangrene, delirium tremens, burns
Decreased in: Loss of muscle mass, late stages of muscular dystrophy

ALDOSTERONE

Normal range: Recumbent: 50-150 ng/L
Upright: 150-300 ng/L
(Highest levels in neonates, decreasing over time to adult levels)
Elevated in: Primary aldosteronism, secondary aldosteronism, pseudoprimary aldosteronism
Decreased in: Patient with hypertension: diabetes mellitus, Turner's syndrome, acute alcohol intoxication, excess secretion of deoxycorticosterone, corticosterone, and 18-hydroxycorticosterone
Patient without hypertension: Addison's disease, hypoaldosteronism resulting from renin deficiency, isolated aldosterone deficiency

ALKALINE PHOSPHATASE (serum)

Normal range: 30-120 U/L (0.5-2 μkat/L [CF: 0.01667; SMI: 0.1 μkat/L])
Elevated in:
LIVER AND BILIARY TRACT ORIGIN
Extrahepatic bile duct obstruction
Intrahepatic biliary obstruction
Liver cell acute injury
Liver passive congestion
Drug-induced liver cell dysfunction
Space-occupying lesions
Primary biliary cirrhosis
Sepsis
BONE ORIGIN (OSTEOBLAST HYPERACTIVITY)
Physiologic (rapid) bone growth (childhood and adolescent)
Metastatic tumor with osteoblastic reaction
Fracture healing
Paget's disease of bone
CAPILLARY ENDOTHELIAL ORIGIN
Granulation tissue formation (active)
PLACENTAL ORIGIN
Pregnancy
Some parenteral albumin preparations
OTHER
Thyrotoxicosis
Benign transient hyperphosphatasemia
Primary hyperparathyroidism
Decreased in: Hypothyroidism, pernicious anemia, hypophosphatemia, hypervitaminosis D, malnutrition

ALPHA-1-FETOPROTEIN (serum); *see* α-1 FETOPROTEIN

ALT; *see* ALANINE AMINOTRANSFERASE

ALUMINUM (serum)

Normal range: 0-6 ng/ml
Elevated in: Chronic renal failure on dialysis, parenteral nutrition, industrial exposure

AMMONIA (serum)

Normal range: 10-80 μg/dl (5-50 μmol/L [CF: 0.5872; SMI: 5 μmol/L])
Elevated in: Hepatic failure, hepatic encephalopathy, Reye's syndrome, portacaval shunt, drugs (diuretics, polymyxin B, methicillin)
Decreased in: Drugs (neomycin, lactulose, tetracycline), renal failure

AMYLASE (serum)

Normal range: 0-130 U/L (0-2.17 μkat/L [CF: 0.01667; SMI: 0.01 μkat/L])
Elevated in: Acute pancreatitis, pancreatic neoplasm, abscess, pseudocyst, ascites, macroamylasemia, perforated peptic ulcer, intestinal obstruction, intestinal infarction, acute cholecystitis, appendicitis, ruptured ectopic pregnancy, salivary gland inflammation, peritonitis, burns, diabetic ketoacidosis, renal insufficiency, drugs (morphine), carcinomatosis (of lung, esophagus, ovary), acute ethanol ingestion, mumps, prostate tumors, post–endoscopic retrograde cholangiopancreatography, bulimia, anorexia nervosa
Decreased in: Advanced chronic pancreatitis, hepatic necrosis, cystic fibrosis

AMYLASE, URINE; *see* URINE AMYLASE

ANA; *see* ANTINUCLEAR ANTIBODY

ANCA; *see* ANTINEUTROPHIL CYTOPLASMIC ANTIBODY

ANGIOTENSIN-CONVERTING ENZYME (ACE level)

Normal range: <40 nmol/ml/min (<670 nkat/L [CF: 16.67; SMI: 10 nkat/L])
Elevated in: Sarcoidosis, primary biliary cirrhosis, alcoholic liver disease, hyperthyroidism, hyperparathyroidism, diabetes mellitus, amyloidosis, multiple myeloma, lung disease (asbestosis, silicosis, berylliosis, allergic alveolitis, coccidioidomycosis), Gaucher's disease, leprosy

ANION GAP

Normal range: 9-14 mEq/L
Elevated in: Lactic acidosis, ketoacidosis (diabetes, alcoholic starvation), uremia (chronic renal failure), ingestion of toxins (paraldehyde, methanol, salicylates, ethylene glycol), hyperosmolar nonketotic coma, antibiotics (carbenicillin)
Decreased in: Hypoalbuminemia, severe hypermagnesemia, IgG myeloma, lithium toxicity, laboratory error (falsely decreased sodium or overestimation of bicarbonate or chloride), hypercalcemia of parathyroid origin, antibiotics (e.g., polymyxin)

ANTICARDIOLIPIN ANTIBODY (ACA)
Normal range: Negative: Test includes detection of IgG, IgM, and IgA antibody to phospholipid, cardiolipin
Present in: Antiphospholipid antibody syndrome, chronic hepatitis C

ANTICOAGULANT; *see* CIRCULATING ANTICOAGULANT

ANTI-DNA
Normal range: Absent
Present in: Systemic lupus erythematosus, chronic active hepatitis, infectious mononucleosis, biliary cirrhosis

ANTIGLOMERULAR BASEMENT ANTIBODY; *see* GLOMERULAR BASEMENT MEMBRANE ANTIBODY

ANTIMITOCHONDRIAL ANTIBODY
Normal range: <1:20 titer
Elevated in: Primary biliary cirrhosis (85% to 95%), chronic active hepatitis (25% to 30%), cryptogenic cirrhosis (25% to 30%)

ANTINEUTROPHIL CYTOPLASMIC ANTIBODY (ANCA)
Positive test: Cytoplasmic pattern (cANCA): positive in Wegener's granulomatosis
Perinuclear pattern (pANCA): positive in inflammatory bowel disease, primary biliary cirrhosis, primary sclerosing cholangitis, autoimmune chronic active hepatitis, crescenteric glomerulonephritis

ANTINUCLEAR ANTIBODY (ANA)
Normal range: <1:20 titer
Positive test: Systemic lupus erythematosus (more significant if titer >1:160), drugs (phenytoin, ethosuximide, primidone, methyldopa, hydralazine, carbamazepine, penicillin, procainamide, chlorpromazine, griseofulvin, thiazides), chronic active hepatitis, age over 60 years (particularly age over 80 years), rheumatoid arthritis, scleroderma, mixed connective tissue disease, necrotizing vasculitis, Sjögren's syndrome, tuberculosis, pulmonary interstitial fibrosis. Table 4-3 describes diseases associated with ANA subtypes. Fig. 4-1 illustrates various fluorescent ANA test patterns.

ANTI-RNP ANTIBODY; *see* EXTRACTABLE NUCLEAR ANTIGEN

ANTI-SM (ANTI-SMITH) ANTIBODY; *see* EXTRACTABLE NUCLEAR ANTIGEN

ANTI-SMOOTH MUSCLE ANTIBODY; *see* SMOOTH MUSCLE ANTIBODY

ANTISTREPTOLYSIN O TITER (Streptozyme, ASLO titer)
Normal range for adults: <160 Todd units
Elevated in: Streptococcal upper airway infection, acute rheumatic fever, acute glomerulonephritis, increased levels of β-lipoprotein
NOTE: A fourfold increase in titer between acute and convalescent specimens is diagnostic of streptococcal upper airway infection regardless of the initial titer.

ANTITHROMBIN III
Normal range: 81% to 120% of normal activity; 17-30 mg/dl
Decreased in: Hereditary deficiency of antithrombin III, disseminated intravascular coagulation, pulmonary embolism, cirrhosis, thrombolytic therapy, chronic liver failure, postsurgery, third trimester of pregnancy, oral contraceptives, nephrotic syndrome, IV heparin >3 days, sepsis, acute leukemia, carcinoma, thrombophlebitis
Elevated in: Warfarin drugs, post–myocardial infarction

ARTERIAL BLOOD GASES
Normal range: Po_2: 75-100 mm Hg
Pco_2: 35-45 mm Hg
HCO_3: 24-28 mEq/L
pH: 7.35-7.45
Abnormal values: Acid-base disturbances (see the following)
METABOLIC ACIDOSIS
Metabolic acidosis with increased AG (AG acidosis)
Lactic acidosis
Ketoacidosis (diabetes mellitus, alcoholic ketoacidosis)
Uremia (chronic renal failure)
Ingestion of toxins (paraldehyde, methanol, salicylate, ethylene glycol)
High-fat diet (mild acidosis)
Metabolic acidosis with normal AG (hyperchloremic acidosis)
Renal tubular acidosis (including acidosis of aldosterone deficiency)
Intestinal loss of HCO_3^- (diarrhea, pancreatic fistula)
Carbonic anhydrase inhibitors (e.g., acetazolamide)
Dilutional acidosis (as a result of rapid infusion of bicarbonate-free isotonic saline)
Ingestion of exogenous acids (ammonium chloride, methionine, cystine, calcium chloride)
Ileostomy
Ureterosigmoidostomy
Drugs: amiloride, triamterene, spironolactone, β-blockers
RESPIRATORY ACIDOSIS
Pulmonary disease (COPD, severe pneumonia, pulmonary edema, interstitial fibrosis)
Airway obstruction (foreign body, severe bronchospasm, laryngospasm)
Thoracic cage disorders (pneumothorax, flail chest, kyphoscoliosis)

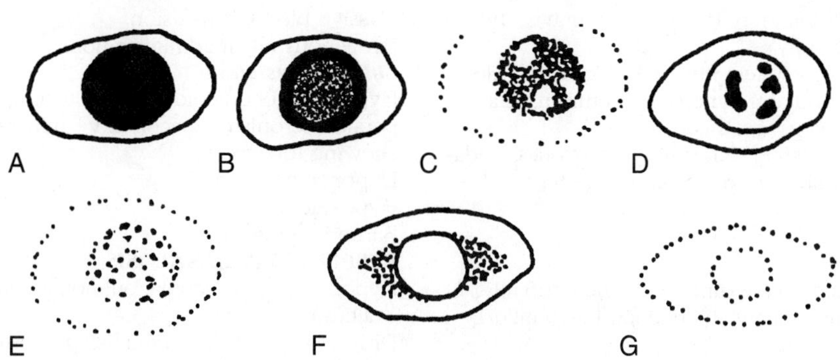

FIGURE 4-1 Fluorescent antinuclear antibody test patterns (HEP-2 cells). A, Solid (homogeneous). **B,** Peripheral (rim). **C,** Speckled. **D,** Nucleolar. **E,** Anticentromere. **F,** Antimitochondrial. **G,** Normal (nonreactive). (From Ravel R [ed]: *Clinical laboratory medicine,* ed 6, St Louis, 1995, Mosby.)

TABLE 4-3 **Disease-Associated ANA Subtypes**

Nuclear Location	Disease(s)
"Native" DNA (dsDNA, or dsDNA/ssDNA complex)	SLE (60%-70%; range, 35%-75%) —also PSS (5%-55%), MCTD (11%-25%), RA (5%-40%), DM (5%-25%), SS (5%)
sNP	SLE (50%) —also other collagen diseases
DNP (DNA-histone complex)	SLE (52%) —also MCTD (8%), RA (3%)
Histones	Drug-induced SLE (95%) —also SLE (30%), RA (15%-24%)
ENA	
Sm	SLE (30%-40%; range, 28%-40%) —also MCTD (0%-8%)
RNP (U1-RNP)	MCTD (in high titer without any other ANA subtype present: 95%-100%) —also SLE (26%-50%), PSS (11%-22%), RA (10%), SS (3%)
SS-A (Ro)*	SS without RA (60%-70%) —also SLE (26%-50%), neonatal SLE (over 95%), PSS (30%), MCTD (50%), SS with RA (9%), PBC (15%-19%)
SS-B (La)	SS without RA (40%-60%) —also SLE (5%-15%), SS with RA (5%)
Scl-70*	PSS (15%-43%)
Centromere*	CREST syndrome (70%-90%; range 57%-96%) —also PSS (4%-20%), PBC (12%)
Nucleolar	PSS (scleroderma) (54%-90%) —also SLE (25%-26%), RA (9%)
RAP (RANA)	SS with RA (60%-76%) —also SS without RA (5%)
Jo-1	Polymyositis (30%)
PM-1	Polymyositis or PMS/PSS overlap syndrome (60%-90%) —also DM (17%)
ssDNA	SLE (60%-70%) —also CAH, infectious mononucleosis, RA, chronic GN, chronic infections, PBC

Cytoplasmic Location	Disease(s)
Mitochondrial	Primary biliary cirrhosis (90%-100%) —also CAH (7%-30%), cryptogenic cirrhosis (30%), acute hepatitis, viral hepatitis (3%), other liver diseases (0%-20%), SLE (5%), SS and PSS (8%)
Microsomal†	Chronic active hepatitis (60%-80%), Hashimoto's thyroiditis (97%)
Ribosomal	SLE (5%-12%)
Smooth muscle‡	Chronic active hepatitis (60%-91%) —also cryptogenic cirrhosis (28%), acute hepatitis, viral hepatitis (5%-87%), infectious mononucleosis (81%), MS (40%-50%), malignancy (67%), PBC (10%-50%)

From Ravel R: *Clinical laboratory medicine,* ed 6, St Louis, 1995, Mosby.
CAH, Chronic active hepatitis; *DM,* dermatomyositis; *GN,* glomerulonephritis; *MS,* multiple sclerosis; *PBC,* primary biliary cirrhosis; *SS,* Sjögren's syndrome.
*Not detected using rat or mouse liver or kidney tissue method.
†Not detected by cultured cell method.
‡Detected by cultured cells but better with rat or mouse tissue.

Defects in muscles of respiration (myasthenia gravis, hypokalemia, muscular dystrophy)
Defects in peripheral nervous system (amyotrophic lateral sclerosis, poliomyelitis, Guillain-Barré syndrome, botulism, tetanus, organophosphate poisoning, spinal cord injury)
Depression of respiratory center (anesthesia, narcotics, sedatives, vertebral artery embolism or thrombosis, increased intracranial pressure)
Failure of mechanical ventilator

METABOLIC ALKALOSIS

It is divided into chloride-responsive (urinary chloride <15 mEq/L) and chloride-resistant forms (urinary chloride level >15 mEq/L)

Chloride-responsive

Vomiting
Nasogastric (NG) suction
Diuretics
Posthypercapnic alkalosis
Stool losses (laxative abuse, cystic fibrosis, villous adenoma)
Massive blood transfusion
Exogenous alkali administration

Chloride-resistant

Hyperadrenocorticoid states (Cushing's syndrome, primary hyperaldosteronism, secondary mineralocorticoidism [licorice, chewing tobacco])
Hypomagnesemia
Hypokalemia
Bartter's syndrome

RESPIRATORY ALKALOSIS

Hypoxemia (pneumonia, pulmonary embolism, atelectasis, high-altitude living)
Drugs (salicylates, xanthines, progesterone, epinephrine, thyroxine, nicotine)
Central nervous system (CNS) disorders (tumor, cerebrovascular accident [CVA], trauma, infections)
Psychogenic hyperventilation (anxiety, hysteria)
Hepatic encephalopathy

Gram-negative sepsis
Hyponatremia
Sudden recovery from metabolic acidosis
Assisted ventilation

ARTHROCENTESIS FLUID

Interpretation of results:

1. **Color:** Normally it is clear or pale yellow; cloudiness indicates inflammatory process or presence of crystals, cell debris, fibrin, or triglycerides.
2. **Viscosity:** Normally it has a high viscosity because of hyaluronate; when fluid is placed on a slide, it can be stretched to a string >2 cm in length before separating (low viscosity indicates breakdown of hyaluronate [lysosomal enzymes from leukocytes] or the presence of edema fluid).
3. **Mucin clot:** Add 1 ml of fluid to 5 ml of a 5% acetic acid solution and allow 1 minute for the clot to form; a firm clot (does not fragment on shaking) is normal and indicates the presence of large molecules of hyaluronic acid (this test is nonspecific and infrequently done).
4. **Glucose:** Normally it approximately equals serum glucose level; a difference of more than 40 mg/dl is suggestive of infection.
5. **Protein:** Total protein concentration is <2.5 g/dl in the normal synovial fluid; it is elevated in inflammatory and septic arthritis.
6. **Microscopic examination for crystals**
   a. Gout: Monosodium urate crystals
   b. Pseudogout: Calcium pyrophosphate dihydrate crystals

ASLO TITER; *see* ANTISTREPTOLYSIN O TITER

ASPARTATE AMINOTRANSFERASE (AST, SGOT)

Normal range: 0-35 U/L (0-0.58 μkat/L [CF: 0.01667, SMI: 0.01 μkat/L])
Elevated in:
HEART
Acute myocardial infarction
Pericarditis (active: some cases)
LIVER
Hepatitis virus, Epstein-Barr, or cytomegalovirus infection
Active cirrhosis
Liver passive congestion or hypoxia
Alcohol or drug-induced liver dysfunction
Space-occupying lesions (active)
Fatty liver (severe)
Extrahepatic biliary obstruction (early)
Drug-induced
SKELETAL MUSCLE
Acute skeletal muscle injury
Muscle inflammation (infectious or noninfectious)
Muscular dystrophy (active)
Recent surgery
Delirium tremens
KIDNEY
Acute injury or damage
Renal infarct
OTHER
Intestinal infarction
Shock
Cholecystitis
Acute pancreatitis
Hypothyroidism
Heparin therapy (60%-80% of cases)

BASOPHIL COUNT

Normal range: 0.4% to 1% of total WBC; 40-100/mm^3
Elevated in: Leukemia, inflammatory processes, polycythemia vera, Hodgkin's lymphoma, hemolytic anemia, after splenectomy, myeloid metaplasia, myxedema
Decreased in: Stress, hypersensitivity reaction, steroids, pregnancy, hyperthyroidism, postirradiation

BILE, URINE; *see* URINE BILE

BILIRUBIN, DIRECT (conjugated bilirubin)

Normal range: 0-0.2 mg/dl (0-4 μmol/L [CF: 17.10; SMI: 2 μmol/L])
Elevated in: Hepatocellular disease, biliary obstruction, drug-induced cholestasis, hereditary disorders (Dubin-Johnson syndrome, Rotor's syndrome)

BILIRUBIN, INDIRECT (unconjugated bilirubin)

Normal range: 0-1.0 mg/dl (2-18 μmol/L [CF: 17.10; SMI: 2 μmol/L])
Elevated in: A. Increased bilirubin production (if normal liver, serum unconjugated bilirubin is usually less than 4 mg/100 ml)

1. Hemolytic anemia
   a. Acquired
   b. Congenital
2. Resorption from extravascular sources
   a. Hematomas
   b. Pulmonary infarcts
3. Excessive ineffective erythropoiesis
   a. Congenital (congenital dyserythropoietic anemias)
   b. Acquired (pernicious anemia, severe lead poisoning; if present, bilirubinemia is usually mild)

B. Defective hepatic unconjugated bilirubin clearance (defective uptake or conjugation)

1. Severe liver disease
2. Gilbert's syndrome
3. Crigler-Najjar type I or II
4. Drug-induced inhibition
5. Portacaval shunt
6. Congestive heart failure
7. Hyperthyroidism (uncommon)

BILIRUBIN, TOTAL

Normal range: 0-1.0 mg/dl (2-18 μmol/L [CF: 17.10, SMI: 2 μmol/L])
Elevated in: Liver disease (hepatitis, cirrhosis, cholangitis, neoplasm, biliary obstruction, infectious mononucleosis), hereditary disorders (Gilbert's disease, Dubin-Johnson syndrome), drugs (steroids, diphenylhydantoin, phenothiazines, penicillin, erythromycin, clindamycin, captopril, amphotericin B, sulfonamides, azathioprine, isoniazid, 5-aminosalicylic acid, allopurinol, methyldopa, indomethacin, halothane, oral contraceptives, procainamide, tolbutamide, labetalol), hemolysis, pulmonary embolism or infarct, hepatic congestion secondary to congestive heart failure

BILIRUBIN, URINE; *see* URINE BILE

BLEEDING TIME (modified Ivy method)

Normal range: 2 to 9½ min
Elevated in: Thrombocytopenia, capillary wall abnormalities, platelet abnormalities (Bernard-Soulier disease, Glanzmann's disease), drugs (aspirin, warfarin, anti-inflammatory medications, streptokinase, urokinase, dextran, β-lactam antibiotics, moxalactam), disseminated intravascular coagulation, cirrhosis, uremia, myeloproliferative disorders, von Willebrand's disease

BRCA ANALYSIS

Description of analysis
Comprehensive BRCA analysis:
BRCA1: Full sequence determination in both forward and reverse directions of approximately 5500 base pairs comprising 22 coding exons and one noncoding exon (exon 4) and approximately 800 adjacent base pairs in the noncoding intervening sequence

(intron). Exon 1, which is noncoding, is not analyzed. The wild-type *BRCA1* gene encodes a protein comprising 1863 amino acids. *BRCA2:* Full sequence determination in both forward and reverse directions of approximately 10,200 base pairs comprising 26 coding exons and approximately 900 adjacent base pairs in the noncoding intervening sequence (intron). Exon 1, which is noncoding, is not analyzed. The wild-type *BRCA2* gene encodes a protein comprising 3418 amino acids.
The noncoding intronic regions of *BRCA1* and *BRCA2* that are analyzed do not extend more than 20 base pairs proximal to the 5′ end and 10 base pairs distal to the 3′ end of each exon.
SINGLE-SITE BRACANALYSIS: DNA sequence analysis for a specified mutation in *BRCA1* and/or *BRCA2*.
MULTISITE 3 BRACANALYSIS: DNA sequence analysis of specific portions of *BRCA1* exon 2, *BRCA1* exon 20 and *BRCA2* exon 11 designed to detect only mutations 187delAG and 5385insC in *BRCA1* and 6174delT in *BRCA2*.
Interpretive Criteria
"POSITIVE FOR A DELETERIOUS MUTATION": Includes all mutations (nonsense, insertions, deletions) that prematurely terminate ("truncate") the protein product of *BRCA1* at least 10 amino acids form the C-terminus, or the protein product of *BRCA2* at least 110 amino acids from the C-terminus (based on documentation of deleterious mutations in *BRCA1* and *BRCA2*). In addition, specific missense mutations and noncoding intervening sequence (IVS) mutations are recognized as deleterious on the basis of data derived from linkage analysis of high-risk families, functional assays, biochemical evidence and/or demonstration of abnormal mRNA transcript processing.
"GENETIC VARIANT, SUSPECTED DELETERIOUS": Includes genetic variants for which the available evidence indicates a likelihood, but not proof, that the mutation is deleterious. The specific evidence supporting such an interpretation will be summarized for individual variants on each such report.
"GENETIC VARIANT, FAVOR POLYMORPHISM": Includes genetic variants for which available evidence indicates that the variant is highly unlikely to contribute substantially to cancer risk. The specific evidence supporting such an interpretation will be summarized for individual variants on each such report.
"GENETIC VARIANT OF UNCERTAIN SIGNIFICANCE": Includes missense mutations and mutations that occur in analyzed intronic regions whose clinical significance has not yet been determined, as well as chain-terminating mutations that truncate *BRCA1* and *BRCA2* distal to amino acid positions 1853 and 3308, respectively.
"NO DELETERIOUS MUTATION DETECTED": Includes nontruncating genetic variants observed at an allele frequency of approximately 1% of a suitable control population (providing that no data suggest clinical significance), as well as all genetic variants for which published data demonstrate absence of substantial clinical significance. Also includes mutations in the protein-coding region that neither alter the amino acid sequence nor are predicted to significantly affect exon splicing, and base pair alterations in noncoding portions of the gene that have been demonstrated to have no deleterious effect on the length or stability of the mRNA transcript.
There may be uncommon genetic abnormalities in *BRCA1* and *BRCA2* that will not be detected by BRCA Analysis. This analysis, however, is believed to rule out the majority of abnormalities in these genes, which are believed responsible for most hereditary susceptibility to breast and ovarian cancer.
"SPECIFIC VARIANT/MUTATION NOT IDENTIFIED": Specific and designated deleterious mutations or variants of uncertain clinical significance are not present in the individual being tested. If one (or rarely two) specific deleterious mutations have been identified in a family member, a negative analysis for the specific mutation(s) indicates that the tested individual is at the general population risk of developing breast or ovarian cancer.

B-TYPE NATRIURETIC PEPTIDE

Normal range: Up to 100 pg/ml
Elevated in: Heart failure. This test is useful to differentiate patients with heart failure from those with chronic obstructive pulmonary disease presenting with dyspnea.

BUN; *see* UREA NITROGEN

C282Y AND H63D MUTATION ANALYSIS

PROCEDURE: Detection of the C282Y and H63D mutations is accomplished by amplification of exons 2 and 4 of the HFE gene on chromosome 6 by polymerase chain reaction (PCR) followed by allele-specific hybridization and chemiluminescent detection of hybridized probes. H63D is viewed by some as a polymorphism rather than a mutation because of its prevalence in the population, because 15% of the individuals affected with hereditary hemochromatosis (HH) are compound heterozygotes for C282Y and H63D and about 1% of patients are H63D homozygotes, which suggests that H63D may be causative in the development of the disorder at reduced penetrance. The test is performed by Quest diagnostics pursuant to a license agreement with Roche Molecular systems, Inc.
INTERPRETATION: Homozygosity for the C282Y mutation has been associated with an increased risk of being affected with hereditary hemochromatosis (HH) compared with the general population. The genotype is observed in 60% to 90% of individuals affected with HH and occurs in less than 1% of the general population. However, approximately 25% of asymptomatic individuals with this genotype do not develop the disorder.
C3; *see* COMPLEMENT C3
C4; *see* COMPLEMENT C4

CALCITONIN (serum)

Normal range: <100 pg/ml (<100 ng/L [CF: 1; SMI: 10 ng/L])
Elevated in: Medullary carcinoma of the thyroid (particularly if level >1500 pg/ml), carcinoma of the breast, apudomas, carcinoids, renal failure, thyroiditis

CALCIUM (serum)

Normal range: 8.8-10.3 mg/dl (2.2-2.58 mmol/L [CF: 0.2495; SMI: 0.02 mmol/L])
Elevated in:
RELATIVELY COMMON
Neoplasia (noncutaneous)
Bone primary
Myeloma
Acute leukemia
Nonbone solid tumors
Breast
Lung
Squamous nonpulmonary
Kidney
Neoplasm secretion of parathyroid hormone-related protein (PTHrP, "ectopic PTH")
Primary hyperparathyroidism
Thiazide diuretics
Tertiary (renal) hyperparathyroidism
Idiopathic
Spurious (artifactual) hypercalcemia
Dehydration
Serum protein elevation
Laboratory technical problem
RELATIVELY UNCOMMON
Neoplasia (less common tumors)
Sarcoidosis

Hyperthyroidism
Immobilization (mostly seen in children and adolescents)
Diuretic phase of acute renal tubular necrosis
Vitamin D intoxication
Milk-alkali syndrome
Addison's disease
Lithium therapy
Idiopathic hypercalcemia of infancy
Acromegaly
Theophylline toxicity

- Table 4-4 describes the laboratory differential diagnosis of hypercalcemia.

DECREASED
Artifactual
Hypoalbuminemia
Hemodilution
Primary hypoparathyroidism
Pseudohypoparathyroidism
Vitamin D–related
Vitamin D deficiency
Malabsorption
Renal failure
Magnesium deficiency
Sepsis
Chronic alcoholism
Tumor lysis syndrome
Rhabdomyolysis
Alkalosis (respiratory or metabolic)
Acute pancreatitis
Drug-induced hypocalcemia
Large doses of magnesium sulfate
Anticonvulsants
Mithramycin
Gentamicin
Cimetidine

- Table 4-5 describes the laboratory differential diagnosis of hypocalcemia.

CALCIUM, URINE; *see* URINE CALCIUM

CANCER ANTIGEN 125

Normal range: Less than 1.4%
The cancer antigen 125 (CA 125) test uses an antibody against antigen from tissue culture of an ovarian tumor cell line. Various published evaluations report sensitivity of about 75%-80% in patients with ovarian carcinoma. There is also an appreciable incidence of elevated values in nonovarian malignancies and in certain benign conditions (see below). Test values may transiently increase during chemotherapy.

MALIGNANT
Epithelial ovarian carcinoma, 75%-80% (range 25%-92%, better in serous than mucinous cystadenocarcinoma)
Endometrial carcinoma, 25%-48% (2%-90%)
Pancreatic carcinoma, 59%
Colorectal carcinoma, 20% (15%-56%)
Endocervical adenocarcinoma, 83%
Squamous cervical or vaginal carcinoma, 7%-14%
Lung carcinoma, 32%
Breast carcinoma, 12%-40%
Lymphoma, 35%

BENIGN
Cirrhosis, 40%-80%
Acute pancreatitis, 38%
Acute peritonitis, 75%
Endometriosis, 88%
Acute pelvic inflammation disease, 33%

TABLE 4-4 Laboratory Differential Diagnosis of Hypercalcemia

	PLASMA TESTS					URINE TESTS			
Diagnosis	**Ca**	**PO_4**	**PTH**	**25(OH)D**	**$1,25(OH)_2D$**	**cAMP**	**TmP/GFR**	**Ca**	**Comments**
Primary hyperparathyroidism	↑	N/↓	↑	N	N/↑	↑	↓	↑	Parathyroid adenoma most common
MEN I									Parathyroid hyperplasia; also includes pituitary and pancreatic neoplasms
MEN IIa									Parathyroid hyperplasia; also includes medullary thyroid carcinoma and pheochromocytoma
MEN IIb									Parathyroid disease uncommon, primarily medullary thyroid carcinoma and pheochromocytoma
FHH	↑	N	N/↑	N	N	N/↑	N/↓	↓↓	Autosomal dominant inheritance; hypercalcemia present within first decade; benign
Malignancy									
Solid tumor—humoral	↑	N/↓	↓	N	N	↑	↓	↑↑	Primarily epidermoid tumors; PTH-related protein(s) is mediator
Solid tumor—osteolytic	↑	N/↑	↓	N	N	↓	↑	↑↑	
Lymphoma	↑	N/↑	↓	N/↓	↑	↓	↑	↑↑	
Granulomatous disease	↑	N/↑	↓	N/↓	↑↑	↓	↑	↑↑	Sarcoid most common etiology
Vitamin D intoxication	↑	N/↑	↓	↑↑	N	↓	↑	↑↑	
Hyperthyroidism	↑	N	↓	N	N	N	N	↑↑	Plasma concentrations of T_4 and/or T_3 are elevated

From Moore WT, Eastman RC: *Diagnostic endocrinology,* ed 2, St Louis, 1996, Mosby.
Ca, Calcium; *cAMP,* cyclic adenosine monophosphate; *FHH,* familial hypocalciuric hypercalcemia; *GFR,* glomerular filtration rate; *MEN,* multiple endocrine neoplasia; *N,* normal; *25(OH)D,* 25 hydroxyvitamin D; *PO_4,* phosphate; *PTH,* parathormone; *T_3,* triiodothyronine; *T_4,* thyroxine; *TmP,* renal threshold for phosphorus.

TABLE 4-5 Laboratory Differential Diagnosis of Hypocalcemia

	PLASMA TESTS					URINE TESTS					
DIAGNOSIS	**Ca**	**PO_4**	**PTH**	**25(OH)D**	**$1,25(OH)_2D$**	**cAMP**	**cAMP AFTER PTH**	**TmP/GFR**	**TmP/GFR AFTER PTH**	**Ca**	**COMMENTS**
Hypoparathyroidism	↓	↑	N/↓	N	↓	↓	↑↑	↑	↓↓	N/↓	Deficiency of PTH
Pseudohypoparathyroidism											
Type I	↓	↑	↑↑	N	↓	↓	NC	↑	↑	N/↓	Resistance to PTH; patients may have Albright's hereditary osteodystrophy and resistance to multiple hormones
Type II	↓	N	↑↑	N	↓	↓	↑	↑	↑	N/↓	Renal resistance to cAMP
Vitamin D deficiency	↓	N/↓	↑↑	↓↓	N/↓	↑	↑	↓	↓	↓↓	Deficient supply (e.g., nutrition) or absorption (e.g., pancreatic insufficiency) of vitamin D
Vitamin D–dependent rickets											
Type I	↓	N/↓	↑↑	N	↓	↑		↓		↓↓	Deficient activity of renal 25(OH)D-1a-hydroxylase
Type II	↓	N/↓	↑↑	N	↑↑	↑		↓		↓↓	Resistance to 1,25(OH)2D

From Moore WT, Eastman RC: *Diagnostic endocrinology,* ed 2, St Louis, 1996, Mosby.

Ca, Calcium; *cAMP,* cyclic adenosine monophosphate; *GFR,* glomerular filtration rate; *NC,* no change or small increase; *(OH)D,* hydroxycalciferol D; *PO_4,* phosphate; *PTH,* parathyroid hormone; *T_4,* thyroxine; *TmP,* renal threshold for phosphorus.

Pregnancy first trimester, 2%-24%
During menstruation (occasionally)
Renal failure (?frequency)
Normal persons, 0.6%-1.4%

CARBAMAZEPINE (Tegretol)

Normal therapeutic range: 4-12 mcg/ml

CARBON MONOXIDE; *see* CARBOXYHEMOGLOBIN

CARBOXYHEMOGLOBIN

Normal range: Saturation of hemoglobin <2%; smokers <9% (coma: 50%; death: 80%)
Elevated in: Smoking, exposure to smoking, exposure to automobile exhaust fumes, malfunctioning gas-burning appliances

CARCINOEMBRYONIC ANTIGEN (CEA)

Normal range: Nonsmokers: 0-2.5 ng/ml (0-2.5 μg/L [CF: 1; SMI: 0.1 μg/L])
Smokers: 0-5 ng/ml (0-5 μg/L [CF: 1; SMI: 0.1 μg/L])
Elevated in: Colorectal carcinomas, pancreatic carcinomas, and metastatic disease (usually produce higher elevations: >20 ng/ml)
Carcinomas of the esophagus, stomach, small intestine, liver, breast, ovary, lung, and thyroid (usually produce lesser elevations)
Benign conditions (smoking, inflammatory bowel disease, hypothyroidism, cirrhosis, pancreatitis, infections) (usually produce levels <10 ng/ml)

CAROTENE (serum)

Normal range: 50-250 μg/dl (0.9-4.6 μmol/L [CF: 0.01863; SMI: 0.1 μmol/L])
Elevated in: Carotenemia, chronic nephritis, diabetes mellitus, hypothyroidism, nephrotic syndrome, hyperlipidemia
Decreased in: Fat malabsorption, steatorrhea, pancreatic insufficiency, lack of carotenoids in diet, high fever, liver disease

CATECHOLAMINES, URINE; *see* URINE CATECHOLAMINES

CBC; *see* COMPLETE BLOOD COUNT

CD4+ T-LYMPHOCYTE COUNT (CD4+ T-Cells)

Calculated as total WBC × % lymphocytes × % lymphocytes stained with CD4.
This test is used primarily to evaluate immune dysfunction in HIV infection and should be done every 3-6 months in all HIV-infected persons. It is useful as a prognostic indicator and as a criterion for initiating prophylaxis for several opportunistic infections that are sequelae of HIV infection. Progressive depletion of CD4+ T-lymphocytes is associated with an increased likelihood of clinical complications (Table 4-6). Adolescents and adults with HIV are classified as having AIDS if their CD4+ lymphocyte count is under 200/μL and/or if their CD4+ T-lymphocyte percentage is less than 14%. HIV-infected patients whose CD4+ count is less than 200/μL and who acquire certain infectious diseases or malignancies are also classified as having AIDS. Corticosteroids decrease CD4+ T-cell percentage and absolute number.

CEA; *see* CARCINOEMBRYONIC ANTIGEN

CEREBROSPINAL FLUID (CSF)

Interpretation of results:

1. Appearance of the fluid
   a. Clear: normal.
   b. Yellow color (xanthochromia) in the supernatant of centrifuged CSF within 1 hour or less after collection is usually the result of previous bleeding (subarachnoid hemorrhage); it may also be caused by increased CSF protein, melanin from meningeal melanosarcomas, or carotenoids.

TABLE 4-6 Relation of CD4 Lymphocyte Counts to the Onset of Certain HIV-Associated Infections and Neoplasms in North America

CD4 Count (Cells/MM³)*	Opportunistic Infection or Neoplasm	Frequency (%)†
>500	Herpes zoster, polydermatomal	5-10
200-500	*Mycobacterium tuberculosis* infection, pulmonary and extrapulmonary	2-20
	Oral hairy leukoplakia	40-70
	Candida pharyngitis (thrush)	40-70
	Recurrent *Candida* vaginitis	15-30 (F)
	Kaposi's sarcoma, mucocutaneous	15-30 (M)
	Bacterial pneumonia, recurrent	15-20
	Cervical neoplasia	1-2 (F)
100-200	*Pneumocystis carinii* pneumonia	15-60
	Herpes simplex, chronic, ulcerative	5-10
	Histoplasma capsulatum infection, disseminated	0-20
	Kaposi's sarcoma, visceral	3-8 (M)
	Progressive multifocal leukoencephalopathy	2-3
	Lymphoma, non-Hodgkin's	2-5
<100	*Candida* esophagitis	15-20
	Mycobacterium avium-intracellulare, disseminated	25-40
	Toxoplasma gondii encephalitis	5-25
	Cryptosporidium enteritis	2-10
	Cytomegalovirus (CMV) retinitis	20-35
	Cryptococcus neoformans encephalitis	2-5
	CMV esophagitis or colitis	6-12
	Lymphoma, central nervous system	4-8

From Andreoli TE (ed): *Cecil essentials of medicine,* ed 5, Philadelphia, 2000, WB Saunders.
F, Exclusively in women; *HIV,* human immunodeficiency virus; *M,* almost exclusively in men.
*Table indicates CD4 count at which specific infections or neoplasms generally begin to appear. Each infection may recur or progress during the subsequent course of HIV disease.
†Even within the United States, great regional differences in the incidence of specific opportunistic infections are apparent. For example, disseminated histoplasmosis is common in the Mississippi River drainage area, but very rare in individuals who have lived exclusively on the East or West Coast.

c. Pinkish color is usually the result of a bloody tap; the color generally clears progressively from tubes 1 to 4 (the supernatant is usually crystal clear in traumatic taps).
d. Turbidity usually indicates the presence of leukocytes (bleeding introduces approximately 1 WBC/500 RBCs into the CSF).

2. CSF pressure: elevated pressure can be seen with meningitis, meningoencephalitis, pseudotumor cerebri, mass lesions, and intracerebral bleeding.
3. Cell count: in the adult the CSF is normally free of cells (although up to 5 mononuclear cells/mm^3 is considered normal); the presence of granulocytes is never normal.
   a. Neutrophils: seen in bacterial meningitis, early viral meningoencephalitis, and early tuberculosis (TB) meningitis.
   b. Increased lymphocytes: TB meningitis, viral meningoencephalitis, syphilitic meningoencephalitis, fungal meningitis.
4. Protein: serum proteins are generally too large to cross the normal blood-CSF barrier; however, increased CSF protein is seen with meningeal inflammation, traumatic tap, increased CNS synthesis, tissue degeneration, obstruction to CSF circulation, and Guillain-Barré syndrome.
5. Glucose
   a. Decreased glucose is seen with bacterial meningitis, TB meningitis, fungal meningitis, subarachnoid hemorrhage, and some cases of viral meningitis.
   b. A mild increase in CSF glucose can be seen in patients with very elevated serum glucose levels.

Table 4-7 describes cerebrospinal fluid findings in central nervous system disorders.

CERULOPLASMIN (serum)

Normal range: 20-35 mg/dl (200-350 mg/L [CF: 10; SMI: 10 mg/L])
Elevated in: Pregnancy, estrogens, oral contraceptives, neoplastic diseases (leukemias, Hodgkin's lymphoma, carcinomas), inflammatory states, systemic lupus erythematosus, primary biliary cirrhosis, rheumatoid arthritis
Decreased in: Wilson's disease (values often <10 mg/dl), nephrotic syndrome, advanced liver disease, malabsorption, total parenteral nutrition, Menkes' syndrome

CHLORIDE (serum)

Normal range: 95-105 mEq/L (95-105 mmol/L [CF: 1; SMI: 1 mmol/L])
Elevated in: Dehydration, excessive infusion of normal saline solution, cystic fibrosis (sweat test), hyperparathyroidism, renal tubular disease, metabolic acidosis, prolonged diarrhea, drugs (ammonium chloride administration, acetazolamide, boric acid, triamterene)
Decreased in: Congestive heart failure, syndrome of inappropriate antidiuretic hormone secretion, Addison's disease, vomiting, gastric suction, salt-losing nephritis, continuous infusion of D_5W, thiazide diuretic administration, diaphoresis, diarrhea, burns, diabetic ketoacidosis

CHLORIDE (sweat)

Normal: 0-40 mmol/L
Borderline/indeterminate: 41-60 mmol/L
Consistent with cystic fibrosis: >60 mmol/L
False low results can occur with edema, excessive sweating, and hypoproteinemia.

CHLORIDE, URINE; *see* URINE CHLORIDE

CHOLESTEROL, HIGH-DENSITY LIPOPROTEIN; *see* HIGH-DENSITY LIPOPROTEIN CHOLESTEROL

CHOLESTEROL, LOW-DENSITY LIPOPROTEIN; *see* LOW-DENSITY LIPOPROTEIN CHOLESTEROL

CHOLESTEROL, TOTAL

Normal range: Varies with age
Generally <200 mg/dl (<5.20 mmol/L [CF: 0.02586; SMI: 0.05 mmol/L])
Elevated in: Primary hypercholesterolemia, biliary obstruction, diabetes mellitus, nephrotic syndrome, hypothyroidism, primary biliary cirrhosis, high-cholesterol diet, pregnancy third trimester, myocardial infarction, drugs (steroids, phenothiazines, oral contraceptives)
Decreased in: Starvation, malabsorption, sideroblastic anemia, thalassemia, abetalipoproteinemia, hyperthyroidism, Cushing's syndrome, hepatic failure, multiple myeloma, polycythemia vera, chronic myelocytic leukemia, myeloid metaplasia, Waldenström's macroglobulinemia, myelofibrosis

CHORIONIC GONADOTROPINS, HUMAN (serum)

Normal range, serum: Female, premenopausal: <0.8 IU/L; postmenopausal <3.3 IU/L
Male: <0.7 IU/L
Elevated in: Pregnancy, choriocarcinoma, gestational trophoblastic neoplasia (including molar gestations), placental site trophoblastic tumors; human antimouse antibodies (HAMA) can produce false serum assay for hCG.
The principal use of this test is to diagnose pregnancy. The concentration of hCG increases significantly during the initial 6 weeks of pregnancy. Peak values approaching 100,000 IU/L occur 60-70 days following implantation.
hCG levels generally double every 1-3 days. In patients with concentration <2000 IU/L, an increase of serum hCG <66% after 2 days is suggestive of spontaneous abortion or ruptured ectopic gestation.

CIRCULATING ANTICOAGULANT (lupus anticoagulant)

Normal: Negative
Detected in: Systemic lupus erythematosus, drug-induced lupus, long-term phenothiazine therapy, multiple myeloma, ulcerative colitis, rheumatoid arthritis, postpartum, hemophilia, neoplasms, chronic inflammatory states, AIDS, nephrotic syndrome
NOTE: The name is a misnomer because these patients are prone to hypercoagulability and thrombosis.

CK; *see* CREATINE KINASE

CLOSTRIDIUM DIFFICILE TOXIN ASSAY (stool)

Normal: Negative
Detected in: Antibiotic-associated diarrhea and pseudomembranous colitis

CO; *see* CARBOXYHEMOGLOBIN

COAGULATION FACTORS; *see* Table 4-8 for characteristics of coagulation factors

Factor reference ranges:
V: >10%
VII: >10%
VIII: 50% to 170%
IX: 60% to 136%
X: >10%
XI: 50% to 150%
XII: >30%

- Table 4-9 describes screening laboratory results in coagulation factor deficiencies.

COLD AGGLUTININS TITER

Normal range: <1:32
Elevated in: Primary atypical pneumonia (mycoplasma pneumonia), infectious mononucleosis, CMV infection
Others: hepatic cirrhosis, acquired hemolytic anemia, frostbite, multiple myeloma, lymphoma, malaria

TABLE 4-7 Cerebrospinal Fluid Findings in Central Nervous System Disorders

Condition	Pressure (mm H_2O)	Leukocytes (mm^3)	Protein (mg/dl)	Glucose (mg/dl)	Comments
Normal	50-80	<5, ≥75% lymphocytes	20-45	>50 (or 75% serum glucose)	
Common Forms of Meningitis					
Acute bacterial meningitis	Usually elevated (100-300)	100-10,000 or more; usually 300-2000; PMNs predominate	Usually 100-500	Decreased, usually <40 (or <66% serum glucose)	Organisms usually seen on Gram stain and recovered by culture. Latex agglutination of CSF usually positive
Partially treated bacterial meningitis	Normal or elevated	5-10,000; PMNs usual but mononuclear cells may predominate if pretreated for extended period of time	Usually 100-500	Normal or decreased	Organisms may be seen on Gram stain. Latex agglutination CSF may be positive. Pretreatment may render CSF sterile
Viral meningitis or meningoencephalitis	Normal or slightly elevated (80-150)	Rarely >1000 cells. Eastern equine encephalitis and lymphocytic choriomeningitis (LCM) may have cell counts of several thousand. PMNs early but mononuclear cells predominate through most of the course	Usually 50-200	Generally normal; may be decreased to <40 in some viral diseases, particularly mumps (15%-20% of cases)	HSV encephalitis is suggested by focal seizures or by focal findings on CT or MRI scans or EEG. Enteroviruses and HSV infrequently recovered from CSF. HSV and enteroviruses may be detected by PCR of CSF
Uncommon Forms of Meningitis					
Tuberculous meningitis	Usually elevated	10-500; PMNs early, but lymphocytes predominate through most of the course	100-3000; may be higher in presence of block	<50 in most cases; decreases with time if treatment is not provided	Acid-fast organisms almost never seen on smear. Organisms may be recovered in culture of large volumes of CSF. *Mycobacterium tuberculosis* may be detected by PCR of CSF
Fungal meningitis	Usually elevated	5-500; PMNs early but mononuclear cells predominate through most of the course. Cryptococcal meningitis may have no cellular inflammatory response	25-500	<50; decreases with time if treatment is not provided	Budding yeast may be seen. Organisms may be recovered in culture. Cryptococcal antigen (CSF and serum) may be positive in cryptococcal infection
Syphilis (acute) and leptospirosis	Usually elevated	50-500; lymphocytes predominate	50-200	Usually normal	Positive CSF serology. Spirochetes not demonstrable by usual techniques of smear or culture; darkfield examination may be positive
Amebic (Naegleria) meningoencephalitis	Elevated	1000-10,000 or more; PMNs predominate	50-500	Normal or slightly decreased	Mobile amebae may be seen by hanging-drop examination of CSF at room temperature

Continued on following page

TABLE 4-7 **Cerebrospinal Fluid Findings in Central Nervous System Disorders** *(Continued)*

Condition	Pressure (mm H_2O)	Leukocytes (mm³)	Protein (mg/dl)	Glucose (mg/dl)	Comments
Brain and Parameningeal Abscesses					
Brain abscess	Usually elevated (100-300)	5-200; CSF rarely acellular; lymphocytes predominate; if abscess ruptures into ventricle, PMNs predominate and cell count may reach >100,000	75-500	Normal unless abscess ruptures into ventricular system	No organisms on smear or culture unless abscess ruptures into ventricular system
Subdural empyema	Usually elevated (100-300)	100-5000; PMNs predominate	100-500	Normal	No organisms on smear or culture of CSF unless meningitis also present; organisms found on tap of subdural fluid
Cerebral epidural abscess	Normal to slightly elevated	10-500; lymphocytes predominate	50-200	Normal	No organisms on smear or culture of CSF
Spinal epidural abscess	Usually low, with spinal block	10-100; lymphocytes predominate	50-400	Normal	No organisms on smear or culture of CSF
Chemical (drugs, dermoid cysts, myelography dye)	Usually elevated	100-1000 or more; PMNs predominate	50-100	Normal or slightly decreased	Epithelial cells may be seen within CSF by use of polarized light in some children with dermoids
Noninfectious Causes					
Sarcoidosis	Normal or elevated slightly	0-100; mononuclear	40-100	Normal	No specific findings
Systemic lupus erythematosus with CNS involvement	Slightly elevated	0-500; PMNs usually predominate; lymphocytes may be present	100	Normal or slightly decreased	No organisms on smear or culture. LE preparation may be positive. Positive neuronal and ribosomal P protein antibodies in CSF
Tumor, leukemia	Slightly elevated to very high	0-100 or more; mononuclear or blast cells	50-1000	Normal to decreased (20-40)	Cytology may be positive

From Behrman RE: *Nelson textbook of pediatrics,* ed 17, Philadelphia, 2004, WB Saunders.
CSF, Cerebrospinal fluid; EEG, electroencephalogram; *HSV,* herpes simplex virus; *PCR,* polymerase chain reaction; *PMN,* polymorphonuclear neutrophils.

TABLE 4-8 Characteristics of Coagulation Factors

Factor	Descriptive Name	Source	Approximate Half-Life (hr)	Function
I	Fibrinogen	Liver	120	Substrate for fibrin clot (CP)
II	Prothrombin	Liver (VKD)	60	Serine protease (CP)
V	Proaccelerin, labile factor	Liver	12-36	Cofactor (CP)
VII	Serum prothrombin conversion accelerator, proconvertin	Liver (VKD)	6	(?) Serine protease (EP)
VIII	Antihemophilic factor or globulin	Endothelial cells and (?) elsewhere	12	Cofactor (IP)
IX	Plasma thromboplastin component, Christmas factor	Liver (VKD)	24	Serine protease (IP)
X	Stuart-Prower factor	Liver (VKD)	36	Serine protease (CP)
XI	Plasma thromboplastin antecedent	(?) Liver	40-84	Serine protease (IP)
XII	Hageman factor	(?) Liver	50	Serine protease contact activation (IP)
XIII	Fibrin-stabilizing factor	(?) Liver	96-180	Transglutaminase (CP)
Prekallikrein	Fletcher factor	(?) Liver	?	Serine protease contact activation (IP)
High-molecular-weight kininogen	Fitzgerald factor, Flaujeac or Williams factor	(?) Liver	?	Cofactor, contact activation (IP)

From Noble J (ed): *Primary care medicine,* ed 3, St Louis, 2001, Mosby.
CP, Common pathway; *EP,* extrinsic pathway; *IP,* intrinsic pathway; *VKD,* vitamin K dependent.

COMPLEMENT

Normal range: C3: 70-160 mg/dl (0.7-1.6 g/L [CF: 0.01; SMI: 0.1 g/L])
C4: 20-40 mg/dl (0.2-0.4 g/L [CF: 0.01; SMI: 0.1 g/L])
Abnormal values:
DECREASED C3: Active SLE, immune complex disease, acute glomerulonephritis, inborn C3 deficiency, membranoproliferative glomerulonephritis, infective endocarditis, serum sickness, autoimmune/chronic active hepatitis
DECREASED C4: Immune complex disease, active SLE, infective endocarditis, inborn C4 deficiency, hereditary angioedema, hypergammaglobulinemic states, cryobulinemic vasculitis
Table 4-10 describes complement deficiency states.

COMPLETE BLOOD COUNT (CBC)

White blood cells 3200-9800 mm^3 ($3.2\text{-}9.8 \times 10^9$/L [CF: 0.001; SMI: 0.1×10^9/L])
Red blood cells
Male: $4.3\text{-}5.9 \times 10^6/mm^3$ ($4.3\text{-}5.9 \times 10^{12}$/L [CF: 0.001; SMI: 0.1×10^{12}/L])
Female: $3.5\text{-}5 \times 10^6/mm^3$ ($3.5\text{-}5 \times 10^{12}$/L [CF: 0.001; SMI: 0.1×10^{12}/L])
Hemoglobin
Male: 13.6-17.7 g/dl (136-172 g/L [CF: 10; SMI: 1 g/L])
Female: 12-15 g/dl (120-150 g/L [CF: 10; SMI: 1 g/L])
Hematocrit
Male: 39% to 49% (0.39-0.49 [CF: 0.01; SMI: 0.01])
Female: 33% to 43% (0.33-0.43 [CF: 0.01; SMI: 0.01])
Mean corpuscular volume (MCV): 76-100 μm^3 (76-100 fL [CF: 1; SMI: 1 fL])
Mean corpuscular hemoglobin (MCH): 27-33 pg (27-33 pg [CF: 1; SMI: 1 pg])
Mean corpuscular hemoglobin concentration (MCHC): 33-37 g/dl (330-370 g/L [CF: 10; SMI: 10 g/L])

TABLE 4-9 Screening Laboratory Results in Coagulation Factor Deficiencies

Deficient Factor	Frequency	PT	PTT	TT
I (fibrinogen)	Rare	↑	↑	↑
II (prothrombin)	Very rare	↑	↑	↑
V 1:1,000,000	↑	↑	NL	
VII	1:500,000	↑	NL	NL
VIII	1:5000 (male)	NL	↑	NL
IX	1:30,000 (male)	NL	↑	NL
X 1:500,000	↑	↑	NL	
XI	Rare*	NL	↑	NL
XII† or HMWK† or PK†	Rare	NL	↑	NL
XIII	Rare	NL	NL	NL

From Andreoli TE (ed): *Cecil essentials of medicine,* ed 5, Philadelphia, 2001, WB Saunders.
↑, Increased over normal range; *HMWK,* high-molecular-weight kininogen; *NL,* normal; *PK,* prekallikrein; *PT,* prothrombin time; *PTT,* partial thromboplastin time; *TT,* thrombin time.
*Except in those of Ashkenazi Jewish descent (approximately 4% are heterozygous for factor XI deficiency).
†Not associated with clinical bleeding.

TABLE 4-10 Complement Deficiency States

Component	Number of Reported Patients	Mode of Inheritance	Functional Defects	Disease Associations
Classic pathway				
C1qrs	31	ACD	Impaired IC handling, delayed C′ activation, impaired immune response	CVD, 48%; infection (encaps bact), 22%; both, 18%; healthy, 12%
C4	21	ACD		
C2	109	ACD		
Alternative pathway				
D	3	ACD	Impaired C′ activation in absence of specific antibody	Infection (meningococcal), 74%; healthy, 26%
P	70	XL		
Junction of classic and alternative pathways				
C3	19	ACD	Impaired IC handling, opson/phag; granulocytosis, CTX, immune response and absent SBA	CVD, 79%; recurrent infection (encaps bact), 71%
Terminal components				
C5	27	ACD	Impaired CTX; absent SBA	Infection (Neisseria, primarily meningococcal), 58%; CVD, 4%
C6	77	ACD	Absent SBA	Both, 1%
C7	73	ACD		Healthy, 25%
C8	73	ACD		
C9	165	ACD	Impaired SBA	Healthy, 91%; infection, 9%
Plasma proteins regulating C′ activation				
C1-INH	Many	AD Acq	Uncontrolled generation of an inflammatory mediator on C′ activation	Hereditary angioedema
H	13	ACD	Uncontrolled AP activation → low C3	CVD, 40%; CVD plus infection (encaps bact), 40%; healthy, 20%
I	14	ACD	Uncontrolled AP activation → low C3	Infection (encaps bact), 100%
Membrane proteins regulating C′ activation				
Decay-accelerating factor Homologous restriction factor CD59	Many	Acq	Impaired regulation of C3b and C8 deposited on host RBC; PMN, platelets → cell lysis	Paroxysmal nocturnal hemoglobinuria
CR3	>20	ACD	Impaired PMN adhesive functions (i.e., margination), CTX, C3bi-mediated opson/phag	Infection (Staphylococcus aureus, Pseudomonas spp.), 100%
Autoantibodies				
C3 nephritic factors	>59	Acq	Stabilize AP, convertase → low C3	MPGN, 41%; PLD, 25%; infection (encaps bact), 16%; MPGN plus PLD, 10%; PLD plus infection, 5%; MPGN plus PLD plus infection, 3%; MPGN plus infection, 2%
C4 nephritic factor		Acq	Stabilize CP, C3 convertase → low C3	Glomerulonephritis, 50%; CVD, 50%

From Mandell GL: *Mandell, Douglas, and Bennett's principles and practice of infectious diseases,* ed 6, New York, 2005, Churchill Livingstone.
ACD, Autosomal codominant; *Acq,* acquired; *AD,* autosomal dominant; *AP,* alternative pathway; *C′,* complement; *CP,* classic pathway; *CTX,* chemotaxis; *CVD,* collagen-vascular disease; encaps bact, encapsulated bacteria; *IC,* immune complex, *MPGN,* membranoproliferative glomerulonephritis; *PLD,* partial lipodystrophy; *PMN,* polymorphonuclear neutrophil; *RBC,* red blood cells; *SBA,* serum bactericidal activity; *XL,* X-linked.

Red blood cell distribution width index (RDW): 11.5% to 14.5%
Platelet count: 130-400 × 10^3/mm^3 (130-400 × 10^9/L [CF: 1; SMI: 5 × 10^9/L])
Differential:
2-6 stabs (bands, early mature neutrophils)
60-70 segs (mature neutrophils)
1-4 eosinophils
0-1 basophils
2-8 monocytes
25-40 lymphocytes

CONJUGATED BILIRUBIN; *see* BILIRUBIN, DIRECT

COOMBS, DIRECT

Normal: Negative
Positive: Autoimmune hemolytic anemia, erythroblastosis fetalis, transfusion reactions, drugs (α-methyldopa, penicillins, tetracycline, sulfonamides, levodopa, cephalosporins, quinidine, insulin)
False positive: May be seen with cold agglutinins

COOMBS, INDIRECT

Normal: Negative
Positive: Acquired hemolytic anemia, incompatible cross-matched blood, anti-Rh antibodies, drugs (methyldopa, mefenamic acid, levodopa)

COPPER (serum)
Normal range: 70-140 μg/dl (11-22 μmol/L [CF: 0.1574, SMI: 0.2 μmol/L])
Decreased in: Wilson's disease, Menkes' syndrome, malabsorption, malnutrition, nephrosis, total parenteral nutrition, acute leukemia in remission
Elevated in: Aplastic anemia, biliary cirrhosis, systemic lupus erythematosus, hemochromatosis, hyperthyroidism, hypothyroidism, infection, iron deficiency anemia, leukemia, lymphoma, oral contraceptives, pernicious anemia, rheumatoid arthritis

COPPER, URINE; *see* URINE COPPER

CORTISOL, PLASMA
Normal range: Varies with time of collection (circadian variation):
8 AM: 4-19 μg/dl (110-520 nmol/L [CF: 27.59; SMI: 10 nmol/L])
4 PM: 2-15 μg/dl (50-410 nmol/L [CF: 27.59; SMI: 10 nmol/L])
Elevated in: Ectopic adrenocorticotropic hormone production (i.e., oat cell carcinoma of lung), loss of normal diurnal variation, pregnancy, chronic renal failure iatrogenic, stress, adrenal, or pituitary hyperplasia or adenomas
Decreased in: Primary adrenocortical insufficiency, anterior pituitary hypofunction, secondary adrenocortical insufficiency, adrenogenital syndromes

C-PEPTIDE
Elevated in: Insulinoma, sulfonylurea administration
Decreased in: Insulin-dependent diabetes mellitus, factitious insulin administration

CPK; *see* CREATINE KINASE

C-REACTIVE PROTEIN
Normal range: 6.8-820 μg/dl (68-8200 μg/L [CF: 10; SMI: 10 μg/L])
Elevated in: Rheumatoid arthritis, rheumatic fever, inflammatory bowel disease, bacterial infections, myocardial infarction, oral contraceptives, pregnancy third trimester (acute phase reactant), inflammatory and neoplastic diseases

C-REACTIVE PROTEIN, HIGH SENSITIVITY (hs-CRP, cardio-CRP)
This is a cardiac risk marker. It is increased in patients with silent atherosclerosis years before a cardiovascular event and is independent of cholesterol level and other lipoproteins. It can be used to help stratify cardiac risk.
Interpretation of results:

Cardio-CRP result (mg/L)	Risk
≤0.6	Lowest risk
0.7-1.1	Low risk
1.2-1.9	Moderate risk
2.0-3.8	High risk
3.9-4.9	Highest risk
≥5.0	Results may be confounded by acute inflammatory disease. If clinically indicated, a repeat test should be performed in 2 or more weeks.

CREATINE KINASE (CK, CPK)
Normal range: 0-130 U/L (0-2.16 μkat/L [CF: 0.01667; SMI: 0.01 μkat/L])
Elevated in: Myocardial infarction, myocarditis, rhabdomyolysis, myositis, crush injury/trauma, polymyositis, dermatomyositis, vigorous exercise, muscular dystrophy, myxedema, seizures, malignant hyperthermia syndrome, IM injections, cerebrovascular accident, pulmonary embolism and infarction, acute dissection of aorta
Decreased in: Steroids, decreased muscle mass, connective tissue disorders, alcoholic liver disease, metastatic neoplasms

CREATINE KINASE ISOENZYMES
CK-BB: Elevated in: cerebrovascular accident, subarachnoid hemorrhage, neoplasms (prostate, gastrointestinal tract, brain, ovary, breast, lung), severe shock, bowel infarction, hypothermia, meningitis
CK-MB: Elevated in: myocardial infarction (MI), myocarditis, pericarditis, muscular dystrophy, cardiac defibrillation, cardiac surgery, extensive rhabdomyolysis, strenuous exercise (marathon runners), mixed connective tissue disease, cardiomyopathy, hypothermia

NOTE: CK-MB exists in the blood in two subforms. MB_2 is released from cardiac cells and converted in the blood to MB_1. Rapid assay of CK-MB subforms can detect MI ($CK\text{-}MB_2 \geq 1.0$ U/L, with a ratio of $CK\text{-}MB_2/CK\text{-}MB_1 \geq 1.5$) within 6 hours of onset of symptoms.
Fig. 4-2 illustrates the time course of CK, AST, troponins, and LDH activity after acute MI.
CK-MM: Elevated in: crush injury, seizures, malignant hyperthermia syndrome, rhabdomyolysis, myositis, polymyositis, dermatomyositis, vigorous exercise, muscular dystrophy, IM injections, acute dissection of aorta

CREATININE (serum)
Normal range: 0.6-1.2 mg/dl (50-110 μmol/L [CF: 88.4; SMI: 10 μmol/L])
Elevated in: Renal insufficiency (acute and chronic), decreased renal perfusion (hypotension, dehydration, congestive heart failure), urinary tract infection, rhabdomyolysis, ketonemia
Drugs (antibiotics [aminoglycosides, cephalosporins], hydantoin, diuretics, methyldopa)
Falsely elevated in: Diabetic ketoacidosis, administration of some cephalosporins (e.g., cefoxitin, cephalothin)
Decreased in: Decreased muscle mass (including amputees and older persons), pregnancy, prolonged debilitation

CREATININE CLEARANCE
Normal range: 75-124 ml/min (1.24-2.08 ml/sec [CF: 0.01667; SMI: 0.02 ml/sec])
Box 4-1 describes a formula for calculation of creatinine clearance. The Cockcroft-Gault formula to calculate creatinine clearance is described in Box 4-2.
Elevated in: Pregnancy, exercise
Decreased in: Renal insufficiency, drugs (cimetidine, procainamide, antibiotics, quinidine)

CREATININE, URINE; *see* URINE CREATININE

CRYOGLOBULINS (serum)
Normal range: Not detectable
Present in: Collagen-vascular diseases, chronic lymphocytic leukemia, hemolytic anemias, multiple myeloma, Waldenström's macroglobulinemia, chronic active hepatitis, Hodgkin's disease

CRYPTOSPORIDIUM ANTIGEN BY EIA (stool)
Normal range: Not detected
Present in: Cryptosporidiosis

CSF; *see* CEREBROSPINAL FLUID

D-DIMER
Normal range: <0.5 mcg/ml
Elevated in: DVT, pulmonary embolism, high levels of rheumatoid factor, activation of coagulation and fibrolytic system from any cause
D-dimer assay by ELISA assists in the diagnosis of DVT and pulmonary embolism. This test has significant limitations because it

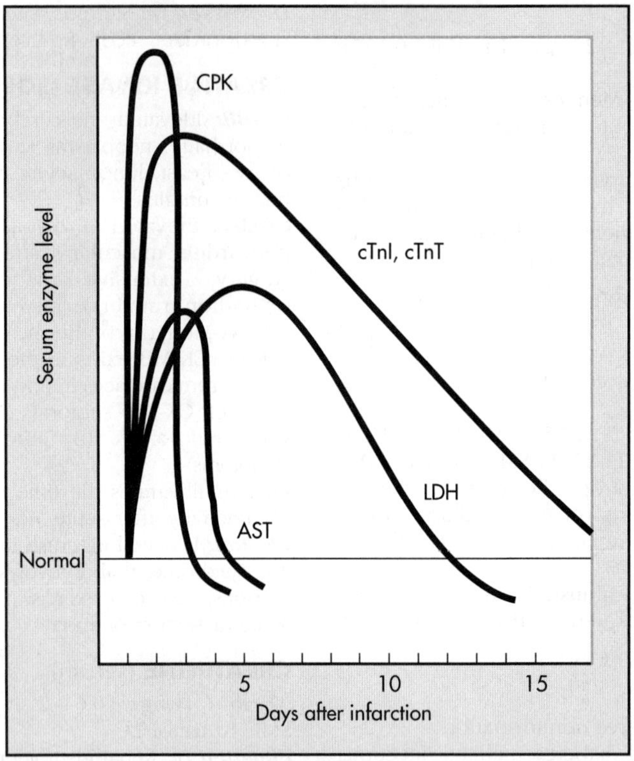

FIGURE 4-2 Evaluation of creatine kinase elevation. *AST,* Aspartate aminotransferase; *cTnI,* cardiac troponin I; *cTnT,* cardiac troponin T; *CPK,* creatine kinase; *LDH,* lactate dehydrogenase. (From Greene HL, Johnson WP, Lemcke D [eds]: *Decision making in medicine,* ed 2, St Louis, 1998, Mosby.)

can be elevated whenever the coagulation and fibrinolytic systems are activated and can also be falsely elevated with high rheumatoid factor levels.

DIGOXIN (LANOXIN)

Normal therapeutic range: 0.5-2 ng/ml
Elevated in: Impaired renal function, excessive dosing, concomitant use of quinidine, amiodarone, verapamil, fluoxetine, nifedipine

DILANTIN; *see* PHENYTOIN

DOPAMINE

Normal range: 0-175 pg/ml
Elevated in: Pheochromocytomas, neuroblastomas, stress, vigorous exercise, certain foods (bananas, chocolate, coffee, tea, vanilla)

D-XYLOSE ABSORPTION

Normal range: 21% to 31% excreted in 5 hr (0.21-0.31 [CF: 0.01; SMI: 0.01])
Decreased in: Malabsorption syndrome

D-XYLOSE ABSORPTION TEST

Normal range:
URINE: ≥4 g/5 hours (5-hour urine collection in adults >12 years [25 g dose])
SERUM: ≥25 mg/dl (adult, I h, 25 g dose, normal renal function)
Normal results: In patients with malabsorption, normal results suggest pancreatic disease as an etiology of the malabsorption.
Abnormal results: Celiac disease, Crohn's disease, tropical sprue, surgical bowel resection, AIDS. False-positives can occur with decreased renal function, dehydration/hypovolemia, surgical blind loops, decreased gastric emptying, vomiting.

ELECTROLYTES, URINE; *see* URINE ELECTROLYTES

ELECTROPHORESIS, HEMOGLOBIN; *see* HEMOGLOBIN ELECTROPHORESIS

ELECTROPHORESIS, PROTEIN; *see* PROTEIN ELECTROPHORESIS

ENA-COMPLEX; *see* EXTRACTABLE NUCLEAR ANTIGEN

BOX 4-1 Calculation of the Creatinine Clearance

$Ccr = U_{cr} \times V/P_{cr}$
where C_{cr} = clearance of creatinine (ml/min)
U_{cr} = urine creatinine (mg/dl)
V = volume of urine (ml/min) (for 24-hr volume: divide by 1440)
P_{cr} = plasma creatinine (mg/dl)

Normal range: 95 to 105 ml/min/1.75m^2

BOX 4-2 Cockroft-Gault Formula to Calculate Creatinine Clearance (Ccr)

$$C_{cr} = \frac{(140 - \text{age in year}) \times (\text{lean body weight in kg})}{S_{cr} \text{ in mg/dl} - 72}$$

For women, multiply final value by 0.85

ENDOMYSIAL ANTIBODIES

Normal: Not detected
Present in: Celiac disease, dermatitis herpetiformis

EOSINOPHIL COUNT

Normal range: 1%-4% eosinophils (0-440/mm^3)
Elevated in:
HELMINTHIC PARASITES
Ascaris lumbricoides (invasive larval stage)
Hookworms (invasive larval stage)
Strongyloides stercoralis (initial infection and autoinfection)
Trichinosis
Filariasis
Echinococcus granulosus and *E. multilocularis*
Toxocara species
Animal hookworms
Angiostrongylus cantonensis and *A.* costaricensis
Schistosomiasis
Liver flukes
Fasciolopsis buski
Anisakiasis
Capillaria philippinensis
Paragonimus westermani
"Tropical eosinophilia" (unidentified microfilariae)
OTHER INFECTIONS/INFESTATIONS
Pulmonary aspergillosis
Severe scabies
ALLERGIES
Asthma
Hay fever
Drug reactions
Atopic dermatitis
AUTOIMMUNE AND RELATED DISORDERS
Polyarteritis nodosa
Necrotizing vasculitis
Eosinophilic fasciitis
Pemphigus
NEOPLASTIC DISEASES
Hodgkin's disease
Mycosis fungoides
Chronic myelocytic leukemia
Eosinophilic leukemia
Polycythemia vera
Mucin-secreting adenocarcinomas
IMMUNODEFICIENCY STATES
Hyperimmunoglobulin E with recurrent infection
Wiskott-Aldrich syndrome
OTHER
Addison's disease
Inflammatory bowel disease
Dermatitis herpetiformis
Toxic/chemical syndrome
Eosinophilic myalgia syndrome, tryptophan, toxic oil syndrome
Hypereosinophilic syndrome (unknown etiology)

EPINEPHRINE, PLASMA

Normal range: 0-90 pg/ml
Elevated in: Pheochromocytomas, neuroblastomas, stress, vigorous exercise, certain foods (bananas, chocolate, coffee, tea, vanilla), hypoglycemia

EPSTEIN-BARR VIRUS SEROLOGY

Normal range: IgG anti VCA <1:10 or negative
Abnormal: IgG anti VCA >1:10 or positive indicates either current or previous infection
IgM anti VCA >1:10 or positive indicates current or recent infection
Anti-EBNA ≥1.5 or positive indicates previous infection
Table 4-11 and Fig. 4-3 describe test interpretation

ERYTHROCYTE SEDIMENTATION RATE (ESR; Westergren)

Normal range: Male: 0-15 mm/hr
Female: 0-20 mm/hr
Elevated in: Collagen-vascular diseases, infections, myocardial infarction, neoplasms, inflammatory states (acute phase reactant), hyperthyroidism, hypothyroidism, rouleaux formation
Decreased in: Sickle cell disease, polycythemia, corticosteroids, spherocytosis, anisocytosis, hypofibrinogenemia, increased serum viscosity

ERYTHROPOIETIN (EP)

Normal: 3.7-16.0 IU/L by radioimmunoassay
Erythropoietin is a glycoprotein secreted by the kidneys that stimulates RBC production by acting on erythroid-committed stem cells.
Increased in: Extremely high: generally seen in patients with severe anemia (Hct <25, <7) such as in cases of aplastic anemia,

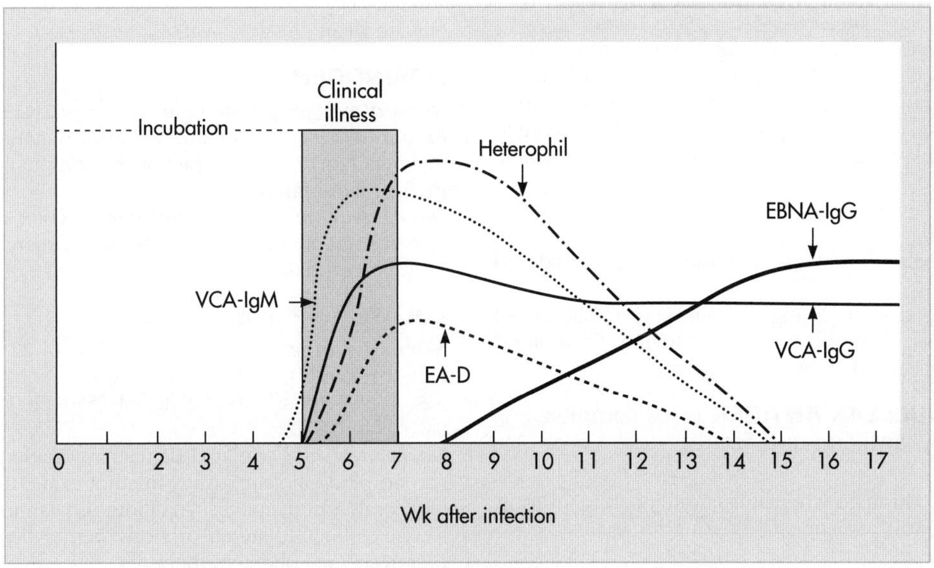

FIGURE 4-3 Tests in Epstein-Barr viral infection. See Table 4-11 for abbreviations. (From Ravel R: *Clinical laboratory medicine*, ed 6, St Louis, 1995, Mosby.)

TABLE 4-11 Antibody Tests in Epstein-Barr Viral Infection

	Appearance	Peak	Disappears
Heterophil Ab	3-5 days after onset of Sx (range, 0-21 days)	During second wk after onset of Sx (1-4 wk)	2-3 mo after onset of Sx (still found at 1 yr in 20% of cases)
VCA-IgM	Beginning of Sx (1 wk before to 1 wk after Sx begins)	During first wk after onset of Sx (0-21 days)	2-3 mo after onset of Sx (1-6 mo)
VCA-IgG	3 days after onset of Sx (0-2 wk)	During second wk after onset of Sx (1-3 wk)	Decline to lower level, then persists for life
EBNA-IgG	3 wk after onset of Sx (1-4 wk)	8 mo after appearance (3-12 mo)	Lifelong
EA-D	5 days after onset of Sx (during first 1-2 wk after onset of Sx)	14-21 days after onset of Sx (1-4 wk)	9 wk after appearance (2-6 mo)
(EBNA-IgM)	(Same as VCA-IgM)	(Same as VCA-IgM)	(Same as VCA-IgM)

From Ravel R: *Clinical laboratory medicine,* ed 6, St Louis, 1995, Mosby.
Ab, Antibody; *EA,* early antigen; *EBNA,* Epstein-Barr virus nuclear antigen; *Sx,* symptoms; *VCA,* viral capsid antigen.

severe hemolytic anemia, hematologic cancers. Very high: patients with mild to moderate anemia (Hct 25-35, Hb 7-10); high: patients with mild anemia (e.g., AIDS, myelodysplasia).
Erythropoietin can be inappropriately elevated in patients with malignant neoplasms, renal cysts, postrenal transplant, meningioma, hemangioblastoma, and leiomyoma.
Decreased in: Renal failure, polycythemia vera, autonomic neuropathy

ESTRADIOL (serum)

Normal range: **FEMALE, PREMENOPAUSAL:** 30-400 pg/ml, depending on phase of menstrual cycle
FEMALE, POSTMENOPAUSAL: 0-30 pg/ml
MALE, ADULT: 10-50 pg/ml
Decreased in: Ovarian failure
Elevated in: Tumors of ovary, testis, adrenal, or nonendocrine sites (rare)

ESTROGEN

Normal range:

Serum:	Males:	20-80 pg/ml
	Females:	Follicular: 60-200 pg/ml
		Luteal: 160-400 pg/ml
		Postmenopausal: <130 pg/ml
Urine:	Males:	4-23 μg/g creatinine
	Females:	Follicular: 7-65 μg/g creatinine
		Midcycle: 32-104 μg/g creatinine
		Luteal: 8-135 μg/g creatinine

Elevated in: Hyperplasia of adrenal cortex, ovarian tumors producing estrogen, granulosa and thecal cell tumors, testicular tumors
Decreased in: Menopause, hypopituitarism, primary ovarian malfunction, anorexia nervosa, hypofunction of adrenal cortex, ovarian agenesis, psychogenic stress, gonadotropin-releasing hormone deficiency

ETHANOL (blood)

Normal range: Negative (values <10 mg/dl are considered negative)
Ethanol is metabolized at 10-25 mg/dl/hour. Levels ≥80 mg/dl are considered evidence of impairment for driving. Fatal blood concentration is considered to be >400 mg/dl.

EXTRACTABLE NUCLEAR ANTIGEN (ENA complex, anti-RNP antibody, anti-Sm, anti-Smith)

Normal: Negative
Present in: Systemic lupus erythematosus, rheumatoid arthritis, Sjögren's syndrome, mixed connective tissue disease

FDP; *see* FIBRIN DEGRADATION PRODUCT

FECAL FAT, QUANTITATIVE (72-hr collection)

Normal range: 2-6 g/24 hr (7-21 mmol/dl [CF: 3.515; SMI: 1 mmol/dl])
Elevated in: Malabsorption syndrome

FERRITIN (serum)

Normal range: 18-300 ng/ml (18-300 μg/L [CF: 1; SMI: 10 μg/L])
Elevated in: Hyperthyroidism, inflammatory states, liver disease (ferritin elevated from necrotic hepatocytes), neoplasms (neuroblastomas, lymphomas, leukemia, breast carcinoma), iron replacement therapy, hemochromatosis, hemosiderosis
Decreased in: Iron deficiency anemia

α-1 FETOPROTEIN

Normal range: 0-20 ng/ml (0-20 μg/L [CF: 1; SMI: 1 μg/L])
Elevated in: Hepatocellular carcinoma (usually values >1000 ng/ml), germinal neoplasms (testis, ovary, mediastinum, retroperitoneum), liver disease (alcoholic cirrhosis, acute hepatitis, chronic active hepatitis), fetal anencephaly, spina bifida, basal cell carcinoma, breast carcinoma, pancreatic carcinoma, gastric carcinoma, retinoblastoma, esophageal atresia

FIBRIN DEGRADATION PRODUCT (FDP)

Normal range: <10 μg/ml
Elevated in: Disseminated intravascular coagulation, primary fibrinolysis, pulmonary embolism, severe liver disease
NOTE: The presence of rheumatoid factor may cause falsely elevated FDP.

FIBRINOGEN

Normal range: 200-400 mg/dl (2-4 g/L [CF: 0.01; SMI: 0.1 g/L])
Elevated in: Tissue inflammation or damage (acute phase protein reactant), oral contraceptives, pregnancy, acute infection, myocardial infarction
Decreased in: Disseminated intravascular coagulation, hereditary afibrinogenemia, liver disease, primary or secondary fibrinolysis, cachexia

FOLATE (folic acid)

Normal range: Plasma: 2-10 ng/ml (4-22 nmol/L [CF: 2.266; SMI: 2 nmol/L])
Red blood cells: 140-960 ng/ml (550-2200 nmol/L [CF: 2.266; SMI: 10 nmol/L])
Decreased in: Folic acid deficiency (inadequate intake, malabsorption), alcoholism, drugs (methotrexate, trimethoprim, phenytoin, oral contraceptives, Azulfidine), vitamin B_{12} deficiency (defective red cell folate absorption), hemolytic anemia
Elevated in: Folic acid therapy

FOLLICLE-STIMULATING HORMONE (FSH)

Normal range: 5-20 mIU/ml
Elevated in: Menopause, primary gonadal failure, alcoholism, castration, Klinefelter's syndrome, gonadotropin-secreting pituitary hormones
Decreased in: Pregnancy, polycystic ovary disease, anorexia nervosa, anterior pituitary hypofunction

FREE T_4; *see* T_4, FREE

FREE THYROXINE INDEX

Normal range: 1.1-4.3

INCREASED THYROXINE OR FREE THYROXINE VALUES

Laboratory error
Primary hyperthyroidism (T_4/T_3 type)
Severe thyroxine-binding globulin elevation
Excess therapy of hypothyroidism
Excessive dose of levothyroxine
Active thyroiditis (subacute, painless, early active Hashimoto's disease)
Familial dysalbuminemic hyperthyroxinemia (some FT_4 kits, especially analog types)
Peripheral resistance to T_4 syndrome
Amiodarone or propranolol
Postpartum transient toxicosis
Factitious hyperthyroidism
Jod-Basedow (iodine-induced) hyperthyroidism
Severe nonthyroid illness
Acute psychosis (especially paranoid schizophrenia)
T_4 sample drawn 2-4 hr after levothyroxine dose
Struma ovarii
Pituitary thyroid-stimulating hormone–secreting tumor
Certain x-ray contrast media (Telepaque and Oragrafin)
Acute porphyria
Heparin effect (some T_4 and FT_4 kits)
Amphetamine, heroin, methadone, and phencyclidine abuse
Perphenazine or 5-fluorouracil
Antithyroid or anti-IgG heterophil (HAMA) autoantibodies
"T_4" hyperthyroidism
Hyperemesis gravidarum; about 50% of patients
High altitudes

DECREASED THYROXINE OR FREE THYROXINE VALUES

Laboratory error
Primary hypothyroidism
Severe nonthyroid illness*
Lithium therapy
Severe thyroxine-binding globulin decrease (congenital, disease, or drug-induced) or severe albumin decrease*
Dilantin, Depakene, or high-dose salicylate drugs*
Pituitary insufficiency
Large doses of inorganic iodide (e.g., saturated solution of potassium iodide)
Moderate or severe iodine deficiency
Cushing's syndrome
High-dose glucocorticoid drugs
Pregnancy, third trimester (low normal or small decrease)
Addison's disease; some patients (30%)
Heparin effect (a few FT_4 kits)
Desipramine or amiodarone drugs
Acute psychiatric illness

FTA-ABS (serum)

Normal: Nonreactive
Reactive in: Syphilis, other treponemal diseases (yaws, pinta, bejel), SLE, pregnancy

GAMMA-GLUTAMYL TRANSFERASE (gGt); *see* γ-GLUTAMYL TRANSFERASE

GASTRIN (serum)

Normal range: 0-180 pg/ml (0-180 ng/L [CF: 1; SMI: 10 ng/L])
Elevated in: Zollinger-Ellison syndrome (gastrinoma), pernicious anemia, hyperparathyroidism, retained gastric antrum, chronic renal failure, gastric ulcer, chronic atrophic gastritis, pyloric obstruction, malignant neoplasms of the stomach, H_2-blockers, omeprazole, calcium therapy, ulcerative colitis, rheumatoid arthritis

GLOMERULAR BASEMENT MEMBRANE (gBm) ANTIBODY

Normal: Negative
Present in: Goodpasture's syndrome

GLUCOSE, FASTING

Normal range: 70-110 mg/dl (3.9-6.1 mmol/L [CF: 0.05551; SMI: 0.1 mmol/L])
Elevated in: Diabetes mellitus, stress, infections, myocardial infarction, cerebrovascular accident, Cushing's syndrome, acromegaly, acute pancreatitis, glucagonoma, hemochromatosis, drugs (glucocorticoids, diuretics [thiazides, loop diuretics]), glucose intolerance
Decreased in: Sulfonylurea therapy, insulin therapy, reactive hypoglycemia (e.g., s/b subtotal gastrectomy), starvation, insulinoma, glycogen storage disorders, severe liver disease or renal disease, ethanol-induced hypoglycemia, mesenchymal tumors that secrete insulin-like hormones

GLUCOSE, POSTPRANDIAL

Normal range: <140 mg/dl (<7.8 mmol/L [CF: 0.05551; SMI: 0.1 mmol/L])
Elevated in: Diabetes mellitus, glucose intolerance
Decreased in: Postgastrointestinal resection, reactive hypoglycemia, hereditary fructose intolerance, galactosemia, leucine sensitivity

GLUCOSE TOLERANCE TEST

Normal values above fasting:
30 min: 30-60 mg/dl (1.65-3.3 mmol/L [CF: 0.05551; SMI: 0.1 mmol/L])
60 min: 20-50 mg/dl (1.1-2.75 mmol/L [CF: 0.05551; SMI: 0.1 mmol/L])
120 min: 5-15 mg/dl (0.28-0.83 mmol/L [CF: 0.05551; SMI: 0.1 mmol/L])
180 min: fasting level or below
Abnormal in: Glucose intolerance, diabetes mellitus, Cushing's syndrome, acromegaly, pheochromocytoma, gestational diabetes

GLUCOSE-6-PHOSPHATE DEHYDROGENASE SCREEN (blood)

Normal: G_6PD enzyme activity detected
Abnormal: If a deficiency is detected, quantitation of G_6PD is necessary; a G_6PD screen may be falsely interpreted as "normal" after an episode of hemolysis because most G_6PD-deficient cells have been destroyed.

γ-GLUTAMYL TRANSFERASE (GGT)

Normal range: 0-30 U/L (0.050 μkat/L [CF: 0.01667; SMI: 0.01 μkat/L])
Elevated in: Chronic alcoholic liver disease, neoplasms (hepatoma, metastatic disease to the liver, carcinoma of the pancreas), systemic lupus erythematosus, congestive heart failure, trauma, nephrotic syndrome, sepsis, cholestasis, drugs (phenytoin, barbiturates)

GLYCATED (GLYCOSYLATED) HEMOGLOBIN (HbA_{1c}) (GLYCOHEMOGLOBIN)

Normal range: 4.0% to 5.9%

Elevated in: Uncontrolled diabetes mellitus (glycated hemoglobin levels reflect the level of glucose control over the preceding 120 days), lead toxicity, alcoholism, iron deficiency anemia, hypertriglyceridemia
Decreased in: Hemolytic anemias, decreased red blood cell survival, pregnancy, acute or chronic blood loss, chronic renal failure, insulinoma, congenital spherocytosis, hemoglobin S, C, and D diseases

HAM TEST (acid serum test)

Normal: Negative
Positive in: Paroxysmal nocturnal hemoglobinuria
False positive in: Hereditary or acquired spherocytosis, recent transfusion with aged red blood cells, aplastic anemia, myeloproliferative syndromes, leukemia, hereditary dyserythropoietic anemia type II

HAPTOGLOBIN (serum)

Normal range: 50-220 mg/dl (0.50-2.2 g/L [CF: 0.01; SMI: 0.01 g/L])
Elevated in: Inflammation (acute phase reactant), collagen-vascular diseases, infections (acute phase reactant), drugs (androgens), obstructive liver disease
Decreased in: Hemolysis (intravascular more than extravascular), megaloblastic anemia, severe liver disease, large tissue hematomas, infectious mononucleosis, drugs (oral contraceptives)

HDL; *see* HIGH-DENSITY LIPOPROTEIN CHOLESTEROL

HELICOBACTER PYLORI (serology, stool antigen)

Normal range: Not detected
Detected in: *H. pylori* infection. Positive serology can indicate current or past infection. Positive stool antigen test indicates acute infection (sensitivity and specificity >90%). Stool testing should be delayed at least 4 weeks after eradication therapy.

HEMATOCRIT

Normal range: Male: 39% to 49% (0.39-0.49 [CF: 0.01; SMI: 0.01])
Female: 33% to 43% (0.33-0.43 [CF: 0.01; SMI: 0.01])
Elevated in: Polycythemia vera, smoking, chronic obstructive pulmonary disease, high altitudes, dehydration, hypovolemia
Decreased in: Blood loss (gastrointestinal, genitourinary) anemia

HEMOGLOBIN

Normal range: Male: 13.6-17.7 g/dl (136-172 g/L [CF: 10; SMI: 1 g/L])
Female: 12.0-15.0 g/dl (120-150 g/L [CF: 10; SMI: 1 g/L])
Elevated in: Hemoconcentration, dehydration, polycythemia vera, chronic obstructive pulmonary disease, high altitudes, false elevations (hyperlipemic plasma, white blood cells >50,000/mm^3), stress
Decreased in: Hemorrhage (gastrointestinal, genitourinary) anemia

HEMOGLOBIN A_{1c}, *see* GLYCATED HEMOGLOBIN

HEMOGLOBIN ELECTROPHORESIS

Normal range:
HbA$_1$: 95%-98%
HbA$_2$: 1.5%-3.5%
HbF: <2%
HbC: absent
HbS: absent

HEMOGLOBIN, GLYCATED; *see* GLYCATED HEMOGLOBIN

HEMOGLOBIN, GLYCOSYLATED; *see* GLYCATED HEMOGLOBIN

HEMOGLOBIN, URINE; *see* URINE HEMOGLOBIN, FREE

HEMOSIDERIN, URINE; *see* URINE HEMOSIDERIN

HEPATITIS A ANTIBODY

Normal: Negative
Present in: Viral hepatitis A; can be IgM or IgG (if IgM, acute hepatitis A; if IgG, previous infection with hepatitis A)
See Fig. 4-4 for serologic tests in HAV infection.

HAV-IGM ANTIBODY

Appearance
About the same time as clinical symptoms (3-4 wk after exposure, range 14-60 days), or just before beginning of AST/ALT elevation (range 10 days before–7 days after)
Peak
About 3-4 wk after onset of symptoms (1-6 wk)

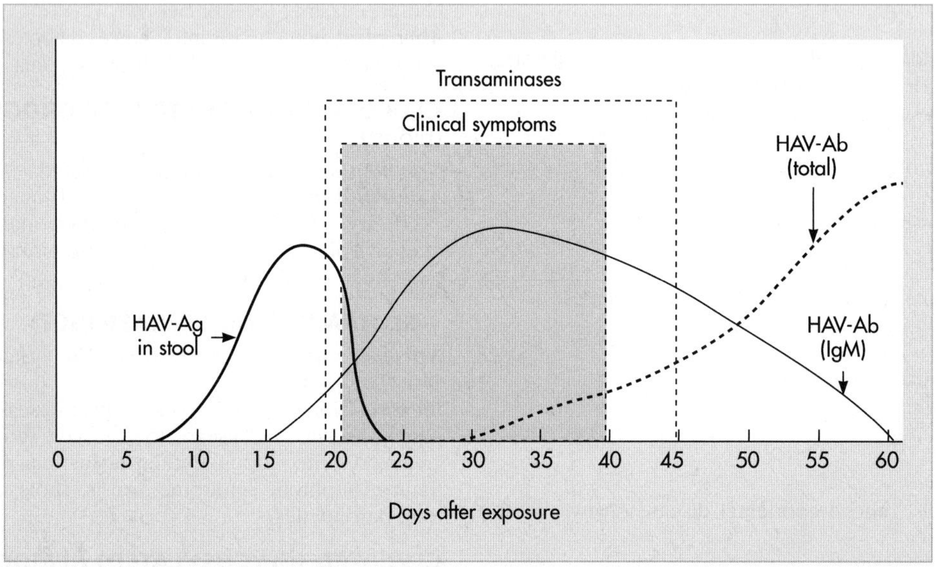

FIGURE 4-4 Serologic tests in hepatitis A virus infection. (From Ravel R: *Clinical laboratory medicine,* ed 6, St Louis, 1995, Mosby.)

Becomes Nondetectable
3-4 mo after onset of symptoms (1-6 mo). In a few cases HAV-IgM antibody can persist as long as 12-14 mo.
HAV-TOTAL ANTIBODY
Appearance
About 3 wk after IgM becomes detectable (therefore about the middle of clinical symptom period to early convalescence)
Peak
About 1-2 mo after onset
Becomes Nondetectable
Remains elevated for life, but can slowly fall somewhat

HEPATITIS A VIRAL INFECTION

Best all-purpose test(s) to diagnose acute HAV infection = HAV-Ab (IgM)
Best all-purpose test(s) to demonstrate past HAV infection/immunity = HAV-Ab (total)

HEPATITIS B SURFACE ANTIGEN (HBsAg)

Normal: Not detected
Detected in: Acute viral hepatitis type B, chronic hepatitis B
Appearance
2-6 wk after exposure (range 6 days–6 mo); 5%-15% of patients are negative at onset of jaundice
Peak
1-2 wk before to 1-2 wk after onset of symptoms
Becomes Nondetectable
1-3 mo after peak (range 1 wk-5 mo)

HEPATITIS B VIRAL INFECTION

Figs. 4-5, 4-6, and 4-7 illustrate antigens and antibodies in Hepatitis B infection.
HB_S
-Ag
HB_SAg: shows current active HBV infection.
Persistence over 6 mo indicates carrier/chronic HBV infection.
HBV nucleic acid probe: present before and longer than HB_SAg. More reliable marker for increased infectivity than HB_SAg and/or HB_eAg.
-Ab
HB_SAb-total: shows previous healed HBV infection and evidence of immunity.
HB_C
-Ab
HB_CAb-IgM: shows either acute or very recent infection by HBV. In convalescent phase of acute HBV, may be elevated when HB_SAg has disappeared (core window).
Negative HB_CAb-IgM with positive HB_SAg suggests either very early acute HBV or carrier/chronic HBV.
HB_CAb-total: only useful to show past HBV infection if HB_SAg and HB_cAb-IgM are both negative.
HB_E
-Ag
HB_e-AbAg: when present, especially without HB_eAb, suggests increased patient infectivity.
HB_eAb-total: when present, suggests less patient infectivity.

I. HB_SAg positive, HB_CAb negative*
   About 5% (range 0%-17%) of patients with early-stage HBV acute infection (HB_CAb rises later)
II. HB_SAg positive, HB_CAb positive, HB_SAb negative
   a. Most of the clinical symptom stage
   b. Chronic HBV carriers without evidence of liver disease ("asymptomatic carriers")
   c. Chronic HBV hepatitis (chronic persistent type or chronic active type)
III. HB_SAg negative, HB_CAb positive,* HB_SAb negative
   a. Late clinical symptom stage or early convalescence stage (core window)
   b. Chronic HBV infection with HB_SAg below detection levels with current tests
   c. Old previous HBV infection
IV. HB_SAg negative, HB_CAb positive, HB_SAb positive
   a. Late convalescence to complete recovery
   b. Old infection

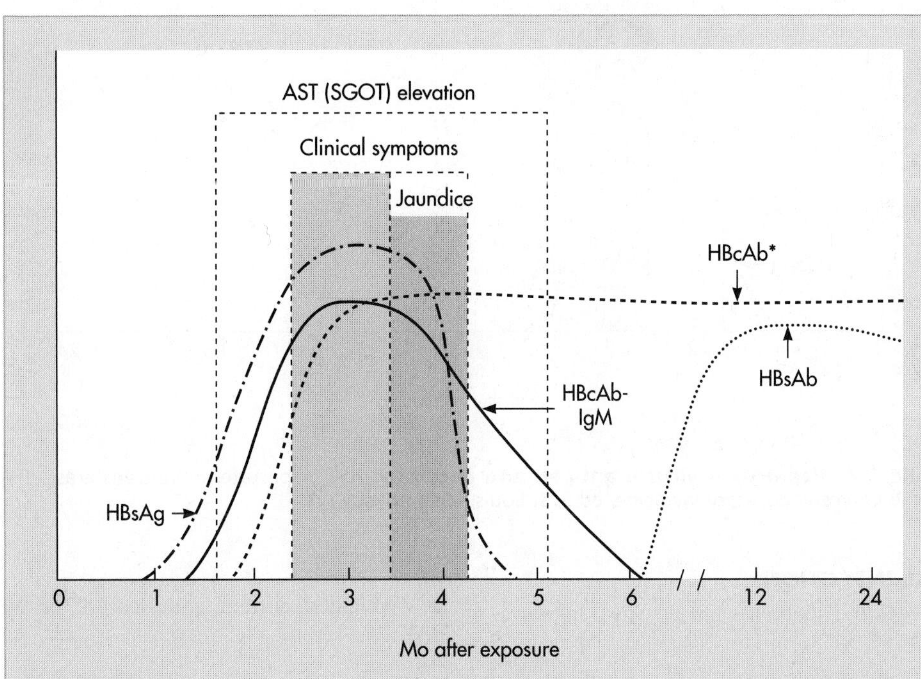

FIGURE 4-5 Hepatitis B virus surface antigen-antibody and core antibodies (note "core window"). *HB_CAb = HB_CAb-IgM + HBCAb-IgG (combined). *AST,* Aspartate aminotransferase. (From Ravel R: *Clinical laboratory medicine,* ed 6, St Louis, 1995, Mosby.)

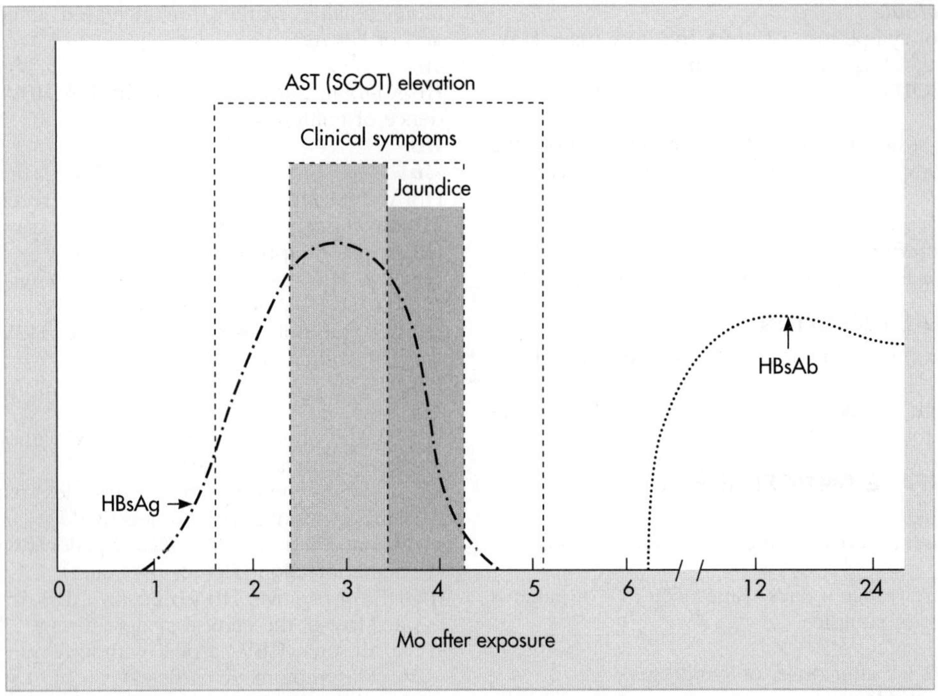

FIGURE 4-6 Hepatitis B virus surface antigen and antibody (HB_sAg and HB_sAb-total). *AST,* Aspartate aminotransferase. (From Ravel R: *Clinical laboratory medicine,* ed 6, St Louis, 1995, Mosby.)

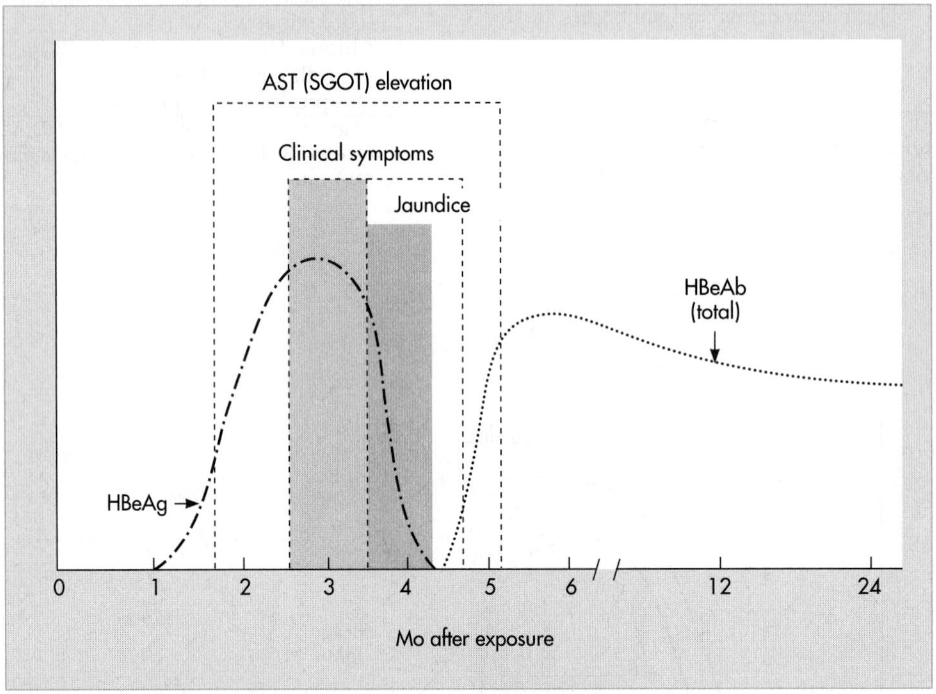

FIGURE 4-7 Hepatitis B virus e antigen and antibody. *AST,* Aspartate aminotransferase. (From Ravel R: *Clinical laboratory medicine,* ed 6, St Louis, 1995, Mosby.)

HEPATITIS C VIRAL INFECTION

Fig. 4-8 illustrates antigens and antibodies in Hepatitis C Infection.

HCV

-Ag

HCV nucleic acid probe: shows current infection by HCV (especially using PCR amplification).

-Ab

HCV-Ab (IgG): current, convalescent, or old HCV infection.

HAV

-Ag

HAV-Ag by EM: shows presence of virus in stool early in infection.

-Ab

HAV-Ab (IgM): current or recent HAV infection.
HAV-Ab (total): convalescent or old HAV infection.

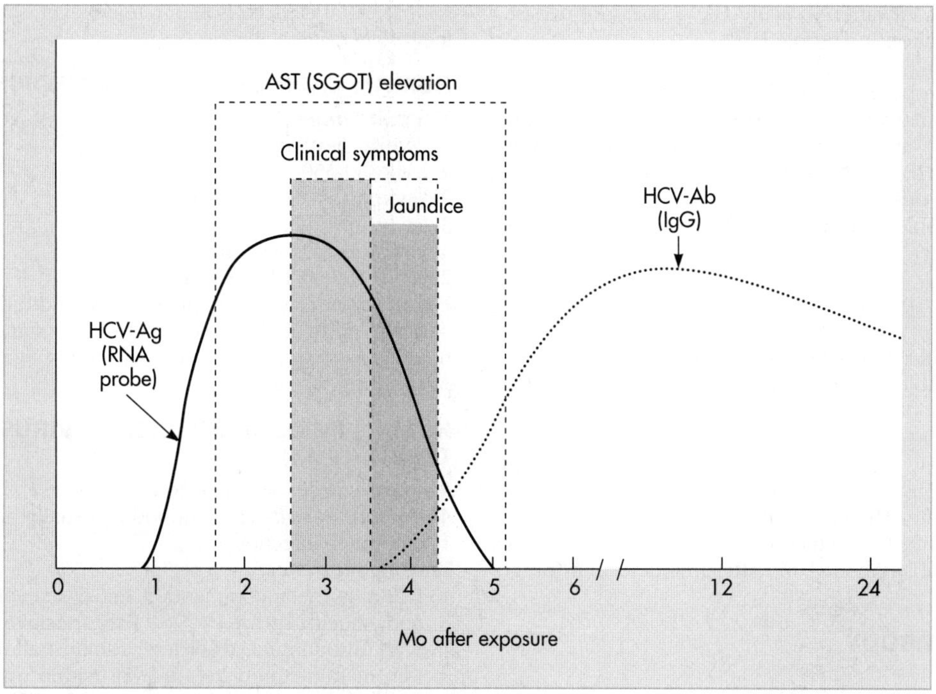

FIGURE 4-8 Hepatitis C virus antigen and antibody. *AST,* Aspartate aminotransferase. (From Ravel R: *Clinical laboratory medicine,* ed 6, St Louis, 1995, Mosby.)

HEPATITIS D VIRAL INFECTION

Fig. 4-9 illustrates antigens and antibodies in Hepatitis D Infection.
Best current all-purpose screening test = ADV-Ab (total)
Best test to differentiate acute from chronic infection = HDV-Ab (IgM)

DELTA HEPATITIS COINFECTION (ACUTE HDV + ACUTE HBV) OR SUPERINFECTION (ACUTE HDV + CHRONIC HBV) HDV

-Ag

HDV-Ag: shows current infection (acute or chronic) by HDV.
HDV nucleic acid probe: detects antigen before and longer than HDV-Ag by EIA.

-Ab

HDV-Ab (IgM): high elevation in acute HDV; does not persist.
Low or moderate elevation in convalescent HDV; does not persist.
Low to high persistent elevation in chronic HDV (depends on degree of cell injury and sensitivity of the assay).

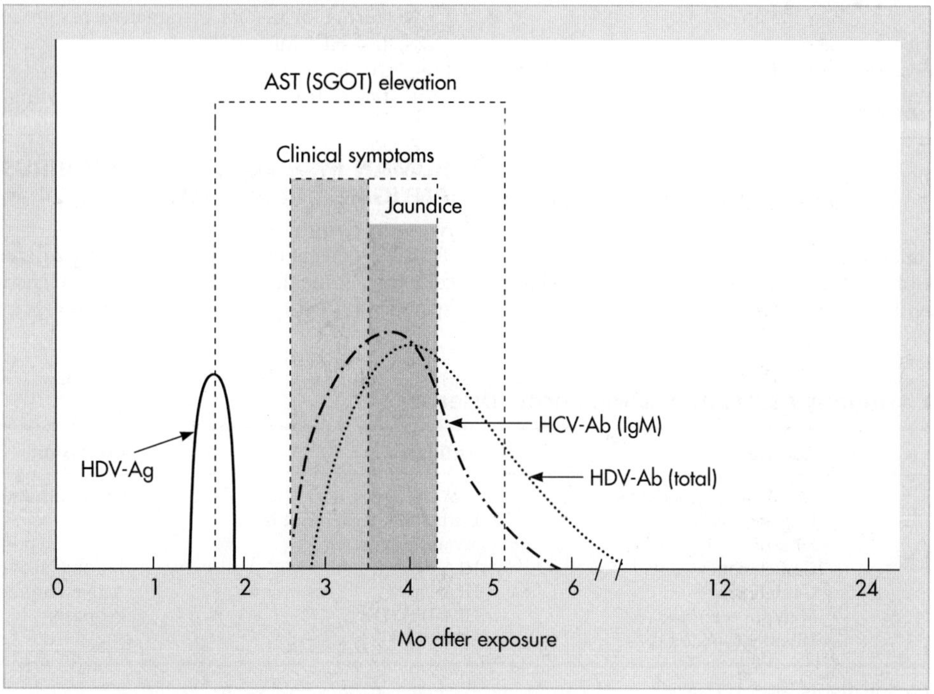

FIGURE 4-9 Hepatitis D virus antigen and antibodies. *AST,* Aspartate aminotransferase. (From Ravel R: *Clinical laboratory medicine,* ed 6, St Louis, 1995, Mosby.)

HDV-Ab (total): high elevation in acute HDV; does not persist. High persistent elevation in chronic HDV.

HDV-AG

Detected by DNA probe, less often by immunoassay

Appearance: Prodromal stage (before symptoms); just at or after initial rise in ALT (about a week after appearance of HB_SAg and about the time HB_CAb-IgM level begins to rise)

Peak: 2-3 days after onset

Becomes nondetectable: 1-4 days (may persist until shortly after symptoms appear)

HDV-AB (IGM)

Appearance: about 10 days after symptoms begin (range 1-28 days)

Peak: about 2 wk after first detection

Becomes nondetectable: about 35 days (range 10-80 days) after first detection (most other IgM antibodies take 3-6 mo to become nondetectable)

HDV-AB (TOTAL)

Appearance: about 50 days after symptoms begin (range 14-80 days); about 5 wk after HDV-Ag (range 3-11 wk)

Peak: About 2 wk after first detection

Becomes nondetectable: about 7 mo after first detection (range 4-14 mo)

HETEROPHIL ANTIBODY

Normal: Negative

Positive in: Infectious mononucleosis

HIGH-DENSITY LIPOPROTEIN (HDL) CHOLESTEROL

Normal range:

Male: 40-70 mg/dl (0.8-1.8 mmol/L [CF: 0.02586; SMI: 0.05 mmol/L])

Female: 50-90 mg/dl (1.1-2.35 mmol/L [CF: 0.02586; SMI: 0.05 mmol/L])

Increased in: Use of gemfibrozil, statins, fenofibrate, nicotinic acid, estrogens, regular aerobic exercise, small (1 oz) daily alcohol intake

Decreased in: Deficiency of apoproteins, liver disease, probucol ingestion, Tangier disease

NOTE: A cholesterol/HDL ratio >4.0 is associated with increased risk of coronary artery disease.

HLA ANTIGENS

Associated disorders: *see* Table 4-12

HOMOCYSTEINE, PLASMA

Normal range:

0-30 years: 4.6-8.1 micromol/L

30-59 years: 6.3-11.2 micromol/L (males), 4-5-7.9 micromol/L (females)

> 59 years: 5.8-11.9 micromol/L

Increased: Thrombophilic states, B_6, B_{12}, folic acid, riboflavin deficiency, pregnancy, homocystinuria

NOTE: An increased homocysteine level is an independent risk factor for atherosclerosis.

HUMAN CHORIONIC GONADOTROPIN (hCG)

Normal range: Varies with gestational stage

1st week: 5-50 mU/ml

1-2 wk: 50-550 mU/ml

2-3 wk: up to 5000 mU/ml

3-4 wk: up to 10,000 mU/ml

4-5 wk: up to 50,000 mU/ml

2-3 mo: 10,000-100,000 mU/ml

Elevated in: Normal pregnancy, hydatidiform mole, choriocarcinoma, germ cell tumors of testicle, some nontrophoblastic neoplasms (e.g., neoplasms of cervix, gastrointestinal tract, ovary, lung, breast)

HUMAN IMMUNODEFICIENCY VIRUS ANTIBODY, TYPE 1 (HIV-1)

Normal range: Not detected

Abnormal result: HIV antibodies usually appear in the blood 1-4 mo after infection.

Testing sequence:

1. ELISA is the recommended initial screening test. Sensitivity and specificity are >99%. False-positive ELISA may occur with autoimmune disorders, administration of immune globulin manufactured before 1985 within 6 wk of testing, presence of rheumatoid factor, presence of DLA-DR antibodies in multigravida female, administration of influenza vaccine within 3 mo of testing, hemodialysis, positive plasma reagin test, certain medical disorders (hemophilia, hypergammaglobulinemia, alcoholic hepatitis)
2. A positive ELISA is confirmed with Western blot. False-positive Western blot may result from connective tissue disorders, human leukocyte antigen antibodies, polyclonal gammopathies, hyperbilirubinemia, presence of antibody to another human retrovirus, or cross reaction with other nonvirus-derived proteins in healthy persons. Undetermined Western blot may occur in AIDS patients with advanced immunodeficiency (caused by loss of antibodies), and in recent HIV infections.
3. Polymerase chain reaction is used to confirm indeterminate Western blot results or negative results in persons with suspected HIV infection.

Fig. 4-10 describes tests in HIV infection.

Indications for plasma HIV RNA testing are described in Table 4-13.

HUMAN IMMUNODEFICIENCY VIRUS TYPE 1 (HIV-1) ANTIGEN (p24), QUALITATIVE (p24 antigen)

Normal range: Negative

This test detects uncomplexed HIV-1 p24 antigen. The core protein p24 is the first detectable protein encoded by the group-specific antigen *(gag)* gene. This protein is a marker for viremia.

TABLE 4-12 HLA Antigens Associated with Specific Diseases

Antigen	Condition	Antigen	Condition
HLA-B27	Ankylosing spondylitis	HLA-B8, Dw3	Celiac disease
Reiter's syndrome	HLA-B8, Dw3	Dermatitis herpetiformis	
Psoriatic arthritis	HLA-B8	Myasthenia gravis	
HLA-A10, B18, Dw2	C2 deficiency	HLA-B8	Chronic active hepatitis in children
HLA-A2, B40, Cw3	C4 deficiency	HLA-Drw4	Active chronic hepatitis in adults
HLA-B7, Dw2	Multiple sclerosis	HLA-B13, Bw17	Psoriasis
HLA-A3	Hemochromatosis		

From Cerra FB: *Manual of critical care,* St Louis, 1987, Mosby.

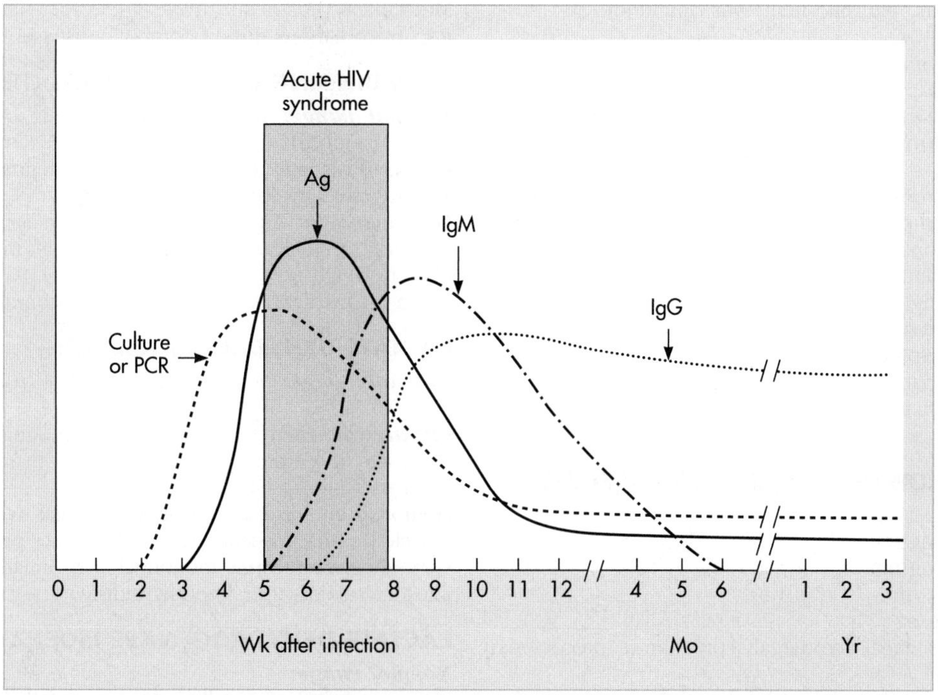

FIGURE 4-10 Tests in HIV-1 infection. *HIV,* Human immunodeficiency virus; *IgG,* immunoglobulin G; *IgM,* immunoglobulin M; *PCR,* polymerase chain reaction. (From Ravel R: *Clinical laboratory medicine,* ed 6, St Louis, 1995, Mosby.)

TABLE 4-13 **Indications for Plasma HIV RNA Testing***

Clinical Indication	Information	Use
Syndrome consistent with acute HIV infection	Establishes diagnosis when HIV antibody test is negative or indeterminate	Diagnosis†
Initial evaluation of newly diagnosed HIV infection	Baseline viral load "set point"	Decision to start or defer therapy
Every 3-4 mo in patients not on therapy	Changes in viral load	Decision to start therapy
4-8 wk after initiation of anti-retroviral therapy	Initial assessment of drug efficacy	Decision to continue or change therapy
3-4 mo after start of therapy	Maximal effect of therapy	Decision to continue or change therapy
Every 3-4 mo in patients on therapy	Durability of antiretroviral effect	Decision to continue or change therapy
Clinical event or significant decline in CD41 T cells	Association with changing or stable	Decision to continue, initiate, or change

From *MMWR,* vol 47, no RR-5, Apr 24, 1998.

*Acute illness (e.g., bacterial pneumonia, tuberculosis, HSV, PCP) and immunizations can cause increase in plasma HIV RNA for 2-4 wk; viral load testing should not be performed during this time. Plasma HIV RNA results should usually be verified with a repeat determination before starting or making changes in therapy. HIV RNA should be measured using the same laboratory and the same assay.

†Diagnosis of HIV infection determined by HIV RNA testing should be confirmed by standard methods (e.g., Western blot serology) performed 2-4 mo after the initial indeterminate or negative test.

This test should not be used in place of HIV-1 antibody testing as a screen for HIV-1 infection. HIV-1 p24 may be detectable in the first month of acute HIV-1 infection and generally falls to undetectable levels during the asymptomatic stage of HIV-1 infection. A negative result does not exclude the possibility of infection or exposure to HIV-1. It is recommended that a negative result be followed with repeat testing at least 8 weeks after the original test. This test is used primarily for screening of donated blood and plasma and as an aid for the prognosis of HIV-1 infection.

HUMAN IMMUNODEFICIENCY VIRUS TYPE 1 (HIV-1) VIRAL LOAD

Normal range: HIV-1 RNA, quant. bDNA 3: less than 50 copies/ml or less than 1.7 log copies/ml

This test should be used only in individuals with documented HIV-1 infection for monitoring the progression of infection, response to antiretroviral therapy, and disease prognosis. It is not indicated for diagnosis of HIV infection.

5-HYDROXYINDOLE-ACETIC ACID, URINE; *see* URINE 5-HYDROXYINDOLE-ACETIC ACID

IMMUNE COMPLEX ASSAY

Normal: Negative

Detected in: Collagen-vascular disorders, glomerulonephritis, neoplastic diseases, malaria, primary biliary cirrhosis, chronic acute hepatitis, bacterial endocarditis, vasculitis

IMMUNOGLOBULINS

Normal range:

IgA: 50-350 mg/dl (0.5-3.5 g/L [CF: 0.01; SMI: 0.01 g/L])
IgD: <6 mg/dl (<60 mg/L [CF: 0.01; SMI: 0.01 g/L])
IgE: <25 μg/dl (<0.00025 g/L [CF: 0.01; SMI: 0.01 g/L])
IgG: 800-1500 mg/dl (8-15 g/L [CF: 0.01; SMI: 0.01 g/L])
IgM: 45-150 mg/dl (0.45-1.5 g/L [CF: 0.01; SMI: 0.01 g/L])

Elevated in:

IgA: lymphoproliferative disorders, Berger's nephropathy, chronic infections, autoimmune disorders, liver disease

IgE: allergic disorders, parasitic infections, immunologic disorders, IgE myeloma
IgG: chronic granulomatous infections, infectious diseases, inflammation, myeloma, liver disease
IgM: primary biliary cirrhosis, infectious diseases (brucellosis, malaria), Waldenström's macroglobulinemia, liver disease
Decreased in:
IgA: nephrotic syndrome, protein-losing enteropathy, congenital deficiency, lymphocytic leukemia, ataxia-telangiectasia, chronic sinopulmonary disease
IgE: hypogammaglobulinemia, neoplasma (breast, bronchial, cervical), ataxia-telangiectasia
IgG: congenital or acquired deficiency, lymphocytic leukemia, phenytoin, methylprednisolone, nephrotic syndrome, protein-losing enteropathy
IgM: congenital deficiency, lymphocytic leukemia, nephrotic syndrome

INSULIN-LIKE GROWTH FACTOR-1 (IGF-1), SERUM

Normal range:
Age 16-24: 182-780 ng/ml
Age 25-39: 114-492 ng/ml
Age 40-54: 90-360 ng/ml
Age $>$ 55: 71-290 ng/ml
Elevated in: Adolescence, acromegaly, pregnancy, precocious puberty, obesity
Decreased in: Malnutrition, delayed puberty, diabetes mellitus, hypopituitarism, cirrhosis, old age

INTERNATIONAL NORMALIZED RATIO (INR)

The INR is a comparative rating of prothrombin time (PT) ratios. The INR represents the observed PT ratio adjusted by the International Reference Thromboplastin. It provides a universal result indicative of what the patient's PT result would have been if measured using the primary World Health Organization International Reference reagent. For proper interpretation of INR values, the patient should be on stable anticoagulant therapy.
Recommended INR ranges:
Proximal deep vein thrombosis: 2-3
Pulmonary embolism: 2-3
Transient ischemic attacks: 2-3
Atrial fibrillation: 2-3
Mechanical prosthetic valves: 3-4.5
Recurrent venous thromboembolic disease: 3-4.5

IRON-BINDING CAPACITY, TOTAL (TIBC)

Normal range: 250-460 μg/dl (45-82 μmol/L [CF: 0.1791; SMI: 1 μmol/L])
Elevated in: Iron deficiency anemia, pregnancy, polycythemia, hepatitis, weight loss
Decreased in: Anemia of chronic disease, hemochromatosis, chronic liver disease, hemolytic anemias, malnutrition (protein depletion)
Table 4-14 describes TIBC and serum iron abnormalities.

LACTATE DEHYDROGENASE (LDH)

Normal range: 50-150 U/L (0.82-2.66 μkat/L [CF: 0.01667; SMI: 0.02 μkat/L])
Elevated in: Infarction of myocardium, lung, kidney
Diseases of cardiopulmonary system, liver, collagen, central nervous system
Hemolytic anemias, megaloblastic anemias, transfusions, seizures, muscle trauma, muscular dystrophy, acute pancreatitis, hypotension, shock, infectious mononucleosis, inflammation, neoplasia, intestinal obstruction, hypothyroidism

LACTATE DEHYDROGENASE ISOENZYMES

Normal range:
LDH_1: 22% to 36% (cardiac, red blood cell) (0.22-0.36 [CF: 0.01, SMI: 0.01])
LDH_2: 35% to 46% (cardiac, red blood cell) (0.35-0.46)
LDH_3: 13% to 26% (pulmonary) (0.15-0.26)
LDH_4: 3% to 10% (striated muscle, liver) (0.03-0.1)
LDH_5: 2% to 9% (striated muscle, liver) (0.02-0.09)
Normal ratios:
$LDH_1 < LDH_2$
$LDH_5 < LDH_4$
Abnormal values:
$LDH_1 > LDH_2$: myocardial infarction (can also be seen with hemolytic anemias, pernicious anemia, folate deficiency, renal infarct)
$LDH_5 > LDH_4$: liver disease (cirrhosis, hepatitis, hepatic congestion)

LAP SCORE; *see* LEUKOCYTE ALKALINE PHOSPHATASE

TABLE 4-14 Serum Iron and Total Iron-Binding Capacity Patterns

SI↓	TIBC↓	Chronic diseases
		Uremia
SI↓	TIBC↑	Chronic iron deficiency anemia
		Pregnancy in third trimester
SI↑	TIBC↓	Hemachromatosis
		Iron therapy overload (TIBC may be normal)
		Hemolytic anemia; thalassemia; lead poisoning; megaloblastic anemia; aplastic, pyridoxine deficiency, or other sideroblastic anemias
SI↑	TIBC↑	Oral contraceptives
		Acute hepatitis (some report TIBC is low normal)
		Chronic hepatitis (some patients)
SI↑	TIBC NL	B12 or folate deficiency
SI↓	TIBC NL	Chronic iron deficiency (some patients)
		Acute infection, surgery, tissue damage
SI NL	TIBC↑	B12/folate deficiency plus iron deficiency

From Ravel R: *Clinical laboratory medicine*, ed 6, St Louis, 1995, Mosby.
NL, Normal; *SI*, serum iron; *TIBC*, total iron-binding capacity.

LDH; *see* LACTATE DEHYDROGENASE

LDL; *see* LOW-DENSITY LIPOPROTEIN CHOLESTEROL

LEGIONELLA TITER

Normal:
Negative
Positive in:
Legionnaire's disease (presumptive: ≥1:256 titer; definitive: fourfold titer increase to ≥1:128)

LEUKOCYTE ALKALINE PHOSPHATASE (LAP)

Normal range: 13-100 (33-188 U)
Elevated in: Leukemoid reactions, neutrophilia secondary to infections (except in sickle cell crisis—no significant increase in LAP score), Hodgkin's disease, polycythemia vera, hairy cell leukemia, aplastic anemia, Down's syndrome, myelofibrosis
Decreased in: Acute and chronic granulocytic leukemia, thrombocytopenic purpura, paroxysmal nocturnal hemoglobinuria, hypophosphatemia, collagen disorders

LEUKOCYTE COUNT; *see* COMPLETE BLOOD COUNT

LIPASE

Normal range: 0-160 U/L (0-2.66 μkat/L [CF: 0.01667; SMI: 0.02 μkat/L])
Elevated in: Acute pancreatitis, perforated peptic ulcer, carcinoma of pancreas (early stage), pancreatic duct obstruction, bowel infarction, intestinal obstruction

LIPOPROTEIN CHOLESTEROL, HIGH-DENSITY; *see* HIGH-DENSITY LIPOPROTEIN CHOLESTEROL

LIPOPROTEIN CHOLESTEROL, LOW-DENSITY; *see* LOW-DENSITY LIPOPROTEIN CHOLESTEROL

LOW-DENSITY LIPOPROTEIN (LDL) CHOLESTEROL

Normal range:
50-130 mg/dl (1.30-1.68 mmol/L [CF: 0.02586; SMI: 0.05 mmol/L])
LDL cholesterol

<70	Optimal in diabetics, prior MI, and patients with cardiac risk factors
100-129	Near or above optimal
130-159	Borderline high
160-189	High
≥190	Very high

LUPUS ANTICOAGULANT; *see* CIRCULATING ANTICOAGULANT

LUTEINIZING HORMONE

Normal range: 5-25 mIU/ml
Elevated in: Postmenopause, pituitary adenoma, primary gonadal dysfunction, polycystic ovary syndrome
Decreased in: Severe illness, anorexia nervosa, malnutrition, pituitary or hypothalamic impairment, severe stress

LYME DISEASE ANTIBODY TITER

Normal range: Negative
Positive result: Fig. 4-11 illustrates the usual serologic response in Lyme disease.
A serologic test is not necessary or helpful for several days after a tick bite, because it is only 40%-50% sensitive in this stage and a negative test does not rule out the diagnosis.

LYMPHOCYTES

Normal range:
15% to 40%: Total lymphocyte count = 800-2600/mm^3
Total T lymphocyte = 800-2200/mm^3
CD4 lymphocytes = ≥400/mm^3
CD8 lymphocytes = 200-800/mm^3
Normal CD4/CD8 ratio is 2.0
Elevated in: Chronic infections, infectious mononucleosis and other viral infections, chronic lymphocytic leukemia, Hodgkin's disease, ulcerative colitis, hypoadrenalism, idiopathic thrombocytopenia
Decreased in: AIDS, bone marrow suppression from chemotherapeutic agents or chemotherapy, aplastic anemia, neoplasms, steroids, adrenocortical hyperfunction, neurologic disorders (multiple sclerosis, myasthenia gravis, Guillain-Barré syndrome)
CD4 lymphocytes are calculated as total white blood cells × % lymphocytes × % lymphocytes stained with CD4. They are decreased in AIDS and other immune dysfunction.
Table 4-15 describes various lymphocyte abnormalities in peripheral blood.

MAGNESIUM (serum)

Normal range: 1.8-3.0 mg/dl (0.80-1.20 mmol/L [CF: 0.4114; SMI: 0.02 mmol/L])
CAUSES OF HYPERMAGNESEMIA
I. Decreased renal excretion
  A. Renal failure—glomerular filtration rate less than 30 ml/min
  B. Hyperparathyroidism

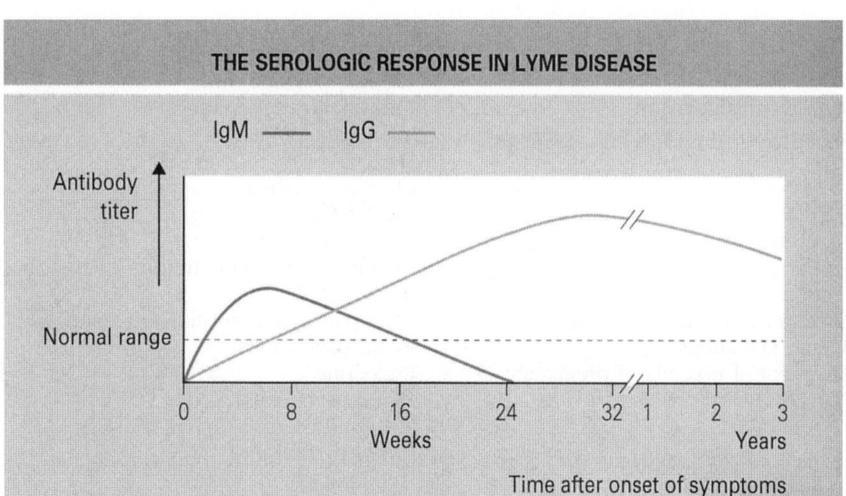

FIGURE 4-11 IgM and IgG response in Lyme disease. *IgG,* Immunoglobulin G; *IgM,* immunoglobulin M.

TABLE 4-15 Differential Diagnosis of Abnormal Lymphocytes in Peripheral Blood

Lymphocyte Type	Usual Disease Association	Cytologic Features	Laboratory Features	Clinical Features
Small lymphocyte	Chronic lymphocytic leukemia	B-cell surface markers with low concentration of surface immunoglobulin, CD5 antigen	Hypogammaglobulinemia in 50%; positive direct Coombs' test in 15%; on node biopsy, diffuse, well-differentiated lymphocytic infiltrate	Elderly adults; presentation runs gamut from asymptomatic with lymphocytosis only to bulky disease with adenopathy, splenomegaly, and "packed" bone marrow
Atypical lymphocyte	Infectious mononucleosis, other viral illnesses	Suppressor T-cell markers	Heterophil agglutinin; positive serology for Epstein-Barr virus, cytomegalovirus, toxoplasma, HBsAg	Pharyngitis, fever, adenopathy, rash, splenomegaly, palatal petechiae, jaundice
Plasmacytoid lymphocyte	Waldenström's macroglobulinemia	Cytoplasmic IgM, periodic acid–Schiff (PAS) positivity	IgM paraprotein, rouleaux, cryoglobulins	Adenopathy, splenomegaly, absence of bone lesions, hyperviscosity syndrome, cryopathic phenomena
Lymphoblast	Acute lymphoblastic leukemia (ALL)	Terminal transferase positivity, common ALL antigen, B- or T-precursor markers	Anemia, granulocytopenia, thrombocytopenia, hyperuricemia, diffuse bone marrow infiltration	Peak incidence in childhood, acute onset, bone pain frequent
Lymphosarcoma cell	Lymphocytic lymphoma	B-cell surface markers with high concentration of monoclonal surface immunoglobulin	Nodular or diffuse, poorly differentiated lymphocytic lymphoma on node biopsy, patchy, peritrabecular bone marrow involvement	Middle-aged to older adults, generalized adenopathy, constitutional symptoms
Sézary cell	Cutaneous lymphomas	T-lymphocyte surface markers	Skin biopsy is diagnostic	Exfoliative erythroderma, cutaneous plaques or tumors
Hairy cell	Hairy cell leukemia	B-lymphocyte markers, cytoplasmic projections, tartrate-resistant acid phosphatase, interleukin-2 receptors, CD11 antigen	Pancytopenia	Middle-aged males, moderate to marked splenomegaly without adenopathy
Prolymphocyte	Prolymphocytic leukemia	B-cell surface markers with high concentration of surface immunoglobulin, CD5 negative	Marked lymphocytosis (frequently $>100 \times 10^9/L$)	Elderly adults, massive splenomegaly, minimum adenopathy, poor response to therapy

From Stein JH (ed): *Internal medicine,* ed 5, St Louis, 1998, Mosby.

C. Hypothyroidism
D. Addison's disease
E. Lithium intoxication
F. Familial hypocalciuric hypercalcemia

II. Other causes: usually in association with decrease in glomerular filtration rate
A. Endogenous loads
1. Diabetic ketoacidosis
2. Severe tissue injury—burns
B. Exogenous loads
1. Gastrointestinal
a. Magnesium-containing laxatives and antacids
b. High-dose vitamin D analogs
2. Parenteral: management of toxemia of pregnancy

CAUSES OF HYPOMAGNESEMIA

Alcoholic abuse
Diuretic use
Renal losses
Acute and chronic renal failure
Postobstructive diuresis
Acute tubular necrosis
Chronic glomerulonephritis
Chronic pyelonephritis
Interstitial nephropathy
Renal transplantation
Gastrointestinal losses
Chronic diarrhea
Nasogastric suctioning
Short bowel syndrome
Protein calorie malnutrition
Bowel fistula
Total parenteral nutrition
Acute pancreatitis
Endocrine
Diabetes mellitus
Hyperaldosteronism
Hyperthyroidism
Hyperparathyroidism
Acute intermittent porphyria
Pregnancy

Drugs
Aminoglycosides
Amphotericin
β-Agonists
Cisplatin
Cyclosporine
Diuretics
Foscarnet
Pentamidine
Theophylline
Congenital disorders
Familial hypomagnesemia
Maternal diabetes
Maternal hypothyroidism
Maternal hyperparathyroidism

MEAN CORPUSCULAR VOLUME (MCV)

Normal range: 76-100 μm³ (76-100 fL) (76-100 fL [CF: 1; SMI: 1 fL])

See Tables 4-16 and 4-17 for descriptions of MCV abnormalities.

METANEPHRINES, URINE; *see* URINE METANEPHRINES

MONOCYTE COUNT

Normal range: 2% to 8%
Elevated in: Viral diseases, parasites, infections, neoplasms, inflammatory bowel disease, monocytic leukemia, lymphomas, myeloma, sarcoidosis
Decreased in: Aplastic anemia, lymphocytic leukemia, glucocorticoid administration

MYOGLOBIN, URINE; *see* URINE MYOGLOBIN

NEUTROPHIL COUNT

Normal range: 50% to 70%
Subsets
Stabs (bands, early mature neutrophils): 2% to 6%
Segs (mature neutrophils): 60% to 70%

TABLE 4-16 Some Causes of Increased Mean Corpuscular Volume (Macrocytosis)

Causes	% of all Macrocytosis Patients*	% of Macrocytosis in Each Disease†
Common		
Folate or B_{12} deficiency	20-30 (5-50)‡	80-90 (4-100)
Chronic liver disease	15-20 (6-28)	25-30 (8-65)
Chronic alcoholism	10-12 (3-15)	60 (26-90)
Cytotoxic chemotherapy	10-15 (2-20)	30-40 (13-82)
Cardiorespiratory abnormality	8 (7-9.5)	?
Reticulocytosis	6-7 (0-15)	Depends on severity
Myelodysplastic syndromes	Frequent over age 40 yr	>60 in RAEB and RARS
Unexplained	25 (22.5-27)	—
Normal newborn		
Less common	<4%	
Noncytotoxic drugs		
Zidovudine		
Phenytoin		30 (14-50)
Azathioprine		
Hypothyroidism		20-30 (8-55)
Chronic leukemia/myelofibrosis		
Radiotherapy for malignancy		
Chronic renal disease (occasional patients)		
Distance-runner macrocytosis (some persons)		
Down syndrome		
Artifactual (e.g., cold agglutinins)		

From Ravel R: *Clinical laboratory medicine,* ed 6, St Louis, 1995, Mosby.
RAEB, Refractory anemia with excessive blasts; *RARS,* refractory anemia with ring sideroblasts (formerly called IASA, or idiopathic acquired sideroblastic anemia).
*Percentage of all patients with macrocytosis.
†Percentage of patients with each condition listed who have macrocytosis.
‡Numbers in parentheses are literature range.

TABLE 4-17 Some Causes of Decreased Mean Corpuscular Volume (Microcytosis)

Common	Less Common
Chronic iron deficiency	Some cases of polycythemia
α- or β-thalassemia (minor)	Some cases of lead poisoning
Anemia of chronic disease	Some cases of congenital spherocytosis
	Some cases of sideroblastic anemia
	Certain abnormal Hbs (Hb E, Hb Lepore)

From Ravel R: *Clinical laboratory medicine,* ed 6, St Louis, 1995, Mosby.

Elevated in: Acute bacterial infections, acute myocardial infarction, stress, neoplasms, myelocytic leukemia
Decreased in: Viral infections, aplastic anemias, immunosuppressive drugs, radiation therapy to bone marrow, agranulocytosis, drugs (antibiotics, antithyroidals, clopidogrel), lymphocytic and monocytic leukemias
- Table 4-18 describes various drugs that can cause neutropenia.

NOREPINEPHRINE

Normal range: 0-600 pg/ml
Elevated in: Pheochromocytomas, neuroblastomas, stress, vigorous exercise, certain foods (bananas, chocolate, coffee, tea, vanilla)

5′-NUCLEOTIDASE

Normal range: 2-16 IU/L (3-27 × 10^8 kat/L [CF: 1.67 × 10^8; SMI: 1 × 10^8 kat/L])
Elevated in: Biliary obstruction, metastatic neoplasms to liver, primary biliary cirrhosis, renal failure, pancreatic carcinoma, chronic active hepatitis

OSMOLALITY (serum)

Normal range: 280-300 mOsm/kg (280-300 mmol/kg [CF: 1; SMI: 1 mmol/kg])
It can also be estimated by the following formula:
2([Na] + [K]) + glucose/18+ BUN/2.8
Elevated in: Dehydration, hypernatremia, diabetes insipidus, uremia, hyperglycemia, mannitol therapy, ingestion of toxins (ethylene glycol, methanol, ethanol), hypercalcemia, diuretics
Decreased in: Syndrome of inappropriate diuretic hormone secretion, hyponatremia, overhydration, Addison's disease, hypothyroidism

OSMOLALITY, URINE; *see* URINE OSMOLALITY

PARACENTESIS FLUID

Testing and evaluation of results:
1. Process the fluid as follows:
   a. Tube 1: LDH, glucose, albumin.
   b. Tube 2: protein, specific gravity.
   c. Tube 3: cell count and differential.
   d. Tube 4: save until further notice.
2. Draw serum LDH, protein, albumin.
3. Gram stain, AFB stain, bacterial and fungal cultures, amylase, and triglycerides should be ordered only when clearly indicated; bedside inoculation of blood-culture bottles with ascitic fluid improves sensitivity in detecting bacterial growth.
4. If malignant ascites is suspected, consider a carcinoembryonic antigen level on the paracentesis fluid and cytologic evaluation.
5. In suspected spontaneous bacterial peritonitis (SBP) the incidence of positive cultures can be increased by injecting 10 to 20 ml of ascitic fluid into blood culture bottles.
6. Peritoneal effusion can be subdivided as exudative or transudative based on its characteristics (see Section III).
7. The serum-ascites albumin gradient (serum albumin level-ascitic fluid albumin level) correlates directly with portal pressure and can also be used to classify ascite. Patients with gradients ≥1.1 g/dl have portal hypertension, and those with gradients <1.1 g/dl do not; the accuracy of this method is >95%.
8. For the differential diagnosis of ascites refer to Section III.
9. An ascitic fluid polymorphonuclear leukocyte count >500/μl is suggestive of SBP.
10. A blood-ascitic fluid albumin gradient.

TABLE 4-18 **Drugs That Cause Neutropenia**

Antiarrhythmics	
	Tocainide, procainamide, propranolol, quinidine
Antibiotics	
	Chloramphenicol, penicillins, sulfonamides, p-aminosalicylic acid (PAS), rifampin, vancomycin, isoniazid, nitrofurantoin
Antimalarials	
	Dapsone, quinine, pyrimethamine
Anticonvulsants	
	Phenytoin, mephenytoin, trimethadione, ethosuximide, carbamazepine
Hypoglycemic agents	
	Tolbutamide, chlorpropamide
Antihistamines	
	Cimetidine, brompheniramine, tripelennamine
Antihypertensives	
	Methyldopa, captopril
Anti-inflammatory agents	
	Aminopyrine, phenylbutazone, gold salts, ibuprofen, indomethacin
Antithyroid agents	
	Propylthiouracil, methimazole, thiouracil
Diuretics	
	Acetazolamide, hydrochlorothiazide, chlorthalidone
Phenothiazines	
	Chlorpromazine, promazine, prochlorperazine
Immunosuppressive agents	
	Antimetabolites
Cytotoxic agents	
	Alkylating agents, antimetabolites, anthracyclines, Vinca alkaloids, cisplatin, hydroxyurea, dactinomycin
Other agents	
	Recombinant interferons, allopurinol, ethanol, levamisole, penicillamine, zidovudine, streptokinase, carbamazepine, clopidogrel, ticlopidine

Modified from Goldman L, Ausiello D (eds): *Cecil textbook of medicine,* ed 22, Philadelphia, 2004, WB Saunders.

PARTIAL THROMBOPLASTIN TIME (PTT), ACTIVATED PARTIAL THROMBOPLASTIN TIME (APTT)

Normal range: 25-41 sec

Elevated in: Heparin therapy, coagulation factor deficiency (I, II, V, VIII, IX, X, XI, XII), liver disease, vitamin K deficiency, disseminated intravascular coagulation, circulating anticoagulant, warfarin therapy, specific factor inhibition (PCN reaction, rheumatoid arthritis), thrombolytic therapy, nephrotic syndrome

NOTE: Useful to evaluate the intrinsic coagulation system.

PH, BLOOD

Normal values:

Arterial: 7.35-7.45

Venous: 7.32-7.42

For abnormal values refer to "Arterial Blood Gases."

PH, URINE; *see* URINE PH

PHENOBARBITAL

Normal therapeutic range: 15-30 mcg/ml for epilepsy control

PHENYTOIN (Dilantin)

Normal therapeutic range: 10-20 mcg/ml

PHOSPHATASE, ACID; *see* ACID PHOSPHATASE

PHOSPHATASE, ALKALINE; *see* ALKALINE PHOSPHATASE

PHOSPHATE (serum)

Normal range: 2.5-5 mg/dl (0.8-1.6 mmol/L [CF: 0.3229; SMI: 0.05 mmol/L])

DECREASED

Parenteral hyperalimentation
Diabetic acidosis
Alcohol withdrawal
Severe metabolic or respiratory alkalosis
Antacids that bind phosphorus
Malnutrition with refeeding using low-phosphorus nutrients
Renal tubule failure to reabsorb phosphate (Fanconi's syndrome; congenital disorder; vitamin D deficiency)
Glucose administration
Nasogastric suction
Malabsorption
Gram-negative sepsis
Primary hyperthyroidism
Chlorothiazide diuretics
Therapy of acute severe asthma
Acute respiratory failure with mechanical ventilation

INCREASED

Renal failure
Severe muscle injury
Phosphate-containing antacids
Hypoparathyroidism
Tumor lysis syndrome

PLATELET COUNT

Normal range: 130-400 × 10^3/mm^3 (130-400 × 10^9/L [CF: 1; SMI: 5 × 10^9/L])

Elevated in:

REACTIVE THROMBOCYTOSIS

Infections or inflammatory states—vasculitis, allergic reactions, etc.
Surgery and tissue damage—myocardial infarction, pancreatitis, etc.
Postsplenectomy state
Malignancy—solid tumors, lymphoma
Iron deficiency anemia, hemolytic anemia, acute blood loss
Uncertain etiology
Rebound effect after chemotherapy or immune thrombocytopenia
Renal disorders—renal failure, nephrotic syndrome

MYELOPROLIFERATIVE DISORDERS

Chronic myeloid leukemia
Primary thrombocythemia
Polycythemia vera
Idiopathic myelofibrosis

Decreased:

A. Increased destruction
   1. Immunologic
      a. Drugs: quinine, quinidine, digitalis, procainamide, thiazide diuretics, sulfonamides, phenytoin, aspirin, penicillin, heparin, gold, meprobamate, sulfa drugs, phenylbutazone, NSAIDs, methyldopa, cimetidine, furosemide, INH, cephalosporins, chlorpropamide, organic arsenicals, chloroquine
      b. Idiopathic thrombocytopenic purpura
      c. Transfusion reaction: transfusion of platelets with platelet antigen HPA-1a (PL^{A1}) in recipients without PL^{A1}
      d. Fetal/maternal incompatibility
      e. Vasculitis (e.g., systemic lupus erythematosus)
      f. Autoimmune hemolytic anemia
      g. Lymphoreticular disorders (e.g., chronic lymphocytic leukemia)
   2. Nonimmunologic
      a. Prosthetic heart valves
      b. Thrombotic thrombocytopenic purpura
      c. Sepsis
      d. Disseminated intravascular coagulation
      e. Hemolytic-uremic syndrome
      f. Giant cavernous hemangioma
B. Decreased production
   1. Abnormal marrow
      a. Marrow infiltration (e.g., leukemia, lymphoma, fibrosis)
      b. Marrow suppression (e.g., chemotherapy, alcohol, radiation)
   2. Hereditary disorders
      a. Wiskott-Aldrich syndrome: X-linked disorder characterized by thrombocytopenia, eczema, and repeated infections
      b. May-Hegglin anomaly: increased megakaryocytes but ineffective thrombopoiesis
   3. Vitamin deficiencies (e.g., vitamin B_{12}, folic acid)
C. Splenic sequestration, hypersplenism
D. Dilutional, secondary to massive transfusion

POTASSIUM (serum)

Normal range: 3.5-5 mEq/L (3.5-5 mmol/L [CF: 1; SMI: 0.1 mmol/L])

CAUSES OF HYPERKALEMIA

I. Pseudohyperkalemia
   A. Hemolysis of sample
   B. Thrombocytosis
   C. Leukocytosis
   D. Laboratory error
II. Increased potassium intake and absorption
   A. Potassium supplements (oral and parenteral)
   B. Dietary—salt substitutes
   C. Stored blood
   D. Potassium-containing medications
III. Impaired renal excretion
   A. Acute renal failure
   B. Chronic renal failure
   C. Tubular defect in potassium secretion
      1. Renal allograft
      2. Analgesic nephropathy
      3. Sickle cell disease

4. Obstructive uropathy
5. Interstitial nephritis
6. Chronic pyelonephritis
7. Potassium-sparing diuretics
8. Miscellaneous (lead, systemic lupus erythematosus, pseudohypoaldosteronism)

D. Hypoaldosteronism
1. Primary (Addison's disease)
2. Secondary
a. Hyporeninemic hypoaldosteronism (type IV RTA)
b. Congenital adrenal hyperplasia
c. Drug-induced
(1) Nonsteroidal anti-inflammatory medications
(2) ACE inhibitors
(3) Heparin
(4) Cyclosporine

IV. Transcellular shifts
A. Acidosis
B. Hypertonicity
C. Insulin deficiency
D. Drugs
1. β-blockers
2. Digitalis toxicity
3. Succinylcholine
E. Exercise
F. Hyperkalemic periodic paralysis

V. Cellular injury
A. Rhabdomyolysis
B. Severe intravascular hemolysis
C. Acute tumor lysis syndrome
D. Burns and crush injuries

CAUSES OF HYPOKALEMIA

I. Decreased intake
A. Decreased dietary potassium
B. Impaired absorption of potassium
C. Clay ingestion
D. Kayexalate

II. Increased loss
A. Renal
1. Hyperaldosteronism
a. Primary
1. Conn's syndrome
2. Adrenal hyperplasia
b. Secondary
1. Congestive heart failure
2. Cirrhosis
3. Nephrotic syndrome
4. Dehydration
c. Bartter's syndrome
2. Glycyrrhizic acid (licorice, chewing tobacco)
3. Excessive adrenal corticosteroids
a. Cushing's syndrome
b. Steroid therapy
c. Adrenogenital syndrome
4. Renal tubular defects
a. Renal tubular acidosis
b. Obstructive uropathy
c. Salt-wasting nephropathy
5. Drugs
a. Diuretics
b. Aminoglycosides
c. Mannitol
d. Amphotericin
e. Cisplatin
f. Carbenicillin

B. Gastrointestinal
1. Vomiting
2. Nasogastric suction
3. Diarrhea
4. Malabsorption
5. Ileostomy
6. Villous adenoma
7. Laxative abuse

C. Increased losses from the skin
1. Excessive sweating
2. Burns

III. Transcellular shifts
A. Alkalosis
1. Vomiting
2. Diuretics
3. Hyperventilation
4. Bicarbonate therapy
B. Insulin
1. Exogenous
2. Endogenous response to glucose
C. β_2-Agonists (albuterol, terbutaline, epinephrine)
D. Hypokalemia periodic paralysis
1. Familial
2. Thyrotoxic

IV. Miscellaneous
A. Anabolic state
B. Intravenous hyperalimentation
C. Treatment of megaloblastic anemia
D. Acute mountain sickness

POTASSIUM, URINE; *see* URINE POTASSIUM

PROCAINAMIDE

Normal therapeutic range: 4-10 mcg/ml

PROLACTIN

Normal range: <20 ng/ml (<20 μg/L [CF: 1; SMI: 1 μg/L])
Elevated in: Prolactinomas (level >200 highly suggestive), drugs (phenothiazines, cimetidine, tricyclic antidepressants, metoclopramide, estrogens, antihypertensives [methyldopa], verapamil, haloperidol), postpartum, stress, hypoglycemia, hypothyroidism

PROSTATE-SPECIFIC ANTIGEN (PSA)

Normal range: 0-4 ng/ml
Table 4-19 describes age-specific reference ranges for PSA.
Elevated in: Benign prostatic hypertrophy, carcinoma of prostate, postrectal examination, prostate trauma
Factors affecting serum PSA are described in Table 4-20.

NOTE: Measurement of free PSA is useful to assess the probability of prostate cancer in patients with normal digital rectal examination and total PSA between 4 and 10 ng/ml. In these patients, the global risk of prostate cancer is 25%; however, if the free PSA is >25%, the risk of prostate cancer decreases to 8%, whereas if the free PSA is <10%, the risk of cancer increases to 56%. Free PSA is also useful to evaluate the aggressiveness of

TABLE 4-19 Age-Specific Reference Ranges for PSA

	SERUM PSA (NG/ML)		
Age (yr)	Whites	Japanese	African American
40-49	0-2.5	0-2.0	0-2.0
50-59	0-3.5	0-3.0	0-4.0
60-69	0-4.5	0-4.0	0-4.5
70-79	0-6.5	0-5.0	0-5.5

From Nseyo UO (ed): *Urology for primary care physicians,* Philadelphia, 1999, WB Saunders.
PSA, Prostate-specific antigen.

TABLE 4-20 **Factors Affecting Serum Prostate-Specific Antigen (PSA)**

Factors Affecting Serum PSA	Duration of Effect
Prostate cell number	Not applicable
Prostate size	Not applicable
Recent ejaculation	6-48 hours
Prostate manipulation	
Vigorous massage	1 week
Cystoscopy	1 week
Prostate biopsy	4-6 weeks
Prostatitis	
Acute	3-6 months
Chronic	Unknown
Prostate cancer	Not applicable
Drugs: finasteride (Proscar)*	3-6 months

From Nseyo UO (ed): *Urology for primary care physicians,* Philadelphia, 1999, WB Saunders.
*Lowers PSA for as long as patient is on the medication.

prostate cancer. A low free PSA percentage generally indicates a high-grade cancer, whereas a high free PSA percentage is generally associated with a slower growing tumor.
Decreased in: Finasteride therapy, dutasteride therapy, saw palmetto use, bedrest, antiandrogens

PROTEIN (serum)

Normal range: 6-8 g/dl (60-80 g/L [CF: 10; SMI: 1 g/L])
Elevated in: Dehydration, multiple myeloma, Waldenström's macroglobulinemia, sarcoidosis, collagen-vascular diseases
Decreased in: Malnutrition, low-protein diet, overhydration, malabsorption, pregnancy, severe burns, neoplasms, chronic diseases, cirrhosis, nephrosis

PROTEIN ELECTROPHORESIS (serum)

Normal range: Albumin: 60% to 75% (0.6-0.75 [CF: 0.01; SMI: 0.01])
α-1: 1.7% to 5% (0.02-0.05)
α-2: 6.7% to 12.5% (0.07-0.13)
β: 8.3% to 16.3% (0.08-0.16)
γ: 10.7% to 20% (0.11-0.2)
Albumin: 3.6-5.2 g/dl (36-52 g/L [CF: 0.01; SMI: 1 g/L])
α-1: 0.1-0.4 g/dl (1-4 g/L)
α-2: 0.4-1 g/dl (4-10 g/L)
β: 0.5-1.2 g/dl (5-12 g/L)
γ: 0.6-1.6 g/dl (6-16 g/L)
Elevated in: Albumin: dehydration
α-1: neoplastic diseases, inflammation
α-2: neoplasms, inflammation, infection, nephrotic syndrome
β: hypothyroidism, biliary cirrhosis, diabetes mellitus
γ: *see* IMMUNOGLOBULINS
Decreased in: Albumin: malnutrition, chronic liver disease, malabsorption, nephrotic syndrome, burns, systemic lupus erythematosus
α-1: emphysema (α-1 antitrypsin deficiency), nephrosis
α-2: hemolytic anemias (decreased haptoglobin), severe hepatocellular damage
β: hypocholesterolemia, nephrosis
γ: *see* IMMUNOGLOBULINS
Fig. 4-12 describes serum protein electrophoretic patterns.

PROTHROMBIN TIME (PT)

Normal range: 10-12 sec
Elevated in: Liver disease, oral anticoagulants (warfarin), heparin, factor deficiency (I, II, V, VII, X), disseminated intravascular coagulation, vitamin K deficiency, afibrinogenemia, dysfibrinogenemia, drugs (salicylate, chloral hydrate, diphenylhydantoin, estrogens, antacids, phenylbutazone, quinidine, antibiotics, allopurinol, anabolic steroids)
Decreased in: Vitamin K supplementation, thrombophlebitis, drugs (glutethimide, estrogens, griseofulvin, diphenhydramine)

PROTOPORPHYRIN (free erythrocyte)

Normal range: 16-36 μg/dl of red blood cells (0.28-0.64 μmol/L [CF: 0.0177; SMI: 0.02 μmol/L])
Elevated in: Iron deficiency, lead poisoning, sideroblastic anemias, anemia of chronic disease, hemolytic anemias, erythropoietic protoporphyria

PSA; *see* PROSTATE-SPECIFIC ANTIGEN

PT; *see* PROTHROMBIN TIME

PTT; *see* PARTIAL THROMBOPLASTIN TIME

RDW; *see* RED BLOOD CELL DISTRIBUTION WIDTH

RED BLOOD CELL (RBC) COUNT

Normal range:
Male: 4.3-5.9 × 10^6/mm^3 (4.3-5.9 × 10^{12}/L [CF: 1; SMI: 0.1 × 10^{12}/L])
Female: 3.5-5 × 10^6/mm^3 (3.5-5 × 10^{12}/L [CF: 1; SMI: 0.1 × 10^{12}/L])
Elevated in: Polycythemia vera, smokers, high altitude, cardiovascular disease, renal cell carcinoma and other erythropoietin-producing neoplasms, stress, hemoconcentration/dehydration
Decreased in: Anemias, hemolysis, chronic renal failure, hemorrhage, failure of marrow production

RED BLOOD CELL DISTRIBUTION WIDTH (RDW)

Measures variability of red cell size (anisocytosis)
Normal range: 11.5-14.5
Normal RDW and:
ELEVATED MEAN CORPUSCULAR VOLUME (MCV): aplastic anemia, preleukemia
NORMAL MCV: normal, anemia of chronic disease, acute blood loss or hemolysis, chronic lymphocytic leukemia (CLL), chronic myelocytic leukemia, nonanemic enzymopathy or hemoglobinopathy
DECREASED MCV: anemia of chronic disease, heterozygous thalassemia
Elevated RDW and:
ELEVATED MCV: vitamin B_{12} deficiency, folate deficiency, immune hemolytic anemia, cold agglutinins, CLL with high count, liver disease
NORMAL MCV: early iron deficiency, early vitamin B_{12} deficiency, early folate deficiency, anemic globinopathy
DECREASED MCV: iron deficiency, red blood cell fragmentation, HbH disease, thalassemia intermedia

RED BLOOD CELL FOLATE; *see* FOLATE

RED BLOOD CELL MASS (volume)

Normal range:
Male: 20-36 ml/kg of body weight (1.15-1.21 L/m^2 body surface area)
Female: 19-31 ml/kg of body weight (0.95-1.00 L/m^2 body surface area)
Elevated in: Polycythemia vera, hypoxia (smokers, high altitude, cardiovascular disease), hemoglobinopathies with high oxygen affinity, erythropoietin-producing tumors (renal cell carcinoma)
Decreased in: Hemorrhage, chronic disease, failure of marrow production, anemias, hemolysis

RED BLOOD CELL MORPHOLOGY; *see* Fig. 4-13

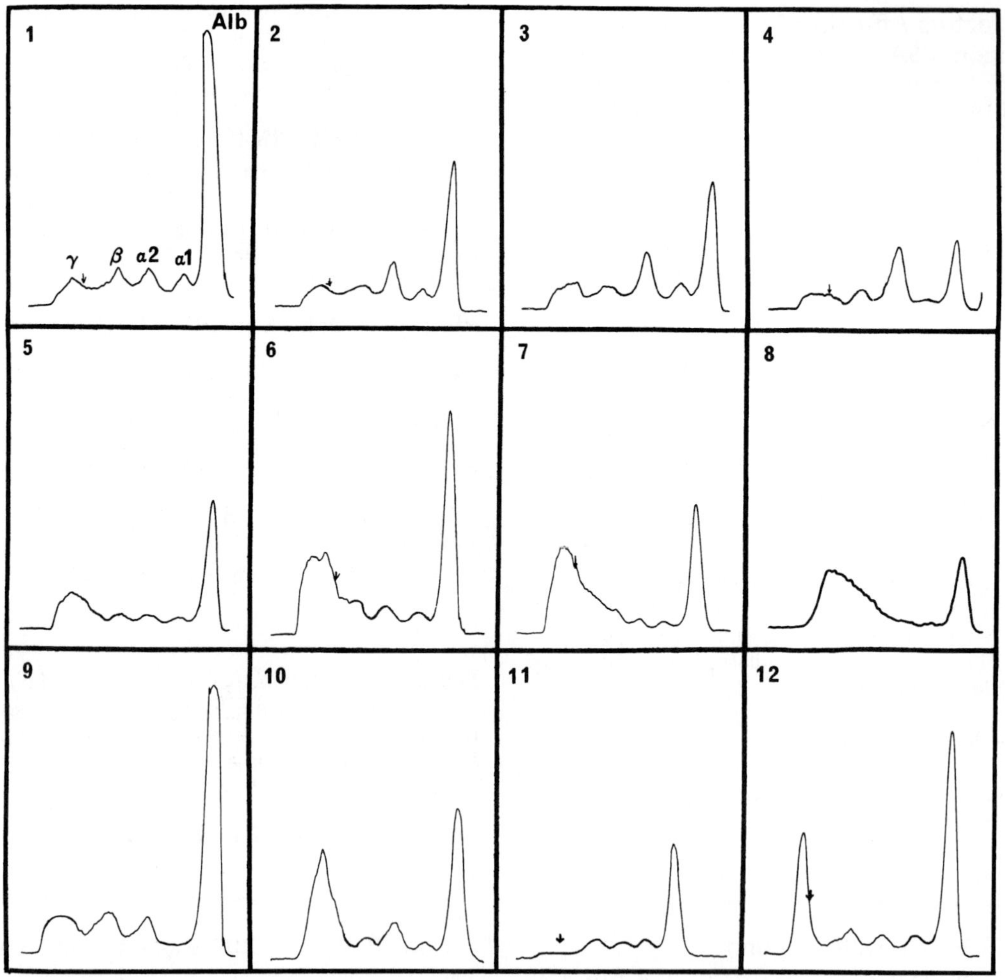

FIGURE 4-12 Typical serum protein electrophoretic patterns. *1,* Normal (*arrow* near γ region indicates serum application point). *2,* Acute reaction pattern. *3,* Acute reaction or nephrotic syndrome. *4,* Nephrotic syndrome. *5,* Chronic inflammation, cirrhosis, granulomatous diseases, rheumatoid-collagen group. *6,* Same as 5, but g elevation is more pronounced. There is also partial (but not complete) β-γ fusion. *7,* Suggestive of cirrhosis but could be found in the granulomatous diseases or the rheumatoid-collagen group. *8,* Characteristic pattern of cirrhosis. *9,* α-1 Antitrypsin deficiency with mild γ elevation suggesting concurrent chronic disease. *10,* Same as 5, but the γ elevation is marked. The configuration of the γ peak superficially mimics that of myeloma, but is more broad-based. There are superimposed acute reaction changes. *11,* Hypogammaglobulinemia or light-chain myeloma. *12,* Myeloma, Waldenström's macroglobulinemia, idiopathic or secondary monoclonal gammopathy. (From Ravel R: *Clinical laboratory medicine,* ed 6, St Louis, 1995, Mosby.)

RENIN (serum)

Elevated in: Drugs (thiazides, estrogen, minoxidil), chronic renal failure, Bartter's syndrome, pregnancy (normal), pheochromocytoma, renal hypertension, reduced plasma volume, secondary aldosteronism

Decreased in: Adrenocortical hypertension, increased plasma volume, primary aldosteronism, drugs (propranolol, reserpine, clonidine)

Table 4-21 describes typical renin-aldosterone patterns in various conditions.

RETICULOCYTE COUNT

Normal range: 0.5% to 1.5%

Elevated in: Hemolytic anemia (sickle cell crisis, thalassemia major, autoimmune hemolysis), hemorrhage, postanemia therapy (folic acid, ferrous sulfate, vitamin B_{12}), chronic renal failure

Decreased in: Aplastic anemia, marrow suppression (sepsis, chemotherapeutic agents, radiation), hepatic cirrhosis, blood transfusion, anemias of disordered maturation (iron deficiency anemia, megaloblastic anemia, sideroblastic anemia, anemia of chronic disease)

RHEUMATOID FACTOR

Normal: Negative

Present in titer >1:20

RHEUMATIC DISEASES

Rheumatoid arthritis
Sjögren's syndrome
Systemic lupus erythematosus
Polymyositis/dermatomyositis
Mixed connective tissue disease
Scleroderma

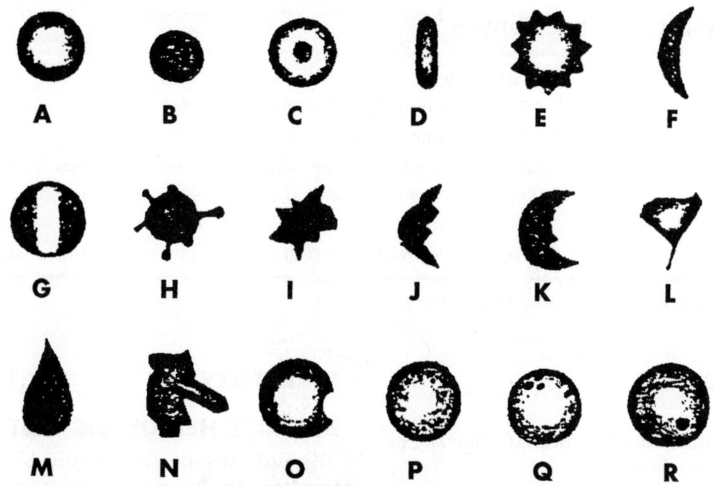

FIGURE 4-13 Abnormal red blood cells (RBCs). A, Normal RBC. **B,** Spherocyte. **C,** Target cell. **D,** Elliptocyte. **E,** Echinocyte. **F,** Sickle cell. **G,** Stomatocyte. **H,** Acanthocyte. **I** to **L,** Schistocytes. **M,** Teardrop RBC. **N,** Distorted RBC with Hb C crystal protruding. **O,** Degmacyte. **P,** Basophilic stippling. **Q,** Pappenheimer bodies. **R,** Howell-Jolly body. (From Ravel R: *Clinical laboratory medicine,* ed 6, St Louis, 1995, Mosby.)

TABLE 4-21 **Typical Renin-Aldosterone Patterns in Various Conditions**

	Plasma Renin	Aldosterone
Primary aldosteronism	Low	High
"Low-renin" essential hypertension	Low	Normal
Cushing's syndrome	Low	Low-normal
Licorice ingestion syndrome	Low	Low
High-salt diet	Low	Low
Oral contraceptives	High	Normal
Cirrhosis	High	High
Malignant hypertension	High	High
Unilateral renal disease	High	High
"High-renin" essential hypertension	High	High
Pregnancy	High	High
Diuretic overuse	High	High
Juxtaglomerular tumor (Bartter's syndrome)	High	High
Low-salt diet	High	High
Addison's disease	High	Low
Hypokalemia	High	Low

From Ravel R: *Clinical laboratory medicine,* ed 6, St Louis, 1995, Mosby.

INFECTIOUS DISEASES
Subacute bacterial endocarditis
Tuberculosis
Infectious mononucleosis
Hepatitis
Syphilis
Leprosy
Influenza
MALIGNANCIES
Lymphoma
Multiple myeloma
Waldenström's macroglobulinemia
Postradiation or postchemotherapy
MISCELLANEOUS
Normal adults, especially the elderly
Sarcoidosis
Chronic pulmonary disease (interstitial fibrosis)
Chronic liver disease (chronic active hepatitis, cirrhosis)
Mixed essential cryoglobulinemia
Hypergammaglobulinemic purpura

RNP; *see* EXTRACTABLE NUCLEAR ANTIGEN

SEDIMENTATION RATE; *see* ERYTHROCYTE SEDIMENTATION RATE

SEMEN ANALYSIS

- Table 4-22 describes semen analysis reference ranges.

SGOT; *see* ASPARTATE AMINOTRANSFERASE

SGPT; *see* ALANINE AMINOTRANSFERASE

TABLE 4-22 **Semen Analysis Reference Ranges**

Color	Grayish white
pH	7.3-7.8 (literature range, 7.0-7.8)
Volume	2.0-5.0 ml (literature range, 1.5-6.0 ml)
Sperm count	20-250 million/ml (literature range for upper limit varies from 100-250 million/ml)
Motility	>60% motile <3 hours after specimen is obtained (literature range, >40% to >70%)
% Normal sperm	>60% (literature range, >60% to >70%)
Viscosity	Can be poured from a pipet in droplets rather than a thick strand

From Ravel R (ed): *Clinical laboratory medicine,* ed 6, St Louis, 1995, Mosby.

SMOOTH MUSCLE ANTIBODY

Normal: Negative
Present in: Chronic acute hepatitis (≥1:80), primary biliary cirrhosis (≤1:80), infectious mononucleosis

SODIUM (serum)

Normal range: 135-147 mEq/L (135-147 mmol/L [CF: 1; SMI: 1 mmol/L])

HYPONATREMIA

A. Sodium and water depletion (deficit hyponatremia)
   1. Loss of gastrointestinal secretions with replacement of fluid but not electrolytes
      a. Vomiting
      b. Diarrhea
      c. Tube drainage
   2. Loss from skin with replacement of fluids but not electrolytes
      a. Excessive sweating
      b. Extensive burns
   3. Loss from kidney
      a. Diuretics
      b. Chronic renal insufficiency (uremia) with acidosis
   4. Metabolic loss
      a. Starvation with acidosis
      b. Diabetic acidosis
   5. Endocrine loss
      a. Addison's disease
      b. Sudden withdrawal of long-term steroid therapy
   6. Iatrogenic loss from serous cavities
      a. Paracentesis or thoracentesis
B. Excessive water (dilution hyponatremia)
   1. Excessive water administration
   2. Congestive heart failure
   3. Cirrhosis
   4. Nephrotic syndrome
   5. Hypoalbuminemia (severe)
   6. Acute renal failure with oliguria
C. Inappropriate antidiuretic hormone (IADH) syndrome
D. Intracellular loss (reset osmostat syndrome)
E. False hyponatremia (actually a dilutional effect)
   1. Marked hypertriglyceridemia*
   2. Marked hyperproteinemia*
   3. Severe hyperglycemia

HYPERNATREMIA

Dehydration is the most frequent overall clinical finding in hypernatremia.

1. Deficient water intake (either orally or intravenously)
2. Excess kidney water output (diabetes insipidus, osmotic diuresis)
3. Excess skin water output (excess sweating, loss from burns)
4. Excess gastrointestinal tract output (severe protracted vomiting or diarrhea without fluid therapy)
5. Accidental sodium overdose
6. High-protein tube feedings

STREPTOZYME; *see* ANTI-STREPTOLYSIN O TITER

SUCROSE HEMOLYSIS TEST (sugar water test)

Normal: Absence of hemolysis
Positive in: Paroxysmal nocturnal hemoglobinuria
False positive: autoimmune hemolytic anemia, megaloblastic anemias
False negative: may occur with use of heparin or EDTA

SUDAN III STAIN (qualitative screening for fecal fat)

Normal: Negative. Test should be preceded by diet containing 100-150 g of dietary fat/day for 1 week, avoidance of high-fiber diet, and avoidance of suppositories or oily material before specimen collection.
Positive in: Steatorrhea, use of castor oil or mineral oil droplets

SYNOVIAL FLUID ANALYSIS

Table 4-23 describes the classification and interpretation of synovial fluid analysis.

T$_3$ (triiodothyronine); *see* Table 4-24 for T$_3$ abnormalities

Normal range: 75-220 ng/dl (1.2-3.4 nmol/L [CF: 0.01536; SMI: 0.1 nmol/L])
Abnormal values:

A. Elevated in hyperthyroidism (usually earlier and to a greater extent than serum T$_4$).
B. Useful in diagnosing:
   1. T$_3$ hyperthyroidism (thyrotoxicosis): increased T$_3$, normal FTI.
   2. Toxic nodular goiter: increased T$_3$, normal or increased T$_4$.
   3. Iodine deficiency: normal T$_3$, possibly decreased T$_4$.
   4. Thyroid replacement therapy with liothyronine (Cytomel): normal T$_4$, increased T$_3$ if patient is symptomatically hyperthyroid.

Not ordered routinely but indicated when hyperthyroidism is suspected and serum free T$_4$ or FTI inconclusive.

T$_3$ RESIN UPTAKE (T$_3$RU)

Normal range:
25% to 35%
Abnormal values:
Increased in hyperthyroidism. T$_3$ resin uptake (T$_3$RU or RT$_3$U) measures the percentage of free T$_4$ (not bound to protein); it does not measure serum T$_3$ concentration; T$_3$RU and other tests that reflect thyroid hormone binding to plasma protein are also known as *thyroid hormone-binding ratios* (THBR).

T$_4$, FREE (free thyroxine)

Normal range: 0.8-2.8 ng/dl
Elevated in: Graves' disease, toxic multinodular goiter, toxic adenoma, iatrogenic and factitious causes, transient hyperthyroidism
Serum free T$_4$ directly measures unbound thyroxine. Free T$_4$ can be measured by equilibrium dialysis (gold standard of free T$_4$

TABLE 4-23 Classification and Interpretation of Synovial Fluid Analysis

Group	Diseases	Appearance	Viscosity	Mucin Clot	WBC/mm³	%PMN	Glucose (mg/dl) (Blood–Synovial Fluid)	Protein (g/dl)
Normal	—	Clear	↑	Firm	<200	<25	<10	<2.5
I (noninflammatory)	Osteoarthritis, aseptic necrosis, traumatic arthritis, erythema nodosum, osteochondritis dissecans	Clear, yellow (may be xanthochromic if traumatic arthritis)	↑	Firm	↑ Up to 10,000	<25	<10	<2.5
II (inflammatory)	Crystal-induced arthritis, rheumatoid arthritis, Reiter's syndrome, collagen-vascular disease, psoriatic arthritis, serum sickness, rheumatic fever	Clear, yellow, turbid	↓	Friable	↑↑ Up to 100,000	40-90	<40	>2.5
III (septic)	Bacterial (staphylococcal, gonococcal, tuberculosis)	Turbid	↓/↑	Friable	↑↑↑ Up to 5 million	40-100	20-100	>2.5

↑, Elevated; ↑↑, markedly high; ↓, decreased; *PMN,* polymorphonuclear leukocytes; *WBC,* white blood cell count. Note that there is considerable overlap in the numbers listed above.

TABLE 4-24 Findings in Thyroid Function Tests in Various Clinical Conditions

Condition	T_4	FT_4I	T_3	FT_3I	TSH	TSI	TRH Stimulation
Hyperthyroidism							
Graves' disease	↑	↑	↑	↑	↓	+	↓
Toxic nodular goiter	↑	↑	↑	↑	↓	–	↓
Pituitary TSH-secreting tumors	↑	↑	↑	↑	↑	–	↓
T_3 thyrotoxicosis	N	N	↑	↑	↓	+, –	↓
T_4 thyrotoxicosis	↑	↑	N	N	↓	+, –	↓
Hypothyroidism							
Primary	↓	↓	↓	↓	↑	+, –	↑
Secondary	↓	↓	↓	↓	↓, N	–	↓
Tertiary	↓	↓	↓	↓	↓, N	–	N
Peripheral unresponsiveness	↑, N	↑, N	↑, N	↑	↑, N	–	N, ↑

From Tilton RC, Barrows A: *Clinical laboratory medicine,* St Louis, 1992, Mosby.
N, Normal; ↑, increased; ↓, decreased; +, – variable.

assays) or by immunometric techniques (influenced by serum levels of lipids, proteins, and certain drugs). The free thyroxine index (FTI) can also be easily calculated by multiplying T_4 times T_3RU and dividing the result by 100; the FTI corrects for any abnormal T_4 values secondary to protein binding: $FTI = T_4 \times T_3RU/100$.
Normal values equal 1.1 to 4.3.

T_4, SERUM T_4, AND FREE (free thyroxine)

Normal range:
0.8-2.8 ng/dl (10-36 pmol/L [CF: 12.87; SMI: 1 pmol/L])
Abnormal values:
Serum thyroxine (T_4)

Elevated in:
1. Graves' disease
2. Toxic multinodular goiter
3. Toxic adenoma
4. Iatrogenic and factitious
5. Transient hyperthyroidism
   a. Subacute thyroiditis
   b. Hashimoto's thyroiditis
   c. Silent thyroiditis
6. Rare causes: hypersecretion of TSH (e.g., pituitary neoplasms), struma ovarii, ingestion of large amounts of iodine in a patient with preexisting thyroid hyperplasia or adenoma (Jod-Basedow phenomenon), hydatidiform mole, carcinoma of thyroid, amiodarone therapy of arrhythmias.

Serum thyroxine test measures both circulating thyroxine bound to protein (represents >99% of circulating T_4) and unbound (free) thyroxine. Values vary with protein binding; changes in the concentration of T_4 secondary to changes in thyroxine-binding globulin (TBG) can be caused by the following:

Increased TBG (↑T_4)	Decreased TBG (↓ T_4)
Pregnancy	Androgens, glucocorticoids
Estrogens	Nephrotic syndrome, cirrhosis
Acute infectious hepatitis	Acromegaly
Oral contraceptives	Hypoproteinemia
Familial	Familial
Fluorouracil, clofibrate, heroin, methadone	Phenytoin, ASA and other NSAIDs, high-dose penicillin, asparaginase
	Chronic debilitating illness

To eliminate the suspected influence of protein binding on thyroxine values, two additional tests are available: T_3 resin uptake and serum free thyroxine.

TEGRETOL; *see* CARBAMAZEPINE

TESTOSTERONE (total testosterone)

Normal range: (Variable with age and sex)

Serum/plasma: Males: 280-1100 ng/dl
Females: 15-70 ng/dl

Urine: Males: 50-135 μg/day
Females: 2-12 μg/day

Elevated in: Testicular tumors, ovarian masculinizing tumors
Decreased in: Hypogonadism

THEOPHYLLINE

Normal therapeutic range: 10-20 mcg/ml

THORACENTESIS FLUID

Testing and evaluation of results:

1. Pleural effusion fluid should be differentiated in exudate or transudate. The initial laboratory studies should be aimed only at distinguishing an exudate from a transudate.
   a. Tube 1: protein, LDH, albumin.
   b. Tubes 2, 3, 4: save the fluid until further notice. In selected patients with suspected empyema, a pH level may be useful (generally ≤ 7.0). See following for proper procedure to obtain a pH level from pleural fluid.

   NOTE: Do not order further tests until the presence of an exudate is confirmed on the basis of protein and LDH determinations (see Section III); however, if the results of protein and LDH determinations cannot be obtained within a reasonable time (resulting in unnecessary delay), additional laboratory tests should be ordered at the time of thoracentesis.
2. A serum/effusion albumin gradient of ≤1.2 g/dl is indicative of exudative effusions, especially in patients with congestive heart failure (CHF) treated with diuretics.
3. Note the appearance of the fluid:
   a. A grossly hemorrhagic effusion can be a result of a traumatic tap, neoplasm, or an embolus with infarction.
   b. A milky appearance indicates either of the following:
      (1) Chylous effusion: caused by trauma or tumor invasion of the thoracic duct; lipoprotein electrophoresis of the effusion reveals chylomicrons and triglyceride levels >115 mg/dl.
      (2) Pseudochylous effusion: often seen with chronic inflammation of the pleural space (e.g., TB, connective tissue diseases).
4. If transudate, consider CHF, cirrhosis, chronic renal failure, and other hypoproteinemic states and perform subsequent workup accordingly.
5. If exudate, consider ordering these tests on the pleural fluid:
   a. Cytologic examination for malignant cells (for suspected neoplasm).
   b. Gram stain, cultures (aerobic and anaerobic), and sensitivities (for suspected infectious process).
   c. AFB stain and cultures (for suspected TB).
   d. pH: a value < 7.0 suggests parapneumonic effusion or empyema; a pleural fluid pH must be drawn anaerobically and iced immediately; the syringe should be prerinsed with 0.2 ml of 1:1000 heparin.
   e. Glucose: a low glucose level suggests parapneumonic effusions and rheumatoid arthritis.
   f. Amylase: a high amylase level suggests pancreatitis or ruptured esophagus.
   g. Perplexing pleural effusions are often a result of malignancy (e.g., lymphoma, malignant mesothelioma, ovarian carcinoma), TB, subdiaphragmatic processes, prior asbestos exposure, and postcardiac injury syndrome.

THROMBIN TIME (TT)

Normal range: 11.3-18.5 sec
Elevated in: Thrombolytic and heparin therapy, disseminated intravascular coagulation, hypofibrinogenemia, dysfibrinogenemia

THYROID-STIMULATING HORMONE (TSH)

Normal range: 2-11 μU/ml (2-11 mU/L [CF: 1; SMI: 1 mU/L])

CONDITIONS THAT INCREASE SERUM THYROID-STIMULATING HORMONE VALUES

Laboratory error
Primary hypothyroidism
Synthroid therapy with insufficient dose
Lithium or amiodarone; some patients
Hashimoto's thyroiditis in later stage
Large doses of inorganic iodide (e.g., SSKI)
Severe nonthyroid illness in recovery phase
Iodine deficiency (moderate or severe)
Addison's disease
TSH specimen drawn in evening (peak of diurnal variation)
Pituitary TSH-secreting tumor
Therapy of hypothyroidism (3-6 wk after beginning therapy [range, 1-8 wk]; sometimes longer when pretherapy TSH is over 100 μU/ml)
Acute psychiatric illness
Peripheral resistance to T_4 syndrome
Antibodies (e.g., HAMA) interfering with monoclonal sandwich method of TSH assay
Telepaque (iopanoic acid) and Oragrafin (ipodate) x-ray contrast media
Amphetamines
High altitudes

CONDITIONS THAT DECREASE SERUM THYROID-STIMULATING HORMONE VALUES

Laboratory error
T_4/T_3 toxicosis (diffuse or nodular etiology)
Excessive therapy for hypothyroidism
Active thyroiditis (subacute, painless, or early active Hashimoto's disease)
Multinodular goiter containing areas of autonomy
Severe nonthyroid illness (especially acute trauma, dopamine, or glucocorticoid)
T_3 toxicosis
Pituitary insufficiency
Cushing's syndrome (and some patients on high-dose glucocorticoid)
Jod-Basedow (iodine-induced) hyperthyroidism

Thyroid-stimulating hormone drawn 2-4 hr after levothyroxine dose
Postpartum transient toxicosis
Factitious hyperthyroidism
Struma ovarii
Radioimmunoassay, surgery, or antithyroid drug therapy for hyperthyroidism 4-6 wk (range 2 wk–2 yr) after the treatment
Interleukin-2 drugs (3%-6% of cases) or α-interferon therapy (1% of cases)
Hyperemesis gravidarum
Amiodarone therapy

THYROXINE (T_4)

Normal range: 4-11 μg/dl (51-142 nmol/L [CF: 12.87; SMI: 1 nmol/L])

TIBC; *see* IRON-BINDING CAPACITY

TRANSFERRIN

Normal range: 170-370 mg/dl (1.7-3.7 g/L [CF: 0.01; SMI: 0.01 g/L])
Elevated in: Iron deficiency anemia, oral contraceptive administration, viral hepatitis, late pregnancy
Decreased in: Nephrotic syndrome, liver disease, hereditary deficiency, protein malnutrition, neoplasms, chronic inflammatory states, chronic illness, thalassemia, hemochromatosis, hemolytic anemia

TRIGLYCERIDES

Normal range: <150 mg/dl (<1.80 mmol/L [CF: 0.01129; SMI: 0.02 mmol/L])
Elevated in: Hyperlipoproteinemias (types I, IIb, III, IV, V), hypothyroidism, pregnancy, estrogens, acute myocardial infarction, pancreatitis, alcohol intake, nephrotic syndrome, diabetes mellitus, glycogen storage disease
Decreased in: Malnutrition, congenital abetalipoproteinemias, drugs (e.g., gemfibrozil, fenofibrate, nicotinic acid, clofibrate)

TRIIODOTHYRONINE; *see* T_3

TROPONINS, SERUM

Normal range: 0-0.4 ng/ml (negative). If there is clinical suspicion of evolving acute MI or ischemic episode, repeat testing in 5-6 hours is recommended.
Indeterminate: 0.05-0.49 ng/ml. Suggest further tests. In a patient with unstable angina and this troponin I level, there is an increased risk of a cardiac event in the near future.
Strong probability of acute MI: ≥0.05 ng/ml
CARDIAC TROPONIN T (CTNT) is a highly sensitive marker for myocardial injury for the first 48 hours after MI and for up to 5-7 days (*see* Fig. 4-2, under "Creatine Kinase Isoenzymes"). It may be also elevated in renal failure, chronic muscle disease, and trauma.
CARDIAC TROPONIN I (CTNI) is highly sensitive and specific for myocardial injury (≥CK-MB) in the initial 8 hours, peaks within 24 hours and lasts up to 7 days. With progressively higher levels of cTnI, the risk of mortality increases because the amount of necrosis increases.

TSH; *see* THYROID-STIMULATING HORMONE

TT; *see* THROMBIN TIME

TUBERCULIN TEST (PPD)

Abnormal results: *see* Boxes 4-3 and 4-4 for interpretation

UNCONJUGATED BILIRUBIN; *see* BILIRUBIN, INDIRECT

UREA NITROGEN, BLOOD (BUN)

Normal range: 8-18 mg/dl (3-6.5 mmol/L [CF: 0.357; SMI: 0.5 mmol/L])
Box 4-5 describes factors affecting BUN level independent of renal function.
Elevated in: Drugs (aminoglycosides and other antibiotics, diuretics, lithium, corticosteroids), dehydration, gastrointestinal bleeding, decreased renal blood flow (shock, congestive heart failure, myocardial infarction), renal disease (glomerulonephritis, pyelonephritis, diabetic nephropathy), urinary tract obstruction (prostatic hypertrophy)

BOX 4-3 PPD Reaction Size Considered "Positive" (Intracutaneous 5 TU Mantoux Test at 48 hr)

5 mm or More
HIV infection or risk factors for HIV
Close recent contact with active TB case
Persons with chest x-ray consistent with healed TB

10 mm or More
Foreign-born persons from countries with high TB prevalence in Asia, Africa, and Latin America
IV drug users
Medically underserved low-income population groups (including Native Americans, Hispanics, and blacks)
Residents of long-term care facilities (nursing homes, mental institutions)
Medical conditions that increase risk for TB (silicosis, gastrectomy, undernourished, diabetes mellitus, high-dose corticosteroids or immunosuppression Rx, leukemia or lymphoma, other malignancies)
Employees of long-term care facilities, schools, child-care facilities, health care facilities

15 mm or More
All others not already listed

HIV, Human immunodeficiency virus; *PPD,* tuberculin test; *Rx,* prescription; *TB,* tuberculosis; *TU,* tuberculin units.

BOX 4-4 Factors Associated with False-Negative Tuberculin Tests

Technical Errors
Improper administration
Inaccurate reading
Loss of potency of antigen

Patient-Related Factors (Anergy)
Age (elderly)
Nutritional status
Medications—corticosteroids, immunosuppressive agents
Severe tuberculosis
Coexisting diseases
- HIV infection
- Viral illness or vaccination
- Lymphoreticular malignancies
- Sarcoidosis
- Solid tumors
- Lepromatous leprosy
- Sjögren's syndrome
- Ataxia telangiectasia
- Uremia
- Primary biliary cirrhosis
- Systemic lupus erythematosus
- Severe systemic disease of any etiology

From Stein JH (ed): *Internal medicine,* ed 4, St Louis, 1994, Mosby.
HIV, Human immunodeficiency virus.

BOX 4-5 Factors Affecting Blood Urea Nitrogen Level Independent of Renal Function

Disproportionate Increase in Blood Urea Nitrogen
Volume depletion "prerenal azotemia"
Gastrointestinal hemorrhage
Corticosteroid or cytotoxic agents
High-protein diet
Obstructive uropathy
Sepsis
Catabolic states tissue breakdown

Disproportionate Decrease in Blood Urea Nitrogen
Low-protein diet
Liver disease

From Andreoli TE (ed): *Cecil essentials of medicine,* ed 5, Philadelphia, 2001, WB Saunders.

Decreased in: Liver disease, malnutrition, pregnancy third trimester, overhydration, acromegaly, celiac disease

URIC ACID (serum)

Normal range: 2-7 mg/dl
Elevated in: Renal failure, gout, excessive cell lysis (chemotherapeutic agents, radiation therapy, leukemia, lymphoma, hemolytic anemia), hereditary enzyme deficiency (hypoxanthine-guanine-phosphoribosyl transferase), acidosis, myeloproliferative disorders, diet high in purines or protein, drugs (diuretics, low doses of ASA, ethambutol, nicotinic acid), lead poisoning, hypothyroidism, Addison's disease, nephrogenic diabetes insipidus, active psoriasis, polycystic kidneys
Decreased in: Drugs (allopurinol, high doses of ASA, probenecid, warfarin, corticosteroid), deficiency of xanthine oxidase, syndrome of inappropriate antidiuretic hormone secretion, renal tubular deficits (Fanconi's syndrome), alcoholism, liver disease, diet deficient in protein or purines, Wilson's disease, hemochromatosis

URINALYSIS

Normal range:
Color: light straw
Appearance: clear
Ketones: absent
pH: 4.5-8 (average, 6)
Protein: absent
Glucose: absent
Specific gravity: 1.005-1.030
Occult blood absent
Microscopic examination:
Red blood cells: 0-5 (high-power field)
White blood cells: 0-5 (high-power field)
Bacteria (spun specimen): absent
Casts: 0-4 hyaline (low-power field)
Abnormalities in the microscopic examination of urine are described in Table 4-25.

URINE AMYLASE

Normal range: 35-260 U Somogyi/hr (6.5-48.1 U/hr [CF: 0.185; SMI: 1 U/hr])
Elevated in: Pancreatitis, carcinoma of the pancreas

URINE BILE

Normal: Absent
Abnormal: Urine bilirubin: hepatitis (viral, toxic, drug-induced), biliary obstruction
Urine urobilinogen: hepatitis (viral, toxic, drug-induced), hemolytic jaundice, liver cell dysfunction (cirrhosis, infection, metastases)

URINE CALCIUM

Normal range: <250 mg/24 hr (<6.2 mmol/dl [CF: 0.02495; SMI: 0.1 mmol/dl])
Elevated in: Primary hyperparathyroidism, hypervitaminosis D, bone metastases, multiple myeloma, increased calcium intake, steroids, prolonged immobilization, sarcoidosis, Paget's disease, idiopathic hypercalciuria, renal tubular acidosis

TABLE 4-25 Microscopic Examination of the Urine

Finding	Associations
Casts	
Red blood cell	Glomerulonephritis, vasculitis
White blood cell	Interstitial nephritis, pyelonephritis
Epithelial cell	Acute tubular necrosis, interstitial nephritis, glomerulonephritis
Granular	Renal parenchymal disease (nonspecific)
Waxy, broad	Advanced renal failure
Hyaline	Normal finding in concentrated urine
Fatty	Heavy proteinuria
Cells	
Red blood cell	Urinary tract infection, urinary tract inflammation
White blood cell	Urinary tract infection, urinary tract inflammation
Eosinophil	Acute interstitial nephritis
(Squamous) epithelial cell	Contaminants
Crystals	
Uric acid	Acid urine, acute uric acid nephropathy, hyperuricosuria
Calcium phosphate	Alkaline urine
Calcium oxalate	Acid urine, hyperoxaluria, ethylene glycol poisoning
Cystine	Cystinuria
Sulfur	Sulfa-containing antibiotics

From Andreoli TE (ed): *Cecil essentials of medicine,* ed 5, Philadelphia, 2001, WB Saunders.

Decreased in: Hypoparathyroidism, pseudohypoparathyroidism, vitamin D deficiency, vitamin D–resistant rickets, diet low in calcium, drugs (thiazide diuretics, oral contraceptives), familial hypocalciuric hypercalcemia, renal osteodystrophy, potassium citrate therapy

URINE CAMP

Elevated in: Hypercalciuria, familial hypocalciuric hypercalcemia, primary hyperparathyroidism, pseudohypoparathyroidism, rickets
Decreased in: Vitamin D intoxication, sarcoidosis

URINE CATECHOLAMINES

Normal range:
Norepinephrine: <100 μg/24 hr (<590 nmol/day [CF: 5.911; SMI: 10 nmol/day])
Epinephrine: <10 μg/24 hr (55 nmol/day [CF: 5.458; SMI: 5 nmol/day])
Elevated in: Pheochromocytoma, neuroblastoma, severe stress

URINE CHLORIDE

Normal range: 110-250 mEq/day (110-250 mmol/day [CF: 1; SMI: 1 mmol/day])
Elevated in: Corticosteroids, Bartter's syndrome, diuretics, metabolic acidosis, severe hypokalemia
Decreased in: Chloride depletion (vomiting), colonic villous adenoma, chronic renal failure, renal tubular acidosis

URINE COPPER

Normal range: <40 μg/24 hr (<0.6 μmol/day [CF: 0.01574; SMI: 0.2 μmol/day])

URINE CORTISOL, FREE

Normal range: 10-110 μg/24 hr (30-300 nmol/day [CF: 2.759; SMI: 10 nmol/day])
Elevated: *see* CORTISOL, PLASMA

URINE CREATININE (24 hr)

Normal range:
Male: 0.8-1.8 g/day (7-16 mmol/day [CF: 8.840; SMI: 0.1 mmol/day])
Female: 0.6-1.6 g/day (5.3-14 mmol/day)

NOTE: Useful test as an indicator of completeness of 24-hr urine collection.

URINE EOSINOPHILS

Normal:
Absent
Present:
Interstitial nephritis, acute tubular necrosis, urinary tract infection, kidney transplant rejection, hepatorenal syndrome

URINE GLUCOSE (qualitative)

Normal: Absent
Present in: Diabetes mellitus, renal glycosuria (decreased renal threshold for glucose), glucose intolerance

URINE HEMOGLOBIN, FREE

Normal: Absent
Present in: Hemolysis (with saturation of serum haptoglobin binding capacity and renal threshold for tubular absorption of hemoglobin)

URINE HEMOSIDERIN

Normal: Absent
Present in: Paroxysmal nocturnal hemoglobinuria, chronic hemolytic anemia, hemochromatosis, blood transfusion, thalassemias

URINE 5-HYDROXYINDOLE-ACETIC ACID (urine 5-HIAA)

Normal range: 2-8 mg/24 hr (10-40 μmol/day [CF: 5.23; SMI: 5 μmol/day])
Elevated in: Carcinoid tumors, after ingestion of certain foods (bananas, plums, tomatoes, avocados, pineapples, eggplant, walnuts), drugs (monoamine oxidase inhibitors, phenacetin, methyldopa, glycerol guaiacolate, acetaminophen, salicylates, phenothiazines, imipramine, methocarbamol, reserpine, methamphetamine)

URINE INDICAN

Normal: Absent
Present in: Malabsorption secondary to intestinal bacterial overgrowth

URINE KETONES (semiquantitative)

Normal: Absent
Present in: Diabetic ketoacidosis, alcoholic ketoacidosis, starvation, isopropanol ingestion

URINE METANEPHRINES

Normal range: 0-2.0 mg/24 hr (0-11.0 μmol/day [CF: 5.458; SMI: 0.5 μmol/day])
Elevated in: Pheochromocytoma, neuroblastoma, drugs (caffeine, phenothiazines, monoamine oxidase inhibitors), stress

URINE MYOGLOBIN

Normal: Absent
Present in: Severe trauma, hyperthermia, polymyositis/dermatomyositis, carbon monoxide poisoning, drugs (narcotic and amphetamine toxicity), hypothyroidism, muscle ischemia

URINE NITRITE

Normal: Absent
Present in: Urinary tract infections

URINE OCCULT BLOOD

Normal: Negative
Positive in: Trauma to urinary tract, renal disease (glomerulonephritis, pyelonephritis), renal or ureteral calculi, bladder lesions (carcinoma, cystitis), prostatitis, prostatic carcinoma, menstrual contamination, hematopoietic disorders (hemophilia, thrombocytopenia), anticoagulants, ASA

URINE OSMOLALITY

Normal range: 50-1200 mOsm/kg (50-1200 mmol/kg [CF: 1; SMI: 1 mmol/kg])
Elevated in: Syndrome of inappropriate antidiuretic hormone secretion, dehydration, glycosuria, adrenal insufficiency, high-protein diet
Decreased in: Diabetes insipidus, excessive water intake, IV hydration with D_5W, acute renal insufficiency, glomerulonephritis

URINE pH

Normal range: 4.6-8 (average 6)
Elevated in: Bacteriuria, vegetarian diet, renal failure with inability to form ammonia, drugs (antibiotics, sodium bicarbonate, acetazolamide)
Decreased in: Acidosis (metabolic, respiratory), drugs (ammonium chloride, methenamine mandelate), diabetes mellitus, starvation, diarrhea

URINE PHOSPHATE

Normal range: 0.8-2.0 g/24 hr
Elevated in: Acute tubular necrosis (diuretic phase), chronic renal disease, uncontrolled diabetes mellitus, hyperparathyroidism, hypomagnesemia, metabolic acidosis, metabolic

alkalosis, neurofibromatosis, adult-onset vitamin D–resistant hypophosphatemic osteomalacia
Decreased in: Acromegaly, acute renal failure, decreased dietary intake, hypoparathyroidism, respiratory acidosis

URINE POTASSIUM

Normal range: 25-100 mEq/24 hr (25-100 mmol/day [CF: 1; SMI: 1 mmol/day])
Elevated in: Aldosteronism (primary, secondary), glucocorticoids, alkalosis, renal tubular acidosis, excessive dietary potassium intake
Decreased in: Acute renal failure, potassium-sparing diuretics, diarrhea, hypokalemia

URINE PROTEIN (quantitative)

Normal range: <150 mg/24 hr (<0.15 g/day [CF: 0.001; SMI: 0.01 g/day])
Elevated in:
Nephrotic syndrome as a result of primary renal diseases
Malignant hypertension
Malignancies: multiple myeloma, leukemias, Hodgkin's disease
Congestive heart failure
Diabetes mellitus
Systemic lupus erythematosus, rheumatoid arthritis
Sickle cell disease
Goodpasture's syndrome
Malaria
Amyloidosis, sarcoidosis
Tubular lesions: cystinosis
Functional (after heavy exercise)
Pyelonephritis
Pregnancy
Constrictive pericarditis
Renal vein thrombosis
Toxic nephropathies: heavy metals, drugs
Radiation nephritis
Orthostatic (postural) proteinuria
Benign proteinuria: fever, heat or cold exposure

URINE SEDIMENT; *see* Fig. 4-14 for evaluation of common abnormalities

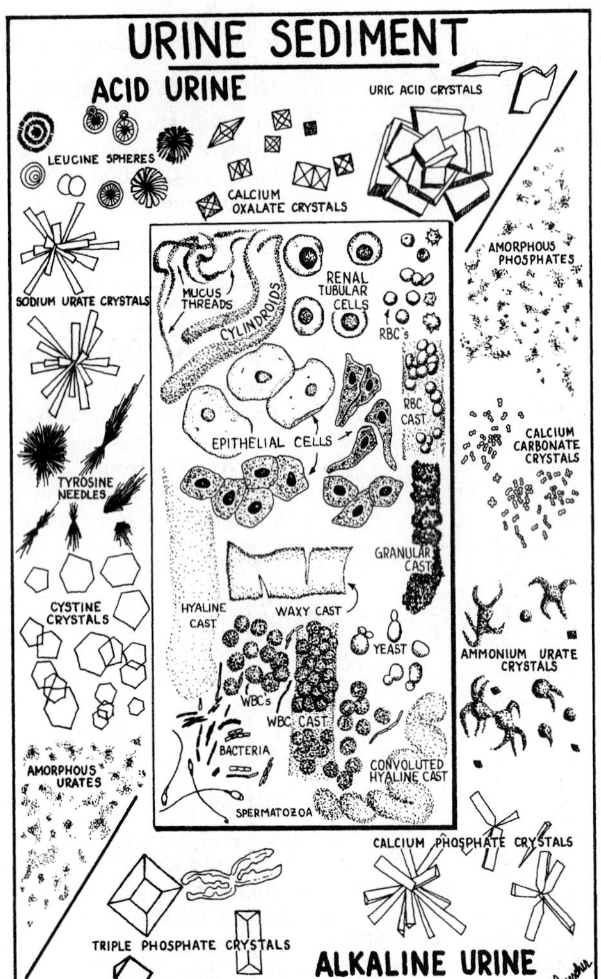

FIGURE 4-14 Microscopic examination of urinary sediment. (From Grigorian Greene M: *The Harriet Lane handbook: a manual for pediatric house officers,* ed 17, St Louis, 2007, Mosby.)

URINE SODIUM (quantitative)

Normal range: 40-220 mEq/day (40-220 mmol/day [CF: 1; SMI: 1 mmol/day])
Elevated in: Diuretic administration, high sodium intake, salt-losing nephritis, acute tubular necrosis, vomiting, Addison's disease, syndrome of inappropriate antidiuretic hormone secretion, hypothyroidism, congestive heart failure, hepatic failure, chronic renal failure, Bartter's syndrome, glucocorticoid deficiency, interstitial nephritis caused by analgesic abuse, mannitol, dextran, or glycerol therapy, milk-alkali syndrome, decreased renin secretion, postobstructive diuresis
Decreased in: Increased aldosterone, glucocorticoid excess, hyponatremia, prerenal azotemia, decreased salt intake

URINE SPECIFIC GRAVITY

Normal range: 1.005-1.03
Elevated in: Dehydration, excessive fluid losses (vomiting, diarrhea, fever), x-ray contrast media, diabetes mellitus, congestive heart failure, syndrome of inappropriate antidiuretic hormone secretion, adrenal insufficiency, decreased fluid intake
Decreased in: Diabetes insipidus, renal disease (glomerulonephritis, pyelonephritis), excessive fluid intake or IV hydration

URINE VANILLYLMANDELIC ACID (VMA)

Normal range: <6.8 mg/24 hr (<35 μmol/day [CF: 5.046; SMI: 1 μmol/day])
Elevated in: Pheochromocytoma, neuroblastoma, ganglioblastoma, drugs (isoproterenol, methocarbamol, levodopa, sulfonamides, chlorpromazine), severe stress, after ingestion of bananas, chocolate, vanilla, tea, coffee
Decreased in: Drugs (monoamine oxidase inhibitors, reserpine, guanethidine, methyldopa)

VDRL

Normal range: Negative
Positive test: Syphilis, other treponemal diseases (yaws, pinta, bejel)

NOTE: A false-positive test may be seen in patients with systemic lupus erythematosus and other autoimmune diseases, infectious mononucleosis, HIV, atypical pneumonia, malaria, leprosy, typhus fever, rat-bite fever, relapsing fever.

NOTE: see Table 4-26 for interpretation of serologic tests for syphilis.

TABLE 4-26 Interpretation of Serologic Tests for Syphilis*

FINDING		
Nontreponemal Tests	**Treponemal Tests**	**Interpretation of Finding: Is Syphilis Present?***
Nonreactive	Nonreactive	Early primary syphilis is not ruled out by negative serologic tests. Early syphilis is present in 13%-30% of patients who have a negative microhemagglutination–Treponema pallidum test; in about 30% of patients who present with chancre but have a nonreactive reagin test; and in about 10% of patients who have a negative FTA-ABS test. Late syphilis is present in a very small fraction of patients. Adequately treated syphilis in remote past may produce these results, but treponemal tests usually remain reactive.
	Reactive	Observed in about 10% of patients with chancre. The treponemal tests may turn positive shortly before the reagin tests. Reagin tests repeated after several days are generally positive. In adequately treated early syphilis, the reagin test may return to nonreactive within 1-2 yr, whereas the treponemal tests generally do not. Late syphilis is not ruled out by a negative reagin test. The sensitivity of the reagin tests is lower than that of treponemal tests in untreated late syphilis. In secondary syphilis, rarely, a highly reactive serum appears negative when tested undiluted with a reagin test because flocculation is inhibited by relative antibody excess. Not reported to occur with treponemal tests. Quantitative reagin tests are positive. False-positive treponemal tests occur in 40% of patients with Lyme disease.
Reactive	Nonreactive	Finding is not diagnostic of syphilis but constitutes a classic biologic false-positive reaction.
	borderline (FTA-ABS)	Not diagnostic of syphilis: most patients (90%) with this pattern do not develop clinical or serologic evidence of syphilis. Repeat test is indicated. Chronic borderline results are associated with a variety of conditions other than syphilis.
	Beaded (FTA-ABS)	Not diagnostic of syphilis. Seen with collagen-vascular disease.
	Reactive	Findings diagnostic of syphilis or other treponemal disease. In adequately treated syphilis, one would expect (1) a sustained fourfold drop in titer of reagin test, although reagin test may remain positive after adequate therapy; (2) treponemal tests remain positive after adequate therapy. Concurrent false-positive results on both nontreponemal and treponemal tests could occur in rare instances. It may be impossible to rule out syphilis in an individual with this test profile.

From Stein JH (ed): *Internal medicine,* ed 4, St Louis, 1994, Mosby.
FTA-ABS, Fluorescent treponemal antibody, absorbed.
*Serologic data must always be interpreted in the light of a total clinical evaluation. Diagnosis based on serologic criteria alone is fraught with error. Serologic tests apparently in conflict with clinical diagnosis should be confirmed by repetition or possibly referral to a reference laboratory.

VISCOSITY (serum)

Normal range: 1.4-1.8 relative to water (1.10-1.22 centipoise)
Elevated in: Monoclonal gammopathies (Waldenström's macroglobulinemia, multiple myeloma), hyperfibrinogenemia, systemic lupus erythematosus, rheumatoid arthritis, polycythemia, leukemia

VITAMIN B_{12}

Normal:
190-900 ng/ml
Causes of Vitamin B_{12} deficiency:
1. Pernicious anemia (antibodies against intrinsic factor and gastric parietal cells)
2. Dietary (strict lacto-ovovegetarians, food faddists)
3. Malabsorption (achlorhydria, gastrectomy, ileal resection, pancreatic insufficiency, drugs [omeprazole, cholestyramine])

Falsely low levels occur in patients with severe folate deficiency, in patients using high doses of ascorbic acid, and when cobalamin levels are measured after nuclear medicine studies (radioactivity interferes with cobalamin radioimmunoassay).
Falsely high or normal levels in patients with cobalamin deficiency can occur in severe liver disease and chronic granulocytic leukemia.
The absence of anemia or macrocytosis does not exclude the diagnosis of cobalamin deficiency.

WBC; *see* COMPLETE BLOOD COUNT

WESTERGREN; *see* ERYTHROCYTE SEDIMENTATION RATE

WHITE BLOOD COUNT; *see* COMPLETE BLOOD COUNT

Section V

Clinical Preventive Services

PART A
THE PERIODIC HEALTH EXAMINATION*

Age-specific charts, 1480

PART B
IMMUNIZATIONS AND CHEMOPROPHYLAXIS

Childhood and adolescent immunizations, 1489

*Data modified from US Preventive Services Task Force: Guide to clinical preventive services: report of the U.S. Preventive Services Task Force, ed 2, Washington, DC, 1996 (revised 2001), U.S. Department of Health and Human Services. Text downloaded from Internet site: http://text.nlm.nih.gov

General recommendations on immunization, 1494

Immunizations for adults, 1509

PART A • THE PERIODIC HEALTH EXAMINATION

Age-Specific Charts

TABLE 5-1 Birth to 10 Years

Interventions considered and recommended for the Periodic Health Examination

Leading causes of death
- Conditions originating in perinatal period
- Congenital anomalies
- Sudden infant death syndrome (SIDS)
- Unintentional injuries (non–motor vehicle)
- Motor vehicle injuries

INTERVENTIONS FOR THE GENERAL POPULATION

Screening

Height and weight
Blood pressure
Vision screen (age 3-4 yr)
Hemoglobinopathy screen (birth)[1]
Phenylalanine level (birth)[2]
T_4 and/or TSH (birth)[3]

Counseling

Injury prevention

Child safety car seats (age <5 yr)
Lap/shoulder belts (age ≥5 yr)
Bicycle helmet; avoid bicycling near traffic
Smoke detector, flame-retardant sleepwear
Hot water heater temperature <120°-130° F
Window/stair guards, pool fence
Safe storage of drugs, toxic substances, firearms, and matches
Syrup of ipecac, poison control phone number
CPR training for parents/caretakers

Diet and exercise

Breast-feeding, iron-enriched formula and foods (infants and toddlers)
Limit fat and cholesterol; maintain caloric balance; emphasize grains, fruits, vegetables (age ≥2 yr)
Regular physical activity*

Substance use

Effects of passive smoking*
Antitobacco message*

Dental health

Regular visits to dental care provider*
Floss, brush with fluoride toothpaste daily*
Advice about baby bottle tooth decay*

Immunizations

Diphtheria-tetanus-pertussis (DTP)[4]
Inactivated poliovirus vaccine (IPV)[5]
Measles-mumps-rubella (MMR)[6]
H. influenzae type b (Hib) conjugate[7]
Hepatitis A vaccine (HR4)
Hepatitis B[8]
Varicella[9]
Pneumococcal vaccine[10]
Influenza[11]
Meningococcal conjugate vaccine (MCV4)[12]

Chemoprophylaxis

Ocular prophylaxis (birth)

INTERVENTIONS FOR HIGH-RISK POPULATIONS

Population	*Potential Interventions (See detailed high-risk definitions)*
Preterm or low birth weight	Hemoglobin/hematocrit (HR1)
Infants of mothers at risk for HIV	HIV testing (HR2)
Low income; immigrants	Hemoglobin/hematocrit (HR1); PPD (HR3)
TB contacts	PPD (HR3)
Native American/Alaska Native	Hemoglobin/hematocrit (HR1); PPD (HR3); pneumococcal vaccine (HR5)
Residents of long-term care facilities	PPD (HR3); hepatitis A vaccine (HR4); influenza vaccine (HR6)
Certain chronic medical conditions	PPD (HR3); pneumococcal vaccine (HR5); influenza vaccine (HR6)
Increased individual or community lead exposure	Blood lead level (HR7)
Inadequate water fluoridation	Daily fluoride supplement (HR8)
Family hx of skin cancer; nevi; fair skin, eyes, hair	Avoid excess/midday sun, use protective clothing* (HR9)

[1]Whether screening should be universal or targeted to high-risk groups will depend on the proportion of high-risk individuals in the screening area, and other considerations. [2]If done during first 24 hr of life, repeat by age 2 wk. [3]Optimally between day 2 and 6, but in all cases before newborn nursery discharge. [4]2, 4, 6, and 12-18 mo; once between age 4-6 yr (DTaP may be used at 15 mo and older). [5]2, 4, 6-18 mo; once between age 4-6 yr. [6]12-15 mo and 4-6 yr. [7]2, 4, 6 and 12-15 mo; no dose needed at 6 mo if PRP-OMP vaccine is used for first 2 doses. [8]Birth, 1 mo, 6 mo; or, 0-2 mo, 1-2 mo later, and 6-18 mo. If not done in infancy: current visit, and 1 and 6 mo later. [9]12-18 mo; or any child without hx of chickenpox or previous immunization. Include information on risk in adulthood, duration of immunity, and potential need for booster doses. Administer a second dose of varicella vaccine at age 4-6 yr. [10]The 7-Valent conjugate vaccine (PCV) can be administered at the same time as the other childhood vaccines at a separate site. [11]Influenza vaccine is recommended in children 6 mo-18 yr of age. [12]Meningococcal conjugate vaccine (MCV4) is preferred to meningococcal polysaccharide vaccine (MPSV4) for children 2-10 yr of age who are at increased risk for meningococcal disease (children traveling to or residents of countries in which the disease is hyperendemic or epidemic, children who have terminal complement component deficiencies, and children who have anatomic or functional asplenia).

*The ability of clinician counseling to influence this behavior is unproven.

HR1: Infants age 6-12 mo who are living in poverty, black, Native American or Alaska Native, immigrants from developing countries, preterm and low birth weight infants, infants whose principal dietary intake is unfortified cow's milk.

HR2: Infants born to high-risk mothers whose HIV status is unknown. Women at high risk include past or present injection drug use; persons who exchange sex for money or drugs, and their sex partners; injection drug–using, bisexual, or HIV-positive sex partners currently or in past; persons seeking treatment for STDs; blood transfusion during 1978-1985.

HR3: Persons infected with HIV, close contacts of persons with known or suspected TB, persons with medical risk factors associated with TB, immigrants from countries with high TB prevalence, medically underserved low-income populations (including homeless), residents of long-term care facilities.

HR4: Hepatitis A vaccine (Hep A) is recommended for all children at 1 yr of age (i.e., 12-23 mo). The two doses in the series should be administered at least 6 mo apart. Children who are not vaccinated by 2 yr of age can be vaccinated at subsequent visits.

HR5: Immunocompetent persons ≥2 yr with certain medical conditions, including chronic cardiac or pulmonary disease, diabetes mellitus, cochlear implant candidates and recipients, and anatomic asplenia. Immunocompetent persons ≥2 yr living in high-risk environments or social settings (e.g., certain Native American and Alaska Native populations).

HR6: Annual vaccination of children ≥6 mo who are residents of chronic care facilities or who have chronic cardiopulmonary disorders, metabolic diseases (including diabetes mellitus), hemoglobinopathies, immunosuppression, or renal dysfunction.

HR7: Children about age 12 mo who: (1) live in communities in which the prevalence of lead levels requiring individual intervention, including residental lead hazard control or chelation, is high or undefined; (2) live in or frequently visit a home built before 1950 with dilapidated paint or with recent or ongoing renovation or remodeling; (3) have close contact with a person who has an elevated lead level; (4) live near lead industry or heavy traffic; (5) live with someone whose job or hobby involves lead exposure; (6) use lead-based pottery; or (7) take traditional ethnic remedies that contain lead.

HR8: Children living in areas with inadequate water fluoridation (<0.6 ppm).

HR9: Persons with a family history of skin cancer, a large number of moles, atypical moles, poor tanning ability, or light skin, hair, and eye color.

TABLE 5-2 Ages 11-24 Years

Interventions considered and recommended for the Periodic Health Examination	Leading causes of death Motor vehicle/other unintentional injuries Homicide Suicide Malignant neoplasms Heart diseases

INTERVENTIONS FOR THE GENERAL POPULATION

Screening
Height and weight
Blood pressure[1]
Papanicolaou (Pap) test[2] (females)
Chlamydia screen[3] (females <25 yr)
HIV screening
Lipid panel (in high-risk young adults only)
Rubella serology or vaccination hx[4] (females >12 yr)
Assess for problem drinking

Counseling

Injury prevention
Lap/shoulder belts
Bicycle/motorcycle/ATV helmets*
Smoke detector*
Safe storage/removal of firearms*

Substance use
Avoid tobacco use
Avoid underage drinking and illicit drug use*
Avoid alcohol/drug use while driving, swimming, boating, etc.*

Sexual behavior
STD prevention: abstinence*; avoid high-risk behavior*; condoms/female barrier with spermicide*
Unintended pregnancy: contraception

Diet and exercise
Limit fat and cholesterol; maintain caloric balance; emphasize grains, fruits, vegetables
Adequate calcium intake (females)
Regular physical activity*

Dental health
Regular visits to dental care provider*
Floss, brush with fluoride toothpaste daily

Immunizations
Tetanus-diphtheria (Td) boosters (11-16 yr), pertussis booster**
Hepatitis B[5]
MMR (11-12 yr)[6]
Varicella (11-12 yr)[7]
Rubella[4] (females >12 yr)
Meningococcal[8]
Human papilloma virus (11-12 yr)[9]
Influenza[10]

Chemoprophylaxis
Multivitamin with folic acid (females)

INTERVENTIONS FOR HIGH-RISK POPULATIONS

Population	*Potential Interventions (See detailed high-risk definitions)*
High-risk sexual behavior	RPR/VDRL (HR1); screen for gonorrhea (female) (HR2), HIV (HR3), chlamydia (female) (HR4); hepatitis A vaccine (HR5)
Injection or street drug use	RPR/VDRL (HR1); HIV screen (HR3); hepatitis A vaccine (HR5); PPD (HR6); advice to reduce infection risk (HR7)
TB contacts; immigrants; low income	PPD (HR6)
Native Americans/Alaska Natives	Hepatitis A vaccine (HR5); PPD (HR6); pneumococcal vaccine (HR8)
Travelers to developing countries	Hepatitis A vaccine (HR5)
Certain chronic medical conditions	PPD (HR6); pneumococcal vaccine (HR8); influenza vaccine (HR9)
Settings where adolescents and young adults congregate	Second MMR (HR10)
Susceptible to varicella, measles, mumps	Varicella vaccine (HR11); MMR (HR12)
Blood transfusion between 1975-1985	HIV screen (HR3)
Institutionalized persons; health care/lab workers	Hepatitis A vaccine (HR5); PPD (HR6); influenza vaccine (HR9)
Family hx of skin cancer; nevi; fair skin, eyes, hair	Avoid excess/midday sun, use protective clothing* (HR13)
Prior pregnancy with neural tube defect	Folic acid 4.0 mg (HR14)
Inadequate water fluoridation	Daily fluoride supplement (HR15)
Pregnancy	HIV screen

[1]Periodic BP for persons aged ≥21 yr. [2]If sexually active at present or in the past: q ≤3 yr. If sexual history is unreliable, begin Pap tests at age 18 yr. [3]If sexually active. [4]Serologic testing, documented vaccination history, and routine vaccination against rubella (preferably with MMR) are equally acceptable alternatives. [5]If not previously immunized: current visit, 1 and 6 mo later. [6]If no previous second dose of MMR. [7]If susceptible to chickenpox. [8]Meningococcal conjugate vaccine can be administered at 11-12 yr visit, at high school entry, or at beginning of college (especially indicated in students living in college dormitories). [9]Quadrivalent human papillomavirus (types 6, 11, 16, 18) recombinant vaccine (Gardasil) should be given to all females aged 13-26 yr who have not been previously vaccinated. The vaccine is indicated for the prevention of cervical cancer and genital warts caused by the human papilloma virus (HPV) 6, 11, 16, or 18. Gardasil is an intramuscular injection for administration to the thigh or upper arm. The schedule consists of three 0.5 ml doses, with the second dose given 2 mo after the first, and the final dose administered 6 mo after the initial dose. [10]Influenza vaccine is recommended for children 6-18 yr.

*The ability of clinician counseling to influence this behavior is unproven.

**Tdap vaccine is recommended for adolescents aged 11-12 yr who have completed the recommended childhood DTP/DTaP vaccination series and have not received a Td booster dose. Adolescents aged 13-18 yr who missed the 11-12 yr Td/Tdap booster dose should also receive a single dose of Tdap if they have completed the recommended childhood DTP/DTaP vaccination series. Subsequent Td boosters are recommended every 10 yr.

HR1: Persons who exchange sex for money or drugs, and their sex partners; persons with other STDs (including HIV); and sexual contacts of persons with active syphilis. Clinicians should also consider local epidemiology.

HR2: Females who have two or more sex partners in the last year; a sex partner with multiple sexual contacts; exchanged sex for money or drugs; or a history of repeated episodes of gonorrhea. Clinicians should also consider local epidemiology.

HR3: Males who had sex with males after 1975; past or present injection drug use; persons who exchange sex for money or drugs, and their sex partners; injection drug–using, bisexual, or HIV-positive sex partner currently or in the past; blood transfusion during 1978-1985; persons seeking treatment for STDs. Clinicians should also consider local epidemiology and consider screening for HIV in general population.

HR4: Sexually active females with multiple risk factors including history of prior STD; new or multiple sex partners; age under 25; nonuse or inconsistent use of barrier contraceptives; cervical ectopy. Clinicians should consider local epidemiology of the disease in identifying other high-risk groups.

HR5: Persons living in, traveling to, or working in areas where the disease is endemic and where periodic outbreaks occur (e.g., countries with high or intermediate endemicity; certain Alaska Native, Pacific Island, Native American, and religious communities); men who have sex with men; injection or street drug users; persons with clotting factor disorders or chronic liver disease. Vaccine may be considered for institutionalized persons and workers in these institutions, military personnel, and day-care, hospital, and laboratory workers. Clinicians should also consider local epidemiology.

HR6: HIV positive, close contacts of persons with known or suspected TB, health care workers, persons with medical risk factors associated with TB, immigrants from countries with high TB prevalence, medically underserved low-income populations (including homeless), alcoholics, injection drug users, and residents of long-term facilities.

HR7: Persons who continue to inject drugs.

HR8: Immunocompetent persons with certain medical conditions, including chronic cardiac or pulmonary disease, diabetes mellitus, cochlear implants candidates and recipients, and anatomic asplenia. Immunocompetent persons who live in high-risk environments or social settings (e.g., certain Native American and Alaska Native populations).

HR9: Annual vaccination of residents of chronic care facilities; persons with chronic cardiopulmonary disorders, metabolic diseases (including diabetes mellitus), hemoglobinopathies, immunosuppression, or renal dysfunction; and health care providers for high-risk patients.

HR10: Adolescents and young adults in settings where such individuals congregate (e.g., high schools and colleges), if they have not previously received a second dose.

HR11: Healthy persons aged ≥13 yr without a history of chickenpox or previous immunization. Consider serologic testing for presumed susceptible persons aged ≥13 yr.

HR12: Persons born after 1956 who lack evidence of immunity to measles or mumps (e.g., documented receipt of live vaccine on or after the first birthday, laboratory evidence of immunity, or a history of physician-diagnosed measles or mumps).

HR13: Persons with a family or personal history of skin cancer, a large number of moles, atypical moles, poor tanning ability, or light skin, hair, and eye color.

HR14: Women with prior pregnancy affected by neural tube defect who are planning pregnancy.

HR15: Persons aged <17 yr living in areas with inadequate water fluoridation (<0.6 ppm).

TABLE 5-3 **Ages 25-64 Years**

Interventions considered and recommended for the Periodic Health Examination	Leading causes of death Malignant neoplasms Heart diseases Motor vehicle and other unintentional injuries Human immunodeficiency virus (HIV) infection Suicide and homicide

INTERVENTIONS FOR THE GENERAL POPULATION

Screening	**Injury prevention**
Blood pressure	Lap/shoulder belts
Height and weight	Motorcycle/bicycle/ATV helmets*
Lipid panel (men age 35-64, women age 45-64)	Smoke detector*
HIV screening	Safe storage/removal of firearms*
Papanicolaou (Pap) test (women)[1]	**Sexual behavior**
Fecal occult blood test[2] and/or colonoscopy (≥50 yr)	STD prevention: avoid high-risk behavior*; condoms/female barrier with spermicide*
Mammogram ± clinical breast exam[3] (women 40-69 yr)	Unintended pregnancy: contraception
Bone density scan in postmenopausal women	**Dental health**
Assess for problem drinking	Regular visits to dental care provider*
Rubella serology or vaccination hx[4] (women of childbearing age)	Floss, brush with fluoride toothpaste daily*
Counseling	*Immunizations*
Substance use	Tetanus-diphtheria (Td) boosters
Tobacco cessation	Rubella[4] (women of childbearing age)
Avoid alcohol/drug use while driving, swimming, boating, etc.*	Influenza vaccine†
Diet and exercise	Human papilloma virus[5]
Limit fat and cholesterol; maintain caloric balance; emphasize grains, fruits, vegetables	Herpes zoster (≥60 yr)[6]
Adequate calcium intake (women)	*Chemoprophylaxis*
Regular physical activity*	Multivitamin with folic acid (women planning or capable of pregnancy)

INTERVENTIONS FOR HIGH-RISK POPULATIONS

Population	*Potential Interventions (See detailed high-risk definitions)*
High-risk sexual behavior	RPR/VDRL (HR1); screen for gonorrhea (female) (HR2), HIV (HR3), chlamydia (female) (HR4); hepatitis B vaccine (HR5); hepatitis A vaccine (HR6)
Injection or street drug use	RPR/VDRL (HR1); HIV screen (HR3); hepatitis B vaccine (HR5); hepatitis A vaccine (HR6); PPD (HR7); advice to reduce infection risk (HR8)
Low income; TB contacts; immigrants; alcoholics	PPD (HR7)
Native Americans/Alaska Natives	Hepatitis A vaccine (HR6); PPD (HR7); pneumococcal vaccine (HR9)
Travelers to developing countries	Hepatitis B vaccine (HR5); hepatitis A vaccine (HR6)
Certain chronic medical conditions	PPD (HR7); pneumococcal vaccine (HR9); influenza vaccine (HR10)
Blood product recipients	HIV screen (HR3); hepatitis B vaccine (HR5); hepatitis C screen
Susceptible to measles, mumps, or varicella	MMR (HR11); varicella vaccine (HR12)
Institutionalized persons	Hepatitis A vaccine (HR6); PPD (HR7); pneumococcal vaccine (HR9); influenza vaccine (HR10)
Health care/lab workers	Hepatitis B vaccine (HR5); hepatitis A vaccine (HR6); PPD (HR7); influenza vaccine (HR10)
Family hx of skin cancer; fair skin, eyes, hair	Avoid excess/midday sun, use protective clothing* (HR13)
Previous pregnancy with neural tube defect	Folic acid 4.0 mg (HR14)
Cardiovascular risk factors	Lipid panel (HR 15)
Pregnancy	HIV screen

[1]Women who are or have been sexually active and who have a cervix: q ≤3 yr. Routine pap smear screening is unnecessary for women who have undergone a complete hysterectomy for benign disease. [2]Annually. [3]Mammogram q1-2 yr, or mammogram q1-2 yr with annual clinical breast examination. [4]Serologic testing, documented vaccination history, and routine vaccination (preferably with MMR) are equally acceptable. [5]Quadrivalent human papillomavirus (types 6, 11, 16, 18) recombinant vaccine (Gardasil) should be given to all females aged 13-26 yr who have not been previously vaccinated. The vaccine is indicated for the prevention of cervical cancer and genital warts caused by the human papilloma virus (HPV) 6, 11, 16, or 18. Gardasil is an intramuscular injection for administration to the thigh or upper arm. The schedule consists of three 0.5 ml doses, with the second dose given 2 mo after the first, and the final dose administered 6 mo after the initial dose. [6]Herpes zoster vaccine (Zostavax) is indicated for prevention of herpes zoster (shingles) in individuals 60 yr or older. Zostavax is administered as a single dose subcutaneously. It is a lyophilic preparation of the Oka/Merck strain of live, attenuated varicella zoster virus (VZV). It should not be administered to individuals with a history of primary or acquired immunodeficiency states, persons on immunosuppressive therapy (including high-dose corticosteroids), those with active untreated tuberculosis, and those who may be pregnant.

*The ability of clinician counseling to influence this behavior is unproven.

†A live attenuated influenza vaccine (LAIV, Flumist) administered intranasally is available for healthy persons 2 to 49 years of age.

HR1: Persons who exchange sex for money or drugs, and their sex partners; persons with other STDs (including HIV); and sexual contacts of persons with active syphilis. Clinicians should also consider local epidemiology.

HR2: Women who exchange sex for money or drugs, or who have had repeated episodes of gonorrhea. Clinicians should also consider local epidemiology.

HR3: Men who had sex with men after 1975; past or present injection drug use; persons who exchange sex for money or drugs, and their sex partners; injection drug–using, bisexual, or HIV-positive sex partner currently or in the past; blood transfusion during 1978-1985; persons seeking treatment for STDs. Clinicians should also consider local epidemiology and consider HIV screening in general population.

HR4: Sexually active women with multiple risk factors including history of STD; new or multiple sex partners; nonuse or inconsistent use of barrier contraceptives; cervical ectopy. Clinicians should also consider local epidemiology.

HR5: Blood product recipients (including hemodialysis patients), persons with frequent occupational exposure to blood or blood products, men who have sex with men, injection drug users and their sex partners, persons with multiple recent sex partners, persons with other STDs (including HIV), travelers to countries with endemic hepatitis B.

HR6: Persons living in, traveling to, or working in areas where the disease is endemic and where periodic outbreaks occur (e.g., countries with high or intermediate endemicity; certain Alaska Native, Pacific Island, Native American, and religious communities); men who have sex with men; injection or street drug users; patients with clotting factor disorders or chronic liver disease. Consider for institutionalized persons and workers in these institutions, military personnel, and day-care, hospital, and laboratory workers. Clinicians should also consider local epidemiology.

HR7: HIV positive, close contacts of persons with known or suspected TB, health care workers, persons with medical risk factors associated with TB, immigrants from countries with high TB prevalence, medically underserved low-income populations (including homeless), alcoholics, injection drug users, and residents of long-term care facilities.

HR8: Persons who continue to inject drugs.

HR9: Immunocompetent institutionalized persons aged ≥50 yr and immunocompetent persons with certain medical conditions, including chronic cardiac or pulmonary disease, diabetes mellitus, cochlear implants candidates and recipients, and anatomic asplenia. Immunocompetent persons who live in high-risk environments or social settings (e.g., certain Native American and Alaska Native populations).

HR10: Annual vaccination of residents of chronic care facilities; persons with chronic cardiopulmonary disorders, metabolic diseases (including diabetes mellitus), hemoglobinopathies, immunosuppression or renal dysfunction; and health care providers for high-risk patients.

HR11: Persons born after 1956 who lack evidence of immunity to measles or mumps (e.g., documented receipt of live vaccine on or after the first birthday, laboratory evidence of immunity, or a history of physician-diagnosed measles or mumps).

HR12: Healthy adults without a history of chickenpox or previous immunization. Consider serologic testing for presumed susceptible adults.

HR13: Persons with a family or personal history of skin cancer, a large number of moles, atypical moles, poor tanning ability, or light skin, hair, and eye color.

HR14: Women with previous pregnancy affected by neural tube who are planning pregnancy.

HR15: Clinicians should consider a fasting serum lipid panel on a case-by-base basis.

TABLE 5-4 Ages 65 and Older

Interventions considered and recommended for the Periodic Health Examination	Leading causes of death Heart diseases Malignant neoplasms (lung, colorectal, breast) Cerebrovascular disease Chronic obstructive pulmonary disease Pneumonia and influenza

INTERVENTIONS FOR THE GENERAL POPULATION

Screening	Regular physical activity*
Blood pressure	**Injury prevention**
Height and weight	Lap/shoulder belts
Fecal occult blood test[1] and/or colonoscopy	Motorcycle and bicycle helmets*
Mammogram ± clinical breast exam[2] (women ≤69 yr)	Fall prevention*
Papanicolaou (Pap) test (women)[3]	Safe storage/removal of firearms*
Bone density scan in postmenopausal patients	Smoke detector*
Vision screening	Set hot water heater to <120°-130° F
Assess for hearing impairment	CPR training for household members
Assess for problem drinking	**Dental health**
Counseling	Regular visits to dental care provider*
Substance use	Floss, brush with fluoride toothpaste daily*
Tobacco cessation	**Sexual behavior**
Avoid alcohol/drug use while driving, swimming, boating, etc.*	STD prevention: avoid high-risk sexual behavior*; use condoms
Diet and exercise	*Immunizations*
Limit fat and cholesterol; maintain caloric balance; emphasize grains, fruits, vegetables	Pneumococcal vaccine
	Influenza[1]
Adequate calcium intake (women)	Tetanus-diphtheria (Td) boosters
	Herpes zoster[4]

INTERVENTIONS FOR HIGH-RISK POPULATIONS

Population	*Potential Interventions (See detailed high-risk definitions)*
Institutionalized persons	PPD (HR1); hepatitis A vaccine (HR2); amantadine/rimantadine (HR4)
Chronic medical conditions; TB contacts; low income; immigrants; alcoholics	PPD (HR1)
Persons ≥75 yr, or ≥70 yr with risk factors for falls	Fall prevention intervention (HR5)
Cardiovascular disease risk factors	Consider lipid screening (HR6)
Family hx of skin cancer; nevi; fair skin, eyes, hair	Avoid excess/midday sun, use protective clothing* (HR7)
Native Americans/Alaska Natives	PPD (HR1); hepatitis A vaccine (HR2)
Travelers to developing countries	Hepatitis A vaccine (HR2); hepatitis B vaccine (HR8)
Blood product recipients	HIV screen (HR3); hepatitis B vaccine (HR8)
High-risk sexual behavior	Hepatitis A vaccine (HR2); HIV screen (HR3); hepatitis B vaccine (HR8); RPR/VDRL (HR9)
Injection or street drug use	PPD (HR1); hepatitis A vaccine (HR2); HIV screen (HR3); hepatitis B vaccine (HR8); RPR/VDRL (HR9); advice to reduce infection risk (HR10)
Health care/lab workers	PPD (HR1); hepatitis A vaccine (HR2); amantadine/rimantadine (HR4); hepatitis B vaccine (HR8)
Persons susceptible to varicella	Varicella vaccine (HR11)
Men aged 65 to 75 who have ever smoked	Ultrasound of abdominal aorta (HR12)

[1]Annually. [2]Mammogram q1-2 yr, or mammogram q1-2 yr with annual clinical breast exam. [3]All women who are or have been sexually active and who have a cervix. Consider discontinuation of testing after age 65 yr if previous regular screening with consistently normal results. [4]Herpes zoster vaccine (Zostavax) is indicated for prevention of herpes zoster (shingles) in individuals age 60 yr or older. Zostavax is administered as a single dose subcutaneously. It is a lyophilic preparation of the Oka/Merck strain of live, attenuated varicella zoster virus (VZV). It should not be administered to individuals with a history of primary or acquired immunodeficiency states, persons on immunosuppressive therapy (including high-dose corticosteroids), those with active untreated tuberculosis, and those who may be pregnant.

*The ability of clinician counseling to influence this behavior is unproven.

HR1: HIV positive, close contacts of persons with known or suspected TB, health care workers, persons with medical risk factors associated with TB, immigrants from countries with high TB prevalence, medically underserved low-income populations (including homeless), alcoholics, injection drug users, and residents of long-term care facilities.

HR2: Persons living in, traveling to, or working in areas where the disease is endemic and where periodic outbreaks occur (e.g., countries with high or intermediate endemicity; certain Alaska Native, Pacific Island, Native American, and religious communities); men who have sex with men; injection or street drug users; persons with clotting factor disorders or chronic liver disease. Consider for institutionalized persons and workers in these institutions, and day-care, hospital, and laboratory workers. Clinicians should also consider local epidemiology and consider HIV screening in the general population.

HR3: Men who had sex with men after 1975; past or present injection drug use; persons who exchange sex for money or drugs, and their sex partners; injection drug–using, bisexual, or HIV-positive sex partner currently or in the past; blood transfusion during 1978-1985; persons seeking treatment for STDs. Clinicians should also consider local epidemiology.

HR4: Consider for persons who have not received influenza vaccine or are vaccinated late; when the vaccine may be ineffective due to major antigenic changes in the virus; for unvaccinated persons who provide home care for high-risk persons; to supplement protection provided by vaccine in persons who are expected to have a poor antibody response; and for high-risk persons in whom the vaccine is contraindicated.

HR5: Persons aged 75 years and older; or aged 70-74 with one or more additional risk factors including use of certain psychoactive and cardiac medications (e.g., benzodiazepines, antihypertensives); use of ≥4 prescription medications; impaired cognition, strength, balance, or gait. Intensive individualized home-based multifactorial fall prevention intervention is recommended in settings where adequate resources are available to deliver such services.

HR6: Clinicians should consider fasting lipid panel screening on a case-by-case basis for persons aged 65-75, especially in those with additional risk factors (e.g., smoking, diabetes, or hypertension).

HR7: Persons with a family or personal history of skin cancer, a large number of moles, atypical moles, poor tanning ability, or light skin, hair, and eye color.

HR8: Blood product recipients (including hemodialysis patients), persons with frequent occupational exposure to blood or blood products, men who have sex with men, injection drug users and their sex partners, persons with multiple recent sex partners, persons with other STDs (including HIV), travelers to countries with endemic hepatitis B.

HR9: Persons who exchange sex for money or drugs and their sex partners; persons with other STDs (including HIV); and sexual contacts of persons with active syphilis. Clinicians should also consider local epidemiology.

HR10: Persons who continue to inject drugs.

HR11: Healthy adults without a history of chickenpox or previous immunization. Consider serologic testing for presumed susceptible adults.

HR12: Consider ultrasound of abdominal aorta to screen for abdominal aortic aneurysm in all men aged 65 to 75 who have ever smoked.

TABLE 5-5 Pregnant Women*

Interventions considered and recommended for the Periodic Health Examination

INTERVENTIONS FOR THE GENERAL POPULATION

Screening

First visit

Blood pressure
Hemoglobin/hematocrit
Hepatitis B surface antigen (HBsAg)
RPR/VDRL
Chlamydia screen (<25 yr)
Rubella serology or vaccination history
D(Rh) typing, antibody screen
Offer CVS (<13 wk)[1] or amniocentesis (15-18 wk)[1] (age ≥35 yr)
Offer hemoglobinopathy screening
Assess for problem or risk drinking
Offer HIV screening[2]

Follow-up visits

Blood pressure
Urine culture (12-16 wk)
Offer amniocentesis (15-18 wk)[1] (age ≥35 yr)
Offer multiple marker testing[1] (15-18 wk)
Offer serum α-fetoprotein[1] (16-18 wk)

Counseling

Tobacco cessation; effects of passive smoking
Alcohol/other drug use
Nutrition, including adequate calcium intake
Encourage breast-feeding
Lap/shoulder belts
Infant safety car seats
STD prevention: avoid high-risk sexual behavior†; use condoms†

Chemoprophylaxis

Multivitamin with folic acid[3]

INTERVENTIONS FOR HIGH-RISK POPULATIONS

Population	*Potential Interventions (See detailed high-risk definitions)*
High-risk sexual behavior	Screen for chlamydia (1st visit) (HR1), gonorrhea (1st visit) (HR2), HIV (1st visit) (HR3); HBsAg (3rd trimester) (HR4); RPR/VDRL (3rd trimester) (HR5)
Blood transfusion 1978-1985	HIV screen (1st visit) (HR3)
Injection drug use	HIV screen (HR3); HBsAg (3rd trimester) (HR4); advice to reduce infection risk (HR6)
Unsensitized D-negative women	D(Rh) antibody testing (24-28 wk) (HR7)
Risk factors for Down syndrome	Offer CVS[1] (1st trimester), amniocentesis[1] (15-18 wk) (HR8)
Prior pregnancy with neural tube defect	Offer amniocentesis[1] (15-18 wk), folic acid 4.0 mg[3] (HR9)

[1]Women with access to counseling and follow-up services, reliable standardized laboratories, skilled high-resolution ultrasound, and, for those receiving serum marker testing, amniocentesis capabilities. [2]Universal screening is recommended. [3]Beginning at least 1 mo before conception and continuing through the first trimester.
*See Tables 5-2 and 5-3 for other preventive services recommended for women of this age group.
†The ability of clinician counseling to influence this behavior is unproven.

HR1: Women with history of STD or new or multiple sex partners. Clinicians should also consider local epidemiology. Chlamydia screen should be repeated in 3rd trimester if at continued risk.

HR2: Women under age 25 with two or more sex partners in the last year, or whose sex partner has multiple sexual contacts; women who exchange sex for money or drugs; and women with a history of repeated episodes of gonorrhea. Clinicians should also consider local epidemiology. Gonorrhea screen should be repeated in the third trimester if at continued risk.

HR3: In areas where universal screening is not performed due to low prevalence of HIV infection, pregnant women with the following individual risk factors should be screened: past or present injection drug use; women who exchange sex for money or drugs; injection drug–using, bisexual, or HIV-positive sex partner currently or in the past; blood transfusion during 1978-1985; persons seeking treatment for STDs.

HR4: Women who are initially HBsAg negative who are at high risk due to injection drug use, suspected exposure to hepatitis B during pregnancy, multiple sex partners.

HR5: Women who exchange sex for money or drugs, women with other STDs (including HIV), and sexual contacts of persons with active syphilis. Clinicians should also consider local epidemiology.

HR6: Women who continue to inject drugs.

HR7: Unsensitized D-negative women.

HR8: Prior pregnancy affected by Down syndrome, advanced maternal age (≥35 yr), known carriage of chromosome rearrangement.

HR9: Women with previous pregnancy affected by neural tube defect.

PART B • IMMUNIZATIONS AND CHEMOPROPHYLAXIS

Childhood and Adolescent Immunizations

TABLE 5-6 Recommended Immunization Schedule for Persons Aged 0-6 Years—United States 2009

Range of Recommended Ages | Certain High-Risk Groups | Catch-Up Immunization

Vaccine ▼ / Age ▶	Birth	1 Month	2 Months	4 Months	6 Months	12 Months	15 Months	18 Months	19-23 Months	2-3 Years	4-6 Years
Hepatitis B[1]	HepB	HepB	HepB	See footnote 1	HepB	HepB	HepB	HepB	HepB Series	HepB Series	HepB Series
Rotavirus[2]			Rota	Rota	Rota						
Diphtheria, tetanus, pertussis[3]			DTaP	DTaP	DTaP		DTaP	DTaP			DTaP
Haemophilus influenzae type b[4]			Hib	Hib	*Hib*[4]	Hib	Hib	Hib	Hib	Hib	Hib
Pneumococcal[5]			PCV	PCV	PCV	PCV	PCV			PCV PPV	PCV PPV
Inactivated poliovirus			IPV	IPV	IPV	IPV	IPV	IPV			IPV
Influenza[6]					Influenza (yearly)	Influenza (yearly)	Influenza (yearly)	Influenza (yearly)	Influenza (yearly)	Influenza (yearly)	Influenza (yearly)
Measles, mumps, rubella[7]						MMR	MMR				MMR
Varicella[8]						Varicella	Varicella				Varicella
Hepatitis A[9]						HepA (2 doses)	HepA (2 doses)	HepA (2 doses)	HepA (2 doses)	HepA Series	HepA Series
Meningococcal[10]										MCV4	MCV4

This schedule indicates the recommended ages for routine administration of currently licensed childhood vaccines, as of December 1, 2007, for children aged 0-6 years. Additional information is available at http://www.cdc.gov/nip/recs/child-schedule.htm. Any dose not administered at the recommended age should be administered at any subsequent visit, when indicated and feasible. Additional vaccines may be licensed and recommended during the year. Licensed combination vaccines may be used whenever any components of the combination are indicated and other components of the vaccine are not contraindicated and if approved by the Food and Drug Administration for that dose of the series. Providers should consult the respective Advisory Committee on Immunization Practices statement for detailed recommendations. Clinically significant adverse events that follow immunization should be reported to the Vaccine Adverse Event Reporting System (VAERS). Guidance about how to obtain and complete a VAERS form is available at http://www.vaers.hhs.gov or by telephone, 800-822-7967.

1. **Hepatitis B vaccine (HepB).** *(Minimum age: birth)*
   At birth:
   - Administer monovalent HepB to all newborns before hospital discharge.
   - If mother is hepatitis surface antigen (HBsAg)-positive, administer HepB and 0.5 ml of hepatitis B immune globulin (HBIG) within 12 hours of birth.
   - If mother's HBsAg status is unknown, administer HepB within 12 hours of birth. Determine the HBsAg status as soon as possible, and if HBsAg-positive, administer HBIG (no later than age 1 week).
   - If mother is HBsAg-negative, the birth dose can be delayed only with physician's order and mother's negative HBsAg laboratory report documented in the infant's medical record.

   After the birth dose:
   - The HepB series should be completed with either monovalent HepB or a combination vaccine containing HepB. The second dose should be administered at age 1-2 months. The final dose should be administered at age ≥24 weeks. Infants born to mothers who are HBsAg-positive should be tested for HBsAg and antibody to HBsAg after completion of ≥3 doses of a licensed HepB series, at age 9-18 months (generally at the next well-child visit).

   4-month dose:
   - It is permissible to administer 4 doses of HepB when combination vaccines are administered after the birth dose. If monovalent HepB is used for doses after the birth dose, a dose at age 4 months is not needed.
2. **Rotavirus vaccine (Rota).** *(Minimum age: 6 weeks)*
   - Administer the first dose at age 6-12 weeks. Do not start the series later than age 12 weeks.
   - Administer the final dose in the series by age 32 weeks. Do not administer a dose later than age 32 weeks.
   - Data on safety and efficacy outside of these age ranges are insufficient.
3. **Diphtheria and tetanus toxoids and acellular pertussis vaccine (DTaP).** *(Minimum age: 6 weeks)*
   - The fourth dose of DTaP may be administered as early as age 12 months, provided 6 months have elapsed since the third dose.
   - Administer the final dose in the series at age 4-6 years.
4. **Haemophilus influenzae type b conjugate vaccine (Hib).** *(Minimum age 6 weeks)*
   - If PRP-OMP (PedvaxHIB or ComVax [Merck]) is administered at ages 2 and 4 months, a dose at age 6 months is not required.
   - TriHiBit (DTaP/Hib) combination products should not be used for primary immunization but can be used as boosters following any Hib vaccine in children aged ≥12 months.
5. **Pneumococcal vaccine.** *(Minimum age: 6 weeks for pneumococcal conjugate vaccine [PCV]; 2 years for pneumococcal polysaccharide vaccine [PPV])*
   - Administer PCV at age 24-59 months in certain high-risk groups. Administer PPV to children aged ≥2 years in certain high-risk groups. See MMWR 49(RR-9):1-35, 2000.
6. **Influenza vaccine.** *(Minimum age: 6 months for trivalent inactivated influenza vaccine [TIV]; 5 years for live, attenuated influenza vaccine [LAIV])*
   - All children aged 6 months-18 years and close contacts of all children aged 6 months-18 years are recommended to receive influenza vaccine according to a recent federal panel of experts.
   - Influenza vaccine is strongly recommended annually for children aged ≥59 months with certain risk factors, health care workers, and other persons (including household members) in close contact with persons in groups at high risk. See MMWR 55(RR-10):1-41, 2006.
   - For healthy persons aged 2-49 years, LAIV may be used as an alternative to TIV.
   - Children receiving TIV should receive 0.25 ml if aged 6-35 months or 0.5 ml if aged ≥3 years.
   - Children aged <9 years who are receiving influenza vaccine for the first time should receive 2 doses (separated by ≥4 weeks for TIV and ≥6 weeks for LAIV)
7. **Measles, mumps, and rubella vaccine (MMR).** *(Minimum age: 12 months)*
   - Administer the second dose of MMR at age 4-6 years. MMR may be administered before age 4-6 years, provided ≥4 weeks have elapsed since the first dose and both doses are administered at age ≥12 months.
8. **Varicella vaccine.** *(Minimum age: 12 months)*
   - Administer the second dose of varicella vaccine at age 4-6 years. Varicella vaccine may be administered before age 4-6 years, provided that ≥3 months have elapsed since the first dose and both doses are administered at age ≥12 months. If second dose was administered ≥28 days following the first dose, the second dose does not need to be repeated.
9. **Hepatitis A vaccine (HepA).** *(Minimum age: 12 months)*
   - HepA is recommended for all children aged 1 year (i.e., aged 12-23 months). The 2-doses in the series should be administered at lest 6 months apart.
   - Children not fully vaccinated by age 2 years can be vaccinated at subsequent visits.
   - HepA is recommended for certain other groups of children, including in areas where vaccination programs target older children. See MMWR 55(RR-7):1-23, 2006.
10. **Meningococcal conjugate vaccine (MCV4).** *(Minimum age: 2 years)*
    - Administer MCV4 to children aged 2-10 years with terminal complement deficiencies or anatomic or functional asplenia and certain other high-risk groups. Use of meningococcal polysaccharide vaccine (MPSV4) is also acceptable. Persons who received MPSV4 3 or more years prior and remain at increased risk for meningococcal disease should be vaccinated with MCV4.

The Recommended Immunization Schedules for Persons Aged 0-18 Years are approved by the Advisory Committee on Immunization Practices (http://wwwcdc.gov/vaccines/recs/acip), the American Academy of Pediatrics (http:www.aap.org), and the American Academy of Family Physicians (http://www.aafp.org).

TABLE 5-7 Recommended Immunization Schedule for Persons Aged 7-18 Years—United States 2009

Range of Recommended Ages | Certain High-Risk Groups | Catch-Up Immunization

Vaccine ▼ / Age ▶	7-10 Years	11-12 Years	13-14 Years	15 Years	16-18 Years
Tetanus, diphtheria, pertussis[1]	*See footnote 1*	Tdap	Tdap		
Human papillomavirus[2]	*See footnote 2*	HPV (3 doses)	HPV Series		
Meningococcal[3]	MPSV4	MCV4	MCV4	MCV4[3] / MCV4	
Pneumococcal[4]	PPV				
Influenza[5]	Influenza (yearly)				
Hepatitis A[6]	HepA Series				
Hepatitis B[7]	HepB Series				
Inactivated poliovirus[8]	IPV Series				
Measles, mumps, rubella[9]	MMR Series				
Varicella[10]	Varicella Series				

This schedule indicates the recommended ages for routine administration of currently licensed childhood vaccines, as of December 1, 2007, for children aged 7-18 years. Additional information is available at http://www.cdc.gov/nip/recs/child-schedule.htm. Any dose not administered at the recommended age should be administered at any subsequent visit, when indicated and feasible. Additional vaccines may be licensed and recommended during the year. Licensed combination vaccines may be used whenever any components of the combination are indicated and other components of the vaccine are not contraindicated and if approved by the Food and Drug Administration for that dose of the series. Providers should consult the respective Advisory Committee on Immunization Practices statement for detailed recommendations. Clinically significant adverse events that follow immunization should be reported to the Vaccine Adverse Event Reporting System (VAERS). Guidance about how to obtain and complete a VAERS form is available at http://www.vaers.hhs.gov or by telephone, 800-822-7967.

1. **Tetanus and diphtheria toxoids and acellular pertussis vaccine (Tdap).** *(Minimum age: 10 years for BOOSTRIX and 11 years for ADACEL)*
   - Administer at age 11-12 years for those who have completed the recommended childhood DTP/DTaP vaccination series and have not received a tetanus and diphtheria toxoids vaccine (Td) booster dose.
   - Adolescents aged 13-18 years who missed the 11-12 year Td/Tdap booster dose should also receive a single dose of Tdap if they have completed the recommended childhood DTP/DTaP vaccination series.
2. **Human papillomavirus vaccine (HPV).** *(Minimum age: 9 years)*
   - Administer the first dose of the HPV vaccine series to females at age 11-12 years.
   - Administer the second dose 2 months after the first dose and the third dose 6 months after the first dose.
   - Administer the HPV vaccine series to females of age 13-18 years if not previously vaccinated.
3. **Meningococcal vaccine.** *Minimum age: 11 years for meningococcal conjugate vaccine [MCV4]; 2 years for meningococcal polysaccharide vaccine [MPSV4])*
   - Administer MCV4 at age 11-12 years and to previously unvaccinated adolescents at age 13-18 years.
   - Administer MCV4 to previously unvaccinated college freshmen living in dormitories; MPSV4 is an acceptable alternative.
   - Vaccination against invasive meningococcal disease is recommended for children and adolescents aged ≥2 years with terminal complement deficiencies or anatomic or functional asplenia and certain other high-risk groups. See MMWR 54(RR-7):1-21, 2005. Use MPSV4 for children aged 2-10 years and MCV4 or MPSV4 for older children.
4. **Pneumococcal polysaccharide vaccine (PPV).** *(Minimum age: 2 years)*
   - Administer for certain high-risk groups. See MMWR 46(RR-8):1-24, 1997; and MMWR 49(RR-9):1-35, 2000.
5. **Influenza vaccine.** *(Minimum age: 6 months for trivalent inactivated influenza vaccine [TIV]; 5 years for live, attenuated influenza vaccine [LAIV])*
   - Influenza vaccine is recommended annually for persons with certain risk factors, health care workers, and other persons (including household members) in close contact with persons in groups at high risk. See MMWR 55 (RR-10):1-41, 2000. A recent federal panel has expanded recommendations for influenza vaccination to all persons from age 6 months-18 years.
   - For healthy persons aged 5-49 years, LAIV may be used as an alternative to TIV.
   - Children aged <9 years who are receiving influenza vaccine for the first time should receive 2 doses (separated by ≥4 weeks for TIV and ≥6 weeks for LAIV).
6. **Hepatitis A vaccine (HepA).** *(Minimum age: 12 months)*
   - The 2 doses in the series should be administered at least 6 months apart.
   - HepA is recommended for certain other groups of children, including in areas where vaccination programs target older children. See MMWR 55(RR-7):1-23, 2006.
7. **Hepatitis B vaccine (HepB).** *(Minimum age: birth)*
   - Administer the 3-dose series to those who were not previously vaccinated.
   - A 2-dose series of Recombivax HB is licensed for children aged 11-15 years.
8. **Inactivated poliovirus vaccine (IPV).** *(Minimum age: 6 weeks)*
   - For children who received an all-IPV or all-oral poliovirus (OPV) series, a fourth dose is not necessary if the third dose was administered at age ≥4 years.
   - If both OPV and IPV were administered as part of a series, a total of 4 doses should be administered, regardless of the child's current age.
9. **Measles, mumps, and rubella vaccine (MMR).** *(Minimum age: 12 months)*
   - If not previously vaccinated, administer 2 doses of MMR during any visit, with ≥4 weeks between the doses.
10. **Varicella vaccine.** *(Minimum age: 12 months)*
    - Administer 2 doses of varicella vaccine to persons without evidence of immunity.
    - Administer 2 doses of varicella vaccine to persons aged <13 years at least 3 months apart. Do not repeat the second dose, if administered ≥28 days after the first dose.
    - Administer 2 doses of varicella vaccine to persons aged ≥13 years at least 4 weeks apart.

The Recommended Immunization Schedules for Persons Aged 0-18 Years are approved by the Advisory Committee on Immunization Practices (http://www.cdc.gov/vaccines/recs/acip), the American Academy of Pediatrics (http://www.aap.org), and the American Academy of Family Physicians (http://www.aafp.org).

TABLE 5-8 Catch-Up Immunization Schedule for Persons Aged 4 Months-18 Years Who Start Late or Who Are ≥1 Month Behind—United States

The table below provides catch-up schedules and minimum intervals between doses for children whose vaccinations have been delayed. A vaccine series does not need to be restarted regardless of the time that has elapsed between doses. Use the section appropriate for the child's age.

Vaccine	Minimum age for Dose 1	Minimum interval between doses			
		Dose 1 to Dose 2	Dose 2 to Dose 3	Dose 3 to Dose 4	Dose 4 to Dose 5
Catch-Up Schedule for Persons Aged 4 Months-6 Years					
Hepatitis B[1]	Birth	4 weeks	8 weeks (and 16 weeks after first dose)		
Rotavirus[2]	6 weeks	4 weeks	4 weeks		
Diphtheria, tetanus, pertussis[3]	6 weeks	4 weeks	4 weeks	6 months	6 months[3]
Haemophilus influenzae type b[4]	6 weeks	**4 weeks** if first dose administered at age <12 months **8 weeks (as final dose)** if first dose administered at age 12-14 months **No further doses needed** if first dose administered at age ≥15 months	**4 weeks[4]** if current age <12 months **8 weeks (as final dose)[4]** if current age ≥12 months and second dose administered at age <15 months **No further doses needed** if previous dose administered at age ≥15 months	**8 weeks (as final dose)** This dose only necessary for children aged 12 months-5 years who received 3 doses before age 12 months	
Pneumococcal[5]	6 weeks	**4 weeks** if first dose administered at age <12 months and current age <24 months **8 weeks (as final dose)** if first dose administered at age ≥12 months or current age 24-59 months **No further doses needed** for healthy children if first dose administered at age ≥24 months	**4 weeks** if current age <12 months **8 weeks (as final dose)** if current age ≥12 months **No further doses needed** for healthy children if previous dose administered at age ≥24 months	**8 weeks (as final dose)** This dose only necessary for children aged 12 months-5 years who received 3 doses before age 12 months	
Inactivated poliovirus[6]	6 weeks	4 weeks	4 weeks	4 weeks[6]	
Measles, mumps, rubella[7]	12 months	4 weeks			
Varicella[8]	12 months	3 months			
Hepatitis A[9]	12 months	6 months			
Catch-Up Schedule for Persons Aged 7-18 Years					
Tetanus, diphtheria/ tetanus, diphtheria, pertussis[10]	7 years[10]	4 weeks	**8 weeks** if first dose administered at age <12 months **6 months** if first dose administered at age ≥12 months	**6 months** if first dose administered at age <12 months	
Human papillomavirus[11]	9 years	4 weeks	12 weeks		
Hepatitis A[9]	12 months	6 months			
Hepatitis B[1]	Birth	4 weeks	**8 weeks** (and 16 weeks after first dose)		
Inactivated poliovirus[6]	6 weeks	4 weeks	4 weeks	4 weeks[6]	
Measles, mumps, rubella[7]	12 months	4 weeks			
Varicella[8]	12 months	**4 weeks** if first dose administered at age ≥13 years **3 months** if first dose administered at age <13 years			

1. **Hepatitis B vaccine (HepB).** *(Minimum age: birth)*
   - Administer the 3-dose series to those who were not previously vaccinated.
   - A 2-dose series of Recombivax HB is licensed for children aged 11-15 years.
2. **Rotavirus vaccine (Rota).** *(Minimum age: 6 weeks)*
   - Do not start the series later than age 12 weeks.
   - Administer the final dose in the series by age 32 weeks. Do not administer a dose later than age 32 weeks.
   - Data on safety and efficacy outside of these age ranges are insufficient.
3. **Diphtheria and tetanus toxoids and acellular pertussis vaccine (DTaP).** *(Minimum age: 6 weeks)*
   - The fifth dose is not necessary if the fourth dose was administered at age ≥4 years.
   - DTaP is not indicated for persons aged ≥7 years.
4. **Haemophilus influenzae type b conjugate vaccine (Hib).** *(Minimum age: 6 weeks)*
   - Vaccine is not generally recommended for children aged ≥5 years.
   - If current age <12 months and the first 2 doses were PRP-OMP (PedvaxHIB or ComVax [Merck]), the third (and final) dose should be administered at age 12-15 months and at least 8 weeks after the second dose.
   - If first dose was administered at age 7-11 months, administer 2 doses separated by 4 weeks plus a booster at age 12-15 months.
5. **Pneumococcal conjugate vaccine (PCV).** *(Minimum age: 6 weeks)*
   - Vaccine is not generally recommended for children aged ≥5 years.
6. **Inactivated poliovirus vaccine (IPV).** *(Minimum age: 6 weeks)*
   - For children who received an all-IPV or all-oral poliovirus (OPV) series, a fourth dose is not necessary if third dose was administered at age ≥4 years.
   - If both OPV and IPV were administered as part of a series, a total of 4 doses should be administered, regardless of the child's current age.
7. **Measles, mumps, and rubella vaccine (MMR).** *(Minimum age: 12 months)*
   - The second dose of MMR is recommended routinely at age 4-6 years but may be administered earlier if desired.
   - If not previously vaccinated, administer 2 doses of MMR during any visit, with ≥4 weeks between the doses.
8. **Varicella vaccine.** *(Minimum age: 12 months)*
   - The second dose of varicella vaccine is recommended routinely at age 4-6 years but may be administered earlier if desired.
   - Do not repeat the second dose in persons aged <13 years if administered >28 days after the first dose.
9. **Hepatitis A vaccine (HepA).** *(Minimum age: 12 months)*
   - HepA is recommended for certain groups of children, including in areas where vaccination programs target older children. See MMWR 55(RR-7):1-23, 2006.
10. **Tetanus and diphtheria toxoids vaccine (Td) and tetanus and diphtheria toxoids and acellular pertussis vaccine (Tdap).** *(Minimum ages: 7 years for Td, 10 years for BOOSTRIX, and 11 years for ADACEL)*
    - Tdap should be substituted for a single dose of Td in the primary catch-up series or as a booster if age appropriate; use Td for other doses.
    - A 5-year interval from the last Td dose is encouraged when Tdap is used as a booster dose. A booster (fourth) dose is needed if any of the previous doses were administered at age <12 months. Refer to ACIP recommendations for further information. See MMWR 55(RR-3), 2006.
11. **Human papillomavirus vaccine (HPV).** *(Minimum age: 9 years)*
    - Administer the HPV vaccine series to females at age 13-18 years if not previously vaccinated.

Information about reporting reactions after immunization is available online at http://www.vaers.hhs.gov or by telephone via the 24-hour national toll-free information line 800-822-7967. Suspected cases of vaccine-preventable diseases should be reported to the state or local health department. Additional information, including precautions and contraindications for immunization, is available from the National Center for Immunization and Respiratory Diseases at http://www.cdc.gov/nip/default.htm or telephone, 800-CDC-INFO (800-232-4636).

QUADRIVALENT HUMAN PAPILLOMAVIRUS (HPV) VACCINE*

SUMMARY OF RATIONALE FOR QUADRIVALENT HPV VACCINE RECOMMENDATIONS*

The availability of a quadrivalent HPV vaccine offers an opportunity to decrease the burden of HPV infection and its sequelae, including cervical cancer precursors, cervical cancer, other anogenital cancers, and genital warts, in the United States. Quadrivalent HPV vaccine is licensed for use among females aged 9 to 26 years. In this age group, clinical trials indicate that the vaccine is safe and immunogenic. Trials among females aged 16 to 26 years indicated the vaccine to be effective against HPV types 6-, 11-, 16-, and 18-related cervical, vaginal, and vulvar cancer precursor and dysplastic lesions and genital warts. HPV 16 and 18 are the cause of approximately 70% of cervical cancers; HPV 6 and 11 are the cause of approximately 90% of genital warts. Because HPV is sexually transmitted and often acquired soon after onset of sexual activity, vaccination should ideally occur before sexual debut. The recommended age for vaccination is 11 to 12 years; vaccine can be administered to females as young as age 9 years. At the beginning of a vaccination program, females aged >12 years will exist who did not have the opportunity to receive vaccine at age 11 to 12 years. Catch-up vaccination is recommended for females aged 13 to 26 years who have not yet been vaccinated.

The recommendation for routine vaccination of females aged 11 to 12 years is based on several considerations, including studies suggesting that quadrivalent HPV vaccine among adolescents will be safe and effective, high antibody titers achieved after vaccination at age 11 to 12 years, data on HPV epidemiology and age of sexual debut in the United States, and the high probability of HPV acquisition within several years of sexual debut. Ideally, HPV vaccine should be administered before sexual debut, and duration of protection should extend for many years, providing protection when exposure through sexual activity might occur. The vaccine has been demonstrated to provide protection for at least 5 years without evidence of waning protection. Long-term follow-up studies are under way to determine duration of protection. The recommendation also considered cost-effectiveness evaluations and the established young adolescent health care visit at age 11 to 12 years recommended by several professional organizations, when other vaccines are also recommended.

Although routine vaccination is recommended at age 11 to 12 years, the majority of females aged 13 to 26 years also can benefit from vaccination. Females not yet sexually active can be expected to receive the full benefit of vaccination. Although sexually active females in this age group might have been infected with one or more vaccine HPV types, type-specific prevalence studies in the United States suggest that a small percentage of sexually active females have been infected with all four of the HPV vaccine types. These data, available from North American females aged 16 to 24 years who participated in the quadrivalent vaccine trials, are from women who were more likely to have ever had sex than similarly aged females in the general U.S. population. Among those sexually active females, the median number of lifetime sex partners (two) was similar in trial participants and females in the general U.S. population. The vaccine does not appear to protect against persistent infection, cervical cancer precursor lesions, or genital warts caused by an HPV type that females are infected with at the time of vaccination. However, females already infected with one or more vaccine HPV types before vaccination would be protected against disease caused by the other vaccine HPV types. Therefore, although overall vaccine effectiveness would be lower when administered to a population of females who are sexually active and would decrease with older age and likelihood of HPV exposure with increasing number of sex partners, the majority of females in this age group will derive at least partial benefit from vaccination.

*From CDC: Quadrivalent human papillomavirus vaccine: recommendations of the Advisory Committee on Immunization Practices (ACIP), *MMWR* 56(RR-2):16-18, 2007.

RECOMMENDATIONS FOR USE OF HPV VACCINE

Recommendations for Routine Use and Catch-Up

Routine Vaccination of Females Aged 11-12 Years

The Advisory Committee on Immunization Practices (ACIP) recommends routine vaccination of females aged 11 to 12 years with 3 doses of quadrivalent HPV vaccine. The vaccination series can be started as young as age 9 years.

Catch-Up Vaccination of Females Aged 13-26 Years

Vaccination also is recommended for females aged 13 to 26 years who have not been previously vaccinated or who have not completed the full series. Ideally, vaccine should be administered before potential exposure to HPV through sexual contact; however, females who might have already been exposed to HPV should be vaccinated. Sexually active females who have not been infected with any of the HPV vaccine types would receive full benefit from vaccination. Vaccination would provide less benefit to females if they have already been infected with one or more of the four vaccine HPV types. However, it is not possible for a clinician to assess the extent to which sexually active persons would benefit from vaccination, and the risk for HPV infection might continue as long as persons are sexually active. Pap testing and screening for HPV DNA or HPV antibody are not needed before vaccination at any age.

Dosage and Administration

The vaccine should be shaken well before administration. The dose of quadrivalent HPV vaccine is 0.5 ml, administered intramuscularly (IM), preferably in the deltoid muscle.

Recommended Schedule

Quadrivalent HPV vaccine is administered in a 3-dose schedule. The second and third doses should be administered 2 and 6 months after the first dose.

Minimum Dosing Intervals and Management of Persons Who Were Incorrectly Vaccinated

The minimum interval between the first and second doses of vaccine is 4 weeks. The minimum recommended interval between the second and third doses of vaccine is 12 weeks. Inadequate doses of quadrivalent HPV vaccine or vaccine doses received after a shorter-than-recommended dosing interval should be readministered.

Interrupted Vaccine Schedules

If the quadrivalent HPV vaccine schedule is interrupted, the vaccine series does not need to be restarted. If the series is interrupted after the first dose, the second dose should be administered as soon as possible and the second and third doses should be separated by an interval of at least 12 weeks. If only the third dose is delayed, it should be administered as soon as possible.

Simultaneous Administration with Other Vaccines

Although no data exist on administration of quadrivalent HPV vaccine with vaccines other than hepatitis B vaccine, quadrivalent HPV vaccine is not a live vaccine and has no components that adversely impact safety or efficacy of other vaccinations. Quadrivalent HPV vaccine can be administered at the same visit as other age-appropriate vaccines, such as the tetanus, diphtheria, pertussis (Tdap) and quadrivalent meningococcal conjugate (MCV4) vaccines. Administering all indicated vaccines together at a single visit increases the likelihood that adolescents and young adults will receive each of the vaccines on schedule. Each vaccine should be administered using a separate syringe at a different anatomic site.

Cervical Cancer Screening among Vaccinated Females

Cervical cancer screening recommendations have not changed for females who receive HPV vaccine. HPV types in the vaccine are responsible for approximately 70% of cervical cancers; females who are vaccinated could subsequently be infected with a carcinogenic HPV type for which the quadrivalent vaccine does not provide protection. Furthermore, those who were sexually active before vaccination could have been infected with a vaccine type HPV before vaccination. Health care providers administering quadrivalent HPV vaccine should educate women about the importance of cervical cancer screening.

Groups for Which Vaccine is Not Licensed

Vaccination of Females Aged <9 Years and >26 Years

Quadrivalent HPV vaccine is not licensed for use among females aged <9 years or those aged >26 years. Studies are ongoing among females aged >26 years. No studies are under way among children aged <9 years.

Vaccination of Males

Quadrivalent HPV vaccine is not licensed for use among males. Although data on immunogenicity and safety are available for males aged 9 to 15 years, no data exist on efficacy in males at any age. Efficacy studies in males are under way.

Special Situations among Females Aged 9-26 Years

Equivocal or Abnormal Pap Test or Known HPV Infection

Females who have an equivocal or abnormal Pap test could be infected with any of approximately 40 high-risk or low-risk genital HPV types. Such females are unlikely to be infected with all four HPV vaccine types, and they might not be infected with any HPV vaccine type. Vaccination would provide protection against infection with HPV vaccine types not already acquired. With increasing severity of Pap test findings, the likelihood of infection with HPV 16 or 18 increases and the benefit of vaccination would decrease. Women should be advised that results from clinical trials do not indicate the vaccine will have any therapeutic effect on existing HPV infection or cervical lesions.

Females who have a positive HC2 High-Risk test conducted in conjunction with a Pap test could have infection with any of 13 high-risk types. This assay does not identify specific HPV types, and testing for specific HPV types is not conducted routinely in clinical practice. Women with a positive HC2 High-Risk test might not have been infected with any of the four HPV vaccine types. Vaccination would provide protection against infection with HPV vaccine types not already acquired. However, women should be advised that results from clinical trials do not indicate the vaccine will have any therapeutic effect on existing HPV infection or cervical lesions.

Genital Warts

A history of genital warts or clinically evident genital warts indicate infection with HPV, most often type 6 or 11. However, these females might not have infection with both HPV 6 and 11 or infection with HPV 16 or 18. Vaccination would provide protection against infection with HPV vaccine types not already acquired. However, females should be advised that results from clinical trials do not indicate the vaccine will have any therapeutic effect on existing HPV infection or genital warts.

Lactating Women

Lactating women can receive HPV vaccine.

Immunocompromised Persons

Because quadrivalent HPV vaccine is a noninfectious vaccine, it can be administered to females who are immunosuppressed as a result of disease or medications. However, the immune response and vaccine efficacy might be less than that in persons who are immunocompetent.

Vaccination during Pregnancy

Quadrivalent HPV vaccine is not recommended for use in pregnancy. The vaccine has not been causally associated with adverse outcomes of pregnancy or adverse events in the developing fetus. However, data on vaccination during pregnancy are limited. Until additional information is available, initiation of the vaccine series should be delayed until after completion of the pregnancy. If a woman is found to be pregnant after initiating the vaccination series, the remainder of the 3-dose regimen should be delayed until after completion of the pregnancy. If a vaccine dose has been administered during pregnancy, no intervention is needed. A vaccine-in-pregnancy registry has been established; patients and health care providers should report any exposure to quadrivalent HPV vaccine during pregnancy (telephone: 800-986-8999).

Precautions and Contraindications

Acute Illnesses

Quadrivalent HPV vaccine can be administered to persons with minor acute illnesses (e.g., diarrhea or mild upper respiratory tract infections with or without fever). Vaccination of persons with moderate or severe acute illnesses should be deferred until after the patient improves.

Hypersensitivity or Allergy to Vaccine Components

Quadrivalent HPV vaccine is contraindicated for persons with a history of immediate hypersensitivity to yeast or to any vaccine component. Data from passive surveillance in Vaccine Adverse Event Reporting System (VAERS) indicates that recombinant yeast-derived vaccines pose a minimal risk for anaphylaxic reactions in persons with a history of allergic reactions to *Saccharomyces cerevisiae* (baker's yeast).

Preventing Syncope after Vaccination

Syncope (i.e., vasovagal or vasodepressor reaction) can occur after vaccination, most commonly among adolescents and young adults. Among reports to VAERS for any vaccine that were coded as syncope during 1990-2004, a total of 35% of these episodes were reported among persons aged 10 to 18 years. Through January 2007, the second most common report to VAERS following receipt of HPV vaccine was syncope (CDC, unpublished data, 2007). Vaccine providers should consider observing patients for 15 minutes after they receive HPV vaccine.

General Recommendations on Immunization

TABLE 5-9 Recommended and Minimum Ages and Intervals between Vaccine Doses of Routinely Recommended Vaccines[a]

Vaccine and Dose Number	Recommended Age for This Dose	Minimum Age for This Dose	Recommended Interval to Next Dose	Minimum Interval to Next Dose
Hepatitis B (HepB)-1[b]	Birth	Birth	1-4 months	4 weeks
HepB-2	1-2 months	4 weeks	2-17 months	8 weeks
HepB-3[c]	6-18 months	24 weeks	—	—
Diphtheria-tetanus-acellular pertussis (DTaP)-1[b]	2 months	6 weeks	2 months	4 weeks
DTaP-2	4 months	10 weeks	2 months	4 weeks
DTaP-3	6 months	14 weeks	6-12 months[d]	6 months[d,e]
DTaP-4	15-18 months	12 months	3 years	6 months[d]
DTaP-5	4-6 years	4 years	—	—
Haemophilus influenzae type b (Hib)-1[b,f]	2 months	6 weeks	2 months	4 weeks
Hib-2	4 months	10 weeks	2 months	4 weeks
Hib-3[g]	6 months	14 weeks	6-9 months[d]	8 weeks
Hib-4	12-15 months	12 months	—	—
Inactivated poliovirus (IPV)-1[b]	2 months	6 weeks	2 months	4 weeks
IPV-2	4 months	10 weeks	2-14 months	4 weeks
IPV-3	6-18 months	14 weeks	3-5 years	4 weeks
IPV-4	4-6 years	18 weeks	—	—
Pneumococcal conjugate (PCV)-1[f]	2 months	6 weeks	2 months	4 weeks
PCV-2	4 months	10 weeks	2 months	4 weeks
PCV-3	6 months	14 weeks	6 months	8 weeks
PCV-4	12-15 months	12 months	—	—
Measles-mumps-rubella (MMR)-1[h]	12-15 months	12 months	3-5 years	4 weeks
MMR-2[h]	4-6 years	13 months	—	—
Varicella (Var)-1[h]	12-15 months	12 months	3-5 years	12 weeks[i]
Var-2[h]	4-6 years	15 months	—	—
Hepatitis A (HepA)-1[b]	12-23 months	12 months	6-18 months[d]	6 months[d]
HepA-2	18-41 months	18 months	—	—
Influenza inactivated[j]	6-59 months	6 months[k]	1 month	4 weeks
Influenza live attenuated[j]	—	5 years	6-10 weeks	6 weeks
Meningococcal conjugate[b]	11-12 years	11 years	—	—
Meningococcal polysaccharide (MPSV)-1	—	2 years	5 years[k]	5 years[l]
MPSV-2[m]	—	7 years	—	—
Tetanus-diphtheria	11-12 years	7 years	10 years	5 years
Tetanus-diphtheria acellular pertussis (Tdap)[n]	≥11 years	10 years	—	—
Pneumococcal polysaccharide (PPV)-1	—	2 years	5 years	5 years
PPV-2[o]	—	7 years	—	—
Human papillomavirus (HPV)-1[p]	11-12 years	9 years	2 months	4 weeks
HPV-2	11-12 years (+2 months)	109 months	4 months	12 weeks
HPV-3	11-12 years (+6 months)	112 months	—	—
Rotavirus (RV)-1[q]	2 months	6 weeks	2 months	4 weeks
RV-2	4 months	10 weeks	2 months	4 weeks
RV-3	6 months	14 weeks	—	—
Zoster[r]	60 years	60 years	—	

TABLE 5-9 Recommended and Minimum Ages and Intervals between Vaccine Doses of Routinely Recommended Vaccines[a] *(Continued)*

From CDC: General recommendations on immunization: recommendations of the Advisory Committee on Immunization Practices (ACIP), *MMWR* 55(RR-15), 2006.

[a]Combination vaccines are available. Use of licensed combination vaccines is preferred over separate injections of their equivalent component vaccines. (Source: CDC: Combination vaccines for childhood immunization: recommendations of the Advisory Committee on Immunization Practices [ACIP], the American Academy of Pediatrics [AAP], and the American Academy of Family Physicians [AAFP], *MMWR* 48[RR-5], 1999.) When administering combination vaccines, the minimum age for administration is the oldest age for any of the individual components; the minimum interval between doses is equal to the greatest interval of any of the individual components.

[b]Combination vaccines containing the hepatitis B component are available (HepB-Hib, DTaP-HepB-IPV, and HepA-HepB). These vaccines should not be administered to infants aged <6 weeks because of the other components (i.e., Hib, DTaP, HepA, and IPV).

[c]HepB-3 should be administered at least 8 weeks after HepB-2 and at least 16 weeks after HepB-1 and should not be administered before age 24 weeks.

[d]Calendar months.

[e]The minimum recommended interval between DTaP-3 and DTaP-4 is 6 months. However, DTaP-4 need not be repeated if administered at least 4 months after DTaP-3.

[f]For Hib and PCV, children receiving the first dose of vaccine at age ≥7 months require fewer doses to complete the series. (Source: CDC: Recommended childhood and adolescent immunization schedule—United States, 2006, *MMWR* 54[51 & 52]:Q1-Q4, 2005.)

[g]If PRP-OMP (Pedvax-Hib, Merck Vaccine Division) was administered at age 2 and 4 months, a dose at age 6 months is not required.

[h]Combination measles-mumps-rubella-varicella (MMRV) vaccine can be used for children aged 12 months-12 years.

[i]The minimum interval from VAR-1 to VAR-2 for persons beginning the series at age ≥13 years is 4 weeks.

[j]Two doses of influenza vaccine are recommended for children aged <9 years who are receiving the vaccine for the first time. Children aged <9 years who have previously received influenza vaccine and persons aged ≥9 years require only 1 dose per influenza season.

[k]The minimum age for inactivated influenza vaccine varies by vaccine manufacturer. Only Fluzone (manufactured by Sanofi Pasteur) is approved for children aged 6-35 months. The minimum age for Fluvirin (manufactured by Novartis) is 4 years. For Fluarix and FluLeval (manufactured by GlaxoSmithKline), the minimum age is 18 years.

[l]Certain experts recommend a second dose of MPSV 3 years after the first dose for persons at increased risk for meningococcal disease.

[m]A second dose of meningococcal vaccine is recommended for persons previously vaccinated with MPSV who remain at high risk for meningococcal disease. MCV4 is preferred when revaccinating persons aged 11-55 years, but a second dose of MPSV is acceptable. (Source: CDC: Prevention and control of meningococcal disease: recommendations of the Advisory Committee on Immunization Practices [ACIP], *MMWR* 54[RR-7], 2005.)

[n]Only 1 dose of Tdap is recommended. Subsequent doses should be administered as Td. If vaccination to prevent tetanus and/or diphtheria disease is required for children aged 7-9 years, Td should be administered (minimum age for Td is 7 years). For one brand of Tdap, the minimum age is 11 years. The preferred interval between Tdap and a previous dose of Td is 5 years. In persons who have received a primary series of tetanus-toxoid-containing vaccine, for management of a tetanus-prone wound, the minimum interval after a previous dose of any tetanus-containing vaccine is 5 years.

[o]A second dose of PPV is recommended for persons at highest risk for serious pneumococcal infection and those who are likely to have a rapid decline in pneumococcal antibody concentration. Revaccination 3 years after the previous dose can be considered for children at highest risk for severe pneumococcal infection who would be aged <10 years of age at the time of revaccination. (Source: CDC: Prevention of pneumococcal disease: recommendations of the Advisory Committee on Immunization Practices [ACIP], *MMWR* 46[RR-8], 1997.)

[p]HPV is approved only for females aged 9-26 years.

[q]The first dose of RV must be administered at age 6-12 weeks. The vaccine series should not be started at age ≥13 weeks. RV should not be administered to children aged ≥33 weeks regardless of the number of doses received at age 6-32 weeks.

[r]Herpes zoster vaccine is approved as a single dose for persons who are aged ≥60 years with a history of varicella.

TABLE 5-10 Guidelines for Spacing of Live and Inactivated Antigens

Antigen Combination	Recommended Minimum Interval between Doses
Two or more inactivated*	Can be administered simultaneously or at any interval between doses
Inactivated and live	Can be administered simultaneously or at any interval between doses
Two or more live intranasal or injectable†	4-week minimum interval if not administered simultaneously

From CDC: General recommendations on immunization: recommendations of the Advisory Committee on Immunization Practices (ACIP), *MMWR* 55(RR-15), 2006.

*Certain experts suggest a 1-month interval between tetanus toxoid, reduced diphtheria toxoid, and reduced acellular pertussis vaccine and quadrivalent meningococcal conjugate vaccine if they are not administered simultaneously.

†Live oral vaccines (e.g., Ty21a typhoid vaccine and rotavirus vaccine) can be administered simultaneously or at any interval before or after inactivated or live injectable vaccines.

TABLE 5-11 Guidelines for Administering Antibody-Containing Products* and Vaccines

Simultaneous Administration

Combination	Recommended Minimum Interval between Doses
Antibody-containing products and inactivated antigen	Can be administered simultaneously at different sites or at any time interval between doses.
Antibody-containing products and live antigen	Should not be administered simultaneously.† If simultaneous administration of measles-containing vaccine or varicella vaccine is unavoidable, administer at different sites and revaccinate or test for seroconversion after the recommended interval.

Nonsimultaneous Administration

Product Administered: First	Product Administered: Second	Recommended Minimum Interval between Doses
Antibody-containing products	Inactivated antigen	Not applicable
Inactivated antigen	Antibody-containing products	Not applicable
Antibody-containing products	Live antigen	Dose-related†§¶
Live antigen	Antibody-containing products	2 weeks†

From CDC: General recommendations on immunization: recommendations of the Advisory Committee on Immunization Practices (ACIP), *MMWR* 55(RR-15), 2006.

*Blood products containing substantial amounts of immunoglobulin include intramuscular and intravenous immune globulin, specific hyperimmune globulin (e.g., hepatitis B immune globulin, tetanus immune globulin, varicella zoster immune globulin, and rabies immune globulin), whole blood, packed red cells, plasma, and platelet products.

†Yellow fever, oral Ty21a typhoid vaccine, and live-attenuated influenza vaccine are exceptions to these recommendations. These live-attenuated vaccines can be administered at any time before, after, or simultaneously with an antibody-containing product without substantially decreasing the antibody response.

§Rotavirus vaccine (RV) should be deferred for 6 weeks after receipt of an antibody-containing product if possible. However, if the 6-week deferral would cause the first dose of RV to be scheduled for age >13 weeks, a shorter deferral interval should be used to ensure the first dose of RV is administered no later than age 13 weeks.

¶The duration of interference of antibody-containing products with the immune response to the measles component of measles-containing vaccine, and possibly varicella vaccine, is dose related.

TABLE 5-12 **Suggested Intervals between Administration of Antibody-Containing Products for Different Indications and Measles-Containing Vaccine and Varicella-Containing Vaccine***

Product/Indication	Dose, Including mg Immunoglobulin G (IgG)/ kg Body Weight*	Recommended Interval before Measles or Varicella-Containing Vaccine Administration (Months)
Respiratory syncytial virus immune globulin (IG) monoclonal antibody (Synagis)†	15 mg/kg intramuscularly (IM)	None
Tetanus IG	250 units (10 mg IgG/kg) IM	3
Hepatitis A IG		
Contact prophylaxis	0.02 ml/kg (3.3 mg IgG/kg) IM	3
International travel	0.06 ml/kg (10 mg IgG/kg) IM	3
Hepatitis B IG	0.06 ml/kg (10 mg IgG/kg) IM	3
Rabies IG	20 international units/kg (22 mg IgG/kg) IM	4
Measles prophylaxis IG		
Standard (i.e., nonimmunocompromised) contact	0.25 ml/kg (40 mg IgG/kg) IM	5
Immunocompromised contact	0.50 ml/kg (80 mg IgG/kg) IM	6
Blood transfusion		
Red blood cells (RBCs), washed	10 ml/kg negligible IgG/kg intravenously (IV)	None
RBCs, adenine-saline added	10 ml/kg (10 mg IgG/kg) IV	3
Packed RBCs (hematocrit 65%)§	10 ml/kg (60 mg IgG/kg) IV	6
Whole blood (hematocrit 35%-50%)§	10 ml/kg (80-100 mg IgG/kg) IV	6
Plasma/platelet products	10 ml/kg (160 mg IgG/kg) IV	7
Cytomegalovirus intravenous immune globulin (IGIV)	150 mg/kg maximum	6
IGIV		
Replacement therapy for immune deficiencies¶	300-400 mg/kg IV¶	8
Immune thrombocytopenic purpura	400 mg/kg IV	8
Postexposure varicella prophylaxis**	400 mg/kg IV	8
Immune thrombocytopenic purpura	1000 mg/kg IV	10
Kawasaki disease	2 g/kg IV	11

From CDC: General recommendations on immunization: recommendations of the Advisory Committee on Immunization Practices (ACIP), *MMWR* 55(RR-15), 2006.

*This table is not intended for determining the correct indications and dosages for using antibody-containing products. Unvaccinated persons might not be fully protected against measles during the entire recommended interval, and additional doses of immune globulin or measles vaccine might be indicated after measles exposure. Concentrations of measles antibody in an immune globulin preparation can vary by manufacturer's lot. Rates of antibody clearance after receipt of an immune globulin preparation also might vary. Recommended intervals are extrapolated from an estimated half-life of 30 days for passively acquired antibody and an observed interference with the immune response to measles vaccine for 5 months after a dose of 80 mg IgG/kg.

†Contains antibody only to respiratory syncytial virus

§Assumes a serum IgG concentration of 16 mg/ml.

¶Measles and varicella vaccinations are recommended for children with asymptomatic or mildly symptomatic human immunodeficiency virus (HIV) infection but are contraindicated for persons with severe immunosuppression from HIV or any other immunosuppressive disorder.

**The investigational product VariZIG, similar to licensed VZIG, is a purified human immune globulin preparation made from plasma containing high levels of antivaricella antibodies (immunoglobulin class G [IgG]). When indicated, health care providers should make every effort to obtain and administer VariZIG. In situations in which administration of VariZIG does not appear possible within 96 hours of exposure, administration of immune globulin intravenous (IGIV) should be considered as an alternative. IGIV also should be administered within 96 hours of exposure. Although licensed IGIV preparations are known to contain antivaricella antibody titers, the titer of any specific lot of IGIV that might be available is uncertain because IGIV is not routinely tested for antivaricella antibodies. The recommended IGIV dose for postexposure prophylaxis of varicella is 400 mg/kg administered once. For pregnant women who cannot receive VariZIG within 96 hours of exposure, clinicians can choose either to administer IGIV or closely monitor the women for signs and symptoms of varicella and institute treatment with acyclovir if illness occurs. (Source: CDC: A new product for postexposure prophylaxis available under an investigational new drug application expanded access protocol, *MMWR* 55 [RR-8]:209-210, 2006.)

TABLE 5-13 Contraindications and Precautions[a] to Commonly Used Vaccines

Vaccine	True Contraindications and Precautions[a]	Untrue (Vaccines Can Be Administered)
General for all routine vaccines, including diphtheria and tetanus toxoids and acellular pertussis vaccine (DTaP); pediatric diphtheria-tetanus toxoid (DT); adult tetanus-diphtheria toxoid (Td); tetanus-reduced-diphtheria toxoid and acellular pertussis vaccine (Tdap), inactivated poliovirus vaccine (IPV); measles, mumps, and rubella vaccine (MMR); *Haemophilus influenzae* type b vaccine (Hib); hepatitis A vaccine; hepatitis B vaccine; varicella vaccine; Rotavirus vaccine, pneumococcal conjugate vaccine (PCV); inactivated influenza vaccine (TIV); live-attenuated influenza vaccine (LAIV) pneumococcal polysaccharide vaccine (PPV); meningococcal conjugate vaccine (MCV4); meningococcal polysaccharide vaccine (MPSV); human papillomavirus vaccine (HPV); and herpes zoster vaccine (HZ)	**Contraindications** Severe allergic reaction (e.g., anaphylaxis) after a previous vaccine dose or to a vaccine component **Precautions** Moderate or severe acute illness with or without fever	Mild acute illness with or without fever Mild-to-moderate local reaction (i.e., swelling, redness, and soreness); low-grade or moderate fever after previous dose Lack of previous physical examination in well-appearing person Current antimicrobial therapy[b] Convalescent phase of illness Preterm birth (hepatitis B vaccine is an exception in certain circumstances)[c] Recent exposure to an infectious disease History of penicillin allergy, other nonvaccine allergies, relatives with allergies, receiving allergen extract immunotherapy Breastfeeding
DTaP	**Contraindications** Severe allergic reaction (e.g., anaphylaxis) after a previous vaccine dose or to a vaccine component Encephalopathy (e.g., coma, decreased level of consciousness; prolonged seizures) not attributable to another identifiable cause within 7 days of administration of previous dose of DTP or DTaP Progressive neurologic disorder, including infantile spasms, uncontrolled epilepsy, progressive encephalopathy: defer DTaP until neurologic status clarified and stabilized **Precautions** Temperature of ≥105° F (≥40.5° C) for ≤48 hours after vaccination with a previous dose of DTP or DTaP Collapse or shocklike state (i.e., hypotonic hyporesponsive episode) ≤48 hours after receiving a previous dose of DTP/DTaP Seizure ≤3 days after receiving a previous dose of DTP/DTaP[d] Persistent, inconsolable crying lasting ≥3 hours within 48 hours after receiving a previous dose of DTP/DTaP Guillain-Barré syndrome (GBS) <6 weeks after previous dose of tetanus-toxoid-containing vaccine Moderate or severe acute illness with or without fever	Temperature of ≤104° F (≤40.5° C), fussiness, or mild drowsiness after a previous dose of diphtheria toxoid-tetanus toxoid-pertussis vaccine (DTP/DTaP) Family history of seizures[d] Family history of sudden infant death syndrome Family history of an adverse event after DTP or DTaP administration Stable neurologic conditions (e.g., cerebral palsy, well-controlled seizure disorder, developmental delay)
DT, Td	**Contraindications** Severe allergic reaction (e.g., anaphylaxis) after a previous vaccine dose or to a vaccine component **Precautions** GBS <6 weeks after previous dose of tetanus-toxoid-containing vaccine Moderate or severe acute illness with or without fever	

TABLE 5-13 **Contraindications and Precautions[a] to Commonly Used Vaccines** *(Continued)*

Vaccine	True Contraindications and Precautions[a]	Untrue (Vaccines Can Be Administered)
Tdap	**Contraindications** Severe allergic reaction (e.g., anaphylaxis) after a previous vaccine dose or to a vaccine component Encephalopathy (e.g., coma, decreased level of consciousness, and prolonged seizures) not attributable to another identifiable cause within 7 days of administration of previous dose of DTP, DTaP, or Tdap **Precautions** Moderate or severe acute illness with or without fever GBS ≤6 weeks after a previous dose of tetanus-toxoid-containing vaccine Progressive or unstable neurologic disorder, uncontrolled seizures or progressive encephalopathy until a treatment regimen has been established and the condition has stabilized History of arthus-type hypersensitivity reactions following a previous dose of tetanus-toxoid-containing vaccine: defer vaccination until at least 10 years have elapsed since the last tetanus-toxoid-containing vaccine	Temperature of >104° F (>40.5° C) for ≤48 hours after vaccination with a previous dose of DTP or DTaP Collapse or shocklike state (i.e., hypotonic hyporesponsive episode) ≤48 hours after receiving a previous dose of DTP/DTaP Seizure ≤3 days after receiving a previous dose of DTP/DTaP[d] Persistent, inconsolable crying lasting ≥3 hours within 48 hours after receiving a previous dose of DTP/DTaP History of extensive limb swelling after DTP/DTaP/Td that is not an arthus-type reaction Stable neurologic disorder Brachial neuritis Latex allergy that is not anaphylactic Breastfeeding Immunosuppression
IPV	**Contraindications** Severe allergic reaction (e.g., anaphylaxis) after a previous vaccine dose or to a vaccine component **Precautions** Pregnancy Moderate or severe acute illness with or without fever	Previous receipt of one or more doses of oral polio vaccine
MMR[e]	**Contraindications** Severe allergic reaction (e.g., anaphylaxis) after a previous vaccine dose or to a vaccine component Pregnancy Known severe immunodeficiency (e.g., hematologic and solid tumors, receiving chemotherapy, congenital immunodeficiency, long-term immunosuppressive therapy,[f] or patients with human immunodeficiency virus [HIV] infection who are severely immunocompromised) **Precautions** Recent (≤11 months) receipt of antibody-containing blood product (specific interval depends on product)[h] History of thrombocytopenia or thrombocytopenic purpura Moderate or severe acute illness with or without fever	Positive tuberculin skin test Simultaneous tuberculosis skin testing[g] Breastfeeding Pregnancy of recipient's mother or other close or household contact Recipient is female of childbearing age Immunodeficient family member or household contact Asymptomatic or mildly symptomatic HIV infection Allergy to eggs
Hib	**Contraindications** Severe allergic reaction (e.g., anaphylaxis) after a previous vaccine dose or to a vaccine component Aged <6 weeks **Precautions** Moderate or severe acute illness with or without fever	

Continued on following page

TABLE 5-13 **Contraindications and Precautions[a] to Commonly Used Vaccines** *(Continued)*

Vaccine	True Contraindications and Precautions[a]	Untrue (Vaccines Can Be Administered)
Hepatitis B	**Contraindication** Severe allergic reaction (e.g., anaphylaxis) after a previous vaccine dose or to a vaccine component **Precautions** Infant weighing <2000 g[c] Moderate or severe acute illness with or without fever	Pregnancy Autoimmune disease (e.g., systemic lupus erythematosis or rheumatoid arthritis)
Hepatitis A	**Contraindications** Severe allergic reaction (e.g., anaphylaxis) after a previous vaccine dose or to a vaccine component **Precautions** Pregnancy Moderate or severe acute illness with or without fever	
Varicella	**Contraindications** Severe allergic reaction (e.g., anaphylaxis) after a previous vaccine dose or to a vaccine component Substantial suppression of cellular immunity Pregnancy **Precautions** Recent (≤11 months) receipt of antibody-containing blood product (specific interval depends on product)[h] Moderate or severe acute illness with or without fever	Pregnancy of recipient's mother or other close or household contact Immunodeficient family member or household contact[i] Asymptomatic or mildly symptomatic HIV infection Humoral immunodeficiency (e.g., agammaglobulinemia)[j]
PCV	**Contraindications** Severe allergic reaction (e.g., anaphylaxis) after a previous vaccine dose or to a vaccine component **Precaution** Moderate or severe acute illness with or without fever	
TIV	**Contraindication** Severe allergic reaction (e.g., anaphylaxis) after a previous vaccine dose or to a vaccine component **Precaution** Moderate or severe acute illness with or without fever	Nonsevere (e.g., contact) allergy to latex or thimerosal Concurrent administration of coumadin or aminophylline
LAIV	**Contraindications** Severe allergic reaction (e.g., anaphylaxis) after a previous vaccine dose or to a vaccine component Pregnancy Known severe immunodeficiency (e.g., hematologic and solid tumors, receiving chemotherapy, congenital immunodeficiency, long-term immunosuppressive therapy,[f] or patients with human immunodeficiency virus [HIV] infection who are severely immunocompromised) Previous history of GBS Certain chronic medical conditions[k] **Precaution** Moderate or severe acute illness with or without fever	

TABLE 5-13 **Contraindications and Precautions[a] to Commonly Used Vaccines** *(Continued)*

Vaccine	True Contraindications and Precautions[a]	Untrue (Vaccines Can Be Administered)
PPV	**Contraindication** Severe allergic reaction (e.g., anaphylaxis) after a previous vaccine dose or to a vaccine component **Precaution** Moderate or severe acute illness with or without fever	History of invasive pneumococcal disease or pneumonia
MCV4	**Contraindications** Severe allergic reaction (e.g., anaphylaxis) after a previous vaccine dose or to a vaccine component **Precautions** Moderate or severe acute illness with or without fever History of GBS (if not at high risk for meningococcal disease)	
MPSV	**Contraindications** Severe allergic reaction after a previous dose or to a vaccine component **Precautions** Moderate or severe acute illness with or without fever	
HPV	**Contraindications** Severe allergic reaction after a previous dose or to a vaccine component **Precautions** Moderate or severe acute illness with or without fever Pregnancy	
Rotavirus	**Contraindications** Severe allergic reaction after a previous dose or to a vaccine component **Precautions** Moderate or severe acute illness with or without fever Immunosuppression Receipt of an antibody-containing blood product within 6 weeks[l] Preexisting gastrointestinal disease Previous history of intussusception	Preterm births Immunosuppression in household contacts Pregnant household contacts

From CDC: General recommendations on immunization: recommendations of the Advisory Committee on Immunization Practices (ACIP), *MMWR* 55(RR-15), 2006.

[a]Events or conditions listed as precautions should be reviewed carefully. Benefits of and risks for administering a specific vaccine to a person under these circumstances should be considered. If the risk from the vaccine is believed to outweigh the benefit, the vaccine should not be administered. If the benefit of vaccination is believed to outweigh the risk, the vaccine should be administered. Whether and when to administer DTaP to children with proven or suspected underlying neurologic disorders should be decided on a case-by-case basis.

[b]Antibacterial drugs and mefloquine might interfere with Ty21a oral typhoid vaccine, and certain antiviral drugs might interfere with varicella-containing and live-attenuated influenza virus vaccine.

[c]Hepatitis B vaccination should be deferred for infants weighing <2000 g if the mother is documented to be hepatitis B surface antigen (HBsAg)-negative at the time of the infant's birth. Vaccination can commence at chronologic age 1 month. For infants born to women who are HBsAg-positive, hepatitis B immunoglobulin and hepatitis B vaccine should be administered at or soon after birth regardless of weight.

[d]Acetaminophen or other appropriate antipyretic can be administered to infants and children with a history of previous seizures at the time of DTaP vaccination and every 4 hours for 24 hours thereafter to reduce the possibility of postvaccination fever. (Source: American Academy of Pediatrics: Active immunization. In Pickering LK, Baker CJ, Long SS, McMillan J (eds): *2006 red book: report of the Committee on Infectious Diseases,* ed 27, Elk Grove Village, IL, 2006, American Academy of Pediatrics.)

[e]MMR and varicella vaccines can be administered on the same day. If not administered on the same day, these vaccines should be separated by at least 28 days.

[f]Substantially immunosuppressive steroid dose is considered to be ≥2 weeks of daily receipt of ≥20 mg or ≥2 mg/kg body weight of prednisone or equivalent.

[g]Measles vaccination might suppress tuberculin reactivity temporarily. Measles-containing vaccine can be administered on the same day as tuberculin skin testing. If testing cannot be performed until after the day of MMR vaccination, the test should be postponed for ≥4 weeks after the vaccination. If an urgent need exists to skin test, do so with the understanding that reactivity might be reduced by the vaccine.

[h]See text for details.

[i]If a vaccinee experiences a presumed vaccine-related rash 7-25 days after vaccination, he or she should avoid direct contact with immunocompromised persons for the duration of the rash if possible.

[j]Vaccine should be deferred for the appropriate interval if replacement IG products are being administered.

[k]For details see CDC: Prevention and control of influenza: recommendations of the Advisory Committee on Immunization Practices (ACIP), *MMWR* 55(RR-10), 2006.

[l]Rotavirus vaccine (RV) should be deferred for 6 weeks after receipt of an antibody-containing product if possible. However, if the 6-week deferral would cause the first dose of RV to be scheduled for age ≥13 weeks, a shorter deferral interval should be used to ensure the first dose of RV is administered no later than age 13 weeks.

TABLE 5-14 **Dose and Route of Administration for Selected Vaccines**

Vaccines	Dose	Route
Diphtheria, tetanus, pertussis (DTaP, DT, Td, Tdap)	0.5 ml	Intramuscular (IM)
Diphtheria, tetanus, acellular pertussis, inactivated polio, hepatitis B vaccine (DTaP-IPV-HepB)	0.5 ml	IM
Diphtheria, tetanus, acellular pertussis, *haemophilus influenza* type b vaccine (DTaP-Hib)	0.5 ml	IM
Haemophilus influenzae type b (Hib)	0.5 ml	IM
Haemophilus influenzae type b–Hepatitis B (Hib-HepB)	0.5 ml	IM
Hepatitis A (HepA)	≤18 years: 0.5 ml ≥19 years: 1.0 ml	IM
HepB	≤19 years: 0.5 ml* ≥20 years: 1.0 ml	IM
HepA/HepB	≥18 years: 1.0 ml	IM
Influenza, live attenuated	0.5 ml	Intranasal spray
Influenza, trivalent inactivated	6-35 months: 0.25 ml ≥3 years: 0.5 ml	IM
Measles, mumps, rubella	0.5 ml	Subcutaneous (SC)
Measles, mumps, rubella, varicella	0.5 ml	SC
Meningococcal conjugate	0.5 ml	IM
Meningococcal polysaccharide	0.5 ml	SC
Pneumococcal conjugate	0.5 ml	IM
Pneumococcal polysaccharide	0.5 ml	IM or SC
Human papillomavirus	0.5 ml	IM
Polio, inactivated	0.5 ml	IM or SC
Rotavirus	2.0 ml	Oral
Varicella	0.5 ml	SC
Zoster	0.7 ml	SC

From CDC: General recommendations on immunization: recommendations of the Advisory Committee on Immunization Practices (ACIP), *MMWR* 55(RR-15), 2006. Adapted from Immunization Action Coalition (http://www.immunize.org).

*Persons aged 11-15 years can be administered Recombivax HB (Merck) 1.0 ml (adult formulation) on a 2-dose schedule.

muscle and only if the skin is stretched flat between thumb and forefinger and the needle inserted at a 90-degree angle to the skin. For toddlers, the anterolateral thigh can be used, but the needle should be at least 1 inch in length.

Adolescents and Adults (Aged >11 Years)

For adults and adolescents, the deltoid muscle is recommended for routine intramuscular vaccinations. The anterolateral thigh also can be used. For men and women weighing <130 lbs (<60 kg) a ⅝- to 1-inch needle is sufficient to ensure intramuscular injection. For women weighing 130 to 200 lbs (60 to 90 kg) and men 130 to 260 lbs (60 to 118 kg), a 1- to 1½-inch needle is needed. For women weighing >200 lbs (>90 kg) or men weighing >260 lbs (>118 kg), a 1½-inch needle is required.

SUBCUTANEOUS INJECTIONS

Subcutaneous injections are administered at a 45-degree angle usually into the thigh for infants aged <12 months and in the upper-outer triceps area of persons aged ≥12 months. Subcutaneous injections can be administered into the upper-outer triceps area of an infant, if necessary. A ⅝-inch, 23- to 25-gauge needle should be inserted into the subcutaneous tissue (Figs. 5-4 and 5-5).

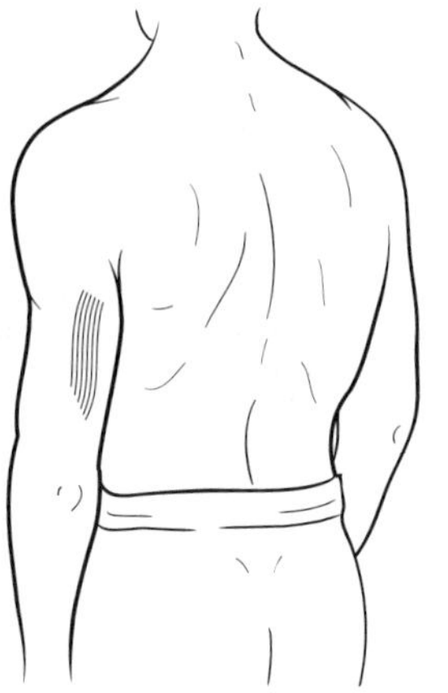

FIGURE 5-4 Subcutaneous site of administration: triceps. (Adapted from Minnesota Department of Health. In CDC: General recommendations on immunization: recommendations of the Advisory Committee on Immunization Practices [ACIP], *MMWR* 55[RR-15]:17, 2006.)

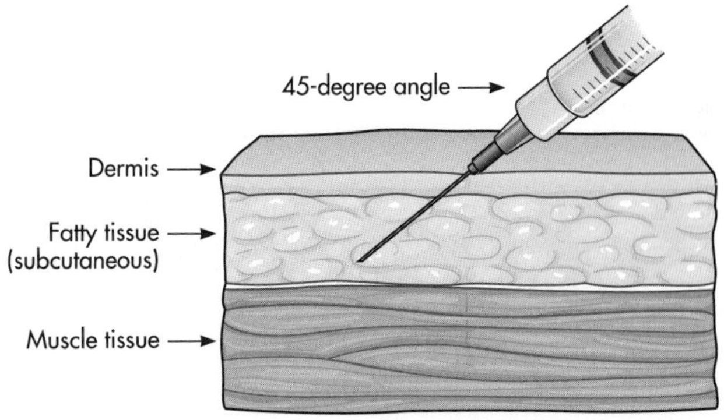

FIGURE 5-5 Subcutaneous needle insertion. (Adapted from California Administration Branch. In CDC: General recommendations on immunization: recommendations of the Advisory Committee on Immunization Practices [ACIP], *MMWR* 55[RR-15]:17, 2006.)

VACCINE ADMINISTRATION*

INFECTION CONTROL AND STERILE TECHNIQUE

Persons administering vaccines should follow appropriate precautions to minimize risk for spread of disease. Hands should be cleansed with an alcohol-based, waterless antiseptic hand rub or washed with soap and water between each patient contact. Occupational Safety and Health Administration (OSHA) regulations do not require that gloves be worn when administering vaccinations unless persons administering vaccinations are likely to come into contact with potentially infectious body fluids or have open lesions on their hands. Needles used for injections must be sterile and disposable to minimize the risk for contamination. A separate needle and syringe should be used for each injection. Changing needles between drawing vaccine from a vial and injecting it into a recipient is not necessary. Different vaccines should never be mixed in the same syringe unless specifically licensed for such use, and no attempt should be made to transfer between syringes.

For all intramuscular injections, the needle should be long enough to reach the muscle mass and prevent vaccine from seeping into subcutaneous tissue but not so long as to involve underlying nerves, blood vessels, or bone. Vaccinators should be familiar with the anatomy of the area into which they are injecting vaccine. Intramuscular injections are administered at a 90-degree angle to the skin, preferably into the anterolateral aspect of the thigh or the deltoid muscle of the upper arm depending on the age of the patient.

Decision on needle size and site of injection must be made for each person on the basis of the size of the muscle, the thickness of adipose tissue at the injection site, the volume of the material to be administered, injection technique, and the depth below the muscle surface into which the material is to be injected (Fig. 5-1). Aspiration before injection of vaccines or toxoids (i.e., pulling back on the syringe plunger after needle insertion before injection) is not required because no large blood vessel exists at the recommended injection sites.

Infants (Aged <12 Months)

For the majority of infants, the anterolateral aspect of the thigh is the recommended site for injection because it provides a large muscle mass (Fig. 5-2). The muscles of the buttock have not been used for administration of vaccines in infants and children because of concern about potential injury to the sciatic nerve, which is well documented after injection of antimicrobial agents into the buttock. If the gluteal muscle must be used, care should be taken to

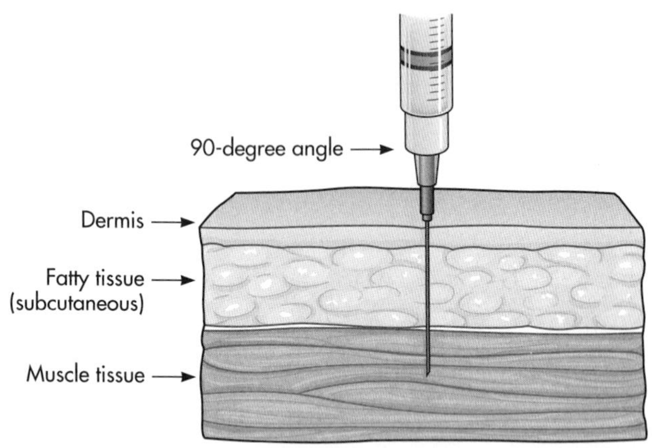

FIGURE 5-1 Intramuscular needle insertion. (Adapted from California Immunization Branch. In CDC: General recommendations on immunization: recommendations of the Advisory Committee on Immunization Practices [ACIP], *MMWR* 55[RR-15]:16 2006.)

*From CDC: General recommendations on immunization: recommendations of the Advisory Committee on Immunization Practices (ACIP), *MMWR* 55(RR-15):14-16, 2006.

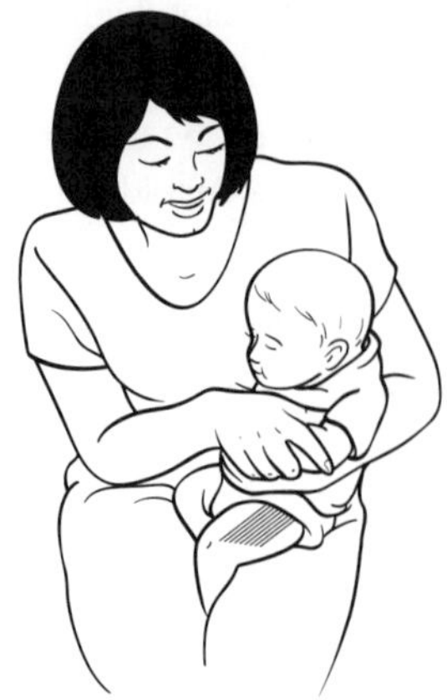

FIGURE 5-2 Intramuscular/subcutaneous site of adi tion: anterolateral thigh. (Adapted from Minnesot ment of Health. In CDC: General recommendations on i tion: recommendations of the Advisory Comm Immunization Practices [ACIP], *MMWR* 55[RR-15]:6, 200

define the anatomic landmarks.† Injection technique i important parameter to ensure efficient intramuscular livery. If the subcutaneous and muscle tissue are bunc mize the chance of striking bone, a 1-inch needle is ensure intramuscular administration in infants. For th infants, a 1-inch, 22- to 25-gauge needle is sufficient muscle in an infant's thigh. For newborn (first 28 day premature infants, a ⅝-inch-long needle usually is ad skin is stretched flat between thumb and forefinger dle inserted at a 90-degree angle to the skin.

Toddlers and Older Children (Aged 12 Month

The deltoid muscle should be used if the muscle quate. The needle size for deltoid site injections c 22 to 25 gauge and from ⅝ to 1 inch on the basis the muscle and the thickness of adipose tissue a site (Fig. 5-3). A ⅝-inch needle is adequate only

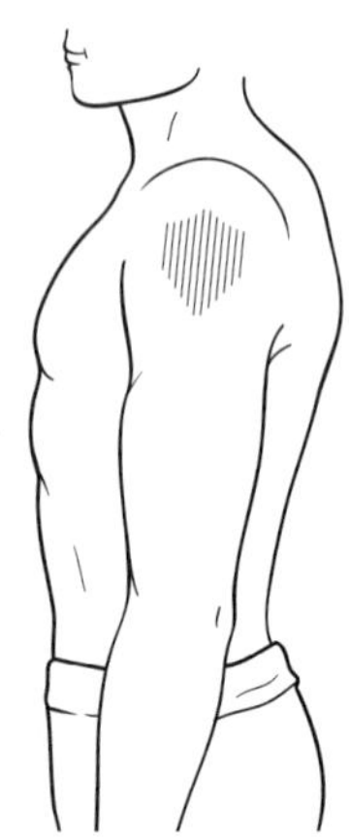

FIGURE 5-3 Intramuscular site of admini (Adapted from Minnesota Department of Hea recommendations on immunization: recomme visory Committee on Immunization Practices [15]:17, 2006.)

†If the gluteal muscle is chosen, injection s lateral and superior to a line between the poste and the greater trochanter or in the ventroglutea angle bounded by the anterior superior iliac sp iliac crest, and the upper border of the greater t

TABLE 5-15 **Treatment of Anaphylaxis with Intramuscular or Oral Pharmaceuticals**

Drug	Dosage
Child	
Primary regimen	
Epinephrine 1:1000 (aqueous) (1 mg/ml)*	0.01 mg/kg up to 0.5 mg (administer 0.01 ml/kg/dose up to 0.5 ml) intramuscularly (IM) repeated every 10-20 minutes up to 3 doses
Secondary regimen	
Diphenhydramine	1-2 mg/kg oral, IM, or intraveneously (IV), every 4-6 hours (maximum single dose: 100 mg)
Hydroxyzine	0.5-1 mg/kg oral, IM, every 4-6 hours (maximum single dose: 100 mg)
Prednisone	1.5-2 mg/kg oral (maximum single dose: 60 mg); use corticosteroids as long as needed
Adult	
Primary regimen	
Epinephrine 1:1000 (aqueous)*	0.01 mg/kg up to 0.5 mg (give 0.01 ml/kg/dose up to 0.5 ml) IM repeated every 10-20 minutes up to 3 doses
Secondary regimen	
Diphenhydramine	1-2 mg/kg up to 100 mg IM or oral every 4-6 hours

From CDC: General recommendations on immunization: recommendations of the Advisory Committee on Immunization Practices (ACIP), *MMWR* 55(RR-15), 2006. Adapted from American Academy of Pediatrics: Passive immunization. In Pickering LK, Baker CJ, Long SS, McMillan J: *Red book: 2006 report of the Committee on Infectious Diseases,* ed 27, Elk Grove, IL, 2006, American Academy of Pediatrics; and Immunization Action Coalition: Medical management of anaphylaxis in adult patients. Available at http://www.immunize.org/catg.d/p3082.pdf, and Mosby's Drug Consult 2005.

*If agent causing anaphylactic reaction was administered by injection, epinephrine can be injected into the same site to slow absorption.

TABLE 5-16 Vaccination of Persons with Primary and Secondary Immune Deficiencies

Category	Specific Immunodeficiency	Contraindicated Vaccines[a]	Risk-Specific Recommended Vaccines[a]	Effectiveness and Comments
		PRIMARY		
B-lymphocyte (humoral)	Severe antibody deficiencies (e.g., X-linked agammaglobulinemia and common variable immunodeficiency)	Oral poliovirus (OPV)[b] Smallpox Live-attenuated influenza vaccine (LAIV) BCG Ty21a (live oral typhoid)	Pneumococcal Influenza (TIV) Consider measles and varicella vaccination	The effectiveness of any vaccine will be uncertain if it depends only on the humoral response; intravenous immune globulin interferes with the immune response to measles vaccine and possibly varicella vaccine
	Less severe antibody deficiencies (e.g., selective IgA deficiency and IgG subclass deficiency)	OPV[b] Other live vaccines appear to be safe	Pneumococcal Influenza (TIV)	All vaccines probably effective; immune response may be attenuated
T-lymphocyte (cell-mediated and humoral)	Complete defects (e.g., severe combined immunodeficiency [SCID] disease, complete DiGeorge syndrome)	All live vaccines[c,d]	Pneumococcal Influenza (TIV)	Vaccines may be ineffective
	Partial defects (e.g., the majority of patients with DiGeorge syndrome, Wiskott-Aldrich syndrome, ataxia-telangiectasia)	All live vaccines[c,d]	Pneumococcal Meningococcal *Haemophilus influenza* type b (Hib) (if not administered in infancy) Influenza (TIV)	Effectiveness of any vaccine depends on degree of immune suppression
Complement	Deficiency of early components (C1, C2, C3, and C4)	None	Pneumococcal Meningococcal Influenza (TIV)	All routine vaccines probably effective
	Deficiency of late components (C5-C9) and C3, properdin, factor B	None	Pneumococcal Meningococcal Influenza (TIV)	All routine vaccines probably effective
Phagocytic function	Chronic granulomatous disease, leukocyte adhesion defect, and myeloperoxidase deficiency	Live bacterial vaccines[c]	Pneumococcal[e] Influenza (TIV) (to decrease secondary bacterial infection)	All inactivated vaccines safe and probably effective Live viral vaccines probably safe and effective

TABLE 5-16 **Vaccination of Persons with Primary and Secondary Immune Deficiencies** *(Continued)*

Category	Specific Immunodeficiency	Contraindicated Vaccines[a]	Risk-Specific Recommended Vaccines[a]	Effectiveness and Comments
		SECONDARY		
	Human immunodeficiency virus/acquired immunodeficiency syndrome (HIV/AIDS)	OPV Smallpox BCG LAIV Withhold MMR and varicella in severely immunocompromised persons	Influenza (TIV) Pneumococcal Consider Hib (if not administered in infancy) and meningococcal vaccination	Measles, mumps, rubella (MMR); varicella; and all inactivated vaccines, including inactivated influenza, might be effective[f]
	Malignant neoplasm, transplantation, immunosuppressive or radiation therapy	Live viral and bacterial, depending on immune status	Influenza (TIV) Pneumococcal	Effectiveness of any vaccine depends on degree of immune suppression
	Asplenia	None	Pneumococcal Meningococcal Hib (if not administered in infancy)	All routine vaccines probably effective
	Chronic renal disease	LAIV	Pneumococcal Influenza (TIV) Hepatitis B	All routine vaccines probably effective

From CDC: General recommendations on immunization: recommendations of the Advisory Committee on Immunization Practices (ACIP), *MMWR* 55(RR-15), 2006. Modified from American Academy of Pediatrics: Passive immunization. In Pickering LK, Baker CJ, Long SS, McMillan J: *Red book: 2006 report of the Committee on Infectious Diseases,* ed 27, Elk Grove, IL, 2006, American Academy of Pediatrics; and CDC: Use of vaccines and immune globulins in persons with altered immunocompetence: recommendations of the Advisory Committee on Immunization Practices (ACIP), *MMWR* 42(RR-4):42, 1993.

[a]Other vaccines that are universally or routinely recommended should be administered if not contraindicated.

[b]OPV is no longer available for routine use in the United States.

[c]Live bacterial vaccines: BCG and Ty21a *Salmonella typhi* vaccine.

[d]Live viral vaccines: MMR, OPV, LAIV, yellow fever, and varicella, including MMRV and HZ vaccine, and vaccinia (smallpox). Smallpox vaccine is not recommended for children or the general public.

[e]Pneumococcal vaccine is not indicated for children with chronic granulomatous disease.

[f]Children infected with HIV should receive IG after exposure to measles and can receive varicella and measles vaccine if CD4+ lymphocyte count is >15%.

TABLE 5-17 Approaches to the Evaluation and Vaccination of Internationally Adopted Children with No or Questionable Vaccination Records

Vaccine	Recommended Approach	Alternative Approach
Measles, mumps, and rubella (MMR)	Revaccinate with MMR	Serologic testing for immunoglobulin G (IgG) antibody to measles, mumps, and rubella
Haemophilus influenzae type b (Hib)	Age-appropriate revaccination	—
Hepatitis A	Age-appropriate revaccination	Serologic testing for IgG antibody to hepatitis A virus
Hepatitis B (Hep B)	Age-appropriate revaccination and serologic testing for HBsAg*	—
Poliovirus	Revaccinate with inactivated poliovirus vaccine (IPV)	Serologic testing for neutralizing antibody to poliovirus types 1, 2, and 3 (limited availability)
Diphtheria and tetanus toxoids and acellular pertussis (DTaP)	Revaccination with DTaP, with serologic testing for specific IgG antibody to tetanus and diphtheria toxins in the event of a severe local reaction	Children whose records indicate receipt of ≥3 doses: serologic testing for specific IgG antibody to diphtheria and tetanus toxins before administering addi tional doses or administer a single booster dose of DTaP, followed by serological testing after 1 month for specific IgG antibody to diphtheria and tetanus toxins with revaccination as appropriate
Varicella	Age-appropriate vaccination of children who lack evidence of varicella immunity	—
Pneumococcal conjugate	Age-appropriate vaccination	—

From CDC: General recommendations on immunization: recommendations of the Advisory Committee on Immunization Practices (ACIP), *MMWR* 55(RR-15), 2006.

*Very rarely, Hep B vaccine can give a false-positive HBsAg result up to 18 days following vaccination; therefore, blood should be drawn to test for HBsAg before vaccinating. (Source: CDC: A comprehensive immunization strategy to eliminate transmission of hepatitis B virus infection in the United States: recommendations of the Advisory Committee on Immunization Practices [ACIP]; Part I: immunization in infants, children, and adolescents, *MMWR* 54[RR-16], 2005.)

Immunizations for Adults

TABLE 5-18 Recommended Adult Immunization Schedule—United States

Vaccine[2,3]	Age group (years) 19-49	50-64	≥65
Tetanus, diphtheria pertussis (Tdap)[4]	1 dose booster every 10 years*	(spans)	(spans)
Human papilloma virus	19-26 years***		
Influenza	1 dose annually†	1 dose annually†	(spans)
Herpes zoster		≥60 years†††	(spans)
Pneumococcal (polysaccharide)	1 dose§¶	(spans)	1 dose§¶
Hepatitis B[4]	3 doses (0, 1-2, 4-6 months)**	(spans)	(spans)
Hepatitis A	2 doses (0, 6-12 months)††	(spans)	(spans)
Measles, mumps, rubella (MMR)[4]	1dose if MMR vaccination history is unreliable; 2 doses for persons with occupational or other indications§§		
Varicella[4]	2 doses (0, 4-8 weeks) for persons who are susceptible¶¶	(spans)	(spans)
Meningococcal (polysaccharide)	1 dose§§§	(spans)	(spans)

For all persons in this age group | For persons with medical/exposure indications | Catch-up on childhood vaccinations

[1] Approved by the Advisory Committee on Immunization Practices and accepted by the American College of Obstetricians and Gynecologists (ACOG) and the American Academy of Family Physicians (AAFP).

[2] This schedule indicates recommended age groups for routine administration of currently licensed vaccines for persons aged ≥19 years. Licensed combination vaccine may be used whenever any components of the combination are indicated and the vaccine's other components are not contraindicated. Health care providers should consult manufacturers' package inserts for detailed recommendations.

[3] Additional information regarding these vaccines and contraindications for vaccination is available from the National Immunization Hotline (telephone, 800-232-2522 [English] or 800-232-0233 [Spanish]) or at http://www.cdc.gov/nip.

[4] Covered by the Vaccine Injury Compensation Program. Information on how to file a claim is available at http://www.hrsa.gov/osp/vicp or by telephone, 800-338-2382. Vaccine injury claims are filed with U.S. Court of Federal Claims, 717 Madison Place, N.W., Washington, D.C. 20005; telephone, 202-219-9657.

*__Tetanus and diphtheria (Tdap).__ Adults, including pregnant women with uncertain histories of a complete primary vaccination series, should receive a primary series of Td. A primary series for adults is 3 doses: the first 2 doses administered at least 4 weeks apart and the third dose, 6-12 months after the second. Administer 1 dose if the person received the primary series and the last vaccination was ≥10 years previously. In addition, information is available regarding administration of Td as prophylaxis in wound management *(1)*. The American College of Physicians Task Force on Adult Immunization supports a second option for Td use in adults: a single Td booster at age 50 years for persons who have completed the full pediatric series, including the teenage/young adult booster. A newly licensed tetanus-diphtheria-acellular-pertussis vaccine is available for adults. The Advisory Committee on Immunization Practices (ACIP) recommends that adults between ages 19 and 64 years receive a single dose of Tdap to replace their next dose of Td booster immunization given for routine vaccination at 10-year intervals.

†**Influenza vaccination.** *Medical indications:* chronic disorders of the cardiovascular or pulmonary systems including asthma; chronic metabolic diseases including diabetes mellitus, renal dysfunction, hemoglobinopathies, or immunosuppression (including immunosuppression caused by medications or by human immunodeficiency virus [HIV]) requiring medical follow-up or hospitalization during the preceding year; women who will be in the second or third trimester of pregnancy during the influenza season. *Occupational indications:* health care workers (HCWs). *Other indications:* residents of nursing homes and other long-term-care facilities; persons likely to transmit influenza to persons at high risk (e.g., in-home caregivers to persons with medical indications; household contact and out-of-home caregivers for children aged ≤23 months, or children with asthma or other indicator conditions for influenza vaccination; household members and caregivers for elderly and adults with high-risk conditions); and anyone who wishes to be vaccinated. For healthy persons age 5-49 years without high-risk conditions, either the inactivated vaccine or the intranasally administered influenza vaccine (FluMist) may be administered *(2,3)*.

§**Pneumococcal polysaccharide vaccination.** *Medical indications:* chronic disorders of the pulmonary system, excluding asthma, cardiovascular diseases, diabetes mellitus, chronic liver diseases (including liver disease as a result of alcohol abuse [e.g., cirrhosis]), chronic renal failure or nephrotic syndrome, functional or anatomic asplenia (e.g., sickle cell disease or splenectomy), immunosuppressive conditions (e.g., congenital immunodeficiency, HIV infection, leukemia, lymphoma, multiple myeloma, Hodgkins disease, generalized malignancy, and organ or bone marrow transplantation), chemotherapy with alkylating agents, antimetabolites, or long-term systemic corticosteroids. *Geographic/other indications:* Alaska Natives and certain American Indian populations. *Other indications:* residents of nursing homes and other long-term-care facilities *(4)*.

¶**Revaccination with pneumococcal polysaccharide vaccine.** One-time revaccination after 5 years for persons with chronic renal failure or nephrotic syndrome, functional or anatomic asplenia (e.g., sickle cell disease or splenectomy), immunosuppressive conditions (e.g., congenital immunodeficiency, HIV infection, leukemia, lymphoma, multiple myeloma, Hodgkins disease, generalized malignancy, and organ or bone marrow transplantation), chemotherapy with alkylating agents, antimetabolites, or long-term systemic corticosteroids. For persons aged ≥65 years, one-time revaccination if they were vaccinated ≥5 years previously and were aged <65 years at the time of primary vaccination *(4)*.

Continued on following page

**Hepatitis B (HepB) vaccine. *Medical indications:* hemodialysis patients, patients who receive clotting-factor concentrates. *Occupational indications:* HCWs and public-safety workers who have exposure to blood in the workplace, persons in training in schools of medicine, dentistry, nursing, laboratory technology, and other allied health professions. *Behavioral indications:* injection-drug users, persons with more than one sex partner during the previous 6 months, persons with a recently acquired sexually transmitted disease (STD), all clients in STD clinics, men who have sex with men (MSM). *Other indications:* household contacts and sex partners of persons with chronic Hepatitis B virus (HBV) infection, clients and staff of institutions for the developmentally disabled, international travelers to countries with high or intermediate prevalence of chronic HBV infection for >6 months, and inmates of correctional facilities *(5)*.

††**Hepatitis A (HepA) vaccine.** For the combined HepA-HepB vaccine, use 3 doses (at 0, 1, and 6 months). *Medical indications:* persons with clotting-factor disorders or chronic liver disease. *Behavioral indications:* MSM, users of injecting and noninjecting illegal drugs. *Occupational indications:* persons working with Hepatitis A virus (HAV)-infected primates or with HAV in a research laboratory setting. *Other indications:* persons traveling to or working in countries that have high or intermediate endemicity of HAV *(6)*.

§§**Measles, mumps, rubella (MMR) vaccination.** *Measles component:* adults born before 1957 might be considered immune to measles. Adults born in or after 1957 should receive at least 1 dose of MMR unless they have a medical contraindication, documentation of at least 1 dose, or other acceptable evidence of immunity. A second dose of MMR is recommended for adults who (1) were exposed recently to measles or were in an outbreak setting, (2) were previously vaccinated with killed measles vaccine, (3) were vaccinated with an unknown vaccine during 1963-1967, (4) are students in postsecondary educational institutions, (5) work in health care facilities, or (6) plan to travel internationally. *Mumps component:* 1 dose of MMR should be adequate for protection. *Rubella component:* Administer 1 dose of MMR to women whose rubella vaccination history is unreliable and counsel women to avoid becoming pregnant for 4 weeks after vaccination. For women of childbearing age, regardless of birth year, routinely determine rubella immunity and counsel women regarding congenital rubella syndrome. Do not vaccinate pregnant women or those planning to become pregnant in the next 4 weeks. If pregnant and susceptible, vaccinate as early in the postpartum period as possible *(7)*.

¶¶**Varicella vaccination.** Recommended for all persons who do not have reliable clinical history of varicella infection, or serologic evidence of varicella zoster virus (VZV) infection who might be at high risk for exposure or transmission. This includes HCWs and family contacts of immunocompromised persons, those who live or work in environments where transmission is likely (e.g., teachers of young children, day-care employees, and residents and staff members in institutional settings), persons who live or work in environments where VZV transmission can occur (e.g., college students, inmates and staff members of correctional institutions, and military personnel) adolescents and adults living in households with children, women who are not pregnant but who might become pregnant in the future, and international travelers who are not immune to infection. Do not vaccinate pregnant women or those planning to become pregnant in the next 4 weeks. If a woman is pregnant and susceptible, vaccinate as early in the postpartum period as possible. Approximately 95% of U.S.-born adults are immune to VZV *(8,9)*. Evidence of immunity to varicella in adults includes any of the following: (1) documented age-appropriate varicella vaccination (i.e., receipt of one dose before age 13 years or receipt of two doses [administered at least 12 weeks apart] after age 13 years), (2) born in the United States before 1980, (3) history of varicella disease based on health care professional or self-report or parental report of typical varicella disease for non-U.S.-born persons born before 1966 and all persons born between 1966 and 1997 (for a patient reporting a history of an atypical, mild case, health care professionals should seek either an epidemiological link with a typical varicella case or evidence of laboratory confirmation, if it was performed at a time of acute disease), (4) history of herpes zoster based on health care professional diagnosis, or (5) laboratory evidence of immunity. Do not vaccinate women who are pregnant or who might become pregnant within 4 weeks of receiving the vaccine. Assess pregnant women for evidence of varicella immunity. Women who do not have evidence of immunity should receive dose 1 of varicella vaccine upon completion or termination of pregnancy and before discharge from the health care facility. Dose 2 should be given 4-8 weeks after dose 1.

***Quadrivalent human papillomavirus (types 6, 11, 16, 18) recombinant vaccine (Gardasil).** Should be given to all adult females aged 19-26 years who have not been previously vaccinated. The vaccine is indicated for the prevention of cervical cancer and genital warts caused by the human papilloma virus (HPV) 6, 11, 16, or 18. Gardasil is an intramuscular injection for administration to the thigh or upper arm. The schedule consists of three 0.5 ml doses, with the second dose given 2 months after the first, and the final dose administered 6 months after the initial dose.

†††**Herpes zoster vaccine (Zostavax).** Indicated for prevention of herpes zoster (shingles) in individuals age 60 years or older. Zostavax is administered as a single dose subcutaneously. It is a lyophilic preparation of the Oka/Merck strain of live, attenuated varicella zoster virus (VZV). It should not be administered to individuals with a history of primary or acquired immunodeficiency states, persons on immunosuppressive therapy (including high-dose corticosteroids), those with active untreated tuberculosis, and those who may be pregnant.

§§§**Meningococcal vaccine (quadrivalent polysaccharide for serogroups A, C, Y, and W-135).** Consider vaccination for persons with medical indications: adults with terminal complement component deficiencies or with anatomic or functional asplenia. Other indications: travelers to countries where meningitis is hyperendemic or epidemic (e.g., the "meningitis belt" of sub-Saharan Africa, Mecca, or Saudi Arabia). Revaccination at 3-5 years may be indicated for persons at high risk for infection (e.g., persons residing in areas in which disease is epidemic). Counsel college freshmen, particularly those who live in dormitories, regarding meningococcal disease and the vaccine so that they can make an educated decision about receiving the vaccination *(10)*. The American Academy of Family Physicians recommends that colleges provide education on meningococcal infection and vaccination and offer it to those who are interested. Physicians need not initiate discussion of the meningococcal quadrivalent polysaccharide vaccine as part of routine medical care.

References

1. CDC: Diphtheria, tetanus, and pertussis: recommendations for vaccine use and other preventive measures. Recommendations of the Immunization Practices Advisory Committee (ACIP), *MMWR* 40(RR-10), 1991.
2. CDC: Prevention and control of influenza: recommendations of the Advisory Committee for Immunization Practices, *MMWR* 52(RR-8), 2003.
3. CDC: Using live, attenuated influenza vaccine for prevention and control of influenza: supplemental recommendations of the Advisory Committee on Immunization Practices (ACIP), *MMWR* 52(RR-13), 2003.
4. CDC: Prevention of pneumococcal disease: recommendations of the Advisory Committee on Immunization Practices (ACIP), *MMWR* 47(RR-8), 1997.
5. CDC: Hepatitis B virus: a comprehensive strategy for eliminating transmission in the United States through universal childhood vaccination. Recommendations of the Immunization Practices Advisory Committee (ACIP), *MMWR* 40(RR-13), 1991.
6. CDC: Prevention of hepatitis A through active or passive immunization: recommendations of the Advisory Committee on Immunization Practices (ACIP), *MMWR* 48(RR-12), 1999.
7. CDC: Measles, mumps, and rubella—vaccine use and strategies for elimination of measles, rubella, and congenital rubella syndrome and control of mumps: recommendations of the Advisory Committee on Immunization Practices (ACIP), *MMWR* 47(RR-8), 1998.
8. CDC: Prevention of varicella: recommendations of the Advisory Committee on Immunization Practices (ACIP), *MMWR* 45(RR-11), 1996.
9. CDC: Prevention of varicella: updated recommendations of the Advisory Committee on Immunization Practices (ACIP), *MMWR* 48(RR-6), 1999.
10. CDC: Prevention and control of meningococcal disease and meningococcal disease and college students: recommendations of the Advisory Committee on Immunization Practices (ACIP), *MMWR* 49(RR-7), 2000.

TABLE 5-19 **Recommended Adult Immunization Schedule for Adults with Medical Conditions—United States**

	Vaccine						
Medical condition	**Tetanus-diptheria (Td)***	**Influenza†**	**Pneumo-coccal (polysac-charide)§¶**	**Hepatitis B****	**Hepatitis A††**	**Measles, mumps, rubella (MMR)§§**	**Varicella¶¶**
Pregnancy		A					
Diabetes, heart disease, chronic pulmonary disease, and chronic liver disease, including chronic alcoholism		B	C		D		
Congenital immunodeficiency, leukemia, lymphoma, generalized malignancy, therapy with alkylating agents, antimetabolites, radiation, or large amounts of corticosteroids			E				F
Renal failure/end-stage renal disease and patients receiving hemodialysis or clotting factor concentrates			E	G			
Asplenia, including elective splenectomy and terminal complement-component deficiencies		H	E,I,J				
Human immunodeficiency virus (HIV) infection			E,K			L	

For all persons in this group — For persons with medical/exposure indications — Catch-up on childhood vaccinations — Contraindicated

From *MMWR Morb Mortal Wkly Rep* 52, 2003.

A. For women without chronic diseases/conditions, vaccinate if pregnancy will be at second or third trimester during influenza season. For women with chronic diseases/conditions, vaccinate at any time during the pregnancy.
B. Although chronic liver disease and alcoholism are not indicator conditions for influenza vaccination, administer 1 dose annually if the patient is aged >50 years, has other indications for influenza vaccine, or requests vaccination.
C. Asthma is an indicator condition for influenza but not for pneumococcal vaccination.
D. For all persons with chronic liver disease.
E. For persons aged <65 years, revaccinate once after ≥5 years have elapsed since initial vaccination.
F. Persons with impaired humoral but not cellular immunity may be vaccinated *(9)*.
G. For hemodialysis patients use special formulation of vaccine (40 μg/ml) or two 1.0 ml 20 μg doses administered at one site. Vaccinate early in the course of renal disease. Assess antibody titers to hepatitis B surface antigen (anti-HBs) levels annually. Administer additional doses if anti-HBs levels decline to ≤10 mIU/ml.
H. No data have been reported specifically on risk for severe or complicated influenza infections among persons with asplenia. However, influenza is a risk factor for secondary bacterial infections that might cause severe disease in asplenics.
I. Administer meningococcal vaccine and consider *Haemophilus influenzae* type b vaccine.
J. In the event of elective splenectomy, vaccinate >2 weeks before surgery.
K. Vaccinate as close to diagnosis as possible when CD4 cell counts are highest.
L. Withhold MMR or other measles-containing vaccines from HIV-infected persons with evidence of severe immunosuppression.

TABLE 5-20 **Immunizations during Pregnancy**

Immuno-biologic Agent	Risk from Disease to Pregnant Woman	Risk from Disease to Fetus or Neonate	Type of Immunizing Agent	Risk from Immunizing Agent to Fetus	Indications for Immunization during Pregnancy	Dose Schedule	Comments
Live Virus Vaccines							
Measles	Significant morbidity, low mortality; not altered by pregnancy	Significant increase in abortion rate; may cause malformations	Live attenuated virus vaccine	None confirmed	Contraindicated (see immune globulins)	Single dose SC, preferably as measles-mumps-rubella*	Vaccination of susceptible women should be part of postpartum care
Mumps	Low morbidity and mortality; not altered by pregnancy	Probable increased rate of abortion in first trimester	Live attenuated virus vaccine	None confirmed	Contraindicated	Single dose SC, preferably as measles-mumps-rubella	Vaccination of susceptible women should be part of postpartum care
Poliomyelitis	No increased incidence in pregnancy, but may be more severe if it does occur	Anoxic fetal damage reported; 50% mortality in neonatal disease	Live attenuated virus (oral polio vaccine [OPV]) and enhanced, potency inactivated virus (e-IPV) vaccine†	None confirmed	Not routinely recommended for women in U.S., except persons at increased risk of exposure	*Primary:* Two doses of e-IPV SC at 4-8 wk intervals and a third dose 6-12 mo after the second dose *Immediate protection:* One dose OPV orally (in out-break setting)	Vaccine indicated for susceptible pregnant women traveling in endemic areas or in other high-risk situations
Rubella	Low morbidity and mortality; not altered by pregnancy	High rate of abortion and congenital rubella syndrome	Live attenuated virus vaccine	None confirmed	Contraindicated	Single dose SC, preferably as measles-mumps-rubella	Teratogenicity of vaccine is theoretic, not confirmed to date; vaccination of susceptible women should be part of postpartum care
Yellow fever	Significant morbidity and mortality; not altered by pregnancy	Unknown	Live attenuated virus vaccine	Unknown	Contraindicated except if exposure is unavoidable	Single dose SC	Postponement of travel preferable to vaccination, if possible

Inactivated Virus Vaccines							
Influenza	Possible increase in morbidity and mortality during epidemic of new antigenic strain	Possible increased abortion rate; no malformations confirmed	Inactivated virus vaccine	None confirmed	Women with serious underlying diseases; public health authorities to be consulted for current recommendation	One dose IM every year	
Rabies	Near 100% fatality; not altered by pregnancy	Determined by maternal disease	Killed virus vaccine	Unknown	Indications for prophylaxis not altered by pregnancy; each case considered individually	Public health authorities to be consulted for indications, dosage, and route of administration	
Hepatitis B	Possible increased severity during third trimester	Possible increase in abortion rate and prematurity; neonatal hepatitis can occur; high risk of newborn carrier state	Recombinant vaccine	None reported	Preexposure and postexposure for women at risk of infection	Three- or four-dose series IM	Used with hepatitis B immune globulin for some exposures; exposed newborn needs vaccination as soon as possible
Inactivated Bacterial Vaccines							
Cholera	Significant morbidity and mortality; more severe during third trimester	Increased risk of fetal death during third-trimester maternal illness	Killed bacterial vaccine	None confirmed	Indications not altered by pregnancy; vaccination recommended only in unusual outbreak situations	Single dose SC or IM, depending on manufacturer's recommendations when indicated	
Plague	Significant morbidity and mortality; not altered by pregnancy	Determined by maternal disease	Killed bacterial vaccine	None reported	Selective vaccination of exposed persons	Public health authorities to be consulted for indications, dosage, and route of administration	
Pneumococcus	No increased risk during pregnancy; no increase in severity of disease	Unknown	Polyvalent polysaccharide vaccine	No data available on use during pregnancy	Indications not altered by pregnancy; vaccine used only for high-risk individuals	In adults, one SC or IM dose only; consider repeat dose in 6 yr for high-risk individuals	
Typhoid	Significant morbidity and mortality; not altered by pregnancy	Unknown	Killed or live attenuated oral bacterial vaccine	None confirmed	Not recommended routinely except for close, continued exposure or travel to endemic areas	*Killed; Primary:* Two injections SC at least 4 wk apart *Booster:* Single dose SC or ID (depending on type of product used) every 3 yr *Oral; Primary:* Four doses on alternate days *Booster:* Schedule not yet determined	

Continued on following page

TABLE 5-20 **Immunizations during Pregnancy** *(Continued)*

Immunobiologic Agent	Risk from Disease to Pregnant Woman	Risk from Disease to Fetus or Neonate	Type of Immunizing Agent	Risk from Immunizing Agent to Fetus	Indications for Immunization during Pregnancy	Dose Schedule	Comments
Toxoids							
Tetanus, diphtheria	Severe morbidity; tetanus mortality 30%, diphtheria mortality 10%; unaltered by pregnancy	Neonatal tetanus mortality 60%	Combined tetanus-diphtheria toxoids preferred: adult tetanus-diphtheria formulation	None confirmed	Lack of primary series, or no booster within past 10 yr	*Primary:* Two doses IM at 1-2 mo interval with a third dose 6-12 mo after the second *Booster:* Single dose IM every 10 yr, after completion of primary series	Updating of immune status should be part of antepartum care
Specific Immune Globulins							
Hepatitis B	Possible increased severity during third trimester	Possible increase in abortion rate and prematurity; neonatal hepatitis can occur; high risk of carriage in newborn	Hepatitis B immune globulin	None reported	Postexposure prophylaxis	Depends on exposure; consult Immunization Practices Advisory Committee recommendations	Usually given with HBV vaccine; exposed newborn needs immediate postexposure prophylaxis
Rabies	Near 100% fatality; not altered by pregnancy	Determined by maternal disease	Rabies immune globulin	None reported	Postexposure prophylaxis	Half dose at injury site, half dose in deltoid	Used in conjunction with rabies killed virus vaccine
Tetanus	Severe morbidity; mortality 21%	Neonatal tetanus mortality 60%	Tetanus immune globulin	None reported	Postexposure prophylaxis	One dose IM	Used in conjunction with tetanus toxoid
Varicella	Possible increase in severe varicella pneumonia	Can cause congenital varicella with increased mortality in neonatal period; very rarely causes congenital defects	Varicella-zoster immune globulin (obtained from the American Red Cross)	None reported	Can be considered for healthy pregnant women exposed to varicella to protect against maternal, not congenital, infection	One dose IM within 96 hr of exposure	Indicated also for newborns of mothers who developed varicella within 4 days before delivery or 2 days after delivery; approximately 90%-95% of adults are immune to varicella; not indicated for prevention of congenital varicella

Standard Immune Globulins							
Hepatitis A	Possible increased severity during third trimester	Probable increase in abortion rate and prematurity; possible transmission to neonate at delivery if mother is incubating the virus or is acutely ill at that time	Standard immune globulin		Postexposure prophylaxis	0.02 ml/kg IM in one dose of immune globulin	Immune globulin should be given as soon as possible and within 2 wk of exposure; infants born to mothers who are incubating the virus or are acutely ill at delivery should receive one dose of 0.5 ml as soon as possible after birth
Measles	Significant morbidity, low mortality; not altered by pregnancy	Significant increase in abortion rate; may cause malformations	Standard immune globulin		Postexposure prophylaxis	0.25 ml/kg IM in one dose of immune globulin, up to 15 ml	Unclear if it prevents abortion; must be given within 6 days of exposure

From *ACOG Technical Bulletin,* No 160, Oct 1991.
ID, Intradermally; *IM,* intramuscularly; *PO,* orally; *SC,* subcutaneously.
*Two doses necessary for adequate vaccination of students entering institutions of higher education, newly hired medical personnel, and international travelers.
†Inactivated polio vaccine recommended for nonimmunized adults at increased risk.

TABLE 5-21 Immunizing Agents and Immunization Schedules for Health Care Workers (HCWs)*

Generic Name	Primary Schedule and Booster(s)	Indications	Major Precautions and Contraindications	Special Considerations
Immunizing Agents Strongly Recommended for Health Care Workers				
Hepatitis B (HB) recombinant vaccine	Two doses IM 4 wk apart; third dose 5 mo after second; booster doses not necessary.	**Preexposure:** HCWs at risk for exposure to blood or body fluids.	Based on limited data no risk of adverse effects to developing fetuses is apparent. Pregnancy should *not* be considered a contraindication to vaccination of women. Previous anaphylactic reaction to common baker's yeast is a contraindication to vaccination.	The vaccine produces neither therapeutic nor adverse effects on HBV-infected persons. Prevaccination serologic screening is not indicated for persons being vaccinated because of occupational risk. HCWs who have contact with patients or blood should be tested 1-2 mo after vaccination to determine serologic response.
Hepatitis B immune globulin (HBIG)	0.06 ml/kg IM as soon as possible after exposure. A second dose of HBIG should be administered 1 mo later if the HB vaccine series has not been started.	**Postexposure prophylaxis:** For persons exposed to blood or body fluids containing HBsAg and who are not immune to HBV infection—0.06 ml/kg IM as soon as possible (but no later than 7 days after exposure).		
Influenza vaccine (inactivated whole-virus and split-virus vaccines)	Annual vaccination with current vaccine. Administered IM.	HCWs who have contact with patients at high risk for influenza or its complications; HCWs who work in chronic care facilities; HCWs with high-risk medical conditions or who are aged ≥65 yr.	History of anaphylactic hypersensitivity to egg ingestion.	No evidence exists of risk to mother or fetus when the vaccine is administered to a pregnant woman with an underlying high-risk condition. Influenza vaccination is recommended during second and third trimesters of pregnancy because of increased risk for hospitalization.
Measles live-virus vaccine	One dose SC; second dose at least 1 mo later.	HCWs† born during or after 1957 who do not have documentation of having received two doses of live vaccine on or after the first birthday **or** a history of physician-diagnosed measles or serologic evidence of immunity. Vaccination should be considered for all HCWs who lack proof of immunity, including those born before 1957.	Pregnancy; immunocompromised persons‡, including HIV-infected persons who have evidence of severe immunosuppression; anaphylaxis after gelatin ingestion or administration of neomycin; recent administration of immune globulin.	MMR is the vaccine of choice if recipients are likely to be susceptible to rubella and/or mumps as well as to measles. Persons vaccinated during 1963-1967 with a killed measles vaccine alone, killed vaccine followed by live vaccine, or with a vaccine of unknown type should be revaccinated with two doses of live measles virus vaccine.

Modified from *MMWR Morb Mortal Wkly Rep* 46(RR-18), 1998.

HBsAg, Hepatitis B surface antigen; *HBV,* hepatitis B virus; *HIV,* human immunodeficiency virus; *IM,* intramuscular; *MMR,* measles, mumps, rubella vaccine; *SC,* subcutaneous.

*Persons who provide health care to patients or work in institutions that provide patient care (e.g., physicians, nurses, emergency medical personnel, dental professionals and students, medical and nursing students, laboratory technicians, hospital volunteers, and administrative and support staff in health care institutions).

†All HCWs (i.e., medical or nonmedical, paid or volunteer, full time or part time, student or nonstudent, with or without patient-care responsibilities) who work in health care institutions (e.g., inpatient and outpatient, public and private) should be immune to measles, rubella, and varicella.

‡Persons immunocompromised because of immune deficiency diseases, HIV infection, leukemia, lymphoma or generalized malignancy or immunosuppressed as a result of therapy with corticosteroids, alkylating drugs, antimetabolites, or radiation.

TABLE 5-21 **Immunizing Agents and Immunization Schedules for Health Care Workers (HCWs)*** *(Continued)*

Generic Name	Primary Schedule and Booster(s)	Indications	Major Precautions and Contraindications	Special Considerations
Mumps live-virus vaccine	One dose SC; second dose at least 1 mo later	HCWs† believed to be susceptible can be vaccinated. Adults born before 1957 can be considered immune.	Pregnancy; immunocompromised persons‡; history of anaphylactic reaction after gelatin ingestion or administration of neomycin	MMR is the vaccine of choice if recipients are likely to be susceptible to measles and rubella as well as to mumps.
Hepatitis A vaccine	Two doses of vaccine either 6-12 mo apart (HAVRIX), or 6 mo apart (VAQTA)	Not routinely indicated for HCWs in the United States. Persons who work with HAV-infected primates or with HAV in a research laboratory setting should be vaccinated.	History of anaphylactic hypersensitivity to alum or, for HAVRIX, the preservative 2-phenoxyethanol. The safety of the vaccine in pregnant women has not been determined; the risk associated with vaccination should be weighed against the risk for hepatitis A in women who may be at high risk for exposure to HAV.	
Meningococcal polysaccharide vaccine (tetravalent A, C, W135, and Y)	One dose in volume and by route specified by manufacturer; need for boosters unknown	Not routinely indicated for HCWs in the United States.	The safety of the vaccine in pregnant women has not been evaluated; it should not be administered during pregnancy unless the risk for infection is high.	
Typhoid vaccine, IM, SC, and oral	IM vaccine: One 0.5-ml dose, booster 0.5 ml every 2 yr. SC vaccine: two 0.5 ml doses, ≥4 wk apart, booster 0.5 ml SC or 0.1 ID every 3 yr if exposure continues *Oral vaccine:* Four doses on alternate days. The manufacturer recommends revaccination with the entire four-dose series every 5 yr	Workers in microbiology laboratories who frequently work with *Salmonella typhi*	Severe local or systemic reaction to a previous dose. Ty21a (oral) vaccine should not be administered to immunocompromised persons† or to persons receiving antimicrobial agents.	Vaccination should not be considered an alternative to the use of proper procedures when handling specimens and cultures in the laboratory.
Vaccinia vaccine (smallpox)	One dose administered with a bifurcated needle; boosters administered every 10 yr	Laboratory workers who directly handle cultures with vaccinia, recombinant vaccinia viruses, or orthopox viruses that infect humans	The vaccine is contraindicated in pregnancy, in persons with eczema or a history of eczema, and in immunocompromised persons† and their household contacts.	Vaccination may be considered for HCWs who have direct contact with contaminated dressings or other infectious material from volunteers in clinical studies involving recombinant vaccinia virus.

Continued on following page

TABLE 5-21 **Immunizing Agents and Immunization Schedules for Health Care Workers (HCWs)*** *(Continued)*

Generic Name	Primary Schedule and Booster(s)	Indications	Major Precautions and Contraindications	Special Considerations
Other Vaccine-Preventable Diseases				
Tetanus and diphtheria (toxoids [Td])	Two IM doses 4 wk apart; third dose 6-12 mo after second dose; booster every 10 yr	All adults	Except in the first trimester, pregnancy is not a precaution. History of a neurologic reaction or immediate hypersensitivity reaction after a previous dose. History of severe local (Arthus-type) reaction after a previous dose. Such persons should not receive further routine or emergency doses of Td for 10 yr.	Tetanus prophylaxis in wound management‡
Pneumococcal polysaccharide vaccine (23 valent)	One dose, 0.5 ml, IM or SC; revaccination recommended for those at highest risk ≥5 yr after the first dose	Adults who are at increased risk of pneumococcal disease and its complications because of underlying health conditions; older adults, especially those age ≥65 who are healthy	The safety of vaccine in pregnant women has not been evaluated; it should not be administered during pregnancy unless the risk for infection is high. Previous recipients of any type of pneumococcal polysaccharide vaccine who are at highest risk for fatal infection or antibody loss may be revaccinated ≥5 yr after the first dose.	
Rubella live-virus vaccine	One dose SC; second dose at least 1 mo later	Indicated for HCWs,† both men and women, who do not have documentation of having received live vaccine on or after their first birthday **or** laboratory evidence of immunity. Adults born before 1957, **except women who can become pregnant,** can be considered immune.	Pregnancy; immunocompromised persons†; history of anaphylactic reaction after administration of neomycin	The risk for rubella vaccine–associated malformations in the offspring of women pregnant when vaccinated or who become pregnant within 3 mo after vaccination is negligible. Such women should be counseled regarding the theoretic basis of concern for the fetus. MMR is the vaccine of choice if recipients are likely to be susceptible to measles or mumps, as well as to rubella.
Varicella zoster live-virus vaccine	Two 0.5-ml doses SC 4-8 wk apart if ≥13 yr of age	Indicated for HCWs† who do not have either a reliable history of varicella or serologic evidence of immunity	Pregnancy, immunocompromised persons,‡ history of anaphylactic reaction following receipt of neomycin or gelatin. Avoid salicylate use for 6 wk after vaccination.	Vaccine is available from the manufacturer for certain patients with acute lymphocytic leukemia (ALL) in remission. Because 71%-93% of persons without a history of varicella are immune, serologic testing before vaccination is likely to be cost-effective.

Modified from *MMWR Morb Mortal Wkly Rep* 46(RR-18), 1998.

*Persons who provide health care to patients or work in institutions that provide patient care (e.g., physicians, nurses, emergency medical personnel, dental professionals and students, medical and nursing students, laboratory technicians, hospital volunteers, and administrative and support staff in health care institutions).

†All HCWs (i.e., medical or nonmedical, paid or volunteer, full time or part time, student or nonstudent, with or without patient-care responsibilities) who work in health care institutions (e.g., inpatient and outpatient, public and private) should be immune to measles, rubella, and varicella.

‡Persons immunocompromised because of immune deficiency diseases, HIV infection, leukemia, lymphoma or generalized malignancy or immunosuppressed as a result of therapy with corticosteroids, alkylating drugs, antimetabolites, or radiation.

TABLE 5-21 **Immunizing Agents and Immunization Schedules for Health Care Workers (HCWs)*** *(Continued)*

Generic Name	Primary Schedule and Booster(s)	Indications	Major Precautions and Contraindications	Special Considerations
Varicella-zoster immune globulin (VZIG)	Persons <50 kg: 125 μ/10 kg IM; persons ≥50 kg: 625 μ§	Persons known or likely to be susceptible (particularly those at high risk for complications, e.g., pregnant women) who have close and prolonged exposure to a contact case or to an infectious hospital staff worker or patient		Serologic testing may help in assessing whether to administer VZIG. If use of VZIG prevents varicella disease, patient should be vaccinated subsequently.
BCG Vaccination				
Bacille Calmette-Guérin (BCG) vaccine (tuberculosis)	One percutaneous dose of 0.3 ml; no booster dose recommended	Should be considered only for HCWs in areas where multidrug tuberculosis is prevalent, a strong likelihood of infection exists, and where comprehensive infection control precautions have failed to prevent TB transmission to HCWs	Should not be administered to immunocompromised persons,‡ pregnant women	In the United States tuberculosis-control efforts are directed toward early identification, treatment of cases, and preventive therapy with isoniazid.
Other Immunobiologics That Are or May Be Indicated for Health Care Workers				
Immune globulin (hepatitis A)	**Postexposure**—One IM dose of 0.02 ml/kg administered ≤2 wk after exposure	Indicated for HCWs exposed to feces of infectious patients	Contraindicated in persons with IgA deficiency; do not administer within 2 wk after MMR vaccine, or 3 wk after varicella vaccine. Delay administration of MMR vaccine for ≥3 mo and varicella vaccine ≥5 mo after administration of IG	Administer in large muscle mass (deltoid, gluteal).

§Some experts recommend 125 μ/10 kg regardless of total body weight.

TABLE 5-22 Recommendations for Persons with Medical Conditions Requiring Special Vaccination Considerations

Condition	Td	MMR	Varicella	HBV	HAV	Pneumovax[a]	Influenza[b]	HbCV	Meningococcal	IPV	Other Live Vaccines[c]	Other Killed Vaccines[d]
HIV infection	Rou	Rou/Contr[e]	Contr[f]	Rou[g]	Rou	Rec	Rec	Cons	Rou	Rou	Contr	Rou
Severe immunocompromise[h]	Rou	Contr	Contr[f]	Rou[g]	Rou	Rec	Rec	Rou[i]	Rou	Rou	Contr	Rou
Renal failure	Rou	Rou	Rou	Rec[g]	Rou	Rec	Rec	Rou	Rou	Rou	Rou	Rou
Diabetes	Rou	Rou	Rou	Rou	Rou	Rec	Rec	Rou	Rou	Rou	Rou	Rou
Chronic liver disease	Rou	Rou	Rou	Rou	Rec	Rec	Rec	Rou	Rou	Rou	Rou	Rou
Cardiac disease	Rou	Rou	Rou	Rou	Rou	Rec	Rec	Rou	Rou	Rou	Rou	Rou
Pulmonary disease	Rou	Rou	Rou	Rou	Rou	Rec	Rec	Rou	Rou	Rou	Rou	Rou
Alcoholism	Rou	Rou	Rou	Rou	Rou	Rec	Rec	Rou	Rou	Rou	Rou	Rou
Functional/anatomic asplenia	Rou	Rou	Rou	Rou	Rou	Rec[j]	Rec	Rec[j]	Rec[j]	Rou	Rou	Rou
Terminal complement deficiency	Rou	Rou	Rou	Rou	Rou	Rou	Rou	Rou	Rec	Rou	Rou	
Clotting factor disorders	Rou	Rou	Rou	Rec	Rec	Rou	Rou	Rou	Rou	Rou	Rou	Rou

Modified and updated from *MMWR Morb Mortal Wkly Rep* 42(RR-4):16 and 17, 1993.

Cons, Consider vaccination; *Contr,* contraindicated; *Rec,* recommended; *Rou,* routine as outlined for all adults.

[a]Pneumovax should be repeated in 5 years for patients in whom vaccine is recommended. Asthma without chronic obstructive pulmonary disease is not an indication for the vaccine.

[b]Influenza vaccine should also be given to caregivers and household members.

[c]Includes bacille Calmette-Guérin, vaccinia, oral typhoid, yellow fever (if exposure cannot be avoided, persons with HIV can be given yellow fever vaccine; see text).

[d]Includes rabies (check postvaccination titers in HIV or severely immunocompromised persons), Lyme, inactivated typhoid, cholera, plague, and anthrax.

[e]For asymptomatic, nonseverely immunocompromised persons with human immunodeficiency virus (HIV), MMR can be used; it is contraindicated in severely immunocompromised persons. MMR can be considered in symptomatic HIV patients without severe immunocompromise.

[f]Varicella can be given to household members and caregivers, but if varicella-like rash develops after vaccination, contact should be avoided.

[g]Recommended for persons with severe chronic renal failure approaching or already receiving dialysis, and higher doses should be given. Antibody titers should be measured after vaccination in these patients and in those with HIV or severe immunocompromise (who may require higher doses) to ensure adequate response. Yearly titers should be measured in dialysis patients.

[h]Severe immunocompromise can result from congenital immunodeficiency, leukemia, lymphoma, malignancy, organ transplant, chemotherapy, radiation therapy, or high-dose corticosteroids.

[i]Only for persons with Hodgkin's disease.

[j]Give at least 2 weeks in advance of elective splenectomy.

TABLE 5-23 **Vaccinations for International Travel**

Disease*	Areas Affected†	Prophylaxis Recommended	Ideal Time between Last Vaccine Dose and Travel
Tetanus	All	All travelers; vaccine series/booster.	Probably 30 days for series Anamnestic response to booster
Measles	All	Born after 1956; ensure immunity by antibody titer, diagnosed measles, or two doses of vaccine.	As MMR, 7-14 days
Rubella	All	Born after 1956 and any female of childbearing age; rubella titer or one dose of vaccine.	As MMR, 7-14 days
Mumps	All	Born after 1956; ensure immunity by antibody titer, diagnosed mumps, or one dose of vaccine.	As MMR, 7-14 days
Varicella	All	All travelers; antibody titer, reported illness, or vaccine series.	7-14 days
Hepatitis B	5%-20% of population are carriers in Africa, Middle East except Israel, all Southeast Asia, Amazon basin, Haiti, and Dominican Republic; 1%-5% of population are carriers in south-central and southwest Asia, Israel, Japan, Americas, Russia, and eastern and southern Europe.	Travelers for more than 6 mo in close contact with population or for less time but with high-risk activities (close household contact, seeking dental or medical care, sex); vaccine series.	Probably 30 days
Hepatitis A	Developing countries.	Travelers to rural areas; eating and drinking in settings of poor sanitation; vaccine or pooled immune globulin (IG).	Vaccine, 30 days Pooled IG, 2 days
Influenza	Tropics throughout the year; southern hemisphere from April to September.	Travelers for whom vaccine is otherwise indicated; give current vaccine and revaccinate in fall as usual.	7-14 days
Meningococcus*	Sub-Saharan Africa "belt" (Senegal to Ethiopia) from December to June; required for pilgrims to Saudi Arabia during Haj; epidemics reported in other African nations, India, Nepal, and Mongolia.	All travelers; vaccine.	7-10 days
Rabies	Endemic dog rabies exists in Mexico, El Salvador, Guatemala, Peru, Colombia, Ecuador, India, Nepal, Philippines, Sri Lanka, Thailand, and Vietnam.	Travelers staying for more than 30 days or at high risk of exposure to domestic or wild animals; vaccine series/booster.	7-14 days
Poliomyelitis	Developing countries not in western hemisphere; at risk all year in tropics; in temperate zones, incidence increases in summer and fall.	All travelers; vaccine series/booster.	Parenteral vaccine series, 28 day (see text) Anamnestic response to booster

Continued on following page

TABLE 5-23 **Vaccinations for International Travel** *(Continued)*

Disease*	Areas Affected†	Prophylaxis Recommended	Ideal Time between Last Vaccine Dose and Travel
Typhoid fever	Many countries in Asia, Africa, Central America, and South America.	Travelers with prolonged stay in rural areas with poor sanitation; vaccine series/booster.	Oral vaccine, 7 days Parenteral vaccine, probably 14 days
Yellow fever*	North and central South America, forest-savannah zones of Africa; some countries in Africa, Asia, and Middle East require travelers from endemic areas to be vaccinated.	All travelers; vaccine/booster at approved yellow fever vaccination center.	10 days
Japanese encephalitis	Seasonally in most areas of Asia, Indian subcontinent, and western Pacific islands; in temperate zones, incidence increases in summer and early fall; in tropics, year-round incidence.	Travelers staying for more than 30 days in high-risk rural areas; staying outdoors during transmission season; vaccine series.	10 days
Cholera*	Certain undeveloped countries.	If required by local authorities, one dose usually suffices; primary series only for those living in high-risk areas under poor sanitary conditions or those with compromised gastric defense mechanisms (achlorhydria, antacid therapy, previous ulcer surgery); booster every 6 mo.	Probably 30 days
Plague	Africa, Asia, and Americas in rural mountainous or upland areas.	Travelers whose research or field activities bring them in contact with rodents; vaccine series/booster; consider taking tetracycline (500 mg four times a day) for chemoprophylaxis (inferred from clinical experience in treating plague).	Probably 30 days

From Noble J: *Primary care medicine,* ed 3, St Louis, 2001, Mosby.

*Only yellow fever vaccine is required for entry by any country; cholera vaccine may be required by some local authorities; and meningococcus vaccine is required for pilgrims to Mecca, Saudia Arabia, during Haj. However, it is important to follow CDC recommendations for all vaccines to prevent disease. If a required vaccine is contraindicated or withheld for any reason, attempts should be made to obtain a waiver from the country's consulate or embassy.

†Because areas affected can change, and for more specific details, consult CDC's traveler's hotline.

Recommendations and Implementation Strategies for Hepatitis B Vaccination of Adults

BOX 5-1 Adults Recommended to Receive Hepatitis B Vaccination

Persons at Risk for Infection by Sexual Exposure
- Sex partners of persons who are hepatitis B surface antigen (HBsAg) positive
- Sexually active persons who are not in a long-term, mutually monogamous relationship (e.g., persons who have had more than one sex partner during the previous 6 months)
- Persons seeking evaluation or treatment for a sexually transmitted disease
- Men who have sex with men

Persons at Risk for Infection by Percutaneous or Mucosal Exposure to Blood
- Current or recent users of injection drugs
- Household contacts of persons who are HBsAg positive
- Residents and staff of facilities for developmentally disabled persons
- Health care and public safety workers with reasonably anticipated risk for exposure to blood or blood-contaminated body fluids
- Persons with end-stage renal disease, including predialysis, hemodialysis, peritoneal dialysis, and home dialysis patients

Others
- International travelers to regions with high or intermediate levels (HBsAg prevalence of ≥2%) of endemic HBV infection
- Persons with chronic liver disease
- Persons with HIV infection
- All other persons seeking protection from HBV infection

From CDC: A comprehensive immunization strategy to eliminate transmission of hepatitis B virus infection in the United States: recommendations of the Advisory Committee on Immunization Practices (ACIP), *MMWR* 55(RR-16):15, 2006.

BOX 5-2 Hepatitis B Vaccine Schedules for Adults (Aged ≥20 Years)*

0, 1, and 6 months
0, 1, and 4 months
0, 2, and 4 months
0, 1, 2, and 12 months†

From CDC: A comprehensive immunization strategy to eliminate transmission of hepatitis B virus infection in the United States: recommendations of the Advisory Committee on Immunization Practices (ACIP), *MMWR* 55(RR-16):15, 2006.

*All schedules are applicable to single-antigen hepatitis B vaccines; Twinrix (combined hepatitis A and hepatitis B vaccine) may be administered at 0, 1, and 6 months.

†A 4-dose schedule of Engerix-B is licensed for all age groups.

TABLE 5-24 Recommended Doses of Currently Licensed Formulations of Adult Hepatitis B Vaccine by Group and Vaccine Type

	Single-Antigen Vaccine				Combination Vaccine	
	RECOMBIVAX HB[a]		ENGERIX-B[b]		TWINRIX[b,c]	
Group	**Dose (μg)[d]**	**Vol. (ml)**	**Dose (μg)[d]**	**Vol. (ml)**	**Dose (μg)[d]**	**Vol. (ml)**
Adults (aged ≥20 years)	10	1.0	20	1.0	20	1.0
Hemodialysis patients and other immunocompromised persons aged ≥20 yrs	40[e]	1.0	40[f]	2.0	—[g]	—

From CDC: A comprehensive immunization strategy to eliminate transmission of hepatitis B virus infection in the United States: recommendations of the Advisory Committee on Immunization Practices (ACIP), *MMWR* 55(RR-16):10, 2006.

[a]Merck & Co., Inc., Whitehouse Station, New Jersey.

[b]GlaxoSmithKline Biologicals, Rixensart, Belgium.

[c]Combined hepatitis A and hepatitis B vaccine, recommended for persons aged >18 years who are at increased risk for both hepatitis B virus and hepatitis A virus infections.

[d]Recombinant hepatitis B surface-antigen protein dose.

[e]Dialysis formulation administered on a 3-dose schedule at 0, 1, and 6 months.

[f]Two 1.0-ml doses administered in 1 or 2 injections on a 4-dose schedule at 0, 1, 2, and 6 months.

[g]Not applicable.

TABLE 5-25 Recommended HIV/AIDS, Sexually Transmitted Disease (STD), and Viral Hepatitis Prevention Services by Risk Population

Risk Population[a]	Recommended Services
High-Risk Heterosexuals	
Persons seeking STD evaluation or treatment	Hepatitis B vaccination Testing for human immunodeficiency virus (HIV) infection[b] Testing for syphilis, gonorrhea, and chlamydia, as clinically indicated[c]
Sexually active men not in a long-term, mutually monogamous relationship	Hepatitis B vaccination Annual testing for HIV infection[b,d]
Sexually active women not in a long-term, mutually monogamous relationship	Hepatitis B vaccination[e] Annual testing for HIV infection[b,d] Annual testing for chlamydia (NOTE: Also recommended for all sexually active females aged <25 yrs)[c]
Men Who Have Sex with Men (MSM)	
All MSM	Hepatitis A vaccination Hepatitis B vaccination[e]
Sexually active MSM not in a long-term, mutually monogamous relationship	Hepatitis A vaccination Hepatitis B vaccination[e] Annual testing for HIV infection[b] Annual testing for syphilis, gonorrhea, and chlamydia[c]
Injection-Drug Users	Hepatitis A vaccination[f] Hepatitis B vaccination Testing for hepatitis C virus infection[g] Annual testing for HIV infection[b] Substance-abuse treatment[h]

From CDC: A comprehensive immunization strategy to eliminate transmission of hepatitis B virus infection in the United States: recommendations of the Advisory Committee on Immunization Practices (ACIP), *MMWR* 55(RR-16):17, 2006.

[a]Testing for HIV infection, chlamydia, gonorrhea, syphilis, and hepatitis B surface antigen also is recommended for pregnant women. (CDC: Revised recommendations for HIV testing of adults, adolescents, and pregnant women in health care settings, *MMWR* 55[RR-14], 2006; CDC: Sexually transmitted diseases treatment guidelines, *MMWR* 55[RR-11], 2006; CDC: A comprehensive immunization strategy to eliminate transmission of hepatitis B virus infection in the United States: recommendations of the Advisory Committee on Immunization Practices [ACIP]. Part 1: immunization of infants, children, and adolescents, *MMWR* 54[RR-16], 2005.)

[b]CDC: Revised recommendations for HIV testing of adults, adolescents, and pregnant women in health care settings, *MMWR* 55(RR-14), 2006.

[c]CDC: Sexually transmitted diseases treatment guidelines 2006, *MMWR* 55(RR-11), 2006.

[d]HIV screening is recommended for all persons aged 13-64 years. Repeat screening is recommended at least annually for persons likely to be at high risk for HIV infection, including MSM or heterosexuals who themselves or whose sex partners have had more than one partner since their most recent HIV test.

[e]Hepatitis B vaccination is recommended for persons who have had more than one sex partner during the previous 6 months.

[f]CDC: Prevention of hepatitis A through active or passive immunization: recommendations of the Advisory Committee on Immunization Practices (ACIP), *MMWR* 55(RR-7), 2006.

[g]CDC: Recommendations for prevention and control of hepatitis C virus (HCV) infection and HCV-related chronic disease, *MMWR* 47(RR-19), 1998. Recommended frequency of testing for hepatitis C virus infection has not been determined.

[h]CDC: Substance abuse treatment for injection drug users: a strategy with many benefits, Atlanta, GA, 2002, U.S. Department of Health and Human Services, CDC. Available at http://www.cdc.gov/idu/facts/treatment.htm.

TABLE 5-26 **Guidelines for Postexposure Prophylaxis* of Persons with Nonoccupational Exposures† to Blood or Body Fluids that Contain Blood by Exposure Type and Vaccination Status**

	TREATMENT	
Exposure	**Unvaccinated Person§**	**Previously Vaccinated Person¶**
HBsAg-Positive Source**		
Percutaneous (e.g., bite or needlestick) or mucosal exposure to HBsAg-positive blood or body fluids	Administer hepatitis B vaccine series and hepatitis B immune globulin (HBIG)	Administer hepatitis B vaccine booster dose
Sex or needle-sharing contact of a person who is HBsAg positive	Administer hepatitis B vaccine series and HBIG	Administer hepatitis B vaccine booster dose
Victim of sexual assault/abuse by a perpetrator who is HBsAg positive	Administer hepatitis B vaccine series and HBIG	Administer hepatitis B vaccine booster dose
Source with Unknown HBsAg Status		
Victim of sexual assault/abuse by a perpetrator with unknown HBsAg status	Administer hepatitis B vaccine series	No treatment
Percutaneous (e.g., bite or needlestick) or mucosal exposure to potentially infectious blood or body fluids from a source with unknown HBsAg status	Administer hepatitis B vaccine series	No treatment
Sexual or needle-sharing contact of person with unknown HBsAg status	Administer hepatitis B vaccine series	No treatment

From CDC: A comprehensive immunization strategy to eliminate transmission of hepatitis B Virus Infection in the United States: recommendations of the Advisory Committee on Immunization Practices (ACIP), *MMWR* 55(RR-16):30, 2006.

*When indicated, immunoprophylaxis should be initiated as soon as possible, preferably within 24 hours. Studies are limited on the maximum interval after exposure during which postexposure prophylaxis is effective, but the interval is unlikely to exceed 7 days for percutaneous exposures or 14 days for sexual exposures. The hepatitis B vaccine series should be completed.

†These guidelines apply to nonoccupational exposures. Guidelines for management of occupational exposures have been published separately and also can be used for management of nonoccupational exposures if feasible.

§A person who is in the process of being vaccinated but has not completed the vaccine series should complete the series and receive treatment as indicated.

¶A person who has written documentation of a complete hepatitis B vaccine series and did not receive postvaccination testing.

**Hepatitis B surface antigen.

TABLE 5-27 **Typical Interpretation of Serologic Test Results for Hepatitis B Virus Infection**

SEROLOGIC MARKER				
HBsAg[a]	**Total Anti-HBc[b]**	**IgM[c] Anti-HBc**	**Anti-HBs[d]**	**Interpretation**
–[e]	–	–	–	Never infected
+[f,g]	–	–	–	Early acute infection; transient (up to 18 days) after vaccination
+	+	+	–	Acute infection
–	+	+	+ or –	Acute resolving infection
–	+	–	+	Recovered from past infection and immune
+	+	–	–	Chronic infection
–	+	–	–	False-positive (i.e., susceptible), past infection, "low-level" chronic infection,[h] or passive transfer of anti-HBc to infant born to mother who is HBsAg positive
–	–	–	+	Immune if concentration is >10 mIU/ml after vaccine series completion;[i] passive transfer after hepatitis B immune globulin administration

From CDC: A comprehensive immunization strategy to eliminate transmission of hepatitis B virus infection in the United States: recommendations of the Advisory Committee on Immunization Practices (ACIP), *MMWR* 55(RR-16):4, 2006.

[a]Hepatitis B surface antigen.

[b]Antibody to hepatitis B core antigen.

[c]Immunoglobulin M.

[d]Antibody to HBsAg.

[e]Negative test result.

[f]Positive test result.

[g]To ensure that an HBsAg-positive test result is not a false-positive, samples with reactive HBsAg results should be tested with a licensed neutralizing confirmatory test if recommended in the manufacturer's package insert.

[h]Persons positive only for anti-HBc are unlikely to be infectious except under unusual circumstances in which they are the source for direct percutaneous exposure of susceptible recipients to large quantities of virus (e.g., blood transfusion or organ transplant).

[i]Milliinternational units per milliliter.

Hepatitis A Prophylaxis

TABLE 5-28 Recommended Dosages of Hepatitis A Immune Globulin

Setting	Duration of Coverage	Dose (ml per kg)
Preexposure prophylaxis	Short term (i.e., less than 3 months)	0.02
	Long term (i.e., 3-5 months)*	0.06
Postexposure prophylaxis	—	0.02

Adapted from CDC: Prevention of hepatitis A through active or passive immunization: recommendations of the Advisory Committee on Immunization Practices (ACIP), *MMWR* 55(RR-07):9, 2006.

NOTE: Immune globulin should be administered intramuscularly into the deltoid or gluteal muscle in children younger than 24 months, it may be administered in the anterolateral thigh muscle.

*Repeat every 5 months if continued exposure to hepatitis A virus occurs.

TABLE 5-29 Licensed Dosages of Hepatitis A Vaccines

Vaccine	Patient's Age	Dose	Volume (ml)	Number of Doses	Schedule (Months)*
Hepatitis A vaccine, inactivated (Havrix)	12 months to 18 years	720 EL.U.	0.5	2	0, 6-12
	19 years or older	1,440 EL.U.	1.0	2	0, 6-12
Hepatitis A vaccine, inactivated (Vaqta)	12 months to 18 years	25 U	0.5	2	0, 6-18
	19 years or older	50 U	1.0	2	0, 6-18
Combined hepatitis A and hepatitis B vaccine (Twinrix)	18 years or older	720 EL.U. of hepatitis A antigen and 20 mcg of hepatitis B surface antigen protein	1.0	3	0, 1, and 6

Adapted from CDC: Prevention of hepatitis A through active or passive immunization: recommendations of the Advisory Committee on Immunization Practices (ACIP), *MMWR* 55(RR-07):10, 2006.

*Zero represents the timing of the initial dose, subsequent numbers represent months after the initial dose.

Influenza Treatment and Prophylaxis

TABLE 5-30 Recommended Daily Dosage of Influenza Antiviral Medications for Treatment and Prophylaxis

	AGE GROUP (YRS)				
Antiviral Agent	**1-6**	**7-9**	**10-12**	**13-64**	**≥65**
Zanamivir*					
Treatment,influenza A and B	–	10 mg (2 inhalations) twice daily	10 mg (2 inhalations) twice daily	10 mg (2 inhalations) twice daily	10 mg (2 inhalations) twice daily
	1-4	**5-9**			
Chemoprophylaxis influenza A and B	–	10 mg (2 inhalations) once daily	10 mg (2 inhalations) once daily	10 mg (2 inhalations) once daily	10 mg (2 inhalations) once daily
Oseltamivir					
Treatment,§ influenza A and B	Dose varies by child's weight¶	Dose varies by child's weight¶	Dose varies by child's weight¶	75 mg twice daily	75 mg twice daily
Chemoprophylaxis influenza A and B	Dose varies by child's weight**	Dose varies by child's weight**	Dose varies by child's weight**	75 mg once daily	75 mg once daily

Modified from *MMWR* 56(RR-6), 2007.

NOTE: Zanamivir is manufactured by GlaxoSmithKline (Relenza—inhaled powder). Zanamivir is approved for treatment of persons ≥7 years and approved for chemoprophylaxis of persons aged ≥5 years. Oseltamivir is manufactured by Roche Pharmaceuticals (Tamiflu—tablet). Oseltamivir is approved for treatment or chemoprophylaxis of persons aged ≥1 year. No antiviral medications are approved for treatment or chemoprophylaxis of influenza among children <1 year. This information is based on data published by the Food and Drug Administration (available at http://www.fda.gov).

*Zanamivir is administered through oral inhalation by using a plastic device included in the medication package. Patients will benefit from instruction and demonstration of correct use of the device. Zanamivir is not recommended for those persons with underlying airway disease.

†Not applicable.

§A reduction in the dose of oseltamivir is recommended for pesons with creatinine clearance <30 ml/min.

¶The treatment dosing recommendation for children weighing ≤15 kg is 30 mg twice a day; for children weighing >15-23 kg, the dose is 45 mg twice a day; for children weighing >23-40 kg, the dose is 60 mg twice a day; and for children weighing >40 kg, the dose is 75 mg twice a day.

**The chemoprophylaxis dosing recommendation for children weighing ≤15 kg is 30 mg once a day; for children weighing >15-23 kg, the dose is 45 mg once a day; for children weighing >23-40 kg, the dose is 60 mg once a day; and for children weighing >40 kg, the dose is 75 mg once a day.

BOX 5-3 Persons for Whom Annual Vaccination Is Recommended

Annual vaccination against influenza is recommended for

- All persons, including school-aged children, who want to reduce the risk of becoming ill with influenza or of transmitting influenza to others
- All children aged 6-59 months (i.e., 6 months-4 years)
- All persons aged ≥50 years
- Children and adolescents (aged 6 months-18 years) receiving long-term aspirin therapy who therefore might be at risk for experiencing Reye's syndrome after influenza virus infection
- Women who will become pregnant during the influenza season
- Adults and children who have chronic pulmonary (including asthma), cardiovascular (except hypertension), renal, hepatic, hematologic or metabolic disorders (including diabetes mellitus)
- Adults and children who have immunosuppression (including immunosuppression caused by medications or by human immunodeficiency virus)
- Adults and children who have any conditions (e.g., cognitive dysfunction, spinal cord injuries, seizure disorders, or other neuromuscular disorders) that can compromise respiratory function or the handling of respiratory secretions or that can increase the risk for aspiration
- Residents of nursing homes and other chronic-care facilities
- Health care personnel
- Healthy household contacts (including children) and caregivers of children aged <5 years and adults aged ≥50 years, with particular emphasis on vaccinating contacts of children aged <6 months
- Healthy household contacts (including children) and caregivers of persons with medical conditions that put them at higher risk for severe complications from influenza

Modified from *MMWR* 56(RR-6), 2007.

TABLE 5-31 **Live, Attenuated Influenza Vaccine (LAIV) Compared with Inactivated Influenza Vaccine (TIV)**

Factor	LAIV	TIV
Route of administration	Intranasal spray	Intramuscular injection
Type of vaccine	Live virus	Killed virus
Number of included virus strains	3 (2 influenza A, 1 influenza B)	3 (2 influenza A, 1 influenza B)
Vaccine virus strains updated	Annually	Annually
Frequency of administration	Annually*	Anually*
Approved age and risk groups§	Healthy persons aged 5-49 years	Persons aged ≥6 mos
Interval between 2 doses recommended for children aged ≥ 6 months-8 years who are receiving influenza vaccine for the first time	6-10 weeks	4 weeks
Can be administered to family members or close contacts of immunosuppressed persons not requiring a protected environment	Yes	Yes
Can be administered to family members or close contacts of immunosuppressed persons requiring a protected environment (e.g., hematopoietic stem cell transplant recipient)	No	Yes
Can be administered to family members or close contacts of persons at high risk but not severely immunosuppressed	Yes	Yes
Can be simultaneously administered with other vaccines	Yes¶	Yes**
If not simultaneously administered, can be administered within 4 weeks of another live vaccine	Prudent to space 4 weeks apart	Yes
If not simultaneously administered, can be administered within 4 weeks of an inactivated vaccine	Yes	Yes

Modified from *MMWR* 56(RR-6), 2007.

*Children aged ≥6 months who have never received influenza vaccine before should receive 2 doses. Those who received only 1 dose in their first year of vaccination should receive 2 doses in the following year.

†LAIV is currently licensed to be administered only to persons aged ≥5 years.

§Annual vaccination against influenza is recommended for (1) all persons, including school-aged children, who want to reduce the risk of becoming ill with influenza or of transmitting influenza to others; (2) all children aged 6-59 months (i.e., 6 months-4 years); all persons aged ≥50 years; (3) children and adolescents (aged 6 months-18 years) receiving long-term aspirin therapy who therefore might be at risk for experiencing Reye's syndrome after influenza virus infection; (4) women who will be pregnant during the influenza season; (5) adults and children who have chronic pulmonary (including asthma), cardiovascular (except hypertension), renal, hepatic, hematologic or metabolic disorders (including diabetes mellitus); (6) adults and children who have immunosuppression (including immunosuppression caused by medications or by human immunodeficiency virus); (7) adults and children who have any condition (e.g., cognitive dysfunction, spinal cord injuries, seizure disorders, or other neuromuscular disorders) that can compromise respiratory function or the handling of respiratory secretions or that can increase the risk for aspiration; (8) residents of nursing homes and other chronic-care facilities; (9) health care workers; (10) healthy household contacts (including children) and caregivers of children aged <5 years and adults aged ≥50 years, with particular focus on vaccinating contacts of children aged <6 months; and (11) healthy household contacts (including children) and caregivers of persons with medical conditions that put them at higher risk for severe complications from influenza. However, no vaccine is approved for children aged <6 months.

¶No data are available regarding effect on safety or efficacy.

**Inactivated influenza vaccine coadministration has been evaluated systematically only among adults with pneumococcal polysaccharide vaccine.

TABLE 5-32 **Approved Influenza Vaccines for Different Age Groups—United States**

Vaccine	Trade Name	Manufacturer	Presentation	Thimerosal Mercury Content (mcg Hg/0.5 ml dose)	Age Group	Number of Doses	Route
TIV[a]	Fluzone	Sanofi Pasteur	0.25-ml prefilled syringe	0	6-35 months	1 or 2[b]	Intramuscular[c]
			0.5-ml prefilled syringe	0	≥36 months	1 or 2[b]	Intramuscular[c]
			0.5-ml vial	0	≥36 months	1 or 2[b]	Intramuscular[c]
			5.0-ml multidose vial	25	≥6 months	1 or 2[b]	Intramuscular[c]
TIV[a]	Fluvirin	Novartis Vaccine	5.0-ml multidose vial	24.5	≥4 years	1 or 2[b]	Intramuscular[c]
TIV[a]	Fluarix	GlaxoSmithKline	0.5-ml prefilled syringe	<1.0	≥18 years	1	Intramuscular[c]
TIV[a]	FluLuval	GlaxoSmithKline	5.0-ml multidose vial	25	≥18 years	1	Intramuscular[c]
LAIV[d]	FluMist[e]	MedImmune	0.2-ml sprayer	0	5-49 years	1 or 2[f]	Intranasal

Modified from *MMWR* 56(RR-6), 2007.

[a]Trivalent inactivated vaccine (TIV). A 0.5-ml dose contains 15 mcg each of A/Solomon Islands/3/2006 (H1N1)-like, A/Wisconsin/67/2005 (H3N2)-like, and B/Malaysia/2506/2004-like antigens.

[b]Two doses administered at least 1 month apart are recommended for children aged 6 months-8 years who are receiving TIV for the first time, and those who only received 1 dose in their first year of vaccination should receive 2 doses in the following year.

[c]For adults and older children, the recommended site of vaccination is the deltoid muscle. The preferred site for infants and young children is the anterolateral aspect of the thigh.

[d]Live, attenuated influenza vaccine (LAIV).

[e]FluMist dosage and storage requirements have changed since the 2007-2008 influenza season. FluMist is now shipped to end users at 35° F-46° F (2° C-8° C). LAIV should be stored at 35° F-46° F (2° C-8° C) upon receipt and should remain at that temperature until the expiration date is reached. The dose is 0.2 ml, divided equally between each nostril.

[f]Two doses administered at least six weeks apart are recommended for children aged 5-8 years who are receiving LAIV for the first time, and those who received only 1 dose in their first year of vaccination should receive 2 doses in the following year.

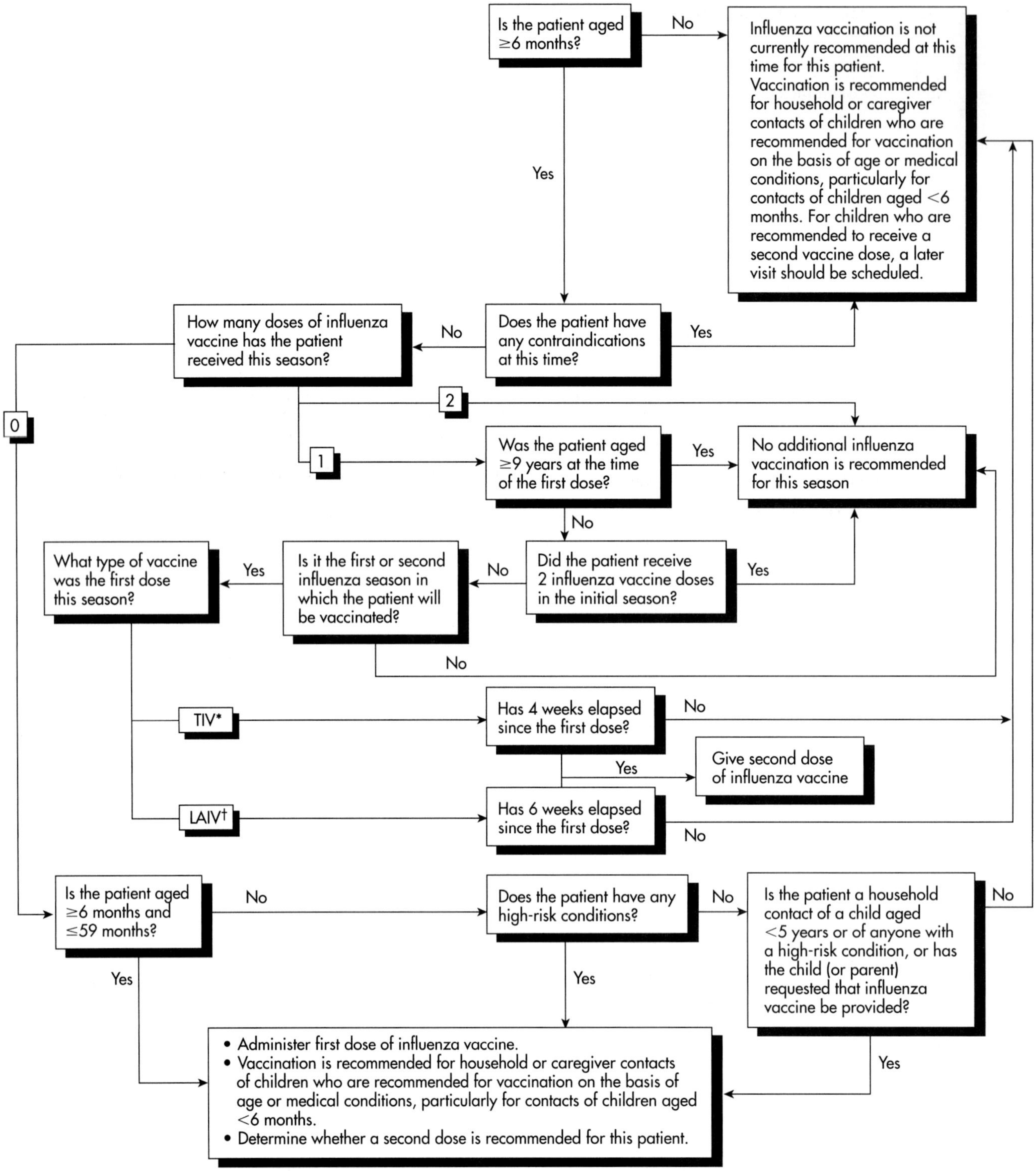

*Trivalent inactivated influenza vaccine.
†Live, attenuated influenza vaccine.

FIGURE 5-6 Algorithm for determining recommended influenza immunization actions for children. (Modified with permission from the American Academy of Pediatrics' Committee on Infectious Diseases: Prevention of influenza: recommendations for influenza immunization of children, 2006-2007, *Pediatrics* 119:846-51.315, 2007.)

HIV Testing and Postexposure Prophylaxis

RECOMMENDATIONS FOR HIV TESTING OF ADULTS, ADOLESCENTS, AND PREGNANT WOMEN

RECOMMENDATIONS FOR ADULTS AND ADOLESCENTS*

CDC recommends that diagnostic human immunodeficiency virus (HIV) testing and opt-out HIV screening be a part of routine clinical care in all health care settings while also preserving the patient's option to decline HIV testing and ensuring a provider-patient relationship conducive to optimal clinical and preventive care. The recommendations are intended for providers in all health care settings, including hospital emergency departments, urgent-care clinics, inpatient services, sexually transmitted disease (STD) clinics or other venues offering clinical STD services, tuberculosis (TB) clinics, substance abuse treatment clinics, other public health clinics, community clinics, correctional health care facilities, and primary care settings. The guidelines address HIV testing in health care settings only; they do not modify existing guidelines concerning HIV counseling, testing, and referral for persons at high risk for HIV who seek or receive HIV testing in nonclinical settings (e.g., community-based organizations, outreach settings, or mobile vans).

SCREENING FOR HIV INFECTION

- In all health care settings, screening for HIV infection should be performed routinely for all patients aged 13-64 years. Health care providers should initiate screening unless prevalence of undiagnosed HIV infection in their patients has been documented to be <0.1%. In the absence of existing data for HIV prevalence, health care providers should initiate voluntary HIV screening until they establish that the diagnostic yield is <1 per 1000 patients screened, at which point such screening is no longer warranted.
- All patients initiating treatment for TB should be screened routinely for HIV infection.
- All patients seeking treatment for STDs, including all patients visiting STD clinics, should be screened routinely for HIV during each visit for a new complaint, regardless of whether the patient is known or suspected to have specific behavior risks for HIV infection.

REPEAT SCREENING

- Health care providers should subsequently test all persons likely to be at high risk for HIV at least annually. Persons likely to be at high risk include users of injection drugs and their sex partners, persons who exchange sex for money or drugs, sex partners of persons who are HIV infected, and men who have sex with men (MSM) or heterosexual persons who themselves or whose sex partners have had more than one sex partner since their most recent HIV test.
- Health care providers should encourage patients and their prospective sex partners to be tested before initiating a new sexual relationship.
- Repeat screening of persons not likely to be at high risk for HIV should be performed on the basis of clinical judgment.
- Unless recent HIV test results are immediately available, any person whose blood or body fluid is the source of an occupational exposure for a health care provider should be informed of the incident and tested for HIV infection at the time the exposure occurs.

CONSENT AND PRETEST INFORMATION

- Screening should be voluntary and undertaken only with the patient's knowledge and understanding that HIV testing is planned.
- Patients should be informed orally or in writing that HIV testing will be performed unless they decline (opt-out screening). Oral or written information should include an explanation of HIV infection and the meanings of positive and negative test results, and the patient should be offered an opportunity to ask questions and to decline testing. With such notification, consent for HIV screening should be incorporated into the patient's general informed consent for medical care on the same basis as are other screening or diagnostic tests; a separate consent form for HIV testing is not recommended.
- Easily understood informational materials should be made available in the languages of the commonly encountered populations within the service area. The competence of interpreters and bilingual staff to provide language assistance to patients with limited English proficiency must be ensured.
- If a patient declines an HIV test, this decision should be documented in the medical record.

DIAGNOSTIC TESTING FOR HIV INFECTION

- All patients with signs or symptoms consistent with HIV infection or an opportunistic illness characteristic of acquired immunodeficiency syndrome (AIDS) should be tested for HIV.
- Clinicians should maintain a high level of suspicion for acute HIV infection in all patients who have a compatible clinical syndrome and who report recent high-risk behavior. When acute retroviral syndrome is a possibility, a plasma RNA test should be used in conjunction with an HIV antibody test to diagnose acute HIV infection.
- Patients or persons responsible for the patient's care should be notified orally that testing is planned, advised of the indication for testing and the implications of positive and negative test results, and offered an opportunity to ask questions and to decline testing. With such notification, the patient's general consent for medical care is considered sufficient for diagnostic HIV testing.

HIV SCREENING FOR PREGNANT WOMEN AND THEIR INFANTS*

Universal Opt-Out Screening

- All pregnant women in the United States should be screened for HIV infection.
- Screening should occur after a woman is notified that HIV screening is recommended for all pregnant patients and that she will receive an HIV test as part of the routine panel of prenatal tests unless she declines (opt-out screening).
- HIV testing must be voluntary and free from coercion. No woman should be tested without her knowledge.
- Pregnant women should receive oral or written information that includes an explanation of HIV infection, a description of interventions that can reduce HIV transmission from mother to infant, and the meanings of positive and negative test results. They should be offered an opportunity to ask questions and to decline testing.
- No additional process or written documentation of informed consent beyond what is required for other routine prenatal tests should be required for HIV testing.
- If a patient declines an HIV test, this decision should be documented in the medical record.

Addressing Reasons for Declining Testing

- Providers should discuss and address reasons for declining an HIV test (e.g., lack of perceived risk, fear of the disease, and concerns regarding partner violence or potential stigma or discrimination).

*From *MMWR* 55(RR-14), 2006.

- Women who decline an HIV test because they have had a previous negative test result should be informed of the importance of retesting during each pregnancy.
- Logistical reasons for not testing (e.g., scheduling) should be resolved.
- Certain women who initially decline an HIV test might accept at a later date, especially if their concerns are discussed. Certain women will continue to decline testing, and their decisions should be respected and documented in the medical record.

Timing of HIV Testing

- To promote informed and timely therapeutic decisions, health care providers should test women for HIV as early as possible during each pregnancy. Women who decline the test early in prenatal care should be encouraged to be tested at a subsequent visit.
- A second HIV test during the third trimester, preferably <36 weeks of gestation, is cost-effective even in areas of low HIV prevalence and may be considered for all pregnant women. A second HIV test during the third trimester is recommended for women who meet one or more of the following criteria:
    - Women who receive health care in jurisdictions with elevated incidence of HIV or AIDS among women aged 15 to 45 years. In 2004, these jurisdictions included Alabama, Connecticut, Delaware, the District of Columbia, Florida, Georgia, Illinois, Louisiana, Maryland, Massachusetts, Mississippi, Nevada, New Jersey, New York, North Carolina, Pennsylvania, Puerto Rico, Rhode Island, South Carolina, Tennessee, Texas, and Virginia.†
    - Women who receive health care in facilities in which prenatal screening identifies at least one pregnant woman who is infected with HIV per 1000 women screened.
    - Women who are known to be at high risk for acquiring HIV (e.g., users of injection drugs and their sex partners, women who exchange sex for money or drugs, women who are sex partners of persons who are infected with HIV, and women who have had a new or more than one sex partner during this pregnancy).
    - Women who have signs or symptoms consistent with acute HIV infection. When acute retroviral syndrome is a possibility, a plasma RNA test should be used in conjunction with an HIV antibody test to diagnose acute HIV infection.

Rapid Testing during Labor

- Any woman with undocumented HIV status at the time of labor should be screened with a rapid HIV test unless she declines (opt-out screening).
- Reasons for declining a rapid test should be explored (see "Addressing Reasons for Declining Testing").
- Immediate initiation of appropriate antiretroviral prophylaxis should be recommended to women on the basis of a reactive rapid test result without waiting for the result of a confirmatory test.

Postpartum/Newborn Testing

- When a woman's HIV status is still unknown at the time of delivery, she should be screened immediately postpartum with a rapid HIV test unless she declines (opt-out screening).
- When the mother's HIV status is unknown postpartum, rapid testing of the newborn as soon as possible after birth is recommended so that antiretroviral prophylaxis can be offered to infants exposed to HIV. Women should be informed that identifying HIV antibodies in the newborn indicates that the mother is infected.
- For infants whose HIV exposure status is unknown and who are in foster care, the person legally authorized to provide consent should be informed that rapid HIV testing is recommended for infants whose biologic mothers have not been tested.
- The benefits of neonatal antiretroviral prophylaxis are best realized when it is initiated ≤ 12 hours after birth.

Confirmatory Testing

- Whenever possible, uncertainties regarding laboratory test results indicating HIV infection status should be resolved before final decisions are made regarding reproductive options, antiretroviral therapy, cesarean delivery, or other interventions.
- If the confirmatory test result is not available before delivery, immediate initiation of appropriate antiretroviral prophylaxis should be recommended to any pregnant patient whose HIV screening test result is reactive to reduce the risk for perinatal transmission.

†A second HIV test in the third trimester is as cost-effective as other common health interventions when HIV incidence among women of childbearing age is ≥ 17 HIV cases per 100,000 person-years. In 2004, in jurisdictions with available data on HIV case rates, a rate of 17 new HIV diagnoses per year per 100,000 women aged 15 to 45 years was associated with an AIDS case rate of at least nine AIDS diagnoses per year per 100,000 women aged 15 to 45 years (CDC, unpublished data, 2005). As of 2004, the jurisdictions listed above exceeded these thresholds. The list of specific jurisdictions where a second test in the third trimester is recommended will be updated periodically based on surveillance data.

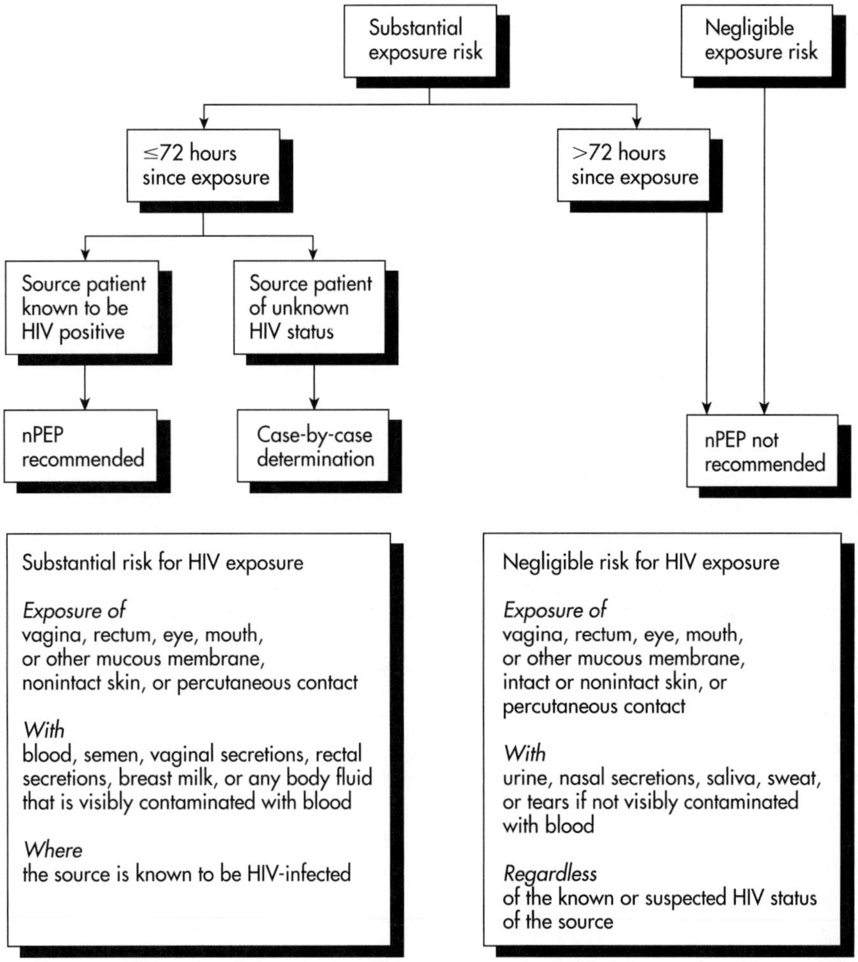

FIGURE 5-7 Algorithm for evaluation and treatment of possible nonoccupational HIV exposure. *nPEP,* Nonoccupational postexposure prophylaxis. (Modified from *MMWR Morb Mort Wkly Rep* 54[RR-2], 2005.)

TABLE 5-33 **HIV Exposure, Estimated Per-Act Risk**

Exposure Route	Risk per 10,000 Exposures to an Infected Source
Blood transfusion	9,000
Needle-sharing injection-drug use	67
Receptive anal intercourse	50
Percutaneous needle stick	30
Receptive penile-vaginal intercourse	10
Insertive anal intercourse	6.5
Insertive penile-vaginal intercourse	5
Receptive oral intercourse	1
Insertive oral intercourse	0.5

Modified from *MMWR Morb Mort Wkly Rep* 54(RR-2), 2005.
Estimates of risk for transmission from sexual exposures assume no condom use.
Source refers to oral intercourse performed on a man.

TABLE 5-34 **Antiretroviral Regimens for Nonoccupational Postexposure Prophylaxis of HIV Infection**

Preferred Regimens	
NNRTI*-based	Efavirenz† plus (lamivudine or emtricitabine) plus (zidovudine or tenofovir)
Protease inhibitor (PI)-based	Lopinavir/ritonavir (co-formulated as Kaletra) plus (lamivudine or emtricitabine) plus zidovudine
Alternative Regimens	
NNRTI-based	Efavirenz plus (lamivudine or emtricitabine) plus abacavrir or didanosine or stavudine§
PI-based	Atazanavir plus (lamivudine or emtricitabine) plus (zidovudine or stavudine or abacavir or didanosine) or (tenofovir plus ritonavir [100 mg/day])
	Fosamprenavir plus (lamivudine or emtricitabine) plus (zidovudine or stavudine) or (abacavir or tenofovir or didanosine)
	Fosamprenavir/ritonavir¶ plus (lamivudine or emtricitabine) plus (zidovudine or stavudine or abacavir or tenofovir or didanosine)
	Indinavir/ritonavir¶** plus (lamivudine or emtricitabine) plus (zidovudine or stavudine or abacavir or tenofovir or didanosine)
	Lopinavir/ritonavir (co-formulated as Kaletra) plus (lamivudine or emtricitabine) plus (stavudine or abacavir or tenofovir or idanosine)
	Nelfinavir plus (lamivudine or emtricitabine) plus (zidovudine or stavudine or abacavir or tenofovir or didanosine)
	Saquinavir (hgc* or sgc*)/ritonavir† plus (lamivudine or emtricitabine) plus (zidovudine or stavudine or abacavir or tenofovir or didanosine)
Triple NRTI*	Abacavir plus lamivudine plus zidovudine (only when an NONRTI- or PI-based regimen cannot or should not be used)

Modified from *MMWR Morb Mort Wkly Rep* 54(RR-2), 2005.
*NNRTI = nonnucleoside reverse transcriptase inhibitor; NRTI = nucleoside reverse transcriptase inhibitor; sgc = soft-gel saquinavir capsule (Fortovase); hgc = hard-gel saquinavir capsule (Invirase).
†Efavirenz should be avoided in pregnant women and women of childbearing potential.
§Higher incidence of lipoatrophy, hyperlipidemia, and mitochondrial toxicities associated with stavudine than with other NRTIs.
¶Low-dose (100–400 mg) ritonavir. See Table 5-31 for doses used with specific PIs.
**Use of ritonavir with indinavir might increase risk for renal adverse events.
Source: U.S. Department of Health and Human Services. Guidelines for the use of antiretroviral agents in HIV-infected adults and adolescents, October 29, 2004 revision. Available at http://www.aidsinfo.nih.gov/guidelines/default_db2.asp?id=50. This document is updated periodically; refer to website for updated versions.

TABLE 5-35 Highly Active Antiretroviral Therapy Medications, Adult Dosage, Cost, and Side Effects

MEDICATION	ADULT DOSAGE*	COST (IN DOLLARS) FOR 4 WEEKS†	SIDE EFFECTS AND TOXICITIES
Combination Tablets			
Lopinavir/ritonavir (Kaletra)§	3 tablets twice daily 400 mg lopinavir/100 mg ritonavir	650	Diarrhea, nausea, vomiting; asthenia; elevated transaminases; hyperglycemia; fat redistribution; lipid abnormalities; possible increased bleeding in persons with hemophilia; and pancreatitis
Zidovudine/lamivudine (Combivir)	1 tablet twice daily 300 mg zidovudine/150 mg lamivudine	640	See following individual medications
Zidovudine/lamivudine/abacavir (Trizivir)	1 tablet twice daily 300 mg zidovudine/150 mg lamivudine/ 300 mg abacavir	1,020	See following individual medications
Lamivudine/abacavir (Epzicom)	1 tablet once daily 300 mg lamivudine/600 mg abacavir	760	See following individual medications
Emtricitabine/tenofovir (Truvada)	1 tablet once daily 200 mg emtricitabine/300 mg tenofovir	800	See following individual medications
Single Agents			
Nucleoside and nucleotide reverse transcriptase inhibitors (Side effects as a class: lactic acidosis, severe hepatomegaly with steatosis, including some fatal cases)			
Abacavir (Ziagen, ABC)§	300 mg twice daily or 600 mg once daily	400	Severe hypersensitivity reaction (can be fatal); nausea; and vomiting
Didanosine (Videx, ddl)§	>60 kg (132 lb) body weight: 200 mg twice daily or 400 mg daily; if with tenofovir, 250 mg/daily <60 kg (132 lb): 125 mg twice daily or 250 mg daily; if with tenofovir, dose not established Do not use with stavudine (d4T, Zerit) during pregnancy; avoid ddl/d4T combination in general because of increased risk for adverse events (e.g., neuropathy, pancreatitis, and hyperlactatemia)	260	Pancreatitis; nausea, diarrhea; and peripheral neuropathy
Emtricitabine (Emtriva, FTC)	200 mg once daily	280	Minimal toxicity; lactic acidosis and hepatic steatosis a rare but possibly life-threatening event
Lamivudine (Epivir, 3TC)§	150 mg twice daily or 300 mg once daily	300	Minimal toxicity; lactic acidosis and hepatic steatosis a rare but possibly life-threatening event
Stavudine (Zerit, d4T)§	>60 kg (132 lb) body weight: 40 mg twice daily <60 kg (132 lb) body weight: 30 mg twice daily Do not use with didanosine (ddl, Videx) during pregnancy; avoid ddl/d4T combination in general because of increased risk for adverse events (e.g., neuropathy, pancreatitis, and hyperlactatemia)	320	Pancreatitis; peripheral neuropathy; rapidly progressive ascending neuromuscular weakness (rare)
Tenofovir (Viread)	300 mg daily	400	Nausea, vomiting, diarrhea; headache; asthenia; flatulence; and renal impairment
Zidovudine (Retrovir, AZT)§	200 mg three times daily or 300 mg twice daily	350	Bone marrow suppression (anemia, neutropenia); gastrointestinal intolerance; headache; insomnia; asthenia; and myopathy

Modified from *MMWR Morb Mortal Wkly Rep* 54(RR-2), 2005.

Continued on following page

TABLE 5-35 **Highly Active Antiretroviral Therapy Medications, Adult Dosage, Cost, and Side Effects** *(Continued)*

MEDICATION	ADULT DOSAGE*	COST (IN DOLLARS) FOR 4 WEEKS†	SIDE EFFECTS AND TOXICITIES
Single Agents			
Nonnucleoside reverse transcriptase inhibitors (Side effects as a class: Stevens-Johnson syndrome)			
Efavirenz (Sustiva)	600 mg daily at bedtime Do not use during known or possible pregnancy	420	Rash; central nervous system symptoms (e.g., dizziness, impaired concentration, insomnia, and abnormal dreams); transaminase elevation; and false-positive cannabinoid test
Protease inhibitors (Side effects as a class: gastrointestinal intolerance, hyperlipidemia, hyperglycemia, diabetes, fat redistribution, and possible increased bleeding in hemophiliacs)			
Atazanavir (Reyataz)	400 mg once daily; if administered with tenofovir plus ritonavir, 300 mg once daily	760	Indirect hyperbilirubinemia; prolonged PR interval (use caution in patients with underlying cardiac conduction defects or on concomitant medications that can cause PR prolongation)
Fosamprenavir (Lexiva)§	1,400 mg twice daily	1,260	Gastrointestinal intolerance, nausea, vomiting, diarrhea; rash; elevated transaminases; and headache
Indinavir (Crixivan)	800 mg every 8 hours With ritonavir (might increase risk for renal adverse events): 800 mg indinavir and 100 mg ritonavir every 12 hours or 800 mg indinavir and 200 mg ritonavir every 12 hours	500	Gastrointestinal intolerance, nausea; nephrolithiasis; headache; asthenia; blurred vision; metallic taste; thrombocytopenia; hemolytic anemia; and indirect hyperbilirubinemia (inconsequential)
Nelfinavir (Viracept)§	750 mg three times daily or 1,250 mg twice daily	600	Diarrhea; and elevated transaminases
Ritonavir (Norvir)§	See doses used in combination with other specific protease inhibitors	700-2,800	Gastrointestinal intolerance; nausea, vomiting, diarrhea; paresthesias; hepatitis; pancreatitis; asthenia; and taste perversion; many drug interactions
Saquinavir (hard-gel capsule) (Invirase)	With ritonavir: 400 mg saquinavir and 400 mg ritonavir twice daily or 1,000 mg saquinavir and 100 mg ritonavir twice daily	270	Gastrointestinal intolerance; nausea, diarrhea; headache; and elevated transaminases
Saquinavir (soft-gel capsule) (Fortavase)	With ritonavir: 400 mg saquinavir and 400 mg ritonavir twice daily or 1,000 mg saquinavir and 100 mg ritonavir twice daily	460	Gastrointestinal intolerance; nausea, diarrhea; abdominal pain; dyspepsia; headache; and elevated transaminases

*For pediatric dosing information, see *Guidelines for Use of Antiretroviral Agents in Pediatric HIV Infection* (available at http://www.aidsinfo.nih.gov/guidelines/default_db2.asp?id=51).
†Available at http://www.cvs.com/CVSApp/cvs/gateway/rxpriceqrequest.
§Pediatric formulation available.
Sources: U.S. Department of Health and Human Services and the Henry J. Kaiser Family Foundation. Guidelines for the use of antiretroviral agents in HIV-infected adults and adolescents. Available at http://www.aidsinfo.nih.gov/guidelines/default_db2.asp?id=50 (refer to website for updated versions). Bartlett JG, Finkbeiner AK: HIV drugs: the guide to living with HIV infection, 2001, 11-13-2001. Available at http://www.thebody.com/jh/bartlett/drugs.html.

TABLE 5-36 **Recommended Laboratory Evaluation of Nonoccupational Prophylaxis (nPEP) of HIV Infection**

Test	Baseline	During nPEP*	4-6 Weeks after Exposure	3 Months after Exposure	6 Months after Exposure
HIV antibody testing	E†, S§		E	E	E
Complete blood count with differential	E	E			
Serum liver enzymes	E	E			
Blood urea nitrogen/creatinine	E	E			
Sexually transmitted diseases screen (gonorrhea, chlamydia, syphilis)	E, S	E¶	E¶		
Hepatitis B serology	E, S		E¶	E¶	
Hepatitis C serology	E, S			E	E
Pregnancy test (for women of reproductive age)	E	E¶	E¶		
HIV viral load	S		E**	E**	E**
HIV resistance testing	S		E**	E**	E**
$CD4^{+}T$ lymphocyte count	S		E**	E**	E**

Modified from *MMWR Morb Mort Wkly Rep* 54(RR-2), 2005.
*Other specific tests might be indicated dependent on the antiretrovirals prescribed. Literature pertaining to individual agents should be consulted.
†E = exposed patient, S = source.
§HIV antibody testing of the source patient is indicated for sources of unknown serostatus.
¶Additional testing for pregnancy, sexually transmitted diseases, and hepatitis B should be performed as clinically indicated.
**If determined to be HIV infected on follow-up testing; perform as clinically indicated once diagnosed.

BOX 5-4 **Situations for Which Expert* Consultation for HIV Postexposure Prophylaxis Is Advised**

- Delayed (i.e., later than 24-36 hr) exposure report
  — the interval after which there is no benefit from postexposure prophylaxis (PEP) is undefined
- Unknown source (e.g., needle in sharps disposal container or laundry)
  — decide use of PEP on a case-by-case basis
  — consider the severity of the exposure and the epidemiologic likelihood of HIV exposure
  — do not test needles or other sharp instruments for HIV
- Known or suspected pregnancy in the exposed person
  — does not preclude the use of optimal PEP regimens
  — do not deny PEP solely on the basis of pregnancy
- Resistance of the source virus to antiretroviral agents
  — influence of drug resistance on transmission risk is unknown
  — selection of drugs to which the source person's virus is unlikely to be resistant is recommended, if the source person's virus is known or suspected to be resistant to ≥1 of the drugs considered for the PEP regimen
  — resistance testing of the source person's virus at the time of the exposure is not recommended
- Toxicity of the initial PEP regimen
  — adverse symptoms, such as nausea and diarrhea are common with PEP
  — symptoms often can be managed without changing the PEP regimen by prescribing antimotility and/or antiemetic agents
  — modification of dose intervals (i.e., administering a lower dose of drug more frequently throughout the day, as recommended by the manufacturer), in other situations, might help alleviate symptoms

HIV, Human immunodeficiency virus.
*Local experts and/or the National Clinicians' Postexposure Prophylaxis Hotline (PEPline [1-888-448-4911]).

BOX 5-5 Occupational Exposure Management Resources

Resource	Contact
National Clinicians' Postexposure Prophylaxis Hotline (PEPline) Run by University of California–San Francisco/San Francisco General Hospital staff; supported by the Health Resources and Services Administration Ryan White CARE Act, HIV/AIDS Bureau, AIDS Education and Training Centers, and CDC.	Phone: (888) 448-4911 Internet: http://www.ucsf.edu/hivcntr
Needlestick! A website to help clinicians manage and document occupational blood and body fluid exposures. Developed and maintained by the University of California, Los Angeles (UCLA), Emergency Medicine Center, UCLA School of Medicine, and funded in part by CDC and the Agency for Healthcare Research and Quality.	Internet: http://www.needlestick.mednet.ucla.edu
Hepatitis Hotline	Phone: (888) 443-7232 Internet: http://www.cdc.gov/ncidod/diseases/hepatitis/index.htm
Reporting to CDC: Occupationally acquired HIV infections and failures of PEP.	Phone: (800) 893-0485
HIV Antiretroviral Pregnancy Registry	Phone: (800) 258-4263 Fax: (800) 800-1052 Address: 1410 Commonwealth Drive Suite 215 Wilmington, NC 28405 Internet: http://www.glaxowellcome.com/preg_reg/antiretroviral
Food and Drug Administration Report unusual or severe toxicity to antiretroviral agents.	Phone: (800) 332-1088 Address: MedWatch HF-2, FDA 5600 Fishers Lane Rockville, MD 20857 Internet: http://www.fda.gov/medwatch
HIV/AIDS Treatment Information Service	Internet: http://www.hivatis.org

BOX 5-6 Management of Occupational Blood Exposures

Provide immediate care to the exposure site:
- Wash wounds and skin with soap and water
- Flush mucous membranes with water

Determine risk associated with exposure:
- Type of fluid (e.g., blood, visibly bloody fluid, other potentially infectious fluid or tissue, and concentrated virus)
- Type of exposure (i.e., percutaneous injury, mucous membrane or nonintact skin exposure, and bites resulting in blood exposure)

Evaluate exposure source:
- Assess the risk of infection using available information
- Test known sources for HBsAg, anti-HCV, and HIV antibodies (consider using rapid testing)
- For unknown sources, assess risk of exposure to HBV, HCV, or HIV infection
- Do not test discarded needles or syringes for virus contamination

Evaluate the exposed person:
- Assess immune status for HBV infection (i.e., by history of hepatitis B vaccination and vaccine response)

Give PEP for exposures posing risk of infection transmission:
- HBV: See Table 5-26
- HCV: PEP not recommended
- HIV: See Tables 5-34, 5-35, and 5-36 and Figure 5-7
  - — Initiate PEP as soon as possible, preferably within hours of exposure
  - — Offer pregnancy testing to all women of childbearing age not known to be pregnant
  - — Seek expert consultation if viral resistance is suspected
  - — Administer PEP for 4 wk if tolerated

Perform follow-up testing and provide counseling:
- Advise exposed persons to seek medical evaluation for any acute illness occurring during follow-up

HBV exposures
- Perform follow-up anti-HBs testing in persons who receive hepatitis B vaccine
  - — Test for anti-HBs 1-2 mo after last dose of vaccine
  - — Anti-HBs response to vaccine cannot be ascertained if HBIG was received in the previous 3-4 mo

HCV exposures
- Perform baseline and follow-up testing for anti-HCV and alanine aminotransferase (ALT) 4-6 mo after exposures
- Perform HCV RNA at 4-6 wk if earlier diagnosis of HCV infection desired
- Confirm repeatedly reactive anti-HCV enzyme immunoassays (EIAs) with supplemental tests

HIV exposures
- Perform HIV-antibody testing for at least 6 mo postexposure (e.g., at baseline, 6 wk, 3 mo, and 6 mo)
- Perform HIV-antibody testing if illness compatible with an acute retroviral syndrome occurs
- Advise exposed persons to use precautions to prevent secondary transmission during the follow-up period
- Evaluate exposed persons taking PEP within 72 hr after exposure and monitor for drug toxicity for at least 2 wk

HBIG, Hepatitis B immune globulin; *HBsAg,* hepatitis B surface antigen; *HBV,* hepatitis B virus; *HCV,* hepatitis C virus; *HIV,* human immunodeficiency virus; *PEP,* postexposure prophylaxis; *RNA,* ribonucleic acid.

Endocarditis Prophylaxis*

TABLE 5-37 Cardiac Conditions Associated with the Highest Risk of Adverse Outcome from Endocarditis for Which Prophylaxis with Dental Procedures is Recommended

Prosthetic cardiac valve

Previous infective endocarditis (IE)

Congenital heart disease (CHD)*

- Unrepaired cyanotic CHD, including palliative shunts and conduits
- Completely repaired congenital heart defect with prosthetic material or device, whether placed by surgery or by catheter intervention, during the first 6 months after the procedure†
- Repaired CHD with residual defects at the site or adjacent to the site of a prosthetic patch or prosthetic device (which inhibit endothelialization)

Cardiac transplantation recipients who develop cardiac valvulopathy

*Except for the conditions listed above, antibiotic prophylaxis is no longer recommended for any other form of CHD.

†Prophylaxis is recommended because endothelialization of prosthetic material occurs within 6 months after the procedure.

TABLE 5-38 Dental Procedures for Which Endocarditis Prophylaxis Is Recommended for Patients in Table 5-37

All dental procedures that involve manipulation of gingival tissue or the periapical region of teeth or perforation of the oral mucosa*

* The following procedures and events do not need prophylaxis: routine anesthetic injections through noninfected tissue, taking dental radiographs, placement of removable prosthodontic or orthodontic appliances, adjustment of orthodontic appliances, placement of orthodontic brackets, shedding of deciduous teeth, and bleeding from trauma to the lips or oral mucosa.

TABLE 5-39 Regimens for a Dental Procedure

		REGIMEN: SINGLE DOSE 30 TO 60 MINUTES BEFORE PROCEDURE	
Situation	**Agent**	**Adults**	**Children**
Oral	Amoxicillin	2 g	50 mg/kg
Unable to take oral medication	Ampicillin	2 g IM or IV	50 mg/kg IM or IV
	OR		
	Cefazolin or ceftriaxone*	1 g IM or IV	50 mg/kg IM or IV
Allergic to penicillins or ampicillin—oral	Cephalexin*†	2 g	50 mg/kg
	OR		
	Clindamycin	600 mg	20 mg/kg
	OR		
	Azithromycin or clarithromycin	500 mg	15 mg/kg
Allergic to penicillins or ampicillin and unable to take oral medicine	Cefazolin or ceftriaxone†	1 g IM or IV	50 mg/kg IM or IV
	OR		
	Clindamycin	600 mg IM or IV	20 mg/kg IM or IV

IM, Intramuscular; *IV,* intravenous.

*Or other first-generation or second-generation oral cephalosporin in equivalent adult or pediatric dosage.

†Cephalosporins should not be used in an individual with a history of anaphylaxis, angiodema, or urticaria with penicillins or ampicillin.

*Prevention of infective endocarditis. Guidelines from the American Heart Association. A guideline from the American Heart Association Rheumatic Fever, Endocarditis, and Kawasaki Disease Committee, Council on Cardiovascular Disease in the Young, and the Council on Clinical Cardiology, Council on Cardiovascular Surgery and Anesthesia, and the Quality of Care and Outcomes Research Interdisciplinary Working Group. *Circulation* published online Apr 19, 2007, DOI: 10.1161/CIRCULATIONAHA.106.183095. Print ISSN: 0009-7322. Online ISSN: 1524-4539.

TABLE 5-40 **Summary of Major Changes in Updated Recommendations**

We concluded that bacteremia resulting from daily activities is much more likely to cause infective endocarditis (IE) than bacteremia associated with a dental procedure.

We concluded that only an extremely small number of cases of IE might be prevented by antibiotic prophylaxis even if prophylaxis is 100% effective.

Antibiotic prophylaxis is not recommended based solely on an increased lifetime risk of acquisition of IE.

Limit recommendations for IE prophylaxis only to those conditions listed in Table 5-37.

Antibiotic prophylaxis is no longer recommended for any other form of CHD, except for the conditions listed in Table 5-37.

Antibiotic prophylaxis is recommended for all dental procedures that involve manipulation of gingival tissues or periapical region of teeth or perforation of oral mucosa only for patients with underlying cardiac conditions associated with the highest risk of adverse outcome from IE (Table 5-37).

Antibiotic prophylaxis is recommended for procedures on respiratory tract or infected skin, skin structures, or musculoskeletal tissue only for patients with underlying cardiac conditions associated with the highest risk of adverse outcome from IE (Table 5-37).

Antibiotic prophylaxis solely to prevent IE is not recommended for GU or GI tract procedures.

The writing group reaffirms the procedures noted in the 1997 prophylaxis guidelines for which endocarditis prophylaxis is not recommended and extends this to other common procedures, including ear and body piercing, tattooing, and vaginal delivery and hysterectomy.

A guide to the clinical preventive services described below is available online at http://www.ahrq.gov/clinic/pocketgd07/.

PART C
GUIDE TO CLINICAL PREVENTIVE SERVICES

1. Cancer

a. Screening for bladder cancer in adults
b. Genetic risk assessment and BRCA mutation testing for breast and ovarian cancer susceptibility
c. Screening for breast cancer
d. Screening for cervical cancer
e. Screening for colorectal cancer
f. Lung cancer screening
g. Screening for ovarian cancer
h. Screening for pancreatic cancer
i. Screening for prostate cancer
j. Counseling to prevent skin cancer
k. Screening for testicular cancer

2. Heart and vascular diseases

a. Screening for abdominal aortic aneurysm
b. Aspirin for the primary prevention of cardiovascular events
c. Screening for coronary heart disease
d. Screening for lipid disorders in adults
e. Screening for peripheral arterial disease

3. Infectious diseases

a. Screening for asymptomatic bacteriuria
b. Screening for chlamydial infection
c. Screening for genital herpes
d. Screening for gonorrhea
e. Screening for hepatitis B virus infection
f. Screening for hepatitis C in adults
g. Screening for syphilis infection

4. Injury and violence

a. Screening for family and intimate partner violence

5. Mental health conditions and substance abuse

a. Screening and behavioral counseling interventions in primary care to reduce alcohol misuse
b. Screening for dementia
c. Screening for depression
d. Screening for suicide risk

6. Counseling to prevent tobacco use and tobacco-caused disease

7. Metabolic, nutritional, and endocrine conditions

a. Behavioral counseling in primary care to promote a healthy diet
b. Hormone therapy for the prevention of chronic conditions in postmenopausal women
c. Screening for obesity in adults
d. Behavioral counseling in primary care to promote physical activity
e. Screening for thyroid disease
f. Screening for type 2 diabetes mellitus in adults

8. Musculoskeletal conditions

a. Primary care interventions to prevent low back pain in adults
b. Screening for osteoporosis in postmenopausal women

9. Vision disorders

a. Screening for glaucoma

Appendix

I. Complementary and Alternative Medicine

II. Primary Care Procedures

Dietary Supplements: What Every Primary Care Provider Should Know

Primary care providers must be knowledgeable regarding the safety, efficacy, and drug interactions associated with common dietary supplements because of the following:

- An estimated 36% of adults ages 18 years and older reported the use of at least one form of complementary and alternative medicine (CAM) according to the National Health Interview Survey in 2004.
- Almost 19% of adults specifically reported the use of dietary supplements, with echinacea (40.3%), ginseng (24.1%), ginkgo (21.1%), and garlic (19.9%) most frequently used.
- Although the use of dietary supplements has plateaued as a result of consumer concerns about effectiveness and potential adverse effects, usage remains common and potentially dangerous.

COMMON TERMINOLOGY

- A *dietary supplement* is defined as an oral product containing vitamins, minerals, herbs, or other botanicals; amino acids; dietary substances used to supplement the diet by increasing the total dietary intake; or a concentrate, metabolite, constituent, extract, or combination.
- *CAM* refers to the broad domain of healing practices that include diverse health systems, modalities, and practices and their accompanying theories and beliefs (see glossary of terms in Appendix Id).
- *Complementary therapies* are those that are used *in addition to* conventional therapies, whereas *alternative therapies* are those that are used *instead of* conventional therapies. Most consumers in the United States use dietary supplements as a complementary therapy.
- *Standardization* refers to the practice of producing dietary supplements with a specific amount of a given compound that may or may not include the actual active ingredient. For example, feverfew has been standardized to its parthenolide content.

LEGISLATION

The U.S. Food and Drug Administration (FDA) is frequently criticized for not closely regulating dietary supplements and monitoring their safety. However, although the agency regulates prescription drugs and over-the-counter (OTC) products, the FDA has limited regulatory authority over dietary supplements. This is because the Dietary Supplement and Health Education Act (DSHEA) of 1994 and its resulting regulations limit the FDA's authority. As a result of DSHEA, the FDA is able to act only when a dietary supplement has been documented to contain a prescription drug, as was the case with glyburide in a natural treatment for diabetes and diazepam in an osteoarthritis preparation. In addition, the FDA can act when safety issues related to a product have been clearly documented, although these cases are frequently challenged in the courts.

HEALTH CLAIMS

Dietary supplements generally are marketed under three types of health claims. The first category is the "nutrient content" claim, in which the product is identified as an excellent source of, typically, a mineral such as calcium, based on recommended daily values. The second type is the "significant scientific agreement" claim; these claims are used when some evidence of the product's efficacy exists (e.g., fish oil supplements). The third and most common type of health claim is called a "structure/function" claim; these claims state that the product has some effect on health—for example, "helps to maintain a healthy heart." However, dietary supplements are not permitted to carry claims stating that they are effective in preventing, treating, or curing diseases.

INFORMATION RESOURCES

Appendix 1b provides a brief overview of common dietary supplements. Until recently, few evidence-based resources on dietary supplements were available. Clinical studies and systematic reviews on dietary supplements are now widely available through PubMed, EMBASE, and the Cochrane Database of Systematic Reviews. Although more information is available, references on specific products vary in their interpretation of the available evidence and may exhibit an unintentional bias, either pro or con, regarding the safety and efficacy of dietary supplements.

"Gold standard" evidence-based databases on dietary supplements (subscription required) include the following:

- Natural Medicines Comprehensive Database (http://www.naturaldatabase.com): This database includes listings for many dietary supplements and is organized in a clinician-friendly manner. Monographs include the different common and scientific names; uses and likely effectiveness for differ-

ent uses; chemical constituents; interactions with drugs, diseases, foods, and laboratory tests; adverse effects; and cautions. The information is extensively referenced and is updated on a daily basis. The primary limitation is that the evaluation of data on clinical effectiveness could be more rigorous.
- Natural Standard (http://www.naturalstandard.com): This database includes listings for dietary supplements and other forms of complementary and alternative medicine. The evidence supporting the assessments in this database is critically evaluated and rigorous in nature. The primary limitation is that many fewer dietary supplements are included in this database.

Evidence-based free websites on dietary supplements include the following:
- National Center for Complementary and Alternative Medicine (NCCAM) (http://nccam.nih.gov)
- Office of Dietary Supplements International Bibliographic Information on Dietary Supplements (http://dietary-supplements.info.nih.gov/Health_Information/IBIDS.aspx)
- Memorial Sloan-Kettering Cancer Center (http://www.mskcc.org/mskcc/html/11570.cfm)

Evidence-based handbooks on dietary supplements include the following:
- *The Professional's Handbook of Alternative & Complementary Medicine,* 3rd edition (C.W. Fetrow & J.R. Avila, eds)
- *Evidence-Based Herbal Medicine* (M. Rotblatt & I. Ziment, eds)
- *Herb Contraindications and Drug Interactions,* 3rd edition (F. Brinker)

Reference books that are of limited clinical usefulness include the following:
- *The Review of Natural Products,* 2006 (A. DerMarderosian & J.A. Beutler). This resource provides information on chemistry and toxicology, but it contains limited information on the actual clinical uses of natural products.
- *Tyler's Honest Herbal,* 1999 (S. Foster & V. Tyler), and *Tyler's Herbs of Choice,* 1999 (J. Robbers & V. Tyler). Although these are classic references and have general information on selected products, they are of limited clinical usefulness and are outdated.
- *Expanded German Commission E Monographs,* 1998 (M. Blumenthal). These were the "gold standard" reference in the past; however, they are now outdated and are not as comprehensive as other resources for primary care providers in the United States.

DRUG INTERACTIONS

Clinically significant interactions have been documented between dietary supplements and prescription or OTC drugs. The challenge for primary care providers is to identify real, clinically relevant interactions versus potential or theoretical interactions. Data on interactions with dietary supplements are usually based on isolated case reports or on studies enrolling healthy volunteers. As with drug-drug interactions, the likelihood of an interaction and its severity are influenced especially by concomitant medical conditions, such as heart failure and presence or absence of impaired kidney and liver function.

Appendix Ic lists interactions between selected natural products and prescription and nonprescription drugs. The following two broad interactions are particularly important in primary care practice:
- St. John's wort, commonly used for depression, is a potent inducer of cytochrome P450 3A4 isoenzymes and has been documented to increase the clearance of many drugs that are metabolized through this (and other) pathways. (For a list of common drugs cleared in this manner, readers should consult http://medicine.iupui.edu/flockhart/clinlist.htm.) In addition, St. John's wort may also induce p-glycoprotein transporter systems that are important for digoxin and some chemotherapeutic agents. St. John's wort has also been associated with the development of serotonin syndrome when used with drugs that have significant serotonergic activity.
- Dietary supplements such as garlic, ginkgo, and feverfew, as well as many others, have been purported to either have antiplatelet activity or have effects on the clotting cascade. This may be important for adults also taking aspirin (and other platelet-active agents) or warfarin.

COUNSELING POINTS

The single most important counseling point related to dietary supplements is always to ask patients about their use of these products and to do so in an open, nonjudgmental manner. The approach should emphasize that many consumers have been interested in vitamins, minerals, herbs, teas, and so on, to maintain their health or to treat illness. If the clinician is unaware of the safety, efficacy, and interactions of a specific product, several websites are available to quickly scan for information. Also, access to drug information centers at colleges of pharmacy is almost always available, and some hospitals now offer programs in integrative medicine.

Patients should be asked about their goals in using the product, as well as how long they have taken it and in what dosage. Allergies to plants should be documented because cross-allergies are common. Clinicians should appreciate that an individual who uses dietary supplements may be interested in making lifestyle changes and potentially decreasing their use of prescription drugs. In addition, if an individual is also consulting an alternative medicine practitioner, clinicians should recognize that some alternative health systems discourage the use of established therapies such as vaccines.

Although problems with safety and efficacy have been identified, many dietary supplements are benign except for their cost. Some patients are at higher risk for adverse outcomes from the use of dietary supplements (e.g., those with chronic kidney and liver disease). Patients should be counseled specifically to avoid purchasing dietary supplements over the Internet.

RESEARCH ISSUES

Many clinical and observational studies of dietary supplements have been published. In the past, clinicians frequently stated that published studies of dietary supplements either did not exist or only a few were available. The reason for this finding was that until recently the National Library of Medicine did not abstract from the peer-reviewed alternative medicine literature. Fortunately, much more research is now readily available. As with all research, the more rigorous the study methodology, the less likely the dietary supplement is to demonstrate clinical benefit.

In evaluating published studies of dietary supplements, the following should be considered:
- Has the correct plant and part of the plant (root, stem, leaf) been used? This critical information may not be known to many clinicians. Consulting a resource such as the National Medicines Comprehensive Database can usually provide the needed information to judge this component of the study.
- Has the content of active ingredients been verified throughout the study? In a recent review of 81 major randomized controlled trials of herbal products, only 12 (15%) reported performing tests to quantify actual contents, and 3 (4%) provided adequate data to compare actual with expected content values of at least one chemical constituent.
- Is the severity of the disease appropriate for study? Negative studies with dietary supplements sometimes inappropriately enroll participants who have moderate-to-severe disease (e.g., those with depression or benign prostatic hyperplasia) when only mild disease would be appropriate.
- Is the duration of the study appropriate? Early studies comparing glucosamine and nonsteroidal anti-inflammatory

agents (NSAIA) demonstrated greater efficacy with the NSAIA because of an inadequate study duration for glucosamine to show any benefit.

- Is a placebo group included? Recent studies with dietary supplements for menopausal symptoms and osteoarthritis have demonstrated placebo responses over 40% to 50%.
- Was the blinding maintained throughout the study? Some dietary supplements, such as saw palmetto, have distinctive odors and tastes that are not easily masked.
- Is the preparation commercially available? Most importantly, when a study with dietary supplements does show benefit, it frequently is difficult to use the product in practice because the specific formulation studied is not commercially available.

AUTHOR: **ANNE L. HUME, PHARM.D.**

Overview of Selected Natural Products

This table includes a few of the common uses and side effects of selected natural products. The evidence supporting the uses and side effects of these products varies considerably and may be based on anecdotal information or theoretical concerns with the natural products.

Natural Products	Common Use(s)	Adverse Effects/Potential Concerns
African plum (Pygeum)	Benign prostatic hyperplasia	Nausea and abdominal pain have been reported, but pygeum is generally well tolerated. Pygeum does not decrease prostate size or influence PSA concentrations.
Andrographis	Prevention and treatment of viral respiratory infections	Headache, fatigue, rash, diarrhea, and vomiting. Products are standardized to 4%-6% andrographolide; this botanical is commonly used in combination products.
Black cohosh	Menopausal symptoms (hot flashes), induction of labor in pregnant women, premenstrual syndrome	Dyspepsia, rash, weight gain, headache, and cramping have been reported. Concern exists that black cohosh causes liver toxicity. The potential development of mild estrogen-like adverse effects, especially endometrial hyperplasia, is of concern.
Butterbur	Prevention of migraine headaches; allergic rhinitis; urinary tract spasms; pain	Diarrhea, stomach upset, fatigue, belching, headache, and drowsiness may occur. Due to concern about hepatotoxicity, butterbur products should be free of pyrrolizidine alkaloids. Products should be standardized to 15% petasin and isopetasin.
Chamomile (German)	Motion sickness, anxiety, insomnia; gastrointestinal spasms; mucositis	Allergic reactions occur on rare occasion. Patients with a ragweed allergy should use chamomile with caution.
Chasteberry	Premenstrual dysphoric disorder, premenstrual syndrome, menopausal symptoms, female infertility, mastalgia	Gastrointestinal upset, headache, rash, acne, weight gain, and menstrual bleeding have been reported.
Chitosan	Weight loss, Crohn's disease, hypercholesterolemia, anemia	Gastrointestinal upset, nausea, flatulence, and constipation have been reported. Patients with a shellfish allergy should avoid the use of chitosan.
Chondroitin sulfate	Osteoarthritis, osteoporosis, hyperlipidemia	Gastrointestinal upset, nausea, diarrhea, constipation, and alopecia. Concern exists that chondroitin may have anticoagulant activity due to its structural similarity to part of heparin.
Cinnamon	Type 2 diabetes mellitus, flatulence, gastrointestinal spasms, anorexia, menopausal symptoms, impotence	Cassia cinnamon is one of three types of cinnamon in commercial food products; this is the only type that may have minor effects to improve blood glucose concentrations.
Coenzyme Q10	Congestive heart failure, angina, dilated cardiomyopathy, statin-induced myopathy, Parkinson's disease, chronic fatigue syndrome, HIV/AIDS	Nausea, vomiting, diarrhea, anorexia, heartburn, and rash have been reported.

AIDS, Acquired immune deficiency disease; *HIV,* human immunodeficiency virus.

Continued on following page

Natural Products and Drug Interactions

This table lists interactions between selected natural products and prescription and nonprescription drugs. Although many of the listed interactions are theoretical in nature and have not been documented to occur in humans, those involving St. John's wort are potentially life threatening in nature, depending on the individual drug. Other interactions are based on small studies of healthy volunteers and use pharmaceutical-quality natural products that may or may not be commercially available.

Natural Products	Drugs	Interaction
Andrographis	Immune suppressants	Andrographis may stimulate immune function, potentially decreasing the effectiveness of drugs such as cyclosporine, tacrolimus, and prednisone.
	Antihypertensive agents	Andrographis may lower blood pressure, potentiating the hypotensive effects of antihypertensive agents.
	Antiplatelet and anticoagulant agents	Andrographis may have antiplatelet activity, potentially increasing the risk of bleeding.
Black cohosh	Hepatotoxic drugs	Concern exists that the risk of hepatotoxicity with black cohosh is increased in the presence of hepatotoxic drugs such as acetaminophen.
	Cisplatin	Animal studies suggest that the efficacy of cisplatin against breast cancer cells may be decreased by black cohosh.
	CYP2D6 substrates	Black cohosh may modestly inhibit CYP2D6 enzyme activity to result in higher drug concentrations.
Butterbur	CYP3A4 inducers (Rifampin, carbamezepine, etc.)	Drugs that induce the activity of CYP3A4 increase the risk of the formation of hepatotoxic metabolites from pyrrolizidine alkaloids from some butterbur products.
Chamomile	CNS depressants (benzodiazepines, opiates, barbiturates, etc.)	Chamomile may have additive CNS depressant effects.
	CYP1A2 substrates	Chamomile may inhibit CYP1A2 enzyme activity to result in higher drug concentrations.
	CYP3A4 substrates	Chamomile may inhibit CYP3A4 enzyme activity to result in higher drug concentrations.
	Estrogens	Chamomile may compete for estrogen receptors.
	Tamoxifen	Chamomile may interfere with the effects of tamoxifen because of its estrogenic effects.
Chaste tree berry	Antipsychotic agents	Chaste tree berry may antagonize the effects of antipsychotic agents through its dopaminergic activity.
	Metoclopramide	Chaste tree berry may antagonize the effects of metoclopramide through its dopaminergic activity.
	Dopamine agonists	Chaste tree berry may possess additive effects to drugs such as levodopa and ropinirole through its dopaminergic activity.
	Oral contraceptives/estrogens	Chaste tree berry may possess additive hormonal effects.
Chondroitin	Warfarin	High-dose chondroitin has structural similarity to a heparinoid and may possess weak anticoagulant effects.

AChE, Acetylcholinesterase; *CCB,* calcium channel blockers; *CNS,* central nervous system; *MAOI,* monoamine oxidase inhibitor; *PPI,* proton pump inhibitors; *SSRI,* selective serotonin reuptake inhibitors.

Continued on following page

Natural Products	Drugs	Interaction
Cinnamon	Hypoglycemic agents	Cinnamon may possess additive effects on blood glucose to those of hypoglycemic agents.
Coenzyme Q10	Antihypertensive agents	Coenzyme Q10 may possess additive effects on blood pressure to those of antihypertensive agents.
	Warfarin	Coenzyme Q10 may lessen the anticoagulant effects of warfarin because of its structural similarity to vitamin K.
	Chemotherapy	The antioxidant effects of coenzyme Q10 may blunt the efficacy of certain chemotherapeutic agents that depend on the formation of free radicals.
Cranberry	CYP2C9 substrates (warfarin)	Cranberry may inhibit CYP2C9 enzyme activity to result in higher drug concentrations; evidence with warfarin is contradictory.
Dehydroepiandrosterone (DHEA)	Tamoxifen and aromatase inhibitors such as anastrozole and exemestane	DHEA may interfere with the antiestrogenic effects of these drugs.
	CYP3A4 substrates	DHEA may slightly inhibit CYP3A4 enzyme activity to result in higher drug concentrations.
Devil's claw	Antihypertensive agents	Devil's claw may possess additive effects on blood pressure to those of antihypertensive agents.
	Hypoglycemic agents	Devil's claw may possess additive effects on blood glucose to those of hypoglycemic agents.
	H_2 antagonists and PPI	Devil's claw may raise gastric pH and blunt the efficacy of H_2 antagonists and PPI.
	CYP3A4 substrates	Devil's claw may inhibit CYP3A4 enzyme activity to result in higher drug concentrations.
	CYP2C9 substrates	Devil's claw may inhibit CYP2C9 enzyme activity to result in higher drug concentrations.
	CYP2C19 substrates	Devil's claw may inhibit CYP2C19 enzyme activity to result in higher drug concentrations.
	Warfarin	Devil's claw may inhibit CYP2C9 enzyme activity to result in higher concentrations of warfarin; purpura has been reported.
Echinacea	Immune suppressants	Echinacea may stimulate immune function, potentially decreasing the effectiveness of drugs such as cyclosporine, tacrolimus, and prednisone.
	CYP3A4 substrates	Echinacea may modestly induce hepatic CYP3A4 enzyme activity to result in lower drug concentrations.
	CYP1A2 substrates	Echinacea may inhibit CYP1A2 enzyme activity to result in higher drug concentrations.
Eleuthero (Siberian ginseng)	CNS depressants (benzodiazepines, opiates, barbiturates, etc.)	Eleuthero may have additive CNS depressant effects.
	Antiplatelet and anticoagulant agents	Eleuthero may have antiplatelet activity, potentially increasing the risk of bleeding.
	CYP3A4 substrates	Eleuthero may inhibit CYP3A4 enzyme activity to result in higher drug concentrations.
	CYP1A2 substrates	Eleuthero may modestly inhibit CYP1A2 enzyme activity to result in higher drug concentrations.
	CYP2C9 substrates	Eleuthero may modestly inhibit CYP2C9 enzyme activity to result in higher drug concentrations.
	CYP2D6 substrates	Eleuthero may inhibit CYP2D6 enzyme activity to result in higher drug concentrations.
	Digoxin	Concentration of digoxin has been reported to increase but without evidence of toxicity.
Evening primrose oil (EPO)	Antiplatelet and anticoagulant agents	EPO may have anticoagulant activity, potentially increasing the risk of bleeding.
Fenugreek	Antiplatelet and anticoagulant agents	Fenugreek may have antiplatelet activity, potentially increasing the risk of bleeding.
	Hypoglycemic agents	Fenugreek may potentially lower blood glucose concentrations and have additive effects with hypoglycemic agents.
Feverfew	Antiplatelet and anticoagulant agents	Feverfew may have antiplatelet activity, potentially increasing the risk of bleeding.
	CYP3A4 substrates	Feverfew may inhibit CYP3A4 enzyme activity to result in higher drug concentrations.
	CYP1A2 substrates	Feverfew may inhibit CYP1A2 enzyme activity to result in higher drug concentrations.
	CYP2C9 substrates	Feverfew may inhibit CYP2C9 enzyme activity to result in higher drug concentrations.
	CYP2C19 substrates	Feverfew may inhibit CYP2C10 enzyme activity to result in higher drug concentrations.

AChE, Acetylcholinesterase; *CCB,* calcium channel blockers; *CNS,* central nervous system; *MAOI,* monoamine oxidase inhibitor; *PPI,* proton pump inhibitors; *SSRI,* selective serotonin reuptake inhibitors.

Natural Products	Drugs	Interaction
Fish oils (omega-3 fatty acids)	Antiplatelet and anticoagulant agents	Fish oils may have antiplatelet activity, potentially increasing the risk of bleeding, although this has not been documented in humans.
	Antihypertensive agents	Fish oils may possess additive effects on blood pressure to those of antihypertensive agents.
	Oral contraceptives	Oral contraceptives may potentially interfere with the triglyceride-lowering effects of fish oil.
Garlic	Antiplatelet and anticoagulant agents	Garlic may have antiplatelet activity, potentially increasing the risk of bleeding.
	CYP3A4 substrates	Garlic may potentially induce CYP3A4 enzyme activity to result in lower drug concentrations; evidence is contradictory.
	CYP2E1 substrates	Garlic may modestly inhibit CYP2E1 enzyme activity to result in higher drug concentrations.
Ginger	Antiplatelet and anticoagulant agents	Ginger may have antiplatelet activity, potentially increasing the risk of bleeding.
	Hypoglycemic agents	Ginger may potentially lower blood glucose concentrations and have additive effects with hypoglycemic agents.
Ginkgo	Antiplatelet and anticoagulant agents	Ginkgo may have antiplatelet activity, potentially increasing the risk of bleeding.
	CYP2C19 substrates	Ginkgo may induce CYP2C19 enzyme activity to result in lower drug concentrations.
	CYP1A2 substrates	Ginkgo may modestly inhibit CYP1A2 enzyme activity to result in higher drug levels.
	CYP2C9 substrates	Ginkgo may modestly inhibit CYP2C9 enzyme activity to result in higher drug concentrations.
	CYP2D6 substrates	Ginkgo may inhibit CYP2D6 enzyme activity to result in higher drug concentrations.
Ginseng (Panax)	Antiplatelet and anticoagulant agents	Panax ginseng may have antiplatelet properties; American ginseng may decrease the effectiveness (international normalized ration [INR]) of warfarin.
	CYP2D6 substrates	Panax ginseng may modestly inhibit CYP2D6 enzyme activity to result in higher drug concentrations.
	Immune suppressants	Panax ginseng may stimulate immune function, potentially decreasing the effectiveness of drugs such as cyclosporine, tacrolimus, and prednisone.
	Hypoglycemic agents	Panax ginseng may potentially lower blood glucose levels and have additive effects with hypoglycemic agents.
Glucosamine	Warfarin	High-dose glucosamine (along with high-dose chondroitin) may have additive effects to those of warfarin because of structural similarity to heparin.
Green tea extract	Antiplatelet agents	Green tea possesses compounds that may have antiplatelet activity, potentially increasing the risk of bleeding.
	Amphetamines	Caffeine in green tea may increase the risk of CNS toxicity.
	Cocaine	Caffeine in green tea may increase the risk of CNS toxicity.
	Oral contraceptives	Oral contraceptives may decrease the clearance of caffeine in green tea.
	Warfarin	Small amounts of vitamin K have been reported to be present in green tea, potentially decreasing the effectiveness of warfarin.
	Theophylline	Caffeine potentially decreases theophylline clearance.
	Verapamil	Verapamil decreases caffeine clearance, resulting in increased concentrations.
	Quinolone antibiotics	Some quinolone antibiotics decrease the clearance of caffeine.
	Hepatotoxic drugs	Concern exists that the risk of hepatotoxicity with green tea is increased in the presence of hepatotoxic drugs such as acetaminophen.
Hawthorn	β-blockers	Hawthorn and β-blockers may have additive effects on blood pressure and heart rate.
	CCB, nitrates	Hawthorn and CCB (or nitrates) may have additive effects due to coronary vasodilation.
	Digoxin	Hawthorn may have additive effects to those of digoxin.
	Phosphodiesterase inhibitors	Hawthorn may have additive vasodilatory and hypotensive effects with sildenafil, tadalafil, and vardenafil.
Horse chestnut seed extract (HCSE)	Antiplatelet and anticoagulant agents	HCSE may have antiplatelet activity, potentially increasing the risk of bleeding.
	Hypoglycemic agents	HCSE may potentially lower blood glucose concentrations and have additive effects with hypoglycemic agents.
Huperzine	AChE inhibitors (donepezil, etc.)	Huperzine may have additive effects when combined with AChE inhibitors.
	Anticholinergic drugs	The effectiveness of huperzine and/or the anticholinergic drug may be decreased by their concomitant administration.
	Cholinergic drugs (bethanechol, neostigmine, etc.)	Huperzine may have additive effects when combined with cholinergic drugs.

Continued on following page

Natural Products	Drugs	Interaction
Kava	CYP3A4 substrates	Kava may inhibit CYP3A4 enzyme activity to result in higher drug concentrations.
	CYP1A2 substrates	Kava may inhibit CYP1A2 enzyme activity to result in higher drug concentrations.
	CYP2C9 substrates, CYP2C19 substrates	Kava may inhibit CYP2C9 and CYP2C19 enzyme activity to result in higher drug concentrations.
	CYP2D6 substrates	Kava may inhibit CYP2D6 enzyme activity to result in higher drug concentrations.
	P-glycoprotein substrates (digoxin; etoposide, paclitaxel, vinblastine, vincristine; itraconazole; diltiazem, verapamil; and many other drugs)	Kava may inhibit P-glycoprotein transporter systems.
	Hepatotoxic drugs	Concern exists that the risk of hepatotoxicity from kava is increased in the presence of hepatotoxic drugs such as acetaminophen.
Melatonin	Antiplatelet and anticoagulant agents	Melatonin may potentiate the effects of antiplatelets and anticoagulants, although the mechanism is unknown.
	CNS depressants	Melatonin may have additive CNS depressant effects.
	Fluvoxamine	Fluvoxamine may increase levels of melatonin.
	Immune suppressants	Melatonin may stimulate immune function, potentially decreasing the effectiveness of drugs such as cyclosporine, tacrolimus, and prednisone.
	Hypoglycemic agents	Melatonin may impair glucose utilization and may decrease the efficacy of hypoglycemic agents.
Milk thistle	Estrogens (and other drugs that undergo glucuronidation)	Silymarin may increase the clearance of estrogens.
	CYP2C9 substrates	Milk thistle may modestly inhibit CYP2C9 enzyme activity to result in higher drug concentrations.
Peppermint oil	H_2 antagonists and proton pump inhibitors	Peppermint oil may raise gastric pH and blunt efficacy of H_2 antagonists and PPI.
	CYP3A4 substrates	Peppermint oil may modestly inhibit CYP3A4 enzyme activity to result in higher drug concentrations.
	CYP1A2 substrates	Peppermint oil may modestly inhibit CYP1A2 enzyme activity to result in higher drug concentrations.
	CYP2C9 substrates, CYP2C19 substrates	Peppermint oil may modestly inhibit CYP2C9 and CYP2C19 enzyme activity to result in higher drug concentrations.
Policosanol	Antiplatelet and anticoagulant agents	Policosanol may have antiplatelet activity, potentially increasing the risk of bleeding.
Probiotics	Antibiotics	Antibiotics may kill the live organisms in different probiotic preparations.
	Immune suppressants	Theoretically, probiotics may cause bacterial or fungal infections in patients who are taking immune suppressants chronically.
Red clover phytoestrogens	Antiplatelet and anticoagulant agents	Theoretically, red clover may possess coumarins, which increase the risk of bleeding with antiplatelet and anticoagulants.
	CYP3A4 substrates	Red clover may inhibit CYP3A4 enzyme activity to result in higher drug concentrations.
	CYP2C9 substrates, CYP2C19 substrates	Red clover may inhibit CYP2C9 and CYP2C19 enzyme activity to result in higher drug concentrations.
	CYP1A2 substrates	Red clover may inhibit CYP1A2 enzyme activity to result in higher drug concentrations.
Red yeast rice	CYP3A4 inhibitors	Drugs that inhibit CYP3A4 may decrease the metabolism of lovastatin in red yeast rice.
	Statins	Red yeast rice contains lovastatin and increases the risk of myopathy (and hepatotoxicity).
	Fibrates and niacin	Fibrates and niacin may increase concentrations of lovastatin in red yeast rice.
S-adenosylmethionine (SAM-e)	Antidepressants (including MAOIs)	Additive effects are possible, and there is potential for toxicity.
	Serotonergic drugs (triptans, SSRIs, tramadol, meperidine, dextromethorphan, etc.)	SAM-e may increase the risk of development of serotonin syndrome when used concomitantly.
Soy phytoestrogens	Antibiotics	Antibiotics may decrease the efficacy of soy because intestinal bacteria convert isoflavones into more active forms.
	Estrogens	Soy potentially may inhibit the effects of estrogen.
	Tamoxifen	Soy's estrogenic effects may antagonize the antitumor effects of tamoxifen.
	MAOIs	Fermented soy products may contain tyramine.

AChE, Acetylcholinesterase; *CCB,* calcium channel blockers; *CNS,* central nervous system; *MAOI,* monoamine oxidase inhibitor; *PPI,* proton pump inhibitors; *SSRI,* selective serotonin reuptake inhibitors.

Natural Products	Drugs	Interaction
St. John's wort	CYP3A4 substrates	St. John's wort strongly induces CYP3A4 enzyme activity to result in lower drug concentrations.
	CYP1A2 substrates	St. John's wort modestly induces CYP1A2 enzyme activity to result in lower drug levels.
	CYP2C9 substrates	St. John's wort induces CYP2C9 enzyme activity to result in lower drug concentrations.
	P-glycoprotein substrates (digoxin; etoposide, paclitaxel, vinblastine, vincristine; itraconazole; diltiazem, verapamil; and other drugs)	St. John's wort induces P-glycoprotein transporter systems.
	Serotonergic drugs (triptans, SSRIs, tramadol, meperidine, dextromethorphan, etc.)	St. John's wort may increase the risk of development of serotonin syndrome when used concomitantly.
Valerian	CNS depressants (benzodiazepines, opiates, barbiturates, alcohol, etc.)	Valerian may increase the sedative effects of CNS depressants.
	CYP3A4 substrates	Valerian may modestly inhibit the CYP3A4 enzyme activity.

EXAMPLES OF DRUGS METABOLIZED BY CYP ENZYMES

The following are example drugs that are metabolized through the different cytochrome P450 isoenzymes:

CYP1A2 substrates: theophylline, imipramine, clozapine, naproxen

CYP2C9 substrates: warfarin, tamoxifen, irbesartan, ibuprofen, glpizide

CYP2C19 substrates: omeprazole and other proton pump inhibitors, phenytoin, phenobarbital, cyclophosphamide

CYP2D6 substrates: S-metoprolol, propafenone, paroxetine, risperidone, tramadol

CYP2E1 substrates: acetaminophen, alcohol

CYP3A4 substrates: most statins, indinavir, amlodipine, verapamil, alprazolam, buspirone

(For a complete list of drugs and their respective metabolic pathways through the cytochrome P450 isoenzyme systems go to http://medicine.iupui.edu/flockhart.)

AUTHOR: **ANNE L. HUME, PHARM.D.**

APPENDIX Id

Definitions of Complementary and Alternative Medicine Terms

Acupuncture Thin needles are inserted superficially on the skin at locations throughout the body. These points are located along "channels" of energy. Heat can be applied by burning (moxibustion), electric current (electroacupuncture), or pressure (acupressure). Healing is proposed by the restoration of a balance of energy flow called *Qi*. Another explanation suggests that, possibly, the stimulation activates endorphin receptors.

Alexander Technique A bodywork technique in which rebalancing of "postural sets" (i.e., physical alignment) is taught by mentally focusing on the way correct alignments should look and feel and through verbal and tactile guidance by the practitioner.

Applied Kinesiology A form of treatment that uses nutrition, physical manipulation, vitamins, diets, and exercise to restore and energize the body. Weak muscles are proposed as a source of dysfunctional health.

Aromatherapy A form of herbal medicine that uses various oils from plants. Route of administration can be through absorption in the skin or inhalation. The aromatic biochemical structures of certain herbs are thought to act in areas of the brain related to past experiences and emotions (e.g., limbic system).

Ayurveda A major health system that originated in India and incorporates the body, mind, and spirit to prevent and treat disease. Includes special types of diets, herbs, and minerals.

Biofeedback A mind-body therapy procedure in which sensors are placed on the body to measure muscle tension, heart rate, and sweat responses or neural activity. Information is provided by visual, auditory, or body-muscle cell activation so as to teach either to increase or decrease physiologic activity, which, when reconstituted, is proposed to improve health problems (e.g., pain, anxiety, or high blood pressure). In some cases, relaxation exercises complement this procedure.

Chelation Therapy Involves the removal—through intravenous infusion of a chelating agent (synthetic amino acid ethylenediamine tetraacetic acid [EDTA])—of heavy metals, including lead, nickel, and cadmium, as a way to treat certain diseases. Ancillary treatments include the use of vitamins, changes in diet, and exercise.

Cognitive Therapy Psychologic therapy in which the major focus is altering and changing irrational beliefs through a type of Socratic dialogue and self-evaluation of certain illogical thoughts. Conditioning and learning are important components of this therapy.

Craniosacral Therapy A form of gentle manual manipulation used for diagnosis and for making corrections in a system made up of cerebrospinal fluid, cranial and dural membranes, cranial bones, and sacrum. This system is proposed to be dynamic, with its own physiologic frequency. Through touch and pressure, tension is proposed to be reduced and cranial rhythms normalized, leading to improvement in health and disease.

Diathermy The use of high-frequency electrical currents as a form of physical therapy and in surgical procedures. The term *diathermy,* derived from the Greek words *dia* and *therma,* literally means "heating through." The three forms of diathermy used by physical therapists are short wave, ultrasound, and microwave.

Eye Movement Desensitization and Reprocessing (EMDR) A technique that proposes to remove painful memories by behavioral techniques. Rhythmic, multisaccadic eye movements are produced by allowing the patient to track and follow a moving object while imagining a stressful memory or event. By using deconditioning, including verbal interaction with the therapist, the painful memory is extinguished and health improved.

Feldenkrais Method A bodywork technique that integrates physics, judo, and yoga. The practitioner directs sequences of movement using verbal or hands-on techniques or teaches a system of self-directed exercise to treat physical impairments through the learning of new movement patterns.

Hatha Yoga The branch of yoga practice that involves physical exercise, breathing practices, and movement. These exercises are designed to have a salutary effect on posture, flexibility, and strength and are intended ultimately to prepare the body to remain still for long periods of meditation.

Hellerwork A bodywork technique that treats and improves proper body alignment through the development of a more complete awareness of the physical body. The goal is to realign fascia for improvement of standing, sitting, and

Modified from Spencer JW: *Complementary/alternative medicine: an evidence-based approach,* St Louis, 1999, Mosby.

breathing using "body energy," verbal feedback, and changing emotions and attitudes.

Homeopathy A form of treatment in which substances (minerals, plant extracts, chemicals, or disease-producing germs), which in sufficient doses would produce a set of illness symptoms in healthy individuals, are given in microdoses to produce a "cure" of those same symptoms. The *symptom* is not thought to be part of the illness but part of a curative process.

Hyperbaric Oxygen A therapy in which 100% oxygen is given at or above atmospheric pressure. An increase in oxygen in the tissue is proposed to increase blood circulation and improve healing and health and influence the course of disease.

Jin Shin Jyutsu An ancient bodywork technique to harmonize body, mind, and spirit by gentle touch that uses specific "healing points" at the body surface. The points are proposed to overlie flowing energy (Qi). The therapist's fingers are used to "redirect, balance, and provide a more efficient energy flow" to and throughout the body.

Light Therapy Natural light or light of specified wavelengths is used to treat disease. This may include ultraviolet light, colored light, or low-intensity laser light. Generally, the eye is the initial entry point for the light because of its direct connection to the brain.

Magnetic Therapy Magnets are placed directly on the skin, theoretically stimulating living cells and increasing blood flow by ionic currents that are created from polarities on the magnets.

Mediterranean Diet A diet that is thought to provide optimal distribution of daily caloric intake of different nutrients and includes 50% to 60% carbohydrates, 30% fats, and 10% proteins. The diet is derived from the eating habits of people in the Mediterranean area, who were shown to have reduced rates of cardiovascular disease.

Mind-Body Therapies A group of therapies that emphasize using the mind or brain in conjunction with the body to assist healing. Mind-body therapies can involve varying degrees of levels of consciousness, including *hypnosis,* in which selective attention is used to induce a specific altered state (trance) for memory retrieval, relaxation, or suggestion; *visual imagery,* in which the focus is on a target visual stimulus; *yoga,* which involves integration of posture and controlled breathing, relaxation, and/or meditation; *relaxation,* which includes lighter levels of altered states of consciousness through indirect or direct focus; and *meditation,* in which there is an intentional use of posture, concentration, contemplation, and visualization.

Muscle Energy Technique A manual therapy in osteopathic medicine that includes both passive mobilization and muscle reeducation. Diagnosis of somatic dysfunction is performed by the practitioner, after which the patient is guided to provide corrective muscle contraction.

Music Therapy The use of music in an either active or passive mode. Used mainly to reduce stress, anxiety, and pain.

Naturopathy A major health system that includes practices that emphasize diet, nutrition, homeopathy, acupuncture, herbal medicine, manipulation, and various mind-body therapies. Focal points include self-healing and treatment through changes in lifestyle and emphasis on health prevention.

Ornish Diet A life-choice program based on eating a vegetarian diet containing less than 10% fat. The diet is high in complex carbohydrates and fiber. Meat and fish are generally avoided.

Oslo Diet An eating plan that emphasizes increased intake of fish and reduced total fat intake. Diet is combined with regular endurance exercise.

Pilates An educational and exercise approach using the proper body mechanics, movements, truncal and pelvic stabilization, coordinated breathing, and muscle contractions to promote strengthening. Attention is paid to the entire musculoskeletal system.

Prayer The use of prayer(s) that are offered to "some higher being" or authority to heal and/or arrest disease. May be practiced by the individual patient, by groups, or by other(s) with or without the patient's knowledge (e.g., intercessory).

Pritikin Diet A weight management plan that is based on a vegetarian framework. Meals are low in fat, high in fiber, and high in complex carbohydrates.

Qi Gong A form of Chinese exercise-stimulation therapy that proposes to improve health by redirecting mental focus, breathing, coordination, and relaxation. The goal is to "rebalance" the body's own healing capacities by activating proposed electrical or energetic currents that flow along meridians located throughout the body. These meridians, however, do not follow conventional nerve or muscle pathways. In Chinese medical training and practice this therapy includes "external Qi," which is energy transmitted from one person to another so as to heal.

Raja Yoga Yoga practice that includes all of the other forms of yoga. The practitioner is instructed to follow moral directives, physical exercises, breathing exercises, meditation, devotion, and service to others to facilitate religious awakening.

Reflexology A bodywork technique that uses reflex points on the hands and feet. Pressure is applied at points that correspond to various body parts, to eliminate blockages thought to produce pain or disease.

Reiki Comes from the Japanese word meaning "universal life force energy." The practitioner serves as a conduit for healing energy directed into the body or energy field of the recipient without physical contact with the body.

Rolfing A bodywork technique that involves the myofascia. The body is realigned by using the hands to apply deep pressure and friction that allows more sufficient posture, movement, and the "release" of emotions from the body.

Shiatsu A Japanese bodywork technique involving finger pressure at specific points on the body mainly to balance "energy" in the body. The major focus is on prevention by keeping the body healthy. The therapy uses more than 600 points on the skin that are proposed to be connected to pathways through which energy flows.

T'ai Chi A technique that uses slow, purposeful motor-physical movements of the body to control and achieve a more balanced physiologic and psychologic state.

Therapeutic Touch A body energy field technique in which hands are passed over the body without actually touching to recreate and change proposed "energy imbalances" for restoring innate healing forces. Verbal interaction between patient and therapist helps maximize effects.

Traditional Chinese Medicine An ancient form of medicine that focuses on prevention and secondarily treats disease with an emphasis on maintaining balance through the body by stimulating a constant, smooth-flowing Qi energy. Herbs, acupuncture, massage, diet, and exercise are also used.

Trager Psychophysical Integration A bodywork technique in which the practitioner enters a meditative state and guides the client through gentle, light, rhythmic, nonintrusive movements. "Mentastics" exercises using self-healing movements are taught to the clients.

AUTHOR: **ANNE L. HUME, PHARM.D.**

Relaxation Techniques

Relaxation Techniques

Relaxation Technique	Summary	Further Resources
Breathing exercise	This is the foundation of most relaxation techniques. Have patients place one hand on the chest and the other on the abdomen. Instruct them to take a slow, deep breath, as if they were sucking in all the air in the room. While doing this, the hand on the abdomen should rise higher than the hand on the chest. This promotes diaphragmatic breathing that increases alveolar expansion in the bases of the lungs. Have them hold the breath for a count of 7 and then exhale. Exhalation should take twice as long as inhalation. Repeat this for a total of five breaths, and encourage patients to do this three times a day.	*Conscious Breathing* by Gay Hendricks is one of many good resources on using breathing for relaxation and health.
Meditation		
Transcendental/The relaxation response	To prevent distracting thoughts, the subject repeats a mantra (a word or sound) over and over again while sitting in a comfortable position. If a distracting thought comes to mind, it is accepted and let go, with the mind focusing again on the mantra.	www.mindbody.harvard.edu or *The Relaxation Response* by Herbert Benson; www.tm.org for information on transcendental meditation.
Mindful meditation	This represents the philosophy of living in the present or in the moment. The *body scan* is one technique where the subject uses breathing to obtain a relaxed state while lying or sitting. The mind progressively focuses on different parts of the body, where it feels any and all sensations intentionally but nonjudgmentally before moving on to another part of the body. A patient with back pain may focus on the quality and characteristics of the pain as if to better understand it and bring it under control.	*Full Catastrophe Living* by Jon Kabat-Zinn describes this technique in full and the program for stress reduction at the University of Massachusetts Medical Center.
Centering prayer	This is a form similar to transcendental meditation that has a more religious foundation. The subject repeats a "sacred word" similar to a mantra. As thoughts come to mind, they are accepted and let go, clearing the mind to become more centered on the spirit within, as if the mind's preoccupied thoughts are the layers of an onion that are peeled away, allowing better understanding of the spirit at the core.	www.Centeringprayer.com; look under "method of centering prayer" for a nondenominational discussion.

From Rakel RE (ed): *Principles of family practice,* ed 6, Philadelphia, 2002, WB Saunders.

Continued on following page

Relaxation Techniques *(Continued)*

Relaxation Technique	Summary	Further Resources
Progressive muscle relaxation (PMR)	A form of relaxation in which the subject is attuned to the difference in feeling when the muscles are tensed and then relaxed. In a comfortable position, start by tensing the whole body from head to toe. While doing this, notice the feelings of tightness. Take a deep breath in and as you let it out, let the tension release and the muscles relax. This is then followed by progressive tension and relaxation throughout the body. One may start by clenching the fists and then tensing the arms, shoulders, chest, abdomen, hips, legs, and so on, with each step followed by relaxation.	www.uaex.edu/publications/pub/fshei28.htm is a good review of PMR as well as other relaxation exercises. It is sponsored by the University of Arkansas. *You Must Relax* is a book by the founder of this technique, Edmund Jacobson.
Visualization/ Self-hypnosis	The subject uses visualization to recruit images that create a relaxed state. For example, if a person is anxious, visualizing images of a place and a time that were peaceful and comforting would help induce relaxation. This is best used in conjunction with a breathing exercise.	There are many audiocassettes that can guide people through a visualization "script" that can result in relaxation. Emmett Miller is one well-known author.
Autogenic training	This induces a physiologic response by using simple phrases. For example, "My legs are heavy and warm" is meant to increase the blood flow to this area, resulting in relaxation. This is done progressively from head to toe with the use of deep breathing and repetition of the phrase. After completing this, focus attention on any body part that may still be tense, and then focus the breath and phrase to that area until the whole body is relaxed.	The British Autogenic Society at www.autogenictherapy.org.uk is a good resource for more information.
Exercise/Movement		
Aerobic	While performing an aerobic exercise, focus attention on a phrase, sound, word, or prayer and passively disregard other thoughts that may enter the mind. Some may focus on their breathing, saying to themselves, "In" with inhalation and "Out" with exhalation, or repeating "one-two, one-two" with each step they take with jogging. Doing this will help the mind focus, preventing other thoughts that may cause tension.	*Beyond the Relaxation Response* by Herbert Benson includes discussion of his research on inducing the relaxation response while exercising.
Yoga	This has been practiced for thousands of years in India. In America, it has been divided into three aspects: breathing (pranayama yoga), bodily postures or asanas (hatha yoga), and meditation to maintain balance and health. Regular practice induces relaxation.	For the following therapies, it is best to encourage patients to take a class at a local community center or gym and to pick up an introductory book at a library or bookstore.
T'ai chi	An ancient Chinese martial art that uses slow, graceful movements combined with inner mindfulness and breathing techniques to help bring balance between the mind and body.	See above.
Qi gong	A traditional Chinese practice that uses movement, meditation, and controlled breathing to balance the body's vital energy force, Qi.	See above.

From Rakel RE (ed): *Principles of family practice,* ed 6, Philadelphia, 2002, WB Saunders.

Primary Care Procedures

Text adapted from Tuggy ML, Garcia J, Newkirk GR (eds): *Pocket procedures* text in *Multimedia primary care procedures,* Philadelphia, 2006, Saunders. Illustrations from Rosen R, Chan TC, Vilke GM, Sternbach G: *Atlas of emergency procedures,* St Louis, 2001, Mosby.

1. ANESTHESIA

A. LOCAL ANESTHESIA

Key Steps

1. Select anesthetic and needle.
2. Provide countertraction.
3. Infiltrate underneath entire lesion.
4. Use field block technique.

Instructions

1. Perform local anesthesia with either direct infiltration or a field block.
2. Block smaller lesions with direct infiltration.
3. Excellent anesthesia may be provided with 1% lidocaine with or without epinephrine.
4. Injection using a 27- or 30-gauge needle is well tolerated.
5. Buffering the lidocaine with bicarbonate suspension reduces the burning associated with infiltration.
6. Applying countertraction to the skin allows for more precise injection into the subcutaneous and dermal layers.
7. Depending on the type of incision, extend the area of infiltration at least 2 to 3 mm beyond the incision that has been planned.
8. Often the area needs several injections for a full block.
9. Perform field blocks by injecting widely around the lesion in a diamond-shaped pattern.
10. Pass the needle at 60-degree angles from one side of the lesion.
11. Perform the same needle passes on the opposite side to completely surround the area with anesthesia.
12. Perform a deep injection below the lesion to ensure that the block is complete in the center of the area.

Indications

- Pain relief for procedures
- Pain relief for trauma or for joint or fracture injection
- Adjunctive pain relief for steroid injection
- Diagnostic to assess origin of pain

Contraindications

- Injecting into a sterile space through superficially infected area
- Attempting to anesthetize areas that are large enough that potential toxicity may occur

CPT and ICD-9 Codes

No appropriate codes

B. TOPICAL ANESTHESIA

Key Steps

1. Cleanse area with alcohol.
2. Apply topical anesthetic.
3. Cover with occlusive dressing.
4. Remove cover in 30 minutes to 2 hours.

Instructions

1. To obtain topical anesthesia of the skin, first wipe the skin with alcohol to remove the surface oils.
2. Apply the topical anesthetic cream to the planned incision area.
3. Use 1 to 2 grams of cream to cover a 3-by-3-cm area.
4. Cover the area with an occlusive dressing for 30 to 120 minutes depending on the topical agent that is chosen and the desired depth of anesthesia.
5. At 30 to 60 minutes, 3-mm depth is usually anesthetized, with an additional 1-mm depth added for every 30 minutes up to 120 minutes total application time.
6. Remove the dressing and perform the procedure.
7. The skin should show some blanching in the area that is anesthetized.
8. For topical anesthesia for mucous membranes, use topical spray lidocaine or benzocaine.
9. Apply the spray; onset of action is under 3 minutes.
10. Start the procedure at that time.

C. DIGITAL BLOCK

Key Steps

1. Cleanse digit with antiseptic.
2. Inject local anesthesia without epinephrine.
3. Inject at 9 to 10 o'clock and at 2 to 3 o'clock.
4. Secondary injections.

Instructions

1. Perform digital blocks by injecting plain lidocaine alongside the base of the digit from 9 to 10 o'clock and from 2 to 3 o'clock to anesthetize the digital nerves.
2. Approximately 1 ml of lidocaine is sufficient to provide adequate anesthesia.
3. In some patients, injecting lidocaine toward the palmar surface may be necessary to obtain complete anesthesia of the digit.
4. In some instances, as with nail removal, a simple tourniquet from a latex drain may be used to minimize bleeding in the field and retain the injected anesthesia agent in vascular digits.

Indications

- Need for local anesthetic that encompasses the digit
- Ingrown nail removal
- Drainage of felon or paronychia
- Management of fracture of phalanx

Contraindications

- Use of epinephrine in the anesthetic is contraindicated
- Patient with hypotension or sepsis leading to peripheral vasoconstriction
- Coagulation defect (either medication related, congenital, or acquired), relative

CPT and ICD-9 Codes

No appropriate codes

2. BIOPSY TECHNIQUES

A. EXCISIONAL SKIN BIOPSY

Key Steps

1. Incise around lesion.
2. Excise lesion.
3. Undermine skin edges.
4. Perform deep layer closure.
5. Perform skin closure.

Instructions

1. Most lesions require an elliptical excision around the lesion.
2. The longitudinal axis of the ellipse should follow the skin lines.
3. Excise the skin through the dermis to obtain a full-thickness biopsy.
4. Once the ellipse is created, completely remove the tissue sample by severing the underlying subcutaneous attachments.
5. To reduce the tension on the wound while it is healing, undermine the tissue along the margins of the excision.
6. Use a subcuticular inverted mattress stitch to close the deep layer prior to placing the cutaneous stitches.
7. Two or three deep stitches are usually adequate to support the closure of small excisions.
8. Deep stitches help to control bleeding and reduce tension on the scar, allowing for improved healing.
9. Perform skin closure using nylon suture material that is appropriate for the size of the lesion and location on the body.
10. Place simple interrupted sutures to bring the wound edges together to allow healing with minimal scarring.
11. Nylon stitches are nonabsorbable and require removal in 5 to 10 days depending on the site.
12. Send the specimen for pathologic review.

Indications

- Skin lesions that appear to be malignant; it is especially important to leave 1- to 2-mm margins beyond the lesion if attempting to cure
- Nevi of uncertain malignant potential—acquired, dysplastic, or atypical in appearance
- Benign growths that cause local irritation (pyogenic granulomas, dermatofibromas)
- Removal of subcutaneous growths (sebaceous cysts, lipomas)

Contraindications

- Local infection at the site of planned biopsy
- Coagulation defect (either medication related, congenital, or acquired)
- Nonexcisional treatment option available and not yet tried
- Patient who is unable to comply with wound care

B. PUNCH BIOPSY

Key Steps

1. Cleanse skin and inject local anesthesia.
2. Perform punch biopsy of lesion.
3. Sever base of punch.
4. Suture or topical hemostasis.

Instructions

1. The punch biopsy allows for a full-depth diagnostic sample to be taken from a lesion in a short period of time.
2. Clean the area with Betadine solution. (First check for iodine allergy.)
3. Then inject 1% lidocaine local anesthetic under the lesion.
4. Here use the 2-mm punch biopsy to create a small plug of tissue that you will excise.
5. Use a pair of Adson's forceps to lift the plug, and use iris scissors to sever the base.
6. Cauterize the open punch with ferrous subsulfate solution (Monsel's solution) on a cotton wick or swab.
7. Punch biopsy sites larger than 3 mm often require stitch closure on keratinized skin or any site where cosmetic result is more critical, such as the face.

Indications

- Skin lesions that appear to be malignant where diagnosis will affect excision of the lesion
- Nevi of uncertain malignant potential: acquired, dysplastic, or atypical in appearance
- Rashes where diagnosis is unclear
- Removal of a small lipoma, which usually requires a large punch biopsy (5 to 6 mm)

Contraindications

- Local infection at the site of planned biopsy
- Coagulation defect (either medication related, congenital, or acquired)
- Nonexcisional treatment option available and not yet tried
- Patient who is unable to comply with wound care

C. SHAVE BIOPSY

Key Steps

1. Cleanse skin.
2. Apply local anesthesia.
3. Shave lesion.
4. Topical hemostasis.

Instructions

1. Perform the shave biopsy in a clean manner, as complete sterile technique is not required for superficial lesions.
2. First, clean the skin with the antiseptic solution.
3. Then inject 1% lidocaine to create a wheal at the base of the lesion.
4. Whether or not epinephrine is used depends on the anatomic location of the lesion that is to be biopsied.
5. Once the lesion has been anesthetized, use a pair of pickups with teeth to raise the lesion and use a 15 blade to shave the lesion off at the dermis.
6. To obtain hemostasis, use ferrous subsulfate solution (Monsel's solution) to chemically cauterize the base of the lesion.
7. Use a simple adhesive bandage to cover the biopsy site.
8. The procedure is now complete.

Indications

- Skin lesions that appear to be benign where cosmetic removal is important
- Nevi of uncertain malignant potential: acquired, dysplastic, or atypical in appearance; complete excision would be required if the lesion is malignant
- Rashes where diagnosis is unclear
- Removal of a small lipoma, usually requiring a large punch biopsy (5 to 6 mm)
- For diagnosis of potential malignant lesions where punch biopsy is not feasible owing to location

Contraindications

- Local infection at the site of planned biopsy
- Coagulation defect (either medication related, congenital, or acquired)
- Nonexcisional treatment option available and not yet tried
- Patient who is unable to comply with wound care

3. SUTURES AND DRESSINGS

A. INSTRUMENT TIE

Key Steps

1. Initiate tie with surgeon's knot.
2. Tighten knot so that it lies flat.
3. Perform second throw in opposite direction.
4. Perform two additional throws to secure knot.

Instructions

1. Initiate the instrument tie with a surgeon's knot.
2. Perform it by wrapping the suture around the needle holder twice before grasping the other end of suture and closing the knot.
3. When the first tie is completed, perform the next wrap of the suture in the opposite direction around the needle holder.
4. Now the knot is locked.
5. Perform two or more separate throws to secure the knot in place.
6. Alternating knot throws in different directions prevents premature unraveling of the knot.

Indications

- Low-tension wound closures
- Deep closure in confined wound space where manual ties would be difficult

Contraindications

- Knots requiring significant tension or sutures applied for hemostasis

B. INVERTED SUBCUTICULAR STITCHES

Key Steps

1. Initial stitch enters deep.
2. Second stitch enters superficially.
3. Tie knot in subcutaneous layer.
4. Repeat for each stitch.

Instructions

1. Use inverted stitches to close deep layers of a wound and allow the knot to be buried in the process.
2. The needle tip enters the deeper layer of the subcutaneous tissue and is then brought upward so that it exits the same side more superficially, often in the subcuticular layer.
3. Bring the needle to the other side of the wound so that it enters in the superficial aspect of the wound at the same level as the first side.
4. Drive the needle deep so that it exits the tissue deep in the wound space where the stitch started.
5. Once that is done, tie the knot.
6. During the tightening of the knot, pull the wound together with the knot lying deep to the subcuticular layers that are brought together by the stitch.
7. Cut the suture short and apply the next stitch elsewhere in the wound to bring about further closure of the wound.
8. For small wounds, one or two inverted knots will close the deep layers well.

Indications

- High-tension wound closures that require deep-layer closure where knots are preferably buried
- Wound closures where external suture punctures would be cosmetically unfavorable
- Wounds that require prolonged support for optimal closure
- Adjunctive closure with subcuticular running stitches

Contraindications

- Knots requiring significant tension or sutures applied for hemostasis

CPT and ICD-9 Codes

No appropriate codes

C. SUBCUTICULAR RUNNING STITCHES

Key Steps

1. Make linear incision under minimal tension.
2. Running suture with knot at each end.
3. Reinforce with Steri-strips or tissue glue.

Instructions

1. Bury subcuticular sutures running horizontal sutures.
2. This technique is useful for wounds that are under minimal tension and in which cosmetic results are important.
3. It is possible to close deeper wounds with deep sutures of subcutaneous sutures first.
4. Begin with a knot beyond one apex of the incision, using polypropylene-coated nylon suture.
5. Place the needle through the skin to emerge in the wound.
6. Run the suture, taking horizontal bites through the superficial papillary dermis, alternating sides so that the exit point of one side matches the entry point of the other.
7. Keep the suture under minimal tension.
8. Emerge at the other end beyond the apex and place a second knot.
9. Reinforce the wound with Steri-strips or tissue glue.

Indications

- Low-tension to moderate-tension wound closures that follow skin lines or wounds partially closed by deeps sutures to support the skin closure
- Wound closures where external suture punctures would be cosmetically unfavorable
- Wounds that require prolonged support for optimal closure

Contraindications

- Knots requiring significant tension or sutures applied for hemostasis

CPT and ICD-9 Codes

No appropriate codes

D. MATTRESS STITCHES

Key Steps

1. Deeply insert needle 0.5 to 1 cm from wound edge.
2. Pass needle deeply across the base of wound.
3. Exit opposite side at same distance.
4. Reinsert at 0.3 cm from edge on same side of wound.
5. Cross wound, exit at same shallow depth, and tie knot.

Instructions

1. Mattress sutures are useful in wounds that are under high or moderate tension and where eversion of wound edges is desired.

2. Vertical mattress sutures are initially a simple deep interrupted suture, with the needle penetrating the skin 0.5 to 1 cm from the wound edge, depending on the location and size of the wound (Fig. AII-1, *A*).
3. Track the suture needle across the wound to 75% of the wound depth, and emerge from the opposite side at the same distance from the skin.
4. Reinsert the needle closer to the wound edge, 0.5 to 0.3 cm from the wound, and to 25% of the wound depth, emerging from the opposite side at the same distance from the wound edge.
5. Tie the knot, keeping the suture in sufficient tension to close the wound but not strangulate the tissue (Fig. AII-1, *B*).
6. Repeat knots about 0.5 to 1 cm apart to close the wound (Fig. AII-1, *C* and *D*).
7. These sutures risk producing cosmetically undesirable marks if left in too long and should be evaluated for removal at 1 week or less, depending on the site.

Indications

- Moderate-tension to high-tension wounds
- Wound closures where external suture punctures would be cosmetically tolerated
- Wounds that require prolonged support for optimal closure
- Wounds in areas where inversion of wound edges is more likely (chest, shoulder, thigh)

Contraindications

- Wound closures where external suture punctures would be cosmetically unfavorable
- Cosmetically sensitive areas where the eversion of the wound may lead to thickened scar

CPT and ICD-9 Codes

No appropriate codes

E. TISSUE GLUE

Key Steps

1. Identify appropriate wound type.
2. Cleanse and dry wound area.
3. Apply three or four layers of tissue glue.
4. Dry between each layer to bond skin edges.

Instructions

1. Tissue glues are useful for low-tension wound closures or for small wounds that need closure for improved hemostasis.
2. First, irrigate, clean, and dry the wound.
3. Crush the applicator ampule and allow the adhesive to fill the tip.
4. Pinch the wound shut and apply the glue to the surface in three or four layers, allowing for drying between each layer.
5. Take care to avoid gluing any unwanted materials or personnel to the patient.
6. Once the glue is dry, you may cover the wound or leave it open depending on the site and risk of contamination.

Indications

- Superficial lacerations
- Nail lacerations
- Superficial closure over deeper tension-reducing sutures
- Repair of lacerated nails or nail beds

Contraindications

- Mucosal lesions
- Wounds under tension
- Contaminated lesions
- Puncture wounds and crush wounds

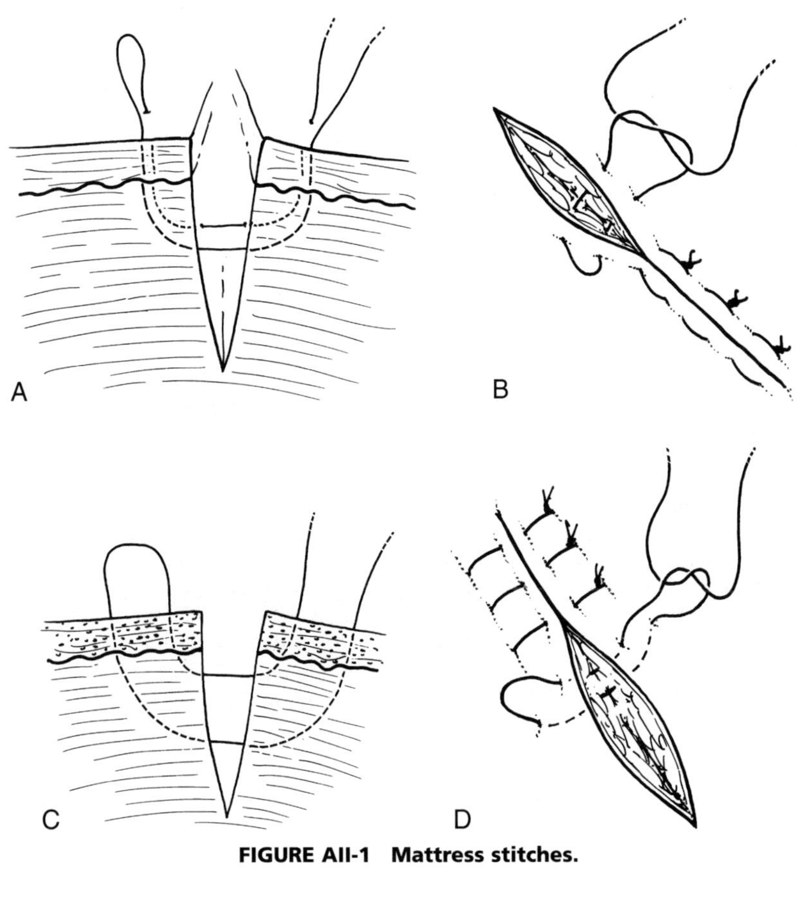

FIGURE AII-1 Mattress stitches.

- Bite wounds
- Complex lacerations
- Lacerations in the axilla

CPT and ICD-9 Codes

Codes are dependent on lesion size and location

F. TOPICAL HEMOSTASIS

Key Steps

1. Perform electrocautery.
2. Silver nitrate may be used.
3. Ferrous subsulfate solution (Monsel's solution) may be used.

Instructions

1. Obtain a topical hemostasis in several ways.
2. Use the Hyfrecator or radiofrequency device to cauterize or coagulate the base of superficial or deep excisions.
3. Silver nitrate sticks are useful for cauterizing superficial lesions, though they may leave a stain in the dermal layer.
4. Ferrous subsulfate solution is an effective topical agent that leaves little residue after its application and is ideal on mucous membranes such as the cervix, vagina, vulva, and penis.

Indications

- For bleeding after cutaneous surgery, especially partial-thickness shave or curetted biopsies
- To treat nail beds after full or partial nail removal
- To treat mucous membrane biopsy sites of the glans penis, vulva, vagina, and cervix

Contraindications

- Allergy to topical agent
- Heavy bleeding, in which case the agent is usually not effective

G. UNNA BOOT APPLICATION

Key Steps

1. Apply moistened Unna boot wrap.
2. Wrap second layer with elastic wrap.
3. Ensure that ankle is at 90 degrees.

Instructions

1. Apply the Unna boot in a manner similar to the application of a cast to the lower leg. The Unna boot is much simpler, however, because it requires only two layers.
2. Place the Unna boot material directly against the skin, wrapping it on the leg.
3. If there are open ulcers or lesions on the foot or lower leg, ensure that the Unna boot covers them well.
4. In areas where there are excess amounts of the wrap owing to changes in the wrapping angle, simply fold in the Unna boot material to allow for compensation of these excess segments of the wrap.
5. Once the Unna boot is applied, wrap a second layer around the entire Unna boot to secure it.
6. Use an elastic wrap material for the second layer.
7. Position the ankle at 90 degrees at the conclusion of wrapping.
8. The Unna boot will dry slowly over the next 24 hours and provide an occlusive dressing to the lower leg and foot that can be left in place for 5 to 7 days.

Indications

- Venous stasis ulcers
- Post–venous thrombosis ulcers
- Severe lower-extremity edema with impending ulceration

Contraindications

- Current venous thrombosis
- Current arterial disease
- Infected ulcers
- Cellulitis
- Allergy to components of the Unna boot

CPT Codes

29580 Unna boot application

ICD-9 Codes

457.1 Lymphedema
707.12 Decubitus ulcers, calf
707.13 Decubitus ulcers, ankle

4. NEEDLE ASPIRATION

A. BREAST CYST ASPIRATION

Key Steps

1. Cleanse skin and palpate nodule.
2. Insert aspiration needle.
3. Multiple passes into nodule.
4. Apply pressure to site.
5. Place aspirate on slide.

Instructions

1. The breast nodule is identified by palpation, and the skin is prepped with antiseptic solution.
2. Fix the cyst to the chest wall between the operator's fingers.
3. Place the needle into the center of the cyst, and then withdraw the plunger to allow for creation of a vacuum.
4. Larger fluid samples can be sent directly to the pathologist.
5. If only a small volume of fluid is obtained, express the contents of the syringe onto a slide and fix with cytology fixative.
6. A second pass may be performed to gather more material for sampling.
7. Apply pressure to the needle insertion site to prevent hematoma formation.
8. Spray the contents of the syringe onto a slide.
9. Use a second slide to gently layer the specimen.
10. Spray cytology fixative onto the slide to prevent drying before fixation.
11. Send the specimen to the laboratory for cytology analysis.

Indications

- Palpable lump in the breast
- Treatment of breast cyst
- Abnormal mammographic findings combine with stereotactic location of biopsy site

Contraindications

- Poorly controlled infection over needle site
- Known malignancy (excisional surgery indicated)

CPT Codes

88170 Fine needle aspirate (FNA) with or without preparation of smears
19100 Biopsy of breast, needle (FNA)

ICD-9 Codes

611.72 Lump or mass in the breast
217 Benign neoplasm of the breast
174.9 Malignant neoplasm of breast (female) unspecified

5. DERMATOLOGY

A. SKIN TAG REMOVAL

Key Steps

1. Inject local anesthesia beneath tag.
2. Make a sharp excision.
3. Cauterize.

Instructions

1. Wipe the skin with antiseptic solution.
2. Treat skin tags with or without anesthesia depending on patient preference and the size of the tag to be removed.
3. Make a small wheal of local anesthetic under each skin tag.
4. Grasp the skin tag with a forceps and trim it at the base with iris scissors.
5. Cauterize the base of the skin tag with either electrical or chemical cautery methods.

Indications

- Symptomatic skin tags in areas of frequent microtrauma, such as the neck line or axilla
- Diagnostic concerns (diagnostic removal)
- Cosmetic concerns

Contraindications

- Local skin infection
- Concern for uncontrollable cosmetic result

CPT Codes

11200 Skin tag removal by excision or destruction 1-15
11201 Each additional tag, up to 10, or portion thereof

ICD-9 Codes

701.9 Skin tags

B. WART TREATMENT

Key Steps

1. Perform cryotherapy: 1-second to 3-second freeze.
2. Refreeze lesions.
3. Use electrocautery method.

Instructions

1. Several options may be used to treat warts.
2. Cryotherapy offers a rapid method of treatment of superficial warts.
3. Cryotherapy is usually effective if the warts are small and the patient either returns for follow-up or continues to use topical medications after the initial treatment.
4. Perform cryotherapy using either a cotton swab dipped in liquid nitrogen and applied to the wart or a liquid nitrogen container equipped with a spray tip to apply the liquid nitrogen directly to the wart.
5. Spray each wart until the entire wart and a 1-mm margin have frozen to form a white disc.
6. Allow this to thaw, then refreeze it.
7. This dual freeze cycle ensures necrosis of the frozen area.
8. Wart cryotherapy also may be done with a nitrous oxide cryotherapy unit fitted with a dermal tip.
9. Often, paring the wart down to skin level improves success with cryotherapy.
10. For persistent or recurrent warts that fail cryotherapy, injecting local anesthetic and using a Hyfrecator to ablate the lesion is an effective way to eradicate the warts.

Indications

- Painful, bleeding, or unsightly warts
- Warts failing to resolve spontaneously (up to 30% of warts disappear without treatment within 6 months)
- Warts have a negative impact on the patient's life (e.g., cosmetic issues, employment issues)
- Warts are growing or multiplying rapidly
- Patient has concerns about spreading the virus

Contraindications

- Poorly controlled local infection, which should be treated prior to the procedure
- Caution in cosmetically sensitive areas such as face, lip, or eyelid

CPT Codes

17110 Destruction of warts 1-14
17111 Greater than 15 warts

ICD-9 Codes

078.19 Plantar warts
078.10 Verruca vulgaris
078.11 Condyloma acuminata

C. ABSCESS INCISION AND DRAINAGE

Key Steps

1. Wear eye protection.
2. Perform field block.
3. Open abscess with incision that follows skin lines.
4. Liberate all areas of abscess.
5. Abrade surface of abscess wall and clear debris from wound.

Instructions

1. Wear eye splash protection. Identify abscess (Fig. AII-2, *A*).
2. Perform a field block by inserting the needle at opposite ends of the area to be anesthetized (Fig. AII-2, *B*).
3. Pass the needle alongside the edge of this region and then withdraw it while anesthesia is injected.
4. Reinsert the needle at 60 to 90 degrees to the initial block at the adjacent aspect of the first injection.
5. After the initial half of the block is completed, anesthetize the opposite side to complete a diamond-shaped field block.
6. Open abscesses with an incision that follows the skin lines (Fig. AII-2, *C*).
7. Use a 15 blade to open the skin and express the material inside the abscess.
8. Use hemostats to break open adhesions or abscess pockets and to ensure that all areas of the abscess are liberated (Fig. AII-2, *D*). Irrigate the abscess cavity (Fig. AII-2, *E*).
9. A sebaceous abscess has a smooth capsular lining that needs to be stripped out to prevent recurrence.
10. Use a curved hemostat to grasp portions of this capsule wall, which may need to be removed piecemeal.
11. In lesions that are not actively inflamed, it may be possible to dissect out the entire wall.
12. Gauze can be used to abrade the surface of the abscess wall and clear debris from within the wound.

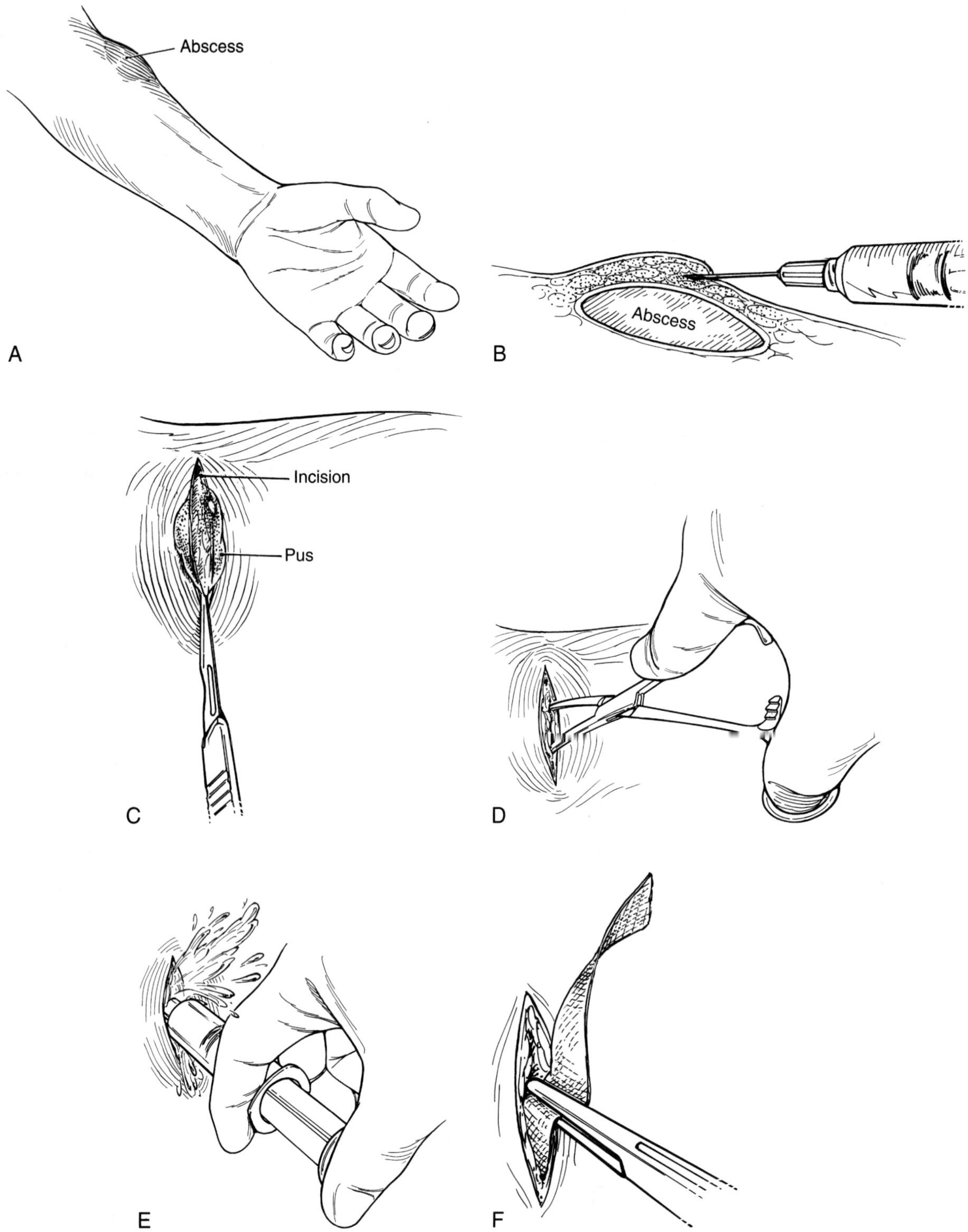

FIGURE AII-2 Abscess incision and drainage.

13. After draining the abscess and removing or disrupting the sebaceous cyst wall, pack iodoform gauze into the wound and leave it in place for 2 to 3 days (Fig. AII-2, *F*).
14. After 2 to 3 days, the wound can be allowed to heal by secondary intention.
15. For larger abscesses, repacking may be necessary to prevent premature closure and abscess reformation.

Indications

- Abscess formation within the cutaneous layers anywhere on the body

Contraindications

- Virtually none, unless the lesion is on the face within the nasolabial triangle and can be treated with warm compresses with a high probability of spontaneous drainage

CPT Codes

10060 I&D, one abscess
10061 I&D, multiple or complex abscess

ICD-9 Codes

682.9 Cellulitis, abscess, NOS

D. BASAL CELL CURETTAGE AND CAUTERY

Key Steps

1. Mark lesion.
2. Inject local anesthesia.
3. Cycles of curettage and cautery.

Instructions

1. Punch biopsy of a suspicious lesion on the patient's arm confirmed basal cell carcinoma.
2. Mark the lesion with a surgical marker to clearly delineate the extent of the superficial cancer.
3. Infiltrate local anesthesia consisting of lidocaine with epinephrine under the lesion.
4. Use a curette to scrape the lesion from the skin surface down into the dermal layer.
5. As curettage is performed, the operator should be able to sense the softness of the basal cell cancer in contrast to the normal dermal layer.
6. Remove all areas of abnormal density tissue.
7. Be especially attentive to the area where the punch biopsy was performed and the prior borders from the surgical marker.
8. Curette the lesion in every direction, performing cautery between each curettage episode.
9. Generally, perform four cycles of curettage and cautery to ensure that the process eradicates any dermal extension of the basal cell cancer.
10. Cover the wound with a simple adhesive bandage on completion of the procedure.
11. Cure is assured by finding normal skin on follow-up examination.

Indications

- Seborrheic and actinic keratoses
- Basal cell carcinoma
- Squamous cell carcinoma
- Condyloma
- Pyogenic granuloma

Contraindications

- Cellulitis and other bacterial infections
- Lesions that require complete excision for diagnosis or treatment
- Pacemakers with electrodesiccation

CPT and ICD-9 Codes

Codes dependent on lesion size and location

E. LIPOMA REMOVAL

Key Steps

1. Inject anesthesia and make incision.
2. Blunt and sharp dissection.
3. Extrude lipoma.
4. Place drain.
5. Close wound.

Instructions

1. The majority of lipoma excisions involve small tumors approximately 3 to 5 cm in size located in the subcutaneous tissues of the trunk or extremities.
2. Occasionally in practice, one will encounter large lipomas that require excisions done in an operating suite under the general anesthesia to avoid lidocaine toxicity.
3. Place the patient under general anesthesia and situate the patient in the right lateral decubitus position.
4. Clean the skin with bactericidal solution and make an incision following the skin lines on the left lateral chest wall.
5. Use blunt dissection to expose the superficial surface of the lipoma using a hemostat to separate the layers of subcutaneous tissues that can moderately adhere to the surface of the lipoma.
6. With larger lesions, more extensive adhesions and subcutaneous fibers may prevent easy extrusion of the tumor.
7. After exposing the initial surface of the lipoma, the dissection continues, using both sharp and blunt dissection to liberate the lipoma from the connective tissue strands holding it to the chest wall.
8. Once the perimeter of the lipoma is fully palpable, use both sharp and manual dissection techniques to lift the lipoma off of the connective tissue overlying the rib cage.
9. After freeing the majority of the lipoma from the adhesions, extrude the mass out of the incision, then lift it to allow sharp dissection of the basal stalk connecting it to the rib cage.
10. Once this has been completed, inspect the wound for any active bleeding and cauterize the necessary vessels.
11. Irrigate and prepare the space for closure.
12. Prior to closing, inject Marcaine local anesthetic into the subcutaneous layer to provide anesthesia for several hours after the procedure.
13. There is significant reduction in pain with use of local anesthetic even in patients who are undergoing surgery with general anesthesia to reduce postoperative pain.
14. Place two deep sutures of 2-0 Vicryl to tack the subcutaneous layer to the connective tissue overlying the rib cage, closing the potential dead space.
15. After removal of a large tumor, place a Penrose drain to prevent accumulation of serous fluid within the potential dead space in the subcutaneous layer.
16. Then use a running subcuticular stitch to close the surface layer of skin and hold the Penrose drain in place.
17. Cover the wound with a sterile dressing and advise the patient to follow up in 48 hours.
18. At the follow-up visit, the patient should have minimal incisional pain, and you should remove the Penrose drain.

Indications

- Large, rapidly growing lipoma, where malignant degeneration is possible
- Lipomas in cosmetically sensitive areas that are visible
- Uncertain diagnosis of subcutaneous mass

Contraindications

- Patient with numerous nonvisible lipomas
- Local infection at the site of planned excision
- Coagulation defect (either medication related, congenital, or acquired)
- Nonexcisional treatment option available and not yet tried
- Patient unable to comply with wound care

F. INGROWN TOENAIL REMOVAL

Key Steps

1. Anesthetize with digital block.
2. Dissect nail.
3. Excise nail.
4. Ablate nail bed.

Instructions

1. Adequately anesthetize the toe with a digital block.
2. Then slip a single blade of the curved iris scissors between the nail and the nail plate along the ingrown area.
3. If the nail tightly adheres to the matrix, a small hemostat can help to separate these structures.
4. Feel a perceptible give when the tip of the scissors has passed the proximal edge of the nail.
5. Once this occurs, use a pair of straight mosquito hemostats to grasp the nail.
6. With firm pressure holding the nail to the nail plate, carefully roll out the affected edge to extract the ingrown portion of the nail out of its compartment.
7. Use bandage scissors to trim off the uplifted nail edge.
8. Take care to ensure that the entire portion of the nail segment to be removed has been excised down to the nail bed.
9. Phenol ablation is the most common method used to cauterize the nail bed to prevent or retard future growth of the unwanted portion of the nail.
10. Form a small plug of cotton by trimming the cotton from the tip of swab and soaking it with phenol.
11. Insert the plug into the opening left by the excised nail edge and push it into the nail bed to cauterize the area.
12. Once the nail bed has been cauterized, remove the plug.
13. Electrosurgical probes have been developed that can ablate the matrix with excellent cosmetic results.

Indications

- Onychocryptosis (ingrown nail)
- Onychomycosis (fungal infection of nail)
- Chronic, recurrent paronychia (inflammation of the nail fold)
- Onychogryposis (deformed curved nail)
- Symptomatic granulation overgrowth of nail fold, especially if recurrent
- Permanently deformed nails after trauma; nail matrix ablation is often performed at the same time

Contraindications

- Noncooperative patient
- Unstable infection, may require pretreatment with antibiotics
- Marginal vascular status of digit; may require clarification prior to injection and surgery

CPT Codes

11730 Nail removal, partial or complete
11750 Permanent nail removal (matrixectomy), partial or complete

ICD-9 Codes

703.0 Ingrown toenail
110.1 Onchomycosis

6. EYE, EARS, NOSE, THROAT

A. NASOPHARYNGOSCOPY

Key Steps

1. Apply decongestant and inspect nares.
2. Apply topical anesthesia.
3. Insert into nasopharynx.
4. Inspect larynx.
5. Withdraw scope.

Instructions

1. The nasopharyngoscope allows the physician to visualize the upper airway precisely in patients who have upper airway complaints.
2. For right-hand-dominant persons, the base of the scope with the direction level is held in the right hand, allowing manipulation of the level by the thumb. The dial on the underside of the scope allows for upward and downward movement of the tip of the scope.
3. This movement, combined with rotation of the scope, allows for 360-degree viewing of the airway.
4. Apply a topical decongestant to allow the nares to open.
5. Inspect the nares to determine which side of the nose is the most patent to pass the nasopharyngoscope through for the examination.
6. Use the tripod technique to hold the nasopharyngoscope on the face while inserting into the nares to avoid any undue trauma.
7. Identify the nasal passage along the floor of the nose, where the scope should be passed to enter the nasopharynx.
8. To prepare for the scope insertion, spray the nares with a decongestant solution.
9. Then anesthetize the throat with a topical anesthetic, followed by application of the anesthetic into the selected side of the nose for scope passage.
10. First, spray the anterior aspect of the nares, then insert the spray tip perpendicular to the plane of the face along the floor of the nose.
11. As the patient holds his or her breath, apply the anesthetic to the deep aspect of the nose as the tip is withdrawn.
12. Now advance the nasopharyngoscope into the nares and along the floor of the nasal passage.
13. The initial structures that are encountered are the palatine tonsils.
14. Rotation of the tip of the scope with flexion laterally to approximately 90 degrees allows one to visualize the Eustachian tube openings and Rosenmuller's fossa.
15. After inspection of these surfaces, advance the scope down into the oropharynx.
16. The key structures of the oropharynx to inspect are the base of the tongue, the vallecula, and the posterior aspect of the tonsils.
17. Having a patient extend the tongue out of the mouth allows one to visualize the vallecula.
18. After inspecting the oropharynx, advance the scope into the hypopharynx, where one visualizes the laryngeal structures and vocal cords.
19. Here, inspect the true cords and false cords and the overlying soft tissue of the laryngeal cartilage.
20. Also inspect the pyriform sinuses on either side of the larynx.
21. The vocal cord movement and symmetry are important to document.
22. One can see clearly the movement of the arytenoid cartilage as the vocal cords are contracted.
23. On finishing the complete inspection, withdraw the scope in neutral position.

Indications

- Epistaxis
- Removal of foreign body
- Chronic rhinorrhea
- Chronic cough evaluation
- Dysphagia
- Chronic or recurrent sinusitis evaluation
- Snoring
- Dysphonia

Contraindications

- Epiglottitis
- Profuse epistaxis

CPT Codes

31231 Nasopharyngoscopy

IDC-9 Codes

472.0 Rhinitis
473.9 Sinusitis, chronic

B. CERUMEN IMPACTION REMOVAL

Key Steps

1. Examine ear canal.
2. Select device for irrigation.
3. Irrigate until cerumen is released.
4. Conduct follow-up examination.

Instructions

1. To remove impacted cerumen, one can use a pulsating water device that allows for pressurized water flow to enter the ear canal.
2. Inject the water along the sidewall of the ear, gently forcing water around the impacted cerumen.
3. Within a few minutes, one can see small fragments of cerumen coming from the ear canal.
4. After several minutes of irrigation, the bulk of the cerumen plug is removed.
5. Other device options include a 20- to 30-ml syringe with a 16- to 20-gauge IV catheter attached to provide directed water flow into the ear canal.
6. Examine the ear after irrigation to ensure that adequate cerumen was removed.

Indications

- Cerumen impaction

Contraindications

- Tympanic membrane perforation

CPT Codes

69210 Cerumen removal

ICD-9 Codes

380.4 Cerumen impaction

7. HAND/DIGIT

A. RING REMOVAL

Key Steps

1. Perform neurovascular examination.
2. Insert tape with hemostat.
3. Wind tape proximal to distal.
4. Do not compromise arterial supply.
5. Pull proximal edge to unwind.

Instructions

1. After careful neurovascular exam demonstrates intact sensation and arterial supply, lubricate the finger (Fig. AII-3, *A*).
2. Carefully insert spooled suture, umbilical tape, or dental floss under the palmar aspect of the ring with a hemostat (Fig. AII-3, *B*).
3. Secure the suture edge to the palm with an adhesive.
4. Proceed to wrap the suture firmly around the finger, starting immediately distal to the ring and moving distally.
5. Wrap the suture tightly enough to compress the edema without producing any arterial compromise (Fig. AII-3, *C*).
6. After relubricating the finger and removing the suture, gently unwind the proximal edge of the suture by pulling distally and circumferentially (Fig. AII-3, *D* and *E*).
7. After removing the ring, repeat the neurovascular exam.

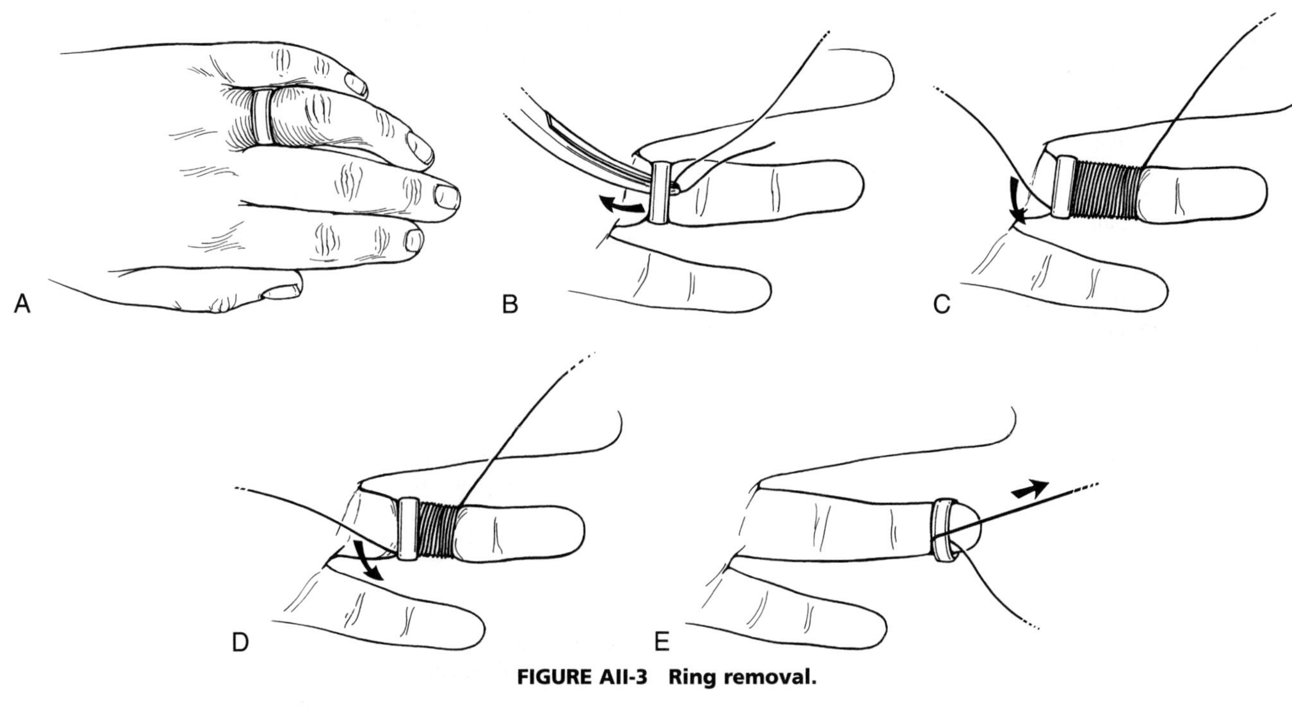

FIGURE AII-3 Ring removal.

Indications

- Distal finger injury with impending swelling of the finger
- Ring finger with signs of vascular compromise due to compression from the ring
- Ring made of conductive or magnetic metal in patient undergoing procedure in which such objects pose a threat to the patient or staff

Contraindications

- Extensive bony injury or swelling where it is clear that cutting the ring is the only option

CPT Codes

20670 Superficial removal of constricting metal band
20680 Deep removal of constricting metal band

ICD-9 Codes

782.3 Traumatic edema

8. ORTHOPEDICS

A. ARTHROCENTESIS—KNEE ASPIRATION

Key Steps

1. Determine best access to effusion.
2. Cleanse skin.
3. Inject local anesthesia at insertion site.
4. Insert needle and aspirate.

Instructions

1. The patient is placed in the supine position.
2. The patient's knee is placed in extension (Fig. AII-4, *A*).
3. Carefully clean the skin with an antiseptic solution.
4. Identify the patella and palpate to determine the effusion size.
5. The ideal location to enter the synovial sac is in the upper outer quadrant of the knee joint space.
6. Local anesthetic injected along the planned trajectory of the arthrocentesis reduces the pain of passing the 18-gauge needle through the joint sac.
7. Pass the needle through the skin and into the palpable effusion.
8. Compress the medial aspect of the knee joint with the opposite hand to push the intraarticular fluid toward the needle and to stabilize the skin for penetration by the needle (Fig. AII-4, *B*).
9. Once the fluid space is entered, obtain a sample for diagnostic purposes.
10. For tense effusions, withdrawing larger volumes of fluid—up to 50 ml at a time—can reduce pain and improve range of motion.
11. After obtaining the desired amount of fluid, withdraw the needle and cover the entry wound.

Indications

- Acute joint effusion
- Acute joint infection
- Joint pain secondary to large effusion (acute or chronic): therapeutic
- Gout

Contraindications

- Local skin infection at the site of joint
- Local bursa infection overlying joint
- Coagulation defect (either medication related, congenital, or acquired), relative
- Artificial joint
- Immunosuppressed patient with noninfected joint
- Sepsis or bacteremia not coming from the joint
- Unstable joint

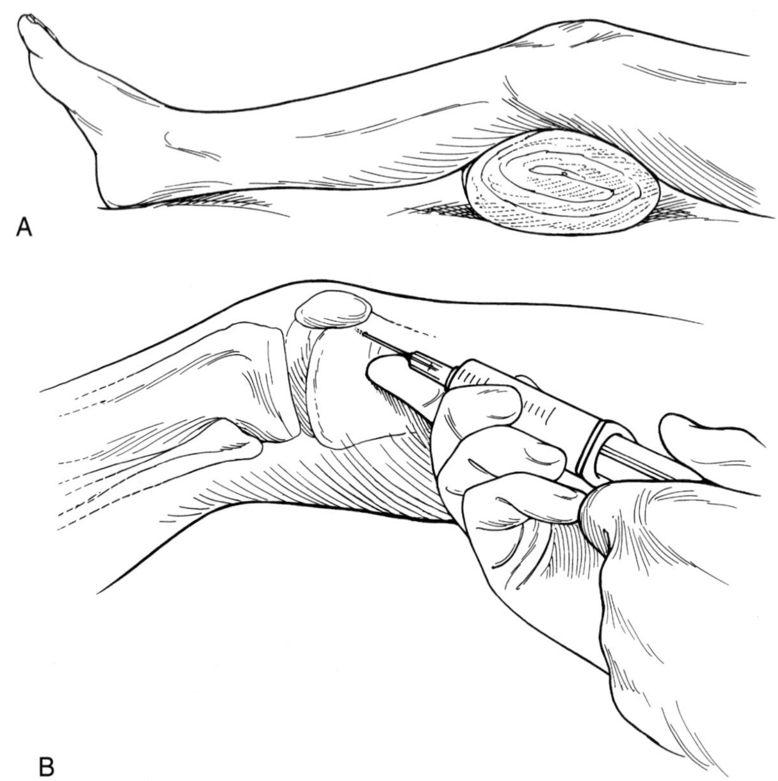

FIGURE AII-4 Knee aspiration.

CPT Codes
20610 Arthrocentesis of the knee

ICD-9 Codes
274.0 Gouty arthropathy
715.16 DJD knee
719.45 Knee pain

B. JOINT INJECTION—SHOULDER

Key Steps
1. Determine injection site. 2. Cleanse skin. 3. Inject local anesthesia. 4. Inject steroid solution.

Instructions
1. Cleanse the area over the acromion and upper deltoid to prepare for the injection.
2. Maintain sterility during the injection process.
3. Identify the space between the acromion and the humerus that is covered by the proximal deltoid attachments.
4. Inject local anesthetic in a wheal on the skin, then deeply along the planned injection path into the subacromial bursa.
5. Draw up 20 mg of methylprednisolone or its equivalent into a 3-ml syringe and mix with 1 to 2 ml of anesthetic solution.
6. Use a 25-gauge needle for injection of the steroid solution.
7. Insert the needle into the subacromial space.
8. Inject the entire volume of the syringe into the joint space.
9. Withdraw the needle and cover the site with a simple adhesive bandage.

Indications
- Tendinitis
- Bursitis
- Rheumatoid arthritis
- Osteoarthritis
- Gout and pseudogout
- Medical conditions with joint manifestations: inflammatory bowel disease, psoriasis, Reiter's syndrome (unless associated with human immunodeficiency virus [HIV]), and ankylosing spondylitis
- Ineffective anti-inflammatory drugs and analgesics

Contraindications
- Acute trauma or fracture
- Metastatic cancer
- Cellulitis over the injection site
- Septic periarticular bursa
- Suspected bacteremia unless the joint is the suspected source
- Broken skin over the injection point
- Primary coagulopathy
- Unstable joints (for steroid injection)
- Joint prosthesis
- Anticoagulant therapy
- Lack of response to two or three prior injections

CPT Codes
20610 Arthrocentesis of shoulder

ICD-9 Codes
274.0 Gouty arthritis
716.91 Arthropathy of shoulder
727.3 Bursitis, unspecified

C. JOINT INJECTION—KNEE

Key Steps
1. Determine injection site. 2. Cleanse skin. 3. Withdraw joint fluid if effusion present. 4. Inject steroid and anesthetic solution.

Instructions
1. Place the patient in the supine position and place the patient's knee in extension.
2. Carefully clean the skin over the upper outer quadrant with an antiseptic solution.
3. Identify the patella and determine the effusion size by palpation.
4. The ideal location to enter the synovial sac is in the upper lateral quadrant of the knee joint space, just above the patella.
5. Mix a solution of steroid, such as 40 mg of methylprednisolone, with bupivacaine to provide short-term anesthesia within the joint space.
6. Pass the needle through the skin and into the joint space.
7. With the opposite hand, compress the medial aspect of the knee joint to push the intraarticular fluid toward the needle.
8. Drain or partially drain any hemorrhagic effusion that is found.
9. After draining the fluid, inject the steroid solution.
10. Withdraw the needle and apply pressure to the site.
11. Cover the injection site with a simple bandage.

Indications
- To rule out septic arthritis
- To rule out crystal or rheumatoid arthritis
- Removal of excessive synovial fluid
- Diagnostic injection of analgesic
- Therapeutic injection of corticosteroid

Contraindications
- Bleeding disorder or excessive anticoagulation
- Superficial infection or cellulites

CPT Codes
20610 Injection of joint
May also charge for office visit

ICD-9 Codes
719.45 Knee pain

D. TRIGGER POINT INJECTION

Key Steps
1. Isolate trigger point by palpation. 2. Cleanse skin. 3. Inject trigger point area. 4. Local massage to disseminate injection.

Instructions
1. Easily inject painful trigger points with a combination of local anesthetics and steroids to obtain immediate and long-term pain relief.
2. Mix 1 ml of bupivacaine with 1.5 ml of lidocaine and the equivalent of 25 mg of hydrocortisone to make up a solution for this injection.
3. Precisely identify the trigger point.
4. Prep the skin with Betadine or alcohol. (First check for iodine allergy.)

5. Insert the needle into the palpable trigger point.
6. Inject the solution in 0.5-ml amounts spread over the region that encompasses the entire trigger point area.
7. After completing the injection, massage the solution into the surrounding soft tissue.
8. Obtain immediate feedback from the patient as the local anesthetics takes effect.

Indications

- Myofascial pain
- Tension headache due to cervical muscle strain
- Chronic neck or back pain due to trigger points
- Fibromyalgia

Contraindications

- Infection at site of trigger point
- Bleeding disorder
- Allergy to any component of injection

CPT Codes

20522 Inject trigger point, one or two sites
20553 Inject trigger points, more than two sites

ICD-9 Codes

729.1 Fibromyalgia

E. LATERAL EPICONDYLE INJECTION

Key Steps

1. Identify focal tenderness over epicondyle.
2. Cleanse skin with antiseptic.
3. Inject steroid/anesthetic solution.
4. Massage injection site.

Instructions

1. Place the elbow in flexion and palpate the focally tender area over the lateral epicondyle.
2. Site of maximal inflammation should be at the proximal attachment of the extensor tendons of the forearm.
3. Cleanse the skin over the epicondyle with an antiseptic solution, maintaining sterility of the injection site.
4. The injection should contain 10 mg of triamcinolone acetate or its equivalent, with 0.5 ml of lidocaine and 0.5 ml of bupivacaine.
5. Insert the needle down to the bony surface of the epicondyle, then withdraw it back 1 to 2 mm.
6. Inject the solution into the area of maximal tenderness and reposition the needle slightly in all directions around this area to distribute the medication into a 1.5-to-2-cm diameter area.
7. Withdraw the needle and massage the area.
8. Cover the site with an adhesive bandage if there is bleeding from the injection.

Indications

- Lateral epicondylitis

Contraindications

- Infection of skin over epicondyle

CPT Codes

20605 Infection of joint
May also charge for office visit

ICD-9 Codes

726.32 Lateral epicondylitis

9. GASTROENTEROLOGY

A. ANOSCOPY

Key Steps

1. Inspect anus.
2. Insert anoscope.
3. Remove obturator.
4. Inspect anorectal mucosa while withdrawing scope.
5. Rotate 90 degrees, reinsert, and inspect.

Instructions

1. The patient is placed in a lateral decubitus position with knees flexed upward toward the chest (Fig. AII-5, *A*).
2. Hold the buttocks apart.
3. Perform a digital exam, allowing for palpation of the anal canal to check for tone, masses, or areas of unusual pain.
4. Lubricate the anoscope with its central guide plug, then slowly insert it past the anal sphincters (Fig. AII-5, *B*).
5. Once the scope is inserted completely, remove the central guide plug for inspection of the distal rectum and the anus (Fig. AII-5, *C* and *D*).
6. Slowly rotate the scope as it is withdrawn to maximize viewing of the mucosa above and below the pectinate line.
7. The operator should be evaluating the mucosa for the presence of mass lesions or hemorrhoids that may be within view (Fig. AII-5, *E*).
8. Masses or polyps that are visible through the scope can be biopsied using a small biopsy forceps.

Indications

- Suspected anorectal malignancy
- Rectal bleeding
- Hemorrhoid evaluation
- Perianal condyloma
- Anal trauma or foreign body, including sexual assault
- Rectal prolapse
- Anorectal pain

Contraindications

- Anal canal stenosis or congenital imperforate anus
- Acute cardiorespiratory compromise

CPT Codes

46600 Diagnostic
46606 Biopsy, single or multiple
46900 Destruction of lesion (e.g., condylomata), chemical
46910 Destruction of lesions, electrodessication

ICD-9 Codes

455.0 Internal hemorrhoids
455.2 Internal hemorrhoids, bleeding
455.3 External hemorrhoid
565.0 Anal fissure
569.0 Anal polyp
698.0 Pruritus ani

B. FLEXIBLE SIGMOIDOSCOPY

Key Steps

1. Insert scope.
2. Advance up the sigmoid.
3. Inspect colon while exiting.
4. Examine rectal vault.

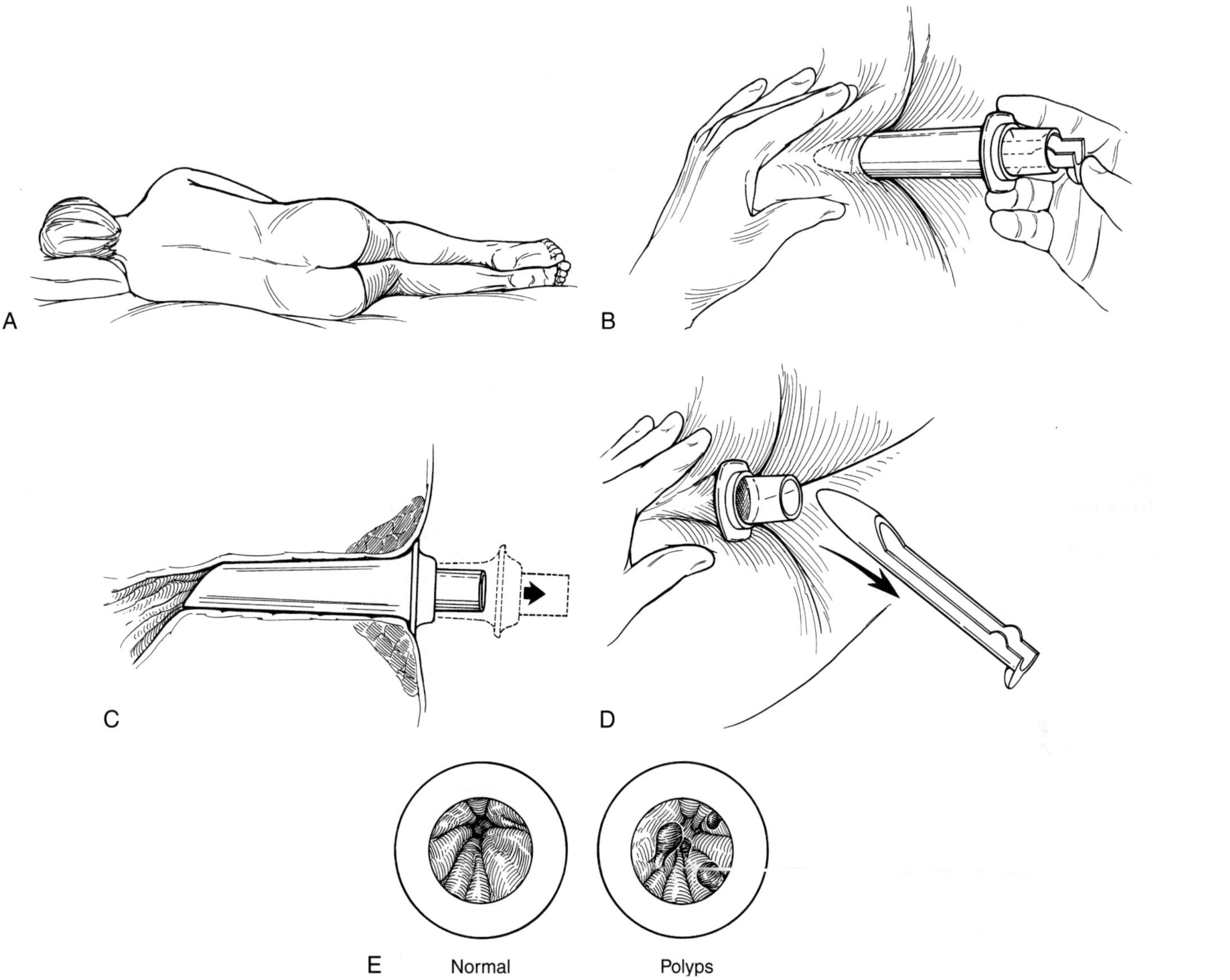

FIGURE AII-5 Anoscopy.

Instructions

1. Anoscopy should be performed in all cases in which palpable abnormality is identified.
2. Place the patient in a left lateral position with knees flexed upward toward the chest.
3. Initial digital rectal examination assists in identifying anal fissures, polyps, and lesions, as well as allowing for initial application of lubricant.
4. Perform anoscopy in all cases in which palpable abnormality is identified.
5. Initially advance the scope at an acute angle with the index finger placed behind the advancing tip.
6. As the anal canal is entered, gently rotate the scope in line with the anal canal as the scope advances into the rectum.
7. Once the scope is inserted approximately 15 cm, insert air to see the rectal vault and find the opening to the lower sigmoid.
8. Easily advance the scope up to the most distal turn of the sigmoid.
9. After passing around the first curve, the operator may need to use one of several techniques to encourage the straightening of the colon around the scope.
10. Once the sigmoid has been traversed, enter the descending colon.
11. Here, the colon has a recognizable abundance of rounded haustra.
12. Once maximal insertion is achieved, slowly withdraw the scope and inspect the colon walls, using the 360-degree view technique, gradually rotating the scope.
13. Take care to inspect behind sharp turns in the sigmoid and behind rectal valves.
14. Once the rectum has been inspected, perform retroflexion to view the inside of the anus and lower rectum from above.
15. Insert the scope to approximately 15 cm and fully rotate the dials to a near maximal rotation to allow the scope to be fully retroflexed.
16. When completed, simple rotation of the shaft of the scope on its axis allows for inspection of the rectum and anus.

Indications

- Rectal bleeding of any type
- Screening for colorectal cancer
- Persons 50 years of age and older, regardless of symptoms
- Unexplained anemia
- Persistent abdominal pain
- Alteration in bowel habits, constipation (particularly unexplained new onset), diarrhea, altered stool diameter
- Unexplained weight loss, fever
- Follow-up of treatment regimens (e.g., for ulcerative colitis, irritable bowel disease)

For the following conditions, colonoscopy may be preferred as first choice to examine the entire colon in patients with higher risk:

- Follow-up for history of polyps or cancer
- Any person with a high-degree risk factor for cancer or other disease in the colon
- Hemoccult-positive stools (positive occult blood)
- Weight loss
- High suspicion of cancer

CPT Codes

45330 Sigmoidoscopy, flexible fiberoptic, diagnostic
45331 Sigmoidoscopy with biopsy
45336 Sigmoidoscopy with ablation of tumor or mucosal lesion

ICD-9 Codes

558.9 Colitis, nonspecific
564.0 Unspecified constipation
564.1 Irritable colon
569.3 Anal hemorrhage
578.1 Melena
789.0 Abdominal pain
V16.0 Family history of colon cancer

C. INTERNAL HEMORRHOID BANDING

Key Steps

1. Prepare banding tool.
2. Perform anorectal inspection.
3. Grasp hemorrhoid with forceps.
4. Release band at base of hemorrhoid.

Instructions

1. Prior to initiation of the banding procedure, prepare the instruments and load the rubber band on the banding forceps.
2. First, place the conical attachment on the banding forceps, slide the rubber band down, and gradually expand it until it fits around the ring portion of the banding forceps.
3. Then adjust the rubber band to the distal edge of the banding forceps so that only a small closure of the forceps will allow the release of the band.
4. Place the patient in a decubitus position, with knees flexed upward toward the chest.
5. Locate the anoscope and insert it into the rectal vault.
6. Prior to banding, ascertain that the hemorrhoid is anesthetized and truly is an internal hemorrhoid.
7. In most instances, identify internal hemorrhoids by their origin proximal to the dentate (or pectinate) line and the fact that they are not sensitive to simple grasping.
8. Insert the grasping forceps through the banding forceps and use it to grasp the body of the hemorrhoid to band.
9. Grasp the hemorrhoid and advance the banding forceps forward.
10. While squeezing the handle, release the rubber band around the proximal end of the hemorrhoid tissue.
11. Painless necrosis of the hemorrhoid will occur within 2 to 3 days, allowing the sloughed tissue to pass in the stool.

Indications

- Symptomatic internal hemorrhoids not responsive to conservative therapy

Contraindications

- Coagulopathy
- Anal infection
- Anal fissure
- Anal tumor
- Pregnancy

CPT Codes

46221 Hemorrhoidectomy by simple ligature, banding

ICD-9 Codes

455.0 Internal hemorrhoids

D. EXTERNAL HEMORRHOID EXCISION

Key Steps

1. Cleanse perianal area.
2. Inject anesthesia.
3. Isolate hemorrhoidal tissue.
4. Excise hemorrhoid.

Instructions

1. The ideal position for anal surgery is to position the patient on the Ritter table with hip and knees flexed in the "bottoms up" position (Fig. AII-6, *A* and *B*).
2. An acceptable alternative is to place the patient in a left lateral position with knees flexed upward toward the chest and with the buttocks held open by an assistant.
3. Clean the anal area with Betadine solution. (First check for iodine allergy.)
4. With an acutely thrombosed hemorrhoid, marked tenderness to palpation is common (Fig. AII-6, *C*).
5. In this case of a chronic recurrent hemorrhoid, the hemorrhoid is nontender; however, the excision technique is the same.
6. Local anesthetic consisting of a combination of lidocaine and bupivacaine provides longer anesthesia and is used to provide a local block (Fig. AII-6, *D*).
7. Prior application of topical 20% benzocaine solution can diminish injection site pain.
8. Inject the hemorrhoid around all aspects of its base to ensure complete anesthesia.
9. Injecting the hemorrhoid itself is not necessary if the base is anesthetized.
10. A single deep injection is also necessary for acute hemorrhoid to allow for extraction of clot within the lesion.
11. Once anesthesia is complete and has been allowed to take effect, test the hemorrhoid for sensation.
12. Once the hemorrhoid is anesthetized, clamp and stabilize it with hemostats and excise the hemorrhoid across the base of the lesion in an elliptical fashion.
13. If there are any visible clots, extract them from the hemorrhoid using the hemostats.
14. Usually, there is minimal bleeding in the wound, which can be left open and allowed to drain while it is healing.
15. Persistent bleeding may require application of Surgicell or Monsel's solution.
16. Proper cleansing of the area postoperatively is important to ensure minimal likelihood of infection.

Indications

- Pain, itching, and burning of thrombosed hemorrhoids
- Poor hygiene and/or difficult stooling secondary to pain
- Failure to respond to local therapy such as sitz baths and topicals

Contraindications

- Poorly characterized bleeding disorder

CPT Codes

46083 Incision and drainage of thrombosed hemorrhoids

ICD-9 Codes

455.3 External hemorrhoids
455.2.1 External hemorrhoids thrombosed

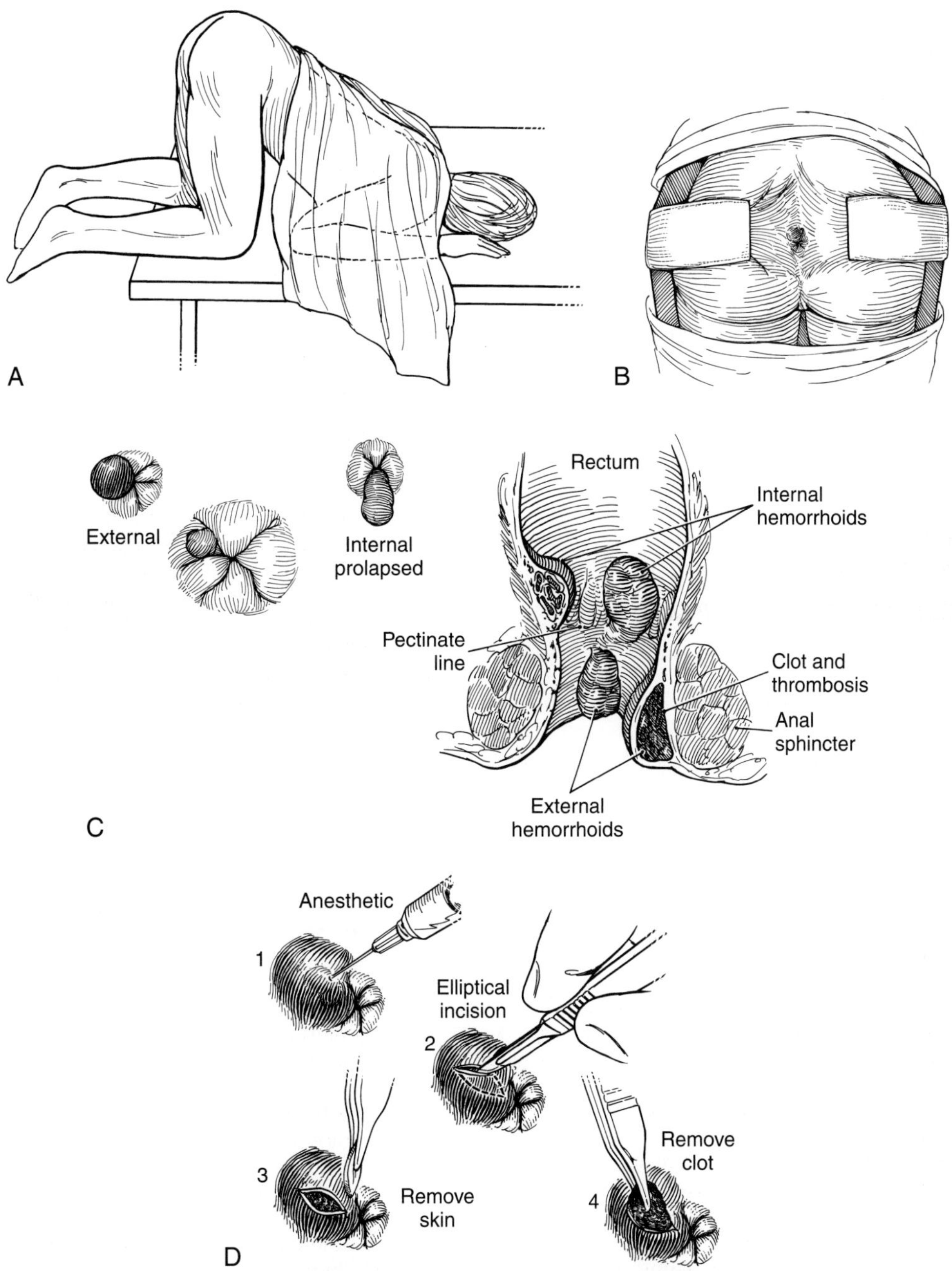

FIGURE AII-6 External hemorrhoid excision.

E. NASOGASTRIC INTUBATION

Key Steps

1. Determine widest nares for insertion.
2. Apply topical anesthetic in nares and throat.
3. Insert tube.
4. Check placement tube.

Instructions

1. Place the patient in a sitting position with the head angled forward in a sniffing posture.
2. Apply topical anesthetic either by spray or gel into the nares selected for insertion.
3. Anesthetizing the back of the throat can also reduce the risk of vomiting during nasogastric (NG) tube insertion.
4. Insert the NG tube along the floor of the nose gently and down the nasopharynx.
5. As the tube approaches the larynx and upper esophagus, the patient should tilt his or her head slightly downward to encourage the tube to pass posteriorly into the esophagus.
6. Advance the tube to the stomach.
7. Test and confirm the tube position by aspiration of gastric contents, which should have a pH of less than 6.
8. If the patient is unconscious or sedated, perform a confirmatory x-ray.
9. If feeding is planned through the tube, confirm its position by x-ray in all patients.

Indications

- Relief of upper gastrointestinal obstruction
- Drainage of gastric contents, bowel rest
- Need for tube-delivered nutrition, dye, or medications

Contraindications

- Facial fractures involving the nose, maxilla, basal bones of the skull, or suspected cervical spine fracture
- Unprotected airway in nonresponsive patient
- Penetrating wound of the neck or chest
- Nasal obstruction
- Esophageal obstruction or anomaly
- Sepsis or bacteremia not coming from the joint
- Placement of percutaneous endoscopic gastrostomy tube would be more appropriate

CPT Codes

43752 Nasogastric or orogastric tube placement necessitating physician's skill
89130 Gastric intubation and aspiration, diagnostic
91105 Gastric intubation and aspiration, therapeutic

ICD-9 Codes

536.2 Vomiting, persistent
537.0 Gastric outlet obstruction
560.1 Ileus, paralytic
561.81 Small bowel obstruction, adhesions
578.0 Hematemesis
578.1 Hematochezia
578.9 GI bleeding, unspecified
787.01 Vomiting, NOS with nausea
977.9 Poisoning, unspecified

10. GYNECOLOGY

A. PAP SMEAR

Key Steps

1. Inspect external genitalia.
2. Insert speculum.
3. Obtain spatula and brush samples.
4. Liquid-based Pap smear sampling.

Instructions

1. Inspect the external genitalia for lesions, then carefully insert the speculum.
2. Advising the patient to relax the perineal musculature can make insertion much less uncomfortable.
3. Clearly visualize the cervix.
4. Perform the Pap smear in several ways.
5. Using a Pap spatula, place the tip of the spatula within the os, and rotate the spatula several times to collect cells on one face.
6. When spreading the spatula over a slide, one must take care that the side that is laden with cells is spread over the glass surface.
7. The cervical brush obtains excellent endocervical samples. It can be used alone, but use it most often in conjunction with the spatula.
8. Commonly use the broom-shaped Pap device with the wet prep and human papillomavirus (HPV) sampling.
9. Place the point of the broom within the os and rotate the brush five times to obtain the sample.
10. Remove the tip of the brush and place it within the wet prep container.
11. Send this sample for both cytology and HPV typing as indicated.

Indications

- Women of reproductive age who are sexually active
- Women who are HIV positive
- Immunocompromised women
- During prenatal care workup

Contraindications

- Active vaginal, cervical, or uterine infection

Relative Contraindication

- Blood contamination, especially if heavy

CPT Codes

87621 HPV sampling—Wet prep Pap
99201-99215 Pap smear and endocervical culture

ICD-9 Codes

795.00 Abnormal Pap
V25.9 Contraceptive management
V70.0 Well adult exam
V72.31 Gynecologic screening exam
V72.32 Follow up abnormal Pap
V13.29 Personal history other genital system and obstetric disorders

B. BARTHOLIN'S MARSUPIALIZATION

Key Steps

1. Determine incision site and anesthetize.
2. Make incision and remove cyst roof.
3. Identify layers for closure.
4. Suture with circumferential stitches.
5. Complete marsupialization.

Instructions

1. The patient is placed in the lithotomy position, and the perineum is washed with antiseptic solution.
2. Palpate the cyst manually to clearly identify its size and location.
3. Outline the incision with a surgical marker at the junction of the vaginal sidewall and labia minora.
4. The incision should be a 2- to 3-cm ellipse whose long axis follows the internal axis of the vaginal side wall, not involving the external labial skin.
5. Use a 15-blade scalpel to create the ellipse to be excised.
6. Enter the vaginal mucosa followed by careful incision through the fascia overlying the cyst.
7. Several layers of fascia and vaginal wall smooth muscles are divided in this process.
8. Open these layers sharply until the cyst wall is entered and drainage occurs.
9. Once the cyst is entered and drained, excise fully the ellipse of tissue, effectively removing the roof of the cyst adjacent to the vaginal sidewall.
10. What remains is the smooth cyst cavity with its distinct edge that must be clearly identified before beginning closure.
11. Use a 3-0 Dexon or Vicryl suture to marsupialize the cyst.
12. Place the initial stitch by passing the needle through the mucosa and then passing through the cyst wall from the submucosal side to open the remaining portion of the cyst.
13. Run the suture continuously around the margin of the incision in small 2- to 3-mm bites.
14. Each stitch must take the vaginal mucosa and cyst wall together.
15. Once the last stitch is placed, overlapping the initial anchoring stitch, tie the suture securely.
16. At the completion of the procedure, one can see that the cyst wall is clearly opened and retracted by the circumferential stitches.
17. Immediately postop, the appearance is that of a small cleft on the side where the surgery was performed.
18. After several days, the repair is barely noticeable as the vaginal wall further contracts.

Indications

- Failed Word catheter treatment in the acute setting
- Recurrent infections or reaccumulation of Bartholin's gland cyst fluid

Contraindications

- Cysts that could be adequately treated with a Word catheter
- Coagulation defect (either medication related, congenital, or acquired) that is uncorrected
- Patient who is unable to comply with wound care

CPT Codes

56440 Bartholin's gland cyst marsupialization

ICD-9 Codes

616.2 Bartholin's cyst
616.3 Bartholin's abscess

C. BARTHOLIN'S CYST WORD CATHETER PLACEMENT

Key Steps

1. Inject local anesthesia.
2. Make incision into abscess.
3. Place catheter.
4. Inflate balloon.

Instructions

1. Place the patient in the lithotomy position and wash the perineum with antiseptic solution.
2. Manually palpate the Bartholin's abscess to clearly identify its size and location (Fig. AII-7, *A*).
3. Identify the incision site at the junction of the vaginal mucosa and the labia minora.
4. Inject local anesthesia of 1% to 2% lidocaine at the incision site.
5. Anesthetize both the skin and deeper fascia overlying the abscess.
6. Test the Word catheter to ensure that it will function properly.
7. Inject 2 to 3 ml of saline into the catheter port, fill, and inspect the balloon.
8. Withdraw the fluid from the catheter prior to insertion.
9. Leave the needle in the catheter port to use promptly after inserting the catheter into the abscess.
10. Use a 15-blade scalpel to incise the wall overlying the abscess; spontaneous drainage of the abscess will occur (Fig. AII-7, *B*).
11. After expressing and draining the entire abscess, insert the Word catheter through the opening (Fig. AII-7, *C*).
12. Take care to insert the tip of the catheter fully into the Bartholin's cyst cavity, not just within the fascia space overlying the cyst.
13. Once the tip is in the infected cyst cavity, inflate the balloon with 3 ml of saline and withdraw the needle from the injection port (Fig. AII-7, *D*).

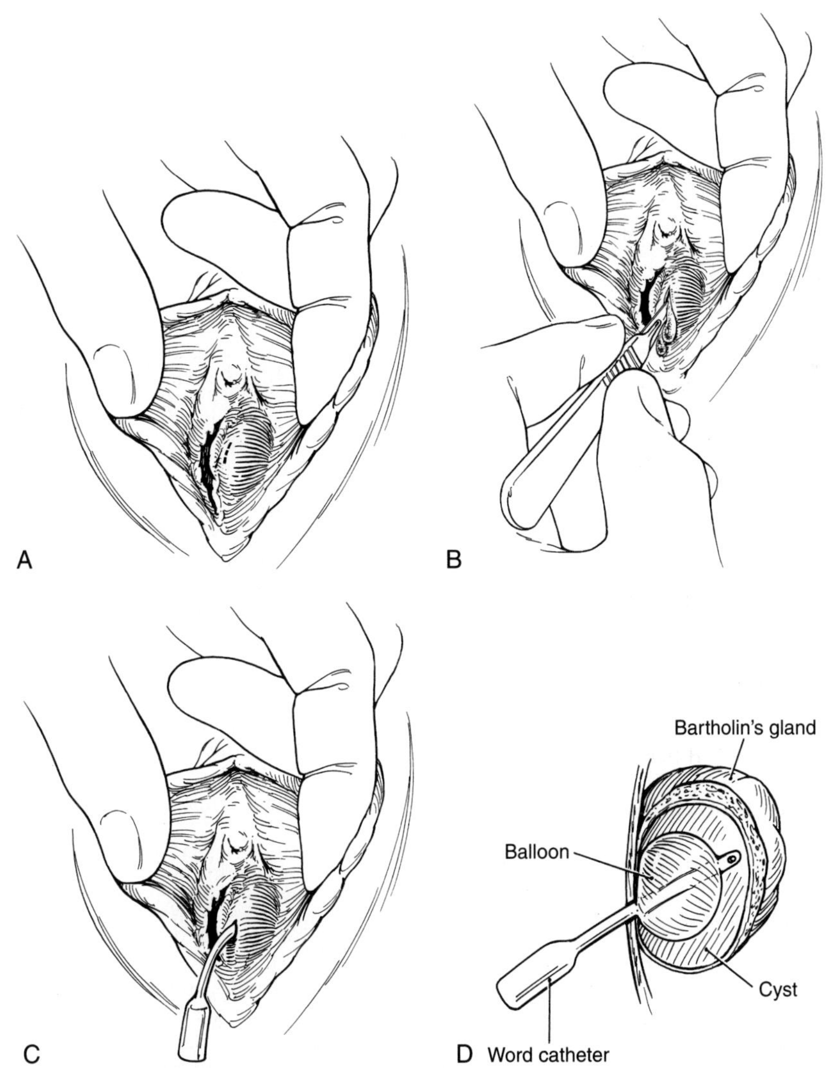

FIGURE AII-7 Bartholin's cyst Word catheter placement.

14. Apply pressure to the syringe to avoid loss of fluid from the catheter.
15. Once the insertion is complete, inspect the area for bleeding.
16. Provide the patient with a perineal pad to collect any further drainage that may occur after the procedure.
17. Recommend postoperative follow-up in 2 to 3 days to ensure that the catheter placement is appropriate and that the abscess continues to drain.
18. Leave the catheter in place for 4 to 6 weeks to induce epithelialization of the cyst and drainage track, preventing further abscess formation.

Indications

- Acute infections
- Pain from cyst enlargement
- Obstructive Bartholin's gland cyst affecting the patient's sexual activity or obstructing the vaginal orifice

Contraindications

- Cysts that should be treated by marsupialization
- Coagulation defect (either medication related, congenital, or acquired) that is uncorrected

CPT Codes

56420 I&D of Bartholin's gland cyst

ICD-9 Codes

616.2 Bartholin's cyst
616.3 Bartholin's abscess

D. VULVAR BIOPSY

Key Steps

1. Evaluate visible lesions.
2. Cleanse skin with antiseptic.
3. Infiltrate with local anesthesia.
4. Biopsy selected area.
5. Perform closure and hemostasis.

Instructions

1. Clean the vulva with Betadine solution. (First check for iodine allergy.)
2. Inject local anesthetic underneath the biopsy site, allowing it to elevate and provide an ideal platform for a punch biopsy.
3. Select a suitably sized punch biopsy to yield a sample through the dermal layer.
4. Excise the core of the punch biopsy using iris scissors and small Adson's forceps.
5. If bleeding is minimal, simple application of Monsel's solution provides adequate hemostasis.
6. If bleeding persists, use a single suture of 5-0 chromic or other absorbable suture.
7. Submit all samples for pathology.

Indications

- Any unidentifiable or concerning lesion
- Lesion that does not respond to conventional therapy
- Pigmented lesions
- Atypical nevi
- Vulvar ulceration of uncertain etiology
- Leukoplakia
- Acetowhite epithelium
- Vulvodynia with acetowhite epithelium (tissue that turns white after the application of vinegar)
- Presumed condylomata that are not responding to conventional therapy (following two treatment attempts of any kind)
- Postmenopausal woman with atrophic vaginitis that does not respond to estrogen therapy and no other cause is evident
- Any skin abnormality requiring definitive diagnosis

Contraindications

- Poorly controlled infection over biopsy site (treat then biopsy)
- Caution with large excisional biopsies with anticoagulation

CPT Codes

56605 Biopsy of vulva
56606 Biopsy of vulva more than one lesion
56820 Colposcopy of vulva
56501 Lesion destruction of vulva

ICD-9 Codes

624.9 Unspecified noninflammatory disorder of vulva and perineum
078.11 Condyloma acuminatum
221.2 Benign vulvar neoplasm
624.8 Vulvar dysplasia

11. INPATIENT MEDICINE

A. LUMBAR PUNCTURE

Key Steps

1. Identify landmarks.
2. Inject local anesthetic at insertion site.
3. Insert spinal needle into cerebrospinal fluid space.
4. Collect cerebrospinal fluid.
5. Remove spinal needle.

Instructions

1. Place the patient in the flexed lateral decubitus position (Fig. AII-8, *A*). Upright position is also acceptable (Fig. AII-8, *B*).
2. Cleanse the skin with antiseptic solution.
3. The iliac crest serves as the landmark that marks the interspace between the third and fourth lumbar vertebrae (Fig. AII-8, *C*).
4. Place a fenestrated drape over this space after it is marked.
5. Anesthetize the skin and deep connective tissue with 1% lidocaine.
6. Insert a 21-gauge spinal needle through the interosseous ligament into the intervertebral space.
7. Advance the needle toward the umbilicus between the L3 and L4 vertebrae, checking periodically if the physician senses that the needle may have entered the dural space (Fig. AII-8, *D*).
8. Usually a "pop" is felt on entering the spinal canal.
9. Once the canal is entered, remove the obturator and allow the spinal fluid to flow out into the collection tube.
10. Normally, collect three or four tubes with 1 to 3 ml of fluid each and label them sequentially for cerebrospinal fluid (CSF) studies.
11. After the collection of fluid is complete, replace the obturator and remove the needle.
12. Place an adhesive bandage over the puncture site.

Indications

- Suspected meningitis or cerebral infection
- Evaluation of CSF or pressures for diagnostic purposes (Guillain-Barré syndrome, lupus, multiple sclerosis, pseudotumor cerebri, suspected central nervous system malignancy)
- Intrathecal or spinal anesthetic
- Imaging procedures where dye infusion into the CSF is necessary

Contraindications

- Local infection at the site of lumbar puncture
- Coagulation defect (either medication related, congenital, or acquired), relative

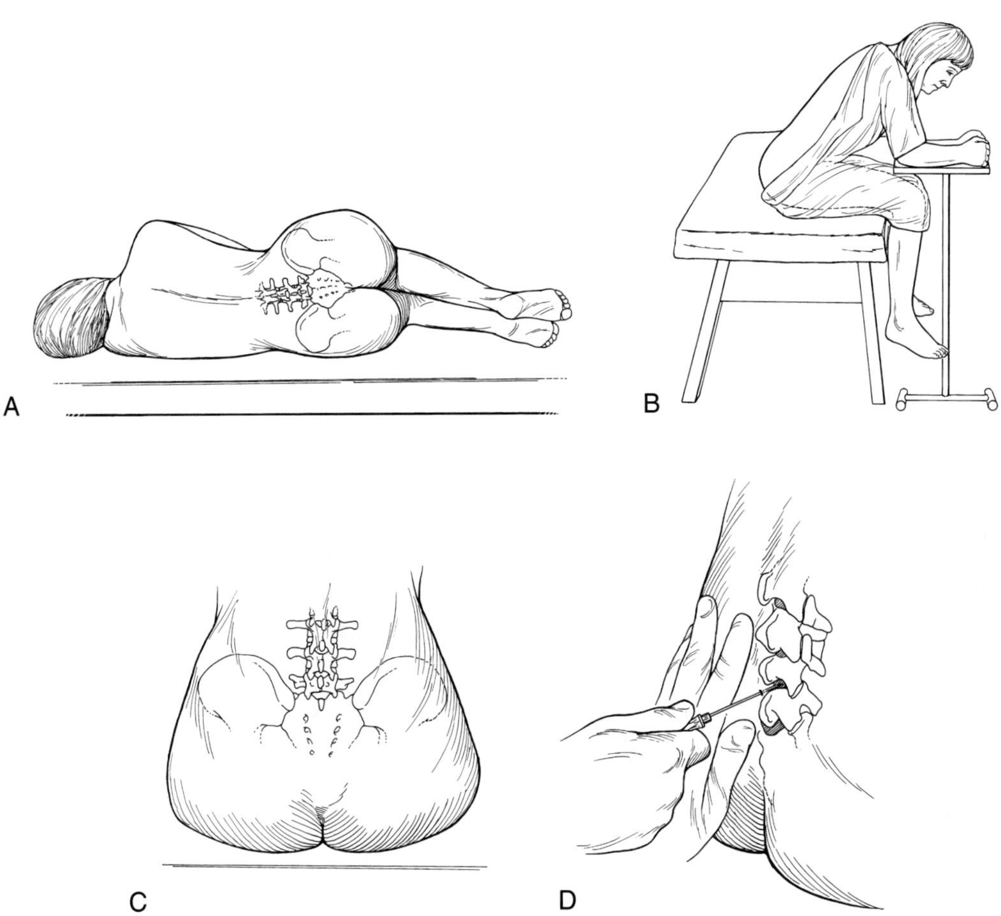

FIGURE AII-8 Lumbar puncture.

- Suspected increased intracranial pressure
- Suspected brainstem herniation

CPT Codes

62270 Spinal puncture, diagnostic
62272 Spinal puncture, therapeutic for drainage of CSF

ICD-9 Codes

322.9 Suspected meningitis
340.00 Multiple sclerosis
348.2 Pseudotumor cerebri
357.0 Guillain-Barré syndrome
710.0 Systemic lupus erythematosus
852.00 Subarachnoid hemorrhage

B. SUBCLAVIAN LINES

Key Steps

1. Identify landmarks.
2. Inject local anesthesia at insertion site.
3. Insert trocar and place wire.
4. Exchange trocar for dilator and catheter over wire.
5. Suture catheter to skin.

Instructions

1. Place the patient in Trendelenburg's position at about 15 degrees and clean, shave, and drape the skin over the midclavicular region.
2. Identify the key landmarks of the midclavicle and the suprasternal notch by palpation.
3. Inject local anesthetic along the planned trajectory of the catheter insertion (Fig. AII-9, *A*), notably anesthetizing the periosteum of the clavicle to avoid pain as the insertion needle passes underneath the clavicle.
4. Insert the introducer trocar at the midclavicular line and pass it under the clavicle, keeping its tip aiming toward the sternal notch (Fig. AII-9, *B*).
5. Retract the syringe plunger to create negative pressure so that when the subclavian vein is entered, a flash is seen in the syringe.
6. Once this occurs, insert the wire through the trocar (Fig. AII-9, *C*), taking care to use the thumb to prevent any air intake into the trocar during transfers.
7. At no time should the operator let go of the wire while it is in the patient (Fig. AII-9, *D*).
8. Insert the wire at least 20 cm.
9. Remove the insertion trocar and incise the skin with an 11 blade to allow the dilator to pass easily (Fig. AII-9, *E*).
10. Pass the catheter and dilator over the wire (Fig. AII-9, *F*).
11. As soon as the wire is visible at the distal end of the catheter, release one hand from the wire proximally and grasp the wire at the distal end.
12. Fully insert the catheter before withdrawing the wire (Fig. AII-9, *G*).
13. Then remove the dilator and test the catheter before securing it to the patient's skin with suture (Fig. AII-9, *H*).
14. Proper venous flow through the catheter suggests proper placement of the catheter.
15. Connect the catheter hub to an IV set (Fig. AII-9, *I*) and obtain a chest x-ray to confirm placement and ensure that a pneumothorax has not occurred due to catheter insertion.

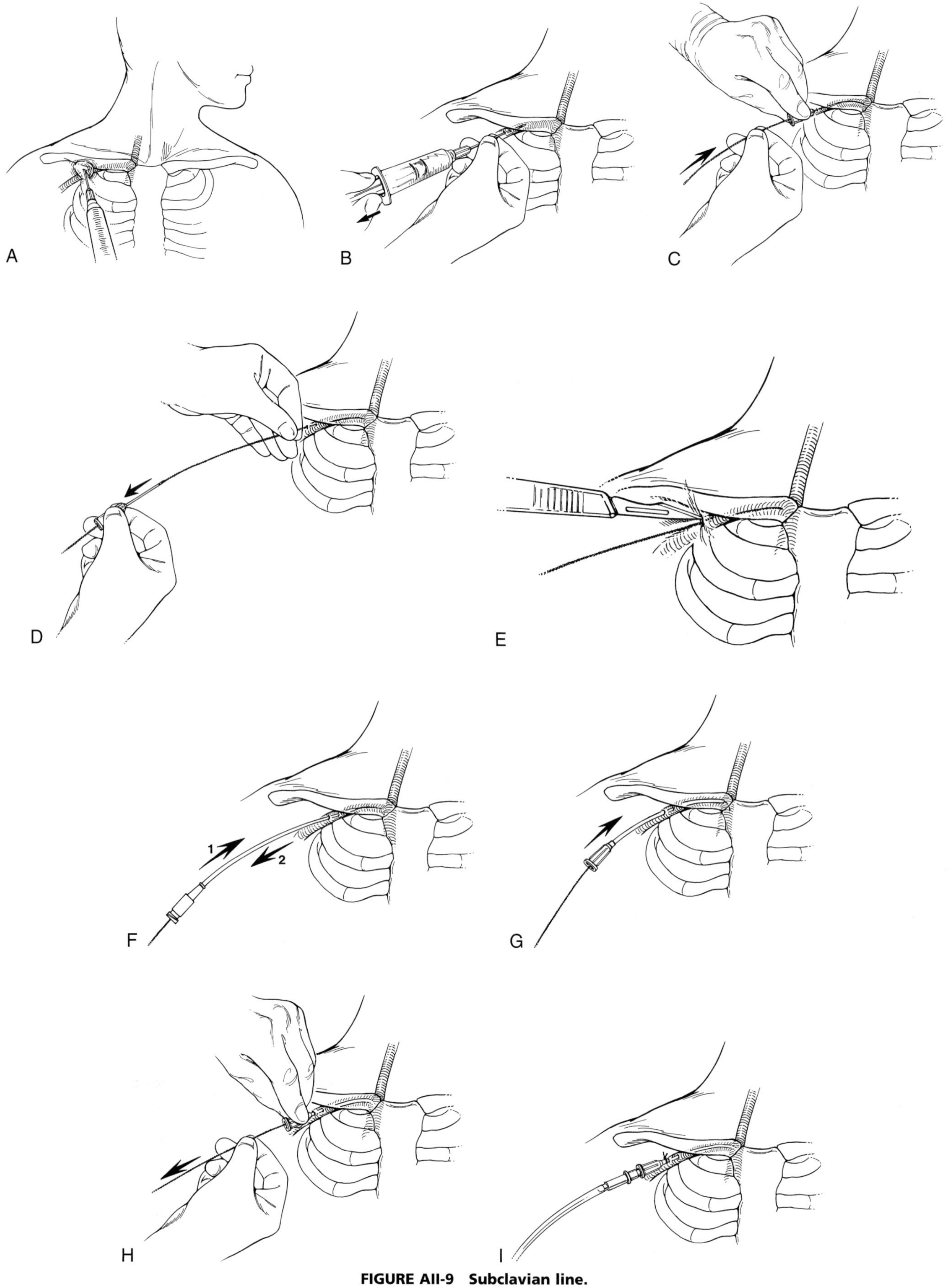

FIGURE AII-9 Subclavian line.

Indications

- Central venous access for fluid resuscitation, hyperalimentation, or delivery of medications in intensive-care situations
- Delivery of medications that may cause sclerosis of smaller veins or necrosis of tissue if leaked from a peripheral vein
- Vascular access for plasmarpheresis, dialysis, pacemakers, or Swan-Ganz catheter placement
- Vascular access for pulmonary or cardiac catheterization

Contraindications

- Chest injury where a pneumothorax on the side of the line placement would compromise patient's survival
- Coagulation defect (either medication related, congenital, or acquired)
- Chest wall deformity or defect, congenital or acquired
- Infection or burn of the chest wall where the line would be placed

CPT Codes

36010 Introduction of catheter, superior or inferior vena cava
36011 Selective catheter placement, venous system, first-order branch, e.g., jugular vein

ICD-9 Codes

276.5 Dehydration
785.5 Shock, unspecified
785.59 Shock (hypovolemic, septic)

C. THORACENTESIS

Key Steps

1. Determine level of effusion.
2. Inject local anesthesia at insertion site.
3. Insert trocar and catheter.
4. Remove catheter.

Instructions

1. Prior to performing a thoracentesis, the operator must determine the level of pleural fluid with the patient sitting in the upright position (Fig. AII-10, *A*).
2. This can be done with percussion of the chest, egophony, or imaging studies.
3. Select an entry site just superior to a rib, along the posterior midclavicular line.
4. Clean the skin with an antiseptic solution and place a sterile drape over the area.
5. Draw up local anesthetic into a syringe using a 23-gauge, 1.5-inch needle to inject the anesthetic.
6. After creating a superficial wheal, pass the needle deep into the intercostal muscle, where 1 ml is injected.
7. Advance the needle 1 cm at a time, injecting 1 ml of anesthetic each time to anesthetize the deep layers superficial to the pleura.
8. Apply negative pressure to the syringe while advancing it.
9. A palpable "pop" can be felt when penetrating the tough, fibrous pleura.
10. Inject 2 ml of anesthetic into the pleural space and then withdraw the needle only slightly to infuse 1 ml more of anesthetic at the pleura.
11. This technique provides superb anesthesia.
12. Carefully insert the trocar just above the rib where the anesthesia has been placed.
13. Apply negative pressure to the syringe so that it is obvious when the pleural space is entered (Fig. AII-10, *B*).
14. Advance the catheter and then withdraw the trocar, leaving the catheter in the pleural space to collect fluid.
15. The catheter is never withdrawn through the trocar as long as either device is in the patient.

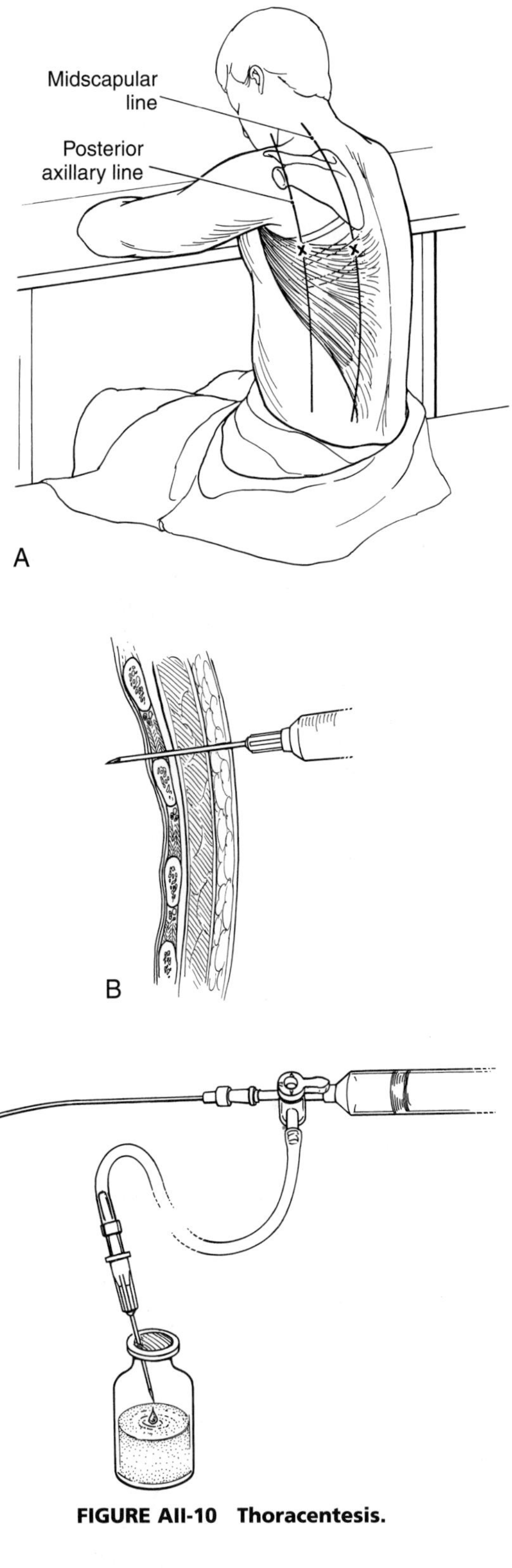

FIGURE AII-10 Thoracentesis.

16. Using a large syringe, withdraw 30 to 60 ml of fluid to send for pathologic studies.
17. If a large effusion is present, then perform a therapeutic thoracentesis during which as much as several liters of fluid can be removed in one setting (Fig. AII-10, *C*).
18. After removing the desired amount of fluid, carefully and quickly withdraw the catheter to avoid an air leak into the chest cavity.
19. Cover the wound with a simple bandage and obtain a post-thoracentesis x-ray.

Indications

- Diagnostic collection of pleural fluid
- Therapeutic extraction of pleural fluid affecting respiratory status
- Relief of spontaneous pneumothorax, though larger-caliber chest tubes are optimal

Contraindications

- Coagulation defect (either medication related, congenital, or acquired), relative
- Suspicion that the lung is adherent to pleura
- Loculated fluid collection in the chest, in which case ultrasound guidance is recommended

CPT Codes

32000 Thoracentesis, puncture of pleural cavity for aspiration, initial or subsequent

ICD-9 Codes

511.9 Pleural effusion
511.1 Bacterial effusion
512.8 Pneumothorax

D. ABDOMINAL PARACENTESIS

Key Steps

1. Cleanse skin site.
2. Inject local anesthesia at entry point.
3. Insert IV or fenestrated catheter.
4. Remove device.

Instructions

1. Place the patient in a supine position rolled toward the left and cleanse the site with antiseptic solution.
2. Select the insertion site on or near the midclavicular line (Fig. AII-11, *A*).
3. Cover the area with a sterile protective drape.
4. Place a local anesthetic block.
5. First, place a wheal in the skin, then advance the needle into the subcutaneous layer and inject 1 ml of solution (Fig. AII-11, *B*).
6. Advance the needle into the muscle and inject the anesthetic into that layer as well.
7. Finally, as the needle is slowly advanced through the peritoneum, maintain suction on the syringe until entering the abdominal cavity (Fig. AII-11, *C*).
8. Once ascitic fluid is obtained, withdraw the needle slowly as 1 to 2 ml of lidocaine is injected to numb the peritoneal layer (Fig. AII-11, *D*).
9. There are two options for draining fluid.
10. For diagnostic paracentesis when removing small volumes, use an IV catheter to obtain a fluid sample.
11. Advance the catheter while applying suction by a syringe until the cavity is entered and fluid enters the syringe.
12. For therapeutic paracentesis, pass a larger catheter through a trocar into the peritoneal cavity.
13. Advance the trocar through the anesthetic area into the peritoneal cavity.
14. Then advance the catheter into the peritoneal cavity through the trocar.
15. Several liters of fluid can be drained from the abdomen using vacuum bottles attached to the catheter system.

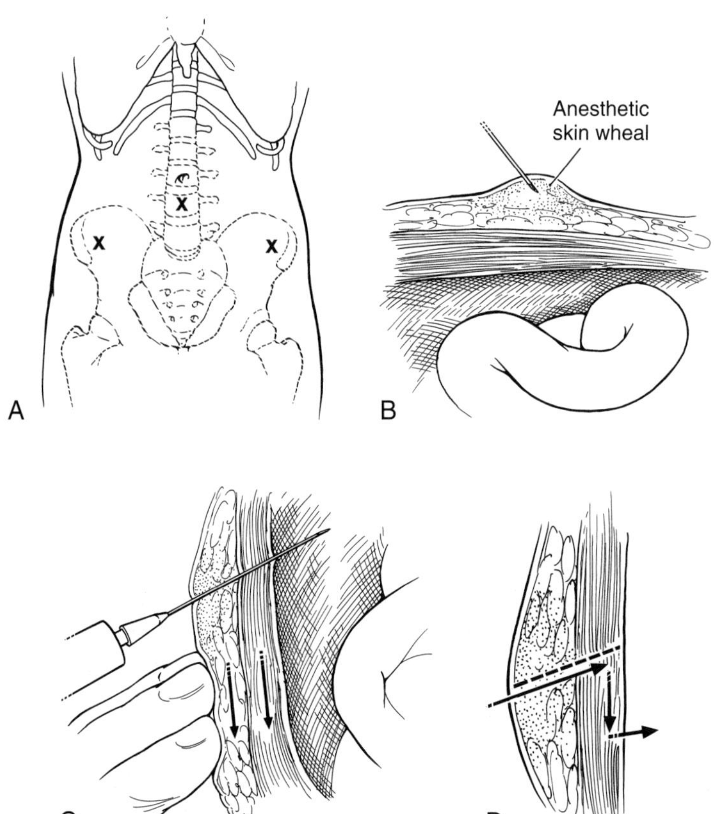

FIGURE AII-11 Abdominal paracentesis.

16. Attach a stopcock system to the catheter.
17. This allows for control of the suction as desired during collection of the fluid.
18. The fluid will flow until the majority of the fluid is removed.
19. At the conclusion of the procedure, remove the needle and catheter.
20. Apply a dressing over the wound in case there is any further fluid leak.

Indications

- Intraabdominal ascites
- Suspected bacterial peritonitis
- Need for tube delivered nutrition, dye, or medications

Contraindications

- Coagulation defect (either medication related, congenital, or acquired)
- Second-trimester or third-trimester pregnancy
- Previous abdominal surgeries (multiple, in which adhesions are more likely)
- Local infection at the site of paracentesis
- Acute abdomen, acute distension (not ascites), or bowel obstruction

CPT Codes

49080 Abdominal paracentesis or peritoneal lavage, initial
49081 Abdominal paracentesis or peritoneal lavage, subsequent

ICD-9 Codes

789.5 Ascites
197.6 Ascites, malignant
567.2 Subacute bacterial peritonitis
014.0 Ascites, tuberculous

12. OBSTETRICS

A. VAGINAL DELIVERY

Key Steps

1. Complete the second stage.
2. Controlled delivery of the head.
3. Delivery of the shoulders.
4. Delivery of the placenta.

Instructions

First Stage of Delivery

1. During the ending of the first stage of delivery, the fetal head engages the maternal pelvis and rotates from a transverse lie to a coronal lie.
2. Normally, the head aligns with the fetal occiput anterior, though occiput posterior may occur approximately 20% of the time.
3. Once the rotation is complete, it allows for easier descent through the pelvic floor through the vagina.
4. Once the patient is fully dilated to 10 cm, she often has a strong urge to push with contractions.
5. Ideally, three or four pushes are done with each contraction, each push lasting 8 to 10 seconds.
6. The propulsive effort of both the uterine contraction and the Valsalva pressure supplied by the abdominal muscles and diaphragm moves the infant's head farther down the vaginal canal.

Second Stage of Delivery

1. The normal second stage of labor is approximately 1 hour for most multiparous patients and up to 2 hours for primiparous patients.
2. As the fetus moves farther down to +3 to +4 station, the infant's head becomes visible as the labia separate with each push (Fig. AII-12, *A*).
3. If tolerated by the infant, allowing the perineum to stretch reduces the degree of tearing as the head is delivered.
4. When the head is crowning, slight counterpressure to the head applied during the delivery process can prevent a rapid expulsion of the head as it passes through the final resistance of the vulva (Fig. AII-12, *B*).
5. Once the head is delivered, the operator tracks a finger along the neck to check for a nucal cord (Fig. AII-12, *C*). If a cord is present, reduce it before the shoulders are delivered. Reduction can be accomplished by slipping the cord over the head in most instances.
6. Apply traction to head and neck in a downward and forward direction to deliver the anterior shoulder. Minimal lateral extension of the neck reduces the risk of traction injury to the brachial plexus (Fig. AII-12, *D*).
7. Immediately after the delivery of the anterior shoulder, raise the head to allow the posterior shoulder to deliver over the posterior fourchette.
8. Place the infant on the operator's lap, suction the airway, and cut the cord (Fig. AII-12, *E* and *F*).

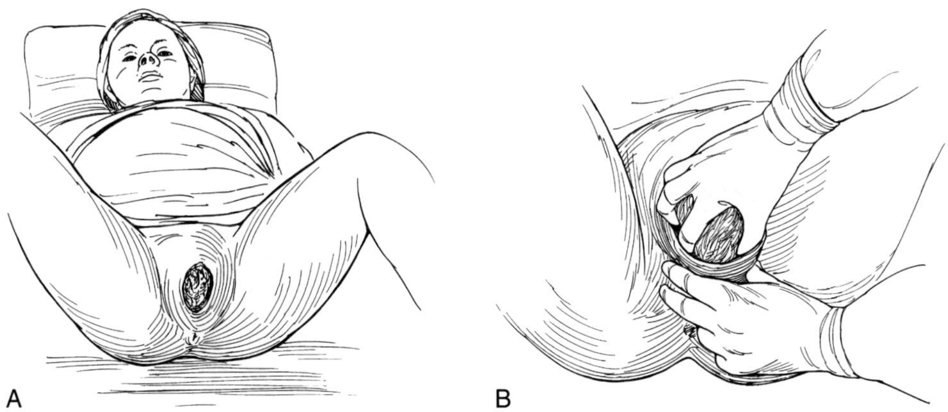

FIGURE AII-12 **Vaginal delivery.**

Continued on following page

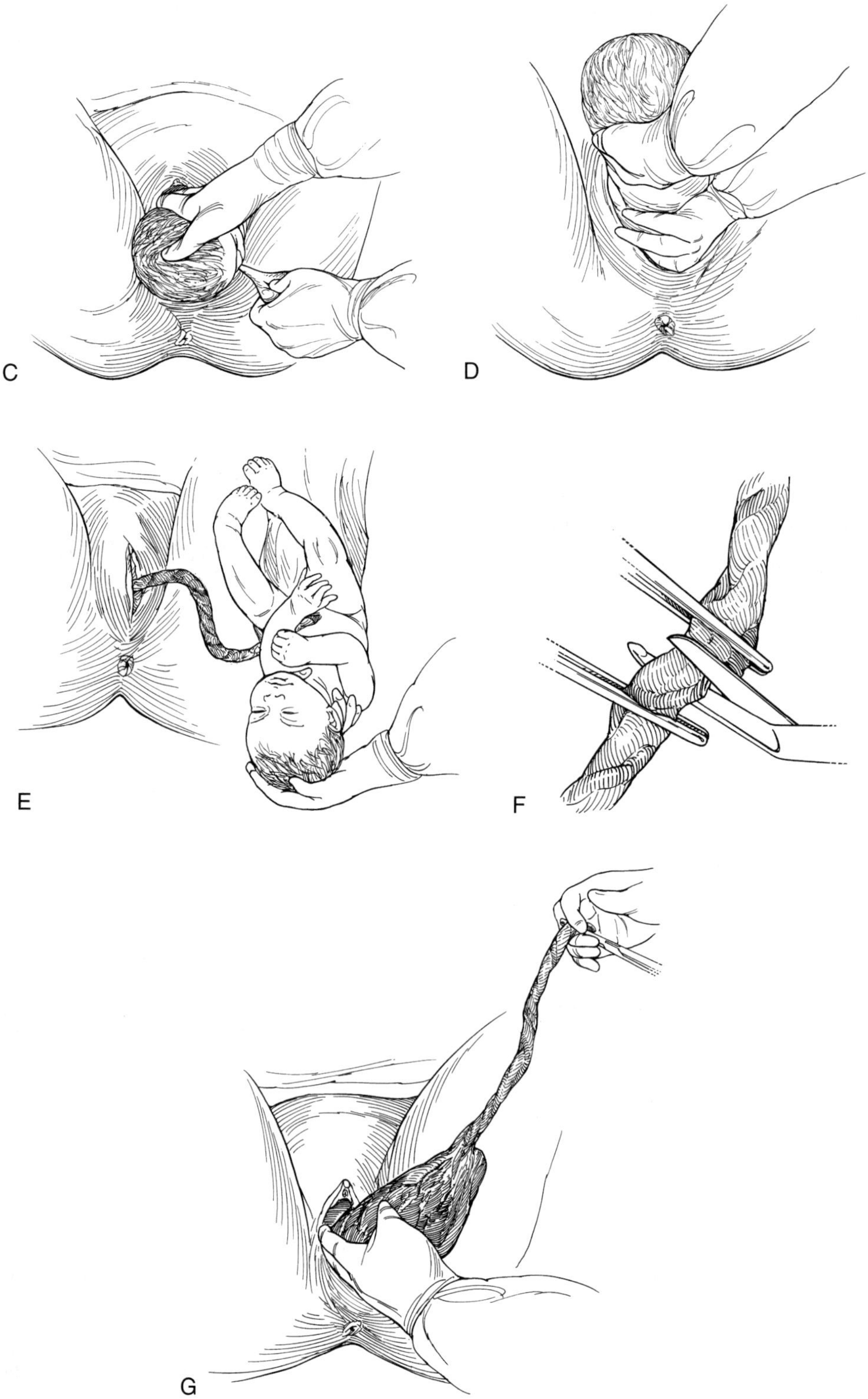

FIGURE AII-12 (Continued) **Vaginal delivery.**

9. Place the stable newborn immediately on the mother to allow for early contact between mother and infant.

Third Stage of Delivery

1. After the infant is delivered, the third stage of labor begins.
2. Cross-clamp the cord with a hemostat to allow gentle traction to be applied to the cord, encouraging the progressive delivery of the placenta.
3. Administer oxytocin at this time to encourage placental delivery. Oxytocin administration in the third stage of labor reduces the risk of maternal hemorrhage at no increased risk of retained placenta.
4. The placenta delivers spontaneously after approximately 10 minutes and is inspected to ensure that there are no missing pieces that may suggest that a remnant of a cotyledon remains in the uterus (Fig. AII-12, *G*).

5. Massage the uterus to encourage contraction and hemostasis.
6. After the patient's bleeding has slowed, inspect the perineum, vaginal orifice, and cervix for lacerations, which may require specific repair to avoid further bleeding and retain appropriate anatomy.

Indications
- Patient in active labor
- Fetus in no distress

Contraindications
- Vasa previa or placenta previa
- Abnormal fetal lie
- Cord prolapse
- Prior classical cesarean section
- Active genital herpes infection
- Fetal deformities

CPT and ICD-9 Codes

Vaginal delivery

CPT and ICD codes depend on many variables of prenatal and postnatal care. Please refer to manuals for appropriate codes.

B. EPISIOTOMY-LACERATION REPAIR

Key Steps

1. Inject anesthesia.
2. Place an anchor stitch and mucosal closure.
3. Perform deep layer closure.
4. Perform perineal subcuticular closure.
5. Place a final anchor stitch.

Instructions
1. To repair a midline laceration or episiotomy, first inspect the area to determine the extent of the laceration.
2. Identify the vaginal apex, posterior fourchette, and perineal apex.
3. It is critical that the two sides of the posterior fourchette are approximated during the repair.
4. Inject local anesthesia along the edges of the laceration to provide a block for the repair.
5. If an epidural is in place with a good block, local anesthesia is not required.
6. The choice of suture varies by operator, but 3-0 chromic, Dexon, or Vicryl absorbable is often selected for closure.
7. Place an anchoring stitch on the inner, or vaginal, aspect of the laceration just above the apex of the tear or episiotomy.
8. Use a continuous running suture to close the internal vaginal portion of the tear to the posterior fourchette.
9. Once near the posterior fourchette, direct the suture deep to begin a deep layer closure of the perineal aspect of the laceration.
10. Run the suture posteriorly in the subcutaneous and deep layers down to the posterior aspect of the tear.
11. Once at the posterior aspect, perform a subcuticular repair in the posterior to anterior direction along the perineal body.
12. Run the suture continuously to the posterior fourchette until the skin is fully closed.
13. Once the external skin is closed, bring the suture up into the vaginal mucosa and anchor it with another stitch along the posterior vaginal wall to bury the knot.
14. After the repair is completed, perform a digital rectal exam to test the integrity of the repair and to ensure that no sutures were placed through the rectal mucosa.
15. In instances in which there is significant tearing toward the anus, perform the rectal examination prior to the repair to ensure adequate layer-by-layer closure.
16. Clean the patient and reevaluate the amount of lochia to ensure that bleeding is well controlled.
17. Control the pain and swelling of the perineum with oral analgesics and ice packs as needed.

Indications
- Instrumented delivery
- Shoulder dystocia
- Perineal barrier to effective delivery
- Fetal prematurity
- Breech presentation

Contraindications
- Extensive vulvar varices

CPT Codes

59300 Episiotomy or laceration repair by other than attending

ICD-9 Codes

664.04 First-degree perineal laceration
664.14 Second-degree perineal laceration

13. REPRODUCTIVE—FEMALE

A. INTRAUTERINE DEVICE (IUD) INSERTION

Key Steps

1. Determine uterine position.
2. Clean cervix with antiseptic solution.
3. Visualize cervix, stabilize with tenaculum if needed.
4. Sound uterus.
5. Mark IUD catheter and insert IUD.
6. Remove catheter, cut strings.

Instructions
1. Before inserting an IUD, the physician must know the position and size of the uterus, which can be determined with a bimanual examination.
2. In most instances, a preprocedure pregnancy test should be performed, and its outcome should be negative.
3. Insert the speculum and clearly visualize the cervix.
4. Clean the cervix with antiseptic solution.
5. Insert the sound and apply pressure to the internal os until it relaxes.
6. A palpable give will be felt when the internal os dilates.
7. It may be necessary to stabilize the uterus with the application of the tenaculum to the cervix.
8. Before being inserted, the IUD must be prepared in a sterile manner.
9. Arm the Paraguard device in a sterile manner within the inner packaging.
10. Retract the Mirena device into the insertion catheter and lock it into position, using the strings at the base of the handle.
11. Set the marker ring on the IUD insertion catheter to match the sound results for both devices.
12. Insert the IUD until the ring is flush to the cervix with the Paraguard device.
13. With the marker ring applied to the cervix, hold the center plunger still while withdrawing the insertion tube out of the cervix.
14. When inserting a Mirena IUD, leave the marker ring 1 cm short of the cervix before releasing the device in the uterus.
15. Pull back the release lever within the handle 1 cm and then advance the catheter up into the uterus so that the marker ring is flush with the cervix.
16. Finally, fully retract the release lever in the handle to free the IUD from the catheter.

17. Withdraw the catheter and see the strings protruding from the os.
18. Trim the strings down to 2 to 3 cm in length.

Indications

- Patient desires reversible, longer-term contraception
- Treatment of dysfunctional uterine bleeding and cramps with progestin-containing IUD
- Emergency contraception if insertion is performed soon after unprotected intercourse (5 days)

Contraindications

- Active pelvic inflammatory disease (PID)
- Active cervical infection
- Nonreducible cervical stenosis, preventing insertion
- Poorly defined uterine position and anatomy as determined by pelvic examination
- Allergy to copper for copper-containing IUD

Relative Contraindications

- Multiple sexual partners, placing patient at risk for PID
- Nulligravida status

CPT Codes

58300 Insertion of IUD (not including device)

ICD-9 Codes

V25.1 Contraceptive management: IUD

B. IUD REMOVAL

Key Steps

1. Visualize cervix, identify IUD strings.
2. Grasp strings with ring forceps.
3. Extract IUD.

Instructions

1. Place the patient in the lithotomy position and insert a speculum to visualize the cervix.
2. Identify the IUD strings.
3. Remove the IUD by firmly grasping the IUD string in the vault, using a ring forceps.
4. With smooth, gentle traction, pull the IUD out of the uterus.

Indications

- Expired IUD (1 to 5 years for progesterone IUD, 10 years for copper IUD)
- Request for removal
- Overall medical condition that warrants removal
- Pregnancy
- Pelvic inflammatory disease
- Lower genital malignancy
- Dyspareunia
- Uterine perforation
- Partial expulsion
- Some precancerous lesions of cervix or endocervical canal to allow for treatment
- High risk for sexually transmitted diseases
- Menopause
- Desire to become pregnant
- Side effects causing significant patient discomfort
- Any condition that makes a woman ineligible for IUD use

Contraindications

- None

CPT Codes

58301 IUD removal

ICD-9 Codes

V25.1 Contraceptive management: IUD
V25.42 IUD removal
996.76 IUD causing menorrhagia

C. DIAPHRAGM INSERTION

Key Steps

1. Place patient in lithotomy position.
2. Measure vaginal vault.
3. Determine size of diaphragm.
4. Gently insert and palpate diaphragm-covered cervix.

Instructions

1. Place the patient in the lithotomy position.
2. With index finger, gently determine the distance from the posterior fornix to the inside of the symphisis pubis, which will be the size of the diaphragm. Most women require a 70-mm to 80-mm size.
3. Apply lubricating jelly to the dome and entire rim of the diaphragm. The patient must understand that effectiveness requires use of spermicidal jelly, not lubricant.
4. With the diaphragm folded in half in one hand and the vulva separated with the other, gently insert the diaphragm into the vagina in the direction of the posterior fornix and gently place the anterior edge under the pubis.
5. Determine correct placement by feeling that the cervix is fully covered by the diaphragm.
6. The diaphragm should be comfortable to the patient.
7. Remove the diaphragm by hooking the anterior rim with the index finger and pulling it out through the introitus.
8. Teach the patient to insert, check position of, and remove the diaphragm; provide written instructions.

Indications

- Desire for self-administered reversible contraception of moderate effectiveness

Contraindications

- When pregnancy must be prevented owing to maternal medical condition, use more effective method
- Inability to tolerate or understand application of self-insertion diaphragm device
- Not to be used for reliable prevention of sexually transmitted disease

CPT Codes

57170 Diaphragm or cervical cap fitting with instructions

ICD-9 Codes

V2509 Family planning advice
V2502 Initiation of other contraceptive measures

14. URINARY

A. BLADDER CATHETERIZATION—FEMALE

Key Steps

1. Position patient.
2. Prepare catheter, check balloon.
3. Cleanse labia and urethral meatus.
4. Insert catheter completely into bladder.
5. Inflate catheter balloon.

Instructions

1. Place the patient in the lithotomy position (Fig. AII-13, *A*).
2. After donning sterile gloves and draping the patient's genitals, prepare the catheter for insertion.
3. Thoroughly cleanse the labia and the urethral meatus with antiseptic solution (Fig. AII-13, *B*).
4. Lubricate the catheter with 2% lidocaine jelly (Fig. AII-13, *C*) and gently insert it through the urethra (Fig. AII-13, *D*).
5. Pass at least 20 cm of the catheter into the urethra to ensure that it is fully within the bladder (Fig. AII-13, *E*).
6. Once urine is obtained, if the catheter is to be left inside, inflate the balloon with 10 ml of sterile water and gently pull the catheter outward to ensure that the balloon is maintaining the catheter in position (Fig. AII-13, *F*).
7. Set up the closed urine collection system and secure the catheter to the patient's thigh with tape.

Indications

- Relief of urinary obstruction
- Monitoring of urine output
- Obtaining a sterile urine specimen
- Instillation of medications or dyes into the bladder
- Incontinence management
- Measurement of post-void residual volumes

Contraindications

- Suspected pubic symphysis fracture (blood at the urethral meatus in trauma patient)
- Known fixed obstruction of the urethra (stricture or malignant fixation of urethra)
- Acute infection of prostate or urethra likely

CPT Codes

53670 Simple catheterization

ICD-9 Codes

598.9 Urethral stricture (nontraumatic)
598.1 Urethral stricture (traumatic)
596.0 Bladder neck obstruction (acquired)
788.20 Urinary retention
788.30 Urinary incontinence

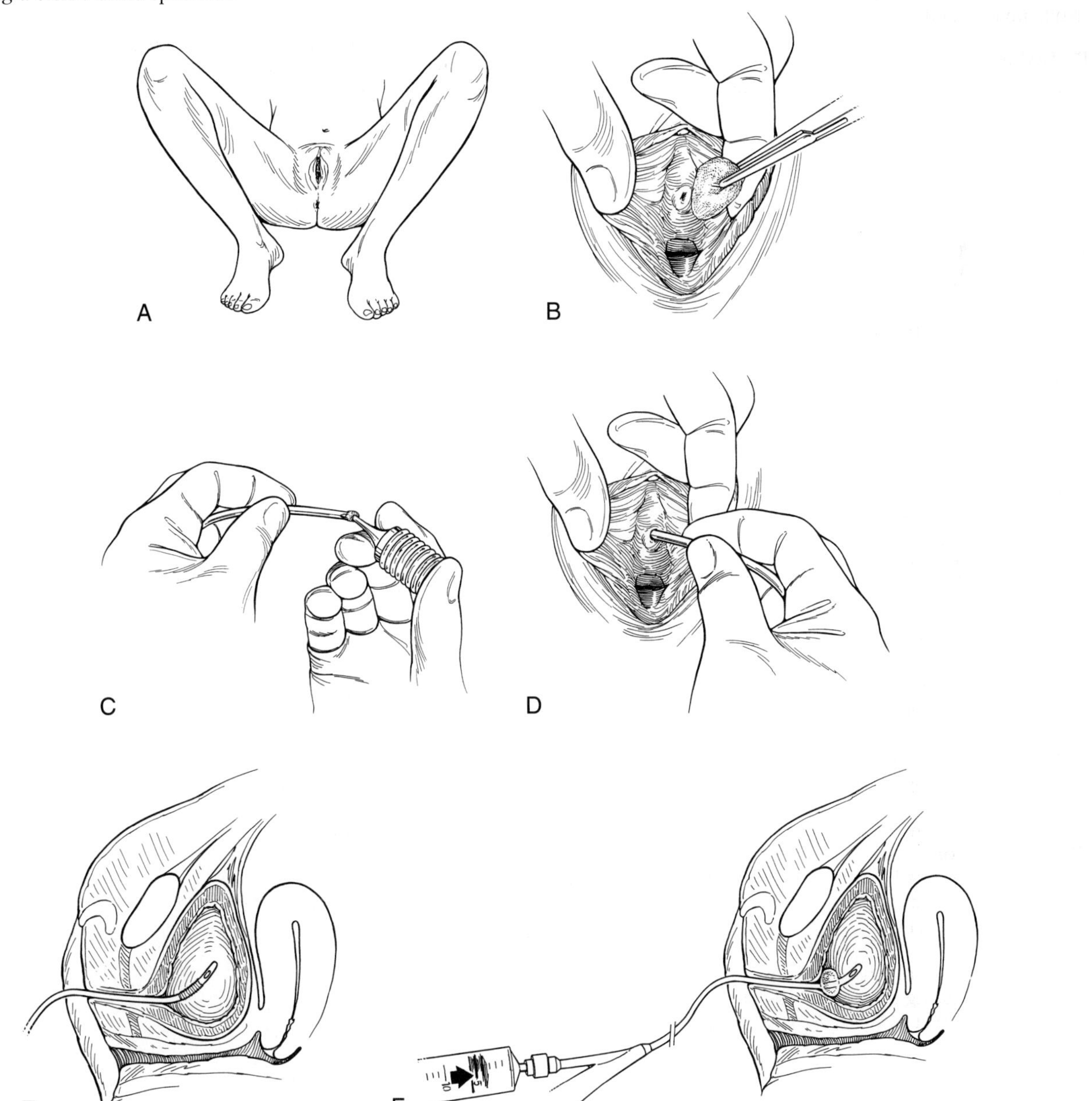

FIGURE AII-13 Bladder catheterization—female.

B. BLADDER CATHETERIZATION—MALE

Key Steps

1. Position and drape patient.
2. Prepare and lubricate catheter.
3. Cleanse urethra.
4. Advance catheter into bladder.
5. Obtain specimen, remove catheter.

Instructions

1. Place the patient in the supine position.
2. Don sterile gloves and drape the patient's genitals.
3. Lubricate the catheter with 2% lidocaine jelly.
4. Thoroughly cleanse the urethral meatus with antiseptic solution (Fig. AII-14, *A*) and lubricate the urethra (Fig. AII-14, *B*).
5. Gently insert the catheter through the urethra (Fig. AII-14, *C*).
6. Pass the entire length of the catheter into the urethra up to the junction of the catheter and the inflation port (Fig. AII-14, *D*).
7. Once urine is obtained, if the catheter is to be left inside, inflate the balloon with 10 ml of sterile water and gently pull the catheter outward to ensure that the balloon is maintaining the catheter in position (Fig. AII-14, *E*).

Indications

- Relief of urinary obstruction
- Monitoring of urine output
- Obtaining a sterile urine specimen
- Instillation of medications or dyes into the bladder
- Incontinence management
- Measurement of post-void residual volumes

Contraindications

- Suspected pubic symphysis fracture (blood at the urethral meatus in trauma patient)
- Known fixed obstruction of the urethra (stricture or malignant fixation of urethra)
- Acute infection of prostate or urethra likely

CPT Codes

53670 Simple catheterization

ICD-9 Codes

600.0 Prostatism
598.9 Urethral stricture (nontraumatic)
598.1 Urethral stricture (traumatic)
596.0 Bladder neck obstruction (acquired)
788.20 Urinary retention
788.30 Urinary incontinence

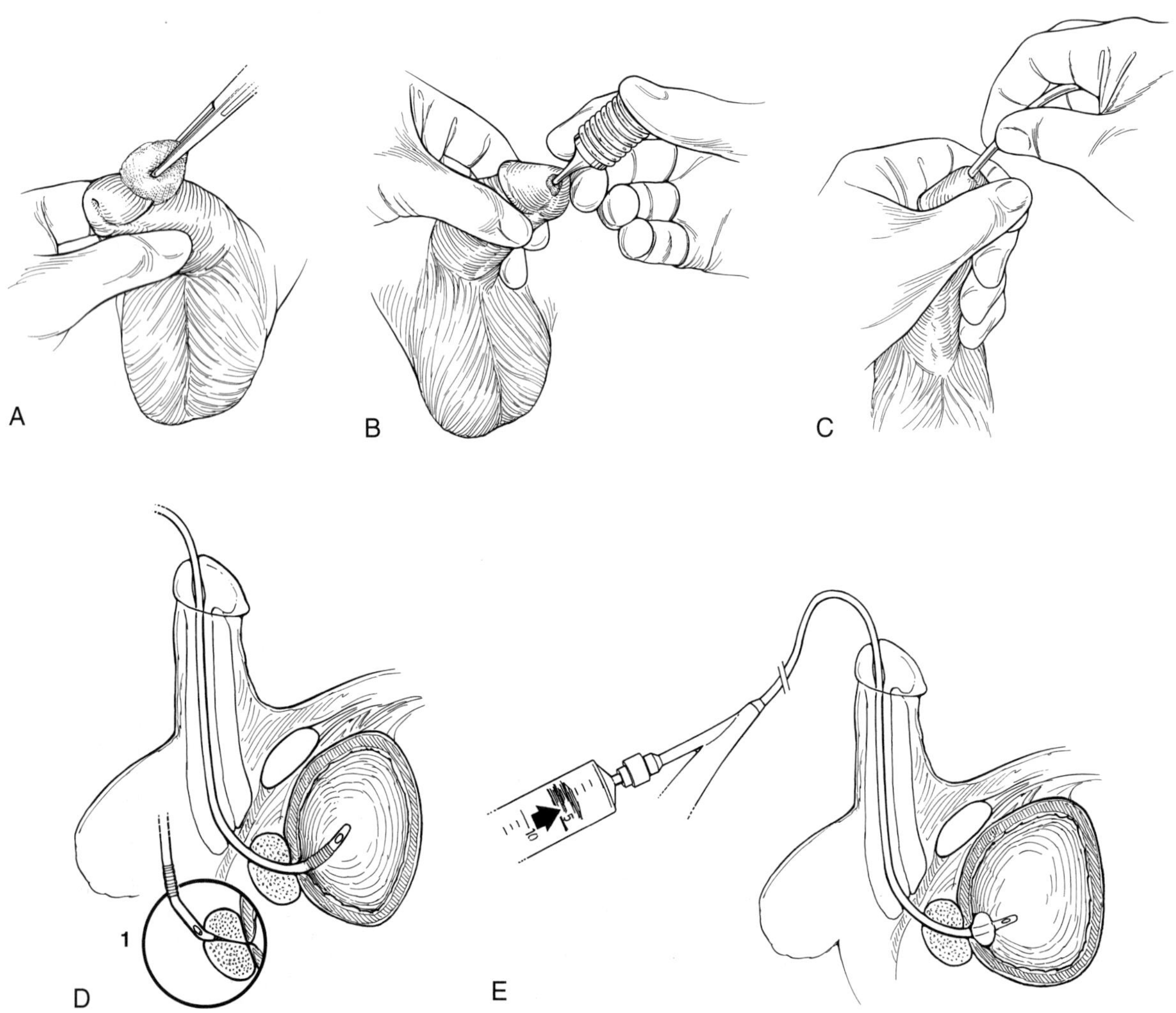

FIGURE AII-14 Bladder catheterization—male.

Index

A

Bolded page numbers indicate principal textual treatment. Page numbers followed by f indicate figures; t, tables; b, boxes.

B

C

D

F

G

H

M

N

O

P

Q

R

S

T

U

V